LIBRARY & INFORMATION SERVICE DRI SDAHT
T13966

KU-308-398

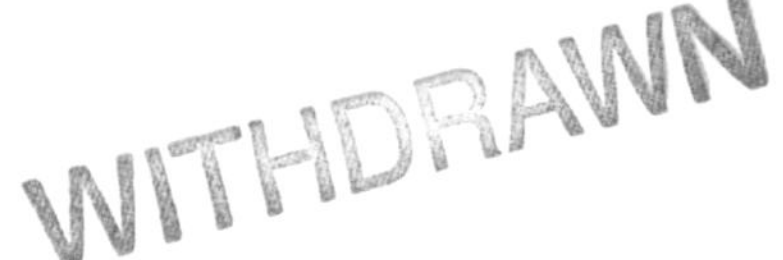
WITHDRAWN

Arthritis and Allied Conditions
A Textbook of Rheumatology

FIFTEENTH EDITION

VOLUME 1

Edited by

William J. Koopman

Professor and Chairman
Department of Medicine
University of Alabama School of Medicine
Birmingham, Alabama

and

Larry W. Moreland

Professor of Medicine
Division of Clinical Immunology and Rheumatology
Department of Medicine
University of Alabama School of Medicine
Birmingham, Alabama

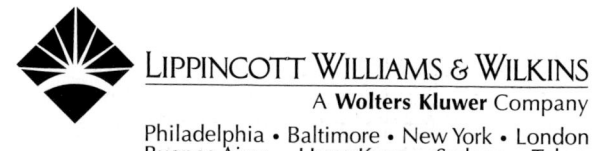

Philadelphia • Baltimore • New York • London
Buenos Aires • Hong Kong • Sydney • Tokyo

Acquisitions Editor: Danette Somers
Managing Editor: Tanya Lazar
Developmental Editor: Nancy Winter
Production Editor: Print Matters, Inc.
Manufacturing Manager: Colin Warnock
Cover Designer: Patricia Gast
Compositor: Compset, Inc.
Printer: Quebecor World Kingsport

530 Walnut Street
Philadelphia, PA 19106 USA
LWW.com

Printed in the USA

Library of Congress Cataloging-in-Publication Data
Arthritis and allied conditions : a textbook of rheumatology.—15th ed. / [edited by]
William J. Koopman, Larry W. Moreland.
p. ; cm.
Includes bibliographical references and index.
ISBN 0-7817-4671-X
1. Arthritis. 2. Rheumatism. I. Koopman, William J. II. Moreland, Larry W.
[DNLM: 1. Arthritis. 2. Rheumatic Diseases. WE 344 A7866 2004]
RC933.A64 2004
616.7′22—dc22

2004048815

Care has been taken to confirm the accuracy of the information presented and to describe generally accepted practices. However, the authors, editors, and publisher are not responsible for errors or omissions or for any consequences from application of the information in this book and make no warranty, expressed or implied, with respect to the currency, completeness, or accuracy of the contents of the publication. Application of this information in a particular situation remains the professional responsibility of the practitioner.

The authors, editors, and publisher have exerted every effort to ensure that drug selection and dosage set forth in this text are in accordance with current recommendations and practice at the time of publication. However, in view of ongoing research, changes in government regulations, and the constant flow of information relating to drug therapy and drug reactions, the reader is urged to check the package insert for each drug for any change in indications and dosage and for added warnings and precautions. This is particularly important when the recommended agent is a new or infrequently employed drug.

Some drugs and medical devices presented in this publication have Food and Drug Administration (FDA) clearance for limited use in restricted research settings. It is the responsibility of the health care provider to ascertain the FDA status of each drug or device planned for use in their clinical practice.

10 9 8 7 6 5 4 3 2 1

Contents

VOLUME 1

Section III: Therapeutic Approaches in the Rheumatic Diseases

Section IV: Surgical Intervention in the Rheumatic Diseases

Section VII: Systemic Rheumatic Diseases

Section VIII: Vasculitis and Related Diseases

Section IX: Miscellaneous Rheumatic Diseases

Section X: Regional Disorders of Joints and Related Structures

Section XI: Osteoarthritis

Section XII: Metabolic Bone and Joint Diseases

Section XIII: Infectious Arthritis

Contributors

Ivona Aksentijevich, M.D.
Staff Scientist
Genetics and Genomics Branch
National Institute of Health
Bethesda, MD

Leena Ala-Kokko, M.D., Ph.D.
Professor
Center for Gene Therapy
Tulane University Health Science Center
New Orleans, LA

Graciela S. Alarcón, M.D., MPH
Jane Knight Lowe Chair of Medicine in Rheumatology
Rheumatologist
Division of Clinical Immunology and Rheumatology
Department of Medicine
University of Alabama at Birmingham
Birmingham, AL

Dirk R. Albrecht, MS
Graduate Student Researcher
Department of Bioengineering
University of California at San Diego
La Jolla, CA

Nancy Bates Allen, M.D.
Professor
Department of Medicine
Duke University Medical Center
Durham, NC

Roy D. Altman, M.D.
Professor
David Geffen School of Medicine
University of California–Los Angeles
Los Angeles, CA

Won C. Bae, Ph.D.
Postdoctoral Fellow
Department of Bioengineering
University of California at San Diego
La Jolla, CA

Dominique Baeten, M.D., Ph.D.
Professor
Department of Rheumatology
Ghent University Hospital
Ghent, Belgium

Gene V. Ball, M.D.
Jane Knight Lowe Professor Emeritus
Division of Clinical Immunology and Rheumatology
Department of Medicine
University of Alabama at Birmingham
Birmingham, AL

Joan M. Bathon, M.D.
Professor
Attending Physician
Department of Medicine
Johns Hopkins Medical Institutions
Johns Hopkins Bayview Medical Center
Baltimore, MD

Michael J. Battistone, M.D.
Assistant Professor
Attending Physician
Division of Rheumatology
Department of Internal Medicine
University of Utah
Salt Lake City, UT

Michael A. Becker, M.D.
Professor
The University of Chicago
Pritzker School of Medicine
University of Chicago Medical Center
Chicago, IL

Nicholas Bellamy, M.D., M.Sc.
Professor
University of Queensland Mayne Medical School
Queensland, Australia

Robert M. Bennett, M.D., FRCP
Professor
Department of Medicine
Oregon Health and Sciences University
Portland, OR

Merrill D. Benson, M.D.
Department of Pathology and Laboratory Medicine
Indiana University School of Medicine
Indianapolis, IN

Christine B. Bernal, M.D.
Pediatric Rheumatology Fellow
Baylor College of Medicine
Houston, TX

Fraser N. Birrell, M.A., M.B., B.Chir, MRCP, Ph.D.
Clinical Senior Lecturer
Department of Rheumatology
University of Newcastle upon Tyne
Wansbeck General Hospital
Newcastle upon Tyne, UK

Warren D. Blackburn, Jr., M.D.
Professor
University of Alabama at Birmingham
Birmingham, AL

Marcy B. Bolster, M.D.
Associate Professor
Division of Rheumatology and Immunology
Medical University of South Carolina
Charleston, SC

Dennis W. Boulware, M.D., FACP
Professor
Attending Physician
Division of Clinical Immunology and Rheumatology
Department of Medicine
University of Alabama at Birmingham
Birmingham, AL

Dimitrios T. Boumpas, M.D.
Department of Rheumatology/Clinical Immunology
Medical School
University of Crete
Heraklion, Greece

Simon J. Bowman, Ph.D., FRCP
Honorary Senior Clinical Lecturer
Consultant Rheumatologist
Department of Rheumatology
Division of Immunity and Infection
University of Birmingham
Birmingham, UK

Laurence A. Bradley, Ph.D.
Division of Clinical Immunology and Rheumatology
Department of Medicine
University of Alabama at Birmingham
Birmingham, AL

S. Louis Bridges, Jr., M.D., Ph.D.
Associate Professor
Division of Clinical Immunology and Rheumatology
Departments of Medicine and Microbiology
University of Alabama at Birmingham
Birmingham, AL

Alan N. Brown, M.D.
Assistant Professor
Medical University of South Carolina
Charleston, SC

Hermine I. Brunner, M.D., M.Sc.
Assistant Professor
Departments of Pediatrics and Rheumatology
University of Cincinnati College of Medicine
Cincinnati Children's Hospital Medical Center
Cincinnati, OH

W. Watson Buchanan, M.D.
Professor Emeritus
McMaster University
Hamilton, ON, Canada

Jane A. Buckner, M.D.
Assistant Member
Clinical Assistant Professor
Department of Medicine
University of Washington
Benaroya Research Institute at Virginia Mason
Seattle, WA

Daniel C. Bullard, Ph.D.
Department of Genetics
University of Alabama at Birmingham
Birmingham, AL

Grant W. Cannon, M.D.
Professor
Associate Chief of Staff
Division of Rheumatology
University of Utah
VA Salt Lake City Health Care Systems
Salt Lake City, UT

Xu Cao, Ph.D.
Associate Professor
Department of Pathology
University of Alabama at Birmingham
Birmingham, AL

Robert H. Carter, M.D.
Professor
Physician
Department of Medicine
University of Alabama at Birmingham
Birmingham VA Medical Center
Birmingham, AL

Rowland W. Chang, M.D., MPH
Professor
Departments of Preventive Medicine, Medicine, and Physical Medicine & Rehabilitation
Director
Arthritis Center
Northwestern University Feinberg School of Medicine
Rehabilitation Institute of Chicago
Chicago, IL

W. Winn Chatham, M.D.
Associate Professor
Division of Clinical Immunology and Rheumatology
Department of Medicine
University of Alabama at Birmingham
Birmingham, AL

Albert C. Chen, Ph.D.
Assistant Project Scientist
Department of Bioengineering
University of California at San Diego
La Jolla, CA

Daniel O. Clegg, M.D.
Professor
Chief, Rheumatology Section
Chief, Division of Rheumatology
Harold J., Ardella T. and Helen T. Stevenson Presidential Chair
University of Utah
George E. Wahlen Department of Veterans Affairs Medical Center
Salt Lake City, UT

Philip L. Cohen, M.D.
Professor
Staff Physician
Department of Medicine
University of Pennsylvania
Philadelphia VA Medical Center
Philadelphia, PA

Andrew L. Concoff, M.D.
Assistant Professor
The University of Texas – Houston Medical School
Houston, TX

Juliet Arambulo Coquia, M.D.
Rheumatology Fellow
Rheumatology Section
UMDNJ-Robert Wood Johnson Medical School
Cooper Hospital/University Medical Center
Camden, NJ

Maripat Corr, M.D.
Associate Professor of Medicine
Division of Rheumatology
University of California – San Diego
San Diego, CA

Mary E. Cronin, M.D.
Associate Professor
Division of Rheumatology
Medical College of Wisconsin
Milwaukee, WI

Bruce N. Cronstein, M.D.
Professor
Director of Clinical Pharmacology
Associate Chairman of Medicine for Research
Division of Clinical Pharmacology
New York University School of Medicine
New York, NY

Mary K. Crow, M.D.
Professor
Senior Scientist
Department of Medicine
Research Division
Weill-Medical College of Cornell University
Hospital for Special Surgery
New York, NY

John M. Cuckler, M.D.
Professor
Surgeon
Department of Surgery
University of Alabama at Birmingham
Birmingham, AL

Catherine Lesko Daniel, M.D.
Assistant Professor
Division of Clinical Immunology and Rheumatology
University of Alabama at Birmingham
Birmingham, AL

Anne Davidson, MBBS, FRACP
Professor
Attending Physician
Departments of Medicine and Microbiology & Immunology
Albert Einstein College of Medicine
Jacobi Hospital
Bronx, NY

John C. Davis, Jr., M.D., MPH, MS
Assistant Professor
University of California – San Francisco
San Francisco, CA

Marietta M. De Guzman, M.D.
Baylor College of Medicine
Texas Children's Hospital
Houston, TX

Filip De Keyser, M.D., Ph.D.
Professor
Head of Clinic
Department of Rheumatology
Ghent University Hospital
Ghent, Belgium

Raphael J. Dehoratius, M.D.
Professor
Division of Rheumatology
Thomas Jefferson University
Philadelphia, PA

Chris T. Derk, M.D.
Senior Clinical Fellow
Division of Rheumatology
Thomas Jefferson University
Philadelphia, PA

D. Scott Devinney, D.O.
Surgeon
Shoulder and Elbow Service
Florida Orthopaedic Institute
Temple Terrace, FL

M. Franklin Dolwick, D.M.D., Ph.D.
Department of Oral and Maxillofacial Surgery
University of Florida College of Dentistry
Shands Teaching Hospital
Gainesville, FL

John P. Donohue, M.D.
Instructor
Department of Rheumatology
Harvard Medical School
Beth Israel Hospital
Boston, MA

N. Lawrence Edwards, M.D.
Professor
Department of Rheumatology and Clinical Immunology
University of Florida
Gainesville, FL

Michael H. Ellman, M.D.
Professor
Department of Medicine
University of Chicago
Chicago, IL

David T. Felson, M.D., MPH
Professor
Chief
Clinical Epidemiology Unit
Boston University School of Medicine
Boston, MA

Barri J. Fessler, M.D.
Assistant Professor
Director, Multidisciplinary Vasculitis Clinic
Division of Clinical Immunology and Rheumatology
University of Alabama at Birmingham
Birmingham, AL

David Fisher, M.D.
Surgeon
Shoulder and Elbow Service
Florida Orthopaedic Institute
Temple Terrace, FL

David A. Fox, M.D.
Professor
Department of Internal Medicine
Chief
Division of Rheumatology
University of Michigan
University of Michigan Hospital
Ann Arbor, MI

Mark A. Frankle, M.D.
Clinical Associate Professor
Chief
Shoulder and Elbow Service
Florida Orthopedic Institute
Temple Terrace, FL

Cem Gabay, M.D.
Associate Professor
Departments of Internal Medicine and Pathology-Immunology
Chief
Division of Rheumatology
University of Geneva School of Medicine
University Hospital of Geneva
Geneva, Switzerland

Renate E. Gay, M.D.
Professor
Chief of Staff
Department of Rheumatology
University of Zurich
University Hospital
Zurich, Switzerland

Steffen Gay, M.D.
Professor
Director, WHO-Center
Department of Rheumatology
University of Zurich
Zurich, Switzerland

Harry K. Genant, M.D.
Professor Emeritus
Department of Radiology
University of California – San Francisco
San Francisco, CA

Edward H. Giannini, M.Sc., Dr.P.H.
Professor
Departments of Pediatrics and Rheumatology
University of Cincinnati College of Medicine
Cincinnati Children's Hospital Medical Center
Cincinnati, OH

Gary S. Gilkeson, M.D.
Professor
Department of Medicine
Medical University of South Carolina
Charleston, SC

Don L. Goldenberg, M.D.
Rheumatology
Newton-Wellesley Hospital
Newton, MA

Tom P. Gordon, M.D., Ph.D.
Professor
Director
Department of Immunology, Allergy and Arthritis
Flinders University
Flinders Medical Centre
Bedford Park, South Australia

Jörg J. Goronzy, M.D.
Professor
Emory University
Atlanta, GA

Jan Tore Gran, M.D., Ph.D.
Professor
Head
Department of Rheumatology
University of Oslo
National Hospital Rikshospitalet
Oslo, Norway

Michele J. Grimm, Ph.D.
Graduate Program in Biomedical Engineering
Wayne State University
Detroit, MI

Barry L. Gruber, M.D.
Professor
Department of Medicine
State University of New York
Northport VA Medical Center
Stony Brook, NY

Nortin M. Hadler, M.D.
Professor
Departments of Medicine and Microbiology/Immunology
University of North Carolina School of Medicine
University of North Carolina Hospitals
Chapel Hill, NC

Paulette C. Hahn, M.D.
Clinical Assistant Professor
Department of Rheumatology and Clinical Immunology
University of Florida
Shands Teaching Hospital
Gainesville, FL

Laura P. Hale, M.D., Ph.D.
Assistant Research Professor
Department of Pathology
Duke University Medical Center
Durham, NC

James T. Halla, M.D.
Spartanburg Rheumatology
Spartanburg, NC

Paul B. Halverson, M.D.
Professor
Department of Internal Medicine
Division of Rheumatology
Medical College of Wisconsin
St. Joseph's Hospital
Milwaukee, WI

Uzma Haque, M.D.
Assistant Professor
Attending Physician
Department of Medicine
Johns Hopkins Medical Institutions
Johns Hopkins Bayview Medical Center
Baltimore, MD

Joe G. Hardin, M.D.
Professor
Department of Internal Medicine
University of South Alabama
University of South Alabama Medical Center
Mobile, AL

John B. Harley, M.D.
Professor
Member
Staff Physician
Departments of Medicine and Internal Medicine
Department of Arthritis and Immunology
University of Oklahoma
Oklahoma Medical Research Foundation
U.S. Department of Veterans Affairs Medical Center
Oklahoma City, OK

Michael Hausman, M.D.
Orthopedic Associates
Leni and Peter W. May Department of Orthopaedics
The Mount Sinai Medical Center
New York, NY

Louis W. Heck, M.D.
Division of Clinical Immunology and Rheumatology
Department of Medicine
University of Alabama at Birmingham
Birmingham, AL

Daniel Holderbaum, Ph.D.
Arthritis Translational Research Program
Case Western Reserve University
Beachwood, OH

James P. Hollowell, M.D.
Integrated Spine Care
Milwaukee, WI

Michele M. Hooper, M.D., M.S.
Arthritis Translational Research Program
Case Western Reserve University
Beachwood, OH

Greg A. Horton, M.D.
Associate Professor
Division of Orthopedic Surgery
University of Kansas Medical Center
Kansas City, KS

Aubrey Johnston Hough, Jr., M.D.
Distinguished Professor
Associate Dean for Special Projects
College of Medicine
University of Arkansas for Medical Sciences
Little Rock, AR

Laura B. Hughes, M.D.
Division of Clinical Immunology and Rheumatology
University of Alabama at Birmingham
Birmingham, AL

Gunnar Husby, M.D., Ph.D.
Professor
Head Physician
Department of Rheumatology
University of Oslo
Rikshospitalet National
Center for Rheumatic Diseases
Oslo, Norway

Elaine M. Husni, M.D.
Instructor
Associate Physician
Division of Rheumatology, Immunology and Allergy
Brigham and Women's Hospital
Harvard Medical School
Boston, MA

Robert D. Inman, M.D., F.R.C.P.C., F.A.C.P., F.R.C.P. Edin.
Professor
Senior Scientist
Department of Medicine and Immunology
University of Toronto
Toronto Western Hospital
Toronto, Ontario

John D. Isaacs, Ph.D., F.R.C.P.
Professor
Consultant Rheumatologist
School of Clinical Medical Sciences
University of Newcastle upon Tyne
Freeman Hospital
Newcastle upon Tyne, UK

Zacharia Isaac, M.D.
Director
Interventional Psychiatry
Orthopedic Arthritis Center
Brigham and Women's Hospital
Boston, MA

Christopher G. Jackson, M.D.
Professor
Staff Physician
Department of Rheumatology
University of Utah
George E. Wahlen Department of Veterans Affairs Medical Center
Salt Lake City, UT

Kyle D. Jadin, M.S.
Graduate Student Researcher
Department of Bioengineering
University of California at San Diego
La Jolla, CA

Hugo E. Jasin, M.D.
Professor
Director
Department of Internal Medicine
Division of Rheumatology and Clinical Immunology
University of Arkansas for Medical Sciences
Little Rock, AR

Meenakshi Jolly, M.D.
Chief
Section of Rheumatology
University of Illinois at Chicago
Advocate Christ Medical Center
Oaklawn, IL

Roland Jonsson, D.M.D., Ph.D.
Professor
Consultant
Department of Rheumatology
Broegelmann Research Laboratory
The Gade Institute
University of Bergen
Haukeland University Hospital
Bergen, Norway

Kenneth C. Kalunian, M.D.
University of California at San Diego
La Jolla, CA

Allen P. Kaplan, M.D.
Professor
Co-Director, Asthma and Allergy Center
Department of Medicine
Medical University of South Carolina
Charleston, SC

Daniel L. Kastner, M.D.
Arthritis Branch
National Institutes of Health
Bethesda, MD

Jeffrey N. Katz, M.D.
Division of Rheumatology
Brigham and Women's Hospital
Boston, MA

Muhammad Asim Khan, M.D., M.A.C.P., F.R.C.P.
Professor
Division of Rheumatology
Department of Medicine
Case Western Reserve University
Cleveland, OH

J. Michael Kilby, M.D.
Associate Professor
Medical Director
Department of Medicine
University of Alabama at Birmingham
Birmingham, AL

Robert P. Kimberly, M.D.
Division of Clinical Immunology and Rheumatology
Department of Medicine
University of Alabama at Birmingham
Birmingham, AL

Lynell W. Klassen, M.D.
Department of Internal Medicine
University of Nebraska Medical Center
Omaha, NE

Travis J. Klein, M.S.
Graduate Student Researcher
Department of Bioengineering
University of California at San Diego
La Jolla, CA

William J. Koopman, M.D.
Chairman
Department of Medicine
Univeristy of Alabama at Birmingham
Birmingham, AL

Joseph H. Korn, M.D.
Arthritis Center
Boston University School of Medicine
Boston, MA

Anita P. Kuan, Ph.D.
Postdoctoral Fellow
Department of Medicine
University of Pennsylvania
Philadelphia, PA

Daniel Lajeunesse, Ph.D.
Associate Professor
Researcher
Department of Medicine
Osteoarthritis Research Unit
University of Montreal
University of Montreal Hospital Centre
Montreal, Quebec

Albert F. Lobuglio, M.D.
Director
Comprehensive Cancer Center
University of Alabama at Birmingham
Birmingham, AL

Michael Dan Lockshin, M.D.
Professor
Attending Physician
Departments of Medicine, Obstetrics-Gynecology, and Rheumatology
Weill-Medical College of Cornell University
Hospital for Special Surgery
New York, NY

Carlos J. Lozada, M.D.
Division of Rheumatology and Immunology
University of Miami School of Medicine
Miami, FL

Stephen E. Malawista, M.D.
Professor
Attending Physician
Department of Internal Medicine
Yale University School of Medicine
Yale-New Haven Medical Center
New Haven, CT

Johanne Martel-Pelletier, Ph.D.
Professor
Director
Department of Medicine
Osteoarthritis Research Unit
University of Montreal
University of Montreal Hospital Centre
Montreal, Quebec

Thomas G. Mason II, M.D.
Department of Medicine
Division of Rheumatology
Mayo Clinic
Rochester, MN

Richard Mayne, Ph.D.
Department of Cell Biology
University of Alabama at Birmingham
Birmingham, AL

Daniel J. McCarty, M.D.
Will and Cara Ross Professor Emeritus
Department of Medicine
Medical College of Wisconsin
Milwaukee, WI

Kevin B. McGowan, M.S.
Graduate Student Researcher
Department of Bioengineering
University of California at San Diego
La Jolla, CA

Thomas A. Medsger, Jr., M.D.
Division of Rheumatology
Department of Medicine
University of Pittsburgh Medical Center
Pittsburgh, PA

Clement J. Michet, M.D., M.P.H.
Mayo Clinic
Rochester, MN

Herman Mielants, M.D., Ph.D.
Professor
Head of Clinic
Department of Rheumatology
Ghent University Hospital
Ghent, Belgium

Mark Mighell, M.D.
Surgeon
Shoulder and Elbow Service
Florida Orthopaedic Institute
Temple Terrace, FL

Ted R. Mikuls, M.D., M.S.P.H.
Assistant Professor
Department of Medicine
University of Nebraska Medical Center
Omaha, NE

Frederick W. Miller, M.D., Ph.D.
Chief, Environmental Autoimmunity Group
Office of Clinical Research
National Institute of Health
Bethesda, MD

Elinor Mody, M.D.
Division of Rheumatology, Immunology and Allergy
Brigham and Women's Hospital
Boston, MA

Gerald F. Moore, M.D.
Professor
Department of Internal Medicine
Section of Rheumatology
University of Nebraska College of Medicine
Omaha, NE

K. David Moore, M.D.
Assistant Professor
Division of Orthopaedic Surgery
University of Alabama at Birmingham
Birmingham, AL

Larry W. Moreland, M.D.
Professor
Division of Clinical Immunology and Rheumatology
Department of Medicine
University of Alabama at Birmingham
Birmingham, AL

Sarah L. Morgan, M.D.
Professor
University of Alabama at Birmingham
Birmingham, AL

Roland W. Moskowitz, M.D.
Professor
Department of Medicine
Case Western Reserve University
Co-Director
Arthritis Translational Research Program
University Hospitals
Cleveland, OH

John D. Mountz, M.D.
Division of Clinical Immunology and Rheumatology
Department of Medicine
University of Alabama at Birmingham
Birmingham, AL

Ulf Müller-Ladner, M.D.
Senior Rheumatology Attendant
CFO, Head Division of Rheumatology and Clinical Immunology
Department of Internal Medicine
University of Regensburg
Regensburg, Germany

Stanley J. Naides, M.D.
Thomas B. Hallowell Professor
Chief
Division of Rheumatology
The Milton S. Hershey Medical Center
Pennsylvania State University College of Medicine
Hershey, PA

Sonali Narain, M.D., M.P.H.
Assistant–IN
Department of Rheumatology and Clinical Immunology
University of Florida
Gainesville, FL

Charles L. Nelson, M.D.
Assistant Professor
Attending Surgeon
Department of Orthopaedic Surgery
University of Pennsylvania
Hospital of the University of Pennsylvania
Philadelphia, PA

Gerald T. Nepom, M.D., Ph.D.
Professor (Affiliate)
Department of Immunology
University of Washington
Director
Benaroya Research Institute at Virginia Mason
Seattle, WA

Gayle E. Nugent, M.S.
Graduate Student Researcher
Department of Bioengineering
University of California at San Diego
La Jolla, CA

Jim C. Oates, M.D.
Assistant Professor
Department of Medicine
Division of Rheumatology and Immunology
Medical University of South Carolina
Charleston, SC

James R. O'Dell, M.D.
Professor
Vice-Chairman
Department of Internal Medicine
Chief
Section of Rheumatology and Immunology
University of Nebraska Medical Center
Omaha, NE

Peter G. Pappas, M.D.
Professor
Department of Medicine
Division of Infectious Diseases
University of Alabama at Birmingham
Birmingham, AL

Bradford O. Parsons, M.D.
Leni and Peter W. May Department of Orthopaedics
The Mount Sinai Medical Center
New York, NY

Mukesh Patel, M.D.
Division of Infectious Diseases
Department of Medicine
University of Alabama at Birmingham
Birmingham, AL

Jean-Pierre Pelletier, M.D.
Professor
Director
Department of Medicine
Osteoarthritis Research Unit
University of Montreal
University of Montreal Hospital Centre
Montreal, Quebec

Maria D. Perez, M.D.
Assistant Professor
Baylor College of Medicine
Texas Children's Hospital
Houston, TX

Andras Perl, M.D., Ph.D.
Professor
Chief of Rheumatology
Department of Medicine
State University of New York
Syracuse, NY

Charles G. Peterfy, M.D., Ph.D.
Chief Medical Officer
Synarc, Inc.
San Francisco, CA

Karin S. Peterson, M.D., Ph.D.
Assistant Professor
Department of Pediatrics
Columbia University
New York, NY

Michelle A. Petri, M.D., M.P.H.
Professor
Director, Lupus Center
Department of Medicine
Division of Rheumatology
Johns Hopkins Medical Institutions
Johns Hopkins Bayview Medical Center
Baltimore, MD

Mark R. Philips, M.D.
Professor
Cell Biology and Pharmacology
NYU Medical Center
New York, NY

A. Robin Poole, Ph.D., D.Sc.
Professor
Director
Departments of Surgery and Medicine
Joint Diseases Laboratory
McGill University
Shriners Hospital for Children
Montreal, Quebec

Gregory J. Przybylski, M.D.
Director of Neurosurgery
The New Jersey Neuroscience Institute at JFK
Edison, NJ

Reed E. Pyeritz, M.D.
Department of Medicine
Division of Medical Genetics
University of Pennsylvania
Philadelphia, PA

Eric L. Radin, M.D.
Adjunct Professor
Department of Orthopaedic Surgery
Tufts-New England Medical Center
Boston, MA

Westley H. Reeves, M.D.
Marcia Whitney Schott Professor
Chief
Department of Rheumatology and Clinical Immunology
University of Florida
Shands Teaching Hospital
Gainesville, FL

Antonio J. Reginato, M.D.*
Division of Rheumatology
UMDNJ-Robert Wood Johnson Medical School
Cooper Hospital/University Medical Center
Camden, NJ

Morris Reichlin, M.D.
George Lynn Cross Research Professor
Vice President of Research, Member Arthritis/Immunology Program
Oklahoma University Health Sciences Center
Head, Clinical Immunology Laboratory
Oklahoma Medical Research Foundation
Oklahoma City, OK

Martin Rodriguez, M.D.
Research Fellow in Medicine
Department of Medicine
Harvard Medical School
Massachusetts General Hospital
Boston, MA

*Deceased

Ann K. Rosenthal, M.D.
Associate Professor
Division of Rheumatology
Department of Medicine
Medical College of Wisconsin
Zablocki VA Medical Center
Milwaukee, WI

Robert A.S. Roubey, M.D.
Associate Professor
Department of Medicine
Division of Rheumatology, Allergy, and Immunology
University of North Carolina School of Medicine
Chapel Hill, NC

Alexander P. Ruggieri, M.D., M.H.S.
Department of Rheumatology
Mayo Clinic
Rochester, MN

Lawrence M. Ryan, M.D.
Division of Rheumatology
Medical College of Wisconsin
Milwaukee, WI

Kenneth G. Saag, M.D., M.Sc.
Associate Professor
Department of Medicine
Division of Clinical Immunology and Rheumatology
University of Alabama at Birmingham
Birmingham, AL

Kenneth E. Sack, M.D.
Professor
Director, Clinical Programs in Rheumatology
Department of Medicine
University of California–San Francisco
San Francisco, CA

Robert L. Sah, M.D., Sc.D.
Professor
Vice-Chair
Department of Bioengineering
University of California at San Diego
La Jolla, CA

Mansoor N. Saleh, M.D.
Professor
Department of Hematology-Oncology
University of Alabama at Birmingham
Birmingham, AL

Charles L. Saltzman, M.D.
Professor
Department of Orthopaedic Surgery
University of Iowa
Iowa City, Iowa

John D. Sandy, Ph.D.
Associate Professor
Senior Investigator
Department of Pharmacology and Therapeutics
Center for Research in Paediatric Orthopaedics
University of South Florida
Shriners Hospital for Children
Tampa, FL

Minoru Satoh, M.D., Ph.D.
Associate Professor
Department of Rheumatology and Clinical Immunology
University of Florida
Gainesville, FL

Amr H. Sawalha, M.D.
Fellow
Department of Medicine
Division of Rheumatology
University of Michigan
Ann Arbor, MI

Allen Dale Sawitzke, M.D.
Associate Professor of Medicine–Clinical
Department of Medicine
University of Utah
Salt Lake City, UT

Tannin A. Schmidt, M.S.
Graduate Student Researcher
Department of Bioengineering
University of California at San Diego
La Jolla, CA

Harry W. Schroeder, Jr., M.D., Ph.D.
Professor
Department of Medicine
University of Alabama at Birmingham
Birmingham, AL

Barbara L. Schumacher, B.S.
Research Associate
Department of Bioengineering
University of California at San Diego
La Jolla, CA

H. Ralph Schumacher, Jr., M.D.
Professor
Department of Medicine
Chief
Division of Rheumatology
University of Pennsylvania
VA Medical Center
Philadelphia, PA

Charles N. Serhan, Ph.D.
Simon Gelman Professor
Director
Departments of Biochemistry, Molecular Pharmacology, Anesthesiology, Perioperative, and Pain Medicine
Center for Experimental Therapeutics and Reperfusion
Harvard Medical School
Brigham and Women's Hospital
Boston, MA

Joseph C. Shanahan, M.D.
Assistant Professor
Department of Medicine
Duke University Medical Center
Durham, NC

Vivian C. Shih, M.D.
Instructor
Department of Physical Medicine and Rehabilitation
Northwestern University Feinberg School of Medicine
Rehabilitation Institute of Chicago
Chicago, IL

Gene P. Siegal, M.D., Ph.D.
Professor and Senior Scientist
Department of Pathology
Director
Division of Anatomic Pathology
UAB Comprehensive Cancer Center and The Center for Metabolic Bone Disease University of Alabama at Birmingham
Birmingham, AL

Joachim Sieper, M.D.
Professor
Department of Rheumatology
Charité University Medicine Berlin
Berlin, Germany

Leonard H. Sigal, M.D.
Department of Medicine
Division of Rheumatology
UMDNJ-Robert Wood Johnson Medical School
Cooper Hospital/University Medical Center
New Brunswick, NJ

Richard M. Silver, M.D.
Professor and Director
Division of Rheumatology and Immunology
Medical University of South Carolina
Charleston, SC

Peter A. Simkin, M.D.
Division of Rheumatology
University of Washington
Seattle, WA

Trent H. Smith, M.D.
Department of Medicine
Mayo Clinic
Rochester, MN

James P. Stannard, M.D.
Associate Professor
Orthopaedic Surgeon
Department of Surgery
University of Alabama at Birmingham
Birmingham, AL

Douglas R. Stewart, M.D.
Division of Medical Genetics
University of Pennsylvania
Hospital of the University of Pennsylvania
Philadelphia, PA

Edward J. Stolarski, M.D.
Department of Orthopaedic Surgery
University of Pennsylvania
Hospital of the University of Pennsylvania
Philadelphia, PA

John H. Stone, M.D., M.P.H.
Associate Professor and Director
Department of Medicine
Johns Hopkins University
Johns Hopkins Bayview Medical Center
Baltimore, MD

John S. Sundy, M.D., Ph.D.
Assistant Professor
Department of Medicine
Division of Rheumatology and Immunology
Duke University Medical Center
Durham, NC

Teresa Kathleen Tarrant, M.D.
Rheumatology, Allergy, Immunology Fellow
Department of Medicine
Duke University Medical Center
Durham, NC

Ioannis Tassiulas, M.D.
Instructor
Assistant Attending Physician
Department of Medicine
Weill-Medical College of Cornell University
Hospital for Special Surgery
New York, NY

Michele M. Temple, M.S.
Graduate Student Researcher
Department of Bioengineering
University of California at San Diego
La Jolla, CA

Robert A. Terkeltaub, M.D.
Professor and Chief
Departments of Medicine and Rheumatology
University of California at San Diego
San Diego VA Medical Center
San Diego, CA

Sergio Miguel Angel Toloza, M.D.
Mary Kirkland Research Fellow
Department of Medicine
Division of Immunology and Rheumatology
University of Alabama at Birmingham
Birmingham, AL

Eric M. Veys, M.D., Ph.D.
Professor and Head
Department of Rheumatology
University of Ghent
Ghent University Hospital
Ghent, Belgium

John E. Volanakis, M.D.
Professor
Division of Clinical Immunology and Rheumatology
Department of Medicine
University of Alabama at Birmingham
Birmingham, AL

Angela A. Wang, M.D.
Assistant Professor
Department of Orthopedics
University of Utah
Salt Lake City, UT

Robert W. Warren, M.D., Ph.D., M.P.H.
Associate Professor
Division of Rheumatology
Baylor College of Medicine
Texas Children's Hospital
Houston, TX

Casey T. Weaver, M.D.
Professor
Staff Pathologist
Departments of Pathology and Microbiology
University of Alabama at Birmingham
Birmingham, AL

Andrew J. Weiland, M.D.
Professor
Orthopedic Surgeon
Weill-Medical College of Cornell University
Hospital for Special Surgery
New York, NY

Cornelia M. Weyand, M.D.
Professor
Emory University
Atlanta, GA

Ronald L. Wilder, M.D., Ph.D.
Vice President, Clinical Development, Immunological and Inflammatory Diseases
Medimmune
Gaithersburg, MD

H. James Williams, M.D.
Professor
Thomas D. and Rebecca E. Jeremy Presidential Endowed Chair for Arthritis Foundation
Attending Physician
Division of Rheumatology
Department of Internal Medicine
University of Utah
Salt Lake City, UT

Robert Winchester, M.D.
Professor
Department of Pediatrics, Medicine, and Pathology
Columbia University
New York, NY

Thomas S. Winokur, M.D.
Associate Professor
University of Alabama at Birmingham
Birmingham, AL

David Wofsy, M.D.
Arthritis/Immunology Unit
VA Medical Center
San Francisco, CA

Anne Woods, Ph.D.
Department of Cell Biology
University of Alabama at Birmingham
Birmingham, AL

Paul H. Wooley, M.D.
Professor
Department of Orthopaedic Surgery
Wayne State University
University Orthopaedics
Detroit, MI

Robert L. Wortmann, M.D.
Chairman
Department of Medicine
University of Oklahoma College of Medicine
Tulsa, OK

Tong Zhou, M.D.
Associate Professor
Division of Clinical Immunology and Rheumatology
Department of Medicine
University of Alabama at Birmingham
Birmingham, AL

Nathan J. Zvaifler, M.D.
Professor Emeritus
Department of Medicine
Division of Rheumatology, Allergy, Immunology
University of California at San Diego
La Jolla, CA

Foreword

As editor emeritus I am pleased to write the foreword for this fifteenth edition. There is surely no better history of rheumatology than this remarkable series of comprehensive texts. Distillation of current knowledge in this ever-burgeoning field into coherent and cohesive text has become ever more challenging. The discipline of rheumatology has expanded exponentially since the pioneering single-authored book by Bernard Isaac Comroe, chief of the arthritis clinic at the hospital of the University of Pennsylvania, appeared in 1940. Although his rank at that time was only Instructor in Medicine, he was clearly destined to become a star in academia like his brother Julius, who laid the scientific foundation of pulmonary medicine. Dr. Comroe based his book largely on information recorded in *Rheumatism Reviews*, a biannual publication begun by Philip S. Hench in 1936.

After Dr. Comroe's tragic death in 1945, Joseph Lee Hollander became chief of the arthritis clinic at the hospital of the University of Pennsylvania and assumed responsibility for the book, titling it *Comroe's Arthritis*. Joe recognized that the rapid growth of new knowledge in rheumatology could now best be presented as a multiauthored work. The fourth to eighth editions were largely written by Joe and his wartime colleagues at the Army Navy General Hospital in Hot Springs, Arkansas. Servicemen with arthritis or other rheumatic diseases were referred to this facility from all branches of the armed forces. Hospital staff included many of the nation's leading academicians and practitioners who later provided much of the impetus for the development of post-bellum rheumatology.

Russell L. Cecil in his foreword to the sixth edition in 1960 called *Arthritis and Allied Conditions* the "Bible of Rheumatology." Robert M. Stecker commented in his forewords to the seventh and eighth editions in 1966 and 1972, respectively, that most physicians treating arthritis patients around the world had gained much of their knowledge from this textbook, which had already been in existence for a quarter century.

I became co-editor of the eighth edition in 1972 and served as editor of editions nine through twelve. Joe Hollander and I felt strongly that each subject should be addressed by the most qualified available author. Our responsibility was to identify the appropriate individuals and to provide the overall style, length, breadth, and depth of treatment of each subject and to keep overlap to a minimum. For coherent results, this requires one, or at most, two editors. Bill Koopman joined me as co-editor of the twelfth edition, and the baton was passed once again.

The quality of the thirteenth and fourteenth editions, under his expert guidance, has been superb. Larry W. Moreland is co-editor of this, the fifteenth edition, and will assume the sole editorship of the sixteenth edition, scheduled to appear in 2009. He will be only the fifth editor in the 70-year history of this book! Both Bill and I are looking forward to the new leadership and fresh vision that he will bring to the task.

In closing, I thank my friends and colleagues for their contributions and suggestions over the years, which have made our textbook preeminent in its field. It remains second to none. I feel privileged to have been a participant in this endeavor for 45 years; as a "galley slave" to the sixth edition when I was a fellow at Penn with Joe Hollander and as a contributor to every volume thereafter. I sometimes wonder, though, if my golf handicap might be lower if I had not undertaken this "labor of love"!

Daniel J. McCarty, M.D.
Milwaukee, WI

Preface

The fifteenth edition of *Arthritis and Allied Conditions* captures the unprecedented advances during the past four years in fundamental insights and clinical knowledge relevant to the rheumatic diseases. The dynamic nature of our discipline is reflected in the changes made in this edition. There are nine chapters addressing new topics (cytokine inhibitors, potential biologic therapies, pain mechanisms and management, vasculitis classification, Wegener's and anti-neutrophil cytoplasmic antibody-associated vasculitis, polyarteritis nodosa and microscopic polyarteritis, hypersensitivity vasculitis, Behcet's syndrome, and other vasculitis syndromes), and 36 chapters authored by new contributors. Comprehensive chapters on the epidemiology of the rheumatic diseases and analytic approaches for their clinical evaluations have been updated. These changes are consistent with the commitment to scholarly excellence and authoritativeness established by our predecessors, Dan McCarty and the late Joe Hollander.

Since the previous edition, substantial progress has been made in understanding of the structure and function of molecular and cellular constituents of the joint; elucidation of the structure and function of cytokines and their receptors, and pathways regulating their expression; mechanisms of inflammation; and the pathogenesis of tissue injury in the rheumatic diseases. A leader in the field, eminently qualified to interpret the significance of these advances, has authored each chapter dealing with the scientific basis of the rheumatic diseases.

New chapters on structure of joints, proteoglycans, and cytokines and their receptors; together with extensively updated chapters on collagen, cartilage, synovial cells, and acute phase reactants, provide contemporary treatments of these important topics. Chapters on cell adhesion molecules, complement, apoptosis, eicosanoids, and nitric oxide capture impressive advances in these important fields, which contribute to the pathogenesis of the rheumatic diseases. The molecular basis of immunoglobulin and T-cell receptor diversity is concisely reviewed. Updated chapters on neutrophils, mast cells and eosinophils, macrophages, lymphrocytes and platelets provide new insights into the cellular basis of inflammation and tissue injury in rheumatic diseases. Rapid progress in delineating the genetic basis of the rheumatic diseases is evident in chapters on the HLA complex and the role of non-HLA genes in disease pathogenesis.

Improved understanding of the pathogenesis of several rheumatic diseases has facilitated the development of several new therapeutic approaches. Chapters on cytokine inhibitors, potential biologic therapies, and immunomodulatory agents record the considerable excitement and promise that these new approaches engender.

Rheumatoid arthritis, as the prototypic chronic inflammatory arthritide, is the focus of the fresh clinical section in this edition. Progress in understanding of the pathology, pathogenesis, clinical expression and treatment of RA is authoritatively captured in new and updated chapters in this section. Progress in surgical approaches for rheumatoid arthritis, as well as osteoarthritis, are extensively covered in a separate section.

Systemic lupus erythemotosis continues to captivate the interest of investigators and clinicians alike. Chapters on pathogenesis, clinical expression, and therapy of SLE capably record evident advances in our understanding of this disease. Progress in delineation of the role of bacteria in triggering the pathogenesis of certain rheumatic diseases is emphasized in chapters on reactive arthritis, enteropathic arthritides, and Lyme disease. An expanded section on vasculitis encompasses a wealth of clinical insights and provides an authoritative perspective for the consulting rheumatologist. An updated comprehensive chapter on osteoporosis capably covers pathogenesis and treatment of this common disorder.

Definitive chapters on pathogenesis, clinical features and therapy of osteoarthritis reflect exciting advances in understanding of this complex disease.

The fifteenth edition of *Arthritis and Allied Conditions* has been capably co-edited by Dr. Larry Moreland, an accomplished clinician and clinical investigator. Dr. Moreland will assume the editorship of the sixteenth edition of this textbook.

I deeply appreciate the outstanding efforts of the many authors who have contributed to this edition and faithfully captured the vitality of our discipline.

William J. Koopman, M.D.
Birmingham, Alabama

Acknowledgments

Our sincere appreciation is acknowledged to Ms. Tanya Lazar, Managing Editor, for her dedicated efforts in coordinating the preparation of this textbook. Her patience and attention to detail were omnipresent. Many thanks for the outstanding efforts of Gloria Purnell and Bettie Stone in keeping this effort on course. We are deeply indebted to our many colleagues, staff and faculty in the Division of Clinical Immunology and Rheumatology for their support and many contributions to this work. We also wish to acknowledge the superb effort of the staff of Lippincott Williams & Wilkins in the production of this textbook.

Above all, we want to thank our beloved wives, Lilliane and Susan, for their patience, love, and support without which this effort would not have been possible. This book is dedicated to them.

SECTION I

Introduction to the Study of the Rheumatic Diseases

CHAPTER 1

Epidemiology of the Rheumatic Diseases

David T. Felson

Epidemiology is the study of how often an illness occurs in populations and the relationship of that illness to characteristics of people and their environments. Epidemiology has a broad mission, which includes describing the distribution of an illness in populations, so that health care can be appropriately allocated; pointing out high rates of disease occurrence in certain locales, suggesting causal factors; studying whether certain prespecified factors might be causes of disease; and even evaluating therapy using clinical trials, an epidemiologic tool. Epidemiology has made major contributions to our understanding of many conditions. Disease prevention efforts, triggered by epidemiologic insights, have led to declines in disease incidence. Among the most important purposes of epidemiologic inquiry is to uncover the cause of a disease by showing, in different groups, a consistent association between a disease and a particular cause. Epidemiologic design strategies are numerous (Table 1.1) (1). There are descriptive studies and analytic studies.

DESCRIPTIVE STUDIES

Descriptive studies are designed to describe the prevalence or impact of a disease in a population and to evaluate whether certain groups have unusually high rates of disease. In addition to studies of disease prevalence, descriptive studies include case reports, case series, or cross-sectional surveys. Lastly, descriptive studies can examine the impact of disease on personal function and on health care use or costs of care.

Differences in the prevalence of disease seen across populations or over time within the same population are often used to generate hypotheses about causal factors. For example, hip osteoarthritis (OA) is much less prevalent in Beijing Chinese than whites in the United States. One postulate is

TABLE 1.1. *Epidemiologic design strategies*

Descriptive studies: observational
Population studies
Case series
Case reports
Cross-sectional surveys
Analytic studies: observational
Case-control studies
Cohort studies
Intervention studies (clinical trials)

From Buring J, Hennekens C. *Epidemiology in medicine.* Boston: Little, Brown, 1987:16–29, with permission.

that the frequency of congenital hip deformities is substantially lower in Chinese (see following discussion). Also, ankylosing spondylitis (AS) is more common in certain Native American populations than in white Americans, a difference accounted for by differences in the prevalence of human leukocyte antigen (HLA)-B27, a risk factor for this disease. The incidence of rheumatoid arthritis (RA) may be decreasing with time (see following discussion), a change that may be accounted for by a decrease in frequency of an as yet unidentified cause.

Case series and case reports can also generate causal hypotheses. When case reports link two uncommon occurrences, which would occur together rarely by chance, then the case series or case report is likely to identify a true association. An example is the cooccurrence of an uncommon disease, systemic lupus erythematosus (SLE), with stroke in young women, a rare phenomenon. A case series is generally more informative than a single case, simply because in case series several individuals show the apparent association. Case series uncovered a previously unappreciated relationship of congenital heart block in babies of mothers with SLE and identified putative disease entities, such as mixed connective tissue disease and eosinophilic fasciitis.

ANALYTIC STUDIES

Analytic studies, including case control and cohort studies, are conducted when there is already a causal hypothesis.

When descriptive studies generate new hypotheses about causes of disease or laboratory or animal work suggest new approaches to disease etiology, analytic studies can be conducted to test these hypotheses (Table 1.2). Intervention studies or clinical trials will not be covered here.

A cohort study compares two or more groups of people free of disease but differing in their extent of exposure to a potential causal agent. The groups are compared with respect to the occurrence of disease on follow-up. For example, a group of runners might be compared with an age-matched sedentary group with respect to the eventual occurrence of knee OA.

In a case control study, those with disease are compared with randomly sampled members of the population from which the cases were drawn. In a case control study, subjects are asked about whether they were exposed to a potential risk factor before the occurrence of disease. In an investigation of whether HLA-DR1 increased the risk for RA, rates of HLA-DR1 carriage could be compared between patients with RA (cases) and controls from the general population.

TABLE 1.2. *Case control and cohort studies*

Study	Defining attribute
Case control	Presence of disease
Cohort	Presence of exposure

INCIDENCE, PREVALENCE, AND THE PROBLEM OF THEIR STUDY IN RHEUMATIC DISEASES

Case control and cohort studies both focus on incident cases. Incidence is the rate of occurrence of new cases of disease during a given period in a defined population. Prevalence is the percentage or proportion of cases that exist in a population at a given time (point prevalence) or the number of cases occurring during a specified interval (period prevalence). Because disease prevalence is a function of both incidence and disease duration, groups of patients with prevalent disease are more likely to be enriched with patients who have disease of long duration. Factors that affect disease duration (e.g., the likelihood of remission or death, age of onset, race, etc.), may affect disease prevalence.

Most population surveys evaluate prevalence of disease; that is, they investigate how many subjects have disease in a population at a given time. To investigate the cause of disease, however, one must know whether a particular exposure occurred before the disease, because many diseases can themselves induce particular sequelae (e.g., OA may induce patients to become sedentary and gain weight, creating a spurious relationship with obesity). It is critical for case control and cohort studies to evaluate subjects with incident disease, those whose disease has just begun. Although epidemiologists studying of other diseases such as myocardial infarction and hip fracture have no trouble finding patients with incident disease, identifying patients with incident rheumatic disease is difficult. Rheumatic diseases start insidiously, and a precise date of onset is often difficult to define.

Several difficulties are common to almost all epidemiologic studies of rheumatic diseases (2). First, case definition is often difficult. Subclinical disease is common, so that, for example, scleroderma spectrum disorders may be highly prevalent, whereas the prevalence of diffuse scleroderma, in which patients meet disease classification criteria, is rare. Diseases, such as OA, may be defined either clinically or radiographically. Disorders that seem easily distinguishable in theory may overlap, such as fibromyalgia and localized soft tissue rheumatism. Second, identification of cases may depend on persons with disease coming to clinical attention, and this may vary depending on how serious the disease is, whether the physicians are attuned to the diagnosis, and whether patients aggressively seek care for symptoms. Third, manifestations of disease may vary with time, so that concepts like point prevalence or even incidence may have artificial meaning. The date of disease onset may be unclear, and whether a particular patient has active prevalent disease at any point may be difficult to clarify. All of these methodologic constraints make epidemiologic investigation of rheumatic diseases more difficult than similar studies of other diseases. Nonetheless, investigators have surmounted these difficulties and produced valuable information about the occurrence of and risk factors for disease.

Natural history studies are an important type of epidemiologic follow-up (cohort) investigaton in which only persons with disease are studied. Patients with a given disease are stratified by factors affecting prognosis, such as age, sex, severity of disease, type of disease onset, and so on, and then followed over time to identify morbidity and mortality. Except for studies of the effect of rheumatic diseases on mortality, this chapter leaves discussion of the course of disease to the chapters covering the individual disease entities.

RHEUMATIC DISEASE CLASSIFICATION CRITERIA

In rheumatic diseases, classification criteria are used to identify and distinguish patients with a specific rheumatic disease from those without this disease. Why are classification criteria needed in rheumatic disease? For fractures and some diseases such as cancer and myocardial infarction, there are clear-cut standards for the presence or absence of the disease. In the case of fracture, a radiographic or imaging study can be performed to indicate that the bone has broken, for example. In most rheumatic diseases, there are no gold standard definitions of the presence or absence of disease. Classification criteria are used to create a uniform definition of disease that has wide applicability to different clinical samples and populations (Table 1.3).

To create classification criteria, committees provide three elements (Table 1.4): cases with disease, controls without disease, and a preliminary set of diagnostic tests or elements that might ultimately be used to define disease (after testing, these will be boiled down to the elements of the classification criteria). The success or failure of the classification criteria depends on the care with which these three components are provided, on how many patients and controls are evaluated, and whether the patients and controls emanate from diverse samples.

TABLE 1.3. *Uses of rheumatic disease classification criteria*

To establish a uniform case definition to evaluate the prevalence/incidence of disease in populations
In clinical studies, to ensure that study subjects have disease and that patient populations are similar across the studies
To teach students the characteristics of a disease (often used inappropriately as diagnostic criteria)

TABLE 1.4. *Classification studies and design issues*

Issue	Recommendations
Selection of cases	Broadly representative of disease patients
Selection of controls	Should be selected with uses of criteria in mind; critical to success of criteria
Selection of potential diagnostic elements	Comprehensive (sample all aspects of disease); define each precisely
Avoiding circularity	Use cases and controls from different clinicians than those who provided a list of potential diagnostic elements
	Test classification criteria in independent sample

From Felson DT, Anderson JJ. Methodological and statistical approaches to criteria development in rheumatic diseases. *Baillieres Clin Rheumatol* 1995;9:253–266, with permission.

Cases should be representative of the broad spectrum of persons with disease from different locales. This will ensure that all of the particular manifestations that might be characteristic of disease are well represented. Classification criteria for a multifaceted disease, such as SLE, in which patients are drawn most heavily from a center that sees primarily patients with kidney involvement, would not be easily generalizable to SLE patients with nonrenal manifestations.

The selection of controls in classification criteria studies is the most critical element. If controls are chosen from the general population, classification criteria are unlikely to accurately distinguish patients with disease from other rheumatic disease patients who have manifestations similar to those with the disease (e.g., SLE and scleroderma). On the other hand, if controls are selected from among patients with other rheumatic diseases (as usually occurs), then the classification criteria may not be useful in differentiating disease patients from those in the general population, compromising the ability of classification criteria to be used in population prevalence studies (an example of this is the OA classification criteria in which controls were drawn primarily from those with RA, and classification criteria exclude those with long-standing morning stiffness, a feature of RA but not a symptom common in the general population).

The diagnostic tests evaluated for classification criteria must be broadly chosen to represent all potential manifestations that might define disease. This is especially relevant in rheumatic diseases, which often affect multiple organs. Lastly, large numbers of both patients and controls need to be studied in not one, but many locations. Even relatively large numbers of patients (e.g., 100 cases vs. 100 controls) do not provide enough information to help distinguish between two diagnostic tests that perform similarly. Lastly, as has occurred for RA and SLE, classification criteria may need to change as our understanding of the disease and diagnostic tests for the disease change.

FREQUENCY, IMPACT, AND COSTS OF RHEUMATIC DISEASES

Diseases of the musculoskeletal system are among the most common human afflictions. Their prevalence is highest among the elderly, but these conditions affect all age groups and frequently cause disability, impairments, handicaps, and job loss. Approximately 33% of adults in the United States are currently affected by musculoskeletal signs or symptoms, such as swelling, limitation of motion, or pain. Among Detroit residents over age 65, musculoskeletal symptoms, including knee trouble, back trouble, and unspecified joint pain, were more common than any other group of symptoms (3). Prevalence rates for self-reported rheumatic disease increase with age, being rare in those under age 18 and common in those 65 years of age and over (4) (Table 1.5). The majority of those 75 years of age and over report having arthritis. Self-reported arthritis is more common in women than men; among racial and ethnic groups, it is more prevalent in American Indians and slightly higher in blacks, and is less prevalent in those of Hispanic ethnicity, compared with whites. Among affected persons, arthritis is more likely to cause activity limitation in older persons, women, and all nonwhite groups than in younger persons, men, and white Americans.

TABLE 1.5. *Prevalence of musculoskeletal disorders: self-reported arthritis*

Characteristic	Prevalence per 100 Crude	Prevalence per 100 Age-adjusged	% with Arthritis Who Have Activity Limitation
Overall	15.0	—	18.4
Age, years			
<25	1.3	—	10.6
25–34	6.6	—	8.7
35–44	12.7	—	11.9
45–54	22.6	—	15.3
55–64	36.5	—	19.4
65–74	45.4	—	21.9
75–84	55.2	—	23.7
≥85	57.1	—	32.3
Sex			
Female	18.0	17.1	20.2
Male	11.7	12.5	15.3
Race			
White	16.0	15.2	17.6
Black	12.3	15.5	24.5
American Indian, Eskimo, Aleut	13.4	17.5	22.6
Asian and Pacific Islander	5.6	7.3	13.0
Other ethnicity	7.8	12.7	17.0
Ethnicity			
Hispanic	6.5	11.3	22.2
Non-Hispanic	15.9	15.3	18.1

Data reflect estimated average annual prevalence of self-reported arthritis and activity limitation attributable to arthritis, by selected characteristics, derived from the National Health Interview Survey–U.S., 1989–1991.

The impact of rheumatic diseases is enormous. Among adults over 65 years of age, these diseases are among the leading causes of visits to physicians. They account for more impairment and functional limitation among middle-aged and older adults than any other disease category (5), as shown for mobility impairment in Fig. 1.1, which summarizes data from a U.S. population survey. This is due to the moderate impact of arthritis and musculoskeletal disease on function, coupled with their extraordinarily high prevalence. These functional limitations and impairments result in substantial work loss, premature retirement, and days spent at home in bed or with restricted activities.

The overall costs of musculoskeletal conditions are high, with estimated costs in 1996 U.S. dollars (the last year available) of $124.8 billion per year (excluding fractures and acute injuries). The costs of musculoskeletal conditions, including arthritis, have been increasing, in part due to the aging of the population and to the better survival of patients with long-term musculoskeletal illnesses. Whereas in the 1960s and 1970s total costs accounted for about 0.7% of the gross domestic product, as of the late 1990s this had increased to 2.4%. In national surveys of patients with arthritis, work loss costs (indirect costs) account for anywhere from 50% to 76.5% of all costs. Nonetheless, as the average age of patients with arthritis increases, and many more individuals of retirement age are affected, direct costs (those due to medical expenditures such as hospitalizations, medications, doctor's visits, etc.) are also rapidly increas-

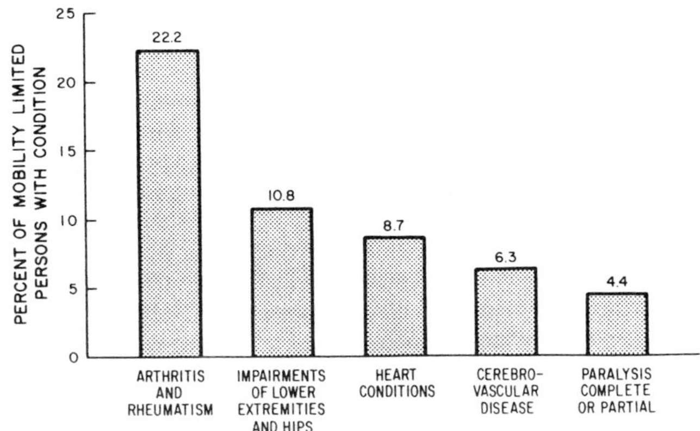

FIG. 1.1. Percentage of persons with mobility limitation who reported selected chronic conditions as the main cause of their limitation. (From Kelsey JL. *Epidemiology of musculoskeletal disorders.* New York: Oxford University Press, 1982, with permission.)

TABLE 1.6. *The most common rheumatic diseases in adults 45 years of age and older*

Extremely common (prevalence >5%)
Low back pain
Osteoarthritis
Tendinitis or bursitis
Common (prevalence 0.5%–5%)
Gout
Fibromyalgia
Rheumatoid arthritis

ing. Studies of costs incurred by patients with the most common rheumatic diseases (RA, OA, and fibromyalgia) suggest that patients with these diseases have much higher than expected direct medical costs, compared with those of similar ages without arthritis. Generally speaking, those with the most severe and disabling disease incur the highest cost (6).

What diseases account for this epidemic of musculoskeletal complaints? The most common musculoskeletal complaints involve regions of the body, most frequently the neck, lower back, knee, hip, or shoulder. Up to 80% of adults experience lower back pain at some point (7). At any given time, as many as 9% of adult men and 12% of adult women experience discomfort in the neck, and up to 35% have a history of neck pain. At least 10% of U.S. adults have experienced knee pain [as reported by the National Health and Nutrition Examination Survey I (NHANES I)] for most days of a month, and 6.7% or more have suffered from shoulder complaints of more than 1 months' duration (NHANES I) (4). Certain rheumatic diseases account for the majority of these regional complaints, most commonly OA, bursitis or tendinitis, and low back pain (Table 1.6). Each of these conditions has a prevalence of 5% or more of the adult population. Other common rheumatic diseases include RA, the seronegative arthritides, and crystal-associated arthritis, including gout and pseudogout. A multitude of less prevalent rheumatic diseases in the aggregate accounts for other common musculoskeletal complaints.

Although it is generally thought that certain rheumatic diseases, such as scleroderma, AS, and SLE, are either uncommon or rare, milder forms of these diseases or illnesses with one or two but not the full panoply of manifestations, are likely to be highly prevalent. Indeed, rheumatic disorders exist that cause pain and disability but in which persons affected do not fulfill classic criteria for the fully manifested rheumatic disease (Table 1.7). In addition, better imaging and more sensitive diagnostic testing has confirmed that persons who have some features of a disease but without florid manifestations, and who do not meet rigorous disease classification criteria, nonetheless may have imaging findings and diagnostic tests suggestive of disease. Thus, the prevalence estimates produced by population studies using rheumatic disease classification criteria may, in many instances, be systematic underestimates of both the prevalence and burden of each of these disease types.

RHEUMATOID ARTHRITIS

Definitions of Disease and Criteria

Rheumatoid arthritis is a chronic inflammatory arthropathy of unknown cause that can affect most joints. The clinical features of RA are described in Chapter 55, and these, rather than diagnostic criteria, best define whether a patient has the disease.

In 1958, a committee of the American Rheumatism Association (ARA) (8) [now called the American College of Rheumatology (ACR)] published diagnostic criteria for RA (Table 1.8) to create more uniform terminology and improve communication by enabling research results from different locations to be compared directly. A patient meeting seven of the criteria is defined as having classic disease; five, definite RA; and three, probable RA. These criteria have been widely used as eligibility criteria for patients in clinical trials (usually restricted to patients having either definite or classic disease) and in epidemiologic studies. To increase the specificity of the ARA criteria, another set of diagnostic criteria was developed in 1966 [the New York criteria (9)] that included symmetry of arthritis and involvement of a distal extremity joint.

The ARA criteria were extremely successful in creating a common language whereby patients with RA could be similarly classified, but there were serious flaws. First, those who met criteria for "probable" disease were unlikely to have clinical RA. In a population-based study in Sudbury, Massachusetts (10), only 15% of cases with probable RA still had disease at a 3- to 5-year follow-up, suggesting that they had a transient problem dissimilar from typical RA. Also, the rate of seropositivity for rheumatoid factor (RF)

TABLE 1.7. *Rheumatic disorders: examples of restrictive vs. broader definitions*

Restrictive definition (prevalence uncommon or rare)	Prevalence in U.S./Europe (per 100,000)	Broader definition (high prevalence)	Maximal prevalence of spectrum disorders (per 100,000)
Scleroderma	25	Scleroderma spectrum disorder	254
Ankylosing spondylitis	200	Spondyloarthropathy	1,800
Systemic lupus erythematosus	24–50	Undifferentiated connective tissue disorder	?

TABLE 1.8. *Criteria for the diagnosis of rheumatoid arthritis*

American Rheumatism Association 1958 criteria[a,b]	American College of Rheumatology 1987 criteria[c,d]
1. Morning stiffness	1. Morning stiffness of at least 1 h in three or more joints
2. Pain on motion or tenderness in at least one joint	2. Arthritis[e] of three or more joint areas
3. Swelling of one joint representing soft tissue or fluid	3. Arthritis[e] of hand joints
4. Swelling of at least one other joint	4. Symmetric arthritis
5. Symmetric joint swelling	5. Rheumatoid nodules
6. Subcutaneous nodules	6. Serum rheumatoid factor positive[f]
7. Typical radiologic arthritic changes	7. Typical radiographic changes in the hand and wrist
8. Positive test for rheumatoid factor in serum	
9. Poor mucin precipitate from synovial fluid	
10. Characteristic histologic changes in synovial membrane	
11. Characteristic histopathology of rheumatoid nodules	

[a]Ropes MS, Bennett GA, Cobb S, et al. 1958 revision of diagnostic criteria for rheumatoid arthritis. *Bull Rheum Dis* 1958;9:175–176.

[b]Classic rheumatoid arthritis (RA), seven criteria needed; definite RA, five criteria needed; probable RA, three criteria needed. Criteria nos. 1–5 require a minimum duration of continuous symptoms and signs.

[c]Arnett FC, Edworthy SM, Block DA, et al. The American Rheumatism Association 1987 revised criteria for the classification of rheumatoid arthritis. *Arthritis Rheum* 1988;24:315–324.

[d]For traditional format, RA is present if at least four of seven criteria are satisfied. Criteria 1–4 must have been present for at least 6 weeks. For classification tree format for RA, can have criteria 2 and 3, 2 and 6, 2 and 7, 4 and 6, or 3 and 6.

[e]Arthritis defined as soft tissue swelling or fluid observed by a physician.

[f]By any method that is positive in <5% of controls.

among those with probable disease was quite low, again dissimilar to typical RA. Another criticism was that a few of the criteria elements (numbers 9, 10, and 11) relied on obsolete tests. The distinction between "definite" and "classic" RA was not useful, because in most studies the two terms were merged. Lastly, the criteria were often not specific, including subjects in the definite or classic category who did not appear clinically to have RA.

The ACR promulgated a new set of criteria (Table 1.8) in 1987 (11); these eliminated multiple diagnostic categories in favor of a single one, better defined morning stiffness (≥1 hour), and eliminated unusual laboratory tests. Also, unlike the old criteria, the new ones did not formally exclude patients with certain other rheumatic diseases. These criteria, presented in either a traditional or classification tree format, demonstrated a sensitivity of 91% to 94% and a specificity of 89% for RA, as compared to control subjects with other rheumatic diseases.

The earlier 1958 criteria have slightly higher sensitivity than the later criteria, but similar specificity. To provide continuity in projections of disease prevalence and incidence, many studies provide rates of RA using both the old and the new criteria.

Because both old and new criteria include rheumatoid factor and other disease features that are frequently absent early in the disease course (like radiographic erosions and nodules), some persons with RA will not meet criteria for disease until later. Thus, criteria have low sensitivity early in disease and may have low sensitivity for mild disease. Because studies can only validly identify etiologic factors before disease onset, there is a need to accurately define disease at an early stage, rather than wait until persons with disease meet conventional criteria. Also, new RA treatments prevent structural deterioration of joints, which could be highly appealing in those with early disease. Lastly, it is likely biologically that risk factors that trigger RA, including environmental factors or infections, may differ from factors that cause its perpetuation (12), and these factors cannot be distinguished unless early disease is defined. Counteracting the need for criteria for early RA is the practical difficulty of identifying persons who are at risk for persistent, disabling disease. Although some risk factors for persistent disease are known, many persons with inflammatory arthritis have it transiently, or their arthritis evolves into a type other than RA. Because of these practical difficulties, there are no current validated tools to define early RA.

Prevalence

The prevalence of RA increases with age in both sexes and, in most populations studied, is most common in the most elderly group studied [often 65 years of age (13) or 70 years of age and over (14)]. Among persons over 60 years of age, prevalence may be highest among those 70 and over and among those with low educational attainment (15). Women have a higher prevalence of disease than men, and RA is uncommon in younger men. RA occurs in all races and in all parts of the world.

Large population surveys over the past 20 years in Europe have produced estimates of RA prevalence ranging from 0.2% (Belgrade) to over 0.8% of adults (Finland). Low prevalence (0.2%–0.4%) has been reported consistently in studies from Southern Europe (Italy, Greece, Yugoslavia), whereas in other European locales, estimates have been more variable. Recent estimates are lower than historical prevalence in England and may reflect a secular decline in disease occurrence. Compared with recent estimates, the prevalence of RA was higher, 1.07% of adults, in Rochester, Minnesota, in 1985 (16).

The prevalence of RA varies across populations throughout the world (Table 1.9). Its prevalence is low in Aborigines and in several rural black African populations, although rates may be higher in urban black Africa. Low prevalence rates of RA have also been reported in urban and rural Chinese and Indonesian communities. On the other hand, RA is extraordinarily common among several well-studied Native American tribes: the Chippewa in Minnesota (17), the Pima in Arizona, and the Alaskan Inupiat, whereas other Native American groups have lower rates of disease (18).

Why are there such population differences in the prevalence of RA? Almost all studies listed in Table 1.9 used ARA definite or classic disease criteria. The differences could be illusory in that different screening strategies were used in different studies. The low rates of disease in the African black populations could be due to underrepresentation of old people or poor survival of those with disease, but this does not completely explain discrepant rates among Native Americans or Chinese. Another possibility is that the small number of cases in each of these studies produces an imprecise prevalence estimate with wide confidence intervals. However, because large studies have found substantial differences, this is unlikely to be the whole explanation. It is therefore likely that real prevalence differences exist, which could be explained by an unequal prevalence across populations of disease susceptibility genes or of infections that may be tied to disease occurrence. Intensive studies of populations with high prevalence rates may reveal such factors.

TABLE 1.9. *Prevalence of definite or classical rheumatoid arthritis in selected adult populations over 30 years of age*

Location (year)	No. of subjects examined	Prevalence (%)
North America (primarily white)		
National (1968)	6,672	1.0
Sudbury, MA (1970)	4,452	0.9
Tecumseh, MI (1967)	6,000	0.5
Rochester, MN (1985)	—	1.1
North America (Native)		
Yupick Eskimos	4,600	0.6
S.E. Alaska Indians	5,169	2.4
Chippewa Indians	205	6.8
Inupiat Eskimo	855	1.4
Europe (primarily white)		
Northern England (1961)	2,234	1.1
Norfolk, England (2002)[a]	—	0.8
Denmark-National (1973)	19,100	0.8
Hanover, Germany (1991)	11,534	0.5
Finland (1989)	8,000	0.8
Oslo, Norway (1997)[a]	10,000	0.4
Italy (1998)[a]	4,456	0.3
Spain (2002)[a]	2,998	0.5
Africa		
Rural Nigeria (1993)	2,000	0
Urban Soweto (1975)	964	0.9
Asia		
Hiroshima/Nagasaki (1971)	11,393	0.6
Rural Kinmen, China (1983)	5,629	0.3
Hong Kong (1993)	2,000	0.3
Rural Indonesia (1993)	4,683	0.2
Urban Indonesia (1993)	1,071	0.3
Kamitonda, Japan (1975)	3,000	0.34
Kamitonda, Japan (1996)	3,000	0.17

[a]Used 1987 ARA criteria for rheumatoid arthritis (the Italian study found the same prevalence for definite or classical rheumatoid arthritis).

Modified from Silman A, Hochberg MC. *Epidemiology of the rheumatic diseases.* Oxford: Oxford University Press, 1993, with permission.

Incidence

Because longitudinal studies are needed to determine incidence rates, incidence has been studied less often than prevalence. Furthermore, because relatively few new cases occur even in large populations, estimates of incidence are often imprecise. Studies from Sudbury, Massachusetts; Norwich, United Kingdom (19); and Finland (20) suggest that the annual incidence of RA is higher in women than men and is between 0.2 and 0.4 cases per 1,000 adults per year. The reported incidence is higher (0.75 per 1,000 adults/year) in Rochester, Minnesota.

Most studies report that the incidence of RA is declining. Long-term studies from the Mayo Clinic (16), from a periodic survey of general practitioners in Great Britain (21), from an ongoing community survey in Japan (22), and from studies of Pima Indians followed over 25 years (23) suggest that the incidence has decreased by 20% to 50%. The proportion of patients with severe disabling disease also may have diminished (24), and the age of disease onset has increased (25). Explanations for these changes in the occurrence of RA include a possible secular change in a causal infectious agent; the increased use of oral contraceptives or other drugs or exposures, which may protect against disease; general improvement in living standards and sanitation, which may somehow affect both disease occurrence and severity; genetic drift with the increasing representation of certain genotypes that protect against RA; and a high rate of RA in a birth cohort exposed to a causal agent and now dying out. Studies from Rochester, Minnesota (16) and from the Pima Indians (the latter with a focus on rheumatoid factor) reported evidence for a birth cohort effect, with a decline in incidence with each subsequent cohort. A decline in RA incidence has paralleled a decline in incidence in other diseases, such as coronary disease and stroke.

Risk Factors

Genetic Factors

Family studies of patients with RA suggest that first-degree relatives have a two to four times higher risk for disease than unrelated individuals. Studies of twins suggest that where one twin has RA there is a 12% to 15% likelihood that a monozygotic twin will develop RA, versus a 3% to 4% likelihood that a dizygotic twin will develop disease. Heritability, the proportion of overall disease explained by genetic factors, is roughly 60%. Disease concordance among twins may be higher in the most severe cases. Despite this prominent inherited component, most individuals closely related to someone with RA do not get the disease. Therefore, the penetrance of disease is relatively low, and environmental factors may be important in disease expression.

RA is associated with the class II major histocompatibility complex (MHC) haplotype HLA-DR4 in whites, in black Africans with disease, and in a Chippewa Indian population with a high rate of RA (26,27). Although DR4 has been the most prominent haplotype associated with RA, only approximately two thirds of patients are DR4 positive compared with about 30% of unaffected controls. DR4 is a broad, serologic specificity defined by alloantisera reactive with class II HLA molecules that are encoded by DR-β and DR-α genes within the HLA complex. DR-β genes are polymorphic, whereas DR-α genes are not. DR-β1 encodes for DR specificities, DR 1 to 14, and five subtypes of HLA-DR4 are defined by the particular DR-α gene. Subtypes DW4 (encoded for by DRB1*0401), DW14 (DRB1*0404), and DW15 (DRB1*0403) are associated with a high risk for RA, whereas persons with other subtypes, such as DW13 (DRB1*0403) and DW10 (DRB1*0402), have no greater rate of disease than in control populations. Although US and European studies report high rates of RA in persons with DW4 and DW14, studies of Israeli Jews, Japanese, and Spaniards show a stronger association of disease with DW15. Furthermore, these DR-β alleles share an oligonucleotide sequence; that is, a shared epitope. Surprisingly, DR4-negative RA patients who express a DR1 haplotype also appear to have a DR-β allele, which shares this critical nucleotide sequence (28,29) (Table 1.10). Of 41 white seropositive RA patients, 35 (85%) carried one or more of these DR-β genes (they were either DR4 or DR1 positive). This shared epitope may account for much, but not all, of the HLA predisposition. Shared epitopes appear to act as codominant genes; therefore, a double dose of the genes further increases the risk for disease (30), and it is possible that carrying two different alleles containing the shared epitope confers a higher risk for RA than carrying two of the same alleles (31) or that one of these DR-β alleles is conferring susceptibility (32). Twins homozygous for the shared epitope have an especially high risk for disease concordance (33). While DR4 subtypes confer disease susceptibility, they also markedly increase the risk for severe disease. Among persons with RA, those with DR4 subtypes are more likely than those without those subtypes to develop radiographic erosions, RF positivity, and nodules (34).

Despite strong association of carriage of the shared epitope with RA, most persons in the population with those genes do not get RA, suggesting that other genes may additionally confer susceptibility. One other susceptibility gene likely lies within the HLA region; evidence for this includes results of a genome scan of a large number of RA multicase families that show a persistent linkage of disease susceptibility to the chromosome 6 site, even after adjusting for the presence of DR-β1 (35). One putative site is in the HLA class III region (36). Strong evidence is emerging (35) for susceptibility sites outside the HLA region, both in linkage and association studies, the latter of which test candidate genes. Among candidates identified is a polymorphism in the gene for tumor necrosis factor (TNF) receptor II (37). It is likely that yet other genes determine clinical aspects of disease expression, such as Felty syndrome.

Hormonal and Reproductive Factors

Much indirect evidence suggests that hormonal factors affect the occurrence or severity of RA: (a) the disease is

TABLE 1.10. *Comparison of the amino acid sequences in the third allelic hypervariable regions of the DRβ chains from susceptible and nonsusceptible haplotypes in rheumatoid arthritis*

Susceptible	DR1 (*0101)	Leu	Leu	Glu	Gln	Arg	Arg	Ala	Ala
Susceptible	DR4 Dw14 (*0404)	—	—	—	—	—	—	—	—
Susceptible	DR4 Dw15 (*0405)	—	—	—	—	—	—	—	—
Susceptible	DR4 Dw4 (*0401)	—	—	—	—	Lys	—	—	—
Not susceptible	DRw10	—	—	—	Arg	—	—	—	—
Not susceptible	DR4 Dw53	—	—	—	Arg	—	—	—	Glu
Not susceptible	DR4 Dw10	gLe	—	—	Asp	Glu	—	—	—
Not susceptible	DR4 Dw13	—	—	—	—	—	—	—	Glu
Not susceptible	DR7	gLe	—	—	Asp	—	—	Gly	Glu
Nucleotide	*0101	CTC	CTG	GAG	CAG	AGG	CGG	GCC	GCG
Sequences	*0401	—	—	—	—	A	—	—	—

Genotypes are susceptible if they share one of two 8–amino acid sequences (starting with leucine). The oligonucleotides of several DRβ genes produce these amino acid sequences, and these genes are associated with rheumatoid arthritis (see bottom).

more common in women than men; (b) RA often spontaneously remits during pregnancy, a time when hormone levels change; and (c) men with RA have low circulating testosterone levels. The relationship of hormonal status to RA has been a subject of intensive inquiry.

Multiple studies have investigated the relationship of RA to oral contraceptive use, and the results have been conflicting. According to a metanalysis (38), studies in which cases were drawn from clinics or hospitals almost uniformly reported a protective effect of oral contraceptives on RA, whereas those that were population based found no such effect. Oral contraceptives may protect against more severe RA (39).

Like studies of oral contraceptives, studies evaluating the effect of postmenopausal estrogen replacement therapy on the risk for RA have yielded conflicting results. Furthermore, there are no consistent differences in endogenous estrogen levels in postmenopausal women with RA versus controls. Although studies suggest women with RA have low fertility rates, these findings may be confounded by the early occurrence of disease, which may cause infertility in women (40).

How does pregnancy affect RA risk? As alluded to previously, RA frequently remits during pregnancy. After delivery, women with preexisting disease are likely to experience flare-ups, and the risk for incident disease is increased, especially within the first 3 months (41). Breast-feeding, especially after the first pregnancy, may further increase risk (42). How can these findings be explained? The levels of cortisol and estrogen, with their antiinflammatory effects, increase during pregnancy and decrease after delivery. A consequent decline in levels of proinflammatory cytokines such as TNF-α occurs during pregnancy, but not afterward (43). High levels of prolactin during breast-feeding may have proinflammatory effects that, unlike pregnancy, are not modulated by high levels of other sex hormones; prolactin, therefore, may increase disease risk.

Nutritional Factors

Increasingly, studies are suggesting that nutritional factors affect RA incidence. This is especially difficult to evaluate because long-term nutrient intakes are not assessed with high accuracy and precision in most epidemiologic studies. Furthermore, individuals may change their diets after disease onset; the most valid studies are therefore cohort studies in which nutrient intake was evaluated before disease occurrence. Even so, there are several nutrients that, because of potential antioxidant, antiinflammatory, or other effects, would be likely to modify disease severity or even its occurrence. The most promising candidates are omega-3 and omega-9 fatty acid–containing foods; vitamin C, E, and other antioxidants such as selenium; and, surprisingly, coffee and tea.

High intake of baked/broiled fish—specifically of oily fish such as salmon or trout, which provide omega-3 fatty acids, lowered the risk for developing RA (44). Evidence regarding the effects of antioxidant vitamins and micronutrients varies: in one large cohort study (45), the intake of cryptoxanthin, a potent antioxidant found in citrus fruits, protected against the development of RA, whereas the effects of vitamin C and E were minimal, at best. In a cohort study from Finland (46), high serum selenium levels protected against RA development, and an increase in serum selenium was hypothesized to be related to the temporal decline in RA incidence.

There is no obvious reason for coffee or tea consumption to be implicated in RA, although tea contains several antioxidants. In one study (47), tea drinkers had a lower risk for RA than nondrinkers. The relationship of coffee to RA is complex and inconsistent across studies. In one study (47), coffee intake increased RA risk; in another, caffeinated coffee was unrelated to risk, but decaffeinated coffee (which at the time of the study contained trace levels of solvents from the caffeine extraction process) was found to increase RA risk. Further studies evaluating all of these nutrients are necessary.

Other Risk Factors

Risk factors for RA are listed in Table 1.11. Individuals with testing positive for RF are at high risk for developing RA, and the magnitude of risk correlates with RF titer (48). A preponderance of evidence suggests that smoking (especially heavy smoking) increases the risk for both RF production and for developing RA (49–51). Smokers get more severe RA than nonsmokers, and the subset of smokers who lack the gene for the enzyme that detoxifies many of the chemicals in smoke may have especially severe disease (52). Smoking has

TABLE 1.11. *Risk factors reported to increase risk for rheumatoid arthritis*

	Strength of Evidence[a]
Rheumatoid factor positivity	a
Carry shared epitope (increases disease occurrence and/or severity)	a
Obesity	a
Postpartum state	a
Breast-feeding	b
Nulliparity	b
Smoking	b
Schizophrenia (lowers risk)	b
Oral contraceptive use (lowers risk)	b
Low serum antioxidants	b
Low levels of consumption of broiled/baked fish	b
Blood transfusion history	b
High serum cholesterol	c
Estrogen use	c

[a]For strength of evidence:
a, At least two incidence studies report association with no conflicting reports (or single conflicting report judged methodologically weaker).
b, In face of conflicting studies, most evidence supports an association, or there is only one incidence study.
c, Conflicting evidence across or within studies.

modest antiestrogenic effects and affects immune competence, both of which may influence RA occurrence.

Finally, patients with RA have very low rates of schizophrenia and vice versa, an association for which there is no clear-cut explanation.

Although no infectious agent has been consistently tied to RA occurrence, the strong likelihood of an environmental trigger and reports of postinfectious arthritis that mimic mild RA leave infection as a strong etiologic candidate. If an infection or environmental toxin caused RA, clustering of disease in space or time might occur. A prospective incidence study of disease in a large area of England has shown no clustering in time, and a modest clustering in space without time/space clustering, suggesting no obvious aggregation of disease pointing to infection or toxin (53).

Rheumatoid Arthritis and Mortality

The prognosis of patients with RA depends on one's point of view. Patients drawn from population studies often have mild disease, with frequent remission of illness (54,55). Many subjects identified from population-screening studies, however, may not have what clinicians would recognize as RA. On the other hand, clinical studies may focus on a biased sample of more severely afflicted patients. Most studies of the long-term prognosis of RA have been clinic based.

Clinic patients with RA experience higher mortality rates than age- and sex-matched controls. Life span is shortened anywhere from 3 to 18 years, and the overall risk for mortality over a 10-year span is increased approximately 1.3- to 2-fold (56). Mortality is especially increased in those with early loss of physical function (57,58), those with severe disease, and those with comorbidities such as cardiovascular disease (59).

Compared with the general population, death in patients with RA is more frequently due to infection (60) and to cardiovascular disease (61). Other prominent causes of death include renal disease (especially in European patients who have a high rate of secondary amyloidosis) and gastrointestinal complications of therapy. Patients with RA do not appear to be at increased risk for malignancy in general, although leukemias and lymphomas occur at higher rates than expected (62), perhaps, in part, because of treatment with alkylating agents. Colon cancer may be reduced in RA because of chronic use of nonsteroidal drugs, which may prevent this cancer (63). Sjögren syndrome, which coexists in many patients with long-standing RA, is associated with a high risk for lymphoma.

JUVENILE IDIOPATHIC ARTHRITIS

Definition of Disease

Many different types of arthritis occur in children. The term *juvenile idiopathic arthritis* has been used to refer to all chronic diseases of unknown cause in children associated with the development of peripheral or axial arthritis. In the United States, the term *juvenile rheumatoid arthritis* (JRA) refers to all juvenile idiopathic peripheral arthritis. In Europe, the term *JRA* refers to a smaller subset, those children who have seropositive RA of childhood onset. Both European League Against Rheumation (EULAR) and ARA diagnostic criteria for juvenile idiopathic arthritis (JIA, but called JRA by the ARA) have been promulgated (see Chapter 61) (64), but the differences in these criteria have created a lack of uniformity. Furthermore, criteria did not accommodate the multiple clinical subsets of disease. Therefore, an international group produced the International League Against Rheumatism (ILAR) criteria for this group of disorders (65) (see Table 61.1). By definition, JIA must have had its onset before age 16, and it must have lasted for at least 6 weeks. Seven different subsets are defined. The performance (sensitivity and specificity) of the ILAR criteria have been preliminarily tested; they have higher sensitivity than the EULAR criteria (66) and may need to be modified to eliminate some exclusions and to add perhaps even more subcategories of disease.

The seven JIA subtypes are as follows: systemic arthritis (Still's), oligoarthritis, polyarthritis (RF negative), polyarthritis (RF positive), psoriatic arthritis, enthesitis-related arthritis (often HLA-B27 positive and may reflect early-onset adult spondyloarthropathy), and "other" (does not fulfill other categories). Among children with polyarthritis, the ILAR criteria differentiate between those with seronegative (RF-negative) disease and others, usually adolescents, who develop seropositive disease that reflects early-onset adult RA. Among those with oligoarticular presentations, there is a large subgroup of predominantly girls with onset under age 10 and a high rate of positive antinuclear antibody (ANA) and iridocyclitis. The multiple diseases subsumed in the JIA category complicate the study of disease epidemiology.

Incidence and Prevalence

Figures derived from referral hospitals or specialty clinics undoubtedly underestimate the occurrence of JIA. Prevalence estimates from such sources suggest there are 0.2 to 1.1 cases per 1,000 individuals under age 16 (67,68) in predominantly white populations in Europe and parts of the United States. Studies from Belgium and Australia suggest that many children with mild JIA are underdiagnosed and that the prevalence of disease may be as high as 4 per 1,000 (69). Evidence suggests annual cyclical incidence (70), but the number of cases in any region is small, and some variability is to be expected. Seasonal variation in rates of systemic onset JIA, reported inconsistently, suggests that environmental or infectious factors may contribute prominently to the occurrence of this JIA subtype.

Oligoarthritis is the most common subtype of JIA. For example, in a Swedish study, oligoarthritis constituted 68% of all cases, whereas 22% were polyarticular (not broken into RF status), with the remainder having systemic arthritis or enthesitis-related (juvenile onset of AS) JIA or other forms. Disease subtype sometimes changes at follow-up.

Reported incidence rates of JIA in studies of primarily white populations range from 3.5 to 22.6 cases per 100,000 children annually (71) and, like prevalence, vary greatly from study to study, perhaps due to differing criteria for disease and source of cases. There is conflicting evidence regarding temporal trends in incidence. African-American children may have a slightly lower incidence than whites (about 6 per 100,000). JIA has been reported among Arab children in the Middle East; among African children in Nigeria, Uganda, and Zambia; and among black and Indian children in South Africa (72). It may be rare among children of Chinese ancestry raised in Europe or the United States, although rates in China are unknown.

JIA exhibits a peak incidence at age 1 to 2 years, mostly accounted for by the high incidence of oligoarthritis in girls at that age (73) (Fig. 1.2). The age of onset for boys shows a bimodal distribution, with a small peak at ages 1 to 2 years and a larger peak just before puberty. This latter peak in boys may be due to the onset of B27-associated arthritis later in childhood. The female/male ratio for JRA ranges from 2:1 to 3:1, but this ratio is influenced both by age of onset and subtype.

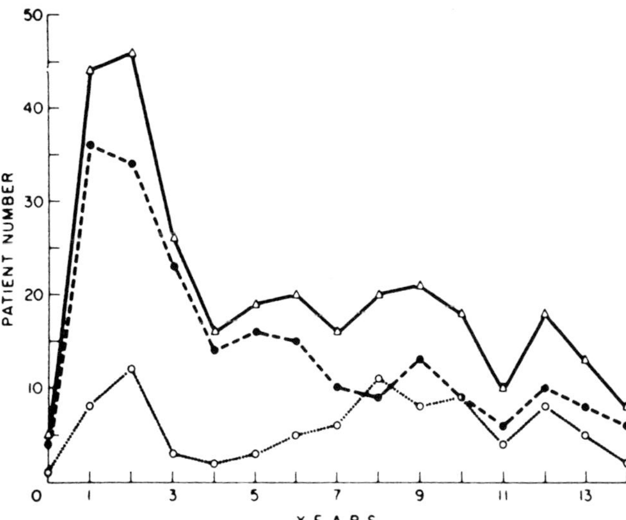

FIG. 1.2. Age of onset (0–14 years) for a group of children with juvenile rheumatoid arthritis (△—△) and for girls (●—●) and boys (○—○) separately. For the total group, a single large peak at 1 to 2 years is observed. Age of onset for boys, however, shows a bimodal distribution, with the first peak at 2 years and the second at 9 years. Age of onset for girls does not clearly show a second peak. No accentuation in frequency of onset was seen in either sex at 10 to 14 years. (From Cassidy JT. Juvenile rheumatoid arthritis. In: Kelley WM, Harris ED, Ruddy S, et al., eds. *Textbook of rheumatology,* 3rd ed. Philadelphia: WB Saunders, 1989:1289–1311, with permission.)

Hereditary Factors

At least 23 families have been reported in which multiple cases of JIA occurred in first-degree relatives (74). Affected family members, including twins, usually share disease subtype. Monozygotic twins have a disease concordance rate of approximately 44%, versus a 4% concordance rate in dizygotic twins (75), providing strong evidence for a hereditary component. The absence of 100% concordance in monozygotic twins suggests variable penetrance. The heritability of oligoarticular JIA may be higher than other subtypes. The absence of large numbers of multiplex families with JIA suggests that interaction of multiple genes (including MHC genes) is necessary to produce disease (76). Some HLA haplotypes may increase the susceptibility, not to JIA per se, but rather to a particular manifestation of the disease. Further non-HLA-linked genetic factors are likely to affect disease susceptibility. Evidence on specific genes predisposing to JIA is reviewed in Chapter 61.

Other Risk Factors

Few nongenetic risk factors for JIA are appreciated. One study has suggested that breast-feeding may prevent JIA (77).

SERONEGATIVE ARTHRITIS

Arthritis Syndromes Related to HLA-B27

HLA-B27 arthritides are generally called the seronegative spondyloarthritides or spondyloarthropathies, characterized by sacroiliitis, peripheral inflammatory arthritis, and the absence of serum RF. Examples of seronegative spondyloarthritides include juvenile and adult AS, acute and chronic reactive arthritis (including those occurring after enteric infection with organisms such as *Yersinia, Shigella, Salmonella,* and *Campylobacter*), spondylitis associated with chronic inflammatory bowel disease, or psoriasis. Certain forms of oligoarticular peripheral arthritis in juveniles or young adults also are included in this category, especially when associated with HLA-B27. All of these disorders share clinical manifestations. The prevalence of sacroiliitis is high, and extraarticular manifestations of disease, including uveitis and occasionally oral ulcers, tend to be similar and frequent among these illnesses.

Classification criteria have defined the clinical features of each spondyloarthropathy. However, because of the overlapping clinical features of these diseases and because many persons may have incomplete forms of one or more of the diseases and could be ignored in disease-specific epidemiologic and clinical studies, both the European Spondyloarthropathy Study Group (78) and Amor proposed classification criteria (Table 1.12) that identify persons with any of these related disorders to distinguish them from symptomatic persons without spondyloarthropathy. These criteria allow for inclusion of both those with primarily spinal disease, such as AS (almost all have spinal pain), and

TABLE 1.12. *Criteria for classification of spondyloarthropathy*

European spondyloarthropathy study group classification criteria for spondyloarthropathy
Inflammatory spinal pain ≥3-month duration (insidious onset of pain at age ≤45, improved by exercise, associated with morning stiffness)
or
Synovitis: asymmetric or predominantly in the lower limbs
and
One or more of the following:
Family history of ankylosing spondylitis, psoriasis, acute uveitis, reactive arthritis, or inflammatory bowel disease
Psoriasis
Inflammatory bowel disease
Nongonococcal urethritis, cervicitis, or acute diarrhea within 1 mo before arthritis
Buttock pain alternating between right and left gluteal areas
Achilles tendonitis or plantar fasciitis
Definite sacroiliitis by radiograph (bilateral grade ≥2 or unilateral grade ≥3 out of 4)

From Dougados M, van der Linden S, Juhlin R, et al. The European Spondyloarthropathy Study Group preliminary criteria for the classification of spondyloarthropathy. *Arthritis Rheum* 1991;34:1218–1227, with permission.

Spondyloarthropathy classification criteria of amor

Parameter	Score
Clinical symptoms or past history of	
Lumbar or dorsal pain at night or morning stiffness of lumbar dorsal spine	1
Asymmetric oligoarthritis	2
Buttock pain	1
or	or
If bilateral or alternating buttock pain	2
Sausagelike toe(s) or digit(s)	2
Heel pain or other well-defined enthesopathic pain	2
Iritis	2
Nongonococcal urethritis or cervicitis within 1 mo before onset of arthritis	1
Acute diarrhea within 1 mo before onset of arthritis	1
Psoriasis, balanitis, or IBD	2
Radiologic findings	
Sacroiliitis (bilateral grade 2 or unilateral grade 3)	2
Genetic background	
Presence of HLA-B27 or family history of ankylosing spondylitis, reactive arthritis, uveitis, psoriasis, or IBD	2
Response to treatment	
Clear-cut, rapid (within 48 h) improvement after NSAID intake or rapid relapse of pain after discontinuation of agent	2

HLA, human leukocyte antigen; IBD, inflammatory bowel disease; NSAID, nonsteroidal antiinflammatory drug.

Diagnosis of spondyloarthropathy requires a score of ≥6.

From Amor B, Dougados M, Mijiyawa M. Critère diagnostique des spondylarthropathies. *Rev Rhum Mal Osteoartic* 1990;57:85–89, with permission.

those with primarily peripheral joint complaints. When tested on 403 patients with spondyloarthropathy, including 109 with unclassified disease who did not meet criteria for any specific disease, the European criteria had a sensitivity of 87%. The criteria also correctly classified most patients with other disorders as not having spondyloarthropathy (specificity 87%). Validation studies have confirmed high sensitivity and specificity (>85%) for both sets of diagnostic criteria (79).

Defined by either of these criteria, the prevalence of spondyloarthropathy is considerably higher than the prevalence of each individual type of spondylitis. This is true largely because many persons with spondyloarthropathy in the population have undifferentiated or reactive disease that does not meet criteria for either AS or reactive arthritis. For example, in Eskimos who are known to have high rates of spondyloarthropathy, more persons had undifferentiated spondyloarthropathy (a milder form of disease that did not meet criteria for any of the specific rheumatic diseases encompassed by this spectrum definition) than had either reactive arthritis or AS. The overall prevalence of spondyloarthropathy in the population may be as high as 1.9% (80), a prevalence much higher than that of AS alone.

A population's prevalence of all of these disorders is directly correlated with its prevalence of HLA-B27, although these conditions do occur in the absence of HLA-B27. The explanation for why HLA-B27 causes these disorders is still uncertain (see Chapters 27 and 64). Except for psoriatic spondylitis, there is increasing evidence that persons with these disorders may have associated enteric inflammation (see Chapters 30, 64, and 66).

Ankylosing Spondylitis

Ankylosing spondylitis, a seronegative inflammatory arthritis of the spine predominant in men, is the prototype HLA-B27-associated seronegative spondylarthritis. Extra-articular manifestations may occur, especially in proximal joints and at entheses (tendon and ligament insertions into bone).

Criteria

Several sets of diagnostic criteria have been promulgated (81) (see Chapter 63). Except for criteria proposed by van der Linden et al. (82) (which have high sensitivity and specificity), their sensitivity and specificity have not been widely assessed, and different epidemiologic studies have used different criteria, unfortunately. Most studies have required definite radiographic sacroiliitis for diagnosis, plus symptoms in the lower back. Physical examination criteria have low sensitivity in patients with AS, especially those with early disease.

The development of diagnostic criteria has been hampered by the broad spectrum of illness. Many subjects have radiographic sacroiliitis but no symptoms. Others have symptoms suggestive of disease and are HLA-B27-positive relatives of patients with AS but do not have radiographic sacroiliitis (83). Also, clinical criteria can distinguish persons with AS from normal individuals, but do not neatly discriminate persons with mechanical low back pain from those with AS. Finally, diagnostic criteria have suffered from lack of reader agreement when radiographs show borderline sacroiliac abnormalities.

Prevalence and Incidence

The prevalence of AS differs markedly among ethnic and racial groups, correlating roughly with the prevalence of HLA-B27 in the population. An exception to this rule has been uncovered in the Fula ethnic group in Gambia where, even among a large number of HLA-B27-positive men, there were no cases of AS. The disease is less prevalent in American blacks than in whites, mostly because the prevalence of HLA-B27 is lower in American blacks. Chinese have a higher prevalence of HLA-B27 than Japanese and a commensurately higher disease prevalence (84). The highest rates of AS occur in Native American groups in whom HLA-B27 carriage is extraordinarily common. For example, 50% of Canadian Haida Indians are HLA-B27 positive, and their prevalence of AS is 4.2% (85–87).

In mixed white populations from Europe and the United States, the HLA-B27 prevalence ranges from 4% to 13%. The prevalence of AS in adults in these populations ranges from 0.1% (88,89) to 0.23% (90). Although the prevalence of chronic back pain in most populations is high, definite sacroiliitis on radiography is rare, leading to a relatively low estimated prevalence of disease. However, the prevalence of AS may be considerably higher than suggested by radiographic studies. A magnetic resonance imaging (MRI)-based study reported that as many as one third of persons in the population with inflammatory symptoms in their back may actually have spondylitis (69), yielding an estimated population prevalence of 0.86%, much higher than previously suggested.

Disease prevalence is highest in those 35 to 64 years of age. The incidence of disease may be highest among those 25 to 34 years of age. AS is more common in men than women, with the sex ratio ranging in different studies from 4:1 to 10:1.

The incidence of AS is extremely difficult to study because its occurrence is rare and onset is often insidious. Studies from the United States and Scandinavia suggest that the incidence rate in adults is approximately 6.9 to 7.3/100,000 per year and has not changed over the period 1935 to 1989.

Other Genetic Issues and Causal Factors

Twenty-three natural variants (subtypes) of HLA-B27 are known, and these are designated B*2701 to B*2723, each one differing from the other in from one to seven amino acid substitutions in the peptide binding groove. Some subtypes are more common in certain racial groups, but all of them, except for HLA-B*2706 and 2709, confer a high risk for AS. Indeed, Chinese who carry a susceptible phenotype of B27 have a higher prevalence of disease than Thais and Indonesians, who tend to carry B*2706 (84). In addition, in some populations in which B27 is rare, such as in West Africa, other HLA-B alleles (e.g., B*14) may increase disease susceptibility. All disease susceptibility alleles appear to share a common peptide motif (91).

The prevalence of AS among those who are HLA-B27 positive varies greatly from population to population. Also, B27-positive relatives of patients with AS have a much higher rate of disease than do B27-positive subjects from the population at large. For example, only 1.3% of HLA-B27-positive individuals drawn from the Dutch population had AS versus 21% of a group of HLA-B27-positive relatives of patients with AS who were of similar age.

Why are there such differences in the prevalence of AS among different groups of HLA-B27-positive individuals? Among HLA-B27-positive twins, the concordance of AS among monozygotic twins is much higher than among dizygotic twins (92), suggesting that genetic susceptibility to disease is not due solely to HLA-B27. Indeed, although these twin studies suggest that over 90% of the variability in occurrence of disease is due to genetic differences, rather than nongenetic or environmental factors, much of this genetic susceptibility is probably conferred by genes other than B27. In fact, at least one other type 1 MHC allele, HLA-B40, enhances susceptibility threefold, independent of HLA-B27 (92). Genome-wide scanning for disease susceptibility genes in affected sibling pairs report linkage of disease to sites both in and outside the MHC (93). Also, genes encoding for TNF-α promoter polymorphisms have been tied to disease occurrence as well as genes outside the MHC locus, such as in the interleukin-1 complex. Definitive studies to identify specific genes will involve larger numbers of cases and controls than have been included to date (94).

Other causal factors may include a high rate of subclinical inflammatory bowel disease in patients with AS as compared with nondisease controls (see Chapter 66). Unlike RA and SLE, women with AS do not appear to have pregnancy-associated lessening of disease activity, nor do they have altered fertility or pregnancy outcomes when compared with normal individuals (95).

Natural History

Prognosis varies with the severity of the disorder and its treatment. A high mortality rate was noted in the past for men with AS treated with radiation therapy. Among men and women who did not receive radiation therapy, there is a 1.5- to 1.9-fold increased mortality rate relative to age- and sex-matched controls (96–98). A variety of causes may contribute to premature mortality, including pneumonia and cardiovascular disease, and some increased mortality may be caused by the development of secondary amyloidosis. Cervical subluxation may also cause premature mortality.

Finally, the natural history of AS is affected by the time of diagnosis. Clear-cut radiographic sacroiliitis may take 10 or more years to evolve in patients with symptoms of disease (99). Therefore, the course of AS may be even more prolonged and insidious than longitudinal clinical studies suggest.

Reactive Arthritis (Formerly Reiter Syndrome)

Reactive arthritis (see Chapter 64) consists of the triad of nongonococcal urethritis, conjunctivitis, and inflammatory arthritis. Like AS and other seronegative arthritides, it is associated with HLA-B27. Although patients with classic Reiter syndrome have at least two of the components of the triad, one of which must be arthritis, many studies now suggest that an incomplete form of reactive arthritis may be as common as the full-blown disease (100). The ARA classification criteria for reactive arthritis include an episode of peripheral arthritis of more than 1 month in duration in association with urethritis or cervicitis.

The sensitivity of the criteria was 84% for the initial attack of arthritis and increased to 97% if the criteria permitted the inclusion of a subsequent attack, during which time many patients experience arthritis associated with other symptoms (101). The specificity of the criteria in differentiating reactive arthritis from other types of arthritis was 98%. The ARA definition of reactive arthritis is somewhat restrictive.

The spectrum of reactive arthritis has been expanded to include another HLA-B27-related syndrome that occurs after an enteric infection and consists of inflammatory arthritis, conjunctivitis, and other peripheral features similar to reactive arthritis. Occasionally, after an epidemic enteric infection, a second epidemic of reactive arthritis will follow, usually concentrated among HLA-B27-positive men. In some, the arthritis is transitory, whereas in others it may be chronic or intermittent. Even if an enteric infection triggered the reactive arthritis, urethritis may occur with relapses of arthritis.

Prevalence and Incidence

Reactive arthritis affects men much more often than women. The highest incidence rates have been observed in young men in the military, in whom it is more common than RA. Among men under age 50 in Rochester, Minnesota, the age-adjusted annual incidence rate was 3.5 per 100,000, with peak age of onset between 25 and 44 years. Reactive arthritis among the young men in this population was less prevalent than AS.

Causal Factors

The cause of reactive arthritis is better characterized than most other rheumatic diseases. A genetic disposition plus a triggering infection are required for disease. No other causal factors are appreciated. The genetic predisposition consists of an HLA-B27 haplotype in approximately 75% of white and about 45% of black patients with the disease. Certain native North American groups, such as the Navajo and Inuit, have high rates of HLA-B27 carriage and correspondingly high rates of reactive arthritis (102). As in AS, other genetic loci may also be tied to disease risk, including polymorphisms of TAP genes.

The infections that trigger reactive arthritis are discussed in more detail in Chapters 30 and 64. There may be a higher than expected rate of reactive arthritis in human immunodeficiency virus (HIV)-positive subjects (103), but this may also be due to the high rate of infectious urethritis and enteric infections in homosexual patients at high risk for HIV infection.

Natural History

Most patients with transitory reactive arthritis after an enteric infection do not develop full-blown chronic reactive arthritis. Up to 25% of patients who fit criteria for the chronic syndrome have complete remission of their illness after their initial episode of arthritis (104,105). On the other end of the spectrum, however, are a large percentage of patients who develop chronic and disabling disease. For example, in one series, 16% of patients had to change jobs at a 5-year follow-up and an additional 11% were unemployable. Presence of pain in the heels may portend a worse prognosis.

Inflammatory Bowel Disease Arthritis

Although only a small proportion of patients with ulcerative colitis or regional enteritis develop spondylitis, their risk is estimated to be 30 times greater than in the general population, and approximately 50% are HLA-B27 positive (106). There are two forms of colitic arthritis: a peripheral form and an axial form. The axial disease, which affects the sacroiliac joints, is strongly associated with HLA-B27 and is unrelated to the activity of the bowel disease, but the peripheral form is not and tends to wax and wane with the activity of the inflammatory bowel disease (see Chapter 66).

Psoriatic Arthritis

Psoriasis is a common skin disease among whites, with a prevalence of 1% to 2%. One impediment to the study of the epidemiology of psoriatic arthritis has been the absence of classification criteria, although attempts to define this entity are gaining strength and include criteria such as absence of RF and presence of psoriasis and dactylitis (swelling of finger or toe) (107). European and American surveys focusing on clinically diagnosed cases suggest a population prevalence ranging from 2.3 to 10.9 per 10,000 (the latter is 0.1%) (108). There are several subtypes of disease, including a peripheral arthritis and a spondyloarthropathy, the latter associated with HLA-B27, although over time, people with peripheral arthritis may develop spine or sacroiliac joint involvement. In studies of clinically diagnosed cases, the incidence of disease has ranged from 6 to 6.7 per 100,000 per year. Incidence was highest in those 45 to 54 years of age (109), with males having slightly higher incidence than females.

Peripheral arthritis is more frequent in those with advanced and severe skin involvement and usually occurs after psoriasis onset (110) (see Chapter 65). Those with psoriasis and only peripheral arthritis have a high rate of carriage of HLA-DR4, which is also associated with seropositive RA. Psoriatic arthritis appears more frequently than expected in siblings of affected patients (111). HIV infection may predispose to psoriatic arthritis (112).

Persons with psoriatic arthritis drawn from population studies do not have an increased risk for mortality compared with those of the same age and gender. However, in patients with psoriatic arthritis drawn from rheumatology clinics, there is a modestly increased risk for mortality, a risk that, nonetheless, is lower than that seen in clinic patients with RA.

CONNECTIVE TISSUE DISEASES

General Concepts

The connective tissue diseases, including RA, share several features:

1. *Host and genetic predisposition.* The impressive body of epidemiologic data described below, and reports of familial occurrence, indicate important underlying predisposing host factors. Similarities in the demographic patterns of these diseases reflect host influences, such as female preponderance and increased incidence with development of sexual maturation, especially in blacks.
2. *Overlapping clinical features.* Clinical and laboratory similarities among the diseases, and difficulty in classifying individual patients, have led investigators to consider them a family of collagen vascular diseases or connective tissue diseases. Some use such terms as *undifferentiated connective tissue disorders* or *mixed connective tissue disease syndrome* to emphasize the overlapping nature of these diseases.
3. *Blood vessels as an important target organ.* Vascular alterations are particularly frequent in these conditions. Arteries, capillaries, or veins of any size may be affected, with a spectrum of changes from noninflammatory intimal proliferative responses to acute necrotizing lesions.
4. *Immunologic correlates.* Immune alterations are often correlated with organ injury, as indicated by the presence of circulating and tissue-localized immunoglobulins, immune complexes, complement components, and changes in cell-mediated immunity. Clinical epidemiologic data suggest that these disorders share important pathogenetic mechanisms, but vary in manifestations, perhaps by virtue of different combinations of predisposing and precipitating factors operating on the major target tissues.

Systemic Lupus Erythematosus

Classification Criteria

In 1982, Tan and co-workers (113) developed classification criteria for SLE to replace earlier criteria that had become outmoded. The 1982 revised ACR criteria are discussed in Chapter 70. Data from analyses such as the ANA, anti-DNA, and anti-Sm tests were added, and later, lupus erythematosus cells were removed and tests used to diagnose the antiphospholipid antibody syndrome were substituted. These are classification criteria, not diagnostic criteria, and are most useful for study purposes, not clinical diagnosis.

Although they identify most patients with active multisystem disease, SLE disease criteria lack the sensitivity to capture many patients with mild or atypical SLE (114). In fact, the prevalence of mild or "incomplete" lupus may be higher than that of fully manifest disease. Furthermore, most persons with mild disease neither develop multisystem disease nor meet disease criteria later (115). Although some researchers have made attempts to define an incomplete lupus syndrome and others have included these patients among those with undifferentiated connective tissue disease, these patients are not generally included in evaluations of the epidemiology of SLE.

Prevalence and Incidence

SLE is an uncommon disease. In the United States and Europe, the prevalence ranges from 0.13 to 0.51 cases per 1,000 population (116). Differences in prevalence estimates could arise from different methods of case ascertainment and from different racial admixtures in populations. Like disease incidence, the prevalence of SLE may be increasing (117).

Reported incidence rates of SLE in the United States and Europe range from 1.8 to 7.6 cases per 100,000 persons per year (118–121). Much higher incidence rates (16.6–27.1 per 100,000) have been found in four Native American populations—the Crow, Arapaho, Sioux, and Alaskan coastal Indians (122,123)—but other Native American groups have incidence rates approximately equal to most U.S. and European rates.

Several studies have suggested there has been a secular increase in SLE incidence. For example, in Olmsted County, Minnesota, SLE incidence tripled from 1.5 per 100,000 in 1950 to 1979 to 5.6 per 100,000 in 1980 to 1992 (117). Part of the increase may be explained by the introduction and widespread use of serologic testing (e.g., ANA) to identify cases.

Among individuals 15 to 64 years of age, women have a 5- to 10-fold higher prevalence and incidence of SLE than men. Less female excess in prevalence and incidence is noted in children and in those 65 and older. The age-specific incidence and prevalence of SLE are highest in women 45 to 64 years of age, although in whites disease incidence remains high among women even after age 65. In men, the incidence and prevalence of disease are highest in those over age 65. Among men under 45 years of age, SLE is rare.

Black women in the United States and Europe have a threefold higher incidence and prevalence of disease than do whites (Table 1.13). Although data on rates of lupus in men are sparse, black men appear to have higher rates than white men. Also, among blacks, SLE begins, on average, at an earlier age.

As for other racial groups, studies suggest a high rate of SLE in U.S. residents of Chinese background (124), but prevalence studies from China do not show the same high prevalence rates (125). High rates of SLE have been reported among Japanese living in Hawaii, but prevalence surveys in Japan again fail to show excess prevalence. A similar high rate of SLE occurs among Indians in England but not those in India (126,127). Other groups reported to have high rates of SLE include those of Polynesian and Filipino extraction.

Thus, for those of Asian extraction, migration to the West is accompanied by an increased prevalence of SLE, a so-called prevalence gradient. For African Americans and Afro-Europeans, there may be a similar gradient (128), but it is hard to be sure, because SLE cases in Africa might not come to medical attention, leading to an underascertainment of disease. This underdiagnosis in the country of origin may also be true for those of Asian extraction, casting doubt on the veracity of the prevalence gradient. If migration to the West does increase disease incidence, the most likely explanation is that there are microbial pathogens or environmental triggers unique to Western countries that act on a susceptible genetic background. This postulate is supported by a study of SLE cases and controls of West African

TABLE 1.13. *Prevalence of systemic lupus erythematosus by sex and race per 100,000 persons*

Investigators	Location	Date	White males	White females	Black males	Black females	Overall
Siegel and Lee[a]	New York	July 1965	3	17	3	56	14.6
Fessel[b]	San Francisco	July 1973	7	71	53	286	50.8
Michet et al.[c]	Rochester, MN	January 1980	19	54	No data	No data	40.0
Hopkinson et al.[d]	Nottingham, UK	April 1990	4	45	No data	No data	24.0
Johnson et al.[e]	Birmingham, UK	April 1995	3	36	61	97	28.0
Molokhia et al[f]	London, UK	May 2001	No data	35	No data	110	No data

[a]Siegel M, Lee SL. The epidemiology of systemic lupus erythematosus. *Semin Arthritis Rheum* 1973;3:1–54.

[b]Fessel WJ. Epidemiology of systemic lupus erythematosus. *Rheum Dis Clin North Am* 1988;14:15–23.

[c]Michet CJ, McKenna CH, Elveback LR, et al. Epidemiology of systemic lupus erythematosus and other connective tissue disease in Rochester, Minnesota, 1950 through 1979. *Mayo Clin Proc* 1985;60:105–113.

[d]Hopkinson ND, Doherty M, Powell RJ. The prevalence and incidence of systemic lupus erythematosus in Nottingham, UK, 1989–1990. *Br J Rheumatol* 1993;32:110–115.

[e]Johnson AE, Gordon C, Palmer RG, et al. The prevalence and incidence of systemic lupus erythematosus in Birmingham, England. Relationship to ethnicity and country of birth. *Arthritis Rheum* 1995;38:551–558.

[f]Molokhia M, McKeigue PM, Cuadrado M, et al. Systemic lupus erythematosus in migrants from west Africa compared with Afro-Caribbean people in the UK. *Lancet* 2001;357:1414–1415.

heritage in the Caribbean showing that the degree of African genetic admixture accounted for most of the high risk for lupus (129).

Risk Factors

Hormonal and Environmental Factors

The high prevalence of SLE in women as opposed to men prompted investigations suggesting that relatively low androgen or high estrogen levels are features of those at risk for disease. For example, reduced androgen levels have been reported in men and women with disease, and heightened 16α-hydroxylation of estradiol producing high estrogenic potential is seen in SLE patients and their relatives. Women on estrogen replacement therapy may be at higher risk for SLE than nonusers (130).

Environmental chemicals implicated as causes of SLE include silica dust and aromatic amines, hydrazines, solvents, and cigarette smoke. Evidence is strongest for association with silica. After ingesting silica particles, alveolar macrophages become activated, producing a variety of cytokines. Studies of workers exposed to silica dust and of those with silicosis suggest high rates of SLE (131), and a large case control study (132) showed a dose-response effect of silica exposure on the risk for SLE for workers in trades or farming.

Smokers may or may not be at increased risk for SLE (114). Although hair dyes contain hydrazines similar to drugs that cause drug-induced lupus, hair dye exposure has, at most, only a modest effect on lupus risk (133). Persons in a community with trichloroethylene water contamination had higher rates of SLE-like symptoms compared with persons from a nonexposed community (134).

The role of nutritional factors is unknown, although alfalfa sprouts (containing the nonessential amino acid L-canavanine) have been reported to cause an SLE-like disease in monkeys and exacerbated disease in one patient.

Dogs of patients with SLE have a tendency to develop positive anti-DNA tests, suggesting a transmissible household agent (135). Also, laboratory personnel working with lupus sera or nucleic acids may be more likely to develop anti-DNA antibodies, but not ANAs, than the general population (136). The role of infectious agents as a potential cause of SLE is reviewed in Chapter 72.

Genetic Factors

First-degree relatives of persons with SLE have higher rates of disease than do controls of similar age and sex, suggesting a strong hereditary contribution to disease (137). Likewise, monozygotic twins have a much higher rate of disease sharing than dizygotic twins (138). However, the concordance rate of SLE among monozygotic twins is 58%, rather than the 100% expected if the disease were entirely genetically transmitted and fully penetrant; 10% to 12% of all cases of SLE occur among families with the disease. Familial inheritance of SLE is more likely if the patient is male or develops the disease at an early age. Patients with SLE are also likely to have relatives with positive serologies or with other connective tissue diseases.

The penetrance of the gene or genes involved in transmitting susceptibility to SLE may vary considerably, depending on environmental or endogenous factors, such as age and sex. Furthermore, the genes predisposing to disease are likely to differ by racial group. Although some rare genetic abnormalities (e.g., CIq deficiency) may be sufficient by themselves to trigger SLE, more often multiple genes may interact to increase disease susceptibility. A detailed discussion of genes predisposing to SLE can be found in Chapters 27, 28, and 72.

Natural History

Survival rates from the time of first diagnosis have improved greatly (117). Early hospital-based studies indicated a 4-year 51% survival rate (139). Clinic-based studies currently show a 90% 5-year survival rate (140) and a 10-year survival rate close to 80%. These improvements in survival are more than expected based on those seen in the general population. Reasons for the improvement might include earlier diagnosis and more frequent diagnosis of mild cases because of the availability of better serologic tests and improved therapies (steroids, immunosuppressive agents, and dialysis and transplantation for those with renal failure).

Most deaths occur within 5 years after SLE diagnosis, but there may be a bimodal curve with a second peak later (141). Early deaths result primarily from infections and less frequently from active disease (142). Gram-negative and fungal infections are increased in frequency as causes of death (143). Late deaths occurring after 10 years of disease may be due to cardiovascular complications of disease or complications of therapy.

As the mortality rate of SLE has diminished, attention has turned to the morbidity of disease and the tempo of disease flares. The development of validated instruments to assess lupus activity (144) will facilitate the measurement of disease activity over time. Several instruments are available that combine information on different organ manifestations of SLE to create a weighted sum that purportedly represents the total amount of lupus activity in a given patient. In long-term studies, lupus appears to be most active at the time of initial diagnosis, and the number of flare-ups decreases dramatically after the first 5 years of disease, and possibly even by year 2 (145,146). Although late reactivation of disease (147) may occur, it seems to be uncommon.

Patients with active renal disease or neuropsychiatric manifestations of disease at the time of diagnosis exhibit high mortality rates and perhaps high morbidity rates (148,149). Renal disease at diagnosis is an important risk factor both for death and for renal failure; however, once renal failure develops, the disease often remits. Other factors reported to be associated with a poor prognosis include

Coombs-positive hemolytic anemia (150), thrombocytopenia (143), and the presence of vasculitis or comorbidities (150). Serologic test results are not consistently predictive of a poor prognosis.

Blacks with SLE have higher case-fatality rates than whites with the disease. This may be partially attributable to their lower average socioeconomic status, a factor linked to poor prognosis (148). However, blacks have more severe disease with higher rates of renal involvement, and even after controlling for socioeconomic status, they have higher fatality rates than whites (143,151).

Older patients are unlikely to have renal disease, and some studies suggest that older patients have a better prognosis than their younger counterparts (151,152).

Polymyositis/Dermatomyositis

Classification Criteria

Poly- and dermatomyositis are a family of similar diseases in which there is idiopathic inflammatory myositis. The best accepted subgroup classification consists of the following disease categories: adult polymyositis, adult dermatomyositis, inflammatory myositis associated with cancer, childhood myositis, and myositis associated with other connective tissue diseases (overlap syndromes). (See Chapter 75 for a discussion of polymyositis and dermatomyositis.) Increasingly, this taxonomy is limited by the recognition of other forms of inflammatory myositis, such as inclusion body myositis, and by the realization that "overlap" syndromes are difficult to define because features of other connective tissue diseases are common in patients with poly- and dermatomyositis.

For epidemiologic purposes, the diagnostic criteria of Bohan and Peter (153) (Table 1.14) are used most frequently. In clinical samples, in which probable and definite disease are combined, these criteria have a sensitivity of 88% for adult poly- and dermatomyositis, and in patients with other connective tissue disorders, specificity is 93% (2). These criteria require combinations of findings including objective proximal muscular weakness, myositis on muscle biopsy, typical electromyographic features, and serum muscle enzyme elevation. Although these criteria are popular, they are imprecise in their definitions of electromyographic changes and may be outmoded by the use of myositis-specific autoantibodies to define disease and its subtypes. Criteria based on the presence of these autoantibodies (154), which are found in many persons with adult poly- and dermatomyositis but infrequently in those with other rheumatic diseases, need further validation.

TABLE 1.14. *Diagnostic criteria for polymyositis/dermatomyositis*

Manifestations

1. Typical skin rash of dermatomyositis
2. Symmetric proximal muscle weakness by history and physical examination
3. Elevation of one or more serum muscle enzymes
4. Myopathic changes on electromyogram
5. Typical polymyositis on muscle biopsy

	Bohan and Peter (153) criteria	
	Dermatomyositis	Polymyositis
Definite criterion	1 + any three of 2, 3, 4, or 5	All four of 2, 3, 4, and 5
Probable criterion	1 + any two of 2, 3, 4, or 5	Any three of 2, 3, 4, or 5
Possible criterion	1 + any one of 2, 3, 4, or 5	Any two of 2, 3, 4, or 5

Incidence and Prevalence

Estimates of the incidence of poly- and dermatomyositis have ranged from 7.4 to 10.2 per million population per year, although some of these estimates may be low because they are based on hospital discharge diagnoses, and many patients may not be hospitalized (153–155). There has been a secular increase in the incidence of this disease, but this may be because of greater awareness of the diagnosis and more widespread availability of serum enzyme muscle tests.

Poly- and dermatomyositis have a bimodal age distribution, with a peak in the 10- to 14-year-old age group, a nadir in the 15- to 24-year-old age group, and a second peak in the 45- to 64-year-old age group. These two peaks correspond to childhood dermatomyositis and adult polymyositis/dermatomyositis. A study from Allegheny County, Pennsylvania, suggests that incidence continues to increase even after age 65 years (156).

As with SLE, disease incidence is about four times greater in blacks than in whites, and both black women and men have higher disease rates than their white counterparts (156). In the Transvaal (South Africa), the incidence of dermatomyositis among the Bantu was nearly 10 times that observed among whites in the same region (157). In adults, polymyositis is the most common form of the illness, whereas, in children, dermatomyositis predominates.

Genetic Factors

Familial aggregation is rare. For studies of histocompatibility antigens, see Chapters 27 and 75.

Environmental Factors and Association with Cancer

Polymyositis occurs in nearly all climates and geographic areas. No association with family income, household crowding, or temporal-spatial clustering has been found (158). In children, a concentration of cases with onset during colder months (158) or with possible exposure to streptococcal diseases (159) has suggested upper respiratory infection as a precipitating factor. High rates of similar antecedent infections have not been found in adult poly-/dermatomyositis. Evidence implicating infections as a cause of poly-/dermatomyositis is reviewed in Chapter 30.

The risk for cancer is increased among middle-aged and older adults with dermatomyositis (160), polymyositis (161,162), and inclusion body myositis (162), although the risk is less pronounced in patients with polymyositis and inclusion body myositis. In dermatomyositis, there is a higher than expected risk for all types of malignancy, whereas in polymyositis, only non-Hodgkin's lymphoma, lung, and bladder cancers are clearly increased (161). Women with dermatomyositis have a markedly high risk for ovarian cancer (161). In dermatomyositis, cancer can occur before myositis diagnosis or as long as several years after it. In polymyositis, cancer occurs concurrent with or in the 2 years after myositis diagnosis. The occurrence of neoplasia before diagnosis of dermatomyositis suggests that it is likely to be a paraneoplastic phenomenon in some patients (161).

Natural History

Patients with polymyositis have survival rates ranging from 53% to 73% at 7 to 8 years (163,164). Those factors consistently associated with a poor prognosis include age at diagnosis over 50 years and more severe disease at onset, including the presence of marked muscle weakness, dysphonia, or cardiac muscle involvement (165). Some studies suggest that dysphagia and aspiration pneumonia, along with failure to respond to initial therapy, are also associated with a poor prognosis.

Mortality may be highest among nonwhite females. Prognosis may be better in rural areas or small towns, although it is possible that the higher mortality rates reported in urban centers may be attributed to the fact that patients with poor prognostic features tend to frequent urban medical centers (165). Survival among patients with childhood poly-/dermatomyositis is 90% or more after 6 years of follow-up.

Scleroderma

The term *scleroderma* encompasses a variety of disorders associated with hardening of the skin (see Chapter 77). The spectrum of scleroderma ranges from classic disease with diffuse cutaneous involvement (systemic sclerosis or diffuse scleroderma), to limited cutaneous disease (the CREST syndrome), in which there is calcinosis, Raynaud phenomenon, esophageal involvement, sclerodactyly, and telangiectasia, to milder variants such as forms of undifferentiated connective disease, including some elements of scleroderma and Raynaud phenomenon. Whereas systemic sclerosis meeting classification criteria is a rare disease, milder forms of disease, which include CREST syndrome and forms of undifferentiated connective tissue disease, in their totality, are much more prevalent than systemic sclerosis itself (Table 1.7). Important clinical and natural history differences between these scleroderma variants suggest that they represent distinct subsets of disease. The association of serum antitopoisomerase and anticentromere antibodies with the diffuse and CREST subsets, respectively, supports this concept.

Classification Criteria

Criteria for classification of definite systemic sclerosis have been proposed by a subcommittee of the ARA based on a multicenter longitudinal evaluation of a large number of patients with systemic sclerosis and patients with other connective tissue diseases (166) (Table 1.15). Using one major criterion, that is, proximal scleroderma (scleroderma proximal to the digits), or at least two of three minor criteria (including sclerodactyly, digital pitting scars, and bilateral basilar pulmonary fibrosis on chest roentgenogram), there was 97% sensitivity for the diffuse form of the disease and 98% specificity. These criteria for definite disease were validated in a clinical population. A validation study performed in a nonclinical population-based sample with relatively mild disease showed considerably lower sensitivity (79%) but high specificity (100%). This suggests that these criteria do not capture patients with early or mild systemic sclerosis very well, and they also are not highly sensitive for limited disease in which systemic involvement or widespread skin disease may be absent. This, in turn, may result in underestimates of disease prevalence in population studies and overrepresentation of those with severe disease in clinical studies. Modifications of the ARA criteria to incorporate new diagnostic tools such as nailfold capillary microscopy and scleroderma specific autoantibodies increase the sensitivity of these criteria for localized disease (167) without adversely affecting specificity.

TABLE 1.15. *American Rheumatism Association: preliminary clinical criteria for systemic sclerosis*[a]

Proximal scleroderma in the single major criterion; sensitivity was 91% and specificity was over 99%
Sclerodactyly, digital pitting scars of fingertips or loss of substance of the distal finger pad, and bibasilar pulmonary fibrosis contributed further as minor criteria in the absence of proximal scleroderma
One major or two or more minor criteria were found in 97% of definite systemic sclerosis patients, but in only 2% of the comparison patients with systemic lupus erythematosus, polymyositis/dermatomyositis, or Raynaud's phenomenon

[a]Excludes localized scleroderma and pseudosclerodermatous disorders.

From Masi AT, Rodnan GP, Medsger TA Jr, et al. Preliminary criteria for the classification of systemic sclerosis (scleroderma). *Arthritis Rheum* 1980;23:581–590, with permission.

Prevalence and Incidence

Early prevalence studies of diffuse scleroderma (systemic sclerosis) were hospital based and therefore missed persons with disease who were not hospitalized or who were not diagnosed. These studies suggested that this disease was rare, with prevalence ranging from 31 to 71 per million persons (Table 1.16). Using the entry point of Raynaud phenomenon, a population survey of South Carolina using several screening strategies to find diffuse scleroderma cases suggested that the disease may be much more common than previously realized, with an estimated prevalence of 286 per million. A comparably high prevalence was found in a Michigan statewide survey of rheumatologists, hospitals, and clinics (242 per million) (168) and in a survey of cases in South Australia (169) (Table 1.16). These studies likely included cases with diffuse and limited disease. Thus, either improved case ascertainment methods have substantially increased estimates of prevalence, or the disease prevalence has actually been increasing. It is also possible that the prevalence of disease is higher in the United States than in Europe, where many earlier studies were conducted. Aggressive therapy for scleroderma renal crisis has lengthened survival, and the prevalence may have increased, in part, because of this.

Incidence studies (Table 1.16) also suggest a secular increase in disease occurrence. A long-term single-center report from Pittsburgh suggests a doubling of incidence between the 1960s and the late 1970s. In England and Wales, despite the improved treatment of scleroderma, mortality rates have increased, providing additional evidence for an actual increase in incidence (170).

Black women have high rates of incident scleroderma, approximately twice as high as white women. Racial differences in incidence are especially notable in cases with onset in childbearing years. Both black and white men have about one third the incidence rate of women, but black men may have a slightly higher incidence of scleroderma than do white men (171,172). Female-to-male incidence ratios are highest for the age range 15 to 44 years and decrease for disease onset after age 45.

The incidence and prevalence of scleroderma increase with age, peaking in the 45- to 64-year-old age group, with no decline in incidence in those over age 65 (171,172). Incident cases occur as late as the seventh and eighth decades. Diffuse scleroderma is rare in children.

TABLE 1.16. *Selected studies of the incidence and prevalence of systemic sclerosis (scleroderma)*

Location	Prevalence per million	Incidence per million/year
Great Britain (1985–1986)	31	3.7
Japan (1988)	38	NA
Iceland (1975–1990)	71	NA
Australia (2001)	230	15
United States		
Olmsted County (1950–1979)	253	13
Pittsburgh[a] (1963–1972)	NA	9.6
Pittsburgh (1973–1982)	NA	18.7
South Carolina (1985)	286	NA
Michigan (1989–91)	242	18.7

[a]Hospitalization cases only.
NA, not available.

Causal Factors

The risk for scleroderma among first-degree family members of patients is 10- to 15-fold higher than the risk in the general population (173). Even so, families with multiple cases of scleroderma are rare, and monozygotic twins often do not share disease. Also, patients with scleroderma frequently have one or more relatives with other related autoimmune diseases, including RA, SLE, Raynaud phenomenon, or positive serologies. Specific genes predisposing to scleroderma are described in Chapters 76 and 77.

Scleroderma occurs more frequently in women than men. Three cases have been found in men with Klinefelter syndrome (174) who have two X chromosomes; all three had low circulating androgen levels relative to estrogens.

Scleroderma resembles graft-versus-host disease and occurs most frequently in parous women. One intriguing finding that may provide clues to disease pathogenesis has been the identification of a high concentration of fetal cells in the blood and organs of female patients with scleroderma and not in normal individuals. This so-called microchimerism involves fetal cells that persist in the maternal circulation after delivery and could serve as the source of disease (175). This topic is further discussed in Chapter 76.

Unusual toxic or environmental exposures may cause scleroderma-like illnesses. These substances, listed in Table 1.17, and their association with disease support the hypothesis that toxins may trigger disease in genetically suscepti-

TABLE 1.17. *Occupational and other agents implicated in causing scleroderma-like illnesses*

Occupational
- Vinyl chloride
- Silica dust
- Organic solvents—aromatic, chlorinated, and aliphatic hydrocarbons
- Biogenic amines—epoxy resins and metaphenylenediamine

Other
- Adulterated rapeseed oil (toxic oil syndrome)
- L-tryptophan (eosinophilia myalgia syndrome)
- Drugs—bleomycin and pentazocine

Modified from Steen VD. Systemic sclerosis. *Rheum Dis Clin North Am* 1990;16:641–654, with permission.

ble hosts. Scleroderma-like cutaneous lesions, Raynaud phenomenon, nailfold capillary changes, and osteolysis of the distal phalanges have been described in workers exposed to vinyl chloride used in the manufacture of plastics (176). Vinyl chloride workers, however, exhibit features of disease uncommon in scleroderma, such as thrombocytopenia and abnormal liver function. Also, workers exposed to silica dust may have high rates of diffuse scleroderma. Organic solvents such as benzene, toluene, and xylene and prolonged exposure to chlorinated aliphatic hydrocarbons (e.g., trichloroethylene) increase the risk for diffuse scleroderma and scleroderma-like illnesses (177). Long-term exposure to paint thinners, which contain several of these organic compounds, also may increase the risk for disease (178). Either all of these environmental chemicals, which tend to have different toxicities, cause scleroderma through some common mechanism, or the recollection of past exposures may be nonspecific, leading scientists to be unable to tease out the causative agent (178).

Nonoccupational exposures also may cause scleroderma-like illnesses. These include eosinophilia myalgia syndrome (EMS), a multiorgan disease with painful skin induration, which was causally linked to contaminated L-tryptophan in the form of di-L-tryptophan. A similar disorder characterized by fever, eosinophilia, and pneumonia and EMS-like skin and neurologic lesions, was reported in Spain among persons who ingested adulterated rapeseed oil. Both of these toxin exposures produce a syndrome more suggestive of eosinophilic fasciitis than scleroderma. Drug-induced scleroderma-like illnesses have also been documented. For example, bleomycin, used to treat cancer, commonly causes Raynaud phenomenon and interstitial pulmonary disease, also a manifestation of scleroderma.

Despite public concerns, evidence from large, well-designed epidemiologic studies indicates that silicone breast implants do not predispose to either scleroderma (179) or other diagnosed rheumatic diseases (180).

Natural History

The course of scleroderma depends mainly on its clinical manifestations. Patients with diffuse disease have relatively poor prognoses, whereas patients with the limited form of disease (such as CREST syndrome) often have a good prognosis. Clinical studies evaluating mostly those with diffuse disease suggest that the 5-year cumulative survival rate from the date of diagnosis ranges from 34% to 86% (181). Many of these studies, however, predate the use of antihypertensive drugs for the treatment of scleroderma renal crisis.

Even after the widespread use of antihypertensives, the age- and gender-adjusted mortality rates for patients with diffuse scleroderma are four- to eightfold higher than in the general population (182). Even those with limited scleroderma have two- to threefold higher mortality rates.

Patients with scleroderma are at increased risk for developing lung cancer. This risk is especially increased in those with pulmonary interstitial fibrosis, and the risk is independent of smoking (183).

Vasculitis

Vasculitis syndromes are characterized by inflammation of arteries, capillaries, or veins (see Chapter 82). These may occur independently of or in association with other rheumatic diseases. The various vasculitis syndromes are often classified according to the type of vessel involved and the histology of the inflammation in the vessel wall. Hypersensitivity vasculitis, affecting small vessels and often occurring after an infection or drug exposure, is the most common and is usually transitory.

Some forms of vasculitis affect certain subsets of the population. For example, Kawasaki syndrome affects infants, especially in Japan and Hawaii. Churg-Strauss vasculitis usually affects adults with a history of asthma. Giant cell (temporal) arteritis (discussed below) occurs most often in older women of Northern European extraction. Behçet syndrome, a vasculitis associated with oral and genital ulceration, is especially frequent in Japan and the Middle East and has a marked male predominance.

Other forms of vasculitis can affect those of either gender and any age. These include Wegener granulomatosus, a granulomatous vasculitis strongly associated with blood test positivity for antineutrophil cytoplasmic antibody. Also, polyarteritis nodosa and variants of it affect muscular arteries and are often caused by hepatitis B infection. Cryoglobulinemia is a form of vasculitis in which antibodies complexed with other molecules precipitate in serum in the cold. Increasing in recognition and frequency, most cases of cryoglobulinemia are caused by hepatitis C infections. In general, HLA and other genetic associations have not been found in vasculitis syndromes, but among patients with Behçet syndrome, there is an increased frequency of HLA-B51.

Because of their rarity, there are few estimates of the incidence and prevalence of different types of vasculitis, and all estimates of each type are based on small numbers of cases. The availability of classification criteria for vasculitis (184,185) has facilitated incidence and prevalence studies. Criteria set developers have used two approaches: one set from the ACR used statistical methods to distinguish different types of vasculitis (184), whereas the other, exemplified by the Chapel Hill Consensus Criteria (185), was developed by experts with an eye toward clinical and pathologic features that defined each syndrome. There are strengths and weaknesses of each approach. The ACR criteria sometimes are not easily applicable to unclassified cases and, because they were developed only among those with diagnosed forms of vasculitis, are not optimal in distinguishing those with vasculitis from those without it (186).

TABLE 1.18. *Annual incidence of systemic vasculitides in Norwich, England, 1988–1994*

Type	Annual incidence per 1,000,000 persons
Wegener granulomatosis	8.5
Churg-Strauss vasculitis	2.4
Microscopic polyarteritis[a]	2.4
Cryoglobulinemia	1.2
Unclassified	4.8

Norwich is an isolated region with a central referral of diseases.

The prevalences of hepatitis B and C (which are strongly associated with risks of polyarteritis and cryoglobulinemia, respectively) are low, and therefore these estimates may be lower than those from a more diverse and heavily urban population.

[a]This category includes many patients with polyarteritis nodosa.

From Watts RA, Carruthers DM, Scott DGI. Epidemiology of systemic vasculitis: changing incidence or definition? *Semin Arthritis Rheum* 1995;25:28–34, with permission.

TABLE 1.19. *Incidence of temporal arteritis: annual rate per 100,000 in persons age 50 and over: from high to low disease rates*

	No. of cases	Rate
Southern Norway, 1987–1994	66	29.0
Iceland, 1984–1990	133	27.0
Ribe County, Denmark, 1982	46	23.3
Denmark (whole country), 1982–1993	—	20.0
Göteberg, Sweden, 1977–1986	284	18.3
Olmsted County, Minnesota, 1950–1991	125	17.8
Göteberg, Sweden, 1973–1975	74	16.8
Jerusalem, Israel, 1980–1991	84	10.2
Lugo, Spain, 1986–1995	93	9.4
Loire-Atlantic, France, 1975–1979	110	9.4
Reggio Emilia, Italy, 1980–1988	41	6.9
Lothian, Scotland, 1964–1977	136	4.2
Shelby County, Tennessee, 1971–1980	26	1.58
Israel, 1960–1978	46	0.49

The latter criteria do not subset patients into mutually exclusive criteria (some patients may meet criteria for more than one) and are not operationalized specifically, so they are hard to apply and may miss some subjects with clear-cut disease.

Excluding temporal arteritis, Wegener granulomatosus has the highest prevalence of the chronic systemic vasculitides. The prevalence of Wegener disease is approximately 3 per 100,000 persons (187). Incidence of different forms of vasculitis is shown in Table 1.18. Clinical and pathologic descriptions of vasculitis can be found in Chapters 83 through 89.

Temporal Arteritis

Temporal (giant cell) arteritis (see Chapter 85) is the most common form of vasculitis in people over age 50. In temporal arteritis, the vascular inflammation predominantly involves the aortic arch and large to medium-sized elastic vessels outside the cranium. Giant cells and other inflammatory cells are noted near the internal elastic lamina in arterial specimens obtained by biopsy or necropsy. Clinical manifestations include headache, scalp tenderness, jaw claudication, visual disturbance, and an elevated erythrocyte sedimentation rate (ESR). Temporal arteritis may produce symptoms of a much more common syndrome called polymyalgia rheumatica (PMR), characterized by proximal muscle aching and stiffness associated with a high ESR in persons over age 50. The overlap between these two disorders is considerable. The percentage of patients with PMR who have coexistent evidence of temporal arteritis either by symptoms or biopsy is 15% to 31% (188). Conversely, approximately one half of patients with temporal arteritis have PMR.

The prevalence of these related disorders has been difficult to study, in part because PMR and temporal arteritis remit and relapse frequently and point prevalence is therefore difficult to estimate. Incidence has been better studied. The incidence rates of temporal arteritis (Table 1.19) are highest among those over 50 in Minnesota (where many are of Scandinavian backgrounds) and in Denmark, Sweden, and Iceland, and rates may be the highest in the world in Southern Norway. Lower rates are reported from France, Italy, Scotland (189,190), Spain (191), and Shelby County, Tennessee, which has a mixed racial population (192). Although the differences in incidence are impressive, studies generating these estimates used different disease criteria and different ascertainment methods. The Shelby County rate is especially low, perhaps because only hospitalized patients were studied. In the United States and Europe, the incidence of temporal arteritis is increasing and this is not fully accounted for just by the aging of the population (191,193).

Polymyalgia rheumatica incidence rates are several times higher than those for temporal arteritis; studies of PMR incidence are generally based on clinically diagnosed cases, and prospective evaluations of elderly populations suggest that the point prevalence may be as high as 2%. If so, many cases go undiagnosed and actual incidence is likely to be higher than reported.

The incidence of temporal arteritis increases with age after age 50. The highest reported rates are among those in their sixties, seventies, and perhaps even eighties (194). In Northern Europe and the United States, there is a female/male predominance of up to 4:1.

Temporal arteritis is an unusually reported diagnosis in Asian populations and in black Africa. In the United States, it is uncommon among blacks (192) and Latinos (195), although it may be more common in U.S. blacks than previously recognized (195). Racial differences do not necessarily account for all of the geographic differences in incidence. For example, the rates among whites in Minnesota appear to be substantially higher than those among whites in Tennessee. It is still not clear whether the incidence of this disease truly varies with geography or with race, but available evidence suggests that both variables are important.

Familial occurrence of temporal arteritis has been noted among siblings, monozygotic twins, and in a father and daughter (190), suggesting that genetic background may confer disease susceptibility. HLA-DR4 increases the risk for both temporal arteritis and polymyalgia rheumatica (2).

Temporal arteritis, especially in women, may be increased in prevalence among smokers (196) and among those with a history of myocardial infarction or peripheral vascular disease (189). The association with vascular disease and smoking may be due to misreading by pathologists of temporal artery biopsy results. For temporal arteritis, long-term studies have reported cyclical peaks in incidence, at a periodicity of 5 to 7 years (197,198) and seasonal variation in incidence (although studies vary as to which season or month marks the highest incidence time). If occurrence follows a periodic pattern, this may implicate an infectious etiology. In one study, peak incidences correlated with epidemics of mycoplasma pneumonia and in another with parvovirus epidemics. Indeed, one study (but not another) has suggested that parvovirus B19 DNA is more often present in temporal artery specimens from those with this disease than controls without it (199,200).

The prognosis of temporal arteritis and polymyalgia rheumatica is generally favorable with a rate of mortality that is either equal to (201) or modestly higher than persons of the same age (190,191). A percentage of patients suffer severe and fatal disease, often before initiation of adequate therapy. Temporal arteritis is treated with high doses of corticosteroids, and morbidity often results from side effects of the treatment.

NONARTICULAR RHEUMATISM AND FIBROMYALGIA

What defines the primary forms of nonarticular rheumatism and fibromyalgia is pain or tenderness in nonarticular areas. Patients with these disorders generally have no clinical or laboratory evidence of inflammation and usually have no frank arthritis. Common and often regional, these disorders include sports-related and occupational soft tissue rheumatism.

Fibromyalgia Syndrome

Fibromyalgia is a disorder consisting of at least two elements: chronic widespread generalized pain, especially in nonarticular areas, and a series of other symptoms such as fatigue, sleep disturbance, cognitive alterations, and psychological distress. In the past, other names have been used for this syndrome, including fibrositis and diffuse myofascial pain. Classification criteria for fibromyalgia have been developed (for further discussion see Chapter 91); the ACR criteria require both chronic widespread pain and multiple "tender points" that consist of tenderness at characteristic sites. The presence of these tender points correlates with evidence of chronic emotional distress such as depression, anxiety, and fatigue (202). Many patients with chronic fatigue syndrome fulfill the criteria for fibromyalgia (203). It must be recognized that pain and nonarticular tenderness occur along a continuum ranging from localized to diffuse. Fibromyalgia is at the extreme of this continuum, and increasingly, evidence suggests that it is associated with a neurologically mediated increase in pain sensitivity. Whether localized nonarticular tenderness (e.g., tendonitis) represents a fundamentally different pathology from diffuse tenderness (e.g., fibromyalgia) is unclear (204). Diffuse complaints are associated more often than local ones with fatigue and depression.

The point prevalence of widespread pain (defined as pain in both sides of the body above and below the waist lasting ≥3 months) is 11% to 12% in mostly white adult populations (205). On the other hand, those identified in the population with chronic widespread pain often do not meet criteria for chronic widespread pain when resurveyed, although they often have regional pain.

Fibromyalgia is present in a subset of those with chronic widespread pain, generally those with evidence of emotional distress (206). Fibromyalgia is one of the most common musculoskeletal disorders affecting adults. In rheumatology clinics, fibromyalgia is either the first or second most prevalent diagnosis (207). Large studies from Europe and the United States of fibromyalgia prevalence in adults have shown rates ranging from 0.7% to 4.8% (Table 1.20). Generally, these population studies initially survey subjects to determine who has widespread pain, and those with pain are examined to see if they have tender points. Differences in estimates occur for one or more of these reasons: different criteria used for the syndrome; different examiners who may have different thresholds for a positive examination; failure of some studies to include a full tender point examination; time elapsed after the survey, since widespread pain (and tender points) may not persist; subjects with different ages; and possibly real differences in fibromyalgia prevalence. The incidence of fibromyalgia is also high, with one report of an incidence of 0.58% per year in women 26 to 55 years of age. Fibromyalgia primarily affects women, with a female/male ratio of at least 2:1, and in many studies 90% of the fibromyalgia subjects are women. Fibromyalgia prevalence appears to increase with age, being most common in women after age 50, but after around age 65 prevalence diminishes both in men and women. Fibromyalgia also commonly occurs in school-age children, in whom the prevalence is 1.2% to 6.2%. Clinic-based studies suggest that whites and Hispanics both have

TABLE 1.20. *Prevalence of fibromyalgia in adults from selected studies*

Country	Prevalence (%)	Age range (yr)	No. of subjects screened	No. of subjects examined
Finland	0.8	≥30	7,217	3,434
Denmark	0.7[a]	≥16	1,595	65
Sweden	1.1	50–56	900	552
Germany	3.0	25–74	541	60
Poland	4.5	Not restricted	1,105	110
Great Britain	4.8	18–75	2,034	177
United States	2.0	Not restricted	3,006	391

[a]Assumes no fibromyalgia cases in persons screened positive yet not contacted. If not correct, prevalence = 1.4%.

Modified from Schochal T, Croft P, Raspe H. The epidemiology of fibromyalgia: Workshop of the Standing Committee on Epidemiology European League Against Rheumatism (EULAR), Bad Sackingen, 19–21, November 1992. *Br J Rheumatol* 1994;33:783–786, with permission.

high prevalence rates, but that the prevalence of fibromyalgia may be lower in blacks (208).

There are several well-known risk factors for fibromyalgia. First, at least in clinic-based settings, fibromyalgia is associated with, and often preceded by, major depression (209). Other associated syndromes include migraine, irritable bowel syndrome, and a variety of sleep disorders. The syndrome often begins after a fall or a car accident or other physical trauma in which the neck or lower back is injured, triggering diffuse pain. Other factors associated with high rates of fibromyalgia include positive ANA test results (210), low educational attainment (211), having a service or manual labor job with high physical stress (211), sleep apnea, hyperprolactinemia, and, possibly, in children, joint hypermobility.

Natural history investigations suggest that fibromyalgia, if diagnosed in the clinic, is chronic with persistent pain, sleep disturbance, and care seeking (212). As noted above, those identified in population surveys may have transitory symptoms. Persons with a traumatic cause may have a more severe clinical course. Current widespread pain may be associated with a heightened risk for mortality.

Soft Tissue Rheumatism

Regional soft tissue disorders constitute the most common forms of rheumatic disease. The pathophysiology of these complaints is often not well understood. For example, an epidemic of chronic upper limb pain occurred among workers in Australia, but an intensive investigation of 229 patients found that only 29 had recognizable rheumatologic diagnoses (213). Regional complaints vary from the easily diagnosable to the enigmatic.

One of the most common sites of musculoskeletal pain is the neck. Approximately 10% of the adult population has neck pain at any given time, and 35% to 60% have experienced episodes of neck pain. Fortunately, severe disability associated with neck pain is uncommon, and approximately 70% of those with pain noted marked symptomatic improvement within a month. The pathophysiology of neck pain is not well understood. Many patients are said to have muscle strain, whereas others may have OA of the cervical spine. Systemic disorders, including RA, can also cause neck pain. Risk factors for neck pain have not been well investigated.

Shoulder pain is also extraordinarily common. Its exact prevalence is hard to estimate because self-reported shoulder pain can be neck pain and vice versa, with an examination required to corroborate the source of the pain. In the NHANES I survey in the United States, 6.75% of the adult population claimed they had suffered from shoulder pain of more than 1 month's duration, but other studies suggest that briefer episodes of shoulder pain are as common as episodes of knee or back pain, occurring in up to 25% of adults (7). The pathophysiology of shoulder pain is generally well understood, usually being ascribed to rotator cuff, bicipital tendinitis, or bursitis, and rarely to arthritis of the shoulder joint itself. Shoulder pain appears to increase with age (214), and in most series is more common in women than men. Also, it tends to affect the right side more frequently than the left, probably because it is the dominant side in most people. Persons with jobs that demand shoulder or arm loading during work, including dentists (215), have a high frequency of shoulder complaints (214). In addition, adult diabetics have a higher rate of shoulder calcification on radiographs than do age- and sex-matched nondiabetic controls, and this may predispose them to a high rate of shoulder tendonitis (216).

Carpal tunnel syndrome consists of median nerve compression in the wrist, causing paresthesias in a distribution corresponding to the area supplied by the nerve. Approximately 55% of patients with carpal tunnel syndrome have bilateral involvement. The dominant hand tends to be involved first and is usually more severely affected. In a population prevalence survey, carpal tunnel syndrome confirmed by tests showing slowed nerve conduction velocity was found in 9.2% of adult women (of whom 3.4% had already been diagnosed) and only 0.6% of men (217). In women, prevalence was highest in those 45 to 74 years of age. Other studies have also reported a high prevalence in women, with female/male ratios ranging from 2:1 to 6.6:1. Interestingly, the prevalence of delayed median nerve conduction across the wrist, depending on how it is defined, may be even more prevalent than diagnosed carpal tunnel syndrome and may be almost as prevalent in men as in women (218). Furthermore, many patients with even classic carpal tunnel symptoms do not appear to have delayed median nerve conduction, and many in the population with documented decreases in nerve conduction have few if any symptoms.

Carpal tunnel syndrome occurs more often than expected in women during pregnancy, after ovariectomy or hysterectomy, and in the early postmenopausal period, and may be more common in women who have used oral contraceptives for at least 5 years than in nonusers (219,220). Furthermore, those whose jobs require repetitive hand motion; prolonged wrist flexion or extension (219); high hand muscle force, especially if applied repetitively; or use of vibratory tools are all at high risk for carpal tunnel syndrome. Although not likely to account for most cases, diabetes and hypothyroidism may predispose to carpal tunnel syndrome, and obesity is also an important risk factor.

LOW BACK PAIN

Chronic impairments of the lower back are the most frequent cause of activity limitations among persons under 45 years of age in the United States, and they rank third as causes of activity limitations in persons age 45 to 64 years (221). The lifetime prevalence of low back pain ranges from 60% to 80%, and in any given month 35% to 37% of adults experience at least one episode of back pain lasting over 24 hours (222). Fortunately, most episodes of low back pain are transitory. Almost half of those seeking care remit within a week; roughly 90% improve within a month. Only 7% have an episode that lasts at least 6 months, but those with a long duration of pain account for most of the economic cost of low back pain. Back pain is often episodic, and recurrences are frequent.

In most patients, specific anatomic lesions causing low back pain cannot be identified. In most cases, neither findings on radiography nor on MRI (223) identify a particular pathologic lesion causing low back pain. Neurologic findings and radicular symptoms along with pain in the sciatic distribution suggest discogenic disease, but most patients do not have any of these symptoms or findings.

The first episodes of low back pain occur most frequently between the ages of 20 and 40 years (221). Women may have a slightly higher prevalence of back pain than men, but back pain leading to workman's compensation is more prevalent in men. Lumbar disc disease, as identified by surgical cases, is more frequent in men (224). The prevalence of back pain remains high throughout adult life, becoming slightly less prevalent after age 75. However, back pain accounts for considerable disability among elders (225).

Cross-sectional and longitudinal studies have identified several characteristics of persons at risk for low back pain. Those in jobs requiring strenuous physical labor, especially ones that require lifting, pushing, or pulling heavy objects and jobs that entail repeated twisting activities, especially during lifting, are at high risk for back pain (221,226). Other occupational features implicated include repeated exposure to vibration. Truck drivers experience the most back injury, with material handlers second, and nurses and nursing aides third (227).

Other occupational factors may increase the risk for low back pain. Ironically, some sedentary jobs may be associated with increased risk, especially if the job requires that the person stay in one position for a long time. Studies suggest that low back pain occurs within a few years after an individual starts the job rather than later on (228).

Modifiable personal factors affect back pain risk, suggesting opportunities for prevention. Smokers are at increased risk for back pain (229), whereas physical fitness may prevent it. Prospective studies have identified weak lumbar extensors (230) and quadriceps (231) as risk factors for incident back pain

Those with severe recurrent low back pain often have typical psychological profiles. They tend to be depressed and anxious, and experience high levels of psychological stress. Even before developing back pain, they are often dissatisfied with their jobs. Adolescents with other somatic symptoms, such as headache and abdominal pain, are at high risk for developing back pain (232). Although psychological stress may make a person vulnerable to back pain, the presence of stress makes an acute back pain sufferer much more likely to develop chronic pain and experience greater levels of disability than those without any psychological abnormalities (233,234).

In industry, training has been successful in preventing low back pain, especially training workers to keep objects close to their body when they lift and to maintain good physical fitness (228). Job modifications ultimately may prevent a substantial proportion of low back pain.

OSTEOARTHRITIS

OA is the most common joint disorder. Pathologic evidence of disease is almost universal in elderly people, and clinical manifestations are common.

Definitions of Disease

The most widely used epidemiologic criteria for OA are the radiographically based Kellgren and Lawrence criteria

(235). In most studies using these criteria, OA cases are defined as those with grade 2 or greater changes (osteophytes with or without joint space narrowing). Other investigators have used a definition of disease that is also radiographic but requires at least joint space narrowing (236). New radiographic grading schemes for OA have been proposed in which osteophytes and joint space narrowing are graded rather than recorded as present or absent (237). Despite these attempts to define disease by radiographs, pathologic lesions in cartilage and other tissues are often advanced by the time radiographs become diagnostic of OA.

An ACR committee has produced diagnostic criteria for hand, knee, and hip OA that focus on clinical disease, not just radiographic changes. These criteria focus on symptomatic disease, usually defined as joint symptoms and radiographic changes of OA in the affected joint. The non-OA group used to develop these criteria had mostly RA, so the criteria are better at distinguishing OA from RA than identifying those with OA in the general population.

Prevalence and Incidence

OA affects some joints and spares others. For example, in the hands, the distal interphalangeal (DIP) joints, proximal interphalangeal (PIP) joints, and carpometacarpal (CMC) joint of the thumb are frequently involved. The cervical and lumbosacral spine, hip, knees, and first metatarsophalangeal (MTP) joint are often affected, whereas the ankle, wrist, elbow, and, to a lesser extent, shoulder are usually spared. OA especially involves weight-bearing lower extremity joints and joints in the hand involved in the pincer grip.

The prevalence of OA varies depending on which joint is being assessed and how disease is defined. Many persons with radiographic disease do not have symptoms, and radiographic OA alone has a much higher prevalence than symptomatic OA (symptoms and radiographic OA). Also, prevalence differs depending on the threshold for symptoms—the prevalence of mild symptoms is high but the prevalence of severe daily symptoms associated with disability is less (238) (Fig. 1.3). As many as 25% of persons age 55 and over have knee pain on most days, but only half of these have radiographic OA, making the prevalence of symptomatic OA in this age group around 12.5%. The prevalence of disabling knee pain is considerably lower, with the proportion of patients in England 35 years and over having severe enough pain and disability to merit a knee replacement being 2.7%.

Regardless of how it is defined, OA prevalence increases strikingly with age. For example, historical data from England suggest that symptomatic hand OA occurs in 2% to 4% of adults. In persons age 70 and over from the Framingham Study, the prevalence was as high as 20% (239). The prevalence of symptomatic knee OA is 6.1% in adults age 30 and over in Framingham, but increases to over 12% to 13% in those age 63 and over. Although symptomatic hip OA is uncommon in young adults, it occurs in 5.5% of men age 55 and over and in 3.6% of women this age (240).

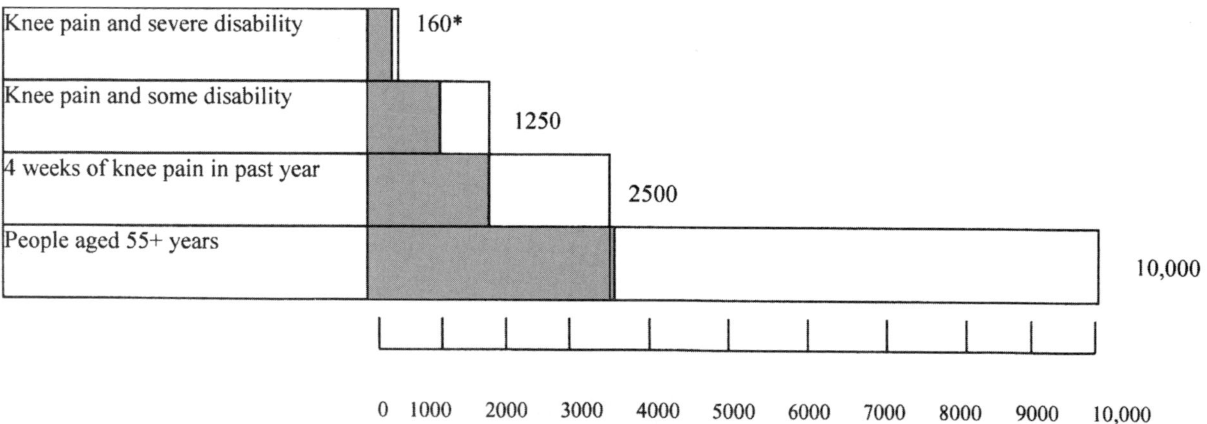

FIG. 1.3. The prevalence of knee pain and osteoarthritis in persons age 55 years and older in England. This "prevalence staircase" shows that the prevalence of knee pain depends on the level of disability and pain, with knee pain and severe disability being uncommon, but frequent knee pain alone being highly prevalent. Shading represents the proportion in each category with radiographic evidence of osteoarthritis. *The proportion with radiographic evidence in this category is not known, although likely to be high. (Adapted from Peat G, McCarney R, Croft P. Knee pain and osteoarthritis in older adults: a review of community burden and current use of primary health care. *Ann Rheum Dis* 2001; 60:91–97, with permission.)

OA occurs more frequently and is more often generalized in women than in men. Under age 45, it occurs with roughly equal frequency in men and women, but after age 50, disease in most joints (especially hands, knees, neck, and lower back) is more common in women. The sex difference in prevalence widens in the elderly (240–242).

Radiographic OA of the hand joints occurs in more than 70% of those age 65 and over (243), but most of these persons do not have symptoms. Radiographic changes in the lumbosacral spine are common, but there is a poor correlation between these changes and back symptoms. In hips and knees, however, the more severe the radiographic disease, the more likely it is to produce symptoms. Furthermore, in knees and hips, symptoms are often disabling.

African Americans appear to have roughly similar rates of knee and hip OA as white Americans, at least in one rural community that is being intensively studied (244,245). Other studies have suggested a very low prevalence of hip OA among black populations in Jamaica, South Africa, Nigeria, and Liberia (1%–4% for radiographic OA) in comparison with European populations (7%–25%).

The prevalence of hip OA is low among Asians. In one study (246), only 1% of Hong Kong residents age 55 and older had hip OA. In a study using uniform methods of ascertainment in the United States and Beijing, the age-adjusted prevalence of radiographic hip OA in China was roughly one tenth of that in the United States, with only one case of symptomatic hip OA seen in 1,500 Chinese elders (247). Furthermore, among those of Asian origin in the United States, hip arthroplasty performed for OA is exceedingly uncommon, suggesting that the low prevalence is not due to environmental factors. Indeed, recent work (248) has found a compelling explanation for the racial difference in anatomic differences in hip structure. Interestingly, knee OA is as prevalent or more prevalent in China compared with the United States, even though Chinese are thinner (249); the daily squatting of Chinese may account for some of their high knee OA prevalence. Hand OA, like hip OA, is less prevalent in China, and given the high heritability of hand OA, the low prevalence may suggest that Chinese do not share some OA susceptibility genes (250).

The incidence of symptomatic OA (Table 1.21) for knee OA is at least twice as great as for either hip or hand disease. For all joints, incidence increases with age and is greater in women than in men, especially after age 50.

TABLE 1.21. *Prevalence and incidence of symptomatic osteoarthritis*

Affected	Prevalence (sources)	Incidence/1,000/ year (sources)
Knee	6.1% (Framingham study)	2 (Olmsted County and Massachusetts)
Hip	0.7% (NHANES I)	0.5–0.74 (Olmsted County and Massachusetts)
Hand	2.4% (Lawrence et al.)[a]	0.9 (Massachusetts)

NHANES, National Health and Nutrition Examination Survey.

From Lawrence JS. *Rheumatism in populations.* Bristol, UK: JW Arrowsmith, 1977:98–155, with permission.

Risk Factors

Malalignment and Local Stressors

Joints become vulnerable to local cartilage and bone injury when they are misshapen or when loading is not uniform across the joint. This causes focal injury within the joint that can lead to high local stresses, further focal injury, and ultimately malalignment or even joint subluxation. Examples include the high prevalence of OA in adults who had congenital or developmental hip diseases, such as congenital hip dysplasia or slipped capital femoral epiphysis. Both of these disorders leave hips misshapen, with excess stress during load on localized areas of cartilage and bone, which then break down. A similar phenomenon occurs when there is malalignment across the knee, imparting varus (medial) or valgus (lateral) stresses. In persons who already have knee OA, varus or valgus malalignment predisposes to rapid cartilage loss (251).

Obesity

Overweight persons more often have knee OA than persons who are not overweight. This is true regardless of how knee OA is defined, whether by symptoms or radiography, and irrespective of whether the focus is on tibiofemoral (252) or patellofemoral (253,254) disease. Longitudinal studies confirm that being overweight increases a person's risk for knee OA, and most studies suggest that the relationship of obesity to knee OA is stronger in women than men (255). Obese persons are at high risk for having bilateral, but not necessarily unilateral, radiographic hip OA (256), and obesity increases the risk for symptomatic hip OA.

Weight change also appears to affect the risk for OA development and progression, perhaps even more dramatically than average weight. In the Framingham Study, a weight loss of 11 pounds in women of medium height was associated with a 50% reduction in the risk for developing symptomatic knee OA. The relationship of increased body weight with hip OA is not as strong as it is with knee OA.

Just why obesity causes OA is unknown. The obvious explanation, increased joint loading, likely accounts for much of the potent effect of obesity on the risk for knee OA and its modest effect on hip OA, but cannot explain why obesity is associated in some, but not all, studies with hand OA, nor does it explain the stronger association of OA with obesity in women. Factors correlated with obesity such as serum lipids, uric acid levels, diabetes, body fat distribution, blood pressure, and high bone density have been investigated, but none was more strongly predictive of OA than obesity itself (257,258).

Acute and Repetitive Joint Injuries

Acute major joint injuries frequently lead to OA (259). Such injuries are common during sports activities and may explain the high rates of knee OA in retired professional athletes. Injury may account for a large proportion of OA cases in joints such as the ankle and shoulder in which OA is otherwise rare.

Stereotyped repetitive joint use in some jobs may lead to OA. The rates of knee and finger OA in shipyard and dockyard workers are high, as are the rates of hand OA in cotton mill workers. In a Virginia textile mill, workers whose jobs required repeated fine pincer grip had higher rates of OA in the DIP joint than control subjects whose jobs did not require such repeated joint use (260). Farmers have much higher than expected rates of hip OA, but the particular farming activities associated with risk for OA are unknown (261). Compared with those in other jobs, workers whose jobs require knee bending and lifting have more than double the prevalence of radiographic knee OA (262). In China, prolonged squatting was associated with an increased risk for tibiofemoral disease.

Most investigations of athletics and OA have compared athletes or former athletes with controls. The effect of the athletics per se is difficult to disentangle from major joint injuries that may occur during sports. Furthermore, it is hard to tease out the effects on joints of endurance, high intensity, and high impact. Even so, studies have consistently indicated that elite athletes are at high risk for later OA, especially in weight-bearing joints. Compared with controls, soccer players have high rates of knee OA (263,264), even those without a history of major injury. Elite runners also are at increased risk for OA in later life (264–273) (Table 1.22).

Intriguingly, the general level of physical activity itself may increase the risk for developing OA, especially in older persons or those whose joints have been previously injured. In elderly Framingham Study subjects without OA followed for 8 years, high levels of physical activity increased the risk for OA threefold compared with a sedentary lifestyle. Those reporting frequent heavy activities were at especially high risk (274). Such activities were generally typified by leisure time walking and gardening. Longitudinal studies of younger subjects have not revealed a link between physical activity and the development of knee OA.

One way to synthesize findings on activities and OA is to distinguish between vulnerable and normal joints. Vulnerable joints are vulnerable to modest loading and stress because mechanisms protecting these joints are impaired. Aging represents the prime cause of vulnerability, but previous injury also provides a model. Physical activity across normal joints is unlikely to result in OA, unless that activity is excessive or injurious, beyond normal protective mechanisms. Studies of workers and elite athletes suggest that excessive repetitive activities damage joints. Framingham Study results indicate that older joints may be more vulnerable to activity-related damage than are younger ones.

TABLE 1.22. *Summary of studies of running and the risk for knee/hip osteoarthritis (OA)*

Elite runners[a] are not at increased risk for knee and hip OA
No increased risk of knee OA has been shown for leisure-time runners
Reports conflict on whether leisure-time runners have heightened risk for hip OA
Major knee injuries increase OA risk and may act synergistically to increase OA risk in runners

This table combines studies of clinical and radiographic OA, as there is no evidence that they differ in results.

[a]Elite runners generally defined as nationally competitive runners or Olympic team members.

Generalized Disease and Heredity

Patients with OA in one joint often have OA elsewhere. They may have generalized OA, which can involve the DIP, PIP, and first CMC joints, joints in the cervical and lumbar spines, knees, first MTP joints, and, occasionally, hips. Generalized OA is more common in women than men.

Many extended families with high rates of early-onset generalized OA have been described (275,276) in which the occurrence of OA has been linked to an autosomal-dominant mutation in type II procollagen. Nonetheless, in the general population, the relationship between type II collagen abnormalities or polymorphisms and the inheritance of OA is not strong (277).

In the hands, greater than 50% of OA occurrence may be associated with inheritance, but for knees this percentage appears to be smaller (278,279), perhaps because knee OA often develops less as a function of inheritance than as a result of repeated mechanical insults or other lifestyle factors. Also, the heritability of OA may be higher in women than men (280). Many genes predisposing to OA may be joint specific and may not confer an increase of generalized disease (281).

Another possible cause of the generalized OA diathesis is crystal deposition. Calcium pyrophosphate dihydrate (CPPD) crystals are found in 18% to 60% of synovial fluids of patients with OA (282). However, radiologic features of CPPD disease differ from those of generalized OA, and the pattern of joint involvement includes the elbow and wrist joints, which are rarely affected by OA. Also, CPPD crystals may be prevalent in patients with OA because both conditions are more common in the aged (283).

Muscle Weakness

Quadriceps muscle weakness is a prominent feature of knee OA, and such weakness may increase knee joint stresses, especially during heel strike. Although this weakness may be, in part, a consequence of disease, in women without knee OA it may increase the risk for developing disease (284). However, the effects of weakness probably differ depending on joint structure. Quadriceps contraction serves as a major source of loading across the knee, and when such contraction occurs in a malaligned knee, the load may impart injurious stresses to a knee, producing progressive disease (285).

Other Risk Factors

A preponderance of evidence supports a protective effect of estrogen use on knee, hip, and hand OA, and although high C-reactive protein (CRP) levels, a marker of inflammation, are associated with a high risk for knee OA progression, this effect seems to be explained by the association of CRP with obesity (286).

Those with low bone density (osteoporosis) have a reduced risk for incident OA (287). Low bone formation may typify those at high OA risk (287). Once OA develops, low bone density, ironically, may protect the joint from progressive disease (288).

Risk Factors for Symptoms

Only 40% to 80% of subjects in population studies with radiographic OA have joint symptoms. Although persons with worse disease are more likely to have symptoms, other structural pathology also predisposes to joint symptoms. Synovitis and joint swelling with fluid are linked to the occurrence of joint symptoms in persons with knee OA (289). Also associated with knee symptoms is the presence on MRI of bone marrow edema, which may be a consequence of repeated bone trauma occurring in malaligned knees (290).

GOUT AND HYPERURICEMIA

Gouty arthritis, recognized since antiquity, remains a common rheumatic disease. It mainly affects men, in contrast to RA, OA, SLE, and most other connective tissue diseases. Gout and RA rarely coexist; the reasons for this remain obscure (291).

Hyperuricemia predisposes to monosodium urate monohydrate (MSU) crystal formation, which in turn precipitates acute gouty inflammation. Elevated serum uric acid levels are seen in at least 90% of patients with gout (292). Not surprisingly, a close correlation exists between factors that influence hyperuricemia and those that contribute to gout.

TABLE 1.23. *Proposed criteria for acute arthritis of gout*

1. More than one attack of acute arthritis
2. Maximum inflammation developed within 1 day
3. Monoarthritis attack
4. Redness observed over joints
5. First metatarsophalangeal joint attack
6. Unilateral first metatarsophalangeal joint attack
7. Unilateral tarsal joint attack
8. Tophus (proved or suspected)
9. Hyperuricemia
10. Asymmetric swelling within a joint on radiograph
11. Subcortical cysts without erosions on radiograph
12. Monosodium urate monohydrate microcrystals in joint fluid during attack
13. Joint fluid culture negative for organisms during attack

From Wallace SL, Robinson H, Masi AT, et al. Preliminary criteria for the classification of the acute arthritis of primary gout. *Arthritis Rheum* 1977;20:895–900, with permission.

Diagnostic Criteria

An ARA subcommittee proposed preliminary criteria for the classification of primary gout (292) (Table 1.23). These performed best when the following diagnostic rules were used:

1. The presence of characteristic urate crystals in the joint fluid (item 12 in Table 1.23), or
2. A tophus proved to contain urate crystals by chemical or polarized light microscopic means, or
3. The presence of 6 of 11 clinical, laboratory, and radiographic features (excluding items 1 and 2 in Table 1.23).

The combined criteria were sensitive (98%) and specific (98% relative to RA and 89% relative to pseudogout and septic arthritis). For population studies in which joint fluid is usually not obtained, criteria were modified slightly, with items 11, 12, and 13 replaced by "complete termination of attack," and monoarthritis (item 3) replaced by "oligoarthritis attack." Six of eleven criteria must be present for a person to be classified as having gout, but without information on synovial fluid, diagnostic test performance deteriorates slightly. Information ascertained during a single visit, by history, or by review of clinic records had a sensitivity for gout of 85% and a specificity of 93% in differentiating gout from pseudogout, with an even higher specificity for other rheumatic diseases.

Prevalence and Incidence

Gout is common, especially in men over age 40. According to the U.S. Health Interview Survey, 2.2 million Americans stated that they have gout (293). Gout was reported more frequently in blacks than whites. Among persons under age 40, gout is uncommon, although in this age group it is much more prevalent in men than women. The low prevalence of gout in premenopausal women is thought to be related to urate-lowering effects of endogenous estrogen. Uric acid levels are increasing secularly and, concomitantly, the incidence of gout has been rising (294,295).

Gout confirmed by physician diagnosis is considerably less prevalent than self-reported gout (296). Definitions of the prevalence of gout have varied from a gout attack in the recent past to a history of any gout attack in a person's life with or without current disease features (such as tophi present), with criteria for gout varying from study to study. Furthermore, studies of gout occurrence have ranged over three decades. Not surprisingly, the prevalence of gout in middle-aged and older adults in the United States and Europe has ranged widely from 0.5% to 2.8% of men (297–299) and from 0.1% to 1.5% of women (297–299).

Estimates of the incidence of gout have also varied across populations. The Veterans Administration Normative Aging Study (295), a cohort study of men 21 to 81 years of age (mean 42 years), found an incidence of gout of 2.8 per 1,000 man-years (0.28% per year). This approximates the gout incidence rate reported in the Framingham Study (299), but is substantially higher than rates reported in other U.S. (296,298) and European (300) studies. The incidence of gout is closely linked to the serum uric acid level (Table 1.24). Nonetheless, even among those with very high serum uric acid levels (>10 mg/dL), the 5-year cumulative incidence was only 30.5%; that is, almost 70% of men did not get a gouty attack.

Population surveys indicate that serum uric acid values (298–301) increase during childhood, irrespective of sex, but starting at 15 to 19 years of age, the average male values are higher, with a maximum difference of almost 1.5 mg/dL in the 20- to 24-year-old age group. The mean female values gradually increase from age 40, reaching within 0.5 mg/dL of the male values after menopause. Levels in men remain essentially constant throughout adulthood, as do those in women from about age 50 (302).

In the United States, most European countries, Japan, and among black Africans, the mean uric acid level among adult men is 5 mg/dL (300,301,303,304). In contrast, some South Pacific populations have mean levels ranging from 6.1 to 7.3 mg/dL (305–307), and in some groups, such as the New Zealand Maoris, Polynesians, and Micronesians, both uric acid levels and rates of gout are higher than elsewhere in the world. Filipinos living in the Philippines have mean levels of 5.2 mg/dL, but levels increase when Filipinos migrate to the United States (308,309), either because of increasing weight after migration or adoption of the Western diet.

TABLE 1.24. *Incidence rates of gouty arthritis in relation to prior serum urate level*

Serum urate level (mg/dL)	Incidence rate (per 1,000 person-years)	5-year cumulative incidence (%)
≤6.0	0.8	0.5
6.0–6.9	0.9	0.6
7.0–7.9	4.1	2.0
8.0–8.9	8.4	4.1
9.0–9.9	43.2	19.8
≥10.0	70.2	30.5

From Campion EW, Glynn RJ, DeLabry LO. Asymptomatic hyperuricemia. Risks and consequences in the normative aging study. *Am J Med* 1987;82:421–426, with permission.

Risk Factors

In addition to increasing age and male gender, risk factors for hyperuricemia include obesity, hypertension, alcohol intake, high serum cholesterol, dietary intake of lead-containing foods, and possibly occupational lead exposure, low levels of physical activity, and low dietary calcium intake. Thiazide and loop diuretics raise serum uric acid, which may account for the association of gout with hypertension (310). The secular increase in serum uric acid levels is attributable in part to the popularity of diuretics, but it may also be due to increased alcohol consumption or a secular increase in weight, at least in the United States (311). The high rate of gout in blacks may be explained by their high rate of diuretic use (312).

Gout and hyperuricemia have been recognized as familial disorders since antiquity. The reported frequency of familial occurrence ranges from 6% to as high as 80% (313). Little of the familiar aggregation of gout is attributable to recognized disorders of purine metabolism, such as Lesch-Nyhan syndrome. Even partial enzyme deficiency states are rarely identified in gouty subjects.

Patients with hyperuricemia or gout are at increased risk for coronary hypertension and heart disease (295,314,315). This increased risk was thought to be due to associated factors, such as hypercholesterolemia and obesity (311). However, several studies suggest that serum uric acid or a history of gout may well be an independent predictor of coronary artery disease risk or it may be a marker for an insulin-resistant state (316).

REFERENCES

1. Buring J, Hennekens C. *Epidemiology in medicine.* Boston: Little, Brown, 1987:16–29.
2. Silman A, Hochberg MC, eds. *Epidemiology of the rheumatic diseases,* 2nd ed. New York: Oxford University Press, 2001.
3. Verbrugge LM. From sneezes to adieux: stages of health for American men and women. *Soc Sci Med* 1986;22:1195–1212.
4. Lawrence RC, Helmick CG, Arnett FC, et al. Estimates of the prevalence of arthritis and selected musculoskeletal disorders in the United States. *Arthritis Rheum* 1998;41:778–799.
5. Haber LD. Disabling effects of chronic disease and impairment—II. Functional capacity limitations. *J Chronic Dis* 1973;26:127–151.
6. Yelin E, Callahan LF. The economic cost and social and psychological impact of musculoskeletal conditions. National Arthritis Data Work Groups. *Arthritis Rheum* 1996;39(11):1931.
7. Hadler NM. *Medical management of the regional musculoskeletal diseases.* Orlando: Grune & Stratton, 1984.
8. Ropes MS, Bennett GA, Cobb S, et al. 1958 revision of diagnostic criteria for rheumatoid arthritis. *Bull Rheum Dis* 1958;9:175–176.

9. Bennett PH, Burch TA. New York symposium on population studies in the rheumatic diseases; new diagnostic criteria. *Bull Rheum Dis* 1967;17:453–458.
10. O'Sullivan JB, Cathcart ES. The prevalence of rheumatoid arthritis. Follow-up evaluation of the effect of criteria on rates in Sudbury, Massachusetts. *Ann Intern Med* 1972;76:573–577.
11. Arnett FC, Edworthy SM, Block DA, et al. The American rheumatism association 1987 revised criteria for the classification of rheumatoid arthritis. *Arthritis Rheum* 1988;24:315–324.
12. Huizinga TWJ, Machold KP, Breedveld FC, et al. Criteria for early rheumatoid arthritis. From Baye's Law revisited to new thoughts on pathogenesis. *Arthritis Rheum* 2002;46:1155–1159.
13. Cathcart ES, O'Sullivan JB. Rheumatoid arthritis in a New England town. A prevalence study in Sudbury, Massachusetts. *N Engl J Med* 1970;282:421–424.
14. Linos A, Worthington JW, O'Fallon WM, et al. The epidemiology of rheumatoid arthritis in Rochester, Minnesota: a study of incidence, prevalence, and mortality. *Am J Epidemiol* 1980;111:87–98.
15. Rasch EK, Hirsch R, Paulose-Ram R, et al. Prevalence of rheumatoid arthritis in persons 60 years of age and older in the United States. *Arthritis Rheum* 2003;48:917–926.
16. Doran MF, Pond GR, Crowson CS, et al. Trends in incidence and mortality in rheumatoid arthritis in Rochester, Minnesota, over a forty-year period. *Arthritis Rheum* 2002;46:625–631.
17. Harvey J, Lotze M, Stevens MB. Rheumatoid arthritis in a Chippewa band. 1. Pilot screening study of disease prevalence. *Arthritis Rheum* 1981;24:717–721.
18. Boyer GS, Templin DW, Cornoni-Huntley JC, et al. Prevalence of spondyloarthropathies in Alaskan Eskimos. *J Rheumatol* 1994:21: 2292–2297.
19. Symmons DPM, Barrett EM, Bankhead CR, et al. The incidence of rheumatoid arthritis in the United Kingdom: results from the Norfolk Arthritis Register. *Br J Rheumatol* 1994;33:735–739.
20. Kaipiainen-Seppanen O, Aho K, Isomaki H, et al. Incidence of rheumatoid arthritis in Finland during 1980–1990. *Ann Rheum Dis* 1996;55:608–611.
21. Hochberg MC. Changes in the incidence and prevalence of rheumatoid arthritis in England and Wales, 1970–1982. *Semin Arthritis Rheum* 1990;19:294–302.
22. Shichikawa K, Inoue, K, Hirota S, et al. Changes in the incidence and prevalence of rheumatoid arthritis in Kamitonda, Wakayama, Japan, 1965–1996. *Ann Rheum Dis* 1999;58:751–756.
23. Jacobsson LTH, Hanson RL, Knowler WC, et al. Decreasing incidence and prevalence of rheumatoid arthritis in Pima Indians over a twenty-five-year period. *Arthritis Rheum* 1994;37:1158–1165.
24. Silman AJ. Trends in the incidence and severity of rheumatoid arthritis. *J Rheumatol* 1992;19(suppl 32):71–73.
25. Kaipiainen-Seppanen, Aho K, Isomaki H, et al. Shift in the incidence of rheumatoid arthritis toward elderly patients in Finland during 1975–1990. *Clin Exp Rheumatol* 1996;14:537–542.
26. Stastny P, Ball EJ, Khan MA, et al. HLA-DR4 and other genetic markers in rheumatoid arthritis. *Br J Rheumatol* 1988;27(suppl 2):132–138.
27. Morel PA, Fathman CG. Immunogenetics of rheumatoid arthritis. *J Rheumatol* 1989;16:421–423.
28. Nepom GT, Byers P, Seyfried C, et al. HLA genes associated with rheumatoid arthritis. *Arthritis Rheum* 1989;32:15–21.
29. Wordsworth P. The immunogenetics of rheumatoid arthritis. *Curr Opin Rheumatol* 1990;2:423–429.
30. Jawaheer D, Thomson W, MacGregor AJ, et al. Homozygosity for the HLA-DR shaped epitope contributes the highest risk for rheumatoid arthritis concordance in identical twins. *Arthritis Rheum* 1994;37: 681–696.
31. McDonagh JE, Dunn A, Ollier WER, et al. Compound heterozygosity for the shared epitope and the risk and severity of rheumatoid arthritis in extended pedigrees. *Br J Rheumatol* 1997;36:322–327.
32. Thomson W, Harrison B, Ollier B, et al. Quantifying the exact role of HLA-DRB1 alleles in susceptibility to inflammatory polyarthritis. Results from a large, population-based study. *Arthritis Rheum* 1999; 42:757–62.
33. Jawaheer D, Rhomson W, MacGregor AJ, et al. "Homozygosity" for the HLA-DR shared epitope contributes the highest risk for rheumatoid arthritis concordance in identical twins. *Arthritis Rheum* 1994;37:681–686.
34. Ollier W, Thomson W. Population genetics of rheumatoid arthritis. *Rheum Dis Clin North Am* 1992;18:741–760.
35. Jawaheer D, Seldin MF, Amos CI, et al. Screening the genome for rheumatoid arthritis susceptibility genes. *Arthritis Rheum* 2003;48: 906–916.
36. Okamato K, Makino S, Yoshikawa Y. Identification of L IκBL as the second major histocompatibility complex-linked susceptibility locus for rheumatoid arthritis. *Am J Hum Genet* 2003;72:303–312.
37. Dieude P, Petit E, Cailleau-Moindrault S, et al. Association between tumor necrosis factor receptor II and familial, but not sporadic, rheumatoid arthritis. Evidence for genetic heterogeneity. *Arthritis Rheum* 2002;46:2039–2044.
38. Spector TD, Hochberg MC. The protective effect of the oral contraceptive pill on rheumatoid arthritis: an overview of the analytic epidemiological studies using meta-analysis. *J Clin Epidemiol* 1990;43: 1221–1230.
39. van Zeben D, Hazes JMW, Vandenbroucke JP, et al. Diminished incidence of severe rheumatoid arthritis associated with oral contraceptives. *Arthritis Rheum* 1990;33:1462–1465.
40. Spector TD, Roman E, Silman AJ. The pill, parity, and rheumatoid arthritis. *Arthritis Rheum* 1990;33:782–789.
41. Silman A, Kay A, Brennan P. Timing of pregnancy in relation to the onset of rheumatoid arthritis. *Arthritis Rheum* 1992;35:152–155.
42. Brennan P, Silman A. Breastfeeding and the onset of rheumatoid arthritis. *Arthritis Rheum* 1994;37:808–813.
43. Kanik KS, Wilder RL. Hormonal alterations in rheumatoid arthritis, including the effects of pregnancy. *Rheum Dis Clin North Am* 2000;24: 805–823.
44. Heliovaara M, Knekt P, Aho K. Serum antioxidants and risk of rheumatoid arthritis. *Ann Rheum Dis* 1994;53:51–53.
45. Cerhan JR, Saag KG, Merlino LA, et al. Antioxidant micronutrients and risk of rheumatoid arthritis in a cohort of older women. *Am J Epidemiol* 2003;157:345–354.
46. Knekt P, Heliovaara M, Aho K, et al. Serum selenium, serum alpha-tocopheral, and the risk of rheumatoid arthritis. *Epidemiology* 2000;11: 402–405.
47. Mikuls TR, Cerhan JR, Criswell LA, et al. Coffee, tea, and caffeine consumption and risk of rheumatoid arthritis. *Arthritis Rheum* 2002; 46:83–91.
48. Del Puente A, Knowler WC, Pettitt DJ, et al. The incidence of rheumatoid arthritis is predicted by rheumatoid factor titer in a longitudinal population study. *Arthritis Rheum* 1988;31:1239–1244.
49. Criswell LA, Merlino LA, Cerhan JR, et al. Cigarette smoking and the risk of rheumatoid arthritis among postmenopausal women: results from the Iowa Women's Health Study. *Am J Med* 2002;112:465–471.
50. Vessey MP, Villard-Mackintosh L, Yeates D. Oral contraceptives, cigarette smoking and other factors in relation to Arthritis. *Contraception* 1987;25:457–464.
51. Heliovaara M, Aho K, Aromaa A, et al. Smoking and risk of rheumatoid arthritis. *J Rheumatol* 1993;20:1830–1835.
52. Mattey DL, Hutchinson D, Dawes PT, et al. Smoking and disease severity in rheumatoid arthritis. Association with polymorphism at the glutathione S-transferase M1 locus. *Arthritis Rheum* 2002;46:640–646.
53. Silman A, Bankhead C, Rowlingson B, et al. Do new cases of rheumatoid arthritis cluster in time or in space? *Int J Epidemiol* 1997; 26: 628–634.
54. Mikkelsen WM, Dodge H. A four-year follow-up of suspected rheumatoid arthritis: the Tecumseh, Michigan, community health study. *Arthritis Rheum* 1969;12:87–91.
55. Isacson J, Allander E, Broström LA. A seventeen-year follow-up of a population survey of rheumatoid arthritis. *Scand J Rheumatol* 1987; 16:145–152.
56. Gabriel SE, Crowson CS, Kremers HM, et al. Survival in rheumatoid arthritis. A population-based analysis of trends over 40 years. *Arthritis Rheum* 2003;48:54–58.
57. Kazis LE, Anderson JJ, Meenan RF. Health status as a predictor of mortality in rheumatoid arthritis: a five-year study. *J Rheumatol* 1990;17:609–613.
58. Pincus T, Callahan LF, Vaughn WK. Questionnaire, walking time and button test measures of functional capacity as predictive markers for mortality in rheumatoid arthritis. *J Rheumatol* 1987;14:240–251.
59. Pincus T, Callahan LF. Taking mortality in rheumatoid arthritis seriously predictive markers, socioeconomic status and comorbidity. *J Rheumatol* 1986;13:841–845.

60. Wolfe F, Mitchell DM, Sibley JT, et al. The mortality of rheumatoid arthritis. *Arthritis Rheum* 1994;37:481–494.
61. Bjornadal L, Baecklund E, Yin L, et al. Decreasing mortality in patients with rheumatoid arthritis: results from a large population based cohort in Sweden, 1964–95. *J Rheumatol* 2002:29:906–912.
62. Isomaüki HA, Hakulinen T, Joutsenlahti U. Excess risk of lymphomas, leukemia and myeloma in patients with rheumatoid arthritis. *J Chronic Dis* 1978;31:691–696.
63. Cibere J, Sibley J, Haga M. Rheumatoid arthritis and the risk of malignancy. *Arthritis Rheum* 1997;40:1580–1586.
64. Cassidy JT, Levinson JE, Brewer EJ Jr. The development of classification criteria for children with juvenile rheumatoid arthritis. *Bull Rheum Dis* 1989;38:1–7.
65. Petty RE, Southwood TR, Baum J, et al. Revision of the proposed classification criteria for juvenile idiopathic arthritis: Durban, 1997. *J Rheumatol* 1998;25:1991–1994.
66. Bernston L, Fasth A, Andersson-Gare B, et al. Construct validity of ILAR and EULAR criteria in juvenile idiopathic arthritis: a population based incidence study from Nordic countries. *J Rheumatol* 2001;28: 2737–2743.
67. Towner SR, Michet CJ, O'Fallon WM, et al. The epidemiology of juvenile arthritis in Rochester, Minnesota 1960–1979. *Arthritis Rheum* 1983;26:1208–1213.
68. Gäre BA, Fasth A. Epidemiology of juvenile chronic arthritis in southwestern Sweden: a 5-year prospective population study. *Pediatrics* 1992;90:950–958.
69. Manners PJ, Diepeveen DA. Prevalence of juvenile chronic arthritis in a population of 12-year-old children in urban Australia. *Pediatrics* 1996;98:84–90.
70. Peterson LS, Mason T, Nelson AM, et al. Juvenile rheumatoid arthritis in Rochester, Minnesota 1960–1993. Is the epidemiology changing? *Arthritis Rheum* 1996;39(8):1385–1390.
71. Kunnamo I, Kallio P, Pelkonen P. Incidence of arthritis in urban Finnish children: a prospective study. *Arthritis Rheum* 1986;28:12–32.
72. Singsen BH. Rheumatic diseases of childhood. *Rheum Dis Clin North Am* 1990;16:581–599.
73. Cassidy JT. Juvenile rheumatoid arthritis. In: Kelley WM, Harris ED, Ruddy S, et al., eds. *Textbook of rheumatology,* 3rd ed. Philadelphia: WB Saunders, 1989:1289–1311.
74. Clemens LE, Albert E, Ansell BM. Sibling pairs affected by chronic arthritis of childhood: evidence for genetic predisposition. *J Rheumatol* 1985;12:108.
75. Howard JF, Sigsbee A, Glass DN. HLA genetics and inherited predisposition to JRA. *J Rheumatol* 1985;12:7–12.
76. Glass DN, Giannini EH. JRA as a complex genetic trait. *Arthritis Rheum* 1999;42:2213–2219.
77. Mason T, Rabinovich CE, Fredrickson DD, et al. Breast feeding and the development of juvenile rheumatoid arthritis. *J Rheumatol* 1995; 22:1166–1169.
78. Dougados M, van der Linden SJEF, Juhlin R, et al. The European Spondylarthritisopathy Study Group preliminary criteria for the classification of spondylarthritisopathy. *Arthritis Rheum* 1991;34:1218–1227.
79. Collantes-Estevez E, Cisnal Del Mazo A, Munoz-Gomariz E. Assessment of 2 systems of spondyloarthritisopathy diagnostic and classification criteria (Amor and ESSG) by a Spanish Multicenter Study. *J Rheumatol* 1995;22:246–251.
80. Braun J, Bollow M, Remlinger G, et al. Prevalence of spondyloarthritisopathies in HLA-B27 positive and negative blood donors. *Arthritis Rheum* 1998;41:58–67.
81. Khan MA, van der Linden SM. Ankylosing spondylitis and other spondyloarthritisopathies. *Rheum Dis Clin North Am* 1990;16:551–579.
82. van der Linden S, Valkenburg HA, Cats A. Evaluation of diagnostic criteria for ankylosing spondylitis. *Arthritis Rheum* 1984;27:361–368.
83. Khan MA, van der Linden SM, Kushner I, et al. Spondylitic disease without radiological evidence of sacroiliitis in relatives of HLA-B27 positive patients. *Arthritis Rheum* 1985;28:40–43.
84. Feltkamp TEW, Mardjuadi A, Huang F, et al. Spondyloopathies in eastern Asia. *Curr Opin Rheumatol* 2001;13:285–290.
85. Gofton JP, Lawrence JS, Bennett PH, et al. Sacroiliitis in eight populations. *Ann Rheum Dis* 1966;25:528–532.
86. Gofton JP, Bennett PH, Smythe HA, et al. Sacroiliitis and ankylosing spondylitis in North American Indians. *Ann Rheum Dis* 1972;31:474–481.
87. Gofton JP, Chalmers A, Price GE, et al. HLA 27 and ankylosing spondylitis in B.C. Indians. *J Rheumatol* 1984;11:572–573.
88. van der Linden SM, Valkenburg HA, de Jongh BM, et al. The risk of developing ankylosing spondylitis in HLA-B27 positive individuals: a comparison of relatives of spondylitis patients with the general population. *Arthritis Rheum* 1984;27;241–249.
89. Carbone LD, Cooper C, Michet CJ, et al. Ankylosing spondylitis in Rochester, Minnesota, 1935–1989. *Arthritis Rheum* 1992;35:1476–1482.
90. Gomor B, Gyodi E, Bakos L. Distribution of HLA B27 and ankylosing spondylitis in the Hungarian population. *J Rheumatol* 1977; 4(suppl 3):33–35.
91. Lopez-Larrea C, Mijiyawa M, Gonzalez S, et al. Association of ankylosing spondylitis with HLA-B* 1403 in a West African population. *Arthritis Rheum* 2002;46:2968–2971.
92. Brown MA, Pile KD, Kennedy G, et al. A genome-wide screen for susceptibility loci in ankylosing spondylitis. *Arthritis Rheum* 1998;41:588–595.
93. Laval SH, Timms A, Edwards S, et al. Whole-genome screening in ankylosing spondylitis: evidence of non-MHC genetic-susceptibility loci. *Am J Hum Genet* 2001:68:918–926.
94. Brown MA, Crane AM, Wordsworth BP. Genetic aspects of susceptibility, severity, and clinical expression in ankylosing spondylitis. *Curr Opin Rheumatol* 2002;14:354–360.
95. Ostensen M, Husby G. A prospective clinical study of the effect of pregnancy on rheumatoid arthritis and ankylosing spondylitis. *Arthritis Rheum* 1983;26:1155–1159.
96. Khan MA, Khan MK, Kushner I. Survival among patients with ankylosing spondylitis: a life-table analysis. *J Rheumatol* 1981;8:86–90.
97. Radford EP, Doll R, Smith PG. Mortality among patients with ankylosing spondylitis not given x-ray therapy. *N Engl J Med* 1977;297: 572–576.
98. Lehtinen K. Mortality and causes of death in 398 patients admitted to hospital with ankylosing spondylitis. *Ann Rheum Dis* 1993;52: 174–176.
99. Mau W, Zeidler H, Mau R, et al. Clinical features and prognosis of patients with possible ankylosing spondylitis. Results of a 10-year follow-up. *J Rheumatol* 1988;15:1109–1114.
100. Arnett FC. Seronegative spondylopathies. *Bull Rheum Dis* 1987;37: 1–12.
101. Willkens RF, Arnett FC, Bitter T, et al. Reiter's syndrome. Evaluation of preliminary criteria for definite disease. *Arthritis Rheum* 1981;24: 844–849.
102. Bardin T, Lathrop GM. Postvenereal Reiter's syndrome in Greenland. *Rheum Dis Clin North Am* 1992;18:81–93.
103. Winchester R, Bernstein DH, Fischer HD, et al. The co-occurrence of Reiter's syndrome and acquired immunodeficiency. *Ann Intern Med* 1987;106:19–26.
104. Fox R, Calin A, Gerber R, et al. The chronicity of symptoms and disability in Reiter's syndrome. An analysis of 131 consecutive patients. *Ann Intern Med* 1979;91:190–193.
105. Butler MJ, Russell AS, Percy JS, et al. A follow-up study of 48 patients with Reiter's syndrome. *Am J Med* 1979;67:808–810.
106. Brewerton DA, James DC. The histocompatibility antigen (HLA 27) and disease. *Semin Arthritis Rheum* 1975;4:191–207.
107. Taylor WJ. Epidemiology of psoriatic Arthritis. *Curr Opin Rheumatol* 2002;14:98–103.
108. Shbeeb M, Uramoto KM, Gibson LE, et al. The epidemiology of psoriatic arthritis in Olmsted County, Minnesota, USA, 1982–1991. *J Rheumatol* 2000;27:1247–1250.
109. Kaipiainen-Seppanen O. Incidence of psoriatic arthritis in Finland. *Br J Rheumatol* 1996;35:1289–1291.
110. Leonard DG, O'Duffy JD, Rogers RS. Prospective analysis of psoriatic arthritis in patients hospitalized for psoriasis. *Mayo Clin Proc* 1978;53:511–518.
111. Stern RS. The epidemiology of joint complaints in patient with psoriasis. *J Rheumatol* 1985;12:315–320.
112. Espinoza LR, Berman A, Vasey FB, et al. Psoriatic arthritis and acquired immunodeficiency syndrome. *Arthritis Rheum* 1988;31: 1034–1040.
113. Tan EM, Cohen AS, Fries JF, et al. The 1982 revised criteria for the classification of systemic lupus erythematosus. *Arthritis Rheum* 1982;25:1271–1277.
114. Hochberg MC. Systemic lupus erythematosus. *Rheum Dis Clin North Am* 1990;16:617–639.

115. Swaak AJG, van de Brink H, Smeenk RJT, et al. Incomplete lupus erythematosus: results of a multicentre study under the supervision of the EULAR Standing Committee on International Clinical Studies including Therapeutic Trials (ESCISIT). *Rheumatology* 2001;40:89–94.
116. Fessel WJ. Epidemiology of systemic lupus erythematosus. *Rheum Dis Clin North Am* 1988;14:15–23.
117. Uramoto KM, Michet CJ Jr, Thumboo J, et al. Trends in the incidence and mortality of systemic lupus erythematosus, 1950–1992. *Arthritis Rheum* 1999;42:46–50.
118. Gudmundsson S, Steinsson K. Systemic lupus erythematosus in Iceland 1975 through 1985. A nationwide epidemiological study in an unselected population. *J Rheumatol* 1990;17:1162–1167.
119. Helve T. Prevalence of mortality rates of systemic lupus erythematosus and causes of death in SLE patients in Finland. *Scand J Rheumatol* 1985;14:43–46.
120. Jonsson H, Nived O, Sturfelt G, et al. Estimating the incidence of systemic lupus erythematosus in a defined population using multiple sources of retrieval. *Br J Rheumatol* 1990;29:185–188.
121. Hopkinson ND, Doherty M, Powell RJ. The prevalence and incidence of systemic lupus erythematosus in Nottingham, UK, 1989–1990. *Br J Rheumatol* 1993;32:110–115.
122. Morton RO, Gershwin ME, Brady C, et al. The incidence of systemic lupus erythematosus in North American Indians. *J Rheumatol* 1976; 3:186–190.
123. Boyer GS, Templin DW, Lanier AP. Rheumatic diseases in Alaskan Indians of the southeast coast: high prevalence of rheumatoid arthritis and systemic lupus erythematosus. *J Rheumatol* 1991;18:1477–1484.
124. Serdula MK, Rhoads GG. Frequency of systemic lupus erythematosus in different ethnic groups in Hawaii. *Arthritis Rheum* 1979;22:328–333.
125. Chou CT, Lee FT, Schumacher RH. Modification of a screening technique to evaluate systemic lupus erythematosus in a Chinese population in Taiwan. *J Rheumatol* 1986;13:806–809.
126. Malaviya AN, Singh RR, Singh YN, et al. Prevalence of systemic lupus erythematosus in India. *Lupus* 1993;2:115–118.
127. Samanta A, Roy S, Feehally J, et al. The prevalence of diagnosed systemic lupus erythematosus in whites and Indian Asian immigrants in Leicester City, UK. *Br J Rheumatol* 1992;31:679–682.
128. Bae S-C, Fraser P, Liang MH. The epidemiology of systemic lupus erythematosus in populations of African ancestry. A critical review of the prevalence gradient hypothesis. *Arthritis Rheum* 1998;41:2091–2099.
129. Molokia M, Hoggart C, Patrick AL. et al. Relations of risk of systemic lupus erythematosus to west African admixture in a Caribbean population. *Hum Genet* 2003;112:310–318.
130. Sanchez-Guerrero J, Liang MH, Karlson EW, et al. Postmenopausal estrogen therapy and the risk of developing systemic lupus erythematosus (SLE). *Ann Intern Med* 1995;122:430–433.
131. Cooper GS, Dooley MA, Treadwell EL, et al. Hormonal, environmental, and infectious risk factors for developing systemic lupus erythematosus. *Arthritis Rheum* 1998;41:1714–1724.
132. Parks CG, Cooper GS, Nylander-French L, et al. Occupational exposure to crystalline silica and risk of systemic lupus erythematosus. A population-based, case-control study in the southeastern United States. *Arthritis Rheum* 2002;46:1840–1850.
133. Cooper GS, Dooley MA, Treadwell EL, et al. Smoking and use of hair treatments in relation to risk of developing systemic lupus erythematosus. *J Rheumatol* 2001;28:2653–2656.
134. Kilburn KH, Warshaw RH. Prevalence of symptoms of systemic lupus erythematosus (SLE) and of fluorescent antinuclear antibodies associated with chronic exposure to trichloroethylene and other chemicals in well water. *Environ Res* 1992;57:1–9.
135. Jones DRE, Hopkinson ND, Powell RJ. Autoantibodies in pet dogs owned by patients with systemic lupus erythematosus. *Lancet* 1992; 339:1378–1380.
136. Hatfield M, Evans M, Suenaga R, et al. Anti-idiotypic antibody against anti-DNA in sera of laboratory personnel exposed to lupus sera or nucleic acids. *Clin Exp Immunol* 1987;70:26–34.
137. Lawrence JS, Martins CL, Drake GL. A family survey of lupus erythematosus I heritability. *J Rheumatol* 1987;14:913–921.
138. Block SR, Winfield JB, Lockshin MC, et al. Studies of twins with systemic lupus erythematosus: a review of the literature and presentation of 12 additional sets. *Am J Med* 1975;59:533–552.
139. Merrell M, Shulman LE. Determination of prognosis in chronic disease, illustrated by systemic lupus erythematosus. *J Chronic Dis* 1955;1:12–32.
140. Bresnihan B. Outcome and survival in systemic lupus erythematosus. *Ann Rheum Dis* 1989;48:443–445.
141. Urowitz MB, Bookman AAM, Koehler BE, et al. The bimodal mortality pattern of systemic lupus erythematosus. *Am J Med* 1976;60:221–225.
142. Rosner S, Ginzler EM, Diamond HS, et al. A multicenter study of outcome in systemic lupus erythematosus; II. Causes of death. *Arthritis Rheum* 1982;25:612–616.
143. Reveille JD, Bartolucci A, Alarcon GS. Prognosis in systemic lupus erythematosus; negative impact of increasing age at onset, black race, and thrombocytopenia, as well as causes of death. *Arthritis Rheum* 1990;33:37–48.
144. Liang MH, Socher SA, Larson MG, et al. Reliability and validity of six systems for the clinical assessment of disease activity in systemic lupus erythematosus. *Arthritis Rheum* 1989;32:1107–1118.
145. Swaak AJG, Bronsveld W, Nieuwenhuyse EJ, et al. Systemic lupus erythematosus. II. Observations on the occurrence of exacerbations in the disease course. Dutch experience with 110 patients studied prospectively. *Ann Rheum Dis* 1989;48:445–460.
146. Jonsson H, Nived O, Sturfelt G. Outcome in systemic lupus erythematosus: a prospective study of patients from a defined population. *Medicine* 1989;68:141–150.
147. Rubin LA, Urowitz MB, Gladman DD. Mortality in systemic lupus erythematosus: the bimodal pattern revisited. *Q J Med* 1985;55:87–98.
148. Ginzler EM, Diamond HS, Weiner M, et al. A multicenter study of outcome in systemic lupus erythematosus. *Arthritis Rheum* 1982;25:601–611.
149. Estes D, Christian CL. The natural history of systemic lupus erythematosus by prospective analysis. *Medicine* 1971;50:85–95.
150. Esdaile JM, Levington C, Federgreen W, et al. The clinical and renal biopsy predictors of long-term outcome in lupus nephritis: a study of 87 patients and review of the literature. *Q J Med* 1989;72:779–833.
151. Studenski A, Allen NB, Calswell DS, et al. Survival in systemic lupus erythematosus: a multivariate analysis of demographic factors. *Arthritis Rheum* 1987;30:1326–1332.
152. Ginzler EM, Schorn K. Outcome and prognosis in systemic lupus erythematosus. *Rheum Dis Clin North Am* 1988;14:67–78.
153. Bohan A, Peter JB. Polymyositis and dermatomyositis. *N Engl J Med* 1975;292:344–347,403–407.
154. Love LA, Leff RL, Fraser DD, et al. A new approach to the classification of idiopathic inflammatory myopathy: myositis-specific autoantibodies define useful homogeneous patient groups. *Medicine* (Baltimore) 70; 1991;6:360–374.
155. Patrick M, Buchbinder R, Jolley D, et al. Incidence of inflammatory myopathies in Victoria, Australia, and evidence of spatial clustering. *J Rheumatol* 1999;26:1094–1100.
156. Oddis CV, Conte CG, Steen VD, et al. Incidence of polymyositis-dermatomyositis: a 20-year study of hospital diagnosed cases in Allegheny County, PA 1963–1982. *J Rheumatol* 1990;17:1329–1334.
157. Findlay GH, Whiting DA, Simson IW. Dermatomyositis in the Transvaal and its occurrence in the Bantu. *S Afr Med J* 1969;43:694–697.
158. Medsger TA Jr, Dawson WN Jr, Masi AT. The epidemiology of polymyositis. *Am J Med* 1970;48:715–723.
159. Koch MJ, Brody JA, Gillespie MM. Childhood polymyositis: a case-control study. *Am J Epidemiol* 1976;104:627–631.
160. Sigurgeirsson B, Lindelof B, Edhag O, et al. Risk of cancer in patients with dermatomyositis or polymyositis: a population-based study. *N Engl J Med* 1992;326:363–367.
161. Hill CL, Zhang Y, Sigurgeirsson B, et al. Frequence of specific cancer types in dermatomyositis and polymyositis: a population-based study. *Lancet* 2001;357:96–100.
162. Buchbinder R, Forbes A, Hall S, et al. Incidence of malignant disease in biopsy-proven inflammatory myopathy. *Ann Intern Med* 2001; 134:1087–1095.
163. Medsger TA Jr, Robinson H, Masi AT. Factors affecting survivorship in polymyositis: a life-table study of 124 patients. *Arthritis Rheum* 1971;14:249–258.
164. Hochberg MC, Feldman D, Stevens MB. Adult onset polymyositis/dermatomyositis: an analysis of clinical and laboratory features and survival in 76 patients with a review of the literature. *Semin Arthritis Rheum* 1986;15:168–178.

165. Hoffman GS, Franck WA, Raddatz DA, et al. Presentation, treatment, and prognosis of idiopathic inflammatory muscle disease in a rural hospital. *Am J Med* 1983;75:433–438.
166. Masi AT, Rodnan GP, Medsger TA Jr, et al. Preliminary criteria for the classification of systemic sclerosis (scleroderma). *Arthritis Rheum* 1980;23:581–590.
167. Lonzetti LS, Joyal R, Jean-Pierre R, et al. Updating the American College of Rheumatology preliminary classification criteria for systemic sclerosis: addition of severe nailfold capillaroscopy abnormalities markedly increases the sensitivity for limited scleroderma. *Arthritis Rheum* 2001;44:735–736.
168. Mayes MD. Scleroderma epidermiology, *Clin N Amer* 1996;22: 751–763.
169. Roberts-Thomson PJ, Jones M, Hakendorf P, et al. Scleroderma in South Australia: epidemiological observations of possible pathogenic significance. *Int Med J* 2001;312:220–229.
170. Silman AJ. Mortality from scleroderma in England and Wales 1968–1985. *Ann Rheum Dis* 1991;50:95–96.
171. Silman A, Jannini S, Symmons D, et al. An epidemiological study of scleroderma in the West Midlands. *Br J Rheumatol* 1988;27: 286–290.
172. Steen VD. Systemic sclerosis. *Rheum Dis Clin North Am* 1990;16: 641–654.
173. Arnett FC, Cho M, Chatterjee S, et al. Familial occurrence frequencies and relative risks for systemic sclerosis (scleroderma) in three United States cohorts. *Arthritis Rheum* 2001;44:1359–1362.
174. De Keyser F, Mielants H, Veys DM. Klinefelter's syndrome and scleroderma. *J Rheumatol* 1990;16:1613–1614.
175. Johnson KL, Nelson JL, Furst DE, et al. Fetal cell microchimerism in tissue from multiple sites in women with systemic sclerosis. *Arthritis Rheum* 2001;44:1848–1854.
176. Black CM, Pereira S, McWhirter A, et al. Genetic susceptibility to scleroderma-like syndrome in symptomatic and asymptomatic workers exposed to vinyl chloride. *J Rheumatol* 1986;13:10–59.
177. Nietert PJ, Sutherland SE, Silver RM, et al. Is occupational organic solvent exposure a risk factor for scleroderma? *Arthritis Rheum* 1998;41:1111–1118.
178. Garabrant DH, James L, Laing TJ, et al. Scleroderma and solvent exposure among women. *Am J Epidemiol* 2003;157:493–500.
179. Hochberg MC, Perlmutter DL, Medsger TA Jr, et al. Lack of association between augmentation mammoplasty and systemic sclerosis (scleroderma). *Arthritis Rheum* 1996;39:1125–1131.
180. Gabriel SE, O'Fallon WM, Kurland LT, et al. Risk of connective tissue diseases and other disorders after breast implantation. *N Engl J Med* 1994;330:1697–1702.
181. Masi AT. Clinical-epidemiological perspective of systemic sclerosis (scleroderma). In: Jayson MIV, Black CM, eds. *Systemic sclerosis: scleroderma.* New York: Wiley, 1988:7.
182. Scussel-Lonzetti, L, Joyal F, Jean-Pierre R, et al. Predicting mortality in systemic sclerosis: analysis of a cohort of 309 French Canadian patients with emphasis on features at diagnosis as predictive factors for survival. *Medicine* 2002;81:154–167.
183. Abu-Shakra M, Guillemin F, Lee P. Cancer in systemic sclerosis. *Arthritis Rheum* 1993:36:460–464.
184. Lightfoot RW Jr, Michel AB, Block DA, et al. The American College of Rheumatology 1990 criteria for the classification of polyarteritis nodosa. *Arthritis Rheum* 1990;33:1088–1093.
185. Jennette JC, Falk RJ, Andrassy K, et al. Nomenclature of systemic vasculitides: proposal of an international consensus conference. *Arthritis Rheum* 1994;37:187–192.
186. Rao JK, Allen NB, Pincus T. Limitations of the 1990 American College of Rheumatology Classification Criteria in the diagnosis of vasculitis. *Ann Intern Med* 1998;129:345–352.
187. Cotch MF, Hoffman GS, Yerg DE, et al. The epidemiology of Wegener's granulomatosus. Estimates of the five-year period prevalence, annual mortality, and geographic disease distribution from population-based data sources. *Arthritis Rheum* 1996;39:87–92.
188. Bengtsson BA, Malmvall BE. The epidemiology of giant cell arteritis including temporal arteritis and polymyalgia rheumatica. *Arthritis Rheum* 1981;24:899.
189. Barrier J, Pion P, Massari R, et al. Epidemiological approach to Horton's disease in the department of Loire-Atlantique: 110 cases in 10 years (1970–1979). *Rev Med Interne* 1983;3:13.
190. Michet CJ. Polymyalgia rheumatica/giant cell arteritis and other vasculitides. *Rheum Dis Clin North Am* 1990;16:667–680
191. Gonzalez-Gay MA, Garcia-Porrua C, Rivas MJ, et al. Epidemiology of biopsy proven giant cell arteritis in northwestern Spain: trend over an 18 year period. *Ann Rheum Dis* 2001;60:367–371.
192. Smith CA, Fidler WJ, Pinals RS. The epidemiology of giant cell arteritis: report of a ten-year study in Shelby County, Tennessee. *Arthritis Rheum* 1983;26:12–14.
193. Machado EBV, Michet CJ, Ballard DJ, et al. Trends in incidence and clinical presentation of temporal arteritis in Olmsted County, Minnesota, 1950–1985. *Arthritis Rheum* 1988;31:745–749.
194. Sonnenblick M, Nesher G, Friedlander Y, et al. Giant cell arteritis in Jerusalem: a 12-year epidemiological study. *Br J Rheumatol* 1994; 33:938–941.
195. Gonzalez EB, Varner WT, Lisse JR, et al. Giant-cell arteritis in the southern United States. *Arch Intern Med* 1989;149:1561–1565.
196. Duhaut P, Pinede L, Demolombe-Rague S, et al. Giant cell arteritis and cardiovascular risk factors. A multicenter, prospective case-control study. *Arthritis Rheum* 1998;41:1960–1965.
197. Elling P, Olsson AT, Elling H. Synchronous variations of the incidence of temporal arteritis and polymyalgia rheumatica in different regions of Denmark; association with epidemics of mycoplasma pneumoniae infection. *J Rheumatol* 1996;23:112–119.
198. Salvarani C, Gabriel SE, O'Fallon WM, et al. The incidence of giant cell arteritis in Olmsted County, Minnesota: apparent fluctuations in a cyclic pattern. *Ann Intern Med* 1995;123:192–194.
199. Gabriel SE, Espy M, Erdman DD, et al. The role of parvovirus B19 in the pathogenesis of giant cell arteritis. *Arthritis Rheum* 1999;42: 1255–1258.
200. Salvarani C, Farnetti E, Casali B, et al. Detection of parvovirus B19 DNA by polymerase chain reaction in giant cell arteritis: a case-control study. *Arthritis Rheum* 2002;46:3099–3101.
201. Matteson EL, Gold KN, Bloch DA, et al. Long-term survival of patients with giant cell arteritis in the American College of Rheumatology giant cell arteritis classification criteria cohort. *Am J Med* 1996;100:193–196.
202. Crofford LJ, Clauw DJ. Fibromyalgia: Where are we a decade after the American College of Rheumatology classification criteria were developed? *Arthritis Rheum* 2002;46:1136–1138.
203. Buchwald D, Goldenberg DL, Sullivan JL, et al. The "chronic, active Epstein-Barr virus infection" syndrome and primary fibromyalgia. *Arthritis Rheum* 1987;30:1132–1136.
204. Croft P, Schollum J, Silman A. Population study of tender point counts and pain as evidence of fibromyalgia. *BMJ* 1994;309:696–699.
205. Croft P, Rigby AS, Boswell R, et al. The prevalence of chronic widespread pain in the general population. *J Rheumatol* 1993;20:710–713.
206. White KP, Nielson WR, Harth M, et al. Chronic widespread musculoskeletal pain with or without fibromyalgia: psychological distress in a representative community adult sample. *J Rheumatol* 2002;29: 588–594.
207. Wolfe F. Fibromyalgia. *Rheum Dis Clin North Am* 1990;16:681–698.
208. Felson DT. Epidemiologic research in fibromyalgia. *J Rheumatol* 1989;16(suppl 19):7–11.
209. Hudson JI, Hudson MS, Pliner LF, et al. Fibromyalgia and major affective disorder. A controlled phenomenology and family history study. *Am J Psychiatry* 1985;142:441–446.
210. Dinerman H, Goldenberg DL, Felson DT. A prospective evaluation of 118 patients with fibromyalgia syndrome: prevalence of Raynaud's phenomenon, Sicca symptoms, ANA, low complement, and Ig deposition at the dermal-epidermal junction. *J Rheumatol* 1986;13:368–373.
211. Makela M, Heliovaara M. Prevalence of primary fibromyalgia in the Finnish population. *BMJ* 1991;203:216–219.
212. Felson DT, Goldenberg DL. The natural history of fibromyalgia. *Arthritis Rheum* 1986;29:1522–1526.
213. Miller MH, Topliss DJ. Chronic upper limb pain syndrome (repetitive strain injury) in the Australian workforce: a systematic cross sectional rheumatological study of 229 patients. *J Rheumatol* 1988; 15:1705–1712.
214. Bjelle A. Epidemiology of shoulder problems. *Baillieres Clin Rheumatol* 1989;3:437–451.
215. Milerad E, Ekenvall L. Symptoms of the neck and upper extremities in dentists. *Scand J Work Environ Health* 1990;16:129–134.
216. Mavrikakis ME, Drimis S, Kontoyannis DA, et al. Calcific shoulder periarthritis (tendinitis) in adult onset diabetes mellitus: a controlled study. *Ann Rheum Dis* 1989;48:211–214.

217. de Krom MCTFM, Knipschild PG, Kester ADM, et al. Carpal tunnel syndrome: prevalence in the general population. *J Clin Epidemiol* 1992;45:373–376.
218. Ferry S, Pritchard T, Keenan J, et al. Estimating the prevalence of delayed median nerve conduction in the general population. *Br J Rheumatol* 1998;37:630–635.
219. Armstrong TJ, Silverstein BA. Upper-extremity pain in the workplace role of usage in causality. In: Hadler NM, ed. *Clinical concepts in regional musculoskeletal illness.* Orlando: Grune & Stratton, 1987:333–354.
220. de Krom MCTFM, Kester ADM, Knipschild PG, et al. Risk factors for carpal tunnel syndrome. *Am J Epidemiol* 1990;132:1102–1110.
221. Kerr MS, Frank JW, Shannon HS, et al. Biomechanical and psychosocial risk factors for low back pain at work. *Am J Public Health* 2001;91:1069–1075.
222. Papageorgiou AC, Croft PR, Ferry S, et al. Estimating the prevalence of low back pain in the general population. Evidence from the South Manchester back pain survey. *Spine* 1995;20:1889–1894.
223. Jarvik JJ, Hollingworth W, Heagerty P, et al. The longitudinal assessment of imaging and disability of the back (LAIDBack) study. *Spine* 2001;26:1158–1166.
224. Spangfort EV. The lumbar disc herniation. A computer-aided analysis of 2504 operations. *Acta Orthop Scand Suppl* 1972;142:1.
225. Edmond SL, Felson DT. Function and back symptoms among older adults. *J Am Geriatr J Am Geriatr Soc* 2003;51:1702–1709.
226. Stevenson J, Weber CL, Smith JT, et al. A longitudinal study of the development of low back pain in an industrial population. *Spine* 2001;26:1370–1377.
227. Macfarlane GJ, Thomas E, Papageorgiou AC, et al. Employment and physical work activities as predictors of future low back pain. *Spine* 1997;22:1143–1149.
228. Snook SH. Low back pain in industry. In: White AA III, Gordon SL, eds. *American Academy of Orthopaedic Surgeons symposium on idiopathic low back pain.* St. Louis: CV Mosby, 1982:23.
229. Bigos SJ, Spengler DM, Martin NA, et al. Back injuries in industry: a retrospective study: II. Injury factors. *Spine* 1986;11:246.
230. Frymoyer JW, Pope MH, Clements JH, et al. Risk factors in low-back pain: an epidemiological survey. *J Bone Joint Surg Am* 1983; 65:215–218.
231. Sjolie AN, Ljunggren AE. The significance of high lumbar mobility and low lumbar strength for current and future low back pain in adolescents. *Spine* 2001;26:2629–2636.
232. Jones GT, Watson KD, Silman AJ, et al. Predictors of low back pain in British schoolchildren: a population-based prospective cohort study. *Pediatrics* 2003;111:822–828.
233. Deyo RA, Tsui-Wu YJ. Functional disability due to back pain: a population-based study indicating the importance of socioeconomic factors. *Arthritis Rheum* 1987;30:1247–1253.
234. Southwick SM. The use of psychological tests in the evaluation of low-back pain. *J Bone Joint Surg Am* 1983;65:560–565.
235. Kellgren JH, Lawrence JS. *Atlas of standard radiographs. The epidemiology of chronic rheumatism,* Vol. 2. Oxford: Blackwell Scientific, 1963.
236. Ahlback S. Osteoarthritis of knee: a radiographic investigation. *Acta Radiol Suppl (Stockh)* 1968;277:7–12.
237. Altman R, Fries JF, Block DA, et al. Radiographic assessment of progression in Osteoarthritis. *Arthritis Rheum* 1987;30:1214–1225.
238. Peat G, McCarney R, Croft P. Knee pain and osteoarthritis in older adults: a review of community burden and current use of primary health care. *Ann Rheum Dis* 2001;60:91–97.
239. Zhang Y, Niu J, Kelly-Hayes M, et al. Prevalence of symptomatic hand osteoarthritis and its impact on functional status among the elderly. *Am J Epidemiol* 2002;156:1021–1027.
240. Lawrence JS. *Rheumatism in populations.* Bristol, UK: JW Arrowsmith, 1977:98–155.
241. Felson DT, Zhang Y. An update on the epidemiology of knee and hip osteoarthritis with a view to prevention. *Arthritis Rheum* 1998;41: 1343–1355.
242. Van Saase JLCM, Van Rommunde LKJ, Cats A, et al. Epidemiology of Osteoarthritis: Zoetermeer survey, comparison of radiological osteoarthritis in a Dutch population with that in 10 other populations. *Ann Rheum Dis* 1989;48:271–280.
243. Engel A. *Osteoarthritis and body measurements.* Series 11, No. 29, U.S. Public Health Service Publication No. 1999. Rockville, MD: National Center for Health Statistics, 1968.
244. Jordan JM, Linder GF, Renner JB, et al. The impact of arthritis in rural populations. *Arthritis Care Res* 1995;8:242–250.
245. Lawrence JS, Sebo M. The geography of osteoarthritis. In: Nuki G, ed. *The aetiopathogenesis of osteoarthritis.* Baltimore: University Park Press, 1980:155–183.
246. Hoaglund FT, Yau ACMC, Wong WL. Osteoarthritis of the hip and other joints in Southern Chinese in Hong Kong. *J Bone Joint Surg Am* 1973;55:545–557.
247. Nevitt MC, Xu L, Zhang Y, et al. Very low prevalence of hip osteoarthritis among Chinese elderly in Beijing, China, compared with whites in the United States. The Beijing Osteoarthritis Study. *Arthritis Rheum* 2002;46:1773–1779.
248. Kim YJ, Zhang Y, Nevitt MC, et al. Morphological differences between Chinese and Caucasian hips in women [Abstract]. *Arthritis Rheum* 2003;49(Suppl):S664.
249. Zhang Y, Xu L, Nevitt MC, et al. Comparison of knee osteoarthritis prevalence between Chinese elderly in Beijing and Caucasians in the U.S.: the Beijing Osteoarthritis Study. *Arthritis Rheum* 2001;44: 2065–2071.
250. Zhang Y, Xu, L, Nevitt MC, Niu J, et al. Lower prevalence of hand osteoarthritis among Chinese subjects in Beijing compared with white subjects in the United States. *Arthritis Rheum* 2003;48:1034–1040.
251. Sharma L, Song J, Felson DT, et al. The role of knee alignment in disease progression and functional decline in knee osteoarthritis. *JAMA* 2001;286:188–195.
252. Felson DT, Anderson JJ, Naimark A, et al. Obesity and knee osteoarthritis: the Framingham Study. *Ann Intern Med* 1988;109:18–24.
253. Cicuttini FM, Bake JR, Spector TD. The association of obesity with osteoarthritis of the hand and knee in women: a twin study. *J Rheumatol* 1996;23:1221–1226.
254. McAlindon T, Zhang Y, Hannan M, et al. Are risk factors for patellofemoral and tibiofemoral knee osteoarthritis different? *J Rheumatol* 1996;23:332–337.
255. Felson DT, Zhang Y, Hannan MT, et al. Risk factors for incident radiographic knee osteoarthritis in the elderly. The Framingham Study. *Arthritis Rheum* 1997;40:728–733.
256. Nevitt M, Lane NE, Scott JC, et al. Relationship of hip osteoarthritis to obesity and bone mineral density in older American women: preliminary results from the Study of Osteoporotic Fractures. *Acta Orthop Scand* 1993;64(suppl):2–5.
257. Davis MA, Ettinger WM, Neuhaus JM. The role of metabolic factors and blood pressure in the association of obesity with osteoarthritis of the knee. *J Rheumatol* 1988;15:1827–1832.
258. Dequeker J, Goris P, Utterhoeven R. Osteoporosis and osteoarthritis (osteoarthrosis): anthropometric distinctions. *JAMA* 1983;249:1448–1451.
259. Felson DT. Epidemiology of hip and knee osteoarthritis. *Epidemiol Rev* 1988;10:1–18.
260. Hadler NM, Gillings DB, Imbus R, et al. Hand structure and function in an industrial setting. *Arthritis Rheum* 1970;21:210–220.
261. Croft P, Coggon D, Cruddas M, et al. Osteoarthritis of the hip: an occupational disease in farmers. *BMJ* 1992;304:1269–1272.
262. Coggon D, Croft P, Kellingray S, et al. Occupational physical activities and osteoarthritis of the knee. *Arthritis Rheum* 2000;43:1443–1449.
263. Kujala UM, Kettunen J, Paananen H, et al. Knee osteoarthritis in former runners, soccer players, weight lifters, and shooters. *Arthritis Rheum* 1995;38:539–546.
264. Roos H, Lindberg H, Gardsell P, et al. The prevalence of gonarthrosis in former soccer players and its relation to meniscectomy. *Am J Sports Med* 1994;22:219–222.
265. Puranen J, Ala-Ketola L, Peltokallio P, et al. Running and primary osteoarthritis of the hip. *BMJ* 1975;2:424–425.
266. Sohn RS, Micheli LJ. The effect on the pathogenesis of osteoarthritis of the hips and knees. *Clin Orthop Rel Res* 1984;198:106–109.
267. Lane NE, Michel B, Bjorkengren A, et al. The risk of osteoarthritis with running and aging: a 5-year longitudinal study. *J Rheumatol* 1993;20:461–468.
268. Panush RS, Hanson CS, Caldwell JR, et al. Is running associated with osteoarthritis? An eight-year follow-up study. *J Clin Rheum* 1994;Oct.
269. Spector TD, Harris PA, Hart DJ, et al. Risk of osteoarthritis associated with long-term weight-bearing sports: a radiographic survey of

the hips and knees in female ex-athletes and population controls. *Arthritis Rheum* 1996;39:988–995.

270. Marti B, Knowbloch M, Tschopp A, et al. Is excessive running predictive of degenerative hip disease? Controlled study of former elite athletes. *BMJ* 1989;299:91–93.
271. Vingard E, Alfredsson L, Goldie I, et al. Sports and osteoarthrosis of the hip: an epidemiologic study. *Am J Sports Med* 1993;21:195–200.
272. Konradsen L, Berg Hansen EM, Sondergaard L. Long distance running and osteoarthritis. *Am J Sports Med* 1990;18:379–381.
273. Kujala UM, Kaprio J, Sarna S. Osteoarthritis of weight bearing joints of lower limbs in former elite male athletes. *BMJ* 1994;308:231–234.
274. McAlindon TE, Wilson PWF, Aliabadi P, et al. Level of physical activity and the risk of radiographic and symptomatic knee osteoarthritis in the elderly: The Framingham Study. *Am J Med* 1999;106:151–157.
275. Ala-Kokko L, Baldwin CT, Moskowitz RW, et al. Single base mutation in the type II procollagen gene (COL2A1) as a cause of primary osteoarthritis associated with a mild chondrodysplasia. *Proc Natl Acad Sci U S A* 1990;87:6565–6568.
276. Palotie A, Ott J, Elim K, et al. Predisposition to familial osteoarthritisosis linked to type II collagen gene. *Lancet* 1989;1:924–927.
277. Ritvaniemi P, Korkko J, Bonaventure J, et al. Identification of COL2A1 gene mutations in patients with chondrodysplasias and familial osteoarthritis. *Arthritis Rheum* 1995;38:999–1004.
278. Spector TD, Cicuttini F, Baker J, et al. Genetic influences on osteoarthritis in women: a twin study. *BMJ* 1996;312:940–944.
279. Felson DT, Couropmitree NN, Chaisson CE, et al. Evidence for a mendelian gene in a segregation analysis of generalized radiographic osteoarthritis: the Framingham Study. *Arthritis Rheum* 1998;41:1064–1071.
280. Kaprio J, Kujala UM, Peltonen L, et al. Genetic liability to osteoarthritis may be greater in women than men [Letter]. *BMJ* 1996;313:232.
281. Hunter DJ, Demissie S, Cupples LA, et al. A new way to think about the genetics of hand osteoarthritis: joint specific phenotypes [Abstract]. The Framingham Study. *Arthritis Rheum* (in press).
282. Schumacher HR, Gordon G, Paul H, et al. Osteoarthritis, crystal deposition, and inflammation. *Semin Arthritis Rheum* 1981;10(suppl 1):116–119.
283. Felson DT, Anderson JJ, Naimark A, et al. The prevalence of chondrocalcinosis in the elderly and its association with knee osteoarthritis: the Framingham Study. *J Rheumatol* 1989;16:1241–1245.
284. Slemenda C, Heilman DK, Brandt KD, et al. Reduced quadriceps strength relative to body weight. A risk factor for knee osteoarthritis in women? *Arthritis Rheum* 1998;41:1951–1959.
285. Sharma L, Dunlop DD, Cahue S, et al. Quadriceps strength and osteoarthritis progression in malaligned and lax knees. *Ann Intern Med* 2003;138:613–619.
286. Nevitt M, Felson, Peterfy C, et al. Inflammation markers (CRP, TNF-α, IL-6) are not associated with radiographic or MRI findings of knee OA in the elderly: the Health ABC Study [Abstract 962]. *Arthritis Rheum* 2002;46(suppl):372.
287. Sowers M, LaChance L, Jamadar D, et al. The associations of bone mineral density and bone turnover markers with osteoarthritis of the hand and knee in pre- and perimenopausal women. *Arthritis Rheum* 1999;42(3):483–489.
288. Zhang Y, Hannan MT, Chaisson CE, et al. Bone mineral density and risk of incident and progressive radiographic knee osteoarthritis in women: the Framingham study. *J Rheumatol* 2000;27:1032–1037.
289. Hill CL, Gale DG, Chaisson CE, et al. Knee effusions, popliteal cysts and synovial thickening: association with knee pain in those with and without Osteoarthritis. *J Rheumatol* 2001;28:1330–1337.
290. Felson DT, Chaisson CE, Hill CL, et al. The association of bone -marrow lesions with pain in knee osteoarthritis. *Ann Intern Med* 2001;134:541–549.
291. McCarty DJ. Coexistent gout and rheumatoid arthritis. *J Rheumatol* 1981;8:253–254.
292. Wallace SL, Robinson H, Masi AT, et al. Preliminary criteria for the classification of the acute arthritis of primary gout. *Arthritis Rheum* 1977;20:895–900.
293. Jack SS. *Current estimates from the national health interview survey: United States, 1979.* Vital and Health Statistics Series 10, No. 136. Washington, DC: U.S. Department of Health and Human Services, 1981.
294. Arromdee E, Michet CJ, Crowson CS, et al. Epidemiology of gout: Is the incidence rising? *J Rheumatol* 2002;29:2403–2406.
295. Campion EW, Glynn RJ, DeLabry LO. Asymptomatic hyperuricemia. Risks and consequences in the Normative Aging Study. *Am J Med* 1987;82:421–426.
296. Roubenoff R. Gout and hyperuricemia. *Rheum Dis Clin North Am* 1990;16:539–550.
297. Mikkelson WH, Dodge HJ, Valkenburg H. The distribution of plasma uric acid values in a population unselected as to gout and hyperuricemia. *Am J Med* 1965;39:242–251.
298. O'Sullivan JB. Gout in a New England town. *Ann Rheum Dis* 1972;31:166–169.
299. Hall AP, Barry PE, Dawber TR, et al. Epidemiology of gout and hyperuricemia. *Am J Med* 1967;42:27–37.
300. Stewart RB, Yost R, Hale W, et al. Epidemiology of hyperuricemia in an ambulatory elderly population. *J Am Geriatr Soc* 1979;27:552–554.
301. Dodge HJ, Mikkelsen WM. Observations on the distribution of serum uric acid levels in participants of the Tecumseh, Michigan, community health studies. *J Chronic Dis* 1970;23:161–172.
302. Yano K, Rhoads GG, Kagan A. Epidemiology of serum uric acid among 800 Japanese-American men in Hawaii. *J Chronic Dis* 1977;30:171–184.
303. Okada M, Veda K, Omae T, et al. Factors influencing the serum uric acid level: a study based on a population survey in Hisayamatown, Kyushu, Japan. *J Chronic Dis* 1980;33:607–612.
304. Akizuki S. A population study of hyperuricemia and gout in Japan—analysis of sex, age and occupational differences in thirty-four thousand people in Nagano prefecture. *Ryumachi* 1982;22:201–208.
305. Prior I. Epidemiology of rheumatic disorders in the Pacific with particular emphasis on hyperuricemia and gout. *Semin Arthritis Rheum* 1981;11:213–229.
306. Healey LA. Epidemiology of hyperuricemia. *Arthritis Rheum* 1975;18:709–712.
307. Darmawan J, Valkenburg HA, Muirden KD, et al. The epidemiology of gout and hyperuricemia in a rural population of Java. *J Rheumatol* 1992;19:1595–1599.
308. Healey LA, Bayani-Sioson PS. A defect in the renal excretion of uric acid in Filipinos. *Arthritis Rheum* 1971;14:721–726.
309. Torralba TP, Bayani-Sioson PS. The Filipino and gout. Semin *Arthritis Rheum* 1975;4:307–320.
310. Gurwitz JH, Kalish SC, Bohn RL, et al. Thiazide diuretics and the initiation of anti-gout therapy. *J Clin Epidemiol* 1997;50:953–959.
311. Gordon T, Kannel WB. Drinking and its relation to smoking, BP, blood lipids, and uric acid. *Arch Intern Med* 1983;143:1366–1374.
312. Hochberg MC, Thomas J, Thomas DJ, et al. Racial differences in the incidence of gout. The role of hypertension. *Arthritis Rheum* 1995;38:628–632.
313. Kelley WN. Inborn errors of purine metabolism—1977. *Arthritis Rheum* 1977;20(suppl):221–227.
314. Levine W, Dyer AR, Shekelle RB, et al. Serum uric acid and 11. 5-year mortality of middle-aged women: findings of the Chicago Heart Association Detection Project in industry. *J Clin Epidemiol* 1989;42:257–267.
315. Abbott RD, Brand FN, Kannel WB, et al. Gout and coronary artery disease: the Framingham Study. *J Clin Epidemiol* 1988;41:237–242.
316. Lee J, Sparrow D, Vokonas PS, et al. Uric acid and coronary heart disease risk: evidence for a role of uric acid in the obesity-insulin resistance syndrome. The Normative Aging Study. *Am J Epidemiol* 1995;142:288–294.

CHAPTER 2

Differential Diagnosis of Arthritis: Analysis of Signs and Symptoms

Daniel J. McCarty

Rational prognosis and therapy require precise diagnosis, and diagnosis depends primarily on skillful history taking and physical examination, with subsequent help from the laboratory, the radiology department, or the surgical staff when indicated. This chapter focuses on the interpretation of those aspects of the clinical history (symptoms) and the physical examination (signs) that relate to the differential diagnosis of arthritis and allied conditions (Table 2.1).

The purpose of the history and physical examination is to classify a patient's problem into one of four broad categories: inflammatory, degenerative-metabolic, functional (including neurotic), or of unknown origin. These categories represent the primary nature of the diseases listed in Table 2.2. This classification does not deny the existence of an inflammatory component in osteoarthritis (OA) or of a degenerative component in inflammatory arthritides such as rheumatoid arthritis (RA) or psoriatic arthritis. There may be an organic component even in those syndromes listed as psychogenic—an organic peg on which is hung a psychoneurotic hat. Conversely, there is often a functional component to most organic illnesses. The "unknown" category is important because of the tendency by many clinicians to force a patient's musculoskeletal complaints into a diagnostic pigeonhole. New syndromes and subsets of old ones are constantly being recognized. At least 10% of patients with musculoskeletal complaints whom I have seen through the years cannot be given a definitive diagnosis. In the remainder, however, a reasonable differential diagnosis could be formulated after the initial examination.

HISTORY

Chief Complaint

Patients consult physicians only for pain, pain equivalent, or anxiety. Pain equivalents include subpainful unpleasant sensations such as itching, aching, stiffness, and nausea. Almost all other complaints are not presented to the doctor unless the patient, or a third party, is concerned or anxious about their presence. Thus, treatment depends on relief of the pain or other unpleasant sensation, an explanation of the pertinent pathophysiology to the patient in lay terms, and a brief explanation of how the prescribed regimen is expected to correct the problem. The history should include detailed inquiry about the patient's motivation in coming to the doctor, especially in the absence of pain or pain equivalent. Why the anxiety? Could the patients with fibromyalgia, making up 28% of new patients in private rheumatologic practice in the United States (1), represent the anxious protruding tip of the iceberg of individuals with tense neck and shoulder muscles? Are patients in a rheumatic disease practice more likely to come to the office with a shopping list of questions written on a slip of paper (*petit morceau de papier* syndrome)? The reason for the anxiety underlying all chief complaints should be probed.

History of Present Illness

In general, the clinician attempts to determine whether the patient has a systemic disease or a purely local condition. A localized condition may affect multiple sites. What joints or other structures are involved? (The word *joint* will be used hereafter, although tendon sheaths and bursae are often involved as well.)

What is the pattern of involvement? In what order did joint involvement occur? How fast did it occur? At what time of the day did it start? If joint involvement is painful, severity can be estimated by whether it interfered with function of the affected extremity or with sleep or work. Was involvement self-limited, migratory, or additive (progressive)? If limited,

TABLE 2.1. *Signs and symptoms useful in differential diagnosis of arthritis*

	Degenerative	Inflammatory	Psychogenic
Symptoms			
Stiffness (duration)	Few minutes; "gelling" after prolonged rest	Hours (often); most pronounced after rest	Little or no variation in intensity with rest or activity
Pain	Follows activity; relieved by rest	Even at rest; nocturnal pain may interfere with sleep	Little or no variation in intensity with rest or activity
Weakness	Present, usually localized and not severe	Often pronounced	Often a complaint; "neurasthenia"
Fatigue	Not usual	Often severe with onset in early afternoon	Often in A.M. on arising
Emotional depression and lability	Not usual	Common; coincides with fatigue; often disappears if disease remits	Often present
Signs			
Tenderness localized over afflicted joint	Usually present	Almost always; the most sensitive indication of inflammation	Tender "all over"; "touch-me-not" attitude; tendency to push away or to grasp the examining hand
Swelling	Effusion common; little synovial reaction	Effusion common; often synovial proliferation and thickening	None
Heat and erythema (skin)	Unusual but may occur	More common	None
Crepitus	Coarse to medium	Medium to fine	None, except with coexistent arthritis
Bony spurs	Common	Sometimes found, usually with antecedent osteoarthritis	None, except with coexistent osteoarthritis

TABLE 2.2. *Examples of diseases in various categories*

Noninflammatory[a]	Inflammatory	Psychogenic/functional
Erosive OA	*Tenosynovitis Calcific (BCP) Other	*Primary figromyalgia
*Primary generalized OA	*Rheumatoid arthritis	*Restless leg syndrome
*Isolated OA, e.g., hip, knee, first CMC lateral patellar facet	*Seronegative polyarthritis	*Hysteria
*Cervical syndrome	*Systemic lupus erythematosus	
*Traumatic arthritis	*Mixed connective tissue disease	
Aseptic (osteo)necrosis	Polyarteritis nodosa	
Amyloid arthropathy	Polymyositis	
*Pseudogout (some types)	Dermatomyositis	
Metabolic arthropathy	Rheumatic fever/poststreptococcal arthritis	
Hemachromatosis	*Reactive arthritis	
Acromegaly	*Psoriatic arthritis	
Hypothyroidism	*Ankylosing spondylitis/spondyloarthropathy	
Hyperparathyroidism	*Juvenile rheumatoid arthritis	
Ochronosis	Inflammatory bowel disease arthritis	
Neuroarthropathy (Charcot)	*Crystal synovitis	
*Enthesopathy	Gout (MSU)	
Tumors	Pseudogout (CPPD)	
Pigmented villondular synovitis; synovial sarcoma	Other (BCP, postcorticosteroid injection flare)	
*Mechanical abnormalities, e.g., torn menisci, tibial torsion	*Polymyalgia rheumatica	
*Reflex sympathetic dystrophies, e.g., shoulder-hand syndrome	*Palindromic rheumatism	
*Periarthritis of shoulder	Viral arthritis (e.g., rubella, mumps, hepatitis B, parvovirus)	
*Tendinitis	Infectious arthritis	
Blood dyscrasias, e.g., hemophilia	Bacterial	
*Benign hypermobility syndrome	Tuberculous	
	Fungal	
	Immune complex arthritis, e.g., cryoglobulinemia, bacterial endocarditis, infected ventriculoatrial shunt	

[a]An inflammatory component may be present intermittently in some of these conditions.
*Common conditions encountered by every clinician.
BCP, basic calcium phosphate; CMC, carpometacarpal; CPPD, calcium pyrophosphate dihydrate; MSU, monosodium urate monohydrate; OA, osteoarthritis.

how long was the episode? *Migratory* means that the process subsided completely in an affected joint while moving to an erstwhile normal joint. *Progressive,* or *additive,* means that the first joint stays afflicted while additional joints are involved by the pathologic process. Was treatment sought? What and how much was given and for how long? What was its effect on the disease? What were the side effects of therapy?

Certain symptoms can be analyzed almost objectively, producing reliable data that should be given much weight diagnostically. The duration of morning stiffness is one such measurement and serves as a convenient clinical yardstick to measure inflammatory activity (see Chapter 3). Patients are often emotional about the magnitude of morning stiffness but not about its duration. Two questions suffice: "What time do you get out of bed?" and "When are you as 'loose' as you are going to get?" The physician then determines the duration of stiffness by subtraction. But if a single question is asked, "How long are you stiff after getting up in the morning?" the patient will provide a time that will nearly always be different (shorter) than that obtained with the two-question technique.

The duration of morning stiffness is directly proportional to the severity of an inflammatory process in an extremity, whether this be arthritis, myositis, bursitis, or sunburn. It signifies, nonspecifically, inflammation. Variations in its duration can be used to quantify inflammation and its response to treatment.

Indeed, morning stiffness is one of the best ways to follow inflammation clinically, and in a world of complex and expensive testing, it is both free of charge and immediately available. It is more precise than the erythrocyte sedimentation rate in following rheumatoid inflammation. True stiffness should be differentiated from the articular "gelling" of OA, which lasts for only a few minutes or even seconds. The hesitant, stiff, first few steps of an elderly person crossing the room to switch television channels are a familiar example of the gelling phenomenon.

The sunburned limb becomes flexible sooner with each passing day, a faithful reflection of the resolution of the thermal injury and the accompanying inflammatory response. The protracted morning stiffness characteristic of polymyalgia rheumatica vanishes completely when low doses of prednisone are given. The average untreated patient with RA is stiff for about 4 hours after arising in the morning. The mechanism of stiffness after immobilization of an inflamed part is unclear, but it may be the subjective perception of increased resistance to motion that has been measured objectively (2), which in turn is probably related to localized tissue edema and accumulation of the metabolic products of inflammation. The milking action of muscular contractions stimulates both lymphatic flow and venous return. Increased stiffness of an inflamed part occurs not only after sleeping, but after any prolonged immobility, such as watching TV.

If a structure is severely inflamed, it is painful on motion, just as sunburned skin over a joint is painful on motion. Overt pain at rest is found only in intense inflammation. Pain is difficult to describe, much less quantify or localize. If trauma, including the microtrauma of motion, is pathogenetically important, then pain will occur on motion and subside with rest. If there is no pattern of pain at all, a psychogenic factor might be involved. In patients with musculoskeletal diseases, pain may arise from stimulation of synovial, capsular, periosteal, ligamentous, or tendinous nerve endings by mechanical irritation or by inflammation; from pressure on entrapped nerves, such as the median nerve in the carpal tunnel at the wrist, the suprascapular in the shoulder, or from nerve roots in the cervical foramina; or from muscle spasm, either directly or, with increased muscle tone, on nerves coursing through tightened muscle. Pain does not arise from cartilage. Electromyographers report little or no evidence of increased muscular contraction (spasm) about inflamed joints at rest, and to differentiate pathologically increased from normally increased electrical activity in contracting muscles is difficult. If a patient complains of parietal pain and has no increased stiffness after prolonged immobility, direct nerve irritation or a psychologic problem is immediately suspected. Elicited pain (tenderness) is much more important clinically and can be localized accurately.

Systemic fatigue, like stiffness, is a subjective phenomenon and is not disease specific. The time of onset of fatigue after arising from bed is inversely proportional to the severity of an inflammatory process. This time is determined by subtracting the point of "bone tiredness" from the time of arising. The average untreated rheumatoid patient has about 3.5 hours before fatigue sets in. The cause of such pathologic fatigue is unknown. Perhaps the products of inflammation, milked from the involved sites by muscular activity, produce tissue effects that subjectively represent fatigue. When asked about fatigue, patients often state that tiredness is present on arising. In the absence of insomnia, anemia, or metabolic disease, such fatigue is of neurotic origin. This sensation usually disappears soon after the patient is up and about. Most of us have had this experience occasionally. Waking unrefreshed may be symptomatic of absence of stage 4 (restorative) sleep, which is common in fibromyalgia patients.

Weakness

Disuse atrophy occurs rapidly, often in a few days, in muscles that move painful joints. In the diffuse systemic rheumatic diseases, direct muscle involvement often occurs as well. With upper extremity involvement, "clumsiness" or weakness of grip may be the complaint, whereas difficulty in rising from a chair or in going up or down stairs may be experienced with lower extremity involvement. This subjective complaint can be verified and quantified by measurement of grip strength or by timing a set task using lower extremity muscles (3).

Depression, Hysteria, and Emotional Lability

Depression may be the most common symptom of our age and is often noted in rheumatologic practice. It is present in patients with fibromyalgia (see Chapter 91) and, often in reactive form, in patients with systemic rheumatic diseases. In RA it often corresponds to the time of onset of pathologic fatigue, when emotional lability (crying, temper tantrums, or withdrawal) also occurs. These symptoms may disappear as the disease remits. Hysteria is less common and is usually dramatic. A patient cannot write clearly and has pain in the fingers (writer's cramp), cannot bend over or straighten up (camptocormia), or cannot straighten a bent extremity. Restless legs syndrome appears to be a hysterical condition or a depressive equivalent. Such patients are inordinately open to suggestion. Almost any medication that is prescribed with conviction will work miraculously but is certain to produce unpleasant side effects; these patients are notorious placebo reactors.

Systems Review

This is part of the routine history and should be performed in all cases.

Past History

A previous account of musculoskeletal or systemic disease may shed light on the current problem. Chorea or "growing pains" in childhood may aid in differentiating rheumatic fever or juvenile rheumatoid arthritis (JRA) in an adult patient. A history of recent exposure to ticks or viral illness may clarify an otherwise obscure arthritis. Even more important is a history of homosexuality or sexual promiscuity in a patient suspected of having gonorrheal arthritis or reactive arthritis.

Family History

A history of diabetes mellitus, hypertension, or heart disease can often be obtained accurately. Diabetes is associated with adhesive capsulitis of the shoulders, Dupuytren contracture, and OA. A family history of arthritis may be obtained in patients with gout, pseudogout, ankylosing spondylitis, and RA, to name a few. I often found it difficult to be sure of the diagnosis of arthritis from the family history, let alone what type of arthritis was actually present. This aspect of history taking may become more important with advances in immunogenetics (see Chapter 27).

Social History

Stability of family life and the stability and type of job are important points to establish because much of the treatment program in arthritis involves them. Avocations should also be recorded because these, too, must often be considered in designing a treatment program. Current drug intake should be listed here, including alcohol and tobacco. The patient's ability to perceive reality and level of emotional maturity should also be ascertained. The finding of Alzheimer's or other dementia in a patient may seriously affect compliance with a needed treatment protocol.

PHYSICAL EXAMINATION

An arthralgia is often an arthritis without a physical examination.

Palpation

Rheumatologists' fingers are their most important diagnostic tool. Although various devices are useful to quantify tenderness, joint swelling, and skin temperature, none supplant the fingers. A working knowledge of topographic anatomy is essential. Examiners must know what structures lie under their hand. This is particularly true when eliciting tenderness, which is the most sensitive sign available, albeit not specific. The neophyte uses too little force when pressing even on superficial structures. I exert sufficient force to blanch my thumbnail (4,5), 74 pounds per square inch, when examining areas that are not obviously inflamed. Of course, one could reduce the rate of return office visits sharply by pressing this hard on red, swollen joints. Common sense must prevail. I use tenderness primarily to exclude disease. If none is present at 74 pounds per square inch, underlying inflammation, in the absence of congenital or acquired insensitivity to pain, is ruled out. If tenderness is present, then either a low pain threshold or pathologic change may be responsible. Fortunately, most tenderness due to an organic cause is accompanied by more specific findings, such as swelling, crepitus, and increased local heat. Tenderness of joints is best elicited by pressure over the areas of synovial reflexion, whereas tendons should be stretched gently and then subjected to pressure. Direct pressure should be exerted on fibrositic areas in every patient. These areas include the lateral neck strap muscles, the belly of the trapezius, the epicondylar area, the buttocks, the medial knee over the collateral ligament and anserine bursa, and the lateral thigh over the tensor fasciae latae (see Chapter 91).

Areas of tenderness can be "controlled" by similar pressure over other nearby areas. A neurotic patient may be tender everywhere on the body. Such patients grasp the examiner's hand or draw the part away from the examiner's grasp—the "touch-me-not" sign. It is important to distinguish tender bones from tender soft tissues. For example, the anterior tibia is tender in most elderly subjects for reasons unknown. Bone tenderness is present in severe osteoporosis and other forms of systemic bone disease. In reflex sympathetic dystrophies, the entire hand (or foot) is tender.

Even allowing for periarticular accentuation of tenderness, tenderness between the joints, over both bone and soft tissue, often suggests this condition rather than a true synovitis (see Chapter 106).

Deep-seated joints, such as the hips, spine, and sacroiliac joints, require even more pressure to elicit tenderness because the intervening pad of soft tissue attenuates the applied force. Here, I exert pressure with the weight of my body against the flat of my hand held over the hip, or over my thumb in the case of spine or sacroiliac joints. It is helpful to drape the patient over the examining table with the legs hanging down and the feet touching the floor, but not bearing weight (Fig. 2.1). The lumbar lordotic curve is flattened in this position. The sacroiliac joints lie between the roof of the sciatic notch and the posteroinferior iliac spine, both of which can be identified easily. Inflammation of the sacroiliac joint is faithfully reflected by localized tenderness. Pressure can be exerted over each vertebral spine separately. The "skip areas" of spinal involvement so common in reactive arthritis, a septic discitis, or the precise level of lumbar degenerative disc disease, can often be mapped out readily with this technique.

A skilled examiner can lay hands on every peripheral joint in the body and can record the presence of tenderness on an appropriate form in about 3 minutes. Examination of the spine requires an additional 3 minutes.

Range of Motion

Passive motion of a joint is an ancillary method of eliciting pain and is also necessary to check for contractures or limitation of motion. When pain is present on passive motion, it is often impossible to determine its origin without further examination. For example, pain on attempting to straighten the elbow to 0 degrees or beyond can arise from intrinsic joint disease such as synovitis, or it may be due to extrinsic causes such as biceps tendinitis. The ability to completely extend the elbow ruled out elbow disease in one study (6). Pain on motion of a hip or shoulder joint is often due to abnormalities in the joint capsule, bursae, or surrounding tendons. It is my practice to examine the anatomic structures about any joint that is painful on passive motion to determine exactly what is and what is not tender. Thus, the absence of pain on passive motion rules out pathologic abnormalities of many structures, but its presence demands further palpatory dissection of the local anatomy in search of its cause.

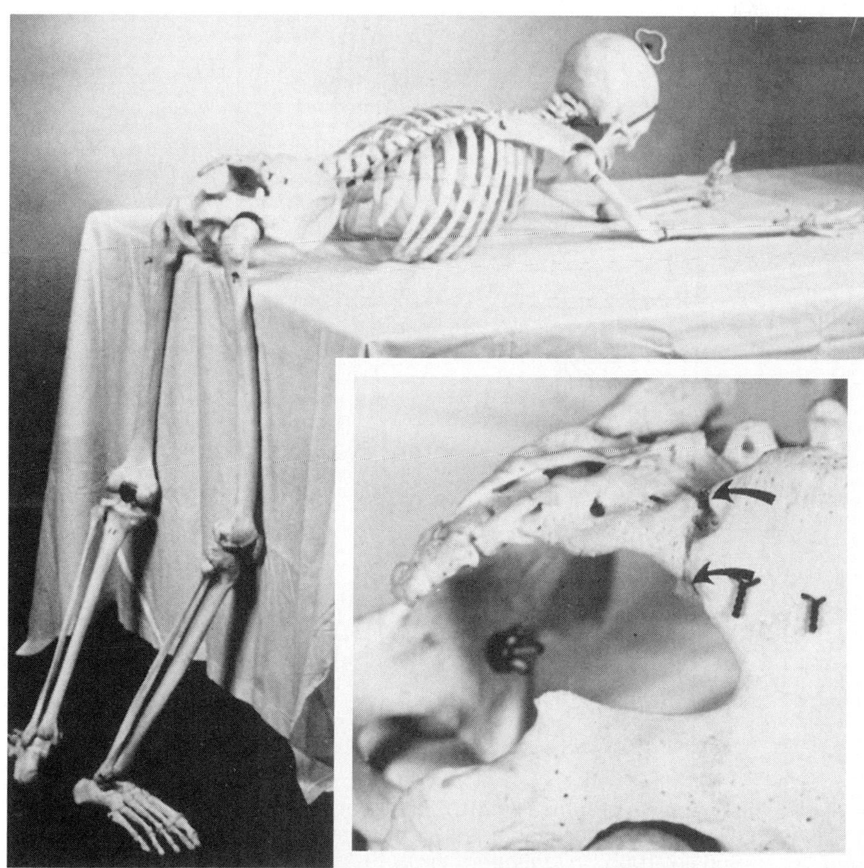

FIG. 2.1. Optimal position for examination of sacroiliac joints and lumbar spine is shown. The posterior aspect of the sacroiliac joints lies between the sciatic notch and the posteroinferior iliac spine (insert, *arrows*).

The range of motion of all joints should be determined while one attempts to elicit tenderness and pain on passive motion (Fig. 2.2). Loss of normal motion can be due to articular changes such as subluxation (partial dislocation), luxation (complete dislocation), capsular contraction, intraarticular adhesion, fibrous ankylosis, a tense effusion, extremely thickened synovium, or an intraarticular loose body. Bony ankylosis occurs commonly in some conditions such as JRA, ankylosing spondylitis, psoriatic arthritis, Reiter disease, and, rarely, in gout, pseudogout, RA, and OA. Extraarticular causes, such as ruptured or dislocated tendons, muscle spasm, tendon inflammation or shortening, or subchondral bony fractures, are perhaps even more common causes of loss of motion.

Abnormal motion of joints should also be noted. The subchondral bony collapse of the medial tibial plateau, so common in OA of the knee, produces a genu varus deformity and an abnormal lateral motion of the unstable knee owing to the slack in the medial collateral ligament. Early loss of lateral stability of the knee should be determined while the knee is flexed to about 25 degrees. Except in carpal or tarsal joints, RA is apt to result in unstable, not fused, joints. Three common examples are the valgus and flexion deformities of laterally unstable knees, sliding at-

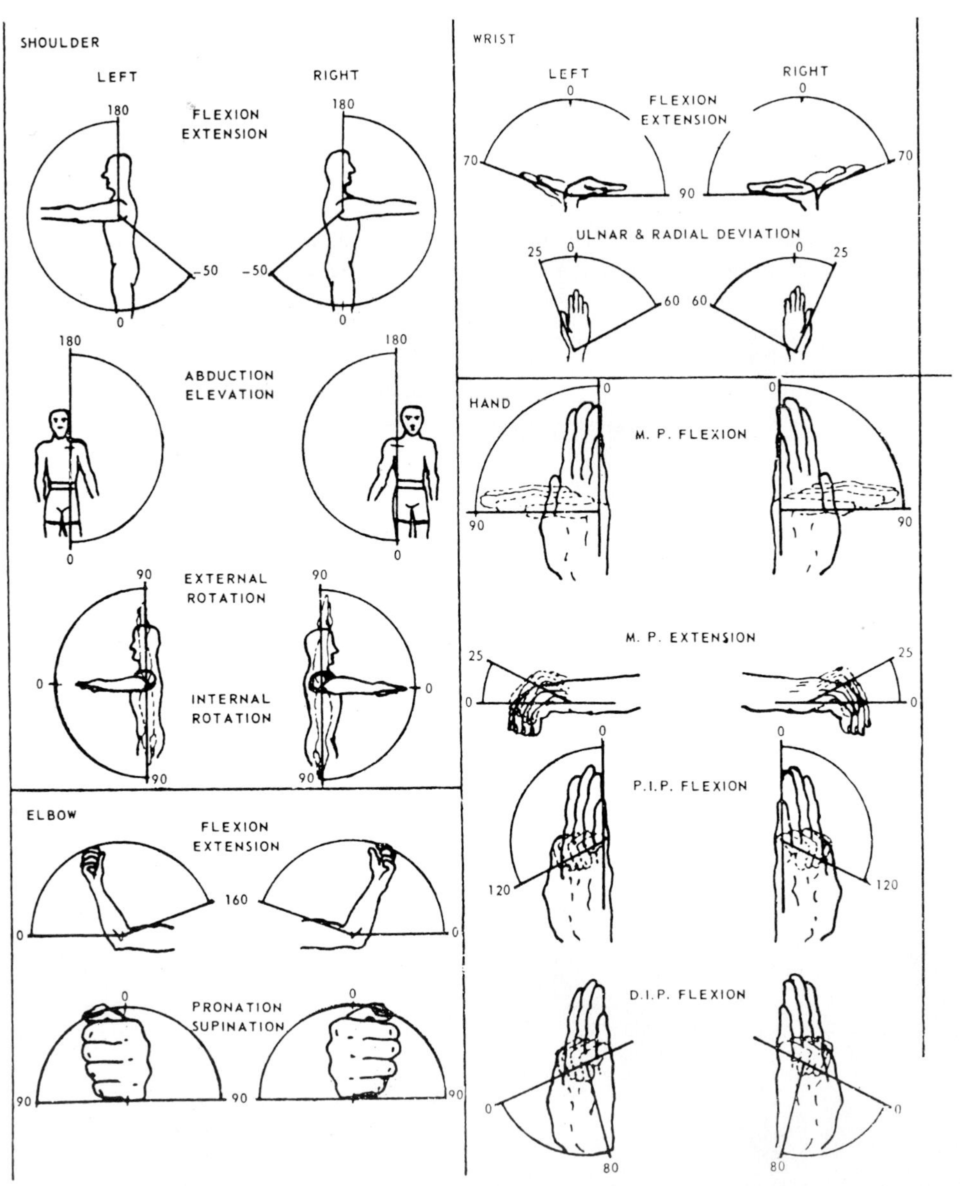

FIG. 2.2. Normal range of motion of all joints is shown graphically. *MCP,* metacarpophalangeal; *PIP,* proximal interphalangeal; *DIP,* distal interphalangeal; *IP,* interphalangeal. (Courtesy of Dr. J. Kenneth Herd, Buffalo Children's Hospital and SUNY-Buffalo, 1965.) *(Continued)*

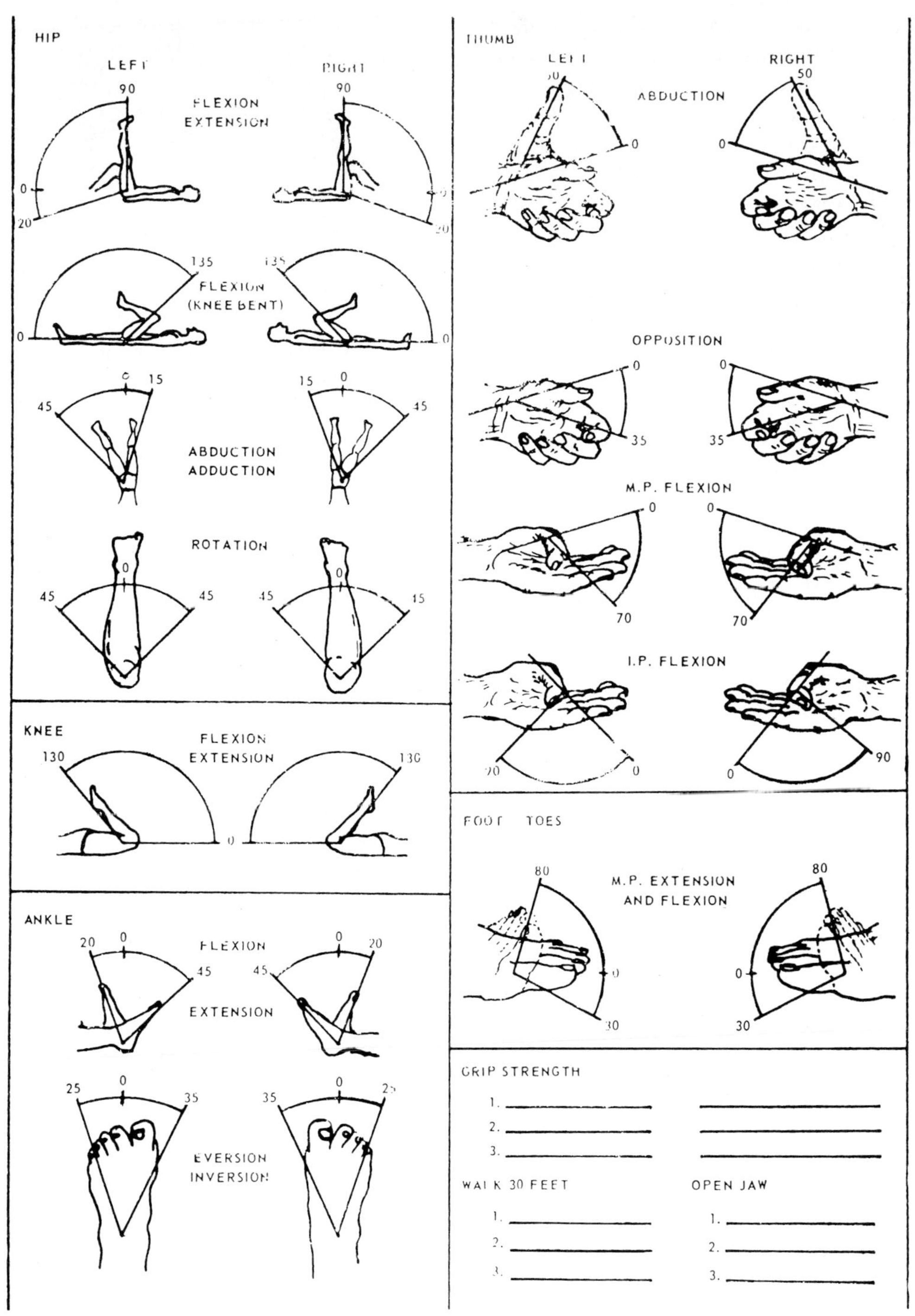

FIG. 2.2. *Continued*

lantoaxial joints, and abnormal lateral motion of the second metacarpophalangeal joint owing to erosion and rupture of its medial collateral ligament. This last should be sought with the joint flexed to 90 degrees, which stretches the collateral ligaments to tautness. Occasionally, in OA, one knee develops a varus, and the other a valgus, deformity, resulting in a "windswept" appearance. Valgus deformities in knees with degeneration are often associated with calcium pyrophosphate dihydrate crystal deposition.

Swelling

Swelling of joints, bursae, and tendons is an important sign that is always abnormal. Unlike tenderness, swelling specifically indicates organic disease. Swelling is most often due to underlying inflammation and can be due to synovial thickening, increased volume of joint fluid, or local edema. Detection of synovial thickening requires a knowledge of the anatomic synovial reflexions. Joints that lie just under the skin, such as the knee, elbow, wrist, metacarpophalangeal (MCP), proximal interphalangeal (PIP), distal interphalangeal (DIP), and metatarsophalangeal (MTP) joints, are particularly suitable. If a pad of thickened tissue is felt, particularly in multiple areas, synovium is probably thickened, owing either to inflammatory proliferation or to storage of abnormal material such as amyloid. The synovia of tendons frequently share in the proliferative process, leading to detectable swelling in the hand with bulging of palmar fat between the tendons (Fig. 2.3). Swelling of the synovium of the MTP joints leads to abnormal separation of the toes—the "window" sign (Fig. 2.4). Synovial thickening in a tendon sheath, common in reactive arthritis or psoriatic arthritis, produces a "sausage finger" or "sausage toe" appearance. In general, synovial swelling is most pronounced on extensor surfaces of joints, where the capsule is more distensible.

Effusions are particularly common in large weight-bearing joints with distensible communicating bursae. Thus, fluid is often found in the knee, is less common in the hip and ankle with their tighter joint capsules, and is much less common in upper extremity joints, where the presence of detectable fluid is related directly to joint size. Fluid is often present in shoulder joints of patients with RA, but these joints are involved in relatively few patients. The wrist has a tight capsule, and fluid is rarely obtained unless the joint is intensely inflamed. Fluid is rarely, if ever, obtained from small hand joints. The importance of detecting fluid lies in its great diagnostic value. (See Chapters 4 and 35 for the techniques of synovianalysis and arthrocentesis.)

Osteophytes also produce a swollen appearance and are easily palpable along the margins of joints or parts of joints that lie just under the skin, such as the MTP, knee, PIP, and DIP. These are hard to the touch and may be tender. They are often more striking on clinical than on radiologic examination.

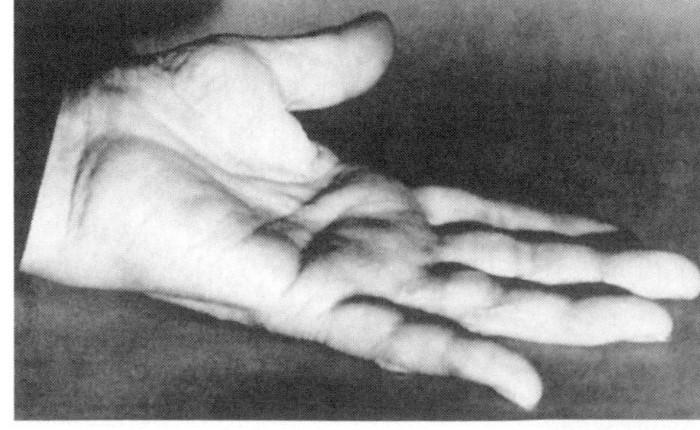

FIG. 2.3. Thickening of the synovium of the flexor digitorum tendons can be felt easily. Displaced tissues produce abnormal bulging between the tendons in the palm.

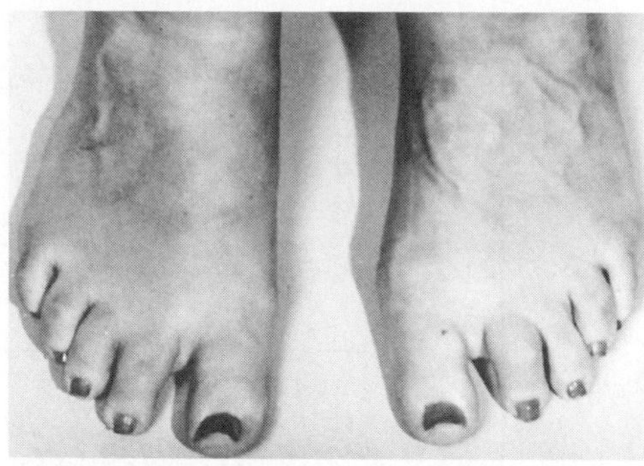

FIG. 2.4. Synovial thickening of the metatarsophalangeal joints spreads the forefoot, separating the toes and producing the "window sign."

Nodular swellings felt over joints or areas exposed to repeated trauma—such as the olecranon, back of the head or heel, ischial tuberosity, external ear, and bridge of the nose in persons wearing eyeglasses—may be due to rheumatoid nodules, gouty tophi, or (rarely) xanthomata or amyloid masses. Clinically, a nodule is only a nodule until its contents are examined microscopically. Most "nodules" over rheumatoid finger joints turn out to be synovium herniated through defects in the joint capsule. Such hernias are usually reducible. Tendon nodules often occur in RA, systemic lupus, and rheumatic fever.

Skin Temperature

Increased warmth of skin overlying an inflamed deeper structure, sometimes accompanied by erythema in individuals with relatively little skin pigment, is common and nonspecific. Differences between the temperature of the skin over an inflamed part and the surrounding skin can be estimated to within 0.5°C using the back of the fingers. This determination is most helpful over large joints for obvious reasons. Unlike tenderness, which is a sensitive parameter because normal structures have none, increased warmth is inherently insensitive because normal parts are normally warm. It is more difficult to be certain of an increase of 0.5°C on a background temperature of 32°C than it is to feel secure that a PIP joint is tender when other PIP joints in the same hand are not.

Crepitus

Crepitus (noise) may be heard or, more often, felt as the joints are put through a range of motion. The coarse crackle in the joints of some individuals is of no pathologic significance. This noise is due to tendons snapping over bony prominences or perhaps to the "cracking" phenomenon (7) (see Chapter 8). Generally, the finer the crepitus, the more significant it is clinically. Crepitus can be felt frequently as a fine vibratory sensation, even when no noise is heard. Crepitus can arise from the grating of roughened cartilages against one another, or from bone rubbing against bone.

A peculiar, fine crepitus can often be felt or heard when a chronically involved rheumatoid joint is moved, especially when loaded, such as in knees or hips on weight bearing. This crepitus is presumably due to friction between destroyed articular cartilages. It always occurs in joints showing severe generalized cartilage loss radiographically, and has been likened to the rubbing together of two sheets of old parchment. Extensive fibrin deposition in certain kinds of trauma or inflammation often gives rise to tendon crepitus. Tendon friction rubs indicate the systemic form of scleroderma with its poorer prognosis (8). The Achilles tendons of the weekend athlete may audibly rebel on Monday. Typically, the latter types of crepitus are prominent after rest and diminish with repetitive movement. They are detected easily by the first, but not the last, student to examine the patient. Some idea of the integrity of the articular cartilages can be obtained by rubbing the distal part of a joint against the firmly anchored proximal part. The patella can be rubbed up and down in its groove as the patient lies supine with the quadriceps muscle relaxed. The humeral head can be grated against the glenoid with the scapula held firmly by the examiner's other hand. The MTP, PIP, and first carpometacarpal joint surfaces can be rubbed together at the same time that stability, range of motion, and tenderness are checked. Thus, the examiner can determine the extent of inflammation that is present and its long-term sequelae: deformity, instability, and cartilage damage.

The mechanism of knuckle cracking has been examined (7). This phenomenon is due to mechanical subluxation of the joint, with intraarticular gas formation due to the accompanying decrease in intraarticular pressure. The accompanying vaporization of joint fluid releases enough free energy to produce an audible crack. Once cracked, a knuckle cannot be cracked again until the gas has been absorbed and the increased space between the bone returns to normal. This process takes about 30 minutes.

Weakness

Atrophy of muscle, especially the extensors, occurs rapidly about an inflamed or injured joint. Such a joint is almost always flexed to midposition, the point of lowest intraarticular pressure and the position of maximum comfort. Muscle strength can be quantified readily by measuring grip with an appropriately rolled blood pressure cuff and by timing a repetitive action involving lower extremity muscles (3). It is often helpful to measure the circumference of the limb at a measured distance above or below a fixed point, such as the olecranon process or patella. Serial measurement provides a method to monitor an exercise program designed to restore missing muscle bulk.

SPECIFIC RHEUMATOLOGIC EXAMINATION

Clinicians should develop a standard, disciplined routine examination of the musculoskeletal system, just as for the abdominal or chest examination. The approach may differ among clinicians, but it should be the same for a given clinician each time a patient is examined. This routine can easily be integrated into the general examination, reference to which is omitted in the following description. Particular attention is given to sites about which the patient specifically complains or those having abnormalities of which the patient is often unaware.

I start at the top with the temporomandibular joints, commonly involved in RA but never in gout. Press over the joint, which lies just below the zygomatic arch in front of the ear. The joint can also be felt by placing a finger in the external auditory canal. Ask the patient to open wide and then bite. The space between the front teeth should accommodate three fingers. Next the range of motion of the cervical spine is examined. Have the patient touch the chin to both shoulders (rotation). Then, with the patient's nose kept in the midline, have the patient attempt to touch first one shoulder and then the other with an ear (lateral flexion). The patient should then place the chin to the chest, and then extend the neck as far as possible. The inion process of the occiput should come within three finger-breadths of the spinous process of C7. The usual fibrositic areas in the neck are pressed at the same time. Arthritic conditions generally produce limitation of rotation or lateral flexion before limitation of flexion or extension occurs. If these last motions are disproportionately restricted, or if they are more painful than attempted, lateral flexion or rotation, a lesion affecting the spinal cord itself, rather than the cervical nerve roots, should be suspected.

Next, apply pressure with the thumb over the acromioclavicular and sternoclavicular joints, which are also examined for synovial thickening. Both are commonly affected by RA, and the acromioclavicular joints often develop osteoarthritic changes. The sternomanubrial cleft and the costal cartilages are next compressed, and the chest expansion measured as an index of costovertebral motion. The lateral motion of the spine is determined as the patient sits. The shoulder joints are then put through a full range of motion, always testing abduction by holding the scapula down with one hand.

The cartilages of the humeral head and glenoid are rubbed together, the fibrous capsule is felt, and the supraspinatus and bicipital tendons are compressed. The last can be "twanged" like a bowstring as it lies in the bicipital groove. The examination of this inherently unstable joint should include an evaluation of its stabilizing structures (9). The extension of the elbows is next examined, and these joints are examined for synovial thickening. The olecranon and proximal ulna are palpated for bursal enlargement and for lumps that might suggest tophi, rheumatoid nodules, xanthoma, or amyloid deposits. The wrist is put through a range of motion and examined for synovial thickening and extensor tenosynovitis or de Quervain's tenosynovitis (extensor tendons of thumb). The radiocarpal joint, the carpal joints, and the ulnar bursa (distal radioulnar joint and contiguous bursa over the distal ulna) are each pressed separately for tenderness. The integrity of the distal radioulnar joint, often eroded by RA with dorsal displacement of the ulna, is assessed. The abnormal vertical motion of the distal ulna has been likened to that of a piano key—thus the "piano key" sign. The extensor carpi ulnaris is compressed. This structure is often involved in RA. The MCP joints are pressed together laterally and are then checked separately if tenderness is elicited. Synovial thickening, range of motion, instability, and cartilage integrity are checked. Tenderness, swelling, and range of motion of all PIP and DIP joints, and of the interphalangeal, MCP, and first carpometacarpal joints of the thumb are assessed. The hand is turned over and is examined for palmar erythema, palmar thickening, and Dupuytren contracture. Each tendon is compressed for tenderness and is felt for thickening when the finger has been fully extended. The flexor carpi radialis and flexor carpi ulnaris tendons are next compressed. The latter tendon has no sheath, but the pisiform bone is incorporated into it as a sesamoid. A synovial sac lies beneath the pisiform.

With the patient supine, each hip is flexed, abducted, and externally rotated (Patrick maneuver). If a flexion contraction is suspected, the opposite hip is held in full flexion to fully flatten the lumbar lordosis, and the hip in question is fully extended. This maneuver prevents disguise of a flexion deformity by an increased lumbar lordosis. The hip joint is compressed from above, and then the tensor fascia lata and trochanteric bursa are compressed from the side.

The range of motion of the knee is determined. The condition of the quadriceps, presence of synovial thickening, foreign bodies, fluid, warmth, osteophytes, stability, and cartilage integrity, especially of the patellofemoral compartment, are determined. Popliteal cysts are sought, and the fat pads under the patellar tendons are compressed. The ankles and subtalar joints are examined separately, as are the posterior and anterior tibialis and peroneal tendons. Synovial thickening at the ankle is often difficult to determine because of the normal increase in the periarticular fibrofatty tissues here in middle age and beyond, especially in women.

The tarsal joints are compressed as a group. The MTP joints are squeezed together laterally and are examined separately if any tenderness ensues. The first MTP joint is felt for osteophytes, range of motion, and cartilage integrity. The bunion bursa and sesamoids in the flexor hallucis tendon are examined. The latter is an extremely common site of symptomatic OA. The position of the metatarsal fat pad, nature's metatarsal support, is checked. This pad often slides forward under the toes in RA and leaves the swollen metatarsal heads just under the skin. The toes are next examined for ankylosis, and for "cock-up" or hammer deformities. The feet should be examined while the patient is weight bearing. Each toe normally touches both the floor and the adjoining toe. Failure to touch the floor may indicate early subluxation of the MTP joint. Spaces between toes, the "window sign" (Fig. 2.4), indicate MTP joint swelling or a spread forefoot. Foot deformities such as pes cavus or pes planus are noted with the patient standing. The spine is examined as already described.

Each of these areas can be examined in greater detail if necessary, with abnormalities pinpointed to specific ligaments, bursae, and tendons. Excellent monographs are available that provide more detailed descriptions and illustrations of the rheumatologic examination (10,11).

DATA SYNTHESIS AND DIFFERENTIAL DIAGNOSIS

The mind of the clinician stores data in much the same way as a computer, but it also does more. It weighs each datum, and weighs each datum differently in each individual. When one is writing about this process, generalizations must be made, but in full recognition of the more subtle analysis actually made in real life. The relative weights of the various signs and symptoms have been indicated in a general way in the foregoing descriptions.

The general category within which a patient's problem falls is usually obvious from the history and physical examination. To pinpoint the diagnosis, however, laboratory examination, including gross and microscopic joint fluid analysis, radiologic study, specialized tests, and, occasionally, biopsy for ordinary or special microscopy, are indicated.

If the process is inflammatory, the diagnostic possibilities differ according to whether it is confined to one joint or is polyarticular and whether it affects the axial (spine, shoulders, hips) or the appendicular (peripheral) joints. The differential diagnosis of some representative common inflammatory conditions is given in Table 2.3 for monoarthritis, Table 2.4 for polyarthritis, Table 2.5 for inflammatory spondyloarthropathy, and Table 2.6 for degenerative and metabolic arthropathy. Such brief vignettes of findings are necessarily superficial and incomplete and are offered here with some diffidence. These tables may be of use to medical students and house staff in their earliest encounters with arthritic patients.

TABLE 2.3. *Differential diagnosis of inflammatory monarthritis*

A. Cystal-induced
  1. Gout—male, lower extremity, previous attack, nocturnal onset, precipitated by medical illness or surgical procedures, response to colchicine, hyperuricemia, sodium urate crystals in joint fluid with neutrophils predominating, and WBC 10,000–60,000/mm^3
  2. Pseudogout—elderly patient, knee or other large joint, previous attack, precipitated by medical illness or surgical procedure, flexion contractures, chondrocalcinosis on radiography, calcium pyrophosphate dihydrate crystals in joint fluid with neutrophils predominating, and WBC 5,000–60,000/mm^3
  3. Calcific tendinitis, bursitis, or periarthritis—extraarticular, tendon or capsule of larger joints, previous attack in same or other area, calcification on radiography, chalky or milky material aspirated from area, neutrophils with phagocytosed ovoid bodies microscopically

B. Palindromic rheumatism
  Middle-aged or elderly male, sudden onset, little systemic reaction, previous attacks, may be positive rheumatoid factor, little or no residual chronic joint inflammation, residual olecranon bursal enlargement; joint fluid rarely obtained; fibrin deposition on biopsy

C. Infectious arthritis
  1. Septic—severe inflammation, primary septic focus, drug or alcohol abuse, joint fluid with neutrophils predominating, WBC 50,000–300,000/mm^3 (pus), infectious agents identified on smear and culture, or bacterial antigens identified in joint fluid
  2. Tubercular—primary focus elsewhere, drug or alcohol abuse, marked joint swelling for long period, joint fluid with neutrophils predominating, acid-fast organisms on smear and culture
  3. Fungal—similar to tuberculosis
  4. Viral—antecedent or concomitant systemic viral illness, joint fluid can be of inflammatory or noninflammatory type, either mononuclear cells or neutrophils may predominate

D. Other
  1. Tendinitis—as in A.3, but without radiologic calcification, antecedent trauma including repetitive motion
  2. Bursitis—as above, but inflamed area is more diffuse, antecedent trauma
  3. Juvenile rheumatoid arthritis—one or both knees swollen in preteen or teenager without systemic reaction, no erosions, mildly inflammatory joint fluid with some neutrophils, and no depression in synovial fluid $C'H_{50}$ levels.

WBC, white blood count.

TABLE 2.4. *Differential diagnosis of inflammatory polyarthritis*

A. RA
  1. Seropositive—female patient, symmetric joint and tendon involvement, synovial thickening, joint inflammation "in phase," nodules, weakness, systemic reaction, erosions on radiogram, rheumatoid factor present, $C'H_{50}$ level depressed in joint fluid that has 5,000–30,000 WBC/mm^3 about 50%–80% neutrophils; possible occurrence in children
  2. Seronegative—either sex, symmetric joint and tendon involvement, joint inflammation "in phase," more bony reaction radiographically (sclerosis, osteophytes, fusion, periostitis), rheumatoid factor absent, $C'H_{50}$ not depressed in joint fluid that has 3,000–20,000 WBC/mm^3 about 20%–60% neutrophils; more asymmetric than in seropositive cases; some cases probably are adult juvenile RA

B. Collagen vascular disease
  1. Systemic lupus erythematosus—female patient, symmetric joint distribution identical to RA, hair loss, mucosal lesions, rash, systemic reaction, visceral organ or brain involvement, leukopenia, positive STS, no erosions radiographically, noninflammatory joint fluid with good viscosity and mucin clot and 1,000–2,000 WBC/mm^3, mostly small lymphocytes; serum, $C'H_{50}$ often depressed, ANA titer elevated, antinative human DNA antibody titer increased, anti-SM antibody increased; anti-SSA (Ro) subset (subacute cutaneous lupus)
  2. Scleroderma—tight skin, Raynaud phenomenon, resorption of digits, dysphagia, constipation, lung, heart or kidney involvement, symmetric tendon contractures, little or no synovial thickening, radiographic calcinosis circumscripta, positive ANA with speckled or nucleolar pattern, anti-SCL-70 (systemic) and anticentromere antibodies (CREST syndrome)
  3. Polymyositis (dermatomyositis)—proximal muscle weakness in pelvic and pectoral girdles, tender muscles, rash, typical nailbed and knuckle pad erythema, symmetric joint involvement, EMG showing combined myopathic and denervation pattern, muscle biopsy abnormal, elevated serum creatinine phosphokinase
  4. Mixed connective tissue disease—swollen hands. Raynaud phenomenon; tight skin, symmetric joint and tendon involvement, possible evidence of joint erosions radiographically, positive ANA speckled pattern, anti-RNP antibody increased, strong response to corticosteroid therapy in antiinflammatory doses
  5. Polyarteritis nodosa—symmetric involvement, diverse clinical picture of systemic disease, histologic or angiographic diagnosis

C. Rheumatic fever
  Young (2–40 years of age), sore throat, group A streptococci, migratory arthritis, rash, pancarditis or pericardial involvement, elevated ASO titers, joint inflammation responds dramatically to aspirin treatment, often no cardiac findings in adults

Continued

TABLE 2.4. *Continued*

D. Juvenile RA
Symmetric joint involvement, rash, fever, absence or rheumatoid factor, radiographic periostitis, erosions late, possibly beginning or recurring in an adult; ANA-positive pauciarticular girls may develop iridocyclitis; B27-positive boys with possible fusion of sacroiliac and spinal joints
E. Psoriatic arthritis
Asymmetric boggy joint and tendon swelling, skin or nail lesions not always prominent or may follow arthritis, DIP joints may be prominently involved, radiologic periostitis or erosions, no rheumatoid factor, $C'H_{50}$ usually not depressed in inflammatory joint fluid with neutrophilic predominance
F. Reactive arthritis
Male patient, homosexual and/or sexually promiscuous, urethritis, iritis, conjunctivitis, asymmetric joints, lower extremity, nonpainful mucous membrane ulcerative lesion, balanitis circinata, keratoderma blennorrhagica, weight loss, $C'H_{50}$ increased in serum and in joint fluid with 5,000–30,000 WBC/mm^3; macrophages in joint fluid with three to five phagocytosed neutrophils ("Reiter" cell); possible sequela of enteric infections or urethritis; syndrome may be incomplete and may affect females
G. Gonorrheal arthritis
Migratory arthritis or tenosynovitis finally settling in one or more joints or tendons, either sex, primary focus urethra, female genitourinary tract, rectum, or oropharynx, skin lesions, vesicles; gram-negative diplococci on smear but not on culture of vesicular fluid, positive culture at primary site, blood, or joint fluid
H. Polymyalgia rheumatica
Elderly patient (>50 years), symmetric pelvic or pectoral girdle complaints without loss of strength, morning stiffness of long duration, prominent fatigue, weight loss, possible joint involvement, especially of shoulders, sternoclavicular joint, knees; sedimentation rate elevated, fibrinogen and β- and τ-globulin elevation, anemia, complete response to low doses (10–20 mg) prednisone, serum CPK normal, elevated alkaline phosphatase (liver)
I. Crystal-induced
1. MSU crystals (gout)—symmetric arthritis, flexion contractures, prior history of acute attacks, tophi, out-of-phase joint inflammation, systemic corticosteroid treatment for RA, hyperuricemia, MSU crystals in joint fluid
2. CPPD crystals (pseudogout)—symmetric arthritis, MCP flexion contractures, as well as of wrist, elbow, shoulder, hip, knees, and ankles, prior acute attacks (sometimes), out-of-phase joint inflammation, CPPD crystals in joint fluid
3. BCP crystals (Milwaukee shoulder)
J. Other
Amyloid arthropathy, peripheral arthritis of inflammatory bowel disease, tuberculosis, SBE, viral or spirochetal arthritis

ANA, antinuclear antibody; ASO, antistreptolysin O; BCP, basic calcium phosphate; CPK, creatinine phosphokinase; CPPD, calcium pyrophosphate dihydrate; CREST syndrome, calcinosis, Raynaud phenomenon, esophageal involvement, sclerodactyly, and telangiectasia; DIP, dorsal interphalangeal; EMG, electromyography; MCP, metacarpophalangeal; MSU, monosodium urate; RA, rheumatoid arthritis; RNP, ribonucleoprotein; SBE, subacute bacterial endocarditis; STS, serologic tests for syphilis; WBC, white blood cell.

TABLE 2.5. *Differential diagnosis of inflammatory spondyloarthropathy*

A. Ankylosing spondylitis—male patient, symmetric sacroilitis clinically and radiologically, limitation of spinal motion, uveitis, smooth symmetric spinal ligamentous calcification, ankylosis (often complete), absence of skip areas, family history, HLA-B27 antigen usually present, good response to NSAIDs
B. Reactive arthritis—sexually promiscuous man with urethritis, skin-eye-heel involvement, asymmetric peripheral joint involvement, sacroilitis often asymmetric and "skip" areas of involvement in spine, coarse asymmetric syndesmophytes in spine, incomplete and asymmetric ankylosis, HLA-B27 often present, equivocal response to NSAIDs
C. Psoriatic spondylitis—skin or peripheral joint involvement, asymmetric sacroilitis, skip areas, possible ankylosis, HLA-B27 often present
D. Inflammatory bowel disease—sacroilitis, often symmetric, ankylosis, possibly silent bowel disease, spinal inflammation; unlike peripheral arthritis, does not vary with and is not responsive to treatment directed at bowel inflammation; HLA-B27 often present
E. Other—infection (bacterial, tuberculous, fungal) osteochondritis, multiple epiphysitis in young adults

Juvenile rheumatoid arthritis spondyloarthropathy occurs almost entirely in HLA-B27–positive boys and is regarded as juvenile ankylosing spondylitis.
NSAID, nonsteroidal antiinflammatory drug.

TABLE 2.6. *Differential diagnosis of degenerative or metabolic arthropathy*

A. Primary generalized "nodal" osteoarthritis
   Heberden nodes in DIP joints; Bouchard nodes in PIP joints; arthritis of first CMC, knee, first MTP joints; symmetric, familial, no systemic reaction; group 1 joint fluid
   Variants
   1. Erosive osteoarthritis—same but with more inflammatory features; possible bony ankylosis
   2. Localized osteoarthritis of DIP, first CMC, first MTP, other joints
B. Nonnodal osteoarthritis
   1. Osteoarthritis localized to one or (usually) both knees—flexion and varus deformities in middle-aged or elderly patient, group 1 joint fluid, subchondral microfractures with collapse of the medial tibial plateau; predominant involvement of medial tibiofemoral compartment
   2. Primary osteoarthritis of hip: (a) unilateral—superior joint space narrowing, long leg on ipsilateral side; (b) bilateral—medial joint space narrowing with medial migration of femoral heads, equal leg lengths
   3. Secondary osteoarthritis—any joint, traumatic origin, slipped epiphysis, mechanical problem, congenital malformation, another antecedent arthritis
   4. Osteoarthritis associated with CPPD or BCP crystals; symmetric involvement, elderly patient, flexion contractures of joints listed in Table 2.4, prior acute attacks, associated metabolic diseases, familial incidence; lateral tibiofemoral and patellofemoral compartments often predominant with valgus deformity and flexion contracture
C. Metabolic
   Diffuse or localized musculoskeletal complaints in patient with endocrine or metabolic disease

BCP, basic calcium phosphate; CMC, carpometacarpal; CPPD, calcium pryrophosphate dihydrate; DIP, distal interphalangeal; MTP, metatarsophalangeal.

REFERENCES

1. ARA Committee on Rheumatologic Practice. A description of rheumatology practice. *Arthritis Rheum* 1977;20:1278–1281.
2. Wright V, Johns RJ. Observation on the measurement of joint stiffness. *Arthritis Rheum* 1960;3:328–340.
3. Csuka ME, McCarty DJ. A rapid method for measurement of lower extremity muscle strength. *Am J Med* 1985;78:77–81.
4. McCarty DJ, Gatter RA, Phelps P. A dolorimeter for quantification of articular tenderness. *Arthritis Rheum* 1965;8:551–559.
5. McCarty DJ, Gatter RA, Steele AD. A twenty pound dolorimeter for quantification of articular tenderness. *Arthritis Rheum* 1968;11:696–698.
6. Docherty MA, Schwab RA, Ma OJ. Can elbow extension be used as a test of clinically significant injury? *South Med J* 2002;95:539–541.
7. Unsworth A, Dowson D, Wright V. Cracking joints. *Ann Rheum Dis* 1971;30:348–358.
8. Steen VD, Medsger TA. The palpable tendon friction rub: an important physical examination finding in patients with systemic sclerosis. *Arthritis Rheum* 1997;40:146–151.
9. Wilk KE, Andrews JR, Arrigo CA. The physical examination of the glenohumeral joint. Emphasis on the stabilizing structures. *J Orthop Sports Phys Ther* 1997;2:380–383.
10. Polley HF, Hunder GG. *Rheumatologic interviewing and physical examination of the joints,* 2nd ed. Philadelphia: WB Saunders, 1978.
11. Doherty M, Doherty J. *Clinical examination in rheumatology.* London: Wolfe, 1992.

CHAPTER 3

Clinical Evaluation in the Rheumatic Diseases

Nicholas Bellamy and W. Watson Buchanan

The evaluation of musculoskeletal patients is often based on a combination of the clinical assessment of symptoms and signs, noninvasive imaging procedures, and the analysis of biologic fluids or tissue (1). This chapter is concerned with clinical evaluation, with special reference to randomized clinical trials of pharmacologic interventions. Readers are referred to other sections of this text for information on structural imaging, and pathologic and biologic aspects of the rheumatic diseases. The methods used in clinical evaluation are variably, and interchangeably, referred to in the literature as tools, instruments, techniques, or tests (2). The major clinical evaluation subtypes are techniques for the assessment of clinical signs and health status instruments used to quantify the severity of symptoms.

The ability to conduct reliable and valid clinical evaluations is a requirement for descriptive research, such as measuring the burden of disease (3), and for predicting current (diagnosis) (4) and future (prognosis) (5) health status. The detection of change over time requires assessment techniques that are also responsive (sensitive). As a consequence, validity, reliability, and responsiveness are the key measurement attributes of techniques used in clinical evaluation in both research and practice environments. Clinical practitioners in particular need to be able to measure whether improvement or deterioration has occurred in a patient's health status and whether the therapeutic goal has been attained.

The application of evaluation techniques is broad and diverse. Applications include epidemiologic research, clinical diagnosis, prognostication, measurement of the consequences of disease for clinical, compensation or litigation purposes, interventional research, performance of health economic analyses, and assessment of the impact of treatment on individual health-care recipients.

In epidemiologic research, the goal is often to define the incidence and prevalence of musculoskeletal disorders and to define the burden of illness in affected individuals. The former requires tools that are robust for differentiating affected from nonaffected individuals, whereas the latter requires instruments that can quantify the impact of disease on affected individuals.

In diagnostic applications, issues of sensitivity, specificity, positive and negative predictive value, and likelihood ratios are paramount, whereas in prognostication the accuracy with which a current measure or combination of measures predicts a future event or health status is the quintessential attribute of the measure.

Reducing the burden of disease is a central theme in the "bone and joint decade" (6). The ability to benchmark the health status of a disease group or individual against normative data (7) is important in defining the gap between health and disease.

In litigation/compensation environments, the consequence of the adverse health event is often factored into the settlement.

The introduction of new pharmacologic interventions into clinical rheumatology is preceded by many years of rigorous evaluation in clinical trials. A comprehensive pharmacodynamic profile of the efficacy, tolerability, acceptability, effectiveness, and cost-effectiveness of a new compound is constructed over time from diverse sources of information, including randomized controlled trials, quasiexperimental studies, case reports and case series, and pharmacoepidemiology and pharmacoeconomic evaluations (1). The aforementioned data are often collated and further evaluated through a systematic review process such as the Cochrane Collaborative Project (8). The Cochrane website can be located at *www.cochrane.org*.

In health economics research, measurement of clinical status is essential to the conduct of cost-effectiveness and cost-utility analyses. Generic measures of health-related quality of life and utility-based instruments are central to the conduct of this type of research (9).

In contrast to applications in research environments, adjudicating the response status of individuals in clinical practice environments requires the use of practical, user-friendly assessment techniques that are brief and simple and make few demands on human or capital resources (10–13).

Evaluation procedures in clinical research are usually conducted within the architecture of a clinical trial design (1). The double-blind, randomized, controlled clinical trial remains the most robust research design for evaluating the pharmacodynamic profile of a new intervention in humans. The sophistication and rigor with which such trials are conducted have evolved progressively over the past half century. However, even today, each new clinical trial is a challenge in design, measurement, and evaluation. A working knowledge of research methods is essential for (a) conducting clinical research projects; (b) critically, but constructively, reviewing the rheumatology literature; and (c) conducting similar evaluations in routine clinical practice.

DESIGN AND INTERPRETATION OF CLINICAL TRIALS

There are eight basic components to a clinical trial, namely (a) research objective; (b) trial design; (c) patient selection; (d) randomization and stratification; (e) intervention, cointervention, contamination, and compliance; (f) outcome assessment; (g) statistical issues; and (h) interpretation and application (1).

Research Objective

In the interests of acquiring knowledge, it is tempting to seek the answers to multiple questions *a priori*, and to dredge data sets *a posteriori*. However, such hypothesis-generating activities should be clearly differentiated from those that test the principal hypothesis. Because different objectives generally impose different, and often very specific methodologic requirements, testing should be restricted to one or, at most, two major hypotheses, for which the trial is adequately powered. At the completion of the trial design, the investigator should reflect on the adequacy of the selected methodology and sample size, not only with regard to rejecting the null hypothesis, if false, but also to accepting it if true within conventional levels of statistical significance.

Trial Design

One of five research designs is generally used in the evaluation of antirheumatic drugs: randomized parallel, randomized crossover, sequential, nonrandomized comparative group, and one-group noncomparative open designs (14). Parallel designs are most commonly used. They offer operational simplicity, but potentially require larger sample sizes than comparable crossover designs and are unable to address issues of preference or within-patient response differences. However, crossover and factorial designs are operationally more complex. Drug interactions and carryover effects may occur, and the statistical and conceptual advantages of the design are frequently outweighed. A special form of the cross-over design is the N-of-1 trial design, which has potential application in the evaluation of individual patient responses to short-acting, but not long-acting, antirheumatic drugs (15,16). Comparison of an active drug against a placebo using an N-of-1 design creates operational challenges that are different from the comparison of two active drugs. In the N-of-1 design, individual responses are determined by the overall outcome of multiple random-ordered pairs of treatment periods. By examining any difference in outcomes from repeated exposures to competing treatment programs, a decision can be made, using clinical or statistical criteria, regarding which treatment program is the most appropriate for an individual patient. In general, nonrandomized comparative group designs and one-group noncomparative open designs (17) lack the necessary rigor essential for the assessment of the relative and absolute efficacy and tolerability of anti-rheumatic compounds. In early trials, where the absolute response to a drug is unknown, it is appropriate to use a placebo control group. In later trials, when the superiority of the compound over placebo has already been demonstrated, it is more appropriate, from both scientific and ethical standpoints, to compare the response to the new compound against one or more standard therapies.

Patient Selection

Most antirheumatic drug trials focus on a single disease; the remainder study groups of patients who differ in their diagnosis. Within a single diagnostic group, "selection" implies that certain patients will be excluded from study, and, therefore, trial results will be only generalizable to patients with characteristics similar to those actually studied (18). Great caution must be exercised in generalizing beyond such obvious limits, because beneficial and adverse responses may vary significantly among subgroups. It should be noted that ineligible patients, as well as eligible patients who decline to participate, are not represented in the study sample, and their exclusion may in itself be a potential source of bias. Indeed, patients who volunteer or consent for clinical studies may differ prognostically from those who do not. In general, selection criteria attempt to increase the homogeneity of the sample with respect to diagnosis, and exclude patients in whom the probability of response is decreased and the probability of an adverse reaction is increased beyond acceptable limits. Therefore, patients who are very young, elderly, or pregnant; have concurrent illness or extremely severe disease; or are receiving other drug therapy are often excluded from early studies of new compounds (1).

The statistical efficiency of studying a relatively homogeneous group of compliant patients with very active and potentially responsive disease needs to be weighed against the more limited generalizability of the study result.

Randomization and Stratification

In a parallel-trial design, the relative effectiveness of two antirheumatic compounds can be determined from the resultant response data only if the two treatment groups are considered to have been prognostically similar. Group comparability can be guaranteed with respect to certain defined variables of potential prognostic importance by the process of stratification (1). In contrast, the process of randomization (of which there are several subtypes) gives no such guarantees, but attempts to increase the probability that undefined variables of potential prognostic importance are evenly distributed between the treatment groups (1). Given that the amount of pain present at baseline is one determinant of the magnitude of the subsequent response to antirheumatic drugs in rheumatoid arthritis (RA) (19) and osteoarthritis (OA) (20) (Table 3.1), comparability in the severity of pain should be addressed either by stratification, or more often, through the randomization process.

Although it is customary to assess group comparability and, therefore, the apparent success of the allocation process by statistical analysis, type II errors can occur in the analysis of randomization variables just as in the analysis of outcome variables. Furthermore, despite randomization and stratification, important prognostic differences can escape statistical detection. Two additional methods of assigning patients to treatment groups are minimization and self-adjusting randomization procedures (1), which attempt to enhance comparability by dynamically minimizing between-group differences during the allocation process.

Intervention, Cointervention, Contamination, and Compliance

Intervention

This term is applied to the use of a specific treatment in a study. The agent tested may be given in a fixed dose or titrated according to a predetermined schedule or to the patient's requirements. Although clinical practice is best simulated by the titration strategy—because it commits patients to neither excessive nor inadequate therapy and thereby minimizes response failures because of either inefficacy or adverse reactions—it renders dose-based comparative analyses difficult, owing to the small residual sample sizes at each dose level (1). In contrast, a fixed-dose strategy allows conclusion about the efficacy and tolerability of a single specified dose, but fails to address the issue of optimal therapy in routine clinical practice.

In either strategy, drug administration may be preceded, punctuated, or followed by a "washout" period. Such periods may require the temporary cessation of one or more classes of antirheumatic drugs, depending on the disease, the objective, and the class of antirheumatic intervention under consideration. It may be single-blinded, double-blinded, triple-blinded, or unblinded. For practical and ethical reasons, analgesia with acetaminophen (usually up to predefined maximum daily levels) is often permitted during washout periods. In contrast, a sudden cessation of systemic corticosteroid therapy is both inappropriate and hazardous, whereas the suspension of disease-modifying drugs is problematic, since the effects of discontinuation will be unapparent for several weeks or months. Washout periods

TABLE 3.1. *Standardized response mean and correlation between initial pain rating and pain relief scores in rheumatoid arthritis and osteoarthritis*

	SRM		Correlation	
Pain Scale	RA	OA	RA	OA
VA	1.08	0.97	0.56	0.49
Numerical	1.08	0.91	0.48	0.48
CCAS	1.04	0.94	0.46	0.43
Likert	0.97	0.84	0.66	0.50
Pain faces 1	0.90	0.78	0.65	0.55
MPQ (total)	0.68	0.74	0.54	0.50
Pain faces 2	0.66	0.70	0.25	0.34
Reversed ladder	0.56	0.50	0.55	0.48

CCAS, Continuous Chromatic Analogue Scale; MPQ, McGill Pain Questionnaire; OA, osteoarthritis; RA, rheumatoid arthritis; SRM, standardized response mean; VA, Veterans Administration.

Adapted from Bellamy N, Campbell J, Syrotuik J. Comparative study of self-rating pain scales in rheumatoid arthritis patients. *Curr Med Res Opin* 1999;15(2):121–127, and Bellamy N, Campbell J, Syrotuik J. Comparative study of self-rating pain scales in osteoarthritis patients. *Curr Med Res Opin* 1999;15(2):113–119, with permission.

are generally restricted, therefore, to the withdrawal of nonsteroidal antiinflammatory drugs (NSAIDs). Because this withdrawal may be poorly tolerated by patients with active joint inflammation, a provision is usually made to advance such patients prematurely ("trap door" provision) to the active treatment phase. Despite these problems, washout periods are advantageous in that they allow assessment of the baseline status of study patients and amplify any subsequent response to active drug therapy, thereby minimizing sample size requirements for detecting statistically significant within-group improvements. Also, they facilitate assessment of patient responsiveness and absolute magnitude of the change, minimize carryover effects from prior treatments, allow clinical baselines to be reestablished in crossover studies, and, when performed at the end of a trial, serve to redefine group comparability and the persistence of patient responsiveness.

Cointervention

Cointervention refers to the administration of another potentially efficacious treatment at the same time as the intervention treatment. It can take many forms, including concomitant analgesic drugs, corticosteroids, or disease-modifying antirheumatic drugs (DMARDs); hospitalization; physiotherapy; and surgery. Because these often have a major biasing effect and confound interpretation of trial results, cointervention should be minimized, monitored, and taken into account in formulating any conclusions (1). Because pain relief is the principal outcome measure in most NSAID trials, such caution is particularly relevant for concomitant analgesics because their use is ubiquitous whether they are officially permitted or not. Thus, unrecognized differential analgesic consumption rates can minimize between-group differences in pain control and lead incorrectly to the assumption that no difference exists. Analgesic consumption is a surrogate measure of pain control and therefore is itself an important end point.

With respect to other classes of antirheumatic compounds, patients taking corticosteroids generally should have been receiving a stable dosage for at least 1 month before entry and during the study, whereas those on slow-acting disease-modifying agents generally should have been taking them at a constant dose level for at least the preceding 3 months. Recommendations regarding cotherapy management can be found in recent guidelines documents (21,22).

Contamination

Contamination is rarely a problem in well-structured, efficiently managed clinical trials of antirheumatic drugs. It occurs when an individual, instead of receiving the intended medication, receives a drug specifically designated for individuals in one of the other treatment groups. Its biasing effects are obvious, and if the effects are unrecognized, patients will be analyzed according to the drug that they were scheduled to receive, rather than that which they truly received (1).

Compliance

Compliance is a measure of the extent to which a patient adheres to the protocol in general and to drug ingestion in particular. It can be measured in four ways: by direct observation, patient report (verbal or diary), pill counting, and plasma drug level monitoring. Each method has its limitations, so noncompliant patients can appear compliant and vice versa. Refinements such as the use of blister packs, or incorporating a microchip in the closure mechanism of the container, cannot address the issue of how many tablets were actually consumed. Measurement of compliance remains less than completely satisfactory. Even when the monitoring procedure is satisfactory, there is no standard definition for any level of compliance beyond which the therapeutic response is significantly compromised (1). In clinical trials, a level of compliance between 80% and 120% is often considered acceptable. Furthermore, because enrollment is entirely voluntary, and because patients are in pain and under close supervision, we believe that compliance levels are generally high, and patient report (by diary) and pill counting are adequate for practical purposes (1).

Outcome Assessment

The timing and nature of outcome assessments should respect both the potential adverse and potential beneficial effects of test compounds. Thus, although adverse reactions to both symptom-modifying antirheumatic drugs (SyMARDs; e.g., NSAIDs, cyclooxygenase-2 inhibitors, analgesics) and structure-modifying antirheumatic drugs (StMARDs; e.g. methotrexate), can occur at any time after administration, the induction-response (efficacy) interval for SyMARDs is much shorter than that for the slower-acting SyMARDs. To avoid bias, neither patients nor assessors should know who is receiving which of the study treatments (double-blinded study). Usually, the test treatments are given in an identical format, either as indistinguishable compounds or using the "double-dummy" technique. When only a single-blinded technique is used, either the patient or, more usually, the assessor can be compromised by an expectation bias that may either enhance or abrogate the clinical result. In a triple-blinded format, not only the patient and assessor are blind, but also a third party (e.g., the data safety monitoring committee), who has responsibility for administering certain aspects of the trial—for example, termination of the study on ethical grounds if adverse reactions or response failures are unexpectedly frequent or severe in one or other treatment group. In a triple-blinded scheme, such decisions can be made without prejudice.

Beneficial Effects

Outcome measures used to assess drug efficacy should be able to detect the smallest clinically important change and, at the same time, should be valid with respect to capturing the dimensionality of the relevant clinical, structural, and biologic responses (2). Fully validated standardized measures are preferred over ad hoc methods.

Adverse Effects

Patient tolerance to the intervention can be monitored by spontaneous patient report or structured open-ended or close-ended questioning. In general, the more rigorous the probe, the greater the incidence of "intolerance" and the more difficult the task of attribution to the studied intervention. Even in a healthy population there is a background level of transient symptoms such as headache, diarrhea, and dyspepsia. For this reason, the term *adverse event* is often used in preference to the term *drug side effect,* and in clinical trials attribution to the study medication is often graded, using such terms as *unrelated, possibly related, probably related,* and *definitely related.* Some adverse effects (e.g., thrombocytopenia) may become more rapidly apparent than others (e.g., some types of anemia) because of physiologic variability in the half-life of the target cells.

For both safety and scientific rigor, patients should be appropriately monitored for both clinical and laboratory tolerance to a drug in accordance with its known pharmacokinetics and pharmacodynamics. Some study assessment points may be necessary to assess toxicity, others to assess efficacy, and still others to assess both.

Statistical Issues

Statistical issues can be subdivided into those relating to sample size calculation and those relevant to statistical analysis of the resulting data. Both should be carefully considered *a priori.*

Sample Size Calculation

The number of patients required for a clinical trial is a function of several factors, including trial design, the magnitude of type I (α) and type II (β) errors, the size of the minimum clinically important difference (MCID) sought (Δ), and the variability (σ) in the underlying data set (23,24). Most antirheumatic drug trials use randomized parallel designs comparing mean values (and/or proportions) of several variables within and between treatment groups. Published reports have increasingly contained detail on methods used in sample size calculation and procedures used to correct the statistical *p* value for multiple comparisons (25). Nevertheless, some recent reports still lack this essential information.

Sample size requirements may be calculated from several standard formulas, which differ depending on trial design and whether the analysis will compare means or proportions (Table 3.2). The type I (α) error (one- or two-tailed) is traditionally set at 0.05; that is, when $\alpha = 0.05$, then the probability that the difference detected has arisen entirely by chance is 1 in 20 or less. There is no such clearly defined level for the type II (β) error, but $\beta = 0.20$ is usually regarded as the minimum and $\beta = 0.10$ as preferable. At the $\beta = 0.10$ level, the investigator accepts a 1 in 10 or less probability that a true difference at a specified level has been overlooked by chance. The power of a study is expressed by the term $1 - \beta$. Thus, when β is set at 0.10, the study has a 90% probability of detecting a postulated difference if one truly exists. It is the quantitative definition of the MCID (Δ) and standard deviation (σ) that creates difficulty for protocol developers.

Although most published reports contain variance estimates (e.g., standard error, standard deviation, confidence limits) there are relatively few published estimates of the MCID. The Outcome Measures in Rheumatology Clinical Trials (OMERACT) group has brought attention to this issue (26,27) and Beaton and colleagues (28,29) have developed a conceptual framework for classifying the difference/change in health status along three dimensions: (a) individual/group; (b) within only/between only/within and between; and (c) type of change (minimum potentially detectable, minimum actually detectable, observed in population, observed in those estimated to have changed, observed in those estimated to

TABLE 3.2. *Standard formulas for calculating sample size*

Comparison of two related means (crossover design)[a]
Number of pairs = $[\sigma_d(Z_\alpha + Z_\beta)/\Delta]^2$
Comparison of two independent means (parallel design)
Number per group = $2\,[\sigma(Z_\alpha + Z_\beta)/\Delta]^2$
Comparison of two related proportions (crossover design)[b]
Number of pairs = $\{Z_\alpha[\pi_0(1 - \pi_0)]^{1/2} + Z_\beta[\pi_1(1 - \pi_1)^{1/2}\}^2(\pi_1 - \pi_0)$
Comparison of two independent proportions (parallel design)[c]
Number per group = $2\{(Z_\alpha + Z_\beta)/[2\sin^{-1}(\pi_1)^{1/2}] - [2\sin^{-1}(\pi_2)^{1/2}]\}^2$

[a] Z_α, the magnitude of the type 1 error; this value expresses the risk the test designer is willing to take that the null hypothesis would be erroneously rejected; Z_β, the magnitude of the type II error; this value expresses the risk that the null hypothesis would be accepted erroneously; Δ, the magnitude of the change in the principal outcome measure; σ, estimate of the expected variance of the principal outcome measure.

[b] π_0 and π_1 (in crossover design) = refer to proportion of patients preferring some new treatment under null and alternate hypothesis, respectively. Usually $\pi_0 = 0.5$ and $\pi_1 > 0.5$.

[c] π_1 and π_2 (in parallel design) = true proportions for a specified outcome in both treatment groups.

have had an important change). Recent observations pertaining to change definitions in osteoporosis (30), RA (31), OA (32), and low back pain (33) can be located in the OMERACT 5 conference proceedings. Interested readers are also directed to a series of studies in ankylosing spondylitis (AS) (34–36), RA (37–39), OA (40–42), and fibromyalgia (FM) (43), which are summarized in a musculoskeletal clinical metrology textbook (2).

When there is a paucity of information regarding the delta and standard deviation, an estimate of effect size may be used to facilitate the calculation (44). Cohen's effect sizes (small, medium, large) are relative and context dependent. The effect size encompasses, in a single number, the relationship between the delta and the standard deviation. The effect size can be factored into the sample size calculation.

It should be noted that sample size requirements vary for different outcome measures. Furthermore, sample size requirements increase as the minimum clinically important difference (Δ) decreases, or the variance increases, or the error constraints are tightened. It is absolutely essential that the sample size be adequate to test the null hypothesis on the primary outcome measure.

Most clinical trials use a variety of outcome measures to capture the multidimensional nature of the response (2). The more outcome variables assessed, however, the more likely that one will achieve a p value of 0.05 because of chance alone (45). Statistical adjustment for multiple comparisons constrains the upper limit for significance and decreases the likelihood of demonstrating a true difference on any single variable. Correction for multiple comparisons might be counterproductive in early exploratory research because, as Feinstein has pointed out, the purpose of a fishing expedition is to catch fish (46). In contrast, in a definitive study, the problem of the type I error in multiple-contrast analyses should be fully addressed by one of several techniques. For example, one could define *a priori* one or two principal outcome measures, relegate the remainder to secondary outcome measure status, and apportion differential type I errors to them. Sample size requirements are clearly speculative, and although Δ and σ may be conveniently fixed, the magnitude of the response may be smaller, and the variance larger, than projected. Furthermore, the calculated number may require augmentation to accommodate a predicted number of patient dropouts.

Statistical Analysis

The results should be analyzed and presented in a way that demonstrates both their clinical importance and their statistical significance. Two types of analytic philosophy, defined *a priori*, are commonly used: explicative, or per protocol, and management, or intention to treat (47). In the explicative approach, all patients failing to complete the study exactly according to protocol are excluded from analysis. In a management trial, all patients entered into the trial are included in the analysis. Although the per protocol strategy is operationally simple, it runs the risk of producing a biased result, usually by eroding wholly or partly any true differences in drug efficacy or tolerability. In the management strategy, patient dropouts, who often represent important drug-dependent events, are included in the analysis. It is often necessary to accommodate for missing values, and readers should be familiar with the various imputation procedures that are available for dealing with discontinuations. These include, but are not limited to, the last observation carried forward, best observation carried forward, worst observation carried forward, and hot deck imputation methods (48).

The intention-to-treat approach is currently the preferred method for analysis in most studies. We recommend that if an explicative strategy is used, the analysis be duplicated using an intention-to-treat approach to establish the stability of the result and the integrity of the conclusions.

Although randomization attempts to achieve group comparability, it does not guarantee a balance of potential confounding variables in each treatment group. If an imbalance is found in factors such as disease severity or duration, response potential, and possibly age, an analytic technique that adjusts for the imbalance should be considered.

Other analytic methods include the use of confidence levels and equivalence testing. Although tests of statistical significance are frequently used, it has been conjectured that significance levels are not appropriate indices of the magnitude or of the clinical importance of between-treatment differences (49). Because it is acknowledged that if the same study is replicated in a different group of patients, the same differences will not be observed, it follows that the true differences are not known with certainty. Those in favor of the use of confidence intervals contend they are a useful supplement to p values because, with a high probability, the interval contains the true difference. The concept of equivalence testing is important because a lack of difference between two treatments is not synonymous with their being exactly the same (1). Debate continues over the relative merits of testing the null hypothesis versus equivalence (1). Indeed, the two approaches may have quite different applications. However, given that most drug development is based on the premise that new agents should be superior in efficacy or tolerability to comparator compounds, and superior in efficacy to placebo, it is not surprising that most statistical comparisons focus on accepting or rejecting the null hypothesis.

Finally, post hoc analyses may be conducted as hypothesis-generating exercises that attempt to extract additional information from the original data set. It is in this setting that statistical correction for multiple comparisons is particularly important. The probability of finding a significant p value is a function of the number of comparisons performed. A Bonferroni correction, where the accepted level for significance is defined by dividing the traditional 0.05 value by the number of comparisons to be performed, is often used in this setting.

Interpretation and Application

Caution is necessary in interpreting the results of a study and in generalizing them to other patients or patient groups that may differ in demographic, disease features, response potential, comorbidity, concomitant therapy, and risk of adverse events than the study population. The results of a trial should be viewed, therefore, in the appropriate clinical context (1). Furthermore, they should be interpreted with respect to other relevant data obtained using different designs. Readers and reviewers should be mindful of the potential for a publication bias, which occurs when positive studies are more likely to be published than negative studies. In a survey of clinical investigators, Dickersin et al. reviewed 271 unpublished and 1,041 published trials among 156 respondents (50). Their analysis suggested the existence of a positive publication bias, nonpublication being largely due to negative results and lack of interest.

The importance of the Cochrane Collaborative Project and other similar systematic review processes that attempt to surface all relevant published and unpublished information on a product are particularly important in gaining an understanding of the efficacy of therapeutic interventions. The first Cochrane center was opened in Oxford in 1992. Through an extensive network of international collaborations, Cochrane centers and their associated research groups around the world actively contribute to the development of an international library of evidence-based medicine. This tremendously important initiative has attracted the international participation of a large number of rheumatologists, as well as health-care professionals in other clinical disciplines. Because of the processes involved, properly conducted systematic reviews of all relevant randomized controlled clinical trials (level 1 evidence) are considered superior in the strengths of evidence hierarchy than evidence obtained from only a single properly designed randomized controlled clinical trial (level 2 evidence) (51). For the practitioner, it is important to note that the results of clinical trials often do correspond fairly well to the experience in the general population (52), notwithstanding the aforementioned issue relating to the impact of restrictive inclusion/exclusion criteria on the generalizability of study results (18).

Clinical Evaluation Methods

Although formalized relatively recently, methods for evaluating a patient's signs and symptoms of musculoskeletal illness doubtless date back to antiquity. More recently, the development and validation of new assessment techniques has been communicated through the rheumatology, orthopaedic, rehabilitation, physical therapy, internal medicine, and related literatures. In rheumatology, a number of agencies and groups—including the World Health Organization (WHO), OMERACT, American College of Rheumatology (ACR), European League of Association of Rheumatologists and its regional bodies, Group for the Respect of Ethics and Excellence in Science, U.S. Food and Drug Administration, Ankylosing Spondylitis Assessment (ASAS) group, Osteoarthritis Society International (OARSI), and the Initiative on Methods, Measurement, and Pain Assessment in Clinical Trials (IMMPACT)—have provided direction in diverse aspects of clinical assessment, including core set outcome measures, responder criteria, and study design. As a result, outcome measurement in clinical research environments has become more standardized.

SELECTION OF OUTCOME MEASURES FOR CLINICAL STUDIES

Decisions regarding what effects to measure and how to measure them can be arrived at by several processes. For several conditions such as RA, OA, and AS, guidelines documents have been developed. Although not in the form of regulations, they do nevertheless represent the international consensus of key stakeholder groups. For situations or conditions where guidelines do not currently exist, the selection of outcome measures can be based on the opinions of key informants and should reflect the nature of the disease, the study population, the pharmacodynamics of the test compounds, and the research hypothesis. Different measures may be required for different patient groups (adults vs. children), conditions (RA vs. OA), and classes of interventions (SyMARDs vs. StMARDs).

It may be useful to conduct the measurement process within a conceptual framework that encompasses key features of health, such as mortality, disability, discomfort, iatrogenic adverse events, and economic impact as popularized by Fries and colleagues (53), or within the WHO framework of impairment, activity, and participation (54). In order to minimize responder burden, there should be close alignment between the measurement battery and the research question. Unnecessary data collection should be avoided.

It is important for readers to be able to differentiate outcome measures from process measures, and hard data from soft data. In recent years, there has been an increasing tendency to consider measures as being of two types: outcome and process. Outcome measures tap into the ultimate clinical consequence of disease, that is, those that can be perceived by the patient and affect everyday life. Process measures include such variables as erythrocyte sedimentation rate and rheumatoid factor, measures that have no intrinsic value to the patient. The terms *hard data* and *soft data* are still sometimes used, albeit inappropriately. In the new discipline of clinical metrology, the terms *hard data* and *soft data* are rarely used, since several of the new health status instruments and quality of life measures (so-called "soft" measures) provide data that have far more robust measurement characteristics than many laboratory data (so-called "hard" measures) (1). Thus, the terms *hard* and *soft* should now be used to refer to the actual strength of the

TABLE 3.3. *Major criteria for selecting assessment techniques for musculoskeletal clinical trials*

1. The measurement process must be ethical.
2. Reliability should be adequate for achieving measurement objectives.
3. Validity (face, content, criterion, and construct) should be adequate for achieving measurement objectives.
4. Responsiveness must be adequate, (i.e., the technique must be able to detect a clinically important statistically significant change in the underlying variable.)
5. The feasibility of data collection and instrument application should not be constrained unduly by time, complexity, or cost.

Adapted from Bellamy N. *Musculoskeletal clinical metrology.* Dordrecht, the Netherlands: Kluwer Academic, 1993, with permission.

measurement characteristics of an instrument, rather than the point of origin of the data.

Irrespective of the specific protocol, the five criteria we consider important for evaluative indices for clinical trials (2) are illustrated in Table 3.3 and discussed below. They are similar to the subsequently proposed "OMERACT filter" for selecting measures for clinical trials (55), differing only on splitting reliability and responsiveness issues, and the specifying of an obligation to meet ethical requirements.

1. *The measurement process must be ethical.* Measurement procedures that are painful, embarrassing, or hazardous to study subjects raise ethical issues. Such issues must be fully disclosed to participants and, if possible, less invasive procedures sought. The necessity for data collection must be carefully weighed against the risks, and the final procedures reviewed by an independent committee versed in judging ethical issues in biomedical research.
2. *Validity should be adequate for achieving measurement objectives.* There are four types of validity: face, content, criterion, and construct (56).

Face Validity

A measure has face validity if informed individuals (investigators and clinicians) judge that it measures part or all of the defined phenomenon. In many instances (e.g., hemoglobin, weight), this decision is self-evident, whereas in others, particularly in subjective measures of functional status, face validity alone may be insufficient, and other forms of validity must also be demonstrated.

Content Validity

An instrument can have face validity but fail to capture the dimension of interest in its entirety. A measure, therefore, has content validity if it is comprehensive; that is, it encompasses all relevant aspects of the defined attributes. Like face validity, content validity is also subjective but can be conferred either by a single individual or by a group of individuals using one of several consensus development techniques. The decision about which items should be included in an instrument and which should be excluded is critical because it defines the nature of the instrument and both guides and constrains the instrument's subsequent applicability. Any subsequent addition or deletion of items creates, in essence, a new instrument requiring revalidation.

Some instruments use only observer-dependent measures, others only observer-independent measures, and still others a combination of both. In general, evaluative instruments for clinical trials should include some measures that comprehensively probe symptoms that occur frequently and are clinically important to patients. The definition of importance can be decided by groups of patients polled to assess the dimensions of their symptoms (57,58), or by clinical investigators whose decision is based on their perception of the patient's symptoms. In our view, the former approach is preferable and avoids issues of paternalism.

Criterion Validity

Criterion validity is assessed statistically by comparing the new instrument against a concurrent independent criterion (Fig. 3.1) or standard (concurrent criterion validity) or against a future standard (predictive criterion validity). It is therefore an estimate of the extent to which a measure agrees with the true value of an independent measure of health status, either present or future. The at-

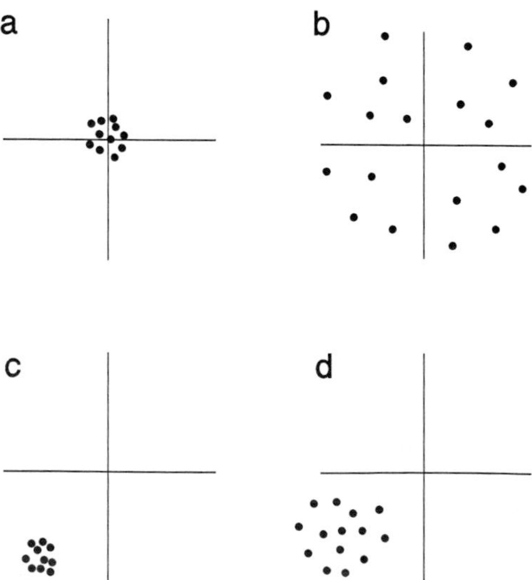

FIG. 3.1. Schematic representation of systematic error (*bias*) and random error (*noise*). A comparison of measurements that are **(A)** valid and reliable, **(B)** valid but *unreliable,* **(C)** reliable but biased, **(D)** biased and unreliable. *Center of the target,* the true value; *black dots,* "measured values" of a single static phenomenon. (Reproduced from Bellamy N. *Musculoskeletal clinical metrology.* Dordrecht, the Netherlands: Kluwer Academic, 1993, with permission.)

tainment of concurrent criterion validity is usually frustrated by the lack of any available standard, whereas predictive criterion validity is not immediately relevant to evaluative objectives.

Construct Validity

Construct validity is of two types: convergent and discriminant. Both represent statistical attempts to demonstrate adherence between instrument values and a theoretic manifestation (construct) or consequence of the attribute. Convergent construct validity testing assesses the correlation between scores on a single health component as measured by two different instruments. If the coefficient is positive and appreciably above zero, the new measure is said to have convergent construct validity. In contrast, discriminant construct validity testing compares the correlation between scores on the same health component as measured by two different instruments (e.g., measures of physical function) and between scores on that health component and each of several other health components (e.g., measures of social and emotional function). A measure has discriminant construct validity if the proposed measure correlates better with a second measure accepted as more closely related to the construct than it does with a third, more distantly related measure (1). Validity, like reliability, has no absolute level, and its adequacy depends on the measurement objective.

To circumvent some of the judgmental requirements of validity testing, several recent multidimensional indices have used multivariate analytic techniques to select items for inclusion and also to evaluate index performance. Although model building should supplement, rather than replace, judgmental activities, these advanced statistical techniques can provide additional useful information regarding validity. In contrast to random error (Fig. 3.1), systematic error (bias) produces invalid results that are not reflected in the standard deviation and cannot be negated by increasing sample size.

3. *Reliability should be adequate for achieving measurement objectives.* Reliability is a synonym for consistency or agreement, and is the extent to which a measurement procedure yields the same result on repeated applications when the underlying phenomenon has not changed (56) (Fig. 3.1). Because repeated measures rarely equal one another exactly, some degree of inconsistency is invariable. This form of measurement error is referred to as noise or random error. Low levels of reliability are reflected in the magnitude of the standard deviation and result in increased sample size requirements for clinical trials using such instruments. In contrast to systematic error (Fig. 3.1), random error can be offset by increasing sample size. Although there is no absolute level for acceptable reliability, reliability coefficients generally should exceed 0.80.

Among methods for assessing reliability, the two most commonly used are test-retest reliability and internal consistency (56). The former, an expression of stability, requires two separate administrations of the test at appropriate intervals. In contrast, internal consistency is determined on a single administration of the test and estimates interitem correlation. In the special case where the measuring instruments are observers, interobserver and intraobserver variability should be assessed and their effects minimized using standardization techniques (34,37,40,43). Depending on the type of scaling, a reliability coefficient can be calculated using intraclass correlation coefficients (e.g., the Cronbach α) or from the variance components of the analysis of variance table (34,37,40,43), or, alternatively, the results expressed to take into account the level of agreement beyond that expected as a result of chance alone using the Cohen kappa statistic (59). There are several methods of calculating the kappa statistic, some of which take into account bias and prevalence (60).

The major sources of measurement error can be divided among the patient, the observer, and the instrument. Patient variability often arises from circadian variation in symptoms (61–64), or from fatigue, poor memory, or inattention. Observers are liable to experience fatigue, particularly if the assessment task is lengthy or complex, or requires judgments based on visual or tactile perception (1). Instruments may also vary as a function of some mechanical component of the device, such as cuff size in a sphygmomanometer or resistance in a dynamometer. Whatever the source of variability, it should be quantitated and, if unacceptably high, should be minimized by design modification of the instrument, training of the assessor (34,37,40,43), or modification of the measurement process to improve patient performance. Such training procedures may have a profound impact on the sample size requirements for a clinical trial (1).

4. *An evaluative index must be responsive to change, that is, capable of detecting differential change in health status occurring in two or more groups of individuals exposed to competing interventions.* This is an absolute prerequisite for an evaluative instrument and requires careful documentation (1). Not only should the instrument be responsive in general, but also it should be specifically responsive in the clinical setting in which it is to be applied. Many factors influence instrument sensitivity, one of the most important being scaling (1). With the exception of the Guttman cumulative scaling techniques, dichotomous scales generally lack the sensitivity required because of the restricted response options they offer. In contrast, 10-cm horizontal visual analogue scales (VAS) (2), numerical rating scales (NRS) (2), and 5-point Likert adjectival scales (2) offer adequate response options. The relative sensitivity of these three types of scales remains controversial, although clearly all are very responsive in RA (19) and OA (20) studies (Table 3.1). In our experience, the VAS appears more

sensitive than the Likert scale (65–67), with the NRS occupying an intermediate position in the response hierarchy (19,20).

There are a number of methods of comparing the relative sensitivity of different assessment techniques. These include the effect size, the standardized response mean, and the relative efficacy statistic (68–70) (Table 3.4). It should be noted that statistical superiority does not necessarily equate with conceptual superiority. However, responsiveness is a key requirement for detecting differences.

5. *The feasibility of data collection should not be unduly constrained by complexity or time.* Measurement procedures that are complex or excessively time consuming run the risk of patient and assessor fatigue, with a resultant decline in data quality. Practicality is particularly important in clinical practice environments.

Musculoskeletal Clinical Metrology

There are three basic decisions in clinical measurement: what to measure, how to measure it, and how to express the resulting data.

What to measure depends on the questions to be addressed. Measurement can be based on clinical examination, clinical performance, or patient report (self-reported or interviewer reported). The measurement process may focus on disease-related variables or outcome-related variables. Finally, the same measurements may be taken on all patients or measurement may be individualized.

How to measure issues are resolved based on a working knowledge of the measurement literature and current and emerging concepts. The reliability, validity, and responsiveness of measurement alternatives is of considerable importance. In general, measurement techniques will be selected from standard tools currently available.

How to express the resulting data is an *a priori* decision and depends on whether the goal is to compare patients at the level of the original data using comparative analyses suitable for continuous data, or to conduct the analysis based on responder criteria using comparative analyses suitable for dichotomous data.

Measurement Strategies

Traditional Strategy

The traditional strategy has been to take measurements on a variety of clinical efficacy and tolerability variables, laboratory variables, and, in some studies, imaging variables (1). The analysis is conducted on a measure-by-measure basis, and from the resulting statistical mosaic, a pronouncement is made on the absolute and relative merits or demerits of the intervention. Often, such studies attempt to gather information simultaneously on the activity, severity, and clinical consequence of disease, as well as monitor aspects of the underlying pathologic process. The traditional strategy requires consideration of two issues: selection of a primary outcome and/or correction of the statistical p value for multiple comparisons in definitive studies, and interpretative procedures defined *a priori* to arbitrate the interpretation when different measures favor different interventions.

Signal Strategy

In the signal strategy, measurement is based on well-defined, individualized targets. The signal may be one or only a few joints (1) or a particular physical activity (or activities) or symptom that the patient regards as particularly important. The criteria for signal selection signal have not been fully explored. In general, however, the signal should be of importance to the patient and should have the potential to change in either direction (i.e., worse or better) to reflect treatment effects. Although this approach tailors the measurement process to the individual, concern has been expressed by clinicians and statisticians that the signal technique is inappropriate because it leads to the evaluation of different disease variables in different patients and reduces statistical comparison to that of "apples with oranges." Nevertheless, the signal strategy has the capacity to accommodate interindividual differences in symptom profiles and preferences. Instruments that use this approach include

TABLE 3.4. *Formulas for calculating effect size, standard response mean and relative efficiency*

Effect size	=	$\dfrac{\text{Mean change in score from baseline}}{\text{Standard deviation of baseline scores}}$
Standardized response mean	=	$\dfrac{\text{Mean change in score between assessments}}{\text{Standard deviation of the change}}$
Relative efficiency	=	$\left[\dfrac{\text{t value for change in instrument 1}}{\text{t value for change in instrument 2}}\right]^2$

the McMaster Toronto Patient Preference Questionnaire (MACTAR) (71).

Analytic Strategies

The data acquired may be analyzed using a number of different strategies: traditional, composite, responder, and state attainment.

Traditional Analysis

The traditional approach is to conduct a variable-by-variable analysis testing the null hypothesis on one or more separate variables. Most often the efficacy analyses are conducted on continuous data, to detect between-group differences based on differential change, and use all original data and in some cases imputed data. In contrast, clinical tolerability analyses are often conducted on discrete data and are based on event rates.

Composite Index Analysis

In contrast to the traditional approach, composite indices can be constructed by statistical or judgmental procedures that allow aggregation of scores assigned to different outcome variables (1). Such variables are generally on different dimensions of health, and are combined using either simple or complex mathematical procedures (72,73). The pooled index (72) and the disease activity score (DAS) (73,74) are examples of composite indices. Composite indices have two advantages over the traditional strategy. First, they provide a basis for combining all relevant end points into a single value. Second, they increase the statistical efficiency of clinical trials by avoiding the issue of p value adjustment for multiple comparisons. Enthusiasm for such weighting and aggregation procedures must be tempered by recognition that the derivation of a single number value from a complex phenomenon does not necessarily imply any greater knowledge about that phenomenon than before. Furthermore, weighting and aggregation can have a profound impact on the perceived efficacy of an intervention (75). For this reason, composite indices require extensive and elaborate *a priori* validation. Of the composite indices, the DAS has attracted particular attention. The DAS index consists of four variables that can be combined into a single value using a nomogram (73). It has found clinical applicability, some popularity (1), and exists in several different forms (74).

Responder Analysis

Determining the response of individual patients to treatment requires a new definition of a clinically important response, that is, response in individual patients rather than a group of patients. Given that patients are treated individually, analysis methods, based on individual patient responses, facilitate extrapolation of clinical trial results to the clinical setting and provide better definition of which patients actually improved and which did not. An expansive list of acronyms is emerging that describe the magnitude of the change produced. It is apparent that change can be classified in several ways, as follows: (a) minimum change potentially detectable (32); (b) minimum percentage change potentially detectable (32); (c) minimum perceptible clinical improvement (76); and (d) minimum clinically important difference (36,39,42,43,77).

The development of responder criteria is predicated on an ability to differentiate a responder from a nonresponder. Several attempts at building responder criteria for RA clinical trials (1) preceded the consensus developed on core set measures by the OMERACT group (78), which subsequently formed the basis for the ACR core set (79) (Table 3.5) and the ACR responder criteria (80) (Table 3.6), that is: 20% improvement in tender and swollen joint counts plus 20% improvement in three of the following five criteria: patient pain, patient global assessment, physical disability,

TABLE 3.5. *Core set outcome measures for rheumatoid arthritis, osteoarthritis, and ankylosing spondylitis clinical trials*

Rheumatoid arthritis	Osteoarthritis	Ankylosing spondylitis
Pain	Pain	Pain[a]
Function	Function	Function[a]
Patient global assessment	Patient global assessment	Patient global assessment[a]
Number of tender joints	Imaging (for studies of ≤ 1 year)	Spinal mobility[a]
Number of swollen joints		Stiffness[a]
Physician global assessment		Peripheral joints and entheses[b]
CRP or ESR		Acute phase reactants[b]
Radiographs (for disease-modifying studies)		Radiograph spine
		Radiograph hips
		Fatigue

[a]Included in all three core sets for DC-ART, SMARD/physical therapy, and clinical recordkeeping.
[b]Included in core sets for DC-ART and clinical recordkeeping.
CRP, C-reactive protein; ESR, erythrocyte sedimentation rate; DC-ART, disease controlling antirheumatic therapy; SMARD, symptom modifying antirheumatic drug.

TABLE 3.6. *Responder criteria for rheumatoid arthritis, osteoarthritis, and ankylosing spondylitis clinical trials*

Rheumatoid Arthritis Required: ≥ 20% improvement in tender joint count ≥ 20% improvement in swollen joint count	and	≥ 20% improvement in three of the following five criteria: Patient pain assessment Patient global assessment Physician global assessment Patient self-assessed disability Acute-phase reactant (ESR or CRP)
Osteoarthritis High improvement in pain or in function ≥50% and absolute change ≥20 nu	or	Improvement in at least 2 two of the three following criteria: Pain ≥20% and absolute change ≥10 nu Function ≥20% and absolute change ≥10 nu Patient's global assessment ≥20% and absolute change ≥10 nu
Ankylosing Spondylitis Improvement of ≥20% and absolute improvement of ≥10 nu (on a scale of 0–100) in at least three of the following four domains: Patient global assessment Pain Function Inflammation	and	Absence of deterioration in the potential remaining domain, where deterioration is defined as a change for the worse of ≥20% and net worsening of ≥10 nu (on a scale of 0–100)

nu, normalized units on a scale of 0–100.

physician global assessment, and levels of an acute-phase reactant. The ACR response criteria (80) are now in common usage. In addition, ACR 50 and ACR 70 criteria based on comparable improvements of 50% and 70%, respectively, may provide a more complete perspective of the therapeutic response but represent a greater therapeutic challenge (81). Analysis of these criteria-based responses supplement traditional forms of analysis based on continuous data.

Consensus for core set measures in OA (Table 3.5) was reached at the OMERACT 3 Conference (82) and were subsequently ratified by the OARSI (22). Thereafter, OARSI proposed a series of responder criteria for different classes of intervention in OA hip and knee studies (83). Recently, these criteria (Table 3.6) have been revised into a single set of criteria that are applicable to either joint and all classes of intervention (84). In contrast to the ACR responder criteria for RA (80), which are based on percentage change, the new OMERACT-OARSI responder criteria are based on a combination of absolute and percentage change (84). It is of note that in OA there appears to be a high level of agreement between the response status assigned to the same patients by the patient-based MPCI, the OARSI criteria, and the opinion of a panel of experts repeatedly exposed to the anonymous opinion of their colleagues (85). Recent subanalyses suggest that the original OARSI responder criteria and the new OMERACT-OARSI criteria may produce similar between-group differentiation (86), and that the Western Ontario and McMaster (WOMAC) 20, 50, and 70 responder criteria might be successfully applied in a similar fashion in OA knee patients (87) as the ACR 20, 50, and 70 responder criteria are applied in RA patients.

Consensus for core set measures in AS has been achieved through the activities of the ASAS group (88). Core set measures for AS differ depending on the application, but for symptom-modifying studies include pain, function, spinal mobility, patient global assessment, and stiffness (Table 3.5). ASAS has also proposed a preliminary definition of short-term improvement in AS (Table 3.6) as follows: improvement by 20% or more, and net improvement by 10 or more normalized units (nu) on a scale of 0 to 100 in each of three domains with no worsening in the fourth, where the domains are physical function, pain, patient global assessment, and inflammation (89).

The acceptability and general usage of response criteria is increasing. They complement rather than replace other forms of statistical analysis, providing a summary of the relative magnitude of the individual, as well as the group responses.

State Attainment Analysis

A novel approach to dissecting the therapeutic response is based not on change from baseline, but on achieving a favorable or preferred clinical state. This favorable state has variably been termed the minimum clinically important state, minimum acceptable clinical severity, low activity clinical state, low disease activity state, patient acceptable symptom severity, and the low intensity symptom severity

(BLISS) index (90,91). With the BLISS approach (91), patients can be classified according to different aspects of the favorable state as follows: (a) ever in the state, (b) time to first being in the state, (c) in the state at termination, (d) percentage time in the state, and (d) number of times in the state. Different cut points can be taken for the LISS index, for example, less than 5nu, less than 10nu, less than 15nu, less than 20nu, and less than 25nu. Collectively, the LISS index provides estimates of the velocity, magnitude and durability of the response. It is of note that similar conclusions have been reached regarding the effectiveness of hylan GF 20 based on a traditional analysis (92), OMERACT-OARSI responder criteria (86), WOMAC 20, 50, 70 (87), and the BLISS index (91). The state attainment approach therefore seems to be a valid additional approach to data analysis. Although experience with the state attainment approach to outcome analysis is limited, further developments can be anticipated in this novel approach to criteria-based response categorization.

Measurement Techniques for Selected Variables of Importance in Outcome Assessment

Outcome Assessment can be based on symptoms, physical signs, and/or physical performance.

Symptom-Based Assessment

Symptom-based assessment can use patient self-report (paper-based, electronic data capture), or interviewer-based report (face-to-face, telephone interview, computer-assisted telephone interview). The instruments used for data capture may be simple unidimensional scales, general arthritis measures, disease-specific health-related quality of life measures, or generic health-related quality of life measures. Pain, physical function and patient global assessment are key measurement domains that have been included in several core set measurement batteries.

Pain

Because pain is the major complaint of the rheumatic sufferer, its measurement becomes extremely important in assessing response to antirheumatic drug medication (1). Pain is an entirely subjective phenomenon and can be measured only by the patient.

Several different methods of scaling the patient's perceived pain level have been developed (Fig. 3.2). The simplest way to assess pain is using single-item pain scales. One of the most popular methods uses the Likert scale (also known as the adjectival or descriptive scale) (1). In this scale, adjectives are used to describe increasing levels of pain severity between none and extreme. Corresponding numerical values can be assigned to the adjectives as follows: 0 = no pain, 1 = mild pain, 2 = moderate pain, 3 = severe pain, and 4 = extreme, or agonizing, pain (Fig. 3.2A). Such a scale is capable of discriminating between the use of NSAIDs and placebo in short-term clinical trials. The scale is simple to administer and easily comprehended, and can be scored quickly.

Another popular method of recording pain is the VAS (1). A line is taken to represent the continuum of pain, the ends defining the extremes of the experience, that is, "no pain" and "extreme pain" (Fig. 3.2B). Patients mark the line at a point corresponding to their estimate of pain, and the distance from zero is taken to represent the severity of pain. Scott and Huskisson showed that the performance of a VAS is profoundly affected by its design (1). Thus, for example, descriptions of pain at intervals along the line result in a clustering of points opposite the descriptions, converting the VAS into a graphic rating scale and resulting in loss of

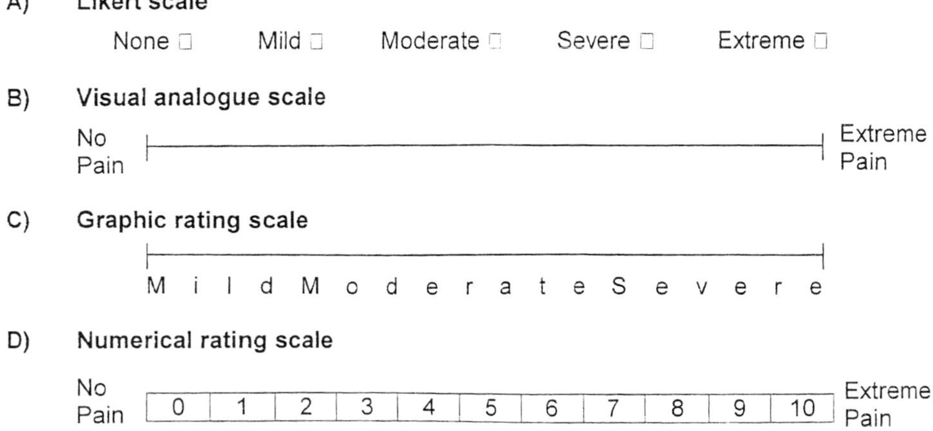

FIG. 3.2. Measurement techniques for symptom-based assessment.

sensitivity (2). Equal spacing of the letters of the pain severity descriptors appears to correct this problem (Fig. 3.2C). A good correlation has been found between horizontal and vertical scales, and there is excellent agreement between repeated measurements of pain using the VAS (1). One of the problems of a VAS is that some patients may have difficulty in understanding the concept, at least initially (2). Very few patients in our experience have difficulty in understanding the concept of a VAS, provided time is taken to carefully explain the nature of the scale. The line should have stops at either end to limit the distribution of results. The conventional length of the line is 10 cm, and it is important to note that this may be altered on photocopying (1). The method has shown good correlation with verbal rating scales, proved sensitive to change (1), and found applicable to patients regardless of ethnic background, as well as to children under 5 years of age (1). The VAS is probably the most responsive scale type (19,20,65–67), but is more complex to administer, may be more difficult to understand, and in paper format takes longer to score. Electronic data capture may greatly facilitate the administration and scoring of various types of scales, but particularly VA scales.

The NRS is often presented as an 11-point box scale (Fig. 3.2D), each box containing a number in ascending order, between 0 and 10. The scale is responsive, simple to administer, provides more response options than the Likert scale, can be scored quickly, and is only slightly less responsive than the VAS (19,20). For this reason, it may be particularly useful in clinical practice environments.

From an administration standpoint, there is controversy in the literature as to whether patients should be given access to their prior pain scores when rating current status (2). Our own observations in OA patients suggest that, in practice, it does not make an important difference (1). Pain in RA and OA varies at different times of the day, and it is therefore wise to standardize the timing of measurements (61–63).

Recent studies in RA and OA (19,20) suggest that Likert, VA, and NRS pain scales are highly responsive. The simpler scales perform at least as well as the more complex (e.g., pain faces scales, continuous chromatic analogue) scales, and the VAS is probably the most responsive, but the Likert and NRS are easier to administer in routine practice.

Two conceptually different approaches to pain assessment are the McGill Pain Questionnaire (MPQ) and Behavioral Observation Methods. The MPQ, developed by Melzack in Montreal, probes sensory, affective, and evaluative qualities of pain (1). Three principal measures can be generated from the MPQ: (a) a pain rating index based on the ranked value of words selected; (b) a rating based on the number of words chosen; and (c) a rating based on present pain intensity. The relative responsiveness of the MPQ has been compared against other pain scales in RA and OA (19,20). Behavioral observation methods attempt to introduce an element of objectivity into pain measurement. A pain behavior is an action displayed by patients communicating to those around them that they are experiencing pain. Such behaviors include sighing, grimacing, and the like. It is unclear whether objectivity is gained, because patients who deviate in scoring on pain scales may also be capable of equal deviance on a performance test (2).

Finally, pain subscales including one or more items may be incorporated into multidimensional health status questionnaires. Specific examples include generic questionnaires such as the SF-36 (93), general arthritis questionnaires such as the Health Assessment Questionnaire (HAQ) (94) and the Arthritis Impact Measurement Scales (AIMS, AIMS2) (95,96), and disease-specific questionnaires such as the Western Ontario and McMaster Osteoarthritis Index (65,66) and the Australian/Canadian Hand Osteoarthritis Index (67). In contrast to the aforementioned Segregated Multidimensional Questionnaires, pain questions are also included in the inventory of Aggregated Multidimensional Questionnaires, such as the Indices of Clinical Severity (97).

Stiffness

The measurement of perceived joint stiffness was formerly commonplace. It has been argued that patients may have difficulty in differentiating stiffness from pain, although this has not been verified. Furthermore, stiffness may be measured in terms of its duration or severity. When questioned regarding the duration of stiffness, the patient must understand whether the question relates to the time of first wakening, the time of getting out of bed, the time of first improvement in stiffness, or the time at which the patient will be as limber as he/she can be for the rest of the day (1). The best indicator of average duration is probably the time from waking to that of maximum improvement (1). Because of difficulty assessing duration, some investigators have preferred to measure stiffness severity. Indeed, Hazes, et al., showed that morning stiffness is better assessed by a severity score than one based on duration (1). It should be noted that even OA patients attribute significant importance to this consequence of their condition (1), and that stiffness measures are included in several OA indices (1,57,58,65–67), and have been retained in the ASAS core set measures for AS (88).

Functional Capacity Indices

The terms *impairment, disability,* and *handicap* in the original WHO classification of the impact of chronic disease (98) have been replaced by a different classification based on impairment, activities, and participation, and recognizes the importance of contextual factors such as the environment and the person (99). Its essence is captured in the recently introduced International Classification of Function (ICF) (100). Impairment is any loss or abnormality of psychological, physiologic, or emotional structure or function.

Activities encompass capabilities in performing activities of daily living. Participation captures the extent to which an individual can participate in society. In essence, therefore, impairment occurs at the organ level, activities at the personal level, and participation at the social level. Disability is a major feature of rheumatic disease and, after pain, is its second most important consequence. Weigl and colleagues have recently linked two disease-specific indices [WOMAC and Index of Clinical Severity (ICS)] to the ICF, an observation that anchors these two questionnaires into the ICF construct (101).

Physical function may be measured in terms of capacity (i.e., what the patient says he or she is capable of) or objectively in terms of performance (i.e., how the patient actually performs on a defined task). A working knowledge of disability indices used to assess physical function is essential for those engaged in evaluative research, and is increasingly important for practicing rheumatologists.

Rheumatoid Arthritis: American College of Rheumatology revised criteria for classification of global functional status in rheumatoid arthritis. The ACR revised criteria (102) are a revision of the original Steinbrocker Functional Grading System (2), adopted by the American Rheumatism Association (ARA). Compared with the original ARA criteria, the ACR criteria show a more uniform distribution, greater use being made of classes I and IV. While providing a simple method of classification, this system provides fewer response options than competing alternatives.

Arthritis impact measurement scales. The AIMS (95) is a widely used instrument that has been extensively validated in different clinical settings, and in several alternate-language forms. It is a multidimensional, self-administered index using 45 items to probe nine separate dimensions of mobility, physical activity, dexterity, social role, social activity, activities of daily living, pain, depression, and anxiety. Within each dimension, items are arranged in Guttman scale order such that patients failing an item also tend to fail all lower items in that same dimension. Each response carries a specific value, a standardization procedure being applied to bring each dimension to a common scale (0–10). Meenan et al. have revised and expanded the instrument, producing a new questionnaire termed AIMS2 (96). These following modifications were made: (a) all items have been produced in a standardized format; (b) the time frame has been standardized to the past 1 month; (c) 35 AIMS items have been left unchanged, four revised, six deleted, and three added; (d) scaling of the overall health status response has been altered from a VAS to a 5-point adjectival scale; (e) three new subscales have been added [(i) arm function, (ii) ability to work, and (iii) support from family and friends]; (f) new names have been given to all revised scales to avoid confusion between AIMS and AIMS2; and (g) three new assessments have been added [(i) satisfaction with current level of function, (ii) specific impact of arthritis on the subject's health status, and (iii) prioritization of three areas in which subjects would most like to see improvement].

Health assessment questionnaire. The HAQ (94), developed by Fries et al., has been extensively validated, is available in multiple alternate-language forms (2), and is widely used. The index has multipurpose applications and is based on a paradigm of five dimensions. The discomfort and disability subscales, both of which are self-administered, are its most familiar elements. Pain is measured using a single 15-cm horizontal VAS with terminal descriptors of "no pain" and "very severe pain." The disability dimension has eight categories: dressing and grooming, arising, eating, walking, hygiene, reach, grip, and activities (each containing two or three items). A 4-point ordinal scale is used to grade responses (to each of 20 questions) from "without any difficulty" to "unable to do." A supplementary section asks the patient to indicate any aids, devices, or assistance used in performing these activities. Scoring rules are used to derive a disability subscale score. In addition to the original form of the HAQ, there are a variety of modifications for use in RA, AS, and in children with juvenile RA (2).

McMaster Toronto arthritis patient preference disability questionnaire. Developed by a collaborative group at McMaster University and the University of Toronto, the MACTAR (71) disability measure uses an approach based on the selection of disability signals by individual patients. In particular, the index quantifies the specific functional priorities of each patient, which are identified by open-ended questioning at the time of initial assessment. Subsequent closed-ended questions probe limitations in other activities. Inquiry is then made to rank disabilities by importance, that is, according to the order in which the patient would most like to be able to perform the listed activities.

Osteoarthritis: Western Ontario and McMaster osteoarthritis index. Developed by Bellamy et al., the WOMAC osteoarthritis index (1,2,65,66,103) is a tridimensional self-administered questionnaire probing pain (5 items), stiffness (2 items), and physical disability (17 items), in patients with OA of either the hip or knee. It has been subject to two major validation studies and numerous other clinimetric evaluations. It is a very responsive measure and is available in 5-point Likert (WOMAC LK), 100-mm visual analogue (WOMAC VA), and 11-point NRS formats. The following clinimetric properties have been evaluated: reliability; validity (face, content, construct); responsiveness; relative efficiency (comparison with other outcome measures); Likert versus VAS; parametric versus nonparametric treatment of the data; Rasch analysis; prior score availability versus blind completion; signal versus aggregate methods of analysis; effect of changing the time frame; weighting and aggregation issues; electronic data capture; and telephone administration (1,2,65,66,103–107). The WOMAC index has been translated into over 65 different alternate-language forms and is used extensively in OA research. Recently WOMAC-based data have been incorporated in the development of OMERACT-OARSI responder criteria (84,86), the WOMAC 20, 50, 70 responder criteria (87), and the BLISS index (91), and can be linked to the ICF

(101). In addition to its traditional evaluative role, the WOMAC index may also have some predictive value (108,109). The WOMAC index is supported by a website (*www.womac.org*), and a user guide (103).

Clinical severity indices (97). Lequesne et al. have developed separate indices of clinical severity (97), one applicable to the hip, the other to the knee. The indices contain three components: pain or discomfort, maximum distance walked, and activities of daily living (a sexual function question included in the hip index is not considered necessary for all types of studies). The two indices are identical with respect to four of the five pain items and maximum distance walked, but differ in the sitting pain and activities of daily living items. In contrast to several other indices, scores on the separate dimensions are ordinarily summated to give a single score. These indices may be self-administered or interviewer administered. Several alternate-language translations are available, and the ICS has been linked to the ICF (101). The ICS score may have predictive value with respect to total hip arthroplasty (110).

Australian-Canadian osteoarthritis hand index (58,67). The Australian-Canadian (AUSCAN) Osteoarthritis Hand Index (58,67) is a tridimensional self-administered questionnaire probing pain (five items), stiffness (one item), and physical disability (nine items) in patients with OA of the hand, and is available in 5-point Likert (AUSCAN LK), 100-mm visual analogue (AUSCAN VA), and 11-point NRS formats. The following clinimetric properties have been evaluated: reliability; validity (face, content, construct), responsiveness, and weighting and aggregation issues (58,67). The AUSCAN index appears to be more responsive than the Functional Index of Hand Osteoarthritis (FIHOA) (67). The AUSCAN index has been translated into over 20 alternate-languages, and is supported by a website (*www.auscan.org*), and a user guide (111).

Algofunctional index (112,113). Developed by Dreiser et al., the Algofunctional Index is a unidimensional questionnaire that probes functional disability in hand OA using a battery of 10 questions (112). Reliability, validity, and responsiveness have been assessed (113). With slight modification, this index has been renamed the FIHOA.

Cochin index (114,115). The Cochin Index, originally developed and validated in RA patients (114), has recently been validated in OA hand patients (115). This index is a disability scale, containing 18 questions on daily activities. Administered by the patient's doctor, responses are recorded on 6-point Likert scales ranging from "done without difficulty" to "impossible." Interobserver reliability is high (ICC = 0.96), and this index exhibits acceptable levels of construct validity and responsiveness. The Cochin Index appears to be more responsive than the FIHOA (115).

Ankylosing Spondylitis: Bath ankylosing spondylitis index (116). The Bath Ankylosing Spondylitis Index is composed of several subindices, including a functional index (BASFI) (117), a disease activity index (118), a metrology index (119), a global index (120), and a radiographic index (121). The indices have grown in popularity. Recent comparative studies suggest that the BASFI may be more sensitive than the HAQ-S and the Dougados Functional Index (DFI) (122), and the HAQ-S more responsive than the DFI (123).

Fibromyalgia: Fibromyalgia impact questionnaire (124). The Fibromyalgia Impact Questionnaire (124) is self-administered and contains 10 questions, the first of which contains 10 subquestions. The item inventory was developed from three sources: patient interactions, FM literature, and existing health status measures. The instrument probes physical functioning, work status, depression, anxiety, sleep, pain, stiffness, fatigue, and well-being. Early work on validity and reliability testing has been encouraging, and more widespread use of this instrument is anticipated.

Arm, Shoulder, and Hand Conditions: Disabilities of Arm, Shoulder, and Hand (DASH) questionnaire (125,126). The DASH is a 30-item self-administered questionnaire, which contains 21 physical function items, 6 symptom items, and 3 social/role function items. Responses are scaled on 5-point Likert scales. A formula can be applied to calculate a DASH global score (0–100), higher scores reflecting higher levels of disability (125,126).

Potential users of the aforementioned instruments should determine which instrument is most suitable for their purpose (2). We recommend contacting the originator when using any health status measure to obtain advice regarding administration, formatting, scoring, and analysis. Furthermore, users' guides are available for several of the commonly used measures. The use of currently available high-performance functional, or health status, measures should be considered mandatory in all future evaluative studies. The use of ad hoc scales that have not been validated should be avoided.

Patient Global Assessment

Patient Global Assessments (PGAs) form part of core set measurements in RA (41,42), OA (22,82), and AS (88). Although commonly used in clinical trials of new therapeutic agents (127–129), there is no international consensus on the wording or preferred scaling format for response to the PGA question. Indeed, the PGA can take several different forms. The PGA question can relate to a joint or symptom, the overall condition, or the person as a whole. It can be phrased as a change question, or can be used to assess health status at a point in time. The process whereby the patient reviews his or her experience, and then selects, weights, and aggregates the information into a single summary response is poorly understood. It seems likely that there is considerable intersubject and even intrasubject variability in the process. Nevertheless, the PGA is considered by many to be an important part of the outcome measurement battery. Further research into the wording, scaling, and placement of the PGA questions is required.

Generic Health Status Measures

The term *generic health status measure* is currently used as a collective term to describe questionnaires that measure various aspects of health-related quality of life (HRQOL) and can be used in a variety of different disorders and patient groups. Few, if any, comprehensively probe all important aspects of the human condition (e.g., personal security, financial well-being, freedom of religion, and nutritional adequacy) and therefore do not measure quality of life in its entirety. Experience with the use of these techniques in evaluative research in arthritis continues to grow. Five instruments of particular importance are the Short-Form 36 Health Status Questionnaire and its variations (SF-12, SF-8) (93,130,131), EuroQoL (132,133), WHOQOL (134), Nottingham Health Profile (135), and the Health Utilities Index (136).

Short-Form 36 Health Status Questionnaire (93). The Short-Form 36 (SF-36) was developed out of the Rand Corporation's health insurance experiment, a comprehensive evaluation of alternative methods of financing health care in the United States. It is a self-administered questionnaire containing 36 items that takes about 5 minutes to complete. It measures three major health attributes (functional status, well-being, and overall evaluation of health) and eight health concepts: (a) limitations in physical activities because of health problems (10 items); (b) limitations in social activities because of physical or emotional problems (2 items); (c) limitations in usual role activities because of physical health problems (4 items); (d) bodily pain (2 items); (e) general mental health (psychologic distress and well-being) (5 items); (f) limitations in usual role activities because of emotional problems (3 items); (g) vitality (energy and fatigue) (4 items); and (h) general health perceptions (5 items). An item regarding health change is part of the questionnaire, but it is not scored. The questionnaire has been constructed for administration by a trained interviewer in person or by telephone. Multiple alternate-language forms of the SF-36 have been developed and widely applied in different disease states. The symptoms reported are not attributed to a particular disease or a particular joint. The measure therefore reflects overall health-related quality of life, and scores may be influenced by various comorbidities. Scores can be reported for each of the eight component domains or summary scores created for the physical (physical component score, or PCS) and mental (mental component score, or MCS) components (93). The SF-36 exists in two versions (versions 1 and 2), normative data being available for some countries. Two short-form versions of this index, termed the SF-12 and SF-8, have also been developed (130,131). For OA clinical trials applications, the SF-36 may be more demanding on sample size than the WOMAC index (137,138). However, it should be noted that these two tools measure two distinct but important aspects of the patient's health (139) and can be strategically applied in combination in OA.

EuroQoL (132,133). EuroQoL is a generic instrument for measuring health-related quality of life (132). It is a short, self-administered questionnaire that classifies the patient into one of 243 health states. It consists of a simple, five-part questionnaire relating to deficits in mobility, self-care, main working activity, social relationships, pain and mood, and a VAS on which patients rate their own health status. It takes only a few minutes to complete and is suitable for use as a postal questionnaire. The instrument generates a single numeric index of health status and therefore can be used as a measure of health outcome in both clinical and economic evaluation. A recent report provides some evidence for the reliability and construct validity of the EuroQoL-5D in OA knee patients (133).

WHOQOL (134). The WHOQOL instrument has been developed as a generic HRQOL measure, having cross-cultural applicability. The pilot WHOQOL contained 236 questions, addressing 29 facets of HRQOL grouped into six major domains. The WHOQOL-100 version has resulted from the collaborative efforts of several centers in diverse cultural settings (134). It contains 100-items encompassing overall quality of life, general health, physical health, psychological state, social relationships, and environment. This instrument has potentially important applications in large-scale international epidemiology studies.

Nottingham Health Profile (135). The Nottingham Health Profile is intended to give brief and simple indications of perceived physical, social, and emotional health problems. The scale contains 38 items that can be grouped into six sections: physical mobility (eight items), pain (eight items), sleep (five items), social isolation (five items), emotional reactions (nine items), and energy level (three items). All items use a yes/no answer format. It is self-administered and requires less than 10 minutes to complete. For scoring purposes, the number of affirmative responses in each of the six sections is counted. Section scores may be presented as a profile, or an overall score may be calculated.

Health Utilities Index (136). This multiattribute health status classification system was developed to provide a comprehensive description of health status. Responses are required to 15 questions that probe aspects of day-to-day health. The system measures eight attributes: vision, hearing, speech, physical mobility, dexterity, cognition, pain and discomfort, and emotion. This self-administered questionnaire takes less than 10 minutes to complete and provides a single, overall summary score. This index is finding application in various settings, including health economics research. The responsiveness of the Health Utilities Index (HUI) in a knee OA environment was recently highlighted in a randomized clinical trial, in which the cost-utility of adding hylan G-F20 to appropriate care was demonstrated (9).

In addition to the aforementioned symptom-based measures, there are opportunities to measure other aspects of health such as coping (140,141), helplessness (142,143), and handicap (144–149) in evaluative research. It is of note that the IMMPACT group recently has developed consensus around core set measurement for future chronic pain trials, including not only measurement of pain, physical function, patient ratings of improvement and satisfaction with treatment, symptoms, and adverse events and patient disposition, but also measurement of emotional function (150). The psychosocial impact of arthritis and musculoskeletal conditions is well recognized (151–156), and tools that can be used to implement this evaluation are available.

Physical Examination-Based Assessment

Assessments based on clinical examination are routine in clinical practice, and have been variably retained in core set measurement recommendations for clinical research. They are retained in the ACR core set measures for RA (79) (number of swollen and tender joints), and the ASAS guidelines (88) (spinal mobility), but not in the OMERACT core set for OA (82) or the IMMPACT core set for chronic pain (150). With few exceptions, concern that examination-based measurement cannot be conducted reliably is not supported by the literature (34,37,40,43). A recent study in OA also suggests that some, but not all, standardized knee examinations can be conducted with acceptable levels of reliability (157). Of greater importance is the consequence to the patient's health-related quality of life of abnormalities discovered on the physical examination. For this reason, it is essential that examination-based assessments be accompanied by symptom-based assessments. The two most important examination-based musculoskeletal assessments are measures of tenderness and swelling.

Musculoskeletal Tenderness: Rheumatoid arthritis. Various methods have been used to score joint tenderness in patients with RA (1). The techniques have differed principally in the joints they encompass, whether they score joints individually or as joint units, and whether they grade the response to firm palpation or use surface area weighting factors. The consequence of these different systems is that the percentage contribution to the total score of individual joint areas when maximally affected is different in different indices. At present, joint tenderness assessment in RA is focused on simple counts of the number of tender joints (1). This approach is recommended in the ACR Preliminary Core Set of Disease Activity Measures for RA Clinical Trials (79). Assessors can be trained to reliably perform joint tenderness counts in RA patients (37).

Several studies have evaluated the role of reduced joint counts. Smolen et al. contend that a 28-joint count is reliable, valid, easier to perform than a full assessment, and evaluates joints that are important in RA (158). Prevoo et al. have demonstrated the successful incorporation of 28-joint counts into a Modified Disease Activity Score (159). The use of reduced counts previously has been challenged (160,161) on the basis that although sensitivity to change may be reduced only slightly, this does not reflect adequately the clinical importance of the excluded joints. However, the ACR Committee on Outcome Measures in RA Clinical Trials has noted that "validated joint counts with as few as 28 joints are equally acceptable in RA clinical trials" (161). Furthermore, van Gestel et al. contend that improvement criteria, which include 28-joint counts, are as valid as improvement criteria using more comprehensive joint counts (162), and Scott et al. have noted that the 28-joint count is becoming the international standard (163).

The inclusion of joint counting in routine practice (163) requires either that the assessor is adequately trained (37) or that the patient self-administer the joint count (1). A recent assessment of the reliability and validity of a self-reported 36-joint count in RA concluded that patients consistently rated their pain/tenderness higher than physicians/trained assistants, and therefore self-report could not replace the standard evaluation method for clinical research purposes (164). In contrast, Houssien et al. have observed adequate agreement between the two different approaches, but note that they are not directly interchangeable (165).

Osteoarthritis. The Doyle Index, a modification of the Ritchie Index, has been configured to have greater relevance to OA patients (1). Each joint, or joint unit, is tested for tenderness on palpation or on passive movement (or, in the case of the lumbar spine, on active movement), and scored according to the Ritchie grading system. The total Doyle score is calculated by summing the component scores. To date, this index has found only limited application, possibly due to the variable and sometimes limited distribution of joint involvement in OA.

Ankylosing spondylitis. Two indices suitable for the assessment of tenderness in AS have been developed (166, 167). Both assess multiple sites of musculoskeletal tenderness, rather than joint-specific tenderness. The Dougados Index (166) assesses 10 sites, whereas the Newcastle Enthesis Index assesses 30 sites (167). Both grade the response according to the Ritchie system (1). These indices may have an important role in evaluative research.

Fibromyalgia. Mechanical dolorimetry, often with the Chatillon dolorimeter, is commonly used in FM clinical trials (1). Standard methods for applying the instrument have been described at acceptable levels of reliability (interobserver reliability = 0.87). In addition to assessing outcomes in clinical trials, dolorimetry may be useful in exploring the determinants of pain threshold in FM (1).

Joint Swelling. The detection of joint swelling is simpler than its gradation and can be accomplished by trained assessors at acceptable levels of reliability (37). Joint swelling assessment in RA has focused on simple accounts of the number of swollen joints (1) and is often based on the same 28 joints included in the tender joint count (163).

The measurement of the circumference of swollen and damaged joints is largely of historic interest and was traditionally accomplished by the use of jewelers rings or a simple plastic arthrocircameter (1).

Performance-Based Assessment

The three most frequently used performance tests in clinical trials have been range of motion, grip strength, and walk time (1).

The range of motion of peripheral joints in normal subjects has been determined by the American Academy of Orthopaedic Surgeons (168). Although goniometry may be performed on most peripheral joints, it is most popular for measurement of knee range of movement. With appropriate training in the method, peripheral joint range of movement in RA and OA can be conducted with adequate levels of reliability (1,37,40,157).

The measurement of spinal movement and chest expansion remains important in the assessment of AS patients. Normal range of spinal movement for different ages in both sexes has been established. Spinal movement has been measured by several methods, the most popular of which are skin distraction techniques and inclinometry (1). Spinal mobility is an ASAS core set measure for AS (88) and can be evaluated with adequate reliability by trained assessors (34).

Other methods of evaluating joint mobility include the Locomotion Score (169), the Gait, Arms, Legs, Spine (GALS) Locomotor Screen (170), and use of an inclinometer (171).

Although previously recommended in international clinical trial guidelines, enthusiasm for the 50-foot walk time and for grip strength measurement has declined (1), possibly due to concerns regarding relevancy and, in the former case, concerns regarding responsiveness (1,2). The walk time is an insensitive measure in OA and of disease activity in RA (1,2). Various instruments have been devised to measure grip strength, but they have failed to provide any advantage over the Davis bag or sphygmomanometer cuff (1). It is important to standardize the time of measurement, patient instructions, and the instrument when evaluating grip strength. The determinants of grip strength are the size of the hand, the strength of the muscles in the forearm and hand, and the pain and degree of joint destruction in the wrist, hand, and finger joints.

ADVERSE DRUG REACTIONS

In contrast to preceding paragraphs, directed at the measurement of potential benefit, it is equally important to use measures directed at assessing potential harm.

Adverse reactions have been defined by Friedman et al. as "any clinical event, sign or symptom that goes in an unwanted direction . . . and has the added dimension of physical findings, complaints, and laboratory results" (172).

Adverse drug reactions (ADRs) are of two types. The first, type A reactions, are due to augmented pharmacologic effects and tend to be common, predictable, and not usually serious. They occur either because of increased tissue or organ sensitivity, or because of slow drug elimination. Type B adverse effects, on the other hand, are unusual, aberrant responses unrelated to the drug's pharmacologic properties, often described as idiosyncratic. Although type B adverse reactions are occasionally fatal, most deaths reported as a result of medicaments are due to the more commonly occurring type A reactions.

The tolerability of an antirheumatic drug may be determined from a combination of sources: (a) controlled clinical trials, (b) pharmacoepidemiologic studies, and (c) case reports or case series.

Definition of an ADR is frequently left to the investigator to describe its occurrence, nature, and causal relationship to the intervention (2). The frequency of ADRs can be affected by the method of ascertainment, drug dosage, the trial strategy (fixed vs. titration), patient selection criteria, duration of follow-up, and the analytic strategy used (intention to treat vs. per protocol).

Because volunteered responses may differ from elicited responses in a manner that is not always consistent, the strategy for eliciting adverse events requires careful consideration (1). Open-ended questioning may elicit a different response than closed-ended questioning. The detection of rare events is problematic in relatively small trials. Although attribution is difficult, when unexpected ADRs are encountered, they should be documented—otherwise they will be erroneously dismissed as unimportant because only one or a few subjects have been affected. We recommend that all events be recorded by occurrence, nature, and severity (mild, moderate, severe) and that the investigator provide a judgment as to whether they are unrelated or related (possibly, probably, or definitely) to the intervention.

The grading of severity is contentious, because physicians vary in their propensity to discontinue study medication. It should not be assumed that all withdrawals from a trial were due to severe side effects, because some ADRs rated as moderate may arouse sufficient concern to result in treatment termination. The converse is less often true, because most severe ADRs result in withdrawal.

ADR outcomes may be reported as the (a) total number of adverse events classified by organ system, (b) number of patients experiencing at least one ADR, (c) number of severe ADRs, or (d) number of patients withdrawn because of ADRs. Clinical and laboratory forms of intolerance may be reported separately or collectively. Some patients experience multiple ADRs, and thus the total number of adverse events may exceed the total number of patients experiencing at least one ADR. Furthermore, the analysis depends on whether only patients with "definite" or "probable" events are included or whether "possible" events or events thought to be "unrelated" are included. It is advisable to plan the analysis *a priori* and avoid post hoc data dredging. In addition to performing between-group comparisons on ADR data, it may be convenient to use survival analysis techniques.

Before a drug is licensed, it will have been studied in clinical therapeutic trials in several hundred or a few thousand patients (1). These sample sizes should be adequate to identify adverse drug reactions occurring with incidences of greater than 1 in 100 or greater than 1 in 1,000, respectively. A rule of thumb is that to be 95% confident of detecting an adverse event, the number of subjects needed is three times that of the estimated frequency of the event—the so-called "rule of three" (1). It should also be noted that clinical therapeutic trials of new medications are conducted on selected patients, such that those potentially at higher risk for adverse events, such as the extremes of age, pregnant woman, those with severe comorbidity, and those receiving specific medications are excluded from study. Clinical trials on such "squeaky-clean" patients can be expected to identify common side effects, such as dyspepsia induced by an NSAID, but are unlikely to identify rare side effects. To do so requires study of patients in the "real world," where different patient groups, comorbidities, and concomitant drug therapy influence the outcome. Large numbers of patients are required, since drugs, contrary to popular belief, are generally relatively innocuous for the majority of recipients (173).

Pharmacoepidemiology offers an opportunity to assess drug toxicity in large numbers of patients across different diseases, age groups, races, geographic areas, and between genders (174). As noted previously, however, systematic error cannot be offset by large numbers. Patients entered into large population databases must represent the target population as a whole and not merely reflect a subset with a greater tendency than usual to either toxicity or tolerability. Voluntary reporting systems have been developed in many countries, including several European countries, Canada, the United States, and Australasia (2). In addition to systems operating locally and nationally, industrial drug surveillance programs are operated by the pharmaceutical industry and by academic institutions (2). Regarding postmarketing surveillance, Strom has noted that no single method was ideal, none was likely to be developed, and the most appropriate method for a particular question should be selected from among competing alternatives (spontaneous ADR reports, aggregate population-based data, computerized databanks of organized medical care, prospective postmarketing surveillance studies, incidental data collected during other ad hoc studies, and *de novo* data deliberately collected to serve a specific purpose) (175). Patient selection criteria, drug dosage schedule, route of administration, concomitant drug therapy, and comorbidity are some factors that may differ between those who are exposed to an antirheumatic drug and develop an ADR that is reported, and those who are exposed but do not develop an ADR, or who develop an ADR that is not reported. The introduction of a new drug may be attended by the Weber effect (176), that is, overreporting of ADRs during the first 2 years after license approval. Finally, it should be noted that spontaneous reporting systems cannot provide incidence rates, only reporting rates (176). The reasons why doctors may fail to report adverse drug reactions include complacency, fear, guilt, ambition, ignorance, diffidence, and lethargy (177).

Finally, it has to be emphasized that case series, which are descriptive and without controls, still provide useful information, at least in the early years of marketing. Also, it must never be forgotten that the initial identification of adverse drug reactions may be signaled by anecdotal reports (e.g., phocomelia due to thalidomide). Indeed, in a review of 18 drugs removed from the market by 1983, Venning noted that 13 were first signaled by anecdotal reports (178–180). Not only are doctors capable of identifying adverse reactions to drugs, but it also seems that patients are capable of discriminating adverse drug reactions and adverse clinical events (1).

In clinical trials environments, different methods of classifying adverse reactions have been used: *The WHO Adverse Reaction Dictionary* (WHO-ART) (181) and *Coding Symbols for Thesaurus of Adverse Reaction Terms* (COSTART) (182). Recently the use of the Medical Dictionary Regulatory Activities preferred terms have been compared with WHO-ART (183). The OMERACT Drug Safety Working Group (184) has proposed further standardization in the assessment of adverse effects in rheumatology clinical trials (185) (Table 3.7). International (186) and national (187) drug monitoring programs have been established by WHO and the Arthritis, Rheumatism, and Aging Medical Information System, respectively, and the establishment of a large multinational cohort proposed for long-term safety monitoring in RA (188). The OMERACT Drug Safety Working Party identified only four patient-based methods of collecting safety data in clinical trials: the Stanford Toxicity Index (STI), Patient-Orientated Symptom Index, Morgan Index, and Juvenile Arthritis Quality of Life Questionnaire (189). The OMERACT Drug Safety Working Party has prioritized the STI and proposed that this index be revised to incorporate missing attributes and then be validated for application in clinical trials (189).

Through a combination of data from controlled clinical trials, pharmacoepidemiologic studies, and case reports or case series, the true safety and tolerability profile of new products eventually emerges.

Pharmacoeconomics

Pharmacoeconomic evaluations are increasingly becoming a part of outcome measurement procedures in antirheumatic drug studies. There are four basic types of analysis: cost-minimization, cost-benefit, cost-effectiveness, and cost-utility (1). Most analyses use one of the latter two

TABLE 3.7. *Severity of symptoms as described in the rheumatology common toxicity criteria*

Mild	Moderate	Severe	Life-Threatening
Asymptomatic	Symptomatic	Prolonged symptoms, reversible	At risk for death
Short duration (<1 wk)	Duration (1–2 wks)	Major functional impairment	Substantial disability, especially if permanent
No change in lifestyle	Alters lifestyle occasionally	Prescription medication/ partial relief	May be hospitalized
No medication or OTC	Prescription medications with relief	May require study drug discontinuation May be hospitalized	May be hospitalized

OTC, over-the-counter medication.

From Woodworth, TG, Furst DE, Strand V, et al. Standardizing assessment of adverse events in rheumatology clinical trials. Status of OMERACT Toxicity Working Group, March 2000: towards a connom understanding of comparative toxity/safety profiles for antirheumatic therapies. *J Rheumatol* 2001;28:1163–1169, with permission.

approaches. Several instruments reviewed earlier in this chapter are suitable for measuring effectiveness (e.g., HAQ, AIMS, WOMAC, etc.), and a few are appropriate for estimating utility values (e.g., HUI and EuroQoL). Several cost-effectiveness and cost-utility studies have been published in recent years (190–195) and tentative guidelines proposed for interpreting economic evaluations and making sound decisions on the adoption and use of new technologies (196). Recent developments have included recommendations from OMERACT 5 (197,198) and OMERACT 6 (199,200) conferences. In particular, 12 key elements of a reference case for economic evaluation have been proposed. The elements include study horizon, duration of therapy, extrapolation beyond trial duration, modeling beyond therapy, synthesis of comparisons where head-to-head trials do not exist, clinical outcome measures, mortality, valuation of health states, resource utilization, discontinuation of therapy, therapeutic sequence, and population risk stratification (199).

Patient Perspective

Recent consideration of the patient's perspective has arisen out of discussions concerning the importance of change and state to consumers (201). Traditionally, although patients may self-report their symptoms, it is often clinicians who use the reports to guide clinical decision making and establish clinical pathways (202). It has been observed that patients and clinicians may have different perspectives on health outcomes (202), and the more direct consideration of the patient's perception, and preferences, is consistent with the principle of shared goal-setting. Carr et al. have noted that some outcomes of importance to patients are not currently measured, and that existing measures need to be calibrated to take account of the differing importance of outcomes at different stages of disease (203). Expectations about future health and satisfaction with health outcomes represent important alternative approaches to outcome assessment (204).

The methods for evaluating the efficacy and tolerability of antirheumatic drugs continue to evolve. There are few international standards, but the development of guidelines by several agencies is a positive step toward harmonization. Future antirheumatic drug studies have an opportunity to use established methodologies, to use fully validated high-performance outcome measures targeting core set variables, and to provide adequate sample size. Weighting and aggregating different outcome measures into a single summary score remains controversial and may be problematic. Specification of a primary outcome measure therefore is extremely important. Because sample size requirements differ for different variables, it is essential that the critical clinical question be addressed with adequate statistical power. Despite these problems, there has been a progressive increase in the sophistication of antirheumatic drug trials in recent years and in the quality of both trials and reports.

RECENT DEVELOPMENTS IN DISEASE-BASED MEASUREMENT

Rheumatoid Arthritis

Agreement on core set measures for RA clinical trials and the emergence of ACR 20, ACR 50, and ACR 70 responder criteria has standardized the measurement process at least from a clinical trials perspective.

Emerging new instruments include a new clinical index of joint damage (Mechanical Joint Score) (205), a brief measure of RA clinical severity not seriously confounded by psychological functioning (Rheumatoid Arthritis Severity Score) (206), a method for scoring irreversible longterm articular damage in RA (Rheumatoid Arthritis Articular Damage Index) (207), a method of measuring parenting function and disability (Parenting Disability Indices) (208), and a Rheumatoid Arthritis Self-Efficacy Scale (209). The HAQ has been the subject of several further studies (210–218), and additional translations have been developed and validated (210,211). Issues relating to the variation between different versions of the HAQ have been addressed (212,213,218), and it has been noted that the original HAQ is better than the MHAQ and the RA-HAQ (213). The HAQ has the potential for monitoring individual patients (214) and for benchmarking (215,216), and may be useful in predicting success in applying for disability benefits (217). In the further validation of existing measures, the validation of the Rheumatoid Arthritis Quality of Life Questionnaire has been extended (219,220). The responsiveness of the Cochin Index has been assessed after RA hand surgery (221), and the psychometric properties of the Dutch-AIMS2-SF evaluated (222). Fransen et al. have confirmed the responsiveness of the Rheumatoid Arthritis Disease Activity Index (RADAI) (223), and Smolen et al. have verified the usefulness of a Simple Disease Activity Index for RA patients (224). In clinical research environments, experience applying the ACR responder criteria (225–229) and the DAS (230–232) has grown considerably. The value of the aforementioned instruments and approaches in evaluating the response to treatment has been noted in trials of leflunomide (233), methotrexate, cyclosporine A, sulphasalazine (234), and infliximab (235), as has their role in target setting in the clinical management of RA patients (236–238). Quantitative evaluation of RA patients has facilitated health status assessment in early RA (239), late-onset RA (240), international comparisons (241), inter-disease comparisons (242), comparisons against population norms (243), and observation of the course of RA in longitudinal observational studies and follow-up studies (244, 245). These developments notwithstanding, the introduction of standardized quantitative measurement into routine care and the routine use of health-related quality of life questionnaires in RA clinical practice remain challenging (246,247).

Osteoarthritis

Agreement on core set measures for OA clinical trials and the emergence of OMERACT-OARSI responder criteria have standardized the measurement process at least from a clinical trials perspective. In addition to instrument developments in OA discussed earlier in this chapter, disease-specific instruments have been compared against one another (248–251) and against generic HRQOL instruments (252, 253). Where differences in responsiveness have been detected, they have generally favored the disease-specific instruments. Korean and Singaporean versions of the WOMAC index have been successfully validated (254,255). The negative effects of socioeconomic status and psychological factors on health status scores have been evaluated (256), but no interracial differences in symptom perception have been observed in the United States (257). The measurement of health status may have important implications for timing joint replacement surgery, since Fortin et al. (258) have noted that those subjects with the worst function and pain at the time of surgery had comparatively worse outcomes postoperatively. This is particularly important because Hawker et al. have noted that, compared with men, women have a higher prevalence of hip or knee arthritis, have worse symptoms and greater disability, and are less likely to have undergone arthroplasty (259).

Ankylosing Spondylitis

Agreement on core set measures for AS clinical trials (88) and the emergence of an ASAS preliminary definition of short-term improvement in AS (89) are important steps toward standardization in AS outcome measurement. Van Tubergen et al. have compared criteria-based responder criteria with response status adjudicated by expert opinion, and concluded that ASAS criteria have an agreement of 70%, sensitivity of 62%, and specificity of 89% (260). Developments in instrumentation have resulted in the emergence of the Ankylosing Spondylitis Quality of Life measure (261,262), and the Patient Generated Index for AS (263), both responsive measures of health-related outcome. In comparative studies, the responsiveness of the EuroQoL VA scale and the SF-12 PCS was strong, but Haywood et al. expressed concern regarding the responsivensss of the EuroQoL-5D scale and the SF-12 MCS in AS patients (264). Eyres et al. have assessed both the BASFI and the Revised Leeds Disability Questionnaire using Rasch analysis and observed both instruments to be unidimensional, but displaying disordered item thresholds (265). The WHO-DAS 11 is considered useful for measuring disability in AS, and is responsive to short-term change (266). Heuft-Dorenbosch et al. have developed and validated the Maastricht Ankylosing Spondylitis Enthesitis Score, although the responsiveness of this tool will need to be confirmed in future studies (267). In concert with observations in RA, self-assessed joint counts in AS are discrepant from joint counts assessed by doctors (268).

Connective Tissue Disease

Progress in developing outcome measurement procedures for complex multisystem disorders such as systemic lupus erythematosus (SLE), systemic sclerosis (SSc), myositis, vasculitis, and Behçet's disease has been considerable.

Systemic Lupus Erythematosus

The Systemic Lupus Activity Measure (269), the Systemic Lupus Erythematosus Disease Activity Index (270), the British Isles Lupus Activity Group Index (271), and the

Systemic Lupus Erythematosus International Collaborating Clinics/American College of Rheumatology Damage Index (SDI) (272,273), are all valid measures of different aspects of this condition (274). Brunner et al. have noted that item weighting of the SDI does not enhance index performance (275). Recent experience with the EuroQoL suggests it is a valid measure of health-related quality of life in SLE patients (276). Consideration has been given to the development of core set measures (277,278) and responder criteria for SLE studies (279).

Systemic Sclerosis

Multiorgan involvement in SSc complicates the development of outcome measurement tools (280–282). Both the HAQ and the AIMS instruments have proven valuable as outcome measures in SSc (283–285). Most recently, the European Scleroderma Study Group has developed separate sets of disease activity criteria for three SSc patient subgroups: SSc patients as a whole, limited SSc patients, and diffuse SSc patients (286).

Vasculitis

The Vasculitis Damage Index (287,288), the Vasculitis Activity Index (289), the Birmingham Vasculitis Activity Score (BVAS) (290), and the Wegener granulomatosis modification of the Birmingham Vasculitis Activity Score (BVAS/WG) (291) are relatively recent additions, and provide measurement opportunities in the systemic vasculitides. In Wegener's granulomatosis, Koldingsnes et al. have noted a relationship between baseline BVAS-1 score and the probability of achieving complete remission (292). Some of the aforementioned tools may have prognostic as well as descriptive and evaluative applications.

Inflammatory Myopathies

The International Myositis Outcome Assessment Collaborative Study Group has recently proposed core set measures for adult and juvenile idiopathic and juvenile inflammatory myopathies (293). The five core set activity domains are global disease activity, muscle strength, physical function, laboratory evaluation, and assessment of extraskeletal muscle involvement (293). Specific instruments and techniques have been recommended based on validity, feasibility, and applicability (293). Alexanderson et al. have developed and validated a self-administered questionnaire termed the Myositis Activities Profile to assess activity limitations in polymyositis/dermatomyositis (294). The Childhood Health Assessment Questionnaire (CHAQ) has been evaluated, and noted to be a valid, reliable, and responsive measure of physical function in juvenile idiopathic inflammatory myopathies (295).

Osteoporosis

Consideration has been given by the OMERACT group to the development of core set measures for osteoporosis studies (296–299). The six core set measures identified by the OMERACT group are as follows: bone mineral density, vertebral and nonvertebral fractures, biochemical markers, pain, quality of life, and height (296–299). In a subsequent evaluation, pain, bone mineral density, and biochemical markers were noted to be the most responsive outcomes (297).

Juvenile Chronic Arthritis

Measurement in children, especially young children, is challenging (300–304). Interested readers are referred to specialty texts on pediatrics and child assessments. The CHAQ is the most widely used functional status measure in childhood (305). Dempster et al. have reported an MCID for improvement of 0.13 and an MCID for deterioration of 0.75 (306). The Paediatric Quality of Life Inventory is a modular instrument designed to measure health-related quality of life (307). The instrument has been validated in a diverse sample of children with rheumatic diseases (307). Further study of the responsiveness of this instrument in particular disease entities, and in different research and clinical practice environments, will be of interest.

Future Perspective

Opportunities are rapidly expanding to conduct health status assessment using tools that are valid, reliable, and responsive. National and international agencies and coalitions are providing strong leadership in defining core set measures and defining response criteria. Clinical research is an environment in which high levels of standardization have been achieved and for which high performance tools are available, many of which are capable of meeting international and multicenter measurement needs. However, the routine clinical practice environment remains challenging due to a combination of culture, rationale, and logistics. It is possible to import outcome measurement techniques, routinely used in clinical research, into clinical practice environments. The impediments may include lack of familiarity with the tools; absence of a requirement to conduct quantitative assessments; uncertainty regarding the value that quantitative measurement brings to decision making and patient outcome; and concern regarding the time and cost requirements of administering, scoring, and interpreting quantitative data. These issues notwithstanding, the emergence of short-form questionnaires, electronic data capture, responder criteria, and low-intensity symptom severity state definitions provides an outstanding opportunity to import quantitative measurement procedures into routine clinical care, an environment receiving increasing attention, and one in which the patient's perspective and shared goal setting are paramount (308–311).

REFERENCES

1. Bellamy N, Buchanan WW. Clinical evaluation in the rheumatic diseases. In: Koopman WJ, ed. *Arthritis and allied conditions,* 14th ed. Philadelphia: Lea & Febiger, 2000:51–82.
2. Bellamy N. *Musculoskeletal clinical metrology.* Dordrecht, the Netherlands: Kluwer Academic, 1993:1–367.
3. Murray CJ, Lopez AD, Jamison DT. The global burden of disease in 1990: summary results, sensitivity analysis and future directions. *Bull WHO* 1994;72(3):495–509.
4. Sackett DL, Haynes RB, Guyatt GH, et al. *Clinical epidemiology: a basic science for clinical medicine,* 2nd ed. Boston: Little, Brown, 1991:1–441.
5. Bellamy N. *Prognosis in the rheumatic diseases.* Lancaster, UK: Kluwer Academic, 1991:11–502.
6. Woolf AD. Leader. The bone and joint decade 2000–2010. *Ann Rheum Dis* 2000;59(2):81–82.
7. Hopman WM, Berger JL, et al. Is there regional variation in the SF-36 scores of Canadian adults. *Can J Public Health* 2002;93(3):233–237.
8. Glasziou AP. Editorial. The Cochrane Library: access for all Australians. *Med J Aust* 2002;177(10):532–533.
9. Torrance GW, Raynauld JP, Walker V, et al. A prospective, randomized, health outcomes trial evaluating the incorporation of hylan G-F 20 into the treatment paradigm for patients with knee osteoarthritis (part 2 of 2): economic results. *Osteoarthritis Cartilage* 2002;10(7): 518–527.
10. Bellamy N, Kaloni S, Pope J, et al. Quantitative rheumatology: a survey of outcome measurement procedures in routine rheumatology outpatient practice in Canada. *J Rheumatol* 1998;25:852–858.
11. Bellamy N, Muirden KD, Brooks PM, et al. Quantitative rheumatology: a survey of outcome measurement procedures in routine rheumatology outpatient practice in Australia. *J Rheumatol* 1999;26:1593–1599.
12. Wolfe F, Pincus T. Data collection in the clinic. *Rheum Dis Clin North Am* 1995;21(2):321–358.
13. Pincus T. Why should rheumatologists collect patient self-report questionnaires in routine rheumatologic care? *Rheum Dis Clin North Am* 1995;21(2):271–319.
14. Feinstein AR. Randomised clinical trials. In: *Clinical epidemiology—the architecture of clinical research.* Philadelphia: WB Saunders, 1985:683–717.
15. Nikles CJ, Glasziou PP, Del Mar CB, et al. N of 1 trials. Practical tools for medication management. *Aust Fam Physician* 2000;29(11):1108–1112.
16. Nikles CJ, Glasziou PP, Del Mar CB, et al. Preliminary experiences with a single-patient trials service in general practice. *Med J Aust* 2000;173(2):100–103.
17. Cook TD, Campbell DT. *Quasi-experimentation: design and analysis issues for field settings.* Boston: Houghton Mifflin, 1979:1–405.
18. Kvien K, Mikkelsen B-Y. Nordvåg editorial. Results from controlled clinical trials: how relevant for clinical practice. *J Rheumatol* 2003: 30(6):1135–1137.
19. Bellamy N, Campbell J, Syrotuik J. Comparative study of self-rating pain scales in rheumatoid arthritis patients. *Curr Med Res Opin* 1999; 15(2):121–127.
20. Bellamy N, Campbell J, Syrotuik J. Comparative study of self-rating pain scales in osteoarthritis patients. *Curr Med Res Opin* 1999;15(2): 113–119.
21. U.S. Food and Drug Administration. Guidance for industry, clinical development, programs for drugs, devices, and biological products for the treatment of rheumatoid arthritis (RA) (Draft). Accessed at *www.fda-gov/cder/guidance/guidance.htm,* January 6, 1997
22. Osteoarthritis Research Society (OARS) Task Force Report. Design and conduct of clinical trials of patients with osteoarthritis: recommendations from a task force of the osteoarthritis research society. *Osteoarthritis Cartilage* 1996;4:217–243.
23. Colton T. Inference on means. In: *Statistics in medicine.* Boston: Little, Brown, 1974:99–150.
24. Colton T. Inference on proportions. In: *Statistics in medicine.* Boston: Little, Brown, 1974:151–188.
25. Gøtzsche PC. Methodology and overt and hidden bias in reports of 196 double-blind trials of nonsteroidal anti-inflammatory drugs in rheumatoid arthritis. *Control Clin Trials* 1989;10:31–56.
26. Wells GA. Minimal clinically important difference module: introduction. *J Rheumatol* 2001;28(2):398–399.
27. Wells G, Anderson J, Beaton D, et al. Minimally clinically important difference module: summary, recommendations, and research agenda. *J Rheumatol* 2001;28(2):452–454.
28. Beaton DE, Bombardier C, Katz JN, et al. Looking for important change/differences in studies of responsiveness. *J Rheumatol* 2001; 28(2):400–405.
29. Wells G, Beaton D, Shea B, et al. Minimal clinically important differences: Review of methods. *J Rheumatol* 2001;28(2):406–412.
30. Cranney A, Welch V, Wells G, et al. Discrimination of changes in osteoporosis outcomes. *J Rheumatol* 2001;28(2):413–421.
31. Felson DT, Anderson JJ. A review of evidence on the discriminant validity of outcome measures in rheumatoid arthritis. *J Rheumatol* 2001;28(2):422–426.
32. Bellamy N, Carr A, Dougados M, et al. Towards a definition of "difference" in osteoarthritis. *J Rheumatol* 2001;28(2):427–430.
33. Bambardier C, Hayden J, Beaton DE. Minimal clinically important difference. Low back pain: outcomes measures. *J Rheumatol* 2001;28 (2):431–438.
34. Bellamy N, Buchanan WW, Esdaile JM, et al. Ankylosing spondylitis antirheumatic drug trials. I. Effects of standardization procedures on observer-dependent outcome measures. *J Rheumatol* 1991;18:1701–1708.
35. Bellamy N, Buchanan WW, Esdaile JM, et al. Ankylosing spondylitis antirheumatic drug trials. II. Tables for calculating sample size for clinical trials. *J Rheumatol* 1991;18:1709–1715.
36. Bellamy N, Buchanan WW, Esdaile JM, et al. Ankylosing spondylitis antirheumatic drug trials. III. Setting the delta for clinical trials of antirheumatic drugs—results of a consensus development (Delphi) exercise. *J Rheumatol* 1991;19:1716–1722.
37. Bellamy N, Anastassiades TP, Buchanan WW, et al. Rheumatoid arthritis antirheumatic drug trials. I. Effects of standardization procedures on observer-dependent outcome measures. *J Rheumatol* 1991;18:1893–1900.
38. Bellamy N, Anastassiades TP, Buchanan WW, et al. Rheumatoid arthritis antirheumatic drug trials. II. Tables for calculating sample size for clinical trials of antirheumatic drugs. *J Rheumatol* 1991;18:1901–1907.
39. Bellamy N, Anastassiades TP, Buchanan WW, et al. Rheumatoid arthritis antirheumatic drug trials. III. Setting the delta for clinical trials of antirheumatic drugs—results of a consensus development (Delphi) exercise. *J Rheumatol* 1991;18:1908–1915.
40. Bellamy N, Carette S, Ford PM, et al. Osteoarthritis antirheumatic drug trials. I. Effects of standardization procedures on observer dependent outcome measures. *J Rheumatol* 1992;19:436–443.
41. Bellamy N, Carette S, Ford PM, et al. Osteoarthritis antirheumatic drug trials. II. Tables for calculating sample size for clinical trials. *J Rheumatol* 1992;19:444–450.
42. Bellamy N, Carette S, Ford PM, et al. Osteoarthritis antirheumatic drug trials. III. Setting the delta for clinical trials—results of a consensus development (Delphi) exercise. *J Rheumatol* 1992;19:451–457.
43. Bellamy N, Bell MJ, Carette S, et al. Estimation of observer reliability and sample size calculation parameters for outcome measures in fibromyalgia clinical trials. *Inflammopharmacology* 1994;2:345–360.
44. Cohen J. *Statistical power analysis for the behavioural sciences,* 2nd ed. New Jersey: Lawrence Erlbaum Associates, 1988:1–567.
45. Armitage P. Comparison of several groups. In: *Statistical methods in medical research.* London: Blackwell Scientific, 1980:202–207.
46. Feinstein AR. Scientific decisions for data and hypothesis. In: *Clinical epidemiology—the architecture of clinical research.* Philadelphia: WB Saunders, 1985:500–529.
47. Sackett DL, Gent M. Controversy in counting and attributing events in clinical trials. *N Engl J Med* 1979;301:1410–1412.
48. Little RJA, Rubin DB. *Statistical analysis with missing data.* Toronto: John Wiley & Sons, 1987.
49. Simon R. Confidence intervals for reporting results of clinical trials. *Ann Intern Med* 1986;105:429–435.
50. Dickersin K, Chan S, Chalmers TC, et al. Publication bias and clinical trials. *Control Clin Trials* 1987;8:343–353.
51. National Health and Medical Research Council (HNHMRC). How to use the evidence: assessment and application of scientific evidence. Biotext, Canberra, Australia, 2000:1–84.

52. Coles LS, Fries JF, Kraines RG, et al. From experiment to experience: side effects of nonsteroidal anti-inflammatory drugs. *Am J Med* 1983; 74:820–828.
53. Fries JF, Bellamy N. Introduction. In: *Prognosis in the rheumatic diseases.* Ed. N Bellamy. Dordrecht, the Netherlands: Kluwer Academic, 1991:1–10.
54. World Health Organization. ICIDH-2. In: *An international classification of impairments, activities and participation.* Geneva: WHO, 1997.
55. Boers M, Brooks PM, Strand V, et al. The OMERACT filter for outcome measures in rheumatology. *J Rheumatol* 1998;25:198–199.
56. Carmines EG, Zeller RA. *Reliability and validity assessment.* Beverly Hills, CA: Sage Publications, 1979.
57. Bellamy N, Buchanan WW. A preliminary evaluation of the dimensionality and clinical importance of pain and disability in osteoarthritis of the hip and knee. *Clin Rheumatol* 1986;5(2):231–241.
58. Bellamy N, Campbell J, Haraoui B, et al. Dimensionality and clinical importance of pain and disability in hand osteoarthritis: development of the Australian/Canadian (AUSCAN) Osteoarthritis Hand Index. *Osteoarthritis Cartilage* 2002;10(11):855–862.
59. Cohen J. A coefficient of agreement for normal scales. *Educ Psych Measurement* 1960;20:27–47.
60. Byrt T, Bishop J, Carlin JB. Bias, prevalence and kappa. *J Clin Epidemiol* 1993;46:423–429.
61. Bellamy N, Sothern RB, Campbell J, et al. Circadian rhythm in pain, stiffness and manual dexterity in rheumatoid arthritis: relation between discomfort and disability. *Ann Rheum Dis* 1991;50:243–248.
62. Bellamy N, Sothern RB, Campbell J. Rhythmic variations in pain perception in osteoarthritis of the knee. *J Rheumatol* 1990;17:364–372.
63. Bellamy N, Sothern RB, Campbell J, et al. Rhythmic variations in pain, stiffness and manual dexterity in hand osteoarthritis. *J Rheumatol* 2002;61(12):1075–1080.
64. Bellamy N, Sothern R, Campbell J. Circadian and circaseptan rhythmicity in pain, stiffness and fatigue in fibromyalgia. *J Rheumatol* 2003 (in press).
65. Bellamy N, Buchanan WW, Goldsmith CH, et al. Validation study of WOMAC: a health status instrument for measuring clinically important patient relevant outcomes to antirheumatic drug therapy in patients with osteoarthritis of the hip or knee. *J Rheumatol* 1988;15:1833–1840.
66. Bellamy N, Buchanan WW, Goldsmith CH, et al. Validation study of WOMAC: a health status instrument for measuring clinically important patient relevant outcomes following total hip or knee arthroplasty in osteoarthritis. *J Orthop Rheumatol* 1988;1:95–108.
67. Bellamy N, Campbell J, Haraoui B, et al. Clinimetric properties of the AUSCAN Osteoarthritis Hand Index: an evaluation of reliability, validity and responsiveness. *Osteoarthritis Cartilage* 2002;10(11):863–869.
68. Davies GM, Watson DJ, Bellamy N. Comparison of the responsiveness and relative effect size of the WOMAC and SF-36 in a randomised clinical trial in patients with osteoarthritis. *Arthritis Care Res* 1999;12(3):172–179.
69. Theiler R, Sangha O, Schaeren S, et al. Superior responsiveness of the pain and function sections of the Western Ontario and McMaster Universities Osteoarthritis Index (WOMAC) as compared to the Lequesne-algofunctional Index in patients with osteoarthritis of the lower extremities. *Osteoarthritis Cartilage* 1999;7:515–519.
70. Griffiths G, Bellamy N, Bailey WH, et al. A comparative study of the relative efficiency of the WOMAC, AIMS and HAQ instruments in evaluating the outcome of total knee arthroplasty. *Inflammopharmacology* 1995;3:1–6.
71. Tugwell P, Bombardier C, Buchanan WW, et al. The MACTAR patient preference disability questionnaire—an individualized functional priority approach for assessing improvement in physical disability in clinical trials in rheumatoid arthritis. *J Rheumatol* 1987;14:446–451.
72. Smythe HA, Helewa A, Goldsmith CH. "Independent assessor" and "pooled index" as techniques for measuring treatment effects in rheumatoid arthritis. *J Rheumatol* 1977;4:144–152.
73. Van der Heijde DMFM, Van't Hof MA, Van Riel PLCM, et al. Judging disease activity in clinical practice in rheumatoid arthritis: first step in the development of a disease activity score. *Ann Rheum Dis* 1990; 49:916–920.
74. Van Riel PLCM, Van Gestel AM. The original "DAS" and the "DAS28" are not interchangeable: comment on the articles by Prevoo et al. *Arthritis Rheum* 1998;41:942–950.
75. Andersson G. Hip Assessment: a comparison of nine different methods. *J Bone Joint Surg [Br]* 1972;54:621–625.
76. Ehrich EW, Davies GM, Watson DJ, et al. Minimal perceptible clinical Improvement with the Western Ontario and McMaster Universities osteoarthritis index questionnaire and global assessments in patients with osteoarthritis. *J Rheumatol* 2000;27(11):2635–2641.
77. Angst F, Aeschlimann A, Michel BA, et al. Minimal clinically important rehabilitation effects in patients with osteoarthritis of the lower extremities. *J Rheumatol* 2002;29:131–138.
78. Boers M, Tugwell P, Felson DT, et al. World Health Organization and International League of Associations for Rheumatology core endpoints for symptom modifying antirheumatic drugs in rheumatoid arthritis clinical trials. *J Rheumatol* 1994;21(suppl 41):86–89.
79. Felson DT, Anderson JJ, Boers M, et al. The American College of Rheumatology Preliminary core set of disease activity measures for rheumatoid arthritis clinical trials. *Arthritis Rheum* 1993;36(6):729–740.
80. Felson DT, Anderson JJ, Boers M, et al. American College of Rheumatology preliminary definition of improvement in rheumatoid arthritis. *Arthritis Rheum* 1995;38:727–735.
81. Felson DT, Anderson JJ, Lange ML, et al. Should improvement in rheumatoid arthritis clinical trials be defined as fifty percent or seventy percent improvement in core set measures, rather than twenty percent? *Arthritis Rheum* 1998;41(9):1564–1570.
82. Bellamy N, Kirwan J, Boers M, et al. Recommendations for a core set of outcome measures for future phase III clinical trials in knee, hip and hand osteoarthritis. Consensus development in OMERACT III. *J Rheumatol* 1997;24:799–802.
83. Dougados M, LeClaire P, van der Heijde D, et al. Response criteria for clinical trials on osteoarthritis of the knee and hip: a report of the Osteoarthritis Research Society International Standing Committee for Clinical Trials Response Criteria Initiative [special article]. *Osteoarthritis Cartilage* 2000;8(6):395–403.
84. Pham T, van der Heijde D, Lassere M, et al. Outcome variables for osteoarthritis clinical trials: the OMERACT-OARSI set of responder criteria. *J Rheumatol* 2003;30(7):1648–1654.
85. Bellamy N, Lybrand SG, Gee T. An evaluation of the convergence between three different methods of response status assignment (RSA) based on the WOMAC Osteoarthritis Index. Abstract from the ACR Annual Scientific Meeting, New Orleans, October 24–29, 2002. *Arthritis Rheum* 2002;336(suppl):159.
86. Bellamy N, Bell MJ, Goldsmith CH, et al. Evaluation of the OARSI and OMERACT-OARSI sets of responder criteria in patients treated with hylan G-F 20 for knee osteoarthritis. *Osteoarthritis Cartilage* 2003;11(suppl A):S80.
87. Bellamy N, Bell MJ, Goldsmith CH, et al. WOMAC 20, 50, 70 response levels in patients treated with hylan G-F 20 for knee osteoarthritis. *Osteoarthritis Cartilage* 2003;11(suppl A):S82.
88. Van der Heijde D, van der Sjef L, Dougados M, et al. Ankylosing spondylitis: plenary discussion and results of voting on selection of domains and some specific instruments. *J Rheumatol* 1999;26:1003–1005.
89. Anderson JJ, Baron G, van der Heijde D, et al. Ankylosing spondylitis assessment group preliminary definition of short-term improvement in ankylosing spondylitis. *Arthritis Rheum* 2001;44(8):1876–1886.
90. Wells G, Anderson J, Boers M, et al. MCID/Low Disease Activity State Workshop: summary, recommendations and research agenda. *J Rheumatol* 2003;30:1115–1118.
91. Bellamy N, Bell MJ, Goldsmith CH, et al. Symptom free response using the WOMAC pain score in patients treated with hylan G-F 20 for knee osteoarthritis. *Osteoarthritis Cartilage* 2003;11(suppl A):S42.
92. Raynauld JP, Torrance GW, Walker V, et al. A prospective, randomized, health outcomes trial evaluating the incorporation of hylan G-F 20 into the treatment paradigm for patients with knee osteoarthritis (part 1 of 2): clinical results. *Osteoarthritis Cartilage* 2002;10(7):506–517.
93. Ware JE Jr, Sherbourne CD. The MOS 36-item Short-Form Health Survey (SF-36). I. Conceptual framework and item selection. *Med Care* 1992;30:473–481.
94. Fries JF, Spitz P, Kraines RG, et al. Measurement of patient outcome in arthritis. *Arthritis Rheum* 1980;23:137–145.
95. Meenan RF, Gertman PM, Mason JH. Measuring health status in arthritis: the arthritis impact measurement scales. *Arthritis Rheum* 1980;23:146–152.
96. Meenan RF, Mason JH, Anderson JJ, et al. AIMS2: the content and properties of a revised and expanded Arthritis Impact Measurement Scales health status questionnaire. *Arthritis Rheum* 1992;35:1–10.

97. Lequesne MG, Mery C, Samson M, et al. Indexes of severity for osteoarthritis of the hip and knee. Validation—value of comparison with other assessment tests. *Scand J Rheumatol* 1987;65(suppl):85–89.
98. Wood PNH. Appreciating the consequences of disease: the international classification of impairments, disabilities and handicaps. *WHO Chronic* 1980;34:376–380.
99. World Health Organization. ICIDH-2. In: *An international classification of impairments, activities and participation.* Geneva: WHO, 1997.
100. World Health Organization. *International Classification of Functioning, Disability and Health.* Geneva: WHO, 2001.
101. Weigl M, Cieza A, Harder M, et al. Linking osteoarthritis-specific health-status measures to the International Classification of Functioning, Disability and Health (ICF). *Osteoarthritis Cartilage* 2003;11: 519–523.
102. Hochberg MC, Chang RW, Dwosh I, et al. The American College of Rheumatology 1991 revised criteria for the classification of global functional status in rheumatoid arthritis. *Arthritis Rheum* 1992;35: 498–502.
103. Bellamy N. WOMAC Osteoarthritis Index—Guide V. 2002. Published by Nicholas Bellamy, Brisbane, Australia.
104. Wolfe F, Kong SX. Rasch analysis of the Western Ontario McMaster Questionnaire (W0MAC) in 2205 patients with osteoarthritis, rheumatoid arthritis, and fibromyalgia. *Ann Rheum Dis* 1999;58: 563–568.
105. Theiler R, Kroesen S, Spielberger J, et al. Validation of the WOMAC 3.0 TS, an audiovisual computerised version of the WOMAC 3.0. *Osteoarthritis Cartilage* 2000;8(2):152–153.
106. Theiler R, Bischoff H, Good M, et al. Rofecoxib improves quality of life in hip and knee OA patients. 10th Asia Pacific League of Associations for Rheumatology Congress, Bangkok, Thailand. Abstract Book 242. 2002:122.
107. Bellamy N, Campbell J, Hill J, et al. A comparative study of telephone versus onsite completion of the WOMAC 3.0 Osteoarthritis Index. *J Rheumatol* 2002;29(4):783–786.
108. Lingard EA, Katz JN, Wright EA, et al. and Kinemax Outcomes Group. Predicting the outcome of total knee arthroplasty from preoperative status. *Arthritis Rheum* 2000;43(9)(suppl):216.
109. Ethgen O, Kahler KH, Kong SX, et al. Are health-related quality of life scores useful in predicting the use of health care services? Exploration in patients with arthritis. *Arthritis Rheum* 2000;43(9)(suppl):163.
110. Dougados M, Gueguen A, Nguyen M, et al. Requirement for total hip arthroplasty: an outcome measure of hip osteoarthritis. *J Rheumatol* 1999;26:855–861.
111. Bellamy N. AUSCAN Osteoarthritis Hand Index—User Guide I. Published by Nicholas Bellamy, 2001.
112. Dreiser R-L, Maheu E, Guillou, et al. Validation of an algofunctional index for osteoarthritis of the hand. *Rev Rheum* 1995;62(suppl 1); 42–53.
113. Maheu E, Dreiser RL, Guillou GB. Functional index for hand osteoarthritis (OA). Sensitivity and discriminant value among other tests in a therapeutic trial (Anstr). *Rheumatology in Europe* 1995;24(suppl 3):195.
114. Duruöz MT, Poiraudeau S, Fermanian J, et al. Development and validation of a Rheumatoid Hand Functional Disability Scale that assesses functional handicap. *J Rheumatol* 1996;23:1167–1172.
115. Poiraudeau S, Chevelier X, Conrozier T, et al. Reliability, validity, and sensitivity to change of the Cochin hand functional disability scale in hand osteoarthritis. *Osteoarthritis Cartilage* 2001;9(6):570–577.
116. Calin A, Nakache J-P, Gueguen A, et al. Defining disease activity in ankylosing spondylitis: is a combination of variables (Bath Ankylosing Spondylitis Disease Activity Index) an appropriate instrument? *Rheumatology* 1999;38:878–882.
117. Calin A, Garrett SL, Whitelock HC, et al. A new approach to defining functional ability in ankylosing spondylitis: the development of the Bath Ankylosing Spondylitis Functional Index (BASFI). *J Rheumatol* 1994;21:2281–2285.
118. Garrett SL, Jenkinson TR, Whitelock HC, et al. A new approach to defining disease status in ankylosing spondylitis: the Bath Ankylosing Spondylitis Disease Activity Index (BASDAI). *J Rheumatol* 1994;21:2286–2291.
119. Jenkinson T, Mallorie PA, Whitelock HC, et al. A defining spinal mobility in ankylosing spondylitis: the Bath Ankylosing Spondylitis Metrology Index (BASMI). *J Rheumatol* 1994;21:1694–1698.
120. Jones SD, Steiner A, Garrett SL, et al. The Bath Ankylosing Spondylitis Global Score (BAS-G). *Br J Rheumatol* 1996;35:66–71.
121. Mackay K, Mack C, Brophy S, et al. The Bath Ankylosing Spondylitis Radiology Index (BASRI): a new validated approach to disease assessment. *Arthritis Rheum* 1998;41:2263–2270.
122. Ruof J, Sangha O, Stucki G. Comparative responsiveness of 3 functional indices in ankylosing spondylitis. *J Rheumatol* 1999;26:1959–1963.
123. Ward MM, Kuzis S. Validity and sensitivity to change of spondylitis-specific measures of functional disability. *J Rheumatol* 1999;26:121–127.
124. Burckhardt CS, Clark Sr, Bennett RM. The Fibromyalgia Impact Questionnaire: development and validation. *J Rheumatol* 1991;18: 728–733.
125. Hudak PL, Amadio PC, Bombardier C. Development of an upper extremity outcome measure: the DASH (disabilities of the arm, shoulder, and hand). *Am J Indust Med* 1996;29:602–608.
126. Navsarikar A, Gladman DD, Husted JA, et al. Validity Assessment of the Disabilities of Arm, Shoulder, and Hand Questionnaire (DASH) for patients with psoriatic arthritis. *J Rheumatol* 1999;26:2191–2194.
127. Geusens PP, Truitt K, Sfikakis P, et al. A placebo and active comparator-controlled trial of rofecoxib for the treatment of rheumatoid arthritis. *Scand J Rheumatol* 2002;31(4):230–238.
128. Kivitz A, Eisen G, Zhao WW, et al. Randomised placebo-controlled trial comparing efficacy and safety of valdecoxib with naproxen in patients with osteoarthritis. *J Fam Pract* 2002;51(6):530–537.
129. Leung AT, Malmstrom K, Gallacher AE, et al. Efficacy and tolerability profile of etoricoxib in patients with osteoarthritis: a randomised, double-blind, placebo and active comparator controlled 12-week efficacy trial. *Curr Med Res Opin* 2002;18(2):49–58.
130. Gandhi SK, Salmon JW, Zhao SZ, et al. Psychometric evaluation of the 12-item short-form health survey (SF-12) in osteoarthritis and rheumatoid arthritis clinical trials. *Clin Ther* 2001;23(7):1080–1098.
131. Burdine JN, Felix MR, Abel AL, et al. The SF-12 as a population health measure: an exploratory examination of potential for application. *Health Serv Res* 2000;35(4):885–904.
132. Hurst NP, Jobanputra P, Hunter M, et al., for the Economic and Health Outcomes Research Group. Validity of EuroQoL—a generic health status instrument—in patients with rheumatoid arthritis. *Br J Rheumatol* 1994;33:655–662.
133. Fransen M, Edmonds J. Reliability and validity of the EuroQoL in patients with osteoarthritis of the knee. *Rheumatology* 1999;38:807–813.
134. The WHOQOL Group. The World Health Organisation quality of life assessment (WHOQOL): development and general psychometric properties. *Soc Sci Med* 1998;46(12):1569–1585.
135. Hunt SM, McKenna SP, McEwen J, et al. The Nottingham Health Profile: subjective health status and medical consultations. *Soc Sci Med* 1981;15A:221–229.
136. Feeny D, Furlong W, Barr RD, et al. A comprehensive multiattribute system for classifying the health status of survivors of childhood cancer. *J Clin Oncol* 1992;10:923–928.
137. March LM, Oh E-S, Cross M, et al. A comparison of WOMAC and MOS SF-36 in OA patients undergoing joint replacement [Abstract 439]. 8th APLAR Congress of Rheumatology, Melbourne, Australia, April 21–26, 1996. Programme and Abstracts (Posters P119).
138. Davies GM, Watson DJ, Bellamy N. Comparison of the responsiveness and relative effect size of the WOMAC and SF-36 in a randomized clinical trial in patients with osteoarthritis. *Arthritis Care Res* 1999;12(3):172–179.
139. Hawker G, Melfi C, Paul J, et al. Comparison of a generic (SF-36) and a disease specific (WOMAC) (Western Ontario and McMaster Universities Osteoarthritis Index) instrument in the measurement of outcomes after knee replacement surgery. *J Rheumatol* 1995;22: 1193–1196.
140. Van Lankveld W, Van't Pad Bosch P, Van De Putte L, et al. Disease-specific stressors in rheumatoid arthritis: coping and well-being. *Br J Rheumatol* 1994;33:1067–1073.
141. Van Lankveld W, Näring G, van't Pad Bosch P, et al. Behavioural coping and physical functioning: the effect of adjusting the level of activity on observed dexterity. *J Rheumatol* 1999;26:1058–1064.
142. DeVellis RF, Callahan LF. A brief measure of helplessness in rheumatic disease: the helplessness subscale of the rheumatology attitudes index. *J Rheumatol* 1993;20:866–869.

143. Nicassio PM, Radojevic V, Weisman MH, et al. The role of helplessness in the response to disease modifying drugs in rheumatoid arthritis. *J Rheumatol* 1993;20:1114–1120.
144. Carr AJ, Thompson PW. Towards a measure of patient-perceived handicap in rheumatoid arthritis. *Br J Rheumatol* 1994;33:378–382.
145. Carr AJ. A patient-centred approach to evaluation and treatment in rheumatoid arthritis: the development of a clinical tool to measure patient-perceived handicap. *Br J Rheumatol* 1996;35:921–932.
146. Harwood RH, Carr AJ, Thompson PW, et al. Handicap in inflammatory arthritis. *Br J Rheumatol* 1996;35:891–897.
147. Carr AJ. Beyond disability: measuring the social and personal consequences of osteoarthritis. *Osteoarthritis Cartilage* 1999;7(2):230–238.
148. Sharpe L, Sensky T, Brewin CR, et al. Characteristics of handicap for patients with recent onset rheumatoid arthritis: the validity of the Disease Repercussion Profile. *Rheumatology* 2001;40:1169–1174.
149. Taylor W, Myers J, McNaughton H, et al. Evidence for inadequate construct validity of the Disease Repercussion Profile in people with rheumatoid arthritis. *Rheumatology* 2001;40:757–762.
150. Turk DC, Dworkin RH, Allen RR, et al. Core outcome domains in chronic pain clinical trials: IMMPACT Recommendations. *Pain* 2003 (in press).
151. Katz PP, Yelin EH. The development of depressive symptoms among women with rheumatoid arthritis. *Arthritis Rheum* 1995;38:49–56.
152. Crotty M, McFarlane AC, Brooks PM, et al. The psychosocial and clinical status of younger women with early rheumatoid arthritis: a longitudinal study with frequent measures. *Br J Rheumatol* 1994; 33:754–760.
153. Dexter P, Brandt K. Distribution and predictors of depressive symptoms in osteoarthritis. *J Rheumatol* 1994;21:279–286.
154. Suurmeijer TP, Waltz M, Moun T, et al. Quality of life profiles in the first years of rheumatoid arthritis results from the EURIDISS longitudinal study. *Arthritis Rheum* 2001;45(2):111–121.
155. Barlow JH, Wright CC, Williams B, et al. Work disability among people with ankylosing spondylitis. *Arthritis Rheum* 2001;45(5): 424–429.
156. Sherman AM. Social relations and depressive symptoms in older adults with knee osteoarthritis. *Soc Sci Med* 2003;56(2):247–257.
157. Cibere J, Bellamy N, Thorne A, et al. Reliability of the knee examination in osteoarthritis: effect of standardization. *Arthritis Rheum* 2004;50(2):458–468.
158. Smolen JS, Breedveld FC, Eberl G, et al. Validity and reliability of the twenty-eight-joint count for the assessment of rheumatoid arthritis activity. *Arthritis Rheum* 1995;38:38–43.
159. Prevoo MLL, Van't Hof MA, Kuper HH, et al. Modified disease activity scores that include twenty-eight-joint counts. *Arthritis Rheum* 1995;38:44–48.
160. Fuchs HA, Pincus T. Reduced joint counts in controlled clinical trials in rheumatoid arthritis. *Arthritis Rheum* 1994;37:470–475.
161. American College of Rheumatology Committee on Outcome Measures in Rheumatoid Arthritis Clinical Trials. Reduced joint counts in rheumatoid arthritis clinical trials [Editorial]. *Arthritis Rheum* 1994; 37:463–464.
162. Van Gestel AM, Haagsma CJ, van Riel PLCM. Validation of rheumatoid arthritis improvement criteria that include simplified joint counts. *Arthritis Rheum* 1998;41:1845–1850.
163. Scott DL, Antoni C, Choy EH, et al. Joint counts in routine practice [Editorial]. *Rheumatology* 2003;42:919–923.
164. Calvo FA, Calvo A, Berrocal A, et al. Self-administered joint counts in rheumatoid arthritis: comparison with stand joint counts. *J Rheumatol* 1999;26:536–539.
165. Houssien DA, Stucki G, Scott DL. A patient-derived disease activity score can substitute for a physician-derived disease activity score in clinical research. *Rheumatology* 1999;38:48–52.
166. Dougados M, Gueguen A, Nakache J-P, et al. Evaluation of a functional index and an articular index in ankylosing spondylitis. *J Rheumatol* 1988;15:302–307.
167. Mander M, Simpson JM, McLellan A, et al. Studies with an enthesis index as a method of clinical assessment in ankylosing spondylitis. *Ann Rheum Dis* 1987;46:197–202.
168. American Academy of Orthopaedic Surgeons. *Joint motion: method of measuring and recording*. Edinburgh: Churchill Livingstone, 1966.
169. Jonsson B, Larsson S-E. Rheumatoid arthritis evaluated by locomotion score. *Scand J Rheumatol* 1990;19:223–231.
170. Doherty M, Dacre J, Dieppe P, et al. The GALS locomotor screen. *Ann Rheum Dis* 1992;51:1165–1169.
171. Green S, Buchbinder R, Forbes A, et al. A standardised protocol for measurement of range of movement of the shoulder using the Plurimeter-V inclinometer and assessment of its intrarater and interrater reliability. *Arthritis Care Res* 1998;11:43–52.
172. Friedman LM, Furberg CD, DeMets DL. Assessment and reporting of adverse events. In: *Fundamentals of clinical trials*. Littleton, MA: PSG Publishing, 1985:147–160.
173. Binns TB. Therapeutic risks in perspective. *Lancet* 1987;25;2(8552): 208–209.
174. Inman WHW. Editor's introduction and commentary. In: Inman WHW, ed. *Monitoring for drug safety*, 2nd ed. Lancaster: MTP Press, 1986:3–11.
175. Strom BL. Overview of different logistical approaches to postmarketing surveillance. *J Rheumatol* 1988;15(suppl 17):9–13.
176. Weber JCP. Epidemiology of adverse reactions to non-steroidal anti-inflammatory drugs. In: Rainsford KD, Velo JP, eds. *Advances in inflammation research*. Vol. 6. New York: Raven, 1984:1–7.
177. Inman WHW, ed. *Monitoring for drug safety*, 2nd ed. Lancaster: MTP Press, 1986:37.
178. Venning GR. Identification of adverse reactions to new drugs: 2. How were 18 important adverse reactions discovered and with what delays? *BMJ* 1983;286:289–293.
179. Venning GR. Identification of adverse reactions to new drugs: 2. Continued: How were 18 important adverse reactions discovered and with what delays? *BMJ* 1983;286:365–368.
180. Venning GR. Identification of adverse reactions to new drugs: 3. Alerting processes and early warning systems. *BMJ* 1983;286:458–547.
181. World Health Organization. *The WHO adverse reaction dictionary*. Uppsala: WHO Collaborating Centre for International Drug Monitoring, 1990.
182. US Department of Commerce, National Technical Information Service. *COSTART: Coding symbols for thesaurus of adverse reaction terms*, 3rd ed. Springfield, IL: US Department of Commerce, National Technical Information Service, 1989.
183. Brown EG. Effects of coding dictionary on signal generation: a consideration of use of MedDRA compared with WHO-ART. *Drug Saf* 2002;25(6):445–452.
184. Brooks PM, Day RO. OMERACT 5 Drug Safety Working Group report: introduction. *J Rheumatol* 2001;28(5):1162.
185. Woodworth TG, Furst DE, Strand V, et al. Standardizing assessment of adverse effects in rheumatology clinical trials. Status of OMERACT Toxicity Working Group, March 2000: Towards a common understanding of comparative toxicity/safety profiles for antirheumatic therapies. *J Rheumatol* 2001;28(5)1163–1169.
186. Lindquist M, Edwards IR. The WHO programme for international drug monitoring, its database and the technical support of the Uppsala Monitoring Center. *J Rheumatol* 2001;28(5):1180–1187.
187. Singh G. Arthritis, Rheumatism and Aging Medical Information System Post-Marketing Surveillance Program. *J Rheumatol* 2001;28(5): 1174–1179.
188. Lipani JA, Strand, Johnson K, et al. A proposal for developing a large patient population cohort for long-term safety monitoring in rheumatoid arthritis. *J Rheumatol* 2001:28(5):1170–1173.
189. Welch V, Singh G, Strand V, et al. Patient based method of assessing adverse events in clinical trials in rheumatology: the Revised Stanford Toxicity Index. *J Rheumatol* 2001;28(5):1181–1191.
190. Ruchlin HS, Elkin EB, Paget SA. Assessing cost-effectiveness analyses in rheumatoid arthritis and osteoarthritis. *Arthritis Care Res* 1997;10:413–421.
191. Rissanen P, Sintonen H, Asikainen K, et al. Costs and cost-effectiveness in hip and knee replacements. *Int J Technol Assess Health Care* 1997;13(4):575–588.
192. Briggs A, Sculpher M, Britton A, et al. The costs and benefits of primary total hip replacement. *Int J Technol Assess Health Care* 1998;14(4):743–761.
193. Givon U, Ginsberg GM, Horoszowski, et al. Cost-utility analysis of total hip arthroplasties. *Int J Technol Assess Health Care* 1998; 14(4):735–742.
194. Lavernia CJ, Guzman JF, Gachupin-Garcia A. Cost effectiveness and quality of life in knee arthroplasty. *Clin Orthop Rel Res* 1997;345: 134–139.

195. Minas T. Chondrocyte implantation in the repair of chondral lesions of the knee: economics and quality of life. *Am J Orthop* 1998;27(11): 739–744.
196. Laupacis A, Feeny D, Detsky AS, et al. How attractive does a new technology have to be to warrant adoption and utilization? Tentative guidelines for using clinical and economic evaluations. *Can Med Assoc J* 1992;146(4):473–481.
197. Gabriel SE. Introduction. OMERACT 5 Economics Working Group Report. *J Rheumatol* 2001;28(3):642–647.
198. Gabriel SE. Summary. OMERACT 5 Economics Working Group: summary, recommendations, and research agenda. *J Rheumatol* 2001;28(3):670–673.
199. Gabriel S, Drummond M, Maetzel A, et al. OMERACT 6 Economics Working Group report: a proposal for a reference case for economic evaluation in rheumatoid arthritis. *J Rheumatol* 2003;30:886–890.
200. Maetzel A, Tugwell P, Boers M, et al. Economic evaluation of programs or interventions in the management of rheumatoid arthritis: defining a consensus-based reference case. *J Rheumatol* 2003;30:891–896.
201. Kirwan J, Heiberg T, Hewlett S, et al. Outcomes from the Patient Perspective Workshop at OMERACT 6. *J Rheumatol* 2003;30:868–872.
202. Hewlett SA. Patients and clinicians have different perspectives on outcomes in arthritis. *J Rheumatol* 2003;30:877–879.
203. Carr A, Hewlett S, Mitchell, et al. Rheumatology outcomes: the patient's perspective. *J Rheumatol* 2003;30:880–883.
204. Kvien TA, Heiberg T. Patient perspective in outcome assessments—perceptions or something more? *J Rheumatol* 2003;30:873–876.
205. Johnson AH, Hassell AB Jones PW, et al. The mechanical joint score: a new clinical index of joint damage in rheumatoid arthritis. *Rheumatology* 2002;41:189–195.
206. Bardwell WA, Nicassio PM, Weisman MH, et al. Rheumatoid Arthritis Severity Scale: a brief, physician-completed scale not confounded by patient self-report of psychological functioning. *Rheumatology* 2002;41:38–45.
207. Zijlstra TR, Moens HJB, Bukhari MAS. The rheumatoid arthritis articular damage score: first steps in developing a clinical index of long term damage in RA. *Ann Rheum Dis* 2002;61(1):20–23.
208. Katz PP, Pasch LA, Wong B. Development of an instrument to measure disability in parenting activity among young women with rheumatoid arthritis. *Arthritis Rheum* 2003;48(4):935–943.
209. Hewlett S, Cockshott Z, Kirwan J, et al. Development and validation of a self-efficacy scale for use in British patients with rheumatoid arthritis (RASE). *Rheumatology* 2001;40:1221–1230.
210. Osiri M, Deesomchok U, Tugwell P. Evaluation of functional ability of Thai patients with rheumatoid arthritis by the use of a Thai version of the Health Assessment Questionnaire. *Rheumatology* 2001;40: 555–558.
211. da Mota Facao D, Ciconelli RM, Ferraz MB. Translation and cultural adaptation of Quality of Life Questionnaires: an evaluation of methodology. *J Rheumatol* 2003;30:379–385.
212. Zandbelt MM, Welsing PMJ, van Gestel AM, et al. Health Assessment Questionnaire modifications: is standardisation needed? *Ann Rheum Dis* 2001;60(9)841–845.
213. Wolfe F. Which HAQ is best? A comparison of the HAQ, MHAQ and RA-HAQ, a difficult 8 item HAQ (DHAQ), and a rescored 20 item HAQ (HAQ20): analyses in 2491 rheumatoid arthritis patients following leflunomide initiation. *J Rheumatol* 2001;28:982–989.
214. Greenwood MC, Doyle DV, Ensor M. Does the Stanford Health Assessment Questionnaire have potential as a monitoring tool for subjects with rheumatoid arthritis? *Ann Rheum Dis* 2001;60(4):344–348.
215. Wolfe F, Choi HK. Leader. Benchmarking and the percentile assessment of RA: adding a new dimension to rheumatic disease measurement. *Ann Rheum Dis* 2001;60(11):994–995.
216. Wiles NJ, Scott DGI, Barrett EM, et al. Benchmarking: the five year outcome of rheumatoid arthritis assessed using a pain score, the Health Assessment Questionnaire, and the Short Form-36 (SF-36) in a community and a clinic based sample. *Ann Rheum Dis* 2001; 60(10):956–961.
217. Memel DS, Kirwan JR, Langley C, et al. Prediction of successful application for disability benefits for people with arthritis using the Health Assessment Questionnaire. *Rheumatology* 2002;41:100–102.
218. Hewlett S, Smith AP, Kirwan JR. Extended report. Measuring the meaning of disability in rheumatoid arthritis: the Personal Impact Health Assessment Questionnaire (PI HAQ). *Ann Rheum Dis* 2002; 61(11):986–993.
219. Tijhuis GJ, de Jong Z, Zwinderman AH, et al. The validity of the Rheumatoid Arthritis Quality of Life (RAQoL) questionnaire. *Rheumatology* 2001;40(10):1112–1119.
220. Neville C, Whalley D, McKenna S, et al. Adaptation and validation of the Rheumatoid Arthritis Quality of Life Scale for use in Canada. *J Rheumatol* 2001;28:1505–1510.
221. Lefevre-Colau MM, Poiraudeau S, Fermanian J, et al. Responsiveness of the Cochin rheumatoid hand disability scale after surgery. *Rheumatology* 2001;40(8):843–850.
222. Taal E, Rasker JJ, Riemsma RP. Psychometric properties of a Dutch short form of the Arthritis Impact Measurement Scales 2 (Dutch-AIMS2-SF). *Rheumatology* 2003;42:427–434.
223. Fransen J, Häuselmann H, Michel BA, et al. Responsiveness of the self-assessed rheumatoid arthritis disease activity index to a flare of disease activity. *Arthritis Rheum* 2001;44(1):53–60.
224. Smolen JS, Breedveld FC, Schiff MH, et al. A simplified disease activity index for rheumatoid arthritis for use in clinical practice. *Rheumatology* 2003;42:244–257.
225. Boers M, Verhoeven AC, van der Linden S. American College of Rheumatology criteria for improvement in rheumatoid arthritis should only be calculated from scores that decrease on improvement. *Arthritis Rheum* 2001;44(5):1052–1055.
226. Pincus T, Strand V, Koch G, et al. An index of the Three Core Data Set Patient Questionnaire Measures distinguishes efficacy of active treatment from that of placebo as effectively as the American College of Rheumatology 20% Response Criteria (ACR20) or the Disease Activity Score (DAS) in a rheumatoid arthritis clinical trial. *Arthritis Rheum* 2003;48(3):625–630.
227. Boers M. Concise communication: demonstration of response in rheumatoid arthritis patients who are nonresponders according to the American College of Rheumatology 20% criteria: the paradox of beneficial treatment effects in nonresponders in the ATTRACT trial. *Arthritis Rheum* 2001;44(11):2703–2704.
228. van Riel PLCM, van Gestel AM. Area under the curve for the American College of Rheumatology improvement criteria: a valid addition to existing criteria in rheumatoid arthritis? [Letters]. *Arthritis Rheum* 2001;44(7):1719–1720.
229. van Riel PLCM, van Gestel AM. Clinical outcome measures in rheumatoid arthritis. *Ann Rheum Dis* 2000;59(suppl 1):i28-i31.
230. den Broeder AA, Creemers MCW, van Gestel AM, et al. Dose titration using the Disease Activity Score (DAS28) in rheumatoid arthritis patients treated with anti-TNF-α. *Rheumatology* 2002;41(6): 638–642.
231. Vrijhoel HJM, Diederiks JPM, Spreeuwenberg C, et al. Applying low disease activity criteria using the DAS28 to assess stability in patients with rheumatoid arthritis [Extended report]. *Ann Rheum Dis* 2003;62:419–422.
232. Welsing PMJ, van Gestel AM, Swinkels HL, et al. The relationship between disease activity, joint destruction, and functional capacity over the course of rheumatoid arthritis. *Arthritis Rheum* 2001;44(9): 2009–2017.
233. Scott DL, Strand V. The effects of disease-modifying anti-rheumatic drugs on the Health Assessment Questionnaire score. Lessons from the leflunomide clinical trials database. *Rheumatology* 2002;41(8): 899–909.
234. Ferraccioli GF, Gremese E, Tomietto P, et al. Analysis of improvements, full responses, remission and toxicity in rheumatoid patients treated with step-up combination therapy (methotrexate, cyclosporin A, sulphasalazine) or monotherapy for three years. *Rheumatology* 2002;41(8):892–898.
235. Russell AS, Conner-Spady B, Mintz A, et al. The responsiveness of Generic Health Status Measures as assessed in patients with rheumatoid arthritis receiving Infliximab. *J Rheumatol* 2003;30:941–947.
236. Capell H, McCarey D, Madhok R, et al. "5D" outcome in 52 patients with rheumatoid arthritis surviving 20 years after initial disease modifying antirheumatic drug therapy. *J Rheumatol* 2002;29:2099–2105.
237. Wells G, Boers M, Shea B, et al. MCID/Low Disease Activity State Workshop: low disease activity state in rheumatoid arthritis. *J Rheumatol* 2003;30:1110–1111.
238. Boers M, Anderson JJ, Felson DT. Deriving an operational definition of low disease activity state in rheumatoid arthritis. *J Rheumatol* 2003;30:1112–1114.
239. Young A, Dixey J, Kulinskaya E, et al. Which patients stop working because of rheumatoid arthritis? Results of five years' follow up in

732 patients from the early RA study (ERAS). *Ann Rheum Dis* 2002;61(4):335–340.
240. Mikuls T, Saag K, Griswell, et al. Health related quality of life in women with elderly onset rheumatoid arthritis. *J Rheumatol* 2003; 30:952–957.
241. Dadoniene J. Uhlig T, Stropuviene S, et al. Disease activity and health status in rheumatoid arthritis: a case-control comparison between Norway and Lithuania. *Ann Rheum Dis* 2003;62:231–235.
242. Sokoll KB, Helliwell PS. Comparison of disability and quality of life in rheumatoid and psoriatic arthritis. *J Rheumatol* 2001;28:1842–1846.
243. Sokka T, Krishnan E, Häkkinen A, et al. Functional disability in rheumatoid arthritis patients compared with a community population in Finland. *Arthritis Rheum* 2003;48(1):59–63.
244. Brekke M, Hjortdahl P, Kvien TK. Self-efficacy and health status in rheumatoid arthritis: a two-year longitudinal observational study. *Rheumatology* 2001;40(4):387–392.
245. Lindqvist E, Saxne T, Geborek P, et al. Ten year outcome in a cohort of patients with early rheumatoid arthritis: health status, disease process, and damage. *Ann Rheum Dis* 2002;60(12):1055–1059.
246. Fransen J, Daneel S, Langenegger T, et al. Rheumatologists' opinions on the feasibility of a measurement feedback system in rheumatoid arthritis and the influence of motivation. *Rheumatology* 2003; 42:924–928.
247. Russak SM, Croft JD, Furst DE, et al. The use of rheumatoid arthritis health-related quality of life patient questionnaires in clinical practice: lessons learned. *Arthritis Rheum* 2003;49(4):574–584.
248. Faucher M, Poiraudeau S, Lefevre-Colau MM, et al. Algo-functional assessment of knee osteoarthritis: comparison of the test-retest reliability and construct validity of the WOMAC and Lequesne Indexes. *Osteoarthritis Cartilage* 2002;10:602–610.
249. Poiraudeau S, Chevalier X, Conrozier T, et al. Reliability, validity and sensitivity to change of the Cochin hand functional disability scale in hand osteoarthritis. *Osteoarthritis Cartilage* 2001;9:570–577.
250. Roos EW, Toksvig-Larsen S. Knee injury and Osteoarthritis Outcome Score (KOOS)—validation and comparison to the WOMAC in total knee replacement. *Health Quality Life Outcomes* 2003;1:17.
251. O'Malley KJ, Suarez-Almazor M, Aniol J, et al. Joint-Specific Multidimensional Assessment of Pain (J-MAP): factor structure, reliability, validity and responsiveness in patients with knee osteoarthritis. *J Rheumatol* 2003;30:534–543.
252. Bachmeier CJM, March LM, Cross MJ, et al. A comparison of outcomes in osteoarthritis patients undergoing total hip and knee replacement surgery. *Osteoarthritis Cartilage* 2001;9:137–146.
253. Angst F, Aeschlimann A, Steiner W, et al. Responsiveness of the WOMAC Osteoarthritis Index as compared with the SF-36 in patients with osteoarthritis of the legs undergoing a comprehensive rehabilitation intervention [Extended reports]. *Ann Rheum Dis* 2001; 60:834–840.
254. Bae S-C, Lee H-S, Yun HR, et al. Cross-cultural adaptation and validation of Korean Western Ontario and McMaster Universities (WOMAC) and Lequesne Osteoarthritis Indices for clinical research. *Osteoarthritis Cartilage* 2001;9(8):746–750.
255. Thumboo J, Chew L-H, Soh C–H. Validation of the Western Ontario and McMaster University Osteoarthritis Index in Asians with osteoarthritis in Singapore. *Osteoarthritis Cartilage* 2001;9:440–446.
256. Thumboo J, Chew L-H, Lewin-Koh S-C. Socioeconomic and psychosocial factors influence pain or physical function in Asian patients with knee or hip osteoarthritis. *Ann Rheum Dis* 2002;61(11): 1017–1020.
257. Ang DC, Ibrahim SA, Burant CJ, et al. Is there a difference in the perception of symptoms between African Americans and whites with osteoarthritis? *J Rheumatol* 2003;30:1305–1310.
258. Fortin PR, Penrod JR, Clark AE, et al. Timing of total joint replacement affects clinical outcomes among patients with osteoarthritis of the hip or knee. *Arthritis Rheum* 2002;46(12):3327–3330.
259. Hawker GA, Wright JG, Coyte PC, et al. Differences between men and women in the rate of use of hip and knee arthroplasty. *N Engl J Med* 2000;342(14):1016–1022.
260. van Tubergen A, van der Heijde D, Anderson J, et al. Comparison of statistically derived ASAS improvement criteria for ankylosing spondylitis with clinically relevant improvement according to an expert panel [Extended report]. *Ann Rheum Dis* 2003;62:215–221.
261. Doward LC, Spoorenberg A, Cook SA, et al. Development of the ASQoL: a quality of life instrument specific to ankylosing spondylitis [Extended report]. *Ann Rheum Dis* 2003;62:20–26.
262. Haywood KL, Garratt AM, Jordan K, et al. Disease-specific, patient-assessed measures of health outcome in ankylosing spondylitis: reliability, validity and responsiveness. *Rheumatology* 2002;41(11): 1295–1302.
263. Haywood KL, Garratt AM, Dziedzic K, et al. Patient centred assessment of ankylosing spondylitis-specific health related quality of life: evaluation of the Patient Generated Index. *J Rheumatol* 2003;30: 764–773.
264. Haywood KL, Garratt AM, Dziedzic K, et al. Generic measures of health-related quality of life in ankylosing spondylitis: reliability, validity and responsiveness. *Rheumatology* 2002;41(12):1380–1387.
265. Eyres S, Tennant A, Kay L, et al. Measuring disability in ankylosing spondylitis: comparison of Bath Ankylosing Spondylitis Functional Index with Revised Leeds Disability Questionnaire. *J Rheumatol* 2002;29:979–986.
266. van Tubergen A, Landewé R, Heuft-Dorenbosch L, et al. Assessment of disability with the World Health Organisation Disability Assessment Schedule II in patients with ankylosing spondylitis. *Ann Rheum Dis* 2003;62:140–145.
267. Heuft-Dorenbosch L, Spoorenberg A, van Tubergen A, et al. Assessment of enthesitis in ankylosing spondylitis [Extended report]. *Ann Rheum Dis* 2003,62:127–132.
268. Spoorenberg A, van der Heijde D, Dougados M, et al. Reliability of self assessed joint counts in ankylosing spondylitis. *Ann Rheum Dis* 2002;61(9):799–803.
269. Liang MH, Socher SA, Larson MG, et al. Reliability and validity of six systems for the clinical assessment of disease activity in SLE. *Arthritis Rheum* 1989;32:1107–1118.
270. Bombardier C, Gladman DD, Chang CH, et al., and the Committee on Prognosis Studies in SLE. Development of the Disease Activity Index: the SLEDAI. *Arthritis Rheum* 1992;35:630–640.
271. Symmons DPM, Coppock JS, Bacon PA, et al. Development and assessment of a computerized index of clinical disease activity in systemic lupus erythematosus. *Q J Med* 1988;69:927–937.
272. Gladman D, Ginzler E, Goldsmith C, et al. Systemic lupus international collaborative clinics: development of a damage index in systemic lupus erythematosus. *J Rheumatol* 1992;19:1820–1821.
273. Stoll T, Seifert N, Isenberg DA. ACR/SLICC Damage Index is a useful predictor of severe outcome in SLE patients and an indicator of morbidity in different ethnic groups. *Br J Rheumatol* 1996;35:248–254.
274. Merrill JT. Measuring disease activity in systemic lupus: progress and problems [Editorial]. *J Rheumatol* 2002;29(11):2256–2257.
275. Brunner HI, Feldman BM, Urowitz MB, et al. Item weighting for the Systemic Lupus International Collaborating Clinics/American College of Rheumatology Disease Damage Index using Rasch Analysis do not lead to an important improvement. *J Rheumatol* 2003;30: 292–297.
276. Wang C, Mayo NE, Fortin PR. The relationship between health related quality of life and disease activity and damage in systemic lupus erythematosus. *J Rheumatol* 2001;28:525–532.
277. Strand V, Gladman D, Isenberg D, et al. Outcome measures to be used in clinical trials in systemic lupus erythematosus. *J Rheumatol* 1999;26:490–497.
278. Smolen JS, Strand V, Cardiel M, et al. Randomized clinical trials and longitudinal observational studies in systemic lupus erythematosus. *J Rheumatol* 1999;26:504–507.
279. Isenberg D, Ramsey-Goldman R. Assessing patients with lupus: towards a drug responder index. *Rheumatology* 1999;38:1045–1049.
280. Medsger Jr TA, Silman AJ, Steen VD, et al. A disease severity scale for systemic sclerosis: development and testing. *J Rheumatol* 1999; 26:2159–2167.
281. Ruof J, Brühlmann P, Michel BA, et al. Development and validation of a self-administered systemic sclerosis questionnaire (SySQ). *Rheumatology* 1999:38(6);535–542.
282. Silman A, Akesson A, Newman J, et al. Assessment of functional ability in patients with scleroderma: a proposed new disability assessment instrument. *J Rheumatol* 1998;25:79–83.
283. Clements PJ, Wong WK, Hurwitz EL, et al. The Disability Index of the Health Assessment Questionnaire is a predictor and correlate of outcome in the high-dose versus low-dose penicillamine in systemic sclerosis trial. *Arthritis Rheum* 2001;44(3):653–661.

284. Merkel PA, Herlyn K, Martin RW, et al. Measuring disease activity and functional status in patients with scleroderma and Raynaud's phenomenon. *Arthritis Rheum* 2002;46(9);2410–2420.
285. Kuwana M, Sato S, Kikuchi K, et al. Evaluation of functional disability using the Health Assessment Questionnaire in Japanese patients with systemic sclerosis. *J Rheumatol* 2003;30:1253–1258.
286. Valentini G, Della Rossa A, Bombardieri S, et al. European multicentre study to define disease activity criteria for systemic sclerosis. II. Identification of disease activity variables and development of preliminary activity indexes. *Ann Rheum Dis* 2001;60(6);592–598.
287. Exley AR, Bacon PA, Luqmani RA, et al. Development and initial validation of the vasculitis damage index for the standardised clinical assessment of damage in the systemic vasculitides. *Arthritis Rheum* 1997;40:371–380.
288. Exley AR, Bacon PA, Luqmani RA, et al. Examination of disease severity in systemic vasculitis from the novel perspective of damage using the vasculitis damage index (VDI). *Br J Rheumatol* 1998;37:57–63.
289. Whiting-O'Keefe QE, Stone JH, Hellmann DB. Validity of a Vasculitis Activity Index for systemic necrotizing vasculitis. *Arthritis Rheum* 1999;42:2365–2371.
290. Luqmani R, Bacon P, Moots R, et al. Birmingham Vasculitis Activity Score (BVAS) in systemic necrotizing vasculitis. *Q J Med* 1994;87:671–678.
291. Stone JH, Hoffman GS, Merkel PA, et al. A disease-specific activity index for Wegener's granulomatosis: modification of the Birmingham Vasculitis Activity Score. *Arthritis Rheum* 2001;44(4):912–920.
292. Koldingsnes W, Nossent JC. Baseline features and initial treatment as predictors of remission and relapse in Wegener's granulomatosis. *J Rheumatol* 2003;30:80–88.
293. Miller FW, Rider LG, Chung Y-L, et al. Proposed preliminary core set measures for disease outcome assessment in adult and juvenile idiopathic inflammatory myopathies [Report]. *Rheumatology* 2001;40(11):1262–1273.
294. Alexanderson H, Lundberg IE, Stenström. Development of the Myositis Activities Profile—validity and reliability of a self-administered questionnaire to assess activity limitations in patients with polymyositis/dermatomyositis. *J Rheumatol* 2002;29:2386–2392.
295. Huber AM, Hicks JE, Lachenbruch PA, et al. Validation of the Childhood Health Assessment Questionnaire in the Juvenile Idiopathic Myopathies. *J Rheumatol* 2001;28:1106–1111.
296. Cranney A, Tugwell P, Cummings S, et al. Osteoporosis clinical trials endpoints: candidate variables and clinimetric properties. *J Rheumatol* 1997;24:1222–1229.
297. Cranney A, Welch V, Tugwell P, et al. Responsiveness of endpoints in osteoporosis clinical trials—an update. *J Rheumatol* 1999;26:222–228.
298. Sambrook PN, Cummings SR, Eisman JA, et al. Workshop report: guidelines for osteoporosis trials. *J Rheumatol* 1997;24:1234–1236.
299. Brooks P, Hochberg M, for ILAR and OMERACT. Outcome measures and classification criteria for the rheumatic diseases. A compilation of data from OMERACT (Outcome Measures for Arthritis Clinical Trials), ILAR (International League of Associations for Rheumatology), regional leagues and other groups [Report]. *Rheumatology* 2001;40(8):896–906.
300. Flatø B, Sørskaar D, Vinje O, et al. Measuring disability in early juvenile rheumatoid arthritis: evaluation of a Norwegian version of the Childhood Health Assessment Questionnaire. *J Rheumatol* 1998;25:1851–1858.
301. Moroldo MB, Giannini EH. Estimates of the discriminant ability of definitions of improvement for juvenile rheumatoid arthritis. *J Rheumatol* 1998;25:986–989.
302. Burgos-Vargas R. Assessment of quality of life in children with rheumatic disease [Editorial]. *J Rheumatol* 1999;26:1432–1435.
303. Ruperto N, Ravelli A, Falcini F, et al. Responsiveness of outcome measures in juvenile chronic arthritis. *Rheumatology* 1999;38:176–180.
304. Giannini EH, Ruperto N, Ravelli A, et al. Preliminary definition of improvement in juvenile arthritis. *Arthritis Rheum* 1997;40:1202–1209.
305. Tennant A, Kearns S, Turner F, et al. Measuring the function of children with juvenile arthritis. *Rheumatology* 2001;40(11):1274–1278.
306. Dempster H, Porepa M, Young N, et al. The clinical meaning of functional outcome scores in children with juvenile arthritis [Research Article]. *Arthritis Rheum* 2001;44(8):1768–1774.
307. Varni JW, Seid M, Smith Knight T, et al. The PedsQL™ in pediatric rheumatology: reliability, validity, and responsiveness of the Pediatric Quality of Life Inventory™ generic core scales and rheumatology module. *Arthritis Rheum* 2002;46(3):714–725.
308. Hewlett SA. Patients and clinicians have different perspectives on outcomes in arthritis. *J Rheumatol* 2003;30:877–879.
309. Carr A, Hewlett S, Hughes R, et al. Rheumatology outcomes: the patient's perspective. *J Rheumatol* 2003;30:880–883.
310. Carr A. Problems in measuring or interpreting change in patient outcomes. *Osteoarthritis Cartilage* 2002;10:503–505.
311. Kirwan J, Heiberg T, Hewlett S, et al. Outcomes from the patient perspective workshop at OMERACT 6. *J Rheumatol* 2003;30:868–872.

CHAPTER 4

Synovial Fluid Analysis

Ted R. Mikuls

Paracelcus, a sixteenth century physician and alchemist, is credited with initial use of the term *synovia* in reference to joint fluid. Synovia, meaning "like egg" (or perhaps more accurately *like egg white*), is a clear and highly viscous fluid that can be found in all normal joints lined by synovium. Synovia, commonly referred to as synovial fluid, is predominantly composed of a plasma dialysate that derives from the microvascular circulation, across both the adjacent subendothelium and the synovium into the joint space. The synovium consists of synoviocytes (synovial lining cells) (see Chapter 8) two to three cell layers thick in normal joints. These cells produce the high-molecular-weight and highly viscous glycosaminoglycan hyaluronate, which can be found in significant concentrations in normal synovial fluid.

In the past 50 years there have been numerous advances in our understanding of the pathophysiology of the normal synovium as well as synovial-based inflammation. Although the direct microscopic examination of diseased synovium may be useful and desirable in certain situations (e.g., research endeavors, synovial malignancies, pigmented villonodular synovitis, granulomatous disease), the routine use of synovial biopsy is limited, given the invasive nature and technical difficulty of this procedure. Synovial tissue samples may be obtained with the use of needles adapted to hollow organ biopsy, a practice that, in large joints such as the knee and shoulder, has largely been replaced by arthroscopy (see Chapter 5). Inflammatory changes involving the synovium and its adjacent subendothelium are routinely reflected in the synovial fluid, pathologic changes that can readily be identified by the diagnostician skilled in both the musculoskeletal examination (see Chapter 3) and arthrocentesis (see Chapter 35). This fact has rendered synovial biopsy of much less practical value than simple synovial aspiration, a practice referred to by McCarty as "liquid biopsy."

In the 1950s, Hollander and colleagues coined the term *synovianalysis*, intentionally drawing parallels between the diagnostic utility of synovianalysis with the more widely performed practice at the time of urinalysis. Like urinalysis, synovial fluid examination can be a powerful diagnostic tool, often supplanting the need for tissue biopsy and narrowing the field of diagnostic possibilities in a given patient with arthritis. The potential diagnostic yield of synovianalysis was further underscored in the 1960s, when McCarty and colleagues characterized the pathognomonic appearance of monosodium urate (MSU) and calcium pyrophosphate dihydrate (CPPD) crystals under polarized microscopy from the synovial fluid of patients with gout and pseudogout, respectively (1,2).

Routine synovianalysis, the focus of much of this chapter, consists of both gross and microscopic examination of joint fluid and allows for the categorization of abnormal joint fluid into one of four categories. Although there is substantial overlap of findings among diagnoses even within different categories, the categorization of abnormal joint fluid (groups I–IV) has practical implications in terms of narrowing the differential diagnosis. In addition to routine synovianalysis, several other laboratory tests have been developed and proposed to play an important role in various clinical situations and will be covered in this chapter. Other special tests, often of theoretical, academic, or historical interest, will be discussed only briefly.

ROUTINE SYNOVIANALYSIS

The types of studies used in synovianalysis are summarized in Table 4.1. Routine synovianalysis, entirely sufficient for the evaluation of a majority of arthritis patients, includes gross and microscopic examination of the synovial aspirate coupled with basic microbiology testing and the measurement of total and differential white blood cell (WBC) counts. These simple test results can aid in classifying joint fluids

TABLE 4.1. *Studies used in synovial fluid analysis*

Routine
- Gross analysis
  - Color
  - Clarity
  - Viscosity
  - Clotting potential
  - Volume measurement
- Microscopic
  - Total leukocyte count
  - Differential leukocyte count
  - Wet smear inspection by polarized and phase contrast microscopy
- Microbiology
  - Gram stain
  - Routine bacterial culture

Special
- Microbiologic
  - Special stains (silver, PAS, Ziehl-Nielsen)
  - Culture for fungi, viruses, or tubercle bacilli
  - Analyses for microbial antigens or nucleic acids (polymerase chain reaction)
- Serologic
  - Total hemolytic complement ($C'H_{50}$)
  - Complement components (e.g., C3 and C4) by immunodiffusion
  - Other antibodies (RF, ANA, Anti-CCP)
- Chemical
  - Glucose
  - Total protein
  - pH
  - pO_2
  - Organic acids (lactic acid and succinic acid)
  - Lactate dehydrogenase

ANA, antinuclear antibody; CCP, cyclic citrullinated peptide; PAS, periodic acid-Schiff; RF, rheumatoid factor.

(Table 4.2) as normal or abnormal (groups I to IV). This classification paradigm has substantial diagnostic implications (Table 4.3). Gross examination, routinely performed at the patient's bedside, includes a precise characterization of synovial fluid clotting potential, volume, viscosity, color, and clarity. To facilitate gross inspection of the synovia, the fluid sample is transferred into a clear glass tube, because commercially available syringes are typically opaque and obscure careful inspection. For the purpose of comprehensive synovianalysis, microscopic examination typically includes standard light microscopy (with 10×, 40×, and 100× oil immersion objectives), compensated polarized microscopy, and phase microscopy.

Gross Examination

Clotting Potential

In contrast to plasma, normal synovial fluid lacks several proteins necessary for clot production, including fibrinogen, prothrombin, factors V and VII, and tissue thromboplastin. Thus, normal synovial fluid does not clot. However, in the context of significant inflammation, the normal "diasylate membrane" of the joint becomes disrupted, and larger plasma proteins, including those involved in clot formation, egress into the joint. Thus, inflammatory fluid, such as that seen in rheumatoid arthritis (RA) or septic arthritis, may clot, and the observed rapidity of clotting has been proposed to correlate with the degree of synovial inflammation. Despite its potential diagnostic utility, clotting may obscure other more important observations, and by "trapping" WBCs within the clot may actually lead to falsely low fluid leukocyte counts. For that reason, the synovia should be transferred into a clear heparinized glass tube (sodium heparin or "brown-top" tube), facilitating both gross fluid examination and accurate cell counts. It should be understood that synovia collected in oxalate and lithium heparin tubes, also used for their anticoagulant properties, may lead to false-positive crystal identification under polarized microscopy (3,4). Likewise ethylenediaminetetraacetic acid tubes can be bacteriostatic and lead to false-negative results if this same fluid is also used to obtain culture and sensitivity data.

Volume

A normal joint usually contains only a small amount of synovial fluid. Even large joints, such as the knee, contain only 3 to 4 mL of synovia, not all of which can be readily aspirated under normal circumstances. In the context of synovitis and the resulting disruption of the articular "dia-

TABLE 4.2. *Use of gross analysis, mucin clot test, and total and differential leukocyte counts in the classification of synovial fluids*

Criteria	Normal	Noninflammatory (group I)	Inflammatory (group II)	Purulent (group III)
Volume (mL)(knee)	<4	Often >4	Often >4	Often >4
Color	Clear to pale yellow	Xanthochromic	Xanthochromic to white	White
Clarity	Transparent	Transparent	Translucent to opaque	Opaque
Viscosity	Very high	High	Low	Very low
Mucin clot[a]	Good	Fair to good	Fair to poor	Poor
Spontaneous clot	None	Often	Often	Often
Leukocytes per mm^3	<50	<3,000	3,000–50,000	50,000–300,000
Polymorphonuclear leukocytes (%)	<25	<25	>70	>90

[a]Recent effusions do not give firm clot because of serum admixture.

TABLE 4.3. *Examples of rheumatic conditions producing different types of synovial fluid*

Noninflammatory (Group I)	Inflammatory[a] (Group II)	Purulent[a] (Group III)	Hemorrhagic (Group IV)
Osteoarthritis	Rheumatoid arthritis	Bacterial infections	Trauma, especially fracture
Early rheumatoid arthritis	Reactive arthritis	Tuberculosis	Neuroarthropathy (Charcot joint)
Trauma	Crystal synovitis, acute (gout, pseudogout, other)	Pseudosepsis	Blood dyscrasia (e.g., hemophilia)
Osteochondritis dissecans	Psoriatic arthritis		Tumor, especially pigmented villonodular synovitis or hemangioma
Osteonecrosis	Arthritis of inflammatory bowel disease		Chrondrocalcinosis
Osteochondromatosis	Viral arthritis		Anticoagulant therapy
Crystal synovitis; chronic or subsiding acute (gout and pseudogout)	Rheumatic fever		Joint prostheses
Systemic lupus erythematosus[b]	Behçet disease		Thrombocytosis
Polyarteritis nodosa[b]	Fat droplet synovitis		Sickle cell trait or disease
Scleroderma	Some bacterial infections, e.g., coagulase negative *Staphylococcus, Neisseria, Borrelia, Moraxella*		Myeloproliferative disease
Amyloidosis (articular)			Milwaukee shoulder syndrome
Polymyalgia rheumatica			
High-dose corticosteroid therapy			

[a]As inflammation in group II and group III fluids abate, the synovial fluid passes through a group I phase before returning to normal.

[b]May occasionally be inflammatory.

sylate membrane," large amounts of fluid can accumulate in the joint space (sometimes more than 100–150 mL in a knee joint). On rare occasions, normal joint fluid has been noted to accumulate in the knee in hypervolemic patients, including those with congestive heart failure, myxedema, and anasarca. Similarly, self-limited, asymptomatic, noninflammatory effusions have been observed to accompany high-dose glucocorticoid therapy (5). Although volume by itself is rarely useful in distinguishing among the different groups of inflammatory and noninflammatory forms of arthritis, noting serial aspirate volumes may be valuable with repeated arthrocenteses as a means of following arthritis treatment because a decrease in fluid volume typically corresponds with clinical improvement.

Viscosity

Normal synovia is highly viscous, owing in large part to its relatively high concentration of polymerized hyaluronate. Hyaluronate or hyaluronic acid is the major hydrodynamic nonprotein component of synovial fluid and appears to play an important role in the boundary lubrication for synovial tissue (6). In inflammatory arthritis, such as RA or joint infection, hyaluronate is broken down or depolymerized, possibly due in part to free radical formation (7–9). Hyaluronate degradation in the context of inflammation, coupled with the dilutional effect of fluid accumulation, leads to a synovial fluid with lower viscosity. Viscosity can be tested satisfactorily using the so-called "string test," which may simply involve observing the fluid during transfer from the aspirating syringe to a glass tube (Fig. 4.1B). Viscous fluid, typically seen with normal and group I synovia, "strings out," often to a length of 7 to 10 cm or greater. The string test may also be performed during transfer of a drop of fluid to a glass slide for microscopic examination by simply lifting the needle (or syringe hub) away from the drop of synovia. Although viscosity can be more formally tested using a viscometer (3), this is only rarely helpful. In patients with hypothyroidism, sometimes observed to have a sluggish bulge sign on knee examination, the synovial fluid may have a formal viscosity value that is higher than what would normally be expected.

As mentioned, viscosity is an indirect measure of synovial fluid hyaluronate concentration. Although mostly of historical interest, the mucin clot test is a formal means of testing polymerized hyaluronate concentration in aspirated synovial fluid samples. The mucin clot test can be performed in one of two ways. The first entails the centrifugation of the fluid sample in a clear glass tube with the subsequent addition of a few drops of glacial acetic acid to the supernatant. With normal synovia, the addition of the acetic acid results in the precipitation of the heavier acid in the bottom of the tube, leaving behind a dense precipitate of protein hyaluronate at the top of the tube. Generally, a "good" clot will remain intact even after the tube is agitated. The clot can be dissolved with the addition of hyaluronidase. A second and perhaps easier way of performing the mucin clot test involves the addition of one part whole synovial fluid to four parts 2% acetic acid. "Good" to "fair" clots are generally seen with normal and group I synovia, whereas "fair" to "poor" clots are more often observed with inflammatory fluids (groups II and III) (Fig. 4.2).

Color and Clarity

Normal synovia is colorless, like water or egg white. In the context of synovial inflammation, both WBCs and red blood cells (RBCs) can be found in increasing quantities in

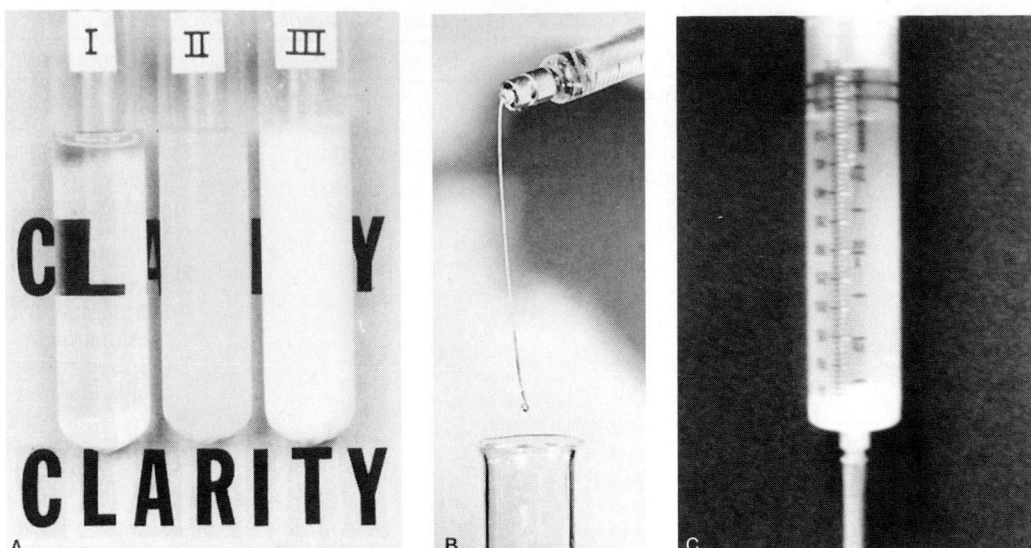

FIG. 4.1. A: Noninflammatory (group I), inflammatory (group II), and purulent (group III) synovial aspirates after transfer to glass tubes for gross inspection. Group I fluids generally lack leukocytes and are transparent, whereas group II and group III fluids have higher total leukocyte concentrations and are opaque. **B:** Viscosity of joint fluid can be tested sufficiently using the "string test." This "string" of fluid is approximately 8 cm long, correlating with a highly viscous aspirate from an osteoarthritic knee. **C:** An inflammatory (group II) fluid taken from a patient with acute pseudogout of the knee is allowed to "settle" over several days. Leukocytes and other fluid debris settle in the bottom of the aspirating syringe, leaving behind a top fluid that is relatively devoid of leukocytes. A similar phenomenon may occur *in vivo* in immobile patients, leading to falsely low total synovial fluid leukocyte counts.

the synovial aspirate. Analogous to what is observed in the cerebral spinal fluid of a patient with a subarachnoid hemorrhage, the breakdown of RBCs within the synovia leads to the release of hemoglobin, which in turn is metabolized into bilirubin, giving group I and inflammatory synovia a yellow (or xanthochromic) color. In contrast, leukocytes confer a white color to the fluid. Thus, with greater levels of inflammation and higher fluid leukocyte counts, the fluid may be white or the "cream color" of pus, as in the case of purulent septic arthritis in which aspirate leukocyte counts often exceed 100,000 to 150,000 per mm^3. Fluid color may also be impacted by chromagens derived from invading organisms. For instance, *Staphylococcus aureus* may add a golden pigment to the synovia, whereas *Serratia marcescens* characteristically adds a reddish hue to the fluid. Other particulate matter, discussed in more detail below, also may impart an abnormal fluid color. Tophaceous MSU crystal deposits within the joint or bursa may lead to a frankly purulent-appearing material, often referred to as "milk of urate" or "gouty pseudosepsis."

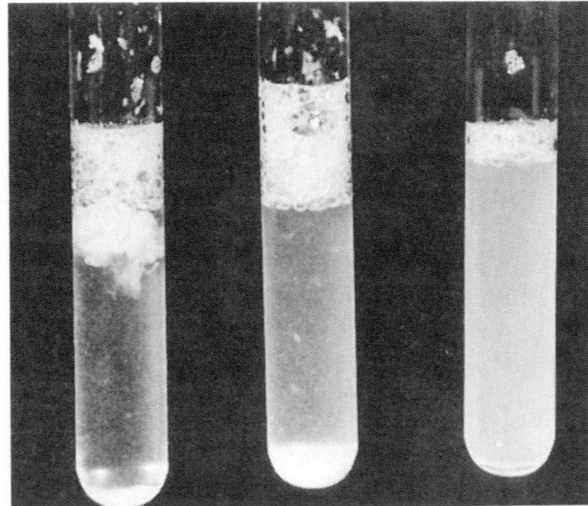

FIG. 4.2. A mucin clot can be produced by adding one part whole joint fluid to four parts 2% acetic acid. A "fair" clot is seen on the left and a "poor" clot can be found in the middle. Treatment of a "good" or "fair" clot with hyaluronidase will abolish the clot (*right*).

The differential diagnosis of hemorrhagic or group IV fluid is reviewed in Table 4.3. Traumatic aspiration or needle-induced trauma represents the most common cause of a bloody joint aspirate. Although truly bloody effusions do not typically clot, hemorrhagic effusions arising from a traumatic tap often do. Additionally, truly bloody effusions are typically homogeneous in character compared with traumatic aspirations, in which the bloody fluid generally enters the arthrocentesis needle in an uneven manner, often appearing only at the beginning or end of the procedure. Truly bloody effusions (blood admixed with synovia) may resemble frank blood with a fluid hematocrit as low as 5% to 10%, making a simple hematocrit test a useful assess-

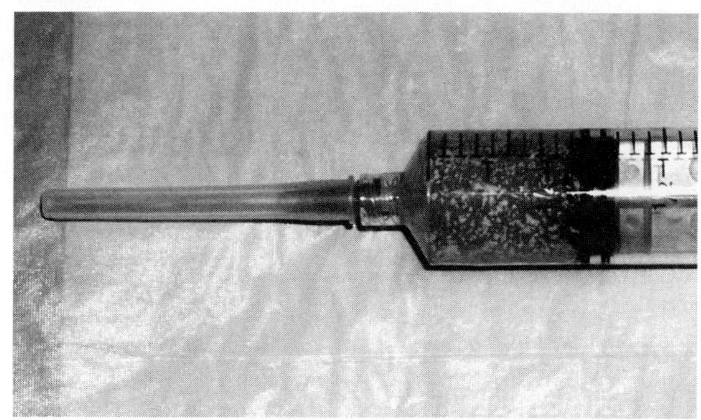

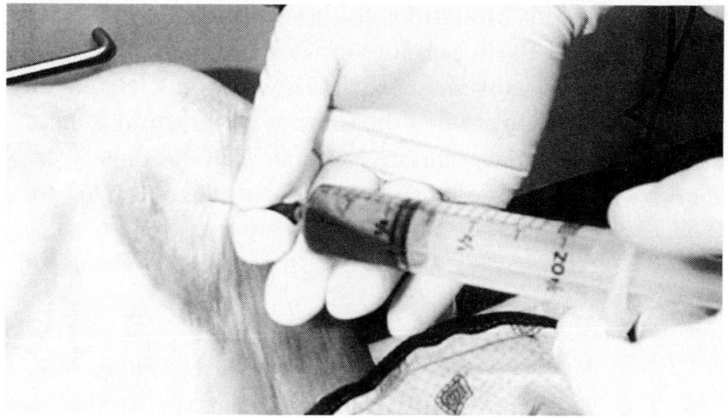

FIG. 4.3. A: Hemorrhagic (group IV) fluid was aspirated from the olecranon bursa of an elderly man with tophaceous gout. In addition to a hemorrhagic fluid, free-floating deposits of monosodium urate can be seen within the aspirate. **B:** A hemorrhagic fluid is aspirated from the shoulder of a woman with an acute-onset inflammatory arthritis. Subsequent examination of the fluid using compensated polarized microscopy revealed numerous intracellular, positively birefringent crystals consistent with calcium pyrophosphate dihydrate.

ment in this clinical situation. With a clinical history of antecedent joint trauma and subsequent joint swelling, the synovial aspirate may be truly bloody with a hematocrit and WBC that mirror that of a simultaneously drawn whole blood specimen. With a truly bloody effusion in the absence of an underlying bleeding diathesis (i.e., hemophilia), a periarticular fracture must be assumed, and appropriate imaging studies should be obtained as part of a more definitive evaluation. A bloody effusion containing fat droplets or elements of bone marrow is highly suggestive of a fracture extending into the joint (4). Crystal-induced arthritis, particularly CPPD crystal and apatite deposition, are frequent and often underrecognized causes of hemorrhagic aspirates (Fig. 4.3A).

Normal and group I fluids are typically clear, and ordinary newsprint can often be read through a clear glass tube containing such synovia (Fig. 4.1A). In contrast, the accumulation of particulate matter, most often leukocytes, renders synovia increasingly opaque. Thus, the opacity of the synovial aspirate routinely correlates with the degree of inflammation as measured by total leukocytes. Other particulate matter, including RBCs (imparting a "smoky" appearance), fat droplets, CPPD and MSU crystal deposits, cholesterol crystals, cartilage fragments, rice bodies, and metal and polyethylene wear particles (from prosthetic joints), may contribute to the opacity of a given sample. Rice bodies, consisting of a collagen core encompassed in fibrin, are small bits of free-floating tissue that resemble "polished white rice" (10) and, although lacking disease specificity, are more commonly encountered in inflammatory effusions (11). Although the number and type of synovial fluid particulate is not routinely diagnostic of a given disorder, there are important exceptions. Aspiration of "chalky" fluid (Fig. 4.4), from a joint, bursa, or subcutaneous nodule is highly characteristic of tophaceous gout, whereas the aspiration of black specks of tissue (so-called "ground pepper" synovia) in the context of otherwise noninflammatory fluid is virtually diagnostic of ochronotic arthropathy (12,13).

Total Leukocyte Count and Differential

The total leukocyte count and WBC differential are helpful in characterizing a given synovial fluid aspirate (Table 4.2). In general, normal synovia contains less than 150 WBCs/mm^3. In contrast, inflammatory group II fluids, characteristic of disorders such as RA and gout, commonly have WBC counts ranging from 3,000 to 50,000 cells/mm^3 with higher counts often indicative of septic arthritis (group III synovia). Although generally helpful in distinguishing noninflammatory from inflammatory arthritis (14–16),

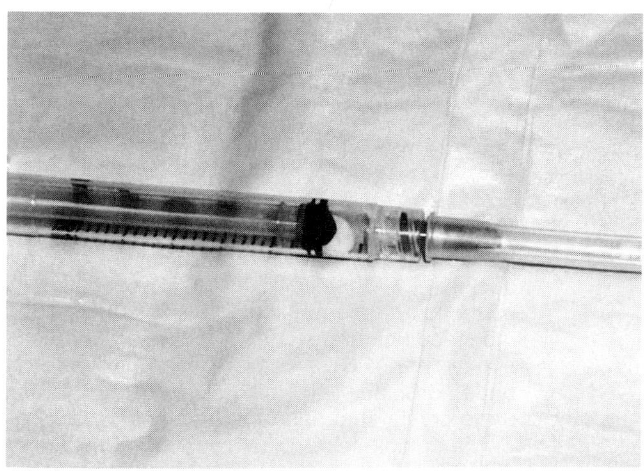

FIG. 4.4. This "chalky" substance was aspirated from a patient's inflamed olecranon bursa, an appearance that is virtually diagnostic of tophaceous gout.

there are important limitations to this simple test that must be considered in its interpretation. Published reports suggest that there is substantial variability in total leukocyte and differential counts when the same synovial fluid is analyzed (17,18). In one such study, total WBC counts from the same synovial fluid were noted to range from 2,467 to 12,000 cells/mm^3 when samples were analyzed in different laboratories (17). Schumacher and colleagues sent aliquots from 30 synovial fluid specimens to four clinical laboratories, comparing the results of the total leukocyte count with that determined by a standard reference laboratory (18). Total WBC counts reported by the four laboratories showed

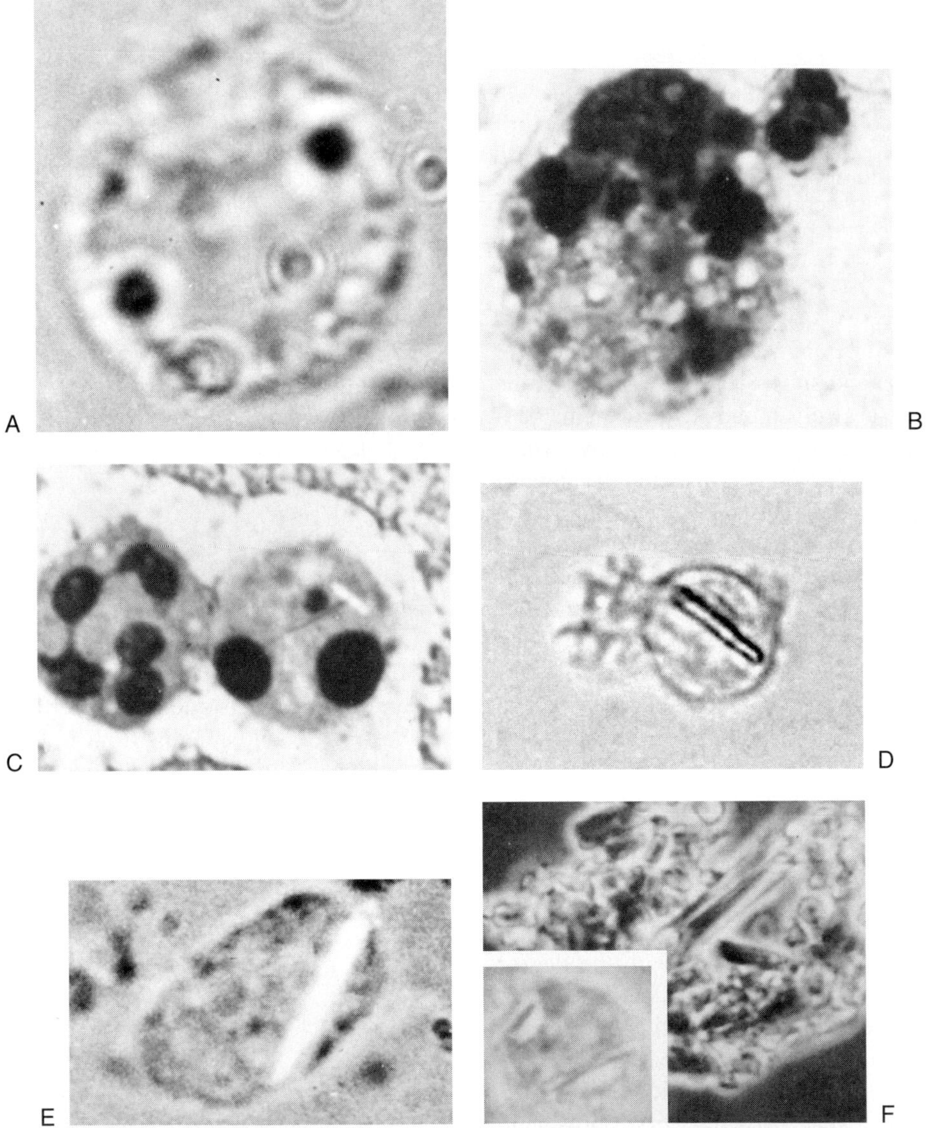

FIG. 4.5. A: An inclusion body cell (*IBC*) seen under ordinary light microscopy (original magnification ×1,250). The cytoplasmic inclusions appear as dark, dense granules. **B:** A cytophagocytic mononuclear (*CPM*) cell or "Reiter cell" seen in a Wright stained smear of synovial fluid from a patient with psoriatic arthritis (original magnification ×1,000). **C:** A Wright stained smear showing a phagocytosed monosodium urate crystal in a polymorphonuclear cell (*PMN*) (polarized light, original magnification ×1,200). **D:** A calcium pyrophosphate dihydrate crystal with rod-shaped morphology as seen under ordinary light microscopy (original magnification ×1,000). **E:** A phagocytosed monosodium urate crystal that appears to extend beyond the outer membrane of a synovial fluid PMN. **F:** Crystals of triamcinolone hexacetonide, a corticosteroid ester, are similar to monosodium urate or calcium pyrophosphate dihydrate crystals in size and shape (phase contrast, original magnification ×1,000; insert phase contrast, original magnification ×800). These crystals are rapidly ingested by synovial fluid PMNs and may appear similar to monosodium urate or calcium pyrophosphate dihydrate crystals under polarized microscopy.

only fair correlation with the reference laboratory (r = 0.76–0.80). Additionally, there were sufficient differences in WBC counts among samples from four patients, causing these fluids to be errantly classified as either noninflammatory or inflammatory. Thus, it is paramount that synovial fluid cell counts are obtained in a standardized fashion by laboratory personnel that are well trained and who fully understand factors that may adversely affect the accuracy of this measure.

Although useful in distinguishing noninflammatory from inflammatory arthritis, total fluid leukocyte counts may be far less helpful in the classification of bursal fluids. In a case series involving 49 episodes of septic bursitis in 45 patients, fluid WBC counts ranged from as low as 350 to over 350,000 cells/mm^3. Moreover, approximately one fourth had total WBC counts less than 5,000 cells/mm^3. However, all fluids showed a predominance of polymorphonuclear leukocytes (PMNs) (>50%), suggesting that the differential WBC count may be of particular importance in distinguishing inflammatory from noninflammatory bursal fluids (19).

Synovial fluid total and differential WBC counts are sometimes obtained using automated cell counters. The use of older generation counters, using particulate size only as its cell marker, may lead to falsely elevated WBC counts by counting extracellular synovial debris (i.e., fat droplets). This phenomenon has been termed "synovial fluid pseudoleukocytosis" (20). Newer generation automated counters, by using both cell size and particle or cell density, may provide more accurate cell counts. However, highly viscous synovia and other fluid particulates may clog the counters and mandate the use of a diluent. In addition to possible inaccuracies caused by technical issues, the "settling phenomenon" may lead to falsely low synovial fluid leukocyte counts (21). Just as leukocytes and other particulates settle over time in an aspirating syringe or glass tube (Fig. 4.1C), synovial fluid leukocytes may "settle" *in vivo,* particularly in a patient who has been rendered immobile by inflammatory polyarticular arthritis. To avoid aspirating the top fluid devoid of WBCs, McCarty has suggested resuspending the "settled" cells prior to arthrocentesis by barbotage or serial aspiration, reinjection, and reaspiration of synovia using the same syringe (21).

Given the technical difficulties associated with the use of automated cell counters, our institution currently performs all synovial fluid cell and differential counts manually. Using plain light microscopy, cell counts are obtained using a hemocytometer with a differential count assessed after the application of Wright stain to the sample. In circumstances when only small amounts (i.e., a single drop) of fluid are obtained by arthrocentesis, the Wright stain can be applied to the same specimen used for wet preparation and crystal analysis. Conversely, crystals may be visualized under polarized microscopy using fluid samples that have already been treated with Wright stain (Fig. 4.5C). If the total WBC count is low, as is often seen with normal and group I fluids, it may be necessary to centrifuge the aspirate, removing the supernatant and reconstituting the sediment with a few drops of remaining supernatant prior to the application of Wright stain. With hemorrhagic fluids, it may be necessary to lyse the RBCs using hypotonic saline (0.3%) prior to examination. Additionally, when numerous RBCs obscure accurate WBC differentiation, the addition of 0.1% methylene blue to the aspirate may help highlight the WBCs, thus differentiating them from erythrocytes.

TABLE 4.4. *Differential diagnosis of synovial fluid eosinophilia*

Rheumatoid arthritis
Rheumatic fever
Parasitic infection
Metastatic adenocarcinoma
Arthrography
Air
Dye
Therapeutic x-irradiation
Urticaria
Acute
Chronic
Idiopathic (eosinophilic synovitis)
Lyme disease
Hypereosinophilic syndrome

In addition to exhibiting higher total WBC counts (>3,000 WBCs/mm^3), inflammatory synovial fluids (groups II and III) are most often characterized by a predominance of PMNs (Table 4.2). In contrast to normal and group I synovia, in which PMNs usually comprise less than 25% of the total WBC count, group II and Group III fluid aspirates contain a much higher percentage of PMNs (>70% PMNs for group II and >90% for group III fluids). There are important caveats to recognize in the interpretation of the WBC differential from synovial fluid samples. For instance, synovial fluid lymphocytosis has been observed in viral-associated arthritis, eosinophilic fasciitis, early RA, serum sickness, and in idiopathic inflammatory arthritis (4). Occasionally, an eosinophilic predominance may be observed in differential leukocyte counts. The differential diagnosis of synovial fluid eosinophilia is shown in Table 4.4 and includes both common (RA, urticaria, Lyme disease) and uncommon conditions (rheumatic fever, parasitic infection, hypereosinophilic syndrome).

Routine Microscopic Examination

Wet Mount and Tissue Sample Preparation

The importance of careful tissue sample and wet mount preparation for the purposes of microscopic examination cannot be overemphasized. For instance, when preparing tissue samples (including synovium or resected nodules) for microscopic crystal examination, it is important to recognize that certain preservatives, such as formaldehyde, dissolve urate crystals, requiring that the sample be examined in frozen section or alternatively placed in an alcohol-based fixative. Once the fluid or tissue sample has been properly prepared, it is essential that a clean glass slide and cover slip that are free of scratches be used, because dust and pieces of cleaning lens paper may have refractile properties and their presence may confuse subsequent crystal analyses. Dust particles, for instance, are positively birefringent and may be readily confused with CPPD crystals. In proper fluid sample preparation, a single drop of synovial fluid is placed on a clean glass slide using either a pipette or sterile wire loop and the slide is then covered with a cover slip. It is of paramount importance that the slide be examined in a timely fashion, since dehydration of the specimen may lead to cellular desiccation and substantial cellular detail may be lost within just a few hours of slide preparation. Given this possibility, many researchers have advocated for the routine use of nail polish placed around the edge of the cover slip as a means of "sealing" the specimen, thus minimizing dehydration and streaming of cells under view, thereby preserving cellular morphology.

Plain Light Microscopy and Basic Cytology

Plain light microscopy is an important component of microscopic synovianalysis and is an often overlooked adjunct to polarized microscopy. Light microscopy (including both plain light and polarized light) is often aided by phase contrast microscopy, which uses a more diffuse (rather than direct) light, allowing for the visualization of far more cellular detail. In addition to WBCs (including PMNs, lymphocytes, monocytes, and eosinophils), plain light microscopy allows for the visualization of synovial lining cells, Reiter cells (cytophagocytic mononuclear cells), lupus erythematosus (LE) cells, and inclusion body cells. Although there has been renewed interest in the role of synovial fluid cytopathology in arthritis diagnosis over recent years (22,23), specialized cytology has not gained wide acceptance as a cost-effective diagnostic tool (24).

Reiter cells, also called cytophagocytic mononuclear cells (CPMs), are mononuclear cells that have engulfed or phagocytized a PMN (Fig. 4.5B). Reiter cells have been noted to constitute up to 2% of all synovial fluid WBCs in acute reactive arthritis (3). Although the name suggests disease specificity, these cells may be found in a variety of inflammatory disorders and, thus, are not of routine diagnostic utility. However, it has been observed that the combination of CPMs and mast cells in the same synovial fluid sample may distinguish the seronegative arthritides (including reactive arthritis, psoriatic arthritis, ankylosing spondylitis, and enteropathic arthritis) from other forms of inflammatory arthritis, including RA (22).

LE cells can be observed on Wright-stained smears in patients with systemic lupus and drug-induced lupus (3,4). As others have noted, the "chance identification" of an LE cell in a synovial aspirate is rarely helpful. The presence of an LE cell in synovial fluid generally reflects the presence of antinuclear antibody (ANA) within the joint, and given the availability of this serologic test (coupled with its low diagnostic yield in this context), the LE test has been relegated to historical interest only.

Similar to the Reiter cell, inclusion body cells (also called "ragocytes" or "raisin cells") are more commonly observed in the context of inflammatory arthritis (25). These cells, originally called "RA cells," represent PMNs that have engulfed cellular debris (immunoglobulins, DNA particles, and fibrin). Under plain light microscopy, the cellular inclusions appear as round or raisin-shaped granules (Fig. 4.5A), whereas they appear as vacuoles using phase contrast microscopy. Freemont and colleagues quantified inclusion body cells in 1,892 patients using cytocentrifuged slide preparations, observing that the percentage of inclusion body cells was substantially higher in patients with inflammatory arthritis (23). In fact, only patients with seropositive arthritis or septic arthritis had more than 65% inclusion body cells. Moreover, a higher percentage of inclusion body cells in serial synovial aspirates was a significant determinant of poor clinical outcome among patients with RA (26).

Compensated Polarized Microscopy

Since the initial descriptions by McCarty and Hollander of MSU and CPPD crystals (1,2), compensated polarized microscopy has become an essential element of routine synovianalysis. Although pathologic crystals, most often MSU or CPPD, may be routinely observed under ordinary light microscopy (Fig. 4.5D), the use of compensated polarized microscopy is needed for the definitive identification of these crystals. Additionally, the observation of small intracellular crystals (often only a few microns in length) may be substantially facilitated by the adjunctive use of phase microscopy, allowing for the visualization of cytoplasmic detail. Under ordinary light microscopy, CPPD crystals may take on a needle-shaped morphology, a characteristic more often attributed to MSU crystals. Only in examining the refractile properties of the crystal (typically done using polarized microscopy) can the crystal be definitively identified. Outfitting an ordinary light microscope with polarizing disks and a makeshift compensator (layers of cellophane tape over a glass slide) has been advocated as an inexpensive means of adapting a microscope for crystal analysis (27).

The lower polarizing plate (or polarizer) of the polarizing microscope orients light into several parallel planes, while the upper plate (analyzer) is placed at a 90-degree angle, effectively blocking all light transmission and creating a dark field when viewed through the eyepiece of the microscope. Any refractile particulate (including MSU or CPPD crystals), when placed on a slide between the two plates, bends or refracts the light sufficiently and as a result appears white on dark-field examination.

Findings on dark-field examination are augmented by the use of a first-order red compensator positioned between the

TABLE 4.5. *Characteristics of monosodium urate (MSU) and calcium pyrophosphate dihydrate (CPPD) crystals using polarized microscopy*

	Crystal	
	MSU	CPPD
Sign of birefringence	Negative	Positive
Strength of birefringence (brightness)	Strong	Weak
Morphology	Rod-shaped, spherule	Rhomboid, rod-shaped
Extinction	Sharp, parallel to plane of polarizer/analyzer	Gradual, oblique to plane of polarizer/analyzer
Size	Submicroscopic, 40 μm	Submicroscopic, 40 μm

polarizing plates. The compensator's axis of slow vibration is oriented at a 45-degree angle from both the analyzer and polarizer. The compensator slows the red component of the light by a one-fourth wavelength, resulting in a red or rose-colored background rather than the dark-field background. Rather than appearing white, MSU and CPPD crystals now appear either blue or yellow, depending on their axis of orientation to the direction of slow vibration of the light in the compensator. Rotating an MSU or CPPD crystal 90 degrees will result in a blue crystal becoming yellow or a yellow crystal turning blue. On most microscopes, the direction of slow vibration is demarcated on the compensator with an arrow, line, or the Greek letter γ. MSU and CPPD crystals are said to be biaxial, meaning that there are two directions in which light can pass through the crystal without being refracted at different speeds.

There are four characteristics of refractile crystals that aid in their identification using polarized microscopy: (a) crystal morphology, including shape and size, (b) the sign of birefringence, (c) the strength of birefringence (or brightness), and (d) the extinction angle. A comparison of polarized microscopy findings for MSU and CPPD crystals is summarized in Table 4.5.

Monosodium Urate Crystals

MSU crystals, diagnostic of gouty arthritis, are typically rod-shaped and range in size from submicroscopic in length to as long as 40 μm (equivalent to the diameter of approximately four WBCs). MSU crystals, in contrast to CPPD crystals, are strongly birefringent, appearing very bright under polarized microscopy (Fig. 4.6). Importantly,

A
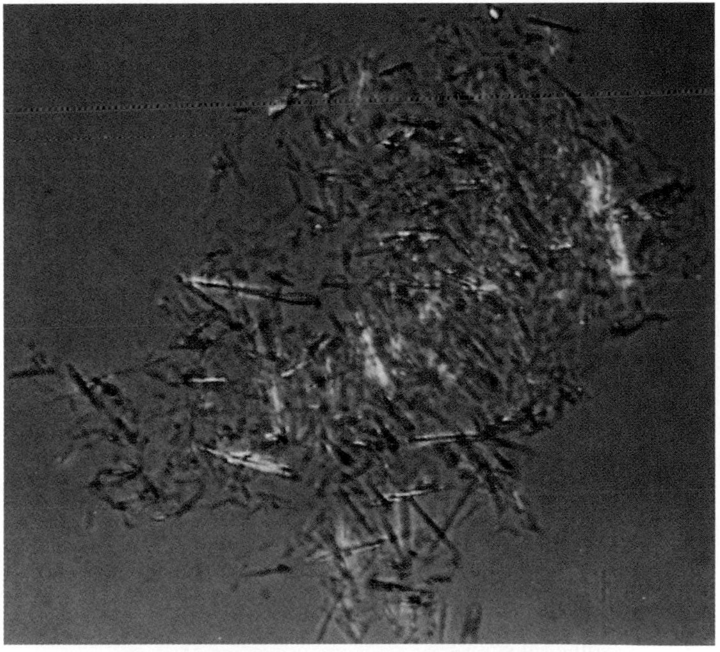

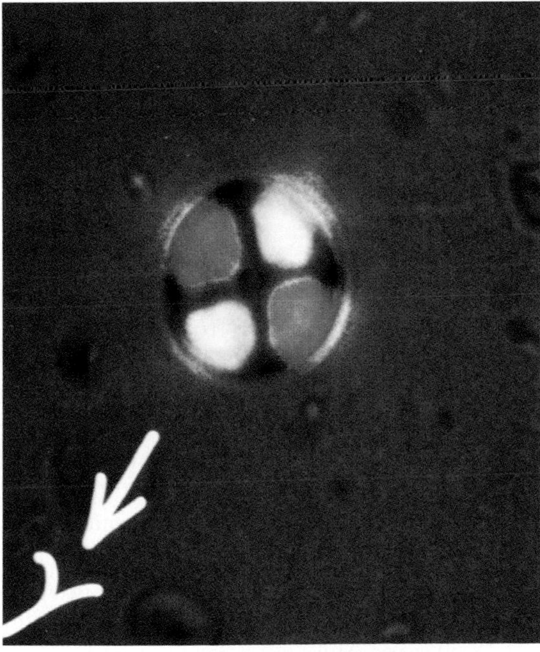

B

FIG. 4.6. A: Numerous monosodium urate crystals in a drop of joint fluid aspirated from a patient with chronic tophaceous gout, viewed by compensated polarized microscopy (original magnification ×500). **B:** A negatively birefringent spherulite in synovial fluid of a patient with gout. These spherulites may rarely present as the only monosodium urate crystalline phase or may be accompanied with more typical rod-shaped needles (original magnification ×1,000). (Reproduced from Fiechtner JJ, Simkin PA. Urate spherulites in gouty synovia. *JAMA* 1981;245:1533–1536, by permission.)

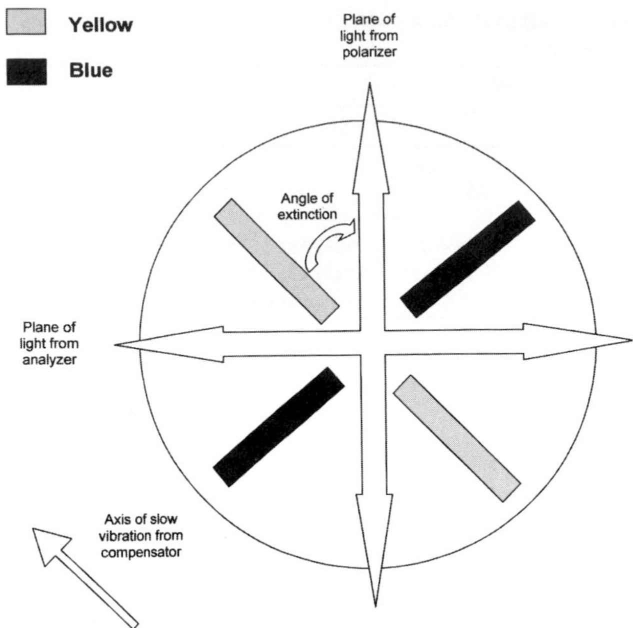

FIG. 4.7. The typical properties of a monosodium urate crystal under compensated polarized microscopy. Monosodium urate crystals are stongly birefringent, appearing yellow when parallel to the axis of slow vibration from the compensator and blue when perpendicular to this axis. The crystal becomes nonrefractile and isotropic with the field when the long axis of the crystal lies parallel to that of the polarizer or analyzer (precisely a 45-degree angle from the positions at which the crystal appears its brightest).

MSU crystals are negatively birefringent (or have a negative elongation angle), appearing yellow when parallel to the axis of slow vibration from the compensator and blue when perpendicular to this axis (Fig. 4.7). In classical gout, MSU crystals are characteristically intracellular and may actually be observed to pierce the outer membrane of the PMN (Fig. 4.5E). MSU crystals display a sharp angle of extinction. Precisely characterizing the extinction angle of refractile material is facilitated by the availability of a rotating microscope stage. When the crystal is orientated at precisely a 45-degree angle from the position at which it appears brightest (or parallel to the axis of light from the polarizer or analyzer), the crystal becomes isotropic with its background (rose colored when the compensator is in position). Although more commonly rod shaped in morphology, MSU crystals may form a spherule (several MSU crystals emanating from a common central axis) (28) (Fig. 4.6). Negatively birefringent MSU spherules display components of both yellow and blue at all times, depending on their orientation to the axis of slow vibration from the compensator. Although rarely needed, the identification of MSU crystals may be augmented by uricase digestion, x-ray diffraction, or electron microscopy (required in rare circumstances when crystals are submicroscopic in size).

Calcium Pyrophosphate Dihydrate Crystals

CPPD crystals, similar in size to MSU crystals, may be rod shaped (Fig. 4.5D) but more commonly appear rhomboidal in shape. In contrast to strongly birefringent MSU crystals, CPPD crystals are only weakly birefringent and as a result may be much more difficult to appreciate for the untrained eye. CPPD crystals are positively birefringent, appearing blue when the long axis of the crystal is parallel to the direction of slow vibration and yellow when perpendicular to this axis. In contrast to MSU crystals, which have a distinct angle of extinction, CPPD crystals have both an oblique and somewhat more gradual extinction angle, becoming isotropic with the field when the crystal is oriented obliquely (20–30 degrees) from the orientation of light from the polarizer or analyzer. As with urate crystals, submicroscopic CPPD crystals may require electron microscopy for detection.

Other Crystals

Increasingly, hydroxyapatite (HA) crystals have been appreciated to play a pathologic role in both joints and periarticular structures (see Chapter 117). Clumps of apatite are not birefringent, and individual crystals are commonly submicroscopic in size (often 70–250 nm in size) and thus require special methods (including stains) for their accurate identification. Individual crystals can only be observed with electron microscopy (29). Clumps of HA crystals may be either extracellular or intracellular (in PMNs) and have been said to appear as "shiny coins" under phase contrast microscopy (30). Although routine polarized microscopy plays a limited role in their identification, the use of Alizarin red S stain, which stains calcium-containing particulate, has been shown in special reference laboratories to be a useful adjunct in the detection of HA crystals (31).

Although their pathologic role remains somewhat speculative, the deposition of calcium hydrogen phosphate dehydrate (brushite) crystals has been reported to result in a destructive synovitis (32). These crystals are rod shaped and display a strongly positive birefringence.

Cholesterol crystals have been observed in joint fluid aspirates in both inflammatory and noninflammatory arthritides and have been said to be characteristic of long-standing effusions (33,34). Cholesterol crystals usually appear as large (often 100 μm or larger), thin, adherent plates and characteristically have "notched corners." Under polarized microscopy, single crystals show a negative elongation angle and are only weakly birefringent and, thus, may be quite difficult to detect. These crystals appear brighter and are easier to see, however, when they are found in typical adherent stacks.

Calcium oxalate crystal deposition has been reported in patients receiving chronic dialysis (35,36). These crystals are typically small in size, intracellular, cuboidal to rhomboidal in shape, and display weakly positive birefringence.

Due to their morphology and positive birefringence, these may be confused with CPPD crystals when polarized microscopy is relied on as the sole technique for crystal identification (35). Calcium oxalate crystals may also represent artifact, forming *in situ* when otherwise normal joint fluid is collected in an oxalate tube.

Other Refractile Particles and Artifacts

Amyloid deposits have been identified in cytocentrifuged synovial fluid specimens from patients with amyloidosis (37). Using Congo red staining, amyloid deposits exhibit "apple green" birefringence under polarized microscopy. Lipid inclusions, which appear as birefringent "maltese crosses" under polarized microscopy, have been observed in cases of inflammatory arthritis (38,39) and in intraarticular fractures. Intraarticular fat droplets may also be seen in cases of pancreatic fat necrosis (40). Talc from older surgical gloves has also been reported to appear as maltese crosses under compensated polarized microscopy. As with calcium oxalate tubes and the formation of calcium oxalate crystals, the use of lithium heparin tubes may lead to the *in situ* formation of lithium crystals. These crystals may be engulfed by activated PMNs and appear as positively birefringent intracellular crystals, in some circumstances closely resembling CPPD crystals.

Corticosteroid preparations may also form crystals within the joint space, which may be present weeks to months after an intraarticular injection (Fig. 4.5F). Corticosteroid crystals display highly variable morphology and birefringent properties, but may closely mimic pathologic crystals, particularly CPPD crystals. Other artifacts, including polyethylene debris (from prosthetic joints), nail polish, immersion oil particulate, dust, collagen fibrils, and other fibers have all been reported to have variable birefringent properties, which may complicate synovial fluid analysis. Nail polish, when used as a sealant, may lead to the formation of numerous positively birefringent crystals along the margin of the cover slip. Crystal particulates found in immersion oils vary both in shape and size, but smaller crystals are often positively birefringent. Birefringent dust and fibers are typically irregular in shape and have a branching morphology, in contrast to the more regularly shaped MSU and CPPD crystals. The effect of dust, fibers, and immersion oil particulates are minimized when the microscope is correctly focused on the plane of aspirate and not on top of the cover slip.

Microbiologic Testing

Stains and Culture

The evaluation, diagnosis, and treatment of septic arthritis is discussed in detail in Chapters 124 through 127, but some salient points are worth reviewing. Given the significant morbidity and mortality associated with septic arthritis, the clinician must have a high index of suspicion for underlying infection, particularly when an inflammatory arthritis occurs concomitantly with a known infection elsewhere in the patient (e.g., endocarditis, pneumonia, bacteremia, cellulitis, or urinary tract infection). In patients with preexisting joint damage (e.g., RA) and those with underlying immunosuppression (e.g., diabetes, posttransplantation) presenting with an inflammatory arthritis, consideration must be given to the potential of an ongoing infectious process.

By definition, the aspiration of group III synovial fluid with a total leukocyte count of greater than 50,000/mm^3 highlights joint infection as a distinct possibility. However, septic arthritis may be seen with synovia that would otherwise be categorized as a group II fluid. Both *Neisseria* and coagulase-negative *Staphylococcus*, for instance, have been frequently associated with relatively low synovial fluid leukocyte counts and a lower percentage of PMNs (21). Conversely, group III fluids with high leukocyte counts can be seen in cases of noninfectious arthritis, such as gout and pseudogout, and these conditions may even coexist with an acute infectious process. In a single case series, half of all fluids from culture-proven septic joints had total WBC counts of less than 28,000 cells/mm^3 (41).

In most instances, Gram stain and routine bacterial culture are sufficient for the purposes of synovianalysis. However, a variety of special stains (Table 4.6) and culture media have been developed that may be helpful in specific clinical situations. For instance, Ziehl-Nielsen and silver stains may be helpful in the identification of acid-fast bacilia (e.g., *Mycobacterium tuberculosis*) and fungal elements, respectively. In cases of Whipple disease, periodic acid-Schiff staining may reveal characteristic deposits within synovial macrophages. *Neisseria gonorrhoeae*, a common cause of septic arthritis, is a highly fastidious organism and is observed in less than one fourth of cases with Gram stain, with positive cultures found in only 30% to 60% of infected patients (42,43). Thus, in suspected cases, chocolate agar or Thayer-Martin media should be inoculated at the bedside (see Chapter 125).

The sensitivity of routine culture can be substantially enhanced through the direct inoculation of blood culture bottles with the synovial fluid aspirate (44,45). Over a 20-year period, von Essen examined 155 culture-positive specimens from 89 patients that were simultaneously cultured in blood culture bottles and on conventional media (44). Over one third of the specimens that were felt to represent true infections were positive by blood culture bottle alone. Recent reports have highlighted the use of pediatric blood culture bottles, which can reliably grow bacteria from smaller inocula than required by conventional blood culture bottle systems (45). Although the use of blood culture bottles may result in an increase in the frequency of isolating bacterial contaminants, the inconvenience arising from these false-positive results has been deemed to be "relatively minor" by investigators (44).

TABLE 4.6. *Stains used in the examination of synovial fluid and associated findings*

Stain	Microscopic findings
Alcian blue	Intracellular mucopolysaccharides
Alizarin red S	Calcium (hydroxyapatite clumps)
Congo red	Amyloid deposits (apple green birefringence using polarized microscopy)
Gram	Intracellular bacteria
Hematoxylin-eosin	Tumor cells and rice bodies[a]
Periodic acid-Shiff	Whipple disease (intracellular deposits[a])
Prussian blue	Iron deposition (hemochromatosis and pigmented villonodular synovitis)
Silver stain	Fungal elements
Sudan black	Large monocytes, lymphoblasts, and synovial lining cells
Von Kossa	Phosphate bound calcium (calcium pyrophosphate dihydrate and hydroxyapatite crystals; purple to brown)
Wright	Differential leukocytes, crystals
Ziehl-Neelsen	Intracellular acid-fast bacilli (e.g., tuberculosis)

[a]Cytocentrifuged specimen.

DNA Amplification

Polymerase chain reaction (PCR) assays of synovial fluid have been advocated to play a role in several diagnostically challenging clinical situations in which septic arthritis is suspected, including *Neisseria* infection (46,47), Lyme-associated arthritis (48–51), infected joint prostheses (52), and Whipple disease (53). It is important to note that a positive PCR assay does not necessarily mean that an active infection is present, but rather denotes the presence of bacterial DNA remnants within the joint space. PCR has been reported to have a sensitivity and specificity of 76% and 96%, respectively (47), in the diagnosis of gonococcal arthritis, results suggesting that PCR may be superior to routine Gram stain and culture in this setting. Investigators have recently reported on the use PCR of synovial fluid in detection of bacterial DNA from *Tropheryma whippelii*, the causative organism in Whipple disease, a notoriously difficult diagnosis to make (53).

Although the detection of bacterial DNA by PCR is increasingly being used in the diagnosis of infectious diseases, caution must be exercised with the routine use of such diagnostic tests, given the fact that these tests are rarely standardized and are not routinely available in most centers.

SYNOVIAL FLUID CHEMISTRIES

Synovial glucose (54), total protein, lactate dehydrogenase (LDH) (55), and organic acids (including lactic acid and succinic acid, often measured by gas-liquid chromatography) (4) have been suggested to play a role in differentiating inflammatory from noninflammatory synovia and, in particular, distinguishing septic arthritis from other inflammatory arthritides. The assessment of synovial fluid glucose level requires that the patient be fasting and that comparisons be made with simultaneous serum levels. Differences [serum glucose value minus synovial fluid value (delta glucose value)] of greater than 40 mg/dL are observed regularly in cases of bacterial and mycobacterial joint infection (54). However, there is substantial overlap in the delta glucose values observed in septic arthritis and nonseptic inflammatory arthritis, limiting the value of synovial fluid glucose measurement.

Synovial fluid lactate and succinic acid have been reported to be markedly elevated in septic arthritis (4,56). Using a cutoff value of 0.05 m*M*, D-lactic acid measurement has been shown to have an overall sensitivity of 85% and a specificity of 96% for the detection of septic arthritis (56). Similar to glucose assessment, however, there has been substantial overlap between values of synovial fluid organic acids among patients with septic arthritis and those with other forms of inflammatory arthritis, limiting the general usefulness of these tests. Additionally, with only modest sensitivity, a negative test result does not rule out the possibility of septic arthritis. Although of little routine diagnostic value in septic arthritis and lacking disease specificity among the nonseptic arthritides, synovial fluid pH, pO_2, and total protein may also be affected by inflammatory stimuli. The pH of normal joint fluid is 7.4 and decreases with inflammation, particularly in cases of septic arthritis (57). Likewise, pO_2 levels decrease with inflammation (58). Oxygen tension also appears to be inversely associated with fluid volume, suggesting a local ischemic effect arising from larger joint effusions. Total synovial fluid protein values, normally averaging 1.8 gm/dL, increase in a nonspecific fashion with inflammation.

In a prospective study involving 100 consecutive synovial fluid aspirates, Shmerling and colleagues examined the utility of several synovial fluid tests in differentiating inflammatory and noninflammatory arthritis (15). Analysis of receiver operator characteristics of the tests revealed that only synovial fluid WBC and PMN percentage contributed independent diagnostic information. In contrast, synovial fluid assessments of glucose, total protein, and LDH (with sensitivities ranging from 20% to 83%) did not provide relevant diagnostic information. Although this study did not examine the measurement of synovial fluid organic acids, the researchers suggested that chemistry studies of synovial fluid aspirates be avoided because they "are likely to provide misleading or redundant information."

Antibiotic Levels

The measurement of antibiotic concentrations may be performed on joint fluid, just as it is done on serum samples. However, high antibiotic concentrations are nearly universally observed in cases of septic arthritis (59), with a highly permeable synovial "diasylate membrane," substantially limiting the value of such testing.

COMPLEMENT

Synovial fluid complement, particularly total hemolytic complement ($C'H_{50}$), has been proposed to be of diagnostic value in the assessment of inflammatory arthritis. Individual complement components (C3 or C4) may also be measured, as may complement degradation products such as C5a (60). In order to measure $C'H_{50}$, synovial fluid specimens must be promptly centrifuged following arthrocentesis and the supernatant stored at −70°C. Synovial fluid $C'H_{50}$ levels appear to be most useful when compared with simultaneous serum values (61). Synovial fluid $C'H_{50}$ values are typically one third to one half of serum values unless there is local complement consumption.

Several early reports showed that $C'H_{50}$ values are reduced in synovial fluid from patients with RA and elevated in fluids from patients with reactive arthritis (62–64), suggesting that this test may be important in differentiating different forms of inflammatory arthritis. Moreover, lower synovial fluid $C'H_{50}$ values have been associated with a more severe disease course in RA and an overall worse disease prognosis (65). Synovial fluid $C'H_{50}$ levels are also decreased in systemic lupus erythematosus (63,66) and elevated in psoriatic arthritis. Subsequent reports have failed to substantiate the early enthusiasm for complement testing. In a retrospective analysis of 174 synovial fluid samples from patients with various arthritides, Kim and colleagues found that synovial fluid $C'H_{50}$ assessment provided little additional diagnostic value to routine synovianalysis (61). For example, synovial fluid $C'H_{50}$ has only modest sensitivity (70%) and specificity (66%) in differentiating rheumatoid from nonrheumatoid effusions. Although comparing synovial fluid $C'H_{50}$ values to simultaneous serum values improved the test's sensitivity (90%), there was no appreciable effect on specificity.

CYTOKINES

Cytokines are small proteins produced by a number of cells, including synovial macrophages and lymphocytes, which play a central role in mediating joint inflammation. The number of cytokines and cytokine inhibitors measured in synovial fluid continues to expand. Although proposed to play a potential role in defining arthritis diagnosis and prognosis (67), complex interactions within the cytokine network, low disease specificity, and the lack of standardized and reproducible assays for their routine measurement have limited the clinical usefulness of assessing synovial fluid cytokine levels. Several proinflammatory cytokines [including interleukin-1 (IL-1), IL-6, IL-8, and tumor necrosis factor-α (TNF-α)] are increased in the synovia of patients with different types of inflammatory arthritis.

Preliminary reports suggest that the measurement of synovial fluid IL-1 and TNF-α may provide valuable information in select circumstances. It has been shown, for instance, that higher levels of synovial IL-1β (>15 pg/mL) differentiate RA from seronegative spondyloarthritis in untreated patients, once septic arthritis and crystal-associated arthritis have been ruled out (68). In a small study of 18 patients with psoriatic monoarthritis, higher baseline values of synovial fluid IL-1 were predictive of disease progression into polyarticular disease over the course of 3 years (68). In a separate study, the measurement of TNF-α and its inhibitor [soluble TNF receptor (sTNFR)] helped to subtype patients with juvenile chronic arthritis (69). Specifically, synovial fluid sTNFR/TNF-α ratios were significantly higher in patients with spondyloarthropathy compared to patients with pauci- and polyarticular arthritis. Despite being shown to decrease with active antiinflammatory therapies (70–73), the measurement of synovial fluid proinflammatory cytokines and their inhibitors remains an unfulfilled promise in predicting therapeutic response.

SEROLOGIES

Several serologies, including rheumatoid factor (RF), ANA, and cryoproteins, have been described in a variety of synovial fluid studies. To date, the measurement of immune complexes in synovial aspirates has not been shown to be a useful diagnostic measure. In most instances, synovial fluid RF titers are identical or similar to simultaneous serum values (3). Moreover, synovial RF appears to have little disease specificity and has been observed in other forms of inflammatory and noninflammatory arthritis (74). Similarly, ANAs and cryoproteins (seen commonly in RA as mixed cryoglobulins) offer little disease specificity and, thus, do not provide additional diagnostic information over serum values.

Although their diagnostic utility in synovianalysis remains to be defined, there has recently been growing interest in the use of serum antibodies directed against filaggrin (filament-aggregating protein) in the diagnosis of RA. These antibodies [which in the past have included antiperinuclear factor and antikeratin antibody (AKA)] bind peptides containing the amino acid citrulline (75). In contrast to RF, which has only modest specificity in RA, use of the cyclic citrullinated peptide (CCP) antigen in enzyme-linked immunosorbent assay has revealed a disease specificity of serum anti-CCP antibodies approaching 95% to 100% (75–77). Notably, the anti-CCP antibodies are produced locally by synovial fluid B lymphocytes (78). In a prior study of 20 patients with RA, immunoglobulin G (IgG) AKAs were detected in both the serum and synovial fluid of 16 (80%) patients. Corrected for the lower immunoglobulin content of synovial fluid, AKAs comprised a higher percentage of the IgG in synovial fluid than in serum. In a separate study involving patients with various forms of inflammatory arthritis, AKAs were found in approximately one half of synovial fluid specimens obtained from patients with RA but were not found in patients with nonrheumatoid diseases (79). Although the precise role of synovial fluid anti-CCP analysis remains to be characterized, preliminary findings suggest that further studies in this area are warranted.

MARKERS OF BONE AND CARTILAGE DEGRADATION

Several synovial fluid biomarkers of bone and cartilage breakdown have been proposed to provide potentially valuable clinical information, particularly in the context of osteoarthritis (OA) diagnosis and management. However, these markers (including proteoglycans, deoxypyridinoline, and N-teleopeptide) do not appear to strongly correlate with clinical findings in either OA (80) or inflammatory arthritis (81). There are several factors that may complicate biomarker measurement, including the use of assays lacking sufficient reproducibility, diurnal variation of serum values, and the dilutional effect of lavage procedures and pathologic effusions. Synovial fluid urea measurement may be a robust and useful method for correcting for the dilutional impact of lavage and effusion in future investigations (82).

Arthrocentesis and synovial fluid analysis clearly play a central role in the assessment of patients with musculoskeletal disease. Continued advances in imaging in addition to genomic and proteomics technologies may soon allow for adjunctive or even alternative methods of assessing diseased synovium and synovial fluid. Recent technologic advances in three-dimensional processing of magnetic resonance imaging (MRI) may represent a noninvasive, albeit more expensive, means of accurately assessing synovial fluid volume (83). In a recent study by Cimmino and colleagues, dynamic MRI allowed for the accurate discrimination of active from inactive disease among patients with RA (84). Computed tomography has been shown to provide specific imaging characteristics of tophaceous deposits in gouty arthritis (85). Separate groups of investigators have reported disease-specific acoustic characteristics of *in vitro* synovial fluid using ultrasonography (86,87), findings that will certainly require *in vivo* confirmation. The growing use of gene microarray systems (88) and synovial protein biochip technology (89) holds promise in synovial fluid analysis, particularly in providing much needed insight into disease pathogenesis and in uncovering potential therapeutic targets.

REFERENCES

1. McCarty DJ, Hollander J. Identification of urate crystals in gouty synovial fluid. *Ann Intern Med* 1961;54:452–460.
2. McCarty DJ, Kohn N, Faires J. The significance of calcium phosphate crystals in the synovial fluid of arthritis patients: the pseudogout syndrome. I. Clinical aspects. *Ann Intern Med* 1962;56:738–745.
3. McCarty DJ. Synovial fluid. In: Koopman W, ed. *Arthritis and allied conditions,* 11th ed. Philadelphia: Lea & Febiger, 1989:69–90.
4. McCarty DJ. Synovial fluid. In: Koopman W, ed. *Arthritis and allied conditions,* 12th ed. Malvern, PA: Lea & Febiger, 1993:63–84.
5. Lally E. High-dose corticosterioid therapy: association with noninflammatory synovial effusions. *Arthritis Rheum* 1983;26:1283–1287.
6. Swann D, Radin E, Nazimiec M, et al. Role of hyaluronic acid in joint lubrication. *Ann Rheum Dis* 1974;33:318–326.
7. Weitz Z, Moak S, Greenwald R. Degradation of hyaluronic acid by neutrophil derived oxygen radicals is stimulus dependent. *J Rheumatol* 1988;15:1250–1253.
8. Uchiyama H, Dobashi Y, Ohkouchi K, et al. Chemical change involved in the oxidative reductive depolymerization of hyaluronic acid. *J Biol Chem* 1990;265:7753–7759.
9. Greenwald R, Moak S. Degradation of hyaluronic acid by polymorphonuclear leukocytes. *Inflammation* 1986;10:15–30.
10. Gatter R. *A practical handbook of joint fluid analysis.* Philadelphia: Lea & Febiger, 1984.
11. Galvez J, Sola J, Ortuno G, et al. Microscopic rice bodies in rheumatoid synovial fluid sediments. *J Rheumatol* 1992;19:1851–1858.
12. Hunter T, Gordon D, Ogryzlo M. The ground pepper sign of synovia fluid: a new diagnostic feature of ochronosis. *J Rheumatol* 1974;1:45–53.
13. Reginato A, Schumacher H, Martinez V. Ochronotic arthropathy with calcium pyrophosphate crystal deposition. A light and electron microscopic study. *Arthritis Rheum* 1973;16:705–714.
14. Shmerling R. Synovial fluid analysis. A critical reappraisal. *Rheum Dis Clin North Am* 1994;20:503–512.
15. Shmerling R, Delbanco T, Tosteson A, et al. Synovial fluid tests. What should be ordered? *JAMA* 1990;264:1009–1014.
16. Kersey R, Benjamin J, Marson B. White blood cell counts and differential in synovial fluid of aseptically failed total knee arthroplasty. *J Arthroplasty* 2000;15:301–304.
17. Hasselbacher P. Variation in synovial fluid analysis by hospital laboratories. *Arthritis Rheum* 1987;30:637–642.
18. Schumacher HJ, Sieck M, Rothfuss S, et al. Reproducibility of synovial fluid analyses. A study among four laboratories. *Arthritis Rheum* 1986;29:770–774.
19. Raddatz D, Hoffman G, Franck W. Septic bursitis: presentation, treatment and prognosis. *J Rheumatol* 1987;14:1160–1163.
20. Vincent J, Korn J, Podewell C, et al. Synovial fluid pseudoleukocytosis. *Arthritis Rheum* 1980;23:1399–1400.
21. McCarty DJ. Synovial fluid. In: Koopman W, ed. *Arthritis and allied conditions*. Vol. 1. Baltimore: Williams & Wilkins, 1997:81–102.
22. Freemont A, Denton J. Disease distribution of synovial fluid mast cells and cytophagocytic mononuclear cells in inflammatory arthritis. *Ann Rheum Dis* 1985;44:312–315.
23. Freemont A, Denton J, Chuck A, et al. Diagnostic value of synovial fluid microscopy: a reassessment and rationalisation. *Ann Rheum Dis* 1991;50:101–107.
24. Swan A, Amer H, Dieppe P. The value of synovial fluid assays in the diagnosis of joint disease: a literature survey. *Ann Rheum Dis* 2002;61:493–498.
25. Hollander J, McCarty DJ, Rawson A. The "R.A. cell," "ragocyte," or "inclusion body cell." *Bull Rheum Dis* 1965;16:382–383.
26. Davis M, Denton J, Freemont A, et al. Comparison of serial synovial fluid cytology in rheumatoid arthritis: delineation of subgroups with prognostic implications. *Ann Rheum Dis* 1988;47:559–562.
27. Owens DJ. A cheap and useful compensated polarizing microscope. *N Engl J Med* 1971;285:1152.

28. Fiechtner J, Simkin P. Urate spherulites in gouty synovia. *JAMA* 1981;245:1533–1536.
29. Schumacher HJ. Crystal-induced arthritis: an overview. *Am J Med* 1996;100(suppl 2A):46–52.
30. McCarty DJ, Gatter R. Recurrent acute inflammation associated with focal apatite crystal deposition. *Arthritis Rheum* 1966;9:804–819.
31. Paul H, Reginato A, Schumacher HJ. Alizarin red S staining as a screening test to detect calcium compounds in synovial fluid. *Arthritis Rheum* 1983;26:191–200.
32. Skinner M, Cohen A. Calcium pyrophosphate dihydrate crystal deposition disease. *Arch Intern Med* 1969;123:636–644.
33. Nye W, Terry R, Rosenbaum D. Two forms of crystalline lipid in "cholesterol" effusions. *Am J Clin Pathol* 1968;49:718–728.
34. Fam A, Pritzker K, Cheng P, et al. Cholesterol crystals in osteoarthritic joint effusions. *J Rheumatol* 1981;8:273–280.
35. Hoffman G, Schumacher HJ, Paul H, et al. Calcium oxalate microcrystalline-associated arthritis in end-stage renal disease. *Ann Intern Med* 1982;97:36–42.
36. Reginato AJ, Ferreiro Seoane JL, Barbazan Alvarez C, et al. Arthropathy and cutaneous calcinosis in hemodialysis oxalosis. *Arthritis Rheum* 1986;29:1387–1396.
37. Gordon D, Pruzanski W, Ogryzlo M. Synovial fluid examination for the diagnosis of amyloidosis. *Ann Rheum Dis* 1973;32:428–430.
38. Reginato A, Schumacher HJ, Allan D, et al. Acute monoarthritis associated with lipid liquid crystals. *Ann Rheum Dis* 1985;44:537–543.
39. Weinstein J. Synovial fluid leukocytosis associated with intracellular lipid inclusions. *Arch Intern Med* 1980;140:560–561.
40. Gibson T, Schumacher HJ, Pascual E, et al. Arthropathy, skin and bone lesions in pancreatic disease. *J Rheumatol* 1975;2:7–13.
41. McCutchan H, Fisher R. Synovial leukocytosis in infectious arthritis. *Clin Orthop* 1990;257:226–230.
42. Scopelitis E, Martinez-Osuna P. Gonococcal arthritis. *Rheum Dis Clin North Am* 1993;19:363–377.
43. O'Brien J, Goldenberg D, Rice P. Disseminated gonococcal infection: a prospective analysis of 49 patients and a review of pathophysiology and immune mechanisms. *Medicine (Baltimore)* 1983;62:395–406.
44. von Essen R. Culture of joint specimens in bacterial arthritis. Impact of blood culture bottle utilization. *Scand J Rheumatol* 1997;26:293–300.
45. Yagupski P, Press J. Use of the isolator 1.5 microbial tube for culture of synovial fluid from patients with septic arthritis. *J Clin Microbiol* 1997;35:2410–2412.
46. Muralidhar B, Rumore P, Steinman C. Use of the polymerase chain reaction to study arthritis due to *Neisseria gonorrhoeae. Arthritis Rheum* 1994;37:710–717.
47. Liebling M, Arkfeld D, Michelini G, et al. Identification of *Neisseria gonorrhoeae* in synovial fluid using the polymerase chain reaction. *Arthritis Rheum* 1994;37:702–709.
48. Nanagara R, Duray P, Schumacher HJ. Ultrastructural demonstration of spirochetal antigens in synovial fluid and synovial membrane in chronic Lyme disease: possible factors contributing to persistence of organisms. *Hum Pathol* 1996;27:1025–1034.
49. Nocton J, Dressler F, Rutledge B, et al. Detection of *Borrelia burgdorferi* DNA by polymerase chain reaction in synovial fluid from patients with Lyme arthritis. *N Engl J Med* 1994;330:229–234.
50. Steere A. Diagnosis and treatment of Lyme arthritis. *Med Clin North Am* 1997;81:179–194.
51. Bradley J, Johnson R, Goodman J. The persistence of spirochetal nucleic acids in active Lyme arthritis. *Ann Intern Med* 1994;120:487–489.
52. Tunney M, Patrick S, Curran M, et al. Detection of prosthetic hip infection at revision arthroplasty by immunofluorescence microscopy and PCR amplification of the bacterial 16S rRNA gene. *J Clin Microbiol* 1999;37:3281–3290.
53. Lange U, Teichmann J. Whipple arthritis: diagnosis by molecular analysis of synovial fluid-current status of diagnosis and therapy. *Rheumatology* 2003;42:473–480.
54. Cohen A, Goldenberg D. Synovial fluid. In: Cohen A, ed. *Laboratory diagnostic procedures in the rheumatic diseases,* 3rd ed. New York: Grune & Stratton, 1985.
55. Pejovic M, Stankovic A, Mitrovic D. Lactate dehydrogenase activity and its isoenzymes in serum and synovial fluid of patients with rheumatoid arthritis and osteoarthritis. *J Rheumatol* 1992;19:529–533.
56. Gratacos J, Vila J, Moya F, et al. D-lactic acid in synovial fluid. A rapid diagnostic test for bacterial synovitis. *J Rheumatol* 1995;22:1504–1508.
57. Ward T, Steigbigel R. Acidosis of synovial fluid correlates with synovial fluid leukocytosis. *Am J Med* 1978;64:933–936.
58. Richman A, Su E, JR. Ho G, Jr. Reciprocal relationship of synovial fluid volume and oxygen tension. *Arthritis Rheum* 1981;24:701–705.
59. Parker R, Schmid F. Antibacterial activity of synovial fluid during therapy of septic arthritis. *Arthritis Rheum* 1971;14:96–104.
60. Jose J, Moss I, Maini R, et al. Measurement of the chemotactic complement fragment C5a in rheumatoid synovial fluids by radioimmunoassay: role of C5a in the acute inflammatory phase. *Ann Rheum Dis* 1990;49:747–752.
61. Kim H, McCarty DJ, Kozin F, et al. Clinical significance of synovial fluid total hemolytic complementary activity. *J Rheumatol* 1980;7:143–152.
62. Fostiropoulos G, Austen K, Bloch K. Total hemolytic complement (CH) and second component of complement (C2) activity in serum and synovial fluid. *Arthritis Rheum* 1965;8:219–232.
63. Hedberg H. The depressed synovial complement activity in adult and juvenile rheumatoid arthritis. *Acta Rheum Scand* 1964;10:109–127.
64. Pekin TJ, Zvaifler N. Hemolytic complement in synovial fluid. *J Clin Invest* 1964;43:1372–1382.
65. Bunch T, Hunder G, Offord K, et al. Synovial fluid complement: usefulness in diagnosis and classification of rheumatoid arthritis. *Ann Intern Med* 1974;81:32–35.
66. Pekin TJ, Zvaifler N. Synovial fluid findings in systemic lupus erythematosus (SLE). *Arthritis Rheum* 1970;13:777–785.
67. Punzi L, Calo L, Plebani M. Clinical significance of cytokine determination in synovial fluid. *Crit Rev Clin Lab Sci* 2002;39:63–88.
68. Punzi L, Bertazzolo N, Pianon M, et al. Value of synovial fluid interleukin-1 beta determination in predicting the outcome of psoriatic monoarthritis. *Ann Rheum Dis* 1996:642–644.
69. Rooney M, Varsani H, Martin K, et al. Tumour necrosis factor alpha and its soluble receptors in juvenile chronic arthritis. *Rheumatology (Oxford)* 2000;39:432–438.
70. Youssef P, Haynes D, Triantafillou S, et al. Effects of pulse methylprednisolone on inflammatory mediators in peripheral blood, synovial fluid, and synovial membrane in rheumatoid arthritis. *Arthritis Rheum* 1997;40:761–767.
71. Yanni G, Nabil M, Farahat M, et al. Intramuscular gold decreases cytokine expression and macrophage numbers in the rheumatoid synovial membrane. *Ann Rheum Dis* 1994;53:315–322.
72. Taylor P, Peters A, Paleolog E, et al. Reduction of chemokine levels and leukocyte traffic to joints by tumor necrosis factor alpha blockade in patients with rheumatoid arthritis. *Arthritis Rheum* 2000;43:38–47.
73. Thomas R, Carroll G. Reduction of leukocyte and interleukin-1 beta concentrations in the synovial fluid of rheumatoid arthritis patients treated with methotrexate. *Arthritis Rheum* 1993;36:1244–1252.
74. Seward C, Osterland C. The pattern of anti-immunoglobulin activities in serum, pleural, and synovial fluids. *J Lab Clin Med* 1973;81:230–240.
75. Schellekens G, Visser H, de Jong B, et al. The diagnostic properties of rheumatoid arthritis antibodies recognizing a cyclic citrullinated peptide. *Arthritis Rheum* 2000;43:155–163.
76. Schellekens G, de Jong B, van den Hoogen F, et al. Citrulline is an essential constituent of antigenic determinants recognized by rheumatoid arthritis-specific autoantibodies. *J Clin Invest* 1998;101:273–281.
77. Vincent C, Simon M, Sebbag M, et al. Immunoblotting detection of autoantibodies to human epidermins filaggrin: a new diagnostic test for rheumatoid arthritis. *J Rheumatol* 1998;25:835–837.
78. Reparon-Schuijt C, van Esch W, van Kooten C, et al. Secretion of anticitrulline-containing peptide antibody by B lymphocytes in rheumatoid arthritis. *Arthritis Rheum* 2000;44:41–47.
79. Youinou P, Le Goff P, Colaco C, et al. Antikeratin antibodies in serum and synovial fluid show specificity for rheumatoid arthritis in a study of connective tissue diseases. *Ann Rheum Dis* 1985;44:450–454.
80. Schmidt-Rohlfing B, Thomsen M, Niedhart C, et al. Correlation of bone and cartilage markers in the synovial fluid with the degree of osteoarthritis. *Rheumatol Int* 2002;21:193–199.
81. Silverman B, Cawston T, Page Thomas D, et al. The sulphated glycosaminoglycan levels in synovial fluid aspirates in patients with acute and chronic joint disease. *Br J Rheumatol* 1990;29:340–344.

82. Kraus V, Heubner J, Fink C, et al. Urea as a passive transport marker for arthritis biomarker studies. *Arthritis Rheum* 2002;46:420–427.
83. Heuck A, Steiger P, Stoller D, et al. Quantification of knee joint fluid volume by MR imaging and CT using three-dimensional data processing. *J Comput Assist Tomogr* 1989;13:287–293.
84. Cimmino M, Innocenti S, Livrone F, et al. Dynamic gadolinium-enhanced magnetic resonance imaging of the wrist in patients with rheumatoid arthritis can discriminate active from inactive disease. *Arthritis Rheum* 2003;48:1207–1213.
85. Gerster J, Landry M, Dufresne L, et al. Imaging of tophaceous gout: computed tomography provides specific images compared with magnetic resonance imaging and ultrasonography. *Ann Rheum Dis* 2002;61:52–54.
86. Farina A, Filippucci E, Grassi W. Sonographic findings for synovial fluid. *Reumatismo* 2002;54:261–265.
87. Wu Y, Wu T, Liu Y, et al. Correlation of acoustic velocity of synovial fluid with markers of inflammation in arthritic patients. *J Formos Med Assoc* 2001;100:631–634.
88. Gu J, Rihl M, Marker-Hermann E, et al. Clues to pathogenesis of spondyloarthropathy derived from synovial fluid mononuclear cell gene expression profiles. *J Rheumatol* 2002;29:2159–2164.
89. Uchida T, Fukawa A, Uchida M, et al. Application of a novel protein biochip technology for detection and identification of rheumatoid arthritis biomarkers in synovial fluid. *J Proteome Res* 2002;1:495–499.

CHAPTER 5

Arthroscopy

Andrew L. Concoff and Kenneth C. Kalunian

Arthroscopic examination of joints enables the clinician to visualize articular cartilage and synovium with minimal operative risk and expense. It can be performed by rheumatologists in an office setting with local anesthesia and conscious sedation. Arthroscopy, which has been applied to most major joints and recently adapted in the form of miniarthroscopy to the small joints of the hands, allows the trained clinician to visualize intraarticular pathology in patients with osteoarthritis (OA) and inflammatory arthritis. As a diagnostic tool, arthroscopy can provide explanations for pain in an individual patient with symptoms that are unresponsive to conventional management and provide physician-scientists with a better understanding of the pathophysiologic mechanisms of arthritis. Arthroscopy also permits treatment of intraarticular abnormalities associated with arthritis, including the removal of loose bodies, débridement of frayed cartilage, and removal of proliferative synovitis. Arthroscopy also may have a role in the identification and treatment of a subset of those with OA of the knee at risk for more rapid cartilage deterioration as a consequence of the presence of proliferative synovitis.

HISTORICAL BACKGROUND

Development of Arthroscopy as a Diagnostic Tool

Arthroscopy was initially developed as an adjunct to physical examination for the diagnosis of joint disorders. Using a cystoscope in 1913, Bircher performed endoscopic examinations of cadaveric knee joints in Switzerland to diagnose meniscal injuries (1). He reported the results of knee arthroscopies in 18 patients, and was able to accurately diagnose abnormalities in 13 cases using subsequent arthrotomy as the standard of comparison (1). He introduced several important principles that are still practiced today, including joint distention for adequate visualization, vascular compression to develop a bloodless field, and the insertion technique for the arthroscope (1). Takagi (2), in 1920, developed an arthroscope in Japan to diagnose early knee tuberculosis. His instrument was large and impractical, but he subsequently incorporated a lens system into a smaller-diameter system. He published the first arthroscopic photographs of the knee in 1932 and introduced an arthroscope that was suitable for obtaining synovial biopsy samples (2). Burman, Finkelstein, and Mayer performed numerous cadaver experiments in New York in the early 1930s, which led to descriptions of various knee arthroscopic approaches (3). Because there were technical deficiencies associated with these approaches, skepticism developed in the orthopedic community, and these descriptions were never published. Watanabe, a student of Takagi, refined arthroscopic techniques and published the *Atlas of Arthroscopy* in 1957 (4). This atlas stimulated international interest in the procedure, but it did not gain widespread application until Watanabe developed several refined arthroscopes in the early 1970s (5).

Development of Arthroscopy as a Therapeutic Tool

Watanabe developed arthroscopy into an interventional tool by removing a suprapatellar pouch tumor under arthroscopic guidance in 1955. He performed the first arthroscopic meniscectomy in 1962 (1). McGinty subsequently introduced video camera–assisted arthroscopy that enabled the projection of intraarticular images onto a television screen. This contribution significantly improved the field of interventional arthroscopy by allowing the operator to perform more varied procedures in less time and with fewer complications (6). By introducing motorized operative instruments and describing arthroscopic procedures directed at cartilage lesions, Johnson provided clinicians with an extensive array of interventional arthroscopic options (7). Interventional arthroscopy has become more cost-effective in recent years and is now associated with less perioperative morbidity, time lost from work, rehabilitation time, and expense compared with similar procedures performed by arthrotomy. It is also associated with improved postoperative range of motion compared with arthrotomy (8). Due to these factors, therapeutic arthroscopy has become the most frequently performed orthopedic operative procedure in North America, with an estimated 1.4 million arthroscopies performed in 1990 (9).

Rheumatologists as Arthroscopists

Rheumatologists have long had an interest in arthroscopy as a diagnostic and therapeutic tool for patients with arthritis. This interest stems from a relative lack of understanding of the pathophysiologic processes responsible for rheumatic diseases and the inadequacy of current management strategies. Rheumatologists used arthroscopic techniques in the 1960s and 1970s to describe the intraarticular anatomy of several chronic rheumatic conditions (10,11). However, it was not until recently that rheumatologists began to use this tool to a significant extent for diagnostic and therapeutic purposes (12,13). Arthroscopy can be performed in an office setting with the patient receiving only local anesthesia and mild systemic sedation (12).

In addition to the potential utility of arthroscopy as a clinical tool, the procedure has importance for the field of rheumatology from an academic perspective. Arthroscopy can provide the physician-scientist with a means of better defining the anatomy and pathophysiology of articular components and can clarify the relationship between clinical signs and symptoms and pathoetiologic mechanisms. Arthroscopy provides the rheumatologist-arthroscopist with the ability to directly inspect intraarticular anatomy and to sample tissues with visual guidance. Tissue sampling by this technique allows the researcher to study histologic characteristics of the synovium and to identify cytokine patterns, disease-associated gene expression "signatures," crystalline particles, and microorganisms in synovium. These findings can then be correlated with intraarticular descriptions to better understand the mechanisms of disease in both inflammatory arthritides and OA.

Rheumatologists have typically avoided sampling articular cartilage via biopsy because of fears of establishing a nidus for cartilage degeneration. Recent research seems to support these concerns, as focal cartilage defects have been identified as an early manifestation of OA (14) and persistent defects in mechanical properties of cartilage have been identified in animal models following harvest of cartilage that mimicked those performed in anticipation of autologous chondrocyte implantation (15). Strict avoidance of cartilage biopsy represents a significant impediment to progress in articular cartilage research, as it necessitates the use of residual tissue from joint replacement, cadaveric tissue, or animal models of OA in order to investigate pathophysiologic processes. However, ethical prohibitions to performing such biopsies are supported by the potential for the focal lesions generated by biopsy to not only fail to heal adequately, but also to initiate events negatively affecting the surrounding cartilage.

In order to describe intraarticular pathology in qualitative and quantitative terms, two instruments for describing and grading cartilage and synovium (16,17) have been developed by rheumatologist-arthroscopists for use in knee OA. The Société Francaise d'Arthroscopie (SFA) system (18–21) has been validated using a global visual analogue scale as the standard of comparison; the instrument has been shown to have significant inter- and intra-rater reliability and is sensitive to change for cartilage damage. A scoring system has been proposed as an adjunct to the SFA instrument for assessing synovial abnormalities in knee OA; validation studies have been conducted (22).

The SFA arthroscopic damage scoring system has been used before and after therapeutic interventions as the primary outcome measure in two longitudinal trials of disease progression in OA (16,17), including a multicenter, international trial of a putatively chondroprotective nonsteroidal antiinflammatory drug (NSAID) (17). In each trial, the arthroscopic scoring system identified changes that were not recognized by plain radiography. Given the recent recognition that no plain radiographic protocol bears adequate validation and clinimetric properties to serve as the primary outcome measure in such trials of cartilage loss in OA over time (23), and the lack of an effective alternative criterion standard, it is difficult to determine whether the SFA scoring is superior to the plain radiographic protocols to which it has been compared or whether the SFA system is "overly sensitive," recognizing clinically irrelevant changes in cartilage appearance.

Two longitudinal studies of knee OA have addressed the utility of magnetic resonance imaging (MRI) versus arthroscopy in following the progression of disease; these two studies have yielded conflicting results (24,25). In the first study (24), arthroscopy was compared with MRI in assessing change over a 1-year time period in patients with knee OA. Results from both arthroscopy and MRI were recorded using the SFA recording system. Only the MRI-based SFA scoring demonstrated statistically significant progression over the course of the 1-year study, suggesting superior responsiveness. Contrary to this finding, the second study (25) used MRI with three-dimensional spoiled gradient-echo sequences with fat suppression and failed to demonstrate any progression after 3 years. Furthermore, observer agreement in MRI-based analysis of cartilage grading in knee OA has been criticized as "slight" or "poor" (26,27), whereas observer agreement in SFA grading of cartilage damage by arthroscopy has been deemed inexact (28). Thus, it is evident that uncertainty persists in the clinimetrics of both arthroscopy-based and MRI-based assessments of cartilage damage for OA, and comparisons between MRI and arthroscopic evaluations of progression appear to be tenuous. Finally, in the absence of long-term follow-up, it is not clear from these studies whether progression to clinically meaningful end points, such as end-stage disease requiring total knee arthroplasty, is better predicted by short-term progression of MRI- or arthroscopic-based cartilage damage scores.

With the support of the American College of Rheumatology (ACR), the ACR/Knee Arthroscopy Osteoarthritis Score (ACR/KAOS) has been developed and validated for intrarater reliability (29); sensitivity to change testing is currently being studied. ACR/KAOS is based on existing systems (29–34) and describes intraarticular knee cartilage and synovial pathology in OA. The SFA and an early version of the ACR/KAOS have been compared with each other and visual analogue scoring systems in terms of their relative interrater reliability in describing knee OA cartilage damage (30). Videotapes of knee arthroscopies on five patients with knee OA of different levels of severity of cartilage damage were analyzed by nine rheumatologist-arthroscopists prior to (pretraining evaluation) and 2 months after a 6-hour training session (posttraining evaluation). At the pretraining evaluation, the SFA grading system provided the highest coefficient of reliability ($r = 0.94$). At the posttraining evaluation, there were observed improvements in the SFA coefficients of reliability; however, improvements were not observed for the ACR system. This prompted changes in the ACR instrument, but subsequent comparative studies have not been conducted. However, the interobserver reliability of the SFA system has also been criticized as a consequence of the results of another trial (28). It appears that scoring changes in damage using serial arthroscopic examinations for an interventional longitudinal clinical study should be performed in such a way that a single observer blindly and randomly reviews all arthroscopie, so that the effect of poor interrater reliability is avoided.

DIAGNOSTIC USES OF ARTHROSCOPY FOR ARTHRITIS PATIENTS

Joint Inspection

The most common diagnostic purpose of arthroscopy is the identification of intraarticular anatomic abnormalities responsible for joint symptoms. Alternatives to diagnostic arthroscopy include arthrography, computed tomography (CT), and MRI.

Despite arthrography being less expensive and more widely available than the other techniques, it is insensitive and nonspecific for many of the intraarticular abnormalities seen in patients with arthritis (35,36). Degenerative meniscal tears, which are common in patients with knee OA, cannot be diagnosed with this technique because the central meniscal edge is not adequately visualized (37). Articular cartilage and synovial lesions are difficult to assess by CT techniques (38).

Diagnostic arthroscopy in recent years has been used less frequently amid reports of the diagnostic accuracy of MRI, which is a less invasive and less expensive procedure (39–43). Studies of the relative accuracies of MRI and arthroscopy have primarily concentrated on mechanical derangements related to athletic injuries in the younger patient. Studies of MRI in this patient population reveal diagnostic accuracies of up to 98% for both meniscal and anterior cruciate ligament abnormalities (44). However, MRI appears to be less accurate when studies use double-blind design and when arthroscopic findings are considered to be the standard of comparison. Raunest et al. (45) noted that MRI had a diagnostic accuracy of 72% for meniscal tears when compared with arthroscopy in a double-blind design in patients suspected of having meniscal disease. The average age of the population studied was 40.9 years. Glashow et al. (46) noted MRI to have a positive predictive value of 75%, a negative predictive value of 90%, a sensitivity of 83%, and a specificity of 84% for meniscal pathology when compared with arthroscopic findings in a double-blind study of patients with a mean age of 36 years. This study noted the sensitivity and specificity of MRI for complete anterior cruciate ligament tears to be 61% and 82%, respectively. Potter et al. (47) compared specialized spin-echo MRI with arthroscopy in 88 patients with clinical injury; the average age of the patients was 38 years (range 23–82 years). Using arthroscopy as the gold standard, MRI had a sensitivity of 87%, a specificity of 94%, an accuracy of 92%, a positive predictive value of 85%, and a negative predictive value of 95% for detection of chondral lesions observed; interobserver variability was minimal. Kreitner et al. (48) prospectively compared 150 patients with proton density–weighted SE-sequence MRI to arthroscopy in patients with traumatic knee lesions. Using arthroscopy as the gold standard, diagnostic accuracy ranged from 77% to 92% for meniscal lesions, 91% to 100% for cruciate ligament lesions, and 73% to 85% for hyaline cartilage defects.

Several studies have addressed the relative accuracies of MRI and arthroscopy in patients with OA. Blackburn et al. (49) compared MRI and small-caliber arthroscopy performed by rheumatologist-arthroscopists for the evaluation of articular cartilage abnormalities in patients with knee OA. The Pearson correlation coefficient of MRI and arthroscopic scores of articular cartilage abnormalities was 0.40, with 32.5% of the MRI cartilage scores being at least two grades less than the corresponding arthroscopic scores, and with 18.8% of the MRI scores indicating normal or grade 1 cartilage lesions when the arthroscopic score indicated severe abnormalities (grades 3 or 4). Drape et al. (50) studied the validity and reliability of T_1-weighted three-dimensional gradient-echo MRI for quantification of articular cartilage damage in knee OA. In 43 patients fulfilling ACR criteria for knee OA, tibiofemoral articular cartilage abnormalities were blindly quantified by MRI and arthroscopic images using the SFA instrument. There was statistically significant correlation between the SFA arthroscopy and SFA MRI scores ($r = 0.83$).

Other recent studies have advocated the use of novel imaging protocols to improve sensitivity and specificity of MRI for articular cartilage (reviewed in references 51 and 52). In general, the discordance between the rapid pace of technologic advances in the field and the slow progress of osteoarthritic cartilage loss has created a recurring theme of new, unvalidated MRI protocols being advocated to displace better-studied but outdated ones. The result has been that no single imaging protocol has been fully validated and accepted for longitudinal use and that MR evaluation of cartilage is a "moving target" with respect to the available arthroscopic scoring systems.

Whereas arthroscopy appears to preferentially detect certain abnormalities associated with knee OA, few studies have compared the relative diagnostic accuracies of MRI and arthroscopy for synovial abnormalities associated with OA. Similarly, few studies have compared the diagnostic capabilities of these two modalities for cartilage, ligament, or synovial abnormalities in other osteoarthritic joints or in other rheumatologic diseases including rheumatoid arthritis (RA) (53) and juvenile RA (JRA) (54). One small study investigated the accuracy of MRI in assessing synovitis as compared with microscopic and intraoperative macroscopic assessments (53). Good correlation (the Spearman $\sigma = 0.55$, $p < 0.001$) was observed between MRI-determined synovial volumes and histologic assessment of synovitis from biopsy, as well as between MRI-assessed synovitis and a qualitative scale (0 = no synovitis, 1 = mild synovitis, 2 = mild synovitis, and 3 = severe synovitis) describing the appearance of the synovium at arthroscopy for synovectomy (n = 9) or arthrotomy for total knee replacement (n = 33) ($\sigma = 0.40$, $p = 0.05$). A similarly strong correlation between MRI-based and arthroscopically assessed synovitis has been reported to exist in juvenile chronic arthritis (reviewed in reference 54). Further studies comparing arthroscopy with newer MRI protocols, including those using contrast agents, are needed. More complete assessments comparing the two modalities using cost-effective and risk-benefit analysis are necessary.

Rheumatologists have reported anatomic descriptions of OA involving the knee during diagnostic knee arthroscopy. The focus of these reports has been on synovial and articular cartilage abnormalities. Ike (55) presented data on 32 knees in 29 patients with OA who had undergone arthroscopy because of chronic pain and sought to define relationships between radiographic, clinical, and intraarticular abnormalities. Meniscal abnormalities were common, with most located in the posterior horn of the medial meniscus, and were associated with degree of articular cartilage damage in the compartment containing the meniscus and with joint space narrowing on weight-bearing knee radiographs. Lateral joint space narrowing on weight-bearing radiographs predicted the presence of chondrocalcinosis as seen by arthroscopy.

Klashman et al. (56) noted the presence of positively birefringent extracellular crystals in the irrigant fluid in 77% of osteoarthritic knees undergoing arthroscopic irrigation for pain refractory to NSAIDs, analgesics, and physical therapy. None of these patients had evidence of chondrocalcinosis on standard radiographs, but several had macroscopic intraarticular evidence of crystalline material

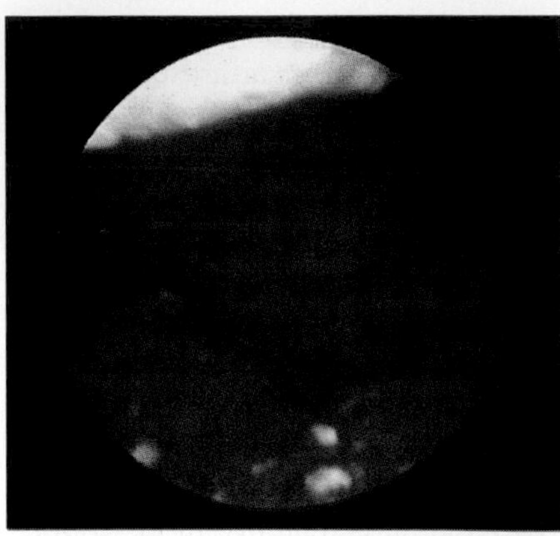

FIG. 5.1. Crystalline material noted in the suprapatellar patch in association with synovial proliferation in a patient with osteoarthritis as visualized with a 2.7-mm office arthroscope.

(Fig. 5.1). All patients with crystalline material in their irrigant fluid had intense synovial proliferation restricted to the area immediately proximal to the femoral trochlea in the suprapatellar pouch (Fig. 5.2), and the patellofemoral articular cartilage was more severely damaged than other articular surfaces of these knees. Patients without crystalline material in the irrigant did not have this synovial proliferation. Studies are underway to characterize the crystalline material and to define its presence in the proliferative synovial matrix.

Synovial Biopsy

Sampling of synovial tissue is another potential diagnostic use for arthroscopy. From a clinical viewpoint, the utility of assessing synovial pathology is controversial, with more frequent use in Europe than in the United States; however, synovial sampling is useful for research purposes. Studies

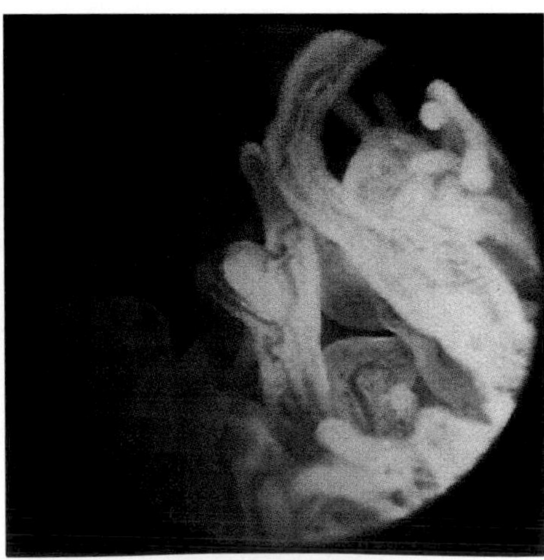

FIG. 5.2. Synovial proliferation proximal to the femoral trochlea in the suprapatellar pouch in a patient with osteoarthritis as visualized with a 2.7-mm office arthroscope.

have used synovial tissue obtained by arthroscopy to assess for the presence of mycoplasma and chlamydia in patients with early RA using culture, immunohistochemistry, *in situ* hybridization, and polymerase chain reaction techniques; to analyze the role of T-cell effector pathways in early versus established RA; and to study the mechanisms of action of biologic therapeutic agents in RA at the tissue level (57). Studies of the suprapatellar synovial proliferative response, seen in the OA patients described by Klashman et al. (56), are using arthroscopically guided synovial tissue sampling techniques. These research studies may identify subsets of arthritis patients who might benefit from therapy that targets specific markers such as microorganisms or crystalline material. It may become clinically important to use synovial sampling to identify these subsets.

Arthroscopic synovial sampling offers several advantages compared to sampling with the closed-needle technique. First, visually guided sampling using arthroscopy allows for the sampling of the region that appears to be most abnormal (33,58). There is a risk for missing significant abnormalities if sampling is performed with a closed-needle technique because synovial pathology is not distributed equally throughout the joint. Lindblad and Hedfors (33) noted the presence of isolated areas of synovial proliferation in OA patients, and Klashman et al. (56) confirmed this finding. Second, visually guided synovial sampling by arthroscopy allows for greater yield. Sampling by closed-needle technique frequently results in an inadequate amount of tissue. Rooney et al. (59) noted that out of 36 synovial tissue samplings by blind closed-needle technique, 7 resulted in inadequate tissue. By contrast, Moreland et al. (60) were successful in obtaining adequate tissue for research protocols with visually guided arthroscopic sampling in 51 consecutive knees. Third, visually guided sampling allows the arthroscopist to assess the extent and macroscopic character of the synovial proliferation and allows a correlative description of corresponding ligament, meniscal, and articular cartilage pathology. Youseff et al. (61) evaluated microscopic measures of inflammation in RA synovial tissue samples selected at arthroscopy compared with those obtained blindly by needle biopsy from the suprapatellar pouch of the same patient. Most microscopic measures of inflammation in synovial tissue samples obtained blindly were similar to those determined in samples obtained at arthroscopy; however, measurements in samples from the suprapatellar pouch may underestimate the intensity of macrophage infiltration in areas more adjacent to cartilage. This finding suggests that arthroscopically directed biopsy may allow sampling of the more intense area of inflammation.

Diagnostic Indications

Diagnostic indications for arthroscopy in patients with arthritis are based on specific clinical situations. Usually these are based on diagnostic uncertainty or symptoms unresponsive to conventional therapeutic modalities. Findings noted during diagnostic arthroscopy can guide the clinician in the development of a therapeutic plan for the patient. Certain surgical therapeutic interventions can be undertaken as part of the arthroscopy, while pharmacologic interventional plans can be based on macroscopic findings noted at arthroscopy or on findings based on synovial biopsy results. Although the clinical indications for diagnostic arthroscopy have not been analyzed from a cost-effectiveness or outcome measurement perspective, the clinical patient subsets that appear to benefit from diagnostic arthroscopy include the following (Table 5.1): (a) OA with symptoms unresponsive to medical management, symptoms disproportionate to clinical findings or effusion, and intermittent catching episodes or transient locking episodes suggestive of the presence of a loose body or meniscal tear (62,63); (b) inflammatory arthritis with symptoms unresponsive to medical management or symptoms disproportionate to clinical findings; (c) acute infectious arthritis with negative cultures by arthrocentesis or signs and symptoms refractory to therapy despite appropriate antibiotic therapy and repeated closed drainage; and (d) inflammatory arthropathy of uncertain diagnosis (38).

OA patients with pain that is unresponsive to conventional therapy or disproportionate to clinical findings account for the majority of arthritis patients for whom diagnostic arthroscopy might be considered (38). The most common finding at arthroscopy in this group of patients is a complex meniscal tear, usually present in the posterior horn of the medial meniscus (39,55,52). This lesion is often associated with adjacent articular cartilage damage and perimeniscal synovitis (53). Meniscal tears may cause intermittent effusion, locking, or catching symptoms (64). In an osteoarthritic population, however, the accuracy with which clinical evaluation correctly identifies meniscal tears is limited (65,66). This is likely a consequence of symptoms elicited during provocative maneuvers being caused by distinct nonmeniscal, arthritis-related pathology (66). Of the clinical evaluations tested in one such study (66), only a positive McMurray test was positively correlated with the presence of an unstable meniscal tear at arthroscopy. In a subsequent study using a different cohort of subjects with

TABLE 5.1. *Suggested indications for needle or conventional arthroscopy in patients with arthritis*

Osteoarthritis
Symptoms unresponsive to medical management
Symptoms disproportionate to clinical findings
Effusion and/or intermittent catching or locking episodes suggestive of a loose body or meniscal tear
Inflammatory arthritis
Symptoms unresponsive to medical management
Symptoms disproportionate to clinical findings
Uncertain diagnosis
Acute infectious arthritis
Negative cultures by arthrocentesis
Symptoms and/or signs refractory to appropriate antibiotic therapy and repeated closed drainage

knee OA refractory to medical management (67), the same group of investigators identified a positive Steinmann test result, medial joint line tenderness, and the presence of an unstable meniscal tear as indicators of a favorable outcome from arthroscopic débridement.

Further complexity regarding the relationship between meniscal pathology and outcomes in OA of the knee was introduced by a recent trial (68) that raises questions concerning whether or not the presence of a meniscal tear by MRI has any relevance to symptoms or functional status. Bhattacharyya et al. (68) evaluated the prevalence of meniscal tears by MRI and the levels of pain by visual analogue scale and functional disability by the Western Ontario and McMaster University Osteoarthritis Index (WOMAC) score, among those with OA of the knee as compared with age-matched controls who presented with other medical problems. Surprisingly, 91% of those with symptomatic arthritis and 76% of the asymptomatic individuals were found to have a meniscal tear by MRI. Furthermore, the results indicated no differences in pain or disability between those with and without meniscal tears. If these results are confirmed, the routine use of MRI to evaluate meniscal integrity in subjects with an exacerbation of OA-related symptoms and the use of MRI-based evidence of meniscal tears as the sole indication for arthroscopy would appear to be inappropriate.

Knee OA is also often associated with the presence of loose bodies, which are fragments of articular cartilage that may cause destruction of intact articular cartilage when they become entrapped in the articulating surfaces (64). Loose bodies characteristically cause intermittent catching or transient episodes. Unlike locking symptoms characteristic of meniscal tears, the locking associated with loose bodies can usually be relieved by positional changes (64). Loose bodies occasionally ossify and can be visualized on standard radiographs; however, MRI or arthroscopy is required for the identification of noncalcified loose bodies (64). Although it appears that the diagnostic accuracy of arthroscopy is superior to MRI for meniscal tears associated with knee OA, studies of the relative diagnostic accuracies of these two modalities for loose bodies associated with OA have not been undertaken. Diagnostic arthroscopy, however, has advantages over MRI because identified loose bodies can be removed during the same procedure (38).

Other arthroscopic findings noted in OA patients with refractory symptoms include the presence of crystalline disease (56), articular cartilage damage that is more severe and extensive than predicted by clinical signs and standard radiographs (38), maltracking of the patella in the femoral trochlear groove (38), cruciate ligament damage (38), and focal areas of synovial proliferation that are usually associated with crystalline disease (56). Before pursuing arthroscopy, extraarticular sources of symptoms, including biomechanical abnormalities, osteochondritis dissecans, and avascular necrosis of bone, should be excluded (38).

Patients with inflammatory arthritis that is unresponsive to medical management or with symptoms disproportionate to clinical findings may have resistant inflammatory disease or intraarticular abnormalities caused by chronic synovitis (38). Chronic inflammation of synovium can tear or destroy adjacent menisci or cruciate ligaments (38). Rice bodies within the joint may cause persistent symptoms, as well as mechanical symptoms of catching and locking (38). Arthroscopic synovectomy is an attractive option to diminish such negative outcomes, particularly in subjects with inflammatory arthropathy that present with a single severely symptomatic large joint with otherwise well-controlled disease. In such cases, arthroscopic synovectomy may obviate the need for disease-modifying antirheumatic drug therapy. Ostergaard et al. (69) studied the accuracy of MRI in evaluating recurrence of synovitis following arthroscopic synovectomy for RA (n = 9) and non-RA (n = 6). MRIs obtained before the procedure and at 1 day, 7 days, 2 months, and 12 months after synovectomy demonstrated persistently reduced synovial burden. Clinical remission was found to correlate inversely with MRI synovial volume at 2 months. Baseline synovial volumes did not correlate with clinical response. Progression of erosion was uncommon and did not correlate with baseline MRI synovial volumes.

Because patients with inflammatory arthritis have a predisposition to infections related to their underlying disease or as a consequence of immunosuppressive therapy, septic arthritis must be considered in patients with persistent inflammation. Chronic septic arthritis may require synovial biopsy for adequate diagnosis (38). Septic arthritis is associated with negative synovial fluid cultures in 15% of cases (70). Diagnostic arthroscopy with visually guided synovial biopsy for culture may be helpful in these patients. If culture of the synovial biopsy tissue is negative, then the patient can be spared a prolonged hospitalization and parenteral antibiotics. Diagnostic arthroscopy may be helpful in identifying alternative explanations for signs and symptoms in patients with negative cultures by synovial biopsy, including crystalline disease, or monoarticular presentations of RA, or a spondyloarthropathy. Patients with septic arthritis noted on arthrocentesis may require diagnostic arthroscopy if there is no clinical response to appropriate antibiotics and repeated closed drainage. Arthroscopy can provide for improved irrigation and débridement of purulent synovial fluid (71) and can identify focal areas of synovial proliferation that may require synovectomy.

For patients with inflammatory arthritis of uncertain diagnosis, diagnostic arthroscopy is perhaps most useful in detecting chronic infections such as tuberculosis and fungal infections using visually guided synovial sampling (38). Diagnostic arthroscopy can also be helpful in this group of patients by establishing the presence of crystalline disease (56).

PROGNOSTIC VALUE OF ARTHROSCOPY IN ARTHRITIS PATIENTS

A recent study (72) suggests that the arthroscopic appearance of synovitis may have value as to the degree of progressive cartilage degradation that occurs over the following year. Upon blinded review of paired videotapes of arthroscopy of the knee in 498 cases, the identification of medial perimeniscal inflammatory synovium, defined as hyperemic, hypertrophic, and/or hypervascular changes, was associated with a significantly increased risk of progression of medial tibiofemoral cartilage damage as assessed by SFA score, defined as an increase of 4.5 units. Among those with inflammatory synovitis, 23.3% demonstrated progression, as compared to 13.1% with normal synovium ($p = 0.02$). This finding is consistent with previous work identifying increased risk for progression in association with a variety of putative biomarkers of inflammation, including ultrasensitive C-reactive protein, hyaluronic acid, and cartilage oligomeric matrix protein (reviewed in reference 73). The direct visualization of inflammatory synovium at arthroscopy may thus have prognostic value and may argue for the use of a regimen of medications with greater antiinflammatory potency, even in the face of a consequent increase in potential for side effects. This provocative interpretation, along with the suggestion that limited synovectomy may be appropriate for such cases to decrease progression, has not been subjected to a longitudinal trial. Efforts are underway to identify synovitis prior to arthroscopy through less invasive means, including ultrasonography with color flow Doppler (74), in order to identify members of the subgroup of patients with more inflammatory OA who might respond more favorably to arthroscopic intervention. A clinical algorithm for use in identifying such patients has been developed retrospectively (75), and a prospective trial to evaluate its performance is underway.

THERAPEUTIC USES OF ARTHROSCOPY FOR ARTHRITIS PATIENTS

Suggested therapeutic uses of arthroscopy for arthritis patients (Table 5.2) have included the removal of loose bodies and the repair of meniscal tears associated with OA; irrigation for removal of debris and/or crystals associated with OA; drainage of purulent material associated with septic arthritis; and débridement for patients with septic arthritis, inflammatory arthritis, and OA. However, these approaches have not been adequately subjected to cost-effectiveness or outcome measurement analysis in these patient populations. Meniscal tears cannot be adequately addressed using small-caliber arthroscopes and require conventional arthroscopic techniques (55,76).

TABLE 5.2. *Suggested therapeutic uses for arthroscopy in patients with arthritis*

Osteoarthritis
Loose body removal
Possibly irrigation in certain subsets of patients (94)
Possibly débridement in certain subsets of patients
Inflammatory Arthritis
Synovectomy
Infectious Arthritis
Irrigation
Synovectomy

Loose Body Removal

Short-term improvement in locking and giving way after arthroscopic removal of loose bodies is typically excellent, although caution must be exercised with arthritic patients regarding their expectations of the procedure. Improvement of the mechanical symptoms should be the goal, as opposed to relieving underlying symptoms, including pain, that are referable to the arthritis itself, rather than the presence of the loose body. No longitudinal studies have investigated the long-term effects of loose body removal on outcomes.

Joint Irrigation

Joint irrigation has been used therapeutically in patients with OA, with relief of pain attributed to the removal of debris from the joint space (3). Joint irrigation is an integral part of all arthroscopies. It is necessary to distend the joint for adequate visualization, and to remove blood and debris that would cloud viewing (77). Indirect evidence supports the concept that irrigation relieves pain in knee OA by removing cartilaginous particles. These indirect supporting data include demonstration of cartilage fragments in synovial fluid (78) and in the synovium (79) of osteoarthritic knees, observations that intraarticular administration of cartilage fragments induced OA in dogs (80) and rabbits (81), and *in vitro* demonstration of protease release from cultured monocytes challenged with cartilage fragments (82). Attempts to duplicate the lavage effect of the irrigation associated with arthroscopy dates to the 1940s with Watanabe's efforts at "articular pumping" (83), in which saline was repeatedly injected, removed, and reinstilled; 58 of 64 patients with knee OA undergoing this procedure had favorable results. Jungmichel et al. (84) noted a response to saline lavage without arthroscopic visualization in patients with knee OA.

Reports by Livesley et al. (85) and Ike et al. (77) support the concept that joint irrigation can be beneficial to patients with knee OA. Livesley compared 44 patients with OA who underwent arthroscopic irrigation using 2 L of saline with 42 patients with OA assigned to a program of physical therapy. Compared with the patients receiving physical therapy, those in the arthroscopic irrigation group experienced significant improvement in three different pain scores that were sustained over 12 months.

Ike et al. (77) evaluated the efficacy of tidal knee irrigation, a technique performed in an ambulatory setting using local anesthesia that involves joint irrigation similar to that accomplished at arthroscopy but without direct visualization. Saline was instilled in a tidal manner (cyclic joint distention followed by evacuation, repeated in small aliquots for a total of 1 L of saline) to disrupt intraarticular adhesions and mobilize debris from the joint. This multicenter single-blind, randomized prospective trial compared tidal knee irrigation and comprehensive medical management (isometric exercises, joint protection, and individually adjusted antiinflammatory or analgesic medications) with comprehensive medical management alone in 77 patients with definite knee OA. Patients fulfilled clinical and radiographic ACR criteria for knee OA, but no patients had severe class IV radiographic disease as defined by Kellgren and Lawrence (86). In this 14-week trial, significant improvements were noted in the following parameters among the patients randomized to irrigation plus medical management compared with patients receiving only medical management: pain after 50-foot walk; pain after four-stair climb; most intense pain in previous day; knee stiffness with inactivity; frequency of morning knee stiffness; knee tenderness; and assessments of therapeutic effectiveness by both patient and physician.

Bradley et al. (87) recently conducted a sham-controlled trial of tidal lavage in knee OA. One hundred eighty subjects were randomized to receive tidal or sham irrigation and were followed for 12 months. In both the sham and the tidal irrigation groups, a 14-gauge needle was inserted through the skin via a lateral suprapatellar portal. The needle was directed either to the level of the joint capsule without passing through it (sham irrigation group) or through the capsule into the suprapatellar pouch (tidal irrigation group). Tidal lavage followed, with surgical drapes obscuring the operative field from the patient's view. Subjects then received either a sham version of the cyclic lavage or the lavage itself, and assessment of the blinding reflected that nearly 90% of each group presumed that they had received the tidal irrigation. Baseline WOMAC scores were worse among those in the treatment arm. However, after adjusting for this difference in baseline level, no differences were noted between those in the sham and tidal lavage groups. Thus, the researchers attributed the observed improvements to the placebo effect, more specifically, the Hawthorne effect, wherein subjects' scores improve over the course of a trial as a consequence of their knowledge that observations are being made.

Three studies have investigated the incremental benefit achieved by combining arthroscopic irrigation with administration of intraarticular medication. Ravaud et al. (88) evaluated the efficacy of joint lavage and intraarticular steroid injection alone and in combinations in the treatment of patients with knee OA. Ninety-eight patients with symptomatic tibiofemoral OA were enrolled in a 24-week prospective, randomized trial. There were four treatment groups: intraarticular placebo, intraarticular corticosteroids, joint lavage and intraarticular placebo, and joint lavage and intraarticular corticosteroids. Patients who underwent joint lavage had significantly improved pain visual analogue scale scores at 6 months; patients treated with only corticosteroids had improvements noted at weeks 1 and 4, but had no long-term benefit. There were no functional improvements noted in any group after week 4.

Conflicting results have been obtained in two trials evaluating the combination of intraarticular hyaluronic acid derivatives and arthroscopic irrigation in OA of the knee (89,90). No differences in Hospital for Special Surgery Knee Scale, Knee Society Clinical Rating System, or a visual analogue pain scale were demonstrated by Edelson et al. (89) following the use of an intraarticular hyaluronic acid derivative or placebo following irrigation in 23 subjects with up to 2-year follow-up. However, Vad et al. (90) found that at an average follow-up of 1.1 years, subjects in the lavage and hyaluronic acid group exhibited significantly more successful outcomes (79.5%) than those receiving only the hyaluronic acid treatment (54%; $p < 0.05$).

Two studies have assessed the role of irrigation in symptomatic knee effusions related to RA (91,92). In a study of 60 knees, Srinivasan et al. (91) randomized patients to receive one of three treatments: intraarticular steroids, joint lavage (without arthroscopy), or joint lavage (without arthroscopy) and intraarticular steroids. All three treatments resulted in a reduction of pain and increased range of movement; however, patients who had joint lavage alone had less improvement compared with the other two groups at 3 months. In a nonrandomized study, Sharma et al. (92) assessed the efficacy of arthroscopic lavage in nine patients with RA exhibiting active knee synovitis; patients received intraarticular steroids through the arthroscope at the end of the procedures. Eight of nine patients had marked improvement in pain and walk time; these effects were maintained for 2 weeks.

Chang et al. (93) compared arthroscopic surgery and tidal knee irrigation in 32 patients with non-end-stage knee OA in a randomized, controlled study. All patients received continuous saline irrigation during the arthroscopic procedure and had interventions performed under arthroscopic guidance as indicated by findings noted at arthroscopy, including débridement of torn menisci and removal of meniscal and cruciate ligament fragments; synovectomy; and excision of loose articular cartilage fragments. Patients randomized to the tidal knee irrigation group received closed-needle lavage as described by Ike et al. (77). Measurements of outcome were made over a 12-month period of follow-up and included clinical parameters as evaluated by physician assessors blinded to treatment group, and subjective outcomes including pain and functional status measures using the Arthritis Impact Measurement Scales (AIMS). At 3 months of follow-up, there were no significant differences between the two treatment groups with regard to pain, either self-reported or observed; functional status; and patient and physician global assessments of disease activity. There were statistically significant improvements in knee tenderness and physician's global assessment scores at 12 months in the arthroscopy group; however, improvements were noted in 29% of patients in the arthroscopy group and 58% of patients in the tidal knee irrigation group at 12 months. Patients with tears involving the lateral meniscus or anterior horn of the medial meniscus were more likely to improve after arthroscopic surgery than were patients with other intraarticular pathology, although this trend did not reach significance in the small group assessed. The researchers concluded that arthroscopically guided removal of abnormal soft tissue did not generally lead to reductions in pain and knee dysfunction associated with non-end-stage knee OA beyond that achieved by closed-joint irrigation and that most patients with non-end-stage knee OA should be treated with nonsurgical approaches. They noted that unless arthroscopic surgery was found to be more effective than closed-needle irrigation in a subset of patients with particular intraarticular lesions and unless reliable diagnostic parameters (including clinical markers, imaging studies, and diagnostic small-caliber office arthroscopic findings) were established to identify this subset of patients, then arthroscopic débridement would not be warranted in patients with non-end-stage OA.

In order to directly evaluate the effect of the volume of irrigant fluid during arthroscopic procedures, Kalunian et al. (94) studied the effectiveness of visually guided arthroscopic irrigation in patients with early knee OA that was unresponsive to conservative management, including analgesics, NSAIDs, and physical therapy. In a large multicenter, prospective randomized study, 90 patients were randomized to receive either arthroscopic irrigation with 3 L of saline or the minimal amount of irrigation (<250 mL) required to perform arthroscopy. The primary outcome variable was aggregate WOMAC score. Although the study did not demonstrate an effect of irrigation on arthritis severity as measured by aggregate WOMAC scores, irrigation with the larger volume did have a significant effect on pain as measured by a visual analogue scale and the WOMAC pain subscale. By 12 months, both patients with and without intraarticular crystals had significant improvements in pain and aggregate WOMAC scores; patients with crystals had statistically greater improvements. The researchers concluded that visually guided irrigation may be a useful therapeutic option for relief of pain in patients with knee OA, particularly in those who have occult intraarticular crystals.

Débridement

Experience with arthroscopic synovectomy in patients with knee OA has been reported by several orthopedic groups; however, the effect of synovectomy on outcome has been difficult to assess because the reports generally have included patients who have undergone several simultaneous interventions, such as partial synovectomy, meniscal débridement, removal of osteophytes and loose bodies, and shaving of eroded articular cartilage. Baumgaertner et al. (95) reported the results of arthroscopic débridement in 48 OA knees. In this study, 67% of patients had knee pain for more than 2 years; no patients had pain for less than 6 months, and all patients had failed conservative treatment, such as NSAIDs, analgesics, and physical therapy. Sixty-five percent of patients had radiographic evidence of tricompartmental disease; severe changes were noted in 69% of these patients, moderate changes were seen in 22%, and 9% had mild changes. Unicompartmental radiographic changes were noted in 35% of patients, of which 59% had severe changes, 35% had moderate changes, and 6% had mild changes. Eighty-six percent of patients had a partial synovectomy, 84% had a partial medial meniscectomy, 31% had osteophyte removal, 18% had a partial lateral meniscectomy, 14% had loose body removal, and 14% had abrasion chondroplasty.

Using symptoms as the outcome measurement, improvement was seen in 52% of patients and was maintained through the 33-month average follow-up period in 40% of the patients. Shorter duration of symptoms, mechanical symptoms, mild-to-moderate radiographic changes, and crystal deposition correlated with improvement; symptoms of longer duration, severe radiographic changes, and malalignment predicted poor outcome. Age, weight, compartment location of arthritis, and preoperative range of motion did not affect outcome.

Hubbard (96) prospectively compared arthroscopic débridement (n = 40) versus irrigation with 3 L of saline (n = 36) in 76 knees with isolated osteoarthritic changes of the medial femoral condyle of grades 3 or 4. The mean follow-up time was 4.5 years in the débridement group and 4.3 years in the irrigation group. At 1 year, 32 knees were pain free in the débridement group compared with 5 in the irrigation group. At 5 years, 19 of a total of 32 survivors were without pain in the débridement group compared with 3 of 26 in the irrigation group. The researchers concluded that arthroscopic débridement was superior to arthroscopic irrigation in knees with lesions of the medial femoral condyle of grades 3 or 5.

Ogilvie-Harris and Fitsialos (97) followed 291 patients for an average of 4 years, who had undergone arthroscopic procedures for knee OA, and separated patient subgroups by type of procedure performed. Partial synovectomy alone had been performed in 238 of the patients, meniscectomy and synovectomy in 148, meniscectomy alone in 18, abrasion chondroplasty alone in 32, and irrigation alone in 4. Using improvement in symptoms lasting greater than 2 years as the outcome measurement, the investigators found that patients who underwent synovectomy of only one compartment had a higher rate of symptom improvement than patients who had synovectomies of two compartments. Of patients who underwent synovectomy of only one compartment, 82% had improvement in symptoms lasting for greater than 2 years, whereas only 58% of patients undergoing synovectomy for two compartments had this response. Patients undergoing meniscectomy alone had the best results; 83% of these patients had improvement in pain lasting for more than 2 years. For all intervention groups, the worst results were noted in patients with chondrocalcinosis and in patients with bicondylar disease; malalignment was associated with poor outcome. Similar outcomes related to malalignment were found by Harwin (98) in a retrospective review of 204 knees with OA débrided arthroscopically and followed far a mean of 7.4 years. Harwin noted that patients with less than 5 degrees of malalignment had better outcomes than patients with greater malalignment. Given the recent work by Sharma et al. (99), the better outcomes after arthroscopy for those with more neutral alignment may actually mirror the underlying disease course rather than relating to a specific response to arthroscopy.

The retrospective design, lack of functional measurements of outcome, and lack of adequate controls, however, make interpretation of these studies difficult. Randomized controlled trials comparing different treatment groups with clinical, functional, and economic outcome measurements are necessary to understand the efficacy of interventions such as synovectomy, meniscectomy, and treatment combinations in OA.

A recent landmark trial has dramatically advanced knowledge of the therapeutic benefits of tidal lavage and arthroscopic irrigation and débridement in OA of the knee. Moseley et al. (100) block randomized 180 patrons of the Houston VA Medical Center, according to the severity of their OA of the knee, to receive either sham arthroscopy, arthroscopy with irrigation alone, or arthroscopy with irrigation and débridement. The lavage group received at least 10 L of fluid and underwent resection of unstable meniscal tears if present. The débridement group was also irrigated with at least 10 L of fluid, and underwent chondroplasty, shaving of tibial spine osteophytes if extension was blocked, and meniscal resection to a stable rim, but not abrasion arthroplasty, microfracture, or synovial resection. A well-designed sham arthroscopy intervention was used that included typical preparation and draping, the surgeon requesting relevant surgical tools and manipulating the knee in standard fashion, the creation of standard arthroscopy portals, and splashing of saline at appropriate times during the case. Outcomes assessed at baseline, 2 weeks, 6 weeks, 3 months, 6 months, 12 months, 18 months, and 24 months included a 12-item, self-reported knee-specific pain scale that was created for the study and was not formally validated, as well as pain and functional sections of the AIMS-2 and the SF-36, among others. No significant differences were noted for pain or function for any of the groups at any time point, because all groups improved to a similar degree, and the benefits noted were attributed to placebo effects. Unfortunately, no assessment of progression of cartilage damage was performed in the trial.

Several limitations are evident in this well-designed trial, many of which have been identified in an accompanying editorial (101). First, OA affects women more often than men, but because the study was performed at a Veterans Administration facility, 93% of those enrolled were men. Although significant differences have been noted in the manifestations of OA among men versus women (102), it is unlikely that a gender difference in response to arthroscopic intervention exists among those with OA of the knee because other, uncontrolled trials have shown no evidence for this possibility (103–105). Additionally, the primary outcome measure used in the trial reported by Moseley et al. (100), the knee-specific pain scale, was not validated prior to publication of the article. Because it is composed of several elements of better validated instruments, and because validated secondary outcome measures revealed no significant treatment effects, this is unlikely to be of great concern. Severity of disease was assessed radiographically according to a modification of the Kellgren and Lawrence system (86) involving summation of compartment scores. According to this system, only 31% of the subjects had mild disease. Given the disparity between arthroscopic and radiographic assessments of severity and the lack of availability of visualization of cartilage from the sham arthroscopy groups, it is unclear whether baseline cartilage damage was similar among the groups studied. Furthermore, the benefits of the lavage treatment may have been limited by failure to resect inflamed synovium or to perform abrasion arthroplasty or microfracture techniques. The study also differs from previous trials (94) that required failure of nonsurgical interventions including physical therapy, widely recognized as first-line therapy for OA of the knee, prior to enrollment. This factor may have increased the magnitude of the placebo effect seen in the sham arthroscopy group. The presence of mechanical symptoms and physical examination findings suggestive of meniscal tears was not assessed in the article. If a discrepancy in the distribution of such findings were present with more in the nondébridement groups, the impact of the débridement would be lessened. Although subjects in this trial all had OA of the knee, it is unclear whether future subgroup analysis (e.g., based on inflammation, obesity, malalignment, age, severity of disease, etc.) will identify those who are apt to exhibit a more robust response to arthroscopic intervention, and whether this response differs from that derived from sham arthroscopy. Finally, because the trial was not designed to assess progression of cartilage damage, structural assessments were not performed and no comment can be made as to the impact of the interventions on disease progression. A recent animal study (106) suggests that chondroplasty may worsen disease progression by adversely affecting the number of viable chondrocytes along the margins of débridement.

Completed studies of the efficacy of synovectomy in patients with inflammatory arthritis have involved limited outcome measurements and inadequate comparison groups. Traditionally, patients with inflammatory arthritis and resistant monoarticular synovitis have been referred to orthopedists for synovectomy by arthrotomy; however, synovectomy using arthroscopic techniques affords several advantages, including less morbidity and improved rehabilitation (12,107). Arthrotomy requires hospitalization, whereas arthroscopy can be performed as an outpatient procedure (107). Whereas patients commonly have arthrofibrosis with an average of 10 to 20 degrees of range of motion loss after arthrotomies, patients have preserved range of motion after arthroscopic synovectomies (8,12). Furthermore, synovectomy by arthrotomy requires both anterior and posterior incisions (8,12).

Cohen and Jones (108) prospectively studied nine patients with RA (10 knees) with chronic knee synovitis who underwent arthroscopic total synovectomy. All the patients had been unresponsive to medical therapy. Mean joint tenderness and swelling significantly improved from preoperative levels and were maintained for 12 months. Knee range of motion improved in all patients (mean 21 degrees). Patients with radiographic grade III or less using the Steinbrocker classification (109) had significant improvements in joint function in daily activity (knee pain with weight bearing, walking, rising from sitting position, climbing stairs, and getting out of bed). Klein and Jensen (8) followed the outcome of 44 knee joints in 43 patients after arthroscopic synovectomy for inflammatory arthritis unresponsive to conservative therapy for greater than 6 months; the mean postoperative follow-up period was 2.7 years. Postoperative pain, swelling, range of motion, walking distance, and patient satisfaction were the outcome measurements studied. Improvements in all clinical parameters were noted, but it is not clear if any of the improvements met statistical significance. Seventy-eight percent of patients were completely satisfied, 7% considered the procedure to be partially successful, and 15% were dissatisfied. Arthrofibrosis was not seen in these patients after the arthroscopic procedures.

Matsui et al. (110) compared the efficacies of arthroscopic synovectomy and synovectomy performed by arthrotomy in patients with RA involving the knee; follow-up periods were greater than 10 years. Patients had similar radiographic grades; however, preoperative clinical comparisons were not noted. After arthroscopic synovectomy, 82.9% of the knees were not painful and had normal function within the first 3 years, but only in 44.7% of the knees were these improvements sustained after 8 years. Similar results were noted in the arthrotomy group. Smiley and Wasilewski (111) studied the effects of arthroscopic synovectomy in 25 knees of 19 patients with inflammatory arthritis. Six months after the procedures, 24 of the 25 knees had good results defined as little or no pain, no effusion, unchanged or increased range of motion, and little or no limitation of activity. These results were maintained in 19 of the 21 knees evaluated at 2 years and in 8 of the 14 knees evaluated at 4 years.

Arnold (112) has noted similar results in 75% of knees of patients with RA undergoing arthroscopic synovectomy. In his series, improvement persisted for over 2 years if the procedure was performed early in the course of the disease; however, radiographic evidence of joint space narrowing (<2 mm in a weight-bearing anteroposterior projection) usually predicted a poor clinical response. Ogilvie-Harris and Basinski (113) have noted significant decreases in pain and synovitis in a study of arthroscopic knee synovectomies in 96 patients with RA followed over 2 to 4 years. Although Ochi et al. (114) have noted that patients with significant erosive disease continue to have radiographic evidence of bony destruction after synovectomy performed by arthrotomy, a large controlled study is needed to address the role of synovectomy as an intervention to prevent erosions in patients with earlier disease.

ARTHROSCOPIC PROCEDURES

Traditional arthroscopes consist of tubes ranging in size from 2.7 to 4.0 mm that contain a glass lens system. Using a high-powered light source delivered through a fiberoptic cable, the joint space is illuminated, and an image is transmitted from the joint space to a camera coupled to the arthroscope eyepiece and projected onto a video monitor (47). Modifications of this system have led to the development of fiberoptic cables that not only transmit light to the joint but also send the image back through the cable to a video camera.

Distention (for purposes of visualization and intraarticular hemostasis) and irrigation can be accomplished by the arthroscopist using a manual hand-held pump system or by using gravity for inflow and suction for outflow. The skin is anesthetized, as are the intraarticular structures; conscious sedation is generally used only when the procedure is performed in an operating room or if an anesthesiologist is present in a procedure room setting. When arthroscopy is performed in an office setting, small-caliber (1.6–1.8 mm) arthroscopes are generally used in order to decrease the incidence of infectious complications, whereas larger-caliber (2.7–4.0 mm) arthroscopes are generally used when the procedures are performed in an operating room setting. There are practicing rheumatologists who currently perform arthroscopy in office settings, others who perform the procedures in operating room settings, and some who perform the procedures in both settings. Small-caliber arthroscopy can accurately detect meniscal, articular cartilage, and synovial abnormalities, but tends to underestimate the severity of these lesions (55). Synovial sampling under visual guidance is accomplished with small-caliber arthroscopy in the office setting; however, resection of pathologic tissues requires the use of motorized shavers and hand-operated cutting and grasping instruments that are not appropriate for the office setting. More stringent precautions against infections are required for the use of these instruments because larger incisions are necessary. This level of sterility is not possible in the office setting.

Joints Examined

Although diagnostic and therapeutic arthroscopy for patients with arthritis has concentrated on the knee, small joints of the hand and feet, as well as olecranon and subacromial bursae, can be visualized with current arthroscopes. Arthroscopy techniques are used to visualize larger joints in patients with arthritis, such as the shoulder and elbow, although application of arthroscopic techniques to these areas requires advanced skills and training.

Complications

Complications of arthroscopy have been detailed in several articles. The rates of these adverse outcomes, when the procedure is performed by rheumatologists are listed in Table 5.3. Minor complications such as tenderness of the arthroscopic portals or postoperative effusion have been reported by Arnold to occur in less than 1% of patients (12). Reflex sympathetic dystrophy, deep venous thrombosis, and peroneal nerve palsies are rare and are usually associated with the use of a tourniquet for hemostasis (115). This form of hemostasis has been supplanted by the automated infusion pumps in operative arthroscopy and is not necessary for office arthroscopy. Postprocedure infection rates are less than 0.1% (115). Hemarthrosis is the most frequent arthroscopic complication, accounting for 23.5% of all complications reported in a survey of members of the Arthroscopy Association of North America (115). It most commonly occurs in procedures involving synovectomy and is rare in diagnostic office arthroscopies (12). Szachnowski et al. (116) retrospectively reviewed the complication rates associated with office arthroscopy in two community-based practices involving 335 arthroscopic procedures performed in 306 patients over a 35-month period. Of the 335 procedures, 131 were diagnostic and 204 were diagnostic and therapeutic. The complication rates for major and minor events were 1.2% and 12.8%, respectively. In another study, Rich et al. (111) addressed the safety of synovial biopsy using needle arthroscopy as performed by rheumatologist-arthroscopists for research purposes in patients with arthritis; there were no complications in 49 knee procedures.

Results from a series of arthroscopies performed at the University of California, Los Angeles (UCLA), by two rheumatologist-arthroscopists were recently reported (117).

TABLE 5.3. *Complications of arthroscopy by rheumatologists*

Minor (<1%)
Tenderness of arthroscopy portals
Effusion
Vasovagal reactions
Rare (probably <0.1%)
Septic arthritis
Hemarthrosis
Reflex sympathetic dystrophy
Deep venous thrombosis
Peroneal nerve palsy
Joint rupture

In their prospective report of complications in consecutive patients having knee arthroscopies performed over an 8-year period, a total of 342 knee arthroscopies were performed with six total complications, including major and minor events (1.8%), consisting of one each of seizure, gout, portal cellulitis, ankle pain, inadequate knee drainage, and vasovagal symptoms. There was no long-term morbidity or mortality secondary to the procedures. The difference between the UCLA complication rate and that reported by Szachnowski et al. may be due to differences in technique; all UCLA patients underwent arthroscopies in a sterile room with laminar flow, whereas the patients in the Szachnowski series underwent the procedures in an office setting. This suggests that knee arthroscopy performed by experienced rheumatologists trained in arthroscopy has a low rate of complications and that this rate may be even further minimized by the performance of the procedures in an operating room rather than an office setting.

Practice of Arthroscopy

Technical considerations require the rheumatologist interested in arthroscopy to acquire adequate training in order to obtain the necessary knowledge and skills to perform the procedure. In 1986, the American Rheumatism Association (ARA) adopted guidelines for the rheumatologist for the training and practice of arthroscopy. These guidelines include recommendations for privileging, training, practice, continuing education, and performance review of rheumatologists performing arthroscopy (Table 5.4). With this document, the ARA recognized the role of the rheumatologist as arthroscopist and established the basis for postfellowship preceptor training programs in arthroscopic techniques for practicing and academic rheumatologists. Based on a model developed at UCLA, the American College of Rheumatology has suggested quality assurance guidelines for use by rheumatologist-arthroscopists.

Research Potential

Rheumatologists trained in the performance of arthroscopy have several major challenges: assessment standards for the description of intraarticular pathology in different forms of arthritis must be further developed and validated, collaborative research efforts need to be expanded, and joints other than the knee need to be examined. Achievement of these goals will enable the rheumatology community to enhance its understanding of disease processes by studies of macroscopic and microscopic pathology. Sophisticated outcome measurement studies designed to understand the role of biologic agents at the tissue level or therapeutic arthroscopic interventions such as débridement or synovectomy may enable the rheumatologist to provide alternatives to conventional arthritis treatment protocols. Studies using arthroscopic techniques for the intraarticu-

TABLE 5.4 *American College of Rheumatology guidelines for the practice of arthroscopy by rheumatologists*

Training

Rheumatologists who perform arthroscopy should have appropriate training and must consistently document their experience. Evidence for adequate training in arthroscopy should include regular attendance of arthroscopic educational courses and successful completion of a fellowship training program in arthroscopy and/or experience with skilled arthroscopists. Experience in any or all of the above should be documented and skills may be demonstrated by observed performance, patient records, and peer review.

Performance

The arthroscopist should:

1. Perform a history and physical examination with specific attention to the joint to be arthroscoped, and summarize the data collected to support the patient's diagnosis, especially those features that may be confirmed or treated at arthroscopy.
2. Document all elements of the comprehensive management program directed at the patient's arthritis, the duration of time that this program has been used, and the specific reasons for performing the arthroscopy.
3. Explain the procedure to the patient, including benefits, possible risks, and complications, and how the arthroscopy will influence the comprehensive management program. For patients undergoing the procedure only for research purposes, the research should be approved by a human use committee. The arthroscopist should explain possible benefits that might accrue from incidental aspects of the procedure (e.g., lavage) and how future management decisions might be affected by the understanding of intraarticular anatomy gained at the procedure.
4. Select any therapeutic arthroscopic procedure to be used with due consideration for the type of arthritis and other therapeutic options available to the patient.
5. Prepare a report of the procedure that includes the interventions performed during the procedure itself and the findings, described in a consistent fashion that permit use of the arthroscopy report as a data source. Whenever possible, the videoarthroscopic portion of the procedure should be recorded.
6. Assure the continuity of the entire comprehensive management program while supervising the rehabilitation in the period following arthroscopy.

Additional Skills

Newly available small-bore arthroscopes ("needle" arthroscopes) can be used with patient undergoing only local anesthesia and mild systemic sedation. Rheumatologists who perform arthroscopy in an outpatient ambulatory setting must be responsible for several aspects of patient management that would be assumed by other specialists were the procedure performed in a conventional operation room setting. The needle arthroscopist should have expertise in these areas:

1. Infection control: including proper sterilization and handling of instruments, institutional guidelines regarding instrumentation that cannot be submitted to standard sterilization procedures, and care and protection of environmental surfaces contacted during the procedure.
2. Conscious sedation: including agents, actions, and institutional policy regarding monitoring of patients receiving these agents.
3. Recovery: including timing of release, instruction on postarthroscopy wound care and follow-up, assurance of transport and guidance home, provision of adequate analgesia, and plans for follow-up.

Continuing Education

The arthroscopist should maintain a high level of expertise in arthroscopy and be aware of the role of arthroscopy in the comprehensive management program for the patient with arthritis. In order to remain informed, the arthroscopist may update his or her knowledge and skill by regular attendance at postgraduate arthroscopic meetings, collaboration with other arthroscopists, and continual review of the current arthroscopic and rheumatologic literature. The arthroscopist should obtain additional necessary training before undertaking a new therapeutic procedure. In addition, the arthroscopist must maintain a high level of expertise in the pharmacologic and rehabilitative aspects of arthritis therapy as well as the latest advances in diagnostic testing for, and classification of, arthritis.

Privileges

The decision to grant and renew hospital privileges in arthroscopy is typically made by individual hospitals with input from medical staff committees and appropriate department chairpersons in accordance with individual hospital and medical staff bylaws, rules, and regulations. It is desirable to include in the decision-making process rheumatologists who have a working knowledge of diagnostic and therapeutic arthroscopy, as well as individuals with board certification in orthopedic surgery. The number of procedures, indications, results, and complications should be made available to appropriate medical staff committees at individual hospitals that are charged with granting, reviewing, and renewing clinical privileges.

lar delivery of agents targeting genetic factors, cartilage growth, and cytokine expression hold promise in revolutionizing the therapeutic approaches to arthritis patients.

REFERENCES

1. Strobel M, Eichhorn J, Schiebler W. *Basic principles of knee arthroscopy: normal and pathologic finds, tips and tricks.* Berlin: Springer-Verlag, 1992:2.
2. Takagi K. Practical experiences using Takagi's arthroscope. *J Jpn Orthop Assoc* 1933;8:132.
3. Burman MS, Finkelstein H, Mayer I. Arthroscopy of the knee joint. *J Bone Joint Surg Am* 1934;16:255–268.
4. Watanabe M, Takeda S, Ikeuchi H. *Atlas of arthroscopy.* 2nd edition. Berlin: Auflage Spinger, 1970.
5. Watanabe M. Arthroscopy: the present state. *Clin Orthop* 1979;10: 503–521.
6. McGinty JB, Friedman PA. Arthroscopy of the knee. *Clin Orthop* 1976;121:173–180.
7. Johnson LL, Becker RL. Arthroscopy, technique and the role of the assistant. *Orthop Rev* 1976;9:31–43.

8. Klein W, Jensen K-U. Arthroscopic synovectomy of the knee joint: indication, technique and follow-up results. *Arthroscopy* 1988;4:63–71.
9. McGinty JB, Johnson LL, Jackson RW, et al. Uses and abuses of arthroscopy: a symposium. *J Bone Joint Surg Am* 1992;74:1563–1577.
10. Jayson MI, Dixon AS. Arthroscopy of the knee in rheumatic diseases. *Ann Rheum Dis* 1968;27:503–511.
11. Altman RD. Arthroscopic findings of the knee in patients with pseudogout. *Arthritis Rheum* 1976;19:286–292.
12. Arnold WJ. Office-based arthroscopy. *Bull Rheum Dis* 1992;41:3–6.
13. Ike RW, O'Rourke KS. Detection of intra-articular abnormalities in osteoarthritis of the knee: a pilot study comparing needle arthroscopy with standard arthroscopy. *Arthritis Rheum* 1993;36:1353–1363.
14. Squires GR, Okouneff S, Ionescu M, et al. The pathobiology of focal lesion development in aging human articular cartilage and molecular matrix changes characteristic of osteoarthritis. *Arthritis Rheum* 2003; 48(5):1261–1270.
15. Lee CR, Grodzinsky AJ, Hsu HP, et al. Effects of harvest and selected cartilage repair procedures on the physical and biochemical properties of articular cartilage in the canine knee. *J Orthop Res* 2000;18(5): 790–799.
16. Listrat V, Ayral X, Patarnello F, et al. Arthroscopic evaluation of potential structure modifying activity of hyaluronan (Hyalgan) in osteoarthritis of the knee. *Osteoarthritis Cartilage* 1997;5:153–160.
17. Ayral X, Mackillop N, Genant HK, et al. Arthroscopic evaluation of potential structure-modifying drug in osteoarthritis of the knee: a multicenter, randomized, double-blind comparison of tenidap sodium vs piroxicam. *Osteoarthritis Cartilage* 2003;11:198–207.
18. Dougados M, Ayral X, Listrat V, et al. The SFA system for assessing articular cartilage lesions at arthroscopy of the knee. *Arthroscopy* 1994;10:69–77.
19. Ayral X, Gueguen A, Listrat V, et al. Simplified arthroscopy system for chondropathy of the knee (revised SFA score). *Rev Rhum* 1994; 61:88–90.
20. Ayral X, Dougados M, Listrat V. Chrondroscopy: a new method for scoring chondropathy. *Semin Arthritis Rheum* 1993;22:289–297.
21. Ayral X, Dougados M, Listrat V, et al. Arthroscopic evaluation of chondropathy in osteoarthritis of the knee. *J Rheumatol* 1996;23:698–706.
22. Ayral X, Mayoux-Benhamou A, Dougados M. Proposed scoring system for assessing synovial membrane abnormalities at arthroscopy in knee osteoarthritis. *Br J Rheumatol* 1996;35(suppl 3):14–17.
23. Brandt KD, Mazzuca SA, Conrozier T, et al. Which is the best radiographic protocol for a clinical trial of a structure modifying drug in patients with knee osteoarthritis? *J Rheumatol* 2002;29:1308–1320.
24. Pessis E, Drape J-L, Ravaud P, et al. Assessment of progression in knee osteoarthritis: results of a 1 year study comparing arthroscopy and MRI. *Osteoarthritis Cartilage* 2003;11:361–369.
25. Gandy SJ, Dieppe PA, Keen MC, et al. No loss of cartilage volume over three years in patients with knee osteoarthritis as assessed by magnetic resonance imaging. *Osteoarthritis Cartilage* 2002;10:929–937.
26. Drape JL, Pessis E, Auleley GR, et al. Quantitative MR imaging evaluation of chondropathy in osteoarthritic knees. *Radiology* 1998; 208(1):49–55.
27. McNicholas MJ, Brooksbank AJ, Walker CM. Observer agreement analysis of MRI grading of knee osteoarthritis. *J R Coll Surg Edinb* 1998;44:31–33.
28. Brismar BH, Wredmark T, Movin T, et al. Observer reliability in the arthroscopic classification of osteoarthritis of the knee. *J Bone Joint Surg Br* 2002;84B:42–47.
29. Klashman DJ, Ike R, Moreland L, et al. Validation of an osteoarthritis data report from for knee arthroscopy. *Arthritis Rheum* 1995;38 (suppl):178.
30. Ayral X, Gueguen A, Ike RW, et al. Inter-observer reliability of the arthroscopic quantification of chondropathy of the knee. *Osteoarthritis Cartilage* 1998;6:160–166.
31. Noyes FR, Stabler CL. A system for grading articular cartilage lesions at arthroscopy. *Am J Sports Med* 1989;17:505–513.
32. Yates DB, Scott JT. Rheumatoid synovitis and joint disease: relationship between arthroscopic and histologic changes. *Ann Rheum Dis* 1975;34:1–6.
33. Lindblad S, Hedfors E. Intra-articular variations in synovitis: local macroscopic and microscopic signs of inflammatory activity are significantly correlated. *Arthritis Rheum* 1985;28:977–986.
34. Paus AC, Pahle JA. Arthroscopic evaluation of the synovial lining before and after open synovectomy of the knee joint in patients with chronic inflammatory joint diseases. *Scand J Rheumatol* 1990;19: 193–201.
35. Bonamo JJ, Shulman G. Double contrast arthrography of the knee: a comparison to clinical diagnosis and arthroscopic findings. *Orthopedics* 1988;11:1041–1046.
36. Hall FM. Pitfalls in assessment of the menisci by knee arthrography. *Radiol Clin North Am* 1981;19:305–328.
37. Ekstrom JE. Arthrography: where does it fit in? *Clin Sports Med* 1990;9:561–566.
38. O'Rourke KS, Ike RW. Diagnostic arthroscopy in the arthritis patient. *Rheum Dis Clin North Am* 1994;20:321–342.
39. Chan WP, Lang P, Stevens MP, et al. Osteoarthritis of the knee: comparison of radiography, CT and MR imaging to assess extent and severity. *AJR* 1991;57:799–806.
40. McAlindon TEM, Watt I, McCrae F, et al. Magnetic resonance imaging in osteoarthritis of the knee: correlation with radiographic and scintigraphic findings. *Ann Rheum Dis* 1991;50:14–19.
41. Martel W, Adler RS, Chan K, et al. Overview: new methods in imaging osteoarthritis. *J Rheumatol* 1991;18(suppl 27):32–37.
42. Stollar DW, Genant HK. Magnetic resonance imaging of the knee and hip. *Arthritis Rheum* 1990;33:441–449.
43. Fischer SP, Fox JM, Del Pizzo W, et al. Accuracy of diagnoses from magnetic resonance imaging of the knee. *J Bone Joint Surg Am* 1991; 73:2–10.
44. Gluckert K, Kladny B, Blank-Schal A, et al. MRI of the knee joint with a 3-D gradient echo sequence: equivalent to diagnostic arthroscopy? *Arch Orthop Trauma Surg* 1992;112:5–14.
45. Raunest J, Oberle K, Lehnert J, et al. The clinical value of magnetic resonance imaging in the evaluation of meniscal disorders. *J Bone Joint Surg Am* 1991;73:11–16.
46. Glashow JL, Katz R, Schneider M, et al. Double-blind assessment of the value of magnetic resonance imaging in the diagnosis of anterior cruciate and meniscal lesions. *J Bone Joint Surg Am* 1989;71: 113–119.
47. Potter HG, Linklater JM, Allen AA, et al. Magnetic resonance imaging of articular cartilage in the knee. *J Bone Joint Surg Am* 1998;80: 1276–1284.
48. Kreitner KF, Hansen M, Schadmand-Fischer S, et al. Low field MRI of the knee joint: results of a prospective, arthroscopically controlled study. *Rofo Fortsch Gebiete Rontgenstrahlen Neuen Bildgebenden Verfahren* 1999;170:35–40.
49. Blackburn WD, Bernreuter WK, Rominger M, et al. Arthroscopic evaluation of knee articular cartilage: a comparison with plain radiographs and magnetic resonance imaging. *J Rheumatol* 1994;21:675–679.
50. Drape HL, Pessis E, Auleley GR, et al. Quantitative MR imaging evaluation of chondroplasty in osteoarthritic knees. *Radiology* 1998;208: 49–55
51. Loeuille D, Oliver P, Mainard D, et al. Magnetic resonance imaging of normal and osteoarthritic cartilage. *Arthritis Rheum* 1998;41(6): 963–975.
52. Waldschmidt JG, Braunstein EM, Buckwalter KA. Magnetic resonance imaging of osteoarthritis. *Rheum Dis Clin North Am* 1999;25 (2):451–465.
53. Ostergaard M, Stoltenberg M, Lovgren-Nielsen P, et al. Magnetic resonance imaging-determined synovial membrane and joint effusion volumes in rheumatoid arthritis and osteoarthritis: comparison with the macroscopic and microscopic appearance of the synovium. *Arthritis Rheum* 1997;40(10):1856–1867.
54. Graham TB, Blebea JS, Gylys-Morin V, Passo MH. Magnetic resonance imaging in juvenile rheumatic arthritis. *Semin Arthritis Rheum* 1997;27(3):161–168.
55. Ike RW. The role of arthroscopy in the differential diagnosis of osteoarthritis of the knee. *Rheum Dis Clin North Am* 1993;19:1–24.
56. Klashman DJ, Moreland LW, Ike RW, et al. Occult presence of CPPD crystals in patients undergoing arthroscopic knee irrigation for refractory pain related to osteoarthritis. *Arthritis Rheum* 1994;37(suppl):240.
57. Rich E, Calvo-Alen J, Koopman WJ, et al. Synovial biopsy by needle arthroscopy: a useful research tool. *Arthritis Rheum* 1995;38(suppl): 237.
58. Ike RW. Refractory knee arthritis: when to consider arthroscopy. *J Musculoskel Med* 1991;8:45–63.

59. Rooney M, Condell D, Quinlan W, et al. Analysis of the histologic variation of synovitis in rheumatoid arthritis. *Arthritis Rheum* 1988; 31:956–963.
60. Moreland LW, Calvo-Alen J, Koopman WJ. Synovial biopsy of the knee joint under direct visualization by needle-arthroscopy. *J Clin Rheumatol* 1995;1:103–109.
61. Youseff PP, Kraan M, Breedveld F, et al. Quantitative microscopic analysis of inflammation in rheumatoid arthritis synovial membrane samples selected at arthroscopy compared with samples obtained blindly by needle biopsy. *Arthritis Rheum* 1998;41:663–669.
62. Rand JA. Role of arthroscopy in osteoarthritis of the knee. *Arthroscopy* 1991;7:358–363.
63. Myers SL, Brandt KD, Ehlich JW, et al. Synovial inflammation in patients with early osteoarthritis of the knee. *J Rheumatol* 1990;17: 1662–1669.
64. Goldberg VM, Kettelkamp DB, Colyer RA. Osteoarthritis of the knee. In: Moskowitz RW, Howell DS, Goldberg VM, et al., eds. *Osteoarthritis: diagnosis and medical/surgical management.* Philadelphia: WB Saunders, 1992:605.
65. Kalunian KC, Arnold WJ, Klashman DJ, et al. Can physical signs or magnetic resonance imaging substitute for diagnostic arthroscopy in knee osteoarthritis patients with suspected internal derangements? A pilot study. *J Clin Rheum* 2000;6(3):123–127.
66. Dervin GF, Stiell IG, Wells GA, et al. Physicians' accuracy and interrater reliability for the diagnosis of unstable meniscal tears in patients having osteoarthritis of the knee. *Can J Surg* 2001;44(4):267–274.
67. Dervin GF, Stiell IG, Rodyt K, et al. Effect of arthroscopic debridement for osteoarthritis of the knee on health-related quality of life. *J Bone Joint Surg Am* 2003;85(1):10–19.
68. Bhattacharyya T, Gale D, Dewire P, et al. The clinical importance of meniscal tears demonstrated by magnetic resonance imaging in osteoarthritis of the knee. *J Bone Joint Surg Am* 2003;85A:4–9.
69. Ostergaard M, Ejberg B, Stoltenberg M, et al. Quantitative magnetic resonance imaging as a marker of synovial membrane regeneration and recurrence of synovitis after arthroscopic knee joint synovectomy: a one year follow up study. *Ann Rheum Dis* 2001;60(3):233–236.
70. Von Essen R, Holtta A. Improved method of isolating bacteria from joint fluids by the use of blood culture bottles. *Ann Rheum Dis* 1986; 45:454–457.
71. Broy SB, Stulberg SD, Schmid FR. The role of arthroscopy in the diagnosis and management of the septic joint. *Clin Rheum Dis* 1986;12:489–499.
72. Ayral X, Pickering EH, Woodworth TG, et al. Synovitis predicts the arthroscopic progression of medial tibiofemoral knee osteoarthritis. *Arthritis Rheum* 2001;44(suppl)(9):101.
73. Poole AR. NIH Osteoarthritis Initiative white paper on biomarkers. Accessed at *www.niams.nih.gov/ne/oi/oabimarwhipap.htm.*
74. Ayral X, personal communication.
75. Concoff AL, Singh R, Klashman D, et al. A clinical algorithm for identifying occult crystalline disease in patients with knee osteoarthritis. *Arthritis Rheum* 1997;40(suppl):239.
76. Ike RW. Arthroscopy in rheumatology: a tool in search of a job. *J Rheumatol* 1994;21:1987–1989.
77. Ike RW, Arnold WJ, Rothschild E, et al., and the Tidal Irrigation Cooperating Group. Tidal irrigation versus conservative medical management in patients with osteoarthritis of the knee: a prospective, randomized study. *J Rheumatol* 1992;19:772–779.
78. Evans CH, Mears DC, McKnight JL. A preliminary ferrographic analysis of the wear particles in human synovial fluid. *Arthritis Rheum* 1981;24:912–918.
79. Horwitz T. Bone and cartilage debris in the synovial membrane. *J Bone Joint Surg Am* 1948;30:579–588.
80. Chrisman OD, Fessel JM, Southwick WO. Experimental production of synovitis and marginal articular exostoses in the knee joints of dogs. *Yale J Biol Med* 1965;37:409–412.
81. Evans CH, Mazzocchi RA, Nelson DD, et al. Experimental arthritis induced by intraarticular injection of allogenic cartilagenous particles into rabbit knees. *Arthritis Rheum* 1984;27:200–207.
82. Evans CH, Mears DC, Cosgrove JL. Release of neutral proteinases from mononuclear phagocytes and synovial cells in response to cartilagenous wear particles *in vitro. Biochem Biophy Acta* 1981;677: 287–294.
83. Watanabe M. Articular pumping. *J Jpn Orthop Assoc* 1949;24:30–42.
84. Jungmichel D, Weber H, Gatzsche L. [Joint washing: treatment possibility in active arthritis.] Gelenkwaschung: eine behandlungsmoglichkeit bei aktivierter arthrose. *Beitr Orthop Traumatol* 1988;35: 512–517.
85. Livesley PJ, Doherty M, Needhoff M, et al. Arthroscopic lavage of osteoarthritis knees. *J Bone Joint Surg Br* 1991;73:922–926.
86. Kellgren JH, Lawrence JS. Radiological assessment of osteoarthritis. *Ann Rheum Dis* 1957;16:494–501.
87. Bradley JD, Heilman DK, Katz BP, et al. Tidal irrigation as treatment for knee osteoarthritis: a sham-controlled, randomized, double-blinded evaluation. *Arthritis Rheum* 2002;46(1):100–108.
88. Ravaud P, Moulinier L, Giraudeau B, et al. Effects of joint lavage and steroid injection in patients with osteoarthritis of the knee: results of a multicenter, randomized, controlled trial. *Arthritis Rheum* 1999; 42:475–482.
89. Edelson R, Burks RT, Bloebaum RD. Short-term effects of knee washout for osteoarthritis. *Am J Sports Med* 1995;23:345–349.
90. Vad VB, Bhat AL, Sculo TP, et al. Management of knee osteoarthritis: knee lavage combined with hylan versus hylan alone. *Arch Phys Med Rehabil* 2003;84(5):634–637.
91. Srinivasan A, Amos M, Webley M. The effects of joint washout and steroid injection compared with either joint washout or steroid injection alone in rheumatoid knee effusion. *Br J Rheumatol* 1995;34: 771–773.
92. Sharma A, Baethge BA, Acebes JC, et al. Arthroscopic lavage treatment in rheumatoid arthritis of the knee. *J Rheumatol* 1996;23: 1872–1874.
93. Chang RW, Falconer J, Stulberg SD, et al. A randomized, controlled trial of arthroscopic surgery versus closed-needle joint lavage for patients with osteoarthritis of the knee. *Arthritis Rheum* 1993;36: 289–296.
94. Kalunian KC, Moreland LW, Klashman DJ, et al. Visually-guided irrigation in patients with early knee osteoarthritis: a multi-center randomized, controlled trial. *Osteoarthritis Cartilage* 2000;8:412–418.
95. Baumgaertner MR, Cannon WD Jr, Vittori JM, et al. Arthroscopic debridement of the arthritic knee. *Clin Orthop Rel Res* 1990;253: 197–202.
96. Hubbard MJS. Articular debridement versus washout for degeneration of the medial femoral condyle. *J Bone Joint Surg Br* 1996;78: 217–219.
97. Ogilvie-Harris DJ, Fitsialos DP. Arthroscopic management of the degenerative knee. *Arthroscopy* 1991;7:151–157.
98. Harwin SF. Arthroscopic debridement for osteoarthritis of the knee: predictors of patient satisfaction. *Arthroscopy* 1999;15:142–146.
99. Sharma L, Song J, Felson D, et al. The role of knee alignment in disease progression and functional decline in knee osteoarthritis. *JAMA* 2001;286(2):188–195.
100. Moseley JB, O'Malley K, Petersen NJ, et al. A controlled trial of arthroscopic surgery for osteoarthritis of the knee. *N Engl J Med* 2002;347(2):81–88.
101. Felson DT, Buckwalter J. Debridement and lavage for osteoarthritis of the knee. *N Engl J Med* 2002;347(2):132–133.
102. Concoff AL. In: DeCherney G, Pregler J, eds. *Osteoarthritis in principles of women's health.* Toronto: BC Decker, 2002.
103. McLaren AC, Blokker CP, Fowler PJ, et al. Arthroscopic debridement of the knee for osteoarthritis. *Can J Surg* 1991;34:595–598.
104. Rand JA. Role of arthroscopy in osteoarthritis of the knee. *Arthroscopy* 1991;7:358–363.
105. Sprague NF. Arthroscopic debridement for degenerative knee joint disease. *Clin Orthop* 1981;160:118–123.
106. Hunziker EB, Quinn TM. Surgical removal of articular cartilage leads to loss of chondrocytes from cartilage bordering the wound edge. *J Bone Joint Surg Am* 2003;85(2):85–92.
107. Arnold WJ, Kalunian K. Arthroscopic synovectomy by rheumatologists: time for a new look. *Arthritis Rheum* 1989;32:108–111.
108. Cohen S, Jones R. An evaluation of the efficacy of arthroscopic synovectomy of the knee in rheumatoid arthritis: 12–24 month results. *J Rheumatol* 1987;14:452–455.
109. Steinbrocker D, Traeger CH, Batterman RC. Therapeutic criteria in rheumatoid arthritis. *JAMA* 1949;140:659–665.
110. Matsui N, Taneda Y, Ohta H, et al. Arthroscopic versus open synovectomy in the rheumatoid knee. *Int Orthop* 1989;13:17–20.
111. Smiley S, Wasilewski SA. Arthroscopic synovectomy. *Arthroscopy* 1990;6:18–23.

112. Arnold WJ. Arthroscopy in the diagnosis and therapy of arthritis. *Hosp Prac* 1992;March 30:43–53.
113. Ogilvie-Harris DJ, Basinski A. Arthroscopic synovectomy of the knee for rheumatoid arthritis. *Arthroscopy* 1991;7:91–97.
114. Ochi T, Iwase R, Kimura T, et al. Effect of early synovectomy on the course of rheumatoid arthritis. *J Rheumatol* 1991;18:1794–1798.
115. Szachnowski P, Wei N, Arnold WJ, et al. Complications of office based arthroscopy of the knee. *J Rheumatol* 1995;22:1722–1725.
116. Rich E, Calvo-Alen J, Koopman WJ, et al. Synovial biopsy by needle arthroscopy: a useful research tool. *Arthritis Rheum* 1995;38(suppl):237.
117. Wollaston S, Brion P, Kumar A, et al. Complications of knee arthroscopy performed by rheumatologists. *J Rheumatol* 2001;28:1871–1873.

CHAPTER 6

Magnetic Resonance Imaging in Arthritis

Charles G. Peterfy and Harry K. Genant

The discovery of the x-ray by Wilhelm Röentgen in 1895 marked a turning point in the history of medicine. This, along with the development of radiopaque contrast material, enabled surgeons for the first time to visualize the interior of a patient without actually cutting the skin. Such a capability could not have been anticipated prospectively by the physicians of that time, as evidenced by the statements of Berkeley George Moynihan of Leeds, one of the forefathers of modern surgery, who at about that same time wrote that with the development of anesthesia and sterile technique he saw little hope for any further discovery in surgery (1).

Soon after Röentgen's pivotal discovery, the first radiographs of osteoarthritic joints were generated, and radiography has remained to this day the mainstay of imaging evaluation of arthritis and related disorders. X-ray-based imaging has seen significant technical advances since then, including the development of more sensitive film-screen combinations, high-resolution optical and geometric magnification imaging (2–5), and computed tomography (CT), but the information provided by these modalities has nevertheless remained fundamentally limited to osseous changes, and therefore has offered only a keyhole view of the complex disease processes involved in arthritis. This inability to noninvasively examine the condition of other important articular tissues has been a principal obstacle to the study of arthritis and its treatment.

The development of magnetic resonance imaging (MRI) approximately 20 years ago represented a conceptual breakthrough that once again provided medicine with a tool of unprecedented capabilities for exploring disease and directing therapy. MRI offers true multiplanar versatility and high spatial resolution without any ionizing radiation. It depicts soft tissue anatomy with unparalleled clarity, and shows a unique potential for differentiating diseased tissues from healthy tissues. Furthermore, the inherent noninvasiveness and generally good patient tolerance of this technique make it possible to obtain frequent serial examinations of even asymptomatic joints. Unlike other imaging modalities, such as radiography, CT, or scintigraphy, MRI is capable of directly visualizing all components of the joint simultaneously. This unique capability is particularly cogent to the current view of arthritis as a disease affecting the joint as a whole organ.

Once considered a relatively inaccessible modality, MRI is now available at almost every major hospital in the world. Moreover, commercial state-of-the-art MRI systems today are capable of performing extremely sophisticated techniques that until only recently were considered exclusively the domain of specialized research facilities. Also, as has been the experience with other maturing technologies, the cost of MRI is continually decreasing and becoming competitive with other routine clinical techniques, such as scintigraphy and CT. Therefore, although the development of MRI for arthritis is still in its infancy, it warrants attention now, because it will undoubtedly play an important role in the development of our understanding of arthritis, as well as in our ability to combat the disease.

TECHNICAL CONSIDERATIONS

Because arthritis is a disease that spans several medical specialties, including orthopedic surgery and rheumatology, many physicians dealing directly with the disease have had relatively little exposure to MRI. For this reason, the following brief review of basic principles and terminology in MRI is provided as an introduction to this chapter. For the interested reader, there are several excellent books and articles that delve deeper into MRI physics and its applications in medicine (6–11).

Comparison of Magnetic Resonance Imaging with Other Imaging Modalities

Unlike radiography or CT, which are based on tissue absorption of radiographs, MRI utilizes no ionizing radiation

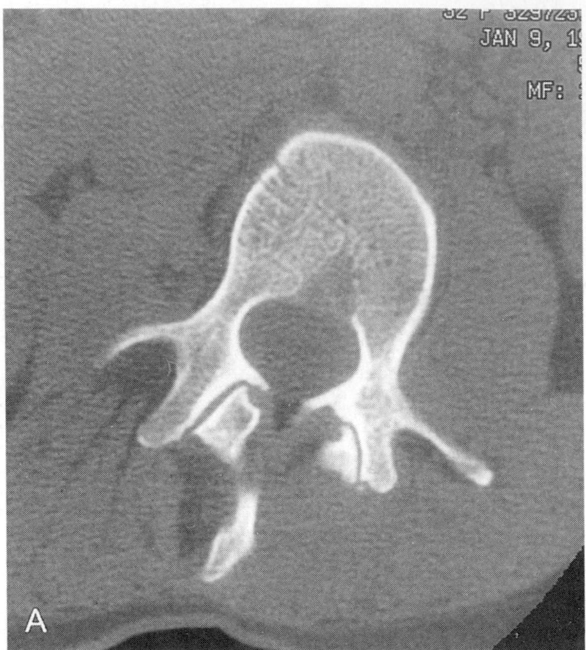

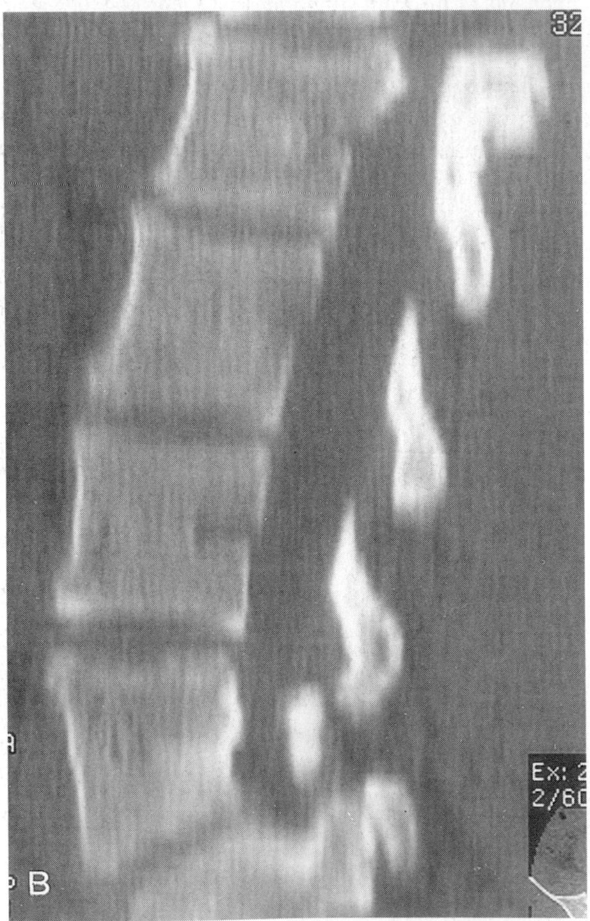

FIG. 6.1. Multiplanar reformatting with computed tomography (CT). **A:** Transverse CT section at the level of the vertebral body of L4 obtained with a 0.3 × 0.3 mm pixel size and 3.0-mm section thickness shows relatively high spatial resolution. **B:** Sagittally reformatted image using the contiguous 3-mm axial CT sections from L1 to S1 shows considerably lower in-plane spatial resolution (3.0 × 0.3 mm pixels).

and is an essentially noninvasive modality. Radiography, particularly with magnification, can provide greater spatial resolution than either CT or MRI, and is therefore potentially better at delineating subtle cortical irregularities or fine soft tissue calcifications. However, because radiography provides only two-dimensional (2D) projections of the three-dimensional (3D) anatomy, structures along the path of the x-ray beam are superimposed. This feature complicates the interpretation of radiographs and can obscure important findings. Both CT and MRI are tomographic techniques and therefore able to spatially separate overlying structures. However, direct sectioning of most large joints by CT is limited to only the transverse (axial) plane; sagittal or coronal tomograms require reformatting of the original transverse data. CT reformations require thinner transverse sections and therefore greater radiation exposure and examination time, and generally show poorer image quality (Fig. 6.1). Although this is less of a problem with spiral CT (12,13), MRI, in contrast, is truly multiplanar and can acquire direct tomograms in virtually any plane. Moreover, MRI's capacity to discriminate among different soft tissues is completely unparalleled. This is also true for bones, in which MRI can detect subtle abnormalities in the marrow space, such as edema and hemorrhage from trauma, exudate from infection or ischemia, and infiltration by neoplasm, with unprecedented sensitivity. CT is capable of differentiating fat from other soft tissues and shows extremely high contrast between calcified structures, such as cortical and trabecular bone, and adjacent soft tissues, but does not approach the scope for tissue discrimination shown by MRI.

Joint scintigraphy has been shown to be more sensitive than physical examination or radiography in identifying articular involvement in patients with inflammatory arthritis (14) and can survey all of the joints in the body during a single examination. Scintigraphy with "bone-seeking" agents, such as technetium 99m methylene diphosphonate, has also been shown to be predictive of radiographic progression in osteoarthritis (OA) (15,16). In a study of 94 patients with established OA of the knee (15), 88% of 32 knees with severe scintigraphic abnormalities progressed radiographically and clinically, whereas none of 55 patients with negative scans at entry showed any progression. In contrast, age, sex, symptom duration, and obesity were not predictive of progression. Although these and more recent results (17) are encouraging, scintigraphy with such bone-seeking agents lacks spatial resolution (Fig. 6.2) and is inherently nonspecific. The question of whether this technique can predict a poor outcome in patients without other evidence of preexisting OA must therefore be examined directly. Gallium 67 citrate and indium 111 chloride are more specific markers for the inflammatory compartment of the joint; however, poor spatial resolution with these high-energy radionuclides compounded by low target-to-background activity ratios limit their utility, particularly in small joints.

Unlike radiography, CT, and scintigraphy, ultrasonography can directly visualize the articular cartilage and synovium (18,19). However, the utility of this modality is

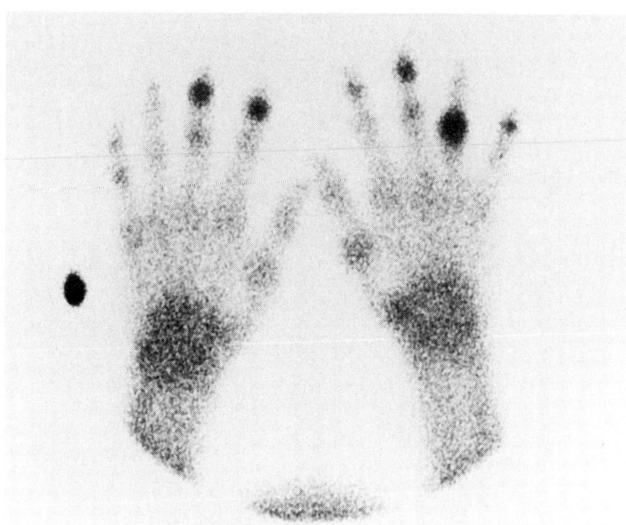

FIG. 6.2. Joint scintigraphy. Scintigraphy with technetium-99m-methylene diphosphonate in a patient with psoriatic arthritis shows asymmetric joint involvement in both hands. Despite the sensitivity and broad coverage provided by this technique, scintigraphy remains relatively nonspecific and offers poor anatomic detail.

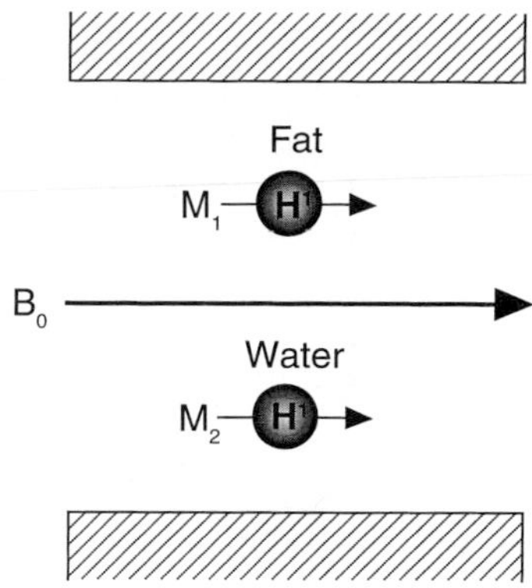

FIG. 6.3. Longitudinal magnetization. Hydrogen protons (H^1) placed within the high magnetic field (B_0) in the bore of a magnetic resonance imaging (*MRI*) magnet align their mean magnetic moments (*M*) along B_0.

limited by the impenetrability of bone to sound waves at the frequency and power ranges used for imaging. As a result, certain regions in most joints are not accessible to inspection. Moreover, ultrasonography offers less scope than MRI for probing the biochemical and biophysical properties of these tissues.

Basic Principles of Magnetic Resonance Imaging

Signal and Tissue Contrast

Conventional MRI is based on the natural magnetization produced by hydrogen nuclei (protons or "spins") as they spin, or more accurately, precess about their axes. The most abundant sources of hydrogen protons in the body are water (H_2O) and fat ($-CH_2-$), and it is from these two substances that MRI derives virtually all of its signal. Calcified tissues, such as cortical bone, in contrast, contain so few hydrogen protons that they usually appear as signal voids on MRI. When the protons within fat- or water-containing tissues, such as bone marrow, are placed within the very high magnetic field (B_0) in the bore of an MRI magnet, they show a net tendency to align their nuclear magnetic moments along this magnetic field, much like a compass needle aligns with the magnetic field of the earth (Fig. 6.3). The vector sum of these individual magnetic moments is known as the bulk magnetization vector (M), and its magnitude is the parameter that is measured in MRI.

The precession frequency (resonant frequency or Larmor frequency) of the protons is directly proportional to the field strength of the magnet, which may vary from 0.1 to 2.0 tesla (T) for clinical MRI scanners. Exposing these protons to an additional alternating or rotating magnetic field tuned to their resonant frequency [i.e., applying a radiofrequency (rf) pulse] causes the protons to resonate and realign with this new field. Thus, an rf pulse oriented perpendicular to the static field (i.e., 90-degree rf pulse) will flip M 90 degrees so that it becomes oriented transverse to the static field (Fig. 6.4). [The term *radiofrequency* in MRI is not to imply that radiowaves are produced or used, but only that the frequency referred to is in the range associated with transmission of radiowaves (typically 10 kHz to 2 GHz). In fact, considerable effort is taken in MRI to ensure that radio waves are neither emitted nor received by the MRI probe or coil (20)].

Precession of M transverse to the static field induces an alternating electrical current in receiver wires in the imaging coil placed near the patient. This current, which is also in the rf range, is then fed to a computer for analysis.

T_1 Relaxation

Immediately after the rf pulse, M gradually tips back to its original longitudinal alignment with the static field of the MRI magnet. Recovery of the longitudinal component of M (M_L) is known as spin-lattice or T_1 relaxation (Fig. 6.4B). Some substances, such as fat, show rapid T_1 relaxation, whereas others, such as water, show slow recovery of M_L. If the relaxing protons in a particular substance are exposed to a second 90-degree rf pulse before M_L has completely recovered [i.e., if the repetition time (TR) is short relative to the T_1 of the substance], only the smaller, recovered portion (i.e., M_L) is available to be flipped transversely, the magnitude of the MRI signal produced is proportionately smaller, and the substance or tissue is said to be partially saturated (Fig. 6.4C). Typically, 128 to 256 repetitions are required to generate a satisfactory MRI image.

Therefore, when a relatively short TR is used (e.g., 500 msec), fat, which has already recovered by this time, shows

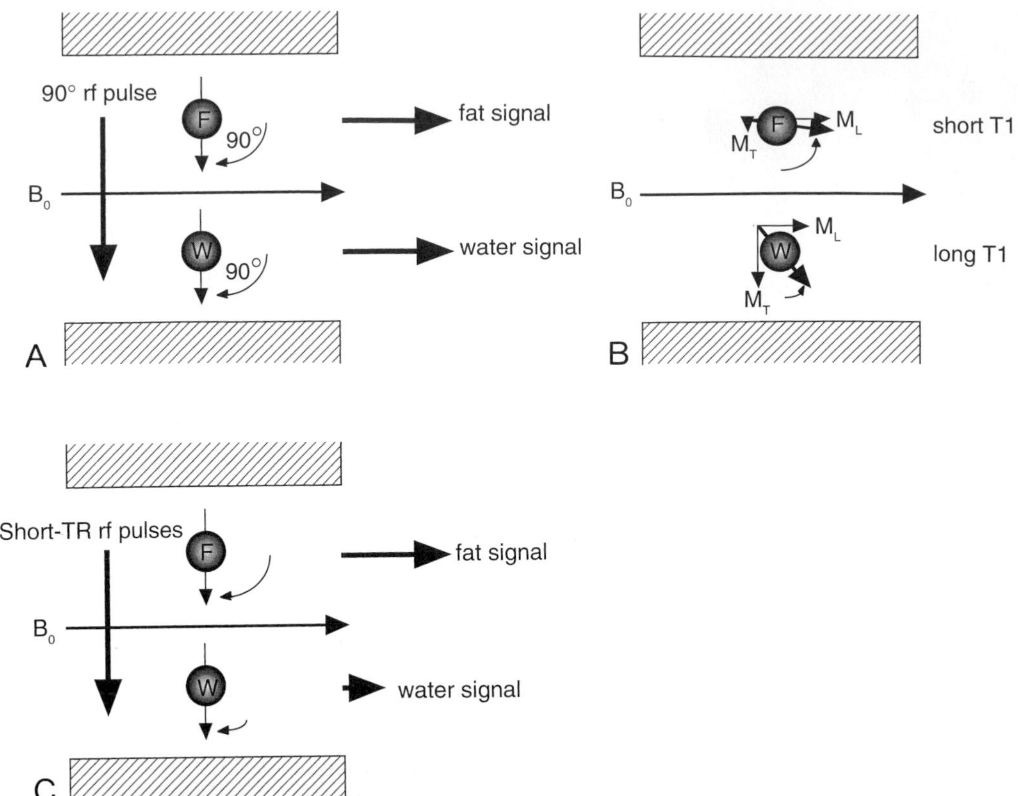

FIG. 6.4. Transverse magnetization and T_1 relaxation. **A:** Exposure of protons within a static magnetic field (B_0) to a second rotating transverse field [90-degree radiofrequency (*rf*) pulse] flips the protons from their original longitudinal orientation into the transverse plane and induces a current in the receiver coil. **B:** Once the transverse field is removed, the protons realign with B_0. This time-dependent recovery of longitudinal magnetization (M_L) is referred to as T_1 relaxation. Fat (*F*) exhibits rapid T_1 relaxation. Water (*W*) shows slow T_1 relaxation. **C:** Repeat exposure of the relaxing protons to additional 90-degree rf pulses before M_L has completely recovered (short-TR sequence) will result in a proportionately smaller magnetic resonance imaging signal.

high signal intensity, whereas water, which is still relatively saturated, shows low signal intensity (Fig. 6.5). If, alternatively, a long TR (e.g., 2,000 msec) is used, permitting both fat and water to almost completely recover their M_L, both substances generate high signal intensity (Fig. 6.5). Paramagnetic substances, such as methemoglobin found in subacute hematomas (Fig. 6.6), and gadolinium-containing MRI contrast agents [e.g., gadolinium–diethylenetriamine pentaacetic acid (Gd-DTPA)] (Fig. 6.7), increase T_1 recovery in adjacent water protons and thereby increase their signal intensity on short-TR (T_1-weighted) images.

T_2 Relaxation

Magnetic resonance imaging signal is also subject to T_2 relaxation, which refers to the loss of transverse magnetization as individual protons fall out of phase with each other (Fig. 6.8). Because the resonant frequency of individual protons is dependent on the field strength of their immediate magnetic environment, microheterogeneities in the field resulting from effects of neighboring proton fields on each other will cause internuclear differences in precession frequency and therefore loss of phase coherence among adjacent protons. Loss of phase coherence of the individual magnetic moments decreases the magnitude of the mean net magnetization vector, M, and therefore the MRI signal observed. The rate of this dephasing (T_2 relaxation) varies from tissue to tissue; highly mobile free water protons, for example, show very slow T_2 relaxation, whereas protons in fat exhibit a more rapid loss of signal (Figs. 6.8 and 6.9). As water protons become more constrained, or bound, as, for example, by the presence of highly ordered collagen molecules in tendons, muscle, or articular cartilage, internuclear effects also increase and the protons dephase more rapidly (i.e., T_2 shortens) and thus lose signal.

MRI signal can be sampled at different times by generating "echoes" with either a 180-degree rephasing rf pulse (spin-echo technique) or a sudden reversal of the polarity of the magnetic gradient used for spatial encoding (gradient-echo technique). The later this echo is acquired [i.e., the longer the echo time (TE)], the greater the degree of dephasing that will have occurred, and thus the smaller the amplitude of the echo. Accordingly, free water, which shows slow T_2 relaxation,

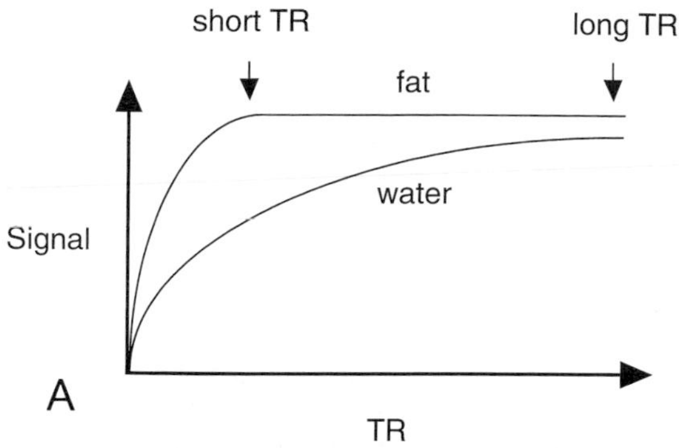

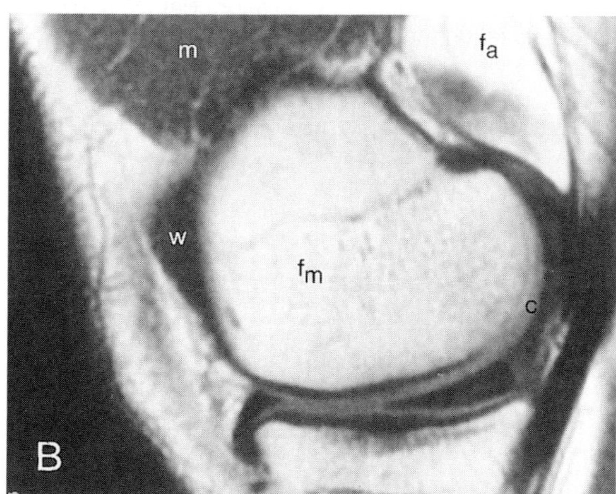

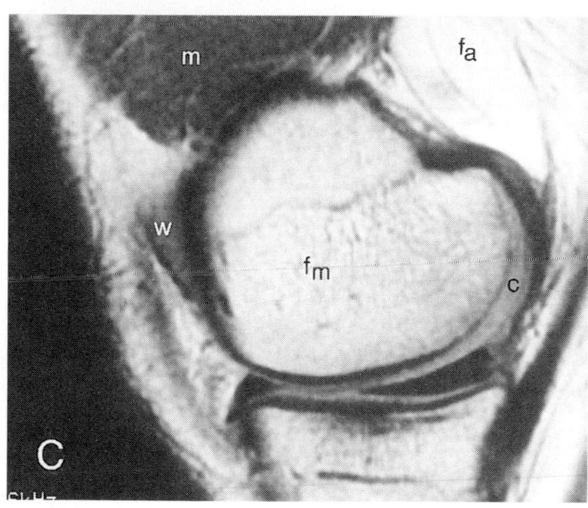

FIG. 6.5. Effect of TR on signal intensity and contrast. **A:** Varying the time interval between successive 90-degree radiofrequency pulses (TR) alters magnetic resonance imaging contrast on the basis of tissue differences in T_1. T_1-weighted sequences use short TR, while proton density–weighted and T_2-weighted images use long TR. **B:** Sagittal T_1-weighted spin-echo image of a normal knee depicts fat in adipose tissue (f_a) and bone marrow (f_m) with high signal intensity, but synovial fluid (*w*), articular cartilage (*c*), and muscle (*m*), which contain primarily water protons, with low signal intensity. **C:** Proton density–weighted image of the same knee again depicts fat (f_a, f_m) with high signal intensity, but because the longer TR allows greater recovery of longitudinal magnetization in water, the signal intensity of cartilage (*c*) and synovial fluid (*w*) is increased.

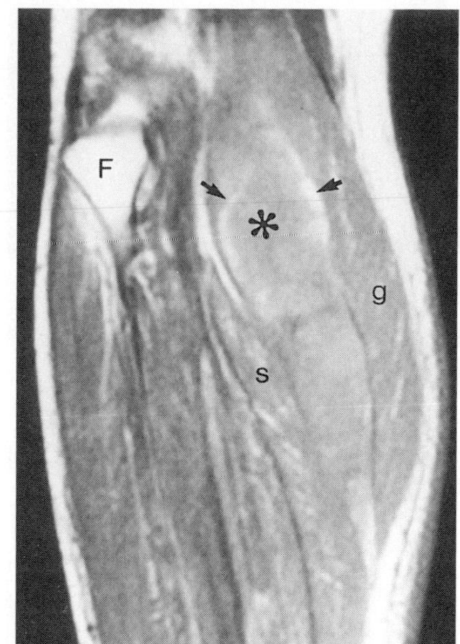

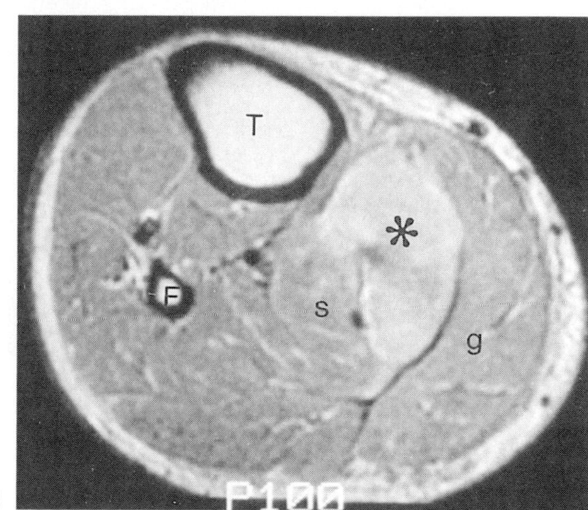

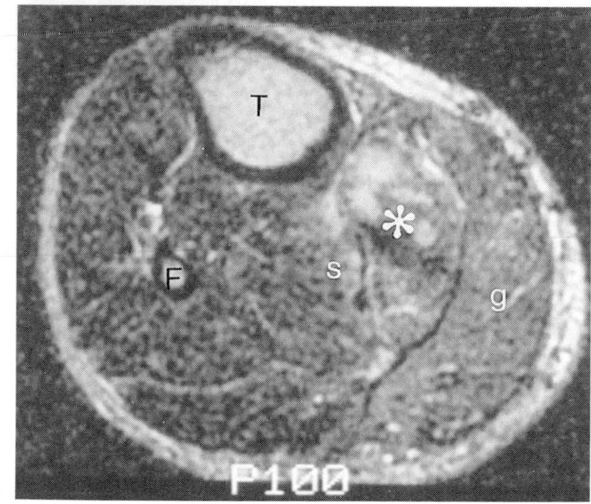

FIG. 6.6. Methemoglobin in subacute hemorrhage shows high signal on T_1-weighted Images. Sagittal **(A)** and transverse **(B)** T_1-weighted spin-echo image of the lower leg of a patient with rheumatoid arthritis (*RA*) shows a large, hemorrhagic Baker cyst (*) dissecting between the gastrocnemius (*g*) and soleus (*s*) muscles. Areas of high signal intensity (*arrows*) in the cyst represent methemoglobin. On T_2-weighted, spin-echo image **(C)**, blood products (deoxyhemoglobin) in the cyst (*) show low signal intensity. *T,* tibia; *F,* fibula.

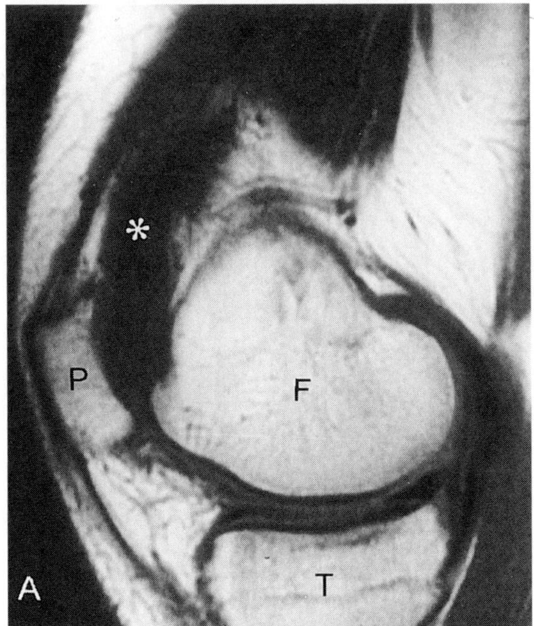

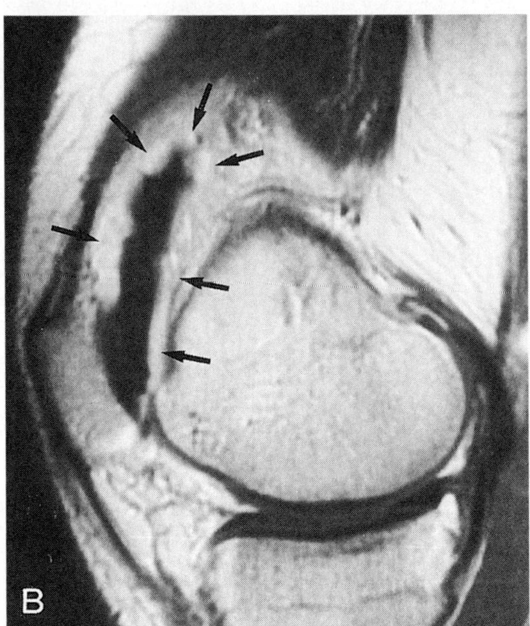

FIG. 6.7. Gadolinium–diethylenetriamine pentaacetic acid (Gd-DTPA)-enhancing tissues show high signal on T_1-weighted images. **A:** Sagittal T_1-weighted spin-echo image of the knee in a patient with RA shows poor discrimination between joint effusion and hypertrophic synovium, both of which show intermediate signal intensity in the distended suprapatellar recess (*). **B:** Following intravenous Gd-DTPA, the hypervascular synovial tissue (*arrows*) shows high signal intensity on the T_1-weighted image, due to the paramagnetic effect of Gd on local water protons. *P,* patella; *F,* femur; *T,* tibia.

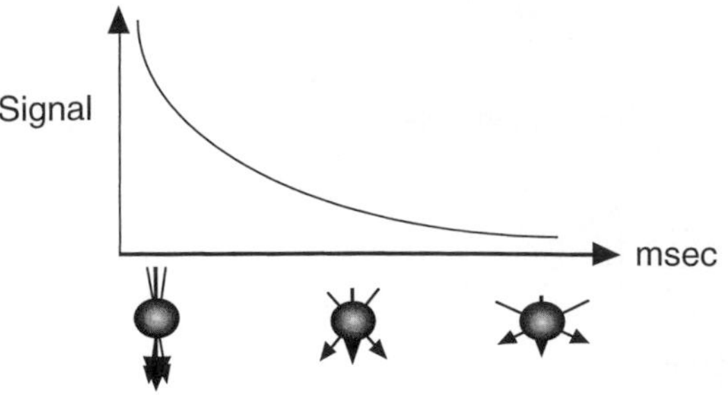

FIG. 6.8. T_2 relaxation (loss of phase coherence). As neighboring protons spinning together in a field influence each other's frequency, they gradually fall out of phase and decrease the net magnetization that is measurable. This exponential decay of Transverse component of M (M_T) (and therefore signal) is called T_2 relaxation. Fat (*F*) shows more rapid T_2 relaxation than does water (*W*).

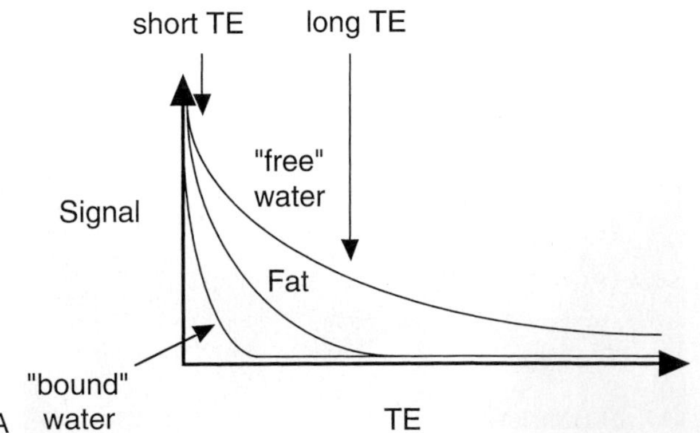

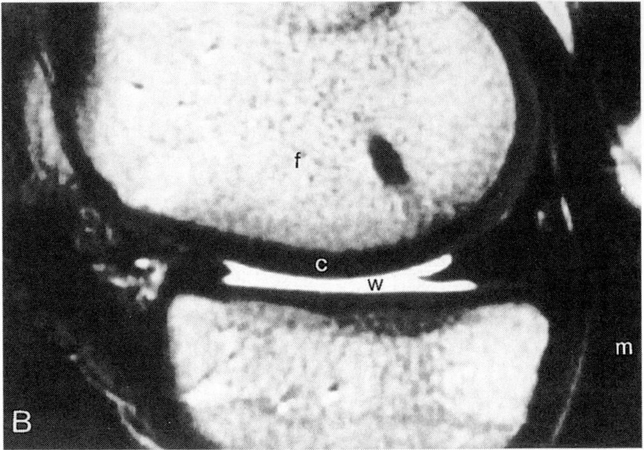

FIG. 6.9. Effect of TE on signal intensity and contrast. **A:** Varying the time between the 90-degree radiofrequency pulse and the acquisition of a spin-echo or gradient-echo image used to measure Transverse component of M (M_T) (TE) alters magnetic resonance imaging (MRI) contrast on the basis of tissue differences in T_2. Longer TE imparts greater T_2 weighting to an MRI. T_2-weighted images are obtained with long TR to minimize T_1 effects, whereas T_1-weighted and proton density–weighted images are acquired with as short a TE as possible to minimize the influence of T_2 relaxation. Free water generally shows very slow T_2 relaxation. However, water protons constrained by collagen or other substances in the microenvironment ("bound" water) can show extremely rapid T_2 relaxation. **B:** Sagittal T_2-weighted spin-echo image of a normal knee shows high signal intensity in joint fluid (*w*) and low signal intensity in other tissues, including fat (*f*). Although both cartilage (*c*) and muscle (*m*) contain primarily water protons, they show low signal intensity because the protons are relatively immobile (bound).

retains relatively high signal intensity on spin-echo images acquired with long (>80 msec) TE, whereas fat and bound water appear dark on the same long-TE images (Fig. 6.9).

Magnetic Susceptibility Effects and T_2 Relaxation*

Warping of the magnetic field at interfaces between substances that have very different magnetic susceptibilities (the degree to which a substance magnetizes when exposed to a magnetic field) also dephases local protons. Magnetic susceptibility effects (Fig. 6.10) are prominent in tissues containing metal (e.g., following surgery) but also occur between trabecular bone and marrow tissue, at the boundary between articular cartilage and subchondral bone, and in tissues containing hemosiderin deposits from chronic hemorrhage. Signal loss resulting from the combination of fixed

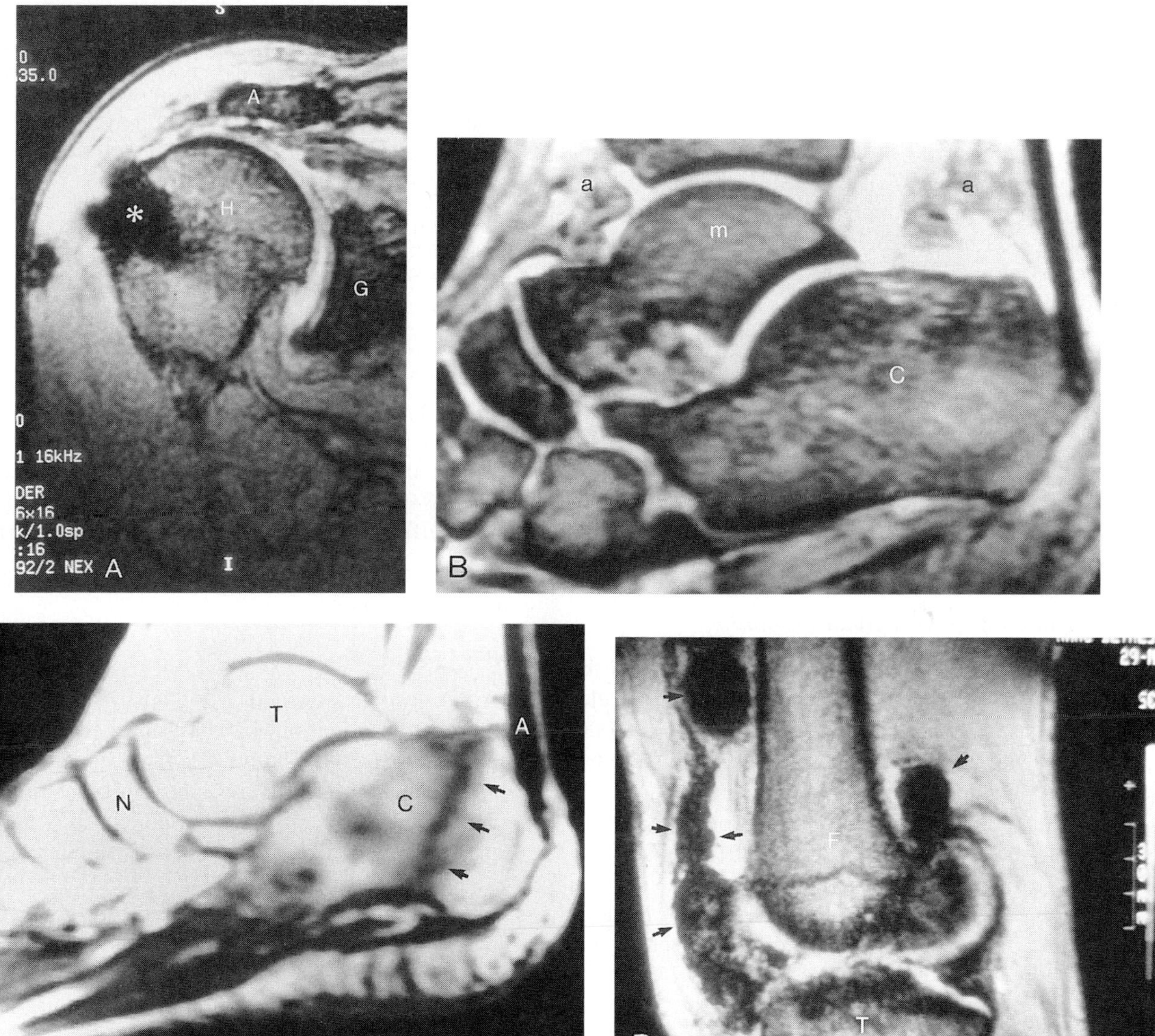

FIG. 6.10. Magnetic susceptibility effects. **A:** Oblique-coronal T_2*-weighted gradient-echo image of a shoulder with prior repair of the supraspinatus tendon. Loss of signal at the site of previous surgery (*) is due to micrometallic fragments implanted in the tissues. *H,* humeral head; *G,* glenoid; *A,* acromion. **B:** Sagittal T_2*-weighted gradient-echo image of the calcaneus (*C*) shows only minor signal heterogeneities in this bone. Note that the signal intensity of fat in the marrow space (*m*) is lower than that in adipose tissue (*a*). This is due to magnetic susceptibility effects in the marrow caused by the presence of trabeculae. **C:** Sagittal T_1-weighted spin-echo image of the same heel clearly shows a vertical band of low signal intensity (*arrows*) in the calcaneus in a pattern that is pathognomonic for fracture. This finding is obscured on the gradient-echo image by local magnetic susceptibility effects but quite salient on the lower-resolution spin-echo image, which took only 52 seconds to acquire. *T,* talus; *N,* navicular; *A,* Achilles tendon. **D:** Sagittal T_2*-weighted gradient-echo image of a knee with pigmented villonodular synovitis and recurrent hemarthrosis shows dramatic signal loss in the synovium (*arrows*) due to magnetic field disturbances caused by the iron in hemosiderin deposits within the synovium. *F,* femur; *T,* tibia.

magnetic heterogeneities (magnetic susceptibility effects) and internuclear interactions (T_2 relaxation) is referred to as T_2^* relaxation. T_2^* is usually considerably shorter than T_2. Spin-echo technique corrects for fixed magnetic heterogeneities and therefore can generate truly T_2-weighted images. Conversely, gradient-echo technique, which does not correct for magnetic susceptibility effects, produces so-called T_2^*-weighted images. This is why the signal intensity of fat in the marrow space, which has a heterogeneous magnetic field, is lower than that of fat in adipose tissue when imaged with gradient-echo technique, while fat in both compartments appears the same with spin-echo imaging (Figs. 6.10B and 6.10C).

Most forms of pathology (e.g., edema, exudate or hemorrhage associated with trauma, ischemia, infection, and neoplasia) are associated with increased free water content and therefore show high signal intensity on long-TE (T_2-weighted) images. An exception to this is when the process is associated with fibrosis (i.e., collagen deposition), hemosiderin deposition, or calcification, all of which increase proton dephasing and signal loss (Fig. 6.10D). The vulnerability of gradient-echo imaging to susceptibility effects in cancellous bone is responsible for its low sensitivity for detecting marrow pathology.

It is important to recognize that T_1, T_2, and T_2^* relaxation occur simultaneously in any tissue during MRI. It is by manipulating imaging parameters, such as TR, TE, and flip angle, and occasionally by the use of MRI contrast agents, that tissues are discriminated by MRI.

Signal-to-Noise Ratio and Spatial Resolution

The total area depicted on an MRI section is called the field of view. It is divided into a matrix of picture elements, or pixels, by spatially encoding the protons on the basis of frequency in one direction and phase in the other (Fig. 6.11). A magnetic gradient is applied in one direction to impart a different frequency to each proton relative to the proton's position along this direction (frequency encoding). A second gradient is transiently applied in the perpendicular direction to vary the phase among protons depending on their position in this direction (phase encoding). A 20-cm field of view divided into a 256 × 192 matrix thus provides pixels measuring 0.8 × 1.0 mm. Multiplying the pixel dimensions by the slice thickness (typically 1–5 mm) defines the voxel size. The spatial resolution of an MRI is determined by the voxel size. The signal intensity of the voxel represents the average of all the signal intensities within it. This is known as volume averaging.

Spatial resolution can be improved by decreasing the voxel size either by reducing the field of view, increasing the matrix, or decreasing the slice thickness. The trade-offs in each of these cases relate to signal-to-noise ratio (S/N) and imaging time. The smaller the voxel size, the greater the S/N required to support it. S/N can be increased by

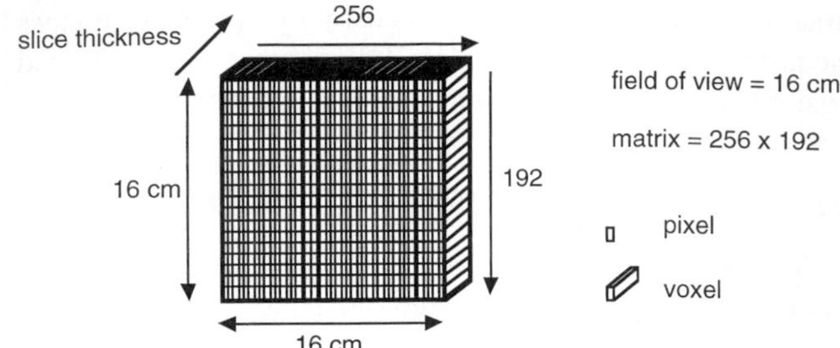

FIG. 6.11. Spatial resolution and signal-to-noise ratio (S/N). A single magnetic resonance imaging slice with a field of view of 16 cm is shown. The image is subdivided in the plane of the section using a matrix produced by frequency encoding in one direction and phase encoding in the other. The field of view divided by the matrix gives the pixel size (in this case 625 × 833 μm), which defines the in-plane resolution of the image. Pixel size multiplied by the slice thickness (e.g., 3 mm) determines the voxel size (625 × 833 × 3,000 μm). As voxel size decreases, spatial resolution improves, but the resolution of an image is ultimately limited by the number of spins each voxel contains (i.e., the S/N).

using a higher field strength magnet (the clinical range is 0.1–3.0 T), increasing the imaging time (i.e., averaging signals from repeated acquisitions), lengthening TR (maximizing T_1 recovery of signal), shortening TE (minimizing T_2 decay of signal), or by using special imaging coils, such as small surface coils, quadrature coils, or phased arrays (21).

Imaging Sequences

Spin Echo

Spin echo has been the workhorse sequence for most clinical applications of MRI. By using a 180-degree rf pulse to rephase the protons following the original 90-degree excitation pulse, it has the advantage of correcting for fixed magnetic heterogeneities and minimizing susceptibility effects. T_1-weighted spin-echo images attempt to separate different tissues on the basis of inherent differences in T_1 relaxation by using short TR. T_2 decay (Fig. 6.5B) is minimized on these images by using short TE. Substances that show high signal intensity on T_1-weighted images (Table 6.1) include fat, methemoglobin in subacute hematomas (Fig. 6.6), and substances exposed to Gd-containing contrast agents (Fig. 6.7). Most other substances appear dark on T_1-weighted images.

T_2-weighted spin-echo technique attempts to discriminate tissues on the basis of inherent differences in T_2 relaxation by using long TE (Fig. 6.9, Table 6.1). Differences in T_1 relaxation are minimized by using long TRs to allow full recovery of M_L. Tissues that show high signal intensity on T_2-weighted images contain significant amounts of free water. This includes most forms of trauma, ischemia, infection, and neoplasia, as well as isolated fluid collections, such as abscesses, hematomas, and cysts. Fibrosis, calcifi-

TABLE 6.1. *Signal behavior of different substances on spin-echo images*[a]

Substance/tissue	T_1-weighted	T_2-weighted
Fat	+++	+
Gadolinium (Gd)-enhanced tissue	+++	(−)[b]
Methemoglobin	+++	+++
Muscle	+	−
Cartilage	+	−
Synovium	+	+++
Effusion	−−	+++
Edematous tissue	−	++/+++
Deoxyhemoglobin	−	−−
Tendon	−−	−−
Meniscus/labrum	−−	−−
Calcification	−−−	−−−
Hemosiderin deposition	−−−	−−−/−−−−

[a]Arranged according to T_1 relaxation.
[b]Gadolinium–diethylenetriamine pentaacetic acid (Gd-DTPA) shortens T_2 mildly.

cation, deoxyhemoglobin from acute hemorrhage, or hemosiderin deposition from chronic hemorrhage tend to decrease signal intensity on T_2-weighted images. T_2-weighted imaging, however, requires relatively long imaging times (because of the long TR) and offers poor S/N (because of signal decay due to T_2 relaxation), which limits the spatial resolution that it can support. Because of this, an earlier echo (short TE) is traditionally collected while waiting for the late echo (long TE) in the sequence. The short-TE images have greater S/N and provide better anatomic detail. Because these images are neither T_1 weighted (because TR is long) nor T_2 weighted (because TE is short), they are referred to as proton density–weighted, and depict both free water and fat with high signal intensity. Because of this poor image contrast between fat and water, abnormalities such as trauma, infection, or neoplasia arising in adipose tissue or the fatty marrow may not be apparent on proton density–weighted images.

Gradient Echo

Gradient-echo technique, which uses partial flip angles (<90 degrees) and collects echoes by gradient reversal rather than 180-degree rf pulses, is faster than spin echo but more vulnerable to magnetic susceptibility effects. These effects can alter tissue contrast and limit the usefulness of gradient-echo imaging following surgery, as well as lower sensitivity for detecting marrow abnormalities (Fig. 6.10). However, the rapid speed with which these images can be obtained makes the use of 3D acquisition feasible. Three-dimensional imaging allows thinner slice thicknesses and improves S/N, but takes longer and is more vulnerable to motion artifacts.

Fast Spin Echo

Fast spin echo is a technique capable of generating heavily T_2-weighted spin-echo images with high spatial resolution and in only a fraction of the time required for conventional spin-echo imaging. Fast spin echo is particularly useful for imaging articular cartilage. However, fat tends to remain high in signal intensity even on relatively long-TE fast spin-echo images and may thus obscure abnormalities in fatty tissue (Fig. 6.12). This often necessitates the use of fat suppression.

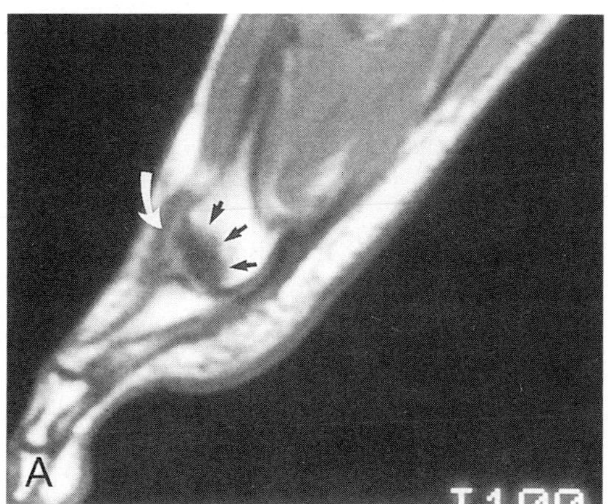

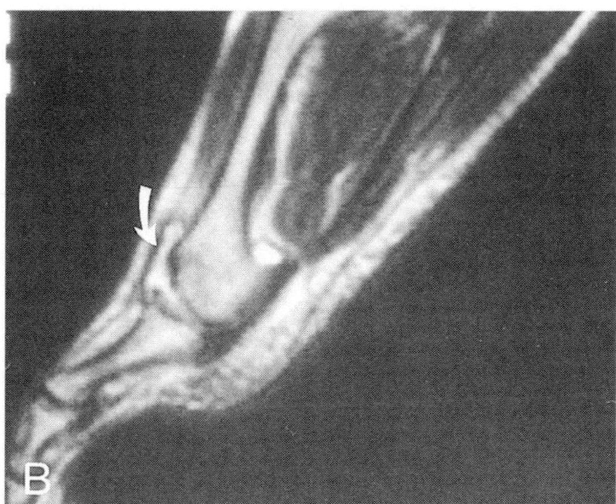

FIG. 6.12. Fast spin-echo imaging. **A:** Sagittal T_1-weighted conventional spin-echo image of the second metatarsophalangeal joint of a patient with a Freiberg infraction shows distention of the joint with a low signal intensity effusion (*curved arrow*) and replacement of the normal high signal intensity marrow fat in the metatarsal head by low signal intensity exudate (*straight arrow*) due to osteonecrosis. **B:** T_2-weighted fast spin-echo image of the same joint shows the joint effusion (*curved arrow*) with high signal intensity, but since both fat and water exhibit relatively high signal with this technique, the marrow abnormality is relatively inconspicuous. *(Continued)*

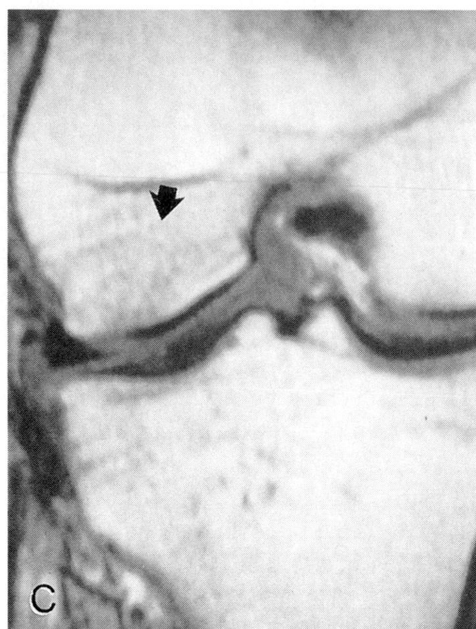

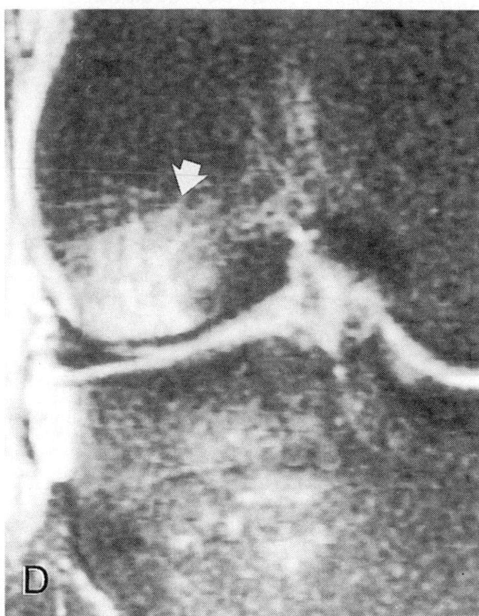

FIG. 6.12. *Continued* **C:** Coronal T_1-weighted conventional spin-echo image of a traumatized knee shows subtle changes of marrow edema (*arrow*) in the medial femoral condyle due to bone contusion. **D:** By suppressing signal from fat (using frequency-selective saturation) on a T_2-weighted fast spin-echo image of the same knee, the bone contusion (*arrow*) is more saliently depicted.

Fat Suppression

The most widely used technique for suppressing signal from fat on MRI is known as frequency-selective presaturation. Because of their different microenvironments, protons in fat precess at a different frequency than those in water. This phenomenon is known as chemical shift. By applying a narrow bandwidth rf saturating pulse tuned to the frequency of fat, fat protons can be selectively saturated without any significant effect on protons in water (Fig. 6.13). This technique applied to a T_2-weighted fast spin-echo sequence generates images in which fat has a low signal intensity while free water has a high signal intensity (Fig. 6.12). Frequency-selective fat saturation can also be used to discriminate high signal intensity methemoglobin or Gd-enhanced tissues from high signal intensity fat on T_1-weighted images.

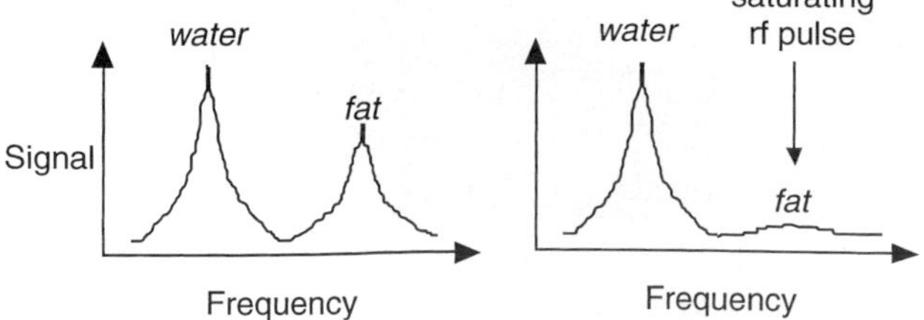

FIG. 6.13. Fat suppression. Because fat and water protons spin at different frequencies (chemical shift phenomenon), fat can be selectively saturated with a frequency-specific radiofrequency pulse without affecting protons in water.

One of the limitations of this approach to fat suppression is that the presaturating pulse adds time to the protocol. An alternative approach is selective excitation of water frequency. This also generates images in which fat shows no signal, but because the technique does not require an additional fat-saturating pulse, it is substantially faster (22). Both of these approaches, however, are vulnerable to heterogeneities in the main magnetic field. These can be caused by metal within or near the tissue or by irregularities in the anatomic shape of the structure being imaged. Since resonant frequency depends on field strength, local heterogeneities in field strength cause heterogeneities in the frequencies of fat and water. Externally applied saturating or exciting frequencies will, accordingly, be ineffective in these locations.

MAGNETIC RESONANCE IMAGING OF THE ARTICULAR CARTILAGE

Effective evaluation of the articular cartilage *in vivo* poses a number of challenges to conventional MRI. Initial efforts to image the cartilage of even large joints, such as the knee, were thwarted by insufficient spatial resolution and inadequate signal contrast between the cartilage and adjacent articular structures, including joint fluid, synovium, and subchondral bone. Recent technical developments, however, have overcome these earlier problems, and MRI now enables unprecedented and unparalleled examination of the articular cartilage of even small joints noninvasively *in vivo*. Improvements in gradient strength and performance and in coil design, and the development of more efficient imaging sequences, have brought spatial resolution on the order of 200 μm to within the reach of routine clinical scanners. Also, by harnessing different relaxation mechanisms in articular cartilage, very high contrast can be generated between the cartilage and its adjacent structures, as well as between areas of diseased and normal cartilage.

Signal Behavior of Normal Cartilage

The signal behavior of articular cartilage on MRI reflects the complex biochemistry and histology of this porovis-coelastic tissue (23–25) (Fig. 6.14). Cartilage can be conceptualized as having a fluid phase composed of water and ions and a solid phase composed of aggregated proteoglycans and fibrous collagen (25). Hydrophilic proteoglycan molecules maintain a high water content (and therefore a high proton density) in cartilage through the Donnan osmotic pressure created by negatively charged glycosaminoglycan (GAG) moieties. These negative charges attract counterions (usually sodium) and thus draw water osmotically into the cartilage. This osmotic pressure, combined with electrostatic repulsion between adjacent GAGs, produces a swelling pressure that keeps the cartilage inflated and the fibrous collagen matrix under tension. The degree of hydration of the cartilage is determined by the balance between this swelling pressure and the resistance to expansion by the collagen meshwork. This high proton density constitutes the potential for generating MRI signal in cartilage. However, equally important as the amount of water protons is their state, and constraint or "binding" of otherwise mobile protons by proteoglycans and collagen promotes T_2 relaxation and speeds up the rate of signal loss (see earlier section on T_2 Relaxation).

This effect of collagen on water protons is particularly important in tendons, ligaments, and meniscal tissue, in which the concentration of collagen is high. T_2 relaxation in these tissues is typically so rapid (<1 msec) (26) that most of the signal decays before it can be sampled by even the shortest TEs attainable with conventional MRI systems (5 msec). For this reason, these structures generally appear low in signal intensity on all pulse sequences (26,27) (Fig. 6.15). The concentration of collagen in articular cartilage is somewhat lower, but nonetheless important, to the signal behavior of this tissue.

The organization of collagen in cartilage varies considerably from the articular surface to the subchondral bone (Fig. 6.14). Differences in T_2 relaxation across the thickness of cartilage correlate with these variations in fibrillar organization (28,29). In the deep radial zone, large bundles of collagen fibrils connected by numerous smaller cross-ties radiate from the subjacent calcified layer toward the articular surface. T_2 relaxation in this zone is relatively rapid, but still slow enough to allow intermediate signal intensity

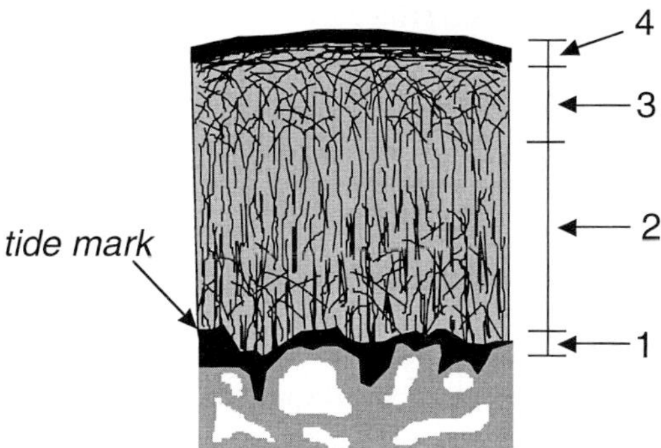

FIG. 6.14. Zonal organization of collagen in articular cartilage. The differing arrangement of collagen fibrils within the various cartilage zones results in heterogeneity of T_2 relaxation and zonal signal behavior on magnetic resonance imaging (MRI). The deepest layer of cartilage is calcified (*1*). Magnetic susceptibility effects and a low proton density in this zone results in low signal intensity on MRI. The calcified zone anchors a relatively parallel array of collagen fibrils that radiate toward the surface through the radial zone (*2*). T_2 relaxation in the radial zone is relatively rapid. The transitional zone (*3*) contains a more disorganized arrangement of collagen and shows slow T_2 relaxation. The most superficial zone (*4*) is composed of a dense network of tangentially arranged collagen fibrils and accordingly exhibits rapid T_2 relaxation. (Modified from Peterfy C, Linares R, Steinbach L. Recent advances in magnetic resonance imaging of the musculoskeletal system. *Radiol Clin North Am* 1994; 32:291–311, with permission.)

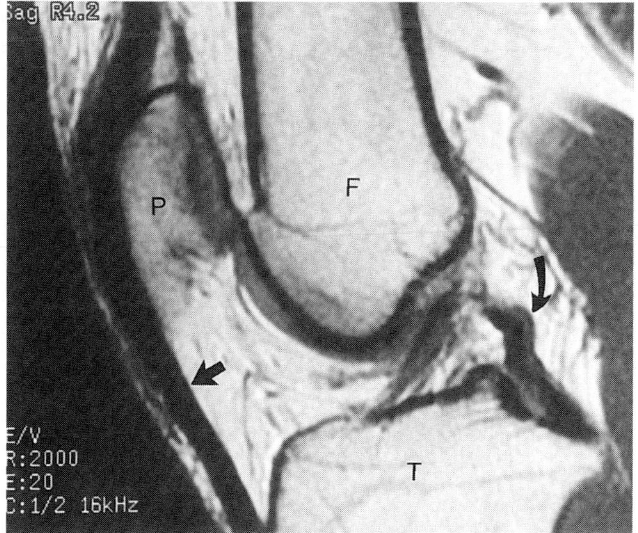

FIG. 6.15. Rapid T_2 relaxation in tendons and ligaments. Sagittal short-TE, proton density–weighted spin-echo image of the knee shows low signal intensity in the patellar tendon (*arrow*) and posterior cruciate ligament (*curved arrow*) due to extremely rapid T_2 relaxation in these structures. *P,* patella; *F,* femur; *T,* tibia.

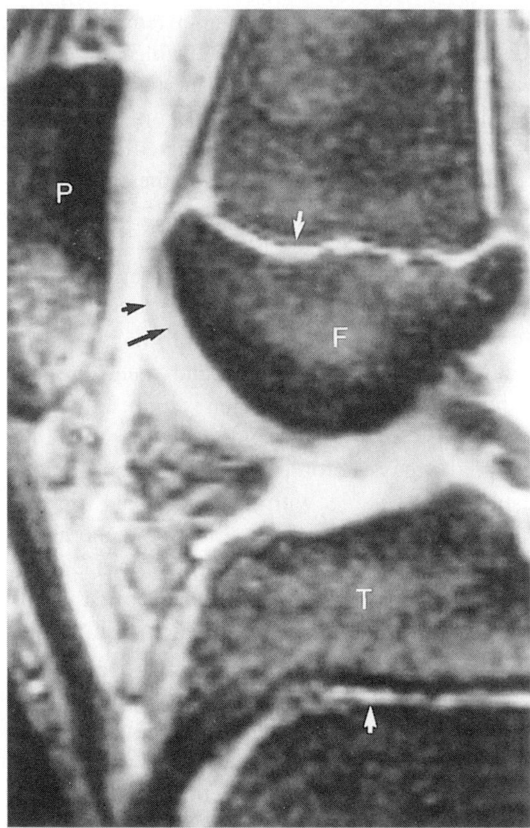

FIG. 6.16. Magnetic resonance imaging appearance of cartilage on short-TE images. Sagittal T_1-weighted spin-echo image of the knee depicts cartilage as a multilaminar structure delimited superficially by a thin band of low signal intensity (*short arrow*) paralleling the articular surface. Just beneath this superficial band is an intermediate signal intensity lamina composed primarily of the transitional zone. Beneath this, midway through the cartilage, is a thin low signal intensity stripe (*long arrow*) corresponding to truncation artifact. The remainder of the radial zone shows intermediate signal intensity. Beneath this, the calcified zone merges with subchondral cortex. Note the open growth plates (*white arrows*) in the femur (*F*) and tibia (*T*) of this knee. *P*, patella.

to be detected on short-TE images (Fig. 6.16). One or more narrow bands of low signal intensity are occasionally seen about midway through the thickness of normal cartilage (30). These bands are due to an artifact called truncation (30) and are less common on high-resolution images. Superficial to the radial zone is the transitional zone, which contains a more disorganized arrangement of collagen and has a correspondingly longer T_2. The most superficial zone of cartilage is called the superficial tangential zone and contains a dense mat of tangentially organized collagen fibrils, which resist tensile forces during compressive loading and form a water-impermeable barrier to interstitial fluid loss during compression (25). Because of the high collagen content of this zone, T_2 relaxation is rapid, and the cartilage surface therefore exhibits a low signal intensity perimeter on short-TE images (Fig. 6.16).

Normal articular cartilage on short-TE images thus typically shows three laminae of alternating intermediate and low signal intensity that correlate loosely with the histologic appearance of this tissue (Fig. 6.16): (a) a low-signal superficial lamina corresponding to the superficial tangential zone; (b) an intermediate-signal lamina incorporating the deep portion of the superficial tangential zone, the entire transitional zone, and the uppermost portion of the radial zone; and (c) a slightly lower-signal band through the remainder of the radial zone. The deep calcified layer of cartilage is typically indistinguishable from the signal void of the subjacent cortex of the subchondral bone on all but ultrashort-TE images. Magnetic susceptibility effects and chemical shift artifact (unless fat suppression is used) may exaggerate the thickness of this deepest lamina (Fig. 6.17A).

As TE is prolonged (i.e., on T_2-weighted images), signal decays from the deep radial lamina, intensifying the trilaminar appearance in cartilage (Fig. 6.17B). With very heavy T_2 weighting, signal also drops out of the transitional lamina, and cartilage becomes homogeneously low in signal intensity (Fig. 6.17C).

Effects of Compositional Changes in Cartilage

Superimposed on this complex MR signal behavior of normal cartilage are changes associated with disease. As proteoglycans are lost from degenerating cartilage, the remaining compressed proteoglycans are allowed to swell and thus expose more negatively charged GAGs to attract cations and water. Loss of collagen decreases the resistance to proteoglycan swelling pressure and thus also increases the water content of cartilage slightly (31). Increased water content raises the proton density of cartilage and thereby increases its signal intensity. This proton density effect, however, is small and would not be expected to be perceptible with conventional MRI. The associated loss of collagen matrix, on the other hand, reduces T_2 decay and thus unmasks more of the water signal (32). Some of the earliest changes in cartilage disease are therefore demonstrable by MRI as increased signal intensity on T_2-weighted images.

Consistent with this, foci of high signal intensity are often seen within the cartilage of knees with OA on T_2-weighted images (Fig. 6.18). These signal changes have been shown to correspond to arthroscopically demonstrable abnormalities (33,34). Patterns of abnormal cartilage signal include superficial, transmural, and deep linear changes (Fig. 6.18). The latter may reflect delamination of the cartilage at the tide mark (35), and is occasionally seen in young patients following trauma. Changes such as these, confined to the deep layers of cartilage, may not be detectable by inspection of the articular surface alone during arthroscopy. We have frequently observed these MRI signal abnormalities in cartilage adjacent to meniscal tears and in patients

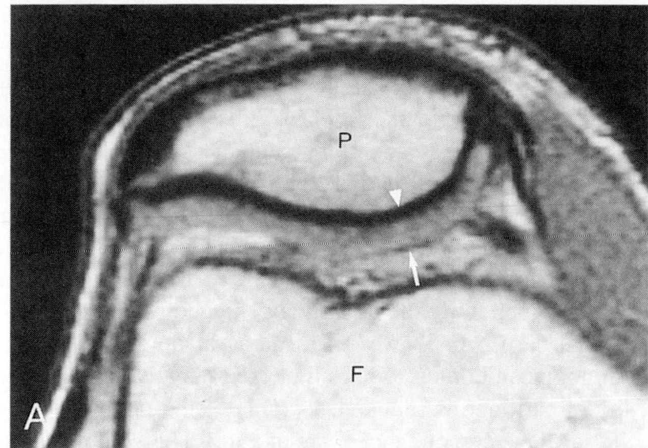

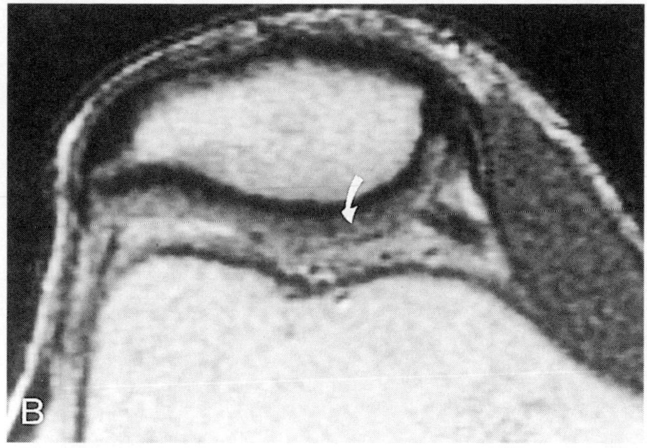

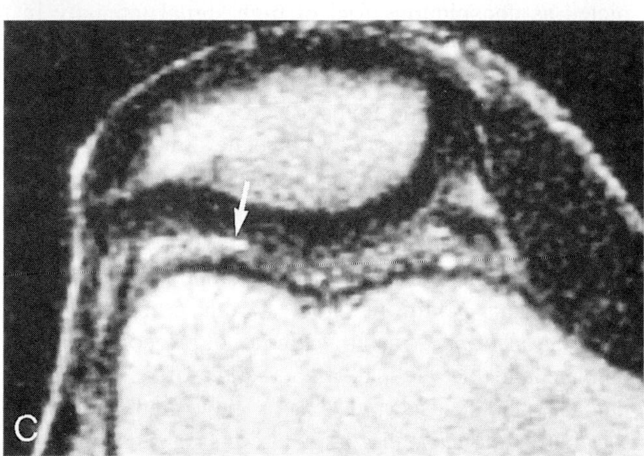

FIG. 6.17. Effect of TE on cartilage signal. **A:** Short-TE (20 msec), proton density–weighted spin-echo image of normal patellar cartilage shows diffuse intermediate signal intensity bounded superficially by a low signal intensity band (*short straight arrow*). Low signal intensity along the cartilage–bone interface (*arrowhead*) is partly due to the combination of deep calcified cartilage and subchondral cortex but may be exaggerated by chemical shift artifact in this case. *P,* patella, *F,* femur. **B:** As TE is lengthened to 40 msec, signal intensity decreases preferentially in the deep cartilage (*curved arrow*). Cartilage just beneath the low signal intensity superficial band remains intermediate in signal. **C:** With further T_2-weighting (TE = 80 msec), the entire cartilage becomes low in signal intensity. Contrast between the cartilage and adjacent joint fluid (*large straight arrow*) is high, but the overall S/N is relatively poor.

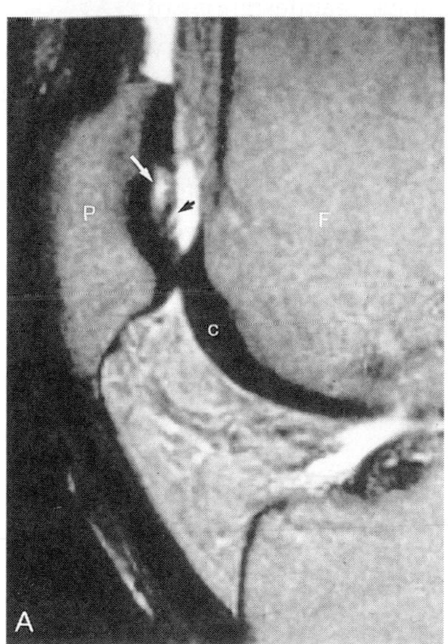

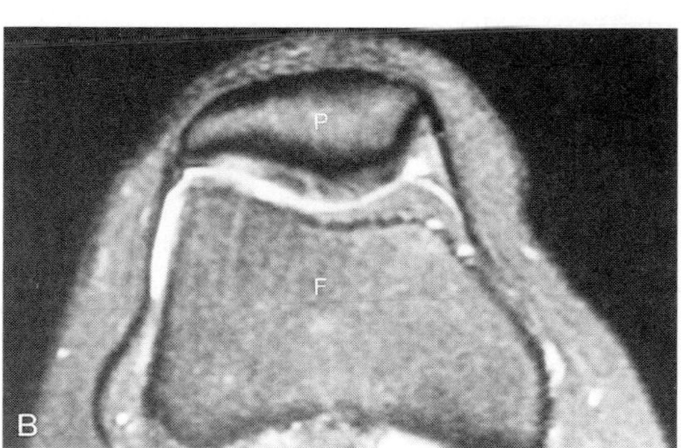

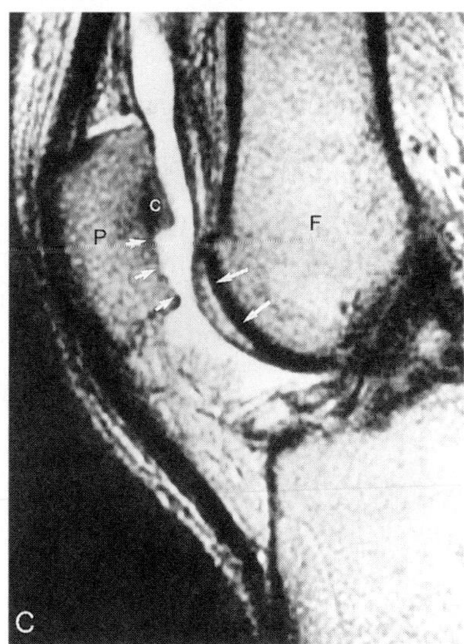

FIG. 6.18. Patterns of signal abnormality in cartilage. **A:** Sagittal T_2-weighted spin-echo image of the knee in a patient with symptoms of chondromalacia patella shows a superficial focus of high signal intensity (*white arrow*) in the otherwise low signal intensity patellar cartilage associated with fissuring of the articular surface (*black arrow*). Note the homogeneous low signal intensity of normal cartilage (*c*) over the femur (*F*). **B:** Transverse, fat-suppressed T_2-weighted fast spin-echo image of a different patella (*P*) shows transmural striations of high signal intensity in the articular cartilage. *F,* femur. **C:** Sagittal, T_2-weighted spin-echo image of the knee of a patient who sustained a direct blow to the anterior aspect of the knee shows full-thickness cartilage loss (*short arrows*) over the inferior pole of the patella (*P*). Note the sharp margin the defect makes with the remaining cartilage (*c*) over the upper pole. Cartilage over the trochlear surface of the femur (*F*) shows normal thickness and an intact articular surface but contains a linear band of high signal intensity at the level of the tide mark (*long arrows*) paralleling the subchondral cortex. This deep signal pattern may reflect early basal delamination of the cartilage resulting from mechanical failure and may not be apparent on arthroscopy.

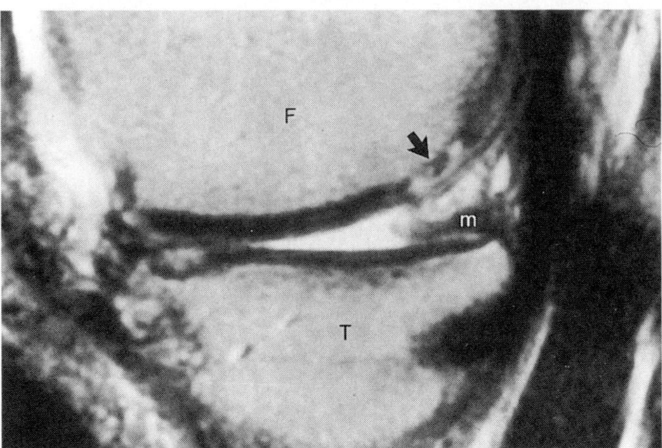

FIG. 6.19. Cartilage defect associated with meniscal tear. Sagittal T_2-weighted fast spin-echo image of the knee shows a focal defect (*arrow*) in the articular cartilage of the medial femoral condyle (*F*) over the torn and macerated posterior horn of the medial meniscus (*m*). *T,* medial tibia.

with established OA (Fig. 6.19), in many cases before surface abnormalities were evident on MRI or arthroscopy. Others have also observed signal abnormalities in cartilage that were not apparent by arthroscopy (34,36,37). All of these studies, however, provided only cross-sectional information. Longitudinal data describing the natural history of these MRI cartilage abnormalities and their association with subsequent cartilage loss and joint failure are currently lacking.

Using more sophisticated research facilities, it is possible to obtain highly detailed information about the composition of articular cartilage. For example, the fractional water content and the diffusion coefficient of water in cartilage can be accurately measured with noninvasive MRI techniques (38,39). Both of these parameters increase with damage to the proteoglycan and collagen matrix in cartilage disease.

Another interesting marker of cartilage matrix integrity is Gd(DTPA2)− uptake (29,40). Gd(DTPA2)− is a widely used MRI contrast agent that enhances T_1 relaxation of water molecules and renders them as a high signal intensity on heavily T_1-weighted images. Under normal circumstances anionic Gd(DTPA2)− introduced into the synovial fluid (either by intravenous or direct intraarticular injection) is repelled by the negatively charged proteoglycans in normal cartilage. However, in areas of decreased glycosaminoglycan content where the fixed negative charge density of cartilage is reduced, Gd(DTPA2)− can diffuse into the cartilage and enhance T_1 relaxation. These areas are depicted as conspicuous foci of high signal intensity in the otherwise low signal intensity cartilage on inversion recovery images. By acquiring the images with different TRs, T_1 can be quantified and mapped across the cartilage. T_1 values determined in this way correlate almost linearly with proteoglycan content in the range normally found in cartilage. However, quantifying T_1 can be time consuming and impractical for most clinical studies. Further work is necessary to establish the optimal method for acquiring these imaging data. Additional studies are also needed to define the relationship between this marker of proteoglycan matrix damage and elevated T_2 as a marker of collagen matrix damage, and to ascertain exactly how predictive each of these are—alone or in combination—for subsequent cartilage loss, the development of other structural features of OA, and ultimately for clinical manifestations of OA.

In addition to the use of Gd(DTPA2)−, proteoglycan content of cartilage can be probed with cationic contrast agents, such as manganese (41,42), or by imaging sodium instead of hydrogen (43).

Magnetization transfer is a specific MRI relaxation mechanism in articular cartilage that can be harnessed to generate additional image contrast (44–47) (Fig. 6.20). This phenomenon reflects the thermodynamic equilibrium that exists between freely mobile protons in tissue water,

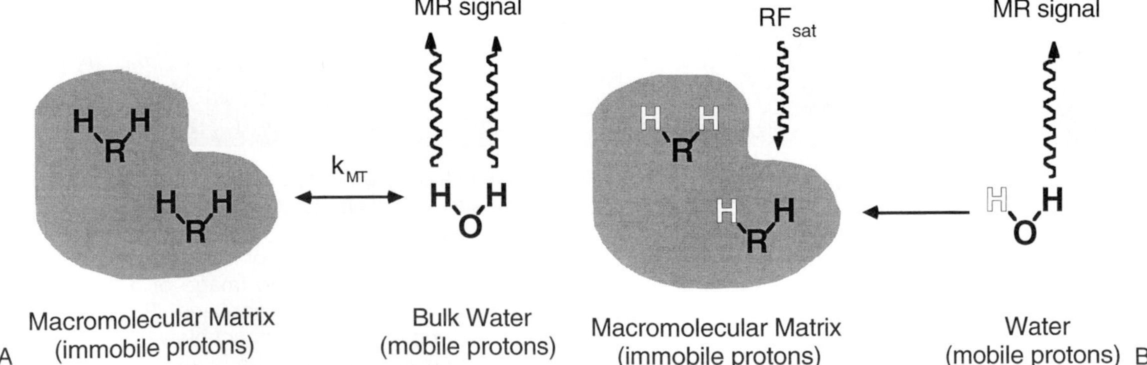

FIG. 6.20. Magnetization transfer phenomenon. **A:** Normal thermodynamic equilibrium between immobile protons [magnetic resonance imaing (MRI)-invisible] associated with macromolecules and mobile protons (MRI-visible) in bulk water. **B:** Selective saturation of the immobile protons results in transfer of longitudinal magnetization (magnetization transfer) from unsaturated water protons to the immobile macromolecular protons to maintain equilibrium, and manifests as a net loss of MRI signal.

and protons constrained by macromolecules within the same tissue. Because the macromolecular protons are relatively immobile, they exhibit an extremely short T_2 relaxation time (<1 msec) and do not contribute directly to the signal on conventional MRI. Selective saturation of this MRI-invisible pool (which can be invoked by a number of different techniques), however, causes a transfer of magnetization (M_L) from the MRI-visible pool of mobile water protons to maintain the equilibrium. This manifests as a loss of signal intensity from the tissue, depending on the rate constant for this equilibrium reaction and the relative proportions of water and macromolecular protons in the tissue. Collagen is a particularly good macromolecular substrate for this reaction (47), and cartilage (44,45), hyperplastic synovium (45), and muscle accordingly exhibit prominent magnetization transfer effect. Fat and joint fluid, on the other hand, do not show any substantial magnetization transfer and thus do not lose signal intensity under conditions in which macromolecular protons are selectively saturated. These tissue-dependent differences in susceptibility to magnetization transfer can be exploited to generate additional image contrast among articular structures (45) (Fig. 6.21). In addition, it may be possible to quantify specific macromolecular constituents of different tissues by measuring the magnetization transfer effect. In cartilage, for example, collagen is the dominant macromolecule

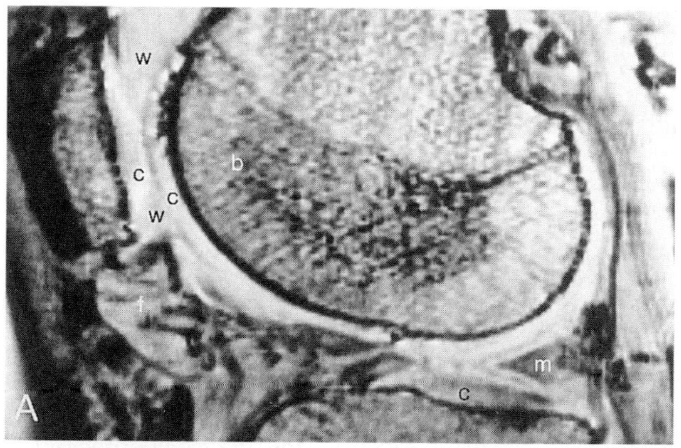

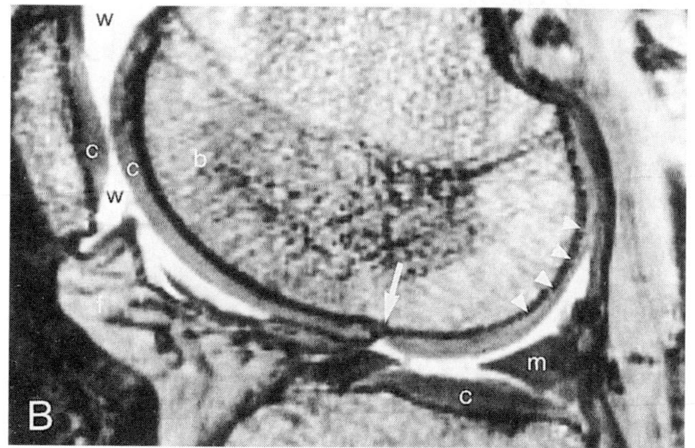

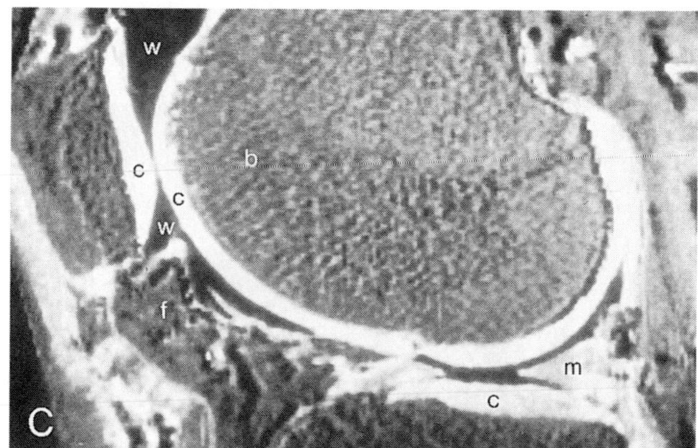

FIG. 6.21. Magnetization transfer in articular cartilage. Sagittal images of an amputated knee following intraarticular injection of 55 mL saline to simulate joint effusion. **A:** T_2*-weighted, three-dimensional gradient-echo image shows poor contrast between cartilage (*c*) and joint fluid (*w*). **B:** Inducing magnetization transfer in the same imaging sequence markedly decreases signal intensity in cartilage (*c*) but has little effect on joint fluid (*w*), bone (*b*), or adipose tissue (*f*). This combines high contrast between cartilage and fluid with sufficient spatial resolution to allow delineation of small surface defects in the cartilage (*long arrow*) as well as more generalized areas of cartilage thinning (*arrowheads*). Contrast at the cartilage–bone interface, however, is decreased. **C:** Magnetization transfer subtraction image (generated by subtracting image **B** from image **A**) maps the spatial distribution of magnetization transfer in the same knee. Hyaline articular cartilage (*c*) is depicted as a high signal intensity structure, whereas effusion (w), bone (b), and adipose (f) are low in signal intensity. Mild magnetization transfer is also evident in the meniscal fibrocartilage (m). Magnetization transfer subtraction images thus provide high contrast at both the cartilage–effusion and cartilage–bone interfaces. (From Peterfy CG, Majumdar S, Lang P, et al. MR imaging of the arthritic knee: improved discrimination of cartilage, synovium and effusion with pulsed saturation transfer and fat-suppressed T_1-weighted sequences. *Radiology* 1994;191:413–419, with permission.)

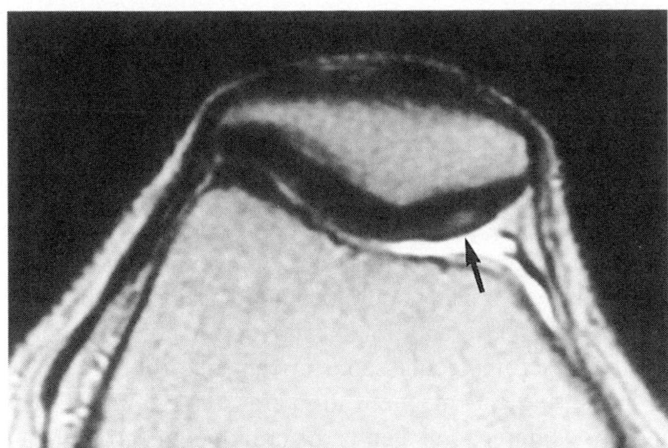

FIG. 6.22. Early chondromalacia patella. Transverse T_2-weighted fast spin-echo image of the knee shows a focus of high signal intensity just beneath the articular surface of the patellar cartilage. The surface at this site is intact but protrudes slightly (*arrow*) as the resistance to swelling pressure is lost.

involved in this phenomenon, with only minor contributions made by proteoglycans and other constituents (47). The prospect of one day quantifying cartilage collagen content by this method is intriguing.

Morphologic Changes in Cartilage

As the compositional and biomechanical properties of articular cartilage continue to deteriorate, substance loss

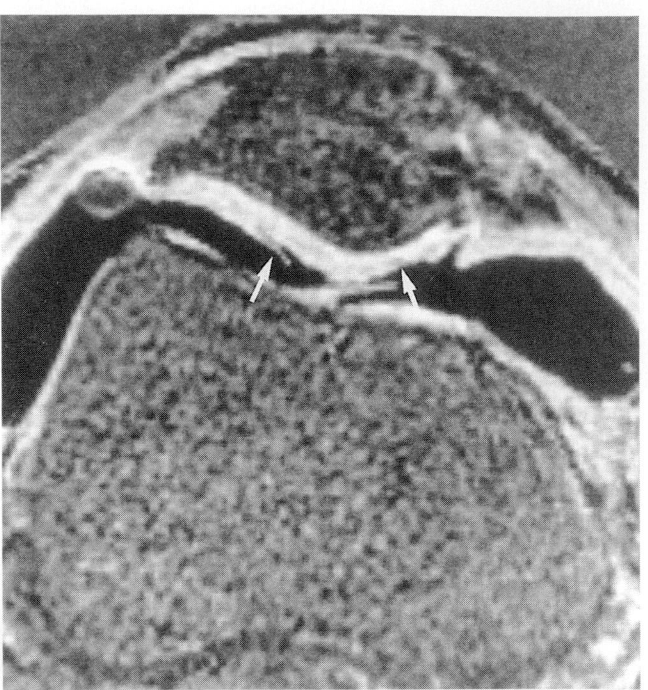

FIG. 6.24. High-resolution imaging of the articular surface with three-dimensional (3D) gradient echo and magnetization transfer subtraction. Transverse, thin-partitioned 3D magnetization transfer subtraction image of the patella delineates small surface irregularities (*arrows*) in the articular cartilage. (From Peterfy CG, Majumdar S, Lang P, et al. MR imaging of the arthritic knee: improved discrimination of cartilage, synovium and effusion with pulsed saturation transfer and fat-suppressed T_1-weighted sequences. *Radiology* 1994;191:413–419, with permission.)

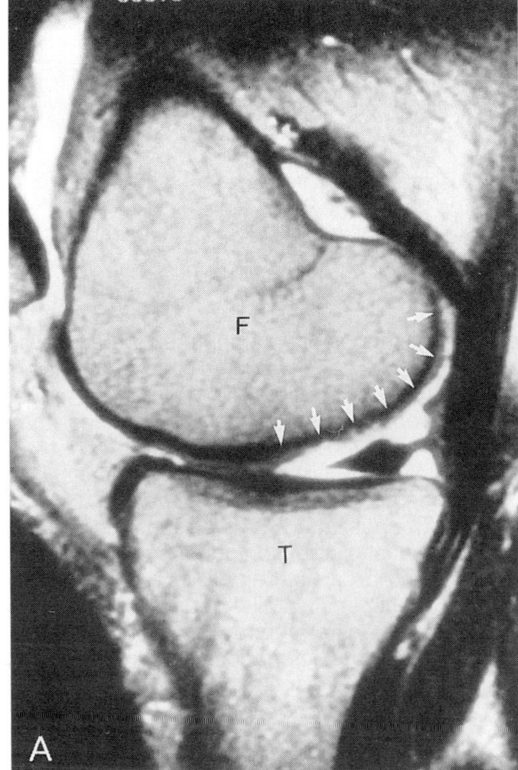

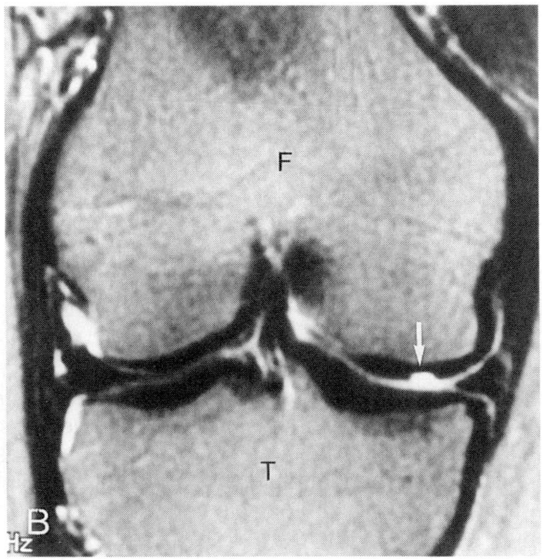

FIG. 6.23. Imaging articular cartilage defects with T_2-weighted spin echo. Sagittal **(A)** and coronal **(B)** T_2-weighted spin-echo images provide sufficient spatial resolution and contrast between articular cartilage and joint fluid to delineate relatively large surface defects (*arrows*). *F,* femur; *T,* tibia.

begins to occur. This may be focal or diffuse, restricted to superficial fraying and fibrillation, or involve the full thickness of cartilage. In some cases, focal swelling or "blistering" of the cartilage may be seen without disruption of the articular surface (48) (Fig. 6.22). Delineation of such morphologic changes, particularly subtle surface fraying, requires both high spatial resolution and high contrast between cartilage and adjacent articular structures, such as joint fluid, synovial tissue, and subchondral bone.

Conventional T_2-weighted spin-echo imaging provides relatively good delineation of large chondral defects (Fig. 6.23). Thinner slices, and therefore higher spatial resolution, can be achieved with three dimensional (3D) MRI, but this technique is currently restricted to gradient-echo sequences, and these generally offer poor contrast between cartilage and adjacent joint fluid (Fig. 6.21A). Additional contrast can be introduced to 3D gradient-echo images with the use of magnetization transfer techniques (49) (Figs. 6.21 and 6.24), or by combining fat suppression with T_1 weighting (45,49,50) (Fig. 6.25). The latter method is easy to use and widely available. It capitalizes on the slightly shorter T_1 of cartilage relative to that of other articular structures. Normally, this minor difference in T_1 is overshadowed by the much greater discrepancy between the short T_1 of fat and that of most other tissues.

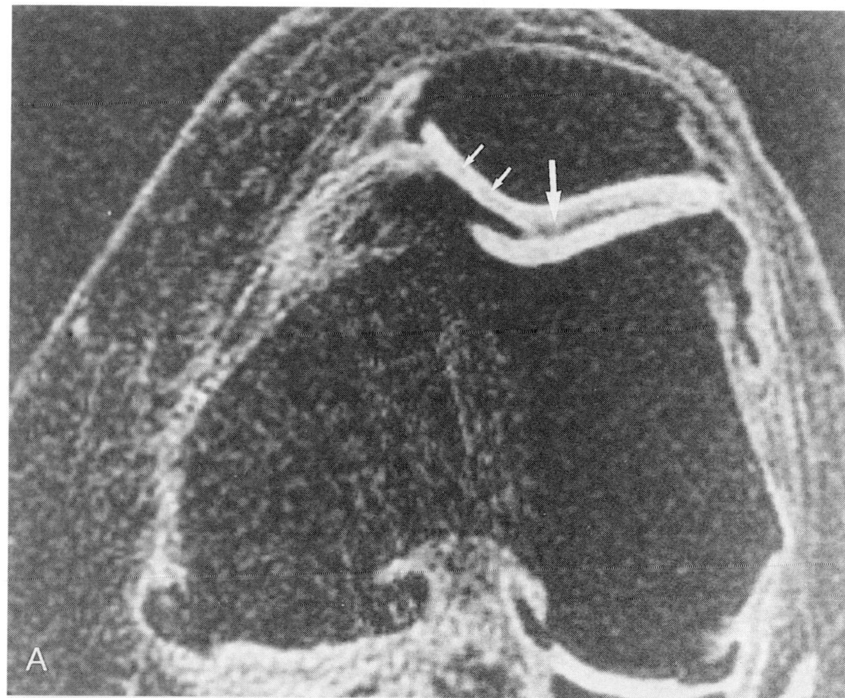

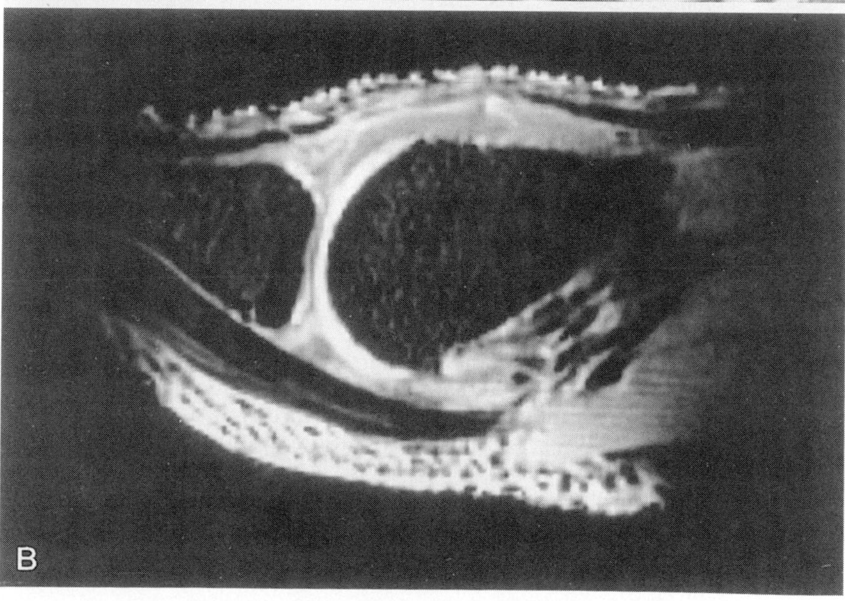

FIG. 6.25. T_1-weighted three-dimensional (3D) gradient-echo imaging with fat suppression. **A:** Transverse, thin-partitioned, fat-suppressed, 3D gradient-echo image through the patella of a 62-year-old man with osteoarthritis (*OA*) delineates the cartilage with high resolution and shows surface fraying and fibrillation of the articular surface (*large arrow*). Note the thin low signal intensity stripe in the femoral and patellar cartilages corresponding to the upper radial zone (*small arrows*). (From Peterfy CG, Majumdar S, Lang P, et al. MR imaging of the arthritic knee: improved discrimination of cartilage, synovium and effusion with pulsed saturation transfer and fat-suppressed T_1-weighted sequences. *Radiology* 1994;191:413–419, with permission.) **B:** Sagittal thin-partitioned, fat-suppressed 3D gradient-echo image of the metacarpophalangeal joint of the index finger depicts the articular cartilage with high contrast and resolution. This image was obtained using a conventional clinical magnetic resonance imaging scanner and commercial imaging software. (From Peterfy CG, van Dijke CF, Lu Y, et al. Quantification of articular cartilage in the metacarpophalangeal joints of the hand: accuracy and precision of 3D MR imaging. *AJR* 1995;165:371–375, with permission.)

Eliminating the high signal from fat on T_1-weighted images, by using fat saturation, increases the dynamic range of signal intensities in the image and increases contrast between cartilage and adjacent structures. Cartilage is accordingly depicted as a band of high signal intensity on such images, whereas adjacent joint fluid, adipose tissue, and subchondral bone show low signal intensity (45). Synovial tissue also generates a relatively high signal intensity with this technique, but the S/N between it and cartilage remains sufficiently high to discriminate these tissues (45). Recht and co-workers (50) have shown this technique to be 96% sensitive and 95% specific for detecting macroscopically visible cartilage defects in cadaveric knees. Disler and co-workers (51) reported a 93% sensitivity and 94% specificity for arthroscopically visible cartilage lesions detected *in vivo* with fat-suppressed 3D MRI. In the same study, conventional T_2-weighted MRI showed a sensitivity of only 53% at a comparable specificity.

Once the cartilage can be isolated from adjacent structures on MRI, a variety of sophisticated analyses can be performed. Shaded 3D surface renderings of the cartilage can be generated using an image processing technique called segmentation (52) (Fig. 6.26). The resulting 3D images accurately depict the surface topography of the cartilage, which does not necessarily correspond to the topography of the underlying cortex. Such images could be used to monitor the distribution and severity of cartilage surface irregularities in patients with arthritis, or to analyze contact areas between articular surfaces in joint malalignment or following surgical procedures, such as patellar realignment, partial meniscectomy, or rotator cuff repair (53).

In addition, by summing the voxels contained within the 3D reconstructed image of the cartilage, the exact volume of this highly complex structure can be determined with great accuracy and precision (22,49,52,54,55) (Fig. 6.27). Using a similar technique, one can map the thickness of cartilage as well. Using conventional MRI of the knee, Cohen et al. (56) achieved an average precision error (root-mean-square standard deviation) of only 0.3 mm for femoral, tibial, and patellar cartilage thickness. Early experience with these techniques suggests that they may be more reliable than conventional radiography for monitoring disease progression and treatment response in patients with arthritis (55,57,58). This method of quantifying volume by MRI applies not only to articular cartilage but also to any structure that can be accurately isolated on MRI (Fig. 6.28). Heuck and co-workers (59) previously demonstrated highly accurate and reproducible quantification of injected joint fluid in cadaveric knees using a similar technique. With sufficient contrast, it would similarly be possible to quantify the amount of hypertrophic synovial tissue in an arthritic joint.

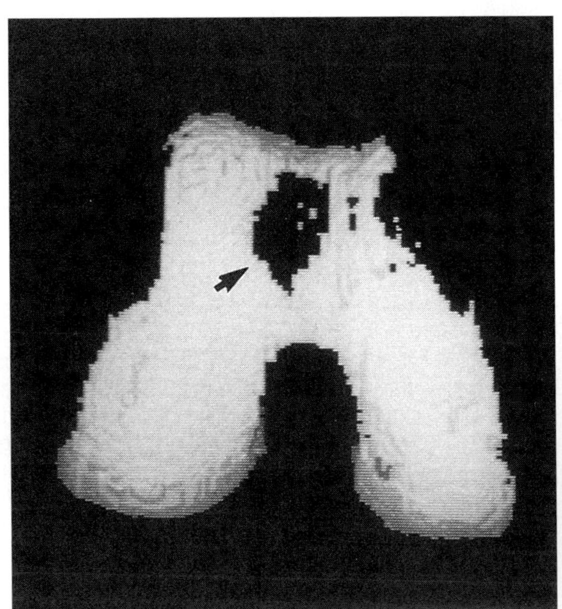

A

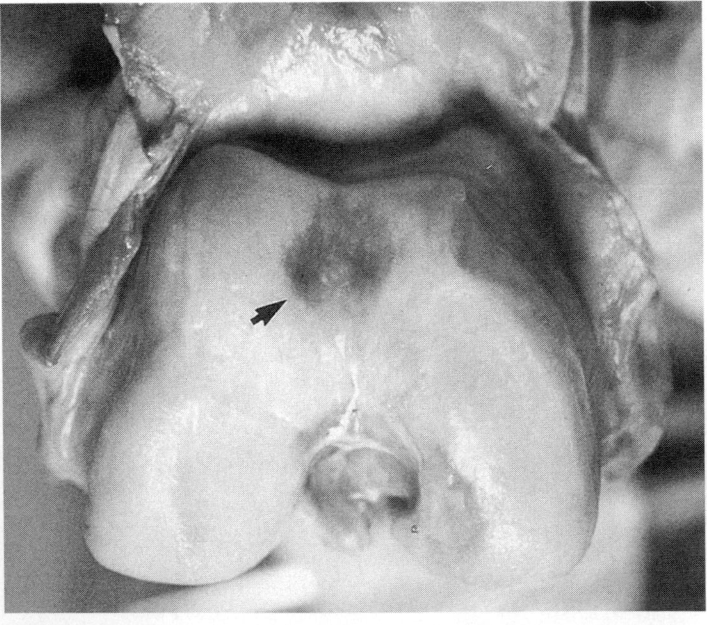

B

FIG. 6.26. Three-dimensional (3D) surface rendering of the femoral cartilage. **A:** Viewed from an anterior vantage point, the 3D rendering from segmented T_1-weighted, fat-suppressed gradient-echo magnetic resonance imaging shows a large focal defect in the trochlear groove (*arrow*). This correlates well with the chondral defect (*arrow*) visible on the gross specimen **(B)**. Adding the voxels contained within the 3D image determines the total volume of femoral cartilage. (From Peterfy CG, van Dijke CF, Janzen DL, et al. Quantification of articular cartilage in the knee by pulsed saturation transfer and fat-suppressed MRI: optimization and validation. *Radiology* 1994;192:485–491, with permission.)

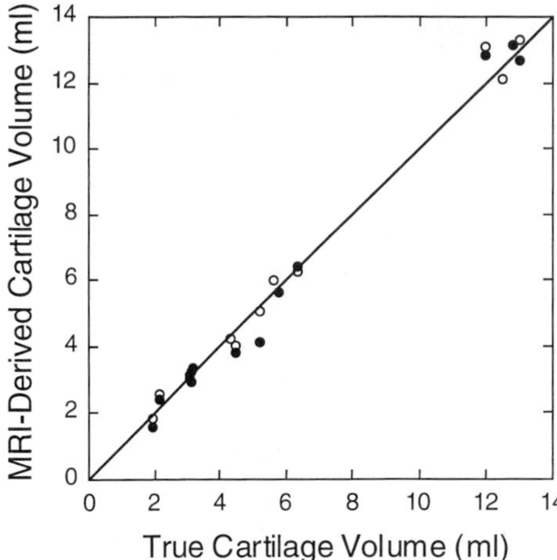

FIG. 6.27. Accuracy of magnetic resonance imaging (MRI) quantification of total articular cartilage volume. The graph depicts cartilage volumes determined by MRI plotted against volumes measured directly by water displacement. A total of 12 cartilage plates (six patellar, three tibial, three femoral) from six knees were included. Line represents theoretic 100% accuracy. (Modified from Peterfy CG, van Dijke CF, Janzen DL, et al. Quantification of articular cartilage in the knee by pulsed saturation transfer and fat-suppressed MRI: optimization and validation. *Radiology* 1994;192:485–491, with permission.)

MAGNETIC RESONANCE IMAGING OF SYNOVIAL TISSUE AND JOINT FLUID

The synovial lining shows a broad spectrum of involvement in various articular disorders, but in the normal joint, it is generally too thin to be delineated with conventional MRI. In many cases, the only sign of synovitis is the presence of a joint effusion. However, the amount of synovial fluid that normally resides in diarthrodial joints varies considerably throughout the body. The ankle in particular may contain a relatively large amount of synovial fluid under normal conditions (60). Exactly what the appropriate threshold is for defining a quantity of joint fluid as abnormal is therefore not known. As discussed above, using 3D reconstruction methods and MRI sequences that provide sufficient contrast between joint fluid and adjacent tissues, it is possible to quantify the amount of free fluid in a joint by MRI with extremely high accuracy and precision (59) (Fig. 6.28). This may be useful for monitoring treatment response in patients with arthritis or for studying the normal role of synovial fluid in joint physiology *in vivo*. As for cartilage imaging, however, the critical issue is whether sufficient contrast can be generated between the joint fluid and adjacent tissues, such as cartilage and synovium.

The signal behavior of nonhemorrhagic joint fluid is dominated by free water and therefore shows slow T_1 recovery

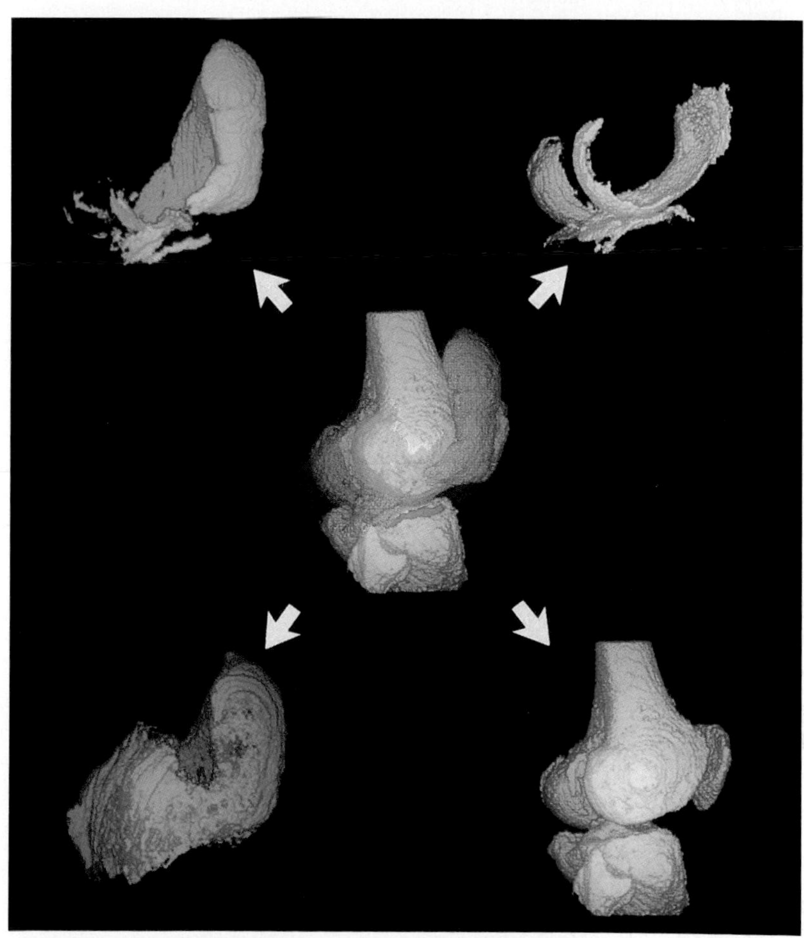

FIG. 6.28. Three-dimensional (3D) imaging of individual articular components. "Exploded" 3D image (posterolateral view) of cartilage (*yellow*), thickened synovium (*transparent red*), effusion (*blue*), and bones (*white*) of an OA knee. The individual articular components are shown surrounding a central composite image. The 3D images were reconstructed using the magnetization-transfer subtraction image data for the knee shown in Fig. 6.21. The volume of each articular component can be determined by summing the voxels within its 3D image. (From Kuettner KE, Goldberg VM, eds. *Osteoarthritic disorders.* Rosemont, IL: American Academy of Orthopaedic Surgeons, 1995, with permission.)

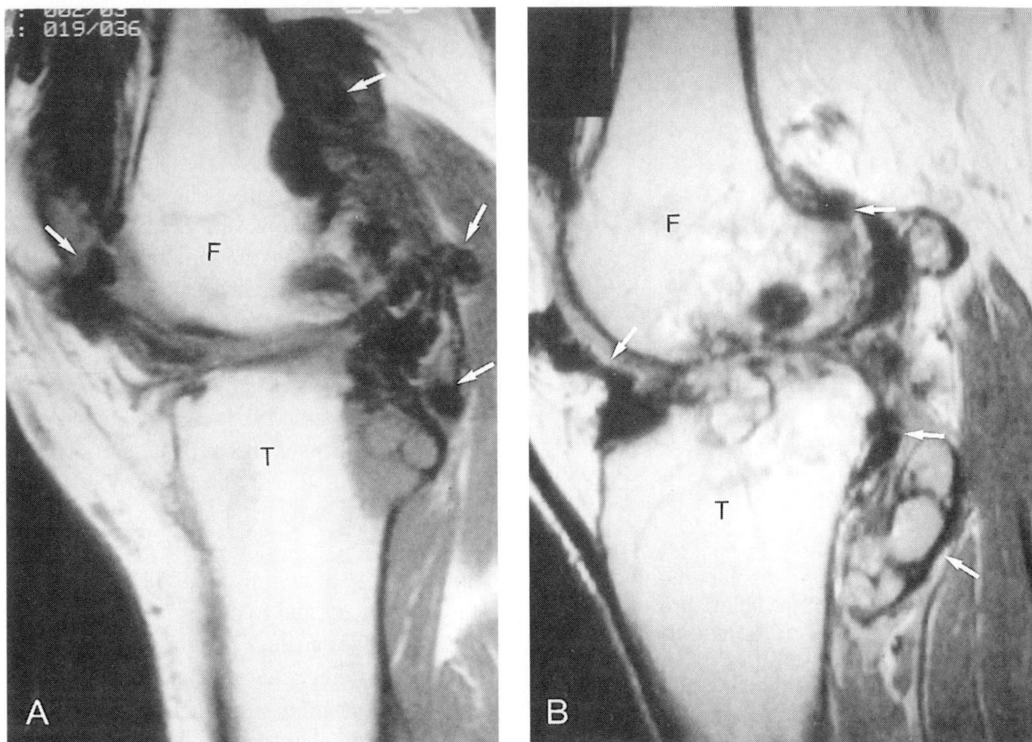

FIG. 6.29. Pigmented villonodular synovitis (PVNS). **A:** Sagittal T_1-weighted spin-echo image of a knee with PVNS shows diffuse synovial thickening with areas of low signal intensity representing hemosiderin deposition (*arrows*). **B:** Sagittal T_1-weighted image of a knee with hemophilic arthropathy shows a similar appearance of synovial thickening and hemosiderin deposition (*arrows*) due to recurrent hemarthrosis. *F,* femur; *T,* tibia.

and slow T_2 decay. Joint effusions accordingly show intensely high signal on T_2-weighted images (Fig. 6.9B). Hemorrhagic effusions, on the other hand, can have the opposite appearance. They may contain methemoglobin, which has a short T_1 and shows high signal intensity on T_1-weighted images (Fig. 6.6A), or deoxyhemoglobin, which shows rapid T_2 relaxation and thus appears low in signal intensity on T_2-weighted images (Fig. 6.6B). A fluid level may be seen in some cases. In chronic recurrent hemarthrosis, hemosiderin accumulation in the synovium may lower signal intensity on both T_1- and T_2-weighted images (Figs. 6.29 and 6.30). Hemorrhage often develops in popliteal cysts as they dissect between the gastrocnemius and soleus muscles of the calf. In these cases, the appearance on T_1-weighted images may resemble a fat-containing neoplasm, such as a liposarcoma (Fig. 6.6), whereas the T_2-weighted images may be suggestive of pigmented villonodular synovitis (Figs. 6.29 and 6.30). Popliteal cysts are also often the repositories for loose intraarticular bodies (Fig. 6.31). Leakage of synovial fluid from ruptured Baker's cysts may produce a feathery pattern of free water signal or Gd-DTPA enhancement along the fascial planes between the muscles behind the knee (61) (Fig. 6.32).

Synovial tissue in the joint can show a variable appearance on MRI. Inflamed, edematous synovium usually exhibits slow T_2 relaxation, reflecting its high interstitial water content. Accordingly, it may be difficult to discriminate

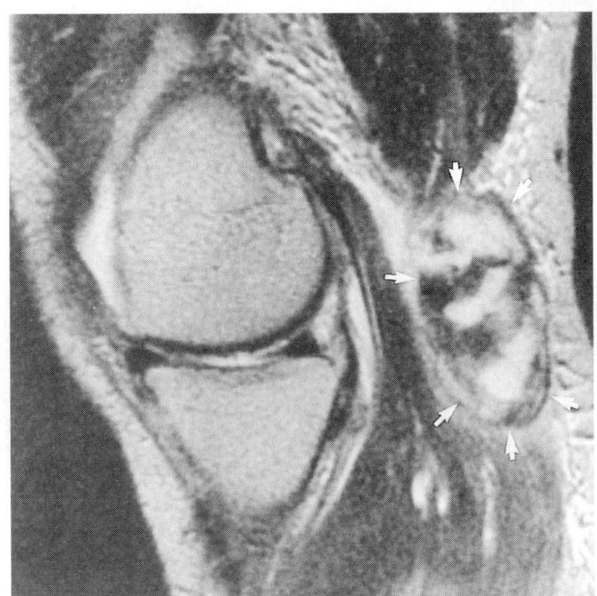

FIG. 6.30. Hemorrhagic Baker's cyst. Sagittal T_2-weighted spin-echo image of the knee of a patient with a hemorrhagic Baker's cyst (*arrows*) containing irregular areas of signal void producing an appearance similar to that of pigmented villonodular synovitis.

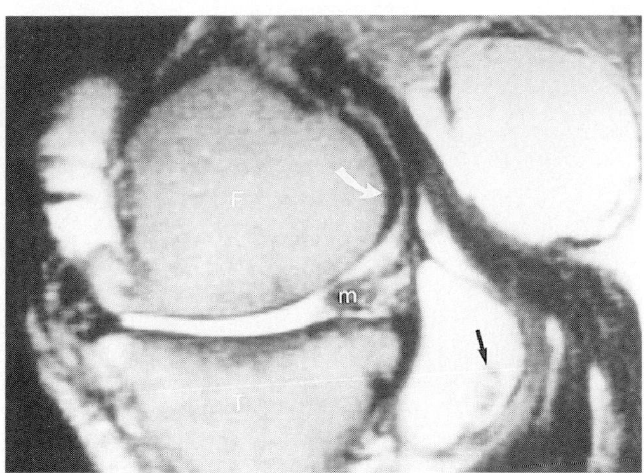

FIG. 6.31. Loose intraarticular body in a Baker's cyst. Sagittal T_2-weighted spin-echo image of a knee with severe osteoarthritis demonstrates a calcified loose body (*straight arrow*) in a popliteal cyst. Cartilage (*curved arrow*) is preserved over the posterior aspect of the femoral condyle (*F*) but is otherwise completely denuded. Note the macerated medial meniscus (*m*). *T*, tibia.

thickened synovial tissue from adjacent joint fluid or cartilage (Fig. 6.33). Hemosiderin deposition or chronic fibrosis can lower the signal intensity of hyperplastic synovial tissue on long-TE images (T_2-weighted) and occasionally even short-TE images (T_1-weighted, proton-density-weighted, most gradient-echo sequences). Most synovial tissue exhibits a slightly shorter T_1 than does joint fluid, but under normal circumstances the contrast on T_1-weighted images is

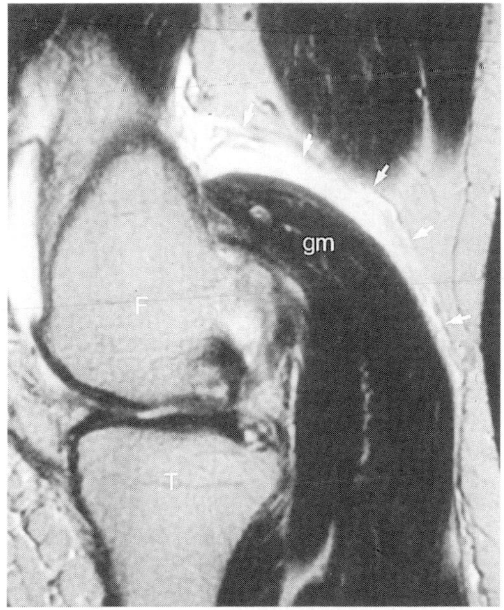

FIG. 6.32. Ruptured Baker's cyst. Sagittal T_2-weighted spin-echo image shows free fluid (*arrows*) from a ruptured Baker cyst tracking along fascial planes deep to the gastrocnemius muscle (*gm*). *F*, femur; *T*, tibia.

relatively poor. Intravenous injection of Gd-DTPA can improve synovial contrast by increasing T_1 recovery and rendering hypervascular synovial tissue high in signal intensity on T_1-weighted images (62–66). Contrast between the high signal intensity synovium and any adjacent high signal intensity adipose tissue can be augmented in this setting by applying fat suppression. However, Gd-DTPA is a relatively small molecule and diffuses rapidly out of even normal capillaries. Accordingly, the Gd-DTPA leaks into the adjacent joint fluid over time (45,67,68) (Figs. 6.34 and 6.35). The rate of equilibration of these two compartments depends on a number of factors, including the degree of hyperemia of the synovium, the relative amounts of synovium and joint fluid, and the degree of mechanical mixing in the joint. In small, intensely inflamed joints in the hand or the temporomandibular joints, for example, this equilibration can be extremely rapid (<5 minutes) (64) (Fig. 6.35). Accordingly, attempts to estimate the amount of Gd-DTPA-enhanced synovial tissue are confounded by a relatively unpredictable accuracy error.

Other approaches to generating contrast between synovial tissue and adjacent structures include the use of magnetization transfer (45). As stated above, selective suppression of the collagenous protons in hypertrophic synovial tissue causes the mobile water protons in the tissue to lose magnetization. The signal intensity of synovial tissue therefore decreases markedly (Fig. 6.36). By subtracting images of the same joint obtained with and without magnetization transfer, images that depict the synovium as a high signal intensity structure can be generated (Fig. 6.36). However, prominent magnetization transfer effects also occur in cartilage, so that it may be difficult to discriminate synovium and adjacent cartilage with this technique. Gd-DTPA tends to suppress magnetization transfer (45,69). Accordingly, intravenous administration of this agent will lower the signal intensity of hypervascular synovial tissue on magnetization transfer subtraction images. However, because Gd-DTPA diffuses slowly, if at all, into articular cartilage, magnetization transfer in this tissue will not be affected, and although the Gd-DTPA will accumulate in the joint fluid, magnetization transfer effects in joint fluid are negligible in the first place (45). The interplay between magnetization transfer in hyperplastic synovial tissue due to collagen content and suppression of this phenomenon by Gd-DTPA may provide a way of noninvasively characterizing this heterogeneous tissue *in vivo*. At present, however, there has been little work in this area.

Gd-DTPA has also been used to grade the severity of synovitis in patients with arthritis (64–66,68–73). Rapid synovial enhancement rate and high maximal enhancement following bolus intravenous injection of Gd-DTPA correlates with severe inflammation and hyperplasia, while sluggish enhancement corresponds to chronic fibrotic synovium. Synovial enhancement rate has been shown to change rapidly with therapy (71,72,74,75). In some cases, changes can be demonstrated within only a few days of initiating therapy. This contrasts sharply with the months of observation typically required to demonstrate disease progression

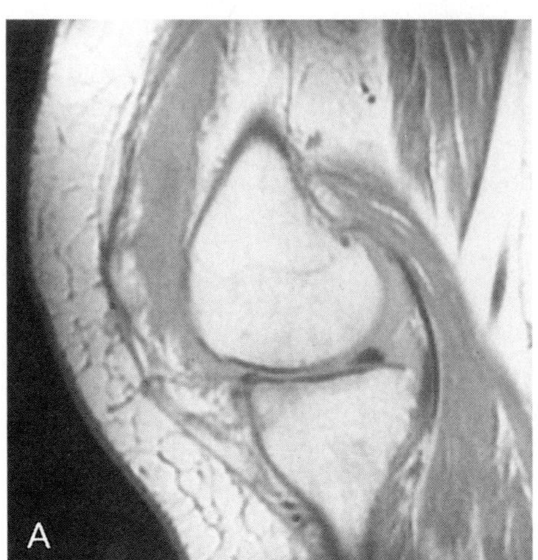

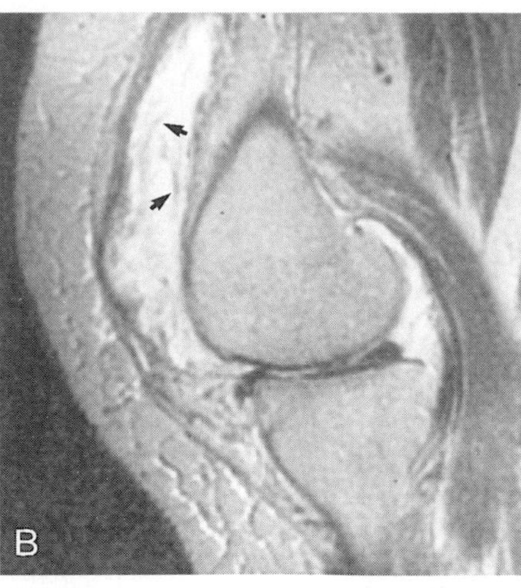

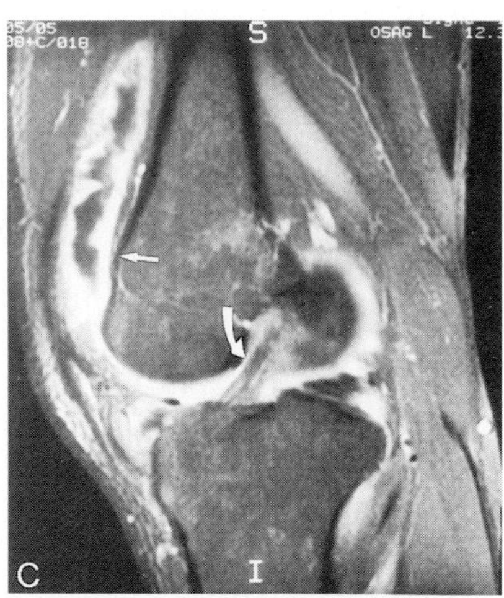

FIG. 6.33. Appearance of synovial tissue on magnetic resonance imaging. **A:** Sagittal T_1-weighted spin-echo image of the knee in a patient with rheumatoid arthritis shows distention of the suprapatellar recess with thickened synovium and effusion. With this technique, both the synovium and effusion show intermediate signal intensity and therefore exhibit poor contrast. **B:** On sagittal T_2-weighted spin-echo images, both synovium and effusion show primarily high signal intensity. Portions of the thickened synovium contain low signal intensity due to hemosiderin deposition (*arrows*), but the majority of the synovium cannot be distinguished from adjacent joint fluid. **C:** Sagittal, fat-suppressed, T_1-weighted spin-echo image of another knee with synovitis shows diffuse enhancement of the hypervascular synovial tissue (*arrow*) following intravenous administration of gadolinium–diethylenetriamine pentaacetic acid. Note the delineation of the intact anterior cruciate ligament (*curved arrow*) by enhancing synovial tissue.

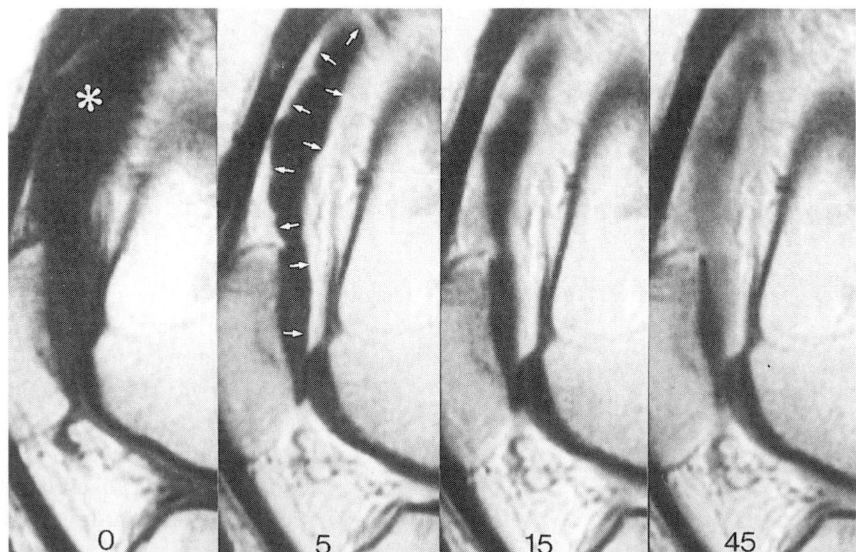

FIG. 6.34. Diffusion of synovial gadolinium–diethylenetriamine pentaacetic acid (Gd-DTPA) into adjacent joint effusion. Sagittal T_1-weighted images of the knee of a patient with nonspecific synovitis obtained at various times (0, 5, 15, and 45 minutes) following intravenous injection of Gd-DTPA. The first panel **(left)** was obtained just prior to injection of Gd-DTPA, and shows poor contrast between hypertrophic synovium and effusion distending the suprapatellar recess (*). Five minutes following injection of Gd-DTPA, the hypervascular synovial tissue exhibits high signal intensity (*arrows*) and high contrast with the adjacent effusion. However, diffusion of Gd into the joint over time (15 and 45 minutes) eventually lowers the contrast between these two compartments and obscures the synovium–effusion boundary.

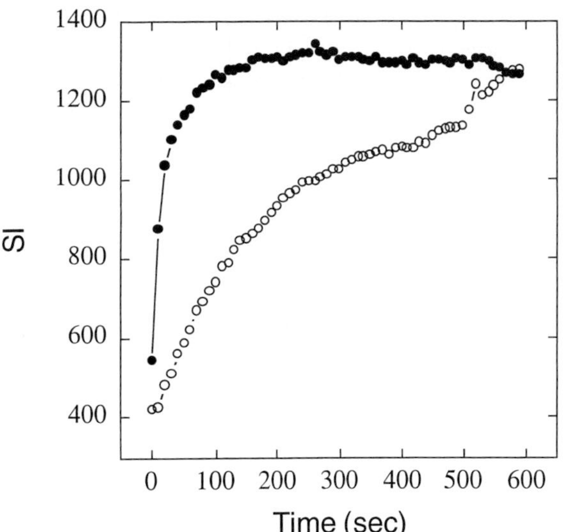

FIG. 6.35. Rapid diffusion of gadolinium–diethylenetriamine pentaacetic acid (Gd-DTPA) from synovium to joint fluid. Graph shows the change in signal intensity (*SI*) in synovial tissue (●) and joint fluid (○) at various times following intravenous injection of Gd-DTPA in the inflamed metacarpophalangeal joint of the thumb of a patient with RA. As shown, SI increases rapidly in both compartments, leading to a loss of tissue contrast in less than 10 minutes.

or treatment response using radiographic bone erosion as the metric. Moreover, high synovial volume in the hand and wrist is predictive of progressive bone erosion in patients with rheumatoid arthritis (RA). In a study by Østergaard and co-workers (72), none of nine patients with less than 5 cm^3 of synovium at baseline showed MRI or radiographic evidence of new bone erosion after 12 months, whereas eight of ten patients with at least 10 cm^3 of synovium at baseline showed progression. Accordingly, MRI measures of synovitis could serve as useful surrogate end points for identifying patients with RA who are likely to develop erosive diseases, as well as for monitoring therapy in these patients. Further work is needed, however, to validate this potential marker as well as to characterize its performance.

An unusual synovial condition that presents with monoarticular hemarthrosis is pigmented villonodular synovitis (76–78). This process typically involves large joints, most commonly the knee. It is closely related to giant cell tumor of the tendon sheath, which is indistinguishable histologically, but as the name implies, it is usually restricted to the synovial lining of tendon sheaths, typically in the digits. Despite their histologic similarities, however, the two lesions have very different MRI appearances. Giant cell tumor of the tendon sheath classically appears as a smoothly marginated mass adjacent to a tendon, with homogeneously low signal intensity on T_2-weighted images (79) (Fig. 6.37). This low signal is due to an abundance

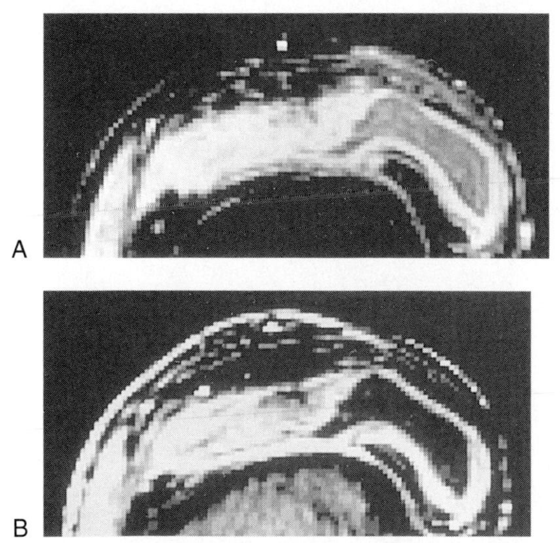

FIG. 6.36. Magnetic resonance imaging of the synovium without gadolinium–diethylenetriamine pentaacetic acid. Transverse images of the knee of a patient with rheumatoid arthritis using magnetization transfer subtraction **(A)** and fat-suppressed T_1-weighted gradient echo **(B)**. Both delineate the thickened synovial tissue with high contrast. (From Peterfy CG, Majumdar S, Lang P, et al. MR imaging of the arthritic knee: improved discrimination of cartilage, synovium and effusion with pulsed saturation transfer and fat-suppressed T_1-weighted sequences. *Radiology* 1994; 191: 413–419, with permission.)

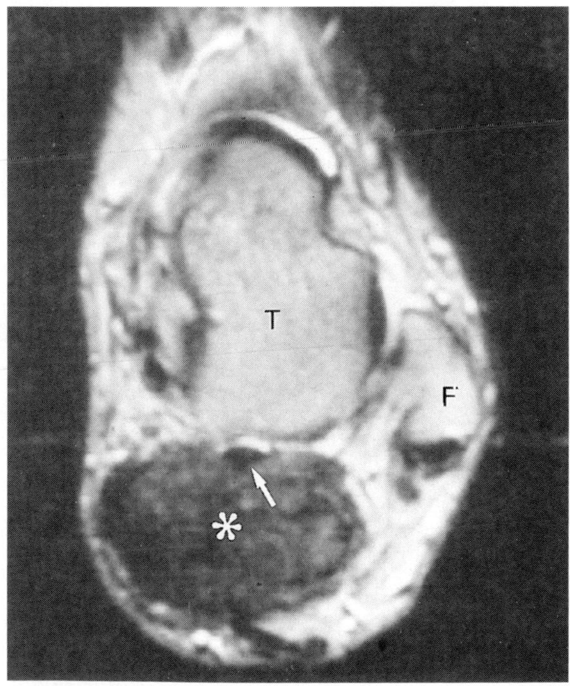

FIG. 6.37. Giant cell tumor of the tendon sheath. Transverse T_2-weighted spin-echo image of the ankle shows a large, homogeneously low signal intensity mass with smooth margins (*) adjacent to the tendon of the flexor hallucis longus (*arrow*). *T*, talus; *F*, fibula.

of collagen and a small amount of hemosiderin within most lesions. Pigmented villonodular synovitis, on the other hand, typically appears as a diffuse, irregular thickening of the synovium with markedly heterogeneous low signal intensity on both long-TE and short-TE images due to extensive hemosiderin deposition from recurrent hemarthrosis (Figs. 6.10D and 6.29). It is completely indistinguishable on MRI from another cause of recurrent hemarthrosis, hemophilia (Fig. 6.29). These two entities are easily differentiated clinically, but their similarity on MRI emphasizes the importance of hemarthrosis to the MRI appearance of pigmented villonodular synovitis. Occasionally, villonodular synovitis arises in a large joint as a discrete nodule without any significant hemarthrosis (Fig. 6.38A). These lesions are usually referred to as focal pigmented villonodular synovitis, but their MRI appearance is virtually identical to that of giant cell tumor of the tendon sheath: round, smoothly marginated, and homogeneously low in signal intensity on T_2-weighted images. Conversely, giant cell tumor of the tendon sheath occasionally presents as a multinodular, hemosiderin-stained lesion (Fig. 6.38B).

Another synovial process that may appear low in signal intensity on MRI is synovial osteochondromatosis (78,80). In this case, the basis for low signal is the presence of calcification, which typically produces a signal void on MRI. Synovial osteochondromatosis begins as a chondroid metaplasia of the synovium. Small chondroid projections may break loose from the synovium and float freely in the joint, where they can grow, nourished by the synovial fluid. These loose intraarticular chondral bodies can reattach to the synovium, develop a vascular supply, and often ossify. Osteochondral bodies are readily detectable by conventional radiography and CT, which also may show associated bone erosions, but these modalities underestimate the sometimes extensive soft tissue component of these lesions (Fig. 6.39). Moreover, in the absence of any significant calcification, these lesions may be completely occult to radiographs. On MRI, noncalcified synovial chondromatosis may be mistaken for loculated fluid collections, such as ganglion cysts or popliteal cysts, unless the fine nodularity of the lesion is identified. There is some speculation that synovial chondromatosis may sometimes undergo malignant transformation to chondrosarcoma (78). However, primary malignancies and even metastatic disease to the synovium, except through direct extension, are exceedingly rare. Even synovial cell sarcomas are almost always extraarticular (81).

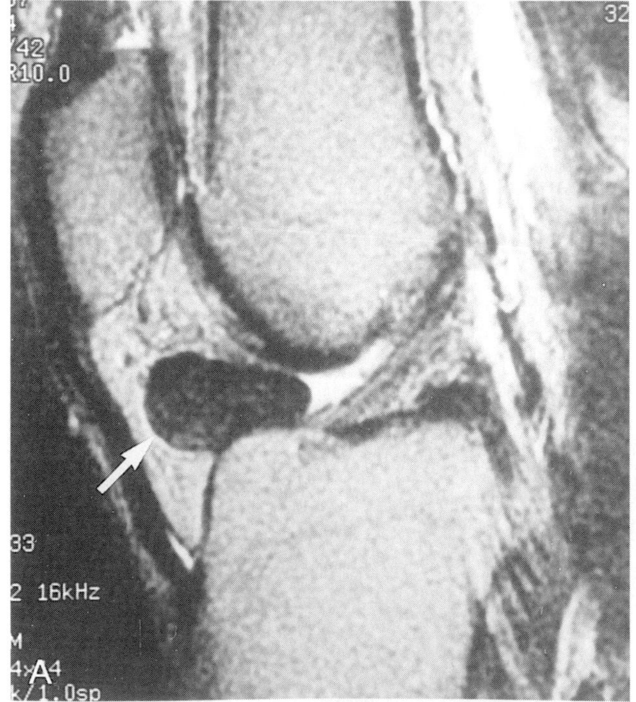

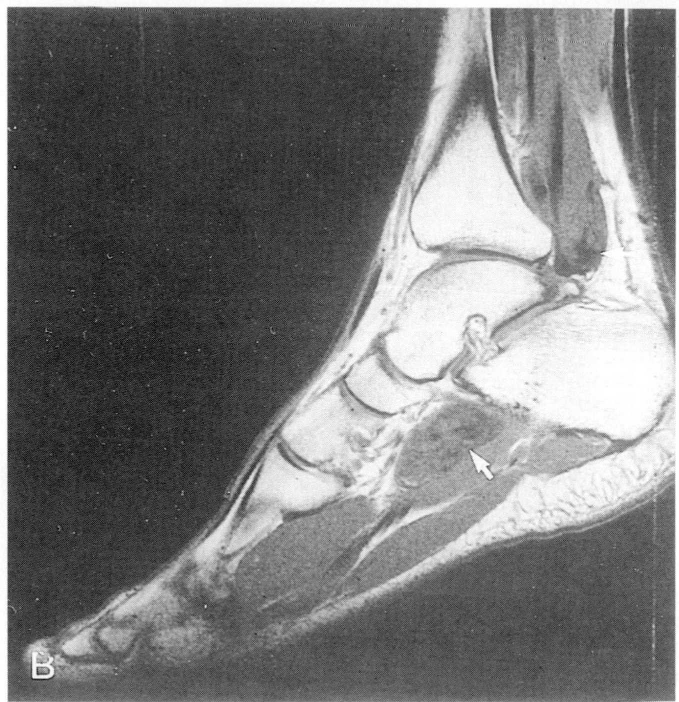

FIG. 6.38. Unusual patterns of villonodular synovitis. **A:** Sagittal T_2-weighted spin-echo image of a knee with focal nodular synovitis shows a homogeneously low signal intensity mass (*arrow*) with smooth margins located in the infrapatellar (Hoffa) fat pad. The lesion exhibits features that are more similar to those of giant cell tumor of the tendon sheath than those of pigmented villonodular synovitis. **B:** Sagittal T_1-weighted spin-echo image of an ankle shows diffuse, intensely hemosiderin-stained villonodular synovitis of the tendon sheath of the flexor hallucis longus (*arrows*). In this case, the process appears more like pigmented villonodular synovitis than giant cell tumor of the tendon sheath.

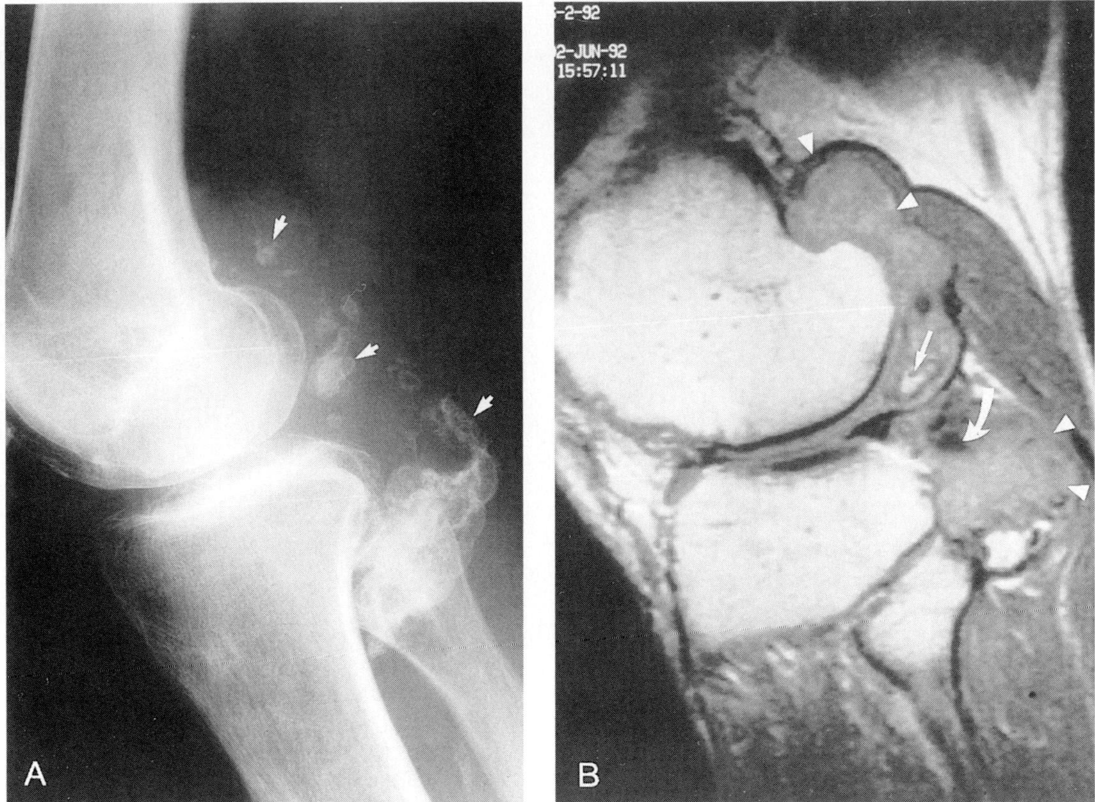

FIG. 6.39. Synovial osteochondromatosis. **A:** Lateral radiograph of the knee shows numerous ossific bodies (*arrows*) within the knee consistent with synovial osteochondromatosis. **B:** On sagittal T_1-weighted spin-echo images of the same knee, some of the ossifications can be seen to contain high signal intensity marrow fat (*straight arrow*), while others appear diffusely low in signal reflecting intense calcification (*curved arrow*). The magnetic resonance image also shows the extensive, noncalcified soft tissue component (*arrowheads*) of this lesion.

MAGNETIC RESONANCE IMAGING OF OTHER ARTICULAR TISSUES

Subarticular Bone

Although it was once felt that MRI had little to offer in musculoskeletal imaging because of its inability to derive signal from calcified structures, in retrospect this could not have been farther from the truth. Today, musculoskeletal applications account for approximately 25% of the clinical use of this modality. Although it is true that calcification and therefore cortical and trabecular bone are depicted as signal voids on MRI, these structures are silhouetted by the intermediate and high signal intensity tissues lining them and therefore are actually well delineated in most cases. Moreover, MRI is unsurpassed in its ability to image the marrow, and it is currently the most sensitive method of detecting bone metastases, osteomyelitis, osteonecrosis, and bone trauma (82). In each of these cases, increased free water, which appears low in signal intensity on T_1-weighted images and high in signal intensity on T_2-weighted images, shows high contrast with the normal marrow fat, which has a high signal intensity on T_1-weighted images and low signal intensity on T_2-weighted images. One exception to this is T_2-weighted fast spin echo, which depicts both fat and water with relatively high signal intensity and therefore necessitates the use of fat suppression to generate contrast between these marrow constituents (see earlier section on Imaging Sequences). It should also be reiterated that gradient-echo techniques are generally insensitive to marrow pathology because of magnetic susceptibility effects in cancellous bone. Bone sclerosis is also visible on MRI and presents a low signal intensity on all pulse sequences due to the presence of dense calcification and fibrosis.

In arthritic joints, MRI delineates osteophytes (Fig. 6.40), erosions (Fig. 6.41), and subchondral cysts with greater sensitivity than does conventional radiography or CT (83). Several studies have found MRI to be at least twice as sensitive as radiography for detecting the presence and progression of bone erosion (72,74,84–86). This is attributable to, among other things, the multiplanar tomographic capability of MRI. In addition, MRI is capable

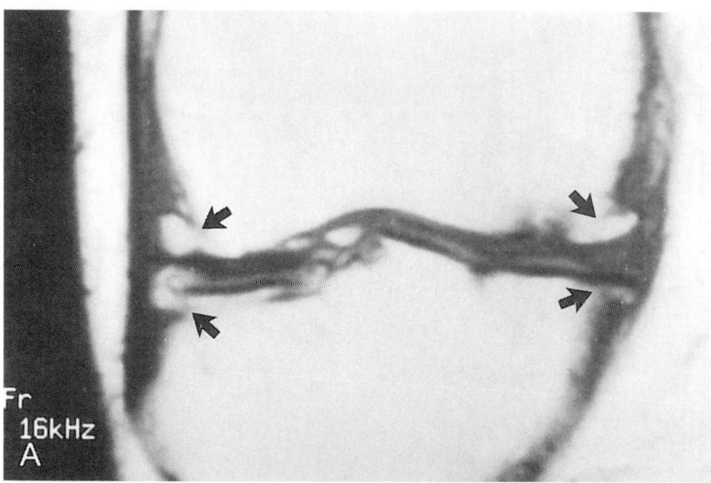

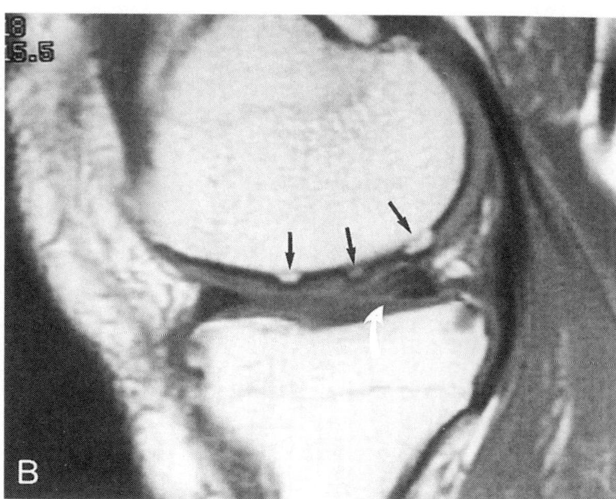

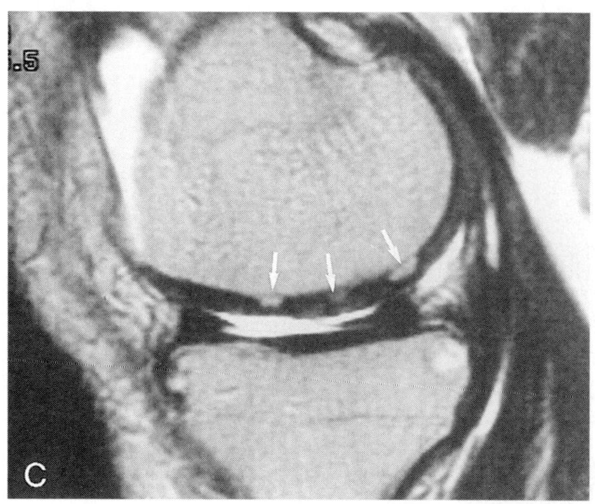

FIG. 6.40. Magnetic resonance imaging appearance of marginal and central osteophytes. **A:** Coronal T_1-weighted spin-echo image of an osteoarthritic knee shows large marginal osteophytes (*arrows*). Sagittal T_1-weighted spin echo **(B)** and T_2-weighted **(C)** fast spin-echo images of a different osteoarthritic knee shows central osteophytes (*arrows*) along the weight-bearing portion of the femoral condyle. These central osteophytes are covered by articular cartilage, although the quality of this cartilage may be abnormal. Note that the meniscal tear (*curved arrow*) visible on the T_1-weighted image is not apparent on the T_2-weighted image.

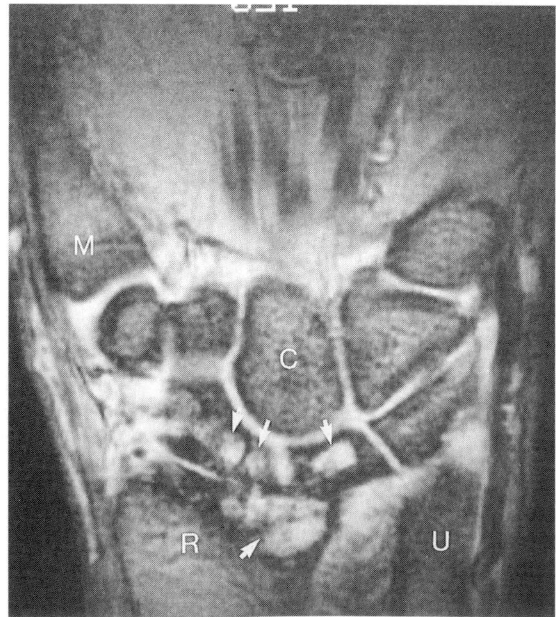

FIG. 6.41. Detection of erosions on magnetic resonance imaging. Coronal T_2*-weighted image of the wrist of a patient with rheumatoid arthritis shows several erosions (*arrows*) in the carpal bones and distal radius (*R*). *U,* ulna; *C,* capitate; *M,* first metacarpal.

of delineating sites of enthesitis (Fig. 6.42) and periostitis and directly visualizing bone marrow edema and inflammation (87–89) (Fig. 6.43). Focal bone marrow edema/inflammation has been reported to precede erosion in RA (88,89). In OA, subarticular marrow edema-like changes are associated with pain (90) and predictive of subsequent cartilage loss (91). Histologically, these areas typically show fibrosis and inflammatory infiltration and probably reflect mechanical injury to the subchondral bone due to biomechanical failure of the overlying cartilage or loss of joint stability.

One important clinical application of MRI of bone is the evaluation of avascular necrosis in arthritis patients treated with steroids (92). MRI is the most sensitive technique for detecting avascular necrosis. The earliest MRI finding of bone marrow ischemia is replacement of the normal fat signal by water signal (Fig. 6.44). The appearance at this stage of avascular necrosis is accordingly nonspecific, and trauma, infection, neoplasm, or transient osteoporosis of the hip must be differentiated on the basis of clinical criteria. As the osteonecrosis matures and the marrow edema subsides, a serpiginous band of reparative

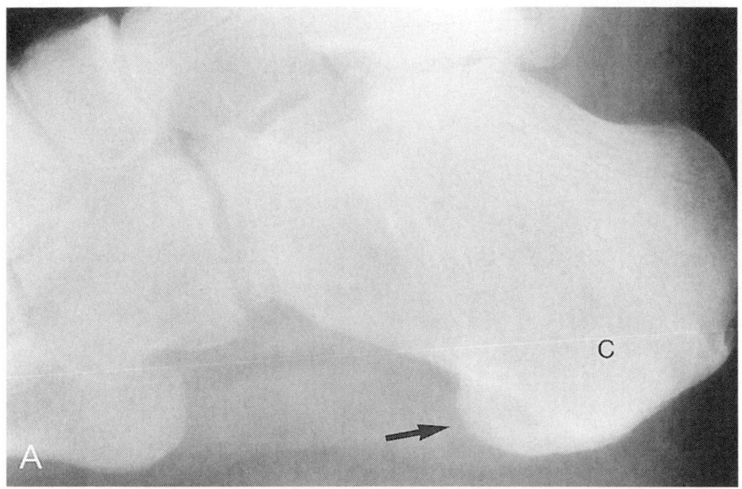

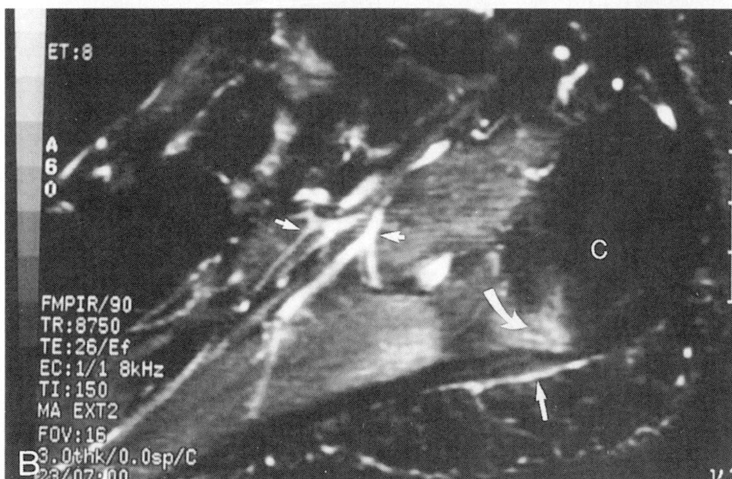

FIG. 6.42. Appearance of enthesitis on magnetic resonance imaging. **A:** Lateral radiograph of the heel of a man with Reiter syndrome shows subtle cortical irregularity at the calcaneal insertion of the plantar aponeurosis (*arrow*). **B:** Sagittal, fast, multiplanar inversion recovery (*FMPIR*) image of the heel depicts water with high signal intensity and fat with low signal intensity, and thus shows edema in the local soft tissues and bone marrow (*curved arrow*) with extremely high sensitivity. Fluid can also be seen tracking along the plantar aponeurosis (*long straight arrow*) (plantar fasciitis). The branching high signal intensity structures (*short straight arrows*) are blood vessels. *C,* calcaneus.

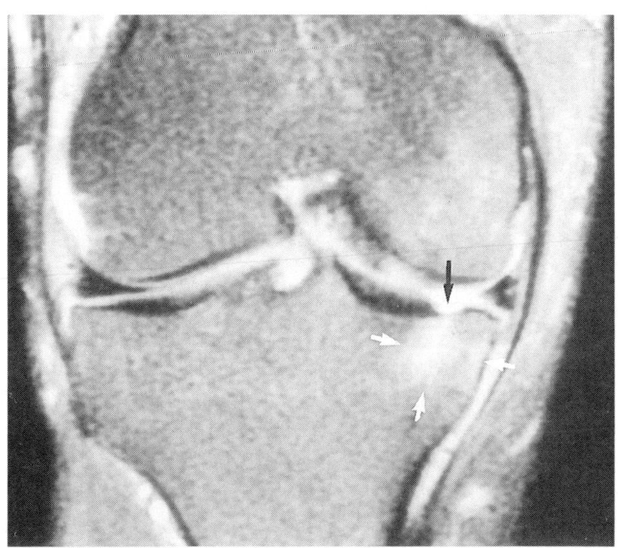

FIG. 6.43. Detecting bone marrow edema in osteoarthritis (OA) using magnetic resonance imaging. Coronal T_2-weighted fast spin-echo image of the knee of a patient with OA shows local marrow edema (*white arrows*) beneath a focal cartilage defect (*black arrow*) in the medial tibial plateau.

tissue eventually forms along the perimeter of the devitalized bone (Fig. 6.44B). This wavy reactive zone typically shows a low signal intensity on T_1-weighted images and a high signal intensity on T_2-weighted images, and is virtually pathognomonic of avascular necrosis. In addition to diagnosing the disorder, MRI is useful for evaluating the extent of bone involvement and identifying subtle deformities of the articular surface that may increase the risk for subsequent OA.

MRI is also the most sensitive technique for detecting stress reactions or insufficiency fractures that may complicate chronic steroid use. In each of these conditions, the normal marrow fat is replaced by water signal, often in a pathognomonic linear configuration (Fig. 6.45).

Articular Ligaments, Menisci, and Labra

Other articular structures that are important in maintaining the functional integrity of diarthrodial joints are the supporting ligaments and meniscal or labral tissue. The ability of MRI to evaluate these structures is well established, and

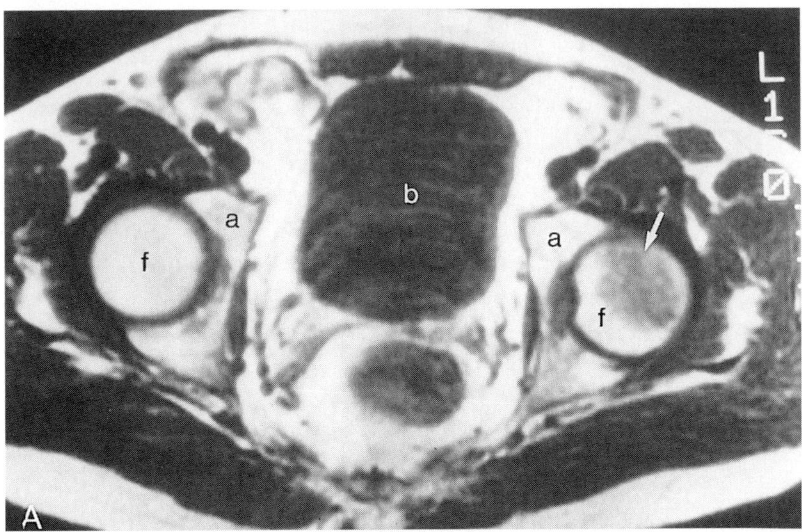

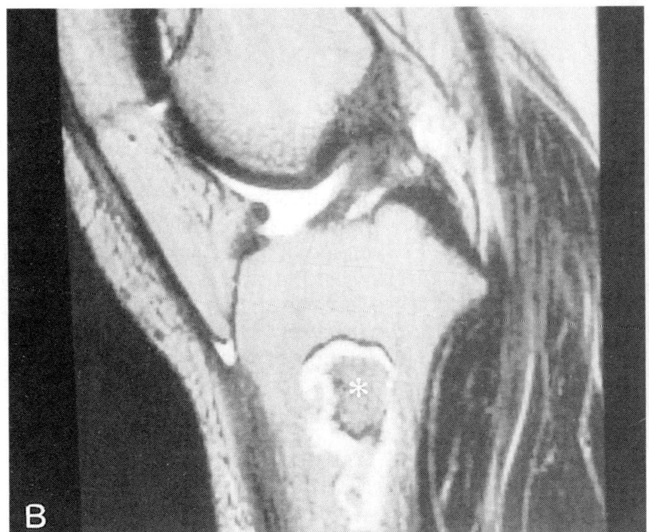

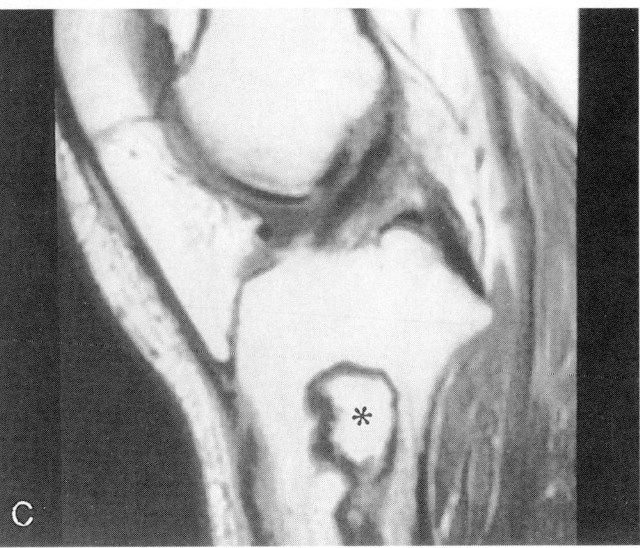

FIG. 6.44. Magnetic resonance imaging appearance of avascular necrosis. **A:** Transverse T_1-weighted image of a patient (supine) with hip pain on long-term steroid therapy for lupus erythematosus shows nonspecific marrow edema (*arrow*) in the left femoral head (*f*). The location and clinical context of this finding are suggestive of avascular necrosis, but the imaging appearance is otherwise nonspecific. *a,* acetabulum; *b,* bladder. Sagittal T_1-weighted **(B)** and T_2-weighted **(C)** spin-echo image of the knee of another patient shows a region of abnormal marrow (*) in the proximal tibia delimited by a serpiginous margin of regenerative tissue in a pattern that is pathognomonic for osteonecrosis.

constitutes a major clinical application of this modality today.

Ligaments

Ligaments are composed primarily of collagen, which provides tensile strength, but also constrains and dephases water protons (see earlier section on T_2 Relaxation) and therefore affects MRI signal behavior. The relative lack of water protons in most normal ligaments compounded by this T_2-shortening effect of collagen explains the extremely low signal intensity of ligaments on most MRIs. Ligaments are, accordingly, most visible on MRI when silhouetted by high signal intensity substances, such as adipose fat or synovial fluid, both of which show greater signal than normal ligaments on proton density–weighted and T_2-weighted spin-echo images or T_2*-weighted gradient-echo images.

Intact ligaments appear as dark bands that can be traced to their insertions (Fig. 6.46). Discontinuity is intuitively a direct sign of ligamentous disruption. However, this may be mimicked by obliquity of the plane

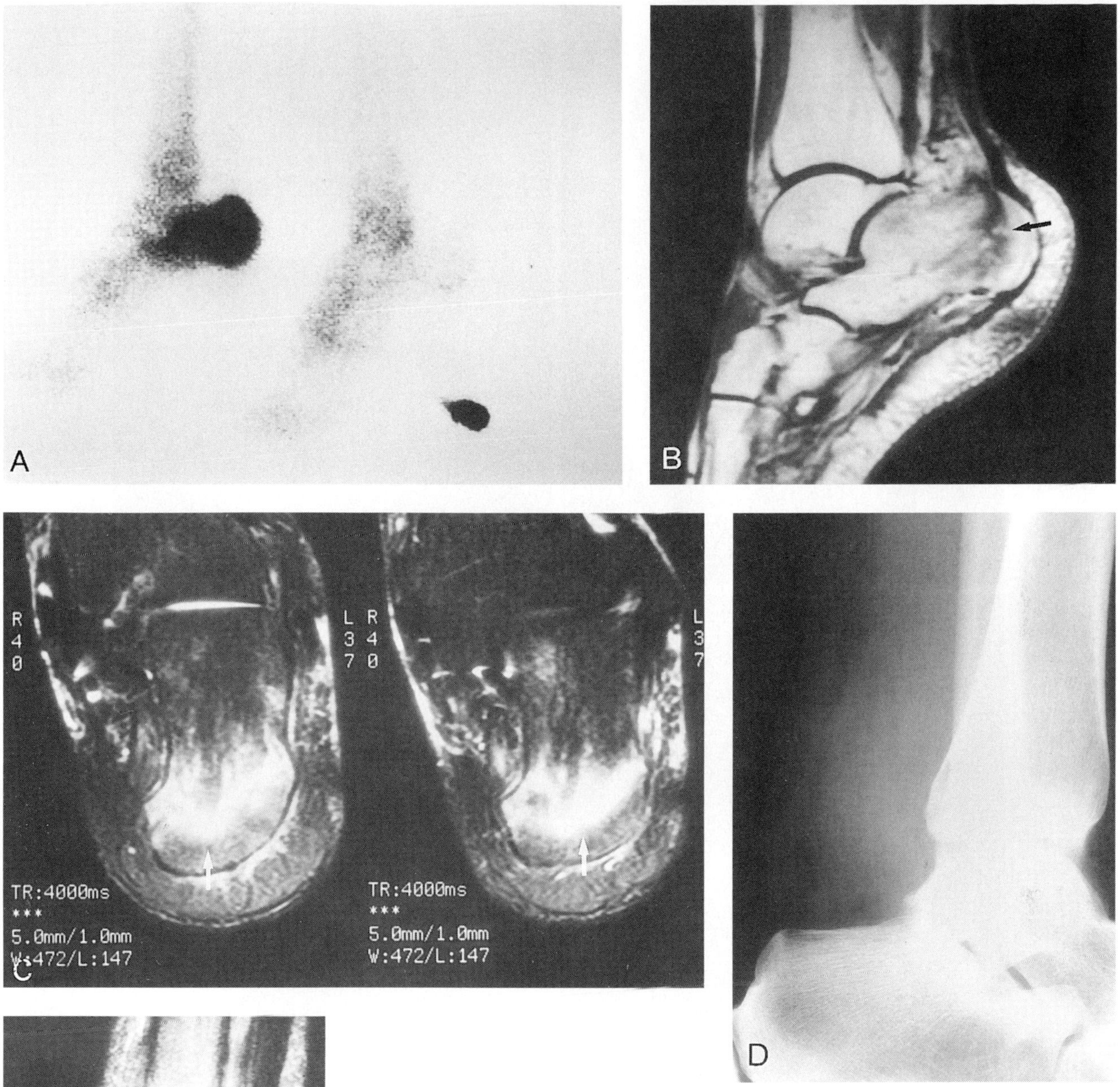

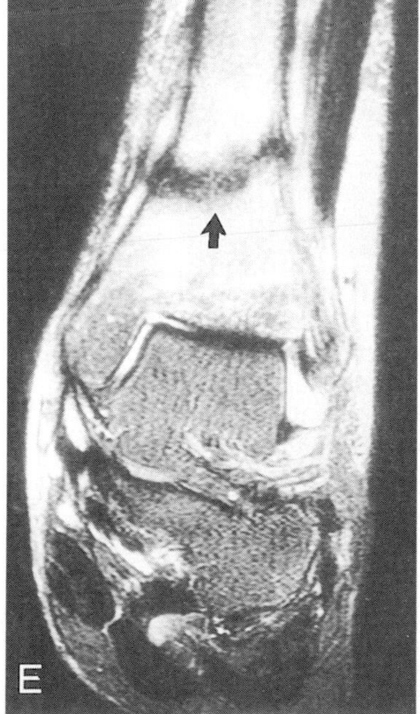

FIG. 6.45. Detection of stress fractures with magnetic resonance imaging. **A:** Lateral bone scintigraphy of the foot of a woman with lung cancer and spontaneous heel pain show increased uptake in the calcaneus but offers no further information about the nature of the process (radiographs were negative). **B:** Sagittal T_1-weighted spin-echo image of the heel shows a vertical band of low signal intensity replacing the normal marrow fat in the calcaneus (*arrow*) in a pattern that is pathognomonic for fracture. **C:** Transverse fat-suppressed T_2-weighted fast spin-echo images of the calcaneus delineate the high signal intensity fracture line (*arrows*). **D:** Lateral radiograph of a patient suspected of posterior tibial tendon rupture shows no abnormalities. **E:** Coronal fat-suppressed, T_2-weighted fast spin-echo image of the same ankle shows a horizontal stress fracture (*arrow*) through the tibia.

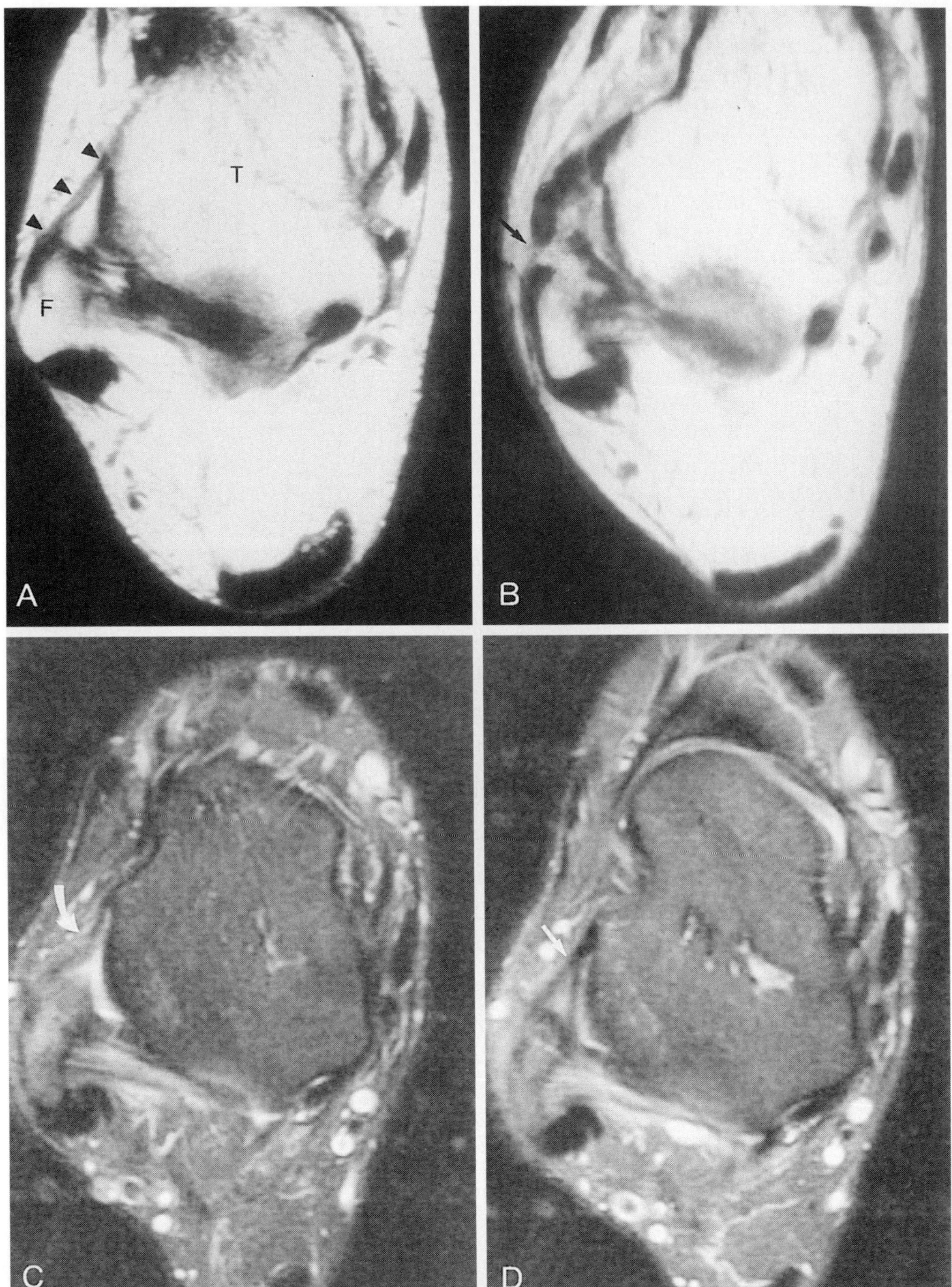

FIG. 6.46. Magnetic resonance images of ligamentous integrity. **A:** Transverse T_1-weighted spin-echo image of the ankle depicts the intact anterior talofibular ligament as a continuous low signal intensity band (*arrowheads*). *T*, talus; *F*, fibula. **B:** Disrupted anterior talofibular ligament (*black arrow*) in another ankle appears thickened and discontinuous. **C:** Transverse fat-suppressed T_2-weighted fast spin-echo imaging of another ankle in plantar flexion results in oblique sectioning and apparent discontinuity of the anterior talofibular ligament (*curved white arrow*). **D:** Repeat examination of the same ankle in dorsiflexion delineates an intact anterior talofibular ligament (*straight white arrow*).

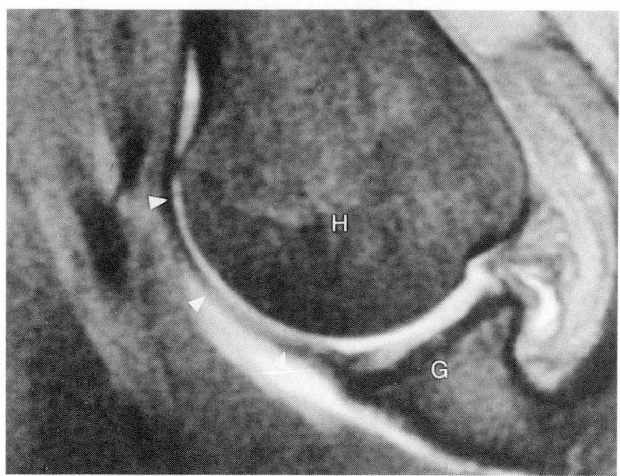

FIG. 6.47. Abducted positioning of the arm for magnetic resonance imaging of the inferior glenohumeral ligament. Fat-suppressed, T_1-weighted spin-echo image acquired with the hand placed behind the head positioning the shoulder in abduction and external rotation puts tension on the inferior glenohumeral ligament (*arrowheads*), which is depicted as a continuous low signal intensity band extending from the inferior glenoid labrum to the humeral neck. In this case, Gd-DTPA was injected directly into the joint to improve delineation of labrocapsular structures. *H,* humeral head; *G,* glenoid.

of section through an intact ligament (Fig. 6.46). Accordingly, special planes may be necessary to delineate certain ligaments. For example, the anterior cruciate ligament in the knee is best seen on oblique sagittal images with the knee in neutral position, or on direct sagittal images with the leg in slight abduction, and the important inferior glenohumeral ligament, which is a principal static stabilizer of the shoulder in abduction, is difficult to visualize unless the shoulder is positioned in abduction and external rotation (93) (Fig. 6.47). With multiplanar reformatting, thorough analysis of ligamentous integrity is possible, regardless of the original plane of image acquisition. Nevertheless, certain ligaments (e.g., the glenohumeral ligaments of the shoulder) continue to elude thorough description by MRI.

Menisci

The menisci in the knee perform important stabilizing and load-distributing functions that are critical to the integrity of that joint. This is evident from the high incidence of OA following partial or complete meniscectomy (94). Accordingly, evaluating meniscal integrity is among the most common clinical indications for MRI.

The menisci are composed of fibrocartilage and contain abundant collagen fibers spatially arranged to withstand the tensile stresses generated during weight bearing. Fiber orientation, as shown by histologic examination, polarized light microscopy, and radiograph diffraction studies, is predominantly circumferential, particularly in the peripheral half of the meniscus. This arrangement accounts for the propensity of tears to run longitudinally, because they follow the split lines between the collagen fibers rather than traversing fibers.

With respect to MRI, this collagen tends to constrain water protons within the meniscal tissue, increasing internuclear interactions and therefore T_2 relaxation. The T_2 of normal meniscal fibrocartilage is in fact so rapid that even the shortest-TE sequences fail to detect substantial signal (Fig. 6.48). If, however, there is focal loss of collagen, as with myxoid or eosinophilic degeneration (which is usually also accompanied by increased local water content), this T_2-shortening effect is diminished and the water signal is unmasked. This manifests as globular or linear areas of intermediate signal intensity within the meniscus on short-TE images (i.e., T_1-weighted or proton density–weighted spin-echo or any gradient-echo sequence) that tend to fade away at longer TEs (Fig. 6.48B). These changes are sometimes referred to as grade 1 or grade 2 signal abnormalities, respectively. They have also been misleadingly called grade 1 or grade 2 "tears," although they are not tears at all and do not, in distinction, violate the articular surfaces of the meniscus.

Tears of the menisci can be associated with gross deformity of the meniscal surface, but most often are only apparent as linear intermediate signal intensity extending to an otherwise smooth articular surface on the short-TE images (Fig. 6.48C). Occasionally, a sufficient amount of joint fluid tracks into a meniscal tear to be visualized on T_2-weighted images, but in most instances, undisplaced tears of the menisci cannot be seen on long-TE images. Short-TE images are thus highly sensitive (>90%) but somewhat nonspecific for meniscal tears, whereas long-TE images are extremely insensitive, though highly specific when present.

Labrum

The glenoid labrum in the shoulder is a somewhat homologous tissue that forms a fibrous cuff around the glenoid margin and plays an important stabilizing function in this inherently unstable joint. As for the meniscus of the knee, the MRI appearance of the glenoid labrum is dominated by its fibrous nature, and when intact, appears as a discrete low signal intensity structure. In the absence of significant capsular distention by joint fluid, however, the labrum is often obscured by adjacent low-signal intensity capsule and glenohumeral ligaments. Intraarticular injection of saline or gadolinium-containing contrast material (i.e., magnetic resonance arthrography) is occasionally necessary to delineate these labrocapsular structures on MRI (93).

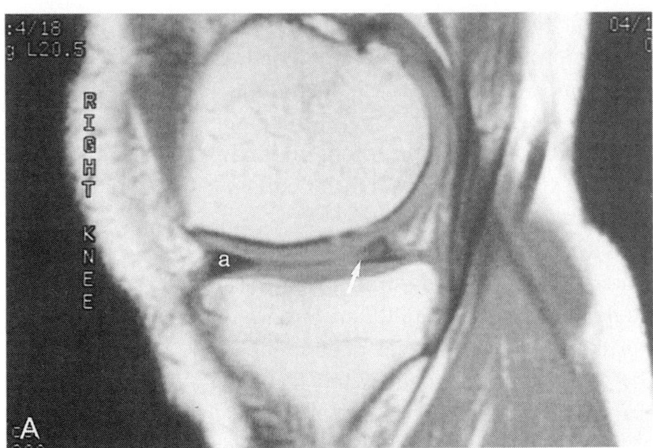

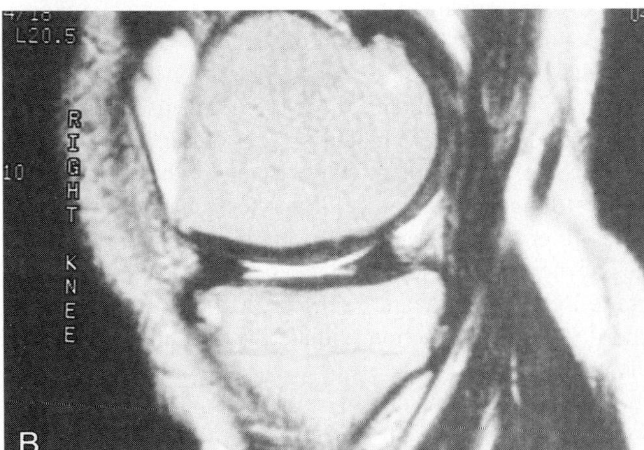

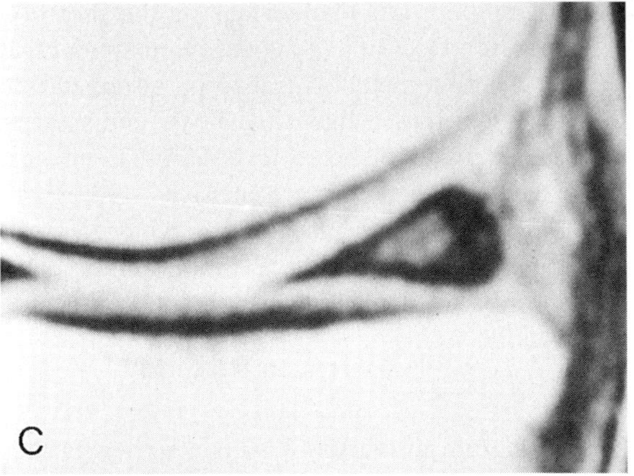

FIG. 6.48. Magnetic resonance imaging of the menisci. **A:** Sagittal T_1-weighted spin-echo image of a medial meniscus depicts the normal anterior (*a*) horn as a diffusely low signal intensity triangular structure. The posterior horn contains linear intermediate signal extending to the inferior articular surface representing a tear (*arrow*). **B:** Sagittal T_2-weighted image of the same knee fails to reveal the tear in the posterior horn. **C:** Myxoid degeneration appears as globular or linear increased intrameniscal signal (*arrow*) on short-TE images (in this case, proton density–weighted spin echo), but does not reach the articular surface.

Tendons and Muscles

Several joints rely heavily on local tendons and muscles for dynamic stability and efficient mechanical loading. Loss of these functions promotes biomechanical wear and, ultimately, joint failure. This is particularly true for the shoulder joint, for which intrinsic instability is the trade-off for its uniquely wide range of motion. Accordingly, tendonitis and rupture of the rotator cuff and long head of the biceps are among the most common causes of pain and disability in the shoulder. Complete rotator cuff tear results in superior subluxation of the humeral head and often leads to OA. Rotator cuff disease is also one of the most frequent referrals for MRI.

Analogous to ligaments and other collagen-containing tissues, normal tendons exhibit low signal intensity on even short-TE MRI because of their high collagen content and correspondingly rapid T_2 decay. Accordingly, high intratendinous signal intensity on T_2-weighted MRI is indicative of tendonitis or tear (Fig. 6.49). Tendon rupture, particularly in the wrist, is a common complication of RA but is often not detected on clinical examination or by the patient (95). Surgical synovectomy, appropriately timed, can prevent an imminent rupture; however, exactly when the critical turning point is reached is not known.

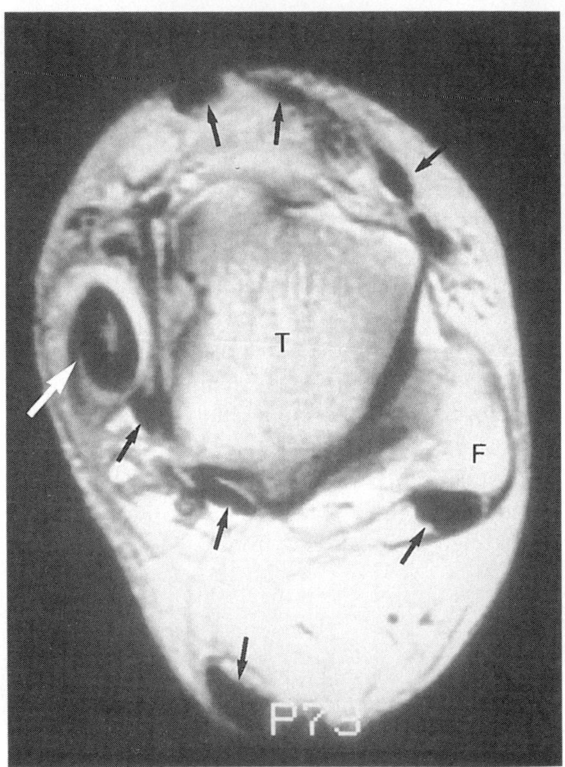

FIG. 6.49. Magnetic resonance imaging of tendon pathology. Transverse T_2-weighted fast spin-echo image of the ankle of a patient with medial ankle pain and flatfoot deformity shows thickening and increased signal intensity of the posterior tibial tendon (*long arrow*) consistent with severe tendonitis. Compare this appearance with that of the normal tendons on the same image (*short arrows*). *T,* talus; *F,* fibula.

Muscles contain somewhat less collagen than tendons and ligaments and therefore exhibit intermediate signal intensity on both T_1- and T_2-weighted images (Fig. 6.50). Muscular inflammation is occasionally seen in association with inflammatory arthritis (Fig. 6.50). On MRI this appears as increased signal intensity on T_2-weighted images both because of elevated water content (i.e., proton density) with interstitial edema, and T_2 prolongation associated with the loss of collagen. Conversely, postinflammatory fibrosis tends to lower signal intensity on T_2-weighted images, whereas fatty atrophy marbles muscles with high signal intensity fat on T_1-weighted images. Typically, muscle

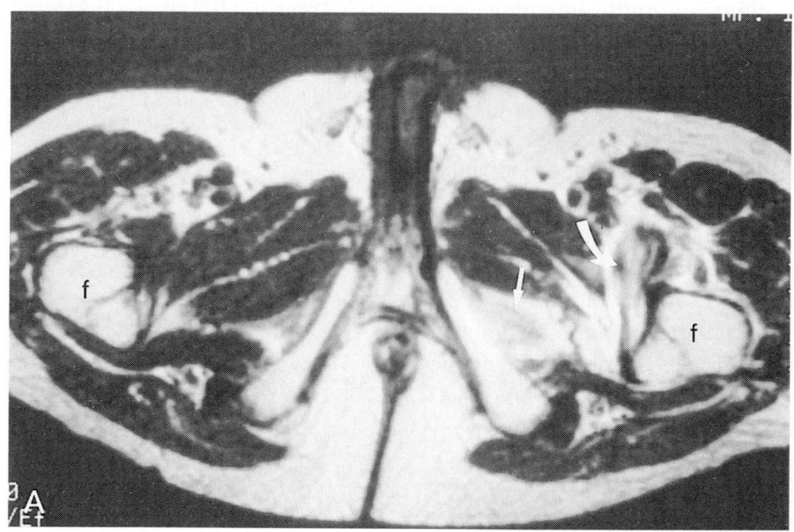

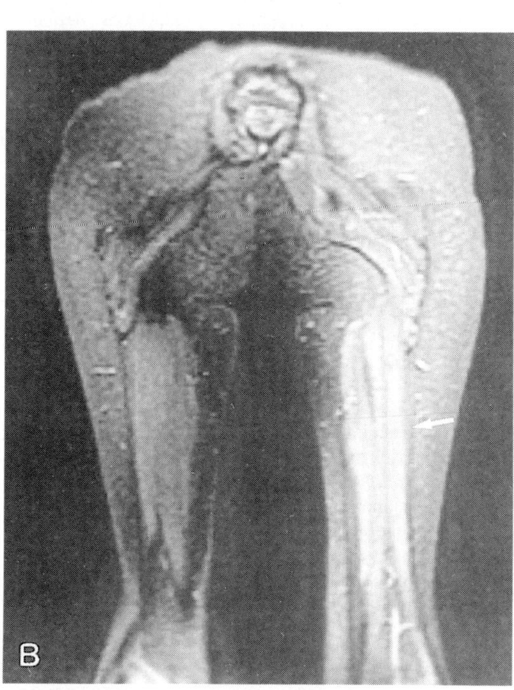

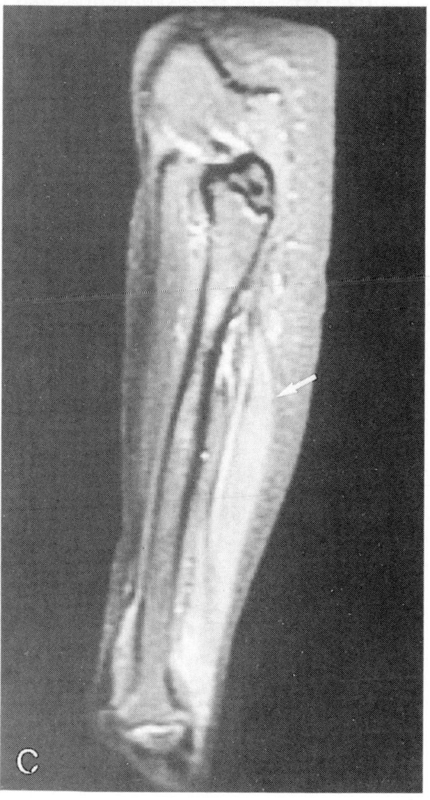

FIG. 6.50. Magnetic resonance images of muscular abnormalities in arthritis. **A:** Transverse T_2-weighted spin-echo image of the hip of a patient with pseudogout shows high signal intensity edema and inflammation in the psoas major (*curved arrow*) and obturator externis (*straight arrow*) muscles. Compare the appearance of these muscles with that of the normal muscle. Coronal **(B)** and sagittal **(C)** fat-suppressed T_2-weighted images of the thigh of a boy with a schwannoma of the sciatic nerve show edema in the hamstring muscles due to denervation (*arrow*).

involvement shows a focal distribution. Therefore, the relationship with symptoms and disability is unpredictable and may vary from case to case. Furthermore, treatment implications may be different from those focused exclusively on synovitis or cartilage loss.

CONCLUSION

Magnetic resonance imaging is rapidly emerging as a tool with unprecedented and unparalleled capabilities for evaluating arthritis and its progression. Not only is it uniquely capable of directly examining all components of a joint simultaneously, it can provide a broad range of morphologic and compositional information about the articular constituents noninvasively. Particularly intriguing is MRI's potential for identifying early changes of joint disease when clinical symptoms may be only minimal or absent. Early detection of patients who are at risk for developing progressive disease may allow appropriate treatment to be initiated earlier, when there may be a greater chance of favorable outcome. MRI can furthermore provide objective and quantitative measures of disease progression and treatment response. This may be useful for titrating specific therapies in individual patients, as well as for testing the efficacy of different treatments in clinical trials. Further work is necessary to thoroughly validate some of these measures, but the evidence thus far is extremely promising.

Although MRI can portray the anatomy with such clarity and detail as to render it intelligible to almost any eye, it must be remembered that this is a highly sophisticated technology and that its proper use requires special expertise. It is important, therefore, that rheumatologists become more familiar with this modality and gain a better sense of what its strengths and weaknesses are, so that they can participate in its development and maximize the potential benefits to rheumatology and its patients.

REFERENCES

1. Medawar P. *The limits of science.* New York: Oxford University Press, 1984:43–54.
2. Genant HK. Methods of assessing radiographic change in rheumatoid arthritis. *Am J Med* 1983;30:35–47.
3. Genant HK, Doi K, Mall JC. Optical versus radiographic magnification for fine detail skeletal radiography. *Invest Radiol* 1975;10:160–172.
4. Buckland-Wright JC, Macfarlane DG, Lynch JA, et al. Joint space width measures cartilage thickness in osteoarthritis of the knee: high resolution plain film and double contrast macroradiographic investigation. *Ann Rheum Dis* 1995;54:263–268.
5. Buckland-Wright JC, Macfarlane DG, Jasani MK, et al. Quantitative microfocal radiographic assessment of osteoarthritis of the knee from weight bearing tunnel and semiflexed standing views. *J Rheum* 1994;21:1734–1741.
6. Abragam A. *The principles of nuclear magnetism.* London: Oxford University Press, 1983.
7. Budinger T, Lauterbur P. Nuclear magnetic resonance technology for medical studies. *Science* 1984;226:288–298.
8. Haacke E, Tkach J. Fast MR imaging: techniques and clinical applications. *AJR* 1990;155:951–964.
9. Pykett I. NMR imaging in medicine. *Sci Am* 1982;246:78–88.
10. Young S. *Magnetic resonance imaging: basic principles.* New York: Raven, 1988.
11. König S, Brown R. Determinants of proton relaxation in tissue. *Magn Reson Imaging* 1984;1:437–449.
12. McEnery KW, Wilson AJ, Murphy WAJ. Comparison of spiral computed tomography versus conventional computed tomography multiplanar reconstructions of a fracture displacement phantom. *Invest Radiol* 1994;29:665–670.
13. Fishman EK, Wyatt SH, Bluemke DA, et al. Spiral CT of musculoskeletal pathology: preliminary observations. *Skel Radiol* 1993;223:253–256.
14. Mottonen TT, Hannonen P, Towanen J, et al. Value of joint scintigraphy in prediction of erosiveness in early rheumatoid arthritis. *Ann Rheum Dis* 1988;47:183–189.
15. Dieppe P, Cushnaghan J, Young P, et al. Prediction of the progression of joint space narrowing in osteoarthritis of the knee by bone scintigraphy. *Ann Rheum Dis* 1993;52:557–563.
16. Hutton CW, Higgs ER, Jackson PC, et al. 99m-Tc-HMDP bone scanning in generalized nodal osteoarthritis. II. The four hour bone scan image predicts radiographic change. *Ann Rheum Dis* 1986;45:622–626.
17. Boegard T, Rudling O, Dahlstrom J, et al. Bone scintigraphy in chronic knee pain: comparison with magnetic resonance imaging. *Ann Rheum Dis* 1999;58(1):20–26.
18. Iagnocco A, Coari G, Zoppini A. Sonographic evaluation of femoral condylar cartilage in osteoarthritis and rheumatoid arthritis. *Scand J Rheumatol* 1992;21:201–203.
19. van Holsbeeck M, van Holsbeeck K, Gevers G, et al. Staging and follow-up of rheumatoid arthritis of the knee. Comparison of sonography, and clinical assessment. *J Ultrasound Med* 1988;7:561–566.
20. Hoult D. The magnetic resonance myth of radio waves. *Concepts Magn Reson* 1989;1:1–5.
21. Kneeland JB, Hyde JS. High-resolution MR imaging with local coils. *Radiology* 1989;171:1–7.
22. Glaser C, Faber S, Eckstein F, et al. Optimization and validation of a rapid high-resolution T1-w 3D FLASH water excitation MRI sequence for the quantitative assessment of articular cartilage volume and thickness. *Magn Reson Imaging* 2001;19:177–185.
23. Hunziker E. Articular cartilage structure in humans and experimental animals. In: Kuettner K, et al., eds. *Articular cartilage and osteoarthritis.* New York: Raven, 1992:183–199.
24. Jeffery AK, Blunn GW, Archer CW, et al. Three-dimensional collagen architecture in bovine articular cartilage. *J Bone Joint Surg Br* 1991;73:795–801.
25. Mow VC, Ratcliffe A, Poole AR. Cartilage and diarthrodial joints as paradigms for hierarchical materials and structures. *Biomaterials* 1992;13:67–97.
26. Fullerton G, Cameron I, Ord V. Orientation of tendons in the magnetic field and its effect on T_2 relaxation times. *Radiology* 1985;155:433–435.
27. Beltran J, Noto AM, Herman LJ, et al. Tendons: high-field strength, surface coil imaging. *Radiology* 1987;162:735–740.
28. Xia Y, Moody JB, Burton-Wurster N, et al. Quantitative *in situ* correlation between microscopic MRI and polarized light microscopy studies of articular cartilage. *Osteoarthritis Cartilage* 2001;9:393–406.
29. Gray ML, Burstein D, Xia Y. Biochemical (and functional) imaging of articular cartilage. *Semin Musculoskel Radiol* 2001;5:329–343.
30. Erickson SJ. High-resolution imaging of the musculoskeletal system. *Radiology* 1997;205(3):593–618.
31. Lehner KB, Rechl HP, Gmeinwieser JK, et al. Structure, function, degeneration of bovine hyaline cartilage: assessment with MR imaging *in vitro. Radiology* 1989;170:495–499.
32. König H, Sauter R, Deimling M, et al. Cartilage disorders: a comparison of spin-echo, CHESS, and FLASH sequence MR images. *Radiology* 1987;164:753–758.
33. Broderick LS, Turner DA, Renfrew DL, et al. Severity of articular cartilage abnormality in patients with osteoarthritis: evaluation with fast spin-echo MR vs arthroscopy. *AJR* 1994;162:99–103.
34. Rose PM, Demlow TA, Szumowski J, et al. Chondromalacia patellae: fat-suppressed MR imaging. *Radiology* 1994;193:437–440.
35. Vener MJ, Thompson RCJ, Lewis JL, et al. Subchondral damage after acute transarticular loading: an *in vitro* model of joint injury. *J Orthop Res* 1992;10:759–769.
36. Yulish BS, Montanez J, Goodfellow DB, et al. Chondromalacia patellae: assessment with MR imaging. *Radiology* 1987;164:763–766.

37. Quinn SF, Rose PM, Brown TR, et al. MR imaging of the patellofemoral compartment. *MRI Clin North Am* 1994;2:425–439.
38. Xia Y, Farquhar T, Burton-Wuster N, et al. Diffusion and relaxation mapping of cartilage-bone plugs and excised disks using microscopic magnetic resonance imaging. *Magn Reson Med* 1994;31: 273–282.
39. Burstein D, Gray ML, Hartman AL, et al. Diffusion of small solutes in cartilage as measured by nuclear magnetic resonance (NMR) spectroscopy and imaging. *J Orthop Res* 1993;11:465–478.
40. Burstein D, Bashir A, Gray ML. MRI techniques in early stages of cartilage disease. *Invest Radiol* 2000;35:622–638.
41. Kusaka Y, Grunder W, Rumpel H, et al. MR microimaging of articular cartilage and contrast enhancement by manganese ions. *Magn Reson Med* 1992;24:137–148.
42. Fujioka M, Kusaka Y, Morita Y, et al. Contrast-enhanced MR imaging of articular cartilage: a new sensitive method for diagnosis of cartilage degeneration. Presented at the 40th Annual Meeting, Orthopaedic Research Society, New Orleans, 1994.
43. Lesperance LM, Gray ML, Burstein D. Determination of fixed charge density in cartilage using nuclear magnetic resonance. *J Orthop Res* 1992;10:1–13.
44. Woolf SD, Chesnick S, Frank JA, et al. Magnetization transfer contrast: MR imaging of the knee. *Radiology* 1991;179:623–628.
45. Peterfy CG, Majumdar S, Lang P, et al. MR imaging of the arthritic knee: improved discrimination of cartilage, synovium and effusion with pulsed saturation transfer and fat-suppressed T_1-weighted sequences. *Radiology* 1994;191:413–419.
46. Hajnal JV, Baudouin CJ, Oatridge A, et al. Design and implementation of magnetization transfer pulse sequences for clinical use. *J Comput Assist Tomogr* 1992;16:7–18.
47. Kim DK, Ceckler TL, Hascall VC, et al. Analysis of water-macromolecule proton magnetization transfer in articular cartilage. *Magn Reson Med* 1993;29:211–215.
48. Hwang WS, Li B, Jin LH, et al. Collagen fibril structure of normal, aging, and osteoarthritic cartilage. *J Pathol* 1992;167:425–433.
49. Peterfy CG, van Dijke CF, Janzen DL, et al. Quantification of articular cartilage in the knee by pulsed saturation transfer and fat-suppressed MRI: optimization and validation. *Radiology* 1994;192:485–491.
50. Recht MP, Kramer J, Marcelis S, et al. Abnormalities of articular cartilage in the knee: analysis of available MR techniques. *Radiology* 1993;187:473–478.
51. Disler DG, McCauley TR, Wirth CR, et al. Detection of knee hyaline articular cartilage defects using fat-suppressed three-dimensional spoiled gradient-echo MR imaging: comparison with standard MR imaging and correlation with arthroscopy. *AJR* 1995;165:377–382.
52. Peterfy CG, van Dijke CF, Lu Y, et al. Quantification of articular cartilage in the metacarpophalangeal joints of the hand: accuracy and precision of 3D MR imaging. *AJR* 1995;165:371–375.
53. Ateshian GA, Cohen ZA, Kwak SD, et al. Determination of *in situ* contact areas in diarthrodial joints by MRI. Presented at the meeting of American Society of Mechanical Engineers, San Francisco, November 1995.
54. Eckstein F, Winzheimer M, Hohe J, et al. Interindividual variability and correlation among morphological parameters of knee joint cartilage plates: analysis with three-dimensional MR imaging. *Osteoarthritis Cartilage* 2001;9:101–111.
55. Raynauld J-P, Pelletier J-P, Beaudoin G, et al. A two-year study in osteoarthritis patients following the progression of the disease by magnetic resonance imaging using a novel quantification imaging system. *Arthritis Rheum* 2002;46(suppl):150.
56. Cohen ZA, McCarthy DM, Kwak SD, et al. Knee cartilage topography, thickness, and contact areas from MRI: *in-vitro* calibration and *in-vivo* measurements. *Osteoarthritis Cartilage* 1999;7(1):95–109.
57. Boegård TL, Rudling O, Petersson IF, et al. Magnetic resonance imaging of the knee in chronic knee pain. A 2-year follow-up. *Osteoarthritis Cartilage* 2001;9:473–480.
58. Nishii T, Sugano N, Tanaka H, et al. Articular cartilage abnormalities in dysplastic hips without joint space narrowing. *Clin Orthop* 2001; 183–190.
59. Heuck AF, Steiger P, Stoller DW, et al. Quantification of knee joint fluid volume by MR imaging and CT using three-dimensional data processing. *J Comput Assist Tomogr* 1989;13:287–293.
60. Schweitzer ME, van Leersum M, Ehrlich SS, et al. Fluid in normal and abnormal ankle joints: amount and distribution as seen on MR images. *AJR* 1994;162:11–114.
61. Eich GF, Hallé F, Hodler J, et al. Juvenile chronic arthritis: imaging of the knees and hips before and after intraarticular steroid injection. *Pediatr Radiol* 1994;24;558–563.
62. Munk P, Vellet AD, Levin MF, et al. Intravenous gadolinium in the evaluation of rheumatoid arthritis of the shoulder. Presented at the meeting of the Society of Magnetic Resonance in Medicine, Berlin, Germany, 1992:457.
63. Björkengren AG, Geborek P, Rydholm U, et al. MR imaging of the knee in acute rheumatoid arthritis: synovial uptake of gadolinium-DOTA. *AJR* 1990;155:329–332.
64. Smith H-J, Larheim TA, Aspestrand F. Rheumatic and nonrheumatic disease in the temporomandibular joint: gadolinium-enhanced MR imaging. *Radiology* 1992;185:229–234.
65. Jevtic V, Watt I, Rozman B, et al. Precontrast and postcontrast (Gd-DTPA) magnetic resonance imaging of hand joints in patients with rheumatoid arthritis. *Clin Radiol* 1993;48:176–181.
66. König H, Sieper J, Wolf KJ. Rheumatoid arthritis: evaluation of hypervascular and fibrous pannus with dynamic MR imaging enhanced with Gd-DTPA. *Radiology* 1990;176:473–477.
67. Winalski CS, Aliabadi P, Wright RJ, et al. Enhancement of joint fluid with intravenously administered gadopentetate dimeglumine: technique, rationale, and implications. *Radiology* 1993;187:197–185.
68. Drapé J-L, Thelen P, Gay-Depassier P, et al. Intraarticular diffusion of Gd-DOTA after intravenous injection in the knee: MR imaging evaluation. *Radiology* 1993;188:227–234.
69. Tanttu JI, Sepponen RE, Lipton MJ, et al. Synergistic enhancement of MRI with Gd-DTPA and magnetization transfer. *J Comput Assist Tomogr* 1992;16:19–24.
70. Yamato M, Tamai K, Yamaguchi T, et al. MRI of the knee in rheumatoid arthritis: Gd-DTPA perfusion dynamics. *J Comput Assist Tomogr* 1993;17:781–785.
71. Østergaard M, Stoltenberg M, Lovgreen-Nielsen P, et al. Quantification of synovitis by MRI: correlation between dynamic and static gadolinium-enhanced magnetic resonance imaging and microscopic and macroscopic signs of synovial inflammation. *Magn Reson Imaging* 1998;16(7):743–754.
72. Østergaard M, Hansen M, Stoltenberg M, et al. Magnetic resonance imaging-determined synovial membrane volume as a marker of disease activity and a predictor of progressive joint destruction in the wrists of patients with rheumatoid arthritis. *Arthritis Rheum* 1999;42 (5):918–929.
73. Klarlund M, Østergaard M, Rostrup E, Skjodt H, Lorenzen I. Dynamic magnetic resonance imaging of the metacarpophalangeal joints in rheumatoid arthritis, early unclassified polyarthritis and healthy controls. *Scand J Rheumatol* 2000;29:108–115.
74. Palmer WE, Rosenthal DI, Schoenberg OI, et al. Quantification of inflammation in the wrist with gadolinium-enhanced MR imaging and PET with 2-(F-18)-fluoro-2-deoxy-D-glucose. *Radiology* 1995; 196(3):647–655.
75. Reece RJ, Kraan MC, Radjenovic A, et al. Comparative assessment of leflunomide and methotrexate for the treatment of rheumatoid arthritis, by dynamic enhanced magnetic resonance imaging. *Arthritis Rheum* 2002;46:366–372.
76. Jelinek JS, Kransdorf MJ, Utz JA, et al. Imaging of pigmented villonodular synovitis with emphasis on MR imaging. *AJR* 1989;152:337–342.
77. Hughes TH, Sartoris DJ, Schweitzer ME, et al. Pigmented villonodular synovitis: MRI characteristics. *Skel Radiol* 1995;24:7–12.
78. Resnick D. Internal derangements of joints. In: Resnick D, ed. *Diagnosis of bone and joint disorders.* Philadelphia: WB Saunders, 1995: 3063–3069.
79. Jelinek JS, Kransdorf MJ, Shmookler BM, et al. Giant cell tumor of the tendon sheath: MR findings in nine cases. *AJR* 1994;162:919–922.
80. Kramer J, Recht M, Deely DM, et al. MR appearance of idiopathic synovial osteochondromatosis. *J Comput Assist Tomogr* 1993;17:772–776.
81. Resnick D. Soft tissues. In: Resnick D, ed. *Diagnosis of bone and joint disorders.* Philadelphia: WB Saunders, 1995:4548.
82. Resnick D, ed. *Diagnosis of bone and joint disorders*, 3rd ed. Philadelphia: WB Saunders, 1995.
83. Chan WP, Lang P, Stevens MP, et al. Osteoarthritis of the knee: comparison of radiography, CT, and MR imaging to assess extent and severity. *AJR* 1991;157:799–806.
84. Peterfy C, Dion E, Miaux Y, et al. Comparison of MRI and X-ray for monitoring erosive changes in rheumatoid arthritis. *Arthritis Rheum* 1998;41(suppl):51.

85. Lindegaard H, Vallö J, Höslev-Petersen K, et al. Low field dedicated magnetic resonance imaging in untreated rheumatoid arthritis of recent onset. *Ann Rheum Dis* 2001;60:770–776.
86. Backhaus M, Burmester GR, Sandrock D, et al. Prospective two year follow up study comparing novel and conventional imaging procedures in patients with arthritic finger joints. *Ann Rheum Dis* 2002;61:895–904.
87. Ahlstrom H, Feltelius N, Nyman R, et al. Magnetic resonance imaging of sacroiliac joint inflammation. *Arthritis Rheum* 1990;33:1763–1769.
88. Peterfy CG. The role of MR imaging in clinical research studies. *Semin Musculoskel Radiol* 2001;5:365–378.
89. McQueen F, Stewart N, Crabbe J, et al. Magnetic resonance imaging of the wrist in early rheumatoid arthritis reveals progression of erosions despite clinical improvement. *Ann Rheum Dis* 1999;58:156–163.
90. Felson DT, Chaisson CE, Hill CL, et al. The association of bone marrow lesions with pain in knee osteoarthritis. *Ann Intern Med* 2001; 134:541–549.
91. Felson D, McLaughlin S, Goggins J, et al. Bone marrow edema (BME) and its relation to x-ray progression in knee osteoarthritis (OA). *Arthritis Rheum* 2003;46(suppl):S558.
92. Tervonen O, Mueller DM, Matteson EL, et al. Clinically occult avascular necrosis of the hip: prevalence in an asymptomatic population at risk. *Radiology* 1992;182:845–847.
93. Tirman PFJ, Bost FW, Garvin GJ, et al. Posterosuperior glenoid impingement: MRI and MR arthrographic findings with arthroscopic correlation. *Radiology* 1994;193:431–436.
94. Lynch MA, Henning CE, Glick KRJ. Knee joint surface changes: long-term follow-up meniscus tear treatment in stable anterior cruciate ligament reconstructions. *Clin Orthop Rel Res* 1983;172:148–153.
95. Rubens DJ, Blebea JS, Totterman SMS, et al. Rheumatoid arthritis: evaluation of wrist extensor tendons with clinical examination versus MR imaging a preliminary report. *Radiology* 1993;187:831–838.

SECTION II

Scientific Basis for the Study of the Rheumatic Diseases

CHAPTER 7

The Structure and Function of Joints

Paul H. Wooley, Michele J. Grimm, and Eric L. Radin

Few examples in nature support the tenant that "form follows function" as closely as the human synovial joint. Evolution has provided humans with superb limb articulation that supports an almost unique ability to move while upright and has an exquisite mixture of efficient force transfer, low friction surfaces, and shock absorption capacity. In this chapter the biochemical, cellular, and biomechanical aspects of joints are discussed and the critical areas of joint physiology important to the performance of the normal joint and the development of the arthritides are addressed. Although all joints are considered, synovial joints and the intervertebral articulations are emphasized because they constitute most joints and are most often involved by the disease processes discussed in this volume.

CLASSIFICATION OF JOINTS

Joints are most often classified according to the type of motion they allow. Three types are recognized: immovable joints (synarthroses), slightly movable joints (amphiarthroses), and movable joints (diarthroses) (1). They can also be classified by the nature of the specialized forms of connective tissue present (1). The two classifications are interrelated because the architecture and tissue construction of the joints determines their relative mobility. Fibrous or cartilaginous membranes (syndesmoses or synchondroses) connect the bony ends of the immovable or slightly movable joints. In contrast, the component bony parts of the movable joints, although covered by hyaline cartilage, are completely enclosed by a joint cavity lined by a synovial membrane (synovial or diarthrodial joints) (1,2).

Synarthroses (nonmovable joints) are generally found in the skull. Here, the bony plate ends that comprise the joints are held together by fibrous or cartilaginous elements. Amphiarthroses are characterized by the presence of broad, flattened discs of fibrocartilage connecting the articulating surfaces. The bony portions of the joint are usually covered by hyaline cartilage, and a fibrous capsule invests the entire structure. Such joints are those between the vertebrae, the distal tibiofibular articulation, the pubic symphysis, and the upper two thirds of the sacroiliac joint. Diarthroses include most of the joints of the extremities. The joint spaces—broad expanses of smooth articular cartilage and loosely applied synovial membranes—allow the wide ranges of motion necessary for locomotion and grasp (1,2).

SYNOVIAL JOINTS

General Structure

Synovial (diarthrodial) joints account for most of the body's articulations and are characterized by wide ranges of almost frictionless movement. The articulating bony surfaces are usually bulbous, sometimes flattened excrescences of cancellous bone, capped by a thin plate of dense cortical bone (the subchondral plate), which is covered by articular cartilage. There is an intermediate layer of calcified cartilage between the subchondral plate and the articular cartilage. Beneath the bony end plate, making up the bulk of the articulating end, lies cancellous bone. In adults, this may contain fatty marrow, whereas in children, it represents the distalmost portion of the epiphysis (growth center) and, thus, frequently contains red (hematopoietic) marrow. The articular cartilage is adherent to the bony end plate and bound by a set of collagen fibers, which run from the articular cartilage into intervening calcified cartilage, and perhaps even into the bone. This hyaline articular cartilage is a specialized form of smooth and resilient connective tissue that serves as the bearing and gliding surface. The joint cavity is a tissue space containing a thin layer of synovial fluid (see Chapters 4 and 8) (Fig. 7.1).

The movement of the cartilaginous surfaces on one another provides the joint with the almost frictionless mobility essential to function. However, to function effectively, joints must be stabilized within their sockets to prevent slipping out of place, with concomitant loss of control. Stability within the joint's bony configuration is primarily the function of the muscles surrounding the joint. (3). The ligaments and capsule mainly act to guide the joint and can act to limit the extent of the motion. However, failure of appropriate concerted and timely muscle action can place the ligaments and capsules under excessive strain, and they can be torn (3). Each joint has a unique configuration that dictates its range of motion. For example, the hip is a ball and socket; the knee is a rounded, condylar, cam-shaped, four-bar linkage that allows flexion and extension, coupled with a small amount of rotation; the ankle is a complexly shaped mortised hinge; and the shoulder is a ball on a disc. The intervertebral segmental articulations are a combination of an amphiarthrosis (bony end plates connected by a fibrocartilaginous disc) and two diarthrodial joints (the intervertebral facet joints), which allow considerable motion but provide great stability.

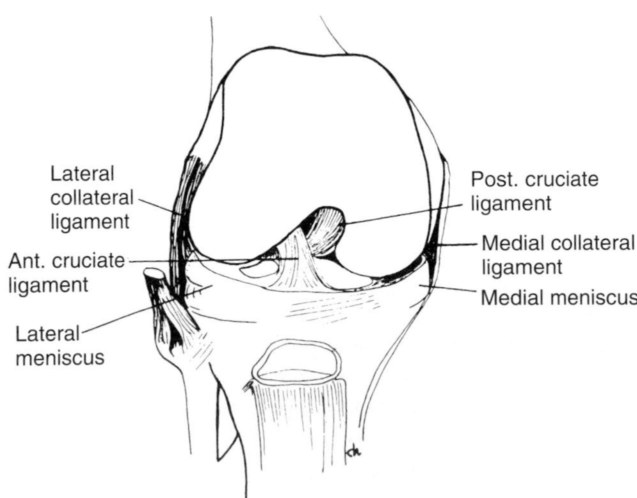

FIG. 7.1. Human knee joint. The patella and capsule have been removed. Note that the distal femur and proximal tibia are covered by hyaline articular cartilage. Affixed to the surface of the tibia are the medial and lateral menisci. The medial and lateral collateral ligaments and stout collagenous bands provide stability in the coronal plane. The cruciate ligaments control stability in the sagittal plane.

The configuration of each individual joint provides an appropriate contact area for the usual positions of loading. This anatomy, combined with appropriate leveraged muscle action, allows for high-efficiency performance (4). The joint contact areas provide for intraarticular stress levels within the tolerance of the tissues involved (~1,000–2,000 kPA or 150–300 psi) (5). Joint design expresses the tradeoff between stability and range of motion. The ankle joints need great stability to provide a platform for a standing or moving body, but for efficient gait, they must also flex and extend. This is accomplished with considerable bony stability, and the distal leg bones create a stirrup or mortise encompassing the talus, essentially forming a hinge joint. The medial malleolus, anterior lip, and posterior margin of the tibia and the fibular malleolus prevent abnormal movement by bony impingement on the talus and provide the stability necessary for normal dorsi and plantar flexion under heavy loads. On the other hand, the shoulder is at the base of the carrying and throwing extremity and, to be effective, needs a wide range of motion. This is accomplished with a shallow, nonrestraining, ball and shallow socket bony configuration, which contributes little to shoulder stability. It is concerted muscle action that provides shoulder stability (6).

Accessory structures that aid in maintaining the integrity of the joint are the fibrous capsule and ligaments (7,8). The fibrous capsule, for most joints, is a firm structure consisting of dense connective tissue that invests the entire joint and usually inserts into the bones close to the articulating surfaces. Within the capsule are thick bands or condensations of parallel collagen fibers known as ligaments. These, too, insert on the bony parts and vary in their tightness between anatomic sites, depending considerably on the position in which the joint is placed.

Within the joint capsule, and defining the intraarticular space is a specialized layer of connective tissue cells, the synoviocytes, that secrete the synovial fluid (9,10). Deep to this layer are varying amounts of highly vascular adipose, fibrous, or areolar tissue supporting the synoviocytes. This allows the sac to be appropriately loose to allow the joint a range of motion without limitation and to keep the synovial folds from becoming entrapped between the joint surfaces (11,12). The synovial sac faithfully replicates the inner surface of the capsule, is reflected at the capsular insertion into the bone, and then extends along the bone to the margin of the articular cartilage (11). The synovial tissue is endowed with a rich blood supply necessary not only to support the synoviocytes, but also to serve as the source of the synovial fluid. The capsule has numerous nerve endings (10) that, along with the spindles in the muscles, ligaments, and tendons, are responsible for keen proprioceptive sense, deep pain perception, and sensation of distention. These afferent stimuli protect the joints and give us a sense of where they are in space (13–15).

Certain joints have within their cavities complete or, more often, incomplete fibrocartilaginous discoid structures known as menisci. The menisci are rudimentary in some areas (e.g., acromioclavicular joint) and highly developed and well defined in others (e.g., knee, temporomandibular joint, and sternoclavicular joints) (1). Synovium does not cover fibrocartilaginous menisci, which are firmly fixed to the joint margin by attachment to bone and to ligaments or capsule, preventing abnormal movement or intraarticular displacement during joint function. As with articular cartilage, menisci are essentially aneural. The function of the menisci varies from site to site, but most authorities feel they primarily contribute to joint stability, shock absorption, and proper tracking of the bony ends during motion. They exist in hinge joints where some rotation is required (16).

Embryology and Development

Recent studies have elucidated the molecular interactions that contribute to the embryonic development of synovial joints. Joint development is considered to take place in three major phases following the appearance of primordial long bones from condensations of mesenchymal tissue. These early bone buds are composed of cartilage precursor cells that eventually branch. Joints first appear at 6 weeks of gestation, when areas of high cell density (interzones) appear. The initial joint demarcation is characterized by a homogeneous interzone created between the chondrifying skeletal elements of the long bones. Next, a three-layered interzone develops that is composed of two chondrogenic layers separated by an intermediate layer.

Cells begin to differentiate away from the prechondrogenic morphology at this stage and mature into densely packed cells with a flattened appearance. This is accompanied by a reduction in the gene expression of type II collagen and other cartilage specific genes. The external mesenchymal tissue forms the joint capsule and tendons, whereas the internal mesenchymal layer forms the synovial membrane and meniscus, typically at 7 weeks. Finally (at around 8 weeks) cavitation occurs to create the articular cavity. Although the initiation of cavitation is independent of articular motion, the final differentiation of the synovial space appears to depend on movement (17,18).

Immobilization of the developing joint through the use of neuromuscular blocking agents resulted in decreased hyaluronan (HA) synthesis and the surface expression of its receptor, CD44, and ultimately, failure of the cavitation process. The expression of HA is central to cavitation, probably through the disruption of cohesion between interzone cells (19), which may trigger apoptosis (programmed cell death) that takes place mainly in the central interzone and partly in the most internal regions of the synovial mesenchymal tissue (20). However, recent studies suggest that the role of apoptosis in cavitations may be restricted to a later time point and only involve hypertrophic chondrocytes in the epiphyseal cartilage and at the growth plate (21).

Although the precise factors that dictate this developmental process remain to be elucidated, a number of key cell signals have been identified that have important regulatory effects. *Wnt14,* a member of the *Wnt* family of cell signaling molecules, appears to exert a critical influence. *Wnt* genes encode locally-acting growth factors, which function to signal cells adjacent to the site of Wnt protein production. Most of the components of the *Wnt* signaling pathway exert an effect on levels and activity of β-catenin, which forms a complex with cadherin that is essential for cell adhesion. The pattern of *Wint14* expression in the embryonic joint suggests that this signaling molecule regulates the segmentation of the mesenchymal condensations (22). High *Wint14* levels appear as prechondrogenic cells differentiate into interzone tissue cells, and this *Wnt14* gene activity is sustained throughout the life of the synovial membrane. The Wnt14 protein regulates downstream gene activity involving *Gdf5* (growth differentiation factor 5, which is also known as cartilage-derived morphogenetic protein 1), autotaxin (an autocrine motility factor), and chordin (an inhibitor of bone morphogenetic proteins), which subsequently block critical differential events in nearby prechondrogenic cells. Thus, the diffusion area of Win14 protein regulates the appearance of the different interzones and may be essential for the correct spacing of the joints. Spitz and Duboule (23) have proposed an attractive hypothesis in which the appearance of the initial joint in an embryonic limb determines the position of the next joint (and so on) via *Win14* expression, although the regulation of the development of the first interzone remains to be explained. However, there are several candidate gene activities for the initial differentiation, including *Cux1* (a homologue of the *Drosophila Cut* gene), which encodes a large transcriptional factor with a single homeodomain and multiple DNA-binding motifs. *Cux1* has been implicated in the formation of the apical ectodermal ridge, which controls the development of the vertebrate limb bud (24) and is precisely expressed in regions of incipient joint formation. *Cux1* activity appears at the time of prechondrogenic cell differentiation into interzone cell tissue, and this gene has been demonstrated to regulate the conversion of chondrocytes into the nonchondrogenic cells characteristic of the interzone (25). In addition, the expression of the *Hox* family genes within the developing limb is critical to the positioning of the joints. The function of this gene family is usually exerted through cell patterning, but there is evidence that *Hox* genes may directly regulate chondrogenesis via changes in chondocyte proliferation or cell adhesion (26).

As the joints develop, the role of bone morphogenetic proteins (BMPs) and their GDF subclass become central. BMPs are part of the transforming growth factor-β superfamily, noted for their ability to induce endochondral bone formation and fracture healing. In the developing embryo, BMPs also control aspects of joint development (27), possibly through their capacity to regulate apoptosis, cell proliferation, and connective tissue matrix production (28). In most situations, BMPs may work together with GDFs, but there is evidence to suggest that the interaction of BMP and GDF-5 varies among different joints. Since these factors may act on the same receptor, differences in the levels of expression may be critical to joint development. Different concentrations and varied complex formations (either homodimers or heterodimers) between these factors may influence whether BMP/GDF production results in proliferation, differentiation, or apoptosis. For instance, the capacity of BMP-7 to promote alkaline phosphatase activity is significantly reduced by the coexpression of GDF-5 (29). BMP and GDF signaling may be modulated at the protein level through interactions with chordin, follistatin, or noggin (all of which antagonize receptor binding) or at the gene regulatory level through the *Smad1* pathway. Noggin appears during early cartilage condensation, becoming restricted to the epiphyseal cartilage (30), whereas chordin expression remains sustained through joint development. These antagonists may control joint formation by preventing the local promotion of chondrogenesis by BMPs and effect regulation simply by differential diffusion rates (between the agonists and antagonists) in the tissue (19). Fibroblast growth factors (FGFs) also regulate BMP activity and may inhibit chondrocyte differentiation and proliferation (31). FGF cell signaling is mediated through the Erk family of MAP kinases and may control phosphorylation of *Smad1*. Mutations in the FGF3 receptor that result in enhanced activation are well recognized to result in the shortened proximal limb bones characteristic of achondroplasia. FGFs are expressed during the early stages of limb formation (32), may inhibit the induction of chondrogenesis by BMPs, and affect chondrogenic pattern formation, resulting in the formation of a cartilaginous mass surrounded by a set of regularly spaced nodules (33). It has been suggested that differential expression of FGF receptors within the developing joint may determine the cell signaling function, with FGF-R1 mediating mesenchymal mitogenesis, FGF-R2 serving as an inhibitory signal, and FGF-R3 upregulating cartilage mitogenesis.

As true cartilage tissue appears, chondroblasts rapidly secrete extracellular matrix and establish the growth plates. Their proliferation acquires unidirectional characteristics, resulting in the hallmark columnar appearance. This differentiation appears to be controlled via *Sox* genes, with *Sox9* expressed from the prechondrytic to the prehypertrophic stage, which serves as an activation factor for cartilage specific genes such as *Col2a1*. *Sox5* and *Sox6* are coexpressed, and may serve as cofactors in the production of type II collagen and aggrecan (34). Furthermore, the transcriptional factor scleraxis may interact and diverge with *Sox9* activity to determine the development of the tendons (35). The development of a bone with articulations at its ends occurs from a cartilaginous anlage at various times for various bones. At birth, the only secondary center of ossification that is radiographically apparent is at the proximal end of the tibia. The rest begin to appear about the third or fourth month of life. A vessel grows into the center of each cartilaginous long bone precursor and forms a marrow cavity, the primary center of ossification. The proximal and distal ends of this cavity form the growth plates (epiphyseal plates) and are responsible for the bone's longitudinal growth, whereas the remaining cartilaginous ends of the bones are invaded in a similar manner by a vessel, which form the secondary centers of ossification responsible for the growth of the articular ends.

STRUCTURE AND COMPONENTS OF THE JOINT'S CONSTITUENT PARTS

Articular Cartilage

The articular cartilages (Fig. 7.2) are the principal surfaces of the diarthrodial joint, and they, and the synovial fluid, are responsible for the almost frictionless movement of the articulating surfaces on each other (36). These specialized connective tissues measure less than 5 mm in thickness in human joints (37), with considerable variation depending on the joint and location within the joint (38,39). Articular cartilage is dense white on gross inspection, tending to become somewhat yellow with age (40). Despite the high water content, cartilage feels semirigid. Contrary to expectations, the surface is not smooth, and a number of studies using the scanning electron microscope have demonstrated gentle undulations and irregular depressions that appear to correspond to the location and shape of cells lying just beneath the surface (37,41,42). These depressions average 20 to 40 μm in diameter and occur with an approximate frequency of 430/mm^2 (43,44) (Fig. 7.3). The irregularities of the surface, evident on scanning electron microscopic studies, may be important in providing a site for attachment of a fine filamentous gliding protein, also known as lubricating glycoprotein (45).

In adults, articular cartilage is aneural, avascular, and alymphatic. The subchondral plate in healthy humans is

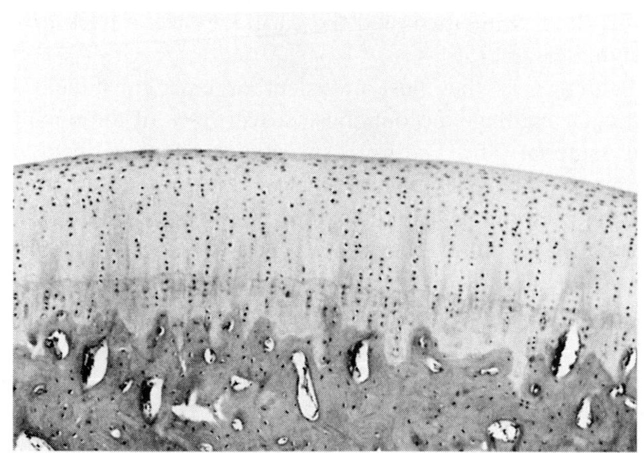

FIG. 7.2. Low-power photomicrograph of adult articular cartilage. Note the zonal distribution of the cells, the calcified layer separated from the radial zone by the tidemark, and the cortical bone of the underlying bony end plate. Articular cartilage is sparsely cellular, and the bulk of the tissue consists of extracellular matrix (hematoxylin and eosin, original magnification ×40).

impervious to blood vessels. Articular cartilage derives its nutrition by a double diffusion system (11,37,46). Because the blood vessels in synovium are situated along the capsular (outer) surface (47), nutrients must first diffuse across the synovial membrane into the synovial fluid and then through the dense matrix of the cartilage to reach the cartilage cells, the chondrocytes (48,49). These are, for the most part, embedded in the cartilage matrix (11,48,49). The diffusion of materials is not simple, in that molecular size, charge, and configuration all play a role in the traverse across the matrix to reach the cell (37). Because there are no nerves in articular cartilage, vertebrates must depend on nerve endings in the capsule, muscles, and subchondral bone for appreciation of pain and proprioception (13–15,50,51). Although articular cartilage exists as a critical part of the joint organ, as in any organ, full function depends on the entire tissue composition.

Histologic and ultrastructural examination of the cartilage demonstrates a preponderance of extracellular matrix and only sparse cellularity (46,52) (Fig. 7.4). The distribution of cells is not random. Three more or less distinct zones have been described (37,53): a tangential or gliding zone, in which elongated fibroblast-like cells lie with their long axes parallel to the surface; a transitional zone, in which the cells are rounded and appear randomly distributed; and a radial zone, in which the cells appear to line up in short, irregular columns. The cells of cartilage are sparse in number and, in adults, are widely separated from one another. There are no bridges, cell–cell interactive systems, or processes that abut, as are commonly seen in other tissues. The asymmetric organization of cells and tissue architecture from the surface to deep layers of articular cartilage reflects the nonuniform distribution of its major macromolecular components, namely collagen and proteoglycans. Biochemical details of these molecules are addressed in Chapters 9, 10, and 11.

The water content in articular cartilage can be almost 80% (53). Most of the water is freely exchangeable with synovial fluid solute and, except for a small component of "bound water" (37), appears to be held in the form of proteoglycan collagen gel (53). The movement of water and,

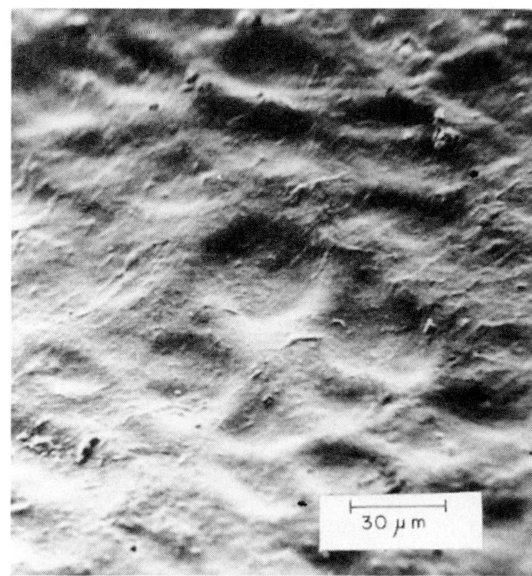

FIG. 7.3. Scanning electron micrograph of the surface of articular cartilage demonstrating irregularly placed rounded or ovoid depressions averaging 20 to 40 μm in diameter (original magnification ×440). (Courtesy of Dr. Ian Clark.)

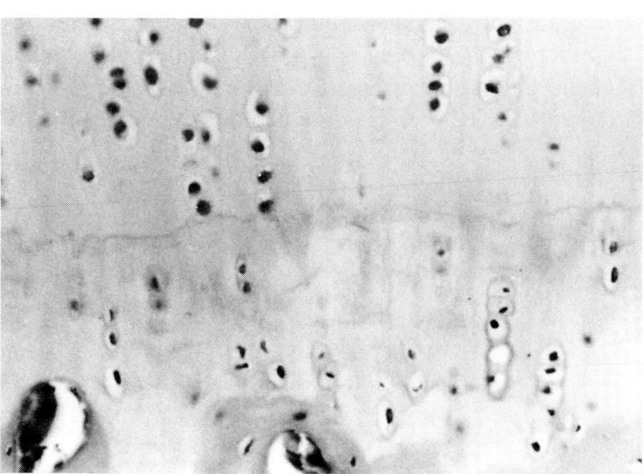

FIG. 7.4. Photomicrograph of mature articular cartilage showing the tidemark, a wavy bluish line (or series of lines) separating the calcified zone below from the radial zone above. The matrix and cells of the calcified zone are heavily encrusted with apatitic salts (hematoxylin and eosin, original magnification ×250).

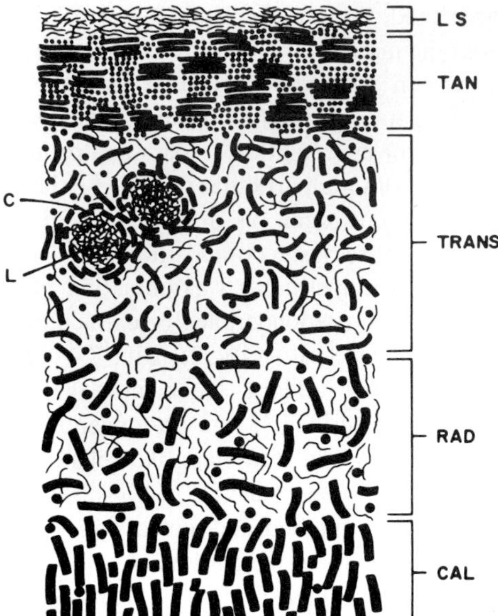

FIG. 7.5. The fibrous architecture of human articular cartilage according to a scheme proposed by Lane and Weiss. The lamina splendens (*LS*) is a layer several microns deep, composed of the fine fibers that cover the articular surface. Beneath this lies the tangential zone (*TAN*), which consists of tightly packed bundles of individual collagen fibers arranged parallel to the articular surface, often at right angles to each other. The collagen fibers in the transitional zone (*TRANS*) are randomly arranged. Collagen fibers of the radial zone (*RAD*) are also randomly arranged, but are of larger diameter, whereas those of the calcified zone (*CAL*) are arranged perpendicular to the articular surface. (From Lane JM, Weiss C. Current comment: review of articular cartilage collagen research. *Arthritis Rheum* 1975;18: 558, with permission.)

more specifically, "weeping" of the cartilage may be essential features of a boundary lubrication system (54,55). Such weeping from the cartilaginous surface, under compression, can cause articular cartilage to temporarily lose up to 20% of its height. When the pressure is removed, water from the joint fluid is imbibed, and the cartilage swells back to its original height (56).

Collagen is the most prevalent organic constituent in articular cartilage, accounting for over 50% of the remaining material (46). The most superficial collagen fibers are arranged in bundles and sheets parallel to the surface of the cartilage, forming a "skin." Vertical fibers extend upward from the subchondral bone (57). These lowermost fibers are perpendicular to the surface and firmly fixed to the underlying bone, thus resisting shear (Fig. 7.5). Collagen in the middle layer appears to be randomly orientated (Fig. 7.6). This appearance belies the overall arcadelike orientation of the articular cartilage collagen, hooplike from the base and arching to just below the surface. These were first described by Benninghoff in 1925 (58,59). The problem with this observation is that collagen fibers are not that long. Electron microscopy finally clarified the situation. The Benninghoff hoops are made up of the basal vertical collagen, the surface horizontal collagen, and the midzone collagen, which is arranged in a more vertical than horizontal way (60). When compressed, however, the midzone collagen lies more horizontal than vertical, the better to resist compressive load (61) (Fig. 7.6). It is a clever engineering construct.

The fibrous collagenous network exhibits mechanical connectivity throughout the tissues. The major component of this network is type II collagen. The fibrils formed are highly cross-linked via the amino groups on lysine residues. Numerous other collagen types are present and serve to modify the nature of the fibril and may providc additional cross-linking of collagen molecules. In addition, matrix macromolecules are present that also interact with collagen, some adding additional cross-links. The spacing and organization of collagen fibrils entrap the proteoglycan aggrecan, preventing its diffusion within and out of the tissue. Aggrecan is over 2 million daltons in molecular weight. Nearly 80% of its mass consists of chondroitin sulfate glycosaminoglycan chains. These chains are polymers of sugars that are negatively charged. Each chain contains about 100 sugars, each sugar containing a negative charge. There

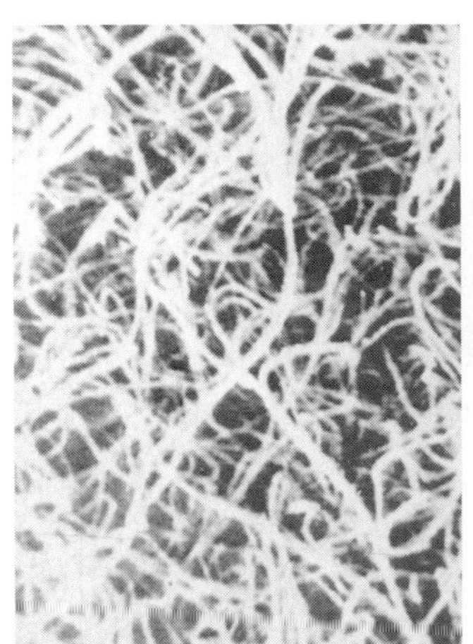
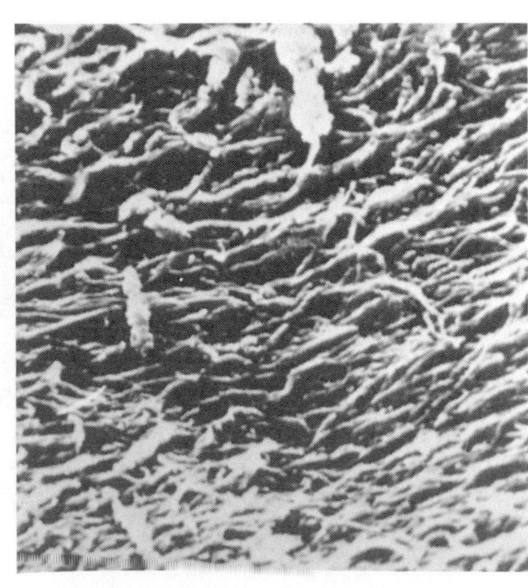

FIG. 7.6. Left: A scanning electron micrograph of the midzone collagen fibers of articular cartilage in the unloaded state. Note the essentially random orientation. **Right:** The same area of the cartilage with compressive load applied. Note how the fibers line up perpendicular to the load. (From McCall J. Load deformation response of the microstructure of articular cartilage. In: Wright V, ed. *Lubrication and wear in joints.* London: Sector, 1969:39–48, with permission.)

are about 100 chains per aggrecan. Each molecule, then, has a charge of about −10,000. These molecules are found in cartilage at concentrations between 50 and 100 mg/mL. Such a concentration of charges results in considerable electrostatic interactions between the fixed proteoglycans and mobile counterions. It is the electrostatic forces between adjacent glycosaminoglycan chains that account for much of the swelling pressure in cartilage (62).

The chemistry of normal articular cartilage varies within each joint and from joint to joint (63). Higher concentrations of proteoglycan and collagen molecules are found in habitually load-bearing areas and are associated with greater interarticular pressures. It is the hydrostatic pressure within the articular cartilage that controls cellular production of cartilage extracellular matrix. Chondrocyte cytoskeletons apparently sense deformation and induce the metabolic changes that determine the tissue's extracellular chemical composition (64). Pauwels, from his analysis of fracture malunions, suggested that cartilage forms from mesenchymal stem cells under hydrostatic pressure, which is the condition in the confined compression of articular cartilage (65–67). This has been verified experimentally (68).

Calcified Cartilage

A layer of calcified cartilage exists in the interface between the articular cartilage and its underlying (subchondral) bone. The articular cartilage and its calcified cartilage bed are separated from the bone by a wavy, irregular bluish line (on hematoxylin and eosin staining) called the tidemark (69,70) (Fig. 7.4). The tidemark is similar in appearance and composition to the cement lines in bone and may act as a limit to calcification (71,72). The collagen in calcified cartilage is type II and it is heavily encrusted with hydroxyapatite. This tissue contains cells that are metabolically active (73). The deep surface of the calcified cartilage merges with the endplate of the underlying bone (70) (Fig. 7.4) in an undulating interface. Redler and co-workers (70) have suggested that this permits a significant increase in resistance to shearing forces and helps to keep the cartilage on its bony bed. The fibers in the lowermost region are perpendicular to the surface and firmly fixed to the underlying calcified subchondral structures, also positioned to resist shear (Fig. 7.5).

Abnormal joint pressures cause remodeling of calcified cartilage, which was once thought to be effite but has more recently been shown to be quite dynamic (74). This tissue appears to heal microdamage by vascular ingrowth (73). In pathologic situations, such as osteoarthrosis, vessels penetrate the subchondral plate and the calcified cartilage (52,75). The calcified cartilage can then act as a source of enchondral calcification, remodeling the subchondral plate and creating a new tidemark (71). After substantial remodeling, as in osteoarthrosis, the tidemark may be duplicated or even appear as multiple lines (76).

Subchondral Bone

Although, at the tissue level, the bone located in the subchondral plate and the cancellous bone that supports it are indistinguishable from bone in other sites, the organization of the subchondral bone is specific. The subchondral plate on which the calcified cartilage lies is thinner than cortical bone in most sites and contains variable numbers of mature haversian systems. These systems run parallel to the joint rather than parallel to the long axis of the bone (Fig. 7.7). The sheets and interconnecting struts of cancellous bone, which support the plate and fill the epiphyseal end of the bone, differ considerably from joint to joint, but are highly ordered and characteristic for any one joint. The major plates are arranged at right angles to the predominating stresses and, together with the subchondral bony plate, are approximately 10 times more deformable than is the cortical bony shaft (77). An increase in this bony structure, so-called subchondral sclerosis, is associated with thickening of the subchondral plate, advance of the tidemark, and thinning of the overlying articular cartilage. These changes are pathognomonic of osteoarthrosis and are deleterious to the function of the joint and the health of the overlying articular cartilage (78,79).

Synovial Membrane

The synovial membrane serves two functions in the adult joint: the provision of nutrients to cells of the articular cartilage and the production of lubricating fluid to ensure the

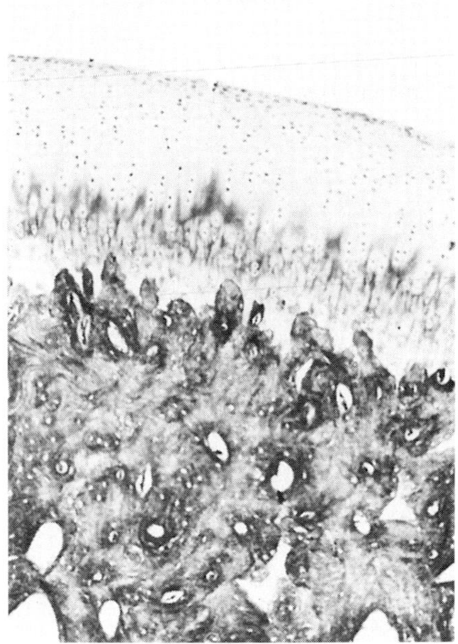

FIG. 7.7. Photomicrograph of distal femur of an adult rabbit showing the subchondral bone. Note the relationship of the bone to the cartilage and the compact nature of the subchondral plate. The Haversian canals appear to be parallel to the joint surface (Masson trichrome, original magnification ×50).

low friction characteristic of joint articulation. The membrane consists of two distinct layers: the thin intimal lining or synovial surface layer, and the subintimal layer of connective tissue that supports both the lining and the blood vessels that supply the membrane. The synovial lining produces synovial fluid and represents the direct interface to the intraarticular cavity. In the normal condition, it is an irregular membrane merely two to three cells thick (Fig. 7.8). In inflammatory disease, this appearance can change dramatically, with both hypertrophy and hyperplasia rapidly developing, resulting in an inflammatory, fibrous membrane. The main cells of the synovial surface layer and its vascular sublining have been historically divided into two distinctive populations, historically termed synovial type A cells and synovial type B cells. Type A cells have a macrophage morphology, whereas type B cells appear fibroblastic. This terminology has fallen from use with the recent recognition that synovial type A cells are actually bone marrow–derived macrophages, which integrate with the resident fibroblast population that comprises the majority of the cells in the synovium. Ultrastructure studies have shown that there is no basement membrane beneath the synovial intima (79), although both laminin and type IV collagen may be found underlying the synovial intima. Subintimal tissue is sparsely populated with cells compared with the intima, and fat cells and blood vessels are integrated within this matrix, which is rich in type I and type III collagen, proteoglycans, and fibronectin (80).

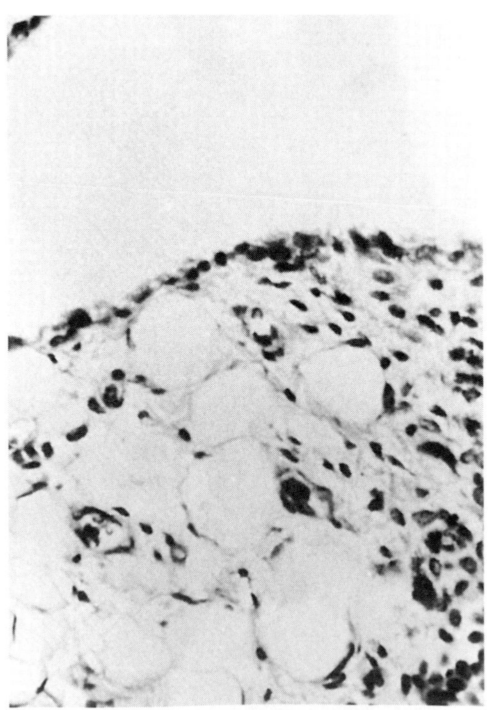

FIG. 7.8. Photomicrograph of normal synovium showing the surface layers of synovial cells and the presence of areolar and fatty synovial tissue (hematoxylin and eosin, original magnification ×225).

Cell Biology of the Synovial Membrane

The cell biology of the synovial lining cells of the intima and the deeper subintimal cells reflect many of the functions ascribed to the distinct layers. Cellular activities and protein production can be examined in great detail using immunohistochemistry, and both the intracellular proteins and cell differentiation markers provide insights into the functions and interactions of the cells that comprise the synovial membrane. Intimal macrophages stain positive for nonspecific esterase, and they can be distinguished by a variety of cell surface markers that vary between the cells resident in the intima and those within the subintima. Synovial macrophages express high levels of CD68, a 110-kd type I transmembrane glycoprotein localized in the cytoplasmic granules of monocytes and macrophages. CD68 is also found in granulocytes, dendritic cells, myeloid progenitor cells, and hematopoietic bone marrow progenitor cells. It is a member of the sialomucin family, and its function has not been fully elucidated. High CD68 expression is relatively consistent on macrophages throughout the synovial tissue, and class II major histocompatibility complex DR antigen expression is also invariant on macrophages throughout the normal joint (81,82). CD14, which is expressed at a higher level on subintimal cells than intimal macrophages, is a glycosylphosphatidylinositol membrane protein, found on neutrophils and B lymphocytes in addition to macrophage/monocyte lineage cells. CD14 is part of the heteromeric lipopolysaccharide (LPS) receptor complex that also contains Toll-like receptor 4 (TLR4), responsible for early innate immune recognition of microorganisms (83). CD14 binds LPS and associates with TLR4, resulting in the transduction of an activation signal (84).

Both synovial lining macrophages and subintimal cells express markers of the lymphocyte function–associated family, which mediate intercellular and cell matrix adhesion interactions. These molecules consist of a common β chain (95 kd) associated with different α chains to produce CD11a, CD11b, or CD11c. Intimal macrophages are essentially restricted to the expression of CD11b, which binds to the complement component iC3b, extracellular matrix proteins, and the third extracellular domain of CD54 intercellular adhesion molecule-1 (ICAM-1). Subintimal macrophages also express CD11a, which mediates a wider variety of leukocyte functions, including interactions with endothelial cells (81).

Synovial macrophages also express all three variants of the receptors for the Fc portion of the immunoglobulin molecule (FcR). However, the ratio of FcγRIII (CD16) to FcγRI (CD64) appears high on intimal macrophages and low on subintimal cells. Fc receptors mediate reactions between cells, antibodies, and immune complexes, and the class of the FcR can determine whether binding leads to an activation signal resulting in phagocytosis, degranulation, or superoxide production, or to an inhibitory signal. Furthermore, the affinity for the different immunoglobulin G subclasses is influenced by polymorphisms within the FcγRIIa, FcγRIIIa, and FcγRIIIb genes (85). It has been observed that the expression of cell surface markers varies between macrophages resident in the intima and the subintimal lining layers. The differences in surface antigen expression may reflect functional differences between the populations, or a maturation of acquired markers as the cells traffic from the circulatory system to the surface of the synovial lining, although the precise significance of the variation remains unknown. Interestingly, synovial macrophages are remarkable for the absence or low expression of markers typically seen on tissue macrophages, notably CD15a (a carbohydrate component of adhesion molecules), CD25 [interleukin-2 (IL-2) receptor], CD34 (a progenitor cell marker), and CD35 (which binds the complement components C3b and C4b) (81).

Cell markers expressed by the synovial fibroblasts allow a clear distinction between the two population of synovial cells using immunohistochemical techniques (Table 7.1). Intimal fibroblasts are characterized by high uridine diphosphoglucose dehydrogenase (UDPGD) activity. This enzyme catalyzes glycosaminoglycan formation, and its expression within the synovial fibroblast appears related to the high level of UDP-glucuronate production, which forms HA by copolymerization with UDP-*N*-acetylglucosamine (86). Synovial fibroblasts also express high levels of CD55, or complement decay accelerating factor (DAF) (87). DAF is an approximately 70-kd transmembrane glycoprotein with a glycosylphosphatidylinositol tail that binds to activated C4b or C3b complement fragments on cell surfaces, and is also a coligand for the G protein–coupled activation antigen CD97. Its action on complement components both prevents the assembly and accelerates the degradation of complement acting in either classical or alternative pathways. The expression of fibroblast DAF may be related to the macrophage expression of FcRγRIIIa and could determine the response to immune complexes that form within the synovial tissue during infection or autoimmune connective tissue disease (88). In addition, synovial fibroblasts produce high levels of cell adhesion molecules, notably the vascular cell adhesion molecule-1 (VCAM-1, or CD106). VCAM-1 expression by normal fibroblasts is unusual, because it is typically considered as the cytokine-activated endothelial cell ligand for very late antigen-1 (VLA-4, or $\alpha_4\beta_1$ of the β_1 integrin family). VCAM-1 facilitates the adhesion of monocytes, lymphocytes, eosinophils, and basophils. ICAM-1, which is a major ligand for the leukocyte β_2 integrins CD11a and CD11b, is also produced by synovial fibroblasts. These adhesion molecules serve to regulate cell trafficking within the synovium, and the detection of E-selectin and ICAM-1 on normal synovial venules serves to emphasize this function. E-selectin expression is most prominent on small superficial venules in synovium, whereas ICAM-1 is most strongly expressed on larger, deep venules (89). Increased expression of cell adhesion molecules in response to exposure to proinflammatory cytokines

TABLE 7.1. *Structure, function, and site of expression for cellular markers expressed by synovial fibroblasts*

Marker	Structure	Function	Expression
CD68	110-kd transmembrane glycoprotein; cell surface and cytoplasmic granules	Unknown	Macrophages Monocytes Lymphocytes
HLA-DR	Covalently bound heterodimers	Antigen presentation	Macrophages Antigen-presenting cells
CD14	GPI-linked glycoprotein	LPS receptor	Macrophages Monocytes
CD11a,b,c	Integrin α chains associated with β_2 integrins	Cell adhesion	Leucocytes
CD16	80-kd transmembrane polypeptide	Low-affinity IgG receptor	Macrophages Natural killer cells
CD64	Fc receptor γRI	High affinity IgG receptor	Macrophages Monocytes
CD54	ICAM-1	Binds to CD11a	Synovial fibroblasts Many tissue types
CD55	DAF	Blocks complement membrane attack	Synovial fibroblasts
CD106	VCAM-1	Binds monocytes and lymphocytes	Synovial fibroblasts Endothelial cells
CD97	G-coupled protein	Activation antigen	Leucocytes
CD49	VLA	Mediate matrix adhesion	Leucocytes

DAF, decay accelerating factor; GPI, glycosylphosphatidylinosital; ICAM-1, intercellular adhesion molecule 1; IgG, immunoglobulin G; VCAM-1, vascular cell adhesion molecule 1; VLA, very late antigens.

such as IL-1β and tumor necrosis factor-α (TNF-α) may result in the up-regulation of ICAM-1 and VCAM-1 and the subsequent recruitment of leukocytes during inflammatory conditions. Several members of the CD49 marker group, including integrin receptors for laminin, types I and IV collagens, fibronectin, and vitronectin are also expressed by synovial fibroblasts. The distribution pattern for CD49 expression mapped closely with the occurrence of laminin and collagen IV within the subintima (90).

Synovial Fluid and Joint Lubrication

Synovial fluid serves multiple roles in the function of the normal joint. It provides nutrients to cells embedded within the cartilage matrix and lubrication to the articulating surfaces of the joint. These functions require a surprisingly low amount of fluid, with an average normal volume of 1.1 mL of fluid and a range of 0.13 to 3.5 mL (91). The control of the normal fluid volume is poorly understood, although the dramatic changes in the properties of the joint fluid during trauma and inflammatory conditions are well recognized. The composition of synovial fluid is similar to that of plasma, but with additional HA, which provides the high viscosity that is characteristic of synovial fluid. HA, a linear, nonbranching polysaccharide, is secreted into the fluid by the fibroblastic cells of the synovial lining and achieves a concentration between 2 and 4 mg/mL (91). HA is a large glycoprotein molecule with an average molecular weight in excess of 1 million daltons, and this molecular size is responsible for the viscous flow characteristics of the synovial fluid. It is thixotropic, in that the more slowly it flows, the more viscous it becomes (92).

The frictional resistance of animal joints lubricated with synovial fluid can be as low as 0.002, which is one half that of rubber on steel and one tenth that of an ice skate on ice (93). Based on observations regarding the thixotropic character of the fluid, it was originally concluded that joints were lubricated by a hydrodynamic system in which the fluid is held between the bearing surfaces by the continuing rotation of one part of the bearing. Joints are poorly suited to this form of lubrication, however, because they oscillate rather than rotate (36). The finding that the coefficient of friction remains unchanged in joints lubricated with hyaluronidase-treated synovial fluid negated this hydrodynamic theory (94). There are two interfaces within synovial joints that benefit from lubrication: cartilage on cartilage and synovium on cartilage or synovium upon itself. Current hypotheses are that two forms of lubrication are provided by synovial fluid: namely, boundary lubrication, which is a property of surface molecule interactions with the articulating surfaces, and fluid film lubrication, which functions to reduce or prevent contact between the surfaces.

Under physiologic circumstances a thin film of fluid separates two hydrated cartilage surfaces under load. There is ample evidence that this fluid is water "squeezed" from the hyperhydrated cartilage (95). Although the major part of water in cartilage is in the form of a proteoglycan collagen gel (53), it is freely exchangeable with synovial fluid, and a significant portion can be liberated by pressure on the cartilage (96). Because, in the adult, there is little or no traverse of water through the subchondral plate and only modest flow through the substance of the cartilage, the water displaced by cartilage compression is expressed onto the surface of the cartilage, preferentially peripheral to the zone of impending contact. Mow and Mansour (97) have concluded that, under the usual circumstances of joint motion, water tends to be pushed out just in front of the contact area. When the compression is released, the matrix within the cartilage contains enough of a fixed charge to osmotically attract the water and small solutes back into the matrix, and the cartilage regains its original height (98). Thus, the fluid film that exists between moving cartilage layers is made up of the cartilaginous interstitial fluid, which is squeezed onto the surface as the cartilage compresses the synovial fluid already trapped in the contact zone. This mechanism of lubrication is referred to as hydrostatic or weeping (95). Within the zone of impending contact, the lubricating film can be thought of as a squeeze film. The secret of the low friction between the cartilage-bearing surfaces is that they never touch (98). This hydrostatic mechanism clearly functions best under substantial loads, because under small loads, there would be little cartilage compression and little weeping of fluid onto the surface. Physiologically, however, joints frequently move under relatively light load. Under such circumstances, a hydrostatic mechanism would not generate a substantial fluid film, particularly at the moment motion begins.

Boundary lubrication of cartilage on cartilage may be achieved through the interaction of surface-active phospholipids (SAPLs) (99) and the glycoprotein lubricin (100) at the cartilage surface, based on *in vitro* tests in loaded animal joints. Hills has suggested that SAPLs, bound via their polar ends to cartilage, generate an external hydrophobic layer that significantly reduces friction (101). Interestingly, HA may serve to protect this layer through inhibition of phospholipase A2 activity within the joint (102). Lubricin is a 227-kd mucinous glycoprotein that has a high homology with vitronectin and superficial zone protein, and a lower homology with hemopexin. Lubricin is approximately 50% O-glycosylated with β(1–3)Gal-GalNAc and nonuniformly capped with NeuAc (103). It is the product of synovial fibroblasts due to transcription of the megakaryocyte stimulating factor (*MSF*) gene, but appears to be the product of *MSF* exons 6 through 9. Posttranslational modification of the exon 6 product appears to account for the lubricating properties of lubricin, based on latex–glass interface *in vitro* studies (103,104). However, the boundary-lubricating properties of lubricin at the cartilage surface have been challenged and await further research.

The lubrication of synovium on cartilage or synovium upon itself is the result of the affinity of HA for synovial surfaces. Thus, HA acts as a boundary lubricant for synovium (105). This is an important component in the ease of motion of joints, because the periarticular soft tissues contribute much more resistance to joint motion than do cartilaginous surfaces (106).

In addition, HA appears to exert a major influence in maintaining the volume of synovial fluid in the joint. HA acts to reduce the volumetric loss that would be expected to occur as fluid pressure increases during joint flexion. This effect has been termed "outflow buffering" by Levick and colleagues (107), and this dynamic resistance to fluid loss may be achieved as a result of the conformation, charge, and osmotic properties of the HA molecules and the ultrafiltration properties of the synovial membrane. As pressure increases, fluid loss is retarded, due to polarized HA accumulation at the interstitial spaces of membrane surface, resulting in elevated osmotic pressure, which retains water molecules within the synovial fluid. HA is resistant to passage through the synovial membrane, due to the formation of large polymer complexes. Polymer interactions between HA and chondroitin sulfate C also appear to enhance the outflow buffering activity (108).

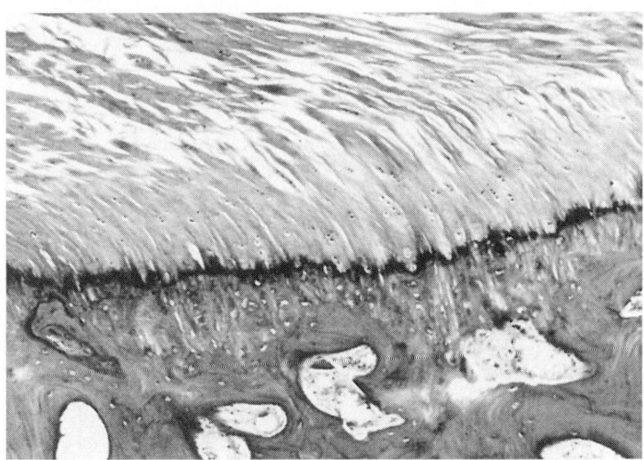

FIG. 7.9. Photomicrograph showing the insertion of a collateral ligament of an interphalangeal ligament into the cortex of the phalanx. Note the parallel bundles of collagen that compose the ligament, becoming first fibrocartilaginous, then calcified, prior to entering the substance of the cortical bond in a fashion similar to Sharpey fibers (hematoxylin and eosin, original magnification ×50).

Ligaments, Tendons, and Capsule

Stability for the joint is provided by the joint capsule, tendons, and ligaments. These structures govern the motion of a joint and distribute the forces that impinge on the joint. Ligaments and tendons are classified as dense connective tissue structures and are generally alike in both structure and function. Ligaments form connections between bones, whereas tendons provide the attachment of muscle to bone.

Ligaments consist of collagen fibrils embedded in a proteoglycan matrix sparsely populated with fibroblastic cells (Fig. 7.9). Cells occur in rows in spaces formed between the type I collagen bundles, which form the dominant constituent of the ligament. The rows of fibroblasts interdigitate with processes extending between the collagen bundles. The microfibril may be considered the basic building block of the ligament derived from the properties of the type I collagen molecule, with its helix of three chains (two α_1 and one α_2 chains) aligned together in a quarter stagger pattern, which provides the strength of the assembly. Five collagen I molecules are bound together in the microfibril, and these units are combined to form subfibrils and, subsequently, fibrils. The fibrils are bound tightly together to form the collagen bundle, and this assembly, with fibroblast-filled spaces and proteoglycan matrix, is bounded by the fascicular membrane (109). The insertion of ligaments into bone can be classified as direct or indirect. Indirect insertions are more common and are characterized by Sharpey fibers, which are oblique anchor points for the deep fibers within bone. Superficial fibers form a contiguous merger directly with the periosteum in indirect attachment. In contrast, the deep fibers involved in direct ligament insertion pass through zones of first uncalcified and then calcified fibrocartilage before integrating with the bone.

Although ligaments may be viewed as resistant to force, whereas tendons actively transfer force, they exhibit the same basic structure. Tendons contain a higher ratio of collagen to proteoglycan matrix than ligaments, and the longitudinal alignment of the collagen fibrils is more polarized in tendons. This reflects the variations in directional loading that impinge on ligaments, as opposed to the unidirectional forces that typically are carried by tendons (42). The proteoglycans (notably decorin) interact with the collagen fibrils to increase tensile strength, and may serve to regulate fibril formation. The distribution of different proteoglycans, particularly decorin and biglycan, can effect a change in response to different *in vivo* mechanical forces exerted by the environment. Proteoglycans can improve the resistance to compressive force, such as that generated when tendons wrap around an articular surface (110). In situations of extreme compression without straight-line motion, tendons are usually protected by a sheath that guides the motion path. Sliding within the sheath is aided by the presence of a fluid that is biochemically indistinguishable from synovial fluid and is probably extruded from the synovial membrane (111,112).

Menisci

As previously noted, menisci normally occur only in the knee and temporomandibular, sternoclavicular, distal radioulnar, and acromioclavicular joints. They consist of complete or incomplete flattened, triangular, or somewhat irregularly shaped fibrocartilaginous discs, firmly attached

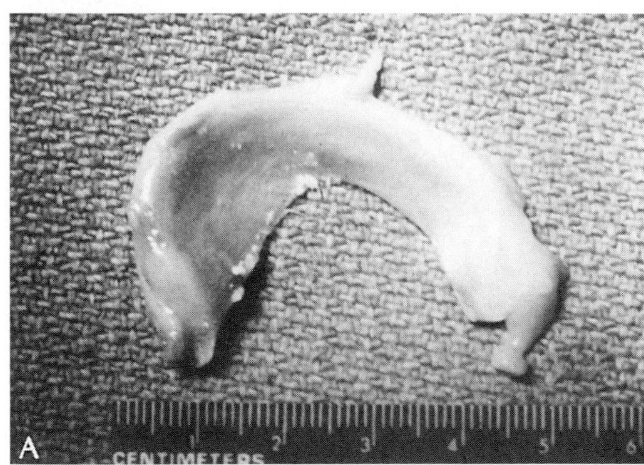
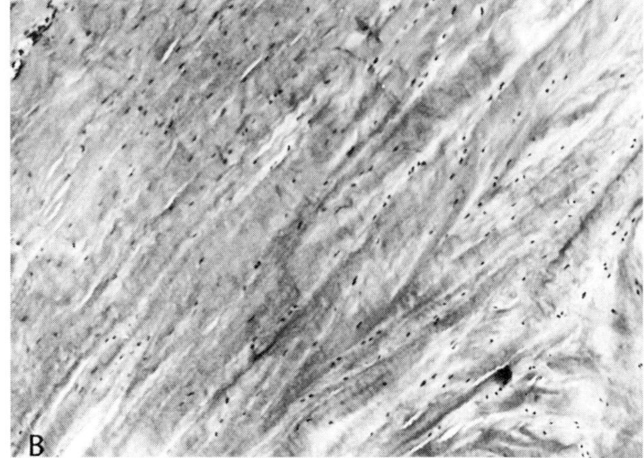

FIG. 7.10. A: Photograph of a normal human medial meniscus. Note the semilunar shape with a thin free edge and considerably thickened marginal attachment site. Menisci increase the stability of the joint and serve as weight-bearing structures in the knee. **B:** Low-power photomicrograph of a fibrocartilaginous human medial meniscus. Note the presence of large numbers of parallel bundles of collagen and the sparse cellularity (hematoxylin and eosin, original magnification ×40).

to the fibrous capsules and often to one of the adjacent bones (1,2) (Fig. 7.10).

The menisci, like articular cartilages, are for the most part, avascular, but at the site of bony attachment, they usually display a surprisingly rich vascular arcade. No nerves or lymphatics have been identified in meniscal tissues. They presumably derive some of their nutrition from synovial fluid, but also by diffusion from vascular plexuses, which are present adjacent to their attachment to bone or fibrous capsule (42). Examination of the menisci of the knee under polarized or light microscopy has shown that meniscal collagen fibers are arranged circumferentially, presumably to withstand the tensile hoop stresses generated during load bearing (113) (Fig. 7.10B). The fibrocartilage of the meniscus has a biochemical composition considerably different from that of articular cartilage (42,113,114). The water content ranges between 70% and 78%. Inorganic ash accounts for approximately 3% of the wet weight. The remainder of the material, the organic solids, are principally collagen, with type I ($2\alpha_1,1\alpha_2$) predominating (114). Collagen accounts for 60% to 90% of the organic solids (42,115–117). Elastin is present in low concentration (<1%). Proteoglycans constitute less than 10% of the dry weight, and the constituent glycosaminoglycans are principally chondroitin sulfates and dermatan sulfate, with keratan sulfate representing only a minor component (118). Meniscal fibrocartilage appears to have a much more sluggish metabolism than hyaline articular cartilage.

THE JOINT AS AN ORGAN

An organ is a biologic construction of several tissues with a unique and specific function. The diarthrodial joints are organs whose purpose is skeletal articulation. The joints enable us to move our bony frame. The joint is composed of articular cartilage, calcified cartilage, a bony subchondral plate and its underlying cancellous bone, capsule, ligaments, synovial membrane, synovial fluid, and, in some joints, menisci. The muscles, which move and stabilize the joints, can be considered an integral part of the construct. As in any organ, the health and function of the component tissues are interrelated. Biologically, what is critical to the health of the tissues that make up the load-bearing structures of a joint is the stress (pressure or force per unit area) to which they are subjected. Similar compressive stresses can occur in the joints of both the upper and lower extremities. Obviously, larger bearing surfaces are required in the major joints of the lower extremity because the total interarticular forces on them are greater. Furthermore, the load on joints is not constant, because activities are intermittent and often create high peak dynamic loads (119). Frequent rapid starts and equally rapid stops, both of which are associated with high rates of loading, characterize joint motion. It is remarkable that under such potentially punishing mechanical conditions, most joints function throughout the life of the individual without evidence of destruction of their major load-bearing areas.

Neuromuscular Control

Historically, the synovium was considered to be denervated tissue, since little or no response to mechanical stimulation could be readily detected. However, immunohistologic techniques have revealed the presence of sympathetic efferent fibers and free nerve endings (nociceptors) with unmyelinated C afferent fibers within the synovial tissue (120). The small-diameter postganglionic sympathetic adrenerginic nerve fibers are generally considered to mediate the response of the vasculature to autonomic and chemical stimuli, and thus, control articular blood flow. However, there is evidence of sensory nerve function in the synovial tissue, with pain responses that can be evoked using hypertonic saline or bradykinin (121). These responses are believed to be mediated via unmyelinated class IV (C) fibers, which are essentially quiescent during normal tissue situations (122). However, these fibers arise from cell bodies in the dorsal root ganglion, where neuropeptides are produced and transported. These neuropeptides, notably substance P, may exert a regulatory role on inflammatory reactions that occur in the joint during arthritic conditions (122,123). In contrast to synovial tissue, the capsule has readily detectable nerve endings that regulate function through proprioreception and maintain the appropriate alignment of the joint to absorb and dissipate the stresses applied during the normal functions of movement (124,125).

Little is known concerning vasoregulation of the sparsely vascularized tendons and ligaments. However, nerve endings in the joint ligaments resemble high-threshold class III (Aδ) cutaneous nociceptors, and sympathetic vasoconstrictor nerve fibers, parasympathetic vasodilator fibers, and small-diameter sensory vasodilator fibers are all present in vessels supplying ligaments and tendons (126). In the meniscus of the knee, nociceptors and mechanoreceptors (Ruffini corpuscles, pacinian corpuscles, and Golgi tendon organ) are distributed throughout the outer body and both the anterior and posterior horns. This distribution is attributed to the requirement for signaling when extreme pressure or tension due to misalignment is exerted on the tissue, evoking mechanical realignment. However, the meniscus may generate proprioceptive information to coordinate movement, velocity, and direction (124).

Biomechanics of Synovial Joints

The mechanical functions of diarthrodial joints require each of the component tissues to play a role in the biomechanics of the joint. Biomechanics is the application of the principles of mechanics, derived from physics and explained through engineering, to the understanding of physiologic function and response. The science of biomechanics examines the forces experienced by a biologic system and the resulting structural, motion, or physiologic responses that occur. In the case of joint function, both the response of the tissues to the load they experience and the motion generated about the joint can be investigated using biomechanics. A joint is a three-dimensional structure and, as such, the forces and responses that it experiences are also three-dimensional. As a result, it is necessary to represent these quantities as vectors. Each vector contains both the magnitude and directional information regarding the force, deformation, velocity, acceleration, or motion of the system. It is extremely important with vector quantities to define a cartesian coordinate system (x, y, and z axes) and to assign positive and negative directions to each axis. In this way, it is possible to track not only the orientation of a vector, but also its sense—whether a force is pushing or pulling on a point, for example. The type of force that is applied to an object is important in understanding how that material responds. Forces are generally applied to surfaces, and they can act in such a way as to push on that surface (compression), pull on the surface (tension), or slide along the surface (shear).

When it comes to assessing the response and function of a joint, several mathematical relationships are important. The first relate to stress, strength, and strain. Stress is the ratio of an applied force to the area over which it is applied. Strength is defined as the maximum stress that a material can sustain before failure occurs. It can depend on the type of load applied, the direction of the load, and the rate at which the load is applied. Strain is the percentage change in length of an object being squeezed or elongated by an applied stress. Separate strains can be calculated for each direction of applied stress.

For any material, the strain that results from an applied stress is related to that material's properties. For an elastic material, like rubber, the relationship between stress and strain is linear, and the elastic modulus defines the slope of the line relating the two quantities. Elastic modulus is independent of the geometry of the object, but it may vary based on the direction of the applied load, the type of load applied, and the rate at which it is applied. For many materials, the variation of strain with stress is nonlinear, and a single elastic modulus cannot be defined. Secondly, when a material is stretched, it extends in the direction of loading and thins in the perpendicular directions. Likewise, a material that is compressed expands in the directions perpendicular to the loading axis (Fig. 7.11). The Poisson ratio defines this behavior, describing the off-axis response as a percentage of the deformation along the axis of loading. Thus, for a material with a Poisson ratio of 0.3 that is stretched an additional 100% of its original length, the cross-sectional thickness will decrease by 30%.

It can be important to distinguish between the material properties of a material, which are independent of the geometry, and the structural properties, which are dependent on both the material and the geometry. For example, steel can be characterized by its material properties, but

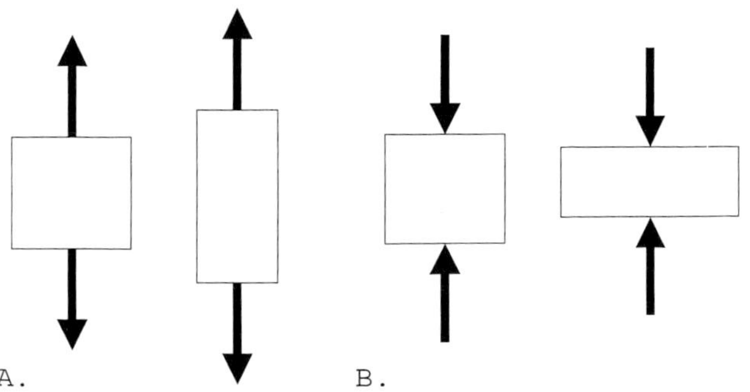

FIG. 7.11. When a load is applied to a piece of material, it deforms both along the axis of the load and perpendicular to it. This behavior is characterized by the material's Poisson ratio.

equally important are the maximum forces that can be sustained when the steel is formed into an I beam that will be used for structural support. Thus, the strength of a tissue or organ is not only dependent on its material properties, derived from its extracellular matrix and its chemical composition, but also on how it is put together.

Of equal interest to how materials respond to a force is how an object may move in space. A force will cause an object to move linearly, or translate, but will not cause it to rotate. In order to rotate an object, a moment (a force applied out of line from an axis of rotation) must be applied. When an object or system of objects is moving or stationary and subjected to forces, the overall response and interaction of the forces, moments, and motion are defined based on Newton's Laws. If a system or an object is not moving, it is in static equilibrium.

Static equilibrium is often referred to as a force and moment balance. Although, in three dimensions, this task can be quite complicated, it can easily be visualized using a seesaw example (Fig. 7.12). If the goal is to balance the seesaw in a horizontal position with a mass on each end, the position of each mass needs to be determined. In this example, there are two masses set on the seesaw and a ground reaction force acting through the supporting structure and axis of the seesaw. Each mass results in a force due to gravity equal to the mass times *g*, acceleration due to gravity. In order to be in equilibrium, both the sum of the forces and the sum of the moments must equal zero. Thus, if the two masses are known, the ground reaction force through the seesaw support can be calculated. The reaction force does not cause a moment as it acts directly through the axis, such that the moment arm of the force is zero. As a result, a smaller force (caused by a smaller mass) must be applied farther away from the axis of rotation to balance an applied moment. Or, conversely, if a force is to be applied close to the axis of rotation of a system, it will have to be of a greater magnitude in order to balance existing moments.

Based on these engineering principles and experimental studies, it is possible to determine how a tissue responds when a load is applied to it and to estimate the forces that occur internally within a joint.

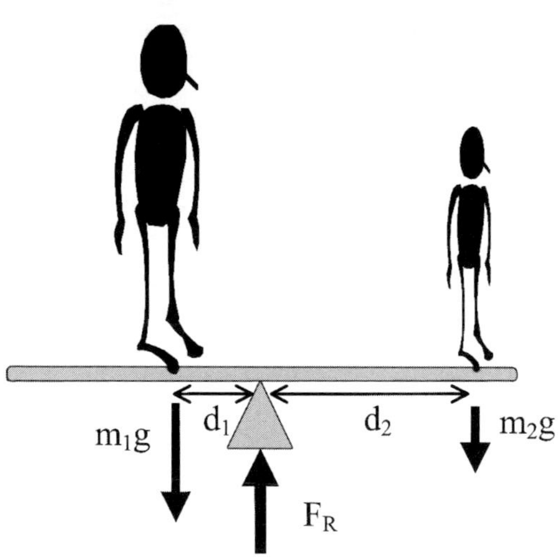

$$\sum \vec{F} = 0 = F_R - m_1 g - m_2 g$$

$$F_R = g(m_1 + m_2)$$

$$\sum M = 0 = m_1 g d_1 - m_2 g d_2 + F_R(0)$$

$$\frac{m_1 g}{m_2 g} = \frac{d_2}{d_1}$$

FIG. 7.12. The principles of force and moment balance are most simply illustrated through a seesaw. In order for the seesaw to balance horizontally, both the sum of the forces and the sum of the moments must equal zero. *F*, force; *M*, moment; *d*, distance; *m*, mass; *g*, acceleration due to gravity; F_R, ground reaction force.

The Biomechanics of Joint Function

The joints of the body transfer a substantial amount of load between bones during all daily activities. Although it is difficult to measure these loads *in vivo*, it has been done using instrumented prostheses (5,127) and estimated based on external measurements. On the basis of such data, models have been constructed using the concepts of both static and dynamic equilibrium (3). Muscles act to move or stabilize the bones of the limbs or spine by generating a moment around the axis of rotation of the joint. These internal moments must balance the external forces caused by the weight of the limbs and items being carried, reaction forces from the ground or other supporting structures, and the inertia due to any motion. Because the distance between the insertion point of the muscle and the joint is significantly smaller than the distance between the line of action of any externally applied forces (3), the force generated by the muscle must be substantially larger than the external forces in order to provide the required moment balance. When this muscular force is included in the calculation of the reaction force within the joint itself, joint force estimates typically range from 2.5 to 10 times the weight of the body or body segment that is supported by the joint (5,127,128).

As an example, the forces transmitted down the spine can be examined for an individual standing erect and also while holding a heavy item in front of them (Fig. 7.13). The weight of the torso is generally assumed to be approximately two thirds of the total body weight. In order to maintain an erect posture, the muscles of the posterior spine, primarily the erector spinae, must provide enough force to balance the moments that result from the action of the torso weight and any items being carried at a distance in front of the spine. When standing erect with arms at the side, the torso weight alone acts through the center of mass of the torso—approximately 10 cm in front of the flexion axis of the spine. For a 75-kg individual, the resulting torso weight (50 kg × *g* = 490 N) creates a moment of 49 N-m tending to flex the spine. In order to balance this moment, the pair

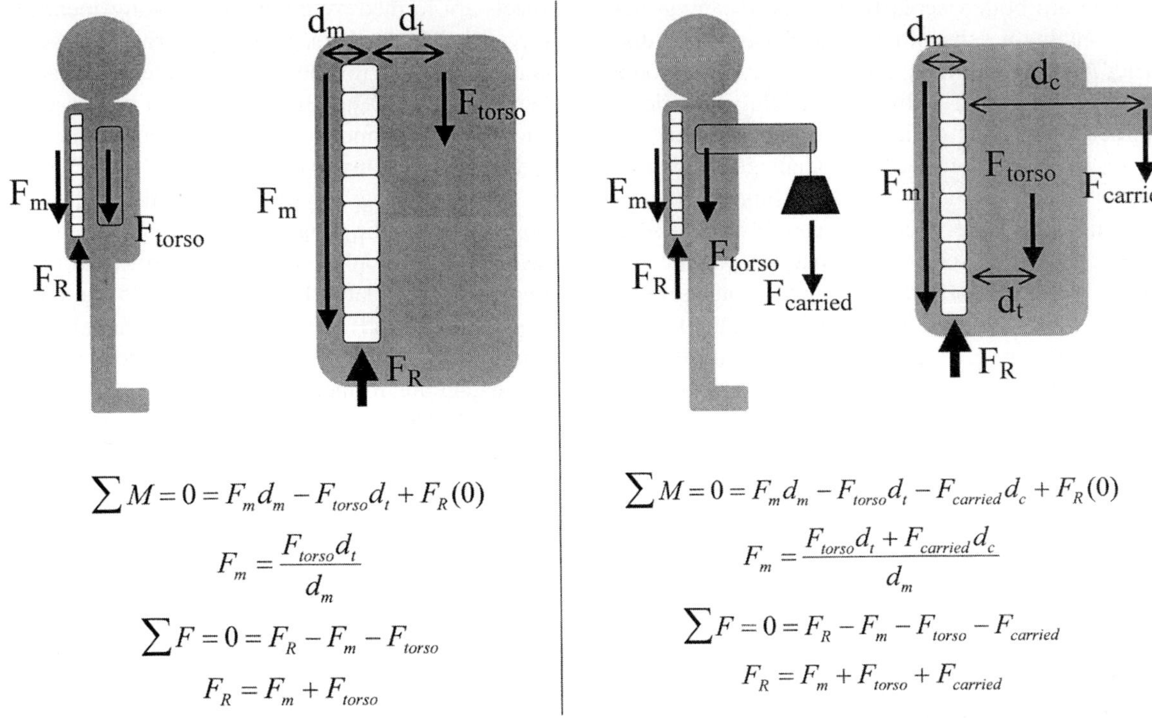

d_m
d_t
F_{torso}
F_m
F_R
d_c
$F_{carried}$
F_{carrie}
$\sum M = 0 = F_m d_m - F_{torso} d_t + F_R(0)$
$F_m = \frac{F_{torso} d_t}{d_m}$
$\sum F = 0 = F_R - F_m - F_{torso}$
$F_R = F_m + F_{torso}$
$\sum M = 0 = F_m d_m - F_{torso} d_t - F_{carried} d_c + F_R(0)$
$F_m = \frac{F_{torso} d_t + F_{carried} d_c}{d_m}$
$\sum F = 0 = F_R - F_m - F_{torso} - F_{carried}$
$F_R = F_m + F_{torso} + F_{carried}$

FIG. 7.13. The principles of equilibrium can be used to estimate the muscular and spinal forces that result when the spine supports either only the weight of the torso **(left)** or the additional weight of a carried object **(right)**. F_m, force generated by the erector spinae; F_R, reaction force along the spine; F_{torso}, weight of the torso; $F_{carried}$, weight of the carried object.

of erector spinae, which acts approximately 3 cm from the flexion axis of the spine, must exert 1,633 N of total force. Then it is important to calculate the total compressive force on the spine, as this will affect pathologies, such as herniated disks, spinal fractures, and low back pain. The reaction force within the spine must balance both the torso weight and the muscle force. In this example, the compressive force that results in the spine is 2,123 N, more than four times the torso weight. When the individual holds a 10-kg mass at arm's length in front of his or her body, this will increase both the muscle moment that must be generated in order to maintain an erect posture and the compressive load experienced by the spine. In this case, the erector spinae must generate 4,083 N of force, and the spinal reaction force is 4,671 N, almost eight times the combination of the torso weight and the carried weight. These interarticular stabilizing forces are far greater than those required for limb motion (3).

This example illustrates the high muscle forces that are required in order to maintain joints in a stable position. Higher internal joint forces result as the distance from an externally applied force to the centerline of the body increases. This is the biomechanical explanation behind recommendations to lift heavy items by bending the knees instead of bending at the back—this keeps the center of gravity of the torso and the item as close to the axis of flexion of the spine as possible.

It is important to remember that the function of a diarthrodial joint is to transfer the load between two adjacent bones during maintenance of posture or limb motion, as well as to allow motion of the parts of the body to occur. In order to do this, most components of the joint must be able to tolerate substantial forces. The subchondral bone and calcified cartilage are subjected primarily to compressive loads through the contact of the joint surfaces. Articular cartilage, on the other hand, sustains both compressive loads (through contact) and shear loads, which result from the motion of the articulating surfaces. Ligaments apply tensile loads to the bones that they connect, resisting forces that would act to separate the bones. The synovial membrane does not serve a substantial load-bearing role; however, it acts to contain the synovial fluid that both lubricates the joint and, during rapid motion, actually forms a film between the articulating surfaces to separate the cartilage and further distribute the load. The muscles, while not a tissue within the joint itself, play an important role in generating forces that maintain posture and move the limbs, transmitting these loads through tendons to the bones.

Biologic tissues that have mechanical functions respond to their loading environment through changes in their microscopic or macroscopic structure. These changes can either be positive, as tissues adapt to an increased stress environment, or negative, as the loading overwhelms the system and causes tissue degradation. Articular cartilage and cancellous bone are both viscolastic tissues, meaning that their matrix contains a substantial fluid phase that is displaced during loading and, thus, absorbs some of the force transmitted. This acts to spare their extracellular matrices. Rapidly applied "impulsive" loads, so fast that the fluid has little time to move, can cause microdamage, which is thought to be a profound trigger for remodeling. As long as the rate of accumulation of microdamage does not exceed the body's ability to heal itself, microdamage is physiologic and can provide a means by which tissue protects itself against future loading. Normal activities subject the tissues of the joint to repetitive, impulsive loading. Substantial damage to the tissue can occur through the resulting accumulation of microdamage if the tissue's ability to heal is overwhelmed by the frequency of this repetitive loading or if the healing processes are impeded as a result of disease or aging.

Injury to one aspect of the musculoskeletal system, whether it is an integral portion of a given joint or simply functioning in the vicinity of the joint, can affect the loading experienced by other tissues in the joints, bones, and muscles. This can initiate a cyclic reaction of tissue adaptation or degeneration that can cause further deviation of physiologic tissue properties and load transfer from the normal state. Thus, it is clinically important to assess the loads on all tissue structures that may result from disease, injury, or clinical intervention. The site-specific changes that occur to the joint in osteoarthrosis are most likely due to these variations in joint loading, be they for anatomic reasons (129) or for neuromuscular control reasons that provoke abnormal, repetitive, impulsive loading (130). However, such determinations are difficult *in vivo*, where they would be most beneficial clinically, due to variations in tissue properties and anatomy between individuals. Novel approaches are now being implemented to determine these parameters by using the experimental data available, as well as more advanced modeling techniques (129).

Biomechanics of Bone

Bone provides the primary structural support for the body. In addition, the relative flexibility of the subchondral bone and underlying cancellous bone is a major factor in allowing for joint congruence under load (131). Failure of these functions will lead to joint failure. Bone is not a simple engineering material, but a living tissue and, as such, it responds to its environment. As a structural material, bone is a composite of organic and inorganic components—namely, collagen and hydroxyapatite. Collagen is a protein with a high tensile strength and viscoelastic properties, while hydroxyapatite is a calcium phosphate compound with properties similar to that of a ceramic. The needle-like hydroxyapatite crystals, with a size of approximately 0.1 nm, are initially embedded in holes between the collagen fibers and, subsequently, in the intermolecular spaces around the collagen fibers (132). At the tissue level, bony sheets are formed by the parallel arrangement of the reinforced collagen fibers, which in turn, are layered in concentric circles with the collagen fiber orientation varying between layers. The dimension about which these concentric layers of composite, or lamellae, are formed depends on the type of bone involved.

The supporting end of the joint, the epiphysis, is composed mainly of spongy, porous bone referred to as cancellous or trabecular bone. It is formed from a series of interconnected plates, beams, and struts (called trabeculae) that are arranged into a three-dimensional structure that mimics the internal skeleton of a modern skyscraper. The trabeculae are formed from layered or wrapped lamellae and are 150 to 300 μm thick. The beams and plates are generally arranged in the direction of primary loading, whereas the struts provide supporting structures in an off-axis direction in order to minimize buckling. Healthy trabecular bone has an improved strength-to-weight ratio compared with cortical bone—it can carry a substantial amount of load while contributing little added weight to the body. Trabecular bone is found in the metaphyseal and epiphyseal regions of long bones, as well as the inner portions of bones, such as the vertebrae of the spine and the carpal bones of the wrist, and plays an important role in the overall load transfer between bones. The subchondral bone, located directly below the calcified cartilage of an articular joint, is less porous than most trabecular bone and has areas that have remodeled around a central blood vessel (haversian canals).

The mechanical properties of trabecular bone have been extensively characterized, and representative properties are listed in Table 7.2.

Bone is a viscoelastic material, as a result of both the collagen component of the tissue microstructure and the marrow that is part of the bone macrostructure. A viscoelastic material is one in which the material properties are dependent on the rate of loading. The more quickly a load is applied, the stiffer bone will become, which means that bone will deform less under a set amount of load when it is applied quickly than when it is applied more slowly. Of great importance is the fact that, unlike traditional engineering materials, the properties of bone are not constant. The strength, modulus, and density can vary between individuals, between anatomic locations (which can be seen as a variation in response to stress), or as a result of age or disease processes. Variations in the properties of bone may be a function of changes in either the material of the tissue (e.g., the properties of the collagen-mineral composite itself) or the structure of the tissue (e.g., how many trabeculae are present and how they are arranged). In healthy tis-

TABLE 7.2. *Representative properties of trabecular bone*

Tissue compressive strength (MPa)	0.5–50
Tissue elastic modulus (MPa)	5–150
Material elastic modulus (GPa)	1–11

See references 100 and 101.

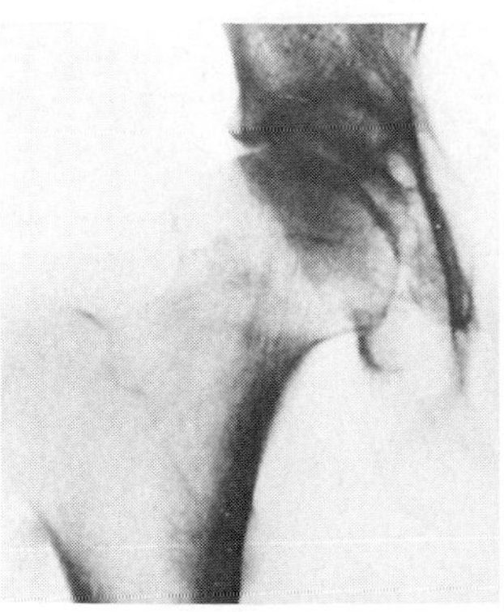
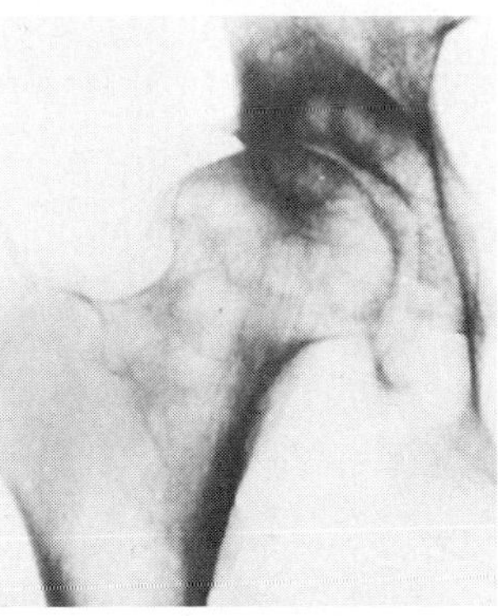

FIG. 7.14. A,B: Radiogram of an osteoarthritic hip that is beginning to sublux laterally. Note the condensation of bone at the lateral rim of the acetabulum and directly across from that area in the femoral head. Where stress is increased above normal, bone becomes sclerotic. If the stress is even greater, cysts will form. Unloaded bone becomes relatively osteopenic.

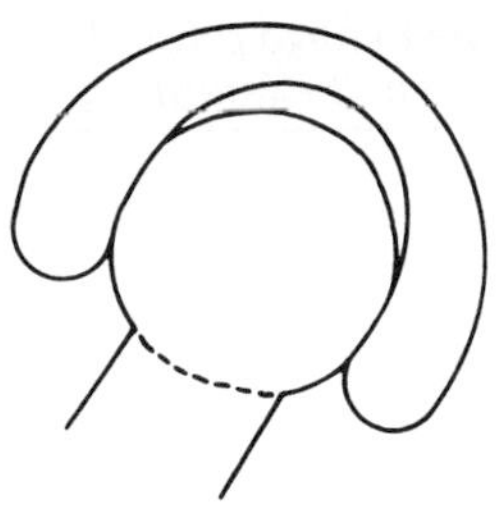
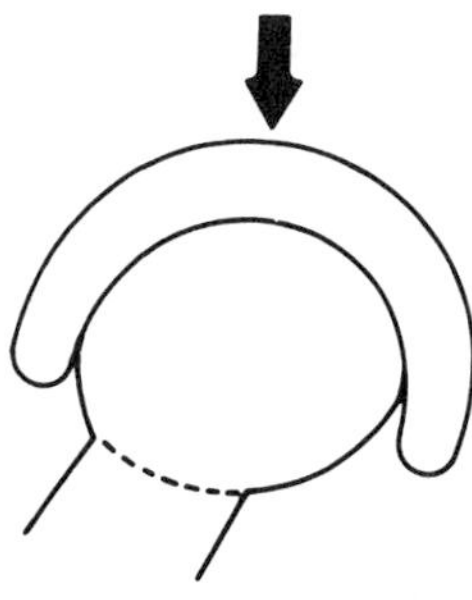

FIG. 7.15. Normally unloaded joints are not completely congruous; under load they become so. It is deformation of the articular cartilage and subchondral bone that allows maximal contact under load. The larger the contact under load, the lower the force per unit area and the consequent stress on these tissues. (From Radin EL, Paul IL, Rose RM, et al. The mechanics of joints as it relates to their degeneration. In: American Academy of Orthopaedic Surgeons. *Symposium on osteoarthritis.* St. Louis: CV Mosby, 1976:41, with permission.)

sue, the bony material changes only minimally, with the mineral density fairly constant at a level of 1.8 to 1.9 g/cm^3 (135) and the mineral to collagen ratio set to about 1:1 by volume. Disease processes can affect the collagen or mineral components of bone and have a profound effect on the underlying properties of the tissue (Fig. 7.14).

The reason for the response of bone to age, disease, and body conditions is that it is a living tissue that responds to its physiologic environment. Two basic processes take place in bone as it responds to physiologic demands. Bone modeling occurs primarily in children and young adults and results in bone growth, both in length and in cross-sectional area. The growth of bones through the addition of material to the endosteum (inner wall of the marrow cavity) or periosteum (outer layer of the bone), the result of the modeling process, can also continue throughout life. Bone remodeling involves the removal, and (in general) replacement, of bone. This process allows for the continual recycling of bone, and in healthy tissue it limits the accumulation of microcracks that could lead to fatigue failure of the structure. The same general processes, on a larger scale, are seen in fracture healing (136,137). In loading-related bone remodeling, the changes in bone mass are due to increases or decreases in the structural arrangement of bone, not a change in the amount of mineral per unit volume of collagen at the material level. The three-dimensional structure of trabecular bone develops in response to the primary tensile and compressive loading axes of the whole bone structure. It has also been suggested that the interconnected plates of subchondral bone, which accurately reflect the stress distribution within the joint, develop so as to provide maximum strength (138).

When a joint is loaded, there is considerable deformation of the epiphyseal and metaphyseal regions, due to the lower stiffness of the subchondral and trabecular bone compared with the cortical diaphysis (131,139). This allows for joint congruence to be maintained (Fig. 7.15). It also allows for a more gradual transition in the stiffness of the loaded tissues in the joint: articular cartilage → calcified cartilage → subchondral and trabecular bone of the epiphyseal/metaphyseal regions → cortical bone of the shaft. This material transition provides for a continuous distribution in the deformation of the overall joint structure and reduces stress concentrations.

Biomechanics of Cartilage

Articular cartilage acts as a smooth, low-friction bearing surface between the bones of a joint. It is a water-filled soft tissue composed of a proteoglycan matrix reinforced with collagen. The orientation of the collagen varies through the thickness of the structure, with fibers oriented perpendicular to the articular surface at the deepest level (farthest from the point of joint contact) and parallel to the surface in the uppermost region (37). The collagen fibers of the deep zone provide mechanical continuity between the articular and the calcified cartilage. In the midregion, the apparently random orientation of the fibrous structure actually reorients itself parallel to the loaded surface under compressive load (61). Because collagen fibers are like ropes and cannot support a compressive load along their length, these arrangements provide a great resistance to both the compressive and shear

TABLE 7.3. *Representative properties of human articular cartilage taken from the lateral condyle of the femur*

Property	Value
Poisson ratio	0.10
Compressive modulus	0.70 MPa
Permeability coefficient	1.18×10^{-15} m^4/Ns

See reference 37.

forces experienced by the cartilage. Cartilage is predominantly loaded in compression and is viscoelastic in nature. Under initial loading, the water within the proteoglycan matrix is extruded, and the stiffness of the material is a function of the tissue permeability. In fact, the fluid pressure within the matrix supports approximately 20 times more load than the underlying material during physiologic loading (37). Under extended, noncyclic loading, the collagen and proteoglycan matrix determines the material behavior after the water has been forced from the tissue. Once a load is removed, the charged nature of the proteoglycan molecules produces an osmotic gradient that draws water back into the cartilage, preparing it for future loading. Table 7.3 shows representative values for cartilage properties.

In addition to providing an optimized articulating surface, cartilage acts with the cancellous bone to improve the fit between the load-bearing, contact surface. This helps to better distribute the load by maximizing the surface contact area (140), preventing stress concentrations from developing in any incongruities that exist in the underlying subchondral bone. Simon and colleagues (141) have shown that cartilage thickness is related to the degree of underlying bony incongruity. Cartilage can be damaged as a result of impacts transmitted through the joints. This typically results in fissures in the tissue that are unlikely to heal. Whether they progress to cartilage loss depends on their location in the joint—habitually loaded cartilage damage will tend to progress; unloaded damage will not (142,143).

Biomechanics of Ligaments

Ligaments, consisting of a combination of collagen and elastin fibers arranged primarily in parallel along the axis of loading, connect bones to each other across a joint. However, in the unloaded state, the fibers are slightly crimped. As a result, initial tensile loading of the structure acts only to straighten out the component fibers, resulting in a region of low stiffness. Once the fibers have been completely straightened, the individual fiber stiffness dictates the overall structural stiffness. The resulting load deformation curve (Fig. 7.16) exhibits a characteristic low-stiffness toe region followed by a region of increasing stiffness. If loading continues, failure of individual fibers within the structure will result in decreasing overall stiffness followed by rupture. Table 7.4 shows typical values for the tensile properties of ligaments. They are viscoelastic in nature (to an even

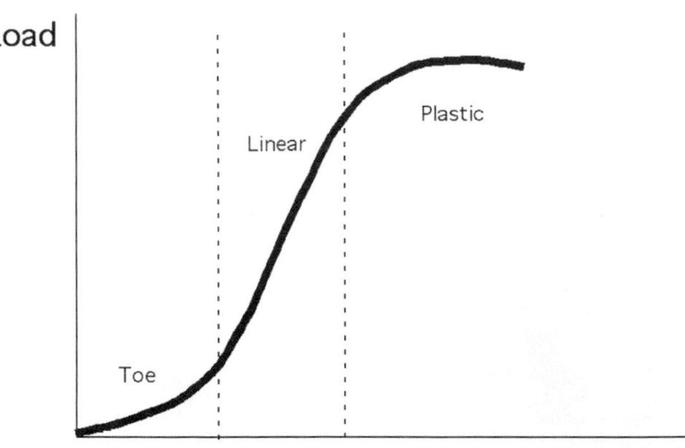

FIG. 7.16. A representative force-deflection curve for a ligament under tensile loading. Notice the first region of very low stiffness, indicative of the straightening of the kinked collagen fibers. This is followed by increasing stiffness as the applied load stretches the parallel fibers of the tissue. Finally, the collagen fibers begin to fail, until final rupture of the ligament body occurs.

greater extent than bone) and will fail at lower extensions when loaded at high rates. This behavior explains why a slow stretch will not injure a ligament, whereas a rapid motion may result in rupture. The properties of ligaments vary based on anatomic location, indicating that the properties develop to match the normal physiologic demands.

Ligaments have a limited blood supply through their insertion sites and only a small population of cells (fibroblasts) within the collagen and elastin fibers. The vascular supply that does exist is necessary for the maintenance of tissue properties. Periods of immobilization, such as occur when a limb is immobilized, result in a decrease in both stiffness and strength in ligaments. The ligament substance can recover in a period of time approximately equal to that of immobilization. However, the strength of the insertion has been seen to reach only 80% to 90% of its original strength after 12 months of recovery following 9 weeks of non–weight bearing (42). Ligaments can be damaged as a result of an excessive load that can rupture some or all of the fibers of the structure. A complete rupture will not properly heal without clinical intervention, because the ligament ends are no longer continuous. Partial ruptures, or sprains,

TABLE 7.4. *Representative properties of ligament under tensile loading as measured for rabbit anterior cruciate ligament with its bony attachments*

Tissue	Property	Value
Ligament	Stiffness (N/mm)	150
	Ultimate load (N)	368
	Energy absorbed to failure (N-mm)	1,330

See references 42 and 109.

will heal, but generally over a substantial period of time due to the limited vascular supply to the tissue.

Biomechanics of Muscles

The function of muscles is to exert a tensile force on tendons that connect the muscles to skeletal structures. In this way, the muscles are able to move limbs, stabilize joints, and change the volume of body cavities. The force-generating unit of a muscle is the combination of actin and myosin fibrils that make up a sarcomere. If it is assumed that each pair of fibrils can generate a maximum amount of force, then the maximum load that can be generated by a whole muscle depends on the number of fibrils in a sarcomere and the number of sarcomeres in the muscle as a whole. Thus, the strength of a muscle is nominally related to its volume. Because the length of a muscle is generally determined based on skeletal anatomy, and is not likely to change in an individual after the point of skeletal maturity, variations in muscle strength in an adult individual can be related to the cross-sectional area of the muscle. Muscles with a higher cross-sectional area can produce a greater force.

Muscle is an active tissue; thus, its properties in its passive state contribute little to the function of the skeletal system. Consequently, the innervation of the muscles plays a substantial role in their performance in postural stability and motion. The stabilization function of muscles may be more important to overall posture and motion that the role of muscles in moving the limbs. This is particularly important in the joints without substantial structural constraint, especially the hip and shoulder. In addition, action of the muscles can act to absorb some of the energy produced by impulse loads through the bones (3).

INTERVERTEBRAL JOINTS

General Structure

The spine is a segmented series of bones that articulate at the intervertebral joints. These joints are composed of two elements: amphiarthrodial, interverterbral disc joints and laterally placed, diarthrodial, interverterbral facet joints. The discs themselves are fibrocartilaginous complexes and separate the vertebral bodies. Motion between any two vertebral segments is limited to a few degrees in any plane by strong ligaments, the amphiarthrodial discs, and the configuration of the intervertebral facet joints, which although diarthrodial, allow little motion. It is the sum of the motion of all of the joints of the entire column that provides the range necessary for the extraordinary mobility of the human spine. Discs from different regions of the spine (cervical, thoracic, and lumbar) vary in size and shape, but are basically identical in their organization (144). The central cartilaginous-like center of the intervertebral discs is constrained on all sides. Its sides are wrapped in a collagenous annulus fibrosus, and its top and bottom surfaces are bordered by the inferior and superior endplates of the adjacent vertebra. (Fig. 7.17).

The water content of the nucleus of the disc tends to be even higher than that of articular cartilage. While under sustained loading (such as prolonged standing), some disc fluid does leak out; however, the permeability of the nucleus and annulus to water is substantially lower than that

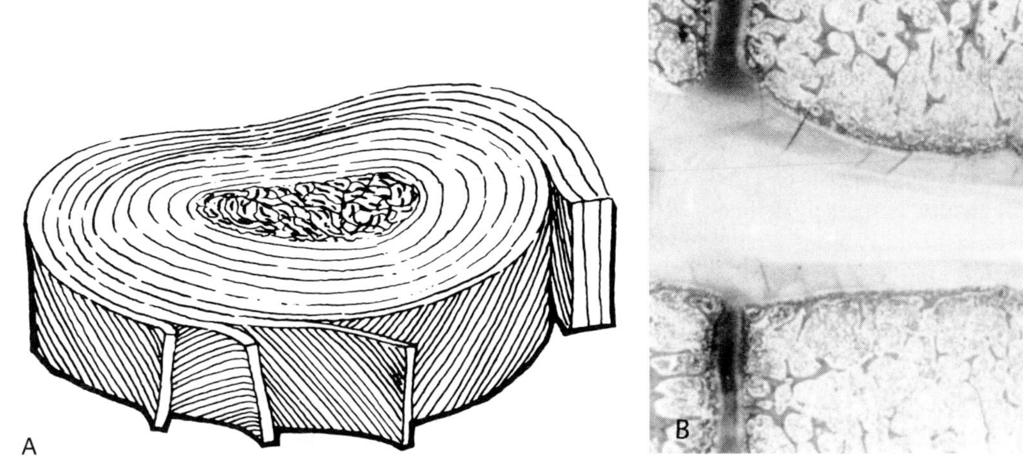

FIG. 7.17. A: Artist's concept of the structure of the intervertebral disc. Note that the concentric layers of the lamina fibrosa show varied orientation of collagen fibers. Centrally placed is the nucleus pulposus, a semifluid mass. **B:** Low-power photomicrograph of the intervertebral disc showing the cartilage plates covering the bony end plates of the vertebral segments. Circumferential rings of fibrous tissue compose the annulus fibrosus, and, in the center, is a poorly staining material, the nucleus pulposus (hematoxylin and eosin, original magnification ×4).

of articular cartilage. The general confinement of the viscous fluid allows the disc to act as a hydrostatic shock absorber. The role of the spine is axial stiffening while allowing flexibilty in almost all planes of motion: flexion-extension, rotation, and tilting. The stability of the interspinal segments is provided by substantial ligamentous structures that envelop the bony parts. Where the ligaments are not continuous, posterolaterally, is where disc herniations occur. The stability of the spinal column is provided by the interspinal muscles, which are substantial and can generate a large force. Paralyze these muscles, and the patients cannot sit or stand without external support (145). The biomechanics of the spine are addressed in the ensuing paragraphs.

As far as the detailed anatomy is concerned, the annulus fibrosus consists of a ring of fibrous lamellae that encases the nucleus and unites the vertebral bodies. This unification is achieved by creating contiguity of the fibrous structure with the margins of the vertebral segments and the investing anterior and posterior longitudinal ligaments (1,144). The fibrous layers of the annulus are approximately 20 μm thick and, on polarized microscopic examination, are organized such that alternating sheets of collagen are set at an angle to each other (146–148). Some flexibility is achieved by random arrangement of the fibers (0.1–0.2 μm in diameter) within the substance of the plates of collagen and by a relatively high proportion of proteoglycan and interstitial fluid in the annulus as compared with the more rigid tendons or ligaments (128,149,150). The annulus is not uniformly thick throughout the structure. The plates in the anterior third of the disc are thickest and most distinct; those in the posterior aspect are more closely packed and somewhat thinner (151).

The second component of the disc is the nucleus pulposus, which occupies the central portion of the disc and is surrounded by the annulus. Actually, the nucleus is not centrally placed within the confines of the annulus, but during erect posture usually lies closer to the posterior margin of the disc (151). The nature of this material and its function in the joint are most evident when, on transverse or sagittal sectioning of the disc, it is found to bulge prominently beyond the plane of the section. The nucleus consists of a viscid fluid structure, which, histologically, is sparsely cellular and consists principally of loose, delicate, fibrous strands embedded in a gelatinous matrix (7). In the central portion of the nucleus, the fibers appear randomly distributed, but as they approach the superior and inferior cartilage plates, they assume an oblique angular orientation to become embedded in the cartilage at the peripheral attachment of the nucleus (146,151,152). The structural interspace between the nucleus and the annulus is difficult to appreciate, and in many older subjects, the two tissues blend imperceptibly (144,146).

The disc is contained superiorly and inferiorly by cartilaginous plates, which are firmly fixed to the bony endplates of the adjacent vertebral segments and differ little in structure from the hyaline articular cartilage seen in diarthrodial joints, except that they have no collagenous "skin," or any discrete superficial surface (144,151). Instead, the cartilage serves as an anchor for the fine filamented fibers of the nucleus pulposus in its central portion and the coarse fibrous plates of the annulus fibrosus peripherally.

Embryology and Development

The development of the intervertebral disc in humans occurs early in fetal life. Following formation of the morula, the mass of primitive cells becomes the blastocyst, which rapidly undergoes proliferation and differentiation into ectoderm and endoderm, which, in turn, combine to form the embryonic disc (153). A primitive streak develops at the caudal end of the dorsum of the embryonic disc. The groove deepens, and at the most caudal portion the primitive node develops. At this site, cells arising from the mesoderm give rise to the notochord, which thickens and rolls up into the neural folds to form the neural tube (154,155). The mesodermal tissues on each side of the notochord form the primitive somites, and, at approximately the third week of gestation, distinct spinal segments can be identified. The central portions of the somite on either side of the notochord form the vertebral column. Mesodermal cells from each side join to form the vertebral bony elements, including not only the cartilaginous endplates, but also the annulus fibrosus and the peripheral portions of the nucleus pulposus (153). The notochord, which originally lies centrally placed in the vertebral body and disc, is compressed as chondrification of the vertebra progresses and, within a short time, is destroyed (155). No notochordal remnants can be found in the vertebral body in the mature fetus or adult (except in an occasional patient who develops a chordoma). The portion of the notochord that lies in the intervertebral disc area, however, becomes the major central portion of the nucleus pulposus (155). The annulus develops early in embryonic life from the densely aggregated cells about each pole of the somitic segment and eventually surrounds the notochord completely. Ossification begins in the vertebral body at the 50- to 60-μm stage (third month) as vessels invade the cartilaginous precursors, but the endplates remain cartilaginous and serve as the attachment site for the adult nucleus pulposus and annulus fibrosus (156).

Biochemistry

The annulus fibrosus is principally collagenous but is relatively hyperhydrated compared with other fibrous tissues, with water estimates ranging between 65% and 70% (148,150). Collagen accounts for approximately 50% to 55% of the dry weight. The remainder of the tissue consists of proteoglycan and the principal glycosaminoglycans, including chondroitin sulfate and keratan sulfate (157,158). A small amount of glycoprotein is present (129,130,159). The nucleus has a much higher water content than the annulus, with estimates for immature animals as high as 88%. The value decreases to about 65% in elderly individuals (126,131,148). Collagen is also present in the nucleus (mostly type II), but accounts for a considerably smaller percentage of the dry weight (20%–30%) than in other joint connective tissues (55,58,59,148,157). Most of the material within the nucleus consists of proteoglycan (149,160–162) and other, as yet poorly defined, proteinaceous materials (159). The distribution of glycosaminoglycans varies considerably, depending on the age of the patient and the amount of degeneration that has occurred, but chondroitin 6-sulfate (~40%), chondroitin 4-sulfate (5%), keratan sulfate (~50%), and hyaluronic acid (<2%) have all been reported (157,158). Pearson and coworkers (159) have described the presence of other proteins, probably glycoproteins, that are believed to be important in maintaining the physical properties of the material. Lysosomal enzymes have been described that presumably play a role in the normal turnover of the proteoglycans (147). Synthetic activity takes place in the outer ring of cells of the nucleus (163).

Function and Biomechanics of the Intervertebral Disc and Spine

The main role of the intervertebral disc is to serve as a load-bearing structure and absorb energy during the compression of the spine (164–166). The resistance to compressive axial loading, one of the predominant mechanisms of spinal force transmission, is mediated through the compressibility of the hyperhydrated nucleus. The nucleus pulposus, in conjunction with the surrounding annulus fibrosus, resists and modifies pressures by "barreling" (losing height while gaining in width) (164,166,167). The application of a force to the disc compresses the nucleus pulposus, which causes the intradiscal pressure to increase and creates a tensile force in the annulus fibrosus. The annulus is designed to absorb most of the barreling of the disc by collagen network stretch.

If an articulated spine is loaded with the weight of a human head, it will buckle. Muscle action is required if the spine is to maintain an erect position (16). These muscle-produced loads on the spine during normal daily activities are thus necessarily higher than body weight, reaching as high as eight times the total supported weight for even a small load carried in front of the body. The spine consists of vertebral bodies and intervertebral discs arranged in series. As a result, a load applied to the end of the spine will result in the same applied force at each level. In reality, the load carried by the vertebrae and discs in the lumbar spine are higher than those of the cervical and thoracic regions, due to the increased percentage of body weight located above each level of interest; spinal loading increases in the caudal direction.

If a healthy spine is loaded in pure compression or compression plus flexion within normal physiologic limits, failure will occur in the vertebral bodies before significant damage occurs to the discs. Rupture of an intervertebral disc requires a combination of compression, flexion, and rotation. Under these circumstances, tearing of the annulus begins at its periphery (164). The biochemical changes associated with aging of the nucleus pulposus would appear to play little role in intervertebral disc rupture (168).

Integrity and congruence of the intervertebral facet joints require the maintenance of the intervertebral disc space. Loss of disc height from rupture and extravasation of disc material, digestion of the nuclear proteoglycans, or surgical excision of the disc will lead to intervertebral space collapse and settling of the intervertebral facet joints, resulting in articular incongruity with diminution of their contact areas (169,170). The disc should not be considered as a separate unit, but rather as an integral part of the intervertebral joint that includes the facet joints and the anterior and posterior longitudinal ligaments. All of these components act together to maintain the axial resistance to compression and stability of the spine (165,171).

HEALING OF SYNOVIAL JOINTS

There is consensus that all the tissues of the joint, except cartilage, can heal. All but cartilage are vascularized and can participate in the usual inflammatory healing phenomenon. In addition, the cells in mature cartilage have limited mobility and are a poor source of cells for healing. But, under certain circumstances, cartilage does heal. The controversy surrounding the healing of articular cartilage is due to the several variables which affect such repair. Articular cartilage repair requires a source of cells, hydrostatic pressure, and physiologic tissue pressures. It initially heals as fibrocartilage and, if that survives, over time, has been reported to mature to hyaline cartilage (172). The cells that heal cartilage come from the synovium or subchondral bone and healing requires motion and reasonable intraarticular pressures (173). Such repair is initially fibrocartilaginous in nature (172,174). There are reports of fibrocartilage evolving over may years to hyaline cartilage (172). The frequently short life of fibrocartilage would appear due to mechanical factors and the difficulty it has bonding with the remaining articular cartilage (172,175). If congruity remains or can be reestablished and the stress concentrations removed, joints can functionally heal, as Pauwels, Coventry, Maquet, and others have shown (172). Meniscal fibrocartilage can undergo repair if the damage is peripheral, in the zone of vascularization (176).

SUMMARY

The major function of the joint is to allow movement of the skeletal frame, which requires transmission of the significant forces generated by muscle action and body weight. Joints are designed to move easily. As in any organ, several tissues play a cooperative role. The articular cartilage and synovial membranes act as lubricating surfaces, both tissues supplying the lubricant. Underlying the articular cartilage is a complicated arrangement of subchondral bone, designed to minimize intraarticular pressure while still allowing transmission of the interarticular load from one bone to the next. The ligaments act mechanically and as proprioceptive sensors to help guide the joint's motion. The muscles control joint movement and act as shock absorbers to dampen impulsive loads. The health of the organ depends on the interrelationship of these various tissues, and failure of one can lead to eventual failure of the whole organ. As discussed in this chapter, the biologic and mechanical factors acting on joints are inseparable. One must understand the relationship between the two to appreciate the physiology of this organ.

In this chapter we have stressed the increased interest in the molecular biology of the tissues of the joint and its relationship to biomechanics. The biphasic model of articular cartilage is still being revised and has become critical for "molecular level" modeling of articular cartilage replacement and predictions of chondrocyte deformation (177). There is finally acceptance that, for the best results, joint structures must be transplanted immediately after injury before remodeling occurs (178) and that establishing proper tension of anterior cruciate ligament grafts is critical for a successful clinical outcome (179). In these days of increasingly aggressive surgical approaches as regards osteoarthrosis, the *Journal of Bone and Joint Surgery* has seen fit almost 50 years later to republish Wally Blount's 1956 editorial, "Don't throw away the cane" (180). We should all be attentive to the lessons of history.

REFERENCES

1. Goss CM, ed. *Gray's anatomy of the human body,* 29th ed. Philadelphia: Lea & Febiger; 1973.
2. Gardner E. The physiology of joints. *J Bone Joint Surg Am* 1963;45: 1061–1066.
3. O'Connor M, Shercliff T, Goodfellow J. The mechanics of the knee in the sagittal plane: mechanics, interactions between muscles, ligaments, and the articular surfaces. In: Muller W, HW, eds. *Surgery and arthroscopy of the knee.* New York: Springer-Verlag, 1988.
4. Neumann DA. Biomechanical analysis of selected principles of hip joint protection. *Arthritis Care Res* 1989;2:146–155.
5. Rydell N. Biomechanics of the hip-joint. *Clin Orthop* 1973;92:6–15.
6. Rothman RH, Marvel JP Jr, Heppenstall RB. Anatomic considerations in glenohumeral joint. *Orthop Clin North Am* 1975;6:341–352.
7. Fithian DC, Kelly MA, Mow VC. Material properties and structure-function relationships in the menisci. *Clin Orthop* 1990:19–31.
8. Kennedy JC, Weinberg HW, Wilson AS. The anatomy and function of the anterior cruciate ligament. As determined by clinical and morphological studies. *J Bone Joint Surg Am* 1974;56:223–235.
9. Mankin HJ, Brandt DK, Moskowitz RW, et al. Biochemistry and metabolism of cartilage in osteoarthritis. In: *Osteoarthritis: diagnosis and management.* 1984:43–79.
10. Revell PA, Mayston V, Lalor P, et al. The synovial membrane in osteoarthritis: a histological study including the characterisation of the cellular infiltrate present in inflammatory osteoarthritis using monoclonal antibodies. *Ann Rheum Dis* 1988;47:300–307.
11. Barnett CH, Davies DV, MacConnail MA. Synovial joints: their structure and mechanics. Synovial joints: 1961.
12. Redler I, Zimny ML. Scanning electron microscopy of normal and abnormal articular cartilage and synovium. *J Bone Joint Surg Am* 1970;52:1395–1404.
13. Peterson HA, Winkelmann RK, Coventry MB. Nerve endings in the hip joint of the cat: their morphology, distribution, and density. *J Bone Joint Surg Am* 1972;54:333–343.
14. Ralston HJ, Miller MR, Kashara M. Nerve endings in human fasciae, tendons, ligaments, periosteum, and joint synovial membrane. *Anat Rec* 1960;136:137–147.
15. Gardner E. Innervation of the knee joint. *Anat Rec* 1948;101:109–130.
16. Radin EL, Rose RM, Blaha JD. *Practical biomechanics for the orthopedic surgeon,* 2nd ed. New York: 1991.
17. Dowthwaite GP, Ward AC, Flannely J, et al. The effect of mechanical strain on hyaluronan metabolism in embryonic fibrocartilage cells. *Matrix Biol* 1999;18:523–532.
18. Pitsillides AA, Skerry TM, Edwards JC. Joint immobilization reduces synovial fluid hyaluronan concentration and is accompanied by changes in the synovial intimal cell populations. *Rheumatology (Oxford)* 1999; 38:1108–1112.
19. Francis-West PH, Parish J, Lee K, et al. BMP/GDF-signalling interactions during synovial joint development. *Cell Tissue Res* 1999;296: 111–119.
20. Edwards JC, Wilkinson LS, Jones HM, et al. The formation of human synovial joint cavities: a possible role for hyaluronan and CD44 in altered interzone cohesion. *J Anat* 1994;185:355–367.
21. Kavanagh E, Abiri M, Bland YS, et al. Division and death of cells in developing synovial joints and long bones. *Cell Biol Int* 2002;26: 679–688.
22. Hartmann C, Tabin CJ. Wnt-14 plays a pivotal role in inducing synovial joint formation in the developing appendicular skeleton. *Cell* 2001;104:341–351.
23. Spitz F, Duboule D. Development. The art of making a joint. *Science* 2001;291:1713–1714.
24. Tavares AT, Tsukui T, Izpisua Belmonte JC. Evidence that members of the Cut/Cux/CDP family may be involved in AER positioning and polarizing activity during chick limb development. *Development* 2000;127:5133–5144.
25. Lizarraga G, Lichtler A, Upholt WB, et al. Studies on the role of Cux1 in regulation of the onset of joint formation in the developing limb. *Dev Biol* 2002;243:44–54.
26. Goff DJ, Tabin CJ. Analysis of Hoxd-13 and Hoxd-11 misexpression in chick limb buds reveals that Hox genes affect both bone condensation and growth. *Development* 1997;124:627–636.
27. Lyons KM, Pelton RW, Hogan BL. Patterns of expression of murine Vgr-1 and BMP-2a RNA suggest that transforming growth factor-beta-like genes coordinately regulate aspects of embryonic development. *Genes Dev* 1989;3:1657–1668.
28. Hogan BL. Bone morphogenetic proteins: multifunctional regulators of vertebrate development. *Genes Dev* 1996;10:1580–1594.
29. Thomas JT, Kilpatrick MW, Lin K, et al. Disruption of human limb morphogenesis by a dominant negative mutation in CDMP1. *Nat Genet* 1997;17:58–64.
30. Merino R, Ganan Y, Macias D, et al. Morphogenesis of digits in the avian limb is controlled by FGFs, TGFbetas, and noggin through BMP signaling. *Dev Biol* 1998;200:35–45.
31. Shimazu A, Nah HD, Kirsch T, et al. Syndecan-3 and the control of chondrocyte proliferation during endochondral ossification. *Exp Cell Res* 1996;229:126–136.
32. Buckland RA, Collinson JM, Graham E, et al. Antagonistic effects of FGF4 on BMP induction of apoptosis and chondrogenesis in the chick limb bud. *Mech Dev* 1998;71:143–150.
33. Moftah MZ, Downie SA, Bronstein NB, et al. Ectodermal FGFs induce perinodular inhibition of limb chondrogenesis *in vitro* and *in vivo* via FGF receptor 2. *Dev Biol* 2002;249:270–282.
34. Smits P, Li P, Mandel J, et al. The transcription factors L-Sox5 and Sox6 are essential for cartilage formation. *Dev Cell* 2001;1:277–290.
35. Asou Y, Nifuji A, Tsuji K, et al. Coordinated expression of scleraxis and Sox9 genes during embryonic development of tendons and cartilage. *J Orthop Res* 2002;20:827–833.
36. Charnley J. Symposium on biomechanics. Institute of Mechanical Engineering 1969.

37. Mankin HJ, Mow VC. Form and function of articular cartilage. In: Simon SR, ed. *Orthopaedic basic science.* Chicago: American Academy of Orthopaedic Surgeons, 1994.
38. Meachim G. Effect of age on the thickness of adult articular cartilage at the shoulder joint. *Ann Rheum Dis* 1971;30:43–46.
39. Simon WH. Scale effects in animal joints. I. Articular cartilage thickness and compressive stress. *Arthritis Rheum* 1970;13:244–256.
40. van der Korst JK, Skoloff L, Miller EJ. Senescent pigmentation of cartilage and degenerative joint disease. *Arch Pathol* 1968;86:40–47.
41. Ghadially FN. Fine structure of joints. In: Sokoloff L, ed. *The joints and synovial fluid.* San Diego: Academic, 1978:105–168.
42. Woo SLY, An KN, Arnoczky SP, et al. Anatomy, biology, and biomechanics of tendon, ligament and meniscus. In: Simon SR, ed. *Orthopaedic basic science.* Chicago: American Academy of Orthopaedic Surgeons, 1994:45–88.
43. Clark IC. Human articular surface contours and related surface depression frequency studies. *Ann Rheum Dis* 1971;20:15–23.
44. Clark IC. Surface characteristics of human articular cartilage—a scanning electron microscope study. *J Anat* 1971;108:23–30.
45. Swann DA, Hendren RB, Radin EL, et al. The lubricating activity of synovial fluid glycoproteins. *Arthritis Rheum* 1981;24:22–30.
46. Mankin HJ. The articular cartilage, cartilage healing, and osteoarthrosis. In: Cruess RL, Rennie WRJ, eds. *Adult orthopaedics.* New York: Churchill Livingstone, 1984:163–270.
47. Davis DV. Blood supply of synovial membrane and interarticular structures. *Ann Coll Surg Engl* 1948;2:156.
48. Brower TD, Orlic PL. Diffusion of dyes through articular cartilage in vivo. *J Bone Joint Surg Am* 1962;44:456–463.
49. McKibben B. The nutrition of immature joint cartilage in the lamb. *J Bone Joint Surg Br* 1966;48:793–803.
50. Gardner E. Physiology of movable joints. *Physiol Rev* 1950;30:127–176.
51. Hogervorst T, Brand RA. Mechanoreceptors in joint function. *J Bone Joint Surg Am* 1998;80:1365–1378.
52. Stockwell RA. *Biology of cartilage cells.* Cambridge: Cambridge University Press, 1979.
53. Mankin HJ, Thrasher AZ. Water content and binding in normal and osteoarthritic human cartilage. *J Bone Joint Surg Am* 1975;57:76–80.
54. McCutchen CW. Boundry lubrication by synovial fluid: demonstration and possible osmotic explanation. *Fed Proc* 1966;25:1061.
55. Torzilli PA. Influence of cartilage conformation on its equilibrium water partition. *J Orthop Res* 1985;3:473–483.
56. Leidy J. On the intimate structure and history of articular cartilage. *Am J Med Sci* 2003;34:277–294.
57. Weiss C, Rosenberg L, Helfet AJ. An ultrastructural study of normal young adult human articular cartilage. *J Bone Joint Surg Am* 1968; 50:663–674.
58. Benninghoff A. Form und Bau der Gelenkknorpel in ihren Beziehungen zur Funktion. I. Die modellierenden und formerhaltenden Faktoren des Knorpelreliefs. *Z Ges Anat* 1925;76:43–63.
59. Benninghoff A. Form und Bau der Gelenkknorpel in ihren Beziehungen zur Gunktion. II. Der Aufbau des Gelenkknorpels in seinen Beziehungen zur Funktion. *Z Zellforsch* 1925;2:783–862.
60. Clark JM, Simonian PT. Scanning electron microscopy of "fibrillated" and "malacic" human articular cartilage: technical considerations. *Microsc Res Tech* 1997;37:299–313.
61. McCall JG. Load-deformation studies of articular cartilage. *J Anat* 1969;105:212–214.
62. Buschmann MD, Grodzinsky AJ. A molecular model of proteoglycan-associated electrostatic forces in cartilage mechanics. *J Biomech Eng* 1995;117:179–192.
63. Cole AA, Kuettner KE. Molecular basis for differences between human joints. *Cell Mol Life Sci* 2002;59:19–26.
64. Guilak F, Jones WR, Ting-Beall HP, et al. The deformation behavior and mechanical properties of chondrocytes in articular cartilage. *Osteoarthritis Cartilage* 1999;7:59–70.
65. Pauwels F. Grundriss einer Biomechanik der Frakturheilung. *Verh Dtsch Orthop Ges* 1940;62.
66. Pauwels F. Eine neue Theorie über den Einfluss mechanisher Reize auf die Differenzierung der Stützgewebe. *Zeitschrift Anat Entwicklungsgeschichte* 1960;121:478–515.
67. Kummer B. *Principles of the biomechanics of the human supporting and locomotor system.* Vienna: Verlag der Wiener Medizinischen Akademie, 1963.
68. Shaw JL, Bassett CA. The effects of varying oxygen concentrations on osteogenesis and embryonic cartilage *in vitro. J Bone Joint Surg Am* 1967;49:73–80.
69. Fawns HT. Histological studies of rheumatic conditions. I. Observations on the fine structure of the matrix of normal bone and cartilage. *Ann Rheum Dis* 2003;12:105–113.
70. Redler I, Mow VC, Zimny ML, et al. The ultrastructure and biomechanical significance of the tidemark of articular cartilage. *Clin Orthop* 1975:357–362.
71. Green WT Jr, Martin GN, Eanes ED, et al. Microradiographic study of the calcified layer of articular cartilage. *Arch Pathol* 1970;90: 151–158.
72. Thompson AM, Stockwell RA. An ultrastructural study of the marginal transitional zone in the rabbit knee joint. *J Anat* 1983;136: 701–713.
73. Burr DB, Schaffler MB. The involvement of subchondral mineralized tissues in osteoarthrosis: quantitative microscopic evidence. *Microsc Res Tech* 1997;37:343–357.
74. Kenzora JE, Yosipovitch Z, Glimcher MJ. The calcified cartilage zone of adult articular cartilage: a viable functional entity. *Orthop Trans* 1978;2:1–20.
75. Bullough PG, Jagannath A. The morphology of the calcification front in articular cartilage. Its significance in joint function. *J Bone Joint Surg Br* 1983;65:72–78.
76. Johnson L. Kinetics of osteoarthritis. *Lab Invest* 1959;8:12–23.
77. Radin EL, Paul IL, Lowy M. A comparison of the dynamic force transmitting properties of subchondral bone and articular cartilage. *J Bone Joint Surg Am* 1970;52:444–456.
78. Radin EL, Wright V. Osteoarthrosis. *Mechanics of human joints: physiology, pathophysiology, and treatment.* New York: Marcel Dekker, 1993:341–354.
79. Barland P, Novikoff AB, Hamerman D. Electron microscopy of the human synovial membrane. *J Cell Biol* 1962;14:207–220.
80. Coleman P, Kavanagh E, Mason RM, et al. The proteoglycans and glycosaminoglycan chains of rabbit synovium. *Histochem J* 1998;30: 519–524.
81. Athanasou NA, Quinn J. Immunocytochemical analysis of human synovial lining cells: phenotypic relation to other marrow derived cells. *Ann Rheum Dis* 1991;50:311–315.
82. Wilkinson LS, Worrall JG, Sinclair HD, et al. Immunohistological reassessment of accessory cell populations in normal and diseased human synovium. *Br J Rheumatol* 1990;29:259–263.
83. Medzhitov R, Preston-Hurlburt P, Janeway CA Jr. A human homologue of the Drosophila Toll protein signals activation of adaptive immunity. *Nature* 1997;388:394–397.
84. Jurk M, Heil F, Vollmer J, et al. Human TLR7 or TLR8 independently confer responsiveness to the antiviral compound R-848. *Nat Immunol* 2002;3:499.
85. de Haas M. IgG-Fc receptors and the clinical relevance of their polymorphisms. *Wien Klin Wochenschr* 2001;113:825–831.
86. Hadler NM, Dourmashkin RR, Nermut MV, et al. Ultrastructure of a hyaluronic acid matrix. *Proc Natl Acad Sci U S A* 1982;79:307–309.
87. Lublin DM, Atkinson JP. Decay-accelerating factor: biochemistry, molecular biology, and function. *Annu Rev Immunol* 1989;7:35–58.
88. Bhatia A, Blades S, Cambridge G, et al. Differential distribution of Fc gamma RIIIa in normal human tissues and co-localization with DAF and fibrillin-1: implications for immunological microenvironments. *Immunology* 1998;94:56–63.
89. Fairburn K, Kunaver M, Wilkinson LS, et al. Intercellular adhesion molecules in normal synovium. *Br J Rheumatol* 1993;32:302–306.
90. Demaziere A, Athanasou NA. Adhesion receptors of intimal and subintimal cells of the normal synovial membrane. *J Pathol* 1992;168: 209–215.
91. Ropes MW, Bauer W. Synovial fluid changes in joint disease. Cambridge, MA: Harvard University Press, 1953.
92. Davies DV. Observations on the volume, viscosity, and nitrogen content of synovial fluid with a note on the histological appearance of synovial membrane. *J Anat* 2003;78:68–78.
93. Radin EL, Paul IL. Response of joints to impact loading. I. *In vitro* wear. *Arthritis Rheum* 1971;14:356–362.
94. Linn FC, Radin EL. Lubrication of animal joints. 3. The effect of certain chemical alterations of the cartilage and lubricant. *Arthritis Rheum* 1968;11:674–682.

95. McCutchen CW. Sponge-hydrostatic and weeping bearings. *Nature* 1959;184:1285–1286.
96. Edwards J. *Lubrication and wear in living and artificial human joints.* London: Institute of Mechanical Engineering, 1967.
97. Mow VC, Mansour JM. The nonlinear interaction between cartilage deformation and interstitial fluid flow. *J Biomech* 1977;10:31–39.
98. Linn FC, Sokoloff L. Movement and composition of interstitial fluid of cartilage. *Arthritis Rheum* 1965;8:481–493.
99. Hills BA, Monds MK. Enzymatic identification of the load-bearing boundary lubricant in the joint. *Br J Rheumatol* 1998;37:137–142.
100. Radin EL, Swann DA, Weisser PA. Separation of a hyaluronate-free lubricating fraction from synovial fluid. *Nature* 1970;228:377–378.
101. Hills BA. Boundary lubrication *in vivo. Proc Inst Mech Eng [H]* 2000;214(1):83–94.
102. Schwarz IM, Hills BA. Surface-active phospholipid as the lubricating component of lubricin. *Br J Rheumatol* 1998;37:21–26.
103. Jay GD, Harris DA, Cha CJ. Boundary lubrication by lubricin is mediated by O-linked beta(1–3)Gal-GalNAc oligosaccharides. *Glycoconj J* 2001;18(10):807–815.
104. Jay GD, Tantravahi U, Britt DE, et al. Homology of lubricin and superficial zone protein (SZP): products of megakaryocyte stimulating factor (MSF) gene expression by human synovial fibroblasts and articular chondrocytes localized to chromosome 1q25. *J Orthop Res* 2001;19(4):677–687.
105. Radin EL, Paul IL, Swann DA, et al. Lubrication of synovial membrane. *Ann Rheum Dis* 1971;30(3):322–325.
106. Johns RJ, Wright V. Relative importance of various tissues in joint stiffness. *J Appl Physiol* 1962;17:284–287.
107. Coleman PJ, Scott D, Mason RM, et al. Role of hyaluronan chain length in buffering interstitial flow across synovium in rabbits. *J Physiol* 2000;526:425–434.
108. Sabaratnam S, Coleman PJ, Badrick E, et al. Interactive effect of chondroitin sulphate C and hyaluronan on fluid movement across rabbit synovium. *J Physiol* 2002;540:271–284.
109. Woo SLY, Livesay GA, Runco TJ, et al. Structure and function of tendons and ligaments. In: Mow VC, Hayes WC, eds. *Basic orthopaedic biomechanics.* Philadelphia: Lippincott-Raven, 1997.
110. Vogel KG, Ordog A, Pogany G, et al. Proteoglycans in the compressed region of human tibialis posterior tendon and in ligaments. *J Orthop Res* 1993;11:68–77.
111. Lundborg G, Myrhage R. The vascularization and structure of the human digital tendon sheath as related to flexor tendon function. An angiographic and histological study. *Scand J Plast Reconstr Surg* 1977;11(3):195–203.
112. Hagberg L, Heinegard D, Ohlsson K. The contents of macromolecule solutes in flexor tendon sheath fluid and their relation to synovial fluid. A quantitative analysis. *J Hand Surg Br* 1992;17(2):167–171.
113. Bullough PG, Munuera L, Murphy J, et al. The strength of the menisci of the knee as it relates to their fine structure. *J Bone Joint Surg Br* 1970;52(3):564–567.
114. Lane JM, Weiss C. Review of articular cartilage collagen research. *Arthritis Rheum* 1975;18(6):553–562.
115. Peters TJ, Smillie IS. Studies on the chemical composition of the menisci of the knee joint with special reference to the horizontal cleavage lesion. *Clin Orthop* 1972;86:245–252.
116. Ghosh P, Taylor TK. The knee joint meniscus. A fibrocartilage of some distinction. *Clin Orthop* 1987(224):52–63.
117. Aspden RM, Yarker YE, Hukins DW. Collagen orientations in the meniscus of the knee joint. *J Anat* 1985;140:371–380.
118. McDevitt CA, Webber RJ. The ultrastructure and biochemistry of meniscal cartilage. *Clin Orthop* 1990;252:8–18.
119. Simon SR, Paul IL, Mansour J, et al. Peak dynamic force in human gait. *J Biomech* 1981;14:817–822.
120. Vilensky JA, O'Connor BL, Fortin JD, et al. Histologic analysis of neural elements in the human sacroiliac joint. *Spine* 2002;27(11): 1202–1207.
121. Kellgren JH, Samuel EP. The sensitivity and innervation of the articular capsule. *J Bone Joint Surg Br* 1950;32:84–92.
122. Mapp PI. Innervation of the synovium. *Ann Rheum Dis* 1995;54(5): 398–403.
123. Elfvin LG, Holmberg K, Johansson J, et al. The innervation of the synovium of the knee joint in the guinea pig: an immunohistochemical and ultrastructural study. *Anat Embryol (Berl)* 1998;197(4):293–303.
124. Kennedy JC, Alexander IJ, Hayes KC. Nerve supply of the human knee and its functional importance. *Am J Sports Med* 1982;10(6): 329–335.
125. Gronblad M, Korkala O, Liesi P, et al. Innervation of synovial membrane and meniscus. *Acta Orthop Scand* 1985;56(6):484–486.
126. Cohen ML. Priciples of pain and pain management. In: Klippel JH, Dieppe PA, eds. *Rheumatology,* 2nd ed. London: CV Mosby, 2003: 3.4.1–3.4.6.
127. Davy DT, Kotzar GM, Brown RH, et al. Telemetric force measurements across the hip after total arthroplasty. *J Bone Joint Surg Am* 1988;70:45–50.
128. Inoue H, Takeda T. Three-dimensional observation of collagen framework of lumbar intervertebral discs. *Acta Orthop Scand* 1975;46(6): 949–956.
129. Herzog W, Clark A, Wu J. Resultant and local loading in models of joint disease. *Arthritis Rheum* 2003;49(2):239–247.
130. Radin EL, Yang KH, Riegger C, et al. Relationship between lower limb dynamics and knee joint pain. *J Orthop Res* 1991;9(3):398–405.
131. Bullough PG, Goodfellow J, O'Conner J. The relationship between degenerative changes and load-bearing in the human hip. *J Bone Joint Surg Br* 1973;55(4):746–758.
132. Tong W, Glimcher MJ, Katz JL, et al. Size and shape of mineralites in young bovine bone measured by atomic force microscopy. *Calcif Tissue Int* 2003;72(5):592–598.
133. An YH. Mechanical properties of bone. In: An YH, ed. *Mechanical testing of bone and the bone–implant interface.* Boca Raton, FL: CRC Press, 2000:41–63.
134. Hayes WC, Bouxsein ML. Biomechanics of cortical and trabecular bone: implications for assessment of fracture risk. In: Mow VC, ed. *Basic orthopaedic biomechanics.* Philadelphia, Lippincott-Raven, 1997.
135. Kaplan FS, Hayes WC, Keaveny TM, et al. Form and function of bone. In: Simon AR, ed. *Orthopaedic basic science.* Chicago: American Academy of Orthopaedic Surgeons, 1994.
136. Frost HM. A brief review for orthopedic surgeons: fatigue damage (microdamage) in bone (its determinants and clinical implications). *J Orthop Sci* 1998;3(5):272–281.
137. Frost HM. The Utah paradigm of skeletal physiology: an overview of its insights for bone, cartilage and collagenous tissue organs. *J Bone Miner Metab* 2000;18(6):305–316.
138. Pugh JW, Rose RM, Radin EL. A possible mechanism of Wolff's law: trabecular microfractures. *Arch Intern Physiol Biochim* 1973; 81(1):27–40.
139. Mital MA. Biomechanical characteristics of the human hip joint [dissertation]. Glasgow, Scotland, University of Strathclyde, 1970.
140. Hayes WC, Mockros LF. Viscoelastic properties of human articular cartilage. *J Appl Physiol* 1971;31(4):562–568.
141. Simon WH, Friedenberg S, Richardson S. Joint congruence. A correlation of joint congruence and thickness of articular cartilage in dogs. *J Bone Joint Surg Am* 1973;55(8):1614–1620.
142. Byers PD, Contepomi CA, Farkas TA. Post-mortem study of the hip joint. III. Correlations between observations. *Ann Rheum Dis* 1976; 35(2):122–126.
143. Meachim G. Cartilage fibrillation at the ankle joint in Liverpool necropsies. *J Anat* 1975;119(3):601–610.
144. Coventry MB. Anatomy of the intervertebral disk. *Clin Orthop* 1969;67:9–15.
145. Radin EL. Mechanically induced periarticular and neuromuscular problems. In: Wright V, Radin EL, eds. Mechanics of human joints. *Physiology, pathophysiology, and treatment.* New York: Marcel Decker, 1993:355–372.
146. Happey F. Studies of the structure of the human intervertebral disc in relation to its functional and aging processes. In: Sokoloff L, ed. *The joints and synovial fluid,* Vol. 2. New York: Academic, 1980:95–136.
147. Naylor A, Happey F, Turner RL, et al. Enzymic and immunological activity in the intervertebral disk. *Orthop Clin North Am* 1975;6(1): 51–58.
148. Naylor A. The biochemical changes in the human intervertebral disc in degeneration and nuclear prolapse. *Orthop Clin North Am* 1971; 2(2):343–358.
149. Skaggs DL, Weidenbaum M, Iatridis JC. Regional variation in tensile properties and biochemical composition of the human lumbar annulus fibrosus. *Spine* 1944;19:1310–1319.

150. Urban JP, McMullin JF. Swelling pressure of the intervertebral disc: influence of proteoglycan and collagen contents. *Biorheology* 1985; 22(2):145–157.
151. Parke WW, Schiff DC. The applied anatomy of the intervertebral disc. *Orthop Clin North Am* 1971;2(2):309–324.
152. Donohue JM, Buss D, Oegema TR Jr, et al. The effects of indirect blunt trauma on adult canine articular cartilage. *J Bone Joint Surg Am* 1983;65(7):948–957.
153. Sherk HH, Nicholson JT. Comparative anatomy and embryology of the cervical spine. *Orthop Clin North Am* 1971;2:325–341.
154. Willis TA. The phylogeny of the intervertebral disk: a pictorial review. *Clin Orthop* 1967;54:215–233.
155. Wolfe HJ, Putschar WGJ VA. Role of the notochord in human intervertebral disk. I. Fetus and infant. *Clin Orthop* 1965;39:205–212.
156. Gardner E. The development and growth of bones. *J Bone Joint Surg Am* 1963;45:856–862.
157. Gower WE, Pedrini V. Age-related variations in proteinpolysaccharides from human nucleus pulposus, annulus fibrosus, and costal cartilage. *J Bone Joint Surg Am* 1969;51(6):1154–1162.
158. Oegema TR Jr, Bradford DS, Cooper KM, et al. Comparison of the biochemistry of proteoglycans isolated from normal, idiopathic scoliotic and cerebral palsy spines. *Spine* 1983;8(4):378–384.
159. Pearson CH, Happey F, Shentall RD, et al. The non-collagenous proteins of the human intervertebral disc. *Gerontologia* 1969;15(2): 189–202.
160. Melrose J, Ghosh P, Taylor TK. Proteoglycan heterogeneity in the normal adult ovine intervertebral disc. *Matrix Biol* 1994;14(1): 61–75.
161. Roberts S, Caterson B, Evans H, et al. Proteoglycan components of the intervertebral disc and cartilage endplate: an immunolocalization study of animal and human tissues. *Histochem J* 1994;26(5):402–411.
162. Brickley-Parsons D, Glimcher MJ. Is the chemistry of collagen in intervertebral discs an expression of Wolff's Law? A study of the human lumbar spine. *Spine* 1984;9(2):148–163.
163. Souter WA, Taylor TK. Sulphated acid mucopolysaccharide metabolism in the rabbit intervertebral disc. *J Bone Joint Surg Br* 1970; 52(2):371–384.
164. Farfan HF. *Mechanical disorders of the low back.* Philadelphia, 1973.
165. Adams MA, Hutton WC. Prolapsed intervertebral disc. A hyperflexion injury 1981 Volvo Award in Basic Science. *Spine* 1982;7(3):184–191.
166. Nachemson A, Morris JM. *In vivo* measurements of intradiscal pressure. *J Bone Joint Surg Am* 1964;46:1077–1092.
167. Broberg KB. On the mechanical behaviour of intervertebral discs. *Spine* 1983;8(2):151–165.
168. Gordon SJ, Yang KH, Mayer PJ, et al. Mechanism of disc rupture. A preliminary report. *Spine* 1991;16(4):450–456.
169. Dunlop RB, Adams MA, Hutton WC. Disc space narrowing and the lumbar facet joints. *J Bone Joint Surg Br* 1984;66(5):706–710.
170. Gotfried Y, Bradford DS, Oegema TR Jr. Facet joint changes after chemonucleolysis-induced disc space narrowing. *Spine* 1986;11(9): 944–950.
171. White AA III, Gordon SL. Synopsis: workshop on idiopathic low-back pain. *Spine* 1982;7(2):141–149.
172. Radin EL, Burr DB. Hypothesis: joints can heal. *Semin Arthritis Rheum* 1984;13(3):293–302.
173. Convery FR, Akeson WH, Keown GH. The repair of large osteochondral defects. An experimental study in horses. *Clin Orthop* 1972;82:253–262.
174. Buckwalter JA. Articular cartilage: injuries and potential for healing. *J Orthop Sports Phys Ther* 1998;28(4):192–202.
175. Buckwalter JA. Articular cartilage injuries. *Clin Orthop* 2002;402: 21–37.
176. Arnoczky SP, Warren RF. The microvasculature of the meniscus and its response to injury. An experimental study in the dog. *Am J Sports Med* 1983;11(3):131–141.
177. Huang CY, Soltz MA, Kopacz M, et al. Experimental verification of the roles of intrinsic matrix viscoelasticity and tension-compression nonlinearity in the biphasic response of cartilage. *J Biomech Eng* 2003;125(1):84–93.
178. Aagaard H, Jorgensen U, Bojsen-Moller F. Immediate versus delayed meniscal allograft transplantation in sheep. *Clin Orthop* 2003(406): 218–227.
179. Heis FT, Paulos LE. Tensioning of the anterior cruciate ligament graft. *Orthop Clin North Am* 2002;33(4):697–700.
180. Blount WP. Don't throw away the cane. 1956. *J Bone Joint Surg Am* 2003;85:380.

CHAPTER 8

Synovial Physiology

Peter A. Simkin

Synovial joints are the bearings through which the human machine accomplishes its work. Surrounding tissues help to maintain, support, and renew these complex living bearings throughout the lifetime of the individual. Principal among these tissues is the synovium, which supports the normal joint in at least three important physiologic ways: (a) provides an unobtrusive, low-friction lining; (b) transports needed nutrients into the joint space while it removes metabolic wastes; and (c) plays an important role in maintaining joint stability. These physiologic functions in health and their alterations in disease are reviewed here. A fourth important role, the provision of biologic lubricants, is discussed in Chapter 7.

SYNOVIAL LINING

Because motion is the business of joints, the synovial lining must be able to adapt to the full range of positions permitted by the surrounding tendons, ligaments, and joint capsule. As a finger flexes, for instance, the palmar synovium of each interphalangeal joint contracts while the dorsal synovium expands. As the finger reextends, the roles are reversed (Fig. 8.1). This expansion and contraction of synovium appears consistent with elements of both an accordion-like process of folding and unfolding and an elastic stretching of the tissue.

Most expansion and contraction of the synovium takes place over unopposed surfaces of articular cartilage. For any joint to flex or extend, there must be a disparity in the opposing surface areas. When the joint moves, the smaller area glides across or around the larger. Cartilage not in contact with opposing cartilage is temporarily covered by synovium, as, for example, are the knuckles of a clenched fist. As the cartilage surfaces move on each other to resume their initial position, an effective lubrication system must prevent pinching of the adjacent, well-vascularized synovial tissue. Were this system to fail, repeated hemarthroses would prove rapidly incapacitating. This lubrication problem has not received the attention devoted to that of cartilage movement on cartilage. Swann and associates have suggested, however, that the hyaluronan molecules that render synovial fluid viscous may play an important physiologic role in lubricating the synovium (1).

The well-lubricated synovium must expand and contract within the confines of the joint capsule. The process is easier when the volume of synovial tissue is at a minimum and is impeded when the volume is excessive. The cellular infiltration, hyperplasia, and edema of active synovitis may thus limit joint motion when the synovium gathers as a mass lesion (2). The problem seems likely to be most acute in full flexion, because the capsule of hinge joints is normally thicker on the flexor surface, and compression of extracapsular soft tissue further compromises the available space. In addition to limiting the range of motion, increased synovial tissue volume may also contribute to the stiffness of many inflamed joints.

Studies of relaxed metacarpophalangeal joints undergoing passive manipulation have found that increased stiffness is readily demonstrable in the hands of patients with rheumatoid arthritis (RA), and this stiffness is greater in flexion than in extension (1). Stiffness in normal joints is a complex phenomenon influenced by the time of day, varying inversely with grip strength, increasing progressively with age, occurring to a greater degree in men than in women, and affected by muscles, tendons, and other periarticular structures, as well as by the capsule and synovium (1). In the more severe stiffness characteristic of the rheumatoid hand, the spondylitic back, or the polymyalgia shoulder, the typical morning pattern with daytime gelling suggests that tissue edema develops during periods of rest and the edematous tissue interferes with free use of the joint. This stiffness may then be relieved by activity because joint motion serves as an effective pump to drive

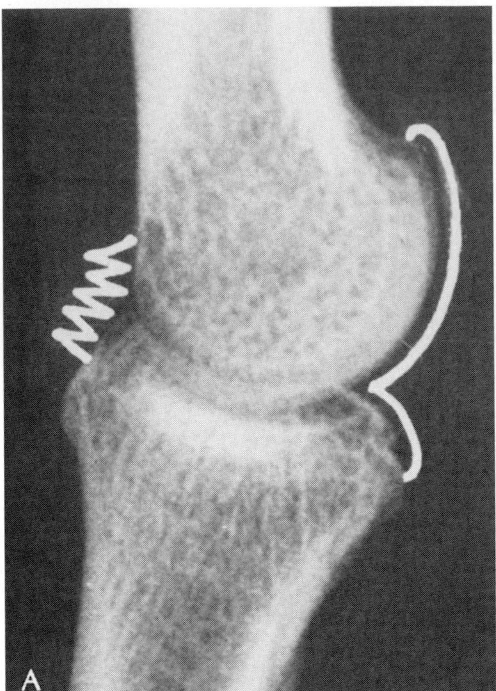

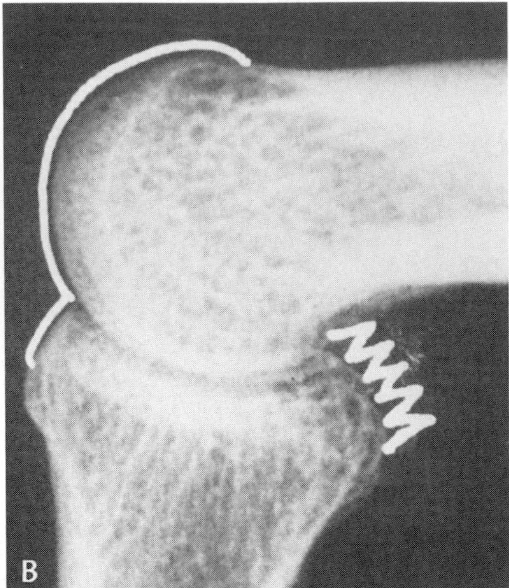

FIG. 8.1. Lateral views of an interphalangeal joint in extension **(A)** and in flexion **(B)**. The greater surface area of proximal articular cartilage permits the distal bone to move around the proximal. Redundant synovium (shown schematically) gathers above the superior margin in extension and below the inferior margin during flexion.

fluid into collecting venules and terminal lymphatics and, thus, to lessen the synovial edema.

SYNOVIAL PERMEABILITY

In their classic studies of synovial effusions, Ropes and Bauer noted that transfer across the synovium "necessitates passage through an endothelial wall as well as diffusion through the intercellular spaces" (1) (Fig. 8.2). Normally, water electrolytes and other small solutes cross the endothelium readily and enter the joint space at rates determined primarily by interstitial diffusion. In contrast, most proteins are retained by the endothelium, and it is this function that fails in the "increased vascular permeability," regarded as a hallmark of inflammation. Then, excessive amounts of protein leak into the interstitium. If this excess is not cleared by a comparable increase in the rate of lymphatic drainage, the extravascular concentration of protein will rise toward the plasma level. The necessary result is a progressive diminution in the colloid osmotic pressure gradient between the two spaces. Because this pressure gradient helps drive venular reabsorption of water, increased vascular permeability to proteins leads to edema in tissues and to effusions in joints. These principles reflect the Starling-Landis concept of microvascular function and underscore the importance of the endothelium in retaining plasma proteins (1).

It would be wrong, however, to infer that increased microvascular permeability to proteins necessarily means a significant increase in synovial permeability to smaller molecules as well. Small solutes normally cross the endothelium not only through the large pores available to proteins, but also through a more abundant and highly permeable small-pore system of microvascular fenestrae that exclude larger molecules. A loss of fenestrae and a lengthened interstitial

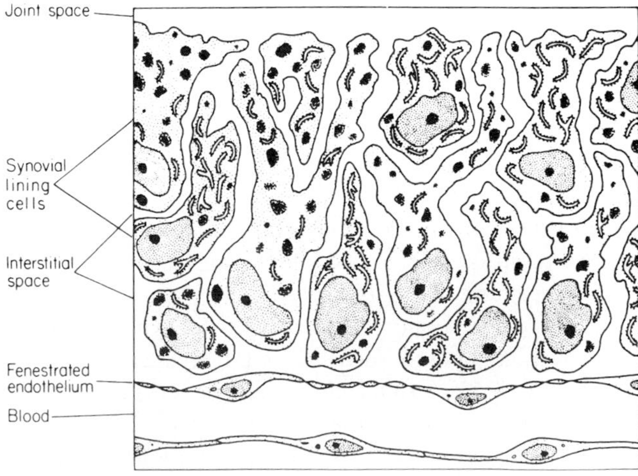

FIG. 8.2. The synovium. Molecules entering or leaving the joint space must traverse both the microvascular endothelium and the interstitial space between synovial cells. The endothelium provides the principal barrier limiting synovial permeability to proteins. The permeability of smaller molecules appears to be limited chiefly by their diffusibility across the synovial interstitium.

diffusion path may restrict small solutes at the same time that more large pores promote protein leakage. Thus, this functional duality permits independent changes in synovial permeability to large and small solutes (3).

Small Molecules

Small physiologic molecules (those under ~10,000 daltons in molecular weight) exist in nearly full equilibration between plasma and synovial fluid. This size range includes oxygen, glucose, carbon dioxide, lactate, and other tissue metabolites. Because articular cartilage has no blood supply of its own, the delivery of nutrients to cartilage and the removal of its wastes are thought to occur primarily through synovial fluid and its nurturing synovial blood supply. The vessels of adjacent, subchondral bone are important in immature individuals but are thought to be less accessible to the chondrocytes of adults. Clearly, then, the mechanisms of synovial transport are vital to the well-being of the most critical tissue in the articular bearing. To study the means by which transynovial exchange functions, one must disturb the normal equilibrium and then measure and interpret the kinetics of the reequilibration process. This may be done in a number of ways (4).

A series of experiments in normal human knees provided the best, early evidence of the normal process of transynovial exchange and supported the critical importance of interstitial diffusion (1). In this model, the knee was injected with a saline solution containing trace amounts of tritiated water, benzyl alcohol, and carbon 14–labeled urea, urate, glucose, or sucrose. Serial samples were then aspirated and assayed for these exogenous tracer compounds, as well as for endogenous urea, urate, glucose, creatinine, and total protein moving from plasma into the saline solution. Over the course of the experiment, the concentration of endogenous molecules progressively rose toward full equilibration with plasma levels, whereas the concentration of exogenous molecules fell toward zero as they were cleared from the joint space. A kinetic analysis of these data then permitted calculation of permeability values analogous to renal clearances, that is, the volume of intrasynovial saline solution equilibrating with plasma per unit time (milliliters per minute).

For most compounds, synovial permeability is inversely related to the dimensions of the molecule. Thus, a plot of observed synovial permeability versus diffusion coefficient (which reflects configuration as well as size) yields a rather linear function (Fig. 8.3). This finding implies that small molecules cross the synovium by free diffusion along relatively long and narrow diffusion paths consistent with the narrow channels between synovial lining cells. (Fig. 8.2). Evolving evidence now shows that not only the dimensions of this pathway but also the matrix components within it are critically important determinants in the transport through this space both of tissue water, and of the solvents dissolved in that water (5,6).

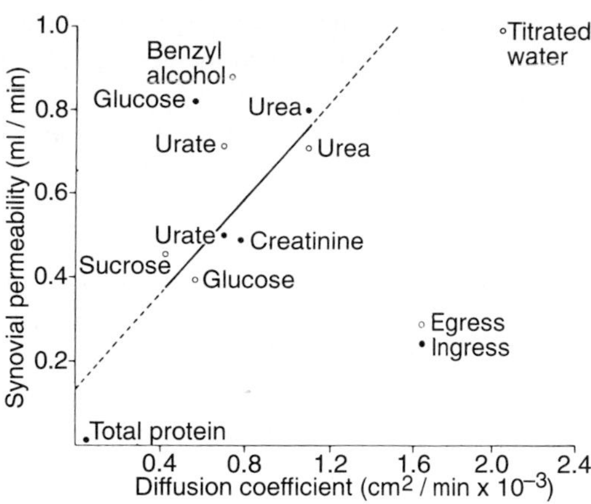

FIG. 8.3. Synovial permeability in normal, resting knees. The permeability is plotted against the diffusion coefficient. Egress and ingress are with respect to the joint space. Most data points are the mean values from 25 studies, but egress values for sucrose, glucose, urate, and urea are based on seven, six, six, and six studies, respectively. Benzyl alcohol leaving and glucose entering the joint space move rapidly because of diffusion into cells and specific transport, respectively. Protein enters slowly because of endothelial pore size limitation. Tritiated water leaves more slowly than predicted by its diffusion coefficient, probably because its egress is limited by effective synovial blood flow. All other small molecules (sucrose, urea, urate, creatinine, and glucose leaving the joint) cross the synovium at rates inversely proportional to their size as predicted by diffusion kinetics.

Additional evidence supporting this concept was found in the high correlation between permeability and intrasynovial volume. Distention of the normal joint space accelerates the transynovial exchange of small molecules as it broadens and shortens the intercellular path and thus facilitates the diffusion process. This finding provides an interesting teleologic explanation for synovial effusions in that the presence of a distending effusion will enhance both the delivery of nutrients and the removal of wastes.

Although the bidirectional permeability of urate ions was symmetric, the egress of other anions from the joint space may be facilitated by a specific transport system. Dick et al. found that potassium perchlorate inhibited clearance of technetium 99m and iodine 131 from dog stifle joints and ^{99m}Tc from human knees (1). These observations are of interest because active export of halide ions would be followed passively by sodium ions and by water. This system may thus be a "pump" capable of moving water out of the joint space.

Several other investigators have also studied the removal of ionic sodium and iodine from human knees (1,4). Sodium 24 and ^{131}I emit gamma rays that pass readily through soft tissues and are easily monitored by external counting. Such tracings characteristically fit a simple exponential function that may be expressed usefully as either a half-life value or a clearance constant. In different series of normal knees, mean clearance constants for ^{24}Na have ranged from 0.022 to 0.051 min^{-1}, whereas similar determinations for ^{131}I have been from 0.022 to 0.055 min^{-1}.

Scholer et al. injected knees with heavy water (D_2O) and either sodium 22 or ^{24}Na, followed the appearance of these isotopes in serial samples of arterial blood, and from these data, calculated clearance constants in the same range as those obtained by external counting over the joint (1). Additionally, the removal of ^{24}Na from the knee was eliminated when Harris and Millard inflated a tourniquet around the thigh to 200 mm Hg (1). These findings demonstrate that isotopic clearance depends on an effective circulation and diffusion into adjacent tissues plays no meaningful role.

The same isotopic technique has been applied to the study of patients with joint diseases. In degenerative joint disease and in RA, ^{24}Na and ^{131}I were cleared at rates that were up to threefold higher than normal. The intrasynovial volume was not determined in these experiments, but clinical impressions suggested a positive correlation between effusion size and isotopic removal rates. Intraarticular steroids led to a lower clearance in repeated studies of a few individuals. In short, these investigators' findings implied that accelerated isotopic clearance reflects enhanced synovial blood flow in active synovitis.

Clinical physiologists have long been interested in accurate determinations of the synovial blood flow (4). The vascular supply, however, is provided by many small vessels and is, in part, shared by the joint capsule, epiphyseal bone, and other perisynovial structures. Thus, it is not possible to isolate and measure that portion of the blood supply specifically destined for synovium, but the synovial blood flow may be indirectly approached by examining the clearance of small marker molecules from the joint space. In the event of full equilibration between synovial fluid and perfusing plasma, the clearance of such a marker would be equal to the synovial blood flow. Using tritiated water as the marker, we estimated a mean synovial blood flow of 1 mL/min in normal knees (1). This value may be higher than the true, resting normal, however, because these knees were distended by 30 mL of normal saline, which contained a mild irritant (0.9% benzyl alcohol). When the same test system was used in inflamed arthritic knees, patients with RA and those with other forms of joint disease had a wide range of values.

The effective blood flow was reexamined using a different experimental method in 11 patients with RA and nine with osteoarthritis (OA) (7,8). In this work, trace amounts of both free ^{123}I- and ^{131}I-labeled human serum albumin were injected into existing knee effusions and both were followed by sequential external counting. The apparent distribution volume was assessed by isotope dilution of the labeled albumin in a synovial fluid specimen aspirated after 24 hours. From the product of the rate constant for removal of free iodide (min^{-1}) and the volume (mL), one can determine a clearance value in mL/min (Table 8.1).

The clearance of free iodide (like that of tritiated water in the previous work), may be taken as an indicator of effective synovial blood flow. The values are generally comparable to those found with tritiated water. Of special interest, however, is the fact that the mean effective blood flow was lower in RA than in OA, and six of the lowest seven values were found in rheumatoid patients. Within the rheumatoid group, the clearance of free iodine correlated significantly with synovial fluid pH ($r = 0.74$), lactate ($r = -0.77$), synovial fluid/serum ratio of glucose ($r = 0.81$), and temperature ($r = 0.88$). The high correlations between blood flow and these metabolic indices of ischemia imply that synovial hypoperfusion may be a common manifestation of RA.

Of necessity, clearance studies of articular blood flow are usually performed in resting joints. As such, they provide a useful baseline, but vascular variables may change dramatically when the joint moves. Because motion is the business of joints, D.J. McCarty, Jr. (9) has tellingly compared synovial studies at rest to cardiologic studies of a stopped heart. Blood flow changes with exercise are most reliably studied with infusions of radiolabeled microspheres, but this method cannot be used in people. In normal dogs, however, the average synovial blood flow to the wrist increased sevenfold, whereas that to the knee increased threefold with modest treadmill exercise (10). This impressive capacity for exercise-induced flow also pertains to the human knee, where evaluations of iodide clearance constants before and after exercise clearly indicate increased synovial flow (11). These observations implicate a substantial vascular reserve capacity in normal articulations, but it is not known whether an inflamed synovium can respond in the same fashion.

Glucose

Because glucose is one of the most important nutrients required by chondrocytes, is easily measured in synovial fluid, and is often low in the synovial fluid of patients with severe synovitis, its transport is of special interest. Ropes, Muller, and Bauer were the first to study this issue in human joints (1). They found that the concentration of glucose in synovial fluid usually was close to that of plasma. Between 3 and 4 hours after meals, however, levels were regularly higher within the joint space than they were in the

TABLE 8.1. *Iodide clearance from rheumatoid and osteoarthritic knees*

	n	Vol (mL)	Rate constant min^{-1}	Clearance (mL/min)
Rheumatoid arthritis	11	106 ± 23	0.018 ± 0.007	1.92 ± 0.98
Osteoarthritis	9	109 ± 105	0.028 ± 0.017	2.40 ± 1.44

perfusing blood. After a series of infusion experiments in people and in cattle, they suggested that a unidirectional transport system might facilitate the transfer of glucose from plasma to synovial fluid.

We used a different experimental approach (described previously) to confirm the presence of asymmetric glucose transport (1). These studies followed serial concentration changes within a saline injectate to compare the egress of ^{14}C-labeled compounds with the ingress of physiologic "cold" molecules in normal human knees. Most small molecules move symmetrically between plasma and synovial fluid in accord with simple diffusion kinetics. In these studies, however, glucose entered the joint space more rapidly than would be expected from its size alone, thus implicating a unidirectional transport system. These studies do not establish whether the specific glucose transport occurs by active (energy requiring) transport or by facilitated diffusion, although the second mechanism appears more likely.

In arthritic joints, the glucose level in synovial fluid may be lower than that in plasma. Although most characteristic of sepsis, this finding is often present in rheumatoid disease (where levels may be undetectably low) and has occasionally been observed in gout, trauma, and other joint afflictions (1). A low level thus offers little or no diagnostic specificity. However, low glucose values may offer valuable insight into the effectiveness of the synovial microcirculation. Specifically, any low value must indicate that the intrasynovial demand for glucose exceeds the supply and suggests that this imbalance may apply for other nutrients as well. For instance, Falchuk, Goetzel, and Kulka found a low glucose concentration in 3 of 15 rheumatoid synovial fluids, and all three had remarkably low partial pressure of oxygen (PO_2), high partial pressure of carbon dioxide (PCO_2), high lactate, and low pH (1). Both increased consumption and impaired delivery appear to be involved in this disruption of the normal equilibration between synovial fluid and plasma, but the specific mechanisms require further study.

Fat-Soluble Solutes

Because fat-soluble solutes can diffuse through, as well as between, cell membranes, their transport is not limited to the path between the lining cells. Instead, the entire surface of the synovium is available for diffusion in or out of the joint space. In our studies of normal knees, this phenomenon was studied with benzyl alcohol, a fat-soluble molecule that left the joint space faster than hydrophilic molecules of equivalent size (1).

Physiologically, the most important fat-soluble molecules are the respiratory gases: oxygen and carbon dioxide. Studies of the synovial fluid content of these crucial metabolites have found that many patients with RA (as well as a smaller number of patients with other joint diseases) have low PO_2 values, and this finding correlates with increased PCO_2, decreased pH, and increased lactate (Fig. 8.4). Despite the high diffusibility of oxygen, its supply is unable to meet synovial demand in such joints. The resultant hypoxia leads synovial cells and chondrocytes to use the metabolically expensive glycolytic pathway, with a consequent increase in consumption of glucose and production of lactic acid. Lactic acid, together with the carbonic acid produced by oxidative metabolism, leads to an intraarticular acidosis with synovial fluid pH values as low as 6.8 (1,12). All these changes reflect a severe circulatory-metabolic imbalance within the inflamed synovium, with the microvasculature unable either to supply sufficient metabolic fuels or to clear the products of their combustion adequately.

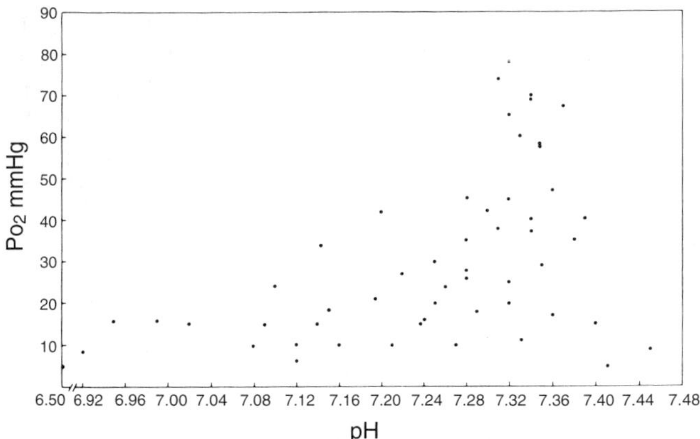

FIG. 8.4. Correlation of oxygen tension (PO_2) with pH in synovial effusion of patients with various joint diseases. The pH varies little with modest local hypoxia, but usually becomes acidotic when the PO_2 falls below 30 mm Hg. (Courtesy of Dr. D.J. McCarty.)

Synovial Ischemia

Synovial ischemia has been studied best in RA, but similar conditions regularly prevail in septic arthritis and are occasionally seen in other forms of joint disease. The significant correlations ($p < 0.005$) we found between effective synovial blood flow and synovial fluid pH, lactate, glucose, and temperature all indicate that insufficient blood supply is largely at fault. The direct relationship between rheumatoid blood flow and temperature is particularly interesting. This finding implies that chronically swollen rheumatoid joints could be more worrisome when they are "cold" than when they are "warm." The significant effusions, cellular response, protein levels, and parallel metabolic indices in these joints all demonstrated that they were not "burned out," but had highly active synovitis.

The clinical implications of synovial ischemia have never been examined in the smaller joints, where RA is most devastating (13). In the knee, however, radiographic evidence of joint damage correlated highly with metabolic

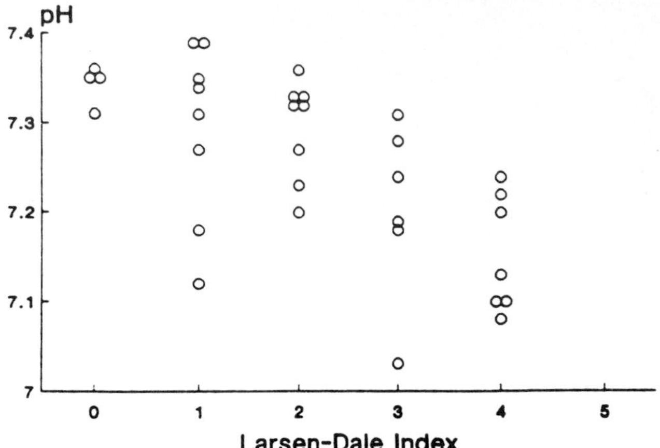

FIG. 8.5. Synovial fluid pH correlates inversely with radiographic evidence of joint destruction in rheumatoid knees ($r = 0.62$, $p < 0.002$). In the Larsen-Dale index, normal cartilage thickness is scored 0 and total loss of cartilage is scored 5. (From Geborek P, Saxne T, Pettersson H, et al. Synovial fluid acidosis correlates with radiological joint destruction in rheumatoid arthritis knee joints. *J Rheumatol* 1989;16:468–472, with permission.)

evidence of ischemia (12) (Fig. 8.5). Analysis of "rice bodies" aspirated from rheumatoid joints showed them to contain collagen types I and III in equal amounts, a proportion identical to that in synovial tissue (1). This observation implies that synovial tissue is periodically sloughed into many rheumatoid joints; the most likely mechanism underlying that process is microinfarction.

Involvement of small blood vessels is recognized as one of the earliest histologic changes in rheumatoid synovitis. As the disease progresses, the vessels can become occluded and drop out with a resultant net loss of vascular support. Morphometric analysis shows that small vessels in the average rheumatoid synovium are deeper and are approximately one third as prevalent as are the vessels of normal synovial tissue (14). Thus, the physiologic evidence of ischemia is consistent with the morphologic evidence of microvascular impairment.

The hypoperfusion of rheumatoid synovium can be exacerbated by vascular compression or tamponade when arthritis is complicated by high-pressure effusions. Resting pressures of up to 80 mm Hg have been recorded in knees, and such synovial hypertension might be more frequent in the firm, rubbery effusions sometimes found in smaller joints (15). The most dramatic pressure changes occur, however, when active muscle contraction or full flexion takes place in an effused joint. Jayson and Dixon recorded a mean pressure of 802 mm Hg with simple passive flexion after 100 mL of saline was instilled into rheumatoid knees (1). More recent studies have used laser Doppler methods to show a significant decrease in synovial blood flow when the articular pressure increases either with prolonged muscle contraction or with sustained flexion (16,17). Complementary evaluations have shown that the same maneuvers exacerbate biochemical evidence of ischemia in rheumatoid synovial fluid (18). Such findings have raised the possibility that normal cyclic joint use could lead to cycles of decreased and increased blood flow that result in reperfusion injury induced by oxygen radicals (17). Conflicting evidence suggests, however, that effective blood supply to rheumatoid knees improves as joints are used and the day goes on (1). It seems premature, therefore, to invoke physiologic arguments against the time-honored premise that rheumatoid joints "should be used but not abused."

Drugs

Physicians treating any form of synovitis are engaged in a battle against inflammation. The principal weapons in this war are drugs intended to eliminate the cause or to ameliorate the effects of the inflammatory process, but how well do these agents reach their target? This question has been posed primarily by examining drug levels in synovial fluid and contrasting them with concurrent concentrations in plasma (19). Although no drug has its site of action in the synovial fluid itself, such studies reasonably presume that drug concentrations in this interstitial fluid provide the best indication of the levels acting on any population of synovial cells.

For any orally-administered drug, plasma levels reflect the sequential, but overlapping, processes of absorption, distribution, and elimination. Peak levels are usually reached within 1 or 2 hours, and the plasma concentration subsequently decreases. The rates of decline of drug concentration can usually be dissected into a rapid, initial phase and a slower, terminal phase. During the rapid phase, metabolism, excretion, or both, begin to eliminate the drug from the bloodstream as it also diffuses into the various tissue compartments. The processes of elimination continue during the terminal phase, but the apparent clearance slows because full equilibration has now occurred with tissue interstitial fluids, and the drug is now beginning to return from those tissue spaces back into the plasma.

The levels in joints are analogous to those in other tissue compartments. Published values characteristically lag behind the rising levels in plasma, reach a later and lower peak, and then begin their own descent. At some point, the downward slopes of both curves usually cross, and subsequently synovial fluid levels are higher than those of plasma (Fig. 8.6). The time required to reach this crossing or equilibration point reflects the half-life of the drug. Short-lived agents, such as aspirin, have the earliest equilibration time, whereas long-lived drugs such as phenylbutazone have the longest, with intermediate agents falling in between (Fig. 8.7).

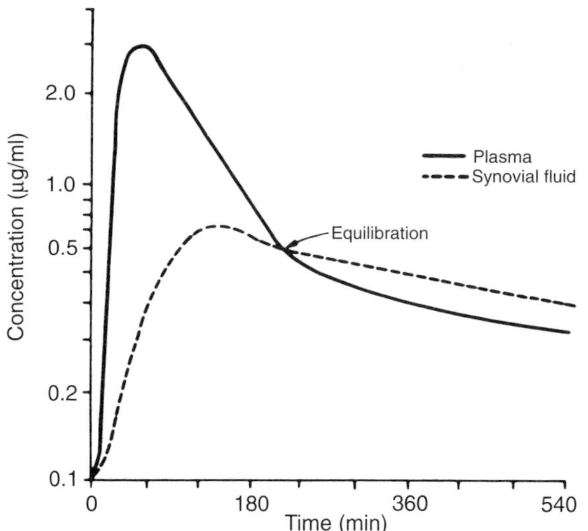

FIG. 8.6. Mean concentrations in serial samples of plasma and synovial fluid after a single oral dose of a therapeutic agent. Plasma levels increase rapidly with gastrointestinal absorption, decrease as the drug is distributed throughout body compartments, and then decline steadily as a result of continuing metabolism and excretion. Synovial fluid levels initially lag behind those in plasma, but then cross over the plasma concentration (at the equilibration point) and eventually decline at a rate comparable with that in plasma. After equilibration, the drug diffuses down the concentration gradient from synovial fluid back into plasma. (Indomethacin data from Emori HW, Champion GD, Bluestone R, Paulus HE. Simultaneous pharmacokinetics of indomethacin in serum and synovial fluid. *Ann Rheum Dis* 1973;32:433–435.)

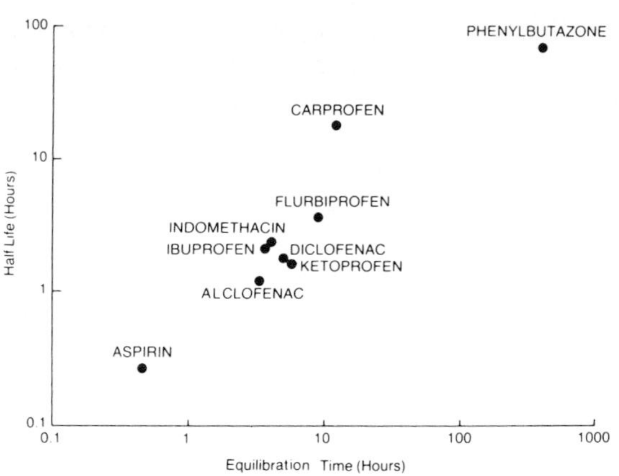

FIG. 8.7. Biologic half-life versus equilibration time for nonsteroidal antiinflammatory drugs. The linear relationship indicates that equilibration occurs early in the case of those agents that are rapidly cleared from plasma and late in those with a long biologic half-life. With usual dosage schedules, short-lived agents are often found with synovial fluid concentrations exceeding the concurrent levels in plasma. (From Wallis WJ, Simkin PA. Antirheumatic drug levels in human synovial fluid and synovial tissue: observations on extravascular pharmacokinetics. *Clin Pharmacokinet* 1983;8:496–522, with permission.)

These experiments are always conducted in pathologic knee effusions, usually in patients with RA. The large distribution volume and modest plasma flow in such joints (for instance 100 mL and 2 mL/min) explain why synovial fluid levels lag well behind during both increasing and decreasing phases of plasma kinetics. In the typical instance cited, full equilibration would require 50 minutes if extraction of the drug were somehow sustained at 100% and plasma levels remained constant. Actual extraction *in vivo* must be considerably lower and serves to prolong the process even more. When articular pharmacokinetics are studied in normal animals with relatively low synovial fluid volumes and albumin concentrations, the synovial fluid curve closely follows the pattern of plasma and never crosses over (20). This is the most likely scenario in people as well when pharmacologic agents are used to treat the majority of clinical conditions that are not associated with large, pathologic effusions.

A second concern in interpreting concentration curves is the high degree of protein binding seen with virtually all nonsteroidal antiinflammatory drugs (NSAIDs). It is the free, rather than the bound, agent that diffuses across the synovial barrier, but it is the total drug level that is measured. Because plasma protein levels are higher, free levels will be in balance when the total level in plasma remains higher than that in synovial fluid. This is why the intrasynovial level begins to decrease well before the crossing point of apparent equilibration. In considering the nature of the binding to plasma proteins, it is important to distinguish between affinity and avidity. Affinity is routinely measured by equilibrium dialysis, is often greater than 99%, and is important in drug distribution as discussed earlier. Avidity, in contrast, is never measured, but is critically important in articular kinetics. Because a large proportion of each NSAID is able to enter the joint in each passage through synovial vessels, the avidity of the binding must be relatively low.

To further examine the mechanism of synovial drug transport, 10 single-dose studies of eight different NSAIDs were analyzed with a simple compartmental model (21). Because all the data were from rheumatoid knees, the synovial plasma flow and articular distribution volume were assumed to have been the same as those measured in rheumatoid knees in Seattle. Basically, the drug mass (concentration times volume) perfusing the knee was taken as a continuous "forcing function" to calculate the rates of drug ingress and egress that would best fit the changing mass in synovial fluid. All 10 data sets fit this model well. The average extraction value of 23% indicates that much protein-bound drug dissociates from albumin and leaves the vasculature during each transit of synovial tissues. Relatively little drug was found to enter with albumin in the bound form, and the clearance of each drug was symmetric in both directions. These findings strongly support the concept that these drugs enter and leave the joint by passive, bidirectional diffusion and that protein binding of NSAIDs has less effect on kinetics than might be expected from the reported high association constants.

Antibiotics constitute a second major class of drugs that has been studied with concurrent plasma and synovial fluid concentration curves. As with the NSAID data, intrasynovial antibiotic concentrations lag somewhat behind plasma concentrations, with a later peak during drug distribution and higher levels during the elimination stage. Effective antibiotic levels are regularly achieved within serial synovial aspirates. It remains possible, and perhaps likely, however, that antibiotic access may be limited in tense, undrained effusions where vascular tamponade may complicate drug delivery. Such conditions, analogous to any other abscess, would be most likely to occur in smaller or less accessible joints in which high-pressure effusions may be most easily overlooked. Therefore, it remains unwise to assume that adequate antibiotic levels are present in any septic joint unless it is regularly aspirated or surgically drained.

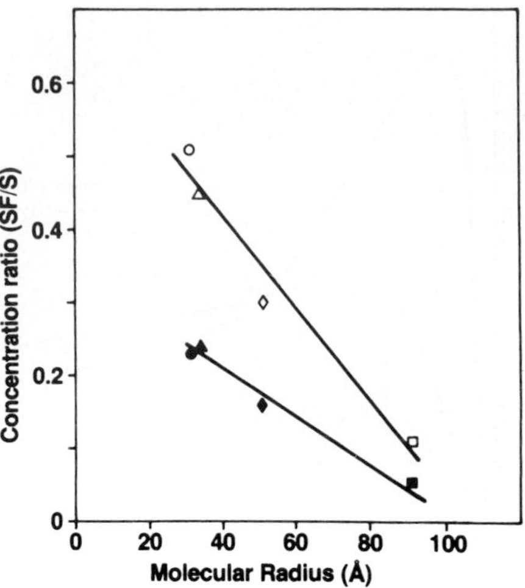

FIG. 8.8. Synovial fluid to serum ratios (*SF/S*) of selected plasma proteins versus molecular radius in clinically normal human hips (*open symbols*) and knees (*closed symbols*). The concentration ratio is inversely related to size in both joints, and hip values are consistently greater than those in the knee. Proteins studied were orosomucoid (*circles*), transferrin (*triangles*), ceruloplasmin (*diamonds*), and α_2-macroglobulin (*squares*). (From Weinberger A, Simkin PA. Plasma proteins in synovial fluids of normal human joints. *Semin Arthritis Rheum* 1989;19:66–76, with permission.)

Protein

All plasma proteins can cross the endothelium, traverse the synovial interstitium, and enter synovial fluid. This transport process, however, is highly size selective: the smaller proteins, like albumin, enter with relative ease, whereas larger molecules such as fibrinogen, macroglobulins, and certain complement components are more restricted. In contrast to this entry mechanism, the clearance or removal of all proteins is by convective lymphatic drainage. This process is unrestricted throughout the size range of almost all plasma proteins. In contrast, larger molecules such as hyaluronan and cartilaginous proteoglycans are now known to be partially restricted in their access to terminal lymphatics (22).

The synovial fluid reflects the balance of ingress and egress, with concentrations of small proteins that are much higher, relative to plasma, than are those of large proteins (23). Mean synovial fluid/serum (SF/S) ratios from normal hip and knee joints are shown in Fig. 8.8. Both joints show the relative exclusion of the largest marker protein, α_2-macroglobulin, and the more ready access of the smallest studied protein, orosomucoid. Transferrin and ceruloplasmin occupy intermediate positions. The normal protein content of hip (and shoulder) synovial fluid is significantly greater than that in knees or in other large peripheral joints, but the qualitative balance of inward and outward transport is obviously similar.

When the knee becomes inflamed, the total protein concentration increases from the normal level of 1.3 g/dL to values that can approach those of plasma. The major change in inflammation is an increase in the normally tiny convective plasma leak. Greater endothelial permeability permits more ready ingress to all proteins, but the most obvious changes are in the larger species. The fluid now clots and complement activity increases (unless intraarticular consumption is present). Mean SF/S values for selected marker proteins in 11 Seattle patients with RA and in 9 with OA are shown in Fig. 8.9. In this series, as in four other closely comparable data sets, the rheumatoid values were not significantly higher than were those in OA. As we will see later, however, these comparable concentrations do not reflect comparable transport kinetics. The size dependence of the ratios remains obvious in all series, thus reflecting the continuing selectivity of much inward transport through small pores in addition to the nonselective, large pore "plasma leak."

Increased endothelial permeability to proteins is not necessarily accompanied by an increased synovial permeability to small solutes. This important differential effect of inflammation is entirely consistent with the double-barrier model of synovial permeability. As previously described, the overall rate of small solute exchange between plasma and synovial fluid is determined by the synovial blood flow and by diffusion through the interstitium. Our short-term equilibration studies showed this duality of pathways clearly. The exchange, for instance, of tritiated water between synovial fluid and plasma was not enhanced by synovitis, whereas the entry of proteins was essentially three times the normal level, both in patients with RA and in those with other miscellaneous forms of

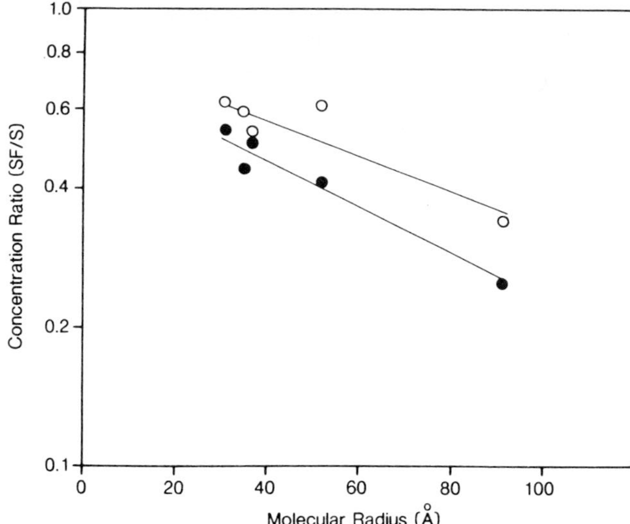

FIG. 8.9. Mean synovial fluid to serum ratios (*SF/S*) as a function of molecular radius for five plasma proteins (transferrin, orosomucoid, albumin, ceruloplasmin, and α_2-macroglobulin) in patients with rheumatoid arthritis (*RA*) (*open circles*) and osteoarthritis (*OA*) (*closed circles*). The concentration ratios differ by a degree that is not statistically significant. (From Wallis WJ, Simkin PA, Nelp WB. Protein traffic in human synovial effusions. *Arthritis Rheum* 1987;30:57–63, with permission.)

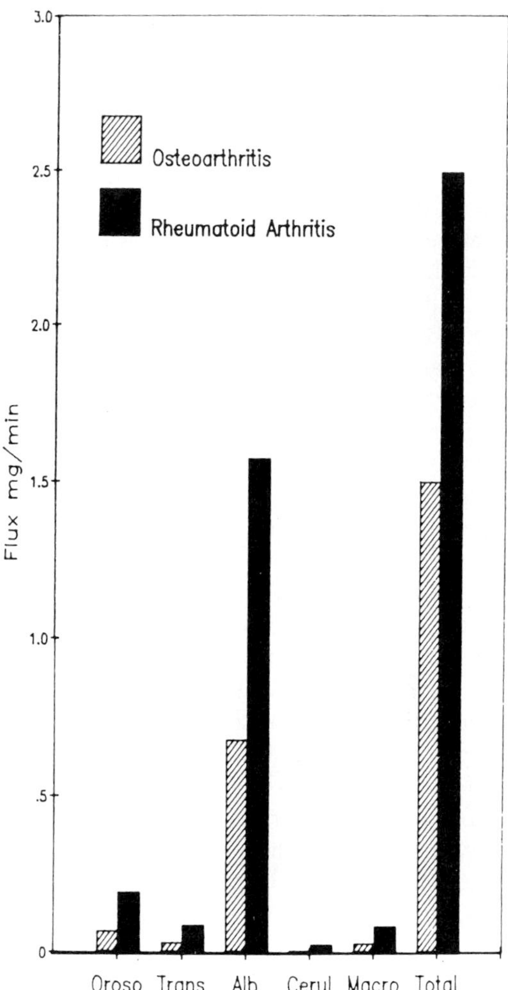

FIG. 8.10. Flux rates, in mg/min, for orosomucoid (*Oroso*), transferrin (*Trans*), albumin (*Alb*), ceruloplasmin (*Cerul*), α_2-macroglobulin (*Macro*), and total protein in knee effusions of patients with osteoarthritis and rheumatoid arthritis. Albumin is the predominant protein traversing the joint space in both diseases.

arthritis (Table 8.2). Thus, the increased vascular permeability of synovial inflammation can lead to striking increases in protein concentration without enhancing the normal microvascular functions of nutrient delivery and metabolic waste removal. In fact, the most ischemic rheumatoid joints had the highest rates of protein entry.

In any stable effusion, the articular flux (in milligrams per minute) of each protein may be determined from the product of its concentration in synovial fluid (milligrams per milliliter) and the effective rate of lymphatic drainage (milliliters per minute). Using the clearance of ^{131}I-labeled human serum albumin to measure lymphatic drainage, flux rates were calculated for total protein and for individual marker proteins in patients with knee effusions (24) (Fig. 8.10). As might be expected, albumin accounts for most of the flux of total protein, whereas minor constituents, such as ceruloplasmin, contribute very little. For every protein, however, the rheumatoid flux is much greater than that in OA, despite comparable SF concentrations. This difference is easily explained. The mean clearance (±SD) from rheumatoid knees (0.071 ± 0.028 mL/min) was significantly greater than that from OA knees (0.039 ± 0.030 mL/min). This essentially twofold difference in lymphatic drainage must enter into any interdisease comparison of synovial fluid proteins (25). Because concentration reflects

TABLE 8.2. *Mean synovial permeability to tritiated water (THO) and total protein*

	n	THO (mL/min)	Protein (mL/min)
Normal	17	1.11 ± 0.05	0.008 ± 0.001
Rheumatoid	13	0.90 ± 0.07	0.021 ± 0.002
Miscellaneous	18	1.11 ± 0.05	0.024 ± 0.003

the balance of ingress/egress, twice as much of any protein must enter the average rheumatoid knee to sustain the same concentration found in the OA knee.

Myers and coworkers (26) used this methodology to study normal dogs with varying degrees of synovitis induced by intraarticular injections of calcium pyrophosphate dihydrate crystals. They found highly significant increases in lymphatic efflux with even low-grade synovitis. Their report emphasizes the profound effect that this accelerated clearance will have on the synovial fluid concentration of the matrix molecules that are now widely studied as indicators of cartilaginous injury in arthritis. For such molecules to serve as true markers of tissue breakdown, it is imperative that their kinetics (25), as well as their concentrations, be examined.

Flux rate is the most valuable means of evaluating plasma protein traffic in synovial effusions. It varies with plasma protein concentration and synovial blood flow, however, and thus, is not a direct measurement of microvascular permeability. To examine permeability directly, we evaluated the fractional extraction of individual proteins from plasma into synovial fluid during a single passage through the articular microvasculature. To do this, we divided the articular flux rate by the vascular delivery of that protein to synovial vessels (calculated in milligrams per minute from the product of the plasma concentration and the effective blood flow). This ratio reflects the fraction of a given protein that leaves the plasma, crosses the synovium, and enters synovial fluid during each passage through the synovial microvasculature. We have termed this value the synovial permeance and, in Fig. 8.11, have recalculated and replotted the SF/S data as permeance values. The disease-dependent differences in permeability are highly significant, but are not apparent from examination of SF/S ratios alone.

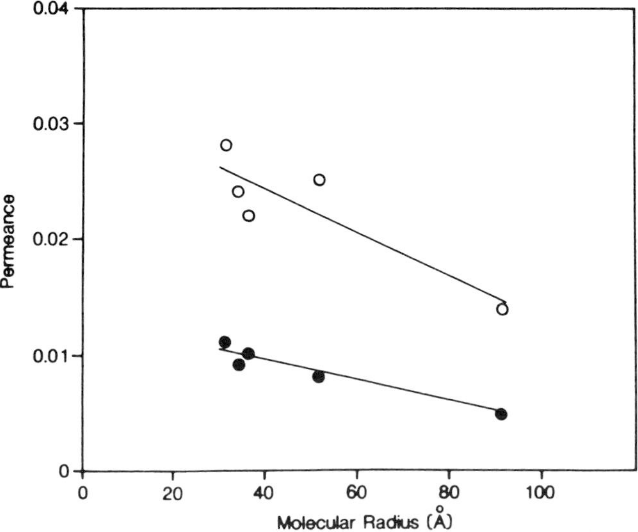

FIG. 8.11. Protein permeance in knee effusions of patients with arthritis. The microvascular escape of each of the five reference proteins is more than twice as great in rheumatoid arthritis (○) as it is in osteoarthritis (●). (From Wallis WJ, Simkin PA, Nelp WB. Protein traffic in human synovial effusions. *Arthritis Rheum* 1987;30:57–63, with permission.)

INTRASYNOVIAL PRESSURE

The humeral head sits snugly in the glenoid fossa, regardless of whether the arm is supported. The hip does not sublux during the swing-through phase of gait. Both at work and at rest, the opposing surfaces of articular cartilage remain in close approximation. This consistent apposition of articulating surfaces reflects a critical stabilizing capacity in normal joint function. Present data indicate that atmospheric pressure and the intercartilaginous film of synovial fluid are important factors in sustaining this apposition.

Pressures in Normal Joints

Only a film of synovial fluid separates the moving surfaces in normal joints. Unlike the distended structure so often depicted in schematic drawings, the articular cavity is primarily a potential space containing so little free fluid that, often, none can be recovered by needle aspiration. Similarly, a microscopic layer of fluid lubricates normal bursae and tendon sheaths. Each of these spaces, then, resembles a collapsed balloon with a wet, slippery inner surface. The state of collapse is apparently maintained by a subatmospheric intracavitary pressure. This concept was introduced by Müller, who found pressures of -8, -8, and -12 cm H_2O in three human knees without effusions and values from -4 to -6 cm H_2O in four additional knees with small effusions (1). Müller also found negative (subatmospheric) intraarticular pressures in anesthetized dogs and in amputated limbs. This finding, implying that resting subatmospheric pressures are generated neither by contraction of skeletal muscles nor by the active pumping of lymphatic vessels, has been confirmed repeatedly in the normal knees of several mammalian species (1). A pressure differential of this magnitude is sufficient to explain the close apposition of synovium on cartilage, sheath on tendon, and bursal lining on itself, but how could these organs maintain such a differential without a specific pumping system and a continuous energy cost?

The exact mechanism of subatmospheric pressures remains controversial, but one reasonable explanation may be drawn from animal experiments using rigid perforated subcutaneous capsules. The pressure in such capsules is consistently subatmospheric by as much as 7 mm Hg. In this model, an equal and opposite colloid osmotic pressure maintains the negative hydrostatic pressure within the capsule (Fig. 8.12). This balance of forces requires fixation of glycosaminoglycans in the gel-like interstitial space of surrounding tissues. The high osmotic pressure of this fixed pericapsular gel "draws" water with a force sufficient to generate a negative pressure within the capsule. Infusions

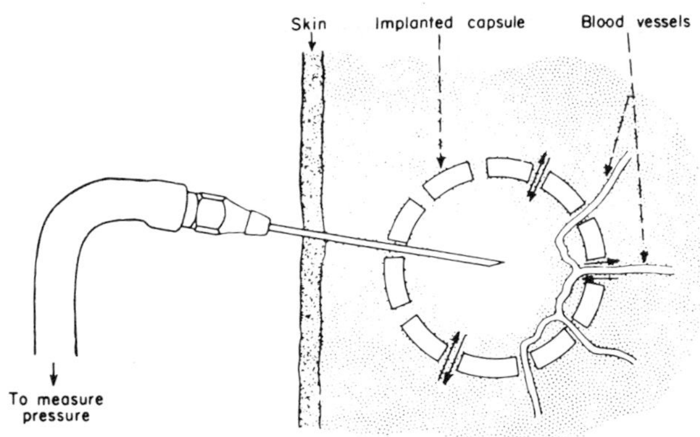

FIG. 8.12. Perforated subcutaneous capsule used in physiologic studies of interstitial fluid. After implantation, the capsule is invested by granulation tissue. The colloid osmotic pressure of this tissue may exceed that of the fluid by an average value of 7 mm Hg, thus generating a subatmospheric pressure within the capsule. A similar discrepancy between colloid osmotic pressures of synovium and synovial fluid would explain the subatmospheric pressures reported in resting normal joints. (From Guyton AC. A concept of negative interstitial pressure based on pressures in implanted perforated capsules. *Circ Res* 1963;12:399–414.)

of either hyaluronidase or collagenase through the capsules disrupt the investing interstitial gel and cause equalization of pressures without and within the capsule (1). This model suggests, then, that an organized matrix of high colloid osmotic pressure acts like a sponge to maintain a negative hydrostatic pressure within an enclosed tissue space. For such a system to remain effective, the synovial "sponge" must be periodically "wrung out," but it is plausible to think that normal joint motion provides sufficient periodic compression to perform this function and thus to sustain the system.

Role in Joint Stability

However achieved, the normal pressure differential may play a significant role in stabilizing joints. In concert with the action of tendons and ligaments, this "suction" draws articulating surfaces into the best possible fit with each other and helps to guide the opposing surfaces as the joint moves through its range of motion. The potential magnitude of these forces was indicated by Jayson and Dixon's studies of normal human knees. With simple isometric contraction of the quadriceps, the mean intraarticular pressure decreased to -107 mm Hg (1). With more severe distractive forces, the guiding mechanism fails, and the pressure falls so low that dissolved tissue gases come out of solution coincident with sudden distraction of the joint surfaces and an audible joint crack. Both the bubble of gas and the distraction of the joint are readily demonstrated by serial radiographs (1). This cavitation or "vacuum" phenomenon has generally been regarded as interesting, but of little practical significance.

The observations are most instructive when assessed from the standpoint of joint stability, as illustrated in the finger. Normally, the extended middle finger may be moved readily throughout a lateral arc of approximately 30 degrees, thus demonstrating laxity in the collateral ligaments of the metacarpophalangeal joint. On applying progressive increments of pull to relaxed third fingers, Unsworth and associates found that a force of 10 kg was required to "crack" the average knuckle (1) (Fig. 8.13). Only at this point did significant distraction occur and did the collateral ligaments accept a significant fraction of the force operating across the joint. At this force, then, an important stabilizing factor has been overcome. A metacarpophalangeal joint surface area is too small for atmospheric pressure alone to explain this 10-kg approximating force. The most likely explanation for the additional increment is the ability of synovial fluid to function as an adhesive, as well as a lubricant. The effective lubrication of normal joints results principally from both boundary layer and hydrodynamic mechanisms (27). The boundary layer is a lubricant that coats each cartilaginous surface, an adherence thought to mainly involve the glycoprotein lubricin (1). Such a boundary layer reduces friction by reducing or eliminating direct contact at the loaded areas where one articular cartilage potentially rubs against its mate. The same adherent layers also bond the opposing surfaces to each other. Such an adhesive bond has been well recognized in other examples of boundary layer lubrication (1). Here, the cohesion of the solvent (water), perhaps enhanced by its viscous solute (hyaluronan), serves as an effective "glue." The functional advantage of such a water bond lies in its high tensile strength with little or no shear strength. Thus, such a system

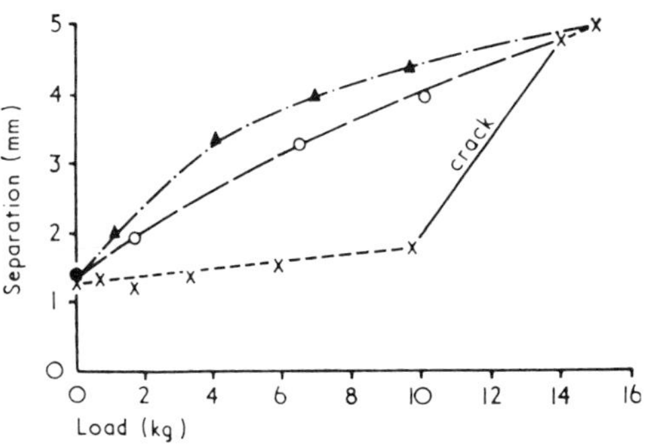

FIG. 8.13. "Cracking" of the third metacarpophalangeal joint. Despite progressive increments of pull of up to 10 kg (lower curve with ×), little separation is seen until the joint cracks with formation of a gas bubble within the joint space. When this happens, the adhesive properties of synovial fluid are overcome, and the load is transferred to the collateral ligaments of the joint. As long as the bubble remains, loading (○) and unloading (▲) of the joint follow the upper curves. (From Unsworth A, Dowson D, Wright V. "Cracking joints": a bioengineering study of cavitation in the metacarpophalangeal joint. *Ann Rheum Dis* 1971;30:348–358, with permission.)

enables opposing surfaces to slide freely across each other but limits their distraction.

When the metacarpophalangeal joint "cracks," the distractive force has fractured the adhesive bond (28). Here, as in other joints, the resultant bubble of intraarticular gas may then be used as a contrast agent for radiographic imaging of articular cartilage and other soft tissues within the joint. A simple comparison of the contact area of metacarpophalangeal joints with that of shoulders, elbows, and knees suggests that forces many times greater than 10 kg would be necessary to distract these joints. Simple atmospheric pressure, aided by adhesive properties of synovial fluid, thus contributes to the stabilization and congruent articulation of large joints. This is especially true in the polyaxial shoulder and hip joints, where ligaments can play only a limited role in maintaining joint stability.

Effect of Effusions

In the presence of effusions, the resting intraarticular pressure becomes positive. The degree of positivity is often 10 to 20 mm Hg, and sometimes much higher, with mechanical consequences that may be profound (10). Effusions eliminate the normal subatmospheric fluid film and substitute, instead, a distending force that increases the stress on the ligaments and joint capsule (Fig. 8.14). The pressures of effusions are greatest in full flexion and extension and lowest around 30 degrees of flexion. The high pressures at extremes of motion cause discomfort and, thus, limit the effective range. They may also cause progressive distention, herniation through the capsule, and rupture of the joint as in

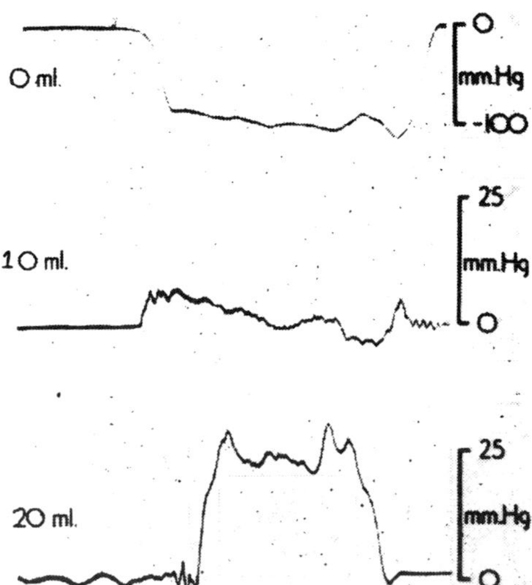

FIG. 8.14. Isometric quadriceps contraction in normal knee containing 0, 10, and 20 mL added saline. With no injection, the intraarticular pressure is subatmospheric. This is no longer seen with 10 mL saline, and the pressure becomes positive with a simulated 20-mL effusion. (From Jayson MIV, Dixon A3tJ. Intraarticular pressure and rheumatoid geodes (bone "cysts"). *Ann Rheum Dis* 1970;29:496–502, with permission.)

Baker cysts of the popliteal fossa. As already discussed, they may also cause tamponade of the synovial microvasculature, thus contributing to the ischemia in chronic rheumatoid synovitis (29). For all these reasons, the high-pressure effusion remains an important problem for investigation and a potentially critical reason for therapeutic intervention.

Articular Variation

Each form of arthritis presented in this text may be characterized by those joints it is most likely to strike, as well as those it will usually spare. For the most part, these patterns are not understood, but it seems reasonable to look at the joints themselves for features that might affect their susceptibility (30). When interarticular physiologic differences are sought, they are invariably found. Thus, the hip versus knee differences in normal synovial fluid protein concentration illustrated in Fig. 8.8 must reflect significant, largely unexplored, differences in the vascular physiology of these joints. In the Starling forces affecting microvascular fluid balance, in the permeability of the vessels, and in the blood flow response to exercise, there are prominent differences between the canine wrist and the knee (9,31,32). Measurements in small, peripheral human joints find pressure values closer to atmospheric levels than those in the knee (33). This field of investigation will become exciting if and when these physiologic differences between joints can be tied into the pathophysiology of each disease to explain its pattern of spared and affected joints.

OPPORTUNITIES IN SYNOVIAL PHYSIOLOGY

Accurate diagnosis and appropriate therapy lie at the heart of good clinical rheumatology. The diagnostic criteria for most rheumatic diseases are broad, resting primarily on clinical observations supported by nonspecific laboratory findings. Within any diagnostic category, as illustrated for RA in Fig. 8.5, there is wide variation in pathophysiologic findings. As yet, however, the implications of this variation have rarely been explored. In which joints is the synovitis most likely to respond to intraarticular corticosteroids? Would the hydrostatic pressure, the lactate level, the pH, the oxygen tension, or some combination of physiologic parameters accurately predict joint destruction? Can such data serve as a useful guide in therapeutic decision making? How well do antibiotics and other medications enter tense effusions? Does the internal milieu of the synovium or of cartilage predispose joints to infection by certain microorganisms? Do unique features of the synovial microvasculature lead to preferred deposition of circulating immune complexes? Do physiologic differences between joints explain characteristic patterns of rheumatic disease, such as the relative sparing by RA of the distal interphalangeal joints that are preferentially involved by OA? Does the subchondral bone share, to some extent, the subatmospheric pressure encountered in working joints? If so, do fluctuations in intraosseous pressure contribute to the lesions of decompression sickness and of other causes of aseptic necrosis? These and many other critical questions remain virtually unexplored. Answers will come only through a new commitment to the problems of articular physiology.

REFERENCES

1. Simkin PA. Synovial physiology. In: McCarty DJ, Koopman WJ, eds. *Arthritis and allied conditions,* 12th ed. Philadelphia: Lea & Febiger, 1993:199–212.
2. Klarlund M, Østergaard M, Lorenzen I. Finger joint synovitis in rheumatoid arthritis: quantitative assessment by magnetic resonance imaging. *Rheumatology* 1999;38:66–72.
3. Simkin PA. Synovial perfusion and synovial fluid solutes. *Ann Rheum Dis* 1995;54:424–428.
4. Simkin PA, Bassett JE, Koh EM. Synovial perfusion in the human knee: a methodologic analysis. *Semin Arthritis Rheum* 1995;25:56–66.
5. Coleman P, Kavanagh E, Mason RM, et al. The proteoglycans and glycosaminoglycan chains of rabbit synovium. *Histochem J* 1998;30: 519–524.
6. Coleman PJ, Scott D, Mason RM, et al. Characterization of the effect of high molecular weight hyaluronan on trans-synovial flow in rabbit knees. *J Physiol* 1999;514:265–282.
7. Wallis WJ, Simkin PA, Nelp WB, et al. Intraarticular volume and clearance in human synovial effusions. *Arthritis Rheum* 1985;28:441–449.
8. Wallis WJ, Simkin PA, Nelp WB. Low synovial clearance of iodide provides evidence of hypoperfusion in chronic rheumatoid synovitis. *Arthritis Rheum* 1985;28:1096–1104.
9. McCarty DJ Jr. Selected aspects of synovial membrane physiology. *Arthritis Rheum* 1974;17:289–296.
10. Simkin PA, Huang A, Benedict RS. Effects of exercise on blood flow to canine articular tissues. *J Orthop Res* 1990;8:297–303.
11. James MJ, Cleland LG, Gaffney D, et al. Effect of exercise on ^{99m}Tc-DTPA clearance from knees with effusions. *J Rheumatol* 1994;21: 501–504.
12. Geborek P, Saxne T, Pettersson H, et al. Synovial fluid acidosis correlates with radiological joint destruction in rheumatoid arthritis knee joints. *J Rheumatol* 1989;16:468–472.
13. Bodamyali T, Stevens CR, Billingham MEJ, et al. Influence of hypoxia in inflammatory synovitis. *Ann Rheum Dis* 1998;57:703–710.
14. Levick JR. Hypoxia and acidosis in chronic inflammatory arthritis: relation to vascular supply and dynamic effusion pressure. *J Rheumatol* 1990;17:576–580.
15. Simkin PA. Feeling the pressure. *Ann Rheum Dis* 1995;54:611–612.
16. Geborek P, Forslind K, Wollheim FA. Direct assessment of synovial blood flow and its relation to induced hydrostatic pressure changes. *Ann Rheum Dis* 1989;48:281–286.
17. Stevens CR, Williams RB, Farrell AJ, et al. Hypoxia and inflammatory synovitis: observations and speculation. *Ann Rheum Dis* 1991;50: 124–132.
18. James MR, Cleland LG, Rofe AM, et al. Intraarticular pressure and the relationship between synovial perfusion and metabolic demand. *J Rheumatol* 1990;17:521–527.
19. Day RO, McLachlan AJ, Graham GC, et al. Pharmacokinetics of nonsteroidal anti-inflammatory drugs in synovial fluid. *Clin Pharmacokinet* 1999;36:191–210.
20. Bengtsson B, Franklin A, Luthman J, et al. Concentrations of sulphadimidine, oxytetracycline and penicillin G in serum, synovial fluid and tissue cage fluid after parenteral administration to calves. *J Vet Pharmacol Ther* 1989;12:37–45.
21. Simkin PA, Wu MP, Foster DM. Articular pharmacokinetics of protein-bound antirheumatic agents. *Clin Pharmacokinet* 1993;25:342–350.
22. Levick JR. A method for estimating macromolecular reflection by human synovium, using measurements of intra-articular half lives. *Ann Rheum Dis* 1998;57:339–344.
23. Weinberger A, Simkin PA. Plasma proteins in synovial fluids of normal human joints. *Semin Arthritis Rheum* 1989;19:66–76.
24. Wallis WJ, Simkin PA, Nelp WB. Protein traffic in human synovial effusions. *Arthritis Rheum* 1987;30:57–63.
25. Simkin PA, Bassett JE. Cartilage matrix molecules in serum and synovial fluid. *Curr Opin Rheumatol* 1995;7:346–351.
26. Myers SL, Brandt KD, Eilam O. Even low-grade synovitis significantly accelerates the clearance of protein from the canine knee—implications for measurement of synovial fluid "markers" of osteoarthritis. *Arthritis Rheum* 1995;38:1085–1091.
27. Simkin PA. Friction and lubrication in synovial joints. *J Rheumatol* 2000;27:567–568.
28. Chen YL, Israelachvili J. New mechanism of cavitation damage. *Science* 1991;252:1157–1160.
29. Funk RHW, Tischendorf R, Bratengeier H. Microendoscopy of the synovial vasculature in the rabbit knee joint. *Microvasc Res* 1995;50: 45–55.
30. Simkin PA. Why this joint and why not that joint? *Scand J Rheumatol* 1995;24(suppl):13–16.
31. Simkin PA, Benedict RS. Hydrostatic and oncotic determinants of microvascular fluid balance in normal canine joints. *Arthritis Rheum* 1990;33:80–86.
32. Simkin PA, Benedict RS. Iodide and albumin kinetics in normal canine wrists and knees. *Arthritis Rheum* 1990;33:73–79.
33. Gaffney K, Williams RB, Jolliffe VA, et al. Intraarticular pressure changes in rheumatoid and normal peripheral joints. *Ann Rheum Dis* 1995;54:670–673.

CHAPTER 9

Collagen Structure and Function

Richard Mayne and Leena Ala-Kokko

Individual collagen fibrils are easily recognized in electron micrographs of connective tissues, and often several fibrils associate laterally to form the highly insoluble fibers that provide the tensile strength of cornea, skin, or tendon (1,2). However, the collagen triple helix is now recognized as a structural motif shared by a wide variety of different proteins, some of which are clearly not collagens, such as acetylcholinesterase or C1q (1). From the recently completed sequence of the human genome, it is now possible to identify all of the proteins that contain a collagenous sequence without any information concerning function. Traditionally, a Roman numeral identifies each new collagen, and there are presently 27 different types of collagens recognized by the Human Gene Nomenclature Committee (*www.gene.ucl.ac.uk/nomenclature/*). Further details of the structure and expression of these collagens can be either found at Online Mendelian Inheritance in Man (*www.ncbi.nlm.nih.gov/omim/*) or at GeneCards (*genecards.weizmann.ac.il/geneloc/*). In addition, numerous collagen-related structural motifs occur in bacterial and viral proteins (3), and it is now possible to describe the evolutionary origins of the unique amino acid sequence that forms the triple helix of collagen (4,5). Many collagen types have well-established structural roles in the extracellular matrix, but this still remains to be convincingly demonstrated for some of the newer proteins that are being called collagens. Indeed, several of the collagens (types XIII, XVII, XXIII, and XXV) are transmembrane proteins and therefore may have functions of a nonstructural nature (6). Individual collagen molecules interact in connective tissues in a remarkable number of ways to form fibrils (types I, II, III, and V/XI), microfibrils (type VI), networks (types IV, VIII, and X), and lateral associations without stagger (type VII) (1,2). Additionally, some collagens (types IX, XII, and XIV) only interact with the surface of collagen fibrils and cannot self-associate. These collagens, which may also include types XVI, XIX, XX, XXI, and XXII collagens are called fibril-associated collagens with interrupted triple helices (FACIT) collagens (7). Two collagens (types XV and XVIII), which are related in primary structure, contain several short collagenous domains interrupted by short noncollagenous sequences (8). The C-terminal noncollagenous domain of type XVIII collagen has been extensively investigated since it acts as an inhibitor of angiogenesis and is called endostatin (8,9). Both types XV and XVIII collagen are largely located in basement membrane zones (10–14). In this chapter, only those collagens that have well-defined structural functions in the extracellular matrix of articular cartilage, bone, and joints will be discussed in detail.

STRUCTURE OF THE TRIPLE HELIX

A remarkable property of the collagen triple helix is its ability to self-assemble in solution to form a triple helix in which every third amino acid is glycine (15) (Figs. 9.1 and 9.2). This makes it possible to synthesize and assemble stretches of triple helix that contain binding sites for collagen-binding macromolecules and to investigate the nature of each interaction in considerable detail. For example, the binding site for both $\alpha_2\beta_1$ and $\alpha_1\beta_1$ integrin was eventually localized to the short sequence, GFOGER, located within the triple helix of type I collagen (16). In subsequent studies, cocrystallization of a triple-helical peptide containing the GFOGER sequence with the recombinant vWA domain (I domain) of the α2 integrin chain was achieved and the molecular nature of the interaction described in detail using x-ray crystallography (17). Synthetic, triple-helical, collagenous peptides have also been crystallized, and their structure has been determined to 1.4 Å resolution (18,19). Such approaches have considerable advantages because specific, known mutations in the collagen triple helix can be created and their effects on the stability and structure of the helix can be directly investigated (20,21). Similar approaches have

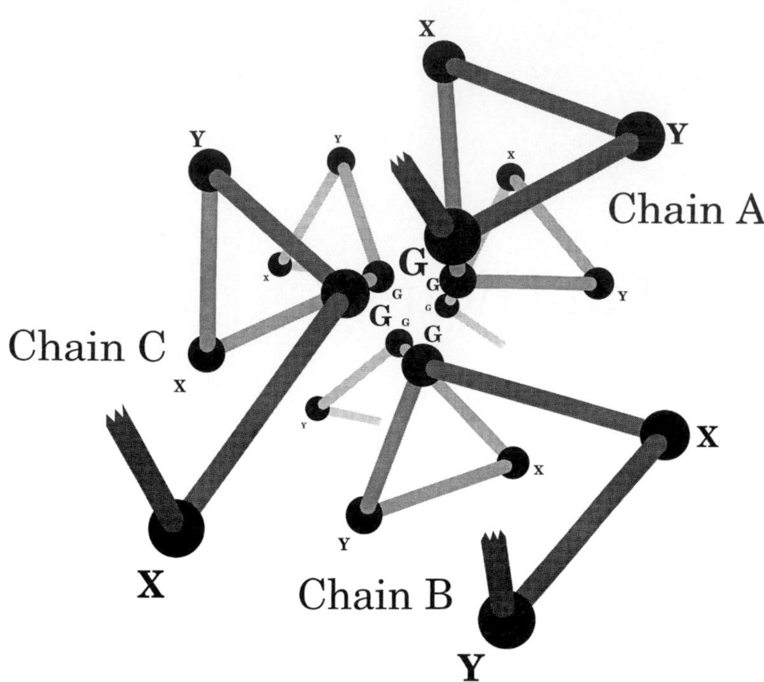

FIG. 9.1. Model for the organization of the three collagen chains to form a triple helix. Note that glycine (*G*) is located at every third amino acid and is present at the center of the helix. Both the X and Y amino acids are located on the surface of the helix such that their side chains (not shown) project away from the molecule. By itself, each chain forms a left-handed helix, but the three chains together form a right-handed superhelix. (Reproduced by permission from Van der Rest M, Garrone R. Collagens as multidomain proteins. *Biochimie* 1990;72: 473–484, with permission.)

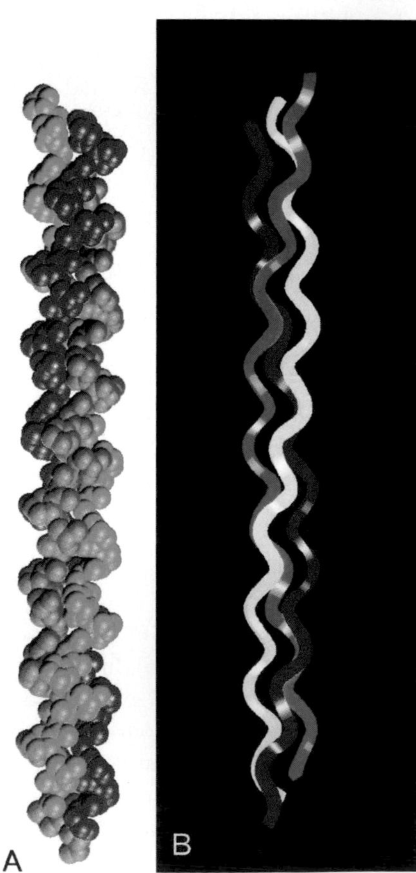

FIG. 9.2. A:. Space-filling model of the collagen triple helix. The three chains lie in parallel with a stagger of one residue. **B:.** Ribbon diagram of native collagen showing the peptide backbone of each collagen chain. (Reproduced by permission from Bella J, Eaton M, Brodsky B, et al. Crystal structure of a collagen-like peptide at 1.9Å resolution. *Science* 1994;266:75–81, with permission.)

also provided model triple-helical substrates for cleavage by matrix metalloproteinases (22). The triple helix is clearly stabilized by conversion of proline to hydroxyproline in the Y position (Fig. 9.1), but the precise mechanism by which this stability is achieved is not well understood (18,23).

FIBRIL-FORMING OR INTERSTITIAL COLLAGENS

Of the 27 different collagen types, only five (types I, II, III, V, and XI) are known to be capable of undergoing the staggered, lateral associations required to form the collagen fibrils observed by electron microscopy (1,24) (Fig. 9.3). Moreover, types V and XI collagens are considered part of a type V/XI family of collagen with a variety of different chain organizations (25,26). Types XXIV and XXVII collagens have recently been cloned and appear related to the interstitial collagens, especially of lower organisms (27–29).

Table 9.1 summarizes the different collagen chains of the fibril-forming or interstitial collagens, together with their molecular organization, chromosomal localizations, and tissue distributions. Type I is the major species found in most connective tissues and forms 80% to 90% of the total collagen in tissues such as bone, dentin, cornea, and tendon. Type III collagen is largely absent from these tissues but is prominent in tissues containing thin collagen fibrils such as kidney, liver, and lymph nodes. Types I and III collagens may form cofibrils in many tissues, and it is proposed that type III collagen plays a key role in limiting fibril diameters (1). It also is possible that type III collagen can form a separate population of thin collagen fibrils and that type III–containing fibrils represent the reticular fibrils of classic histology.

Type II collagen forms the thin fibrils of both embryonic cartilages and the vitreous of the eye (26). Analysis of fibril

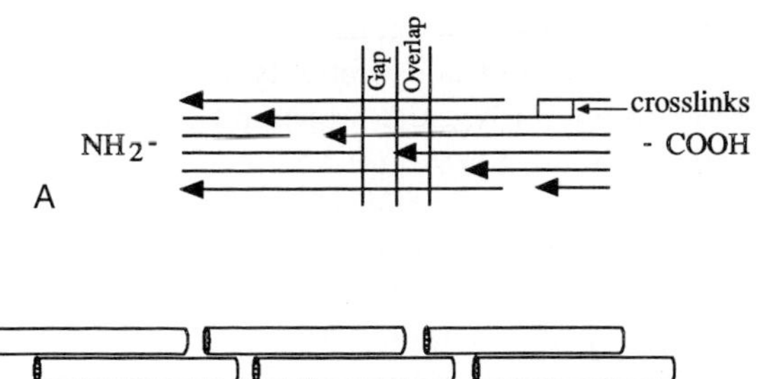

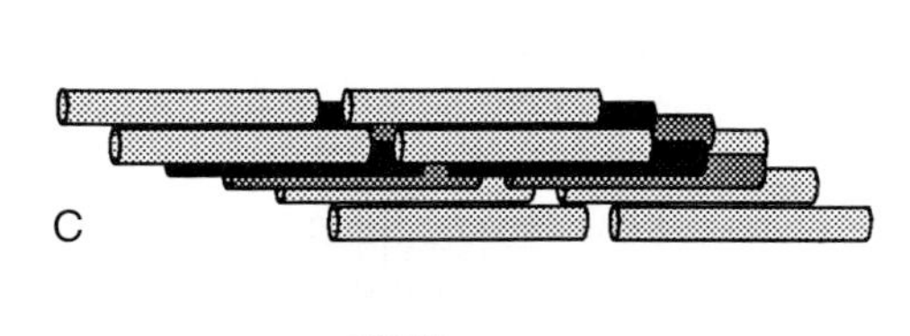

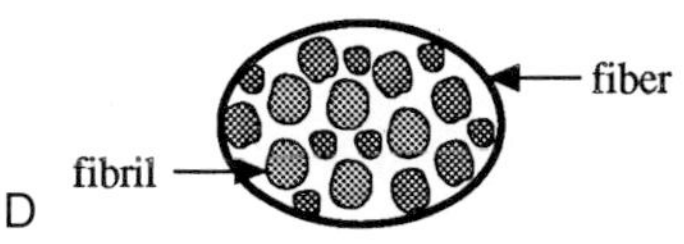

FIG. 9.3. Models for the organization of interstitial collagens to form a fiber. **A:** Organization of individual molecules to form a fibril. Note the staggered arrangement of molecules giving rise to a "gap" and "overlap" region. Additionally, the location of the major lysine-derived cross-links between molecules is shown. **B:** Lateral association of individual molecules. **C:** Three-dimensional organization of molecules to form a fibril. **D:** Organization of several fibrils in tendon to form a fiber. Note that between each fibril there is considerable space, which contains proteoglycans and noncollagenous proteins.

formation *in vitro* strongly suggests that types II, IX, and XI collagens are all required to form thin fibrils (30,31). In articular cartilage of adult animals, however, the collagen fibrils are much thicker and consist almost entirely of type II collagen (32). Further experiments suggest that these differences arise from the hydroxylysine content and hence glycosylation of the collagen molecule (33).

Members of the type V/XI collagen family are present in variable amounts (usually 10% or less) in all connective tissues (25). However, molecules of chain organization $[\alpha1(V)]_2\ \alpha2(V)$ constitute approximately 20% of the total collagen of the chicken cornea (34), which possesses the most highly organized fibrillar array of all tissues. The function of this family of collagens remains somewhat obscure, although analyses suggest that these molecules are involved in determining fibril diameters as well as establishing the overall organization of the collagen fibrils within the matrix (35).

Gene Structure

The genes for the interstitial collagens are widely distributed on different chromosomes (Table 9.1) and are usually large, with many short exons often interspersed with large introns (36). The organization of a typical collagen gene is shown in Fig. 9.4, which represents the human $\alpha1(I)$ gene, consisting of a total of 18 kb of nucleotide sequence. Each bar reflects a single exon, which in the triple helix is usually a multiple of 54 bp, occasionally with the deletion of 9 bp, resulting in 45 or 99 bp. In the noncollagenous amino-termini and carboxy-termini, the exons are much larger. These results suggest that 54 bp may represent a primordial gene unit for collagenous molecules (37), but this cannot be the case for all collagens since the triple helix of type X collagen is encoded by a single, large exon (38).

Gene Regulation

Transcriptional regulation of the interstitial collagen genes remains poorly understood and often controversial despite extensive experimentation involving the transfection of promoter constructs either into cells in culture or, more recently, expression of promoter constructs incorporated into the genome of

TABLE 9.1. *Molecular organization of interstitial collagens*

Type	Chain	Molecular organization	Gene	Chromosomal localization	Occurrence
I	$\alpha1(I)$	$[\alpha1(I)]_2\ \alpha2(I)$	COL1A1	17q21.3-q22	Most connective tissues: blood vessels, bone, cornea, dentin, skin, tendon
	$\alpha2(I)$	$[\alpha1(I)]_3$ (rare)	COL1A2	7q21.3	
II	$\alpha1(II)$	$[\alpha1(II)]_3$	COL2A1	12q13.11	Hyaline cartilage, vitreous
III	$\alpha1(III)$	$[\alpha1(III)]_3$	COL3A1	2q32.2	Blood vessels, kidney, liver, lung
V/XI	$\alpha1(V)$	$[\alpha1(V)]_2\ \alpha2(V)$	COL5A1	9q34.2-q34.3	Ubiquitous (small amounts in most tissues): blood vessels, bone, cartilage, cornea, tendon, vitreous, etc.
	$\alpha2(V)$	$\alpha1(V)\alpha2(V)\alpha3(V)$	COL5A2	2q14-q32	
	$\alpha3(V)$		COL5A3	19p13.2	
	$\alpha1(XI)$	$\alpha1(XI)\alpha2(XI)\alpha3(XI)$	COL11A1	1p21	
	$\alpha2(XI)$	$[\alpha1(XI)]_2\ \alpha2(V)$	COL11A2	6p21.3	
	$\alpha3(XI)$[a]		COL11A3	12q13.11	
XXIV	$\alpha1(XXIV)$	unknown	COL24A1	1p22.3	Widespread: bone, cornea, retina, skin, tendon
XXVII	$\alpha1(XXVII)$	unknown	COL27A1	9q32	Widespread: cartilage, colon, ear, eye, lung

[a]Derived from the same gene as the $\alpha1(II)$ chain

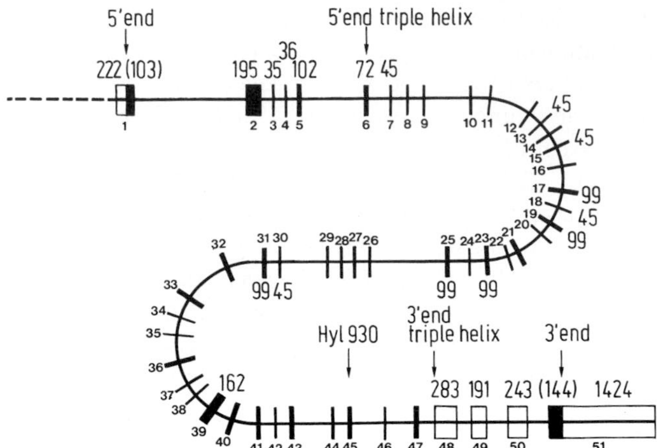

FIG. 9.4. Exon/intron organization of the human α1(I) collagen gene. The gene is 18 kb in length and contains 51 exons. In the 5′ and 3′ noncollagenous regions, the length of each exon is indicated. In the triple helical domain, the *thin bars* designate exons with 54 nucleotides, and the *thick bars* designate exons of 108 bp. Additionally, exons of length of 45, 99, and 162 bp are shown. The same organization of exons, particularly for the triple helical domain, is found for types I, II, and III collagen. (Reproduced by permission from Kühn, K. In: Mayne R, Burgeson RE, eds. *Structure and function of collagen types.* Orlando: Academic Press, 1987:30.)

transgenic mice (39–41). It is clear that short upstream sequences act as minimal promoters for the collagen genes (42), but there are also upstream and downstream elements that have considerable enhancer/promoter activity (39). One of the unexplained features of the control of expression of type I collagen is the number of different tissues that are able to express both the α1(I) and α2(I) genes at high levels. Considerable effort has been expended to identify tissue-specific elements of the promoter (43). At present, regions promoting specific expression in bone (40,41) and tendon (44) have been identified. Part of the difficulty in the past in identifying control elements may have arisen from a failure to appreciate that remote upstream elements (at least 10 kb upstream) may play important roles in transcription for both the α1(I) (45) and α2(I) (46,47) genes. Despite the limited progress and the variable results from different laboratories, such analyses of transcriptional regulation of type I collagen are important to understand both the transcriptional activity of growth factors such as TGF-β in up-regulating collagen biosynthesis (48,49) and the potential loss of regulatory control during fibrosis of tissues (50,51).

In contrast to the transcriptional control of the α1(I) and α2(I) collagen genes, considerable progress has been made in identifying short enhancer sequences required for cartilage-specific expression of the α1(II) and α2(XI) collagen genes (52). The results show that a transcription factor called SOX9 binds to these sites, where it serves as a potent activator (52,53). In cartilage, SOX9 is coexpressed with other SOX genes (called L-SOX5 and SOX6), which also bind cooperatively to the enhancer element (54). Importantly, cells prepared by homologous recombination that are Sox9 −/− are unable to enter the cartilage lineage of chimeric mice (55), and a conditional, limb-specific, knockout of Sox9 results in failure of cartilage formation, specifically in the limbs (56). However, it is also clear that Sox9 is not the only transcription factor involved in chondrogenesis, and recently a helix-loop-helix protein called DEC1 has been described that induces type II expression (57). Other transcription factors have been described that apparently interact with Sox9 (58,59) and therefore will potentially provide insight into the mechanism by which Sox9 functions. Interestingly, the type II collagen gene also appears to be under negative control, and recently, two transcription repressors of the *Snail* family have been identified, which appear to down-regulate type II collagen expression during hypertrophy (60).

Biosynthesis of Procollagens

After synthesis of the primary transcript, the interstitial collagens must undergo extensive splicing before the processed transcript is secreted from the nucleus. Biosynthesis of individual chains then occurs on the rough endoplasmic reticulum with subsequent chain assembly occurring within the cisternae (1,2). For the interstitial collagens, chain assembly occurs from the noncollagenous carboxy-terminus and proceeds to the amino-terminus with the establishment of interchain and intrachain disulfide bridges (Fig. 9.5). Prior to triple helix assembly, however, the important posttranslational modifications of proline and lysine to hydroxyproline and hydroxylysine, respectively, occur as a result of the activity of the enzymes prolyl hydroxylase and lysyl hydroxylase located within the cisternae of the rough endoplasmic reticulum (1,2). Subsequently, the collagen molecules are transported to the Golgi apparatus and, at least in some tissues such as the developing tendon or cultured fibroblasts, are packaged into distinct vacuoles prior to secretion (61–65). It is likely that chaperone proteins are involved both in promoting the formation and passage of correctly folded triple-helical collagen molecules through the secretory pathway and in targeting incorrectly folded molecules for rapid degradation. Intriguingly, the β subunit of prolyl-4-hydroxylase is identical to protein disulfide isomerase, which catalyzes the rearrangement of disulfide bonds in a variety of proteins (2), and a chaperone-like function for this enzyme was proposed (66). It also appears that some chaperone proteins, such as protein disulfide isomerase or binding protein, are involved in the recognition of the C-propeptide and, potentially, the retention of incorrectly folded collagen molecules within the cell (67–69). However, the major collagen-binding protein of the rough endoplasmic reticu-

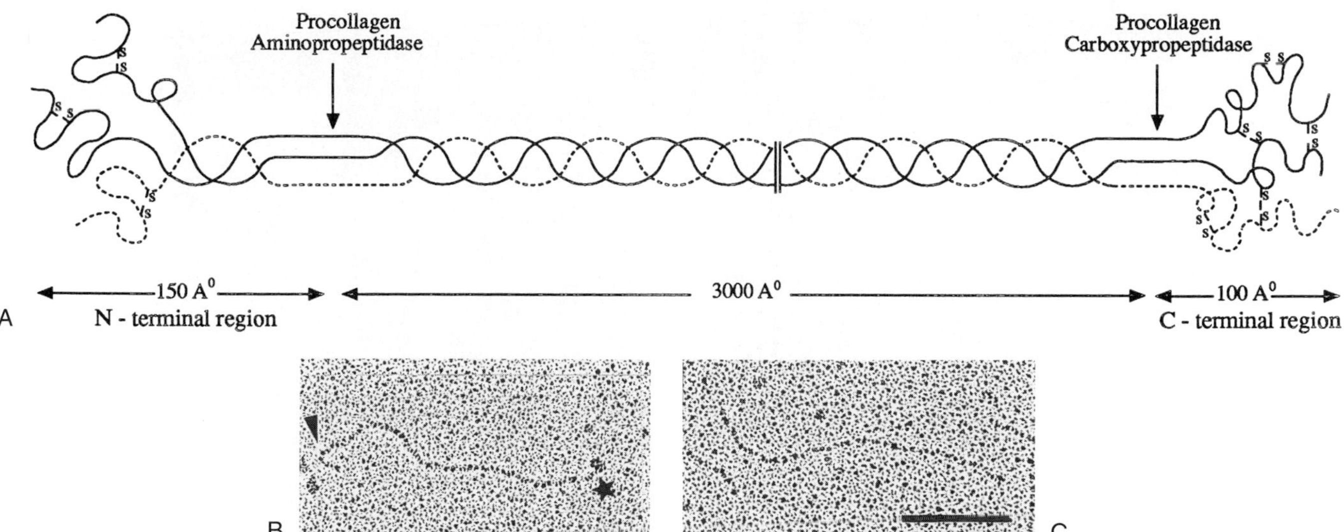

FIG. 9.5. A: Structure of type I or II procollagen showing the cleavage sites for procollagen aminopropeptidase and procollagen carboxypropeptidase. Note the presence of interchain disulfide bonds in the carboxy-terminus but not in the amino-terminus. Also, note the presence of a short collagenous triple helix in the aminopropeptide. (Reproduced and redrawn by permission from Burgeson RE, Nimni ME. Collagen types. Molecular structure and tissue distribution. *Clin Orthop Rel Res* 1992;282: 250–272, with permission.) **B:** Rotary shadowing of type II procollagen. *Arrowhead* indicates the aminopropeptide, and *star* indicates the carboxypropeptide. **C:** Rotary shadowing of a type II collagen molecule after processing. Bar = 100 nm. (**B** and **C** are reproduced by permission from Mayne R, Brewton RG. Extracellular matrix of cartilage: collagen. In: Woessner JF, Howell DS, eds. *Joint cartilage degradation.* New York: Marcel Dekker, 1993:85, with permission.)

lum is called variously HSP47, gp46, or colligin (70–76). It is proposed that this protein also has chaperone-like functions and acts in a coordinated manner with other chaperones during passage from the rough endoplasmic reticulum to the Golgi apparatus. Although the roles of different chaperones in collagen biosynthesis still remain poorly understood in normal cells, these proteins are clearly important in quality control of type I collagen production. Such quality control is likely to be especially important for the interstitial collagens that require precise alignment of individual molecules without interruption of the triple helix for (a) ordered fibril formation, (b) successful cleavage of procollagen molecules, and (c) precise formation of lysine-derived cross-links (1,2).

In some tissues, such as the developing tendon, cornea, or odontoblasts, individual procollagen molecules apparently align in parallel arrays without stagger and are secreted within discrete vacuoles that appear to arise from the Golgi apparatus (63) (Fig. 9.6). It still is not clearly established, however, that formation of large secretory vacuoles occurs in all tissues that secrete interstitial collagens. For example, in developing chondrocytes that synthesize predominantly type II collagen, secretory vacuoles cannot be easily identified by electron microscopic analysis, and most of the intracellular type II procollagen molecules are located in the rough endoplasmic reticulum and not in the Golgi apparatus (77,78). In contrast, both secretion and concentration of aggrecan in the Golgi apparatus were clearly demonstrated in the same cells.

Fibril Formation

In the developing tendon, but not in other tissues, individual collagen fibrils are apparently assembled in deep recesses within the cell (Fig. 9.6). This unique mechanism is likely to reflect the specific interactions necessary for morphogenesis and remodeling of tendons in which all fibrils eventually form a highly organized parallel array (79–80). Before fibril formation can occur, however, the noncollagenous extensions of individual procollagen molecules must be cleaved both at their amino-termini and carboxy-termini by procollagen proteinases (81) (Fig. 9.5). Considerable progress has been made in identifying and characterizing the enzymes required for procollagen cleavage both at the C-terminus (82–86) and at the N-terminus (81,87). It appears that these enzymes have several other processing functions within the cell, cleaving several collagenous (88–90) and noncollagenous proteins (91,92). However, it is poorly understood for most tissues how collagen fibrils first form and whether fibril formation is always closely associated with the cells. In many tissues, such as cornea or embryonic tendon, both the diameter of individual fibrils and their organization are carefully controlled (93). How this

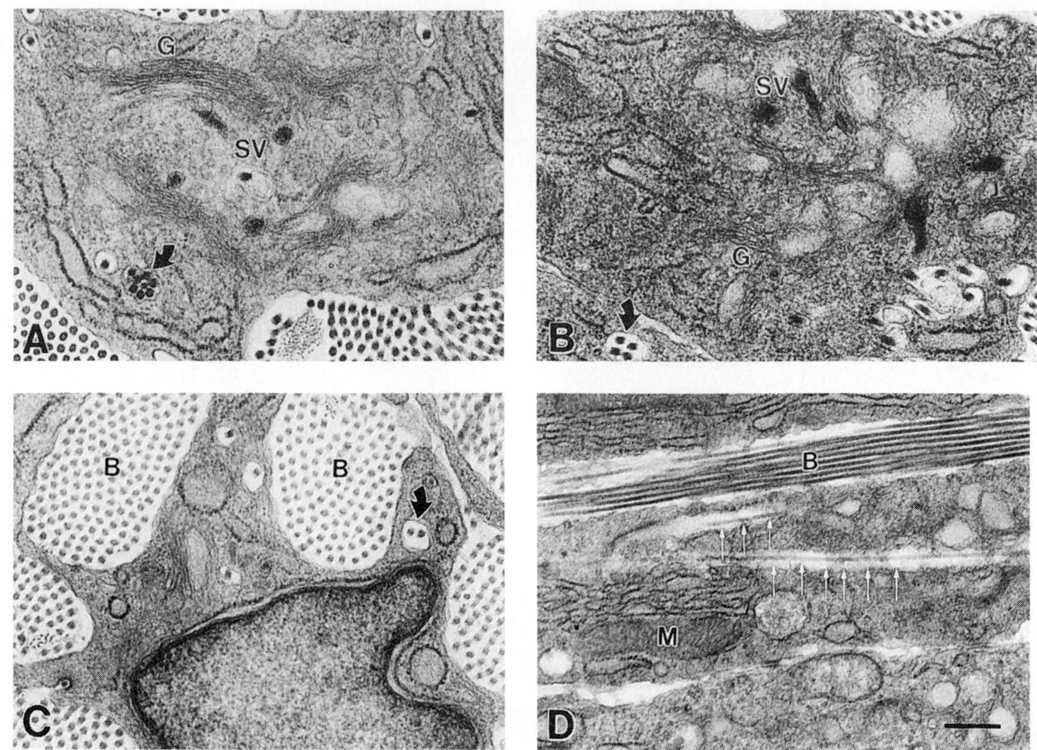

FIG. 9.6. A, B, C, and **D:** Electron micrographs of developing chick tendon showing the formation and organization of collagen fibrils. **A, B,** and **C** are cross sections showing collagen fibrils apparently located within foldings of the cell membrane (*black arrows*). **D** is a longitudinal section showing a single collagen fibril (*white arrows*). *G* = Golgi; *SV* = secretory vesicles; *B* = bundle of collagen fibrils; *M* = mitochondrion.

occurs is still poorly understood, although members of the type V/XI collagen family are thought to play a role (1, 94). Finally, collagen fibrils are stabilized by the formation of lysine-derived cross-links between individual molecules at the locations depicted in Fig. 9.3. This requires the enzyme lysyl oxidase that recognizes lysine and hydroxylysine residues at specific sites and forms highly reactive aldehydic groups that subsequently react with neighboring lysine residues in other molecules (95).

In addition to the well-established collagens described above, two new collagenous molecules called types XXIV and XXVII have recently been identified and are listed in Table 9.1. At present, nothing is known about the function of these collagens, although it is speculated that they are related to the collagens of invertebrates. Type XXIV is found in a variety of tissues, whereas type XXVII is primarily found in cartilage.

Genetic Diseases Involving Interstitial Collagens

Table 9.2 lists the genetic diseases of connective tissues that are known to involve mutations in the interstitial collagens or other collagens described later in this chapter (1,2). Useful models for some of these diseases have also arisen spontaneously in a variety of animals or can be studied in knockout mice (96).

Single base substitutions that convert a codon for the obligatory glycine in a Gly-X-Y triplet to a codon for a larger amino acid are the most common mutations found in the collagen genes. Because glycine is required as every third amino acid for triple helix formation (Fig. 9.1), its substitution can affect collagen biosynthesis in two ways. If folding is prevented by a glycine substitution, the partially assembled procollagen molecules are quickly degraded by a process known as "procollagen suicide." If molecular assembly is not prevented, glycine substitution can result in an interruption in the triple helix and lead to the formation and secretion of structurally and functionally abnormal procollagen molecules that interfere with fibril assembly. Splicing mutations and other mutations that result in small in-frame deletions or insertions can also have a similar effect on triple helix formation. All these mutations are considered to be dominant negative, since the mutated pro-α chains interfere with the assembly of the normal pro-α chains. Mutations that decrease the total amount of collagen synthesized are also relatively common in these genes. These mutations typically result in milder phenotypes than

TABLE 9.2. *Human genetic diseases involving collagen mutations*

Gene	Disease
COL1A1; COL1A2	Osteogenesis imperfecta Ehlers-Danlos syndrome type VIIA, VIIB (Osteoporosis)
COL2A1	Several chondrodysplasias Achondrogenesis and hypochondrogenesis Spondyloepiphyseal dysplasia Kniest syndrome Stickler syndrome type 1 (Osteoarthritis)
COL3A1	Ehlers-Danlos syndrome type IV (Familial aortic aneurysms)
COL4A3; COL4A4	Alport syndrome, autosomally inherited forms
COL4A5	Alport syndrome, X-linked form
COL4A5 and COL4A6	Alport syndrome with diffuse esophageal leiomyomatosis, X-linked
COL6A1; COL6A2; COL6A3	Bethlem myopathy, Ullrich syndrome
COL7A1	Epidermolysis bullosa, dystrophic forms
COL8A2	Fuchs corneal endothelial dystrophy, posterior polymorphous corneal dystrophy
COL9A1	Multiple epiphyseal dysplasia
COL9A2; COL9A3	Multiple epiphyseal dysplasia, intervertebral disc disease
COL10A1	Schmid metaphyseal chondrodysplasia
COL11A1	Stickler syndrome type 2
COL11A2	Stickler syndrome, non-ocular form, type 3
COL17A1	Junctional epidermolysis bullosa
COL18A1	Knobloch syndrome
Type I collagen aminopropeptidase	Ehlers-Danlos syndrome VIIC
Lysyl hydroxylase	Ehlers-Danlos syndrome VI

the dominant negative mutations, because all collagen is structurally and functionally normal (97).

Type I Collagen

Type I collagen is found in most connective tissues, but mutations in either COL1A1 or COL1A2 usually manifest themselves as brittle bones or osteogenesis imperfecta (OI) (98). The inheritance is almost exclusively autosomal dominant. Linkage and mutation studies have clearly established that over 90% of all patients with OI have a mutation in one or more of the type I collagen genes (2,98). OI is a clinically heterogeneous disorder, and although type I collagen is the major collagen of many tissues, this disease is always characterized by bone fragility. The number of fractures can vary from a few to over 200. Most patients with OI also have eyes with blue sclerae. Hearing loss and dentinogenesis imperfecta can also be present. Short stature and deformities are typical in the severe forms. OI is divided into four main types, I through IV (98). Type I is the mildest form, and it is characterized by bone fractures that may be few or numerous. The patients do not develop deformities, and they have a normal to near-normal stature. OI type II, the perinatally lethal variant, is the most severe form. Affected infants have a typical facial appearance, dark sclera, and a soft calvarium. Fractures are rare, because the bone is soft. OI type III is a progressively deforming variant in which the patients already have fractures *in utero*. They typically have a high fracture rate, short stature, and develop pronounced deformities later in life. Type IV is a mildly deforming variant that is clinically similar, but milder, than type III.

Mutations that decrease the production of type I collagen are the most common causes for type I OI. All such mutations, which include (a) point mutations that change codons to termination codons, (b) out-of-frame deletions or insertions, and (c) splicing mutations that decrease messenger RNA (mRNA) levels have all been identified in COL1A1. Structural mutations, such as mutations causing glycine substitutions in COL1A1 or COL1A2, can also cause OI type I, although these mutations are more rare than null mutations. Glycine substitutions; mutations causing exon skipping, small deletions, or duplications; and multiexon rearrangements in either of the type I collagen genes are found in OI types II, III, and IV. These mutations result in the failure to form or fold the collagen triple helix correctly.

In one extensively investigated case of lethal OI, the glycine at position 748 of the $\alpha 1(I)$ chain was shown to be mutated to a cysteine (99). This resulted in a visible kink in the molecule as observed in the electron microscope after rotary shadowing and failure to form organized fibrils during fibrillogenesis with normal type I collagen *in vitro* (100). Instead, fractal-like structures were formed, clearly demonstrating that the mutation directly interfered with the lateral associations of individual molecules during fibril assembly. This mutation appears to be exceptional, however, and further investigation of fibril formation using type I collagen with substitution of cysteine for glycine at different locations resulted in thicker fibrils without the formation of fractal-like structures (101). Several attempts have been made to equate the site of mutation along the triple helix with the severity of OI, which can vary from a phenotype that is lethal at birth to a mild phenotype in the adult with only an occasional broken bone (102,103). In general, for glycine to cysteine substitutions, the phenotype becomes milder when the mutation occurs toward the amino-terminus (102,104). However, the results are often difficult to interpret because mutations that interfere with fibril assembly may also alter the triple-helical structure of individual molecules in such a manner that cleavage by the aminopropeptidase occurs more slowly (105) (Fig. 9.5). Some OI patients with mutations in type I collagen have a mild phenotype, and a small percentage (1%–3%) of patients diagnosed as having postmenopausal osteoporosis may also harbor mutations in type I collagen (106). There is evidence that a polymorphism in the Sp1 binding site of COL1A1 is associated with decreased bone density and osteoporotic fractures (107–109).

Ehlers-Danlos syndrome (EDS) types VIIA and VIIB also involve type I collagen but usually arise from a mutation within exon 6 or at a splicing site for exon 6 such that this exon is missing from the final transcript (2,110) (see also Chapter 96). Exon 6 encodes the aminopropeptidase cleavage site so that the bulky aminopropeptide is retained after secretion with such mutations and interferes with fibril formation. EDS can also arise, however, from defective synthesis of the aminopropeptidase itself, in which case it is called EDS type VIIC or dermatosparaxis (110). This disease is rare and presents with marked joint hypermotility, multiple joint dislocations, and congenital hip dislocation. In many cases, fibrils of a hieroglyphic appearance are observed in tissues. These fibrils are considered to originate from the incorporation of molecules containing uncleaved and globular aminopropeptides onto the surface of the fibrils. Mutations in another collagen-modifying enzyme, lysyl hydroxylase, have been shown to cause EDS type VI, characterized by muscular hypotonia, kyphoscoliosis, osteoporosis, microcornea, and ruptures of arteries and the eye globe (110,111). These mutations almost completely abolish the enzyme activity and result in diminished hydroxylysine content of collagens, reduced number of cross-links derived from hydroxylysine aldehydes, and eventually to mechanical weakness of the connective tissues.

Animal Models of Diseases Arising from Genetic Defects in Type I Collagen

In general, any modification of type I collagen synthesis, either in transgenic mice or as a naturally occurring mutation in animals, manifests itself by brittle bones in a manner similar to that of human OI. A good example is the *oim* mouse, in which a failure to synthesize proα2(I) chains results in molecules with a chain organization of $[\alpha 1(I)]_3$ (112). A similar failure to synthesize α2(I) was described earlier in a human patient with OI (113). Transgenic mice were obtained that expressed a "minigene" of human COL1A1 in which 41 exons encoding for the central region of the molecule were deleted (114). It was proposed that expression of the minigene with its normal carboxy-terminus resulted in association with normal α1(I) chains during chain assembly, thus leading to procollagen suicide. Transgenic mice that expressed high levels of the minigene displayed phenotypes that closely resemble a severe form of OI (114), although considerable variability was encountered (115).

Type II Collagen

A large number of different chondrodysplasias are recognized clinically, and it is now known that mutations in type II collagen are one cause of many of these cartilage disorders (116,117) (Table 9.2). Because type II collagen is important for skeletal development and growth, most of these phenotypes are severe, either being lethal or resulting in dwarfism. Mutations that lead to these phenotypes are usually located in the triple helix of the type II molecule and are therefore likely to result either in procollagen suicide or structurally and functionally abnormal molecules through a dominant negative effect, as described for type I collagen above. Less is usually known concerning the phenotypic effects of mutations in type II collagen on the macromolecular and ultrastructural organization of cartilage, unless cartilagenous tissue can be obtained at surgery or from a biopsy. It seems likely that slightly defective type II collagen molecules, if incorporated into fibrils, will additionally affect interactions with types XI and IX collagens, resulting in a poorly organized matrix. As with type I collagen, it has been difficult to correlate the site and type of mutation with the severity of the clinical condition, although a large number of mutations in type II collagen have now been identified (118). Of special interest is the Stickler syndrome, which represents a relatively mild COL2A1 phenotype. It is characterized by extensive eye involvement, including high myopia, vitreoretinal degeneration, and retinal detachment. Other findings include cleft palate, typical facial features, hearing loss, and early onset osteoarthritis (116,119). A subset of these patients have mutations in COL2A1 that always involve a premature termination codon so that only one half of the normal type II collagen will be synthesized in the heterozygotes (116). However, mutations that introduce stop codons in exon 2 of COL2A1 result in predominantly ocular Stickler syndrome (120–122). Type II procollagen is synthesized in two different forms as a result of alternative splicing of exon 2 (123). The long form contains a large cysteine-rich domain in the aminopropeptide encoded by exon 2, whereas the short form lacks this domain. The long form is predominant in prechondrogenic cells, and the short form replaces it during the maturation of chondrocytes (124,125). Unlike adult cartilage, adult bovine vitreous has been shown to contain the long form (126,127), possibly explaining the predominant ocular findings in the patients with the exon 2 mutations. The fibrils of the vitreous humor are mainly type II collagen, and an insufficient amount of this collagen may be available during vitreous formation for the proper assembly of fibrils to incorporate type IX and type XI collagen correctly. In the vitreous, this may eventually lead to the collapse of the gel, resulting in retinal detachment. Not all patients with Stickler syndrome show linkage to COL2A1 (119,128), and present estimates suggest that less than half of families have mutations in type II collagen (128). Recently, Stickler syndrome was split into three types (Online Mendelian Inheritance in Man #108300). Type 1 Stickler syndrome involves mutations in type II collagen as described above, whereas type 2 involves mutations in the α1(XI) chain (118,119,129,130). Type 3 involves mutations in the α2(XI) chain, and patients with this condition present with a Stickler-like phenotype but without eye involvement (131–133). This is the predicted result, because the vitreous does not contain the α2(XI) chain, which is replaced by the α2(V) chain. However, there are also patients in whom mutations in α1(II), α1(XI), and α2(XI) cannot be found, suggesting the presence of at least one additional locus for Stickler syndrome. It also has been suggested that milder forms of chondrodysplasia may present clinically as a familial and premature form of osteoarthritis that involves mutations in type II collagen (134,135). In extensive investigations, mutations of type II collagen specifically involving $arg^{519} \rightarrow$ cys and $arg^{75} \rightarrow$ cys were found to give rise to early onset osteoarthritis with a mild chondrodysplasia in several unrelated families (135). Even though results from some linkage and association studies have suggested COL2A1 as a locus for generalized osteoarthritis (136–138), COL2A1 is unlikely to be a major susceptibility locus (139,140).

Animal Models of Diseases Arising from Mutations in Type II Collagen

Several transgenic mice have been obtained that either overexpress type II procollagen molecules that are truncated in the triple helix (141) or contain specific mutations or deletions at different sites in the triple helix (142). In general, the phenotype of these animals resembles a relatively mild chondrodysplasia with (a) disorganized growth plates, (b) shorter limbs with a poorly organized cartilage matrix containing thick collagen fibrils, and (c) chondrocytes with a greatly expanded rough endoplasmic reticulum. More recently, knockout mice have been obtained for type II collagen, and, as expected, the heterozygotes showed a relatively mild phenotype with a disorganized growth plate and mild chondrodysplasia (143,144). The homozygotes died *in utero*. The transgenic and knockout mice are likely to provide good models for the human chondrodysplasias caused by various mutations in COL2A1.

Type III Collagen

Mutations in COL3A1 form the biochemical basis of a rare clinical condition called Ehlers-Danlos syndrome type IV (EDS IV), which involves the skin, blood vessels, colon, and rupture of the gravid uterus (2,103) (see also Chapter 96). These tissues all contain a high proportion of type III collagen, and, in the same manner as OI, mutations with clinical consequences involve (a) replacement of glycine residues in the triple helix, (b) exon-skipping mutations, or (c) multiple exon deletions often accompanied by a failure to secrete normal amounts of type III procollagen. EDS IV is inherited in an autosomal-dominant fashion so that mutated molecules have a dominant negative effect on triple-helical formation, secretion, and subsequent fibril formation. The collagen fibrils in tissues are smaller and lack organization, and, often, fibroblastic cells are observed with extended rough endoplasmic reticulum. It has been suggested that there may be clinical overlap between EDS IV and familial aortic aneurysms such that both will involve mutations in type III collagen (145). Extensive investigation involving DNA sequencing of type III procollagen from many unrelated patients showed that mutations in COL3A1 are the likely cause of only 2% of aortic aneurysms (146). Interestingly, in mice in which the type III collagen gene has been inactivated, the primary cause of death is rupture of the major blood vessels (147).

Type V/XI Collagen

Although members of this family of collagens are considered to play key functions in the organization of connective tissues (25), it is only recently that the phenotypic consequences of mutations in these chains have begun to be described. Several mutations have now been described in both COL5A1 (148–151) and COL5A2 (152) that give rise to EDS type I or type II. EDS type I is characterized by marked skin hyperextensibility, joint laxity, and complications related to tissue fragility and joint laxity, such as hernias and joint dislocations (103). EDS type II is similar to type I but milder. These findings are complemented by experiments with transgenic mice in which an abnormal α2(V) collagen chain was expressed as a result of homologous recombination. Morphologic analysis of these mice revealed disorganized collagen fibrils in a variety of tissues (153).

Even though types V and XI collagens are structurally related and the α chains of types V and XI collagens can replace each other, type V collagen is mainly found in tissues that express type I collagen, such as skin, bone, tendon, and ligament. Type XI collagen mainly resides in tissues that express type II collagen, such as hyaline cartilage and the vitreous of the eye. For this reason, mutations in the COL11A1 and COL11A2 genes result in similar phenotypes as COL2A1 mutations. Dominant negative mutations in COL11A1 can cause type II Stickler syndrome as discussed above (119,128–130). Splicing mutations, which involve 54-bp exons in the 3′ half of the gene, result in a related phenotype designated Marshall syndrome (119). Patients with Marshall syndrome usually have more pronounced hearing problems and less severe eye findings than patients with Stickler syndrome. Interestingly, as mentioned before, families with Stickler-like syndrome, but without eye involvement, were found to have mutations in COL11A2 (131–133). Otospondylomegaepiphyseal dysplasia (OSMED) represents the severe end of the COL11A2 mutation spectrum (131, 154). The clinical findings consist of sensorineural hearing loss, enlarged epiphyses, disproportionate shortness of the limbs, abnormalities in the vertebral bodies, and typical facial features, including midface hypoplasia with a short upturned nose, depressed nasal bridge, and small mandible and cleft palate. OSMED is a recessive disorder, and most of the mutations lead to loss of function of COL11A2 (154). Surprisingly, COL11A2 haploinsufficiency does not result in a phenotype. The phenotype of Col11a2 knockout mice was similar to that of nonocular Stickler syndrome and OSMED, in that the mice had small body sizes, receding snouts, and deafness (155). Nonsyndromic hearing loss represents the mild end of the spectrum of diseases caused by COL11A2 mutations. Two large families, presenting with only nonsyndromic sensorineural hearing loss (DFNA13), have been described with heterozygous missense mutations in the COL11A2 gene (156).

The clinical phenotypes are most likely explained by the effect of the mutations either on fibril formation, fibril diameter, or fibril-fibril interactions. This is supported by findings from *in vitro* fibril formation studies (31), as well as Col11a2 knockout mice (155) and *cho* mice, which both have disorganized fibrils in the cartilage matrix with the presence of some very thick fibrils. The phenotype of the *cho* mice is known to arise from a premature stop codon in Col11a1 (157).

NONFIBRILLAR COLLAGENS

A wide variety of different collagen types cannot form staggered fibrils characteristic of the interstitial collagens (1,6,158). Their structure and chromosomal localizations are described in Table 9.3 with appropriate references. It is not possible to describe the known properties of all of these collagens; interested readers are directed to the references provided in this table. Only those nonfibrillar collagens specifically located in cartilage will be discussed further.

Fibril-Associated Collagens

Several members of this family have been described, including types IX, XII, and XIV collagens (1,159) (Fig. 9.7).

TABLE 9.3. *Molecular organization of nonfibrillar collagens*

Type	Chain	Molecular organization	Gene	Chromosomal localization	Occurrence	References
FACIT (fibril-associated collagen with interrupted triple-helix) and FACIT-like						
IX	α1(IX)	α1(IX) α2(IX) α3(IX)	COL9A1	6q13	Cartilage, vitreous	159
	α2(IX)		COL9A2	1p34.2		
	α3(IX)		COL9A3	20q13.33		
XII	α1(XII)	$[\alpha1(XII)]_3$	COL12A1	6q13	Widespread	158
XIV	α1(XIV)	$[\alpha1(XIV)]_3$	COL14A1	8q24.12	Widespread	158
XVI	α1(XVI)		COL16A1	1p35.2	Fibroblasts, keratinocytes	160
XIX	α1(XIX)		COL19A1	6q13		161, 162
XX	α1(XX)		COL20A1	20q13.33		163
XXI	α1(XXI)		COL21A1	6p12.1		164–166
XXII	α1(XXII)		COL22A1	8q24.23		167
Basement membrane						
IV	α1(IV)	$[\alpha1(IV)]_2\ \alpha2(IV)$	COL4A1	13q34	All basement membranes	168
	α2(IV)		COL4A2	13q34	All basement membranes	
	α3(IV)	α3(IV) α4(IV) α5(IV)	COL4A3	2q36.3	Glomerular basement membrane	
	α4(IV)		COL4A4	2q36.3	Glomerular basement membrane	
	α5(IV)		COL4A5	Xq22.3	Glomerular basement membrane	
	α6(IV)		COL4A6	Xq22.3	Bowman's capsule/distal tubule	

Continued

TABLE 9.3. *Continued*

Type	Chain	Molecular organization	Gene	Chromosomal localization	Occurrence	References
Short chain						
VIII	α1(VIII)	[α1(VIII)]$_3$	COL8A1	3q12.1	Descemet's membrane, blood vessel endothelium	1
	α2(VIII)	[α2(VIII)]$_3$	COL8A2	1p34.3		
X	α1(X)	[α1(X)]$_3$	COL10A1	6q22.1	Hypertrophic cartilage	1
Microfibril						
VI	α1(VI)	α1(VI) α2(VI) α3(VI)	COL6A1	21q22.3	Most tissues	1,169
	α2(VI)	(other combinations?)	COL6A2	21q22.3		
	α3(VI)		COL6A3	2q37.3		
Epithelium-associated						
VII		[α1(VII)]$_3$	COL7A1	3p21.31	Anchoring fibrils	1
XVII		[α1(XVII)]$_3$	COL17A1	10q25.1	Hemidesmosome-associated	1
Multiplexin						
XV			COL15A1	9q22.33	Widespread	8
XVIII			COL18A1	21q22.3	Liver, kidney, placenta	8, 9, 170
Transmembrane						
XIII			COL13A1	10q22	Widespread	6
XXIII	α1(XXIII)		COL23A1	5q35.3	Prostate tumor cells	6, 171
XXV	α1(XXV)		COL25A1	4q25	Amyloid plaques	6, 172
Other						
XXVI[a]	α1(XXVI)		COL26A1	7q22.1	Ovary, testis	173, 174

[a]Type XXVI is also called emu2 (173); a closely related gene called emu1 (174) has also been described.
All chromosome locations were derived from the following website: http://*www.cse.ucsc.edu/~kent/*.

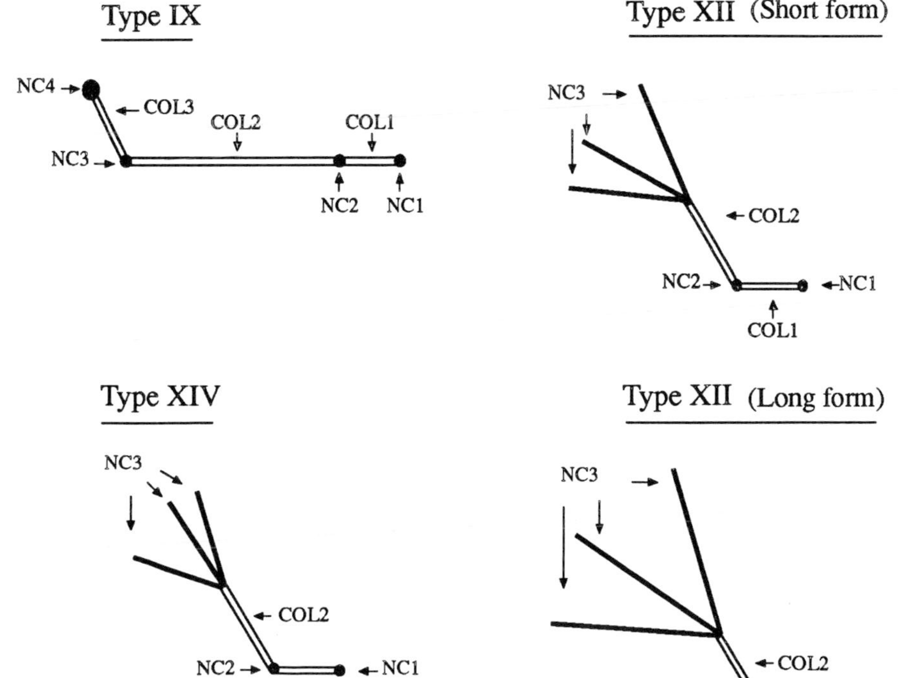

FIG. 9.7. Models to show the structure of types IX, XII, and XIV collagens. Type IX contains three collagenous domains (COL1–COL3) and four noncollagenous domains (NC1–NC4). Types XII and XIV share similar COL1 domains but have longer NC3 domains. The short- form and long- form of type XII arise from differential splicing (see reference 158).

Additionally, types XVI, XIX, XX, XXI, and XXII collagens share common structural motifs with these collagens and may also be members of the FACIT family. Types XX, XXI, and XXII collagens have not been extensively investigated. However, type XVI appears to be located close to microfibrils and collagen fibrils (160), and type XIX is apparently concentrated at basement membrane zones (161,162).

Type IX Collagen

As shown in Fig. 9.7, this molecule consists of three collagenous domains (COL1 → COL3) and four noncollagenous domains (NC1 → NC4) that are numbered from the carboxy-terminus. It is assembled from three different chains to give a single molecule with a chain organization of α1(IX) α2(IX) α3(IX). In many tissues, including hyaline cartilage, a single chondroitin sulfate chain is located at the NC3 domain of the α2(IX) chain (26). Additionally, the use of an alternative promoter can give rise to two variants of the α1(IX) chain in which the NC4 domain is present or absent. Type IX collagen molecules in hyaline and articular cartilage largely consist of the longer form of the molecule (26). Rotary shadowing observations of collagen fibrils from embryonic chicken hyaline cartilage clearly show that molecules of type IX collagen are associated with the surface of fibrils (Figs. 9.8 and 9.9). Additionally, analyses of the location of lysine-derived cross-links between types IX and II collagens strongly suggest that type IX molecules are organized antiparallel to type II collagen (175,176) as shown in Fig. 9.9. Type IX collagen therefore provides a mechanism for potentially limiting fibril diameter in hyaline cartilage or for the interaction of fibrils with other extracellular matrix components. The NC4 domains, which project away from the surface of the fibrils, might potentially interact with other molecules of cartilage matrix, including proteoglycans (177,178).

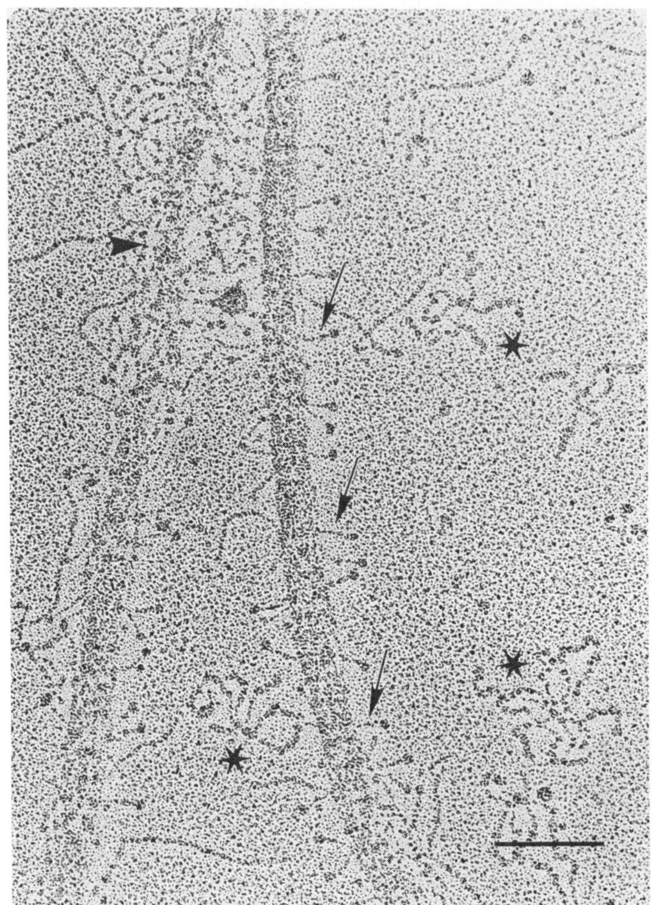

FIG. 9.8. Rotary shadowing of a collagen fibril from hyaline cartilage to show the location of type IX collagen (*arrows*) on the surface of the fibrils such that the COL3 and NC4 domains (see Fig. 9.7) project away from the surface. Also note the presence of numerous molecules of tenascin in the preparation (*stars*) and that one fibril is slightly unraveled (*arrowhead*). Bar = 100 nm. (Reproduced by permission from Vaughan L, Mendler M, Huber S, et al. D-periodic distribution of collagen type IX along cartilage fibrils. *J Cell Biol* 1988;106:991–997, by permission.)

It seems likely that type IX collagen plays only a subtle role in the organization of cartilage matrix, since the knockout of the α1(IX) chain did not result in detectable developmental changes in homozygous mice (179). Instead, in later life, the mice developed degeneration of their articular cartilage in a manner resembling human osteoarthritis and could therefore serve as a good model for studying this disease. Subsequent studies using these mice showed that lack of α1(IX) could not be compensated for and resulted in the failure to form an intact type IX collagen molecule (180). In a form of human chondrodysplasia designated multiple epiphyseal dysplasia (MED), mutations were identified in the COL3 domain of the α1(IX), α2(IX), and α3(IX) chains (181–187). However, not all patients with MED have mutations in type IX collagen. Linkage of this condition, as well as the related pseudoachondroplasia, to chromosome 19 occurs with mutations being identified in cartilage oligomeric matrix protein (COMP) (188). It was recently demonstrated that mutations in the MATN3 gene that encodes for matrilin 3 could also cause MED (188). In addition, mutations in the solute carrier member 26, member 2 gene (SLC26A2), have been found in patients who have a recessively inherited form of MED (189).

The role of type IX collagen in maintaining tissue integrity is also supported by recent findings that two amino acid substitutions, Gln326Trp in the α2(IX) chain and Arg103Trp in the α3(IX) chain, predispose to a common musculoskeletal disorder, intervertebral disc disease, which is characterized by sciatica, disc herniation, and degeneration (190–192).

Types VIII and X Collagens

For type VIII collagen, two chains designated α1(VIII) and α2(VIII) have been identified and found to be closely related in structure and sequence to the α1(X) chain of type X collagen (193). Each molecule of type VIII or X collagen consists

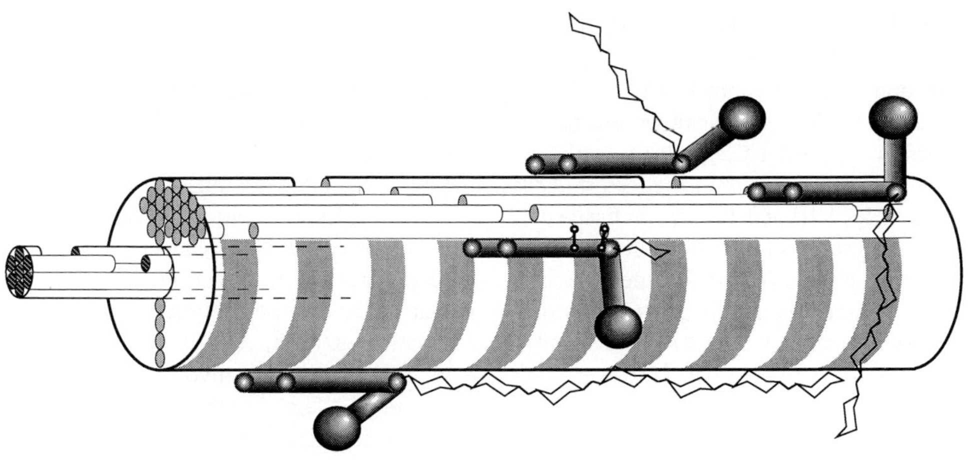

FIG. 9.9. Model for the structure of a collagen fibril from embryonic chick cartilage. Note the presence of numerous type IX molecules on the surface of the fibril, which are organized in an antiparallel manner to the type II molecules and have a single chondroitin sulfate chain attached to the NC3 domain (see Fig. 9.7). (Reproduced by permission from Bruckner P, van der Rest M. Structure and function of cartilage collagens. *Microscop Res Tech* 1994;28:378–384, by permission.)

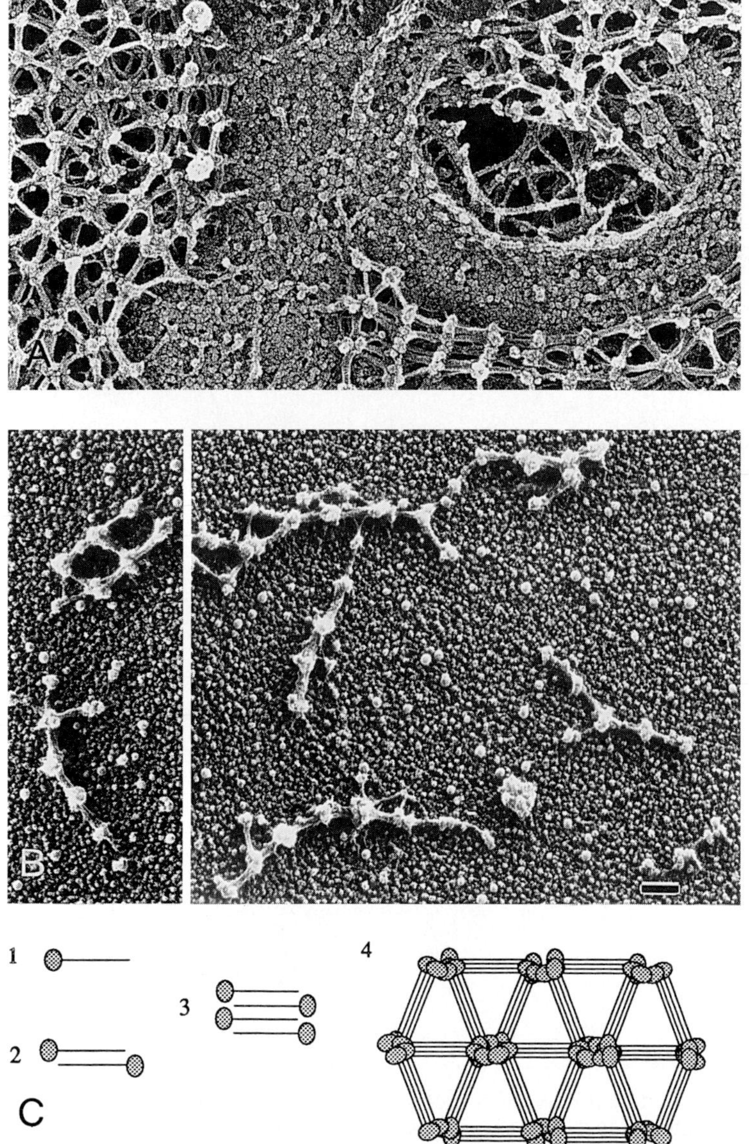

FIG. 9.10. A. Freeze-etch replica view of hexagonal lattices formed from type VIII collagen by bovine corneal endothelial cells in cell culture in the presence of β-aminopropionitrile (see reference 194). Bar = 100 nm. **B:** Freeze- etch replica of a 1-day culture in which an early stage of lattice production is shown. Bar = 100 nm. **C:** Potential antiparallel assembly of individual type VIII molecules. *1,* monomer; *2,* dimer; *3,* tetramer; *4,* hexagonal lattice.

of a short collagenous domain approximately half the length of the interstitial collagens with noncollagenous extensions both at the amino-terminus (called NC2) and the carboxy-terminus (called NC1). They are therefore called short-chain collagens, and although types VIII and X differ in tissue distribution, they are thought to serve similar functions.

Type VIII is a major constituent of Descemet membrane of the corneal endothelium, where it is considered to be a structural component of the hexagonal lattice observed in electron micrographs of the tissue (194) (Fig. 9.10). However, type VIII is widely distributed in different tissues and is prominently found in blood vessels, where it is synthesized by both smooth muscle and endothelial cells (195). Disease-causing mutations have been recently found in the COL8A2 gene in familial and sporadic cases of Fuchs endothelial corneal dystrophy and posterior polymorphous corneal dystrophy (196).

Type X collagen is uniquely found in hypertrophic cartilage (Fig. 9.11) where it is the major collagen that is synthesized and may form a temporary scaffold for the matrix (197). Although hexagonal-like structures have been observed for isolated type X collagen after rotary shadowing (198), a similar organization has not been clearly demonstrated in hypertrophic cartilage *in vivo* (discussed further in reference 197). Instead, it appears from electron microscopic immunolocalization that type X forms pericellular mats and is also closely associated with the fibrils of type II collagen (197). Other studies have suggested that type X collagen may be involved in the calcification of hypertrophic cartilage, but this has not been clearly demonstrated. In articular cartilage, type X collagen is detected at the calcification front and in the calcified zone, whereas synthesis of type X collagen in osteoarthritic cartilage is detected in some cells above the tidemark (199–201). It appears from these and other studies performed with cultures of embryonic chick chondrocytes (202) that all chondrocytes have the potential to undergo hypertrophy and initiate the synthe-

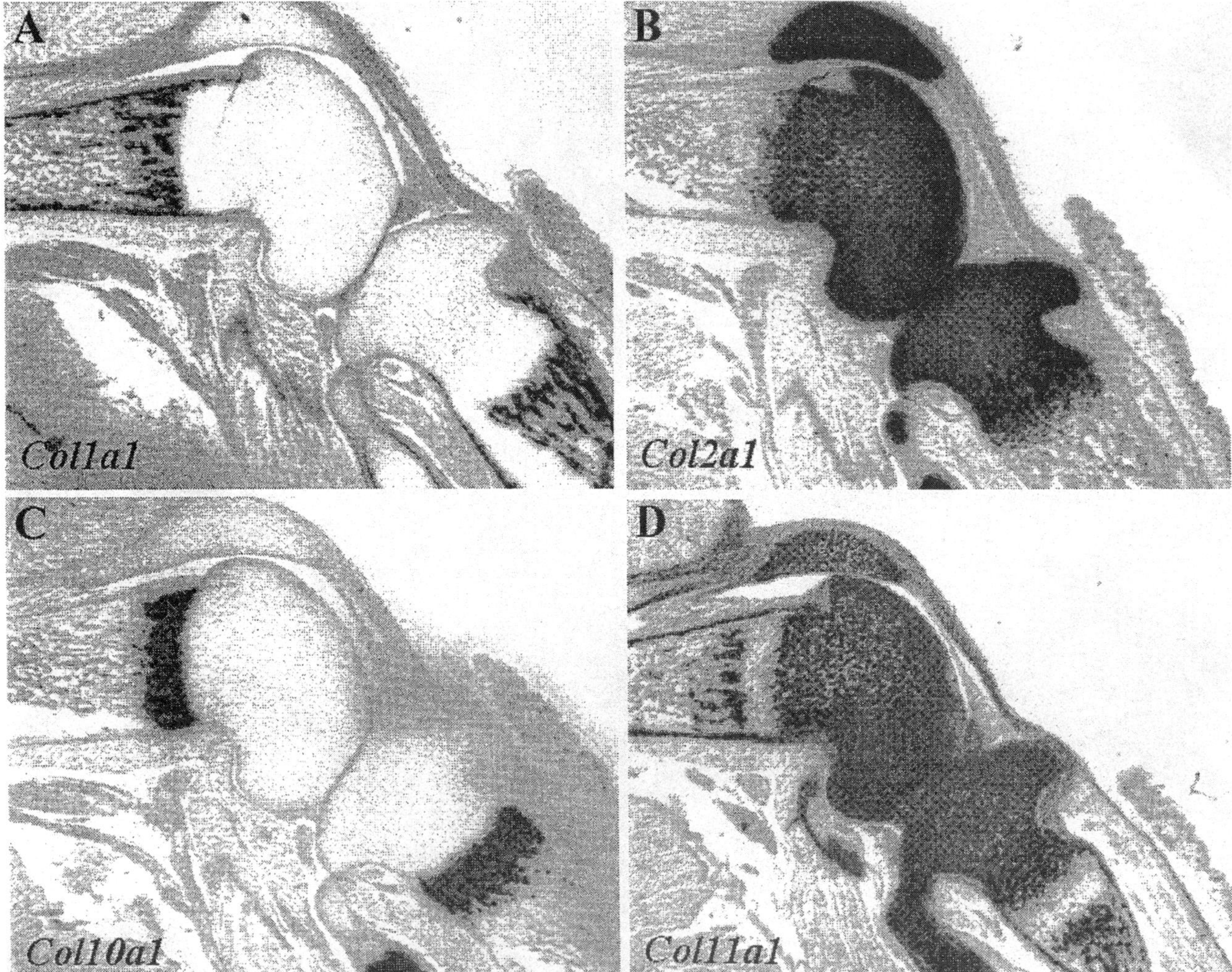

FIG. 9.11. *In situ* hybridization of the hind knee joint of a new born mouse. **A:** Col1a1. **B:** Col2a1. **C:** Col10a1. **D:** Col11a1. Note the contrast in distribution of Col1a1 (bone and tendon) and Col2a1 (cartilage). Also note that Col10a1 is found specifically in hypertrophic cartilage where expression of Col11a1 is missing. Interestingly, expression of Col11a1 can be detected in both cartilage and bone.

sis of type X collagen regardless of whether this ever occurs *in vivo*.

Mutations in the human α1(X) gene result in Schmid metaphyseal chondrodysplasia (203,204). These mutations almost exclusively arise at sites in the noncollagenous carboxy-terminus (NC1 domain) that are required for initiation of the assembly of the three chains prior to triple helix formation (204). It appears that strong hydrophobic interactions play a key role in the recognition process (205). If the three chains cannot associate correctly, then the formation of the triple helix does not occur. Thus, it is believed that expression of mutated type X chains in heterozygotes has a dominant negative effect and results in a clinically distinct chondrodystrophy. These results suggest that type X collagen plays a key role in the structure of hypertrophic cartilage, and it was therefore surprising that a knockout of type X collagen resulted in normal or modest effects on long bone growth in mice (206,207). The most likely explanation is that the dominant negative effect is created by overexpression of incompletely folded molecules in the rough endoplasmic reticulum (208,209). Such molecules are targeted by chaperones for removal but may also accumulate and interfere with the normal secretion of other macromolecules required for growth of hypertrophic cartilage. With a knockout or null mutation of type X collagen, this does not occur. This hypothesis, however, has been questioned recently. It was demonstrated that at least in some patients with premature translation termination codon mutations, the mutant mRNAs were subjected to complete nonsense-mediated mRNA decay in chondrocytes, resulting in haploinsufficiency (210).

Type VI Collagen

Type VI collagen assembles in a unique manner to form microfibrils that are located between the larger collagen fibrils of most tissues (211). The Type VI collagen microfibrils differ from the elastin microfibrils, which are also found in most connective tissues. The latter are usually present as bundles and appear to be involved in the deposition of elastin (212).

The initial model for the structure of type VI microfibrils was largely derived from rotary shadowing observations of isolated monomers, dimers, and tetramers (Fig. 9.12).

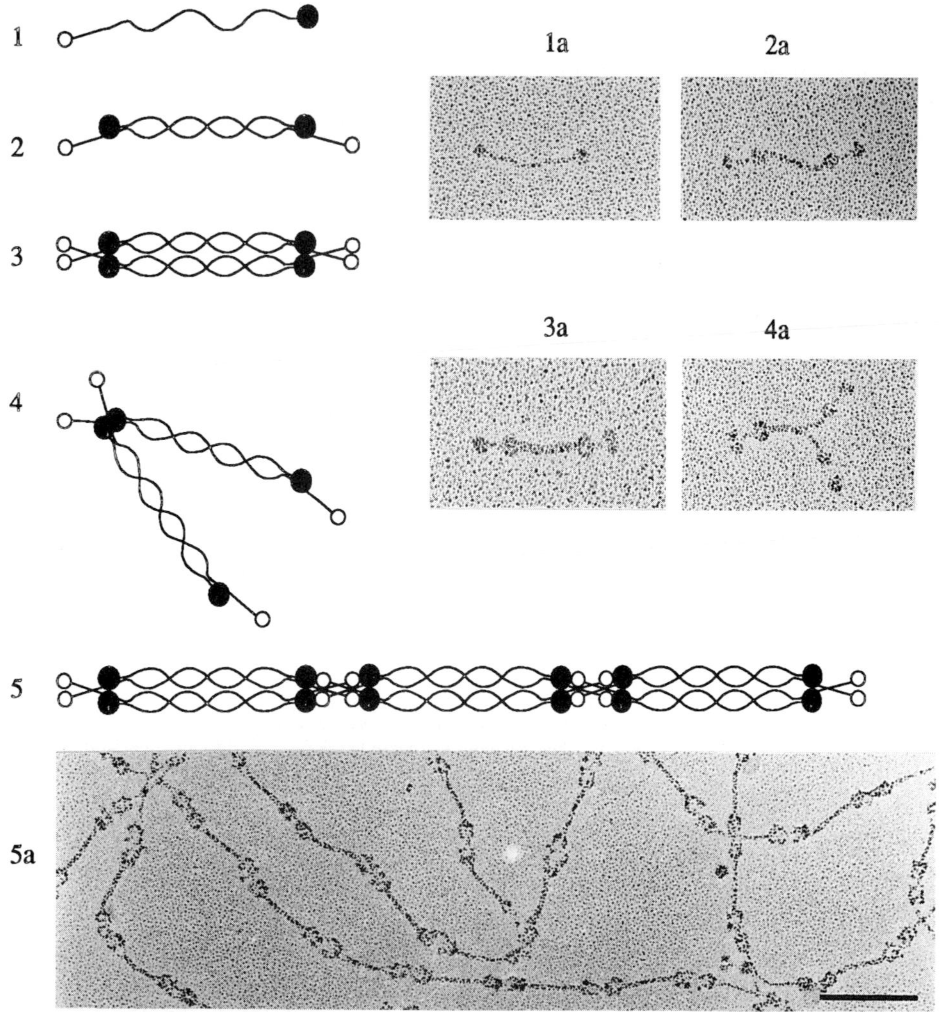

FIG. 9.12. Organization of fibrils of type VI collagen. Panels 1 and 1a show a monomer both diagrammatically and after rotary shadowing. Panels 2 and 2a show a dimer. This subsequently forms tetramers that may be completely associated, (3 and 3a) or only partially associated (4 and 4a). The tetramers are secreted from the cell and associate end to end to form a fibril (5 and 5a). (Rotary shadowing in 5a is reproduced by permission from Kielty C, Whittaker SP, Grant ME, et al. Type VI collagen microfibrils: evidence for a structural association with hyaluronan. *J Cell Biol* 1992;118:979–990.)

Each molecule appears to be assembled from three different chains called α1(VI), α2(VI), and α3(VI), and two molecules are assembled in an antiparallel arrangement, as shown in Fig. 9.12. Finally, a tetramer is formed within the cell followed by secretion and end-to-end association of tetramers to form the microfibrils, which possess a characteristic appearance after rotary shadowing (Fig. 9.12). Remarkably, type VI collagen does not contain lysine-derived cross-links, and depolymerization to tetramers occurs in acidic conditions (212). Despite extensive investigation, the function of the type VI microfibril is still not clearly understood. Molecular cloning of the three chains has provided detailed structural information and shown that the α3(VI) chain is much longer than the other chains, with noncollagenous domains at both the amino-termini and carboxy-termini (211,213). Binding of type VI microfibrils to interstitial collagen fibrils, hyaluronan, and type IV collagen may all occur (214,215). In addition, a membrane-associated chondroitin sulfate proteoglycan called NG2 is also reported to interact with type VI collagen (216). In articular cartilage, numerous fibrils of type VI collagen have a unique pericellular location around the chondrocytes. The general conclusion from all these studies is that type VI collagen may act as a bridging molecule between the cell surface and the collagen fibrils of the extracellular matrix. Although type VI collagen is found in most connective tissues, the only genetic diseases associated with the molecule are rare forms of muscular dystrophies, dominantly inherited Bethlem myopathy (217,218), and Ullrich syndrome, a recessive disorder (219). Mice in which the Col6a1 gene has been inactivated by targeted gene disruption also show only a myopathy involving fiber necrosis and phagocytosis and are considered to be good animal models for the myopathies (220).

SUMMARY

Many different collagenous molecules have now been described that can self-assemble into a variety of structures. The newly identified collagens do not form fibrils of classic morphology, but, rather, they form a variety of other structures in which the collagen triple helix provides stability. Each collagen chain undergoes a series of post-translational processing events that must be completed successfully before secretion can occur. For the assembly of a macromolecular structure, further processing events may also be necessary. It might be anticipated that a wide variety of human genetic diseases would result from mutations in the different collagen types. It is now clearly established that many, and often rare, genetic disorders of connective tissues involve mutations in the different collagen types. However, careful examination of more common disorders that possess a familial component such as osteoporosis, aortic aneurysms, and osteoarthritis has consistently failed to show extensive involvement of mutated collagens.

ACKNOWLEDGMENTS

We thank Ionut Radu for his assistance in the preparation of this manuscript. We also thank David Birk, Barbara Brodsky, Peter Bruckner, Rachel Kramer, Hajime Sawada, Masamine Takanosu, Rupert Timpl, Michel van der Rest, Lloyd Vaughan, and Hanna Wiedemann for contributing drawings, electron micrographs, and results from *in situ* hybridization. This article is dedicated to the memory of Rupert Timpl.

REFERENCES

1. Kielty CM, Grant ME. The collagen family: structure, assembly, and organization in the extracellular matrix. In: *Connective tissue and its heritable disorders*. New York: Wiley-Liss, 2002:159–221.
2. Myllyharju J, Kivirikko KI. Collagens and collagen-related diseases. *Ann Med* 2001;33:7–21.
3. Rasmussen M, Jacobsson M, Björck L. Genome-based identification and analysis of collagen-related structural motifs in bacterial and viral proteins. *J Biol Chem* 2003;278:32313–32316.
4. Exposito J, Cluzel C, Garrone R, et al. Evolution of collagens. *Anat Rec* 2002;268:302–316.
5. Boot-Hanford RP, Tuckwell DS. Fibrillar collagen: the key to vertebrate evolution? A tale of molecular incest. *Bioessays* 2003;25:142–151.
6. Franzke C, Tasanen K, Schumann H, et al. Collagenous transmembrane proteins: collagen XVII as a prototype. *Matrix Biol* 2003;22:299–309.
7. Shaw LM, Olsen BR. FACIT collagens: diverse molecular bridges in extracellular matrices. *Trends Biochem Sci* 1991;16:191–194.
8. Rehn M, Pihlajaniemi T. Type XV and XVIII collagens, a new subgroup within the family of collagens. *Semin Cell Dev Biol* 1996;7:673–679.
9. Zatterstrom UK, Felbor U, Fukai N, et al. Collagen XVIII/endostatin structure and functional role in angiogenesis. *Cell Struct Funct* 2000;25:97–101.
10. Myers JC, Dion AS, Abraham V, et al. Type XV collagen exhibits a widespread distribution in human tissues but a distinct localization in basement membrane zones. *Cell Tissue Res* 1996;286:493–505.
11. Halfter W, Dong S, Schurer B, et al. Collagen XVIII is a basement membrane heparan sulfate proteoglycan. *J Biol Chem* 1998;273:25404–25412.
12. Tomono Y, Naito I, Ando K, et al. Epitope-defined monoclonal antibodies against multiplexin collagens demonstrate that type XV and XVIII collagens are expressed in specialized basement membranes. *Cell Struct Funct* 2002;27:9–20.
13. Miosge N, Simniok T, Sprysch P, et al. The collagen type XVIII endostatin domain is co-localized with perlecan in basement membranes *in vivo*. *J Histochem Cytochem* 2003;51:285–296.
14. Oh SP, Warman ML, Seldin MF, et al. Cloning of cDNA and genomic DNA encoding human type XVII collagen and localization of the alpha1(XVIII) collagen gene to mouse chromosome 10 and human chromosome 21. *Genomics* 1994;19:494–499.
15. Piez KA. Molecular and aggregate structures of the collagens. In: Piez KA, Reddi AH, eds. *Extracellular matrix biochemistry*. New York: Elsevier, 1984:1–39.
16. Knight CG, Morton LF, Peachey AR, et al. The collagen-binding A-domains of integrins alpha(1)beta(1) and alpha(2)beta(1) recognize the same specific amino acid sequence GFOGER, in native (triple-helical) collagens. *J Biol Chem* 2000;275:35–40.
17. Emsley J, Knight CG, Farndale RW, et al. Structural basis of collagen recognition by integrin $\alpha_2\beta_1$. *Cell* 2000;101:47–56.
18. Berisio R, Vitagliano L, Mazzarella L, et al. Crystal structure of a collagen-like polypeptide with repeating sequence pro-hyp-gly at 1.4Å resolution: implications for collagen hydration. *Biopolymers* 2001;56:8–13.
19. Berisio R, Vitagliano L, Mazzarella L, et al. Recent progress on collagen triple helix structure, stability, and assembly. *Protein Pept Lett* 2002;9:107–116.
20. Bella J, Eaton M, Brodsky B, et al. Crystal and molecular structure of a collagen-like peptide at 1.9Å resolution. *Science* 1994;266:75–81.

21. Baum J, Brodsky B. Folding of peptide models of collagen and misfolding in disease. *Curr Opin Struct Biol* 1999;9:122–128.
22. Lauer-Fields JL, Sritharan T, Stack MS, et al. Selective hydrolysis of triple-helical substrates by matrix metalloproteinase-2 and -9. *J Biol Chem* 2003;278:18140–18145.
23. Holmgren SK, Taylor KM, Bretscher LE, et al. Code for collagen's stability deciphered. *Nature* 1998;392:666–667.
24. Hulmes DJS. Building collagen molecules, fibrils, and suprafibrillar structures. *J Struct Biol* 2002;137:2–10.
25. Fichard A, Kleman J-P, Ruggiero F. Another look at collagen V and XI molecules. *Matrix Biol* 1994;14:515–531.
26. Brewton RG, Mayne R. Heterotypic type II, IX, and XI fibrils: comparison of vitreous and cartilage forms. In: Yurchenco PD, Birk DE, Mecham RP, eds. *Extracellular matrix assembly and structure*. San Diego: Academic, 1994:129–170.
27. Koch M, Laub F, Zhou P, et al. Collagen XXIV, a vertebrate fibrillar collagen with structural features of invertebrate collagens: selective expression in developing cornea and bone. *J Biol Chem* 2003;278: 43236–43244.
28. Pace JM, Corrado M, Missero C, et al. Identification, characterization, and expression analysis of a new fibrillar collagen gene, COL27A1. *Matrix Biol* 2003;22:3–14.
29. Boot-Handford RP, Tuckwell DS, Plumb DA, et al. A novel and highly conserved collagen [proα1(XXVII)] with a unique expression pattern and unusual molecular characteristics establishes a new clade within the vertebrate fibrillar collagen family. *J Biol Chem* 2003;278:31067–31077.
30. Mendler M, Eich-Bender SG, Vaughan L, et al. Cartilage contains mixed fibrils of collagen types II, IX, and XI. *J Cell Biol* 1989;108: 191–197.
31. Blaschke UK, Eikenberry EF, Hulmes DJ, et al. Collagen XI nucleates self-assembly and limits lateral growth of cartilage fibrils. *J Biol Chem* 2000;275:10370–10378.
32. Eyre DR, Wu JJ, Apone S. A growing family of collagens in articular cartilage: identification of 5 genetically distinct types. *J Rheumatol* 1987;14(suppl 14):25–27.
33. Notbohm H, Nokelainen M, Myllyharju J, et al. Recombinant human type II collagens with low and high levels of hydroxylysine and its glycosylated forms show marked differences in fibrillogenesis *in vitro*. *J Biol Chem* 1999;274:8988–8992.
34. McLaughlin JS, Linsenmayer TF, Birk DE. Type V collagen synthesis and deposition by chicken embryo corneal fibroblasts in vitro. *J Cell Sci* 1989;94:371–379.
35. Marchant JK, Hahn RA, Linsenmayer TF, et al. Reduction of type V collagen using a dominant-negative strategy alters the regulation of fibrillogenesis and results in the loss of corneal-specific fibril morphology. *J Cell Biol* 1996;135:1415–1426.
36. Sandell LJ, Boyd CD. Conserved and divergent sequence and functional elements within collagen genes. In: Sandell LJ, Boyd CD, eds. *Extracellular matrix genes*. San Diego: Academic, 1990:1–56.
37. Yamada Y, Avvedimento VE, Mudryj M, et al. The collagen gene: evidence for its evolutionary assembly by amplification of a DNA segment containing an exon of 54 bp. *Cell* 1980;22:887–892.
38. Ninomiya Y, Gordon M, van der Rest M, et al. The developmentally regulated type X collagen gene contains a long open reading frame without introns. *J Biol Chem* 1986;261:5041–5050.
39. Rossert J, de Crombrugghe B. Type I collagen: structure, synthesis, and regulation. In: *Principles of bone biology,* 2nd ed. San Diego: Academic, 2002:189–210.
40. Kalajzic I, Kalajzic Z, Kaliterna M, et al. Use of type I collagen green fluorescent protein transgenes to identify subpopulations of cells at different stages of the osteoblast lineage. *J Bone Miner Res* 2002;17: 15–25.
41. Dacquin R, Starbuck M, Schinke T, et al. Mouse α1(I)-collagen promoter is the best known promoter to drive efficient Cre recombinase expression in osteoblast. *Dev Dyn* 2002;224:245–251.
42. Riquet FB, Tan L, Choy BK, et al. YY1 is a positive regulator of transcription of the *Col1a1* gene. *J Biol Chem* 2001;276:38665–38672.
43. Sokolov B, Ala-Kokko L, Dhulipala R, et al. Tissue-specific expression of the gene for type I procollagen (COL1A1) in transgenic mice. *J Biol Chem* 1995;270:9622–9629.
44. Terraz C, Brideau G, Ronco P, et al. A combination of *cis*-acting elements is required to activate the pro-α1(I) collagen promoter in tendon fibroblasts of transgenic mice. *J Biol Chem* 2002;277:19019–19026.
45. Terraz C, Toman D, Delauche M, et al. δEF1 binds to a far upstream sequence of the mouse pro-α1(I) collagen gene and represses its expression in osteoblasts. *J Biol Chem* 2001;276:37011–37019.
46. Antoniv TT, De Val S, Wells D, et al. Characterization of an evolutionary conserved far-upstream enhancer in the human α2(I) collagen (COL1A2) gene. *J Biol Chem* 2001;276:21754–21764.
47. De Val S, Ponticos M, Antoniv TT, et al. Identification of the key regions within the mouse *pro-α2(I)* collagen gene far-upstream enhancer. *J Biol Chem* 2002;277:9286–9292.
48. Zhang W, Ou J, Inagaki Y, et al. Synergistic cooperation between Sp1 and Smad3/Smad4 mediates transforming growth factor β1 stimulation of α2(I)-collagen (COL1A2) transcription. *J Biol Chem* 2000; 275:39237–39245.
49. Poncelet A-C, Schnaper HW. Sp1 and Smad proteins cooperate to mediate transforming growth factor-β1-induced α2(I) collagen expression in human glomerular mesangial cells. *J Biol Chem* 2001; 276:6983–6992.
50. Ramirez F, Rifkin DB. Cell signaling events: a view from the matrix. *Matrix Biol* 2003;22:101–107.
51. Cutroneo KR. How is type I procollagen synthesis regulated at the gene level during tissue fibrosis. *J Cell Biochem* 2003;90:1–5.
52. Lefebvre V, Huang W, Harley VR, et al. SOX9 is a potent activator of the chondrocyte-specific enhancer of the pro a1(II) collagen gene. *Mol Cell Biol* 1997;17:2336–2346.
53. Bridgewater LC, Walker MD, Miller GC, et al. Adjacent DNA sequences modulate Sox9 transcriptional activation at paired Sox sites in three chondrocyte-specific enhancer elements. *Nucleic Acids Res* 2003;31:1541–1553.
54. Lefebvre V, Li P, de Crombrugghe B. A new long form of Sox5 (L-Sox5), Sox6, and Sox9 are coexpressed in chondrogenesis and cooperatively activate the type II collagen gene. *EMBO J* 1998;17: 5718–5733.
55. Bi W, Deng JM, Zhang Z, et al. Sox9 is required for cartilage formation. *Nat Genet* 1999;22:85–89.
56. Akiyama H, Chaboissier MC, Martin JF, et al. The transcription factor Sox9 has essential roles in successive steps of the chondrocyte differentiation pathway and is required for expression of Sox5 and Sox6. *Genes Dev* 2002;16:2813–2828.
57. Shen M, Yoshida E, Yan W, et al. Basic helix-loop-helix protein DEC1 promotes chondrocyte differentiation at the early and terminal stages. *J Biol Chem* 2002;277:50112–50120.
58. Huang W, Lu N, Eberspaecher H, et al. A new long form of c-Maf cooperates with Sox9 to activate the type II collagen gene. *J Biol Chem* 2002;277:50668–50675.
59. Tsuda M, Takahashi S, Takahashi Y, et al. Transcriptional co-activators CREB-binding protein and p300 regulate chondrocyte-specific gene expression via association with Sox9. *J Biol Chem* 2003;278: 27224–27229.
60. Seki K, Fujimori T, Savagner P, et al. Mouse *Snail* family transcription repressors regulate chondrocyte, extracellular matrix, type II collagen, and aggrecan. *J Biol Chem* 2003;278:41862–41870.
61. Stephens DJ, Pepperkok R. Imaging of procollagen transport reveals COPI-dependent cargo sorting during ER-to-Golgi transport in mammalian cells. *J Cell Sci* 2002;115:1149–1160.
62. Mironov AA, Mironov AA Jr, Beznoussenko GV, et al. ER-to-Golgi carriers arise through direct en bloc protrusion and multistage maturation of specialized ER exit domains. *Dev Cell* 2003;5:583–594.
63. Birk DE, Silver FH, Trelstad RL. Matrix assembly. In: Hay ED, ed. *Cell biology of extracellular matrix,* 2nd ed. New York: Plenum, 1991: 221–254.
64. Bonfanti L, Mironov AA Jr, Martínez-Menárguez JA, et al. Procollagen traverses the Golgi stack without leaving the lumen of cisternae: evidence for cisternal maturation. *Cell* 1998;95:993–2003.
65. Mironov AA, Beznoussenko GV, Nicoziani P, et al. Small cargo proteins and large aggregates can traverse the Golgi by a common mechanism without leaving the lumen of cisternae. *J Cell Biol* 2001;155:1225–1238.
66. Wilson R, Lees JF, Bulleid NJ. Protein disulfide isomerase acts as a molecular chaperone during the assembly of procollagen. *J Biol Chem* 1998;273:9637–9643.
67. Chessler SD, Byers PH. BiP binds type I procollagen proα chains with mutations in the carboxyl-terminal propeptide synthesized by cells from patients with osteogenesis imperfecta. *J Biol Chem* 1993;268: 18226–18233.
68. Lamandé SR, Chessler, SD, Golub SB, et al. Endoplasmic reticulum-mediated quality control of type I collagen production by cells from

osteogenesis imperfecta patients with mutations in the proα1(I) chain carboxyl-terminal propeptide which impair subunit assembly. *J Biol Chem* 1995;270:8642–8649.
69. Bottomley MJ, Batten MR, Lumb RA, et al. Quality control in the endoplasmic reticulum: PDI mediates the ER retention of unassembled procollagen C-propeptides. *Curr Biol* 2001;11:1114–1118.
70. Nagata K. Hsp47: a collagen-specific molecular chaperone. *Trends Biochem Sci* 1996;21:22–26.
71. Tasab M, Batten MR, Bulleid NJ. Hsp47: a molecular chaperone that interacts with and stabilizes correctly-folded procollagen. *EMBO J* 2000;19:2204–2211.
72. Hendershot LM, Bulleid NJ. Protein-specific chaperones: the role of hsp47 begins to gel. *Curr Biol* 2000;10:R912–R915.
73. Tasab M, Jenkinson L, Bulleid NJ. Sequence-specific recognition of collagen triple helices by the collagen-specific molecular chaperone hsp47. *J Biol Chem* 2002;277:35007–35012.
74. Koide T, Takahara Y, Asada S, et al. Xaa-arg-gly triplets in the collagen triple helix are dominant binding sites for the molecular chaperone hsp47. *J Biol Chem* 2002;277:6178–6182.
75. Macdonald JR, Bachinger HP. Hsp47 binds cooperatively to triple helical type I collagen but has little effect on the thermal stability or rate of refolding. *J Biol Chem* 2001;276:25399–25403.
76. Dafforn TR, Della M, Miller AD. The molecular interactions of heat shock protein 47 (hsp47) and their implications for collagen biosynthesis. *J Biol Chem* 2001;276:49310–49319.
77. Vertel BM, Velasco A, LaFrance S, et al. Precursors of chondroitin sulfate proteoglycan are segregated within a subcompartment of the chondrocyte endoplasmic reticulum. *J Cell Biol* 1989;109:1827–1836.
78. Iozzo RV, Pacifici M. Ultrastructural localization of the major proteoglycan and type II collagen in organelles and extracellular matrix of cultured chondroblasts. *Histochemistry* 1986;86:113–122.
79. Birk DE, Linsenmayer TF. Collagen fibril assembly, deposition, and organization into tissue specific matrices. In: Yurchenco PD, Birk DE, Mecham RP, eds. *Extracellular matrix assembly and structure*. San Diego: Academic, 1994:91–128.
80. Canty EG, Kadler KE. Collagen fibril biosynthesis in tendon: a review and recent insights. *Comp Biochem Physiol* 2002;133:979–985.
81. Prockop DJ, Sieron AL, Li SW. Procollagen N-proteinase and procollagen C-proteinase. Two unusual metalloproteinases that are essential for procollagen processing probably have important roles in development and cell signaling. *Matrix Biol* 1997/98;16:399–408.
82. Kessler E, Takahara K, Biniaminov L, et al. Bone morphogenetic protein-1: the type I procollagen C-proteinase. *Science* 1996;271:360–362.
83. Lee S, Solow-Cordero DE, Kessler E, et al. Transforming growth factor-β regulation of bone morphogenetic protein-1/procollagen C-proteinase and related proteins in fibrogenic cells and keratinocytes. *J Biol Chem* 1997;272:19059–19066.
84. Pappano WN, Steiglitz BM, Scott IC, et al. Use of Bmp1/Tll1 doubly homozygous null mice and proteomics to identify and validate *in vivo* substrates of bone morphogenetic protein 1/tolloid-like metalloproteinases. *Mol Cell Biol* 2003;23:4428–4438.
85. Sieron AL, Tretiakova A, Jameson BA, et al. Structure and function of procollagen C-proteinase (mTolloid) domains determined by protease digestion, circular dichroism, binding to procollagen type I, and computer modeling. *Biochemistry* 2000;39:3231–3239.
86. Hartigan N, Garrigue-Antar L, Kadler KE. Bone morphogenetic protein-1 (BMP-1): identification of the minimal domain structure for procollagen C-proteinase activity. *J Biol Chem* 2003;278:18045–18049.
87. Colige A, Sieron AL, Li SW, et al. Human Ehlers-Danlos syndrome type VII C and bovine dermatosparaxis are caused by mutations in the procollagen I N-proteinase gene. *Am J Hum Genet* 1999;65:308–317.
88. Wang WM, Lee S, Steiglitz BM, et al. Transforming growth factor-β induces secretion of activated ADAMTS-2. *J Biol Chem* 2003;278:19549–19557.
89. Rattenholl A, Pappano WN, Koch M, et al. Proteinases of the bone morphogenetic protein-1 family convert procollagen VII to mature anchoring fibril collagen. *J Biol Chem* 2002;277:26372–26378.
90. Unsöld C, Pappano WN, Imamura Y, et al. Biosynthetic processing of the pro-α1(V)$_2$pro-α2(V) collagen heterotrimer by bone morphogenetic protein-1 and furin-like proprotein convertases. *J Biol Chem* 2002;277:5596–5602.
91. Veitch DP, Nokelainen P, McGowan KA, et al. Mammalian tolloid metalloproteinase, and not matrix metalloprotease 2 or membrane type I metalloprotease, processes laminin-5 in keratinocytes and skin. *J Biol Chem* 2003;278:15661–15668.
92. Scott IC, Imamura Y, Pappano WN, et al. Bone morphogenetic protein-1 processes probiglycan. *J Biol Chem* 2000;275:30504–30511.
93. Ruggeri A, Motta PM, eds. In: *Ultrastructure of the connective tissue matrix*. Boston: Kluwer, 1984.
94. Linsenmayer TF, Gibney E, Igoe F, et al. Type V collagen: molecular structure and fibrillar organization of the chicken α1(V) NH2-terminal domain, a putative regulator of corneal fibrillogenesis. *J Cell Biol* 1993;121:1181–1189.
95. Bailey AJ. Molecular mechanisms of ageing in connective tissues. *Mech Ageing Dev* 2001;122:735–755.
96. Gustafsson E, Fassler R. Insights into extracellular matrix functions from mutant mouse models. *Exp Cell Res* 2000;261:52–68.
97. Prockop DJ, Kivirikko KI. Collagens: molecular biology, diseases, and potentials for therapy. *Annu Rev Biochem* 1995;64:403–434.
98. Byers PH, Cole WG. Osteogenesis imperfecta. In: Royce PM, Steinmann B, eds. *Connective tissue and its heritable disorders*, 2nd ed. New York: Wiley-Liss, 2002:385–430.
99. Vogel BE, Doelz R, Kadler KE, et al. A substitution of cysteine for glycine 748 of the α1 chain produces a kink at this site in the procollagen I molecule and an altered N-proteinase cleavage site over 225nm away. *J Biol Chem* 1988;263:19249–19255.
100. Kadler KE, Torre-Blanco A, Adachi E, et al. A type I collagen with substitution of a cysteine for glycine-748 in the α1(I) chain copolymerizes with normal type I collagen and can generate fractal-like structures. *Biochemistry* 1991;30:5081–5088.
101. Torre-Blanco A, Adachi E, Romanic AM, et al. Copolymerization of normal type I collagen with three mutated type I collagens containing substitutions of cysteine at different glycine positions in the α1(I) chain. *J Biol Chem* 1992;267:4968–4973.
102. Starman BJ, Eyre D, Charbonneau H, et al. Osteogenesis imperfecta. The position of substitution for glycine by cysteine in the triple helical domain of the proα1(I) chains of type I collagen determines the clinical phenotype. *J Clin Invest* 1989;84:1206–1214.
103. Byers PH. Mutations in collagen genes: biochemical and phenotypic consequences. In: Sandell LJ, Boyd CD, eds. *Extracellular matrix genes*. San Diego: Academic, 1990:251–263.
104. Shapiro JR, Stover ML, Burn VE, et al. An osteopenic nonfracture syndrome with features of mild osteogenesis imperfecta associated with the substitution of a cysteine for glycine at triple helix position 43 in the proα1(I) chain of type I collagen. *J Clin Invest* 1992;89:567–573.
105. Lightfoot SJ, Holmes DF, Brass A, et al. Type I procollagens containing substitutions of aspartate, arginine, and cysteine for glycine in the proα1(I) chain are cleaved slowly by N-Proteinase, but only the cysteine substitution introduces a kink in the molecule. *J Biol Chem* 1992;267:25521–25528.
106. Spotila LD, Colige A, Sereda L, et al. Mutation analysis of coding sequences for type I procollagen in individuals with low bone density. *J Bone Miner Res* 1994;9:923–932.
107. Grant SF, Reid DM, Blake G, et al. Reduced bone density and osteoporosis associated with a polymorphic Sp1 binding site in the collagen type I alpha 1 gene. *Nat Genet* 1996;14:203–205.
108. Langdahl BL, Ralston SH, Grant SF, et al. An Sp1 binding site polymorphism in the COL1A1 gene predicts osteoporotic fractures in both men and women. *J Bone Miner Res* 1998;13:1384–1389.
109. Mann V, Hobson EE, Li B, et al. A COL1A1 Sp1 binding site polymorphism predisposes to osteoporotic fracture by affecting bone density and quality. *J Clin Invest* 2001;107:899–907.
110. Steinmann B, Royce PM, Superti-Furga A. The Ehlers-Danlos syndrome. In: Royce PM, Steinmann B, eds. *Connective tissue and its heritable disorders*, 2nd ed. New York: Wiley-Liss, 2002:431–523.
111. Hyland J, Ala-Kokko L, Royce P, et al. A homozygous stop codon in the lysyl hydroxylase gene in two siblings with Ehlers-Danlos syndrome type VI. *Nat Genet* 1992;2:228–231.
112. Chipman SD, Sweet HO, McBride DJ Jr, et al. Defective proα2(I) collagen synthesis in a recessive mutation in mice: a model of human osteogenesis imperfecta. *Proc Natl Acad Sci U S A* 1993;90:1701–1705.
113. Nicholls AC, Osse G, Schloon HG, et al. The clinical features of homozygous alpha 2(I) collagen deficient osteogenesis imperfecta. *J Med Genet* 1984;21:257–262.
114. Khillan JS, Olsen AS, Kontusaari S, et al. Transgenic mice that express a mini-gene version of the human gene for type I procollagen

(COL1A1) develop a phenotype resembling a lethal form of osteogenesis imperfecta. *J Biol Chem* 1991;266:23373–23379.
115. Pereira R, Halford K, Sokolov B, et al. Phenotypic variability and incomplete penetrance of spontaneous fractures in an inbred strain of transgenic mice expressing a mutated collagen gene (COL1A1). *J Clin Invest* 1994;93:1765–1769.
116. Vikkula M, Metsäranta M, Ala-Kokko L. Type II collagen mutations in rare and common cartilage diseases. *Ann Med* 1994;26:107–114.
117. Mundlos S, Olsen BR. Heritable diseases of the skeleton. Part II: Molecular insights into skeletal development-matrix components and their homeostasis. *FASEB J* 1997;11:227–233.
118. Horton WA, Hecht JT. Chondrodysplasias: disorders of cartilage matrix proteins. In: Royce PM, Steinmann B, eds. *Connective tissue and its heritable disorders,* 2nd ed. New York: Wiley-Liss, 2002:909– 937.
119. Annunen S, Körkkö J, Czarny M, et al. Splicing mutations of 54 bp exons in the COL11A1 gene cause Marshall syndrome but other mutations cause overlapping Marshall/Stickler phenotypes. *Am J Hum Genet* 1999;65:974–983.
120. Richards AJ, Martin S, Yates JR, et al. COL2A1 exon 2 mutations: relevance to the Stickler and Wagner syndromes. *Br J Ophthalmol* 2000;84:364–371.
121. Donoso LA, Edwards AO, Frost AT, et al. Identification of a stop codon mutation in exon 2 of the collagen 2A1 gene in a large stickler syndrome family. *Am J Ophthalmol* 2002;134:720–727.
122. Parma ES, Korkko J, Hagler WS, et al. Radial perivascular retinal degeneration: a key to the clinical diagnosis of an ocular variant of Stickler syndrome with minimal or no systemic manifestations. *Am J Ophthalmol* 2002;134:728–734.
123. Ryan MC, Sandell LJ. Differential expression of a cysteine-rich domain in the amino-terminal propeptide of type II (cartilage) procollagen by alternative splicing of mRNA. *J Biol Chem* 1990;265: 10334–10339.
124. Sandell LJ, Nalin AM, Reife RA. Alternative splice form of type II procollagen mRNA (IIA) is predominant in skeletal precursors and non-cartilaginous tissues during early mouse development. *Dev Dyn* 1994;199:129–140.
125. Lui VC, Ng LJ, Nicholls J, et al. Tissue-specific and differential expression of alternatively spliced alpha 1(II) collagen mRNAs in early human embryos. *Dev Dyn* 1995;203:198–211.
126. Reardon A, Sandell L, Jones CJ, et al. Localization of pN-type IIA procollagen on adult bovine vitreous collagen fibrils. *Matrix Biol* 2000;19:169–173.
127. Bishop PN, Reardon AJ, McLeod D, et al. Identification of alternatively spliced variants of type II procollagen in vitreous. *Biochem Biophys Res Commun* 1994;203:289–295.
128. Snead MP, Payne SJ, Barton DE. Stickler syndrome: correlation between vitreoretinal phenotypes and linkage to COL2A1. *Eye* 1994;8: 609–614.
129. Richards AJ, Yates JRW, Williams R, et al. A family with Stickler syndrome type 2 has a mutation in the COL11A1 gene resulting in the substitution of glycine 97 by valine in α1(XI) collagen. *Hum Mol Genet* 1996;5:1339–1343.
130. Griffith AJ, Sprunger LK, Sirko-Osadsa DA, et al. Marshall syndrome associated with a splicing defect at the COL11A1 locus. *Am J Hum Genet* 1998;62:816–823.
131. Vikkula M, Mariman ECM, Lui VCH, et al. Autosomal dominant and recessive osteochondrodysplasias associated with the COL11A2 locus. *Cell* 1995;80:431–437.
132. Sirko-Osadsa DA, Murray MA, Scott JA, et al. Stickler syndrome without eye involvement is caused by mutations in COL11A2, the gene encoding the α2(XI) chain of type XI collagen. *J Pediatr* 1998; 132:368–371.
133. Pihlajamaa T, Prockop DJ, Faber J, et al. Heterozygous glycine substitution in the COL11A2 gene in the original patient with the Weissenbacher-Zweymüller syndrome demonstrates its identity with heterozygous (OSMED) (Nonocular Stickler Syndrome). *Am J Med Genet* 1998;80:115–120.
134. Prockop DJ, Ala-Kokko L, McLain DA, et al. Can mutated genes cause common osteoarthritis? *Br J Rheumatol* 1997;36:827–830.
135. Holderbaum D, Haqqi TM, Moskowitz RW. Genetics and osteoarthritis: exposing the iceberg. *Arthritis Rheum* 1999;42:397–405.
136. Palotie A, Vaisanen P, Ott J, et al. Predisposition to familial osteoarthrosis linked to type II collagen gene. *Lancet* 1989;1:924–927.
137. Loughlin J, Irven C, Athanasou N, et al. Differential allelic expression of the type II collagen gene (COL2A1) in osteoarthritic cartilage. *Am J Hum Genet* 1995;56:1186–1193.
138. Meulenbelt I, Bijkerk C, De Wildt SC, et al. Haplotype analysis of three polymorphisms of the COL2A1 gene and associations with generalised radiological osteoarthritis. *Ann Hum Genet* 1999;63:393–400.
139. Loughlin J, Irven C, Fergusson C, et al. Sibling pair analysis shows no linkage of generalized osteoarthritis to the loci encoding type II collagen, cartilage link protein or cartilage matrix protein. *Br J Rheumatol* 1994;33:1103–1106.
140. Ritvaniemi P, Korkko J, Bonaventure J, et al. Identification of COL2A1 gene mutations in patients with chondrodysplasias and familial osteoarthritis. *Arthritis Rheum* 1995;38:999–1004.
141. Helminen H, Kiraly K, Pelttari A, et al. An inbred line of transgenic mice expressing an internally deleted gene for type II procollagen (COL2A1). *J Clin Invest* 1993;92:582–595.
142. De Crombrugghe B, Katzenstein P, Mukhopadhyay K, et al. Transgenic mice with deficiencies in cartilage collagens: possible models for gene therapy. *J Rheumatol* 1995;22(suppl 43):140–142.
143. Li S-W, Prockop DJ, Helminen H, et al. Transgenic mice with targeted inactivation of the Col2a1 gene for collagen II develop a skeleton with membranous and periosteal bone but no endochondral bone. *Genes Dev* 1995;9:2821–2830.
144. Aszódi A, Chan D, Hunziker E, et al. Collagen II is essential for the removal of the notochord and the formation of intervertebral discs. *J Cell Biol* 1998;143:1399–1412.
145. Kuivaniemi H, Tromp G, Prockop DJ. Genetic causes of aortic aneurysms. *J Clin Invest* 1991;88:1441–1444.
146. Tromp G, Wu Y, Prockop DJ, et al. Sequencing of cDNA from 50 unrelated patients reveals that mutations in the triple-helical domain of type III procollagen are an infrequent cause of aortic aneurysms. *J Clin Invest* 1993;91:2539–2545.
147. Liu X, Wu H, Byrne M, et al. Type III collagen is crucial for collagen I fibrillogenesis and for normal cardiovascular development. *Proc Natl Acad Sci U S A* 1997;94:1852–1856.
148. Toriello HV, Glover TW, Takahara K, et al. A translocation interrupts the *COL5A1* gene in a patient with Ehlers-Danlos syndrome and hypomelanosis of Ito. *Nat Genet* 1996;13:361–365.
149. Wenstrup RJ, Langland GT, Willing, MC, et al. A splice-junction mutation in the region of *COL5A1* that codes for the carboxyl propeptide of pro α1(V) chains results in the *gravis* form of the Ehlers-Danlos syndrome (type I). *Hum Mol Genet* 1996;5:1733–1736.
150. De Paepe A, Nuytinck L, Hausser I, et al. Mutations in the COL5A1 gene are causal in the Ehlers-Danlos syndromes I and II. *Am J Hum Genet* 1997;60:547–554.
151. Burrows NP, Nicholls AC, Richards AJ, et al. A point mutation in an intronic branch site results in aberrant splicing of COL5A1 and in Ehlers-Danlos syndrome type II in two British families. *Am J Hum Genet* 1998;63:390–398.
152. Michalickova K, Susic M, Willing MC, et al. Mutations of the α2(V) chain of type V collagen impair matrix assembly and produce Ehlers-Danlos syndrome type I. *Hum Mol Genet* 1998;7:249–255.
153. Andrikopoulos K, Liu X, Keene DR, et al. Targeted mutation in the col5a2 gene reveals a regulatory role for type V collagen during matrix assembly. *Nat Genet* 1995;9:31–36.
154. Melkoniemi M, Brunner HG, Manouvrier S, et al. Autosomal recessive disorder otospondylomegaepiphyseal dysplasia is associated with loss-of-function mutations in the COL11A2 gene. *Am J Hum Genet* 2000;66:368–377.
155. Li SW, Takanosu M, Arita M, et al. Targeted disruption of Col11a2 produces a mild cartilage phenotype in transgenic mice: comparison with the human disorder otospondylomegaepiphyseal dysplasia (OSMED). *Dev Dyn* 2001;222:141–152.
156. McGuirt WT, Prasad SD, Griffith AJ, et al. Mutations in COL11A2 cause non-syndromic hearing loss (DFNA13). *Nat Genet* 1999;23: 413–419.
157. Li Y, Lacerda DA, Warman ML, et al. A fibrillar collagen gene, Col11a1, is essential for skeletal morphogenesis. *Cell* 1995;80:423–430.
158. Ricard-Blum S, Dublet B, van der Rest M. In: Sheterline P, ed. *Unconventional collagens: types VI, VII, VIII, IX, X, XII, XIV, XVI and XIX.* Oxford, UK: Oxford University Press, 2000.
159. Olsen BR. Collagen IX. *Int J Biochem Cell Biol* 1997;29:555–558.

160. Kassner A, Hansen U, Miosge N, et al. Discrete integration of collagen XVI into tissue-specific collagen fibrils or beaded microfibrils. *Matrix Biol* 2002;22:131–143.
161. Myers JC, Li D, Bageris A, et al. Biochemical and immunohistochemical characterization of human type XIX defines a novel class of basement membrane zone collagens. *Am J Pathol* 1997;151:1729– 1740.
162. Myers JC, Li D, Amenta PS, et al. Type XIX collagen purified from human umbilical cord is characterized by multiple sharp kinks delineating collagenous subdomains and by intermolecular aggregates via globular, disulfide-linked, and heparin-binding amino termini. *J Biol Chem* 2003;278:32047–32057.
163. Koch M, Foley JE, Hahn R, et al. α1(XX) collagen, a new member of the collagen subfamily, fibril-associated collagens with interrupted triple helices. *J Biol Chem* 2001;276:23120–23126.
164. Fitzgerald J, Bateman JF. A new FACIT of the collagen family: COL21A1. *FEBS Lett* 2001;505:275–280.
165. Tuckwell D. Identification and analysis of collagen α1(XXI), a novel member of the FACIT collagen family. *Matrix Biol* 2002;21:63–66.
166. Chou M-Y, Li H-C. Genomic organization and characterization of the human type XXI collagen (*COL21A1*) gene. *Genomics* 2002;79: 395–401.
167. Koch M, Jin W, Ashworth T, et al. Alpha 1(XXII) collagen, a new member of the collagen subfamily. *NCBI Sequence Viewer* 2001. *www.ncbi.nlm.nih.gov/.*
168. Hudson BG, Tryggvason K, Sundaramoorthy M, et al. Alport's syndrome, Goodpasture's syndrome, and type IV collagen. *N Engl J Med* 2003;348:2543–2556.
169. Timpl R, Chu M-L. Microfibrillar collagen type VI. In: Yurchenco PD, Birk DE, Mecham RP, eds. *Extracellular matrix assembly and structure*. San Diego: Academic, 1994:207–242.
170. Sertie AL, Sossi V, Camargo AA, et al. Collagen XVIII, containing an endogenous inhibitor of angiogenesis and tumor growth, plays a critical role in the maintenance of retinal structure and in neural tube closure (Knobloch syndrome). *Hum Mol Genet* 2000;9:2051–2058.
171. Banyard J, Bao L, Zetter BR. Type XXIII collagen, a new transmembrane collagen identified in metastatic tumor cells. *J Biol Chem* 2003;278:20989–20994.
172. Hashimoto T, Wakabayashi T, Watanabe A, et al. CLAC: a novel Alzheimer amyloid plaque component derived from a transmembrane precursor, CLAC-P/collagen type XXV. *EMBO J* 2002;21: 1524–1534.
173. Sato K, Yomogida K, Wada T, et al. Type XXVI collagen, a new member of the collagen family, is specifically expressed in the testis and ovary. *J Biol Chem* 2002;277:37678–37684.
174. Leimeister C, Steidl C, Schumacher N, et al. Developmental expression and biochemical characterization of emu family members. *Dev Biol* 2002;249:204–218.
175. Wu JJ, Woods PE, Eyre DR. Identification of cross-linking sites in bovine cartilage type IX collagen reveals an antiparallel type II-type IX molecular relationship and type IX to type IX bonding. *J Biol Chem* 1992;267:23007–23014.
176. Eyre DR, Pietka T, Weis MA, et al. Covalent cross-linking of the NC1 domain of collagen type IX to collagen type II in cartilage. *J Biol Chem* 2004;279:2568–2574.
177. Vaughan L, Mendler M, Huber S, et al. D-periodic distribution of collagen type IX along cartilage fibrils. *J Cell Biol* 1988;106:991– 997.
178. Pihlajamaa T, Perälä M, Vuoristo MM, et al. Characterization of recombinant human type IX collagen. *J Biol Chem* 1999;274:22464–22468.
179. Fässler R, Schnegelsberg PNJ, Dausman J, et al. Mice lacking α1(IX) collagen develop noninflammatory degenerative joint disease. *Proc Natl Acad Sci U S A* 1994;91:5070–5074.
180. Hagg R, Hedbom E, Möllers U, et al. Absence of the α1(IX) chain leads to a functional knock-out of the entire collagen IX protein in mice. *J Biol Chem* 1997;272:20650–20654.
181. Muragaki Y, Mariman ECM, van Beersum SEC, et al. A mutation in the gene encoding the α2 chain of the fibril-associated collagen IX, COL9A2, causes multiple epiphyseal dysplasia (EDM2). *Nat Genet* 1996;12:103–105.
182. Holden P, Canty EG, Mortier GR, et al. Identification of novel pro-α2(IX) collagen gene mutations in two families with distinctive oligo-epiphyseal forms of multiple epiphyseal dysplasia. *Am J Hum Genet* 1999;65:31–38.
183. Paassilta P, Lohiniva J, Annunen S, et al. *COL9A3*: a third locus for multiple epiphyseal dysplasia. *Am J Hum Genet* 1999;64:1036– 1044.
184. Bonnemann CG, Cox GF, Shapiro F, et al. A mutation in the alpha 3 chain of type IX collagen causes autosomal dominant multiple epiphyseal dysplasia with mild myopathy. *Proc Natl Acad Sci U S A* 2000;97:1212–1217.
185. Lohiniva J, Paassilta P, Seppanen U, et al. Splicing mutations in the COL3 domain of collagen IX cause multiple epiphyseal dysplasia. *Am J Med Genet* 2000;90:216–222.
186. Spayde EC, Joshi AP, Wilcox WR, et al. Exon skipping mutation in the COL9A2 gene in a family with multiple epiphyseal dysplasia. *Matrix Biol* 2000;19:121–128.
187. Czarny-Ratajczak M, Lohiniva J, Rogala P, et al. A mutation in COL9A1 causes multiple epiphyseal dysplasia: further evidence for locus heterogeneity. *Am J Hum Genet* 2001;69:969–980.
188. Briggs MD, Chapman KL. Pseudoachondroplasia and multiple epiphyseal dysplasia: mutation review, molecular interactions, and genotype to phenotype correlations. *Hum Mutat* 2002;19:465–478.
189. Superti-Furga A, Neumann L, Riebel T, et al. Recessively inherited multiple epiphyseal dysplasia with normal stature, club foot, and double layered patella caused by a DTDST mutation. *J Med Genet* 1999; 36:621–624.
190. Annunen S, Paassilta P, Lohiniva J, et al. An allele of COL9A2 associated with intervertebral disc disease. *Science* 1999;285:409–412.
191. Paassilta P, Lohiniva J, Gorin HH, et al. Identification of a novel common genetic risk factor for lumbar disk disease. *JAMA* 2001;285: 1843–1849.
192. Ala-Kokko L. Genetic risk factors for lumbar disc disease. *Ann Med* 2002;34:42–47.
193. Shuttleworth CA. Molecules in focus: type VIII collagen. *Int J Biochem Cell Biol* 1997;29:1145–1148.
194. Sawada H, Konomi H, Hirosawa K. Characterization of the collagen in the hexagonal lattice of Descemet's membrane: its relation to type VIII collagen. *J Cell Biol* 1990;110:219–227.
195. MacBeath JRE, Kielty CM, Shuttleworth CA. Type VIII collagen is a product of vascular smooth-muscle cells in development and disease. *Biochem J* 1996;319:993–998.
196. Biswas S, Munier FL, Yardley J, et al. Missense mutations in COL8A2, the gene encoding the alpha2 chain of type VIII collagen, cause two forms of corneal endothelial dystrophy. *Hum Mol Genet* 2001;10:2415–2423.
197. Linsenmayer TF, Long F, Nurminskaya M, et al. Type X collagen and other up-regulated components of the avian hypertrophic cartilage program. *Prog Nucleic Acid Res Mol Biol* 1998;60:79–109.
198. Kwan APL, Cummings CE, Chapman JA, et al. Macromolecular organization of chicken type X collagen *in vitro*. *J Cell Biol* 1991;114: 597–604.
199. Oegema TR, Thompson RC Jr. The zone of calcified cartilage: its role in osteoarthritis. In: Kuettner KE, ed. *Articular cartilage and osteoarthritis*. New York: Raven, 1992:319–331.
200. Hoyland JA, Thomas JT, Donn R, et al. Distribution of type X collagen mRNA in normal and osteoarthritic human cartilage. *Bone Miner* 1991;15:151–163.
201. Girkontaite I, Frischholz S, Lammi P, et al. Immunolocalization of type X collagen in normal fetal and adult osteoarthritic cartilage with monoclonal antibodies. *Matrix Biol* 1996;15:231–238.
202. Castagnola P, Dozin B, Moro G, et al. Changes in the expression of collagen genes show two stages in chondrocyte differentiation *in vitro*. *J Cell Biol* 1988;106:461–467.
203. Warman ML, Abbott M, Apte SS, et al. A type X collagen mutation causes Schmid metaphyseal chondrodysplasia. *Nat Genet* 1993;5: 79–82.
204. Chan D, Jacenko L. Phenotypic and biochemical consequences of collagen X mutations in mice and humans. *Matrix Biol* 1998;17:169–184.
205. Marks DS, Gregory CA, Wallis, GA, et al. Metaphyseal chondrodysplasia type Schmid mutations are predicted to occur in two distinct three-dimensional clusters within type X collagen NC1 domains that retain the ability to trimerize. *J Biol Chem* 1999;274:3632–3641.
206. Rosati R, Horan GSB, Pinero GJ, et al. Normal long bone growth and development in type X collagen-null mice. *Nat Genet* 1994;8:129– 135.
207. Kwan KM, Pang MKM, Zhou S, et al. Abnormal compartmentalization of cartilage matrix components in mice lacking collagen X: implications for function. *J Cell Biol* 1997;136:459–471.
208. Chan D, Freddi S, Weng YM, et al. Interaction of collagen α1(X) containing engineered NC1 mutations with normal α1(X) *in vitro*. *J Biol Chem* 1999;274:13091–13097.

209. Dublet B, Vernet T. van der Rest M. Schmid's metaphyseal chondrodysplasia mutations interfere with folding of the C-terminal domain of human collagen X expressed in *Escherichia coli*. *J Biol Chem* 1999;274:18909–18915.
210. Bateman JF, Freddi S, Nattrass G, et al. Tissue-specific RNA surveillance? Nonsense-mediated mRNA decay causes collagen X haploinsufficiency in Schmid metaphyseal chondrodysplasia cartilage. *Hum Mol Genet* 2003;12:217–225.
211. Kielty CM, Cummings C, Whittaker SP, et al. Isolation and ultrastructural analysis of microfibrillar structures from foetal bovine elastic tissues. *J Cell Sci* 1991;99:797–807.
212. Spissinger T, Engel J. Type VI collagen beaded microfibrils from bovine cornea depolymerize at acidic pH, and depolymerization and polymerization are not influenced by hyaluronan. *Matrix Biol* 1994; 14:499–505.
213. Baldock C, Sherratt MJ, Shuttleworth CA, et al. The supramolecular organization of collagen VI microfibrils. *J Mol Biol* 2003;330:297–307.
214. Keene DR, Ridgway CC, Iozzo RV. Type VI microfilaments interact with a specific region of banded collagen fibrils in skin. *J Histochem Cytochem* 1998;46:215–220.
215. Kuo H-J, Maslen CL, Keene DR, et al. Type VI collagen anchors endothelial basement membranes by interacting with type IV collagen. *J Biol Chem* 1997;272:26522–26529.
216. Burg MA, Tillet E, Timpl R, et al. Binding of the NG2 proteoglycan to type VI collagen and other extracellular matrix molecules. *J Biol Chem* 1996;271:26110–26116.
217. Jöbsis GJ, Keizers H, Vreijling JP, et al. Type VI collagen mutations in Bethlem myopathy, and autosomal dominant myopathy with contractures. *Nat Genet* 1996;14:113–115.
218. Lamandé SR, Bateman JF, Hutchison W, et al. Reduced collagen VI causes Bethlem myopathy: a heterozygous *COL6A1* nonsense mutation results in mRNA decay and functional haploinsufficiency. *Hum Mol Genet* 1998;7:981–989.
219. Camacho Vanegas O, Bertini E, Zhang RZ, et al. Ullrich scleroatonic muscular dystrophy is caused by recessive mutations in collagen type VI. *Proc Natl Acad Sci USA* 2001;98:7516–7521.
220. Bonaldo P, Braghetta P, Zanetti M, et al. Collagen VI deficiency induces early onset myopathy in the mouse: an animal model for Bethlem myopathy. *Hum Mol Genet* 1998;7:2135–2140.

CHAPTER 10

Structure, Function, and Metabolism of Cartilage Proteoglycans

Anne Woods

Cellular interactions with extracellular matrix regulate several basic biologic processes, including development, homeostasis, and disease. When different tissues are examined, such as bone, skin, or cartilage, it is evident that there is exquisite organization to generate a three-dimensional structure of cells and extracellular matrix that allows for the specialized function of differentiated tissues. Although this architecture may change during development and disease, several basic components remain in place. From the early days of microscopy, these were separated into those visible as fibers (collagens and elastic fibers) and those believed to be amorphous (ground substance, composed of structural glycoproteins and proteoglycans/glycosaminoglycans). However, more recent studies have indicated that most extracellular matrix components do have structure, and that this structure provides integrity to the tissue. In this chapter, the proteoglycans of cartilage will be described. Cartilage is unique, with its major function being to absorb pressure and act as a "shock absorber." In addition, cartilage and synovial fluid allow the two articular surfaces to move against each other without continual destruction. The properties of cartilage are dependent on the correct presence and amounts of their extracellular matrix components. In turn, this is dependent on the correct functioning of the chondrocytes within cartilage and the synoviocytes. Alterations in their homeostasis result in joint dysfunction, particularly the cartilage degradation seen in arthritis. In light of this, cartilage has been well studied. Many proteoglycans of both the extracellular matrix and the cell surface have been identified, together with some mechanisms of control of matrix synthesis, assembly, and degradation.

Proteoglycans consist of a protein core to which one or more glycosaminoglycan chains [chondroitin (CS), heparan (HS), dermatan (DS), or keratan sulfate (KS)] are covalently attached (1–5). The structures of these glycosaminoglycan chains are shown in Fig. 10.1. Proteoglycans are unusual because the long unbranched polysaccharide chains of the glycosaminoglycans often play a more significant role than their core proteins. Proteoglycans are present in most extracellular matrices, on cell surfaces, and in intracellular organelles in some cells (3–8). They are grouped into families on the basis of their core proteins (e.g., aggregating proteoglycans that bind hyaluronate), the transmembrane family of syndecans, the leucine-rich proteoglycans, and others (Table 10.1). To date, over 40 genes encoding proteoglycan core proteins have been identified. Some of these also exist as nonglycanated proteins, and have been termed "part-time" proteoglycans (e.g., betaglycan, which is also the type III transforming growth factor receptor).

The structures of proteoglycans are complex. They can vary by alteration of the number of glycosaminoglycan chains/core protein, and the type of glycosaminoglycan chain attached (HS, CS, DS, or KS). Synthesis of HS, CS, and DS proteoglycans begins by stepwise addition of xylose, galactose, and glucuronate residues to form a linkage tetrasaccharide at serine residues on the core protein, followed by the action of *N*-acetylglucosaminyltransferase (for HS) or *N*-acetylgalactosaminlytransferase (for CS). KS glycosaminoglycans are initiated by the addition of *N*-acetylglucosamine to serine or threonine (O-linked) or to asparagine (N-linked), and two types of stem structures link to the disaccharide repeats. The extent of chain elongation determines the length of the glycosaminoglycan. Even while chain elongation is continuing, existing monosaccharides are modified by interdependent enzymatic reactions. This results in variable degrees of epimerization, and variable levels of sulfation, as indicated in Fig. 10.1. Many of the enzymes involved in glycosaminoglycan synthesis and modification have now been cloned, and knockout technology is determining their crucial roles in development and disease

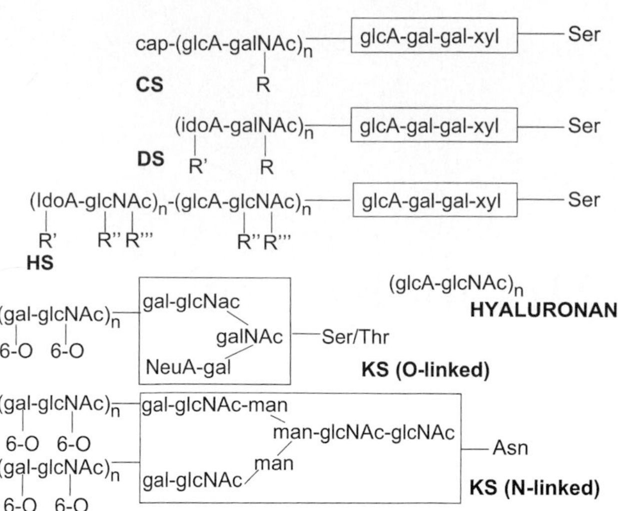

FIG. 10.1. Glycosaminoglycan structures. Stem structures attached to the core proteins are boxed. The structure of heparon sulfate (*HS*) disaccharides is variable and complex; the extent of sulfation and uronic acid epimerization varies along a single chain, but is tightly regulated. *Ser*, serine; *Thr*, threonine; *Asn*, asparagine; *xyl*, xylose; *gal*, galactose; *glcA*, glucuronic acid; *idoA*, iduronic acid; *galNAc*, *N*-acetyl galactosamine; *glcNAc*, *N*-acetyl glucosamine; *man*, mannose; *NeuA*, neuraminic acid; *R*, galNAc (may be unsulfated, 4- or 6-sulfated); *R′*, idoA (may be unsulfated or 2-sulfated); *R″*, glcNAc (may be 6-sulfated or, less commonly, 3-sulfated); *R‴*, glcNAc (may be *N*-sulfated, infrequently glucosamine residues may be present that are not *N*-acetylated); *6-O*, 6-O sulfation; KS, keratin sulfate; CS, chondroitin sulfate; cap, terminal 4,6-disulfated galactosamine residue.

(9–24). Two glycosyltransferases (EXT1 and EXT2) are putative tumor suppressors, particularly for cartilagenous tumors (18,19). Although progress is being made, there remains a lot to be learned concerning proteoglycan biology, particularly the regulated assembly of extracellular matrix, its homeostasis, and the degradation of cartilage during disease. The major proteoglycan in cartilage is aggrecan (25), the most abundant component of cartilage matrix. Aggrecan has a large core protein to which hundreds of glycosaminoglycan chains are attached. The glycosaminoglycan chains are mainly CS, but KS chains are also attached, and the

TABLE 10.1. *Cartilage proteoglycans*

Proteoglycan group	Examples
Aggregating (hyalectans)	Aggrecan, versican
Small leucine-rich (SLRPs)	Decorin, biglycan, epiphycan, chondroadherin, osteoadherin, opticin
Basement membrane	Perlecan
Cell surface	Syndecans 1–4, developmentally regulated
Others	SZP, lubricinj, PRG4

SZP, cartilage superficial zone protein/proteoglycan; PRG4, proteoglycan 4.

amounts of each type, their length and degree of sulfation have been shown to vary with mechanical loading, aging, and disease (26–38). The protein core of aggrecan interacts with hyaluronan, which is itself a glycosaminoglycan, and many aggrecan molecules bind to one hyaluronan chain. The association of aggrecan with hyaluronan is stabilized by a third component, link protein, which binds to both aggrecan core protein and hyaluronan (39–41). This results in a large molecular complex, termed the cartilage proteoglycan aggregate, which endows cartilage with its biophysical properties. Degradation of cartilage, particularly articular cartilage, occurs in several diseases [e.g., rheumatoid arthritis (RA) and osteoarthritis (OA)].

AGGRECAN: THE MAJOR PROTEOGLYCAN OF CARTILAGE

Aggrecan is the major proteoglycan in cartilage and is interspersed within the fibers of collagen type II, which comprise up to 40% of its dry weight. Aggrecan is a large molecule (Figs. 10.2 and 10.3) and is not found as a monomer. It is always associated with hyaluronan, with as many as 200 aggrecan molecules being linked noncovalently to a hyaluronan molecule. This leads to proteoglycan aggregates being 3 to 4 μm long, approximately half the diameter of a red blood cell. Due to the negative charge on the hyaluronan and the sulfation of the aggrecan proteoglycans, cations bind to the aggregate, and this, in turn, leads to binding of water. Indeed, up to 80% of the wet weight of cartilage is water. This allows the tissue to act as a shock absorber, releasing water when compressed, and to resilience, returning to its previous size and shape rapidly when compression is relieved. Aggrecan binding to hyaluronan distinguishes it as a member of the small family of aggregating proteoglycans; other members are versican, neurocan, and brevican (2,7,24,42,43). Although versican is

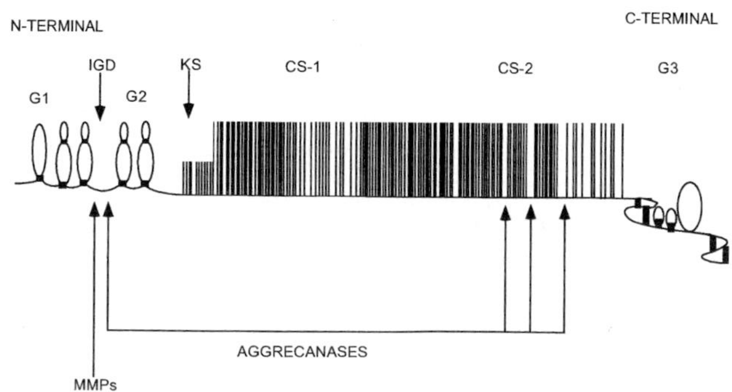

FIG. 10.2. Overall structure of aggrecan. Each domain is indicated, together with sites of susceptibility to matrix metalloproteinases (*MMPs*) and aggrecanases. The three globular (*G*) domains of the core protein are indicated, together with domains substituted with keratan sulfate (*KS*) and chondroitin sulfate (*CS-1* and *CS-2*). The interglobular domain (*IGD*) is particularly sensitive to proteolysis.

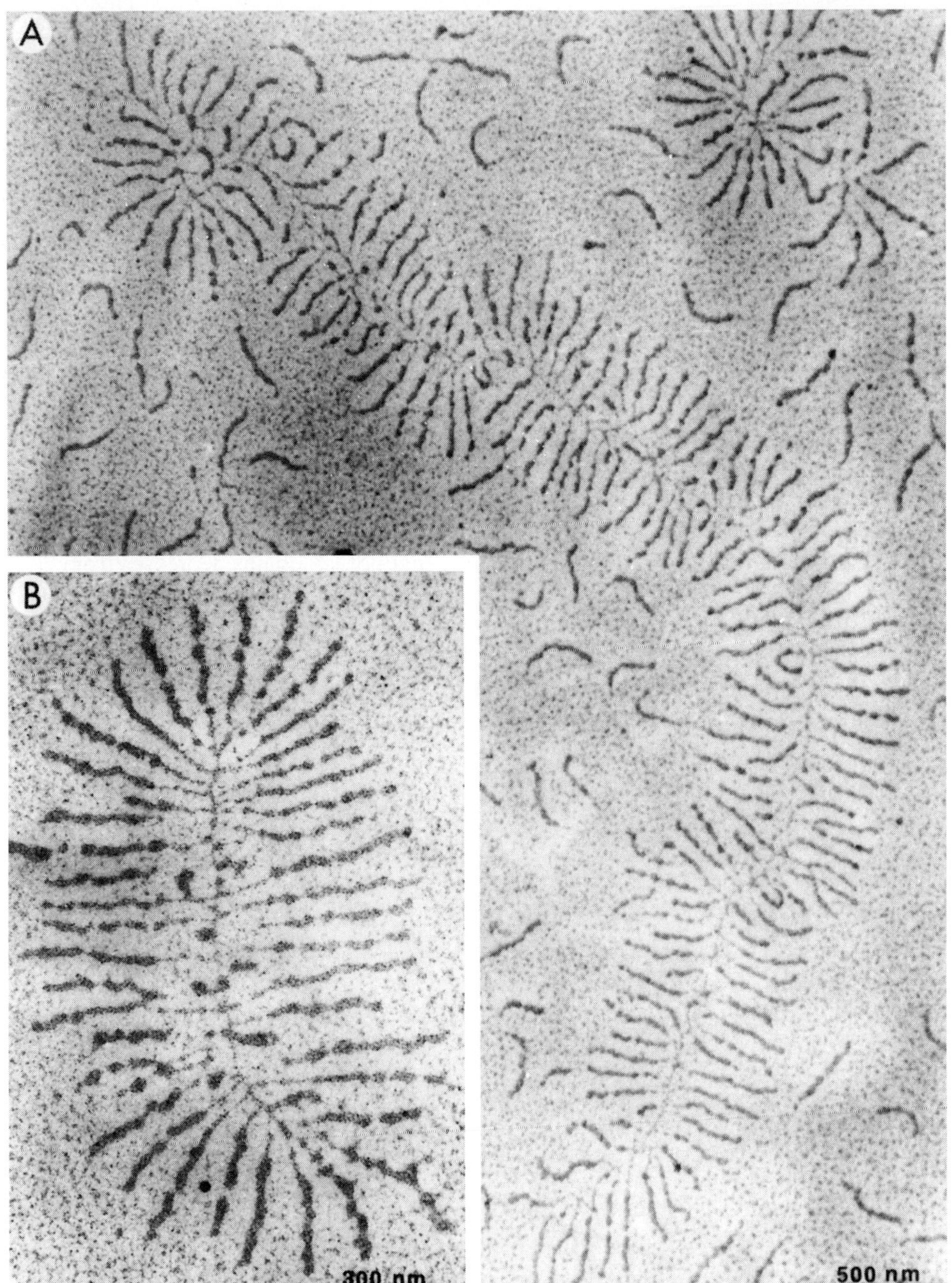

FIG. 10.3. A, B: Electron micrograph of aggrecan aggregates from bovine fetal epiphyseal cartilage. The size of an individual aggregate is determined mainly by the length of the hyaluronan central filament. Chondroitin sulfate (CS) chains condense along the protein core, so the CS region appears as a homogeneous, dense, widened area (*thick segment*). The centrally located *thin segment* near the hyaluronan is devoid of CS chains and contains the G2, IGD, and G1 domains. (Reproduced from Buckwalter JA, Rosenberg LC. Structural changes during development in bovine fetal epiphyseal cartilage. II. Electron microscopic studies of proteoglycan monomers and aggregates. *Coll Relat Res* 1983; 3:489–504, with permission.)

the major proteoglycan in developing cartilage, aggrecan predominates in mature cartilage (24,42).

The core protein of aggrecan is approximately 220 kd in molecular weight and contains several distinct domains (44,45). The G1 domain is at the N-terminus, and consists of an immunoglobulin (Ig)-like repeat and two link modules. In aggrecan, but not versican, there is a second globular domain that contains two further repeats. These two globular domains are separated by an interglobular domain (IGD), which can be cleaved by metalloproteinases. Following the G2 domain is the KS glycosaminoglycan substitution domain, which precedes a large region that is substituted with CS glycosaminoglycans. The C-terminus comprises another globular domain (G3). The G3 domain contains three subdomains: two alternately spliced EGF-like repeats that flank a central lectinlike structure, and a terminal complement regulatory protein module. The gene for aggrecan is approximately 80 kb long, with four exons encoding G1, three encoding G2, six encoding G3, and single exons that encode the IGD, the KS region, and the CS region. Glycosaminoglycan chains attach to serine residues that are present in two sets (CS-1 and CS-2) of repeating serine-glycine residues (44). The CS-1 region is polymorphic in humans (46), because the number of CS chains attached may vary widely. Since there is some genetic predisposition to OA (47), it is possible that the variability in CS substitution may play a role in disease susceptibility.

Aggrecan functions as part of the proteoglycan aggregate formed by association with hyaluronan (Fig. 10.3). This aggregate can have a mass of over 200 million, dependent on how many aggrecan monomers bind to the hyaluronan backbone. This, in turn, may depend on the length of the hyaluronan. The G1 domain of aggrecan binds to approximately five disaccharides of hyaluronan (48), and this interaction is stabilized by link protein. Link protein has similarities to the G1 domain of aggrecan and forms a ternary complex with both aggrecan and hyaluronan that occupies approximately 25 disaccharides within hyaluronan (39–41). Interestingly, each component of the proteoglycan aggregate (hyaluronan, aggrecan, and link protein) is secreted individually, with assembly occurring outside the cell. Assembly is slow (49) taking up to 24 hours. This allows for some diffusion of individual components away from the site of secretion and may explain the different composition of the territorial (pericellular) and interterritorial matrix. The former, which comprises a zone approximately 50 μm wide, is richer in CS than collagen, whereas the interterritorial matrix is richer in collagen with reduced proteoglycan content. Despite these minor differences, the matrices are similar with a highly distensible proteoglycan aggregate intertwined within the more rigid framework provided by fibers of collagen type II. Because the linkage to hyaluronan is through the G1 domain of aggrecan, it is probably not surprising that specific cleavage of the IGD of aggrecan can result in arthritis due to the loss of cartilage proteoglycan. The G1 domain of aggrecan is essential for cartilage formation and function. The gene for aggrecan in the cmd/cmd (cartilage matrix deficiency) mouse has a point mutation that results in premature truncation of the G1 domain (50,51). This results in gross abnormalities in cartilage due to the absence of aggrecan. Moreover, the cmd/+ mouse exhibits dwarfism and vertebral misalignment (52).

Functions of the other regions of aggrecan core protein remain elusive. The G2 domain does not bind hyaluronan or link protein. The region bearing KS chains may interact with collagen type II, but the affinity is low, and KS chains are not required for normal cartilage function (53). The G3 domain interacts with fucose and galactose (54), leading to this class of proteoglycans also being termed hyalectans. The G3 domain of versican has been shown to interact with tenascin-R (55), which is restricted to neuronal tissue, although there is a cartilage homologue, tenascin-C (56). Indeed, recent studies have shown that aggrecan, versican, and brevican lectin domains bind fibulin-2 through the same site that binds tenascin-R (57). A second possible role for the G3 region is in intracellular trafficking of aggrecan, because a truncated mutant form is retained in the endoplasmic reticulum (43).

The CS chains of aggrecan are essential for cartilage function, and loss of CS is accompanied by alterations in chondrocyte metabolism, matrix degradation and arthritis (26–29,36,58). It is increasingly clear that cartilage structure, especially the extracellular matrix, differs with age, particularly in the years prior to age 20 (29–31). This is mainly due to changes in aggrecan, in which the average length of CS chains decreases from 20 to 8 kd and the ratio of CS-6 to CS-4 increases (31). The CS content also varies with disease. For example, CS-4,6 disulfate is present at 60% of the nonreducing termini of CS chains in normal cartilage, but this is reduced to 30% in cartilage from patients with OA (32).

It is likely that changes in the extracellular matrix exert reciprocal influences on the chondrocytes, and vice versa. For example, a reduction in CS content would decrease the "shock absorber" effectiveness of the matrix, subjecting chondrocytes to increased stress on application of pressure. This could then lead to alterations in matrix synthesis, export, organization, and degradation. All extracellular matrices are remodeled, albeit at different rates, and the overall homeostasis of the extracellular matrix is crucial in cartilage. The matrix of cartilage is linked to the chondrocyte through the glycoprotein CD44, the principal hyaluronan receptor. In turn, the hyaluronan binds aggrecan, providing the means by which the chondrocytes can retain proteoglycans in the pericellular matrix and, thereby, organize the territorial and interterritorial matrix. Moreover, CD44 interacts with the actin cytoskeleton and these interactions are crucial for matrix retention by chondrocytes in culture (59).

Many studies have investigated the metabolism of aggrecan, both in normal tissue homeostastis and in aging and disease (Fig. 10.4). The G3 domain, particularly, is subject to cleavage and release in mature cartilage. In contrast, the G1 domain is trapped and retained by hyaluronan, whereas other degraded fragments are released into the matrix (Fig. 10.4). A large number of proteases can cleave aggrecan, with cleavage occurring in the IGD, KS, and CS domains (42,60–74). Members of the matrix metalloproteinase family (MMP), including MMPs 1 through 3 and 7 through 9, can cleave aggrecan within the IGD. This occurs in both inflammatory and noninflammatory arthritis and can be monitored with monoclonal antibodies that detect new epitopes generated by the cleavage. Since these cleavage products are often released into the synovium, this allows the severity of the degradation to be monitored (67–70,75). Although the MMPs cleave between Asn and Phe, the major-

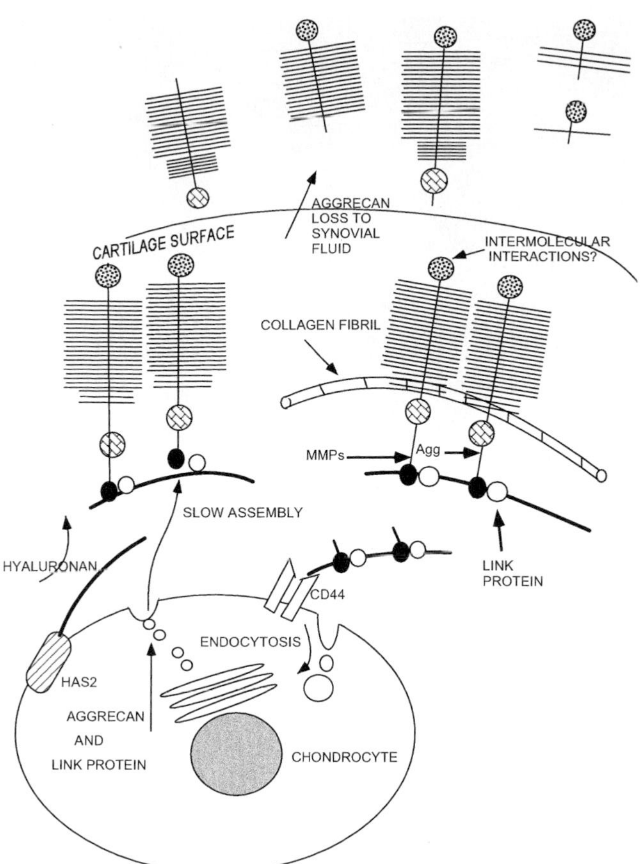

FIG. 10.4. Simplified diagram of aggrecan metabolism. Chondrocyte synthesis of aggrecan, link protein, and hyaluronan is followed by assembly in the extracellular environment. Catabolic events center around cleavage by aggrecanases (*Agg*) and metalloproteinases (*MMPs*), with loss of aggrecan fragments to the synovial fluid, and uptake of hyaluronan by the chondrocytes. *CD44*, hyaluronan receptor.

ity of detected released products were cleaved between Glu^{373} and Ala^{374} of the IGD (69–72,75), suggesting additional proteases. These products were detected not only in cartilage from patients with OA and RA, but also in healthy individuals, suggesting that degradation of aggrecan occurs as a part of normal homeostasis (69–72). Additional cleavage occurs in the CS domain (71–75), and this activity was ascribed to an aggrecanase capable of cleaving in both the IGD and the CS domain (73,74). Further immunohistochemical analysis indicated that MMP-induced neoepitopes were found in damaged cartilage, whereas aggrecanase-induced neoepitopes were present in normal tissue (69–75). Aggrecanases 1 and 2 were originally cloned by cDNA techniques and are metalloproteinases with special features. The purified proteins are members of the ADAMTS (a disintegrin and metalloproteinase with thrombospondin motifs) family. Aggrecanases 1 and 2 cleave aggrecan at multiple sites and are now termed ADAMTS4 and ADAMTS5 (73–78). These aggrecanases degrade cartilage during inflammatory disease and exhibit more restricted substrate specificity than the MMP family members. Further detailed studies are needed to determine the time sequence of degradation and the factors that induce specific protease synthesis and release or activation.

HYALURONAN

Hyaluronan is a linear chain consisting of repeating disaccharides of glucuronic acid and *N*-acetylglucosamine. Unlike other glycosaminoglycans, hyaluronan exists as independent glycosaminoglycan chains that are not attached to a core protein. In addition, hyaluronan differs from KS, CS, and HS in that it is not sulfated. Hyaluronan is crucial for cartilage matrix structure, maintenance, and function. It is the ligand for CD44 glycoprotein, which is a transmembrane receptor that transmits forces from the extracellular matrix to the cytoskeleton (59,79) and also controls hyaluronan turnover (80). Interestingly, CD44 itself is a "part-time" proteoglycan that can be substituted with CS, DS, or HS.

Hyaluronan can have over 30,000 repeating disaccharides with a mass of 10^7 daltons (81). It is produced by chondrocytes in cartilage and type A synoviocytes in the synovial tissue. Due to its viscosity, it acts as a lubricant in the joint. Exogenous hyaluronan has been used as a clinical treatment, particularly in horses (82), to counteract the reduced amount and length of synovial hyaluronan in arthritis. Hyaluronan is unusual because it is synthesized at the cell surface by hyaluronan synthases (HAS proteins) and released directly into the extracellular matrix. HAS proteins have multiple membrane-spanning domains but intracellular N- and C-termini. Recent studies have shown that recombinant HAS1 can synthesize oligosaccharides in an *in vitro* system (83). Three mammalian HAS proteins have been identified (21,22,83–86), and each appears to generate a different size of hyaluronate (21). The tissue expression patterns of HAS proteins are highly regulated (22), and a "knockout" of HAS2 is embryonically lethal due to cardiovascular effects. The latter observation emphasizes the critical role of hyaluronan in development, probably through its effects on cell migration (23,84–86), as well as cartilage matrix function (87,88). Moreover, there is now much interest in HAS expression during tumorigenesis (23 and references therein). The expression of each HAS gene differs, with HAS2 gene expression being high in synovial membrane and articular cartilage, whereas HAS3 is lowest in these tissues (22). In addition, proinflammatory cytokines regulate the gene expression of HAS messenger RNAs (mRNAs) in cultured synoviocytes (88). This is a relatively new area of research, but detailed knowledge of the control of HAS protein expression and activity may well lead to new interventional therapies for arthritic diseases.

SMALL LEUCINE-RICH PROTEOGLYCANS

The class of proteoglycans and glycoproteins that contain leucine-rich domains (Fig. 10.5) is also referred to as

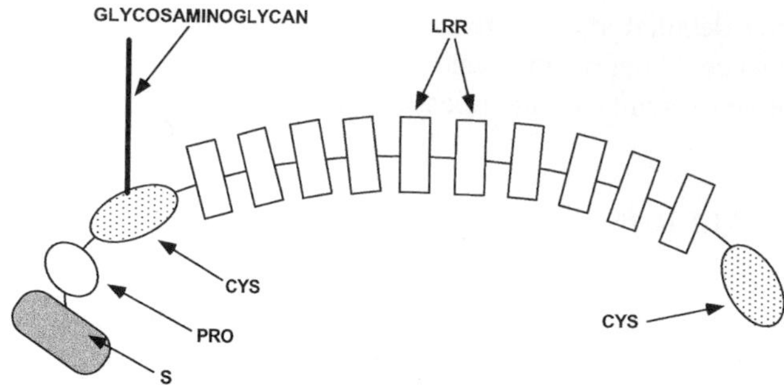

FIG. 10.5. Schematic structure of decorin, a small leucine-rich proteoglycan. At the N-terminus is a signal peptide (*S*), followed by a propeptide (*PRO*) and a cysteine-rich repeat (*CYS*), which may be glycanated, in the case of decorin, usually by a single chondroitin sulfate or dermatan sulfate chain. A series of 10 leucine-rich repeats (*LRR*) follows, with a C-terminal second cysteine-rich repeat.

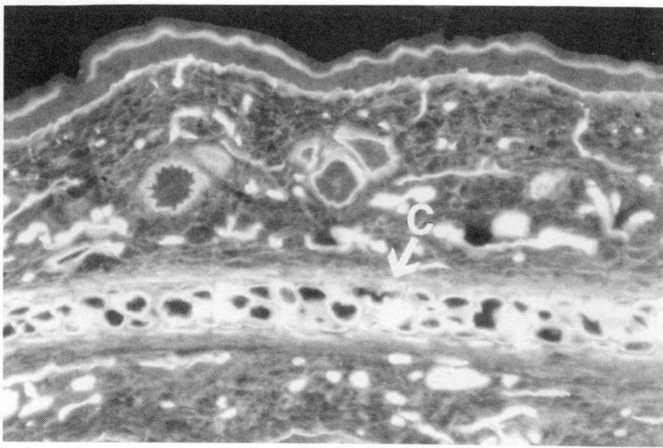

FIG. 10.6. Perlecan is present in basement membranes and is a cartilage (*C*) component (*arrow*). (Courtesy of Dr. A. Ljubimov, Cedars-Sinai Medical Center, Los Angeles, CA.)

"horseshoe" proteoglycans (89–94). They consist of a signal peptide, a propeptide that may control glycosaminoglycan substitution, a cysteine-rich region that can be tyrosine-sulfated or substituted with glycosaminoglycans, and a large stretch of leucine-rich repeats, ending with another cysteine-rich region. The leucine-rich motif is LXXLXLXXNXL/I, where L is leucine, I is isoleucine, and N is asparagine. This motif is not only present in matrix proteins, but also in intracellular proteins, and may be a common protein/protein interaction motif. Indeed, the horseshoe designation derives from the crystal structure of ribonuclease inhibitor (95). This class of proteins includes decorin, epiphycan, and biglycan, which have just one or two CS or DS chains, fibromodulin, lumican and keratocan, and others that are not proteoglycans, including proline/arginine-rich end leucine-rich repeat protein (PRELP) and osteoglycin. Decorin and biglycan can regulate the assembly of collagen fibrils in cartilage (96–99). This activity seems to be due to protein/protein interactions because removal of glycosaminoglycan chains does not affect function. Knockouts for several of these molecules have been generated; none dramatically affect cartilage matrix, despite both decorin and biglycan being cartilage components. This may be due to redundancy with other small leucine-rich proteins. There is still much to learn concerning the roles of individual small leucine-rich proteoglycans in normal and diseased cartilage. This is emphasized by the interaction of biglycan, fibromodulin, and decorin with members of the transforming growth factor-β family (100–102), which have important roles in cartilage development and repair.

PERLECAN

Perlecan is a basement membrane proteoglycan, but it is also present in cartilage (Fig. 10.6), particularly in articular cartilage and the growth plate. It is synthesized by proliferating chondrocytes and by synoviocytes, and is a matrix proteoglycan of the synovium (103–107). A large proteoglycan, perlecan is substituted with both HS and CS chains in cartilage (104). The human perlecan gene encodes a core protein of approximately 470 kd, consisting of five domains (I–V), with each having homology to other proteins (108) (Fig. 10.7). Domain I is the main glycosaminoglycan substitution site and has a cluster of three potential attachment sites together with an SEA (sperm protein, enterokinase, agrin) module (109). This domain has the main chondrogenic activity, possibly through growth factor binding (107); domain II has homology to the low-density lipoprotein receptor; and domain III, which has overall homology to laminin α1, comprises three globular domains dispersed between four cysteine-rich repeat modules. The latter domain (in mice, but not in humans) contains the sequence Arg-Gly-Asp, which may promote cell adhesion through recognition by integrin receptors, although integrin-independent adhesion has also been reported (110,111). Domain IV is the largest and comprises 21 Ig modules in the human, most closely resembling Ig modules occurring in neural cell adhesion molecule, which is involved in cell-cell adhesion. Domain V at the C-terminus also has homology to laminin α subunits, and contains three globular regions connected by epidermal growth factor (EGF)-like repeats. This domain also has been suggested to function in cell adhesion, self-association, and interaction with other matrix components, and it can be glycanated with both HS and CS (111,112).

Perlecan is crucial for cartilage development and ossification. Perlecan knockout mice show a high degree of embryonic death and severe skeletal abnormalities. In addition, mutations in the perlecan 2 gene (HSPG2) are associated with two classes of skeletal disorders: Schwartz-Jampel syndrome (chondrodystrophic myotonia), which is relatively mild (113), and Silverman-Handmaker syndrome, which is a severe neonatal lethal dysplasia (114). Perlecan interacts through its core protein with other base-

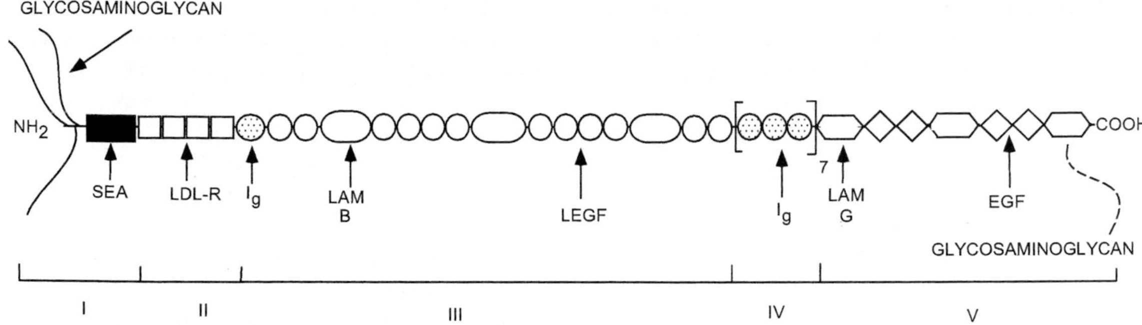

FIG. 10.7. Schematic structure of perlecan. Domains I through V are shown, but domain IV is abbreviated for clarity. In the human, there are 21 immunoglobulin repeats in this domain. Modules with homology to laminin, laminin-1 epidermal growth factor (EGF)-like (*LEGF*), and C-terminal EGF-like (*EGF*) repeats, and the low-density lipoprotein receptor (*LDL-R*) are shown. Glycosaminoglycan substitution is mainly in domain I, but may also occur in domain V.

ment components, including laminin, type IV collagen, and entactin, and with other matrix glycoproteins such as fibronectin. These interactions appear crucial for initial primordial cartilage formation (24,105,113–115). *In vitro* studies have also shown that perlecan can prevent dedifferentiation of chondrocytes and promote chondrogenesis (104,105).

SYNDECANS

There are four mammalian syndecans with cell type and developmentally-specific expression (Fig. 10.8). The syndecans are a family of transmembrane proteoglycans (4,6, 116–119) that possess small core proteins whose ectodomains are divergent, except for the three to four sites of glycosaminoglycan substitution (predominantly HS). Syndecan transmembrane domains are highly homologous, and their short cytoplasmic domains bear regions of high homology proximal (C1 subdomain) and distal (C2 subdomain) to the membrane. Each family member exhibits a unique (V) intervening region and has a C-terminal Phe-Tyr-Ala amino acid sequence that interacts with proteins that contain PDZ (PSD95/DLG/ZO-1) domains. PDZ domain–containing proteins have been postulated to function as linkers to form protein-protein networks (120), or as trafficking molecules (121). Binding partners for syndecan cytoplasmic domains are now being identified and the role(s) of their interactions determined (122–127).

Syndecan-1 is the major syndecan in epithelial tissues, and its down-regulation leads to loss of epithelial phenotype. Syndecan-2 is the major syndecan in mesenchymal cells, and it is present in chondrocytes (128). It is expressed in high amount in macrophages from the synovial fluid of patients with a variety of diseases, including RA, systemic lupus erythematosus, and psoriatic arthritis (129). The levels of syndecan-2 are increased by interleukin-1 (IL-1), and

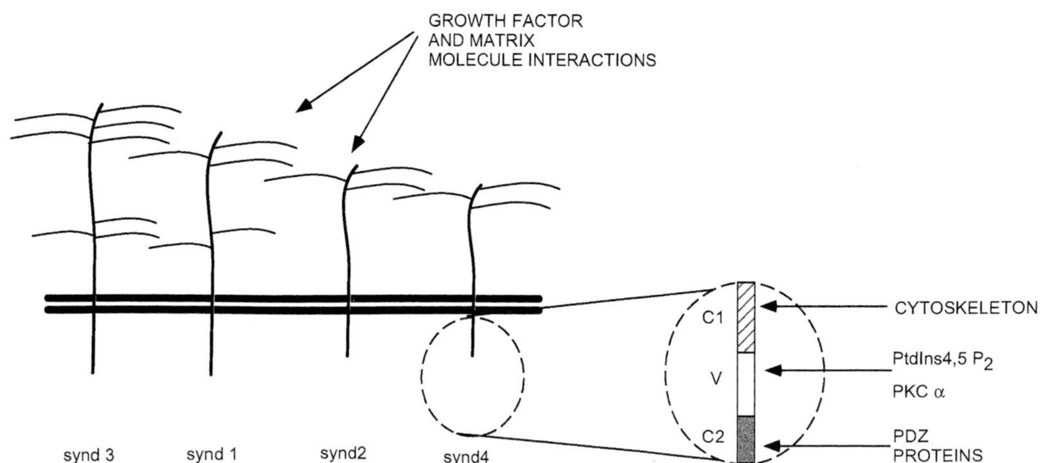

FIG. 10.8. Diagram of the four mammalian syndecans. Each bears glycosaminoglycans on the ectodomain, and has a cytoplasmic domain consisting of two conserved regions (*C1* and *C2*) flanking a central variable (*V*) region. Interaction sites for protein kinase Cα (*PKCα*), phosphatidylinositol 4,5 bisphosphate, and PDZ domain proteins are shown.

syndecan-2 can bind and present fibroblast growth factor-2 (FGF-2) to cells (129), so it may be involved in growth factor signaling in response to inflammation. Syndecan-2 plays a critical role in matrix assembly by fibroblasts (130), but possible roles in cartilage assembly have not yet been investigated. Syndecan-3 is the major syndecan in neuronal tissue, but is also present in developing cartilage (131–135). The expression of syndecan-3 in chondrocytes is increased by FGF-2, and this correlates with increased growth (136). In contrast, syndecan-3 is not expressed in mature cartilage (131). Syndecan-4 is unusual in that it is normally a minor component in cells, but it is present in many cell lineages that show stable adhesion to extracellular matrix (137). The role of syndecan-4 in cell adhesion is becoming clearer (4,6,116–119,138). It acts in concert with integrins to generate stable adhesion, with the formation of specialized areas of cell-matrix adhesion (focal adhesions). These structures represent the interface between the matrix and the cytoskeleton and consist of a multicomponent complex that regulates adhesion, cell cycle progression, apoptosis, and gene expression. The cytoplasmic domain of syndecan-4 associates with the actin cross-linker α-actinin (125), and its V region binds and directly activates protein kinase Cα (PKC-α) (126). The activation of PKC-α by syndecan-4 requires oligomerization of the syndecan, which is promoted by phosphatidylinositol 4,5 bisphosphate (139), which in turn is increased when integrin receptors bind ligand. Interestingly, oligomerization of syndecan can be regulated by serine phosphorylation upstream of the V region by FGF, allowing the convergence of growth factor and adhesion-mediated signaling (140). In general, syndecans are coreceptors for matrix molecules, growth factors, and cytokines. Thus, they may regulate matrix formation, cell adhesion, and cell proliferation, all involved in cartilage development, homeostasis, and disease. Elucidation of the precise roles of syndecans should be a fertile area for future research.

PROTEOGLYCAN EXPRESSION IN CARTILAGE DEVELOPMENT AND DISEASE

Several proteoglycans have been shown to differ in expression in cartilage during development and disease. Much of the current knowledge has come from genetic analysis and knockout technology. There are now over 11 skeletal defects in animal models, or in humans that have been attributed to abnormal proteoglycan synthesis or processing (24). It is not possible here to discuss these in detail, but several are embryonically lethal or result in pronounced chondrodystrophies, emphasizing the role of proteoglycans in cartilage development and stability. Responsible genetic defects range from mutations in core proteins that result in nonsecretion (e.g., perlecan and aggrecan) to mutations in proteins involved in glycosaminoglycan sulfation [e.g., phosphoadenosine phosphosulfate (PAPS) synthetase and sulfate transporter gene] or elongation (e.g., glycosyltransferase). Indeed, it is now clear that glycosaminoglycan processing plays a crucial role in development (20,24). Heparan sulfate biosynthetic enzymes known to affect cartilage development and disease include EXT1 and EXT2, which are associated with multiple exostosis and have glucuronyl-transferase and *N*-acetylglucosaminyl-transferase activity (18,19). Knockout studies (18,19) show that heterozygous mice have reduced HS production, and homozygous mice die at gastrulation. Perlecan-deficient embryos either die at day 10 to 12 due to rupture of cardiac basement membranes, or die perinatally. The embryos also exhibit chondrodysplasia, consistent with the suggestion that perlecan protects cartilage matrix from degradation (115). Other studies emphasize that perlecan is essential for cartilage development (114,115). One particular perlecan gene mutation results in dyssegmental dysplasia, Silverman-Handmaker type, through synthesis of an unstable perlecan that is not secreted into the matrix, while another results in chondrodystrophic myotonia.

Direct studies of developing cartilage have also indicated changing patterns of proteoglycan expression. There are three phases of cartilage formation. The first is characterized by epithelial-mesenchymal interactions that precede condensation, the second is cellular condensation, and the third is differentiation (132). Stage 1 is characterized by high syndecan-1 gene expression and the presence of versican and perlecan, stage 2 by high syndecan-3 (131) and versican, and stage 3 by aggrecan and hyaluronan (132). Versican and aggrecan appear to have opposite expression patterns: versican is present in the early limb bud, but later disappears as cartilage differentiation progresses and aggrecan predominates (24). The importance of syndecan-3 expression in high amounts during condensation is emphasized by *in vitro* studies that demonstrate that antibodies to syndecan-3 core protein reduce mRNAs for cartilage-specific genes, such as collagen type II and aggrecan core protein (134). Proliferating immature cartilage from chick embryo tibia and sternum have higher amounts of syndecan-3 mRNA than mature hypertrophic cartilage (133). Immunolocalization confirmed the restriction of syndecan-3 to immature proliferating chondrocytes, and *in vitro* studies confirmed that the high gene expression of syndecan-3 in immature proliferating chondrocytes was markedly reduced following induction of maturation by vitamin C.

Changes in cartilage proteoglycans in aging and disease have also been demonstrated. When mRNAs for six cell surface proteoglycans were analyzed in freshly isolated articular chondrocytes from juveniles and adults, similar results were seen with cells from both ages (34). The most abundant messages were for syndecan-4 (amphiglycan) and CD44, with low levels for syndecan-2 (fibroglycan), glypican and betaglycan. Syndecan-1 mRNA was not detectable. There are also reports (37) of no significant changes in collagen type II or glycosaminoglycan content in human ankle cartilage after 30 years of age. Interestingly, however, fetal bovine chondrocytes grown in alginate cultures produce more cell-associated matrix than young or adult cells (38), and more was released with age. In addition, there was an increase in the ratio of hyaluronan to proteoglycan in cells from adult animals, while the length of the HA molecules decreased. Other studies have monitored the stability of cartilage by determining the ease of extraction of its components (36) with increasingly chaotropic conditions. High amounts of aggrecan, link protein, and hyaluronan were extracted from immature human articular cartilage by saline solution, but extraction from adult cartilage required harsher conditions. There are also differences in aggrecan sulfation and structure with respect to the CS chains. From 10 to 20 years of age, the level of 6-sulfation of *N*-acetylgalactosamine in the linkage region increases, then remains reasonably stable, until a slight reduction is seen beyond 40 years of age (35); the chain length decreases with age in the first 20 years of life, while the ratio of 6-sulfated to 4-sulfated CS increases (43).

Much attention has been directed to changes in proteoglycans that correlate with RA or OA. The major proteoglycan, aggrecan, is depleted in arthritic cartilage due to increased proteolytic cleavage of the core protein. The MMPs mainly cleave Asn^{341}-Phe^{342} in the IGD, whereas the aggrecanases cleave between Glu^{373}-Ala^{374} in the IGD. Aggrecan IGD cleavage by MMPs occurs during the late stage of degradation, with MMP C-terminal catabolism and the generation of CS-deficient aggrecan monomers occurring earlier (141). Aggrecan fragments in both inflammatory and OA synovial fluid show the ^{374}ARGS neoepitope indicative of aggrecanase activity (64–73,142,143). ADAMTS4 also cleaves at four other sites in the CS-rich region (Glu^{1545}-Gly^{1546}, Glu^{1714}-Gly^{1715}, Glu^{1819}-Ala^{1820}, and Glu^{1919}-Leu^{1920}), and fragments from cleavage at these sites have been found after IL-1α treatment of bovine articular cartilage. Normal synovial fluid has at least 10 fragment species, 9 resulting from ADAMTS-dependent cleavage. Aggrecan from cartilage of patients with late-stage OA is similar to normal, but synovial fluid aggrecan is more fragmented, suggesting excessive ADAMTS activity. ADAMTS4 is specifically induced in OA cartilage, whereas ADAMTS5 is constitutively expressed, with increased expression of both being a hallmark of human inflammatory disease–associated cartilage degradation (143). Inhibition of ADAMTS4 and 5 prevents aggrecan degradation in human OA cartilage (142), suggesting a basis for future intervention. Prevention of aggrecan degradation may have broader effects, since the aggrecan deficiency in *cmd/cmd* mouse fetuses is accompanied by changes in link protein, syndecan-3, and several collagens (144), indicating that the overall integrity of the matrix depends on aggrecan.

Other proteases known to be active in cartilage degradation are the cathepsins. Cathepsin D cleavage of aggrecan in the IGD and CS-rich region may contribute to the proteolytic processing of aggrecan in articular cartilage (145). In addition, cathepsin K–positive synovial fibroblasts were consistently found at sites of cartilage and bone degradation in RA patients and in cultured synovial fibroblasts from patients. Cathepsin K has a potent aggrecan degrading activity, and the cleavage products potentiate the collagenolytic activity of cathepsin K (146).

In contrast to aggrecan, changes in other proteoglycans with disease have not been widely studied. Syndecan-1 mRNA is reduced in heavily damaged areas of OA cartilage in comparison with that in healthy-appearing areas, but syndecan-4 levels were increased (147). Syndecan-3 increases in OA, particularly in the upper zone of severely affected cartilage (136), and the levels of decorin and biglycan message (and protein) are also upregulated (148). Proinflammatory cytokines increase HAS2 mRNA expression, resulting in accumulation and fragmentation of hyaluronan (88). Intact aggrecan can be released from cartilage, consistent with hyaluronan degradation. Indeed, IL-1β and retinoic acid both induce hyaluronan degradation in cartilage (149); thus, hyaluronan synthesis and turnover, in addition to that of aggrecan, may regulate matrix stability.

CONCLUSIONS

The current time is one of rapidly expanding knowledge of cartilage components and their developmental control, homeostasis, and degradation. Most of the major components have probably been identified, and in the postgenomic era, their biologic properties will be determined and correlated with genetic defects. This will allow determination of the roles of specific components in maintaining cartilage and the synovium. More detailed knowledge of the proteases responsible for cartilage degradation should allow the introduction of new therapeutic agents to prevent or, hopefully, reverse inflammatory and arthritic changes. Similarly, the recent advances in identifying, cloning, and expressing enzymes involved in glycosaminoglycan synthesis and posttranslational modification form the basis for a detailed understanding of proteoglycan biology, the prospect of *in vitro* synthesis of proteoglycans or glycosaminoglycans crucial for joint health, and their eventual use in a new era in the practice of rheumatology.

ACKNOWLEDGMENTS

Some of the work described here was supported by National Institutes of Health Grants GM50194 and DK54605 to the author. Dr. John R. Couchman is gratefully acknowledged for some figures.

REFERENCES

1. Gallagher JT. Structure-activity relationship of heparan sulphate. *Biochem Soc Trans* 1997;25:1206–1209.
2. Hascall VC, Heinegård DK, Wight TN. Proteoglycans: metabolism and pathology. In: Hay ED, ed. *Cell biology of extracellular matrix*. New York: Plenum, 1991:149–175.

3. Lindahl U, Kusche-Gullberg M, Kjellén L. Regulated diversity of heparan sulphate. *J Biol Chem* 1998;273:24979–24982.
4. Tumova S, Woods A, Couchman JR. Heparan sulfate proteoglycans on the cell surface: versatile coordinators of cellular function. *Int J Biochem Cell Biol* 2000;32:269–288.
5. Iozzo RV. Matrix proteoglycans: from molecular design to cellular function. *Annu Rev Biochem* 1998;67:609–652.
6. Bernfield M, Gotte M, Park PW, et al. Functions of cell surface heparan sulfate proteoglycans. *Annu Rev Biochem* 1999;68:729–778.
7. Iozzo RV. *Proteoglycans: structure, biology and molecular interactions*. New York: Marcel Dekker, 2000.
8. Matsumoto R, Sbreve A, Ghildyal N, et al. Packaging of proteases and proteoglycans in the granules of mast cells and other hematopoietic cells. *J Biol Chem* 1995;270:19524–19531.
9. Fukuta M, Inazawa J, Torri T, et al. Molecular cloning and characterization of human keratan sulfate gal-6-sulfotransferase. *J Biol Chem* 1997;272:32321–32328.
10. Habuchi H, Kobayashi M, Kimata K. Molecular characterization and expression of heparan-sulfate 6-sulfotransferase. *J Biol Chem* 1998; 273:9208–9213.
11. Uchimura K, Muramasu H, Kadomatsu K, et al. Molecular cloning and characterization of an *N*-acetylglucosamine-6-*O*-sulfotransferase. *J Biol Chem* 1998;273:22577–22583.
12. Ong E, Hey J-C, Ding Y, et al. Expression cloning of a human sulfotransferase that directs the synthesis of the HNK-1 glycan on the neural cell adhesion molecule and glycolipids. *J Biol Chem* 1998;273: 5190–5195.
13. Kobayashi M, Sugumaran G, Liu J, et al. Molecular cloning and characterization of a human uronyl 2-sulfotransferase that sulfates iduronyl and glucuronyl residues in dermatan/chondroitin sulfate. *J Biol Chem* 1999;274:10474–10480.
14. Kusche-Gullberg M, Eriksson I, Pikas DS, et al. Identification and expression in mouse of two heparan sulfate glucosaminyl *N*-deacetylase/*N*-sulfotransferase genes. *J Biol Chem* 1998;273:11902–11907.
15. Aikawa J, Esko JD. Molecular cloning and expression of a third member of the heparan sulfate/heparin GlcNAc *N*-deacetylase/*N*-sulfotransferase family. *J Biol Chem* 1999;274:2690–2695.
16. Shworak NW, Liu J, Petros L, et al. Multiple isoforms of heparan sulfate D-glucosaminyl 3-*O*-sulfotransferase: isolation, characterization, and expression of human cDNAs and identification of distinct genomic loci. *J Biol Chem* 1999;274:5170–5184.
17. Wei G, Bai X, Sarkar AK, et al. Formation of HNK-1 determinants and the glycosaminoglycan tetrasaccharide linkage region by UDP-GlcUA:galactose β1,3-glucuronosyltransferase. *J Biol Chem* 1999; 274:7857–7864.
18. Lind T, Tufaro F, McCormick C, et al. The putative tumor suppressors EXT1 and EXT2 are glycosyltransferases required for the biosynthesis of heparan sulfate. *J Biol Chem* 1998;273:26265–26268.
19. Kitagawa H, Shimakawa H, Sugahara K. The tumor suppressor EXT-like gene EXTL2 encodes a 1, 4-*N*-acetylhexosaminyltransferase that transfers *N*-acetylgalactosamine and *N*-acetylglucosamine to the common glycosaminoglycan-protein linkage region. *J Biol Chem* 1999; 274:13933–13937.
20. Forsberg E, Kjellén, L. Heparan sulfate: lessons from knockout mice. *J Clin Invest* 2001;108:175–180.
21. Itano N, Sawai T, Yoshida M, et al. Three forms of mammalian hyaluronan synthases have distinct enzymatic properties. *J Biol Chem* 1999;274:23085–25092.
22. Ohno S, Tanimoto K, Fujimoto K, et al. Molecular cloning of rabbit hyaluronic acid synthases and their expression patterns in synovial membrane and articular cartilage. *Biochim Biophys Acta* 2002;1520: 71–78.
23. Toole B. Hyaluronan is not just a goo! *J Clin Invest* 2000;106:335–336.
24. Schwartz NB, Dominowicz M. Chondrodyplasias due to proteoglycan defects. *Glycobiology* 2002;12:57R–68R.
25. Watanabe H, Yamada Y, Kimata K. Roles of aggrecan, a large chondroitin sulfate proteoglycan, in cartilage structure and function. *J Biochem* 1998;124:687–693.
26. Lohmander LS, Ionescu M, Jugessur H. Changes in joint cartilage aggrecan after knee injury and in osteoarthritis. *Arthritis Rheum* 1999; 42:534–544.
27. Carney SL, Billingham ME, Caterson B, et al. Changes in proteoglycan turnover in experimental canine osteoarthritic cartilage. *Matrix* 1992;12:137–147.
28. Rizkalla G, Reiner A, Bogoch E, et al. Studies of the articular cartilage proteoglycan aggrecan in health and osteoarthritis: evidence for molecular heterogeneity and extensive molecular changes in disease. *J Clin Invest* 1992;90:2268–2277.
29. Thonar EJ-MA, Bjornsson K, Kuettner KE. Age-related changes in cartilage proteoglycans. In: Kuettner KE, Schleyerbach R, Hascall VC, eds. *Articular cartilage biochemistry.* New York: Raven, 1986: 273–288.
30. Plaas AH, Wong-Palms S, Roughley PJ, et al. Chemical and immunological assay of the nonreducing terminal residues of chondroitin sulfate from human aggrecan. *J Biol Chem* 1997;272:20603–20610.
31. Bayliss MT, Osborne D, Woodhouse S, et al. Sulfation of chondroitin sulfate in human articular cartilage. *J Biol Chem* 1999;274:15892–15900.
32. Plaas AHK, West LA, Wong-Palms S, et al. Glycosaminoglycan sulfation in human osteoarthritis. *J Biol Chem* 1998;273:12642–12649.
33. DeGroot J, Bank RA, Tchetverikov I, et al. Molecular markers for osteoarthritis: the road ahead. *Curr Opin Rheumatol* 2002;14:585–589.
34. Grover J, Roughley PJ. Expression of cell-surface proteoglycan mRNA by human articular chondrocytes. *Biochem J* 1995;309:963–968.
35. Lauder RM, Huckerby TN, Brown GM, et al. Age-related changes in the sulfation of the chondroitin sulfate linkage region from human articular cartilage aggrecan. *Biochem J* 2001;358:523–528.
36. Wells T, Davidson C, Morgelin M, et al. Age-related changes in the composition, the molecular stoichiometry and the stability of proteoglycan aggregates extracted from human articular cartilage. *Biochem J* 2003;370:69–79.
37. Aurich M, Poole AR, Reiner A, et al. Matrix homeostasis in aging normal human ankle cartilage. *Arthritis Rheum* 2002;46:2903–2910.
38. Kamada H, Masuda K, D'Souza AL, et al. Age-related differences in the accumulation and size of hyaluronan in alginate culture. *Arch Biochem Biophys* 2002;408:192–199.
39. Neame PJ, Christner JE, Baker JR. The primary structure of link protein from rat chondrosarcoma proteoglycan aggregate. *J Biol Chem* 1986;261:3519–3535.
40. Doege K, Hassell JR, Caterson B, et al. Link protein cDNA sequence reveals a tandemly repeated protein structure. *Proc Natl Acad Sci U S A* 1986;83:3761–3765.
41. Goetinck PF, Stirpe NS, Tsonis PA, et al. The tandemly repeated sequences of cartilage link protein contain the sites for interaction with hyaluronic acid. *J Cell Biol* 1987;105:2403–2408.
42. Lee V, Chen L, Paiwand F, et al. Cleavage of the carboxyl tail from the G3 domain of aggrecan but not versican and identification of the amino acids involved in the degradation. *J Biol Chem* 2002;277: 22279–22288.
43. Knudson CB, Knudson W. Cartilage proteoglycans. *Semin Cell Dev Biol* 2001;12:69–78.
44. Doege KJ, Sasaki M, Kimura T, et al. Complete coding sequence and deduced primary structure of the human cartilage large aggregating proteoglycan, aggrecan: human-specific repeats, and additional alternatively spliced forms. *J Biol Chem* 1991;266:894–902.
45. Valhmu WB, Palmer GD, Rivers PA, et al. Structure of the human aggrecan gene: exon-intron organization and association with the protein domains. *Biochem J* 1995;309:535–542.
46. Doege KJ, Coulter SN, Meek LM, et al. A human-specific polymorphism in the coding region of the aggrecan gene. *J Biol Chem* 1997; 272:13974–13979.
47. Jimenez SA, Dharmavaram RM. Genetic aspects of familial osteoarthritis. *Ann Rheum Dis* 1994;53:789–797.
48. Nieduszynski IA, Sheehan JK, Phelps CF, et al. Equilibrium-binding studies of pig laryngeal cartilage proteoglycans with hyaluronate oligosaccharide fractions. *Biochem J* 1980;185:107–114.
49. Sandy JD, O'Neill JO, Ratzlaff L. Acquisition of hyaluronate binding affinity by newly synthesized proteoglycans *in vivo*. *Biochem J* 1989; 258:875–880.
50. Rittenhouse E, Dunn LC, Cookingham J, et al. Cartilage matrix deficiency (*cmd*): a new autosomal recessive lethal mutation in the mouse. *J Embryol Exp Morphol* 1978;43:71–84.
51. Watanabe H, Kimata K, Lin S, et al. Mouse cartilage matrix deficiency (CMD) caused by a 7 bp deletion in the aggrecan gene. *Nat Genet* 1994;7:154–157.
52. Watanabe H, Nakata K, Kimata K, et al. Dwarfism and age-associated spinal degeneration of heterozygote cmd mice defective in aggrecan. *Proc Natl Acad Sci U S A* 1997;94:6943–6947.

53. Hedlund H, Hedbom E, Heinegård D, et al. Association of the aggrecan keratan sulfate-rich region with collagen in bovine articular cartilage. *J Biol Chem* 1999;274:5777–5781.
54. Halberg DF, Proulx G, Doege K, et al. A segment of the cartilage proteoglycan core protein has lectin-like activity. *J Biol Chem* 1988;263: 9486–9490.
55. Aspberg A, Miura R, Bourdoulous S, et al. The C-type lectin domains of lecticans: a family of aggregating chondroitin sulfate proteoglycans, bind tenascin-R by protein-protein interactions independent of carbohydrate moiety. *Proc Natl Acad Sci U S A* 1997;94:10116–10121.
56. Mackie EJ, Murphy LI. The role of tenascin-C and related glycoproteins in early chondrogenesis. *Microsc Res Tech* 1998;43:102–110.
57. Olin AI, Morgelin M, Sasaki T, et al. The proteoglycans aggrecan and versican form networks with fibulin-2 through their lectin domain binding. *J Biol Chem* 2001;276:1253–1261.
58. Hardingham TE, Fosang AJ. The structure of aggrecan and its turnover in cartilage. *J Rheumatol* 1995;43:86–90.
59. Nofal GA, Knudson CB. Latrunculin and cytochalasin decrease chondrocyte matrix retention. *J Histochem Cytochem* 2002;50:1313–1323.
60. Fosang AJ, Neame PJ, Hardingham TE, et al. Cleavage of cartilage proteoglycan between G1 and G2 domains by stromelysins. *J Biol Chem* 1991;266:15579–15582.
61. Flannery CR, Lark MW, Sandy JD. Identification of a stromelysin cleavage site within the interglobular domain of human aggrecan: evidence for proteolysis at this site *in vivo* in human articular cartilage. *J Biol Chem* 1992;267:1008–1014.
62. Fosang AJ, Neame PJ, Last K, et al. The interglobular domain of cartilage aggrecan is cleaved by PUMP, gelatinases, and cathepsin B. *J Biol Chem* 1992;267:19470–19474.
63. Fosang AJ, Last K, Knauper V, et al. Fibroblast and neutrophil collagenases cleave at two sites in the cartilage aggrecan interglobular domain. *Biochem J* 1993;295:273–276.
64. Fosang AJ, Last K, Neame PJ, et al. Neutrophil collagenase (MMP-8) cleaves at the aggrecanase site E373-A374 in the interglobular domain of cartilage aggrecan. *Biochem J* 1994;304:347–351.
65. Arner EC, Decicco CP, Cherney R, et al. Cleavage of native cartilage aggrecan by neutrophil collagenase (MMP-8) is distinct from endogenous cleavage by aggrecanase. *Am Soc Biochem Mol Biol* 1997;272: 9294–9299.
66. Fosang AJ, Last K, Knauper V, et al. Degradation of cartilage aggrecan by collagenase-3 (MMP-13). *FEBS Lett* 1996;380:17–20.
67. Fosang AJ, Last K, Maciewicz RA. Aggrecan is degraded by matrix metalloproteinases in human arthritis. *J Clin Invest* 1996;98:2292–2299.
68. Lark MW, Bayne EK, Flanagan J, et al. Aggrecan degradation in human cartilage. *J Clin Invest* 1997;100:93–106.
69. Lohmander LS, Neame PJ, Sandy JD. The structure of aggrecan fragments in human synovial fluid: evidence that aggrecanase mediates cartilage degradation in inflammatory joint disease, joint injury and osteoarthritis. *Arthritis Rheum* 1993;36:1214–1222.
70. Sandy JD, Flannery CR, Neame PJ, et al. The structure of aggrecan fragments in human osteoarthritic synovial fluid: evidence for the involvement in osteoarthritis of a novel proteinase which cleaves the glu 373-ala 374 bond of the interglobular domain. *J Clin Invest* 1992; 89:1512–1516.
71. Ilic MZ, Robinson HC, Handley CJ. Characterization of aggrecan retained and lost from the extracellular matrix of articular cartilage. *J Biol Chem* 1998;273:17451–17458.
72. Sandy JD, Neame PJ, Boynton RE, et al. Catabolism of aggrecan in cartilage explants: identification of a major cleavage site within the interglobular domain. *J Biol Chem* 1991;266:8683–8685.
73. Arner EC, Pratta MA, Trzaskos JM, et al. Generation and characterization of aggrecanase: a soluble, cartilage-derived aggrecan-degrading activity. *J Biol Chem* 1999;274:6594–6601.
74. Rodriguez-Manzaneque JC, Westling J, Thai SNM, et al. ADAMTS1 cleaves aggrecan at multiple sites and is differentially inhibited by metalloproteinase inhibitors. *Biochem Biophys Res Commun* 2002; 293:501–508.
75. Hughes CE, Caterson B, Fosang AJ, et al. Monoclonal antibodies that specifically recognize neoepitope sequences generated by "aggrecanase" and matrix metalloproteinase cleavage of aggrecan: application to catabolism *in situ* and *in vitro*. *Biochem J* 1995;305:799–800.
76. Tortorella MD, Burn TC, Pratta MA, et al. Purification and cloning of aggrecanase-1: a member of the ADAMTS family of proteins. *Science* 1999;284:1664–1666.
77. Abbaszade I, Liu R, Yang F, et al. Cloning and characterization of ADAMTS11, and aggrecanase from the ADAMTS family. *J Biol Chem* 1999;274:23443–23450.
78. Flannery CR, Little CB, Hughes CE, et al. Expression of ADAMTS homologues in articular cartilage. *Biochem Biophys Res Commun* 1999;260:318–322.
79. Knudson CB. Hyaluronan receptor-directed assembly of chondrocyte pericellular matrix. *J Cell Biol* 1993;120:825–834.
80. Hua Q, Knudson CB, Knudson W. Internalization of hyaluronan by chondrocytes occurs via receptor-mediated endocytosis. *J Cell Sci* 1993;106:365–375.
81. Weigel PH, Hascall VC, Tammi M. Hyaluronan synthases. *J Biol Chem* 1997;272:13997–14000.
82. Balazs EA, Denlinger JL. Viscosupplementation: a new concept in the treatment of osteoarthritis. *J Rheumatol* 1993;395:3–9.
83. Yoshida, M, Itano N, Yamada Y, et al. *In vitro* synthesis of hyaluronan by a single protein derived from mouse HAS1 gene and characterization of amino acid residues essential for its activity. *J Biol Chem* 2000;275:497–506.
84. Toole BP. Hyaluronan and its binding proteins, the hyaladherins. *Curr Opin Cell Biol* 1990;2:839–844.
85. Toole BP. Hyaluronan in morphogenesis. *J Intern Med* 1997;42:35–40.
86. Laurent T-C, Laurent U-B, Fraser J-R. The structure and function of hyaluronan: an overview. *Immunol Cell Biol* 1996;74:A1–A7
87. Nishida Y, Knudson CB, Nietfeld JJ, et al. Antisense inhibition of hyaluronan synthase-2 in human articular chondrocytes inhibits proteoglycan retention and matrix assembly. *J Biol Chem* 1999;274: 21893–21899.
88. Tanimoto K, Ohno S, Fujimoto K, et al. Proinflammatory cytokines regulate the gene expression of hyaluronic acid synthetase in cultured rabbit synovial membrane cells. *Connect Tiss Res* 2001;42:187–195.
89. Iozzo RV. The biology of the small leucine-rich proteoglycans. *J Biol Chem* 1999;274:18843–18846.
90. Fisher LW, Termine JD, Young MF. Deduced protein sequence of bone small proteoglycan I (biglycan) shows homology with proteoglycan II (decorin) and several nonconnective tissue proteins in a variety of species. *J Biol Chem* 1989;264:4571–4576.
91. Johnson HJ, Rosenberg L, Chois HU, et al. Characterization of epiphycan, a small proteoglycan with a leucine-rich repeat core protein. *J Biol Chem* 1997;272:18709–18717.
92. Bengtsson E, Neame PJ, Heinegård D, et al. The primary structure of a basic leucine-rich repeat protein, PRELP, found in connective tissues. *J Biol Chem* 1995;270:25639–25644.
93. Corpus LM, Funderburgh JL, Funderburgh ML, et al. Molecular cloning and tissue distribution of keratocan. *J Biol Chem* 1996;271: 9759–9763.
94. Plaas AH, Neame PJ, Nivens, et al. Identification of the keratan sulfate attachment sites on bovine fibromodulin. *J Biol Chem* 1990;265: 20634–20640.
95. Kobe B, Deisenhofer J. Crystal structure of porcine ribonuclease inhibitor: a protein with leucine-rich repeats. *Nature* 1993;366:751–756.
96. Schönherr E, Hausser H, Beavan L, et al. Decorin-type I collagen interaction: presence of separate core protein-binding domains. *J Biol Chem* 1995;270:8877–8883.
97. Svensson L, Heinegård D, Oldberg A. Decorin-binding sites for collagen type I are mainly located in leucine-rich repeats. *J Biol Chem* 1995;270:20712–20716.
98. Hedbom E, Heinegård D. Binding of fibromodulin and decorin to separate sites on fibrillar collagens. *J Biol Chem* 1993;268:27307–27312.
99. Rada JA, Cornuet PK, Hassell R. Regulation of corneal collagen fibrillogenesis *in vitro* by corneal proteoglycan (lumican and decorin) core proteins. *Exp Eye Res* 1993;56:635–648.
100. Yamaguchi Y, Mann DM, Ruoslahti E. Negative regulation of transforming growth factor-beta by the proteoglycan decorin. *Nature* 1990;346:281–284.
101. Takeuchi Y, Kodama Y, Matsumoto T. Bone matrix decorin binds transforming growth factor-beta and enhances its bioactivity. *J Biol Chem* 1994;269:32634–32638.
102. Hildebrand A, Romaris M, Rasmussen LM, et al. Interaction of the small interstitial proteoglycans biglycan, decorin and fibromodulin with transforming growth factor beta. *Biochem J* 1994;302:527–534.
103. Dodge GR, Boesler EW, Jimenez SA. Expression of the basement membrane heparan sulfate proteoglycan (perlecan) in human synovium and in cultured human synovial cells. *Lab Invest* 1995;73: 649–657.

104. SundarRaj N, Fite D, Ledbetter S, et al. Perlecan is a component of cartilage matrix and promotes chondrocyte attachment. *J Cell Sci* 1995;108:1–10.
105. French MM, Smith SE, Akanbi K, et al. Expression of the heparan sulfate proteoglycan, perlecan, during mouse embryogenesis and perlecan chondrogenic activity *in vitro*. *J Cell Biol* 1999;145:1103–1115.
106. Melrose J, Smith S, Knox S, et al. Perlecan, the multidomain HS-proteoglycan of basement membranes, is a prominent pericellular component of ovine hypertrophic vertebral growth plate and cartilagenous endplate chondrocytes. *Histochem Cell Biol* 2002;118: 269–280.
107. French MM, Gomes RR, Timpl R, et al. Chondrogenic activity of the heparan sulfate proteoglycan perlecan maps to the N-terminal domain I. *J Bone Miner Res* 2002;17:48–55.
108. Kallunki P, Tryggvason K. Human basement membrane heparan sulfate proteoglycans core protein: a 467-kD protein containing multiple domains resembling elements of the low density lipoprotein receptor, laminin, neural cell adhesion molecules and epidermal growth factor. *J Cell Biol* 1992;116:559–571.
109. Bork P, Patthy L. The SEA module: a new extracellular domain associated with O-glycosylation. *Protein Sci* 1995;4:1421–1425.
110. Hayashi K, Madri JA, Yurchenco PD. Endothelial cells interact with the core protein of basement membrane perlecan through β_1 and β_3 integrins: an adhesion modulated by glycosaminoglycan. *J Cell Biol* 1992;119:945–959.
111. Brown JC, Sasaki T, Göhring W, et al. The C-terminal domain V of perlecan promotes β_1 integrin-mediated cell adhesion, binds heparin, nidogen and fibulin-2 and can be modified by glycosaminoglycans. *Eur J Biochem* 1997;250:39–46.
112. Yurchenco PD, Cheng YS, Ruben GC. Self-assembly of a high molecular weight basement membrane heparan sulfate proteoglycan into dimers and oligomers. *J Biol Chem* 1987;262:17688–17676.
113. Arikawa-Hirasawa E, Le AH, Nishino I, et al. Structural and functional mutations of the perlecan gene cause Schwartz-Jampel syndrome, with myotonic myopathy and chondrodysplasia. *Am J Hum Genet* 2002;70:1368–1375.
114. Arikawa-Hirasawa E, Wilcox WR, Yamada Y. Dyssegmental dysplasia, Silverman-Handmaker type: unexpected role of perlecan in cartilage development. *Am J Med Genet* 2001;106:254–257.
115. Costell M, Gustafsson E, Aszodi A, et al. Perlecan maintains the integrity of cartilage and some basement membranes. *J Cell Biol* 1999;147:1109–1122.
116. Carey DJ. Syndecans: multifunctional cell-surface co-receptors. *Biochem J* 1997;327:1–16.
117. Woods A, Couchman JR. Syndecans: synergistic activators of cell adhesion. *Trends Cell Biol* 1998;8:189–192.
118. Rapraeger AC, Ott VL. Molecular interactions of the syndecan core proteins. *Curr Opin Cell Biol* 1998;10:620–628.
119. Woods A. Syndecans: transmembrane modulators of adhesion and matrix assembly. *J Clin Invest* 2001;107:935–941.
120. Fanning AS, Anderson J. Protein-protein interactions: PDZ domain networks. *Curr Biol* 1996;6:1385–1388.
121. Fialka I, Steinlein P, Ahorn H, et al. Identification of syntenin as a protein of the apical early endocytic compartment in Madin-Darby canine kidney cells. *J Biol Chem* 1999;274:26233–26239.
122. Grootjans JJ, Zimmerman P, Reekmans G, et al. Syntenin: a PDZ protein that binds syndecan cytoplasmic domains. *Proc Natl Acad Sci U S A* 1997;94:13683–13688.
123. Cohen AR, Woods DF, Marfatia SM, et al. Human CASK/LIN-2 binds syndecan-2 and protein 4.1 and localizes to the basolateral membrane of epithelial cells. *J Cell Biol* 1998;142:129–138.
124. Baciu PC, Saoncella S, Lee SH, et al. Syndesmos, a protein that interacts with the cytoplasmic domain of syndecan-4, mediates cell spreading and actin cytoskeletal organization. *J Cell Sci* 2000;113: 315–324.
125. Greene DK, Tumova S, Couchman JR, et al. Syndecan-4 associates with α-actinin. *J Biol Chem* 2003;278:7617–7623.
126. Oh ES, Woods A, Couchman JR. Syndecan-4 proteoglycan regulates the distribution and activity of protein kinase C. *J Biol Chem* 1997; 272:8133–8136.
127. Granes F, Urena JM, Rocamoro N, et al. Ezrin links syndecan-2 to the cytoskeleton. *J Cell Sci* 2000;113:1267–1276.
128. David G, Bai XM, Van der Schueren B, et al. Spatial and temporal changes in the expression of fibroglycan (syndecan-2) during mouse embryonic development. *Development* 1933;119:841–854.
129. Clasper S, Vekeman S, Fiore M, et al. Inducible expression of the cell surface heparan sulfate proteoglycan syndecan-2 (fibroglycan) on human activated macrophages can regulate fibroblast growth factor action. *J Biol Chem* 1999;274:24113–24123.
130. Klass CM, Couchman JR, Woods A. Control of extracellular matrix assembly by syndecan-2 proteoglycan. *J Cell Sci* 2000;113:493–506.
131. Gould SE, Upholt WB, Kosher RA. Syndecan-3: a member of the syndecan family of membrane-intercalated proteoglycans that is expressed at high amounts at the onset of chicken limb cartilage differentiation. *Proc Natl Acad Sci U S A* 1992;89:3271–3275.
132. Hall BK, Miyak T. Divide, accumulate, differentiate: cell condensation in skeletal development revisited. *Int J Dev Biol* 1995;39:881–893.
133. Shimazu A, Nah HD, Kirsch T, et al. Syndecan-3 and the control of chondrocyte proliferation during endochondral ossification. *Exp Cell Res* 1996;229:126–136.
134. Seghatoleslami MR, Kosher RA. Inhibition of *in vitro* cartilage differentiation by syndecan-3 antibodies. *Dev Dyn* 1996;207:114–119.
135. Koyama E, Leatherman JL, Shimazu A, et al. Syndecan-3, tenascin-C, and the development of cartilagenous skeletal elements and joints in chick limbs. *Dev Dyn* 1995;203:152–162.
136. Pfander D, Swoboda B, Kirsch T. Expression of early and late differentiation markers (proliferating cell nuclear antigen, syndecan-3, annexin VI and alkaline phosphatase) by human osteoarthritic chondrocytes. *Am J Pathol* 2001;159:1777–1783.
137. Woods A, Couchman JR. Syndecan 4 heparan sulfate proteoglycan is a selectively enriched and widespread focal adhesion component. *Mol Biol Cell* 1994;5:183–192.
138. Couchman JR, Woods A. Syndecan-4 and integrins: combinatorial signaling in cell adhesion. *J Cell Sci* 1999;112:3415–3420.
139. Oh ES, Woods A, Lim St, et al. Syndecan-4 proteoglycan cytoplasmic domain and phosphatidylinositol 4,5-bisphosphate coordinately regulate protein kinase C activity. *J Biol Chem* 1998;273:10624–10629.
140. Horowitz A, Simons M. Phosphorylation of the cytoplasmic tail of syndecan-4 regulates activation of protein kinase Cα. *J Biol Chem* 1998;273:25548–25551.
141. Little CB, Hughes CE, Curtis CL, et al. Matrix metalloproteinases are involved in C-terminal and interglobular domain processing of cartilage aggrecan in late stage cartilage degradation. *Matrix Biol* 2002;21:271–288.
142. Malfait AM, Liu RQ, Ijiri K, et al. Inhibition of ADAM-TS4 and ADAM-TS5 prevents aggrecan degradation in osteoarthritic cartilage. *J Biol Chem* 2002;277:22201–22208.
143. Arner EC. Aggrecanase-mediated cartilage degradation. *Curr Opin Pharmacol* 2002;2:322–329.
144. Wai AW, Ng LJ, Watanabe H, et al. Disrupted expression of matrix genes in the growth plate of the mouse cartilage matrix deficiency (cmd) mutant. *Dev Genet* 1998;22:349–358.
145. Handley CJ, Mok MT, Ilic MZ, et al. Cathepsin D cleaves aggrecan at unique sites within the interglobular domain and chondroitin sulfate attachment regions that are also cleaved when cartilage is maintained at acid pH. *Matrix Biol* 2001;20:543–553.
146. Hou WS, Li Z, Gordon RE, et al. Cathepsin k is a critical protease in synovial fibroblast-mediated collagen degradation. *Am J Pathol* 2001;159:2167–2177.
147. Barre PE, Redini F, Boumediene K, et al. Semiquantitative reverse transcription-polymerase chain reaction analysis of syndecan-1 and -4 messages in cartilage and cultured chondrocytes from osteoarthritic joints. *Osteoarthritis Cartilage* 2000;8:34–43.
148. Bock HC, Michaeli P, Bode C, et al. The small proteoglycans decorin and biglycan in human articular cartilage of late-stage osteoarthritis. *Osteoarthritis Cartilage* 2001;9:654–663.
149. Sztrolovics R, Recklies AD, Roughley PJ, et al. Hyaluronate degradation as an alternative mechanism for proteoglycan release from cartilage during interleukin-1β-stimulated catabolism. *Biochem J* 2002; 362:473–479.

CHAPTER 11

Cartilage in Health and Disease

A. Robin Poole

Cartilage is a highly specialized skeletal tissue that is elaborated at sites where a semisolid architecture is required to provide shape and form, yet to ensure strength, deformability, and durability. Its metabolism, like that of other musculoskeletal tissues, is regulated chemically and mechanically. It acts as an intermediate tissue in bone growth and repair, being present in the anlage in embryonic development and in the epiphyses, primary and secondary growth plates, and fracture repair. In growth and aging, articular cartilage is essential for articulation but can degenerate and be destroyed in arthritis, leading to a loss of joint function. Nonarticular cartilages play critical roles throughout the body, such as in nasal septa, the ears, larynx, bronchioles, and costal cartilages. Specialized cartilages constitute the intervertebral discs.

This chapter examines hyaline cartilage formation, development, structure, and degeneration and how these are regulated. In the adult, emphasis is placed on articular cartilage. The structure, composition, and organization of cartilage at the tissue and molecular levels is described, as is the function of the extensive extracellular matrix, which is elaborated by chondrocytes. The turnover of this matrix is regulated by chondrocytes that are under the control and influence (in health and disease) of growth factors, cytokines, and mechanical stimuli. These regulatory factors and the changes that occur in disease are described. The mechanisms of cartilage degradation, how this occurs in arthritis, and how cartilage may act as a source of autoantigens to drive inflammatory arthritides such as rheumatoid arthritis (RA) also are discussed. Finally, the tumors of cartilage and cartilage transplantability are briefly discussed.

CHONDROGENESIS IN EMBRYONIC AND POSTNATAL STATES

Chondroblasts (a newly differentiated cell that is maturationally immature) and chondrocytes (mature fully differentiated cells) develop from mesenchymal chondroprogenitor cells. In development, avascular mesenchymal cell aggregates (blastema) precede cartilage formation both *in vivo* (1) and in high–cell density cell cultures (2) (Fig. 11.1). They are characterized by high expression of fibronectin and laminin, receptors for these molecules (3), and the chondroblast/chondrocyte transcription factors homeoprotein 1 (4) and Sox9 (5). The latter is required for type II collagen expression and is essential for chondrogenesis (6). Type IIA procollagen mRNA, expressed in mesenchymal condensations, is unlike type IIB collagen in that it contains the product of expression of exon 2, which encodes a 70–amino acid, cysteine-rich, globular domain in the aminopropeptide (7,8). When chondrocytes develop, exon 2 (i.e., type IIA collagen) is transcribed for a while with type IIB collagen. With further development, expression is restricted to type IIB. The type IIA aminopropeptide can bind the growth and differentiation factors transforming growth factor (TGF)-β_1 and bone morphogenetic protein (BMP)-2 (9). The large aggregating cartilage proteoglycan aggrecan is also first detectable at this time (10). After condensation, type II collagen and aggrecan increase in content.

The perichondrium, from which cartilage forms during development (as in the embryonic epiphysis, nasal cartilage, and cartilages of the ear), retains chondrogenic potential in the adult (11), as does periosteum (12). Cartilage can occasionally form by metaplasia in the synovial membranes of joints and in bursae or tendon sheaths, but some secondary calcification of cartilage usually occurs, associated with expression of the hypertrophic phenotype (13).

The differentiation of mesenchyme into chondrocytes involves a superfamily of regulatory molecules called BMPs, also known as osteogenic proteins (OPs) (14) (Fig. 11.1). TGF-β is perhaps the best known member. OP-1 (BMP-7), BMP-2B, TGF-β_1, and TGF-β_2 can each induce cartilage formation. BMP-2, BMP-4, BMP-5, and BMP-7 are expressed in perichondrial cells surrounding cartilage elements. Disruption of BMP-5 in the short-ear mouse mutant results

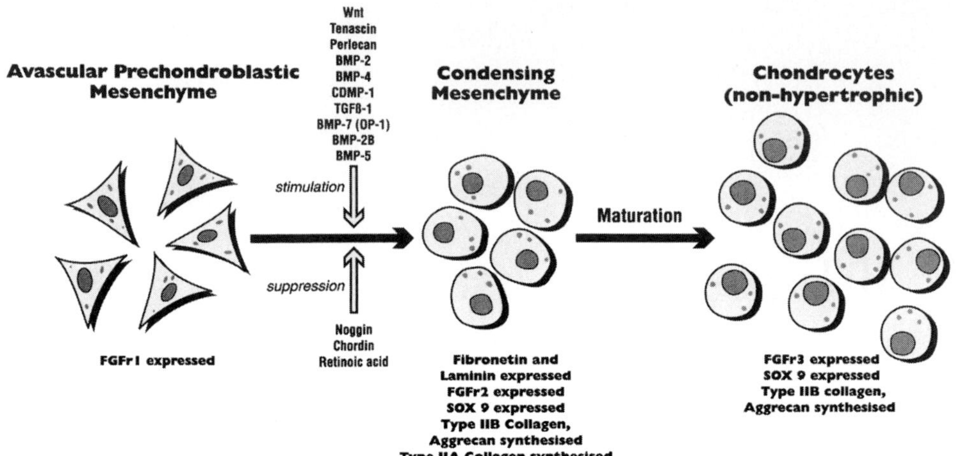

FIG. 11.1. Chondrocyte differentiation from mesenchyme. Some of the molecules that regulate this process are shown. Maturation involves cell proliferation and the establishment of an extensive extracellular matrix. The transcriptional factor SOX9 is required for type II collagen synthesis, without which the chondrocytic phenotype is not expressed. *BMP*, bone morphogenetic protein; *CDMP*, cartilage-derived morphogenetic protein; *FGF*, fibroblast growth factor; *TGF*, transforming growth factor.

in loss of chondrocyte condensations (15), demonstrating its requirement for cellular differentiation. Overexpression of BMP-2 and BMP-4 in chicks (16) and cartilage-derived morphogenetic protein-1 (CDMP-1; also known as growth/differentiation factor-5) in mice (17) results in overgrowth of cartilage and accelerated chondroprogenitor cell development, respectively. Null mutations in BMP-7 in mice result in abnormal skeletal development (18).

BMP signaling can be antagonized by Noggin or Chordin, each of which can directly bind BMPs, preventing them from binding to their receptors. In mice lacking Noggin, cartilage condensations develop normally but exhibit hyperplasia. Initiation of joint development also is prevented (19). Chordin overexpression suppresses chondrocyte maturation in developing skeletal elements (20). Retinoic acid or a constitutively active retinoic acid receptor can inhibit mesenchymal differentiation (21,22). Inhibition of retinoid signaling induces Sox9 expression, the transcription factor that is a "master switch" for chondroblast differentiation (23).

Fibroblast growth factors (FGFs) play a key role in mesenchymal differentiation, as indicated by the essential requirement for FGF-10 in limb bud outgrowth (24). Whereas FGF receptor 1 (FGFr1) is expressed mainly in undifferentiated proliferating mesenchyme, FGFr2 is found in precartilage condensations, and FGFr3, in differentiated cartilage nodules (25).

MATURATION OF CHONDROCYTES TO EXPRESS HYPERTROPHIC AND NONHYPERTROPHIC PHENOTYPES

The chondrocytes of hyaline cartilage formed from chondroblasts continue to divide under the control of specific cell cycle genes (26). They synthesize and secrete type II collagen and aggrecan, and elaborate an extensive extracellular matrix that usually lasts for the life of the animal. Such cartilages are typified by articular and nasal cartilages. Chondrocytes can also synthesize and secrete elastin

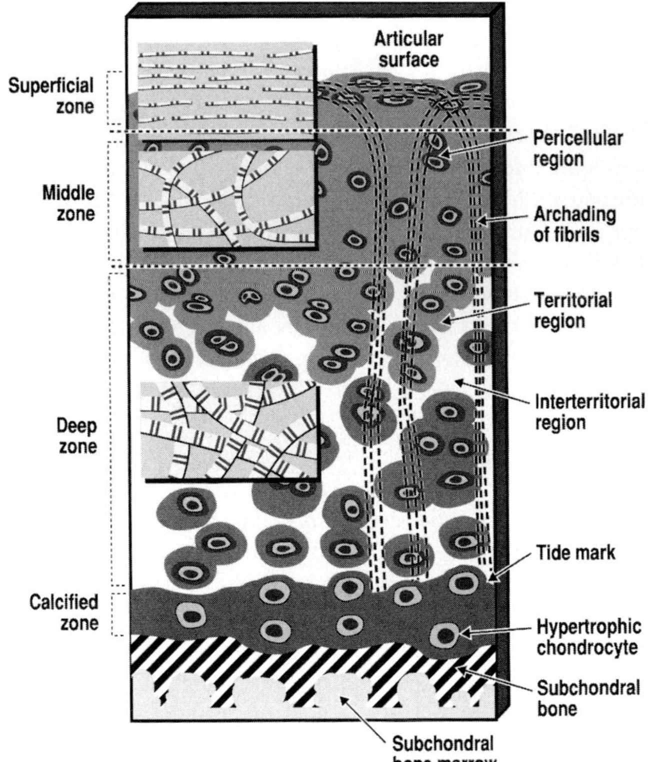

FIG. 11.2. Regional organization of articular cartilage based on studies in adult cattle and humans. The ultrastructural organization of the territorial, interterritorial, and pericellular regions is different (180). The pericellular region contains a high concentration of aggrecan, the proteoglycan decorin, and type VI collagen. The superficial zone contains thin collagen fibrils arranged in parallel with the articular surfaces. The partly calcified cartilage of the calcified zone is indicated. The interterritorial zone is first recognizable at about 17 years of age in humans, based on changes in the distribution of aggrecan and link protein. The relative sizes and organization of collagen fibrils are shown as inserts. These are not to scale. The arcading of collagen fibrils is also shown by the broken lines.

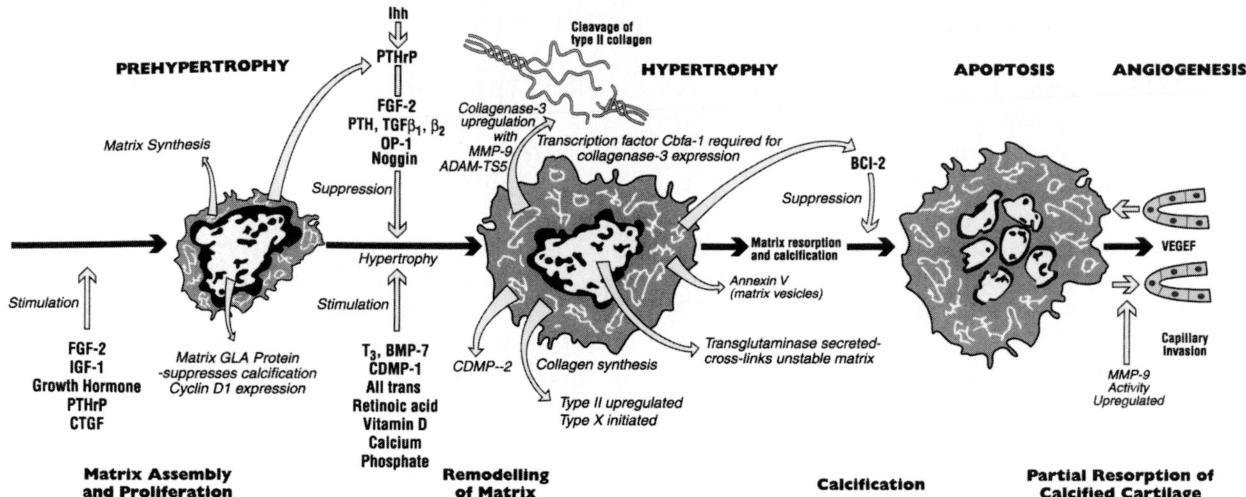

FIG. 11.3. Chondrocyte maturation and its regulation. Starting from the proliferating, matrix-synthesizing, prehypertrophic chondrocyte; cellular hypertrophy occurs, followed by mineralization of the extensive extracellular matrix, culminating in apoptosis of the hypertrophic chondrocyte, which is closely linked to angiogenesis. Some of the principal events and regulatory molecules are shown. *ADAM-TS,* a distintegrin and metalloproteinase with thrombospondin motifs; *BMP,* bone morphogenetic protein; *CDMP,* cartilage-derived morphogenetic protein; *CTGF,* connective tissue growth factor; *FGF,* fibroblast growth factor; *IGF,* insulin-like growth factor; *Ihh,* Indian hedgehog; *MMP,* matrix metalloproteinase; *OP,* osteogenic protein; *PTHrP,* parathyroid hormone–related peptide; T_3, triioclothyronine; *TGF,* transforming growth factor; *VEGF,* vascular endothelial growth factor.

to provide the matrix with greater flexibility; such elastic cartilages are typified by the auricular cartilage and the cartilages of the epiglottis. These cartilages do not ordinarily calcify, although a partly calcified cartilage layer may be seen, as observed in articular cartilage, at the interface with subchondral bone. Its upper limit is delineated by the tidemark (Fig 11.2).

In contrast, chondroblasts in developing bones, growth plates, and fracture callus differentiate to form hypertrophic chondrocytes that then calcify their extracellular matrix (27) (Figs. 11.3 and 11.4). The calcified cartilage acts as a scaffold upon which the formation of woven bone takes place. Osteoblasts settle on the remaining calcified trabecular cartilage and deposit osteoid that calcifies. This bone is subsequently resorbed, together with the core of calcified cartilage, and is replaced by trabecular, lamellar, or cortical bone, according to the location. Chondroblasts isolated from growth plate cartilages and chick sterna (where there is progressive maturation of chondroblasts to form hypertrophic chondrocytes) display a preprogrammed cellular maturation leading to the expression of the hypertrophic phenotype, provided they are maintained in a permissive environment (28,29).

The factors regulating differentiation of chondroblasts to the hypertrophic phenotype are complex. Hypertrophy follows the cessation of chondrocyte proliferation and is characterized by synthesis of type X collagen. This proliferation and matrix assembly requires growth hormone (GH) that generates insulin-like growth factor-1 (IGF-1) synthesis and autocrine/paracrine receptor–mediated activation of the chondrocytes (see later section on Molecules that Regulate

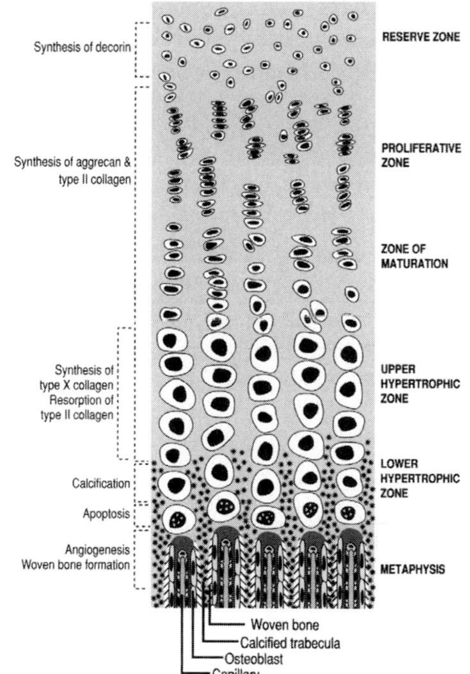

FIG. 11.4. Primary mammalian (bovine) growth plate showing progressive development of chondroblasts from the proliferative zone to the lower hypertrophic zone, where matrix synthesis stops, and the extracellular matrix is calcified. As part of the angiogenic response, capillaries grow into and erode uncalcified transverse septa and erode some of the calcified longitudinal septa. (Modified and reproduced from Poole AR. The growth plate: cellular physiology, cartilage assembly and mineralization. In: Hall BK, Newman S, eds. *Cartilage: molecular aspects.* Boca Raton, FL: CRC Press, 1991:179–211, with permission.)

Chondrocyte Metabolism). FGF-2 and its receptor, the cell surface proteoglycan syndecan-3, are required for chondrocyte proliferation (30), as is integrin-linked kinase (ILK), inactivation of which leads to a reduction of proliferation and impairment of binding to type II collagen (31).

Thyroxine (T_4) and, more potently, triiodothyronine (T_3), induce rapid maturation of these immature chondrocytes (32). Vitamin D, both 1,25-dihydroxycholecalciferol and 24, 25-dihydroxycholecalciferol, are required to ensure complete maturation, matrix calcification, and vascular invasion (see later section on Molecules that Regulate Chondrocyte Metabolism).

Chondrocytes that become hypertrophic selectively upregulate expression of the retinoic acid receptor γ (RARγ) gene (33). Retinoids are present in chondrocytes and, particularly, in neighboring perichondrial cells that produce BMPs. Retinoids are required for hypertrophy. Their antagonists inhibit hypertrophy, whereas all-*trans*-retinoic acid induces terminal differentiation (33,34). Retinoic acid stimulates annexin-mediated Ca^{2+} influx into growth plate chondrocytes. Specific annexin Ca^{2+} channel blockers prevent hypertrophy (35), pointing to the importance of Ca^{2+} uptake during chondrocyte differentiation. Phosphate is also required for hypertrophy (28).

BMPs, such as CDMP-1, accelerate maturation to hypertrophy (17). In contrast, Noggin, a potent BMP antagonist (36), suppresses hypertrophy. Other BMPs, namely OP-1 (BMP-7) (37) and TGF-$\beta_{1,2}$ (38,39), suppress hypertrophy. Chondrocytes also express these BMPs. However, CDMP-2 expression is restricted to hypertrophic chondrocytes (40). Suppression of hypertrophy also is caused by FGFs such as FGF-2 (39,41). Although FGF-2 is a strong suppressor of hypertrophy, mature hypertrophic chondrocytes fail to respond to FGF-2 because of loss of the receptor (42). Disruption of the FGFr3 gene produces severe and progressive bone dysplasia in mice, with increased proliferation and an expanded hypertrophic zone (43). Other alterations in FGF receptors, such as constitutive activation, lead to skeletal dysplasias associated with accelerated apoptosis of hypertrophic chondrocytes but unchanged proliferation (44) (Table 11.1).

Another key molecule in the regulation of hypertrophy is parathyroid hormone–related peptide (PTHrP). PTHrP is produced in prehypertrophic chondrocytes as well as in perichondrium. It stimulates proliferation of prehypertrophic chondrocytes (45) through its receptor PTHrP, together with TGFβ_1, by activating cyclin D1 expression (46). Furthermore, PTHrP suppression of hypertrophy involves downregulation of expression of the transcription factor Cbfa1 (Runx2) (47). If PTHrP or its receptor is deleted, premature hypertrophy results (48,49). Overexpression of PTHrP also suppresses hypertrophy (50). Peptides derived from PTHrP (1–34) and PTH (1–34) can both reverse expression of the hypertrophic phenotype *in vitro* (51).

TABLE 11.1. *Genetically determined molecular defects of chondrocytes that result in abnormal human skeletal development*

Condition	Gene
Camptodactyly-arthropathy coxa vara-pericarditis syndrome	Superficial zone protein
Kniest dysplasia	COL2A1
Achondrogenesis II	COL2A1
Hypochondrogenesis	COL2A1
Spondyloepiphyseal dyslasia	COL2A1 COL9A2
Stickler syndrome	COL2A1
Marshall syndrome	COL11A2
Schmid-type metaphyseal dysplasia	COL10A1
Multiple epiphyseal dysplasia (EDMI)	Cartilage oligomeric protein
Pseudoachondroplasia	Cartilage oligomeric protein
Marfan syndrome	Fibrilin-1
Diastrophic dysplasia	Sulfate transporter
Achondrogenesis 1B	Sulfate transporter
Atelosteogenesis II	Sulfate transporter
Hypophosphatasia	Alkaline phosphatase
Keutel syndrome	Matrix Gla protein
Achondroplasia	Fibroblast growth factor receptor 3
Thanatotrophic dysplasias types I and II	Fibroblast growth factor receptor 3
Jansen-type metaphyseal dysplasia	PTH-PTHrP receptor
Acromesomelic chondrodysplasia, Hunter-Thompson type	CDMP-1 growth factor (Gdf-5)
Campomelic dysplasia	SOX9 transcription factor
Dyssegmental dysplasia, Silverman-Handmaker type	Perlecan
Brachydactyly type A-1	Indian hedgehog

CDMP, cartilage-derived morphogenetic protein; PTH, parathyroid hormone; PTHrP, parathyroid hormone-related peptide.

PTHrP can be induced in prehypertrophic cells by a protein designated Indian hedgehog (Ihh), the receptor for which is called Patched. Hedgehog controls hypertrophy by operating upstream of PTHrP (52,53). TGF-β_2 mediates the effects of Hedgehog on hypertrophy and PTHrP expression (54). A lack of expression of Ihh results in reduced chondrocyte proliferation and premature hypertrophy (55). Ihh also up-regulates BMP-2 and BMP-4 expression, in addition to Noggin and Chordin (36). Full expression of hypertrophy is dependent on the activity of the transcription factor osf2/Cbfa1 (Runx2) without which collagenase-3/matrix metalloproteinase 13 (MMP-13) is not expressed (56–58). This is the collagenase that is used by hypertrophic chondrocytes to resorb neighboring extracellular matrix before and during its calcification (59,60). Inhibition of this proteolysis prevents chondrocyte hypertrophy (60). Aggrecanase-2/ADAM-TS5 (a disintegrin and metalloproteinase with thrombospondin motifs 5) expression (61) and proteoglycan degradation mediated by aggrecanases and MMPs occur as part of this maturational process. Up-regulation of expression of the proteinase MMP-9 accompanies chondrocyte hypertrophy (62). When MMP-9 is not expressed, hypertrophy is arrested and calcification becomes disorganized and is premature (63).

Members of the Wnt family also play an important role in cartilage development. The Wnt proteins are paracrine/autocrine signaling molecules. They bind to receptors called frizzled on the cell surface. Proteins with Wnt antagonistic properties include Frzb-1. The latter exerts a strong influence on limb skeletogenesis and can modulate chondrocyte maturation (64). Wnt5a and Wnt5b promote early chondrogenesis *in vitro* while inhibiting terminal (hypertrophic) differentiation *in vivo* (65). Delta-1 is a transmembrane ligand expressed on hypertrophic cells. Its receptor (Notch-2) is expressed in chondrocytes at all stages of development. These molecules are involved in determining cell differentiation. If Delta-1 is misexpressed, prehypertrophic cells form but do not differentiate into hypertrophic cells (66).

Apoptosis represents the end stage in the hypertrophic process. Expression of Bcl-2, a protein that negatively regulates programmed cell death (67), is reduced in hypertrophic chondrocytes as they undergo apoptosis.

There is an absolute requirement for angiogenesis in skeletal development. This involves invasion by blood vessels into chondrocyte lacunae, occupied by dying apoptotic chondrocytes. Hypertrophy of chondrocytes precedes vessel ingrowth (68). These hypertrophic cells produce two principal splice variants of vascular endothelial cell growth factor (VEGF) (69,70). The receptors for VEGF (KDR and FLT-1) are present on endothelial cells of vessels growing into hypertrophic cartilage (70).

Connective tissue growth factor (CTGF) is also now recognized as an essential requirement for normal growth plate development. Null mice for CTGF exhibit impaired chondrocyte proliferation, decreased expression of matrix components and MMPs, and expanded hypertrophic zones where angiogenesis (decreased VEGF expression) and calcification are impaired (71). Some of these regulatory molecules are summarized in Fig. 11.3.

Matrix Changes and Mineral Formation in Hypertrophy and Endochondral Ossification

Unlike articular cartilage, the cartilaginous growth plate (physis) and fracture callus are transient tissues committed to provision of a calcified cartilage scaffold on which woven bone is formed by osteoblasts (Fig. 11.4). The cellular and matrix changes that are involved in this process can be observed in primary growth plates. Here, a reserve zone of chondrocytes can be clearly identified that resides in an extensive extracellular matrix. This gives rise to a proliferative zone in which proliferating cells are arranged in longitudinal columns separated by transverse and longitudinal septa. Matrix synthesis is active (29). As cells mature from the lower proliferative to the hypertrophic zone, matrix is resorbed. This involves the selective cleavage, denaturation, and removal of type II collagen by collagenase (72,73), which accompanies hypertrophy. As discussed above, this resorptive process results from the activity of collagenase-3 (MMP-13), and other proteinases, which include MMP-9 and aggrecanases. Matrix resorption is accompanied by the formation of cross-links in the extracellular matrix catalyzed by transglutaminase activity (74). Extracellular matrix synthesis continues undiminished, if not at an accelerated rate, early in hypertrophy. Type X collagen synthesis is initiated as the chondrocytes enlarge and become hypertrophic (75,76), as is the synthesis of a lipocalin called extracellular fatty acid binding protein (77). Alkaline phosphatase synthesis also increases (78).

The loss of type II collagen contrasts with the retention of aggrecan (72,73,79). Type X collagen interacts with the collagen fibrillar network (76), but it is also cleaved (80). In the lower hypertrophic zone, when matrix volume is minimal and aggrecan content is maximal within the extracellular matrix (72,79), matrix synthesis is arrested. Calcification is initiated in focal sites between collagen fibrils where the C-propeptide of type II procollagen (an apatite- and calcium-binding protein) is concentrated (27,81).

Mineral formation also occurs in matrix vesicles (82) (Fig. 11.5). These are small (100-nm diameter) vesicular products of projections of the plasma membrane that are rich in alkaline phosphatase (82) and annexin V (83). Annexins II, V, and VI, stimulated by retinoic acid, mediate Ca^{2+} uptake in vesicles, promoting nucleation (83,84,85). Whether these vesicles act as the principal nucleators of the major mineralization events that occur in the lower hypertrophic zone remains controversial. Focal sites of mineralization often do not coincide with matrix vesicles

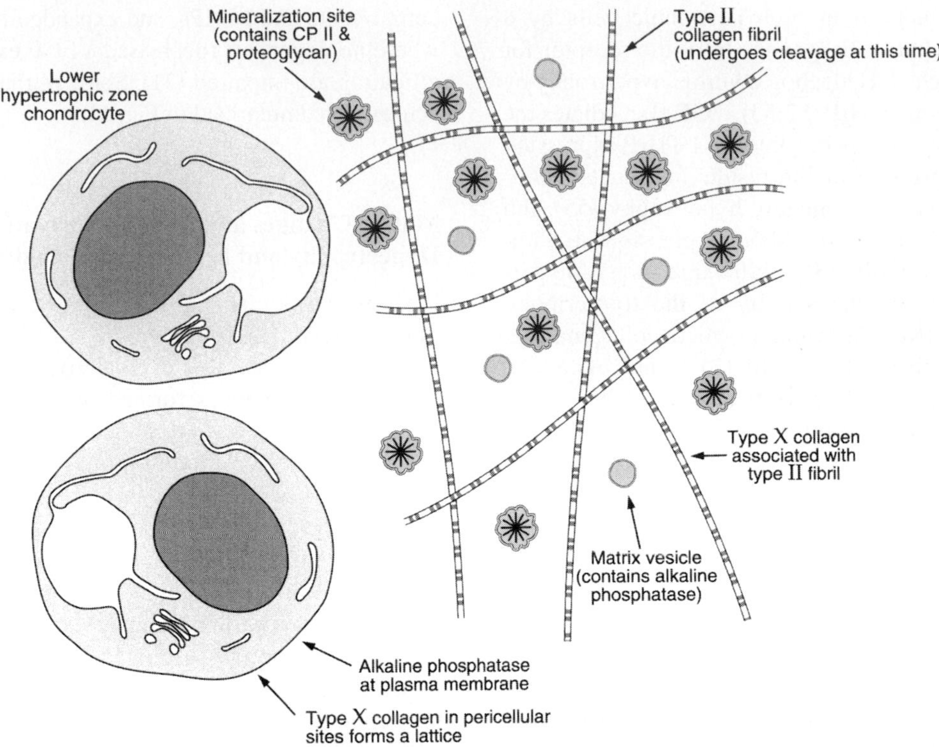

FIG. 11.5. Primary mineralization sites in extracellular matrix of the hypertrophic zone of growth plate, which contains elevated concentrations of the proteoglycan aggrecan and the C-propeptide of type II collagen (CPII). Mineralization also is initiated in matrix vesicles. (Reproduced from Poole AR. The growth plate: cellular physiology, cartilage assembly and mineralization. In: Hall BK, Newman S, eds. *Cartilage: molecular aspects.* Boca Raton, FL: CRC Press, 1991:179–211, with permission.)

(76,86–88), although they exist adjacent to each other (Fig. 11.5).

A high concentration of alkaline phosphatase is always found in calcifying cartilages (72,89). The activity of this enzyme is essential (see Table 11.1) for the production of inorganic phosphate that is required for hypertrophy and the formation of mineral in the presence of inorganic calcium (27,28). Pyrophosphate, a substrate of alkaline phosphatase, which is an inhibitor of mineralization, is elaborated by prehypertrophic cells and is regulated by a transmembrane protein called Ank (90). TGF-β, which suppresses hypertrophy, stimulates the expression of Ank (91).

A local increase in phosphate concentration (provided by the action of alkaline phosphatase on organic substrates) can displace calcium, leading to the formation of a calcium phosphate known as hydroxyapatite (27,28). Proteoglycans can act as focal nucleators of calcification (92,93). The presence of a focal concentration of the C-propeptide of type II procollagen (chondrocalcin) (94) in sites of mineral formation (81) probably results from the hydroxyapatite-binding properties of this molecule (95), which could influence mineral growth. The lack of mineral formation on collagen fibrils might relate to the presence of type X collagen (76) and the extensive denaturation and cleavage of type II collagen (73). In the growth plates, the process of matrix formation and calcification is rapid, requiring about 3 to 5 days from the time that cells first appear in the upper proliferative zone to the completion of cartilage calcification (96). Calcification itself is even more rapid (about 12–24 hours) (96,97). Therefore, the maturation of chondroblasts and mineral growth must be regulated with extreme care so that the events of cell proliferation, matrix formation, selective matrix degradation, reorganization, and calcification are carefully organized and balanced by the angiogenic process of invasive ingrowth of capillaries from the metaphysis, which results in the removal of uncalcified cartilage and some of the calcified cartilage. Matrix γ-carboxyglutamic acid (GLA) protein appears to play a key role in this regulation, in that mice deficient in this protein exhibit calcification of various cartilages including premature calcification in the growth plate in the proliferative zone, leading to short stature (98).

The Calcified Layer of Articular Cartilage

This represents the terminal product of growth involving the secondary center of ossification. Thus, it involves an endochondral calcification of cartilage of the kind described earlier. Chondrocytes express type X collagen, but vascular invasion terminates with cessation of growth. Hyaline cartilage is not normally invaded. It contains troponin 1, an inhibitor of angiogenesis (99). Whether this is absent from growth plate cartilages is not known. It is likely that traumatic compressive damage to articular cartilage, leading to the formation of microfractures within the bone and calcified layer and the development of osteoarthritis (OA), can lead to the formation of new tidemarks (demarcation lines between noncalcified and calcified cartilage). This results from reinitiation of the endochondral process in the adjacent previously uncalcified cartilage. These changes might relate to increased subchondral bone formation seen in OA when there is onset of vascular invasion of the calcified layer and the tidemark (100), as in RA. Cells immediately above the tidemark often stain intensely for alkaline phosphatase (101), indicating that they are undergoing hypertrophy.

Chondrodysplasias, Skeletal Abnormalities, and Arthritis

These are a heterogeneous group of heritable cartilage disorders that are associated with abnormalities of skeletal development. They frequently display pronounced growth plate abnormalities and disproportionately short stature. Table 11.1 presents a list of some of these skeletal dysplasias, which are identifiable either at birth or in later life.

Premature OA is commonly observed in the chondrodysplasias. This is often associated with defects in cartilage-associated collagen genes.

These and other skeletal abnormalities resulting from genetic mutations are reviewed elsewhere (102,103) (see Chapters 9 and 96).

STRUCTURAL ORGANIZATION OF ARTICULAR CARTILAGE AND ITS EXTRACELLULAR MATRIX

Articular cartilage is organized in a manner that reflects the tensile and compressive forces and shear stresses acting on this tissue. Its regional organization is shown in Fig. 11.2. In the superficial zone (also called the tangential zone), the cells are flattened. Whereas in the ankle the superficial zone chondrocytes are arranged in tightly packed clusters of 2 to 13 cells, such clusters are not normally seen in the knee (104). The significance of this is unclear. Superficial cells have matrix biosynthetic capacity different from that of other chondrocytes. This is a region in which the tissue is maximally exposed to the shearing, compressive, and tensile forces of articulation. Not surprisingly, the tensile properties are highest here (105). Interestingly, the collagen fibrils throughout the more superficial matrix are much thinner, but are arranged parallel to each other and to the articular surface. The small proteoglycan decorin is most concentrated at the surface (106,107), being closely associated with the collagen fibrils: the large proteoglycan aggrecan is present at its lowest concentration in the superficial zone, but its concentration increases with depth in contrast to collagen content, which is the reverse. The superficial zone contains unique molecules, such as superficial zone protein and Del 1.

The midzone (also called the intermediate or transitional zone) consists of rounded cells surrounded by an extensive extracellular matrix. In the deep zone (also called the radial or radiate zone), cell volume is at its lowest; cells in this zone are often grouped in clusters and resemble the hypertrophic chondrocytes of the growth plate. Cell density is at its highest at the articular surface and is progressively reduced in the mid and deep zones to about half to one third that of the superficial zone (108,109). Cell density also decreases with increasing age (110,111).

Cells of articular cartilage vary in their responses to cytokines and probably also growth factors. For example, superficial cells are more susceptible to interleukin-1 (IL-1)-induced damage than chondrocytes in deeper layers (112).

The cartilage matrix consists of distinct regions that can be identified by structural differences revealed at the electron microscopic level and by histochemical and immunochemical staining for proteoglycans and link protein (113,114) (Fig. 11.2). All chondrocytes are surrounded by a thin pericellular matrix of up to 2 mm thick that contains few well-defined collagen fibrils, appears amorphous in the electron microscope, and consists mainly of filamentous and fine fibrillar material. It is rich in the filament/microfibril-forming cartilage matrix proteins, type VI collagen and fibrilin-1; decorin is also concentrated here. The chondrocyte and its pericellular matrix have been called a chondron (115,116). In superficial, mid, and deep zones, there is a well-defined territorial region that exists around the pericellular regions and between this and the interterritorial region (where this is present). The interterritorial zone is ordinarily clearly recognizable only in the deep zone in mature articular cartilage, where it is well demarcated from the territorial region by differences in proteoglycan aggrecan structure and composition (113) (Fig. 11.2). The interterritorial region represents that part of the matrix that is most remote from chondrocytes. In adult human articular cartilage, it stains poorly for chondroitin sulfate, keratan sulfate, and the aggregating proteoglycan (aggrecan), compared with the territorial and pericellular regions. The interterritorial zone is recognizable in humans only when growth ceases at about age 17 years. Thus, there may be significant changes in turnover of the extracellular matrix in the deep zone at this time, when cell density has decreased.

Adjacent to the deep zone is the calcified zone. The junction is defined by a boundary called the tidemark, which can most clearly be observed in sections stained with hematoxylin and eosin. The calcified layer no doubt provides an effective interface with the subchondral bone: it likely has mechanical properties intermediate between those of cartilage and bone.

Composition of the Extracellular Matrix of Cartilage

The extracellular matrix contains 65% to 80% water depending on the cartilage. Water content is maximal in the superficial zone and is progressively reduced with increasing depth in the adult (117). Type II collagen, and types IX and XI collagens, are organized in fibrils that endow cartilage with its tensile properties (Figs. 11.2 and 11.6). The collagens (principally type II) account for about 15% to 25% of the wet weight and about half the dry weight, except in the superficial zone, where they account for most of the dry weight (118). The proteoglycan glucosaminoglycan content (mainly that of the very large molecule called aggrecan) accounts for the compressive stiffness of cartilage (its resistance to deformation). It is responsible for up to 10% of the wet weight or about one fourth of the dry weight. Because these glycosaminoglycan chains can bind up to 50 times their weight of water (although they are never normally fully hydrated), they account for much of the water content. Aggrecan degradation products, which accumulate with age and consist mainly of the G1 globular domain (119), and G1 and G2 domains together with the keratan sulfate–rich region (120) (Fig. 11.7), account for a significant part of the remaining dry weight in adult articular cartilage.

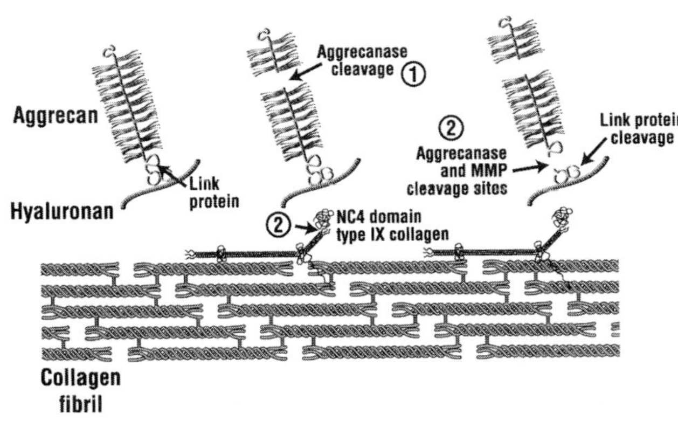

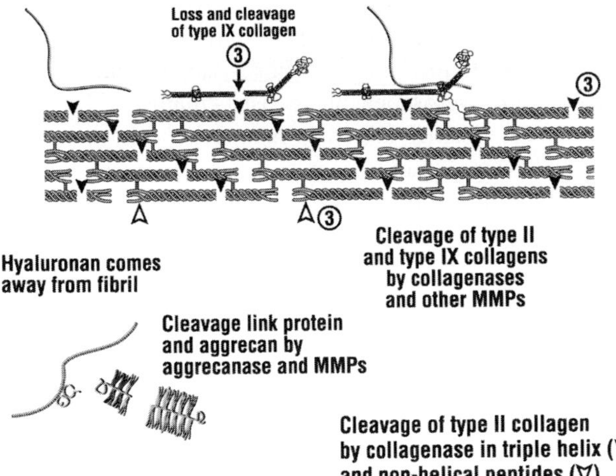

FIG. 11.6. Diagrammatic representation of part of the structure of a collagen microfibril to show the cross-linked triple helical molecules of type II collagen. **Top:** The fibril is seen associated with hyaluronan to which aggrecan and link protein are bound. Type IX collagen is covalently bound to the fibril surface in an antiparallel periodic manner. **Bottom:** Sites of cleavage of type II collagen by collagenase are shown as *solid arrowheads*. *Open arrowheads* indicate sites of cleavage in the telopeptide domains of collagen. Aggrecan cleavage (*arrows*) occurs in the G1–G2 interglobular domain and at sites in the chondroitin sulfate–rich region. The likely order of cleavage of these molecules, based on studies of the growth plate (73) and *in vitro* experiments (unpublished), are indicated numerically. *MMP,* matrix metalloproteinase. (Modified and reproduced from Mort JS, Poole AR. Mediators of inflammation, tissue destruction and repair. D. Proteases and their inhibitors. In: Klippel JH ed. *Primer on the rheumatic diseases,* 12th ed. Atlanta: Arthritis Foundation, 2001:72–81, with permission.)

Collagens

Collagens are described in detail in Chapter 9. Therefore, only selected aspects of their structure and organization in cartilage are discussed here.

The Collagen Fibril

Type II Collagen

In the mid and deep zones, collagen fibrils appear to be organized randomly, but there is a macromolecular organization of fibrils contributing to an arcading at right angles to the articular surface (115) (Fig. 11.2). The fibrils contain 300-nm long type II tropocollagen molecules (each of which contains a triple helix of three identical α chains), with nonhelical amino- and carboxyl-terminal telopeptide domains (Fig. 11.6). These are arranged in a quarter stagger as the fibril forms. In the adult, these collagen molecules are joined by hydroxypyridinium (pyridinoline) cross-links (121,122). In adult articular cartilage, collagen fibrils are usually of larger diameter (~75 nm) in the middle and deep zones than in the superficial zone (30 nm) (123). The turnover of type II collagen in adult articular cartilage is usually considered to be very limited (124,125) except in pericellular sites, where there is evidence for active type II cleavage (126,127) and synthesis (128).

Type II collagen is synthesized as a high-molecular-weight precursor. The amino (N) and carboxy (C) propeptides are required for the correct alignment of procollagen molecules during fibril assembly. They are removed by specific N- and C-proteinases. The C-propeptide remains transiently within cartilage matrix after cleavage (128). It can also bind Ca^{2+} (129) and may influence mineral growth (28).

The alternative splicing of the N-propeptide in COL2A1 collagen was discussed in the earlier section on Chondrogenesis in Embryonic and Postnatal States.

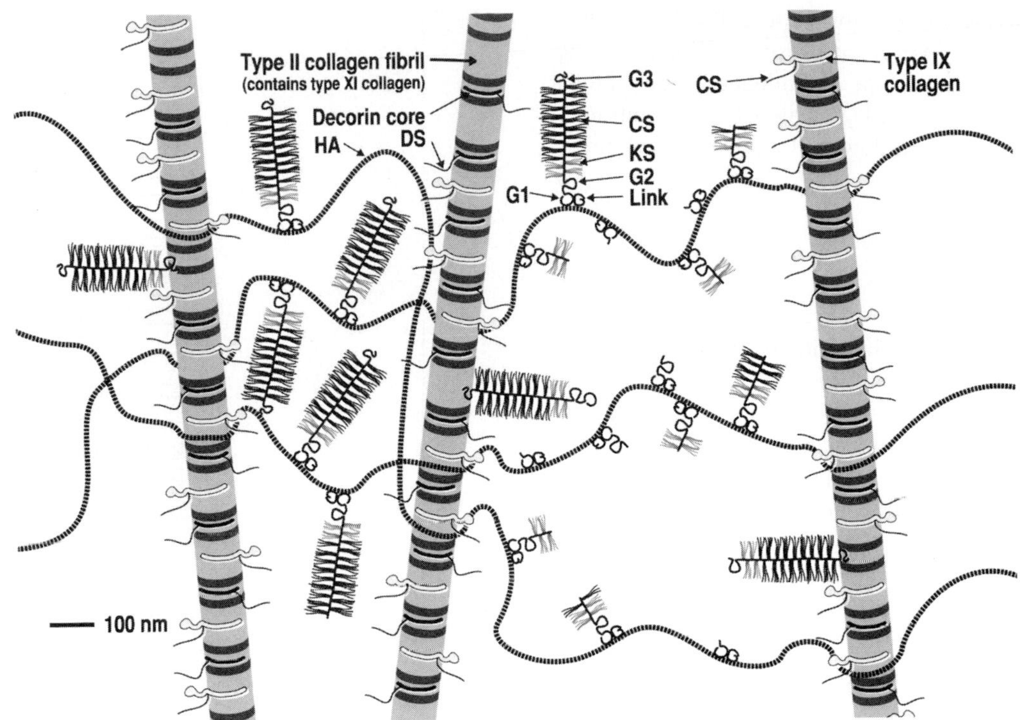

FIG. 11.7. Organization of type II collagen fibrils and aggrecan [bound to hyaluronic acid (HA)] in the extracellular matrix of articular cartilage. HA interacts directly or indirectly with collagen fibrils in a periodic manner. It might bind to the basic NC4 domain of type IX collagen (shown as a globular terminal component). This collagen is covalently bound to type II collagen. Decorin also binds to type II collagen through its core protein in a periodic manner and has a dermatan sulfate (*DS*) side chain. Intact aggrecan molecules (on the left side of the figure) contain a G3 globular domain at the C-terminus. They are attached to HA through a globular G1 N-terminal domain. The G2 globular domain has no known function. Keratan sulfate (*KS*) and chondroitin sulfate (*CS*) are bound to core protein as shown. Link protein stabilizes the interaction of G1 with HA. Some aggrecan molecules bind directly/indirectly to collagen. Degradation products of aggrecan (right side of figure) accumulate with age because they remain bound to HA through the functional G1 domain. The nature of the direct association of aggrecan with collagen fibrils remains to be established. This figure depicts adult human cartilage matrix and is drawn approximately to scale.

Type VI Collagen

Type VI collagen resembles types IX and X collagens in that it is a "shorter-chain" collagen than type II. It is present mainly within the pericellular matrix (130). It consists of α chains that form a highly branched filamentous network based on the formation of tetramers (130). The formation of these networks probably involves binding to hyaluronan (131,132).

Type IX Collagen

Type IX collagen is composed of three distinct gene products: the α_1, α_2, and α_3 chains that each contain collagenous and noncollagenous domains. It is covalently bound to type II collagen on the surfaces of fibrils in an antiparallel fashion. Cross-links bind the N-terminal and C-terminal nonhelical telopeptide domains to type II collagen (Fig. 11.6). When present, it has a periodic distribution along the fibril of approximately 67 nm. The globular NC4 domain at the N-terminus of the α_1(IX) chain extends out from the fibril. Because it is basic, the NC4 domain might act as a binding site for glycosaminoglycans such as hyaluronic acid and chondroitin sulfate (Fig. 11.7). Type IX collagen is also a proteoglycan because it has a single chondroitin sulfate chain bound to the α_2(IX) chain. The fact that mice lacking type IX collagen develop a degenerative arthritis demonstrates its importance in fibril–matrix organization (133). Moreover, human defects in type IX collagen genes also can result in chondrodysplasias (Table 11.1).

Type X Collagen

This is another shorter-chain collagen. It is not present in healthy articular cartilages. Type X collagen is ordinarily synthesized only by hypertrophic chondrocytes and is the principal phenotypic marker for these cells. It is synthesized and secreted before calcification and interacts with itself and with fibrils of type II collagen in pericellular sites and throughout the cartilage matrix (76). Mutations in the type X gene result in abnormal skeletal development (Table 11.1).

Type XI Collagen

Type XI collagen is present within and at the surface of collagen fibrils (134). It contains three collagenous α chains, of which α_3 is a product of the COL2A1 gene. The function of this collagen also is unknown, but its importance in development and cartilage integrity is indicated by the development of skeletal abnormalities and familial OA in patients with genetic mutations in this molecule (Table 11.1).

Types XII and XIV Collagen

These collagens resemble type IX in sequence and structure, having collagenous and noncollagenous domains. Type XII is associated with early chondrocyte maturation. Both collagens are proteoglycans, in that they may contain chondroitin sulfate chains (135).

Proteoglycans

Although these molecules are discussed in detail in Chapter 10, some aspects of their properties and organization relevant to this chapter are reviewed here.

Aggrecan and Link Protein

The primary proteoglycan of cartilage matrix is a very large molecule (designated aggrecan) that aggregates with hyaluronic acid (Figs. 11.6 and 11.7). Its detailed structure is shown in Fig. 11.8.

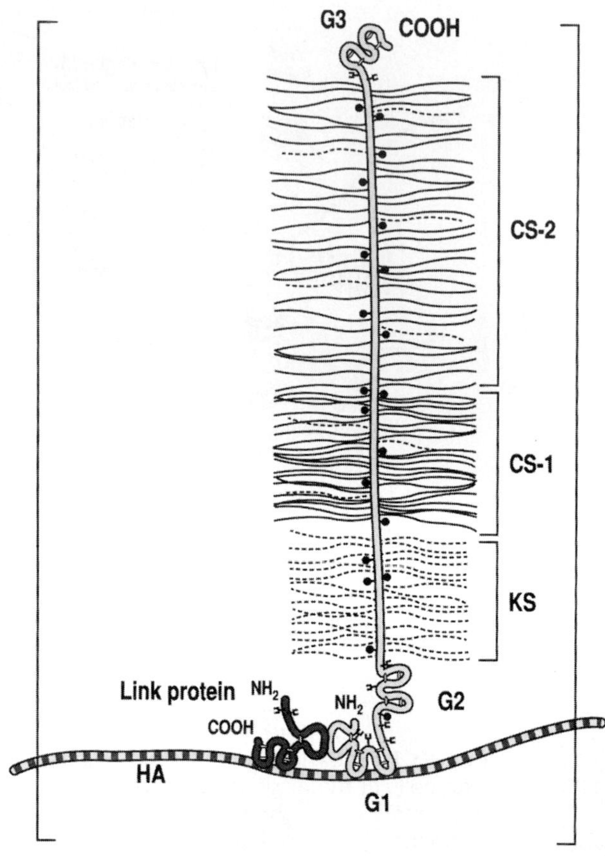

FIG. 11.8. Structures of the large adult human proteoglycan aggrecan and link protein, which bind to each other and to hyaluronan through the G1 globular domain of aggrecan. Keratan sulfate chains also are present on the G1 and G2 domains and in the interglobular G1–G2 domain.

Aggrecan is retained primarily in cartilage matrix as a result of its binding to hyaluronic acid through its G1 globular domain. Human aggrecan contains a protein core that features three globular domains (136) (Fig. 11.8). In the adult, the region immediately carboxy-terminal to the G2 domain contains a high concentration of about 30 keratan sulfate chains. The keratan sulfate–rich region can bind to type II collagen (137). The core protein in this region contains a hexapeptide motif that repeats 11 times (138). The chondroitin sulfate attachment region in human aggrecan consists of two subregions, CS-1 and CS-2 (136). A 19–amino acid sequence in the CS-1 region repeats 19 times. Up to 100 chondroitin sulfate chains are present in the CS-1 and CS-2 regions.

Aggrecan creates a highly hydrated matrix, but hydration and swelling are constrained by the collagen fibrillar network (Fig. 11.7). Thus, aggrecan is only partially hydrated and exhibits a swelling pressure (139). This property endows cartilage with its compressive stiffness and ability to resist deformation and dissipate load (see later section on Mechanical and Physical Properties of the Extracellular Matrix of Cartilage). In adult human articular cartilage, the concentration of aggrecan increases with increasing depth. The inverse relationship between the water content and fixed charge density of articular cartilage with depth (117) indicates that aggrecan molecules located in the deep zone might be the least hydrated in articular cartilage. Moreover, they are concentrated primarily in the territorial region of the deep zone, whereas a more even distribution is seen elsewhere, except in the superficial zone, where there are fewer molecules. Aggrecan is often concentrated in pericellular regions (140). This would theoretically provide further protection for the chondrocyte against compressive forces.

The interaction of each of these molecules with hyaluronic acid is stabilized by the presence of a single link protein (141). Link protein binds directly to the G1 domain of aggrecan and to hyaluronan (142). Its importance is demonstrated by the severe skeletal changes that its absence produces during development (143). The G3 globular domain contains a lectin-like sequence that binds to fucose and galactose (144), which might be of importance in binding to other molecules in the extracellular matrix. Within this domain, alternative transcription (exon use) occurs (136).

Versican

This large proteoglycan is also expressed by chondrocytes (145), but it may not always be detectable as protein (146). It binds to hyaluronan through a G1 globular domain similar to that of aggrecan. Although the G2 domain is absent, a carboxy-terminal G3 domain is present, as in aggrecan. A number of chondroitin sulfate chains are bound to the core protein. The G3 domain can inhibit mesenchymal chondrogenesis (147). Whether this has implications for repair of cartilage is not known.

The Small Leucine-Rich Proteoglycans

Biglycan and Decorin

These proteoglycans are both found in fetal, developing, and mature cartilages (148). In adult human articular cartilage, their contents are similar (107). There are about as many decorin or biglycan molecules as aggrecan molecules. Decorin and biglycan are often codistributed in adult human cartilage, being most concentrated just under the articular surface and in pericellular sites. They are least concentrated in the deep zone (107). Decorin binds to forming fibrils and is closely associated with collagen fibrils near the d and e bands in the D period. The binding of the core protein of decorin to forming type I collagen fibrils limits fibril diameter (149). In the decorin null mouse (−/−), fibril assembly is disorganized, and tensile properties of skin are markedly reduced (150). This clearly demonstrates a role for decorin in determining fibril organization and its tensile properties. Decorin also binds to type XIV collagen (151). There is no evidence, however, for a type II collagen fibril defect in biglycan null (−/−) mice (152).

The core proteins of these molecules are similar in size and structure and consist of a series of tandem repeats of a leucine-rich consensus sequence, as in related molecules. Whereas in articular cartilage, biglycan has two dermatan sulfate chains, decorin has only one (153).

Fibromodulin

This has a core protein similar in size to those of decorin and biglycan (154), but up to four N-linked keratan sulfate chains may be attached (155). Fibromodulin also can bind to collagen types I and II and influence fibrillogenesis (156).

Lumican

Like fibromodulin, lumican contains keratan sulfate chains. It also is present in cartilage (157), where it is likely to be associated with collagen fibrils, as in the cornea. Expression of lumican is at its highest in adult cartilage, where it exists in a form lacking keratan sulfate. Lumican regulates collagen fibril assembly, because in its absence, fibril diameter is excessive in various tissues (158). Unlike fibromodulin, decorin, and biglycan, lumican is absent from the growth plate (159).

Other Proteoglycans

Perlecan

This cell-associated proteoglycan was originally thought to be present only in basement membranes. It is present in developing cartilage (160) and in hyaline cartilages (161). It has a core protein of 260 kd and contains both heparan sulfate and chondroitin sulfate side chains. Perlecan promotes chondrogenesis of mesenchymal or pluripotential cells (160). If perlecan is not expressed, cartilage development is severely impaired with the creation of a degenerate matrix and lack of cartilage calcification (162), suggesting that it plays an important role in chondrocyte signaling.

Syndecan-3

Four isoforms of syndecan-3 have been identified. There is a single-pass transmembrane domain and a long extended extracellular domain bearing heparan sulfate chains. The intracellular domain is involved in signal transduction. This proteoglycan is expressed on proliferative cells. It mediates FGF-2 induction of cell proliferation (163).

Superficial Zone Protein Proteoglycan

This 345-kd molecule is expressed by the superficial zone chondrocytes of articular cartilage as well as by synovial cells (164,165). It is also known as megakaryocyte-stimulating factor and was originally called lubricin. It appears to play an essential role in the surface lubrication of cartilage and synovium. Genetic defects in this molecule result in early joint destruction (166) (Table 11.1).

For a general review of proteoglycans, see Iozzo (167).

Other Matrix Molecules

Developmental Endothelial Locus-1 (Del 1)

This 52-kd protein contains three epidermal growth factor (EGF) repeats, an arginine-glycine-aspartate (RGD) motif, and two discoidin 1–like domains. It binds the $\alpha_v\beta_3$

integrin and mediates endothelial cell attachment and migration. Because it may inhibit or promote angiogenesis, it is of interest that it is expressed in the superficial zone of cartilage (168), a site where pannus formation and vascular overgrowth is seen in RA and sometimes in OA. Its role in cartilage remains to be established.

Fibulin-1

Expressed in a variety of tissues where versican is present, fibulin-1 is also found in developing cartilage. It binds to the G3 lectin domains of versican and aggrecan by a central calcium-binding EGF-like domain (169).

Cartilage Matrix Protein (CMP)/Matrilin-1

This is a member of the matrilin family, all of which contain von Willebrand factor A domains (170). Absent from healthy articular cartilage (only seen in OA), it is present in nasal, tracheal, and other cartilages (171,172). It is a compact trimer of identical ellipsoid subunits assembled through C-terminal extension domains in a coiled-coil α helix (170). CMP binds through one of its subunits to aggrecan core protein in the chondroitin sulfate–rich region. Binding of CMP to aggrecan increases with age (173). In cartilage, it also forms a noncollagenous filamentous network in pericellular sites that extend from the chondrocyte surface (174). In the presence of type II collagen, CMP is a potent adhesion protein for chondrocytes, binding to the $\alpha_1\beta_1$ integrin (175). CMP is also important in type II collagen fibrillogenesis, as evidenced by abnormalities observed in the growth plates of matrilin-1 null mice (176).

Cartilage Oligomeric Protein

This 524-kd protein consists of five subunits (177,178). It is a member of the thrombospondin family and is present in hyaline cartilages (179). It can act as a cell-binding protein and may play a role in cell/matrix interactions (180). It exhibits high-affinity zinc-dependent binding to type II collagen (181).

Cartilage Intermediate Layer Protein (Cilp)

This large secreted glycoprotein (182) is increased in content with aging and is up-regulated in early OA (183). Its expression is induced by TGF-β, whereas IGF-1 suppresses CILP expression (184). Contrary to earlier belief, CILP has no nucleotide pyrophosphatase phosphodiesterase activity, but is an IGF-1 antagonist (185).

TSG-6

This protein belongs to the hyaladherin family, which includes the CD44 receptor, cartilage link protein, aggrecan, and versican. It is a 35-kd secretory glycoprotein that contains a single link module that binds hyaluronic acid (186, 187) and aggrecan (187). It potentiates plasmin inhibition by inter-α-inhibitor and exerts a strong antiinflammatory effect *in vivo* (188). In healthy cartilage, it is absent, but is induced by IL-1β, tumor necrosis factor (TNF)-α, TGF-β, and platelet-derived growth factor AA (189).

Fibronectin

Fibronectin is a component of articular cartilage of young and older animals (190,191) but is absent from healthy human articular cartilage (192). Its function in cartilage is unknown, although it is well established that fibronectin can bind to collagen and heparan sulfate proteoglycans by a specific binding site and to cell-surface receptors through the RGD sequence (193). As a result of alternative splicing of pre-mRNA, chondrocytes synthesize different splice variants, some of which are cartilage specific (194–196). Their functional significance is unclear.

Matrix γ-Carboxyglutamic Acid Protein

This 79-residue protein contains five GLA residues (197). It probably arose by duplication of the gene that gave rise to osteocalcin, which also is known as bone Gla protein. It is present in a wide variety of cartilages, including articular and growth plate (198). Its deletion in mice leads to premature calcification of cartilage, including the growth plate (98). Chondrocytes also develop in the arterial media and become hypertrophic, calcifying the vessel walls.

Tenascin

Tenascin is a large extended "octopus-like" molecule in which six arms radiate out from a central point. Each arm has a molecular weight of 200 kd and consists of a single polypeptide chain. Multiple forms of this subunit have been observed that are probably products of alternative mRNA splicing (199). The domain structure is consistent with that of a molecule that interacts with multiple ligands (200). It can interact, directly or indirectly, with a variety of cartilage matrix molecules (201). Although present in chondrogenesis and embryonic cartilage, it is absent in developing and mature healthy cartilages, although present in perichondrium (202). Its presence is closely associated with chondrogenic, as well as osteogenic, differentiation, and it promotes chondrogenesis *in vitro* (203).

Fibrilin-1

Fibrilin-1 is found in the eye, blood vessels, and cartilage. It is a 350-kd glycoprotein that is the major component of microfibrils, which may be associated with elastin. The monomers readily form aggregates. It appears in cartilage matrix during fetal development and forms banded fibrils in pericellular sites (204–206). Defects in this gene cause Marfan syndrome (205) (Table 11.1)

Elastin

By definition, elastin occurs only in elastic cartilages such as the pinnae of the ears and the epiglottis. Its structure and the considerable alternative splicing that is observed in elastin mRNA have been reviewed (207,208). Elastin constitutes the amorphous component of the elastic fiber end and is responsible for its elastic properties. Individual elastin polypeptide chains (tropoelastin) are extensively covalently cross-linked, producing an insoluble protein, and presumably forming a random coil-like structure.

Hyaluronan (Hyaluronic Acid)

The macromolecular organization and retention of aggrecan in the extracellular matrix is determined by hyaluronan. It binds directly or indirectly to the collagen fibrillar network (Fig. 11.7). Hyaluronan has a molecular weight of approximately 2,000 kd in immature cartilage, but is reduced to 300 kd in the adult. This reduction in size must occur in the extracellular matrix because the molecular mass of newly synthesized molecules is very high (209). Hyaluronan concentrations increase approximately fivefold in the adult (209,210), which is similar to the increased concentration observed in the hypertrophic zone of the growth plate as compared with the proliferative zone (72).

A listing of some of the matrix components is provided in Table 11.2.

MECHANICAL AND PHYSICAL PROPERTIES OF THE EXTRACELLULAR MATRIX OF CARTILAGE

The structural organization of articular cartilage matrix endows this tissue with special physical properties that enable it (a) to absorb and dissipate loads and, (b) in the presence of synovial fluid, to provide an almost frictionless articulating surface. Its rigidity provides shape and substance to structures such as embryonic limbs, the nose, pinnae of the ears, and auditory bones, as well as the trachea, bronchioles, and articular cartilage.

The tensile properties of cartilage are determined primarily by the collagenous fibrillar network, the backbone of which is the type II collagen fibril. In adult articular cartilage, tensile properties are greatest in the superficial zone, where fibrils are aligned parallel to each other and to the articular surface (105). Removal of proteoglycan does not affect the intrinsic tensile stiffness and strength of cartilage (211). However, the proteoglycan component (mainly aggrecan) likely retards the rate of stretch and alignment of collagen when a tensile load is suddenly applied; the proteoglycan also protects the collagen network from mechanical damage (211–213). Cleavage of collagen by a collagenase leads to a loss of tensile stiffness and strength (212). Cartilage in high weight–bearing areas contains an increased content of proteoglycan, but is not as stiff as cartilage in low weight–bearing areas, which contain less proteoglycan (214). Because large tensile loop stresses probably exist at

TABLE 11.2. *Structural macromolecules of adult articular cartilage matrix*

Molecule	Size structure/organization	Distribution/comments	Function
Collagens			
Type II	Forms banded fibrils; 80%–90% of total collagen	Throughout matrix	Tensile strength
Type VI	Forms microfibrils in pericellular sites	Pericellular, mid, and deep zones	Unknown
Type IX	Cross-linked to type II; has single CS or DS-chain; hence a proteoglycan	Throughout matrix	Tensile properties of type II fibril?
Type X	Associated with type II fibrils and in pericellular network	Pericellular, territorial, hypertrophic cartilage	Unknown
Type XI	Present in type II fibrils	Throughout cartilage	Tensile properties of type II fibril?
Types XII and XIV	Both are homotrimeric; resemble type IX in structure and sequence; both are proteoglycans if chondroitin sulfate chains are present	Each is present in distinct sites in association with collagen fibrils	Unknown
Proteoglycans			
Aggrecan	3×10^6 kd; largest proteoglycan; binds to hyaluronic acid through G1 globular domain; forms majority (by mass) of cartilage proteoglycans	Throughout matrix, but deficient at articular surface	Provides compressive stiffness through hydration of high fixed charged density
Biglycan	Mr = 76.3 kd; Mr core = 38 kd, two DS chains in articular cartilage	Most concentrated under articular surface; codistributed with decorin	Unknown

Continued

TABLE 11.2. *Continued*

Molecule	Size structure/organization	Distribution/comments	Function
Decorin	Mr = 76 kd; Mr core = 36.5 kd; one CS or DS chain	Codistributed with biglycan. Binds to collagen fibril	Regulates formation
Fibromodulin	Mr = 58 kd; has up to 4 N-linked KS chains	Absent from prehypertrophic and hypertrophic cartilage	Regulates collagen fibril formation
Lumican	Mr = 58 kd; has up to 4 N-linked KS chains	Unknown	Regulates collagen II fibril formation.
Other molecules			
Cartilage matrix protein (Matrilin-1)	3 subunits each of Mr = 54 kd linked via disulfide bridges	Absent from healthy articular cartilage and intervertebral disc	Unknown
Cartilage oligomeric protein	Five subunits of 100–115 kd, disulfide bonded	Cartilage is primary location	Unknown but defect produces pseudoachondroplasia
Link Protein	Mr = 38.6 kd (protein sequence)	Throughout matrix binds to aggrecan and hyaluronan	Stabilizes attachment of aggrecan/versican to HA via G1 domain
Chondroadherin	Mr = 38 kd	Cell surface	Promotes attachment of chondrocytes to matrix
Annexin V	Mr = 34 kd (protein sequence); also called anchorin CII	Cell surface/matrix vesicles	Receptor for type II collagen
Fibronectin	Mr = 440 kd (2 subunits each of 220 kd)	Mainly in fetal and diseased cartilages	Promotes attachment of cells; interacts with collagen and glycosaminoglycans
Matrix γ-carboxyglutamic acid (gla) protein (MGP)	84-residue protein	Pericellular (adult), diffuse (fetal)	Inhibits calcification
Tenascin	Six 200-kd subunits forming a six-armed glycoprotein	Might be absent from mature cartilage	Involved in chondrogenesis
Fibrilin-1	350-kd glycoprotein; forms banded microfibrils	Interfibrillar pericellular sites	Forms microfibrillar network
Elastin	Found only in elastic cartilages such as ear and epiglottis	Throughout elastic cartilages	Elasticity of cartilage
Hyaluronic acid	Mr = 1,000–3,000 kd	Interacts directly or indirectly with collagen fibrils; aggrecan and versican bind to it via G1 domain	Retention of aggrecan and versican in matrix

CS, chondroitin sulfate; DS dermatan sulfate, HA hyaluronic acid, KS, keratan sulfate.

the periphery of highly loaded regions, a higher tensile stiffness is required in low weight–bearing sites (214).

Compression of the highly charged cartilage matrix, within physiologic ranges, leads to the production of electrical streaming potentials. These are created by fluid convection of counterions, which separates these ions from the oppositely charged matrix molecules, giving rise to a voltage gradient or "streaming potential" in the direction of fluid flow. An electrokinetic surface probe has been developed to apply small sinusoidal currents to the surface of articular cartilage to measure the current-generated stress with a piezoelectric sensor (215). This may be of value in detecting local structural changes reflective of degradation or repair, if used in conjunction with arthroscopic techniques.

During growth, tensile strength and stiffness increase with increasing depth from the articular surface. In the adult, the opposite occurs (105,216). Methods have been developed to measure the Young modules of the pericellular matrix or chondron in healthy cartilage. It is similar throughout articular cartilage; but is significantly decreased in OA cartilage (217). In both growing and adult articular cartilages, the distribution with depth of the proteoglycan decorin [greatest at the articular surface (107)] generally directly correlates with tensile strength and stiffness. Work on the decorin null mouse has demonstrated that decorin plays a key role in determining tensile properties of skin (150), because in its absence, these are markedly depressed. The same probably applies to cartilage.

Chondrocytes in articular cartilages respond to shear stresses, as well as strains. The collagen–proteoglycan matrix is more viscoelastic and dissipative in shear than is collagen alone. Thus, the stiffness and energy-dissipative properties in shear are provided by the combined organization of aggrecan and collagen fibrils. Articular cartilage is subjected to considerable compressive forces. Whether these are more pronounced in male subjects, in whom articular cartilage volume is significantly greater (218), is unclear.

The ability to resist compression results from the compressive stiffness of the cartilage, which is determined by its content of aggrecan and the swelling pressure it generates (219–221). Swelling is balanced by the tensile forces in the collagen fibrils. The loss of proteoglycan results in a decrease in the compressive modulus (212,220), without influencing the inherent stiffness of the collagen network (222).

Intraarticular Pressures Acting on Cartilage

In vitro studies of patellofemoral contact pressures have revealed that *in vivo* pressures may reach a contact force of 65 times body weight or 10 megapascals (MPa) (223). An *in vivo* analysis of a patient with an instrumented femoral head prosthesis recorded pressures up to 18 MPa (224). Pressures varied within the joint, depending on the site. Moreover, rapid changes were recorded with activities such as stair climbing, in which maximal increases as high as 107 MPa per second occurred.

Mechanical Pressure Influences Chondrocyte-Mediated Matrix Turnover, Cell Viability, and Matrix Integrity

Chondrocyte proteoglycan synthesis is selectively stimulated or inhibited by cyclic loading. Proteoglycan and collagen synthesis can be stimulated for up to 2 hours by very brief (20-second) applications of hydrostatic pressure in the physiologic 5- to 15-MPa range. At greater than 20 MPa, synthesis decreases (225). Clearly, chondrocytes respond sensitively to their mechanical environment.

Static compressive loading (and increased osmotic pressure) results in a decreased water content, but increases the concentrations of sulfate and carboxyl group counterions—K^+, H^+, Na^+, and Ca^{2+}—and decreases the concentration of free SO_4^{2-}. This can inhibit proteoglycan synthesis. Compressive forces promote SOX9, type II collagen, and aggrecan expression but inhibit IL-1β expression (226). Cyclic strain of chondrocytes also can induce matrix degradation through enhanced gene expression of MMPs and IL-1 (227).

Shear stress favors apoptosis via up-regulation of nitric oxide (NO), which is associated with reduced expression of the antiapoptotic molecule Bcl-2 (228).

The collagen fibrillar network is sensitive to direct damage when exposed to excessive mechanical forces, such as those that can cause and promote OA (229). Excessive cyclic stresses stimulate collagen cleavage by collagenase, leading to denaturation and even cell death in more superficial cartilage (230). Damage to collagen stimulates the swelling of cartilage caused by increased hydration of proteoglycans (231).

Integrin receptors on the cell surface may mediate mechanically induced signaling that involves changes in membrane potential and a role for cell surface mechanoreceptors (232) (Fig. 11.9). Mechanically induced $\alpha_5\beta_1$ integrin activation

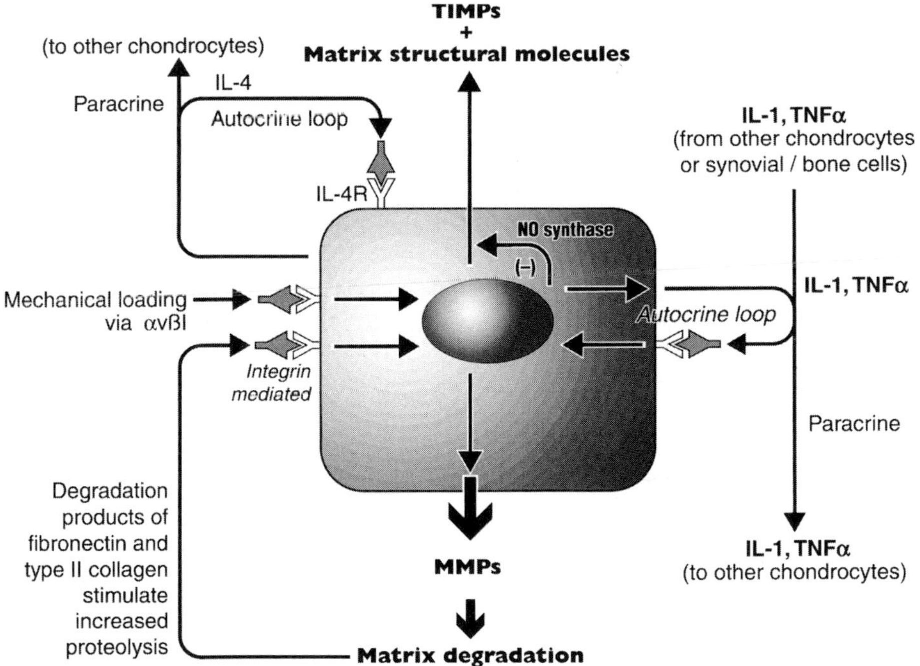

FIG. 11.9. The manner whereby a chondrocyte may communicate with its extracellular environment and how this may regulate gene expression and matrix turnover is shown. Cytokines such as interleukin-1 (*IL-1*) and tumor necrosis factor-α (*TNF-α*) may be derived from remote sites, such as synovium or bone, and activate chondrocytes. Chondrocytes also produce these cytokines, which are used in signaling in both an autocrine and paracrine manner. Matrix degradation products can, through cell surface receptors and IL-1 signaling, regulate gene expression. Receptors bound to matrix molecules (e.g., integrins) can sense changes in mechanical loading and signal through cytokines such as IL-4. Nitric oxide (*NO*) synthesis induced by IL-1 can suppress (−) matrix synthesis. *IL-4R,* interleukin-4 receptor; *TIMP,* tissue inhibitor of metalloproteinases. (Modified and reproduced with permission from Poole AR, Howell DS. Etiopathogenesis of osteoarthritis. In: Moskowitz R, Goldberg V, Howell DS, et al., eds. *Osteoarthritis: diagnosis and medical/surgical management,* 3rd ed. Philadelphia: WB Saunders, 2001:29–47.)

requires the production of IL-4 and a signaling pathway involving tyrosine kinases (233). Repetitive cyclic loading can stimulate the expression and activation of MMP-2 and MMP-9 without any effect on tissue inhibitors of these proteinases (234). Constant or static compression that suppresses matrix synthesis in cartilage involves the generation of IL-1α and IL-1β, as well as NO synthase expression. Inhibition of IL-1 by IL-1 receptor antagonist protein can negate this suppression of synthesis (235).

The neuropeptide receptor neurokinin 1 and its ligand substance P are also involved in mechanotransduction (236). The protein Ihh maintains chondrocytes in a mitotic cycle and prevents hypertrophy (see earlier section on Maturation of Chondrocytes to Express Hypertrophic and Nonhypertrophic Phenotypes). Cyclic mechanical stress (stretching) greatly enhances Ihh expression. Inhibition of Ihh activity prevents the stimulation of proliferation caused by stretching (237). The activity of Ihh is BMP mediated since Noggin (a BMP antagonist) inhibits the stimulation of proliferation.

In Vivo Responses to Alterations in the Mechanical Environment

The formation of osteophytes (composed of hyaline cartilage covering bony protuberances) in marginal regions of unstable diarthrodial joints in human OA and in experimental OA may in part result from abnormal cyclic loading of periosteum, leading to osteophyte formation through an endochondral process. The deeper layers calcify and form bone as part of a process of endochondral ossification. A "cap" of uncalcified hyaline articular cartilage that remains to cover the osteophyte demonstrates the distinction between calcified and noncalcified cartilages, as well as the capacity to form new cartilage in the adult.

The influence of mechanical forces on the differentiation of tissues to form cartilage during skeletal development is of special interest (238,239). In the adult, cyclic loading of smooth muscle cells of the media of arterial vessels, caused by the introduction of a solid wire, induces the formation of a sheath of hyaline cartilage as the cyclic pulsating arterial pressure stimulates these cells to express a chondroblastic phenotype (240). Similarly, injection of carrageenan into the media also induces cartilage formation.

When a tendon is relocated so that it abnormally contacts a solid surface such as bone, the tendon cells in this region come under abnormal compressive load (probably cyclic because of movement) and synthesize aggrecan, although they might continue to synthesize type I collagen (241). Thus, they differentiate into fibrochondroblasts.

Chondrocytes respond to mechanical stimuli *in vivo*. The proteoglycan content of habitually unloaded canine femoral condylar cartilage is lower than that in habitually loaded regions, even though synthesis is similar (242). Eight weeks of immobilization of the hind leg of the dog in flexion also leads to a reversible arrest of proteoglycan synthesis and loss of cartilage (243). Increased weight bearing in the contralateral limb leads to an increase in uncalcified cartilage thickness and proteoglycan content (up to 35%) in all but the superficial zone (244). Excessive exercise can lead to cartilage damage (245,246).

That exercise can be protective, if it is not excessive, is revealed by the observation that passive exercise (on a treadmill) over a 3-month period can protect against the degeneration of articular cartilage observed in sedentary unexercised hamsters (247).

MOLECULES THAT REGULATE CHONDROCYTE METABOLISM

Chondrocytes are exposed to a complex array of environmental molecules that can have opposite concentration-dependent effects on proliferation, matrix synthesis, and degradation. Some of these are shown in Fig. 11.10. There are clear indications that growth plate cells respond differently to articular chondrocytes. Articular chondrocytes differ in their responses according to whether they come from knee or ankle cartilages (248). The interactions of chondrocytes with their environment involve receptor-mediated mechanisms that can involve structural molecules or soluble mediators, some of which may be structural degradation products.

Cell Surface Receptors

These include the integrins, which may vary in cartilage according to its type, development, and disease. A variety of integrin α and β chains have been described (249–252). The α_v subunit is expressed more in the superficial zone; in osteoarthritic cartilage, the α_2, α_4, and β_2 subunits also are expressed (253). The β_1 integrin is required for type X collagen deposition in matrix and cartilage growth. Antibody binding to the β_1 chain induces apoptosis (253). β_1 integrins can mediate attachment to type II collagen and fibronectin (254). Whereas the RGD integrin recognition sequence inhibits attachment to fibronectin, it has no effect on type II collagen attachment (250). There is a specific receptor for type II collagen called annexin V (255). It binds to the telopeptide region of type II collagen (256). Annexin V exhibits extensive homology with the calcium-binding proteins calpactin, lipocortin, and protein II. It also binds to type X collagen, as well as to the C-propeptide of type II procollagen (257).

Chondrocytes have calcium-mobilizing purine receptors that may mediate adenosine-5-triphosphate-induced up-regulation of prostaglandin E_2 (258). The CD44 receptor for hyaluronan is expressed by chondrocytes. Its down-regulation results in a loss of the proteoglycan aggrecan, associated with increased cleavage of aggrecan by an "aggrecanase" (259).

Chondrocytes possess estrogen receptors and display marked metabolic differences in matrix synthesis and degradation in male versus female subjects (260). Estrogen

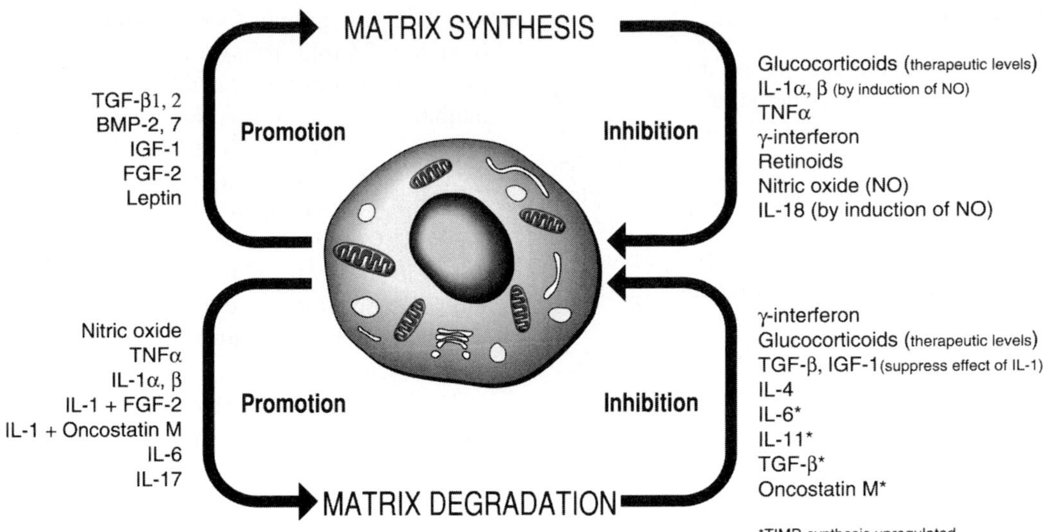

FIG. 11.10. Effects of cytokines/growth factors and other molecules that favor either cartilage matrix synthesis or degradation. Synergistic and antagonistic effects are shown. *BMP,* bone morphogenetic protein; *FGF,* fibroblast growth factor; *IGF,* insulin-like growth factor; *IL,* interleukin; *TGF,* transforming growth factor; *TNF,* tumor necrosis factor.

replacement therapy increases chondrocyte synthesis of proteoglycans and IGF binding protein 2 (IGFBP-2), indicating that estrogen can have a direct effect on adult articular cartilage (261). Whether this may have relevance to the development and the degeneration of cartilage in diseases such as RA and OA, which are more common in female subjects, remains to be elucidated.

Chondrocytes have receptors for histamine (H_2) (262) and bradykinin (263). Neurokinin 1 (NK1), a neuropeptide receptor for substance P, is expressed by articular chondrocytes together with substance P and preprotachykinin, from which substance P and other neuropeptides are generated by alternate splicing (236). The functional significance of this remains to be established, although there is evidence for the involvement of substance P in mechanotransduction via the NK1 receptor (236).

Oxygen

Because chondrocytes are usually not close to blood vessels, they normally experience reduced oxygen tensions. They generate their energy through aerobic glycolysis, which results in the conversion of one molecule of glucose to two molecules of pyruvate and two of ATP. Hypoxia-inducible factor (HIF-1) is centrally involved in the transcriptional response to hypoxia. The α subunit, HIF-1α, confers oxygen responsiveness by translocating to the nucleus under hypoxic conditions, binding to HIF-1β to form a heterodimer that binds to cis-acting promoter regions of hypoxia-responsive genes. The loss of HIF-1α induces apoptosis in growth plate chondrocytes (264). HIF-1α null mice are unable to maintain ATP levels in hypoxia. This results in a reduction in aggrecan and type II collagen expression and content compared with wild-type chondrocytes, which selectively increase type II content (265).

Insulin-Like Growth Factor 1

Insulin alone is much less potent than IGF-1 in stimulating matrix synthesis (266). IGF-1 is a potent inducer of collagen and proteoglycan synthesis *in vitro* (267,268). These effects are receptor mediated (269,270). In the growth plate, proliferative cells (267,271) are most responsive in terms of stimulation of matrix assembly and cell division. IGF-1 can stimulate chondrocyte proliferation *in vitro* (272,273) and physeal growth in the growth plate *in vivo* (274,275). IGF-1 is synthesized by chondrocytes (276,277), appears to be bound to cartilage matrix (278), and functions in a paracrine/autocrine manner. It can sustain proteoglycan synthesis at a rate equivalent to that observed with fetal calf serum (279). In addition to stimulating synthesis, IGF-1 also can maintain homeostasis and decrease cytokine-induced catabolism (278, 280,281) through suppression of MMP expression (282,283) and expression of IL-1 receptor II (IL-1RII) (284). In synovial fluid, IGF-1 is the major stimulant of proteoglycan synthesis (285). Cartilage obtained from inflamed murine joints does not respond to IGF-1 (286). This may be because IL-1 and TNF-α can stimulate an increase in IGFBP-3 in chondrocytes (287), thereby neutralizing IGF-1.

IGF-1 levels are elevated in the serum (288) and urine (289) of patients with acromegaly. In pituitary insufficiency, urinary IGF-1 is reduced (289).

Insulin-Like Growth Factor 2

IGF-2 exhibits considerable homology to IGF-1 and human proinsulin in the A and B domains (290). IGF-2 stimulates DNA and RNA synthesis (291) and is more potent than IGF-1 in stimulating clonal growth in fetal cells, whereas IGF-1 is more effective on adult chondrocytes. IGF-2 can stimulate proteoglycan synthesis but, like insulin, is much less effective than IGF-1. A separate receptor for IGF-2 exists, in addition to the IGF-1 receptor (270).

Growth Hormone

Parenteral administration of GH can stimulate localized growth plate development *in vivo* (292,293). Hypophysectomy leads to disappearance of IGF-1 in growth plate chondrocytes, indicating a cessation of synthesis (276). Conversely, treatment with GH, systemically or locally, results in the reappearance of IGF-1 (278) and of normal growth rates (271). IGF-1 and, to a lesser extent, IGF-2 can stimulate growth in the absence of GH (271,290). Thus, GH increases synthesis of IGF-1, which appears to be responsible for the growth effects of this hormone.

TGF-β and Bone Morphogenetic Proteins

TGF-β is a homodimeric polypeptide, of which five different isoforms have been identified. It stimulates expression of the chondrogenic phenotype (see earlier section on Chondrogenesis in Embryonic and Postnatal States). It is produced by articular chondrocytes (isoforms 1–4) as well as by other cells. IL-6 induces synthesis of TGF-β_1, whereas IL-1β induces TGF-β_3 synthesis (294).

Like IGF-1, TGF-β can preserve proteoglycan homeostasis in articular chondrocytes by increasing general protein synthesis, including collagen, and decreasing proteoglycan degradation (295,296) and, in the case of TGFβ_1, cytokine-induced collagen cleavage (281). It can protect against IL-1-induced degradation (297) and inhibition of synthesis, but TGF-β_1 can only protect in young animals (298). This may favor overactivity of IL-1 in aging.

The importance of the TGF-β family in cartilage homeostasis has been clearly demonstrated under circumstances in which a nonfunctional TGF-β-receptor II was overexpressed (299) and the SMAD signaling pathway was disrupted (300). In both cases, cartilage degeneration was observed in these mice. This was accompanied by chondrocyte hypertrophy, demonstrating the importance of the TGF-β family in the suppression of hypertrophy in articular cartilage. Specifically, TGF-β_1 can down-regulate MMP-1 and MMP-13 expression and reduce gene expression of IL-1RI, IL-1RII, TNF receptor I (TNFR-I), and TNFR-II, as well as levels of proinflammatory cytokines (301).

FGF-2 (basic FGF) can induce production of TGF-β (302). Like FGF-2, TGF β stimulates chondrocyte replication. The two growth factors exhibit synergism, resulting in up to a 73-fold increase in cell division (303). Whereas FGF-2 stimulates IGF-1 synthesis by chondrocytes, TGF-β inhibits both IGF-1 production and the action of FGF-2 (304). Although TGF-β and FGF-2, individually or together, suppress transcription of type II collagen mRNA in growth plate chondrocytes, TGF-β stimulates collagen synthesis by articular chondrocytes (296). This is probably due to its ability to inhibit IL-1 receptor expression (305). Thus, clear differences exist between the responsiveness of growth plate and non–growth plate chondrocytes to these growth factors.

The BMPs or the osteogenins are members of the TGF-β superfamily. They play key roles in development (see sections on Chondrogenesis and Maturation) and also can regulate the effects of proinflammatory cytokines on cartilage (reviewed in references 14, 306, and 307). Interestingly, nuclear factor κB (NFκB) can activate BMP-2 gene expression in growth plate chondrocytes (308). Because NFκB is also a transcriptional activator of proinflammatory molecules, this would suggest a regulatory linkage between matrix catabolism and anabolism. BMP-7 (309) and BMP-2 (310) *in vitro* and BMP-2 *in vivo* (311) can potently stimulate proteoglycan and collagen synthesis in cartilage. *In vitro,* BMP-7 or OP-1 can suppress the inhibition of proteoglycan synthesis caused by low doses of IL-1β (312) and suppress cartilage damage and MMP-13 expression (283), as well as enhance proteoglycan synthesis (313). CDMP-1 and CDMP-2 are the respective human homologues of mouse growth differentiation factors 5 and 6. They are expressed by chondrocytes in health and disease and can stimulate proteoglycan synthesis as observed with OP-1 (314).

Epidermal Growth Factor

Epidermal growth factor (EGF) has no effect on chondrocyte proliferation, but it can stimulate proteoglycan synthesis, although less potently than IGF-1 (266,268,315). Together with insulin, EGF synergistically stimulates proteoglycan synthesis and induces proliferation of chondrocytes (268).

Fibroblast Growth Factors

A potent chondrocyte mitogen, FGF-2 (basic FGF) stimulates proteoglycan synthesis in the growth plate (303), whereas it can stimulate hyaluronan synthesis and inhibit proteoglycan synthesis in fetal articular cartilage (304). It appears to function additively with IGF-1 in adult articular cartilage. FGF-2 and IGF-1 synergistically stimulate mitosis and proteoglycan synthesis (268). *In vivo,* FGF-2 potently stimulates chondrocyte proliferation and extracellular matrix formation (316). Like TGF-β, FGF-2 can inhibit terminal differentiation of hypertrophic chondrocytes, which lose their receptors for FGF-2 (42,317). This might explain how FGF-2 stimulates cartilage formation *in vivo* in the absence of calcification (316).

High levels of the precursor of FGF-1 (acidic FGF) have been detected in RA and, to a lesser degree, in OA synovia (318). FGF-1 stimulates cartilage enlargement and inhibits chondrocyte gene expression during fracture healing (319).

FGF-2 acts synergistically with IL-1 to increase prostanoid production and enhances IL-1-induced protease release from chondrocytes (320). FGF-2 up-regulates receptors for IL-1, although IL-1 blocks the mitogenic effects of FGF-2 (321). FGF and its various receptors play key roles in chondrogenesis. The latter is discussed in the section on chondrogenesis. Overactivity of FGF receptors due to mutations cause chondrodysplasias (Table 11.1).

Cytokines and Nitric Oxide

IL-1 decreases the synthesis of proteoglycans (322,323) and types II, IX, and XI collagens (324–326) at much lower concentrations (10–100 times) than those required to induce synthesis and secretion of metalloproteinases and matrix degradation (327,328). IL-1β is more potent than IL-1α (329). IL-1 also inhibits cartilage synthesis *in vivo* (330) and induces the synthesis of IL-6 by human chondrocytes, the levels of which are comparable with those found in synovial fluids of patients with RA (331). IL-1 in combination with oncostatin M can more effectively induce collagen degradation than either cytokine alone (332). ADAM-TS4 or aggrecanase-1 is up-regulated by the combination, whereas ADAM-TS5 is stimulated by IL-1α alone (333).

Reports that IL-6 mediates IL-1-induced inhibition of proteoglycan synthesis (331) have been disputed by other reports that claim that IL-6 has no effect on proteoglycan synthesis in human cartilage (334). Others have shown that IL-6 can induce synthesis of MMP-1 and MMP-13 in OA chondrocytes (301). In contrast, IL-6 has been reported to block IL-1-induced collagenolytic activity (335). Induction of aggrecan degradation by IL-1 or TNF-α can be enhanced by IL-6 or its soluble receptor (336). This is dependent on aggrecanases, not MMPs.

NO, which is produced by chondrocytes after stimulation by IL-1α (337), IL-1β, or TNF-α (338), inhibits proteoglycan synthesis and may be the primary mediator of matrix synthesis inhibition by these cytokines. IL-1β also down-regulates the expression of glucuronosyltransferase 1, a key enzyme priming glycosaminoglycan synthesis (339). This can be prevented by glucosamine. NO also induces apoptosis in chondrocytes (340) but only under conditions in which other reactive oxygen species are generated (341).

Apoptosis in chondrocytes can also be induced by TNF-related apoptosis ligand (TRAIL) (342), IL-1α, TNF-α, and interferon (IFN)-γ (343).

Although excessive generation of IL-1β and NO is usually considered to result in pathologic changes, these molecules are also important at lower concentration in the maintenance of normal homeostasis. Thus, in null mice lacking IL-1β, IL-1 converting enzyme (which generates IL-1β), and inducible NO synthase, there is an acceleration in the development of experimental knee OA (344).

TNF-α can inhibit the synthesis of type II collagen (345), although it is less potent than IL-1β and IL-1α. Synergistic inhibition is seen with IL-1 and TNF-α (345). IFN-γ can inhibit type II collagen synthesis (346). Chondrocytes at the articular surface are more sensitive to inhibition by IL-1 and exhibit more receptors (112). The most potent inhibitor of proteoglycan synthesis in cartilage *in vivo* that is associated with intraarticular inflammation is clearly IL-1 (347). The stimulation of degradation by IL-1 is discussed in the later section on Articular Cartilage Degradation: Mechanisms and Regulation.

The induction of cartilage degradation by IL-1 and TNF-α can be inhibited by IL-4 (348). *In vivo* IL-4 overexpression prevents cartilage destruction in type II collagen–induced arthritis (349). Thus, IL-4 is an important regulatory cytokine that can protect against cartilage damage. IL-17, a T cell–derived cytokine, is increased in RA and can stimulate proinflammatory cytokine expression in chondrocytes (350) and can alone and in combination with other cytokines promote type II collagen and proteoglycan degradation mediated by these cells (351). IL-17 also augments NO generation in OA cartilage via NFκB activation, which is independent of IL-1β signaling (352). Inhibition of proteoglycan synthesis induced by IL-17 can be reduced by IL-4 (353).

A study of the differential capacity of IL-17, IL-1β, and TNF-α to stimulate the generation of different chemokines from human chondrocytes reveals that IL-8 is potently generated by IL-17, IL-1β, or TNF-α, the same cytokines that induce monocyte chemoattractant protein 1 (MCP-1) and GRO-α. RANTES (regulated upon activation normal T cell expressed and secreted) is stimulated by IL-1β or TNF-α (354). IL-18 is also produced by chondrocytes, and the active molecule is secreted following stimulation with IL-1. It inhibits TGF-β-induced proliferation and enhances NO production and expression and synthesis of inducible NO synthase, cyclooxygenase, IL-6, and MMP-3 (355).

Leptin

A leptin receptor is expressed by chondrocytes. Stimulation of chondrocytes with leptin results in enhanced proliferation and matrix synthesis (356). The significance of this needs to be established.

Chondromodulin 1

This 25-kd molecule that is found in cartilage is capable of stimulating chondrocyte proliferation and proteoglycan synthesis. More interestingly, it is an inhibitor of angiogenesis, which is absent from calcifying cartilage where angiogenesis occurs (357).

Human Cartilage Glycoprotein 39

This is a member of the chitinase family, which lacks chitinase activity. It is a major secreted product of activated chondrocytes in OA and synovial cells and macrophages in inflammation. It can potently stimulate the growth of synovial cells, as well as fibroblasts in a dose similar to IGF-1 (358). It also synergizes with IGF-1.

Vitamin D

Vitamin D deficiency disrupts endochondral ossification, arrests calcification, and produces a lengthened hypertrophic zone and impaired angiogenesis, resulting in rickets. Receptors for 1,25$(OH)_2$ vitamin D_3 are present on growth plate chondrocytes, with receptor density being highest in hypertrophic cells in association with an elevated content of alkaline phosphatase (78). In healthy rats, both 1,25$(OH)_2$ and 24,25$(OH)_2$ vitamin D_3 are required to stimulate growth plate cartilage calcification maximally *in vitro* (359). However, in rachitic (vitamin D–deficient) rats, 24,25$(OH)_2$ vitamin D_3 alone is required to stimulate calcification. Together, 1,25 $(OH)_2$ and 24,25 $(OH)_2$ vitamin D_3 maximally stimulate type II procollagen synthesis in healthy rat growth plate cells in culture, as reflected by enhanced synthesis of type II collagen (359).

A summary of how some of these molecules influence chondrocyte metabolism is shown in Fig. 11.10.

Matrix Degradation Products

Matrix degradation products can potently regulate chondrocyte gene expression and matrix turnover. Fibronectin fragments stimulate matrix degradation. These fragments include those containing the RGD sequence (360), alternatively spliced transcripts (361), and the carboxy-terminal heparin-binding region (362,363). IL-1 signaling appears to be involved in this effect (360,362,364) (Fig. 11.9). Low concentrations of one fibronectin fragment can in fact stimulate matrix synthesis (365).

A 16-residue amino-terminal fragment of link protein in the adult that may be naturally generated can stimulate synthesis of proteoglycan (366) and types II and IX collagens (367). There is also evidence that a mixture of degradation products of type II collagen can induce matrix degradation as well as inhibit collagen synthesis (368). A 24 residue synthetic peptide based on an intrahelical sequence can selectively induce collagenases, leading to digestion of type II collagen but not aggrecan (369). In contrast, intact type II collagen is essential for maintaining expression of the chondrocyte phenotype.

Circadian Rhythm of Matrix Synthesis

Rates of matrix synthesis in growth plate and articular cartilages are not necessarily constant during the day and are not synchronous. In rats, mice, and rabbits, cartilage formation in growth plates peaks during the day (370). The reasons for these cyclic differences might be related to hormonal changes, physical activity, and possibly feeding.

ARTICULAR CARTILAGE DEGRADATION: MECHANISMS AND REGULATION

Degradation of cartilage matrix involves the extracellular cleavage of matrix molecules, primarily by proteases, but probably also by free radicals released from chondrocytes (371). When degradation is induced in healthy cartilage (e.g., by IL-1), the proteoglycan aggrecan is lost rapidly (372,373). Subsequently type II collagen is degraded (374) (Fig. 11.6). The delay observed in type II collagen cleavage in culture, following, for example, addition of IL-1 (374), is related to a delay in the activation of procollagenases, which are rapidly induced but slowly activated (375). The collagen fibril–associated proteoglycans (decorin, biglycan, and lumican) are resistant to degradation and may play a protective role. In contrast, fibromodulin is degraded early (376). Degradation products can remain in the extracellular matrix, either because they are part of a larger macromolecular structure such as a collagen fibril (where they can be covalently retained) or because they represent a molecule that remains bound, such as that part of the aggrecan monomer that remains bound (by the G1 domain) to hyaluronan. Aggrecan fragments lacking the G1 domain, which are released from the macromolecular complex, are free to diffuse through matrix, where they can be locally endocytosed by chondrocytes or enter synovial fluid and the lymphatics. Degradation products of type II collagen (377) and the proteoglycan aggrecan, including the G1 domain, can be detected in synovial fluid (378) (see earlier section on Monitoring Cartilage Metabolism *In Vivo*: Detection of Molecular Synthetic and Degradation Products of Cartilage in Body Fluids).

The degradation of matrix molecules is an integral feature of remodeling during growth and development and matrix turnover in the adult. Thus, it is not just a feature of pathology. It is ordinarily carefully regulated by cytokines, growth factors, and hormones that regulate the synthesis of proteinases, their inhibitors, and structural matrix molecules (Fig. 11.11). Excessive proteolysis can occur as a result of an imbalance between the relative concentrations of a proteinase and its inhibitor. This can be physiologically

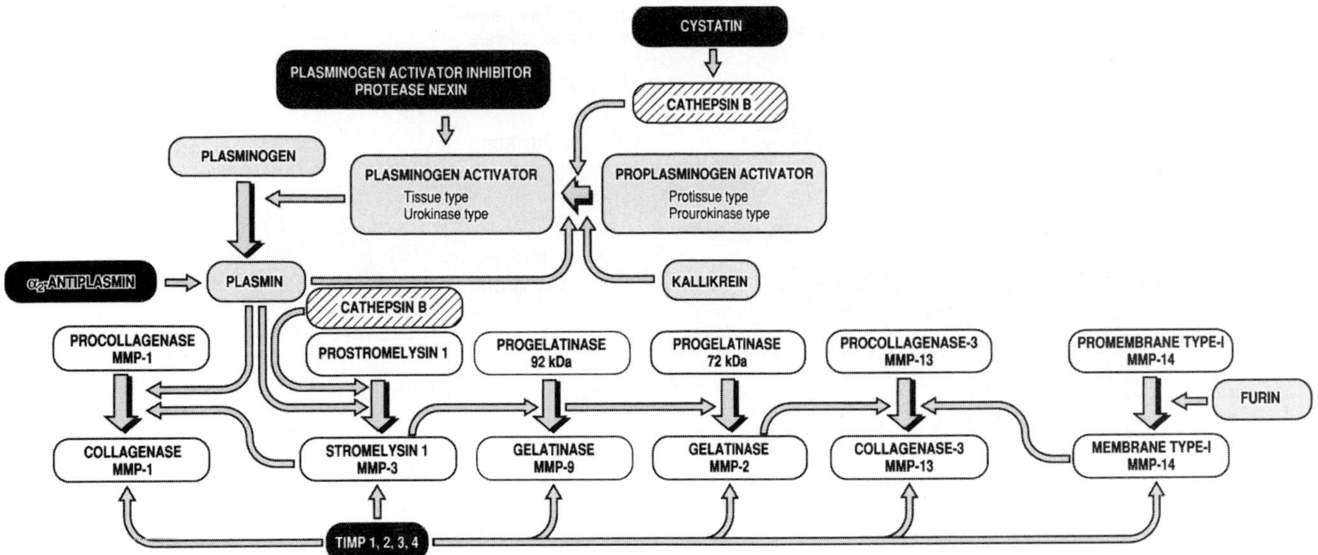

FIG. 11.11. Examples of interactions of proteinases, their activators, and their inhibitors. Inhibitors are shown in dark boxes. Serine proteinases are shown in gray boxes and matrix metalloproteinases (*MMPs*) in open boxes. Cathepsin B, a cysteine proteinase, is also shown in a hatched box. Activations of latent metalloproteinases by other proteinases are indicated. *TIMP,* tissue inhibitor of metalloproteinases

regulated, as in the growth plate, or it can be a pathologic event, such as in arthritis. Ordinarily, the synthesis and degradation of matrix molecules are finely balanced, particularly in cartilages that will survive, such as articular cartilages. In contrast, growth plate cartilages are transient, and their matrix is short lived; this is reflected in the structure of the matrix. In this section, mechanisms of degradation as well as their regulation are discussed.

Cellular Changes Involved in Articular Cartilage Degradation

With the onset of arthritis, chondrocytes exhibit changes characteristic of chondrocytes undergoing hypertrophy. There is, for example, increased expression of type X collagen in RA (379) and of type X collagen (380), PTHrP (381), and annexins II and V (382) in OA. All of these molecules are expressed by immediately prehypertrophic or hypertrophic chondrocytes. This is associated with apoptosis (383,384) and matrix calcification (385,386). These changes occur in association with excessive cleavage of type II collagen, as seen in the growth plate (127). If growth plate–mediated matrix degradation, including collagen cleavage, is arrested by a synthetic MMP-13 (collagenase-3) inhibitor, chondrocyte hypertrophy is also arrested (60). Moreover, collagenase treatment of healthy cartilage induces apoptosis (379). Therefore, it is believed that the excessive collagen degradation observed in OA cartilage matrix may trigger these cellular changes. Apoptosis is also observed much more frequently in articular cartilage in RA (380). Thus, similar mechanisms of chondrocyte differentiation may occur in different types of arthritis with degeneration of the extracellular matrix. The chondrocyte undergoes a fundamental change in its behavior, which is apparently not reversible. This is a point of no return that leads to the inability of the chondrocyte to repair the damage. By then it is incapable of proliferation and is heading toward its own death.

Proteinases Involved in Cartilage Degradation

The cysteine proteinase cathepsin K, which is generated by osteoclasts and plays a key role in bone resorption, is expressed in increased amounts within chondrocytes in OA (387). Although it is active at neutral pH and the pH decreases progressively with matrix damage to pH 5.5 in OA, there is no direct evidence to implicate cathepsin K at this time in the pathology of OA (387). In fact, there is no convincing evidence that proteinases other than MMPs are involved in the direct cleavage of molecules within the extracellular matrix of cartilage. Other proteinases such as serine proteinases (e.g., plasmin) and MMPs (MMP-3 and MMP-14) can activate these MMPs (Fig. 11.11). In health and arthritis, the proteinases originate primarily from chondrocytes and destroy their surrounding matrix (388,389). In RA, at the articular surface, cartilage–pannus junction, and elsewhere, proteinases may also originate from polymorphonuclear leukocytes and synovial cells (328,390,391), as well as from chondrocytes (Fig. 11.12).

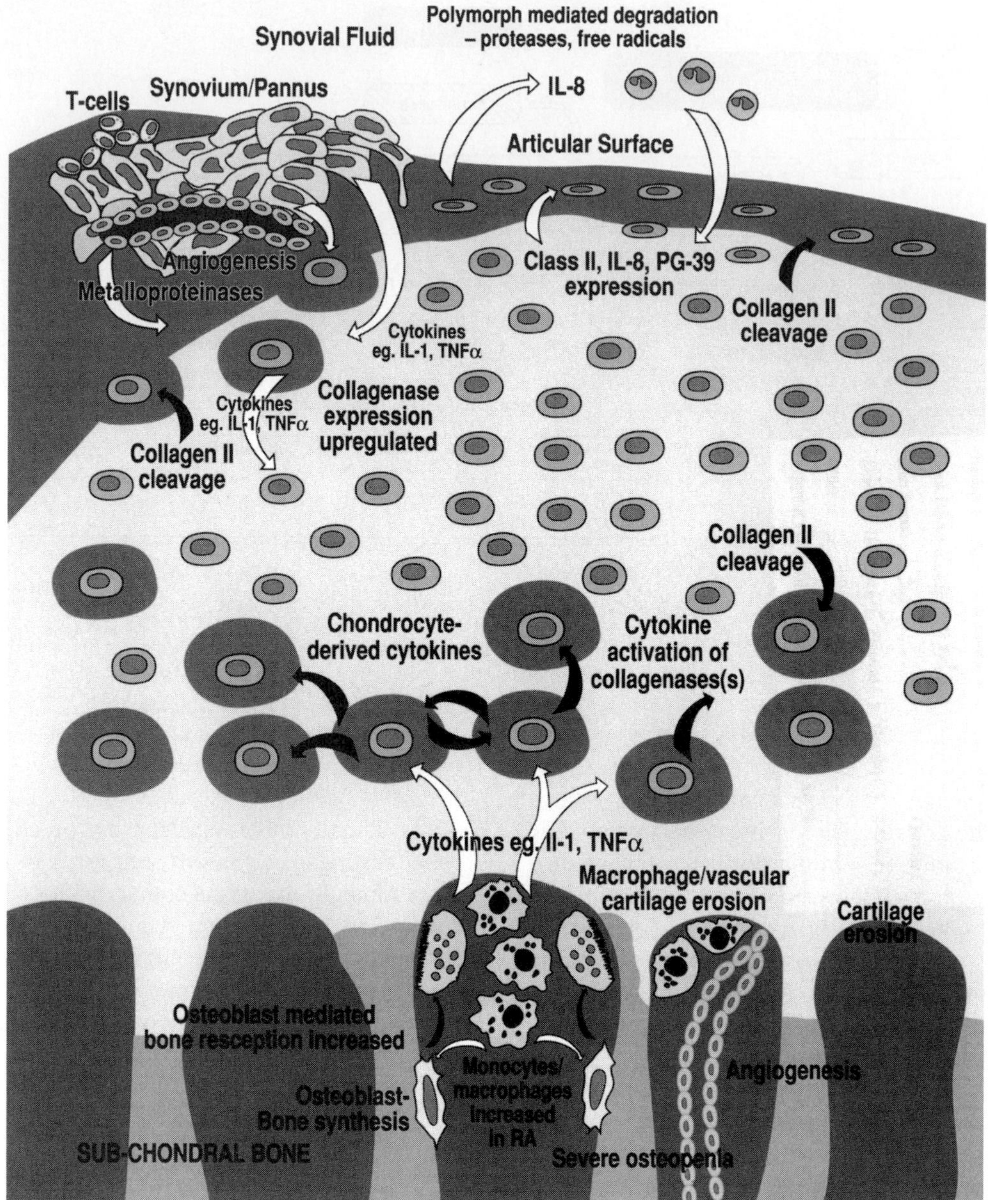

FIG. 11.12. The influence of synovium/pannus and inflamed bone on cartilage degradation in rheumatoid arthritis. The darkly shaded matrix identifies sites of type II collagen degradation. This is observed adjacent to pannus, at the articular surface, and adjacent to subchondral bone, where extensive osteopenia is seen. At the latter junction, vascular invasion and monocytic erosion of cartilage are observed in association with excessive osteoclast-mediated resorption of subchondral bone that causes osteopenia. Chondrocytes respond to interleukin-1 (*IL-1*) and tumor necrosis factor-α (*TNF-α*) and produce these same cytokines. Polymorphonuclear leukocytes and synovial cells can produce matrix metalloproteins (*MMPs*) that may directly damage cartilage or cytokines that activate chondrocytes to degrade their matrix. *GP-39,* human cartilage glycoprotein 39. (Modified and reproduced from Poole AR, Alini M, Hollander AP. Cellular biology of cartilage degradation. In: Henderson B, Pettifer R, Edwards J, eds. *Mechanisms and models in rheumatoid arthritis.* London: Academic, 1995:163–204, with permission.)

Proteinases and their substrates found in the extracellular matrix of cartilage are shown in Table 11.3.

The MMPs exhibit considerable structural homology (392). They are secreted as latent proenzymes, which are activated extracellularly. MMPs contain one atom of zinc in the active site, ligated by histidine residues, as in collagenase-1 (MMP-1). Here, a second structural zinc atom is present, together with structural calcium (393). A cysteine residue, eight residues from the cleavage site for conversion of proenzyme to active enzyme, is thought to be normally bound to the zinc atom (394,395), thereby endowing the protein with latency. Activation is believed to involve the dissociation of cysteine

TABLE 11.3. *Proteinases, substrates, and natural inhibitors*

Proteinase classes and names	Activator	Cartilage substrates
Metallo proteinases		
Collagenase-1 (interstitial or MMP-1)	Stromelysin-1, plasmin, kallikrein, cathepsin B	Collagen types I, II, III, X, IX; denatured type II; aggrecan.
Collagenase-3 (MMP-13)	MMP-14, MMP-2, plasmin	Prefers type II collagen
Collagenase-2 (neutrophil or MMP-8)	Probably same as interstitial collagenase	Collagen type II
Membrane type 1 MMP (MMP-14)	Furin (intracellular), urokinase, plasmin	Type II (weak activity), aggrecan
Gelatinase A (72-kd gelatinase, MMP-2)	Plasmin, elastase MMP-14	Denatured type II, aggrecan
Gelatinase B (92-kd gelatinase, MMP-9)	Urokinase type plasminogen activator, MMP-2 and MMP-14, stromelysin-1	General proteolysis
Stromelysin-1 (MMP-3)	Plasmin, cathepsin B	Aggrecan, fibronectin, type IX and XI collagens, procollagens, link protein, decorin, elastin
Stromelysin-2 (MMP-10)	Same as stromelysin-1?	Same as stromelysin 1?
Stromelysin-3 (MMP-11)	Furin (intracellular), plasmin	General proteolysis
Matrilysin (MMP-7)	Same as stromelysin-1?	Aggrecan
Macrophage Metalloelastase (MMP-12)	Unknown	Elastin
Aggrecanase-1, (ADAMTS-4)	Not known	Aggrecan at Glu^{373}–Ala^{374}
Aggrecanase-2 (ADAMTS-11)	Not known	Aggrecan at Glu^{373}–Ala^{374}
Serine proteinases		
Plasmin (from plasminogen)	Plasminogen activators (UPA, TPA), plasmin, cathepsin B, kallikrein	Prometalloproteinases
Tissue plasminogen activator (from pro TPA)	Cathepsin B, kallikrein	Plasminogen
Urokinase-type plasminogen activator (from pro UPA)	Cathepsin B	
Elastase[a]	None	Type II, IX, X, XI collagens; aggrecan; fibronectin
Cathepsin G[1]	None	TIMP, aggrecan, elastin, type II collagen
Kallikrein (from plasma)	Factor XII_a, XII_f	Procollagenase, prostromelysin (?), progelatinase (?)
Cysteine proteinases		
Cathepsin B	None	Procollagen, type II collagen (telopeptides)
Cathepsin L	None	Link protein, elastin, type II collagen (telopeptides), aggrecan
Cathepsin K	None	Type II collagen (intrahelical) aggrecan
Aspartate proteinases		
Cathepsin D	None	Aggrecan, denatured type II collagen

MMP and serine proteinase activities are at neutral pH whereas cathepsins operate at acidic pH.
[a]From polymorphonuclear leukocytes (neutrophils).
ADAMTS, a disintegrin and metalloproteinase with thrombospondin motifs; MMP, matrix metalloproteinase; TIMP, tissue inhibitor of metalloproteinases; TPA, tissue plasminogen activator; UPA, urinary plasminogen activator.

from the active-site zinc atom and its replacement with water, resulting in the exposure and activation of the active site, switching the role of zinc from a noncatalytic to a catalytic function. This conversion and activation can be induced chemically by aminophenol mercuriacetate. Activation is naturally accompanied by removal of the propiece (395).

Stromelysin-1 (MMP-3) is a superactivator of interstitial procollagenase (MMP-1) (396,397). Cleavage of type II collagen by collagenase-3 (MMP-13) is not observed in antigen-induced arthritis in the stromelysin-1 null mouse (in contrast to the wild type), providing strong evidence in support of a role for stromelysin-1 in procollagenase-3 activation in the mouse (only collagenase-3 has been demonstrated in murine articular cartilage) (398). Stromelysin-1 (MMP-3) also can degrade aggrecan. Aggrecan cleavage also is arrested in stromelysin-1 null mice (398). MMP-3 can cleave collagen types II, IX, and XI in nonhelical sites (399). Thus, it might play an important role in degradation of matrix collagen fibrils. Although MMP-3 is viewed as a degradative proteinase, its presence is important in cartilage since in MMP-3 null mice there is enhanced damage to cartilage in experimental OA (344).

The serine proteinases plasmin (derived from plasminogen by the activity of plasminogen activators) and kallikrein, as well as the cysteine proteinase cathepsin B (400), can each activate procollagenase (MMP-1) and are probably capable of activating other metalloproteinases (Fig. 11.11). An inhibitor of urokinase-type plasminogen activator can potently inhibit IL-1 and TNF-α-stimulated proteoglycan release in nasal and articular cartilages, directly implicating this enzyme (401). Serine proteinase inhibitors can partially block collagen breakdown in nasal cartilage (375), thereby implicating these proteinases in the activation of procollagenase. Cathepsin B activates proplasminogen activator at neutral pH (402), procollagenase, and prostromelysin (328), and degrades proteoglycans like most proteinases. Inhibition of cysteine proteinases can arrest proteoglycan degradation in cartilage (403), probably as a consequence of inhibition at the level of pro-MMP activation. Membrane type I MMP (MMP-14) and gelatinase A (MMP-2) each can activate procollagenase-3 (404); collagen cleavage by fibroblasts in MMP-14 null mice is impaired (405), but cartilage resorption in development appears unimpaired except at the level of angiogenesis at the secondary center of ossification.

Aggrecan Cleavage

Degradation of the protein core of aggrecan *in situ* involves cleavage between the G1 and G2 domains (Fig. 11.6) at Glu373-Ala374 (aggrecanase cleavage site) and Asn341-Phe342 (MMP cleavage site) (406,407). Cathepsin B also can act on this MMP cleavage site after an initial cleavage three residues carboxy-terminal to the MMP site (408). Other cleavages occur in the chondroitin sulfate–rich region and the G3 domain (409). The ADAM-TS (a disintegrin and metalloproteinase-1 with thrombospondin motif) proteinases are also known as aggrecanases in view of their involvement in the degradation of this molecule (410,411). They are synthesized as proenzymes requiring activation like other MMPs and are inhibited by tissue inhibitor of metalloproteinases (TIMP)-1. Aggrecanase-1 (ADAM-TS4) and aggrecanase-2 (ADAM-TS5) are both thought to be of importance, although aggrecan is susceptible to cleavage by many proteinases. ADAM-TS5 is probably constitutively expressed, whereas ADAM-TS4 is induced by IL-1 and TNF-α treatment (412) and by IL-1 in combination with oncostatin M (333). Aggrecanase cleavage is observed early after induction of experimental inflammatory arthritis, whereas there is less evidence for aggrecanase activity later when MMP cleavage is observed (413). This is presumably because the MMP cleavage site preferentially remains available because it is closer to the G1 domain that remains bound to hyaluronic acid.The G1 domain remains attached to hyaluronan after cleavage of aggrecan in the G1–G2 interglobular domain, resulting in a large accumulation of this complex in aging articular cartilage (119). This is reflective of ongoing proteolysis in the extracellular matrix. Link protein cleavage in human articular cartilage that occurs both *in situ* and *in vitro* involves a primary cleavage site between residues 16 and 17. This cleavage can be effected by MMP-3 or stromelysin-1 (414).

Collagen Cleavage

Type II collagen cleavage is selectively inhibited by carboxylate and hydroxamate inhibitors of MMPs in bovine and human articular cartilages (374,415). These observations point to a primary role for MMPs in the cleavage of this matrix molecule.

The degradation of fibrillar collagens usually involves a primary cleavage by collagenases in the triple helix at Gly775-Leu776 (in type II), although multiple proteases can cleave in the non-helical telopeptide domain of the type II collagen α chain (Fig. 11.6). However, little is known about cleavage in these telopeptide sites. Helical cleavage results in the denaturation of the triple helix with subsequent cleavage of the α chains by gelatinases and stromelysins, as well as by collagenases. Of these collagenases, collagenase-3/MMP-13, which is involved in chondrocyte hypertrophy, is the most efficient at cleaving type II collagen, and it is an excellent gelatinase (416,417). Collagenase-1/MMP-1 does not play a rate-limiting role in collagen II cleavage in mature bovine articular cartilages induced by IL-1α (374), but rather collagenase-3 (and/or -2) is involved. Similar results have been obtained for the increased degradation of collagen observed in cultured human articular cartilage (in the absence of a stimulant) taken from OA joints (415). However, there is evidence for the involvement of collagenase-1 in the degradation of type II collagen in nonarticular cartilages such as nasal cartilage (374), and in the degradation of newly synthesized collagen in OA (415).

The cleavage and denaturation of type II collagen is first observed in pericellular sites in aging and arthritis (127). Much of our understanding of proteolysis in cartilage has been made possible by the detection of site-specific cleavages in matrix molecules by use of an immunochemical approach. Antibodies have been made to specific neoepitopes generated at cleavage sites in link protein (418) and aggrecan (419,420), as well as collagen (421). These antibodies also have been used extensively in studies of arthritic cartilages where there is evidence for both MMP and aggrecanase cleavage of aggrecan. In murine inflammatory arthritis, they have been used to study the relative contributions of MMPs and aggrecanases to aggrecan cleavage (413). Antibodies to intrachain epitopes in type II collagen (126,421) have been developed to identify the denaturation of type II collagen *in situ,* to quantify it, and to localize it (126,422), revealing increased damage in OA and RA. In addition, antibodies to the collagenase cleavage site have provided a means to detect cleavage of type II collagen by collagenases and have shown that collagenase cleavage of type II collagen also is enhanced in OA (127,415,421).

Proteinase Inhibition

Proteinase inhibitors are listed in Table 11.3. There are four tissue inhibitors of metalloproteinases, commonly known as TIMP-1, TIMP-2, TIMP-3, and TIMP-4. TIMPs are deficient (compared with proteinase activity) in the growth plate in the hypertrophic zone (423), where selective and pronounced degradation of type II collagen mediated by hypertrophic chondrocytes prepares the matrix for calcification (72). There is a reported deficiency of TIMPs (with respect to collagenase) in OA cartilage (424,425), where proteolysis is excessive, yet TIMP-4 gene expression is increased (426). Neither TIMP-1 nor TIMP-2 can arrest the degradation of aggrecan in cartilage induced by IL-1, although either molecule can arrest collagen degradation (427). Inhibitors of the serine proteinases include protease nexin-1, plasminogen activator inhibitor-1, and α_1-proteinase inhibitor (Fig. 11.11). Inhibitors of plasmin and kallikrein, which can regulate the activation of prometalloproteinases (Fig. 11.11), also are deficient in osteoarthritic cartilage (425), although TSG-6, which potentiates inhibition by inter-α inhibitor, is reportedly increased in OA and probably also in RA cartilages (187). The cystatins, which are inhibitors of cysteine proteinases (428), are also present in cartilage. TGF-β_1 (429) and IL-6 (430), as well as oncostatin M (431), stimulate TIMP synthesis in chondrocytes (Fig. 11.10). IL-6 may exert its effect through induction of TGF-β (294). IL-11, which is inducible in human articular chondrocytes by IL-1β and TGF-β, also can stimulate TIMP-1 synthesis in chondrocytes (432). TIMP-3 is retained in the extracellular matrix, where it may more effectively regulate proteolysis mediated by metalloproteinases. Clearly cytokines, growth factors, hormones, and pharmacologic compounds have the potential to shift the balance between proteinases and their inhibitors, producing either net degradation or net synthesis (Fig. 11.10).

Mechanisms of Regulation of Gene Expression of Metalloproteinases

The AP-1 (activator protein-1) binding site is present within the promoter region of all the metalloproteinases, except gelatinase A (MMP-2). TNF-α, which induces collagenase (MMP-1) and IL-1 synthesis, produces a prolonged increase of c-*jun* as well as *fos* expression, contrasting with the transient increase elicited by phorbol ester (432). IL-1 also activates an AP-1 site (433,434) and transiently induces both c-*jun* and c-*fos* expression. Induction of MMP-13 by TNF-α is mediated by mitogen-activated protein (MAP) kinases and NFκB transcription factors in articular chondrocytes (435). MMP-13 induction by IL-1β requires p38 signaling, c-*jun* N-terminal kinase, and NFκB translocation (436). In OA, induction of MMP-1 gene expression is regulated by the inflammation responsive transcription factor SAF-1 (437).

Reactive oxygen species, the production of which is induced by cytokines such as IL-1, TNF-β, and basic FGF, mediate induction of c-*jun* (438) and c-*fos* (439) expression in chondrocytes. In addition, the specific interactions of AP-1 with other *cis*-acting elements such as PEA3 sites is required (440).

The transcription factor *Cbfa1,* also known as Run X2, regulates collagenase-3 gene expression in hypertrophic chondrocytes. Its absence in null mice often results in a lack of collagenase expression (57,58).

The AP-1 site also plays a dominant role in repression of MMPs by TGF-β and glucocorticoids (440). TGF-β inhibits stromelysin gene expression through an upstream sequence in the stromelysin promoter referred to as the TGF-β inhibitory element. This sequence binds a nuclear protein complex that contains *fos*. Induction of c-*fos* expression is required for the inhibitory effect. All-*trans*-retinoic acid also inhibits IL-1 and phorbol ester induction of collagenase, but inhibits induction only of *fos*, not of c-*jun,* gene expression (434).

The importance of members of the TGF-β family in preventing cartilage degradation has been demonstrated by several studies. Expression of a truncated, kinase-defective TGF-β type II receptor promotes chondrocyte terminal differentiation and onset of OA (299,441). Likewise, impairment of the SMAD signaling pathway, which is important for TGF-β signaling, also leads to cartilage degeneration and hypertrophy (300).

CARTILAGE CHANGES IN AGING AND ARTHRITIS

Aging

As human articular cartilage ages, the proliferative responses of chondrocytes to serum and growth factors decreases progressively (441). The mitotic potential and telomere length are both diminished in chondrocytes of older people, pointing to the importance of telomerase in maintaining replicative capacity (442). This is associated with a decrease with age in response of chondrocytes to TGF-β, IL-1 (298), and IGF-1 (443). There is a decrease in overall proteoglycan synthesis. An increase is observed in the accumulation of pentosidine, a cross-link formed by lysine, a sugar, and arginine (444,445). This nonenzymatic glycation results from a spontaneous reaction of reducing sugars, such as glucose, with free amino groups of proteins. The glycation involves mainly collagen molecules (445). The content of pentosidine can increase 50-fold in human cartilage from age 20 to 80 years (446). With increased formation of these advanced glycation end products on collagen, the fibril becomes stiffer. This may predispose toward OA (447). The increase in pentosidine in the matrix is inversely correlated with a decrease in MMP-mediated degradation measured as glycosaminoglycan release (448). Thus, glycation may also be a protective mechanism.

Progressive extracellular degradation of aggrecan also occurs, resulting in a reduction in its molecular size. Intact molecules containing the G3 globular domain are less commonly seen in aging (449,450), whereas smaller keratan sulfate–rich molecules appear in increasing numbers (120) (Fig. 11.7). The G1 globular domain (hyaluronan-binding region) increases considerably in content. Most of this exists as the G1 domain bound to hyaluronan in the absence of the remainder of the molecule (119). This complex reflects proteolytic cleavage between the G1 and G2 globular domains of aggrecan. These degradation products accumulate in the deep zone (451,452), remote from the chondrocytes in the interterritorial matrix where glycosaminoglycan staining is reduced. The half-life of the G1 domain has been estimated at 19 to 25 years (445,453), whereas that of the whole molecule is only 3.4 years (454). Link protein also is progressively reduced in molecular size during development and aging, as a result of cleavage close to the N-terminus (455). The accumulation of these breakdown products reflects progressive damage to the extracellular matrix over time and a lack of turnover and replacement of these damaged molecules.

The superficial zone of the knee articular cartilage exhibits an increase in tensile strength up to the third decade of life, after which it decreases markedly with age (456). Degradation of type II collagen in aging healthy adult human articular cartilage is usually confined to pericellular sites and the articular surface (126,127,388). The basal turnover is probably restricted to these sites. In the knee, the deep zone also exhibits a progressive decrease in tensile strength with increasing age (456), although total collagen content does not decrease (457). These changes in tensile properties in aging also are seen in the hip (458); in contrast, the articular cartilage of the talus of the ankle joint exhibits little or no reduction in tensile properties (459). Whereas OA commonly develops in the knee and the hip with increasing age, it is uncommon in the ankle joint. This points to a relationship between the loss of the tensile properties of cartilage and the development of OA. In contrast, analyses of compressive tests have revealed only a marginal decrease in the equilibrium modulus of human patella cartilage with age; this decrease is associated with surface degeneration (459). These observations indicate that there are clearly degenerative tensile changes in joints predisposed to OA. These must reflect changes in the structural organization of cartilage with aging that, if sufficiently developed, can predispose cartilage to traumatic damage and alterations in the mechanical loading of chondrocytes that would induce changes in matrix turnover. These changes are associated with thinning of articular cartilage as detected by magnetic resonance imaging. Patellar cartilage is thinner in older women and femoral cartilage is thinner in both sexes, whereas tibial cartilage exhibits no significant changes (460). Deformability is also reduced in patellar cartilages. This may relate to the accumulation of advanced glycation end products. Visibly degenerate human femoral condylar cartilage (105) and OA cartilage (214) both exhibit reduced tensile stiffness compared with normal cartilage. Experimentally induced canine OA also is accompanied by a reduction in compressive and tensile properties (461). These changes are particularly pronounced in the superficial cartilage, where tensile stiffness may be reduced by almost half, accompanied by a marked decrease in collagen and proteoglycan content and a decrease in hydroxypyridinium cross-link density (462). This is likely due to damage to the collagen network, which leads to increased water uptake and a reduction in proteoglycan concentration and increased deformation (232).

As aging progresses, damage to type II collagen is seen in knee femoral articular cartilages in about 25% of specimens at 30 to 40 years, but after 40 years, it is always observed at the histochemical level (127,388). It is initiated at the articular surface and extends progressively into the underlying cartilage. This damage, although similar in appearance to that in early OA, is less than the denaturation (421) and cleavage of type II collagen by collagenase (463) observed in OA. In ankle cartilage where tensile properties do not decrease, there is no clear evidence for a change in collagen and proteoglycan content, nor is there evidence of significant damage to the collagen network (463).

Osteoarthritis

Proteinase expression and activity in cartilage increases in OA and most proteinase inhibitors decrease in content (328), except TIMP-4 (425) (Table 11.4), resulting in net proteinase activity. Evidence for this comes from an examination of the changes in the structure, content, distribution, and degradation of matrix molecules (464) (summarized in Table 11.4). There is increased cleavage of aggrecan by MMPs and the aggrecanases ADAM-TS4 and ADAM-TS5 (389,465). In these same sites early in disease development, collagen damage is observed (126). Local loss of the proteoglycan aggrecan (388), decorin, and biglycan (107) from the articular surface, and sometimes around chondrocytes, is seen in early human and experimentally induced OA. In advanced disease, above Mankin grade 6, aggrecan molecules are larger, and glycosaminoglycans are chemically and immunochemically different (464) (Table 11.4). This pattern is indicative of a loss of preexisting molecules and their replacement with newly synthesized proteoglycans, a fraction of which are partly degraded. There is increased expression of other proteoglycans and induction of synthesis of a variety of molecules previously seen only in chondrogenesis, such as tenascin and type IIA collagen (Table 11.4).

In OA, when collagen damage is extensive, with resultant deep fibrillation, there is a net loss of type II collagen aggrecan and hyaluronan (466,467). This is reflected by the extensive loss of staining for proteoglycan in OA cartilage. Damage to type II collagen is initiated around chondrocytes at the articular surface and progressively involves deeper cells as the disease progresses (126). The tensile properties of the cartilage collagen are lost (105,214). The increased swelling and instantaneous deformation of osteoarthritic cartilage is highly correlated with collagen degradation

TABLE 11.4. *Changes associated with moderate early degeneration of articular cartilage (limited or no fibrillation) in the development of osteoarthritis*

Item	Change	Item	Change
Chondrocytes		**Matrix proteins**	
Size and cloning	+	**Collagens**	
Expression of hypertrophic phenotype		Type IIB content	−
Type X collagen	+	Denaturation	+
Annexin II and V	+	Cleavage by collagenase	+
PTHrP	+	Synthesis	+
Apoptosis	+	Type IIA	+
Alkaline phosphatase	+	Type III	+
NO/cytokines/growth factors		Type VI	+
Inducible NO synthase	+	Type X	+
IL-1β, TNF-α, IL-6, IL-8	+		
p55 TNF-α receptor	+	**Proteoglycans**	
IL-1 receptors	+	Aggrecan synthesis (+ overall);	+/−
IGF-1, IGF-2, GP-39	+	content (−) at surface	
IGFBP-3	+	Altered sulfation of chondroitin sulfate	+/−
		Decorin and biglycan contents	−
Chondrocytes and matrix		Decorin and biglycan expression	+
metalloproteinases		Fibromodulin and lumican expression	+
Collagenases-1, 2, 3 (MMP-1, 8, 13)	+	Link protein expression	+
Stromelysin-1 (MMP-3)	+	**Other proteins**	
Gelatinases A and B (MMP-2, 9)	+	Clusterin	+
Matrilysin (MMP-7)	+	Cartilage oligomeric protein	+
MT1-MMP (MMP-14)	+	Tenascin	+
Aggrecanase (ADAMTS family)	+	Fibronectin	+
Serine proteinases		Cartilage matrix protein induced	+
Plasminogen activitors (PA)	+	SPARC (osteonectin)	+
(urokinase or tissue PA)		TSG-6	+
Serine proteinases	+	Cartilage intermediate layer protein	+
Cysteine proteinase		**Hydroxyapatite**	+
Cathepsin B	+		
Cathepsin K	+		
Proteinase, inhibitors			
TIMPs	−		
Plasminogen activitor inhibitor-1	−		

Changes indicated by increases (+) and decreases (−).

ADAMTS, a disintegrin and metalloproteinase with thrombospondin motifs; GP, glycoprotein; IGF, insulin-like growth factor; IL, interleukin; MMP, matrix metalloproteinase; PTHrP, parathyroid hormone-related peptide; TNF, tumor necrosis factor.

(231). Increased type II collagen degradation occurs early after anterior cruciate ligament rupture and precedes clinical onset of posttraumatic OA (468).

Where collagen II cleavage and denaturation occurs around chondrocytes is also where the Young modulus is reduced (217). Together this damage involves changes in the mechanical environment of the cartilage in the superficial zone that can lead to abnormal mechanical loading on chondrocytes, resulting in progressive net degradation mediated both directly and through the chondrocyte. Degradation of type II collagen can result from abnormal loading *in vitro* and *in vivo* (see earlier section on Mechanical and Physical Properties of the Extracellular Matrix of Cartilage).

Lesions form focally, as seen in aging mice (469) and at autopsy (466). Degradation of extracellular matrix is pronounced, especially involving type II collagen cleavage by collagenases. Analyses of these focal sites and the surrounding cartilage reveal that the lesions probably start focally and then progressively enlarge in size (466).

The degradation of type II collagen involving excessive collagenase activity, is probably mainly due to MMP-13 (415), which is expressed in the same sites as the cleavage (126).

These degenerative changes in OA cartilages are accompanied by marked changes in growth factor and cytokine/receptor expression (Table 11.4), implicating these molecules in disease pathogenesis. IL-1 and TNF-α expression are markedly up-regulated in OA chondrocytes (470). TNF-α receptor (p55) (471–473) and, to a lesser degree, IL-1 receptors (470,474) are up-regulated. When canine articular cartilage is traumatized and OA develops, there is an early increase in IL-1β and TNF-α, as well as stromelysin-1 (MMP-3) (475).

The susceptibility of chondrocytes to the degradative effects of concentrations of IL-1β and TNF-α found in arthritic joints varies within an OA joint, pointing to regional differences in the pathology (476). IL-1β can induce the secretion of IGF-1 and IGF-binding proteins by chondrocytes, as well as up-regulating receptor number, but has no effect on IGF-1 mRNA expression (477). Moreover, IGF-1 can counteract the activity of IL-1 by inducing expression of soluble IL-1 receptor II protein (284). There is increased synthesis and increased expression of IGF-1 (a potent stimulator of matrix synthesis) in OA cartilages (277,478), which accompanies an increase in receptor binding (479). Thus, it seems that catabolic cytokines can induce anabolic responses in chondrocytes to regulate the catabolic stimulus. In response to this increase in IGF-1 there is up-regulation of IGFBP-3 content in OA cartilage (480). Osteopontin expression is markedly up-regulated in OA cartilage (481) and can also modulate degradation by inhibiting spontaneous and IL-1β-induced NO and PGE_2 production (481). How this is achieved remains unclear. However osteopontin, as well as pyrophosphate, can also suppress the deposition of hydroxyapatite that occurs in OA (482). The involvement of cytokines and growth factors in OA has been reviewed (483).

The loss of matrix molecules is partially compensated by increases in the content of type II collagen, aggrecan, decorin, and biglycan deeper in the cartilage (Table 11.4), a consequence of increased synthesis. But whereas the deeper, healthier cartilage is the site of much of this increased synthesis, the more superficial cartilage remains badly damaged. The changes in the deeper cartilage can be profound, because an increase in its tensile properties may occur (105).

Overall, degradation prevails, with net loss of cartilage matrix. Newly synthesized collagen molecules are degraded in OA, unlike in healthy cartilage (415). The multiplicity of these and other changes in OA are summarized in Table 11.4. For a review of the changes that occur in OA, see reference 484.

With the degradation of articular cartilage, vascular invasion from subchondral bone is often seen. In fact experimental studies of angiogenesis using the chick embryo chorioallantoic membrane have shown that OA cartilage loses its ability to resist invasion (485), suggesting that angiogenic molecules are generated, such as VEGF. These probably originate from hypertrophic chondrocytes.

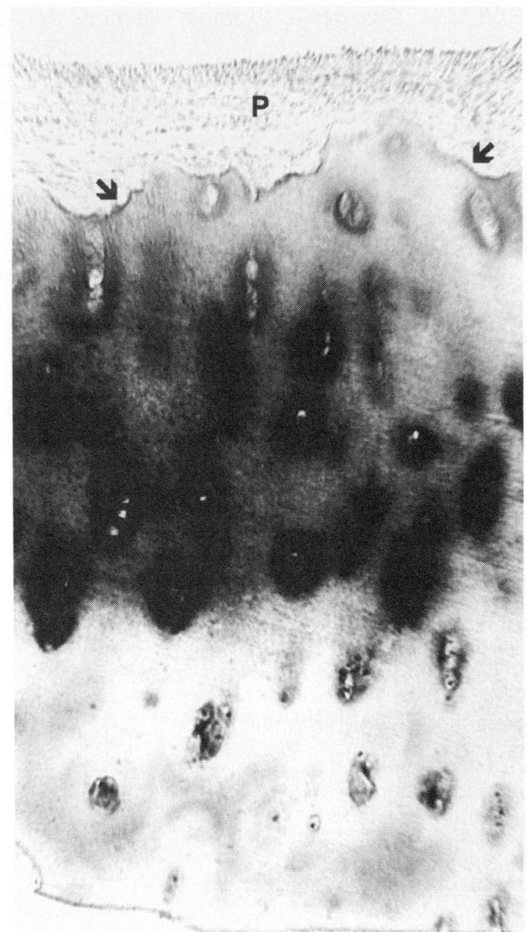

FIG. 11.13. The pannus (*P*) and articular cartilage junction in rheumatoid arthritis stained to show sites of cleavage of type II collagen by collagenases. Notice that this is most concentrated around chondrocytes. This band of increased cleavage is observed only adjacent to the pannus that is eroding the cartilage, the junction of which is indicated (*arrows*). (From Poole AR, Pidoux I, Billinghurst RC. Unpublished observations.)

Rheumatoid Arthritis

In RA, the combined actions of free radicals and proteinases released from polymorphonuclear leukocytes probably contribute to the damage seen at the articular surface. Free radicals released from these cells can activate latent collagenases (486). However, there is evidence of damage to type II collagen fibrils around chondrocytes in the territorial matrix of the deep zone of articular cartilage next to subchondral bone (126) (Fig. 11.12), as well as adjacent to pannus tissue (328) (Figs. 11.12 and 11.13). This is closely associated with proinflammatory cytokine expression (IL-1, TNF-α) by adjacent bone cells, synovial cells, and macrophages. In antigen-induced arthritis in rabbits (a model for RA), TNF-α has been detected in deep-zone chondrocytes (487), as observed in rheumatoid articular cartilages (488). The pericellular pattern of destruction of cartilage adjacent to both pannus (390,391) and bone suggests that this is likely a result of degradation by MMPs generated by activated chondrocytes (126) (Figs 11.12 and 11.13), as well by synovial cells (392). Cytokines no doubt activate these chondrocytes to degrade matrix. Most of the type II collagen throughout the cartilage is eventually damaged in RA (126), as in OA. Thus, the main distinction between articular cartilage damage in these two types of arthritis is no doubt the result of the massive generation of prodegradative cytokines, such as IL-1 and TNF-α, by synovial cells, macrophages, and cells in the inflamed subchondral bone. Thus, there is an attack on cartilage from all sides in RA (Fig. 11.12).

Although cytokines can induce cartilage degradation, inhibition of individual cytokines can have profound effects. Inhibition of TNF-α can markedly suppress inflammatory changes in patients, as well as in animals, demonstrating its importance in inflammation. Suppression of inflammation may, however, have little or no effect on aggrecan degradation, as revealed when TNF-α is neutralized by antibodies in experimental models (487,489). Whereas TNF-α neutralization has little effect on the suppression of proteoglycan synthesis, neutralization of IL-1 can totally prevent this suppression (489) and protect against cartilage damage. Other studies also have revealed that IL-1 blockade can prevent cartilage destruction in murine inflammatory arthritis, whereas TNF-α blockade only ameliorates joint inflammation (490). This suppression of aggrecan synthesis by IL-1 is, as described earlier, mediated by generation of NO. In mice that lack inducible NO synthase 2, the inhibition of proteoglycan synthesis is prevented in experimental joint inflammation. Responsiveness to IGF-1 also is restored, and net proteoglycan depletion is markedly reduced, demonstrating a role for NO in inflammation-induced damage to articular cartilage (491). The capacity of IL-4 to protect against cartilage damage in inflammatory arthritis in the mouse (349) demonstrates the potential of this cytokine to regulate this degradative process. As in OA, there are likely many matrix changes that result from cartilage damage, although in general they have been much less studied. Moreover, cartilage matrix protein (matrilin-1) synthesis is induced (492), and the expression of proinflammatory cytokines is up-regulated (470). Apoptosis also is up-regulated in articular cartilage in RA (as in OA), and this is associated with a decrease in *Bcl*-2 expression (380), which also is observed in association with apoptosis in the growth plate (see earlier section on Maturation of Chondrocytes to Express Hypertrophic and Nonhypertrophic Phenotypes).

MONITORING CARTILAGE METABOLISM *IN VIVO*: DETECTION OF MOLECULAR SYNTHETIC AND DEGRADATION PRODUCTS OF CARTILAGE IN BODY FLUIDS

The introduction of specific immunoassays for molecules found mainly or exclusively within cartilage has permitted a variety of new *in vivo* studies of cartilage matrix metabolism by analyses of synovial fluids, sera/plasma, and urine (Fig. 11.14). The concentrations of the cartilage proteoglycan aggrecan are, as expected, higher in synovial fluid of arthritic joints than in serum (377,493). These molecules generally represent degradation products of synthetic or degradative processes. The largest breakdown products include the keratan sulfate–rich domain and the G1 and G2 globular domains of aggrecan (378). Traumatic injury in humans (494) causing joint instability rapidly results in a persistent increase of aggrecan and other products in synovial fluids of affected joints. These increases may have prognostic value because they are likely to be indicative of the establishment of progressive degenerative joint disease. In inflammatory joint disease, high levels of aggrecan in joint fluids may be prognostic for increased joint destruction in RA.

Studies of joints of RA patients also have revealed that in early disease, where little damage is observed radiographically, predominantly glycosaminoglycan-rich aggrecan fragments are released. This contrasts to more advanced disease in which there has been more proteoglycan degradation, and the hyaluronan-binding region (G1 globular domain) and associated aggrecan components predominate (495), probably as a result of their preferential retention in cartilage matrix as a result of hyaluronan binding.

A chondroitin sulfate epitope, 846, present only on the largest aggrecan molecules that exhibit complete aggregation with hyaluronic acid (464), is released in close association with aggrecan synthesis (Fig. 11.14), and is present in increased concentration in synovial fluids after joint injury (496) and in joint fluid of patients with OA (493,496). This reflects the increased content of this molecule in OA cartilage (464). Serum levels are reduced in patients with early aggressive RA (497), in contrast to those with chronic or less rapidly progressive disease (493,497). In both types of arthritis, joint fluid analyses have revealed inverse correlations between the 846 epitope and a keratan sulfate epitope, which is present mainly on aggrecan degradation products (493). These studies point to the potential use of markers of aggrecan synthesis (846 epitope) and degradation to study the effects of inflammation on the turnover of this molecule in hyaline cartilages.

Elevations of serum cartilage proteoglycans bearing keratan sulfate have been observed in OA, suggesting enhanced degradation (466,498). Others have been unable to confirm these observations in humans (493,499). In RA, the level of the circulating keratan sulfate epitope is generally decreased (493,500), suggesting that the decreased levels of serum keratan sulfate might reflect changes in systemic aggrecan synthesis, which is inhibited by inflammatory mediators such as IL-1 and TNF-α (see section on Molecules that Regulate Chondrocyte Metabolism). Significant inverse correlations between levels of a serum keratan sulfate epitope and the duration of morning stiffness and levels of orosomucoid (500,501) and TNF-α (501) (as measures of inflammation) support this conclusion.

As suggested earlier, by measuring these epitopes in sera of patients with early RA, it may be possible to distinguish at presentation between those with rapidly and slowly progressive erosive joint disease. In patients with reduced levels of the 846 epitope (the probable rapid erosion group), cartilage oligomeric matrix protein (COMP) levels are increased (497). In patients with OA, elevations of COMP (502,503) and persistent elevations of hyaluronic acid (502, 504,505) are associated with disease progression. Hyaluronic acid levels also correlate with joint space changes

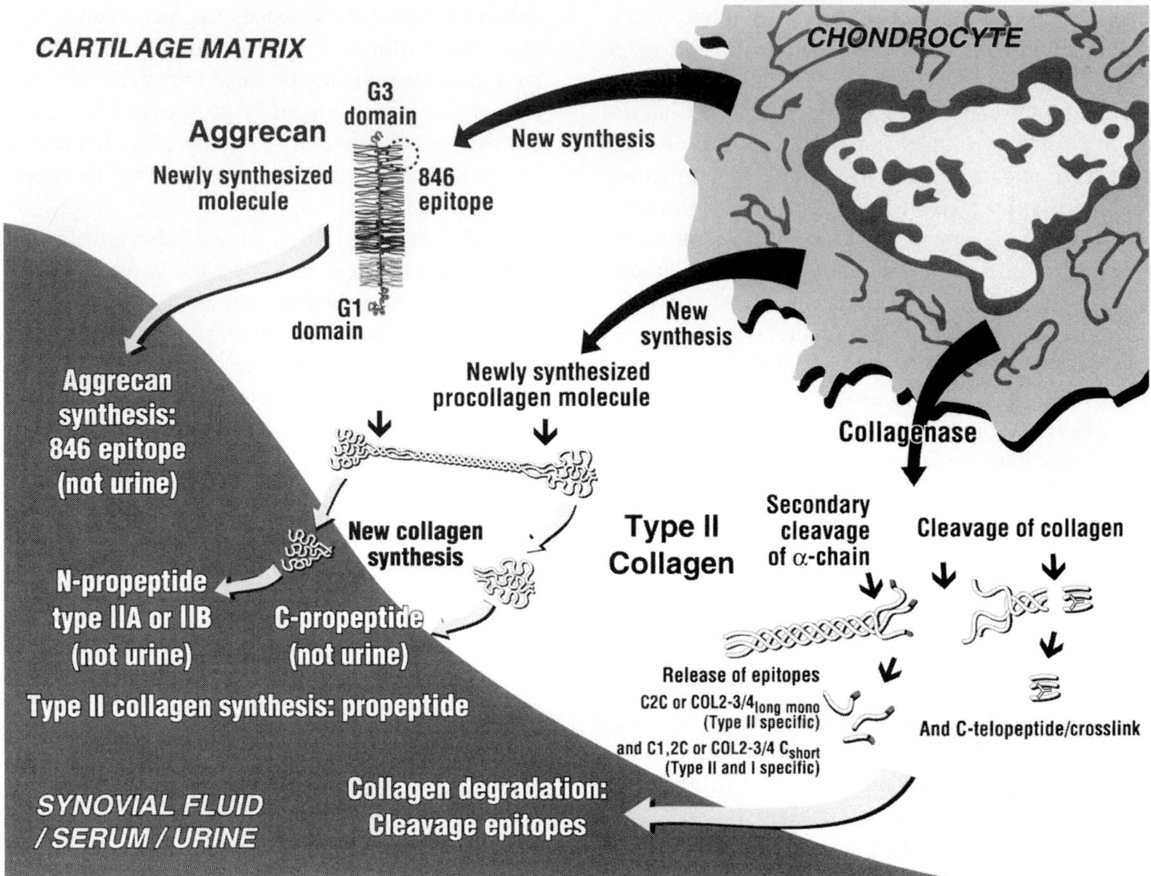

FIG. 11.14. Biomarkers of cartilage turnover. Products of proteoglycan aggrecan synthesis/turnover (846 epitope), type II procollagen synthesis (N- and C-propeptides), and type II collagen degradation cleavage epitopes are shown that are released into body fluids where they can be detected by immunoassay. (Reproduced from Poole AR. Biochemical/immunochemical biomarkers of osteoarthritis: utility for prediction of incident or progressive osteoarthritis. *Rheum Dis Clin North Am* 2003;29:803–818, with permission.)

(504,505). These elevations may well signify the presence of a synovitis that contributes to disease progression in OA, because serum hyaluronic acid levels have been shown to correlate with joint involvement in RA (reviewed in 506), and COMP also is synthesized and secreted by activated synovial cells (507). Separate studies have revealed that COMP levels are increased in OA compared with control populations (508).

Recently, methods have been developed to detect cleavage (509–512) and synthesis of type II collagen (Fig. 11.14). In a model of RA in the rat, serum levels of a collagenase cleavage product of type II collagen correlated closely with joint damage (509). Such an assay may prove of value in human studies. The C-propeptide of type II procollagen is an indicator of the synthesis of this molecule (128) (Fig. 11.14). Marked serum elevations are observed in patients with early RA, irrespective of progression rates, in contrast to the decreased levels of the aggrecan biosynthesis marker epitope 846 (497). Thus, the synthesis or release of cartilage molecules can be influenced differently by inflammation. Cartilage matrix protein (matrilin-1), which is found only in healthy nonarticular cartilage, is increased in the sera of patients with RA, but not reactive arthritis (513), presumably as a result of induction of its synthesis in both noninvolved and involved joints in RA (492).

Cross-sectional studies of the levels of C-propeptide of type II collagen in the sera of patients with OA have revealed significant decreases compared with nonarthritic controls (126). Similar results have been obtained for the aminopropeptide of type IIA collagen, which reappears in OA cartilage (514). In contrast, the cleavage of type II collagen, reflected by release of its carboxytelopeptide into urine, is increased in OA (510,514). When the ratio of synthesis to degradation is examined, it is apparent that in patients with knee OA, when degradation is high and synthesis is low, progression of joint destruction is enhanced (514). These results may relate to differences in the systemic turnover of type II collagen in persons that develop OA: the changes may not simply be a consequence of the disease. In patients with familial OA caused by the $Arg^{519}Cys$ mutation in type II collagen, the C-propeptide is more often elevated in these individuals than in mutation-negative persons. The same applies to a keratan sulfate epitope and to cartilage oligomeric protein, the latter two differences being significant (515). These changes reflect more general alterations in cartilage turnover caused by abnormalities in the structure of the triple helix of type II collagen that lead to the early development of a degenerative arthritis. In patients with RA, type II collagen degradation is also increased, more so than in OA (510). The greater the increase, the more this is correlated with disease progression (516,517). The proteoglycan aggrecan (detected by a keratan sulfate epitope assay) is increased in sera of children in early growth, reaching a peak between ages 4 and 12 years (518). It then decreases markedly (518,519). Treatment with GH increases serum levels in children with GH deficiency (520). When keratan sulfate epitope levels decrease during growth, at about 12 years, the circulating concentration of the C-propeptide of type II collagen increases (521). Because the latter increase is seen during the growth spurt, it would seem that these serum changes in cartilage components may reflect this increased growth, particularly because much of the C-propeptide is thought to originate from the growth plates. The analysis of these molecules may therefore be of value in determining the more immediate effects of therapy in children with growth defects and the effects of arthritis, inflammation, and therapy on growth and cartilage metabolism.

IMMUNITY TO CARTILAGE: IMPLICATIONS FOR JOINT DESTRUCTION IN THE INFLAMMATORY ARTHRITIDES

Cartilage is an avascular tissue that has previously been considered "immunologically privileged" and, like the cornea, transplantable as an allograft. Cartilage is, in fact, an immunologically reactive tissue eliciting both humoral and cellular immunity. The extracellular matrix, however, plays an important protective role in shielding chondrocytes from immune damage, such as that caused by cytotoxic ($CD8^+$) T lymphocytes and antibodies. Most of the extracellular matrix of articular cartilage is ordinarily impermeable to antibodies and complement components (522, 523). This is attributable to the presence of high concentrations of the proteoglycan aggrecan. Only at the articular surface is the concentration of aggrecan low enough to permit antibody penetration (523). As proteoglycans are lost in disease, the cartilage becomes increasingly permeable to these molecules. Likewise, the damage results in the release of cellular and extracellular components that may stimulate the immune system.

Interest in the importance of immunity to cartilage components in the pathogenesis of inflammatory arthritis has been stimulated by the common observation that following arthroplasty of rheumatoid joints in which articular cartilage is removed, synovial inflammation is reduced. Recently it was shown that there is a reduction in lymphocyte infiltration and activation in the rheumatoid synovial membrane following arthroplasty (524). Human chondrocytes in the superficial zone express class II major histocompatibility complex (MHC) antigens in arthritis (525) and therefore may subserve an antigen presentation function. These can be induced by IFN-γ (526).

Antibodies to Cartilage Collagens

Circulating antibodies to type II and other cartilage collagens are commonly detected in patients with rheumatic diseases. Immunity is generally directed to denatured type II collagen and type XI collagen (527,528). This is to be expected because fragmented collagens are probably released from cartilage and recognized by the immune system. Individual epitopes have been detected in the cyanogen bromide (CB) 11 domain (529). Recognition of this epitope varies among patients. The presence of circulating antibodies to type II collagen is correlated with the presence of polyarthritis in psoriasis (530) and ankylosing spondylitis (AS) (531). The antibodies never precede the clinical onset of RA (532), appearing after damage to articular cartilage. B cells, producing antibodies to type II collagen, are present in rheumatoid synovia (533,533a,534). Antibodies to a specific sequence in the type II collagen α chain are elevated in sera of RA patients. Monoclonal antibodies directed against this epitope can induce (in combination with a second monoclonal antibody) arthritis in BALB/c mice (535). Moreover, antibodies to type II collagen, isolated from the serum of a patient with RA, caused transient arthritis when injected into mice (536). Antibodies to type II collagen also are found in relapsing polychondritis, in which there is widespread cartilage destruction associated with inflammation of cartilage (537–539). In Ménière disease and otosclerosis, damage to auditory cartilage is accompanied by the appearance of antibodies to type II collagen (540). Thus, immunity to cartilage collagen mediated by antibodies may contribute to tissue damage.

Cellular Immunity to Type II Collagen

This is commonly observed in patients with most inflammatory arthritides and is often directed against denatured type II collagen (541,542). Immunity to native type II collagen is frequently observed in juvenile RA (JRA) and systemic lupus erythematosus, but is uncommon in patients with AS (542). $CD4^+$ T-cell clones that recognize type II collagen have been isolated from rheumatoid synovia (543). Only if psoriasis patients have an erosive arthritis do they exhibit cellular immunity to type II collagen (530). If this immunity is expressed *in vivo,* it could induce connective tissue destruction.

Humoral and Cellular Immunity to Aggrecan, Link Protein, and Glycoprotein-39

Aggrecan is also an immunogen. Antibodies to aggrecan have been reported in patients with RA in only one study (544).

In contrast, cellular immunity to aggrecan, involving CD4+ T cells, has been detected in patients with AS, JRA, and RA (541,542,545). It also has been reported in patients with relapsing polychondritis (546,547). In RA, it is directed to the G1 domain, which binds to hyaluronic acid (548). It also is observed in patients with OA, together with immunity to link protein (549). Link protein shares homology with the G1 domain. Immunity to link protein also is observed in JRA (550).

Immunity to these cartilage proteoglycans and related molecules can result in cross-reactions with epitopes shared by proteoglycans (e.g., versican, which has a similar G1 domain as aggrecan) found in other tissues such as sclera, ligaments, entheses, and arterial vessels (551–554), as well as to link protein, which is present in these other tissues in association with versican. It is of interest that aortitis is often observed in relapsing polychondritis (555) and AS (556), where immunity is observed. Scleritis is sometimes seen in RA (557), but more commonly in relapsing polychondritis (555,558). There have been unconfirmed reports of cross-reactive T-cell immunity between heat-shock protein and aggrecan in human and animal arthritis (559,560). At present, there is no direct evidence for this in humans, because clonal T-cell populations have not been examined.

Induction of Erosive Arthritis by Experimental Induction of Immunity to Cartilage Components

The expression of cellular immunity to collagens types II, IX, and XI in the inflammatory arthritides, as well as to aggrecan, might be causally related to the pathogenesis of these diseases, or, like humoral immunity, could be an epiphenomenon (immunity that develops secondary to and as a consequence of the primary pathogenesis). However, pivotal observations that injections of type II collagen (561), type XI collagen [α_3(XI) chain, which is the same gene product as α_1(II)] (562), and type IX and XI collagens (563); aggrecan (specifically the G1 globular domain) (564,565); link protein (566); and gp39 (567) can each induce an inflammatory erosive arthritis in animals indicates that these immune responses might be causally related to the pathogenesis of these erosive arthritides. In contrast, spondylitis and sacroiliitis are features of AS and not of RA. Only experimental immunity to aggrecan or versican can induce these pathologies (554,565,568), although an axial ossifying enthesopathy has been described in chronic arthritis induced by injection of type II collagen in rats (569). Immunization of Lewis rats with syngeneic nucleus pulposus in incomplete Freund adjuvant produces a spondylodiscitis when the nucleus of the intervertebral disc of these rats is ruptured, exposing autoantigen (570).

Immunity to the proteoglycan aggrecan is directed mainly at the G1 globular domain (564,568). If keratan sulfate is present on G1 and the interglobular G1–G2 domain, immune reactivity is suppressed, and the development of arthritis is prevented (564,571). Interestingly, the content of keratan sulfate in aggrecan is increased with development and aging (232,572), and this may be protective against the development of immunity. The immunity to aggrecan in BALB/c mice involves cross-reactive recognition of a T-cell epitope and several B-cell epitopes in mouse aggrecan. T cells specific for a single epitope can home to joints (where the relevant peptide epitope has been injected) and induce arthritis (572). In contrast, immunity to versican only involves cross-reactive antibodies (554).

Extraarticular pathology of the kind seen in rheumatic diseases also can develop in animals immunized with other molecules ordinarily only found in nonarticular cartilages. Thus, rats immunized with cartilage matrix protein (matrilin-1) develop a relapsing polychondritis–like condition (573). A proportion of patients with relapsing polychondritis have antibodies to matrilin-1 which bind to tracheolaryngeal cartilage and correlate with respiratory symptoms in 69% of cases (574). Chronic inflammation of the middle ear, associated with damage to the cartilaginous bones, is also seen in rats immunized with type II collagen (575, 576). This may have relevance to the pathogenesis of otosclerosis and Ménière disease.

Transplantation and Repair of Cartilage

Many experimental studies have revealed that whereas allografts of animal cartilages show some resistance to immune rejection, this will eventually occur (577,578). Rejection is associated with the local production of antibodies to cartilage allografts and synovium/pannus-mediated resorption (579). Many plasma cells and large lymphocytes are seen in the invading synovial/pannus tissue covering and eroding the graft. Only autografts and histocompatibility-matched allografts survive, and then synovial changes are minimal. The cellular events that underlie synovium/pannus-mediated cartilage rejection strikingly resemble those seen in RA, suggesting that immunity to cartilage is in part a causative factor in this disease, as discussed earlier. There is tissue invasion of the cartilage graft, heavy mononuclear cell infiltration, and extensive formation of pannus tissue growing over and into the graft. It is known that cartilage slices can survive in a joint until they become adherent to synovium, at which time they are destroyed (580). This probably occurs both by direct proteolytic attack and by the production of cytokines such as IL-1 by the invading synovial tissue with subsequent activation of chondrocytes to degrade their local extracellular matrix.

Antibodies reactive with chondrocytes can, in the presence of complement, destroy chondrocytes in intact articular cartilage (581,582), presumably because chondrocytes can rapidly replace their lost proteoglycans, which limit access of antibodies and complement components. Only when soft connective tissue (e.g., synovium) is present (as a source of cytokines such as IL-1) will cartilage destruction and resorption result (583,584).

In contrast to experiences in animals, allografts of fresh and frozen cartilage can be successfully transplanted in humans (585,586). However, results in cases of OA, osteonecrosis, and osteochondritis desiccans are generally disappointing, probably as a result of the degenerative changes already present in the recipient cartilage. This could be due to immunity to chondrocytes and matrix molecules discussed previously. The best results are seen in patients with traumatic injuries whose cartilage is healthy (587–589), and the immune response seems to be more theoretical than an actual problem. Indeed, immune responses often are never detected in these cases (590–592). Successful allografting of human menisci is well documented (593). The apparent discrepancies with animal studies might be related to the fact that class II MHC antigens are only weakly expressed on human chondrocytes compared with those of animals.

The repair of articular cartilage is an uncommon event in the adult, yet in children with JRA, reduction in disease activity may be accompanied by restoration of articular cartilage, with an increase in joint space, as revealed by radiographic examination (594,595). Isolated autologous chondrocytes from unloaded regions of knee articular cartilages are now being used, after expansion in culture, to fill defects in cartilage (596). Although good success is claimed, outcome data are limited. Periosteal flaps are used to contain the chondrocytes. It is not clear how important the contribution of the periosteum is, in the human studies, to the production of new cartilage. Experimental studies of the repair of cartilage have demonstrated that it is possible to use periosteum as a source of chondroprogenitor cells to repair defects in articular cartilage (597–599). The cartilage that is formed is a hyaline cartilage containing type II collagen. In contrast to fracture callus and the growth plate, this cartilage is formed under cyclic loading because of its location within the joint. Cyclic loading probably prevents cellular hypertrophy and cartilage calcification, which ordinarily occur only adjacent to subchondral bone. Containment of transplanted isolated chondrocytes in a suitable biodegradable matrix is another important approach to promoting effective repair. Some experimental approaches use fibrous polyglycolic acid scaffolds (600) (see Chapter 112). A recent review of this area of research is provided in reference 601.

TUMORS OF CARTILAGE AND TRANSFORMED CHONDROCYTE CELL LINES

There are several types of cartilage tumors (602–604). The osteochondromas, cartilage-capped bony masses that arise in the metaphyses of bones, account for about 50% of all benign tumors. They often arise after radiation therapy. Multiple osteochondromas develop in the autosomal-dominant condition designated multiple osteocartilaginous exostosis. Enchondromas form in the medullary cavity of a cartilaginous bone, usually in a long bone. They account for about 10% of all the benign tumors of bone. Chondrosarcomas are malignant neoplasms in which no osteoid is produced (as in an osteosarcoma), but they often partly calcify. They arise from a healthy bone or from a benign cartilaginous neoplasm. Clear cell and mesenchymal chondrosarcomas are histologically recognizable variants. Chondrosarcomas account for about 10% of the malignant tumors of cartilage (603). Experimentally induced overexpression of c-*fos* and Fos protein leads to the development of chondrogenic tumors (605). Chondrosarcomas have been histologically classified on the basis of nuclear size, cellular appearance (chondroid or myxoid), mitoses, and general cellularity. Grade 1 tumors are hyaline-like, resembling normal cartilage. They can be invasive, but are nonmetastatic. The prognosis is good, with 83% survival at 10 years (602). Grade III chondrosarcomas often are very myxoid in appearance, with nuclear aberrations and high mitotic rates. Those of lowest grade contain a normal adult content of keratan sulfate, whereas high-grade tumors contain little or no keratan sulfate (606).

Several immortalized chondrocyte cell lines are of value in ongoing research. Retrovirus encoding the SV40 large T antigen has been used to transform mouse (607) and human (608) chondrocytes. These cells produce a variety of matrix proteins, including type II collagen and aggrecan.

CONCLUSION

The development and physiology of cartilage is regulated in a precise manner by a combination of chemical and mechanical factors. Cartilage can survive and form a permanent tissue, as in the case of articular cartilage, or the cells can become hypertrophic and calcify their matrix. Calcified matrix can act as a template on which osteoblasts settle and form woven bone as part of the process of endochondral ossification. Abnormal development of cartilage and bone can result from mutations in chondrocyte genes, producing recognizable chondrodysplasias. Cartilage contains an extensive extracellular matrix that is synthesized by the chondrocytes. The functions of many of these matrix molecules remain to be identified. Chondrocytes can remodel or destroy this matrix in response to a changing chemical and mechanical environment. This occurs in OA and RA and is characterized by increased turnover of matrix and net loss of cartilage. Degradation products of cartilage molecules can be detected *in vivo*. They can stimulate matrix degradation mediated by chondrocytes and act as autoantigens and stimulate immunity directed against cartilage. The repair of cartilage is very problematic in the adult, but there is progress in this area.

This overview of cartilage is intended to focus attention on the considerable increase in our knowledge of this important tissue in recent years and the fact that there is the potential now to use this information to promote cartilage formation and protect it from damage in disease.

ACKNOWLEDGMENTS

I thank Dorothy Redhead for her assistance with the compilation of this chapter, and Mark Lepik and Guylaine Bedard for their help in preparing the figures. My work has been funded by the Shriners Hospitals for Children, the Canadian Institutes of Health Research, the Canadian Arthritis Network, and the National Institute of Aging, National Institutes of Health.

REFERENCES

1. Fell HB. The histogenesis of cartilage and bone in the long bones of the embryonic fowl. *J Morphol* 1925;40:417–451.
2. Caplan AI, Syftestad G, Osdoby P. The development of embryonic bone and cartilage in tissue culture. *Clin Orthop* 1983;174:243–263.
3. Tavella S, Bellese G, Castagnola P, et al. Regulated expression of the fibronectin, laminin, and related integrin receptors during the early chondrocyte differentiation. *J Cell Sci* 1997;110:2261–2270.
4. Zhao G-Q, Zhou X, Eberspaecher H, et al. Cartilage homeoprotein 1: a homeoprotein selectively expressed in chondrocytes. *Proc Natl Acad Sci U S A* 1993;90:8633–8637.
5. Lefebvre V, deCrombrugghe B. Toward understanding SOX9 function in chondrocyte differentiation. *Matrix Biol* 1998;16:529–540.
6. Bi W, Deng JM, Zhang Z, et al. Sox9 is required for cartilage formation. *Nat Genet* 1999;22:85–89.
7. Sandell LJ, Morris N, Robbins JR, Goldring MB. Alternatively spliced type II procollagen mRNAs define distinct populations of cells during vertebral development: differential expression of the amino-propeptide. *J Cell Biol* 1991;114:1307–1319.
8. Nah H-D, Upholt WB. Type II collagen mRNA containing alternatively spliced exon predominates in the chick limb prior to chondrogenesis. *J Biol Chem* 1991;266:23446–23452.
9. Zhu J, Organesian A, Keene DR, et al. Type IIA procollagen containing the cysteine-rich amino propeptide is deposited in the extracellular matrix of prechondrogenic tissue and binds to TGF-β_1 and BMP-2. *J Cell Biol* 1999;144:1069–1080.
10. Kosher RA, Gay SW, Kamanitz JR, et al. Cartilage proteoglycan core protein gene expression during limb cartilage differentiation. *Dev Biol* 1986;118:112–117.
11. Bulstra S, Homminga GN, Buurman WA, et al. The potential of adult human perichondrium to form hyaline cartilage. *J Orthop Res* 1990; 8:328–335.
12. Fell HB. The osteogenic capacity *in vitro* of periosteum and endosteum isolated from the limb skeleton of fowl embryos and young chicks. *J Anat* 1932;66:157–185.
13. Maurice H, Crone M, Watt I. Synovial chondromatosis. *J Bone Joint Surg Br* 1988;70:807–811.
14. Wozney JM, Rosen V. Bone morphogenetic protein and bone morphogenetic protein gene family in bone formation and repair. *Clin Orthop Res* 1998:346:26–37.
15. King JA, Marker PC, Seung KJ, et al. BMP5 and the molecular, skeletal and soft tissue alterations in short ear mice. *Dev Biol* 1994;166:112–122.
16. Duprez D, Bell EJ, Richardson MK, et al. Overexpression of BMP-2 and BMP-4 alters the size and shape of developing skeletal elements in the chick limb. *Mech Dev* 1996;57:145–157.
17. Tsumaki N, Tonaka K, Arikawa-Hirasawa E, et al. Role of CDMP-1 in skeletal morphogenesis: promotion of mesenchymal cell recruitment and chondrocyte differentiation. *J Cell Biol* 1999;144:161–173.
18. Jena N, Martøn-Seisdedos C, McCue P, et al. BMP7 null mutation in mice: developmental defects in skeleton, kidney, and eye. *Exp Cell Res* 1997;230:28–37.
19. Brunet LJ, McMahon JA, McMahon AP, et al. Noggin, cartilage morphogenesis, and joint formation in the mammalian skeleton. *Science* 1998;280.1455–1457.
20. Zhang D, Ferguson CM, O'Keefe RJ, et al. A role for the BMP antagonist chordin in endochondral ossification. *J Bone Miner Res* 2002;17: 293–300.
21. Cash DE, Bock CB, Schughart K, et al. Retinoic acid receptor α function in vertebrate limb skeletogenesis: a modulator of chondrogenesis. *J Cell Biol* 1997;136:445–457.
22. Iwamoto M, Golden EB, Adams SL, et al. Responsiveness to retinoic acid changes during chondrocyte maturation. *Exp Cell Res* 1993;205: 213–224.
23. Hoffman LM, Weston AD, Underhill TM. Molecular mechanisms regulating chondroblast differentiation. *J Bone Joint Surg Am* 2003;85A (suppl 2):124–132.
24. Sekine K, Ohuchi H, Fujiwara M, et al. Fgf10 is essential for limb and lung formation. *Nat Genet* 1999;21:138–141.
25. Szebenyi G, Savage MP, Olwin BB, et al. Changes in the expression of fibroblast growth factor receptors mark distinct stages of chondrogenesis *in vitro* and during chick limb skeletal patterning. *Dev Dyn* 1995;204:446–456.
26. Beier F, Leask TA, Hague S, et al. Cell cycle genes in chondrocyte proliferation and differentiation. *Matrix Biol* 1999;18:109–120.
27. Poole AR. The growth plate: cellular physiology, cartilage assembly and mineralization. In: Hall BK, Newman S, eds. *Cartilage: molecular aspects.* Boca Raton, FL: CRC Press, 1991:179–211.
28. Alini M, Carey D, Hirata S, et al. Cellular and matrix changes before and at the time of calcification in the growth plate studied *in vitro*: arrest of type X collagen synthesis and net loss of collagen when calcification is initiated. *J Bone Miner Res* 1994;9:1077–1087.
29. Mwale F, Billinghurst RC, Ionescu M, et al. The assembly and degradation of types II and IX collagens associated with expression of the hypertrophic phenotype. *Dev Dyn* 2000;218:648–662
30. Shimazu A, Nah HD, Kirsch T, et al. Syndecan-3 and the control of chondrocyte proliferation during endochondral ossification. *Exp Cell Res* 1996;229:126–136.
31. Terpstra L, Prud'homme J, Arabian A et al. Reduced chondrocyte proliferation and chondrodysplasia in mice lacking the integrin-linked kinase in chondrocytes. *J Cell Biol* 2003;162:139–148.
32. Alini M, Kofsky Y, Wu W, et al. In serum-free culture thyroid hormones can induce full expression of chondrocyte hypertrophy leading to matrix calcification. *J Bone Miner Res* 1996;11:105–113.
33. Koyama E, Golden EB, Kirsch T, et al. Retinoid signalling is required for chondrocyte maturation and endochondral bone formation during limb skeletogenesis. *Dev Biol* 1999;208:375–391.
34. Underhill TM, Western AD. Retinoids and their receptors in skeletal development. *Microsc Res Tech* 1998;43:137–155.
35. Wang W, Xu J, Kirsch T. Annexin-mediated Ca^{2+} influx regulates growth plate chondrocyte maturation and apoptosis. *J Biol Chem* 2003; 278:3762–3769.
36. Pathi S, Rutenberg JB, Johnson RL, et al. Interaction of Ihh and BMPB/Noggin signalling during cartilage differentiation. *Dev Biol* 1999;209:239–253.
37. Chen P, Vukicevic S, Sampath TK, et al. Bovine articular chondrocytes do not undergo hypertrophy when cultured in presence of serum and osteogenic protein-1. *Biochem Biophys Res Commun* 1993;197: 1253–1259.
38. Kato Y, Iwamoto M, Koike T, et al. Terminal differentiation and calcification in rabbit chondrocyte cultures grown in centrifuge tubes: regulation by transforming growth factor β and serum factors. *Proc Natl Acad Sci U S A* 1988;85:9552–9556.
39. Böhme K, Winterhalter KK, Brückner P. Terminal differentiation of chondrocytes in culture is a spontaneous process and is arrested by transforming growth factor-β2 and basic fibroblast growth factor. *Exp Cell Res* 1995;216:191–198.
40. Chang SC, Hoang B, Thomas JT, et al. Cartilage-derived morphogenetic proteins: new members of the transforming growth factor-β superfamily predominantly expressed in long bones during human embryonic development. *J Biol Chem* 1994;269:28227–28234.
41. Iwamoto M, Shimazu A, Pacifici M. Regulation of chondrocyte maturation by fibroblast growth factor-2 and parathyroid hormone. *J Orthop Res* 1995;13:838–845.
42. Iwamoto M, Shimazu A, Nakashima K, et al. Reduction in basic fibroblast growth factor receptor is coupled with terminal differentiation of chondrocytes. *J Biol Chem* 1991;266:461–467.
43. Deng C, Wynshaw-Boris A, Zhou F, et al. Fibroblast growth factor receptor 3 is a negative regulator of bone growth. *Cell* 1996;84:911–921.

44. Legeai-Mallet L, Benoist-Lasselin B, Debezoide A-L, et al. Fibroblast growth factor receptor 3 mutations promote apoptosis but do not alter chondrocyte proliferation in the thanatophoric dysplasia. *J Biol Chem* 1998;273:13007–13014.
45. Loveys LS, Gelb D, Hurwitz SR, et al. Effects of parathyroid hormone-related peptide on chick growth plate chondrocytes. *J Orthop Res* 1993;11:884–891.
46. Beier F, Ali Z, Mok D et al. TGFβ and PTHrP control chondrocyte proliferation by activating cyclin D1 expression. *Mol Biol Cell* 2001; 12:3852–3863.
47. Iwamoto M, Kitagaki J, Tamamara Y, et al. Run X2 expression and action in chondrocytes are regulated by retinoid signalling and parathyroid hormone-related peptide (PTHrP). *Osteoarthritis Cartilage* 2003; 11:6–15.
48. Amizuka N, Warshawsky H, Henderson JE, et al. Parathyroid hormone-related peptide depleted mice show abnormal epiphyseal cartilage development and altered endochondral bone formation. *J Cell Biol* 1994;126:1611–1623.
49. Chung U-I, Lanske B, Lee K, et al. The parathyroid hormone/parathyroid hormone-related peptide receptor coordinates endochondral bone development by directly controlling chondrocyte differentiation. *Proc Natl Acad Sci U S A* 1998;95:13030–13035.
50. Weir EC, Philbrick WM, Amling M, et al. Targeted overexpression of parathyroid hormone-related peptide in chondrocytes causes chondrodysplasia and delayed endochondral bone formation. *Proc Natl Acad Sci U S A* 1996;93:10240–10245.
51. Zerega B, Cermelli S, Bianco P, et al. Parathyroid hormone [PTH(1–34)] and parathyroid hormone-related protein [PTHrP(1–34)] promote reversion of hypertrophic chondrocytes to a prehypertrophic proliferating phenotype and prevent terminal differentiation of osteoblast-like cells. *J Bone Miner Res* 1999;14:1281–1289.
52. Lanske B, Karapalis AC, Lee K, et al. PTH/PTHrP receptor in early development and Indian hedgehog-regulated growth. *Science* 1996; 273;663–666.
53. Vortkamp A, Lee K, Lanske B, et al. Regulation of cartilage differentiation by Indian hedgehog and PTH-related protein. *Science* 1996;273: 613–622.
54. Alvarez J, Sohn P, Zeng X et al. $TGF\beta_2$ mediates the effects of Hedgehog on hypertrophic differentiation and PTHrP expression. *Development* 2002;129:1913–1924.
55. St-Jacques B, Hammerschmidt M, McMahon AP. Indian hedgehog signalling regulates proliferation and differentiation of chondrocytes and is essential for bone formation. *Genes Dev* 1999;13:2072–2086.
56. Komori T, Yagi H, Nomura S, et al. Targeted disruption of Cbfa1 results in a complete lack of bone formation owing to a maturational arrest of osteoblasts. *Cell* 1997;89:755–764.
57. Jiménez MJG, Balbín M, López JM, et al. Collagenase-3 is a target of Cbfa1, a transcription factor of the runt gene family involved in bone formation. *Mol Cell Biol* 1999;19:4431–4442.
58. Inada M, Yasui T, Nomura S, et al. Maturational disturbance of chondrocytes in Cbfa1-deficient mice. *Dev Dyn* 1999;214:279–290.
59. Johansson N, Saarialho-Kere U, Airola K, et al. Collagenase-3 (MMP-13) is expressed by hypertrophic chondrocytes, periosteal cells, and osteoblasts during human fetal bone development. *Dev Dyn* 1997;208:387–397.
60. Wu W, Tchetina E, Mwale F et al. Proteolysis involving MMP-13 (collagenase-3) and the expression of the chondrocyte hypertrophic phenotype. *J Bone Miner Res* 2002;17:639–651.
61. Makihira S, Yan W, Murakami H, et al. Thyroid hormone enhances aggrecanase-2/ADAMTS-5 expression and proteoglycan degradation in growth plate cartilage. *Endocrinology* 2003;144:2480–2488.
62. Lee ER, Lamplugh L, Davoli MA, et al. Enzymes active in the areas undergoing cartilage resorption during the development of the secondary ossification center in the tibial of rats ages 0–21 days: two groups of proteinases cleave the core protein of aggrecan. *Dev Dyn* 2001;222: 52–70.
63. Vu TH, Shipley JM, Bergers G, et al. MMP-9/gelatinase B is a key regulator of growth plate angiogenesis and apoptosis of hypertrophic chondrocytes. *Cell* 1998;93:411–422.
64. Enomoto-Iwamoto M, Kitagaki J, Koyama E, et al. The Wnt antagonist Frzb-1 regulates chondrocyte maturation and long bone development during limb skeletogenesis. *Dev Biol* 2002;251;142–156.
65. Church V, Nohno T, Linker C, et al. Wnt regulation of chondrocyte differentiation. *J Cell Sci* 2002;115:4809–4818.
66. Crowe R, Zikherman J, Niswander L. Delta-1 negatively regulates the transition from prehypertrophic chondrocytes during cartilage formation. *Development* 1999;126:987–998.
67. Amiling M, Neff L, Tonaka S, et al. Bcl-2 lies downstream of the parathyroid hormone-related peptide in a signalling pathway that regulates chondrocyte maturation during skeletal development. *J Cell Biol* 1997;136:205–213.
68. Floyd WE, Zaleske DJ, Schiller AL, et al. Vascular events associated with the appearance of the secondary center of ossification in the murine distal femoral epiphysis. *J Bone Joint Surg Am* 1987;69:185–190.
69. Gerber HP, Vu TH, Ryan AM, et al. VEGF couples hypertrophic cartilage remodelling, ossification and angiogenesis during endochondral bone formation. *Nat Med* 1999;5:623–628.
70. Petersen W, Tsokos M, Pufe T. Expression of $VEGF_{121}$ and $VEGF_{165}$ in hypertrophic chondrocytes of the human growth plate and epiphyseal cartilage. *J Anat* 2002;201:153–157.
71. Ivkrovic S, Yoon BS, Popoff SN, et al. Connective tissue growth factor coordinates chondrogenesis and angiogenesis during skeletal development. *Development* 2003;130:2779–2791.
72. Alini M, Matsui Y, Dodge GR, et al. The extracellular matrix of cartilage in the growth plate before and during calcification: changes in composition, and degradation of type II collagen. *Calcif Tissue Int* 1992;50:327–335.
73. Mwale F, Tchetina E, Poole AR. The assembly and remodelling of the extracellular matrix in the growth plate in relationship to mineral deposition and cellular hypertrophy: an *in situ* study of collagens II and IX and proteoglycan. *J Bone Miner Res* 2002;17:275–283.
74. Aeschlimann D, Kaupp O, Paulsson M. Transglutaminase-catalyzed matrix cross-linking in differentiating cartilage: identification of osteonectin as a major glutaminyl substrate. *J Cell Biol* 1995;129:881–892.
75. Gibson GJ, Bearman CH, Flint MH. The immunoperoxidase localization of type X collagen in chick cartilage and lung. *Coll Rel Res* 1986; 6:163–184.
76. Poole AR, Pidoux I. Immunoelectron microscopic studies of type X collagen in endochondral ossification. *J Cell Biol* 1989;109:2547–2554.
77. Cancedda FD, Malpeli M, Gentili C, et al. The developmentally regulated avian Ch21 lipocalin is an extracellular fatty acid-binding protein. *J Biol Chem* 1996;271:20163–20169.
78. Iwamoto M, Sato K, Nakashima K, et al. Hypertrophy and calcification of rabbit permanent chondrocytes in pelleted cultures: synthesis of alkaline phosphatase and 1,25-dihydroxycholecalciferol receptor. *Dev Biol* 1989;136:500–507.
79. Matsui Y, Alini M, Webber C, et al. Characterization of aggregating proteoglycans from the proliferative, maturing hypertrophic and calcifying zones of the cartilage physes (growth plate). *J Bone Joint Surg Am* 1991;73:1064–1074.
80. Cole AA, Boyd T, Lucherne L, et al. Type X collagen degradation in long-term serum-free culture of the embryonic chick tibia following production of active collagenase and gelatinase. *Dev Biol* 1993;159: 528–534.
81. Poole AR, Pidoux I, Reiner A, et al. Association of an extracellular protein (chondrocalcin) with the calcification of cartilage in endochondral bone formation. *J Cell Biol* 1984;98:54–65.
82. Anderson HC. Mechanisms of mineral formation in bone. *Lab Invest* 1989;60.320–330.
83. Kirsch T, Nah HD, Shapiro IM, Pacifici M. Regulated production of mineralization-competent matrix vesicles in hypertrophic chondrocytes. *J Cell Biol* 1997;137:1149–1160.
84. Kirsch T, Nah HD, Demuth DR, et al. Annexin V-mediated calcium flux across membranes is dependent on the lipid composition: implications for cartilage mineralization. *Biochemistry* 1997;36:3359–3367.
85. Wang W, Kirsch T. Retinoic acid stimulates annexin-mediated growth plate chondrocyte mineralization. *J Cell Biol* 2002;157:1061–1069.
86. Shepard N, Mitchell N. Ultrastructural modifications of proteoglycans coincident with mineralization in local regions of rat growth plate. *J Bone Joint Surg Am* 1985;67:455–464.
87. Landis WJ, Glimcher MJ. Electron optical and analytical observations of rat growth plate cartilage prepared by ultramicrotomy: the failure to detect a mineral phase in matrix vesicles and the identification of heterodispersed particles as the initial solid phase of calcium phosphate deposited in the extracellular matrix. *J Ultrastruct Res* 1982;78: 227–268.

88. Thyberg J. Electron microscopic studies on the initial phases of calcification in guinea pig epiphyseal cartilage. *J Ultrastruct Res* 1974; 46:206–218.
89. Fell HB, Robison R. The growth, development and phosphatase activity of embryonic avian femora and limb-buds activated *in vitro*. *Biochem J* 1929;23:767–784.
90. Ho AM, Johnson MD, Kingsley DM. Role of mouse ank gene in control of tissue calcification and arthritis. *Science* 2000;289:265–270.
91. Sohn P, Crowley M, Statlery E, et al. Developmental and TGF-β-mediated regulation of Ank mRNA expression in cartilage and bone. *Osteoarthritis Cartilage* 2002;10:482–490.
92. Hunter GK. Role of proteoglycan in the provisional calcification of cartilage: a review and reinterpretation. *Clin Orthop* 1991;262:256–280.
93. Hunter GK. An ion exchange mechanism of cartilage calcification. *Connect Tissue Res* 1987;16:111–120.
94. van der Rest M, Rosenberg LC, Olsen BR, et al. Chondrocalcin is identical with the C-propeptide of type II procollagen. *Biochem J* 1986;237:923–925.
95. Choi HO, Tang L-H, Johnson TL, et al. Isolation and characterization of a 35,000 molecular weight subunit fetal cartilage matrix protein. *J Biol Chem* 1983;258:655–661.
96. Hunziker EB, Schenk RK, Cruz-Orive L-M. Quantitation of chondrocyte performance in growth plate cartilage during longitudinal bone growth. *J Bone Joint Surg Am* 1987;69:162–173.
97. Luder HU, Leblond CP, von der Mark K. Cellular stages in cartilage formation as revealed by morphometry, radioautography and type II collagen immunostaining of the mandibular condyle from weanling rats. *Am J Anat* 1988;182:197–214.
98. Luo G, Ducy P, McKee MD, et al. Spontaneous calcification of arteries and cartilage in mice lacking matrix GLA protein. *Nature* 1997; 6:78–81.
99. Moses MA, Wiederschain D, Wu I, et al. Troponin 1 is present in human cartilage and inhibits angiogenesis. *Proc Natl Acad Sci U S A* 1999;96:2645–2650.
100. Mankin HJ, Dorfman H, Lippiello L, et al. Biochemical and metabolic abnormalities in articular cartilage from osteoarthritic hips. II. Correlation of morphology with biochemical and metabolic data. *J Bone Joint Surg Am* 1971;53:523–537.
101. Rees JA, Ali SY. Ultrastructural localisation of alkaline phosphatase activity in osteoarthritic human articular cartilage. *Ann Rheum Dis* 1998;47:747–753.
102. Zelzer E, Olsen BR. The genetic basis for skeletal diseases. *Nature* 2003;423;343–348.
103. Superfiti-Furga A, Bonafé L, Rimoin DL. Molecular pathogenetic classification of genetic disorders of the skeleton. *Am J Med Gen* 2001;106:282–293.
104. Schumacher BL, Su J-L, Lindley KM et al. Horizontally oriented clusters of multiple chondrosis in the superficial zone of ankle, but not knee articular cartilage. *Anat Rec* 2002;266:241–248.
105. Kempson GE, Muir H, Pollard C, et al. The tensile properties of the cartilage of human femoral condyles related to the content of collagen and glycosaminoglycans. *Biochim Biophys Acta* 1973;297:465–472.
106. Poole AR, Webber C, Pidoux I, et al. Localization of a dermatan sulfate proteoglycan (DS-PGII) in cartilage and the presence of an immunologically related species in other tissues. *J Histochem Cytochem* 1986;34:619–625.
107. Poole AR, Rosenberg LC, Reiner A, et al. Contents and distribution of the proteoglycans decorin and biglycan in normal and osteoarthritic human articular cartilage. *J Orthop Res* 1996;14:681–689.
108. Stockwell RA, Meachim G. The chondrocytes. In: Freeman MAR, ed. *Adult articular cartilage,* 2nd ed. Tunbridge Wells, UK: Pitman Medical, 1979:69–144.
109. Mitrovic D, Quintero M, Stankovic A, et al. Cell density of adult human femoral condylar articular cartilage: joints with normal and fibrillated surfaces. *Lab Invest* 1983;49:309–316.
110. Stockwell R. The interrelationship of cell density and cartilage thickness in mammalian articular cartilage. *J Anat* 1971;109:411–421.
111. Evans C. An inverse relationship between mammalian lifespan and cartilage cellularity. *Exp Gerontol* 1983;18:137–138.
112. Haüselmann HJ, Flechtenmacher J, Michal L, et al. The superficial layer of human articular cartilage is more susceptible to interleukin-1 induced damage than the deeper layers. *Arthritis Rheum* 1996;39: 478–488.
113. Poole AR, Pidoux I, Reiner A, et al. An immunoelectron microscope study of the organization of proteoglycan monomer, link protein, and collagen in the matrix of articular cartilage. *J Cell Biol* 1982;93: 921–937.
114. Poole AR, Pidoux I, Reiner A, et al. Localization of proteoglycan monomer and link protein in the matrix of bovine articular cartilage: an immunohistochemical study. *J Histochem Cytochem* 1980;28: 621–635.
115. Benninghoff A. Form und Bau der Gelenkknorpel in ihren beziehunger zur funktion. Zweiter Tiel. Der aufbau des Gelenkknorpels in seinen beziehungen zur funktion. *Z Zellforsch Mikrosk Anat* 1925;2: 783–862.
116. Poole CA, Flint MH, Beaumont BW. Chondrons in cartilage: ultrastructural analysis of the pericellular microenvironments in adult human articular cartilages. *J Orthop Res* 1987;5:509–522.
117. Brocklehurst R, Bayliss M, Maroudas A, et al. The composition of normal and osteoarthritic articular cartilage from human knee joints. *J Bone Joint Surg Am* 1984;66:95–106.
118. Muir IHM. Biochemistry. In: Freeman MAR, ed. *Adult articular cartilage,* 2nd ed. Tunbridge Wells, UK: Pitman Medical, 1979:145–214.
119. Roughley PJ, White RJ, Poole AR. Identification of a hyaluronic acid-binding protein that interferes with the preparation of high-buoyant density proteoglycan aggregates from adult human articular cartilage. *Biochem J* 1985;231:129–138.
120. Webber C, Glant TT, Roughley PJ, et al. The identification and characterization of two populations of aggregating proteoglycans of high buoyant density isolated from post-natal human articular cartilages of different ages. *Biochem J* 1987;248:735–740.
121. Wu J-J, Eyre D. Identification of hydroxypyridinium cross-linking sites in type II collagen of bovine articular cartilage. *Biochemistry* 1984;23:1850–1857.
122. Eyre DR, Paz MA, Gallop PM. Cross-linking in collagen and elastin. *Annu Rev Biochem* 1984;53:717–748.
123. Ratcliffe A, Fryer PR, Hardingham TE. The distribution of aggregating proteoglycans in articular cartilage: comparison of quantitative immunoelectron microscopy with radioimmunoassay and biochemical analysis. *J Histochem Cytochem* 1984;32:193–201.
124. Repo RU, Mitchell N. Collagen synthesis in mature articular cartilage of the rabbit. *J Bone Joint Surg Br* 1971;53:541–548.
125. Eyre DR, McDevitt CA, Billingham MEJ, et al. Biosynthesis of collagen and other matrix proteins by articular cartilage in experimental osteoarthrosis. *Biochem J* 1980;188:823–837.
126. Dodge GR, Poole AR. Immunohistochemical detection and immunochemical analysis of type II collagen degradation in human normal, rheumatoid and osteoarthritic articular cartilage and in explants of bovine articular cartilage cultured with interleukin 1. *J Clin Invest* 1989;83:647–661.
127. Wu W, Billinghurst RC, Pidoux I, et al. Sites of collagenase cleavage and denaturation of type II collagen in articular cartilage in ageing and osteoarthritis and their relationship to the distribution of the collagenases MMP-1 and MMP-13. *Arthritis Rheum* 2002;46:2087–2094.
128. Nelson F, Dahlberg L, Reiner A, et al. The synthesis of type II procollagen is markedly increased in osteoarthritic cartilage in vivo. *J Clin Invest* 1998;102:2115–2125.
129. Kirsch T, von der Mark K. Ca^{2+} binding properties of type X collagen. *FEBS Lett* 1991;294:149–152.
130. Keene DR, Engvall E, Glanville RW. Ultrastructure of type VI collagen in human skin and cartilage suggests an anchoring function for this filamentous network. *J Cell Biol* 1988;107:1995–2006.
131. Kielty CM, Whittaker SP, Grant ME, et al. Type VI collagen microfibrils: evidence for a structural association with hyaluronan. *J Cell Biol* 1992;118:979–990.
132. McDevitt CA, Marcelino J, Tucker L. Interaction of intact type VI collagen with hyaluronan. *FEBS Lett* 1991;294:167–170.
133. Fässler R, Schnegelsberg PNJ, Dansman J, et al. Mice lacking a_1(IX) collagen develop noninflammatory degenerative joint disease. *Proc Natl Acad Sci U S A* 1994;91:5070–5074.
134. Mendler M, Eich-Bender SG, Vaughan L, et al. Cartilage contains mixed fibrils of collagen types II, IX and XI. *J Cell Biol* 1989;108: 191–197.
135. Watt SL, Lunstrum GP, McDonough AM, et al. Characterization of collagen types XII and XIV from fetal bovine cartilage. *J Biol Chem* 1992;267:20093–20099.

136. Doege KJ, Sasaki M, Kimura T, et al. Complete coding sequence and deduced primary structure of the human cartilage large aggregating proteoglycan aggrecan: human-specific repeats and additional alternatively spliced forms. *J Biol Chem* 1991;266:894–902.
137. Hedland H, Hedbom E, Heinegård D, et al. Association of the aggrecan keratan sulfate-rich region with collagen in bovine articular cartilage. *J Biol Chem* 1999;274:5777–5781.
138. Antonsson P, Heinegård D, Oldberg Å. The keratan sulfate-enriched region of bovine cartilage proteoglycan consists of a consecutively repeated hexapeptide motif. *J Biochem* 1989;264:16170–16173.
139. Maroudas A. Physical chemistry of articular cartilage and the intervertebral disc. In: Sokoloff L, ed. *The joints and synovial fluid.* Vol II. New York: Academic, 1980:239–291.
140. Shepard N, Mitchell N. Simultaneous localization of proteoglycan by light and electron microscopy using toluidine blue O: a study of epiphyseal cartilage. *J Histochem Cytochem* 1976;24:621–629.
141. Tang L-H, Rosenberg L, Reiner A, et al. Proteoglycans from bovine nasal cartilage: properties of a soluble form of link protein. *J Biol Chem* 1979;254:10523–10531.
142. Mörgelin M, Paulsson M, Hardingham TE, et al. Cartilage proteoglycans: assembly with hyaluronate and link protein as studied by electron microscopy. *Biochem J* 1988;253:175–185.
143. Watanabe H, Yamada Y. Mice lacking link protein develop dwarfism and craniofacial abnormalities. *Nat Genet* 1999;21:225–229.
144. Halberg DF, Proulx G, Doege K, et al. A segment of the cartilage proteoglycan core protein has lectin-like activity. *J Biol Chem* 1988;263: 9486–9490.
145. Grover J, Roughley PJ. Versican gene expression in human articular cartilage and comparison of mRNA splicing variation with aggrecan. *Biochem J* 1993;291:361–367.
146. Shi S, Ciurli C, Cartman A, et al. Experimental immunity to the G1 domain of the proteoglycan versican induces spondylitis, sacroiliitis and enthesitis in BALB/c mice without peripheral polyarthritis. *Arthritis Rheum* 2003;48:2903–2915.
147. Zhang Y, Cao K, Kiani CG, et al. The G3 domain of versican inhibits mesenchymal chondrogenesis via the epidermal growth factor-like motifs. *J Biol Chem* 1998;273:33054–33063.
148. Rosenberg LC, Choi H-U, Tang L-H, et al. Isolation of dermatan sulfate proteoglycans from mature bovine articular cartilages. *J Biol Chem* 1985;260:6304–6313.
149. Vogel K, Trotter JA. The effect of proteoglycans on the morphology of collagen fibrils formed in vitro. *Coll Rel Res* 1987;7:105–114.
150. Danielson KG, Baribault H, Holmes DF, et al. Targeted disruption of decorin leads to abnormal collagen fibril morphology and skin fragility. *J Cell Biol* 1997;136:729–743.
151. Ehnis T, Dieterich W, Bauer M, et al. Localization of a binding site for the proteoglycan decorin on collagen XIV (undulin). *J Biol Chem* 1997;272:20414–20419.
152. Xu T, Bianco P, Fisher LW, et al. Targeted disruption of the biglycan gene leads to an osteoporosis-like phenotype in mice. *Nat Genet* 1998;20:78–82.
153. Choi H-U, Johnson TL, Pal S, et al. Characterization of the dermatan sulfate proteoglycans, DS-PGI and DS-PGII, from bovine articular cartilage and skin isolated by octyl-Sepharose chromatography. *J Biol Chem* 1989;264:2876–2884.
154. Oldberg A, Antonsson P, Lindblom K, Heinegård D. A collagen-binding 58kD protein (fibromodulin) is structurally related to the small interstitial proteoglycans PG-S1 and PG-S2 (decorin). *EMBO J* 1989;8:2601–2604.
155. Plaas AHK, Neame PJ, Nivens CM, Reiss L. Identification of the keratan sulfate attachment sites on bovine fibromodulin. *J Biol Chem* 1990;265:20634–20640.
156. Hedbom E, Heinegård D. Binding of fibromodulin and decorin to separate sites on fibrillar collagens. *J Biol Chem* 1993;268:27307–27312.
157. Grover J, Chen X-N, Korenberg JR, Roughley PJ. The human lumican gene: organization, chromosomal location and expression in articular cartilage. *J Biol Chem* 1995;270:21942–21949.
158. Chakravarti S, Magnuson T, Lass JH, et al. Lumican regulates collagen fibril assembly: skin fragility and corneal opacity in the absence of lumican. *J Cell Biol* 1998;141:1277–1286.
159. Alini M, Roughley PJ. Changes in leucine-rich repeat proteoglycans during maturation of the bovine growth plate. *Matrix Biol* 2001;19: 805–813.
160. French MM, Smith SE, Akanbi K, et al. Expression of the heparan sulfate proteoglycan, perlecan, during mouse embryogenesis and perlecan chondrogenic activity *in vitro*. *J Cell Biol* 1999;145:1103–1115.
161. Sundarhaj N, Fite D, Ledbetter S, et al. Perlecan is a component of cartilage matrix and promotes chondrocyte attachment. *J Cell Sci* 1995;108:2663–2672.
162. Costell M, Gustafsson E, Aszodi A, et al. Perlecan maintains the integrity of cartilage and some basement membranes. *J Cell Biol* 1999; 147:1109–1122.
163. Kirsch T, Koyama E, Liu M, et al. Syndecan-3 is a selective regulator of chondrocyte proliferation. *J Biol Chem* 2002;277:42171–42177.
164. Schumacher BL, Block JA, Schmid TM, et al. A novel proteoglycan synthesized and secreted by chondrocytes of the superficial zone of articular cartilage. *Arch Biochem Biophys* 1994;311:144–152.
165. Schumacher BL, Hughes CE, Kuettner KE, et al. Immunodetection and partial cDNA sequence of the proteoglycan, superficial zone protein, synthesized by cells lining synovial joints. *J Orthop Res* 1999; 17:110–120.
166. Warman ML. Human genetic insights into skeletal development, growth, and homeostasis. *Clin Orthop* 2000;37a(suppl):540–554.
167. Iozzo RV. Matrix proteoglycans: from molecular design to cellular function. *Annu Rev Biochem* 1998;67:609–652.
168. Pfister BE, Aydelotte MB, Burkhart W, et al. Del 1: a new protein in the superficial layer of articular cartilage. *Biochem Biophys Res Commun* 2001;286:268–273.
169. Aspberg A, Adam S, Kostka G, et al. Fibulin-1 is a ligand for the c-type lectin domains of aggrecan and versican. *J Biol Chem* 1999; 274:20444–20449.
170. Deak F, Wagener R, Kiss I, et al. The matrilins: a novel family of oligomeric extracellular matrix proteins. *Matrix Biol* 1999;18:55–64.
171. Franzen A, Heinegård D, Solursh M. Evidence for sequential appearance of cartilage matrix proteins in developing mouse limbs and in cultures of mouse mesenchymal cells. *Differentiation* 1987;36:199–210.
172. Paulsson M, Heinegård D. Radioimmunoassay of the 148-kilodalton cartilage protein: distribution of the protein among bovine tissues. *Biochem J* 1982;207:207–213.
173. Hauser N, Paulsson M, Heinegård D, and Mörgelin M. Interaction of cartilage matrix protein with aggrecan: increased covalent cross-linking with tissue maturation. *J Biol Chem* 1996;271:32247–32252.
174. Chen Q, Zhang, Y, Johnson DM, et al. Assembly of a novel cartilage matrix protein filamentous network: molecular basis of differential requirements of von Willebrand factor A domains. *Mol Biol Cell* 1999;10:2149–2162.
175. Makihira S, Yan W, Ohno S, et al. Enhancement of cell adhesion and spreading by a cartilage specific noncollagenous protein cartilage matrix protein, (CMP/matrilin-1) via integrin $\alpha_1\beta_1$. *J Biol Chem* 1999;274:11417–11423.
176. Hunag X, Birk DE, Goetinck kPF. Mice lacking matrilin-1 (cartilage matrix protein) have alterations in type II collagen fibrillogenesis and fibril organization. *Dev Dyn* 1999;216:434–441.
177. Oldberg A, Antonsson P, Lindblom K, et al. COMP (cartilage oligomeric matrix protein) is structurally related to the thrombospondins. *J Biol Chem* 1992;267:22346–22350.
178. Newton G, Weremowicz S, Morton CC, et al. Characterization of human and mouse cartilage oligomeric matrix protein. *Genomics* 1994;24:435–439.
179. Hedbom E, Antonsson P, Hjerpe A, et al. Cartilage matrix proteins: an acidic oligomeric protein (COMP) detected only in cartilage. *J Biol Chem* 1992;267:6132–6136.
180. DiCesare PE, Mörgelin M, Mann K, et al. Cartilage oligomeric matrix protein and thrombospondin 1: purification from articular cartilage, electron microscopic structure and chondrocyte binding. *Eur J Biochem* 1994;223:927–937.
181. Rosenberg K, Olsson H, Mörgelin M, et al. Cartilage oligomeric matrix protein shows high affinity zinc-dependent interaction with triple helical collagen. *J Biol Chem* 1998;273:20397–20403.
182. Lorenzo P, Neame P, Sommarin Y, et al. Cloning and deduced amino acid sequence of a novel cartilage protein (CILP) identifies a proform including a nucleotide-pyrophosphohydrolase. *J Biol Chem* 1998;273:23469–23475.
183. Lorenzo P, Bayliss MT, Heinegård D. A novel cartilage protein (CILP) present in the mid-zone of human articular cartilage increases with age. *J Biol Chem* 1998;273:23463–23468.

184. Hirose J, Masuda I, Ryan LM. Expression of cartilage intermediate layer protein/nucleotide pyrophosphohydrolase parallels the production of extracellular inorganic pyrophosphate in response to growth factors and with aging. *Arthritis Rheum* 2000;43:2703–2711.
185. Johnson K, Farley D, Hu, S-I, et al. One of two chondrocyte-expressed isoforms of cartilage intermediate-layer protein functions is an insulin-like growth factor 1 antagonist. *Arthritis Rheum* 2003; 48:1302–1314.
186. Lee TH, Wisniewski HG, Vilcek J. A novel secretory tumor necrosis-factor-inducible protein (TSG-6) is a member of the family of hyaluronate binding proteins closely related to the adhesion receptor CD44. *J Cell Biol* 1992;116:545–550.
187. Parkar AA, Kahmann JD, Howat SLT, et al. TSG-6 interacts with hyaluronan and aggrecan in a pH-dependent manner via a common functional element: implications for its regulation in inflamed cartilage. *FEBS Letts* 1998;428:171–176.
188. Wisniewski H-G, Hua J-C, Poppers DM, et al. TNF/IL-1-inducible protein TSG-6 potentiates plasmin inhibition by inter-α-inhibitor and exerts a strong anti-inflammatory effect *in vivo*. *J Immunol* 1996; 156:1609–1615.
189. Maier R, Wisniewski H-G, Vilcek J, et al. TSG-6 expression in human articular chondrocytes: possible implications in joint inflammation and cartilage degradation. *Arthritis Rheum* 1996;39: 552–559.
190. Weiss RF, Reddi AM. Appearance of fibronectin during the differentiation of cartilage, bone and bone marrow. *J Cell Biol* 1981;88: 630–636.
191. Wurster NB, Lust G. Synthesis of fibronectin in normal and osteoarthritic articular cartilage. *Biochim Biophys Acta* 1984;800:52–58.
192. Jones KL, Brown M, Ali SY, et al. An immunohistochemical study of fibronectin in human osteoarthritic and disease free articular cartilage. *Ann Rheum Dis* 1987;46:809–815.
193. Hakomori S, Fukuda M, Sekiguchi K, et al. Fibronectin, laminin and other extracellular glycoproteins. In: Piez KA, Reddi AH, eds. *Extracellular matrix biochemistry.* New York: Elsevier, 1984:229–275.
194. Bennett VD, Pallante KM, Adams SL. The splicing pattern of fibronectin mRNA changes during chondrogenesis resulting in an unusual form of the mRNA in cartilage. *J Biol Chem* 1991;266:5918–5924.
195. Zhang D-W, Burton-Wurster N, Lust G. Alternative splicing of ED-A and ED-B sequences of fibronectin pre-mRNA differs in chondrocytes from different cartilaginous tissues and can be modulated by biological factors. *J Biol Chem* 1995;270:1817–1822.
196. Parker AE, Boutell J, Carr A, et al. Novel cartilage-specific splice variants of fibronectin. *Osteoarthritis Cartilage* 2002;10:528–534.
197. Price PA, Williamson MK. Primary structure of bovine matrix Gla protein: a new vitamin K-dependent bone protein. *J Biol Chem* 1985; 260:14971–14975.
198. Loesser R, Carlson CS, Tulli H, et al. Articular cartilage matrix g-carboxyglutamic acid-containing protein characterization and immunolocalization. *Biochem J* 1992;282:1–6.
199. Weller A, Beck S, Ekblom P. Amino acid sequence of mouse tenascin and differential expression of two tenascin isoforms during embryogenesis. *J Cell Biol* 1991;112:355–362.
200. Nies DE, Hemesath JJ, Kim J-H, et al. The complete cDNA sequence of human hexabrachion (tenascin): a multidomain protein containing unique epidermal growth factor domains. *J Biol Chem* 1991;266: 2818–2823.
201. Vaughan L, Huber S, Chiquet M, Winterhalter KH. A major six-armed glycoprotein from embryonic cartilage. *EMBO J* 1987;6:349–353.
202. Väkevä L, Mackie E, Kantomaa T, et al. Comparison of the distribution of patterns of tenascin and alkaline phosphatase in developing teeth, cartilage, and bone of rats and mice. *Anat Rec* 1990;228:69–76.
203. Mackie EJ, Thesleff I, Chiquet-Ehrismann R. Tenascin is associated with chondrogenic and osteogenic differentiation *in vitro*. *J Cell Biol* 1987;105:2569–2579.
204. Corson GM, Chalberg SC, Dietz HC, et al. Fibrillin binds calcium and is coded by cDNAs that reveal a multidomain structure and alternatively spliced exons at the 58 end. *Genomics* 1993;17:476–484.
205. Pereira L, D'Alessio M, Ramirez F, et al. Genomic organization of the sequence coding for fibrilin: the defective gene product in Marfan syndrome. *Hum Mol Genet* 1993;2:961–968.
206. Keene DR, Jordan CD, Reinhardt DP, et al. Fibrilin-1 in human cartilage: developmental expression and formation of special banded fibers. *J Histochem Cytochem* 1997;45:1069–1082.
207. Gosline JM, Rosenbloom J. Elastin. In: Piez KA, Reddi AH, eds. *Extracellular matrix biochemistry.* Amsterdam: Elsevier, 1984:191–227.
208. Indik Z, Yeh H, Ornstein-Goldstein N, et al. Structure of the elastin gene and alternative splicing of elastin mRNA: implications for disease. *Am J Med Genet* 1989;34:81–90.
209. Holmes WA, Bayliss MT, Muir H. Hyaluronic acid in human articular cartilage: age related changes in content and size. *Biochem J* 1988;250:435–441.
210. Thonar EJ-MA, Sweet MBE, Immelman AR, et al. Hyaluronate in articular cartilage: age-related changes. *Calcif Tissue Res* 1978;26: 19–21.
211. Schmidt MB, Mow VC, Chun LE, Eyre DR. Effects of proteoglycan extraction on the tensile behaviour of articular cartilage. *J Orthop Res* 1990;8:353–363.
212. Kempson GE, Tuke MA, Dingle JT, et al. The effects of proteolytic enzymes on the mechanical properties of adult human articular cartilage. *Biochim Biophys Acta* 1976;428:741–760.
213. Mow VC, Howell DS, Buckwalter JA. Structure and function relationships of articular cartilage and the effects of joint instability and trauma on cartilage function. In: Brandt KD, ed. *Cartilage changes in osteoarthritis.* Indianapolis: Indiana School of Medicine, Ciba-Geigy Corporation, 1990:22–42.
214. Akizuki S, Mow VC, Muller F, et al. Tensile properties of human knee joint cartilage. 1. Influence of ionic conditions, weight-bearing, and fibrillation on the tensile modulus. *J Orthop Res* 1986;4:379–392.
215. Berkenblit SI, Frank EH, Salant EP, Grodzinsky AJ. Nondestructive detection of cartilage degeneration using electromechanical surface spectroscopy. *J Biomech Eng* 1994;116:384–392.
216. Roth V, Mow VC. The intrinsic tensile behaviour of the matrix of bovine articular cartilage and variation with age. *J Bone Joint Surg Am* 1980;62:1102–1117.
217. Alexopoulos LG, Haider MA, Vail TP, Guilak F. Alterations in the mechanical properties of the human chondrocyte pericellular matrix with osteoarthritis. *J Biomech Eng* 2003;125:323–333.
218. Cicuttini F, Forbes A, Morris K, et al. Gender differences in knee cartilage volume as measured by magnetic resonance imaging. *Osteoarthritis Cartilage* 1999;7:265–271.
219. Kempson GE, Muir H, Freeman MAR, et al. Correlations between the compressive stiffness and chemical constituents of human articular cartilage. *Biochim Biophys Acta* 1970;215:70–77.
220. Kempson GE. Mechanical properties of articular cartilage. In: Freeman MAR, ed. *Adult articular cartilage.* Tunbridge Wells, UK: Pitman Medical, 1979:333–414.
221. Urban JPG, Maroudas A, Bayliss MT, et al. Swelling pressures of proteoglycans at the concentrations found in cartilaginous tissues. *Biorheology* 1979;16:447–464.
222. Basser PJ, Schneidermann R, Bank RA, et al. Mechanical properties of the collagen network in human articular cartilage as measured by osmotic stress technique. *Arch Biochem Biophys* 1998;351:207–219.
223. Huberti HH, Hayes WC. Patellofemoral contact pressures: the influence of Q-angle and tendofemoral contact. *J Bone Joint Surg Am* 1984;66:715–724.
224. Hodge WA, Fijan RS, Carlson KL, et al. Contact pressures in the human hip joint measured *in vivo*. *Proc Natl Acad Sci U S A* 1986; 83:2879–2883.
225. Hall AC, Urban JPG, Gehp KA. The effects of hydrostatic pressure on matrix synthesis in articular cartilage. *J Orthop Res* 1991;9:1–10.
226. Takahashi I, Nuckolls GH, Takahashi K, et al. Compressive force promotes SOX9, type II collagen and aggrecan and inhibits IL-1β expression resulting in chondrogenesis in mouse embryonic limb bud mesenchymal cells. *J Cell Sci* 1998;111:2067–2076.
227. Fujisawa T, Hattori J, Takahashi K, et al. Cyclic mechanical stress induces extracellular matrix degradation in cultured chondrocytes via gene expression of matrix metalloproteinases and interleukin-1. *J Biochem* 1999;125:966–975.

228. Lee M, Frindade MCD, Ikenoue T, et al. Regulation of nitric oxide and Bcl-2 expression by shear stress in human osteoarthritic chondrocytes *in vitro*. *J Cell Biochem* 2003;90:80–86.
229. Thibault M, Poole AR, Buschmann MD. Cyclic compression of cartilage/bone explants *in vitro* leads to physical weakening, mechanical breakdown of collagen and release of matrix fragments. *J Orthop Res* 2002;20:1285–1273.
230. Chen C-T, Bhargava M, Lin PM, et al. Time, stress, and location dependent chondrocyte death and collagen damage in cyclically loaded articular cartilage. *J Orthop Res* 2003;21:888–898.
231. Bank RA, Soudry M, Maroudas A, et al. The increased swelling and instantaneous deformation of osteoarthritic cartilage is highly correlated with collagen degradation. *Arthritis Rheum* 2000;43:2202–2210.
232. Wright MO, Nishida K, Bavington C, et al. Hyperpolarization of cultured human chondrocytes follows cyclical pressure-induced strain: evidence of a role for $\alpha_5\beta_1$ integrin as a chondrocyte mechanoreceptor. *J Orthop Res* 1997;15:742–747.
233. Millward SJ, Wright MO, Lee H-S, et al. Integrin-regulated secretion of interleukin 4: a novel pathway of mechanotransduction in human articular chondrocytes. *J Cell Biol* 1999;145:183–189.
234. Blain EJ, Gilbert SJ, Wardale RJ, et al. Upregulation of matrix metalloproteinase expression and activation following cyclical compressive loading of articular cartilage *in vitro*. *Arch Biochem Biophys* 2001;396;49–55.
235. Murata M, Bonassar LJ, Wright M, et al. A role for the interleukin-1 receptor in the pathway linking static mechanical compression to decreased proteoglycan synthesis in surface articular cartilage. *Arch Biochem Biophys* 2003;413:229–235.
236. Millward-Sadler SJ, Mackenzie A, Wright MO, et al. Tachykinin expression in cartilage and function in human articular chondrocyte mechanotransduction. *Arthritis Rheum* 2003;48:146–156.
237. Wu QY, Zhang Y, Chen Q. Indian hedgehog is an essential component of mechanotransduction complex to stimulate chondrocyte proliferation. *J Biol Chem* 2001;276:35290–35296.
238. Carter DR. Mechanical loading history and skeletal development. *J Biomech* 1987;20:1095–1109.
239. Carter DR, Orr TE, Fyhrie DP, ET AL. Influences of mechanical stress on prenatal and postnatal development. *Clin Orthop* 1987;219: 237–250.
240. Rodbard S. Negative feedback mechanism in the architecture and function of the connective and cardiovascular tissues. *Perspect Biol Med* 1970;13:507–527.
241. Gillard GC, Reilly HC, Bell-Booth PG, et al. The influence of mechanical forces on the glycosaminoglycan content of the rabbit flexor digitorum profundus tendon. *Connect Tissue Res* 1979;7:37–46.
242. Slowman SD, Brandt KD. Composition and glycosaminoglycan metabolism of articular cartilage from habitually loaded and habitually unloaded sites. *Arthritis Rheum* 1986;29:88–94.
243. Palmoski MJ, Perricone E, Brandt KD. Development and reversal of a proteoglycan aggregation defect in normal canine knee cartilage after immobilization. *Arthritis Rheum* 1979;22:508–517.
244. Kiviranta I, Jurvelin J, Tammi M, et al. Weight bearing controls glycosaminoglycan concentration and articular cartilage thickness in the knee joints of young beagle dogs. *Arthritis Rheum* 1983;30:801–809.
245. Säämänen A-M, Tammo M, Kiviranta I, et al. Maturation of proteoglycan matrix in articular cartilage under increased and decreased joint loading: a study in young rabbits. *Connect Tissue Res* 1987;16: 163–175.
246. Vasan N. Effects of physical stress on the synthesis and degradation of cartilage matrix. *Connect Tissue Res* 1983;12:49–58.
247. Otterness IG, Eskra JD, Bliven ML, et al. Exercise protects against articular cartilage degeneration in the hamster. *Arthritis Rheum* 1998; 41:2068–2076.
248. Eger W, Schumacher BL, Mollenhauer J, et al. Human knee and ankle explants: catabolic differences. *J Orthop Res* 2002;20:526–534.
249. Salter DM, Godolphin JL, Gowlay MS. Chondrocyte heterogeneity: immunohistologically defined variation of integrin expression at different sites in human fetal knees. *J Histochem Cytochem* 1995;43: 447–457.
250. Loesser RF. Integrin-mediated attachment of articular chondrocytes to extracellular matrix proteins. *Arthritis Rheum* 1993;36:1103–1110.
251. Woods VL Jr, Schreck PJ, Gesink DS, et al. Integrin expression by human articular chondrocytes. *Arthritis Rheum* 1994;37:537–544.
252. Ostergaard K, Salter DM, Petersen J, et al. Expression of α and β subunits of the integrin superfamily in articular cartilage from macroscopically normal and osteoarthritic human femoral heads. *Ann Rheum Dis* 1998;57:303–308.
253. Hirsch MS, Lunsford LE, Trinkaus-Randall V, Svoboda KKH. Chondrocyte survival and differentiation *in situ* are integrin mediated. *Dev Dyn* 1997;210:249–263.
254. Enomoto M, Leboy PS, Menko AS, et al. β_1 Integrins mediate chondrocyte interaction with type I collagen, type II collagen and fibronectin. *Exp Cell Res* 1993;205:276–285.
255. Turnay J, Pfannmüller E, Lizarbe MA, et al. Collagen binding activity of recombinant and N-terminally modified annexin V (archorin CII). *J Cell Biochem* 1995;58:208–220.
256. Fernandez MP, Selmin O, Martin GR, et al. The structure of anchorin CII: a collagen binding protein isolated from chondrocyte membrane. *J Biol Chem* 1988;263:5921–5925.
257. Kirsch T, Pläffle M. Selective binding of anchorin cII (annexin V) to type II and X collagen and to chondrocalcin (C-propeptide of type II procollagen): implications for anchoring function between matrix vesicles and matrix proteins. *FEBS Lett* 1992;310:143–147.
258. Koolpe M, Benton HP. Calcium-mobilizing purine receptors on the surface of mammalian articular chondrocytes. *J Orthop Res* 1997;15: 204–213.
259. Chow G, Nietfeld JAAP, Knudson CB, et al. Antisense inhibition of chondrocyte CD44 expression leading to cartilage chondrolysis. *Arthritis Rheum* 1998;41:1411–1419.
260. Da Silva JAP, Willoughby DA. The influence of sex in arthritis: is cartilage an overlooked factor? *J Rheumatol* 1994;21:791–796.
261. Richmond RS, Carlson CS, Register TC, et al. Functional estrogen receptors in adult articular cartilage: estrogen replacement therapy increases chondrocyte synthesis of proteoglycans and insulin-like growth factor binding protein 2. *Arthritis Rheum* 2000;43:2081–2090.
262. Taylor DJ, Yoffe JR, Woolley DE. Histamine H_2 receptors on fetal-bovine articular chondrocytes. *Biochem J* 1983;212:517–520.
263. Benton HP, Jackson TR, Hanley MR. Identification of a novel inflammatory stimulant of chondrocytes: early events in cell activation by bradykinin receptors on pig articular chondrocytes. *Biochem J* 1989;258:861–867.
264. Schipani E, Ryan ME, Didrrickson S, et al. Hypoxia in cartilage: HIF-1α is essential for chondrocyte growth arrest and survival. *Genes Dev* 2001;15:2865–2876.
265. Pfander D, Cramer T, Schipani E, et al. HIF-1α controls extracellular matrix synthesis by epiphyseal chondrocytes. *J Cell Sci* 2003;116: 1819–1826.
266. Prins APA, Lipman JM, McDevitt CA, et al. Effect of purified growth factors on rabbit articular chondrocytes in monolayer culture. II. Sulfated proteoglycan synthesis. *Arthritis Rheum* 1982;25: 1228–1238.
267. Guenther HL, Guenther HE, Froesch ER, et al. Effect of insulin-like growth factor on collagen and glycosaminoglycan synthesis by rabbit articular chondrocytes in culture. *Experientia* 1982;38:979–980.
268. Osborn KD, Trippel SB, Mankin HJ. Growth factor stimulation of adult articular cartilage. *J Orthop Res* 1989;7:35–42.
269. Watanabe N, Rosenfeld RG, Hintz RL, et al. Characterization of a specific insulin-like growth factor-I/somatomedin-C receptor on high density, primary monolayer cultures of bovine articular chondrocytes: regulation of receptor concentration by somatomedin, insulin and growth hormone. *J Endocrinol* 1985;107:275–283.
270. Trippel SB, Chernausek SD, Van Wyk JJ, et al. Demonstration of type I and type II somatomedin receptors on bovine growth plate chondrocytes. *J Orthop Res* 1988;6:817–826.
271. Hunziker E, Wagner J, Zapf J. Differential effects of insulin-like growth factor 1 and growth hormone on developmental stages of rat growth plate chondrocytes *in vivo*. *J Clin Invest* 1994;93:1078–1086.
272. Vetter U, Zapf J, Heit W, et al. Human fetal and adult chondrocytes: effect of insulin-like growth factors I and II, insulin and growth hormone on clonal growth. *J Clin Invest* 1986;77:1903–1908.
273. Makower A-M, Wroblewski J, Pawlowski A. Effects of IGF-1, rGF, FGF, EGF and NCS on DNA-synthesis, cell proliferation and morphology of chondrocytes isolated from rat rib growth cartilage. *Cell Biol Int Rep* 1989;13:259–270.

274. Schoenle E, Zapf J, Humbel RE, et al. Insulin-like growth factor 1 stimulates growth in hypophysectomized rats. *Nature* 1982;296:252–253.
275. Schoenle E, Zapf J, Hauri C, et al. Comparison of *in vivo* effects of insulin-like growth factor I and II and of growth hormone in hypophysectomised rats. *Acta Endocrinol* 1985;108:167–174.
276. Nilsson A, Isgaard J, Lindahl A, et al. Regulation by growth hormone of number of chondrocytes containing IGF-1 in rat growth plate. *Science* 1986;233:571–574.
277. Middleton JFS, Tyler JA. Upregulation of insulin-like growth factor 1 gene expression in the lesions of osteoarthritic human articular cartilage. *Ann Rheum Dis* 1992;51:440–447.
278. Luyten FP, Hascall VC, Nissley SP, et al. Insulin-like growth factors maintain steady state metabolism of proteoglycans in bovine articular cartilage explants. *Arch Biochem Biophys* 1988;267:416–425.
279. McQuillan DJ, Handley CJ, Campbell MA, et al. Stimulation of proteoglycan biosynthesis by serum and insulin-like growth factor-1 in cultured bovine articular cartilage. *Biochem J* 1986;240:423–430.
280. Tyler JA. Insulin-like growth factor 1 can decrease degradation and promote synthesis of proteoglycan in cartilage exposed to cytokines. *Biochem J* 1989;260:543–548.
281. Hui W, Cawston T, Rowan AD. Transforming growth factor β1 and insulin-like growth factor 1 block collagen degradation induced by oncostatin M in combination with tumour necrosis factor from bovine cartilage. *Ann Rheum Dis* 2003;62:172–174.
282. Hui W, Rowan AD, Cawston T. Insulin-like growth factor 1 blocks collagen release and down regulates matrix metalloproteinase-1, -3, -8, and -13 in RNA expression in bovine nasal cartilage stimulated with oncostatin M in combination with interleukin 1α. *Ann Rheum Dis* 2001;60:254–261.
283. Im H-J, Pacione C, Chubinskaya S, et al. Inhibitory effects of insulin-like growth factor-1 and osteogenic protein-1 on fibronectin fragment and interleukin-1β stimulated matrix metalloproteinase-13 expression in human chondrocytes. *J Biol Chem* 2003;278:25386–25394.
284. Wang J, Elewant D, Veys EM, et al. Insulin-like growth factor-1 induced interleukin-1 receptor II overrides the activity of interleukin-1 and controls the homeostasis of the extracellular matrix of cartilage. *Arthritis Rheum* 2003;48:1281–1291.
285. Schalkwijk J, Joosten LAB, van den Berg WB, et al. Insulin-like growth factor stimulation of chondrocyte proteoglycan synthesis by human synovial fluid. *Arthritis Rheum* 1989;32:66–71.
286. Schalkwijk J, Joosten LAB, van den Berg WB, et al. Chondrocyte nonresponsiveness to insulin-like growth factor I in experimental arthritis. *Arthritis Rheum* 1989;32:894–900.
287. Olney RC, Wilson DM, Mohtai M, et al. Interleukin-1 and tumor necrosis factor-α increase insulin-like growth factor binding protein-3 (IGFBP-3) production and IGFBP-3 protease activity in human articular chondrocytes. *J Endocrinol* 1995;146:279–286.
288. Rieu M. Evaluation of insulin-like growth factor (somatomedin) levels in acromegaly. *Hormone Res* 1986;24:112–115.
289. Yokoya S, Suwa S, Maesaka H, Tanaka T. Immunoreactive somatomedin C/insulin-like growth factor I in urine from normal subjects, pituitary dwarfs, and acromegalics. *Pediatr Res* 1988;23:151–154.
290. Zapf J, Froesch ER. Insulin-like growth factors/somatomedins: structure, secretion, biological actions and physiological role. *Horm Res* 1986;24:121–130.
291. Sessions CM, Emiler CA, Schalch DS. Interaction of insulin-like growth factor II with rat chondrocytes: receptor binding, internalization and degradation. *Endocrinology* 1987;120:2108–2116.
292. Isaksson OGP, Jansson J-O, Gause IAM. Growth hormone stimulates longitudinal bone growth directly. *Science* 1982;216:1237–1239.
293. Russell SM, Spencer EM. Local injections of human or rat growth hormone or purified somatomedin-C stimulate unilateral tibial epiphyseal growth in hypophysectomized rats. *Endocrinology* 1985;116:2563–2567.
294. Villiger PM, Kusari AB, ten Dijke P, et al. IL-1β and IL-6 selectively induce transforming growth factor-β isoforms in human articular chondrocytes. *J Immunol* 1993;151:3337–3344.
295. Morales TI, Roberts AB. Transforming growth factor β regulates the metabolism of proteoglycans in bovine cartilage organ cultures. *J Biol Chem* 1988;263:12828–12831.
296. Redini F, Galera P, Mauviel A, et al. Transforming growth factor β stimulates collagen and glycosaminoglycan biosynthesis in cultured rabbit articular chondrocytes. *FEBS Lett* 1988;234:172–176.
297. Chandrasekhar S, Harvey AK. Transforming growth factor-β is a potent inhibitor of IL-1 induced protease activity and cartilage proteoglycan degradation. *Biochem Biophys Res Commun* 1988;157:1352–1359.
298. Scharstuhl A, van Beuningen HM, Vitters EL et al. Loss of transforming growth factor counteraction on interleukin-1 mediated effects in cartilage of old mice. *Ann Rheum Dis* 2002;61:1095–1098.
299. Serra R, Johnson M, Filvaroff EH, et al. Expression of a truncated, kinase-defective TGF-β type II receptor in mouse skeletal tissue promotes terminal chondrocyte differentiation and osteoarthritis. *J Cell Biol* 1997;134:541–552.
300. Yang X, Chen L, Xu X, et al. TGFβ/Smad3 signals repress chondrocyte hypertrophic differentiation and are required for maintaining articular cartilage. *J Cell Biol* 2001;153:35–46.
301. Shlopov BV, Gunanovskaya ML, Hasty KA. Autocrine regulation of collagenase 3 (matrix metalloproteinase 13) during osteoarthritis. *Arthritis Rheum* 2000;43:195–205.
302. Gelb DE, Rosier R, Puzas JE. The production of transforming growth factor-β by chick growth plate chondrocytes in short term monolayer culture. *Endocrinology* 1990;127:1941–1947.
303. Crabb ID, O'Keefe RJ, Puzas JE, Rosier RN. Synergistic effect of transforming growth factor β and fibroblast growth factor on DNA synthesis in chick growth plate chondrocytes. *J Bone Miner Res* 1990;5:1105–1112.
304. Elford PR, Lamberts SWJ. Contrasting modulation by transforming growth factor-b1 of insulin-like growth factor-1 production in osteoblasts and chondrocytes. *Endocrinology* 1990;127:1635–1639.
305. Harvey AK, Hrubey PS, Chandrasekhar S. Transforming growth factor-β inhibition of interleukin-1 activity involves down-regulation of interleukin-1 receptors on chondrocytes. *Exp Cell Res* 1991;195:376–385.
306. Hogan BLM. Bone morphogenetic proteins: multifunctional regulators of vertebrate development. *Genes Dev* 1996;10:1580–1594.
307. Schmidt JM, Hwang K, Winn SR, et al. Bone morphogenetic proteins: an update on basic biology and clinical relevance. *J Orthop Res* 1999;17:269–278.
308. Feng JQ, Xing L, Zhang JH, et al. NF-kβ specifically activates BMP-2 gene expression in growth plate chondrocytes *in vivo* and in a chondrocyte cell line *in vitro*. *J Biol Chem* 2003;278:29130–29135.
309. Flechtenmacher J, Huch K, Thonar EJ-MA, et al. Recombinant human osteogenic protein 1 is a potent stimulator of the synthesis of cartilage proteoglycans and collagens by human articular chondrocytes. *Arthritis Rheum* 1996;39:1896–1904.
310. Sailor LZ, Hewick RM, Morris EA. Recombinant human bone morphogenetic protein-2 maintains the articular chondrocyte phenotype in long-term culture. *J Orthop Res* 1996;14:937–945.
311. Glansbeek HL, van Beuningen HM, Vitters EL, et al. Bone morphogenetic protein 2 stimulates articular cartilage proteoglycan synthesis *in vivo* but does not counteract interleukin-1α effects on proteoglycan synthesis and content. *Arthritis Rheum* 1997;40:1020–1028.
312. Huch K, Wilbrink B, Flechtenmacher J, et al. Effects of recombinant human osteogenic protein 1 on the production of proteoglycan, prostaglandin E_2 and interleukin-1 receptor antagonist by human articular chondrocytes cultured in the presence of interleukin-1β. *Arthritis Rheum* 1997;40:2157–2161.
313. Koepp HE, Sampath KT, Kuettner KE, et al. Osteogenic protein-1 (OP-1) blocks cartilage damage caused by fibronectin fragments and promotes repair by enhancing proteoglycan synthesis. *Inflamm Res* 1999;48:199–204.
314. Bobacz K, Gruber R, Soleiman A, et al. Cartilage-derived morphogenetic proteins-2 and -2 are endogenously expressed in healthy and osteoarthritic human articular chondrocytes and stimulate matrix synthesis. Osteoarthritis Cartilage 2002;10:394–401.
315. Makower A-M, Wroblewski J, Pawlowski A. Effects of IGF-1, EGF and FGF on proteoglycans synthesized by fractionated chondrocytes of rat rib growth plate. *Exp Cell Res* 1988;179:498–506.
316. Cuevas P, Burgos J, Baird A. Basic fibroblast growth factor (FGF) promotes cartilage repair *in vivo*. *Biochem Biophys Res Commun* 1988;156:611–618.
317. Kato Y, Iwamoto M. Fibroblast growth factor is an inhibitor of chondrocyte terminal differentiation. *J Biol Chem* 1990;265:5903–5909.
318. Sano H, Forough R, Maier JAM, et al. Detection of high levels of heparin binding growth factor-1 (acidic fibroblast growth factor) in inflammatory arthritic joints. *J Cell Biol* 1990;110:1417–1426.

319. Jinguishi S, Heydemann A, Kana SK, et al. Acidic fibroblast growth factor (aFGF) injection stimulates cartilage enlargement and inhibits cartilage gene expression in rat fracture healing. *J Orthop Res* 1990; 8:364–371.
320. Phadke K. Fibroblast growth factor enhances the interleukin-1 mediated chondrocyte protease release. *Biochem Biophys Res Commun* 1987;142:448–453.
321. Chin JE, Hatfield CA, Krzesicki RF, et al. Interactions between interleukin-1 and basic fibroblast growth factor on articular chondrocytes: effects on cell growth, prostanoid production and receptor modulation. *Arthritis Rheum* 1991;34:314–324.
322. Tyler JA. Articular cartilage cultured with catabolin (pig interleukin 1) synthesizes a decreased number of normal proteoglycan molecules. *Biochem J* 1985;227:869–878.
323. Morales TI, Hascall VC. Specificity of action of lipopolysaccharide on bovine articular cartilage metabolism: a comparison with interleukin-1. *Connect Tissue Res* 1989;19:255–275.
324. Tyler JA, Benton HP. Synthesis of type II collagen is decreased in cartilage cultured with interleukin-1 while the rate of extracellular degradation remains unchanged. *Coll Rel Res* 1988;8:393–405.
325. Goldring MB, Birkhead J, Sandell LJ, et al. Interleukin-1 suppresses expression of cartilage-specific types II and IX collagens and increases types I and III collagens in human chondrocytes. *J Clin Invest* 1988; 82:2026–2037.
326. Lefebvre V, Peeters-Joris C, Vaes G. Modulation by interleukin-1 and tumor necrosis factor α of production of collagenase, tissue inhibitor of metalloproteinases and collagen types in differentiated and dedifferentiated articular chondrocytes. *Biochim Biophys Acta* 1990; 1052:366–378.
327. Arner EC, Pratta MA. Independent effects of interleukin-1 on proteoglycan breakdown, proteoglycan synthesis and prostaglandin E_2 release from cartilage in organ culture. *Arthritis Rheum* 1989;32: 288–297.
328. Poole AR, Alini M, Hollander AP. Cellular biology of cartilage degradation. In: Henderson B, Pettifer R, Edwards J, eds. *Mechanisms and models in rheumatoid arthritis*. London: Academic, 1995: 163–204.
329. Yaron I, Meyer FA, Dayer J-M, et al. Some recombinant human cytokines stimulate glycosaminoglycan synthesis in human synovial fibroblasts cultures and inhibit it in human articular cartilage cultures. *Arthritis Rheum* 1989;32:173–180.
330. van de Loo AAJ, van Beuningen HM, van Lent PLEM, et al. Direct effect of murine IL-1 on cartilage metabolism *in vivo*. *Agents Actions* 1989;26:153–155.
331. Nietfeld JJ, Duits AJ, Tilanus MGJ, et al. Antisense oligonucleotides: a novel tool for the control of cytokine effects on human cartilage: focus on interleukin-1 and 6 and proteoglycan synthesis. *Arthritis Rheum* 1994;37:1357–1362.
332. Cawston TE, Curry VA, Summers CA, et al. The role of oncostatin M in animal and human connective tissue collagen turnover and its localization within the rheumatoid joint. *Arthritis Rheum* 1998;41: 1760–1771.
333. Koshy PJT, Lundy CJ, Rowan AD, et al. The modulation of matrix metalloproteinase and ADAM gene expression in human chondrocytes by interleukin-1 and oncostatin M. A time course study using real-time quantitative reverse transcription-polymerase chain reaction. *Arthritis Rheum* 2002;46:961–967.
334. Seckinger P, Yaron I, Meyer FA, et al. Modulation of the effects of interleukin-1 on glycosaminoglycan synthesis by the urine-derived interleukin-1 inhibitor, but not by interleukin-6. *Arthritis Rheum* 1990;33:1807–1814.
335. Silacci P, Dayer J-M, Desgeorges A, et al. Interleukin (IL)-6 and its soluble receptor induce TIMP-1 expression in synoviocytes and chondrocytes and block IL-1 induced collagenolytic activity. *J Biol Chem* 1998;273:13625–13629.
336. Flannery CR, Little CB, Hughes CE, et al. IL-6 and its soluble receptor augment aggrecanase-mediated proteoglycan catabolism in articular cartilage. *Matrix Biol* 2000;19:549–553.
337. Häuselmann HJ, Oppliger L, Michel BA, et al. Nitric oxide and proteoglycan biosynthesis by human articular chondrocytes in alginate culture. *FEBS Lett* 1994;352:361–364.
338. Taskiran D, Stefanovic-Racic M, Georgescu H, et al. Nitric oxide mediates suppression of cartilage proteoglycan synthesis by interleukin-1. *Biochem Biophys Res Commun* 1996;200:142–148.
339. Gouze J-N, Bordji K, Gulberti S, et al. Interleukin-1β downregulates the expression of glucuronosyltransferase 1, a key enzyme priming glycosaminoglycan biosynthesis. Influence of glucosamine on interleukin-1β-mediated effects in rat chondrocytes. *Arthritis Rheum* 2001;44:351–360.
340. Blanco FJ, Ochs RL, Schwarz H, Lotz M. Chrondocyte apoptosis induced by nitric oxide. *Am J Pathol* 1995;146:75–85.
341. Del Carlo M Jr, Loesser RF. Nitric-oxide-mediated chondrocyte cell death requires the generation of additional reactive oxygen species. *Arthritis Rheum* 2002;46:394–403.
342. Pettersen I, Figenschau Y, Olsen E, et al. Tumor necrosis factor–related apoptosis-inducing ligand induces apoptosis in human articular chondrocytes *in vitro*. *Biochem Biophys Res Commun* 2002;296: 671–676.
343. Schwerwegh AJ, Dombrecht EJ, Stevens WJ, et al. Influence of proinflammatory (IL-1α, IL-6, TNF-α, IFN-γ) and anti-inflammatory (IL-4) cytokines on chondrocyte function. *Osteoarthritis Cartilage* 2003;11:681–687.
344. Clements KM, Price JS, Chambers MG, et al. Gene deletion of either IL-1β, ICE; Nos or SLN-1 accelerates the development of knee osteoarthritis in mice after surgical transection of the medial collateral ligament and partial medial meniscectomy. *Arthritis Rheum* 2003;48: 3452–3463.
345. Goldring MB, Birkhead J, Sandell LJ, et al. Synergistic regulation of collagen gene expression in human chondrocytes by tumor necrosis factor-α and interleukin-1β. *Ann NY Acad Sci* 1990;580: 536–539.
346. Goldring MB, Sandell LJ, Stephenson ML, et al. Immune interferon suppresses levels of procollagen in mRNA and type II collagen synthesis in cultured human articular and costal chondrocytes. *J Biol Chem* 1986;261:9049–9056.
347. Fons AJ, van de Loo J, Joosten LAB, et al. Role of interleukin-1, tumor necrosis factor α and interleukin-6 in cartilage proteoglycan metabolism and destruction. *Arthritis Rheum* 1995;38:164–172.
348. Yeh LA, Augustine AJ, Lee P, et al. Interleukin-4, an inhibitor of cartilage breakdown in bovine articular cartilage explants. *J Rheumatol* 1995;22:1740–1746.
349. Lubberts E, Joosten LA, van Den Bersselaar L, et al. Adenoviral vector-radiated overexpression of IL-4 in the knee joint of mice with collagen-induced arthritis prevents cartilage destruction. *J Immunol* 1999;163:4546–4556.
350. Shalon-Barak T, Quach J, Lotz M. Interleukin-17 induced gene expression in articular chondrocytes is associated with activation of mitogen-activated protein kinases and NF-κB. *J Biol Chem* 1998; 273:27467–27473.
351. Koshy PJ, Henderson N, Logan C, et al. Interleukin-17 induces cartilage collagen breakdown: novel synergistic effects in combination with proinflammatory cytokines. *Ann Rheum Dis* 2002;61:704–713.
352. Attur MG, Patel RN, Abramson SB, et al. Interleukin-17 upregulation of nitric oxide production in human osteoarthritis cartilage. *Arthritis Rheum* 1997;40:1050–1053.
353. Lubberts E, Joosten LAB, van de Loo FAJ, et al. Reduction of interleukin-17 induced inhibition of chondrocyte proteoglycan synthesis in intact murine articular cartilages by interleukin-4. *Arthritis Rheum* 2000;43:1300–1306.
354. Honorati MC, Bovara M, Cattini L, et al. Contribution of interleukin 17 to human cartilage degradation and synovial inflammation in osteoarthritis. *Osteoarthritis Cartilage* 2002;10:799–807.
355. Olec T, Hashimoto S, Quach J, et al. IL-18 is produced by articular chondrocytes and induces proinflammatory and catabolic responses. *J Immunol* 1999;162:1096–1100.
356. Figenschau Y, Knutsen G, Shahazeydi S, et al. Human articular chondrocytes express functional leptin receptors. *Biochem Biophys Res Commun* 2001;287:190–197.
357. Hirak Y, Inoue H, Iyama K-I, et al. Identification of chondromodulin 1 as a novel endothelial cell growth inhibitor. Purification and its localization in the avascular zone of epiphyseal cartilage. *J Biol Chem* 1997;272:32419–32426.
358. Recklies AD, White C, Ling H. The chitinase-3 like protein human cartilage glycoprotein 39 (HC-gp39) stimulates proliferation of human connective-tissue cells and activates both extracellular signal-regulated kinase and protein kinase B–mediated signalling pathways. *Biochem J* 2002;365:119–126.

359. Hinek A, Poole AR. The influence of vitamin D metabolites on the calcification of cartilage matrix and the C-propeptide of type II collagen (chondrocalcin). *J Bone Miner Res* 1988;3:421–429.
360. Homandberg GA, Hui F, Wen C, et al. Fibronectin-fragment induced cartilage chondrolysis is associated with release of catabolic cytokines. *Biochem J* 1997;321:751–757.
361. Peters JH, Loredo GA, Benton HP. Is osteoarthritis a fibronectin-integrin imbalance disorder? *Osteoarthritis Cartilage* 2002;10:831–835.
362. Yasuda T, Poole AR. A fibronectin fragment induces type II collagen degradation by collagenase through an interleukin-1 mediated pathway. *Arthritis Rheum* 2002;46:138–148.
363. Yasuda T, Poole AR, Shimizu M, et al. Involvement of CD44 in induction by a carboxyterminal heparin-binding fibronectin domain of matrix metalloproteinases in human articular cartilage in culture. *Arthritis Rheum* 2003;48:1271–1280.
364. Arner EC, Tortorella MD. Signal transduction through chondrocyte integrin receptors induces matrix metalloproteinase synthesis and synergizes with interleukin-1. *Arthritis Rheum* 1995;38:1304–1314.
365. Homandberg GA, Wen C. Exposure of cartilage to a fibronectin fragment amplifies catabolic processes while also enhancing anabolic processes to limit damage. *J Orthop Res* 1998;16:237–246.
366. McKenna LA, Liu H, Sansom P, et al. A N-terminal peptide from link protein stimulates proteoglycan biosynthesis in human articular cartilage *in vivo*. *Arthritis Rheum* 1998;41:157–162.
367. Mwale F, Demers CN, Petit A, et al. A synthetic peptide of link protein stimulates the biosynthesis of collagens II, IX and proteoglycan by cells of the intervertebral disc. *J Cell Biochem* 2003;88:1202–1213.
368. Jennings L, Wu L, King KB, et al. The effects of collagen fragments on the extracellular matrix metabolism of bovine and human chondrocytes. *Connect Tissue Res* 2001;42:71–86.
369. Yasuda T, Wu W, Poole AR. A fragment of type II collagen can induce collagenase-mediated cleavage of type II collagen: identification of a positive degradative feedback loop in cartilage resorption. *Arthritis Rheum* (In press).
370. Simmons DJ, Whitesidc LA, Whitson SW. Biorhythmic profiles in the rat skeleton. *Metab Bone Dis Rel Res* 1979;2:49–64.
371. Tiku ML, Liesch JB, Robertson FM. Production of hydrogen peroxide by rabbit articular chondrocytes: enhancement by cytokines. *J Immunol* 1990;145:690–696.
372. Dingle JT, Horsfield P, Fell HB, et al. Breakdown of proteoglycan and collagen induced in pig articular cartilage in organ culture. *Ann Rheum Dis* 1975;34:303–311.
373. Cawston TE, Ellis AJ, Lean E, et al. Interleukin-1 and oncostatin M in combination promote the release of collagen fragments from bovine nasal cartilage in culture. *Biochem Biophys Res Commun* 1995;215:377–385.
374. Billinghurst RC, Wu W, Ionescu M, et al. Comparison of the degradation of type II collagen and proteoglycan in nasal and articular cartilages induced by interleukin-1 and the selective inhibition of type II collagen cleavage by collagenase. *Arthritis Rheum* 2000;43:664–672.
375. Milner JM, Elliott S-F, Cawston TE. Activation of procollagenases is a key control point in cartilage collagen degradation. Interaction of serine and metalloproteinase pathways. *Arthritis Rheum* 2001;44: 2084–2096.
376. Sztrolovics R, White RJ, Poole AR, et al. Resistance of small leucine rich repeat proteoglycans to proteolytic during interleukin-1 stimulated cartilage. *Biochem J* 1999;339:571–577.
377. Cheung HS, Ryan LM, Kozin F, et al. Identification of collagen subtypes in synovial fluid sediments from arthritic patients. *Am J Med* 1980;68:73–79.
378. Witter J, Roughley PJ, Webber C, et al. The immunological detection and characterization of cartilage proteoglycan degradation products in synovial fluids of patients with arthritis. *Arthritis Rheum* 1987; 30:519–526.
379. Kim HA, Song YW. Apoptotic chondrocyte death in rheumatoid arthritis. *Arthritis Rheum* 1999;42:1528–1537.
380. Von der Mark K, Kirsch T, Nerlich A, et al. Type X collagen synthesis in human osteoarthritic cartilage: induction of chondrocyte hypertrophy. *Arthritis Rheum* 1992;35:806–811.
381. Terkeltaub R, Lotz M, Johnson K, et al. Parathyroid hormone-related protein is abundant in osteoarthritic cartilage, and the parathyroid hormone-related protein 1–173 isoform is selectively induced by transforming growth factor beta in articular chondrocytes and suppresses generation of extracellular inorganic pyrophosphate. *Arthritis Rheum* 1998;41:2152–2164.
382. Kirsch T, Swoboda B, Nah HD. Activation of annexin II and V expression, terminal differentiation, mineralization and apoptosis in human osteoarthritic cartilage. *Osteoarthritis Cartilage* 2000;8:294–302.
383. Hashimoto H, Ochs RL, Komiya S, et al. Linkage of chondrocyte apoptosis and cartilage degradation in human osteoarthritis. *Arthritis Rheum* 1998;41;1632–1638.
384. Blanco FJ, Guitan R, Vazquez-Martel E, et al. Osteoarthritis chondrocytes die by apoptosis: a possible pathway for osteoarthritis pathology. *Arthritis Rheum* 1998;41:284–289.
385. Gordon GV, Villanueva T, Schumacher HR, et al. Autopsy study correlating degree of osteoarthritis, synovitis and evidence of articular calcification. *J Rheumatol* 1984;11:681–686.
386. Ohira T, Ishikawa K. Hydroxyapatite deposition in osteoarthritic articular cartilage of the proximal femoral head. *Arthritis Rheum* 1987; 30:651–660.
387. Konttinen YT, Mordelin J, Li T-F, et al. Acidic endoproteinase cathepsin K in the degeneration of the superficial articular hyaline cartilage in osteoarthritis. *Arthritis Rheum* 2002;46:953–960.
388. Hollander AP, Pidoux I, Reiner A, et al. Damage to type II collagen in ageing and osteoarthritis: starts at the articular surface, originates around chondrocytes and extends into the cartilage with progressive degeneration. *J Clin Invest* 1995;96:2859–2869.
389. Lark MW, Bayne EK, Flanagan J, et al. Aggrecan degradation in human cartilage: evidence for both matrix metalloproteinase and aggrecanase activity in normal osteoarthritic, and rheumatoid joints. *J Clin Invest* 1997;100:93–106.
390. Woolley D, Crossley MJ, Evanson J. Collagenase at sites of cartilage erosion in the rheumatoid joint. *Arthritis Rheum* 1977;20:1231–1239.
391. Kobayashi I, Ziff M. Electron microscopic studies of the cartilage-pannus junction in rheumatoid arthritis. *Arthritis Rheum* 1975;18: 475–483.
392. Mort JS, Poole AR. Mediators of inflammation, tissue destruction and repair. D. Proteases and their inhibitors. In: Klippel JH ed. *Primer on the rheumatic diseases,* 12th ed. Atlanta: Arthritis Foundation, 2001:72–81.
393. Lovejoy B, Hassell AM, Luther MA, et al. Crystal structures of recombinant 19-kDa human fibroblast collagenase complexed to itself. *Biochemistry* 1994;33:8207–8217.
394. Van Wart HE, Birkedal-Hansen H. The cysteine switch: a principle of regulation of metalloproteinases activity with potential applicability to the entire matrix metalloproteinase gene family. Proc Natl Acad Sci U S A 1990;87:5578–5582.
395. Springman EB, Angleton EL, Birkedal-Hansen H, et al. Multiple modes of activation of latent human fibroblast collagenase: evidence for the role of a Cys^{73} active-site zinc complex in latency and a "cysteine switch" mechanism for activation. *Proc Natl Acad Sci U S A* 1990;87:364–368.
396. Murphy G, Cockett MI, Stephens PE, et al. Stromelysin is an activator of procollagenase: a study with natural and recombinant enzymes. *Biochem J* 1987;248:265–268.
397. Brinckerhoff CE, Suzuki K, Mitchell TI, et al. Rabbit procollagenase synthesized and secreted by a high yield mammalian expression vector requires stromelysin (matrix metalloproteinase-3) for maximal activation. *J Biol Chem* 1990;265:22262–22269.
398. van Meurs J, van Lent P, Stoop R. et al. Cleavage of aggrecan at the ASN^{341}-PHE^{342} site coincides with the initiation of collagen damage in murine antigen-induced arthritis. *Arthritis Rheum* 1999;42:2074–2084.
399. Wu J-J, Lark M, Chun LE, Eyre DR. Sites of stromelysin cleavage in collagen types II, IX, X, and XI of cartilage. *J Biol Chem* 1991;266: 5625–5628.
400. Eeckhout Y, Vaes G. Further studies on the activation of procollagenase, the latent precursor of bone collagenase: effects of lysosomal cathepsin B, plasmin and kallikrein and spontaneous activation. *Biochem J* 1977;166:21–31.
401. Bryson H, Bunning RAD, Feltell R, et al. A serine proteinase inactivator inhibits chondrocyte-mediated cartilage proteoglycan breakdown occurring in response to proinflammatory cytokines. *Arch Biochem Biophys* 1998;355:15–25.

402. Kobayashi H, Schmitt M, Goretzki L, et al. Cathepsin B efficiently activates the soluble and the tumor cell receptor-bound form of the proenzyme urokinase type plasminogen activator (Pro-uPA). *J Biol Chem* 1991;266:5147–5152.
403. Buttle DJ, Handley CJ, Ilic MZ, et al. Inhibition of cartilage proteoglycan release by a specific inactivator of cathepsin B and an inhibitor of matrix metalloproteinases: evidence for two converging pathways of chondrocyte mediated proteoglycan degradation. *Arthritis Rheum* 1993;36:1709–1717.
404. Knäuper V, Will H, López-Otin C, et al. Cellular mechanisms for human procollagenase-3 (MMP-13) activation: evidence that MT1-MMP (MMP-14) and gelatinase A (MMP-2) are able to generate active enzyme. *J Biol Chem* 1996;271:17124–17131.
405. Holmbeck K, Bianco P, Caterina J, et al. MT1-MMP-deficient mice develop dwarfism, osteopenia, arthritis, and connective tissue disease due to inadequate collagen turnover. *Cell* 1999;99:81–92.
406. Flannery CR, Lark MW, Sandy JD. Identification of a stromelysin cleavage site within the interglobular domain of human aggrecan: evidence for proteolysis at this site *in vivo* in human articular cartilage. *J Biol Chem* 1992;267:1008–1014.
407. Sandy JD, Neame PJ, Boyton RE, et al. Catabolism of aggrecan in cartilage explants: identification of a major cleavage site within the interglobular domain. *J Biol Chem* 1991;266:8683–8685.
408. Mort JS, Magny M-C, Lee ER. Cathepsin B an alternative protease for the generation of an aggrecan "metalloproteinase" cleavage neoepitope. *Biochem J* 1998;335:491–494.
409. Ilic MZ, Robinson HC, Hudley CJ. Characterization of aggrecan retained and lost from the extracellular matrix of articular cartilage: involvement of carboxyl-terminal processing in the catabolism of aggrecan. *J Biol Chem* 1998;273:17451–17458.
410. Tortorella MD, Burn TC, Pratta MA, et al. Purification and cloning of aggrecanase-1: a member of the ADAMTS family of proteins. *Science* 1999;284:1664–1666.
411. Abbaszade I, Liu R-Q, Yang F, et al. Cloning characterization of ADAMTS 11, an aggrecanase from the ADAMTS family. *J Biol Chem* 1999;274:23443–23450.
412. Tortorella MD, Malfait A-M, Deccico C, et al. The role of ADAM-TS4 (aggrecanase-1) and ADAM-TS5 (aggrecanase-2) in a model of cartilage degradation. *Osteoarthritis Cartilage* 2001;9:539–552.
413. van Meurs JB, van Lent PL, Holthuysen AE, et al. Kinetics of aggrecanase- and metalloproteinase-induced neoepitopes in various stages of cartilage destruction in murine arthritis. *Arthritis Rheum* 1999;42: 1128–1139.
414. Nguyen Q, Murphy G, Roughley PJ, et al. Degradation of proteoglycan aggregate by a cartilage metalloproteinase. *Biochem J* 1989;259: 61–67.
415. Dahlberg L, Billinghurst RC, Manner P, et al. Collagenase-mediated cleavage of resident type II collagen is selectively enhanced in cultured osteoarthritic cartilage and can be arrested with a synthetic inhibitor which spares collagenase-1 (MMP-1). *Arthritis Rheum* 2000; 43:673–682.
416. Knäuper V, Lopez-Otin C, Smith B, et al. Biochemical characterization of human collagenase-3. *J Biol Chem* 1996;271:1544–1550.
417. Mitchell PH, Magna HA, Reeves LM, et al. Cloning, expression, and type I collagenolytic activity of matrix metalloproteinase-13 from human osteoarthritic cartilage. *J Clin Invest* 1996;97:761–768.
418. Hughes CE, Caterson B, White RJ, et al. Monoclonal antibodies recognizing protease-generated neoepitopes from cartilage proteoglycan degradation: application to studies of human link protein cleavage by stromelysin. *J Biol Chem* 1992;267:16011–16014.
419. Hughes CE, Caterson B, Fosang AJ, et al. Monoclonal antibodies that specifically recognize neoepitope sequences generated by "aggrecanase" and matrix metalloproteinase cleavage of aggrecan: application to catabolism *in situ* and *in vitro*. *Biochem J* 1995;305:799–804.
420. Singer IJ, Kawka DW, Bayne EK, et al. VDIPEN, a metalloproteinase-generated neoepitope, is induced and immunolocalized in articular cartilage during inflammatory arthritis. *J Clin Invest* 1995; 95:2178–2186.
421. Billinghurst RC, Dahlberg L, Ionescu M, et al. Enhanced cleavage of type II collagen by collagenases in osteoarthritic articular cartilage. *J Clin Invest* 1997;99:1534–1545.
422. Hollander A, Heathfield TF, Webber C, et al. Increased damage to type II collagen in osteoarthritic cartilage detected by a new immunoassay. *J Clin Invest* 1994;93:1722–1732.
423. Dean DD, Muniz OE, Woessner JF Jr, et al. Production of collagenase and tissue inhibitor of metalloproteinases by rat growth plates in culture. *Matrix* 1990;10:320–330.
424. Dean DD, Martel-Pelletier J, Pelletier JP, et al. Evidence for metalloproteinase and metalloproteinase inhibitor imbalance in human osteoarthritic cartilage. *J Clin Invest* 1989;84:678–685.
425. Yamada H, Nakagawa T, Stephens RW, et al. Proteinases and their inhibitors in normal and osteoarthritic articular cartilage. *Biomed Res* 1987;8:289–300.
426. Huang W, Li WQ, Dehnade F, et al. Tissue inhibitor of metalloproteinase-4 (TIMP-4) gene expression is increased in human osteoarthritic femoral head cartilage. *J Cell Biochem* 2002;85:295–303.
427. Ellis AJ, Curry VA, Powell EK, et al. The prevention of collagen breakdown in bovine nasal cartilage by TIMP, TIMP-2 and a low molecular weight synthetic inhibitor. *Biochem Biophys Commun* 1994;201:94–101.
428. Barrett AJ. The cystatins: a new class of peptidase inhibitors. *TIPS* 1987;12:193–196.
429. Günther M, Haubeck H-D, Van de Leur E, et al. Transforming growth factor β1 regulates tissue inhibitor of metalloproteinases-1 expression in differentiated human articular chondrocytes. *Arthritis Rheum* 1994;37:395–405.
430. Lotz M, Guerne P-A. Interleukin-6 induces the synthesis of tissue inhibitor of metalloproteinases-1/erythroid potentiating activity (TIMP-1/EPA). *J Biol Chem* 1991;266:2017–2020.
431. Nemoto O, Yamada H, Mukaida M, et al. Stimulation of TIMP-1 production by oncostatin M in human articular cartilage. *Arthritis Rheum* 1996;39:560–566.
432. Maier R, Ganu V, Lotz M. Interleukin-11, an inducible cytokine in human articular chondrocytes and synoviocytes, stimulates the production of the tissue inhibitor of metalloproteinases. *J Biol Chem* 1993;268:21527–21532.
433. Brenner DA, O'Hara M, Angel P, et al. Prolonged activation of jun and collagenase genes by tumour necrosis factor α. *Nature* 1989;337: 661–663.
434. Lafyatis R, Kim S-J, Angel P, et al. Interleukin-1 stimulates and all-*trans*-retinoic acid inhibits collagenase gene expression through its 58 activator protein-1-binding site. *Mol Endocrinol* 1990;4:973–980.
435. Liacini A, Sylvester J, Li WQ, et al. Induction of matrix metalloproteinase-13 gene expression by TNFα is mediated by MAP kinases, AP-1, and NF-κB transcription factors in articular chondrocytes. *Exp Cell Res* 2003;288:208–217.
436. Mengshol JA, Vincenti MP, Coon CI, et al. Interleukin-1 induction of collagenase 3 (matrix metalloproteinase 13) gene expression in chondrocytes requires p38, C-JUN N-terminal kinase and nuclear factor Kβ. *Arthritis Rheum* 2000;43:801–811.
437. Ray A, Kwoki K, Cook JL et al. Induction of matrix metalloproteinase gene expression is regulated by inflammation-responsive transcription factor SAF-1 in osteoarthritis. *Arthritis Rheum* 2003;48:134–145.
438. Lo YYC, Wong JMS, Cruz TF. Reactive oxygen species mediate cytokine activation of c-Jun NH_2-terminal kinases. *J Biol Chem* 1996;271:15703–15707.
439. Lo YYC, Cruz TF. Involvement of reactive oxygen species in cytokine and growth factor induction of c-*fos* expression in chondrocytes. *J Biol Chem* 1995;270:11727–11730.
440. Benbow U, Brinckerhoff CE. The AP-1 site and MMP gene regulation: what is all the fuss about? *Matrix Biol* 1997;15:519–526.
441. Guerne P-A, Blanco F, Kadin A, et al. Growth factor responsiveness of human articular chondrocytes in aging and development. *Arthritis Rheum* 1995;38:960–968.
442. Martin JA, Buckwalter JA. Telomere erosion and senescence in human articular cartilage chondrocytes. *J Gerontol A Biol Sci Med Sci* 2001;56:B172–179.
443. Loesser RF, Shanker G, Carlson CS, et al. Reduction in the chondrocyte response to insulin-like growth factor 1 in ageing and osteoarthritis. Studies in a non-human primate model of naturally occurring disease. *Arthritis Rheum* 2000;43:2110–2120.
444. De Groot J, Verzijl N, Bank RA, et al. Age-related decrease in proteoglycan synthesis of human articular chondrocytes: the role of nonenzymatic glycation. *Arthritis Rheum* 1999;42:1003–1009.
445. Verzijl N, DeGroot J, Bank RA, et al. Age-related accumulation of the advanced glycation end product pentosidine in human articular cartilage aggrecan: the use of pentosidine levels as a quantitative measure of protein turnover. *Matrix Biol* 2001;20:409–417.

446. Bank RA, Bayliss MT, Lafeber F-PJG, et al. Ageing and zonal variation in posttranslational modification of collagen in normal human articular cartilage. *Biochem J* 1998;330:345–351.
447. Verzijl N, DeGroot J, Ben ZC, et al. Crosslinking by advanced glycation end products increases the stiffness of the collagen network in human articular cartilage: a possible mechanism through which age is a risk factor for osteoarthritis. *Arthritis Rheum* 2002;46:114–123.
448. DeGroot J, Verzijl N, Wentig-van Wijk MJG, et al. Age-related decrease in susceptibility of human articular cartilage to matrix metalloproteinase-mediated degradation. The role of advanced glycation end products. *Arthritis Rheum* 2001;44:2562–2571.
449. Dudhia J, Davidson CM, Wells TM, et al. Age-related changes in the content of the C-terminal region of aggrecan in human articular cartilage. *Biochem J* 1996;303:933–940.
450. Paulsson M, Morgelin M, Wiedemann H, et al. Extended and globular proteins domains in cartilage proteoglycans. *Biochem J* 1987;245:763–772.
451. Franzen A, Inerot S, Hejderup S-O, et al. Variations in the composition of bovine hip articular cartilage with distance from the articular surface. *Biochem J* 1981;195:535–543.
452. Bayliss MT, Ali SY. Age-related changes in the composition and structure of human articular-cartilage proteoglycans. *Biochem J* 1978;176:683–693.
453. Maraoudas A, Bayliss MT, Uchitel-Kaushansky N, et al. Aggrecan turnover in human articular cartilage: use of asparitic acid racemization as a marker of molecular age. *Arch Biochem Biophys* 1998;350:61–71.
454. Maroudas A, Bayliss MT, Uchitel-Kaushansky N, et al. Aggrecan turnover in human articular cartilage: use of aspartic acid racemization as a marker of molecular age. *Arch Biochem Biophys* 1998;350:61–71.
455. Nguyen Q, Liu J, Roughley PJ, et al. Link protein as a monitor of endogenous proteolysis in adult human articular cartilage. *Biochem J* 1991;278:143–147.
456. Kempson GE. Relationship between the tensile properties of articular cartilage from the human knee and age. *Ann Rheum Dis* 1982;41:508–511.
457. Venn MF. Variation of chemical composition with age in human femoral head cartilage. *Ann Rheum Dis* 1978;37:168–174.
458. Kempson GE. Age-related changes in the tensile properties of human articular cartilage: a comparative study between the femoral head of the hip joint and the talus of the ankle joint. *Biochim Biophys Acta* 1991;1075:223–230.
459. Armstrong CG, Mow VC. Variations in the intrinsic mechanical properties of human articular cartilage with age, degeneration and water content. *J Bone Joint Surg Am* 1982;64:88–94.
460. Hudelmaier M, Glaser C, Hohe J, et al. Age-related changes in the morphology and deformational behaviour of knee joint cartilage. *Arthritis Rheum* 2001;44:2556–2561.
461. Setton LA, Mow VC, Müller FJ, et al. Mechanical properties of canine articular cartilage are significantly altered following transection of the anterior cruciate ligament. *J Orthop Res* 1994;12:451–463.
462. Guilak F, Ratcliffe A, Lane N, et al. Mechanical and biochemical changes in the superficial zone of articular cartilage in canine experimental osteoarthritis. *J Orthop Res* 1994;12:474–484.
463. Aurich M, Poole AR, Reiner A, et al. Matrix homeostasis in aging normal ankle cartilage. *Arthritis Rheum* 2002;46:2903–2910.
464. Rizkalla G, Bogoch ER, Poole AR. Studies of the articular cartilage proteoglycan aggrecan in health and osteoarthritis: evidence for molecular heterogeneity and extensive molecular changes in disease. *J Clin Invest* 1992;90:2268–2277.
465. Malfait A-M, Liu R-Q, Ijiri K, et al. Inhibition of ADAM-TS4 and ADAM-TS5 prevents aggrecan degradation in osteoarthritic cartilage. *J Biol Chem* 2002;277:22201–22208.
466. Squires G, Okouneff S, Ionescu M, et al. Pathobiology of focal lesion development in aging human articular cartilage reveals molecular matrix changes characteristic of osteoarthritis. *Arthritis Rheum* 2003;48:1261–1270.
467. Sweet M, Thonar E, Immelman A, et al. Biochemical changes in progressive osteoarthrosis. *Ann Rheum Dis* 1977;36:387–398.
468. Price JS, Bickerstaff DR, Bayliss MT, et al. Degradation of cartilage type II collagen precedes the onset of osteoarthritis following anterior cruciate ligament rupture. *Arthritis Rheum* 1999;42:2390–2398.
469. Stoop, R, van der Kraan PM, Buma P, et al. Type II collagen degradation in spontaneous osteoarthritis in C57/Bl/6 and BALB/c mice. *Arthritis Rheum* 1999;42:2381–2389.
470. Melchiorri C, Meliconi R, Frizziero L, et al. Enhanced and coordinated in vivo expression of inflammatory cytokines and nitric oxide synthase by chondrocytes from patients with osteoarthritis. *Arthritis Rheum* 1998;41:2165–2174.
471. Westacott CI, Sharif M. Cytokines in osteoarthritis: mediators or markers of joint destruction. *Semin Arthritis Rheum* 1996;25:254–272.
472. Westacott CI, Atkins RM, Dieppe PA, et al. Tumor necrosis factor-α receptor expression on chondrocytes isolated from human articular cartilage. *J Rheumatol* 1994;21:1710–1715.
473. Webb GR, Westacott CI, Elson CJ. Chondrocyte tumor necrosis factor receptors and focal loss of cartilage in osteoarthritis. *Osteoarthritis Cartilage* 1997;5:427–437, 543.
474. Martel-Pelletier J, McCollum R, DiBattista JA, et al. The interleukin-1 receptor in normal and osteoarthritic human articular chondrocytes: identification as the type I receptor and analysis of binding kinetics and biologic function. *Arthritis Rheum* 1992;35:530–540.
475. Pickvance EA, Oegema J-R Jr, Thompson RC Jr. Immunolocalization of selected cytokines and proteases in canine articular cartilage transarticular loading. *J Orthop Res* 1993;11:313–323.
476. Barakat AF, Elson CJ, Westacott CI. Susceptibility to physiological concentrations of IL-1β varies in cartilage at different anatomical locations on human osteoarthritic knee joints. *Osteoarthritis Cartilage* 2002;10:264–269.
477. Matsumoto T, Tsukazaki T, Enomoto H, et al. Effects of interleukin-1β on insulin-like growth factor-1 autocrine/paracrine axis in cultured rat articular chondrocytes. *Ann Rheum Dis* 1994;53:128–133.
478. Schneiderman R, Rosenberg N, Hiss J, et al. Concentration and size distribution of insulin-like growth factor-2 in human normal and osteoarthritic synovial fluid and cartilage. *Arch Biochem Biophys* 1995;324:173–188.
479. Doré S, Pelletier J-P, DiBattista JA, et al. Human osteoarthritic chondrocytes possess an increased number of insulin-like growth factor 1 binding sites but are unresponsive to its stimulation: possible role of IGF-1 binding proteins. *Arthritis Rheum* 1994;37:253–263.
480. Morales TI. The insulin-like growth factor binding proteins in uncultured human cartilage. Increases in insulin-like growth factor binding proteins during osteoarthritis. *Arthritis Rheum* 2002;46:2358–2367.
481. Attur MG, Dave MN, Stuchin S, et al. Osteopontin: an intrinsic inhibitor in cartilage. *Arthritis Rheum* 2001;44:578–584.
482. Johnson K, Goding J, Van Etten D, et al. Linked deficiencies in extracellular PP(i) and osteopontin mediate pathologic calcification associated with defective PC-1 and ANK expression. *J Bone Miner Res* 2003;18:994–1004.
483. Goldring MB. The role of the chondrocyte in osteoarthritis. *Arthritis Rheum* 2000;43:1916–1926.
484. Poole AR, Howell DS. Etiopathogenesis of osteoarthritis. In: Moskowitz R, Goldberg V, Howell DS, et al., eds. *Osteoarthritis: diagnosis and medical/surgical management*, 3rd ed. Philadelphia: WB Saunders, 2001:29–47.
485. Fenwick SA, Gregg PJ, Rooney P. Osteoarthritic cartilage loses its ability to remain avascular. *Osteoarthritis Cartilage* 1999;7:441–452.
486. Burkhardt H, Schwingel M, Menninger H, et al. Oxygen radicals as effectors of cartilage destruction: direct degradative effect on matrix components and indirect action via activation of latent collagenase from polymorphonuclear leukocytes. *Arthritis Rheum* 1986;29:379–387.
487. Lethwaite J, Blake S, Hardingham T, et al. Role of TNF-α in the induction of antigen induced arthritis in the rabbit and the anti-arthritic effect of species specific TNF-α neutralizing monoclonal antibodies. *Ann Rheum Dis* 1995;54:366–374.
488. Chu CQ, Field M, Allard S, et al. Detection of cytokines at the cartilage/pannus junction in patients with rheumatoid arthritis: implications for the role of cytokines in cartilage destruction and repair. *Br J Rheumatol* 1992;31:653–661.
489. van Loo FAJ, Joosten LAB, van Lent PLEM, et al. Role of interleukin-1, tumor necrosis factor α, and interleukin-6 in cartilage proteoglycan metabolism and destruction: effect of *in situ* blocking in murine antigen and zymosan induced arthritis. *Arthritis Rheum* 1995;38:164–172.
490. Joosten LA, Helsen MM, Saxne T, et al. IL-1 alpha beta blockade prevents cartilage and bone destruction in murine type II collagen-induced arthritis whereas TNF-alpha blockade only ameliorates joint inflammation. *J Immunol* 1999;163:5049–5055.

491. van den Berg WB, van de Loo F, Joosten LA, et al. Animal models of arthritis in NOS2-deficient mice. *Osteoarthritis Cartilage* 1999;7: 413–415.
492. Okimura A, Okada Y, Makihira S, et al. Enhancement of cartilage matrix protein synthesis in arthritic cartilage. *Arthritis Rheum* 1997; 40:1029–1036.
493. Poole AR, Ionescu M, Swan A, et al. Changes in cartilage metabolism in arthritis are reflected by altered serum and synovial fluid levels of the cartilage proteoglycan aggrecan: implications for pathogenesis. *J Clin Invest* 1994;94:25–33.
494. Lohmander LS, Dahlberg L, Ryd L, et al. Increased levels of proteoglycan fragments in knee joint fluid after injury. *Arthritis Rheum* 1989;32:1434–1442.
495. Saxne T, Heinegaärd D. Synovial fluid analysis of two groups of proteoglycan epitopes distinguishes early and late cartilage lesions. *Arthritis Rheum* 1992;35:385–390.
496. Lohmander LS, Ionescu M, Jugessur H, et al. Changes in joint cartilage aggrecan after knee injury and in osteoarthritis. *Arthritis Rheum* 1999;42:534–544.
497. Månsson B, Carey D, Alini M, et al. Cartilage and bone metabolism in rheumatoid arthritis: differences between rapid and slow progression of disease identified by serum markers of cartilage metabolism. *J Clin Invest* 1995;95:1071–1077.
498. Poole AR. Can osteoarthritis as a disease be distinguished from ageing by skeletal and inflammation markers? Implications for "early" diagnosis, monitoring skeletal changes and effects of therapy. In: Hamerman D, ed. *Osteoarthritis and the ageing population.* Baltimore: Johns Hopkins University Press, 1997:187–214.
499. Spector TD, Woodward L, Hall GM, et al. Keratan sulphate in rheumatoid arthritis, osteoarthritis and inflammatory diseases. *Ann Rheum Dis* 1992;51:1134–1137.
500. Poole AR, Witter J, Roberts N, et al. Inflammation and cartilage metabolism in rheumatoid arthritis: studies of the blood markers hyaluronic acid, orosomucoid and keratan sulfate. *Arthritis Rheum* 1990; 33:790–799.
501. Manicourt D-A, Troki R, Fukuda K, et al. Levels of circulating tumor necrosis factor α and interleukin-6 in patients with rheumatoid arthritis: relationship to serum levels of hyaluronan and antigenic keratan sulfate. *Arthritis Rheum* 1993;36:490–499.
502. Sharif M, Saxne T, Shepstone L, et al. Relationship between serum cartilage oligomeric matrix protein levels and disease progression in osteoarthritis of the knee joint. *Br J Rheumatol* 1995;34:306–310.
503. Peterson IF, Boegsrd T, Svensson B, et al. Changes in cartilage and bone metabolism identified by serum markers in early osteoarthritis of the knee joints. *Br J Rheumatol* 1998;37:46–50.
504. Sharif M, George E, Shepstone L, et al. Serum hyaluronic acid level as a predictor of disease progression in osteoarthritis of the knee. *Arthritis Rheum* 1995;38:760–767.
505. Sharma L, Hurwitz DE, Thonar EJ-MA, et al. Knee adduction moment, serum hyaluronan level, and disease severity in medial tibiofemoral osteoarthritis. *Arthritis Rheum* 1998;41:1233–1240.
506. Poole AR, Dieppe P. Biological markers in rheumatoid arthritis. *Semin Arthritis Rheum* 1994;23:17–31.
507. Recklies AD, Baillargeon L, White C. Regulation of cartilage oligomeric matrix protein synthesis in human synovial cells and articular chondrocytes. *Arthritis Rheum* 1998;41:997–1006.
508. Clark AG, Jordan JM, Vilim V, et al. Serum cartilage oligomeric matrix protein reflects osteoarthritis presence and severity. *Arthritis Rheum* 1999;42:2356–2364.
509. Song X-Y, Zeng L, Jin W, et al. Secretory leukocyte protease inhibitor suppresses the inflammation and joint damage of bacterial and wall-induced arthritis. *J Exp Med* 1999;190:535–542.
510. Christgau S, Garnero P, Filedelius C, et al. Collagen type II c-telopeptide fragments as an index of cartilage degradation. *Bone* 2001;29:209–215.
511. Downs JT, Lane CL, Nestor NB, et al. Analysis of collagenase cleavage of type II collagen using a neoepitope ELISA. *J Immunol Methods* 2001;247:25–34.
512. Poole AR. Biochemical/immunochemical biomarkers of osteoarthritis: Utility for prediction of incident or progressive osteoarthritis. *Rheum Dis Clin North Am* 2003;29:803–818.
513. Saxne T, Heinegård D. Involvement of nonarticular cartilage, as demonstrated by release of a cartilage-specific protein in rheumatoid arthritis. *Arthritis Rheum* 1989;32:1080–1086.
514. Garnero P, Ayral X, Rousseau J-C, et al. Uncoupling of type II collagen synthesis and degradation predicts progression of joint damage in patients with knee osteoarthritis. *Arthritis Rheum* 2002;46:2613–2624.
515. Bleasel JF, Poole AR, Heinegård D, et al. Changes in serum cartilage marker levels indicate altered cartilage metabolism in families with the osteoarthritis-related type II collagen gene COL2A1 mutation. *Arthritis Rheum* 1999;42:39–45.
516. Garnero P, Gineyts E, Christian S, et al. Association of urinary glycosyl-galactosyl-pyridinoline and type II collagen C-telopeptide with progression of joint destruction in patients with early rheumatoid arthritis. *Arthritis Rheum* 2002;46:21–30.
517. Garnero P, Landewé R, Boers M, et al. Association of baseline levels of markers of bone and cartilage degradation with long-term progression of joint damage in patients with early rheumatoid arthritis. The Cobra Study. *Arthritis Rheum* 2002;46:2843–2856.
518. Saxne T, Castro F, Rydholm U, et al. Cartilage derived proteoglycans in body fluids of children: inverse correlation with age. *J Rheumatol* 1989;16:1341–1344.
519. Thonar EJM, Pachman LM, Lenz ME, et al. Age related changes in the concentration of serum keratan sulfate in children. *J Clin Chem Clin Biochem* 1988;26:57–63.
520. Pachman LM, Green OC, Lenz ME, et al. Increase in serum concentrations of keratan sulfate after treatment of growth hormone deficiency with growth hormone. *J Pediatr* 1990;116:400–403.
521. Carey D, Alini M, Poole AR, et al. Serum content of the C-propeptide of the cartilage molecule type II collagen in children. *Clin Exp Rheumatol* 1997;15:325–328.
522. Maroudas A. Transport of solutes through cartilage, permeability to large molecules. *J Anat* 1976;122:335–347.
523. Poole AR, Barratt MEJ, Fell HB. The role of soft connective tissue in the breakdown of pig articular cartilage in the presence of complement-sufficient antiserum to pig erythrocytes. II. Distribution of immunoglobulin G (IgG). *Int Arch Allergy Appl Immunol* 1973;44:469–488.
524. Konttinen YT, Li T-F, Lassus J, et al. Removal of hyaline articular cartilage reduces lymphocyte infiltration and activation in rheumatoid synovial membrane. *J Rheumatol* 2001;28:2184–2189.
525. Burmester GR, Menche D, Merryman P, et al. Application of monoclonal antibodies to the characterization of cells eluted from human articular cartilage: expression of Ia antigen in certain diseases and identification of an 85-kD cell surface molecule accumulated in the pericellular matrix. *Arthritis Rheum* 1983;26:1187–1195.
526. Jahn B, Burmester GR, Schmid HJ, et al. Changes in cell surface antigen expression on human articular chondrocytes induced by γ-interferon. *Arthritis Rheum* 1987;30:64–74.
527. Boissier MC, Chiocchia G, Texier B, et al. Pattern of humoral reactivity to type II collagen in rheumatoid arthritis. *Clin Exp Immunol* 1989;78:177–183.
528. Morgan K, Clague RB, Collins I, et al. Incidence of antibodies to native and denatured cartilage collagens (types II, IX and XI) and to type I collagen in rheumatoid arthritis. *Ann Rheum Dis* 1987;46: 902–907.
529. Worthington J, Turner S, Brass A, et al. Epitopes on the CB-11 peptide of type II collagen recognized by antibodies from patients with rheumatoid arthritis. *Br J Rheumatol* 1993;32:658–662.
530. Trentham DE, Kammer GM, McCune WJ, et al. Autoimmunity to collagen: a shared feature of psoriatic and rheumatoid arthritis. *Arthritis Rheum* 1981;24:1363–1369.
531. Clague RB, Shaw MJ, Holt PJL. Incidence of serum antibodies to native type I and type II collagens in patients with inflammatory arthritis. *Ann Rheum* 1980;39:201–206.
532. Möttönen T, Hannonen P, Oka M, et al. Antibodies against native type II collagen do not precede the clinical onset of rheumatoid arthritis. *Arthritis Rheum* 1988;31:776–779.
533. Andriopoulos NA, Mestecky J, Miller EJ, et al. Antibodies to human native and denatured collagens in synovial fluids of patients with rheumatoid arthritis. *Clin Immunol Immunopathol* 1976; 6:209–212.
533a. Mestecky J, Miller EJ. Presence of antibodies specific to cartilage-type collagen in rheumatoid synovial tissue. *Clin Exp Immunol* 1975; 22:453–456.
534. Tarkowski A, Klareskog L, Carlsten H, et al. Secretion of antibodies to types I and II collagen by synovial tissue cells in patients with rheumatoid arthritis. *Arthritis Rheum* 1989;32:1087–1092.

535. Burkhardt H, Koller T, Engstrom A, et al. Epitope-specific recognition of type II collagen by rheumatoid arthritis antibodies is shared with recognition by antibodies that are arthritogenic in collagen-induced arthritis in the mouse. *Arthritis Rheum* 2002;46:2339–2348.
536. Wooley PH, Luthra HS, Singh SK, et al. Passive transfer of arthritis to mice by injection of human anti-type II collagen antibody. *Mayo Clin Proc* 1984;59:737–743.
537. Foidart JM, Abe S, Martin GR, et al. Antibodies to type II collagen in relapsing polychondritis. *N Engl J Med* 19789;299:1203–1207.
538. Ebringer R, Rook G, Swana GT, et al. Autoantibodies to cartilage and type II collagen in relapsing polychondritis and other rheumatic diseases. *Ann Rheum Dis* 1981;40:473–479.
539. Meyer O, Cyna J, Dryll A, et al. Relapsing polychondritis-pathogenic role of anti-native collagen type II antibodies. *J Rheumatol* 1981;8: 820–824.
540. Yoo T, Stuart JM, Kang AH, et al. Type II collagen autoimmunity in otosclerosis and Meniere's disease. *Science* 1982;217:1153–1155.
541. Golds EE, Stephen IBM, Esdaile JM, et al. Lymphocyte transformation to connective tissue antigens in adult and juvenile rheumatoid arthritis, osteoarthritis, ankylosing spondylitis, systemic lupus erythematosus and non-arthritic control populations. *Cell Immunol* 1983;82: 196–209.
542. Stuart JM, Postlethwaite AZ, Townes AS, et al. Cell mediated immunity to collagen and collagen a chains in rheumatoid arthritis and other rheumatic diseases. *Am J Med* 1980;69:13–18.
543. Londei M, Savill CM, Verhoef A, et al. Persistence of collagen type II-specific T cell clones in the synovial membrane of a patient with rheumatoid arthritis. *Proc Natl Acad Sci U S A* 1989;86:636–640.
544. Glant T, Csongar J, Szucs T. Immunopathologic role of proteoglycan antigens in rheumatoid joint disease. *Scand J Immunol* 1980;11:247–252.
545. Mikecz K, Glant TT, Baron M, et al. Isolation of proteoglycan specific T lymphocytes from patients with ankylosing spondylitis. *Cell Immunol* 1988;112:55–63.
546. Rajapakse D, Bywaters E. Cell mediated immunity to cartilage proteoglycans in relapsing polychondritis. *Clin Exp Immunol* 1974;16: 497–502.
547. Herman J, Dennis M. Immunopathologic studies in relapsing polychondritis. *J Clin Invest* 1973;52:549–588.
548. Guerassimov A, Zhang Y, Banerjee S, et al. Cellular immunity to the G1 domain of cartilage proteoglycan aggrecan is enhanced in patients with rheumatoid arthritis but only after removal of keratan sulfate. *Arthritis Rheum* 1998;41:1019–1025.
549. Guerassimov A, Zhang Y, Cartman A, et al. Immune responses to cartilage link protein and the G1 domain of proteoglycan aggrecan in patients with osteoarthritis. *Arthritis Rheum* 1999;42:527–533.
550. Guerassimov A, Duffy C, Banerjee S, et al. Immunity to cartilage link protein is observed in patients with juvenile rheumatoid arthritis. *J Rheumatol* 1997;27:959–964.
551. Poole AR, Pidoux I, Reiner A, et al. Mammalian eyes and associated tissues contain molecules that are immunologically related to cartilage proteoglycan and link protein. *J Cell Biol* 1982;93:910–920.
552. Cöster L, Rosenberg LC, van der Rest M, et al. The dermatan sulfate proteoglycans of bovine sclera and their relationship to those of articular cartilage: an immunological and biochemical study. *J Biol Chem* 1985;260:6020–6025.
553. Poole AR. The histopathology of ankylosing spondylitis: are there unifying hypotheses? *Am J Med Sci* 1998;316:228–233.
554. Shi S, Ciurli C, Cartman A, et al. Experimental immunity to the G1 domain of the proteoglycan versican induces spondylitis and sacroiliitis of a kind seen in human spondyloarthropathies. *Arthritis Rheum* 2003;48:2903–2915.
555. Dolan DL, Lemmon GB, Teitelbaum SL. Relapsing polychondritis: analytical review and studies on pathogenesis. *Am J Med* 1966;41: 285–299.
556. Calin A. Ankylosing spondylitis. In: Kelley WN, Harris ED Jr, Ruddy S, et al., eds. *Textbook of rheumatology,* 2nd ed. Philadelphia: WB Saunders, 1989:1021–1037.
557. Tessler HH. The eye in rheumatic diseases. *Bull Rheum Dis* 1985; 35:1–8.
558. McKay DAR, Watson PG, Lyne AJ. Relapsing polychondritis and eye disease. *Br J Ophthalmol* 1974;58:600–605.
559. Van Eden W, Holoshitz J, Nevo Z, et al. Arthritis induced by a T-lymphocyte clone that responds to *Mycobacterium tuberculosis* and to cartilage proteoglycans. *Proc Natl Acad Sci U S A* 1985;82: 5117–5120.
560. Van Eden W, Thole JER, van der Zee R, et al. Cloning of the mycobacterial epitope recognized by T lymphocytes in adjuvant arthritis. *Nature* 1988;331:171–173.
561. Trentham DE, Townes AS, Kang AH. Autoimmunity to type II collagen: an experimental model of arthritis. *J Exp Med* 1977;146: 857–868.
562. Cremer MA, Terato K, Seyer JM, et al. Immunity to type XI collagen in mice: evidence that the α3(XI) chain of type XI collagen and the α1(II) chain of type II collagen share arthritogenic determinants and induce arthritis in DBA/1 mice. *J Immunol* 1991;146:4130–4137.
563. Boissier M-C, Chiocchia G, Ronziere M-C, et al. Arthritogenicity of minor cartilage collagens (types IX and XI) in mice. *Arthritis Rheum* 1990;33:1–8.
564. Leroux J-Y, Poole AR, Webber C, et al. Characterization of proteoglycan-reactive T cell lines and hybridomas from mice with proteoglycan-induced arthritis. *J Immunol* 1992;148:2090–2096.
565. Glant T, Mikecz K. Antigenic profiles of human, bovine and canine articular chondrocytes. *Cell Tissue Res* 1986;244:359–369.
566. Zhang Y, Guerassimov A, Leroux J-Y, et al. Induction of arthritis in BALB/c mice by cartilage link protein: the involvement of distinct regions recognized by T and B lymphocytes. *Am J Pathol* 1998;153: 1283–1291.
567. Verheijden GFM, Rijnders AWM, Bos E, et al. Human cartilage glycoprotein-39 as a candidate autoantigen in rheumatoid arthritis. *Arthritis Rheum* 1997;40:1115–1125.
568. Leroux J-Y, Guerassimov A, Cartman A, et al. Immunity to the G1 domain of the cartilage proteoglycan aggrecan can induce inflammatory erosive polyarthritis and spondylitis on BALB/c mice but immunity to G1 is inhibited by covalently bound keratan sulfate *in vitro* and *in vivo. J Clin Invest* 1996;97:621–632.
569. Gillet P, Bannwarth B, Charriere G, et al. Studies on type II collagen induced arthritis in rats: an experimental model of peripheral and axial ossifying enthesopathy. *J Rheumatol* 1989;16:721–728.
570. Takenaka Y, Kahan A, Amor B. Experimental autoimmune spondylodiscitis in rats. *J Rheumatol* 1986;13:397–499.
571. Zhang Y, Guerassimov A, Leroux J-Y, et al. Arthritis induced by proteoglycan aggrecan G1 domain in BALB/c mice: evidence for T-cell involvement and the immunosuppressive influence of keratan sulfate on recognition of T and B cell epitopes. *J Clin Invest* 1998;101: 1678–1686.
572. Glant TT, Mikecz K, Roughley PJ, et al. Age-related changes in protein-related epitopes of human articular cartilage proteoglycans. *Biochem J* 1986;236:71–75.
573. Hansson A-S, Heinegård D, Holmdahl R. A new animal model for relapsing polychondritis, induced by cartilage matrix protein (matrilin-1). *J Clin Invest* 1999;104:589–598.
574. Hansson A-S, Heinegård D, Piette J-C, et al. The occurrence of autoantibodies to matrilin-1 reflects a tissue specific response to cartilage of the respiratory tract in patients with relapsing polychondritis. *Arthritis Rheum* 2001;44:2402–2412.
575. Huang CC, Saporta D, Abramson M. Type II collagen induced bone resorption in the temporal bone of rats: histological and immunohistochemical studies. *Arch Otorhinolaryngol* 1985;242:183–188.
576. Huang CC, Saporta D, Abramson M. Immunologically induced salpingitis in rats. *Am J Otolaryngol* 1985;6:368–372.
577. Stevenson S. The immune response to osteochondral allografts in dogs. *J Bone Joint Surg Am* 1989;69:573–582.
578. Stevenson S, Dannucci GA, Sharkey NA, et al. The fate of articular cartilage after transplantation of fresh and cryopreserved tissue-antigen-matched and mismatched osteochondral allografts in dogs. *J Bone Joint Surg Am* 1989;71:1297–1307.
579. Yablon IG, Brandt KD, Deheblis R, et al. Destruction of joint homografts: an experimental study. *Arthritis Rheum* 1977;20:1526–1537.
580. Sengupta S. The fate of transplants of articular cartilage in the rabbit. *J Bone Joint Surg Br* 1974;56:167–177.
581. Millroy SJ, Poole AR. Pig articular cartilage in organ culture: effect of enzymatic depletion of the matrix on response of chondrocytes to complement-sufficient antiserum against pig erythrocytes. *Ann Rheum Dis* 1974;33:500–508.

582. Fell HB, Barratt MEJ, Welland H, et al. The capacity of pig articular cartilage in organ culture to regenerate after breakdown induced by complement-sufficient antiserum to pig erythrocytes. *Calcif Tissue Res* 1976;20:3–21.
583. Fell HB, Barratt MEJ. The role of soft connective tissue in the breakdown of pig articular cartilage cultivated in the presence of complement-sufficient antiserum to pig erythrocytes. I. Histological changes. *Int Arch Allergy* 1973;44:441–468.
584. Fell HB, Jubb RW. The effect of synovial tissue on the breakdown of articular cartilage in organ culture. *Arthritis Rheum* 1977;20:1359–1371.
585. Gross AE, Silverstein EA, Falk J, et al. The allotransplantation of partial joints in the treatment of osteoarthritis of the knee. *Clin Orthop* 1975;108:7–14.
586. Parrish FF. Allograft replacement of all or part of the end of a long bone following excision of a tumor: report of twenty-one cases. *J Bone Joint Surg Am* 1973;55:1–22.
587. McDermott AGP, Langer F, Pritzker kPH, Gross AE. Fresh small-fragment osteochondral allografts: long-term follow-up study on first 100 cases. *Clin Orthop* 1985;197:96–102.
588. Czitrom AA, Langer F, McKnee N, et al. Bone and cartilage allotransplantation: a review of 14 years of research and clinical studies. *Clin Orthop* 1985;208:141–145.
589. Gross AE, Garel A, Langer F, et al. Analysis of the histopathology of failed fresh osteochondral allografts. *Orthop Trans* 1984;8:399.
590. Zukor DJ, Gross AE. Osteochondral allograft reconstruction of the knee. Part I: a review. *Am J Knee Surg* 1989;2:139–149.
591. Mankin HJ, Gebhardt MC, Tomford WW. The use of frozen cadaveric allografts in the management of patients with bone tumors of the extremities. *Orthop Clin North Am* 1987;18:275–289.
592. Zukor DJ, Oakeshott RD, Gross AE. Osteochondral allograft reconstruction of the knee. Part 2: Experience with successful and failed fresh osteochondral allografts. *Am J Knee Surg* 1989;2:182–191.
593. Zukor DJ, Cameron JC, Brooks PJ, et al. The fate of human meniscal allografts. In: Ewing JW, ed. *Articular cartilage and knee joint function: basic science and arthroscopy.* New York: Raven, 1990:147–152.
594. Bernstein B, Forrester D, Singsen B, et al. Hip joint restoration in juvenile rheumatoid arthritis. *Arthritis Rheum* 1977;20:1099–1104.
595. Garcia-Morteo O, Babini JC, Maldonado-Cocco JA, et al. Remodelling of the hip joint in juvenile rheumatoid arthritis. *Arthritis Rheum* 1981;24:1570–1574.
596. Brittberg M, Lindahl A, Nilsson A, et al. Treatment of deep cartilage defects in the knee with autologous chondrocyte transplantation. *N Engl J Med* 1994;331:889–895.
597. O'Driscoll SW, Salter RB. The induction of neochondrogenesis in free intra-articular periosteal autografts under the influence of continuous passive motion: an experimental investigation in the rabbit. *J Bone Joint Surg Am* 1984;66:1248–1257.
598. O'Driscoll SW, Keeley FW, Salter RB. Durability of regenerated articular cartilage produced by free autogenous periosteal grafts in major full-thickness defects in joint surfaces under the influence of continuous passive motion: a follow-up report at one year. *J Bone Joint Surg Am* 1988;70:595–606.
599. O'Driscoll SW, Keeley FW, Salter RB. The chondrogenic potential of free autogenous periosteal grafts for biological resurfacing of major full-thickness defects in joint surfaces under the influence of continuous passive motion: an experimental investigation in the rabbit. *J Bone Joint Surg Am* 1986;68:1017–1035.
600. Freed LE, Grande DA, Lingbin Z, et al. Joint resurfacing using allograft chondrocytes and synthetic biodegradable polymer-scaffolds. *J Biomed Mater Res* 1994;28:891–899.
601. Buckwalter JA, Mankin HJ. Articular cartilage repair and transplantation. *Arthritis Rheum* 1998;41:1331–1342.
602. Wright BA, Cohen MM Jr. Tumors of cartilage. In: Hall BH, ed. *Cartilage.* Vol 3. Orlando: Academic, 1983:143–163.
603. Dahlin DC, Unni KK. *Bone tumors: general aspects and data on 8,542 cases*, 4th ed. Springfield, IL: Charles C Thomas, 1986.
604. Aigner T. Towards a new understanding and classification of chondrogenic neoplasias of the skeleton-biochemistry and cell biology of chondrosarcoma and its variants. *Virchows Arch* 2002;441:219–230.
605. Wang ZQ, Grigoriadis AE, Mohle-Steinlein U, et al. A novel target cell for c-fos-induced oncogenesis: development of chondrogenic tumours in embryonic stem cell chimeras. *EMBO J* 1991;10:2437–2450.
606. Pal S, Strider W, Margolis R, et al. Isolation and characterization of proteoglycans from human chondrosarcomas. *J Biol Chem* 1978; 253:1279–1289.
607. Mallein-Gerin F, Olsen BR. Expression of simian virus 40 large T (tumor) oncogene in mouse chondrocytes induces cell proliferation without loss of the differentiated phenotype. *Proc Natl Acad Sci U S A* 1993;90:3289–3293.
608. Goldring MB, Birkhead JR, Suen L-F, et al. Interleukin-1β-modulated gene expression in immortalized human chondrocytes. *J Clin Invest* 1994;94:2307–2316.

CHAPTER 12

Structure and Function of Synoviocytes

Ulf Müller-Ladner, Renate E. Gay, and Steffen Gay

During the past decade, molecular biology has provided new insights into the role and function of synovial cells in rheumatoid arthritis (RA). The synovial fibroblast (SF), also referred to as fibroblast-like synoviocyte, previously considered a rather nondescript hyaluronic acid–producing lubricating cell, is now recognized as a pivotal pathogenic cell that mediates joint destruction in RA. In particular, the activated synoviocytes, initially described as "transformed-appearing" by Fassbender (1), or the activated SFs, are thought to be the cellular component of this destructive process.

The rapid accumulation of new data concerning these cells, facilitated by molecular analyses (2–4), has resulted in the recognition of at least two cellular pathways involved in rheumatoid joint destruction (5). Besides T cell–dependent pathways, the molecular and cellular characterization of T cell–independent pathways has emerged (6). Regarding the latter, the expression of certain protooncogenes (2,7), the attachment to articular cartilage, and the up-regulation of matrix-degrading metalloproteinases and cathepsins at sites of synovial attachment mediate the invasive and destructive growth of these cells (6).

Functional changes occurring in the rheumatoid synovium include an imbalance between synovial cell proliferation and apoptosis. In the absence of human T cells, the aggressive behavior of the rheumatoid SF is maintained for more than 220 days in the severe combined immunodeficiency (SCID) mouse model of RA involving coimplantation of RA synovium with normal human cartilage under the kidney capsule of these animals (8). In addition to cytokine-dependent pathways mediated by p38α and -β, evidence for a cytokine-independent activation pathway of SFs includes expression of endogenous L1 elements in these cells, leading to the up-regulation of p38δ, a strong inducer of matrix metalloproteinase-1 (MMP-1) (9). Moreover, evidence for cytokine-independent induction of chemokine secretion by SFs via Toll-like receptor 2 (TLR-2) indicates that SFs are part of the innate immune system and likely play an important role in the induction of inflammation in the synovium (10). Both key pathways are illustrated in Fig. 12.1.

In this chapter the specific properties of RA SFs are compared with other fibroblasts and synovial cells. These properties have led to the designation of these cells as "transformed aggressors" (11,12) or simply activated SFs.

CLASSIFICATION, MORPHOLOGY, AND NORMAL FUNCTION OF SYNOVIOCYTES

In normal, healthy synovium, synoviocytes are the predominant cell type of the terminal layer lining the joint cav-

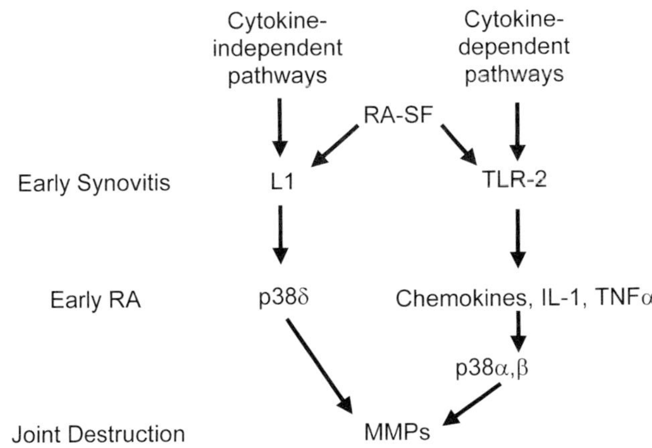

FIG. 12.1. Cytokine-dependent and -independent activation mechanisms in rheumatoid synovial fibroblasts. The figure illustrates the potential involvement of different activation mechanisms for an extended period of time. Cytokine-independent stimulation leads to an upregulation of the L1 element (9) in early arthritis followed by activation of the p38δ mitogen-activated protein (MAP) kinase resulting in production of matrix metalloproteinases (MMPs) and joint destruction. The second, cytokine-driven pathway acts via Toll-like receptor (TLR)-2, followed by synthesis of interleukin-1 and tumor necrosis factor-α (TNFα), and subsequent p38α and β MAP kinase, also followed by MMP production in the rheumatoid joint.

ity. In the sublining, fibroblasts, macrophages, mast cells, vascular cells, and lymphatic cells are found. Although all of these cell types comprise the synovium and vary considerably in number (13), only two distinct cells are regarded as synoviocytes. These two cell types form the lining layer, usually one to three cells deep, and are not separated from the underlying connective tissue by a basement membrane. Based on their morphology and molecular surface markers, type A synoviocytes resemble tissue macrophages, whereas type B synoviocytes bear the characteristics of fibroblasts (14,15). The exact origin of both synovial cells is controversial (16). About two thirds of the synovial lining cells exhibit ultrastructural characteristics of type A synoviocytes, and one third those of type B. Intermediate cell types also have been described but not classified (17). These may represent a developmental stage of synoviocytes, but the possibility that they have distinct functions cannot yet be excluded.

Macrophage-like type A synoviocytes resemble tissue macrophages. Their shape varies, sometimes forming dendritic extensions. The nucleus is rich in heterochromatin, and they have numerous cytoplasmic vacuoles, a prominent Golgi apparatus, and little endoplasmic reticulum. Type B cells, with a bipolar shape, are synoviocytes that resemble tissue fibroblasts. Their endoplasmic reticulum is prominent, and the Golgi apparatus is well developed. Their nucleus is pale and usually exhibits a number of nucleoli. The shape of synoviocytes does not necessarily remain constant during their lifetime. In various diseases, synoviocytes frequently alter their morphologic appearance and undergo either proliferation or programmed cell death (apoptosis). The major functions of the synoviocytes forming the synovial membrane are to provide the joint cavity and the adjacent cartilage of the two articulating bones (and the resident chondrocytes) with lubricant molecules, such as hyaluronic acid, as well as oxygen and nutrients. Although sharing a common tissue location, the two types of synoviocytes have different biologic and molecular functions.

Macrophage-like type A synoviocytes express various cell surface macrophage markers, including CD11b, CD14, CD33, and CD68, although this characterization is limited by the variation in expression of CD antigens with different stages of activation (14,18,19). Type A synoviocytes, in addition to their typical phagocytic activity that is responsible for removal of debris from the joint cavity, possess antigen-processing properties. They express Fc receptors, estrogen and androgen receptors (reviewed in reference 20), as well as major histocompatibility complex (MHC) class II antigens [human leukocyte antigens (HLA) DR and DQ] (21,22). Another distinct population are the CD14/33-positive cells, sometimes designated dendritic cells (23), which appear to be associated with radiographic joint destruction in RA (24). These cells function as potent antigen-presenting cells (25). Another characteristic of type A synoviocytes that might contribute to inflammation in the synovium is their capability of generating prostaglandins in their lysosomes (26). Synovial macrophages drive the amplification of proinflammatory and matrix-degrading signals, which still leaves the question unanswered, whether these cells are a "mastermind" or a "workhorse" (27).

The production of hyaluronic acid for joint lubrication is one of the major properties of type B fibroblast-like synoviocytes. These cells also synthesize numerous matrix components, including collagen. Conversely, they are equipped with a variety of enzymes, which are capable of degrading cartilage and bone. Type B synoviocytes lack specific HLA DR marker molecules and cannot yet be detected by specific antibodies. Both types of synoviocytes, however, interact with each other and other cells by complementary adhesion molecules and through release of cytokines, growth factors, and chemokines, as outlined below. In further discussions of the biologic and functional properties of the two distinct types of synoviocytes, the type A synoviocytes are hereafter designated as synovial macrophages, and the type B synoviocytes as SFs.

Synoviocytes: Part of Synovial Histopathology

In general, the absolute number of every cell type is increased in the inflamed synovium. In inflammatory arthritides, infiltrations by blood-borne or bone marrow–derived cells, including T and B lymphocytes, as well as monocytes, are observed in the synovium. In early RA, although initial events are unknown and may even occur before inflammation is evident, a few lymphocytes accumulate in areas around terminal vessels (28). A prominent feature is the impressive increase of synoviocytes in the lining layer, including activated fibroblasts. The latter cells exhibit an activated phenotype and appear to destroy adjacent cartilage and bone invasively (5,6). They are characterized by large, pale nuclei containing prominent nucleoli and an abundant cytoplasm, therefore, to some extent, resembling transformed-appearing malignant cells (1). Activation of these cells is accompanied by enhanced expression of enzymes and signaling molecules (2). Synovial macrophages, on the other hand, may display various shapes and also contribute to the destructive characteristics of the RA synovium through up-regulation of cytokines and proteolytic enzymes. In contrast, fibrosis in rheumatoid synovium appears to be mediated by differentiation of certain SFs into myofibroblast-like cells when stimulated by transforming growth factor (TGF)-β (29).

ACTIVATION OF SYNOVIOCYTES

Possible Triggers for the Activation of Synoviocytes

As outlined above, activated synoviocytes are a pathohistologic feature of RA (5,6,11,12). Although these cells exhibit properties of activation or even of malignant cells, these properties do not imply uncontrolled proliferation but, rather, describe a state of metabolic cellular activation. Activated SFs are characterized by a dense, rough endoplasmic reticulum, numerous irregular nuclei, and changes in the normally spindle-shaped cell skeleton. Oncogene- or virus-derived gene sequences incorporated into the SF DNA, as demonstrated in an experimental model (30,31), might be the primary triggers for such an appearance. In rheumatic diseases, retroviruses have been repeatedly proposed as an etiologic factor for the induction of autoimmunity and cellular activation (32). In the context of a possible role for a retrovirus in these diseases, the reports describing the association of human T-cell lymphotropic virus type I (HTLV-I) with the development of a chronic arthropathy are of interest (33). On the other hand, cellular activation requires at least two cooperating oncogenes (34,35). A prototype model for a retrovirus-induced activation is the *tax* transgenic mouse model. These *tax*-transfected animals develop severe RA-like arthritis (36). Of interest, *tax,* a part of the HTLV-I genome, has been detected in murine SFs (37). Consistent with the known trans-activation of the c-*fos* promotor by *tax* (38), messenger RNA (mRNA) for c-*fos*, interleukin-1β (IL-1β), and IL-6 were up-regulated in specific clones of these *tax*-expressing SFs (39). However, there is, at present, no evidence for a transactivation mediated by the HTLV-I *tax* in human RA. Additional evidence for a cytokine-independent activation of SFs is provided by the expression of endogenous L1 elements in these cells leading to the up-regulation of p38δ, a strong inducer of the MMP-1 protease (9).

Animal Models Reveal Details of Synoviocyte Activation

Several animal models have provided novel insights into the pathways that likely lead to joint destruction (40). The most thoroughly examined model of spontaneous arthritis in animals was the MRL-*lpr/lpr* mouse. In homozygous animals, the mutation of a single gene (*lpr*) leads to severe autoimmune disease (41). These mice developed a lymphoproliferative disorder with the production of rheumatoid factors, as well as an RA-like symmetric polyarthritis (42). Interestingly, the initial disease in these animals was characterized by increased numbers of synovial cells exhibiting a transformed appearance, as observed by Fassbender (1) in human RA. Subsequently, these cells attached to cartilage and bone and progressively invaded these tissues. The expression of the proliferation-associated protooncogenes *ras* and *myc* in these cells has been shown to be associated with the expression of cathepsins B and L, as well as MMP-1 (43,44). It was striking that, at this early stage, inflammatory cells was absent. After the initial stage of cartilage destruction, however, inflammatory cells appeared in the subsynovial tissue, resembling the rheumatoid synovium in the human joint (42,45). The genomic mutation site in these animals is located in the *Fas* apoptosis gene (41). This *lpr* mutation is the result of a retrotransposon (endogenous retrovirus) insertion within the *Fas* gene (46,47). However, puzzling is the fact that MRL-lpr/lpr mice do not develop destructive arthritis anymore, possibly through out breeding.

Development of a model permitting the direct study of synoviocytes and synovial tissue *in vivo* within a living organism, but without the influence of its immune system, was important to explore the role of synoviocytes in cartilage destruction. First, experiments were performed with thymus-deficient nude mice, in which SFs derived from RA patients formed a pannus-like tissue (48). A second model was established based on the observation that synovium can be implanted in SCID mice (49). The latter model consisted of coimplanting normal human cartilage and RA synovium under the kidney capsule of SCID mice. These grafts survived for at least 220 days, and the synovium invaded progressively into the cartilage (8). The resulting cartilage erosions resembled those observed in RA (Fig. 12.2). Characterization of this early stage of RA-like synovial growth revealed production of mRNA encoding matrix-degrading proteinases in SFs at the site of cartilage destruction. The critical role of the SF in this model was supported by the implantation of cultured SFs with human normal cartilage. Most strikingly, RA SFs, but not skin fibroblasts or synoviocytes from patients with osteoarthritis (OA), were able to invade the cartilage and elaborate cathepsins at the site of attachment without the apparent involvement of T cells (50). This model resembles features of joint destruction observed in c-*fos* transgenic mice, in which the virtual absence of T cells in articular lesions suggests that synovial hyperplasia can occur independent of overt T-cell influence (51).

Taken together, these data provide strong evidence for SFs as pivotal players in the destruction of joints in RA. In

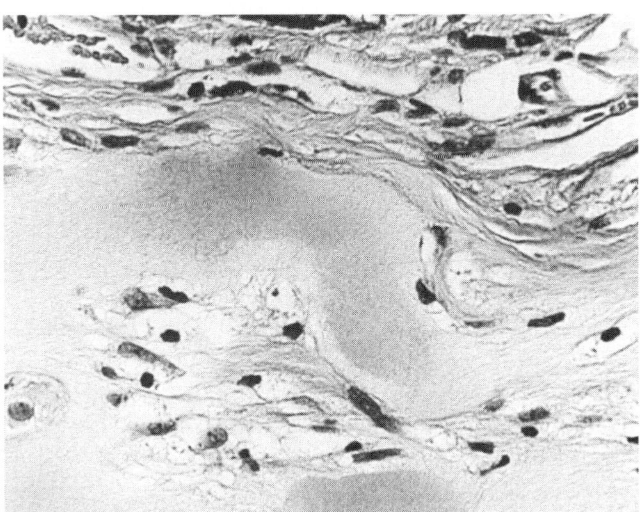

FIG. 12.2. Capability of rheumatoid arthritis synovium (*S*) to invade normal human cartilage (*C*) when coimplanted under the renal capsule of severe combined immunodeficiency (*SCID*) mice. In this environment, human lymphocytes and other mononuclear cells are completely lacking. Note the transformed-appearing shape of the synovial fibroblasts at the site of destruction.

this regard, an unfortunate experiment of nature provided a link between model and reality. An acquired immunodeficiency syndrome (AIDS) patient with long-term RA showed progressive joint destruction, despite lacking synovial or peripheral blood CD4+ T cells (52). Progression of joint destruction was associated with the production of matrix-degrading proteinases, including cathepsins B and L, by SFs at the site of invasion. Interestingly, there were no clinical features of inflammation in the examined joints. These observations support the concept that T cell–independent pathways, mediated by resident SFs (6), may persist in RA in the absence of overt inflammation, which is supported by radiographic observations that articular destruction can progress independently of local and systemic inflammation (53,54).

The Impact of Gene Transcription, Protooncogenes, and Intracellular Signaling

Evidence suggests that the observed cellular and metabolic alterations of synoviocytes in RA are mediated by up-regulated transcription of protooncogenes (2,7,55), involved in the regulation of the cell cycle. Both early growth response genes and proliferation-associated protooncogenes have been implicated in contributing to the pathogenesis of RA (7,55). Although the precise events leading to the induction of fibroblast growth in RA are unclear, the c-*sis*/platelet-derived growth factor (PDGF) system is one of the few examples of a chain of defined events capable of stimulating synovial growth. PDGF is produced mainly in platelets and macrophages. SFs are responsive to the mitogenic effect of PDGF (56).

Early-response genes appear to be involved in the initial steps of synovial cell activation. The early-response gene *egr-1*, also named zinc finger gene *Z-225* (57), was found to be significantly up-regulated in RA SFs (58), and increased expression of *egr-1* persisted over numerous passages (59). By *in situ* hybridization, mRNA of *egr-1* was detected in numerous cells of the rheumatoid synovium. *Egr-1* regulates not only the expression of other oncogenes (such as *sis* and *ras*), which are overexpressed in RA synovium (43), but also the expression of collagen and tissue inhibitor of metalloproteinases 1 (TIMP-1) (60).

The c-*fos* oncogene in mammalian cells, which has a counterpart in the murine sarcoma virus gene v-*fos*, is another gene activated in SFs in RA (58,61). A major effect of the translated Fos proteins is the control of the activation of tissue-degrading molecules such as MMP-1 (62) and MMP-3 (63). Therefore, it is not surprising that the expression of *fos* and *egr-1* is correlated with the expression of MMP-1 at sites of synovial invasion in rheumatoid joint destruction (58). Fos proteins dimerize with Jun proteins to form AP-1 (64), a transcriptional activator exhibiting enhanced DNA binding activity in RA synovium (65). Various cytokines and growth factors [epidermal growth factor (EGF), fibroblast growth factor (FGF), PDGF, tumor necrosis factor (TNF), and IL-1] mediate the cellular production of the transcription factors (c-*fos*/c-*jun*), which bind to the AP-1 promoter element (66), and *fos*/*jun* then triggers the expression of several other genes such as MMP-1 and MMP-3. On the other hand, glucocorticoid receptors can interact with AP-1. This interaction might explain one of the effects of steroids in RA: the inhibition of MMP-1 production (67). As synthesis of proteins is dependent on intact mRNA, inhibition of relevant protooncogenes by antisense oligonucleotides is an attractive therapeutic approach to inhibit protooncogene-dependent cellular pathways. It is of interest that c-*fos* antisense oligonucleotides are able to inhibit the expression of AP-1 protein and SF proliferation (68). Moreover, the transformed appearance of SFs is associated with the expression of the protooncogenes *myc* and *ras* in RA synovium (69). It is known that transcribed *myc* sequences may rescue cells from senescence and cooperate with *ras* in cell activation (70). *Myc* gene product expression could be demonstrated in SFs at sites of cartilage and bone destruction in RA (43,71). Similarly, the oncogene *ras* was expressed mainly in the synovial lining layer and modulates the proliferative response of rheumatoid synovial cells to TNF-α and TGF-α (72). Moreover, *ras* was associated with the expression of the proteolytic enzyme cathepsin L at sites of invasive growth (43).

Another important regulator of gene transcription is the nuclear factor κB (NFκB), which is expressed by RA SFs and triggered by retroviral infection such as HTLV-I (73), as well as by proinflammatory cytokines such as IL-1 (74). Both subunits of NFκB can be detected in RA synovium, especially in synovial lining cells (75–77). With regard to proinflammatory pathways, NFκB can increase cyclooxygenase-2 protein expression in RA SFs (76). In chronic inflammation, gene transcription of NFκB can be altered significantly by cytokines and growth factors and results in general cell activation.

When exposed to TNF-α, SFs show an increased proliferation and decreased contact inhibition (78). These effects are related to TNF-α-dependent induction of *egr-1* (79) and NFκB (80). In spontaneously IL-6-producing rheumatoid SF cell lines, significantly higher activity of NFκB and CBF1 (Epstein-Barr virus C–promoting factor 1) could be detected, as compared with low IL-6-producing clones (81,82).

With regard to NFκB signaling, RANK (receptor activator of nuclear factor κB), a member of the TNF receptor family, appears to be one of the most important membrane receptors. In rheumatoid synovium, RANK initiates a bone-degrading pathway via its binding partner RANK ligand (RANKL), which can also be bound by a soluble decoy receptor named osteoprotegerin/osteoclast differentiation factor (OPG/ODF). RANKL/ODF is expressed at sites of bone erosion, as well as by RA SFs (83) involved substantially in osteoclastogenesis and bone destruction (84–86). Figure 12.3 illustrates RANK/RANKL-dependent signaling pathways. Of interest, rheumatoid SFs expressing higher levels

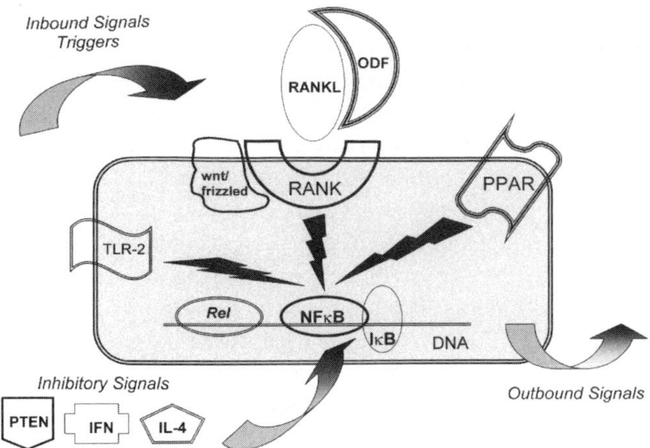

FIG. 12.3. Summary of the in- and outbound pericellular mechanisms operative in rheumatoid arthritis (RA) synovium that stimulate or result from nuclear factor κB (NFκB) activation. NFκB is expressed by RA synovial fibroblasts and triggered by a number of extracellular stimuli, including retroviruses and proinflammatory cytokines, usually resulting in cell activation, whereas inhibitory signals to counteract this activation are lacking. In general, NFκB activation in RA synovial fibroblasts leads to the synthesis of other proinflammatory and matrix-degrading molecules, but distinct pathways appear to be specifically associated with RA. Of these, the receptor activator of nuclear factor-κB RANK initiates a bone-degrading pathway via its binding partner RANK ligand (*RANKL*), which can also be bound by a soluble decoy receptor named osteoprotegerin/osteoclast differentiation factor (*OPG/ODF*). RANKL/ODF is involved in osteoclastogenesis and bone destruction. Moreover, Toll-like receptors [e.g., Toll-like receptor 2, (*TLR-2*)] have been shown to translocate NFκB and induce inflammation, and peroxisome proliferator-activated receptor (*PPAR*) appears to mediate another mechanism of activation of NFκB. IκB, inhibitor of (nuclear factor) κB; *IFN*, interferon; *PTEN*, phosphatase and tensin homologue deleted on chromosome 10.

of RANKL/ODF induced a larger number of osteoclast-like cells than did RA SFs expressing only low levels of RANKL/ODF (85). Moreover, Toll-like receptors, especially TLR-2, have been shown to mediate translocation of NFκB and induce inflammation, including IL-1 (10).

That targeting of NFκB-dependent pathways is a potentially useful therapeutic approach in RA has been supported by the NFκB-inhibiting effects of glucocorticoids through up-regulation of the inhibitor of κB (IκB) (87). IκB activity is regulated by two kinases, IκB kinases-1 and -2, also named IKK1 and IKK2. The presence of IκB as well as IKK1 and IKK2 was demonstrated in RA synovium (88). Because TNF-α and IL-1 were found to be key inducers of activation of NFκB (88), most likely another key element of this pathway includes the known inactivation of IκB by cytokine-dependent phosphorylation and ubiquitination. In addition, IKK-2 dominant negative mutant cell populations exhibited resistance to TNF-α-triggered NFκB nuclear translocation, whereas lack of IKK1 did not affect this pathway (89). In addition, antagonizing NFκB mRNA by using antisense oligonucleotides resulted in decreased binding of NFκB to the cyclooxygenase gene promoter (76). TNF-α appears to be important for the regulation of NFκB in RA SFs, because inhibition of TNF-α activity by the antioxidant *N*-acetylcysteine not only reduced TNF-α/NFκB-dependent gene expression, but also synovial proliferation considerably (78).

Overexpression of accessory proteins that bind to nuclear receptors and, subsequently, suppress gene transcription and intracellular signaling kinases may play an important role in proinflammatory and autoimmune mechanisms (90), and in the activation of synoviocytes (91). For example, the nuclear receptor cofactor SMRT (silencing mediator for retinoid and thyroid hormone receptors), which is present in SFs, suppresses MMP-1 promoter activity (92).

Expression of genes in RA fibroblasts is further modulated through mRNA stabilization. In this regard, it has been demonstrated that IL-6 gene expression is regulated by p38 mitogen-activated protein kinase (MAPK), which enhances the stability of IL-6 mRNA (93). That p38 MAPK also regulates proinflammatory pathways in RA SFs is suggested by the observation that inhibition of p38 MAPK inhibited IL-1-dependent up-regulation of prostaglandin E_2 and cycloooxygenase-2 (91). Similar to NFκB, intracellular MAPK cascades such as p38 MAPK and c-*jun* kinases (JNKs) appear to be among the key mechanisms involved in the regulation of matrix degradation in rheumatoid synovium, because activation of p38 MAPK inhibited *Ras*/*Raf*-induced MMP-1 gene expression (94) and JNK modulates IL-1-dependent MMP-1 gene expression (95).

Recently, a novel ligand-dependent transcriptional factor, the peroxisome proliferator-activated receptor-γ (PPAR-γ), has been identified as playing a role in synoviocyte pathophysiology. Stimulation of PPAR-γ results in inhibition of transcription activity of nuclear transcription factors and down-regulation of proinflammatory cytokines. In RA SFs, stimulation of PPAR-γ induces negative regulation of NFκB and AP-1, followed by down-regulation of expression of numerous cytokines, including TNF-α, IL-1, IL-6, and IL-8, as well as of matrix metalloproteinases such as MMP-1 and MMP-3 (96–98).

Long-Term Dysregulation of the Cell Cycle: Proliferation and Apoptosis

Increasing evidence indicates that the proliferation of SFs and their invasive growth is due to an impaired regulation of the cell cycle [i.e., the balance between proliferation and programmed cell death (apoptosis)]. In this regard, it is important to note that activated RA SFs do not exhibit an increased rate of proliferation *in vitro* (59,99) or *in vivo* (100), a property that can only be circumvented by manipulation of growth-regulating genes, such as homeobox genes

(101). In contrast, apoptosis is triggered by ligation of surface receptors, such as the *Fas* receptor or the TNF-α receptor, and results in intracellular degradation of cellular DNA and phagocytosis of the dying cell. A potent inhibitor of apoptosis is the protooncogene *Bcl-2* (102), located in the inner mitochondrial membrane, the endoplasmic reticulum, and the nuclear membrane (103). *Bcl-2* inhibits one of the terminal steps of apoptosis. In RA synovium, less than 3% of the activated SFs are undergoing overt apoptosis (104,105), and mRNA for the apoptosis gene *Fas* is detected mainly in cells associated with terminal vessels (106). Recent findings indicate that the regulation of *Bcl-2* [and *Bcl-x(L)*] expression is related to the degree of autocrine activation of IL-15 receptors by SF–derived antiapoptotic IL-15 (107). Of interest, other members of the *Bcl* family are also involved in RA pathophysiology. *Bcl-3,* a known regulator of NFκB activity, is involved in IL-1-dependent synthesis of MMP-1 via NFκB (108).

Another factor contributing to net proliferation of RA SFs might be defective or deficient tumor-suppressor genes such as p53, phosphatase and tensin homologue deleted on chromosome 10 (PTEN) (109), or sentrin (110). Although the role of p53, which is expressed in RA SFs and synovial tissue (111,112), has not been completely elucidated, its presence and activity appear to be influenced by distinct, but varying, environmental factors and genomic mutations (113,114). Accumulation of intracellular p53 following treatment with proteasome inhibitors can prevent PDGF-stimulated synovial cells from progressing into the S phase of the cell cycle (115). Conversely, in the collagen-induced arthritis model, p53-deficient mice showed an increased severity of arthritis, with synovial cell apoptosis being virtually absent (116). Finally, inhibition of endogenous p53 significantly enhanced the destructiveness of RA SFs toward normal cartilage in the SCID mouse model (117).

PTEN, on the other hand, is a tumor suppressor with tyrosine phosphatase activity found to promote the development of malignancies when mutated. In RA, the absence of PTEN in the synovial lining and at sites of invasive growth could enhance the longevity of activated SFs at sites of cartilage destruction (109). This might be explained by the PTEN-dependent effect on IκB/NFκB and other nuclear factors such as akt/protein kinase B, as observed in cancer cells (118–120). The serine/threonine kinase akt appears to be crucial in TNF-dependent regulation of synoviocyte proliferation (121). Sentrin, a novel protein that protects against *Fas*- and TNF-induced cell death (122), has also been shown to be expressed intensively in RA synovium (110).

These alterations of cell cycle regulation favoring proliferation have prompted researchers to examine the effect of enhanced apoptosis in RA synovium induced by treatment with anti-*Fas* antibody (123). In the HTLV-I *tax* transgenic mouse model, which exhibits an RA-like destructive arthritis, intraarticular application of anti-*Fas* antibody improved joint swelling and arthritis within a few days. Immunohistologic examination of the joints revealed that the effect was most likely attributable to induction of apoptosis, consistent with previous observations demonstrating functional *Fas* expression in RA synovium (124). However, RA SFs appear relatively resistant to *Fas*-induced apoptosis by anti-*Fas* antibodies, despite the fact that *Fas* is expressed. This resistance might be due—at least in part—to the up-regulation of *Fas*-like IL-1 converting enzyme (FLICE) inhibitory protein (FLIP), which exerts an antiapoptotic effect through inhibition of the apoptosis-triggering intracellular enzyme FLICE (caspase 8), in the synovial lining (125). Targeted induction of apoptosis in SFs represents a promising therapeutic approach that warrants further investigation.

Growth Factors

TGF-β, FGF, and PDGF induce cell proliferation and, therefore, form a subfamily of growth factors. TGF-β is abundantly expressed in synovial tissue and synovial fluid and is produced predominantly by synovial macrophages. Whether it induces pro- or antiinflammatory effects depends on its location and concentration. In animals, TGF-β induces proliferation of the synovial lining when injected directly into the joint cavity (126) and stimulates collagen production by SFs. TGF-β also exhibits a synergistic effect in stimulating both IL-1 and MMP-1 synthesis (127). Of interest, recent data indicate that the effects of TGF-β are directly linked to antiapoptotic pathways through modulation of the activity of phosphatidylinositol 3 kinase and akt in rheumatoid SFs (128). TGF-β also is a potent inhibitor of T cells, apparently through interference with the IL-1 receptor (129). FGF is an autocrine growth factor for synoviocytes and vascular epithelium. SFs not only proliferate in response to FGF, but also can produce FGF, thus triggering local fibroblast growth (130). Present in the synovial lining, PDGF is a highly potent stimulator of synovial growth (131). PDGF also is one of the few cytokines for which a direct protooncogene-triggered activation of synovial cells has been demonstrated (56).

Intensive vascularization is one of the prerequisites for sustained synovial proliferation and joint destruction. One of the key mechanisms in this process is the up-regulation of the proangiogenic growth factor, vascular endothelial growth factor (VEGF). VEGF mRNA and protein, as well as its relevant receptor Flt-1 (KDR), are present in rheumatoid synovium (132,133) and cocultivation experiments of fibroblast-like synoviocytes with polymorphonuclear neutrophils demonstrate that both VEGF synthesis, as well as neovascularization, is triggered by this interaction (132).

Cytokines

Cytokines known to be produced by various synovial cells, either spontaneously or after stimulation, include IL-1α, IL-1β, IL-6, IL-8, IL-10, IL-11, IL-15, IL-16, IL-17, IL-18, IL-21R, interferon-γ (IFN-γ), and TNF-α, as well as (pleiotropic) growth factors with cytokine functions, such as epidermal growth factor (EGF), VEGF, TGF, insulin-like growth factor-1 (IGF-1) and IGF-2, granulocyte-macrophage colony-stimulating factor (GM-CSF), and macrophage colony-stimulating factor (M-CSF) (131,134–145). Most of these cytokines induce synoviocytes to produce other cytokines and matrix-degrading enzymes, and the effects of even the major proinflammatory cytokines, such as TNF-α, can be further enhanced by costimulatory cytokines such as TNF-like weak inducer of apoptosis (TWEAK) (146). In addition to the examination of the presence of cytokines in the synovial lining and the measurement of the amount of individual cytokines produced by synoviocytes, the most important questions involve the role of these molecules in cytokine-synoviocyte-cytokine pathways and in the crosstalk between different cytokine-dependent signaling cascades (147).

The production of cytokines, however, is not limited to RA synoviocytes. Synovial membranes derived from patients with OA demonstrate a cytokine expression pattern similar to those from patients with RA. The only difference observed was the significantly higher amounts of IL-1, IL-6, GM-CSF, TNF-α, and EGF produced by synoviocytes in RA synovial membranes, presumably due to the higher cellularity in RA synovial specimens (148). The inflammation-suppressing cytokine IL-10 also is expressed in both RA and OA (149). The addition of recombinant IL-10 to cultures of RA synovial membranes considerably diminished the levels of proinflammatory cytokines, suggesting a potential therapeutic role for this cytokine in RA. Inhibitors of the macrophage-derived inflammatory cytokine TNF-α, including its soluble receptor (150), are among the recently established new therapeutic modalities for RA (151,152).

Interestingly, little is known of the cytokine pattern expressed by synoviocytes in reactive arthritis, although studies on T cells revealed an up-regulation of IFN-γ and IL-4 (150). All experiments concerning cytokine production by synoviocytes *in vitro* are difficult to evaluate, however, because the rate of synthesis varies considerably, depending on sites of retrieval of tissue samples and culture conditions (153–155).

Prostaglandins

Proinflammatory prostaglandin pathways also contribute to synovial inflammation and joint destruction in RA (156). Cyclooxygenases (COX-1 and COX-2) catalyze the enzymatic activation of arachidonic acid to prostaglandins, which are potent mediators of inflammation. COX-1 is found in the majority of human tissues, whereas COX-2 expression is limited to distinct tissues (e.g., brain and kidney). In RA synovium, COX-2 can be detected in synovial lining cells, lymphocytes, and endothelial cells (157). The source of COX-2 in the synovial lining appears to be predominantly SFs (76), because only a few COX-2-expressing synovial lining cells bear the macrophage marker CD68 (158), and inhibition experiments revealed a direct link between SFs and COX-2 synthesis (91). In addition, selective COX-2 inhibitors appear also to exert proapoptotic effects on SFs, since celecoxib was able to inhibit proliferation of SFs by induction of PPAR-γ-independent apoptosis (159). Of interest, nonsteroidal antiinflammatory drugs (NSAIDs) that inhibit cyclooxygenase pathways have only a limited effect on the generation of another important arachidonic acid–derived group of mediators, the leukotrienes. Thus, inhibition of both leukotriene and prostaglandin synthesis (through the use of a combination of lipoxygenase and cyclooxygenase inhibitors) might be an effective approach (160–162).

INTERACTIONS AND COMMUNICATIONS

Short-Range Interaction with Other Cells and Matrices

The direct interaction of cells with other cells and their surrounding matrix is mediated by cell adhesion molecules. Within this group of communication ligands and receptors, the large majority of adhesion molecules can be conveniently grouped into the integrin, selectin, and immunoglobulin supergene families (163) (Chapter 20). Knowledge of the functional aspects of adhesion molecules in RA synovium itself is largely limited to T-cell interactions (164–167) and interactions of several cell types with endothelial cells (168,169). Less is known about the expression and the functional role of adhesion molecules expressed on RA synoviocytes. Interesting data indicate that certain members of the immunoglobulin gene superfamily are expressed on SFs. Abundant expression of vascular cell-adhesion molecule-1 (VCAM-1) was found in the lining layer of proliferating RA synovium and, to a lesser extent, in OA synovium (170). Double-labeling with antibodies against macrophage-specific CD68 antigen revealed that, in particular, the SFs, which are prone to attach to and invade articular cartilage, expressed VCAM-1 (171). Therefore, VCAM-1 likely supports multiple, crucial adhesion functions, especially in RA synovium. In the synovial microvasculature, VCAM-1 binds to the lymphocyte membrane very late activation antigen-4 (VLA-4). VLA-4, on the other hand, serves also as ligand for an alternatively spliced form of fibronectin, designated CS-1, which is involved in multidirectional interaction between SFs, matrices, and lymphocytes (172). Figure 12.4 illustrates this interactive network.

Proinflammatory cytokines such as TNF-α and IL-1β enhance VCAM-1 expression on SFs, and most recent data can demonstrate that IL-18 appears to play a key role in up-regulation of VCAM-1 in SFs through at least three different intracellular activation pathways (173,174). Of interest, activation of the IL-18/IL-18 receptor-dependent pathways in SFs appears to require cellular interaction with T cells (175). In addition, some of the antiinflammatory effects of glucocorticoids may be mediated by inhibition of VCAM-1 expression on RA SFs, resulting in a reduced binding to

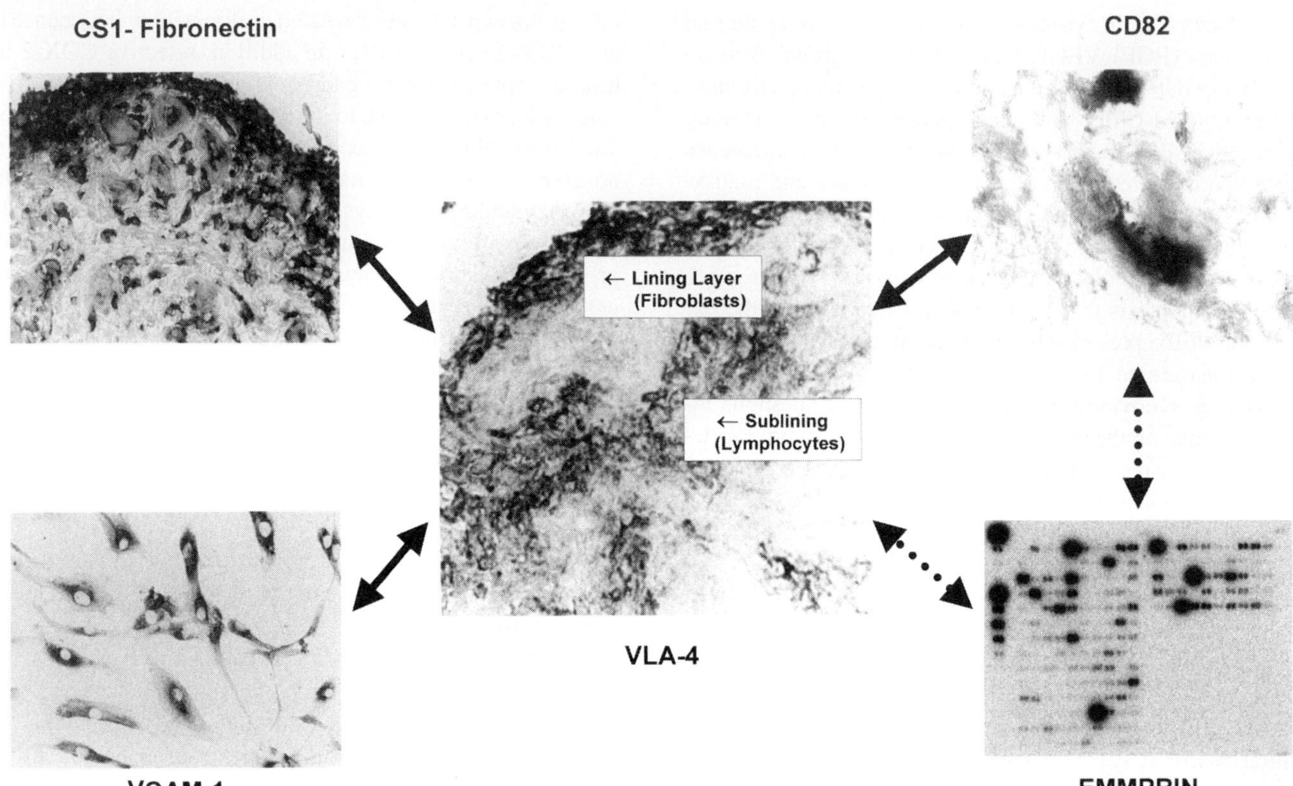

FIG. 12.4. Multidirectional interaction network in rheumatoid synovium connecting matrix to fibroblasts and inflammatory cells to matrix-degrading enzymes. Matrix components such as fibronectin *CS-1* can bind to integrin very late antigen-4 (*VLA-4*) expressed on lymphocytes and synovial fibroblasts which, in turn can bind to the adhesion molecule vascular cell adhesion molecule-1 (*VCAM-1*). VLA-4 most likely can also link to CD82 on synovial fibroblasts, with the latter having a potential modulatory effect on matrix metalloproteinase inducers such as extracellular matrix metalloproteinase inducer (*EMMPRIN*).

VLA-4-expressing lymphocytes (176). The bidirectional VCAM ↔ CS-1 ↔ VLA-4 relationship might also be important in the binding of the activated synovium to cartilage, because previous studies have demonstrated a higher concentration of fibronectin in superficial layers of cartilage than in deeper layers (177). Thus, distinct adhesion molecules might not only be a marker for the RA synovium, but also contribute to the pathogenesis of the disease.

The integrin $\alpha_5\beta_1$ (CD49e), a ligand for fibronectin, is up-regulated in cultured RA SFs, indicating the potential of these cells to adhere to other matrix components (178). Similar results were obtained for integrin receptors for collagen type IV, laminin, and tenascin (178). In addition, invasion of RA SFs into bovine cartilage can be inhibited by antibodies to α_4 integrins (179). Besides cell-to-cell signaling, adhesion molecules facilitate migration of proinflammatory cells into the rheumatoid synovium. VLA-4 and -5 enhance monocyte migration through a SF barrier (180). Interestingly, blockade of the ligand for VCAM-1 inhibited only transendothelial migration but not migration through SFs (180). It is of interest that rheumatoid SFs express mRNA for the sensory neuropeptide substance P (181), which enhances the effect of proinflammatory cytokines on VCAM-1 expression (182).

Synovial macrophages express high levels of ICAM-1 (164,168,176). ICAM-1, which binds to its integrin counterreceptor on different leukocytes [leukocyte function–associated antigen-1 (LFA-1)], is expressed on RA and normal synoviocytes (164) and represents an adhesion molecule that is induced by cytokines. On cultured SFs, ICAM-1 is expressed at low levels. When stimulated with various cytokines such as IFN-γ, IL-1, or TNF-α, the expression of ICAM-1 on these cells is markedly increased (183). Another interaction likely to be important is the communication of RA SFs with T lymphocytes through binding of ICAM-1 to LFA-1. By immunohistochemistry, it has been demonstrated that ICAM-1-positive SFs are surrounded by LFA-1-positive T lymphocytes, associated with up-regulation of IL-1 expression by SFs (184). A role for ICAM-1 in the pathogenesis of RA is suggested by previous clinical trials in which short-term treatment with monoclonal antibodies to ICAM-1 in RA patients resulted in clinical improvement without serious side effects in about half of the patients (185). Interestingly, pulse methylprednisolone was shown to reduce considerably the expression of synovial lining ICAM-1 (186). ICAM-3, another counterreceptor for the leukocyte receptor LFA-1, also is present on synovial macrophages and lymphocytes, but its functions relative to other cell adhesion molecules remains to be determined (187,188).

Clearly, the expression of adhesion molecules on synoviocytes provides a mechanism for binding to inflammatory cells, such as lymphocytes and monocytes/macrophages. In addition, cell-matrix adhesion mechanisms not only facilitate the binding of synoviocytes to articular matrix, but they also reveal distinct differences between macrophages and SFs. For example, the laminin receptor ($\alpha_6\beta_1$ integrin) is expressed only by SFs and not by synovial macrophages (189). On the other hand, another member of the immunoglobulin supergene family, CD31, which is structurally similar to CD4 and ICAM-1, is expressed by both synovial macrophages and fibroblasts, and a general "adhesive" role within the RA synovium has been postulated for this molecule (190). E-selectin, L-selectin, and P-selectin also are present in RA synovium, and because their function appears to be predominantly related to adhesive interactions between endothelial cells and mononuclear cells in the synovial microvasculature (190), they represent a target for therapeutic interventions. In addition, other observations indicate that the production and release of matrix-degrading enzymes (e.g., MMP-1) by SFs is triggered by integrin/matrix interactions (191). In addition, IL-1β is able to enhance integrin expression on RA SFs (192).

Long-Range Interactions: The Role of Chemokines

Fibroblasts can also be regarded as "sentinel cells" (193) enhancing (chemo)attraction of leukocytes. For example, after stimulation of the CD40 ligand/CD40 system, fibroblasts can release several chemoattractant molecules, such as the chemokines macrophage inflammatory protein (MIP), monocyte chemoattractant protein (MCP), and RANTES (regulated upon activation normal T cell expressed and secreted) (194). Similarly, SFs are able to express MIP-3α after stimulation with IL-1β and TNF-α, and this mechanism appears to be operative specifically in (perivascular) chemoattraction of mononuclear cells (195). In addition, release of the chemokine MCP-1 by SFs is stimulated by oncostatin M (196). In RA synovium, oncostatin M is produced mainly by cells of the monocyte-macrophage type and is able to increase the production of matrix metalloproteinases. Influx of proinflammatory $CD4^+$ lymphocytes is also promoted by SFs because of the production of considerable amounts of chemoattractive IL-16 (134). The amount of IL-16 elaborated by RA SFs correlates with the resultant chemoattractant activity. Conversely, the $CD4^+$ T cell–derived cytokine IL-17 can induce cytokine production in rheumatoid SFs, and therefore stimulate the proinflammatory interaction cascade (135). Of interest, modulation of chemokine and chemokine production by synoviocytes appears to be through both autocrine and paracrine pathways (197). These pathways include CCL-2/MCP-1-dependent up-regulation of extracellular signal–related kinases (erk)-1 and -2 (197).

The importance of chemokine-related pathways for synovial pathophysiology is illustrated by the fact that there are costimulatory links to cellular adhesion mechanisms. Although SFs constitutively express the chemokine stromal cell-derived factor-1 (SDF-1), which can be further enhanced by hypoxia (198), B-cell pseudoemperipolesis could only be achieved after IL-4-dependent up-regulation of VCAM-1 (199). Thus, blockade of chemokine receptors and receptor-dependent intracellular mechanisms might constitute attractive targets for RA therapy. IL-10, on the other hand, is involved in the down-regulation of proinflammatory chemokines (200) and might be a pluripotent molecule in the inhibition of RA joint destruction, a view supported by the fact that after retrovirus-based IL-10 gene transfer, alone or in combination with IL-1, the invasive growth of RA SFs could be completely inhibited (30,201). However, more recent data demonstrate that activation of SFs via the TLR-2 expressed on these cells (10) leads to the induction of potent chemokines, including MCP-2 (202). This novel observation proves that SFs are part of the innate immune system and play a pivotal role in the induction of inflammation in the rheumatoid joint.

THE ROLE OF SYNOVIOCYTES IN JOINT DESTRUCTION

Matrix Metalloproteinases

Numerous proteolytic enzymes contribute to the destructive potential of RA synovium. Key players in this concert are MMPs and cathepsins. MMPs belong to a growing family of zinc-containing enzymes including collagenases, stromelysin, gelatinases, and membrane-type (MT) MMPs. At present, MMPs 1 through 24 have been characterized. Numerous intracellular signaling pathways operative in the regulation of MMP synthesis have been examined in recent years (203,204). MMPs are capable of cleaving connective tissue matrix components such as collagens, glycoproteins, and proteoglycans. In RA synovium, the number of MMP-1-producing cells and the net excess of MMP-1 compared with their natural inhibitors TIMPs 1 through 3 (tissue inhibitors of metalloproteinases 1–3) are correlated with the degree of synovial inflammation (205–208). Recent data indicate that at least part of the production of MMPs is due to the presence of the extracellular MMP inducer (EMMPRIN) (209), which not only increases the destructive potential of fibroblasts (210), but also appears to be specifically up-regulated in rheumatoid synovium both at the mRNA as well as the protein level (2). Moreover, evaluation of the invasiveness of SFs in an artificial matrix indicates that the invasive properties of these cells are correlated with a distinct MMP profile, including expression of MMP-1, MMP-3, and MMP-10 (99). Of interest, direct cellular contacts and interactions within the synovial compartment appear to regulate the secretion of MMPs. Part of this regulation is due to the functional integrity of gap junctions between synoviocytes (211).

The best characterized member of the MMP family is MMP-1, also referred to as collagenase-1. MMP-1 cleaves collagens I, II, VII, and X. MMP-1 is the most prominent MMP, but most other MMPs also have been detected in RA synovium. SFs at sites of invasion, or within the synovial lining layer, are a major source of these enzymes (212) and MMPs are most likely one of the driving forces in RA joint destruction (213). Another MMP known to cleave predominantly cartilage collagen type II rather than proteoglycan is MMP-13, also named collagenase-3. MMP-13 was shown to be expressed both at the mRNA and the protein level in the synovial lining of patients with rheumatoid joint destruction (214). A pleiotropic member of the MMP family, MMP-9 (or gelatinase B) is a marker for inflammation rather than being specific for RA. This finding is supported by the fact that MMP-9 is not restricted to SFs, but is also synthesized by endothelial cells, macrophages, and leukocytes (215,216).

In the past decade, other members of the MMP family, the membrane-type MMPs, have been described and associated with tissue destruction. Of these, MT1-MMP (MMP-14) and MT3-MMP (MMP-16) are of particular interest because they are capable of cleaving extracellular matrix components as well as activating other MMPs. In RA synovium, abundant expression of MT1-MMP and MT3-MMP was observed, with MT3-MMP being expressed by SFs, and MT1-MMP both by SFs and CD68-positive osteoclasts and macrophages (217,218). In addition, proteolytic activity at sites of synovium/cartilage interactions appears to be mediated by a complex consisting of MT1-MMP, TIMP-2, and MMP-2. Furthermore, the important role of MT1 and MT3-MMP in joint destruction was suggested by their abundant expression in RA synovium in contrast to MT2-MMP (MMP-15) and MT4-MMP (MMP-17), which are expressed in only limited amounts (218).

Cathepsins

A second important family of proteolytic enzymes in RA synovium are cathepsins. The expression of these matrix-degrading enzymes is linked to the activation of numerous protooncogenes observed in SFs. Studies have shown that the transfection of *ras* oncogene into fibroblasts leads to cellular activation and the induction of cathepsin L (219,220). Indeed, the expression of cathepsin L correlates with both the extent of *ras* expression and the metastatic potential of cells (221). Because cathepsin L is capable of degrading collagen types I, II, IX, and XI (222), as well as proteoglycans (223), the up-regulation of this cysteine proteinase in activated synovial cells is thought to play a major role in cartilage destruction in RA (43,55,224). At sites of bone erosions, cathepsin L is released from CD68-positive macrophage-like synovial cells (225), whereas CD68-positive osteoclasts show only limited expression of cathepsin L. Convincing data indicate that the major contribution of CD68-positive osteoclasts and CD68-negative SFs to cartilage and bone degradation might be through the production of cathepsin K (226).

It should be stressed that the increased number of matrix-degrading enzyme–producing synoviocytes in RA versus OA largely reflects the hypercellularity characteristic of RA. The most important difference between the diseases, however, is that in RA, the activated synoviocytes become attached to cartilage and the osseous matrix. It is therefore presumed that the proteolytic enzymes released by attached synoviocytes in RA may degrade matrix without encountering the inhibitors present in synovial fluid.

A promising approach directed toward inhibiting the destructive activity of invasive synovium in the "hot zone," the synovium-cartilage/bone junction, is the development of inhibitors of cathepsins. A class of such inhibitors, the fluoromethylketones, not only inhibited cathepsin B and L activity *in vivo,* but also reduced joint destruction in an animal model of arthritis when administered orally (227). Similar experiments are being performed to test inhibitors of MMP-1. Chlorotaurine, a chloramine generated by neutrophils during their oxidative burst, was found to decrease the degradative effect of bacterial collagenase on collagen (228).

Another system of matrix destruction is the plasminogen activation system, centered around the serine proteinase plasmin. Plasmin can activate matrix metalloproteinases and has direct proteolytic properties. Both RA and OA SFs synthesize high amounts of urokinase-plasminogen activator *in vitro,* and the receptor of this activator is also expressed on the surface of fibroblasts (229). Of interest, part of the matrix-degrading capabilities of RA SFs appears to be mediated by plasmin, as shown by gene transfer of a plasmin inhibitor (230), supporting the hypothesis of a substantial role for the plasminogen activation system in rheumatoid synovium. Most recent evidence has shown that activated SFs do not only contribute to osteoclastogenesis (85) but also appear to degrade bone by the expression of a proton pump (231,232).

In summary, the majority of matrix-degrading enzymes are expressed predominantly by activated SFs at sites of invasion of the activated synovium into adjacent cartilage and bone. Inhibition of this deleterious process is an attractive strategy for the treatment of RA. In this regard, it is important to note that a family of antagonizing molecules exists in the rheumatoid synovium: the TIMPs. TIMP-1 mRNA and protein is present in the synovial lining (233,234), but its occurrence is not limited to RA synovium. Cytokines such as IL-1 and TNF-α do not influence TIMP-1 gene expression significantly (235), but its production in synoviocytes and chondrocytes is considerably diminished by IL-1 (129). On the other hand, gene transfer experiments

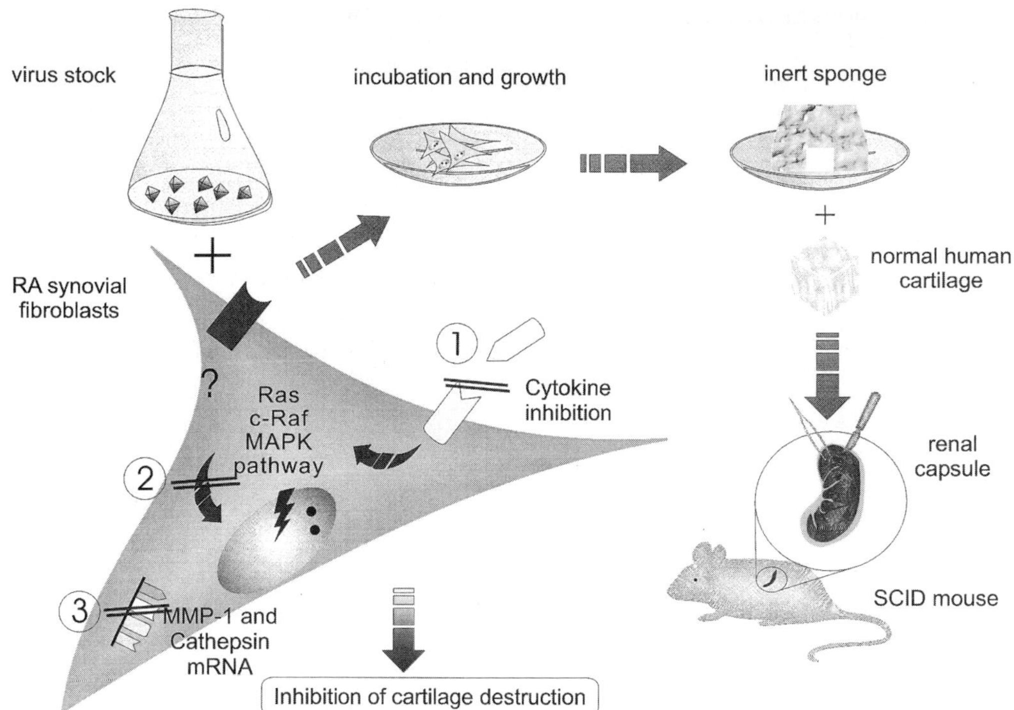

FIG. 12.5. Molecular targets of gene transfer in rheumatoid synoviocytes. The figure shows how the severe combined immunodeficiency (SCID) mouse model is being used for assessment of potential molecular targets of gene transfer in the treatment of rheumatoid arthritis (RA). RA synovial fibroblasts transduced with a retroviral vector encoding inhibitors of (*1*) inflammatory cytokines; (*2*) the Ras-Raf-MAPK (mitogen-activated protein kinase) pathway; and (*3*) matrix-degrading enzymes can be engrafted with cartilage into SCID mice. Subsequent cartilage degradation and invasive growth of fibroblasts into the cartilage are then assessed. *MMP-1*, matrix metalloproteinase-1. (Reproduced from Jorgensen C, Gay S. Gene therapy in osteoarticular diseases: Where are we? *Immunol Today* 1998;9:387–391, with permission.)

have shown that both TIMP-1 and TIMP-3, which is also an inhibitor of TACE (236), a molecule that contributes to TNF synthesis in RA synovium, can significantly inhibit the SF-mediated destruction of cartilage in the SCID mouse model (237).

FUTURE OUTLOOK

Key cellular and molecular events distinguish RA from other arthritides. It appears that the activated SF, which is acted on by a network of activating factors, plays a pivotal role in joint destruction in RA and is a logical target for the development of novel therapeutic interventions, including gene transfer. As outlined in more detail in Chapter 37 and illustrated in Fig. 12.5, adenoviral and retroviral constructs have been developed for *in vivo* gene transfer into synovial cells. This approach has been very successful in developing novel therapeutic strategies. In this regard it has been shown that gene transfer of IL-1RA, IL-10, in raf and *myc*, TIMP-1 to -3, and plasmin inhibitor into human SFs alters key pathways involved in joint destruction (238). In this regard, it needs to be stressed that gene transfer has not only become feasible to evaluate the regulation of specific signaling pathways but also as "proof of principle" for future drug targets.

ACKNOWLEDGMENTS

The work was supported by the German Research Society (DFG Mu 1383/1–3 and 3–4) and the Swiss National Science Foundation (SNF 3200–64142.00).

REFERENCES

1. Fassbender HG. Histomorphologic basis of articular cartilage destruction in rheumatoid arthritis. *Coll Rel Res* 1983;3:141–155.
2. Neumann E, Kullmann F, Judex M, et al. Identification of differentially expressed genes in rheumatoid arthritis by a combination of complementary DNA array and RNA arbitrarily primed-polymerase chain reaction. *Arthritis Rheum* 2002;46:52–63.
3. Watanabe N, Ando K, Yoshida S, et al. Gene expression profile analysis of rheumatoid synovial fibroblast cultures revealing the overexpression of genes responsible for tumor-like growth of rheumatoid synovium. *Biochem Biophys Res Commun* 2002;294:1121–1129.
4. Judex M, Neumann E, Lechner S, et al. Laser-mediated microdissection facilitates analysis of area-specific gene expression in rheumatoid synovium. *Arthritis Rheum* 2003;48:97–102.

5. Gay S, Gay RE, Koopman WJ. Molecular and cellular mechanisms of joint destruction in rheumatoid arthritis: two cellular mechanisms explain joint destruction? *Ann Rheum Dis* 1993;52(suppl):39–47.
6. Franz JK, Pap T, Müller-Ladner U, Gay RE, et al. T cell-independent joint destruction. In: Miossec P, van den Berg WB, Firestein GS, eds. *T cells in arthritis.* Basel, Switzerland: Birkhäuser Verlag, 1998:55–74.
7. Müller-Ladner U, Kriegsmann J, Gay RE, Gay S. Oncogenes in rheumatoid arthritis. *Rheum Dis Clin North Am* 1995;21:675–690.
8. Geiler T, Kriegsmann J, Keyszer G, et al. A new model for rheumatoid arthritis generated by engraftment of rheumatoid synovial tissue and normal human cartilage into SCID mice. *Arthritis Rheum* 1994;37:1664–1671.
9. Neidhart M, Rethage J, Kuchen S, et al. Retrotransposable L1 elements expressed in rheumatoid arthritis synovial tissue: association with genomic DNA hypomethylation and influence on gene expression. *Arthritis Rheum* 2000;43:2634–2447.
10. Seibl R, Birchler T, Loeliger S, et al. Expression and regulation of toll-like receptor 2 in rheumatoid arthritis synovium. *Am J Pathol* 2003; 162:1221–1227.
11. Firestein GS. Invasive fibroblast-like synoviocytes in rheumatoid arthritis: passive responders or transformed aggressors? *Arthritis Rheum* 1996;39:1781–1790.
12. Firestein GS, Zvaifler NJ. How important are T cells in chronic rheumatoid synovitis ? II. T cell-independent mechanisms from beginning to end. *Arthritis Rheum* 2002;46:298–308.
13. Rooney M, Condell D, Quinlan W, et al. Analysis of the histologic variation of synovitis in rheumatoid arthritis. *Arthritis Rheum* 1988; 31:956–963.
14. Wilkinson LS, Pitsillides AA, Worrall JG, et al. Light microscopic characterization of the fibroblast-like synovial intimal cell (synoviocyte). *Arthritis Rheum* 1992;35:1179–1184.
15. Graabaek PM. Ultrastructural evidence for two distinct types of synoviocytes in rat synovial membrane. *J Ultrastruct Res* 1982;78:321–339.
16. Edwards JCW. Structure of synovial lining. In: Henderson B, Edwards JCW, eds. *The synovial lining in health and disease.* London: Chapman & Hall, 1987:17–40.
17. Ghadially FN. Fine structure of joints. In: Sokoloff L, ed. The joints and synovial fluid. New York: Academic, 1978:110–120.
18. Bröker BM, Edwards JCW, Fanger M, et al. The prevalence and distribution of macrophages bearing FcγRI, FcγRII, and FcγRIII in synovium. *Scand J Rheumatol* 1990;19:123–135.
19. Sack U, Stiehl P, Geiler G. Distribution of macrophages in rheumatoid synovial membrane and its association with basic activity. *Rheumatol Int* 1994;13:181–186.
20. Cutolo M, Sulli A, Barone A, et al. Macrophages, synovial tissue and rheumatoid arthritis. Clin Exp Rheumatol 1993;11:331–339.
21. Klareskog L, Forsum U, Kabelitz D, et al. Immune functions of human synovial cells: phenotypic and T cell regulatory properties of macrophage-like cells that express HLA-DR. *Arthritis Rheum* 1982; 25:488–501.
22. Burmester GR, Jahn B, Rohwer P, et al. Differential expression of Ia antigens by rheumatoid synovial lining cells by rheumatoid synovial lining cells. *J Clin Invest* 1987;80:595–604.
23. Van Dinther-Janssen ACHM, Pals ST, Scheper RJ, et al. Dendritic cells and high endothelial venules in the rheumatoid synovial membrane. *J Rheumatol* 1990;17:11–17.
24. Yanni G, Whelan A, Feighery C, et al. Synovial tissue macrophages and joint erosion in rheumatoid arthritis. *Ann Rheum Dis* 1994;53: 39–44.
25. Thomas R, Davis LS, Lipsky PE. Rheumatoid synovium is enriched in mature antigen-presenting dendritic cells. *J Immunol* 1994;152:2613–2623.
26. Fujii I, Shingu M, Nobunaga M. Monocyte activation in early onset rheumatoid arthritis. *Ann Rheum Dis* 1990;49:497–503.
27. Burmester GR, Stuhlmüller B, Keyszer G, et al. Review: mononuclear phagocytes and rheumatoid synovitis: mastermind or workhorse in arthritis? *Arthritis Rheum* 1997;40:5–18.
28. Schumacher HR Jr, Bautista BB, Krauser RE, et al. Histological appearance of the synovium in early rheumatoid arthritis. *Semin Arthritis Rheum* 1994;23(suppl 2):3–10.
29. Mattey DL, Dawes PT, Nixon NB, et al. Transforming growth factor β_1 and interleukin 4 induced a smooth muscle actin expression and myofibroblast-like differentiation in human synovial fibroblasts *in vitro*: modulation by basic fibroblast growth factor. *Ann Rheum Dis* 1997;56:426–431.
30. Neumann E, Judex M, Kullmann F, et al. Inhibition of cartilage destruction by double gene transfer of IL-1ra and IL-10 is mediated by the activin pathway. *Gene Ther* 2002;9:1508–1519.
31. Lemaire R, Flipo R-M, Monte D, et al. Synovial fibroblast-like cell transfection with the SV40 large T antigen induces a transformed phenotype and permits transient tumor formation in immunodeficient mice. *J Rheumatol* 1994;21:1409–1419.
32. Gay S, Kalden JR. Retroviruses and autoimmune rheumatic diseases. *Clin Exp Immunol* 1994;98:1–5.
33. Nishioka K, Nakajima T, Hasunuma T, et al. Rheumatic manifestations of human leukemia virus infection. *Rheum Dis Clin North Am* 1993;19:489–503.
34. Carson DA, Ribeiro JM. Apoptosis and disease. *Lancet* 1993;341: 1251–1254.
35. Land H, Parada LF, Weinberg RA. Tumorigenic conversion of primary fibroblasts requires at least two cooperating oncogenes. *Nature* 1983; 304:596–602.
36. Iwakura Y, Tosu M, Yoshida E, et al. Introduction of inflammatory arthropathy resembling rheumatoid arthritis in mice transgenic for HTLV-I. *Science* 1991;253:1026–1028.
37. Kitajima I, Yamamoto K, Sato K, et al. Detection of human T cell lymphotropic virus type I proviral DNA and its gene expression in synovial cells in chronic inflammatory arthropathy. *J Clin Invest* 1991;88: 1315–1322.
38. Fujii M, Sassone-Corsi P, Verma IM. C-*fos* promoter trans-activation by the tax1 protein of human T-cell leukemia virus type I. *Proc Natl Acad Sci U S A* 1988;85:8526–8530.
39. Nakajima T, Aono H, Hasunuma T, et al. Overgrowth of human synovial cells driven by the human T cell leukemia virus type I *tax* gene. *J Clin Invest* 1993;92:186–193.
40. O'Sullivan FX, Gay RE, Gay S. Spontaneous arthritis models. In: Henderson B, Pettipher R, Edwards J, eds. *Mechanisms and models in rheumatoid arthritis.* London: Academic, 1995:471–483.
41. Watanbe-Fukunaga R, Brannan CI, Copeland NG, et al. Lymphoproliferation disorder in mice explained by defects in *Fas* antigens that mediate apoptosis. *Nature* 1992;356:314–317.
42. O'Sullivan FX, Fassbender HG, Gay S, et al. Etiopathogenesis of the rheumatoid arthritis-like disease in MRL/l mice. I. The histomorphologic basis of joint destruction. *Arthritis Rheum* 1985;28: 529–536.
43. Trabandt A, Aicher WK, Gay RE, et al. Expression of the collagenolytic and *ras*-induced cysteine protease cathepsin L and proliferation-associated oncogenes in synovial cells of MRL/l mice and patients with rheumatoid arthritis. *Matrix* 1990;10:349–361.
44. Trabandt A, Gay RE, Fassbender HG, et al. Cathepsin B in synovial cells at the site of joint destruction in rheumatoid arthritis. *Arthritis Rheum* 1991;34:1444–1451.
45. Tanaka A, O'Sullivan FX, Koopman WJ, et al. Etiopathogenesis of the rheumatoid arthritis-like disease in MRL/l mice: II. Ultrastructural basis of joint destruction. *J Rheumatol* 1988;15:10–16.
46. Wu J, Zhou T, He J, et al. Autoimmune disease in mice due to integration of an endogenous retrovirus in an apoptosis gene. *J Exp Med* 1993;178:461–468.
47. Chu J-L, Drappa J, Parnassa A, et al. The defect in *Fas* mRNA expression in MRL/lpr mice is associated with insertion of the retrotransposon. *J Exp Med* 1993;178:723–730.
48. Brinckerhoff CE, Harris ED. Survival of rheumatoid synovium implanted into nude mice. *Am J Pathol* 1981;103:411–419.
49. Rendt KE, Barry TS, Jones DM, et al. Engraftment of human synovium into severe combined immune deficient (SCID) mice: migration of human peripheral blood T-cells to engrafted human synovium and to mouse lymph nodes. *J Immunol* 1993;151:7324–7336.
50. Müller-Ladner U, Kriegsmann J, Franklin BN, et al. Synovial fibroblasts of patients with rheumatoid arthritis attach to and invade normal human cartilage when engrafted into SCID mice. *Am J Pathol* 1996; 149:1607–1615.
51. Shiozawa S, Tanaka Y, Fujita T, et al. Destructive arthritis without lymphocyte infiltration in H2-c-*fos* transgenic mice. *J Immunol* 1992; 148:3100–3104.
52. Müller-Ladner U, Kriegsmann J, Gay RE, et al. Progressive joint destruction in a HIV-infected patient with rheumatoid arthritis. *Arthritis Rheum* 1995;38:1328–1332.

53. Mulherin D, Fitzgerald O, Bresnihan B. Clinical improvement and radiological deterioration in rheumatoid arthritis: evidence that the pathogenesis of synovial inflammation and articular erosion may differ. *Br J Rheumatol* 1996;35:1263–1268.
54. McQueen FM, Stewart N, Crabbe J, et al. Magnetic resonance imaging of the wrist in early rheumatoid arthritis reveals progression of erosions despite clinical improvement. *Ann Rheum Dis* 1999;58:156–163.
55. Trabandt A, Gay RE, Gay S. Oncogene activation in rheumatoid synovium. *APMIS* 1992;100:861–875.
56. Lafyatis R, Remmers EF, Roberts AB, et al. Anchorage independent growth regulation of synoviocytes from arthritic and normal joints: stimulation by exogenous platelet-derived growth factor and inhibition by transforming growth factor-beta and retinoids. *J Clin Invest* 1989;83:1267–1276.
57. Wright JJ, Gunter KC, Mitsuya H, et al. Expression of a zinc finger gene in HTLV-I and HTLV-II transformed cells. *Science* 1990;248:588–591.
58. Trabandt A, Aicher WK, Gay RE, et al. Spontaneous expression of immediately-early response genes c-*fos* and *egr-1* in collagenase-producing rheumatoid synovial fibroblasts. *Rheumatol Int* 1992;12:53–59.
59. Aicher WK, Heer AH, Trabandt A, et al. Overexpression of zinc-finger transcription factor Z-225/*egr-1* in synoviocytes from rheumatoid arthritis patients. *J Immunol* 1994;152:5940–5948.
60. Aicher WK, Alexander D, Haas C, et al. Transcription factor early growth response gene 1 activity up-regulates expression of tissue inhibitor of metalloproteinases in human synovial fibroblasts. *Arthritis Rheum* 2003;48:348–359.
61. Krane SM, Conca W, Stephenson ML, et al. Mechanisms of matrix degradation in rheumatoid arthritis. *Ann NY Acad Sci* 1990;580:350–354.
62. Schönthal A, Herrlich P, Rahmsdorf HJ, et al. Requirement for *fos* gene expression in the transcriptional activation of collagenase by other oncogenes and phorbol esters. *Cell* 1988;54:325–344.
63. Mauviel A. Cytokine regulation of metalloproteinase gene expression. *J Cell Biochem* 1993;53:288–295.
64. Angel P, Karin M. The role of *Jun*, *Fos* and the AP-1 complex in cell proliferation and activation. *Biochim Biophys Acta* 1991;1072:129–157.
65. Asahara H, Fujisawa K, Kobata T, et al. Direct evidence of high DNA binding activity of transcription factor AP-1 in rheumatoid arthritis synovium. *Arthritis Rheum* 1997;40:912–918.
66. Muegge K, Durum SK. From cell code to gene code: cytokines and transcription factors. *New Biol* 1989;1:239–247.
67. Jonat C, Rahmsdorf HJ, Park KK, et al. Antitumor promotion and anti-inflammation: down-modulation of AP-1 (*Fos/Jun*) activity by glucocorticoid hormone. *Cell* 1990;62:1189–1204.
68. Morita Y, Kashihara N, Yamamura M, et al. Antisense oligonucleotides targeting c-*fos* mRNA inhibit rheumatoid synovial fibroblast proliferation. *Ann Rheum Dis* 1998;57:122–124.
69. Gay S, Gay RE. Cellular basis and oncogene expression of rheumatoid joint destruction. *Rheumatol Int* 1989;9:105–113.
70. Sorrentino V, Drozdoff V, McKinney MD, et al. Potentiation of growth factor activity by exogenous c-*myc* expression. *Proc Natl Acad Sci U S A* 1986;83:8167–8171.
71. Case JP, Lafyatis R, Remmers EF, et al. Transin/stromelysin expression in rheumatoid synovium: a activation-associated metalloproteinase secreted by phenotypically invasive synoviocytes. *Am J Pathol* 1989;135:1064.
72. Kitasato H, Noda M, Akahoshi T, et al. Activated *ras* modifies the proliferative response of rheumatoid synovial cells to TNF-α and TGF-α. *Inflamm Res* 2001;50:592–597.
73. Mori N, Shirakawa F, Abe M, et al. Human T-cell leukemia virus type I *tax* transactivates the interleukin-6 gene in human rheumatoid synovial cells. *J Rheumatol* 1995;22:2049–2054.
74. Inoue H, Takamori M, Nagata N, et al. An investigation of cell proliferation and soluble mediators induced by interleukin-1β in human synovial fibroblasts: comparative response in osteoarthritis and rheumatoid arthritis. *Inflamm Res* 2001;50:65–72.
75. Handel ML, McMorrow LB, Gravallese EM. Nuclear factor κB in rheumatoid synovium: localization of p50 and p65. *Arthritis Rheum* 1995;38:1762–1770.
76. Crofford LJ, Tan B, McCarthy CJ, et al. Involvement of nuclear factor κB in the regulation of cyclooxygenase-2 expression by interleukin-1 in rheumatoid synoviocytes. *Arthritis Rheum* 1997;40:226–236.
77. Asahara H, Asanuma M, Ogawa N, et al. High DNA-binding activity of transcription factor NFκB in synovial membranes of patients with rheumatoid arthritis. *Biochem Mol Biol Int* 1995;37:827–832.
78. Fujisawa K, Aono H, Hasunuma T, et al. Activation of transcription factor NFκB in human synovial cells in response to tumor necrosis factor-α. *Arthritis Rheum* 1996;39:197–203.
79. Grimbacher B, Aicher WK, Peter HH, et al. TNF-α induces the transcription factor *Egr-1*, pro-inflammatory cytokines and cell proliferation in human skin fibroblasts and synovial lining cells. *Rheumatol Int* 1998;17:185–192.
80. Gerritsen ME, Shen C-P, Perry A. Synovial fibroblasts and the sphingomyelinase pathway: sphingomyelin turnover and ceramide generation are not signaling mechanisms for the actions of tumor necrosis factor-α. *Am J Pathol* 1998;152:505–512.
81. Miyazawa K, Mori A, Yamamoto K, et al. Constitutive transcription of the human interleukin-6 gene by rheumatoid synoviocytes: spontaneous activation of NF-κB and CBF-1. *Am J Pathol* 1998;152:793–803.
82. Miyazawa K, Mori A, Yamamoto K, et al. Transcriptional roles of CCAAT/enhancer binding protein-β nuclear factor-κB, and C-promoter binding factor 1 in interleukin (IL)-1β-induced IL-6 synthesis by human rheumatoid fibroblast-like synoviocytes. *J Biol Chem* 1998;273:7620–7627.
83. Gravallese EM, Manning C, Tsay A, et al. Synovial tissue in rheumatoid arthritis is a source of osteoclast differentiation factor. *Arthritis Rheum* 2000;43:250–258.
84. Takayanagi H, Iizuka H, Juji T, et al. Involvement of receptor activator of nuclear factor κB ligand/osteoclast differentiation factor in osteoclastogenesis from synoviocytes in rheumatoid arthritis. *Arthritis Rheum* 2000;43:259–269.
85. Shigeyama Y, Pap T, Künzler P, et al. Expression of osteoclast differentiation factor in rheumatoid arthritis. *Arthritis Rheum* 2000;43:2523–2530.
86. Romas E, Gillespie MT, Martin TJ. Involvement of receptor activator of NFκB ligand and tumor necrosis factor-α in bone destruction in rheumatoid arthritis. *Bone* 2002;30:340–346.
87. Boumpas DT. A novel action of glucocorticoids: NFκB inhibition. *Br J Rheumatol* 1996;35:709–710.
88. Aupperle KR, Bennett BL, Boyle DL, et al. NF-κB regulation by IκB kinase in primary fibroblast-like synoviocytes. *J Immunol* 1999;163:427–433.
89. Aupperle KR, Bennett BL, Han Z, et al. NF-κB regulation by IκB kinase-2 in rheumatoid arthritis synoviocytes. *J Immunol* 2001;166:2705–2711.
90. Johnson GL, Lapadat R. Mitogen-activated protein kinase pathways mediated by ERK, JNK, and protein kinases. *Science* 2002;298:1911–1912.
91. Faour WH, He Y, He QW, et al. Prostaglandin E(2) regulates the level and stability of cyclooxygenase-2 mRNA through activation of p38 mitogen-activated protein kinase in interleukin-1β treated human synovial fibroblasts. *J Biol Chem* 2001;276:31720–31731.
92. Schroen DJ, Chen JD, Vincenti MP, et al. The nuclear receptor corepressor SMRT inhibits interstitial collagenase (MMP-1) transcription through an HRE-independent mechanism. *Biochem Biophys Res Commun* 1997;237:52–58.
93. Miyazawa K, Mori A, Miyata H, et al. Regulation of interleukin-1β-induced interleukin-6 gene expression in human fibroblast-like synoviocytes by p38 mitogen-activated protein kinase. *J Biol Chem* 1998;273:24832–24838.
94. Westermarck J, Li SP, Kallunki T, et al. p38 mitogen-activated protein kinase-dependent activation of protein phosphatases 1 and 2A inhibits MEK1 and MEK2 activity and collagenase 1 (MMP-1) gene expression. *Mol Cell Biol* 2001;21:2373–2383.
95. Han Z, Boyle DL, Chang L, et al. c-*Jun* N terminal kinase is required for metalloproteinase expression and joint destruction in inflammatory arthritis. *J Clin Invest* 2001;108:73–81.
96. Fahmi H, Pelletier JP, Di Battista JA, et al. Peroxisome proliferator-activated receptor γ activators inhibit MMP-1 production in human synovial fibroblasts likely by reducing the binding of the activator protein 1. *Osteoarthritis Cartilage* 2002;10:100–108.
97. Yamasaki S, Nakashima T, Kawakami A, et al. Functional changes in rheumatoid fibroblast-like synovial cells through activation of peroxisome proliferator-activated receptor γ-mediated signalling pathway. *Clin Exp Immunol* 2002;129:379–384.

98. Ji JD, Cheon H, Jun JB, et al. Effects of peroxisome proliferator-activated receptor-γ (PPAR-γ) on the expression of inflammatory cytokines and apoptosis induction in rheumatoid synovial fibroblasts and monocytes. *J Autoimmun* 2001;17:215–221.
99. Tolboom TC, Pieterman E, van der Laan WH, et al. Invasive properties of fibroblast-like synoviocytes: correlation with growth characteristics and expression of MMP-1, MMP-3, and MMP-1. *Ann Rheum Dis* 2002;61:975–980.
100. Mohr W, Beneke K, Mohing W. Proliferation of synovial lining cells and fibroblasts. *Ann Rheum Dis* 1975;34:219–224.
101. Khoa ND, Nakazawa M, Hasunuma T, et al. Potential role of HOXD9 in synoviocyte proliferation. *Arthritis Rheum* 2001;44:1013–1021.
102. Yang E, Zha J, Jockel J, et al. Bad, a heterodimeric partner for Bcl-xL and *Bcl-2*, displaces Bax and promotes cell death. *Cell* 1995;80:285–291.
103. Hockenbery D, Nunez G, Milliman C, et al. *Bcl-2* is an inner mitochondrial membrane protein that blocks programmed cell death. *Nature* 1990;348:334–336.
104. Nakajima T, Aono H, Hasunuma T, et al. Apoptosis and functional *Fas* antigen in rheumatoid arthritis synoviocytes. *Arthritis Rheum* 1995;38:485–491.
105. Matsumoto S, Müller-Ladner U, Gay RE, et al. Ultrastructural demonstration of apoptosis, *Fas* and *Bcl-2* expression of rheumatoid synovial fibroblasts. *J Rheumatol* 1996;23:1345–1352.
106. Müller-Ladner U, Kriegsmann J, Gay RE, et al. Upregulation of *Bcl-2* and *fas* mRNA in synovium of patients with rheumatoid arthritis (RA). *Arthritis Rheum* 1994;37(suppl):163.
107. Kurowska M, Rudnicka W, Kontny E, et al. Fibroblast-like synoviocytes from rheumatoid arthritis patients express functional IL-15 receptor complex: endogenous IL-15 in autocrine fashion enhances cell proliferation and expression of *Bcl-x(L)* and *Bcl-2*. *J Immunol* 2002;169:1760–1767.
108. Elliott SF, Coon CI, Hays E, et al. Bcl-3 is an interleukin-1-responsive gene in chondrocytes and synovial fibroblasts that activates transcription of the matrix metalloproteinase 1 gene. *Arthritis Rheum* 2002;46:3230–3239.
109. Pap T, Franz JK, Hummel KM, et al. Activation of synovial fibroblasts in rheumatoid arthritis: lack of expression of the tumour suppressor PTEN at sites of invasive growth and destruction. *Arthritis Res* 2000;2:59–64.
110. Franz JK, Pap T, Hummel KM, et al. Expressions of sentrin, a novel anti-apoptopic molecule at sites of synovial invasion in rheumatoid arthritis. *Arthritis Rheum* 2000;43:544–607.
111. Firestein GS, Nguyen K, Aupperle KR, et al. Apoptosis in rheumatoid arthritis: p53 overexpression in rheumatoid arthritis synovium. *Am J Pathol* 1996;149:2143–2151.
112. Yamanishi Y, Boyle DL, Rosengren S, et al. Regional analysis of p53 mutations in rheumatoid arthritis synovium. *Proc Natl Acad Sci U S A* 2002;99:10025–10030.
113. Firestein GS, Echeverri F, Yeo M, et al. Somatic mutations in the p53 tumor suppressor gene in rheumatoid arthritis synovium. *Proc Natl Acad Sci U S A* 1997;94:10895–10900.
114. Kullmann F, Judex M, Neudecker I, et al. Analysis of the p53 tumor suppressor gene in rheumatoid arthritis synovial fibroblasts. *Arthritis Rheum* 1999;42:1594–1600.
115. Migita K, Tanaka F, Yamasaki S, et al. Regulation of rheumatoid synoviocyte proliferation by endogenous p53 induction. *Clin Exp Immunol* 2001;126:334–338.
116. Yamanishi Y, Boyle DL, Pinkoski MJ, et al. Regulation of joint destruction and inflammation by p53 in collagen-induced arthritis. *Am J Pathol* 2001;160:123–130.
117. Pap T, Aupperle KR, Gay S, et al. Invasiveness of synovial fibroblasts is regulated by p53 in the SCID mouse *in vivo* model of cartilage invasion. *Arthritis Rheum* 2001;44:676–681.
118. Gustin JA, Maehama T, Dixon JE, et al. The PTEN tumor suppressor protein inhibits tumor necrosis factor-induced nuclear factor-κB activity. *J Biol Chem* 2001;276:27740–27744.
119. Koul D, Yao Y, Abbruzzese JL, et al. Tumor suppressor MMAC/PTEN inhibits cytokine-induced NFκB activation without interfering with the IκB degradation pathway. *J Biol Chem* 2001;276:11402–11408.
120. Pianetti S, Arsura M, Romieu-Mourez R, et al. Her-2/neu overexpression induces NF-κB via a PI3-kinase/Akt pathway involving calpain-mediated degradation of IκB-α that can be inhibited by the tumor suppressor PTEN. *Oncogene* 2001;20:1287–1299.
121. Zhang HG, Wang Y, Xie JF, et al. Regulation of tumor necrosis factor α-mediated apoptosis of rheumatoid arthritis synovial fibroblasts by the protein kinase akt. *Arthritis Rheum* 2001;44:1555–1567.
122. Okura T, Gong L, Kamitani T, et al. Protection against *Fas*/APO-1-and tumor necrosis factor-mediated cell death by a novel protein, sentrin. *J Immunol* 1997;157:4277–4281.
123. Fujisawa K, Asahara H, Okamoto K, et al. Therapeutic effect of the anti-*Fas* antibody on arthritis in HTLV-I *tax* transgenic mice. *J Clin Invest* 1996;98:271–278.
124. Hoa TTM, Hasunuma T, Aono H, et al. Novel mechanisms of selective apoptosis in synovial T cells of patients with rheumatoid arthritis. *J Rheumatol* 1996;23:1332–1337.
125. Schedel J, Gay RE, Künzler P, et al. FLICE-inhibitory protein expression in synovial fibroblasts and at sites of cartilage and bone erosion in rheumatoid arthritis. *Arthritis Rheum* 2002;46:1512–1518.
126. Allen JB, Manthey CL, Hand AR, et al. Rapid onset synovial inflammation and hyperplasia induced by transforming growth factor beta. *J Exp Med* 1990;171:231–247.
127. Cheon H, Yu SJ, Yoo DH, et al. Increased expression of pro-inflammatory cytokines and metalloproteinase-1 by TGF-β1 in synovial fibroblasts from rheumatoid arthritis and normal individuals. *Clin Exp Immunol* 2002;127:547–552.
128. Kim G, Jun B, Elkon KB. Necessary role of phosphatidylinositol 3-kinase in transforming growth factor β-mediated activation of akt in normal and rheumatoid arthritis synovial fibroblasts. *Arthritis Rheum* 2002;46:1504–1511.
129. Wahl SM, Allen JB, Wong HL, et al. Antagonistic and agonistic effects of transforming growth factor-beta and IL-1 in rheumatoid synovitis. *J Immunol* 1990;145:2514–2519.
130. Melnyk VO, Shipley GD, Sternfeld MD, et al. Synoviocytes synthesize, bind, and respond to basic fibroblast growth factor. *Arthritis Rheum* 1990;33:493–500.
131. Kumkumian GK, Lafyatis R, Remmers EF, et al. Platelet-derived growth factor and IL-1 interactions in rheumatoid arthritis: regulation of synoviocyte proliferation, prostaglandin production, and collagenase transcription. *J Immunol* 1989;143:833–837.
132. Kasama T, Shiozawa F, Kobayashi K, et al. Vascular endothelial growth factor expression by activated synovial leukocytes in rheumatoid arthritis: critical involvement of the interaction with synovial fibroblasts. *Arthritis Rheum* 2001;44:2512–2524.
133. Giatromanolaki A, Sivridis E, Athanassou N, et al. The angiogenic pathway "vascular endothelial growth factor/flk-1(KDR)-receptor" in rheumatoid arthritis and osteoarthritis. *J Pathol* 2001;194:101–108.
134. Franz JK, Kolb SA, Hummel KM, et al. Interleukin-16, produced by synovial fibroblasts, mediates chemoattraction for CD4+ T lymphocytes in rheumatoid arthritis. *Eur J Immunol* 1998;28:2661–2671.
135. Chabaud M, Fossiez F, Taupin J-L, Miossec P. Enhancing effect of IL-17 on IL-1-induced IL-6 and leukemia inhibitory factor production by rheumatoid arthritis synoviocytes and its regulation by Th2 cytokines. *J Immunol* 1998;161:409–414.
136. Maier R, Ganu V, Lotz M. Interleukin-11, an inducible cytokine in human articular chondrocytes and synoviocytes, stimulates the production of the tissue inhibitor of metalloproteinases. *J Biol Chem* 1993;268:21527–21532.
137. McInnes IB, Liew FY. Interleukin-15: a proinflammatory role in rheumatoid arthritis synovitis. *Immunol Today* 1998;19:75–79.
138. Firestein GS, Alvaro-Gracia JM, Maki R. Quantitative analysis of cytokine gene expression in rheumatoid arthritis. *J Immunol* 1990;144:3347–3353.
139. Brennan FM, Field M, Chu CQ, et al. Cytokine expression in rheumatoid arthritis. *Br J Rheumatol* 1991;30:76–80.
140. Gracie JA, Forsey RJ, Chan WL, et al. A proinflammatory role in rheumatoid arthritis synovitis. *Immunol Today* 1998;19:75–79.
141. Koch AE, Kunkel SL, Burrows JC, et al. Synovial tissue macrophage as a source of the chemotactic cytokine IL-8. *J Immunol* 1991;147:2187–2195.
142. Keyszer GM, Heer AH, Kriegsmann J, et al. Detection of insulin-like growth factor I and II in synovial tissue specimens of patients with rheumatoid arthritis and osteoarthritis by in situ hybridization. *J Rheumatol* 1995;22:275–281.

143. Lotz M, Guerne PA. Interleukin-6 induces the synthesis of tissue inhibitor of metalloproteinases-1/erythroid potentiating activity (TIMP-1/EPA). *J Biol Chem* 1991;266:2017–2020.
144. Alvaro-Gracia JM, Zvaifler NJ, Firestein GS. Cytokines in chronic inflammatory arthritis. V. Mutual antagonism between interferon-gamma and tumor necrosis factor-alpha on HLA-DR expression, proliferation, collagenase production, and granulocyte-macrophage colony-stimulating factor production by rheumatoid arthritis synoviocytes. *J Clin Invest* 1990;86:1790–1798.
145. Hirth A, Distler O, Seibl R, et al. Interleukin-21 receptor is expressed in synovial lining cells of patients with rheumatoid arthritis. *Arthritis Rheum* 2001;44(suppl):164.
146. Chicheportiche Y, Chicheportiche R, Sizing I, et al. Proinflammatory activity of TWEAK on human dermal fibroblasts and synoviocytes: blocking and enhancing effects of anti-TWEAK monoclonal antibodies. *Arthritis Res* 2002;4:126–133.
147. Deon D, Ahmed S, Tai K, et al. Cross-talk between IL-1 and IL-6 signaling pathways in rheumatoid arthritis synovial fibroblasts. *J Immunol* 2001;167:5395–5403.
148. Farahat MN, Yanni G, Poston R, Panayi GS. Cytokine expression in synovial membranes of patients with rheumatoid arthritis and osteoarthritis. *Ann Rheum Dis* 1993;52:870–875.
149. Katsikis PD, Chu C, Brennan FM, et al. Immunoregulatory role of interleukin-10 in rheumatoid arthritis. *J Exp Med* 1994;179:1517–1527.
150. Taylor DJ. Cytokine combinations increase p75 tumor necrosis factor receptor binding and stimulate receptor shedding in rheumatoid synovial fibroblasts. *Arthritis Rheum* 1994;37:232–235.
151. Maini RN. Testing immunological concepts by clinical trials in rheumatoid arthritis. *Immunologist* 1994;2:147–176.
152. Furst DE, Breedveld FC, Kalden JR, et al. Updated consensus statement on biological agents for the treatment of rheumatoid arthritis and other rheumatic diseases (May 2002). *Ann Rheum Dis* 2002; 61(suppl 2):2–7.
153. Simon AK, Seipelt E, Sieper J. Divergent T-cell cytokine patterns in inflammatory arthritis. *Proc Natl Acad Sci U S A* 1994;91:8562–8566.
154. Fong K-Y, Boey M-L, Koh W-H, et al. Cytokine concentrations in the synovial fluid and plasma of rheumatoid arthritis patients: correlation with bony erosions. *Clin Exp Rheumatol* 1994;12:55–58.
155. Eberhard BA, Laxer RM, Andersson U, et al. Local synthesis of both macrophage and T cell cytokines by synovial fluid cells from children with juvenile rheumatoid arthritis. *Clin Exp Immunol* 1994; 96:260–266.
156. Müller-Ladner U, Gay RE, Gay S. Signaling and effector pathways. *Curr Opin Rheumatol* 1999;1:194–201.
157. Kang RY, Freire-Moar J, Sigal E, et al. Expression of cyclooxygenase-2 in human and an animal model of rheumatoid arthritis. *Br J Rheumatol* 1996;35:711–718.
158. Franz JK, Hummel KM, Aicher WK, et al. *In-situ* detection of cyclooxygenase (COX) 1 and 2 mRNA in rheumatoid arthritis (RA) and osteoarthritis (OA) synovium. *Arthritis Rheum* 1996;39(suppl):197.
159. Kusunoki N, Yamazaki R, Kawai S. Induction of apoptosis in rheumatoid synovial fibroblasts by celecoxib, but not by other selective cyclooxygenase 2 inhibitors. *Arthritis Rheum* 2002;46:3159–3167.
160. Nickerson-Nutter CL, Medvedeff E. The effect of leukotriene synthesis inhibitors in models of acute and chronic inflammation. *Arthritis Rheum* 1996;39:515–521.
161. Laufer SA, Augustin J, Dannhardt D, Kiefer W. (6,7-Diarydihydropyrrolizin-5-yl)acetic acids: a novel class of potent dual inhibitors of both cyclooxygenase and 5-lipoxygenase. *J Med Chem* 1994;12: 1894–1897.
162. Gay RE, Neidhart M, Pataky F, et al. Dual inhibition of 5-lipoxygenase and cyclooxygenases 1 and 2 by ML3000 reduces joint destruction in adjuvant arthritis. *J Rheumatol* 2001;28:2060–2065.
163. Springer TA. Adhesion receptors of the immune system. *Nature* 1990;346:425–433.
164. Hale LP, Martin ME, McCollum DE, et al. Immunohistologic analysis of the distribution of cell adhesion molecules within the inflammatory synovial microenvironment. *Arthritis Rheum* 1989;32:22–30.
165. Oppenheimer-Marks N, Lipsky PE. The role of cell adhesion in the evolution of inflammatory arthritis. In: Wegner CD, ed. *Adhesion molecules.* San Diego: Academic, 1994:141–161.
166. Springer TA. Traffic signals for lymphocyte recirculation and leucocyte emigration: the multistep paradigm. *Cell* 1994;76:301–314.
167. Pitzalis C, Kingsley G, Panayi G. Adhesion molecules in rheumatoid arthritis: role in the pathogenesis and prospects for therapy. *Ann Rheum Dis* 1994;53:278–288.
168. Koch AE, Burrows JC, Haines GK, et al. Immunolocalization of endothelial and leukocyte adhesion molecules in human rheumatoid and osteoarthritic synovial tissues. *Lab Invest* 1991;64:313–320.
169. Kriegsmann J, Keyszer GM, Geiler T, et al. Expression of endothelial leukocyte adhesion molecule-1 (ELAM-1) mRNA and protein in rheumatoid arthritis (RA). *Arthritis Rheum* 1995;38:750–754.
170. Morales-Ducret J, Wayner E, Elices MJ, et al. Alpha 4/beta 1 integrin (VLA-4) ligands in arthritis: vascular cell adhesion molecule in synovium and on fibroblast-like synoviocytes. *J Immunol* 1992;149: 1424–1431.
171. Kriegsmann J, Keyszer GM, Geiler T, Bräuer R, et al. Expression of vascular cell adhesion molecule-1 mRNA and protein in rheumatoid arthritis synovium demonstrated by *in situ* hybridization and immunohistochemistry. *Lab Invest* 1995;72:209–213.
172. Müller-Ladner U, Kriegsmann J, Stahl D, at al. Expression of alternatively spliced CS-1 fibronectin isoform and its counter-receptor VLA-4 in rheumatoid arthritis synovium. *J Rheumatol* 1997;24: 1873–1880.
173. Morel JC, Park CC, Woods JM, et al. A novel role for interleukin-18 in adhesion molecule induction through NFκB and phosphatidylinositol (PI) 3-kinase-dependent signal transduction pathways. *J Biol Chem* 2001;276:37069–37075.
174. Morel JC, Park CC, Zhu K, et al. Signal transduction pathways involved in rheumatoid arthritis synovial fibroblast interleukin-18-induced vascular cell adhesion molecule-1 expression. *J Biol Chem* 2002;277:34679–34691.
175. Möller B, Kessler U, Rehart S, et al. Expression of interleukin-18 receptor in fibroblast-like synoviocytes. *Arthritis Res* 2002;4:139–144.
176. Tessier PA, Cattaruzzi P, McColl SR. Inhibition of lymphocyte adhesion to cytokine-activated synovial fibroblasts by glucocorticoids involves the attenuation of vascular cell adhesion molecule 1 and intercellular adhesion molecule 1 gene expression. *Arthritis Rheum* 1996;39:226–234.
177. Hayashi T, Abe E, Jasin HE. Fibronectin synthesis in superficial and deep layers of normal articular cartilage. *Arthritis Rheum* 1996;39: 567–573.
178. Rinaldi N, Schwarz-Eywill M, Leppelmann-Jansen P, et al. Increased expression of integrins on fibroblast-like synoviocytes from rheumatoid arthritis in vitro correlates with enhanced binding to extracellular matrix proteins. *Ann Rheum Dis* 1997;56:45–51.
179. Wang AZ, Wang JC, Fisher GW, et al. Interleukin-1β-stimulated invasion of articular cartilage by rheumatoid synovial fibroblasts is inhibited by antibodies to specific integrin receptors and by collagenase inhibitors. *Arthritis Rheum* 1997;40:1298–1307.
180. Shang X-Z, Lang BJ, Issekutz AC. Adhesion molecule mechanisms mediating monocyte migration through synovial fibroblast and endothelium barriers: role for CD11/CD18, very late antigen-4 (CD49d/CD29), very late antigen-5 (CD49e/CD29), and vascular cell adhesion molecule-1 (CD106). *J Immunol* 1998;160:467–474.
181. Sakai K, Matsuno H, Tsuji H, et al. Substance P receptor (NK1) gene expression in synovial tissue in rheumatoid arthritis and osteoarthritis. *Scand J Rheumatol* 1998;27:135–141.
182. Lambert N, Lescoulié PL, Yassine-Diab B, et al. Substance P enhances cytokine-induced vascular cell adhesion molecule-1 (VCAM-1) expression on cultured rheumatoid fibroblast-like synoviocytes. *Clin Exp Immunol* 1998;113:269–275.
183. Chin JE, Winterrowd GE, Krzesicki RF, et al. Role of cytokines in inflammatory synovitis: the coordinate regulation of intercellular adhesion molecule 1 and HLA class I and class II antigens in rheumatoid synovial fibroblasts. *Arthritis Rheum* 1990;33:1776–1786.
184. Nakatsuka K, Tanaka Y, Hubscher S, et al. Rheumatoid synovial fibroblasts are stimulated by the cellular adhesion to T cells through lymphocyte function associated antigen-1/intercellular adhesion molecule-1. *J Rheumatol* 1997;24:458–464.
185. Kavanaugh AF, Davis SL, Nichols LA, et al. Treatment of refractory rheumatoid arthritis with a monoclonal antibody to intercellular adhesion molecule 1. *Arthritis Rheum* 1994;37:992–999.
186. Youssef PP, Triantafillou S, Parker A, et al. Effects of pulse methylprednisolone on cell adhesion molecules in the synovial membrane

in rheumatoid arthritis: reduced E-selectin and intercellular adhesion molecule 1 expression. *Arthritis Rheum* 1996;39:1970–1979.
187. El-Gabalawy H, Gallatin M, Vazeux R, et al. Expression of ICAM-R (ICAM-3): a novel counter-receptor for LFA-1 in rheumatoid and non-rheumatoid synovium. *Arthritis Rheum* 1994;37:846–854.
188. Skezanecz Z, Haines GK, Lin TR, et al. Differential distribution of intercellular adhesion molecules (ICAM-1, ICAM-2, and ICAM-3) and the MS-1 antigen in normal and diseased human synovia. *Arthritis Rheum* 1994;37:221–231.
189. Pirila L, Aho H, Roivainen A, et al. Identification of α6β1 integrin positive cells in synovial lining layer as type B synoviocytes. *J Rheumatol* 2001;28:478–484.
190. Johnson BA, Haines GK, Harlow LA, et al. Adhesion molecule expression in human synovial tissue. *Arthritis Rheum* 1993;36:137–146.
191. Riikonen T, Westermarck J, Koivisto L, et al. Integrin α2β1 is a positive regulator of collagenase [MMP-1] and collagen α1[1] gene expression. *J Biol Chem* 1995;270:13548–13352.
192. Pirilä L, Heino J. Altered integrin expression in rheumatoid synovial lining type B cells: *in vitro* cytokine regulation of α1β1, α6β1, αvβ5 integrins. *J Rheumatol* 1996;23:1691–1698.
193. Smith RS, Smith TJ, Blieden TM, et al. Fibroblasts as sentinel cells: synthesis of chemokines and regulation of inflammation. *Am J Pathol* 1997;151:317–322.
194. Liu MF, Chao SC, Wang CR, et al. Expression of CD40 and CD40 ligand among cell populations within rheumatoid synovial compartment. *Autoimmunity* 2001;34:107–113.
195. Matsui T, Akahoshi T, Namai R, et al. Selective recruitment of CCR6-expressing cells by increased production of MIP-3α in rheumatoid arthritis. *Clin Exp Immunol* 2001;125:155–161.
196. Langdon C, Leith J, Smith F, et al. Oncostatin M stimulates monocyte chemoattractant protein-1- and interleukin-1-induced matrix metalloproteinase-1 production by human synovial fibroblasts *in vitro. Arthritis Rheum* 1997;40:2139–2136.
197. Nanki T, Nagasaka K, Hayashida K, et al. Chemokines regulate IL-6 and IL-8 production by fibroblast-like synoviocytes from patients with rheumatoid arthritis. *J Immunol* 2001;167:5381–5385.
198. Hitchon C, Wong K, Ma G, et al. Hypoxia-induced production of stromal cell-derived factor 1 (CXCL12) and vascular endothelial growth factor by synovial fibroblasts. *Arthritis Rheum* 2002;46: 2587–2597.
199. Burger JA, Zvaifler NJ, Tsukada N, et al. Fibroblast-like synoviocytes support B-cell pseudoemperipolesis via a stromal cell-derived factor-1-and CD106 (VCAM-1)-dependent mechanism. *J Clin Invest* 2001;107:305–315.
200. Kunkel SL, Lukacs N, Kasama T, et al. The role of chemokines in inflammatory joint disease. *J Leukoc Biol* 1996;59:6–12.
201. Müller-Ladner U, Evans CH, Franklin BN, et al. Gene transfer of cytokine inhibitors into human synovial fibroblasts in the SCID mouse model. *Arthritis Rheum* 1999;42:490–497.
202. Pierer M, Kyburz D, Rethage J, et al. TLR2 dependent upregulation of chemokines in RA-SF. *Arthritis Rheum* 2002;46(suppl):553.
203. Vincenti MP, Brinckerhoff CE. Transcriptional regulation of collagenase (MMP-1, MMP-13) genes in arthritis: integration of complex signaling pathways for the recruitment of gene-specific transcription factors. *Arthritis Res* 2002;4:157–164.
204. Smolian H, Aurer A, Sittinger M, et al. Secretion of gelatinases and activation of gelatinase A (MMP-2) by human rheumatoid synovial fibroblasts. *Biol Chem* 2001;382:1491–1499.
205. Maeda S, Sawai T, Uziki M, et al. Determination of interstitial collagenase (MMP-1) in patients with rheumatoid arthritis. *Ann Rheum Dis* 1995;54:970–975.
206. Clark IM, Powell LK, Ramsey S, et al. The measurement of collagenase, TIMP, and collagenase-TIMP complex in synovial fluids from patients with osteoarthritis and rheumatoid arthritis. *Arthritis Rheum* 1993;36:372–380.
207. Konttinen YT, Ceponis A, Takagi M, et al. New collagenolytic enzymes/cascade identified at the pannus-hard tissue junction in rheumatoid arthritis: destruction from above. *Matrix Biol* 1998;17: 585–601.
208. Kozaci LD, Buttle DJ, Hollander AP. Degradation of type II collagen, but not proteoglycan, correlates with matrix metalloproteinase activity in cartilage explant cultures. *Arthritis Rheum* 1997;40:164–174.
209. Tomita T, Nakase T, Kaneko M, et al. Expression of extracellular matrix metalloproteinase inducer and enhancement of the production of matrix metalloproteinases in rheumatoid arthritis. *Arthritis Rheum* 2002;46:373–378.
210. Zucker S, Hymowitz M, Rollo EE, et al. Tumorigenic potential of extracellular matrix metalloproteinase inducer. *Am J Pathol* 2001;158: 1921–1928.
211. Kolomytkin OV, Marino AA, Waddell DD, et al. IL-1β-induced production of metalloproteinases by synovial cells depends on gap junction conductance. *Am J Physiol Cell Physiol* 2002;282:C1254–C1260.
212. Gravallese EM, Darling JM, Ladd AL, et al. *In situ* hybridization studies on stromelysin and collagenase mRNA expression in rheumatoid synovium. *Arthritis Rheum* 1991;34:1071–1084.
213. Müller-Ladner U, Gay S. MMPs and rheumatoid synovial fibroblasts: Siamese twins in joint destruction? *Ann Rheum Dis* 2002;61: 957–959.
214. Lindy O, Konttinen YT, Sorsa T, et al. Matrix metalloproteinase 13 (collagenase 3) in human rheumatoid synovium. *Arthritis Rheum* 1997;40:1391–1399.
215. Ahrens D, Koch AE, Pope RM, et al. Expression of matrix metalloproteinase 9 (96-kd gelatinase B) in human rheumatoid arthritis. *Arthritis Rheum* 1996;39:1576–1587.
216. Gruber BL, Sorbi D, French DL, et al. Markedly elevated serum MMP-9 (gelatinase B) levels in rheumatoid arthritis: a potentially useful laboratory marker. *Clin Immunol Immunopathol* 1996:78: 161–171.
217. Mitsui H, Nishimura A, Yoshimura K, et al. Expression of membrane type matrix metalloproteinases in the synovial tissue from patients with rheumatoid arthritis. *Arthritis Rheum* 1998;42(suppl):1710.
218. Pap T, Shigeyama Y, Kuchen S, et al. Differential expression pattern of membrane-type matrix metalloproteinases in rheumatoid arthritis. *Arthritis Rheum* 2000;43:1226–1232.
219. Joseph L, Lapid S, Sukhatme VP. The major *ras* induced protein in NIH 3T3 cells is cathepsin L. *Nucleic Acid Res* 1987;15:3186–3192.
220. Mason RW, Wilcox D, Wikstrom P, et al. The identification of active forms of cysteine proteinases in Kirsten virus transformed mouse fibroblasts by use of a specific radiolabelled inhibitor. *Biochem J* 1989;257:125–129.
221. Denhardt DT, Greenberg AH, Egan SE, et al. Cysteine proteinase cathepsin L expression correlates closely with the metastatic potential of H-*ras*-transformed murine fibroblasts. *Oncogene* 1987;2:55–59.
222. Maciewicz RA, Wotton SF, Etherington DJ, et al. Susceptibility of the cartilage collagens type II, IX and XI to degradation by the cysteine proteinases, cathepsin D and L. *FEBS Lett* 1990;269:189–193.
223. Nguyen Q, Mort JS, Roughley PJ. Cartilage proteoglycan aggregate is degraded more extensively by cathepsin L than by cathepsin B. *Biochem J* 1990;266:569–573.
224. Keyszer GM, Heer AH, Kriegsmann J, et al. Comparative analysis of cathepsin L, cathepsin D and collagenase mRNA expression in synovial tissues of patients with rheumatoid arthritis and osteoarthritis by *in situ* hybridization. *Arthritis Rheum* 1995;38:976–984.
225. Iwata Y, Mort JS, Tateishi H, et al. Macrophage cathepsin L: a factor in the erosion of subchondral bone in rheumatoid arthritis. *Arthritis Rheum* 1997;40:499–509.
226. Hummel KM, Petrow PK, Jeisy E, et al. Cathepsin K mRNA is expressed in synovium of patients with rheumatoid arthritis (RA) at sites of bone destruction. *J Rheumatol* 1998;25:1887–1894.
227. Esser RE, Angelo RA, Murphey MD, et al. Cysteine proteinase inhibitors decrease articular cartilage and bone destruction in chronic inflammatory arthritis. *Arthritis Rheum* 1994;37:236–247.
228. Davies JMS, Horwitz DA, Davies KJA. Inhibition of collagenase activity by N-chlorotaurine: a product of activated neutrophils. *Arthritis Rheum* 1994;37:424–427.
229. Matucci Cerinic M, Generini S, Partsch G, et al. Synoviocytes from osteoarthritis and rheumatoid arthritis produce plasminogen activators and plasminogen activator inhibitor-1 and display u-PA receptors on their surface. *Life Sci* 1998;63:441–453.
230. Van der Laan WH, Pap T, Ronday HK, et al. Cartilage degradation and and invasion by rheumatoid synovial fibroblasts is inhibited by gene transfer of a cell surface-targeted plasmin inhibitor. *Arthritis Rheum* 2000;43:1710–1718.
231. Pap T, Claus A, Ohtsu S, et al. Osteoclast-independent bone resorption by fibroblast-like cells. *Arthritis Res* 2003;5:R163–R173.

232. Ohtsu S, Pap T, Shigeyama Y, et al. Identification of a novel splice variant of an osteoclast-like v-ATPase BETA-1 subunit in activated fibroblasts. *Arthritis Rheum* 2000;43(suppl):165.
233. Firestein GS, Paine M. Expression of stromelysin and TIMP in rheumatoid arthritis synovium. *Am J Pathol* 1992;1401309–1314.
234. Okada Y, Gonoij Y, Nakanishi I, et al. Immunohistochemical demonstration of collagenase and tissue inhibitor of metalloproteinases (TIMP) in synovial lining cells of rheumatoid synovium. *Virchows Arch B Cell Pathol* 1990;59:305–312.
235. MacNaul KL, Chartrain N, Lark M, et al. Discoordinate expression of stromelysin, collagenase, and tissue inhibitor of metalloproteinases-1 in rheumatoid human synovial fibroblasts: synergistic effects interleukin-1 and tumor necrosis factor-α on stromelysin expression. *J Biol Chem* 1990;265:17238–17245.
236. Ohta S, Harigai M, Tanaka M, et al. Tumor necrosis factor-α (TNF-α) converting enzyme contributes to production of TNF-α in synovial tissues from patients with rheumatoid arthritis. *J Rheumatol* 2001;28: 1756–1763.
237. Van der Laan WH, Quax PH, Seemayer CA, et al. Cartilage degradation and invasion by rheumatoid synovial fibroblasts is inhibited by gene transfer of TIMP-1 and TIMP-3. *Gene Ther* 2003;10:234–242.
238. Neumann E, Judex M, Kullmann, et al. Inhibition of cartilage destruction by double gene transfer of IL-1Ra and IL-10 involves the active pathway. *Gene Ther* 2002;9:1508–1519.

CHAPTER 13

Immunoglobulins and Their Genes

Harry W. Schroeder, Jr.

Immunoglobulin (Ig) molecules are responsible for two major functions: (a) a receptor function that entails the recognition of foreign antigens, such as toxins, viruses, and exposed molecules on the surface of pathogenic organisms, and (b) an effector function that results in the elimination or inactivation of the foreign antigen or of the cell that is marked by the presence of that antigen (1). The portion of the antigen bound by the antibody is termed the epitope. The V (or variable) domain of the antibody demonstrates the molecular heterogeneity necessary to allow differentiation between antigens. Thus, it is the V domain that encodes the receptor function, thereby defining the specificity of the antibody. In contrast, it is the C (or constant) domain of the Ig heavy (H) chain that triggers the effector functions of the antibody after the V region binds the antigen. Effector functions are generally inflammatory reactions and include complement fixation, complement activation, and binding to Fc receptors on the cell surface of basophils, monocytes, platelets, and other components of the immune response.

Immunization of heterologous species with monoclonal antibodies (or a restricted set of immunoglobulins) revealed that immunoglobulins contain both common and individual antigenic determinants. Individual determinants, termed idiotypes, are contained within the V portion of the antibodies used for immunization. Common determinants, termed isotypes, are specific for the constant portion of the antibody and first allowed grouping of immunoglobulins into recognized classes, each class defining an individual type of C domain. Determinants common to subsets of individuals within a species, yet differing between other members of that species, are termed allotypes and define inherited polymorphisms that result from allelic forms of immunoglobulin genes (2).

Several general features of the immunoglobulins deserve mention here in the context of our understanding of this system in relation to rheumatologic diseases. First, the various classes and subclasses of immunoglobulins have special functions that relate to immunologic defense mechanisms. For example, immunoglobulin A (IgA), the major class of immunoglobulin present in all external secretions, is responsible for protecting mucosal surfaces from the primary attack of exogenous substances. A second general consideration is that cross-reactivities or alterations of antigens that are presented to the immune system of the host, unique genetic rearrangements of immunoglobulin genes, or abnormal immune responses to self antigen can lead to the production of antibodies that are reactive with self constituents (3). Such aberrations in the immune response are most often encountered in rheumatoid arthritis (RA), in systemic lupus erythematosus (SLE), and in related disorders. As discussed in other chapters of this text, these immunologic reactions appear to play a significant role in the pathogenesis of some of the manifestations of these diseases (4).

STRUCTURE OF AN ANTIBODY MOLECULE

The basic structure of all immunoglobulins is the same. Immunoglobulins consist of two types of polypeptide chains (Fig. 13.1). The larger is called the heavy (H) chain; the smaller is designated the light (L) chain. Each immunoglobulin subunit contains two identical H and two identical L chains, thus the basic molecular formula is H_2L_2 (5). The disulfide bonds joining the H and L chains connect the carboxyl termini of the L chains to the H chains. The interchain disulfide bridges in the H chain range in number from 1 to 11 for the different classes, and are generally located in the center of the molecule in a region known as the "hinge." The molecular weight of the L chain is about 25,000 daltons; that of the H chain varies between 50,000 and 65,000 daltons. The differences in size are related to differences in the structure of the "hinge," or to the presence of an extra domain in μ and ϵ H chains. The hinge in the γ3 constant region, for example, is four times as long as the hinge in γ1 and is heavily enriched for cysteine and proline residues.

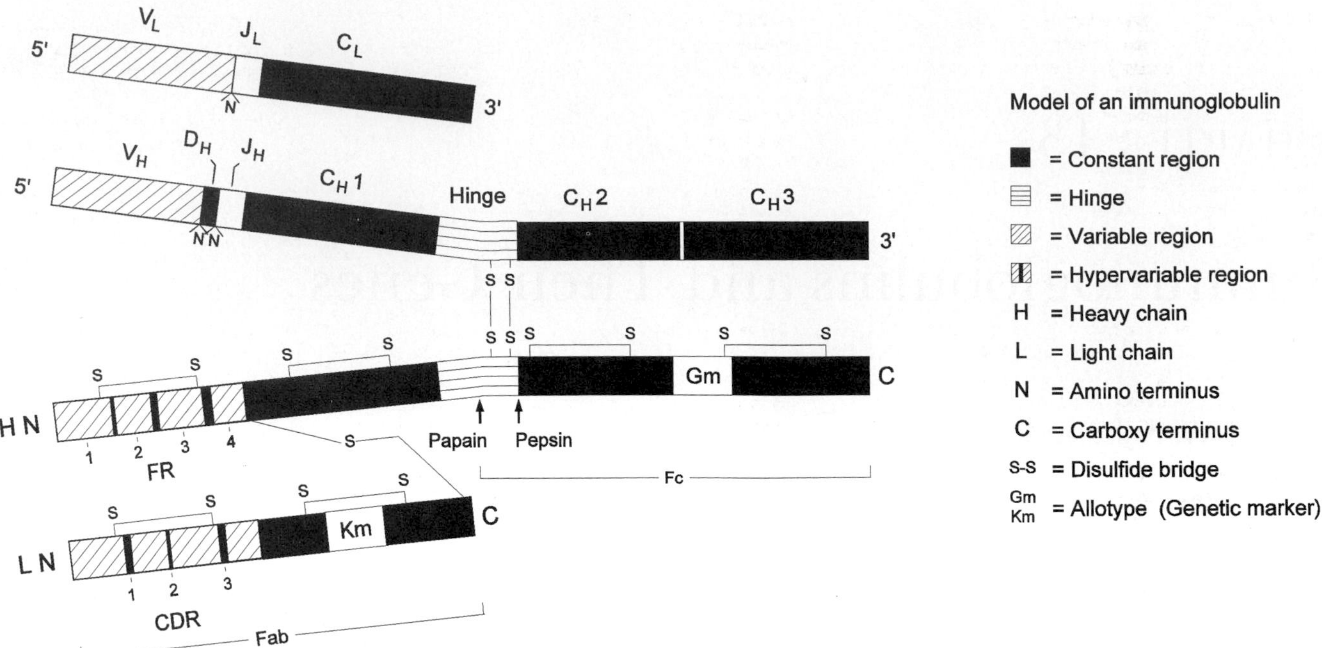

FIG. 13.1. Two-dimensional model of the immunoglobulin molecule.

Comparison of the amino acid sequences of a large number of homogeneous immunoglobulins has documented that the H and L chains, like the intact antibody molecule, can be divided structurally and functionally into V and C regions. The V region, which is the most diverse, is encoded by the first 110 to 120 amino terminal residues. The remaining half of the L chain and three fourths of the H chain are known as the C regions because their structure is virtually the same for all molecules belonging to a single immunoglobulin class or subclass.

Each polypeptide chain can also be divided into a series of globular subunits or domains, each of which are about 110 to 120 residues in length and are characterized by a highly conserved intrachain disulfide bridge spanning about 60 residues and making the domain compact (Fig. 13.1). Analysis of sequence and similarities in gene organization suggest that these domains are the result of a series of gene duplications that occurred during the evolution of the vertebrate kingdom. In those classes and subclasses in which functional localization of various biologic properties has been achieved, it would appear that individual domains may have evolved to serve different biologic functions (6). The central portion of each C domain consists of two antiparallel β-pleated sheets, one consisting of three strands and the other consisting of four strands. This compact form confers great stability to the immunoglobulin fold. The V domain differs from C domains in that it has two additional strands that form an extra loop. These strands and their associated loop help to stabilize the interaction between V_H and V_L, which together create the antigen-binding site (7–9).

Each V domain contains four intervals containing relatively conserved sequence that are termed frameworks (FRs) and are separated from each other by three intervals of hypervariable sequence (8–10). The three hypervariable intervals, termed complementarity-determining regions (CDRs), encode the β loops that connect the antiparallel strands of the β-pleated sheets of the central portion of the V domain. These flexible loops demonstrate minimal constraints regarding peptide composition. The three CDRs of the H chain and the three CDRs of the L chain are juxtaposed to form the antigen binding site (Fig. 13.2). These hypervariable intervals are intimately involved in forming the idiotypic determinants of the antibody, and antibodies with the same specificity may have similar, if not identical, CDRs. In turn, the framework regions primarily encode the β-pleated sheets that form the structural scaffold holding the V_H and V_L domains together.

The constant portion of the L chain contains only one C domain, whereas the H chain may contain either three or four C domains. In antibodies of the IgG, IgD, and IgA classes, the constant portion of the H chain also contains an interdomain region in the center of the molecule that is termed the hinge. Comparison of the structure of the constant portions of the different classes and subclasses of H chains demonstrates striking homologies among those domains that occupy the same relative position in the molecule (11). The structural features of the homologous C_H domains determine the biologic functions that distinguish the different classes and subclasses of immunoglobulins from each other. These features of the C_H domains can also influence the localization and sites of action of the different immunoglobulin classes. For example, the IgG C_H2 and C_H3 domains and their homologues are important for the interaction of the immunoglobulin with class-specific Fc recep-

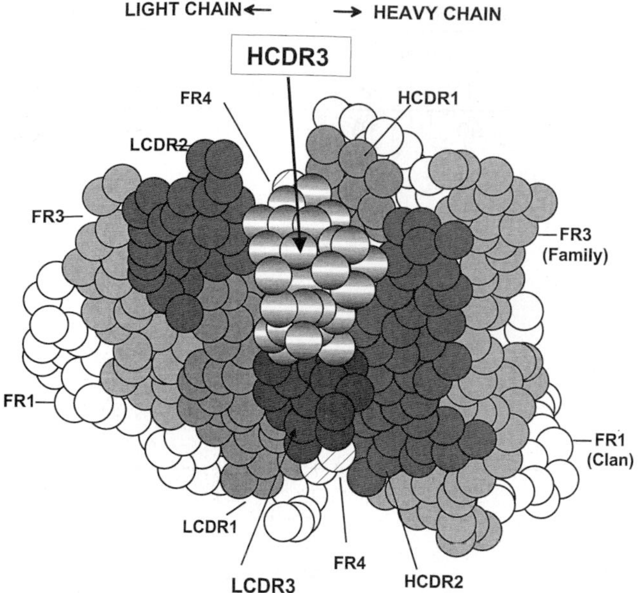

FIG. 13.2. The antigen-binding site is created by the juxtaposition of the three complementarity determining regions (CDRs) of the H chain and the three CDRs of the light chain. The view is looking into the binding site as an antigen would see the CDRs. The VH domain is on the right side. The central location of the CDR3 intervals is readily apparent.

tors on the surface of effector cells (12–14), such as neutrophils, monocytes, lymphocytes, mast cells, and endothelial cells. Complement fixation is focused on the C_H2 domain, although the interface between C_H2 and C_H3 can play a critical role (15,16). Both of these interactions are important in initiating the process of phagocytosis, in allowing certain subclasses to traverse the placenta, and in influencing the biologic functions of lymphocytes, platelets, and other cells. Similarly, regulation of the catabolic properties of the antibody requires an appropriate conformation of the C_H2 and C_H3 interface, which is controlled in part by the hinge region (17,18).

Although the H and L chains are the true structural subunits of immunoglobulins, a simple way of obtaining biologically-active fragments with differing biologic properties is by proteolytic digestion, which occurs preferentially at the exposed hinge region (19). The products obtained differ for different enzymes. Classically, papain yields an Fc and two Fab fragments, whereas pepsin degrades the Fc fragment and yields the two Fab fragments still joined by a disulfide bridge: $(Fab')_2$. These proteolytic fragments, which generally include one or more intact domains, have provided much useful biologic information, because Fab fragments (Fig. 13.1) can combine with antigen, and the Fc fragment can be used to study the secondary biologic properties of immunoglobulins.

CLASSES AND SUBCLASSES

The C domains of the H chain define the class and subclass of the antibody. Although these C domains appear to be derived from a common ancestral sequence, they have evolved different structures and, consequently, have different effector function. In humans, two L-chain classes exist, κ and λ (11). Two of the five major H-chain classes, α and γ, have undergone duplication (11). For example, IgG1, IgG2, IgG3, and IgG4 all have the same basic structural design and differ only in the primary sequence of their constant regions and in the location of their interchain disulfide bonds. The H chain in each of these subclasses is referred to as γ1, γ2, etc. Similarly, IgA consists of the two subclasses α1 and α2. Differences in the C_H domains of the subclasses can significantly influence functional affinity for multivalent antigen in an epitope density-dependent fashion (20). Table 13.1 lists the five major classes of immunoglobulins in humans and describes some of their physical and chemical features. Table 13.2 compares the four subclasses of IgG, the two of IgA, and the classes of IgM, IgD, and IgE from the standpoint of their biologic functions.

IgM

IgM exists in two primary forms (19). One is the basic subunit, the 8S 180,000-dalton IgM with the molecular formula μ_2L_2. This is a minor fraction in serum, but in its transmembrane form is a major component of B-lymphocyte surfaces. The major form in serum is the 19S, 900,000-dalton pentameric IgM $(\mu_2L_2)_5$, in which five subunits are linked by disulfide bridges and generally contain one molecule of an additional polypeptide chain, the J chain, which joins two of

TABLE 13.1. *Selected properties of immunoglobulin classes*

	IgG	IgA	IgM	IgD	IgE
Molecular weight	160,000	170,000 or polymer	900,000	160,000	180,000
Sedimentation constant	7S	7S (9, 11, 13)	19S	7S	8S
Approximate concentration of serum (mg/dL)	1,000–1,500	250–300	100–150	0.3–30	0.0015–0.2
Valence	2	2 (monomer)	10 (small antigen) 5 (large antigen)	2	2
Molecular formula	γ_2L_2	$(\alpha_2L_2)_N$	$(\mu_2L_2)_5$	δ_2L_2	ε_2L_2
Half-life (days)	23	6	5	3	2.5
Special property	Placental passage	Secretory Ig	Primary response lymphocyte surface	Lymphocyte surface	Reagin

TABLE 13.2. *Selected biologic properties of classes and subclasses of immunoglobulins*

	IgG				IgA				
	1	2	3	4	1	2	IgM	IgD	IgE
Percentage of total (%)	65	20	10	5	90	10			
Complement fixation	++	+	++	−	−	−	++	−	−
Complement fixation (alternative)			+	+	+/−	+/−			
Placental passage	+	+	+	+	−	−	−	−	−
Fixing to mast cells or basophils	−	−	−	−	−	−	−	−	+
Binding to									
Macrophages	+	±	+	±	−	−	−	−	−
Neutrophils	+	+	+	+	+	+	−	−	−
Platelets	+	+	+	+	−	−	−	−	−
Lymphocytes	+	+	+	+	−	−	+	−	−
Reaction with *Staphylococcus A*	+	+	−	+	−	−	−	−	−
Half-life (days)	23	23	8–9	23	6	6	5	3	2.5
Synthesis mg/kg/day	25	?	3.5	?	24	?	7	0.4	0.02

+, Positive; ++, Highly Positive; −, Negative; ±, Equevical.

the subunits by a disulfide bridge. This 15,000-dalton molecule appears to be important in initiating the disulfide-bonded polymer formation and can be found in IgA as well (21).

IgM is the predominant immunoglobulin produced during the primary immune response. Occasionally, as in the case of rheumatoid factors, cold agglutinins, and isohemagglutinins, it can remain the major or sole antibody class for long periods. It differs from most other immunoglobulins in having an H chain that is larger, owing to the presence of an extra domain. IgM avidly fixes complement, and studies suggest that this property is influenced by the μ C_H2 and C_H4 domains, but is focused in C_H3, the IgG C_H2 homologue (22). Although the valence of each μ_2L_2 subunit is 2, when binding to large protein antigens, 5 of the 10 antigen-binding sites in the pentameric form of IgM appear blocked due to steric hindrance. As a consequence, the valence for large antigens is five. Thus, IgM rheumatoid factor can exist in serum in the form of a 22S complex $(\mu_2L_2)_5$-$(IgG)_5$.

Immunoglobulin G

IgG, the major immunoglobulin class, accounts for the bulk of antibody activity in response to most antigens. The four IgG subclasses are numbered in relation to their levels in serum relative to each other, with IgG_1 the predominant subclass and IgG4 the least common. The subclasses play unique roles. IgG1 and IgG3 fix complement (23) and bind phagocyte Fcγ receptors well, whereas IgG_2 fixes complement (24) and binds Fcγ receptors to a lesser extent (25). IgG4 does not fix complement effectively in the native state, but has been reported to do so after proteolytic cleavage. The sequence and structure of the C_H2 domains define the ability of the IgG subclass to fix complement (24).

IgG1 and IgG3 are most frequently elicited by viral antigens (26), IgG2 by carbohydrates (27), and IgG4 by helminthic parasites (28). Although the presence of these isotypes is not required for humoral protection from their associated antigens, individuals that lack such antibodies appear more susceptible to specific types of infectious organisms (29). For example, individuals that lack IgG2 appear more likely to suffer from infections with encapsulated organisms, but there is no evidence that IgG4-deficient individuals (1% of normal males and 9% of normal females) are more susceptible to parasites. The Fc fragments of all four IgG subclasses can interact with rheumatoid factors.

Immunoglobulin A

In the serum, IgA generally exists in a monomeric form (α_2L_2). On occasion, and especially in patients with myeloma, IgA can appear as a polymer $(\alpha_2L_2)_{2,3}$-J. Although second in concentration to IgG in serum, its major role is as the predominant form of immunoglobulin in mucosal secretions (30).

Secretory IgA has several unique properties (31). First, it is synthesized largely by plasma cells located in, or originating from, the lymphoid tissues in the intestinal tract. In the secretions, the molecule usually exists in an alternative polymeric form with two subunits in association with the 70,000-dalton secretory component $(\alpha_2L_2)_2$-SC (Fig. 13.3). SC is synthesized by the epithelial cells that line the lumen of the gut. The complete function of SC remains uncertain, but it appears to serve as a receptor for IgA and may play a role in attracting IgA-bearing lymphocytes to the gut and other organs of secretion (32). It may also attract circulating IgA to the surface of the epithelial cells within which the molecule combines with the secretory component. A second function may be to render the secretory IgA complex more resistant to proteolytic digestion by delaying cleavage in the hinge/Fc region of the α chain (33).

The importance of the mucosal immune system in the host cannot be overestimated. Most infectious agents enter through the gastrointestinal and respiratory tracts and initiate a humoral/mucosal immune response involving, primarily, the IgA class (see also Chapter 66). Consequently,

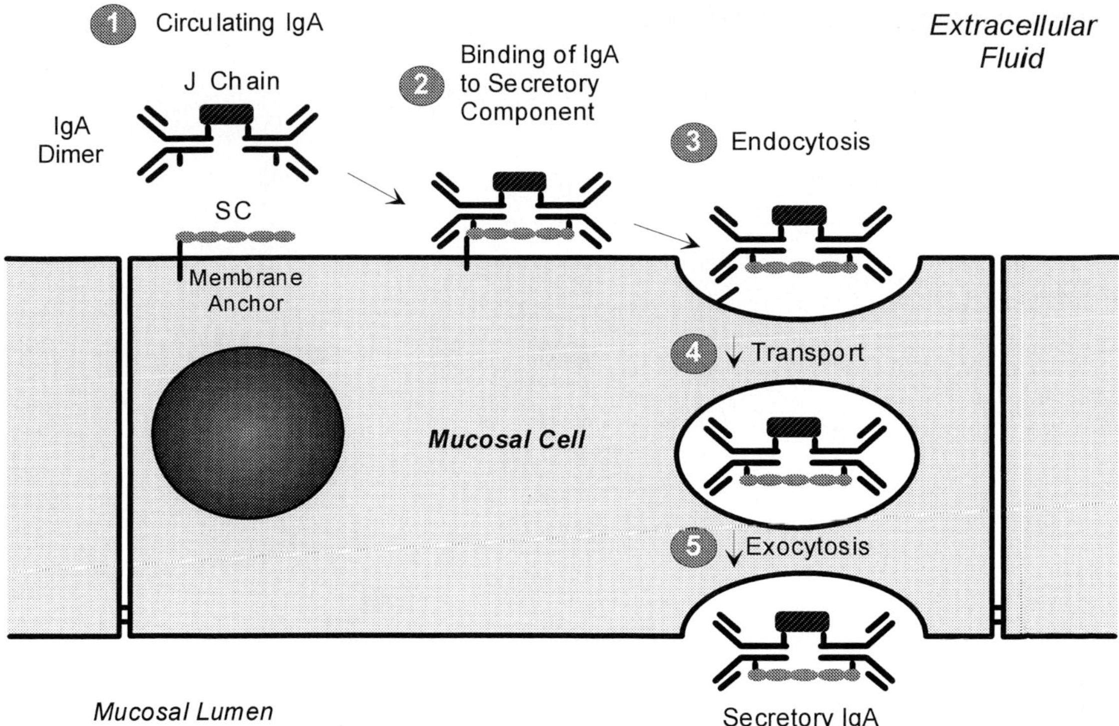

FIG. 13.3. Generation and active transport of secretory immunoglobulin A (IgA) across the mucosal barrier. Secretory IgM is generated in a similar fashion.

as demonstrated in the polio vaccination program, oral vaccinations for these types of agents can be more effective than those administered by the systemic route. It seems likely that the mucosal immune system also plays a major role in the genitourinary, lacrimal, salivary, and respiratory systems. It may also be the primary defense against a variety of environmental pathogens, even though IgA is relatively weak with regard to activation of the complement system or initiation of phagocytosis.

Immunoglobulin E

The distribution of IgE is largely extravascular, and its plasma turnover is rapid, with a half-life of about 2 days. The major type of antibody associated with IgE is the reaginic antibody, which plays a role in a variety of allergic conditions. Through their interaction with Fcϵ receptors on mast cells and basophils, IgE reaginic antibodies, in the presence of antigens, induce the release of histamine and various other vasoactive substances, which are responsible for clinical manifestations of various allergic states (Chapter 17) (29). IgE antibodies may play a protective role in numerous parasitic infections, perhaps by increasing vascular permeability, thus permitting other types of antibodies to be active.

Immunoglobulin D

Although the H chain of IgD can undergo alternative splicing to a secretory form (34), IgD serum antibodies in humans are uncommon and are absent in the serum of mice and primates. Instead, IgD typically is found in association with IgM on the surface of mature lymphocytes (35). The appearance of IgD is associated with the transition of a B lymphocyte from a cell that can be tolerized to antigen to a cell that will respond to antigen with the production of antibody. The role of IgD in this transition is poorly understood. Free IgD differs from other immunoglobulins in its unusual susceptibility to proteolysis.

Gm Allotype System

A series of serologically-defined genetic markers of the C domains of both H and L chains have been termed Gm for the gammaglobulin fraction of the serum in which they were first identified (36). Different allelic forms have been defined for C domains of the γ1, γ2, γ3, γ4, α2, and ϵ H chains, and for the κ L chain. Associations between certain Gm allotypes and predisposition to develop certain autoimmune diseases have been reported (2,36). At present, it is unclear whether this association reflects the direct contribution of variant C alleles to immunoglobulin function or if the allotype is a marker for the presence of linked genes located near the C region locus, including alleles of individual V gene segments.

IMMUNOGLOBULIN GENE ORGANIZATION

The H chains and the two types of L chains, κ and λ, are each encoded by a separate multigene family (37,38). The variability of the V region of a single immunoglobulin

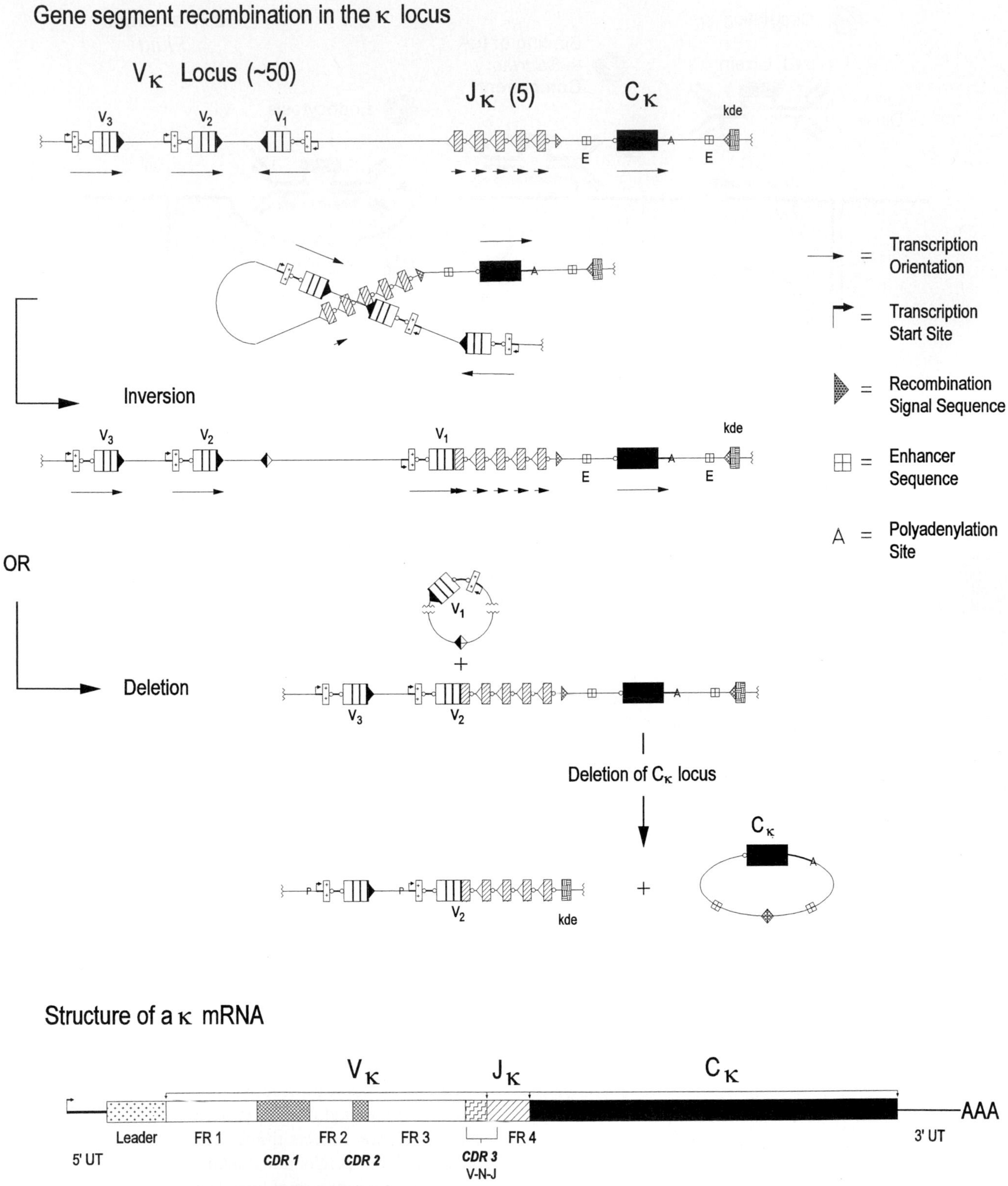

Gene segment recombination in the κ locus

V_κ Locus (~50)

J_κ (5)

C_κ

V_3 V_2 V_1 kde

E E

Transcription Orientation

Transcription Start Site

Recombination Signal Sequence

Enhancer Sequence

A = Polyadenylation Site

Inversion

V_3 V_2 V_1 kde

E E

OR

V_1

Deletion

V_3 V_2

Deletion of C_κ locus

C_κ

V_2 kde

Structure of a κ mRNA

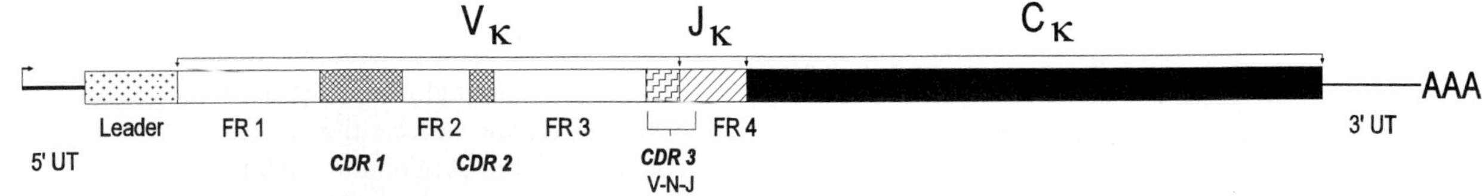

FIG. 13.4. Genetic events involved in gene segment organization and messenger RNA splicing during the rearrangement of a human κ light chain gene. V, variable region; J, joining region; C, constant region of the κ light chain. See text for further description.

polypeptide chain, in conjunction with a nearly invariable constant region, gave rise to the concept that the functionally-distinct V and C regions of these polypeptides are encoded by independent genetic elements, or gene segments, within each gene family. That is, more than one gene is required to encode a single polypeptide chain (39).

Confirmation of the two gene/one polypeptide hypothesis came from nucleotide sequence analysis of immunoglobulin genes. For example, a single gene segment encoding the κ C domain is located in the κ locus on human chromosome 2 (40). In contrast, the V domain is created by the splicing together of two discrete gene segments ($V_κ$ and $J_κ$) (Fig. 13.4A). Each $V_κ$ gene segment contains its own promoter, a leader exon, an intervening intron of approximately 100 nucleotides, an exon that encodes the first three framework regions (FR 1, 2, and 3), the first two complementarity-determining regions in their entirety, the amino terminal portion of CDR 3, and a recombination signal sequence. A $J_κ$ (J for joining) element begins with its own recombination signal, the remaining portion of CDR 3, and the complete FR 4 (Fig. 13.4B).

Use of the same abbreviation (V) for both the complete variable domain of an immunoglobulin peptide chain and for the gene segment that encodes only a portion of that same variable domain is the result of historic precedent. It is unfortunate that the reader must depend on the context of the surrounding text in order to determine which V region of the antibody is being discussed.

Recombination signal sequences (RSS) contain a strongly conserved seven–base pair, or heptamer, sequence (e.g., CACAGTG), which is separated from a less well-conserved nine–base pair, or nonamer, sequence (e.g., ACAAAACCC), by either a 12– (one-turn) or 23– (two-turn) base pair spacer. For example, $V_κ$ gene segments have a 12–base pair spacer and $J_κ$ elements have a 23–base pair spacer. These spacers place the heptamer and nonamer sequences on the same side of the DNA molecule, separated by either one or two turns of the DNA helix. A one-turn recombination signal sequence will preferentially recognize a two-turn signal sequence. In this way, wasteful V-V or J-J rearrangements are kept to a minimum. Depending on the transcriptional orientation of the $V_κ$ gene segment, rearrangement can proceed through either inversion or deletion of the intervening DNA (Fig. 13.4A). In both cases, the two palindromic recombination signals and the coding regions of the V and J gene segment are juxtaposed; however, the products of inversion remain in the DNA of the cell, whereas in the case of deletion, the intervening DNA is discarded.

Immunoglobulin gene rearrangement may be viewed as a specialized form of site-specific cleavage followed by nonhomologous DNA end joining (41,42). The RSS provide recognition sites for the binding of the lymphoid-specific RAG1 and RAG2 proteins, which cooperate to make double-strand breaks at the heptamer termini of the RSS. Broken ends are then processed and joined with the help of several factors also involved in repair of radiation-damaged DNA, including the DNA-dependent protein kinase (DNA-PK) and the Ku70, Ku80, Artemis, DNA ligase IV, and Xrcc4 proteins. Other proteins, including histone H2AX, the Mre11/Rad50/Nbs1 complex, and HMG1 and 2, may also be involved. V(D)J recombination is strongly regulated by limiting access to RSS sites within chromatin, so that particular sites are available only in certain cell types and developmental stages.

The noncoding ends, which contain the RSS, are typically blunt-end joined. In contrast, the neighboring coding DNA is converted to a hairpin during breakage, connecting the 3′ end of one strand to the 5′ end of the antiparallel strand of DNA. The hairpin can be clipped in the middle or several bases down from the hairpin terminus. When clipped asymmetrically, the hairpin leaves a staggered cut end. Exonuclease activity results in loss of terminal sequence. However, polymerase repair of a staggered end yields a palindromic duplication of the terminal nucleotide sequence that is termed a P junction (43). Terminal deoxynucleotidyl transferase (TdT), if present, can add nucleotides at random to the 3′ terminus of the cut end (44), termed N nucleotides. Variation in the sequence of the heptamer and nonamer and the intervening sequence have been shown to influence rearrangement frequency in the TCR locus and likely contribute to differences in gene utilization in the Ig locus as well (45).

Juxtaposition of the $V_κ$ promoter to the two enhancers that flank the $C_κ$ exon allows high-frequency transcription of the locus. After transcription, the intervening introns are spliced away, yielding a mature messenger RNA (mRNA) of 1.2 kilobases. The leader peptide, which is removed from the mature polypeptide, directs the light-chain protein into the secretory pathway (Fig. 13.4B).

There are five $J_κ$ and 75 $V_κ$ gene segments upstream of $C_κ$ (Fig. 13.5). One third of the $V_κ$ gene segments are pseudogenes that contain frameshift mutations or stop codons that preclude them from forming functional protein (46). The 28 $V_κ$ gene segments that have been found in the expressed repertoire can be grouped into six different families (40,47, 48) composed of gene segments that share extensive sequence and structural similarity (9). The sizes of these families vary, ranging from the $V_κ1$ family with approximately 14 active members, to the $V_κ4$ and $V_κ5$ families, with only a single member each (40,48).

Each of the 28 active $V_κ$ gene segments has the potential to rearrange to any one of the five $J_κ$ elements, generating a potential repertoire of more than 140 distinct VJ combinations. Even more diversity is created at the site of gene segment joining. The terminus of each rearranging gene segment can undergo an exonucleolytic loss of one to five nucleotides during the recombination process, and N nucleotides can be inserted in addition to the original germline sequence (49). The random insertion of N nucleotides is attributed to the action of TdT. Each codon created by N region addition increases the potential diversity of the repertoire 20-fold. Thus, the initial diversification of the κ repertoire is focused at the VJ junction that defines CDR3.

The λ locus, on chromosome 22, contains seven different $C_λ$ constant domains, of which only four are functional. Each $C_λ$ is associated with its own $J_λ$ (50) (Fig. 13.6). The $V_λ$ genes are arranged in three distinct clusters, each containing

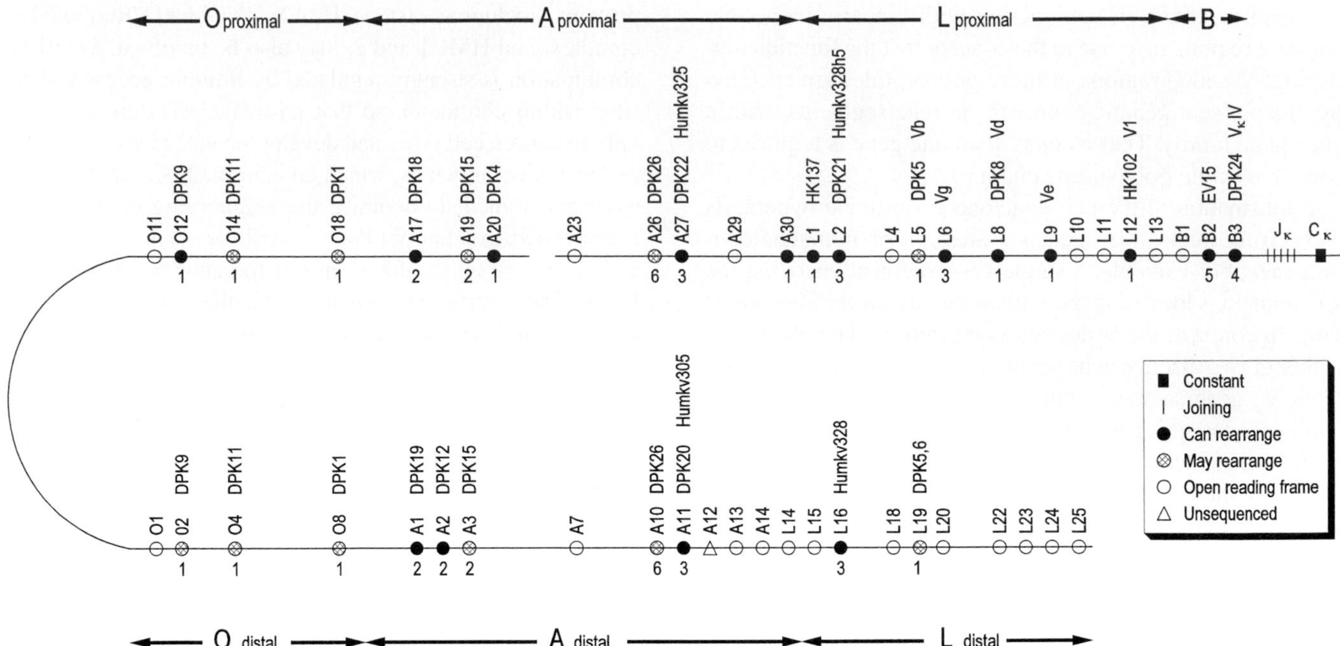

FIG. 13.5. Schematic representation of the human immunoglobulin κ locus on chromosome 2. Only the Vκ gene segments with open reading frames, or which have yet to be sequenced, are shown. *Dark circles* represent gene segments that are known to rearrange. *Shaded circles* represent gene segments with duplicates that are so close in sequence that rearranged sequences cannot be assigned to segments of the distal or proximal region (e.g., L5 and L19). The gene segments are identified by their Zachau (*O, A, L,* or *B*) and Winter (*DPK*) designations, or by other trivial names where appropriate. The Vκ family is identified beneath the appropriate circle for each of the gene segments known to be expressed or believed to be expressed. The portion of the Vκ locus distal to Jκ (distal O, A, and L) is an inverted duplicate of a portion of the locus proximal to Jκ (proximal O, A, and L).

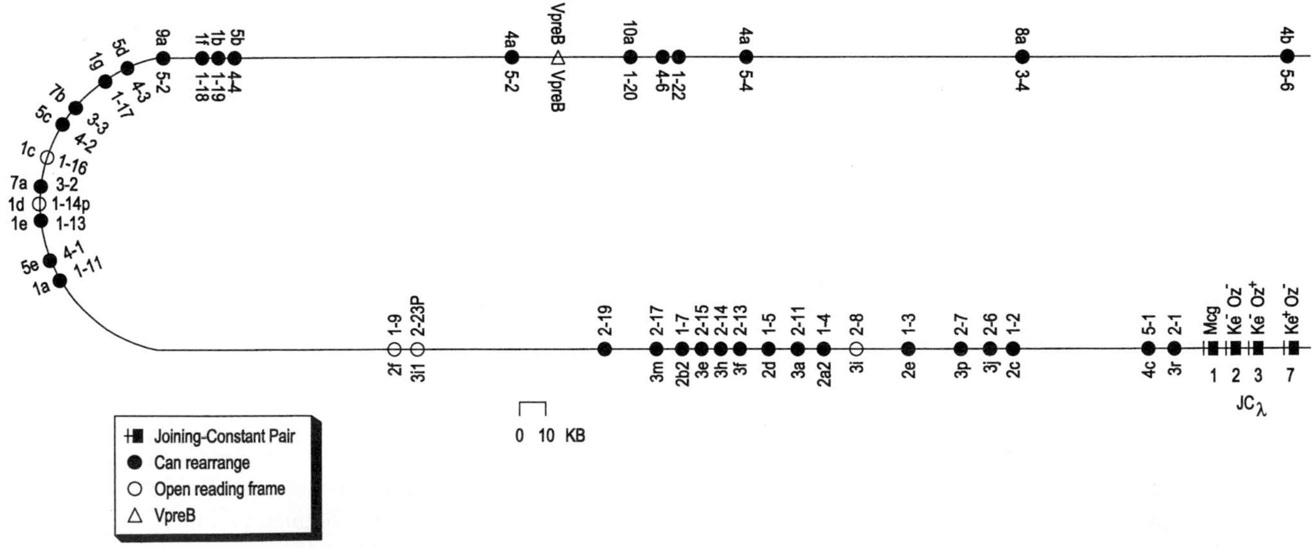

FIG. 13.6. Schematic representation of the human immunoglobulin λ locus on chromosome 22. Only the Vκ gene segments with open reading frames, or which have yet to be sequenced, are shown. *Dark circles* represent gene segments that are known to rearrange. The gene segments are identified by their Shimizu (inner circle) and Winter (outer circle) designations. The four constant regions, identified by their allotypic markers, each have their own associated J element.

members of different V_λ families (51). Depending on the haplotype, there are approximately 30 to 36 potentially functional V_λ gene segments and an equal number of pseudogenes.

H chains can also form a complex with unconventional λ L chains, known as surrogate or pseudo light chains (ΨLC) (50). The genes encoding the ΨLC proteins, 14.1 and V_{preB}, are located within the λ light-chain locus on chromosome 22 (Fig. 13.6). These genes show considerable homology to conventional λ L chains, the λ14.1 gene containing J_λ and C_λ-like sequences and the V_{preB} gene, including a V_λ-like sequence. A critical difference between conventional and ΨLC genes is that 14.1 and V_{preB} gene rearrangement is not required for ΨLC expression, thus mRNA encoding the ΨLC can be detected in the earliest B-cell precursors prior to the onset of Ig gene rearrangement.

The H-chain locus, coding as it does for both the receptor and effector functions of the antibody, is considerably more complex than the κ and λ loci (11,38,52). There are approximately 90 V_H gene segments near the telomere of the long arm of chromosome 14 (53,54). Of these, approximately 50 are functional and can be grouped into seven different families of related gene segments (9,55). Adjacent to the most centromeric V_H, V6–1, are 27 D_H (D for diversity) gene segments (56) (Fig. 13.7) and six functional J_H gene segments

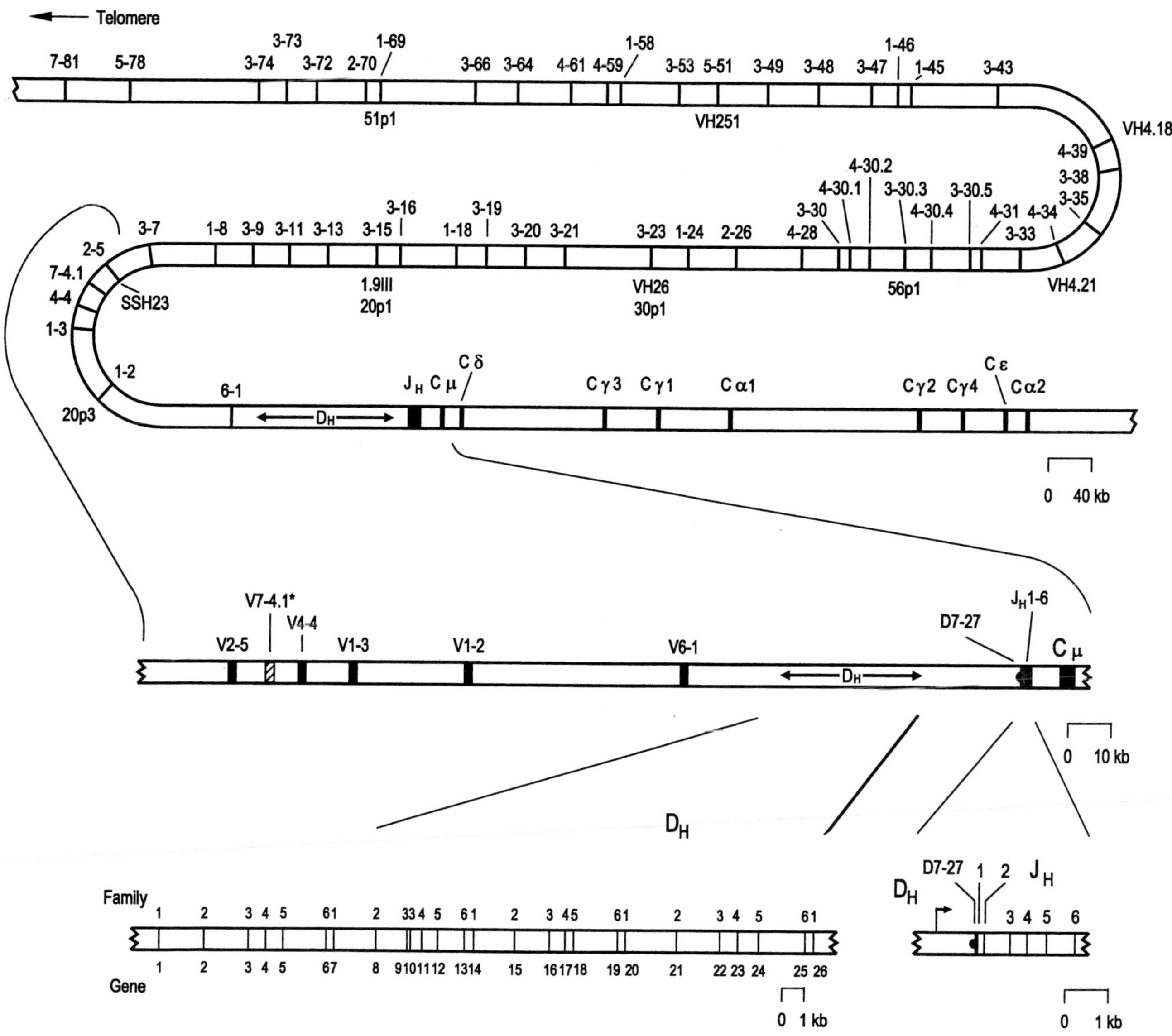

FIG. 13.7. Germline organization of the human H chain locus on chromosome 14q32. **Top:** Fifty-three VH gene segments found in a typical human VH haplotype and the associated DH, JH, and CH gene segments. Each VH gene segment is identified by its family and its location relative to the downstream DH, JH, and CH loci. Also shown are the trivial names by which some clinically significant VH gene segments are also known. **Middle:** An expanded view of the six most JH proximal VH gene segments and the DH and JH loci. An asterisk marks the V7–4.1 gene segment, which is absent in some haploid genomes. **Bottom:** An expanded view of the DH locus, and an expanded view of the JH locus that includes the highly conserved D7–27 (DHQ52) gene segment, which is primarily used in fetal life.

(57). Each V_H and J_H gene segment is associated with a two-turn recombination signal sequence, which prevents direct V→J joining. A pair of one-turn recombination signal sequences flanks each D_H. D-D joins are possible, but rare. Recombination begins with the joining of a D_H to a J_H gene segment, followed by the joining of a V_H element to the amino-terminal end of the DJ intermediate. The V_H gene segment contains FR1, -2, and -3, CDR1 and -2, and the amino-terminal portion of CDR3; the D_H gene segment forms the middle of CDR3; and the J_H element contains the carboxyl terminus of CDR3 and FR4 in its entirety (Fig. 13.8). Random assortment of one of approximately 50 V_H and one of 27 D_H with one of the six J_H gene segments can generate up to 10^4 different VDJ combinations.

Although combinatorial joining of individual V, D, and J gene segments creates diversity, the major source of variation in the pre-immune repertoire is the VDJ join itself. First, D_H gene segments can rearrange by either inversion or deletion, and thus have the potential to be read backward as well as forward. Moreover, each D_H gene segment can be spliced and translated in each of the three potential reading frames. Thus, each D_H gene segment essentially encodes six different peptide fragments. Second, the terminus of each rearranging gene segment can undergo a loss of one or more nucleotides during the recombination process. This imprecision of the joining process creates additional diversity. Third, non–germ line–encoded nucleotides (N regions) can replace some or all of the lost nucleotides or be included in addition to the original germ line sequence. Every codon that is added by N region addition increases the potential diversity of the repertoire 20-fold. N regions can be inserted both between the V and the D, and between the D and the J. Fourth, P junctions (43) can also be incorporated into the junction between the rearranging gene segments, further enhancing diversity. In total, potentially more than 10^{10} different H-chain VDJ junctions, or CDR3s, can be generated at the time of gene segment rearrangement. Finally, because any L chain can theoretically associate with any H chain, random combination of the H- and L-chain partners yields a potential preimmune antibody repertoire of greater than 10^{16} different immunoglobulins.

Located downstream of the VDJ loci are nine functional C region gene segments (11) (Fig. 13.7). The C genes consist of a series of exons, each encoding a separate domain, hinge, or terminus (Fig. 13.9). All of the H-chain genes can undergo alternative splicing to generate two different types of carboxyl termini: either a membrane terminus that anchors immunoglobulin on the B-lymphocyte surface, or a secreted terminus that occurs in the soluble form of the immunoglobulin (11). Each C_H1 constant region, except for $C_H1\delta$, is preceded by both an exon that cannot be translated (an I exon) and a region of repetitive DNA termed the switch (S). Through the activation-induced cytidine deaminase (AID or AICDA) catalyzed recombination between the Cμ switch region and one of the switch regions of the seven other H-chain constant regions (a process termed class switching), the same VDJ heavy-chain V domain can be juxtaposed to any of the H-chain classes (11,58,59) (Fig. 13.10). Class switching requires direct T-cell/B-cell interaction through the binding of CD40 on the B cell to CD40 ligand (CD40L) on the T cell. It also requires transcription of the individual switch region, which is regulated by cytokines produced by specific

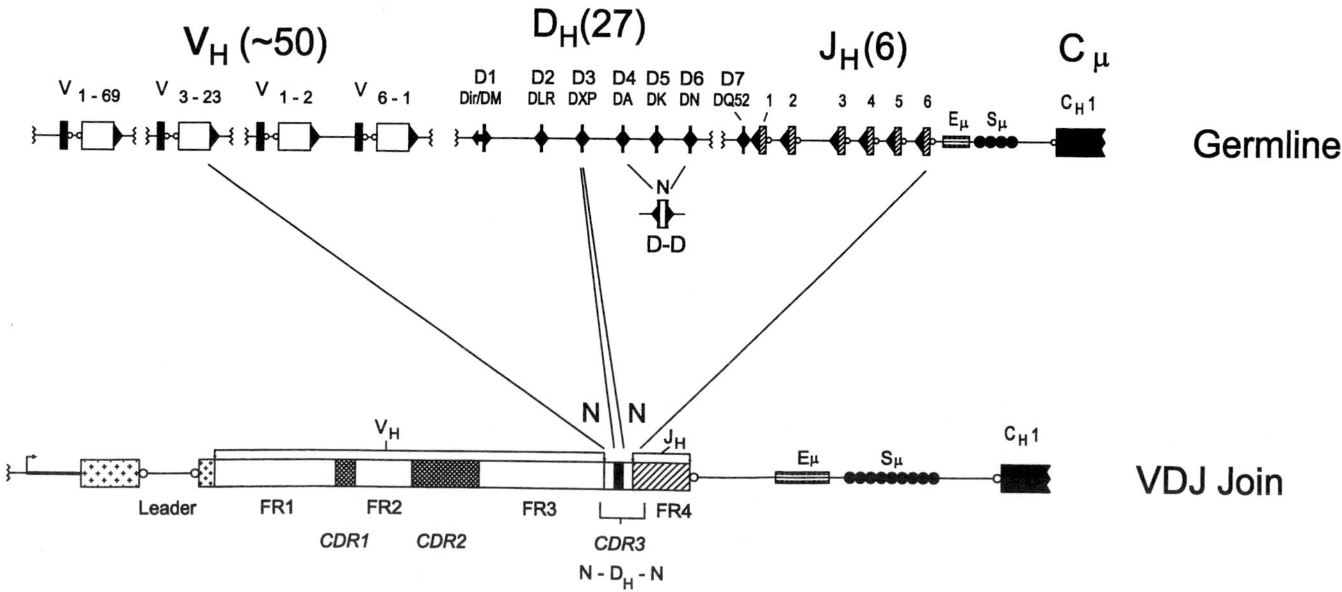

FIG. 13.8. Recombination in the heavy-chain variable region. Previous designations for the DH gene segment families are also shown. Although most VDJ joins contain only a single D gene segment, D-D fusion can occur.

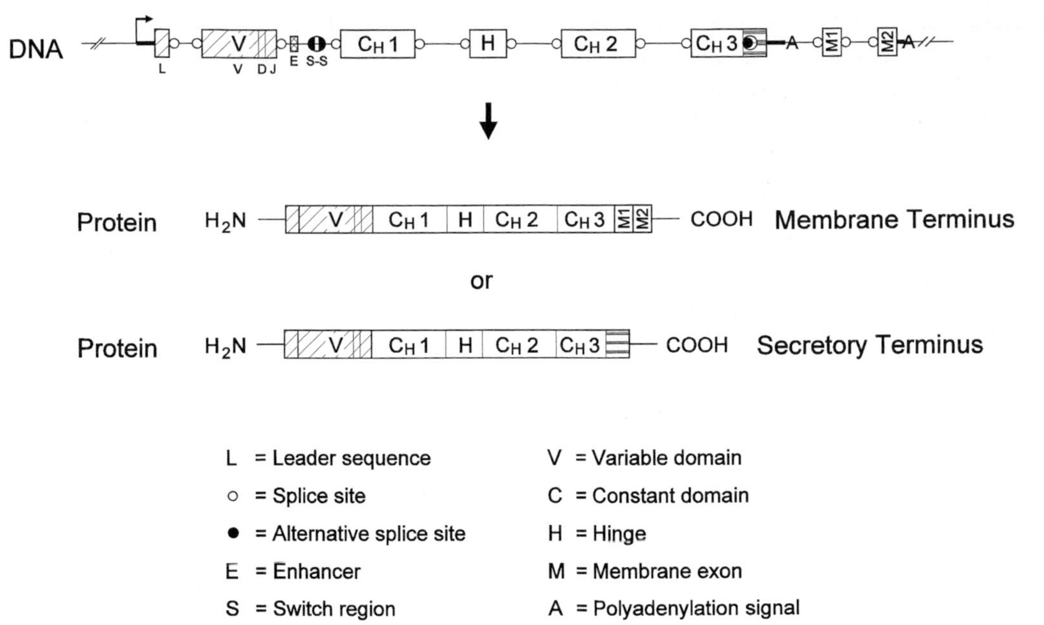

FIG. 13.9. Molecular events involved in alternative gene segment splicing for the constant region domains of the heavy chain.

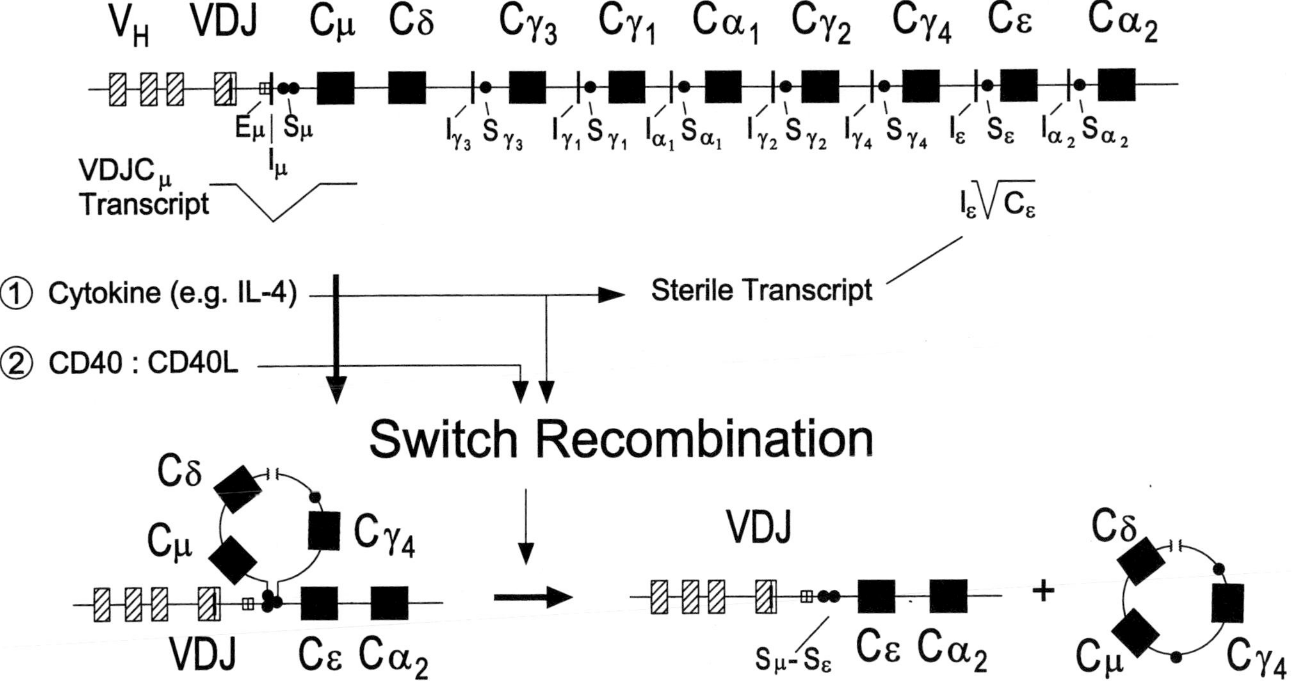

FIG. 13.10. Immunoglobulin H chain class switching in humans (only the functional elements are shown). The molecular events involved in switching from expression of one class of immunoglobulin to another are depicted. **Top:** Gene organization during μ chain synthesis. **Bottom:** Switch region recombination event resulting in a deletion of the intervening DNA, which is necessary for ultimate expression of the ϵ polypeptide chain. Exposure to the appropriate cytokine or T cell–B cell interaction through the CD40:CD40L pathway results in activation of the I exon that yields a sterile epsilon transcript (Iϵ-Cϵ). The CD40:CD40L interaction is necessary for the subsequent replacement of Cμ by another constant gene (in this case, Cϵ). The S loci indicate switch-specific recombination signals. Both somatic hypermutation and switch recombination are catalyzed by activator-induced cytosine deaminase (*AID*).

T helper cell subsets. For example, exposure to interleukin-4 (IL-4) produced by T_H2 cells activates the I exon promoters upstream of the $C_\gamma 4$ and C_ϵ switch regions inducing transcription and permitting switching to IgG4 and IgE. In this way, the system can tailor both the receptor and the effector ends of the antibody molecule to meet a specific need.

The complexity of the system can best be understood by correlating molecular events with the development of the B lymphocyte (60) (Fig. 13.11). The immunoglobulin loci begin in embryonic form in the first B-cell progenitor. In the presence of TdT, first a D_H gene segment rearranges to a J_H; then a V_H is juxtaposed to the DJ intermediate. Only one in three possible splices will result in a VDJ join with both the V_H and the J_H in the same reading frame. Failure to generate a translatable H chain on the first H-chain locus is followed by attempted rearrangement on the second. Successful rearrangement terminates recombination in the H-chain locus, a process termed allelic exclusion because it prevents the cell from generating two functional H chains with different binding sites. Production of a functional H chain in the presence of the λ pseudo light chain (ΨLC) allows expression of small amounts of IgM on the surface of the pre–B cell.

Although H-chain rearrangement is not required, rearrangement of a κ or λ L chain typically occurs after generation of a functional H chain (60). Cells expressing λ chains may delete the C_κ domain as a result of rearrangement between the κ deleting element (kde) located 3′, or downstream, of C_κ and a recombination signal located either in the J-C intron or at the 3′ terminus of a V_κ (61) (Fig. 13.4). After production of a conventional L-chain protein, the immature B lymphocyte is now able to express a fully functional IgM on its cell surface. Exposure to antigen at this stage can result in further L chain rearrangement, termed receptor editing (62), anergy of the B cell, or even cell death. In this way, B cells expressing self-reactive antibodies can be modulated.

Alternate splicing of the V domain to the C_H1 exon of either the C_μ or C_δ genes allows the mature B lymphocyte to express both IgM and IgD on the cell surface. At this stage, exposure to antigen and to the appropriate cytokine in conjunction with T-cell help that includes signaling through the CD40-CD40L pathway can result in class switching or differentiation into a plasma cell that can secrete massive quantities of antibody.

Following exposure to antigen and T-cell help, the V domain genes of germinal center lymphocytes undergo mutation at a rate of up to 10^{-3} changes per base pair per cell cycle (63), a process termed somatic hypermutation. Somatic

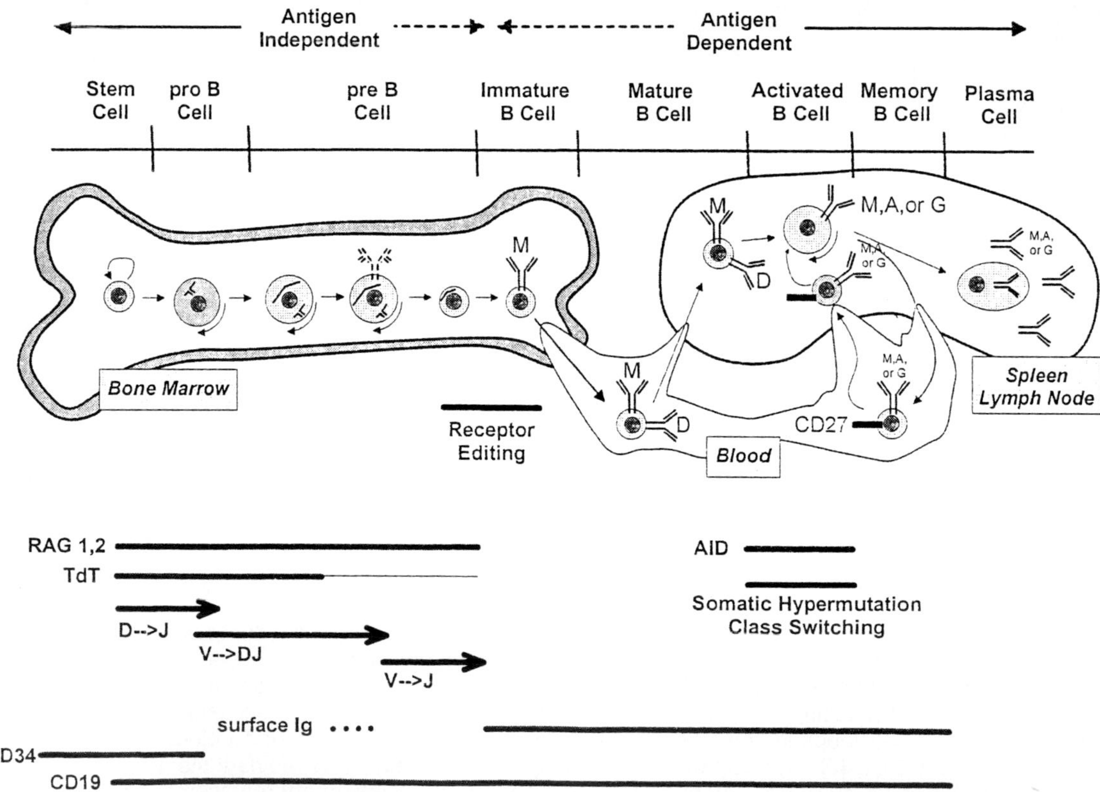

FIG. 13.11. Simplified pathway of B-cell differentiation in humans (49). Although not shown, many mature B cells, memory B cells, and plasma cells circulate back into the bone marrow. Curved arrows adjacent to the cell indicate cell replication. Other arrows indicate the direction of maturation. D→J, V→DJ, and V→J indicate rearrangements. *RAG*, recombinase; *SIg*, surface immunoglobulin; *TdT*, terminal deoxynucleotidyl transferase.

hypermutation allows affinity maturation of the antibody repertoire in response to repeated immunization or exposure to antigen.

Somatic hypermutation requires transcription of the locus and expression of AID (59,64,65). The activity of AID appears to depend on its interaction with various cofactors. It was previously hypothesized that at least two separate mechanisms were involved in somatic hypermutation. The first targeted mutation hot spots with the RGYW (purine/G/pyrimidine/A) motif (66) and the second incorporated an error-prone DNA synthesis that would lead to a nucleotide mismatch between the original template and the mutated DNA strand (67). Recent work suggests that mutations in the RGYW hot spot are due to AID deamination of the cytosine on the strand opposite of the guanosine, which is then repaired in an error-prone way. In contrast, mutations of adenine and thymine away from the initial deamination result from the effects of translesional DNA polymerases, such as polymerases η, ι, and ζ, which are typically recruited to repair the DNA.

In theory, the effect of combinatorial rearrangement of gene segments, combinatorial association of H and L chains, flexibility in the site of gene segment joining, N region addition, P junctions, somatic hypermutation, and class switching can create an antibody repertoire that is limited only by the total number of B cells in circulation at any one time. In practice, there appear to be significant constraints on both the structure and sequence of the antibody repertoire.

The representation of individual V gene elements is nonrandom. Among V_κ and V_H elements, half of the potentially functional V gene elements contribute minimally to the expressed repertoire (46,48,68). These restrictions are even greater among V_λ elements, where only three gene segments contribute to half of the expressed repertoire (69).

Particular patterns of amino acid composition in the sequences of the V domains create canonical structures for several of the hypervariable regions. In κ chains, CDR2 encodes a single canonical structure, whereas CDR1 creates one of four structures (70). In the H chain, germ line CDR1 and CDR2 elements encode one of three or one of five distinct canonical structures, respectively (71). The canonical structures selected during the primary response are conserved during affinity maturation: the key residues that determine the conformations of the antigen binding loops are unmutated or undergo conservative mutation.

The enhanced sequence diversity of the CDR3 region is mirrored by its structural diversity. In κ chains, although 70% of the rearranged sequences correspond to one of three known canonical structures, the remaining 30% can be quite variable. Canonical structures have been defined for the base of CDR-H3 (72), but few such structures have been defined for the loop. At the sequence level, there is a preference for serine, tyrosine, and glycine residues in CDR-H3. This preference manifests in the nonrandom representation of amino acids among the six reading frames of D_H elements (73,74). Each reading frame encodes either a series of hydrophobic residues, a series of charged residues, or a neutral reading frame containing the aforementioned serine, tyrosine, and glycine residues. This reading frame, known as reading frame 1, is used preferentially in the expressed repertoire (70,74).

Although affinity maturation often preserves the canonical structure of the CDR, the distribution of diversity differs between the primary and antigen-selected repertoire (75). In the primary repertoire, diversity is focused at the center of the binding site in CDR3. With somatic hypermutation, diversity spreads to the CDR1 and CDR2 regions at the periphery of the binding site.

CLINICAL SIGNIFICANCE

The need to be able to respond to a highly divergent array of potential antigens led vertebrates to develop an elegant system for the generation of a diverse array of antibodies, as described earlier. Inherent in the nature of the system is the potential to generate autoreactive molecules whose overproduction can result in disease, especially rheumatic disease (3).

The nature of the diversification process has certain specific implications for our understanding of how exposure to the same antigen can yield dissimilar antibody responses in different individuals, some of which are perhaps more likely to result in disease. For example, because of the random nature of the rearrangement events, only a small subset of the potential antibody repertoire is available for use at any one time, and this repertoire changes with time. Thus, even identical twins exposed to the same infectious agent can produce quite different antibody responses.

Through the use of monoclonal antibody technology, it has been possible to generate antiidiotypic antibodies against paraproteins and other immunoglobulins with self-reactivity. Similarly, through advanced techniques of cellular immunology, it has been possible to isolate and immortalize B cells from the tissues of patients with RA, SLE, and other rheumatic disorders that express self-reactive antibodies (76–79). Although a wide variety of gene segments, especially after they have undergone somatic mutation, can be used in pathogenic autoantibodies, certain self-specificities can be associated with the use of specific germ line gene elements (77,78). For example, paraproteins with rheumatoid factor activity are enriched for use of the L chain κ gene segments Humkv325 and Humkv328 and for H chains that share homology with a member of the V_H1 family, V1–69 (51p1) (78). Antibodies directed against the I/i red cell antigen are commonly encoded by antibodies that contain the V4–34 (VH4.21) gene segment (80). The anti-DNA 8.12 idiotype is encoded by members of the $V_\lambda2$ gene family (81). Similarly, the anti-DNA 16.6 idiotype is associated with a member of the V_H3 family, V3–23 (30p1,VH26) (77,82).

Animal models have indicated that the presence or absence of specific V gene segments can influence the manifestations of rheumatic disease; for example, the development and age of onset of glomerulonephritis in certain mouse strains (83). Similarly, it is conceivable that abnormal regulation of the expression of critical immunoglobulin gene segments or gene sequence could result in disease. To test these hypotheses, investigators have analyzed the extent of variation, or polymorphism, in germline V gene segments and their associated regulatory sequences. These studies have shown that some V regions, notably the rheumatoid factor–associated V_κ Humvk325 and Humkv328 segments (78), exhibit little sequence polymorphism; whereas others, such as the V_H gene segments V1–69 and V7–4.1, which can also encode rheumatoid factor (84), are highly polymorphic (85,86).

The individual first develops the ability to distinguish self from nonself during fetal life. During this developmental process, the ability to respond to specific antigens unfolds in a programmed, stepwise fashion (87). Associated with this programmed appearance of antigen responsiveness is control of the diversity of the antibody repertoire through preferential use of a limited set of V, D, and J gene segments (88). Although it would seem logical that developmentally-regulated V gene segments would be unlikely to react with self, included among them are some of the autoreactive antibody-associated V_κ and V_H gene segments described above, that is, V3–23 and Humkv325 (77,78). The preferential use of these potentially pathologic gene segments would suggest that they play such an important role in the development of the immune response that the benefits derived from their presence far outweigh the risk for generating self-reactive antibodies.

One possible biologic role for V3–23 is suggested by studies of human antibodies directed against the capsular polysaccharide of *Haemophilus influenzae* type b (Hib PS), a developmentally-controlled antigen specificity (89). A number of these antibodies contain sequences highly similar to V3–23. The fact that V3–23 is a major component of the fetal repertoire, yet encodes antibodies with antibacterial specificities to which a normal infant will not respond until the second year of life, as well as potentially pathogenic anti-DNA specificity, suggests that factors other than V_H utilization must play a role in the programmed development of the humoral immune response, as well as in diseases of immune function.

In addition to V_H, the antigen binding site is the product of the light-chain repertoire, the varied combinations that can be made between heavy and L chains, somatic hypermutation, and the composition of HCDR3. Considerable evidence suggests that control of somatic mutation can play a major role in controlling the diversity of the antibody repertoire (90). For example, through somatic mutation, an otherwise benign or protective V domain can become a pathogenic antibody (91).

The composition of the antibody repertoire varies greatly according to the age of the individual. In the fetus, few sequences contain somatic mutations, hence the outside border of the antigen binding site is essentially limited to germline sequence. HCDR3, which contributes to the center of the antigen binding site (Fig. 13.2), contains somatic variation due to combinatorial joining of V, D, and J gene segments and N region addition. D_H and J_H utilization and N addition are controlled during early human life (88), yielding an HCDR3 repertoire that varies from the adult in length distribution, gene segment content, and amino acid representation. Superimposed on this genetic regulation of the repertoire is a selection for length that is first exerted when immunoglobulin is expressed on the surface of the developing B cell. Pressure is also exerted on the sequence composition of CDR3. Through selection during evolution, each D_H reading frame has been shaped to exhibit a characteristic hydropathicity profile: neutral, charged, or hydrophobic. Neutral reading frames enriched for glycine, serine, and tyrosine are preferred in all species examined to date (74). Anti-DNA binding antibodies, however, often contain charged amino acids in CDR3 that have been introduced by use of alternative D_H reading frames, N addition, or somatic mutation (3,92). Thus, control of the structure and sequence composition of CDR3 may play a major role in limiting or controlling the self-reactivity of nascent V gene domains that are potentially autoreactive.

In older individuals, B-cell production in the bone marrow diminishes (93), enriching the repertoire for antibodies that have been shaped by previous exposure to antigens and that include numerous somatic mutations. Mechanisms of peripheral control of the repertoire thus take on added importance. The contribution of the accumulation with age of antigen-selected and somatically mutated B cells to the development of autoreactive antibodies remains unclear.

These and other aspects of the immune system are areas of active investigation. As the mechanisms by which the antibody repertoire is regulated at the molecular level are better understood, and the manner in which inherited or acquired perturbations in these regulatory processes can influence the development of disease is elucidated, it should be possible to apply the appropriate knowledge to reverse pathologic alterations of the immune response.

REFERENCES

1. Schroeder HW Jr. Immunoglobulins and their genes. In: Koopman WJ, ed. *Arthritis and allied conditions: a textbook of rheumatology.* Baltimore: Williams & Wilkins, 2001:301–316.
2. Jazwinska EC, Dunckley H, Propert DN, et al. GM typing by immunoglobulin heavy chain gene RFLP analysis. *Am J Hum Genet* 1988; 43:175–181.
3. Marion TN, Krishnan MR, Desai DD, et al. Monoclonal anti-DNA antibodies: structure, specificity, and biology. *Methods* 1997;11:3–11.
4. Jang YJ, Stollar BD. Anti-DNA antibodies: aspects of structure and pathogenicity. *Cell Mol Life Sci* 2003;60:309–320.
5. Edelman GMN. Antibody structure and molecular immunology. *Science* 1973;180:830–840.

6. Yasmeen D, Ellerson JR, Dorrington KJ, et al. The structure and function of immunoglobulin domains. IV. The distribution of some effector functions among the Cgamma2 and Cgamma3 homology regions of human immunoglobulin G1. *J Immunol* 1976;116:518–526.
7. Amzel LM, Poljak RJ. Three-dimensional structure of immunoglobulins. *Annu Rev Biochem* 1979;48:961–997.
8. Padlan EA. Anatomy of the antibody molecule. *Mol Immunol* 1994; 31:169–217.
9. Kirkham PM, Schroeder HW Jr. Antibody structure and the evolution of immunoglobulin V gene segments. *Semin Immunol* 1994;6:347–360.
10. Kabat EA, Wu TT, Perry HM, et al. *Sequences of proteins of immunological interest.* Bethesda: U.S. Department of Health and Human Services, 1991:1–2387.
11. Honjo T. Immunoglobulin genes. *Annu Rev Immunol* 1983;1:499–528.
12. Weng Z, Gulukota K, Vaughn DE, et al. Computational determination of the structure of rat Fc bound to the neonatal Fc receptor. *J Mol Biol* 1998;282:217–225.
13. Maxwell KF, Powell MS, Hulett MD, et al. Crystal structure of the human leukocyte Fc receptor, Fc gammaRIIa. *Nature Struct Biol* 1999;6:437–442.
14. Herr AB, Ballister ER, Bjorkman PJ. Insights into IgA-mediated immune responses from the crystal structures of human FcalphaRI and its complex with IgA1-Fc. *Nature* 2003;423:614–620.
15. Duncan AR, Winter G. The binding site for C1q on IgG. *Nature* 1988;332:738–740.
16. Okada M, Utsumi S. Role for the third constant domain of the IgG H chain in activation of complement in the presence of C1 inhibitor. *J Immunol* 1989;142:195–201.
17. Kim JK, Tsen MF, Ghetie V, et al. Evidence that the hinge region plays a role in maintaining serum levels of the murine IgG1 molecule. *Mol Immunol* 1995;32:467–475.
18. Medesan C, Matesoi D, Radu C, et al. Delineation of the amino acid residues involved in transcytosis and catabolism of mouse IgG1. *J Immunol* 1997;158:2211–2217.
19. Davie DR, Metzger H. Structural basis of antibody function. *Annu Rev Immunol* 1983;1:87–117.
20. Cooper LJ, Robertson D, Granzow R, et al. Variable domain-identical antibodies exhibit IgG subclass-related differences in affinity and kinetic constants as determined by surface plasmon resonance. *Mol Immunol* 1994;31:577–584.
21. Koshland ME. The coming of age of the immunoglobulin J chain. *Annu Rev Immunol* 1985;3:425–453.
22. Chen FH, Arya SK, Rinfret A, et al. Domain-switched mouse IgM/IgG2b hybrids indicate individual roles for C mu 2, C mu 3, and C mu 4 domains in the regulation of the interaction of IgM with complement C1q. *J Immunol* 1997;159:3354–3363.
23. Bruggeman MG, Williams GT, Bindon CI, et al. Comparison of the effector functions of human immunoglobulins using a matched set of chimeric antibodies. *J Exp Med* 1987;166:1351–1361.
24. Sensel MG, Kane LM, Morrison SL. Amino acid differences in the N-terminus of C(H)2 influence the relative abilities of IgG2 and IgG3 to activate complement. *Mol Immunol* 1997;34:1019–1029.
25. Waldmann H. Manipulation of T cell responses with monoclonal antibodies. *Annu Rev Immunol* 1989;7:407–444.
26. Skvaril F, Schilt U. Characterization of the subclass and light chain types of IgG antibodies to rubella. *Clin Exp Immunol* 1984;55:671–676.
27. Barrett DJ, Ayoub EM. IgG2 subclass restriction of antibody to pneumococcal polysaccharides. *Clin Exp Immunol* 1986;63:127–134.
28. Otteson EA, Skvaril F, Tripathy SP, et al. Prominence of IgG4 in the IgG antibody response to human filiariasis. *J Immunol* 1985;134: 2707–2712.
29. Preudhomme JL, Hanson LA. IgG subclass deficiency. *Immunodef Rev* 1990;2:129–149.
30. Goldblum RM. The role of IgA in local immune protection [discussion]. *J Clin Immunol* 1990;10(suppl):64–70.
31. Underdown BJ, Schiff JM. Immunoglobulin A: strategic defense initiative at the mucosal surface. *Annu Rev Immunol* 1986;4:389–417.
32. Crago SS, Kulhavy R, Prince SJ, et al. Secretory component of epithelial cells is a surface receptor for polymeric immunoglobulins. *J Exp Med* 1978;147:1832–1837.
33. Crottet P, Corthesy B. Secretory component delays the conversion of secretory IgA into antigen-binding competent F(ab′)2: a possible implication for mucosal defense. *J Immunol* 1998;161:5445–5453.
34. Blattner FR, Tucker PW. The molecular biology of immunoglobulin D. *Nature* 1984;307:417–422.
35. Cooper MD, Kuritani T, Chen C-L, et al. Expression of IgD as a function of B-cell differentiation. *Ann NY Acad Sci* 1982;399:146–156.
36. Grubb R. Immunogenetic markers as probes for polymorphism, gene regulation and gene transfer in man—the Gm system in perspective. *APMIS* 1991;99:199–209.
37. Leder P. The genetics of antibody diversity. *Sci Am* 1982;246:102–115.
38. Tonegawa S. Somatic generation of antibody diversity. *Nature* 1983; 302:575–581.
39. Dreyer WJ, Bennett JC. The molecular basis of antibody formation: a paradox. *Proc Natl Acad Sci U S A* 1965;54:864–869.
40. Zachau HG. The human immunoglobulin kappa genes. In: Honjo T, Alt FW, Rabbitts PH, eds. *Immunoglobulin genes.* London: Academic, 1995:173.
41. Bassing CH, Swat W, Alt FW. The mechanism and regulation of chromosomal V(D)J recombination. *Cell* 2002;109(suppl):45–55.
42. Gellert M. V(D)J recombination: RAG proteins, repair factors, and regulation. *Annu Rev Biochem* 2002;71:101–132.
43. Lafaille JJ, DeCloux A, Bonneville M, et al. Junctional sequences of T cell receptor γδ genes: implications for γδ T cell lineages and for a novel intermediate of V-(D)-J joining. *Cell* 1989;59:859–870.
44. Desiderio SV, Yancopoulos GD, Paskind M, et al. Insertion of N regions into heavy-chain gene is correlated with expression of terminal deoxytransferase in B cells. *Nature* 1984;311:752–755.
45. Bassing CH, Alt FW, Hughes MM, et al. Recombination signal sequences restrict chromosomal V(D)J recombination beyond the 12/23 rule. *Nature* 2000;405:583–586.
46. Klein R, Jaenichen H-R, Zachau HG. Expressed human immunoglobulin kappa genes and their hypermutation. *Eur J Immunol* 1993;23: 3248–3271.
47. Brodeur PH, Riblet RJ. The immunoglobulin heavy chain variable region (IgH-V) locus in the mouse. I. One hundred Igh-V genes comprise seven families of homologous genes. *Eur J Immunol* 1984;14:922–930.
48. Cox JPL, Tomlinson IM, Winter G. A directory of human germ-line Vk segments reveals of strong bias in their usage. *Eur J Immunol* 1994;24:827–836.
49. Lee SK, Bridges SL Jr, Koopman WJ, et al. The immunoglobulin kappa light chain repertoire expressed in the synovium of a patient with rheumatoid arthritis. *Arthritis Rheum* 1992;35:905–913.
50. Blomberg BB, Solomon A. The murine and human lambda light chain immunoglobulin loci: organization and expression. In: Herzenberg LA, Weir DM, Blackwell C, eds. *Weir's handbook of experimental immunology.* Oxford: Blackwell Science, 1996:10.1–10.26.
51. LeBien TW, Bollum FJ, Yasmineh WG, et al. Phorbol ester-induced differentiation of a non-T, non-B leukemic cell line: model for human lymphoid progenitor cell development. *J Immunol* 1982;128:1316–1320.
52. Yancopoulos GD, Alt FW. Regulation of the assembly and expression of variable region genes. *Annu Rev Immunol* 1986;4:339–368.
53. Cook GP, Tomlinson IM, Walter G, et al. A map of the human immunoglobulin VH locus completed by analysis of the telomeric region of chromosome 14q. *Nature Genet* 1994;7:162–168.
54. Matsuda F, Ishii K, Bourvagnet P, et al. The complete nucleotide sequence of the human immunoglobulin heavy chain variable region locus. *J Exp Med* 1998;188:2151–2162.
55. Pallares N, Lefebvre S, Contet V, et al. The human immunoglobulin heavy variable genes. *Exp Clin Immunogenet* 1999;16:36–60.
56. Corbett SJ, Tomlinson IM, Sonnhammer EL, et al. Sequence of the human immunoglobulin diversity (D) segment locus: a systematic analysis provides no evidence for the use of DIR segments, inverted D segments, "minor" D segments or D-D recombination. *J Mol Biol* 1997;270:587–597.
57. Ravetch JV, Siebenlist U, Korsmeyer SJ, et al. Structure of human immunoglobulin mu locus: characterization of embryonic and rearranged J and D genes. *Cell* 1981;27:583–591.
58. Manis JP, Tian M, Alt FW. Mechanism and control of class-switch recombination. *Trends Immunol.* 2002;23:31–39.
59. Ta V-H, Nagaoka H, Catalan N, et al. AID mutant analyses indicate requirement for class-switch-specific cofactors. *Nature Immunol* 2003; 4:843–848.
60. Burrows PD, Schroeder HW Jr, Cooper MD. B-cell differentiation in humans. In: Honjo T, Alt FW, eds. *Immunoglobulin genes.* London: Academic, 1995:3–32.

61. Selsing E, Daitch LE. Immunoglobulin lambda genes. In: Honjo T, Alt FW, eds. *Immunoglobulin genes.* London: Academic, 1995:193–204.
62. Tiegs SL, Russell DM, Nemazee D. Receptor editing in self-reactive bone marrow B cells. *J Exp Med* 1993;177:1009–1020.
63. Shlomchik MJ, Marshak-Rothstein A, Wolfowicz CB, et al. The role of clonal selection and somatic mutation in autoimmunity. *Nature* 1987;328:805–811.
64. Fukita Y, Jacobs H, Rajewsky K. Somatic hypermutation in the heavy chain locus correlates with transcription. *Immunity* 1998;9:105–114.
65. Reynaud CA, Aoufouchi S, Faili A, et al. What role for AID: mutator, or assembler of the immunoglobulin mutasome? [Review]. *Nat Immunol* 2003;4:631–638.
66. Dorner T, Foster SJ, Farner NL, et al. Somatic hypermutation of human immunoglobulin heavy chain genes: targeting of RGYW motifs on both DNA strands. *Eur J Immunol* 1998;28:3384–3396.
67. Rada C, Ehrenstein MR, Neuberger MS, et al. Hot spot focusing of somatic hypermutation in MSH2-deficient mice suggests two stages of mutational targeting. *Immunity* 1998;9:135–141.
68. Cook GP, Tomlinson IM. The human immunoglobulin VH repertoire. *Immunol Today* 1995;16:237–242.
69. Ignatovich O, Tomlinson IM, Jones PT, et al. The creation of diversity in the human immunoglobulin V(lambda) repertoire. *J Mol Biol* 1997; 268:69–77.
70. Tomlinson IM, Cox JP, Gherardi E, et al. The structural repertoire of the human V kappa domain. *EMBO J* 1995;14:4628–4638.
71. Chothia C, Lesk AM, Gherardi E, et al. Structural repertoire of the human VH segments. *J Mol Biol* 1992;227:799–817.
72. Shirai H, Kidera A, Nakamura H. H3-rules: identification of CDR-H3 structures in antibodies. *FEBS Lett* 1999;455:188–197.
73. Schroeder HW Jr, Ippolito GC, Shiokawa S. Regulation of the antibody repertoire through control of HCDR3 diversity. *Vaccine* 1998; 16:1363–1368.
74. Ivanov I, Link JM, Ippolito GC, et al. Constraints on hydropathicity and sequence composition of HCDR3 are conserved across evolution. In: Zanetti M, Capra JD, eds. *The antibodies.* London: Taylor & Francis, 2002:43–67.
75. Tomlinson IM, Walter G, Jones PT, et al. The imprint of somatic hypermutation on the repertoire of human germline V genes. *J Mol Biol* 1996;256:813–817.
76. Randen I, Thompson KM, Pascual V, et al. Rheumatoid factor V genes from patients with rheumatoid arthritis are diverse and show evidence of an antigen-driven response [Review]. *Immunol Rev* 1992;128:49–71.
77. Dersimonian H, Schwartz RS, Barrett KJ, et al. Relationship of human variable region heavy chain germ-line genes to genes encoding anti-DNA autoantibodies. *J Immunol* 1987;139:2496–2501.
78. Carson DA, Chen PP, Kipps TJ. New roles for rheumatoid factor. *J Clin Invest* 1991;87:379–383.
79. Schrohenloher RE, Accavitti MA, Bhown AS, et al. Monoclonal antibody 6B6.6 defines a cross-reactive kappa light chain idiotope on human monoclonal and polyclonal rheumatoid factors. *Arthritis Rheum* 1990; 33:187–198.
80. PascualV, Capra JD. VH 4.21, a human V_H gene segment over represented in the autoimmune repertoire. *Arthritis Rheum* 1992;34:11–18.
81. Paul E, Iliev AA, Livneh A, et al. The anti-DNA associated idiotype 8.12 is encoded by the V lambda II gene family and maps to the vicinity of light chain CDR1. *J Immunol* 1992;149:3588–3595.
82. Schroeder HW Jr, Hillson JL, Perlmutter RM. Early restriction of the human antibody repertoire. *Science* 1987;238:791–793.
83. Datta SK. A search for the underlying mechanisms of systemic autoimmune disease in the NZB x SWR model. *Clin Immunol Immunopathol* 1989;51:141–156.
84. Randen I, Thompson KM, Pascual V, et al. Rheumatoid factor V genes from patients with rheumatoid arthritis are diverse and show evidence of an antigen-driven response [Review]. *Immunol Rev* 1992;128:49–71.
85. Matsuda F, Shin EK, Nagaoka H, et al. Structure and physical map of 64 variable segments in the 3′ 0.8-megabase region of the human immunoglobulin heavy-chain locus. *Nat Genet* 1993;3:88–94.
86. Sasso EH, Willems van Dijk K, Bull AP, et al. A fetally expressed immunoglobulin VH1 gene belongs to a complex set of alleles. *J Clin Invest* 1993;91:2358–2367.
87. Silverstein AM. Ontogeny of the immune response: a perspective. In: Cooper MD, ed. *Development of host defense.* New York: Raven, 1977:1–10.
88. Zemlin M, Schelonka RL, Bauer K, et al. Regulation and chance in the ontogeny of B and T cell antigen receptor repertoires [Review]. *Immunol Res* 2002;26:265–278.
89. Adderson EE, Shackelford PG, Quinn A, et al. Restricted Ig H chain V gene usage in the human antibody response to Haemophilus influenzae type b capsular polysaccharide. *J Immunol* 1991;147:1667–1674.
90. Meffre E, Catalan N, Seltz F, et al. Somatic hypermutation shapes the antibody repertoire of memory B cells in humans. *J Exp Med* 2001; 194:375–378.
91. Giusti AM, Chien NC, Zack DJ, et al. Somatic diversification of S107 from an antiphosphocholine to an anti-DNA autoantibody is due to a single base change in its heavy chain variable region. *Proc Natl Acad Sci U S A* 1987;84:2926–2930.
92. Shlomchik MJ, Mascelli MA, Shan H, et al. Anti-DNA antibodies from autoimmune mice arise by clonal expansion and somatic mutation. *J Exp Med* 1990;171:265–297.
93. Nunez C, Nishimoto N, Gartland GL, et al. B cells are generated throughout life in humans. *J Immunol* 1996;156:866–872.

CHAPTER 14

Structure and Function of Macrophages and Other Antigen-Presenting Cells

Mary K. Crow

Cells of the mononuclear phagocyte system are ubiquitous throughout the organism and are involved at all stages of immune and inflammatory responses, from the first recognition of a foreign microorganism or toxin to the final effector functions that mediate sequestration, clearance, or death of the invader. Although these cells do not express the exquisite antigen specificity of lymphoid cells and their immunoglobulin products, their regulation is at least as sophisticated as that of their lymphocyte partners, and they are, in turn, responsible for coordination of virtually all inflammatory responses. In the absence of their antigen recognition and presentation functions, cellular and humoral immune responses would fail to be recruited to battle. Thus, the complement of cellular activities performed by the mononuclear phagocytes and their related antigen-presenting cells (APCs) is central to host defense. When the full differentiative capacity of mononuclear phagocytes is considered, the impact of those cells is extended to the removal of senescent, apoptotic, and necrotic cells and tissue; wound healing; and tissue remodeling. It is not surprising that cells with such wide-ranging and centrally important functions can be primary mediators of disease pathogenesis when their regulation goes awry.

INNATE AND ADAPTIVE IMMUNE RESPONSES

The cells and molecules that mediate host defense against foreign invaders can be generally classified, with some overlap, into two systems: the innate and adaptive immune responses. Phylogenetically, the innate response is observed before the adaptive immune response, but both are required for efficient protection of a human from microorganisms. Both innate and adaptive immune responses can contribute to disease when overactive. Each is characterized by mechanisms that confer recognition, amplification, and effector processes.

Phagocytes are the first line of defense and include macrophages and neutrophils. These cells work, together with serum proteins such as complement, to clear invading organisms. In the process of doing so, they produce new cell surface and soluble proteins that result in inflammation and recruit the more sophisticated adaptive immune response, if their efforts are not sufficient to rid the host of the microbe. So the key functions of mononuclear phagocytes are to engulf and digest foreign microbes, as well as senescent or apoptotic host cells, and to activate the adaptive immune response through antigen presentation and secretion of soluble mediators. A fascinating, and as yet poorly understood, aspect of these key functions is that the phagocyte is somehow able to differentiate foreign and self products, so that ingestion of a foreign microbe results in effective T-cell activation while ingestion of self products apparently does not.

ANTIGEN RECOGNITION AND PRESENTING CELLS

Considering the singular role of mononuclear phagocytes as the sentinel cells that recognize microbial pathogens, or dangerous situations of any kind, it is no wonder that they must be the "wandering cells" that Metchnikoff first observed (1). Although some of those cells are fairly stationary, situated in skin, mucosa, and epithelial linings that are most likely to come in contact with invaders, many of the monocyte/macrophages, as well as the "veiled cells" that are the specialized antigen recognition cells of lymph, are usually in motion, wandering from organ to organ, acting as sentries, and providing the first defense against infectious agents. The readily visible pseudopods that constantly extend and retract, amoeba-like, permit movement in a set direction, when necessary, and act almost as "sense organs" to sample the cellular environment. Although monocytes are the most abundant antigen recognition cells that mediate innate immune system activation, the more specialized dendritic cells play an essential role in recruiting the adaptive immune response. Activated B lymphocytes, once triggered by interaction with antigen and antigen-activated T helper cells, can also function as highly specific APCs to expand and perpetuate the adaptive immune response.

Monocytes

The cells of the mononuclear phagocyte system are derived from bone marrow stem cell precursors that undergo myelopoiesis under the influence of granulocyte-macrophage colony-stimulating factor (GM-CSF) and M-CSF, enter the blood as monocytes, and further differentiate into macrophages under the influence of cytokines and tissue matrix components (2). The cellular and molecular structure of the monocyte-macrophage at each stage of its differentiation reflects its function, with a decreasing nucleus/cytoplasm ratio and increased expression of enzyme-containing organelles and cell surface receptors paralleling the maturation process. The bone marrow monoblast has a high nucleus/cytoplasm ratio, is esterase positive, and begins to develop a ruffled membrane. Promonocytes, the form that leaves bone marrow to join the circulating pool, have more active cytoplasm, are peroxidase positive, and have some proliferative capacity. Those cells have many of the cell surface receptors characteristic of mature monocytes, such as CD14, and once in the circulation, complete differentiation to the mature monocyte stage, fully competent to respond to microbe invasion or tissue injury with a broad range of effector functions. Stimulation by host or foreign factors induces circulating monocytes to increase cell surface expression of adhesion molecules, resulting in their capacity to stop on an endothelial cell surface, jump along the endothelium, move between endothelial cells in a process termed diapedesis, and finally, to digest their way through connective tissue matrix to move toward a site of tissue disruption (3). The half-life of a circulating monocyte is about 22 hours. Once present in the tissue, those cells complete differentiation to macrophages and have little capacity to undergo proliferation, but maintain increased effector function for an extended period of time. Among the fully differentiated cells of the monocyte lineage are peritoneal macrophages and those in other serosal spaces, Kupffer cells in liver, alveolar macrophages in the lung, microglial cells in the brain, histiocytes in connective tissue, osteoclasts in bone, and type A synovial lining cells in the synovial membrane.

Dendritic Cells

Dendritic cells are the most potent APCs and are especially enriched at sites of potential host invasion: the skin, gut, and respiratory epithelium (4). The many studies addressing the hematopoietic origin of dendritic cells have not completely resolved the contribution of myeloid versus lymphoid precursors to the generation of these important APCs (5,6). The issue is complicated by the presence of several classes of dendritic cells at different locations in the body, each with a somewhat distinct phenotype. Among these, so-called myeloid dendritic cells can be generated from common myeloid precursor cells or from monocytes *in vitro*. Plasmacytoid dendritic cells, the major source of type I interferon, can probably derive from either lymphoid or myeloid precursors, and Langerhans cells, present in the epidermis, are likely to be derived from a myeloid precursor but may require a signal from transforming growth factor-β (TGF-β) to develop their characteristic phenotype (6–8). At least *in vitro,* differentiation of dendritic cells from bone marrow–derived precursors or peripheral blood monocytes is induced by the cytokines GM-CSF and interleukin-4 (IL-4), and further maturation signals are provided by tumor necrosis factor-α (TNF-α) (9,10).

The Langerhans cells in the epidermis are specialized to "drink in" antigen through a process called macropinocytosis. Those cells then move from the skin to lymph nodes via lymphatic channels. The interdigitating cells in the T cell–rich areas of secondary lymphoid tissue are somewhat more differentiated and active than Langerhans cells. They have lost much of their capacity to ingest material, but have developed potent T-cell stimulatory activity (7,9). A current paradigm suggests that dendritic cells are as important for the maintenance of tolerance to self antigens as they are for induction of immunity to foreign antigens (7,11). Dendritic cells bearing self antigens associated with major histocompatibility complex (MHC) molecules are likely to be mature but quiescent because they require so-called "danger" signals for activation. Interaction between those cells and T cells is proposed to generate either inadequate T-cell activation or induction of regulatory T cells that inhibit immune system activation. In contrast, dendritic cells that have encountered foreign antigens become activated via signals from conserved pattern recognition receptors and effectively induce naïve T-cell activation and a panoply of effector T-cell functions. The high cell surface density of MHC class II molecules, and of costimulatory and adhesion molecules, contributes to the specialized functions of dendritic cells. Another category of dendritic cell, the follicular dendritic cell, is not bone marrow derived, but is essential for presentation of antigens to B cells (12). The follicular dendritic cells use complement receptors to trap antigens associated with antibody and complement components in immune complexes and display those complexes on their surface for sampling by B-cell antigen receptors.

Activated B Cells

Because each B cell bears on its surface a specific receptor for antigen, those cells can bind that antigen, ingest it, and generate potentially immunogenic peptides in intracellular vesicles, which can then be presented to T cells in the antigen-binding groove of MHC class II molecules. After having received activation signals through surface immunoglobulin (the B-cell antigen receptor), stimulation of B cells with constituents of the microbe [such as lipopolysaccharide (LPS) or cytosine phosphate guanosine (CpG) oligodeoxynucleotide motifs in microbial DNA] through Toll-like receptors (TLR), or by interaction with T helper cells, confers a high level of expression of the same costimulatory and adhesion molecules that support such active APC function on dendritic cells.

MONONUCLEAR PHAGOCYTE FUNCTION IN THE INNATE IMMUNE RESPONSE

Recognition

Stimuli

The innate immune system is geared for rapid response and must distinguish potentially threatening insults by invading microorganisms from the physiologic fluxes in the host's internal milieu that should not trigger immune system activity (13). Some of the immunostimulatory components of microorganisms have been known for decades, an example being LPS, an important virulence factor of gram-negative bacteria. It is only recently that a much wider spectrum of microbe-derived immune system stimuli have been characterized and understood to have in common pathogen-associated molecular patterns (PAMPs) that are rapidly recognized by cell receptors and then signal an insult from outside the host (14,15).

The cell envelope of bacteria is a complex structure, composed of peptidoglycan, phospholipids, LPS, and lipoproteins in the case of gram-negative bacteria, and of many peptidoglycan layers in the case of gram-positive organisms. Components of these bacterial coats contain some of the pattern recognition motifs that are among the first stimuli for the innate immune response (13). LPS initiates an inflammatory cascade by interacting with LPS-binding protein and then binding to the monocyte-macrophage CD14 cell surface receptor (14). Although dendritic cells do not express cell surface CD14, they are stimulated to produce cytokines and increased cell surface costimulatory and adhesion molecules by LPS, through a proposed soluble CD14-dependent pathway (15). Muramyldipeptide, lipoteichoic acid, lectins, and *N*-formylated di- and tripeptides made by bacteria can trigger monocyte activation. These latter peptides can be distinguished from self peptides that do not bear a formyl group at the N-terminus. The synthetic *N*-formyl-methionyl-leucyl-phenylalanine (f-met-leu-phe) tripeptide is often used as a potent monocyte stimulant in *in vitro* studies.

The CpG oligodeoxynucleotide motifs of bacterial and viral DNA are among the microbe-derived molecules recognized by the mammalian immune system as distinct from self (16–18). The CpG DNA sequences are a particularly intriguing example of the fundamental alterations through evolution in the molecular composition of organisms that have resulted in the ability of one class of organism to signal its presence to another class of organism. CpG or immunostimulatory motifs are unmethylated nucleotides with a core sequence that most typically includes two purines, a cytosine, a guanine, and two pyrimidines (17). Such a pattern is significantly more common in virus and bacterial genomes than it is in vertebrate genomes, and higher organisms have developed a recognition system that is triggered by the presence of these immunostimulatory motifs. Krieg et al. have performed extensive studies to determine the optimal DNA sequence that activates mononuclear cells and have identified GTCGTT as highly effective (17,19). The specific cellular receptor for CpG motifs has been identified as Toll-like receptor-9 (TLR9), one member of the TLR family (20). The uptake of TLR9-bound DNA stimulatory motifs into the intracellular compartment is required for activation of the kinases, including interleuxin 1-associated receptor kinase (IRAK), tumor necrosis factor receptor-associated factor (TRAF6), nuclear factor κB (NFκB), and mitogen activated protein (MAP) kinase, that mediate new gene transcription.These CpG nucleotides activate B cells and monocytes, trigger production of reactive oxygen species, and promote the activation of cellular immune responses. Knowledge of the special adjuvant properties of CpG motifs is being used to develop gene vectors containing such motifs that will preferentially stimulate T helper 1 (T_H1)-type T-cell responses (18). Beyond the role of immunostimulatory DNA sequences, the double-stranded RNA (dsRNA) characteristic of many viruses can also stimulate the innate immune response. Polyriboinosinic polyribocytidylic acid [poly(I:C)] is a synthetic mimic of dsRNA that has been shown to induce differentiation of immature dendritic cell precursors to fully competent mature dendritic cells with potent APC activity. Poly(I:C) is also a potent stimulus for secretion of interferon-α (IFN-α), a cytokine that promotes natural killer (NK) cell activity (21). TLR3 is now known to be responsible for recognition of dsRNA (22).

Particulate stimuli, like microbe-derived products, can induce an activated monocyte profile. For example, β-1,3-glucan triggers the respiratory burst and production of cytokines. It also induces the phosphatidylserine receptor that binds apoptotic cells. Silica and latex particles can also be phagocytosed by monocyte-macrophages (23).

Many host proteins synergize with microbe-derived factors to activate the innate immune response (13). Complement activation products, such as C5a, activate the arachidonic acid pathway, generating leukotrienes (24). The acute-phase protein serum amyloid A acts as a chemoattractant for phagocytes (25). Heat shock proteins (HSPs) and cleavage products of fibronectin and hyaluronan are also recognized to activate the immune response after binding to TLR (19,26,27). Among the most effective innate immune system activators are immune complexes formed from excess antibody binding its antigen and solubilized by serum complement, as well as larger particles that are opsonized, or coated, with antibody. These immune complexes or opsonized particles can bind to several isoforms of Fc receptors (FcR), together with complement receptors, to trigger a variety of phagocyte functions (28–31). The stimulatory activity of immune complexes containing microbial antigens, soluble mediators of the innate immune response (complement), and the highly specific products of the adaptive immune response (antibody) demonstrates the central role of the mononuclear phagocyte and the value of the coordinated actions of innate and adaptive immunity in host defense.

In contrast to these activating stimuli, host-derived components that must be cleared by phagocytic cells usually fail to trigger innate immune system activation (32). Apoptotic cells and their debris, as well as senescent cells, are rapidly removed from the host without inducing immune system activity. Although the mechanisms that account for this failure to stimulate cell function are not fully understood, complement components and C-reactive protein contribute to the efficient and safe removal of debris by the mononuclear phagocyte system (33). The interaction of self components with monocytes does have biochemical and functional consequences. Phagocytosis of apoptotic cells induces synthesis of some cytokines, but they may be more immunosuppressive than activating, permitting the adaptive immune system to maintain immune ignorance of these host components (22). TGF-β is implicated in the inhibitory effects of apoptotic cell clearance on immune system activity (33).

Mononuclear Phagocyte Receptors

Each of these extracellular foreign and host stimuli must interact with the phagocyte through its cell surface, most often as ligands for cell surface glycoprotein receptors (Table 14.1). Some of these receptors are constitutively expressed on the mature monocyte surface, as is the case with the TLRs, and some are induced following the initial cell activation events. Among the latter are receptors for cytokines, the key modulators of the effector

TABLE 14.1. *Mononuclear phagocyte receptors*

Receptor	Ligands
Pattern recognition and Toll-like receptors	
TLR-2	Lipoarabinomannan; mycolylarabinogalactin–peptidoglycan complex; lipoteichoic acid; zymosan
TLR-3	dsRNA
TLR-4	LPS; HSP60; HSP70; fibronectin EDA domain; hyaluronic acid; polysaccharide fragments of heparan sulfate
TLR-5	Flagellin
TLR-7	Imidazoquinolines; R-848
TLR-9	Unmethylated CpG DNA
CD14	LPS/LPS-binding protein complex
Receptors mediating phagocytosis	
FcR: FcγRI (CD64); FcγRIIa (CD32); FcγRIIb2 (CD32); FcγRIII (CD16)	Fc fragment of IgG
FcεRII (CD23)	Fc fragment of IgE
Mannose-6-phosphate receptor	Mannose-6-phosphate
Macrophage scavenger receptors (I and II)	Acetylated low-density lipoproteins
MARCO	Uteroglobin-related protein 1
DC-SIGN	*Candida albicans*; HIV gp120
Complement receptors	
CR1 (CD 35)	C3b; C4b
CR2 (CD21; on follicular dendritic and B cells)	C3d
CR3 (CD11b)	C3bi; fibrinogen
CR4 (CD11c)	C3bi
C1q receptor	C1q

Continued

TABLE 14.1. *Continued*

Receptor	Ligands
Receptors for clearance of apoptotic or senescent cells	
CD36	Phosphatidylserine; thrombospondin
$\alpha_v\beta_3$ (monocytes)	Apoptotic cells; vitronectin
$\alpha_v\beta_5$ (dendritic cells)	Apoptotic cells
Sialoadhesin receptor	Erythrocytes
Receptor for advanced glycation end products (RAGE)	AGE products
Cytokine receptors	
TGF-β receptor	TGF-β
p55 and p75 TNF-α receptor	TNF-α
Interferon-α receptor	Interferon-α
Interferon-γ receptor	Interferon-γ
M-CSF receptor (c-fms)	M-CSF
GM-CSF receptor	GM-CSF
IL-1, IL-3, IL-4, IL-6, IL-10, IL-15, IL-18 receptors	Cytokines indicated
Chemokine and other seven-transmembrane G-protein-coupled receptors	
FPR-1 (high affinity)	*N*-formyl peptides
FPRL-1 (low affinity)	*N*-formyl peptides; amyloid A protein; lipoxin A4
C5a receptor	C5a; C5a-des-arg
PAF receptor	PAF
LTB_4 receptor	LTB_4
Substance P receptor	Substance P
C-C (β) chemokine receptor 1	MIP-1α; MIP-1β; RANTES; MCP-1
IL-8 receptor α	IL-8
IL-8 receptor β	IL-8; other β chemokines
Adrenergic receptor	Adrenergic neurotransmitters
Opioid receptor	Endogenous and exogenous opioids
Hormone receptors	
Glucocorticoid receptor	Glucocorticoids
Vitamin D receptor	Vitamin D_3
Adhesion receptors	
Integrins	
CD18 family of β_2 integrins	
LFA-1 (CD11a)	ICAM-1
Mac-1 (CD11b; CR3)	C3bi; β-glucans; ICAM-1
P150,95 (CD11c; CR4)	Fibrinogen; ICAM-1
β_1 integrins	
VLA4 ($\alpha_4\beta_1$)	VCAM-1; fibronectin
Adhesion molecules of immunoglobulin superfamily	
ICAM-1 (CD54)	LFA-1
ICAM-2 (CD102)	LFA-1, MAC-1
LFA-3 (CD58)	CD2
PECAM (CD31)	PECAM; $\alpha_v\beta_3$ integrin
L-selectin; E-selectin	Sialyl Lewis x
Leukocyte endothelial cell adhesion molecule (CD44)	Hyaluronan
Receptors active in adaptive immune response	
MHC class I	Antigenic peptide; CD8; TCR
MHC class II	Antigenic peptide; CD4; TCR
CD1	αGal-ceramide
B7.1 (CD80); B7.2 (CD86)	CD28; CTLA-4
B7h	ICOS
B7-H1	PD-1
Triggering receptors expressed by myeloid cells	
TREM1	?
TREM2	?

FPR, formyl peptide receptor; FPRL, formyl peptide receptor–like; GM-CSC, granulocyte-macrophage colony-stimulating factor; ICAM, intercellular adhesion molecule; Ig, immunoglobulin; IL, interleukin; LFA, leukocyte function antigen; LPS, lipopolysaccharide; LTB_4, leukotriene B_4; MARCO, macrophage scavenger receptor with collagenous structure; MCP, monocyte chemoattractant protein; MHC, major histocompatibility complex; MIP, macrophage inhibitory protein; PAF, platelet-activating factor; PECAM, platelet endothelial cell adhesion molecule; RANTES, regulated upon activation normal T cell expressed and secreted; TCR, T-cell receptor; TGF, transforming growth factor; TNF, tumor necrosis factor; TLR, Toll-like receptor; TREM, triggering receptors expressed by myeloid cells; VCAM, vascular cell adhesion molecule; VLA, very late activation.

programs mediated by both innate and adaptive immune system cells.

Pattern Recognition and Toll-Like Receptors

The mechanisms of innate immune response activation by microbial products have recently reached a new level of understanding with the elucidation of the TLR family (14,15,19,26,27,34–39). The identification of sequence homology between this family of signaling molecules in *Drosophila* and human IL-1 receptors, both of which activate components of NFκB transcription factors, led to the cloning of a new family of mammalian receptors, the TLRs, which play a central role in the recognition of microbial invasion by mononuclear phagocytes (34). There are 10 members of the human TLR family, and recent studies have expanded the list of their ligands. Among these are bacterial and fungal lipoproteins and glycolipids, demethylated CpG DNA motifs, dsRNA, host proteins such as HSPs, and synthetic chemicals. Reports available to date indicate that TLR4 mediates monocyte activation by gram-negative bacteria and cooperates with CD14, the previously identified receptor for LPS, to trigger macrophage effector function (35,37,38). Among the ligands for TLR4 are LPS, as well as several host proteins that may be candidates as inflammatory stimuli in rheumatic diseases. HSP60, HSP70, the type III repeat extracellular domain A of fibronectin, and fragments of hyaluronic acid, heparan sulfate, and fibrinogen have all been identified as TLR4 ligands. TLR2 mediates innate immune system activation by yeast, gram-positive bacteria, *Mycobacterium tuberculosis,* and spirochetes (35–39). Mycobacterial cell wall lipoarabinomannan and the mycolylarabinogalactin–peptidoglycan complex, *Staphylococcus aureus*–derived lipoteichoic acid, and yeast-derived zymosan are some of the microbial components recognized by TLR2. As noted above, TLR3 mediates cell activation by dsRNA, and TLR9 has been identified as required for cell activation by demethylated CpG DNA (20,22). The microbial or host ligands for TLR7 have not yet been identified, but this TLR has been shown to be involved in the effects of several synthetic chemicals, including the antiviral agent imiquimod, with structures related to nucleic acids (19). Heterodimers composed of TLR2 and either TLR1 or TLR6 have also been described and likely confer even broader capacity for recognition of microbial products (19). The current concept of the role of TLRs in the coordinated activation of innate immunity is that pathogens bind to general pattern recognition receptors, such as CD14 or mannose receptor, but that additional ligand specificity is conferred by the TLRs. The microbial ligands are internalized, and the TLRs, now on the surface of the phagocytic vacuole, activate adaptor molecules to drive the various signaling cascades that result in new gene expression and production of proinflammatory mediators. One such adaptor molecule is MyD88, which is required for TLR signaling (40). In addition, an MyD88-independent pathway has been identified that is used by TLR3 and TLR4 to induce activation of interferon regulatory factor-3 (IRF3), a transcription factor that is important for transcription of type 1 interferon (41,42). Intracellular adaptor molecules bearing sequence homology to MyD88, called Mal and TRIF (or TICAM-1), have recently been identified as participants in the MyD88 signaling pathways (Fig. 14.1). Recent data indicate that TLRs trigger pathways, leading to production of TNF-α, IL-12, inducible nitric oxide synthase, and nitric oxide, as well as interferon-β (IFN-β) and downstream IFN-regulated genes (36). The complexity of the TLR family is amplified by the differential distribution of TLR on various cell types. It is already clear that macrophages and dendritic cells have a much more sophisticated system for distinguishing "self" and "other" than was previously imagined. In fact, the TLR receptors could be considered to be the specific antigen receptors of the innate immune system. It might be predicted that the failure of TLRs to detect their specific ligands in a phagocytic vacuole containing debris from apoptotic host cells might account for the maintenance of self tolerance under those circumstances.

A family of innate immune receptors distinct from the TLRs has recently been described, with their ligands as yet uncharacterized. These triggering receptors expressed by myeloid cells (TREMs) are encoded in the MHC on human chromosome 6p21 and include both stimulatory and inhibitory receptors (43). TREM1 is expressed on neutrophils

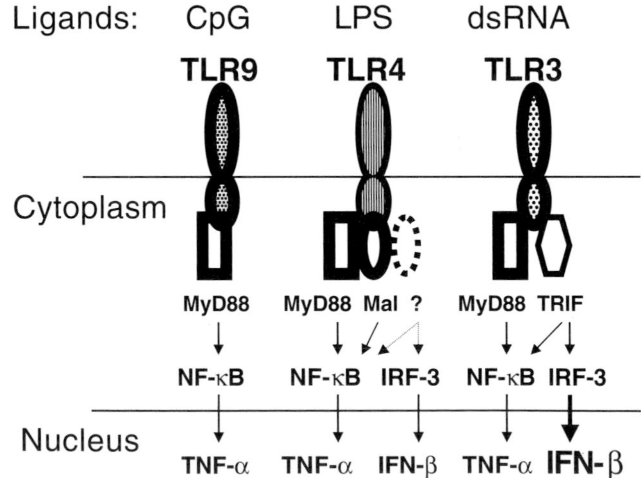

FIG. 14.1. Toll-like receptor (TLR)-mediated mononuclear cell signaling. Representative TLR receptors and their currently proposed signaling pathways are shown. TLR-9-mediated signals are dependent on the adaptor MyD88, activate nuclear factor κB (NF-κB), and result in transcription of tumor necrosis factor-α, interleukin-1, and other cytokines. TLR-4-mediated signals use the MyD88 and Mal adaptor molecules to activate NF-κB and may also use an additional adaptor to activate interferon regulatory factor-3 (IRF-3). TLR-3-mediated signals may use the MyD88-dependent pathway but also use the TIR domain containing adaptor (TRIF or TICAM-1) to activate IRF-3 and induce interferon-β gene transcription.

and some monocyte/macrophages and, when triggered, promotes production of chemokines and release of myeloperoxidase. It also appears to contribute to the differentiation of some monocytes into dendritic cells with augmented capacity to activate the T_H1 subset of T cells. TREM2 is expressed on immature dendritic cells, as well as on microglia and osteoclasts, and when ligated induces partial dendritic cell maturation.

Phagocytic Receptors

FcRs are immunoglobulin (Ig) superfamily members that are expressed on cells of the innate immune system and bind the constant segment (Fc) of immunoglobulin molecules (28–30) (see Chapter 25). When bound by their ligands, the FcRs both transduce activation signals to the phagocyte and mediate phagocytosis of the particle to which the Ig is bound. The human FcR family of receptors for IgG comprises three subfamilies: FcγRI, II, and III. FcγRI is a high-affinity receptor that binds monomeric IgG. FcγRII and FcγRIII are low-affinity receptors that only bind IgG complexes. The FcγRII family includes both activating (FcγRIIa) and inhibitory (FcγRIIb) receptors, based on variability in the amino acid sequence of the intracytoplasmic tails of those receptors, with the activating receptors bearing an immunoreceptyrosine-based activation motif (ITAM) and inhibitory receptors bearing an immunoreceptyrosine-based inhibiting motif (ITIM) (29,44). After ligation of the activating receptors, actin and other components of the cytoskeleton rearrange to promote phagocytosis of the complex bound to the receptor (45). Intracellular calcium is released, and cellular kinases, such as Lyn protein tyrosine kinase, are activated; they phosphorylate cytoplasmic adaptor molecules and trigger new gene transcription. The result is removal of antibody-opsonized particles and immune complexes, generation of antigens for activation of the adaptive immune response, and production of cytotoxic mediators, such as reactive oxygen species and cytokines (28–30). Genetic polymorphisms in the nucleotide sequence of several of these FcRs confer structural and functional variability, and both FcγRII and FcγRIII polymorphisms have been associated with an increased occurrence of lupus nephritis (46,47). Although the basis of the increased nephritis in patients with an FcγRII allele is postulated to be attributable to impaired phagocytosis and clearance of immune complexes, increased macrophage activation through the FcR, with its many biochemical and immunologic sequelae, or more efficient processing of antigens, could also confer altered disease susceptibility or severity based on FcR structural differences.

The mannose-6-phosphate receptor can directly recognize molecules, including microbial components, expressing that sugar, and can mediate uptake and targeting of these mannose-bearing particles to intracellular compartments (13,48). TLR may then sample phagosome contents for the presence of their ligands (35). Molecules phagocytosed by the mannose-6-phosphate receptor can also be processed for presentation on MHC class II molecules (49). Type I and II macrophage scavenger receptors mediate endocytosis of modified (acetylated) low-density lipoproteins, generating foam cells, and contributing to development of atherosclerotic lesions (23).

Complement Receptors

Complement receptors work together with Fc receptors to promote the clearance of pathogens by phagocytes (31,50,51). C3b can bind directly to bacteria, and C1q binds to Ig that opsonizes bacteria (see Chapter 21). Complement receptor 1 (CR1) on phagocytes binds C3b and C4b; CR2 on follicular dendritic (and B) cells binds C3d; CR3 and CR4, integrins expressed on phagocytes, bind C3bi, a complement degradation product; and the C1q receptor can directly bind C1q-associated bacteria. Although complement receptors and FcRs each promote the activity of the other, data suggest that without the FcRs, most of the complement receptors are unable to independently induce phagocytosis of the complex or particle. Together, the complement and Fc receptors stimulate biochemical pathways in the phagocyte that result in new gene expression and toxic mediator production.

Receptors for Clearance of Apoptotic or Senescent Cells

The cells that compose most tissues have a finite life span. Senescent cells, and those that are undergoing programmed cell death (apoptosis), must be efficiently removed but must not trigger the inflammatory cascade initiated by phagocytosis of foreign microbes (33). One of the earliest events in apoptosis is the flipping of the plasma membrane structure to expose phospholipids ordinarily not present on the external face of the membrane. Exposure of phosphatidylserine may serve as a marker for apoptotic cells, because it triggers phagocytic removal of such cells. CD36, a monocyte cell surface receptor, has been shown to specifically bind phosphatidylserine vesicles and is likely to be important for initiating the phagocytosis of apoptotic cells (52,53). Under other conditions of monocyte-macrophage activation, the $\alpha_v\beta_3$ integrin has been shown to mediate recognition and phagocytosis of apoptotic cells (54). On dendritic cells, the $\alpha_v\beta_5$ integrin mediates uptake of apoptotic cells (55). Red blood cells (RBCs) bind to macrophages by the sialoadhesin receptor, and sickled or otherwise malformed RBCs are active triggers of monocyte phagocytosis (56). Another type of monocyte receptor, the receptor for advanced glycation end products (RAGE), is a member of the immunoglobulin family of cell surface molecules and mediates clearance of various products of cellular stress, including those generated in the setting of diabetes and amyloidosis (57,58). RAGE is likely to contribute to disease pathogenesis by inducing production of TNF-α.

Cytokine Receptors

Although space does not permit an extensive review of the cytokine receptors relevant to monocyte and dendritic cell function, it is clear that regulation of the cell surface expression of, and signaling by, the receptors for each of the proinflammatory, immunomodulatory, and inhibitory cytokines is at least as carefully programmed as the induction of the cytokine proteins themselves. Some cytokine receptors, such as those for TNF-α, are constitutively present on the cell surface, but most are increased in their expression after cell triggering through phagocytosis or membrane interaction with proinflammatory triggers. The biochemical signaling pathways used by cytokine receptors generally fall into several classes. The Janus kinase signal transducer and activator of transcription (Jak-STAT) pathway of kinases and adaptor molecules is used by many cytokines, including the prototypes IFN-α and IFN-γ (59). The highly proinflammatory transcription factor NFκB is activated by a number of cytokine receptors, with the TNF-α receptor being a prototype (60). And the TGF-β receptor triggers yet another set of intracellular adaptor proteins (61). Whatever the pathway used by each of the cytokine receptors, they all result in the activation of transcription factors that bind to their respective DNA binding motifs in the promoter regions of genes and induce transcription and translation of proteins that control the next phase of inflammation and adaptive immune system activation.

Chemokine and Other Seven-Transmembrane G-Protein-Coupled Receptors

Macrophages express receptors for chemoattractants, which recruit cells based on a concentration gradient (62–65). As a group, these chemoattractants bind to receptors with a common overall structure, the seven-transmembrane G-protein-coupled receptors. Ligation of these receptors activates guanosine triphosphate (GTP)-binding regulatory proteins that stimulate intracellular biochemical signaling pathways. A family of soluble host mediators called chemokines acts as cell type–specific chemoattractants. The chemokine receptors bind T cell-derived RANTES (regulated upon activation normal T cell expressed and secreted), migration inhibition factor (MIF), and monocyte-derived monocyte chemoattractant protein-1 (MCP-1). The recent discoveries that a coreceptor for human immunodeficiency virus-1 is the receptor for a β-chemokine (CC-CKR-5 or CCR5) and that the β-chemokines RANTES, macrophage inhibitory protein-1α (MIP-1α), and MIP-1β suppress the macrophage trophic strains of HIV demonstrate the facility with which microbial pathogens use host molecules to their own devices, and suggest new approaches for antiviral therapy (66,67).

In addition to acting as receptors for host chemokines, members of the seven-transmembrane, G-protein-coupled receptor family bind other chemoattractants, whether host or microbe derived. The formylated bacterial chemotactic peptide f-met-leu-phe binds to either a high-affinity receptor (formyl peptide receptor) or a low-affinity receptor [formyl peptide receptor-like 1 (FPRL-1)] to induce chemotaxis and calcium flux in phagocytes (64,66). Several other chemoattractants also utilize FPRL-1, including serum amyloid A protein and lipoxin A4 (25). Several important macrophage receptors of this class bind either C5a or its degradation product, C5a-des-arg (50).

Less clearly defined are several families of opiate-alkaloid receptors, some of which are G-protein coupled (68). Both endogenous and pharmacologic opiates bind to these receptors, expressed on monocytes and granulocytes, and have a generally negative effect on inflammatory responses by inhibiting chemokine-induced chemotaxis. Ligation of opioid receptors may also modulate cytokine secretion, with IFN-γ being decreased and TGF-β increased.

Hormone Receptors

Cellular receptors for glucocorticoid hormones are constitutively present in the cytoplasm of many cells, including monocytes, and after binding of their ligand, migrate into the nucleus where they bind to hormone responsive elements in gene promoters (69–71). Some specific effects of glucocorticoids on monocyte function are described below. Vitamin D is a well-studied inducer of macrophage activation that acts through its specific cytoplasmic receptor (50).

Amplification

Movement

Movement is a characteristic feature of mononuclear phagocytes, with extending and retracting of pseudopods mediating motion along a matrix or chemoattractant gradient. The activation of the intracellular skeleton, formed from actin and gelsolin, provides a structure on which the plasma membrane moves (45). A number of chemoattractant proteins, particularly the chemokines, act on monocyte/macrophages to initiate movement across a concentration gradient. The complement activation product C5a and its degradation product C5a-des-arg, often generated by immune complexes, are early mediators of macrophage and neutrophil chemotaxis to a site of tissue injury and increase the adherence of phagocytes to endothelial cells.

Adherence

Spreading of monocytes and macrophages is readily observed *in vitro* and reflects similar events that are triggered by matrix components *in vivo.* Interaction of the macrophage membrane with collagen, proteoglycans, elastin, and hyaluronic acid through binding to receptors such as CD44 mediates migration of those cells after exit from the vascular space.

Recruitment

After activation by bacterial constituents, macrophages produce cytokines that initiate vascular dilatation and recruitment of the innate immune system cells. Localization of immune and inflammatory cells to the site of invasion or injury comprises several discrete steps: (a) rolling on endothelial cells, mediated by selectins; (b) firm attachment to endothelium with arrested movement, mediated by integrins; (c) extravasation across the endothelial barrier, or diapedesis, involving integrins and adhesion molecules of the immunoglobulin superfamily; and (d) movement of phagocytes through the subendothelial tissue matrix to the site of infection or injury, with concentration gradients of chemokines directing the migration (72) (Fig. 14.2).

Selectins and integrins are expressed on the surface of activated monocytes and neutrophils, as well as other cell types, and mediate interaction between immune system cells and the cells they encounter on the way to sites of infection (72). L-selectin is the major phagocyte selectin, and it binds to carbohydrates, such as sialyl Lewis^x, on the endothelial cell surface. A reverse interaction also occurs, with sialyl Lewis^x on the phagocyte mediating reversible binding to P- or E-selectin on the endothelial cells (73). The endothelial selectins are expressed in response to bacterial

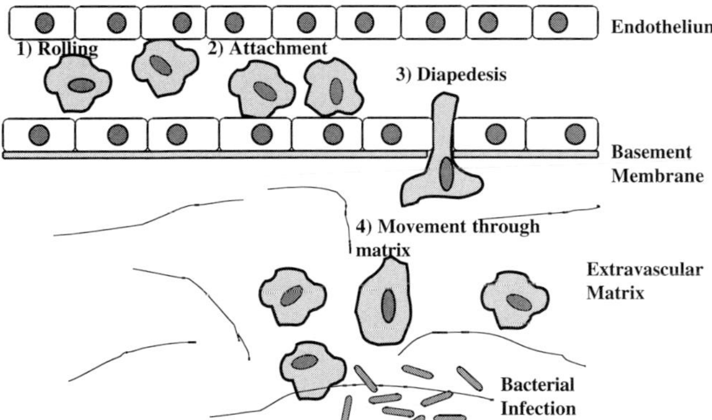

FIG. 14.2. Recruitment of mononuclear phagocytes to sites of infection or tissue injury. Activation of the innate immune response initiates a carefully orchestrated series of events that results in movement of mononuclear phagocytes from the circulation to the site of tissue invasion. This process can be characterized as having four phases: *1,* rolling of mononuclear phagocytes on the vascular endothelium; *2,* attachment of mononuclear phagocytes to the vascular endothelium; *3,* diapedesis, or extravasation of mononuclear phagocytes, between adjacent endothelial cells; and *4,* movement through the subendothelial tissue matrix toward the damaged site. The key molecules that mediate these events are cell surface selectins, integrins, and members of the immunoglobulin superfamily. Soluble chemokines attract the mononuclear phagocytes across a concentration gradient.

products (LPS), complement activation products (C5a), or products of phagocytes, including a leukotriene (LTB_4) and TNF-α. The interaction of these selectins with carbohydrates on the phagocyte cell surface produces reversible adherence and rolling of the phagocyte along the blood vessel surface.

The integrins are an important class of cell surface adhesion molecules that are constitutively present on monocytes, but undergo "inside-out" signaling to acquire a conformation with increased capacity for interaction with their ligands after monocyte activation by IL-8 or other stimuli (72,73). The best described of the integrins are included in the CD18 family, which includes at least three glycoprotein molecular complexes comprising a β subunit paired with either CD11a [leukocyte function–associated antigen-1 (LFA-1)], CD11b (Mac-1), or CD11c (p150/95) (31,72). Both LFA-1 and p150,95 (CR4) are integrins expressed on monocytes and dendritic cells. The ligand for LFA-1 is intercellular adhesion molecule-1 (ICAM-1), present on endothelial cells and most leukocytes. MAC-1 is a receptor (CR3) for the C3bi component of the complement system and helps to bind and mediate phagocytosis of particles opsonized with C3bi. Other ligands of MAC-1 include lectins such as β-glucans and ICAMs. The ICAMs are cell surface adhesion molecules with structures that include the immunoglobulin-like domain. They are found on dendritic cells, lymphocytes, and activated endothelium and promote APC/T-cell interactions. These immunoglobulin superfamily members include ICAM-1 (CD54), ICAM-2 (CD102), and LFA-3 (CD58). ICAM-1 is induced on the endothelial cell surface by the proinflammatory cytokine TNF-α. Diapedesis of phagocytes is mediated by the integrins, as well as by the immunoglobulin family member platelet endothelial cell adhesion molecule (CD31), which is expressed on the phagocyte, as well as on the surface of endothelial cells, at the points where they abut each other.

Invasion

Once through the basement membrane underlying the vascular endothelium, phagocytes must make their way through the connective tissue matrix to arrive at the site of tissue disruption. Adhesion molecules on the phagocyte cell surface interact with components of extracellular matrix, such as fibronectin, while cell surface and secreted proteolytic enzymes induce sufficient matrix degradation to allow cell movement. Macrophage plasminogen activator converts inactive plasminogen to plasmin. Among the proteolytic actions of plasmin that facilitate tissue invasion is digestion of extracellular matrix. At the same time, plasmin contributes to the early inflammatory response through cleavage of C3 to C3a, an anaphylatoxin, and activation of latent TGF-β, which acts as a chemotactic factor for neutrophils and monocytes. Collagenase and elastase are also secreted by monocytes in response to stimulation by LPS or cytokines, and cell surface matrix metalloproteinases may contribute to cell invasion of matrix (74). However, macrophages closely regulate these potentially damaging activities through their concurrent production of antiproteases, such as α_2-macroglobulin and α_1-antiprotease, which inhibit elastase.

Effector Function

Phagocytosis

Phagocytosis of immune complexes, opsonized particles, and apoptotic cells is mediated through many of the receptors already mentioned, depending on the particle being cleared (23). Opsonized particles, including bacteria, bind FcR, while apoptotic cells and debris are cleared by binding to phosphatidylserine and other receptors (33,53–56,75). The ingested material is enclosed in a lipid membrane, derived from the plasma membrane, with subsequent fusion with enzyme-containing lysosomes to form a phagolysosome. Ingestion of organisms triggers the phagocyte to produce a host of mediators that are toxic and can directly or indirectly kill the microorganism. The lysosomal enzymes include acid hydrolases and proteases, which can act within a phagolysosome or can be secreted into the extracellular environment. Because the substrates for these enzymes are not restricted to microbes, but include host connective tissues as well, lysosomal enzymes can mediate tissue damage. Lysozyme is constitutively secreted and can degrade bacterial cell walls by hydrolyzing *n*-acetylmuramic-β1–4-*n*-acetyl glucose linkages. Most of the neutral proteases and lysosomal enzymes have been detected at inflammatory sites, including rheumatoid synovium, and it is presumed that they play an important role in cartilage degradation.

Although phagocytosis of apoptotic debris also results in its degradation in phagolysosomes, the cellular activation induced is much more limited compared with that triggered by engulfment of foreign material. Ingestion of host debris does not usually induce increased expression of costimulatory molecules, and so is not immunogenic for T cells, does not activate the respiratory burst, and only induces a limited panel of cytokines, predominantly those that are inhibitory to inflammatory processes (32).

Secretion

Arachidonic Acid Metabolites

Macrophage activation stimulates the function of cellular phospholipases that act on plasma membrane phospholipids to undergo enzymatic generation of arachidonic acid (see Chapter 23). The end products of cyclooxygenase or lipoxygenase cleavage of arachidonic acid include prostaglandins (PGs), thromboxanes, and leukotrienes (76). Through its activation of 3′,5′-cyclic adenosine monophosphate (cAMP), prostaglandin E_2 (PGE_2) is generally inhibitory to many lymphocyte functions and induces fever and hyperalgesia (77). On the other hand, prostaglandins stimulate osteoclasts and bone resorption. Leukotrienes C and D (slow-reacting substance of anaphylaxis) mediate smooth muscle contraction, and LTB_4 is a chemoattractant for neutrophils and macrophages. Thromboxanes act as vasoconstrictors.

Cytokines

The cytokines secreted by phagocytes after interaction with microbial products or immune system stimuli are central to the amplification of the inflammatory response and to the initiation of the more specific adaptive immune response (Table 14.2). Production of cytokines requires activation and translocation of transcription factors to the cell nucleus, and new gene transcription. Most cytokines have multiple cell sources and are pleiotropic, acting on a wide range of cell targets. After binding to specific cell surface receptors, many of the cytokines activate members of the family of intracellular adaptor proteins, the Jak-STAT proteins, which then trigger the transcription of various genes encoding effector molecules (59). Other cytokines regulate proteins that control progression through the cell cycle and cell division. Among the most important cytokines produced by macrophages and dendritic cells are IFN-α, TNF-α, IL-1, IL-6, IL-12, IL-15, and IL-18 (48,78–89). IFN-α, the first cytokine studied more than 40 years ago (90), is now known to be produced by plasmacytoid dendritic cells (8,78,79). Its most significant trigger is dsRNA, a key component of viruses. Once it is produced, this type 1 IFN directly inhibits viral replication and acts on components of the immune system to combat viral infection (91–93). IFN-α not only promotes the cytotoxic activity of NK cells against virus-infected cells or tumor cells, but also inhibits T-cell proliferation. The former activity may be important in the therapeutic efficacy of IFN-α in patients with hepatitis B or C infection or in patients with melanoma, Kaposi sarcoma, or other malignancies (94).

TNF-α is one of the most essential cytokines produced by mononuclear phagocytes for handling infection by microbial pathogens, yet it is also the cytokine with the most potential for mediating host tissue damage. TNF-α synthesis and secretion are triggered by most of the microbial stimuli discussed above. Activation of TLR by LPS, CpG motifs, or other stimuli and phagocytosis of immune complexes by FcR all induce TNF-α production. The essential role of TNF-α in controlling infection is demonstrated by the shortened life span in murine models, in which TNF-α is knocked out or anti-TNF-α antibodies are administered to neutralize the cytokine, followed by infection of the animals with bacteria (95,96). Thus, TNF-α is required for mobilizing phagocytes to destroy, and failing that, to wall off a nidus of infection. If this effort fails, the host is placed in considerable jeopardy, because it not only is subject to hematogenous dissemination of the bacteria from its initial site to the rest of the organism, but also must suffer the consequences of systemic exposure to the highly proinflamma-

TABLE 14.2. *Cytokines and chemokines secreted by mononuclear phagocytes*

Mediator	Functional property
Colony-stimulating factors	
GM-CSF	Differentiation of granulocytes and macrophages
M-CSF	Differentiation of mononuclear phagocytes and osteoclasts
G-CSF	Differentiaton of granulocytes
Interferons	
Interferon-α	Promotes natural killer cell function; induces dendritic cell differentiation and macrophage iNOS production; inhibits T-cell proliferation
Interleukins	
IL-1α and IL-1β	Induction of cytokines, metalloproteinases, acute-phase reactants; T-cell proliferation
IL-6	Induction of acute-phase reactants; B-cell differentiation
IL-10	Inhibits macrophage co-stimulatory function; augments B-cell differentiation
IL-12	Promotes Th1 effector function
IL-15	Induction of T-cell activation through IL-2 receptor
IL-18	Induction of GM-CSF, TNF-α, and iNOS
Other Cytokines	
TNF-α	Induction of proinflammatory cytokines and mediators; promotes bone resorption
BLyS	B-cell survival factor
TGF-β	Chemotactic factor; immunosuppressive; profibrotic
Platelet-derived growth factor	Induction of MCP-1; mitogenic and chemotactic for vascular smooth muscle cells
Fibroblast growth factor	Induction of MCP-1; chemotactic for endothelial cells; promotes osteoblast survival
Insulin-like growth factor	Induction of ICAM-1 and TNF-α; promotes osteoblast survival
Chemokines	
IL-8	Chemotactic for neutrophils
MIP-1α	Chemotactic for neutrophils
MCP-1	Chemotactic for monocytes and memory T cells; activates respiratory burst

BlyS, B lymphocyte stimulator; GM-CSF, granulocyte macrophage colony-stimulating factor; iNOS, inducible nitric oxide synthase; MCP, monocyte chemoattractant protein; MIP, macrophage inhibitory protein; TGF, transforming growth factor; Th1, T helper 1 subset; TNF, tumor necrosis factor.

tory cytokines that are present in increasing concentrations and that are also dispersed throughout the body. The result is shock and all of its detrimental consequences. When present chronically, as in the anatomic space defined by the synovial membrane in rheumatoid arthritis (RA), TNF-α is the important inducer of many pro-inflammatory mediators (97). TNF-α stimulates collagenase and PGE_2 production by synovial fibroblasts and stimulates bone resorption, contributing to cartilage damage and periarticular osteopenia. The notable efficacy of TNF-α blockade in RA supports the key pathogenic role of that cytokine in chronic inflammation (98,99). Endogenous soluble TNF-α receptors, acting to adsorb excess soluble TNF-α, may provide a physiologic regulator of TNF-α that is comparable in its mechanism to one of these new pharmacologic agents.

B-lymphocyte stimulator (BLyS) is another member of the TNF family that is produced by myeloid cells, including monocytes and dendritic cells. BLyS binds to receptors on B cells and promotes their survival. Inhibition of BLyS in murine lupus models results in decreased production of some autoantibodies. The potential of blockade of the BLyS pathway as a therapeutic approach in autoimmune and inflammatory diseases is currently being tested.

IL-1 is another monocyte-macrophage product that is induced by many of the microbial and host monocyte stimuli and has pleiotropic effects (82). Among its most productive actions is its support for activation of T cells and induction of cytokine synthesis. It also promotes many of the systemic manifestations of uncontrolled microbial infection, such as fever, neutrophilia, and production of acute phase proteins. Along with TNF-α, IL-1 contributes to synoviocyte activation, collagenase production, proteoglycan degradation, and bone resorption, events that are pathologic in the rheumatoid joint. In view of the highly damaging potential of IL-1, it is not surprising that there is a natural inhibitor (82). IL-1 receptor antagonist (IL-1RA) is a product of monocytes that, when present in marked excess to the concentration of IL-1, inhibits binding of IL-1 to its cell surface receptor and many IL-1-mediated effector functions. IL-1RA has served as the first test modulator of joint inflammation in animal trials of a gene therapy approach to treatment of RA (100).

IL-6 is produced by monocytes and by T_H2 cells. It is an important factor for terminal B-cell differentiation to the plasma cell stage, and it induces secretion of numerous acute-phase reactants by hepatocytes. IL-12, a heterodimer that includes 35- and 40-kd subunits, is produced by monocytes and dendritic cells and plays a key role in the induction of a dominant T_H1 response by T cells (83,84). Two other cytokines, IL-15 and IL-18, may have important activity in RA pathogenesis. IL-15 is a monocyte-derived cytokine that mediates T-cell activation through the IL-2 receptor (85–88). One of its important effects is the induction of T-cell-dependent TNF-α and chemokine synthesis by monocytes. It has been proposed that IL-15 plays an important role in generating the T-cell phenotype observed in RA synovial tissues (85,101). IL-18 receptors are present on synovial lymphocytes and macrophages, and IL-18 messenger RNA (mRNA) and protein are seen in RA synovial tissue samples (89). IL-18 induces production of GM-CSF, TNF-α, and nitric oxide by macrophages. IL-12, IL-15, and IL-18 may work together to perpetuate the T_H1-dominant phenotype and macrophage activation that occurs at the site of disease in RA.

Other cytokines produced by monocytes are less clearly proinflammatory, but play a more dominant role in terminating immune responses. TGF-β, while a chemotactic factor early on after the activation of monocytes, is generally suppressive of T-cell proliferation and promotes fibrosis and wound healing as an immune response is winding down (102). IL-10, an important immunomodulatory cytokine produced by macrophages and T_H2 T cells, acts on monocytes to inhibit their APC capacity and cytokine production (103,104). However, IL-10 is important as a B-lymphocyte activator, serving to increase the level of B-cell proliferation and Ig class switching induced by antigen binding to surface Ig and CD40 ligation by activated T helper cells (105).

Chemokines

Chemokines are soluble proteins produced by many cell types in response to microbial products (LPS), physical agents, or endogenous proinflammatory cytokines, including TNF-α or IL-1, and act to regulate the recruitment of immune and inflammatory cells to sites of infection or tissue injury. Among the most important of these relevant to phagocytes are members of the α (CXC) chemokine family (e.g., IL-8) and members of the β (CC) chemokine family (MCP-1, RANTES, and MIP-1α). IL-8 is produced by monocytes and acts on neutrophils to bring them into the inflammatory site, whereas MCP-1 and MIP-1α attract both monocytes and memory T cells (67,86). RANTES is produced by activated T cells and attracts monocytes, as well as granulocytes and lymphocytes. A concentration gradient of the chemokines on an extracellular matrix or endothelial cell substrate is detected by cells expressing specific receptors. The chemokines can also activate their target cells to generate toxins, such as nitric oxide, that are damaging to microbes. IL-8 also stimulates release of lysosomal enzymes.

Neutral Proteases

These enzymes are secreted upon macrophage stimulation, and some are also found on the cell membrane (74,106). Collagenase and elastase may assist movement of macrophages through connective tissue, but also contribute to tissue damage when produced in excess. Other enzymes, such as those in the adamalysin family that contain a disintegrin and metalloproteinase domain (ADAMs), convert inactive cytokine precursors to their active form. For example, the TNF-α convertase enzyme mediates enzymatic cleavage of cell surface TNF-α to produce the soluble form (106). Another neutral protease is plasminogen activator, which, as discussed above, triggers complement activation and fibrin degradation. Antiproteases produced by macrophages limit the destructive potential of those enzymes.

Others

Monocyte-macrophages are among the cells that produce complement components. Platelet-activating factor is a phosphorylcholine derivative produced by macrophages that is chemotactic for macrophages and neutrophils and induces bronchoconstriction.

Cytotoxicity

Reactive Oxygen Products of the Respiratory Burst

A number of monocyte stimuli, as a final common pathway, trigger the biochemical reactions of the respiratory burst (107). In this reaction, oxygen is consumed and reduced nicotinamide-adenine dinucleotide phosphate (NADPH) oxidase, a membrane-associated enzyme, is activated, converting the oxygen into supcroxide anion (O_2^-) in the reaction: $NADPH + H^+ + 2O_2 = NADP^+ + 2H^+ + -2O_2^-$. In a subsequent reaction, the enzyme superoxide dismutase generates the formation of hydrogen peroxide (H_2O_2), and in the presence of iron, hydrogen peroxide forms hydroxyl radical (·OH) and singlet oxygen (·O_2). Finally, myeloperoxidase, together with a halide such as Cl^-, converts singlet oxygen to hypochlorous acid (HOCl). NADPH oxidase is not a single protein, but a complex whose components have recently been defined, leading to new insights into immune deficiency states. Two cytosolic factors, p47-phox and p67-phox, a membrane-associated flavoprotein, and heterodimeric cytochrome b_{558}, comprising p22-phox and gp91-phox proteins, make up this complex. Chronic granulomatosis disease can occur due to mutations and functional defects in any of these proteins (108,109).

All of these oxidizing agents—hydrogen peroxide, superoxide anion, singlet oxygen, hydroxyl radical, and hypochlorous ion—can inactivate the sulfhydryl groups of enzymes or proteins and can result in killing of parasites or tumor cells. Oxidizing agents can also inactivate chemoattractants or antiproteases by oxidation of methionine to sulfoxides. Induction of these toxic mediators is increased by IFN-γ and, through the activation of protein kinase C, by chemoattractants.

The production of toxic metabolites, potentially destructive to host tissue, by the phagocyte is at least partially regulated by the generation in the same cells of chemicals that neutralize these dangerous products. Superoxide dismutase converts superoxide anion to hydrogen peroxide, and catalase metabolizes hydrogen peroxide.

Reactive Nitrogen Products

In addition to the reactive oxygen products of activated macrophages, studies have demonstrated an important role for the induction of nitric oxide synthase and its product, nitric oxide, in the antimicrobial, and tissue-destructive, potential of the innate immune response (110–114).

ANTIGEN-PRESENTING CELL FUNCTION IN THE ADAPTIVE IMMUNE RESPONSE

Recognition

The dendritic cell is the most important APC for initiation of an adaptive immune response and is enriched in the T-cell areas of lymph nodes and spleen as interdigitating cells (4,7). These dendritic cells mostly derive from circulating lymph or from skin, where they are termed Langerhans cells. Macrophages can also present processed antigen to T cells, and B cells that have received activation signals and have increased their surface expression of costimulatory molecules, such as CD80 and CD86, are potent APCs, because their cell surface antigen receptor specifically picks up the antigen relevant to the adaptive immune response (115).

MHC Class I Antigen-Processing Pathway

Antigen-processing pathways differ in their mechanisms, depending on the type of antigen involved. Intracellular microbes, particularly viruses, generate immunostimulatory peptides through the MHC class I antigen-processing pathway (116) (Fig. 14.3A). A virus, for example, might become integrated into the host cell genome, allowing

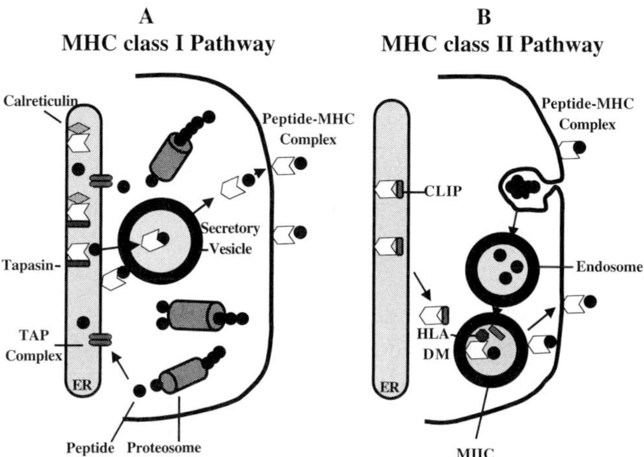

FIG. 14.3. Antigen processing by mononuclear phagocytes. **A:** Major histocompatibility complex (MHC) class I pathway. **B:** MHC class II pathway.

transcription and translation of viral proteins by that host cell. After synthesis, some of those proteins can be degraded in the cytosol by the proteosome, with peptides of appropriate size then actively transported into the endoplasmic reticulum (ER) by host proteins called TAP1 and TAP2 (transporter associated with antigen presentation) (117–122). The peptides are then available to load onto newly formed MHC class I molecules, composed of a 45-kd glycosylated α-chain protein and an associated nonglycosylated 12-kd β_2-microglobulin chain, and held in a conformation conducive to binding proteins by the chaperons calnexin, calreticulin, and tapasin. Once loaded with either foreign or self peptide, the class I molecule leaves the ER and moves to the cell membrane. Peptide bound to MHC class I molecules preferentially interacts with $CD8^+$ T cells, because CD8 binds to the nonpolymorphic region of class I molecules, stabilizing the interaction between APC and T cell. Of potential interest for understanding genetic predisposition to autoimmune disease is allelic variability in the TAP molecules that may confer selective transport of certain peptides to the MHC class I binding compartment (123).

MHC Class II Antigen-Processing Pathway

In contrast to the path followed by intracellular organisms, extracellular pathogens, such as bacteria and some parasites, are taken into an APC through phagocytosis or endocytosis, entering a series of intracellular compartments that lead to an MHC class II–rich vesicle (the MIIC) (117, 118) (Fig. 14.3B). After degradation of the antigenic particle by enzymes that include the cathepsins, peptides from the particle can be loaded onto the nascent MHC class II molecules and expressed on the APC surface, ready to interact with a T cell through its T-cell receptor (TCR), should a TCR with a good molecular fit for the peptide bound in the MHC class II binding groove be available. The MHC class II molecules are heterodimeric glycoproteins consisting of a 33-kd α chain and a 29-kd β chain (124). As in the case of the class I molecule, the binding groove for antigen is formed by two polymorphic domains, although in contrast to MHC class I, where both of these domains are part of the α chain, in the MHC class II molecules, the α and β chains each contribute part of the binding groove. The mechanisms that allow antigenic peptide to bind to the cleft of the MHC class II molecule have been recently elucidated. On emerging from the endoplasmic reticulum as DR, DQ, or DP α and β chains [the products of three human leukocyte antigen (HLA)-D gene loci], the newly formed peptide-binding groove is occupied by a temporary ligand, the invariant chain. After being sorted into the endocytic pathway of cytoplasmic vesicles, the class II molecule enters the acidic, peptide-rich MIIC. In the MIIC, the invariant chain is trimmed until only the segment bound in the MHC class II groove remains, a peptide termed CLIP, or class II–associated invariant chain peptide (125). CLIP can then be displaced from the binding groove, an event promoted by the HLA-related molecule DM, permitting insertion of a foreign antigen–derived peptide in the cleft and transport of the peptide–MHC complex to the cell surface (126). The T cell, in the case of MHC class II–presented peptides, is a $CD4^+$ cell, because the CD4 molecule has the capacity to bind to the nonpolymorphic region of MHC class II and to stabilize the binding of the APC to the T cell.

It should be noted that MHC molecules not only bind foreign peptides. In fact, most cell surface class I and II molecules express self protein–derived peptides. There is some experimental suggestion that various MHC alleles may differ in their capacity to bind self peptides (127,128). The more promiscuous peptide-binding capacity of several of the RA-associated MHC class II alleles, such as DRB1*0401, may be of pathogenic significance. It has also been proposed that RA-associated alleles may confer a conformation on cell surface MHC class II that promotes direct interactions with the TCR, regardless of the peptide bound (129). The failure to trigger an immune response to self antigens in healthy individuals must depend on the failure of APC to express costimulatory molecules in the absence of an invading microbe, and the relative paucity of strongly self-reactive T cells in the immune repertoire.

Nonclassic Antigen-Processing Pathways

Nonpeptide antigens can also be processed and presented to T cells on the surface of macrophages. The CD1 molecular family is genetically related to the classic MHC class I and II molecules, but is encoded outside of the MHC (130–134). The crystal structure of CD1 demonstrates its generally similar molecular structure to the classic antigen-binding proteins, but in the case of CD1, lipids and glycolipids, rather than peptides, are bound (135). Among the clinically important microbial antigens presented to T cells by CD1 family molecules are mycobacterial lipid antigens, such as mycolic acid. Antigen presentation by CD1 nicely complements the antigen-presenting capacities of MHC class I and II molecules to permit more extensive targeting of components of pathogenic microorganisms by the adaptive immune response.

Costimulation

Costimulation refers to the requirement of T or B cells of the adaptive immune system for a second signal, in addition to that through the cell surface antigen receptor, in order to undergo full activation (115,136). In the case of T-cell activation by the antigenic peptide–MHC complex on the APC, several costimulatory pathways have been described. B7.1 (CD80) and B7.2 (CD86) are the best characterized and likely most important APC cell surface molecules that mediate T-cell costimulation through their CD28 ligand (115,137). An additional costimulatory pathway has been documented recently, in which a B7-related molecule, which is inducible by TNF-α, interacts with the T cell–inducible costimulator (ICOS) molecule, providing an activating signal to T cells (138–141). The B7 molecules are expressed as homodimers and are members of the immunoglobulin supergene family. They are present in low density, or not at all, on the surface of monocytes, but after stimulation of those cells following interaction with microbes, the expression of B7 molecules is induced. Bacterial proteins, enriched in adjuvant properties, are particularly active in inducing costimulatory molecule expression, a property that contributes to their immunogenicity. When APC-bearing peptide–MHC complexes interact with an antigen-specific T cell in the absence of costimulatory molecule expression, the T cell can be anergized, conferring a relatively refractory state on reexposure to the same antigenic peptide (142). Thus, costimulatory molecule expression on APC is a key point of regulation of the adaptive immune response. In addition to these positive costimulatory molecular pairs, inhibitory receptor-ligand pairs help to modulate T-cell activation and contribute to termination of an immune response (143). CTLA4 and PD-1 are two such negative costimulatory molecules. As CTLA4 shares the B7 ligands with CD28 and binds them with high affinity, a soluble form of CTLA4 can effectively block CD28-B7 interaction, a therapeutic approach that is under investigation.

Cross-Priming

Although the classic route for processing of antigens presented to $CD8^+$ T cells is, as described above, through the entry of cytoplasmic peptides into the ER with subsequent loading onto MHC class I molecules, an alternative mechanism has been noted (53). In the event termed cross-priming, apoptotic cells and any foreign antigens they might contain are engulfed by dendritic cells, their contents processed, and then presented on MHC class I molecules to $CD8^+$ T cells. This mechanism differs from the rule that MHC class I–presented peptides do not derive from extracellular material. In this case, the antigens are phagocytosed, as is typical for class II–presented peptides. This pathway permits viral antigens in one host cell, that may not express adequate costimulatory molecules for T-cell stimulation, to trigger the adaptive immune response by presentation on another host APC.

Amplification and Modulation of the Adaptive Immune Response by Mononuclear Phagocytes

Through their production of and response to cytokines and other immunomodulatory molecules, APCs modulate the magnitude and effector cell programs expressed by T lymphocytes.

Cytokines

One of the most important roles of APCs is to mold the functional activities of responding T cells by virtue of the cytokines that those APCs produce. Both monocytes and dendritic cells secrete IL-12 that binds to activated T cells and NK cells. When bound to CD4 T cells, IL-12 supports the differentiation of those cells to secretion of IL-2 and IFN-γ (83). When IL-12 binds to its receptor on $CD8^+$ T cells, differentiation to cytotoxic effector cells is supported. In contrast to this positive effect on the generation of cellular immunity, inhibitory cytokines, particularly IL-10 and TGF-β, are produced by macrophages. Both of these cytokines inhibit T-cell proliferation, either directly or by decreasing the expression of costimulatory molecules on APC (102–104).

Prostaglandins

PGE_2, one of the important products of the arachidonic acid pathway, is generally suppressive of T-cell proliferation and effector function. PGE_2 increases cAMP levels, an effect that blunts intracellular signaling pathways in the T cell (76,77).

Mononuclear Phagocyte Effector Function in the Adaptive Immune Response

Antibody-Mediated Cellular Cytotoxicity

Once antigen-specific antibody has been produced by the humoral immune response, that antibody can bridge antigen-expressing target cells and cytotoxic effector cells to which the antibody is bound via the FcR. Antibody-mediated cellular cytotoxicity is a mechanism by which the adaptive immune response makes use of the cells of the innate immune system to mediate effector function. This killing mechanism is promoted by both GM-CSF and M-CSF, growth factors produced by activated T cells and other cells that induce monocyte maturation.

Killing of Intracellular Organisms

Many macrophage effector mechanisms depend on, or are more efficient, when the macrophage has been activated by T lymphocytes triggered by their specific antigens (144, 145). Intracellular bacteria, including tuberculosis and leprosy, and parasites, such as leishmania, take up residence in phagocytic cells, where they reproduce and protect themselves from the host immune response. Microbial products have evolved to foil the macrophages' capacity to digest the microorganism, so the adaptive immune response is called on to mediate defense against these organisms. T_H1 cell surface proteins and cytokines, particularly IFN-γ and TNF-α, activate macrophages to directly kill the microbes. The molecules that mediate this cytotoxic function include nitric oxide, oxygen radicals, and the contents of the phagocyte lysosome. The same cellular pathways can also be recruited to kill tumor cells. These destructive mechanisms, so effective against invading microorganisms, can mediate extensive host tissue damage if not controlled.

Granuloma Formation

Granulomas, the typical histopathologic manifestation of chronic infection with many intracellular microbes, represent an attempt of the immune system to wall off and limit the pathogenic potential of microorganisms that are not successfully killed and degraded. The center of the granuloma is formed from fused macrophages, resulting in cells with a multinucleated appearance, surrounded by lymphocytes and a palisade of fibroblastoid cells. Microorganisms can sometimes be seen in the central region of the granuloma. T-cell and fibroblast-derived cytokines, particularly IFN-γ and TNF-α, promote the formation of these infection-induced granulomas.

Regulation of Antigen-Presenting Cells

Regulation by Cytokines

Important points of regulation of mononuclear phagocytes occur at the level of maturation from bone marrow precursors and at the time of differentiation of mature monocytes (or dendritic cells) into the terminally differentiated phenotype (as discussed above) (2). Among the cytokines that stimulate progenitor cells are T cell–derived IL-3, IL-6, and GM-CSF; B cell–derived IL-6; and the macrophage products GM-CSF, M-CSF, and IL-6. After $CD4^+$ T_H1 cells have undergone antigen-specific activation, IFN-γ and TNF-α are produced and modulate macrophage activity (Fig. 14.4). After binding its specific cell surface receptor, IFN-γ, through the Jak-STAT pathway, triggers many of the effector programs of macrophages. The enzymes of the respiratory burst are generated, and cell surface expression of MHC class I and II molecules is increased, promoting macrophage cytotoxic and APC function. Production of IFN-γ is not an exclusive property of the adaptive immune response, because NK cells also secrete it after activation by IFN-α. Other cytokines, including GM-CSF and M-CSF, promote monocyte production of cytokines and increase cell surface expression of adhesion molecules.

Monocyte Activation Through Cell-Cell Interactions

After antigen-specific activation, T cells produce cell surface, as well as soluble, molecules that activate phagocytes and other APCs. Ligation of cell surface CD40 by T-cell CD40 ligand (CD40L) induces increased costimulatory molecule expression, and production of TNF-α and nitric oxide, in the case of macrophages, and IL-12 by dendritic cells (146). The activation profile induced by CD40L/CD40

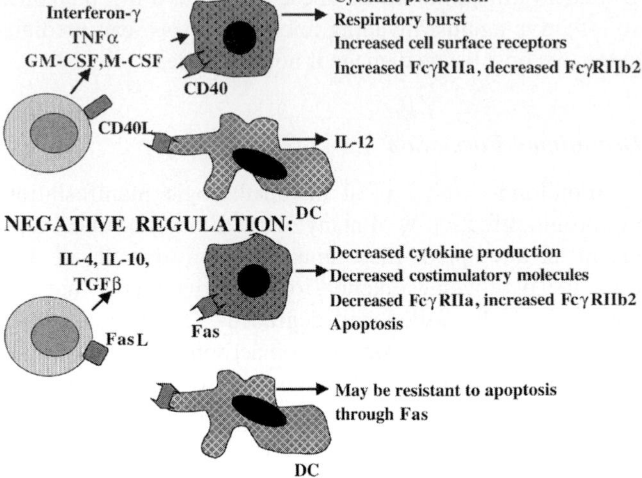

FIG. 14.4. Regulation of antigen-presenting cells (APCs). After mononuclear phagocytes and other APCs initiate the activation of the adaptive immune response, activated T cells, in turn, regulate the APCs. T cell–mediated regulation occurs through cytokines and cell surface interaction molecules. Regulation has both positive and negative effects on the mononuclear phagocytes.

interactions prepares the monocytes to more effectively provide costimulation for the generation of antigen-specific $CD8^+$ cytotoxic cells, and promotes T-cell differentiation along the T_H1 cytokine pathway.

Down-Regulation of Monocyte and Dendritic Cell Function by Soluble Mediators and Cell Surface Interactions

In contrast to IFN-γ and other monocyte-activating cytokines, IL-4, an important cytokine product of Th2 T cells, inhibits macrophage activation (144). Recent data indicate that, among the macrophage targets differentially regulated by IFN-γ and IL-4, are two isoforms of the macrophage FcγRII. The activating form of the receptor, FcγRIIa, is increased in expression by IFN-γ and decreased by IL-4, while the inhibitory form of the receptor, FcγRIIb2, is decreased by IFN-γ and increased by IL-4 (44). Two pleiotropic cytokines, produced by T_H2 cells and monocytes, IL-10 and TGF-β, are generally inhibitory to monocyte activation (103,104,147). IL-10 decreases costimulatory molecule expression and, for that reason, can blunt the antigen-presenting function of the monocytes. Other soluble mediators produced in the context of both innate and adaptive immune responses suppress monocyte differentiation. PGE_1 and PGE_2 are generated by monocytes, but also inhibit their function.

As CD40L/CD40 interactions between activated T helper cells and macrophages promote macrophage activation (146), other members of the same molecular families, Fas ligand and Fas receptor, regulate macrophage viability by inducing apoptosis through the Fas pathway (148). An interesting recent observation is that while macrophages and B cells can be induced to undergo apoptosis after ligation of Fas under some conditions, dendritic cells are relatively resistant to Fas-mediated apoptosis, perhaps reflecting their important role in mediating induction of the adaptive immune response (149).

CLINICAL SYNDROMES OF PHAGOCYTE OR ANTIGEN-PRESENTING CELL DEFICIENCY

The critical role of the mononuclear phagocyte system in host defense is demonstrated by the experiments of nature defined by deficiencies in several of the macrophage effector cell pathways. Deficiency of components of the plasma membrane-associated NADPH oxidase complex accounts for impaired generation of superoxide characteristic of chronic granulomatous disease (108,109). An autosomal-recessive form is characterized by alterations in p67-phox or p47-phox cytosolic proteins or the p22-phox subunit of cytochrome b_{558}. The most frequent form is x-linked and is based on defects in the gp91-phox cytochrome b_{558} component. Children with this disorder fail to adequately clear catalase-positive bacteria and have severe chronic infections contributing to granuloma formation. Treatment with IFN-γ, which promotes increased macrophage function, together with antibiotic prophylaxis, has been efficacious (150).

Myeloperoxidase acts on H_2O_2 to produce HOCl, a potent antioxidant that is highly toxic for microorganisms and tumor cells. The relatively common deficiency in myeloperoxidase, in contrast to the much rarer NADPH oxidase deficiency, has few clinical consequences (151). Several of the other phagocyte mechanisms for handling microbial infection are increased in activity and compensate for the impaired generation of HOCl.

In an autosomal-recessive syndrome called leukocyte adhesion deficiency, mutation of the common integrin β_2 chain (CD18) confers impaired function of all three integrins that use this chain (Mac-1, LFA-1, and p150,95) (152). These patients have impaired macrophage function and poor formation of pus, leading to life-threatening bacterial infections, presumably due to impaired migration of phagocytes across the vascular endothelium. The degree of the common β_2-chain deficiency and severity of the clinical state is variable, based on whether the chain fails to be produced at all in the case of the severe deficiency, or whether it is either made at lower than normal levels or is impaired in its capacity to appropriately assemble, resulting in cell surface adhesion molecule expression that is less than 10% of the normal level. There are no effective treatments for leukocyte adhesion deficiency at this time, other than bone marrow transplantation, although gene therapy might be an appropriate approach (152).

MONONUCLEAR PHAGOCYTES IN RHEUMATOID ARTHRITIS

Consideration of the functional properties of monocytes and dendritic cells reviewed in this chapter draws attention to the pathogenic potential, as well as the key host defense functions, of those cells. Analysis of the cells, cytokines, chemokines, and other soluble mediators present in the rheumatoid synovial membrane and fluid supports the central role of the mononuclear phagocyte system in this prototype rheumatic disease. Virtually every proinflammatory and antigen-presenting activity discussed is in evidence in the inflamed RA joint (89,114,153).

Macrophages compose a significant proportion of the mononuclear cells infiltrating the synovial membrane stroma, and the macrophage-derived type A synoviocytes that expand to form a multilayered lining for the pannus are viewed by some as expressing some of the earliest phenotypic changes at the initiation of the arthritic process (154,155). While macrophages are the dominant APC in the tissue, synovial fluid from RA patients is highly enriched in dendritic cells (156).

Although investigators hold differing views regarding the relative importance of T cells and macrophages in the pathogenesis of inflammation and cartilage destruction in the rheumatoid joint (157), a balanced view might implicate many components of both innate and adaptive immune responses in the chronic inflammatory process that feeds on itself in the confined anatomic space of the diarthrodial joint in RA. Whatever the initiating or etiologic trigger for immune system activation, it is clear that the site of pathology includes abundant T cells that are relatively restricted in their TCR sequences, compared with peripheral blood T cells, indicating that those T cells are selected by either an antigen, a panel of antigens, or, less likely, a superantigen (158). Some of those T cells are CD40L$^+$, giving them the potential to directly stimulate the activation of macrophages and dendritic cells through CD40 (159). The RA joint is swimming in products of mononuclear phagocytes, including complement degradation products, cytokines (TNF-α, IL-1, IL-6, IL-12, IL-15, IL-18, and others), chemokines (IL-8 and MIP-1α), reactive oxygen species, nitric oxide, leukotrienes (LTB_4), lysozymes, and neutral proteases.

The balance of proinflammatory and antiinflammatory mediators, many macrophage derived, is clearly skewed toward an inflammatory profile. Although it could be postulated that an intrinsic genetic defect in macrophage regulatory function could account for this highly active and destructive environment, such a defect is not a requirement for the development of the pathologic scenario observed. In the absence of information on the primary triggering mechanisms, our knowledge of the proinflammatory cells and mediators present in the RA joint provides many rational targets for interruption of the vicious cycle of activation events that perpetuate joint disease.

THERAPEUTIC MANIPULATION OF THE MONONUCLEAR PHAGOCYTE SYSTEM

Knowledge that macrophages and their products are abundant in the rheumatoid synovial membrane and fluid elucidates the clear efficacy of three classes of therapeutic agents in RA.

Glucocorticoids

Glucocorticoids (GCs) are the mainstay of treatment in many rheumatic diseases, despite their considerable toxicity, because of their profound antiinflammatory effects on all components of the immune system (160). It is only in recent years that progress in elucidating mechanisms of intracellular biochemical signaling and gene transcription has provided the groundwork for understanding some of the most important pharmacologic actions of GC (161). The GC receptor, constitutively present in the cytoplasm of macrophages and many other cell types, is basically a hormone-activated transcriptional regulator. It moves to the nucleus after binding to its ligand, and when bound to a GC response element in gene promoters in dimeric form, it serves as a substrate for assembly of proteins that promote formation of the transcription initiation complex (69–71). When present in the nucleus as a monomer, the GC receptor is more likely to bind corepressor proteins and inhibit gene activation. Most investigators agree that the important proinflammatory transcription factor NFκB is a prime target of GC action (162–165). Dimeric GC receptor promotes transcription of a molecule, IκBα, that inhibits the translocation of NFκB to its site of activity in the nucleus, contributing to impaired transcription of NFκB-dependent genes, many of which are proinflammatory. GCs inhibit transcription of many cytokine genes by inhibiting the activity of other transcription factors, such as AP-1, that are required for cytokine promoter activity (166–168). GCs also induce production of lipocortin-1 (also called lipomodulin or annexin-1), an inhibitor of phospholipase A_2 activity (169–172). As phospholipase A_2 generates arachidonic acid, lipocortin-1 decreases arachidonic acid production, with a consequent decrease in levels of prostaglandins, leukotrienes, and oxygen radicals.

Among the many actions of GC are effects on monocyte-macrophages and APCs. GCs decrease the expression of cell surface MHC class II molecules and selectively decrease costimulatory molecules, with B7.1 (CD80), but not B7.2 (CD86), expression on human macrophages affected (173). Glucocorticoids increase IFN-γ-induced FcγRI expression (174). Consistent with these data, intravenous methylprednisolone treatment increased binding and phagocytosis of IgG-sensitized erythrocytes by human monocytes, suggesting both increased Fc receptor expression and function after GC exposure (175). GCs inhibit the secretion of certain macrophage cytokines, including IL-1β and IL-6, and decrease production of chemotactic factors induced by either IL-1 or TNF-α (176). TNF-α secretion by LPS-stimulated human monocytes is also inhibited (177). GCs also abrogate macrophage support of T_H1 responses by inhibiting their secretion of IL-12, required for the T_H1 effector response. Dexamethasone has produced a dose-dependent (0.001–1.0 m*M*) decrease in the activity of inducible nitric oxide synthase in an LPS-treated monocyte cell line, suggesting a mechanism that may, in part, account for early observations of impaired killing of intracellular microbial organisms by macrophages treated with GC (178).

Interesting recent data define a negative regulatory pathway by which GC down-regulate their own function. GCs induce MIF production in LPS-activated macrophages and T cells (179). This cytokine is proinflammatory and overrides GC-mediated inhibition of secretion of other cytokines *in vitro* and endotoxin-induced lethality *in vivo.* MIF overcomes GC inhibition of TNF-α, IL-1β, IL-6, and IL-8 secretion by LPS-activated monocytes. Anti-MIF antibodies potentiate the inhibitory effects of dexamethasone, supporting the important role of MIF in down-regulating GC actions.

In addition to their effects on macrophages, GC also alter the antigen-processing and -presenting functions of dendritic cells and decrease dendritic cell viability (180–182). Dexamethasone (10^{-8} *M*) has been shown to impair full maturation of DC from monocytes cultured with GM-CSF and IL-4. Molecules that mediate antigen uptake and cell adhesion were increased, and endocytic capacity was augmented. In contrast, glucocorticoids decrease expression of costimulatory molecules on the dendritic cell surface, including CD86, thereby impairing their capacity for antigen presentation to T cells (182).

This brief review of the macrophage and dendritic cell–directed actions of GC explicates the dramatic anti-inflammatory response of patients with RA to steroid therapy. The negative side of this therapy, however, is clear, and is reviewed in Chapter 34.

TNF-α and IL-1 Blockade

TNF-α, a macrophage-derived cytokine, has been deemed a proximal activator of the inflammatory cascade in the rheumatoid joint, based on the decreased concentration and activity of many other cytokines when TNF-α activity is inhibited (97). TNF-α promotes the production of IL-1, activates metalloproteinase secretion by synoviocytes, and mediates bone resorption. The efficacy of soluble TNF-α receptors, monoclonal antibodies to TNF-α, and soluble IL-1-RA in therapy of RA is reviewed in Chapter 39 (98,99).

Adenosine

A role for the macrophage-derived product adenosine in the antiinflammatory effects of several of the therapeutics used clinically in RA has been supported by data from several laboratories (183,184). By binding to adenosine A2 receptors, adenosine increases cAMP and protein kinase A, cellular signaling events that inhibit IL-12 and increase IL-10 production in monocytes. It appears that several anti-inflammatory drugs may work through this pathway. Methotrexate, sulfasalazine, and aspirin all increase adenosine release at sites of inflammation and decrease inflammation through subsequent binding of adenosine to the A2 receptors.

REFERENCES

1. De Kruif P. *Microbe hunters.* New York: Harcourt Brace, 1926.
2. Metcalf D. The molecular control of cell division, differentiation commitment and maturation in hemopoietic cells. *Nature* 1989;339:27–30.
3. Harlan JM. Leukocyte-endothelial interactions. *Blood* 1985;65:513–525.
4. Steinman RM. The dendritic cell and its role in immunogenicity. *Annu Rev Immunol* 1993;9:271–296.
5. Hume DA, Ross IL, Himes SR, et al. The mononuclear phagocyte system revisited. *J Leukoc Biol* 2002;72:621–627.
6. Ardavin C. Origin, precursors and differentiation of mouse dendritic cells. *Nature Rev* 2003;3:1–9.
7. Shortman K, Liu Y-J. Mouse and human dendritic cell subtypes. *Nature Rev* 2002;2:151–161.
8. Colonna M, Krug A, Cella M. Interferon-producing cells: on the front line in immune responses against pathogens. *Curr Opin Immunol* 2002;14:373–379.
9. Pickl WF, Majdic O, Kohl P, et al. Molecular and functional characteristics of dendritic cells generated from highly purified CD14+ peripheral blood monocytes. *J Immunol* 1996;157:3850–3859.
10. Sallusto F, Lanzavecchia A. Efficient presentation of soluble antigen by cultured human dendritic cells is maintained by granulocyte/macrophage colony-stimulating factor plus interleukin-4 and downregulated by tumor necrosis factor. *J Exp Med* 1994;179:1109–1118.
11. Steinman RM, Howiger D, Nussenzweig MC: Tolerogenic dendritic cells. *Ann Rev Immunol* 2003;21:685–711.
12. Humphrey JH, Grennan D, Sundaram V. The origin of follicular dendritic cells in the mouse and the mechanism of trapping of immune complexes on them. *Eur J Immunol* 1984;14:859–864.
13. Fearon DT. Seeking wisdom in innate immunity. *Nature* 1997;388: 323–324.
14. Medzhitov R, Janeway CA Jr. Decoding the patterns of self and non-self by the innate immune system. *Science* 2002;296:298–300.
15. Verhasselt V, Buelens C, Willems F, et al. Bacterial lipopolysaccharide stimulates the production of cytokines and the expression of costimulatory molecules by human peripheral blood dendritic cells. *J Immunol* 1997;158:2929–2925.
16. Messina JP, Gilkeson GS, Pisetsky DS. Stimulation of *in vitro* murine lymphocyte proliferation by bacterial DNA. *J Immunol* 1991;147: 1759–1764.
17. Krieg AM, Yi AK, Matson S, et al. CpG motifs in bacterial DNA trigger direct B-cell activation. *Nature* 1995;374:546–549.
18. Weiner GJ, Liu H-M, Wooldridge JE, et al. Immunostimulatory oligodeoxynucleotides containing the CpG motif are effective as immune adjuvants in tumor antigen immunization. *Proc Natl Acad Sci U S A* 1997;94:10833–10837.
19. Akira S, Hemmi H. Recognition of pathogen-associated molecular patterns by TLR family. *Immunol Lett* 2003;85:85–95.
20. Hemmi H, Takeuchi O, Kawai T, et al. A Toll-like receptor recognizes bacterial DNA. *Nature* 2000;408:740–745.
21. Verdijk RM, Mutis T, Esendam B, et al. Polyriboinosinic polyribocytidylic acid (poly(I:C)) induces stable maturation of functionally active human dendritic cells. *J Immunol* 1999;163:57–61.
22. Alexopoulou L, Holt AC, Medzhitov R, Flavell RA. Recognition of double-stranded RNA and activation of NF-kappaB by Toll-like receptor 3. *Nature* 2001;413:732–738.
23. Aderem A, Underhill DM. Mechanisms of phagocytosis in macrophages. *Annu Rev Immunol* 1999;17:593–623.

24. Snyderman R, Phillips JK, Mergenhagen SE. Biological activity of complement in vivo: role of C5 in the accumulation of polymorphonuclear leukocytes in inflammatory exudates. *J Exp Med* 1971;134: 1131–1134.
25. Su SB, Gong W, Gao JL, et al. A seven-transmembrane, G protein-coupled receptor, FPRL1, mediates the chemotactic activity of serum amyloid A for human phagocytic cells. *J Exp Med* 1999;189:395–402.
26. Armant M, Fenton MJ. Toll-like receptors: a family of pattern-recognition receptors in mammals. *Gen Biol* 2002;3:3011.1–3011.6.
27. Takeda K, Kaisho T, Akira S. Toll-like receptors. *Annu Rev Immunol* 2003;21:335–376.
28. Ravetch JV, Kinet J. Fc receptors. *Annu Rev Immunol* 1993;9:457–492.
29. Ravetch JV. Fc receptors: rubor redux. *Cell* 1994;78:553–560.
30. Ravetch JV, Clynes RA. Divergent roles for Fc receptors and complement in vivo. *Annu Rev Immunol* 1998;16:421–432.
31. Carroll MC. The role of complement and complement receptors in induction and regulation of immunity. *Annu Rev Immunol* 1998;16: 545–568.
32. McDonald PP, Fadok VA, Bratton D, et al. Transcriptional and translational regulation of inflammatory mediator production by endogenous TGF-beta in macrophages that have ingested apoptotic cells. *J Immunol* 1999;163:6164–6172.
33. Savill J, Dransfield I, Gregory C, Haslett C. A blast from the past: clearance of apoptotic cells regulates immune responses. *Nature Rev* 2002;2:965–975.
34. Rock FL, Hardiman G, Timans JC, et al. A family of human receptors structurally related to Drosophila Toll. *Proc Natl Acad Sci U S A* 1998;95:588–593.
35. Underhill DM, Ozinsky A, Hajjar AM, et al. The Toll-like receptor 2 is recruited to macrophage phagosomes and discriminates between pathogens. *Nature* 1999;401:811–815.
36. Underhill DM, Ozinsky A, Smith KD, et al. Toll-like receptor-2 mediates mycobacteria-induced proinflammatory signaling in macrophages. *Proc Natl Acad Sci U S A* 1999;96:14459–14463.
37. Takeuchi O, Hoshino K, Kawai T, et al. Differential roles of TLR2 and TLR4 in recognition of gram-negative and gram-positive bacterial cell wall components. *Immunity* 1999;11:443–451.
38. Hirschfeld M, Kirschning CJ, Schwandner R, et al. Cutting edge: inflammatory signaling by *Borrelia burgdorferi* lipoproteins is mediated by toll-like receptor 2. *J Immunol* 1999;163:2382–2386.
39. Brightbill HD, Libraty DH, Krutzik SR, et al. Host defense mechanisms triggered by microbial lipoproteins through Toll-like receptors. *Science* 1999;285:732–736.
40. Takeuchi O, Takeda K, Hoshino K, et al. Cellular responses to bacterial cell wall components are mediated through MyD88-dependent signaling cascades. *Int Immunol* 2000;12:113–117.
41. O'Neill LAJ. Toll-like receptor signal transduction and the tailoring of innate immunity: a role for Mal. *Trends Immunol* 2002;23:296–300.
42. O'Neill LAJ, Fitzgerald KA, Bowie AG. The Toll-IL-1 receptor adaptor family grows to five members. *Trends Immunol* 2003;24:286–289.
43. Colonna M. TREMs in the immune system and beyond. *Nature Rev* 2003;3:1–9.
44. Pricop L, Redecha P, Teillaud J-L, et al. Differential modulation of stimulatory and inhibitory Fc gamma receptors on human monocytes by Th1 and Th2 cytokines. *J Immunol* 2001;166:531–537.
45. Hartwig JH, Chambers KA, Stossel TP. Association of gelsolin with actin filaments and cell membranes of macrophages and platelets. *J Cell Biol* 1989;108:467–479.
46. Salmon JE, Millard S, Schachter LA, et al. Fc gamma RIIA alleles are heritable risk factors for lupus nephritis in African Americans. *J Clin Invest* 1996;97:1348–1354.
47. Wu J, Edberg JC, Redecha PB, et al. A novel polymorphism of FcγRIIIa (CD16) alters receptor function and predisposes to autoimmune disease. *J Clin Invest* 1997;100:1059–1070.
48. Milone MC, Fitzgerald-Bocarsly P. The mannose receptor mediates induction of IFN-alpha in peripheral blood dendritic cells by enveloped RNA and DNA viruses. *J Immunol* 1998;161:2391–2399.
49. Parra-Lopez CA, Lindner R, Vidavsky I, et al. Presentation on class II MHC molecules of endogenous lysozyme targeted to the endocytic pathway. *J Immunol* 1997;158:2670–2679.
50. Zahn S, Zwirner J, Spengler HP, et al. Chemoattractant receptors for interleukin-8 and C5a: expression on peripheral blood leukocytes and differential regulation on HL-60 and AML-193 cells by vitamin D3 and all-trans retinoic acid. *Eur J Immunol* 1997;27:935–940.
51. Crass T, Raffetseder U, Martin U, et al. Expression cloning of the human C3a anaphylatoxin receptor (C3aR) from differentiated U-937 cells. *Eur J Immunol* 1996;26:1944–1950.
52. Tait JF, Smith C. Phosphatidylserine receptors: role of CD36 in binding of anionic phospholipid vesicles to monocytic cells. *J Biol Chem* 1999;274:3048–3054.
53. Albert ML, Sauter B, Bhardwaj N. Dendritic cells acquire antigen from apoptotic cells and induce class I-restricted CTLs. *Nature* 1998; 392:86–89.
54. Finnemann SC, Rodriguez-Boulan E. Macrophages and retinal pigment epithelium phagocytosis: apoptotic cells and photoreceptors compete for alpha$_v$beta$_3$ and alpha$_v$beta$_5$ integrins, and protein kinase C regulates alpha$_v$beta$_5$ binding and cytoskeletal linkage. *J Exp Med* 1999;190:861–874.
55. Inaba K, Turley S, Yamaide F, et al. Efficient presentation of phagocytosed cellular fragments on the major histocompatibility complex class II products of dendritic cells. *J Exp Med* 1998;188:2163–2173.
56. Crocker PR, Kelm C, Dubois B, et al. Purification and properties of sialoadhesin, a sialic acid binding receptor of murine tissue macrophages. *EMBO J* 1991;10:1661–1669.
57. Miyata T, Hori O, Zhang J, et al. The receptor for advanced glycation end products (RAGE) is a central mediator of the interaction of AGE-beta$_2$microglobulin with human mononuclear phagocytes via an oxidant-sensitive pathway. Implications for the pathogenesis of dialysis-related amyloidosis. *J Clin Invest* 1996;98:1088–1094.
58. Schmidt AM, Yan SD, Wautier JL, et al. Activation of receptor for advanced glycosylation end products: a mechanism for chronic vascular dysfunction in diabetic vasculopathy and atherosclerosis. *Circ Res* 1999;84:489–497.
59. Ivashkiv LB. Cytokines and STATs: how can signals achieve specificity? *Immunity* 1995;3:1–4.
60. Kopp E, Ghosh S. Inhibition of NF-κB by sodium salicylate and aspirin. *Science* 1994;165:956–959.
61. Pick E, Heldin CH, Ten Dijke P. Specificity, diversity, and regulation in TGF-beta superfamily signaling. *FASEB J* 1999;13:2105–2124.
62. Holmes WE, Lee J, Kuang WJ, et al. Structure and functional expression of a human interleukin-8 receptor. *Science* 1991;253:1278–1280.
63. Kavelaars A, Broeke D, Jeurissen F, et al. Activation of human monocytes via a non-neurokinin substance P receptor that is coupled to Gi protein, calcium, phospholipase D, MAP kinase, and IL-6 production. *J Immunol* 1994;153:3691–3699.
64. Le Y, Gong W, Li B, et al. Utilization of two seven-transmembrane, G protein-coupled receptors, formyl peptide receptor-like 1 and formyl peptide receptor, by the synthetic hexapeptide WKYMVm for human phagocyte activation. *J Immunol* 1999;163:6777–6784.
65. Denecke B, Meyerdierks A, Bottger EC. RGS1 is expressed in monocytes and acts as a GTPase-activating protein for G-protein-coupled chemoattractant receptors. *J Biol Chem* 1999;274:26860–26868.
66. Deng X, Ueda H, Su SB, et al. A synthetic peptide derived from human immunodeficiency virus type 1 gp120 downregulates the expression and function of chemokine receptors CCR5 and CXCR4 in monocytes by activating the 7 transmembrane G-protein-coupled receptor FPRL1/LXA4R. *Blood* 1999;94:1165–1173.
67. Cocchi F. Identification of RANTES, MIP-1 alpha, and MIP-1 beta as the major HIV-suppressive factors produced by CD8$^+$ T cells. *Science* 1995;270:1811–1815.
68. Grimm MC, Ben-Baruch A, Taub DD, et al. Opiates transdeactivate chemokine receptors: δ and μ opiate receptor-mediated heterologous desensitization. *J Exp Med* 1998;188:317–325.
69. Tsai M-J, O'Malley B. Molecular mechanisms of action of steroid/thyroid receptor superfamily members. *Annu Rev Biochem* 1994;63: 451–486.
70. Schmid W, Strahle U, Schutz G, et al. Glucocorticoid receptor binds cooperatively to adjacent recognition sites. *EMBO J* 1989;8:2257–2263.
71. Westin S, Kurokawa R, Nolte RT, et al. Interactions controlling the assembly of nuclear-receptor heterodimers and co-activators. *Nature* 1998;395:199–202.
72. Springer TA. Traffic signals on endothelium for lymphocyte recirculation and leukocyte emigration. *Annu Rev Physiol* 1995;57:827–872.
73. Ebnet K, Kaldjian EP, Anderson AO, et al. Orchestrated information transfer underlying leukocyte endothelial interactions. *Annu Rev Immunol* 1996;14:155–177.
74. Rittner HL, Kaiser M, Brack A, et al. Tissue-destructive macrophages in giant cell arteritis. *Circ Res* 1999;84:1050–1058.

75. Karakawa WW, Sutton A, Scheerson R, et al. Capsular antibodies induce type-specific phagocytosis of capsulated *Staphylococcus aureus* by human polymorphonuclear leukocytes. *Infect Immun* 1986;56:1090–1095.
76. Bachwich PR, Chensue SW, Larrick JW, et al. Tumor necrosis factor stimulates interleukin-1 and prostaglandin E_2 production in resting macrophages. *Biochem Biophys Res Commun* 1986;136:94–101.
77. Kammer GM. The adenylate cyclase-cAMP-protein kinase A pathway and regulation of the immune response. *Immunol Today* 1988;9:222–229.
78. Ferbas JJ, Toso JF, Logar AJ, et al. CD4+ blood dendritic cells are potent producers of IFN-alpha in response to in vitro HIV-1 infection. *J Immunol* 1994;152:4649–4662.
79. Siegal FP, Kadowaki N, Shodell M, et al. The nature of the principal type I interferon-producing cells in human blood. *Science* 1999;284:1835–1837.
80. Munoz Fernandez MA, Fernandez MA, Fresno M. Synergism between tumor necrosis factor-alpha and interferon-γ on macrophage activation for the killing of intracellular *Trypanosoma crusi* through a nitric oxide-dependent mechanism. *Eur J Immunol* 1992;22:301–307.
81. Kinler V, Sappino A-P, Grau GE, et al. The inducing role of tumor necrosis factor in the development of bactericidal granulomas during BCG development. *Cell* 1989;56:731–740.
82. Arend WP, Malyak M, Cuthridge CJ, et al. Interleukin-1 receptor antagonist: role in biology. *Annu Rev Immunol* 1998;16:27–55.
83. Avice MN, Demeure CE, Delespesse G, et al. IL-15 promotes IL-12 production by human monocytes via T cell-dependent contact and may contribute to IL-12–mediated IFN-γ secretion by CD4+ T cells in the absence of TCR ligation. *J Immunol* 1998;161:3408–3415.
84. Link AA, Kino T, Worth JA, et al. Ligand-activation of the adenosine A2a receptors inhibits IL-12 production by human monocytes. *J Immunol* 2000;164:436–442.
85. McInnes IB, Leung BP, Sturrock RD, et al. Interleukin-15 mediates T cell-dependent regulation of tumor necrosis factor-alpha production in rheumatoid arthritis. *Nat Med* 1997;3:189–195.
86. Badolato R, Ponzi AN, Millesimo M, et al. Interleukin-15 (IL-15) induces IL-8 and monocyte chemotactic protein 1 production in human monocytes. *Blood* 1997;90:2804–2809.
87. Musso T, Calosso L, Zucca M, et al. Human monocytes constitutively express membrane-bound, biologically active, and interferon-γ-upregulated interleukin-15. *Blood* 1999;93:3531–3539.
88. Carson WE, Ross ME, Baiocchi RA, et al. Endogenous production of interleukin 15 by activated human monocytes is critical for optimal production of interferon-gamma by natural killer cells in vitro. *J Clin Invest* 1995;96:2578–2582.
89. Gracie JA, Forsey RJ, Chan WL, et al. A proinflammatory role for IL-18 in rheumatoid arthritis. *J Clin Invest* 1999;104:1393–1401.
90. Pfeffer LM, Dinarello CA, Herberman RB, et al. Biologic properties of recombinant α-interferons: 40th anniversary of the discovery of the interferons. *Cancer Res* 1998;58:2489–2499.
91. Trinchieri G, Santoli D. Antiviral activity induced by culturing lymphocytes with tumor-derived or virus-transformed cells. Enhancement of natural killer cell activity by interferon and antagonistic inhibition of susceptibility of target cells to lysis. *J Exp Med* 1978;147:1314–1333.
92. Herberman RB, Ortaldo JR, Bonnard GD. Augmentation by interferon of human natural and antibody-dependent cell-mediated cytotoxicity. *Nature* 1979;277:221–223.
93. Lindahl-Magnuson P, Leary P, Gresser I. Interferon inhibits DNA synthesis induced in mouse lymphocyte suspensions by phytohaemagglutinin or by allogeneic cells. *Nature New Biol* 1972;237:120–121.
94. Appasamy R, Bryant J, Hassanein T, et al. Effects of therapy with interferon-α on peripheral blood lymphocyte subsets and NK activity in patients with chronic hepatitis C. *Clin Immunol Immunopathol* 1994;73:350–357.
95. Douni E, Akassoglou K, Alexopoulou L, et al. Transgenic and knockout analysis of the role of TNF in immune regulation and disease pathogenesis. *J Inflamm* 1995–1996;47:27–38.
96. Rayhane N, Lortholary O, Fitting C, et al. Enhanced sensitivity of tumor necrosis factor/lymphotoxin-α-deficient mice to *Cryptococcus neoformans* infection despite increased levels of nitrite/nitrate, interferon-gamma, and interleukin-12. *J Infect Dis* 1999;180:1637–1647.
97. Brennan FM, Maini RN, Feldmann M. TNF α—a pivotal role in rheumatoid arthritis. *Br J Rheumatol* 1992;31:293–298.
98. Maini RN, Breedveld FC, Kalden JR, et al. Therapeutic efficacy of multiple intravenous infusions of anti-tumor necrosis factor alpha monoclonal antibody combined with low-dose weekly methotrexate in rheumatoid arthritis. *Arthritis Rheum* 1998;41:1552–1563.
99. Moreland LW, Schiff MH, Baumgartner SW, et al. Etanercept therapy in rheumatoid arthritis. A randomized, controlled trial. *Ann Intern Med* 1999;130:478–486.
100. Ghivizzani SC, Lechman ER, Kang R, et al. Direct adenovirus-mediated gene transfer of interleukin 1 and tumor necrosis factor alpha soluble receptors to rabbit knees with experimental arthritis has local and distal anti-arthritic effects. *Proc Natl Acad Sci U S A* 1998;95:4613–4618.
101. Sebbag M, Parry SL, Brennan FM, et al. Cytokine stimulation of T lymphocytes regulates their capacity to induce monocyte production of tumor necrosis factor-α, but not interleukin-10: possible relevance to pathophysiology of rheumatoid arthritis. *Eur J Immunol* 1997;27:624–632.
102. DelGiudice G, Crow MK. Role of transforming growth factor beta (TGF β) in systemic autoimmunity. *Lupus* 1993;2:213–220.
103. Ding L, Shevach EM. IL-10 inhibits mitogen-induced T cell proliferation by selectively inhibiting macrophage costimulatory function. *J Immunol* 1992;148:3133–3139.
104. Malefyt RDW, Yssel H, de Vries J. Direct effects of IL-10 on subsets of human CD4+ T cell clones and resting T cells. Specific inhibition of IL-2 production and proliferation. *J Immunol* 1993;150:4754–4765.
105. Zan H, Cerutti A, Dramitinos P, et al. Induction of Ig somatic hypermutation and class switching in a human monoclonal IgM+ IgD+ B cell line in vitro: definition of the requirements and modalities of hypermutation. *J Immunol* 1999;162:3437–3447.
106. Patel IR, Attur MG, Patel RN, et al. TNF-alpha convertase enzyme from human arthritis-affected cartilage: isolation of cDNA by differential display, expression of the active enzyme, and regulation of TNF-alpha. *J Immunol* 1998;160:4570–4579.
107. Nathan CF. Secretion of oxygen intermediates: role in effector functions of activated macrophages. *Fed Proc* 1982;41:2206–2211.
108. Noack D, Rae J, Cross AR, et al. Autosomal recessive chronic granulomatous disease caused by novel mutations in NCF-2, the gene encoding the p67-phox component of phagocyte NADPH oxidase. *Hum Genet* 1999;105:460–467.
109. Leusen JH, Meischl C, Eppink MH, et al. Four novel mutations in the gene encoding gp91-phox of human NADPH oxidase: consequences for oxidase assembly. *Blood* 2000;95:666–673.
110. Sharara AI, Perkins DJ, Misukonis MA, et al. Interferon (IFN)-α activation of human blood mononuclear cells *in vitro* and *in vivo* for nitric oxide synthase (NOS) type 2 mRNA and protein expression: possible relationship of induced NOS2 to the anti-hepatitis C effects of IFN-α in vivo. *J Exp Med* 1997;186:1495–1502.
111. Snell JC, Chernyshev O, Gilbert DL, et al. Polyribonucleotides induce nitric oxide production by human monocyte-derived macrophages. *J Leukoc Biol* 1997;62:369–373.
112. Grabowski PS, Wright PK, Van't Hof RJ, et al. Immunolocalization of inducible nitric oxide synthase in synovium and cartilage in rheumatoid arthritis and osteoarthritis. *Br J Rheumatol* 1997;36:651–655.
113. St Clair EW, Wilkinson WE, Lang T, et al. Increased expression of blood mononuclear cell nitric oxide synthase type 2 in rheumatoid arthritis patients. *J Exp Med* 1996;184:1173–1178.
114. Borderie D, Hilliquin P, Hernvann A, et al. Nitric oxide synthase is expressed in the lymphomononuclear cells of synovial fluid in patients with rheumatoid arthritis. *J Rheumatol* 1999;26:2083–2088.
115. Lenschow DJ, Walunas JA, Bluestone JA. CD28/B7 system of T cell costimulation. *Annu Rev Immunol* 1996;14:233–258.
116. Pamer E, Cresswell P. Mechanisms of MHC class I-restricted antigen processing. *Annu Rev Immunol* 1998;16:323–358.
117. Morrison LA, Lukacher AE, Brachiale VL, et al. Differences in antigen presentation to MHC class I– and class II–restricted influenza virus–specific cytolytic T-lymphocyte clones. *J Exp Med* 1986;163:903–921.
118. Germain RN. MHC-dependent antigen processing and peptide presentation: providing ligands for T lymphocyte activation. *Cell* 1994;76:287–299.
119. Song R, Harding CV. Roles of proteosomes, transporter for antigen presentation (TAP), and β_2-microglobulin in the processing of bacte-

rial or particulate antigens via an alternate class I MHC processing pathway. *J Immunol* 1996;156:4182–4190.
120. Shepard JC, Schumacher TNM, Ashton-Rickardt P, et al. TAP1-dependent peptide translocation *in vitro* is ATP-dependent and peptide-selective. *Cell* 1993;74:577–584.
121. Lehner PJ, Cresswell P. Processing and delivery of peptides presented by MHC class I molecules. *Curr Opin Immunol* 1996;8:59–67.
122. Germain RN, Castellino F, Han RE, et al. Processing and presentation of endocytically acquired protein antigens by MHC class I and class II molecules. *Immunol Rev* 1996;151:5–30.
123. Foley PJ, Lympany PA, Puscinska E, et al. Analysis of MHC encoded antigen-processing genes TAP1 and TAP2 polymorphisms in sarcoidosis. *Am J Respir Crit Care Med* 1999;160:1009–1014.
124. Fremont DH, Hendrickson WA, Marrack P, et al. Structures of an MHC class II molecule with covalently bound single peptides. *Science* 1996;272:1001–1004.
125. Cresswell P, Denzin LK. HLA-DM induces CLIP dissociation from MHC class II α:β dimers and facilitates peptide loading. *Cell* 1995; 82:155–165.
126. Morris P, Shaman J, Attaya M, et al. An essential role for HLA-DM in antigen presentation by class II major histocompatibility molecules. *Nature* 1994;368:551–554.
127. Carmichael P, Copier J, So A, et al. Allele-specific variation in the degeneracy of major histocompatibility complex (MHC) restriction. *Hum Immunol* 1997;54:21–29.
128. Hammer J, Gallazi F, Bono E, et al. Peptide binding specificity of HLA-DR4 molecules: correlation with rheumatoid arthritis association. *J Exp Med* 1995;181:1847–1855.
129. Penzotti JE, Doherty D, Lybrand TP, et al. A structural model for TCR recognition of the HLA class II shared epitope sequence implicated in susceptibility to rheumatoid arthritis. *J Autoimmun* 1996;9:287–293.
130. Porcelli SA, Modlin RL. The CD1 system: antigen-presenting molecules for T cell recognition of lipids and glycolipids. *Annu Rev Immunol* 1999;17:297–329.
131. Blumberg RS, Gerdes D, Chott A, et al. Structure and function of the CD1 family of MHC-like cell surface proteins. *Immunol Rev* 1995; 147:5–29.
132. Porcelli SA, Morita ST, Modlin RL. T cell recognition of non-peptide antigens. *Curr Opin Immunol* 1996;8:510–516.
133. Beckman EM, Melian A, Behar SM, et al. CD1c restricts responses of mycobacteria-specific T cells. Evidence for antigen presentation by a second member of the human CD1 family. *J Immunol* 1996;157: 2795–3803.
134. Moody DB, Besra GS, Wilson IA, et al. The molecular basis of CD1-mediated presentation of lipid antigens. *Immunol Rev* 1999;172:285–296.
135. Zeng Z, Castano AR, Segelke BW, et al. Crystal structure of mouse CD1: an MHC-like fold with a large hydrophobic binding groove. *Science* 1997;277:339–345.
136. Liu Y, Janeway CA Jr. Cells that present both specific ligand and co-stimulatory activity are the most efficient inducers of clonal expansion of normal CD4 T cells. *Proc Natl Acad Sci* 1992;89:3845–3949.
137. Razi-Wolf Z, Freeman GJ, Galvin F, et al. Expression and function of the murine B7 antigen, the major co-stimulatory molecule expressed by peritoneal exudate cells. *Proc Natl Acad Sci U S A* 1992;89:4210–4214.
138. Yoshinaga SK, Whoriskey JS, Khare SD, et al. T-cell co-stimulation through B7RP-1 and ICOS. *Nature* 1999;402:827–832.
139. Swallow MM, Wallin JJ, Sha WC. B7h, a novel costimulatory homolog of B7.1 and B7.2, is induced by TNF-α. *Immunity* 1999;11: 423–432.
140. Okazaki T, Iwai Y, Honjo T. New regulatory co-receptors: inducible co-stimulator and PD-1. *Curr Opin Immunol* 2002;14:779–782.
141. Sharpe AH, Freeman GJ. The B7-CD28 family. *Nature Rev Immunol* 2002;2:116–126.
142. Mueller DL, Jenkins MK. Molecular mechanisms underlying functional T-cell unresponsiveness. *Curr Opin Immunol* 1995;7:375–381.
143. Greenwald RJ, Latchman YE, Sharpe AH. Negative co-receptors on lymphocytes. *Curr Opin Immunol* 2002;14:391–396.
144. Stout R, Bottomly K. Antigen-specific activation of effector macrophages by interferon-γ producing (Th1) T-cell clones: failure of IL-4 producing (Th2) T-cell clones to activate effector functions in macrophages. *J Immunol* 1989;142:760–765.
145. Paulnock DM. Macrophage activation by T cells. *Curr Opin Immunol* 1992;4:344–349.
146. Banchereau J, Bazan F, Blanchard F, et al. The CD40 antigen and its ligand. *Annu Rev Immunol* 1994;12:881–922.
147. Tsunawaki S, Sporn M, Ding A, et al. Deactivation of macrophages by transforming growth factor-β. *Nature* 1988;334:260–262.
148. Suda T, Takahashi T, Goldstein P, et al. Molecular cloning and expression of the Fas ligand, a novel member of the tumor necrosis factor family. *Cell* 1993;75:1169–1178.
149. Ashany D, Savir A, Bhardwaj N, et al. Dendritic cells are resistant to apoptosis through the Fas (CD95/APO-1) pathway. *J Immunol* 1999; 163:5303–5311.
150. Conte D, Fraquelli M, Capsoni F, et al. Effectiveness of IFN-γ for liver abscesses in chronic granulomatous disease. *J Interferon Cytokine Res* 1999;19:705–710.
151. DeLeo FR, Goedken M, McCormick SJ, et al. A novel form of hereditary myeloperoxidase deficiency linked to endoplasmic reticulum/proteosome degradation. *J Clin Invest* 1998;101:2900–2909.
152. Bauer TR, Schwartz BR, Conrad Liles W, et al. Retroviral-mediated gene transfer of the leukocyte integrin CD18 into peripheral blood CD34+ cells derived from a patient with leukocyte adhesion deficiency type I. *Blood* 1998;91:1520–1526.
153. Al-Mughales J, Blyth TH, Hunter JA, et al. The chemoattractant activity of rheumatoid synovial fluid for human lymphocytes is due to multiple cytokines. *Clin Exp Immunol* 1996;106:230–236.
154. Burmester GR, Dimitriu-Bona A, Waters SJ, et al. Identification of three major synovial cell lining populations by monoclonal antibodies directed to Ia antigens and antigens associated with monocytes/macrophages and fibroblasts. *Scand J Immunol* 1983; 17:69–82.
155. Holmdahl R, Jonsson R, Larsson P, et al. Early appearance of activated CD4+ T lymphocytes and class II antigen-expressing cells in joints of DBA/1 mice immunized with type II collagen. *Lab Invest* 1988;58:53–60.
156. Tsai V, Bergroth V, Zvaifler NJ. Synovial dendritic cells and T cells in rheumatoid arthritis. *Scand J Rheumatol* 1988;74:79–88.
157. Firestein GS, Zvaifler NJ. How important are T cells in chronic rheumatoid synovitis. *Arthritis Rheum* 1990;33:768–773.
158. Li Y, Sun GR, Tumang JR, et al. CDR3 sequence motifs shared by oligoclonal rheumatoid arthritis synovial T cells. Evidence for an antigen-driven response. *J Clin Invest* 1994;94:2525–2531.
159. Wagner UG, Kurtin PJ, Wahner A, et al. The role of CD8+ CD40L+ T cells in the formation of germinal centers in rheumatoid synovitis. *J Immunol* 1998;161:6390–6397.
160. Hench PS. The reversibility of certain rheumatic and nonrheumatic conditions by the use of cortisone or of the pituitary adrenocorticotrophic hormone. *Ann Intern Med* 1952;36:1–38.
161. Crow MK. Mechanism of glucocorticoid action on the immune system and in inflammation. In: Lin AN, Paget SA, eds. *Principles of corticosteroid therapy.* New York: Arnold, 2002.41–65.
162. Auphan N, DiDonato JA, Rosette C, et al. Immuno-suppression by glucocorticoids: inhibition of NF-κB activity through induction of IkB synthesis. *Science* 1995;270:286–290.
163. Scheinman RI, Cogswell PC, Lofquist AK, et al. Role of transcriptional activation of IκBa in mediation of immunosuppression by glucocorticoids. *Science* 1995;270:283–286.
164. De Vera ME, Taylor BS, Wang Q, et al. Dexamethasone suppresses iNOS gene expression by upregulating I-κ B-a and inhibiting NF-κ B. *Am J Physiol* 1997;273:G1290–G1296.
165. De Bosscher K, Schmitz ML, Vanden Berghe W, et al. Glucocorticoid-mediated repression of nuclear factor-κB-dependent transcription involves direct interference with transactivation. *Proc Natl Acad Sci U S A* 1997;94:13504–13509.
166. Kerppola TK, Luk D, Curran T. Fos is a preferential target of glucocorticoid receptor inhibition of AP-1 activity *in vitro. Mol Cell Biol* 1993;13:3782–3791.
167. Heck S, Bender K, Kullman M, et al. I-κBα-independent downregulation of NF-kappaB activity by glucocorticoid receptor. *EMBO J* 1997;16:4698–4707.
168. Scheinman RI, Gualberto A, Jewell CM, et al. Characterization of mechanisms involved in transrepression of NF-κ B by activated glucocorticoid receptors. *Mol Cell Biol* 1995;15:943–953.

169. Blackwell GJ, Carnuccio R, DiRosa M, et al. Macrocortin: a polypeptide causing the anti-phospholipase effect of glucocorticoids. *Nature* 1980;287:147–149.
170. Flower RJ, Blackwell GJ. Anti-inflammatory steroids induce biosynthesis of a phospholipase A2 inhibitor which prevents prostaglandin generation. *Nature* 1979;278:456–459.
171. Crompton MR, Moss SE, Crumpton MJ. Diversity in the lipocortin/calpactin family. *Cell* 1988;55:1–3.
172. Wallner BP, Mattaliano RJ, Hession C, et al. Cloning and expression of human lipocortin, a phospholipase A2 inhibitor with potential anti-inflammatory activity. *Nature* 1986;320:77–81.
173. Girndt M, Sester U, Kaul H, et al. Glucocorticoids inhibit activation-dependent expression of costimulatory molecule B7-1 in human monocytes. *Transplantation* 1998;66:370–375.
174. Pan L, Mendel DB, Zurlo J, et al. Regulation of the steady state level of Fcγ R1 mRNA by IFN-γ and dexamethasone in human monocytes, neutrophils, and U-937 cells. *J Immunol* 1990;145:267–275.
175. Salmon JE, Kapur S, Meryhew NL, et al. High-dose, pulse intravenous methylprednisolone enhances Fcγ receptor-mediated mononuclear phagocyte function in systemic lupus erythematosus. *Arthritis Rheum* 1989;32:717–725.
176. Amano Y, Lee SW, Allison AC. Inhibition by glucocorticoids of the formation of interleukin-1 α, interleukin-1 β, and interleukin-6: mediation by decreased mRNA stability. *Mol Pharmacol* 1993;43:176–182.
177. Waage A, Bakke O. Glucocorticoids suppress the production of tumour necrosis factor by lipopolysaccharide-stimulated human monocytes. *Immunology* 1988;63:299–302.
178. Di Rosa M, Radomski M, Carnuccio R, et al. Glucocorticoids inhibit the induction of nitric oxide synthase in macrophages. *Biochem Biophys Res Commun* 1990;172:1246–1252.
179. Calandra T, Bernhagen J, Metz CN, et al. MIF as a glucocorticoid-induced modulator of cytokine production. *Nature* 1995;377:68–71.
180. Holt PG, Thomas JA. Steroids inhibit uptake and/or processing but not presentation of antigen by airway dendritic cells. *Immunology* 1997;91:145–150.
181. Piemonti L, Monti P, Allavena P, et al. Glucocorticoids affect human dendritic cell differentiation and maturation. *J Immunol* 1999;162:6473–6481.
182. Moser M, De Smedt T, Sornasse T, et al. Glucocorticoids down-regulate dendritic cell function *in vitro* and *in vivo*. *Eur J Immunol* 1995;25:2818–2824.
183. Gadangi P, Longaker M, Naime D, et al. The anti-inflammatory mechanism of sulfasalazine is related to adenosine release at inflamed sites. *J Immunol* 1996;156:1937–1941.
184. Cronstein BN, Montesinos MC, Weissmann G. Salicylates and sulfasalazine, but not glucocorticoids, inhibit leukocyte accumulation by an adenosine-dependent mechanism that is independent of inhibition of prostaglandin synthesis and p105 of NFκB. *Proc Natl Acad Sci U S A* 1999;96:6377–6381.

CHAPTER 15

Structure and Function of Lymphocytes

Robert H. Carter and Casey T. Weaver

Lymphocytes are responsible for the adaptive immune response. The world around us is swarming with pathogens whose growth depends on evading our immune systems. Viruses and bacteria can mutate more rapidly than can humans. If our immune system were hard wired, new pathogens would evolve to circumvent it. In contrast to innate immunity, lymphocytes provide a mechanism for adjusting the immune response according to the environmental exposures encountered over the course of a lifetime. This is accomplished by the generation of an enormous diversity of lymphocytes by recombinatorial events involving the genes for the antigen receptors. This leads to two problems. Highly reactive lymphocytes must be selected out of the array of clones generated from progenitor cells. Conversely, the recombinatorial events at the genetic level give rise to lymphocytes whose receptors react with the body's own tissues, and these lymphocytes must be tightly regulated or eliminated.

Disease occurs when these processes go awry. Self-reactive clones, rather than being eliminated or suppressed, proliferate and attack, causing tissue injury. The damage may occur directly, such as with the production of anti-hematopoietic cell antibodies, or as part of a multicellular inflammatory response.

This chapter emphasizes the mechanisms of generation of diversity, clonal selection, and control of autoreactivity at the molecular level, because these mechanisms hold potential keys to new therapies for many rheumatic diseases. Knowledge of lymphocyte regulation has exploded over the past decade, especially in the area of control of cells by surface receptors. Nevertheless, our understanding of the role of these cells in most diseases seen by rheumatologists is remarkably poor. Several therapies targeting lymphocytes, developed from our growing knowledge of the basic biology of these cells, are now in early stages of testing in humans (see Chapter 40). Such therapies may not only improve patients' lives but also may teach us about the pathophysiology of disease. Knowing how these therapies work requires an understanding of lymphocyte structure and function.

We start with an overview of how lymphocytes interact to develop an immune response, stressing the anatomic structure of lymphoid organs. The development and function of T, B, and natural killer (NK) cells are described. Finally, we focus on the molecular events that control lymphocytes, potential targets for future treatments of rheumatic diseases.

OVERVIEW OF LYMPHOCYTE BIOLOGY

Lymphocyte progenitor cells circulate in the blood. Early B cells continue to develop in the bone marrow, whereas early T cells migrate to the thymus. Precursors of both types of cells undergo gene rearrangements to generate antigen receptors. The B and T cell antigen receptors are both heterodimers, consisting of two different, disulfide-linked chains, whose binding properties are determined by the protein sequence resulting from the recombination that occurred at the genetic level. The part of the antigen receptor that will bind to antigen is generated from two or three gene fragments: the variable, diversity, and joining segments. The genes for the antigen receptors contain multiple variants of each of these segments. Combining one variant of each of these segments generates the array of different receptors. The resulting fragment encoding the antigen-binding portion of the receptor (variable domain) is spliced with a constant domain, which encodes the part of the protein that connects the binding domain to the cell and is responsible for signal transduction across the cell membrane. In general, a particular lymphocyte generally expresses only one antigen receptor at a given time, and thus has a single antigen specificity (there are exceptions). In B cells, the same heavy-chain gene is alternatively spliced at the RNA level to give rise, in combination with a light chain, to both the transmembrane form of immunoglobulin that serves as the antigen receptor and the secreted immunoglobulin. The structure of immunoglobulin has been described in detail for B cells in Chapter 13. Recombination in T cells is similar and is described later.

Once an immature lymphocyte undergoes successful recombination to produce an antigen receptor, the B and T cells undergo selection in the bone marrow and thymus, respectively. Positive selection is the process whereby only those cells that express functional receptors survive. Negative selection refers to the elimination of autoreactive cells. If a B or T cell passes these tests, it leaves the bone marrow or thymus and enters the periphery as a mature lymphocyte, but these cells are naïve in that they have yet to encounter antigen.

A fundamental distinction between B and T cells is in the manner in which these cells bind and "recognize" antigen. The membrane form of immunoglobulin (see Chapter 13), which serves as the B-cell antigen receptor, can bind fluid phase, deposited, or cell surface–associated molecules, as long as the portion of the molecule (the epitope) that is bound by the immunoglobulin is exposed in the correct configuration. In contrast, the T cell receptor (TCR) binds only to fragments of proteins that have either been taken up or produced and degraded inside cells and presented on the cell surface by major histocompatibility complex (MHC) molecules (see Chapter 27). In either case, if the binding is sufficiently strong, then the antigen receptor becomes engaged. However, the consequence of this binding is determined by the context in which antigen is recognized. Binding of the antigen receptor alone does not lead to an effective response. Other coreceptors on the lymphocyte surface also must be engaged. The immune system has evolved such that ligands for these coreceptors are available only in the context when an immune response to antigen is appropriate. If the antigen receptor is engaged but necessary coreceptors are not, the result is not only failure to respond to this engagement, but the cell is rendered anergic, unable to respond if the antigen is reencountered. Thus, in addition to the elimination of autoreactive cells by negative selection at the immature stage, there is a mechanism for maintenance of unresponsiveness (tolerance) in the periphery, either to self antigens not encountered at the immature stage or after further mutation in the antigen receptor genes in mature B cells. This process has tremendous implications for both the pathophysiology and the treatment of autoimmune disease.

If the lymphocyte is successfully activated, it then undergoes clonal expansion. As a first approximation, lymphocytes with different antigen receptors compete for binding to antigen. The lymphocytes with receptors that bind more tightly survive and proliferate, whereas those with less avid binding do not. B lymphocytes undergo somatic hypermutation, a high frequency of point mutations along the gene encoding the binding domain of the immunoglobulin receptor. As a result of these mutations, certain of the progeny will have receptors with higher affinity than the parental cells. These higher-affinity cells are selected and proliferate. The result is a population of lymphocytes with greater numbers and higher affinity than was present before the encounter with the pathogen.

Once an immune response has effectively eliminated a pathogen, the response must be turned off. As a result of additional coreceptors, most responding cells undergo programmed cell death, or apoptosis (see Chapter 26). However, a percentage of the progeny of the responding cells survive to become memory cells. Even after resolution of an infection, an expanded pool of higher affinity cells persists. Moreover, these cells are primed and respond more rapidly and effectively if they re-encounter antigen, compared with the response of naïve cells. The result is immune memory, whereby the system is able to eliminate more effectively pathogens that have been encountered previously, whether by infection or vaccination.

ANATOMY OF THE IMMUNE SYSTEM

Organs of the Lymphoid System

Anatomic structure is just as critical for the function of the lymphoid system as it is for other organs (Fig. 15.1). In

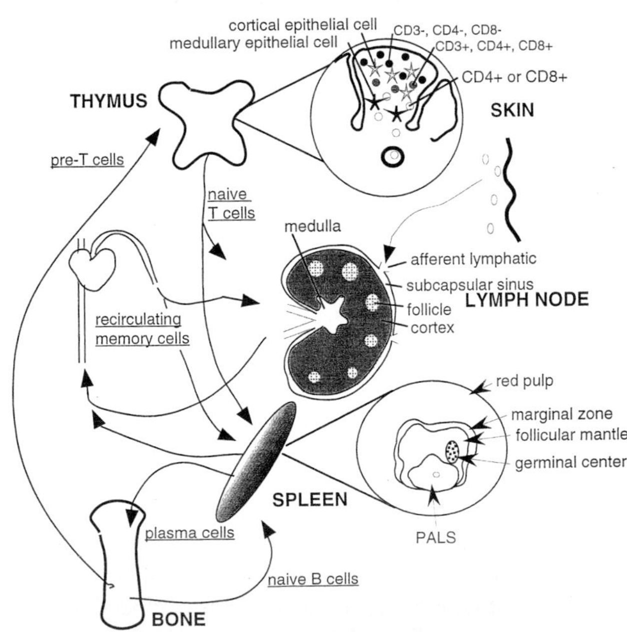

FIG. 15.1. Anatomy of the lymphoid system. Maturation and selection of B and T cells occur in primary lymphoid organs, the bone marrow and thymus, respectively. Mature but antigen-naïve cells travel from these to the secondary lymphoid organs, the spleen and lymph nodes. Memory cells circulate through these and the blood and are available for recruitment into the tissues. Dendritic cells in the skin carry antigen to regional lymph nodes. *PALS*, periarteriolar lymphoid sheath.

an immune response, cell-cell contact must occur at the right time and place in order to engage lymphocyte surface receptors properly. Different microenvironments within primary and secondary lymphoid organs contain highly specialized cells. The interactions between these cells form the basis of immune regulation. However, the immune system is different from other organ systems; lymphocytes can move out of the lymphoid structures and into any place in the body, if sometimes pathologically. In this section, we consider first the various lymphoid structures and then how lymphocytes circulate.

Bone Marrow

The bone marrow is a primary lymphoid organ and is the site of differentiation of hematopoietic stem cells into B cell precursors in association with local stromal cells. The developing B cells undergo recombination of germ line genes to produce immunoglobulin heavy and light chains. The processes of positive and negative selection ensure that development only proceeds once a productive surface immunoglobulin is expressed, but one which does not react strongly to self antigens. The bone marrow also is collectively the largest site of antibody production, except for secretory immunoglobulin A (IgA) in the gut. Finally, a pool of recirculating mature lymphocytes also can be found in the bone marrow (1).

Thymus

The thymus is a primary lymphoid organ that specializes in support of T cell development. It is in the thymus that developing T cells rearrange their antigen-receptor genes and the T cell repertoire is selected. The thymus is fully developed before birth and maintains a high output of mature T cells until puberty, after which progressive involution occurs, and T cell output declines. The thymic stromal elements are critical for support and selection of the developing T cell repertoire and are organized into distinct compartments that correlate with their function. The outer region of the thymus, the cortex, contains the large majority of thymocytes and is the site for both TCR gene rearrangements and repertoire selection. The outer zone of the cortex contains rapidly dividing immature thymocytes, whereas the inner cortex contains primarily nondividing cells undergoing selection. The cortical thymic epithelium is highly branched to facilitate contact with the densely packed thymocytes and is responsible for positive selection. The central region of the thymus, the medulla, contains primarily mature T cells ready for export to the periphery. It also contains medullary epithelial cells and bone marrow–derived macrophages and dendritic cells that are thought to be important in the process of negative selection (see later section on T Cell Development).

The Skin

Langerhans cells in the skin serve as sentinels for the immune system. They take up antigen by macropinocytosis and binding of molecules to a surface mannose receptor. The antigens are processed efficiently, but in the skin, the ability of these cells to present antigen is limited. However, in the presence of inflammatory cytokines released in infections, these cells leave the skin, migrate to lymph nodes, and up-regulate not only MHC molecules but also costimulatory molecules (2). Thus, the antigens taken up in the skin are carried to the lymph nodes and presented in a highly efficient manner to lymphocytes.

Lymph Nodes

Lymph nodes are secondary lymphoid structures with anatomic features that are uniquely adapted for their role as sites for primary activation of naïve B and T cells. They are immunologic crossroads where circulating B and T cells arrive from the bloodstream and meet macrophages and dendritic cells carrying antigens originating from the extracellular tissue spaces via lymphatic vessels. The lymph node consists of a subcapsular sinus, cortex, and medulla. The subcapsular sinus is continuous with the afferent lymphatics and receives lymph and cells from the extracellular tissue spaces. The cortex consists of B cell follicles that are distributed peripherally and paracortical T cell areas that surround them. The medulla consists of collections of macrophages and plasma cells that line draining sinuses that connect to the efferent lymphatic vessels. Circulating B and T cells enter the paracortical zones through postcapillary venules that are lined by a specialized endothelium (high endothelial venules), which selectively binds naïve lymphocytes. B cells migrate to the follicles, whereas the T cells are retained in the paracortical areas. It is in the paracortex that naïve B and T cells meet incoming macrophages and dendritic cells and scan them for their specific antigen. In the absence of antigen recognition, B and T cells emigrate from the lymph node through the medulla and return to the bloodstream through the efferent lymphatics. B or T cells that encounter antigen during their migration through the lymph node are retained and activated to undergo proliferation and differentiation there.

Spleen

The spleen functions both as a surveillance mechanism for blood-borne antigens and as a reservoir for lymphocytes. Lymphocyte activation occurs in the white pulp (3). The vasculature of the white pulp of the spleen consists of a central arteriole with projecting terminal branches. The lymphoid follicles are intimately related to these structures. Immediately around the central arteriole is a region rich in T cells, the periarteriolar lymphoid sheath (PALS) region.

Around the PALS region is a collection of B cells in the follicular mantle. The terminal branches from the arterioles form sinusoids, the marginal sinus, around the outer edge of the follicular mantle. Macrophages line the sinusoids. Between the sinusoids and the red pulp is another region rich in B cells, termed the marginal zone. During an immune response, a novel structure, called the germinal center, forms at the interface of the PALS and the follicular mantle, and is composed of B and T cells and follicular dendritic cells (FDCs).

Gut

The intestinal tract contains the largest fraction of immune cells in the body, organized into secondary lymphoid structures that are collectively referred to as the gut-associated lymphoid tissues (GALT) (4). The GALT includes the tonsils, adenoids, appendix, small intestinal Peyer patches, and colonic lymphoid follicles. The GALT is uniquely exposed to a tremendous load of ingested food antigens, as well as bacterial antigens derived from commensal organisms of the intestinal flora. The mechanisms that maintain immune homeostasis in the face of such chronic antigenic challenge are only just beginning to be understood.

The B-1 subpopulation of B cells is found predominantly in the peritoneal cavity. These cells often express a membrane immunoglobulin that is unmutated and has broad reactivity, including to self antigens, with relatively low affinity. Current evidence suggests that continual low-level binding to the antigen receptor leads to this pattern of differentiation. As a result of the nature of the antibody they express, these cells provide the body with a reservoir of antibody that can bind a broad range of antigens, at low affinity but sufficient to help trigger complement activation and a full immune response. The continuous "tickling" by self antigen may prime these cells to react more rapidly to a challenge (5).

Lymphocyte Homing

The frequencies of individual specificities in the B- and T-cell repertoires are small (1×10^{-5} to 1×10^{-6}), and the anatomic surfaces across which pathogenic antigens can penetrate is large. Lymphocytes must be mobile and capable of surveillance over relatively vast territories. The adaptive immune system has therefore evolved sophisticated mechanisms for trafficking between different anatomic compartments and for homing to sites of infection to permit efficient interactions with antigens. Chemokines and adhesion molecules regulate lymphocyte localization. Chemokines provide a signal to move; adhesion molecules provide a means of attachment. This is an area of rapidly evolving research, particularly with the demonstration that chemokine receptors play a crucial role in internalization of human immunodeficiency virus and determine virus tropism.

The chemokines are small proteins with characteristic intrachain disulfide bonds linking cysteine residues. In one class (CC chemokines), two cysteines are adjacent, whereas in another class (CXC), they are separated by one amino acid. Each class of chemokine binds to a particular class of receptor (CCR or CXCR). The system is complex, since one chemokine may bind more than one receptor, and cells may secrete more than one chemokine and express more than one receptor, but both secretion and receptor expression are regulated (6).

In lymphocytes, chemokines are important in bone marrow development, lymphoid follicle formation, and inflammation. Bone marrow stromal cells and thymic dendritic cells express chemokines (SDF-1 and TECK, respectively) that attract B and T lymphocyte progenitors, respectively. Spleen and lymph node cells also express the chemokine BCA-1, which binds to CXCR5, which is preferentially expressed on B cells. In mice lacking CXCR5, the B cells develop normally but are unable to enter the B-cell zones in lymph nodes and the spleen. Dendritic cells at different stages of differentiation express a range of chemokines that attract different T cell subsets into different areas of the lymphoid follicle. The expression of chemokine receptors on mature T cells is particularly complex. Some are present on most T cells, some only on subsets. The expression of particular receptors is determined by the prior activation history of the T cell (naïve vs. memory), the differentiation path of the T cell [helper T cell subset 1 (T_H1) vs. T_H2], and the nature of stimulation (exposure to inflammatory cytokines vs. triggering of the T cell antigen receptor or particular costimulatory molecules). Some chemokine receptors will bind chemokines that are produced locally, and T cells that express these will remain, for example, in a lymphoid follicle. In some cases, these receptors will be down-modulated, and presumably, these cells will leave the follicle and enter the recirculating pool. If these cells have up-regulated receptors for chemokines that are being produced in sites of inflammation in tissues, these T cells will migrate into such regions. Thus, T cells that have been activated in different ways are recruited to different sites (7).

Adhesion molecules assist in the attachment of lymphocytes to each other, to antigen-presenting cells (APCs), to endothelial cells, and to the extracellular matrix (see Chapter 20). There are four categories of adhesion molecules. Some adhesion molecules, including intercellular adhesion molecules (ICAMs), vascular cell adhesion molecules (VCAMs), CD2, and leukocyte function–associated antigen-3 (LFA-3), contain extracellular folds characteristic of the immunoglobulin family of proteins. These are found on lymphocytes, APCs, and endothelial cells and bind proteins on other cells, including other members of this same family, or integrins. The integrins consist of two subunits (α and β chains) and are expressed on a wide variety of leukocytes. These bind to adhesion molecules on other cells (including those of the immunoglobulin family), to matrix proteins, and to polysaccharide-containing proteins. The selectins are found on leukocytes and endothelial cells and have lectin domains that bind particular modified oligosaccharides on glycoproteins. The addressins are found on different endothelial cells and have polysaccharide side chains that bind to the selectins or integrins. For a lymphocyte traveling through the blood, the initial contact is typically between a selectin on the lymphocyte and a polysaccharide on the endothelial cell. This tethers the lymphocyte so that it appears to roll along the endothelial cell. Endothelial cells in different anatomic locations express different polysaccharides and, hence, tether lymphocytes that have differentiated to express different selectins or integrins. Tight attachment follows and is usually mediated by binding of integrins on the lymphocyte to ICAMs or VCAMs on the endothelial cells. Diapedesis is controlled by yet another integrin binding to other ICAM or VCAM molecules on the endothelial cell. Once the cell reaches the site of inflammation (or a lymphoid follicle), interactions between lymphocytes and APCs are mediated by integrins and ICAMs, CD2, or LFA-3. Blocking these interactions inhibits antigen presentation. Not only do these molecules tighten the binding of the cells, but their ligation also triggers an activating signal in the lymphocyte (in particular, LFA-1 and CD2 on T cells) (8).

LYMPHOCYTE DEVELOPMENT AND FUNCTION

B Cells

B Cell Development

Recent advances have linked expression of particular surface markers on early B-lineage cells with discrete stages of maturation. The different steps of B-cell development can be dissected (9). The important considerations for this chapter are the rearrangement and expression of immunoglobulin genes and the selection of B cells for maturation. These processes are particularly important in the generation and control of autoreactive B cells.

After lineage commitment occurs, the first step is rearrangement of the immunoglobulin heavy-chain genes. This process involves a breaking of the germline chromosome and joining of V_H, D_H, and J_H segments (described in the earlier overview and in Chapter 13), first linking one D_H to one J_H and then linking one V_H to the DJ_H to form a VDJ_H cassette. Diversity is generated by the selection of different V, D, and J segments. However, the breaking and joining process is inexact, so one or more flanking DNA bases may or may not be included in the product, further increasing diversity. Finally, terminal deoxytransferase (TdT), expressed in cells undergoing rearrangement, adds extra bases to the ends of the fragments before recombination, providing a third mechanism for diversity. The result is a huge diversity of immunoglobulin genes in different B-cell progenitors. The bases that have been added or subtracted in the joining process will result in some genes that contain shifts in the downstream reading frame, so that no mature protein can be made. In this case, the cell attempts to rearrange the second heavy-chain allele on the other chromosome. In cells that successfully produce a heavy-chain protein, this joins with a pair of molecules that form the surrogate light-chain complex and is expressed on the cell surface (10). Expression of a heavy-chain–surrogate light-chain complex, which requires successful heavy-chain recombination, signals the cell to stop rearranging heavy-chain genes and to move on to rearrange the light-chain gene (11). Thus, surface expression of a heavy-chain protein is a first checkpoint in B-cell development and is required for progression beyond the pre–B cell stage (12).

The rearrangement of light-chain genes is similar except that there are no D regions. Rearrangement occurs first at the κ locus. If successful, a light-chain protein is produced that associates with the heavy chain present in the cells to form an immunoglobulin molecule, which moves to the cell surface, and the cell progresses to the immature B-cell stage. If the rearranged κ locus is unable to produce a protein, or the light chain that is produced is unable to pair with the particular heavy chain, then no immunoglobulin molecule is expressed, and the cell proceeds to attempt rearrangement of the other κ alleles and then the λ loci. This represents a second checkpoint, for the cell must produce a light chain that can pair with the heavy chain to proceed in development.

The heavy-chain–surrogate light-chain complex on the pre–B cell and the complete immunoglobulin molecule on the immature B cell associate with a pair of transmembrane proteins termed Igα and Igβ. These are the signaling molecules that are required for the positive selection of B cells to pass these checkpoints (13). The formation of a complete surface complex in itself could result in a low but sufficient signal. In some instances, low-affinity binding to self antigens appears to select cells positively (14). Thus, positive selection of B cells in the bone marrow either could be simply satisfied by formation of a surface immunoglobulin complex or could be determined by actual binding ability.

In some cases, the immunoglobulin on the surface of the immature B cell is strongly self-reactive and binds tightly to the body's native molecules in the bone marrow. Cells expressing such immunoglobulin are not normally found in the periphery. It had been assumed that these cells were negatively selected and eliminated by programmed cell death in the bone marrow. For example, in mice carrying a transgene encoding for a high-affinity antibody such as an anti-DNA antibody or a high-affinity rheumatoid factor, early, immature B cells expressing the immunoglobulin could be detected, but there were no corresponding mature B cells. However, we now know that instead of dying, such cells can undergo a process of "receptor editing" to make a new immunoglobulin (15). High-affinity, anti-self antibodies trigger reexpression of a set of enzymes that are similar to those that participate in the initial recombination of the heavy- and light-chain genes. The terminal segments of the gene that are still present on the chromosome are used to replace the V-(D)-J segments that formed the first, self-reactive immunoglobulin. If this secondary rearrangement is successful, a new immunoglobulin molecule is expressed. If the new immunoglobulin does not bind to self molecules with high affinity, the genes for the recombinase enzymes are turned off, and rearrangement ceases. This puts an interesting twist on the clonal selection theory—rather than simply being selected to survive or not, lymphocytes can change the immunoglobulin they express (16). One hypothesis to explain the escape from negative selection that occurs in autoimmunity is that, rarely, both the initially expressed, self-reactive antibody and the new antibody may be expressed, but the level of expression of the self-reactive antibody is low and escapes selection. Such cells, if activated, may be able to produce the self-reactive antibody.

B Cell Differentiation

The cells that survive the selection process exit the bone marrow as newly formed, mature B cells and travel to the spleen and enter the PALS region. It is possible to label such cells, but they are difficult to detect after 3 days. It had been assumed that there was competition between these newly formed cells and that only a small percentage were selected to enter the pool of long-lived B cells, but their fate is not well understood (17).

When antigen is carried through the blood into the spleen, it enters the white pulp through the marginal sinuses and is taken up and presented by the nearby macrophages, which are rich in scavenger receptors. The first lymphocytes to be triggered are the marginal zone B cells, which are specialized in that they tend to respond to nonprotein antigens like polysaccharides on bacteria and do so very rapidly, initiating the differentiation into antibody-secreting cell in hours. Antigen is carried into the PALS region, where T cells are stimulated and T cell–B cell contact occurs. The marginal zone B cells then move into the red pulp and differentiate into plasmablasts, providing a rapid, initial antibody response to the pathogen. Other T and B cells move to form a germinal center. Here, a complicated dance occurs involving T cells, B cells, and FDCs. The latter hold immune complexes containing antigens on the surface of long processes by receptors that bind the complement and antibody in the immune complex (2). The antigen receptor on the B cells recognizes this antigen. However, the B cells also must interact with activated T cells. The B cells present antigen to the T cells via the MHC class II molecules on the B cells (see Chapter 27). Additional coreceptors on the B and T cells have counterreceptors on the other, which provide additional signals that are crucial for a productive immune response. The B cells that are properly activated proliferate and undergo somatic hypermutation, with introduction of mutations in the variable regions of the rearranged immunoglobulin gene (18). In the early stages of germinal center formation, B cells from different clonal origins are present. Clones of B cells that initially have relatively low affinity can form a germinal center. Later, only a few clones are present, and these often contain selected mutations that allow one to trace their development from the cells present in the germinal center (19). Mutation in immunoglobulin genes may result in a receptor that has either higher or lower affinity than the parental B cell clone. The receptors with higher affinity bind more strongly. This leads to increased signaling and results in greater proliferation (20). The clones with mutations that result in higher affinity are "selected" to survive.

Class switching from IgM to IgG or other classes also occurs in the germinal center. Isotype switching by the B cell is controlled by the costimulatory signals received from helper T cells, depending on binding of CD40 and secretion of certain cytokines (21). IL-4 and other cytokines secreted by T_H2 cells, which target extracellular pathogens largely by antibody-directed mechanisms, induce switching to IgG1 and IgE. The former fixes complement and opsonizes pathogens for phagocytosis, whereas the latter activates allergic mechanisms, providing obvious advantages against such pathogens. Recent evidence also suggests that interferon-γ (IFN-γ) and tumor necrosis factor (TNF), usually associated with T_H1-type cell-mediated attack on intracellular antigens, can induce switching to IgG2 isotypes. Collaboration between T and B cells and the differentiation of T_H1 versus T_H2 cells are covered in more detail below.

Some of the high affinity, switched cells migrate to the red pulp or to the bone marrow as plasma cells and secrete the selected, high-affinity immunoglobulins. Others survive as a pool of high-affinity cells for the immunizing antigens, providing an expanded reservoir of memory cells able to respond more rapidly and with higher affinity should the same antigen be encountered again (22).

What happens to the cells that are not selected? Cells whose accessory receptors are bound, as would happen in the milieu of activated B and T cells, but receive an inadequate signal through the antigen receptor due to low affinity, undergo programmed cell death. Recently, a different fate also has been suggested. Some of the enzymes that promote rearrangement of genes in the bone marrow, including recombinase genes, also are expressed in germinal centers. B cells that lose in the competition for antigen receptor binding may undergo rearrangement of the immunoglobulin genes in the germinal center, as occurred in the bone marrow, to produce an entirely new antigen receptor (16). However, the importance of this has yet to be established (23). A second problem is that, in the course of hypermutation, a new receptor may be produced that now binds to self molecules. Thus, there must be a mechanism that prevents expansion of cells that have developed autoreactivity through mutation in the periphery. Such cells would be exposed to self antigen without binding of the accessory receptors that are only induced in inflammation. The antigen receptor signal that occurs in the absence of the accessory signals leads to anergy. This helps eliminate cells carrying mutations in the immunoglobulin genes that lead to autoreactive antigen receptors (24). Perhaps autoreactive cells are rescued from anergy when they recognize self, but in the presence of inflammation produced by some other mechanism, with induction of the accessory receptors. Another interesting possibility is that self-reactive cells might undergo selection outside of the germinal center, thereby escaping the normal mechanisms for negative selection.

B Cell Effector Functions

Peripheral B cells carry out two functions. First, B cells can activate T cells by antigen presentation, regulated by secretion of cytokines and expression of cell-surface molecules by the B cell. Second, differentiated B cells secrete antibody either locally in tissues or into the plasma.

The avidity of the immunoglobulin on the surface of the B cell serves to concentrate antigen for presentation. As an approximation, one can think of B cells as scavenging antigen from their milieu. Binding of antigen triggers rapid internalization of the surface immunoglobulin, carrying the antigen with it. The antigen–immunoglobulin complex is carried to a special internal compartment and degraded into peptide fragments. In this same compartment, MHC class II molecules are released from chaperone proteins. The binding site of the MHC molecules becomes available for binding of the peptide fragments. Newly formed complexes of snippets of antigen bound to MHC class II molecules are then transported back to the cell surface for presentation to the antigen receptors on T cells (Fig. 15.2).

Antigen processing and presentation are both regulated (25). In addition to the enhancement of internalization, binding of antigen to membrane immunoglobulin also activates the formation of the structures inside the cell necessary for antigen degradation. Activation of the B cell also increases the amount of MHC class II expressed on the cell surface. All of these steps increase the efficiency of the uptake and presentation of antigen. However, the ability of the B cell to activate the T cell, as opposed to simply binding the TCR, depends on the expression of costimulatory molecules on the surface of the B cell in addition to the MHC–peptide complex. A B cell that has received no stimulus other than binding of antigen is a poor activator of T cells. Such antigen presentation in the absence of other signals may, in fact, render the T cell anergic—unable to respond properly if presented with the same antigen even with proper costimulation. However, prior activation of the B cell by stimulatory cytokines or by other activated cells leads to expression of new proteins on the B-cell surface (the molecules involved in collaboration between B and T cells are covered in depth later, but those that alter antigen presentation will be included here). Previously activated B cells can express CD80 or CD86 (B7.1 or B7.2). Such a B cell can now deliver two signals to the T cell—one by binding of the T cell antigen receptor to the MHC class II–peptide complex on the B cell, and the other by binding of CD28 on the T cell by CD80 and CD86 on the B cell. Such two-signal activation leads to high levels of secretion of interleukin-2 (IL-2) and proliferation of the T cell. The effector function of the T cell depends on the type of stimulus it receives, as discussed in the later section on T-Cell Differentiation. This subject is complex, because the differentiation of the T cell depends on the engagement of different costimulatory molecules, cytokines, and the activation history of the T cell. The expression of CD80 versus CD86 and the secretion of different cytokines by B cells can alter the differentiation of the T cell after antigen presentation. The shift between T_H1 and T_H2 can have profound effects on the manifestations of autoimmunity, as well as on recovery from infections. In this regard, B cells can play an important role in altering the balance between the two.

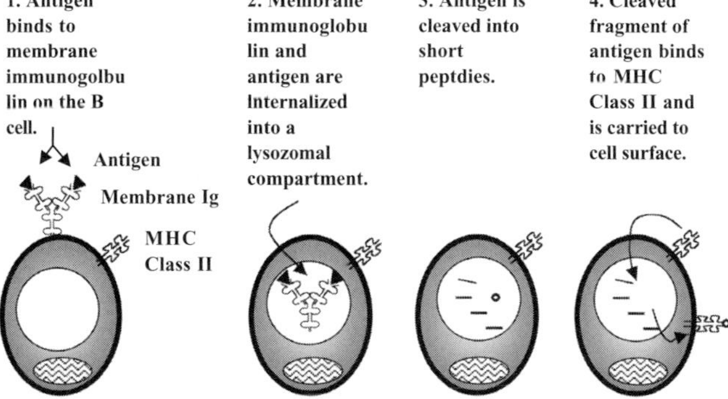
1. Antigen binds to membrane immunogolbu lin on the B cell.
Antigen
Membrane Ig
MHC Class II
2. Membrane immunoglobu lin and antigen are Internalized into a lysozomal compartment.
3. Antigen is cleaved into short peptdies.
4. Cleaved fragment of antigen binds to MHC Class II and is carried to cell surface.

FIG. 15.2. Antigen presentation by B cells. After antigen binds to membrane immunoglobulin (*Membrane Ig*) (*1*), the complex is internalized (*2*) and cleaved into peptides in a lysosomal compartment (*3*). Major histocompatibility complex (MHC) class II molecules also are carried to this compartment, where they bind fragments of the antigen. The MHC class II–peptide complex is transported to the cell surface for presentation to T cells (*4*).

Antigen presentation of self antigen by B cells also may play a critical role in autoimmunity. Compared with B cells, autoreactive T cells are more tightly controlled—it is harder to get a T cell to react to a self protein than a B cell. However, a B cell that has taken up self antigen and received a second stimulatory signal can present that antigen along with appropriate costimulatory signals to the T cell. This can overcome the T cell tolerance and lead to T-cell responsiveness to the self antigen. Studies in animal models have suggested that presentation of self antigen by B cells to T cells is necessary for the development of autoimmunity (26).

After sufficient stimulation, B cells differentiate to plasma cells and produce predominantly secreted immunoglobulin. The initial antibody produced after initial vaccination with antigen is predominately IgM of relatively low affinity. Two subsets of B cells, the B1 subpopulation and marginal zone cells, express more broadly reactive IgM and appear to require a low level of continuous stimulation, perhaps provided by self antigens (5). Perhaps as a result of this low-level stimulation, these cells respond more rapidly when a higher-level stimulus is received. Newly formed B cells also may contribute to the IgM response. In the spleen, most of the IgM antibody–secreting cells are found in the PALS and red pulp. During the first week after immunization, germinal centers form, and cells of higher affinity emerge. B cells also undergo isotype switching, and IgG becomes predominant. Most memory cells also are switched. The function of the secreted immunoglobulins is covered in Chapter 13.

T Cells

T Cell Development

Subsequent to the earliest stages of T cell lineage commitment, T cell development can be divided into two additional stages: specificity selection and functional differentiation. Specificity selection occurs in the thymus and determines the range of antigenic specificities recognized by the mature T cell repertoire. Unlike the B cell, the T cell does not undergo somatic hypermutation of its antigenic receptor, and its antigenic specificity is therefore fixed once selected during thymic "education." Also, the TCR does not recognize native or intact antigenic structures, as does the B-cell receptor (BCR), but recognizes fragments of antigens that are bound to MHC molecules. Hence, specificity selection in the thymus is shaped by both antigenic and self-MHC specificities. Functional differentiation of T cells occurs in extrathymic, or peripheral, lymphoid tissues (e.g., spleen and lymph nodes) after thymic emigration and entry into the recirculating lymphocyte pool. This process is initiated by interactions with antigen-bearing dendritic cells in the T cell zones of secondary lymphoid structures. Prior to antigen recognition, mature, recirculating T cells are referred to as naïve T cells and must divide and differentiate into cells with enhanced functional capabilities, so-called effector T cells, to participate in adaptive immunity. Because the T cell exerts the principal regulatory control of the immune response, the process of effector cell differentiation is central to effective immunity, and the transition from naïve to effector T cell is a critical checkpoint in immune regulation. Accordingly, dysregulated effector T cell differentiation plays an important role in many forms of autoimmunity.

Like B cells, T cells derive from a common lymphoid precursor (CLP) that develops from hematopoietic stem cells in the bone marrow. Unlike B cells, which complete most of their development within the bone marrow, T cells primarily develop in the thymus from CLP-like cells that migrate there from the bone marrow; hence the name, thymus-dependent, or T lymphocytes. It is in the thymus that developing T cells undergo antigen receptor gene rearrangements and selection to generate a single antigenic specificity (27,28). As a consequence of the recognition of antigen in the form of a complex of peptide bound to highly polymorphic MHC molecules, thymic selection is a two-step process. In the first step, thymocytes that have successfully rearranged and expressed the genes encoding the antigenic receptor are positively selected for recognition of self-MHC molecules. In the second step, those thymocytes that react strongly to self antigens are eliminated by negative selection. Through the combined processes of positive and negative selection, a mature T-cell repertoire that is both self-MHC restricted and self tolerant is generated (Fig. 15.3).

The successive stages of thymocyte maturation can be defined by distinct expression patterns of several cell surface proteins. The principal developmental stages are defined by expression of the TCR and the CD4 and CD8 coreceptors (Fig. 15.3). Immature thymocytes (pro–T cells) recently arrived from the bone marrow are devoid of these cell surface markers. Owing to the absence of CD4 and CD8 expression, these cells are referred to as "double-negative" thymocytes. It is at this stage that TCR gene rearrangement begins. This process shares many features with that of early B cell development, except that developing thymocytes initiate gene rearrangements for two different sets of TCR genes that ultimately define two distinct T cell lineages: αβ and γδ TCRs. γδ T cells develop from the same immature thymic precursors ($CD3^-CD4^-CD8^-$) as αβ cells, but their specificities, pattern of coreceptor expression, and function are

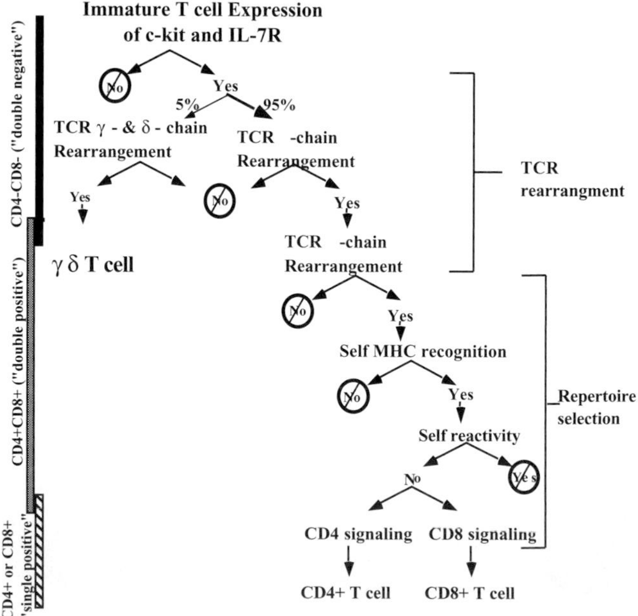

FIG. 15.3. Thymic development. As immature T cells develop in the thymus, they must pass a series of restriction points. The first requirements involve successful recombination of the genes for the T cell receptor chains. If successful, the cell must then undergo positive and negative selection. Failure at any of these tests leads to cell death. *IL-7R*, interleukin-7 receptor.

distinct from those of the αβ T cell lineage. Commitment to either the γδ or αβ T cell lineages is probably stochastic and is determined by which receptor set is the first to be successfully rearranged and functionally expressed. The γδ T cells comprise approximately 5% of the developing T cells in the thymus, but do not appear to require an intact thymus for maturation. The αβ lineage predominates in the thymus and is considered in more detail.

Rearrangement of the genes that encode the β chain of the TCR are initiated in the double negative ($CD3^-CD4^-CD8^-$) thymocyte population and are analogous to heavy-chain rearrangement of the BCR. D_β to J_β rearrangement is followed by V_β to $D_\beta J_\beta$ rearrangement. The mechanisms for generation of diversity parallel those for the immunoglobulin heavy chain: variable utilization of V-, D-, or J-chain segments, inexact splicing of D segments, and TdT-mediated nucleotide additions at splice joints. The β-chain gene contains two clusters of D_β and J_β segments, each of which is paired with its own constant, or C_β segment. This permits a second attempt at rearrangement on each of the β-chain alleles if the first rearrangement is unsuccessful. Thus, the double-negative pre–T cell can make four attempts to rearrange the β-chain gene segments, increasing the chance that a productive rearrangement will occur. In the minority of cases (<20%), in which neither allele is successfully rearranged, the cell dies at the double-negative stage. Once there is productive β-chain rearrangement, the β-chain protein pairs with a pre-Tα chain and is assembled with CD3 components to generate a functional pre-TCR (29). Signaling through this receptor halts additional β-chain rearrangement (allelic exclusion) and stimulates active proliferation to increase the numbers of clonal progeny. This is accompanied by sequential expression of CD8 and CD4, and the expanded clone then exits the cell cycle as $CD3^+CD4^+CD8^+$ "double-positive" T cells.

Rearrangement of TCR α -chain genes follows successful β-chain rearrangement early in the double-positive stage of thymic maturation. Just as β-chain rearrangement resembles B-cell heavy-chain rearrangement, α-chain rearrangement resembles light-chain rearrangement. Like the genes that encode the κ and λ light-chain components of the BCR, TCR α-chain genes lack D segments, and first rearrange a V_α to J_α. If a productive $V_\alpha J_\alpha$ join is made, a full-length $V_\alpha J_\alpha C_\alpha$ transcript is produced and tested for pairing with newly synthesized β chains. If a productive $V_\alpha J_\alpha$ join is not made, sequential $V_\alpha J_\alpha$ rearrangements continue until a productive transcript is produced. Unlike the β chain, each α-chain allele contains only a single $V_\alpha J_\alpha$ cluster and a single C_α segment. However, there are a large number of V_α and J_α gene segments (~70 and 50, respectively), and multiple, sequential recombinations can occur. Also, unlike the β chain, the α chain does not undergo allelic exclusion, and rearrangements can continue on the second allele even after productive rearrangement of the first allele. Hence, productive α-chain rearrangement seldom, if ever, fails. A by-product of this strategy for successful α-chain rearrangement is that a significant fraction of the developing thymocytes expresses two TCRs with a common β chain, but distinct α chains (dual-receptor T cells) (30). However, because positive selection eliminates the large majority of developing thymocytes (~95% of functional TCRs fail positive selection), and negative selection removes self-reactive TCRs, the probability that a single mature T cell will express two functional TCRs is low (31). Therefore, most of the circulating, mature T cells that express two TCR specificities (30% of mature T cell repertoire) are functionally monospecific.

Successful α-chain rearrangement stimulates a second burst of proliferation to expand the clonal population before selection. The double-positive ($CD3^+CD4^+CD8^+$) cells therefore constitute the largest thymocyte population (~80%). These cells are tested for binding to self-MHC class I– and II–peptide complexes on thymic cortical epithelial cells (thymic nurse cells). Double-positive thymocytes expressing TCRs that bind with sufficient avidity to self-MHC/self-peptide complexes (~5%) are protected from programmed cell death and are positively selected; those that do not bind (~95%) are "neglected" and undergo apoptotic cell death (32). During positive selection, cells that express TCRs that bind preferentially to class I MHC molecules down-regulate CD4 to become $CD3^+CD4^-CD8^+$. Conversely, those cells whose receptors bind class II MHC become $CD3^+CD4^+CD8^-$ ("single-positive" stage) (33). The ratio of $CD4^+CD8^-$ to $CD4^-CD8^+$ cells is approximately 2:1. Positively selected cells that bind self-MHC plus peptide too strongly are stimulated to undergo cell death by suicide, and are thus negatively selected (34). Negative selection may occur through interactions with bone marrow–derived APCs (macrophages or dendritic cells) or medullary epithelial cells in the thymic medulla (35). Remaining viable cells at the single-positive stage are nondividing and constitute approximately 15% of thymocytes. These cells are exported to the periphery as mature, but antigen-naïve T cells.

Effector T Cell Differentiation and Memory

$CD4^+$ and $CD8^+$ T cells enter a long-lived, recirculating pool after their emigration from the thymus. Prior to antigen recognition, the pattern of adhesion molecules and chemokine receptors that they express directs them to continuously circulate between the blood, secondary lymphoid tissues (e.g., spleen and lymph nodes), and back to blood (8,36). The anatomic organization of the secondary lymphoid structures is such that the circulating T-cell pool is regularly brought into contact with antigen-bearing dendritic cells that migrate there through the afferent lymphatics or blood from tissue sites where they ingest and process antigens (37). Dendritic cells are a diverse lineage of hematopoietically derived cells that reside in most tissues in an immature state. These cells have highly active receptor-independent (macropinocytotic) and receptor-mediated mechanisms for the uptake of pathogens, and are readily induced to migrate to draining lymphoid tissues upon engulfment of microbes. Coordinate with their activation and migration, dendritic cells mature into potent APCs that express high levels of MHC molecules bearing processed antigenic fragments poised for T cell recognition (38) (Fig. 15.4).

Before their first encounter with antigen in the secondary lymphoid tissues, naïve CD4+ and CD8+ T cells have limited functional capabilities. Antigen recognition on activated, mature dendritic cells stimulates a proliferative burst and initiates a program of differentiation that arms the T cell for heightened functional responses for the elimination of pathogens. There is significant plasticity in the range of differentiation pathways available to the naïve T cell. Thus, naïve T cells of identical antigenic specificity may differentiate into distinct functional effector phenotypes (e.g., T_H1 or T_H2 cells) depending on the environmental cues that are received during the initial stimulation by antigen. Costimulatory molecules expressed by antigen-bearing dendritic cells are one important class of signals that are integrated with those from the antigen receptor to initiate effector T cell differentiation. Another class of "second signals" is proinflammatory cytokines that are released by cells of the innate immune system (e.g., macrophages, NK cells) that have recognized microbes at sites of infection. Unlike B and T cells, cells of the innate immune system lack receptors for specific antigen, but express receptors for conserved microbial structures that stimulate their elaboration of inflammatory products, such as cytokines, that control the differentiation of naïve T cells into functional effectors. In this manner, microbes exert a form of "secondary education" of naïve T cells, instructing them, through indirect effects exerted by the cells of the innate immune system, to differentiate into an appropriate type of cell to effect their elimination. Three general programs of effector cell differentiation have evolved to eliminate pathogens whose survival strategies are dependent on different microanatomic niches: intracytoplasmic, intravesicular (e.g., phagosomes and lysosomes), and extracellular pathogens.

Peptide fragments derived from infectious agents that replicate intracellularly in the cytoplasm of their cellular hosts, such as viruses and certain bacteria, are transported into the endoplasmic reticulum and bound in the antigen-binding cleft of newly synthesized MHC class I molecules (39). The MHC class I–peptide complex is transported to the cell surface where it can be recognized by CD8+ T cells. Because these pathogens are best eliminated by destruction of the infected host cell, CD8+ effector cell differentiation is dominated by the development of cytolytic mechanisms that destroy cells bearing MHC–peptide complexes that they recognize. Pathogens that are adapted for intravesicular or extracellular survival produce antigens that are processed in special lysosomal vesicles in APCs. MHC class II molecules also traffic into these vesicles. After removal of the invariant chain in antigen-processing vesicles,

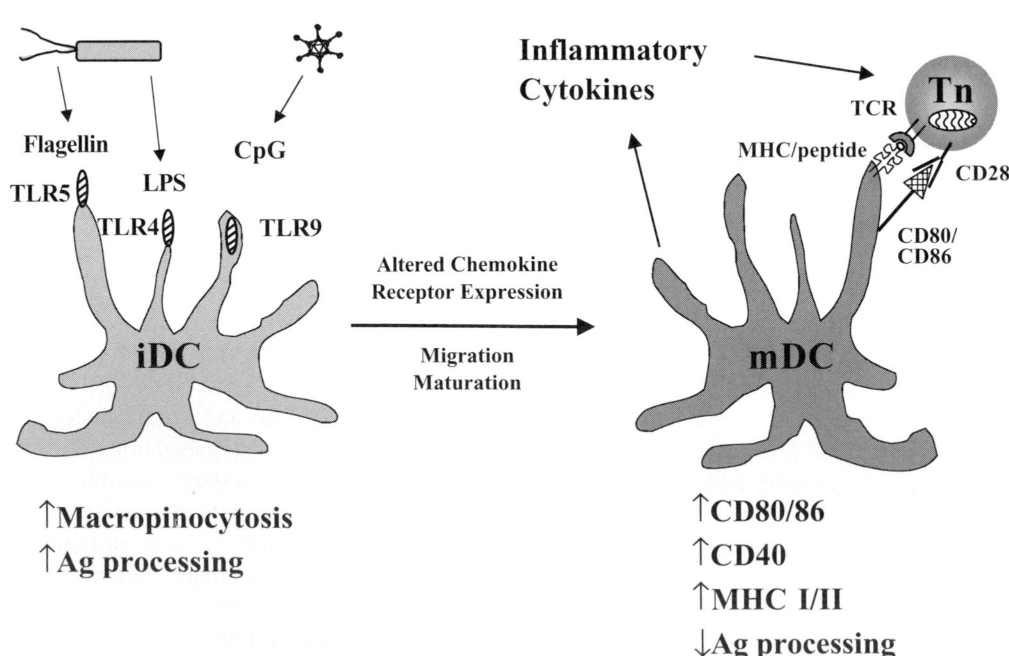

FIG. 15.4. Activation of Toll-like receptors (*TLR*) links dendritic cell maturation/activation to naïve T cell activation and effector cell differentiation. *CpG*, bacterial CpG-rich DNA; *iDC*, immature dendritic cell; *LPS*, bacterial lipopolysaccharide; *mDC*, mature dendritic cell; *TCR*, T cell receptor; *Tn*, naïve T cell; *TCR*, T cell receptor.

the class II molecules are freed to bind peptides that have been proteolytically cleaved from pathogen-associated proteins. These MHC class II–peptide complexes also are transported to the cell surface, where they are recognized by CD4+ T cells. Certain pathogens that replicate within the phagocytic vesicles of macrophages (e.g., *Mycobacterium* and *Leishmania* species), or that must be targeted to phagocytic vesicles to be destroyed, are preferentially eliminated by specialized CD4+ T cells that produce cytokines that activate macrophages for intracellular killing: T_H1 cells. T_H1 cells also provide help to B cells that favors the production of opsonizing IgG2 and IgG3 antibodies that target the antigen for phagocytosis and intracellular killing. Pathogens that are free living and replicate in the extracellular environment also generate antigens that are handled by the class II pathway and activate CD4+ T cells. These antigens preferentially stimulate the differentiation of T_H2 cells, which are especially adapted for helping B cells to produce complement-activating and opsonizing IgG1 antibodies and IgE antibodies that arm mast cells and basophils. Thus, effector CD4+ T cells, either T_H1 or T_H2 cells, generate effector responses primarily by activating other immune cells such as macrophages or B cells to heightened function.

Most naïve CD8+ T cells appear destined to differentiate into cytolytic cells, whose effector function is primarily mediated by cell-cell contact (40). CD8+ T cell differentiation is marked by the development of lytic granules. These are modified lysosomes in which are packaged effector molecules that initiate programmed cell death, or apoptosis, in cells targeted for destruction by the display of specific antigen. Two classes of proteins unique to differentiated CD8+ T cells function together to kill target cells. Perforin is a pore-forming protein that polymerizes in the target cell membrane to breach its cell membrane, much in the same way that the attack complex of complement does. Several cytotoxic serine proteases called granzymes are released through the perforin pore into the target cell, where they activate intracellular caspases that initiate the apoptotic cascade. Differentiated CD8+ cells also express members of the TNF superfamily, including Fas ligand (FasL), TNF-α, and TNF-β, that are induced by antigen recognition and may also stimulate apoptosis of infected target cells. The importance of these mechanisms relative to the perforin-granzyme system is not yet clear, but presumably reflects an adaptation for elimination of different types of cytosolic pathogens.

The differentiation of naïve CD4+ cells into either T_H1 or T_H2 effector cells also reflects the unique class of pathogens that each phenotype has evolved to eliminate. T_H1 and T_H2 cells are distinguished by the patterns of cytokines they produce when activated by antigen (41) (Fig. 15.5). T_H1 cells produce IFN-γ, a cytokine that is effective at activating macrophages and stimulating B-cell switching that favors production of opsonizing antibodies. T_H1 cells also can express FasL and kill infected targets through activation of the Fas death cascade. T_H2 cells produce IL-4, IL-5,

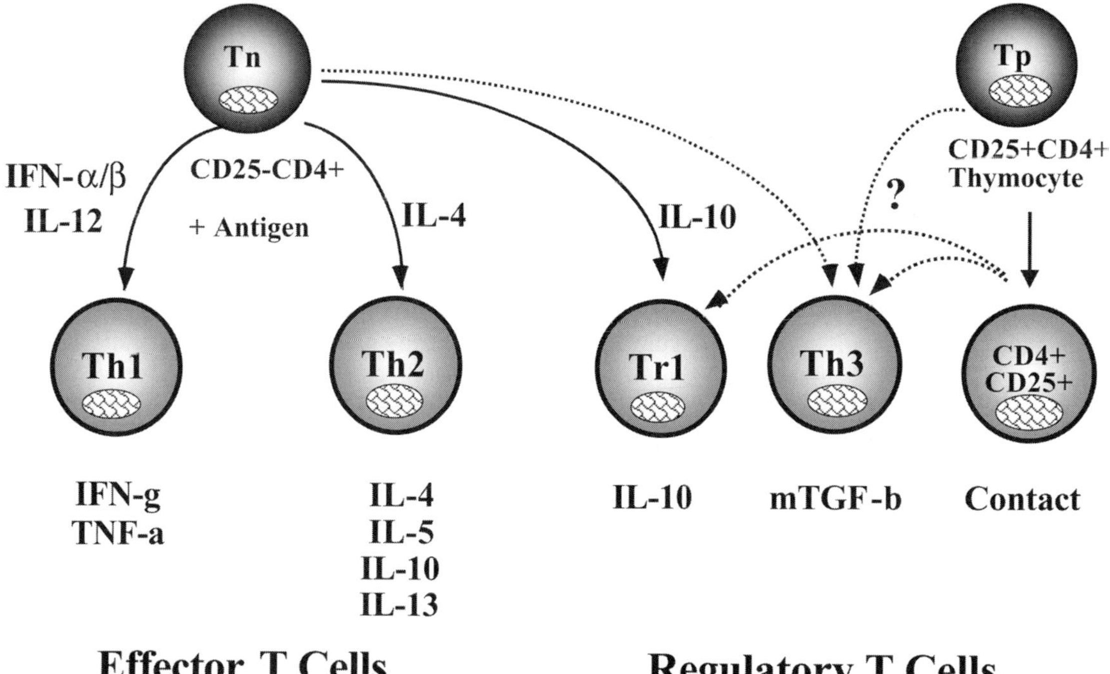

FIG. 15.5. Effector and regulatory CD4+ T cells. CD4+ T cells may differentiate into distinct lineages of effector or regulatory cells. Arrows denote established (*solid arrows*) and putative (*dashed arrows*) lineage relationships. T-helper 1 (*Th1*), T-helper 2 (*Th2*), and T regulatory 1 (*Tr1*) cells can develop from mature, naïve precursors (Tu, naïve T cell). Lineage relationships between CD25+ regulatory T cells (Treg) and other regulatory T cells are less clearly defined, but CD25+ T negs develop from T cell percursors (TP) during interthymic development.

IL-10, and IL-13, potent activators of B-cell differentiation (see Chapter 19). Importantly, T_H1 and T_H2 cytokines are counterregulatory (42). That is, T_H1 cytokines act on APCs and developing naïve CD4+ T cells to induce T_H1 differentiation and suppress T_H2 differentiation. Conversely, T_H2 cytokines promote T_H2 differentiation and suppress T_H1 differentiation. Thus, factors that favor the development of either differentiation pathway tend to be self-reinforcing, and lead to phenotype stability. Although all of the factors that determine whether an antigen-activated, naïve CD4+ cell will differentiate into a T_H1 or T_H2 cell are not completely understood, a principal determinant is the presence of specific cytokines that are elicited by the pathogens to which a response is directed. T_H1 differentiation is primarily induced by IL-12 and IFN-γ, whereas T_H2 differentiation is induced by IL-4 (43,44). Differentiated T_H1 or T_H2 cells could themselves contribute some of these cytokines in a recall response, but their principal source early in a primary antigenic response appears to be cells of the innate immune system. Macrophages, dendritic cells, and NK cells can each be activated by microbial products to produce IL-12, which, in turn, stimulates production of IFN-γ (45). The cellular source of IL-4 that directs T_H2 development is not well understood, but a unique class of primitive T cells, Natural Killer T (NKT) cells, are capable of producing large amounts of IL-4 in response to some microbial stimuli and may produce IL-4 that contributes to T_H2 development.

The actions of IL-12 and IL-4 in the regulation of T_H1 and T_H2 cell differentiation, respectively, are now understood in some detail (46) (Fig. 15.6A). Antigen-activated naïve T cells express components of receptors for each of these cytokines. Both receptors are multicomponent signaling complexes that regulate effector T-cell differentiation subsequent to antigen-induced TCR signaling. The IL-12 receptor is composed of two chains, IL-12R β1 and IL-12R β2. Both subunits are required for high-affinity binding of IL-12, whereas the β2 chain is primarily responsible for signal transduction. The cytoplasmic tail of IL-12R β2 contains tyrosine residues that are phosphorylated by a receptor-associated Janus kinase (Jak) after ligand binding. IL-12R β2 chain phosphorylation leads to recruitment of the signal transducer and activator of transcription 4 (STAT4), which is in turn activated by Jak phosphorylation. STAT4 activation is important for T_H1 development, because STAT4-deficient mice produce limited T_H1 responses. Interestingly, expression of the IL-12R β2 chain in antigen-activated, naïve T cells is regulated by IFN-γ-induced STAT1. STAT1 signaling induces expression of the transcription factor T-bet, which is required for stable expression of IL-12R β2 chain in developing and established T_H1 cells. T-bet also acts to facilitate expression of the gene that encodes IFN-γ. IL-12 signaling, in turn, induces high-level expression of IFN-γ and induces expression of the IL-18 receptor, signaling through which amplifies IFN-γ expression. Thus, IFN-γ and IL-12 act sequentially and coordinately to initiate and stabilize the T_H1 differentiation program. Through mechanisms that are not yet understood, STAT4 signaling suppresses the induction of IL-4 expression in developing T cells.

In contrast, IL-4R signaling during the initial stages of naïve T cell activation blocks the expression of the IL-12R β2 subunit, thereby extinguishing IL-12 signaling and the T_H1 program of differentiation in developing T_H2 cells (47). The IL-4 receptor is a heterodimer composed of a unique IL-4R α chain that pairs with the γ_c chain on IL-4 binding (48). The γ_c chain is common to the type I cytokine receptor family that also includes the IL-2, IL-7, and IL-15 receptors. IL-4 binding to its receptor stimulates Jak-mediated phosphorylation and activation of STAT6, which is required for T_H2 differentiation. STAT4 and STAT6 are therefore lineage-specific signaling intermediates that play central roles in differentiation of T_H1 and T_H2 cells, respectively (49). IL-4R signaling through STAT6 induces expression of GATA3, and subsequently cMAF, transcription factors that are selectively expressed in T_H2 cells and important for their differentiation and maintenance.

A hallmark of the adaptive immune response is the generation of a more rapid and robust response to antigen after the initial exposure. This capacity for "memory" of previous antigen encounters is held at the cellular level (40). T cell memory reflects quantitative and qualitative adaptations of the T cell that are both dependent on antigen-driven differentiation: increased frequency of antigen-specific cells and enhanced responsiveness of previously stimulated cells. The exact nature of memory has been more difficult to define for T cells than for B cells, partially because T cells do not undergo somatic hypermutation. Accordingly, it is difficult to measure changes in the T cell's functional efficiency directly. Nevertheless, it is clear that, in addition to the increases in clonal T cell frequency that accompany antigenic stimulation, T cells also recognize antigen more efficiently in a secondary, or recall, response. Hence, secondary T cells are activated at approximately 100-fold lower levels of antigen than are primary T cells. Because there are no changes in the affinity of the TCR as a consequence of antigenic stimulation, the basis for increased antigenic sensitivity must reside in non-TCR recognition structures or more effective coupling of antigen binding of the TCR to intracellular signaling pathways.

Expression of several cell surface molecules is modulated during antigen-driven T cell differentiation, and these changes correlate with T cell memory or effector function (50). Among these, several are adhesion molecules, such as L-selectin (CD62L) and LFA-3, changes in expression of which affect T cell trafficking or adhesive interactions with APCs. Similarly, the cell membrane–associated tyrosine phosphatase CD45 undergoes differentiation-dependent changes in expression of different isoforms that are generated by alternative splicing of exons coding portions of its extracellular domain (51). CD45 regulates the responsiveness of the TCR to antigenic signaling through action of its intracellular phosphatase domain, but how different splice

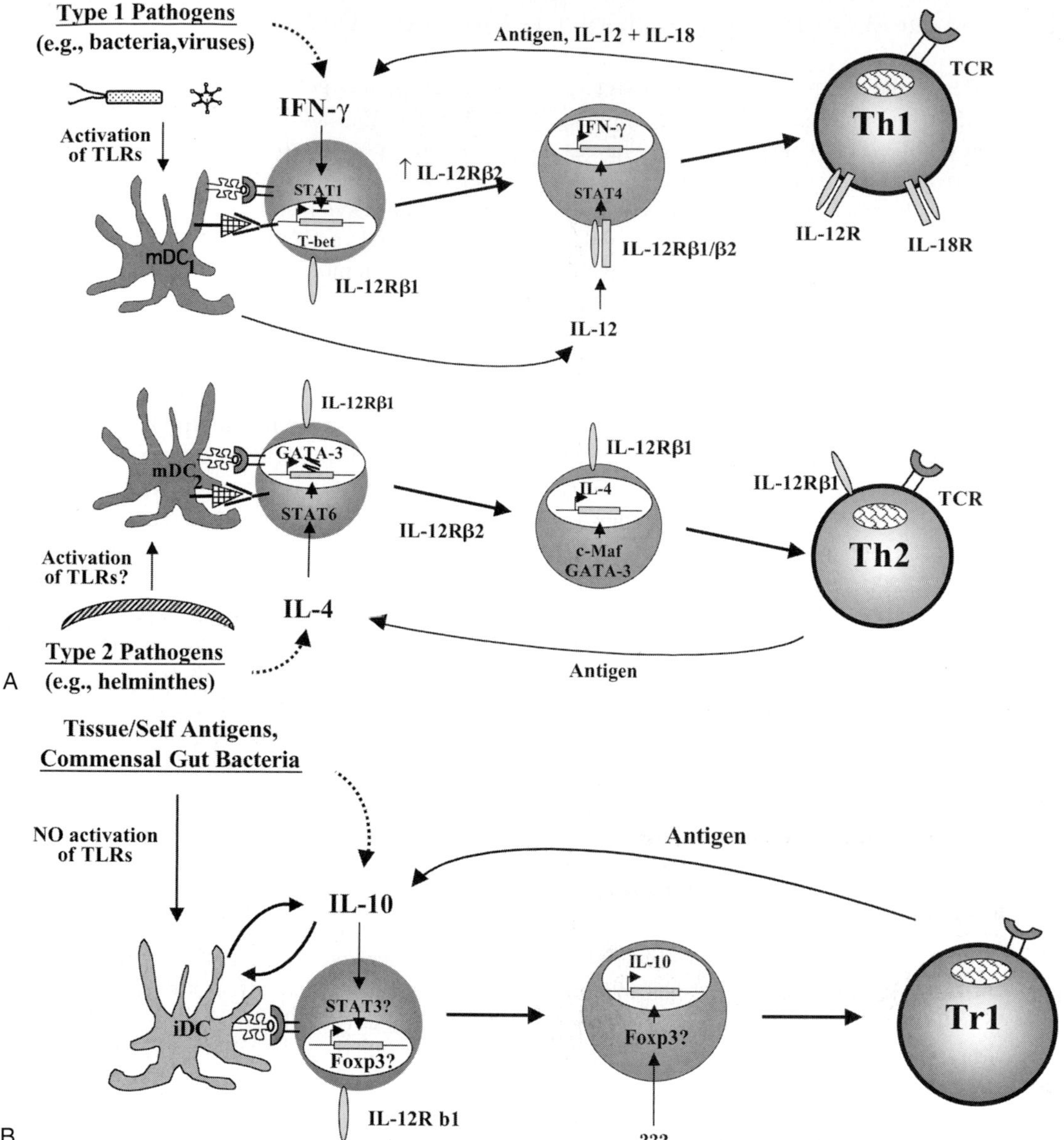

FIG. 15.6. Pathways of effector and regulatory T cell (Treg) differentiation. **A:** T-helper 1 (Th1) and Th2 effector cell differentiation. Uptake of type 1 or type 2 pathogens induces the migration, maturation, and activation of distinct populations of dendritic cells (mDC1 and mDC2, respectively). Th1 and Th2 development from naïve T-cell precursors is initiated by recognition of these antigen-loaded dendritic cells in secondary lymphoid tissues. Mature, activated DCs that have processed type 1 pathogens induce antigen-specific naïve T cells to undergo Th1 effector cell differentiation through cytokines/factors produced directly by the DC [e.g., interleukin-12 (IL-12)] and cytokines produced by other cells of the innate immune system [e.g., interferon-γ (IFN-γ) produced by natural killer cells], or previously differentiated Th1 cells. IFN-γ receptor signaling through STAT1 (signal transducer and activator of transcription 1) in coordination with T cell receptor (*TCR*) signaling induces the transcription factor T-bet, which in turn induces expression of the β_2 chain of the IL-12 receptor (*IL-12Rβ_2*), rendering it competent for signaling through STAT4. IL-12-induced STAT4 in turn cooperates with additional transcription factors to initiate expression of the IFN-γ gene, setting up a possible positive feedback loop for Th1 differentiation. Th2 differentiation is distinguished by IL-4-induced signaling through the STAT6 pathway to induce the transcription factor GATA-3, which inhibits expression of the IL-12Rβ_2 chain, thus preventing IL-12 signaling. Alternatively, the absence of IFN-γ and IL-12 signaling may lead to GATA-3 expression as a default pathway. Both T-bet and GATA-3 autoamplify their own expression through positive feedback, and may inhibit each other's expression, thereby stabilizing the distinct differentiation programs once initiated. **B:** Treg differentiation. Although less is known regarding the molecular pathways involved in Treg differentiation, it now appears that at least one lineage of Tregs, Tr1 cells, can develop from naïve CD4 precursors through a program initiated by recognition of cognate antigen presented on immature dendritic cells (*iDC*). Analogous to IFN-γ/IL-12 and IL-4 for Th1 and Th2 development, respectively, IL-10 appears to be critical for Tr1 development. The transcription factor Foxp3 may be a "master regulator" of Treg development, comparable to T-bet and GATA-3 for Th1 and Th2 lineages. Note that these pathways are shown for CD4 T cells; comparable pathways may exist for CD8 T cells, but are less well characterized.

variants of CD45 differ in their regulation of T cell signaling is unclear. Anti-CD45 monoclonal antibodies recognize a determinant present on all CD45 splice variants, whereas anti-CD45R (for "restricted") antibodies recognize epitopes encoded by one of the alternatively spliced exons. Both CD4+ and CD8+ cells can be divided into two subpopulations based on their expression of CD45 isoforms. Naïve T cells typically express a high-molecular-weight form of CD45 that includes the "A" exon (CD45RA), whereas memory T cells typically express the low-molecular-weight form of CD45 (CD45RO) that has spliced out all variable exons. Stimulation of CD45RA cells leads to a loss of CD45RA and expression of CD45RO (52). These observations have given rise to the designation of CD45RA and CD45RO as naïve and memory markers, respectively. Recent studies in rodents suggest that this association is not absolute, however, because CD45RO T cells may revert to CD45RA over time. Thus, the precise relationship between CD45 isoform expression and T cell differentiation and memory remains incompletely defined. Similar changes in cell surface molecules on effector T cells and antigen-stimulated cells with limited effector function have stimulated debate over the lineage relations between memory and effector cells. It is presently unclear if memory T cells arise from effector T cells or represent a distinct differentiation pathway.

T Cell Tolerance

The positive and negative selection processes that occur during T cell development in the thymus balance the requirements for self restriction and lack of self reactivity. Developing clones that are positively selected, but that bind autoantigens too strongly in the thymus are deleted during the process of negative selection, so-called central tolerance. It has been recognized for some time that many autoantigens that are uniquely expressed in extrathymic tissues can contribute to central tolerance through their uptake and transport to the thymus by tissue macrophages and dendritic cells. Recognition of these tissue-specific antigens by developing thymocytes affects their deletion, thereby eliminating potentially autoreactive T cells. Because antigens taken up by macrophages or dendritic cells are readily presented by MHC class II molecules and recognized by developing CD4+ T cells, intrathymic deletion of this subset by negative selection on specialized APCs of hematopoietic origin occurs. Since antigens processed into the pathway for presentation by MHC class I molecules are not efficiently handled in this manner, it has been less clear how tissue-specific antigens could contribute to the intrathymic deletion of developing CD8+ T cells. Recently, however, it has been shown that many "tissue-specific" antigens are expressed at low levels by specialized epithelial cells in the thymic medulla (thymic medullary epithelial cells, or MECs), under control of the transcription factor AIRE (autoimmune regulator) (53). Many proteins that are ectopically expressed by MECs are target antigens for well-defined autoimmune diseases (e.g., insulin, type 1 diabetes; myelin basic protein, multiple sclerosis; thyroglobulin, thyroiditis). Humans with defects in the *Aire* gene develop a multiorgan autoimmune syndrome, autoimmune polyendocrine syndrome type 1, and mice with an induced mutation of the *Aire* gene demonstrate defective negative selection of high-affinity T cell clones, providing a link between defective negative selection on MECs and autoimmunity (54–56).

Thymic selection is very efficient, but is not fail-safe, at least in part because not all self antigens are present in the thymus to contribute to negative selection or because low-affinity T cell clones may escape intrathymic deletion. This is particularly true for autoantigens that are anatomically sequestered in sites of "immune privilege" (e.g., central nervous system and testes), but also includes tissue-specific antigens that are not normally expressed at sufficient levels to contribute to thymic deletion, or antigens that may not be expressed until late in development (e.g., neoantigens expressed during puberty). The extrathymic T cell repertoire therefore contains a fraction of clones that express TCRs that can recognize autoantigens. Several mechanisms have evolved to silence-autoreactive clones in the periphery: immune ignorance, clonal anergy, immune suppression, and peripheral deletion. Collectively referred to as peripheral tolerance, the circumstances under which these processes are invoked differ depending on the nature of the autoantigen and the stage in T cell differentiation that they must act (i.e., naïve T cells vs. effector or memory T cells), and may not be mutually exclusive.

A prerequisite for T cell activation is binding of antigenic peptide fragments to self-MHC molecules and the simultaneous engagement of a sufficient number of TCRs to initiate the signaling cascade that induces cell cycle entry and differentiation. Below an antigenic threshold required for signaling, the T cell "ignores" antigen, and no response occurs. Tolerance to many autoantigens probably occurs by this process of immune ignorance, due either to lack of binding of antigenic peptide fragments to self-MHC or to lack of sufficient quantities of antigen to exceed the threshold for T cell activation. In several anatomic sites, such as the brain, testis, or anterior chamber of the eye, there is limited or no lymphatic or blood drainage of tissue antigens to sites of immune induction, and immune ignorance is therefore a consequence of the sequestration of autoantigens. For autoantigens that are present in sufficient levels to stimulate T cells that recognize them, other mechanisms are needed to prevent autoimmunity.

In addition to the requirement for a minimal TCR signaling threshold, the naïve T cell requires additional signals to initiate effector cell differentiation (57). Principal among these is cosignaling through the CD28 receptor (Fig. 15.4). The ligands for CD28 [CD80 (B7–1) and CD86 (B7–2)] are referred to as costimulators, and are expressed by APCs. Although effector and memory CD4+ T cells may be activated by antigen presented by one of several professional

APCs and comparable CD8+ cells can be activated by antigen presented on most MHC class I–bearing cells (including non-APCs), antigen-naïve CD4+ and CD8+ T cells are only activated by antigen presented by bone marrow-derived dendritic cells. These APCs express high levels of CD80 and CD86 following their activation by stimulation of Toll-like receptor (TLR) signaling or inflammatory cytokines. TLRs are a diverse family of highly evolutionarily conserved molecules, each member of which recognizes a conserved molecular structure uniquely associated with microbes. Collectively, these microbial structures are termed pathogen-associated molecular patterns (PAMPs) and include bacterially-associated proinflammatory agents such as lipopolysaccharide, peptidoglycans, or bacterial flagellin, and virally-associated structures such as double-stranded RNA (58). The recognition of PAMPs by TLRs stimulates a signaling cascade linked to activation of the nuclear factor κB (NFκB) and mitogen-activated protein kinase (MAPK) pathways through the common adaptor protein MyD88. MyD88, and related adaptor proteins (e.g., Trif) that associate with only certain TLR family members, bind a common motif (Toll/IL-1 receptor, or TIR domain) in the cytoplasmic portion of all TLRs to initiate TLR signaling (59). The induction of an inflammatory response by TLR recognition of PAMPs represents a highly evolutionary conserved mechanism for signaling the host about the presence of a pathogen. TLR-linked induction of costimulator and proinflammatory cytokine expression on dendritic cells, each of which participates in effector T-cell differentiation, represents an important mechanism by which the adaptive immune response is guided by the innate immune response.

T cell recognition of innocuous antigens, such as tissue antigens, which fail to activate TLR or inflammatory signaling and thus lack costimulator-inducing properties, fail to stimulate effector cell development and may induce a limited program of T cell activation referred to as anergy (60,61). Anergic T cells are deficient in IL-2 production and fail to undergo significant proliferation. As a consequence, they do not undergo effector differentiation. It is unclear whether anergized T cells persist and differentiate into a regulatory population that has antigen-specific suppressive functions, or rather undergo deletion by a mechanism akin to the removal of thymocytes that fail positive selection. In any case, these autospecific clones are functionally silenced. Costimulator expression by APCs, which is contingent on the recognition of TLR-activating microbial structures, is therefore a critical checkpoint for self/nonself discrimination in the periphery. Given their unique role as the sole APCs capable of activating naïve T cells, the linkage of TLR signaling on dendritic cells with requirement for activation of effector T cell differentiation positions the dendritic cell as the "gatekeeper" of immune tolerance in the periphery (62).

In addition to immune ignorance and anergy, immune suppression is an important mechanism by which peripheral tolerance to self antigens is normally maintained. Recent studies have identified distinct lineages of differentiated CD4+ T cells that can down-regulate or suppress the differentiation of effector T cells from naïve T cell precursors, and may actively suppress existing T effectors and memory cells as well (Fig. 15.5). These cells express a pattern of cytokines and surface markers that are distinct from T_H1 and T_H2 effectors, and are collectively referred to as regulatory T cells, or Treg cells. The best characterized of these cells are within the CD4+ T cell lineage, although CD8+ Tregs likely exist.

Three types of CD4+ Tregs have been described to date: CD25+CD4+ Treg cells; Tr1 (T regulatory 1) cells; and T_H3 cells (63–65) (Fig. 15.5). CD25+CD4+ Tregs are so called because they constitutively express the CD25 marker, the high-affinity component (IL-2R α chain) of the IL-2 receptor complex that is normally expressed only on recently activated T cells. These cells also express CTLA-4, an inhibitory receptor for the B7–1 and B7–2 costimulators. CD25+CD4+ Tregs appear to develop during positive selection in the thymus through recognition of certain tissue-specific antigens. CD25+CD4+ Tregs act in the periphery to block activation of self-reactive naïve T cells by inhibiting the maturation and activation of dendritic cells that might otherwise stimulate effector differentiation of naïve T cell precursors (66) (Fig. 15.7). The mechanism by which CD25+CD4+ Tregs suppress activation of dendritic cells is unclear, but requires cell-cell contact between the Treg and dendritic cell and prevents induction of costimulator expression. Insights into the molecular mechanisms that control the development of CD25+CD4+ Treg cells have been gained through studies that have linked an aggressive autoimmune syndrome in humans, IPEX (immune dysregulation, polyendocrinopathy, enteropathy, X-linked syndrome) or XLAAD (X-linked autoimmunity-allergic dysregulation syndrome), with defects in the gene that encodes the Foxp3 transcription factor (67,68). Mice with mutations in the *Foxp3* gene that lead to deficiency of Foxp3 expression fail to develop CD25+CD4+

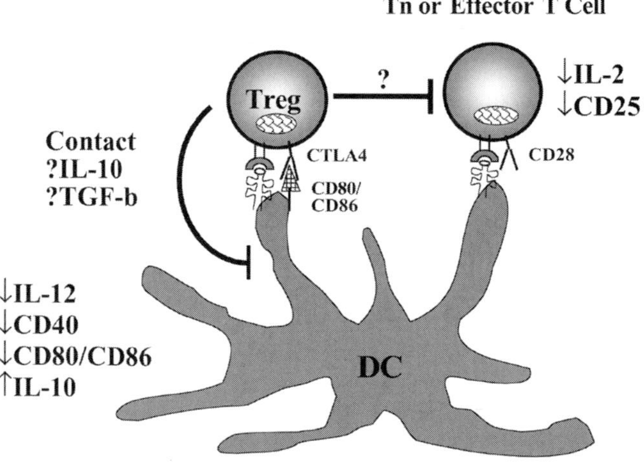

FIG. 15.7. Mechanisms of immunosuppression mediated by regulatory T cells.

Tregs and exhibit a clinical syndrome with similarities to the human disease, implicating a central role for this factor in CD25+CD4+ Treg cell development.

Tr1 cells are derived from naïve CD4 T cell precursors activated by dendritic cells that have matured under the influence of IL-10 (69,70) (Fig. 15.6B). Unlike CD25+CD4+ Tregs, Tr1 cells appear to develop extrathymically. Antigen-activated Tr1 cells are characterized by their production of high levels of IL-10, with modest IFN-γ and no IL-4 or IL-13 (65). IL-10 produced by Tr1 cells blocks the production by dendritic cells and macrophages of proinflammatory cytokines, such as IL-12 and IL-6, which are important for effector T-cell differentiation. T_H3 cells were originally isolated from lymph nodes draining the intestines of mice fed antigen, and are distinguished by their production of high levels of the immunosuppressive cytokine, transforming growth factor-β1 (64). Details of the conditions that lead to the development of T_H3 cells and the mechanisms by which they may contribute to peripheral tolerance are not well understood. It is postulated that they develop in tissue sites rich in immunosuppressive cytokines, such as the intestinal tract, or that they may develop from poorly activated, anergized precursors.

A general feature of tolerance mediated by regulatory T cells is that reactivity of these cells to their cognate antigen can suppress tissue injury mediated by effector T cells reactive to an independent antigen, a phenomenon referred to as bystander suppression (71). Whether mediated by cell-cell contact (e.g., CD25+CD4+ Treg cells) or cytokines (e.g., Tr1 cells), this may ultimately permit therapeutic interventions that specifically down-regulate disease-causing effector T cells in the absence of global immune suppression. It also holds promise for interventions that might suppress preexisting disease. Unfortunately, recent attempts to ameliorate human autoimmune diseases (e.g., multiple sclerosis and rheumatoid arthritis) through the induction of regulatory T cells by antigen feeding has met, at best, with limited success.

An important regulatory process for editing clonal specificities from the peripheral T cell repertoire is the process of activation-induced cell death (AICD). AICD provides an active mechanism for deleting antigen-activated lymphocytes and is mediated by the cell suicide mechanism, apoptosis. Although apoptosis of lymphocytes may be initiated through several mechanisms, the best characterized involves the interactions of the Fas receptor (CD95) with Fas ligand (FasL) (72). Fas and FasL are members of the TNF receptor and ligand superfamilies, respectively (73). Fas is expressed by many cell types, including resting and activated B and T cells, whereas FasL is expressed primarily by activated T_H1 cells. Fas signaling appears to be coupled to an apoptotic suicide response in effector, but not naïve T cells. Similarly, FasL is expressed by activated effector cells, particularly CD8+ cytolytic cells and T_H1 cells. The expression of Fas and FasL by antigen-activated effector T cells provides a mechanism by which these cells may initiate their own elimination during an immune response (74). There remains controversy, however, over the physiologic setting in which this pathway is activated. Less controversial is the role that Fas/FasL interactions play in the elimination of effector T cells in certain immunologically privileged tissue sites. FasL is constitutively expressed by nonlymphoid cells in the eye and testis, tissue sites in which inflammatory T cell responses might be severely crippling or block reproductive capability, respectively. The expression of FasL in these sites stimulates AICD in infiltrating effector cells, and provides a back-up mechanism to maintain self-tolerance in these tissues (75). There is considerable interest in harnessing the physiologic mechanisms that mediate AICD, either through Fas or related members of the TNF receptor superfamily, such as death receptor 4 or 5, to eliminate autoreactive cells.

Natural Killer Cells

NK cells constitute a third class of lymphoid cell that mediates genetically unrestricted, antigen nonspecific cytotoxicity of selected cellular targets without the need for prior activation or immunization (76). NK cells therefore constitute an important component of the innate immune system. Constituting 5% to 20% of circulating lymphocytes in adults, NK cells may form a first line of defense against viral infection and malignancy. NK cells contain large intracellular granules that contain perforin and granzymes. The cytotoxic potential of these cells is analogous to that of CD8+ effector cells, although the signals that stimulate cytotoxic activity are distinct. Two general types of cell surface receptors regulate the cytolytic activity of NK cells: Fc receptors and MHC class I–specific receptors (77). Most NK cells express CD16 (FcγRIII), the low-affinity IgG Fc receptor (also found on neutrophils), and as such, these cells can mediate antibody-dependent cellular cytotoxicity through IgG bound to cellular targets. Although NK cells lack most components of the CD3–TCR complex, they express the CD3 ζ chain, which forms a complex with CD16 and mediates signal transduction through this receptor. NK cells do not express the remaining CD3 chains on the cell surface or rearrange TCR genes, and therefore lack the clonally-restricted antigenic specificities of T cells. Accordingly, NK cells do not require a thymus for development. NK cells resemble certain types of γ/δ T cells that populate epithelial surfaces, which do express a complete complement of CD3 signaling components, but use a single, monospecific rearranged TCR for target recognition.

NK cells recognize MHC class I molecules through two different families of receptors: CD94 and its homologues, and the killer inhibitory receptors (78). These receptors contain immunoreceptor tyrosine activation motifs (ITIMs) in their cytoplasmic tails, and thus, transmit a negative signal to the NK cell when they bind class I MHC molecules on potential targets. Cells that lose class I expression are targeted for NK-mediated cytotoxicity by loss of this inhibitory signaling. This "missing self" strategy affords the immune system a mechanism to destroy cells infected with certain pathogens that suppress class I expression as a means to subvert their recognition by CD8+ T cells. Similarly, this permits the elimination of malignant cells that may otherwise escape immune surveillance by down-regulating class I MHC molecules. The cytolytic function of NK cells can be greatly augmented by their activation with IL-2, IL-12, or type 1 (IFN-α and IFN-β) and type 2 (IFN-γ) interferons. Little is known about NK cell precursors, but these cells are believed to develop primarily in the bone marrow.

In addition to their cytolytic activity, NK cells contribute to the immune response through noncytolytic mechanisms (79). For example, under the influence of IL-12 and TNF-α, these cells secrete large amounts of IFN-γ, which can activate other effector cells of the innate immune system and facilitate T_H1 cell differentiation. Recently, NK cells have also been reported to play a critical role in the differentiation of CD8+ cytotoxic effector T cells through mechanisms not yet understood.

MOLECULAR REGULATION OF LYMPHOCYTE FUNCTION

Cell Surface Receptors and Cell-Cell Interactions

Both B and T cells require more than simple antigen receptor ligation for effective activation. At rest, neither expresses the appropriate counterreceptor necessary to bind the accessory molecules on the other. A resting, unprimed B cell, even if it has taken up and processed an appropriate antigen, fails to activate a T cell productively. Conversely, a resting T cell fails to provide help for B-cell activation. However, with activation, both cell types increase the levels of appropriate counterreceptors and can stimulate the other for a maximal response.

Lymphocytes that encounter antigen outside of the context of an inflammatory response do not receive a signal from the accessory receptors and are not productively activated, protecting the host from attack on their own tissues. However, in inflammation, cytokines such as TNF and IL-1 can induce the necessary counterreceptors on APCs, signaling the lymphocyte that antigens encountered in this context are likely to be dangerous. The accessory receptors and their counterligands have added importance, because they are likely to be clinically useful in therapeutic up- or down-regulation of immune responses.

The site of contact with antigen may provide an initial activation context. In a lymph node draining a site of infection, dendritic cells are activated by inflammatory cytokines and become very efficient APCs for T cells (2). A blood-borne antigen will filter through the marginal zone of the spleen, activating primed B cells residing there, which also are effective at presenting antigen to T cells. The activated T cell can now interact with an appropriate B cell in a cooperative activation (Fig. 15.8). As discussed previously,

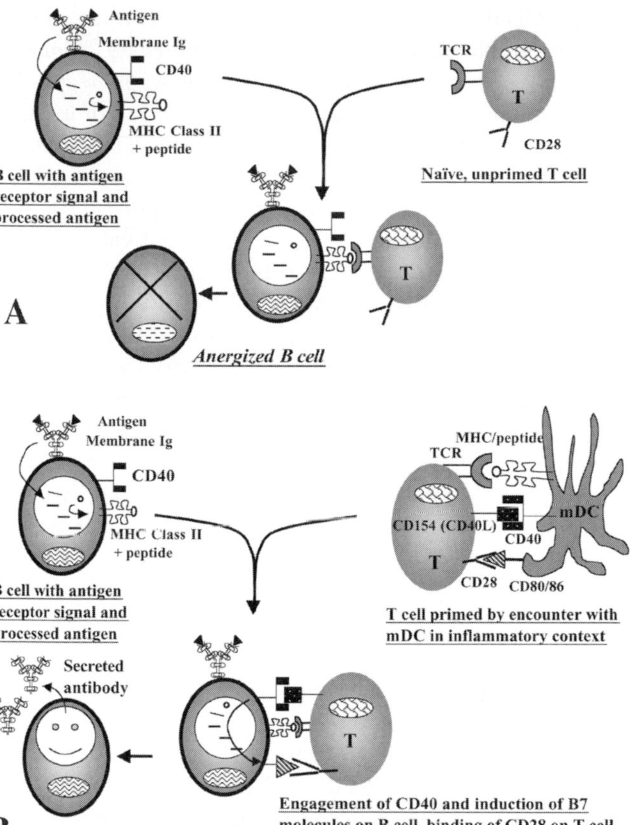

FIG. 15.8. T and B cell collaboration. If a B cell encounters an appropriate antigen, this binds the membrane immunoglobulin (*Ig*) on the surface of the B cell, which triggers antigen receptor signaling. As illustrated in Fig. 15.2, the antigen is taken up, degraded, and brought back to the B cell surface in a complex with major histocompatibility complex (MHC) class II. The peptide–MHC complex may be recognized by a T cell expressing an appropriate T cell receptor. **A:** If the T cell has not been previously activated, then the T cell will not express the surface coreceptors required for productive activation of the B cell. Binding of the B cell antigen receptor, membrane Ig, in the absence of additional signals from coreceptors results in B cell anergy. **B:** In contrast, previous exposure of the T cell to an activated antigen-presenting cell results in new expression of CD154 (CD40L) on the T cell. If the B cell, which has bound and processed antigen, is recognized by a primed T cell, the CD154 on the T cell binds the CD40 on the B cell, and the B cell is productively activated. In addition, the B cell is now induced to express CD80/86 (B7) on its surface, which binds CD28 on the T cell. B and T cells both require signals from both their antigen receptors and from coreceptors for productive activation.

the type of initial stimulus the T cell receives helps determine what type of effector cell that cell becomes. In either case, the T cell becomes activated and expresses a new cell surface molecule, CD154, also known as gp39 or CD40L (80). This is the counterreceptor for CD40, a member of the TNF receptor superfamily, which is present on resting B cells. The CD154 on the activated T cell is now available to bind CD40 on the B cell. Binding of CD40 provides a viability signal so that the B cell is protected from programmed cell death, induces switching to IgG and IgE immunoglobulin isotypes, and favors induction of memory B cells over differentiation to plasma cells. The combination of binding of antigen to the membrane immunoglobulin and of CD154 to CD40 also induces expression of new molecules on the surface of the B cell. One of these is CD80 (B7.1). This is the counterreceptor for CD28, which is expressed on T cells (81). Binding of CD28 on the T cell now sends a signal to the T cell that acts in synergy with the TCR to induce a large increase in cytokine production by the T cell, particularly IL-2 (82). Thus, effective T cell/B cell collaboration requires induction of expression of new counterligands on the surface of both cell types that bind their reciprocal accessory receptors on the respective cells. Once this occurs, the accessory receptors, in concert with the antigen receptors, activate the cells to carry out their effector functions.

Other regulated receptor ligand couples are also induced. Binding of CD40 on the B cell induces expression of another molecule on the B cell, CD95 ligand (CD154, Fas ligand). This binds to CD95 (Fas) on T cells. Normally, binding of CD95 ligand induces cell death. However, B cells that have received a signal from their antigen receptor as well as through CD40 are protected—but if not, they die. This provides a mechanism for prevention of activation of B cells that are not triggered by antigen. At a latter stage in activation, binding of CD28 sends a message to the T cell to express CD152 (CTLA-4). This also binds CD80, but with even higher affinity than CD28. For this reason, a soluble CTLA4 fusion protein, CTLA4-Ig, is in clinical development as an inhibitor of the interaction of B7 and CD28. Unlike CD28, CD152 provides a negative signal to the T cell (83). This provides a way to shut down the immune response after productive collaboration has occurred.

Recently, additional, inducible costimulatory molecules of both the TNF receptor superfamily and the B7 family have been described. These appear more important in the later phases of immune responses. This makes them attractive targets for clinical intervention, with the goal of blocking the effector arm of the immune system that is responsible for disease manifestations in autoimmunity. Among the TNF receptor family are death receptor 5, OX40, and 4–1BB. Additional B7 family ligands are ICOS and PD-1. Specific members of either family can act as either positive or negative regulators. Evidence for effectiveness in animal models of autoimmunity has been presented for each of these (84,85).

Signal Transduction: Overview

B and T lymphocytes share common mechanisms of signal transduction that can be summarized by three themes (Fig. 15.9). First, recognition of antigen by the antigen receptor (surface Ig on B cells or the TCR on T cells) induces the phosphorylation of cytosolic proteins and membrane glycolipids. Second, activation triggers second messenger molecules, with current interest focused on calcium and lipid intermediates. Third, phosphorylation and second messenger molecules regulate the assembly of macromolecular complexes that lead to downstream effects. Ultimately, these processes control the translocation of proteins from the cytosol to the nucleus, where they regulate gene transcription.

Kinases and Phosphatases

Kinases are enzymes that transfer phosphate groups [most commonly from adenosine triphosphate (ATP)] to hydroxyl groups on either tyrosines, or serines and threonines, or glycolipids. The phosphorylation of proteins can regulate enzymatic activity directly or control protein/protein interactions. Phosphorylation of glycolipids can regulate their use as substrates for generation of second messengers and also can regulate interactions with proteins.

Many cytoplasmic signaling proteins have regions called src homology-2 (SH2) domains (named because they share a sequence similar to a portion of the src kinase). The SH2 domains bind to phosphorylated tyrosines. The precise sequence of the SH2 domains from different proteins varies. Different SH2 domains bind with higher affinity to phosphorylated tyrosines flanked by particular amino acids. Thus, SH2 domains from different proteins will bind to different phosphotyrosines, providing a specificity to the interaction. Activation leads to tyrosine phosphorylation of multiple substrates, providing docking sites for SH2-containing proteins. By this means, activation leads to the regulated formation of multimeric protein complexes, the precise members of which are determined by the sequences within different SH2 domains and the amino acids flanking different phosphotyrosines.

None of the lymphocyte receptors considered here are themselves kinases. However, the B and T cell antigen receptors associate with CD79 and CD3, respectively, both of which can bind cytosolic kinases. CD3 and CD79 contain tyrosines with common flanking amino acids and a common spacing. This sequence is called the immunoreceptor tyrosine activation motif (ITAM) and is responsible for binding of tyrosine kinases to the antigen receptor complex in activated cells. Certain accessory receptors contain tyrosines within a different but related sequence, called an ITIM, which, when phosphorylated, binds SH2 domains of phosphatases. These, in general, down-regulate signaling by removing phosphate groups. Thus, lymphocytes are controlled by the different receptors that regulate the balance of cytosolic kinases, which add phosphate groups and promote the formation of protein complexes, and phosphatases, which remove them. This is one of the mechanisms by which antigen receptor and accessory receptor signals are integrated to determine the fate of the cell.

The lipid kinases add phosphate groups to the inositol carbohydrate ring attached to the phosphatidylinositol

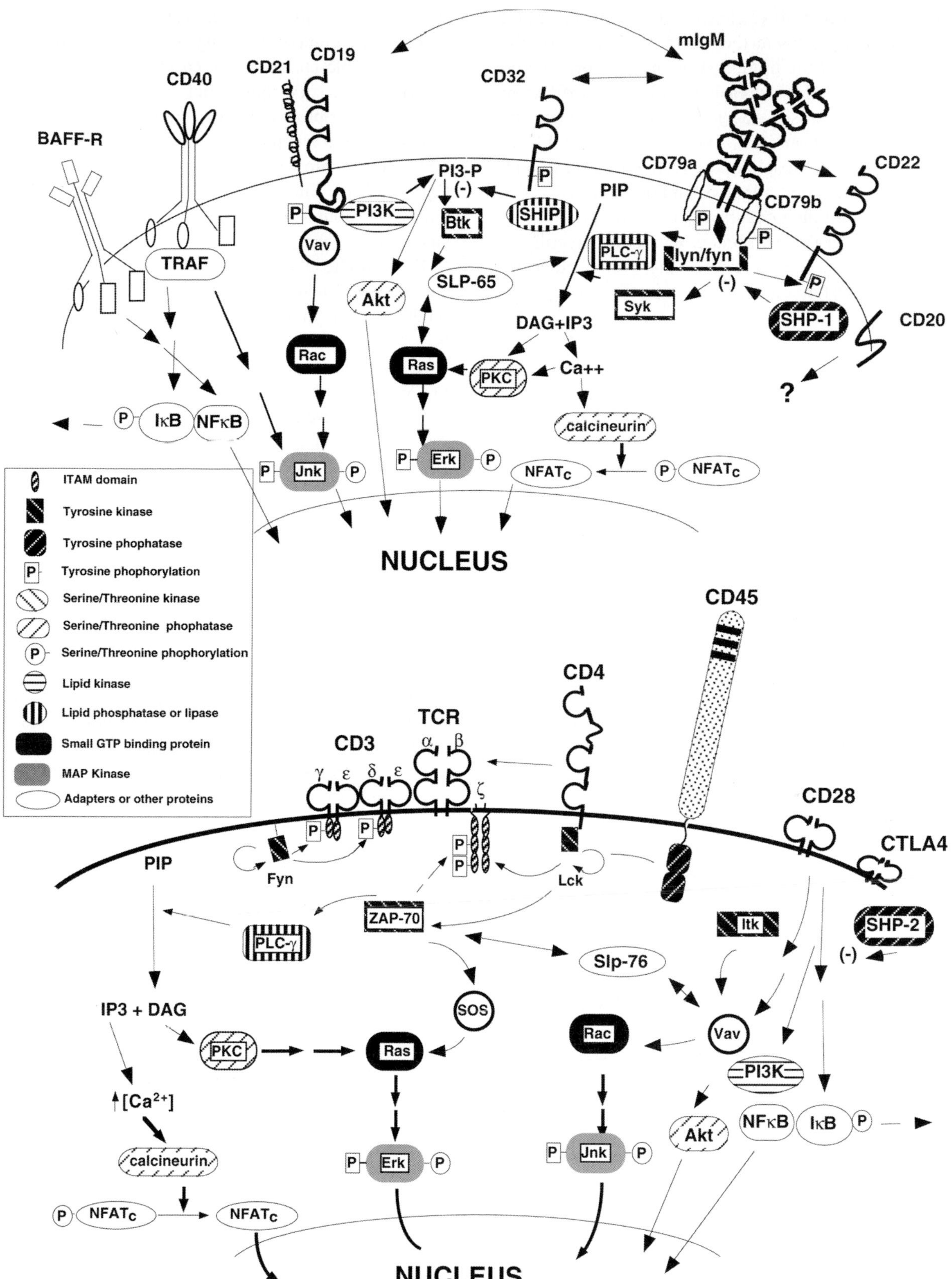

FIG. 15.9. Signal transduction in B and T cells. Different signaling molecules are illustrated according to their class. Only selected protein phosphorylation is shown. *DAG*, diacylglycerol; *IP3*, inositol trisphosphate; *mIgM*, membrane immunoglobulin; *PIP3*, phosphatidylinositol trisphosphate; ↔, associations between proteins.

glycolipids. Phospholipase C cleaves phosphatidylinositol that has phosphate groups at the 4 and 5 positions on the inositol ring. Some of the lipid kinases increase production of this substrate, thereby increasing signaling. A different kinase, phosphatidylinositol 3-kinase, phosphorylates the inositol at the 3 position (86). These products no longer serve as substrates for phospholipase C, but are able to bind to a protein domain called a Pleckstrin homology (PH) domain. This type of binding occurs as part of the assembly of protein complexes at the membrane, where the glycolipids are found, and can directly activate kinases and other enzymes containing PH domains.

Second Messengers

Phospholipase C acts on one of the lipids in the plasma membrane—phosphatidylinositol 4,5-bisphosphate—and cleaves it into two products: inositol phosphate and diacylglycerol. The former opens channels in the endoplasmic reticulum, releasing stores of sequestered calcium into the cytoplasm. The increase in calcium has several effects. Binding of calcium to calmodulin controls the translocation of a transcription factor, nuclear factor of activated T cells, into the nucleus (this is the pathway regulated by cyclosporine). Calcium and diacylglycerol activate a type of serine kinase, protein kinase C, of which there are multiple isoforms, which regulate multiple signaling pathways linked to regulation of other transcription elements.

Assembly of Protein Complexes

Among the molecules that are first phosphorylated on tyrosine after T- or B-cell antigen receptor ligation are the adapter proteins, SLP-76 and SLP-65, respectively (87,88). These cytoplasmic molecules have no enzymatic activity themselves, but contain tyrosines and SH2 and other protein-binding domains. The phosphorylated tyrosines and SH2 domains on the adapter bind SH2 domains and phosphorylated tyrosines, respectively, on other molecules. These interactions, regulated by the phosphorylation of the tyrosines, lead to the assembly of complexes of proteins. The adapters act as scaffolding for this assembly, which results in activation of the associated proteins. For example, adapters bring together kinases, such as zap-70 or syk and their substrates. The adapters also may control the intracellular localization of these assemblies. For some enzymes, being near the plasma membrane is important for their activation, and this is controlled by adapters.

Antigen Receptor Signal Transduction

Although the nature of the antigenic structures recognized by the B and T cell antigen receptors are distinct, they share important structural and functional features. Both are multisubunit complexes comprising two functional components: variable chains involved in antigen recognition and invariant accessory chains that are required both for transport of the receptors to the cell surface and for the signaling function of the receptor (Fig. 15.9). The membrane immunoglobulin component of the BCR associates with CD79 (Igα and Igβ). The α/β heterodimer of the TCR associates with CD3 subunits (CD3δ, CD3ϵ, CD3γ, and CD3ζ). Tyrosine kinases can constitutively associate with CD3 and CD79 in a phosphorylation-independent manner in unactivated cells. When the TCR or membrane immunoglobulin binds antigen, there is clustering of receptor complexes, bringing multiple CD3 or CD79 and associated kinases together. The kinases phosphorylate the tyrosines in the ITAMs on nearby CD3 or CD79 subunits. These form the hub for the assembly of an activated signaling complex. The phosphorylated ITAMs on CD3 and CD79 on T and B cells recruit and activate the related cytosolic tyrosine kinases, zap-70 and syk, respectively (89). These phosphorylate tyrosines on other cytoplasmic molecules that are not part of the antigen receptor complex. The targets for phosphorylation by zap-70 or syk include adapter proteins, cytosolic enzymes, or transmembrane molecules (90,91).

The increase in the tyrosine phosphorylation of cytosolic proteins is dramatic and occurs within seconds of aggregation of lymphocyte antigen receptors. SLP-65 and SLP-76 are phosphorylated by the syk and zap-70 kinases activated by the B and T cell antigen receptor complexes, respectively. These provide the scaffolding for the formation of a signaling complex that includes other adapter molecules, phospholipase C, and kinases. The complexes are critical for the activation of phospholipase C. As described earlier, activation of phospholipase C leads to the release of the second messengers diacylglycerol and inositol phosphate. The resulting increase in calcium peaks after approximately 1 minute, but remains elevated for a prolonged plateau phase.

Another set of enzymes regulated by lymphocyte antigen receptors through adapter molecules are the small guanosine triphosphate (GTP)-binding proteins, the most well known of which is Ras (92). These control, through association, a series of downstream kinases, collectively known as MAPKs, including extracellular signal response kinase (ERK) and Jun N-terminal kinase (JNK). The presence of a series of enzymatic steps allows amplification of signal. The final enzymes in the cascades, once activated, move to the nucleus, where they phosphorylate nuclear transcription factors, particularly members of the AP-1 complex that is associated with many genes that are turned on quickly after lymphocyte activation.

Thus, these various signaling pathways, activated by B and T cell antigen receptor signaling, regulate the activation of new gene transcription that leads to later cellular responses. However, the pathways also are controlled by the lymphocyte accessory receptors. By controlling these signal transduction pathways, the accessory receptors control genes turned on in response to antigen, according to the context in which antigen is bound.

Accessory Receptor Function

Antigen binding by the B cell or TCR is insufficient for activation of a complete program of B or T cell responses. Indeed, antigen receptor binding in the absence of activation of secondary or accessory signaling pathways is an important mechanism for lymphocyte inactivation. We consider here the function of several B cell and T cell accessory receptors, some of which were introduced above. Many other surface molecules have been described, including some with important roles in regulating antigen receptor signaling (93).

B-Cell Accessory Receptor Function

CD19/CD21

CD19 and CD21 are found together on the surface of the B cell. Deficiency of either results in decreased survival of B cells in the germinal center reaction and poor antibody responses to protein antigens (94,95). The physical association and their common physiologic function have led to the hypothesis that they function together, although this has yet to be proven definitively. CD21 binds to the cleavage fragment of the complement protein C3 that becomes covalently linked to antigen in immune complexes. If a B cell encounters an immune complex containing an antigen that binds to the antigen receptor on that cell, and CD21 binds to the C3dg fragment covalently linked to the immune complex, then the immune complex would physically bridge the antigen receptor with CD21. *In vitro,* such cross-linking of CD21 and the antigen receptor provides a powerful enhancement of B-cell activation. However, CD21 has a relatively short cytoplasmic tail, whereas that of CD19 has a relatively long cytoplasmic domain. CD19 may function as a signal transduction subunit for the CD19–CD21 complex, although each also may be independently competent for certain functions.

The cytoplasmic domain of CD19 contains nine tyrosine residues and acts like an adapter molecule, except that it is regulated by extracellular events (96). The tyrosines become phosphorylated when the B-cell antigen receptor is bound. The phosphorylated tyrosines bind to SH2 domains of cytoplasmic proteins, including phosphatidylinositol 3-kinase and Vav. As described earlier, phosphatidylinositol 3-kinase, like other kinases, transfers a phosphate group from ATP to the 3 position on the inositol sugar head group on the plasma membrane glycolipid phosphatidylinositol, which then binds proteins that contain PH domains. Such binding can result in a shift of cytosolic proteins to the plasma membrane, where the phosphatidylinositol 3-phosphate groups are located. The range of signaling pathways regulated by phosphatidylinositol 3-kinase, directly or indirectly, includes tyrosine kinases (Btk), serine kinases (protein kinase C and Akt), and MAPKs. The other cytosolic protein that binds to CD19, Vav, regulates small GTP-binding proteins and is important in the generation of calcium fluxes and MAPK activation.

CD32 (Fc Receptor)

CD32 binds the Fc portion of IgG molecules. The affinity is relatively low, so significant binding occurs only when IgG is present on a fixed array, such as in an immune complex. If the B cell binds to antigen in an immune complex that contains IgG, CD32 and the antigen receptor will be effectively bridged. CD32 has a cytoplasmic tyrosine in an ITIM motif that becomes phosphorylated only on such coligation with the antigen receptor. A cytosolic phosphatase, SHIP, binds to this phosphotyrosine. SHIP removes phosphate groups from inositol and thereby down-regulates cellular activation (97,98). CD32 dampens the responses of B lymphocytes to antigens that are already coated with IgG.

CD40

Unlike the accessory receptors described earlier, CD40 can function independent of the antigen receptor (21). Its role in regulation of B-cell activation, T-cell/B-cell collaboration, germinal center formation, and antibody class switching were described earlier. CD40 is a member of the TNF receptor family. These have no intrinsic enzymatic activity (CD40 does not even have cytoplasmic tyrosines). When members of this family bind their ligands, they form trimers. This favors association with cytoplasmic signaling molecules called TNF receptor–associated factors (TRAFs). At least four of these bind CD40, but they are linked to different downstream signaling pathways (99). These include the MAPK pathways previously described (the ERK, JNK, and p38 families) and NFκB. The latter is a nuclear transcription factor that is held in the cytoplasm by an inhibitory factor, IκB. Phosphorylation of IκB, which is regulated in part by a TRAF associated with CD40, leads to the degradation of IκB. NFκB then is free to move to the nucleus and regulate gene transcription. Other members of the TNF receptor superfamily, discussed in relation to B cell differentiation and effector functions, signal through similar pathways.

T-Cell Accessory Receptors

An important feature distinguishing TCRs and BCRs is recognition by the former of a complex of antigenic peptide and MHC molecules displayed by the APC. Recognition of the MHC–antigenic peptide complex alone by the TCR is a poor stimulus for T cell activation. Engagement of the coreceptor molecules CD4 or CD8 on MHC class II– or class

I–restricted T cell lineages, respectively, is critical for efficient signal transduction through the TCR. In addition, costimulatory receptors for ligands expressed on the APC modulate the effects of T cell antigen recognition through the generation of "second signals" that control T-cell activation and differentiation.

CD4 and CD8

CD4 and CD8 cell surface proteins are differentially expressed by the two predominant lineages of αβ T cells (100). CD4 is a single-chain molecule composed of four extracellular Ig-like domains and a cytoplasmic domain that associates with the tyrosine kinase Lck. The extracellular portion of CD4 binds an invariant portion of the MHC class II molecule away from the antigenic peptide binding site, and thus associates with the MHC–antigenic peptide/TCR complex during T cell antigen recognition. The recruitment of CD4 into the TCR complex is required to bring Lck into proximity to its ITAM phosphorylation targets on the intracytoplasmic domains of the TCR complex (CD3 subunits and ζ-chain homodimer) (101). The exact targets for Lck phosphorylation on the antigen-activated TCR complex are not clear, because the Fyn kinase also participates in the early phosphorylation of ITAMs in the TCR complex. However, CD4-asssociated Lck appears to be the principal kinase that phosphorylates the ZAP-70 kinase after its recruitment to phosphotyrosines on the ζ chain. Thus, the CD4 coreceptor plays a critical role in the initiation and propagation of signaling through the TCR complex. It has been estimated that the participation of the CD4 coreceptor enhances TCR signaling approximately 100-fold. Accordingly, antibodies that block the interaction of CD4 with MHC class II strongly inhibit CD4 T cell activation.

Although the structure of CD8 is different from CD4, its function in TCR signaling parallels that of CD4. CD8 is typically a heterodimer composed of α and β chains, each containing a single Ig-like extracellular domain. Some T cells, particularly those that are resident in epithelial surfaces such as the gut, may express a homodimer of CD8 α chains in the absence of CD8 β chains. The extracellular domain of CD8 contains a binding site for an invariant region of MHC class I molecules homologous to that of the CD4 binding site on MHC class II. Like CD4, CD8 binds Lck through the cytoplasmic tail of the α chain, and thus recruits Lck to the TCR signaling complex during antigenic activation. The phosphorylation targets for CD4- and CD8-associated Lck appear to be the same, and the enhancement of TCR signaling imparted by CD8 cosignaling parallels that of CD4.

CD28 and CD152 (CTLA-4)

In addition to the specific signal generated by binding of the TCR and CD4 or CD8 to an MHC–peptide complex, naïve or primary T cells have a strict requirement for costimulatory signaling through additional cell surface receptors for complete activation (57). The best-studied costimulatory molecules are CD80 and CD86 (B7–1 and B7–2) (102). These are structurally-related homodimeric glycoproteins that are expressed on activated APCs. B7–1 and B7–2 are ligands for the CD28 receptor, which is constitutively expressed by unactivated T cells. Both B7 molecules bind CD28 with comparable affinity, so it is unclear whether these two family members have distinct functional effects. However, their expression patterns differ according to APC type and the signals that induce their expression (103). B7 expression is up-regulated either directly by signals derived from recognition of TLR binding ligands, such as endotoxin, or indirectly by inflammatory mediators such as IL-1.

Signaling through CD28 on T cells shares some features with the B-cell coreceptor complex, CD19/CD21 (104). B7 binding to CD28 recruits and activates the guanine-nucleotide exchange factor Vav, which, in turn, binds and activates the small G protein Rac. Rac activation initiates an MAPK cascade distinct from that activated by the TCR complex. The terminal kinase in this pathway is JNK, which when phosphorylated enters the nucleus and activates the transcription factor Jun. Jun complexes with Fos to form a functional AP-1 transcriptional complex that is required for optimal transcriptional initiation of a number of B- and T-cell gene products.

A second receptor for B7, CD152 (CTLA-4), is induced on antigen-activated T cells and is constitutively expressed by certain Tregs (105,106). CD152 is structurally related to CD28, but has a significantly higher affinity for B7–1 and B7–2. Unlike CD28, signaling through CD152 delivers an inhibitory signal to the activated T cell (107). Given the higher affinity of CD152 for B7–1 and B7–2, and its delayed expression relative to CD28, CD152 probably plays an important role in the termination of T-cell activation. In essence, CD152 provides a molecular brake to the T cell response. CTLA-4 signaling by $CD25^+CD4^+$ Tregs is required for their inhibitory function. The details of the signaling cascade initiated by binding of B7 to CD152 have yet to be defined, but the cytoplasmic tail of CD152 is highly conserved between species, and contains an ITIM motif that binds the tyrosine phosphatase SHP-2 as well as activating serine phosphatases. Thus, CD152 appears to preferentially bind B7 late in the T-cell activation process to activate phosphatases that down-regulate T cell activation. Other members of the B7/CD28/CTLA-4 family, ICOS/B7h and PD-1/PD-L, also control B and T cell differentiation, and may signal similarly (108).

REFERENCES

1. Paramithiotis E, Cooper M. Memory B lymphocytes migrate to bone marrow in humans. *Proc Natl Acad Sci U S A* 1997;94:208.
2. Banchereau J, Steinman RM. Dendritic cells and the control of immunity. *Nature* 1998;392:245.
3. MacLennan ICM. Germinal centers. *Annu Rev Immunol* 1994;12:117.

4. McGhee JR. The mucosal immune system. In: Paul WE, ed. *Fundamental immunology.* Philadelphia: Raven, 1999:909.
5. Lam K-P, Rajewsky K. B cell antigen receptor specificity and surface density together determine B-1 versus B-2 cell development. *J Exp Med* 1999;190:471.
6. Baggiolini M. Chemokines and leukocyte traffic. *Nature* 1998;392:565.
7. Ward SG, Bacon K, Westwick J. Chemokines and T lymphocytes: more than an attraction. *Immunity* 1998;9:1.
8. Butcher EC, Picker LJ. Lymphocyte homing and homeostasis. Science 1996;272:60.
9. Ghia P, ten Boekel E, Rolink AG, et al. B-cell development: a comparison between mouse and man. *Immunol Today* 1998;19:480.
10. Loffert D, Ehlich A, Muller W, et al. Surrogate light chain expression is required to establish immunoglobulin heavy chain allelic exclusion during early B cell development. *Immunity* 1996;4:133.
11. ten Boekel E, Melchers F, Rolink AG. Precursor B cells showing allelic inclusion display allelic exclusion at the level of pre-B cell receptor surface expression. *Immunity* 1998;8:199.
12. Melchers F. Fit for life in the immune system? Surrogate L chain tests H chains that test L chains. *Proc Natl Acad Sci U S A* 1999;96:2571–2573.
13. Rolink AG, Brocker T, Bluethmann H, et al. Mutations affecting either generation or survival of cells influence the pool size of mature B cells. *Immunity* 1999;10:619.
14. Hayakawa K, Asano M, Shinton SA, et al. Positive selection of natural autoreactive B cells. *Science* 1999;285:113.
15. Retter MW, Nemazee D. Receptor editing occurs frequently during normal B cell development. *J Exp Med* 1998;188:1231.
16. Nussenzweig M. Immune receptor editing: revise and select. *Cell* 1998;95:875.
17. Pillai S. The chosen few: positive selection and the generation of naive B lymphocytes. *Immunity* 1999;10:493.
18. Wagner SD, Neuberger MS. Somatic hypermutation of immunoglobulin genes. *Annu Rev Immunol* 1996;14:441.
19. Kuppers R, Zhao M, Hansmann ML, et al. Tracing B cell development in human germinal centres by molecular analysis of single cells picked from histological sections. *EMBO J* 1993;12:4955–4967.
20. Batista FD, Neuberger MS. Affinity dependence of the B cell response to antigen: threshold, a ceiling, and the importance of off-rate. *Immunity* 1998;8:751.
21. Vogel LA, Noelle RJ. CD40 and its crucial role as a member of the TNFR family. *Semin Immunol* 1998;10:435.
22. Rajewsky K. Clonal selection and learning in the antibody system. *Nature* 1996;381:751.
23. Schatz DG. Developing B-cell theories. *Nature* 1999;400:614–615, 617.
24. Kench JA, Russell DM, Nemazee D. Efficient peripheral clonal elimination of B lymphocytes in MRL/lpr mice bearing autoantibody transgenes. *J Exp Med* 1998;188:909–917.
25. Aluvihare VR, Khamlichi AA, Williams GT, et al. Acceleration of intracellular targeting of antigen by the B-cell antigen receptor: importance depends on the nature of the antigen-antibody interaction. *EMBO J* 1997;16:3553–3562.
26. Chan OT, Hannum LG, Haberman AM, et al. A novel mouse with B cells but lacking serum antibody reveals an antibody-independent role for B cells in murine lupus. *J Ext Med* 1999;189:1639.
27. Janeway CA, Travers P, Walport M, et al. The thymus and the development of T lymphocytes. In: Janeway CA, Travers P, Walport M, et al., eds. *Immunobiology: the immune system in health and disease.* New York: Garland Publishing, 1999:227.
28. Medzhitov R, Janeway CA Jr. Innate immunity: impact on the adaptive immune response. *Curr Opin Immunol* 1997;9:4–9.
29. von Boehmer H, Fehling HJ. Structure and function of the pre-T cell receptor. *Annu Rev Immunol* 1997;15:433.
30. Padovan E, Casorati G, Dellabona P, et al. Expression of two T cell receptor alpha chains: dual receptor T cells. *Science* 1993;262:422.
31. Hardardottir F, Baron JL, Janeway CA Jr. T cells with two functional antigen-specific receptors. *Proc Natl Acad Sci U S A* 1995;92:354.
32. Jameson SC, Hogquist KA, Bevan MJ. Positive selection in the thymus. *Ann Rev Immunol* 1995;13:93.
33. Ellmeier W, Sawada S, Littman DR. The regulation of CD4 and CD8 coreceptor gene expression during T cell development. *Annu Rev Immunol* 1999;17:523.
34. Bevan MJ. In thymic selection, peptide diversity gives and takes away. *Immunity* 1997;7:175.
35. Sprent J, Webb SR. Intrathymic and extrathymic clonal deletion of T cells. *Curr Opin Immunol* 1995;7:196.
36. Ford WL, Gowans JL. The traffic of lymphocytes. *Semin Hematol* 1969;6:67.
37. Picker LJ, Siegelman MH. Lymphoid tissues and organs. In: Paul WE, ed. *Fundamental immunology.* Philadelphia: Raven, 1999;479.
38. Mellman I, Steinman RM. Dendritic cells: specialized and regulated antigen processing machines. *Cell* 2001;106:255.
39. Pamer E, Cresswell P. Mechanisms of MHC class I–restricted antigen processing. *Annu Rev Immunol* 1998;16:323.
40. Ahmed R, Gray D. Immunological memory and protective immunity: understanding their relation. *Science* 1996;272:54.
41. Mosmann TR, Coffman RL. T_H1 and T_H2 cells: different patterns of lymphokine secretion lead to different functional properties. *Annu Rev Immunol* 1989;7:145.
42. Fiorentino DF, Bond MW, Mosmann TR. Two types of mouse T helper cell. IV. Th2 clones secrete a factor that inhibits cytokine production by Th1 clones. *J Exp Med* 1989;170:2081.
43. O'Garra A, Murphy K. Role of cytokines in determining T-lymphocyte function. *Curr Opin Immunol* 1994;6:458.
44. Paul WE, Seder RA. Lymphocyte responses and cytokines. *Cell* 1994; 76:241–251.
45. Abbas AK, Murphy KM, Sher A. Functional diversity of helper T lymphocytes. *Nature* 1996;383:787.
46. Murphy KM. T lymphocyte differentiation in the periphery. *Curr Opin Immunol* 1998;10:226.
47. Szabo SJ, Jacobson NG, Dighe AS, et al. Developmental commitment to the Th2 lineage by extinction of IL-12 signaling. *Immunity* 1995;2: 665–675.
48. Nelms K, Keegan AD, Zamorano J, et al. The IL-4 receptor: signaling mechanisms and biologic functions. *Annu Rev Immunol* 1999;17:701.
49. Leonard WJ. STATs and cytokine specificity. *Nat Med* 1996;2:968.
50. Sprent J. T and B memory cells. *Cell* 1994;76:315–322.
51. Trowbridge IS, Thomas ML. CD45: an emerging role as a protein tyrosine phosphatase required for lymphocyte activation and development. *Annu Rev Immunol* 1994;12:85–116.
52. Mason D, Powrie F. Memory CD4+ T cells in man form two distinct subpopulations, defined by their expression of isoforms of the leucocyte common antigen, CD45. *Immunology* 1990;70:427–133.
53. Derbinski J, Schulte A, Kyewski G, et al. Promiscuous gene expression in medullary thymic epithelial cells mirrors the peripheral self. *Nat Immunol* 2001;2:1032–1039.
54. Bjorses P, Aaltonen J, Horelli-Kuitunen N, et al. Gene defect behind APECED: a new clue to autoimmunity. *Hum Mol Genet* 1998;7: 1547–1553.
55. Anderson MS, Venanzi ES, Klein L, et al. Projection of an immunological self shadow within the thymus by the aire protein. *Science* 2002;298:1395–1401.
56. Liston A, Lesage S, Wilson J, et al. Aire regulates negative selection of organ-specific T cells. *Nat Immunol* 2003;4:350.
57. Schwartz RH. Costimulation of T lymphocytes: the role of CD28, CTLA-4, and B7/BB1 in interleukin-2 production and immunotherapy. *Cell* 1992;71:1065.
58. Medzhitov R, Janeway CA Jr. Decoding the patterns of self and nonself by the innate immune system. *Science* 2002;296:298.
59. Hoebe K, Du X, Georgel P, et al. Identification of Lps2 as a key transducer of MyD88-independent TIR signalling. *Nature* 2003;424: 743.
60. Mueller DL, Jenkins MK, Schwartz RH. An accessory cell-derived costimulatory signal acts independently of protein kinase C activation to allow T cell proliferation and prevent the induction of unresponsiveness. *J Immunol* 1989;142:2617.
61. Schwartz RH. T cell anergy. *Annu Rev Immunol* 2003;21:305.
62. Matzinger P. Tolerance, danger, and the extended family. *Annu Rev Immunol* 1994;12:991.
63. Sakaguchi S. Regulatory T cells: key controllers of immunologic selftolerance. *Cell* 2000;101:455.
64. Chen Y, Kuchroo VK, Inobe J, et al. Regulatory T cell clones induced by oral tolerance: suppression of autoimmune encephalomyelitis. *Science* 1994;265:1237.
65. Groux H, O'Garra A, Bigler M, et al. A CD4+ T-cell subset inhibits antigen-specific T-cell responses and prevents colitis. *Nature* 1997; 389:737.
66. Shevach EM. Regulatory T cells in autoimmmunity. *Annu Rev Immunol* 2000;18:423.

67. Hori S, Nomura T, Sakaguchi S. Control of regulatory T cell development by the transcription factor Foxp3. *Science* 2003;299:1057–1061.
68. Fontenot JD, Gavin MA, Rudensky AY. Foxp3 programs the development and function of CD4+CD25+ regulatory T cells. *Nat Immunol* 2003;4:330.
69. Groux H. Type 1 T-regulatory cells: their role in the control of immune responses. *Transplantation* 2003;75(suppl):8.
70. Wakkach A, Fournier N, Brun V, et al. Characterization of dendritic cells that induce tolerance and T regulatory 1 cell differentiation *in vivo*. *Immunity* 2003;18:605.
71. Weiner HL, Friedman A, Miller A, et al. Oral tolerance: immunologic mechanisms and treatment of animal and human organ-specific autoimmune diseases by oral administration of autoantigens. *Ann Rev Immunol* 1994;12:809.
72. Nagata S, Golstein P. The Fas death factor. *Science* 1995;267:1449.
73. Smith CA, Farrah T, Goodwin RG. The TNF superfamily of cellular and viral proteins: activation, costimulation, and death. *Cell* 1994;76: 959–962.
74. Crispe N. Fatal attractions: Fas-induced apoptosis of mature T cells. *Immunity* 1994;1:347.
75. Griffith TS, Ferguson TA. The role of FasL-induced apoptosis in immune privilege. *Immunol Today* 1997;18(5):240.
76. Yokoyama WM. Natural killer cells. In: Paul WE, ed. *Fundamental immunology.* Philadelphia: Raven, 1999:575.
77. Lanier LL. Natural killer cells: from no receptors to too many. *Immunity* 1997;6:371.
78. Lanier LL. NK cell receptors. *Annu Rev Immunol* 1998;16:359.
79. Biron CA, Nguyen KB, Pien GC, et al. Natural killer cells in antiviral defense: function and regulation by innate cytokines. *Annu Rev Immunol* 1999;17:189.
80. Grewal I, Flavell R. CD40 and CD154 in cell-mediated immunity. *Annu Rev Immunol* 1998;16:111.
81. Lenschow DJ, Walunas TL, Bluestone JA. CD28/B7 system of T cell costimulation. *Annu Rev Immunol* 1996;14:233–258.
82. Daikh D, Wofsy D, Imboden JB. The CD28-B7 costimulatory pathway and its role in autoimmune disease. *J Leukoc Biol* 1997;62:156.
83. Boussiotis VA, Freeman GJ, Gribben JG, et al. The role of B7–1/B7–2:CD28/CLTA-4 pathways in the prevention of anergy, induction of productive immunity and down-regulation of the immune response. *Immunol Rev* 1996;153:5.
84. Nurieva RI, Treuting P, Duong J, et al. Inducible costimulator is essential for collagen-induced arthritis. *J Clin Invest* 2003;111:701.
85. Foell J, Strahotin S, O'Neil SP, et al. CD137 costimulatory T cell receptor engagement reverses acute disease in lupus-prone NZB × NZW F1 mice. *J Clin Invest* 2003;111:1505.
86. Fruman DA, Snapper SB, Yballe CM, et al. Impaired B cell development and proliferation in absence of phosphoinositide 3-kinase p85alpha. *Science* 1999;283:393.
87. Fu C, Turck CW, Kurosaki T, et al. BLNK: a central linker protein in B cell activation. *Immunity* 1998;9:93.
88. Clements JL, Yang B, Ross-Barta SE, et al. Requirement for the leukocyte-specific adapter protein SLP-76 for normal T cell development. *Science* 1998;281:416.
89. Jiang A, Craxton A, Kurosaki T, et al. Different protein tyrosine kinases are required for B cell antigen receptor-mediated activation of extracellular signal-regulated kinase, c-Jun NH2-terminal kinase 1, and p38 mitogen-activated protein kinase. *J Exp Med* 1998;188:1297.
90. Reth M, Wienands J. Initiation and processing of signals from the B cell antigen receptor. *Annu Rev Immunol* 1997;15:453.
91. Cantrell D. T cell antigen receptor signal transduction pathways. *Annu Rev Immunol* 1996;14:259.
92. Hashimoto A, Okada H, Jiang A, et al. Involvement of guanosine triphosphatases and phospholipase C-gamma2 in extracellular signal-regulated kinase, c-Jun NH2-terminal kinase, and p38 mitogen-activated protein kinase activation by the B cell antigen receptor. *J Exp Med* 1998;188:1287.
93. Janeway CA, Travers P, Walport M, et al. *Immunobiology: the immune system in health and disease.* New York: Garland Publishing, 1999.
94. Carroll MC. The role of complement and complement receptors in induction and regulation of immunity. *Annu Rev Immunol* 1998;16:545.
95. Tedder T, Inaoki M, Sato S. The CD19-CD21 complex regulates signal transduction thresholds governing humoral immunity and autoimmunity. *Immunity* 1997;6:107.
96. Fearon DT, Carter RH. The CD19/CR2/TAPA-1 complex of B lymphocytes: linking natural to acquired immunity. *Annu Rev Immunol* 1995;13:127.
97. Ono M, Okada H, Bolland S, et al. Deletion of SHIP or SHP-1 reveals two distinct pathways for inhibitory signaling. *Cell* 1997;90:293.
98. Pearse RN, Kawabe T, Bolland S, et al. SHIP recruitment attenuates Fc gamma RIIB-induced B cell apoptosis. *Immunity* 1999;10:753.
99. Lee HH, Dempsey PW, Parks TP, et al. Specificities of CD40 signaling: involvement of TRAF2 in CD40-induced NF-kappaB activation and intercellular adhesion molecule-1 up-regulation. *Proc Natl Acad Sci U S A* 1999;96:1421–1426.
100. Bierer BE, Sleckman BP, Ratnofsky SE, et al. The biologic roles of CD2, CD4, and CD8 in T-cell activation. *Ann Rev Immunol* 1989;7:579.
101. Qian D, Weiss A. T cell antigen receptor signal transduction. *Curr Opin Cell Biol* 1997;9:205.
102. Liu Y, Linsley PS. Costimulation of T-cell growth. *Curr Opin Immunol* 1992;4:265–270.
103. Thompson CB. Distinct roles for the costimulatory ligands B7–1 and B7–2 in T helper cell differentiation? *Cell* 1995;81:979–982.
104. Rudd CE. Upstream-downstream: CD28 cosignaling pathways and T cell function. *Immunity* 1996;4:527.
105. Linsley PS, Brady W, Urnes M, et al. CTLA-4 is a second receptor for the B cell activation antigen B7. *J Exp Med* 1991;174:561–569.
106. Takahashi T, Tagami T, Yamazaki S, et al. Immunologic self-tolerance maintained by CD25(+)CD4(+) regulatory T cells constitutively expressing cytotoxic T lymphocyte-associated antigen 4. *J Exp Med* 2000;192:303–310.
107. Thompson CB, Allison JP. The emerging role of CTLA-4 as an immune attenuator. *Immunity* 1997;7:445.
108. Frauwirth KA, Thompson CB. Activation and inhibition of lymphocytes by costimulation. *J Clin Invest* 2002;109:295.

CHAPTER 16

Structure and Function of Neutrophils

Mark R. Philips and Bruce N. Cronstein

In addition to describing phagocytosis in the closing years of the nineteenth century, Metchnikoff (1) proposed that phagocytic leukocytes may liberate substances that are capable of damaging adjacent tissues. It remained until the middle years of the twentieth century for the demonstration of the critical role of neutrophils in immune-mediated tissue injury. The first experimental proof came in the study of the Arthus reaction: depletion of neutrophils by either nitrogen mustard or heterologous antineutrophil antisera inhibited the Arthus reaction in several species (2). Despite the expected deposition of antigen, antibody, and complement components in the vessels of antiserum-treated animals, no microscopic evidence of vascular injury could be found (3–7). Other experimental models of immunologic injury have been shown to depend on the neutrophil for tissue damage. These models include the necrotizing arteritis of experimental serum sickness in rabbits (8), the proteinuria associated with acute nephrotoxic vasculitis in rats and rabbits (9), and arthritis in rabbits induced by an intraarticular reversed passive Arthus reaction (10). In the last of these experimental systems, intraarticular injections of purified suspensions of neutrophils reconstituted the immunologic lesions in neutrophil-depleted rabbits. Thus, neutrophils, histologically the hallmark of acute inflammation, are important mediators of the inflammatory tissue injury observed in rheumatic diseases.

MYELOPOIESIS AND NEUTROPHIL STRUCTURE

Polymorphonuclear leukocytes (PMNs), also known as granulocytes, are postmitotic, terminally-differentiated phagocytes that constitute the first line of cell-mediated host defense against microorganisms. Three types of granulocytes (neutrophils, eosinophils, and basophils) can be readily distinguished in blood by the staining characteristics of their cytoplasmic granules. Ninety-five percent of granulocytes are neutrophils, which are the most abundant leukocyte in the peripheral circulation. Fifty-five percent to 60% of the hematopoietic capacity of the normal bone marrow is dedicated to the production of neutrophils, which are delivered to the peripheral circulation at a rate of 10^{11} per day (11). This flux can increase dramatically under conditions of stress, such as infection.

Like monocytes, megakaryocytes, and erythrocytes, granulocytes are derived from myeloid stem cells that populate the bone marrow. The first cell committed to granulocyte differentiation is the myeloblast, which differentiates into the neutrophilic promyelocyte, the first dedicated precursor of the neutrophil. Neutrophilic promyelocytes differentiate sequentially into neutrophilic myelocytes, metamyelocytes, band cells, and, finally, mature neutrophils (11). Like all aspects of hematopoiesis, neutrophil differentiation is controlled by a specific set of cytokines and hematopoietic growth factors, the best characterized of which include granulocyte colony stimulating factor (G-CSF) and granulocyte/macrophage colony stimulating factor (GM-CSF) (12,13). Both of these growth factors are now available in recombinant form and have dramatically reduced the mortality associated with cancer chemotherapy by hastening myeloid recovery. Retinoic acid also plays an important role in activating transcriptional programs responsible for neutrophil maturation (14). Clinically, all *trans*-retinoic acid is effective in treating promyelocytic leukemia because of its ability to promote differentiation of leukemic cells. The genes that are activated by cytokines and retinoid acid to promote granulocytic differentiation are under active investigation (15).

Neutrophil precursors through the myelocyte stage undergo mitoses, but once they reach the metamyelocyte stage, they stop dividing. The mitotic and postmitotic stages of neutrophil differentiation in the bone marrow each last approximately 7 days. Once released into the peripheral circulation, the neutrophil half-life is only 6 hours, however (11).

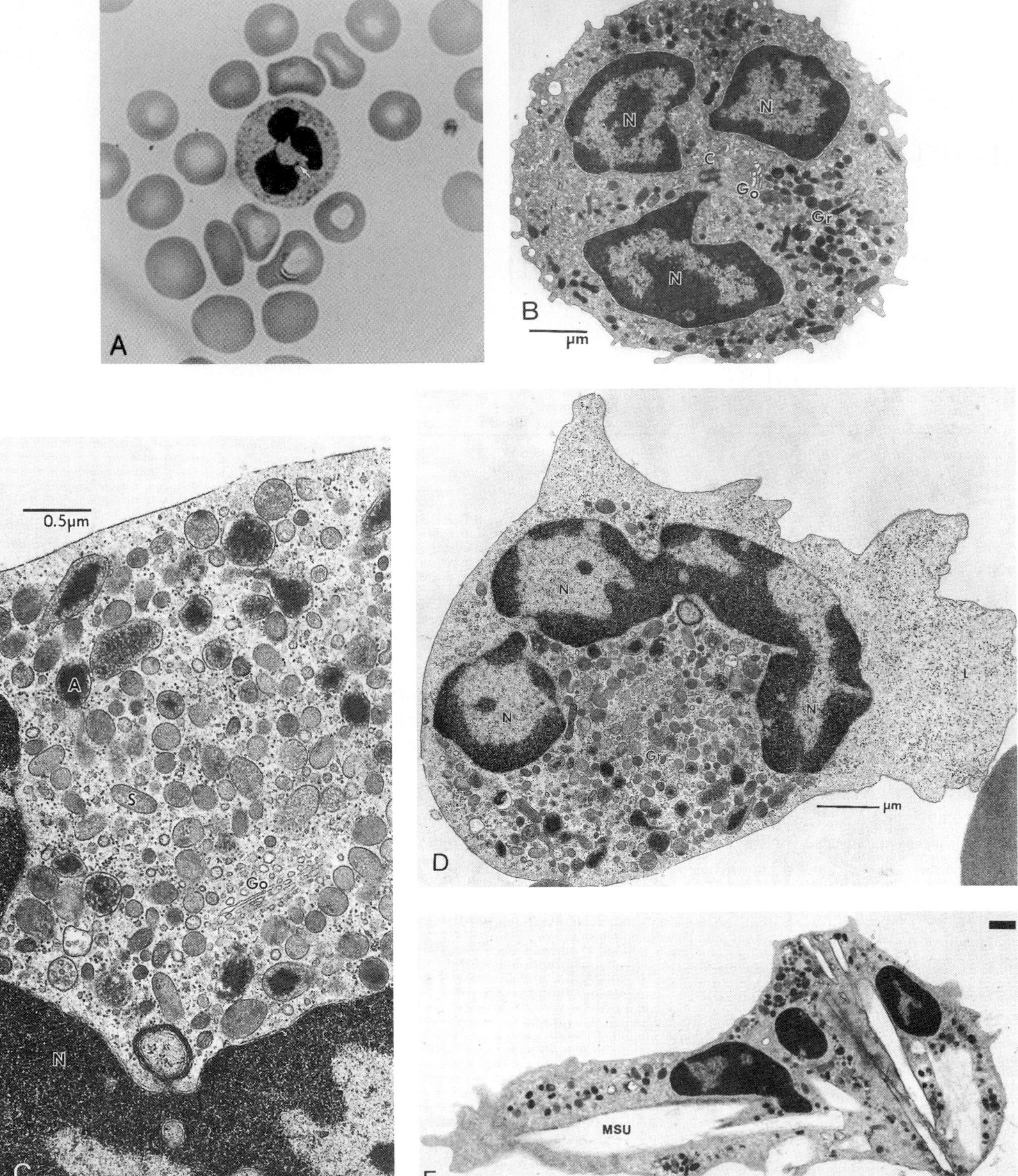

FIG. 16.1. Neutrophil morphology. **A:** Wright-stained smear of human peripheral blood showing a neutrophil surrounded by erythrocytes. The multilobed nucleus and polychromatic cytoplasmic granulations are evident. *Arrow,* Barr body, an appendage of the chromatin that contains the inactive X chromosome of a female subject. **B:** Transmission electron photomicrograph of a neutrophil. **C:** Higher magnification electron photomicrograph of neutrophil cytoplasm revealing granule morphology. **D:** Electron photomicrograph of a polarized neutrophil spreading on a surface, revealing the lamelli podium, or leading edge, which excludes cytoplasmic granules by virtue of its meshwork of actin filaments (not resolved). **E:** Electron photomicrograph of a neutrophil that has ingested monosodium urate crystals (*MSU*) (¥7,600). Markers show 0.5 or 1 mm, as indicated. *A*, azurophilic granule; *C*, centriole; *Go*, Golgi; *Gr*, granules; *L*, lamellipodium; *N,* nucleus; *S*, specific granule. (Photomicrographs in **B–D** courtesy of Dr. Dorothea Zucker-Franklin; photomicrograph in **E** courtesy of Dr. Abby Rich.)

It has recently been appreciated that senescent neutrophils, like appropriately stimulated mitotic cells, undergo a process of programmed cell death known as apoptosis (16). The bulk of apoptotic neutrophils are removed by the reticuloendothelial system (17). The half-life of the small pool of neutrophils that traverse blood vessels and enter tissues, particularly those attracted to sites of inflammation, is unknown.

The most prominent feature of a polychromatically stained (e.g., Wright-stained) neutrophil is its multilobed nucleus containing condensed heterochromatin (Fig. 16.1A). In some neutrophils from females, the inactive X chromosome can be seen attached to one nuclear lobe as a "drumstick" appendage known as a Barr body (arrow in Fig. 16.1A). Relative to mononuclear leukocytes, mature neutrophils are biosynthetically quiescent, consistent with their condensed chromatin, lack of nucleoli, and relative dearth of endoplasmic reticulum. Recent studies have demonstrated that neutrophils are both transcriptionally and translationally active, however, synthesizing gene products that include interleukin (IL)-1α, IL-1β (18), IL-8 (19), tumor necrosis factor (TNF)-α, G-CSF, GM-CSF (20), cRaf-1 (21), complement receptor 1 (CR1), CD11a, immunoglobulin constant region receptor (FcγR), actin, and class I major histocompatibility complex (MHC) molecules (22).

The most prominent feature of neutrophil cytoplasm is the abundance of cytoplasmic granules (Fig. 16.1A–C). These granules serve two critical functions. Their lumina contain a broad spectrum of antimicrobial enzymes and peptides critical for host defense (23), and their membranes contain a mobilizable pool of surface proteins that regulate the inflammatory response (24). Based on morphology and histochemical staining, two types of granules can be distinguished in human neutrophils (Fig. 16.1C). These are the azurophilic and specific granules, named for their staining characteristics and specificity for neutrophilic granulocytes, respectively. Azurophilic granules are specialized lysosomes that are peroxidase positive on electron microscopic analysis. Because azurophilic granules develop first, at the promyelocyte stage, they are also referred to as primary granules. Specific granules are formed during the myelocyte stage of differentiation and are referred to as secondary granules (11). Subcellular fractionation techniques that can readily separate the denser azurophilic granules from specific granules have permitted a detailed analysis of the molecular content of each type of granule (Table 16.1). More recent studies using immunogold electron microscopy to subcategorize peroxidase-negative granules (25) and high-voltage, free-flow electrophoresis to separate plasma membrane from copurifying vesicles (26) have defined four types of neutrophil vesicles that undergo stimulated exocytosis: secretory vesicles (27,28), gelatinase granules (29,30), specific granules, and azurophilic granules. The secretory vesicles are characterized by their endocytosis-derived content of plasma proteins, their copurification with plasma membrane on conventional density gradients, and their extreme lability when isolated neutrophils are warmed or stimulated. The physiologic importance of this newly defined compartment appears to be that it serves as the most important reservoir for surface glycoproteins such as complement receptor 1 (31), CD11b/CD18 (32), cytochrome b_{558} (33), and the formyl peptide receptor (34) that can be rapidly upregulated on the surface of neutrophils exposed to inflammatory stimuli. In addition to serving as a reservoir for surface glycoproteins, secretory vesicles, as well as specific and gelatinase granules, provide an intracellular pool of membrane that can be used to expand the surface area of the cell rapidly as lamellipodia are formed (Fig. 16.2), a process critical for phagocytosis.

Neutrophils are motile and move both randomly and in a directed fashion toward a source of chemoattractant. When a particulate stimulus is encountered by a neutrophil, it is phagocytosed. Both the motile and phagocytic functions of neutrophils depend on the dynamic nature of the actin cytoskeleton. Indeed, cytochalasin B, a fungal metabolite that inhibits actin polymerization, blocks neutrophil motility and phagocytosis. Actin microfilaments are 6 nm in diameter and, in association with myosin, constitute the contractile system of the cell. Microfilaments are prominent in areas of the cell involved in adhesion, motility, and particle ingestion (35). The neutrophil contractile system bears a striking resemblance to that of skeletal muscle. Actin, myosin [with actin-activated Mg^{2+} adenosine triphosphatase (ATPase) activity], actin-binding protein, and a cofactor that allows actin to activate the Mg^{2+} ATPase have all been isolated from phagocytic cells (3). Like most ameboid cells, neutrophils in motion are polarized with a dense meshwork of subplasmalemmal actin filaments at the leading edge, or lamellipodium, that excludes cytoplasmic granules (Fig. 16.1D). The cytoplasmic domains of adhesion molecules of the integrin class serve as organizing centers for actin polymerization, thus linking the extracellular matrix with the intracellular cytoskeleton. Structures formed at the junction of integrins and actin filaments are known as focal adhesion plaques (36) and consist of several actin-associated molecules, including vinculin, talin, and α-actinin (37). In addition to promoting ameboid motion, filamentous webs of actin mediate phagosome formation. During normal phagocytosis, contractions occur in two directions. Contraction occurs under the particle to form an invagination. Because submembranous actin meshworks form a "zone of exclusion" for cytoplasmic granules, the dynamic nature of actin polymerization is critical for degranulation. A second type of actin-mediated movement critical for phagocytosis involves lateral movement of the plasma membrane, which serves to close the phagocytic vacuole, like a purse string.

In addition to actin microfilaments, the neutrophil cytoskeleton is composed of microtubules. Microtubules are polymers of tubulin, a 55-kd protein. The centrioles, located between the Golgi apparatus and the nucleus (Fig.

TABLE 16.1. *Neutrophil granules and their contents*

Constituent classification	Organelle (from least to most readily mobilized for exocytosis)			
	Azurophilic (primary) granule	Specific (secondary) granule	Gelatinase (tertiary) granule	Secretory vesicle
Antimicrobial enzymes	5′-Nucleotidase α-Fucosidase α-Manosidase Acid phosphatase Arylsulfatase Azurocidin β-Glucosaminadase β-Glucuronidase β-Glycerophosphatase **Cathepsins** **Elastase** Lysozyme **Myeloperoxidase** Neuraminadase Phospholipase A **Proteinase 3** Sialidase	**Collagenase** **Heparanase** Histaminase Lysozyme Plasminogen activator Sialidase	Acetyltransferase **Gelatinase**	
Antimicrobial proteins/peptides	Bacterial/permeability-inducing protein Defensins Ubiquitin	hCap 18 Lactoferrin Vitamin B_{12}–binding protein		
Other macromolecules	Chondroitin sulfate Glycosaminoglycans Heparin-binding protein Heparin sulfate	β_2-Microglobulin		
Endocytosis-derived plasma proteins				Albumin Immunoglobulins Transferrin
Membrane-associated proteins	CD63 CD68	CD11b/CD18 CD66 CD67 Cytochrome b_{558} Fibronectin receptor Formyl peptide receptor G protein α subunit Laminin receptor rap1/2 Thrombospondin receptor Tumor necrosis factor receptor Vitronectin receptor	CD11b/CD18 DAG-deacylating enzyme Formyl peptide receptor	Alkaline phosphatase CD11b/CD18 Complement receptor 1 Cytochrome b_{558} Formyl peptide receptor Uroplasminogen activating receptor

Bolded constituents have been implicated in inflammatory tissue damage.

16.1B), have an electron-dense organizing center from which microtubules originate. The microtubules then radiate outward, passing very close to and appearing to graze membrane-bound organelles such as granules (38). The "assembly" and "disassembly" of microtubules are controlled in a variety of ways, both *in vitro* and *in vivo.* Calcium ions promote dissolution of polymerized tubulin, as does decreased pH or osmolality (39). Cyclic guanosine monophosphate (cGMP) and agents that elevate its intracellular levels, such as phorbol myristate acetate and carbamylcholine, promote assembly of tubulin, whereas cyclic 3′,5′-adenosine monophosphate (cAMP) and agents that elevate its intracellular levels, such as prostaglandin E_1 (PGE_1) and isoproterenol, promote disassembly (40). The redox state of the cells also may regulate assembly of microtubules (41). Micromolar concentrations of the plant alkaloids colchicine and vinblastine induce reversible dissolution of microtubules. Studies done with the aid of these

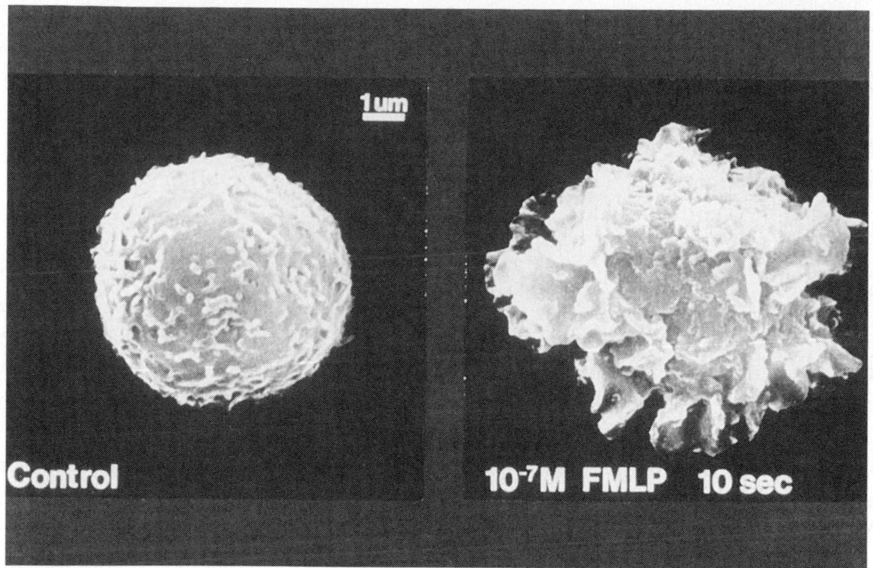

FIG. 16.2. Scanning electron photomicrograph of a human neutrophil in a resting state **(left)** or stimulated with the chemoattractant *N*-formyl-methionyl-leucyl-phenylalanine (*FMLP*) **(right)**, revealing the marked increase in surface area resulting from extensive lamellipodia formation.

agents, especially colchicine, suggest that microtubules play a critical role in degranulation (42).

NEUTROPHIL FUNCTION

Neutrophil function can be divided into early and late events. Early events are those that lead to the recruitment of neutrophils into inflammatory sites. These include adhesion, diapedesis, and chemotaxis. The past 15 years has witnessed a virtual explosion in our understanding of these events, as several classes of adhesion molecules have been characterized at the molecular level. Adding to the excitement of these discoveries is the hope that the earliest adhesive events will serve as targets for new generations of antiinflammatory drugs less likely to affect noninflammatory cells. Late events constitute the effector functions of phagocytosis, degranulation, respiratory burst, and elaboration of inflammatory mediators. Underlying both early and late events are mechanisms of signal transduction, whereby neutrophils sense their environment through surface receptors and respond in an appropriate fashion.

Adherence, Diapedesis, and Chemotaxis

To arrive at inflamed or infected sites (Fig. 16.3), neutrophils must first adhere to the vascular endothelium (margination), roll along endothelial surfaces to areas of altered endothelium (loose adhesion), stick and spread on endothe-

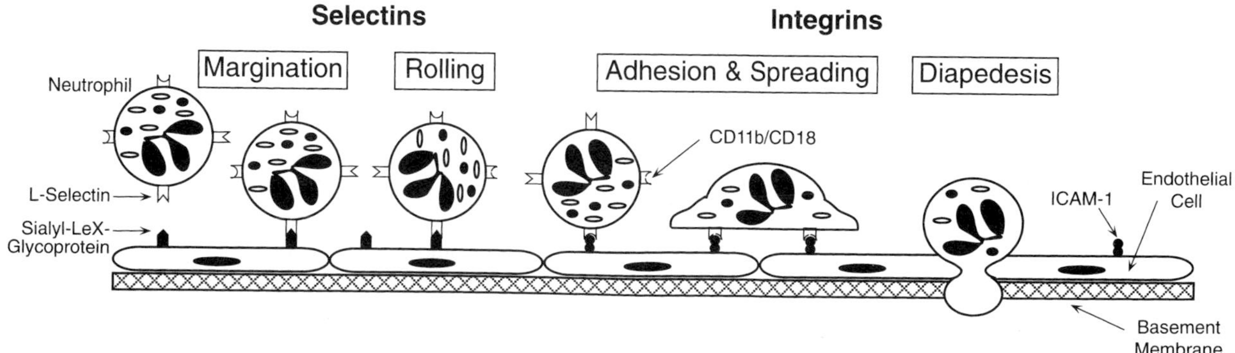

FIG. 16.3. Mechanisms of neutrophil-endothelium adhesion mediating recruitment of neutrophils into sites of inflammation.

lium adjacent to inflamed tissue (tight adhesion), crawl between the endothelial cells into the extravascular space (diapedesis), and finally navigate the extracellular matrix toward the source of inflammation (chemotaxis). This process is choreographed by vascular and leukocyte adhesion molecules, the biology and regulation of which have been the focus of intense investigation over the past decade. Both the endothelium and neutrophils are capable, on appropriate stimulation, of increasing their adhesiveness for each other by regulating adhesion molecules (see Chapter 20).

Three major families of proteins are expressed on the surface of either leukocytes or endothelium that play a role in leukocyte–endothelium interactions. The integrins are a large family of heterodimeric adhesive proteins expressed on leukocytes and other cell types. All leukocytes express one or more of the β_2 integrins, a group of related heterodimeric adhesive proteins that share a common β chain (CD18), but differ with respect to their α chains (CD11a,b,c). The integrins bind to a specific amino acid motif in their counterligands, and peptides containing this sequence of amino acids (RGD or arginine-glycine-aspartate) block many integrin-dependent functions. The integrins bind to proteins on the surface of the endothelium (and other cells) that belong to the immunoglobulin superfamily, namely intracellular adhesion molecule (ICAM)-1 and -2 and constitute a second major family of adhesion molecules. A third family of adhesive proteins (selectins) binds to carbohydrate residues on glycoproteins and glycolipids. Three distinct molecules compose the selectin family: P-selectin, E-selectin, and L-selectin. P-selectin is expressed on stimulated platelets and endothelium, L-selectin on leukocytes (neutrophils, monocytes, and a subset of lymphocytes), and E-selectin on stimulated endothelium. The genes encoding these molecules are all located on chromosome 1 and appear to have arisen from a single ancestral gene. The selectins share an extracellular C-type (Ca^{2+}-dependent) lectin domain (responsible for binding to their cognate ligands), an epidermal growth factor (EGF)-related domain of unknown function, and variable numbers of short consensus repeats (complement regulatory protein domains) in their extracellular portions, a hydrophobic transmembrane domain and a short cytoplasmic tail. E-selectin and P-selectin both bind to glycoproteins and glycolipids that contain sialyl Lewis X antigen (a complex carbohydrate). Sialyl Lewis X antigen is expressed predominantly on the surface of neutrophils (43–46).

The interaction between neutrophils and the vascular endothelium is mediated by the sequential interaction of the specific adhesion molecules on the neutrophil and endothelial surface. L-selectin is involved in the initial adhesion of neutrophils to the endothelium and then, after prolonged adhesion of neutrophils to endothelium or neutrophil stimulation by chemoattractants, is shed from the surface of the neutrophil (47). The β_2 integrin CD11b/CD18 on the neutrophil is then activated by a mechanism that is not completely understood, and becomes responsible for strengthening adhesion and promoting transendothelial migration (48–52). At sites of acute inflammation, the endothelium expresses P-selectin and E-selectin, which interact with specific glycosyl residues on the surface of the neutrophils (46,53). Thus, neutrophils may be drawn into inflamed sites as a result of stimulated alterations of the surface of neutrophils, or endothelium, or both.

Once adherent to the vascular surface of the endothelium, neutrophils find their way to the intercellular junctions between endothelial cells, where they emigrate from the vasculature in a process known as diapedesis. The cells then traverse the vascular basement membrane by a process that most likely involves local proteolysis. These processes appear to depend on the sequential activation and inactivation of CD11b/CD18 and the interaction of this integrin with ICAM-1 (54).

Neutrophils express receptors for a number of agents elaborated at inflamed or infected sites. Because neutrophils are capable of moving in a directed fashion along a gradient of these molecules, they are referred to as chemoattractants. Among inflammatory chemoattractants are complement activation products (C3a, C5a), chemokines (e.g., IL-8), arachidonic acid metabolites (leukotriene B_4), lipids [platelet-activating factor (PAF)], growth factors [transforming growth factor (TGF)-β], and *N*-formylated peptides derived from bacteria. Although chemoattractants constitute a diverse group of compounds, chemoattractant receptors comprise a set of closely related glycoproteins with a distinctive seven-transmembrane-spanning domain structure. Chemoattractant receptors are expressed in greatest density at the front of the neutrophil, the lamellipodia, where they encounter chemoattractants ("headlight phenomenon"). Once the receptor has bound its ligand, it is swept toward the rear of the cell, where it clusters with other bound receptors and is internalized (55–57).

The act of neutrophil chemotaxis involves ameboid motion. This requires coordinated actin remodeling to create both membrane protrusions at the leading edge (lamellipodia) and retraction at the tail (uropod). Interestingly, both processes have been shown to be regulated by the monomeric guanosine triphosphatase (GTPase) rac1 (58). Chemotaxis is an ancient cellular process that evolved in the most primitive eukaryotes, and recently the mechanisms of molecular control have been found to be remarkably conserved. Critical to chemotaxis in both cellular slime molds and leukocytes is a gradient of phosphoinositides established by the spatial regulation of the relevant lipid kinases [phosphatidylinositol-3 kinase (PI3k)] and phosphatase and tensin homologue deleted on chromosome 10 (PTEN) (59).

Phagocytosis

Once they arrive at the inflamed site, neutrophils ingest microorganisms and other particles. For particles to be efficiently phagocytosed, however, they must be opsonized (from the Greek "to prepare for the table"). The classic opsonins are immunoglobulins and complement, both derived from plasma. Neutrophils express on their surface receptors for these opsonins: two types of receptors for the constant region of immunoglobulins, FcγRII and FcγRIII (60), and two types of receptors for complement fragments, CR1 (for C3b and C4b) and CR3 (for iC3b) (61). In addition to mediating adhesion of opsonized particles to neutrophils, the opsonin receptors transduce signals into the cell. Whereas ligation of FcγRs is sufficient to promote phagocytosis, ligation of complement receptors requires a second stimulus to promote particle ingestion (62).

Phagocytosis is an active process that requires the expenditure of energy and is mediated, in part, by remodeling of the actin cytoskeleton. Neutrophils invaginate their surface membranes at the point of contact and surround the particle. The resulting intracellular vacuole, called a phagosome or phagocytic vesicle, pinches off from the surface of the cell and becomes completely internalized within the cytoplasm (63,64). After phagocytosis, the cells become rounded and have less available surface membrane. Despite its relatively large and expandable surface area (Fig. 16.2), the neutrophil's membrane content is finite, and limitations in availability of surface membrane may limit the number of particles that can be ingested by a single cell. Fusion of granule membranes with those of the phagosome begins the process of digestion of the phagocytosed particles. The lysosomal granules discharge their contents into the phagosome in a process known as degranulation (65–67). The phagosome, now called a phagolysosome, is actively acidified and contains a wide array of microbicidal proteins and degradative enzymes.

The molecular basis of phagocytosis has been difficult to approach experimentally in neutrophils because they are resistant to culture and genetic manipulation. However, it is likely that much of the knowledge gained from the recent explosion of molecular analysis of phagocytosis in macrophages (68,69) will pertain to neutrophils as well. Among the recent discoveries made in the field of macrophage phagocytosis is the observation that the mechanism of FcγR-mediated phagocytosis differs from that mediated by complement receptors, the former involving a zippering mechanism of cellular extensions that is regulated by the small GTPases rac1 and cdc42hs and leads to elaboration of proinflammatory mediators, with the latter involving pulling the opsonized particle into the cell, a process that depends on the GTPase rhoA and does not produce inflammatory mediators (70). Localized remodeling of phosphoinositides by type Iα phosphatidylinositol phosphate kinase to produce 4,5-PIP_2 appears to be one important way that the phagosome membrane is differentiated from that of the plasma membrane (71). One of the most intriguing recent advances in the understanding of phagocytosis is the discovery that the vast reserve of cellular membranes represented by the endoplasmic reticulum serves as an important source of phagosome membrane (72).

Degranulation

Degranulation is defined as the morphologic loss of cytoplasmic granules that is observed in activated neutrophils. Phagosome–lysosome fusion, the defining event in degranulation, is an area of intense investigation that is as yet poorly understood. Among the factors controlling membrane–membrane apposition and fusion is the dissolution of the "zone of organelle exclusion" afforded by the mesh of filamentous actin required to form the phagosome. As in other exocytic cells, the annexin family of calcium-dependent phospholipid binding proteins may be involved in regulating neutrophil degranulation (73). The observations that specific granules fuse with phagosomes earlier than azurophilic granules (74) and that incomplete secretagogues such as phorbol myristate acetate stimulate specific, but not azurophilic, granule discharge (75), suggest that mobilization of different granule compartments is differentially regulated, a conclusion concordant with the observation that different populations of neutrophil granules are associated with distinct small GTPases (76).

Neutrophil granules contain a wide array of macromolecules (Table 16.1), including enzymes (e.g., proteases, esterases, nucleotidases, carbohydrate hydrolases, and peroxidases), nonenzymatic proteins (e.g., lactoferrin and vitamin B_{12}–binding protein), glycosaminoglycans, and antimicrobial peptides (e.g., defensins and bacterial/permeability-inducing protein). Whereas some of these products are of obvious utility in neutralizing microorganisms (e.g., lysozyme and defensins), the role of others (e.g., lactoferrin and chondroitin sulfate) is unclear. Among the proteins unique to neutrophil granules is myeloperoxidase, a constituent of azurophilic granules that accounts for the yellow-green color of pus. Myeloperoxidase plays a critical role in host defense by converting the moderately microbicidal products of the neutrophil respiratory burst, superoxide anion (O_2^-) and H_2O_2, into the potent antimicrobial compound hypochlorous acid (chlorine bleach) (77).

Although many of the granular enzymes are potentially destructive to host tissues, their activities are kept in check by sequestration within the membrane-enclosed organelles, by requiring the acid microenvironment of the phagolysosome for full activity, and by inactivation with extracellular inhibitors abundant in plasma. Nevertheless, it is clear that neutrophil granular enzymes do play an important role in the tissue destruction associated with inflammatory processes such as those seen in rheumatic diseases. This paradox has been resolved by the recognition that dying neutrophils release their lysosomal contents and, more importantly, that neutrophils secrete specific and azurophilic granule contents by forming phagosomes not yet closed to the extracellular space (78).

Until 30 years ago, it was thought that granular contents could be released into the extracellular space only by the necrosis of neutrophils, as was often observed histologically in such conditions as leukocytoclastic vasculitis. It is now clear that viable neutrophils actively secrete granular contents (79).

The secretory vesicles and, to some extent, the gelatinase-containing tertiary granules are easily mobilized and release their contents through plasma membrane–targeted exocytosis in response to soluble stimuli such as C5a and LTB_4 (27). In this capacity, they not only secrete their soluble content but also serve as a rapidly mobilizable pool of membrane that at once expands surface area and delivers new surface proteins (24). In contrast, lactoferrin-containing specific granules and azurophilic granules release their content *in vitro* only in response to particulate stimuli, although they can be pharmacologically provoked to secrete in response to soluble agonists in the presence of cytochalasin B (79). Electron microscopic studies have revealed that specific and azurophilic granules are targeted only to the phagosome membrane (74). The process of phagosome–lysosome fusion begins well before the phagosome is closed, however, allowing escape of granular content proteins in a process referred to as "regurgitation while eating" (78).

Several hypotheses have been proposed to explain how proteases secreted from neutrophils at sites of inflammation escape inactivation by protease inhibitors, such as α_1-antitrypsin and β_2-macroglobulin. The reactive oxygen species and hypochlorous acid produced by activated neutrophils have been shown to inactivate antiproteases (80). A role for a microenvironment inaccessible to plasma antiproteases has been proposed in the model of "frustrated phagocytosis," wherein a neutrophil endeavors to phagocytose foreign substances embedded in a surface that it cannot encompass, such as occurs in the rheumatoid synovium where rheumatoid factor–containing immune complexes become embedded in the hyaline cartilage (81,82). Among the granular hydrolases that are the most destructive to the connective tissues at sites of inflammation are elastase, collagenase, and cathepsin G. Elastase is a neutral protease abundantly expressed in neutrophils that can degrade elastin in tendons, blood vessels, and lung tissue and also behaves as a broad-spectrum serine protease. Neutrophil collagenase is a metalloproteinase that degrades type I collagen found in cartilage and bone, but must first be activated by proteolytic cleavage, a function fulfilled by elastase. Cathepsin G is a broad-spectrum chymotrypsin-like enzyme that is fully active at neutral pH.

Respiratory Burst

Phagocytic leukocytes are uniquely efficient in their capacity to reduce molecular oxygen and produce reactive oxygen species critical for host defense against microorganisms. The enzyme responsible for the single electron reduction of molecular oxygen is known as the "respiratory burst" or reduced nicotinamide adenine dinucleotide phosphate (NADPH) oxidase. The former designation reflects the discovery in 1959 by Sbarra and Karnovsky that, on phagocytosis, neutrophils dramatically increase their oxygen consumption in a cyanide-insensitive reaction known as the respiratory burst (83). The latter, and more frequently used, designation reflects the discovery 5 years later that NADPH, largely derived from the hexose monophosphate shunt, is the electron donor for the phagocyte oxidase (84). The initial product of the NADPH oxidase is O_2^-, which serves as the precursor for more toxic species that include singlet oxygen, H_2O_2, and hypochlorous acid. The importance of the NADPH oxidase to the human immune system is dramatically illustrated by patients with chronic granulomatous disease (CGD), a heritable disorder characterized by the absence of NADPH oxidase activity associated with recurrent life-threatening pyogenic infections universally fatal in the preantibiotic era. It is now known that CGD, a genetically heterogeneous group of disorders, results from defects in one of four genes that encode components of the NADPH oxidase complex. Although the oxidizing species generated during the respiratory burst are antibacterial in and of themselves, recent work indicates that the major role of the respiratory burst is to maintain an acidic pH in the phagolysosome, thereby ensuring optimal antibacterial activity of the granular enzymes and proteins secreted into the phagolysosome (85).

The NADPH oxidase is latent in resting neutrophils but is rapidly activated in the membrane of the phagolysosome (86). The molecular nature of the NADPH oxidase complex has been the subject of intense investigation over the past two decades (Fig. 16.4). Studies of patients with the most common X-linked form of CGD permitted the identification of the first component of the oxidase, cytochrome b_{558} (87), a heterodimeric glycoprotein intrinsic to the neutrophil plasma membrane that contains two heme groups and binding domains for both flavin adenine dinucleotide (FAD) and NADPH (88). Over the last two decades, the development of cell-free systems for studying NADPH oxidase activation (89–92) has permitted the identification of other proteins associated with the oxidase (93). The minimal complement of proteins required to assemble an active NADPH oxidase in a fully recombinant system include cytochrome b_{558} and three cytosolic factors designated $p47^{phox}$, $p67^{phox}$, and $p21^{rac}$ (94). A third cytosolic factor was identified as $p40^{phox}$ (95). Both $p40^{phox}$ and $p47^{phox}$ contain src homology 3 (SH3) domains that bind proline-rich regions of interacting proteins. They also possess a recently recognized PX domain that has been shown to bind phosphoinositides (96). Activation of the latent NADPH oxidase is regulated by phosphorylation and involves translocation of the cytosolic factors to the plasma or phagosome membrane (Fig. 16.4). $p47^{phox}$, $p40^{phox}$, and $p67^{phox}$ appear to be structural components of the oxidase, although their role in electron transport is not established. Although $p21^{rac1}$ is a ubiquitously expressed member of the ras superfamily of regulatory GTPases, $p21^{rac2}$ is myeloid

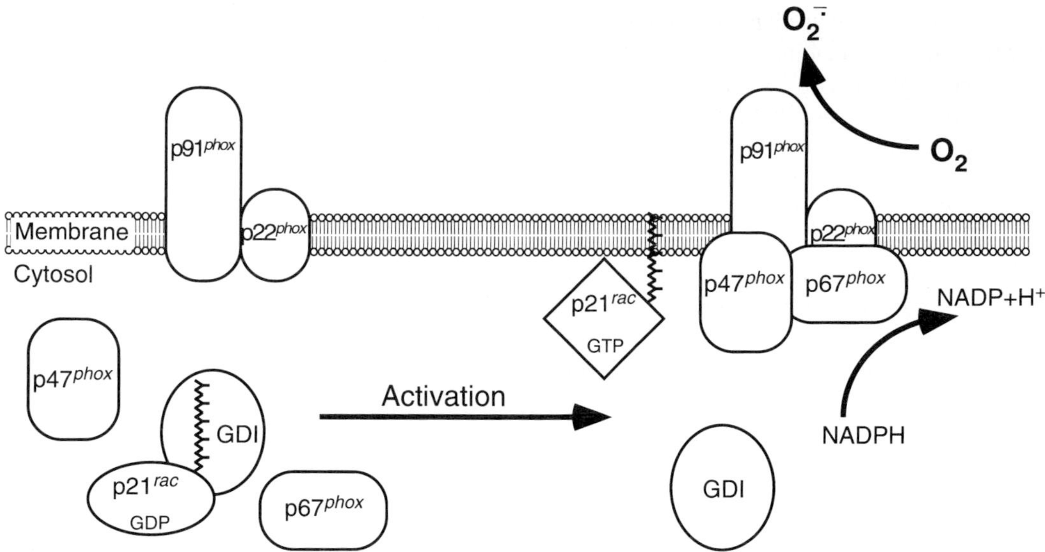

FIG. 16.4. Multimolecular assembly of the neutrophil nicotinamide adenine dinucleotide phosphate oxidase complex.

restricted. Whereas targeted disruption of p21^{rac1} in mice is embryonic lethal, disruption of the gene for p21^{rac2} is tolerated and causes only a minor defect in neutrophil NADPH oxidase, suggesting that p21^{rac1} can substitute for p21^{rac2} (97). Interestingly, neutrophils from p21^{rac2}-null mice manifest several defects in chemoattractant signaling, suggesting a role for p21^{rac2} in neutrophil processes other than the oxidase. Like other members of the rho subfamily of ras-related GTPases, p21^{rac} is involved in signaling for actin cytoskeleton remodeling, specifically for the formation of lamellipodia (97). The role of p21^{rac} in NADPH oxidase assembly is under intense investigation (98).

Synthesis and Secretion of Inflammatory Mediators

Neutrophils both participate in and amplify the inflammatory process. By synthesizing and releasing a variety of soluble mediators, neutrophils can recruit more cells to an inflamed site and can activate those cells once they have arrived. Two general classes of mediators are secreted by neutrophils: cytokines, which are generally small proteins and peptides (molecular weight <20,000 daltons), and lipid-derived mediators, including the eicosanoids and leukotrienes.

Cytokines

Neutrophils secrete several proteins that are important in the pathogenesis of inflammation. When studied *in vitro,* neutrophils secrete IL-1α, TNF-α, IL-6, and IL-8 in response to inflammatory stimuli such as opsonized bacteria, yeast, or crystals (e.g., monosodium urate) (99–104). Moreover, recent studies demonstrate that secretion of cytokines by neutrophils also occurs *in vivo* (104). Interestingly, resting neutrophils also secrete a specific IL-1 inhibitor recently identified as IL-1 receptor antagonist (IL-1RA) (105,106). Thus, in the resting state, neutrophils secrete antiinflammatory cytokines, but once activated, secrete proinflammatory cytokines that amplify and prolong the inflammatory response. Neutrophils also release IL-6 receptor, which acts as a sponge for IL-6 at inflamed sites and, like IL-1RA, acts as an endogenous regulator of inflammation (107,108).

Eicosanoids and Leukotrienes

Neutrophils release activated products of arachidonate when exposed to phagocytic stimuli. These include products of the cyclooxygenase (COX) pathway, prostaglandins (PGs), and thromboxanes (TXs), and products of the lipoxygenase (LO) pathway, the leukotrienes (LTs). The exact role and interaction of these compounds with each other and other mediators of inflammation is not completely understood. Additionally, these compounds appear to have both anti- and proinflammatory effects (see Chapter 23).

On stimulation, arachidonic acid is released from the sn-2 position of membrane phospholipids through activation of phospholipase A_2 (PLA_2). This step is inhibited by antiinflammatory corticosteroids. Arachidonic acid, a 20-carbon polyunsaturated fatty acid, can interact with reactive oxygen species generated during the respiratory burst (109,110). More important, several enzymes transform arachidonic acid into lipid mediators by introducing oxygen at specific bonds. The two best studied of these enzymes, COX (also called prostaglandin H synthase) and 5-LO, are expressed in neutrophils and produce eicosanoids (prostaglandins and thromboxanes) and leukotrienes, respectively.

Two isoforms of COX have been identified, a constitutive enzyme (COX1) and an inducible enzyme (COX2), which differ in their susceptibility to inhibition by various nonsteroidal antiinflammatory drugs (NSAIDs) (reviewed in reference 111; see also Chapter 31). The fatty acid endoperoxides formed by COX-mediated metabolism of arachidonate (the PGG and PGH series) are weak potentiators of edema caused by bradykinin and histamine (112) and serve as intermediates in the formation, through isomerization, of the more stable PGs and TXs. Of these, PGE_2 and PGI_2 appear to be the primary mediators of inflammation because they cause local vasodilatation and edema when injected and act synergistically with bradykinin and histamine; their injection into the midbrain of experimental animals causes fever; and they sensitize nerve endings to painful stimuli. These compounds are present in elevated concentrations in inflammatory exudates, and their synthesis is inhibited by most antiinflammatory drugs (113). Conversely, there is also evidence that PGs can be antiinflammatory. The PGE series can stimulate cAMP production and thereby suppress immediate hypersensitivity reactions and reactions associated with cellular immunity such as lectin-induced T-cell mitogenesis (114) and neutrophil degranulation (115).

The products of the LO pathway have been elucidated, and their role in inflammation is becoming increasingly evident. The predominating pathway of LT metabolism depends on the cell type: the 12-LO in platelets, the 15-LO in T lymphocytes, and the 5-LO in neutrophils. Arachidonic acid metabolism through the 5-LO pathway is depicted in Fig. 16.5. LO is not inhibited by the NSAIDs. 5-LO catalyzes the formation of 5-HETE, which is converted to the unstable epoxide LTA_4 (116), which then is either enzymatically hydrolyzed to LTB_4 or acted on through glutathione 5-transferase to form LTC_4. The latter can be further modified by glutamyl transpeptidase to form LTD_4 and LTE_4 (117,118).

LTB_4 is a neutrophil autocoid in that it is both released from and acts on the neutrophil. Nanomolar concentrations of LTB_4 are chemotactic for neutrophils (119) and stimulate adhesion to endothelial cells and other neutrophils (120). Thus, neutrophil-derived LTB_4 acts to amplify an acute inflammatory response by recruiting other neutrophils. At higher concentrations, LTB_4 causes degranulation, superoxide anion generation, and mobilization of membrane-associated calcium (121,122). These observations suggest the importance of LTB_4 in the pathogenesis of tissue injury during inflammation and have prompted the development of agents that inhibit either the synthesis or the action of LTB_4 for use in the treatment of inflammatory diseases.

The cysteine-containing leukotrienes (LTC_4, LTD_4, and LTE_4), produced by macrophages and basophils, consti-

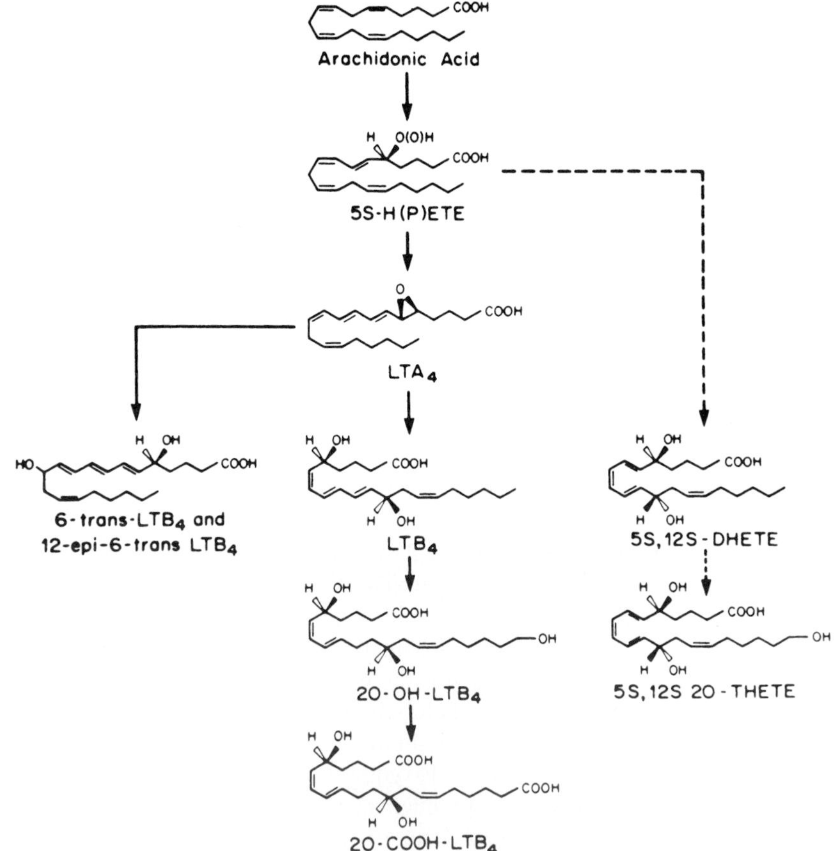

FIG. 16.5. Arachidonic acid metabolism in neutrophils by the 5-lipoxygenase pathway. *DHETE*, dihydroxytetraenoic acid; *H(P)ETE*, hydroperoxyeicosatetraenoic acid; *LTB_4*, leukotriene B_4.

tute the immunologically-mediated "slow reactive substance of anaphylaxis" (SRS-A). Among their diverse biologic effects is a dose-dependent vascular contraction, most marked in terminal arterioles. Although the vasoconstriction is short lived, it is followed by a dose-dependent, reversible leakage of macromolecules at the postcapillary venules (123). Thus, with PGE_2 and PGI_2, SRS-A contributes to edema formation.

Signal Transduction

Like all cells, neutrophils respond to their environment by sensing signaling molecules through surface receptors. Unlike the lymphoid arm of the immune system that depends on mitogenic signaling (hours to days), neutrophils depend on rapid signaling (seconds to minutes) to protect the host adequately from infection. Indeed, the critical neutrophil functions described earlier are initiated, and in some cases completed, within minutes of encountering an inflammatory stimulus. It is, therefore, not surprising that neutrophils, like neuroendocrine cells, are endowed with a wide variety of G protein–linked receptors that rapidly transduce signals often leading to immediate responses.

Chemoattractant Receptors

Both the classic chemoattractants [formyl-methionyl-leucyl-phenylalanine tripeptide (FMLP), C5a, LTB_4, and PAF] and the more recently recognized chemoattractant cytokines (IL-8, GRO, NAP-2, ENA-78, and GCP-2) bind to molecules on neutrophils that are members of a large family of receptors that interact with G proteins. Complementary DNAs (cDNAs) for the receptors for formyl peptides, C5a, IL-8, and PAF have been reported recently (124–128). Molecular analyses of these cDNAs revealed that each receptor contains seven hydrophobic α helices, predicted to form seven-transmembrane-spanning domains, and a series of extracellular and cytoplasmic loops, analogous to the deduced structure of the best studied receptor of this class, the β-adrenergic receptor. In addition to the chemoattractant receptors, other receptors of this class that are expressed on neutrophils include receptors for β-adrenergic agents, PGE, and adenosine.

G Proteins

Guanine nucleotide regulatory binding proteins, or G proteins, are αβγ heterotrimeric proteins associated with the inner leaflet of the plasma membrane that transduce signals from transmembrane receptors to effector molecules by cycling between a guanosine diphosphate (GDP)-bound, inactive, and GTP-bound, active, conformation (Fig. 16.6). Receptor occupancy leads to a conformational change that allows the receptor to interact with a G protein and, thereby, stimulate the dissociation of GDP from G_a, the GTP-binding subunit. GTP then binds, leading to a dissociation of G_α

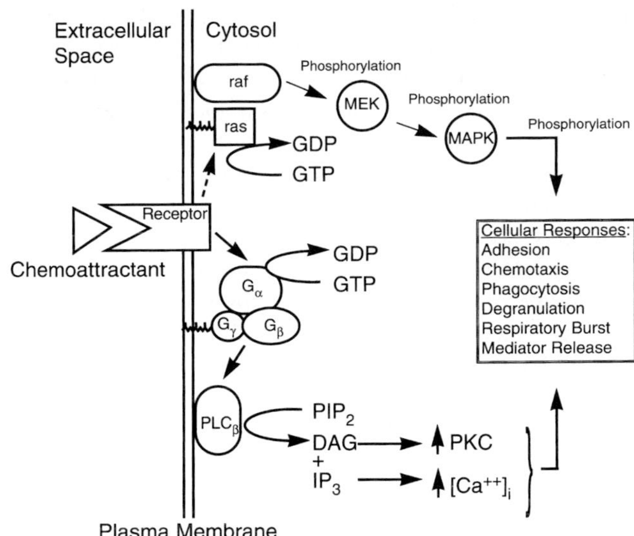

FIG. 16.6. Chemoattractant-stimulated signal transduction in neutrophils.

from $G_{\beta/\gamma}$, each of which plays a role in activating effector molecules. The signal is terminated by the intrinsic GTPase activity of G_α. At least 16 α, as well as multiple β and γ subunits, have been identified (129,130). Some of the α subunits serve as substrates for the adenosine diphosphate ribosyl transferases contained in pertussis and cholera toxins. Human neutrophil plasma membranes contain substrates for both pertussis and cholera toxins (131). Because pertussis toxin inhibits much, but not all, of FMLP-stimulated neutrophil function, it has been deduced that neutrophils contain both pertussis-sensitive and -insensitive G proteins. Immunoblot analysis with subunit-specific antisera have identified $G_{\alpha i1,2}$, $G_{\alpha 8}$ (132), $G_{\beta 1,2}$ (133), and $G_{\gamma 2}$ (134) in human neutrophil membranes. A considerable body of evidence supports the involvement of $G_{\alpha i2}$ in chemoattractant-stimulated neutrophil activation (135).

Effectors and Second Messengers

The most extensively characterized effector molecule for G protein signaling in neutrophils is a polyphosphoinositide-specific phospholipase C (PLC) that is stimulated by chemoattractants (Fig. 16.6). Both PLC-β_1 and PLC-β_2 are activated by $G_{\alpha i}$, whereas only the latter isoform is activated by $G_{\beta/\gamma}$ (136). PLC catalyzes the hydrolysis of phosphatidylinositol 4,5-biphosphate (PIP_2), a minor phospholipid constituent of the plasma membrane, into the second messengers diacylglycerol (DAG) and inositol 1,4,5-triphosphate (IP_3). DAG activates protein kinase C, an enzyme that phosphorylates serine and threonine residues on a wide variety of cellular proteins, and IP_3 releases Ca^{2+} from intracellular stores, which in turn regulates a wide variety of Ca^{2+}-dependent proteins. Whereas the early increase in DAG can be attributed to PLC activity, sustained increases in DAG have been attributed to the subsequent activation of a phosphatidylcholine-specific phospholipase D, which is regulated by protein kinase C (PKC), Ca^{2+}, and ADP ribosylation factor (ARF) (137). Chemoattractants, β-adrenergic agents, prostaglandins of the E series, and adenosine all stimulate increases in neutrophil intracellular cAMP (138) indicating that, like in most cells, adenyl cyclase is a G protein–stimulated effector and cAMP is an important second messenger. Neither the subtype of adenyl cyclase nor the relevant G proteins have been elucidated in neutrophil signaling. Increases in intracellular cAMP generally have inhibitory effects on neutrophil function, although the mechanism is unresolved (139). Recent evidence demonstrating that cAMP, acting through protein kinase A, inhibits neutrophil mitogen-activated protein kinase (MAPK) at the level of Raf-1 (140,141) suggests a molecular mechanism for cAMP-mediated down-regulation of neutrophil activation (142). Other effector molecules implicated in neutrophil signal transduction include a novel phosphoinositide 3 kinase that is activated by $G_{\beta/\gamma}$ (143) and PLA_2 that releases arachidonate from the sn-2 position of glycerophospholipids (144). Arachidonate both has direct effects on neutrophils (144) and serves as the precursor of a wide variety of eicosanoids that have both pro- and antiinflammatory effects.

Monomeric GTPases

In addition to the heterotrimeric G proteins, a second superfamily of regulatory GTPases related to the protooncogene product $p21^{ras}$ controls a wide variety of cellular processes (145,146). Ras-related GTPases are monomeric GTP-binding proteins that undergo conformational changes when they cycle between their GDP-bound, inactive, and GTP-bound, active, states. The ras superfamily of GTPases can be divided into the ras family involved in signal transduction for growth and differentiation, the rho family involved in signaling for actin cytoskeleton remodeling, and the rab and ARF families involved in regulating vesicular trafficking. Members of each of these families have been identified in human neutrophils. Notable examples are $p21^{rac}$, which activates the NADPH oxidase (147,148); $p21^{rap1}$, which is associated with cytochrome b_{558}, but is not required for *in vitro* NADPH oxidase activity (149); $p21^{rho}$ (76,150), which is involved in actin stress fiber formation in fibroblasts (151); $p21^{CDC42}$ (150), which activates a specific kinase (152); and ARF, which activates phospholipase D (137), whose product, phosphatidic acid, may be involved in vesicular fusion. Chemoattractants activate $p21^{ras}$, Raf-1, and MAPK in neutrophils (153–155), although the pathway(s) coupling G protein–linked receptors to the $p21^{ras}$ signaling pathway are undefined (Fig. 16.6). Both ras-related GTPases and heterotrimeric G proteins are intrinsically hydrophilic proteins that exert their biologic effects at membranes. Both ras-related proteins and the γ subunit of G proteins are targeted to membranes by a series of posttranslational modifications of their carboxyl termini that involves prenylation (addition of a 15- or 20-carbon polyisoprene lipid), proteolysis, and carboxyl methylation (156). Carboxyl methylation, the only reversible step in this processing, is associated with neutrophil activation and may play a regulatory role in signal transduction (150).

Non–G Protein–Linked Receptors

In addition to the G protein–linked receptors discussed earlier, neutrophils express a wide variety of other classes of receptors. These include receptors for opsonins [complement receptors and receptors for the constant regions of immunoglobulins (FcγRs)], receptors for intracellular adhesion molecules and extracellular matrix (integrins), and receptors for cytokines and several members of the Toll-like receptor family (TLR 1,2,4,5) involved in pattern recognition of pathogen-associated molecular patterns (157). Like T-cell receptors, FcγRs appear to signal through tyrosine activation domains on the cytoplasmic portions of aggregated receptor complexes that, in turn, activate src family tyrosine kinases such as $p72^{syk}$ (158). Interestingly, FcγRIIIB, which is abundantly expressed on neutrophils, has a glycosylphosphatidylinositol anchor that lacks a cytoplasmic domain, and, therefore, must signal through an accessory molecule, perhaps the ξ homodimer associated with the T-cell receptor and FcγRIIIA, a transmembrane isoform (158). Similarly, signaling from the extracellular matrix through integrins involves protein tyrosine phosphorylation, although the other integrin-mediated functions, including cell-cell adhesion and actin cytoskeleton organization, may be regulated independently (159). The Toll-like receptors signal through activation and translocation of nuclear factor κB (NFκB) to the nucleus, where it regulates transcription of a large number of genes involved in the inflammatory response (160). The best studied of the TLRs expressed on neutrophils is TLR4, the ligand for which is bacterial endotoxin (bound to its accessory molecules lipopolysaccharide binding protein and CD14). Like bacterial lipopolysaccharide, the cytokines TNF-α, GM-CSF, and interferon-γ (IFN-γ) do not themselves stimulate neutrophil responses, but they prime neutrophils to respond to lower concentrations of chemoattractants, a biologic activity that is likely of great physiologic relevance. Signaling from cytokine receptors in mitotic cells involves hetero-oligomerization of the receptors with signaling molecules such as members of the JAK and STAT families that lead to transcription of specific sets of genes (161), but cytokine signaling in neutrophils has not been extensively studied. Most of the classic protein tyrosine kinase receptors, such as platelet-derived growth factors that homodimerize on ligation with mitogens (162) and transduce signals to the nucleus via $p21^{ras}$, Raf-1, and MAPK (163), have not been described on neutrophils.

NEUTROPHILS IN RHEUMATIC DISEASE

Because the etiology of many of the rheumatic diseases is believed to be autoimmune, much research in this area has focused on the lymphocyte. Although neutrophils, acting alone, do not have the capacity to distinguish self from nonself; as a potent effector arm of the immune system, they play a central role in the pathophysiology of rheumatic diseases by mediating much of the tissue destruction.

Mechanisms of Tissue Injury

Neutrophils may injure tissues, such as the synovium in arthritis or the microvasculature in vasculitis, by several mechanisms. First, as described earlier, neutrophils stimulated by chemoattractants, immune complexes, or cytokines release a variety of potentially toxic metabolites of oxygen (O_2^-, H_2O_2, HOCl). These reactive oxygen species can oxidize membrane phospholipids, cause mutations in DNA, and deplete target cells of essential metabolites (e.g., ATP). Although both cells and extracellular fluids contain antioxidants and free radical scavengers (e.g., glutathione and ceruloplasm), these systems can be overwhelmed in areas of intense inflammation, allowing tissue damage by reactive oxygen species.

Second, neutrophils may actively release the contents of their granules, which can dislodge cells from their substrates, destroy matrix proteins, and directly injure cells. As is the case for reactive oxygen species, the extracellular space is endowed with some protection against neutrophil proteases (i.e., protease inhibitors such as α_1-antitrypsin and α_2-macroglobulin). However, several mechanisms have been proposed to account for the action of neutrophil-derived proteases at inflammatory sites. Among these mechanisms are sequestration of proteases in closed spaces between neutrophils and target cells or extracellular matrix and inactivation of antiproteases by HOCl (80). Studies performed by Vartio et al. (164) have demonstrated that proteinases from neutrophil granules (e.g., cathepsin G) may degrade matrix proteins into peptides, some of which are chemotactic for other neutrophils and other inflammatory cells. These peptides can attract other inflammatory cells into the area and thereby amplify the inflammatory process. Harlan et al. (165), using human neutrophils activated with serum-treated zymosan, demonstrated endothelial cell detachment caused by neutral protease digestion of endothelial cell surface proteins, including fibronectin. There are several mechanisms by which the proteases and other lysosomal constituents are released from the neutrophil and gain access to their substrates.

Necrosis

One mechanism by which neutrophils may release their lysosomal contents at an inflamed site is simply cell death. When neutrophils are exposed to toxins (e.g., phospholipases in snake venom or materials that could be encountered in some forms of septic arthritis), injury to the plasma membrane is an early consequence, and all intracellular materials are released *pari passu* from the injured cell, including those ordinarily sequestered within lysosomes. Biologic detergents, such as the amphipath melittin, act in this manner to cause primary lysis of the cell membrane and, only subsequently, disruption of lysosomes (78). Under these circumstances, cytoplasmic enzymes, potassium, and other cellular constituents, in addition to lysosomal hydrolases, are directly released into the surrounding tissues.

Apoptosis

Neutrophils are short-lived cells and, like other cells, when they reach the end of their useful life or after receiving appropriate stimuli, undergo a form of programmed cell death known as apoptosis (166) (see Chapter 26). Neutrophils that undergo apoptosis may also release their granule contents into the surrounding milieu, although apoptotic neutrophils are more often cleared from the circulation by the reticuloendothelial system and from inflamed sites by local macrophages. Macrophages phagocytose apoptotic (but not healthy) neutrophils by a process dependent on thrombospondin, the thrombospondin receptor (CD36), and the vitronectin receptor ($\alpha_5\beta_3$) (167). Recognition and phagocytosis of apoptotic neutrophils by macrophages has been documented to occur in synovial fluid, among other inflamed sites. Removal of dying neutrophils with their complement of destructive proteolytic enzymes is essential for limiting damage due to leakage of granule enzymes from dying neutrophils at an inflamed site and for terminating the inflammatory process (168).

Perforation from Within

Under some circumstances, phagocytosed material can directly cause rupture of lysosomal membranes in a process known as perforation from within. Damage to the organelles leads to autolysis of cytoplasmic structures and ultimately rupture of the cell with concomitant release of both lysosomal and cytoplasmic enzymes. Crystalline substances, such as monosodium urate and silica, act on phagocytic cells in this fashion (169). Hence, this form of lysosomal enzyme release is a primary promoter of inflammation in gout (see Chapter 115).

Whereas these first three mechanisms of lysosomal enzyme release involve death of the neutrophil, two additional mechanisms involving intact, viable neutrophils also have been recognized. Both are relevant to the pathogenesis of immune tissue injury and have proven to be influenced by several pharmacologic agents, particularly those that affect the state of assembly of cytoplasmic microtubules or the level of cyclic nucleotides within cells.

Regurgitation While Feeding

Under some circumstances, for example, during the ingestion by neutrophils of insoluble immune complexes, as encountered in synovial fluid in rheumatoid arthritis (RA), or of other particulates, neutrophil granules begin to fuse with the forming phagosome before it is closed to the extracellular space. Thus, regurgitation of lysosomal hydrolases occurs, and inflammatory materials are released into the surrounding tissues without associated phagocytic cell death or release of cytoplasmic enzymes (78). Biochemical and morphologic evidence for this mechanism, called regurgitation while feeding, has been presented for a variety of systems involving particle ingestion by phagocytic cells. Ohlsson (170) has shown that the neutral proteases, elastase and collagenase, are regurgitated by this mechanism. This appears to be a common mechanism of tissue injury in a variety of disease states.

Exocytosis

Another related mechanism of selective lysosomal enzyme secretion from viable neutrophils is exocytosis. In this process, material previously stored within granules is exported to the external milieu in the absence of a forming phagosome. For example, cells that encounter immune complexes or aggregated immunoglobulins deposited on solid surfaces, such as millipore filters or collagen membranes, that cannot be ingested ("frustrated phagocytosis") adhere to these surfaces and selectively release their lysosomal constituents (171). Under these circumstances, enzyme release appears to occur through an exocytic pathway that has been termed reverse endocytosis. Fusion of granules with the plasma membrane results in discharge of lysosomal enzymes directly to the outside of the cell rather than into a phagocytic vacuole. The viability of the adherent neutrophil is not altered. This mechanism of enzyme release is involved in the pathogenesis of tissue injury when immune complexes are deposited on cell surfaces or extracellular structures, such as vascular basement membranes. For example, the nephritis of systemic lupus erythematosus (SLE) may be generated by this form of granule enzyme release, stimulated by the surface deposition of immune complexes (DNA–anti-DNA IgG) and complement activation products.

Exocytosis is an active process stimulated by several distinct inflammatory ligands. These include Fc regions of IgG molecules that have undergone a conformational change as a result of combining with antigen (FcγR stimulus), fragments of the third component of complement (C3b and C3bi receptor stimulus), and the soluble, low-molecular-weight complement component C5a. For example, immune complexes prepared by reacting IgG with rheumatoid factor or heat-aggregated IgG alone, either in suspension or deposited on nonphagocytizable surfaces, can provoke the selective discharge of lysosomal constituents from human neutrophils by reverse endocytosis (78,172–175). Neutrophils exposed to fragments of C3 fixed on nonphagocytizable surfaces (in the absence of IgG) respond in a similar manner. C5a, generated by activation of either the classic or alternative complement pathways, can interact with neutrophils in the absence of particles (or immunoglobulins) to stimulate membrane fusion between lysosomal granules and the plasma membrane (174). Both cytochalasin B and the adherence of neutrophils to surfaces augment the secretory response to C5a (175).

Exocytosis involves all four classes of cytoplasmic vesicles. However, whereas the secretory granules and, to some extent, gelatinase granules are relatively easily mobilized (e.g., by heating neutrophils *in vitro*), release of specific and azurophilic granule contents requires the special circumstances discussed earlier. Nevertheless, markers for both specific and azurophilic granules (e.g., lactoferrin and β-glucuronidase) are readily detected in the supernatants of appropriately stimulated neutrophils (78,172–175). Most inflammatory stimuli, such as formylated peptides and complement components, are known as complete secretagogues because they stimulate secretion of both specific and azurophilic granule contents. Interestingly, some nonimmune stimuli appear to provoke selective discharge of specific granule constituents and are therefore known as incomplete secretagogues. Such stimuli include the tumor promoter phorbol myristate acetate (176,177) and concanavalin A (178). These observations, together with the reported sequential degranulation during phagocytosis (74), indicate that the exocytosis of specific and azurophilic granules is differentially controlled (76). Having considered the capacity of neutrophils to injure host tissues, it is important to note that neutrophils are the most abundant cells in synovial fluids from patients with rheumatoid, crystal-induced, and seronegative arthritides. Neutrophils are also the predominant cell type present in several different types of vasculitis. The localization of neutrophils to inflamed areas in patients with the rheumatic diseases suggests that these cells contribute to tissue destruction in the rheumatic diseases.

Neutrophils in Rheumatoid Arthritis

RA is generally considered a T cell–driven disease with an autoimmune etiology. Indeed, the rheumatoid synovium contains activated T cells, as well as autoantibody-secreting plasma cells, but few neutrophils. In contrast, the synovial fluid from a rheumatoid joint, which can yield up to 100,000 white blood cells per mm^3, contains almost exclusively neutrophils. Moreover, the flux of neutrophils in a 30-mL rheumatoid knee effusion can reach 10^9 cells/day (179), a formidable number of potentially destructive cells. The presence of neutrophils within the joint space is not surprising because a number of different chemoattractants for neutrophils are present in the synovial fluid (180). The differential mechanisms by which lymphocytes remain in the synovial tissue are unknown, whereas neutrophils, also derived from transmigration through synovial vessels, quickly traverse the synovial tissue and enter the synovial space. These observations suggest a role for the neutrophil in the tissue destruction characteristic of RA. Within the synovial fluid, neutrophils generate toxic oxygen metabolites and other substances that may degrade hyaluronan, the major lubricating component of joint fluid. The degradation of hyaluronan leads to a marked diminution in the viscosity of joint fluid and may abrogate the capacity of hyaluronan to protect cartilage from injury by stimulated neutrophils (82). Besides their abundance in the rheumatoid joint, a role for neutrophils in the pathogenesis of RA also may be inferred from the fact that many drugs effective in treating rheumatoid inflammation profoundly affect neutrophil recruitment or function.

Neutrophils in Gout

Like RA, gouty arthritis is characterized by an intense neutrophilic infiltrate in the synovial space, sometimes greater than 100,000 cells per mm^3. Unlike in RA, neutrophils are the only type of inflammatory cell required in the pathogenesis of gouty arthritis. Monosodium urate crystals, usually coated with plasma proteins such as IgG or complement, are potent phagocytic stimuli for neutrophils and induce the secretion of inflammatory mediators (181). One of these mediators, IL-1, mediates the signs of systemic inflammation occasionally seen in gout (182). Studies performed in knockout mice indicate that IL-8 is critical for recruitment of neutrophils to the joint space during attacks of acute gouty arthritis (183).

Metabolites of arachidonic acid may contribute to the pathogenesis of gouty arthritis (see Chapter 113). Monosodium urate crystals stimulate the formation of arachidonate metabolites by neutrophils and platelets. Neutrophils exposed to nonlytic quantities of monosodium urate generate hydroxy-eicosatetraenoic acid (5-HETE), LTB_4 (and its nonenzymatically formed isomers 6-*trans*-LTB_4, 12-epi-6-*trans*-LTB_4), and 20-COOH-LTB_4 through the 5-LO pathway. Neutrophils treated with colchicine are unable to form LTA_4 from 5-HETE after addition of monosodium urate crystals, and thus do not form LTB_4 and its isomers. This shifts metabolism of arachidonate to other metabolites such as 5*S*,12*S*-DiHETE, which antagonize the action of LTB_4 (184). These effects are observed at high concentrations of colchicine, concentrations that may be achieved only after large doses of colchicine are administered. More recent studies demonstrated that high concentrations of colchicine diminish neutrophil expression of L-selectin, rendering these cells less able to adhere to vascular endothelium and, therefore, less likely to emigrate into the acutely inflamed gouty joint (185). More strikingly, at the very low concentrations of colchicine that are achieved with prophylactic doses of the drug, endothelial adhesive molecules are rendered nonsticky for neutrophils (185). This observation suggests, for the first time, a mechanism for the prophylactic effects of colchicine at doses used to prevent gouty arthritis (see Chapter 113).

Neutrophils in Glomerulonephritis and Vasculitis

Neutrophilic infiltrates are characteristic in rapidly progressive glomerulonephritis and in vasculitis. *In vivo* experiments demonstrate that neutrophils are responsible for tissue destruction in some forms of glomerulonephritis and many forms of vasculitis (1–10). Leukocytoclastic angiitis, named for the histologic appearance of fragments of broken neutrophils, is a form of vasculitis characterized by neutrophil infiltration and destruction of the blood vessel wall, usually in response to deposition of immune complexes within the vessel wall. Although it is generally accepted that intravascular activation of neutrophils leads to glomerular and vascular injury by neutrophils, recent studies suggest that the vascular endothelium plays an active role in recruiting neutrophils to these inflamed areas of the vasculature by expressing adhesive molecules for neutrophils (186,187).

Several forms of vasculitis and glomerulonephritis are associated with circulating autoantibodies reactive with components of neutrophil cytoplasm and are referred to as antineutrophil cytoplasmic antibodies (ANCAs). The two immunohistologic staining patterns originally described as C-ANCA and P-ANCA have now been determined to result from autoantibodies to proteinase-3 and myeloperoxidase, respectively. The demonstration that autoantibodies to neutrophil granule constituents are strongly associated with Wegener granulomatosis, microscopic polyarteritis, and idiopathic necrotizing glomerulonephritis, has led to the suggestion that these antibodies may play a role in the pathogenesis of these diseases. According to this hypothesis, ANCAs may bind to the surface of neutrophils, particularly after neutrophils have been primed by cytokines to secrete and adsorb granular enzymes, and thereby activate neutrophils, resulting in injury to vascular and glomerular endothelium (188) (see Chapter 83). This hypothesis is supported by the demonstration that a polymorphism in a subset of neutrophil Fc receptors (FcRII) associated with increased IgG binding activity is associated with greatly increased susceptibility to development of glomerulonephritis in Wegener granulomatosis (189). An alternative hypothesis is that ANCAs are markers of the disease process and do not play a pathophysiologic role.

PHARMACOLOGIC CONTROL OF NEUTROPHIL FUNCTION

There are two general pharmacologic approaches to the prevention of neutrophil-mediated tissue injury. The first strategy involves the prevention of neutrophil accumulation at an inflamed site. The second approach is to diminish the capacity of neutrophils to release harmful substances (granule contents or oxygen metabolites) once they have entered an inflamed site. Most currently available antiinflammatory agents have been shown to have both activities, but also have significant side effects. New agents are being developed that specifically block either neutrophil accumulation or function.

Antiinflammatory Agents Inhibit Neutrophil/Endothelium Interactions

A great deal of effort has been expended in developing agents that interact specifically with the molecules involved in adhesion. Antibodies directed against neutrophil adhesive molecules (CD11b/CD18, L-selectin) or endothelial adhesive molecules (E-selectin, ICAM-1) may indeed be useful in the treatment of acute inflammation (190). Soluble receptors, peptides, and sugars that interfere with selectin-mediated interactions also may be effective therapeutic agents for preventing or treating acute inflammation (191). In addition to newly developed antiinflammatory drugs, recent reports suggest that many of the agents currently in use for the treatment of inflammatory conditions may act, at least in part, by inhibiting leukocyte/endothelium interactions, thereby preventing the accumulation of neutrophils in inflamed tissues. NSAIDs, such as aspirin (see Chapter 31), modulate the capacity of stimulated neutrophils to adhere to endothelium *in vitro* (192,193). Inhibition of arachidonic acid metabolism in endothelial cells by NSAIDs may lead to the production of chemorepellants for neutrophils (194). Moreover, some, but not all, NSAIDs modulate the expression of adhesion molecules (L-selectin) on neutrophils, both *in vitro* and *in vivo* (195). Other studies demonstrate that one of the first changes seen in synovial tissue from patients treated with gold salts is a reduction in E-selectin expression on the synovial microvasculature (196) (see Chapter 42). Studies performed *in vitro* also demonstrate a direct and selective effect of gold salts on the stimulated endothelial expression of adhesive molecules (197). The capacity of glucocorticoids to diminish the expression of adhesion molecules on cytokine-stimulated endothelium may explain the potent antiinflammatory and immunosuppressive properties of this class of agent as well (198). We have recently found that, by disrupting microtubules, colchicine induces the shedding of L-selectin from the surface of the neutrophil and alters the capacity of E-selectin to mediate adhesion of neutrophils to endothelial cells, thus diminishing the capacity of synovial endothelium to recruit neutrophils to the site of gouty inflammation (185). In other studies, we have demonstrated that methotrexate inhibits neutrophil adhesion to endothelial cells by virtue of its capacity to induce increased adenosine release (199). The local increase in adenosine release resulting from treatment with methotrexate also leads to diminished neutrophil accumulation in an *in vivo* model of acute inflammation (200).

Antiinflammatory Agents Inhibit Release of Mediators from Neutrophils

Much attention has been given to pharmacologic inhibition of neutrophil lysosomal enzyme release and O_2^- generation. In general, two major types of compounds have been studied for their effect on granular enzyme secretion: those that directly affect microtubule assembly and those that influence the intracellular level of the cyclic nucleotides, cAMP and cGMP. Exogenous cAMP (in the presence of phosphodiesterase inhibitors), as well as agents that elevate intracellular levels of cAMP (e.g., PGE_1 or isoproterenol), reduce enzyme release (174). Exogenous cGMP and agents that elevate levels of cGMP (e.g., serotonin or carbamylcholine) enhance lysosomal enzyme release (174). Similarly, agents that promote disassembly of microtubules (e.g., colchicine or vinblastine) reduce and agents that promote microtubule assembly (e.g., deuterium oxide) enhance, lysosomal enzyme release. For some of these agents, such as colchicine, which specifically inhibits LTB_4 production by neutrophils, alternative mechanisms of action may exist (186).

Although NSAIDs, including aspirin, share the property of inhibiting PG synthesis, which may explain their antipyretic, analgesic, and antithrombotic effects, their antiinflammatory effects cannot be explained by this mode of action (201,202). NSAIDs, at antiinflammatory doses, have a variety of effects on neutrophil function (203). Aspirin and piroxicam inhibit neutrophil degranulation, aggregation, and superoxide anion generation. Ibuprofen inhibits only aggregation and degranulation, and indomethacin inhibits only aggregation (204). Among the possible prostaglandin-independent modes of action of NSAIDs on neutrophils is an effect on signaling through G protein–linked receptors (205). Salicylates also inhibit activation of MAPK, a downstream signaling molecule, leading to diminished adhesion by stimulated neutrophils (206).

Other work in our laboratory suggests that a potent endogenous modulator of neutrophil function is adenosine. This purine engages receptors on the surface of neutrophils that selectively inhibit the generation of O_2^- and other toxic oxygen metabolites while still permitting degranulation. Surprisingly, adenosine and its analogues modulate neutrophil function in response to some (e.g., C5a, FMLP, and opsonized zymosan particles), but not other (immune complexes) stimuli. A seemingly paradoxic observation is that engagement of adenosine receptors promotes neutrophil chemotaxis (207–213). Thus, adenosine, released from damaged tissue, may promote migration of neutrophils to sites of infection or tissue damage while preventing the activated neutrophils from damaging healthy tissues along the way. Recent studies from our laboratory demonstrate that methotrexate promotes adenosine release from injured tissues and that the adenosine released at these inflamed sites inhibits the accumulation of neutrophils (see Chapter 32). Thus, adenosine may mediate the antiinflammatory effects of methotrexate (201,202). Similarly, high-dose salicylates also induce adenosine release with a marked reduction in neutrophil accumulation in response to an inflammatory stimulus (214). In addition to adenosine, nitric oxide (NO) may be an endogenous downmodulator of neutrophil function because NO has been shown to inhibit neutrophil adhesion and O_2^- generation, suggesting that agents that promote NO synthesis may be antiinflammatory (215).

HERITABLE DISORDERS

As discussed earlier, neutrophil function is regulated by a multitude of extrinsic and intrinsic factors, disruption of any one of which can lead to malfunction. Defects that lead to impaired neutrophil function result in an immunocompromised host, whereas defects that interfere with mechanisms that turn off inflammation contribute to inflammatory diseases such as RA, SLE, and the adult respiratory distress syndrome. At least 15 primary (probably heritable) defects of neutrophil function have been identified (216). Additionally, neutrophils isolated from patients with autoimmune diseases such as RA and SLE have been found to have secondarily impaired functions (217). Abnormalities of neutrophil function can be classified in terms of their major responses to inflammatory stimuli: defects of receptor coupling, chemotaxis, adherence, phagocytosis, degranulation, respiratory burst oxidase, or specific defects in nonoxidative bactericidal mechanisms. Although most heritable defects of neutrophil function are exceedingly rare, studies of defective neutrophils have provided critical insights into normal neutrophil function.

Chronic Granulomatous Disease

The disorder of neutrophil function that is best characterized at the molecular level is CGD. CGD is a rare inherited disorder (prevalence estimated at 1 in 500,000) that is seen in early childhood with recurrent life-threatening pyogenic infections, particularly of the skin, lungs, and gastrointestinal tract, and associated granulomas that can become obstructive (218). Thus, CGD is a disease with impaired neutrophil function associated with an abnormal inflammatory response. Biochemically, CGD is characterized by a complete, or near complete, absence of the respiratory burst in neutrophils and macrophages due to a defect in one of the components of the NADPH oxidase (218,219). Interestingly, the clinical spectrum of disease is broad, sometimes even within a given family, suggesting that other factors play a role in the clinical expression of disease. The most common pathogens include catalase-positive *Staphylococcus aureus,* gram-negative organisms including *Pseudomonas cepacia, Nocardia* species, and fungi such as *Candida albicans, Torulopsis glabrata,* and *Pseudallescheria boydii.* The narrow spectrum of pathogens causing the worst morbidity and mortality in CGD is somewhat surprising. Two hypotheses have been offered to explain this narrow spectrum (218). The first hypothesis derives from the observation that most pathogens are catalase positive and proposes that these pathogens therefore have a mechanism to destroy microorganism-derived H_2O_2 in the phagosome before it can be used by neutrophil myeloperoxidase. The second hypothesis is that these microorganisms represent a subset of pathogens that are poorly killed by the neutrophil's nonoxidative microbicidal systems.

Sixty-five percent of CGD patients have the X-linked form of the disease that has now been attributed to defects in the gene for the large subunit of cytochrome b_{558}, $p91^{phox}$, located at Xp21.1. The remaining 35% of cases display an autosomal-recessive mode of inheritance. Among these patients, most (23% of all patients) have been found to have a defect in the $p47^{phox}$ gene located at 7q11.23. The remainder is evenly split between defects in the $p67^{phox}$ gene located at 1q25 and the $p22^{phox}$ gene located at 16p24 that encodes the small subunit of cytochrome b_{558}. Deletions, insertions, and point mutations leading to stop codons, amino acid substitutions, or splice site defects have all been reported in these genes, and most CGD patients studied have mutations specific to their families. Of note, no patients with defective $p21^{rac}$ have been reported, suggesting that such a defect might be lethal, which is consistent with the observation that $p21^{rac1}$ is an essential gene that can apparently substitute *in vivo* for $p21^{rac2}$ (97).

Until recently, therapy for CGD consisted of aggressive treatment of infections with antibiotics. IFN-γ has now been shown to be efficacious in decreasing the frequency and severity of infections in CGD patients (220,221), although the mechanism of action, particularly in patients with complete deletions of genes for NADPH oxidase components, remains unknown. The recent development by homologous recombination of two knockout mice defective in either $p91^{phox}$ (222) or $p47^{phox}$ (223) has provided an animal model with which future therapies can be tested. Research aimed at treating CGD by the emerging techniques of gene-transfer therapy is currently underway (224). Although the immunocompromised state of CGD mice is relatively mild, as is that of mice lacking inducible nitric oxide synthase, when both systems are disrupted, the mice are severely immunocompromised, demonstrating the redundancy of reactive oxygen and reactive nitrogen species in host defense (225). The intensive investigation into the molecular basis of CGD over the past 15 years has resulted not only in an unusually profound understanding of a human immunodeficiency syndrome, but has also proven essential in the elucidation of the biochemistry of the NADPH oxidase.

Leukocyte Adhesion Deficiency

In addition to CGD, another inherited disorder of neutrophil function, known as leukocyte adhesion deficiency (LAD), has recently been characterized at the molecular level. There are two types of LAD, and like CGD, both forms of LAD are characterized clinically by recurrent bacterial and fungal infections, particularly of the skin and mucosa, but without granuloma formation. Unlike CGD, LAD type 1 is associated with impaired wound healing, delayed severing of the umbilical cord in affected neonates, gingivitis, and persistent granulocytosis (226). Clinically severe and moderate forms of LAD have been recognized. Neutrophils from patients with LAD have a normal respiratory burst, but display impaired mobility and phagocytosis. Early reports of an absent surface glycoprotein in LAD neutrophils led to the discovery that leukocytes from patients with LAD lacked all three forms of the β_2 integrins [Mac-1, leukocyte function–associated antigen-1 (LFA-1), and gp150/95] that mediate many of the adhesive events critical for leukocyte function (227). Because all three of these heterodimers share a common β chain, CD18, a defect in the expression of this molecule was sought and found. As currently understood, LAD results from any one of a number of mutations in the gene for CD18, located at 21q22.3, that results in either diminished expression of CD18 or impaired ability of mutant CD18 to combine with its three cognate α chains, CD11a, CD11b, or CD11c. Failure to form a proper heterodimer in the endoplasmic reticulum prevents the molecule from trafficking to the cell surface, and it is, instead, degraded (228). The molecular basis for the clinical heterogeneity is not understood, but clinical severity has been shown to correlate with surface expression of β_2 integrins (229). LAD type II results from a defect in the synthesis of appropriate glycoprotein ligands for selectins due to a generalized defect in fucosylation (230,231). Like CGD, LAD is an attractive candidate disease for gene-transfer therapy, and pilot studies using retroviral vectors have already been reported (232). Analogous to the role played by CGD in elucidating the biochemistry of the neutrophil NADPH oxidase, the study of the molecular basis of LAD has played an essential role in unraveling the biology of leukocyte adhesion molecules.

Chédiak-Higashi Syndrome

One of the most intriguing of the heritable neutrophil defects is a rare autosomal recessive disorder designated Chédiak–Higashi syndrome. This syndrome is characterized by neutrophils that have large, bizarre cytoplasmic granules. Because these granules are peroxidase positive, and there is a dearth of normal azurophilic granules, the large granules are believed to arise from fusion of azurophilic granules. Chédiak-Higashi neutrophils display defective migration and degranulation and are deficient in cathepsin G, although they have a normal respiratory burst. Clinical features of Chédiak-Higashi syndrome include oculocutaneous albinism, photophobia, nystagmus, progressive peripheral neuropathy, gingivitis, neutropenia, and recurrent pyogenic infections out of proportion to the degree of neutropenia. Although the molecular basis of Chédiak-Higashi syndrome is unknown, biochemical defects observed in neutrophils from affected patients include abnormal cyclic nucleotide metabolism and disordered microtubule assembly (233). Several animal models for Chédiak-Higashi syndrome have been characterized, including the beige mouse, and it has been postulated that the *bg* mutation giving rise to this strain may be the homologue of the Chédiak-Higashi gene (234).

Specific Granule Deficiency

Another rare disorder of neutrophils is specific granule deficiency (235,236). Neutrophils from patients with this syndrome display bilobed nuclei, and ultrastructural and cell fractionation studies (237) reveal a dearth of specific granules. Biochemical markers of specific granules (e.g., lactoferrin and vitamin B_{12}–binding protein) are either absent or markedly reduced (237). Patients with specific granule deficiency have depressed inflammatory responses and recurrent bacterial infections without predilection for specific pathogens. The peripheral blood neutrophil count is normal, as is the respiratory burst. The molecular basis of this disorder is unknown, and the few reported cases suggest that the disorder is inherited in an autosomal-recessive fashion. Neutrophils from patients with thermal injury (238) and from normal neonates (239) also display relative specific granule deficiency and functional impairment similar to neutrophils from patients with specific granule deficiency.

Myeloperoxidase Deficiency

Myeloperoxidase deficiency is a relatively common heritable defect of neutrophils (prevalence, 1 in 2,000) (213, 236,240,241). Fortunately, myeloperoxidase deficiency is of little clinical consequence in that it does not predispose to bacterial infection, perhaps because neutrophils from affected individuals make excessive amounts of H_2O_2. Myeloperoxidase deficiency is an autosomal-recessive trait consistent with the localization of the gene for myeloperoxidase at 7q21 (240).

REFERENCES

1. Metchnikoff E. Sur la lutte des cellules de l'organisme contre l'invasion des microbes. *Ann Inst Pasteur* 1886;1:321.
2. Cochrane CG, Weigle WO, Dixon FJ. The role of polymorphonuclear leukocytes in the initiation and cessation of the Arthus vasculitis. *J Exp Med* 1959;110:481–494.
3. Boxer LA, Stossel TP. Interactions of actin, myosin, and an actin-binding protein of chronic myelogenous leukemia leukocytes. *J Clin Invest* 1976;57:964–976.
4. DeShazo CV, McGrade MP, Henson PM, et al. The effect of complement depletion on neutrophil migration in acute immunologic arthritis. *J Immunol* 1972;108:1414–1419.
5. Humphrey JH. The mechanism of Arthus reactions. I. The role of polymorphonuclear leucocytes and other factors in reversed passive Arthus reactions in rabbits. *Br J Exp Pathol* 1955;36:268–282.
6. Parish WE. Effects of neutrophils on tissues: experiments on the Arthus reaction, the flare phenomenon, and post-phagocytic release of lysosomal enzymes. *Br J Dermatol* 1969;81:28–35.

7. Stetson CA. Similarities in the mechanisms determining the Arthus and Shwartzman phenomena. *J Exp Med* 1951;94:347–358.
8. Kniker WT, Cochrane CG. Pathogenic factors in vascular lesions of experimental serum sickness. *J Exp Med* 1965;122:83–98.
9. Cochrane CG, Unanue ER, Dixon FJ. A role of polymorphonuclear leukocytes and complement in nephrotoxic nephritis. *J Exp Med* 1965; 122:99–116.
10. DeShazo CV, Henson PM, Cochrane CG. Acute immunologic arthritis in rabbits. *J Clin Invest* 1972;51:50–57.
11. Bainton DF, Ullyot JL, Farquhar MG. The development of neutrophilic polymorphonuclear leukocytes in human bone marrow. *J Exp Med* 1971;134:907–934.
12. Crosier PS, Clark SC. Basic biology of the hematopoietic growth factors. *Semin Oncol* 1992;19:349–361.
13. Golde DW, Baldwin GC. Myeloid growth factors. In: Gallin JI, Goldstein IM, Snyderman R, eds. *Inflammation: basic principles and clinical correlates.* New York: Raven, 1992:291–301.
14. Lawson ND, Berliner N. Neutrophil maturation and the role of retinoic acid. *Exp Hematol* 1999;27:1355–1367.
15. Berliner N. Molecular biology of neutrophil differentiation. *Curr Opin Hematol* 1998;5:49–53.
16. Squier MK, Sehnert AJ, Cohen JJ. Apoptosis in leukocytes. *J Leukoc Biol* 1995;57:2–10.
17. Homburg CH, Roos D. Apoptosis of neutrophils. *Curr Opin Hematol* 1996;3:94–99.
18. Lord PCW, Wilmoth LMG, Mizel SB, et al. Expression of interleukin-1α and β genes by human blood polymorphonuclear leukocytes. *J Clin Invest* 1991;87:1312–1321.
19. Cassatella MA, Bazzoni F, Ceska M, et al. IL-8 production by human polymorphonuclear leukocytes: the chemoattractant formyl-methionyl-leucyl-phenylalanine induces the gene expression and release of IL-8 through a pertussis toxin–sensitive pathway. *J Immunol* 1992;148: 3216–3220.
20. Lindermann A, Riedel D, Oster W, et al. Granulocyte-macrophage stimulating factor induces cytokine secretion by human polymorphonuclear leukocytes. *J Clin Invest* 1989;83:1308–1312.
21. Colotta F, Polentarutti N, Mantovani A. Differential expression of Raf-1 protooncogene in resting and activated human leukocyte populations. *Exp Cell Res* 1991;194:284–288.
22. Jack R, Fearon D. Selective synthesis of mRNA and proteins by human peripheral blood neutrophils. *J Immunol* 1988;140:4286–4293.
23. Spitznagel JK. Antibiotic proteins of human neutrophils. *J Clin Invest* 1990;86:1381–1386.
24. Borregaard N, Kjeldsen L, Lollike K, et al. Granules and vesicles of human neutrophils: the role of endomembranes as source of plasma membrane proteins [Review]. *Eur J Hematol* 1993;51:318–322.
25. Kjeldsen L, Bainton DF, Sengelov H, et al. Structural and functional heterogeneity among peroxidase-negative granules in human neutrophils: identification of a distinct gelatinase-containing granule subset by combined immunocytochemistry and subcellular fractionation. *Blood* 1993;82:3183–3191.
26. Sengelov H, Mielsen MH, Borregaard N. Separation of human neutrophil plasma membrane from intracellular vesicles containing alkaline phosphatase and NADPH oxidase activity by free flow electrophoresis. *J Biol Chem* 1992;167:14912–14917.
27. Borregaard N, Christensen L, Bejerrum OW, et al. Identification of a highly mobilizable subset of human neutrophil intracellular vesicles that contains tetranectin and latent alkaline phosphatase. *J Clin Invest* 1990;85:408–416.
28. Borregaard N, Miller LJ, Springer TA. Chemoattractant-regulated mobilization of a novel intracellular compartment in human neutrophils. *Science* 1987;237:1204–1206.
29. Dewald B, Bretz U, Baggiolini M. Release of gelatinase from a novel secretory compartment of human neutrophils. *J Clin Invest* 1982;70: 518–525.
30. Kjeldsen L, Bjerrum OW, Askaa J, et al. Subcellular localization and release of human neutrophil gelatinase, confirming the existence of separate gelatinase-containing granules. *Biochem J* 1992;287:603–610.
31. Sengelov H, Kjeldsen L, Kroeze W, et al. Secretory vesicles are the intracellular reservoir of complement receptor 1 in human neutrophils. *J Immunol* 1994;153:804–810.
32. Sengelov H, Kjeldsen L, Diamond MS, et al. Subcellular localization and dynamics of mac-1 ($a_m b_2$) in human neutrophils. *J Clin Invest* 1993;92:1467–1476.
33. Calafat J, Kuijpers TW, Janssen H, et al. Evidence for small intracellular vesicles in human blood phagocytes containing cytochrome b_{558} and the adhesion molecule CD11b/CD18. *Blood* 1993;81:3122–3129.
34. Sengelov H, Boulay F, Kjeldsen L, Borregaard N. Subcellular localization and translocation of the receptor for *N*-formylmethionyl-leucyl-phenylalanine in human neutrophils. *Biochem J* 1994;299: 473–479.
35. Reaven EP, Axline SG. Subplasmalemmal microfilaments and microtubules in resting and phagocytizing cultivated macrophages. *J Cell Biol* 1976;59:12–27.
36. Samuelsson SJ, Luther PW, Pumplin DW, et al. Structures linking microfilament bundles to the membrane at focal contacts. *J Cell Biol* 1993;122:485–496.
37. Turner CE, Burridge K. Transmembrane molecular assemblies in cell–extracellular matrix interactions. *Curr Opin Cell Biol* 1991;3: 849–853.
38. Weissmann G, Korchak HM, Perez HD, et al. The secretory code of the neutrophil. *J Res Soc* 1979;26:687–701.
39. Rich AM, Hoffstein S. Inverse correlation between neutrophil microtubule numbers and enhanced random migration. *J Cell Sci* 1981;48: 181–191.
40. Reibman J, Haines K, Weissmann G. Alterations in cyclic nucleotides and the activation of neutrophils. In: Grinstein S, Rotstein O, eds. *Current topics in membranes and transport.* Vol. 35. Mechanisms of leukocyte activation. New York: Academic, 1990:399–424.
41. Mellon MG, Rebhun LI. Sulfhydryls and the *in vitro* polymerization of tubulin. *J Cell Biol* 1976;70:226–238.
42. Malawista SE. Microtrobules and the mobilization of hisosomes in phagocytizing human leukocytes. *Ann NY Acad Sci* 1975;253: 738–749.
43. Osborn L. Leukocyte adhesion to endothelium in inflammation. *Cell* 1990;62:3–6.
44. Paulson JC. Selectin/carbohydrate-mediated adhesion of leukocytes. In: Harlan JM, Liu DY, eds. *Adhesion: its role in inflammatory disease.* New York: WH Freeman, 1992:19–42.
45. Lobb RR. Integrin-immunoglobulin superfamily interactions in endothelial-leukocyte adhesion. In: Harlan JM, Liu DY, eds. *Adhesion: its role in inflammatory disease.* New York: WH Freeman, 1992:1–18.
46. Cronstein BN, Weissmann G. The adhesion molecules of inflammation. *Arthritis Rheum* 1993;36:147–157.
47. Smith CW, Kishimoto TK, Abbass O, et al. Chemotactic factors regulate lectin adhesion molecule 1 (LECAM-1)-dependent neutrophil adhesion to cytokine-stimulated endothelial cells *in vitro*. *J Clin Invest* 1881;87:609–618.
48. Smith CW, Rothlein R, Hughes BJ, et al. Recognition of an endothelial determinant for CD18-dependent human neutrophil adherence and transendothelial migration. *J Clin Invest* 1988;82:1746–1756.
49. Smith CW, Marlin SD, Rothlein R, et al. Cooperative interactions of LFA-1 and Mac-1 with intracellular adhesion molecule-1 in facilitating adherence and transendothelial migration of human neutrophils *in vitro*. *J Clin Invest* 1991;83:2008–2017.
50. Schwartz BR, Ochs HD, Beatty PG, et al. A monoclonal antibody-defined membrane antigen complex is required for neutrophil-neutrophil aggregation. *Blood* 1985;65:1553–1556.
51. Wallis WJ, Hiekstein DD, Schwartz BR, et al. Monoclonal antibody-defined functional epitopes on the adhesion-promoting glycoprotein complex (CD18) of human neutrophils. *Blood* 1986;67:1007–1013.
52. Harlan JM, Killen PD, Senecal FM, et al. The role of neutrophil membrane glycoprotein GP-150 in neutrophil adherence to endothelium *in vitro*. *Blood* 1985;66:167–178.
53. Springer TA. Traffic signals for lymphocyte recirculation and leukocyte emigration: the multistep paradigm. *Cell* 1994;76:301–314.
54. Smith CW, Marlin SD, Rothlein R, et al. Cooperative interactions of LFA-1 and Mac-1 with intercellular adhesion molecule-1 in facilitating adherence and transendothelial migration of human neutrophils *in vitro*. *J Clin Invest* 1991;83:2008–2017.
55. Jesaitis AJ, Naemura JR, Sklar LA, et al. Rapid modulation of *N*-formyl chemotactic peptide receptors on the surface of human granulocytes: formation of high affinity ligand-receptor complexes in transient association with cytoskeleton. *J Cell Biol* 1984;98:1378–1387.
56. Jesaitis AJ, Tolley JO, Bokoch GM, et al. Regulation of chemoattractant receptor interaction with transducing proteins by organizational control in the plasma membrane of human neutrophils. *J Cell Biol* 1989;109:2783–2790.

57. Weinbaum DL, Sullivan JA, Mandell GL. Orientation of membrane receptors on the neutrophil. In: Weissmann G, ed. *Advances in inflammation research.* New York: Raven, 1982:95–108.
58. Gardiner EM, Pestonjamasp KN, Bohl BP, et al. Spatial and temporal analysis of Rac activation during live neutrophil chemotaxis. *Curr Biol* 2002;12:2029–2034.
59. Iijima M, Huang YE, Devreotes P. Temporal and spatial regulation of chemotaxis. *Dev Cell* 2002;3:469–478.
60. Unkeless JC. Function and heterogeneity of human Fc receptors for immunoglobulin G. *J Clin Invest* 1989;83:355–361.
61. Ross GD, Medoff ME. Membrane complement receptors specific for bound fragments of C3. *Adv Immunol* 1985;37:217–267.
62. Wright SD, Silverstein SC. Tumor-promoting phorbol esters stimulate C3b and C3b8 receptor-mediated phagocytosis in cultured human monocytes. *J Exp Med* 1982;156:1149–1164.
63. Korn ED, Weisman RA. Phagocytosis of latex beads by *Acanthamoeba.* II. Electron microscopic study of the initial events. *J Cell Biol* 1969;34:219–227.
64. Mudd J, McCutcheon M, Lucke B. Phagocytosis. *Physiol Rev* 1934; 14:210–275.
65. Zucker-Franklin D, Hirsch JG. Electron microscope studies on the degranulation of rabbit peritoneal leukocytes during phagocytosis. *J Exp Med* 1964;120:569–576.
66. Cohn ZA, Hirsch JG. The influence of phagocytosis on the intracellular distribution of granule-associated components of polymorphonuclear leucocytes. *J Exp Med* 1960;112:1015–1022.
67. Ohlsson K, Olsson I, Spitznagel JK. Localization of chymotrypsin-like cationic protein, collagenase, and elastase in azurophil granules of human neutrophilic polymorphonuclear leukocytes. *Hoppe Seylers Z Physiol Chem* 1977;358:361–366.
68. Allen LH, Aderem A. Mechanisms of phagocytosis. *Curr Opin Immunol* 1996;8:36–40.
69. Desjardins M. ER-mediated phagocytosis: a new membrane for new functions. *Nature Rev Immunol* 2003;3:280–291.
70. Caron E, Hall A. Identification of two distinct mechanisms of phagocytosis controlled by different rho GTPases. *Science* 1998;282:1717–1721.
71. Botelhoa RJ, Teruele M, Dierckmanb R, et al. Localized biphasic changes in phosphatidylinositol-4,5-bisphosphate at sites of phagocytosis. *J Cell Biol* 2000;151:1353–1368.
72. Gagnon E, Duclos S, Rondeau C, et al. Endoplasmic reticulum-mediated phagocytosis is a mechanism of entry into macrophages. *Cell* 2002;110:119–131.
73. Sjolin C, Stendahl O, Dahlgren C. Calcium-induced translocation of annexins to subcellular organelles of human neutrophils. *Biochem J* 1994;300:325–330.
74. Bainton DF. Sequential degranulation of the two types of polymorphonuclear leukocyte granules during phagocytosis of microorganisms. *J Cell Biol* 1973;58:249–264.
75. Smolen JE, Weissmann G. Stimuli which provoke secretion of azurophil enzymes from human neutrophils induce increments in adenosine cyclic 38–58-monophosphate. *Biochim Biophys Acta* 1981;672:197– 206.
76. Phillips MR, Agramson SB, Kolasinki SL et al. Low molecular weight GTP binding protein S in.
77. Klebanoff SJ. Myeloperoxidase: contribution to the microbicidal activity of intact leukocytes. *Science* 1972;169:1095–1097.
78. Zurier RB, Hoffstein S, Weissmann G. Mechanisms of lysosomal enzyme release from human leukocytes. *J Cell Biol* 1973;58:27–48.
79. Zurier RB, Hoffstein S, Weissmann G. Cytochalasin B: effect on lysosomal enzyme release from human leucocytes. *Proc Natl Acad Sci U S A* 1973;70:844–848.
80. Weiss SJ. Tissue destruction by neutrophils. *N Engl J Med* 1989;320: 365–376.
81. Ugai K, Ishikawa H, Hirohata K, et al. Interaction of polymorphonuclear leukocytes with immune complexes trapped in rheumatoid articular cartilage. *Arthritis Rheum* 1983;26:1434–1441.
82. Sbarra AJ, Karnovsky ML. The biochemical basis of phagocytosis. 1. Metabolic changes during the ingestion of particles by polymorphonuclear leukocytes. *J Biol Chem* 1959;234:1355–1362.
83. Rossi F. The O_2^--forming NADPH oxidase of the phagocytes: nature, mechanisms of activation and function. *Biochim Biophys Acta* 1986; 853:65–89.
84. Morel F, Doussiere J, Vignais PV. The superoxide-generating oxidase of phagocytic cells: physiological, molecular and pathological aspects. *Eur J Biochem* 1991;201:523–546.
85. Reeves EP, Lu H, Jacobs HL, et al. Killing activity of neutrophils is mediated through activation of proteases by K^+ flux. *Nature* 2002; 416:291–297.
86. Segal AW, Jones OTG, Webster D, et al. Absence of a newly described cytochrome b from neutrophils of patients with chronic granulomatous disease. *Lancet* 1978;2:446–449.
87. Rotrosen D, Yeung CL, Leto TL, et al. Cytochrome b_{558}: the flavin-binding component of the phagocyte NADPH oxidase. *Science* 1992; 256:1459–1462.
88. Bromberg Y, Pick E. Activation of NADPH-dependent superoxide production in a cell-free system by sodium dodecyl sulfate. *J Biol Chem* 1985;260:13539–13545.
89. Curnutte JT. Activation of human neutrophil nicotinamide adenine dinucleotide phosphate, reduced (triphosphopyridine nucleotide, reduced) oxidase by arachidonic acid in a cell-free system. *J Clin Invest* 1985;75:1740–1743.
90. McPhail LC, Shirley PS, Clayton CC, et al. Activation of the respiratory burst enzyme from human neutrophils in a cell-free system: evidence for a soluble factor. *J Clin Invest* 1985;75:1735–1739.
91. Bromberg Y, Pick E. Unsaturated fatty acids stimulate NADPH-dependent superoxide production by cell-free system derived from macrophages. *Cell Immunol* 1984;88:213–221.
92. Segal AW, Abo A. The biochemical basis of the NADPH oxidase of phagocytes. *Trends Biochem Sci* 1993;18:43–47.
93. Rotrosen D, Yeung CL, Katkin JP. Production of recombinant cytochrome b_{558} allows reconstitution of the phagocyte NADPH oxidase solely from recombinant proteins. *J Biol Chem* 1993;268:14256–14260.
94. Roberts AW, Kim C, Zhen L, et al. Deficiency of the hematopoietic cell-specific rho family GTPase rac2 is characterized by abnormalities of neutrophil function and host defense. *Immunity* 1999;10: 183–196.
95. Wientjes FB, Hsuan JJ, Totty NF, et al. p40phox, a third cytosolic component of the activation complex of the NADPH oxidase to contain src homology 3 domains. *Biochem J* 1993;296:557–561.
96. Xu Y, Hortsman H, Seet L, et al. SNX3 regulates endosomal function through its PX-domain-mediated interaction with PtdIns(3)P. *Nat Cell Biol* 2001;3:658–666.
97. Nobes C, Hall A. Rho, Rac and Cdc42 GTPases regulate the assembly of multimolecular focal complexes associated with actin stress fibers, lamellipodia, and filopodia. *Cell* 1995;81:53–62.
98. Philips MR, Feoktistov A, Pillinger MH, et al. Translocation of p21rac2 from cytosol to plasma membrane is neither necessary nor sufficient for neutrophil NADPH oxidase activity. *J Biol Chem* 1995; 270:11514–11521.
99. Tiku K, Tiku ML, Skosey JL. Interleukin-1 production by human polymorphonuclear neutrophils. *J Immunol* 1986;136:3677–3685.
100. Arnold R, Scheffer J, Konig B, et al. Effects of *Listeria monocytogenes* and *Yersinia enterocolitica* on cytokine gene expression and release from human polymorphonuclear granulocytes and epithelial (HEp-2) cells. *Infect Immunol* 1993;61:2545–2552.
101. Roberge CJ, Grassi J, de Medicis R, et al. Crystal-neutrophil interactions lead to interleukin-1 synthesis. *Agents Actions* 1991;34:38–41.
102. Fujishima S, Hoffman AR, Vu T, et al. Regulation of neutrophil interleukin-8 gene expression and protein secretion by LPS, TNF-alpha, and IL-1 beta. *J Cell Physiol* 1993;154:478–485.
103. Kusaka Y, Cullen RT, Donaldson K. Immunomodulation in mineral dust-exposed lungs: stimulatory effect and interleukin-1 release by neutrophils from quartz-elicited alveolitis. *Clin Exp Immunol* 1990; 80:293–298.
104. Takeichi O, Saito I, Tsurumachi T, et al. Human polymorphonuclear leukocytes derived from chronically inflamed tissue express inflammatory cytokines in vivo. *Cell Immunol* 1994;156:296–309.
105. Tiku K, Tiku ML, Liu S, et al. Normal human neutrophils are a source of a specific interleukin 1 inhibitor. *J Immunol* 1986;136: 3686–3692.
106. Re F, Mengozzi M, Muzio M, et al. Expression of interleukin-1 receptor antagonist (IL-1ra) by human circulating polymorphonuclear cells. *Eur J Immunol* 1993;23:570–573.
107. Marin V, Montero-Julian F, Gres S, et al. Chemotactic agents induce IL-6Ralpha shedding from polymorphonuclear cells: involvement of a metalloproteinase of the TNF-alpha-converting enzyme (TACE) type. Eur J Immunol 2002;32:2965–2970.
108. Hurst SM, Wilkinson TS, McLoughlin RM, et al. IL-6 and its soluble receptor orchestrate a temporal switch in the pattern of leukocyte re-

cruitment seen during acute inflammation. *Immunity* 2001;14: 705–714.
109. Perez HD, Weksler B, Goldstein I. A new mechanism for the generation of biologically active products from arachidonic acid. *Clin Res* 1979;27:464a.
110. Vane J. Towards a better aspirin. *Nature* 1994;367:215–216.
111. Kuehl FA Jr, Humes JL, Egan RW, et al. Role of prostaglandin endoperoxide PGG_2 in inflammatory processes. *Nature* 1977;265:170–172.
112. Robinson DR, Curran DP, Hamer PJ. Prostaglandins and related compounds in inflammatory rheumatic diseases. In: Ziff M, Velo G, Gorini S, eds. *Advances in inflammation research.* New York: Raven, 1982.
113. Goodwin JS, Bankhurst AD, Messner RP. Suppression of human T-cell mitogenesis by prostaglandin: existence of a prostaglandin-producing suppressor cell. *J Exp Med* 1971;146:1719–1734.
114. Smolen JE, Korchak HM, Weissmann G. Increased levels of cyclic adenosine 38,58-monophosphate in human polymorphonuclear leukocytes after surface stimulation. *J Clin Invest* 1980;65:1077–1085.
115. Radmark O, Malmsten C, Samuelsson B, et al. Leukotriene A: stereochemistry and enzymatic conversion to leukotriene B. *Biochem Biophys Res Commun* 1980;92:954–961.
116. Hammarstrom S. Metabolism of leukotriene C_2 in the guinea pig: identification of metabolites formed by the lung, liver, and kidney. *J Biol Chem* 1981;256:9573–9578.
117. Hammarstrom S. Rapid *in vivo* metabolism of LTB C_3 in the monkey, *Macaca irus. Biochem Biophys Res Commun* 1981;101:1109–1115.
118. Smith MJ, Ford-Hutchinson AW, Bray MA. Leukotriene B: a potential mediator of inflammation. *J Pharm Pharmacol* 1980;32:517–518.
119. Dahlen S-E, Hedqvist P, Hammarstrom S, et al. Leukotrienes are potent constrictors of human bronchi. *Nature* 1980;288:484–486.
120. Feinmark SJ. Stimulation of human leukocyte degranulation by leukotriene B_4 and its omega-oxidized metabolites. *FEBS Lett* 1981; 136:141–144.
121. Serhan CN, Fridovich J, Goetzl EJ, et al. Leukotriene B_4 and phosphatidic acid are calcium ionophores: studies employing arsenazo III in liposomes. *J Biol Chem* 1982;257:4746–4752.
122. Samuelsson B. Leukotrienes: mediators of immediate hypersensitivity reactions and inflammation. *Science* 1983;220:568–575.
123. Boulay F, Tardif M, Brouchon L, et al. The human *N*-formylpeptide receptor: characterization of two cDNA isolates and evidence for a new subfamily of G-protein-coupled receptors. *Biochemistry* 1990; 29:11123–11133.
124. Gerard NP, Gerard C. The chemotactic receptor for human C5a anaphylatoxin. *Nature* 1991;349:614–617.
125. Murphy PM, Tiffany HL. Cloning of complementary DNA encoding a functional human interleukin-8 receptor. *Science* 1991;253:1280–1283.
126. Boulay F, Mery L, Tardif M, et al. Expression cloning of a receptor for C5a anaphylatoxin on differentiated HL-60 cells. *Biochemistry* 1991;30:2993–2999.
127. Honda Z, Nakamura M, Miki I, et al. Cloning by functional expression of platelet-activating factor receptor from guinea-pig lung. *Nature* 1991;349:342–346.
128. Neer EJ. Heterotrimeric G proteins: organizers of transmembrane signals. *Cell* 1995:80:249–257.
129. Simon MI, Strathmann MP, Gautam N. Diversity of G proteins in signal transduction. *Science* 1991;252:802–808.
130. Volpp BD, Nauseef WM, Clark RA. Two cytosolic neutrophil oxidase components absent in autosomal chronic granulomatous disease. *Science* 1988;242:1295–1297.
131. Goldsmith P, Gierschik P, Milligan G, et al. Antibodies directed against synthetic peptides distinguish between GTP-binding proteins in neutrophil and brain. *J Biol Chem* 1987;30:14683–14688.
132. Gierschik P, Sidiropoulous D, Spiegel A, et al. Purification and immunochemical characterization of the major pertussis toxin-sensitive guanine nucleotide binding protein in bovine neutrophil membranes. *Eur J Biochem* 1987;165:185–194.
133. Philips MR, Staud R, Pillinger M, et al. Activation-dependent carboxyl methylation of neutrophil G-protein a subunit. *Proc Natl Acad Sci U S A* 1995;92:2283–2287.
134. Polakis PG, Uhing RJ, Snyderman R. The formylpeptide chemoattractant receptor copurifies with a GTP-binding protein containing a distinct 40-kDa pertussis toxin substrate. *J Biol Chem* 1988;263: 4969–4976.
135. Camps M, Carozzi A, Schnabel P, et al. Isozyme-selective stimulation of phospholipase C-b_2 by G protein bg-subunits. *Nature* 1992; 360:684–686.
136. Cockcroft S, Thomas GMH, Fensome A, et al. Phospholipase D: a downstream effector of ARF in granulocytes. *Science* 1994;263:523–526.
137. Smolen JE, Korchak HM, Weissmann G. Increased levels of cyclic adenosine-38,58-monophosphate in human polymorphonuclear leukocytes after surface stimulation. *J Clin Invest* 1980;79:1077–1085.
138. Zurier RB, Weissmann G, Hoffstein S, et al. Mechanisms of lysosomal enzyme release from human leukocytes. II. Effects of cAMP and cGMP, autonomic agonists, and agents which affect microtubule function. *J Clin Invest* 1974;53:297–309.
139. Cook SJ, McCormick F. Inhibition by cAMP of ras-dependent activation of Raf. *Science* 1993;262:1069–1072.
140. Wu J, Dent P, Jelinek T, et al. Inhibition of the EGF-activated MAP kinase signaling pathway by adenosine 38,58-monophosphate. *Science* 1993;262:1065–1068.
141. Pillinger MH, Philips MR, Feoktistov A, et al. Crosstalk in signal transduction via EP receptors: prostaglandin E_1 inhibits chemoattractant-induced mitogen-activated protein kinase activity in human neutrophils. In: Samuelsson B, ed. *Advances in prostaglandin, thromboxane, and leukotriene research.* New York: Raven, 1995:23:311–316.
142. Stephens L, Smrcka A, Cooke FT, et al. A novel phosphoinositide 3 kinase activity in myeloid-derived cells is activated by G protein bg subunits. *Cell* 1994;77:83–93.
143. Forehand JR, Johnston RB Jr, Bomalaski JS. Phospholipase A_2 activity in human neutrophils: stimulation by lipopolysaccharide and possible involvement in priming for an enhanced respiratory burst. *J Immunol* 1993;151:4918–4925.
144. Abramson SB, Leszczynska-Piziak J, Weissmann G. Arachidonic acid as a second messenger: interactions with a GTP-binding protein of human neutrophils. *J Immunol* 1991;147:231–236.
145. Hall A. The cellular functions of small GTP-binding proteins. *Science* 1990;249:635–640.
146. Abo A, Pick E, Hall A, et al. Activation of the NADPH oxidase involves the small GTP-binding protein $p21^{rac1}$. *Nature* 1992;353: 668–670.
147. Knaus UG, Heyworth PG, Evans T, et al. Regulation of phagocyte oxygen radical production by the GTP-binding protein Rac 2. *Science* 1991;254:1512–1515.
148. Quinn MT, Parkos CA, Walker L, et al. Association of a ras-related protein with cytochrome b of human neutrophils. *Nature* 1989;342: 198–200.
149. Philips MR, Abramson SB, Kolasinski SL, et al. Low molecular weight GTP-binding proteins in human neutrophil granule membranes. *J Biol Chem* 1991;266:1289–1298.
150. Philips MR, Pillinger MH, Staud R, et al. Carboxyl methylation of ras-related proteins during signal transduction in neutrophils. *Science* 1993;259:977–980.
151. Ridley AJ, Hall A. The small GTP-binding protein rho regulates the assembly of focal adhesions and actin stress fibers in response to growth factors. *Cell* 1992;70:389–399.
152. Martin GM, Bollag G, McCormick F, et al. A novel serine kinase activated by rac1/CDC42Hs-dependent autophosphorylation is related to PAK65 and STE20. *EMBO J* 1995;14:1970–1978.
153. Torres M, Hall FL, O'Neill K. Stimulation of human neutrophils with formyl-methionyl-leucyl-phenylalanine induces tyrosine phosphorylation and activation of two distinct mitogen-activated protein-kinases. *J Immunol* 1993;150:1563–1578.
154. Worthen GS, Avdi N, Buhl AM, et al. FMLP activates Ras and Raf in human neutrophils: potential role in activation of MAP kinase. *J Clin Invest* 1994;94:815–823.
155. Buhl AM, Avdi N, Worthen GS, Johnson GL. Mapping of the C5a receptor signal transduction network in human neutrophils. *Proc Natl Acad Sci U S A* 1994;91:9190–9194.
156. Clarke S. Protein isoprenylation and methylation at carboxyl terminal cysteine residues. *Annu Rev Biochem* 1992;61:355–386.
157. Muzio M, Bosisio D, Polentarutti N, et al. Differential expression and regulation of toll-like receptors (TLR) in human leukocytes: selective expression of TLR3 in dendritic cells. *J Immunol* 2000;164: 5998–6004.
158. Ravetch JV. Fc receptors: rubor redux. *Cell* 1994;78:553–560.

159. Miyamoto S, Akiyama SK, Yamada KM. Synergistic roles for receptor occupancy and aggregation in integrin transmembrane function. *Science* 1995;267:883–885.
160. Sabroe I, Prince LR, Jones EC, et al. Selective roles for Toll-like receptor (TLR)2 and TLR4 in the regulation of neutrophil activation and life span *J Immunol* 2003;170:5268–5275.
161. Kishimoto T, Taga T, Akira S. Cytokine signal transduction. *Cell* 1994;76:253–262.
162. Heldin CH. Dimerization of cell surface receptors in signal transduction. *Cell* 1995;80:213–223.
163. Crews CM, Erikson RL. Extracellular signals and reversible protein phosphorylation: what to Mek of it all. *Cell* 1993;74:215–217.
164. Vartio T, Seppa H, Vaheri A. Susceptibility of soluble and matrix fibronectin to degradation by tissue proteinases, mast cell chymase and cathepsin G. *J Biol Chem* 1981;256:471–477.
165. Harlan JM, Killen PD, Harker LA, et al. Neutrophil-mediated endothelial injury *in vitro*: mechanisms of cell detachment. *J Clin Invest* 1981;68:1394–1403.
166. Savill JS, Wylie AH, Henson JE, et al. Macrophage phagocytosis of aging neutrophils in inflammation: programmed cell death in the neutrophil leads to its recognition by macrophages. *J Clin Invest* 1989;83:865–875.
167. Savill J, Hogg N, Ren Y, et al. Thrombospondin cooperates with CD36 and the vitronectin receptor in macrophage recognition of neutrophils undergoing apoptosis. *J Clin Invest* 1992;90:1513–1522.
168. Haslett C. Resolution of inflammation and the role of apoptosis in the tissue fate of granulocytes. *Clin Sci* 1992;83:639–647.
169. Rich AM, Giedd KN, Cristello P, et al. Granules are necessary for death of neutrophils after phagocytosis of crystalline monosodium urate. *Inflammation* 1985;9:221–232.
170. Ohlsson K. Granulocyte collagenase and elastase and their interactions with alpha 1-antitrypsin and alpha 2-macroglobulin. In: Reich DB, Shaw E, eds. *Proteases and biological control.* New York: Cold Spring Harbor Laboratory, 1975.
171. Herlin T, Petersen CS, Esmann V. The role of calcium and cyclic adenosine 38,58-monophosphate in the regulation of glycogen metabolism in phagocytozing human polymorphonuclear leukocytes. *Biochim Biophys Acta* 1978;542:63–76.
172. Zurier RB, Weissmann G, Hoffstein S, et al. Mechanisms of lysosomal enzyme release from human leukocytes. II. Effects of cAMP and cGMP, autonomic agonists, and agents which affect microtubule function. *J Clin Invest* 1974;53:297–309.
173. Malmsten CL, Palmblad J, Uden AM, et al. Leukotriene B_4: a highly potent and stereospecific factor stimulating migration of polymorphonuclear leukocytes. *Acta Physiol Scand* 1980;110:449–451.
174. Goldstein IM, Hoffstein S, Gallin JI, et al. Mechanisms of lysosomal enzyme release from human leukocytes: microtubule assembly and membrane fusion induced by a component of complement. *Proc Natl Acad Sci U S A* 1973;70:2916–2920.
175. Zurier RB, Hoffstein S, Weissmann G. Cytochalasin B: effect of lysosomal enzyme release from human leukocytes. *Proc Natl Acad Sci U S A* 1973;70:844–848.
176. Goldstein IM, Hoffstein S, Weissmann G. Mechanisms of lysosomal enzyme release from human polymorphonuclear leukocytes. *J Cell Biol* 1975;66:647–652.
177. Wolfson M, McPhail LC, Nasrallah VN, et al. Phorbol myristate acetate mediates redistribution of protein kinase C in human neutrophils: potential role in the activation of the respiratory burst enzyme. *J Immunol* 1985;135:2057–2062.
178. Hoffstein S, Soberman R, Goldstein I, et al. Concanavalin A induces microtubule assembly and specific granule discharge in human polymorphonuclear leukocytes. *J Cell Biol* 1976;68:781–787.
179. Hollingsworth JW, Siegel ER, Creasey WA. Granulocyte survival in synovial exudate of patients with rheumatoid arthritis and other inflammatory joint diseases. *Yale J Biol Med* 1967;39:289–296.
180. Koch AE, Kunkel SL, Strieter RM. Cytokines in rheumatoid arthritis. *J Invest Med* 1995;43:28–38.
181. Terkeltaub RA. Gout and mechanisms of crystal-induced inflammation. *Curr Opin Rheum* 1993;5:510–516.
182. di Giovine FS, Malawista SE, Thornton E, et al. Urate crystals stimulate production of tumor necrosis factor alpha from blood monocytes and synovial cells: cytokine mRNA and protein kinetics, and cellular distribution. *J Clin Invest* 1991;87:1375–1381.
183. Terkeltaub R, Baird S, Sears P, et al. The murine homolog of the interleukin-8 receptor CXCR-2 is essential for the occurrence of neutrophilic inflammation in the air pouch model of acute urate crystal-induced gouty synovitis. *Arthritis Rheum* 1998;41:900–909.
184. Serhan CN, Lundberg U, Weissmann G, et al. Formation of leukotrienes and hydroxy acids by human neutrophils and platelets exposed to monosodium urate. *Prostaglandins* 1984;274:563–581.
185. Cronstein BN, Molad Y, Reibman J, et al. Colchicine alters the quantitative and qualitative display of selectins on endothelial cells and neutrophils. *J Clin Invest* 1995;96:994–1002.
186. Lozada C, Levin RI, Huie M, et al. Identification of C1q as the heat-labile serum co-factor required for immune complexes to stimulate endothelial expression of the adhesion molecules E-selectin, ICAM-1 and VCAM-1. *Proc Natl Acad Sci U S A* 1995;92:8378–8392.
187. Mulligan MS, Varani J, Dame MK, et al. Role of endothelial-leukocyte adhesion molecule 1 (ELAM-1) in neutrophil-mediated lung injury in rats. *J Clin Invest* 1991;88:1396–1406.
188. Jennette JC, Falk RJ. Pathogenic potential of anti-neutrophil cytoplasmic autoantibodies. *Adv Exp Med Biol* 1993;336:7–15.
189. Edberg JC, Wainstein E, Wu J, et al. Analysis of FcgRII gene polymorphisms in Wegener's granulomatosis. *Exp Clin Immunogenet* 1997;14:183–195.
190. Kavanaugh AF, Davis LS, Nichols LA, et al. Treatment of refractory rheumatoid arthritis with a monoclonal antibody to intercellular adhesion molecule 1. *Arthritis Rheum* 1994;37:992–999.
191. Cronstein BN. Adhesion molecules in inflammation: current research and new therapeutic targets. *Clin Immunol* 1994;1:323–326.
192. Buchanan MR, Vasquez MJ, Gimbrone MAJ. Arachidonic acid metabolism and the adhesion of human polymorphonuclear leukocytes to cultures vascular endothelial cells. *Blood* 1983;62:889–895.
193. Cronstein BN, Van de Stouwe M, Druska L, et al. Nonsteroidal antiinflammatory agents inhibit stimulated neutrophil adhesion to endothelium: adenosine dependent and independent mechanisms. *Inflammation* 1994;18:323–335.
194. Buchanan MR, Haas T, Lagarde M, et al. 13-Hydroxyoctadecadienoic acid is the vessel wall chemorepellant. *J Biol Chem* 1986; 260:16056–16059.
195. Diaz-Gonzalez F, Gonzalez-Alvaro I, Campanero MR, et al. Prevention of *in vitro* neutrophil endothelial attachment through shedding of L-selectin by nonsteroidal anti-inflammatory drugs. *J Clin Invest* 1995;95:1756–1765.
196. Corkill MM, Kirkham BW, Haskard DO, et al. Gold treatment of rheumatoid arthritis decreases synovial expression of the endothelial leukocyte adhesion receptor ELAM-1. *J Rheumatol* 1991;18:1453–1460.
197. Newman PM, To SST, Robinson BG, et al. Effect of gold sodium thiomalate and its thiomalate component on *in vitro* expression of endothelial cell adhesion molecules. *J Clin Invest* 1994;94:1864–1871.
198. Cronstein BN, Kimmel SC, Levin RI, et al. A mechanism for the antiinflammatory effects of corticosteroids: the glucocorticoid receptor regulates leukocyte adhesion to endothelial cells and expression of ELAM-1 and ICAM-1. *Proc Natl Acad Sci U S A* 1992;89:9991–9996.
199. Cronstein BN, Eberle MA, Gruber HE, et al. Methotrexate inhibits neutrophil function by stimulating adenosine release from connective tissue cells. *Proc Natl Acad Sci U S A* 1991;88:2441–2445.
200. Cronstein BN, Naime D, Ostad E. The anti-inflammatory mechanism of methotrexate: increased adenosine release at inflamed sites diminishes leukocyte accumulation in an *in vivo* model of inflammation. *J Clin Invest* 1993;92:2675–2682.
201. Abramson SB, Korchak H, Ludewig R, et al. Modes of action of aspirin-like drugs. *Proc Natl Acad Sci U S A* 1985;82:7227–7231.
202. Weissmann G. Aspirin. *Sci Am* 1991;264:84–90.
203. Abramson SB, Cherksey B, Gude D, et al. Nonsteroidal anti-inflammatory drugs exert differential effects on neutrophil function and plasma membrane viscosity: studies in human neutrophils and liposomes. *Inflammation* 1990;14:11–30.
204. Kaplan HB, Edelson HS, Korchak HM, et al. Effects of non-steroidal anti-inflammatory agents on human neutrophil functions *in vitro* and *in vivo*. *Biochem Pharmacol* 1984;33:371–378.
205. Abramson SB, Leszczynska-Piziak J, Haines KA, et al. Nonsteroidal anti-inflammatory drugs: effects on a GTP binding protein within the neutrophil plasma membrane. *Biochem Pharmacol* 1991; 41:1567–1573.

206. Pillinger MH, Capodici C, Rosenthal P, et al. Modes of action of aspirin-like drugs: salicylates inhibit erk activation and integrin-dependent neutrophil adhesion. *Proc Natl Acad Sci U S A* 1998;94:14540–14545.
207. Cronstein BN, Rosenstein ED, Kramer SB, et al. Adenosine: a physiological modulator of superoxide anion generation by human neutrophils. II. Adenosine acts via an A_2 receptor on human neutrophils. *J Immunol* 1985;135:1366–1371.
208. Cronstein BN, Leven RL, Belanoff J, et al. Adenosine: an endogenous inhibitor of neutrophil mediated injury to endothelial cells. *J Clin Invest* 1986;78:760–770.
209. Cronstein BN, Kubersky SM, Weissmann G, et al. Engagement of adenosine receptors inhibits H_2O_2 release by activated human neutrophils. *Clin Immunol Immunopathol* 1987;42:76–85.
210. Cronstein BN, Kramer SB, Rosenstein ED, et al. Engagement of adenosine receptors raises cAMP alone and in synergy with engagement of the FMLP receptor and inhibits membrane depolarization but does not affect stimulated Ca^{++} fluxes. *Biochem J* 1988;252:709–715.
211. Rose FR, Hirschhorn R, Weissmann G, et al. Adenosine promotes chemotaxis. *J Exp Med* 1988;167:1186–1194.
212. Cronstein BN, Levin RI, Hirschhorn R, et al. The opposing effects of adenosine A_1 and A_2 receptor occupancy on stimulated neutrophil (PMN) adherence. *J Clin Invest* 1992;148:2201–2206.
213. Cronstein BN, Kramer SB, Weissmann G, et al. Adenosine: a physiological modulator of superoxide anion generation by human neutrophils. *J Exp Med* 1983;153:1160–1177.
214. Cronstein BN, Montesinos MC, Weissmann G. Salicylates and sulfasalazine, but not glucocorticoids, inhibit leukocyte accumulation by an adenosine-dependent mechanism that is independent of inhibition of prostaglandin synthesis and p105 of NfkappaB. *Proc Natl Acad Sci U S A* 1999;96:6377–6381.
215. Clancy RM, Leszczynska-Piziak J, Abramson SB. Nitric oxide, an endothelial cell relaxation factor, inhibits neutrophil activation via a direct action on the NADPH oxidase. *J Clin Invest* 1992;90:1116–1121.
216. Gallin JI. Disorders of phagocytic cells. In: Gallin JI, Goldstein IM, Snyderman R, eds. *Inflammation: basic principles and clinical correlates.* New York: Raven, 1992:859–874.
217. Casimir C, Chetty M, Bohler MC, et al. Identification of the defective NADPH-oxidase component in chronic granulomatous disease: a study of 57 European families. *Eur J Clin Invest* 1992;22:403–406.
218. Curnutte JT. Chronic granulomatous disease: the solving of a clinical riddle at the molecular level. *Clin Immunol Immunopathol* 1993;67 (suppl):2–15.
219. Vojtek AB, Cooper JA. Rho family members activators of MAP kinase cascades. *Cell* 1995;82:527–529.
220. Sechler JM, Malech HL, White CJ, et al. Recombinant human interferon-gamma reconstitutes defective phagocyte function in patients with chronic granulomatous disease of childhood. *Proc Natl Acad Sci U S A* 1988;85:4874–4878.
221. Ezekowitz RA, Dinauer MC, Jaffe HS, et al. Partial correction of the phagocyte defect in patients with X-linked chronic granulomatous disease by subcutaneous interferon gamma. *N Engl J Med* 1988;319: 146–151.
222. Pollock JD, Williams DA, Gifford MA, et al. Mouse model of X-linked chronic granulomatous disease, an inherited defect in phagocyte superoxide production. *Nat Genet* 1995;9:202–209.
223. Jackson SH, Gallin JI, Holland SM. The $p47^{phox}$ mouse knock-out model of chronic granulomatous disease. *J Exp Med* 1995;182: 751–758.
224. Dinauer MC, Li LL, Bjorgvinsdottir H, et al. Long-term correction of phagocyte NADPH oxidase activity by retroviral transfer in murine X-linked chronic granulomatous disease. *Blood* 1999;94: 914–922.
225. Shiloh MU, MacMicking JD, Nicholson S, et al. Phenotype of mice and macrophages deficient in both phagocyte oxidase and inducible nitric oxide synthase. *Immunity* 1999;10:29–38.
226. Springer TA, Thompson WS, Miller LJ, et al. Inherited deficiency of the Mac-1, LFA-1 and gp150/95 glycoprotein family and its molecular basis. *J Exp Med* 1984;160:1901–1918.
227. Anderson DC, Springer TA. Leukocyte adhesion deficiency: an inherited defect in the Mac-1, LFA-1 and p150/95 glycoproteins. *Annu Rev Med* 1987;38:175–194.
228. Arnaout MA. Leukocyte adhesion molecules deficiency: its structural basis, pathophysiology and implications for modulating the inflammatory response. *Immunol Rev* 1990;114:145–180.
229. Anderson DC, Schmalstieg FC, Finegold MJ, et al. The severe and moderate phenotypes of heritable Mac-1, LFA-1 deficiency: their quantitative definition and relation to leukocyte dysfunction and clinical features. *J Infect Dis* 1985;152:668–689.
230. Etzioni A, Harlan JM, Pollack S, et al. Leukocyte adhesion deficiency (LAD) II: a new adhesion defect due to absence of sialyl Lewis X, the ligand for selectins. *Immunodeficiency* 1993;4:307–308.
231. Marquardt T, Brune T, Luhn K, et al. Leukocyte adhesion deficiency II syndrome, a generalized defect in fucose metabolism. *J Pediatr* 1999;134:681–688.
232. Wilson JM, Ping AJ, Krauss JC, et al. Correction of CD18-deficient lymphocytes by retrovirus-mediated gene transfer. *Science* 1990; 248:1413–1416.
233. Nath J, Flavin M, Gallin JI. Tubulin tyrosinolation in human polymorphonuclear leukocytes: studies in normal subjects and in patients with the Chédiak-Higashi syndrome. *J Cell Biol* 1982;95:519–526.
234. Rotrosen D, Gallin JI. Disorders of phagocyte function. *Annu Rev Immunol* 1987;5:127–150.
235. Gallin JI. Neutrophil specific granule deficiency. *Annu Rev Med* 1985;36:263–274.
236. Malech HL, Gallin JI. Neutrophils in human disease. *N Engl J Med* 1987;317:687–694.
237. Gallin JI, Fletcher MP, Seligmann BE, et al. Human neutrophil specific granule deficiency: a model to assess the role of neutrophil specific granules in the evolution of the inflammatory response. *Blood* 1982;59:1317–1329.
238. Davis JM, Dineen P, Gallin JI. Neutrophil degranulation and abnormal chemotaxis after thermal injury. *J Immunol* 1980;124:1467–1471.
239. Ambruso DR, Bentwood B, Henson PM, et al. Oxidative metabolism of cord blood neutrophils: relationship to content and degranulation of cytoplasmic granules. *Pediatr Res* 1984;18:1148–1153.
240. Nauseef WM, Root RK, Malech HL. Biochemical and immunological analysis of hereditary myeloperoxidase deficiency. *J Clin Invest* 1983;71:1297–1307.
241. Nauseef WM. Myeloperoxidase deficiency. *Hematol Pathol* 1990;4: 165–178.

CHAPTER 17

Mast Cells, Eosinophils, and Rheumatic Diseases

Barry L. Gruber and Allen P. Kaplan

MAST CELLS

Mast cells, historically recognized for their contribution in immediate-type hypersensitivity reactions, have more recently been assigned critical protective and homeostatic functions, particularly in the expression of innate immunity (1–3). In addition, our understanding of the potential contribution of mast cells in pathologic settings and, specifically, rheumatic diseases has progressed, although the precise role of mast cells in these settings remains to be further defined. Abundant evidence indicates that mast cells are frequently found, often in striking quantity, in affected tissues from a spectrum of rheumatic disorders. Because the density of mast cells within a given tissue under normal conditions is tightly regulated and remarkably constant, the finding of localized mast cell hyperplasia has been taken as evidence toward participation in disease pathogenesis. This assumption is bolstered by detecting activated mast cell products released within involved tissues, as noted in synovial fluid (4,5). In addition, ultrastructural studies in diseases such as scleroderma (6) and rheumatoid arthritis (RA) (7,8) frequently detect activated (or secretory) mast cell phenotypes. Perhaps more specific evidence for mast cell involvement in rheumatologic disorders emerges from microscopic analyses revealing mast cell clusters at precise sites of tissue injury, as recorded at the leading edge of pannus eroding into subchondral bone (9,10). It is now widely recognized that mast cells are capable of synthesizing an array of inflammatory substances, growth factors, and cytokines (11). Many of these mediators have been implicated in the evolution of rheumatic diseases. Nonetheless, it remains conceivable that mast cells may be recruited nonspecifically and merely serve as relatively innocent bystanders in a complex chronic inflammatory process (12).

Thus, the more knowledge that is gathered concerning the basic biology of mast cells, the closer we come to grasping an understanding of its potential role in chronic inflammatory conditions. Mast cells are distributed widely throughout connective tissue, particularly in vascularized regions. In fact, mast cells are often referred to as gatekeepers of the microvasculature since they are strategically located on the periphery of small venules. This location facilitates regulation of the microcirculation by releasing rapidly diffusable mediators such as histamine, nitric oxide, and arachidonic acid metabolites such as prostaglandin D_2 (PGD_2), leukotriene B_4 (LTB_4), and leukotriene C_4 (LTC_4), all which profoundly affect vascular permeability and leukocyte trafficking. Histamine, for example, incites endothelial cells to transiently express P-selectin, thereby causing leukocytes to slow their transit through the microvasculature (13). Other mast cell derived mediators likewise modulate endothelial cells to facilitate leukocyte adhesion. Mast cell degranulation results in endothelial cell surface expression of E-selectin, intercellular adhesion molecule-1 (ICAM-1), and vascular cell adhesion molecule-1 (VCAM-1), chiefly as a result of secreted tumor necrosis factor-α (TNF-α) (14–16). Consequently, after an initial wheal and flare, mast cells stimulate leukocyte emigration, leading to what is termed a late-phase inflammatory reaction. Thus, mast cell products enhance vascular permeability, promote adhesion of circulating cells to microvascular endothelium, and induce transmigration of inflammatory cells into tissue sites. In certain settings, these proinflammatory effects may assist the host in defense, for example, against invasion by some parasitic or bacterial pathogens (17). Recent evidence indicates that mast cells may participate in innate immune responses by directly recognizing products of bacterial infection through several surface receptor proteins and in response release biologically active phlogistic molecules to limit the spread of the bacterial infection and facilitate host repair (1,3,18,19). *In vitro* studies suggest that the spectrum of microbes capable of eliciting a mast cell response is quite broad and includes common respiratory viruses, mycoplasma, coliforms, and even products of tissue injury such as nucleotides (2). The mast cells recognize the microbial products via several surface receptors, including Toll-like receptor 4 and specific complement receptors (20–22). Helper T cell subset 2 (T_H2)-polarized inflammation elicits a reactive hyperplasia of mast cells at the involved mucosal surfaces. Several T_H2 cytokines [interleukin-3 (IL-3), IL-4, IL-5, and IL-9] appear to act synergistically with stem cell factor (SCF) to facilitate mast cell proliferation (2). IL-4 may additionally prime mast cells to express critical inflammation-associated genes, such as LTC_4 synthase, FcεRI, and several cytokines.

The concept that mast cells may also contribute to tissue reparative processes is supported by finding numerous degranulating mast cells during wound repair or in the vicinity of a healing bone fracture (23). The tissue sequelae of chronic inflammation, including angiogenesis and connective tissue matrix remodeling, may be modulated by mast cells directly or via the recruitment of inflammatory cells. Mast cells may well serve dual roles: amplifying tissue responses to evoke acute inflammatory reactions (e.g., innate immune responses) and chronically orchestrating tissue reorganization, neovascularization, and matrix remodeling. This may involve mast cell–derived release of proinflammatory cytokines (11), serine proteases capable of activating latent matrix metalloproteases (24,25), and products that recruit and stimulate fibroblast and endothelial cell proliferation (26,27). In the setting of tumorigenesis, recent experimental evidence supports a pivotal role for mast cells in up-regulating and sustaining angiogenesis and reorganizing the surrounding stroma (28).

The fact that mast cell hyperplasia is common to a variety of chronic diseases argues for a fundamental role in tissue biologic responses surrounding injury/repair, complex processes potentially modulated by mast cell products or processes that become dysregulated in the evolution of many rheumatologic diseases. This chapter reviews the mast cell in the context of current concepts about the pathogenesis of certain rheumatic disorders. A brief review of mast cell biology and mediators is presented first.

Mast Cell Morphology

Certain features characteristic of mast cells constitute the basis for their identification within tissues. Most prominent is the brightly violaceous granules observed throughout the cytoplasm, often masking the appearance of the nucleus. Hence, Paul Ehrlich originally coined the term *mast zellen,* "well fed" cell, more than a century ago. The granules acquire this bright color following exposure to basic aniline stains, a property termed metachromasia. Metachromasia, in essence, is a color change resulting from the dye molecules aligning themselves with the cloud of negative charges imparted by the proteoglycan core of the granules. Basophils likewise stain with metachromasia, rendering it difficult at times to differentiate these cells in tissue specimens. However, basophils are circulating cells that are considerably smaller and rarely enter tissues in the absence of inflammation.

Identifying mast cells in tissues is accomplished routinely with aniline dyes such as toluidine blue or Giemsa. Alternatively, the compound berberine can be used, which forms a stable complex with heparin and causes the granules to brightly fluoresce (29,30). Investigators later noted that heparin also binds tightly to unconjugated avidin, which then can be tagged for easy detection of mast cells (31). Immunoperoxidase techniques using specific monoclonal antibodies directed to unique mast cell membrane antigens [e.g., immunoglobulin E (IgE), c-*kit*] or granule protease constituents such as tryptase and chymase have been used for investigative purposes (32,33). By combining several techniques on the same specimen, highly activated mast cells that lose their distinctive metachromatic granules can be detected *in situ* and, in this regard, have been referred to as phantom mast cells (34).

Electron microscopy offers an alternative approach to the identification of tissue mast cells and for monitoring their state of activation (30). However, considerable expertise may be required, because mast cells may undergo dramatic structural alterations with degranulation (31,32). In the resting state, cytoplasmic granules may acquire a highly ordered internal structure, giving the appearance of scrolls, particles, or crystals. It has been suggested that a particular appearance of the granular infrastructure comprises a basis for subtyping different mast cells, because these patterns reflect discrete protease profiles (33). The cytoplasm also contains numerous oval lipid bodies that appear electron dense and are usually larger than the granules. The surface of mast cells is covered with multiple, thin projections, and the plasma membrane often has prominent folds. Following degranulation, one of the earliest recognized alterations is loss of electron denseness with disorganization of granule infrastructure, followed by subsequent fusion of individual granules into large degranulation sacs. These then fuse with the plasma membrane, and granule contents are extruded. Studies performed *in situ* with dermal explants demonstrate that the granule contents assume an amorphous fibrillar appearance outside the perimeter of the cell and may be observed in apposition with neighboring pericytes or smooth muscle cells (34). Alternatively, the activation of tissue mast cells results in granules appearing as "moth-eaten," in a process termed piecemeal necrosis (30,35). These activated states may vary with the particular stimulus that induces degranulation.

Origin and Distribution

Both mast cells and basophils, which share some but not all properties, arise from bone marrow–derived hematopoietic precursors (41–43). It seems unlikely, from evidence to date, that these two cells stem from a common progenitor. Basophils reach full differentiation in the bone marrow and then enter the circulation, representing approximately 0.5% of the total granulocyte pool. Mast cells, on the other hand, presumably circulate briefly and mature peripherally in the tissues. Basophils, like eosinophils, rarely leave the circulation other than during an inflammatory response, such as in contact dermatitis (44) and are, therefore, not found within tissues under normal conditions. The recruitment of these cells is dependent on the expression and interaction of specific membrane adhesion molecules. Activation of basophils and eosinophils leads to leukocyte functional antigen-1 (LFA-1) (CD11a/18) expression, and these cells then home to sites where vascular endothelial cells display counterligand receptors such as ICAM-1, molecules of the integrin superfamily that mediate adhesion (32,45). Additionally, eosinophils utilize the expression of very late antigen-4 (VLA-4) to bind to microvasculature expressing VCAM-1 and polysaccharide receptors to bind vascular E-selectin (46,47). This process may be regulated by mast cells via the release of mediators that stimulate the expression of these endothelial cell adhesion molecules. Several investigators have demonstrated that degranulating dermal mast cells up-regulate the endothelial expression of E-selectin and ICAM-1, presumably by release of mast cell–derived TNF-α (15,48). Data from our laboratory indicate that endothelial cells express high levels of VCAM-1 and ICAM-1 in response to mast cell–secreted products (16), and we observed similar effects on fibroblasts and keratinocytes (49). The net result is to incite inflammatory cell transmigration through the vascular basement membrane and retention in the subendothelial compartment as facilitated by adhesion to activated tissue fibroblasts. This further allows for close interaction between mast cells and tissue fibroblasts, which results in up-regulation of procollagen synthesis and myofibroblast transformation (50–53).

Mast cells arise from committed precursors in the bone marrow that are distinct from the monocyte/macrophage precursors and may form a unique cell lineage (43,54). In the peripheral blood, the mast cell–committed precursor has been identified as a sparsely granulated CD34$^+$ mononuclear cell (55). In contrast to basophils and eosinophils, mature mast cells are, in essence, never observed in the circulation. The CD34$^+$ mononuclear precursor mast cell will further differentiate following ligation of the tyrosine kinase transmembrane receptor c-*kit* (56–58). Other cell surface markers indicate that mast cells do not arise directly from monocytes (54) and have a unique phenotype distinct from other myeloid lineages (59). The precursor cells populate the perivascular tissue compartments, where they undergo terminal differentiation, regulated by permissive factors yet to be fully characterized within the microenvironment of peripheral tissues (60). Virtually every organ contains mast cells, with higher densities noted within mucosal tissues, lung parenchyma, skin, and throughout the gastrointestinal tract, usually situated around blood vessels, lymphatics, and nerves. Detailed anatomic studies reveal that mast cells are frequently intertwined with fibroblasts or neuronal cells (61,62). Mast cells may be involved in promoting lymphocyte-fibroblast adhesion, as supported by ultrastructural studies of the lung that demonstrate tight apposition of fibroblasts, mast cells, and lymphocytes (63).

The efficient mechanism by which mast cell precursors transmigrate and rapidly home to specific tissue compartments has similarities to T lymphocytes, as suggested by detailed analyses in mice (64). Integrin receptors have been described on purified and cultured human mast cells (65, 66), which may engage vascular addressins to facilitate this homing process. The recruitment of mast cell precursors into tissues is governed at least in part by surface integrin and matrix interactions that promote binding to basement membrane components, such as laminin and fibronectin (67–69). Mast cells may also contribute to the formation of basement membrane components, such as laminin and type IV collagen (70). The perivascular localization of mast cells may be governed by endothelial cells expressing c-*kit* ligand (71). Recently, it has been shown that precursor mast cells transiently express not only CD34 but also CD38, a molecule involved in regulation of leukocyte adhesion to endothelial cells (59,72). These observations provide insight into understanding how mast cells migrate and localize to perivascular sites.

Interestingly, rodent mast cells synthesize messenger RNA (mRNA), which encodes α and β chains (α_4, β_1, and β_7) of the lymphocyte Peyer patch adhesion molecule-1 (LPAM-1) and LPAM-2 lymphocyte homing receptors (73,74). The $\alpha_4\beta_7$ integrin is known to promote binding of lymphocytes to the mucosal addressin cell adhesion molecule-1 (MAdCAM-1) (75) and governs trafficking into intestinal lymphoid tissue (76). Further analysis reveals that the ratio of α_4 chains to $\beta_{1,7}$ chains expressed differs among rodent mast cells collected from connective tissue sites compared with bone marrow (the latter reflecting the phenotype of mucosal mast cells). Changes in expression of these integrin chains can be modulated *in vitro* by exposing bone marrow–derived mast cells to c-*kit* ligand, IL-3, or combinations of these factors (73). Similar studies of β integrins in human mast cells disclose that LTB_4 up-regulates expression and homotypic cell aggregation (77). Therefore, localization of mast cells to mucosal or connective tissue may be regulated by differential expression of distinct integrin chains and subsequent changes in cell adhesive properties. These integrins thus play a critical role in determining the final destination of mast cell residence. Other adhesion molecules have been described on human mast cells dispersed from different organs using flow cytometry, with slight differences depending on the site of derivation. Human lung and uterine mast cells express ICAM-1 (CD54), uterine mast cells also express CD11c and the β_2 subunit (CD18) as well as vitronectin receptors (CD51 and CD61) $\alpha_v\beta_3$ and VLA-4 ($\alpha_4\beta_1$) (CD49d and CD29) (reviewed in references 78 and 79). Other researchers have documented the presence of CD29, CD43 (leukosialin), CD44 (Pgp-1), CD45, CD49d, CD49e, CD117 (c-*kit*), and, of course, FcϵRI (32,65,80,81). More recently, expression of a functional high-affinity IgG receptor, FcγRI, has been demonstrated on human mast cells and noted to be up-regulated by interferon-γ_{1b} (IFN-γ_{1b}) (82,83). Additional receptors characterized on murine mast cells of considerable interest including Fas antigen (CD95, APO-1), and receptors for transforming growth factor-β (TGF-β), hepatocyte growth factor (c-*met*), and nerve growth factor (NGF) (Trk-A) (84–87). These latter receptors may be engaged in cell signaling pathways critical for development and survival.

Mast cell trafficking into peripheral tissues may also be influenced by the presence of chemotactic factors for mast cells. Even fully mature mast cells appear capable of directed migration if exposed to appropriate signals. For example, the ligand for c-*kit* facilitates mast cell migration in modified Boyden chambers (88,89). In addition, certain cytokines, such as IL-3 and TGF-β, and the β-chemokine RANTES (regulated upon activation normal T cell expressed and secreted) may function as chemotactic factors for mast cells (86,89,90). These factors signal mast cells to rapidly mobilize their cytoskeletal elements, resulting in remarkable shape changes to a polarized morphology in preparation for migration. Growth factors, especially angiogenic factors such as fibroblast growth factor (FGF), platelet-derived growth factor (PDGF), vascular endothelial growth factor (VEGF), and platelet-derived endothelial cell growth factor (PDECGF), all appear capable of stimulating mast cell directed migration, at least *in vitro* (91). More recently, chemokine receptors CXCR1 and CXCR2 have been noted on human mast cells with a functional chemotactic response to IL-8 and related neutrophil-activating peptide-2 (NAP-2) (92,93). These important observations may well explain the frequent clustering of mast cells near sites of active inflammation, angiogenesis, and fibrosis.

After precursor mast cells arrive in the tissue, their proliferation, differentiation, and maturation is governed by interactions with c-*kit* and its cognate ligand (and IL-3 in rodents). The protooncogene c-*kit* encodes a receptor that possesses intrinsic protein tyrosine kinase activity essential for triggering signal transduction and mast cell proliferation. The c-*kit* ligand (also termed mast cell growth factor, SCF, steel locus factor, and steel factor) is expressed in two alternatively spliced forms: one is soluble and secreted while the other remains cell associated. Adhesion of mast cells to mesenchymal cells within tissues may be a consequence of direct binding of the cell-associated ligand and c-*kit* on mast cell surfaces (94), although this has not been confirmed by other researchers (95). IL-4 and c-*kit* ligand have the capacity to regulate adhesion to extracellular matrix proteins (96). In murine mast cells, IL-3 is an additional mast cell maturation and differentiation factor; this is not an analogous situation in humans since mature mast cells lack IL-3 receptors (97,98). However, it is possible that human mast cell precursors transiently express IL-3 receptors and respond to this factor (99). Other cytokines that may modulate maturation, growth, or differentiation of murine mast cells include IL-4, IL-9, IL-10, and NGF. For example, cultured mature rat peritoneal mast cells die within 6 days by apoptosis; however, in the presence of NGF the apoptotic death is markedly delayed, presumably related to induction of c-*fos* (100). Similar observations have been described showing that c-*kit* ligand may also suppress apoptosis (101). Thus, determinants of mast cell numbers within a given tissue are complex and include unique homing mechanisms and extrinsic factors that modulate directional migration, and permissive tissue factors that influence the balance between mast cell survival and apoptosis (102–104).

Studies of human mast cell ontogeny have evolved from earlier observations showing that fibroblasts modulate mast cell differentiation, growth, and survival (105–107). Experimental research has demonstrated that human mature mast cells can be propagated directly from cord blood mononuclear cells or dispersed fetal liver cells if cocultured with 3T3 fibroblasts (108,109). The putative growth factor provided by the transformed 3T3-fibroblasts is principally membrane-bound c-*kit* ligand or SCF; cultures treated with soluble recombinant SCF added directly to cord blood develop, albeit into less mature mast cells, raising the intriguing possibility of a second accessory cell present in cord blood necessary for full mast cell maturation (41,110). Another group of investigators has identified a cell strain from a patient with mastocytosis that may promote full maturity in cultivated mast cells (111). Other cytokines that promote differentiation or survival include IL-3, IL-4, IL-5, and IL-6 (99). In general, however, cultured mast cells proliferate for only a limited time, usually several weeks at most, and viability has been too difficult to sustain thereafter. Thus, other factors yet to be characterized must be operative in the permissive microenvironment *in vivo* to prevent cell death and sustain survival. At present, maintaining human mast cells long term *in vitro* and, hence, cultivating large numbers for experimental research, remains a technical obstacle for investigators. Most researchers have relied on rodent mast cells or an immature transformed human mast cell line (HMC-1) for study purposes (112). Interestingly, this cell line has a gain-of-function mutation of c-*kit* that seems critical for proliferation and survival (113).

Rodent mast cells can be readily subdivided into distinct subsets based on phenotypic appearances, biochemical differences, and possibly functional heterogeneity (60). The study of mast cell–deficient mice has proven an excellent resource to unravel the mechanism of differentiation into distinct mast cell subsets (114). Mast cell–deficient mice injected with competent mast cell precursors (e.g., bone marrow) will become replete with mast cells, the phenotype of which will be largely determined by the site of residence (i.e., connective tissue or mucosal) (60). The most widely studied mast cell–deficient mice have mutations at the white spotting or *W* locus, such as the W/W^v strain. These mice also display a macrocytic anemia, sterility, albinism, and an absence of interstitial cells of Cajal, which generate intestinal pacemaker activity (115). The genetic basis of W/W^v mice was determined to be a mutation localized to chromosome 5, at a locus allelic with the c-*kit* protooncogene (116,117).

Another strain of mast cell–deficient mice has genetic defects at the steel locus (*Sl/Sl*^{d}). By crossover experiments, it has been known for some time that the defect in *Sl/Sl*^{d} mice involves a critical microenvironmental factor, whereas the defect in the *W/W*^{v} mice involves the stem cell itself (60). Further understanding emerged as a result of molecular cloning of these loci (57,118). The *Sl* locus was found to encode for the ligand of the c-*kit* receptor, explaining the complementary nature of these phenotypic abnormalities noted in the *W* and *Sl* mutants (119). The *Sl* gene, cloned from rats, mice, and humans, transcribes two alternatively spliced products, 220 and 248 amino acids in length, which may be proteolytically cleaved to either a soluble, secreted, or a cell-associated glycoprotein, variably termed steel factor, mast cell growth factor (MGF), c-*kit* ligand (KL), or SCF. This protein appears to have a remarkable range of biologic activities (119). Synergizing with other growth factors, SCF has profound effects on inducing survival, proliferation, and differentiation in early myeloid, lymphoid, and erythroid cells (120). SCF is capable of correcting the anemia and mast cell deficiency in *Sl/Sl*^{d} mice, and cultured mucosal-type mast cells are transformed to a connective tissue phenotype by this peptide (121). The mast cell is unique among hematopoietic lineages in that *kit* receptor expression is retained into maturity; thus, responsiveness to SCF is manifested throughout its life span. SCF has many biologic effects on mast cells analyzed *in vitro*, including survival, chemotaxis, proliferation, differentiation, alterations of phenotype and mediator content, promotion of degranulation, or synergizing with other factors to secrete mediators and alter expression of other receptors (120,122). Membrane-bound SCF can be cleaved into a soluble and biologically-active peptide at a novel site by mast cell chymase, suggesting a potential amplification loop for mast cell signaling (123). As mentioned above, human SCF also promotes the development of mast cells from hematopoietic progenitor cells, and recurrent administration to patients with advanced breast carcinoma in clinical trials resulted in generalized mast cell hyperplasia and markedly increased levels of circulating mast cell α-tryptase (124).

It is speculated that fibroblast/mast cell interactions are governed largely by interactions of these cognate cell surface receptors (SCF-*kit*), although it remains unproven if the relatively short intracytoplasmic domain of SCF within fibroblasts can actually induce signal transduction following ligation to implicate bidirectional cell activation (125). Within any given tissue, factors that up-regulate the expression of membrane SCF or alter the secretion of the soluble form may lead to alterations in the size of mast cell populations. *In vitro* studies have recently begun to define factors that potentially stimulate mRNA expression for SCF, typically in a setting of inflammation (126). As predicted, clinical disorders of mastocytosis have been associated with either "gain-of-functions" mutations of c-*kit* or elevated tissue levels of SCF (127–129). Furthermore, the local decrease in mast cell populations observed following exposure to glucocorticoids may reflect suppression of regional SCF production (130).

Studies of human mast cells have been less definitive than in rodents in establishing distinct subclasses of mast cells. A comparable lymphocyte-dependent (or IL-3-dependent) subset of mast cells cultured from bone marrow cells has not been clearly defined in humans (102). An alternative classification system has been devised for human mast cells, one based primarily on differences in protease content of cytoplasmic granules (131). Two of the major granule-associated enzymes in mast cells are tryptase and chymase. Mast cells located in connective tissue, intestinal submucosa, breast parenchyma, synovium, and lymph nodes contain both of these enzymes. Mast cells in mucosal tissue and lung have been found to be deficient in chymase (hence, the current proposed nomenclature involves the use of the terms MC_{TC} and MC_{T} mast cells) (132). With further scrutiny, at least two other proteases, carboxypeptidase A and a cathepsin G–like protease, have been localized within the MC_{TC} mast cell population (133,134). A third population of mast cells deficient in tryptase but containing chymase may exist (MC_{C}), although some debate surrounds this finding (135).

The exact relevance and importance of cellular heterogeneity within a population of mast cells is difficult to determine at this time. An intriguing finding in settings of T-lymphocyte deficiencies (such as acquired immunodeficiency syndrome and severe combined immunodeficiency disease) was that biopsies of mucosal tissues show a paucity of MC_{T} mast cells (136). These data suggest that certain human mast cells (i.e., MC_{T}) are lymphocyte dependent, analogous to mice, and may be identifiable by their protease profile. Current concepts suggest that T cell–dependent mast cells (MC_{T}) are termed responsive and are largely involved with innate immune responses as might occur at mucosal surfaces, whereas T cell–independent mast cells (MC_{TC}) are referred to as constitutive and are principally involved in tissue remodeling (2). The effect of T cell–dependent mast cells in disease states remains to be defined. Studies, for example, in scleroderma tissue revealed that mast cells in the fibrotic dermis appear to be largely of the tryptase (MC_{T}) variety, unlike that seen in normal skin, where essentially all mast cells are the MC_{TC} phenotype (137). It is tempting to speculate that these MC_{T} mast cells have specialized or distinct functional properties, and their mere presence outside their normal boundary is a clue toward further understanding the complex pathophysiology of scleroderma (138).

Activation and the Degranulation Process

Both basophils and mast cells are uniquely associated with the allergic response through their capacity to bind IgE by environmental antigens and, subsequently, degranulate. However, in the past decade, a number of additional pathways to induce degranulation in these cells have been described. These will be briefly discussed later in this section. The IgE/antigen-dependent system was the first recognized and remains the most thoroughly studied. This pathway is accomplished with great efficiency because each mast cell expresses up to 200,000 IgE receptors (FcεRI), which are expressed as a tetramer, ($\alpha\beta\gamma_2$) and have extremely high affinity for the Fc portion of IgE molecules (affinity constant 10^{-9} *M*) (139,140). FcεRI may also be expressed as a trimer ($\alpha\gamma_2$) on antigen-presenting cells, such as monocytes, Langerhans cells, and peripheral blood dendritic cells (140). IgE may alternatively bind with a much lower affinity to alternate receptors (FcεRII) expressed on a variety of cells, including lymphocytes, neutrophils, platelets, monocytes, dendritic cells, and possibly eosinophils (141). The function of these low-affinity receptors is not entirely clear. The high-affinity receptor generates a transmembrane signal when a multivalent allergenic substance contacts the mast cell surface. If the substance is the appropriate size, neighboring IgE molecules bind the allergen, resulting in FcεRI receptor clustering within the plasma membrane, and an activating signal is initiated. Much knowledge has recently been gained concerning the regulation of IgE synthesis, and the reader is referred to several comprehensive reviews (140,142). The presence and specificity of IgE molecules in an individual thereby determines the potential for a cellular response to a particular foreign substance. On the other hand, mast cells (and basophils) are responsible for propagation and expression of the inflammatory response. In autoimmune diseases, IgE may be directed to self-antigens and, therefore, initiate an inflammatory response without exposure to a foreign substance (143,144). Autoantibodies directed to high-affinity IgE receptors have been described in patients afflicted with chronic urticaria, suggesting an autoimmune basis for this disorder (145).

The intracellular response to an activation signal is mediated by a complex cascade of reactions, which begin within the lipid bilayer of the cell membrane (reviewed in references 146–148). The early events lead within minutes to a series of membrane and cytoskeletal alterations causing secretion and within hours to cytokine production. The reactions involve a series of amplification steps, initiated by aggregating two or more FcεRI receptors with multivalent ligands (149). FcεRI is a member of the multisubunit immune response receptor (MIRR) family of cell surface receptors that lack intrinsic enzymatic activity but transduce signals through association with cytoplasmic tyrosine kinases (148,150). The earliest detectable event following receptor aggregation entails phosphorylation of tyrosine residues of the FcεRI α chain, within a conserved motif that is common to activation receptors on B and T cells, termed immunoreceptor tyrosine-based activation motif (ITAM) (151). This has been shown to be a critical step for FcεRI-induced degranulation and defines receptor activation. The phosphorylation of ITAM residues is mediated by Lyn, a member of the Src family of protein tyrosine kinases, which tend to constitutively associate with FcεRI at specific sites within the β subunit (152,153). The phosphorylated ITAMs within these subunits lead to conformational changes that then serve as scaffolds for additional signaling molecules to aggregate, some with their own additional binding sites and others with catalytic domains such as Syk (ZAP-70) (151). Recruitment and activation of Syk by Lyn and via other pathways appears to be a pivotal step to propagate further tyrosine phosphorylations and downstream signaling events (148). These later events ultimately regulate skeletal reorganization with polymerization and redistribution of actin, changes in cell surface morphology and adhesiveness, gene activation, and degranulation/secretion (151).

A series of intermediary signaling pathways related to tyrosine kinases have been described, including the activation of different classes of mitogen-activated protein (MAP) kinases, such as ERK1 and ERK2, JNK/SAPK, and other guanine triphosphatases that are mediated by activation and recruitment of $P21^{ras}$ and are critical for nuclear translocation of several transcription factors such as nuclear factor κB (NFκB) that regulate synthesis of cytokines and chemokines (148,154,155). Other important second messengers in FcεRI signaling pathways include the products of activated enzymes such as phosphatidylinositol-3 (PI-3) kinase and γ_1 and γ_2 isoforms of phospholipase C (PLC) (156). The activation of these enzymes is a major downstream target of FcεRI-mediated signaling and is mediated by activated Syk and Bruton's tyrosine kinase (Btk). The interplay between PI-3 kinase and PLC isoforms is exceedingly complex and tightly regulated (157). Mobilization and activation of PLC γ_1 catalyzes lipid products to form inositol 1,4,5-triphosphate (IP_3) and diacylglycerol (DAG). IP_3 then facilitates calcium release from internal stores and DAG activates protein kinase C (PKC). While these intracellular intermediate events are evolving, external calcium channels open, allowing Ca^{2+} influx and membrane current fluctuations, crucial for antigen-induced secretion to facilitate granule or vesicle fusion to the plasma membrane and release of granular contents. The generation of this voltage-independent calcium influx, a process highly regulated by intracellular intermediates (PI-3 kinase) and other signal pathways (157), is critical for secretion because absence of extracellular calcium will abort release of cytoplasmic components (158). Precise details of the IgE-mediated Ca^{2+} entry pathway and linkage of Ca^{2+} channels with FcεRI receptors are still not clear. Evidence has suggested that metabolism of sphingomyelin (SM) pathways and, specifically, activation of a sphingosine kinase, rather than the traditionally implicated PLC, may be the key calcium mobilizer leading to exocytosis of granule constituents in mast cells (159,160).

These second messengers belonging to SM pathways or PLC itself regulate small membrane-associated G proteins that link receptor activation to the PLC pathways and directly facilitate the exocytotic fusion event. Calcium mobilization and PKC activation then coordinate downstream activation of certain transcription factors, including MAP kinases and nuclear factor of activated T cells, which directly regulate gene expression of newly formed products, including mast cell–derived cytokines (161). Other pathways converge downstream to also modulate cytokine production, such as ligation of c-*kit* receptor with resultant enhancement of TNF-α production (162). A description of these complex series of events is reviewed in greater detail elsewhere (148,163) and schematically shown in Fig. 17.1.

In brief, engagement of FcεRI receptors by an allergen leads to cell activation, as manifested by degranulation and mediator release. As soon as activation occurs, cell energy

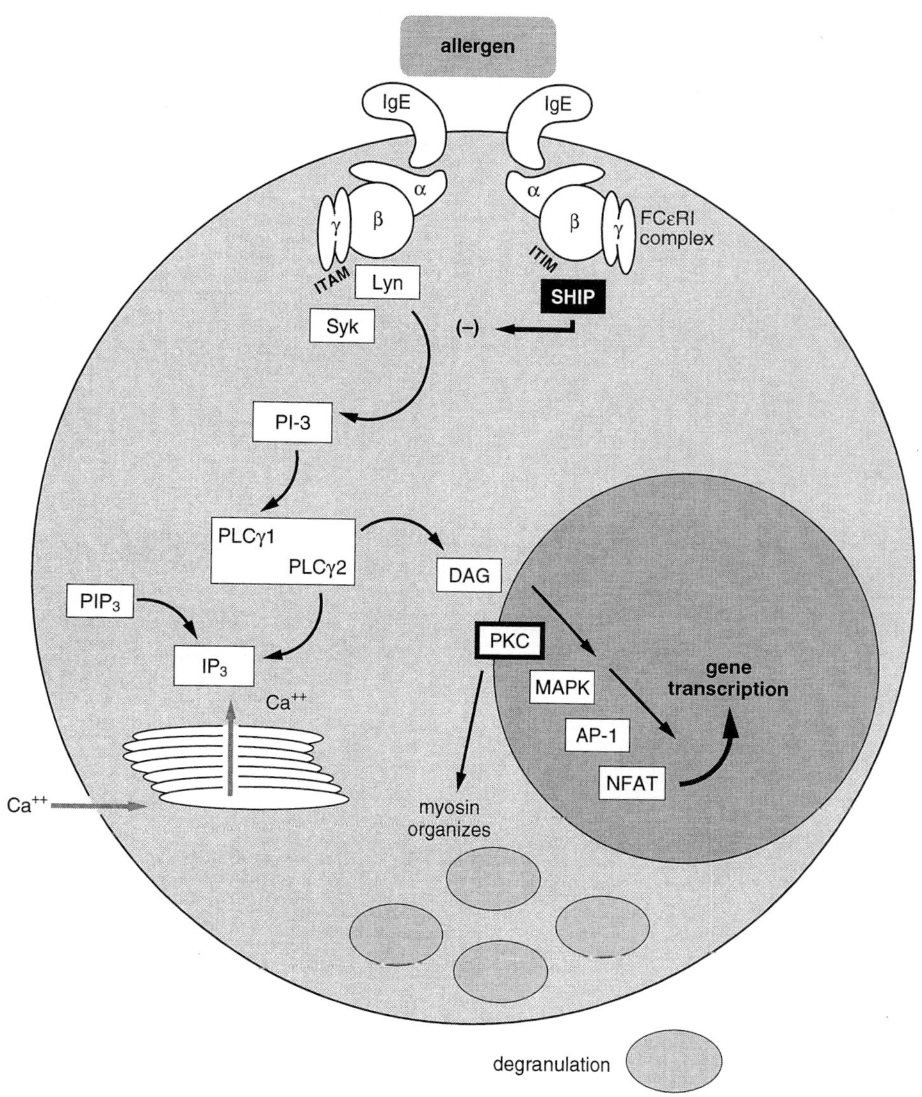

FIG. 17.1. Schema of mast cell activation. Following exposure to an allergen, immunoglobulin E (*IgE*) is clustered and receptor activation rapidly proceeds as shown. A series of intracytoplasmic tyrosine kinase signaling molecules are activated by phosphorylation, initially at specific sites [immunoreceptor tyrosine-based activation motif (*ITAM*)] within the subunits of the FcεRI receptor. This subsequently leads to a cascade of kinase assembly and activation, culminating with voltage-independent calcium entry and degranulation. Simultaneously, downstream signal transduction pathways proceed and regulate gene transcription to promote cytokine production such as tumor necrosis factor-α (*TNF-α*). Concurrent with receptor activation, negative regulators acting via inhibitory receptors, such as FcγIIRB containing immunoreceptor tyrosine-based inhibition motif (*ITIM*), allow assembly and activation of phosphatases [e.g., src homology-2-containing inositol phosphatase (*SHIP*)] at specific sites within the FcεRI receptor to dephosphorylate intermediates and effectively dampen the overall cellular response. Btk, Bruton's tyrosine kinase; DAG, diacylglycerol; IP_3, inositol 1,4.5-triphosphate; MAPK, mitogen-activated protein kinase; NFAT, nuclear factor of activated T cells; PI-3, phosphotidyl inositol 3-kinase; PIP_3, phosphotidyl inositol 3,4.5-triphosphate; PKC, protein kinase C; PLC, phospholipase C.

is expended to turn the activation signals from on to off. It seems sensible that mast cells, as part of our immune response repertoire, react to foreign organisms or specific substances in an immediate but short-lived fashion. Downregulation of activation pathways involves a growing family of structurally similar cell surface receptors known as the inhibitory receptor superfamily (IRS) (148). All members of the IRS contain at least one copy of a conserved sequence termed immunoreceptor tyrosine-based inhibition motifs (ITIMs) and are common to other immune effector cells (148,164). These transmembrane receptors, as exemplified by the FcγRIIB receptor, coaggregate with the activating receptors (e.g., FcϵRI), which leads to rapid phosphorylation of the ITIM tyrosine and provides a docking site for the src homology 2 (SH2) domain–containing protein tyrosine phophatases SHP-1 and SHP-2 and the inositol 5-phosphatases SH2-containing inositol phosphatase (SHIP) and SHIP2 (148). These proteins, which bind to ITIM, become activated and inhibitory basically by their ability to dephosphorylate activation pathway molecules, as shown schematically in Fig. 17.1. It has been of considerable interest to note that these negative signaling molecules generally bind to the β subunit, whereas the activating proteins such as Syk bind to the γ subunit, which lacks the consensus region ITIM (148,151). An example of this type of gatekeeper of mast cell degranulation has been the recently described SHIP. The function of this molecule was elegantly demonstrated in a knockout mouse model with subsequent massive degranulation observed in response to IgE aggregates (165). The mechanism by which SHIP abrogates mast cell degranulation is not entirely clear, but likely relates to its ability to hydrolyze phosphatidylinositol 3,4,5-triphosphate (PIP_3) and interfere with entry of extracellular calcium (165). Another recently described novel membrane IRS receptor has been termed mast cell function-associated antigen and is unique in that aggregation alone generates inhibitory signals (148). Further research unraveling the pathways that abrogate or dampen an allergic response is of significant commercial interest to pharmacologically design novel approaches based on mimicking or stimulating these negative regulators (166).

It should be emphasized that alternative means exist to activate mast cells, pathways independent of classic IgE bound by multivalent ligands or autoantibodies. Examples of this type of activation include neurotransmitters, such as substance P; proinflammatory peptides secreted by granulocytes (167), platelets, and mononuclear cells; as well as complement components and certain proteases that stimulate mast cell secretion. Many of these substances have been defined based on their *in vitro* ability to release histamine from basophils, hence the term *histamine-releasing factors* (HRFs) (168). Subsequently, most of these factors have been characterized and identified as either interleukins, chemokines, or a unique IgE-dependent factor. Certain interleukins and hematopoietic factors have the ability to either potentiate or directly induce histamine release, in an IgE-independent manner (169). For example, high concentrations of IL-3, IL-8, and granulocyte-macrophage colony-stimulating factor (GM-CSF) release histamine from basophils *in vitro* (IL-1 is also weakly positive), whereas low concentrations of IL-3, IL-5, and GM-CSF are not direct agonists but appear to prime basophils for histamine release (169,170). IL-1, IL-6, and IL-7 may do so as well (169). The only cytokine-like molecule that clearly primes and initiates secretion by mast cells is SCF (171, 172). Mast cells, derived from mouse bone marrow and exposed to IL-4, were found to be functionally responsive to endothelin-1 (173).

Another group of cell-derived peptides with IgE-independent histamine-releasing activity is the chemokines, which are chemotactic cytokines (174). These peptides are members of a superfamily of proteins with a molecular weight range of 6,000 to 14,000 daltons and are classified into four subgroups according to the position of cysteine residues within their sequence (175). The first two cysteines may have a single intervening amino acid (C-X-C) characteristic of the α subgroup, or these two cysteines may be adjacent (C-C), as is seen in the β subgroup. Two other minor subgroups have recently been described. Members from both α and β subgroups have been shown to release histamine from basophils (HRF activity), although, in general, the C-C chemokines such as monocyte chemotactic proteins (MCP-1, -2, -3, and -4) are more active as stimuli (176–178). MCP-1 is the most potent and plentiful in this respect, whereas MCP-3 is equipotent, but less plentiful. The remaining ones in decreasing potency are MCP-4, RANTES, MCP-2, and macrophage inflammatory proteins (MIP-1α, and MIP-1β) (178). Mast cells are far less responsive to these agents than are basophils, and although MIP-1 α is active on rodent mast cells (178) and both MIP-1 α and RANTES have been shown to induce murine mast cell chemotaxis (93), their effects on human mast cells are uncertain. Indeed, one study has shown no effect of chemokines on human mast cells from lung, uterus, skin, or tonsils (179).

Mast cells are also responsive to complement-derived peptides C3a, C4a, and C5a; certain proteases such as trypsin and chymotrypsin; bacterial cell wall products; kinins; parathyroid hormone (PTH); and arachidonic acid products (180–184). Of potential relevance in rheumatic diseases is the finding that collagen degradation products may stimulate mast cell secretion (185). Recent evidence also suggests that activated T cells, which often reside in close apposition with tissue mast cells, can induce mast cell degranulation or enhance FcϵRI-dependent secretion (186,187). This mechanism appears to involve an independent activation pathway involving cell surface LFA-1/ICAM interaction and heterotypic aggregation of these cells (186). The accumulation of T lymphocytes in mast cell–mediated inflammation may be facilitated by release of the $CD4^+$ lymphocyte chemoattractant IL-16 by mast cells (188).

In summary, it appears that numerous pathways exist that might initiate mast cell secretion in addition to the classic IgE allergen–coupled mechanism (Table 17.1). Many, if not most, of these activators, do not transmit their signal via aggregating FcεRI receptors. Furthermore, evidence suggests that the classic anaphylactic cellular response seen in allergic settings characterized by extensive cytoplasmic degranulation may in fact be an uncommon mechanism of mediator release; exchange of products may ensue upon cell-cell contact in a process termed transgranulation (61) or by selective release of specific preformed mediators.

At present, the details of these varying cellular responses still require further elaboration. From a morphologic perspective, the changes during degranulation noted by electron microscopy are vivid (35,36,189,190). Minutes after mast cells are exposed *in vitro* to a stimulus, there is detectable swelling of individual granules, reduction of electron density of the granule matrix, and then fusion of several granules. These fused granules grow progressively larger, and the matrix becomes more fibrillar in appearance. Eventually, within approximately 10 minutes, these giant altered granules contact the plasma membrane and extrude their granule contents through a pore. At this point they appear as empty channels in the cytoplasm (Fig. 17.2). These cytoplasmic alterations are quite specific for mast cells (37), since stimulation of basophils results in a different cytoplasmic pattern with fusion of individual granule membranes with the plasma membrane. The contents of the granules are released through multiple narrow communications to the exterior surface. As in mast cells, the granules appear hypodense with the release of mediators. It is assumed that exocytosis occurs at this time as the granule matrix solubilizes upon exposure to the exterior environment.

TABLE 17.1. *Mast cell activators*

Acquired immune responses
IgE-dependent pathways
Multivalent allergens
IgE complexes
Anti-IgE antibodies
IgE rheumatoid factors
Anti-FcεRI antibodies
IgE-dependent HRF
IgE-independent pathways
Other FcR receptor ligation (e.g., FcγRI)
Chemokines: MCP-1, MCP-2, MCP-3, RANTES, MIP-1α, MIP-1β
Endothelin-1
Complement-derived peptides: C3a, C4a, C5a
TNF-α, IL-12
Proteases: trypsin, chymotrypsin
Stem cell factor
Kinins
Parathormone
Collagen degradation products
Eosinophil-derived major basic protein
Substance P
Cell-cell contact (T cells, fibroblasts)
Innate immune responses (Toll-like receptors)
Bacterial products
Lipopolysaccharide
Fimbriae
Hemolysins
Toxins
Parasites
Schistosoma mansoni
Viruses
Influenza A

HRF, histamine releasing factor; IgE, immunoglobulin E; IL, interleukin; MCP, monocyte chemoattractant protein; MIP, macrophage inhibitory protein; RANTES, regulated upon activation normal T cell expressed and secreted; TNF, tumor necrosis factor.

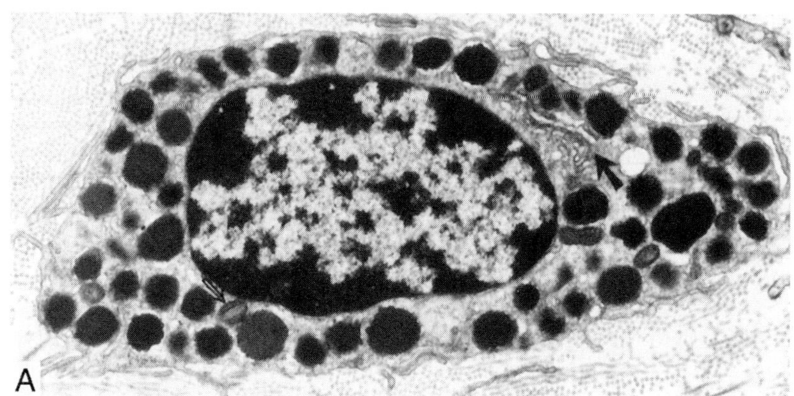

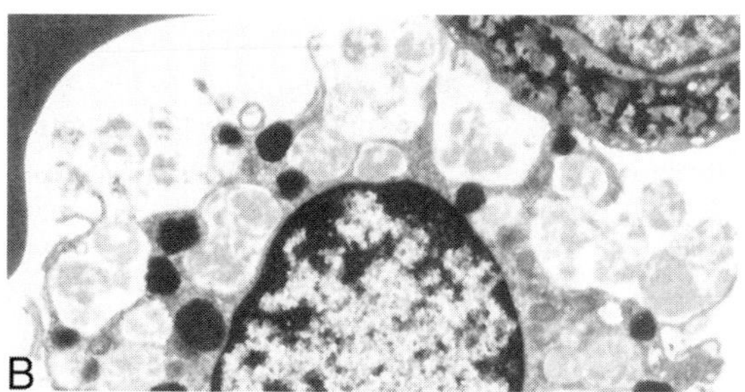

FIG. 17.2. A: Human skin mast cell from a patient with breast adenoma showing a monolobed nucleus with partially condensed chromatin, small golgi area (*solid arrow*), numerous membrane-bound dense granules with peripheral scrolls, and mitochondria, one of which has a crystalline matrix inclusion (*open arrow*) (original magnification ×16,500). (Courtesy of Ann M. Dvorak.) **B:** Human skin mast cell 3 minutes after stimulation with anti–immunoglobulin E. Note the multiple cytoplasmic channels with altered granule matrix material, some of which is being extruded through the cell membrane. A few unaltered granules remain in the cytoplasm (original magnification ×17,000). *Continued*

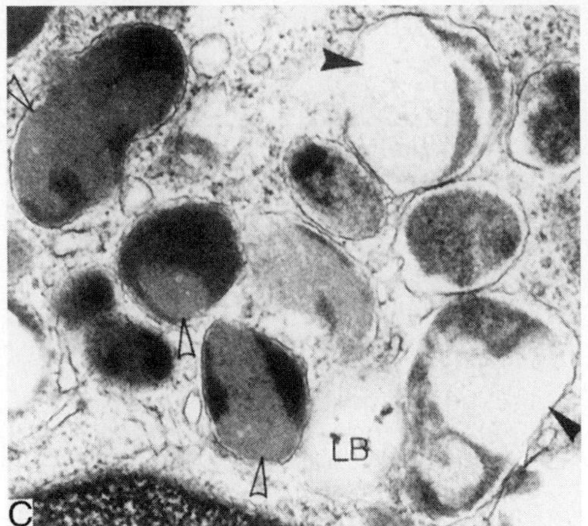

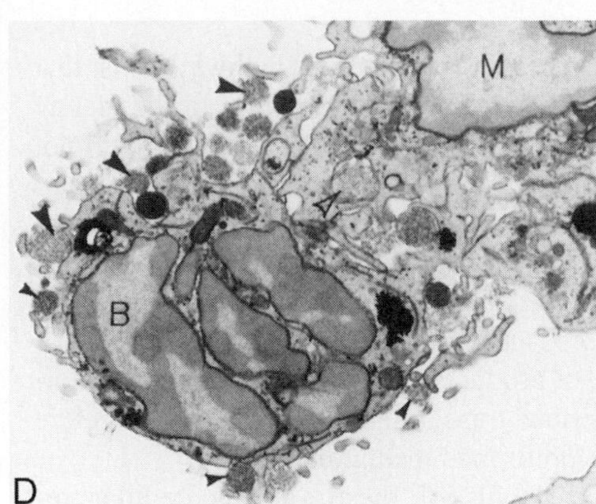

FIG. 17.2. *Continued* **C:** High magnification of the cytoplasm from a human skin mast cell obtained from lesional skin of a patient with bullous pemphigoid showing focal, geographic piecemeal losses from some granules (*solid arrows*). Other granules demonstrate some crystalline content (*open arrow*). A lipid body (*LB*) is seen (original magnification ×72,000). **D:** Basophil "B" 1 minute following stimulation with formyl methionine leucine phenylalanine tripeptide (*FMLP*). Note the extruding membrane-free granules (*closed arrows*) through multiple openings in the plasma membrane and adjacent monocyte (*M*) in close contact, which has phagocytosed a granule (*open arrow*) (original magnification ×20,500). (Courtesy of Ann M. Dvorak.)

As indicated above, cross-linkage of IgE receptors induces the release of the membrane-associated unsaturated fatty acid arachidonic acid. Metabolism of this compound then leads to the formation of products of the cyclooxygenase (prostaglandins) and lipoxygenase (leukotrienes) pathways, as well as the potent platelet-activating factor (PAF) (191). As discussed below, these are mast cell products that are formed in the process of cell activation and not stored in the granules.

Mediators

The mast cell is replete with substances that have the capacity to regulate vascular permeability, control cell trafficking into tissues, potentiate neural pathways, constrict smooth muscles, and exert effects on surrounding cells to stimulate angiogenesis and extracellular matrix turnover. The classic mediators released by mast cells are categorized into three groups: preformed/easily eluted, preformed/granule associated, and newly generated (for more extensive reviews of mast cell–derived mediators, see reference 192). In addition, mast cells synthesize a plethora of cytokines (11). Many of these mast cell–derived substances have potential relevance to rheumatic disease and will be briefly discussed (Tables 17.2 and 17.3).

Histamine

The granule-associated amine that has been subject to classic investigation with regard to its role in the allergic response is histamine. Mast cells and basophils contain approximately 1 to 5 mg of histamine per 10^6 cells. This accounts for 5% to 10% of the weight of granules. Within the granules, histamine is bound to the core proteoglycan. Essentially all histamine in

TABLE 17.2. *Human mast cell mediators*

Preformed and easily eluted
Histamine
Eosinophil chemotactic factors
Neutrophil chemotactic factors
Superoxide
Arylsulfatase A
Elastase
β-Hexosaminidase
β-Glucosonidase
β-Galactosidase
Kallikrein-like enzyme
Preformed and granule associated
Heparin/chondroitin sulfate E
Tryptase [α, βI, βII, βIII, δ, and transmembrane form (TMT)]
Chymase
Carboxypeptidase
Cathepsin G
Superoxide dismutase, catalase (rodents)
Arylsulfatase B
Procollagenase
Newly generated
Leukotrienes (LTC_4, LTD_4, LTE_4)
Platelet-activating factor
Prostaglandins (PGD_2)
Mast cell-derived chemokines
RANTES
MCP-1
MIP-1β, MIP-1α
Mast cell-derived cytokines and potential fibrogenic factors
Interleukins-1β, -3, -4, -5, -6, -8, -13, -14, -16
Granulocyte-macrophage colony-stimulating factor (GM-CSF)
Tumor necrosis factor-α (TNF-α)
Platelet-derived growth factor (PDGF)
Interferon-γ
Vascular endothelial growth factor
Fibroblast growth factor (basic)
Nerve growth factor
Transforming growth factor-β
Endothelin-1
Stem cell factor (mast cell growth factor, c-*kit* ligand)

TABLE 17.3. *Action of mast cell products*

Selected mediators	Actions
Histamine	Triple response of Lewis (vasodilation, endothelial cell contraction, and increased vascular permeability, axon reflex) (H1), pruritus (H1), gastric acid secretion (H2), lymphocyte suppression (H2), chondrocyte activation (H2), regulation of synovial microcirculation (H2), chemoattraction (eosinophils), induction of substance P release, fibroblast proliferation, induction of P-selectin on endothelial cells
Heparin	Anticoagulation, anticomplementary (Clq binding; C4, C2, C3 activation; C3bBb convertase), stimulation of angiogenesis, enhancement of elastase activity, modulation of parathyroid hormone calcitonin to induce osteoporosis, stimulation of collagenase synthesis, inhibition of activated collagenase, stabilization of tryptase, potentiation of fibronectin binding to collagen, fibroblast proliferation, potentiation of fibroblast growth factors
Tryptase	Cleavage of trypsin substrates, inactivation of fibrinogen and high-molecular-weight kininogen, activation of urinary-type plasminogen activator, activation of latent synovial collagenase via conversion of prostromelysin, degradation of vasoactive intestinal peptide (VIP)-canine, bronchoconstriction Cellular effects (presumably by cleavage of N-terminus of protease activated receptor, PAR-2): stimulation of fibroblast chemotaxis, proliferation, collagen synthesis, myofibroblast transformation, COX-2 expression, induction of epithelial cell proliferation, IL-8 release, expression of ICAM-1, promotion of endothelial cell migration and vascular tube formation, eosinophil activation and release of IL-6 and IL-8
Chymase	Cleavage of chymotrypsin substrates, conversion of angiotensin I to II, cleavage of basement membrane substances (laminin, type IV collagen, fibronectin, and elastin), cleavage of dermal–epidermal junction, degradation of neuropeptides VIP and substance P, augmentation of histamine-induced wheal and flare, conversion of pro-IL-1β to active IL-1β, conversion of big endothelin-1 to vasoactive endothelin-1, liberation of latent TGF-β, activation of progelatinase B (MMP-9), enhancement of mucosal gland secretion, cleavage of membrane-associated stem cell factor
Prostaglandins (PGD_2)	Bronchoconstriction, chemoattraction, inhibition of platelet aggregation, vasodilation, potentiation of LTC_4 on vasculature
Leukotrienes (LTC_4, LTD_4, LTE_4)	Slow-reacting substances of anaphylaxis, smooth muscle contraction, vasodilation, endothelial cell activation
Platelet-activating factor (PAF)	Activation of neutrophils, platelets, smooth muscle contraction, vasopermeability, chemotaxis for eosinophils and neutrophils, induction of immune complex–mediated vasculitis
Kallikrein-like enzyme	Generation of bradykinin
Cytokines	Immunologic effects and connective tissue effects described elsewhere in text

ICAM, intracellular adhesion molecule; COX, cyclooxygenase; IL, interleukin; TGF, transforming growth factor; VIP, vasoactive intestinal polypeptide.

humans is contained or released from mast cells or basophils, although platelets contain small amounts.

Elevated circulating plasma histamine levels have been reported in systemic sclerosis, including cases with limited and diffuse involvement (193), and idiopathic pulmonary fibrosis (194,195). Histamine content has been reported to be increased in keloid tissue and hypertrophic scars (196). *In vitro*, histamine has been shown to enhance fibroblast proliferation, collagen synthesis (179–199), and release of the cytokine IL-11 (200). Histamine has also been shown to rapidly up-regulate endothelial cell adhesion molecules such as P-selectin (201,202), forcing leukocytes to roll (203) within the microvasculature as they initiate egress to inflammatory sites.

Clinically, the release of histamine in skin causes edema, flushing, and pruritus, collectively referred to as the wheal and flare or triple response of Lewis. At least a portion of this response is due to the simultaneous release of the neuropeptide substance P (204). Histamine is responsible for the release of substance P from type C unmyelinated nerve fibers, which results in the flare and also feeds back to mast cells, causing further degranulation. Many scleroderma patients complain of pruritus; whether this is related to histamine release or secondary neuropeptide release remains to be determined.

Platelet-Activating Factor

Originally described by its ability to aggregate platelets following IgE-mediated basophil release, this molecule possesses extraordinarily potent biologic activities at concentrations below 10^{-10} *M* (205). In addition to being the most effective platelet aggregator known, it also aggregates neutrophils and monocytes. Neutrophils are particularly sensitive to the actions of PAF through a specific receptor and will respond with directed migration, an oxidative burst, and the production of lipoxygenase products. Injected into skin, PAF causes a wheal-and-flare response that can be associated with leukocyte infiltration, particularly eosinophils (206). The presence of eosinophils is often observed in conjunction with mast cell–mediated reactions; release of PAF may be contributory. The relevance of eosinophils in fibrotic reactions is discussed later in this chapter. Suffice it to say that eosinophils appear rich in fibrogenic peptides such as TGF-α and TGF-β, which may potentiate sclerosing reactions (207,208). PAF has been implicated as a major mediator of immune complex–mediated vasculitis in animal models (209). Its possible role as a significant mediator of human forms of vasculitis warrants further study.

Arachidonic Acid Metabolites

Elsewhere in this text is presented a complete discussion of the distinct pathways leading to formation of prostaglandins and the sulfidopeptide leukotrienes (see Chapter 23). At least two major phopholipases A_2 (PLA_2) are involved in mast cell mobilization of arachidonatic acid: a high-molecular-weight inducible cytosolic ($cPLA_2$) and a secreted low-molecular-weight ($sPLA_2$) (210). Human mast cells (from lung, heart, and gut) are unique in synthesizing PGD_2 (211) by both immediate pathways involving prostaglandin synthase-1 and delayed pathways by generation of prostaglandin synthase-2 (212). This particular compound, when injected intracutaneously, produces an asymptomatic wheal and flare, followed by progressive dermal edema lasting more than 2 hours. Accompanying this, a perivenular neutrophilic infiltrate peaks in a biphasic manner at 30 minutes and 6 hours. Some evidence suggests that the flushing and hypotension, occurring in patients with systemic mastocytosis, is a result of excess circulating PGD_2 (213).

The lipoxygenase pathway in mast cells is rich in enzymes that generate hydroperoxy products of the hydroperoxyeicosatetraenoic acid (HPETE) group, which are rapidly metabolized to 5-hydroxyeicosatetraenoic (5-HETE). It has been recently appreciated that regulation of this pathway in mast cells may be modulated by T cell–derived (T_H2) cytokines such as IL-4 (2). Once mast cells are activated, 5-lipoxygenase (5-LO) is translocated to the nuclear membrane, where it interacts with an 18-kd protein known as 5-LO-activating protein (FLAP), which serves to stabilize binding of arachidonate to 5-LO in order to generate LTA_4 and its subsequent metabolites (214). HPETE is transformed into LTB_4, LTC_4, LTD_4, and LTE_4. It is not clear whether human mast cells are a source of LTB_4, but the latter three compounds (LTC_4, LTD_4, and LTE_4) compose a group of mast cell products previously designated as slow-reacting substances of anaphylaxis (SRS-A). This term reflects the biologic activities of these substances. Injection into the skin generates a burning, erythematous wheal and flare that persists for 4 hours. Microscopically, one finds dermal edema, dilatation of venules and capillaries, and endothelial cell activation (as reflected by alterations in morphology). Inhalation studies using LTD_4 have demonstrated reversible constriction of peripheral airways, with a potency 100- to 1,000-fold that of histamine. In general, the sulfidopeptides have similar activities to histamine, but are much more potent on a molar basis and are longer lasting. Both PAF and the leukotrienes are considered prime candidates as mediators of asthma. Recent evidence from a mouse model of allergic airway disease suggests that leukotrienes may elicit bronchial smooth muscle hyperplasia and submucosal collagen deposition, critical features of airway remodeling and with broader implications for potential mast cell involvement in rheumatic diseases (215). Several leukotriene inhibitors are now available for clinical use for atopic conditions, specifically bronchial asthma, with promising results for leukotriene receptor inhibitors as well as lipoxygenase antagonists.

Chemotactic Factors

A number of mast cell products have been identified that mediate migration of granulocytes and mononuclear cells. Neutrophil chemotactic factors [e.g., high-molecular-weight (HMW-NCF)] are released in the circulation shortly after mast cell activation (216). The release of HMW-NCF can be demonstrated in asthmatics in response to antigen challenge and is accompanied by transient leukocytosis. As mentioned above, the arachidonic acid metabolites (particularly LTB_4) and PAF are chemotactic for human neutrophils. HMW-NCF has a molecular weight of approximately 500,000 daltons and is contained in mast cell granules; its structure is unknown.

In the low-molecular-weight region of mast cell supernatants, an eosinophilic chemotactic factor has been identified following antigen challenge. This factor, termed eosinophil chemotactic factor of anaphylaxis, was originally thought to explain the observed eosinophilic infiltrates or eosinophilia associated with allergic responses (217). Some of this activity is attributed to two synthetic tetrapeptides, val-gly-ser-glu and ala-gly-ser-glu. Clearly, these compounds are much less potent as eosinophilic factors than PAF, or the relevant β-chemokines such as eotaxin, MCP-3, and RANTES.

Other factors have been identified that modulate T- and B-lymphocyte trafficking, some of which inhibit while others promote directed migration. In addition, many mononuclear cell functions are modulated by leukotrienes, prostanoids, and biogenic amines released by mast cells. Several members of the chemokine family and specific cytokines (e.g., IL-8 and IL-16) have been identified within mast cells, as described in further detail below (188,218). These molecules are potent chemotactic factors (175). Other mast cell–derived peptides are capable of inducing nonhematopoietic cell migration, as exemplified by the release of VEGF (26).

Enzymes

The vast majority of the granule proteins in human mast cells can be accounted for by neutral proteases. The most prominent enzyme found in mammalian mast cells is tryptase. This tryptic protease comprises approximately

25% of the dry weight of mast cells (219,220). It is stabilized in an active tetrameric conformation with a molecular weight of 134 kd by forming a tight complex with heparin (221). Human basophils contain a trace amount of tryptase; no other human cell has convincingly been shown to produce this enzyme other than mast cells. Thus, tryptase has become an extremely important marker for identifying mast cells in tissue specimens (132). Furthermore, the detection of elevated levels of tryptase is the most specific and reliable clinical indicator of mast cell–dependent events (222,223). Mast cells express a group of closely related tryptases, designated transmembrane tryptase, β/I, β/II, β/III, α and γ, all encoded by genes on chromosome 16p13.3 (224–228). The β-tryptases are considered to be the major functional enzymes released with degranulation, whereas α-tryptase having a more restricted substrate specificity as a result of a single amino acid variation in its substrate-binding cleft, is released constitutively in an inactive form (227).

Tryptase is an endopeptidase at neutral pH and can be quantified by monitoring hydrolysis of synthetic substrates, such as tosyl-L-arginine methyl ester (TAMe) or specific nitroanilides, or more conveniently by immunoassays (220,229,230). Immunoassay has become a commercially available method used to quantify this enzyme in clinical settings (222); it is more specific for mast cells than histamine levels that reflect the contributions of both basophils and mast cells. Clinical settings, in which the role of mast cells has been subject to controversy, can be investigated by quantitating tryptase levels. As an example, provocative assertions implicating mast cells in the pathogenesis of sudden infant death syndrome were supported by such data (231).

The structural conformation of tryptase's catalytic site is unique, rendering it relatively resistant to native antiproteases, that is, compounds that have an essential capacity to inhibit all active proteases found in the circulation or within tissues and yet have no apparent effect on tryptase (232). Another intriguing feature about this enzyme is that the major target or natural substrate *in vivo* remains essentially unknown. Certainly, the substrate specificity of both β-tryptase and α-tryptase appears very restricted (233). However, it remains puzzling that despite being the most abundant mast cell product secreted and a substance that has been subjected to detailed molecular cloning and careful structural analysis, a definitive biologic function has not been defined. In the *in vitro* setting, tryptase metabolizes high-molecular-weight kininogen and partially degrades fibrinogen (192). The capacity to rapidly degrade fibrinogen may be physiologically important to prevent fibrin clots and allow granulocyte extravasation at sites of mast cell–mediated edema and inflammation. Tryptase can also cleave and activate the latent metalloproteinase prostromelysin (proMMP-3), which in turn degrades several matrix components and activates procollagenase (24). In this manner, mast cells conceivably function to assist in connective tissue degradation. Tryptase has been shown to activate urinary-type plasminogen activator (u-PA or pro-urokinase), which would also promote extracellular matrix proteolysis (234). In addition, canine tryptase has been shown to catalyze degradation of the neuropeptide vasoactive intestinal polypeptide (VIP) (235), and human tryptase degrades calcitonin gene–related peptide (236), suggesting a neuroregulatory role by inactivating bronchodilatory feedback mechanisms.

The focus of research involving tryptase has recently concentrated on its ability to specifically cleave the N-terminus of protease-activated receptors (PARs), allowing tryptase to function as a cell signaling effector molecule analogous to thrombin. In fact, tryptase is more potent on a molar basis than thrombin in stimulating thymidine uptake and cell proliferation in some studies (237,238). The cytokine-like effect of tryptase on different cell types has now been extended beyond its mitogenic effects (239). Microvascular endothelial cells migrate and assemble into tubes reminiscent of an angiogenic response to tryptase (240) (Fig. 17.3). Fibroblasts respond by migration, proliferation, and production of procollagen (51,241). Epithelial cells proliferate, express ICAM-1, and produce IL-8 in response to tryptase (242). The role of tryptase (and chymase) in stimulating angiogenesis and stromal remodeling during tumorigenesis has been elegantly demonstrated recently in a transgenic model of squamous carcinoma (28).

The mechanism by which tryptase induces paracrine cellular effects has not been fully elucidated, although substantial loss of "cytokine-like" activity upon pharmacologic blockade of its catalytic site supports the notion that cleavage of a specific protease activated receptor is involved. Although the protease-activated receptor specific for thrombin (PAR-1) is insensitive to tryptase, as reflected by the lack of calcium mobilization, insensitivity to pertussis toxin, and absence of PLC activation (237,238), other proteolytic-activated receptors within this family (243) may be activated by tryptase (244–247). Investigators have characterized PAR-2 as a potential target for tryptase on mesenchymal cells, with important implications in mast cell–mediated tissue remodeling (228,239,248,249). If these studies are confirmed, future directions will likely include specifically identifying and characterizing the cellular effects following ligation of these tryptase-specific receptors. Considering the abundance of tryptase released from human mast cells and the previous difficulty in finding susceptible isolated substrates, it is anticipated that this new avenue of investigation will be the upcoming focus for some time. Potent selective noncytotoxic pharmacologic inhibitors of human tryptase have been developed (250, 251) that should further facilitate delineating the role of tryptase in disease states (248).

Chymase, the next most abundant human mast cell neutral protease defined by its chymotryptic-like specificity, has been purified from dermal mast cells and is characterized as a monomer of 28 kd. Human chymase has been cloned from skin, placenta, tonsils, and myocardial tissue

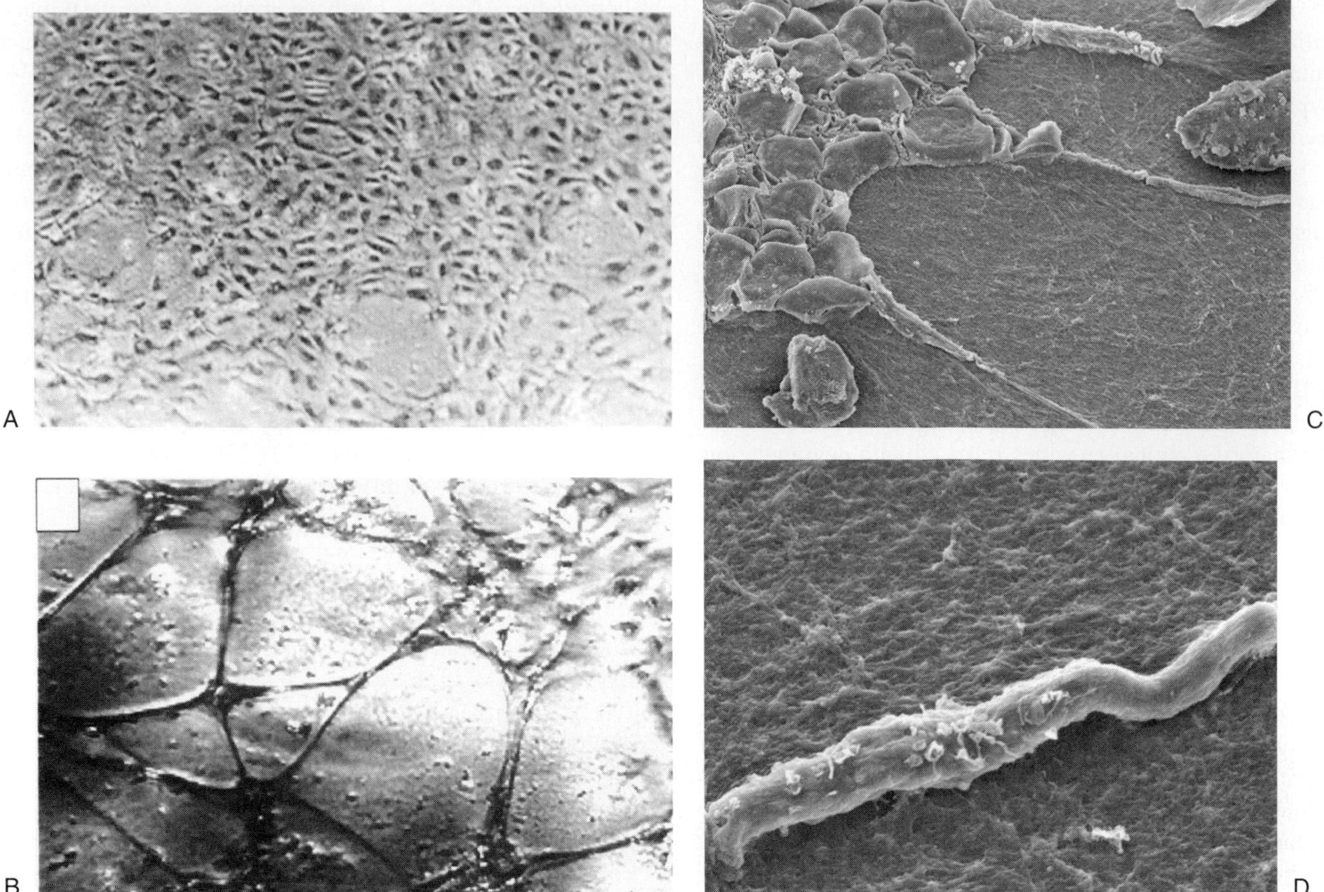

FIG. 17.3. Mast cell tryptase induces angiogenesis. Cultured dermal microvascular endothelial cells on Matrigel are shown prior to stimulation in a random monolayer growth pattern **(A)** and contrasted to the growth pattern following exposure to mast cell–derived tryptase **(B)**. Note assembly into rudimentary cylinder-shaped vascular tubes following exposure to tryptase, suggesting a proangiogenic effect of tryptase. In the lower panels are shown scanning electron micrographs of these endothelial cells following exposure to tryptase. Note the typical cobblestone appearance of the endothelial cells **(C)** rapidly changing and reorganizing into tubelike structures **(D)**.

(252,253). Its primary structure has been determined, using mast cells derived from urticaria pigmentosa lesions (254). Chymase and a closely related protease, cathepsin G, are both produced by MC_{TC} mast cells and can be mapped to a gene cluster on chromosome 14 that includes granzyme B and H/cathepsin G/chymase (253). Chymase displays considerably less substrate specificity than tryptase. *In vitro*, chymase can convert angiotensin I to angiotensin II, inactivate bradykinin, metabolize thrombin, and degrade extracellular matrix components of basement membranes, including laminin and type IV collagen (255–259). The latter finding may explain the dermal-epidermal separation observed when fragments of human skin are incubated with chymase (260). The major angiotensin-converting enzyme in heart tissue, presumably serving an important role in vasoconstriction, has proven to be human chymase (252). In addition, canine-derived chymase degrades neuropeptides VIP and substance P, enhances mucosal gland secretion, and may augment the histamine-induced wheal-and-flare reaction (180,235). Chymase has the capacity to cleave membrane-bound SCF to an active soluble product, establishing a possible autocrine amplification loop for mast cell activation (123). Chymase was recognized as a converting enzyme for the inactive proform of IL-1 to yield an active molecule (261). Of further potential importance when considering the vascular abnormalities in scleroderma, chymase can process big endothelin-1 to the vasoactive form of endothelin-1 (262). In addition, latent TGF-β may be activated by chymase from cell surfaces leading to a fibrotic tissue response (263). The findings that chymase can serve as an activator of progelatinase B and can directly cleave interstitial collagen are of considerable relevance to the potential degradative nature of mast cells in joint diseases (25,264) and in promoting angiogenesis (28). Carboxypeptidase has also been shown to be produced by human mast cells of the MC_{TC} phenotype (265). Whether mast cells themselves are capable of synthesizing metalloproteinases remains unknown, although some evidence suggests that mast cells may be at least a major storage site for procollagenase (266).

Proteoglycans

The core of the secretory granules of both mast cells and basophils is composed of oversulfated proteoglycan molecules (267). The predominant proteoglycan in human mast cells is heparin, the most acidic molecule in the entire body (268). Bone marrow–derived rodent mast cells and human basophils contain mostly chondroitin sulfate; however, the mast cells synthesize an oversulfated form termed chondroitin sulfate E (267,269). The protein core is identical in these proteoglycans; the difference in structure is found in their glycosaminoglycan side chains, with heparin consisting of uronic acids linked to glucosamine while chondroitin sulfate E is composed of uronic acid linked to galactosamine. These molecules are relatively resistant to proteases, mainly because of the dense distribution of these side chains.

Proteoglycans, as they exist in the mast cell granules, have many functions, one of which is to bind and stabilize other stored active substances such as proteases. This may protect the cell as well as provide conformational stability to the proteases. For example, if heparin is dislodged from tryptase, the tetrameric structure rapidly dissociates into monomers with subsequent loss of catalytic activity (221). The ability of proteoglycans to serve as important modulators of growth factors is well appreciated (270,271). In addition, heparin as a secreted product (or a commercial product as isolated from porcine gut) has many diverse biologic activities (272). A clinically-relevant example is the inhibition of blood coagulation by potentiating the activity of antithrombin III. Other miscellaneous effects include increasing the enzymatic activity of elastase, promoting the release of plasminogen activator from endothelial cells, and enhancing collagen binding to fibronectin (273). Heparin also appears to potentiate endothelial cell–derived and other angiogenic growth factors by inducing their release, prolonging their half-life by binding and protecting these factors from protease degradation, and enhancing their effects on other cells (274–277). In fact, preliminary studies demonstrate that mast cell–derived heparin can activate FGF by displacing bound FGF from a heparin matrix *in vitro*, thus allowing FGF to engage its cellular receptor (278). Heparin inhibits the proliferation and migration of smooth muscle cells; the mechanism may involve the modulation of oncogene expression. Certain oncogenes, such as c-*myc* and c-*fos*, are requisite for cells to enter the growth cycle, and heparin may inhibit their expression (279). Heparin acts on arterial smooth muscle cells in another manner, inhibiting induction of several metalloproteinases, including collagenase, stromelysin, and gelatinase B (280). Heparin also interacts with the complement cascade by inhibiting C1q binding to immune complexes, C1s activation of C4 and C2, the amplification convertase C3bBb, and zymosan-dependent activation of C3 (281,282). On the other hand, C1 inhibitor activity appears to be enhanced in the presence of heparin. Heparin has also been shown to induce osteoporosis, when administered as an anticoagulant for prolonged periods of time (283). This may be the result of a synergistic effect of PTH and heparin on osteoblasts, although *in vitro* studies have yielded conflicting results (284–287). Alternatively the mechanism may involve activation of collagenase (288), although this also has not been confirmed (266). An effect of heparin on the proliferation of fibroblasts has also been reported (199,289), perhaps partly related to inhibition of cell attachment to collagen substrata (290).

Cytokines

One of the exciting developments in mast cell biology was the recognition that mast cells can synthesize a rich array of cytokines. Monokines including TNF-α, IL-1 α, IL-1β, and IL-6; chemokines including RANTES, MCP-1, MIP-1 α, and MIP-1β; hematologic growth factors including IL-3, IL-4, IL-5, IL-6, IL-8, GM-CSF, and SCF; immunomodulating cytokines including IL-10, IL-13, and IFN-γ; and mesenchymal growth factors including TGF-β, basic fibroblast growth factor (bFGF), and NGF have all been detected; the majority of studies indicate gene expression following cross-linkage of IgE in murine mast cells (11,291–295). TGF-β is constitutively expressed (292) and TNF-α appears to be stored in mast cell granules, features unique among mammalian cells (296). Human studies have been limited, although investigators have employed immunohistologic techniques using different tissues or, alternatively, focused on the HMC-1 cell line, originally derived from a patient with mast cell leukemia (112,297). From these efforts, it appears that at least TNF-α, IL-8, other IL-8-related chemokines, and probably IL-1β, -3, -4, -5, -6, -13, and -16, and TGF-β can be produced by human mast cells (155,188,218,293,297–304). It seems, from available studies, that, although the array of cytokines elaborated by mast cells is quite broad, individual cells may differentially express a specific subset or profile of cytokines. Under some circumstances, the cytokine secretion is independent of histamine release, as observed with IL-6 in rodent mast cells (305). Activation signal pathways may specifically affect gene transcription of cytokines (and other peptide products) independently of histamine release, as noted following mast cell stimulation with NGF (306) or SCF (162). Studies have investigated the role of nuclear factor of activated T-cells (NFAT-1) and related proteins in regulating cytokine transcriptional expression (307) in response to IgE cross-linking or SCF. In addition, it appears that NFκB, c-Fos, and c-Jun (components of activator protein 1 or AP-1) are critical for human mast cell cytokine transcription (155).

As might be predicted from these findings, stimulation of mast cells in organ explants or *in vivo* results in microvascular endothelial cell activation, as reflected by increased expression of E-selectin and ICAM-1 (14,15). This endothelial cell activation can be greatly suppressed by prior addition of neutralizing antibodies to TNF-α (15). Several studies have now confirmed that human mast cells are an important source of TNF-α, perhaps the major source in dermal tissue under physiologic conditions (296,308,309). Overall, the finding that mast cells may readily release significant quantities of cytokines is fundamental to understanding the extent of potential paracrine effects of activated mast cells. Prior speculation about mast cells in a number of acute and chronic immune responses is substantiated by these findings. Additional data indicate that mast cells, including human mast cells, synthesize, store, and release VEGF and bFGF (26, 310), which may provide insight as to how mast cells contribute to connective tissue remodeling. In addition, mast cells have been implicated in diseases often accompanied by neovascularization.

Mast cells are also capable of expressing class II major histocompatibility antigens on their surface, as well as accessory molecules such as ICAM-1 (32,311). These surface molecules may allow for productive interactions between lymphocytes and mast cells (186). Thus, it is likely that with further delineation of human mast cell–derived cytokine profiles, we will better comprehend the potential for mast cells to participate in a variety of biologic responses related to growth, repair, and inflammation, with subsequent impact in many areas of human disease.

Mast Cells in Specific Rheumatic Disorders

Mast Cells in Arthritis

The precise pathogenic role of mast cells in inflammatory arthritides remains speculative (312–314). Unlike rodents, no human is completely devoid of mast cells, and no drug exists that specifically targets and nullifies mast cells. Therefore, a full understanding of its contribution cannot be realized at this time in humans. However, genetic mutations leading to mast cell deficiency in mice provide a unique opportunity to gain insight into the function of mast cells in experimentally induced arthritis (114). In a recently described experimental model of chronic erosive inflammatory arthritis induced by transfer of arthritogenic sera from the K/BxN mice, an inbred strain of mice that lack mast cells [*W/W*^{v} (c-*kit*) and *Sl/Sl*^{d} (c-*kit* ligand) deficient mutants] demonstrated nearly complete resistance to developing arthritis as compared with control littermates (315). If the mast cells were restored by engraftment, inflammatory arthritis promptly developed (315). Furthermore, mast cells were noted to degranulate prior to neutrophil recruitment as well as during the chronic phase, suggesting a pivotal role in orchestrating the histopathology in this model of RA (316). Other murine models of arthritis support this conclusion. In an experimental model of adjuvant arthritis in the *W/W*^{v} (c-*kit*) mutant mouse strain, disease severity was monitored and compared with normal +/+ littermates (317). The early acute inflammatory phase of synovitis was indistinguishable between the two groups. In contrast, however, chronic changes, involving matrix depletion within articular cartilage as well as chondrocyte death, were more severe in animals replete with mast cells. Furthermore, when a flare of acute arthritis was experimentally induced during the chronic persistent stage of disease, the presence of mast cells significantly augmented this response.

Another animal model of arthritis, induced by injecting a purified arthritogenic factor isolated from type II collagen-primed lymphocytes, revealed an acute mast cell degranulation in association with edema, dense inflammatory infiltration, and fibrin deposition (318). Presumably, the injected purified lymphokine was capable of directly stimulating mast cell degranulation while at the same time inducing arthritis. Similar findings were noted following intraarticular administration of TGF-β, that is, acute and chronic synovitis with marked recruitment of mast cells (86,319). These observations are consistent with other experiments using Lewis rats injected with streptococcal polysaccharide (320). Marked degranulation of periarticular mast cells was noted 30 minutes following intravenous injection. This led to an increase in microvascular permeability that facilitated the deposition of peptidoglycan and persistent chronic synovitis. The fibrinlike deposition characteristic of chronic synovitis may be mediated by mast cell activation, as suggested by earlier findings in experimentally induced cutaneous inflammation comparing mast cell–deficient animals to normal littermates (321).

Previous studies of adjuvant-induced arthritis demonstrated the prompt appearance of numerous mast cells in perisynovial tissues within the first week prior to onset of inflammation. These mast cells subsequently degranulate, and an intense mononuclear cell infiltration leads to an overt synovitis (322). A cleverly designed variation of these experimental models allowed direct activation of synovial mast cells *in vivo* using specific IgE-mediated stimulation after presensitizing the animals (323). This model elegantly demonstrated the potential for producing an acute, transient arthritis by first activating synovial mast cells. The pattern of arthritis noted in this animal model, with marked edema, granulocyte extravasation, but generally nonerosive inflammation, resembled that seen clinically in lupus or intermittent hydrarthrosis, an observation further bolstered by the finding of extremely high levels of synovial mast cells and histamine during arthritic flares in a patient with systemic lupus erythematosus (SLE) (4,323,324). It is conceivable that IgE rheumatoid factors, anti-IgE autoantibodies, or antibodies to FcεRI noted in the circulation of patients with autoimmune diseases may serve as synovial mast cell activators (143,144,325–327), because experiments *in vitro* demonstrate that IgE rheumatoid factor sensitizes and induces degranulation of human synovial mast cells (143). Whether patients also synthesize antibodies to the high-affinity IgE receptor, as described in individuals with chronic urticaria (145), is still unknown and may be another potential mechanism for mast activation in rheumatic diseases (328).

These findings implicate mast cells in mediating connective tissue damage during chronic stages of arthritis, as well as amplifying or coordinating the acute inflammatory responses. These findings are consonant with morphologic observations in human arthritic conditions. A consistent feature in both RA and osteoarthritis (OA) has been mast cell hyperplasia (4,329–335). Descriptions of the regional localization of mast cells within rheumatoid synovium (7,331,336) and additional characterization has indicated a phenotype with functional properties similar to mast cells in other organs, although surface expression of C5a receptors (CD88) appears up-regulated (337) and responses to other specific secretagogues implies a degree of uniqueness to these mast cells (338). The recruitment of mast cells to synovial tissue in RA has been attributed to elevated levels of mast cell chemoattractants, including TFG-β and SCF or c-*kit* ligand—the latter may be released by TNF-stimulated synovial fibroblasts (339–341).

Mast Cell Degranulation in Arthritis

The extent and nature of synovial mast cell activation has also been the subject of study (5). By assaying synovial fluid for mast cell–derived products, α-tryptase, β-tryptase, and histamine are detectable in the majority of patients with RA, seronegative spondyloarthritis, and OA (5). The greatest degree of mast cell degranulation, as reflected by the levels of these products in the joint cavity, was noted in OA, despite the relative lack of apparent inflammation (5). A particular subset of mast cell expansion was noted in specimens from OA synovium, which were depicted as containing tryptase but lacking chymase (MC_T) (342). Additional studies of mast cell subsets in RA indicate a mixed population of MC_T and MC_{TC}, with MC_T mast cell expansion correlating more with degree of synovial inflammation and MC_{TC} associated with underlying matrix damage or fibrous tissue (7,336,343–345). These observations suggest that mast cells in rheumatoid synovium may possess distinct functions, contributing to different aspects of the spectrum of inflammatory events (344).

The detection of histamine and tryptase in synovial fluid or extracellular tissue indicates mast cell activation predominantly (5,7), as does earlier ultrastructural evidence documenting mast cells degranulating in synovial tissue (4,8,346), although recently it has been noted that chondrocytes also have the capacity to decarboxylate histidine to histamine (314). The increased mast cells residing within the synovium correlate with disease activity (329,332). Furthermore, during the course of detailed morphologic studies to determine the cell types that accumulate at pannus–cartilage junctions in RA, an unexpected finding was mast cells predominating and often forming aggregates at this site (10,347) (Fig. 17.4). Traditionally, this junction is viewed as the invasive front of the chronic synovial inflammatory process exhibiting matrix dissolution, forming the

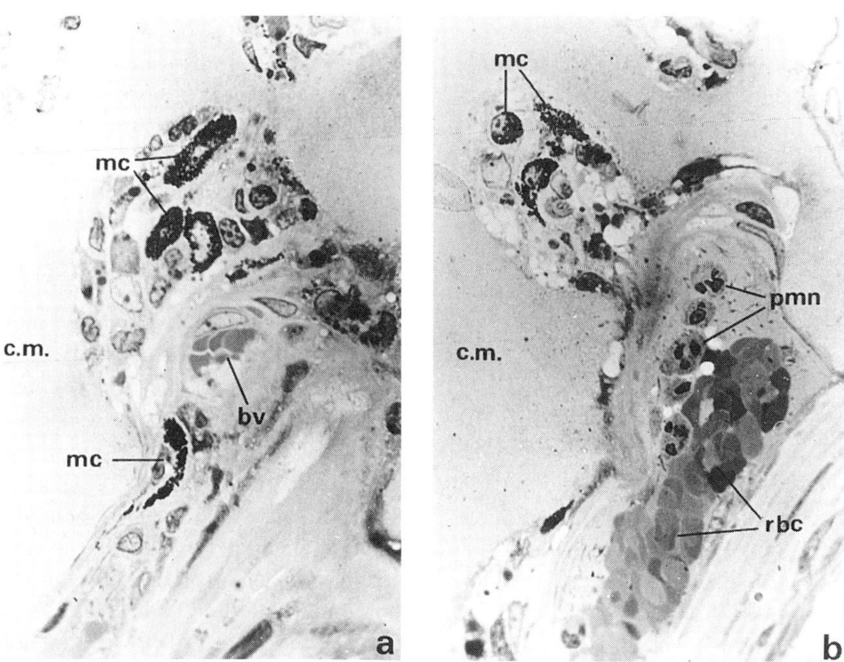

FIG. 17.4. A, B: Two views of advancing pannus tissue invading subchondral bone in rheumatoid arthritis. Note the cluster of mast cells (*mc*) at the advancing edge into the cartilage matrix (*cm*), just a short distance from a blood vessel (*bv*) containing red blood cells (*rbc*) and polymorphonuclear leukocytes (*pmn*), as indicated (original magnification ×825).

basis of the characteristic cartilage erosions in RA (348). The finding of mast cells at this site raises issues as to their degradative capacity (349), and studies have demonstrated mast cell–derived proteases at sites of cartilage erosion (7,350). Mast cell products such as tryptase or chymase, capable of activating members of the latent metalloprotease family (24,25,351), may directly contribute to this destructive process (24,352,353). Interstitial collagenase (matrix metalloproteinase-1) has been recently demonstrated as synthesized and released by human mast cells (354). Certain mast cell products may also stimulate production and release of matrix-degrading metalloproteinases (355). These observations are consistent with the findings of diminished cartilage depletion in the setting of mast cell–deficient animals, as mentioned above (317). Mast cells have also been implicated in promoting the loosening of prosthetic joints by similar proteolytic mechanisms (356).

IgE antibodies synthesized against structural components of the synovial microenvironment can induce mast cell degranulation in arthritic diseases. An example would be the formation of IgE against cartilage collagens (357,358). Alternatively, synovial plasma cells might synthesize IgE with rheumatoid factor–like activity. The IgE would become mast cell membrane–bound via the high-affinity IgE receptor. Upon contact with IgG aggregates in the joint, the mast cell is triggered. Considerable data have accumulated to support this mechanism, including the presence of IgE rheumatoid factors as well as their ability *in vitro* to induce synovial mast cell degranulation (143,326,327,359,360). Along similar lines, IgE with antinuclear, anti-DNA, or anti-RNA activity might be biologically relevant in a tissue with a high cell turnover such as the rheumatoid synovium (361,362).

The IgE molecule itself may induce an immune response in either an antiidiotypic fashion or as the target of rheumatoid factors (anti-IgE autoantibodies). Evidence exists to support both of these possibilities, along with the *in vitro* demonstration of histamine release as a result (143,144, 363–367). Furthermore, IgE immune complexes formed by any of the above mechanisms may activate cells that have low-affinity IgE receptors (368,369), such as monocytes, platelets, eosinophils, and stimulated B lymphocytes.

Mast Cells in Bone Disease

Mast cells have received relatively little attention as important effector cells in bone disease. Yet these cells are strategically located within the collagenous matrix and the hematopoietic compartments of skeletal tissue and accumulate at sites of active bone resorption and turnover. Bone turnover or remodeling is central to an understanding of potential mast cell influences. First, normal healing or reparative processes associated with bone remodeling have concomitant transient mast cell hyperplasia as noted in callus formation (370,371). Furthermore, the disorder of mastocytosis generally affects bone more than any other organ, with a rather characteristic pattern. The uncontrolled growth of mast cells in systemic mastocytosis invariably leads to alterations in both axial and appendicular skeletal tissues in over 70% of cases, as reflected by skeletal surveys (372). The most common presentation is diffuse osteopenia, but poorly demarcated sclerotic and lucent areas are also encountered, as are well-defined circumscribed lesions, either osteoporotic or blastic in nature. Generalized osteopenia has been appreciated in this setting, at times with pathologic fractures. Some believe that mastocytosis is underestimated in the differential diagnosis of idiopathic osteoporosis (372,373), with one recent large survey indicating an overall prevalence of 1.25% and even higher in younger individuals (374). Furthermore, it has been appreciated, of late, that some patients with systemic mastocytosis may present with rather indolent or smoldering disease (375). Examination of bone in age-related and postmenopausal osteoporosis reveals a consistent increase in mast cell numbers (376,377). Bone scintigraphy in mastocytosis detects abnormalities not often appreciated with skeletal surveys. Histomorphometric analyses of trabecular bone in this disorder reveals accelerated remodeling, characterized by excessive osteoid lined by numerous osteoblasts and peritrabecular fibrosis (373,378). Peritrabecular granulomas consisting of mast cell clusters are associated with both large excavated resorption zones and areas of new bone formation. Descriptions of the marrow cavity in many of these patients reveal mast cell infiltration with variable degrees of fibrosis and trabecular sclerosis. It seems likely that mast cell products stimulate or modulate bone remodeling. In the setting of mastocytosis, the histologic studies support enhanced osteoclastic activity (374). This would result in areas of radiographic lucency, representing increased bone resorption juxtaposed with sclerosis, reflecting coupled new bone formation.

Many years ago, Urist and McLean (379) observed that numerous mast cells accumulated on the endosteal surface in experimentally induced secondary hyperparathyroidism and rickets. These experiments involved several hundred rats weaned on a diet deficient in calcium and vitamin D. The rats were sustained on this regimen for up to 105 days before being sacrificed. Analysis of bone revealed, as anticipated, that ricketic features developed early and were followed by manifestations of hyperparathyroidism. This included an increase in osteoclast cell number and proliferation of fibrous tissue. Concomitantly, vast numbers of mast cells accumulated on the endosteal surface and in the marrow interspersed within the fibrous tissue. The number of mast cells correlated with duration of the diet. Administration of vitamin D corrected the mineralization defect, reversed the osteitis fibrosa, and normalized the mast cell counts. This association between PTH and mast cell accumulation has been confirmed by others (380). A recent experimental model of parathyroid bone disease induced by constant infusion of parathormone indicated increased osteoclastic activity and elevated immunostaining for PDGF-A (381). Interestingly, the PDGF-A was localized entirely to mast cells, providing data to postulate a mechanistic scheme for mast cell participation in hyperparathyroid-related bone disease (381). In humans with primary hyperparathyroidism, the bone marrow cavity contains excess mast cells, as does the marrow of patients with renal osteodystrophy (382). McKenna and Frame (383) described one case with mast cells contiguous with the resorptive sites. In this specimen, the high resorptive activity was not associated with increased osteoclastic activity but rather with a marked increase in mast cells, suggesting that mast cells themselves were responsible for matrix resorption.

What mast cell products might contribute to bone remodeling? Heparin is well known for its bone-resorptive properties, both from the standpoint of clinical experience and from *in vitro* observations. The laboratory evidence suggests that a major effect of heparin is to augment PTH-mediated resorption, consistent with the histomorphometric observations described above (286,384). However, heparin has many biologic effects, as mentioned earlier, including its ability to act as a cofactor and stabilize certain growth factors (e.g., FGF) and to directly influence the proliferation of connective tissue cells (199,289). Heparin also confers stability to the functional tetrameric structure of mast cell granule-associated protease tryptase, which may have a multifunctional role in bone turnover. Other mast cell–derived mediators that may promote resorption include PGD_2, peroxidases, kinin-generating factors, and cytokines such as TNF-α, IL-1, and IL-6.

Studies of bone remodeling cycles in W/W^v mast cell–deficient mice have been performed to study the influence of mast cells (385). In a series of experiments designed to stimulate alveolar bone remodeling either by molar extraction or chronic foreign body–induced periodontitis, a delay in the early activation phase and subsequent diminished bone matrix formation is observed in mast cell–deficient animals. No mineralization defect was detected using relatively crude methods. In the chronic periodontitis model, transient alveolar bone loss was observed in the control mice followed by a repair process involving new bone formation. In the mast cell–deficient animals, greater bone loss occurred followed by diminished bone formation during the reparative phase. These studies provide persuasive evidence that the mast cell is involved in bone remodeling. It is not clear whether this involves recruitment, differentiation, or activation of osteoblasts or osteoclasts. Because redundancy likely exists in these cellular processes, the absence of mast cells only partially alters the biologic outcome. Hence, the bones of the naive W/W^v mast cell–deficient mice appear essentially normal. This is in contrast to another species of mast cell–deficient mice, *mi/mi*. These latter mice develop osteopetrosis due to a defect in both osteoclast and mast cell progenitor cells. The relationship of the mast cells to the osteopetrosis in these animals is not clear.

The implication of these studies for physiologic bone turnover or remodeling is likely influenced by mast cell products. When mast cells accumulate above the normal quantity in diseases such as in mastocytosis, then excess remodeling may occur that significantly affects the delicate balance of coupled resorption-formation within osseous multifunctional units. Further support for this contention stems from a study in which a mast cell secretagogue (compound 48/80) proved to be a potent inhibitor of bone resorption induced by PTH (386). This is somewhat in contrast to findings of other investigators (387), who administered a mast cell antagonist to beagles with periodontal disease and observed an inhibition of concomitant bone loss. Nonetheless, these observations point to a measurable effect of mast cell products on the control of bone turnover.

The precise role of mast cells in modulating the regulation of bone growth and remodeling awaits further elucidation. There is a paucity of information concerning mast cells and the important osteoclast receptor activator of NFκB (RANK), its ligand (RANKL), and the soluble decoy receptor osteoprotegerin, all of which are pivotal in controlling osteoclastic differentiation and activity (388). Clearly, more investigation is needed to define the mast cell contribution in normal physiologic states and specific bone diseases. Little information is available concerning the latter, although the possibility that mast cells play an effector role in osteoporosis, osteomalacia, and osteitis fibrosa is supported by experimental animal data and the limited available clinical studies.

Mast Cells in Scleroderma

It is well appreciated that an inflammatory infiltrate occurs in the dermis during the early stages of scleroderma (389). Less well recognized is the large numbers of mast cells also present in involved tissues (390–393). The work of several investigators has directed considerable attention to mast cells as potential effector cells in the development of fibrosis (53,228), both experimentally and in scleroderma (6,12,356,394–396). Mast cells have been previously implicated in related clinical problems, such as hypertrophic scarring, pulmonary fibrosis, eosinophilic fasciitis, and neurofibromas (371,397–401).

The concept that mast cells contribute to the development of fibrosis has been supported by experimental animal studies. Direct repetitive stimulation of mesenteric or dermal mast cells in rodents resulted in proliferation of neighboring mesenchymal cells (402,403). The thickened dermis seen in the genetically predisposed tight skin (Tsk) mice reveals microscopic evidence of numerous degranulating mast cells (404). Perhaps the most intriguing line of investigation involves the graft-versus-host disease model of scleroderma in rodents (34,396,405). In this setting, Claman and co-workers (396) noted a loss of mast cell granules occurring immediately prior to developing fibrosis. These

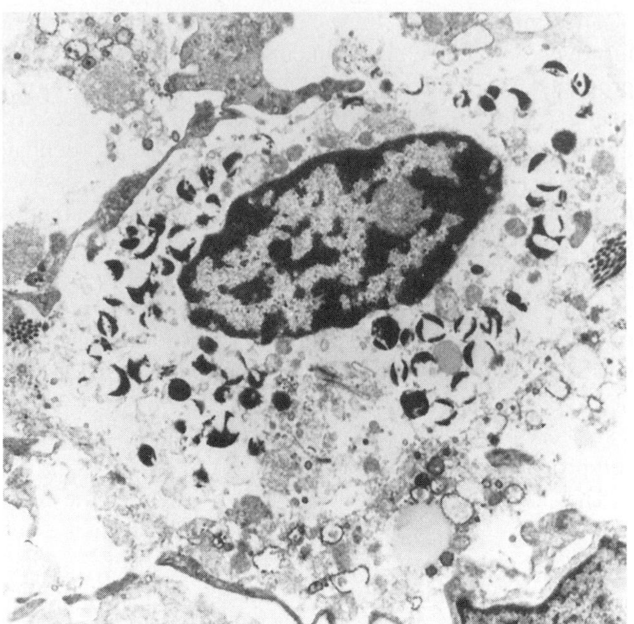

FIG. 17.5. Human mast cell from a patient with aggressive diffuse scleroderma. Note the edematous appearance and the loss of the outer cell membrane. The nucleus is intact, but the cytoplasm reveals fragmentation of the granule structure and a "moth-eaten" appearance, suggestive of piecemeal degranulation (original magnification ×10,300). (Courtesy of Henry N. Claman.)

mast cells were difficult to recognize using the standard histologic techniques relying on the presence of intact metachromatic cytoplasmic granules; hence, they were termed phantom cells (Fig. 17.5). Such cells were noted in a case of fatal scleroderma, in which ultrastructural studies were performed on the involved skin (395). These phantom cells were also observed in myocardial tissue as well as in the dermis of patients with scleroderma (393,406).

The pathogenesis of scleroderma is undoubtedly complex, involving a series of upstream events and numerous amplification pathways. The clinical data suggest that activation of endothelial cells is an early event leading to platelet aggregation, which results in the release of a number of cytokines and PDGFs. These factors contribute to the recruitment and activation of fibroblasts. During this process, connective tissue mast cells accumulate. Platelet products such as TGF-β may induce the local recruitment of mast cells (86,319). Recently, investigators have demonstrated increased c-*kit* ligand (SCF) in the dermis and serum of patients with scleroderma (407). Platelet-derived products may also be instrumental in causing mast cell degranulation (174). Activated mast cells then release products such as TNF-α, which induce endothelial cells to strongly express adhesion molecules, further promoting a local inflammatory response. Mast cells and fibroblasts themselves interact in ways still only partially understood, leading to a state of sustained fibroblast activity with resultant fibrosis. Alterations in the behavior and phenotype of mast cells likewise result from coculturing with fibroblasts (106). In addition, an increase in the metabolic activity and proliferation of fibroblasts may be mediated by mast cell–secreted products, not only cytokines but also mast cell–derived proteases such as tryptase (51,241,408,409). It has been observed from coculture studies that mast cells attach to fibroblasts; the adherence mechanism is not yet completely understood, although both SCF and cadherin receptors with counterligands, as well as surface connexins, have been implicated (94,95,410). After this heterotypic cell-cell contact is established, the fibroblast proliferation rate increases, which has been attributed to mast cell–derived IL-4 as a critical signaling molecule (411).

The role of the mast cell in fibrosis has also been investigated by using mast cell–deficient mice in experimental models that incite varying degrees of organ fibrosis (412–414). The most compelling report indicates that mast cell–deficient mice, when compared with mast cell–intact mice, were less apt to develop silica-induced pulmonary inflammation, especially granulomatous lesions and alveolar thickening (415). These mice were then reconstituted with mast cells, and the degree of inflammatory pathologic changes was restored to that observed in control mice (415). Bronchial alveolar fluid was analyzed and, similar to the tissue histology, considerably less neutrophilia developed in mast cell–deficient mice. In a later model of mast cell deficiency, mice were bred to hybridize with the tight-skin genetic mutation (416) in order to study the effect of mast cells on disease expression. The investigators noted that mast cells were not absolutely required for the development of fibrosis but did enhance its evolution (417). Thus, these experiments represent examples of how mast cells may modulate tissue remodeling, either directly or indirectly, by participating in the inflammatory response and the later development of fibrosis.

Specific mast cell mediators, once released, have demonstrable *in vitro* effects on fibroblasts and endothelial cells that may be relevant to the pathogenesis of scleroderma. Histamine stimulates collagen synthesis under certain experimental conditions, and heparin potentiates important endothelial cell–derived growth factors and FGFs (274, 275,277,418–420). FGF is also synthesized by mast cells (310,421). The relevance to scleroderma is obvious. Other fibrogenic cytokines released by mast cells have been delineated by several investigators (422,423). On the other hand, a series of studies have focused on the ability of mast cell–derived tryptase to promote fibroblast activation (51, 237,241). More specifically, tryptase stimulates fibroblast chemotaxis, proliferation, and production of type I procollagen (51,237,241,424). The capacity of mast cells to enhance contraction of stromal tissue has been supported by a series of investigations that demonstrate that mast cells mediate fibroblast transformation to a myofibroblast phenotype (52,425,426). In a clinical setting, the role of tryptase released by mast cells has been defined recently in the development of renal interstitial fibrosis (424).

An important question remains regarding the extent to which activated mast cells contribute to a disease such as scleroderma. One approach to unravel this question is by administering mast cell–stabilizing agents and following the clinical course of this disease (427). At this time, few drugs (if any) are available that adequately stabilize mast cell degranulation. Some encouraging results were provided by experiments using cromolyn sodium and ketotifen in the Tsk mouse model (428). However, either the bioavailability or the potency of these currently available agents in stabilizing mast cells remains a practical barrier in their usage (429).

Mast Cells in Other Rheumatic Disorders

Histologic studies in a number of other connective tissue diseases have reported a prominent mast cell hyperplasia. This includes tissue specimens from Sjögren syndrome, Lyme synovitis, toxic oil syndrome, eosinophilic fasciitis, eosinophilic myalgia syndrome, familial acroosteolysis, and Behçla;et disease, to mention just a few (397, 430–434). It is difficult to define a specific role of the mast cell in each of these disparate conditions. It is more likely that chronic inflammation, often in association with eosinophils, is common to these disorders and creates a microenvironment conducive to mast cell hyperplasia. The contribution of the mast cells after their accumulation remains speculative, although considerable experimental evidence discussed throughout this chapter implicates mast cells as potent effector cells rather than mere innocent bystanders (313,435).

In addition to the above diseases, in which mast cells have been guilty by association, mast cell–derived vasoactive products have long been assigned a role in the development of immune complex–mediated vasculitis. The classic model to study this phenomenon has been serum sickness, both in humans and experimental animals (436,437). The vascular lesion in this setting can be abrogated if the animals are pretreated with drugs that antagonize mast cell products (436). A role for histamine is suggested by the finding that cutaneous injection of histamine can induce local leukocytoclastic vasculitis following immune complex deposition (438). In addition to histamine, which enhances vascular permeability (439), studies reveal that leukocyte adhesiveness to the endothelium and granulocyte extravasation is enhanced by activated mast cells (15,16,440).

We can now begin to appreciate what will be required to solve the age-old riddle regarding the generic role of mast cells in human pathology (441). In recent years, it has been shown that mast cells are unique in their remarkably high content of biologically active constituents. Specifically, the rapidly expanding inventory of mast cell–derived cytokines and growth factors, along with a new appreciation for the biologic effects of mast cell proteases, opens new avenues of investigation to unravel the contribution of mast cells in rheumatic diseases. The evidence points to an active role for mast cells in normal healing processes, host defense mechanisms, acute and chronic inflammation, angiogenesis, and pathologic fibrosis. Because many skeletal disorders and connective tissue diseases evolve from an undefined tissue injury with a resultant imbalance in reparative processes, the participation of mast cells at some level is perhaps not surprising. Unfortunately, despite the rapid advances in available information regarding mast cell constituents, no clear formulation can be advanced to establish a more definitive role of mast cells in these processes. This requires further basic studies and, as new modalities of therapy become available that better target mast cells, further clinical studies. In a mouse model of RA, a mast cell–stabilizing drug appeared beneficial (442). Parenthetically, it has been known for some time that gold inhibits mast cell mediator release (443). Nonetheless, more specific agents will be required if we are to surmise the magnitude of this cell's contribution to rheumatic conditions.

EOSINOPHILS

Eosinophils were named by Paul Ehrlich in 1979 because of their intense cytoplasmic staining with the acidic dye eosin. They are derived from bone marrow granulocytes and normally contribute up to 5% of circulating white blood cells, with a much larger reserve (about 100-fold) located within tissues (444). Eosinophils are mobilized to sites of inflammation (or infection) and may increase within the vasculature in a variety of disorders, including allergic diseases, helminthic parasite infections, some autoimmune and vasculitic disorders, and a number of idiopathic syndromes (445). Eosinophils can be activated by many inflammatory substances, including peptides, lipids, or small proteins and are capable of secreting a very large array of inflammatory substances, including cytokines and chemokines. The mechanisms by which activation and secretion occurs is an area of continuing investigation, and considerable progress has been made in recent years.

Eosinophil Differentiation, Kinetics, and Distribution

The development and differentiation of eosinophils within the bone marrow are promoted by cytokines such as GM-CSF, IL-3, and IL-5 (445), as well as the chemokine RANTES (446). IL-3 acts on $CD34^+$ stem cells to expand virtually all bone marrow elements, with eosinophil colonies accounting for about 10% of the total. GM-CSF acts on a more mature precursor population to yield colonies of eosinophils, neutrophils, and monocytes, with eosinophil colonies increasing to 25% of the total. The progenitor cell of each of these appears to be different, whereas a single progenitor can yield colonies of basophils plus eosinophils or pure colonies of each. IL-5 is a more specific cytokine and acts on the eosinophil/basophil precursor to yield pure eosinophil colonies (447), whereas TGF-β mediates the switch to basophil commitment (448). IFN-α inhibits multipotential colony formation, including eosinophil progenitors (449).

Once released into the blood, the circulating half-life of eosinophils is about 8 hours and their residence within tissues is 2 to 5 days, but the cytokines can increase that to 14 days. Rapid increases within the circulation can occur in acute allergic reactions or certain helminth infections; their recruitment into tissues is dependent on priming within the circulation, margination along the vascular endothelium (rolling and adherence), and transendothelial migration in response to a chemotactic gradient to enter tissues.

IL-5 is the cytokine most closely related to eosinophil mobilization, and IL-5 levels are actually increased in some (but not all) disorders associated with eosinophilia such as *Onchocerca volvulus* infection, recombinant IL-2 therapy, episodic angioedema associated with eosinophilia, and T cell–dependent idiopathic hypereosinophilic syndrome (450).

Eosinophil Structure and Constituents

The eosinophil has a diameter of 12 to 17 μm on blood films, which is slightly larger than a neutrophil. It has a bilobed nucleus with distinctive specific (secondary) granules composed of an electron-dense core and an electron-lucent matrix. Primary granules are round, uniformly electron dense, and are mainly seen in eosinophilic promyelocytes. There is also a third group of small granules, which possess enzymes such as aryl sulfatase and acid phosphatase. Another cytoplasmic structure, distinct from granules, are lipid bodies. They are globular, can be minute or large, lack a limiting membrane, and are positive for osmium fixation due to their lipid content. They can serve as repositories for esterified arachidonic acid and can therefore serve as sites of prostaglandin and leukotriene formation (445,451).

The crystalloid core of the specific granule contains major basic protein (MBP), whereas the secondary matrix contains other cationic proteins such as eosinophil cationic protein (ECP), eosinophil peroxidase (EPO), and eosinophil-derived neurotoxin (EDN) as well as the enzyme β-glucuronidase. MBP accounts for 55% of the granule protein, has an isoelectric point of 11, and is rich in arginine residues. It is derived from a pre pro MBP with an N-terminus rich in glutamic acid and aspartic acid so that the precursor has a much lower isoelectric point of 6.2. MBP is also found in basophils, attesting to the common precursor origin of these cells, and is seen in some subpopulations of mast cells. MBP binds directly to the membrane of schistosomula of *Schistosoma mansoni*, causes membrane disruption, and can be released from eosinophils when in contact with antibody-coated schistosomula. It is toxic to a variety of other helminths as well. MBP can directly release histamine from basophils, cause superoxide and lysosome release from neutrophils, and stimulate platelet serotonin secretion. MBP inhibits activation of the classical complement pathway and causes ciliostasis and exfoliation of epithelial respiratory cells. It can thereby contribute to the bronchial hyperreactivity associated with asthma.

ECP, like EDN, has RNAse activity (ratio of 1:100), and the two proteins share 89% sequence hemology. One monoclonal antibody (EG1) recognizes stored ECP, whereas another (EG2) recognizes conformations associated with activation (although with some limitations in distinguishing quiescent from activated eosinophils) (452). ECP is 10-fold more toxic to schistosomula than MBP, but is far less abundant; it is also toxic to the larvae of *Trichinella spiralis* and microfilaria of *Brugia malayi*. Like MBP, it binds and neutralizes heparin and shortens the partial thromboplastin time, apparently by activating factor XII (Hageman factor).

EDN damages myelinated neurons and may relate to the neuropathic changes observed in the hypereosinophilic syndrome or Churg-Strauss syndrome. It is homologous to pancreatic RNAse (and ECP).

EPO differs from neutrophil or monocyte myeloperoxidase by absorption spectra and the heme prosthetic group. In the presence of H_2O_2 plus halide it yields hypohalous acids, but in this instance prefers bromide ions to chloride. Serum also contains thiocyanate, a pseudohalide, which reacts with EPO to form hypothiocyanous acid, the major oxidant produced by EPO in biologic fluids.

Another protein that is associated with the eosinophil is the Charcot Leyden crystal protein, which was originally described as hexagonal bipyramidal crystals found in the sputum of asthmatics. The crystal is derived from an enzyme, lysophospholipase (453), estimated to represent 7% to 10% of total eosinophil protein. It is a membrane-bound protein in a subpopulation of eosinophil granules. Its function is unknown, but it may degrade surfactant lysophospholipid and contribute to the development of atelectasis. Small amounts are also detected in basophils but not other cells. Eosinophils have arylsulfatase B and acid phosphatase in small granules and also contain the enzymes β-glucuronidase, lysozyme, neutrophil elastase (which may be ingested rather than synthesized), a collagenase, and a 92-kd metalloproteinase corresponding to one of the gelatinases.

The lipid bodies are a source of esterified arachidonic acid that can be cleaved by phospholipase A_2 to liberate arachidonic acid, which can then be metabolized by cyclooxygenases or 5-lipoxygenase plus FLAP into prostaglandins and leukotrienes, respectively, as well as lipoxins and 5-HETE. Eosinophils produce large quantities of LTC_4 (from which LTD_4 and LTE_4 can be generated) and 5-HETE, whereas only small amounts of LTD_4 or LTE_4 are secreted. PAF, in the form of 1-alkyl 2-lyso-sn-glycero-3 phosphocholine is produced by acetylating the 2-position after arachidonate is liberated. Its role in disease is not

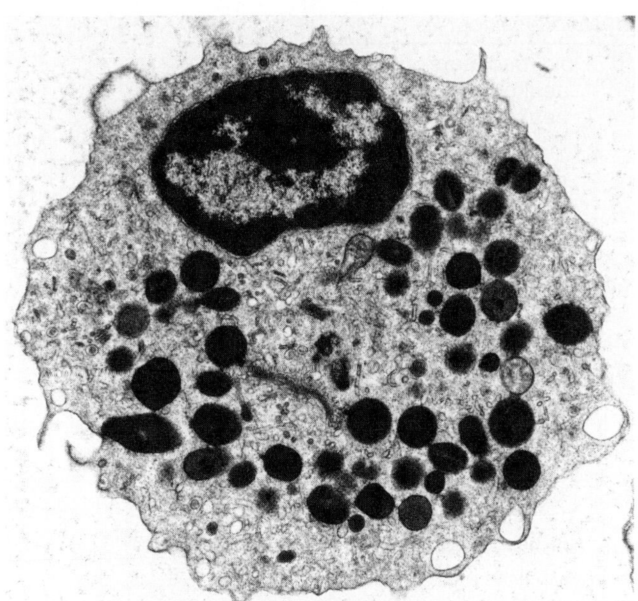

FIG. 17.6. Peripheral blood eosinophil from a patient with the hypereosinophilic syndrome. A single nuclear lobe with condensed chromatin is seen. Cytoplasmic granules include many membrane-bound, large, dense, spherical, crystalloid-containing granules; less numerous large, dense, spherical crystalloid-free granules; small dense granules; and tubulovesicular structures. [From Dvorak AM, Letourneau L, Logan GR, et al. Ultrastructural localization of the Charcot-Leyden crystal protein (lysophospholipase) to a distinct crystalloid-free granule population in mature human eosinophils. *Blood* 1988;72:150–158, with permission.]

yet clear, although it increases vascular permeability and causes bronchoconstriction, and is an eosinophil chemoattractant when studied *in vitro* (Fig 17.6 is an electron micrograph of the eosinophil).

Eosinophils have cell surface receptors that interact with immunoglobulins or endothelial cell counter ligands, which are critical for migration into tissues. There are receptors for IgG, IgA, and IgE. The major IgG receptor is the low-affinity FcγRII (CD32), although FcγRIII (CD16) can be induced by IFN-γ. The low-affinity IgE receptor FcϵRII (CD23) is present and eosinophils may also express the high-affinity FcϵRI, as is seen in basophils and mast cells, but this remains controversial (454,455). An IgA receptor is present that is particularly avid for secretory IgA. Eosinophils have complement receptors, including receptors for C1q, C3b/C4b (CR1), iC3b (CR3), C3a, and C5a. Prominent chemokine receptors are CCR1 (binds MIP-1α, MCP-3, and RANTES) and CCR3 (binds MCP-3, MCP-4, eotaxin I and II, and RANTES). There are receptors for cytokines involved in eosinophilopoiesis that also inhibit eosinophil apoptosis, thereby increasing eosinophil presence in tissues, namely receptors for IL-3, IL-5, and GM-CSF. There are also receptors for IL-1α, IL-2, IL-4, IL-8, IFN-α and -γ, TNF-α, and IL-16, as well as receptors for PAF and LTB_4. IL-16 stimulates eosinophils via CD4, which is unique. PAF and LTB_4 stimulate chemotaxis, eosinophil degranulation, and a respiratory burst. Eosinophils have intracellular estrogen and glucocorticoid receptors, and express membrane proteins for cell/cell interactions, including CD40, CD40 ligand, CD28, and CD86. They can also be stimulated to express major histocompatibility complex class II antigens.

Eosinophils also produce a variety of cytokines. TGF-α and TGF-β in particular may contribute to fibrosis and basement membrane thickening. Eosinophils produce IL 3, IL-5, and GM-CSF, each of which can prime eosinophils and inhibit apoptosis. Eosinophil production of GM-CSF has been documented in nasal polyposis (456). Bronchoalveolar lavage eosinophils from asthmatics are positive for IL-5 and GM-CSF mRNA (457), and by *in situ* hybridization, IL-5 mRNA has been found in intestinal tissue of celiac disease (458) and hypereosinophilic syndrome (449). Eosinophils have the capacity to produce IL-4 when stimulated, but basophils do so more prominently. Eosinophil production of IL-6, IL-8, IL-10, TNF-α, MIP-1α, RANTES, and IL-16 have all been reported. Table 17.4 summarizes the secretory products of eosinophils.

Migration of Eosinophils

Preferential accumulation of eosinophils at sites of inflammation is the result of adhesive interactions with endothelial cells and transmigration into tissues caused by chemotactic factors. Cells are initially slightly adherent to the endothelium and roll along its surface. This is followed by leukocyte activation with development of a higher-affinity adherence and then transmigration proceeds. Eosinophil rolling is mediated by L-selectin, which interacts with endothelial cell sialoglycoproteins. Endothelial cell P-selectin and E-selectin interact with eosinophil P-selectin glycoprotein ligand-1 (459) and sialyl-dimeric Lewis^x, respectively, whereas eosinophil VLA-4 interacts with endothelial cell VCAM-1 (460). Eosinophils express several integrins that bind to immunoglobulin family receptors on endothelial cells and to components of extracellular matrix with much stronger affinity than the selectin/carbohydrate interaction. This binding is associated with inside-out signaling in which receptors convert from low-affinity states to high-affinity states. Eosinophil CD11a/CD18 (LFA-1) binds to endothelial cell ICAM-1 and ICAM-2; CD11b/CD18 (MAC-1) binds to ICAM-1; and eosinophil VLA-4 ($\alpha_4\beta_1$) binds to endothelial cell VCAM-1. Eosinophils also express $\alpha_4\beta_7$, which interacts with the gut MAdCAM-1 and to a lesser degree VCAM-1. These interactions are facilitated by IL-1, TNF-α, IL-4, and IL-13, which stimulate endothelial cells. IL-3, IL-5, GM-CSF, and PAF stimulate eosinophils. These factors prime the cells to augment their responsiveness by increasing ligand number or affinity. These same substances facilitate transmigration of eosinophils through the endothelial cell barrier, but it is the

TABLE 17.4. *Secretory products of eosinophils*

Granule proteins	Lipid mediators
Major basic protein	Leukotriene B_4 (small amount)
Eosinophil peroxidase	Leukotriene C_4
Eosinophil cationic protein	Leukotriene C_5
Eosinophil-derived neurotoxin	5-HETE
β-Glucuronidase	5.15- and 8.15-diHETE
Acid phosphatase	5-oxo-15-hydroxy 6,8,11,13-ETE
Arylsulfatase B	Prostaglandins E_1 and E_2
	6-keto-prostaglandin F_1
Cytokines	Thomboxane B_2
IL-1	PAF
IL-3	Enzymes
IL-4	Elastase (questionable)
IL-5	Charcot-Leyden crystal protein
IL-6	Collagenase
IL-8	92-kd gelatinase
IL-10	Reactive oxygen intermediates
IL-16	Superoxide radical anion
GM-CSF	H_2O_2
RANTES	Hydroxy radicals
TNF-α	
TGF-α	
TGF-β_1	
MIP-1α	

HETE, hydroxyeicosatetraenoic acid; ETE, eicosatetraenoic acid; diHETE, dihydroxy-eicosatetraenoic acid; TNF, tumor necrosis factor; TGF, transforming growth factor; MIP, macrophage inflammatory protein; PAF, platelet-activating factor.

From Kita H, Gleich GJ. The eosinophil structure and functions. In: Kaplan AP, ed. *Allergy,* 2nd ed. Philadelphia: WB Saunders, 1997:153, with permission.

presence of chemotactic factors that stimulate cells to migrate into tissues, and some of them also enhance adhesion and migration through the endothelium. A partial list of these is given in Table 17.5. Both complement C3a and C5a are chemotactic for eosinophils, but C3a is more selective, because it does not stimulate neutrophil migration (461). Of the chemokines, eotaxins 1, 2, and 3 have the most restricted specificity (462–464) and act via the CCR3 chemokine receptor (465), which is also present on basophils and some T_H2 cells. Chemokines, MCP-3, MCP-4, and RANTES also act via CCR3 but interact with other chemokine receptors as well. They contribute significantly to eosinophil chemotaxis and vary with the particular disease process. Histamine has chemotactic and chemokinetic properties for eosinophils *in vitro,* with considerable selectivity (466), yet it is not a major eosinophilotactic agent *in vivo.* LTB_4 is chemotactic for both neutrophils and eosinophils, whereas LTD_4 is selectively chemotactic for eosinophils at physiologic concentrations (467), as are other lipoxygenase products such as the diHETES (468). PAF is another potent eosinophilotactic factor and, when injected into skin, elicits eosinophils if the recipient is atopic, but elicits neutrophils in nonatopic individuals (469). Of the CXC chemokines, IL-8 is chemotactic for primed eosinophils, but the aforementioned C-C chemokines appear to be most important (470).

TABLE 17.5. *Eosinophil chemoattractants*

Chemokines	Eotaxin
	Eotaxin 2
	Eotaxin 3
	MCP 2, MCP 3, MCP 4
	RANTES
	MIP 1 α
	IL-8
Cytokines	IL-16, IL-2
Primers	IL-3, IL-5, GM-CSF
Humoral mediators	PAF
	C5a
	C3a
	LTB_4
	LTD_4
	DiHETES
	Histamine

DiHETE, dihydroxy-eicosatetraenoic acid; GM-CSF, granulocyte-macrophage colony-stimulating factor; IL, interleukin; LTD_4, leukotriene D_4; MCP, monocyte chemoattractant protein; MIP, macrophage inhibitory protein; PAF, platelet-activating factor; RANTES, regulated upon activation normal T cell expressed and secreted.

Although IL-5, IL-3, and GM-CSF (particularly IL-5) are critical for eosinophil migration, none, including IL-5, is a potent chemotactic factor when tested *in vitro.* It is the maturation of eosinophils, mobilization from bone marrow, priming of eosinophils to render them more responsive to other chemotactic factors, and antiapoptotic effects that are most critical. IL-5 therefore appears to be require for tissue eosinophil accumulation to occur, even though its chemotactic activity is weak and eosinophils are the only peripheral blood cells with IL-5 receptors. At the endothelial cell level, ICAM-1 is activated by IL-1 and TNF-α, whereas IL-4 and IL-13 stimulate VCAM-1 (471).

Activation of Eosinophils

There is a large body of literature regarding the generation of "hypodense" eosinophils, previously thought to represent an activated phenotype. However, these cells appear to represent a primed or partially activated cell, released from the bone marrow prematurely. On the other hand, activated eosinophils are not necessarily hypodense. CD69 represents an early activation antigen, and HLA-DR, as well as receptors such as CD11b and CD11c, are upregulated, while L-selectin is down-regulated. Eosinophils stimulated with C5a or PAF do not produce LTC_4, but they will do so if pretreated with IL-5, IL-3, or GM-CSF. This is a classic example of priming leading to a partially activated state. IL-5 stimulates integrin-dependent adhesion of eosinophils to fibronectin or laminin, and stimulates superoxide generation, phagocytosis, and IgG-dependent degranulation. It activates a variety of kinases such as JaK-2, lyn, Ras, Raf-1, and MAP kinases, as well as induction of the DNA-binding complex containing STAT-1 protein (472–474).

A striking feature of eosinophil-rich tissues is the deposition of granule proteins. This can result from three different processes, namely, cell injury, regulated secretion, or piecemeal degranulation. Cell injury is associated with plasma membrane and organelle membrane damage, and chromatolysis of nuclei. "Regulated secretion" is associated with fusion of individual granule membranes with the plasma membrane at the cell periphery with extrusion of specific granule matrix and core elements through degranulation pores. Piecemeal degranulation is characterized by vesicular transport of granule constituents with partially empty granule chambers in the cytoplasm. The role of each of these in particular disease states is not well understood, and all may, to some degree, be present. Their distinctive regulation or signal transduction mechanisms are not well delineated. When secretion does occur, however, there is not a burst reaction, as is seen with mast cells or basophils (halftime about 30 seconds to 3 minutes, depending on the stimulus) but a gradual release of constituents starting a few minutes after the stimulus and continuing for 1 to 2 hours. Many of the stimulants for cell activation and chemotaxis also lead to degranulation. Eosinophils will degranulate when exposed to IL-5 but need to be cultured with this cytokine for 4 days, whereas GM-CSF includes degranulation after several hours. Opsonized particles (coated with immunoglobulin and complement) cause degranulation, as do mediators such as PAF, if the cells are adherent to a matrix with engagement of receptors such as MAC-1. The C-C chemokines, such as RANTES and eotaxins, cause degranulation of primed cells with maximal release *in vitro* in 1 to 2 hours (475,476).

Eosinophils and Rheumatic Disease

Eosinophilic infiltration of tissues or an elevated blood eosinophil count may occasionally be seen in many rheumatic diseases, but it is most characteristic of Churg-Strauss syndrome (allergic angiitis and granulomatosis) (see Chapter 88). A necrotizing vasculitis involving small arteries and venules is seen associated with small necrotizing granulomas composed of a central eosinophilic core surrounded radially by macrophages and epitheloid giant cells. Eosinophils predominate early in the course, neutrophils and lymphocytes are present in varying but smaller numbers, and macrophages and giant cells predominate in more chronic lesions. There may be a prodrome with an allergic background of rhinitis and asthma, followed by tissue infiltration (e.g., eosinophilic pneumonitis, or Loffler syndrome) or gastroenteritis, and then vasculitis. The chemotactic factors mediating this accumulation of eosinophils are not clear, but because the subjects are atopic, chemokines such as RANTES, eotaxin 1, 2, or 3, or MCP-3 or -4 may be operative. Any vasculitis with complement activation and liberation of C5a and C3a can lead to accumulation of neutrophils, eosinophils, and monocytes; neutrophils typically predominate, reflecting the blood differential. Eosinophilic fasciitis and eosinophilic-myalgia syndrome, associated with contaminated L-tryptophan, are other predominantly eosinophilic disorders. In selected cases, however, eosinophilia may be associated with RA and Sjögren's syndrome.

REFERENCES

1. Galli J, Maurer M, Lantz CS. Mast cells as sentinels of innate immunity. *Curr Opin Immunol* 1999;11:53–59.
2. Boyce JA. Mast cells: beyond IgE. *J Allergy Clin Immunol* 2003;111:1–15.
3. Mekori YA, Metcalfe DD. Mast cells in innate immunity. *Immunol Rev* 2000;173:131–140.
4. Malone DA, Irani AM, Schwartz LB, et al. Mast cell numbers and histamine levels in synovial fluids from patients with diverse arthritides. *Arthritis Rheum* 1986;29:956–963.
5. Buckley MG, Walters C, Wong WM, et al. Mast cell activation in arthritis: detection of alpha- and beta-tryptase, histamine and eosinophil cationic protein in synovial fluid. *Clin Sci* 1997;93:363–370.
6. Claman HN. On scleroderma: mast cells, endothelial cells, and fibroblasts. *JAMA* 1989;262:1206–1209.
7. Tetlow LC, Woolley DE. Distribution, activation and tryptase/chymase phenotype of mast cells in the rheumatoid lesion. *Ann Rheum Dis* 1995;54:549–555.
8. DePaulis A, Marino I, Ciccarelle A, et al. Human synovial mast cells: ultrastructural *in situ* and *in vitro* immunologic characterization. *Arthritis Rheum* 1996;39:1222–1233.
9. Dabbous MK, Walker R, Haney L, et al. Mast cells and matrix degradation at sites of tumor invasion in rat mammary adenocarcinoma. *Br J Cancer* 1986;54:459–465.
10. Bromley M, Fischer WD, Woolley DE. Mast cells at the site of cartilage erosion in the rheumatoid joint. *Ann Rheum Dis* 1984;43:76–79.
11. Atkins FM, Clark RAF. Mast cells and fibrosis. *Arch Dermatol* 1987;123:191–193.

12. Galli SJ. New concepts about the mast cell. *N Engl J Med* 1993;328: 257–265.
13. Osborn L. Leukocyte adhesion to endothelium in inflammation. *Cell* 1990;62:3–6.
14. Kyan-Aung U, Haskard DO, Poston RN, et al. Endothelial leukocyte adhesion molecule-1 mediate the adhesion of eosinophils to endothelial cells *in vitro* and are expressed by endothelium in allergic cutaneous inflammation *in vivo*. *J Immunol* 1991;146:521–528.
15. Klein LM, Lavker RM, Matis WL, et al. Degranulation of human mast cells induces an endothelial antigen central to leukocyte adhesion. *Proc Natl Acad Sci U S A* 1989;86:8972–8976.
16. Meng H, Tonnesen MG, Marchese MJ, et al. Mast cells are potent regulators of endothelial cell adhesion molecule ICAM-1 and VCAM-1 expression. *J Cell Physiol* 1995;165:40–53.
17. Brown SJ, Galli SJ, Gleich GJ, et al. Ablation of immunity to Amblyomma americanum by anti-basophil serum: cooperation between basophils and eosinophils in expression of immunity to extoparasites (ticks) in guinea pigs. *J Immunol* 1982;129:790–796.
18. Malaviya R, Ross E, Jakschik BA, et al. Mast cell degranulation induced by type 1 fimbriated *Escherichia coli* in mice. *J Clin Invest* 1994;93:1645–1653.
19. Wershil BK, Theodos CM, Stephen JG, et al. Mast cells augment lesion size and persistence during experimental Leishmania major infection in the mouse. *J Immunol* 1994;152:4563–4570.
20. Supajatura J, Ushio H, Nakao A, et al. Differential responses of mast cell Toll-like receptors 2 and 4 in allergy and innate immunity. *J Clin Invest* 2002;109:1351–1359.
21. Gommerman JL, Oh DY, Zhou X, et al. A role for CD21/CD35 and CD19 in responses to acute septic peritonitis: a potential mechanism for mast cell activation. *J Immunol* 200;165:6915–6921.
22. Supajatura V, Ushio H, Nakao A, et al. Protective roles of mast cells against enterobacterial infection are mediated by Toll-like receptor 4. *J Immunol* 2001;167:2250–2256.
23. Gruber BL. Mast cells: accessory cells which potentiate fibrosis. *Intern Rev Immunol* 1995;12:259–279.
24. Gruber BL, Marchese MJ, Suzuki K, et al. Synovial procollagenase activation by human mast cell tryptase dependence upon matrix metalloproteinase 3 activation. *J Clin Invest* 1989;84:1657–1662.
25. Fang K, Raymond W, Blount J, et al. Dog mast cell alpha-chymase activates progelatinase B by cleaving the Phe88-Gin89 and Phe91-Glu92 bonds of the catalytic domain. *J Biol Chem* 1997;1997:25628–25635.
26. Grutzkau A, Kruger-Krasagakes S, Baumeister H, et al. Synthesis, storage, and release of vascular endothelial growth factor/vascular permeability factor (VEGF/VPF) by human mast cells: implications for the biological significance of VEGF-206. *Mol Biol Cell* 1998;9: 875–884.
27. Kanbe N, Kurosawa M, Nagata H, et al. Cord blood-derived human cultured mast cells produce transforming growth factor β. *Clin Exp Allergy* 1999;29:105–113.
28. Coussens LM, Raymond WW, Bergers G, et al. Inflammatory mast cells up-regulate angiogenesis during squamous epithelial carcinogenesis. *Genes Dev* 1999;13:1382–1397.
29. Dimlich RVW, Meineke HA, Reilly FD, et al. The fluorescent staining of heparin in mast cells using berberine sulfate: compatibility with paraformaldehyde or *o*-pthalaldehyde induced fluorescence and metachromasia. *Stain Technol* 1980;55:217–223.
30. Enerbäck L. Berberine sulfate binding to mast cell polyanions: a cytofluorometric method for the quantitation of heparin. *Histochemistry* 1974;42:301–313.
31. Bergstresser PR, Tigelaar, RE, Tharp MD. Conjugated avidin identifies cutaneous rodent and human mast cells. *J Invest Dermatol* 1984; 83:214–218.
32. Valent P, Majdic O, Maurer D, et al. Further characterization of surface membrane structures expressed on human basophils and mast cells. *Int Arch Allergy Appl Immunol* 1990;91:198–203.
33. Schwartz LB. Monoclonal antibodies against human mast cell tryptase demonstrate shared antigenic sites on subunits of tryptase and selective localization of the enzyme to mast cells. *J Immunol* 1985;134: 526–531.
34. Claman HN. Mast cell depletion in murine chronic graft-versus-host disease. *J Invest Dermatol* 1985;84:246–248.
35. Dvorak AM. New aspects of mast cell biology. *Int Arch Allerg Immunol* 1997;114:1–9.
36. Galli SJ, Dvorak AM, Dvorak HF. Basophils and mast cells: morphologic insights into their biology, secretory patterns and function. *Prog Allergy* 1984;34:1–141.
37. Dvorak AM, Galli SJ, Schulman L, et al. Basophil and mast cell degranulation ultrastructural analysis of mechanisms of mediator release. *Fed Proc* 1983;42:2510–2515.
38. Craig SS, Schechter NM, Schwartz LB. Ultrastructural analysis of maturing human T and TC mast cells *in situ*. *Lab Invest* 1989;60:147.
39. Kaminer MS, Lavker RM, Walsh RM, et al. Extracellular localization of human connective tissue mast cell granule contents. *J Invest Dermatol* 1991;96:857–863.
40. Dvorak AM. *Basophil and mast cell degranulation and recovery*. New York: Plenum, 1991.
41. Valent P, Spanblochl E, Sperr WR, et al. Induction of differentiation of human mast cells from bone marrow and peripheral blood mononuclear cells by recombinant human stem cell factor/*kit*-ligand in long-term culture. *Blood* 1992;80:2237–2245.
42. Denburg JA. Basophil and mast cell lineages *in-vitro* and *in-vivo*. *Blood* 1992;79:846–860.
43. Fodinger M, Fritsch G, Winkler K, et al. Origin of human mast cells: development from the transplanted hematopoietic stem cells after allogenic bone marrow transplantation. *Blood* 1994;84:2954–2959.
44. Dvorak AM, Newball HH, Dvorak HF. Degranulation of basophilic leukocytes in allergic contact dermatitis reactions in man. *J Immunol* 1976;116:687–695.
45. Bochner BS, Peachell PT, Brown KE, et al. Adherence of human basophils to cultured umbilical vein endothelial cells. *J Clin Invest* 1988; 81:1355–1364.
46. Weller PF, Rand TH, Goelz SE, et al. Human eosinophil adherence to vascular endothelium mediated by binding to vascular cell adhesion molecule 1 and endothelial leukocyte adhesion molecule 1. *Proc Natl Acad Sci U S A* 1991;88:7430–7433.
47. Bochner BS, Luscinskas FW, Gimbrone MA Jr, et al. Adhesion of human basophils, eosinophils, and neutrophils to IL-1 activated human vascular endothelial cells: contributions of endothelial cell adhesion molecules. *J Exp Med* 1991;173:1553–1557.
48. Leung YM, Pober JS, Cotran RS. Expression of endothelial-leukocyte adhesion molecule-1 in elicited late phase allergic reactions. *J Clin Invest* 1991;87:1805–1809.
49. Meng H, Marchese MJ, Garlick JA, et al. Mast cells induce T-cell adhesion to human fibroblasts by regulating ICAM-1 and VCAM-1 expression. *J Invest Dermatol* 1995;105:789–796.
50. Gordon JR, Galli SJ. Promotion of mouse fibroblast collagen gene expression by mast cells stimulated via the FcεRI. Role for mast cell–derived transforming growth factor-β and tumor necrosis factor-α. *J Exp Med* 1994;180:2027–2037.
51. Gruber BL, Kew RR, Jelaska A, et al. Human mast cells activate fibroblasts: tryptase is a fibrogenic factor stimulating collagen messenger ribonucleic acid synthesis and fibroblast chemotaxis. *J Immunol* 1997;158:2310–2317.
52. Gailit J, Marchese MJ, Kew RR, et al. Mast cells stimulate fibroblast transformation to a myofibroblast morphology and functional state. *J Invest Dermatol* 2001;117:1113–1119.
53. Gruber BL. Mast cells in the pathogenesis of fibrosis. *Curr Rheum Rep* 2003;5:147–153.
54. Agis H, Wilheim M, Sperr WR, et al. Monocytes do not make mast cells when cultured in the presence of SCF. Characterization of the circulating mast cell progenitor as a c-*kit*+, CD34+, Ly−, CD14−, CD17−, colony forming cell. *J Immunol* 1993;15:4221–4227.
55. Kirshenbaum AS, Goff JP, Semere T, et al. Demonstration that mast cells arise from a progenitor cell population that is CD34+, c-*kit*+, and expresses aminopeptidase N (CD-13). *Blood* 1999;94:2333–2342.
56. Kirshenbaum AS, Kessler SW, Goff JP, et al. Demonstration of the origin of human mast cells from CD34+ bone marrow progenitor cells. *J Immunol* 1991;146:1410–1415.
57. Galli SJ, Tsai M, Wershil BK. The c-*kit* receptor, stem cell factor, and mast cells. What each is teaching us about the others. *Am J Pathol* 1993;142:965–974.
58. Rottem M, Okada T, Goff JP, et al. Mast cells cultured from the peripheral blood of normal donors and patients with mastocytosis originate from a CD34/FcRI− cell population. *Blood* 1994;84:2489–2496.
59. Kempuraj D, Saito H, Kaneko A, et al. Characterization of mast cell–committed progenitors present in human umbilical cord blood. *Blood* 1999;93:3338–3346.

60. Galli SJ. New insights into "The riddle of the mast cells": microenvironmental regulation of mast cell development and phenotypic heterogeneity. *Lab Invest* 1990;62:5–33.
61. Greenberg G, Burnstock G. A novel cell-to-cell interaction between mast cells and other cell types. *Exp Cell Res* 1983;147:1–13.
62. Baraniuk JN, Kowalski ML, Kaliner MA. Relationships between permeable vessels, nerves, and mast cells in rat cutaneous neurogenic inflammation. *J Appl Physiol* 1990;68:2305–2311.
63. Heard BE, Dewar A, Corrin B. Apposition of fibroblasts to mast cells and lymphocytes in normal human lung and in cryptogenic fibrosing alveolitis—ultrastructure and cell perimeter measurements. *J Pathol* 1992;166:303–310.
64. Smith T, Weis J. Mucosal T cells and mast cells share common adhesion receptors. *Immunol Today* 1996;17:60–64.
65. Guo CB, Kageysobotka A, Lichtenstein LM, et al. Immunophenotyping and functional analysis of purified human uterine mast cells. *Blood* 1992;79:708–712.
66. Shimizu Y, Irani A, Brown E, et al. Human mast cells derived from fetal liver cells cultured with stem cell factor express a functional CD51/CD61 (avB3) integrin. *Blood* 1995;86:930–939.
67. Dastych J, Costa JJ, Thompson HL, et al. Mast cell adhesion to fibronectin. *Immunology* 1991;73:478–484.
68. Thompson HL, Burbelo PD, Yamada Y, et al. Mast cells chemotax to laminin with enhancement after IgE-mediated activation. *J Immunol* 1989;143:4188–4192.
69. Thompson HL, Burbelo PD, Metcalfe DD. Regulation of adhesion of mouse bone-marrow derived mast cells to laminin. *J Immunol* 1990; 145:3425–3431.
70. Thompson HL, Burbelo PD, Yamada Y, et al. Mast cells synthesize basement membrane components: a potential role in early fibrosis. *Clin Res* 1990;38:448A.
71. Weiss RR, Whitaker-Menezes D, Longley J, et al. Human dermal endothelial cells express membrane-associated mast cell growth factor. *J Invest Dermatol* 1995;104:101–106.
72. Deaglio S, Morra M, Mallone R, et al. Human CD38 (ADP-ribosyl cyclase) is a counter-receptor of CD31, an Ig superfamily member. *J Immunol* 1998;160:395–401.
73. Ducharme LA, Weis JH. Modulation of integrin expression during mast cell differentiation. *Eur J Immunol* 1992;22:2603–2607.
74. Gurish MF, Bell AM, Smith TJ, et al. Expression of murine β_7, α_4 and β_1 integrin genes by rodent mast cells. *J Immunol* 1992;149:1964–1972.
75. Berlin C, Berg EL, Briskin MJ, et al. $\alpha_4\beta_7$ integrin mediates lymphocyte binding to the mucosal vascular addressin MAdCAM-1. *Cell* 1993;74:185–195.
76. Gurish MF, Tao H, Abonia JP, et al. Intestinal mast cell progenitors require CD49 $\delta\beta_7(\alpha_4\beta_7$ integrin) for tissue specific homing. *J Exp Med* 2001;194:1243–1252.
77. Weber S, Babina M, Feller G, et al. Human leukemic (HMC-1) and normal mast cells express beta 2-integrins: characterization of beta 2-integrins and ICAM-1 on HMC-1 cells. *Scand J Immunol* 1997;45:471–481.
78. Metcalfe DD, Costa JJ, Burd PR. Mast cells and basophils. In: Goldstein JIG, Goldstein IM, eds. *Inflammation: basic principles and clinical correlates.* New York: Raven, 1992:709–725.
79. Hamawy MM, Mergenhagen SE, Siraganian RP. Adhesion molecules as regulators of mast cell and basophil function. *Immunol Today* 1994; 15:62–66.
80. Weber S, Ruh B, Dippel E, et al. Monoclonal antibodies to leucosialin (CD43) induce homotypic aggregation of the human mast cell line HMC-1: characterization of leucosialin on HMC-1 cells. *Immunology* 1994;82:638–644.
81. Metcalfe D, Baram D, Mekori Y. Mast cells. *Physiol Rev* 1997;77: 1033–1079.
82. Okayama Y, Kirshenbaum AS, Metcalfe DD. Expression of a functional high-affinity IgG receptor, Fc gamma RI, on human mast cells: regulation of IFN-gamma. *J Immunol* 2000;164:4332–4339.
83. Tkaczyk C, Okayama Y, Woolhiser M, et al. Activation of human mast cells through the high affinity IgG receptor. *Mol Immunol* 2002;38: 1289–1294.
84. Nilsson G, Forsberg-Nilsson K, Xiang Z. Human mast cells express functional TrkA and are a source of nerve growth factor. *Eur J Immunol* 1997;27:2295–2301.
85. Hartmann K, Wagelie-Steffen A, von Stebut E, et al. Fas (CD95, APO-1) antigen expression and function in murine mast cells. *J Immunol* 1997; 159:4006–4014.
86. Gruber BL, Marchese MJ, Kew R. Transforming growth factor-β1 mediates chemotaxis of mast cells. *J Immunol* 1994;152:5860–5867.
87. Yano K, Nakao K, Sayama K, et al. The HMC-1 human mast cell line expresses the hepatocyte growth factor receptor c-*met*. *Biochem Biophys Res Commun* 1997;239:740–745.
88. Meininger CJ, Yano H, Rottapel R, et al. The c-*kit* receptor ligand functions as a mast cell chemoattractant. *Blood* 1992;79:958–963.
89. Nilsson G, Butterfield JH, Nilsson K, et al. Stem cell factor is a chemotactic factor for human mast cells. *J Immunol* 1994;153:3717–3723.
90. Matsuura N, Zetter BR. Stimulation of mast cell chemotaxis by interleukin 3. *J Exp Med* 1989;170:1421–1425.
91. Gruber BL, Marchese MJ, Kew RR. Angiogenic factors stimulate mast cell migration. *Blood* 1995;86:2488–2493.
92. Lippert U, Artuc M, Grutzkau A, et al. Expression and functional activity of the IL-8 receptor type CXCR1 and CXCR2 on human mast cells. *J Immunol* 1998;161:2600–2608.
93. Taub D, Dastych J, Inamura N, et al. Bone marrow-derived murine mast cells migrate, but do not degranulate, in response to chemokines. *J Immunol* 1995;154:2393–2402.
94. Adachi S, Ebi Y, Nishikawa SI, et al. Necessity of extracellular domain of W(c-*kit*) receptors for attachment of murine cultured mast cells to fibroblasts. *Blood* 1992;79:650–656.
95. Trautmann A, Feuerstein B, Ernst N, et al. Heterotypic cell-cell adhesion of human mast cells to fibroblasts. *Arch Dermatol Res* 1997; 289:194–203.
96. Lorentz A, Schuppan D, Gebert A, et al. Regulatory effects of stem cell factor and interleukin-4 on adhesion of human mast cells to extracellular matrix proteins. *Blood* 2002;99:966–972.
97. Rennick D, Lee FD, Yokota T, et al. A cloned MCGF cDNA encodes a multilineage hematopoietic growth-factor: multiple activities of interleukin 3. *J Immunol* 1985;134:910–914.
98. Ihle JN, Keller J, Oroszlan S, et al. Biological properties of homogeneous interleukin 3. I. Demonstration of WEHI-3 growth-factor activity, mast cell growth-factor activity, P cell-stimulating factor activity and histamine-producing factor activity. *J Immunol* 1983;131: 282–287.
99. Li L, Zhang X, Krilis SA. Factors that affect human mast cell and basophil growth. In: Razin E, Rivera J, eds. *Signal transduction in mast cells and basophils.* New York: Springer-Verlag, 1999:54–65.
100. Horigome K, Bullock ED, Johnson EM. Effects of nerve growth factor on rat peritoneal mast cells. *J Biol Chem* 1994;269:2695–2702.
101. Yee NS, Paek I, Besmer P. Role of *kit*-ligand in proliferation and suppression of apoptosis in mast cells: basis for radiosensitivity of white spotting and steel mutant mice. *J Exp Med* 1994;179:1777–1787.
102. Kirshenbaum AS, Goff JP, Kessler SW, et al. Effect of IL-3 and stem cell factor on the appearance of human basophils and mast cells from CD34+ pluripotent progenitor cells. *J Immunol* 1992;148:772–777.
103. Swieter M, Mergenhagen SE, Siraganian RP. Microenvironmental factors that influence mast cell phenotype and function. *Proc Soc Exp Biol Med* 1992;199:22–33.
104. Mekori YA, Harmann K, Metcalfe DD. Mast cell apoptosis. In: Razin E, Rivera J, eds. *Signal transduction in mast cells and basophils.* New York: Springer-Verlag, 1999:85–96.
105. Davidson S, Mansour A, Gallily R, et al. Mast cell differentiation depends on T cells and granule synthesis on fibroblasts. *J Immunol* 1983;48:439–452.
106. Levi-Schaffer F, Austen KF, Gravallese PM, et al. Coculture of interleukin 3-dependent mouse mast cells with fibroblasts results in a phenotypic change of the mast cells. *Proc Natl Acad Sci U S A* 1986; 83:6485–6488.
107. Levi-Schaffer F, Austen KF, Caulfield JP, et al. Fibroblasts maintain the phenotype and viability of the rat heparin-containing mast cell *in vitro*. *J Immunol* 1985;135:3454–3461.
108. Furitsu T, Saito H, Dvorak AM, et al. Development of human mast cells in vitro. *Proc Natl Acad Sci U S A* 1989;86:10039–10043.
109. Irani AA, Craig SS, Nilsson G, et al. Characterization of human mast cells developed *in vitro* from fetal liver cells cocultured with murine 3T3 fibroblasts. *Immunology* 1992;77:136–143.
110. Irani AM, Nilsson G, Miettinen U, et al. Recombinant human stem cell factor stimulates differentiation of mast cells from dispersed human fetal liver cells. *Blood* 1992;80:3009–3021.
111. Li L, Macpherson JJ, Adelstein S, et al. Conditioned media from a cell strain derived from a patient with mastocytosis induces preferential development of cells that possess high affinity IgE receptors and

the granule protease phenotype of mature cutaneous mast cells. *J Biol Chem* 1995;270:2258–2263.
112. Butterfield JH, Weiler D, Dewald G, et al. Establishment of an immature mast cell line from a patient with mast cell leukemia. *Leukoc Res* 1988;12:345–355.
113. Kanakura Y, Furitsu T, Tsujimura T, et al. Activating mutations of the c-*kit* proto-oncogene in a human mast cell leukemia cell line. *Leukemia* 1994;8(suppl):18–22.
114. Galli SJ. New approaches for the analysis of mast cell maturation, heterogeneity, and function. *Fed Proc* 1987;46:1906–1914.
115. Huizinga H, Thuneberg L, Kluppel M, et al. *W/Kit* gene required for interstitial cells of Cajal and for intestinal pacemaker activity. *Nature (Lond)* 1995;373:347–349.
116. Chabot B, Stephenson DA, Chapman VM, et al. The protooncogene c-*kit* encoding a transmembrane tyrosine kinase receptor maps to the mouse W locus. *Nature* 1988;335:88–89.
117. Geissler EN, Ryan MA, Housman DE. The dominant-white spotting (W) locus of the mouse encodes the c-*kit* proto-oncogene. *Cell* 1988; 55:185–192.
118. Galli SJ, Zsebo KM, Geissler EN. The *kit* ligand, stem cell factor. *Adv Immunol* 1994;55:1–96.
119. Witte ON. Steel locus defines new multipotent growth factor: minireview. *Cell* 1990;63:5–6.
120. Broudy VC. Stem cell factor and hematopoiesis. *Blood* 1997;90: 1345–1364.
121. Tsai M, Takeishi T, Thompson H, et al. Induction of mast cell proliferation, maturation, and heparin synthesis by the rat c-*kit* ligand, stem cell factor. *Proc Natl Acad Sci U S A* 1991;88:6382–6386.
122. Galli SJ, Zsebo KM, Geissler EN. The *kit* ligand, stem cell factor. *Adv Immunol* 1994;55:1–96.
123. Longley BJ, Tyrrell L, Ma Y, et al. Chymase cleavage of stem cell factor yields a bioactive, soluble product. *Proc Natl Acad Sci U S A* 1997;94:9017–9021.
124. Costa JJ, Demetri GD, Harrist TJ, et al. Recombinant human stem cell factor (*kit* ligand) promotes human mast cell and melanocyte hyperplasia and functional activation *in vivo*. *J Exp Med* 1996;183: 2681–2686.
125. Flanagan JG, Leder P. The *kit* ligand: a cell surface molecule altered in steel mutant fibroblasts. *Cell* 1990;63:185–194.
126. Aye MT, Hashemi S, Leclair B, et al. Expression of stem cell factor and c-*kit* messenger RNA in cultured endothelial cells, monocytes and cloned human bone marrow stromal cells (CFU-RF). *Exp Hematol* 1992;20:523–527.
127. Longley BJ, Tyrrell L, Zu SZ, et al. Somatic c-*kit* activating mutation in urticaria pigmentosa and aggressive mastocytosis: establishment of clonality in a human mast cell neoplasm. *Nat Genet* 1996;12: 312–314.
128. Longley BJ, Morganroth GS, Tyrrell L, et al. Altered metabolism of mast cell growth factor (c-*kit* ligand) in cutaneous mastocytosis. *N Engl J Med* 1993;328:1302–1307.
129. Hirota S, Nomura S, Asada H, et al. Possible involvement of c-*kit* receptor and its ligand in increase of mast cells in neurofibroma tissues. *Arch Pathol Lab Med* 1993;117:996–999.
130. Finotto S, Mekori YA, Metcalfe DD. Glucocorticoids decrease tissue mast cell number by reducing the production of the c-*kit* ligand, stem cell factor, by resident cells: *in vitro* and *in vivo* evidence in murine systems. *J Clin Invest* 1997;99:1721–1728.
131. Welle M. Development, significance, and heterogeneity of mast cells with particular regard to the mast cell–specific proteases chymase and tryptase. *J Leukoc Biol* 1997;61:233–245.
132. Irani AM, Schechter NM, Craig SS, et al. Two types of human mast cells that have distinct neutral protease compositions. *Proc Natl Acad Sci U S A* 1986;83:4464–4468.
133. Schechter NM, Irani AM, Sprows JL, et al. Identification of a cathepsin G-like proteinase in the MCTC of human mast cell. *J Immunol* 1990;145:2652–2661.
134. Irani AM, Goldstein SM, Wintroub BU, et al. Human mast cell carboxypeptidase: selective localization to MCTC cells. *J Immunol* 1991;147:247–253.
135. Weidner N, Austen KF. Heterogeneity of mast cells at multiple body sites: fluorescent determination of avidin binding and immunofluorescent determination of chymase, tryptase, and carboxypeptidase content. *Pathol Res Pract* 1993;189:156–162.
136. Irani AMA, Craig SS, DeBlois G, et al. Deficiency of the tryptase-positive, chymase-negative mast cell type in gastrointestinal mucosa of patients with defective T lymphocyte function. *J Immunol* 1987; 138:4381–4386.
137. Irani AA, Gruber BL, Kaufman LD, et al. Mast cell changes in scleroderma. Presence of MCt cells in the skin and evidence of mast cell activation. *Arthritis Rheum* 1992;35:933–939.
138. Gruber BL. The mast cell in the pathogenesis of scleroderma. *Clin Dermatol* 1994;12:397–406.
139. Metzger H, Alcaraz G, Hohman RJ, et al. The receptor with high affinity for immunoglobulin E. *Annu Rev Immunol* 1986;4:419–470.
140. Prussin C, Metcalfe DD. The immune system. IgE, mast cells, basophils, and eosinophils. *J Allergy Clin Immunol* 2003;111:1–17.
141. Speigelberg HL. Structure and function of Fc receptors for IgE for lymphocytes, monocytes, and macrophages. *Adv Immunol* 1984;35: 61–88.
142. Verelli D. The regulation of IgE synthesis. *J Clin Allergy Immunol* 2002;16:179–196.
143. Gruber BL, Ballan D, Gorevic PD. IgE rheumatoid factors: quantification in synovial fluid and ability to induce synovial mast cell histamine release. *Clin Exp Immunol* 1988;71:289–294.
144. Gruber BL, Kaufman LD, Marchese M, et al. Anti-IgE autoantibodies in systemic lupus erythematosus: prevalence and functional significance. *Arthritis Rheum* 1988;31:1000–1006.
145. Hide M, Francis DM, Grattan CEH, et al. Autoantibodies against the high-affinity IgE receptor as a cause of histamine release in chronic urticaria. *N Engl J Med* 1993;328:1599–1604.
146. Holowka D, Baird B. Antigen-mediated IgE receptor aggregation and signaling: a window on cell surface structure and dynamics. *Annu Rev Biophys Biomol Struct* 1996;25:79–112.
147. Tkaczyk C, Gilfillan AM. FcεRI-dependent signaling pathways in human mast cells. *Clin Immunol* 2001;99:198–210.
148. Ott VL, Cambier JC. Molecular mechanisms in allergy and clinical immunology. Activating and inhibitory signaling in mast cells: new opportunities for therapeutic intervention? *J Allergy Clin Immunol* 2000;106:1–16.
149. Ishizaka T, Ishizaka K. Triggering of histamine release from rat mast cells by divalent antibodies against IgE-receptors. *J Immunol* 1978; 120:800–805.
150. Kinet JP. The high-affinity IgE receptor (Fc epsilon RI): from physiology to pathology. *Ann Rev Immunol* 1999;17:931–972.
151. Siraganian RP. Signaling pathways that regulate effector function: perspectives. In: Razin E, Rivera J, eds. *Signal transduction in mast cells and basophils.* New York: Springer-Verlag, 1999:181–190.
152. Cambier JC. Antigen and Fc receptor signaling. *J Immunol* 1995;15: 3281–3285.
153. Eisman E, Bolen JB. Engagement of the high affinity IgE receptor activates src protein-related tyrosine kinases. *Nature (Lond)* 1992; 355:78–80.
154. Suzuki H, Takei M, Yanagida M, et al. Early and late events in FcεRI signal transduction in human cultured mast cells. *J Immunol* 1997; 159:5881–5888.
155. Lorentz A, Klopp I, Gebhardt T, et al. Role of activator protein 1, nuclear factor κ-B, and nuclear factor of activated T-cells in IgE-receptor-mediated cytokine expression in mature human mast cells. *J Allergy Clin Immunol* 2003;111:1–10.
156. Wilson BS, Barker SA, Graham TE, et al. Phosphoinositide-derived second messengers in FcεR1 signaling: PI-3 kinase products control membrane topography and the translocation and activation of PLC-γ1 in antigen-stimulated mast cells. In: Razin E, Rivera J, eds. *Signal transduction in mast cells and basophils.* New York: Springer-Verlag, 1999:191–206.
157. Barker SA, Lujan D, Wilson BS. Multiple roles for PI 3-kinase in the regulation of PLCγ activity and Ca^{2+} mobilization in antigen-stimulated mast cells. *J Leukoc Biol* 1999;65:321–329.
158. McCloskey MA. New perspectives on Ca^{2+} influx in mast cells. In: Razin E, Rivera J, eds. *Signal transduction in mast cells and basophils.* New York: Springer-Verlag, 1999:227–246.
159. Choi OH, Kim J-H, Kinet J-P. Calcium mobilization via sphingosine kinase in signalling by the FcεRI antigen receptor. *Nature (Lond)* 1996;380:634–636.
160. Beaven MA. Calcium signaling: sphingosine kinase versus phospholipase C? *Curr Biol* 1996;6:798–801.

161. Baumruker T, Prieschl EE. FcεRI-mediated activation of NF-AT. In: Razin E, Rivera J, eds. *Signal transduction in mast cells and basophils.* New York: Springer-Verlag, 1999:328–336.
162. Ishizuka T, Kawasome H, Terada N, et al. Stem cell factor augments FcεRI-mediated TNF-α production and stimulates MAP kinases via a different pathway in MC/9 mast cells. *J Immunol* 1998;161:3624–3630.
163. Razin E, Rivera J. *Signal transduction in mast cells and basophils.* New York: Springer-Verlag, 1999.
164. Cambier JC. Inhibitory receptors abound? *Proc Natl Acad Sci U S A* 1997;94:5993–5995.
165. Huber M, Helgason C, Damen J, et al. The src homology 2 containing inositol phosphatase (SHIP) is the gatekeeper of mast cell degranulation. *Proc Natl Acad Sci U S A* 1998;95:11330–11335.
166. Moriya K, Rivera J, Odom S, et al. ER-27319, an acridone-related compound, inhibits release of antigen-induced allergic mediators from mast cells by selective inhibition of Fc-epsilon receptor I-mediated activation of Syk. *Proc Natl Acad Sci U S A* 1997;94: 12539–12544.
167. White MV, Baer H, Kubota Y, et al. Neutrophils and mast cells: characterization of cells responsive to neutrophil-derived histamine-releasing activity (HRA-N). *J Allergy Clin Immunol* 1989;84:773–780.
168. MacDonald SM. Histamine releasing factors. In: Razin E, Rivera J, eds. *Signal transduction in mast cells and basophils.* New York: Springer-Verlag, 1999:390–401.
169. Liao T-N, Hsieh K-H. Characterization of histamine-releasing activity: role of cytokines and IgE heterogeneity. *J Clin Immunol* 1992;12: 248–258.
170. Kirai K, Yamaguchi M, Misaki Y, et al. Enhancement of human basophil histamine release in basophils triggered by interleukin 5. *J Exp Med* 1990;172:1525–1528.
171. Bischoff SC, Dahinden CA. 1992 c-*kit* ligand: a unique potential for mediator release by human lung mast cells. *J Exp Med* 1992;175: 237–244.
172. Columbo M, Horowitz EM, Botana LM, et al. The human recombinant c-*kit* receptor ligand, rhCSF, induces mediator release from human cutaneous mast cells and enhances IgE-dependent mediator release from both skin mast cells and peripheral blood basophils. *J Immunol* 1992;599–608.
173. Egger D, Gueenich S, Denzlinger C, et al. IL-4 renders mast cells functionally responsive to endothelin-1. *J Immunol* 1995;154:1830–1837.
174. Baeza ML, Reddigari SR, Kornfeld D, et al. Relationship of one form of human histamine releasing factor (HRF) to connective tissue activating peptide-III (CTAP-III). *J Clin Invest* 1990;85:1516–1521.
175. Hedrick JA, Zlotnik A. Chemokines and lymphocyte biology. *Curr Opin Immunol* 1996;8:343–347.
176. Kuna P, Reddigari SR, Rucinski D, et al. Monocyte chemotactic and activating factor is a potent histamine-releasing factor for human basophils. *J Exp Med* 1992;175:489–493.
177. Kuna P, Reddigari SR, Schall TJ, et al. RANTES, A monocyte and T lymphocyte chemotactic cytokine releases histamine from human basophils. *J Immunol* 1992;149:636–642.
178. Alam R, Forsythe PA, Stafford S, et al. Macrophage inflammatory protein Ia activates basophils and mast cells. *J Exp Med* 1992;176: 781–786.
179. Fureder W, Agis H, Semper H, et al. Differential response of human basophils and mast cells to recombinant chemokines. *Ann Hematol* 1995;70:251–258.
180. Johnson AR, Erdos EG. Release of histamine from mast cells by vasoactive peptides. *Proc Soc Exp Biol Med* 1973;142:1252–1256.
181. Rubinstein I, Nadel JA, Graf PD, et al. Mast cell chymase augments histamine-induced wheal formation in allergic dog skin. *FASEB J* 1990;4:A1939.
182. West GB. Thoughts on mast cells, histamine release and immunoglobulin E. *Int Arch Allergy Appl Immunol* 1985;78:221–223.
183. Lagunoff D, Chi EY, Wan H. Effects of chymotrypsin and trypsin on rat peritoneal mast cells. *Biochem Pharmacol* 1975;24:1573–1578.
184. Schulman ES, Post TP, Henson PM, et al. Differential effects of the complement peptides, C5a and C5a des arg on human basophil and lung mast cell histamine release. *J Immunol* 1988;81:918–923.
185. Wize J, Wojtecka-Lukasik E, Maslinski S. Collagen-derived peptides release mast cell histamine. *Agents Actions* 1986;18:262–265.
186. Inamura N, Mekori Y, Bhattacharyya S, et al. Induction and enhancement of FcεRI-dependent mast cell degranulation following coculture with activated T cells: dependency on ICAM-1- and leukocyte function-associated antigen (LFA)-1-mediated heterotypic aggregation. *J Immunol* 1998;160:4026–4033.
187. Bhattacharyya SP, Drucker I, Reshef T, et al. Activated T lymphocytes induce degranulation and cytokine production by human mast cells following cell-to-cell contact. *J Leukoc Biol* 1998;63:337–341.
188. Rumsaeng V, Cruikshank W, Foster B, et al. Human mast cells produce the CD4+ T lymphocyte chemoattractant factor, IL-16. *J Immunol* 1997;159:2904–2910.
189. Dvorak AM, Schulman ES, Peters SP, et al. Immunoglobulin E-mediated degranulation of isolated human lung mast cells. *Lab Invest* 1985;53:45–56.
190. Dvorak A, Costa J, Monahan-Earley R, et al. Ultrastructural analysis of human skin biopsy specimens from patients receiving recombinant human stem cell factor: subcutaneous injection of rhSCF induces dermal mast cell degranulation and granulocyte recruitment at the injection site. *J Allergy Clin Immunol* 1998;101:793–806.
191. MacGlashan DWJ, Schleimer RP, Peters SP, et al. Generation of leukotrienes by purified human lung mast cells. *J Clin Invest* 1982;70: 747–752.
192. Schwartz LB, Huff T. Biology of mast cells and basophils. In: Middleton EJ, ed. *Allergy: principles and practice.* St. Louis: CV Mosby, 1993:135–168.
193. Falanga V, Soter NA, Altman RD, et al. Elevated plasma histamine levels in systemic sclerosis (scleroderma). *Arch Dermatol* 1990;126: 336–338.
194. Haslam PL, Cromwell O, Dewar A, et al. Evidence of increased histamine levels in lung lavage fluids from patients with cryptogenic fibrosing alveolitis. *Clin Exp Immunol* 1981;44:587–591.
195. Casale TB, Trapp S, Zehr B, et al. Bronchoalveolar lavage fluid histamine levels in interstitial lung diseases. *Am Rev Respir Dis* 1988; 138:1604–1609.
196. Hakanson R, Owman C, Sjoberg NO, et al. Direct histochemistry demonstration of histamine in cutaneous mast cells. *Experientia* 1969;25:854–855.
197. Russell JD, Russell SB, Trupin KM. The effect of histamine on the growth of cultured fibroblasts isolated from normal and keloid tissue. *J Cell Physiol* 1977;93:389–393.
198. Hatamochi A, Ono M, Arakawa M, et al. Analysis of collagen gene expression by cultured fibroblasts in morphea. *Br J Dermatol* 1992; 126:216–221.
199. Kalenderian R, Gruber BL, Simon S, et al. Effects of histamine and heparin on human lung fibroblasts. *Am Rev Respir Dis* 1990;42: A499.
200. Zheng T, Nathanson M, Elias J. Histamine augments cytokine-stimulated IL-11 production by human lung fibroblasts. *J Immunol* 1994;153:4742.
201. Asako H, Kurose I, Wolf R, et al. Role of H1 receptors and P-selectin in histamine-induced leukocyte rolling and adhesion in postcapillary venules. *J Clin Invest* 1994;93:1508–1513.
202. Gaboury JP, Johnston B, Niu X-F, et al. Mechanisms underlying acute mast cell–induced leukocyte rolling and adhesion *in vivo. J Immunol* 1995;154:804–813.
203. Kubes P, Kanwar S. Histamine induces leukocyte rolling in post-capillary venules. *J Immunol* 1994;152:3570–3577.
204. Church MK, Lowman MA, Rees PH, et al. Plenary lecture. Mast cells, neuropeptides and inflammation. *Agents Actions* 1989;27:8–16.
205. Pinckard RN, McManus LM, Hanahan DJ. Chemistry and biology of acetylglyceryl ether phosphorylcholine (platelet activating factor). In: Weismann G, ed. *Advances in inflammation research.* Vol. 4. New York: Raven, 1982:147–160.
206. Archer CB, Page CP, Roubin R, et al. Inflammatory characteristics of platelet-activating factor (Paf-acether) in human skin. *Br J Dermatol* 1984;110:45–51.
207. Wong DTW, Donoff BR, Yang J, et al. Sequential expression of transforming growth factors alpha and beta1 by eosinophils during cutaneous wound healing in the hamster. *Am J Pathol* 1993;143:130–142.
208. Costa JJ, Matossian K, Resnick MB, et al. Human eosinophils can express the cytokines tumor necrosis factor-alpha and macrophage inflammatory protein-1 alpha. *J Clin Invest* 1993;91:2673–2684.

209. Warren JS, Mandel DM, Johnson KJ, et al. Evidence for the role of platelet-activating factor in immune complex vasculitis in the rat. *J Clin Invest* 1989;83:669–678.
210. Dennis EA. The growing phospholipase A_2 superfamily of signal transduction enzymes. *Trends Biochem Sci* 1997;2:1–2.
211. Heavy DJ, Ernst PB, Stevens RL, et al. Generation of leukotriene B_4, leukotriene C_4, and prostaglandin D_2 by immunologically activated rat intestinal mucosa mast cells. *J Immunol* 1988;140:1953–1957.
212. Reddy S, Herschman HR. Prostaglandin synthase-1 and prostaglandin synthase-2 are coupled to distinct phospholipases for their generation of prostaglandin D_2 in activated mast cells. *J Biol Chem* 1997; 272:3231–3237.
213. Roberts LJ, Sweetman BJ, Lewis RA, et al. Increased production of prostaglandin D_2 in patients with systemic mastocytosis. *N Engl J Med* 1980;303:1400–1404.
214. Brock TG, Paine IR, Peters-Golden M. Localization of 5-lipoxygenase to the nucleus of unstimulated rat basophilic leukemic cells. *J Biol Chem* 1994;269:361–368.
215. Henderson WR Jr, Tang LO, Chu SJ, et al. A role for cysteinyl leukotrienes in airway remodeling in a mouse asthma model. *Am J Respir Crit Care Med* 2002;165:108–116.
216. Atkins PC, Norman M, Weiner H, et al. Release of neutrophil chemotactic activity during immediate hypersensitivity reactions in humans. *Ann Intern Med* 1977;86:415–418.
217. Goetzl EJ, Austen KF. Purification and synthesis of eosinophilotactic tetrapeptides of human lung tissue: identification as eosinophil chemotactic factor of anaphylaxis (ECF-A). *Proc Natl Acad Sci U S A* 1975;72:4123–4127.
218. Moller A, Lippert D, Lessman D, et al. Human mast cells produce IL-8. *J Immunol* 1993;151:3261–3266.
219. Schwartz LB, Lewis RA, Seldin D, et al. Acid hydrolases and tryptase from secretory granules of dispersed human lung mast cells. *J Immunol* 1981;126:1290–1294.
220. Schwartz LB, Lewis RA, Austen KF. Tryptase from human pulmonary mast cells: purification and characterization. *J Biol Chem* 1981; 256:11939–11943.
221. Schwartz LB, Bradford TR. Regulation of tryptase from human lung mast cells by heparin: stabilization of the active tetramer. *J Biol Chem* 1986;261:7372–7379.
222. Schwartz LB. Tryptase: a clinical indicator of mast cell–dependent events. *Allergy Proc* 1994;15:119–123.
223. Hogan AD, Schwartz LB. Markers of mast cell degranulation. *Methods* 1997;13:43–52.
224. Miller JS, Westin EH, Schwartz LB. Cloning and characterization of complementary DNA for human tryptase. *J Clin Invest* 1989;84: 1188–1195.
225. Miller JS, Moxley G, Schwartz LB. Cloning and characterization of a second complementary DNA for human tryptase. *J Clin Invest* 1990; 86:864–870.
226. Vanderslice P, Ballinger SM, Tam EK, et al. Human mast cell tryptase—multiple cDNAs and genes reveal a multigene serine protease family. *Proc Nat Acad Sci U S A* 1990;87:3811–3815.
227. Huang C, Li L, Krilis SA, et al. Human tryptases α and β/II are functionally distinct due, in part, to a single amino acid difference in one of the surface loops that form the substrate-binding cleft. *J Biol Chem* 1999;274:19670–19676.
228. Abraham WM. Tryptase: a potential role in airway inflammation and remodeling. *Am J Physiol Lung Cell Mol Physiol* 2002;24:158–161.
229. Smith TJ, Houghland MW, Johnson DA. Human lung tryptase, purification and characterization. *J Biol Chem* 1984;259:11046–11051.
230. Schwartz LB, Bradford TR, Rouse C, et al. Development of a new, more sensitive immunoassay for human tryptase: use in systemic anaphylaxis. *J Clin Immunol* 1994;14:190–204.
231. Platt MS, Yunginger JW, Sekulat-Perlman A, et al. Involvement of mast cells in sudden infant death syndrome. *J Allergy Clin Immunol* 1994;94:250–256.
232. Alter SC, Kramps JA, Janoff A, et al. Interactions of human mast cell tryptase with biological protease inhibitors. *Arch Biochem Biophys* 1990;276:26–31.
233. Schwartz LB. Mast cells: function and contents. *Curr Opin Immunol* 1994;6:91–97.
234. Stack MS, Johnson DA. Human mast cell tryptase activates single-chain urinary-type plasminogen activator (pro-urokinase). *J Biol Chem* 1994;269:9416–9419.
235. Caughey GH, Leidig F, Viro NF, et al. Substance P and vasoactive intestinal peptide degradation by mast cell tryptase and chymase. *J Pharmacol Exp Ther* 1988;244:133–137.
236. Walls AF, Brain SD, Desai A, et al. Human mast cell tryptase attenuates the vasodilator activity of calcitonin gene-related peptide. *Biochem Pharmacol* 1992;43:1243–1248.
237. Ruoss SJ, Hartmann T, Caughey GH. Mast cell tryptase is a mitogen for cultured fibroblasts. *J Clin Invest* 1991;88: 493–499.
238. Hartmann T, Ruoss SJ, Raymond WW, et al. Human tryptase as a potent, cell-specific mitogen: role of signaling pathways in synergistic responses. *Am J Physiol* 1992;262:L528–L534.
239. Levi-Schaeffer F, Piliponsky AM. Tryptase, a novel link between allergic inflammation and fibrosis. *Trends Immunol* 2003;24:158–161.
240. Blair RJ, Meng H, Marchese MJ, et al. Human mast cells stimulate vascular tube formation: tryptase is a novel, potent angiogenic factor. *J Clin Invest* 1997;99:2691–2700.
241. Cairns JA, Walls AF. Mast cell tryptase stimulates the synthesis of type I collagen in human lung fibroblasts. *J Clin Invest* 1997;99: 1313–1321.
242. Cairns JA, Walls AF. Mast cell tryptase is a mitogen for epithelial cells: stimulation of IL-8 production and intercellular adhesion molecule-1 expression. *J Immunol* 1996;156:275–283.
243. Dery O, Corvera CU, Steinhoff M, et al. Proteinase-activated receptors: novel mechanisms of signaling by serine proteases. *Am J Physiol* 1998;274:C1429–C1452.
244. Schechter NM, Brass LF, Lavker RM, et al. Reaction of mast cell proteases tryptase and chymase with protease activated receptors (PARs) on keratinocytes and fibroblasts. *J Cell Physiol* 1998;176:365–373.
245. Corvera C, Dery O, McConalogue K, et al. Mast cell tryptase regulates rat colonic myocytes through proteinase-activated receptor 2. *J Clin Invest* 1997;100:1383–1393.
246. Mirza H, Schmidt VA, Derian SK, et al. Mitogenic responses mediated through the proteinase-activated receptor-2 are induced by expressed forms of mast cell alpha- or beta-tryptases. *Blood* 1997;90: 3914–3922.
247. Molino M, Barnathan DS, Numerof R, et al. Interactions of mast cell tryptase with thrombin receptors and PAR-2. *J Biol Chem* 1997;272: 4043–4049.
248. Lan RS, et al. Role of protease-activated receptors in airway function: a target for therapeutic intervention? *Pharmacol Ther* 2002;95: 239–257.
249. Frungieri MB, et al. Proliferative action of mast cell tryptase is mediated by PAR-2, COX2, prostaglandins and PPARγ: possible relevance to human fibrotic disorders. *Proc Natl Acad Sci U S A* 2002; 99:15072–15077.
250. Burgess LE, Newhouse BJ, Ibrahim P, et al. Potent selective nonpeptidic inhibitors of human lung tryptase. *Proc Natl Acad Sci U S A* 1999;96:8348–8352.
251. Clark JM, Abraham WM, Fishman CE, et al. Tryptase inhibitors block allergen-induced airway and inflammatory responses in allergic sheep. *Am J Respir Crit Care Med* 1995;152:2076–2083.
252. Urata H, Kinoshita A, Perez DM, et al. Cloning of the gene and cDNA for human heart chymase. *J Biol Chem* 1991;266:17173–17179.
253. Caughey GH, Schaumberg TH, Zerweck EH, et al. The human mast cell chymase gene (CMA1): mapping to the cathepsin G/granzyme gene cluster and lineage-restricted expression. *Genomics* 1993;15: 614–620.
254. Schechter NM, Wang ZM, Blacher RW, et al. Determination of the primary structures of human skin chymase and cathepsin G from cutaneous mast cells of urticaria pigmentosa lesions. *J Immunol* 1994;152:4062–4069.
255. Vartio T, Seppa H, Vaheri A. Susceptibility of soluble and matrix fibronectins to degradation by tissue proteinases, mast cell chymase and cathepsin G. *J Biol Chem* 1981;256:471–476.
256. Wintroub BU, Schechter NM, Lazarus GS, et al. Angiotensin I conversion by human and rat chymotryptic proteinases. *J Invest Dermatol* 1984;83:336–339.
257. Sayama S, Iozzo RV, Lazarus GS, et al. Human skin chymotrypsin-like proteinase chymase. *J Biol Chem* 1987;262:6808–6815.
258. Gunnar P, Karlstrom A. Thrombin is inactivated by mast cell secretory granule chymase. *J Biol Chem* 1993;268:11817–11822.
259. Schechter NM, Choi JK, Slavin DA, et al. Identification of a chymotrypsin-like proteinase in human mast cells. *J Immunol* 1986; 137:962–970.

260. Briggaman RA, Schechter NM, Fraki J, et al. Degradation of the epidermal-dermal junction by proteolytic enzymes from human skin and human polymorphonuclear leukocytes. *J Exp Med* 1984;160:1027–1042.
261. Mizutani H, Schechter N, Lazarus G, et al. Rapid and specific conversion of precursor interleukin 1b (IL-1b) to an active IL-1 species by human mast cell chymase. *J Exp Med* 1991;174:821–825.
262. Wypij DM, Nichols JS, Novak PJ, et al. Role of mast cell chymase in the extracellular processing of big-endothelin-1 to endothelin-1 in the perfused rat lung. *Biochem Pharmacol* 1992;43:845–853.
263. Taipale J, Lohi J, Saarinen J, et al. Human mast cell chymase and leukocyte elastase release latent transforming growth factor-β1 from the extracellular matrix of cultured human epithelial and endothelial cells. *J Biol Chem* 1995;270:4689–4696.
264. Saarinen J, Kalkkinen N, Welgus H, et al. Activation of human interstitial procollagenase through direct cleavage of the Leu83-Thr84 bond by mast cell chymase. *J Biol Chem* 1994;269:18134–18140.
265. Natsuaki M, Stewart CB, Vanderslice P, et al. Human skin mast cell carboxypeptidase: functional characterization, cDNA cloning, and genealogy. *J Invest Dermatol* 1992;99:138–145.
266. Krejci NC, Knapp DM, Rudd RJ, et al. Dermal mast cell granules bind interstitial procollagenase and collagenase. *J Invest Dermatol* 1992;98:748–752.
267. Stevens RL, Fox CC, Lichtenstein LM, et al. Identification of chondroitin sulfate E proteoglycans and heparin proteoglycans in the secretory granules of human lung mast cells. *Proc Natl Acad Sci U S A* 1988;85:2284–2287.
268. Metcalfe DD, Lewis RA, Silbert JE, et al. Isolation and characterization of heparin from human lung. *J Clin Invest* 1979;64:1537–1543.
269. Razin E, Stevens RL, Akiyama F, et al. Culture from mouse bone marrow of a subclass of mast cells possessing a distinct chondroitin sulfate proteoglycan with glycosaminoglycans rich in *N*-acetylgalactosamine-4, 6-disulfate. *J Biol Chem* 1982;257:7229–7236.
270. Ruoslahti E. Proteoglycans in cell regulation. *Cell* 1989;264:13369–13372.
271. Yamaguchi Y, Mann DM, Ruoslahti E. Negative regulation of TGF-β by the proteoglycan decorin. *Nature* 1990;346:281–284.
272. Rosenberg RD. Biological actions of heparin. *Semin Hematol* 1977; 14:427–440.
273. Lonky SA, Marsh J, Wohl H. Stimulation of human granulocyte elastase by platelet factor 4 and heparin. *Biochem Biophys Res Commun* 1978;85:1113–1118.
274. Gajdusek C. Release of endothelial cell-derived growth factor (ECDGF) by heparin. *J Cell Physiol* 1984;121:13–21.
275. Gospodarwicz D, Cheng J. Heparin protects basic and acidic FGF from inactivation. *J Cell Physiol* 1986;128:475–484.
276. McCaffrey TA, Falcone DJ, Brayton CF, et al. Transforming growth factor-beta activity is potentiated by heparin via dissociation of the transforming growth factor-beta/alpha 2-macroglobulin inactive complex. *J Cell Biol* 1989;109:441–448.
277. Schreiber AB, Kenney J, Kowalski WJ, et al. Interaction of endothelial cell growth factor with heparin: characterization by receptor and antibody recognition. *Proc Natl Acad Sci U S A* 1985;82:6138–6142.
278. Meininger CJ, Sherwood SJ, Hawker JR. Mast cell heparin displaces with basic fibroblast growth factor from endothelial cell matrix [Abstract]. *J Cell Biochem* 1991;15(suppl):232.
279. Wright TCJ, Pukac LA, Castellot JJJ, et al. Heparin suppresses the induction of c-*fos* and c-*myc* mRNA in murine fibroblasts by selective inhibition of a protein kinase C-dependent pathway. *Proc Natl Acad Sci U S A* 1989;86:3199–3203.
280. Kenagy RD, Nikkari ST, Welgus HG, et al. Heparin inhibits the induction of three matrix metalloproteinases (stromelysin, 92-kD gelatinase, and collagenase) in primate smooth muscle cells. *J Clin Invest* 1994;93:1987–1993.
281. Weiler JM, Yurt RW, Fearon DT, et al. Modulation of the formation of the amplification convertase of complement, C3b, Bb, by native and commercial heparin. *J Exp Med* 1978;147:409–421.
282. Kazatchkine MD, Fearson DT, Silbert JE, et al. Surface-associated heparin inhibits zymosan-induced activation of the human alternative complement pathway by augmenting the regulatory action of the control proteins on particle-bound C3b. *J Exp Med* 1979;150:1202–1215.
283. Avioli LV. Heparin induced osteopenia: an appraisal. *Adv Exp Med Biol* 1975;52:375–387.
284. Crisp AJ, Wright JK, Hazleman BL. Effects of heparin, histamine, and salmon calcitonin on mouse calvarial bone resorption. *Ann Rheum Dis* 1986;45:422–427.
285. Glowacki J. The effects of heparin and protamine on resorption of bone particles. *Life Sci* 1983;33:1019–1024.
286. Goldhaber P. Heparin enhancement of factors stimulating bone resorption in tissue culture. *Science* 1965;147:407–408.
287. Hurley MM, Gronowicz G, Kream BE, et al. Effect of heparin on bone formation in cultured fetal rat calvaria. *Calcif Tissue Int* 1990; 46:183–188.
288. Sakamoto S, Sakamoto M, Goldhaber P, et al. Studies on the interaction between heparin and mouse bone collagenase. *Biochim Biophys* 1975;385:41–50.
289. Yamashita Y, Nakagomi K, Hasegawa S, et al. Effect of heparin on proliferation of pulmonary fibroblasts. *Am Rev Respir Dis* 1990;42:A912.
290. Sanantonio JD, Lander AD, Wright TC, et al. Heparin inhibits the attachment and growth of BALB/c-3T3 fibroblasts on collagen substrata. *J Cell Physiol* 1992;150:8–16.
291. Burd PR, Rogers HW, Gordon JR, et al. Interleukin 3-dependent and -independent mast cells stimulated with IgE and antigen express multiple cytokines. *J Exp Med* 1989;170:245–254.
292. Tsai M, Gordon JR, Galli SJ. Mast cells constitutively express transforming growth factor-beta mRNA. *FASEB J* 1990;4:A1944.
293. Gordon JR, Burd PR, Galli SJ. Mast cells as a source of multifunctional cytokines. *Immunol Today* 1990;11:458–464.
294. Plaut M, Pierce JH, Watson CJ, et al. Mast cell lines produce lymphokines in response to cross-linkage of Fc epsilon RI or to calcium ionophores. *Nature* 1989;339:64–67.
295. Young J, Lice CC, Butler G, et al. Identification, purification, and characterization of a mast cell–associated cytolytic factor related to tumor necrosis factor. *Proc Natl Acad Sci U S A* 1987;84:9175–9179.
296. Ohkawara Y, Yamauchi K, Tanno Y, et al. Human lung mast cells and pulmonary macrophages produce tumor necrosis factor-alpha in sensitized lung tissue after IgE receptor triggering. *Am J Respir Cell Mol Biol* 1992;7:385–392.
297. Moller A, Henz BM, Grutzkau A, et al. Comparative cytokine gene expression: regulation and release by human mast cells. *Immunology* 1998;93:289–295.
298. Bradding P, Okayama Y, Howarth PH, et al. Heterogeneity of human mast cells based on cytokine content. *J Immunol* 1995;155:297–307.
299. Bradding P. Human mast cell cytokines. *Clin Exp Allergy* 1996;26: 13–19.
300. Kruger-Krasagakes S, Moller S, Kolde G, et al. Production of interleukin-6 by human mast cells and basophil cells. *J Invest Dermatol* 1996;106:75–79.
301. Galli SJ, Gordon JR, Wershil BK. Mast cell cytokines in allergy and inflammation. *Agents Actions Suppl* 1993;43:209–220.
302. Selvan RS, Butterfield JH, Krangel MS. Expression of multiple chemokine genes by human mast cell leukemia. *J Biol Chem* 1994; 269:13893–13898.
303. Bradding P, Feather IH, Howarth PH, et al. Interleukin 4 is localized to and released by human mast cells. *J Exp Med* 1992;176:1381–1386.
304. Ying S, Durham SRJ, Jacobson MR, et al. T lymphocytes and mast cells express messenger RNA for IL-4 in the nasal mucosa in allergen-induced rhinitis. *Immunology* 1994;82:200–206.
305. Leal-Berumen I, Conlon P, Marshall JS. IL-6 production by rat peritoneal mast cells is not necessarily preceded by histamine release and can be induced by bacterial lipopolysaccharide. *J Immunol* 1994; 152:5468–5475.
306. Bullock E, Johnson E. Nerve growth factor induces the expression of certain cytokine genes and bcl-2 in mast cells: potential role in survival promotion. *J Biol Chem* 1996;271:27500–27508.
307. Rao A. A transcription factor required for the co-ordinate induction of several cytokine genes. *Immunol Today* 1994;15:274–281.
308. Steffen M, Abboud M, Potter GK, et al. Presence of tumor necrosis factor or related factor in human basophil/mast cells. *Immunology* 1989;66:445–450.
309. Walsh LJ, Trinchieri G, Waldorf HA, et al. Human dermal mast cells contain and release tumor necrosis factor a, which induces endothelial leukocyte adhesion molecule 1. *Proc Natl Acad Sci U S A* 1991; 88:4220–4224.
310. Qu Z, Liebler JM, Powers MR, et al. Mast cells are a major source of basic fibroblast growth factor in chronic inflammation and cutaneous hemangioma. *Am J Pathol* 1995;147:564–573.

311. Banovac K, Neylan D, Leone J, et al. Are the mast cells antigen presenting cells? *Immunol Invest* 1989;18:901–906.
312. Wasserman SI. Current comment: the mast cell and synovial inflammation. What's a nice cell like you doing in a joint like this? *Arthritis Rheum* 1984;27:841–844.
313. Marone G. Mast cells in rheumatic disorders: mastermind or workhorse? *Clin Exp Rheumatol* 1998;16:245–249.
314. Woolley DE. Mast cell in inflammatory arthritis. *N Engl J Med* 2003; 348:1709–1711.
315. Lee DM, Friend DS, Gurish MF, et al. Mast cells: a cellular link between autoantibodies and inflammatory arthritis. *Science* 2002;297: 1689–1692.
316. Benoist C, Mathis C. Mast cells in autoimmune diseases. *Nature* 2002;420:875–878.
317. van den Broek MF, van den Berg WB, van de Putte LBA. The role of mast cells in antigen induced arthritis in mice. *J Rheumatol* 1988;15: 544–551.
318. Caulfield JP, Hein A, Helfgott SM, et al. Intraarticular injection of arthritogenic factor causes mast cell degranulation, inflammation, fat necrosis, and synovial hyperplasia. *Lab Invest* 1988;59:82–95.
319. Allen JB, Manthey CL, Hand AR, et al. Rapid onset synovial inflammation and hyperplasia induced by transforming growth factor beta. *J Exp Med* 1990;171:231–247.
320. Dalldorf FG, Anderle SK, Brown RR, et al. Mast cell activation by a group A streptococcal polysaccharide in the rat and its role in experimental arthritis. *Am J Pathol* 1988;132:258–264.
321. Wershil BK, Mekori YA, Murakami T, et al. 125-I fibrin deposition in IgE-dependent immediate hypersensitivity reactions in mouse skin. *J Immunol* 1987;139:2605–2614.
322. Gryfe A, Sanders PM, Gardner DL. The mast cell in early rat adjuvant arthritis. *Ann Rheum Dis* 1971;30:24–29.
323. Malone DG, Metcalfe DD. Demonstration and characterization of a transient arthritis in rats following sensitization of synovial mast cells with antigen-specific IgE and parenteral challenge with specific antigen. *Arthritis Rheum* 1988;31:1063–1067.
324. Malone DG, Metcalfe DD. Mast cells and arthritis. *Ann Allergy* 1988;61:27–30.
325. De Clerck LS, Struyf NJ, Bridts CH, et al. IgE-containing immune complexes in synovial fluid of patients with rheumatoid arthritis. *Clin Rheumatol* 1990;9:176–181.
326. Zuraw BL, O'Hair CH, Vaughan JH, et al. Immunoglobulin E-rheumatoid factor in the serum of patients with rheumatoid arthritis, asthma and other diseases. *J Clin Invest* 1981;68:1610–1613.
327. Merity K, Falus A, Erhardt CC, et al. IgE and IgE-rheumatoid factors in circulating immune complexes in rheumatoid arthritis. *Ann Rheum Dis* 1984;43:246–250.
328. Marone G. The anti-IgE/anti-Fc epsilon RI alpha autoantibody network in allergic and autoimmune diseases. *Clin Exp Allergy* 1999;29: 17–27.
329. Crisp A, Chapman J, Clifford M, et al. Articular mastocytosis in rheumatoid arthritis. *Arthritis Rheum* 1984;27:845–850.
330. Godfrey HP, Ilardi C, Engber W, et al. Quantification of human synovial mast cells in rheumatoid arthritis and other rheumatic diseases. *Arthritis Rheum* 1984;27:851–854.
331. Gruber BL, Gorevic PD, Kaplan AP, et al. Rheumatoid synovial mast cells: functional studies. *J Allergy Clin Immunol* 1985;75:202.
332. Malone DG, Wilder RC, Saavedra-Delgado AM, et al. Mast cell numbers in rheumatoid synovial tissues: correlation with quantitative measure of lymphocytic infiltration and modulation by anti-inflammatory therapy. *Arthritis Rheum* 1987;30:130–138.
333. Okada J. The mast cell in synovial membrane of patients with joint diseases. *Jpn J Orthop Surg* 1973;47:657.
334. Fremont AJ, Denton J. Disease distribution of synovial fluid mast cells and cytophagocytic mononuclear cells in inflammatory arthritis. *Ann Rheum Dis* 1984;44:312–315.
335. Sajveiya K. Synovial mast cells. *Ind J Pathol Microbiol* 1983;26: 111–115.
336. Irani AM, Golzar N, Deblois G, et al. Distribution of mast cell subsets in rheumatoid arthritis and osteoarthritis synovia. *Arthritis Rheum* 1987;30:566.
337. Kiener H, Baghestanian M, Dominkus M, et al. Expression of the C5a receptor (CD88) on synovial mast cells in patients with rheumatoid arthritis. *Arthritis Rheum* 1998;41:233–245.
338. de Paulis A, Marino I, Ciccarelli A, et al. Human synovial mast cells. I. Ultrastructural *in situ* and *in vitro* immunologic characterization. *Arthritis Rheum* 1996;39:1222–1233.
339. Carsons SE. Detection and quantitation of stem cell factor (*kit* ligand) in the synovial fluid of patients with rheumatic disease. *J Rheumatol* 2000;27:2798–2800.
340. Olsson N. Demonstration of mast cell chemotactic activity in synovial fluid from rheumatoid patients. *Ann Rheum Dis* 2001;60:187–193.
341. Keiner HP. Tumor necrosis factor alpha promotes the expression of stem cell factor in synovial fibroblasts and their capacity to induce mast cell chemotaxis. *Arthritis Rheum* 2000;43:164–174.
342. Buckley M, Gallagher P, Walls A. Mast cell subpopulations in the synovial tissue of patients with osteoarthritis: selective increase in numbers of tryptase-positive, chymase-negative mast cells. *J Pathol* 1998;186:67–74.
343. Gotis-Graham I, McNeil HP. Mast cell responses in rheumatoid synovium. Association of the MCTC subset with matrix turnover and clinical progression. *Arthritis Rheum* 1997;40:479–489.
344. Gotis-Graham I, Smith M, Parker A, et al. Synovial mast cell responses during clinical improvement in early rheumatoid arthritis. *Ann Rheum Dis* 1998;57:664–671.
345. McNeil HP. Human mast cell subsets—distinct functions in inflammation? *Inflamm Res* 2000;49:3–7.
346. Gruber BL, Pozansky M, Boss E, et al. Characterization and functional studies of rheumatoid synovial mast cells: activation by secretagogues, anti-IgE and histamine-releasing lymphokine. *Arthritis Rheum* 1986;29:944–955.
347. Bromley M, Woolley DE. Histopathology of the rheumatoid lesion: identification of cell types at sites of cartilage erosion. *Arthritis Rheum* 1984;27:857–863.
348. Woolley DE, Crossley MJ, Evanson JM. Collagenase at the site of cartilage erosion in the rheumatoid joint. *Arthritis Rheum* 1977;20: 1231–1239.
349. Gruber BL, Schwartz LB. The mast cell as an effector of connective tissue degradation: a study of matrix susceptibility to human mast cells. *Biochem Biophys Res Commun* 1990;171:1272–1278.
350. Tetlow LC, Woolley DE. Mast cells, cytokines, and metalloproteinases at the rheumatoid lesion: dual immunolocalisation studies. *Ann Rheum Dis* 1995;54:896–903.
351. Johnson J, Jackson C, Angelini G, et al. Activation of matrix-degrading metalloproteinases by mast cell proteases in atherosclerotic plaques. *Arterioscler Thromb Vasc Biol* 1998;18:1707–1715.
352. Gruber BL, Schwartz LB, Ramamurthy NS, et al. Activation of latent rheumatoid synovial collagenase by human mast cell tryptase. *J Immunol* 1988;140:3936–3942.
353. Yoffe J, Taylor DJ, Woolley DE. Mast cell products stimulate collagenase and prostaglandin E production by cultures of adherent rheumatoid synovial cells. *Biochem Biophys Res Commun* 1984;122: 270–276.
354. DiGirolamo N. *In vitro* and *in vivo* expression of interstitial collagenase/MMP-1 by human mast cells. *Dev Immunol* 2000;7:131–142.
355. Zhang J, Nie G, Jian W, et al. Mast cell regulation of human endometrial matrix metalloproteinases: a mechanism underlying menstruation. *Biol Reprod* 1998;59:693–703.
356. Solovieva SA, Ceponis A, Konttinen YT, et al. Mast cells in loosening of totally replaced hip joints. *Clin Orthop Rel Res* 1996;322: 158–165.
357. Bartholomew JS, Evanson JM, Woolley DE. Serum IgE anti-cartilage antibodies in rheumatoid patients. *Rheumatol Int* 1991;11: 37–40.
358. Cooper AL, Snowden N, Woolley DE. IgE antibodies specific for cartilage collagens type II, IX, and XI in rheumatic diseases. *Scand J Rheumatol* 1993;22:207–214.
359. Chatpar PC, Muller D, Gruber BL, et al. Prevalence of IgE rheumatoid factor (IgE RF) in mixed cryoglobulinemia and rheumatoid arthritis. *Clin Exp Rheum* 1986;4:313–317.
360. Permin H, Egeskjold EM. IgE anti-IgG antibodies in patients with juvenile and adult rheumatoid arthritis including Felty's syndrome. *Allergy* 1982;37:421–427.
361. Permin H, Stahl Skov P, Norn S, et al. Basophil histamine release by RNA, DNA and aggregated IgG examined in rheumatoid arthritis and systemic lupus erythematosus. *Allergy* 1978;33:15–23.

362. Permin H, Stahl Skov P, Norn S. Basophil histamine release induced by leukocyte nuclei in patients with rheumatoid arthritis. *Allergy* 1983;38:273–281.
363. Magnusson CGM. Detection of anti-IgE autoantibodies. In: Shakib F, ed. *Monographs in allergy.* Vol. 26. Basel, Switzerland: S Karger, 1989:18–26.
364. Gruber BL. Activation of rheumatoid synovial mast cells: role of IgE-associated antiglobulins. In: Shakib F, ed. *Monographs in allergy.* Vol. 26. Basel, Switzerland: S Karger, 1989:120–134.
365. Johansson S. Anti-IgE antibodies in human serum. *J Allergy Clin Immunol* 1986;77:555–557.
366. Nawata Y, Koike T, Yanagisawa T, et al. Anti-IgE autoantibody in patients with bronchial asthma. *Clin Exp Immunol* 1984;58:348–356.
367. Nawata Y, Koike T, Hosokawa H, et al. Anti-IgE autoantibodies in patients with atopic dermatitis. *J Immunol* 1985;135:478–482.
368. Rouzer CA, Scott WA, Hamill AL, et al. Secretion of leukotriene C and other arachidonic acid metabolites by macrophages challenged with immunoglobulin E immune complexes. *J Exp Med* 1982;156: 1077–1086.
369. Paganelli R, Quinti I. Pathological significance of circulating IgG anti-IgE complexes. In: Shakib F, ed. *Monographs in allergy.* Vol. 26. Basel, Switzerland: S Karger, 1989:184–197.
370. Lindholm OR, Lindholm PS, Liukko HP, et al. The mast cell as a component of healing fractures in callus. *J Bone Joint Surg* 1969;51: 148–155.
371. Severson AR. Mast cells in areas of experimental bone resorption and remodelling. *Br J Exp Pathol* 1969;50:17–21.
372. Rafii M, Firooznia H, Golimbu C, et al. Pathologic fracture in systemic mastocytosis. Radiographic spectrum and review of the literature. *Clin Orthop* 1983;180:260–267.
373. Fallon MD, Whyte MP, Teitelbaum SL. Systemic mastocytosis associated with generalized osteopenia. *Hum Pathol* 1981;12:813–820.
374. Delling G. Histological characteristics and prevalence of secondary osteoporosis in systemic mastocytosis. A retrospective analysis of 158 cases. *Pathologe* 2001;22:132–140.
375. Tharp MD. Mastocytosis. *Dermatol Clin* 2001;19:679–696.
376. Fallon MD, Whyte MP, Craig BJ, et al. Mast cell proliferation in postmenopausal osteoporosis. *Calcif Tissue Int* 1983;35:29–31.
377. Frame B, Nixon RK. Bone marrow mast cells in osteoporosis of aging. *N Engl J Med* 1968;279:626–630.
378. Hills E, Dunstan CR, Evans RA. Bone metabolism in systemic mastocytosis. *J Bone Joint Surg Am* 1981;63:665–669.
379. Urist MR, McLean FC. Accumulation of mast cells in endosteum of bones of calcium-deficient rats. *Arch Pathol* 1957;63:239- 251.
380. Rockoff SD, Armstrong JD. Parathyroid hormone as a stimulus to mast cell accumulation in bone. *Calcif Tissue Res* 1970;5:41–55.
381. Lotinun S. Triazolopyrimidine (trapidil), a platelet-derived growth factor antagonist, inhibits parathyroid bone disease in an animal model for chronic hyperthryoidism. *Endocrinology* 2003;144:2000–2007.
382. Ellis HA, Peart KM. Iliac bone marrow mast cells in relation to the renal osteodystrophy of patients treated by haemodialysis. *J Clin Pathol* 1976;29:502–516.
383. McKenna MJ, Frame B. The mast cell and bone. *Clin Orthop* 1985; 200:226–233.
384. Crisp AJ, Roelke MS, Goldring SR, et al. Heparin modulates intracellular cyclic cAMP in human trabecular bone cells and adherent rheumatoid synovial cells. *Ann Rheum Dis* 1984;43:628–634.
385. Rosenstein R, Greenberg G, Melnick M, et al. Mast cells in bone remodeling—using a genetically defined mouse model as a clue to human disease. *Craniofac Struct Connect Tissue Disord* 1990;25:15–25.
386. Greenberg G, Pokress S, Minkin C. Inhibition of bone resorption *in vitro* by Compound 48/80. *Calcif Tissue Int* 1985;37:447–449.
387. Jeffcoat MK, Williams RC, Johnson HG. Treatment of periodontal disease in beagles with iodoxamide ethyl, an inhibitor of mast cell release. *J Periodont Res* 1985;20:532–541.
388. Bell NH. Rank ligand and the regulation of skeletal remodeling. *J Clin Invest* 2003;111:1120–1122
389. Fleischmajer R, Perlish JS, Reeves JRT. Cellular infiltrates in scleroderma skin. *Arthritis Rheum* 1977;20:975–984.
390. Nishioka K, Kobayashi Y, Katayama I, et al. Mast cell numbers in diffuse scleroderma. *Arch Dermatol* 1987;123:205–208.
391. Hawkins RA, Claman HN, Clark RAF, et al. Increased dermal mast cell populations in progressive systemic sclerosis: a link in chronic fibrosis? *Ann Intern Med* 1985;102:182–186.
392. Takeda K, Hatamochi A, Ueki H. Increased number of mast cells accompany enhanced collagen synthesis in linear localized scleroderma. *Arch Dermatol Res* 1989;281:288–290.
393. Lichtbroun AS, Sandhaus LM, Giorno RC, et al. Myocardial mast cells in systemic sclerosis: a report of three fatal cases. *Am J Med* 1990;89:372–376.
394. Claman HN. Mast cells, T cells and abnormal fibrosis. *Immunol Today* 1985;6:192–194.
395. Claman HN. Mast cell changes in a case of rapidly progressive scleroderma: ultrastructural analysis. *J Invest Dermatol* 1989;92:290–295.
396. Claman HN, Lee Choi K, Sujansky W, et al. Mast cell "disappearance" in chronic murine graft-vs-host disease (GVHD)—ultrastructural demonstration of "phantom mast cells." *J Immunol* 1986;137:2009–2013.
397. Kirkpatrick CJ, Curry A. Interaction between mast cells and perineural fibroblasts in neurofibroma: new insights into mast cell function. *Pathol Res Pract* 1988;183:453–458.
398. Kawanami O, Ferrans VJ, Fulmer JD, et al. Ultrastructure of pulmonary mast cells in patients with fibrotic lung disorders. *Lab Invest* 1979;40:717–734.
399. Gabrielli A, DeNictolis M, Campanati G, et al. Eosinophilic fasciitis: a mast cell disorder? *Clin Exp Rheumatol* 1983;1:75–78.
400. Kirscher CW, Bailey JF. The mast cell in hypertrophic scars. *Tex Rep Biol Med* 1972;30:327–338.
401. Walls AF, Bennett AR, Godfrey RC, et al. Mast cell tryptase and histamine concentrations in bronchoalveolar lavage fluid from patients with interstitial lung disease. *Clin Sci* 1991;81:183–188.
402. Norrby K, Arnqvist HJ, Bergstrom S, et al. Augmented mitogenesis in normal connective tissue cells following mast cell secretion in diabetic rats. *Virchows Arch (Cell Pathol)* 1982;39:137–144.
403. Norrby K. Intradermal mast-cell secretion causing cutaneous mitogenesis. *Virchows Arch (Cell Pathol)* 1983;42:263–269.
404. Walker MA, Harley R, Maise J, et al. Mast cells and their degranulation in the Tsk mouse model of scleroderma. *Proc Soc Exp Biol Med* 1985;180:323–328.
405. Claman HN, Jaffee BD, Huff JC, et al. Chronic graft-versus-host disease (GVHD) as a model for scleroderma. II: Mast cell depletion with deposition of immunoglobulins in the skin and fibrosis. *Cell Immunol* 1985;94:73–84.
406. Seibold JR, Giorno RC, Claman HN. Dermal mast cell degranulation in systemic sclerosis. *Arthritis Rheum* 1990;33:1702–1709.
407. Kihira C. Increased cutaneous immunoreactive stem cell factor expression and serum stem cell factor level in systemic scleroderma. *J Dermatol Sci* 1999;20:72–78.
408. Levi-Schaeffer F, Kupietzky A. Mast cells enhance migration and proliferation of fibroblasts into an *in vitro* wound. *Exp Cell Res* 1990; 188:42–49.
409. Subba Rao PV, Friedman MM, Atkins FM, et al. Phagocytosis of mast cell granules by cultured fibroblasts. *J Immunol* 1983;130:341–349.
410. Vliagoffis H, Hutson AM, Mahmudi-Azer S, et al. Mast cells express connexins on their cytoplasmic membrane. *J Allergy Clin Immunol* 1999;103:656–662.
411. Trautmann A, Krohne G, Brocker E, et al. Human mast cells augment fibroblast proliferation by heterotypic cell-cell adhesion and action of IL-4. *J Immunol* 1998;160:5053–5057.
412. Groto T, Befus D, Low R, et al. Mast cell heterogeneity and hyperplasia in bleomycin-induced pulmonary fibrosis in rats. *Am Rev Respir Dis* 1984;130:797–802.
413. Horuchi T, Ohta K, Yamaguchi M, et al. Mast cell involvement in bleomycin induced lung injury of mice. *Am Rev Respir Dis* 1990;42:A498.
414. O'Brien-Ladner A, Wesselius LJ, Stechshulte DJ. Decreased lung collagen deposition in mast cell deficient mice after bleomycin. *Am Rev Respir Dis* 1990;42:A499.
415. Suzuki N, Horiuchi T, Ohta K, et al. Mast cells are essential for the full development of silica-induced pulmonary inflammation: a study with mast cell–deficient mice. *Am J Respir Cell* 1993;9:475–483.
416. Siracusa LD, Christner P, McGrath R, et al. The tight skin (Tsk) mutation in the mouse, a model for human fibrotic diseases, is tightly linked to the beta 2-microglobulin (B2m) gene on chromosome 2. *Genomics* 1993;17:748–751.

417. Everett ET, Pablos JL, Harley RA, et al. The role of mast cells in the development of skin fibrosis in tight-skin mutant mice. *Comp Biochem Physiol [A]* 1995;110:159–165.
418. Cohen IK, Beaven MA, Horakova K, et al. Histamine and collagen synthesis in keloid and hypertrophic scars. *Surg Forum* 1972;23:509–510.
419. Hatamochi A, Fujiwara K, Ueki H. Effects of histamine on collagen synthesis by cultured fibroblasts derived from guinea pig skin. *Arch Dermatol Res* 1985;277:60–64.
420. Barzu T, Molho P, Tobelem G, et al. Binding and endocytosis of heparin by human endothelial cells in culture. *Biochim Biophys Acta* 1985;845:196–203.
421. Qu Z, Planck SR, Rosenbaum JT. Mast cells rather than macrophages or synoviocytes are the major source of basic fibroblast growth factor in arthritic joints. *Arthritis Rheum* 1994;37(suppl):305.
422. Kanbe N. Production of fibrogenic cytokines by cord blood-derived cultured human mast cells. *J Allergy Clin Immunol* 2000;106(suppl): 91–98.
423. Li CY, Baek JY. Mastocytosis and fibrosis: role of cytokines. *Int Arch Allergy Immunol* 2002;127:123–126.
424. Kondo S. Role of mast cell tryptase in renal interstitial fibrosis. *J Am Soc Nephrol* 2001;12:1668–1676.
425. Yamamato T. Mast cells enhance contraction of three-dimensional collagen lattices by fibroblasts by cell-cell interaction: role of stem cell factor/c-*kit*. *Immunology* 2000;99:435–439.
426. Skold CM. Co-cultured human mast cells stimulate fibroblast mediated contraction of collagen gels. *Inflammation* 2001;25:47–51.
427. Gruber BL, Kaufman LD. Remission in progressive early diffuse scleroderma induced by ketotifen: evidence for the role of mast cells in disease pathogenesis. *Am J Med* 1990;89: 392–395.
428. Walker MA, Harley RA, LeRoy EC. Inhibition of fibrosis in Tsk mice by blocking mast cell degranulation. *J Rheumatol* 1987;14:299–301.
429. Gruber BL, Kaufman LD. A double-blind randomized controlled trial of ketotifen versus placebo in early diffuse scleroderma. *Arthritis Rheum* 1990;34:362–366.
430. Fonseca E, Solis J. Mast cells in the skin: progressive systemic sclerosis and the toxic oil syndrome. *Ann Intern Med* 1985;102:864–865.
431. Konttinen YT, Tuominen S, Segerbergkonttinen M, et al. Mast cells in the labial salivary glands of patients with Sjögren's syndrome—a histochemical, immunohistochemical, and electron microscopical study. *Ann Rheum Dis* 1990;49:685–689.
432. Lichtig C, Haim S, Gilhar A, et al. Mast cells in Behçet's disease: ultrastructural and histamine content studies. *Dermatologica* 1981; 162:167–174.
433. Kaufman LD, Seidman RJ, Philips ME, et al. Cutaneous manifestations of L-tryptophan associated eosinophilic-myalgia syndrome: a spectrum of sclerodermatous skin disease. *J Am Acad Dermatol* 1990;23:1063–1069.
434. Johnston YE, Duray PH, Steere AC, et al. Lyme arthritis: spirochetes found in synovial microangiopathic lesions. *Am J Pathol* 1985;118: 26–34.
435. Gruber BL, Kaplan AP. Mast cells and rheumatic diseases. In: McCarty DJ, Koopman WJ, eds. *Arthritis and allied conditions*. Philadelphia: Lea & Febiger, 1993:417–436.
436. Cochrane CG, Koffler D. Immune complex disease in experimental animals and man. *Adv Immunol* 1973;16:185–264.
437. Bielory L, Gascon P, Lawley T, et al. Human serum sickness: a prospective analysis of 35 patients treated with equine anti-thymocyte globulin for bone marrow failure. *Medicine* 1988;67:40–57.
438. Braverman IM, Yen A. Demonstration of immune complexes in spontaneous and histamine-induced lesions and in normal skin of patients with leukocytoclastic angiitis. *J Invest Dermatol* 1975;64: 105–112.
439. Majno G, Shea SM, Leventhal M. Endothelial contraction induced by histamine-type mediators. *J Cell Biol* 1969;42:647–659.
440. Van Haaster C, Derhaag J, Engels W, et al. Mast cell–mediated induction of ICAM-1, VCAM-1 and E-selectin in endothelial cells *in vitro*: constitutive release of inducing mediators but no effect of degranulation. *Pflugers Arch* 1997;435:137–144.
441. Riley JF. Pharmacology and functions of mast cells. *Pharmacol Rev* 1955;7:267–277.
442. Kobayashi Y. Mast cells as a target of rheumatoid arthritis treatment. *Jpn J Pharmacol* 2002;90:7–11.
443. Takaishi T, Morita Y, Kudo K, et al. Auranofin, an oral chrysotherapeutic agent, inhibits histamine release from human basophils. *J Allergy Clin Immunol* 1984;74:296–301.
444. Rytomaa T. Organ distribution and histochemical properties of eosinophil granulocytes in the rat. *Acta Pathol Microbiol Scand* 1960; 50(suppl 140):1–118.
445. Kita H, Adolphson CR, Gleich GJ. Biology of eosinophils. In: *Allergy—principles and practice,* Eds. Adkinson NF, Yunginger, Busse WW et al. Mosby 2003 6th edition, pp. 305–332.
446. Paltraman RI, Collins PD, Williams TJ, et al. Eotaxin induces a rapid release of eosinophils and their progenitors from the bone marrow. *Blood* 1998;91:2240–2248.
447. Sanderson CJ. Control of eosinophilia. *Int Arch Allergy Appl Immunol* 1991;94:122–126.
448. Sillaber C, Geissler K, Scherrer R, et al. Type beta transforming growth factors promote interleukin-3 (IL-3)-dependent differentiation of human basophils but inhibit IL-3-dependent differentiation of human eosinophils. *Blood* 1992;80:634–641.
449. Butterfield JH, Gleich GJ. Interferon gamma treatment of six patients with the idiopathic hypereosinophilic syndrome. *Ann Intern Med* 1994;121:648–653.
450. Cogan E, Schandene L, Crusiaux A, et al. Brief report: Clinical proliferation of type 2 helper T cells in a man with the hypereosinophilic syndrome. *N Eng J Med*1994;330:535–538.
451. Weller P. Eosinophil structure and function. In: Koopman WJ, ed. *Arthritis and allied conditions.* Vol. I. Philadelphia: Lippincott Williams & Wilkins, 2001:383–392.
452. Jahnsen FL, Brandtzaeg P, Halstensen TS. Monoclonal antibody EG2 does not provide reliable immunohistochemical discrimination between resting and activated eosinophils. *J Immunol Methods* 1994;175:23–36.
453. Ackerman SJ, Corrette SE, Rosenberg HF. Molecular cloning and characterization of human eosinophil Charcot-Leyden crystal protein (lysophospholipase). *J Immunol* 1993;156:456–468.
454. Gounni AS, Lamkhioued B, Ochiai K, et al. High-affinity IgE receptor on eosinophils is involved in defense against parasites. *Nature* 1994;367:183–186.
455. Kita H, Kaneko M, Bartemes KR, et al. Does IgE bind to and activate eosinophils from patients with allergy? *J Immunol* 1999;162:6901–6911.
456. Ohno I, Lea R, Finotto S, et al. Granulocyte/macrophage colony stimulating factor (GM-CSF) gene expression by eosinophils in nasal polyposis. *Am J Respir Cell Mol Biol* 1991;5:505–510.
457. Broide DH, Paine MM, Firestein GS. Eosinophils express interleukin 5 and granulocyte macrophage-colony stimulating factor mRNA at sites of allergic inflammation in asthmatics. *J Clin Invest* 1992;90: 1414–1424.
458. Desreumaux P, Janin A, Colombel JF, et al. Interleukin 5 messenger RNA expression by eosinophils in the intestinal mucosa of patients with cochliac disease. *J Exp Med* 1992;175:293–296.
459. Symon FA, Lawrence MB, Williamson MI, et al. Functional and structural characterization of the eosinophil P-selectin ligand. *J Immunol* 1996;157:1711–1719.
460. Walsh GM, Symon FA, Lazarovites AI, et al. Integrin alpha 4 beta 6 mediates human eosinophil interaction with MAdCAM 1, VACM-1 and fibronectin. *Immunology* 1996;89:112–119.
461. Daffern PJ, Pfeifer PH, Ember JA, et al. C3a is a chemotaxin for human eosinophils but not for neutrophils. I, C3a stimulation of neutrophils is secondary to eosinophil activation. *J Exp Med* 1995;171:2119–2127.
462. Ponath PD, Qin S, Ringler DJ, et al. Cloning of the human eosinophil chemoattractant, eotaxin. Expression, receptor binding, and functional properties suggest a mechanism for the selective recruitment of eosinophils. *J Clin Invest* 1996;97:604–612.
463. Forssmann U, Ugoccioni M, Loetscher P, et al. Eotaxin-2, a novel CC chemokine that is selective for the chemokine receptor CCR3, and acts like eotaxin on human eosinophil and basophil leukocytes. *J Exp Med* 1997;185:2171–2176.
464. Shinkai A, Yoshisue H, Koike M, et al. A novel human CC chemokine, eotaxin-3, which is expressed in IL-4-stimulated vascular endothelial cells, exhibits potent activity toward eosinophils. *J Immunol* 1999;163:1602–1610.
465. Heath H, Qin S, Rao P, et al. Chemokine receptor usage by human eosinophils. The importance of CCR3 demonstrated using an antagonistic monoclonal antibody. *J Clin Invest* 1997;99:178–184.
466. Clark RAF, Gallin JI, Kaplan AP. The selective eosinophil chemotactic activity of histamine. *J Exp Med* 1975;142:1462–1476.
467. Spada CS, Nieves AL, Krauss AH-P, et al. Comparison of leukotriene B4 and D4 effects on human eosinophil and neutrophil motility *in vitro*. *J Leukoc Biol* 1994;55:183–191.

468. Sehmi R, Cromwell O, Taylor GW, et al. Identification of guinea pig eosinophil chemotactic factor of anaphylaxis as leukotriene B4 8(S), 15(S)-dihydroxy-5, 9, 11, 13 (Z.E.Z.E.)-eicosatetraenoic acid. *J Immunol* 1991;147:2276–2283.
469. Sigal CE, Valone FH, Holtzman J, et al. Preferential human eosinophil chemotactic activity of the platelet activating factor (PAF): 1–0-hexadecyl-2-acetyl-sn-glyceryl-3-phosphocholine (AGEPC). *J Clin Immunol* 1987;7:179–184.
470. Shute J. Interleukin-8 is a potent eosinophil chemoattractant [Editorial]. *Clin Exp Allergy* 1994;24:203–206.
471. Bochner BS. Cellular adhesion and its antagonism. *J Allergy Clin Immunol* 1997;100:581–585.
472. Pazdrak K, Stafford S, Alam R. The activation of the JAK-STAT 1 signaling pathway by IL-5 in eosinophils. *J Immunol* 1995;155:397–402.
473. Pazdak K, Schreiber D, Forsythe P, et al. The intracellular signal transduction mechanism of interleukin 5 in eosinophils—the involvement of Lyn tyrosine kinase and the Ras-Raf-1-Mek-microtubule-associated protein kinase pathway. *J Exp Med* 1995;181:1827–1834.
474. van der Bruggen T, Caldenhoven E, Kanters D, et al. Interleukin-5 signaling in human eosinophils involves JAK2 tyrosine kinase and STAT1-alpha. *Blood* 1995;85:1442–1448.
475. Kaplan AP, Kuna P, Reddigari SR. Chemokines: Chemotactic factors that activate basophils (histamine releasing factor) and eosinophils. In: Johansson SGO, ed. *Progress in allergy and clinical immunology.* Gottingen, Germany: Hogrefe & Huber, 1995:30–37.
476. Kaplan AP, Iyer M, Simone J, et al. Studies of the activation of eosinophils by RANTES. *Int Arch Allergol Clin Immunol* 1995;1: 4–11.

CHAPTER 18

Platelets in Rheumatic Diseases

Mansoor N. Saleh and Albert F. Lobuglio

Platelets are minute cytoplasmic fragments produced by bone marrow megakaryocytes under the regulatory influence of a host of cytokines, humoral growth factors, and the total platelet mass (1–8). The physiologic role of platelets is to form an initial plug at the site of tissue injury, both external and internal. Subendothelial collagen is a potent platelet activator and triggers a chain of events leading to platelet-plug formation and, ultimately, to the development of a hemostatic clot at the site of injury (9,10). Platelet activation is accompanied by degranulation and release of platelet granule contents into the immediate surroundings (11). These substances are stimuli for a variety of cellular processes, including those leading to tissue inflammation and wound healing (12–14). Rheumatic diseases are frequently accompanied by processes that can serve as stimuli for platelet activation (15–17). Platelet activation under these circumstances can potentially contribute to and potentiate the inflammatory response associated with rheumatic disorders (11,18–20). In addition, a number of quantitative, as well as qualitative, disorders of platelets have been associated with rheumatic diseases, and platelet function is often altered by medications prescribed for the treatment of rheumatic disorders. This chapter reviews this dual relationship between platelets and rheumatic diseases.

THROMBOPOIESIS

Pluripotent hematopoietic stem cells under the influence of appropriate cytokines can differentiate into multipotent myeloid progenitors (1,6–8,21,22). A variety of factors, including total platelet mass and cytokines, influence platelet production *in vitro* and *in vivo*. In 1994, five different investigator groups, using three distinct laboratory approaches, simultaneously cloned the elusive platelet growth and maturation factor (23–28). Thrombopoietin (TPO), also designated c-Mpl ligand or megakaryocyte growth and development factor (MGDF), induces megakaryocyte differentiation and platelet production (22,26–30). Early clinical trials have used two independently produced forms of TPO: a truncated version of TPO covalently bound to polyethylene glycol to achieve a longer half-life (PEG-rHuMGDF) (31) and a full-length glycosylated recombinant molecule (rhTPO) (6). In placebo-controlled trials, PEG-rHuMGDF enhanced platelet recovery in a dose-dependent manner when administered either before or after chemotherapy (32–34). Reversible thrombocytosis occurred in occasional patients. More disconcerting was the development of neutralizing antibody, which was associated with thrombocytopenia. Early clinical trials of rhTPO demonstrated attenuation of both the degree and duration of thrombocytopenia associated with high-dose chemotherapy (35, 36). As with PEG-rHuMGDF, thrombocytosis was observed in some patients treated with rhTPO and was reversible. The concern over the unexpected immunogenicity of the recombinant molecules and the associated thrombocytopenia has stalled further clinical development of these two molecules.

The only platelet colony-stimulating factor (CSF) to receive U.S. Food and Drug Administration (FDA) approval to date is recombinant human interleukin-11 (IL-11), a pleiotrophic hematopoietic growth factor that acts on different stages in the platelet development process both on the level of the stem cell and the megakaryocyte (6). In randomized, placebo-controlled trials, rhIL-11 has been found to be safe and effective in reducing chemotherapy-induced thrombocytopenia and the need for platelet transfusions (37–41). Toxicity included fluid retention requiring diuretics, as well as atrial arrhythmias (42). The discovery of TPO and IL-11 has led to the redefinition of the role of other cytokines and growth factors such as IL-3, IL-6, stem cell factor, and granulocyte-monocyte CSF (GM-CSF) in the overall growth and maturation of megakaryocytes and platelet production (31, 43–46). Although the clinical effects of platelet stimulatory cytokines studied to date show promise, the general clinical utility of these reagents has yet to be demonstrated.

Megakaryocyte maturation in the marrow generally takes 4 to 5 days (2,5,9). Mature megakaryocytes possess a distinguishing demarcation membrane system that partitions the cytoplasm into platelet territories containing mitochondria and cytoplasmic dense granules (47). Channels of the open canalicular system perforate through the platelet territories, provide access to the extracellular plasma, and facilitate endocytosis of plasma components. Platelets are apparently released when mature megakaryocytes rupture, leaving gaps in this open canalicular system. This results in the release of packets of membrane-bound cytoplasmic particles. The concept of platelets "budding" from the megakaryocyte membrane, as had been previously accepted, may not be accurate. Platelets, however, may be "secreted" from cytoplasmic processes emanating from marrow megakaryocytes (47).

Platelet-labeling studies demonstrate platelet survival to be approximately 9 days. Following intravenous administration, platelets distribute into the vascular pool (~70%) and the splenic pool (~30%), which are in equilibrium with each other (2,3,48). Platelet volume is generally inversely proportional to the platelet count because platelets released during late polyploid megakaryocyte maturation apparently originate from smaller platelet territories and, thus, are morphologically smaller than those released prematurely during stress thrombopoiesis (49).

PLATELET STRUCTURE

This topic has been the subject of numerous reviews (4, 47,50). Platelets are approximately 1.5- to 3-μm discoid cytoplasmic fragments enclosed by a plasma membrane and originating from mature megakaryocytes, which contain an array of diverse platelet granules (9,47,50,51) (Fig. 18.1). The cells have no nucleus and, therefore, cannot perform nuclear DNA- or RNA-dependent protein synthesis. Platelets do, however, possess a rich supply of glycogen, which, together with cytoplasmic mitochondria, provides for metabolic energy. The exterior coat of the platelet membrane bears a variety of surface glycoproteins and phospholipids (50). The distribution of platelet membrane phospholipids is similar to that seen in other hematopoietic cells with hydrophobic choline phospholipids located on the outer coat and the hydrophilic acidic phospholipids primarily exposed on the cytoplasmic side of the inner plasma membrane (52). The platelet surface phospholipids play an important role in coagulation (53), as well as in the production of arachidonic acid derivatives such as thromboxane, a potent platelet-aggregating agent (54) (see Chapter 23). Platelet surface glycoproteins, on the other hand, have been shown to possess specific ligand-binding properties that are central to the platelet's role in adhesion and platelet aggregation (10,20,55–61). Clinical syndromes associated with the inheritable absence of such glycoproteins have been described and generally present with a bleeding diathesis (61–67). The associated platelet functional defect can be characterized by platelet aggregation studies. Studies using readily available murine monoclonal antibodies to specific surface glycoproteins can be used to confirm the absence of the specific membrane component (67,68). Several surface glycoproteins have also been implicated as target antigens in autoimmune thrombocytopenias (69–74). In addition to inducing thrombocytopenia, platelet-directed autoantibodies may, under certain but as yet not completely understood circumstances, promote platelet degranulation and release of proinflammatory mediators that subsequently contribute to inflammation (75).

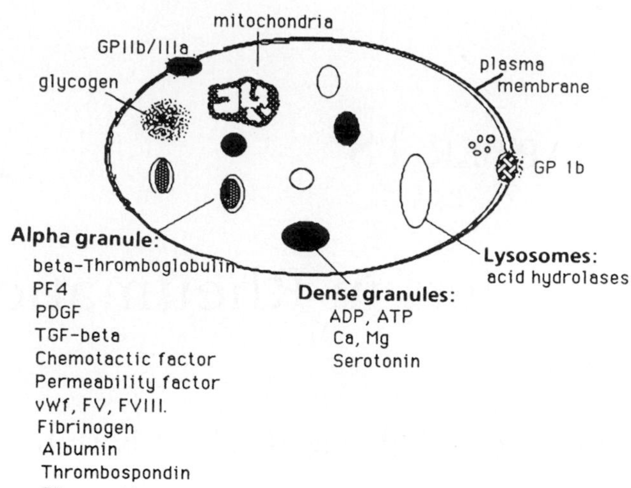

FIG. 18.1. Platelet with its inventory of granular content. *ADP,* adenosine diphosphate; *ATP,* adenosine triphosphate; *FV,* factor V; *GPIb,* platelet surface glycoprotein Ib; *PDGF,* platelet-derived growth factor; *VEGF,* vascular endothelial growth factor; *PF4,* platelet factor 4; *TGF-β,* transforming growth factor-β; *vWf,* von Willebrand factor.

The platelet cytoplasm contains a variety of organelles, most prominent of which are three types of storage granules: α granules, dense granules, and lysosomes. Under the influence of appropriate excitatory stimuli, platelet granular contents, especially those of α granules, which are destined for release during platelet activation at sites of tissue injury, are secreted into the environment, and lead to changes that contribute to the activation of other platelets as well as surrounding cellular elements (76,77). A number of bleeding disorders stemming from abnormalities in the storage and release of platelet granular content have been described (storage pool deficiency) (61,62,67,78).

PLATELET FUNCTION IN HEMOSTASIS

The physiologic role of platelets is to form a platelet plug upon activation (Fig. 18.2). Such a plug can subsequently serve as a matrix for the formation of a hemostatic clot (9,10,77,79). On exposure to subendothelial collagen, platelets are rapidly transformed into sticky cellular elements adhering to the underlying surface (adherence).

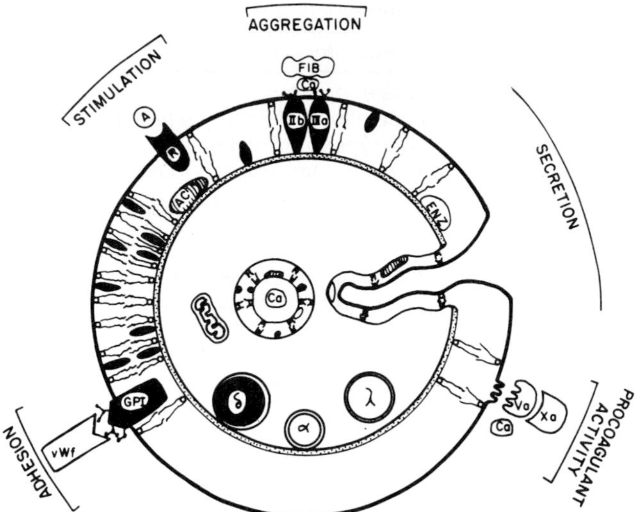

FIG. 18.2. Platelet structure and function. The platelet membrane contains clothespin-shaped phospholipids in a bilayer 8 nm thick with polar head groups *(white circles)* oriented to the aqueous environment and each pair of flexible fatty acid chains *(wavy lines)* oriented toward the hydrophobic middle of the bilayer. Interspersed are cholesterol *(small black ellipsoids)*, proteins, and glycoproteins. Protruding from the surface membrane is platelet surface glycoprotein I (*GPI*), to which von Willebrand factor (*vWf*) binds in the process of adhesion. Platelet aggregation and secretion are initiated by the binding of agonists (*A*), such as thrombin, epinephrine, or adenosine diphosphate (*ADP*), to specific receptors (*R*). In the presence of extracellular Ca^{2+} (*Ca*), aggregation is induced by binding of fibrinogen (*FIB*) to the GPIIb-IIIa complex spanning the membrane. Platelet secretion requires prostaglandin synthesis and other reactions that take place on the membrane of the cell, the open canalicular system, and the dense tubular system *(center)*. These synthetic reactions require enzymes (*ENZ*) such as phospholipase A_2 and cyclooxygenase. Release requires transfer of calcium from nucleated calcium stores into the cytosol, an event that triggers secretion from δ, α, and λ granules. The procoagulant activity of platelets is initiated by binding of factor Va to its surface receptors, and Va in the presence of Ca^{2+} acts as the receptor for factor Xa, thereby activating prothrombin at the cell surface. Platelet function is partially autoregulated by membrane adenylate cyclase enzyme complex (*AC*); this enzyme, plus 3′,5′-cyclic adenosine monophosphate (cAMP)-dependent phosphodiesterases, determines the platelet content of cAMP, an inhibitor of platelet function. (From Shattil SJ, Bennett JS. Platelets and their membrane in hemostasis: physiology and pathophysiology. *Ann Intern Med* 1981;94: 108–118, with permission.)

Platelet adherence is mediated by binding of subendothelial von Willebrand factor (vWf) to the platelet surface glycoprotein Ib (gpIb). Additionally, naturally-occurring plasma adhesive proteins have been implicated in this initial platelet/ surface interaction. This process is followed by shape change and platelet/platelet interaction (aggregation) resulting from the fibrinogen-mediated cross-linking of activated platelets via the surface glycoprotein gpIIb/IIIa. Activated platelets can also bind vWf via gpIIb/IIIa. Simultaneously, and in concert with aggregation, platelets release their intracellular granular contents (secretion). These include vasoactive amines, adenosine diphosphate, platelet-derived growth factor (PDGF), vascular endothelial growth factor (VEGF), transforming growth factor (TGF)-β, β-thromboglobulin, and platelet factor 4 (PF4) (10,20,60,76,79). This process leads to the recruitment of additional circulating platelets (amplification). The final outcome is the formation of a platelet plug and triggering of the coagulation cascade leading to thrombin activation and fibrin clot formation. The coordinated and balanced interplay between platelet activation and inhibition signals is pivotal to physiologic platelet function. Imbalances in either process can lead to pathologic platelet plug formation, as in the case of systemic lupus erythematosus (SLE)-associated antiphospholipid antibodies, which induce platelet activation and contribute to arterial and venous thrombi (75,80–86) (see Chapter 74). Conversely, defective platelet function, as in the case of storage pool defect, results in loss of normal platelet hemostasis and a subsequent bleeding diathesis (62,65,76). At the biochemical level, platelet activation or inhibition is triggered when extracellular ligands interact with specific receptors on the platelet surface (56–59,61,79,87). Extracellular signals are transmitted through the plasma membrane by transducer G proteins (57,88,89). Intracellular platelet response is mediated by a second messenger system. In a delicately balanced, but as yet not fully understood process, the activation signal pathway appears to be mediated by inositol 1,4,5-triphosphate and sn-1,2-diacylglycerol, whereas inhibitory signals use 3′,5′-cyclic adenosine monophosphate (cAMP) as the second messenger (57,61).

ROLE OF PLATELETS IN THE PATHOGENESIS OF RHEUMATIC DISEASE

There is substantial evidence indicating that platelets play an important role in processes other than hemostasis (12,13,20,60,90,91). Platelets have been implicated in the pathophysiology of several cellular processes, including atherosclerosis (91–93), rheumatoid arthritis (RA) (18,94), inflammatory bowel disorders (95), and tumor metastasis (96–99). Activation of platelets results in the release of a number of factors, many of which have the capacity to contribute toward a tissue inflammatory response (18,20,60) (Table 18.1). Platelet activation at the site of inflammatory injury has been demonstrated (18,100), and the protective effect of platelet depletion has been reported for some forms of immunologic injury associated with allergic reactions (101). The evidence for the involvement of platelets in the pathogenesis of human rheumatic diseases, however, remains indirect and circumstantial. This section reviews some of the laboratory data implicating platelets and platelet products in tissue inflammation and provides some basis

TABLE 18.1. *Major platelet-derived mediators of tissue inflammatory response*

Platelet-derived factor (source)	Inflammatory response
Thromboxane A_2 (cyclooxygenase dependent)	Vasoconstriction, platelet aggregation
12L-hydroperoxyeicosatetraenoic acid (lipoxygenase dependent)	Vasoconstriction, stimulation of leukocyte leukotriene B_4 synthesis, cyclooxygenase inhibition
12L-hydroxyeicosatetraenoic acid (lipoxygenase dependent)	Chemotaxis, stimulation of monocyte procoagulant activity
Adhesive glycoproteins: thrombospondin, fibronectin (α granules)	Cell adhesion
Platelet-specific proteins: β-thromboglobulin, PF4 (α granules)	Platelet aggregation, chemotaxis
Growth factors: PDGF, VEGF, TGF-β (α granules)	Chemotaxis, fibrogenesis, chondrogenesis, angiogenesis
Cationic proteins: chemotactic factor, permeability factor (α granules)	Chemotaxis, vascular permeability, histamine release
Acid hydrolases (lysosomes)	Tissue digestion
Serotonin (dense granule)	Vasoconstriction, vascular permeability, fibrogenesis

PDGF, platelet-derived growth factor; PF4, platelet factor 4; TGF-β, transforming growth factor-β, VEGF, vascular endothelial growth factor.

for understanding the role of platelets in human rheumatic diseases.

PDGF has been extensively studied and shown to specifically stimulate the proliferation of fibroblasts, smooth muscle cells, and connective tissue *in vitro* (102,103). PDGF is potentially one of the most important cytokines involved in the complex biologic responses associated with inflammation and wound healing (20,60,104,105). Recent evidence suggests that platelet surface molecules, in concert with platelet granule constituents, mediate the ability of platelets to cross-talk with other inflammatory cells. PDGF derived from platelet α granules, and P-selectin expressed on the platelet surface, together with histamine released from platelets at the site of inflammation, play an important role in this process (20). Platelet-derived VEGF has also been implicated in angiogenesis during physiologic wound healing (105,106), as well as in restenosis following percutaneous coronary revascularization (91), atherosclerosis, and even tumor growth and metastasis (105). Similarly, TGF-β induces chondrogenesis in mesenchymal cells (107, 108). Secretion of acid hydrolases from platelet lysosomes has been demonstrated to contribute to the digestion of extracellular matrix in model systems. Serotonin, permeability factor, and chemotactic factor derived from platelet α granules have been shown to increase vascular permeability and promote chemotaxis (51). Thus, it is evident that secretory products of platelet activation are capable of participating in an inflammatory reaction. Under physiologic conditions, such processes might contribute toward wound healing and tissue repair (104,109). On the other hand, under the influence of excessive stimulatory signals (56,57), such as IL-1, TNF, or products of leukocyte activation, such a process could lead to uncurbed inflammation such as that associated with rheumatic disorders. The megakaryocyte and platelet stimulatory cytokine IL-11 has been shown to play a protective role in the inflammatory joint process, presumably through the induction of tissue inhibitor of matrix metalloproteinases (TIMP), which counteracts the increased metalloproteinase activity associated with rheumatic diseases (110).

Rheumatic diseases can thus be viewed as diseases in which platelets are exposed to a multitude of activating factors, leading to platelet activation and propagation of the primary inciting pathologic stimulus. A number of examples illustrate this point. Increased plasma levels of platelet-derived connective tissue activating peptide III have been found in a significant proportion of patients with RA, systemic sclerosis, and SLE (19,111,112). Deposition and partial processing of such peptides in the synovium, spleen, and kidney could potentially induce neutrophil and fibroblast activation, and thus contribute to the inflammatory process. Gliostatin/platelet-derived endothelial cell growth factor is elevated in the sera of patients with RA, originating from stimulated platelets as well as cytokine-stimulated synovial cells, and is a useful marker of clinical disease (113). Antibody-mediated endothelial damage has been demonstrated in several autoimmune collagen vascular diseases, including SLE (114,115) and Kawasaki syndrome (116), and serves as a potent platelet activator at the site of endothelial injury, thereby promoting the inflammatory process (20,60,117–121). Circulating immune complexes have been implicated in the pathogenesis of a number of rheumatic conditions (122–125) and may bind directly to platelets via the low-affinity platelet immunoglobulin G (IgG) Fc receptors (FcγRII) (126) and lead to aggregation and platelet activation. Platelet activation can also occur via binding of immune complexes to the Clq receptor (112,127). IgE antibody-mediated platelet activation (128) has been described in asthma (129) and cold urticaria (130), but it is unclear whether IgE-mediated processes occur in rheumatic diseases. Radiolabeled platelets have been shown to localize to regions of active inflammation but not to quiescent joints in patients with RA (100,131), and platelet-specific proteins have been demonstrated in rheumatoid synovial fluid, as well as in sera of patients with active RA (131). Thus, there is substantial indirect evidence implicating the contribution of platelets to the pathogenesis of rheumatic disorders.

ABNORMALITIES OF PLATELET NUMBER IN RHEUMATIC DISEASES

Thrombocytopenia

Low platelet counts are not infrequently encountered in patients with rheumatic diseases. In the absence of an obvious underlying etiology, the differential diagnosis should include decreased platelet production (132), altered platelet distribution (133), or accelerated platelet destruction (133–136).

Megakaryocytic hypoplasia in rheumatic diseases is most frequently caused by drug-induced bone marrow suppression. The offending drugs are generally immunosuppressive agents used in the treatment of recalcitrant disease (e.g., cytoxan, methotrexate, azathioprine). All myelosuppressive drugs are capable of suppressing megakaryocyte replication, depending on the dose and duration of exposure. A clue to the diagnosis may be the concomitantly low white blood cell count. The bone marrow aspirate is generally diagnostic, and platelet counts recover on cessation of drug therapy. The time to recovery may depend on the duration of immunosuppressive therapy. A few cases of autoantibody-mediated megakaryocytic hypoplasia in SLE have been described (137–140). In these cases, the autoantibody may react with antigens shared by platelets as well as megakaryocytes (141). In the absence of any offending drug, the diagnosis is suspected when thrombocytopenia is associated with elevated levels of platelet-bound IgG (142) and a decreased number of bone marrow megakaryocytes.

A second potential cause of thrombocytopenia in rheumatic diseases is altered platelet distribution as a result of splenomegaly. An enlarged spleen may contain 50% to 80% of the circulating platelet mass, resulting in platelet sequestration and peripheral thrombocytopenia without associated platelet destruction (hypersplenism) (133). This type of thrombocytopenia is encountered in Felty syndrome, SLE, juvenile rheumatoid arthritis (JRA), and other rheumatic disorders (133). The associated thrombocytopenia is generally not severe, and patients are usually asymptomatic. The enlarged spleen suggests the diagnosis, although other causes of thrombocytopenia must be excluded. The possibility of a malignant B-cell process localized to the spleen (splenic marginal zone lymphoma) (143,144) should also be considered in patients with isolated splenomegaly. Clinical history, physical findings, and staging workup are generally sufficient to differentiate between a malignant process versus benign hypersplenism.

A third mechanism of thrombocytopenia is immune-mediated accelerated platelet destruction (134,136,145). Immune thrombocytopenic purpura (ITP) is encountered in nearly 15% to 25% of patients with SLE, although only about a third of these cases are symptomatic and require active intervention (146–150). Females are more frequently afflicted, and there appears to be an association with the human leukocyte antigen (HLA)-DRw2. On the one hand, the clinical course of SLE-associated immune thrombocytopenia may be independent of other manifestations of SLE, and thus, may behave much like *de novo* ITP (145, 149–152). On the other hand, the severe thrombocytopenia that occurs during episodes of systemic vasculitis has a more complex pathogenesis, a worse clinical course, and poorer outcome (85,147,149,152,153). Patients generally have abundant marrow megakaryocytes. In the absence of another cause of platelet consumption (e.g., sepsis, disseminated intravascular coagulopathy, or active vasculitis), thrombocytopenia is presumably due to the binding of IgG autoantibodies to platelet surface antigens with subsequent macrophage Fc receptor–mediated phagocytosis of the opsonized platelets (154). Nonspecific binding of IgG-containing immune complexes via the platelet FcγRII can also occur. Quantitation of platelet-bound antibody using radiolabeled monoclonal anti-IgG reagents is generally useful in differentiating between immune and nonimmune causes of thrombocytopenia (142). Platelet-specific autoantibodies bind to the target antigens via the Fab region, and various investigators have identified the putative platelet surface antigens (155,156). However, monoclonal antibodies derived from the fusion of myeloma cell lines with lymphocytes from patients with SLE (157,158) have often shown cross-reactivity with single- and double-stranded DNA and cytoskeletal, as well as cytoplasmic, antigens, in addition to platelet surface antigens (158–161). The primary inciting antigen and the role of these autoantibodies in the pathogenesis of SLE remain to be clarified.

Immune-mediated platelet destruction may be drug induced (133,134,162–165). A variety of drugs used in the treatment of rheumatic diseases, including gold salts and certain antiinflammatory agents, have been implicated in drug-induced immune thrombocytopenias (163,166–170). Nearly 5% of patients receiving intramuscular gold salts for the treatment of RA develop thrombocytopenia (170–172). The development of thrombocytopenia is insidious and may be accompanied by pancytopenia. HLA-DRw3 appears to predispose to this complication. The pathogenesis of this toxicity has not been clearly defined, although evidence appears to implicate drug-induced antibodies (163,164, 171–174). More recently, antibodies directed against platelet-associated gpV have been implicated in the pathogenesis of gold-induced immune thrombocytopenia (166). Interestingly, platelet surface glycoprotein–specific antibodies have also been implicated in rare cases of drug-dependent immune thrombocytopenia following ingestion of naproxen and acetaminophen (168). Treatment of choice is withdrawal of the causative drug and, in general, platelet counts return to pretreatment levels following cessation of therapy, although long-term persistence of thrombocytopenia has been described. Treatment with corticosteroids is seldom indicated unless the patient has symptomatic thrombocytopenia (167–169,175)

Circulating immune complexes binding to the platelet surface via FcγRII can also cause thrombocytopenia. Platelet destruction may be macrophage Fc receptor-mediated or may involve the activation of complement and lysis of platelets by the membrane attack complex. Complement components have been detected on the surface of circulating platelets that have escaped the full lytic process (176).

Therapy of antibody-mediated thrombocytopenia associated with rheumatic diseases varies slightly from that of *de novo* immune thrombocytopenic purpura (134,145,168, 170,177). Therapy is generally initiated with corticosteroids. Splenectomy, the treatment of choice for steroid refractory *de novo* immune thrombocytopenic purpura, is generally not recommended initially for the treatment of thrombocytopenia associated with rheumatic diseases (178). Patients with immune complex or IgM-mediated thrombocytopenia frequently do not respond to splenectomy. Additionally, splenectomy in a patient population that is frequently on long-term immunosuppressive therapy carries an increased risk for sepsis. Vincristine, another drug that is frequently used in the treatment of *de novo* immune thrombocytopenic purpura, produces responses in a small proportion of patients. The use of this agent has to be advocated with great caution in view of the associated drug-induced peripheral neuropathy. Intravenous γ-globulin (IVIgG) has been advocated in patients already receiving steroid therapy or in those who are refractory. IVIgG therapy appears to induce responses in some patients (177, 179) with SLE-associated thrombocytopenia. The precise mechanism of action of IVIgG remains to be elucidated, although recent data suggest a critical role for host FcγR genetic polymorphisms (180). Additionally, suppression of autoantibody production (antiidiotype activity) (181) and Fc receptor blockade (182) have also been implicated. Danazol, a synthetic androgen, has been used with some measure of clinical efficacy and without much toxicity (183). The treatment of thrombocytopenia associated with systemic vasculitis is more difficult, and response is linked to the clinical course of the primary process (119,121). Pulses of high-dose steroid, intermittent cyclophosphamide, or combined immunosuppressive therapy are generally recommended (184–187). Finding the appropriate therapeutic regimen for patients with refractory rheumatic diseases and concomitant immune thrombocytopenia often presents a challenge to the clinician. Immunoadsorption columns using *Staphylococcus* protein A has been approved for the treatment of refractory ITP and have been successfully used in the treatment of immune thrombocytopenia associated with rheumatologic conditions (188–192). The treatment should be reserved for recalcitrant cases, since it is cumbersome both technically as well as from the patient standpoint. The chimeric anti-CD20 monoclonal antibody effectively depletes B cells and has been found to effectively treat autoimmune cytopenias (193–197) and should be considered for the treatment of immune thrombocytopenia associated with rheumatologic disorders. Depletion of peripheral B-cell occurs within a week of the first infusion, and recovery takes nearly 4 to 6 months (198,199). Peripheral B-cell depletion is generally not associated with an increased infection rate, and immunoglobulin levels generally are maintained, albeit slightly depressed (199).

Thrombocytosis

Platelet counts are often elevated in patients with active RA (131). The degree of thrombocytosis appears to correlate with the extent of joint inflammation and with several acute-phase plasma proteins (200), as well as serum levels of platelet stimulatory cytokines (201–203). The underlying cause of this phenomenon is not well understood, although reactive thrombocytosis that is due to the chronic inflammatory process has been postulated and is supported by increased cytokine levels observed *in vivo*. Interestingly, platelet-labeling studies demonstrate significant localization of platelets preferentially at sites of joint inflammation (131). The observation that platelet counts are elevated, despite this localized sequestration, underscores the complex nature of this phenomenon. The associated thrombocytosis generally is not associated with any morbidity and rarely requires treatment. Platelet counts above $10^6/\mu L$ should trigger a workup for a myeloproliferative disorder and require hematologic intervention.

ABNORMALITIES OF PLATELET FUNCTION IN RHEUMATIC DISEASES

Platelet Activation

Between 5% and 10% of patients with SLE develop antiphospholipid antibodies that interfere with *in vitro* coagulation tests (lupus anticoagulant) (133,204–206) (see Chapter 74). The presence of a lupus anticoagulant is recognized by the prolongation of phospholipid-dependent coagulation tests. This clinical entity is commonly associated with a prolonged partial thromboplastin time and prothrombin time, even though most patients do not have associated bleeding abnormalities. Paradoxically, affected patients are at risk for arterial, as well as venous, thrombotic disease (81,85,86,207–211), and a syndrome of recurrent abortions and intrauterine fetal death has been described in women (212–214). The pathophysiologic mechanisms underlying these observations have not been fully elucidated. Lupus anticoagulants are autoantibodies that presumably inhibit the release of prostaglandin I_2 (PGI_2), a potent platelet inhibitory factor, from vascular endothelium (215), thereby promoting platelet aggregation. In addition, binding of the antibodies to platelet surface phospholipids can itself induce platelet aggregation and degranulation, thus contributing to the pathologic process and promoting thrombosis (75,216–218). Nearly 50% of patients with SLE and circulating lupus anticoagulant experience thrombotic events compared with only 10% of patients with SLE without lupus anticoagulant. Approximately one third of patients with lupus anticoagulant not associated with SLE experience similar complications. Patients with recurrent arterial or venous thrombotic phenomena in the absence of specific risk factors should be evaluated for the presence of the lupus anticoagulant in addition to studies to detect other causes of the hypercoagulable state. Such individuals often express other autoantibodies (anti-DNA, anticardiolipin). There is a significant correlation between the presence of anticardiolipin antibodies, lupus anticoagulant, and recurrent thrombosis (219,220). The presence of lupus anticoagulant should be suspected in patients in whom phospholipid-dependent *in vitro* coagulation tests (partial thromboplastin time, prothrombin time, tissue thromboplastin inhibition test, diluted Russell venom viper time) are abnormally prolonged in the absence of any known cause and a negative bleeding history. The laboratory abnormality is not corrected by mixing with normal plasma, but does correct after premixing with plasma containing excess platelet phospholipids. Whether corticosteroids combined with platelet antiaggregating agents [e.g., acetylsalicylic acid (ASA)] diminish the risk for thrombotic episodes is unclear. Recently, the use of chronic anticoagulation using low-molecular-weight heparin plus aspirin has been advocated, especially in women suffering from thrombosis and recurrent fetal loss syndrome (220,221,222).

Inhibition of Platelet Function

Nonsteroidal antiinflammatory drugs (NSAIDs) are generally the mainstay of treatment in rheumatic disorders. Drugs that do not selectively inhibit cyclooxygenase-2 (COX-2) interfere with platelet aggregation and secretion (223,224). An important example of a nonselective COX inhibitor is ASA, which induces irreversible acetylation and inactivation of the pivotal enzyme COX. The inhibition of COX has two opposing effects on platelets and vascular endothelium (225). Inhibition of platelet COX prevents formation of the arachidonic acid metabolite thromboxane A_2, a potent platelet-aggregating agent. Vascular endothelial COX is also inhibited by ASA, with resulting inhibition of formation of the antiaggregating agent prostacyclin (PGI_2). Inhibition of COX by ASA extends through the duration of the platelet life span (up to 9 days) because platelets lack the ability to synthesize additional enzyme. Inhibition of endothelial COX, on the other hand, is rapidly corrected by replacement of inactivated enzyme. Other nonselective NSAIDs, such as indomethacin, ibuprofen, and phenylbutazone, reversibly impair platelet function by competitively inhibiting platelet COX (224,225). Unlike ASA, the effect of these drugs depends on their plasma half-lives and is reversible on cessation of drug therapy. Platelet dysfunction secondary to NSAID use is associated with petechiae and easy bruisability, and has been associated with increased risk for gastrointestinal bleeding as well as development of peptic ulcer disease (226–229). Patients with preexisting gastrointestinal lesions (ulcers, polyps, cancer) are more prone to bleed while receiving NSAID agents. *In vitro*, the bleeding time is prolonged, and platelet function studies demonstrate characteristic abnormalities.

Newly developed specific COX-2 inhibitors have been shown to possess antiinflammatory properties with less gastrointestinal toxicity and alteration of platelet function (230–234). Whether this holds true with the widespread prescription of these new agents remains to be demonstrated (235). Whereas normal platelet function promotes hemostasis and wound healing, it is often useful to specifically inhibit platelet activation at sites of iatrogenic procedures, such as coronary angioplasty. A new class of specific platelet function inhibitors has been developed as antithrombotic agents (236–238). *In vivo*, the platelet glycoprotein gpIIb/IIIa binds circulating adhesive proteins, primarily fibrinogen, leading to platelet–platelet bridging and cohesion (230–240). Monoclonal antibodies directed at gpIIb/IIIa have been shown to inhibit platelet aggregation and recruitment at sites of vascular injury (236,239,241–243). In a prospective randomized double-blind study, administration of Fab fragments of a chimeric anti-gpIIb/IIIa antibody (c7E3), following high-risk angioplasty, demonstrated a significant reduction in acute vascular closure and restenosis (244,245). As expected, treatment was associated with an increased risk for bleeding (244) due to the associated iatrogenically-induced platelet function abnormality. Additionally, both true as well as pseudothrombocytopenia has been associated with the use of c7E3. Whether this novel agent can be used in preventing vascular thrombi associated with platelet activation in other disorders (e.g., vasculitis) has yet to be established (246).

CONCLUSION

Platelets play a central role in hemostasis via a delicate balance between activators and inhibitors of platelet function. Rheumatic disorders, in turn, are frequently associated with abnormalities of platelet number, with thrombocytopenia being much more frequent than thrombocytosis. Additionally, a variety of platelet function abnormalities have been associated with rheumatic disorders, some of which are related to the primary disease process while others are caused by antiinflammatory drugs. A number of mediators of inflammation are associated with platelet activation *in vitro*, and there is evidence to suggest that the response of platelets to such stimuli *in vivo* may play an important role in promoting the tissue inflammation associated with rheumatic disorders. Much has been learned about the possible linkage between platelets and rheumatic disorders, including mediators that influence both. A better understanding of the reciprocal role of platelets in human inflammatory diseases will pave the way toward better therapeutic manipulation of both.

ACKNOWLEDGMENTS

We gratefully acknowledge the help of Alfreda Lewis in preparing the manuscript.

REFERENCES

1. Hoffman R. Regulation of megakaryocytopoiesis. *Blood* 1989;74: 1196–1212.
2. Harker LA, Finch CA. Thrombokinetics in man. *J Clin Invest* 1969; 48:963–974.
3. Corash L, Chen HY, Levin J, et al. Regulation of thrombopoiesis: effects of the degree of thrombocytopenia on megakaryocyte ploidy and platelet volume. *Blood* 1987;70:177–185.
4. Penington DG. Formation of platelets. In: Gordon JL, ed. *Platelets in biology and pathology.* Vol. 2. Amsterdam: Elsevier/North-Holland 1981:19–42.
5. Han ZC, Bellucci S, Caen JP. Megakaryocytopoiesis: characterization and regulation in normal and pathologic states. *Int J Hematol* 1991; 54:3–14.
6. Prow D, Vadhan-Raj S. Thrombopoietin: biology and potential clinical applications. *Oncology* 1998;12:1597–1608.
7. Kuter DJ. Thrombopoietin: biology and clinical applications. *Oncologist* 1996;1:98–106.
8. Gewirtz AM. Megakaryocytopoiesis: the state of the art. *Thromb Haemost* 1995;74:204–209.
9. Lichtman MA, Brennan JK. Platelet production and destruction. In: Colman RW, Hirsh J, Marder VJ, et al., eds. *Hemostasis and thrombosis: basic principles and clinical practice,* 2nd ed. Philadelphia: JB Lippincott 1987:395–824.
10. Lind SE. The hemostatic system. In: Handin RI, Lux SE, Stossel TP, eds. *Principles and practice of hematology.* Philadelphia: JB Lippincott 1995:949–972.
11. Skaer RJ. Platelet degranulation. In: Gordon JL, ed. *Platelets in biology and pathology.* Vol. 2. Amsterdam: Elsevier/North-Holland 1981:321–348.
12. Gentry PA. The mammalian blood platelet. Its role in haemostasis, inflammation and tissue repair. *J Comp Pathol* 1992;107:243–270.
13. Chung KF. Platelet-activating factor in inflammation and pulmonary disorders. *Clin Sci* 1992;83:127–138.
14. Steed DL. The role of growth factors in wound healing. *Surg Clin North Am* 1997;77:575–586.
15. Jefferies WM. The etiology of rheumatoid arthritis. *Med Hypotheses* 1998;51:111–114.
16. Hermann JA, Hall MA, Maini RN, et al. Important immunoregulatory role of interleukin-11 in the inflammatory process in rheumatoid arthritis. *Arthritis Rheum* 1998;41:1388–1397.
17. Feldmann M, Brennan FM, Maini RN. Role of cytokines in rheumatoid arthritis. *Annu Rev Immunol* 1996;14:397–440.
18. Ginsberg MH. Role of platelets in inflammation and rheumatic disease. *Adv Inflamm Res* 1986;2:53–71.
19. Castor CW, Andrews PC, Swartz RD, et al. Connective tissue activation. XXXVI. The origin, variety, distribution, and biologic fate of connective tissue activating peptide-III isoforms: characteristics in patients with rheumatic, renal and arterial disease. *Arthritis Rheum* 1993;36:1142–1153.
20. Mannaioni PF, Di Bello MG, Masini E. Platelets and inflammation: role of platelet-derived growth factor, adhesion molecules and histamine. *Inflamm Res* 1997;46:4–18.
21. Clark SC, Kamen R. The human hematopoietic colony stimulating factors. *Science* 1987;236:1229–1237.
22. Mazur EM. Megakaryocytopoiesis and platelet production: a review. *Exp Hematol* 1987;15:340–350.
23. Sohma Y, Akahori H, Seki N, et al. Molecular cloning and chromosomal localization of the human thrombopoietin gene. *FEBS Lett* 1994;353:57–61.
24. de Sauvage FJ, Haas PE, Spencer SD, et al. Stimulation of megakaryocytopoiesis and thrombopoiesis by the c-Mpl ligand. *Nature* 1994; 369:533–538.
25. Lok S, Kaushansky K, Holly RD, et al. Cloning and expression of murine thrombopoietic cDNA and stimulation of platelet production *in vivo*. *Nature* 1994;369:565–568.
26. Bartley TD, Bogenberger J, Hunt P, et al. Identification and cloning of a megakaryocyte growth and development factor that is a ligand for the cytokine receptor Mpl. *Cell* 1994;77:1117–1124.
27. Kaushansky K, Lok S, Holly RD, et al. Promotion of megakaryocyte progenitor expansion and differentiation by the c-Mpl ligand thrombopoietin. *Nature* 1994;369:568–571.
28. Kuter DJ, Beeler DL, Rosenberg RD. The purification of megapoietin: a physiological regulator of megakaryocyte growth and platelet production. *Proc Natl Acad Sci U S A* 1994;91:11104–11108.
29. Wendling F, Maraskovsky E, Debili N, et al. c-Mpl ligand a humoral regulator of megakaryocytopoiesis. *Nature* 1994;369:571–574.
30. Kaushansky K. Thrombopoietin: the primary regulator of platelet production. *Blood* 1995;86:419–431.
31. Choi ES, Hokom MM, Chen JL, et al. The role of megakaryocyte growth and development factor in terminal stages of thrombopoiesis. *Br J Haematol* 1996;95:227–233.
32. Fanucchi M, Glaspy J, Crawford J, et al. Effects of polyethylene glycol-conjugated recombinant human megakaryocyte growth and development factor on platelet counts after cancer. *N Engl J Med* 1997;336: 404–409.
33. Basser RL, Rasko JE, Clarke K, et al. Randomized, blinded, placebo-controlled phase I trial of pegylated recombinant human megakaryocyte growth and development factor with filgrastim after dose-intensive chemotherapy in patients with advanced cancer. *Blood* 1997;89:3118–3128.
34. Basser RL, Rasko JE, Clarke K, et al. Thrombopoietic effects of pegylated recombinant human megakaryocyte growth and development factor (PEG-rHuMGDF) in patients with advanced cancer. *Lancet* 1996;348:1279–1281.
35. Vadhan-Raj S. Recombinant human thrombopoietin: clinical experience and in vivo biology. *Semin Hematol* 1998;35:261–268.
36. Vadhan-Raj S, Murray LJ, Bueso-Ramos C, et al. Stimulation of megakaryocyte and platelet production by a single dose of recombinant human thrombopoietin in patients with cancer. *Ann Intern Med* 1997;126:673–681.
37. Vredenburgh JJ, Hussein A, Fisher D, et al. A randomized trial of recombinant human interleukin-11 following autologous bone marrow transplantation with peripheral blood progenitor cell support in patients with breast cancer. *Biol Blood Marrow Transplant* 1998;4:134–141.
38. Isaacs C, Robert NJ, Bailey FA, et al. Randomized placebo-controlled study of recombinant human interleukin-11 to prevent chemotherapy-induced thrombocytopenia in patients with breast cancer receiving dose-intensive cyclophosphamide and doxorubicin. *J Clin Oncol* 1997;15:3368–3377.
39. Kaye JA. Clinical development of recombinant human interleukin-11 to treat chemotherapy-induced thrombocytopenia. *Curr Opin Hematol* 1996;3:209–215.
40. Tepler I, Elias L, Smith JW II, et al. A randomized placebo-controlled trial of recombinant human interleukin-11 in cancer patients with severe thrombocytopenia due to chemotherapy. *Blood* 1996;87:3607–3614.
41. Gordon MS, McCaskill-Stevens WJ, Battiato LA, et al. A phase I trial of recombinant human interleukin-11 (neumega rhIL-11 growth factor) in women with breast cancer receiving chemotherapy. *Blood* 1996;87:3615–3624.
42. Kuter DJ, Cebon J, Harker LA, et al. Platelet growth factors: potential impact on transfusion medicine. *Transfusion* 1999;39:321–332.
43. Quesenberry PJ, Ihle JN, McGrath E. The effect of interleukin-3 and GM-CSA-2 on megakaryocyte and myeloid clonal colony formation. *Blood* 1985;65:214–217.
44. Ishibashi T, Kimura H, Uchida T, et al. Human interleukin-6 is a direct promoter of maturation of megakaryocytes *in vitro*. *Proc Natl Acad Sci U S A* 1989;86:5953–5957.
45. Ikebuchi K, Wong GG, Clark SC, et al. Interleukin-6 enhancement of interleukin-3 dependent proliferation of multipotential hemopoietic progenitors. *Proc Natl Acad Sci U S A* 1987;84:9035–9039.
46. Teramura M, Kobayashi S, Hoshino S, et al. Interleukin-11 enhances human megakaryocytopoiesis *in vitro*. *Blood* 1992;79:327–331.
47. Zucker-Franklin D, Greaves MF, Grossi CE, et al. *Atlas of blood cells: function and pathology,* 2nd ed. Philadelphia: Lea & Febiger, 1988.
48. Aster RH, Jandl JM. Platelet sequestration in man. I. Methods. *J Clin Invest* 1964;43:843–855.
49. Paulus J-M. Platelet size in man. *Blood* 1975;46:321–336.

50. Isenberg WH, Bainton DF. Megakaryocyte and platelet structure. In: Hoffman R, Benz EJ Jr, Shattil SJ, et al., eds. *Hematology: basic principles and practice.* New York: Churchill Livingstone, 1994:1516–1524.
51. Holmsen H. Platelet secretion. In: Colman RW, Hirsch J, Marder VJ, et al., eds. *Hemostasis and thrombosis: basic principles and clinical practice,* 2nd ed. Philadelphia: JB Lippincott 1987:606–617.
52. Chap HJ, Zwall RF, van Deenan LL. Action of highly purified phospholipids on blood platelets. Evidence for an asymmetric distribution of phospholipids in the surface membrane. *Biochem Biophys Acta* 1977;467:146.
53. Shattil SJ, Bennett JS. Platelets and their membrane in hemostasis: physiology and pathophysiology. *Ann Intern Med* 1981;94:108–118.
54. Roth GJ. Platelet arachidonate metabolism and platelet-activating factor. In: Phillips DR, Shuman MA, eds. *Biochemistry of platelets.* San Diego: Academic, 1986:69.
55. Phillips DR, Shuman MA, eds. *Biochemistry of platelets.* San Diego: Academic, 1986.
56. Siess W. Molecular mechanisms of platelet activation. *Physiol Rev* 1989;69:58–178.
57. Knoll MH, Schafer AI. Biochemical mechanisms of platelet activation. *Blood* 1989;74:1181–1195.
58. Nurden AT, Caen JP. Membrane glycoproteins and human platelet function. *Br J Haematol* 1978;38:155–160.
59. Phillips DR, Jennings LK, Edwards HH. Identification of membrane proteins mediating the interaction of human platelets. *J Cell Biol* 1980;86:77–86.
60. Lukaszyk A, Bodzenta-Lukaszyk A, Aksiucik A, et al. The role of epidermal growth factor in platelet-endothelium interactions. *J Physiol Pharmacol* 1998;49:229–239.
61. Handin RI. Platelet membrane proteins and their disorders. In: Handin RI, Lux SE, Stossel TP, eds. *Blood: principles and practice of hematology.* Philadelphia: JB Lippincott, 1995:1049–1068.
62. Weiss HJ. Congenital disorders of platelet-function. *Semin Hematol* 1980;17:228–241.
63. Bellucci S, Tobelem G, Caen JP. Inherited platelet disorder. *Prog Hematol* 1983;13:223–263.
64. Grottum KA, Hovig T, Holmsen H, et al. Wiskott-Aldrich syndrome: qualitative platelet defects and short platelet survival. *Br J Haematol* 1969;17:373–388.
65. Bick RL. Platelet function defects: a clinical review. *Semin Thromb Hemost* 1992;18:167–185.
66. Sham RL, Francis CW. Evaluation of mild bleeding disorders and easy bruising. *Blood* 1994;8:98–104.
67. Bennett JS, Kolodziej MA. Disorders of platelet function. *Dis Mon* 1992;38:577–631.
68. George JN, Nurden AT, Phillips DR. Molecular defects in interaction of platelets with the vessel wall. *N Engl J Med* 1984;311:1084–1098.
69. Niessner H, Clemetson KJ, Panzer S, et al. Acquired thrombasthenia due to GP IIb-IIIa-specific auto-antibodies. *Blood* 1986;68:571–576.
70. Devine DV, Currie MS, Rosse WF, et al. Pseudo-Bernard-Soulier syndrome: thrombocytopenia caused by autoantibody to platelet glycoprotein Ib. *Blood* 1987;70:428–431.
71. Lynch DM, Howe SE. Antigenic determinants in idiopathic thrombocytopenic purpura. *Br J Haematol* 1986;63:301–308.
72. Beardsley DS, Spiegal JE, Jacobs MM, et al. Platelet membrane glycoprotein IIIa contains target antigens that bind anti-platelet antibodies in immune thrombocytopenia. *J Clin Invest* 1985;74:1701–1707.
73. Woods VL Jr, Oh EH, Mason D, et al. Autoantibodies against the platelet glycoprotein IIb/IIIa complex in patients with chronic ITP. *Blood* 1984;63:368–375.
74. Beer JH, Rabaglio M, Berchtold P, et al. Autoantibodies against the platelet glycoproteins (GP) IIb/IIIa, Ia/IIa, and IV and partial deficiency in GPIV in a patient with a bleeding disorder and a defective platelet collagen interaction. *Blood* 1993;82:820–829.
75. Deckmyn H, Vanhoorelbeke K, Peerlinck K. Inhibitory and activating human antiplatelet antibodies. *Baillieres Clin Haematol* 1998;11:343–359.
76. Shaefer AI. The platelet life cycle: normal function and qualitative disorders. In: Handin RI, Lux SE, Stossel TP, eds. *Blood: principles and practice of hematology.* Philadelphia: JB Lippincott 1995:1095–1126.
77. Harrison P, Savidge GF, Cramer EM. The origin and physiological relevance of alpha-granule adhesive proteins. *Br J Haematol* 1990;74:125–130.
78. Weiss HJ, Witte JD, Kaplan KL, et al. Heterogeneity in storage pool deficiency: studies on granule-bound substrates in 18 patients including variant deficient in α-granules, platelet factor 4, β-thromboglobulin and platelet derived growth factor. *Blood* 1979;54:1296–1319.
79. Caen JP, Rosa JP. Platelet-vessel wall interaction: from the bedside to molecules. *Thromb Haemost* 1995;74:18–24.
80. Colaco CB, Elkon KB. The lupus anticoagulant. A disease marker in antinuclear antibody negative lupus that is cross-reactive with autoantibodies to double-stranded DNA. *Arthritis Rheum* 1995;28:67–74.
81. Mueh JR, Herbst KD, Rapaport SI. Thrombosis in patients with the lupus anticoagulant. *Ann Intern Med* 1980;92:156–159.
82. McNeil HP, Chesterman CN, Krilis SA. Immunology and clinical importance of antiphospholipid antibodies. *Adv Immunol* 1991;49:193–280.
83. Galli M, Bevers EM, Comfurius P, et al. Effect of antiphospholipid antibodies on procoagulant activity of activated platelets and platelet-derived microvesicles. *Br J Haematol* 1993;83:466–472.
84. Wiener HM, Vardinon N, Yust I. Platelet antibody binding and spontaneous aggregation in 21 lupus anticoagulant patients. *Vox Sang* 1991;61:111–121.
85. Rauch J. Platelet phospholipid antigen-antibody interactions: detection and biological relevance. *Transfusion Med Rev* 1990;4:110–114.
86. Eisenberg PR, Ghigliotti G. Platelet-dependent and procoagulant mechanisms in arterial thrombosis. *Int J Cardiol* 1999;68(suppl 1):3–10.
87. Michelson AD, Furman MI. Laboratory markers of platelet activation and their clinical significance. *Curr Opin Hematol* 1999;6:342–348.
88. Brass LF, Manning DR, Shattil SJ. GTP-binding proteins and platelet activation. *Prog Hemost Thromb* 1990;10:127–174.
89. Neer EJ, Clapham DE. Roles of G protein subunits in transmembrane signaling. *Nature* 1988;333:129–134.
90. Arnaout MA. Cell adhesion molecules in inflammation and thrombosis: status and prospects. *Am J Kidney Dis* 1993;21:72–76.
91. Le Breton H, Plow EF, Topol EJ. Role of platelets in restenosis after percutaneous coronary revascularization. *J Am Coll Cardiol* 1996;28:1643–1651.
92. Lassila R. Inflammation in atheroma: implications for plaque rupture and platelet-collagen interaction. *Eur Heart J* 1993;14(suppl K):94–97.
93. Ross R. The pathogenesis of atherosclerosis: an update. *N Engl J Med* 1986;314:488–500.
94. DeLisser HM, Newman PJ, Albelda SM. Platelet endothelial cell adhesion molecule (CD31). *Curr Topics Microbiol Immunol* 1993;184:37–45.
95. Collins CE, Cahill MR, Newland AC, et al. Platelets circulate in an activated state in inflammatory bowel disease. *Gastroenterology* 1994;106:840–845.
96. Honn KV, Tang DG, Chen YQ. Platelets and cancer metastasis: more than an epiphenomenon. *Semin Thromb Hemost* 1992;18:392–415.
97. Poggi A, Stella M, Donati MB. The importance of blood cell-vessel wall interactions in tumour metastasis. *Baillieres Clin Haematol* 1993;6:731–752.
98. Honn KV, Tang DG, Crissman JD. Platelets and cancer metastasis: a causal relationship? *Cancer Met Rev* 1992;11:325–351.
99. Weiss L. Overview of the metastatic cascade. In: Honn KV, Sloan BF, eds. *Hemostatic mechanisms and metastasis.* Boston: Martinus Nijhoff, 1984:15.
100. Oxholm P, Winther K. Thrombocyte involvement in immune inflammatory reaction. *Allergy* 1986;41:1–10.
101. Terkeltaub RA, Ginsberg MH. Platelets in rheumatic disease. In: McCarthy DJ, ed. *Arthritis and allied conditions,* 11th ed. Philadelphia: Lea & Febiger, 1989.
102. Kohler M, Lipton A. Platelets as a source of fibroblast growth promoting activity. *Exp Cell Res* 1974;87:297–301.
103. Ross R, Raines EW, Bowen-Pope DF. The biology of platelet-derived growth factor. *Cell* 1986;46:155–169.
104. Deuel TF, Kawahara RS, Mustoe TA, et al. Growth factors and wound healing: platelet-derived growth factor as a model cytokine. *Annu Rev Med* 1991;42:56–584.
105. Wartiovaara U, Salven P, Mikkola H, et al. Peripheral blood platelets express VEGF-C and VEGF which are released during platelet activation. *Thromb Haemost* 1998;80:171–175.
106. Assoian RK, Grotendorst GR, Miller DM, et al. Cellular transformation by coordinated action of three peptide growth factors from human platelets. *Nature* 1984;309:804–806.

107. Sporn MB, Roberts AB, Wakefield LM, et al. Transforming growth factor-beta: biological function and chemical structure. *Science* 1986;233:532–534.
108. Assoian RK, Komoriya A, Meyers CA, et al. Transforming growth factor beta in human platelets: identification of major storage site, purification and characterization. *J Biol Chem* 1983;258:7155–7160.
109. Zucker-Franklin D, Drosenberg L. Platelet interaction with modified articular cartilage: its possible relevance to joint repair. *J Clin Invest* 1977;59:641–651.
110. Trontzas P, Kamper EF, Potamianou A, et al. Comparative study of serum and synovial fluid interleukin-11 levels in patients with various arthritides. *Clin Biochem* 1998;31:673–679.
111. Ertenli I, Kiraz S, Arici M, et al. P-selectin as a circulating molecular marker in rheumatoid arthritis with thrombocytosis. *J Rheumatol* 1998;25:1054–1058.
112. Vollertsen RS, Conn DL. Vasculitis associated with rheumatoid arthritis. *Rheum Dis Clin North Am* 1990;16:445–461.
113. Waguri Y, Otsuka T, Sugimura I, et al. Gliostatin/platelet-derived endothelial cell growth factor as a clinical marker of rheumatoid arthritis and its regulation in fibroblast-like synoviocytes. *Br J Rheumatol* 1997;36:315–321.
114. Cines DB, Lyss AP, Reeber M, et al. Presence of complement fixing anti-endothelial cell antibodies in systemic lupus erythematosus. *J Clin Invest* 1984;73:611–625.
115. LeRoux GL, Wautier MP, Guillerin L, et al. IgG binding to endothelial cells in systemic lupus erythematosus. *Thromb Haemost* 1986; 56:144–146.
116. Leung DY, Collins T, Lapierre LA, et al. IgM antibodies present in the acute phase of Kawasaki's syndrome lyse cultured vascular endothelial cells stimulated by gamma interferon. *J Clin Invest* 1986;77: 1428–1435.
117. Kuryliszyn-Moskal A, Bernacka K, Klimiuk PA. Circulating intercellular adhesion molecule 1 in rheumatoid arthritis: relationship to systemic vasculitis and microvascular injury in nailfold capillary microscopy. *Clin Rheumatol* 1996;15:367–373.
118. Bacons PA, Kitas GD. The significance of vascular inflammation in rheumatoid arthritis. *Ann Rheum Dis* 1994;53:621–623.
119. Goronzy JJ, Weyand CM. Vasculitis in rheumatoid arthritis. *Curr Opin Rheumatol* 1994;6:290–294.
120. van der Zee JM, Heurkens AH, van der Voort EA, et al. Characterization of anti-endothelial antibodies in patients with rheumatoid arthritis complicated by vasculitis. *Clin Exp Rheumatol* 1991;9:589–594.
121. Vollertsen RS, Conn DL. Vasculitis associated with rheumatoid arthritis. *Rheum Dis Clin North Am* 1990;16:445–461.
122. Jarvis JN, Pousak T, Krenz M, et al. Complement activation and immune complexes in juvenile rheumatoid arthritis. *J Rheumatol* 1993;20:114–117.
123. Oleesky DA, Daniels RH, Williams BD, et al. Terminal complement complexes and C1/C1 inhibitor complexes in rheumatoid arthritis and other arthritic conditions. *Clin Exp Immunol* 1991;84:250–255.
124. Goronzy JJ, Weyand CM. Vasculitis in rheumatoid arthritis. *Curr Opin Rheumatol* 1994;6:290–294.
125. Moulds JM, Krych M, Holers VM, et al. Genetics of the complement system and rheumatic diseases. *Rheum Dis Clin North Am* 1992;18: 893–914.
126. Stuart SG, Simister NE, Clarkson SB, et al. The low affinity Fc receptor for human IgG (hFcRII) exists as multiple isoforms. *EMBO J* 1989;8:3657–3666.
127. Peerschke EI, Ghebrehiwet B. Human blood platelets possess specific binding sites for Clq. *J Immunol* 1987;138:1537–1541.
128. Joseph M, Capron A, Amiesen J-C, et al. The receptor for IgE on blood platelets. *Eur J Immunol* 1986;16:306–312.
129. Krauer KA. Platelet-activation during antigen induced airway reactions in asthmatic subjects. *N Engl J Med* 1981;304:1404–1406.
130. Grandel KE, Farr RS, Wanderer AA, et al. Association of platelet activating factor with primary acquired cold urticaria. *N Engl J Med* 1985;313:405–409.
131. Farr M, Scott DL, Constable TJ, et al. Thrombocytosis of active rheumatoid disease. *Ann Rheum Dis* 1983;42:545–549.
132. Burstein SA. Thrombocytopenia due to decreased platelet production. In: Hoffman R, Benz EJ Jr, Shattil SJ, et al., eds. *Hematology: basic principles and practice.* New York: Churchill Livingstone, 1995:1870–1878.
133. Warkentin TE, Trimble MS, Kelton JG. Thrombocytopenia due to platelet destruction and hypersplenism. In: Hoffman R, Benz EJ Jr, Shattil SJ, et al., eds. *Hematology: basic principles and practice.* New York: Churchill Livingstone, 1995:1889–1909.
134. Bussel J, Cines D. Immune thrombocytopenic purpura, neonatal alloimmune thrombocytopenia, and post-transfusion purpura. In: Hoffman R, Benz EJ Jr, Shattil SJ, et al., eds. *Hematology: basic principles and practice.* New York: Churchill Livingstone, 1995: 1849–1870.
135. Franck H, Rau R, Herborn G. Thrombocytopenia in patients with rheumatoid arthritis on long-term treatment with low dose methotrexate. *Clin Rheumatol* 1997;16:429–430.
136. McCrae KR, Bussel JB, Mannucci PM, et al. Platelets: an update on diagnosis and management of thrombocytopenic disorders. *Hematology* 2001;282–305.
137. Kaplan C, Champeix P, Blanchard D, et al. Platelet antibodies in systemic lupus erythematosus. *Br J Haematol* 1987;67:89–93.
138. Griner PF, Hoyer LW. Amegakaryocytic thrombocytopenia in systemic lupus erythematosus. *Arch Intern Med* 1970;125:328–332.
139. Nagasawa T, Sakurai T, Kashiwagi H, et al. Cell-mediated amegakaryocytic thrombocytopenia associated with systemic lupus erythematosus. *Blood* 1986;67:479–483.
140. Hasegawa Y, Nagasawa T, Kamoshita M, et al. Effects of antiplatelet glycoprotein Ib and/or IIb/IIIa autoantibodies on the size of megakaryocytes in patients with immune thrombocytopenia. *Eur J Haematol* 1995;55:152–157.
141. Stahl CP, Zucker-Franklin D, McDonald TP. Incomplete antigenic cross-reactivity between platelets and megakaryocytes: relevance in ITP. *Blood* 1986;67:421–428.
142. Court WS, Bozeman JM, Soong S-J, et al. Platelet surface-bound IgG in patients with immune and nonimmune thrombocytopenia. *Blood* 1987;69:278–283.
143. Franco V, Florena AM, Iannitto E. Splenic marginal zone lymphoma [Review]. *Blood* 2003;101:2464–2472.
144. Thieblemont C, Felman P, Callet-Bauchu E, et al. Splenic marginal-zone lymphoma: a distinct clinical and pathological entity. *Lancet* 2003;4:95–103.
145. Sutor AH, Gaedicke G. Acute autoimmune thrombocytopenia. *Baillieres Clin Haematol* 1998;11:381–389.
146. Doan CA, Bouroncle BA, Wiseman BK. Idiopathic and secondary thrombocytopenic purpura: clinical study and evaluation of 381 cases over a period of 28 years. *Ann Intern Med* 1960;53:861–876.
147. Nossent JC, Swaak AJG. Prevalence and significance of haematological abnormalities in patients with systemic lupus erythematosus. *Q J Med* 1991;80:605–612.
148. Gladman DD, Urowitz MB, Tozman EC, et al. Haemostatic abnormalities in systemic lupus erythematosus. *Q J Med* 1983;52:424–433.
149. Pistiner M, Wallace DJ, Nessim S, et al. Lupus erythematosus in the 1980s: a survey of 570 patients. *Semin Arthritis Rheum* 1991;21: 55–64.
150. Rabinowitz Y, Dameshek W. Systemic lupus erythematosus after acute "idiopathic" thrombocytopenic purpura: a review. *Ann Intern Med* 1960;52:1–28.
151. Alger M, Alarcon-Segovia D, Rivero SJ. Hemolytic anemia and thrombocytopenic purpura: two related subsets of systemic lupus erythematosus. *J Rheumatol* 1977;4:351–357.
152. Miller MH, Urowitz MB, Gladman DD. The significance of thrombocytopenia in systemic lupus erythematosus. *Arthritis Rheum* 1983; 26:1181–1186.
153. Reveille JD, Bartolucci A, Alarcon GS. Prognosis in systemic lupus erythematosus. Negative impact of increasing age at onset, black race, and thrombocytopenia, as well as causes of death. *Arthritis Rheum* 1990;33:37–48.
154. Saleh MN, Moore DL, Lee JY, et al. Monocyte-platelet interaction in immune and non-immune thrombocytopenia. *Blood* 1989;74:1328–1331.
155. van Leeuwen EF, van der Ven JT, Engelfriet CP, et al. Specificity of autoantibodies in autoimmune thrombocytopenia. *Blood* 1982;59:23–26.
156. Woods VL, Kurata Y, Montgomery RR, et al. Autoantibodies against platelet glycoprotein Ib in patients with chronic immune thrombocytopenic purpura. *Blood* 1984;64:156–160.
157. Shoenfeld Y, Hsu-Lin SC, Gabriels JE, et al. Production of autoantibodies by human-human hybridomas. *J Clin Invest* 1982;70:205–208.
158. Nugent DJ. Human monoclonal antibodies in the characterization of platelet antigens. In: Kunicki TJ, George JN, eds. *Platelet immunobiology: molecular and clinical aspects.* Philadelphia: JB Lippincott, 1989:273–290.

159. Asano T, Furie BC, Furie B. Platelet binding properties of monoclonal lupus autoantibodies produced by human hybridomas. *Blood* 1985;66:1254–1260.
160. Andre-Schwartz J, Datta SK, Shoenfeld Y, et al. Binding of cytoskeletal proteins by monoclonal anti-DNA lupus autoantibodies. *Clin Immunol Immunopathol* 1984;31:261–271.
161. Fabris F, Steffan A, Cordiano I, et al. Specific antiplatelet autoantibodies in patients with antiphospholipid antibodies and thrombocytopenia. *Eur J Haematol* 1994;53:232–236.
162. Dixon RH, Rosse WF. Platelet antibody in autoimmune thrombocytopenia. *Br J Haematol* 1975;31:129–134.
163. Lerner W, Caruso R, Faig D, et al. Drug-dependent and non-drug-dependent antiplatelet antibody in drug-induced immunologic thrombocytopenic purpura. *Blood* 1985;66:306–311.
164. Aster RH. Drug-induced immune thrombocytopenia: an overview of pathogenesis. *Semin Hematol* 1999;36(suppl 1):2–6.
165. Hegde UM. Platelet antibodies in immune thrombocytopenia. *Blood Rev* 1992;6:34–42.
166. Burgess JK. Molecular mechanisms of drug-induced thrombocytopenia. *Curr Opin Hematol* 2001;8:294–298.
167. Greinacher A, Eichler P, Lubenow N, et al. Drug-induced and drug-dependent immune thrombocytopenias. *Rev Clin Exp Hematol* 2001;5:166–200.
168. Bougie D, Aster R. Immune thrombocytopenia resulting in sensitivity to metabolites of naproxen and acetaminophen. *Blood* 2001;97: 3846–3850.
169. Aster RH. Drug-induced immune thrombocytopenia: an overview of pathogenesis. *Semin Hematol* 1999;36:2–6.
170. Aster RH. The immunologic thrombocytopenias. In: Kunicki TJ, George JN, eds. *Platelet immunobiology: molecular and clinical aspects*. Philadelphia: JB Lippincott, 1989:387–435.
171. Adachi JD, Bensen WG, Kassam Y, et al. Gold induced thrombocytopenia: 12 cases and a review of the literature. *Semin Arthritis Rheum* 1987;16:287–293.
172. Walker DJ, Saunders P, Griffiths ID. Gold induced thrombocytopenia. *J Rheumatol* 1986;13:225–227.
173. Kelton JG, Meltzer D, Moore J, et al. Drug-induced thrombocytopenia is associated with increased binding of IgG to platelets both *in vivo* and *in vitro*. *Blood* 1981;58:524–529.
174. von dem Borne AE, Pegels JG, van der Stadt RJ, et al. Thrombocytopenia associated with gold therapy: a drug-induced autoimmune disease? *Br J Haematol* 1986;63:509–516.
175. Saleh MN, Dhodaphar N, Allen K, et al. Quinidine-induced immune thrombocytopenia. *Henry Ford Hospital Med J* 1989;37:28–43.
176. Sims PJ. Interaction of human platelets with the complement system. In: Kunicki TJ, George JN, eds. *Platelet immunobiology: molecular and clinical aspects*. Philadelphia: JB Lippincott, 1989:354–383.
177. Mobini N, Sarela A, Ahmed AR. Intravenous immunoglobulins in the therapy of autoimmune and systemic inflammatory disorders. *Ann Allergy Asthma Immunol* 1995;74:119–128.
178. Rivero SJ, Alger M, Alcarcon-Segovia D. Splenectomy for hemocytopenia in systemic lupus erythematosus. A controlled appraisal. *Arch Intern Med* 1979;139:773–776.
179. Maier WP, Gordon DS, Howard RF, et al. Intravenous immunoglobulin therapy in systemic lupus erythematosus-associated thrombocytopenia. *Arthritis Rheum* 1990;33:1233–1239.
180. Binstadt BA, Geha RS, Bonilla FA. IgG Fc receptor polymorphisms in human disease: implications for intravenous immunoglobulin therapy. *J All Clin Immunol* 2003;111:697–703.
181. Sultan Y, Kazatchkine MD, Maisonneuve P, et al. Anti-idiotypic suppression of autoantibodies to factor VIII (antihaemophilic factor) by high-dose intravenous gammaglobulin. *Lancet* 1984;2: 757–767.
182. Bussel JB, Kimberly RP, Inman RD, et al. Intravenous gammaglobulin treatment of chronic idiopathic thrombocytopenic purpura. *Blood* 1983;62:480–486.
183. Blanco R, Martinez-Taboada VM, Rodriguez-Valverde V, et al. Successful therapy with danazol in refractory autoimmune thrombocytopenia associated with rheumatic diseases. *Br J Rheumatol* 1997; 36:1095–1099.
184. Warner M, Kelton JG. High-dose pulsed dexamethasone for immune thrombocytopenia. *N Engl J Med* 1997;337:425–427.
185. Busto MJ, Llamas P, Cabrera R, et al. Pulsed high-dose dexamethasone in the treatment of refractory immune thrombocytopenia. *Br J Haematol* 1996;93:738–739.
186. Lurie DP, Kahaleh MB. Pulse corticosteroid therapy for refractory thrombocytopenia in systemic lupus erythematosus. *J Rheumatol* 1982;9:311–314.
187. Mackworth-Young CG, Walport MJ, Hughes GR. Thrombocytopenia in a case of systemic lupus erythematosus: repeated administration of "pulse" methyl prednisolone. *Br J Rheumatol* 1984;23:298–300.
188. Matic G, Bosch T, Ramlow W. Background and indications for protein A-based extracorporeal immunoadsorption. *Ther Apher* 2001;5: 394–403.
189. Hughes LB, Moreland LW. New therapeutic approaches to the management of rheumatoid arthritis. *Biodrugs* 2001;15:379–393.
190. Furst D, Felson D, Thoren G, et al. Immunoadsorption for the treatment of rheumatoid arthritis: final results of a randomized trial. *Ther Apher* 2000;4:363–373.
191. Blanchette V, Freedman Jd, Garvey B. Management of chronic immune thrombocytopenic purpura in children and adults. *Semin Hematol* 1998; 35:36–51.
192. Schneider M, Gaubitz M, Pernoik A. Immunoadsorption in systemic connective tissue diseases and primary vasculitis. *Ther Apher* 1997; 1:117–120.
193. Silverman GJ, Weisman S. Rituximab therapy and autoimmune disorders: prospects for anti-B cell therapy. *Arthritis Rheum* 2003;48: 1484–1492.
194. Saleh MN, Gutheil J, Moore M, et al. A pilot study of the anti-CD20 monoclonal antibody rituximab in patients with refractory immune thrombocytopenia. *Semin Oncol* 2000;27:99–103.
195. Vose JM. Therapeutic uses of MAbs directed against CD20. *Cytotherapy* 2000;2:455–461.
196. Ratanatharathorn V, Carson E, Reynolds C, et al. Anti-CD20 chimeric monoclonal antibody treatment of refractory immune-mediated thrombocytopenia in a patient with chronic graft-versus-host disease. *Ann Intern Med* 2000;133:275–279.
197. Arzoo K, Sadeghi S, Liebman HA. Treatment of refractory antibody mediated autoimmune disorders with an anti-CD20 monoclonal antibody (rituximab). *Ann Rheum Dis* 2002;61:922–924.
198. Grillo-Lopez AJ, White CA, Varns C, et al. Overview of the clinical development of rituximab: first monoclonal antibody approved for the treatment of lymphoma. *Semin Oncol* 1999;26(suppl 14): 66–73.
199. Maloney DG. Preclinical and phase I and II trials of rituximab. *Semin Oncol* 1999;26(suppl 14):74–78.
200. Dixon JS, Martin MFR, Bird HA, et al. A comparison of platelet count and acute phase proteins in the measurement of disease activity in rheumatoid arthritis. *Br J Rheumatol* 1983;22:233–238.
201. Ertenli I, Haznedaroglu IC, Kiraz S, et al. Cytokines affecting megakaryocytopoiesis in rheumatoid arthritis with thrombocytosis. *Rheumatol Int* 1996;16:5–8.
202. Crilly A, Madhok R. Relationship between interleukin-6 levels and platelet counts in systemic juvenile rheumatoid arthritis. *Arthritis Rheum* 1992;35:840.
203. de Benedetti F, Massa M, Robbioni P, et al. Correlation of serum interleukin-6 levels with joint involvement and thrombocytosis in systemic juvenile rheumatoid arthritis. *Arthritis Rheum* 1991;34: 1158–1163.
204. Anonymous. Lupus anticoagulant. *Lancet* 1984;1:1157- 1158.
205. Morgan M, Downs K, Chesterman CN, et al. Clinical analysis of 125 patients with the lupus anticoagulant. *Aust N Z J Med* 1993;23:151–156.
206. Soltesz P, Veres K, Lakos G, et al. Evaluation of clinical and laboratory features of antiphospholipid syndrome: a retrospective study of 637 patients. *Lupus* 2003;12:302–307.
207. Elias M, Eldor A. Thromboembolism in patients with the "lupus"-type circulating anticoagulant. *Arch Intern Med* 1984;144:510–515.
208. Gladman DD, Urowitz MB, Tozman EC, et al. Haemostatic abnormalities in systemic lupus erythematosus. *Q J Med* 1983;52:424–433.
209. Rand JH. The antiphospholipid syndrome. *Ann Rev Med* 2003;54: 409–424.
210. Somers E, Magder LS, Petri M. Antiphospholipid antibodies and incidence of venous thrombosis in a cohort of patients with systemic lupus erythematosus. *J Rheumatol* 2002;29:2531–2536.
211. Galli M, Luciani D, Bertolini G, et al. Lupus anticoagulants are stronger risks factors for thrombosis than anticardiolipin antibodies in the antiphospholipid syndrome: a systematic review of the literature. *Blood* 2003;101:1827–1832.

212. Firkin BG, Howard MA, Radford N, et al. Possible relationship between lupus inhibitor and recurrent abortion in young women. *Lancet* 1980;2:366.
213. Scott JS. Immunological factors and recurrent fetal loss. *Lancet* 1984;1:1122.
214. Branch DW, Khamashta MA. Antiphospholipid syndrome: obstetric diagnosis, management, and controversies. *Obstet Gynecol* 2003; 101:1333–1344.
215. Carreras LO, Defreyn G, Mackin SJ. Arterial thrombosis, intrauterine death and "lupus" anticoagulant: detection of immunoglobulin interfering with prostacyclin formation. *Lancet* 1981;1:244–246.
216. Dorsch CA, Meyerhoff J. Mechanisms of abnormal platelet aggregation in systemic lupus erythematosus. *Arthritis Rheum* 1982;25: 966–973.
217. Weissbart E, Baruth B, Mielke H, et al. Platelets as target cells in rheumatoid arthritis and systemic lupus erythematosus: a platelet specific immunoglobulin inducing the release reaction. *Rheumatol Int* 1982;2:67–73.
218. Deckmyn H, Vanhoorelbeke K, Peerlinck K. Inhibitory and activating human antiplatelet antibodies. *Baillieres Clin Haematol* 1998;11: 343–359.
219. Hardin JA, Cronlund M, Haber E, et al. Activation of blood clotting in patients with systemic lupus erythematosus. *Am J Med* 1978;65: 430–436.
220. Harris EN, Asherson RA, Gharavi AE, et al. Thrombocytopenia in SLE and related autoimmune disorders. Association with anticardiolipin antibodies. *Br J Haematol* 1985;59:227–230.
221. Triolo G, Ferrante A, Ciccia F, et al. Randomized study of subcutaneous low molecular weight heparin plus aspirin versus intravenous immunoglobulin in the treatment of recurrent fetal loss associated with antiphospholipid antibodies. *Arthritis Rheum* 2003;48:728–731.
222. Von Dadelszen P, Kent N. Antiphospholipid syndrome in pregnancy: a randomized, controlled trial of treatment. *Obstet Gynecol* 2002;100: 408–413.
223. O'Brien JR. Effect of anti-inflammatory agents on platelets. *Lancet* 1968;1:894–895.
224. McQueen EG, Facoory B, Faed JM. Non-steroidal anti-inflammatory drugs and platelet function. *N Engl J Med* 1986;99:358–360.
225. Weksler BB, Pett SB, Alonso D, et al. Differential inhibition by aspirin of vascular and platelet prostaglandin synthesis in atherosclerotic patients. *N Engl J Med* 1983;308:800–805.
226. Ferraris VA, Swanson E. Aspirin usage and perioperative blood loss in patients undergoing unexpected operations. *Surg Gynecol Obstet* 1983;156:439–442.
227. Ferraris VA, Ferraris SP, Lough FC, et al. Preoperative aspirin ingestion increases operative blood loss after coronary artery bypass grafting. *Ann Thorac Surg* 1988;45:71–74.
228. Garcia Rodriguez LA. Variability in risk of gastrointestinal complications with different nonsteroidal anti-inflammatory drugs. *Am J Med* 1998;104(suppl):30–34.
229. Henry D, Lim LL, Garcia Rodriguez LA, et al. Variability in risk of gastrointestinal complications with individual non-steroidal anti-inflammatory drugs: results of a collaborative meta-analysis. *BMJ* 1996;312:1563–1566.
230. Simon LS. Role and regulation of cyclooxygenase-2 during inflammation. *Am J Med* 1999;106(suppl):37–42.
231. Dubois RN, Abramson SB, Crofford L, et al. Cyclooxygenase in biology and disease. *FASEB J* 1998;12:1063–1073.
232. Simon LS, Lanza FL, Lipsky PE, et al. Preliminary study of the safety and efficacy of SC-58635, a novel cyclooxygenase 2 inhibitor: efficacy and safety in two placebo-controlled trials in osteoarthritis and rheumatoid arthritis, and studies of gastrointestinal and platelet effects. *Arthritis Rheum* 1998;41:1591–1602.
233. Lipsky PE. Specific COX-2 inhibitors in arthritis, oncology and beyond: where is the science headed? *J Rheumatol* 1999;26(suppl 56): 25–30.
234. Geis GS. Update on clinical developments with celecoxib, a new specific COX-2 inhibitor: what can we expect? *J Rheumatol* 1999; 26(suppl 56):31–36.
235. Lipsky PE, Isakson PC. Outcome of specific COX-2 inhibition in rheumatoid arthritis. *J Rheumatol* 1997;24(suppl 49):9–14.
236. Harker LA, Maraganore JM, Hirsh J. Novel antithrombotic agents. In: Colman RW, Hirsh J, Marder VJ, et al., eds. *Hemostasis and thrombosis: basic principles and clinical practice.* Philadelphia: JB Lippincott, 1994:1638–1660.
237. Antiplatelet Trialists' Collaboration. Collaborative overview of randomized trials of antiplatelet therapy. I. Prevention of death, myocardial infarction, and stroke by prolonged antiplatelet therapy in various categories of patients. *BMJ* 1994;308:81–106.
238. Conti CR. Glycoprotein IIb/IIIa platelet receptor blockers: are they ready for prime time in patients with unstable coronary artery disease? *Clin Cardiol* 1999;22:57–58.
239. Coller BS, Peerschke EI, Scudder LE, et al. A murine monoclonal antibody that completely blocks the binding of fibrinogen to platelets produces a thrombasthenic-like state in normal platelets and binds to glycoprotein IIb and/or IIIa. *J Clin Invest* 1983;72:325–338.
240. Phillips DR, Charo IF, Scarborough RM. GPIIb-IIIa: the responsive integrin. *Cell* 1991;65:359–362.
241. Frelinger AL III, Cohen I, Plow EF, et al. Selective inhibition of integrin function by antibodies specific for ligand-occupied receptor conformers. *J Biol Chem* 1990;265:6346–6352.
242. Gawaz M, Ruf A, Neumann FJ, et al. Effect of glycoprotein IIb-IIIa receptor antagonism on platelet membrane glycoproteins after coronary stent placement. *Thromb Haemost* 1998;80:994–1001.
243. Madan M, Berkowitz SD, Tcheng JE. Glycoprotein IIb/IIIa integrin blockade. *Circulation* 1998;98:2629–2635.
244. EPIC (Evaluation of 7E3 for the Prevention of Ischemic Complications) Study Group. Use of a monoclonal antibody directed against the platelet glycoprotein IIb/IIIa receptor in high-risk coronary angioplasty. *N Engl J Med* 1994;330:956–961.
245. Harker LA. Platelets and vascular thrombosis. *N Engl J Med* 1994;330:1006–1007.
246. Futterman LG, Lemberg L. Harnessing the platelet. *Am J Crit Care* 1997;6:406–414.

CHAPTER 19

Cytokines and Cytokine Receptors

Cem Gabay

Cytokines regulate cell differentiation, replication, survival, and death during development, while maintaining homeostasis in the mature organism during host defense responses to injury. In the mature organism, cytokine action is successful when the cellular responses are integrated into a sequence of events that proceeds from initiation through effector phases to restoration of function at the level of the affected organ, as well as the entire organism. The regulation of a cell function by a cytokine can be reduced *in vitro* to the interaction of a specific cytokine with its receptor, intracellular signaling events, and resulting cell responses. *In vivo*, cytokines are components of a large, complex signaling network. Cytokines operate both as a cascade and as a network. Some cytokines stimulate the production of other cytokines and receptors. In addition, cells are seldom exposed to only a single cytokine. Instead, combinations of mediators convey biologically-relevant information. The effect of cytokines on target cells may be inhibited or enhanced by other cytokines, receptor antagonists, and soluble receptors. Combinations of cytokines have been found to exhibit additive, synergistic, or inhibitory effects. These general principles that govern physiologic responses of cells to cytokine stimulation provide a framework for the understanding of pathogenic mechanisms and the identification of targets or tools for therapeutic intervention. Many of the recent advances in the development of new treatments are based on progress in research on the biology of cytokines and their receptors.

The first part of this chapter reviews general aspects of cytokine biology. The second part discusses individual cytokine families and summarizes molecular characteristics, biologic activities *in vitro* and *in vivo*, expression in rheumatic diseases, information on pathogenesis, and therapeutic interventions that are based on cytokines or their receptors.

GENERAL OVERVIEW ON CYTOKINE FAMILIES

Cytokines can be classified according to common structural characteristics that correlate, to some degree, with functional relatedness. However, some cytokine families include molecules with distinct and sometimes antagonistic effects on cell function. Conversely, members of distinct cytokine families can have similar effects on cell function. The conserved structures within cytokine families represent motifs for receptor binding. Correspondingly, receptor families are characterized by extracellular, structurally-similar motifs for ligand recognition and, in addition, by intracellular domains that are responsible for the activation of similar signal transduction pathways. The cytokines are listed in Table 19.1 with their corresponding receptor families in Table 19.2.

The three interleukin-1 (IL-1) ligands are structurally related, but include two agonistic (IL-1α and IL-1β) and one specific antagonistic cytokine, the IL-1 receptor antagonist (IL-1Ra). Novel members of the IL-1 family of cytokines have been recently cloned, but their functions *in vivo* are still unknown. The IL-1 receptors were the first identified members of cytokine receptors that have immunoglobulin-like structure. The recently identified Toll-like receptor (TLR) family is part of the IL-1R superfamily. TLRs have intracellular domains that are homologous to the IL-1R. However, the extracellular domains of the receptors are distinct and consist of leucine-rich motifs. TLRs play an important role in host responses to infectious agents and constitute a link between innate and adaptive immune responses. The tumor necrosis factor (TNF) receptor family has the common structure of repeated cysteine-rich motifs in the extracellular domains of the receptors.

The next three families constitute the superfamily of hematopoietic cytokines. All three of these families utilize structurally-related receptors, the hematopoietic cytokine receptors. These receptors consist of at least two distinct subunits in which the β or γ chains activate signal transduction and can combine with different α chains that determine ligand specificity. The family of cytokines that utilizes the

TABLE 19.1. *Cytokine families*

Family	Members
TNF	TNF-α, LT-α, LT-β, CD40L, FasL, BAFF, APRIL, TRAIL, RANKL, NGF, CD27
IL-1	IL-1α, IL-1β, IL-1Ra, IL-18, IL-1F5 to IL-1F10
IL-6	IL-6, LIF, OSM, IL-11, CNTF, CT-1, CLC
Cytokines binding the common γ chain	IL-2, IL-4, IL-7, IL-9, IL-15, IL-21
IL-10	IL-10, IL-19, IL-20, IL-22, IL-24, IL-26, IL-28, IL-29
IL-12	IL-12, IL-23, IL-27
IL-17	IL-17A to IL-17F, IL-25
Hematopoietic cytokines	SCF, IL-3, TPO, EPO, GM-CSF, G-CSF, M-CSF
Interferon (IFN)	IFN-α subfamily, IFN-β, IFN-γ
CXC chemokines	CXCL1 to CXCL16
CC chemokines	CCL1 to CCL28
C chemokines	XCL1, XCL2
CX3C chemokine	CX3CL1
TGF-β superfamily	TGF-β, BMP family, activin, inhibin, MIS, nodal, leftys
Growth factors	PDGF, EGF, PGF, IGF, VEGF

APRIL, a proliferation-inducing ligand; BAFF, B cell–activating factor; BMP, bone morphogenetic protein; CLC, cardiotrophin-like cytokine; CNTF, ciliary neurotrophic factor; CT, cardiotrophin; EGF, epidermal growth factor; ENA, epithelial neutrophil activating peptide; EPO, erythropoietin; FGF, fibroblast growth factor; G-CSF, granulocyte colony-stimulating factor; GM-CSF, granulocyte-macrophage colony-stimulating factor; IFN, interferon; IGF, insulin-like growth factor; IL, interleukin; IL-1Ra, interleukin-1 receptor antagonist; L, ligand; LIF, leukemia inhibitory factor; LT, lymphotoxin; M-CSF, monocyte colony-stimulating factor; MIS, müllerian inhibiting substance; NGF, nerve growth factor; OSM, oncostatin M; PDGF, platelet-derived growth factor; RANK, receptor activator of nuclear factor κB; SCF, stem cell factor; TGF, transforming growth factor; TNF, tumor necrosis factor; TPO, thrombopoietin; TRAIL, TNF-related apoptosis-inducing ligand; VEGF, vascular endothelial cell growth factor.

TABLE 19.2. *Cytokine receptor families*

Receptor family	Members	Common features
IL-1R	IL-1RI, IL-1RII, IL-1RAcP, IL-18Rα, IL-18Rβ, T1/ST2, IL-1Rrp2	Ig-like extracellular domains
Toll-like R	TLR 1-10	Leucine-rich extracellular domains
TNFR	TNFRI, TNFRII, Fas, CD27, CD30, LTβR, NGFR, RANK, BAFFR, BCMA, TACI, TRAILR1,2,3	Cysteine-rich extracellular domains
Hematopoietin R	IL-2R, IL-3R, IL-4R, IL-5R, IL-6R, IL-7R, IL-9R, IL-13R IL-15R, G-CSFR, GM-CSFR, EPOR, TPOR	C-terminal W-S-X-W-S motifs
IFNR	IFN-α/βR, IFN-γR, IL-10R, IL-19R, IL-20R, IL-22R, IL-24R	Clustered four cysteines
Chemokine R	CXCR1–4; CCR1–8, CR, C3XCR	Seven transmembrane–spanning domains
TGF-β R	TGF-βRI, TGF-βRII, BMPR, ActivinR	Serine-threonine kinase
Growth factor R	EGFR, PDGFR, FGFR, M-CSFR (c-*fms*), SCFR (c-*kit*)	Tyrosine kinase

BAFF, B cell–activating factor; BCMA, B-cell maturation antigen; BMP, bone morphogenetic protein; EGF, epidermal growth factor; EPO, erythropoietin; FGF, fibroblast growth factor; G-CSF, granulocyte colony-stimulating factor; GM-CSF, granulocyte-macrophage colony-stimulating factor; IL, interleukin; IL-1RacP, IL-1R accessory protein; IL-1Rrp2, IL-1R related protein 2; M-CSF, monocyte colony-stimulating factor; NGF, nerve growth factor; PDGF, platelet-derived growth factor; RANK, receptor activator of nuclear factor κB; SCF, stem cell factor; TACI, transmembrane activator and calcium modulator and cyclophilin ligand interactor; TGF, transforming growth factor; TLR, Toll-like receptor; TNF, tumor necrosis factor; TPO, thrombopoietin; TRAIL, TNF-related apoptosis-inducing ligand.

common IL-2 receptor γ chain for signal transduction includes IL-2, IL-4, IL-7, IL-15, and IL-21. The cytokines IL-6, leukemia inhibitory factor (LIF), oncostatin M (OSM), IL-11, and ciliary neurotrophic factor (CNTF) utilize glycoprotein 130 (gp130) or LIFR as signal transducer. Granulocyte-macrophage colony-stimulating factor (GM-CSF), granulocyte colony-stimulating factor (G-CSF), and IL-5 activate cells via the GM-CSF β chain.

The interferon (IFN) family includes three major subtypes. The α and β IFNs (also termed type I IFN) are more closely related functionally and use the same receptor. IFN-γ (also known as type II IFN) functions are quantitatively and qualitatively different. The IFN-γ receptor is related to the type I IFN receptor, and each receptor utilizes different members of the same families of intracellular signal transducers and activators of transcription (STAT) factors. IL-10 and its related cytokines, IL-19, IL-20, IL-22, IL-24, IL-26, IL-28, and IL-29, bind to receptors related to the IFN receptor family.

The chemokines share common structures, and the spacing of the first two cysteines distinguishes the subfamilies. Chemokines bind to seven transmembrane domain receptors that utilize G proteins for signal transduction. The transforming growth factor-β (TGF-β) superfamily includes the TGF-βs, the bone morphogenetic proteins (BMP), activin, and inhibin. The receptors for the different members of this cytokine family have serine-threonine kinase activity. Platelet-derived growth factors (PDGFs), insulin-like growth factors (IGFs), epidermal growth factor (EGF), and fibroblast growth factors (FGFs) activate cells via receptors that have intracellular domains with intrinsic tyrosine kinase activity. The receptors for monocyte colony-stimulating factor (M-CSF) and stem cell factor (SCF) are also part of this family.

In addition to this structural classification, cytokines can also be grouped according to their cellular sources. The major distinction is between cytokines that are predominantly products of T lymphocytes, also termed lymphokines, and those that are produced by cells from different lineages. Cytokines with the broadest tissue distribution are the type I IFNs, IL-6, IL-1, several members of the TNF family, and the chemokine and CSF families. TGF-βs are produced by almost all normal cell types. Cytokines that are predominantly or exclusively produced by lymphocytes are IL-2, IL-3, IL-4, IL-5, IL-13, IL-17, and IFN-γ. Subsets of T helper (T_H) cells can be distinguished by the profile of cytokines they produce. Cytokines produced by T_H1 cells include IL-2, IFN-γ, and lymphotoxin (LT), whereas major T_H2-derived cytokines are IL-4, IL-5, IL-9, IL-10, and IL-13. IL-10 is a potent inhibitor of IFN-γ production by T_H1 cells. IL-4, IL-10, and IL-13 inhibit cytokine production by monocytes. In contrast, IL-12 and IL-18 are potent stimuli of IFN-γ production and promote T_H1 responses. Attempts to reveal distinct cytokine profiles has not produced clear associations for most autoimmune diseases. In rheumatoid arthritis (RA), synovial macrophages and fibroblasts are the major cytokine-producing cell types, at least in patients with established disease.

REGULATION OF CYTOKINE EXPRESSION

During homeostasis, most cytokines are either not expressed or are expressed only at low levels. Increased expression of cytokines in response to cell activation *in vitro* or during host defense responses *in vivo* occurs transcriptionally, posttranscriptionally, translationally, and through the conversion of latent precursors to biologically-active forms. Cytokines regulate the expression of cytokine receptors, and soluble forms of cytokine receptors and receptor antagonists are involved in the modulation of cytokine activity.

In response to injury, such as trauma or infection, stimuli are generated that trigger the induction of cytokine gene transcription. Cytokine inducers can be microbial antigens, fragments of degraded extracellular matrix, or products resulting from the activation of humoral mediator systems, such as the complement components C3a and C5a or kinins. Neuropeptides are also involved in the early activation phase since they are preformed, released immediately following tissue injury, and act on cells in the blood vessel wall and on leukocytes and stromal cells.

The binding of cytokine inducers to cell surface receptors stimulates intracellular signals, including protein kinases or phosphatases (Fig. 19.1), leading to the activation of transcription factors. These DNA-binding proteins recognize specific regions in the promoters of cytokine genes, including binding sites for AP-1; nuclear factor κB (NFκB); NF-IL-6; 3′,5′-cyclic adenosine monophosphate (cAMP) response element binding protein (CREB); STATs; SP-1; and IFN regulatory element-1 (IRF1). Protein binding to several of these sites is required for high levels of cytokine gene expression. The DNA binding proteins act additively or synergistically for the induction of cytokine expression.

Upon activation of the essential transcription factors or inhibition of negative transcriptional regulators, cytokine mRNA synthesis is initiated. Cytokine expression can also be influenced by the rate and duration of transcription and by posttranscriptional mechanisms. In the case of IL-1 expression in human monocytes, lipopolysaccharide (LPS) primarily increases the rate of transcription, whereas preincubation of the cells results in increased messenger RNA (mRNA) levels via longer duration of transcription and increased mRNA stability (1,2). The production of TNF-α is regulated both at the transcriptional and posttranscriptional level. Many cytokines, including IL-1, TNF-α, and GM-CSF, share UAUUAU or AUUA motifs in their 3′-untranslated region (UTR), which are responsible for rapid mRNA degradation (3). The importance of these AU-rich elements in the TNF-α gene is underscored by the severe phenotype of genetically-modified mice having a mutation in these regulatory regions. These animals produce high amounts of TNF-α and develop spontaneous inflammatory bowel disease and arthritis (4). The presence of cytokine mRNA does not necessarily result

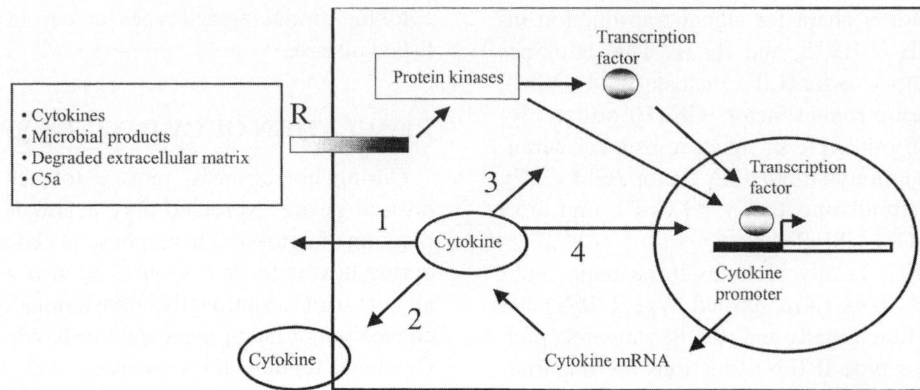

FIG. 19.1. Regulation of cytokine expression. Different stimuli induce intracellular signal transduction pathways after binding to cell surface receptors (*R*). Activation of cytoplasmic and nuclear transcription factors by proteins kinases stimulates cytokine gene transcription. Cytokines are released from cells through classical and nonclassical pathways (1), are expressed as membrane-anchored proteins (2), remain in the cytoplasm (3), or migrate into the nucleus (4).

in the production of protein. Translational regulation is important in the expression of several cytokines. Examples of this include IL-1 and TNF-α. The mRNA of these cytokines can be induced by monocyte adherence, but protein is only produced upon further stimulation of the cells with activators such as LPS (2,5). Some cytokines are secreted, others are stored in large quantities intracellularly, with additional stimuli are required to trigger secretion, and finally, some cytokines remain inside cells where they exert specific intracellular functions. The secreted cytokines contain a hydrophobic signal sequence at the N-terminal region and follow the classical endoplasmic reticulum to Golgi pathway of secretion. However, some cytokines such as IL-1α, IL-1β, IL-16, and IL-18 lack this consensus secretory signal sequence and are transported out of the cells through other pathways. When secreted from the cell, most cytokines are biologically active. In contrast, some cytokines (e.g., TGF-β) are secreted in a biologically inactive or latent form and require further extracellular processing by proteases to become biologically active (6).

Cytokines can be membrane associated or secreted. TNF-α and most other members of this cytokine family are expressed as membrane-anchored proteins. These membrane-bound cytokines are biologically active and, in some cellular responses, are more potent than the secreted forms (7). TNF-α is cleaved from the cell surface by TNF-α converting enzyme (TACE), an ADAM (a disintegrin and metalloproteinase) family matrix metalloproteinase. Approximately 10% to 15% of the IL-1α is myristoylated, transported to the cell surface, and expressed as a membrane-bound protein. IL-1α and TNF-α expressed as membrane-bound proteins are able to stimulate human fibroblasts and endothelial cells upon direct cell-cell contact.

Cytokines interact in the regulation of their expression. Cytokines that can induce their own expression include IL-1, IL-2, IL-6, LIF, and TGF-β. Autoinduction represents a potent amplification mechanism. IL-1, TNF-α, LIF, IL-17, and IL-18 induce each other's expression and that of a series of other cytokines, including IL-2, IL-6 family cytokines, chemokines, and CSFs.

Inhibition of cytokine expression represents an important regulatory mechanism by which potentially detrimental cytokine activities are controlled. TGF-β, IL-4, IL-10, and IL-13 are the best characterized inhibitors of cytokine production (8,9). TGF-β can inhibit IL-1 or LPS-induced TNF-α or IL-6 synthesis in monocytes (10). IL-4 is a potent inhibitor of monocyte activation and interferes with the production of IL-1, TNF-α, IL-6, and IL-8 (11). Furthermore, IL-4 is able to stimulate the production of IL-1Ra. IL-10 is a cytokine that has been discovered on the basis of its ability to inhibit IFN-γ production by T lymphocytes (12). It is also a monocyte deactivator, which is produced in relatively large quantities by monocytes, and inhibits synthesis of several cytokines by monocytes. A further important negative regulatory control of cytokine expression is provided by glucocorticoids. During the acute-phase response, circulating levels of endogenous glucocorticoids are enhanced. Inflammation-associated cytokines stimulate the production of corticotropin-releasing hormone, with consequent stimulation of corticotropin and cortisol release. Most cytokine promoters contain glucocorticoid response elements that bind ligand-occupied glucocorticoid receptors (13). Glucocorticoids are potent inhibitors of the expression of diverse cytokines induced by proinflammatory stimuli (14).

CYTOKINE POSTRECEPTOR SIGNALING PATHWAYS

Membrane-bound and secreted cytokines bind to cell surface receptors, soluble receptors, or carrier proteins and associate with matrix components. The activation of postreceptor signal transduction defines the different cellular responses to cytokines. The tissue distribution of the receptor for a specific cytokine defines the spectrum of biologic activities of its ligand. Variations in the levels of cytokine receptors represent another mechanism to control cellular responses to cytokines. Some receptors are constitutively expressed at high levels, whereas the expression of others is regulated by agents that induce cytokine production and by cytokines themselves. IL-1 contributes to the up-regulation of IL-2 receptors, and IL-2 is a potent inducer of its own receptor. TGF-β has been shown, in some cell types, to inhibit the expression of IL-1 receptors, and this may represent one mechanism by which it interferes with the biologic effects of IL-1. In addition, cytokines can stimulate the cleavage of cell surface receptors, thereby inhibiting cellular responses.

The diversity of cell functions that are regulated by cytokines is reflected by the utilization of structurally-different receptors that activate different postreceptor signaling pathways. Protein phosphorylation is a common mechanism of cell signaling. Protein kinases are enzymes that covalently attach phosphate to the side chain of either serine, threonine, or tyrosine of specific proteins inside cells. Such phosphorylation controls their enzymatic activities (cascade of intracellular kinase activity), their location inside cells (translocation in the nucleus), and their degradation by intracellular proteases. Mitogen-activated protein kinases (MAPKs) are a family of signaling proteins that phosphorylate specific serines and threonines on substrate proteins and regulate different cellular activities in response to cytokines and other stimuli (15). MAPKs are the substrates of other kinases, MAPK kinases (MKK), which are also activated by upstream kinases, MKK kinases (MKKK). In multicellular organisms, MAPKs are divided into three subfamilies, including extracellular signal-regulated kinases (ERK)1 and ERK2 (previously termed p42/44), c-Jun N-terminal kinases (JNK1, 2, 3), and p38 MAPK. Substrates for these kinases include other protein kinases, transcription factors, and cytoskeletal proteins. The different MAPKs are involved in cellular responses to cytokines and in the regulation of cytokine expression at the transcriptional level. In addition, p38 MAPK has been shown to play a major role in enhancing the expression of TNF-α at the posttranscriptional level by increasing mRNA stability. JNKs are activated by inflammation-associated cytokines, including TNF-α, IL-1, and IL-6. JNKs bind and phosphorylate c-Jun, a component of the transcription factor AP-1. This pathway plays an important role in cell proliferation and in controlling cell death. In addition, JNKs may be specifically involved in mechanisms of joint damage in arthritis by up-regulating matrix melloproteinase (MMP) expression. There are four p38 MAPKs: α, β, γ, and δ. IL-1 and TNF-α are major activators of p38α and p38β. Because p38 MAPKs are involved in the regulation of proinflammatory cytokines and in cellular responses to cytokines, they are considered as key factors in inflammatory diseases. Administration of p38 MAPK inhibitors had antiinflammatory effects in experimental models of arthritis and of lupus nephritis (16). Clinical trials with p38 MAPK inhibitors in RA patients are in progress.

NFκB is a family of ubiquitously-expressed transcription factors that regulate the expression of different gene products involved in innate and adaptive immune responses. NFκB is present as homo- or heterodimers in the cytoplasm of cells. Many of these NFκB-regulated genes are important in cellular responses to stress, injury, and inflammation. TNF-α, IL-1, products of infectious agents, and proapoptotic and necrotic stimuli activate NFκB. Five members of the NFκB family have been identified in mammalian cells, including p65/RelA, c-Rel, RelB, p50, and p52, but the predominant species in many cell types is p50/p65 heterodimer. Each member of the NFκB family has a conserved N-terminal region termed the Rel homology domain that contains the DNA-binding and dimerization domains, and the nuclear localization signal. NFκB has noncovalent interactions with a class of inhibitors called IκBs that mask its nuclear localization signal and retain NFκB in the cytoplasm. The IκB family includes IκB-α, IκB-β, IκB-γ, IκB-ε, Bcl-3, p100, and p105. Mice with an engineered deletion in the IκB-α gene exhibit perinatal lethality with multiorgan inflammation, suggesting that some of these inhibitors play an important role in maintaining body homeostasis (17,18). Recently, two pathways of NFκB activation have been delineated. One pathway targets most of the NFκB dimers, particularly those containing p65, and is based on the inducible phosphorylation of IκB at two specific serines located in the N-terminal region. IκB phosphorylation is followed by ubiquitination-dependent degradation, thereby allowing NFκB dimers to be translocated into the nucleus (Fig. 19.2). The other pathway is based on inducible processing of p52/p100 precursor. Both pathways depend on the components of the IκB kinase (IKK) complex, which is composed of two catalytic domains (IKK-α and IKK-β) and a regulatory domain IKK-γ (also termed NEMO). IKK-β and IKK-γ are required for IκB phosphorylation and subsequent degradation in response to inflammatory signals, whereas IKK-α is primarily involved in the inducible p100 processing (19). NFκB-inducing kinase (NIK) is not involved in response to inflammatory stimuli, such as TNF-α and IL-1, but is selectively required for gene transcription induced through ligation of LT-β receptors. NIK knockout mice display abnormalities in lymphoid tissue development and antibody responses (20).

The Janus kinase (JAK)/STAT pathway is involved in the cellular signals induced by numerous cytokines, growth factors, and hormones (21). Cytokine receptors lacking catalytic domains mediate ligand-induced activation of protein tyrosine phosphorylation through their association with members of the JAK family of protein kinases, including JAK1, JAK2, JAK3, and TYK2. The activated JAKs phosphorylate specific tyrosine residues of the receptor cytoplasmic domains, thereby creating docking sites for src

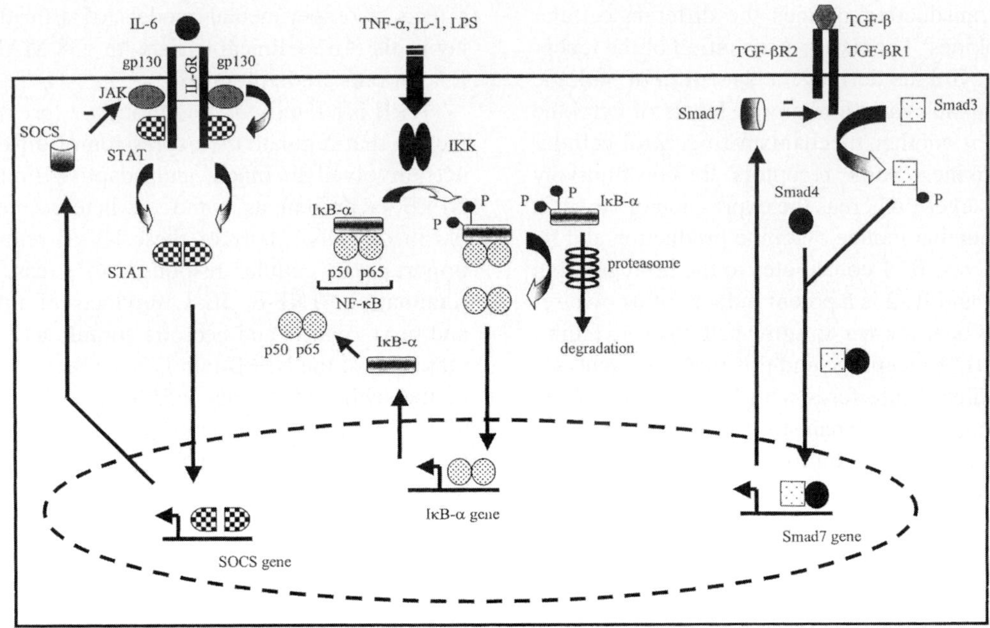

FIG. 19.2. Three examples of induction of intracellular inhibitory pathways. Upon IL-6 binding, the heterodimerization of gp130 induces the tyrosine phosphorylation of JAK, of the cytoplasmic domain of gp130, and of STATs. STAT3 dimers are translocated into the nucleus, where they bind to the promoter region of SOCS and other target genes. SOCS3 inhibits the phosphorylation of JAK and functions as a natural inhibitor of the JAK-STAT cascade. Nuclear factor κB (NFκB) is maintained in the cytoplasm by IκB. Upon cell activation by interleukin-1, tumor necrosis factor-α, lipopolysaccharide, and other inducers, the IκB kinase complex is activated, leading to the phosphorylation of IκB-α. Then, IκB-α is ubiquinated and degraded. Free NFκB migrates into the nucleus and stimulates the expression of IκB-α and other genes. Newly synthesized IκB-α binds to free NFκB in the cytoplasm, leading to the termination of NFκB effects. Transforming growth factor-β (TGF-β) binds to TGF-β receptor type II, leading to the recruitment and phosphorylation of TGF-β receptor type I. Smad3 is phosphorylated by TGF-β receptor type I and binds to Smad4. The Smad complex migrates into the nucleus. Smad7 expression is activated by TGF-β, and Smad7 inhibits TGF-β signaling by blocking the interaction between Smad3 and TGF-β receptor type I.

homology 2 (SH2)-containing signaling proteins. The STAT proteins are a family of transcription factors that contain SH2-binding domains and are recruited to the receptor complex to be phosphorylated. Tyrosine phosphorylation of STATs induces their homo- or heterodimerization and rapid translocation of the dimer into the nucleus (Fig. 19.2). Several STATs also undergo serine phosphorylation. Phosphorylation of Ser727 is of particular interest because it is a potential site for MAPK phosphorylation, thus allowing some cross-talk between STATs and MAPK pathways. In addition to STATs, tyrosine phosphorylation of cytokine receptors can activate other intracellular signals, including the Ras/Raf/MAPK, phosphatidyl-inositol-3 (PI3) kinase, and phospholipase C-γ (PLCγ). The STAT family consists of seven members. STAT1 is primarily involved in responses to IFN. STAT4 is activated by IL-12 and mediates the effect of IL-12 on CD4+ T-cell differentiation along the T_H1 pathway. STAT4-deficient mice exhibit virtually the same phenotype as IL-12 knockout mice. STAT6 is activated by IL-4 and IL-13 and plays a critical role in the development of T_H2 responses. STAT6-deficient mice lack most of the functions induced by IL-4, including the differentiation of T_H2 cells and the ability to produce IgE. STAT3 is stimulated by IL-6-related cytokines, IL-10, and leptin. STAT3 gene deletion results in embryonic lethality. STAT5a and STAT5b are stimulated by a variety of cytokines (IL-2, IL-3, IL-5, IL-7, IL-9, IL-15, and IL-21), CSFs (thrombopoietin, erythropoietin, and GM-CSF), growth factors, and hormones (platelet-derived growth factor, epidermal growth factor, growth hormone, prolactin, and insulin). The phenotypes of STAT5a and STAT5b knockout mice are limited to impaired growth hormone and prolactin signaling as well as IL-2-dependent T-cell functions.

Recently, much attention has been directed toward endogenous signal inhibitors. By gene targeting experiments, it has been possible to demonstrate that these inhibitory signals play an important role in maintaining homeostasis. Overexpression of these inhibitors provided important insight on the role of some signaling pathways in the pathophysiology of rheumatic diseases. Some signals stimulate the production of their own inhibitors (Fig 19.2). Expression of IκB-α is up-regulated in response to NFκB activation, leading to the termination of NFκB effects on gene transcription. Levels of inhibitory Smads, which down-regulate TGF-β signaling, are enhanced in response to TGF-β. The mechanisms regulating the JAK-STAT cascade have been particularly well studied. The suppressors of cytokine signaling (SOCS) family demonstrates a novel mechanism of negative feedback regulation. These inhibitors are also designated cytokine-inducible SH2 (CIS) proteins or STAT-induced STAT inhibitors (SSIs). The eight members of the SOCS family contain an SH2 domain. IL-6 induces the expression of SOCS1, erythropoietin induces SOCS2, TNF-α- and IL-6-related cytokines induce SOCS3, whereas IFN-γ is a potent inducer of all three family members. SOCS1 and SOCS3 play an important role in the regulation of cytokine signals. SOCS1 knockout mice exhibit unbridled IFN-γ signaling with widespread myelomonocytic infiltration of several organs. Blocking IFN-γ can eliminate much of the pathologic phenotype of SOCS1 knockout mice. Expression of SOCS3 was up-regulated in the colon tissue of patients with inflammatory bowel diseases and has been shown to play an important regulatory role in an experimental model of colitis (22). SOCS3 mRNA expression was also enhanced in the synovial samples of RA patients. Forced expression of SOCS3 by adenoviral gene transfer was efficacious both in the prevention and treatment of two experimental models of arthritis (23).

SOLUBLE RECEPTORS

In addition to membrane-associated cytokine receptors, soluble forms have been described for the IL-2R, the TNF receptor (TNFR), IL-6R, IFN-γR, IL-4R, IL-7R, IL-9R, IL-22, GM-CSFR, and Fas. Soluble receptors are generated either by cleavage of the membrane-associated proteins or are products of differentially-spliced mRNAs. Soluble receptors are generated in response to cell activation *in vitro* and may correlate with disease activity in conditions that are associated with activated immune or inflammatory responses (24). Soluble TNFRs bind TNF-α and block its biologic activity (25). In contrast, soluble IL 6Rα binds IL-6, and then the IL-6/sIL-6Rα complex associates with gp130 to activate cellular responses. Soluble forms of cytokine receptors that can inhibit cytokine activity are being tested for therapeutic efficacy. Etanercept, a fusion molecule containing the extracellular portion of TNFR p75, is already approved for the treatment of RA and juvenile idiopathic arthritis (JIA) (see Chapter 39).

CYTOKINES AND THE RHEUMATIC DISEASES

Cytokines are important in rheumatic diseases as mediators of pathogenesis, as markers of pathogenetic mechanisms, in some cases as markers of disease activity, and as tools or targets for new therapeutic interventions. Several control mechanisms protect against pathogenic cytokine effects: (a) transient expression and short half-life of the cytokines and their receptors; (b) the production of antagonistic cytokines or cytokine inhibitors; and (c) negative feedback mechanisms with inhibitors of intracellular signals. Local and systemic manifestations of the rheumatic diseases are the consequence of cytokine-mediated cell activation of inappropriate intensity or duration.

Cytokines and Pathogenesis

Inflammation, destruction of extracellular matrix and parenchymal cells, and the formation of functionally-inadequate repair tissues represent the common local manifestations of rheumatic diseases. Cytokines translate diverse etiologic factors into pathogenic responses and maintain the chronic phase of inflammation and tissue destruction. Using cartilage as an example, mechanisms of cytokine-mediated tissue destruction are summarized in Table 19.3. IL-1 and TNF-α have received the most attention as cytokines that can promote tissue degradation (26). Both cytokines induce the expression of a series of proteases and inhibit the formation of extracellular matrix or stimulate excessive matrix accumulation. IL-1 is also an inhibitor of chondrocyte proliferation and induces in chondrocytes the production of high levels of nitric oxide (NO) (see Chapter 24). NO not only inhibits chondrocyte proliferation, but also inhibits proteoglycan synthesis and induces apoptosis in cultured chondrocytes (27). Cartilage destruction is, in part, the consequence of synovitis in the inflammatory arthropathies and related to chondrocyte-derived catabolic factors in osteoarthritis (OA). As cartilage extracellular matrix is resorbed, there is an attempt at cartilage repair by the remaining chondrocytes, which does not lead to successful restoration of cartilage, but to the production of repair tissue and osteophytes. This latter process is at least partially driven by anabolic factors such as TGF-β. Locally-produced cytokines that reach detectable plasma levels are responsible for the induction of the acute-phase response.

Cytokines and the Treatment of Rheumatic Diseases

Cytokines are targets and tools for therapeutic interventions in rheumatic diseases. The central role of TNF-α and IL-1 in the pathogenesis of rheumatic diseases is now well

TABLE 19.3. *Catabolic effects of interleukin-1 on cartilage*

Induction of	Inhibition of
Proteases	Collagen II synthesis
Prostaglandin E_2	Proteoglycan synthesis
Nitric oxide	Chondrocyte proliferation
Oxygen radicals	
Proinflammatory cytokines	

demonstrated. The results of *in vitro* and *in vivo* experiments indicate that additional cytokines, including IL-6, IL-7, IL-15, and IL-18, also contribute to the pathophysiology of rheumatic diseases. In contrast, some cytokines, such as IL-4, TGF-β, IL-10, and IL-13, are considered antiinflammatory cytokines. However, the function of cytokines in the maintenance of body homeostasis and in the pathogenic mechanisms of rheumatic diseases is complex, and the separation between deleterious and protective cytokines is artificial. TNF-α, IL-18, and IL-1 exert proinflammatory activities in RA but also have important functions in host responses against infections. In addition, as demonstrated in animal models and in patients treated with TNF-α inhibitors, TNF-α controls the development of autoimmunity. IL-10 has been shown to play an important role in the pathophysiology of systemic lupus erythromatosus (SLE). TGF-β and other growth factors play a critical role in the progression of skin and organ fibrosis in systemic sclerosis (SSc). TGF-β exerts a protective effect on articular cartilage, but stimulates the development of osteophytes.

Currently, TNF-α and IL-1 are the most prominent targets for inhibition of cytokine function as an antirheumatic therapy. Cytokine-based therapeutic interventions can be directed toward using cytokines therapeutically or inhibiting their production or activities (Table 19.4). Problems in using cytokines or soluble cytokine receptors in the treatment of chronic diseases are the relatively short half-life of the administered proteins. Novel approaches, such as using fusion proteins containing some of the extracellular binding motifs of cytokines coupled to the Fc fraction of human immunoglobulin IgG, may overcome this problem (28). Gene therapy also provides a potential approach to achieve prolonged increases in circulating or local levels of cytokines (see Chapter 37). However, technical problems regarding the duration of cytokine expression and safety issues should be solved before adopting the clinical use of gene transfer in the treatment of rheumatic diseases. A potential problem in inhibiting specific cytokines as a therapeutic approach for chronic rheumatic diseases relates to the overlapping biologic activities of different cytokines. This problem can possibly be addressed by simultaneously using inhibitors of different cytokines. Alternatively, it appears possible to target intracellular messengers, such as p38 MAPK, NFκB, or JNK pathways, that are commonly used by several pathogenic cytokines.

TABLE 19.4. *Inhibition of cytokine activity*

Monoclonal antibody to ligand
Monoclonal antibody to receptor
Soluble receptor
Immunoglobulin/receptor fusion protein
Antisense oligonucleotides
Ribozymes, RNAi
Peptides corresponding to sites of ligand binding to receptor
Nonpeptide inhibitors of cell signaling
Inhibitors of cytokine processing enzymes

RNAi, interference RNA

TUMOR NECROSIS FACTOR AND RELATED CYTOKINES

The TNFs are part of what is now known as a large family of functionally-diverse cytokines. The members of the TNF receptor family regulate a large number of cellular functions that are closely involved in the pathogenesis of inflammatory disorders, including immune-mediated diseases and infectious conditions. The number of receptors and corresponding ligands has rapidly expanded during the past decade. The identification of their biologic function has already led to the development of different strategies targeting TNF family members in the treatment of autoimmune diseases. Among these approaches, the use of TNF-α inhibitors is now widely accepted in the treatment of a variety of inflammatory conditions, including RA, spondyloarthropathies, and inflammatory bowel diseases.

The family of TNFRs and ligands share several common structural features. All the receptors are type I transmembrane proteins with conserved, cysteine-rich motifs and a certain degree of extracellular homology. In contrast, no significant homology exists in the intracellular domains. A certain number of receptors, including Fas, TNF-α receptor p55, some TRAIL receptors (DR4 and DR5), DR3, and DR6, have a cytoplasmic death domain that is responsible for transducing the apoptosis signal (29,30). In addition, despite the lack of cytoplasmic death domain, the Hodgkin antigen DR30 can also act as a proapoptosis receptor (31).

All the members of the ligand family are type II transmembrane proteins that are expressed both as membrane-bound and soluble forms. Oligomerization of the receptor as a consequence of ligand binding is required to induce intracellular responses. Immune cells can express at their surface either the ligand, the receptor, or both. Thus, the interactions between ligands and their cognate receptors can mediate either paracrine or autocrine effects. In addition to cell membrane–bound receptors, within this family, soluble forms have been described for the low-affinity nerve growth factor (NGF) receptor, two TNF-α receptors (p55 and p75), CD27, and Fas. Soluble TNFRs appear to be generated by proteolytic cleavage of the membrane-associated forms since for each of these receptors only a single mRNA species has been detected. In contrast, a soluble form of the Fas molecule originates from an RNA splice variant. Osteoprotegerin (OPG) is produced as a secreted protein and acts as a decoy receptor for the receptor activator of NFκB ligand (RANKL) (32). The soluble forms of TNF-α receptors (p55 and p75) bind to their ligand, TNF-α, and prevent its interaction with cell surface receptors, thus acting as natural inhibitors. The soluble form of Fas is also biologically active and inhibits apoptosis induced by an agonistic antibody. The use of recombinant forms of the soluble receptors that contain the entire extracellular regions, or parts thereof, has provided important tools in characterizing the biologic functions of their ligands.

The members of TNF receptor superfamily can deliver signals leading to cell death or to survival and proliferation. Some of the receptors, such as TNFR p55, LT-β receptor, and DR3, are able to transduce both types of signals (30,33). Differentiation between apoptosis and survival signals are dependent on cell type and functional status. Stimulation of cells through the TNFR p55 and Fas can induce apoptosis through the use of cytoplasmic death domain and activation of the enzymatic caspase cascade. One of the most important functions of death receptors is the maintenance of tolerance through the activation-induced cell death of immune cells. Activated T cells express Fas and its ligand (FasL), thereby enabling apoptosis in an autocrine fashion. Defective expression of Fas or FasL leads to the development of lymphoid proliferation and autoimmune manifestations (34,35). In contrast, the stimulatory signals are mediated through activation of the NFκB pathway.

Function of Tumor Necrosis Factor and Related Cytokines

TNF-α primarily originates from mononuclear phagocytes, and its production can be induced by similar stimuli. TNF-α is synthesized as a 27-kd transmembrane protein that is cleaved from the cell surface by TACE to generate a secreted 17-kd mature form (36,37). Biologic effects of TNF-α that are relevant to rheumatic diseases include activation of macrophages and polymorphonuclear (PMN) leukocytes, stimulation of T- and B-cell proliferation, stimulation of proinflammatory cytokines in different cell types, NO release, enhancement of fibroblast proliferation, secretion of collagenase and prostaglandin E_2 (PGE_2) by fibroblasts, and the resorption of bone and cartilage (26). Systemic effects of TNF-α are similar to those of IL-1. It also contributes to stimulation of acute-phase responses, including weight loss, fever, metabolic changes, and anemia. Peripheral blood mononuclear cell (PBMC) supernatants from anemic RA patients suppressed erythropoiesis, which was almost completely neutralized by antibodies to TNF-α (38). TNF-α effects on energy metabolism in RA have been suggested on the basis of correlations between elevated TNF-α plasma levels and reduced lean body mass.

LT-α, LT-β, and TNF-α are structurally related and are encoded by genes located within the major histocompatibility complex (MHC) genes on chromosome 6. The genes encoding LT and TNF-α are highly homologous and apparently derive from an ancestor gene (39). Although TNF-α is predominantly produced by monocytes and macrophages, LT-α and LT-β expression is restricted to activated lymphocytes, natural killer (NK) cells, and a subset of $CD4^+$ $CD3^-$ cells (40,41). LT-α lacks a transmembrane domain and is secreted as a homotrimer (LT3-α) or interacts with membrane-bound LT-β to form a heterotrimer, LT-α1β2. LT-α has only approximately 30% sequence homology with TNF-α, but it binds to the same receptors and has similar effects *in vitro*. In contrast, LT-α1β2 signals through a distinct receptor (LT-βR). Studies with gene-targeted mice showed that TNF-α plays a major role in host defense and regulation of inflammatory responses, and is also involved in the formation of germinal centers and in the maturation of the humoral immune response (42). LT-βR signaling is essential in the development of lymph nodes, Peyer patches, and the organization of the white pulp of the spleen (43). The deletion of the entire TNF/LT locus by gene targeting supported that TNF-α and LT exhibit essentially nonredundant functions *in vivo* (44).

Tumor Necrosis Factor-α and Experimental Models of Arthritis

Several studies in experimental models of arthritis suggested that TNF-α and IL-1 might exert different effects. TNF-α plays an important role in the induction of synovial inflammation, whereas IL-1 could be predominantly involved in the mechanisms leading to cartilage destruction (45). Intraarticular injection of TNF-α into rabbit knees induced infiltration of leukocytes, but did not cause significant proteoglycan loss from cartilage. The nature of the leukocytic infiltrate induced by TNF-α was predominantly monocytic, compared with the mixed PMN/monocytic infiltrate induced by IL-1. On a molar basis, TNF-α was significantly less active than IL-1 in causing cell accumulation in the joint. Injection of submaximal doses of IL-1 and TNF-α resulted in a marked synergy with respect to PMN accumulation. Transgenic mice carrying a TNF-α transgene developed chronic inflammatory polyarthritis, which was completely prevented by treatment with a monoclonal antibody against TNF-α. The therapeutic value of inhibiting TNF-α activity has been examined in experimentally-induced arthritis. In mice with collagen-induced arthritis (CIA), TNF-α receptor Fc fusion protein or anti-TNF-α antibody significantly reduced both the incidence and the severity of arthritis, when administered during the induction of the disease. Varying results were obtained with respect to effects on established disease and anticollagen antibody production (46,47).

Tumor Necrosis Factor-α Expression in Rheumatoid Arthritis

RA synovial fluids (SFs) contain TNF-α and soluble TNFRs that inhibit TNF activity in cytolytic assays (48,49). LT was not detected in any RA sera or SFs. RA patients with detectable TNF-α had higher erythrocyte sedimentation rates and SF leukocyte counts. TNF-sR55 and TNF-sR75 were present in SF, and their concentrations were higher in SF from patients with seropositive RA than in patients with other inflammatory arthritides (50). The SF levels of soluble TNFR were higher than levels in serum, suggesting local production in the joint (51). TNF-α was secreted by SF mononuclear cells and tissues from patients with various forms of arthropathies. By immunohistochemistry, TNF-α was localized to mononuclear cells in the lining layer, sublining, and perivascular areas of synovial tissue (52). TNF-α and TNFRs have a similar distribution, suggesting that TNF-α has the potential for autocrine and paracrine activity in the joint (53), which was demonstrated in freshly isolated cells from SF or synovial membrane. These cultures showed prolonged expression of IL-1α and IL-1β mRNA, which was reduced by anti-TNF-α but not anti-LT antibody, suggesting that TNF-α may be a main inducer of IL-1. In transgenic mice overexpressing human TNF-α, the administration of antibodies blocking IL-1 signaling completely prevented the development of arthritis, suggesting that IL-1 mediated the effects of TNF-α in this animal model. TNF-α is also able to induce the expression of IL-6, IL-8, and GM-CSF in different experimental systems. These results led to the hypothesis that a cytokine network is present in rheumatoid synovium with TNF-α at its apex. Indeed, TNF-α is the first cytokine for which successful cytokine-directed intervention has been demonstrated in human arthritis. The results of clinical trials in RA patients are reviewed in detail in Chapter 39.

Tumor Necrosis Factor-α and Systemic Lupus Erythematosus

Presently available data do not permit a clear assessment of the role of TNF-α in human SLE or in murine models of SLE. Evidence has been presented to indicate involvement of TNF-α in the genetic predisposition to murine SLE (54). This concept was based on unexpected initial findings in the New Zealand black (NZB) × New Zealand white (NZW) F1 mouse. The severe form of the disease found in F1 mice is due in part to dominant NZW genes mapping within the murine MHC, where the TNF-α gene is located. A restriction fragment length polymorphism in the TNF-α gene was identified, and it correlated with reduced levels of TNF-α produced by these mice (55). Replacement therapy with recombinant TNF-α significantly delayed the development of lupuslike nephritis. However, there is also evidence of a role for TNF-α in local manifestations of murine lupus, such as in the development of autoimmune pulmonary inflammation. TNF-α mRNA levels in lung preparations of lupus-prone mice were elevated, and antibodies to TNF-α prevented the development of pulmonary lesions (56). Furthermore, the findings obtained from (NZB × NZW) F1 mice also differed from MRL-*lpr/lpr* mice, which produce increased levels of TNF-α as the disease progresses (57).

Several studies examined TNF-α production by cells from patients with SLE. One report suggested that *in vitro* activated monocytes from patients with SLE produced significantly lower amounts of TNF-α mRNA and protein than normal monocytes (58). However, spontaneous synthesis of TNF-α in nonstimulated cultures was increased in the SLE patients (59). Circulating TNF-α does not appear to be depressed in human SLE, although elevated serum levels of TNF-α were observed in only 29% of patients with SLE as compared to 46% of patients with RA (60). In SLE patients with infection, the level of TNF-α in the circulation increased (61). The mean concentrations of both the p55 (type I) and p75 (type II) soluble TNFR were significantly higher in SLE patients than in controls and correlated with disease activity (62). The concentrations of soluble TNFR present in SLE serum effectively inhibit TNF-α bioactivity and, thus, represent an additional variable that determines available levels of biologically-active TNF-α.

The use of TNF-α inhibitors in clinical practice has shed some light on the potential role of TNF-α in the regulation of autoimmunity and in downstream inflammatory events. In clinical trials, the presence of antinuclear and anti–double stranded DNA antibodies was detected in a larger percentage of treated patients with RA or ankylosing spondylitis than in those receiving a placebo. In addition, a limited number of patients developed clinical signs of lupuslike syndrome that disappeared after discontinuation of TNF-α inhibitors (63). However, TNF-α also plays an important role in the inflammatory processes that are present in target organs, as exemplified by the positive results obtained following the administration of antibody to TNF-α to patients with severe lupus nephritis (64).

Tumor Necrosis Factor-α and Spondyloarthropathies

Elevated levels of TNF-α were detected in the circulation and SF of some patients with spondyloarthropathies. In addition, the presence of TNF-α messenger RNA and protein was detected in sacroiliac joints at the site of inflammation (65). These findings provided a rationale for the use of TNF inhibitors, such as thalidomide, which is thought to decrease the production of TNF-α, and biologic agents blocking TNF-α. The results of clinical trials with TNF-blocking agents in ankylosing spondylitis and psoriatic arthritis have further substantiated the importance of TNF-α in these diseases (66). Treatment of ankylosing spondylitis with a monoclonal antibody to TNF-α (infliximab) or with a soluble TNFR (etanercept) led to significant improvements in clinical and serologic evidence of active disease in the axial skeleton (66–69). In a similar fashion, patients with psoriasis and active peripheral arthritis exhibited significant responses to treatment with etanercept (70).

Nerve Growth Factor

NGF levels are increased in the synovium of patients with RA and in the synovium of animals with experimentally induced arthritis. Transgenic mice with the human

TNF gene also express elevated levels of NGF. The levels of NGF in mice were enhanced by the intraarticular injection of TNF-α and IL-1 (71). On the other hand, NGF regulates the production of TNF-α in experimental models of arthritis (72). Subcutaneous injection of NGF antibodies attenuated the loss of body weight caused by the development of disease in these mice. Increased numbers of synovial mast cells occurred in the transgenic mice and suggest a functional link between NGF and mast cells (73). Interestingly, rapid healing of vasculitic ulcers was observed in RA patients treated with topical NGF. This effect may be related to the activity of NGF on neoangiogenesis and keratinocyte proliferation (74).

Fas (CD95)/APO-1

Fas/APO-1 was discovered as a cell membrane receptor that, upon activation by specific antibody, triggered cell death by apoptosis. The *lpr* mutation in the MRL strain of mice is caused by the insertion of a transposable element in the Fas gene. The insertion causes a decrease in Fas mRNA expression, and the Fas protein is not expressed on resting or activated lymphocytes from MRL *lpr/lpr* mice. Fas may play a role in both thymic selection and T-cell survival in the periphery, and the accelerated autoimmunity in MRL *lpr/lpr* mice likely results from a defect in these pathways (75).

FasL is a transmembrane protein that induces apoptosis in Fas-expressing target cells. FasL is expressed on activated splenocytes and thymocytes, consistent with its involvement in T cell–mediated cytotoxicity (76). The MRL mouse strain with generalized lymphadenopathy (*gld*) develops autoimmune manifestations similar to those of the *lpr* strain. The *gld* mutation is a point mutation in the FasL gene that abolishes binding to its receptor (Fas). Because wild-type MRL mice also develop mild forms of autoimmune disease, it appears that the *lpr* and *gld* mutations lead to a more severe and accelerated manifestation of an underlying predisposition to autoimmune disease. Mutations of the Fas gene can result in a rare and severe autoimmune lymphoproliferative syndrome (Canale-Smith syndrome) in humans (77). In addition, defective Fas-mediated apoptosis secondary to the presence of mutations of the Fas gene can also represent a risk factor for lymphoma (78). A potential association between impairment in the induction of apoptosis and SLE has been suggested. PBMCs from SLE patients produced increased levels of a soluble form of Fas. This soluble receptor competes for binding with FasL and protects cells from apoptosis (79). The potential role of defective apoptosis can also contribute to the development of synovial pannus in RA. FasL is present at the surface of synovial fibroblasts (80). Naturally-processed, soluble FasL is present in high amounts in the SF of patients with RA. As opposed to its membrane-bound form, soluble form FasL did not induce apoptosis (80). Thus, the accumulation of soluble FasL in rheumatoid joints may exert a protective effect against Fas-induced apoptosis.

CD40 and CD40 Ligand

The interaction of CD40 ligand (CD40L; or CD154) on activated T cells with CD40 on B cells induces B-cell proliferation and formation of germinal centers. Within germinal centers, further CD40/CD40L interactions lead to B-cell maturation through immunoglobulin isotype class switching, somatic mutation, clonal expansion of specific B cells, and terminal differentiation to plasma cells. CD40 ligation on memory B lymphocytes is also required for their activation and terminal differentiation during secondary antibody responses (81). CD40L/CD40 interaction promoted the differentiation of dendritic cells (82). It was suggested that CD40L could participate in the perpetuation of RA (83). Interactions of CD40 and CD40L activated production of IL-1, IL-6, IL-8, and TNF-α from monocytes, dendritic cells, and fibroblasts and augmented the expression of adhesion molecules and metalloproteinase (84–88). CD40 engagement stimulated the production of vascular endothelial growth factor (VGEF) by synovial fibroblasts, thereby promoting the neovascularization of the synovial pannus (89). Administration of CD40L antibodies reduced severity of CIA in mice with an associated decrease in the titers of antibodies to type II collagen (90). Both human and murine SLE are characterized by aberrantly increased expression of CD40L on T cells and production of autoreactive B cells (91,92). Studies in experimental models of SLE demonstrated that administration of antibodies against CD40L was effective in delaying the onset of disease and ameliorating the course of established nephritis (93,94). In patients with SLE, a brief period of treatment with a humanized monoclonal anti-CD40L antibody resulted in improvement of serologic markers (levels of anti-DNA antibodies) and hematuria. However, the occurrence of severe side effects, including myocardial infarctions and thromboembolic events, led to the premature cessation of the trial (95). In contrast, the result of a recent trial with another humanized monoclonal anti-CD40L antibody in SLE patients was not associated with thrombotic events but demonstrated no significant effect on disease activity (96). Thus, further studies are needed to further explore the efficacy of targeting CD40/CD40L interactions in the treatment of autoimmune diseases.

RANK Ligand and Osteoprotegerin

RANKL regulates osteoclast differentiation and activity through binding to its receptor RANK (97). RANKL is also known as osteoprotegerin ligand (OPGL), TNF-related activation-induced cytokine (TRANCE), and osteoclast differentiating factor (ODF). RANK is expressed on osteoclast progenitors and mature osteoclasts. RANKL can activate mature osteoclasts and promote osteoclastogenesis in the presence of CSF-1. It is expressed by osteoblasts and can be up-regulated by the bone-resorbing factors vitamin D_3, IL-11, PGE_2, and parathyroid hormone (98). Mice with a disrupted RANKL gene show severe osteopetrosis and a complete lack of osteoclasts (99). In addition, RANKL regulates lymph node development and interactions between dendritic cells and lymphocytes (99). RANKL expression is up-regulated in T cells following antigen receptor engagement. It is detected at the surface of activated, but not resting, T lymphocytes. RANKL is also released by activated T cells, suggesting that activated T cells may regulate bone metabolism through activation of RANK signaling. Systemic activation of T cells *in vivo* leads to a RANKL-mediated increase in osteoclastogenesis and bone loss (100). Upon ligand binding, RANK recruits adapter protein TRAF6, thereby leading to the activation of NFκB and c-Jun N-terminal kinase pathways. Mice deficient in TRAF6 have osteopetrosis, indicating that TRAF6 plays an essential role in RANK signaling (101).

OPG was originally identified by sequence homology as a new member of the TNF receptor family (32). OPG does not contain a transmembrane domain and is secreted as a soluble decoy receptor. OPG binds OPGL and, thereby, prevents this cytokine from activating the RANK.

Synovial fibroblasts and T cells from the rheumatoid synovium express RANKL, suggesting that this cytokine plays an important role in the development of bone erosions. The best support for the role of RANKL in the development of articular erosions was obtained with the use of its inhibitor. The administration of recombinant OPG to rats with adjuvant-induced arthritis had minimal effect on synovial inflammation but almost completely abolished the development of bony erosions (100). Similar findings were observed in CIA in the rat and in TNF-α transgenic mice (102,103).

B-Cell Activating Factor of the Tumor Necrosis Factor Family and Related Molecules

B-cell activating factor of the TNF family (BAFF) is a novel member of the TNF family and an essential component of B-cell homeostasis. BAFF can be found in the literature under several other names, such as BlyS (B-lymphocyte stimulator), TALL-1 (TNF- and ApoL-related leukocyte-expressed ligand 1), THANK (TNF homologue that activates apoptosis, NFκB, and JNK), TNFSF13B (TNF-superfamily member 13B), and zTNF4. BAFF is a homotrimer that is found at the cell surface or as a soluble protein that binds three different receptors, including BCMA (B-cell maturation antigen), TACI (transmembrane activator and calcium-modulator and cyclophilin ligand interactor), and BAFF-R (BAFF receptor) (104). BAFF-R is the only receptor that specifically binds BAFF. These receptors are expressed primarily on the B-cell lineage but also to a lesser extent on T-cells. Dendritic cells, macrophages, and monocytes produce BAFF, and its expression is up-regulated by IFN-γ and IL-10 (105–107). BAFF is a crucial mediator for survival of transitional and mature B cells. In contrast, BAFF overexpression leads to B-cell hyperplasia and to the development of autoimmune manifestations suggestive of an SLE-like disease, including anti-DNA antibodies and renal deposition of immune complexes (108,109). As BAFF transgenic mice get older, they develop a condition similar to human Sjögren's syndrome. Elevated circulating levels of BAFF can be detected in patients with SLE, RA, and primary Sjögren's syndrome (30). In RA patients, BAFF levels in the SF greatly exceeded the levels in the blood (110). In addition, BAFF was also highly expressed in the rheumatoid synovium and in salivary glands of patients with Sjögren's syndrome (111).

APRIL (a proliferation-inducing ligand) is closely related to BAFF and is expressed as a secreted protein. APRIL binds to TACI and BCMA, but in contrast to BAFF, the biologic function of APRIL is still not clear. Overexpression of transgenic TACI-Ig, an inhibitor of APRIL, does not modify the B-cell compartment. Overexpression of APRIL in T-cells enhanced their survival *in vitro* and *in vivo*, and enhanced the T-independent type 2 humoral response (112). As is the case with all of the different members of the TNF family, APRIL is generally expressed as a homotrimer. However, APRIL and BAFF can also form heterotrimeric molecules, which are capable of inducing B-cell proliferation *in vitro*. Elevated levels of these heterotrimers were detected in the circulation of patients with inflammatory rheumatic diseases, suggesting that BAFF/APRIL heterotrimers may play a role in the development of autoimmunity (113).

TNF-related apoptosis-inducing ligand (TRAIL), also known as Apo2 ligand, is a transmembrane protein. Like other members of the TNF ligand family, TRAIL induces apoptosis in a variety of cell types (114,115). In particular, TRAIL limits its activities to tumor cells. A variety of immune cells such as CD4$^+$ T cells, NK cells, macrophages, and dendritic cells express TRAIL. TRAIL could play a substantial role in suppressing tumor metastasis and in the control of virus-induced diseases. Recent findings have indicated that TRAIL is expressed on salivary gland–infiltrating T cells and thus may be involved in the pathology of Sjögren's disease (116). TRAIL, like FasL, may also play a role in preventing the development of autoimmunity. Blocking TRAIL in mice enhances the proliferation of autoreactive lymphocytes, leading to arthritis and joint destruction (117).

INTERLEUKIN-1 AND RELATED CYTOKINES

Interleukin-1 Family Members

The IL-1 family of cytokines includes three different members: two agonists, IL-1α and IL-1β, and a natural inhibitor, IL-1Ra. IL-1α and IL-1β are encoded by two different genes and share 26% amino acid homology. Both forms are synthesized as 31-kd precursor peptides (pro-IL-1α and pro-IL-1β), which are specifically cleaved to generate 17-kd mature IL-1α and IL-1β. IL-1β is primarily produced by macrophages and is primarily secreted after cleavage of its proform by IL-1β-convertase enzyme

(ICE, also termed caspase 1). In addition, pro-IL-1β can be processed by other enzymes in the absence of ICE. IL-1β is produced without a hydrophobic leader peptide and, thus, does not follow the typical secretion pathway. Recently, it has become apparent that IL-1β can be secreted either through the exocytosis of endoplasmic vesicles or can be rapidly released by microvesicles budding off the cell membrane (118,119). In contrast, IL-1α is expressed as a 31-kd intracellular or membrane-bound protein in the human. An important distinction between these two molecules is that pro-IL-1β is biologically inactive, whereas both pro-IL-1α and mature IL-1α exhibit full receptor binding activity. In addition to its biologic effects following receptor binding, IL-1α exerts other functions inside cells. Intracellular IL-1α can regulate cell migration, cell proliferation, and cytokine production (120–122). The IL-1α 16-kd amino-terminal propiece contains a nuclear localization sequence, and this 16-kd propiece migrates into the nucleus where it can act as a transforming oncoprotein or induce the apoptosis of malignant but not of normal cell lines (123,124).

IL-18 has structural similarities with the IL-1 family of proteins. In addition, six additional novel IL-1 members have recently been identified, which expand the IL-1 family to 10 different members. The recently proposed nomenclature for the IL-1 family is IL-1F1 (IL-1α), IL-1F2 (IL-1β), IL-1F3 (IL-1Ra), IL-1F4 (IL-18), IL-1F5 (IL-1H3, IL-1Hy1, FIL1δ, IL-1RP3, IL-1L1, IL-1δ), IL-1F6 (FIL1ϵ), IL-1F7 (IL-1H4, FIL1ζ, IL-1RP1, IL-1H), IL-1F8 (IL-1H2 and FILη) IL-1F9 (IL-1H1, IL-1RP2, IL-1ϵ), and IL-1F10 (IL-1Hy2 and FKSG75) (125). The genes encoding for IL-1α, IL-1β, IL-1Ra, and the six novel members form a cluster on the long arm of chromosome 2. IL-18 and its binding protein are located on chromosome 11.

IL-1R antagonist (IL-1Ra) is the third member of the IL-1 family. IL-1Ra binds to cell surface IL-1 receptors with the same affinity as IL-1, but does not stimulate any intracellular response. IL-1Ra competitively prevents the interactions between IL-1 and its target cells. However, a large amount of IL-1Ra is necessary to block the biologic effects of IL-1 because binding of only a few molecules of IL-1 per cell suffices to stimulate a full biologic response. IL-1Ra is produced as four different isoforms. One isoform has a hydrophobic leader peptide and is secreted (sIL-1Ra), whereas the three others are intracellular (icIL-1Ra1, 2, 3). These different IL-1Ra peptides are produced from the same gene by the use of alternate first exons, alternative mRNA splicing, or alternative translation initiation (126).

Interleukin-1 Receptor Family Members

Three types of IL-1 receptors exist as both membrane-bound and soluble forms, including IL-1 receptor type I (IL-1RI), IL-1RII, and IL-1R accessory protein (IL-1RAcP). The extracellular domains of the three types of IL-1 receptors belong to the immunoglobulin (Ig) superfamily and share some amino-acid sequence homology. In addition, the cytoplasmic domains of three types of IL-1 receptors exhibit a sequence homology with Toll-like receptors. The most striking structural difference between IL-1RI and IL-1RII is the short cytoplasmic domain of IL-1RII (29 amino acids), whereas IL-1RI possesses a cytoplasmic tail of 213 residues. After ligand binding, intracellular signaling occurs only through IL-1RI. IL-1RI binds to IL-1α with highest affinity, and IL-1RII binds to IL-1β with highest affinity. IL-1Ra binds to IL-1R with the same affinity as IL-1α; thus, when both receptors are expressed at the cell surface, IL-1Ra will preferentially bind to IL-1RI (127).

IL-1 treatment of cells induces the formation of a complex of high affinity containing IL-1RI and IL-1RAcP. Cells that express IL-1RI but lack IL-1RAcP are not responsive to IL-1, indicating that the IL-1 signal transduction machinery is dependent on the presence of IL-1RAcP (128). IL-1 activates cells through the NF-κB, JNK/AP-1, p38 MAPK, and ERK1/ERK2 transduction pathways. After formation of the complex between IL-1, IL-1RI, and IL-1RAcP, the intracellular domains of IL-1RI and IL-1RAcP recruit two cytosolic adapter proteins: myeloid differentiation factor 88 (MyD88) and Tollip (129,130). These molecules recruit IL-1R-associated kinases (IRAK), a family of serine-threonine kinases, which are then phosphorylated at the receptor complex and dissociate to interact with TRAF6 (131). IRAK includes four different homologous proteins, namely IRAK-1, IRAK-2, IRAK-M, and IRAK-4. IRAK-4 has recently been shown to be indispensable for the responses to IL-1R and other Toll-like receptors (132). To activate the NFκB pathway, TRAF6 stimulates IKK activity. However, TRAF6 also activates the JNK/AP-1 pathway through a different domain, which does not require TRAF6 phosphorylation (130). Evidence of tyrosine kinase activation by IL-1 has been provided in several cell systems, including T lymphocytes and chondrocytes. Pharmacologic inhibitors of tyrosine kinases interfered with the induction of most IL-1-responsive genes in chondrocytes (133). New approaches to inhibit pathogenic effects of IL-1 by interfering with intracellular signaling events are currently under investigation. Promising results for therapy in humans have been obtained by using pharmacologic inhibitors of NFκB and JNK/AP-1 pathways in animal models of arthritis (134,135).

IL-1RII may exist on the cell surface or in a soluble form as a decoy molecule (136). Soluble IL-1RII is found in biologic fluids in a variety of pathophysiologic conditions. Glucocorticoids, IL-4, LPS, and TNF-α stimulate expression or release of IL-1RII. Soluble IL-1RII can be generated by proteolysis of the extracellular domain by matrix metalloproteases (137) or by alternative splicing of a primary transcript leading to a secreted protein (138). Soluble IL-1RII binds IL-1β with high avidity and prevents its interaction with cell surface IL-1RI. Thus, soluble IL-1RII acts as a naturally-occurring IL-1 inhibitor. Adenovirally transduced chondrocytes and synovial fibroblasts expressing IL-1RII were resistant to IL-1β-stimulated production of IL-6, CXCL8/IL-8, PGE_2, and NO (139). In contrast, soluble IL-1RII binds IL-1Ra with a much lower affinity than IL-1β and may supplement the antiinflammatory effects of IL-1Ra (140). In addition, membrane-bound IL-1RII also has an inhibitory effect on IL-1 responses, which is probably related to a ligand sink function (141).

In addition to IL-1R and IL-18 receptors, five other members of the IL-1R family are known, including T1/ST2, IL-1R rp2, APL, TIGIRR (or APL-2), and SIGIRR. T1/ST2 and IL-1R rp2 have a structural homology with the members of the IL-1R and IL-18R complexes. APL, TIGIRR, and SIGIRR contain additions of approximately 100 amino acids on their carboxyl-terminal tail. The other structural variation is the presence of a single Ig domain in the extracellular region of SIGIRR rather than the usual three (142). Limited information is available regarding the function and the putative ligands of the IL-1R homologues. In Jurkat cells transfected with IL-1R rp2, IL-1F9 can activate NFκB, and this effect is inhibited by IL-1F5 (143). T1/ST2 is expressed on T-helper type 2 (T_H2) lymphocytes, and some evidence indicates that T1/ST2 plays an important role in T_H2 responses (IL-4, IL-5, IgE production) (144). IL-7Fb binds to IL-18Rα but fails to recruit IL-18Rβ and thus, does not exhibit any agonist or antagonist activity. However, IL-1F7b binds to IL-18 binding protein and forms a molecular complex with IL-18Rβ, thus inhibiting IL-18 activity (145).

Function of Interleukin-1

IL-1 is an important regulator of host defense responses. Monocytes and macrophages are the primary sources of IL-1, but it is expressed in different tissues during different types of inflammatory responses. Most cells that produce IL-1 also produce its antagonist, IL-1Ra. The balance between IL-1 and IL-1Ra has important functional consequences. Interestingly, IL-1 has been shown to induce the synthesis of IL-1Ra in different models, thus producing a negative feedback mechanism that actively regulates the inflammatory response. In addition, the biologic effects of IL-1 reflect direct effects on target cells and indirect effects that are also regulated by other mediators, including a large number of cytokines.

Immune Response and Inflammation

IL-1 is an important regulator of immune function. It serves as a monocyte-derived costimulatory molecule in T-cell activation and enhances B-cell proliferation in response to antigens or antibodies to cell surface immunoglobulin. In monocytes, IL-1 can induce its own synthesis and that of a large number of other cytokines. IL-1 is known to activate mature neutrophils and enhance superoxide (O_2^-) release, chemotaxis, and degranulation (146–150). IL-1 also promotes neutrophil spreading and prolongs neutrophil survival (151).

An additional important effect in the early phases of proinflammatory responses is the IL-1 activation of endothelial cells with the induction of adhesion molecules, cytokine production, NO, tissue plasminogen activator production (152), and increased vascular permeability (153). IL-1 induces phospholipase A_2 activity and the expression of cyclooxygenase-2 with consequent production of PGE_2.

Systemic Effects of Interleukin-1

In addition to its local effects at the site of tissue injury, IL-1 mediates systemic effects on the bone marrow, liver, and central nervous system (CNS) (127). IL-1 induces somnolence, depression, anorexia, and neuroendocrine changes and stimulates the release of corticotropin-releasing hormone, with consequent stimulation of corticotropin and cortisol production. IL-1 regulates the central control of food intake in the hypothalamus. Humans injected with IL-1 experienced fever, myalgia, headache, and arthralgias, each of which was reduced by the administration of cyclooxygenase (COX) inhibitors, indicating that these effects were mediated by PGE_2. IL-1β induces COX-2 in the CNS, which then contributes to pain hypersensitivity. This phenomenon may play an important role in the generalized illness behavioral syndrome of infectious diseases and in the occurrence of hyperalgesia secondary to central sensitization (154). IL-1 causes a dose-dependent decrease in systolic blood pressure, probably due to induction of NO. IL-1 directly, and indirectly through the stimulation of other cytokines including IL-6 family members, stimulates the production of acute-phase proteins. IL-1 has direct and indirect effects on hematopoiesis, resulting in anemia in chronic inflammatory diseases, neutrophilia, and thrombocytosis. Moreover, IL-1 contributes to cachexia that is present in chronic diseases, including decreases in skeletal muscle, fat tissue, as well as bone loss (155).

The Balance Between Interleukin-1 and Interleukin-1 Receptor Antagonist

The balance between IL-1 and IL-1Ra plays a critical role in the course of a variety of inflammatory diseases, including inflammatory bowel disease, sepsis, fulminant hepatitis, and liver graft rejection. The physiologic function of endogenous IL-1Ra has been further demonstrated in several studies by using blocking antibodies against IL-1Ra and with IL-1Ra gene knockout mice. Mice lacking the expression of IL-1Ra were more susceptible to endotoxin-induced lethality. In contrast, transgenic mice overexpressing IL-1Ra were protected from endotoxin-induced lethality but were more susceptible to *Listeria* infection, indicating that the IL-1/IL-1Ra ratio plays an important role in host defense (156). IL-1Ra knockout mice had a significantly earlier onset of CIA and more severe synovitis, often accompanied by bony erosions (157). Most interestingly, the absence of IL-1Ra by gene deletion in BALB/cA mice was associated with the spontaneous development of chronic polyarthritis with the presence of autoantibodies, thus reproducing some of the clinical and biologic features of RA (158). An arterial inflammatory disease resembling polyarteritis nodosa spontaneously developed in IL-1Ra knockout mice bred on an MFI × 129 background (159). The IL-1β/IL-1Ra ratio is elevated in the synovium of mice with CIA, and this ratio correlates with the severity of joint scores. In contrast, the IL-1β/IL-1Ra ratio decreases at later time points, coincident with a progressive reduction in the levels of inflammatory activity in the joints (160).

An important antiinflammatory role for endogenous IL-1Ra in arthritis was also suggested by a study that compared the clinical course of knee arthritis in patients with Lyme disease. Patients with high concentrations of SF IL-1Ra and low concentrations of IL-1β had rapid resolution of acute attacks of arthritis, whereas patients with the reverse pattern of cytokine concentrations had a more protracted course (161).

Expression of Interleukin-1 and Interleukin-1 Receptor Antagonist in Rheumatic Diseases

SFs from a large number of patients with different rheumatic diseases contained IL-1α, IL-1β, and IL-1Ra. Correlations between IL-1 levels in SF or plasma and measures of disease were variable (162). In patients treated with methotrexate who showed significant clinical improvement, the number of leukocytes and the concentration of IL-1β in the SF were reduced (163). Neutrophils may be the major source of IL-1Ra in SFs, although these cells produced relatively less IL-1Ra and more IL-1β than did peripheral blood neutrophils (164,165). SF mononuclear cells, as well as synovial tissue macrophages, are also potential sources of IL-1Ra (166).

In the rheumatoid synovium, IL-1Ra mRNA and protein were found mainly in the sublining and perivascular areas and were present at lower levels in the intimal lining layer (167,168). The production of IL-1Ra by cultured rheumatoid synovial cells was relatively low in comparison with IL-1. Up to 90% of the cells at the cartilage–pannus interface in the rheumatoid synovium stained for IL-1α, but fewer than 10% of these cells expressed IL-1Ra protein (167).

The expression of IL-1α is elevated in the skin of patients with SSc. The presence of IL-1α in dermal fibroblasts contributes to the phenotype of SSc fibroblasts by the induction of cytokines and procollagen type I (121,122).

Serum levels of IL-1 are generally undetectable. In contrast, elevated serum levels of IL-1Ra were found in various inflammatory rheumatic diseases, including RA, SLE, and myositis, and in individuals with severe infections or trauma. Recent findings suggest that serum IL-1Ra may be derived primarily from hepatocytes in response to stimulation with IL-1β and IL-6 as an acute-phase protein (169,170).

Potential Role of Interleukin-1 in the Pathophysiology of Rheumatoid Arthritis

The results of several studies indicate that local effects of IL-1 play an important role in the pathophysiology of RA. IL-1 induces the chemotaxis of neutrophils, lymphocytes, and monocytes by increasing the expression of both chemokines and adhesion molecules, enhances the proliferation of fibroblasts leading to pannus formation, and stimulates the production of PGE_2. IL-1 also contributes to the destruction of cartilage, bone, and periarticular tissues through effects on both synovial fibroblasts and chondrocytes. The effects of IL-1 on cartilage include an increase in proteoglycan degradation, through inducing the production of neutral metalloproteinases such as collagenase and stromelysin, and a decrease in proteoglycan synthesis by articular chondrocytes. IL-1 decreases the production of collagen type II, the main constituent of cartilage, and stimulates the production of collagen type I. IL-1 has a catabolic effect on bone, primarily through the maturation and activation of osteoclasts. This effect may be mediated in part by up-regulating the expression of RANKL. In addition, IL-1 induces osteoclast activation through a RANKL-independent pathway.

Studies in experimental animal models of arthritis offer further evidence that IL-1 is an important contributor to pathophysiologic events in RA. IL-1 injected into animal joints induced the chemotaxis of neutrophils, followed by the attraction of mononuclear cells. In addition, IL-1 injection led to similar metabolic changes in cartilage, as seen in RA, such as loss of proteoglycans. The administration of IL-1 in animal models of inflammatory arthritis markedly accentuated both pannus formation and cartilage destruction. Transgenic mice overexpressing IL-1α develop a severe form of arthritis characterized by a marked infiltration of neutrophils and macrophages in the synovium (171). The lack of susceptibility of IL-1β and ICE knockout mice to CIA further supports an important role for IL-1 in the pathophysiology of inflammatory arthritis (127). Transgenic mice overexpressing sIL-1Ra or icIL-1Ra1 were protected from developing CIA (172). IL-1Ra, administered either as a recombinant protein or by local gene delivery, was able to reduce the severity of arthritis in different experimental models of arthritis and to prevent the development of joint damage (173).

Taken together, these results supported the role of IL-1 in the pathogenic mechanisms of articular inflammation and joint damage occurring in RA and, thus, provided a strong rationale to target IL-1 in the treatment of RA. As described in detail in Chapter 39, the administration of recombinant human IL-1Ra, alone or in combination with other disease modifying antirheumatic drugs to RA patients, was efficacious, both in improving clinical parameters of disease activity and in preventing the radiologic progression of articular damage.

Toll-like Receptors

TLRs represent a recently identified subset of the IL-1 receptor superfamily. In *Drosophila,* the Toll receptor signaling pathway is required for embryonic dorsoventral patterning and, at later developmental stages, for innate immune responses (174). These receptors recognize a wide array of microbial components and play a major role in the innate immune response in different organisms, including humans, mice, and flies. Cloning of the first human homologue of *Drosophila* Toll receptor also identified it as a type I transmembrane protein with an extracellular domain consisting of a leucine-rich repeat domain that is distinct from the Ig-like domains of the IL-1 receptors and a cytoplasmic domain homologous to the cytoplasmic domain of the human IL-1R (175). To date, 10 TLRs (TLR1–10) have been cloned, and all have in common leucine-rich extracellular repeats and intracellular domains homologous to the IL-1R, the Toll/IL-1R homology (TIR) domains.

As the receptor for gram-negative bacterial LPS, TLR4 is the best characterized member of the TLR family. Cloning of the *lps* gene in the LPS hyporesponsive C3H/HeJ mouse revealed a missense mutation in the third exon, causing the replacement of histidine by proline in the signaling domain of TLR4. In addition, deletion of the TLR4 gene in knockout mice confirmed the role of this receptor in the inflammatory response to LPS (176,177). In addition, MD2, an extracellular accessory protein, interacts with TLR4 and is required for the detection of LPS (178). TLR4 is also involved in the recognition of other exogenous and self ligands, including Taxol, a plant antimitotic compound; the fusion protein F of the respiratory syncytial virus *Mycobacterium tuberculosis*; both microbial and human heat-shock protein 60; the extra domain A of fibronectin; and fibrinogen (179–185). TLR2, in combination with TLR6 or other TLRs, binds and is activated by a wide array of molecules, including bacterial lipopeptides, peptidoglycans, zymosan, leptospiral LPS, and glycolipids of mycobacteria (186). The agent of Lyme disease, *Borrelia burgdorferi,* stimulated nuclear translocation of NFκB and cytokine production via TLR2. These data indicate that TLR2 facilitates the inflammatory events associated with Lyme arthritis (187). TLR5 recognizes bacterial flagellin (188), TLR9 binds to unmethylated CpG DNA motifs (which are found primarily in microbial DNA) (189), and TLR3 is implicated in the recognition of double-stranded RNA produced during viral infection (190).

The signaling pathways activated by TLRs share much in common with IL-1R owing to their conserved TIR. Activation through TIR stimulates the recruitment of MyD88, Tollip, IRAK and TRAF6, leading to the activation of downstream signals responsible for the changes in gene expression. In addition to the MyD88-IRAK pathway, there is growing evidence that additional signaling pathways are required. TLRs provide a link between innate and adaptive immune responses. The maturation of dendritic cells, including production of cytokines (TNF-α and IL-12), chemokine receptors, and expression of costimulatory molecules (CD40, CD80, CD86), can be induced by TLR signaling in response to various microbial products. Mature dendritic cells migrate from peripheral tissue to lymph nodes, where they stimulate the T-cell responses. In addition, activation of different TLRs may elicit different cytokine responses.

TLRs can be important in bacterial arthritis, characterized by prominent joint inflammation and rapid cartilage destruction. The expression of TLRs may be increased in arthritic tissues and render these cells more sensitive to activation by microbial components. The occurrence of flares in established RA could be the result of subclinical infections and TLR-mediated cell stimulation. In addition, the activation of TLR signaling pathways by self molecules released in damaged tissues such as HSP 60, fibronectin, and fibrinogen may participate in the perpetuation of inflammatory responses in arthritic joints.

Interleukin-18

IL-18 has structural similarities with the IL-1 family of proteins. IL-18 is also synthesized as a 23-kd, biologically-inactive precursor and subsequently cleaved by ICE (191). The human IL-18 receptor is also remarkably similar to the IL-1R complex. The binding chain is termed IL-18Rα, and its sequence was found to be identical to the previously identified IL-1R-related protein. A signaling peptide, IL-18Rβ (also termed accessory protein–like), is related to IL-1RAcP. IL-18Rβ itself does not bind IL-18, but is recruited to form a high-affinity heterotrimeric complex with IL-18Rα and the ligand. This high-affinity complex recruits the same intracellular adapter molecules (MyD88, IRAK, and TRAF6) and results in similar responses (NFκB, JNK, p38 MAP kinase), as does IL-1 (192).

IL-18 was originally identified as an IFN-γ-inducing factor (IGIF) that circulated during endotoxinemia in mice primed with *Propionibacterium acnes.* Pro-IL-18 is expressed in macrophages, dendritic cells, Kupffer cells, keratinocytes, chondrocytes, synovial fibroblasts, and osteoblasts. The IL-18R complex is present on naïve T cells, mature T_H1 lymphocytes, NK cells, macrophages, neutrophils, and chondrocytes. IL-18 acts in synergy with IL-12 to enhance IFN-γ gene expression (193). IL-18 is thus a cytokine that, together with IL-12, promotes differentiation of T_H1 cells. Consistent with this concept, the IL-18 receptor is expressed on T_H1 but not on T_H2 lymphocytes (194). IL-18, as observed with IL-12, augments NK cell activity (195,196). IL-18 also induces the expression of cytokines, including GM-CSF, TNF-α, and IL-1β, as well as chemokines such as IL-8 (197). It enhances FasL expression in T cells and NK cells and induces apoptosis in Fas-expressing cells (198). Moreover, IL-18 has T cell–chemoattractant properties *in vitro* and *in vivo* (199).

In addition to its effect on IFN-γ production, IL-18 is also able to stimulate T_H2 responses. In combination with IL-2, IL-18 enhances the production of IL-13 by cultured T lymphocytes and NK cells. IL-18 can potentially induce IgG1, IgE, and T_H2 cytokines such as IL-4, IL-5, and IL-10 production in murine experimental models. Transgenic mice overexpressing IL-18 produced high levels of both T_H1 and T_H2 cytokines and of IgE and IgG1 (200).

Interleukin-18 Binding Protein

Methods of purification of cytokine-binding molecules from human urine led to the identification of a 38-kd IL-18 binding protein (IL-18BP). Although IL-18BP represents the extracellular domain of a cytokine binding chain receptor, no transmembrane domain and cytoplasmic domain of IL-18BP has been found. Thus, IL-18BP is expressed as a secreted binding protein. IL-18BP binds IL-18 and prevents its interaction with cell surface receptors, and thus acts as a natural inhibitor. IL-18BP inhibits both human and murine IL-18 (201).

The human IL-18BP gene encodes for four different isoforms (IL-18BPa, b, c, and d) produced by alternative mRNA splicing. These isoforms differ primarily in their carboxy-terminal region. IL-18BPa exhibits the greatest affinity for IL-18 with a dissociation constant of 399 pM. IL-18BPc shares the same immunoglobulin domain as IL-18BPa except for 29 amino acids in the carboxy-terminal region. IL-18BPc has 10 times less binding affinity than IL-18BPa. IL-18a and c neutralize greater than 95% of IL-18 at a molar excess of 2. IL-18BPb and d lack a complete immunoglobulin domain and do not have the ability to bind or inhibit IL-18 (202).

The circulating level of IL-18BP in healthy individuals ranges from 0.5 to 7 ng/mL. In general, the molar excess of IL-18BP to IL-18 is on the order of 20- to 30-fold. Given the high binding affinity of IL-18BP for IL-18, IL-18BP represents an important regulator of the immune and inflammatory response in IL-18-associated diseases.

Potential Role of Interleukin-18 in Arthritis

IL-18 mRNA and protein were expressed in RA synovial tissues in significantly higher levels than in OA tissues. IL-18 receptor expression was detected on synovial lymphocytes and macrophages. Together with IL-12 or IL-15, IL-18 induced IFN-γ production by synovial tissues *in vitro*. IL-18 independently promoted GM-CSF and NO production, and it induced significant TNF-α synthesis by macrophages. IL-18 production in synovial cultures and purified synovial fibroblasts was up-regulated by TNF-α and IL-1β (203).

IL-18 is also produced by articular chondrocytes. Chondrocytes produced the IL-18 precursor and in response to IL-1 stimulation secreted the mature form of IL-18. Studies regarding IL-18 effects on chondrocytes showed that it inhibits cell proliferation and enhances NO production. IL-18 stimulated the production of stromelysin, IL-6, and COX-2. Treatment of normal human articular cartilage with IL-18 increased the release of glycosaminoglycans. IL-18 is thus a cytokine that exerts a catabolic effect on cartilage (204). In contrast, IL-18 may have a protective effect on bone erosions. Osteoblastic stromal cells produce IL-18, which inhibits osteoclast formation, apparently through the release of GM-CSF by T cells (205).

In vivo studies have confirmed the role of IL-18 in the pathogenesis of arthritis. IL-18 administration to mice with CIA facilitated the development of an erosive, inflammatory arthritis, suggesting that IL-18 can be proinflammatory *in vivo* (203). In contrast, IL-18 knockout mice have a reduced frequency and severity of CIA (206). The administration of anti-IL-18 antibodies or IL-18BP significantly reduced the clinical severity of CIA. Attenuation of disease severity was associated with reduced cartilage destruction on histology (207).

INTERLEUKIN-6 AND RELATED CYTOKINES

IL-6 is part of a cytokine family that includes LIF, OSM, CNTF, IL-11, cardiotrophin, and cardiotrophin-like cytokine. IL-6 plays a prominent role in the coordinated systemic host defense response to injury, because it regulates immune and inflammatory responses, hepatic acute-phase protein synthesis, hematopoiesis, and bone metabolism. A broad spectrum of cell types, including epithelial cells, endothelial cells, smooth muscle cells, mesangial cells, hepatoma cells, fibroblasts, chondrocytes, synoviocytes, osteoblasts, osteoclasts, glial cells, and astrocytes, can be activated to express IL-6. Among bone marrow–derived cells, mononuclear phagocytes are an important source of IL-6, but neutrophils, eosinophils, and mast cells can also express this cytokine.

The high-affinity human IL-6R complex consists of IL-6 and two membrane-associated receptor components, the IL-6R α subunit and the high-affinity converter and signal-transducing molecule gp130 β subunit. The 80-kd IL-6 ligand-binding chain has a short 82–amino acid intracellular portion that is not required for signal transduction. A soluble form of IL-6R (sIL-6Rα) has been detected in serum and urine of healthy individuals, and its levels are increased in patients with multiple myeloma and human immunodeficiency virus infection. sIL-6Rα can be generated either by shedding of the membrane-anchored receptor by a mechanism involving TACE or by mRNA splicing resulting in a peptide lacking the cytoplasmic and transmembrane domains. Elevated levels are also detected in the SF of patients with inflammatory rheumatic diseases. SF levels of sIL-6Rα correlated with leukocyte numbers. Hepatocytes may be a major source of circulating sIL-6Rα (208). Circulating complexes of IL-6 with its soluble receptor can induce cellular responses by associating with membrane-bound gp130. A soluble form of gp130 is also detected in the human serum. Soluble gp130 was able to block the stimulatory effects of IL-6/sIL-6Rα complexes on gp130 signaling and should, therefore, be considered as a natural IL-6 inhibitor. Administration of gp130-Fc fusion protein caused marked suppression of colitis in an animal model of Crohn disease (209).

In addition to the IL-6R α subunit, gp130 interacts with several different receptor chains and functions as a common signal transducer for IL-6, OSM, LIF, CNTF, and IL-11. CNTF, LIF, OSM, and IL-6 initiate signaling by inducing either the β signal–transducing receptor component gp130 (in the case of IL-6) or heterodimerization between gp130 and the gp130-related LIFR-β (in the case of CNTF, LIF, and OSM) or between gp130 and OSMR-β (in the case of OSM). Anti-gp130 monoclonal antibodies blocked the biologic responses induced by all of these factors (210,211). Binding of cytokines to gp130 activates JAK1, JAK2, and TYK2, which phosphorylate tyrosine residues in the cytoplasmic domains of gp130. The transcription factor STAT3 is recruited and activated. Dimerized STAT3 is then translocated in the nucleus, where it exerts its regulatory effects on gene transcription. Besides the JAK-STAT pathway, the ERK MAP kinase pathway is also activated through the recruitment and phosphorylation of SHP2 on the tyrosine residue at position 759 (Y759) of gp130. Several experiments *in vitro* have indicated the SHP2- and STAT3-mediated signals are involved in cell growth and gene expression (212). By using mice with knock-in mutations directed on STAT3 or SHP2 binding sites, it was possible to demonstrate that these two pathways exert important regulatory effects on each other. Mutation of the Y759 SHP2 binding site showed that SHP2 negatively regulated the biologic effects of STAT3 *in vivo.* In contrast, deletion of gp130 STAT binding sites resulted in sustained SHP2/ras/ERK activation (213). The mutation in the SHP2 binding site resulted in enhanced acute-phase response, increased T_H1 cytokine production and IgG2a and IgG2b levels, splenomegaly, and lymphadenopathy. Furthermore, these mice develop late-onset arthritis with marked joint destruction and autoantibody production resembling that of RA (213,214). In contrast, mutations in the tyrosine residues responsible for STAT3 activation led to decreased T_H1 cytokine production and IgG2a and IgG2b levels. Deletion of the STAT binding sites resulted in impaired mucosal immune response and acute-phase protein production. In addition, these mice developed gastrointestinal ulcerations and a severe arthropathy characterized by degradation of articular cartilage and chronic synovitis (215).

Interleukin-6 Function

IL-6 Regulates the Inflammatory and Acute-Phase Responses

IL-6 is one of the most potent hepatocyte stimulators. IL-6 regulates the production of acute-phase proteins, a set of plasma proteins the levels of which vary during various inflammatory conditions (see Chapter 22). The production of some acute-phase proteins is enhanced (positive acute-phase proteins), whereas the levels of others decrease (negative acute-phase proteins). In addition, acute-phase proteins vary largely according to the kinetics and magnitude of their levels following an inflammatory stimulation. Serum amyloid A and C-reactive protein (CRP) are considered major acute-phase proteins because their levels can increase up to 1,000-fold in inflammatory conditions. Other positive, acute-phase proteins include fibrinogen, α_1-antitrypsin, α_1-acid glycoprotein, haptoglobin, C1 esterase inhibitor, and tissue inhibitor of metalloproteinases (TIMP). Negative, acute-phase proteins include albumin and apolipoprotein A_1 (155). A similar set of acute-phase proteins is induced by LIF, IL-11, and OSM. IL-6 is considered as the major stimulator of acute-phase protein synthesis, whereas IL-1 and TNF-α induce only a limited number of acute-phase reactants. *In vivo,* administration of IL-6 to rats caused the production of the same set of acute-phase proteins that is induced in experimental models of inflammation. In most diseases or experimental systems in which IL-6 was overexpressed, there was a hepatic acute-phase response and a good correlation between the levels of circulating IL-6 and levels of hepatic acute-phase proteins. Levels of IL-6 also correlate positively with levels of acute-phase proteins in some inflammatory rheumatic disease. Experiments using IL-6 knockout mice have indicated very interesting results regarding the role of IL-6 in the production of APP. In IL-6 knockout mice, the hepatic acute-phase response after tissue damage or infection was severely compromised, but it was only moderately affected after challenge with LPS (216,217), suggesting that the pattern of circulating cytokines varies according to the type of stimulation.

Effects on the nervous system are also part of the role of IL-6 as a coordinator of host defense responses to injury. IL-6 induces fever through a PGE_2-dependent mechanism (218) and activates the hypothalamic-pituitary-adrenal axis. Intravenous administration of IL-6 induced the release of adrenocorticotropic hormone, probably through the induction of corticotropin-releasing hormone, which is consistent with a protective negative feedback as adrenal steroids inhibit inflammatory responses and synergize with IL-6 in the stimulation of hepatic acute-phase proteins.

To address the role of IL-6 in host defense, in view of the overlapping activities with other members of this cytokine family, the IL-6 gene was disrupted by homologous recombination. IL-6-deficient mice developed normally. Defective control of infection with vaccinia virus and *Listeria monocytogenes* was demonstrated in IL-6 knockout mice. The T-cell-dependent antibody response against vesicular stomatitis virus was impaired.

An important and distinct biologic activity of IL-6 is the reduction of LPS-induced expression of TNF-α, IL-1, and chemokines (219). From these studies, it appears that, in contrast to the monocyte-activating properties of other cytokines, IL-6 is primarily directed at differentiation and the down-regulation of certain pro-inflammatory responses in monocytes. This potential antiinflammatory activity of IL-6 was observed in a model of lethal endotoxemia, where IL-6 pretreatment improved survival and reduced TNF-α production (220). In contrast, levels of TNF-α were increased in IL-6-deficient mice injected with LPS. Some of the anti-inflammatory effects of IL-6 may be mediated by its effect on the release of TNF soluble receptor and IL-1Ra. In addition, IL-6 induces acute-phase proteins, at least some of which may also have antiinflammatory properties *in vivo* (221,222).

Recent findings indicate that IL-6 plays a major role in the transition from neutrophil to monocyte infiltrate during inflammation. Levels of neutrophils were significantly higher in IL-6 knockout mice after administration of LPS. In wild-type mice, the local infiltrate of acute peritonitis was primarily made of neutrophils followed by monocytes, whereas neutrophils were the only cells present in the peritoneal fluid of IL-6-deficient mice. The administration of IL-6/sIL-6Rα restored the presence of monocytes in IL-6 knockout mice (223).

Interleukin-6 and Hematopoiesis

IL-6 is expressed by bone marrow stromal fibroblasts and may contribute to the maintenance of normal, basal hematopoiesis *in vivo*. Tissue injury is often associated with high circulating levels of IL-6, which promotes the formation of platelets and leukocytes. Thus, IL-6 represents one of the stimuli that regulates this adaptive response (224). In its effects on thrombocytopoiesis, IL-6 also synergized with IL-3 and increased the number of megakaryocyte colonies induced by IL-3 *in vitro* and in primates *in vivo* (225). LIF and IL-11 have similar effects on thrombocytopoiesis. However, IL-6 and related cytokines are not the major stimuli of platelet formation. This is the function of the recently identified cytokine thrombopoietin, the inducer of megakaryocytopoiesis and maturation.

Bone Metabolism

Maintenance of bone mass is a function of bone formation by osteoblasts and resorption by osteoclasts. Giant cell tumors of bone produce high levels of IL-6, and neutralizing antibodies to IL-6 inhibited bone resorption by these cells (226). Enhanced levels of IL-6 have been observed in different conditions associated with excessive bone loss, including periodontal disease, Paget disease, multiple myeloma, RA, and hyperparathyroidism. IL-6 is produced in response to parathyroid hormone stimulation. In the presence of sIL-6Rα, IL-6 induced osteoclast-like multinucleated cell formation. IL-6 can stimulate RANKL expression in stromal cells/osteoblasts by a mechanism involving gp130 and STAT3 activity. In addition, other IL-6 family members, such as IL-11, LIF, and OSM, have been shown to stimulate RANKL production with consequent osteoclast maturation and bone resorption. Through the differentiation of osteoclasts, IL-6 has been suggested to be involved in the pathogenesis of osteoporosis after estrogen loss. Estrogens inhibit the production of IL-6, and the increase in osteoclasts after ovariectomy was prevented by antibody to IL-6 (227). These data suggest that IL-6 may act as both an autocrine and a paracrine factor for human osteoclasts and that IL-6 may play an important role in the bone-resorbing capacity of these cells. Recently, two promoter polymorphisms located at −572 and −174 have been shown to influence IL-6 activity. The presence of either the −572 C or −174 G alleles was associated with increased levels of C-terminal cross-links of type I collagen, a marker of bone resorption, and circulating CRP levels but had no influence on osteocalcin, a marker of bone formation. The presence of both alleles had an additive effect. Individuals carrying these alleles had lower bone mineral density values at the lumbar spine (228).

B-Cell Response

IL-6 was first recognized as a B cell–activating factor. The role of IL-6 in promoting differentiation of B lymphocytes into antibody-secreting cells has been demonstrated in various experimental systems *in vitro* and *in vivo*. IL-6 is necessary for plasma cell survival and maturation and has been suggested to induce B-cell hyperreactivity. One of the most supportive examples for a role of IL-6 in the production of autoantibodies is cardiac myxoma, a tumor that produces high levels of IL-6. Surgical removal of the tumor usually results in a decline in autoantibodies, hypergammaglobulinemia, and the hepatic acute-phase response (229).

IL-6 is elevated systemically, or at least at local sites of disease manifestations, in spontaneously-occurring autoimmune disorders such as RA, SLE, type I diabetes, and experimental models of autoimmune disease. It appears likely that IL-6 contributes to the production of autoantibodies in these diseases. Under conditions in which autoantibodies are directly pathogenic or form pathogenic immune complexes, IL-6 may contribute to autoimmune pathogenesis. Excessive B-cell function, including autoantibody production, is a common feature of SLE and considered to be associated with spontaneous cytokine secretion. SLE B cells express IL-6Rs and secrete IL-6 without *in vitro* stimulation. Anti-IL-6R antibody inhibits spontaneous production of polyclonal Ig and anti-DNA autoantibodies (230). Studies involving patients and experimental models of autoimmune disease clearly show a prominent role of IL-6 in autoantibody formation. Neutralization of IL-6 may thus be of therapeutic value in experimental models of lupus. In (NZB × NZW) F1 mice, neutralizing antibody to IL-6 prevented production of anti-dsDNA, significantly reduced proteinuria, and prolonged life (231). Administration of neutralizing anti-IL-6 antibodies to MRL mice decreased the production of anti-dsDNA antibodies and the development of renal damage (232).

Dysregulated IL-6 expression in transgenic mice initially resulted in polyclonal hypergammaglobulinemia and, at later stages, IgG1 plasmacytosis, the development of autoantibodies, activation of acute-phase response genes, and increased numbers of megakaryocytes in the spleen and bone marrow. Although these animals did not develop specific organ-specific autoimmune manifestations, they developed mesangial proliferative glomerulonephritis that was similar to that seen in human SLE (233,234).

T-Cell Responses

IL-6 stimulates proliferation of thymocytes and peripheral blood T cells and represents one of the monocyte-derived cofactors that are required for T-cell activation (235).

IL-6 can also be considered as an important link between the innate and the adaptive immune responses. IL-6 stimulated differentiation of human monocytes to more efficient antigen-presenting cells. $CD4^+$ $CD25^+$ regulatory T cells exert a suppressive effect on effector T-cell activation upon interaction with antigen-presenting cells. Interestingly, this effect of regulatory T cells can be overcome by IL-6, which is released by activated antigen-presenting cells (236). Thus, IL-6 can represent a good therapeutic target in inflammatory conditions with participation of activated effector T cells.

Interleukin-6 Expression in Rheumatic Diseases

Rheumatoid Arthritis

In RA synovial membranes, cells containing IL-6 reside in the thickened lining layer and also in a perivascular distribution in the deeper synovium. Macrophages are the major cells of the immune system in which IL-6 can be localized in RA. High levels of IL-6 are present in SF from patients with arthritis, and there is a good correlation with the intensity of the inflammatory response. IL-6 levels in SF are higher in samples from patients with inflammatory arthropathies as compared to those with OA. Comparative studies in patients with RA of IL-6 levels in SF and serum showed up to 1,000-fold higher concentrations in the joint. SF IL-6 levels correlate with serum IL-6, suggesting that the joint is the source of circulating IL-6. In general, good correlations have been found between IL-6 levels in serum and levels of acute-phase proteins (237).

Systemic Lupus Erythematosus

Most SLE sera contain higher than normal levels of IL-6, and concentrations correlate with disease activity. Several investigators have noted that elevated IL-6 is not, as expected, associated with increased levels of CRP or other acute-phase proteins, such as fibrinogen. This lack of a correlation between IL-6 and CRP in SLE suggests that there may be a defect in the hepatocyte responses to this cytokine in this disease (238). IL-6 may contribute to pathogenesis of mesangial proliferative glomerulonephritis, since it stimulates mesangial cell proliferation. In 50% of patients with this disorder, urine IL-6 levels were elevated and mesangial cells were shown to be at least one cellular source of IL-6 (239). Cerebrospinal fluid IL-6 levels were elevated in 10 of 14 patients with CNS lupus (240). All patients showed increased cerebrospinal fluid Ig levels. Only one of nine SLE patients without CNS involvement had moderately increased IL-6. Cerebrospinal fluid IL-6 levels markedly decreased during therapy as symptoms improved. Serum IL-6 levels in lupus patients with CNS involvement did not correlate with those in cerebrospinal fluids.

Other Rheumatic Diseases

Patients with polymyalgia rheumatica and giant cell arteritis have a strong hepatic acute-phase response, and in a series of 15 untreated patients, all had high serum IL-6 levels. However, there was no correlation with therapy and the hepatic acute-phase response. Interestingly, six of the patients continued to have increased IL-6 levels 6 months after steroid therapy, although hepatic acute-phase proteins had decreased (241). In giant cell arteritis, IL-6-expressing macrophages are primarily located in the adventitia (242).

JIA patients with systemic-onset disease exhibited significantly elevated serum IL-6 levels, and these decreased during remission (243). Serum IL-6 levels also correlated with the extent and severity of arthritis and with thrombocytosis. Patients with systemic-onset JIA demonstrate a rapid increase and decrease of serum IL-6 levels that parallel the profile of the fever. Elevated levels of IL-6 can partially explain the presence of impaired growth in children with JIA (244). Sequence analysis of the IL-6 gene promoter region revealed that young patients (<5 years) had a reduced frequency of the potentially protective −174 C genotype. The finding that this allele is associated with a higher transcriptional activity may contribute to the pathogenesis of systemic-onset JIA (245).

Inflammatory microcrystals, including monosodium urate and calcium pyrophosphate dihydrate but not hydroxyapatite crystals, induce the secretion of IL-6 from mononuclear phagocytes and synoviocytes, and high concentrations of IL-6 can be found in SFs from patients with gout and pseudogout (246).

Interleukin-6 Targeting in the Treatment of Rheumatoid Arthritis

The consequence of IL-6 inhibition was also examined in several animal models of arthritis. A blocking IL-6R antibody inhibited the development of CIA. The antibody-treated mice exhibited lower serum levels of IgG anti-collagen type II antibody and reduced responsiveness of lymphocytes to collagen type II. These results substantiated a role for IL-6 in the development of immunity to collagen type II (247). Consistent with these findings, knockout mice lacking IL-6 were protected from CIA (248). IL-6-

deficient mice developed only a mild form of antigen-induced arthritis (AIA). Safranin O staining demonstrated that articular cartilage was well preserved in IL-6-deficient mice, whereas it was destroyed completely in IL-6-producing mice. This study suggested that IL-6 may play a key role not only in the inductive but also in the effector phase of arthritis (249). In contrast to this apparent pathogenic role of IL-6 in AIA and CIA, the spontaneous arthritis observed in TNF-α transgenic mice was not affected by inactivation of the IL-6 gene (248).

In non–immunologically-mediated, zymosan-induced arthritis, acute joint inflammation in IL-6-deficient mice was comparable with that in wild-type mice during the first week, but only wild-type mice developed chronic inflammation. However, suppression of chondrocyte proteoglycan synthesis and induction of proteoglycan degradation were higher in the IL-6-deficient mice, which resulted in more striking proteoglycan depletion. Injection of recombinant IL-6 into the joint space significantly reduced cartilage destruction (250).

These findings from various animal models of arthritis suggest that IL-6 is an important factor in the development of autoimmunity to type II collagen and chronic joint inflammation. However, IL-6 does not appear to be a direct pathogenic factor in connective tissue degradation. In contrast, IL-6 may exert a protective effect on extracellular matrix degradation by stimulating the production of TIMP-1 and TGF-β (251–253). A small, open-label study targeted IL-6 in five patients with RA. Anti-IL-6 monoclonal antibody was given intravenously for 10 consecutive days. No side effects were noted. Clinical improvement and a reduction in CRP levels were observed. However, clinical improvement was only transient (254). Recently, a randomized, double-blind, placebo-controlled, dose escalation trial with a monoclonal anti-IL-6R antibody was conducted in 45 patients with active RA. The patients were divided into four groups to receive a single intravenous dose of either 0.1, 1, 5, or 10 mg/kg monoclonal anti-IL-6R antibody or placebo. After two weeks, five of nine patients treated with a single dose of 5 mg/kg of the antibody achieved an American College of Rheumatology (ACR)20 response, whereas no statistical difference was observed between other doses of anti-IL-6R antibody and placebo (255). There were no serious adverse events related to the study drug. The results of a 12-week, randomized, double-blind, placebo-controlled study without other disease-modifying antirheumatic drugs confirmed the efficacy and safety of monoclonal anti-IL-6R antibody in the treatment of RA (256).

Leukemia Inhibitory Factor, Oncostatin M, and Interleukin-11

LIF is present in SF from patients with OA and at higher concentrations in samples from patients with RA (257,258). Cultured human synoviocytes and articular chondrocytes produced biologically-active LIF after stimulation with IL-1 (257). An LIF effect that potentially contributes to disease pathogenesis is the activation of monocytes (259). LIF increases the stimulatory effect of TNF-α on PGE_2 production by synovial fibroblasts and, thus, can participate in the inflammatory manifestations of RA. IL-11 is expressed by synoviocytes and chondrocytes and, similar to IL-6 and OSM, it induces the production of TIMP (260). IL-11 is present in the SF of RA patients, but its presence in the serum is variable. Exogenous addition of IL-11 inhibited the production of TNF-α, MMP-1, and MMP-3 by RA synovium (261). IL-11 is produced by the synovium of mice with CIA. The administration of recombinant human IL-11 after the onset of CIA significantly reduced the severity of arthritis and the progression of joint damage (262). A phase I/II randomized, dose-escalating, double-blind, placebo-controlled trial with recombinant human IL-11 was conducted in patients with active RA. A total of 91 patients were randomized in five groups to receive subcutaneous injections of either 2.5 to 7.5 μg or placebo twice a week or 5 to 15 μg or a placebo once per week. After 12 weeks, the patients treated with 15 μg IL-11 once per week had a significant reduction of the number of tender joints, but did not achieve a significant improvement of the ACR20 response as compared with the placebo group. Injection site reaction was the only adverse event clearly associated with IL-11 (263).

OSM exerts proinflammatory effects in different experimental models. OSM stimulates the expression of adhesion molecules by endothelial cells and increased neutrophil migration through the endothelial cell layer. OSM stimulates the expression of proinflammatory mediators (264). Intra-articular injection of adenovirus-encoding murine OSM induces a severe articular inflammation with synovial hyperplasia, mononuclear cell infiltration, pannus formation, and cartilage degradation (265). In contrast, OSM favors periosteal bone deposition rather than resorption *in vivo* (266). OSM mRNA was detected in the joints of mice with CIA. The administration of neutralizing anti-OSM antibodies after the onset of CIA resulted in marked reduction of joint inflammation and cartilage damage (267), suggesting that targeting OSM may be of potential value for the treatment of RA.

INTERLEUKIN-2 AND RELATED CYTOKINES

IL-2 is the major T-cell growth factor. IL-2 receptors are expressed on lymphocytes and mononuclear phagocytes and occur in different combinations of three subunit chains with different affinities for IL-2. IL-2Rα binds IL-2 with low affinity. Intermediate affinity is a function of IL-2Rβ and IL-2Rγ complexes, and high-affinity receptors contain all three components. The IL-2 receptor α chain is shed from lymphocytes and monocytes in response to cell activation *in vitro*. The IL-2Rγ chain is required for signal transduction. It is also the signal transducing component of IL-4R, IL-7R, IL-9R, IL-15R, and IL-21R. The shared use of the same signal-transducing receptor component explains the similarities in the biologic activities of these cytokines. IL-2Rγ mutations result in X-linked severe combined immunodeficiency (XSCID) in humans, a disease characterized by the presence of few or no T cells. In contrast, SCID patients with IL-2 deficiency and IL-2-deficient mice have normal numbers of T cells, suggesting compensation by the other cytokines that activate the IL-2Rγ chain.

Within this family, IL-4 and IL-13 are closely related, because they both have antiinflammatory effects on mononuclear phagocytes. Besides this, they share with all other members of this cytokine family a role in the regulation of B- and T-lymphocyte function. IL-15 is functionally similar to IL-2, but in contrast to the lymphocyte-restricted expression of IL-2, diverse cell types, including macrophages and fibroblasts, produce IL-15. IL-21 is closely related to IL-2 and IL-15. IL-21 is produced by activated T lymphocytes and promotes the proliferation of T and B cells, and the proliferation and maturation of NK cells.

Interleukin-2

The expression of IL-2, induction of its multiple receptor subunits, and subsequent ligand receptor interactions are critical events in T-cell activation. IL-2 also serves as an important regulator for B lymphocytes, NK cells, and lymphokine-activated killer cells (268). IL-2 is a 15.5-kd single-chain glycoprotein. T lymphocytes are its major cell source. IL-2 expression is dependent on activation of the T-cell receptor (TCR)–CD3 complex and is enhanced by cytokines and other receptors that mediate interactions between antigen-presenting cells and T lymphocytes. Mice with a disrupted IL-2 gene had normal T-cell development. *In vitro,* T-cell proliferation was inducible but reduced as compared with normal mice. B-cell differentiation was impaired with an increase in IgG1 and IgE levels. At 6 weeks of age, these mice developed inflammatory bowel disease as the result of an abnormal immune response to normal enteric antigens (269).

Expression of Interleukin-2 and Interleukin-2 Receptors in Rheumatic Diseases

Although IL-2 is a major cytokine in the induction of immune responses, its role in the pathogenesis of human autoimmune diseases has not been clearly established. This is partially based on unexpectedly low levels of IL-2 expression in tissue or body fluids from patients with autoimmune diseases. Furthermore, only a small number of studies have targeted IL-2 in the treatment of experimental models of arthritis or lupus. The aspect of IL-2 that has received the most attention is the presence of soluble forms of the IL-2 receptor α chain (CD25) in body fluids.

Only a few studies were able to detect IL-2-like biologic activities or immunoreactivities in SF or serum from patients with rheumatic diseases (270). IL-2 mRNA expression in tissues from patients with rheumatic diseases was detectable, but low (271). In contrast to the difficulties in detecting IL-2 expression, the soluble form of the IL-2 receptor α chain (sIL-2Rα) was readily detectable, and a large number of studies have addressed the value of measuring soluble IL-2 receptors in diverse rheumatic disorders. The soluble form of the IL-2 receptor was first discovered in culture supernatants of activated lymphocytes. The 45-kd sIL-2Rα is generated by proteolytic cleavage of the 55-kd membrane-associated IL-2Rα subunit (272). The function of this soluble receptor in the regulation of T-cell responses is not clear. It inhibits the biologic activity of IL-2 only at high concentrations, probably related to its relatively low affinity for IL-2.

Soluble Interleukin-2 Receptor α in Rheumatoid Arthritis

Earlier studies on relatively small patient populations suggested a correlation between disease activity and sIL-2Rα in RA. Although later studies confirmed increased levels in RA, the correlations with disease activity were less clear. The sIL-2Rα levels of 148 patients with refractory RA were determined during a prospective, randomized, placebo-controlled trial of methotrexate. The mean sIL-2Rα level in all RA patients was markedly elevated compared with that in normal control subjects, and decreased significantly during the trial. There was no correlation of sIL-2Rα levels with joint pain or tenderness, and the level of sIL-2Rα did not predict the response to methotrexate (273). The levels of sIL-2Rα were determined in a cohort of 155 patients with early RA to examine its potential use in predicting the development of erosions. After a follow-up of 2 years, the results did not show any significant association between serum sIL-2R levels and erosive changes (274).

A few studies have examined soluble sIL-2Rα in JIA. Levels were increased in sera from patients as compared with healthy controls, and the highest titers were found in the subset with systemic-onset disease. In a study of 16 children treated with oral methotrexate, there was a good correlation between sIL-2Rα and therapeutic response (275).

Soluble Interleukin-2 Receptor in Systemic Lupus Erythematosus

In a large number of SLE patients, even in the absence of active disease, sIL-2Rα levels were higher than in healthy controls. As compared with other rheumatic diseases, serum levels of sIL-2Rα were higher in SLE (276). Exacerbations of SLE were preceded by a significant increase in sIL-2Rα and correlated with levels of anti-dsDNA, C3, and C4. Levels of sIL-2Rα decreased following treatment (277). In a prospective study, all 62 of the SLE patients had significantly higher sIL-2Rα levels than did normal controls. During a lupus nephritis flare, 9 of 10 patients showed significant elevations of sIL-2Rα, whereas only 6 of 10 patients showed either elevation of anti-DNA antibody or decrease in hemolytic complement ($C'H_{50}$). sIL-2Rα correlated with histologic activity and chronicity indices and IgG and C3 deposition, whereas anti-DNA antibody and $C'H_{50}$ levels did not (278). Similar observations were obtained in a longitudinal study of SLE patients where changes in sIL-2Rα and anti-dsDNA antibody measurements did not correlate (279). Serum sIL-2Rα concentrations were higher in patients with nephritis before treatment and decreased significantly 6 months after treatment (280). Cerebrospinal fluid levels of IL-1β, TNF-α, IL-2, and sIL-2Rα were measured in 20 young adults with a first episode of stroke. The levels of sIL-2Rα were significantly higher in 5 patients who developed SLE during the follow-up, suggesting that sIL-2Rα determination may be useful to differentiate immunologically mediated vascular process in the CNS from stroke of other origins (281). In response to infection, sIL-2Rα increased significantly in patients with either active or inactive SLE (282). Additional studies are required to determine whether longitudinal measurements are a generally useful marker for disease exacerbation.

Soluble Interleukin-2 Receptor in Other Rheumatic Diseases

In Wegener granulomatosis, sIL-2Rα levels were increased in patients with active disease as compared to those in remission. In patients with disease exacerbation, sIL-2Rα levels increased earlier than CRP and cytoplasmic antineutrophil cytoplasmic antibody levels. In addition, patients with active disease, but low CRP and antineutrophil cytoplasmic antibodies, had increased sIL-2Rα. This study, which analyzed 102 patients, thus suggested that sIL-2Rα may be a good marker of disease activity and an early sign of imminent relapse in Wegener granulomatosis (283).

A good correlation was observed in patients with polymyositis between levels of sIL-2Rα and response to corticosteroid therapy. In addition, sIL-2Rα levels increased prior to other laboratory markers in patients who developed relapse of their disease. In Sjögren syndrome, SSc (284), and localized scleroderma (285), the highest levels of sIL-2Rα were an indicator of disease activity, prognosis, and overall disease severity.

In Vivo *Administration of Interleukin-2 and Interleukin-2 Antagonists*

With respect to the development of therapeutic interventions, the IL-2/IL-2R system has been studied primarily in the treatment of malignancies. Agents that inhibit IL-2 synthesis and action provide new approaches for the treatment of autoimmune disorders, but only limited data are available. Recombinant IL-2 has been administered to tumor patients, and a small number of cases have been reported in which this reactivated RA (286) or resulted in the development of inflammatory arthritis (287).

A fusion protein, in which the receptor binding domain of diphtheria toxin was replaced with IL-2, binds to T cells expressing the high-affinity IL-2 receptor and induces cytotoxicity of activated T cells by inhibition of protein synthesis. Results from a phase I trial showed that 9 of 19 patients treated with a high- or medium-dose of the fusion protein had rapid clinical benefit (288). Further controlled studies did not confirm the efficacy of this approach in the treatment of RA. The prophylactic and therapeutic effect of daclizumab, a humanized monoclonal antibody against IL-2Rα, was recently tested in rhesus monkeys with CIA. Administration of daclizumab reduced the development of arthritis in immunized animals and also proved effective in decreasing articular inflammation and joint damage in arthritic monkeys (289). These results are promising but should be confirmed in clinical trials.

Interleukin-4 and Interleukin-13

IL-4 was initially recognized on the basis of its effects on B lymphocytes. It stimulates B-cell proliferation and production of IgG and IgM by activated B cells, and increases expression of CD23, the low-affinity receptor for IgE. IL-4 is predominantly a product of T_H2 cells and inhibits the production of IL-2 and IFN-γ by T_H1 cells. In addition, IL-4 also suppresses the synthesis of inflammatory cytokines in monocytes. In cultures of RA synovium, IL-4 inhibits *in vitro*–induced production of IL-1 and TNF-α and the spontaneous production of IL-6, TNF-α, LIF, and PGE_2. Furthermore, IL-4 inhibits growth factor–induced synoviocyte proliferation *in vitro*. Some of these antiinflammatory effects of IL-4 (and IL-13) may be mediated by an inhibitory effect on NFκB activation in macrophages (290). In contrast, IL-4 had no effect on NFκB activity in synovial fibroblasts (291). IL-4 also induces the production of antiinflammatory mediators. IL-4 stimulates the secretion of IL-1Ra by LPS-stimulated PBMCs and by rheumatoid synovial explants (292,293). Moreover, IL-4 enhances the stimulatory effects of IL-1 on IL-1Ra production by cultured human hepatocytes and increases the release of IL-1Ra by TNF-α-stimulated neutrophils in culture (294, 295). IL-4 also stimulates the expression of soluble IL-1RII and TNFRs. Taken together, all these properties suggest a potential antiinflammatory role for IL-4. However, in other systems, IL-4 may exert proinflammatory effects by increasing the stimulatory effects of IL-1 on production of monocyte chemotactic protein and IL-6 by endothelial (296) and of IL-6 by synovial fibroblasts (291). IL-4 can also enhance the inducing effect of TNF-α on vascular cell adhesion molecule-1 (VCAM-1) expression by endothelial cells (297) and on IL-8 expression by synovial fibroblasts (298). IL-4 may have chondroprotective activity because it prevents and possibly even reverses cartilage degradation. Intraarticular injection of adenovirus expressing IL-4 into the knee joints of mice with CIA prevented chondrocyte apoptosis and cartilage erosion (299). IL-4 can also prevent the progression of bone destruction. Overexpression of IL-4 in the joints of mice with CIA suppressed the expression of RANKL and prevented the formation of osteoclast-like cells and development of bone erosions. *In vitro* studies with bone explants from RA patients cultured in the presence of IL-4 revealed consistent suppression of type I collagen breakdown (300). Interestingly, the protective effects of IL-4 on cartilage and bone were observed, despite the persistence of severe articular inflammation and of synovial fibroblast expansion. These findings may be related to an antiapoptotic effect of IL-4 (301).

Notably, IL-4 was not detected in RA SF and tissue (293). This lack of IL-4 could contribute to the uneven T_H1/T_H2 balance and the chronic nature of RA. Studies in animal models of arthritis supported this characterization of IL-4 as a cytokine with antiarthritic potential. IL-4-deficient mice have a more chronic relapsing form of CIA (302). In proteoglycan-induced arthritis, immunization of mice lacking IL-4 or STAT6 led to a more severe arthritis with a significant increase in production of IL-12, TNF-α, and IFN-γ than in wild-type animals, indicating that endogenous IL-4 plays an important regulatory role in determining the magnitude of articular inflammation (303). In arthritis induced by streptococcal cell wall fragments, daily treatment with IL-4 had a minimal effect on the acute phase. However, IL-4 suppressed the chronic, destructive phase; decreased the influx of inflammatory cells; and eliminated pannus and erosions. In CIA, IL-4 synergized with IL-10 in the protection against cartilage degradation (304).

IL-13 shares biologic activities with IL-4. Their genes are closely linked in both the human and mouse genomes, and their protein sequences are homologous (305,306). However, IL-4 can induce unique responses in certain cells such as T cells that do not respond to IL-13 (9). These specific effects of IL-4 can be explained by the presence of different receptor subunits. Three types of functional receptors have been described in different cellular contexts. Type I IL-4 receptor, which consists of IL-4Rα and the common γ chain, is found in T cells and NK cells. Type II receptor, which contains IL-4Rα and IL-13Rα1, is present in nonhematopoietic cells. Type III IL-4R, a heterotrimer containing IL-4Rα, IL-13Rα1, and the common γ chain, is found in B cells and monocytes.

IL-13 is secreted by activated T_H2 cells and modulates monocyte and B-cell functions. IL-13 mediates its effect by binding to a complex receptor system comprising IL-4Rα and two IL-13 binding proteins, IL-13Rα1 and IL-13Rα2. IL-13 receptors are expressed on human B cells, basophils, eosinophils, mast cells, endothelial cells, fibroblasts, monocytes/macrophages, respiratory epithelial cells, and smooth muscle cells. IL-13 enhances CD23/Fcε receptor and MHC class II expression on B lymphocytes. It costimulates B-cell proliferation by anti-Ig and anti-CD40 and induces IgE synthesis. In monocytes, IL-13 inhibits LPS-induced production of IL-1, IL-6, IL-8, IL-10, IL-12, TNF, and NO, but enhances the production of IL-1Ra (307). These inhibitory effects on macrophage function lead to a suppression of T_H1 cell–mediated responses. IL-13 treatment of mice with CIA reduced disease severity and lowered TNF-α levels.

Following the encouraging results observed with the administration of IL-4 in animal models of arthritis, a phase I dose-escalating, double-blind, placebo-controlled safety study of recombinant human IL-4 was conducted in RA patients. Treatment did not produce significant benefit, but was well tolerated (308).

Expression in Rheumatic Diseases

Elevated serum levels of IL-4, IL-6, and IL-10 were found in patients with SLE. These results suggested that SLE should be considered as a T_H2-driven disease. In addition, the presence of B-cell hyperreactivity and hyperglobulinemia supported this hypothesis. However, results of experimental models regarding the role of IL-4 in SLE led to contradictory results. Treatment of MRL-*lpr/lpr* mice with anti-IL-4 antibodies reduced mortality and disease activity (309). Conversely, IL-4 was shown not to be necessary in the BxSB male lupus model (310). Transgenic mice overexpressing IL-4 either exhibited a lupus-like disease or had a protective effect according to the background (311,312). Elevated levels of IL-4 and IL-13 were also detected in patients with SSc (313,314). IL-4 stimulated the production of collagen by normal and SSc fibroblasts at the level of transcription and mRNA stability (315), suggesting a potential role for IL-4 in the pathophysiology of scleroderma. However, multiple other cytokines and growth factors are also involved.

Interleukin-7, Interleukin-15, and Interleukin-21

IL-7 shares many activities with IL-2, including stimulation of T-cell proliferation, induction of cytotoxic effector cells and NK cells, stimulation of B cells and immunoglobulin production, and prevention of T-cell apoptosis. These common activities are related to the use of the same γ chain of the IL-2 receptor. In addition, IL-7 has a specific IL-7Rα chain receptor that is expressed by T cells and monocytes/macrophages. Unlike IL-2, production of IL-7 is not restricted to activated T lymphocytes but is also detected in resting T cells. In addition, IL-7 mRNA has been found in various tissues and cell types, including spleen, thymus, keratinocytes, and intestinal epithelial cells. The results of different studies indicate that, in contrast to IL-2, the production of which is primarily regulated at the level of transcription, IL-7 synthesis is also regulated at the level of translation. Several recent findings indicate that IL-7 can be considered as a proinflammatory cytokine and may thus contribute to the pathogenesis of inflammatory rheumatic diseases. IL-7 induced the production of TNF-α, IL-1β, IL-6, and IL-8 by monocytes/macrophages (316). Serum levels of IL-7 were significantly higher in patients with systemic JIA as compared with healthy children. Elevated IL-7 levels correlated with the presence of persistent systemic symptoms (317). Circulating levels of IL-7 were elevated in RA patients as compared with healthy controls and correlated positively with CRP concentrations (318). Freshly isolated cells from RA synovium spontaneously express IL-7 mRNA and protein in greater amounts than cells from OA patients. Isolated synovial fibroblasts, but not macrophages or T cells, produced low levels of IL-7 protein, and IL-1β and TNF-α enhanced this production. IL-7 stimulated both the proliferation of synovial tissue T cells (319) and TNF-α production by SF mononuclear cells. SF $CD4^+$ T cells expressed IL-7Rα chain receptor at their cell surface and IL-7 stimulated the production of TNF-α and IFN-γ by $CD4^+$ T cells. In contrast, IL-7 had no influence on IL-4 production, indicating that IL-7 specifically promoted T_H1 responses. This effect of IL-7 on T_H1 responses was mediated by the release of IL-12 from antigen-presenting cells including macrophages. In contrast to IFN-γ, the release of TNF-α was independent of IL-12 and may be a direct effect on T cells or through interactions between activated T cells and macrophages (318). Analysis of cytokine expression in cartilage from RA, OA, and control joints showed that IL-7 mRNA was exclusively expressed in RA cartilage (320). IL-7 also participates in bone loss and possibly in the development of joint erosions by the induction of RANKL by T cells (321).

As with IL-7, IL-15 is produced by a wide variety of tissues and cell types, including macrophages, fibroblasts, keratinocytes, and skeletal muscle. In macrophages, IL-15 production is induced by IFN-γ, LPS, bacteria, and viruses. IL-15 is produced in two different isoforms, which differ in size of the signal sequence, cellular localization, and tissue distribution (322,323). One isoform has a 48–amino acid long leader peptide and is expressed both as a transmembrane and a secreted protein. The shorter isoform has a 21–amino acid leader sequence and is found in the nucleus or as a cytosolic peptide. As with other cytokines, such as TNF-α and IL-1α, transmembrane IL-15 is biologically active (324). Overexpression of the transmembrane and secreted isoform led to an increased number of memory $CD8^+$ T cells in lymph nodes, enhanced IFN-γ production, and protection against *Salmonella* infection, whereas transgenic mice overexpressing the intracellular isoform exhibited impaired IFN-γ production upon TCR engagement and were susceptible to *Salmonella* infection. These results suggest that the balance between the two isoforms may play an important role in the regulation of host defense and in inflammatory conditions (325). IL-15 interacts with a heterotrimeric receptor including IL-2Rβ and the common γ chain, but does not require the β chain. The third component is the IL-15-specific IL-15Rα binding receptor. In contrast to IL-2Rα, which is exclusively present on activated T cells, IL-15Rα is expressed on different cells, including T cells, neutrophils, mast cells, myoblasts, synovial fibroblasts, endothelial cells, and human neural cells. IL-1β and TNF-α stimulate the expression of IL-15Rα mRNA and protein by synovial fibroblasts (326).

IL-15 can readily be detected in RA, but not in OA, SF. Immunostaining identified IL-15-positive cells in RA synovium, mainly macrophages and some fibroblast-like cells. IL-15 can induce TNF-α production in monocytes through activation of synovial T cells via a cell contact–dependent mechanism (327). IL-15 also induces the production of other proinflammatory cytokines, including IL-1β, IL-8, and IL-17. IL-15 acts as a T cell–chemotactic and –antiapoptotic factor, shares biologic activities with IL-2, and stimulates T-cell proliferation, induces IFN-γ production, and inhibits apoptosis. It also promotes B-cell proliferation and differentiation and activates NK cells. Recently, neutrophil activation and protection from apoptosis by IL-15 has been described, as has induction of mast cell proliferation. IL-15 stimulates the proliferation of RA synovial fibroblasts in culture and the expression of antiapoptotic Bcl-2 and Bcl-x_L. The addition of IL-15 mutant/Fcγ2a, an IL-15Rα antagonist, to cultured synovial fibroblasts reduced the endogenous expression of Bcl-2 and Bcl-x_L and synoviocyte proliferation and was associated with increased apoptosis (326). IL-15 also exerted antiapoptotic effects on synovial vascular endothelial cells *in vitro*, thus potentially contributing to the angiogenic process within the synovial membrane (328). In addition, IL-15 stimulated the differentiation of osteoclast progenitors into preosteoclasts, and this effect was independent of TNF-α, IL-2, or IL-7 (329). The results of these studies suggest that IL-15 plays an important role both in the initiation and in the perpetuation of articular inflammation, as well as in the mechanisms leading to joint damage. Administration of recombinant IL-15 during priming of mice with type II collagen in incomplete Freund's adjuvant reproduces the arthritis obtained in mice immunized with complete Freund's adjuvant (330). The administration of a soluble fragment of the mouse IL-15Rα chain after immunization markedly suppressed the development of CIA. This effect was accompanied *in vitro* by marked reductions in antigen-specific proliferation and IFN-γ synthesis by spleen cells from treated mice as compared with control mice and *in vivo* by a significant reduction in serum levels of anti–type II collagen antibody (331). In addition, a soluble fragment of human IL-15Rα could also suppress the development of CIA in monkeys (330). Collectively, the results of *in vitro* and *in vivo* studies suggest that antagonists to IL-15 may have therapeutic potential in RA. Recently, the safety and efficacy of a fully human monoclonal antibody against IL-15 (HuMax-IL-15) was examined in a randomized, double-blind, dose-escalating, placebo-controlled clinical trial in 30 RA patients. Preliminary data suggested that administration of HuMax-IL-15 is safe and efficacious for the treatment of RA patients (332).

IL-21 is a recently described cytokine that is expressed by activated $CD4^+$ T lymphocytes. IL-21 is capable of costimulating T- and B-cell proliferation and regulating NK cell activation and expansion. IL-21 shares sequence homologies with the cytokines IL-2, IL-4, and IL-15 and mediates its effects through a heterodimeric receptor, including a novel class I receptor IL-21 and the common γ cytokine receptor chain. IL-21R is expressed on T, B, and NK cells (333,334). Binding to both IL-21R and the common γ receptor chain are necessary to transduce intracellular signals. The mutation of the γ chain is associated in humans with X-linked SCID disease. The absence of response to IL-2, IL-7, and IL-15 can explain the absence of T and NK cells, but not the B-cell defect. By using IL-21R gene knockout mice, IL-21 was shown to cooperate with IL-4 and to play a critical role in the production of immunoglobulin following immunization. These results suggest that the absence of response to IL-4 and IL-21 is responsible for the B-cell defect in X-linked SCID (335). IL-21 is also a growth and survival factor for myeloma cells, and this effect may be mediated by the activation of JAK-STAT and ERK1/2 signaling pathways (336).

Using different systems, IL-21 has been shown to stimulate both T_H1 and T_H2 responses. *In vivo* studies indicate that IL-21 is required to modulate a T_H1 response. Previously, immunized IL-21R −/− mice mounted a much stronger footpad inflammatory reaction than wild-type mice in response to specific antigen injection. This increased delayed-type hypersensitivity correlated with a marked increase in IFN-γ production by isolated lymph node T cells (337). According to these findings, IL-21 may exert a protective effect in diseases with an excessive T_H1 response, such as RA.

Interleukin-9

IL-9 is expressed by activated T cells and is considered a T_H2 cytokine. IL-9 interacts with its specific receptor (IL-9Rα) and the common γ chain. After ligand binding, both JAK-STAT and MAP kinase ERK pathways are activated (338). IL-9 and IL-4 have been implicated in immune responses against extracellular parasites and in asthma. Transgenic mice overexpressing IL-9 develop mastocytosis, and expansion of B1 lymphocytes and eosinophils. Some of the phenotypic manifestations of IL-9 transgenic mice, including eosinophilia, bronchial hyperresponsiveness, elevated IgE levels, and mucus secretion, suggest that this cytokine is involved in the pathogenic mechanisms of asthma (339).

INTERLEUKIN-10 AND RELATED CYTOKINES

Interleukin-10

IL-10 was originally termed cytokine synthesis inhibitory factor and was identified as a T_H2 cell–derived factor that inhibited production of IFN-γ by T_H1 cells. IL-10 is produced by monocytes and T and B lymphocytes. Its expression in monocytes is stimulated by LPS and reduced by IFN-γ. In contrast to many other cytokines, IL-10 transcription can be regulated by transcription factors Sp1 and Sp3, which are expressed constitutively by many cell types (340,341). In addition, IL-10 mRNA levels are also controlled at the posttranscriptional level by alteration of mRNA stability (342). Several polymorphisms within the IL-10 gene 5′ flanking region have been described. The −1082 (G) allele was associated with higher ConA-induced IL-10 production (343). Possible linkage of IL-10 promoter haplotypes with disease susceptibility has been reported in SLE patients. This association may be of importance because elevated IL-10 levels may predispose to disease.

The inhibitory effect of IL-10 on T cells and NK cells was found to be indirect, via the inhibition of accessory cell (macrophages/monocyte) function. Indeed, IL-10 reduces the production of IL-1, TNF-α, IL-6, IL-8, NO, and reactive oxygen species by monocytes in response to LPS and IFN-γ. IL-10 inhibits the production of a variety of both C-C and C-X-C chemokines by activated monocytes (344–347). In addition, IL-10 also interferes with the expression of class II MHC and costimulatory molecules such as CD80/CD86 (348). IL-10 inhibited PGE_2 through downregulation of COX-2 expression by monocytes. IL-10 inhibited the ability of monocytes/macrophages to degrade the extracellular matrix by its inhibitory effect on MMP production and its ability to enhance the production of TIMP (349). IL-10 also exerts antiinflammatory effects through the stimulation of IL-1Ra production by monocytes and neutrophils (295,350). Mice rendered deficient in IL-10 had normal immune system development, but manifested chronic enterocolitis due to uncontrolled immune responses to enteric pathogens (351). In addition, by using other experimental models, IL-10 −/− mice exhibited other exaggerated inflammatory responses, indicating that IL-10 exerts critical *in vivo* functions to limit inflammatory responses (352,353). Both transcriptional and posttranscriptional mechanisms have been implicated in the inhibitory effects of IL-10 on cytokine and chemokine production (354,355).

The IL-10 receptor consists of two subunits that are members of the IFN receptor family. IL-10R1 is the ligand-binding subunit. IL-10R1 was detected in all IL-10-responsive cells, and neutralization of IL-10R1 by monoclonal antibodies blocked the effects of IL-10. IL-10R1 is expressed on hematopoietic and nonhematopoietic cells. Its expression is up-regulated in activated monocytes and in LPS-stimulated fibroblasts (356). IL-10R2 is an accessory subunit for signaling and is constitutively expressed in most cells and tissues. IL-10R2 contributes little to IL-10 binding, but its main function appears to be the recruitment of JAK kinases in the signaling complex (357,358). IL-10 activates STAT3, STAT1, and STAT5. However, STAT3 has been shown to be of prime importance for IL-10 signaling in all IL-10-responsive cells.

Based on the ability to suppress cytokine synthesis in monocytes, IL-10 was tested in LPS-induced shock. A single injection of IL-10 reproducibly protected mice from a lethal intraperitoneal injection of endotoxin. The protective effect of IL-10 correlated with a substantial decrease in endotoxin-induced TNF-α release (359). Intravenous administration of IL-10 inhibited LPS-induced increases in temperature and release of cytokines in healthy human volunteers (360).

Interleukin-10 and Rheumatoid Arthritis

IL-10 mRNA and protein were spontaneously produced in RA and OA synovial membrane cultures. In RA and OA synovial membrane biopsies, IL-10 was present in monocytes and T cells in the mononuclear cell aggregates. Neutralization of endogenously produced IL-10 in RA synovial membrane cultures increased TNF-α and IL-1β secretion, but IL-6 and IL-8 levels were not affected. Exogenous IL-10 decreased the spontaneous levels of TNF-α and IL-1β (361). T-cell clones derived from RA do not produce large amounts of T_H1 cytokines. The presence of IL-10 in the synovium is one possible explanation for the relative lack of IL-2 and IFN-γ.

Systemic administration of IL-10 was protective in animal models of RA. When administered before or after the induction of disease, IL-10 reduced joint swelling, synovial infiltration, cytokine production, and cartilage degradation in collagen- and streptococcal cell wall–induced arthritis (304,362–365). Neutralization of IL-10 with antibodies increased disease severity in these models (366). A viral homologue of IL-10 shares most of the biologic effects of IL-10, but it does not induce MHC class II expression on B cells and does not act as a costimulatory molecule in T-cell activation. Systemic adenoviral delivery of IL-10 had modest antiarthritic effects. However, periarticular delivery of viral IL-10 by adenoviral gene transfer resulted in strong and persistent suppression of CIA (367).

The efficacy and safety of daily injections of recombinant human IL-10 was evaluated in a 28-day phase I randomized, double-blind, placebo-controlled clinical trial in RA patients. During therapy, a reversible dose-dependent thrombocytopenia was observed with a trend toward improvement of disease activity. Circulating levels of soluble TNFRs p55 and p75, as well as IL-1Ra, were significantly increased at the highest doses, and *ex vivo* production of IL-1 and TNF in response to stimulation with phytohemagglutinin and LPS tended to decrease (368). IL-10 was well tolerated. However, the lack of efficacy in subsequent studies resulted in discontinuation of development. A double-blind, dose-escalating, placebo-controlled phase II clinical trial was performed in patients with psoriatic arthritis. The administration of IL-10 was safe; however, whereas a positive response to treatment with IL-10 was observed for psoriasis, psoriatic arthritis did not improve (369).

Interleukin-10 and Systemic Lupus Erythematosus

Elevated serum levels of IL-10 are present in SLE patients and correlate with disease activity and anti-dsDNA antibody levels (370). IL-10 enhances the survival of normal B cells, which correlates with expression of the anti-apoptotic protein bcl-2 (371). IL-10 is also a potent cofactor for proliferation of mature B cells activated by IgM or CD40 cross-linking. IL-2 and IL-4 further enhance this effect. PBMC from SLE patients produce high amounts of IL-10. Transfer of PBMC from SLE patients to SCID mice results in high titers of anti-dsDNA antibodies, which are almost completely abolished by anti-IL-10 antibodies (372). Immune complexes from SLE sera induce the production of IL-10 by an FcγRII mechanism, thus leading to the maintenance of B-cell hyperactivity (373). Anti-IL-10 antibodies delay the onset of disease in (NZB × NZW) F1 mice. This protection against autoimmunity appears to be due to an anti-IL-10-induced up-regulation of endogenous TNF-α, because anti-IL-10-protected mice rapidly develop autoimmunity when neutralizing anti-TNF-α antibodies are introduced. Consistent with the protective role of anti-IL-10 treatment in these experiments, administration of IL-10 accelerates the onset of autoimmunity (374). In an open-label clinical trial, the administration of a murine monoclonal anti–human IL-10 antibody to six patients for 21 days achieved a long-lasting reduction of most criteria of disease activity in five of six patients, thus supporting a role for IL-10 in the pathogenesis of SLE (375).

Interleukin-10–Related Cytokines

Five novel cytokines, including IL-19, IL-20, IL-22, IL-24, and IL-26, demonstrating limited primary sequence homology with IL-10, have recently been identified (376, 377). These cellular cytokines, in addition to viral homologues of IL-10, form a family of IL-10-related cytokines. As with IL-10, all of these novel cytokines require two distinct receptor subunits for signaling. In addition, these cytokines also share some common receptor subunits. IL-10R2 is a common subunit for IL-10 and IL-22. IL-19, IL-20, and IL-24 can bind IL-20R1 and IL-20R2. Upon ligand binding, heterodimerization of various R1 and R2 chains induce the activation of the JAK/STAT system. STAT3 is the predominant STAT molecule activate by IL-10-related cytokines. IL-22BP is the only soluble receptor from this class of receptors. The coding sequence of IL-22BP lacks the cytoplasmic and transmembrane regions. Thus, IL-22BP is released as a secreted protein, specifically binds IL-22, and acts as a natural IL-22 antagonist (378).

Some of these IL-10-related cytokines may be involved in skin development and homeostasis. IL-20 transgenic mice develop hyperproliferation of keratinocytes resembling psoriasis, but without the common T-cell infiltrate in the dermis (379). IL-24 is expressed in normal skin and its expression is up-regulated during wound healing (380). Immune cells produce IL-19, IL-20, and IL-24 in response to different stimuli. The expression of IL-26 is expressed by virally transformed T cells and in freshly isolated PBMCs from healthy donors (377). In contrast to IL-10, activated

T_H1, rather than T_H2, CD4+ cells produced mouse and human IL-22 (381). Some evidence suggests that IL-22 may be potentially involved in inflammatory processes. IL-22 is able to induce the production of acute-phase proteins by the HepG2 hepatoma cell line (382). IL-22 was produced in response to LPS in various organs. However, in contrast to IL-10, IL-22 does not inhibit the production of TNF-α, IL-1, and IL-6 by LPS-stimulated monocytes (383). It had no effect on IFN-γ production, but had a modest inhibitory effect on IL-4 production by T_H2 CD4+ cells (383). Interestingly, IL-22BP mRNA, the IL-22 antagonist, was detected by *in situ* hybridization in mononuclear cells of inflammatory infiltrates in several tissues (383).

Three novel cytokines, IL-28A, IL-28B, and IL-29, with antiviral activity were recently described. These cytokines are expressed by virally-infected PBMCs and bind to a heterodimeric receptor that consists of IL-10R2 and a novel receptor chain, IL-28Rα, which has 23% amino acid sequence identity with IL-22Rα (384).

INTERLEUKIN-12 AND RELATED CYTOKINES

Interleukin-12

IL-12 is a 70-kd heterodimeric cytokine consisting of two covalently-linked chains, p40 and p35. Although it does not have sequence homology with IL-2, the three-dimensional structure of the two cytokines appears to be similar. In addition, the p35 gene has homologies with class I cytokines such as IL-6 and G-CSF. Interestingly, p40 has homologies with the extracellular domains of the 80-kd IL-6R α chain and the CNTF receptor (385). IL-12 was originally isolated from Epstein-Barr virus–transformed B lymphocytes. Both p40 and p35 are produced by *in vitro*–activated peripheral blood adherent cells and probably by B cells (386). Although p35 mRNA is detected in many cells, free p35 protein is not secreted. In contrast, production of IL-12 by activated macrophages and dendritic cells results in the release of a large excess of monomeric or dimeric p40. Homodimeric p40 can act as a receptor antagonist of IL-12. However, other experiments have demonstrated that treatment of IL-12p35/p40 −/− mice with homodimeric p40 restored the delayed-type hypersensitivity, indicating that p40 exerts agonist activity in the absence of p35. p40 is a chemoattractant for macrophages and can induce the expression of inducible nitric oxide synthase (iNOS). It is possible that the antagonist and agonist activities of dimeric p40 are mediated through its binding to the β1 subunit of IL-12R (387).

IL-12 stimulates the production of T_H1-associated cytokines, particularly IFN-γ by T cells and NK cells. IL-12, originally termed NK cell–stimulating factor, inhibits T_H2-associated cytokine production and binds to a high-affinity receptor composed of two subunits, β1 and β2. Both β1 and β2 are closely related to the family of gp130 and LIF receptors. These receptors are expressed on T and NK cells and are required for IL-12 bioactivity. The β2 subunit plays an important role in signal transduction by providing a binding site for STAT4, which mediates the effects of IL-12.

IL-12 and Arthritis

The role of IL-12 has been examined in experimental models of arthritis. The administration of IL-12 to mice immunized with type II collagen and incomplete Freund adjuvant resulted in the occurrence of a high incidence of arthritis. In addition, IL-12 enhanced the severity of arthritis, the production of collagen-specific IgG2a and IgG2b antibodies, and the production of IFN-γ. Neutralization of IFN-γ prevented the effect of IL-12 on the development of arthritis (388). In addition, other investigators showed that IL-12 stimulated the development of CIA independently of its ability to induce IFN-γ (389). The incidence and severity of CIA was significantly reduced in mice treated with neutralizing anti-IL-12 antibodies and in IL-12 −/− mice (390–392). In contrast to its effect during immunization or at the time around arthritis onset, IL-12 seems to exert a protective effect in established arthritis. The administration of anti-IL-12 antibodies induced an exacerbation of established arthritis with enhanced expression of IL-1β and TNF-α (393). The administration of mouse recombinant IL-12 resulted in a profound suppression of arthritis (394). The antiinflammatory effect of IL-12 in established CIA was mediated by the stimulation of IL-10 production (393).

IL-12p40 mRNA was detected in SF mononuclear cells of RA patients with early and late disease. Levels of IL-12 protein were increased in RA SF as compared with the levels in the serum of RA patients and controls. In addition, IL-12 p40 mRNA was detected in the synovial tissue of RA patients. Cells isolated from the rheumatoid synovium spontaneously produced IL-12. By immunohistochemistry, IL-12 was detected in the sublining layer and mostly expressed by CD68+ cells (395). IL-12 mRNA and protein was also identified in rheumatoid nodules (396).

Interleukin-23 and Interleukin-27

IL-23 is a novel, heterodimeric molecule consisting of p40 and p19, which form a disulfide-bridge complex. IL-23 binds to IL-12Rβ1 and IL-23R. IL-23R is responsible for intracellular signaling and has a cytoplasmic STAT4-binding site (397). Similar to IL-12 p35, coexpression of p19 and p40 in the same cell is necessary for expression of IL-23. IL-23 is produced by activated dendritic cells and stimulates the proliferation of memory T cells and has a modest effect on IFN-γ production as compared with IL-12 (398). Transgenic mice overexpressing p19 exhibit multiorgan inflammatory disease with premature death, suggesting that IL-23 exerts proinflammatory effects (399).

IL-27 is a heterodimeric protein consisting of Epstein-Barr virus–induced gene 3 (EBI3), a p40-related protein, and p28, a novel p35-related peptide. IL-27 is produced by activated antigen-presenting cells and induces the proliferation of naïve CD4+ T cells. IL-27 and IL-12 induce the production of IFN-γ in a synergistic manner (400). IL-27 binds to TCCR, a novel receptor chain with some homology to IL-12Rβ2, and to gp130. TCCR is expressed on naïve T cells, and its expression is decreased on differentiated T_H1 or T_H2 cells (401). In addition, TCCR is required for the early initiation of T_H1 differentiation, but is not necessary for the maintenance of a T_H1 response. These findings suggest that IL-27 and IL-12 act sequentially in initiating and maintaining T_H1 responses, respectively (387).

INTERLEUKIN-16

IL-16 is produced by CD8+, but not CD4+, T cells. This cytokine is not a member of the chemokine family but exerts a chemoattractant activity for CD4+ T lymphocytes, monocytes, and eosinophils. IL-16 is produced as a 631-amino acid precursor without an N-terminal signal peptide. Pro-IL-16 is processed and released in the extracellular compartment (402). IL-16 binds to CD4 and can downregulate the activity of CD4-expressing cells (403). Serum and SF concentrations of IL-16 are elevated in RA and are significantly higher than in OA (404,405). IL-16 mRNA and protein is also detected in RA synovial tissues (404, 406). *In situ* hybridization studies revealed that it is expressed by synovial fibroblasts and within inflammatory infiltrates. IL-16 protein was also detected in CD8+ cells within the rheumatoid synovium (406). Serum and SF levels of IL-16 do not correlate with biologic and clinical markers of disease activity (404,405).

Adoptive transfer of syngeneic CD8+ T cells induced a marked reduction in production of IFN-γ and macrophage-derived proinflammatory cytokines, including IL-1β and TNF-α, in a model of rheumatoid synovial tissue implantation in SCID mice. The use of neutralizing anti-IL-16 antibodies and of recombinant IL-16 demonstrated that the antiinflammatory effect of transferred CD8+ T cells was mediated by IL-16 (406).

Elevated circulating levels of IL-16 were detected in SLE patients and were higher in patients with severe disease and correlated with disease activity index (407,408).

INTERLEUKIN-17 AND RELATED CYTOKINES

The complementary DNA encoding human IL-17 was cloned from a CD4+ T-lymphocyte library. IL-17 is a 155–amino acid peptide containing an N-terminal leader sequence. It exhibits 72% amino acid identity with HVS13, an open reading frame from *Herpesvirus saimiri*, and 63% with murine CTLA8. IL-17 is produced primarily by activated CD4+ lymphocytes and secreted as a homodimeric molecule (409). Results obtained from T-cell lines allowed the classification of IL-17 as a T_H1 cytokine (410). IL-17 binds to its cell surface receptor IL-17R, which is expressed on most cells; consequently, IL-17 is biologically active in different tissues. IL-17, IL-1, and TNF-α stimulate common intracellular signaling pathways, including p38 MAPK and NFκB (411,412). Consequently, these cytokines share many activities. IL-17 stimulates the production of IL-6, IL-8, and intercellular adhesion molecule-1 (ICAH-1) in human fibroblasts. In addition, IL-17 stimulates the production of TNF-α and IL-1 by monocytes/macrophages (413).

SF levels of IL-17 were higher in RA than in OA. IL-17 mRNA was detected in the synovial tissue of RA but not of OA patients (414). IL-17 expression was restricted to a minor subset of infiltrating lymphocytes around blood vessels (415). The proinflammatory effects of IL-17 suggest that it participates in the pathogenic mechanisms of RA and other inflammatory diseases. In synovial fibroblasts, IL-17 stimulated the production of IL-6, IL-8, LIF, and PGE_2 (416). Although IL-1 was more potent in stimulating these responses, IL-17 could act in synergy with IL-1 and TNF-α to induce the production of cytokines and MMP (416). IL-17 stimulated the migration of dendritic cells and the recruitment of T cells by inducing the production of macrophage inflammatory protein 3α (MIP-3α, also termed CCL20) (415). IL-17 also contributes to the development of articular damage by inducing the production of MMP-3 and by decreasing the synthesis of proteoglycans by articular chondrocytes (417). T cells producing IL-17 contribute to the development of bony erosions. Indeed, IL-17 stimulates osteoclastogenesis by increasing the expression of RANKL and the RANKL/OPG ratio (418). The role of IL-17 in the pathogenic mechanisms of RA was further supported by the results of *in vivo* experiments. The intraarticular administration of IL-17 in normal mouse joints induced cartilage degradation (419). This effect of IL-17 was independent of IL-1 (420). Overexpression of IL-17 in the joints of mice with CIA promoted severe bone destruction accompanied by marked osteoclast activity and RANKL expression (418). The production and biologic effect of IL-17 can be decreased by T_H2 cytokines (415). The administration of IL-4 to mice with CIA prevented the development of erosions and decreased the number of osteoclasts. IL-4 decreased the levels of RANKL and IL-17 mRNA (300).

Serum levels of IL-17 were significantly increased in SSc patients as compared with healthy controls. IL-17 mRNA was detected in the skin as well as in bronchoalveolar lavage lymphocytes. IL-17 was particularly present at the early stages of SSc, suggesting a role of IL-17 in the early events of SSc. IL-17 induced the proliferation of cultured dermal fibroblasts from healthy donors and SSc patients, and the expression of adhesion molecules, IL-1β, and IL-6 by endothelial cells (421). Levels of IL-17 were also elevated in SLE patients (422).

More recently, other peptides were identified with some sequence homology with IL-17. Each of these IL-17 family members shares four highly conserved cysteine residues that may be involved in interchain disulfide linkages. These homologues are now designated as IL-17B to IL-17F and also include IL-25. As opposed to IL-17, IL-25 is produced by T_H2 cells and mast cells, and stimulates the production of IL-4, IL-5, IL-13, and eotaxin (423). Administration of IL-25 induces a marked eosinophilia and is thus probably involved in allergic diseases (424).

COLONY-STIMULATING FACTORS

This section discusses cytokines that are primarily regulators of hematopoiesis. Three aspects relevant to rheumatic diseases are highlighted: the role of these cytokines in hematopoiesis and on mature hematopoietic cells, which may contribute to inflammation and tissue damage; their expression in rheumatic diseases; and the potential therapeutic use of CSFs in patients with rheumatic diseases.

Regulation of Hematopoiesis and Effect on Mature Cells

Most of the CSFs and their receptors are members of the hematopoietin family. The receptor for M-CSF (c-*fms*) and SCF receptor (c-*kit*) have intrinsic receptor tyrosine kinase activity. The major growth factor for $CD34^+$ hematopoietic stem cells is SCF. IL-3 stimulates multipotential hematopoietic progenitors, as well as cells that are committed to the granulocyte, macrophage, eosinophil, mast cell, megakaryocytic, or erythroid lineage. IL-3 is, therefore, also referred to as multi-CSF. GM-CSF stimulates not only the formation of granulocyte and macrophage precursors, but also more immature progenitors and other lineages. IL-5 has a major role in eosinophil development and, in contrast to its effects on B-cell differentiation in mice, it does not appear to regulate human B lymphocytes. G-CSF generates granulocytes by inducing clonal proliferation and differentiation of progenitor cells.

Erythropoietin (Epo) is produced in response to hypoxia in the kidney and in fetal liver. It circulates to hematopoietic tissues, inhibits programmed death, and stimulates proliferation and differentiation of committed erythroid progenitor cells (425). In contrast to most other hematopoietic cytokines, Epo is restricted to peritubular interstitial cells as the single site of production in the mature organism, and it is specific, as it has little effect on other cells.

Two activities are required for megakaryocytopoiesis: one induces the proliferation and differentiation of megakaryocyte progenitors, and the second causes megakaryocyte maturation. Both activities are now known to be a function of the same molecule, termed thrombopoietin. This cytokine is closely related to erythropoietin and binds to the c-*mpl*-encoded receptor, a member of the hematopoietic cytokine receptor family (426).

In addition to regulating hematopoietic cell development, CSFs also can activate mature cells. IL-3 and IL-5 stimulate secretory responses in mature human basophils and eosinophils, whereas GM-CSF is an important activator of mature human monocytes. The latter induces MHC class II antigens on synovial tissue cells (427) and the expression of plasminogen activator by monocytes. M-CSF stimulates cytokine synthesis and promotes survival of macrophages. M-CSF deficiency is responsible for the lack of osteoclasts and macrophages in osteopetrotic mice, which can be corrected by the administration of M-CSF (428). M-CSF also acts on mature osteoclasts. It is chemotactic, induces cell spreading, and promotes osteoclast survival. G-CSF and GM-CSF activate and prime neutrophil secretory responses. GM-CSF enhances the constitutive production of IL-1Ra, which is the major *de novo*–synthesized product of activated neutrophils. Neutrophils isolated from RA SF also responded to GM-CSF with increased IL-1Ra synthesis (429). Administration of G-CSF to healthy volunteers caused immediate neutrophil activation with FcγRIII up-regulation, intravascular release of specific granules, and elevated plasma levels of elastase (430).

Colony-Stimulating Factor Expression in Rheumatic Diseases

Synovial fibroblasts are a significant cell source of different CSFs. GM-CSF and G-CSF are induced by IL-1 and TNF-α (431,432). Cyclooxygenase inhibitors potentiate the action of IL-1 on GM-CSF synthesis but suppress G-CSF synthesis. Stimulation of synovial cells with IL-1β, TNF-α, IFN-γ, or IL-4 also increases M-CSF production. M-CSF may be particularly important for sustaining long-term influx, activation, and survival of mononuclear phagocytes at sites of inflammation. GM-CSF is produced spontaneously, both by RA synovial cells and, to a lesser extent, by OA synovial cells in the absence of extrinsic stimuli. Neutralizing antibodies to TNF-α reduce spontaneous GM-CSF production in RA synovial cell cultures. Articular chondrocytes also produce these three CSFs in response to the same inducers as synoviocytes.

The plasma GM-CSF levels of patients with severe or moderate RA and of patients with SLE are elevated, but plasma levels in patients with spondyloarthropathy were not increased. GM-CSF concentrations as high as 1,300 pg/mL were detected in RA SF. Serum levels of G-CSF were elevated in RA patients with active disease and correlated significantly with morning stiffness and the number of swollen joints (433). The serum level of IL-3, as determined by ELISA, was higher in patients with SLE than in healthy controls (434).

The role of GM-CSF in the pathogenesis of arthritis was examined in CIA. Administration of neutralizing anti-GM-CSF antibodies at the time of antigen challenge was effective in ameliorating the ensuing disease. The administration of anti-GM-CSF antibodies decreased the level of articular inflammation, SF IL-1β and TNF-α, and subsequent joint damage in established CIA, but was devoid of effect on humoral and cellular response to type II collagen (435).

Colony-Stimulating Factor in the Treatment of Rheumatic Diseases

Anemia of chronic disease (ACD) is a frequent problem in patients with inflammatory rheumatic diseases. The pathogenesis of ACD includes decreased responsiveness of erythrocyte precursors to Epo, decreased production of Epo, and impaired mobilization of iron stores from macrophages (436). Treatment with Epo in patients with RA and ACD resulted in a significant increase of hemoglobin values and an improvement of disease activity (437,438).

GM-CSF and G-CSF have been applied in the treatment of drug-induced agranulocytosis and cause significantly faster recovery of the peripheral blood granulocytes and reduced mortality rates. No difference in granulocyte recovery was observed in patients treated with GM-CSF or G-CSF (439).

G-CSF inhibitors may participate in the pathogenesis of neutropenia in autoimmune diseases. IgG anti-G-CSF antibodies were detected in patients with Felty syndrome and in SLE patients with neutropenia, but not in control RA patients. The presence of these antibodies was associated with elevated G-CSF levels and low neutrophil counts. A neutralizing effect of these antibodies on its target molecule was found in some patients with neutropenia (440). Studies on large patient populations that address the value of CSF in treating hematopoietic deficiencies in autoimmune diseases are not available, although case reports consistently have demonstrated beneficial effects. G-CSF improved granulocytopenia in Felty syndrome (441) and may also be effective in the treatment of lupus neutropenia (442). A case of Felty syndrome with infectious complications due to severe neutropenia responded to short-term treatment with GM-CSF. Leukocyte counts rose and granulocyte function improved (443).

INTERFERONS

Interferons (IFNs) are a family of naturally-secreted proteins with immunomodulatory functions. They enhance the ability of macrophages to eliminate tumor cells, viruses, and bacteria. IFNs are divided into two types: type 1 IFNs including IFN-α and IFN-β, and type 2 IFN consists of IFN-γ alone. There are numerous genes for IFN-α, but only single genes for IFN-β and IFN-γ. IFN-γ differs structurally from the two other types of IFN and in its cellular origin. Essentially, all types of leukocytes produce IFN-α; IFN-β is predominantly of fibroblast origin. IFN-γ production is restricted to T lymphocytes and NK cells. All types of $CD8^+$ cells, T_H1 cells, and more immature T_H0 subsets of $CD4^+$ cells produce IFN-γ. In contrast to IFN-α and IFN-β, IFN-γ is not induced by virus infection, but rather by antigenic or mitogenic stimulation of lymphocytes. The regulation of IFN-γ production by lymphocytes is an important aspect of the differentiation of immune responses and is controlled by other cytokines. IL-12 and IL-18 stimulate IFN-γ production in T lymphocytes and NK cells, whereas IL-10 is an inhibitor of IFN-γ production.

IFN receptors constitute a distinct cytokine receptor family. The gene structures of IFN-α and IFN-β are similar and, despite a low degree of overall amino acid sequence homology, bind to the same receptor. The IFN-γ receptor is distinct from the receptor for IFN-α and IFN-β. Both IFN receptors contain long, intracellular domains and activate common and distinct members of the same families of signal transduction molecules. Most cell types express IFN receptors.

Interferon Function

The antiviral activities of IFNs are related to the induction of proteins and enzymes that inhibit viral RNA and protein synthesis. IFNs are also potent growth inhibitors for a broad spectrum of cell types and play a major role in the regulation of immune responses. IFNs can modulate mesenchymal cell functions and exhibit antiangiogenic effects.

Immunomodulatory Effects of Interferons

IFN-α stimulates the maturation of dendritic cells, favors a T_H1 response, and potentiates the activation of monocytes/macrophages (444). IFN-α also exerts antiinflammatory effects. Administration of IFN-α to healthy humans increased the production of IL-1Ra and decreased the stimulatory effect of IL-1 on IL-8 production (445). IFN-α enhanced the release of IL-1Ra and soluble TNFR p55 by mononuclear cells isolated from synovial tissue from OA and RA patients. In addition, IFN-α induced the synthesis of OPG but had no effect on the production of RANKL, IL-1β, and TNF-α by SF mononuclear cells from RA patients (446). IFN-β can exert antiinflammatory effects by decreasing the release of TNF-α and IL-1β and enhancing the production of IL-10 and IL-1Ra. IFN-β also enhanced T-cell cytotoxicity, inhibited T-cell proliferation and migration, enhanced IL-2 production by T_H1 cells, up-regulated the expression of TGF-β and of its receptor on peripheral monocytes, decreased the expression of MHC class II on virally infected and tumor cells, and decreased expression of several adhesion molecules (447). The immunomodulatory effects of IFN-γ include induction of MHC class I and II antigens and the activation of monocytes. IFN-γ also regulates antigen processing by stimulating the production of enzymes and peptide transporters in antigen-presenting cells. As a macrophage-activating factor, IFN-γ stimulates cell surface expression of Fc and complement receptors; enhances the ability of macrophages to kill intracellular pathogens; and increases their tumoricidal activity. IFN-γ enhances cytokine synthesis in response to other factors such as LPS. In murine macrophages, it stimulates the production of NO and stimulates the synthesis of complement components and C1 esterase inhibitor in monocytes (448). In macrophages, IFN-γ decreases LPS-stimulated production of the latent forms of 92- and 72-kd type IV gelatinase (449), collagenase, and stromelysin (450). The suppression of collagenase production by IFN-γ is related to its ability to reduce PGE_2 levels, which is a consequence of a reduction in membrane-bound phospholipase activity in IFN-γ-treated monocytes (451).

Effect of Interferons on Mesenchymal Cells

IFNs have effects on mesenchymal cells that are distinct from those of the catabolic factors, IL-1 and TNF-α, and differ from the anabolic effects of TGF-β. Administration of recombinant IFN-β to RA patients resulted in decreased MMP and IL-1β levels in synovial tissues (452). IFN-β enhanced the effect of IL-1 on IL-1Ra production by cultured articular chondrocytes and synovial fibroblasts (453). In addition, IFN-β plays a critical role in bone homeostasis by modulating the effect of RANKL on osteoclastogenesis through a negative feedback mechanism. IFN-β expression in osteoclast precursors is induced by RANKL via the transcription factor c-Fos. Following its induction, IFN-β then binds to its own receptors on osteoclasts and decreases the expression of c-Fos , an essential factor for the maturation of osteoclasts (454).

IFN-γ inhibits synovial cell proliferation and transcription for types I and III collagen (455,456). It also constitutively reduces increased collagen synthesis characteristic of fibroblasts derived from lesions of patients with scleroderma. IL-1- or TNF-α-induced PGE_2 and collagenase production in human synovial fibroblasts is depressed by IFN-γ (457). In contrast, the production of hyaluronic acid is moderately increased by IFN-γ. The IFN-γ inhibition of collagenase activity is not due to inhibition of procollagenase protein or mRNA expression, but is related to reduced production of stromelysin, the activator of procollagenase (458). In articular chondrocytes, IFN-γ decreases the expression of the genes for types II, IX, and XI collagens and collagen biosynthesis (459,460). As with IFN-β, IFN-γ suppresses the formation of osteoclasts by interfering with the RANKL signaling pathway. IFN-γ induces rapid degradation of TRAF6, resulting in the inhibition of NFκB and JNK activation (461).

Interferon Levels in Rheumatic Diseases

Sera from patients with SLE, Sjögren's syndrome, and RA contain IFN activity as measured in a biologic cytopathic effect inhibition assay (462). IFN titers correlate with disease activity and levels of autoantibodies and complement, as well as with response to therapy (463). Elevated serum levels of IFN-α detected in SLE patients may participate in the pathogenic mechanisms of autoimmunity. Indeed, experiments with neutralizing antibodies indicated that circulating IFN-α in SLE patients induced monocytes to differentiate into dendritic cells (464). Such dendritic cells may capture apoptotic cells and nucleosomes present in SLE patient's blood and induce the expansion of autoreactive $CD4^+$ T-cell clones followed by differentiation of autoantibody-producing B cells (465). PBMCs from pediatric patients with SLE have alterations in gene transcription that are attributable to changes induced by IFN-α (466). Consistent with these findings, the frequency of autoimmune disorders in patients undergoing treatment with IFN-α is increased and ranges from 0.15% to19% (467). The incidence of autoimmune disorders varies according to the underlying disease, treatment regimen, and duration of therapy.

IFN-α levels in cerebrospinal fluid from patients with CNS lupus were increased, particularly in patients with lupus psychosis, as compared with other manifestations of CNS lupus such as seizures. IFN-γ immunoreactivity and mRNA were detected in neurons. IFN-γ produced within the CNS may contribute to the development of lupus psychosis and perhaps may become a useful test in the differential diagnosis of psychosis in patients with SLE (468). Serum levels of IL-18, an inducer of IFN-γ production, were elevated in SLE patients and correlated with disease activity and IFN-γ levels (469). By flow cytometry, the T_H1/T_H2 ratio was elevated in patients with renal lupus, with particularly high values in those patients with diffuse proliferative lupus nephritis (470).

IFN-α levels in RA SF are very low. Increased concentrations are found in approximately 25% of RA SF, but the majority of the samples were below the detection limit of the assay (471). IFN-γ was either not detected or was found to be present at low levels in arthritic joints (472). This correlated with an absence of IFN-γ mRNA in RA synovial tissue (471).

Interferon in Experimental Models of Autoimmune Disease

Models of Systemic Lupus Erythematosus

The pathogenic role of type I IFN in lupus was investigated in murine models of SLE. IFN-α/IFN-β inducers [poly (I:C)] accelerated autoimmunity in (NZB × NZW) F1 mice (473). Glomerulonephritis induced in normal mice infected by lymphocytic choriomeningitis virus was inhibited by anti-IFN antibodies (474). Experiments performed in NZB mice lacking the α chain of the IFN-α/β receptor further supported the role of type I IFN in the pathogenesis of lupus. As opposed to their wild-type littermates, homozygous IFN-α/βR −/− mice exhibited a significant reduction in autoantibodies, kidney disease, and mortality (475). IFN-γ may play an important role in lupus models. The importance of IFN-γ in (NZB × NZW) F1 mice was suggested by acceleration of renal disease after administration of IFN-γ, whereas mice receiving neutralizing IFN-γ antibodies at an early stage exhibited significantly delayed onset (476). In addition, significant reduction in serologic abnormalities and extended survival was observed in MRL-*lpr/lpr* mice in which the IFN-γ or IFN-γ receptor genes had been deleted (477–479).

Models of Rheumatoid Arthritis

The effect of IFN-β was examined in CIA. Syngeneic fibroblasts were infected *in vitro* with retroviruses expressing

IFN-β and injected intraperitoneally before the onset of arthritis. The mice injected with IFN-β-expressing fibroblasts developed less severe disease. A beneficial effect was also observed when IFN-β-producing fibroblasts were injected in established CIA. Histologic analysis showed a significant reduction in joint destruction in mice treated with IFN-β. Anti–type II collagen IgG2a levels decreased, whereas anti-type II collagen IgG1 levels increased in mice receiving IFN-β-expressing fibroblasts. These results indicated that IFN-β induced a switch toward a T_H2 response (480). In a subsequent study in mice with CIA, daily injection of recombinant IFN-β decreased articular inflammation and had a protective effect on joint damage (481). Recombinant IFN-β was also tested in monkeys with CIA. Three monkeys with established arthritis received daily subcutaneous injection of IFN-β for 1 week. Two of them exhibited significant clinical improvement with a marked decrease in CRP levels (482).

The role of IFN-γ signaling in CIA led to conflicting results. In two reports, an IFN-γR knockout bred onto the DBA/1 background developed an accelerated form of arthritis, more severe articular inflammation, and subsequent joint damage (483,484). In CIA, the levels of anti–type II collagen IgG, particularly the IgG2a isotype, were significantly lower in IFN-γR −/− mice as compared with IFN-γR +/+ mice (484). In contrast, other investigators observed that IFN-γR −/− mice had a milder form of CIA (485).

Interferon Treatment of Rheumatoid Arthritis

An open phase I clinical trial with IFN-β was performed in 12 RA patients. Three different doses of IFN-β (22, 44, or 66 μg) were administered subcutaneously three times per week. The treatment was well tolerated. There was a significant but limited improvement in tender and swollen joint counts, patient assessment of pain, and patient and doctor global assessment (482). Expression of IL-1β, IL-6, MMP-1, and TIMP was significantly decreased in the synovial tissue of patients treated with IFN-β (452).

Several controlled trials using IFN-γ in RA have been performed. A large controlled phase III trial with 249 RA patients showed a significantly higher response rate after 3 months of treatment in the IFN-γ group (486). However, follow-up studies showed that the beneficial effect of IFN-γ tended to decrease and that the main cause of discontinuation was lack of clinical benefit (487). The results of a 24-week, multicenter, randomized, double-blind, placebo-controlled clinical trial in 197 RA patients demonstrated that IFN-γ had no more therapeutic value than placebo (488). In addition, as in multiple sclerosis, different studies suggest that IFN-γ may lead to exacerbation of autoimmune diseases (489–491). A recent study suggested that treatment with antibodies against IFN-γ might be a more appropriate therapeutic strategy for RA (492).

Interferon Treatment of Scleroderma

Based on their inhibitory effects on fibroblast proliferation and collagen production, IFNs were tested in patients with SSc. Intramuscular administration of IFN-α improved or stabilized the skin score in 10 of 14 patients with diffuse cutaneous SSc. However, it had no significant effect on grip strength, digital contractures, respiratory function, or visceral involvement. Type I collagen synthesis was significantly reduced in fibroblasts cultured from clinically uninvolved skin, but not in those from lesional skin (493). IFN-γ administered subcutaneously to nine scleroderma patients for 12 months produced a significant improvement in total skin score and blood gas analysis. Other clinical parameters were not altered significantly, but no serious adverse effects were noted (494). A total of 44 patients with SSc were enrolled in a multicenter, randomized, placebo-controlled clinical trial; 27 received subcutaneous injections of IFN-γ and 17 were in the control group. The results showed that IFN-γ had only a mild beneficial effect on skin sclerosis and was not associated with improvement in quality of life parameters. Organ involvement improved in 8 of 18 treatment patients and in 3 of 11 control patients. It worsened in 3 of 18 treatment patients and in 4 of 11 control patients. IFN-γ treatment was well tolerated, except for the occurrence of influenza-like adverse events (495).

Treatment of other Rheumatic Diseases

In Behçet disease, the subcutaneous administration of IFN-α (3 million units thrice a week) was associated with an improvement of ocular inflammation (496). In a randomized, double-blind clinical trial, patients received either 6 million units IFN-α-2a thrice a week or placebo injections. IFN-α-2a was efficacious for the management of the mucocutaneous lesions and was associated with an improvement in severity and frequency of ocular attacks (497). Two randomized, double-blind, placebo-controlled trials showed that oral administration of IFN-α in patients with Sjögren syndrome increased the production of saliva and improved the symptoms of xerostomia (498,499). In one of these studies, there was also an improvement in symptoms of xerophthalmia (499).

CHEMOKINES

Chemokines are 8- to 10-kd cytokines whose major biologic activity is to exert chemotactic activity toward neutrophils, monocytes, and lymphocytes, as well as basophils and eosinophils. In addition, a number of these chemokines are also involved in angiogenesis and induction of other cytokines. This superfamily of cytokines now contains nearly 50 ligands and at least 19 receptors. The identification of chemokines by different laboratories meant that they have often been given different names, leading to much confusion. Recently, a systematic nomenclature for chemokines and receptors has been adopted (500). Chemokines have been classified into at least four different families according to their structural homology regarding the location of two or four cysteine residues. These chemokine and chemokine receptor families are designated as C-X-C, C-C, C and C-X3-C, and CXCR, C-CR, CR and CX3CR, respectively (500).

In C-X-C chemokines, the cysteines are separated by an intervening amino acid. This chemokine family (CXCL1 to CXCL16) includes, among others, CXCL-1 or growth-related oncogene (gro)α, CXCL4 or platelet factor-4, CXCL5 or epithelial-neutrophil activating protein (ENA)-78, CXCL6 or connective tissue activating peptide (CTAP)-III, CXCL8 or IL-8, CXCL9 or monokine induced by IFN-γ (MIG), CXCL10 or IFN-γ-inducible protein (IP-10), and CXCL12 or stromal-derived factor (SDF)-1. In general, C-X-C chemokines are involved in the chemotaxis of neutrophils. The C-C chemokines have two adjacent conserved cysteine residues. The C-C chemokine family (CCL1 to CCL28) includes CCL2 or monocyte chemoattractant protein (MCP)-1, CCL3 or MIP-1α, CCL5 or RANTES (regulated upon activation normally T cell expressed and secreted), and CCL20 or MIP-3α. These chemokines mainly exert their chemoattractant activities toward monocytes. Some members of this family of chemokines are also chemotactic for subsets of T lymphocytes, NK cells, basophils, and eosinophils (501). The C family (XCL1 and XCL2) has a single cysteine, and the C-X3-C family has three intervening noncysteines. The CL family includes XCL1 or lymphotactin, which is involved in T-lymphocyte migration to inflammatory sites (502). CX3CL1 or fractalkine is expressed on cytokine-activated endothelial cells and is chemotactic for lymphocytes and monocytes (503, 504).

Chemokines are the only cytokines to act on G protein-coupled, seven-transmembrane spanning receptors. This is a class of receptors for which it has been easy to find small molecules with agonist or antagonist activities, thus representing interesting targets for therapy (505).

Chemokine receptors exhibit a nonspecific affinity for their chemokine ligand. C-X3-C has its own receptor (503,504). Chemokine receptors may influence the type of cell infiltrate during inflammation. CCR3 is expressed on T_H2 but not T_H1 lymphocytes. Accordingly, CCR3 is expressed in allergic infiltrates. In contrast, CCR5 is expressed on most T_H1 lymphocytes and has been detected in RA synovial fluid and tissue (506). The CXCL8/IL-8 receptors (CXCR1 and CXCR2) bind CXCL1/groα and CXCL5/ENA-78 (507). The sequence of the CXCL8/IL-8 receptors is homologous to receptors for the other neutrophil chemoattractants, fMet-Leu-Phe and C5a. The Duffy blood group antigen (also termed Duffy antigen receptor for chemokines), a receptor for the malarial parasite *Plasmodium vivax,* is the erythrocyte chemokine receptor and binds CXCL8/IL-8, CXCL1/groα, and CXCL5/ENA-78 (508).

Function of Chemokines

C-X-C Chemokines

The C-X-C chemokines not only are chemotactic for neutrophils, but also activate neutrophil secretory responses. CXCL8/IL-8 stimulates release of lysosomal enzymes, activates the respiratory burst, and increases expression of complement and adhesion receptors (509). CXCL8/IL-8 is also a chemoattractant for T cells and basophils (510). Some C-X-C chemokines stimulate, whereas others inhibit, angiogenesis. In general, chemokines carrying the glutamyl-leucyl-arginyl (ELR) motif, such as CXCL8/IL-8, CXCL1/groα, CXCL5/ENA-78, and CTAP-III/CXCL6 promote angiogenesis, whereas chemokines lacking ELR inhibit neovascularization. As an exception, CXCL12/SDF-1 lacks the ELR residues and is angiogenic (511–513). CXCL8/IL-8 was angiogenic when implanted in the rat cornea and induced proliferation and chemotaxis of human umbilical vein endothelial cells. Neutralizing antibody to CXCL8/IL-8 blocked some of the angiogenic activity present in the conditioned media of rheumatoid synovial macrophages, suggesting that CXCL8/IL-8 may contribute to the angiogenesis-dependent synovial hyperplasia in arthritis (514).

CXCL1/groα is a mitogenic protein secreted by melanoma cells that corresponds to the polypeptide encoded by the human gro gene. Two additional isoforms, groβ and groγ, share 90% and 86% amino acid sequence identity with groα, respectively. CXCL8/IL-8 and CXCL1/groα have several common biologic activities. IL-8 can act as a growth factor for human melanoma cells (515). Purified CXCL1/groα competes with CXCL8/IL-8 for binding to neutrophils and exhibits neutrophil chemotactic activity equivalent to that of CXCL8/IL-8 (516). CXCL1/groα induces chemotaxis, exocytosis of elastase, and changes in cytosolic-free calcium similar to CXCL8/IL-8. However, CXCL1/groα is considerably less potent than CXCL8/IL-8 in inducing the respiratory burst in neutrophils. Intradermal injections of CXCL1/groα in rats resulted in a massive accumulation of neutrophils. CXCL1/groα and CXCL8/IL-8, but not C-C chemokines, decreased the expression of interstitial collagens by rheumatoid synovial fibroblasts. This was not related to effects on MMPs or TIMPs and suggests that CXCL1/groα and CXCL8/IL-8 may be involved in the regulation of collagen turnover (517).

C-C Chemokines

The C-C chemokines are potent chemoattractants of monocytes and lymphocytes, as well as activators and attractants of eosinophils and basophils. CCL2/MCP-1 and other members of the C-C subfamily (CCL5/RANTES, CCL3/MIP-1α, and CCL7/MCP-3) stimulate arachidonic acid release in human monocytes. CCL8/MCP-2 and CCL7/MCP-3 have high sequence similarity with CCL2/MCP-1. Nevertheless, CCL8/MCP-2 differed considerably from CCL2/ MCP-1 and

CCL7/MCP-3 in its potency to stimulate arachidonate and calcium mobilization, and in its capacity to compete with labeled CCL2/MCP-1 (518). CCL3/MIP-1α and CCL4/MIP-1β are chemoattractants of activated, but not resting, human T lymphocytes. CD4+ T cells migrate in response to CCL4/MIP-1β, whereas CCL3/MIP-1α induces chemotaxis of predominantly CD8+ T cells (518). CCL5/RANTES causes the selective migration of human blood CD4+ T lymphocytes involved in memory T-cell function (519). CCL2/MCP-1 induced angiogenesis both *in vitro* and *in vivo* (520). Cell migration from blood into tissue depends on integrin-mediated adhesion to endothelium. Adhesion requires not only integrin ligands on the endothelium, but also activation of relevant T-cell integrins. CCL3/MIP-1β induces both chemotaxis and adhesion of T cells and augments adhesion of CD8+ T cells to VCAM-1. CCL4/MIP-1β is immobilized on endothelial cells by binding to a proteoglycan and induces binding of T cells to VCAM-1. Through this mechanism, these heparin-binding cytokines can be presented by endothelial cell proteoglycans and trigger adhesion (521).

Chemokine Expression in Arthritis

Studies regarding the expression of chemokines in joint tissues have demonstrated that many of these cytokines are expressed by synovial fibroblasts, macrophages, and chondrocytes (522). Some of the chemokines are expressed constitutively by cells from arthritic tissues. The most potent chemokine inducers *in vitro* are IL-1, TNF-α, and LPS. Dexamethasone inhibits chemokine RNA and protein synthesis. A number of chemokines are involved in the pathogenesis of RA, including CXCL8/IL-8, CXCL5/ENA-78, groα/CXCL1, CXCL6/CTAP-III and CXCL12/SDF-1, whereas others such as CXCL10/IL-10, CXCL4/PF4 and CXCL9/MIG exert antiinflammatory and antiangiogenic effects (507).

CXCL8/IL-8 is detected in large quantities in the circulation, SF, and tissue of RA patients (523–525). Spontaneous production of IL-8 was observed in RA PBMCs and, at higher levels, in SF mononuclear cells as compared with controls. IL-8 production was enhanced by LPS, rheumatoid factor–containing immune complexes, zymosan, and IL-1. Cultured synovial fibroblasts produced IL-8 in response to IL-1 or TNF-α stimulation. IL-4 further enhanced, whereas IFN-γ decreased, IL-8 synthesis (298). Monosodium urate crystals stimulated IL-8 release from monocytes. IL-8 was increased in SFs from patients with gout, relative to OA SFs, and may be an important factor in neutrophil recruitment in crystal-induced inflammation (526). CXCL5/ENA-78 is detected in large amounts in the SF and tissue of RA patients (527). Both SF mononuclear cells and synovial fibroblasts produce CXCL5/ENA-78. The rheumatoid synovium contains chemotactic activity for neutrophils, and approximately equal parts were neutralized by antibodies to IL-8 or ENA-78 (527). CXCL1/groα is expressed by lining and sublining macrophages in the rheumatoid synovial tissue and stimulates fibroblast growth and angiogenesis. In contrast to findings with most other cytokines, the majority of synovial fibroblast cell lines from OA or noninflammatory synovia showed a relative increase in the constitutive expression of CXCL1/groα and groβ, when compared with rheumatoid synovial fibroblasts (523). CXCL6/CTAP-III has anabolic effects on synovial fibroblasts and simulates proliferation and proteoglycan production by human synovial fibroblasts (512,528). CXCL6/CTAP-III levels were increased in the plasma of patients with RA, SSc, and SLE (528).

CCL2/MCP-1 levels in SF were significantly higher in RA as compared with OA. Elevated CCL2/MCP-1 levels were also present in RA sera (529). CCL3/MIP-1α was higher in RA SF compared with other forms of arthritis, including OA. RA synovial tissue macrophages and SF produced CCL2/MCP-1 (529), CCL3/MIP-1α (530), and CCL5/RANTES (523). The production of these chemokines by RA synovial fibroblasts is stimulated by IL-1 and TNF-α. Anti– CCL3/MIP-1α antibodies neutralized 36% of the chemotactic activity for macrophages in RA SF (530). CCL20/MIP-3α has chemotactic activity toward memory T cells, B cells, monocytes, and immature dendritic cells. Elevated levels of CCL20/MIP-3α were detected in RA SF and tissue. This chemokine is present in the synovial lining layer and in infiltrating macrophages. Its production by synovial fibroblasts is induced by IL-1, TNF-α, and IL-17 stimulation (415).

CX3CL1/fractalkine is present in high amounts in the SF of RA patients and exerts chemotactic activity toward monocytes and lymphocytes. SF monocytes and synovial tissue macrophages, fibroblasts, endothelial cells, and dendritic cells produce CX3CL1/fractalkine.

Chemokine receptors were examined in peripheral blood, SF, and tissue monocytes/macrophages of RA patients. RA peripheral blood monocytes expressed CCR1, CCR2, CCR3, CCR4, and CCR5, whereas in the SF, monocytes expressed CCR3 and CCR5. In synovial tissue, CCR1, CCR2, and CCR5 were detected on macrophages. These results suggest that some chemokine receptors are involved in the recruitment of monocytes in the joints and others in monocyte retention in the inflamed synovium (531).

Chemokines in the Modulation of *In Vivo* Models of Inflammation and Arthritis

The involvement of chemokines in the pathogenesis of arthritis was studied by using different experimental models. Injection of CXCL8/IL-8 into the rabbit knee joint resulted in the development of articular inflammation with histologic features resembling RA (525). Injection of CCL2/MCP-1 stimulated the recruitment of macrophages into the synovial tissue (532). Increased cellular sensitivity to chemokines has been demonstrated in a model involving preexisting inflammation. It was associated with an increase of chemokine receptors and altered leukocyte recruitment profiles in response to CCL2/MCP-1 (533). Increased levels of CCL5/RANTES and CCL3/MIP-1α were detected in the joints of mice with CIA (534). In animals with adjuvant-induced arthritis, the levels of CCL5/RANTES were increased in peripheral blood and in the joint. CCL3/MIP-1α was unchanged. A polyclonal antibody to CCL5/RANTES greatly ameliorated symptoms of inflammation. Polyclonal antibodies to CCL3/MIP-1α were ineffective (535). The production of CXCL5/ENA-78 in joint homogenates and levels in sera of rats with AIA showed very early increases, even before the onset of overt signs of arthritis. Anti–human CXCL5/ENA-78 polyclonal antibodies administered before disease onset modified the severity of AIA, whereas administration of anti–CXCL5/ENA-78 antibodies after clinical onset of AIA did not modify the disease, indicating that this chemokine is primarily involved in early phases of the disease (536). In contrast, CCL2/MCP-1 may be involved mostly in later phase of AIA (362). These early findings suggest that inhibition of single chemokines is of limited efficacy in the treatment of arthritis, because a large number of chemokines and their receptors are up-regulated and activated.

TRANSFORMING GROWTH FACTOR-β SUPERFAMILY

The TGF-β superfamily is a large group of secreted cytokines controlling many aspects of development, wound repair, tissue fibrosis, cell growth, cell death or apoptosis, and cellular differentiation. This family of cytokines consists of more than 35 members in vertebrates, including TGF-βs, BMPs, growth differentiation factors (GDFs), activins, inhibins, müllerian inhibiting substance (MIS), Nodal, and Leftys. The TGF-β superfamily members are translated as prepropeptide precursors with an N-terminal signal peptide followed by a prodomain and the mature domain. The common structural characteristics of cytokines in the TGF-β superfamily are six to nine conserved cysteine residues in the mature domain forming intra- and intermolecular disulfide bonds (537,538). Three different genes encode the TGF-β isoforms found in mammals, including TGF-β1, TGF-β2, and TGF-β3. TGF-βs are secreted as latent, biologically-inactive precursors, where the activity of the mature domain is masked by the propeptide latency associated peptide (LAP). Dissociation of LAP activates TGF-β subfamily ligands. Release from this complex with activation of TGF-β can be induced *in vitro* by exposure to acidic or alkaline milieus. Extracellular matrix proteins, including thrombospondin 1 and integrin $\alpha_v\beta_6$, mediate TGF-β activation in physiologic conditions (539,540). In addition, various proteases, including plasmin, thrombin, cathepsin D, and plasma transglutaminase have been implicated as TGF-β activators. In the case of TGF-β1, the precursor is a 390–amino acid protein. Mature TGF-β1, TGF-β2, and TGF-β3 proteins are 25-kd homodimers consisting of 112–amino acid monomers released from this complex.

The TGF-β superfamily ligands bind to a family of transmembrane serine/threonine kinases known as the TGF-β receptor superfamily. On the basis of their structural properties, the TGF-β receptors are divided into three subfamilies. Type I and type II receptors are glycoproteins of approximately 55 and 70 kd, respectively. The two receptors are coexpressed by most cell types. Initiation of signaling requires binding to the TGF-β receptor type II, a constitutively active serine/threonine kinase, resulting in the recruitment and phosphorylation of TGF-β receptor type I. The formation of this heterodimeric complex results in the activation of a downstream signaling cascade. Type I receptors have a conserved region between the transmembrane and kinase domains containing a conserved SGSGSG motif, termed the GS domain. Serine/threonine phosphorylation of the GS domain is essential for TGF-β signaling (541–543). For TGF-β and activins, ligands directly bind type II receptors, and then type I receptors are recruited. In contrast, BMPs bind to both type I and type II receptors. Type I receptors are thought to determine the specificity of intracellular signals, whereas type II receptors are thought to be responsible for ligand specificity (541,544). TGF-β type I receptor alone is unable to bind the ligand and type II receptor is unable to transduce signal without type I receptor (541). Another type of cell surface receptor, called type III receptor because of its higher molecular weight compared with type I and type II receptors, binds ligands with high affinity and facilitates their interaction with type II receptors, but is unable to transduce signal (545). Betaglycan and endoglin are two examples of type III receptors. Betaglycan can also act as a naturally occurring inhibitor of signaling. Indeed, the betaglycan extracellular region can be shed by cells into the medium. Recombinant soluble betaglycan can bind TGF-β and has been shown to inhibit TGF-β binding to membrane receptors. Soluble betaglycan, which is also present in serum, is thus a TGF-β antagonist (546). Betaglycan can also bind to inhibin and promote its interaction with activin type II receptors, thus acting as an inhibitor of activin signaling (547).

Smad proteins are intracellular components of the TGF-β superfamily signal transduction pathways. Smads are the vertebrate homologues of MAD and Sma, which were first identified in *Drosophila melanogaster* and *Caenorhabditis elegans,* respectively (548–550). At least 10 different Smad proteins were identified in vertebrates. Mutations in Smads were associated with human tumors, suggesting that these proteins may function as tumor suppressors. TGF-β receptor type I phosphorylates the ligand-specific receptor-associated Smad (R-Smad). R-Smads include Smad1, Smad5, Smad8 downstream of BMPs, and Smad2 and Smad3 downstream of TGF-β and activin. Phosphorylation of R-Smads occurs principally on serine residues within the C terminus. Upon phosphorylation by TGF-β type I receptors, R-Smads form a heterodimeric complex with Smad4, which is then translocated into the nucleus and functions as a transcription factor (551). Inhibitory Smad proteins include Smad6 and Smad7 in vertebrates. Smad6 preferentially inhibits BMP signaling, whereas Smad7 can inhibit both TGF-β and BMP signaling. The mechanisms of action of inhibitory Smads are slightly different (552). Smad7 inhibits the phosphorylation of R-Smads by occupying the binding site of type I receptors for BMPs, TGF-β, and activin. Smad6 inhibits BMP signaling by competing with Smad4 for its interaction with receptor-activated Smad1. Levels of inhibitory Smads are enhanced in response to BMPs, TGF-β, and activin signaling, suggesting that they function as negative feedback controls. In addition, other extracellular signals stimulate Smad7 expression, including TNF-α, IFN-γ, ultraviolet light, and ligation of the CD40 receptor (553–556).

Immunomodulatory Effects of Transforming Growth Factor-β

TGF-β has diverse immunoregulatory activities that range from the regulation of lymphohematopoiesis to the modulation of differentiation and effector functions of mature cells. Overall, TGF-β effects on immune function are inhibitory. However, there are some stimulatory effects, most notably its chemotactic activity for monocytes. *In vitro*, TGF-β inhibits T-cell proliferation, differentiation, and activation of cytotoxic cells. Similarly, B-cell proliferation and antibody formation are inhibited by TGF-β, with the exception of IgA production. TGF-β is an important stimulant of IgA production by the mucosal immune system. TGF-β effects on mononuclear phagocytes are complex. Direct chemotactic activity for monocytes has been demonstrated extensively *in vitro* and *in vivo*. Furthermore, TGF-β stimulation of synoviocytes increases CCL2/MCP-1 production, providing an indirect mechanism for monocyte recruitment (557). Other potentially proinflammatory monocyte functions that are activated by TGF-β include induction of the third receptor for the constant region of Ig (FcγRIII, CD16), which can trigger release of superoxide anion (558). TGF-β was the first cytokine used to establish the concept of monocyte deactivation. TGF-β pretreatment of monocytes inhibited LPS-stimulated production of IL-1 and TNF-α. Cytokine production was not inhibited if the addition of TGF-β occurred after the inducing stimulus (559). Disruption of the TGF-β1 gene by homologous recombination led to a pronounced mononuclear leukocyte infiltration in multiple organs, followed by cachexia and, eventually, death (560).

The outcome of TGF-β administration *in vivo* is dependent on the site of injection and the preexisting condition of the tissues or experimental animals. Intraarticular injections of TGF-β almost uniformly induced proinflammatory changes. In contrast, the intraperitoneal injection of TGF-β in animals with experimentally-induced autoimmune diseases was associated with suppression of inflammation and reduced tissue destruction.

Intraarticular injection of TGF-β1 or TGF-β2 into normal rabbit joints induced synovial inflammation and hyperplasia with a predominantly mononuclear phagocyte infiltrate (561,562). Proinflammatory effects of intraarticular injections of TGF-β were also documented in experimental models of arthritis. When injected into ankle joints of rats after immunization with bovine type II collagen, TGF-β1 induced sustained, clinically-obvious inflammation (563). Intraarticular injection of neutralizing antibody to TGF-β reduced inflammatory cell accumulation and tissue pathology in streptococcal cell wall–induced arthritis (564).

Systemic administration of TGF-β1 had immunosuppressive and antiinflammatory effects. Intraperitoneally injected TGF-β1 significantly ameliorated arthritis, even when started at the time of arthritis development, although it did not reverse established disease (565). Systemic administration of TGF-β1 similarly inhibited the development of streptococcal cell wall–induced polyarthritis. TGF-β1 treatment reduced inflammatory cell infiltration, pannus formation, and joint erosion (566). Systemic TGF-β also had beneficial effects in relapsing experimental allergic encephalomyelitis (EAE), the animal model of multiple sclerosis (567). Suppression of EAE can be induced by oral administration of myelin basic protein. This suppression is mediated by $CD8^+$ T cells that adoptively transfer protection and is mediated by the release of TGF-β. EAE is self-limited, and TGF-β is also involved in the naturally occurring spontaneous recovery of the disease (568). In CIA, TGF-β mRNA levels increased at late time points and coincided with the resolution of articular inflammation (534).

Transforming Growth Factor-β and Extracellular Matrix

Members of the TGF-β superfamily are important regulators of mesenchymal cell differentiation and connective tissue development (569). TGF-β is physiologically associated with matrix formation and tissue repair. It is released at sites of tissue injury from the α granules of platelets and synthesized by inflammatory cells and mesenchymal cells. *In vivo,* it stimulates the formation of granulation tissue and promotes subcutaneous and dermal wound healing. Chemotactic activity for monocytes and fibroblasts provides an additional indirect mechanism important in connective tissue repair. The important role of TGF-β in tissue repair is demonstrated by the markedly delayed healing of wounds in TGF-β knockout mice (570).

Tissue fibrosis can be defined as a complex process involving proliferation of fibroblasts and production of elevated quantities of extracellular matrix (ECM). One of the most potent profibrotic stimuli to fibroblasts is TGF-β. Recent studies have demonstrated that a synergistic action of Smad and Sp1 is required for the stimulatory effect of TGF-β on collagen production (571). TGF-β increases the production of inhibitors of matrix-degrading enzyme, thus further increasing the accumulation of ECM. Moreover, TGF-β enhances the production of TIMP-1 (572), plasminogen activator inhibitor 1 (573,574), and collagenase/MMP-1 (575).

Some of the effects of TGF-β on fibrosis are also partly mediated by the induction of connective tissue growth factor (CTGF), a 36- to 38-kd cysteine-rich peptide. CTGF belongs to the CCN (CTGF, cysteine rich 61/cef 10, nephroblastoma overexpressed protein) family of growth factors. TGF-β increases the production of CTGF by human fibroblasts. The stimulatory effect of TGF-β on CTGF production is dependent on Smad3 and Smad4 (576). In addition to Smads, the Ras/MEK/ERK signaling pathway contributes to TGF-β-induced CTGF production (577). CTGF was reported to have mitogenic effects on fibroblasts and to stimulate the production of ECM. CTGF enhances the mRNA levels of α1(I) collagen, fibronectin, and α5 integrin in fibroblasts (578). CTGF can enhance the biologic effects of TGF-β1 by increasing its binding activity to TGF-β receptors (579).

The role of TGF-β and CTGF in the pathogenesis of skin fibrosis was investigated by subcutaneous injections in newborn mice. TGF-β, alone, did not result in persistent fibrosis. Injections of CTGF after TGF-β caused fibrotic tissue formation that persisted for up to 14 days, although injections were discontinued on day 7. In contrast, injections of CTGF before TGF-β did not cause any significant change in comparison with TGF-β alone. Injections of basic FGF and CTGF resulted in similar effects on tissue fibrosis. These results suggest that TGF-β plays an important role in the induction of fibrosis and that CTGF is important in maintaining fibrosis (580).

Transforming Growth Factor-β Signaling in Experimental Models of Fibrosis

The possible role of TGF-β in the pathogenesis of disease-associated fibrosis was examined in experimental models. The central pathologic feature of human kidney disease that leads to kidney failure is the accumulation of extracellular matrix in glomeruli. Mice transgenic for TGF-β1 spontaneously develop renal fibrosis (581).

TGF-β has been studied extensively in bleomycin-induced lung fibrosis. Increased production of TGF-β appears to have an important role in the pathophysiology of this process. Administration of TGF-β2 antibody reduces bleomycin-induced accumulation of lung collagen (582). More recent studies demonstrated the role of TGF-β signaling in the development of tissue fibrosis. Overexpression of dominant negative TGF-β receptor type II prevents liver fibrosis in rats (583). Bleomycin-treated mice deficient in Smad3 had a reduced accumulation of collagen in lungs as compared with wild-type mice and showed attenuation of fibrotic changes. However, the development of fibrosis was not completely prevented by the absence of Smad3, suggesting that other Smads and other signaling pathways may also be involved. Inhibition of TGF-β signaling by adenoviral transfer of Smad7 prevented the development of experimentally induced lung and renal fibrosis in rodents (584,585).

Systemic Sclerosis

SSc is characterized by the development of tissue fibrosis. Excessive production of type I, III, V, VI, and VII collagens, as well as fibronectin and proteoglycans, is a consistent finding in the skin of SSc patients. Due to their role in the pathogenesis of fibrosis, the presence of TGF-β and CTGF was examined in patients with SSc. TGF-β2 levels in skin biopsies from patients with SSc were increased and colocalized with pro-α1(I) collagen around dermal blood vessels (586). The increased expression of type VII collagen in the skin of SSc patients was accompanied by elevated expression of TGF-β1 and TGF-β2 (587). In Raynaud phenomenon, endothelial cells in skin biopsy samples exhibited intracellular and extracellular TGF-β. The role of TGF-β in the pathogenesis of fibrosis is supported by the ability of neutralizing anti-TGF-β antibodies to down-regulate elevated collagen production by SSc fibroblasts (588). TGF-β1 expression was also examined in lung biopsies from patients with SSc and interstitial lung disease. In cryptogenic fibrosing alveolitis, alveolar macrophages, bronchial epithelium, and pneumonocytes expressed intracellular TGF-β1, and extracellular TGF-β1 was found in the fibrous tissue. Spontaneous increase of TGF-β mRNA expression and TGF-β production was also observed in bronchoalveolar mononuclear cells of patients with systemic autoimmune diseases affecting the lung (589). CTGF mRNA has been detected in fibroblasts of sclerotic lesions in SSc patients (590). A correlation between CTGF mRNA levels and fibrosis was found in sclerotic lesions (591). Serum CTGF levels are elevated in SSc patients and correlated with the extent of skin sclerosis and the degree of pulmonary fibrosis, suggesting that CTGF plays an important role in the development of scleroderma (592). Prostacyclin suppresses the production of CTGF in fibroblasts and in the skin of SSc patients (577). This antifibrotic effect of prostacyclin is mediated by the activation of protein kinase A, which is able to block TGF-β-induced Ras/MEK/ERK signaling in fibroblasts. Taken together, the presence of TGF-β and CTGF in scleroderma lesions and their role in the progression of ECM deposition suggest that therapies targeting these cytokines may prove of potential value for the treatment of SSc and other fibrosis-associated conditions.

Transforming Growth Factor-β Expression in Arthritis

SFs from patients with RA or other inflammatory joint diseases contained high levels of both active and latent TGF-β (558,593). Freshly isolated RA synovial cells express mRNA for TGF-β1 and secrete latent TGF-β protein. TGF-β1 is one of the fibroblast mitogenic factors that is constitutively produced by fibroblasts cultured from rheumatoid and other inflammatory arthropathies, but not OA synovia (594). Abundant expression of TGF-β1, as well as TGF-β receptor type II, was seen in most actively proliferating synovial intimal cells (595). TGF-β1 protein was detected in the synovial tissue and cartilage/pannus junction from a majority of RA patients. It was found predominantly in the thickened synovial lining layer in RA in monocyte/macrophages, as well as the type B synovial lining cells (596).

Cartilage Repair

Cartilage repair is a major concern in the treatment of traumatic and inflammatory lesions that may progress to OA. Growth factors play an important role in cartilage metabolism. Insulin-like growth factor (IGF)-1 is a major homeostatic factor controlling matrix synthesis and degradation. IGF-1, present in the SF, exhibited a significant role in the maintenance of normal cartilage turnover (597). Other growth factors, including members of the TGF-β superfamily, such as BMPs and TGF-β, are involved in cartilage metabolism.

IGF-1 stimulated chondrocyte proliferation and proteoglycan production. Osteoarthritic chondrocytes and cartilage from inflamed joints display a state of nonresponsiveness to IGF-1, thereby limiting the application of IGF-1 for cartilage repair (598). TGF-β is one of the most important anabolic factors in articular cartilage. TGF-β promoted collagen type II and IX (599) and proteoglycan synthesis (600). It did not stimulate the production of metalloproteases, but increased the expression of TIMP in chondrocytes (601). Among the known growth factors, TGF-β appears to be the most potent stimulus of chondrocyte proliferation, and all three isoforms of TGF-β show similar effects on differentiated chondrocytes (602). Osteoarthritic chondrocytes displayed an enhanced sensitivity to TGF-β. Prolonged exposure of normal chondrocytes to TGF-β also induced an enhanced responsiveness. This effect is probably linked to shifts in receptor expression and intracellular signal transduction.

IL-1 exerts a major catabolic effect on articular cartilage. Results in different experimental models of arthritis and osteoarthritis have demonstrated that IL-1 is involved in cartilage destruction. In many connective tissue cell responses, TGF-β is a functional IL-1 antagonist. In rabbit articular chondrocytes, TGF-β reduced IL-1-induced synthesis of collagenase and stromelysin by reducing steady-state mRNA levels. In addition, TGF-β also down-regulated IL-1R, which may be one mechanism by which it antagonizes IL-1 activity on chondrocytes (603). There are some conditions, however, in which TGF-β may also potentiate IL-1 effects. Expression of the serine proteinase, urokinase-type plasminogen activator (u-PA) is often correlated with tissue remodeling. In rheumatoid synovial fibroblasts, TGF-β stimulated u-PA activity similar to IL-1 (604).

TGF-β and BMP-2 exerted anabolic effects on articular cartilage. However, BMP-2 induced a rapid and transient effect, whereas TGF-β had a delayed and sustained mode of action (605,606). In addition, TGF-β, but not BMP-2, counteracted the inhibitory effect of IL-1 on proteoglycan synthesis. Experiments in iNOS-deficient mice indicated that BMP-2 maintained its anabolic effect in the presence of IL-1, suggesting that NO interferes with BMP-2 signaling. In contrast to BMP-2, BMP-7 could counteract the activities of IL-1 *in vitro* (607). The role of endogenous TGF-β in cartilage repair was examined in arthritis models. Administration of soluble TGF-β receptor type II in mice with zymosan-induced arthritis significantly worsened proteoglycan loss in the articular cartilage (608).

In addition to its effects on chondrocyte proliferation and gene expression, TGF-β also promotes responses that lead to calcification of extracellular matrix and bone formation (609) and can thus contribute to the development of osteophytes in OA joints. Intraarticular injections of TGF-β alone, or in combination with IL-1, in zymosan-induced arthritis stimulated the formation of osteophytes at the joint margins (606,610). By using TGF-β inhibitors in the papain-induced model of OA, it was possible to demonstrate that endogenous TGF-β is involved in the formation of osteophytes (605). As with TGF-β, BMP-2 was also able to induce the development of osteophytes but with some difference in their location (608). These results indicate that, despite their positive effect on articular cartilage, growth factors contribute to serious side effects in other joint tissues, limiting their application in the treatment of cartilaginous lesions.

REFERENCES

1. Arend WP, Gordon DF, Wood WM, et al. IL-1 beta production in cultured human monocytes is regulated at multiple levels. *J Immunol* 1989;143:118–126.
2. Haskill S, Johnson C, Eierman D, et al. Adherence induces selective mRNA expression of monocyte mediators and proto-oncogenes. *J Immunol* 1988;140:1690–1694.
3. Malter JS. Identification of an AUUUA-specific messenger RNA binding protein. *Science* 1989;246:664–666.
4. Kontoyiannis D, Pasparakis M, Pizarro TT, et al. Impaired on/off regulation of TNF biosynthesis in mice lacking TNF AU-rich elements:

implications for joint and gut-associated immunopathologies. *Immunity* 1999;10:387–398.
5. Schindler R, Clark BD, Dinarello CA. Dissociation between interleukin-1 beta mRNA and protein synthesis in human peripheral blood mononuclear cells. *J Biol Chem* 1990;265:10232–10237.
6. Myazono K, Heldin CH. The mechanism of action of transforming growth factor-beta. *Gastroenterol Jpn* 1993;28:81–85; discussion 86–87.
7. Macchia D, Almerigogna F, Parronchi P, et al. Membrane tumour necrosis factor-alpha is involved in the polyclonal B-cell activation induced by HIV-infected human T cells. *Nature* 1993;363:464–466.
8. Bogdan C, Nathan C. Modulation of macrophage function by transforming growth factor beta, interleukin-4, and interleukin-10. *Ann NY Acad Sci* 1993;685:713–739.
9. Zurawski G, de Vries JE. Interleukin 13, an interleukin 4-like cytokine that acts on monocytes and B cells, but not on T cells. *Immunol Today* 1994;15:19–26.
10. Ruscetti FW, Dubois CM, Jacobsen SE, et al. Transforming growth factor beta and interleukin-1: a paradigm for opposing regulation of haemopoiesis. *Baillieres Clin Haematol* 1992;5:703–721.
11. Banchereau J, Briere F, Galizzi JP, et al. Human interleukin 4. *J Lipid Mediat Cell Signal* 1994;9:43–53.
12. Howard M, O'Garra A. Biological properties of interleukin 10. *Immunol Today* 1992;13:198–200.
13. Ray A, LaForge KS, Sehgal PB. On the mechanism for efficient repression of the interleukin-6 promoter by glucocorticoids: enhancer, TATA box, and RNA start site (Inr motif) occlusion. *Mol Cell Biol* 1990;10:5736–5746.
14. Amano Y, Lee SW, Allison AC. Inhibition by glucocorticoids of the formation of interleukin-1 alpha, interleukin-1 beta, and interleukin-6: mediation by decreased mRNA stability. *Mol Pharmacol* 1993;43:176–182.
15. Johnson GL, Lapadat R. Mitogen-activated protein kinase pathways mediated by ERK, JNK, and p38 protein kinases. *Science* 2002;298:1911–1912.
16. Iwata Y, Wada T, Furuichi K, et al. p38 Mitogen-activated protein kinase contributes to autoimmune renal injury in MRL-Fas(lpr) mice. *J Am Soc Nephrol* 2003;14:57–67.
17. Beg AA, Sha WC, Bronson RT, et al. Constitutive NF-kappa B activation, enhanced granulopoiesis, and neonatal lethality in I kappa B alpha-deficient mice. *Genes Dev* 1995;9:2736–2746.
18. Klement JF, Rice NR, Car BD, et al. IkappaBalpha deficiency results in a sustained NF-kappaB response and severe widespread dermatitis in mice. *Mol Cell Biol* 1996;16:2341–2349.
19. Ghosh S, Karin M. Missing pieces in the NF-kappaB puzzle. *Cell* 2002;109(suppl):81–96.
20. Yin L, Wu L, Wesche H, et al. Defective lymphotoxin-beta receptor-induced NF-kappaB transcriptional activity in NIK-deficient mice. *Science* 2001;291:2162–2165.
21. Ihle JN. The Stat family in cytokine signaling. *Curr Opin Cell Biol* 2001;13:211–217.
22. Suzuki A, Hanada T, Mitsuyama K, et al. CIS3/SOCS3/SSI3 plays a negative regulatory role in STAT3 activation and intestinal inflammation. *J Exp Med* 2001;193:471–481.
23. Shouda T, Yoshida T, Hanada T, et al. Induction of the cytokine signal regulator SOCS3/CIS3 as a therapeutic strategy for treating inflammatory arthritis. *J Clin Invest* 2001;108:1781–1788.
24. Rubin LA. The soluble interleukin-2 receptor in rheumatic disease. *Arthritis Rheum* 1990;33:1145–1148.
25. Wallach D, Engelmann H, Nophar Y, et al. Soluble and cell surface receptors for tumor necrosis factor. *Agents Actions Suppl* 1991;35:51–57.
26. van den Berg WB, Joosten LA, van de Loo FA. TNF alpha and IL-1 beta are separate targets in chronic arthritis. *Clin Exp Rheumatol* 1999;17:105–114.
27. Lotz M. The role of nitric oxide in articular cartilage damage. *Rheum Dis Clin North Am* 1999;25:269–282.
28. Economides AN, Carpenter LR, Rudge JS, et al. Cytokine traps: multi-component, high-affinity blockers of cytokine action. *Nat Med* 2003;9:47–52.
29. Smith CA, Farrah T, Goodwin RG. The TNF receptor superfamily of cellular and viral proteins: activation, costimulation, and death. *Cell* 1994;76:959–962.
30. Zhou T, Mountz JD, Kimberly RP. Immunobiology of tumor necrosis factor receptor superfamily. *Immunol Res* 2002;26:323–336.
31. Amakawa R, Hakem A, Kundig TM, et al. Impaired negative selection of T cells in Hodgkin's disease antigen CD30-deficient mice. *Cell* 1996;84:551–562.
32. Simonet WS, Lacey DL, Dunstan CR, et al. Osteoprotegerin: a novel secreted protein involved in the regulation of bone density. *Cell* 1997;89:309–319.
33. Liu ZG, Hsu H, Goeddel DV, et al. Dissection of TNF receptor 1 effector functions: JNK activation is not linked to apoptosis while NF-kappaB activation prevents cell death. *Cell* 1996;87:565–576.
34. Watanabe-Fukunaga R, Brannan CI, Copeland NG, et al. Lymphoproliferation disorder in mice explained by defects in Fas antigen that mediates apoptosis. *Nature* 1992;356:314–317.
35. Takahashi T, Tanaka M, Brannan CI, et al. Generalized lymphoproliferative disease in mice, caused by a point mutation in the Fas ligand. *Cell* 1994;76:969–976.
36. Black RA, Rauch CT, Kozlosky CJ, et al. A metalloproteinase disintegrin that releases tumour-necrosis factor-alpha from cells. *Nature* 1997;385:729–733.
37. Moss ML, Jin SL, Milla ME, et al. Cloning of a disintegrin metalloproteinase that processes precursor tumour-necrosis factor-alpha. *Nature* 1997;385:733–736.
38. Katevas P, Andonopoulos AP, Kourakli-Symeonidis A, et al. Peripheral blood mononuclear cells from patients with rheumatoid arthritis suppress erythropoiesis *in vitro* via the production of tumor necrosis factor alpha. *Eur J Haematol* 1994;53:26–30.
39. Locksley RM, Killeen N, Lenardo MJ. The TNF and TNF receptor superfamilies: integrating mammalian biology. *Cell* 2001;104:487–501.
40. Ware CF, Crowe PD, Grayson MH, et al. Expression of surface lymphotoxin and tumor necrosis factor on activated T, B, and natural killer cells. *J Immunol* 1992;149:3881–3888.
41. Mebius RE, Rennert P, Weissman IL. Developing lymph nodes collect $CD4^{+}CD3^{-}$ $LTbeta^{+}$ cells that can differentiate to APC, NK cells, and follicular cells but not T or B cells. *Immunity* 1997;7:493–504.
42. Pasparakis M, Alexopoulou L, Episkopou V, et al. Immune and inflammatory responses in TNF alpha-deficient mice: a critical requirement for TNF alpha in the formation of primary B cell follicles, follicular dendritic cell networks and germinal centers, and in the maturation of the humoral immune response. *J Exp Med* 1996;184:1397–1411.
43. Rennert PD, James D, Mackay F, et al. Lymph node genesis is induced by signaling through the lymphotoxin beta receptor. *Immunity* 1998;9:71–79.
44. Kuprash DV, Alimzhanov MB, Tumanov AV, et al. Redundancy in tumor necrosis factor (TNF) and lymphotoxin (LT) signaling *in vivo*: mice with inactivation of the entire TNF/LT locus versus single-knockout mice. *Mol Cell Biol* 2002;22:8626–8634.
45. van den Berg WB. Joint inflammation and cartilage destruction may occur uncoupled. *Springer Semin Immunopathol* 1998;20:149–164.
46. Wooley PH, Dutcher J, Widmer MB, et al. Influence of a recombinant human soluble tumor necrosis factor receptor FC fusion protein on type II collagen-induced arthritis in mice. *J Immunol* 1993;151:6602–6607.
47. Williams RO, Feldmann M, Maini RN. Anti-tumor necrosis factor ameliorates joint disease in murine collagen-induced arthritis. *Proc Natl Acad Sci U S A* 1992;89:9784–9788.
48. Neale ML, Williams BD, Matthews N. Tumour necrosis factor activity in joint fluids from rheumatoid arthritis patients. *Br J Rheumatol* 1989;28:104–108.
49. Di Giovine FS, Nuki G, Duff GW. Tumour necrosis factor in synovial exudates. *Ann Rheum Dis* 1988;47:768–772.
50. Roux-Lombard P, Punzi L, Hasler F, et al. Soluble tumor necrosis factor receptors in human inflammatory synovial fluids. *Arthritis Rheum* 1993;36:485–489.
51. Cope AP, Aderka D, Doherty M, et al. Increased levels of soluble tumor necrosis factor receptors in the sera and synovial fluid of patients with rheumatic diseases. *Arthritis Rheum* 1992;35:1160–1169.
52. Yocum DE, Esparza L, Dubry S, et al. Characteristics of tumor necrosis factor production in rheumatoid arthritis. *Cell Immunol* 1989;122:131–145.

53. Deleuran BW, Chu CQ, Field M, et al. Localization of tumor necrosis factor receptors in the synovial tissue and cartilage-pannus junction in patients with rheumatoid arthritis. Implications for local actions of tumor necrosis factor alpha. *Arthritis Rheum* 1992;35:1170–1178.
54. Jacob CO. Studies on the role of tumor necrosis factor in murine and human autoimmunity. *J Autoimmun* 1992;5(suppl A):133–143.
55. Jacob CO, McDevitt HO. Tumour necrosis factor-alpha in murine autoimmune "lupus" nephritis. *Nature* 1988;331:356–358.
56. Deguchi Y, Kishimoto S. Tumour necrosis factor/cachectin plays a key role in autoimmune pulmonary inflammation in lupus-prone mice. *Clin Exp Immunol* 1991;85:392–395.
57. Magilavy DB, Rothstein JL. Spontaneous production of tumor necrosis factor alpha by Kupffer cells of MRL/lpr mice. *J Exp Med* 1988; 168:789–794.
58. Mitamura K, Kang H, Tomita Y, et al. Impaired tumour necrosis factor-alpha (TNF-alpha) production and abnormal B cell response to TNF-alpha in patients with systemic lupus erythematosus (SLE). *Clin Exp Immunol* 1991;85:386–391.
59. Malave I, Searles RP, Montano J, et al. Production of tumor necrosis factor/cachectin by peripheral blood mononuclear cells in patients with systemic lupus erythematosus. *Int Arch Allergy Appl Immunol* 1989;89:355–361.
60. Maury CP, Teppo AM. Tumor necrosis factor in the serum of patients with systemic lupus erythematosus. *Arthritis Rheum* 1989;32:146–150.
61. Maury CP, Teppo AM. Cachectin/tumour necrosis factor-alpha in the circulation of patients with rheumatic disease. *Int J Tissue React* 1989;11:189–193.
62. Gabay C, Cakir N, Moral F, et al. Circulating levels of tumor necrosis factor soluble receptors in systemic lupus erythematosus are significantly higher than in other rheumatic diseases and correlate with disease activity. *J Rheumatol* 1997;24:303–308.
63. Shakoor N, Michalska M, Harris CA, et al. Drug-induced systemic lupus erythematosus associated with etanercept therapy. *Lancet* 2002; 359:579–580.
64. Aringer M, Zimmermann C, Graninger WB. TNF-alpha is an essential mediator in lupus nephritis. *Arthritis Rheum* 2002;46:LB08.
65. Braun J, Bollow M, Neure L, et al. Use of immunohistologic and *in situ* hybridization techniques in the examination of sacroiliac joint biopsy specimens from patients with ankylosing spondylitis. *Arthritis Rheum* 1995;38:499–505.
66. Braun J, Sieper J. Therapy of ankylosing spondylitis and other spondyloarthritides: established medical treatment, anti-TNF-alpha therapy and other novel approaches. *Arthritis Res* 2002;4:307–321.
67. Brandt J, Haibel H, Cornely D, et al. Successful treatment of active ankylosing spondylitis with the anti-tumor necrosis factor alpha monoclonal antibody infliximab. *Arthritis Rheum* 2000;43:1346–1352.
68. Braun J, Brandt J, Listing J, et al. Treatment of active ankylosing spondylitis with infliximab: a randomised controlled multicentre trial. *Lancet* 2002;359:1187–1193.
69. Gorman JD, Sack KE, Davis JC Jr. Treatment of ankylosing spondylitis by inhibition of tumor necrosis factor alpha. *N Engl J Med* 2002; 346:1349–1356.
70. Mease PJ, Goffe BS, Metz J, et al. Etanercept in the treatment of psoriatic arthritis and psoriasis: a randomised trial. *Lancet* 2000; 356:385–390.
71. Aloe L, Tuveri MA. Nerve growth factor and autoimmune rheumatic diseases. *Clin Exp Rheumatol* 1997;15:433–438.
72. Manni L, Aloe L. Role of IL-1 beta and TNF-alpha in the regulation of NGF in experimentally induced arthritis in mice. *Rheumatol Int* 1998;18:97–102.
73. Aloe L, Probert L, Kollias G, et al. The synovium of transgenic arthritic mice expressing human tumor necrosis factor contains a high level of nerve growth factor. *Growth Factors* 1993;9:149–155.
74. Tuveri M, Generini S, Matucci-Cerinic M, et al. NGF, a useful tool in the treatment of chronic vasculitic ulcers in rheumatoid arthritis. *Lancet* 2000;356:1739–1740.
75. Drappa J, Brot N, Elkon KB. The Fas protein is expressed at high levels on CD4+CD8+ thymocytes and activated mature lymphocytes in normal mice but not in the lupus-prone strain, MRL lpr/lpr. *Proc Natl Acad Sci U S A* 1993;90:10340–10344.
76. Suda T, Takahashi T, Golstein P, et al. Molecular cloning and expression of the Fas ligand, a novel member of the tumor necrosis factor family. *Cell* 1993;75:1169–1178.
77. Drappa J, Vaishnaw AK, Sullivan KE, et al. Fas gene mutations in the Canale-Smith syndrome, an inherited lymphoproliferative disorder associated with autoimmunity. *N Engl J Med* 1996;335:1643–1649.
78. Straus SE, Jaffe ES, Puck JM, et al. The development of lymphomas in families with autoimmune lymphoproliferative syndrome with germline Fas mutations and defective lymphocyte apoptosis. *Blood* 2001;98: 194–200.
79. Cheng J, Zhou T, Liu C, et al. Protection from Fas-mediated apoptosis by a soluble form of the Fas molecule. *Science* 1994;263:1759–1762.
80. Hashimoto H, Tanaka M, Suda T, et al. Soluble Fas ligand in the joints of patients with rheumatoid arthritis and osteoarthritis. *Arthritis Rheum* 1998;41:657–662.
81. Arpin C, Banchereau J, Liu YJ. Memory B cells are biased towards terminal differentiation: a strategy that may prevent repertoire freezing. *J Exp Med* 1997;186:931–940.
82. Noelle RJ. CD40 and its ligand in host defense. *Immunity* 1996;4: 415–419.
83. MacDonald KP, Nishioka Y, Lipsky PE, et al. Functional CD40 ligand is expressed by T cells in rheumatoid arthritis. *J Clin Invest* 1997; 100:2404–2414.
84. Malik N, Greenfield BW, Wahl AF, et al. Activation of human monocytes through CD40 induces matrix metalloproteinases. *J Immunol* 1996;156:3952–3960.
85. Yellin MJ, Winikoff S, Fortune SM, et al. Ligation of CD40 on fibroblasts induces CD54 (ICAM-1) and CD106 (VCAM-1) up-regulation and IL-6 production and proliferation. *J Leukoc Biol* 1995;58: 209–216.
86. Kiener PA, Moran-Davis P, Rankin BM, et al. Stimulation of CD40 with purified soluble gp39 induces proinflammatory responses in human monocytes. *J Immunol* 1995;155:4917–4925.
87. Caux C, Massacrier C, Vanbervliet B, et al. Activation of human dendritic cells through CD40 cross-linking. *J Exp Med* 1994;180: 1263–1272.
88. Sekine C, Yagita H, Miyasaka N, et al. Expression and function of CD40 in rheumatoid arthritis synovium. *J Rheumatol* 1998;25: 1048–1053.
89. Cho CS, Cho ML, Min SY, et al. CD40 engagement on synovial fibroblast up-regulates production of vascular endothelial growth factor. *J Immunol* 2000;164:5055–5061.
90. Durie FH, Fava RA, Foy TM, et al. Prevention of collagen-induced arthritis with an antibody to gp39, the ligand for CD40. *Science* 1993; 261:1328–1330.
91. Koshy M, Berger D, Crow MK. Increased expression of CD40 ligand on systemic lupus erythematosus lymphocytes. *J Clin Invest* 1996; 98:826–837.
92. Desai-Mehta A, Lu L, Ramsey-Goldman R, et al. Hyperexpression of CD40 ligand by B and T cells in human lupus and its role in pathogenic autoantibody production. *J Clin Invest* 1996;97:2063–2073.
93. Mohan C, Shi Y, Laman JD, et al. Interaction between CD40 and its ligand gp39 in the development of murine lupus nephritis. *J Immunol* 1995;154:1470–1480.
94. Kalled SL, Cutler AH, Datta SK, et al. Anti-CD40 ligand antibody treatment of SNF1 mice with established nephritis: preservation of kidney function. *J Immunol* 1998;160:2158–2165.
95. Boumpas DT, Furie R, Manzi S, et al. A short course of BG9588 (anti-CD40 ligand antibody) improves serologic activity and decreases hematuria in patients with proliferative lupus glomerulonephritis. *Arthritis Rheum* 2003;48:719–727.
96. Kalunian KC, Davis JC Jr, Merrill JT, et al. Treatment of systemic lupus erythematosus by inhibition of T cell costimulation with anti-CD154: a randomized, double-blind, placebo-controlled trial. *Arthritis Rheum* 2002;46:3251–3258.
97. Lacey DL, Timms E, Tan HL, et al. Osteoprotegerin ligand is a cytokine that regulates osteoclast differentiation and activation. *Cell* 1998;93:165–176.
98. Yasuda H, Shima N, Nakagawa N, et al. Osteoclast differentiation factor is a ligand for osteoprotegerin/osteoclastogenesis-inhibitory factor and is identical to TRANCE/RANKL. *Proc Natl Acad Sci U S A* 1998; 95:3597–3602.
99. Kong YY, Yoshida H, Sarosi I, et al. OPGL is a key regulator of osteoclastogenesis, lymphocyte development and lymph-node organogenesis. *Nature* 1999;397:315–323.

100. Kong YY, Feige U, Sarosi I, et al. Activated T cells regulate bone loss and joint destruction in adjuvant arthritis through osteoprotegerin ligand. *Nature* 1999;402:304–309.
101. Lomaga MA, Yeh WC, Sarosi I, et al. TRAF6 deficiency results in osteopetrosis and defective interleukin-1, CD40, and LPS signaling. *Genes Dev* 1999;13:1015–1024.
102. Romas E, Sims NA, Hards DK, et al. Osteoprotegerin reduces osteoclast numbers and prevents bone erosion in collagen-induced arthritis. *Am J Pathol* 2002;161:1419–1427.
103. Redlich K, Hayer S, Maier A, et al. Tumor necrosis factor alpha-mediated joint destruction is inhibited by targeting osteoclasts with osteoprotegerin. *Arthritis Rheum* 2002;46:785–792.
104. Mackay F, Schneider P, Rennert P, et al. BAFF and APRIL: a tutorial on B cell survival. *Annu Rev Immunol* 2003;21:231–264.
105. Schneider P, MacKay F, Steiner V, et al. BAFF, a novel ligand of the tumor necrosis factor family, stimulates B cell growth. *J Exp Med* 1999;189:1747–1756.
106. Shu HB, Hu WH, Johnson H. TALL-1 is a novel member of the TNF family that is down-regulated by mitogens. *J Leukoc Biol* 1999; 65:680–683.
107. Nardelli B, Belvedere O, Roschke V, et al. Synthesis and release of B-lymphocyte stimulator from myeloid cells. *Blood* 2001;97:198–204.
108. Khare SD, Sarosi I, Xia XZ, et al. Severe B cell hyperplasia and autoimmune disease in TALL-1 transgenic mice. *Proc Natl Acad Sci U S A* 2000;97:3370–3375.
109. Mackay F, Woodcock SA, Lawton P, et al. Mice transgenic for BAFF develop lymphocytic disorders along with autoimmune manifestations. *J Exp Med* 1999;190:1697–1710.
110. Cheema GS, Roschke V, Hilbert DM, et al. Elevated serum B lymphocyte stimulator levels in patients with systemic immune-based rheumatic diseases. *Arthritis Rheum* 2001;44:1313–1319.
111. Groom J, Kalled SL, Cutler AH, et al. Association of BAFF/BLyS overexpression and altered B cell differentiation with Sjögren's syndrome. *J Clin Invest* 2002;109:59–68.
112. Stein JV, Lopez-Fraga M, Elustondo FA, et al. APRIL modulates B and T cell immunity. *J Clin Invest* 2002;109:1587–1598.
113. Roschke V, Sosnovtseva S, Ward CD, et al. BLyS and APRIL form biologically active heterotrimers that are expressed in patients with systemic immune-based rheumatic diseases. *J Immunol* 2002;169: 4314–4321.
114. Baetu TM, Hiscott J. On the TRAIL to apoptosis. *Cytokine Growth Factor Rev* 2002;13:199–207.
115. Renshaw SA, Parmar JS, Singleton V, et al. Acceleration of human neutrophil apoptosis by TRAIL. *J Immunol* 2003;170:1027–1033.
116. Matsumura R, Umemiya K, Kagami M, et al. Expression of TNF-related apoptosis inducing ligand (TRAIL) on infiltrating cells and of TRAIL receptors on salivary glands in patients with Sjögren's syndrome. *Clin Exp Rheumatol* 2002;20:791–798.
117. Song K, Chen Y, Goke R, et al. Tumor necrosis factor-related apoptosis-inducing ligand (TRAIL) is an inhibitor of autoimmune inflammation and cell cycle progression. *J Exp Med* 2000;191: 1095–1104.
118. MacKenzie A, Wilson HL, Kiss-Toth E, et al. Rapid secretion of interleukin-1beta by microvesicle shedding. *Immunity* 2001;15: 825–835.
119. Andrei C, Dazzi C, Lotti L, et al. The secretory route of the leaderless protein interleukin 1beta involves exocytosis of endolysosome-related vesicles. *Mol Biol Cell* 1999;10:1463–1475.
120. Garfinkel S, Haines DS, Brown S, et al. Interleukin-1 alpha mediates an alternative pathway for the antiproliferative action of poly(I.C) on human endothelial cells. *J Biol Chem* 1992;267:24375–24378.
121. Kawaguchi Y, Hara M, Wright TM. Endogenous IL-1alpha from systemic sclerosis fibroblasts induces IL-6 and PDGF-A. *J Clin Invest* 1999;103:1253–1260.
122. Higgins GC, Wu Y, Postlethwaite AE. Intracellular IL-1 receptor antagonist is elevated in human dermal fibroblasts that overexpress intracellular precursor IL-1 alpha. *J Immunol* 1999;163:3969–3975.
123. Stevenson FT, Turck J, Locksley RM, et al. The N-terminal propiece of interleukin 1 alpha is a transforming nuclear oncoprotein. *Proc Natl Acad Sci U S A* 1997;94:508–513.
124. Pollock AS, Turck J, Lovett DH. The prodomain of interleukin 1alpha interacts with elements of the RNA processing apparatus and induces apoptosis in malignant cells. *FASEB J* 2003;17:203–213.
125. Sims JE, Nicklin MJ, Bazan JF, et al. A new nomenclature for IL-1-family genes. *Trends Immunol* 2001;22:536–537.
126. Arend WP, Malyak M, Guthridge CJ, et al. Interleukin-1 receptor antagonist: role in biology. *Annu Rev Immunol* 1998;16:27–55.
127. Dinarello CA. Biologic basis for interleukin-1 in disease. *Blood* 1996;87:2095–2147.
128. Wesche H, Korherr C, Kracht M, et al. The interleukin-1 receptor accessory protein (IL-1RAcP) is essential for IL-1-induced activation of interleukin-1 receptor–associated kinase (IRAK) and stress-activated protein kinases (SAP kinases). *J Biol Chem* 1997;272: 7727–7731.
129. Wesche H, Henzel WJ, Shillinglaw W, et al. MyD88: an adapter that recruits IRAK to the IL-1 receptor complex. *Immunity* 1997;7: 837–847.
130. Li X, Commane M, Jiang Z, et al. IL-1-induced NFkappa B and c-Jun N-terminal kinase (JNK) activation diverge at IL-1 receptor-associated kinase (IRAK). *Proc Natl Acad Sci U S A* 2001;98: 4461–4465.
131. Cao Z, Xiong J, Takeuchi M, et al. TRAF6 is a signal transducer for interleukin-1. *Nature* 1996;383:443–446.
132. Suzuki N, Suzuki S, Duncan GS, et al. Severe impairment of interleukin-1 and Toll-like receptor signalling in mice lacking IRAK-4. *Nature* 2002;416:750–756.
133. Geng Y, Maier R, Lotz M. Tyrosine kinases are involved with the expression of inducible nitric oxide synthase in human articular chondrocytes. *J Cell Physiol* 1995;163:545–554.
134. Sagot Y, Sattonet-Roche P, Bhagwat SS, et al. Two IKK2 inhibitors are orally active small molecules decreasing severity of collagen-induced arthritis in DBA/1 mice. *Arthritis Rheum* 2001;44:368.
135. Han Z, Boyle DL, Chang L, et al. c-Jun N-terminal kinase is required for metalloproteinase expression and joint destruction in inflammatory arthritis. *J Clin Invest* 2001;108:73–81.
136. Colotta F, Dower SK, Sims JE, et al. The type II "decoy" receptor: a novel regulatory pathway for interleukin 1. *Immunol Today* 1994; 15:562–566.
137. Orlando S, Sironi M, Bianchi G, et al. Role of metalloproteases in the release of the IL-1 type II decoy receptor. *J Biol Chem* 1997;272: 31764–31769.
138. Liu C, Hart RP, Liu XJ, et al. Cloning and characterization of an alternatively processed human type II interleukin-1 receptor mRNA. *J Biol Chem* 1996;271:20965–20972.
139. Attur MG, Dave MN, Leung MY, et al. Functional genomic analysis of type II IL-1beta decoy receptor: potential for gene therapy in human arthritis and inflammation. *J Immunol* 2002;168:2001–2010.
140. Burger D, Chicheportiche R, Giri JG, et al. The inhibitory activity of human interleukin-1 receptor antagonist is enhanced by type II interleukin-1 soluble receptor and hindered by type I interleukin-1 soluble receptor. *J Clin Invest* 1995;96:38–41.
141. Neumann D, Kollewe C, Martin MU, et al. The membrane form of the type II IL-1 receptor accounts for inhibitory function. *J Immunol* 2000;165:3350–3357.
142. Sims JE. IL-1 and IL-18 receptors, and their extended family. *Curr Opin Immunol* 2002;14:117–122.
143. Debets R, Timans JC, Homey B, et al. Two novel IL-1 family members, IL-1 delta and IL-1 epsilon, function as an antagonist and agonist of NF-kappa B activation through the orphan IL-1 receptor–related protein 2. *J Immunol* 2001;167:1440–1446.
144. Townsend MJ, Fallon PG, Matthews DJ, et al. T1/ST2-deficient mice demonstrate the importance of T1/ST2 in developing primary T helper cell type 2 responses. *J Exp Med* 2000;191:1069–1076.
145. Bufler P, Azam T, Gamboni-Robertson F, et al. A complex of the IL-1 homologue IL-1F7b and IL-18-binding protein reduces IL-18 activity. *Proc Natl Acad Sci U S A* 2002;99:13723–13728.
146. Yagisawa M, Yuo A, Kitagawa S, et al. Stimulation and priming of human neutrophils by IL-1 alpha and IL-1 beta: complete inhibition by IL-1 receptor antagonist and no interaction with other cytokines. *Exp Hematol* 1995;23:603–608.
147. Brandolini L, Bertini R, Bizzarri C, et al. IL-1 beta primes IL-8-activated human neutrophils for elastase release, phospholipase D activity, and calcium flux. *J Leukoc Biol* 1996;59:427–434.
148. Ferrante A, Nandoskar M, Walz A, et al. Effects of tumour necrosis factor alpha and interleukin-1 alpha and beta on human neutrophil migration, respiratory burst and degranulation. *Int Arch Allergy Appl Immunol* 1988;86:82–91.

149. Sullivan GW, Carper HT, Sullivan JA, et al. Both recombinant interleukin-1 (beta) and purified human monocyte interleukin-1 prime human neutrophils for increased oxidative activity and promote neutrophil spreading. *J Leukoc Biol* 1989;45:389–395.
150. Dularay B, Elson CJ, Clements-Jewery S, et al. Recombinant human interleukin-1 beta primes human polymorphonuclear leukocytes for stimulus-induced myeloperoxidase release. *J Leukoc Biol* 1990;47: 158–163.
151. Colotta F, Re F, Polentarutti N, et al. Modulation of granulocyte survival and programmed cell death by cytokines and bacterial products. *Blood* 1992;80:2012–2020.
152. Schleef RR, Bevilacqua MP, Sawdey M, et al. Cytokine activation of vascular endothelium. Effects on tissue-type plasminogen activator and type 1 plasminogen activator inhibitor. *J Biol Chem* 1988;263: 5797–5803.
153. Royall JA, Berkow RL, Beckman JS, et al. Tumor necrosis factor and interleukin 1 alpha increase vascular endothelial permeability. *Am J Physiol* 1989;257:L399–410.
154. Samad TA, Moore KA, Sapirstein A, et al. Interleukin-1beta-mediated induction of Cox-2 in the CNS contributes to inflammatory pain hypersensitivity. *Nature* 2001;410:471–475.
155. Gabay C, Kushner I. Acute-phase proteins and other systemic responses to inflammation. *N Engl J Med* 1999;340:448–454.
156. Hirsch E, Irikura VM, Paul SM, et al. Functions of interleukin 1 receptor antagonist in gene knockout and overproducing mice. *Proc Natl Acad Sci U S A* 1996;93:11008–11013.
157. Ma Y, Thornton S, Boivin GP, et al. Altered susceptibility to collagen-induced arthritis in transgenic mice with aberrant expression of interleukin-1 receptor antagonist. *Arthritis Rheum* 1998;41: 1798–1805.
158. Horai R, Saijo S, Tanioka H, et al. Development of chronic inflammatory arthropathy resembling rheumatoid arthritis in interleukin 1 receptor antagonist-deficient mice. *J Exp Med* 2000;191:313–320.
159. Nicklin MJ, Hughes DE, Barton JL, et al. Arterial inflammation in mice lacking the interleukin 1 receptor antagonist gene. *J Exp Med* 2000;191:303–312.
160. Gabay C, Marinova-Mutafchieva L, Williams RO, et al. Increased production of intracellular interleukin-1 receptor antagonist type I in the synovium of mice with collagen-induced arthritis: a possible role in the resolution of arthritis. *Arthritis Rheum* 2001;44:451–462.
161. Miller LC, Lynch EA, Isa S, et al. Balance of synovial fluid IL-1 beta and IL-1 receptor antagonist and recovery from Lyme arthritis. *Lancet* 1993;341:146–148.
162. di Giovine FS, Poole S, Situnayake RD, et al. Absence of correlations between indices of systemic inflammation and synovial fluid interleukin 1 (alpha and beta) in rheumatic diseases. *Rheumatol Int* 1990;9:259–264.
163. Thomas R, Carroll GJ. Reduction of leukocyte and interleukin-1 beta concentrations in the synovial fluid of rheumatoid arthritis patients treated with methotrexate. *Arthritis Rheum* 1993;36: 1244–1252.
164. Malyak M, Swaney RE, Arend WP. Levels of synovial fluid interleukin-1 receptor antagonist in rheumatoid arthritis and other arthropathies. Potential contribution from synovial fluid neutrophils. *Arthritis Rheum* 1993;36:781–789.
165. Malyak M, Smith MF Jr, Abel AA, et al. Peripheral blood neutrophil production of interleukin-1 receptor antagonist and interleukin-1 beta. *J Clin Immunol* 1994;14:20–30.
166. Firestein GS, Boyle DL, Yu C, et al. Synovial interleukin-1 receptor antagonist and interleukin-1 balance in rheumatoid arthritis. *Arthritis Rheum* 1994;37:644–652.
167. Deleuran BW, Chu CQ, Field M, et al. Localization of interleukin-1 alpha, type 1 interleukin-1 receptor and interleukin-1 receptor antagonist in the synovial membrane and cartilage/pannus junction in rheumatoid arthritis. *Br J Rheumatol* 1992;31:801–809.
168. Firestein GS, Berger AE, Tracey DE, et al. IL-1 receptor antagonist protein production and gene expression in rheumatoid arthritis and osteoarthritis synovium. *J Immunol* 1992;149:1054–1062.
169. Gabay C, Smith MF, Eidlen D, et al. Interleukin 1 receptor antagonist (IL-1Ra) is an acute-phase protein. *J Clin Invest* 1997;99:2930–2940.
170. Gabay C, Gigley J, Sipe J, et al. Production of IL-1 receptor antagonist by hepatocytes is regulated as an acute-phase protein *in vivo*. *Eur J Immunol* 2001;31:490–499.
171. Niki Y, Yamada H, Seki S, et al. Macrophage- and neutrophil-dominant arthritis in human IL-1 alpha transgenic mice. *J Clin Invest* 2001;107: 1127–1135.
172. Palmer G, Talabot-Ayer D, Szalay-Quinodoz L, et al. Mice transgenic for intracellular interleukin-1 receptor antagonist type 1 are protected from collagen-induced arthritis. *Eur J Immunol* 2003;33: 434–440.
173. Gabay C. IL-1 inhibitors: novel agents in the treatment of rheumatoid arthritis. *Expert Opin Invest Drugs* 2000;9:113–127.
174. Wright SD. Toll, a new piece in the puzzle of innate immunity. *J Exp Med* 1999;189:605–609.
175. Medzhitov R, Preston-Hurlburt P, Janeway CA Jr. A human homologue of the *Drosophila* Toll protein signals activation of adaptive immunity. *Nature* 1997;388:394–397.
176. Poltorak A, He X, Smirnova I, et al. Defective LPS signaling in C3H/HeJ and C57BL/10ScCr mice: mutations in Tlr4 gene. *Science* 1998;282:2085–2088.
177. Hoshino K, Takeuchi O, Kawai T, et al. Cutting edge: Toll-like receptor 4 (TLR4)-deficient mice are hyporesponsive to lipopolysaccharide: evidence for TLR4 as the Lps gene product. *J Immunol* 1999; 162:3749–3752.
178. Shimazu R, Akashi S, Ogata H, et al. MD-2, a molecule that confers lipopolysaccharide responsiveness on Toll-like receptor 4. *J Exp Med* 1999;189:1777–1782.
179. Kawasaki K, Akashi S, Shimazu R, et al. Mouse toll-like receptor 4.MD-2 complex mediates lipopolysaccharide-mimetic signal transduction by Taxol. *J Biol Chem* 2000;275:2251–2254.
180. Kurt-Jones EA, Popova L, Kwinn L, et al. Pattern recognition receptors TLR4 and CD14 mediate response to respiratory syncytial virus. *Nat Immunol* 2000;1:398–401.
181. Means TK, Wang S, Lien E, et al. Human toll-like receptors mediate cellular activation by *Mycobacterium* tuberculosis. *J Immunol* 1999; 163:3920–3927.
182. Ohashi K, Burkart V, Flohe S, et al. Cutting edge: heat shock protein 60 is a putative endogenous ligand of the Toll-like receptor-4 complex. *J Immunol* 2000;164:558–561.
183. Bulut Y, Faure E, Thomas L, et al. Chlamydial heat shock protein 60 activates macrophages and endothelial cells through Toll-like receptor 4 and MD2 in a MyD88-dependent pathway. *J Immunol* 2002; 168:1435–1440.
184. Okamura Y, Watari M, Jerud ES, et al. The extra domain A of fibronectin activates Toll-like receptor 4. *J Biol Chem* 2001;276: 10229–10233.
185. Smiley ST, King JA, Hancock WW. Fibrinogen stimulates macrophage chemokine secretion through toll-like receptor 4. *J Immunol* 2001;167:2887–2894.
186. Underhill DM, Ozinsky A. Toll-like receptors: key mediators of microbe detection. *Curr Opin Immunol* 2002;14:103–110.
187. Hirschfeld M, Kirschning CJ, Schwandner R, et al. Cutting edge: inflammatory signaling by *Borrelia burgdorferi* lipoproteins is mediated by Toll-like receptor 2. *J Immunol* 1999;163:2382–2386.
188. Hayashi F, Smith KD, Ozinsky A, et al. The innate immune response to bacterial flagellin is mediated by Toll-like receptor 5. *Nature* 2001; 410:1099–1103.
189. Hemmi H, Takeuchi O, Kawai T, et al. A Toll-like receptor recognizes bacterial DNA. *Nature* 2000;408:740–745.
190. Alexopoulou L, Holt AC, Medzhitov R, et al. Recognition of double-stranded RNA and activation of NF-kappaB by Toll-like receptor 3. *Nature* 2001;413:732–738.
191. Gu Y, Kuida K, Tsutsui H, et al. Activation of interferon-gamma inducing factor mediated by interleukin-1beta converting enzyme. *Science* 1997;275:206–209.
192. Thomassen E, Bird TA, Renshaw BR, et al. Binding of interleukin-18 to the interleukin-1 receptor homologous receptor IL-1Rrp1 leads to activation of signaling pathways similar to those used by interleukin-1. *J Interferon Cytokine Res* 1998;18:1077–1088.
193. Dinarello CA. IL-18: a TH1-inducing, proinflammatory cytokine and new member of the IL-1 family. *J Allergy Clin Immunol* 1999;103: 11–24.
194. Xu D, Chan WL, Leung BP, et al. Selective expression and functions of interleukin 18 receptor on T helper (Th) type 1 but not Th2 cells. *J Exp Med* 1998;188:1485–1492.
195. Hyodo Y, Matsui K, Hayashi N, et al. IL-18 up-regulates perforin-mediated NK activity without increasing perforin messenger RNA

expression by binding to constitutively expressed IL-18 receptor. *J Immunol* 1999;162:1662–1668.
196. Takeda K, Tsutsui H, Yoshimoto T, et al. Defective NK cell activity and Th1 response in IL-18-deficient mice. *Immunity* 1998;8:383–390.
197. Puren AJ, Fantuzzi G, Gu Y, et al. Interleukin-18 (IFNgamma-inducing factor) induces IL-8 and IL-1beta via TNFalpha production from non-CD14+ human blood mononuclear cells. *J Clin Invest* 1998;101:711–721.
198. Faggioni R, Cattley RC, Guo J, et al. IL-18-binding protein protects against lipopolysaccharide- induced lethality and prevents the development of Fas/Fas ligand-mediated models of liver disease in mice. *J Immunol* 2001;167:5913–5920.
199. Komai-Koma M, Gracie JA, Wei XQ, et al. Chemoattraction of human T cells by IL-18. *J Immunol* 2003;170:1084–1090.
200. Hoshino T, Kawase Y, Okamoto M, et al. Cutting edge: IL-18-transgenic mice: *in vivo* evidence of a broad role for IL-18 in modulating immune function. *J Immunol* 2001;166:7014–7018.
201. Novick D, Kim SH, Fantuzzi G, et al. Interleukin-18 binding protein: a novel modulator of the Th1 cytokine response. *Immunity* 1999; 10:127–136.
202. Kim SH, Eisenstein M, Reznikov L, et al. Structural requirements of six naturally occurring isoforms of the IL-18 binding protein to inhibit IL-18. *Proc Natl Acad Sci U S A* 2000;97:1190–1195.
203. Gracie JA, Forsey RJ, Chan WL, et al. A proinflammatory role for IL-18 in rheumatoid arthritis. *J Clin Invest* 1999;104:1393–1401.
204. Olee T, Hashimoto S, Quach J, et al. IL-18 is produced by articular chondrocytes and induces proinflammatory and catabolic responses. *J Immunol* 1999;162:1096–1100.
205. Horwood NJ, Udagawa N, Elliott J, et al. Interleukin 18 inhibits osteoclast formation via T cell production of granulocyte macrophage colony-stimulating factor. *J Clin Invest* 1998;101:595–603.
206. Wei XQ, Leung BP, Arthur HM, et al. Reduced incidence and severity of collagen-induced arthritis in mice lacking IL-18. *J Immunol* 2001;166:517–521.
207. Plater-Zyberk C, Joosten LA, Helsen MM, et al. Therapeutic effect of neutralizing endogenous IL-18 activity in the collagen-induced model of arthritis. *J Clin Invest* 2001;108:1825–1832.
208. Desgeorges A, Gabay C, Silacci P, et al. Concentrations and origins of soluble interleukin 6 receptor-alpha in serum and synovial fluid. *J Rheumatol* 1997;24:1510–1516.
209. Atreya R, Mudter J, Finotto S, et al. Blockade of interleukin 6 trans signaling suppresses T-cell resistance against apoptosis in chronic intestinal inflammation: evidence in Crohn disease and experimental colitis *in vivo*. *Nat Med* 2000;6:583–588.
210. Nishimoto N, Ogata A, Shima Y, et al. Oncostatin M, leukemia inhibitory factor, and interleukin 6 induce the proliferation of human plasmacytoma cells via the common signal transducer, gp130. *J Exp Med* 1994;179:1343–1347.
211. Zhang XG, Gu JJ, Lu ZY, et al. Ciliary neurotropic factor, interleukin 11, leukemia inhibitory factor, and oncostatin M are growth factors for human myeloma cell lines using the interleukin 6 signal transducer gp130. *J Exp Med* 1994;179:1337–1342.
212. Taga T, Kishimoto T. Gp130 and the interleukin-6 family of cytokines. *Annu Rev Immunol* 1997;15:797–819.
213. Ohtani T, Ishihara K, Atsumi T, et al. Dissection of signaling cascades through gp130 *in vivo*: reciprocal roles for STAT3- and SHP2-mediated signals in immune responses. *Immunity* 2000;12:95–105.
214. Atsumi T, Ishihara K, Kamimura D, et al. A point mutation of Tyr-759 in interleukin 6 family cytokine receptor subunit gp130 causes autoimmune arthritis. *J Exp Med* 2002;196:979–990.
215. Ernst M, Inglese M, Waring P, et al. Defective gp130-mediated signal transducer and activator of transcription (STAT) signaling results in degenerative joint disease, gastrointestinal ulceration, and failure of uterine implantation. *J Exp Med* 2001;194: 189–203.
216. Kopf M, Baumann H, Freer G, et al. Impaired immune and acute-phase responses in interleukin-6-deficient mice. *Nature* 1994;368: 339–342.
217. Fattori E, Cappelletti M, Costa P, et al. Defective inflammatory response in interleukin 6–deficient mice. *J Exp Med* 1994;180: 1243–1250.
218. Dinarello CA, Cannon JG, Mancilla J, et al. Interleukin-6 as an endogenous pyrogen: induction of prostaglandin E_2 in brain but not in peripheral blood mononuclear cells. *Brain Res* 1991;562:199–206.
219. Aderka D, Le JM, Vilcek J. IL-6 inhibits lipopolysaccharide-induced tumor necrosis factor production in cultured human monocytes, U937 cells, and in mice. *J Immunol* 1989;143:3517–3523.
220. Barton BE, Jackson JV. Protective role of interleukin 6 in the lipopolysaccharide-galactosamine septic shock model. *Infect Immun* 1993;61:1496–1499.
221. Tilg H, Dinarello CA, Mier JW. IL-6 and APPs: anti-inflammatory and immunosuppressive mediators. *Immunol Today* 1997;18:428–432.
222. Szalai AJ, Nataf S, Hu XZ, et al. Experimental allergic encephalomyelitis is inhibited in transgenic mice expressing human C-reactive protein. *J Immunol* 2002;168:5792–5797.
223. Hurst SM, Wilkinson TS, McLoughlin RM, et al. IL-6 and its soluble receptor orchestrate a temporal switch in the pattern of leukocyte recruitment seen during acute inflammation. *Immunity* 2001;14: 705–714.
224. Ogawa M. IL6 and haematopoietic stem cells. *Res Immunol* 1992; 143:749–751.
225. Asano S, Okano A, Ozawa K, et al. *In vivo* effects of recombinant human interleukin-6 in primates: stimulated production of platelets. *Blood* 1990;75:1602–1605.
226. Ohsaki Y, Takahashi S, Scarcez T, et al. Evidence for an autocrine/paracrine role for interleukin-6 in bone resorption by giant cells from giant cell tumors of bone. *Endocrinology* 1992;131:2229–2234.
227. Jilka RL, Hangoc G, Girasole G, et al. Increased osteoclast development after estrogen loss: mediation by interleukin-6. *Science* 1992; 257:88–91.
228. Ferrari SL, Ahn-Luong L, Garnero P, et al. Two promoter polymorphisms regulating interleukin-6 gene expression are associated with circulating levels of C-reactive protein and markers of bone resorption in postmenopausal women. *J Clin Endocrinol Metab* 2003; 88:255–259.
229. Strassmann G, Fong M, Windsor S, et al. The role of interleukin-6 in lipopolysaccharide-induced weight loss, hypoglycemia and fibrinogen production, *in vivo. Cytokine* 1993;5:285–290.
230. Nagafuchi H, Suzuki N, Mizushima Y, et al. Constitutive expression of IL-6 receptors and their role in the excessive B cell function in patients with systemic lupus erythematosus. *J Immunol* 1993;151: 6525–6534.
231. Finck BK, Chan B, Wofsy D. Interleukin 6 promotes murine lupus in NZB/NZW F1 mice. *J Clin Invest* 1994;94:585–591.
232. Kiberd BA. Interleukin-6 receptor blockage ameliorates murine lupus nephritis. *J Am Soc Nephrol* 1993;4:58–61.
233. Suematsu S, Matsusaka T, Matsuda T, et al. Generation of plasmacytomas with the chromosomal translocation t(12;15) in interleukin 6 transgenic mice. *Proc Natl Acad Sci U S A* 1992;89:232–235.
234. Woodroofe C, Muller W, Ruther U. Long-term consequences of interleukin-6 overexpression in transgenic mice. *DNA Cell Biol* 1992;11:587–592.
235. Lotz M, Jirik F, Kabouridis P, et al. B cell stimulating factor 2/interleukin 6 is a costimulant for human thymocytes and T lymphocytes. *J Exp Med* 1988;167:1253–1258.
236. Pasare C, Medzhitov R. Toll pathway-dependent blockade of CD4+CD25+ T cell-mediated suppression by dendritic cells. *Science* 2003;299:1033–1036.
237. Vreugdenhil G, Lowenberg B, van Eijk HG, et al. Anaemia of chronic disease in rheumatoid arthritis. Raised serum interleukin-6 (IL-6) levels and effects of IL-6 and anti-IL-6 on *in vitro* erythropoiesis. *Rheumatol Int* 1990;10:127–130.
238. Gabay C, Roux-Lombard P, de Moerloose P, et al. Absence of correlation between interleukin 6 and C-reactive protein blood levels in systemic lupus erythematosus compared with rheumatoid arthritis. *J Rheumatol* 1993;20:815–821.
239. Horii Y, Muraguchi A, Iwano M, et al. Involvement of IL-6 in mesangial proliferative glomerulonephritis. *J Immunol* 1989;143:3949–3955.
240. Hirohata S, Miyamoto T. Elevated levels of interleukin-6 in cerebrospinal fluid from patients with systemic lupus erythematosus and central nervous system involvement. *Arthritis Rheum* 1990;33: 644–649.
241. Dasgupta B, Panayi GS. Interleukin-6 in serum of patients with polymyalgia rheumatica and giant cell arteritis. *Br J Rheumatol* 1990; 29:456–458.

242. Wagner AD, Goronzy JJ, Weyand CM. Functional profile of tissue-infiltrating and circulating CD68+ cells in giant cell arteritis. Evidence for two components of the disease. *J Clin Invest* 1994;94: 1134–1140.
243. de Benedetti F, Massa M, Robbioni P, et al. Correlation of serum interleukin-6 levels with joint involvement and thrombocytosis in systemic juvenile rheumatoid arthritis. *Arthritis Rheum* 1991;34: 1158–1163.
244. De Benedetti F, Alonzi T, Moretta A, et al. Interleukin 6 causes growth impairment in transgenic mice through a decrease in insulin-like growth factor-I. A model for stunted growth in children with chronic inflammation. *J Clin Invest* 1997;99:643–650.
245. Fishman D, Faulds G, Jeffery R, et al. The effect of novel polymorphisms in the interleukin-6 (IL-6) gene on IL-6 transcription and plasma IL-6 levels, and an association with systemic-onset juvenile chronic arthritis. *J Clin Invest* 1998;102:1369–1376.
246. Guerne PA, Terkeltaub R, Zuraw B, et al. Inflammatory microcrystals stimulate interleukin-6 production and secretion by human monocytes and synoviocytes. *Arthritis Rheum* 1989;32:1443–1452.
247. Takagi N, Mihara M, Moriya Y, et al. Blockage of interleukin-6 receptor ameliorates joint disease in murine collagen-induced arthritis. *Arthritis Rheum* 1998;41:2117–2121.
248. Alonzi T, Fattori E, Lazzaro D, et al. Interleukin 6 is required for the development of collagen-induced arthritis. *J Exp Med* 1998;187: 461–468.
249. Ohshima S, Saeki Y, Mima T, et al. Interleukin 6 plays a key role in the development of antigen-induced arthritis. *Proc Natl Acad Sci U S A* 1998;95:8222–8226.
250. van de Loo FA, Kuiper S, van Enckevort FH, et al. Interleukin-6 reduces cartilage destruction during experimental arthritis. A study in interleukin-6-deficient mice. *Am J Pathol* 1997;151: 177–191.
251. Lotz M, Guerne PA. Interleukin-6 induces the synthesis of tissue inhibitor of metalloproteinases-1/erythroid potentiating activity (TIMP-1/EPA). *J Biol Chem* 1991;266:2017–2020.
252. Villiger PM, Kusari AB, ten Dijke P, et al. IL-1 beta and IL-6 selectively induce transforming growth factor-beta isoforms in human articular chondrocytes. *J Immunol* 1993;151:3337–3344.
253. Silacci P, Dayer JM, Desgeorges A, et al. Interleukin (IL)-6 and its soluble receptor induce TIMP-1 expression in synoviocytes and chondrocytes, and block IL-1-induced collagenolytic activity. *J Biol Chem* 1998;273:13625–13629.
254. Wendling D, Racadot E, Wijdenes J. Treatment of severe rheumatoid arthritis by anti-interleukin 6 monoclonal antibody. *J Rheumatol* 1993;20:259–262.
255. Choy EH, Isenberg DA, Garrood T, et al. Therapeutic benefit of blocking interleukin-6 activity with an anti-interleukin-6 receptor monoclonal antibody in rheumatoid arthritis: a randomized, double-blind, placebo-controlled, dose-escalation trial. *Arthritis Rheum* 2002;46: 3143–3150.
256. Nishimoto N, Yoshizaki K, Miyasaka N, et al. A multi-center, randomized, double-blind, placebo-controlled trial of humanized anti-interleukin-6 (IL-6) receptor monoclonal antibody (MRA) in rheumatoid arthritis (RA). *Arthritis Rheum* 2002;46:559.
257. Lotz M, Moats T, Villiger PM. Leukemia inhibitory factor is expressed in cartilage and synovium and can contribute to the pathogenesis of arthritis. *J Clin Invest* 1992;90:888–896.
258. Waring P, Wycherley K, Cary D, et al. Leukemia inhibitory factor levels are elevated in septic shock and various inflammatory body fluids. *J Clin Invest* 1992;90:2031–2037.
259. Villiger PM, Geng Y, Lotz M. Induction of cytokine expression by leukemia inhibitory factor. *J Clin Invest* 1993;91:1575–1581.
260. Maier R, Ganu V, Lotz M. Interleukin-11, an inducible cytokine in human articular chondrocytes and synoviocytes, stimulates the production of the tissue inhibitor of metalloproteinases. *J Biol Chem* 1993;268:21527–21532.
261. Hermann JA, Hall MA, Maini RN, et al. Important immunoregulatory role of interleukin-11 in the inflammatory process in rheumatoid arthritis. *Arthritis Rheum* 1998;41:1388–1397.
262. Walmsley M, Butler DM, Marinova-Mutafchieva L, et al. An anti-inflammatory role for interleukin-11 in established murine collagen-induced arthritis. *Immunology* 1998;95:31–37.
263. Moreland L, Gugliotti R, King K, et al. Results of a phase-I/II randomized, masked, placebo-controlled trial of recombinant human interleukin-11 (rhIL-11) in the treatment of subjects with active rheumatoid arthritis. *Arthritis Res* 2001;3:247–52.
264. Modur V, Feldhaus MJ, Weyrich AS, et al. Oncostatin M is a proinflammatory mediator. *In vivo* effects correlate with endothelial cell expression of inflammatory cytokines and adhesion molecules. *J Clin Invest* 1997;100:158–168.
265. Langdon C, Kerr C, Hassen M, et al. Murine oncostatin M stimulates mouse synovial fibroblasts *in vitro* and induces inflammation and destruction in mouse joints *in vivo*. *Am J Pathol* 2000;157: 1187–1196.
266. de Hooge AS, van de Loo FA, Bennink MB, et al. Adenoviral transfer of murine oncostatin M elicits periosteal bone apposition in knee joints of mice, despite synovial inflammation and up-regulated expression of interleukin-6 and receptor activator of nuclear factor-kappa B ligand. *Am J Pathol* 2002;160:1733–1743.
267. Plater-Zyberk C, Buckton J, Thompson S, et al. Amelioration of arthritis in two murine models using antibodies to oncostatin M. *Arthritis Rheum* 2001;44:2697–2702.
268. Waldmann TA. The IL-2/IL-15 receptor systems: targets for immunotherapy. *J Clin Immunol* 2002;22:51–56.
269. Sadlack B, Merz H, Schorle H, et al. Ulcerative colitis-like disease in mice with a disrupted interleukin-2 gene. *Cell* 1993;75:253–261.
270. Tebib JG, Boughaba H, Letroublon MC, et al. Serum IL-2 level in rheumatoid arthritis: correlation with joint destruction and disease progression. *Eur Cytokine Netw* 1991;2:239–243.
271. Firestein GS, Xu WD, Townsend K, et al. Cytokines in chronic inflammatory arthritis. I. Failure to detect T cell lymphokines (interleukin 2 and interleukin 3) and presence of macrophage colony-stimulating factor (CSF-1) and a novel mast cell growth factor in rheumatoid synovitis. *J Exp Med* 1988;168:1573–1586.
272. Rubin LA, Galli F, Greene WC, et al. The molecular basis for the generation of the human soluble interleukin 2 receptor. *Cytokine* 1990;2:330–336.
273. Polisson RP, Dooley MA, Dawson DV, et al. Interleukin-2 receptor levels in the sera of rheumatoid arthritis patients treated with methotrexate. *Arthritis Rheum* 1994;37:50–56.
274. Camilleri JP, Amos N, Williams BD, et al. Serum soluble interleukin 2 receptor levels and radiological progression in early rheumatoid arthritis. *J Rheumatol* 2001;28:2576–2578.
275. Rose CD, Fawcett PT, Gibney K, et al. Serial measurements of soluble interleukin 2 receptor levels (sIL2-R) in children with juvenile rheumatoid arthritis treated with oral methotrexate. *Ann Rheum Dis* 1994;53:471–474.
276. Raziuddin S, al-Janadi MA, al-Wabel AA. Soluble interleukin 2 receptor levels in serum and its relationship to T cell abnormality and clinical manifestations of the disease in patients with systemic lupus erythematosus. *J Rheumatol* 1991;18:831–836.
277. ter Borg EJ, Horst G, Limburg PC, et al. Changes in plasma levels of interleukin-2 receptor in relation to disease exacerbations and levels of anti-dsDNA and complement in systemic lupus erythematosus. *Clin Exp Immunol* 1990;82:21–26.
278. Laut J, Senitzer D, Petrucci R, et al. Soluble interleukin-2 receptor levels in lupus nephritis. *Clin Nephrol* 1992;38:179–184.
279. Ward MM, Dooley MA, Christenson VD, et al. The relationship between soluble interleukin 2 receptor levels and antidouble stranded DNA antibody levels in patients with systemic lupus erythematosus. *J Rheumatol* 1991;18:235–240.
280. Davas EM, Tsirogianni A, Kappou I, et al. Serum IL-6, TNFalpha, p55 srTNFalpha, p75srTNFalpha, srIL-2alpha levels and disease activity in systemic lupus erythematosus. *Clin Rheumatol* 1999;18: 17–22.
281. Gilad R, Lampl Y, Eshel Y, et al. Cerebrospinal fluid soluble interleukin-2 receptor in cerebral lupus. *Br J Rheumatol* 1997;36: 190–193.
282. Wong KL, Wong RP. Serum soluble interleukin 2 receptor in systemic lupus erythematosus: effects of disease activity and infection. *Ann Rheum Dis* 1991;50:706–709.
283. Schmitt WH, Heesen C, Csernok E, et al. Elevated serum levels of soluble interleukin-2 receptor in patients with Wegener's granulomatosis. Association with disease activity. *Arthritis Rheum* 1992; 35:1088–1096.
284. Manoussakis MN, Papadopoulos GK, Drosos AA, et al. Soluble interleukin 2 receptor molecules in the serum of patients with autoimmune diseases. *Clin Immunol Immunopathol* 1989;50:321–332.

285. Uziel Y, Krafchik BR, Feldman B, et al. Serum levels of soluble interleukin-2 receptor. A marker of disease activity in localized scleroderma. *Arthritis Rheum* 1994;37:898–901.
286. Lavelle-Jones M, al-Hadrani A, Spiers EM, et al. Reactivation of rheumatoid arthritis during continuous infusion of interleukin 2: evidence of lymphocytic control of rheumatoid disease. *BMJ* 1990;301: 97.
287. Massarotti EM, Liu NY, Mier J, et al. Chronic inflammatory arthritis after treatment with high-dose interleukin-2 for malignancy. *Am J Med* 1992;92:693–697.
288. Sewell KL, Parker KC, Woodworth TG, et al. DAB486IL-2 fusion toxin in refractory rheumatoid arthritis. *Arthritis Rheum* 1993;36: 1223–1233.
289. Brok HP, Tekoppele JM, Hakimi J, et al. Prophylactic and therapeutic effects of a humanized monoclonal antibody against the IL-2 receptor (DACLIZUMAB) on collagen-induced arthritis (CIA) in rhesus monkeys. *Clin Exp Immunol* 2001;124:134–141.
290. Lentsch AB, Shanley TP, Sarma V, et al. *In vivo* suppression of NF-kappa B and preservation of I kappa B alpha by interleukin-10 and interleukin-13. *J Clin Invest* 1997;100:2443–2448.
291. Donnelly RP, Crofford LJ, Freeman SL, et al. Tissue-specific regulation of IL-6 production by IL-4. Differential effects of IL-4 on nuclear factor-kappa B activity in monocytes and fibroblasts. *J Immunol* 1993;151:5603–5612.
292. Allen JB, Wong HL, Costa GL, et al. Suppression of monocyte function and differential regulation of IL-1 and IL-1ra by IL-4 contribute to resolution of experimental arthritis. *J Immunol* 1993;151:4344–4351.
293. Miossec P, van den Berg W. Th1/Th2 cytokine balance in arthritis. *Arthritis Rheum* 1997;40:2105–2115.
294. Gabay C, Porter B, Guenette D, et al. Interleukin-4 (IL-4) and IL-13 enhance the effect of IL-1beta on production of IL-1 receptor antagonist by human primary hepatocytes and hepatoma HepG2 cells: differential effect on C-reactive protein production. *Blood* 1999;93:1299–1307.
295. Marie C, Pitton C, Fitting C, et al. IL-10 and IL-4 synergize with TNF-alpha to induce IL-1ra production by human neutrophils. *Cytokine* 1996;8:147–151.
296. Colotta F, Sironi M, Borre A, et al. Interleukin 4 amplifies monocyte chemotactic protein and interleukin 6 production by endothelial cells. *Cytokine* 1992;4:24–28.
297. Iademarco MF, Barks JL, Dean DC. Regulation of vascular cell adhesion molecule-1 expression by IL-4 and TNF-alpha in cultured endothelial cells. *J Clin Invest* 1995;95:264–271.
298. Rathanaswami P, Hachicha M, Sadick M, et al. Expression of the cytokine RANTES in human rheumatoid synovial fibroblasts. Differential regulation of RANTES and interleukin-8 genes by inflammatory cytokines. *J Biol Chem* 1993;268:5834–5839.
299. Lubberts E, Joosten LA, van Den Bersselaar L, et al. Adenoviral vector-mediated overexpression of IL-4 in the knee joint of mice with collagen-induced arthritis prevents cartilage destruction. *J Immunol* 1999;163:4546–4556.
300. Lubberts E, Joosten LA, Chabaud M, et al. IL-4 gene therapy for collagen arthritis suppresses synovial IL-17 and osteoprotegerin ligand and prevents bone erosion. *J Clin Invest* 2000;105:1697–1710.
301. Joosten LA, Lubberts E, Helsen MM, et al. Protection against cartilage and bone destruction by systemic interleukin-4 treatment in established murine type II collagen-induced arthritis. *Arthritis Res* 1999;1:81–91.
302. Svensson L, Nandakumar KS, Johansson A, et al. IL-4-deficient mice develop less acute but more chronic relapsing collagen-induced arthritis. *Eur J Immunol* 2002;32:2944–2953.
303. Finnegan A, Grusby MJ, Kaplan CD, et al. IL-4 and IL-12 regulate proteoglycan-induced arthritis through STAT-dependent mechanisms. *J Immunol* 2002;169:3345–3352.
304. Joosten LA, Lubberts E, Durez P, et al. Role of interleukin-4 and interleukin-10 in murine collagen-induced arthritis. Protective effect of interleukin-4 and interleukin-10 treatment on cartilage destruction. *Arthritis Rheum* 1997;40:249–260.
305. McKenzie AN, Culpepper JA, de Waal Malefyt R, et al. Interleukin 13, a T-cell-derived cytokine that regulates human monocyte and B-cell function. *Proc Natl Acad Sci U S A* 1993;90:3735–3739.
306. Minty A, Chalon P, Derocq JM, et al. Interleukin-13 is a new human lymphokine regulating inflammatory and immune responses. *Nature* 1993;362:248–250.
307. de Waal Malefyt R, Figdor CG, Huijbens R, et al. Effects of IL-13 on phenotype, cytokine production, and cytotoxic function of human monocytes. Comparison with IL-4 and modulation by IFN-gamma or IL-10. *J Immunol* 1993;151:6370–6381.
308. Van den Bosch F, Russell A, Keystone EC. rHu IL-4 in subjects with active rheumatoid arthritis (RA): a phase I dose escalating safety study. *Arthritis Rheum* 1998;41:56.
309. Schorlemmer HU, Dickneite G, Kanzy EJ, et al. Modulation of the immunoglobulin dysregulation in GvH- and SLE-like diseases by the murine IL-4 receptor (IL-4-R). *Inflamm Res* 1995;44:194–196.
310. Kono DH, Balomenos D, Park MS, et al. Development of lupus in BXSB mice is independent of IL-4. *J Immunol* 2000;164:38–42.
311. Erb KJ, Ruger B, von Brevern M, et al. Constitutive expression of interleukin (IL)-4 *in vivo* causes autoimmune-type disorders in mice. *J Exp Med* 1997;185:329–339.
312. Santiago ML, Fossati L, Jacquet C, et al. Interleukin-4 protects against a genetically linked lupus-like autoimmune syndrome. *J Exp Med* 1997;185:65–70.
313. Needleman BW, Wigley FM, Stair RW. Interleukin-1, interleukin-2, interleukin-4, interleukin-6, tumor necrosis factor alpha, and interferon-gamma levels in sera from patients with scleroderma. *Arthritis Rheum* 1992;35:67–72.
314. Hasegawa M, Fujimoto M, Kikuchi K, et al. Elevated serum levels of interleukin 4 (IL-4), IL-10, and IL-13 in patients with systemic sclerosis. *J Rheumatol* 1997;24:328–332.
315. Lee KS, Ro YJ, Ryoo YW, et al. Regulation of interleukin-4 on collagen gene expression by systemic sclerosis fibroblasts in culture. *J Dermatol Sci* 1996;12:110–117.
316. Alderson MR, Tough TW, Ziegler SF, et al. Interleukin 7 induces cytokine secretion and tumoricidal activity by human peripheral blood monocytes. *J Exp Med* 1991;173:923–930.
317. De Benedetti F, Massa M, Pignatti P, et al. Elevated circulating interleukin-7 levels in patients with systemic juvenile rheumatoid arthritis. *J Rheumatol* 1995;22:1581–1585.
318. van Roon JA, Glaudemans KA, Bijlsma JW, et al. Interleukin 7 stimulates tumour necrosis factor alpha and Th1 cytokine production in joints of patients with rheumatoid arthritis. *Ann Rheum Dis* 2003; 62:113–119.
319. Harada S, Yamamura M, Okamoto H, et al. Production of interleukin-7 and interleukin-15 by fibroblast-like synoviocytes from patients with rheumatoid arthritis. *Arthritis Rheum* 1999;42:1508–1516.
320. Leistad L, Ostensen M, Faxvaag A. Detection of cytokine mRNA in human, articular cartilage from patients with rheumatoid arthritis and osteoarthritis by reverse transcriptase-polymerase chain reaction. *Scand J Rheumatol* 1998;27:61–67.
321. Toraldo G, Roggia C, Qian WP, et al. IL-7 induces bone loss *in vivo* by induction of receptor activator of nuclear factor kappa B ligand and tumor necrosis factor alpha from T cells. *Proc Natl Acad Sci U S A* 2003;100:125–130.
322. Tagaya Y, Kurys G, Thies TA, et al. Generation of secretable and nonsecretable interleukin 15 isoforms through alternate usage of signal peptides. *Proc Natl Acad Sci U S A* 1997;94:14444–14449.
323. Gaggero A, Azzarone B, Andrei C, et al. Differential intracellular trafficking, secretion and endosomal localization of two IL-15 isoforms. *Eur J Immunol* 1999;29:1265–1274.
324. Musso T, Calosso L, Zucca M, et al. Human monocytes constitutively express membrane-bound, biologically active, and interferon-gamma-upregulated interleukin-15. *Blood* 1999;93:3531–3539.
325. Nishimura H, Yajima T, Naiki Y, et al. Differential roles of interleukin 15 mRNA isoforms generated by alternative splicing in immune responses *in vivo*. *J Exp Med* 2000;191:157–170.
326. Kurowska M, Rudnicka W, Kontny E, et al. Fibroblast-like synoviocytes from rheumatoid arthritis patients express functional IL-15 receptor complex: endogenous IL-15 in autocrine fashion enhances cell proliferation and expression of Bcl-x(L) and Bcl-2. *J Immunol* 2002;169:1760–1767.
327. McInnes IB, Leung BP, Sturrock RD, et al. Interleukin-15 mediates T cell-dependent regulation of tumor necrosis factor-alpha production in rheumatoid arthritis. *Nat Med* 1997;3:189–195.
328. Yang L, Thornton S, Grom AA. Interleukin-15 inhibits sodium nitroprusside-induced apoptosis of synovial fibroblasts and vascular endothelial cells. *Arthritis Rheum* 2002;46:3010–3014.

329. Ogata Y, Kukita A, Kukita T, et al. A novel role of IL-15 in the development of osteoclasts: inability to replace its activity with IL-2. *J Immunol* 1999;162:2754–2760.
330. Liew FY, McInnes IB. Role of interleukin 15 and interleukin 18 in inflammatory response. *Ann Rheum Dis* 2002;61:100–102.
331. Ruchatz H, Leung BP, Wei XQ, et al. Soluble IL-15 receptor alpha-chain administration prevents murine collagen-induced arthritis: a role for IL-15 in development of antigen-induced immunopathology. *J Immunol* 1998;160:5654–5660.
332. Baslund B, Tvede N, Danneskiold-Samsoe B, et al. First use of a human monoclonal antibody against IL-15 (HUMAX-IL15) in patients with active rheumatoid arthritis (RA): results of a double-blind, placebo-controlled phase i/ii trial. *Ann Rheum Dis* 2003;62:66.
333. Ozaki K, Kikly K, Michalovich D, et al. Cloning of a type I cytokine receptor most related to the IL-2 receptor beta chain. *Proc Natl Acad Sci U S A* 2000;97:11439–11444.
334. Parrish-Novak J, Dillon SR, Nelson A, et al. Interleukin 21 and its receptor are involved in NK cell expansion and regulation of lymphocyte function. *Nature* 2000;408:57–63.
335. Ozaki K, Spolski R, Feng CG, et al. A critical role for IL-21 in regulating immunoglobulin production. *Science* 2002;298:1630–1634.
336. Brenne AT, Baade Ro T, Waage A, et al. Interleukin-21 is a growth and survival factor for human myeloma cells. *Blood* 2002;99:3756–3762.
337. Wurster AL, Rodgers VL, Satoskar AR, et al. Interleukin 21 is a T helper (Th) cell 2 cytokine that specifically inhibits the differentiation of naive Th cells into interferon gamma-producing Th1 cells. *J Exp Med* 2002;196:969–977.
338. Demoulin JB, Louahed J, Dumoutier L, et al. MAP kinase activation by interleukin-9 in lymphoid and mast cell lines. *Oncogene* 2003;22:1763–1770.
339. Soussi-Gounni A, Kontolemos M, Hamid Q. Role of IL-9 in the pathophysiology of allergic diseases. *J Allergy Clin Immunol* 2001;107:575–582.
340. Brightbill HD, Plevy SE, Modlin RL, et al. A prominent role for Sp1 during lipopolysaccharide-mediated induction of the IL-10 promoter in macrophages. *J Immunol* 2000;164:1940–1951.
341. Tone M, Powell MJ, Tone Y, et al. IL-10 gene expression is controlled by the transcription factors Sp1 and Sp3. *J Immunol* 2000;165:286–291.
342. Powell MJ, Thompson SA, Tone Y, et al. Posttranscriptional regulation of IL-10 gene expression through sequences in the 3′-untranslated region. *J Immunol* 2000;165:292–296.
343. Turner DM, Williams DM, Sankaran D, et al. An investigation of polymorphism in the interleukin-10 gene promoter. *Eur J Immunogenet* 1997;24:1–8.
344. Berkman N, John M, Roesems G, et al. Inhibition of macrophage inflammatory protein-1 alpha expression by IL-10. Differential sensitivities in human blood monocytes and alveolar macrophages. *J Immunol* 1995;155:4412–4418.
345. Rossi DL, Vicari AP, Franz-Bacon K, et al. Identification through bioinformatics of two new macrophage proinflammatory human chemokines: MIP-3alpha and MIP-3beta. *J Immunol* 1997;158:1033–1036.
346. Marfaing-Koka A, Maravic M, Humbert M, et al. Contrasting effects of IL-4, IL-10 and corticosteroids on RANTES production by human monocytes. *Int Immunol* 1996;8:1587–1594.
347. Kopydlowski KM, Salkowski CA, Cody MJ, et al. Regulation of macrophage chemokine expression by lipopolysaccharide *in vitro* and *in vivo*. *J Immunol* 1999;163:1537–1544.
348. Kubin M, Kamoun M, Trinchieri G. Interleukin 12 synergizes with B7/CD28 interaction in inducing efficient proliferation and cytokine production of human T cells. *J Exp Med* 1994;180:211–222.
349. Lacraz S, Nicod LP, Chicheportiche R, et al. IL-10 inhibits metalloproteinase and stimulates TIMP-1 production in human mononuclear phagocytes. *J Clin Invest* 1995;96:2304–2310.
350. Cassatella MA, Meda L, Gasperini S, et al. Interleukin 10 (IL-10) upregulates IL-1 receptor antagonist production from lipopolysaccharide-stimulated human polymorphonuclear leukocytes by delaying mRNA degradation. *J Exp Med* 1994;179:1695–1699.
351. Kuhn R, Lohler J, Rennick D, Rajewsky K, Muller W. Interleukin-10-deficient mice develop chronic enterocolitis. *Cell* 1993;75:263–274.
352. Berg DJ, Kuhn R, Rajewsky K, et al. Interleukin-10 is a central regulator of the response to LPS in murine models of endotoxic shock and the Shwartzman reaction but not endotoxin tolerance. *J Clin Invest* 1995;96:2339–2347.
353. van der Poll T, Marchant A, Buurman WA, et al. Endogenous IL-10 protects mice from death during septic peritonitis. *J Immunol* 1995;155:5397–5401.
354. Kim HS, Armstrong D, Hamilton TA, et al. IL-10 suppresses LPS-induced KC mRNA expression via a translation-dependent decrease in mRNA stability. *J Leukoc Biol* 1998;64:33–39.
355. Kishore R, Tebo JM, Kolosov M, et al. Cutting edge: clustered AU-rich elements are the target of IL-10-mediated mRNA destabilization in mouse macrophages. *J Immunol* 1999;162:2457–2461.
356. Weber-Nordt RM, Meraz MA, Schreiber RD. Lipopolysaccharide-dependent induction of IL-10 receptor expression on murine fibroblasts. *J Immunol* 1994;153:3734–3744.
357. Kotenko SV, Krause CD, Izotova LS, et al. Identification and functional characterization of a second chain of the interleukin-10 receptor complex. *EMBO J* 1997;16:5894–5903.
358. Spencer SD, Di Marco F, Hooley J, et al. The orphan receptor CRF2–4 is an essential subunit of the interleukin 10 receptor. *J Exp Med* 1998;187:571–578.
359. Howard M, Muchamuel T, Andrade S, et al. Interleukin 10 protects mice from lethal endotoxemia. *J Exp Med* 1993;177:1205–1208.
360. Pajkrt D, Camoglio L, Tiel-van Buul MC, et al. Attenuation of proinflammatory response by recombinant human IL-10 in human endotoxemia: effect of timing of recombinant human IL-10 administration. *J Immunol* 1997;158:3971–3977.
361. Katsikis PD, Chu CQ, Brennan FM, et al. Immunoregulatory role of interleukin 10 in rheumatoid arthritis. *J Exp Med* 1994;179:1517–1527.
362. Kasama T, Strieter RM, Lukacs NW, et al. Interleukin-10 expression and chemokine regulation during the evolution of murine type II collagen-induced arthritis. *J Clin Invest* 1995;95:2868–2876.
363. Tanaka Y, Otsuka T, Hotokebuchi T, et al. Effect of IL-10 on collagen-induced arthritis in mice. *Inflamm Res* 1996;45:283–288.
364. van Roon JA, van Roy JL, Gmelig-Meyling FH, et al. Prevention and reversal of cartilage degradation in rheumatoid arthritis by interleukin-10 and interleukin-4. *Arthritis Rheum* 1996;39:829–835.
365. Walmsley M, Katsikis PD, Abney E, et al. Interleukin-10 inhibition of the progression of established collagen-induced arthritis. *Arthritis Rheum* 1996;39:495–503.
366. Persson S, Mikulowska A, Narula S, et al. Interleukin-10 suppresses the development of collagen type II-induced arthritis and ameliorates sustained arthritis in rats. *Scand J Immunol* 1996;44:607–614.
367. Whalen JD, Lechman EL, Carlos CA, et al. Adenoviral transfer of the viral IL-10 gene periarticularly to mouse paws suppresses development of collagen-induced arthritis in both injected and uninjected paws. *J Immunol* 1999;162:3625–3632.
368. Keystone E, Wherry J, Grint P. IL-10 as a therapeutic strategy in the treatment of rheumatoid arthritis. *Rheum Dis Clin North Am* 1998;24:629–639.
369. McInnes IB, Illei GG, Danning CL, et al. IL-10 improves skin disease and modulates endothelial activation and leukocyte effector function in patients with psoriatic arthritis. *J Immunol* 2001;167:4075–4082.
370. Grondal G, Gunnarsson I, Ronnelid J, et al. Cytokine production, serum levels and disease activity in systemic lupus erythematosus. *Clin Exp Rheumatol* 2000;18:565–570.
371. Itoh K, Hirohata S. The role of IL-10 in human B cell activation, proliferation, and differentiation. *J Immunol* 1995;154:4341–4350.
372. Llorente L, Zou W, Levy Y, et al. Role of interleukin 10 in the B lymphocyte hyperactivity and autoantibody production of human systemic lupus erythematosus. *J Exp Med* 1995;181:839–844.
373. Ronnelid J, Tejde A, Mathsson L, et al. Immune complexes from SLE sera induce IL10 production from normal peripheral blood mononuclear cells by an FcgammaRII dependent mechanism: implications for a possible vicious cycle maintaining B cell hyperactivity in SLE. *Ann Rheum Dis* 2003;62:37–42.
374. Ishida H, Muchamuel T, Sakaguchi S, et al. Continuous administration of anti-interleukin 10 antibodies delays onset of autoimmunity in NZB/W F1 mice. *J Exp Med* 1994;179:305–310.
375. Llorente L, Richaud-Patin Y, Garcia-Padilla C, et al. Clinical and biologic effects of anti-interleukin-10 monoclonal antibody administration in systemic lupus erythematosus. *Arthritis Rheum* 2000;43:1790–1800.

376. Moore KW, de Waal Malefyt R, Coffman RL, et al. Interleukin-10 and the interleukin-10 receptor. *Annu Rev Immunol* 2001;19:683–765.
377. Kotenko SV. The family of IL-10-related cytokines and their receptors: related, but to what extent? *Cytokine Growth Factor Rev* 2002; 13:223–240.
378. Kotenko SV, Izotova LS, Mirochnitchenko OV, et al. Identification, cloning, and characterization of a novel soluble receptor that binds IL-22 and neutralizes its activity. *J Immunol* 2001;166:7096–7103.
379. Blumberg H, Conklin D, Xu WF, et al. Interleukin 20: discovery, receptor identification, and role in epidermal function. *Cell* 2001; 104:9–19.
380. Soo C, Shaw WW, Freymiller E, et al. Cutaneous rat wounds express c49a, a novel gene with homology to the human melanoma differentiation associated gene, mda-7. *J Cell Biochem* 1999;74:1–10.
381. Pittman DD, Goad B, Lambert AJ, et al. IL-22 is a tightly-regulated IL10-like molecule that induces an acute-phase response and renal tubular basophilia. *Genes Immunol* 2001;2:172.
382. Dumoutier L, Van Roost E, Colau D, et al. Human interleukin-10-related T cell-derived inducible factor: molecular cloning and functional characterization as an hepatocyte-stimulating factor. *Proc Natl Acad Sci U S A* 2000;97:10144–10149.
383. Xie MH, Aggarwal S, Ho WH, et al. Interleukin (IL)-22, a novel human cytokine that signals through the interferon receptor-related proteins CRF2–4 and IL-22R. *J Biol Chem* 2000;275:31335–31339.
384. Sheppard P, Kindsvogel W, Xu W, et al. IL-28, IL-29 and their class II cytokine receptor IL-28R. *Nat Immunol* 2003;4:63–68.
385. Gearing DP, Cosman D. Homology of the p40 subunit of natural killer cell stimulatory factor (NKSF) with the extracellular domain of the interleukin-6 receptor. *Cell* 1991;66:9–10.
386. D'Andrea A, Rengaraju M, Valiante NM, et al. Production of natural killer cell stimulatory factor (interleukin 12) by peripheral blood mononuclear cells. *J Exp Med* 1992;176:1387–1398.
387. Brombacher F, Kastelein RA, Alber G. Novel IL-12 family members shed light on the orchestration of Th1 responses. *Trends Immunol* 2003;24:207–212.
388. Germann T, Szeliga J, Hess H, et al. Administration of interleukin 12 in combination with type II collagen induces severe arthritis in DBA/1 mice. *Proc Natl Acad Sci U S A* 1995;92:4823–4827.
389. Matthys P, Vermeire K, Mitera T, et al. Anti-IL-12 antibody prevents the development and progression of collagen-induced arthritis in IFN-gamma receptor-deficient mice. *Eur J Immunol* 1998;28: 2143–2151.
390. McIntyre KW, Shuster DJ, Gillooly KM, et al. Reduced incidence and severity of collagen-induced arthritis in interleukin-12-deficient mice. *Eur J Immunol* 1996;26:29332938.
391. Butler DM, Malfait AM, Maini RN, et al. Anti-IL-12 and anti-TNF antibodies synergistically suppress the progression of murine collagen-induced arthritis. *Eur J Immunol* 1999;29:2205–2212.
392. Malfait AM, Butler DM, Presky DH, et al. Blockade of IL-12 during the induction of collagen-induced arthritis (CIA) markedly attenuates the severity of the arthritis. *Clin Exp Immunol* 1998;111:377–383.
393. Joosten LA, Lubberts E, Helsen MM, et al. Dual role of IL-12 in early and late stages of murine collagen type II arthritis. *J Immunol* 1997;159:4094–4102.
394. Hess H, Gately MK, Rude E, et al. High doses of interleukin-12 inhibit the development of joint disease in DBA/1 mice immunized with type II collagen in complete Freund's adjuvant. *Eur J Immunol* 1996;26:187–191.
395. Morita Y, Yamamura M, Nishida K, et al. Expression of interleukin-12 in synovial tissue from patients with rheumatoid arthritis. *Arthritis Rheum* 1998;41:306–314.
396. Hessian PA, Highton J, Kean A, et al. Cytokine profile of the rheumatoid nodule suggests that it is a Th1 granuloma. *Arthritis Rheum* 2003;48:334–338.
397. Parham C, Chirica M, Timans J, et al. A receptor for the heterodimeric cytokine IL-23 is composed of IL-12Rbeta1 and a novel cytokine receptor subunit, IL-23R. *J Immunol* 2002;168:5699–5708.
398. Oppmann B, Lesley R, Blom B, et al. Novel p19 protein engages IL-12p40 to form a cytokine, IL-23, with biological activities similar as well as distinct from IL-12. *Immunity* 2000;13:715–725.
399. Wiekowski MT, Leach MW, Evans EW, et al. Ubiquitous transgenic expression of the IL-23 subunit p19 induces multiorgan inflammation, runting, infertility, and premature death. *J Immunol* 2001;166: 7563–7570.
400. Pflanz S, Timans JC, Cheung J, et al. IL-27, a heterodimeric cytokine composed of EBI3 and p28 protein, induces proliferation of naive CD4(+) T cells. *Immunity* 2002;16:779–790.
401. Chen Q, Ghilardi N, Wang H, et al. Development of Th1-type immune responses requires the type I cytokine receptor TCCR. *Nature* 2000;407:916–920.
402. Center DM, Kornfeld H, Cruikshank WW. Interleukin 16 and its function as a CD4 ligand. *Immunol Today* 1996;17:476–481.
403. Theodore AC, Center DM, Nicoll J, et al. CD4 ligand IL-16 inhibits the mixed lymphocyte reaction. *J Immunol* 1996;157:1958–1964.
404. Blaschke S, Schulz H, Schwarz G, et al. Interleukin 16 expression in relation to disease activity in rheumatoid arthritis. *J Rheumatol* 2001;28:12–21.
405. Kageyama Y, Ozeki T, Suzuki M, et al. Interleukin-16 in synovial fluids from cases of various types of arthritis. *Joint Bone Spine* 2000; 67:188–193.
406. Klimiuk PA, Goronzy JJ, Weyand CM. IL-16 as an anti-inflammatory cytokine in rheumatoid synovitis. *J Immunol* 1999;162:4293–4299.
407. Matsushita M, Hayashi T, Ando S, et al. Changes of CD4/CD8 ratio and interleukin-16 in systemic lupus erythematosus. *Clin Rheumatol* 2000;19:270–274.
408. Lard LR, Roep BO, Verburgh CA, et al. Elevated IL-16 levels in patients with systemic lupus erythematosus are associated with disease severity but not with genetic susceptibility to lupus. *Lupus* 2002; 11:181–185.
409. Yao Z, Painter SL, Fanslow WC, et al. Human IL-17: a novel cytokine derived from T cells. *J Immunol* 1995;155:5483–5486.
410. Aarvak T, Chabaud M, Miossec P, et al. IL-17 is produced by some proinflammatory Th1/Th0 cells but not by Th2 cells. *J Immunol* 1999;162:1246–1251.
411. Kehlen A, Thiele K, Riemann D, et al. Expression, modulation and signalling of IL-17 receptor in fibroblast-like synoviocytes of patients with rheumatoid arthritis. *Clin Exp Immunol* 2002;127: 539–546.
412. Shalom-Barak T, Quach J, Lotz M. Interleukin-17-induced gene expression in articular chondrocytes is associated with activation of mitogen-activated protein kinases and NF-kappaB. *J Biol Chem* 1998;273:27467–27473.
413. Jovanovic DV, Di Battista JA, Martel-Pelletier J, et al. IL-17 stimulates the production and expression of proinflammatory cytokines, IL-beta and TNF-alpha, by human macrophages. *J Immunol* 1998; 160:3513–3521.
414. Kotake S, Udagawa N, Takahashi N, et al. IL-17 in synovial fluids from patients with rheumatoid arthritis is a potent stimulator of osteoclastogenesis. *J Clin Invest* 1999;103:1345–1352.
415. Chabaud M, Page G, Miossec P. Enhancing effect of IL-1, IL-17, and TNF-alpha on macrophage inflammatory protein-3alpha production in rheumatoid arthritis: regulation by soluble receptors and Th2 cytokines. *J Immunol* 2001;167:6015–6020.
416. Miossec P. Interleukin-17 in rheumatoid arthritis: if T cells were to contribute to inflammation and destruction through synergy. *Arthritis Rheum* 2003;48:594–601.
417. Lubberts E, Joosten LA, van de Loo FA, et al. Reduction of interleukin-17-induced inhibition of chondrocyte proteoglycan synthesis in intact murine articular cartilage by interleukin-4. *Arthritis Rheum* 2000;43:1300–1306.
418. Lubberts E, Van Den Bersselaar L, Oppers-Walgreen B, et al. IL-17 promotes bone erosion in murine collagen-induced arthritis through loss of the receptor activator of NF-kappaB ligand/osteoprotegerin balance. *J Immunol* 2003;170:2655–2662.
419. Dudler J, Renggli-Zulliger N, Busso N, et al. Effect of interleukin 17 on proteoglycan degradation in murine knee joints. *Ann Rheum Dis* 2000;59:529–532.
420. Lubberts E, Joosten LA, Oppers B, et al. IL-1-independent role of IL-17 in synovial inflammation and joint destruction during collagen-induced arthritis. *J Immunol* 2001;167:1004–1013.
421. Kurasawa K, Hirose K, Sano H, et al. Increased interleukin-17 production in patients with systemic sclerosis. *Arthritis Rheum* 2000; 43:2455–2463.
422. Wong CK, Ho CY, Li EK, et al. Elevation of proinflammatory cytokine (IL-18, IL-17, IL-12) and Th2 cytokine (IL-4) concentra-

tions in patients with systemic lupus erythematosus. *Lupus* 2000; 9:589–593.
423. Fort MM, Cheung J, Yen D, et al. IL-25 induces IL-4, IL-5, and IL-13 and Th2-associated pathologies *in vivo*. *Immunity* 2001;15: 985–995.
424. Hurst SD, Muchamuel T, Gorman DM, et al. New IL-17 family members promote Th1 or Th2 responses in the lung: *in vivo* function of the novel cytokine IL-25. *J Immunol* 2002;169:443–453.
425. Nissenson AR. Erythropoietin overview—1993. *Blood Purif* 1994; 12:6–13.
426. Foster DC, Sprecher CA, Grant FJ, et al. Human thrombopoietin: gene structure, cDNA sequence, expression, and chromosomal localization. *Proc Natl Acad Sci U S A* 1994;91:13023–13027.
427. Alvaro-Gracia JM, Zvaifler NJ, Firestein GS. Cytokines in chronic inflammatory arthritis. IV. Granulocyte/macrophage colony-stimulating factor-mediated induction of class II MHC antigen on human monocytes: a possible role in rheumatoid arthritis. *J Exp Med* 1989;170: 865–875.
428. Kodama H, Yamasaki A, Nose M, et al. Congenital osteoclast deficiency in osteopetrotic (op/op) mice is cured by injections of macrophage colony-stimulating factor. *J Exp Med* 1991;173:269–272.
429. McColl SR, Paquin R, Menard C, et al. Human neutrophils produce high levels of the interleukin 1 receptor antagonist in response to granulocyte/macrophage colony-stimulating factor and tumor necrosis factor alpha. *J Exp Med* 1992;176:593–598.
430. de Haas M, Kerst JM, van der Schoot CE, et al. Granulocyte colony-stimulating factor administration to healthy volunteers: analysis of the immediate activating effects on circulating neutrophils. *Blood* 1994;84:3885–3894.
431. Hamilton JA, Piccoli DS, Cebon J, et al. Cytokine regulation of colony-stimulating factor (CSF) production in cultured human synovial fibroblasts. II. Similarities and differences in the control of interleukin-1 induction of granulocyte-macrophage CSF and granulocyte-CSF production. *Blood* 1992;79:1413–1419.
432. Alvaro-Gracia JM, Zvaifler NJ, Brown CB, et al. Cytokines in chronic inflammatory arthritis. VI. Analysis of the synovial cells involved in granulocyte-macrophage colony-stimulating factor production and gene expression in rheumatoid arthritis and its regulation by IL-1 and tumor necrosis factor-alpha. *J Immunol* 1991;146:3365–3371.
433. Nakamura H, Ueki Y, Sakito S, et al. High serum and synovial fluid granulocyte colony stimulating factor (G-CSF) concentrations in patients with rheumatoid arthritis. *Clin Exp Rheumatol* 2000;18:713–718.
434. Fishman P, Kamashta M, Ehrenfeld M, et al. Interleukin-3 immunoassay in systemic lupus erythematosus patients: preliminary data. *Int Arch Allergy Immunol* 1993;100:215–218.
435. Cook AD, Braine EL, Campbell IK, et al. Blockade of collagen-induced arthritis post-onset by antibody to granulocyte-macrophage colony-stimulating factor (GM-CSF): requirement for GM CSF in the effector phase of disease. *Arthritis Res* 2001;3:293–298.
436. Means RT Jr. Pathogenesis of the anemia of chronic disease: a cytokine-mediated anemia. *Stem Cells* 1995;13:32–37.
437. Peeters HR, Jongen-Lavrencic M, Vreugdenhil G, et al. Effect of recombinant human erythropoietin on anaemia and disease activity in patients with rheumatoid arthritis and anaemia of chronic disease: a randomised placebo controlled double blind 52 weeks clinical trial. *Ann Rheum Dis* 1996;55:739–744.
438. Kaltwasser JP, Kessler U, Gottschalk R, et al. Effect of recombinant human erythropoietin and intravenous iron on anemia and disease activity in rheumatoid arthritis. *J Rheumatol* 2001;28:2430–2436.
439. Sprikkelman A, de Wolf JT, Vellenga E. The application of hematopoietic growth factors in drug-induced agranulocytosis: a review of 70 cases. *Leukemia* 1994;8:2031–2036.
440. Hellmich B, Csernok E, Schatz H, et al. Autoantibodies against granulocyte colony-stimulating factor in Felty's syndrome and neutropenic systemic lupus erythematosus. *Arthritis Rheum* 2002;46: 2384–2391.
441. Bhalla K, Ross R, Jeter E, et al. G-CSF improves granulocytopenia in Felty's syndrome without flare-up of arthritis. *Am J Hematol* 1993; 42:230–231.
442. Euler HH, Schwab UM, Schroeder JO. Filgrastim for lupus neutropenia. *Lancet* 1994;344:1513–1514.
443. Kaiser U, Klausmann M, Kolb G, et al. Felty's syndrome: favorable response to granulocyte-macrophage colony-stimulating factor in the acute phase. *Acta Haematol* 1992;87:190–194.
444. Hermann P, Rubio M, Nakajima T, et al. IFN-alpha priming of human monocytes differentially regulates gram-positive and gram-negative bacteria-induced IL-10 release and selectively enhances IL-12p70, CD80, and MHC class I expression. *J Immunol* 1998;161:2011–2018.
445. Reznikov LL, Puren AJ, Fantuzzi G, et al. Spontaneous and inducible cytokine responses in healthy humans receiving a single dose of IFN-alpha2b: increased production of interleukin-1 receptor antagonist and suppression of IL-1-induced IL-8. *J Interferon Cytokine Res* 1998;18:897–903.
446. Wong T, Majchrzak B, Bogoch E, et al. Therapeutic implications for interferon-alpha in arthritis: a pilot study. *J Rheumatol* 2003;30: 934–940.
447. van Holten J, Plater-Zyberk C, Tak PP. Interferon-beta for treatment of rheumatoid arthritis? *Arthritis Res* 2002;4:346–352.
448. Lotz M, Zuraw BL. Interferon-gamma is a major regulator of C1-inhibitor synthesis by human blood monocytes. *J Immunol* 1987;139: 3382–3387.
449. Xie B, Dong Z, Fidler IJ. Regulatory mechanisms for the expression of type IV collagenases/gelatinases in murine macrophages. *J Immunol* 1994;152:3637–3644.
450. Shapiro SD, Campbell EJ, Kobayashi DK, et al. Immune modulation of metalloproteinase production in human macrophages. Selective pretranslational suppression of interstitial collagenase and stromelysin biosynthesis by interferon-gamma. *J Clin Invest* 1990;86:1204–1210.
451. Wahl LM, Corcoran ME, Mergenhagen SE, et al. Inhibition of phospholipase activity in human monocytes by IFN-gamma blocks endogenous prostaglandin E_2-dependent collagenase production. *J Immunol* 1990;144:3518–3522.
452. Smeets TJ, Dayer JM, Kraan MC, et al. The effects of interferon-beta treatment of synovial inflammation and expression of metalloproteinases in patients with rheumatoid arthritis. *Arthritis Rheum* 2000; 43:270–274.
453. Palmer G, Mezin F, Juge-Aubry CE, et al. Interferon-B stimulates interleukin-1 receptor antagonist production in human articular chondrocytes and synovial fibroblasts. *Ann Rheum Dis* 2004;63: 43–49
454. Takayanagi H, Kim S, Matsuo K, et al. RANKL maintains bone homeostasis through c-Fos-dependent induction of interferon-beta. *Nature* 2002;416:744–749.
455. Narayanan AS, Whithey J, Souza A, et al. Effect of gamma-interferon on collagen synthesis by normal and fibrotic human lung fibroblasts. *Chest* 1992;101:1326–1331.
456. Meyer FA, Yaron I, Yaron M. Synergistic, additive, and antagonistic effects of interleukin-1 beta, tumor necrosis factor alpha, and gamma-interferon on prostaglandin E, hyaluronic acid, and collagenase production by cultured synovial fibroblasts. *Arthritis Rheum* 1990;33:1518–1525.
457. Nakajima H, Hiyama Y, Tsukada W, et al. Effects of interferon gamma on cultured synovial cells from patients with rheumatoid arthritis: inhibition of cell growth, prostaglandin E_2, and collagenase release. *Ann Rheum Dis* 1990;49:512–516.
458. Unemori EN, Bair MJ, Bauer EA, et al. Stromelysin expression regulates collagenase activation in human fibroblasts. Dissociable control of two metalloproteinases by interferon-gamma. *J Biol Chem* 1991; 266:23477–23482.
459. Goldring MB, Fukuo K, Birkhead JR, et al. Transcriptional suppression by interleukin-1 and interferon-gamma of type II collagen gene expression in human chondrocytes. *J Cell Biochem* 1994;54: 85–99.
460. Reginato AM, Sanz-Rodriguez C, Diaz A, et al. Transcriptional modulation of cartilage-specific collagen gene expression by interferon gamma and tumour necrosis factor alpha in cultured human chondrocytes. *Biochem J* 1993;294:761–769.
461. Takayanagi H, Ogasawara K, Hida S, et al. T-cell-mediated regulation of osteoclastogenesis by signalling cross-talk between RANKL and IFN-gamma. *Nature* 2000;408:600–605.
462. Hooks JJ, Moutsopoulos HM, Geis SA, et al. Immune interferon in the circulation of patients with autoimmune disease. *N Engl J Med* 1979;301:5–8.
463. Preble OT, Black RJ, Friedman RM, et al. Systemic lupus erythematosus: presence in human serum of an unusual acid-labile leukocyte interferon. *Science* 1982;216:429–431.

464. Blanco P, Palucka AK, Gill M, et al. Induction of dendritic cell differentiation by IFN-alpha in systemic lupus erythematosus. *Science* 2001;294:1540–1543.
465. Hardin JA. Directing autoimmunity to nucleoprotein particles: the impact of dendritic cells and interferon alpha in lupus. *J Exp Med* 2003;197:681–685.
466. Bennett L, Palucka AK, Arce E, et al. Interferon and granulopoiesis signatures in systemic lupus erythematosus blood. *J Exp Med* 2003; 197:711–723.
467. Ronnblom LE, Alm GV, Oberg KE. Autoimmunity after alpha-interferon therapy for malignant carcinoid tumors. *Ann Intern Med* 1991;115:178–183.
468. Shiozawa S, Kuroki Y, Kim M, et al. Interferon-alpha in lupus psychosis. *Arthritis Rheum* 1992;35:417–422.
469. Amerio P, Frezzolini A, Abeni D, et al. Increased IL-18 in patients with systemic lupus erythematosus: relations with Th-1, Th-2, pro-inflammatory cytokines and disease activity. IL-18 is a marker of disease activity but does not correlate with pro-inflammatory cytokines. *Clin Exp Rheumatol* 2002;20:535–538.
470. Akahoshi M, Nakashima H, Tanaka Y, et al. Thl/Th2 balance of peripheral T helper cells in systemic lupus erythematosus. *Arthritis Rheum* 1999;42:1644–1648.
471. Hopkins SJ, Meager A. Cytokines in synovial fluid: II. The presence of tumour necrosis factor and interferon. *Clin Exp Immunol* 1988; 73:88–92.
472. Buchan G, Barrett K, Fujita T, et al. Detection of activated T cell products in the rheumatoid joint using cDNA probes to Interleukin-2 (IL-2) IL-2 receptor and IFN-gamma. *Clin Exp Immunol* 1988;71:295–301.
473. Carpenter DF, Steinberg AD, Schur PH, et al. The pathogenesis of autoimmunity in New Zealand mice. II. Acceleration of glomerulonephritis by polyinosinic-polycytidylic acid. *Lab Invest* 1970;23: 628–634.
474. Gresser J, Morel-Maroger L, Verroust P, et al. Anti-interferon globulin inhibits the development of glomerulonephritis in mice infected at birth with lymphocytic choriomeningitis virus. *Proc Natl Acad Sci U S A* 1978;75:3413–3416.
475. Santiago-Raber ML, Baccala R, Haraldsson KM, et al. Type-I interferon receptor deficiency reduces lupus-like disease in NZB mice. *J Exp Med* 2003;197:777–788.
476. Jacob CO, van der Meide PH, McDevitt HO. *In vivo* treatment of (NZB X NZW)F1 lupus-like nephritis with monoclonal antibody to gamma interferon. *J Exp Med* 1987;166:798–803.
477. Balomenos D, Rumold R, Theofilopoulos AN. Interferon-gamma is required for lupus-like disease and lymphoaccumulation in MRL-lpr mice. *J Clin Invest* 1998;101:364–371.
478. Haas C, Ryffel B, Le Hir M. IFN-gamma receptor deletion prevents autoantibody production and glomerulonephritis in lupus-prone (NZB × NZW)F1 mice. *J Immunol* 1998;160:3713–3718.
479. Schwarting A, Wada T, Kinoshita K, et al. IFN-gamma receptor signaling is essential for the initiation, acceleration, and destruction of autoimmune kidney disease in MRL-Fas(lpr) mice. *J Immunol* 1998; 161:494–503.
480. Triantaphyllopoulos KA, Williams RO, Tailor H, et al. Amelioration of collagen-induced arthritis and suppression of interferon-gamma, interleukin-12, and tumor necrosis factor alpha production by interferon-beta gene therapy. *Arthritis Rheum* 1999;42:90–99.
481. Holten VJ, Sattonet-Roche P, Siegfried C, et al. Treatment with recombinant interferon beta slows cartilage destruction and reduces inflammation in the collagen-induced arthritis model of rheumatoid arthritis. *Arthritis Rheum* 2000;43:231.
482. Tak PP, Hart BA, Kraan MC, et al. The effects of interferon beta treatment on arthritis. *Rheumatology (Oxford)* 1999;38:362–369.
483. Vermeire K, Heremans H, Vandeputte M, et al. Accelerated collagen-induced arthritis in IFN-gamma receptor-deficient mice. *J Immunol* 1997;158:5507–5513.
484. Manoury-Schwartz B, Chiocchia G, Bessis N, et al. High susceptibility to collagen-induced arthritis in mice lacking IFN-gamma receptors. *J Immunol* 1997;158:5501–5506.
485. Kageyama Y, Koide Y, Yoshida A, et al. Reduced susceptibility to collagen-induced arthritis in mice deficient in IFN-gamma receptor. *J Immunol* 1998;161:1542–1548.
486. Group GLS. Double blind controlled phase III multicenter clinical trial with interferon gamma in rheumatoid arthritis. German Lymphokine Study Group. *Rheumatol Int* 1992;12:175–185.
487. Cannon GW, Emkey RD, Denes A, et al. Prospective 5-year followup of recombinant interferon-gamma in rheumatoid arthritis. *J Rheumatol* 1993;20:1867–1873.
488. Veys EM, Menkes CJ, Emery P. A randomized, double-blind study comparing twenty-four-week treatment with recombinant interferon-gamma versus placebo in the treatment of rheumatoid arthritis. *Arthritis Rheum* 1997;40:62–68.
489. Graninger WB, Hassfeld W, Pesau BB, et al. Induction of systemic lupus erythematosus by interferon-gamma in a patient with rheumatoid arthritis. *J Rheumatol* 1991;18:1621–1622.
490. Machold KP, Smolen JS. Interferon-gamma induced exacerbation of systemic lupus erythematosus. *J Rheumatol* 1990;17:831–832.
491. Seitz M, Franke M, Kirchner H. Induction of antinuclear antibodies in patients with rheumatoid arthritis receiving treatment with human recombinant interferon gamma. *Ann Rheum Dis* 1988;47:642–644.
492. Sigidin YA, Loukina GV, Skurkovich B, et al. Randomized, double-blind trial of anti-interferon-gamma antibodies in rheumatoid arthritis. *Scand J Rheumatol* 2001;30:203–207.
493. Stevens W, Vancheeswaran R, Black CM. Alpha interferon-2a (Roferon-A) in the treatment of diffuse cutaneous systemic sclerosis: a pilot study. UK Systemic Sclerosis Study Group. *Br J Rheumatol* 1992;31:683–689.
494. Hein R, Behr J, Hundgen M, et al. Treatment of systemic sclerosis with gamma-interferon. *Br J Dermatol* 1992;126:496–501.
495. Grassegger A, Schuler G, Hessenberger G, et al. Interferon-gamma in the treatment of systemic sclerosis: a randomized controlled multicentre trial. *Br J Dermatol* 1998;139:639–648.
496. Wechsler B, Bodaghi B, Huong DL, et al. Efficacy of interferon alfa-2a in severe and refractory uveitis associated with Behçet's disease. *Ocul Immunol Inflamm* 2000;8:293–301.
497. Alpsoy E, Durusoy C, Yilmaz E, et al. Interferon alfa-2a in the treatment of Behçet disease: a randomized placebo-controlled and double-blind study. *Arch Dermatol* 2002;138:467–471.
498. Ship JA, Fox PC, Michalek JE, et al. Treatment of primary Sjögren's syndrome with low-dose natural human interferon-alpha administered by the oral mucosal route: a phase II clinical trial. IFN Protocol Study Group. *J Interferon Cytokine Res* 1999;19:943–951.
499. Khurshudian AV. A pilot study to test the efficacy of oral administration of interferon-alpha lozenges to patients with Sjögren's syndrome. *Oral Surg Oral Med Oral Pathol Oral Radiol Endod* 2003; 95:38–44.
500. Zlotnik A, Yoshie O. Chemokines: a new classification system and their role in immunity. *Immunity* 2000;12:121–127.
501. Szekanecz Z, Strieter RM, Kunkel SL, et al. Chemokines in rheumatoid arthritis. *Springer Semin Immunopathol* 1998;20(1–2):115–32.
502. Borthwick NJ, Akbar AN, MacCormac LP, et al. Selective migration of highly differentiated primed T cells, defined by low expression of CD45RB, across human umbilical vein endothelial cells: effects of viral infection on transmigration. *Immunology* 1997;90:272–280.
503. Bazan JF, Bacon KB, Hardiman G, et al. A new class of membrane-bound chemokine with a CX3C motif. *Nature* 1997;385:640–644.
504. Ruth JH, Volin MV, Haines GK 3rd, et al. Fractalkine, a novel chemokine in rheumatoid arthritis and in rat adjuvant-induced arthritis. *Arthritis Rheum* 2001;44:1568–1581.
505. Proudfoot AE, Power CA, Rommel C, et al. Strategies for chemokine antagonists as therapeutics. *Semin Immunol* 2003;15:57–65.
506. Loetscher P, Uguccioni M, Bordoli L, et al. CCR5 is characteristic of Th1 lymphocytes. *Nature* 1998;391:344–345.
507. Szekanecz Z, Kim J, Koch AE. Chemokines and chemokine receptors in rheumatoid arthritis. *Semin Immunol* 2003;15:15–21.
508. Horuk R, Chitnis CE, Darbonne WC, et al. A receptor for the malarial parasite *Plasmodium vivax*: the erythrocyte chemokine receptor. *Science* 1993;261:1182–1184.
509. Baggiolini M, Dewald B, Moser B. Interleukin-8 and related chemotactic cytokines—CXC and CC chemokines. *Adv Immunol* 1994;55: 97–179.
510. Larsen CG, Anderson AO, Appella E, et al. The neutrophil-activating protein (NAP-1) is also chemotactic for T lymphocytes. *Science* 1989;243:1464–1466.
511. Szekanecz Z, Koch AE. Chemokines and angiogenesis. *Curr Opin Rheumatol* 2001;13:202–208.
512. Strieter RM, Polverini PJ, Kunkel SL, et al. The functional role of the ELR motif in CXC chemokine-mediated angiogenesis. *J Biol Chem* 1995;270:27348–27357.

513. Moore BB, Keane MP, Addison CL, et al. CXC chemokine modulation of angiogenesis: the importance of balance between angiogenic and angiostatic members of the family. *J Invest Med* 1998;46: 113–120.
514. Koch AE, Polverini PJ, Kunkel SL, et al. Interleukin-8 as a macrophage-derived mediator of angiogenesis. *Science* 1992;258: 1798–1801.
515. Schadendorf D, Moller A, Algermissen B, et al. IL-8 produced by human malignant melanoma cells *in vitro* is an essential autocrine growth factor. *J Immunol* 1993;5:2667–2675.
516. Balentien E, Han JH, Thomas HG, et al. Recombinant expression, biochemical characterization, and biological activities of the human MGSA/gro protein. *Biochemistry* 1990;29:10225–10233.
517. Unemori EN, Amento EP, Bauer EA, et al. Melanoma growth-stimulatory activity/GRO decreases collagen expression by human fibroblasts. Regulation by C-X-C but not C-C cytokines. *J Biol Chem* 1993;268:1338–1342.
518. Taub DD, Conlon K, Lloyd AR, et al. Preferential migration of activated CD4+ and CD8+ T cells in response to MIP-1 alpha and MIP-1 beta. *Science* 1993;260:355–358.
519. Schall TJ, Bacon K, Toy KJ, et al. Selective attraction of monocytes and T lymphocytes of the memory phenotype by cytokine RANTES. *Nature* 1990;347:669–671.
520. Salcedo R, Ponce ML, Young HA, et al. Human endothelial cells express CCR2 and respond to MCP-1: direct role of MCP-1 in angiogenesis and tumor progression. *Blood* 2000;96:34–40.
521. Tanaka Y, Adams DH, Hubscher S, et al. T-cell adhesion induced by proteoglycan-immobilized cytokine MIP-1 beta. *Nature* 1993;361: 79–82.
522. Villiger PM, Terkeltaub R, Lotz M. Monocyte chemoattractant protein-1 (MCP-1) expression in human articular cartilage. Induction by peptide regulatory factors and differential effects of dexamethasone and retinoic acid. *J Clin Invest* 1992;90:488–496.
523. Hogan M, Sherry B, Ritchlin C, et al. Differential expression of the small inducible cytokines GRO alpha and GRO beta by synovial fibroblasts in chronic arthritis: possible role in growth regulation. *Cytokine* 1994;6:61–69.
524. Koch AE, Kunkel SL, Burrows JC, et al. Synovial tissue macrophage as a source of the chemotactic cytokine IL-8. *J Immunol* 1991;147: 2187–2195.
525. Endo H, Akahoshi T, Takagishi K, et al. Elevation of interleukin-8 (IL-8) levels in joint fluids of patients with rheumatoid arthritis and the induction by IL-8 of leukocyte infiltration and synovitis in rabbit joints. *Lymphokine Cytokine Res* 1991;10:245–252.
526. Terkeltaub R, Zachariae C, Santoro D, et al. Monocyte-derived neutrophil chemotactic factor/interleukin-8 is a potential mediator of crystal-induced inflammation. *Arthritis Rheum* 1991;34:894–903.
527. Koch AE, Kunkel SL, Harlow LA, et al. Epithelial neutrophil activating peptide-78: a novel chemotactic cytokine for neutrophils in arthritis. *J Clin Invest* 1994;94:1012–1018.
528. Castor CW, Andrews PC, Swartz RD, et al. Connective tissue activation. XXXVI. The origin, variety, distribution, and biologic fate of connective tissue activating peptide-III isoforms: characteristics in patients with rheumatic, renal, and arterial disease. *Arthritis Rheum* 1993;36:1142–1153.
529. Koch AE, Kunkel SL, Harlow LA, et al. Enhanced production of monocyte chemoattractant protein-1 in rheumatoid arthritis. *J Clin Invest* 1992;90:772–779.
530. Koch AE, Kunkel SL, Harlow LA, et al. Macrophage inflammatory protein-1 alpha. A novel chemotactic cytokine for macrophages in rheumatoid arthritis. *J Clin Invest* 1994;93:921–928.
531. Katschke KJ Jr, Rottman JB, Ruth JH, et al. Differential expression of chemokine receptors on peripheral blood, synovial fluid, and synovial tissue monocytes/macrophages in rheumatoid arthritis. *Arthritis Rheum* 2001;44:1022–1032.
532. Akahoshi T, Wada C, Endo H, et al. Expression of monocyte chemotactic and activating factor in rheumatoid arthritis. Regulation of its production in synovial cells by interleukin-1 and tumor necrosis factor. *Arthritis Rheum* 1993;36:762–771.
533. Johnston B, Burns AR, Suematsu M, et al. Chronic inflammation upregulates chemokine receptors and induces neutrophil migration to monocyte chemoattractant protein-1. *J Clin Invest* 1999;103: 1269–1276.
534. Thornton S, Duwel LE, Boivin GP, et al. Association of the course of collagen-induced arthritis with distinct patterns of cytokine and chemokine messenger RNA expression. *Arthritis Rheum* 1999;42: 1109–1118.
535. Barnes DA, Tse J, Kaufhold M, et al. Polyclonal antibody directed against human RANTES ameliorates disease in the Lewis rat adjuvant-induced arthritis model. *J Clin Invest* 1998;101:2910–2919.
536. Halloran MM, Woods JM, Strieter RM, et al. The role of an epithelial neutrophil-activating peptide-78-like protein in rat adjuvant-induced arthritis. *J Immunol* 1999;162:7492–7500.
537. Massague J. TGF-beta signal transduction. *Annu Rev Biochem* 1998; 67:753–791.
538. Padgett RW, Savage C, Das P. Genetic and biochemical analysis of TGF beta signal transduction. *Cytokine Growth Factor Rev* 1997;8:1–9.
539. Schultz-Cherry S, Lawler J, Murphy-Ullrich JE. The type 1 repeats of thrombospondin 1 activate latent transforming growth factor-beta. *J Biol Chem* 1994;269:26783–26788.
540. Munger JS, Huang X, Kawakatsu H, et al. The integrin alpha v beta 6 binds and activates latent TGF beta 1: a mechanism for regulating pulmonary inflammation and fibrosis. *Cell* 1999;96:319–328.
541. Wrana JL, Attisano L, Wieser R, et al. Mechanism of activation of the TGF-beta receptor. *Nature* 1994;370:341–347.
542. Souchelnytskyi S, ten Dijke P, Miyazono K, et al. Phosphorylation of Ser165 in TGF-beta type I receptor modulates TGF-beta1-induced cellular responses. *EMBO J* 1996;15:6231–6240.
543. Wieser R, Wrana JL, Massague J. GS domain mutations that constitutively activate T beta R-I, the downstream signaling component in the TGF-beta receptor complex. *EMBO J* 1995;14:2199–2208.
544. Attisano L, Wrana JL, Lopez-Casillas F, et al. TGF-beta receptors and actions. *Biochim Biophys Acta* 1994;1222:71–80.
545. Lopez-Casillas F, Payne HM, Andres JL, et al. Betaglycan can act as a dual modulator of TGF-beta access to signaling receptors: mapping of ligand binding and GAG attachment sites. *J Cell Biol* 1994; 124:557–568.
546. Lopez-Casillas F, Wrana JL, Massague J. Betaglycan presents ligand to the TGF beta signaling receptor. *Cell* 1993;73:1435–1444.
547. Lewis KA, Gray PC, Blount AL, et al. Betaglycan binds inhibin and can mediate functional antagonism of activin signalling. *Nature* 2000;404:411–414.
548. Sekelsky JJ, Newfeld SJ, Raftery LA, et al. Genetic characterization and cloning of mothers against dpp, a gene required for decapentaplegic function in *Drosophila melanogaster. Genetics* 1995;139: 1347–1358.
549. Savage C, Das P, Finelli AL, et al. *Caenorhabditis elegans* genes sma-2, sma-3, and sma-4 define a conserved family of transforming growth factor beta pathway components. *Proc Natl Acad Sci U S A* 1996;93:790–794.
550. Derynck R, Gelbart WM, Harland RM, et al. Nomenclature: vertebrate mediators of TGFbeta family signals. *Cell* 1996;87:173.
551. Chang H, Brown CW, Matzuk MM. Genetic analysis of the mammalian transforming growth factor-beta superfamily. *Endocr Rev* 2002;23:787–823.
552. Ishisaki A, Yamato K, Hashimoto S, et al. Differential inhibition of Smad6 and Smad7 on bone morphogenetic protein- and activin-mediated growth arrest and apoptosis in B cells. *J Biol Chem* 1999; 274:13637–13642.
553. Bitzer M, von Gersdorff G, Liang D, et al. A mechanism of suppression of TGF-beta/SMAD signaling by NF-kappa B/RelA. *Genes Dev* 2000;14:187–197.
554. Ulloa L, Doody J, Massague J. Inhibition of transforming growth factor-beta/SMAD signalling by the interferon-gamma/STAT pathway. *Nature* 1999;397:710–713.
555. Quan T, He T, Voorhees JJ, et al. Ultraviolet irradiation blocks cellular responses to transforming growth factor-beta by down-regulating its type-II receptor and inducing Smad7. *J Biol Chem* 2001;276: 26349–26356.
556. Patil S, Wildey GM, Brown TL, et al. Smad7 is induced by CD40 and protects WEHI 231 B-lymphocytes from transforming growth factor-beta–induced growth inhibition and apoptosis. *J Biol Chem* 2000;275:38363–38370.
557. Villiger PM, Terkeltaub R, Lotz M. Production of monocyte chemoattractant protein-1 by inflamed synovial tissue and cultured synoviocytes. *J Immunol* 1992;149:722–727.
558. Wahl SM, Allen JB, Welch GR, et al. Transforming growth factor-beta in synovial fluids modulates Fc gamma RII (CD16) expression on mononuclear phagocytes. *J Immunol* 1992;148:485–490.

559. Brennan FM, Chantry D, Turner M, et al. Detection of transforming growth factor-beta in rheumatoid arthritis synovial tissue: lack of effect on spontaneous cytokine production in joint cell cultures. *Clin Exp Immunol* 1990;81:278–285.
560. Shull MM, Ormsby I, Kier AB, et al. Targeted disruption of the mouse transforming growth factor-beta 1 gene results in multifocal inflammatory disease. *Nature* 1992;359:693–699.
561. Allen JB, Manthey CL, Hand AR, et al. Rapid onset synovial inflammation and hyperplasia induced by transforming growth factor beta. *J Exp Med* 1990;171:231–247.
562. Elford PR, Graeber M, Ohtsu H, et al. Induction of swelling, synovial hyperplasia and cartilage proteoglycan loss upon intra-articular injection of transforming growth factor beta-2 in the rabbit. *Cytokine* 1992;4:232–238.
563. Cooper WO, Fava RA, Gates CA, et al. Acceleration of onset of collagen-induced arthritis by intra-articular injection of tumour necrosis factor or transforming growth factor-beta. *Clin Exp Immunol* 1992; 89:244–250.
564. Wahl SM, Allen JB, Costa GL, et al. Reversal of acute and chronic synovial inflammation by anti-transforming growth factor beta. *J Exp Med* 1993;177:225–230.
565. Thorbecke GJ, Shah R, Leu CH, et al. Involvement of endogenous tumor necrosis factor alpha and transforming growth factor beta during induction of collagen type II arthritis in mice. *Proc Natl Acad Sci U S A* 1992;89:7375–7379.
566. Brandes ME, Allen JB, Ogawa Y, et al. Transforming growth factor beta 1 suppresses acute and chronic arthritis in experimental animals. *J Clin Invest* 1991;87:1108–1113.
567. Kuruvilla AP, Shah R, Hochwald GM, et al. Protective effect of transforming growth factor beta 1 on experimental autoimmune diseases in mice. *Proc Natl Acad Sci U S A* 1991;88:2918–2921.
568. Khoury SJ, Hancock WW, Weiner HL. Oral tolerance to myelin basic protein and natural recovery from experimental autoimmune encephalomyelitis are associated with downregulation of inflammatory cytokines and differential upregulation of transforming growth factor beta, interleukin 4, and prostaglandin E expression in the brain. *J Exp Med* 1992;176:1355–1364.
569. Hill DJ, Logan A. Peptide growth factors and their interactions during chondrogenesis. *Prog Growth Factor Res* 1992;4:45–68.
570. Crowe MJ, Doetschman T, Greenhalgh DG. Delayed wound healing in immunodeficient TGF-beta 1 knockout mice. *J Invest Dermatol* 2000;115:3–11.
571. Zhang W, Ou J, Inagaki Y, et al. Synergistic cooperation between Sp1 and Smad3/Smad4 mediates transforming growth factor beta1 stimulation of alpha 2(I)-collagen (COL1A2) transcription. *J Biol Chem* 2000;275:39237–39245.
572. Verrecchia F, Chu ML, Mauviel A. Identification of novel TGF-beta/Smad gene targets in dermal fibroblasts using a combined cDNA microarray/promoter transactivation approach. *J Biol Chem* 2001; 276:17058–17062.
573. Hua X, Miller ZA, Wu G, et al. Specificity in transforming growth factor beta-induced transcription of the plasminogen activator inhibitor-1 gene: interactions of promoter DNA, transcription factor muE3, and Smad proteins. *Proc Natl Acad Sci U S A* 1999;96:13130–13135.
574. Stroschein SL, Wang W, Luo K. Cooperative binding of Smad proteins to two adjacent DNA elements in the plasminogen activator inhibitor-1 promoter mediates transforming growth factor beta–induced smad-dependent transcriptional activation. *J Biol Chem* 1999;274:9431–9441.
575. Yuan W, Varga J. Transforming growth factor-beta repression of matrix metalloproteinase-1 in dermal fibroblasts involves Smad3. *J Biol Chem* 2001;276:38502–38510.
576. Holmes A, Abraham DJ, Sa S, et al. CTGF and SMADs, maintenance of scleroderma phenotype is independent of SMAD signaling. *J Biol Chem* 2001;276:10594–10601.
577. Stratton R, Rajkumar V, Ponticos M, et al. Prostacyclin derivatives prevent the fibrotic response to TGF-beta by inhibiting the Ras/MEK/ERK pathway. *FASEB J* 2002;16:1949–1951.
578. Frazier K, Williams S, Kothapalli D, et al. Stimulation of fibroblast cell growth, matrix production, and granulation tissue formation by connective tissue growth factor. *J Invest Dermatol* 1996;107:404–411.
579. Abreu JG, Ketpura NI, Reversade B, et al. Connective-tissue growth factor (CTGF) modulates cell signalling by BMP and TGF-beta. *Nat Cell Biol* 2002;4:599–604.
580. Takehara K. Hypothesis: pathogenesis of systemic sclerosis. *J Rheumatol* 2003;30:755–759.
581. Schiffer M, Bitzer M, Roberts IS, et al. Apoptosis in podocytes induced by TGF-beta and Smad7. *J Clin Invest* 2001;108:807–816.
582. Giri SN, Hyde DM, Hollinger MA. Effect of antibody to transforming growth factor beta on bleomycin induced accumulation of lung collagen in mice. *Thorax* 1993;48:959–966.
583. Qi Z, Atsuchi N, Ooshima A, et al. Blockade of type beta transforming growth factor signaling prevents liver fibrosis and dysfunction in the rat. *Proc Natl Acad Sci U S A* 1999;96:2345–2349.
584. Nakao A, Fujii M, Matsumura R, et al. Transient gene transfer and expression of Smad7 prevents bleomycin-induced lung fibrosis in mice. *J Clin Invest* 1999;104:5–11.
585. Terada Y, Hanada S, Nakao A, et al. Gene transfer of Smad7 using electroporation of adenovirus prevents renal fibrosis in post-obstructed kidney. *Kidney Int Suppl* 2002;61:94–98.
586. Kulozik M, Hogg A, Lankat-Buttgereit B, et al. Co-localization of transforming growth factor beta 2 with alpha 1(I) procollagen mRNA in tissue sections of patients with systemic sclerosis. *J Clin Invest* 1990;86:917–922.
587. Rudnicka L, Varga J, Christiano AM, et al. Elevated expression of type VII collagen in the skin of patients with systemic sclerosis. Regulation by transforming growth factor-beta. *J Clin Invest* 1994;93: 1709–1715.
588. Ihn H, Yamane K, Kubo M, et al. Blockade of endogenous transforming growth factor beta signaling prevents up-regulated collagen synthesis in scleroderma fibroblasts: association with increased expression of transforming growth factor beta receptors. *Arthritis Rheum* 2001;44:474–480.
589. Deguchi Y. Spontaneous increase of transforming growth factor beta production by bronchoalveolar mononuclear cells of patients with systemic autoimmune diseases affecting the lung. *Ann Rheum Dis* 1992;51:362–365.
590. Igarashi A, Nashiro K, Kikuchi K, et al. Significant correlation between connective tissue growth factor gene expression and skin sclerosis in tissue sections from patients with systemic sclerosis. *J Invest Dermatol* 1995;105:280–284.
591. Igarashi A, Nashiro K, Kikuchi K, et al. Connective tissue growth factor gene expression in tissue sections from localized scleroderma, keloid, and other fibrotic skin disorders. *J Invest Dermatol* 1996;106: 729–733.
592. Sato S, Nagaoka T, Hasegawa M, et al. Serum levels of connective tissue growth factor are elevated in patients with systemic sclerosis: association with extent of skin sclerosis and severity of pulmonary fibrosis. *J Rheumatol* 2000;27:149–154.
593. Lotz M, Kekow J, Carson DA. Transforming growth factor-beta and cellular immune responses in synovial fluids. *J Immunol* 1990;144: 4189–4194.
594. Bucala R, Ritchlin C, Winchester R, et al. Constitutive production of inflammatory and mitogenic cytokines by rheumatoid synovial fibroblasts. *J Exp Med* 1991;173:569–574.
595. Taketazu F, Kato M, Gobl A, et al. Enhanced expression of transforming growth factor-beta s and transforming growth factor-beta type II receptor in the synovial tissues of patients with rheumatoid arthritis. *Lab Invest* 1994;70:620–630.
596. Chu CQ, Field M, Abney E, et al. Transforming growth factor-beta 1 in rheumatoid synovial membrane and cartilage/pannus junction. *Clin Exp Immunol* 1991;86:380–386.
597. Schalkwijk J, Joosten LA, van den Berg WB, et al. Insulin-like growth factor stimulation of chondrocyte proteoglycan synthesis by human synovial fluid. *Arthritis Rheum* 1989;32:66–71.
598. Schalkwijk J, Joosten LA, van den Berg WB, et al. Chondrocyte nonresponsiveness to insulin-like growth factor 1 in experimental arthritis. *Arthritis Rheum* 1989;32:894–900.
599. Bradham DM, in der Wiesche B, Precht P, et al. Transrepression of type II collagen by TGF-beta and FGF is protein kinase C dependent and is mediated through regulatory sequences in the promoter and first intron. *J Cell Physiol* 1994;158:61–68.
600. Galera P, Redini F, Vivien D, et al. Effect of transforming growth factor-beta 1 (TGF-beta 1) on matrix synthesis by monolayer cultures of rabbit articular chondrocytes during the dedifferentiation process. *Exp Cell Res* 1992;200:379–392.
601. Gunther M, Haubeck HD, van de Leur E, et al. Transforming growth factor beta 1 regulates tissue inhibitor of metalloproteinases-1 expres-

sion in differentiated human articular chondrocytes. *Arthritis Rheum* 1994;37:395–405.

602. Guerne PA, Sublet A, Lotz M. Growth factor responsiveness of human articular chondrocytes: distinct profiles in primary chondrocytes, subcultured chondrocytes, and fibroblasts. *J Cell Physiol* 1994;158: 476–484.
603. Harvey AK, Hrubey PS, Chandrasekhar S. Transforming growth factor-beta inhibition of interleukin-1 activity involves down-regulation of interleukin-1 receptors on chondrocytes. Exp Cell Res. 1991;195: 376–385.
604. Hamilton JA, Piccoli DS, Leizer T, et al. Transforming growth factor beta stimulates urokinase-type plasminogen activator and DNA synthesis, but not prostaglandin E_2 production, in human synovial fibroblasts. *Proc Natl Acad Sci U S A* 1991;88:7180–7184.
605. van den Berg WB, van der Kraan PM, Scharstuhl A, et al. Growth factors and cartilage repair. *Clin Orthop* 2001:244–250.
606. Glansbeek HL, van Beuningen HM, Vitters EL, et al. Bone morphogenetic protein 2 stimulates articular cartilage proteoglycan synthesis in vivo but does not counteract interleukin-1alpha effects on proteoglycan synthesis and content. *Arthritis Rheum* 1997;40:1020–1028.
607. Huch K, Wilbrink B, Flechtenmacher J, et al. Effects of recombinant human osteogenic protein 1 on the production of proteoglycan, prostaglandin E_2, and interleukin-1 receptor antagonist by human articular chondrocytes cultured in the presence of interleukin-1beta. *Arthritis Rheum* 1997;40:2157–2161.
608. van de Loo FA, Arntz OJ, van Enckevort FH, et al. Reduced cartilage proteoglycan loss during zymosan-induced gonarthritis in NOS2-deficient mice and in anti-interleukin-1-treated wild-type mice with unabated joint inflammation. *Arthritis Rheum* 1998;41: 634–646.
609. Roberts AB, Sporn MB. Physiological actions and clinical applications of transforming growth factor-beta (TGF-beta). *Growth Factors* 1993;8:1–9.
610. van Beuningen HM, van der Kraan PM, Arntz OJ, et al. Transforming growth factor-beta 1 stimulates articular chondrocyte proteoglycan synthesis and induces osteophyte formation in the murine knee joint. *Lab Invest* 1994;71:279–290.

CHAPTER 20

Cell Adhesion Molecules in the Rheumatic Diseases

Casey T. Weaver and Daniel C. Bullard

Adhesion molecules are multifunctional cell surface proteins that mediate both cell/cell and cell/matrix interactions. In addition to their role in the maintenance of tissue structure and integrity, these proteins participate in active cellular processes, such as motility, signaling, and activation. For example, adhesion molecule–mediated interactions are critical for the development of many different inflammatory and immune responses, including leukocyte emigration from the vasculature into tissue following an inflammatory stimulus, immune surveillance and homing, phagocytosis, and leukocyte/endothelial activation. A large number of adhesion molecules have now been described, and many can be grouped into families based on similarities in structure and function, including the selectin, integrin, cadherin, CD44, and immunoglobulin families of adhesion proteins.

Considerable experimental evidence suggests that these proteins also play an active role in the pathogenesis of inflammatory diseases, including rheumatoid arthritis (RA), systemic lupus erythematosus (SLE), and vasculitic syndromes (reviewed in references 1–9). Much of this information has been derived from analyses of adhesion molecule expression in affected patients, inhibitory studies in animal models, and from *in vitro* adhesion assays using frozen tissues or cell lines. This chapter gives a brief overview of the structure and functions of the major adhesion molecule families and their members, and discusses their potential roles in the development of rheumatic diseases.

SELECTINS

The selectin family of adhesion molecules consists of three structurally-similar proteins: E-selectin, P-selectin, and L-selectin. Together, these proteins facilitate leukocyte rolling, the initial step in leukocyte recruitment from the vascular lumen to the extravascular tissue. Selectin-dependent rolling on the endothelium allows the leukocyte to "survey" the endothelium for chemokines that activate the leukocyte for enhanced binding of integrins, which then mediate firm adhesion necessary to permit transmigration of the leukocyte across the endothelium into adjacent tissue spaces. The selectins were first discovered through the use of monoclonal antibodies that inhibited leukocyte homing (L-selectin), inhibited leukocyte binding to endothelial cells (E-selectin), or bound to activated platelets (P-selectin) (10–13). P-selectin was also later identified in endothelial cells (14). All three selectins were cloned and sequenced in the late 1980s (15–20).

The selectins are highly homologous with 40% and 60% homology at the nucleic acid and protein level, respectively (21). The selectin structure consists of a short cytoplasmic domain, a transmembrane domain, a series of short consensus repeat (SCR) domains, a single epidermal growth factor (EGF)-like domain, and a C-type Ca^{2+}-dependent lectin binding domain at the amino-terminus (Fig. 20.1A). The cytoplasmic portion appears to be involved in intracellular signaling and can be phosphorylated on tyrosine, threonine, and serine residues (22). The role of selectin phosphorylation is still under investigation, but it may be important in ligand binding, secretion, or signal transduction (23–27). The number of SCR domains varies between the selectins, with L-selectin, E-selectin, and P-selectin containing two, six, and nine domains, respectively. SCR domain-swapping studies done between the various selectins demonstrated that they could functionally substitute for each other (28, 29). The SCR domains may also be involved in the maintenance of protein structure and the enhancement of ligand binding (30,31). The EGF-like domain is quite homologous among all selectins and appears to be involved in cell adhesion through stabilization of the lectin binding conformation or through direct interaction with ligand (29,31–33).

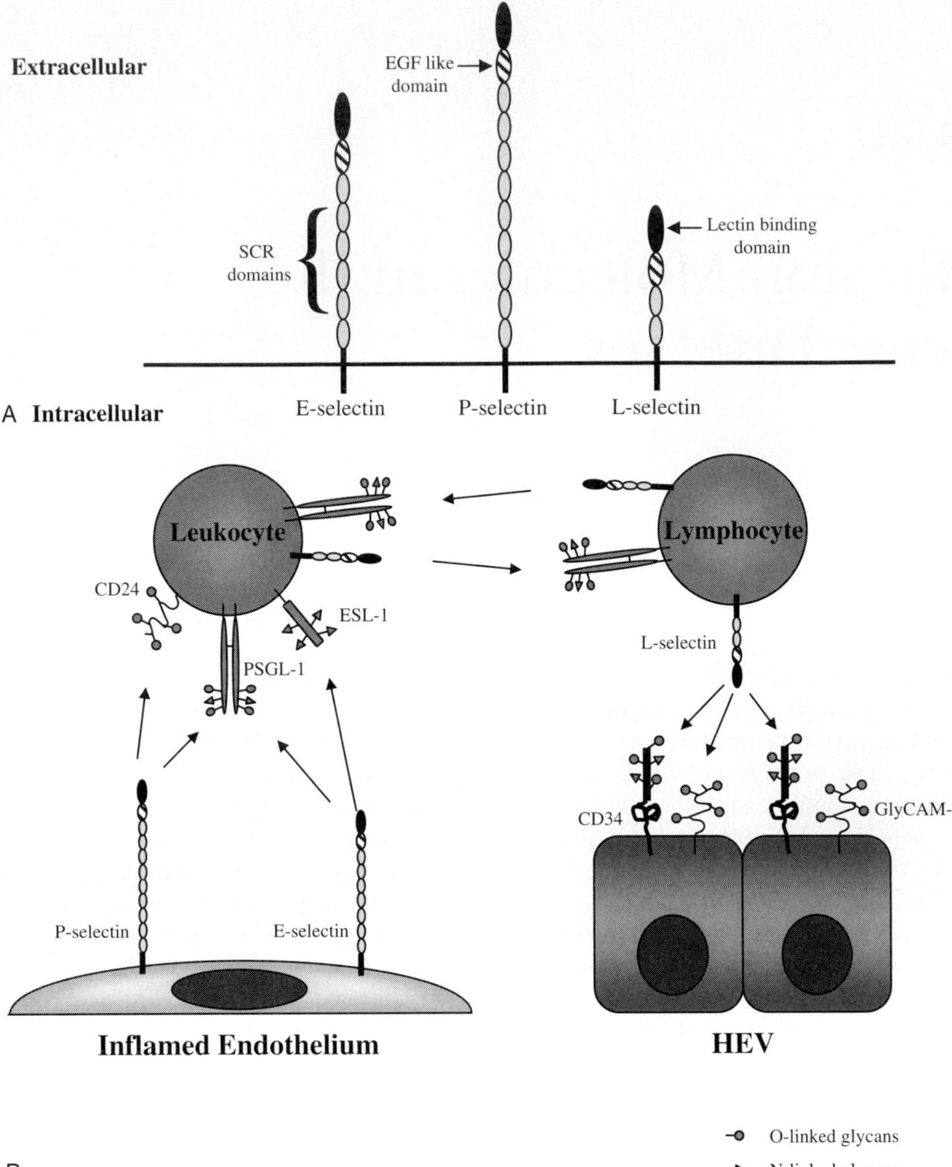

FIG. 20.1. Selectin protein structure. **A:** All of the selectin family members have three general structural motifs: short consensus repeats (*SCR*), an epidermal growth factor (*EGF*)-like domain, and a lectin-binding domain. The selectin family members differ in the number of SCR domains. **B:** Representative P-, E-, and L-selectin ligands and cell types that express them.

Deletion of either the SCR or EGF domains abolished ligand binding, suggesting these regions are important for selectin interactions (31).

P-selectin (CD62P) is expressed by both platelets and endothelial cells, whereas E-selectin (CD62E) is restricted to endothelium. Both E- and P-selectin facilitate leukocyte rolling on the endothelial cell surface, whereas P-selectin also facilitates platelet aggregation and adhesion to other cells (34–38). P-selectin is stored in Weibel-Palade bodies of endothelial cells or α-granules of platelets (14, 39–42) and is rapidly mobilized to the cell surface following cell activation with inflammatory mediators, such as histamine or thrombin (13,14,40,43,44). E-selectin, like P-selectin, is induced by a number of different inflammatory cytokines such as tumor necrosis factor-α (TNF-α), interleukin-1 (IL-1), or bacterial lipopolysaccharide (LPS) (15,45). Maximal levels of E-selectin expression generally appear on the endothelial cell surface within several hours (15). Unlike P- and E-selectin, which are expressed by activated endothelium or platelets, L-selectin (CD62L) is expressed by essentially all granulocytes and monocytes, and the majority of lymphocytes and natural killer (NK) cells (46). L-selectin expression by lymphocytes is primarily limited to antigen-naïve B and T cells; it is rapidly shed from the leukocyte surface following activation (47,48), and is not reexpressed by most effector or memory cells (49,50). L-selectin is the principal mediator of lymphocyte homing to secondary lymphoid tissues, such as peripheral lymph nodes and Peyer patches, but it may also contribute to leukocyte rolling on endothelium of nonlymphoid tissue that has been activated by an inflammatory stimulus (10,51–53).

The most critical domain for selectin function is the Ca^{2+}-dependent lectin binding domain, which governs ligand-binding properties of the selectins (28,54). Each of the selectins binds glycan structures that are attached to glycoproteins through the actions of glycosyltransferases. The dominant glycan structures recognized by selectins are O-linked glycans attached to serine or threonine residues of protein backbones, with a lesser contribution by N-linked glycans attached to asparagine residues (38,55). The tetrasaccharide structure sialyl Lewis^x (sLex) was the first glycan to be described as a selectin ligand and, to date, is the best characterized carbohydrate motif bound by selectins (56–60). P-, E-, and L-selectins demonstrate significant overlap in the repertoire of glycoproteins that bear glycans that they recognize, but there appears to be a hierarchy of preferred ligands, depending on the tissue site. The dominant glycoprotein recognized by P-selectin is P-selectin glycoprotein ligand-1 (PSGL-1), a homodimeric sialomucin rich in O-linked glycans that is expressed by most leukocytes (38,55,61,62) (Fig. 20.1B). CD24 is an additional ligand for P-selectin that appears to contribute a relatively minor role in adhesion of leukocytes that express both PSGL-1 and CD24 (38,55). PSGL-1 is also a ligand for E-selectin, although E-selectin additionally recognizes a distinct ligand termed E-selectin ligand-1 (ESL-1). E-selectin may also bind certain glycolipids and even appropriately-glycosylated L-selectin (38,55).

The ligands recognized by L-selectin include a family of molecules that are expressed by the specialized endothelium that lines the high endothelial venules (HEVs) of secondary lymphoid tissues (Fig. 20.1B). Originally referred to as peripheral lymph node addressin (PNAd), it is now appreciated that this is, in fact, a complex of several L-selectin ligands that are constitutively expressed by the HEV (38, 63). Included in this complex are glycosylated cell adhesion molecule-1 (GlyCAM-1), mucosialin (CD34), podocalyxin, endomucin, endoglycan, and, in Peyer patches of the gut, mucosal addressin cell adhesion molecule-1 (MAdCAM-1) (63–65). Each of these ligands is a sialomucin, expressing a predominance of O-linked carbohydrates. Interestingly, L-selectin can also bind PSGL-1, thereby mediating leukocyte/leukocyte, in addition to endothelial/leukocyte, interactions (55).

As implied by the foregoing discussion, display of appropriate ligands for the selectins, whether on leukocytes (e.g., PSGL-1 and ESL-1), endothelium of HEV (e.g., GlyCAM-1 and CD34), or platelets (e.g., PSGL-1), is dependent on the expression by these cells of the corresponding glycosyl-, sialyl-, and sulfotransferases required for their biosynthesis (38). Although further work is necessary to precisely identify and characterize all of the enzymes that contribute to the biosynthesis of the *in vivo* ligands involved in selectin function, several key enzymes have now been identified. Principal among these are the core 2 β1-6-N glucosaminyltransferase I (C2GlcNAcT-I), which generates a core glycan that is acted on by subsequent modifying enzymes to form P- and E-selectin, and some L-selectin ligands (66); the α-1,3 fucosyltransferases, predominantly FucT-VII, with lesser contribution by FucT-IV, which contribute the critical fucose residues in the capping groups (e.g., sLex) of selectin ligands (67–69); the glycan O-sulfotransferase, GST-3, which sulfates glycosyl residues in the capping groups (38); and an α2–3 sialyltransferase, which sialylates the penultimate galactose residue in the sLex structure (38,66, 69–73). Variable cellular expression of critical glycosyltransferases that modify the glycan expression profile of selectin ligands provides a mechanism for altering recruitment of inflammatory cells. An important example is the differential expression of α-1,3 fucosyltransferase, FucT-VII, during the development of T_H1 and T_H2 lymphocytes, which may produce efficient P- and E-selectin binding by the former but not the latter (74,75).

INTEGRINS

The integrins comprise a family of 24 heterodimeric proteins formed by various combinations of 18 α- and eight β-subunit genes (76,77). These proteins are critical for cell-cell (leukocyte–endothelial cell adhesion) and cell-matrix adhesion (hemidesmosome and focal contacts) in both vertebrates and invertebrates (78). Integrins are also involved in cytoskeletal organization and signal transduction (79). Integrin expression is ubiquitous, with every cell expressing multiple integrin proteins. The α and β subunits are encoded by separate genes, and individual members do not typically show coordinate transcriptional regulation (80). The subunits appear to have evolved in higher organisms such that many α subunits can noncovalently interact with multiple β subunits (Fig. 20.2A). Many different integrin ligands have been identified and include members of the immunoglobulin superfamily, as well as extracellular matrix proteins, such as fibronectin, collagen, and laminin (81).

The extracellular portion of integrins consists of a head region attached by two legs (77,82) (Fig. 20.2B). Based on crystallography studies, the head region of integrins appears to consist of a seven-bladed β-propeller fold in the α subunit that is complexed with a von Willebrand factor A domain or βA domain in the β subunit (77,82,83). Cross-linking studies demonstrate that ligand recognition occurs in the head portions of both of the α and β subunits, which also contain divalent cation (e.g., Ca^{+2} and Mg^{+2}) binding regions (84–86). Half of the α- subunit proteins also contain an inserted domain (I or βA domain) formed by exon shuffling that can influence ligand specificity (87,88). This alternative splic-

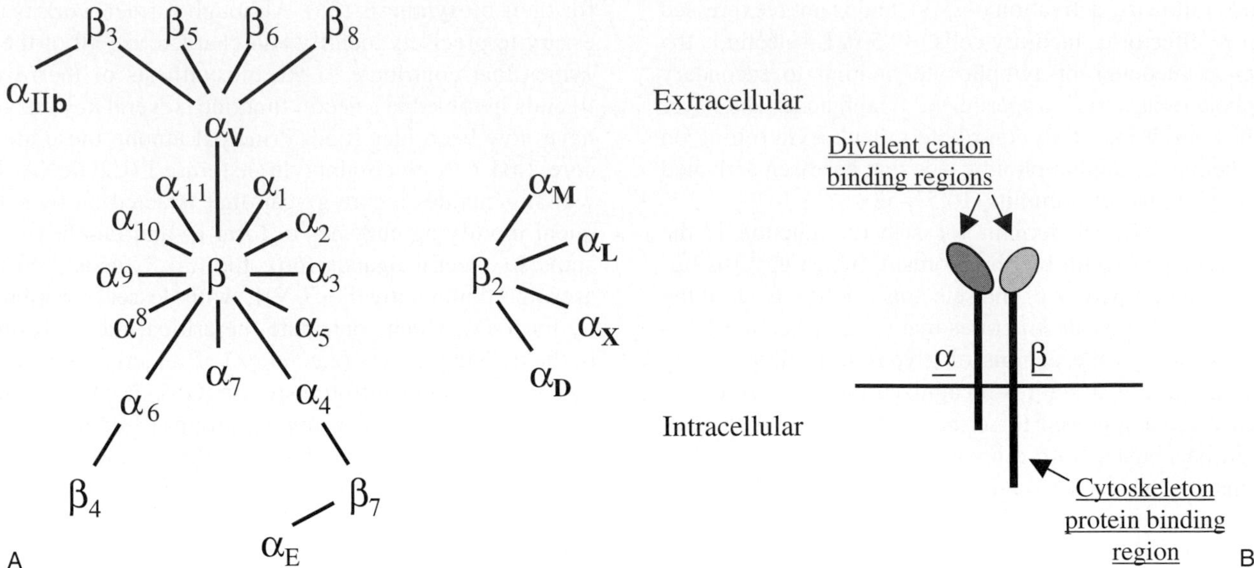

FIG. 20.2. Integrin subunit associations and structure. **A:** Some of the various α and β subunit combinations. **B:** The basic structure of both the α and β subunits. The divalent cation binding region is located in the globular heads of the α and β subunits, whereas the cytoskeletal-associated protein binding region is found in the cytoplasmic tail of the β subunit.

ing results in the addition of an approximately 200–amino acid sequence in the third portion of the amino-terminus (81). In the α subunit, the region proximal to the transmembrane domain is referred to as the leg domain and contains three β sandwich domains (calf 1, calf 2, and thigh) (76). The β -subunit leg contains several different structures with homologies to other proteins, including a hybrid or immunoglobulin fold domain, a plexin-semaphorin-integrin (PSI) domain, four epidermal growth factor–like repeats, and a β tail domain (77,82,83). Both the α and β subunits contain short, cytoplasmic tails (except for β_4) and a single transmembrane domain (Fig. 20.2B). The cytoplasmic tail of the β subunit is involved in linking the integrin complex to the cytoskeleton through various linker proteins such as vinculin, talin, and α-actinin (89).

Integrin-mediated cell adhesion is controlled through multiple mechanisms, including alterations in surface density of the protein, clustering of integrins at the cell surface, and changes in receptor affinity. Increased surface expression levels of several integrins can be induced by various extracellular stimuli (90). For example, cytokines and chemokines facilitate leukocyte adhesion during inflammatory responses through increased integrin gene expression and mobilization of integrin protein from intracellular stores (91). Many integrins can also undergo conformational changes or cluster at the cell surface upon activation, events that augment the ability of the integrin to bind ligand (79,92). Finally, the expression patterns of integrins on a particular cell type may change during differentiation or in response to environmental signals (81). Thus, the dynamic expression patterns of integrins can regulate the specific adhesive interactions between cells and influence their functional properties.

The elucidation of integrin functions has benefited from the discovery and characterization of two different diseases that result from integrin mutations: leukocyte adhesion deficiency type 1 (LAD-1) and Glanzmann thrombasthenia. LAD-1 results from mutations in the β subunit of the β_2 integrins, and has been described in humans and cattle. Loss of β_2 integrin expression results in increased susceptibility to infections, impaired neutrophil emigration, leukocytosis, delayed wound healing, and phagocytosis defects (93,94). Glanzmann thrombasthenia is a heterogeneous disease that results from mutations in either the α_{II} or β_3 integrin subunits (95). These mutations lead to platelet defects that result in increased susceptibility to bleeding in affected individuals.

IMMUNOGLOBULIN SUPERFAMILY

The members of the immunoglobulin superfamily of adhesion molecules share a similar structure, characterized by extracellular IgG-like domains that mediate ligand binding (96). The primary structure of these proteins consists of a cytoplasmic domain, a transmembrane domain, and IgG-like regions with disulfide bridged loops and α-antiparallel β-pleated sheets (Fig. 20.3). IgG adhesion family members participate in a wide variety of cellular responses, including immune surveillance, leukocyte activation, and leukocyte emigration. The proteins include adhesion molecules such as intercellular adhesion molecules -1, -2, and -3 (ICAM-1, -2, and -3), vascular cell adhesion molecule-1 (VCAM-1),

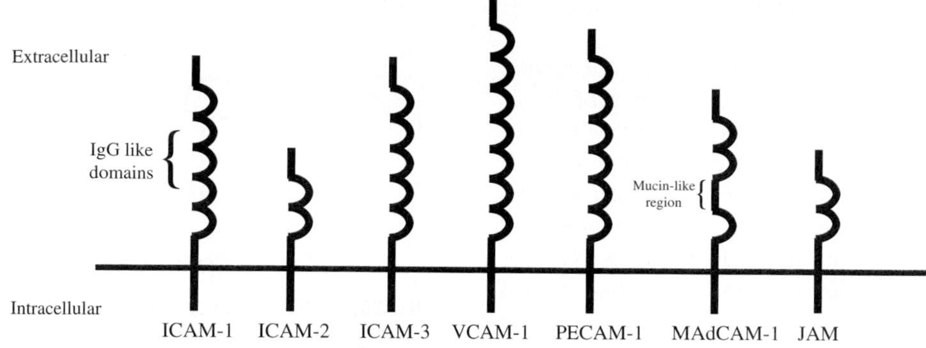

FIG. 20.3. Structural features of the immunoglobulin superfamily proteins. The extracellular portion of immunoglobulin superfamily proteins contains the IgG-like domain repeats. The number of the IgG repeats is variable between different molecules within the superfamily.

platelet endothelial cell adhesion molecule-1 (PECAM-1), MAdCAM-1, and junctional adhesion molecules 1, 2, and 3 (JAM-1, -2, and -3).

ICAM-1 was originally identified as a ligand for the β_2 integrin lymphocyte function-associated antigen-1 (LFA-1) (97). Since its discovery, ICAM-1 has been shown to bind to many different ligands, including the β_2 integrins Mac-1 and p150/95, hyaluronan, and fibrinogen (98–100). ICAM-1 is constitutively expressed on many different cell types and can be up-regulated by various inflammatory mediators, such as TNF-α and LPS (97,101). ICAM-1 participates in a wide variety of leukocyte and endothelial responses, including leukocyte firm adhesion and emigration through the endothelium, leukocyte-leukocyte aggregation, and leukocyte activation (97,102–105). These cellular events are facilitated by ICAM-1 interactions with the β_2 integrins, which stimulate outside-in signaling pathways (91,96). Cross-linking of ICAM-1 activates signal transduction cascades through intracellular Ca^{2+} release and mitogen-activated protein (MAP) kinase activation, causing increased expression of other members of the immunoglobulin superfamily (106).

ICAM-2 was identified through expression cloning, using a monoclonal antibody that inhibited LFA-1-mediated leukocyte adhesion and emigration on resting endothelium (107). ICAM-2 is constitutively expressed on the cell surface and is primarily observed on endothelial cells, antigen-presenting cells, and some intestinal epithelial cells (108). Unlike ICAM-1, ICAM-2 is not inducible by inflammatory mediators, suggesting that ICAM-2 is important for normal immune surveillance (108). ICAM-3 was identified in 1992 and is expressed on all resting leukocytes (109,110). This molecule binds to LFA-1 and is important in leukocyte aggregation and activation (109–111). The three ICAMs differ in the number of IgG-like domains on the extracellular surface. ICAM-1 and -3 both have five IgG-like domains, whereas ICAM-2 has only two (Fig. 20.3).

VCAM-1 was first identified through its ability to mediate lymphocyte adhesion (112). VCAM-1 gene expression is increased by inflammatory cytokines and cross-linking of ICAM-1 (106,113). A major ligand for VCAM-1 is the $\alpha_4\beta_1$ integrin [very late antigen-4 (VLA-4)], which is important for monocyte and lymphocyte firm adhesion and emigration, as well as for lymphocyte stimulation. VCAM-1 has also been reported to bind to the integrins $\alpha_4\beta_7$, $\alpha_9\beta_1$, and $\alpha_d\beta_2$ (91,114,115). Alternative splicing of the VCAM-1 messenger RNA results in two distinct protein isoforms. The larger VCAM-1 protein consists of seven IgG-like domains, whereas the shorter molecule is lacking IgG domain 4 (112). Domain 1, and possibly domain 4, largely mediate VCAM-1/ligand interactions. Antibody-blocking studies have shown that domain 1 is involved in leukocyte adhesion of both splice variant forms, and that the lack of domain 4 in the smaller VCAM-1 isoform may result in differential adhesion properties (96).

PECAM-1 was initially identified by serologic characterization of surface proteins on vascular endothelium and is localized to the intercellular junctions of endothelial cells (116,117). Anti-PECAM-1 antibodies were also shown to prevent leukocyte emigration across endothelial monolayers (118). PECAM-1 is also expressed on platelets, monocytes, neutrophils, NK cells, and certain T-cell subsets (119, 120). More recent data also suggest that PECAM-1 may be involved in angiogenic processes, cell migration, macrophage phagocytosis, and apoptosis (121,122).

The PECAM-1 protein contains six IgG-like domains, a transmembrane domain, and a cytoplasmic domain (Fig. 20.3). The cytoplasmic domain contains immunoreceptor tyrosine inhibitory motifs, exhibits differential phosphorylation of both serine and tyrosine, and can undergo alternative splicing (120–122). PECAM-1 signaling has been shown to be important for normal endothelial monolayer integrity and activation of leukocyte β_2 integrins (123). PECAM-1 adhesion is mediated by homophilic interactions, although some experimental evidence suggests that this adhesion molecule can interact with other heterophilic ligands (122). Antibodies to domains 1 and 2 have been shown to block PECAM-1 homophilic interactions and also prevent PECAM-1-mediated leukocyte activation (117, 119,123).

MAdCAM-1 was initially identified by a monoclonal antibody that stained high endothelial venules of Peyer patches and mesenteric lymph nodes (124,125). Further characterization of MAdCAM-1 expression in tissues revealed constitutive expression in mucosal tissues (124, 126). MAdCAM-1 expression can also be up-regulated by TNF-α (127). This adhesion molecule mediates lymphocyte adhesion and emigration in high endothelial venules in secondary lymphoid organs. MAdCAM-1 contains three extracellular IgG-like domains. A mucin-like region, located between domains 2 and 3, is involved in ligand binding (Fig. 20.3). MAdCAM-1 ligands include the $\alpha_4\beta_7$ integrin and L-selectin that bind to domain 1 and the mucin-like region of the MAdCAM-1 protein, respectively (53).

JAM family members (JAM-1, -2, and -3) are all expressed in endothelial cells, but can also be found in epithelial cells, leukocytes, and platelets (128–131). This is a relatively new family of adhesion molecules, and additional members will likely be identified in the near future. These proteins are localized to intercellular regions of endothelial cells and are enriched at tight junctions (132,133). JAM molecules contain two extracellular IgG domains, a single transmembrane domain, and a short cytoplasmic tail (133) (Fig. 20.3). JAM members participate in leukocyte transendothelial migration as well as in the regulation of permeability (128,134). The ligand specificities for each JAM adhesion molecule have not been completely characterized, and are still under investigation. JAM-1 shows homophilic dimerization at interendothelial junctions, but can also bind in a heterophilic fashion to the β_2 integrin LFA-1, and is a receptor for reovirus (135–137). JAM-2 can interact with JAM-3, as well as the β_1 integrin VLA-4, whereas JAM-3 on platelets can bind to the β_2 integrin Mac-1 (138–140).

CD44

CD44 is a heavily glycosylated adhesion protein originally identified on neuronal cells, leukocytes, and erythrocytes (141,142). Since its initial description and identification, CD44 has been shown to participate in many different cellular processes. These include mediating lymphocyte/endothelial cell interactions and extracellular matrix rearrangement and remodeling (143). The diverse functions of CD44 are believed to be due to the different glycoprotein isoforms that are generated through alternative splicing. CD44 is a type I membrane glycoprotein that consists of a cytoplasmic tail, a transmembrane domain, and an extracellular region containing a globular domain located at the amino-terminus (Fig. 20.4). The amino-terminal globular domain contains disulfide bonds of critical cysteine residues that are important for ligand binding (144,145). However, given the significant amount of glycosylation, other extracellular regions may also participate in

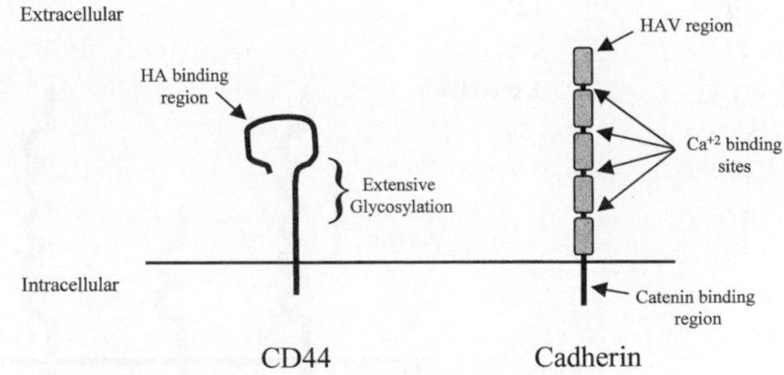

FIG. 20.4. CD44 and cadherin structural features. The CD44 molecule can be extensively glycosylated throughout most of the extracellular portion of the protein. The hyaluronan (*HA*) binding region is found in the globular head of the extracellular region. The classic cadherins typically contain 5 extracellular domains (*EC 1–5*) separated by Ca^{+2} binding sites. The last extracellular domain contains the histidine, alanine, valine (*HAV*) motif that mediates cadherin homotypic interaction. The cadherin cytoplasmic domain contains the catenin-binding region that is important for cytoskeletal association.

ligand binding. The major physiologic CD44 ligand has been shown to be hyaluronic acid (HA) (146). Inflammatory stimuli such as TNF-α and IL-1β have been shown to increase endothelial HA expression (147). *In vitro* studies have also shown that other components of the extracellular matrix may bind CD44 as well (e.g., fibronectin, laminin, and collagen type I) (148,149).

Early studies of CD44 function showed that this molecule was involved in lymphocyte homing, since monoclonal antibodies blocked peripheral blood lymphocyte adhesion to mucosal high endothelial venules (150). *In vivo* injection of CD44 antibodies has also been shown to inhibit edema and cellular infiltration in early stages of delayed-type hypersensitivity reactions (151). DeGrendele et al. showed that CD44 was important for activated T-cell extravasation into inflammatory sites (143,152). *In vitro,* CD44 has been shown to facilitate lymphocyte rolling on endothelium, and CD44/HA interactions also potentiate the expression of proinflammatory cytokines by leukocytes (143,153). Although it is clear that CD44/HA interactions are involved in lymphocyte adhesion and emigration during inflammation, more studies are necessary to further define the role of CD44 in inflammatory responses in different tissues.

CADHERINS

The cadherins were originally identified as cell surface proteins with characteristic calcium sensitivities (154). To date, over 80 different cadherins have been described in vertebrates. Cadherins are typically involved in homotypic adhesion of specific cell types, such as epithelial, endothelial, and neuronal cells. In addition to these structural functions, cadherins also function in cell growth and differentiation

(154). Homotypic interactions of these cells can be mediated by a single cadherin; however, cells may also express many other types of cadherins. For example, E-cadherin is primarily involved in epithelial cell-cell adhesion yet these cells can express other cadherins such as N- and P-cadherin (155). Cadherins have also been shown to participate in heterophilic interactions. For example, T lymphocytes can adhere to intestinal epithelial cells through E-cadherin interactions with the $\alpha_E\beta_7$ integrin (156).

Cadherin proteins generally consist of three major structural regions: a cytoplasmic domain, a transmembrane domain, and an amino-terminal extracellular domain (Fig. 20.4). The cytoplasmic domain is highly conserved between different cadherin species (154). This region is critical in that the catenin family of proteins is associated with the cytoplasmic tail of cadherins (157–160). Catenins link the cadherin molecule to the actin cytoskeleton, resulting in the formation of adherens junctions and desmosomes seen in epithelial and endothelial cells. The extracellular region of the classic cadherins consists of five repeat motifs referred to as extracellular domains 1 through 5 (EC1–5) (160). The amino-terminal end of the extracellular portion also contains the HAV (histidine, alanine, and valine) region that mediates cadherin homophilic interactions (159, 160). Site-directed mutagenesis and chimeric constructions of different cadherins show that amino acids adjacent to the HAV region may also be important for specificity of cadherin homophilic interactions (160).

MECHANISMS OF LEUKOCYTE/ENDOTHELIAL ADHESION

Leukocyte/endothelial interactions are essential for the development of both normal inflammatory responses and inflammatory diseases. The adhesive interactions that occur during leukocyte extravasation have been actively studied and shown to require the cooperative binding of many different adhesion molecules. Recruitment of leukocytes into extravascular tissues occurs through a concerted, multistep process involving leukocyte rolling, adhesion, and emigration across the vasculature (96,161). The majority of evidence supporting these mechanisms has come from both intravital observations of postcapillary venules and from studies of *in vitro* model systems using isolated leukocytes and endothelial cells. Leukocyte adhesion can also be observed in arterial vessels under certain pathologic conditions, such as transplantation rejection, vasculitis, and atherosclerosis (7,162). The mechanisms of leukocyte adhesion at the postcapillary level are well known; however, relatively little is known regarding leukocyte/arterial adhesive pathways. Figure 20.5 presents a general overview of the leukocyte adhesion cascade.

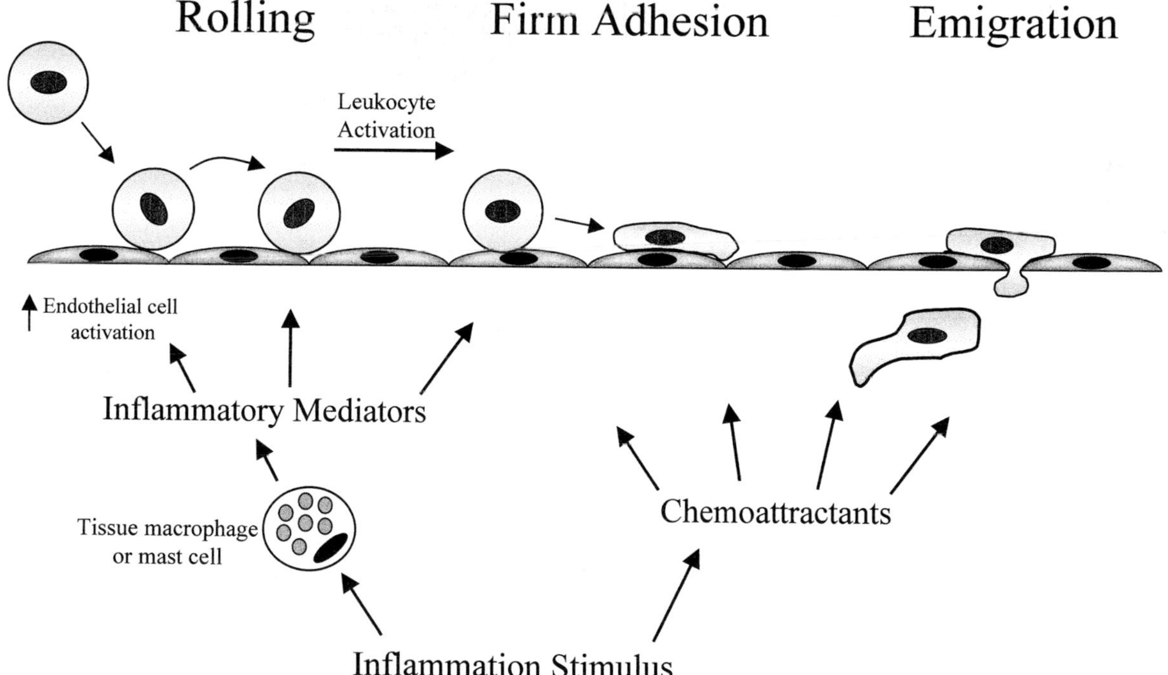

FIG. 20.5. Mechanisms of leukocyte adhesion and emigration. Leukocyte extravasation involves three major steps: leukocyte rolling, firm adhesion, and emigration. Inflammatory stimuli initiate these events through activation of resident leukocytes and other cell types. These cells then release inflammatory mediators that lead to endothelial cell activation. Inflammatory stimuli can also stimulate the release of chemoattractants that facilitate leukocyte emigration across the endothelium and through extravascular tissue.

Both leukocytes and endothelium can exist in an activated or nonactivated state. Efficient leukocyte recruitment during an inflammatory response requires activation of both of these cell types, which results in increased expression and receptor affinity changes in adhesion molecules. Many inflammatory stimuli, such as infectious agents and tissue damage, can activate postcapillary venular endothelium and facilitate leukocyte adhesion and extravasation (163,164). Activation of endothelial cells and leukocytes can also occur within the vascular lumen and promote leukocyte/endothelial cell interactions. This mechanism may be important in the development of lesions in several different vasculitic diseases (7). Table 20.1 lists many of the ligand/receptor interactions between leukocytes and endothelial cells during the adhesion and emigration process.

The initial step of the leukocyte adhesion cascade involves leukocyte margination and rolling along the vascular endothelium (36). As leukocytes exit the capillary lumen and empty into the postcapillary venule, hemodynamic forces cause an outward movement of leukocytes toward the venular endothelium. Margination is largely due to erythrocytes overwhelming leukocytes as they exit the capillary lumen and pushing them toward the vessel wall. With the leukocyte in close proximity to the venular endothelium, low affinity (weak) cell/cell interactions occur and initiate leukocyte rolling. Adhesion molecules that can directly mediate leukocyte rolling include the selectins, VLA-4, $\alpha 4/\beta 7$, VCAM-1, MAdCAM-1, and CD44 (36,143,165). Rolling results in increased leukocyte transit time on the endothelial cell surface and allows high affinity (strong) cell/cell interactions to occur. Other adhesion molecules also contribute to this process, although they cannot directly mediate leukocyte rolling along the vascular wall. For example, interactions between the β_2 integrins LFA-1 and Mac-1 and their endothelial ligands have been shown to modulate or decrease neutrophil rolling velocity (166). This has been termed slow rolling and appears to be one of the critical factors for promoting efficient stationary or firm adhesion.

High-affinity interactions occur following activation of rolling leukocytes by chemokines as well as other endothelial-derived mediators. These mediators stimulate L-selectin shedding, changes in integrin protein conformation, and release of integrin proteins such as Mac-1 from intracellular stores (48,91,167). These events help prime the β_2 integrins for binding to members of the immunoglobulin superfamily and are critical for subsequent leukocyte firm adhesion. LFA-1, Mac-1, ICAM-1 and -2, MAdCAM-1, and VCAM-1 have all been shown to mediate firm adhesion of one or more leukocyte subtypes (163). Firmly-adherent leukocytes then begin to flatten and spread across the endothelial cell surface. The leukocyte extends microvilli between adjacent endothelial cells to begin the process of transmigration across the postcapillary venule.

Many different adhesion molecules, with the exception of the selectins, have been shown to participate in transendothelial migration. On endothelial cells, PECAM-1, JAM-1, -2, and -3, and VE-cadherin are all concentrated at the lateral borders and aid in leukocyte emigration between adjacent endothelial cells (120,128,132). On leukocytes, several integrins, including LFA-1 and VLA-4, have also been shown to mediate this process through interactions with different members of the immunoglobulin superfamily (105,135). More work is necessary to determine the specific adhesion pathways used by different leukocyte subtypes during transendothelial migration, as well as the cellular events that regulate this process.

TABLE 20.1. *Leukocyte/endothelial cell adhesion molecule interactions*

Interaction	Endothelial adhesion molecule	Leukocyte adhesion molecule
Rolling	E-selectin	ESL-1[a]
	P-selectin	PSGL-1
	HA	CD44
	Unknown[b]	L-selectin
	VCAM-1	VLA-4
Firm adhesion	ICAM-1	LFA-1, Mac-1
	ICAM-2	LFA-1
	VCAM-1	VLA-4
	HA	CD44
Emigration	ICAM-1	LFA-1, Mac-1
	ICAM-2	LFA-1
	VCAM-1	VLA-4
	PECAM-1	PECAM-1, others?
	JAM	Multiple Ligand

[a]ESL-1 has not yet been shown to bind to E-selectin and mediate rolling *in vivo.*

[b]The physiologic L-selectin ligands that are involved in inflammatory leukocyte recruitment have not yet been identified.

ESL, E-selectin ligand; HA, hyaluronan; ICAM, intercellular adhesion molecule; JAM, junctional adhesion molecule; LFA, lymphocyte function-associated antigen; PECAM, platelet endothelial cell adhesion molecule; PSGL, P-selectin glycoprotein ligand; VCAM, vascular cell adhesion molecule; VLA, very late antigen.

ADHESION MOLECULES IN THE PATHOGENESIS OF RHEUMATIC DISEASES

The pathogenic mechanisms that lead to the development of many different rheumatic diseases are still poorly understood. However, there is a substantial body of evidence that now suggests that adhesion-molecule expression is a critical determinant for the development of tissue inflammation in these disorders. In rheumatoid arthritis (RA), for example, adhesion molecules appear to mediate many different cellular interactions during disease progression, including leukocyte entry into synovial tissue and fluid, synovial proliferation and pannus formation, adhesion of leukocytes to cartilage, adhesion of pannus tissue to cartilage and bone, and angiogenic activity in synovial tissue (reviewed in references 1–6). During the development of vasculitic disorders, adhesion molecules also appear to be crucial for leukocyte interactions with endothelium and smooth muscle and leukocyte activation events leading to blood vessel destruction (7–9).

Strong support for an active role of adhesion molecules in disease pathogenesis has been derived from studies of patients with various rheumatic disorders. Reports have demonstrated increased expression of specific adhesion molecules, including E-selectin, ICAM-1, VCAM-1, E-cadherin, and various members of the β_1 and β_2 integrins on peripheral blood leukocytes or in inflamed tissues from patients with many different rheumatic diseases (1,3,7,168). In addition, increased levels of soluble adhesion molecules in serum have also been reported, and may be indicative of chronic leukocyte and endothelial activation (3,169). Finally, many of the currently used therapeutic agents such as corticosteroids, methotrexate, and cyclosporine A, have been shown to down-regulate adhesion molecule expression. Thus, decreased expression of adhesion proteins may be one pathway by which these agents act (3).

Other, more indirect evidence comes from studies in both animal models and *in vitro* experimental adhesion systems. For example, many of the inflammatory mediators associated with rheumatic disorders, such as infectious agents, cytokines, immune complexes, complement proteins, and autoantibodies, have been shown to up-regulate expression of specific adhesion molecules on leukocytes or in other tissues (5,7,163,164,170). This mechanism may be responsible for both the initiation and establishment of inflammation during disease development. Animal model systems for RA and vasculitis have been used to more specifically define the function of particular adhesion molecules. Loss or inhibition of P-selectin, ICAM-1, VLA-4, CD44, and several β_2 integrins has been shown to inhibit the development of joint inflammation in several different rodent arthritis models (171–175). Also, mice genetically deficient in ICAM-1 were shown to have a significant reduction in the development of vasculitis in the MRL/MpJ/*Fas*^{lpr} lupus model system (176). Taken together, these studies provide support for the concept that adhesion molecules actively participate in the initiation and progression of rheumatic diseases. However, further investigation is necessary to identify the precise role of individual adhesion molecules in the development of these different diseases.

Therapeutic strategies designed to inhibit adhesion molecule interactions have now been successfully used for the treatment of chronic inflammatory diseases, although few studies have used anti–adhesion molecule therapy in RA or related disorders (177–181). Previously, treatment of RA patients with a murine monoclonal antibody against ICAM-1 was shown to reduce disease activity (182). However, repeated courses of therapy with this antibody were associated with adverse effects, and clinical efficacy was less than that observed in the initial trial (183). This was most likely due to the immunogenicity of this murine antibody. Recently, humanized monoclonal antibodies against LFA-1, a major ligand for ICAM-1, have shown promising results in clinical trials involving psoriasis patients (178,179). In addition, humanized antibodies against the α_4 integrins showed significant clinical benefit in both inflammatory bowel disease and multiple sclerosis (180,181). More work is necessary to test the efficacy of these, as well as other, anti–adhesion molecule therapeutics, in the treatment of patients with RA, and other diseases.

ACKNOWLEDGMENTS

This work was supported by a Young Investigator Grant to D.C.B. from the Arthritis Foundation.

REFERENCES

1. McMurray RW. Adhesion molecules in autoimmune disease. *Semin Arthritis Rheum* 1996;25:215.
2. Oppenheimer-Marks N, Lipsky PE. Adhesion molecules in rheumatoid arthritis. *Springer Semin Immunopathol* 1998;20:95.
3. Mojcik CF, Shevach EM. Adhesion molecules; a rheumatologic perspective. *Arthritis Rheum* 1997;40:991.
4. Liao H-X, Haynes BF. Role of adhesion molecules in the pathogenesis of rheumatoid arthritis. *Rheumatoid Arthritis* 1995;21:715.
5. Szekanecz Z, Szegedi G, Koch AE. Cellular adhesion molecules in rheumatoid arthritis: regulation by cytokines and possible clinical importance. *J Invest Med* 1996;44:124.
6. Szekanecz Z, Szegedi G, Koch AE. Angiogenesis in rheumatoid arthritis: pathologic and clinical significance. *J Invest Med* 1998;46:27.
7. Kevil CG, Bullard DC. Roles of leukocyte/endothelial cell adhesion molecules in the pathogenesis of vasculitis. *Am J Med* 1999;106:677.
8. Cid MC. New developments in the pathogenesis of systemic vasculitis. *Curr Opin Rheum* 1996;8:1.
9. Sundy JS, Haynes BF. Pathogenic mechanisms of vessel damage in vasculitis syndromes. *Rheum Dis Clin North Am* 1995;21:861.
10. Gallatin WM, Weissman IL, Butcher EC. A cell-surface molecule involved in organ-specific homing of lymphocytes. *Nature* 1983;304:30.
11. Bevilacqua MP, Pober JS, Mendrick DL, et al. Identification of an inducible endothelial-leukocyte adhesion molecule. *Proc Natl Acad Sci U S A* 1987;84:9238.
12. Hsu-Lin S-C, Berman CL, Furie BC, et al. A platelet membrane protein expressed during platelet activation and secretion. *J Biol Chem* 1984;259:9121.
13. McEver RP, Martin MN. A monoclonal antibody to a membrane glycoprotein binds only to activated platelets. *J Biol Chem* 1984;259:9799.
14. McEver RP, Beckstead JH, Moore KL, et al. GMP-140, a platelet alpha granule membrane protein, is also synthesized by vascular endothelial cells and is localized in Weibel-Palade bodies. *J Clin Invest* 1989;84:92.
15. Bevilacqua MP, Stengelin S, Gimbrone MAJ, et al. Endothelial leukocyte adhesion molecule 1: an inducible receptor for neutrophils related to complement regulatory proteins and lectins. *Science* 1989;243:1160.
16. Camerini D, James SP, Stamenkovic I, et al. Leu-8/TQ1 is the human equivalent of the Mel-14 lymph node homing receptor. *Nature* 1989;342:78.
17. Johnston GI, Cook RG, McEver RP. Cloning of GMP-140, a granule membrane protein of platelets and endothelium: sequence similarity to proteins involved in cell adhesion and inflammation. *Cell* 1989;56:1033.

18. Lasky LA, Singer MS, Yednock TA, et al. Cloning of a lymphocyte homing receptor reveals a lectin domain. *Cell* 1989;56:1045.
19. Siegelman MH, Van De Rijn M, Weissman IL. Mouse lymph node homing receptor cDNA clone encodes a glycoprotein revealing tandem interaction domains. *Science* 1989;243:1165.
20. Tedder TF, Isaacs CM, Ernst TJ, et al. Isolation and chromosomal localization of cDNAs encoding a novel human lymphocyte cell surface molecule, LAM-1. *J Exp Med* 1989;170:123.
21. Huang KS, Graves BJ, Wolitzky BA. Functional analysis of selectin structure. In: Vestweber D, ed. *The selectins: initiators of leukocyte endothelial adhesion.* Vol. 3. Amsterdam: Harwood Academic, 1997:1.
22. Crovello CS, Furie BC, Furie B. Rapid phosphorylation and selective dephosphorylation of P-selectin accompanies platelet activation. *J Biol Chem* 1993;268:14590.
23. Weyrich AS, McIntyre TM, McEver RP, et al. Monocyte tethering by P-selectin regulates monocyte chemotactic protein-1 and tumor necrosis factor-α secretion. Signal integration and NF-κB translocation. *J Clin Invest* 1995;95:2297.
24. Waddell TK, Fialkow L, Chan CK, et al. Potentiation of the oxidative burst of human neutrophils. A signaling role for L-selectin. *J Biol Chem* 1994;269:18485.
25. Waddell TK, Fialkow L, Chan CK, et al. Signaling functions of L-selectin. Enhancement of tyrosine phosphorylation and activation of MAP kinase. *J Biol Chem* 1995;270:15403.
26. Laudanna C, Constantin G, Baron P, et al. Sulfatides trigger increase of cytosolic free calcium and enhanced expression of tumor necrosis factor-alpha and interleukin-8 mRNA in human neutrophils. Evidence for a role of L-selectin as a signaling molecule. *J Biol Chem* 1994; 269:4021.
27. Simon SI, Burns AR, Taylor AD, et al. L-selectin (CD62L) cross-linking signals neutrophil adhesive functions via the Mac-1 (CD11b/CD18) beta 2-integrin. *J Immunol* 1995;155:1502.
28. Kansas GS, Spertini O, Stoolman LM, et al. Molecular mapping of functional domains of the leukocyte receptor for endothelium, LAM-1. *J Cell Biol* 1991;114:351.
29. Kansas GS, Saunders KB, Ley K, et al. A role for the epidermal growth factor-like domain of P-selectin in ligand recognition and cell adhesion. *J Cell Biol* 1994;124:609.
30. Watson SR, Imai Y, Fennie C, et al. The complement binding-like domains of the murine homing receptor facilitate lectin activity. *J Cell Biol* 1991;115:235.
31. Li SH, Burns DK, Rumberger JM, et al. Consensus repeat domains of E-selectin enhance ligand binding. *J Biol Chem* 1994;269:4431.
32. Pigott R, Needham LA, Edwards RM, et al. Structural and functional studies of the endothelial activation antigen endothelial leukocyte adhesion molecule-1 using a panel of monoclonal antibodies. *J Immunol* 1991;147:130.
33. Spertini O, Kansas GS, Reinmann KA, et al. Functional and evolutionary conservation of distinct epitopes on the leukocyte adhesion molecule (LAM-1) that regulate leukocyte migration. *J Immunol* 1991;147: 942.
34. Hamburger SA, McEver RP. GMP-140 mediates adhesion of stimulated platelets to neutrophils. *Blood* 1990;75:550.
35. Larsen E, Celi A, Gilbert GE, et al. PADGEM protein: a receptor that mediates the interaction of activated platelets with neutrophils and monocytes. *Cell* 1989;59:305.
36. Ley K. The selectins as rolling receptors. In: Vestweber D, ed. *The selectins—initiators of leukocyte endothelial adhesion.* Vol. 3. Amsterdam: Harwood Academic, 1997:63.
37. Johnson RC, Mayadas TN, Frenette PS, et al. Blood cell dynamics in P-selectin-deficient mice. *Blood* 1995;86:1106.
38. Lowe JB. Glycosylation in the control of selectin counter-receptor structure and function. *Immunol Rev* 2002;186:19.
39. Stenberg PE, McEver RP, Shuman MA, et al. A platelet alpha-granule membrane protein (GMP-140) is expressed on the plasma membrane after activation. *J Cell Biol* 1985;101:880.
40. Hattori R, Hamilton KK, Fugate RD, et al. Stimulated secretion of endothelial von Willebrand factor is accompanied by rapid redistribution to the cell surface of the intracellular granule membrane protein GMP-140. *J Biol Chem* 1989;264:7768.
41. Bonfanti R, Furie BC, Furie B, et al. PADGEM (GMP140) is a component of Weibel-Palade bodies of human endothelial cells. *Blood* 1989;73:1109.
42. Berman CL, Yeo EL, Wencel-Drake JD, et al. A platelet alpha granule membrane protein that is associated with the plasma membrane after activation. *J Clin Invest* 1986;78:130.
43. Hattori R, Hamilton KK, McEver RP, et al. Complement proteins C5b-9 induce secretion of high molecular weight multimers of endothelial von Willebrand factor and translocation of granule membrane protein GMP-140 to the cell surface. *J Biol Chem* 1989;264:9053.
44. Kubes P, Kanwar S. Histamine induces leukocyte rolling in postcapillary venules. A P-selectin-mediated event. *J Immunol* 1994;152:3570.
45. Cotran RS, Gimbrone MAJ, Bevilacqua MP, et al. Induction and detection of a human endothelial activation antigen *in vivo*. *J Exp Med* 1986;164:661.
46. Lewinsohn DM, Bargatze RF, Butcher EC. Leukocyte-endothelial cell recognition: evidence of a common molecular mechanism shared by neutrophils, lymphocytes, and other leukocytes. *J Immunol* 1987;138: 4313.
47. Jung TM, Gallatin WM, Weissman IL, et al. Down-regulation of homing receptors after T cell activation. *J Immunol* 1988;141:4110.
48. Kishimoto TK, Jutila MA, Berg EL, et al. Neutrophil Mac-1 and MEL-14 adhesion proteins inversely regulated by chemotactic factors. *Science* 1989;245:1238.
49. Kansas GS, Wood GS, Fishwild DM, et al. Functional characterization of human T lymphocyte subsets distinguished by monoclonal anti-Leu-8. *J Immunol* 1985;134:2995.
50. Picker LJ, Treer JR, Ferguson-Darnell B, et al. Control of lymphocyte recirculation in man. I. Differential regulation of the peripheral lymph node homing receptor L-selectin on T cells during the virgin to memory cell transition. *J Immunol* 1993;150:1105.
51. Bradley LM, Watson SR, Swain SL. Entry of naive CD4 T cells into peripheral lymph nodes requires L-selectin. *J Exp Med* 1994;180: 2401.
52. Arbones ML, Ord DC, Ley K, et al. Lymphocyte homing and leukocyte rolling and migration are impaired in L-selectin-deficient mice. *Immunity* 1994;1:247.
53. Bargatze RF, Jutila MA, Butcher EC. Distinct roles of L-selectin and integrins $\alpha_4\beta_7$ and LFA-1 in lymphocyte homing to Peyer's patch-HEV in situ: the multistep model confirmed and refined. *Immunity* 1995;3:99.
54. Erbe DV, Watson SR, Presta LG, et al. P- and E-selectin use common sites for carbohydrate ligand recognition and cell adhesion. *J Cell Biol* 1993;120:1227.
55. Patel KD, Cuvelier SL, Wiehler S. Selectins: critical mediators of leukocyte recruitment. *Semin Immunol* 2002;14:73.
56. Phillips ML, Nudelman E, Gaeta FCA, ET AL. ELAM-1 mediates cell adhesion by recognition of a carbohydrate ligand, Sialyl-Le^x. *Science* 1990;250:1130.
57. Polley MJ, Phillips ML, Wayner E, et al. CD62 and endothelial cell-leukocyte adhesion molecule 1 (ELAM-1) recognize the same carbohydrate ligand, sialyl-Lewis X. *Proc Natl Acad Sci U S A* 1991;88:6224.
58. Foxall C, Watson SR, Dowbenko D, et al. The three members of the selectin receptor family recognize a common carbohydrate epitope, the sialyl Lewis^x oligosaccharide. *J Cell Biol* 1992;117:895.
59. Zhou Q, Moore KL, Smith DF, et al. The selectin GMP-140 binds to sialylated, fucosylated lactosaminoglycans on both myeloid and nonmyeloid cells. *J Cell Biol* 1991;115:557.
60. Kansas GS. Selectins and their ligands: current concepts and controversies. *Blood* 1996;88:111.
61. Sako D, Chang X-J, Barone KM, et al. Expression cloning of a functional glycoprotein ligand for P-selectin. *Cell* 1993;75:1179.
62. Moore KL, Patel KD, Breuhl RE, et al. P-selectin glycoprotein ligand-1 mediates rolling of human neutrophils on P-selectin. *J Cell Biol* 1995; 128:661.
63. Fieger CB, Sassetti CM, Rosen SD. Endoglycan, a member of the CD34 family, functions as a L-selectin ligand through modification with tyrosine sulfation and sialyl Lewis x. *J Biol Chem* 2003;278: 27390–27898.
64. Lasky LA, Singer MS, Dowbenko D, et al. An endothelial ligand for L-selectin is a novel mucin-like molecule. *Cell* 1992;69:927.
65. Puri KD, Finger EB, Gaudernack G, et al. Sialomucin CD34 is the major L-selectin ligand in human tonsil high endothelial venules. *J Cell Biol* 1995;131:261.
66. Ellies LG, Tsuboi S, Petryniak B, et al. Core 2 oligosaccharide biosynthesis distinguishes between selectin ligands essential for leukocyte homing and inflammation. *Immunity* 1998;9:881.

67. Erdmann I, Scheidegger EP, Koch FK, et al. Fucosyltransferase VII-deficient mice with defective E-, P-, and L-selectin ligands show impaired CD4+ and CD8+ T cell migration into the skin, but normal extravasation into visceral organs. *J Immunol* 2002;168:2139.
68. Homeister JW, Thall AD, Petryniak B, et al. The alpha(1,3)fucosyltransferases FucT-IV and FucT-VII exert collaborative control over selectin-dependent leukocyte recruitment and lymphocyte homing. *Immunity* 2001;15:115.
69. Knibbs RN, Craig RA, Maly P, et al. a1,3-fucosyltransferase VII dependent synthesis of P- and E-selectin ligands on cultured T lymphoblasts. *J Immunol* 1998;161:6305.
70. Knibbs RN, Craig RA, Natsuka S, et al. The fucosyltransferase FucT-VII regulates E-selectin ligand synthesis in human T cells. *J Cell Biol* 1996;133:911.
71. Maly P, Thall AD, Petryniak B, et al. The a (1,3) fucosyltransferase FucT-VII controls leukocyte trafficking through an essential role in L-, E-, and P-selectin ligand biosynthesis. *Cell* 1996;86:643.
72. Wagers AJ, Stoolman LM, Kannagi R, et al. Expression of leukocyte fucosyltransferases regulates binding to E-selectin. Relationship to previously implicated carbohydrate epitopes. *J Immunol* 1997;159: 1917.
73. Kumar R, Camphausen RT, Sullivan FX, et al. Core 2 b-1, 6-N-acetylglucosaminyltransferase enzyme activity is critical for P-selectin glycoprotein ligand-1 binding to P-selectin. *Blood* 1996;88:3872.
74. Lim YC, Henault L, Wagers AJ, et al. Expression of functional selectin ligands on Th cells is differentially regulated by IL-12 and IL-4. *J Immunol* 1999;162:3193.
75. Wagers AJ, Waters CM, Stoolman LM, et al. Interleukin 12 and interleukin 4 control T cell adhesion to endothelial selectins through opposite effects on alpha1, 3-fucosyltransferase VII gene expression. *J Exp Med* 1998;188:2225.
76. Hynes RO. Integrins: bidirectional, allosteric signaling machines. *Cell* 2002;110:673.
77. Humphries MJ, McEwan PA, Barton SJ, et al. Integrin structure: heady advances in ligand binding, but activation still makes the knees wobble. *Trends Biochem Sci 2003;28:313.*
78. Burke RD. Invertebrate Integrins: structure, function, and evolution. *Int Rev Cytol* 1999;191:257.
79. Liddington RC, Ginsberg MH. Integrin activation takes shape. *J Cell Biol* 2002;158:833.
80. Hughes AL. Coevolution of the vertebrate integrin alpha and beta chain genes. *Mol Biol Evolution* 1992;9:216.
81. Shimizu Y, Rose DM, Ginsberg MH. Integrins in the immune system. *Adv Immunol* 1999;72:325.
82. Arnaout MA. Integrin structure: new twists and turns in dynamic cell adhesion. *Immunol Rev* 2002;186:125.
83. Xiong JP, Stehle T, Diefenbach B, et al. Crystal structure of the extracellular segment of integrin alpha Vbeta3. *Science* 2001;294:339.
84. D'Souza SE, Ginsberg MH, Burke TA, et al. Localization of an Arg-Gly-Asp recognition site within an integrin adhesion receptor. *Science* 1998;242:91.
85. Smith JW, Cheresh DA. The Arg-Gly-Asp binding domain of the vitronectin receptor. Photoaffinity cross-linking implicates amino acid residues 61–203 of the β-subunit. *J Biol Chem* 1988;263:18726.
86. Smith JW, Cheresh DA. Integrin ($\alpha_v\beta_3$)-ligand interaction. Identification of a heterodimeric RGD binding site on the vitronectin receptor. *J Biol Chem* 1990;265:2168.
87. Fleming JC, Pahl HL, Gonzalez DA, et al. Structural analysis of the CD11b gene and phylogenetic analysis of the X alpha-integrin gene family demonstrate remarkable conservation of genomic X organization and suggest early diversification during evolution. *J Immunol* 1993;150:480.
88. Larson RS, Corbi AL, Berman L, et al. Primary structure of the leukocyte function-associated molecule-1a subunit: an integrin with an embedded domain defining a protein superfamily. *J Cell Biol* 1989;108: 703.
89. Hynes RO. Integrins: versatility, modulation, and signaling in cell adhesion. *Cell* 1992;69:11.
90. Larson RS, Springer TA. Structure and function of leukocyte integrins. *Immunol Rev* 1990;114:181.
91. Springer TA. Adhesion receptors of the immune system. *Nature* 1990; 346:425.
92. Takagi J, Springer TA. Integrin activation and structural rearrangement. *Immunol Rev* 2002;186:141.
93. Anderson DC, Schmalsteig FC, Finegold MJ, et al. The severe and moderate phenotypes of heritable Mac-1, LFA-1 deficiency: their quantitative definition and relation to leukocyte dysfunction and clinical feature. *J Infect Dis* 1985;152:668.
94. Anderson DC, Springer TA. Leukocyte adhesion deficiency: an inherited defect in the Mac-1, LFA-1 and p150,95 glycoproteins. *Annu Rev Med* 1987;38:175.
95. Kato A. The biologic and clinical spectrum of Glanzmann's thrombasthenia: implications of integrin $\alpha_{IIb}\beta_3$ for its pathogenesis. *Crit Rev Oncol Hematol* 1997;26:1.
96. Carlos TM, Harlan JM. Leukocyte-endothelial adhesion molecules. *Blood* 1994;84:2068.
97. Rothlein R, Dustin ML, Marlin SD, et al. A human intercellular adhesion molecule (ICAM-1) distinct from LFA-1. *J Immunol* 1986;137: 1270.
98. Diamond MS, Staunton DE, Marlin SD, et al. Binding of the integrin Mac-1 (CD11b/CD18) to the third immunoglubulin-like domain of ICAM-1 (CD54) and its regulation by glycosylation. *Cell* 1991;65: 961.
99. McCourt PAG, Ek B, Forsberg N, et al. Intercellular adhesion molecule-1 is a cell surface receptor for hyaluronan. *J Biol Chem* 1994; 269:30081.
100. Languino LR, Duperray A, Joganic KJ, et al. Regulation of leukocyte-endothelium interaction and leukocyte transendothelial migration by intercellular adhesion molecule 1-fibrinogen recognition. *Proc Natl Acad Sci USA* 1995;92:1505.
101. Dustin ML, Rothlein R, Bhan AK, et al. Induction by IL-1 and interferon, tissue distribution, biochemistry, and function of a natural adherence molecule (ICAM-1). *J Immunol* 1986;137:245.
102. Makgoba MW, Sanders ME, Ginther Luce GE, et al. ICAM-1: a ligand for LFA-1-dependent adhesion of B, T and myeloid cells. *Nature* 1988;331:86.
103. Fischer H, Gjorloff A, Hedlund G, et al. Stimulation of human naive and memory T helper cells with bacterial superantigen; naive CD4+45RA+ T cells require a costimulatory signal mediated through the LFA-1/ICAM-1 pathway. *J Immunol* 1992;148:1993.
104. Kuhlman P, Moy VT, Lollo BA, et al. The accessory function of murine intercellular adhesion molecule-1 in T lymphocyte activation. *J Immunol* 1991;146:1773.
105. Issekutz AC, Rowter D, Springer TA. Role of ICAM-1 and ICAM-2 and alternate CD11/CD18 ligands in neutrophil transendothelial migration. *J Leukoc Biol* 1999;65:117.
106. Lawson C, Ainsworth M, Yacoub M, et al. Ligation of ICAM-1 on endothelial cells leads to expression of VCAM-1 via a nuclear factor-κB-independent mechanism. *J Immunol* 1999;162:2990.
107. Staunton DE, Dustin ML, Springer TA. Functional cloning of ICAM-2, a cell adhesion ligand for LFA-1 homologous to ICAM-1. *Nature* 1989; 339:61.
108. de Fougerolles AR, Stacker SA, Schwarting R, et al. Characterization of ICAM-2 and evidence for a third counter-receptor for LFA-1. *J Exp Med* 1991;174:253.
109. de Fougerolles AR, Springer TA. Intercellular adhesion molecule 3, a third adhesion counter-receptor for lymphocyte function-associated molecule 1 on resting lymphocytes. *J Exp Med* 1992;175:185.
110. Vazeux R, Hoffman PA, Tomita J, et al. Cloning and characterization of a new intercellular adhesion molecule ICAM-R. *Nature* 1992;360: 485.
111. de Fougerolles AR, Qin X, Springer TA. Characterization of the function of intercellular adhesion molecule (ICAM)-3 and comparison with ICAM-1 and ICAM-2 in immune responses. *J Exp Med* 1994;179:619.
112. Osborn L, Hession C, Tizard R, et al. Direct expression cloning of vascular cell adhesion molecule 1, a cytokine-induced endothelial protein that binds to lymphocytes. *Cell* 1989;59:1203.
113. Kalogeris TJ, Kevil CG, Laroux FS, et al. Differential monocyte adhesion and adhesion molecule expression in venous and arterial endothelial cells. *Am J Physiol* 1999;276:L9–L19.
114. Taooka Y, Chen J, Yednock T, et al. The integrin $\alpha_9\beta_1$ mediates adhesion to activated endothelial cells and transendothelial neutrophil migration through interaction with vascular cell adhesion molecule-1. *J Cell Biol* 1999;145:413.
115. Vieren MVd, Crowe DT, Hoekstra D, et al. The leukocyte integrin alpha D beta 2 binds VCAM-1: evidence for a binding interface between I domain and VCAM-1. *J Immunol* 1999;163:1984.

116. Newman PJ, Berndt MC, Gorski J, et al. PECAM-1 (CD31) cloning and relation to adhesion molecules of the immunoglobulin gene superfamily. *Science* 1990;247:1219.
117. Newman PJ. The role of PECAM-1 in vascular cell biology. *Ann NY Acad Sci* 1994;714:165.
118. Muller WA. The role of PECAM-1 (CD31) in leukocyte emigration: studies *in vitro* and *in vivo*. *J Leukoc Biol* 1995;57:523.
119. DeLisser HM, Newman PJ, Albelda SM. Molecular and functional aspects of PECAM-1/CD31. *Immunol Today* 1994;15:490.
120. Newman PJ. Perspectives series: cell adhesion in vascular biology; the biology of PECAM-1. *J Clin Invest* 1997;100(suppl):25.
121. Bird IN, Taylor V, Newton JP, et al. Homophilic PECAM-1 (CD31) interactions prevent endothelial cell apoptosis but do not support cell spreading or migration. *J Cell Sci* 1999;112:1989.
122. Jackson DE. The unfolding tale of PECAM-1. *FEBS Lett* 2003; 540:7.
123. Elias CG, Spellberg JP, Karan-Tamir B, et al. Ligation of CD31/PECAM-1 modulates the function of lymphocytes, monocytes and neutrophils. *Eur J Immunol* 1998;28:1948.
124. Nakache M, Berg EL, Streeter PR, et al. The mucosal vascular addressin is a tissue-specific endothelial cell adhesion molecule for circulating lymphocytes. *Nature* 1989;337:179.
125. Briskin MJ, McEvoy LM, Butcher EC. MAdCAM-1 has homology to immunoglobulin and mucin-like adhesion receptors and to IgA1. *Nature* 1993;363:461.
126. Streeter PR, Berg EL, Rouse BTN, et al. A tissue-specific endothelial cell molecule involved in lymphocyte homing. *Nature* 1988;331:41.
127. Connor EM, Eppihimer MJ, Morise Z, et al. Expression of mucosal addressin cell adhesion molecule-1 (MAdCAM-1) in acute and chronic inflammation. *J Leukoc Biol* 1999;65:349.
128. Martin-Padura I, Lostaglio S, Schneemann M, et al. Junctional adhesion molecule, a novel member of the immunoglobulin superfamily that distributes at intercellular junctions and modulates monocyte transmigration. *J Cell Biol* 1998;142:117.
129. Aurrand-Lions M, Duncan L, Ballestrem C, et al. JAM-2, a novel immunoglobulin superfamily molecule, expressed by endothelial and lymphatic cells. *J Biol Chem* 2001;276:2733.
130. Palmeri D, van Zante A, Huang CC, et al. Vascular endothelial junction-associated molecule, a novel member of the immunoglobulin superfamily, is localized to intercellular boundaries of endothelial cells. *J Biol Chem* 2000;275:19139.
131. Arrate MP, Rodriguez JM, Tran TM, et al. Cloning of human junctional adhesion molecule 3 (JAM3) and its identification as the JAM2 counter-receptor. *J Biol Chem* 2001;276:45826.
132. Muller WA. Leukocyte-endothelial-cell interactions in leukocyte transmigration and the inflammatory response. *Trends Immunol* 2003;24: 327.
133. Luscinskas FW, Ma S, Nusrat A, et al. The role of endothelial cell lateral junctions during leukocyte trafficking. *Immunol Rev* 2002;186:57.
134. Johnson-Leger CA, Aurrand-Lions M, Beltraminelli N, et al. Junctional adhesion molecule-2 (JAM-2) promotes lymphocyte transendothelial migration. *Blood* 2002;100:2479.
135. Ostermann G, Weber KS, Zernecke A, et al. JAM-1 is a ligand of the beta(2) integrin LFA-1 involved in transendothelial migration of leukocytes. *Nat Immunol* 2002;3:151.
136. Bazzoni G, Martinez-Estrada OM, Mueller F, et al. Homophilic interaction of junctional adhesion molecule. *J Biol Chem* 2000;275:30970.
137. Barton ES, Forrest JC, Connolly JL, et al. Junction adhesion molecule is a receptor for reovirus. *Cell* 2001;104:441.
138. Liang TW, Chiu HH, Gurney A, et al. Vascular endothelial-junctional adhesion molecule (VE-JAM)/JAM 2 interacts with T, NK, and dendritic cells through JAM 3. *J Immunol* 2002;168:1618.
139. Cunningham SA, Rodriguez JM, Arrate MP, et al. JAM2 interacts with alpha4beta1. Facilitation by JAM3. *J Biol Chem* 2002;277: 27589.
140. Santoso S, Sachs UJ, Kroll H, et al. The junctional adhesion molecule 3 (JAM-3) on human platelets is a counterreceptor for the leukocyte integrin Mac-1. *J Exp Med* 2002;196:679.
141. Lucas MG, Green AM, Telen MJ. Characterisation of the serum In (Lu)-related antigen: identification of a serum protein related to erythrocyte p80. *Blood* 1989;73:596.
142. Telen MJ, Rogers I, Letarte M. Further characterisation of erythrocyte p80 and the membrane protein defect of In (Lu) Lu (a-b-) erythrocytes. *Blood* 1987;70:1475.
143. DeGrendele HC, Estess P, Picker LJ, et al. CD44 and its ligand hyaluronate mediate rolling under physiologic flow: a novel lymphocyte-endothelial cell primary adhesion pathway. *J Exp Med* 1996;183:1119.
144. Ponta H, Wainwright D, Herrlich P. The CD44 protein family. *Int J Biochem Cell Biol* 1998;30:299.
145. Borland G, Ross JA, Guy K. Forms and functions of CD-44. *Immunology* 1998;93:139.
146. Lesley J, Hyman R, English N, et al. CD44 in inflammation and metastasis. *Glycoconjugate J* 1997;14:611.
147. Mohamadzadeh M, DeGrendele H, Arizpe H, et al. Proinflammatory stimuli regulate endothelial hyaluronan expression and CD44/HA-dependent primary adhesion. *J Clin Invest* 1998;101:97.
148. Jalkanen S, Jalkanen M. Lymphocyte CD44 binds the COOH-terminal heparin-binding domain of fibronectin. *J Cell Biol* 1992;116:817.
149. Wayner EA, Carter WG. Identification of multiple cell adhesion receptors for collagen and fibronectin in human fibrosarcoma cells possessing unique alpha and distinct beta subunits. *J Cell Biol* 1987; 105:1873.
150. Jalkanen S, Bargatze RF, de la Toyos J, et al. Lymphocyte recognition of high endothelium: antibodies to distinct epitopes of an 85–95kD glycoprotein antigen differentially inhibit lymphocyte binding to lymph node, mucosal, or synovial endothelial cells. *J Cell Biology* 1987;105:983.
151. Camp RL, Scheynius A, Johansson C, et al. CD44 is necessary for optimal contact allergic responses but is not required for normal leukocyte extravasation. *J Exp Med* 1993;178:497.
152. De Grendele HC, Estess P, Siegelman MH. Requirement for CD44 in activated T cell extravasation into an inflammatory site. *Science* 1997;278:672.
153. McKee CM, Penno MB, Cowman M, et al. Hyaluronan fragments induce chemokine gene expression in alveolar macrophages: the role of HA size and CD44. *J Clin Invest* 1996;98:2403.
154. Yagi T, Takeichi M. Cadherin superfamily genes: functions, genomic organization, and neurologic diversity. *Genes Dev* 2000;14:1169.
155. Johnson KR, Lewis JE, Li D, et al. P- and E-cadherin are in separate complexes in cells expressing both cadherins. *Exp Cell Res* 1993; 207:252.
156. Cepek KL, Shaw SK, Parker CM, et al. Adhesion between epithelial cells and T lymphocytes mediated by E-cadherin and the $a^E B_7$ integrin. *Nature* 1994;372:190.
157. Gumbiner BM. Cell adhesion: the molecular basis of tissue architecture and morphogenesis. *Cell* 1996;84:345.
158. Magee AI, Buxton RS. Transmembrane molecular assemblies regulated by the greater cadherin family. *Curr Opin Cell Biol* 1991;3:854.
159. Takeichi M. Cadherins: a molecular family important in selective cell-cell adhesion. *Annu Rev Biochem* 1990;59:237.
160. Takeichi M. Morphogenetic roles of classic cadherins. *Curr Opin Cell Biol* 1995;7:619.
161. Springer TA. Traffic signals for lymphocyte recirculation and leukocyte emigration: the multistep paradigm. *Cell* 1994;76:301.
162. Price DT, Loscalzo J. Cellular adhesion molecules and atherogenesis. *Am J Med* 1999;107:85.
163. Harlan JM, Winn RK, Vedder NB, et al. *Adhesion: its role in inflammatory disease*. New York: WH Freeman, 1992.
164. Granger DN, Kvietys PR, Perry MA. Leukocyter endothelial cell adhesion induced ischemia and reperfusion. *Can J Physiol Pharmacol* 1993;71:67–75.
165. Berlin C, Bargatze RF, Campbell JJ, et al. $\alpha 4$ Integrins mediate lymphocyte attachment and rolling under physiologic flow. *Cell* 1995; 80:413.
166. Dunne JL, Ballantyne CM, Beaudet AL, et al. Control of leukocyte rolling velocity in TNF-alpha-induced inflammation by LFA-1 and Mac-1. *Blood* 2002;99:336.
167. Landis RC, Bennett RI, Hogg N. A novel LFA-1 activation epitope maps to the I domain. *J Cell Biol* 1993;120:1519.
168. Trollmo C, Nilsson I-M, Sollerman C, et al. Expression of the mucosal lymphocyte integrin $\alpha^E\beta_7$ and its ligand E-cadherin in the synovium of patients with rheumatoid arthritis. *Scand J Immunol* 1996;44:293.
169. Tervaert JWC, Kallenberg CGM. Cell adhesion molecules in vasculitis. *Curr Opin Rheum* 1997;9:16.
170. Westlin WF, Gimbrone MAJ. Neutrophil-mediated damage to human vascular endothelium. Role of cytokine activation. *Am J Pathol* 1993; 142:117.

171. Bullard DC, Hurley LA, Lorenzo I, et al. Reduced susceptibility to collagen-induced arthritis in mice deficient in intercellular adhesion molecule-1. *J Immunol* 1996;157:3153.
172. Issekutz AC, Ayer L, Miyasaka M, et al. Treatment of established adjuvant arthritis in rats with monoclonal antibody to CD18 and very late activation antigen-4 integrins suppresses neutrophil and T-lymphocyte migration to the joints and improves clinical disease. *Immunology* 1996:88:569–576.
173. Barbadillo C, G-Arroyo A, Salas C, et al. Anti-integrin immunotherapy in rheumatoid arthritis: protective effect of anti-α4 antibody in adjuvant arthritis. *Springer Semin Immunopathol* 1995;16:427.
174. Mikecz K, Brennan FR, Kim JH, et al. Anti-CD44 treatment abrogates tissue oedema and leukocyte infiltration in murine arthritis. *Nat Med* 1995;1:558.
175. Schimmer RC, Schrier DJ, Flory CM, et al. Streptococcal cell wall-induced arthritis. Requirements for neutrophils, P-selectin, intercellular adhesion molecule-1, and macrophage-inflammatory protein-2. *J Immunol* 1997;159:4103.
176. Bullard DC, King PD, Hicks MJ, et al. Intercellular adhesion molecule-1 deficiency protects MRL/MpJ-Fas^{lpr} mice from early lethality. *J Immunol* 1997;159:2058.
177. Cornejo CJ, Winn RK, Harlan JM. Anti-adhesion Therapy. *Adv Pharmacol* 1997;39:99.
178. Gottlieb A, Krueger JG, Bright R, et al. Effects of administration of a single dose of a humanized monoclonal antibody to CD11a on the immunobiology and clinical activity of psoriasis. *J Am Acad Dermatol* 2000;42:428.
179. Gottlieb AB, Krueger JG, Wittkowski K, et al. Psoriasis as a model for T-cell-mediated disease: immunobiologic and clinical effects of treatment with multiple doses of efalizumab, an anti-CD11a antibody. *Arch Dermatol* 2002;138:591.
180. Ghosh S, Goldin E, Gordon FH, et al. Natalizumab for active Crohn's disease. *N Engl J Med* 2003;348:68.
181. Miller DH, Khan OA, Sheremata WA, et al. A controlled trial of natalizumab for relapsing multiple sclerosis. *N Engl J Med* 2003; 348:15.
182. Kavanaugh AF, Davis LS, Nichols LA, et al. Treatment of refractory rheumatoid arthritis with a monoclonal antibody to intercellular adhesion molecule-1. *Arthritis Rheum* 1994;37:992.
183. Kavanaugh AF, Schulze-Koops H, Davis LS, et al. Repeat treatment of rheumatoid arthritis patients with a murine anti-intercellular adhesion molecule 1 monoclonal antibody. *Arthritis Rheum* 1997;40:849.

CHAPTER 21

Molecular Biology of the Complement System

John E. Volanakis

The relationship of the complement system to rheumatic diseases is severalfold: it mediates acute inflammatory reactions in response to triggering by immune complexes, plays a major role in the clearance of immune complexes and apoptotic cells, and regulates immune responses (1). The molecular bases for these functions of the complement system are either already known or are rapidly being clarified, and potential therapies based on these molecular principles are at the stage of development or of clinical trials. This chapter presents the background necessary to understand the role of complement in rheumatic diseases.

MOLECULAR BIOLOGY OF COMPLEMENT PROTEINS

The complement system consists of more than 35 plasma or membrane-associated proteins that participate in the activation or regulation of the system or serve as cellular receptors for biologically active products of complement activation (Table 21.1). Proteins participating in activation of complement act as recognition molecules, enzymes, enzyme cofactors, or precursors of biologically-active fragments. Regulatory proteins control the rate and extent of activation by regulating proteolytic enzymes or inactivating active products. Additionally, cell membrane–associated regulatory proteins protect host cells from complement-mediated damage (2).

C3, the most abundant complement protein in blood, is clearly the central and most versatile molecule of the complement system. It serves as the precursor for numerous fragments with diverse biologic activities and as a cofactor for several intrinsic complement enzymes. All other complement proteins appear to have evolved in order to ensure efficient and controlled production and utilization of the multiple biologically active fragments derived from C3 and from its structurally homologous protein, C5. This view is supported by available phylogenetic, functional, and structural data.

C3 is encoded as a single polypeptide chain, which, during posttranslational processing, is cleaved into two disulfide-linked chains (α and β) of 110 and 75 kd, respectively. An additional posttranslational event leads to the formation of a functionally important thioester bond between Cys1010 and Gln1013 of the α chain. The primary structure of C3 is similar to that of C5 and of the two isotypes of C4 (C4A and C4B), although C5 has no thioester bond. It seems likely that the genes encoding these four proteins represent gene duplication products, having evolved from an ancestral gene encoding a single host defense protein (3). In blood, under physiologic conditions, the internal thioester bond of C3 is relatively stable, being hydrolyzed at very slow rates, estimated at 7.2% of the plasma pool per day. C3, with a hydrolyzed thioester bond, is termed $C3_{H2O}$ and has the ability to initiate the assembly of an unstable enzyme, called initiation C3-convertase (2). This enzyme can cleave native C3 into two fragments: C3a, a small peptide; and C3b, a large two-polypeptide chain fragment. Formation of this enzyme proceeds through the binding of $C3_{H2O}$ to factor B and the subsequent cleavage of factor B by factor D, a serine proteinase, to generate the $C3_{H_2O}Bb$ complex, which is the initiation C3-convertase. The series of reactions starting with the hydrolysis of the thioester bond of C3 and concluding with the cleavage of C3 into C3a and C3b by the initiation C3-convertase is considered to occur continuously at slow rates and has been termed "C3 tickover." Thus, a supply of freshly generated C3b is always available in blood. Under normal conditions, the initiation convertase and the products of its catalytic action, C3a and C3b, are efficiently inactivated by regulatory proteins, and do not produce pathophysiologic effects.

Cleavage of C3 into C3a and C3b results in a change of the conformation of C3b associated with an extremely reactive (metastable) form of the thioester bond, which reacts avidly with nucleophiles in its immediate vicinity. Reaction with H_2O generates fluid-phase C3b, which similarly to $C3_{H_2O}$ can form an unstable initiation C3-convertase,

TABLE 21.1. *Proteins participating in the activation and regulation of the complement system*

	Approximate molecular mass (kd)	Polypeptide chains	Serum concentration (mg/mL)	Cleavage fragments
Enzymes				
Clr	80	(A, B)[a]	50	
Cls	87	(A, B)[a]	50	
MASP-1	93	(H, L)[a]	6	
MASP-2	76	(H, L)[a]	ND	
MASP-3	90	(H, L)[a]	ND	
Factor D	24	Single	2	
C2	100	Single	20	C2a, C2b
Factor B	90	Single	180	Ba, Bb
Factor I	88	H, L	35	
Recognition proteins, enzyme cofactors, and substrates				
Clq	460	$(A, B, C)_6$	100	
MBL	200–600	$(\text{homotrimer})_{2–6}$	1	
Ficolin L	387–827	$(\text{homotrimer})_{4–8}$	2–12	
Ficolin H	650	$(\text{homotrimer})_6$	7–23	
C4 (C4A and C4B)	209	α, β, γ	600	C4a, C4b, C4c, C4d
C3	190	α, β	1,300	C3a, C3b, C3bi, C3c, C3dg, C3d, C3e
C5	191	α, β	75	C5a, C5b
Cytolytic proteins				
C6	128	Single	45	
C7	95	Single	90	
C8	153	α, β, γ	80	
C9	71	Single	60	
Regulatory proteins				
C1 INH	105	Single	150	
C4 binding protein (C4bp)	540	$(a)_7b$	200	
Factor H	155	Single	520	
Factor P (properdin)	110–220	$(\text{Single})_{2–4}$	5	
S-protein (vitronectin)	80	Single	600	
Clusterin	80	α, β	50	
Decay accelerating factor (DAF, CD55)	70	Single	Membrane-associated	
Membrane cofactor protein (MCP, CD46)	51–68	Single	Membrane-associated	
CD59 (membrane inhibitor of reactive lysis, MIRL)	18	Single	Membrane-associated	
Receptors				
Complement receptor type I (CR1, CD35)	210–290	Single		
Complement receptor type II (CR2, CD21)	145	Single		
Complement receptor type III (CR3, CD11b/CD18)	165 (a) 95 (b)	α, β		
p150/95 (CR4, CD11c/CD18)	150 (a) 95 (b)	α, β		
Clq receptor (ClqRp, CD93)	126	Single		
C3a receptor (C3aR)	54	Single		
C5a receptor (C5aR, CD88)	40	Single		

Nomenclature for complement proteins follows two conventions. Proteins originally described as components of the classical pathway are symbolized with a capital C and a number. Proteins described as part of the alternative pathway are referred to as factors and symbolized with a capital letter. Cleavage fragments are symbolized with lower case letters. Regulatory proteins are usually symbolized with the initials of their descriptive names. For polypeptide chains, parentheses indicate stoichiometry.

[a]Clr, Cls, MASP-1, MASP-2, and MASP-3 are cleaved into two polypeptide chain molecules during their activation.

C1 INH, C1 inhibitor; MASP, mannose binding lectin-associated serine protease; MBL, mannose binding lectin; ND, not determined.

and, thus, can contribute to the continuous, slow-rate cleavage of native C3. Reaction of the metastable thioester bond with free hydroxyl (-OH) groups on the surface of cells, proteins, or protein complexes results in the covalent attachment of C3b to these surfaces through ester bonds (4). The fate and function of covalently-attached C3b depends on the chemical properties of the surface. Among the multiple functions of this fragment are formation of intrinsic complement enzymes that cleave C3 and C5, activation of cellular functions through interaction with specific cellular receptors, and generation of additional biologically-active fragments by the catalytic action of proteolytic enzymes.

Most of the remaining complement proteins are characterized by extensive structural similarities with conservation of a small number of structural modules or domains, indicating that multiple exon shuffling and gene duplication events marked the evolution of the system (reviewed in reference 5) (Fig. 21.1).

The nine complement enzymes, C1r, C1s, MASP-1 [mannose-binding lectin (MBL)-associated serine proteinase-1], MASP-2, MASP-3, C2, and factors B, D, and I, which are responsible, either directly or indirectly, for the production of biologically-active fragments, have in common a catalytic domain structurally similar to that found in all members of the large chymotrypsin family of serine proteinases (6). With the exception of factor D, complement enzymes have additional structural domains, derived from other gene superfamilies, which apparently provide them with protein/protein interactive sites. All complement enzymes are characterized by extremely restricted substrate specificity.

Two important complement receptors, CR1 and CR2, and four regulatory proteins, factor H, C4b binding protein (C4bp), membrane cofactor protein (MCP), and decay accelerating factor (DAF), consist almost entirely of a repeating structural motif termed short consensus repeat (SCR)

Enzymes

SP Factor D
CUB EG CUB CP CP SP MASPs/C1r/C1r
CP CP CP VA SP Factor B/C2
FM SR LA LA SP Factor I

Cytolytic

TI TI LA MACPF EG TI CP CP FM FM C6
TI LA MACPF EG TI CP CP FM FM C7
TI LA MACPF EG TI C8α/C8β
TI LA MACPF EG C9

Receptors and Regulatory

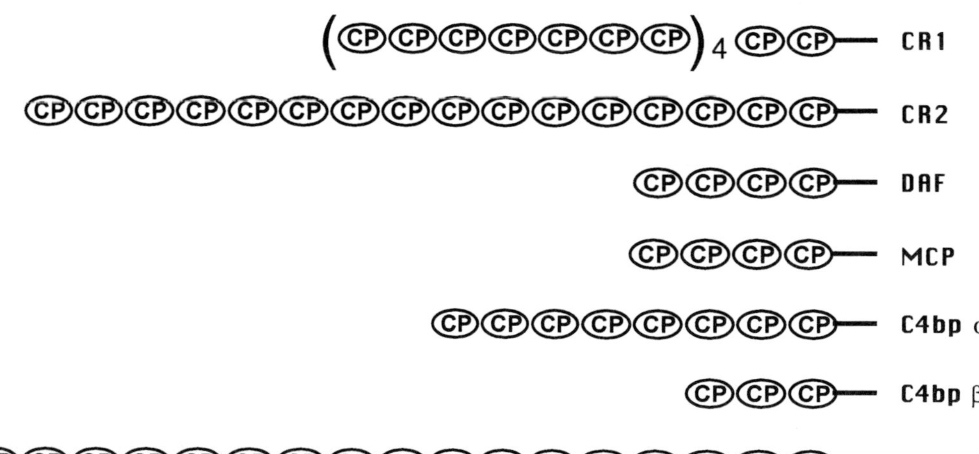

FIG. 21.1. Modular structure of complement proteins. *SP,* serine protease domain. Module designation: *CP,* complement control protein; *CUB,* first found in C1r, C1s, uEGF, bone morphogenic protein; *EG,* epidermal growth factor (EGF)-like; *FM,* factor I/membrane attack complex proteins C6/C7 (FIMAC); *LA,* low-density lipoprotein-receptor class A, (LDLRA); *MACPF,* membrane attack complex proteins/perforin; *SR,* scavenger receptor cysteine-rich; *T1,* thrombospondin type-1; *VA,* von Willebrand factor type A.

(7) or complement control protein (CCP) module. Two copies of the same structural motif are also found in C1r, C1s, MASP-1, MASP-2, MASP-3, C6, and C7, and three copies in C2 and factor B, as well as a variable number of copies in several noncomplement proteins. Functionally, SCRs provide complement proteins with a suitable structural framework for binding sites for fragments of C3, C4, and C5.

The five polypeptide chains, C6, C7, C8α, C8β, and C9, which interact with C5b and with each other to form lytic lesions on cell membranes, share a common structural domain that is also present in perforin, the cytolytic molecule of natural killer cells and cytolytic T cells (8).

Additional structural motifs for complement proteins have been derived from a variety of protein families unrelated to the complement system. A domain present in three copies in von Willebrand factor constitutes the middle domain of C2 and factor B, providing additional protein-binding sites (9). This domain is also present in single copies in two complement receptors, CR3 (10) and p150/95 (CR4), as well as in many noncomplement proteins (11). Properdin consists almost entirely of six copies of a structural motif first described in thrombospondin (12). This structural motif is also present in one or two copies in all cytolytic proteins, except C5. A cysteine-rich domain of epidermal growth factor (EGF) is present in single copies in C1r, C1s, MASP-1, MASP-2, and MASP-3, as well as in cytolytic complement proteins. A module of the low-density lipoprotein (LDL) receptor is found in single copies in cytolytic complement proteins and in two copies in factor I (13). The recognition proteins C1q, MBL, and ficolins L and H consist of collagen-like and globular protein domains (14). Finally, C1 inhibitor (C1INH) is structurally and functionally homologous to the group of serine proteinase inhibitors (serpins).

Thus, most complement proteins have a modular structure, which obviously contributes to their exquisite specificity. The genes encoding these proteins have apparently evolved from a relatively small pool of exons or exon clusters through multiple duplication events.

COMPLEMENT ACTIVATION

Activation is necessary for expression of biologic activities by the complement system. Complement activation is initiated by a wide variety of substances and proceeds through two main stages. The first stage includes a series of highly specific protein/protein interactions and proteolytic cleavages that culminate in the assembly of intrinsic complement proteinases termed C3-convertases. The proteolytic activity of these enzymes is restricted to the cleavage of a single peptide bond on the α chain of C3. Depending on the nature of the complement activator, one of three available pathways, termed classical, lectin, and alternative, is predominantly activated to yield a C3-convertase. The three activation pathways use different proteins to form

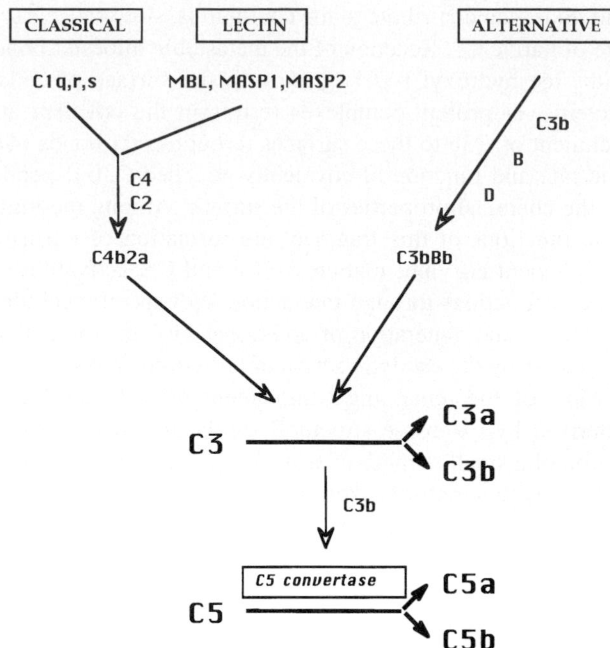

FIG. 21.2. Complement-activation pathways.

C3-convertases. All C3-convertases, however, cleave the same peptide bond of C3, giving rise to the same two fragments, C3a and C3b (Fig. 21.2). The second stage of complement activation proceeds through either of two effector pathways. The first involves successive proteolytic cleavages of surface-bound C3b and results in the generation of additional biologically active fragments. The second is initiated by the assembly of C5-convertases and concludes with the formation of large potentially cytolytic protein–protein complexes.

Assembly of C3-Convertases

In the classical pathway, the most extensively studied mechanism for assembly of the C3-convertase is the one initiated by immunoglobulin G (IgG) or IgM antibodies in complex with their respective antigens. Many other substances, including C-reactive protein (CRP) complexes, apoptotic cells, certain viruses, and gram-negative bacteria, can also initiate formation of a C3-convertase through this mechanism. Activators are recognized by C1q. In the blood of healthy individuals, C1q circulates in complex with two molecules of C1r and two molecules of C1s. This large complex, called C1, is held together by Ca^{2+}. C1q carries an activator-binding site in each of its six globular domains. In the case of immune complexes, these sites recognize structural elements in the Fc regions of antibody molecules. Binding of two or more recognition sites induces a conformational change in C1q that causes the autoactivation of proenzyme C1r to enzymatically active C1r, which in turn cleaves proenzyme C1s, converting it to active C1s (15). Next, C1s cleaves C4, resulting in the covalent attachment of its major fragment, C4b, to the surface of the activator. Attachment of C4b is accomplished through a transacylation reaction involving the thioester bond, similar to that leading to covalent binding of C3b to cell and protein surfaces. Of the two C4 isotypes, C4A preferentially forms amide linkages, whereas C4B preferentially forms ester linkages (16). In the next step of the activation sequence, C2 binds to C4b and is also cleaved by C1s into two fragments, the larger of which, C2a, remains bound to C4b, completing the assembly of the C4b2a complex, which is the C3-convertase of the classical pathway.

In the lectin pathway, recognition of pathogens is carried out by MBL and the serum ficolins L and H (14,17). All three proteins are pattern recognition lectins consisting of collagen and globular lectin domains. They are oligomers of homotrimeric subunits in which the collagen regions form a triple helix. In MBL, the lectin is a C-type carbohydrate recognition domain, whereas in the ficolins it is a fibrinogen domain. MBL has binding specificity for mannose, glucose, fucose, *N*-acetylmannosamine, and *N*-acetylglucosamine. The ficolins have specificity for *N*-acetylglucosamine. Their lectin specificity endows these proteins with the ability to bind to a variety of gram-positive and gram-negative bacteria. In blood, all three proteins circulate as complexes with homodimers of MASP-1, -2, or -3. Binding of the lectin to a bacterial cell surface leads to activation of MASP through a currently unknown mechanism. Activated MASP-2 can then sequentially activate C4 and C2 to form the C4b2a C3-convertase (18,19) (Fig. 21.2). MASP-1 has weak C3-cleaving activity (19), whereas the function of MASP-3, an alternative splicing product of the MASP-1/MASP-3 gene, remains unknown. MBL complexes also contain an additional, low-molecular-weight protein, MAP19, a product of alternative splicing of the MASP-2 transcript (20). The role of MAP19 also remains unknown.

Several mechanisms ensure that the extent of classical and lectin pathway activation is proportional to the amount and duration of presence of their activators. C1INH binds to and inhibits C1r, C1s, MASP-1, and MASP-2, regulating their activation and action. The C4b2a convertase has a short half-life; it decays as a result of dissociation of C2a in an inactive form. C4bp, DAF, and CR1 bind to C4b, blocking the binding of C2 or accelerating the dissociation of bound C2a. C4bp, MCP, and CR1 act as cofactors for factor I, a serine protease, which cleaves C4b into inactive fragments.

The alternative pathway is activated by a variety of cellular surfaces, including those of certain bacteria, viruses, fungi, and parasites (21,22). Antibodies, particularly in the form of large, insoluble complexes with antigen, can also activate this pathway. Assembly of the C3-convertase is initiated by the covalent attachment of metastable C3b to the surface of the activator. The chemical nature of the activator surface allows factor B to form a complex with C3b. Factor B bound to C3b is then cleaved by factor D into two fragments, the largest of which, Bb, remains attached to C3b. The resulting C3bBb complex is the C3-convertase of the alternative pathway. This complex has a short half-life, but it is stabilized by the binding of properdin and is usually termed the amplification C3-convertase, because it generates many C3b fragments and, thus, additional C3-convertase complexes. Metastable C3b cannot discriminate between activators and nonactivators of the alternative pathway. Thus, C3b can become covalently attached to any cell or protein surface in its vicinity, including cells of the host. However, C3b, covalently attached to the surface of a nonactivator of the alternative pathway, cannot initiate the assembly of an amplification C3-convertase, because the chemical composition of the nonactivating surface endows it with a 100-fold higher affinity for factor H than factor B (23). By comparison, C3b on the surface of a cell or particle that activates the alternative pathway has about equal affinity for factors B and H. Factor H, bound to C3b, acts as a cofactor for factor I, which cleaves C3b, thus preventing the formation of a C3-convertase. A biochemical feature determining whether a surface can function as an activator is the relative amount of sialic acid present in membrane-associated glycoproteins and glycolipids. The presence of sialic acid on a cell surface increases the affinity of C3b for factor H, which prevents the formation of the C3-convertase.

In addition to sialic acid, several membrane-associated proteins prevent the formation of an amplification C3-convertase on the surface of cells of the host. DAF and CR1 bind C3b, preventing the binding of factor B or dissociating C3b-bound Bb, causing the decay of the convertase (24). CR1 and MCP serve as cofactors for the cleavage of C3b by factor I. Each of these proteins has similar effects on the C3-convertase of the classical pathway. Thus, these regulatory proteins protect the host from the harmful potential of complement activation.

Effector Pathways of Complement Activation

A C3-convertase assembled on the surface of a complement activator can catalyze the cleavage of numerous C3 molecules. A portion of the resulting metastable C3b binds covalently to the surface of the activator around the C3-convertase site. Such C3b molecules can initiate the assembly of the amplification C3-convertase, can be recognized by CR1 receptors, or serve as precursors for smaller C3 fragments with distinct biologic functions (Fig. 21.3). Initially, factor I cleaves two neighboring peptide bonds on the α chain of C3b, resulting in the release of a small peptide, C3f, and the generation of iC3b, which remains attached to the activator surface. Both of these proteolytic cleavages require an obligatory cofactor, factor H, CR1, or MCP. iC3b cannot form a C3-convertase but reacts preferentially with CR3 and p150/95 receptors (25) and is also recognized by CR2 receptors. In the presence of CR1, factor I cleaves an additional peptide bond on the α chain of iC3b. This cleavage results in the release into the fluid phase of a large fragment, termed C3c, which consists of three polypeptide chains. The remainder of the α chain of

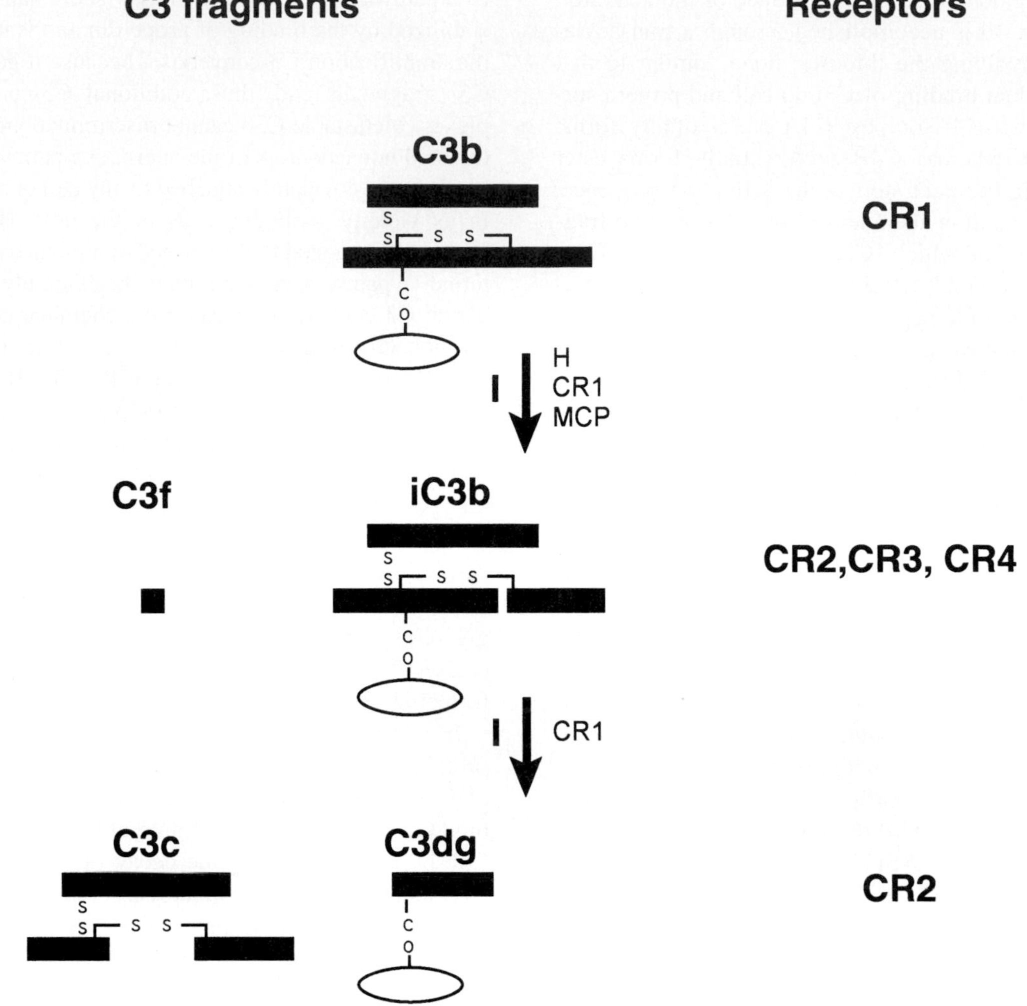

FIG. 21.3. Major cleavage fragments generated from C3b. C3b and its biologically active fragments are shown attached to an activating surface through an ester bond.

iC3b, termed C3dg, remains attached to the activator surface. C3dg is the principal ligand for CR2 receptors. Trypsin, and possibly certain serum enzymes, can cleave C3dg into two small peptides, C3g, which is released in the fluid phase, and C3d, which remains attached to the surface and is also recognized by CR2 receptors.

Metastable C3b, generated by the action of C3-convertases, can also react with nucleophiles on the noncatalytic subunits, C4b or C3b, of C3-convertases. Attachment of C3b to a C3-convertase results in the formation of a trimolecular complex, C4b2a3b or $(C3b)_2Bb$, respectively (26,27). Both of these complexes express C5-convertase proteolytic activity, which is restricted to the cleavage of the same single-peptide bond on the α chain of C5. Cleavage of C5 by a C5-convertase thus generates two fragments, C5a, a small peptide, and C5b, a large two-polypeptide chain fragment. C5b can initiate the assembly of a large protein–protein complex, termed membrane attack complex (MAC), by interacting sequentially with single molecules of C6, C7, and C8, and with 6 to 12 molecules of C9 (8). During these sequential interactions, hydrophobic regions of the participating proteins become exposed on the surface of the complex. Assembly of the complex on the surface of a biologic membrane favors interactions of these hydrophobic regions with the fatty acid chains of phospholipids. The complex becomes gradually inserted into the lipid bilayer and eventually forms a transmembrane channel, which can elicit cellular functions (28) or lead to the killing of susceptible cells. This process is regulated by several proteins. The serum proteins vitronectin and clusterin inhibit the formation of the MAC, precluding its interaction with lipid bilayers (29,30). The cell-associated protein, CD59 (29), inhibits the formation of the MAC on cell membranes of the host by binding to the cytolytic complex at the C5b678 step.

BIOLOGY OF THE COMPLEMENT SYSTEM

The generation of ligands, mainly from C3 and C5, for various cellular receptors (Tables 21.2 and 21.3) enables the complement system to alter the function of cells in-

TABLE 21.2. *Soluble mediators of complement biology*

Mediator	Biologic response
C3a	Anaphylatoxin (histamine release; smooth muscle contraction), chemotaxin for eosinophils
C5a	Anaphylatoxin; chemotaxin and secretagogue for myelomonocytic cells; secretagogue for mast cells and basophils; augmented expression of CR1 and CR3 on myelomonocytic cells; costimulant for LTC_4 production with IL-3 and IL-5 production in basophils; production of tumor necrosis factor and IL-1 by monocyte/macrophages
C3e	Leukocytosis

IL, interleukin; LTC_4, leukotriene C_4.

volved in inflammatory and immune reactions. Inflammation is the phylogenetically older of these two biologic functions, and complement participation is relatively well understood, whereas complement's role in the immune response, which connects these otherwise independent recognition systems, probably evolved later and has only recently begun to approach a molecular level of characterization (31,32). The biology of complement will be reviewed in relation to these two functions and their involvement in human disease.

Complement and Acute Inflammation

The acute inflammatory response is the principal means of host defense against infection by pyogenic bacteria. The microbicidal reactions of inflammation interfere with basic biologic requirements that are shared by prokaryotes and eukaryotes so that this process causes human disease when it is excessive or misdirected against host tissue. The complement system can elicit all aspects of acute inflammation and frequently is activated in inflammatory diseases of autoimmune or unknown etiology.

Acute inflammation is a stereotypical series of reactions that includes microvascular changes and the selective accumulation of myelomonocytic cells, whose function is regulated by locally formed mediators. Three products of complement activation (C3a, C5a, and the C5b-9 MAC) elicit vascular changes characteristic of inflammation. C3a and C5a diffuse locally from the site of complement activation to interact with their respective receptors, C3aR (33) and C5aR (34), on either mast cells or basophils, causing the release of vasoactive mediators, such as histamine and leukotrienes (35). The C5b-9 complex can cause drastic changes in the microvasculature when formed on endothelial cells, by creating transient calcium channels at the plasma membrane (36,37). The resulting increase in intracellular calcium induces a secretory response involving endothelial intracellular granules, the Weibel-Palade bodies, which contain von Willebrand factor and factor V of the coagulation pathway and whose perigranular membrane expresses GMP-140, a selectin that promotes the attachment of leukocytes. In terms of host antimicrobial defense, the consequences of this secretory reaction are the recruitment of cells with bactericidal capability and the formation of a clot to "wall off" the area and prevent the intravascular dissemination of bacteria. This process may also lead to ischemic necrosis of host tissue.

Studies on animal models of ischemia-reperfusion injury have provided evidence that complement activation is initiated by natural IgM antibodies reacting with epitopes on the surface of injured endothelial cells (reviewed in reference 38). Presumably, the normal, noncomplement-activating state of endothelial cells, which is maintained by the expression of DAF, MCP, and CD59, membrane proteins with complement regulatory functions, is overcome by the activation of the classical pathway. When excessive, these proinflammatory changes on the surface of the endothelium, coupled with thc attachment of C3b and iC3b, which further promote the adherence of leukocytes (39), can lead to extensive damage to host tissue. A florid example of C5b-9-mediated endothelial changes is the hemorrhagic necrosis occurring with hyperacute allograft and xenograft rejection, reactions that are caused by antiendothelial antibodies that activate complement.

TABLE 21.3. *Receptors for complement proteins that are bound to activators*

Receptor	Ligand	Cells
CR1	C3b; C4b	Erythrocytes; myelomonocytic cells; B and some T cells; follicular dendritic cells; glomerular podocytes
CR2	C3bi; C3dg	B and some T cells; some thymocytes; follicular dendritic cells
CR3	C3bi and several noncomplement ligands	Myelomonocytic
CR4	C3bi and C3dg	Neutrophils; platelets
ClqRp	Clq	Myelomonocytic cells; endothelial cells; platelets

The complement system also induces fundamental changes in myelomonocytic cells that lead to their accumulation at sites of complement activation. Leukocytes must engage in at least three distinct reactions for this process to occur: adherence to endothelial cells; passage between endothelial cells and across the underlying basement membrane; and movement toward the site of infection. C5a can mediate all three reactions, and intradermal injection of this peptide causes the rapid perivascular infiltration of neutrophils. C5a regulates neutrophil function by binding to its receptor (C5aR), which has a structure typical of seven-transmembrane domain, G protein–coupled, rhodopsin family receptors (34). Engagement of the receptor triggers the rapid up-regulation of CR1 and CR3 on myelomonocytic cells and increases the avidity of CR3 for its counterreceptor on vascular endothelial cells, intracellular adhesion molecule-1 (ICAM-1) (40), which causes leukocyte-endothelial interaction (Chapter 20). The importance of CR3, which is a member of the leukocyte integrin family of proteins, for the process of leukocyte accumulation at sites of bacterial infection is emphasized by the inability of cells from patients with an inherited deficiency in this family of proteins to adhere to natural and artificial substrata and to appear at tissue sites of infection (reviewed in reference 41).

Neutrophils and monocytes that have adhered to endothelial cells then respond to C5a by migrating between endothelial cells and across the basement membrane, without causing a disruption of the vessel wall. Only if complement activation is occurring in the vessel wall, as with immune complex–induced vasculitis and ischemia-reperfusion injury, does damage to this structure ensue. When the myelomonocytes reach the interstitial tissues, they respond by migrating along the gradient of C5a in a process termed chemotaxis and, in this manner, become concentrated at the site of complement activation. C5a also increases the proinflammatory potential of these cells by inducing a respiratory burst and the secretion of tumor necrosis factor (42). The C5a peptide, in the presence of interleukin-3 (IL-3) (43) and IL-5 (44), also causes basophils to synthesize and secrete large amounts of leukotriene C_4 (LTC_4).

The purpose for which myelomonocytic cells accumulate in tissue is the phagocytosis and intracellular killing of bacteria. Phagocytosis by these cells requires that receptors be engaged by ligands on the bacteria, and complement provides two relevant ligands by virtue of the covalent attachment of C3b and iC3b. CR1 and CR3 mediate the cellular binding of particles bearing these C3 fragments, which greatly enhances phagocytosis triggered by Fc receptors. Induction of phagocytosis by CR1 and CR3 requires that the cells be activated by chemotactic peptides, such as C5a, or by proteins present in the intercellular matrix. Furthermore, phagocytosis mediated solely by CR1 or CR3 differs fundamentally from that caused by Fc receptors in that it does not induce a respiratory burst. There are circumstances for which it is advantageous to clear certain complement-activating substances without eliciting the full repertoire of bactericidal functions of these cells. A consequence of this "quiet" phagocytosis is that certain intracellular pathogens have usurped this pathway to gain entry into macrophages without inducing a microbicidal response.

Soluble CR1: A Model Inhibitor of Complement-Dependent Inflammation

Acute inflammation, although necessary for the elimination of microorganisms, can lead to the destruction of normal tissue when the infectious source cannot be eliminated (e.g., abscesses); when initiated by physically injured tissues (e.g., ischemia, burn, or crush injury); or when initiated by antigen–antibody complexes that have formed in tissue, the antigen being from foreign or host origin. Examples of animal models of human diseases in which the complement system has been shown to play a pathogenetic role are listed in Table 21.4 and include diseases affecting many organ systems. These studies have been based on determining whether disease occurs in rats or mice rendered deficient in C3 and C5 by treatment with cobra venom factor, or in mice having a genetically engineered or naturally inherited deficiency of a complement component or receptor. Conclusions regarding the role of complement in the human counterparts of these animal models are based on indirect evidence, because it has not been possible to regulate activation of complement in humans. However, the finding in 1990 that a soluble, recombinant form of human CR1 is an effective inhibitor of complement in rats indicates that complement inhibition in humans may soon be possible (45).

CR1 was first recognized functionally as an entity on erythrocytes and neutrophils that mediated the adherence of C3b-coated particles and enhanced the phagocytosis of particles also bearing IgG (reviewed in references 7 and 46). It is now evident that the role of CR1 in the complement system is more complex and may be summarized as the capture of complement-activating complexes followed by the processing of the complexes to a noncomplement-activating state and the transfer of the complexes to other receptors. CR1 is a cofactor for the factor I–mediated cleavage of C4b and C3b to fragments that no longer bind to CR1, or interact at a markedly lower affinity, so that

TABLE 21.4. *Animal models of human diseases in which tissue injury is complement dependent*

Autoimmune model	Nonspecific tissue injury
Myasthenia gravis	Burns
Experimental allergic encephalitis	Myocardial ischemia
Experimental allergic neuritisd	
Heymann nephritis	
Immune complex–induced vasculitis	
Anti-GPI antibody–induced arthritis	
Collagen-induced arthritis	

the receptor releases these ligands rather than maintaining a stable ligand–receptor complex. Furthermore, these fragments of C4b and C3b have lost the complement-activating functions of their parent molecules, and two fragments, iC3b and C3dg, are ligands for the other C3 receptors, CR2 and CR3. Therefore, although CR1 has been shown to have certain biologic functions on myelomonocytes and B lymphocytes, its unique role in the complement system may be to suppress further complement activation by antigen–antibody complexes, once sufficient C3b has been bound to such complexes to mediate cellular uptake, and to participate in the processing of C3b into iC3b and C3dg, forms capable of ligating other receptors with signal-transducing capability.

This view of CR1 is consistent with the receptor being a member of the regulators of complement activation (RCA) family of complement proteins. The extracytoplasmic domain of CR1 is a filamentous structure made up entirely of 30 tandemly aligned SCRs. The SCR, also termed CCP, has an elongated β-barrel structure with the long axis running between the amino (N)- and carboxy (C)-termini. It consists of a central anti-parallel β-sheet with two extended loops flanked by short antiparallel β sheets (47). There is a single membrane-spanning region and a cytoplasmic domain of 43 amino acids. Twenty-eight of the SCRs are divided into four long homologous repeats (LHRs), termed LHR-A, -B, -C, and -D, each having seven SCRs. The LHRs are considered to have arisen by duplication of genomic segments containing the eight exons encoding the seven SCRs because the SCRs occupying corresponding positions in the LHRs are 60% to 100% identical. As shown in Fig. 21.4, LHR-A binds C4b, and LHR-B and -C each have a C3b-/C4b-binding site; LHR-D does not bind either complement protein and may serve to extend the ligand-binding domains from the plasma membrane. Analysis of deletion mutants and chimeric constructs has shown that the first three SCRs of LHR-B and -C account for all of the C3b-binding functions of these LHRs (48,49). The C4b-binding domain of CR1 consists of the first three SCRs of LHR-A. The fifth through seventh SCRs of the first three LHRs perhaps serve as a spacer between the ligand-binding domains to permit multivalent interaction of the receptor with complexes bearing multiple molecules of C3b and C4b. The structural features of CR1 account for its bispecificity and multivalency and contribute to its complement-inhibitory function being greater than the other members of the RCA family. CR1 is a cofactor for the cleavage by factor I of both C3b and C4b, and it decay-dissociates the classical, lectin, and alternative pathway C3/C5-convertases, a composite of functions achieved only by both plasma RCA proteins, H and C4bp, and by both membrane proteins, DAF and MCP. The multivalency of CR1 allows it to bind to dimers and higher order oligomers of C3b and C4b at least bivalently, yielding dissociation constants in the nanomolar range rather than the micromolar range of monovalent interactions (45). Most importantly, CR1 binds to C3b on alternative pathway activating and nonactivating surfaces

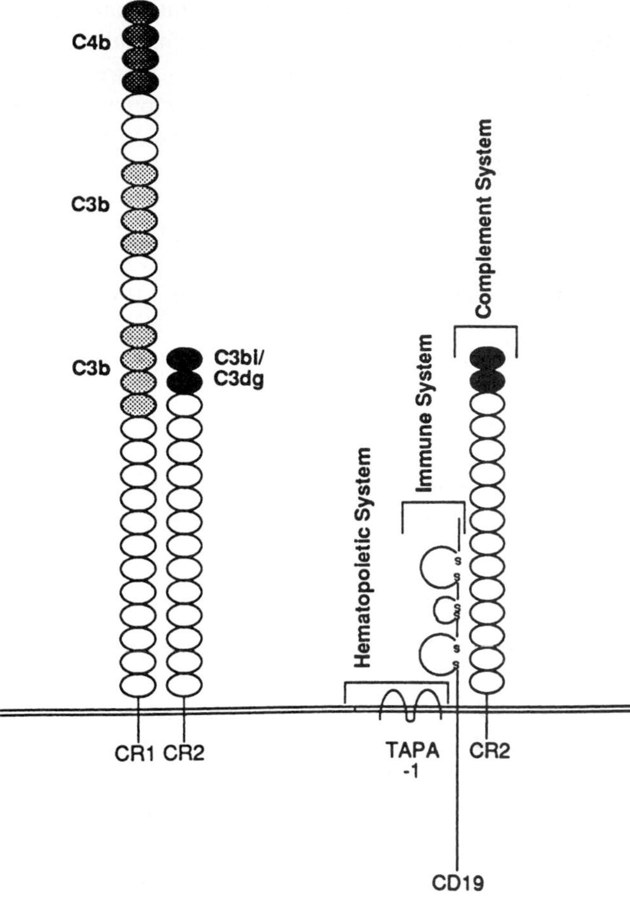

FIG. 21.4. CR1 and CR2, the location of their ligand-binding sites, and their participation in molecular complexes on B lymphocytes. *TAPA-1,* target of an antiproliferative antibody-1.

with equivalent affinities and is equally effective at suppressing complement activation on either surface, whereas H and DAF (50) are less effective inhibitors of alternative pathway activators because their functions are restricted by these surfaces.

CR1 does not have a significant complement inhibitory role *in vivo,* relative to the other RCA proteins, because of its limited tissue distribution (Table 21.3). However, a soluble form of the receptor that was genetically engineered by deleting the cytoplasmic and transmembrane domains was at least 100-fold more effective than the endogenous RCA proteins, H and C4bp, in suppressing complement activation by the classical and alternative pathways and blocked complement activation in rat models of myocardial reperfusion injury (45), hyperacute allograft (51), and xenograft rejection (52). These studies suggested that the marked complement inhibitory functions of CR1, which permit this membrane protein to capture and process C3b-bearing complexes, can be used for therapy of human inflammatory diseases mediated by complement activation.

During the past decade, efforts to develop effective and safe therapeutic agents to prevent or reduce complement activation *in vivo* have multiplied. Several products have been shown beneficial in animal models of inflammatory and autoimmune diseases and a few are in clinical trials (reviewed in 53 and 54). Among these products are modified soluble CR1 constructs, including a recombinant form of CR1 expressing sialyl Lewis^x tetrasaccharide groups (55). This modification allows targeting the receptor at the endothelium by binding to P-, E-, and L-selectins. Other anticomplement agents include monoclonal anti-C5 antibodies that inhibit activation of C5 and have been shown to inhibit a variety of mouse and rat models of inflammatory disease, including collagen-induced arthritis in mice and to delay the onset of glomerulonephritis in systemic lupus erythematosus (SLE)-prone NZB/W F1 mice (56). Finally, a cyclic peptide that is a potent antagonist of the C5a receptor has been shown to reduce the severity of various rat models of inflammatory disease, including antigen-induced arthritis (57). This peptide has the advantage of being active orally.

Complement and the Processing of Immune Complexes

Complement has a paradoxic relationship with immune complex–mediated diseases, especially SLE. On the one hand there is evidence for complement participation in the pathogenesis of tissue injury in many of these diseases, and on the other hand genetic deficiencies of proteins of the classical pathway are strongly associated with SLE. Characteristically, the prevalence of SLE among individuals with C1q deficiency is 93% and it declines gradually in deficiency of C1r, C1s, C4, and C2. This association suggests a role of the classical pathway in protecting against the development of SLE (58). Several non–mutually exclusive mechanisms have been proposed for the protective action of complement. Included are the role of complement in the clearance of immune complexes and apoptotic cells, and its contribution to the regulation of immune responses.

The complement system alters the distribution and clearance of antigen–antibody complexes by two mechanisms: maintaining the solubility of immune complexes and directing the clearance of intravascular complexes to the reticuloendothelial system. These effects of complement on the metabolism of immune complexes may decrease their deposition in tissues and lessen the possibility of their causing inflammatory tissue damage and activation of B cells.

The formation of insoluble aggregates of antigen and antibody is suppressed by the classical pathway through the binding of C1q, C4b, and C3b to antibody in the complexes. Maintenance of the solubility of immune complexes permits clearance mechanisms to capture these complexes and prevent their deposition in tissues. Complement also provides a means by which preformed insoluble immune complexes can be solubilized through the alternative pathway. Although most soluble antigen–antibody complexes cannot activate the alternative pathway, large insoluble aggregates have this capability. The marked generation of C3b and binding of this protein to antibody solubilizes the antigen–antibody complexes. Complementing these reactions that create soluble immune complexes is a process for the clearance of intravascular C3b-containing complexes that involves the erythrocyte (reviewed in reference 59). Human erythrocytes express a genetically regulated low number of CR1, ranging from approximately 100 to 1,000 per cell, but the large quantity of erythrocytes in blood constitutes an important reservoir of immune complex binding activity, and, as long as complexes remain attached to CR1 on erythrocytes, they cannot deposit in tissues. When erythrocytes pass through the major reticuloendothelial organ, the liver, the bound complexes are released, probably transferred to Kupffer cells. The transfer may involve the capacity of CR1 to mediate the cleavage by factor I of bound C3b to iC3b, resulting in a 100-fold decrease in binding to CR1; Kupffer cells express both CR3, which binds iC3b, and Fc receptors for the IgG component of the immune complexes, and should bind the antigen–antibody complexes as they are released from the erythrocytes. A defect in this clearance mechanism may accentuate immune complex–mediated disease processes.

Complement and the Clearance of Apoptotic Cells

Keratinocytes that undergo apoptosis after exposure to ultraviolet light or following viral infection generate subcellular structures termed surface blebs, which are rich in nuclear antigens frequently targeted by autoantibodies in SLE (60). It has been demonstrated that normal mice injected with apoptotic cells develop antinuclear autoantibodies, including anti-single-stranded DNA (ssDNA) and antiphospholipid antibodies (61). It was shown that C1q binds specifically and directly to the surface blebs of apoptotic keratinocytes (62) and mice rendered C1q deficient (C1q$^{-/-}$) by gene targeting develop glomerulonephritis characterized by immune deposits and multiple apoptotic cell bodies (63,64). C1q$^{-/-}$ mice also develop autoantibodies. The combined data indicate that complement, specifically C1q, is necessary for the clearance of apoptotic cells, which have the potential to cause autoantibody production and immune complex tissue injury.

Complement and the Immune Response

Recognition of foreign antigens by the complement system involves a developmentally simple, relatively nonpolymorphic system of plasma proteins and cellular receptors, which contrasts with the complex developmental process that selects highly polymorphic cellular antigen receptors involved in recognition by the immune system. The complement and immune systems are also distinguished by the absence of shared structural motifs. Nevertheless, the complement and immune systems intersect at two points. The Fc region of IgM and IgG antibody binds the C1q subunit of C1 to initiate activation of the classical pathway, and CR2 associates with CD19 (65), a member of the immunoglobulin superfamily that is expressed only on B lymphocytes and has an essential role in B-cell activation by

T cell–dependent antigens as well as in the maturation of B cells into the memory compartment (66).

The absence of C3 or C4 in gene-targeted mice is associated with an impaired primary antibody response to limited, but not high, concentrations of T cell–dependent antigens (67). Humans who have inherited deficiencies of C1q, C4, C2, or C3 have low constitutive serum levels of IgG4 (68), suggesting that complement has a role in isotype switching. The enhancement of the primary antibody response by antigen-specific IgM is dependent on the capacity of the IgM to activate complement and on the presence of C3. Complement enhances immune responses by attaching C3 fragments to antigen, either following binding of polyspecific IgM and activation of the classical pathway, or by the lectin or the alternative pathway if the antigen has the appropriate surface characteristics. The presence of C3b, iC3b, or C3dg on the antigen facilitates localization of antigen to two cell types involved in the primary antibody response: B lymphocytes, which express CR1 and CR2; and follicular dendritic cells, which express CR1, CR2, and CR3, and are involved more in the development of memory B lymphocytes than in primary responses. Follicular dendritic cells retain antigen for interaction with germinal center B cells, a function necessary for the generation of normal immune responses and especially for vigorous secondary antibody responses (69,70). On B cells, complement receptors are involved in transduction of signals that are important for the regulation of their responses.

Of the two complement receptors on B lymphocytes, CR1 and CR2, the latter mediates the enhancing effect of complement on the primary antibody response. Human CR2 is similar structurally to CR1 in that it contains an extracytoplasmic domain of 16 SCRs, one of which is alternatively spliced with no known functional consequences, a single membrane-spanning region, and a 34–amino acid, carboxy-terminal cytoplasmic domain. The ligand-binding site for iC3b and C3dg is made up by the two amino-terminal SCRs, which also mediate binding of the Epstein-Barr virus (71,72). CR2 probably does not directly transmit signals to B cells but is a ligand-binding subunit of two distinct membrane protein complexes: a bimolecular complex of CR2 and CR1 (73), and a CR2-CD19-TAPA-1 complex (65,74) (Fig. 21.4). The CR2–CR1 complex has no signal-transducing capability and its primary purpose probably is to capture antigen coated with C3b and facilitate processing of C3b to iC3b and C3dg, thus allowing the antigen–C3dg complex to transfer to the CR2 component of the complex, which may then diffuse away to become associated with CD19.

The CR2–CD19–TAPA-1 complex is probably the critical site at which the complement and immune systems interact. CR2 associates directly with CD19, a member of the immunoglobulin superfamily restricted to cells of the B lineage, being expressed from the earliest recognizable stage of B-cell development through mature B cells and memory B cells. CR2 is expressed predominantly on mature B cells, so that this membrane protein complex lacks CR2 through most of the developmental stages of the B cell. The two immunoglobulin-like domains in the extracytoplasmic portion of CD19 are linked to a large cytoplasmic region of approximately 247 amino acids, which interacts with cytosolic components involved in signal transduction. CD19 associates with TAPA-1 (74), which is not specific for lymphocytes, is homologous to the leukocyte antigen, CD37, and the ME491 melanoma-associated antigen, and is distinctive in having four membrane-spanning regions (75). CR1 is not present in the complex despite its capacity to associate with CR2, indicating that an individual CR2 molecule associates either with CR1 or CD19, but not both at the same time.

CR2 serves as a ligand-binding subunit of the complex linking the complement system to this signal transduction complex of the immune system. CD19 also is likely to have a ligand-binding function because it is the only component of the complex that is unique to the B lymphocyte and is present throughout the B lineage. Recently, IgM and heparin/heparan sulfate were recognized as ligands of CD19 (76). Obviously, antigen-bound IgM could cross-link CD19 to the antigen receptor on B cells, although the role of heparin/heparan sulfate is less clear. CD19 may be involved in signal transduction by two mechanisms: its large cytoplasmic domain suggests a capacity for interaction with cytosolic proteins, and its association with TAPA-1 links it to cellular reactions triggered by this protein. TAPA-1 is expressed on non-B cells, and antibodies to this protein cause cellular aggregation.

The CR2–CD19–TAPA-1 complex couples to cytosolic effectors through the cytoplasmic domain of CD19 (77), including lyn, phosphatidylinositol 3-kinase (PI3 kinase), and Vav. Lyn is an *src*-related protein tyrosine kinase with which CD19 associates constitutively. PI3 kinase and Vav contain src homology 2 (SH2) domains that mediate their binding to CD19 after the latter is tyrosine phosphorylated when membrane Ig (mIg) is ligated. PI3 kinase phosphorylates phosphatidylinositol-4,5-bisphosphate (PIP_2) to generate PIP_3. Although the mechanisms are not clarified, PIP_3 is a second messenger that may account for the important role of PI3 kinase in several cellular responses, including cytoskeletal organization, endocytosis, vesicular trafficking, and proliferation. Vav is a protooncogene whose function has not yet been defined; however, interruption of Vav expression in mice impairs the development and function of B and T cells.

Functional studies of the CR2/CD19/TAPA-1 complex indicate that it synergizes with mIg for B-cell activation (78). Cross-linking CR2 or CD19 to mIg in model systems enhances the generation of inositol triphosphate (IP_3) and the release of free intracellular Ca^{2+}, and lowers by two orders of magnitude the number of mIg molecules that must be ligated to induce B-cell proliferation. The immunizing dose of hen egg lysozyme (HEL) required to induce the production of IgG1 anti-HEL and memory B cells in mice is reduced by 1,000- to 10,000-fold when three copies of C3d are attached to the antigen (79). This effect of C3d is blocked by the coadministration of antibody either to CR2 or CD19, suggesting that it is mediated by the cross-linking of the complex to mIg on B cells. Thus, the CR2–CD19–TAPA-1 complex can reset the threshold at which the immune system responds to an antigen, a function that probably evolved to promote the immunologic recognition of microorganisms, but which may lead to autoimmunity when self-antigen is coated with C3dg.

In the mouse, CR1 and CR2 are alternatively spliced products of the same gene, termed *Cr2*. Mice made *Cr2*$^{-/-}$ deficient by gene targeting have severe defects in antibody responses to T-cell-dependent antigens (80) and in the number, size, and persistence of germinal centers within specific follicles (81). They also have a reduction in the population of peritoneal CD5^{+} B-1 cells (82). A similar although more profound phenotype is seen in CD19$^{-/-}$ mice (66,83), which supports the contention that the CR2 and CD19 are members of the same signal-transducing complex. It is relevant that overexpression of CD19 in transgenic mice is associated with high levels of autoantibodies (84,85). Therefore, it appears that CD19 has an important regulatory function for the balance between peripheral tolerance and autoimmunity. Experiments using *Cr2*$^{-/-}$ mice have indicated that CR2 also plays a similar role in maintaining peripheral tolerance (86).

These combined studies have produced important insights into the possible participation of complement in the pathogenesis of autoimmune diseases and have provided clues about future therapeutic approaches.

REFERENCES

1. Walport MJ. Complement. *N Engl J Med* 2001;344:1058–1066, 1140–1144.
2. Volanakis JE. Overview of the complement system. In: Volanakis JE, Frank MM, eds. *The human complement system in health and disease.* New York: Marcel Dekker, 1998:9–32.
3. Sunyer JO, Zarkadis IK, Lambris JD. Complement diversity: a mechanism for generating immune diversity? *Immunol Today* 1998;19:519–523.
4. Gadjeva M, Dodds AW, Taniguchi-Sidle A, et al. The covalent binding reaction of complement component C3. *J Immunol* 1998;161:985–990.
5. Campbell RD, Law SKA, Reid KBM, et al. Structure, organization, and regulation of the complement genes. *Annu Rev Immunol* 1988;6:161–195.
6. Arlaud G, Volanakis JE, Thielens NM, et al. The atypical serine proteases of the complement system. *Adv Immunol* 1998;69:249–307.
7. Ahearn JM, Fearon DT. Structure and function of the complement receptors CR1 (CD35) and CR2 (CD21). *Adv Immunol* 1989;46:183–219.
8. Plumb ME, Sodetz JM. Proteins of the membrane attack complex. In: Volanakis JE, Frank MM, eds. *The human complement system in health and disease.* New York: Marcel Dekker, 1998:119–148.
9. Tuckwell DS, Xu Y, Newham P, et al. Surface loops adjacent to the cation-binding site of the complement factor B von Willebrand factor type A module determine C3b binding specificity. *Biochemistry* 1997;36:6605–6613.
10. Lee J-O, Rieu P, Arnaout MA, et al. Crystal structure of the A domain from the a subunit of integrin CR3(CD11b/CD18). *Cell* 1995;80:631–638.
11. Perkins SJ, Smith KF, Williams SC, et al. The secondary structure of the von Willebrand factor type A domain in factor B of human complement by Fourier transform infrared spectroscopy. *J Mol Biol* 1994;238:104–119.
12. Goundis D, Reid KBM. Properdin, the terminal complement components, thrombospondin and the circumsporozite protein of malaria parasites contain similar sequence motifs. *Nature* 1988;335:82–85.
13. Catteral CF, Lyons A, Sim RB, et al. Characterization of the primary amino acid sequence of human complement control protein factor I from an analysis of cDNA clones. *Biochem J* 1987;242:849–856.
14. Holmskov U, Thiel S, Jensenius JC. Collectins and ficolins: humoral lectins of the innate immune system. *Ann Rev Immunol* 2003;21:547–578.
15. Gregory LA, Thielens NM, Arlaud GJ, et al. X-ray structure of the Ca^{2+}-binding interaction domain of C1s: insights into the assembly of the C1 complex of complement. *J Biol Chem* 2003;278:32157–32164.
16. Law SK, Dodds AW. The internal thioester and the covalent binding properties of the complement proteins C3 and C4. *Protein Sci* 1997;6:263–274.
17. Matsushita M, Fujita T. Ficolins and the lectin complement pathway. *Immunol Rev* 2001;180:78–85.
18. Thiel S, Vorup-Jensen T, Stover TM, et al. A second serine protease associated with mannan-binding lectin that activates complement. *Nature* 1997;386:506–510.
19. Rossi V, Cseh S, Bally I, et al. Substrate specificities of recombinant mannan-binding lectin-associated serine proteases-1 and -2. *J Biol Chem* 2001;276:40880–40887.
20. Stover CM, Thiel S, Thelen M, et al. Two constituents of the initiation complex of the mannan-binding lectin activation pathway of complement are encoded by a single structural gene. *J Immunol* 1999;162:3481–3490.
21. Fearon DT, Austen KF. The alternative pathway of complement: a system for host defense of microbial infection. *N Engl J Med* 1980;303:259–263.
22. Pangburn MK, Müller-Eberhard HJ. The alternative pathway of complement. *Springer Semin Immunopathol* 1984;7:163–192.
23. Fearon DT. Regulation by membrane sialic acid of β1H-dependent decay-dissociation of amplification C3 convertase of the alternative complement pathway. *Proc Natl Acad Sci U S A* 1978;75:1971–1975.
24. Liszewski MK, Atkinson JP. Regulatory proteins of complement. In: Volanakis JE, Frank MM, eds. *The human complement system in health and disease.* New York: Marcel Dekker, 1998:149–165.
25. Ross GD, Medof ME. Membrane complement receptors specific for bound fragments of C3. *Adv Immunol* 1985;37:217–267.
26. Takata Y, Kinoshita T, Kozono H, et al. Covalent association of C3b with C4b within C5 convertase of the classical complement pathway. *J Exp Med* 1987;165:1494–1507.
27. Kinoshita T, Takata Y, Kozono H, et al. C5 convertase of the alternative complement pathway: covalent linkage between two C3b molecules within the trimolecular complex enzyme. *J Immunol* 1988;141:3895–3901.
28. Rus HG, Niculescu FI, Shin ML. Role of the C5b-9 complement complex in cell cycle and apoptosis. *Immunol Rev* 2001;180:49–55.
29. Morgan BP. Regulation of the complement membrane attack pathway. *Crit Rev Immunol* 1999;19:173–198.
30. Turnberg D, Botto M. The regulation of the complement system: insights from genetically-engineered mice. *Mol Immunol* 2003;40:145–153.
31. Carroll MC. The role of complement and complement receptors in induction and regulation of immunity. *Annu Rev Immunol* 1998;16:545–568.
32. Fearon DT. The complement system and adaptive immunity. *Semin Immunol* 1998;10:355–361.
33. Ames RS, Li Y, Sarau HM, et al. Molecular cloning and characterization of the human anaphylatoxin C3a receptor. *J Biol Chem* 1996;271:20231–20234.
34. Gerard NP, Gerard C. The chemotactic receptor for human C5a anaphylatoxin. *Nature* 1991;349:614–617
35. Ember JA, Jagels MA, Hugli TE. Characterization of complement anaphylatoxins and their biological responses. In: Volanakis JE, Frank MM, eds. *The human complement system in health and disease.* New York: Marcel Dekker, 1998:241–284.
36. Hattori R, Hamilton KK, McEver RP, et al. Complement proteins C5b-9 induce secretion of high molecular weight multimers of endothelial von Willebrand factor and translocation of granule membrane protein GMP-140 to the cell surface. *J Biol Chem* 1989;264:9053–9060.
37. Hamilton KK, Hattori R, Esmon CT, et al. Complement proteins C5b-9 induce vesiculation of the endothelial plasma membrane and expose catalytic surface for assembly of the prothrombinase enzyme complex. *J Biol Chem* 1990;265: 3809–3814.
38. Barrington R, Zhang M, Fisher M, Carroll MC. The role of complement in inflammation and adaptive immunity. *Immunol Rev* 2001;180:5–15.

39. Marks RM, Todd RF III, Ward PA. Rapid induction of neutrophil-endothelial adhesion by endothelial complement fixation. *Nature* 1989;339:314–317.
40. Diamond MS, Staunton DE, Marlin SD, et al. Binding of the integrin Mac-1 (CD11b/CD18) to the third immunoglobulin-like domain of ICAM-1 (CD54) and its regulation by glycosylation. *Cell* 1991;65: 961–971.
41. Springer TA. The sensation and regulation of interactions with the extracellular environment: the cell biology of lymphocyte adhesion receptors. *Annu Rev Cell Biol* 1990;6:359–402.
42. Okusawa S, Yancey KB, van der Meer JWM, et al. C5a stimulates secretion of tumor necrosis factor from human mononuclear cells *in vitro*. Comparison with secretion of interleukin 1 beta and interleukin 1 alpha. *J Exp Med* 1988;168:443–448.
43. Kurimoto Y, de Weck AL, Dahinden CA. Interleukin 3-dependent mediator release in basophils triggered by C5a. *J Exp Med* 1989;170:467–479.
44. Bischoff SC, Brunner T, de Weck AL, et al. Interleukin 5 modifies histamine release and leukotriene generation by human basophils in response to diverse agonists. *J Exp Med* 1990;172:1577–1582.
45. Weisman HF, Bartow T, Leppo MK, et al. Soluble human complement receptor type 1: *in vivo* inhibitor of complement suppressing post-ischemic myocardial inflammation and necrosis. *Science* 1990;249: 146–151.
46. Hourcade D, Holers VM, Atkinson JP. The regulators of complement activation (RCA) gene cluster. *Adv Immunol* 1989;45:381–416.
47. Smith BO, Mallin RL, Krych-Goldberg M, et al. Structure of the C3b binding site of CR1 (CD35), the immune adherence receptor. *Cell* 2002;108:769–780.
48. Kalli KR, Hsu P, Bartow TJ, et al. Mapping of the C3b-binding site of CR1 and construction of a (CR1)2-F(ab8)2 chimeric complement inhibitor. *J Exp Med* 1991;174:1451–1460.
49. Krych-Goldberg M, Atkinson JP. CR1 and CR1-like: the primate immune adherence receptors. *Immunol Rev* 2001;180:112–122.
50. Pangburn MK. Reduced activity of DAF on complement enzymes bound to alternative pathway activators. Similarity with factor H. *Immunology* 1990;71:598–600.
51. Pruitt SK, Bollinger RR. The effect of soluble complement receptor type 1 on hyperacute allograft rejection. *J Surg Res* 1991;50:350–355.
52. Xia W, Fearon DT, Moore FD Jr, et al. Prolongation of guinea pig cardiac xenograft survival in rats by soluble human complement receptor type 1. *Transplantation* 1991;254:102–105.
53. Makrides SC. Therapeutic inhibition of the complement system. *Pharmacol Rev* 1998;50:59–87.
54. Morgan BP, Harris CL. Complement therapeutics; history and current progress. *Mol Immunol* 2003;40:159–170.
55. Rittershaus CW, Thomas LJ, Miller DP, et al. Recombinant glycoproteins that inhibit complement activation and also bind the selectin adhesion molecules. *J Biol Chem* 1999;274:11237–11244.
56. Wang Y, Hu Q, Madri JA, et al. Amelioration of lupus-like autoimmune disease in NZB/W F_1 mice after treatment with a blocking monoclonal antibody specific for complement component C5. *Proc Natl Acad Sci U S A* 1996;93:8563–8568.
57. Woodruff TM, Strachan AJ, Dryburg N, et al. Antiarthritic activity of an orally active C5a receptor antagonist against antigen-induced monoarticular arthritis in the rat. *Arthritis Rheum* 2002;46:2476–2485.
58. Pickering MC, Walport MJ. Links between complement abnormalities and systemic lupus erythematosus. *Rheumatology* 2000;39:133–141.
59. Davies KA, Walport MJ. Processing and clearance of immune complexes by complement and the role of complement in immune complex diseases. In: Volanakis JE, Frank MM, eds. *The human complement system in health and disease.* New York: Marcel Dekker, 1998:423–453.
60. Casciola-Rosen L, Anhalt G, Rosen A. Autoantigens targeted in systemic lupus erythematosus are clustered in two populations of surface structures on apoptotic keratinocytes. *J Exp Med* 1994;179:1317–1330.
61. Mevorach D, Zhou JL, Song X, et al. Systemic exposure to irradiated apoptotic cells induces autoantibody production. *J Exp Med* 1998;188: 387–392.
62. Korb LC, Ahearn JM. C1q binds directly and specifically to surface blebs of apoptotic human keratinocytes. Complement deficiency and systemic lupus erythematosus revisited. *J Immunol* 1997;158:4525–4528.
63. Botto M, Dell'Agnola C, Bygrave AE, et al. Homozygous C1q deficiency causes glomerulonephritis associated with multiple apoptotic bodies. *Nat Genet* 1998;19:56–59.
64. Mitchell DA, Taylor PR, Cook HT, et al. Cutting edge: C1q protects against the development of glomerulonephritis independently of C3 activation. *J Immunol* 1999;162:5676–5679.
65. Matsumoto AK, Kopicky-Burd J, Carter RH, et al. Intersection of the complement and immune systems: a signal transduction complex of the B lymphocyte-containing complement receptor type 2 and CD19. *J Exp Med* 1991;173:55–64.
66. Rickert RC, Rajewsky K, Roes J. Impairment of T-cell-dependent B-cell responses and B-1 cell development in CD19-deficient mice. *Nature* 1995;376:352–355.
67. Fischer MB, Ma M, Goerg S, et al. Regulation of B cell response to T-dependent antigens by classical pathway complement. *J Immunol* 1996;157:549–556.
68. Bird P, Lachman PJ. The regulation of IgG subclass production in man: low serum IgG4 in inherited deficiencies of the classical pathway of C3 activation. *Eur J Immunol* 1988;18:1217–1222.
69. Fang Y, Xu C, Fu Y-X, et al. Expression of complement receptors 1 and 2 on follicular dendritic cells is necessary for the generation of a strong antigen-specific IgG response. *J Immunol* 1998;160:5273–5279.
70. Qin D, Wu J, Carroll MC, et al. Evidence for an important interaction between a complement-derived CD21 ligand on follicular dendritic cells and CD21 on B cells in the initiation of IgG responses. *J Immunol* 1998;161:4549–4554.
71. Lowell CA, Klickstein LB, Carter RH, et al. Mapping of the Epstein-Barr virus and C3dg binding sites to a common domain on complement receptor type 2. *J Exp Med* 1989;170:1931–1946.
72. Carel JC, Myones BL, Frazier B, et al. Structural requirements for C3d,g/Epstein-Barr virus receptor (CR2/CD21) ligand binding, internalization, and viral infection. *J Biol Chem* 1990;265:12293–12299.
73. Tuveson DA, Ahearn JM, Matsumoto AK, et al. Molecular interactions of complement receptors on B lymphocytes: a CR1/CR2 complex distinct from the CR2/CD19 complex. *J Exp Med* 1991;173: 1083–1089.
74. Bradbury LE, Kansas GS, Levy S, et al. The CD19/CD21 signal transducing complex of human B lymphocytes includes the target of antiproliferative antibody-1 and Leu-13 molecules. *J Immunol* 1992;149: 2841–2850.
75. Oren R, Takahashi S, Doss C, et al. TAPA-1, the target of an antiproliferative antibody, defines a new family of transmembrane proteins. *Mol Cell Biol* 1990;10:4007–4015.
76. de Fougerolles AR, Batista F, Johnsson E, et al. IgM and stromal cell-associated heparan sulfate/heparin as complement-independent ligands for CD19. *Eur J Immunol* 2001;31:2189–2199.
77. Wang Y, Brooks SR, Li X, et al. The physiologic role of CD19 cytoplasmic tyrosines. *Immunity* 2002;17:501–514.
78. Fearon DT, Carter RH. The CD19/CR2/TAPA-1 complex of B lymphocytes: linking natural to acquired immunity. *Annu Rev Immunol* 1995;13:127–150.
79. Dempsey PW, Allison MED, Akkaraju S, et al. C3d of complement as a molecular adjuvant: bridging innate and acquired immunity. *Science* 1996;271:348–350.
80. Molina H, Holers VM, Li B, et al. Markedly impaired humoral immune response in mice deficient in complement receptors 1 and 2. *Proc Natl Acad Sci U S A* 1996;93:3357–3361.
81. Croix DA, Ahearn JM, Rosengard AM, et al. Antibody response to a T-dependent antigen requires B cell expression of complement receptors. *J Exp Med* 1996;183:1857–1864.
82. Ahearn JM, Fischer MB, Croix D, et al. Disruption of the Cr2 locus results in a reduction of B-1a cells and in an impaired B cell response to T-dependent antigen. *Immunity* 1996;4:251–262.
83. Sato S, Steeber DA, Tedder TF. The CD19 signal transduction molecule is a response regulator of B-lymphocyte differentiation. *Proc Natl Acad Sci U S A* 1995;92:11558–11562.
84. Sato S, Ono N, Steeber DA, et al. CD19 regulates B lymphocyte signaling thresholds critical for the development of B-1 lineage cells and autoimmunity. *J Immunol* 1996;157:4371–4378.
85. Inaoki M, Sato S, Weintraub BC, et al. CD19-regulated signaling thresholds control peripheral tolerance and autoantibody production in B lymphocytes. *J Exp Med* 1997;186:1923–1931.
86. Prodeus AP, Goerg S, Shen LM, et al. A critical role for complement in maintenance of self-tolerance. *Immunity* 1998;9:721–731.

CHAPTER 22

Acute-Phase Proteins in Rheumatic Disease

John E. Volanakis

The term *acute phase* was introduced in 1941 to describe sera obtained from patients acutely ill with infectious diseases (1). Eleven years earlier, Tillett and Francis (2) had shown that such sera contained C-reactive protein (CRP). Later, it became apparent that high plasma concentrations of CRP are associated not only with the acute phase of infectious diseases, but also with all other forms of tissue injury, including trauma, ischemia, malignancy, and hypersensitivity reactions. It also became evident that the plasma concentration of several other proteins increases following tissue injury. These proteins are collectively referred to as acute-phase proteins (APPs). Increases in the plasma concentration of these proteins constitute an integral part of the acute-phase response or acute-phase reaction of the host to tissue injury. Fever, leukocytosis, and changes in fat, carbohydrate, and trace metal metabolism are also features of the response (3). The plasma concentration of APPs returns to normal with restoration of tissue structure and function. In many rheumatic diseases, inflammatory processes are a major feature of tissue pathology, and levels of APP often parallel clinical activity.

This chapter provides an overview of the structure and function of the major human APPs and then briefly discusses the regulation of their synthesis and their clinical utility, particularly in rheumatic diseases.

OVERVIEW OF ACUTE-PHASE PROTEINS

Human plasma APPs can be categorized into three main functional groups: proteins participating in host defense against pathogens, inhibitors of serine proteinases, and transport proteins with antioxidant activity (Table 22.1). Collectively, these proteins perform several important functions. First, they participate in the recognition and elimination of pathogens. Second, they limit damage to host tissues by proteolytic enzymes and oxygen metabolites produced during acute inflammatory reactions. Third, they "turn off" the inflammatory reaction and participate in the restoration of the normal architecture of injured tissues (Table 22.1).

HOST DEFENSE ACUTE-PHASE PROTEINS

CRP is the prototype human APP and the most extensively studied. On the basis of its structure and Ca^{2+}-dependent binding specificities, CRP is classified as a pentraxin. Pentraxins (from the Greek πεγτε, five, and ραξ, berry) (4) constitute a phylogenetically ancient family of proteins exhibiting remarkable conservation of structure and binding reactivities. The most ancient member of the family is the major protein in the hemolymph of the invertebrate *Limulus polyphemus* (horseshoe crab). All pentraxins consist of subunits arranged in pentagonal or, rarely, hexagonal cyclic symmetry. They all bind Ca^{2+} ions, which are necessary for the expression of ligand-binding activity. In vertebrates, there are two main branches of the pentraxin family. CRP-like members bind phosphocholine (PCh), whereas serum amyloid P–like members bind carbohydrate moieties. Not all pentraxins are APPs. The stable conservation of structure and binding specificities, through an extremely long evolutionary time estimated at more than 500 million years, suggests an important biologic function for pentraxins.

The structure of CRP determined by x-ray crystallography at 3.0 Å resolution comprises five protomers, each of 206 amino acids, in cyclic symmetry (5). Protomers have a flattened, jellyroll appearance, and each consists of antiparallel β strands arranged into two β sheets. Two calcium ions are ligated, in close proximity to each other, to side chains and main chain carbonyls of each protomer (5,6). They are integral structural elements of the PCh-binding site and are all located on the same face of the CRP pentamer (7). On the opposite face, each protomer has an unusual extended deep cleft, which contains the C1q- and probably also the Fcγ receptor binding site (8). Results of *in vitro* and *in vivo* experiments indicate that the function of CRP relates to its

TABLE 22.1. *Functional properties of human acute phase proteins*

Functional group	Protein	Function
Host defense proteins	C-reactive protein (CRP)	Complement activation, opsonization
	Mannan-binding lectin (MBL)	Complement activation, opsonization
	Lipopolysaccharide (LPS)-binding protein (LBP)	LPS transfer protein
	Complement proteins C3, C4, C5 Factor B, C9 Factor H, C4bp	Increased vascular permeability, opsonization, bacterial killing
	Fibrinogen	Formation of hemostatic plugs, wound healing
Proteinase inhibitors	α_1-Proteinase inhibitor (α_1-PI)	Control of extracellular matrix degradation
	α_1-Antichymotrypsin (α_1-Achy)	Control of extracellular matrix degradation
	α_2-Antiplasmin (α_2-AP)	Control of plasmin
	C1 inhibitor (C1 INH)	Control of complement and contact system activation
Antioxidants	Ceruloplasmin	Inhibition of oxyradical formation
	Hemopexin (Hx)	Binding of heme, inhibition of lipid peroxidation
	Haptoglobin (Hp)	Binding of hemoglobin, inhibition of lipid peroxidation
Function uncertain	Serum amyloid A (SAA)	
	Secretory phospholipase A_2 group IIA (sPLA$_2$-IIA)	
	Interleukin-1 receptor antagonist (IL-1Ra)	
	α_1-Acid glycoprotein (AGP)	

ability to bind microbial pathogens and damaged and apoptotic cells of the host and to initiate their elimination by recruiting the complement system and phagocytic cells (reviewed in reference 9). Additional data indicate that CRP plays a role in regulating the intensity and extent of the acute inflammatory reaction.

The first described binding reactivity of CRP, which led to its discovery and naming, was with the C-polysaccharide of the cell wall of pneumococci (PnC) (2). The reaction resulted in precipitation, but could be differentiated from antigen-antibody reactions because it required Ca^{2+} ions. It was subsequently shown that PCh residues of PnC are the major ligand for CRP binding (10). The binding specificity for PCh endows CRP with the ability to bind to a variety of cell wall and capsular polysaccharides of bacterial and fungal pathogens as well as to PCh-containing phospholipids of cell membranes and lipoproteins. A disturbance of the normal architecture of the lipid bilayer of cell membranes is required for binding of CRP, however (11). *In vitro,* membrane alteration allowing CRP binding can be induced by sublytic concentrations of lysolecithin or by treatment of cells with snake phospholipase A_2, which catalyzes hydrolysis of phospholipids in the membrane, resulting in the production of lysolecithin (12). *In vivo,* CRP has been shown to bind to damaged cells at inflammatory sites (13) and to apoptotic cells (14). It has been proposed that hydrolysis of phospholipids by the acute phase secretory phospholipase A_2 is responsible for these reactivities (15). A similar mechanism has been proposed for the observed binding of CRP to oxidized low-density lipoprotein (LDL) (16). Several additional binding specificities have been described. Of particular biologic interest is the binding of CRP to nuclear constituents, such as histones (17) and small nuclear ribonucleoproteins (18,19). Finally, CRP has been shown to bind to a variety of cationic substances (20). These combined binding specificities enable CRP to recognize a variety of pathogens, as well as membranes and nuclear constituents of damaged or necrotic cells of the host.

Following binding to one of its ligands, CRP exhibits two important effector functions: complement activation and signaling through Fcγ receptors. Activation of complement by CRP proceeds through the classical pathway (21) and results in deposition of C3 and C4 cleavage fragments on both CRP and the ligand (22). Similarly to immune aggregates, insoluble CRP–PnC complexes are solubilized by complement, apparently as a result of the covalent binding of C3 and C4 fragments (23). These data indicate that CRP-initiated activation of the classical pathway of complement leads to the assembly of an effective C3-convertase, and it seems reasonable to assume that it results in the generation of host defense–related complement fragments, including the anaphylatoxin C3a and the opsonins C3b and iC3b (see Chapter 21). However, complement activation by complexed CRP does not lead to the formation of an efficient amplification convertase of the alternative pathway nor to a C5-convertase, due to direct binding of the complement regulatory protein factor H to CRP (24,25). Thus, complement activation by CRP effectively recruits the opsonic function of the system, but not its proinflammatory and membrane-damaging effects, which require cleavage of C5 and generation of C5a and C5b.

Initial evidence indicating that CRP is an opsonin was provided in 1944 by Löfström (26). Subsequent studies demonstrated opsonization of a variety of gram-positive and gram-negative pathogens by CRP (27). The relevance of the *in vitro* opsonic properties of CRP to its *in vivo* function has been demonstrated in a murine pneumococcal infection model. Unlike human CRP, mouse CRP is expressed at low levels and is not an acute-phase reactant. Thus, human CRP-transgenic mice (CRPtg) provide an excellent model for the *in vivo* study of the biologic activities of human CRP, which is expressed in these animals as an APP. Compared to their wild-type (wt) littermates, CRPtg mice experimentally infected with *Streptococcus pneumoniae* lived longer and had significantly lower mortality (28). The increased resistance to infection was associated with a 10- to 400-fold reduction in bacteremia. It was also shown that the protective effects of CRP are mainly mediated via activation of the complement system (29). However, a weak complement-independent CRP-mediated protective effect could also be demonstrated. *In vitro* experiments indicate that this effect is mediated by interactions of CRP with Fcγ receptors (30). Indeed, CRP has been shown to bind to the FcγRI and FcγRIIA receptors on phagocytic cells (31,32). In addition to phagocytosis, interaction of CRP with Fcγ receptors on monocytes results in multiple proinflammatory effects, including a respiratory burst (33), production of hydrogen peroxide (34), and secretion of interleukin (IL)-1 and tumor necrosis factor (TNF)-α (35). In contrast to monocytes, the net effect of the interaction of CRP with Fcγ receptors on neutrophils appears to be downregulation of inflammation. Thus, CRP has been reported to inhibit chemotactic responses of neutrophils (36) in association with reduced p38 kinase activity (37), to cause cleavage and shedding of L-selectin, leading to decreased adhesion of neutrophils to endothelial cells (38), and to induce shedding of IL-6 receptor, resulting in modulation of IL-6 proinflammatory effects (39). *In vivo* correlates of these activities are provided by the CRP-induced inhibition of experimental C5a-induced alveolitis (40) and by the protection of mice from lethal endotoxin shock (41). The latter effect has been shown to be mediated by interaction with Fcγ receptors (42).

Mannose-binding lectin (MBL) belongs to the collectin family of proteins and has binding specificity for terminal mannose, glucose, L-fucose, *N*-acetylmannosamine, and *N*-acetylglucosamine (reviewed in reference 43). MBL is an APP exhibiting up to threefold increases in serum concentration during the acute phase (44). However, genetic variation in its serum concentration is much larger. MBL is found in the plasma in several oligomeric forms, containing 9 to 18 identical polypeptide chains. Each 31-kd polypeptide chain consists of a short NH_2-terminal region involved in interchain disulfide bonds, followed by a collagen-like region of about 60 amino acids, and a globular C-type carbohydrate recognition domain (45). The collagenous regions of three chains form a collagen triple helix, which makes MBL structurally similar to other collectins, such as lung surfactant proteins A and D and conglutinins, all of which have similar globular and collagen domains (43). Its lectin specificity endows MBL with the ability to bind to a variety of pathogens displaying the appropriate terminal sugar residues. Ligand-bound MBL functions as a complement activator and perhaps also as an opsonin, thus mediating elimination of pathogens. Activation of complement by ligand-bound MBL proceeds through the "lectin pathway," which also includes serine-proteinases termed MASP (MBL-associated serine proteinases). There are three MASPs in blood, and homodimers of each one form complexes with MBL. MASP2 is apparently responsible for the sequential activation of C4 and C2, which leads to the formation of a C4b2a C3-convertase (46,47). It has been reported that MBL can also activate the alternative pathway of complement (48), leading to direct killing and opsonization of pathogens. Complement activation appears to be the main effector mechanism for MBL, although the protein also interacts with the widely distributed C1q phagocytic receptor.

Lipopolysaccharide (LPS)-binding protein (LBP) is a 60-kd acute-phase glycoprotein that induces monomerization of LPS aggregates and binds to LPS monomers through the lipid A moiety (49,50). LBP acts as a lipid transfer protein, catalytically transferring LPS to soluble or membrane-associated CD14 (51). CD14 is the major high-affinity receptor for LPS and is expressed preferentially on monocytes, macrophages, and neutrophils. It is attached to the cell membrane through a glycosylphosphatidylinositol anchor and is part of a large LPS receptor complex, comprising the signal-transducing Toll-like receptor 4 (TLR4) and myeloid differentiation protein 2 (MD2) (52). Binding of LPS–LBP complexes to the receptor complex induces several genes encoding inflammatory cytokines, defensins, adhesive proteins, and enzymes that produce low-molecular-weight mediators (53). The products of these inducible genes participate in host defense reactions that help eliminate gram-negative bacteria. LBP also transfers LPS into lipoproteins, where LPS is functionally neutralized (54,55). Through its ability to enhance cellular activation by LPS, LBP also seems to play a role in the pathogenesis of septic shock, although it has been reported that the high concentrations of LBP during the acute-phase response play a major role in inhibiting LPS activity (56). Studies using two independently-derived strains of LBP gene-targeted mice ($LBP^{-/-}$) produced conflicting results, perhaps due to different genetic backgrounds of the mice. One study failed to demonstrate differences in TNF-α production between $LBP^{-/-}$ and wt mice challenged with LPS, suggesting an alternative mechanism for transferring LPS to its receptor complex (57). The other study, demonstrated that LBP$^{-/-}$ mice challenged with *Salmonella typhimurium* failed to mount a TNF-α response and in contrast to their wt counterparts did not survive the infection (58,59).

Complement is a major effector system of host defense against invading pathogens. It comprises more than 30 proteins that, on activation, elaborate protein fragments and protein–protein complexes that interact with specific cellular receptors or directly with cell membranes to mediate acute inflammatory reactions, clearance of foreign cells and molecules, and killing of pathogenic microorganisms. Complement proteins exhibit extensive structural homologies among themselves with remarkable conservation of a small number of repeated structural motifs, indicating that multiple gene-duplication events marked the evolution of the system. A detailed description of the biology and pathophysiology of the complement system is presented in Chapter 21. Most of the serum-soluble complement proteins are synthesized in the liver, and almost all of these have been reported to be APPs. Table 22.1 lists the best documented complement APPs. C3 is the pivotal protein of the complement system, serving multiple functions in the activation sequences and serving as a substrate for the production of several fragments with important host defense functions. Biologic activities are also produced during activation of C5. C4 and factor B are constituents of the C3 and C5 convertases of the classical and the alternative pathway, respectively. C9 is a major structural constituent of the complement attack complex, which is responsible for lysis and death of serum-sensitive pathogens. Finally, factor H and C4b-binding protein (C4bp) participate in the regulation of complement convertases. Additionally, factor H serves as a cofactor for factor I, an enzyme that generates biologically active fragments from C3b, the major activation fragment of C3.

Fibrinogen is an abundant plasma protein that plays a major role in hemostasis and probably also in tissue repair and wound healing (60). It is an extended, multidomain molecule about 450 Å long with an molecular mass of 340,000 daltons. The molecule consists of two identical disulfide-linked subunits. Each subunit contains three disulfide-linked polypeptide chains termed Aα, Bβ, and γ. Thrombin-catalyzed cleavage of fibrinogen results in the release of two small fibrinopeptides and the polymerization of the remaining molecule. The polymer is stabilized by cross-linking of the γ chains of neighboring molecules by factor XIII, resulting in the formation of a strong fibrin clot. In addition, fibrinogen, through recognition domains on the Aα and γ chains, binds to the glycoprotein IIb/IIIa (GPIIb/IIIa) receptor complex on activated platelets (61), forming interplatelet bridges. Thus, fibrinogen is an essential structural element of effective platelet-fibrin hemostatic plugs that restore the structural integrity of injured blood vessels (62) (see Chapter 18). Several observations indicate that fibrinogen and fibrin can also interact with endothelial cells, promoting adhesion, motility, and cytoskeletal organization of these cells (63). The interaction is mediated through receptors on endothelial cells that are immunologically and biochemically related to the GPIIb/IIIa receptors on platelets (64). At sites of vascular injury, fibrin deposition on the subendothelium promotes adhesion, spreading, and proliferation of endothelial cells, leading to tissue repair and wound healing (65).

ACUTE-PHASE PROTEINASE INHIBITORS

All acute-phase proteinase inhibitors belong to the *ser*ine *p*roteinase *in*hibitor (serpin) family of proteins. Under physiologic conditions, serpins control a variety of important homeostatic events, including extracellular matrix turnover, fibrinolysis, contact and complement system activation (66). Their role becomes critical following tissue injury, because the resulting acute inflammatory reaction involves the activation of multiple plasma serine proteinases and the release of additional ones from phagocytic cells. Effective control of these enzymes is essential for the protection of the structural integrity of host tissues. All serpins inhibit serine proteinases by forming stoichiometric complexes with their target enzymes (67).

Human α_1-proteinase inhibitor (α_1PI), also termed α_1-antitrypsin, is a 53-kd single-polypeptide chain glycoprotein (68). Although it has been shown to inactivate a large number of serine proteinases, the primary function of α_1PI is to control the activity of neutrophil elastase. The significance of this activity is demonstrated by the pathophysiology of the clinical syndrome associated with deficiency of α_1PI. Deficient individuals develop pulmonary emphysema at an early age as a result of increased turnover of pulmonary extracellular matrix proteins, particularly elastin. During acute inflammatory reactions, neutrophils release large amounts of elastase, which presents a threat to the integrity of the extracellular matrix. The need for effective control of this enzyme is obvious.

α_1-Antichymotrypsin (α_1-Achy) is a 68-kd single-polypeptide chain glycoprotein (69). It is a specific inhibitor of chymotrypsin-like serine proteinases and is a particularly potent inhibitor of neutrophil cathepsin G. The latter enzyme is also released from neutrophils during acute inflammation and has the potential to degrade proteoglycan and fibronectin (70). An additional potential role for α_1-Achy is suggested by its ability to inhibit mast cell chymase. Both chymase and cathepsin G act as effective angiotensin-converting enzymes (71) generating angiotensin II, which mediates smooth muscle contraction and aldosterone release. α_2-Antiplasmin (α_2-AP) is a 65-kd single-chain glycoprotein (72). It is an extremely efficient inhibitor of plasmin, particularly when the enzyme is free in solution. α_2-AP also inhibits several other serine proteases, but at significantly slower rates than plasmin.

C1 inhibitor (C1INH) is a 104-kd single-chain glycoprotein (73). It is the only known inhibitor of C1r and C1s, and thus an important control protein of the classical pathway of complement activation. C1INH prevents the spontaneous autoactivation of C1r through a reversible interaction with native C1, and it also inactivates activated C1 by forming stable complexes with C1r and C1s. These complexes are dissociated from C1 in the form of a tetramolecular, C1INH-C1r-C1s-C1INH complex. C1INH is also the major plasma inhibitor of kallikrein, an enzyme having two major functions: generation of bradykinin from kininogen and amplification of the early phase of the intrinsic pathway of blood coagulation. Finally, C1INH is also important for the control of factors XIIa and XIIf, accounting for approximately 90% of the inactivation of both (73). The physiologic importance of C1INH for the control of effector systems of inflammation in the blood is underlined by the clinical syndrome associated with its deficiency. C1INH deficiency is transmitted as an autosomal-dominant trait and is associated with hereditary angioedema, characterized by recurrent attacks of circumscribed edema of the skin or mucosa.

TRANSPORT PROTEINS WITH ANTIOXIDANT ACTIVITY

The third group of human APPs (Table 22.1) includes three important plasma antioxidants: ceruloplasmin, hemopexin, and haptoglobin (74). These three proteins play an important role in protecting host tissues from the damaging potential of toxic oxygen metabolites released during acute inflammatory reactions from phagocytic cells. Reactive oxygen metabolites are important in bacterial killing, but if unchecked, they can lead to host cell injury and death through peroxidation of membrane lipids (75). Additionally, oxidants can also damage proteins, carbohydrates, and DNA.

Ceruloplasmin is a 132-kd single-polypeptide chain copper-containing ferroxidase circulating in the blood as a holoprotein with six atoms of copper incorporated during biosynthesis (76). It plays a critical role in iron metabolism and participates in many biologic processes, including tissue angiogenesis, copper transport, and antioxidant defense (77). The antioxidant properties of ceruloplasmin depend mainly on its ferroxidase activity, which allows it to inhibit iron ion-dependent lipid peroxidation and hydroxyl radical (◊OH) formation from H_2O_2. Ceruloplasmin also inhibits copper ion–stimulated formation of reactive oxidants and scavenges H_2O_2 and superoxide (O_2^-).

Hemopexin (Hx) is a 60-kd single-chain serum glycoprotein containing 20% carbohydrate (78). Its primary structure is characterized by the presence of a structural motif of about 45 amino acids, which is repeated 10 times. Hx binds heme released from damaged heme-containing proteins with high affinity. Hx-heme complexes react with specific receptors on hepatocytes, resulting in the uptake of heme and the release of Hx, which returns to the circulation. This mechanism is important for the conservation of body iron stores. Additionally, because free heme represents a reactive form of iron able to participate in oxygen-radical reactions, its binding by Hx results in protection of host tissues (79).

Haptoglobin (Hp) is a 104-kd polymorphic glycoprotein, consisting of two α and two β disulfide-linked polypeptide chains (80). Hp binds hemoglobin, released during hemolysis, through distinct binding sites on the α and β chains (81). Hp–hemoglobin complexes are recognized by the scavenger receptor CD163 and are removed quickly from the circulation (82). CD163 is expressed exclusively on monocytes and macrophages and is up-regulated by IL-6 during the acute phase. Free hemoglobin can accelerate lipid peroxidation by two mechanisms involving the production of either oxo-iron species or hydroxyl radicals (◊OH) (74). Binding by Hp prevents these reactions, thereby serving as a protective mechanism. In addition, Hp plays a role in wound healing by stimulating angiogenesis (83).

ACUTE-PHASE PROTEINS OF UNCERTAIN FUNCTION

This last group includes additional APPs whose functions have not been fully defined: serum amyloid A (SAA), secretory phospholipase A_2 group IIA (sPLA$_2$-IIA), IL-1 receptor antagonist (IL-1Ra), and α_1-acid glycoprotein (AGP). SAA is a major APP, the concentration of which increases by as much as 1,000-fold in acute inflammatory conditions (84). Initially considered a single protein, SAA has been shown to comprise a family of differentially expressed isomorphs (reviewed in reference 85). In humans, the SAA family consists of three members, only two of which are APPs. SAA is the precursor of amyloid A protein, the principal component of secondary amyloid deposits. During the acute phase, SAA associates predominantly with the HDL3 fraction of high-density lipoprotein (HDL), replacing apolipoprotein A-1. It has been proposed that, during inflammatory states, SAA is mainly involved in lipid transport and cholesterol metabolism (86). A host defense function has been suggested for SAA by experiments demonstrating that it is chemotactic for human neutrophils, monocytes, and T lymphocytes (87,88). Its effects on myeloid cells are mediated through a seven-transmembrane, G protein–coupled receptor that also binds *N*-formyl-methionyl-leucyl-phenylalanine with low affinity (89). SAA induces production of extracellular matrix–degrading enzymes, including collagenase, stromelysin, and matrix metalloproteinases 2 and 3, all of which are important for repair processes after tissue damage (90); it also enhances the catalytic activity of sPLA$_2$-IIA (91).

In humans, secretory phospholipases A_2 comprise nine closely related isozymes that hydrolyze the acyl group at the *sn*-2 position of phospholipids, resulting in the release of arachidonic acid and lysophospholipid. sPLA$_2$-IIA, a widely distributed isozyme, is highly up-regulated during the acute phase, with levels in blood and extracellular fluids increasing by several hundred fold (92). Multiple functions have been ascribed to sPLA$_2$-IIA. They include enhanced stimulus-coupled release of arachidonic acid and prostaglandin generation (93), hydrolysis of phospholipids of LDL and acute-phase HDL (91), and defense against bacteria. The antibacterial activity of $sPLA_2$-IIA has been demonstrated both *in vitro* (94) and *in vivo* using transgenic mice (95) and is directed primarily against *Staphylococcus aureus* and other gram-positive bacteria.

IL-1Ra, a member of the IL-1 cytokine family (96), binds to the IL-1 receptor but cannot initiate signaling and thus acts as a competitive inhibitor of IL-1 (97). Secretory IL-1Ra is an APP and it serves to modulate the proinflammatory effects of IL-1 (98). The antiinflammatory activity of IL-1Ra has been demonstrated by gene targeting in mice, although the observed phenotypes were diverse and depended on the genetic background of the animals. Thus, IL-1Ra$^{-/-}$ mice on the BALB/cA background develop a chronic inflammatory polyarthritis resembling rheumatoid arthritis (RA) (99), those on the MF1x129/Ola background exhibit a lethal arterial inflammatory disease with features of giant cell arteritis and polyarteritis nodosa (100), those on the DBA1 background demonstrate increased susceptibility to collagen-induced arthritis (101), whereas on the C57BL/6J background, the deficient mice manifest decreased body weight and increased susceptibility to lethal endotoxemia (102).

AGP, also termed orosomucoid, is a 41- to 43-kd polymorphic single-chain, heavily glycosylated protein containing 45% carbohydrate. During the acute phase, the serum concentration of AGP rises two- to fivefold and its glycosylation pattern changes (reviewed in references 103 and 104). Changes in glycan composition and, particularly, the expression of sialyl Lewis X structures during the acute phase have been shown to influence the activities of the protein. Although the exact biologic function of AGP is not clear, several *in vitro* and *in vivo* antiinflammatory and immunomodulatory activities have been described. AGP has been shown to inhibit chemotactic responses and superoxide production by neutrophils as well as platelet aggregation and release reaction. It has also been reported to induce cytokine release from monocytes, including IL-1β, IL-6, IL-12, TNFα, and IL-1 receptor antagonist and soluble TNF receptor (104). *In vivo*, AGP has been shown to protect mice from TNF-induced lethal shock and against lethal challenge with *Klebsiella pneumoniae* (105). It also has beneficial effects in septic peritonitis and in ischemia/reperfusion mice models. These effects have been attributed to interaction of AGP with the endothelium and the resulting decreased capillary permeability (106).

REGULATION OF SYNTHESIS OF ACUTE-PHASE PROTEINS

An increased plasma concentration in response to tissue injury is the shared feature of all APPs. However, significant differences exist among individual APPs in terms of the kinetics, magnitude, and duration of the response. Elevated plasma concentrations of CRP and SAA can be measured 4 hours after tissue injury, and peak levels are attained within 24 to 72 hours. Depending on the nature and intensity of the stimulus, acute-phase levels of CRP and SAA can be up to 1,000-fold higher than normal. On the other hand, the plasma concentration of fibrinogen increases by only two- to threefold, and peak levels are seen 7 to 10 days after injury. Similarly, C3 levels increase by about 50% 5 to 7 days after injury. Despite these differences, which reflect differential regulation, gene expression of most APPs is regulated primarily by shared mechanisms affecting the rates of transcription. These mechanisms, including participating cytokines and their receptors, signaling pathways, and transcription factors, have been largely elucidated and are summarized briefly here.

A relatively small number of cytokines characterized by functional pleiotropy and redundancy are responsible for induction of acute-phase proteins. They include IL-6, IL-1β, TNF-α, interferon-γ (IFN-γ), and IL-8 (3,107). The action of these cytokines is modulated by growth factors, including insulin and transforming growth factor-β (TGF-β), and by glucocorticoids. Following tissue injury, activated macrophages initially release IL-1β and TNF-α, which trigger the next wave of local cytokine production from macrophages and stromal cells. This secondary wave includes, in addition to IL-1β and TNF-α, IL-6 and the chemotactic chemokines IL-8 and monocyte chemotactic protein, which in turn recruit additional macrophages to the site of injury (108). IFN-γ is probably produced by γδ T cells stimulated by a combination of IL-12 and IL-1β (109). Locally-produced cytokines are transferred through the bloodstream to the liver, where they bind to specific receptors expressed on the surface of hepatocytes. This binding triggers a series of reactions that lead to transcriptional activation of APP genes.

The best described IL-1β-dependent signaling cascade is initiated by the formation of a ternary complex of IL-1β, IL-1 receptor type 1 (IL-1R1) and IL-1R accessory protein (IL-1RAcP) (110). IL-1R1 and IL-1RAcP belong to the Toll/IL-1 receptor (TIR) family of evolutionary conserved transmembrane proteins that are critically involved in innate immunity from plants to humans (111). The TIR family is subdivided into the IL-1R and the TLR groups. In mammals, the IL-1R group of receptors binds cytokines and mediate inflammatory and immune responses, whereas TLRs recognize conserved molecular patterns of bacterial pathogens and are important components of innate immunity. The two groups have different ligand recognition extracellular domains, but share a conserved intracellular domain, the TIR domain. Signaling through the TIR domain leads to activation of transcription factors nuclear factor κB (NFκB), AP-1, and ATF-2, which induce transcription of genes encoding for cytokines, chemokines, and APPs (112). The cascade initiated by binding of IL-1β to the extracellular recognition domain of IL-1R can be summarized briefly as follows. In a first step, the adapter protein MyD88 is recruited as a dimer to the signaling TIR domains of IL-1R and IL-1RAcP. MyD88, in turn, mediates the recruitment of the serine/threonine kinase IRAK (IL-1R associated kinase). which dissociates from its silencer protein Tollip and interacts with MyD88. IRAK dimers are then auto- or cross-phosphorylated, which leads to their dissociation from the active receptor complex and their interaction with the adapter protein TNF receptor–activated factor 6 (TRAF6) (113). IRAK activates TRAF6 by a poorly understood mechanism, which leads to polyubiquitination and oligomerization of three or more TRAF6 molecules (114).

NFκB is a ubiquitous, evolutionarily-conserved transcription factor rapidly activated in response to external stimuli. It consists of heterodimers comprising a DNA-binding subunit (p50 or p52) and a transcription-activating subunit (p65 or RelB). The dimers reside in the cytoplasm in the form of an inactive complex with IκB (inhibitor of κB). Activation of NFκB requires degradation of IκBs achieved through a complex process initiated by activated TRAF6 and involving a large number of proteins. It proceeds through the activation of the IκB kinase (IKK) complex, which in turn phosphorylates the IκBs, leading to their polyubiquitination and rapid degradation by the 26S proteasome (reviewed in reference 115). Once freed from IκB, NFκB translocates to the nucleus to activate gene transcription. Recent data indicate that IKK-β, one of three proteins in the IKK complex, is actually responsible for IκB phosphorylation, whereas activated IKK-α moves into the nucleus where it associates with the promoters of target genes and phosphorylates a histone protein, thus promoting NFκB transcriptional activity (116,117). Although NFκB activation is a complex, multistep process, it occurs rapidly, making it ideal for transduction of injurious stimuli requiring immediate host responses.

Activated polyubiquinated TRAF6 oligomers also mediate activation of the mitogen activated protein kinases (MAPK) c-Jun amino (N)-terminal kinase (JNK) and p38 kinase, which in turn activate transcription factors, including cJun, ELK-1, and ATF-2 (118,119). JNK activation proceeds through activation of the MAPK kinase TAK1 in the context of a complex with IRAK, TRAF6, and the adapter proteins TAB1 and TAB2 (120,121). Activated TAK1 then phosphorylates the MAPK kinase, MKK6, leading to the activation of the JNK-p38 kinase pathways (122).

Another major signaling pathway used mainly by IL-6 and IFN-γ to activate transcription of APP genes employs Janus kinases (JAK) and signal transducers and activators of transcription (STAT) (123–127). The JAK/STAT pathway is conserved from invertebrates to mammals and is remarkably simple for membrane-to-nucleus signaling, therefore being ideally suited for APP production. The pathway is activated by all members of the large hematopoietin family of cytokines, and it has apparently evolved to regulate host responses to exogenous stresses, especially infection (128). There are four JAKs and seven STATs. Specificity is attained by the diversity of structure and tissue distribution of the STATs. IL-6 activates the JAK/STAT pathway by binding to its cognate receptor IL-6R. IL-6R forms a signal-transducing complex with a 130-kd transmembrane protein, termed gp130, also used as a signal transducer by the receptors of other cytokines, including leukemia inhibitory factor, oncostatin M, IL-11, IL-12, and IL-23 (129). Formation of the IL-6/IL-6R/gp130 complex results in conformational changes in the cytoplasmic portion of gp130, which dimerizes and brings into apposition the associated JAK1s. The JAK1s then catalyze phosphorylation of themselves and of gp130 at tyrosine residues. STAT3 dimers recognize the phosphorylated motifs through their src homology 2 (SH2) domains, are recruited to gp130, and are themselves activated by JAK-catalyzed tyrosine phosphorylation. Activated STAT3s dissociate from gp130 and form new-type "classical" dimers that translocate to the nucleus where they recognize γ-activated site (GAS) enhancers on APP genes. Binding of STAT3 to the GAS enhancer results in striking increases in transcriptional rates of target genes. However, within hours the activated STAT signals decay as a result of multi-layered regulatory mechanisms, including protein tyrosine phosphatases (130,131), inactivators of JAKs, termed SOCS (suppressors of cytokine signaling) (132), and protein inhibitors of activated STATs (133). IFN-γ also induces APP genes through the JAK-STAT pathway. The dimeric IFN-γ receptor uses JAK1 and 2 and STAT1 to transduce signals.

In summary, the main transcriptional factors activated by APP-inducing cytokines are NFκB, STAT1, STAT3, AP-1, and ATF-2. The *cis*-acting elements for these proteins are present in different combinations in most APP genes. As with other genes, these transcription factors do not function in isolation. Instead, they form supramolecular complexes of gene-specific combinations of transcription factors and *cis*-DNA elements, which are termed enhaceosomes and interact with promoters of inducible genes to enhance their expression (134).

CLINICAL ASSESSMENT OF THE ACUTE-PHASE RESPONSE

For the past 75 years, the erythrocyte sedimentation rate (ESR), one of the most frequently used clinical tests, has been the major tool for assessing the magnitude of the acute-phase response. For several reasons, summarized by Deodhar (135) and Kushner (136), it now seems desirable to substitute quantitative CRP measurements for ESR in assessing the activity of inflammatory diseases. In the absence of immunoglobulin and erythrocyte abnormalities, ESR increases mainly reflect elevated plasma fibrinogen concentrations. As mentioned earlier, fibrinogen is an APP, but its concentration in plasma rises slowly after injury, requiring several days to attain levels two- to threefold higher than normal. In contrast, levels of CRP start rising within a few hours after tissue injury, reaching peak levels within 24 to 72 hours and returning promptly to normal with resolution of the inflammatory reaction. More importantly, the magnitude of the CRP response correlates closely with the extent of injury, and peak levels can be as much as 1,000 times higher than normal. Thus, it seems obvious that direct measurement of CRP concentration is a more sensitive index of inflammation than indirect estimates of fibrinogen by the ESR.

The clinical value of CRP measurement in a variety of diseases caused by infectious agents, hypersensitivity reactions, ischemia and tissue necrosis, and surgical trauma has been well documented (137). In these conditions, CRP levels in the range of 10 to 200 μg/mL, or even higher, accurately reflect clinical activity, and in certain cases, can be used in differential diagnosis. CRP levels have been reported to be of value in differentiating cystitis from pyelonephritis (138), sarcoidosis from tuberculosis (139), Crohn disease from ulcerative colitis (140), and viral from bacterial meningitis (141). Additionally, CRP measurements are of value in suggesting the presence of bacterial infections in patients with malignancies (142) and systemic lupus erythematosus (SLE) (143).

In recent years, slightly elevated levels of CRP, in the range of 1 to 10 μg/mL, previously considered to be within the normal range, have emerged as one of the most powerful predictors of risk for vascular disease. Several prospective studies have shown that such levels of CRP are associated with an increased risk for myocardial infarction (144,145), stroke (146,147), sudden death from cardiac causes (148), and peripheral arterial disease (149). Elevated CRP levels were shown to be a stronger predictor of cardiovascular events than LDL cholesterol (150) and to be strongly related to the long-term risk for death in unstable coronary artery disease (151). At present, it is not clear whether elevated CRP is simply a sensitive marker of underlying low-level inflammation or a participant in the pathogenesis of atherosclerotic lesions.

CLINICAL VALUE OF C-REACTIVE PROTEIN MEASUREMENTS IN RHEUMATIC DISEASES

Acute inflammatory processes constitute a major component of the pathology of most rheumatic diseases. It follows that changes in the concentration of APPs and, particularly, of CRP would accurately reflect disease activity, providing a useful objective measure for the follow-up and management of patients with rheumatic diseases. Indeed, a substantial number of clinical studies demonstrate a correlation between clinical activity and CRP plasma concentrations in many rheumatic diseases (Table 22.2). The main exception to this general rule is SLE, where CRP levels remain low, despite clinical and laboratory indications of inflammatory disease activity.

In patients with gout (Chapter 113), CRP levels correlate well with the number of involved joints, temperature, and ESR. CRP concentration returns promptly to normal with treatment and clinical response (152). In RA (see Chapter 57), CRP levels can be used to establish the diagnosis, particularly to differentiate RA from osteoarthritis (153). It also has been reported that high levels of CRP in early RA are associated with a relatively poor prognosis and progressive erosive disease (154). Several studies have shown a good correlation between effective treatment of RA with either nonsteroidal antiinflammatory drugs or disease-modifying antirheumatic drugs and levels of CRP (155). Finally, a correlation has been established between high CRP levels over time and radiologic progression of RA (156).

TABLE 22.2. *Rheumatic diseases in which elevated C-reactive protein levels may occur*

Gout
Rheumatoid arthritis
Juvenile rheumatoid arthritis
Psoriatic arthritis
Ankylosing spondylitis
Reactive arthritis
Polymyalgia rheumatica–giant cell arteritis
Systemic vasculitis
Wegener granulomatosis
Behçet syndrome
Systemic lupus erythematosus

In juvenile RA, elevated concentrations of CRP have been reported to be associated with systemic or polyarticular, but not pauciarticular, onset (157). Remission of symptoms correlates with a decrease in CRP levels, except in patients who develop amyloidosis within 5 years from onset. Elevated levels of CRP, correlating with the clinical index of disease activity, have also been reported in psoriatic arthritis, whereas patients with psoriasis alone had normal CRP levels (158).

In ankylosing spondylitis (AS) (see Chapter 63), elevated CRP levels are observed, particularly in patients with peripheral arthritis or iritis (159). A correlation between CRP concentration and disease activity has been demonstrated in both AS and reactive arthritis (160). Markedly elevated concentrations of CRP are observed in polymyalgia rheumatica–giant cell arteritis (see Chapter 85). One study reported that serum CRP levels decline to normal at a rate that precisely reflects clinical improvement during induction of remission with prednisone (161). In another study, however, it was found that CRP concentration was not a good index of clinical activity in this disease (162). Elevated concentrations of CRP, which declined rapidly in association with clinical remission induced by immunosuppression, were also observed in patients with Wegener granulomatosis (163) and various types of systemic vasculitis (164). Finally, CRP was found to be elevated in Behçet syndrome, particularly when arthritic, neurologic, or ocular manifestations were present (165).

Several studies indicate that the serum concentration of CRP is normal or only modestly elevated in SLE, even in patients with clinically-active disease and high ESR (143,166,167). In contrast to CRP, IL-6 levels are significantly elevated in active SLE and correlate with disease activity (168). Interestingly, intercurrent bacterial infections in SLE are associated with high CRP levels, and it has been suggested that CRP can be a valuable aid in the diagnosis of infections in SLE (137). Elevated concentrations of serum CRP also can be seen in patients with active SLE in the presence of synovitis (169) or acute serositis (170). In contrast to SLE, CRP levels are elevated in mixed connective tissue syndrome (171).

REFERENCES

1. MacLeod CM, Avery OT. The occurrence during acute infections of a protein not normally present in the blood: II. Isolation and properties of the reactive protein. *J Exp Med* 1941;73:183–190.
2. Tillett WS, Francis T Jr. Serological reactions in pneumonia with a non-protein somatic fraction of pneumococcus. *J Exp Med* 1930;52: 561–571.
3. Gabay C, Kushner I. Acute-phase proteins and other systemic responses to inflammation. *N Engl J Med* 1999;340:448–454.
4. Osmand AP, Friedenson B, Gewurz H, et al. Characterization of C-reactive protein and the complement subcomponent C1t as homologous proteins displaying cyclic pentameric symmetry (pentraxins). *Proc Natl Acad Sci U S A* 1977;74:739–743.
5. Shrive AK, Cheetham GMT, Holden D, et al. Three dimensional structure of human C-reactive protein. *Nature Struct Biol* 1996;3: 346–354.
6. Thompson D, Pepys MB, Wood SP. The physiological structure of C-reactive protein and its complex with phosphocholine. *Structure* 1999;7:169–177.
7. Agrawal A, Lee S, Carson M, et al. Site-directed mutagenesis of the phosphocholine-binding site of human C-reactive protein. Role of Thr76 and Trp67. *J Immunol* 1997;158:345–350.
8. Agrawal A, Shrive AK, Greenhough TJ, et al. Topology and structure of the C1q-binding site on C-reactive protein. *J Immunol* 2001;166: 3998–4004.
9. Volanakis JE. Human C-reactive protein: expression, structure, and function. *Mol Immunol* 2001;38:189–197.
10. Volanakis JE, Kaplan MH. Specificity of C-reactive protein for choline phosphate residues of pneumococcal C-polysaccharide. *Proc Soc Exp Biol Med* 1971;136:612–614.
11. Volanakis JE, Wirtz KWA. Interaction of C-reactive protein with artificial phosphatidyl-choline bilayers. *Nature* 1979;281:155–157.
12. Narkates AJ, Volanakis JE. C-reactive protein binding specificities: artificial and natural phospholipid bilayers. *Ann NY Acad Sci* 1982; 389:172–182.
13. Kushner I, Kaplan MH. Studies of acute phase protein: I. An immunohistochemical method for the localization of C-reactive protein in rabbits: association in local inflammatory lesions. *J Exp Med* 1961;114: 961–974.
14. Gershov D, Kim S, Brot N, et al. C-reactive protein binds to apoptotic cells, protects the cells from assembly of the terminal complement components, and sustains an anti-inflammatory innate immune response: implications for systemic autoimmunity. *J Exp Med* 2000;192: 1353–1363.
15. Hack EC, Wolbink GJ, Schalkwijk C, et al. A role for secretory phospholipase A_2 and C-reactive protein in the removal of injured cells. *Immunol Today* 1997;18:111–115.
16. Chang MK, Binder CJ, Torzewski M, et al. C-reactive protein binds to both oxidized LDL and apoptotic cells through recognition of a common ligand: phosphorylcholine of oxidized phospholipids. *Proc Natl Acad Sci U S A* 2002;99:13043–13048.
17. DuClos TW, Zlock LT, Rubin RL. Analysis of the binding of C-reactive protein to histones and chromatin. *J Immunol* 1988;141: 4266–4270.
18. DuClos TW. C-reactive protein reacts with the Ul small nuclear ribonucleoprotein. *J Immunol* 1989;143:2553–2559.
19. Pepys MB, Booth SE, Tennent GA, et al. Binding of pentraxins to different nuclear structures: C-reactive protein binds to small nuclear ribonucleoprotein particles, serum amyloid P binds to chromatin and nucleoli. *Clin Exp Immunol* 1994;97:152–157.
20. DiCamelli R, Potempa LA, Siegel J, et al. Binding reactivity of C-reactive protein for polycations. *J Immunol* 1980;125:1933–1938.
21. Kaplan MH, Volanakis JE. Interaction of C-reactive protein complexes with the complement system: I. Consumption of human complement associated with the reaction of C-reactive protein with pneumococcal C-polysaccharide and with the choline phosphatides, lecithin and sphingomyelin. *J Immunol* 1974;112:2135–2147.
22. Volanakis JE, Narkates AJ. Binding of human C4 to C-reactive protein-pneumococcal C-polysaccharide complexes during activation of the classical complement pathway. *Mol Immunol* 1983;20:1201–1207.
23. Volanakis JE. Complement-induced solubilization of C-reactive protein-pneumococcal C-polysaccharide precipitates: evidence for covalent binding of complement proteins to C-reactive protein and to pneumococcal C-polysaccharide. *J Immunol* 1982;128:2745–2750.
24. Berman S, Gewurz H, Mold C. Binding of C-reactive protein to nucleated cells leads to complement activation without cell lysis. *J Immunol* 1986;136:1354–1359.
25. Jarva H, Jokiranta TS, Hellwage J, et al. Regulation of complement activation by C-reactive protein: targeting the complement inhibitory activity of factor H by an interaction with short consensus repeat domains 7 and 8–11. *J Immunol* 1999;163:3957–3962.
26. Löfström G. Comparison between the reactions of acute phase serum with pneumococcus C-polysaccharide and with pneumococcus type XXVII. *Br J Exp Pathol* 1944;25:21–26.
27. Kindmark CO. Stimulating effect of C-reactive protein on phagocytosis of various species of pathogenic bacteria. *Clin Exp Immunol* 1971;8:941–948.
28. Szalai AJ, Briles DE, Volanakis JE. Human C-reactive protein is protective against fatal *Streptococcus pneumoniae* infection in transgenic mice. *J Immunol* 1995;155:2557–2563.
29. Szalai AJ, Briles DE, Volanakis JE. The role of complement in C-reactive protein mediated protection of mice from *Streptococcus pneumoniae*. *Infect Immun* 1996;64:4850–4853.
30. Mold C, Gresham H, Du Clos TW. Serum amyloid P component and C-reactive protein mediate phagocytosis through murine FcγRs. *J Immunol* 2001;166:1200–1205.
31. Marnell LL, Mold C, Volzer MA, et al. C-reactive protein binds to FcγRI in transfected COS cells. *J Immunol* 1995;155:2185–2193.
32. Bharadwaj D, Stein M-P, Volzer M, et al. The major receptor for C-reactive protein on leukocytes is Fc receptor II. *J Exp Med* 1999; 190:585–590.
33. Zeller JM, Landay AL, Lint TF, et al. Enhancement of human peripheral blood monocyte respiratory burst activity by aggregated C-reactive protein. *J Leukoc Biol* 1986;40:769–783.
34. Tebo JM, Mortensen RF. Internalization and degradation of receptor-bound C-reactive protein by U-937 cells: induction of H_2O_2 production and tumoricidal activity. *Biochim Biophys Acta* 1991;1095: 210–216.
35. Galve-de Rochemonteix B, Wiktorowiz K, Kushner I, et al. C-reactive protein increases production of IL-1 alpha, IL-1 beta, and TNF alpha, and expression of mRNA by human alveolar macrophages. *J Leukoc Biol* 1993;53:439–445.
36. Zhong W, Zen Q, Tebo J, et al. Effect of human C-reactive protein on chemokine and chemotactic factor-induced neutrophil chemotaxis and signaling. *J Immunol* 1998;161:2533–2540.
37. Heuertz RM, Tricomi SM, Ezekiel UR, et al. C-reactive protein inhibits chemotactic peptide-induced p38 mitogen-activated protein kinase activity and human neutrophil movement. *J Biol Chem* 1999; 274:17968–17074.
38. Zouki C, Beauchamp M, Baron C, et al. Prevention of *in vitro* neutrophil adhesion to endothelial cells through shedding of L-selectin by C-reactive protein and peptides derived from C-reactive protein. *J Clin Invest* 1997;100:522–529.
39. Jones SA, Novick D, Horiuchi S, et al. C-reactive protein: a physiological activator of interleukin 6 receptor shedding. *J Exp Med* 1999; 189:599–604.
40. Heuertz RM, Xia D, Samols D, et al. Inhibition of C5a des Arg-induced neutrophil alveolitis in transgenic mice expressing C-reactive protein. *Am J Physiol* 1994;266:L649–L654.
41. Xia D, Samols D. Transgenic mice expressing rabbit C-reactive protein are resistant to endotoxemia. *Proc Natl Acad Sci U S A* 1997;94: 2575–2580.
42. Mold C, Rodriguez W, Rodic-Polic B, et al. C-reactive protein mediates protection from lipopolysaccharide through interactions with FcγR. *J Immunol* 2002;169:7019–7025.

43. Holmskov U, Thiel S, Jensenius JC. Collectins and ficollins: humoral lectins of the innate immune defense. *Annu Rev Immunol* 2003;21: 547–578.
44. Ezekowitz RAB, Day LE, Herman GA. A human mannose-binding protein is an acute-phase reactant that shares sequence homology with other vertebrate lectins. *J Exp Med* 1988;167:1034–1086.
45. Drickamer KM, Dordal MS, Reynolds L. Mannose-binding proteins isolated from rat liver contain carbohydrate-recognition domains linked to collagenous tails. *J Biol Chem* 1986;261:6878–6886.
46. Matsushita M, Fujita T. Activation of the classical complement pathway by mannose-binding protein in association with a novel C1s-like serine protease. *J Exp Med* 1992;176:1497–1502.
47. Thiel S, Vorup-Jensen T, Stover CM, et al. A second serine protease associated with mannan-binding lectin that activates complement. *Nature* 1997;386:506–510.
48. Schweinle JE, Ezekowitz RA, Tenner AJ, et al. Human mannose-binding protein activates the alternative complement pathway and enhances serum bactericidal activity on a mannose-rich isolate of *Salmonella*. *J Clin Invest* 1989;84:1821–1829.
49. Tobias P, Soldau K, Ulevitch R. Isolation of a lipopolysaccharide-binding acute-phase reactant from rabbit serum. *J Exp Med* 1986;164: 777–793.
50. Grube BJ, Cochrane CG, Ye RD, et al. Cytokine and dexamethasone regulation of lipopolysaccharide binding protein (LBP) expression in human hepatoma (HepG2) cells. *J Biol Chem* 1994;269:8477–8482.
51. Hailman E, Lichenstein HS, Wurfel MM, et al. Lipopolysaccharide (LPS)-binding protein accelerates the binding of LPS to CD14. *J Exp Med* 1994;179:269–277.
52. Takeda K, Kaisho T, Akira S. Toll-like receptors. *Annu Rev Immunol* 2003;21:335–376.
53. Ulevitch RJ, Tobias PS. Receptor-dependent mechanisms of cell stimulation by bacterial endotoxin. *Annu Rev Immunol* 1995;13:437–457.
54. Vreugdenhil ACE, Snoek AMP, van't Veer C, et al. LPS-binding protein circulates in association with apoB-containing lipoproteins and enhances endotoxin-LDL/VLDL interaction. *J Clin Invest* 2001;107: 225–234.
55. Wurfel MM, Kunitake ST, Lichenstein H, et al. Lipopolysaccharide (LPS)-binding protein is carried on lipoproteins and acts as cofactor in the neutralization of LPS. *J Exp Med* 1994;180:1025–1035.
56. Zweigner J, Gramm H-J, Singer OC, et al. High concentrations of lipopolysaccharide-binding protein in serum of patients with severe sepsis or septic shock inhibit the lipopolysaccharide response in human monocytes. *J Clin Invest* 2001;98:3800–3808.
57. Wurfel MM, Monks BG, Ingalls RR, et al. Targeted deletion of the lipopolysaccharide (LPS)-binding protein gene leads to profound suppression of LPS responses *ex vivo,* whereas *in vivo* responses remain intact. *J Exp Med* 1997;186:2051–20568.
58. Heinrich J-M, Bernheiden M, Minigo G, et al. The essential role of lipopolysaccharide-binding protein in protection of mice against a peritoneal *Salmonella* infection involves the rapid induction of an inflammatory response. *J Immunol* 2001;167:1624–1628.
59. Jack RS, Fan X, Bernheiden M, et al. Lipopolysaccharide-binding protein is required to combat a murine Gram-negative bacterial infection. *Nature* 1997;389:742–745.
60. Fuller GM. Fibrinogen: a multifunctional acute phase protein. In: Mackiewicz A, Kushner I, Baumann H, eds. *Acute phase proteins.* Boca Raton, FL: CRC Press, 1993:169–183.
61. Bennett JS. Platelet-fibrinogen interactions. *Ann NY Acad Sci* 2001; 936:340–354.
62. Bloom AL. Physiology of blood coagulation. *Haemostasis* 1990; 20(suppl 1):14–29.
63. Dejana E, Zanetti A, Conforti G. Biochemical and functional characteristics of fibrinogen interaction with endothelial cells. *Haemostasis* 1988;18:262–272.
64. Newman PJ, Kawai Y, Montgomery RR, et al. Synthesis by cultured umbilical vein endothelial cells of two proteins structurally and immunologically related to platelet membrane glycoproteins IIb and IIIa. *J Cell Biol* 1986;103:81–86.
65. Colvin RB. Wound healing processes in haemostasis and thrombosis. In: Gimbrone MA, ed. *Vascular endothelium in haemostasis and thrombosis.* New York: Churchill Livingstone, 1986:220–241.
66. Potempa J, Korzus E, Travis J. The serpin superfamily of proteinase inhibitors: structure, function, and regulation. *J Biol Chem* 1994;269: 15957–15960.
67. Silverman GA, Bird PI, Carrell RW, et al. The serpins are an expanding superfamily of structurally similar but functionally diverse proteins. Evolution, mechanism of inhibition, novel functions, and a revised nomenclature. *J Biol Chem* 2001;276:33293–33296.
68. Kurachi K, Chandra T, Degen SJ, et al. Cloning and sequence of cDNA for alpha 1-antitrypsin. *Proc Natl Acad Sci U S A* 1981;78: 6826–6830.
69. Baumann U, Huber R, Bode W, et al. Crystal structure of cleaved human alpha 1-antichymotrypsin at 2. 7 Å resolution and its comparison with other serpins. *J Mol Biol* 1991;218:595–606.
70. Vartio T, Seppa H, Vaheri A. Susceptibility of soluble and matrix fibronectin to degradation by tissue proteinases, mast cell chymase and cathepsin G. *J Biol Chem* 1981;256:471–477.
71. Gaffar SA, Princler GL, McIntire KR, et al. A human lung tumor-associated antigen cross-reactive with alpha 1-antichymotrypsin. *J Biol Chem* 1980;255:8334–8339.
72. Holmes WE, Nelles L, Lijnen HR, et al. Primary structure of human alpha 2-antiplasmin, a serine protease inhibitor (serpin). *J Biol Chem* 1987;262:1659–1664.
73. Davis AE III. C1 inhibitor gene and hereditary angioedema. In: Volanakis JE, Frank MM, eds. *The human complement system in health and disease.* New York: Marcel Dekker, 1998:455–480.
74. Halliwell B, Gutteridge JMC. The antioxidants of human extracellular fluids. *Arch Biochem Biophys* 1990;280:1–8.
75. Fantone JC, Ward PA. Polymorphonuclear leukocyte-mediated cell and tissue injury: oxygen metabolites and their relations to human disease. *Hum Pathol* 1985;16:973–978.
76. Hellman NE, Gitlin JD. Ceruloplasmin metabolism and function. *Annu Rev Nutr* 2002;22:439–458.
77. Samokyszyn VM, Miller DM, Reif DW, et al. Inhibition of superoxide and ferritin-dependent lipid peroxidation by ceruloplasmin. *J Biol Chem* 1989;264:21–26.
78. Altruda F, Poli V, Restagno G, et al. The primary structure of human hemopexin deduced from cDNA sequence: evidence for internal, repeating homology. *Nucleic Acids Res* 1985;13: 3841–3859.
79. Gutteridge JM, Smith A. Antioxidant protection by haemopexin of haem-stimulated lipid peroxidation. *Biochem J* 1988;256:861–865.
80. Haugen TH, Hanley JM, Heath EC. Haptoglobin. A novel mode of biosynthesis of a liver secretory glycoprotein. *J Biol Chem* 1981;256: 1055–1057.
81. McCormick DJ, Atassi MZ. Hemoglobin binding with haptoglobin: delineation of the haptoglobin binding site on the alpha chain of human hemoglobin. *J Protein Chem* 1990;9:735–742.
82. Kristiansen M, Graversen JH, Jacobsen C, et al. Identification of the hemoglobin scavenger receptor. *Nature* 2001;409:198–201.
83. Cid MC, Grant DS, Hoffman GS, et al. Identification of haptoglobin as an angiogenic factor in sera from patients with systemic vasculitis. *J Clin Invest* 1993;91:977–985.
84. Malle E, De Beer FC. Human serum amyloid A (SAA) protein: a prominent acute-phase reactant for clinical practice. *Eur J Clin Invest* 1996;26:427–435.
85. Uhlar CM, Whitehead AS. Serum amyloid A, the major vertebrate acute-phase reactant. *Eur J Biochem* 1999;265:501–523.
86. Banka CL, Yuan T, de Beer MC, et al. Serum amyloid A (SAA): influence on HDL-mediated cellular cholesterol efflux. *J Lipid Res* 1995; 36:1058–1065.
87. Badolato R, Wang JM, Murphy WJ, et al. Serum amyloid A is a chemoattractant: induction of migration, adhesion, and tissue infiltration of monocytes and polymorphonuclear leukocytes. *J Exp Med* 1994;180:203–209.
88. Xu L, Badolato R, Murphy WJ, et al. A novel biologic function of serum amyloid A. Induction of T lymphocyte migration and adhesion. *J Immunol* 1995;155:1184–1190.
89. Su SB, Gong W, Gao J-L, et al. A seven-transmembrane, G protein-coupled receptor, FPRL1, mediates the chemotactic activity of serum amyloid A for human phagocytic cells. *J Exp Med* 1999;189:395–402.
90. Migita K, Kawabe Y, Tominaga M, et al. Serum amyloid A protein induces production of matrix metalloproteinases by human synovial fibroblasts. *Lab Invest* 1998;78:535–539.
91. Pruzanski W, Stefanski E, de Beer FC, et al. Lipoproteins are substrates for human secretory group IIA phospholipase A_2: preferential hydrolysis of acute phase HDL. *J Lipid Res* 1998;39:2150–2160.
92. Pruzanski W, Vadas P. Phospholipase A_2—a mediator between proximal and distal effectors of inflammation. *Immunol Today* 1991;12:143–146.

93. Murakami M, Koduri RS, Enomoto A, et al. Dinstict arachidonate-releasing functions of mammalian secreted phospholipase A_2s in human embryonic kidney 293 and rat mastocytoma RBL-2H3 cells through heparan sulfate shuttling and external plasma membrane mechanisms. *J Biol Chem* 2001;276:10083–10096.
94. Weinrauch Y, Abad C, Liang NS, et al. Mobilization of potent plasma bactericidal activity during systemic bacterial challenge. Role of group IIA phospholipase A2. *J Clin Invest* 1998;102:633–638.
95. Laine VJO, Grass DS, Nevalainen TJ. Protection by group II phospholipase A2 against *Staphylococcus aureus*. *J Immunol* 1999;162:7402–7408.
96. Carter DB, Deibel MR Jr, Dunn CJ, et al. Purification, cloning, expression and biological characterization of an interleukin-1 receptor antagonist protein. *Nature* 1990;344:633–638.
97. Dripps DJ, Brandhuber BJ, Thompson RC, et al. Interleukin-1 (IL-1) receptor antagonist binds to the 80-kDa IL-1 receptor but does not initiate IL-1 signal transduction. *J Biol Chem* 1991;266:10331–10336.
98. Gabay C, Smith MF Jr, Eidlen D, et al. Interleukin 1 receptor antagonist (IL-1Ra) is an acute-phase protein. *J Clin Invest* 1997;99:2930–2940.
99. Horai R, Saijo S, Tanioka H, et al. Development of chronic inflammatory arthropathy resembling rheumatoid arthritis in interleukin 1 receptor antagonist-deficient mice. *J Exp Med* 2000;191:313–320.
100. Nicklin MJH, Hughes DE, Barton JL, et al. Arterial inflammation in mice lacking the interleukin 1 receptor antagonist gene. *J Exp Med* 2000;191:303–311.
101. Ma Y, Thornton S, Boivin GP, et al. Altered susceptibility to collagen-induced arthritis in mice with aberrant expression of interleukin-1 receptor antagonist. *Arthritis Rheum* 1998;41:1798–1805.
102. Hirsch E, Irikura VM, Paul SM, et al. Functions of interleukin 1 receptor antagonist in gene knockout and overproducing mice. *Proc Nat Acad Sci U S A* 1996;93:11008–11013
103. Fournier T, Medjoubi-N N, Porquet D. Alpha-1-acid glycoprotein. *Biochim Biophys Acta* 2000;1482:157–171.
104. Hochepied T, Berger FG, Baumann H, Libert C. α_1-Acid glycoprotein: an acute phase protein with inflammatory and immunomodulating properties. *Cytokine Growth Factor Rev* 2003;14:25–34.
105. Hochepied T, Van Molle W, Berger FG, et al. Involvement of the acute phase protein α_1-acid glycoprotein in nonspecific resistance to a lethal gram-negative infection. *J Biol Chem* 2000;275:14903–14909.
106. Schnitzer JE, Pinney E. Quantitation of specific binding of orosomucoid to cultured microvascular endothelium: role in capillary permeability. *Am J Physiol* 1992;263:H48–H55.
107. Wigmore SJ, Fearon KCH, Maingay JP, et al. Interleukin-8 can mediate acute-phase protein production by isolated human hepatocytes. *Am J Physiol* 1997;273:E720–E726.
108. Baumann H, Gauldie J. The acute phase response. *Immunol Today* 1994;15:74–80.
109. Skeen MJ, Ziegler HK. Activation of $\gamma\delta$ T cells for production of IFN-γ is mediated by bacteria via macrophage-derived cytokines IL-1 and IL-12. *J Immunol* 1995;154:5832–5841.
110. Jensen LE, Kmuzio M, Mantovani A, Whitehead AS. IL-1 signaling cascade in liver cells and the involvement of a soluble form of the IL-1 receptor accessory protein. *J Immunol* 2000;164:5277–5286
111. Janeway CA Jr, Medzhitov R. Innate immune recognition. *Annu Rev Immunol* 2002;20:197–216.
112. Akira S, Takeda K, Kaisho T. Toll-like receptors: critical proteins linking innate and acquired immunity. *Nature Immunol* 2001;2:675–680.
113. Martin MU, Wesche H. Summary and comparison of the signaling mechanisms of the Toll/interleukin-1 receptor family. *Biochim Biophys Acta* 2002;1592:265–280.
114. Boch JA, Yoshida Y, Koyama Y, et al. Characterization of a cascade of protein interactions initiated at the IL-1 receptor. *Biochem Biophys Res Commun* 2003;303:525–531.
115. Karin M, Delhase M. The IκB kinase (IKK) and NF-κB: key elements of proinflammatory signaling. *Semin Immunol* 2000;12:85–98.
116. Yamamoto Y, Verma UN, Prajapati S, et al. Histone H3 phosphorylation by IKK-α is critical for cytokine-induced gene expression. *Nature* 2003;423:655–659.
117. Anest V, Hanson JL, Cogswell PC, et al. A nucleosomal function for IκB kinase-α in NF-κB-dependent gene expression. *Nature* 2003;423:659–663.
118. Baud V, Liu ZG, Bennett B, et al. Signaling by proinflammatory cytokines: oligomerization of TRAF2 and TRAF6 is sufficient for JNK and IKK activation and target gene induction via an amino-terminal effector domain. *Genes Dev* 1999;13:1297–1308.
119. Davis RJ. Signal transduction by the JNK group of MAP kinases. *Cell* 2000;103:239–252.
120. Takaeshu G, Kishida S, Hiyama A, et al. TAB2, a novel adaptor protein, mediates activation of TAK1 MAPKKK by linking TAK1 to TRAF6 in the IL-1 signal transduction pathway. *Mol Cell* 2000;5:649–658.
121. Jiang Z, Ninomiya-Tsuji J, Qian Y, et al. Interleukin-1 (IL-1) receptor-associated kinase-dependent IL-1-induced signaling complexes phosphorylate TAK1 and TAB2 at the plasma membrane and activate TAK1 in the cytosol. *Mol Cell Biol* 2002;22:7158–7167.
122. Wang C, Deng L, Hong M, et al. TAK1 is a ubiquitin-dependent kinase of MKK and IKK. *Nature* 2001;412:346–351.
123. Darnell JE Jr, Kerr IM, Stark GR. Jak-STAT pathways and transcriptional activation in response to IFNs and other extracellular signaling proteins. *Science* 1994;264:1415–1421.
124. Kisseleva T, Bhattacharya S, Braunstein J, et al. Signaling through the JAK/STAT pathway, recent advances and future challenges. *Gene* 2002;285:1–24.
125. O'Shea JJ, Gadina M, Schreiber RD. Cytokine signaling in 2002: new surprises in the Jak/Stat pathway. *Cell* 2002;109(suppl):121–131.
126. Aaronson DS, Horvath CM. A road map for those who don't know JAK/STAT. *Science* 2002;296:1653–1655.
127. Heinrich PC, Behrmann I, Haan S, et al. Principles of interleukin (IL) IL-6-type cytokine signaling and its regulation. *Biochem J* 2003;374:1–20.
128. Schindler CW. JAK-STAT signaling in human disease. *J Clin Invest* 2002;109:1133–1137.
129. Naka T, Nishimoto N, Kishimoto T. The paradigm of IL-6: from basic science to medicine. *Arthritis Res* 2002;4(suppl):233–242.
130. Irie-Sasaki J, Sasaki T, Matsumoto W, et al. CD45 is a JAK phosphatase and negatively regulates cytokine receptor signaling. *Nature* 2001;409:349–354.
131. Haspel RL, Salditt-Georgieff M, Darnell JE Jr. The rapid inactivation of nuclear tyrosine phosphorylated Stat1 depends upon protein tyrosine phosphatase. *EMBO J* 1996;15:6262–6268.
132. Krebs DL, Hilton DJ. SOCS proteins: negative regulators of cytokine signaling. *Stem Cells* 2001;19:378–387.
133. Shuai K. Modulation of STAT signaling by STAT-interacting proteins. *Oncogene* 2000;19:2638–2644.
134. Merika M, Thanos D. Enhaceosomes. *Curr Opin Gen Dev* 2001;11:205–208.
135. Deodhar SD. C-reactive protein: the best laboratory indicator available for monitoring disease activity. *Cleve Clin J Med* 1989;56:126–130.
136. Kushner I. C-reactive protein in rheumatology. *Arthritis Rheum* 1991;34:1065–1068.
137. Pepys MB, de Beer FC, Dyck RF, et al. Clinical measurement of serum C-reactive protein in monitoring and differential diagnosis of inflammatory diseases and tissue necrosis and in the recognition and management of intercurrent infection. *Ann NY Acad Sci* 1982;389:459–460.
138. Hellerstein S, Duggan E, Welchert E, et al. Serum C-reactive protein and the site of urinary tract infections. *J Pediatr* 1982;100:21–25.
139. Hind CRK, Flint KC, Hudspith BN, et al. Serum C-reactive protein concentration in patients with pulmonary sarcoidosis. *Thorax* 1987;42:332–335.
140. Fagan EA, Dyck RF, Maton PN, et al. Serum levels of C-reactive protein in Crohn's disease and ulcerative colitis. *Eur J Clin Invest* 1982;12:351–359.
141. Gray BM, Simmons DR, Mason H, et al. Quantitative levels of C-reactive protein in cerebrospinal fluid in patients with bacterial meningitis and other conditions. *J Pediatr* 1986;108:665–670.
142. Venditti M, Brandimarte C, Trobiani P, et al. Serial study of C-reactive protein for the diagnosis of bacterial and fungal infections in neutropenic patients with hematologic malignancies. *Haematologica* 1988;73:285–291.
143. Becker GJ, Waldburger M, Hughes GR, et al. Value of serum C-reactive protein measurement in the investigation of fever in systemic lupus erythematosus. *Ann Rheum Dis* 1980;39:50–52.

144. Koenig W, Sund M, Frohlich M, et al. C-reactive protein a sensitive marker of inflammation predicts future risk of coronary heart disease in initially healthy middle-aged men: results from the MONICA (Monitoring Trends and Determinants in Cardiovascular Disease) Augsburg Cohort Study, 1984 to 1992. *Circulation* 1999;99:237–242.
145. Albert M, Glynn RJ, Ridker PM. Plasma concentration of C-reactive protein and the calculated Framingham coronary heart disease risk score. *Circulation* 2003;108:161–165.
146. Rost NS, Wolf PA, Kase CS, et al. Plasma concentration of C-reactive protein and risk of ischemic stroke and transient ischemic attack: the Framingham study. *Stroke* 2001;32:2575–2579.
147. Cao JJ, Thach C, Manolio TA, et al. C-reactive protein, carotid intima-media thickness, and incidence of ischemic stroke in the elderly. The cardiovascular health study. *Circulation* 2003;108:166–170.
148. Albert CM, Ma J, Rifai N, et al. Prospective study of C-reactive protein, homocysteine, and plasma lipid levels as predictors of sudden cardiac death. *Circulation* 2002;105:2595–2599.
149. Ridker PM, Stampfer MJ, Rifai N. Novel risk factors for systemic atherosclerosis: a comparison of C-reactive protein, fibrinogen, homocysteine, lipoprotein(a) and standard cholesterol screening as predictors of peripheral arterial disease. *JAMA* 2001;285:2481–2485.
150. Ridker PM, Rifai N, Rose L, et al. Comparison of C-reactive protein and low-density lipoprotein cholesterol levels in the prediction of first cardiovascular events. *N Engl J Med* 2002;347:1557–1565.
151. Lindahl B, Toss H, Siegbahn A, et al. Markers of myocardial damage and inflammation in relation to long-term mortality in unstable coronary artery disease. *N Engl J Med* 2000;343:1139–1147.
152. Roseff R, Wolgethan JR, Sipe JD, et al. The acute phase response in gout. *J Rheumatol* 1987;14:974–977.
153. Sukenik S, Henkin J, Zimlichman S, et al. Serum and synovial fluid levels of serum amyloid A protein and C-reactive protein in inflammatory and noninflammatory arthritis. *J Rheumatol* 1988;15:942–945.
154. Amos RS, Constable TJ, Crockson RA, et al. Rheumatoid arthritis: relation of serum C-reactive protein and erythrocyte sedimentation rate to radiographic changes. *BMJ* 1977;1:195–197.
155. Cush JJ, Lipsky PE, Postlethwaite AE, et al. Correlation of serologic indicators of inflammation with the effectiveness of nonsteroidal antiinflammatory drug therapy in rheumatoid arthritis. *Arthritis Rheum* 1990;33:19–28.
156. Plant MJ, Williams AL, O'Sullivan MM, et al. Relationship between time-integrated C-reactive protein levels and radiologic progression in patients with rheumatoid arthritis. *Arthritis Rheum* 2000;43:1473–1477.
157. Gwyther M, Schwarz H, Howard A, et al. C-reactive protein in juvenile chronic arthritis: an indicator of disease activity and possibly amyloidosis. *Ann Rheum Dis* 1982;41:259–262.
158. Laurent MR, Panayi GS, Shepherd P. Circulating immune complexes, serum immunoglobulins, and acute phase proteins in psoriasis and psoriatic arthritis. *Ann Rheum Dis* 1983;40:524–528.
159. Laurent MR, Panayi GS. Acute-phase proteins and serum immunoglobulins in ankylosing spondylitis. *Ann Rheum Dis* 1983;42:524–528.
160. Nashel DJ. C-reactive protein: a marker for disease activity in ankylosing spondylitis and Reiter's syndrome. *J Rheumatol* 1986;13:364–367.
161. Mallya RK, de Beer FC, Berry H, et al. Serum C-reactive protein in polymyalgia rheumatica. A prospective serial study. *Arthritis Rheum* 1985;28:383–387.
162. Kyle V, Cawston TE, Hazleman BL. Erythrocyte sedimentation rate and C-reactive protein in the assessment of polymyalgia rheumatica/giant cell arteritis as presentation and during followup. *Ann Rheum Dis* 1989;48:667–671.
163. Hind CR. Objective monitoring of activity in Wegener's granulomatosis by measurement of serum C-reactive protein concentration. *Clin Nephrol* 1984;21:341–345.
164. Hind CR, Winearls CG, Pepys MB. Correlation of disease activity in systemic vasculitis with serum C-reactive protein measurement. A prospective study of thirty-eight patients. *Eur J Clin Invest* 1985;15: 89–94.
165. Lehner T, Adinolfi M. Acute phase proteins, C9, factor B, and lysozyme in recurrent oral ulceration and Behçet's syndrome. *J Clin Pathol* 1980;33:269–275.
166. Pereira Da Silva JA, Elkon KB, Hughes GR, et al. C-reactive protein levels in systemic lupus erythematosus. A classification criterion? *Arthritis Rheum* 1980;23:770–771.
167. Sitton NG, Dixon JS, Bird HA, et al. Serum biochemistry in rheumatoid arthritis seronegative arthropathies, osteoarthritis, SLE, and normal subjects. *Br J Rheum* 1987;26:131–135.
168. Stuart RA, Littlewood AJ, Maddison PJ, et al. Elevated serum interleukin-6 levels associated with active disease in systemic connective tissue disorders. *Clin Exp Rheumatol* 1995;13:17–22.
169. ter Borg EJ, Horst G, Limburg PC, et al. C-reactive protein levels during disease exacerbations and infections in systemic lupus erythematosus. A prospective longitudinal study. *J Rheumatol* 1990;17: 1642–1648.
170. Moutsopoulos HM, Mavridis AK, Acritidis NC, et al. High C-reactive protein response in lupus polyarthritis. *Clin Exp Rheumatol* 1983;1: 53–55.
171. Bakri Hassan A, Ronnelid J, Gunnarsson I, et al. Increased serum levels of immunoglobulins, C-reactive protein, type 1 and type 2 cytokines in patients with mixed connective tissue disease. *J Autoimmun* 1998;11:503–508.

CHAPTER 23

Eicosanoids and Related Compounds

Charles N. Serhan

Acute inflammation is characterized by pain, redness, swelling, heat, and eventual loss of function of the affected area. These events, namely the "cardinal signs of inflammation," as well as other physiologic processes, are mediated in part by lipid-derived mediators, such as the eicosanoids and platelet-activating factor (PAF) that serve as local chemical autacoids (Fig. 23.1). Several new drugs have been launched targeting these mediators, emphasizing their importance in human disease, particularly rheumatoid arthritis (RA). These mediators/modulators are biosynthesized from the membrane lipids of a wide range of cell types and can serve intracellular roles within their cell type of origin or can be released to the extracellular milieu to act as either paracrine or autocrine signals, namely local mediators (1).

Eicosanoids are 20-carbon, bioactive oxygenation products biosynthesized from arachidonic acid and are the most thoroughly studied of the now many known classes of lipid mediators. The eicosanoids are generated by the actions of three major classes of intracellular enzymes: cyclooxygenases (COX) [prostaglandins (PGs)], lipoxygenases (LOs) [leukotrienes (LTs) and lipoxins (LX)], and P450 epoxygenases (epoxyeicosatrienoic acids) (Table 23.1 and Fig. 23.1). Because our understanding of the role of epoxygenase-derived products in the pathogenesis of inflammation is still evolving (2–4), this chapter focuses on the biosynthesis and actions of the COX- and LO-derived eicosanoids and related new bioactive compounds produced from essential ω-3 fatty acids termed resolvins and docosatrienes that are of interest in the pathophysiology and treatment of arthritis and related diseases.

After several decades of intense investigation, we are now poised to appreciate the diversity in eicosanoid signaling systems and the impact of drugs in these biochemical and signaling circuits. In particular, with the discovery of (a) new isozymes (COX-1, -2, and the recently added COX-3), (b) new bioactive compounds, and (c) identified and cloned relevant receptors as well as the heightened appreciation of the role and importance of cell/cell interactions that enable transcellular biosynthesis to enhance the repertoire of eicosanoids relevant in inflammation and host defense.

Most attention has focused on arachidonic-derived compounds because of their potent nanomolar to micromolar bioactions in almost all human tissues and the finding that aspirin blocks the formation of prostanoids.

Investigations along these lines began in the 1930s with the observations of von Euler and Goldblatt of substances in semen that cause smooth muscle contractions. It required almost 30 years of work by Sune Bergström, Bengt Samuelsson, and colleagues at the Karolinska Institute, Stockholm, to elucidate the structures of these bioactive substances, termed prostaglandins (5). In the 1960s and 1970s, the detailed biosynthesis of these potent lipid mediators from arachidonic acid was established by Samuelsson and colleagues. These studies also opened the way for the structural elucidation of thromboxane (also known as rabbit aorta contracting substance) (Figs. 23.1 and 23.2) as well as the structural elucidation of the slow reaction substance of anaphylaxis, originally noted in 1938 by Kellaway (6) and termed leukotrienes in 1979. Hence, the investigative origin of the eicosanoids lies within their potent bioactions and a cross-disciplinary union of small-molecule structural elucidation, organic chemistry, cell biology, structural immunology, and pathophysiology.

Our appreciation of the information conveyed by these small-lipid mediators continues to evolve rapidly, and because we know little about the information within lipids per se, the lessons learned from the eicosanoids provide important direction. The discovery of the PGs and their biosynthetic link to fatty acids resulted in a paradigm shift and challenged the dogma of the time that lipids serve only structural roles in biologic systems (5,7). It is now clear that eicosanoids play key roles in several physiologic and pathophysiologic settings: they act on smooth muscle in both intestine and uterus; regulate kidney function, including water

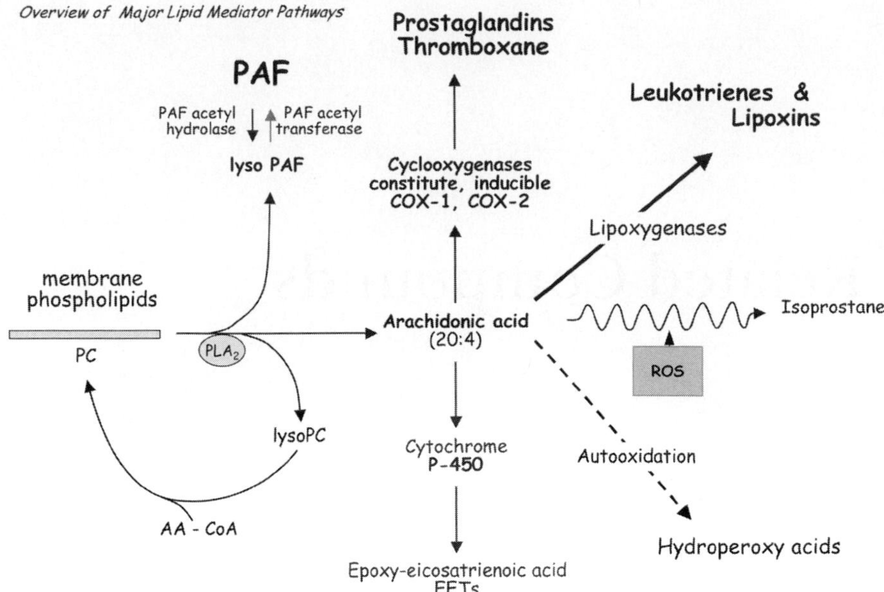

FIG. 23.1. Lipid mediators: overview of eicosanoids and platelet-activating factor (PAF). Epoxy-eicosatetranoic acids (EETs) are p450 products (141) and isoeicosanoids are generated via nonenzymatic, free radical mechanisms (142). Arachidonic acid possesses 20 carbons [carbon 1 is at the carboxylic acid end, and C20 denotes the omega end (ω)] and four double bonds (Δ5, Δ8, Δ11, Δ14) that are not conjugated and are 1,4-*cis*-pentadiene units. *AA,* arachidonic acid; *PC,* phosphocholine; *PLA*$_2$*,* phospholipase A$_2$; *ROS,* reactive oxygen species.

balance and Na^{2+} excretion; influence the hemodynamics affecting blood pressure; affect platelet/endothelial cell interactions; and contribute to the resolution of inflammation. In this regard, eicosanoids play key roles in host defense and pain and evoke the cardinal signs of inflammation (Table 23.2), responses that are of special importance to rheumatologists.

The elucidation of the PG biosynthetic pathway enabled Sir John Vane and colleagues in 1971 to uncover the action of aspirin and related antiinflammatory drugs as inhibitors of PGs (8). These discoveries and the important role of eicosanoids in human health and disease led to the 1982 Nobel Prize in Physiology or Medicine awarded to Bergström, Samuelsson, and Vane for their contributions, and a Nobel Prize in Chemistry in 1990 awarded to Dr. E.J. Corey for his contribution to the total organic synthesis of these molecules, which enabled the elucidation of their biologic properties (9). This proved to be a key component to understanding the biologic importance of this system, because eicosanoids are generated in only small amounts in human tissues (nanogram to microgram range) and are rapidly inactivated, which limited their assessments after isolation. Total organic synthesis of larger quantities of eicosanoids of defined stereochemistry permitted unambiguous evaluation of their biologic roles.

It is clear that different eicosanoids within a class [i.e., prostaglandin E_2 (PGE_2) vs. $PGF_{2\alpha}$] can exert opposing actions, such as constriction and dilatory effects or prothrombotic and antithrombotic effects (see actions of thromboxane and prostacyclin, Fig. 23.2B). Counterregulatory effects of products generated from a common precursor, such as arachidonic acid, are also evident within

TABLE 23.1. *Glossary and acronyms*

ATL	Aspirin-triggered lipoxin; 15-epi-LX
COX	Cyclooxygenase (1 and 2 or 3) or endoperoxide synthase (PGH synthase)
Leukotrienes (LT)	5-LO products containing conjugated triene structure
LTA_4 hydrolase	Catalyzes the enzymatic production of LTB_4 from LTA_4
LTC_4 synthase	Catalyzes the conjugation of LTA_4 with reduced glutathione to form LTC_4
Lipoxins (LX)	Lipoxygenase interaction products; contain 20 carbons and four conjugated double bonds (tetraene structure)
Lipoxygenase (LO)	Catalyzes the insertion of molecular oxygen into polyunsaturated fatty acids
5-Lipoxygenase (5-LO)	Initial enzyme of the leukotriene pathway; catalyzes the insertion of molecular oxygen into the C-5 of arachidonic acid
NSAIDs	Nonsteroidal antiinflammatory drugs
Peptido-leukotrienes	Originally the slow-reacting substance of anaphylaxis; LTC_4, LTD_4, LTE_4
Prostaglandin (PG)	A 20-carbon fatty acid containing a five-carbon ring
Thromboxanes	20 carbons with a six-member oxirane ring

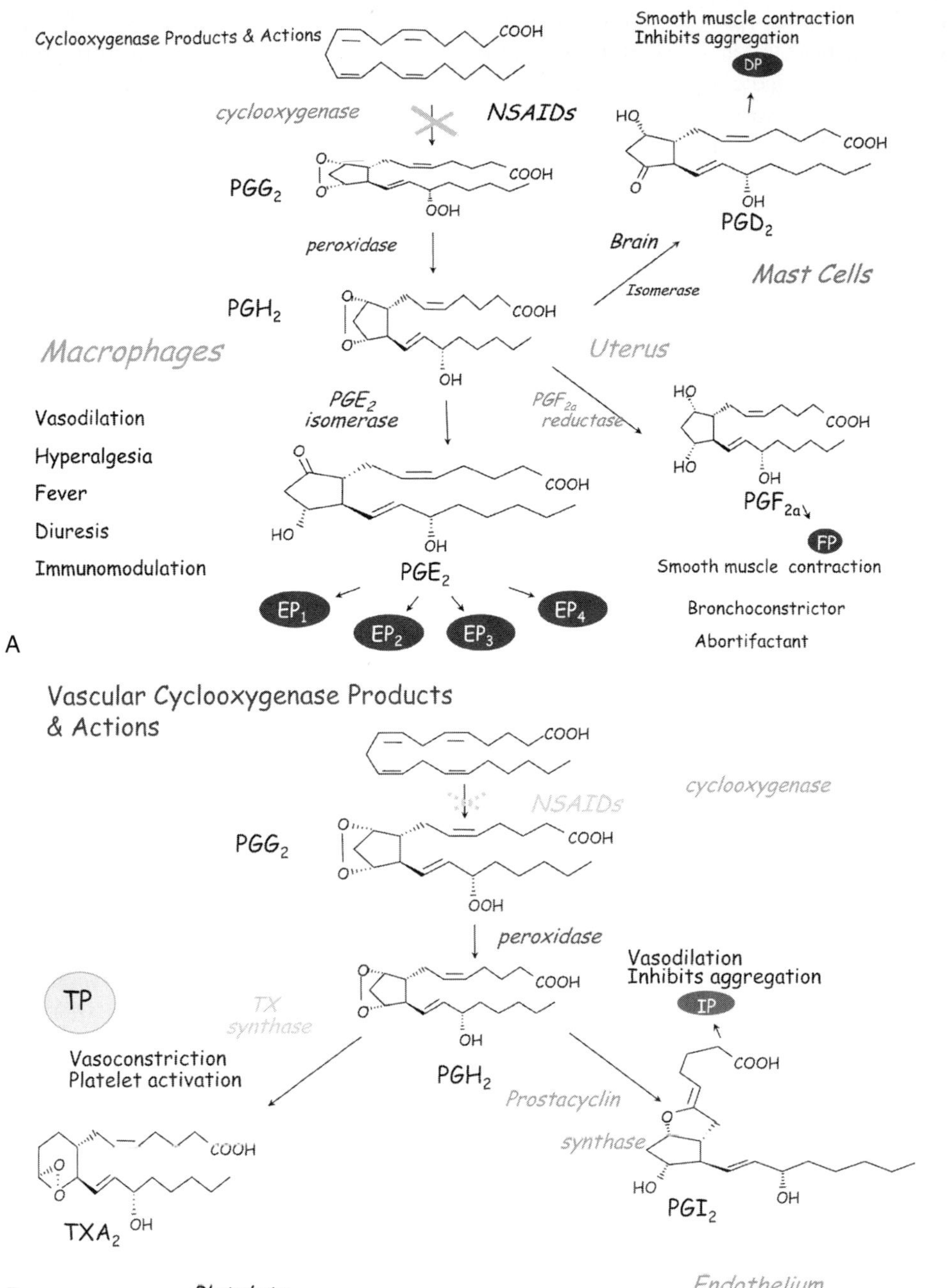

FIG. 23.2. Cyclooxygenase products and actions. **A:** Cyclooxygenase products and their actions. Filled circles denote cloned receptors (i.e., FP, EP, TP). **B:** Vascular cyclooxygenase products and actions. *NSAIDs,* nonsteroidal anti-inflammatory drugs (e.g., aspirin, indomethacin); *TX,* thromboxane; *PG,* prostaglandin.

TABLE 23.2. *Actions of lipid-derived molecules in inflammation*

Cardinal sign	Lipid mediator	Endogenous inhibitor
Pain and hyperalgesia	PGE_2, LTB_4, PAF	
Redness (vasodilation)	PGE_2, PGI_2, LTB_4, LXA_4, PAF	
Heat (local and systemic fever)	PGE_2, PGI_2, LXA_4, PAF	
Edema (swelling)	PGE_2, LTB_4, LTC_4, LTD_4, LTE_4, PAF	Lipoxins, ATL

ATL, aspirin-triggered lipoxin; LT, leukotriene; LX, lipoxin; PAF, platelet activating factor; PG, prostaglandin.

inflammation with the LO products leukotrienes (proinflammatory) and LX (anti-inflammatory) (see Fig. 23.1 and Table 23.2). Recently, results from my laboratory indicate that aspirin, in addition to its ability to block PG formation, is also capable of triggering the biosynthesis of the 15-epimers of LX (1) and additional novel aspirin-triggered mediators termed resolvins (10–12). These mimic the anti-inflammatory actions of the native LX and resolvins, hence appearing to at least partially mediate some of aspirin's antiinflammatory therapeutic impact (13–15). Given the contribution of eicosanoids and other autacoid mediators derived from lipids to inflammation and newly uncovered mechanisms in endogenous antiinflammation and resolution, these pathways have been the focus of the pharmaceutical industry to develop new classes of drugs (selective inhibitors, mimetics, and antagonists) acting within this system. Several new drugs have reached the rheumatology clinic with disease-modifying action (16) (see also Chapters 16 and 31). Hence, knowledge of new lipid mediators and the eicosanoid biosynthetic pathways continues to provide unique therapeutic opportunities and novel strategies for rheumatologists that will likely continue well into the next century. The goal of this chapter is to succinctly update our appreciation of the roles of eicosanoids and related compounds in inflammation and highlight our progress toward uncovering new compounds and signaling processes relevant in inflammation and its resolution.

SIGNALS FOR THE FORMATION OF LIPID MEDIATORS

Table 23.2 summarizes some of the key inflammatory actions known for the major series of eicosanoids and PAF. Many of these compounds stimulate the cardinal signs of inflammation (pain, heat, redness, and swelling) and, thus, have the potential to serve as proinflammatory mediators. It is also now clear that LX and their aspirin-triggered C15 epimers serve as agonists of resolution of inflammation by activating the uptake of apoptotic polymorphonuclear leukocytes (PMNs) by macrophages, an important process in resolution of acute inflammatory events (1,17).

In general, most lipid-derived mediators are not stored by cells, but rather their *de novo* biosynthesis from cellular precursors is evoked by various stimuli. Arachidonic acid is a fatty acid derived from dietary sources or is synthesized in the body from an essential fatty acid, linoleic acid. It is stored in lipid bilayers of cell membranes and is esterified predominantly to phospholipids such as phosphatidylcholine, phosphatidylethanolamine, and phosphatidylinositol. Hence, a major rate-limiting step in eicosanoid biosynthesis is the release or deacylation of arachidonic acid from esterified sources (i.e., membrane storage sites) by specific phospholipases (PLs). One such enzyme is PLA_2 (Table 23.3). This particular phospholipase cleaves the ester bond covalently linking arachidonate to the glycerol backbone of the phospholipid precursor. In many cell types, PLA_2 is membrane associated and Ca^{2+} dependent. Hence, eicosanoid biosynthesis can be initiated by a wide variety of stimuli that increase the levels of intracellular Ca^{2+} and may occur via specific receptor-mediated signal transduction mechanisms (e.g., hormones and autacoids) or through disruption of cell membrane integrity (physical, chemical, or immunologic trauma), events that lead to phospholipase activation. Two main classes of human PLA_2 have been cloned: secretory PLA_2 ($sPLA_2$) (14–18 kd) and cytosolic PLA_2 ($cPLA_2$) (31–110 kd) (Table 23.3). The cytosolic form appears to be key in regulated C20:4 release in human immune cells. As many as 17 related enzymes have been cloned to date, and their role, for the most part, remains to be elucidated (18).

TABLE 23.3. *Phospholipase A_2 characteristics*

Phospholipase A_2	Molecular weight (kd)	Ca^{2+}	Regulation	Substrate specificity
Secreted				
$sPLA_2$				
Group I (pancreatic)	14	m*M*	Posttranslational	Lacks specificity
Group II (synovial fluid/platelets)	14	m*M*	Transcriptional	Lacks specificity
PAF-acetylhydrolase (plasma)	45	None		sn-2 short chain
Nonsecreted cytosolic				
$cPLA_2$	85	m*M*	Transcriptional/ phosphorylation	sn-2 arachidonic acid
$iPLA_2$ (myocardium)	40	None	ATP	Plasmalogen sn-2-arachidonic acid
$iPLA_2$ (macrophage)	80	None	ATP	Lacks specificity for arachidonic acid but can release several other PUFAs

ATP, adenosine triphosphate; $cPLA_2$, cytosolic phospholipase A_2; $iPLA_2$, calcium-independent phospholipase A_2; $sPLA_2$, secretory phospholipase A_2.

ENZYMATIC CONVERSION OF ARACHIDONIC ACID TO UNIQUE CLASSES OF BIOACTIVE AUTACOIDS

The fate of unesterified arachidonic acid (denoted C20:4), once released from membrane phospholipid storage sites, is cell specific and initially depends on the presence of specific arachidonic acid–converting enzymes, such as COX-1 or COX-2 or 5- or 15-LO, and then on the presence of specific synthases that convert LO- and COX-generated intermediates into biologically-active products. Arachidonic acid is converted to PGs by the initial action of COX, whereas LT and LX are formed from the initial action of LO (Fig. 23.1). Other fatty acids, such as linoleic acid (C18:2 or 9,12-octadecadienoic acid), are also substrates for some of these enzymes that give rise to different series of oxygenated compounds, some with reduced potencies (19), whereas other newly isolated compounds have increased potencies compared with their substrate (i.e., resolvins and docosatrienes) (11,12). Arachidonic acid appears to be the preferred substrate in most human cell types, but can be replaced by dietary supplementation with fish oils (ω-3 fatty acids). PAF is also formed *de novo* from precursors found in membrane phospholipids. Again PLA_2 plays a critical role in this biosynthetic scheme. PLA_2 causes the release of a precursor molecule, termed lyso-PAF, from alkylacylglycerophosphorylcholine in cell membranes (Table 23.3).

MAJOR PHOSPHOLIPASES INVOLVED IN EICOSANOID SIGNALING

Each major group of phospholipase contains multiple family members that carry out a similar reaction but are regulated by different mechanisms. Each PLA_2 is thought to act on different substrates, thus providing several alternative pathways for the highly controlled process of phospholipid degradation, membrane remodeling, and eicosanoid biosynthesis.

Phospholipases

Secreted Phospholipase A_2

The products of PLA_2 actions on phospholipids are free fatty acids and lysophospholipids that are themselves also regulatory molecules. Mammalian cells contain multiple, structurally-diverse PLA_2 enzymes (Table 23.3). The most well characterized are the secretory, low-molecular-weight PLA_2 enzymes ($sPLA_2$) that are structurally similar to the two groups of $sPLA_2$ found in snake venoms. The two groups can be distinguished by differences in primary structure and the distribution of disulfide bonds. Mammalian pancreatic $sPLA_2$ is a Group I enzyme, whereas Group II $sPLA_2$, which was first identified in synovial fluid and platelets, is found in a variety of cell types. The $sPLA_2$s require millimolar Ca^{2+} for catalytic activity and do not show acyl-chain substrate specificity. There is considerable interest in Group II $sPLA_2$ because of its increased levels in serum and inflammatory exudates during diseases such as septic shock and RA. Group II PLA_2 is implicated as an acute-phase protein that may play a role in microbial defense (20). Cytokines, such as interleukin-1 (IL-1), tumor necrosis factor (TNF), and IL-6, induce increased expression of Group II $sPLA_2$ that correlates with increased PG production, both of which can be suppressed by glucocorticoids. The mechanism whereby Group II $sPLA_2$ mediates arachidonic acid release is not elucidated, yet results suggest that it may act as an extracellular enzyme on membranes that are altered or on neighboring cell types (21). Of interest, this enzyme may carry information without its catalytic activity (22), possibly acting as a ligand at cell surface receptors.

Cytosolic Phospholipase A_2

The 85-kd cytosolic PLA_2 ($cPLA_2$), the first arachidonic acid–selective PLA_2 identified, is an important enzyme mediating agonist-induced arachidonic acid release (18). In addition, $cPLA_2$ exhibits relatively high lysophospholipase activity and can completely deacylate diacylphospholipids. The active site serine at position 228 (Ser228) of $cPLA_2$ is essential for both PLA_2 and lysophospholipase catalytic activities. $cPLA_2$ contains an N-terminal, Ca^{2+}, and phospholipid binding (CaLB) domain that is responsible for Ca^{2+}-dependent membrane association (reviewed in references 1 and 18).

$cPLA_2$ is regulated posttranslationally by both serine phosphorylation and Ca^{2+}. Phosphorylation of $cPLA_2$ occurs in a variety of cell types by diverse agonists, such as mitogens, thrombin, adenosine triphosphate (ATP), zymosan, endotoxin, TNF-α, IL-1, calcium ionophore, phorbol ester, and okadaic acid, and results in an increase in PLA_2 activity and a decrease in electrophoretic mobility (gel shift) on sodium dodecyl sulfate gels. Phosphorylation of $cPLA_2$ by ERK1 and ERK2 mitogen activated protein (MAP) kinases at Ser505 induces a gel shift and increases PLA_2 activity. Overexpression of $cPLA_2$ in Chinese hamster ovary (CHO) cells increases arachidonic acid release. However, overexpression of a mutated $cPLA_2$ in which Ser505 is replaced with an alanine prevents release, thereby implicating a role for MAP kinases in the signal transduction pathway.

In platelets treated with the thrombin receptor agonist peptide SFLLRN, phosphorylation of $cPLA_2$ and a gel shift occurs without activating ERK1 and ERK2, suggesting the involvement of alternate kinase pathways. In many cell types, phosphorylation of $cPLA_2$ along with an increase in intracellular Ca^{2+} is necessary for full activation of the enzyme. The calcium-mobilizing agonists IgE/antigen and A23187 induce $cPLA_2$ translocation to the nuclear envelope in rat basophilic leukemia (RBL) mast cells. In CHO cells overexpressing $cPLA_2$, A23187-induced translocation of

$cPLA_2$ to endoplasmic reticulum and the nuclear envelope is dependent on the CaLB domain but not dependent on phosphorylation at Ser505. The mechanisms involved in specific targeting of $cPLA_2$ to the nuclear membrane or other membranes remain to be established. Colocalization of $cPLA_2$, 5-LO, 5-lipoxygenase activating protein (FLAP), and PG endoperoxide H synthase 2 on the nuclear envelope represents another level of coordinate regulation of enzymes involved in eicosanoid production (see Fig. 23.6). Gene disruption of cytosolic PLA_2 demonstrated several anticipated important physiologic roles for this enzyme (23,24). Most relevant to inflammation is the finding that $cPLA_2$-deficient mice give reduced eicosanoid release (LTs, PGs) and, upon challenge, show reduced allergic responses (reviewed in reference 25).

Calcium-Independent Phospholipase A_2

Mammalian cells also contain calcium-independent forms of PLA_2 ($iPLA_2$) (Table 23.2). Myocardium is rich in $iPLA_2$, and the purified enzyme is a 40-kd protein that exhibits specificity for plasmalogen substrates, the predominant form of phospholipid in myocardium. This $iPLA_2$ exists as a high-molecular-weight complex composed of the 40-kd catalytic subunit and an 85-kd regulatory subunit homologous to phosphofructokinase. ATP enhances PLA_2 activity of the complex, but has no effect on the purified 40-kd subunit. Results with inhibitors suggest that $iPLA_2$ catalyzes arachidonic acid release in smooth muscle and pancreatic islet cells and maybe macrophages. However, additional results are needed to evaluate the potential role of $iPLA_2$ in inflammation and arthritis.

Given the diversity in lipid-derived mediator networks, the pathways of biosynthesis and actions of each class of lipid mediators are introduced separately.

BIOSYNTHESIS AND CELL SOURCES OF PROSTAGLANDINS

The basic structure of a PG molecule is a 20-carbon carboxylic acid containing a cyclopentane ring between carbons 9, 10, 11, and 12 and a hydroxyl group at carbon 15 (Fig. 23.2). This backbone structure was termed prostanoic acid or a prostanoid. PGs are divided into series that differ in the oxygen substitution in the cyclopentane ring as coded by a letter (PGD, PGE, PGF, PGG, PGH). The subscript numeral in PG nomenclature indicates the number of double bonds present in the compound. In general, PGs in the 1 series are derived from the precursor linoleic acid (which is also a substrate for these enzymes), whereas compounds in the 2 series are derived from arachidonic acid. PGs are formed from arachidonic acid by the initial action of COX (PG endoperoxide G/H synthase) (Fig. 23.2).

COX is a heme-containing enzyme that is most abundant in the endoplasmic reticulum and catalyzes two distinct reactions: (a) cyclization of arachidonic acid to form PGG_2 and (b) hydroperoxidation of PGG_2 to yield PGH_2. The latter is a relatively unstable compound that has a half-life of seconds and is a common intermediate that is converted to biologically-active products, including thromboxane (TXA_2), prostacyclin (PGI_2), PGD_2, PGE_2, and $PGF_{1\alpha}$, in a cell-specific manner. Figure 23.2 presents an overview of the pathways for PG biosynthesis, the major cell sources of the individual compounds, and the predominant actions of key products. PGH_2 is converted to PGE_2 by an enzyme termed PGE_2 isomerase. This enzyme is expressed by a wide range of cell types, including phagocytic cells such as neutrophils and macrophages. PGD_2 isomerase, an enzyme that is particularly abundant in the brain and certain inflammatory cells, such as mast cells, converts PGH_2 to PGD_2. PGF reductase converts PGH_2 to $PGF_{2\alpha}$. This enzyme is abundant, for example, in uterine tissue.

Figure 23.2B illustrates important eicosanoids of the vessel wall that control thromboregulation (26). Prostacyclin synthase and thromboxane synthase convert PGH_2 to prostacyclin and thromboxane, respectively. Prostacyclin is a main arachidonic acid product generated by vascular endothelial cells. Thromboxane is formed by platelets and macrophages. These two compounds (TXA_2 and PGI_2) play critical roles in hemostasis, as well as inflammation, and have opposing actions. Each COX product acts at specific receptors, many of which have been cloned and characterized.

Cyclooxygenases

COX converts C20:4 to endoperoxide-containing intermediates that are transformed to PG and TX. COX activity is inhibited by nonsteroidal antiinflammatory drugs (NSAIDs; this class of drugs includes aspirin) and is the subject of extensive investigations aimed toward achieving more selective drugs. In the past several years it has been recognized that "COX activity" is not a single enzyme but rather represents two (Fig. 23.3) and perhaps more isoforms that await elucidation (16,27–30). COX-2 expression is inhibited by corticosteroids (classic antiinflammatory agents with many side effects), whereas COX-1 (e.g., the "original" enzyme present in platelets) is not sensitive to these agents. COX-2 is induced by lipopolysaccharides in macrophages and is associated with differentiation in monocytic cell lines (Fig. 23.3). Within the vasculature *in vivo*, it is now appreciated that COX-2 is expressed in endothelial cells in response to physiologic flow and shear force (31). Most COX-derived products from endothelial cells appear to be generated by endothelial cell COX-2 *in vivo* (32). The ability of COX-2 to generate the bulk of PGI_2 *in vivo* leads to apparent increased thrombogenicity with the use of COX-2 inhibitors (32). The production of COX-2-derived PGI_2 apparently is an important role for vascular COX-2. Because COX-2 selective inhibitors block PGI_2 formation, more selective PG inhibitors, such as those recently directed to the new target $mPGE_2$ synthase (33), may prove to

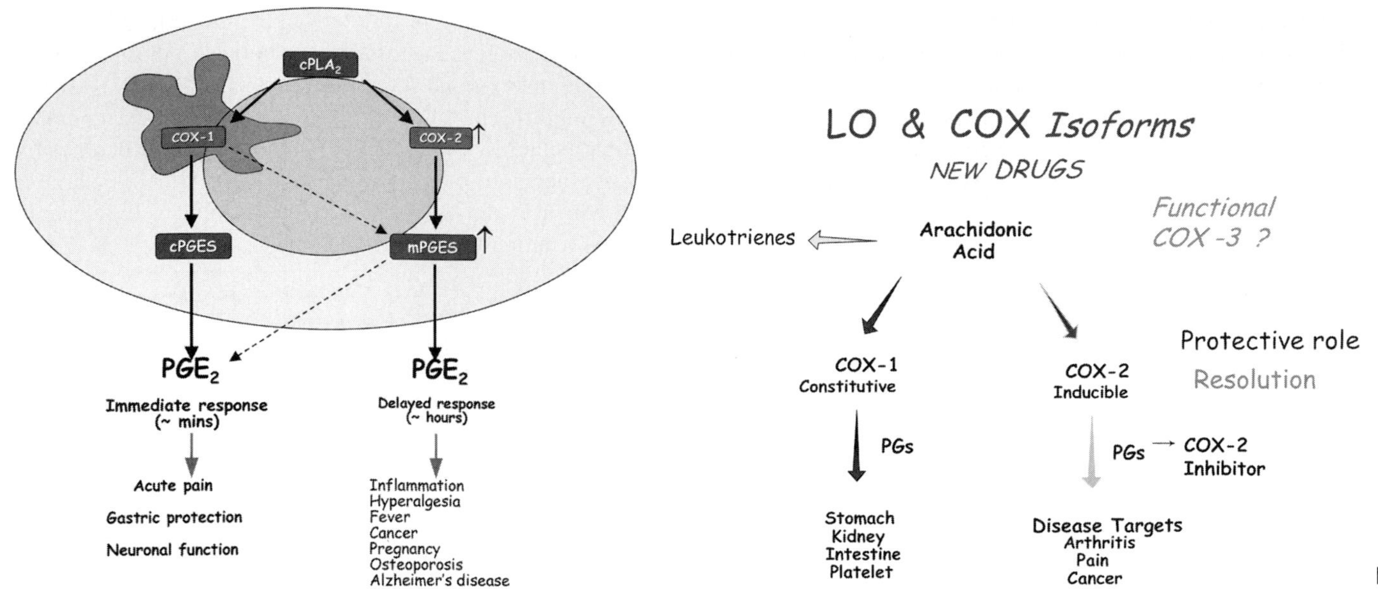

FIG. 23.3. Lipoxygenase and cyclooxygenase (COX) isoforms: separate systems and opportunities for improved drugs. **A:** Topography and relationship between COX-1 and COX-2. **B:** Potential new targets.

be valuable future therapeutic agents in RA and related arthritic diseases (34).

A functional third form of the enzyme, denoted COX-3 was proposed to play a role in resolution rather than initiation of inflammation because inhibitors of COX-2 delayed resolution in experimental models of inflammation (29). This and other results raise concern as to the unwanted side effects of selective COX-2 inhibition. In addition to potential COX-3 isoforms, Simmons and colleagues also described several other COX-related proteins denoted P-COX. Their role in PG formation remains to be established. A functional form of COX also denoted as COX-3 has been assigned an antiinflammatory role (35,36). Recently, a structural third isoform, also called COX-3, was identified from brain and is held to be the long sought after paracetamol-sensitive COX activity that might be important in fever regulation (30,37). This isoform appears to be a truncated version of the COX-like structure that raises concern regarding the nomenclature of these new forms of COX. However, because the putative COX-3 nucleotide sequence was obtained initially from canine tissues, it has recently been questioned whether such an isoform is present in human tissues (38). Further research is needed to clarify whether additional functional isoforms are present that might be relevant in the generation of prostanoids during the pathogenesis of arthritic diseases.

Functionally-Separate Prostanoid Biosynthetic Systems: the Simplicity of "Good COX" Versus "Bad COX"

COX-1 and COX-2 are membrane-bound enzymes; however, in murine 3T3 cells and in human and bovine endothelial cells, COX-2 is twice as abundant in the nuclear envelope as compared with the endoplasmic reticulum, whereas COX-1 is found in equal amounts in the two compartments. COX-1 is mostly functional in the endoplasmic reticulum, whereas COX-2 activity is mainly detected in the nucleus (39,40). These findings, in conjunction with the differences in gene expression and earlier observations that COX-1 and COX-2 utilize different subcellular sources of arachidonate, suggest that the two isozymes represent separate and independently operating PG biosynthetic systems (Fig. 23.3). According to this hypothesis, COX-1 produces PG constitutively for secretion as extracellular mediators and COX-2 would be active only in certain circumstances to produce PG within the nucleus to possibly influence processes such as cell division, growth, and differentiation (41).

Mouse lines that do not express either COX-1 or COX-2 were developed by targeted gene disruption (42,43; and reviewed in reference 25). COX-1 (−/−) mice exhibit reduced fertility, platelet aggregability, and sensitivity to arachidonic acid–induced ear inflammation. Interestingly, COX-2–deficient mice give normal inflammatory responses with exogenous arachidonic acid but exhibit an increased incidence of suppurative peritonitis (42). Although some of these exciting results should be interpreted with caution, they do agree with the view that COX-1 and COX-2 are two distinct prostanoid biosynthetic systems with separate biologic functions for their products. Further studies with these transgenic animals may help clarify the role of these enzymes in physiologic and pathologic processes.

As illustrated in Fig. 23.3A, both COX-1 and COX-2 enzymes colocalize in endoplasmic reticulum and share common catalytic and product transport features, although they are distinct in primary structure (39). Discovery of COX-2 inspired swift development of new selective COX inhibitors that preferentially act on COX-1 versus COX-2 and further distinguish their roles in inflammation. Also, COX-3 is thought to be sensitive to acetaminophen (30,44). Several NSAIDs inhibit functional responses of PMN, including generation of reactive oxygen species, degranulation, and LTB_4 release. However, their effects in these responses are independent of their impact on the COX system (45–47).

Actions of Prostaglandins Relevant to Inflammation

The major actions of PGs in humans are also summarized in Fig. 23.2. PGs act locally (autacoids), have short half-lives, and are further metabolized rapidly in the circulation or local environment for inactivation. PGE_2 is a potent vasodilator. $PGF_{1\alpha}$, in contrast, causes vasoconstriction, whereas PGD_2 inhibits platelet aggregation and evokes contraction of smooth muscle. Prostacyclin and thromboxane have opposing actions on vascular tone and platelet aggregability. Although prostacyclin is a potent vasodilator that also inhibits platelet aggregation, TXA_2 causes vasoconstriction and promotes platelet aggregation. Hence, the balance between these opposing forces is critical in the control of vascular tone and blood coagulability in health and disease (7,8).

This balance between PGI and thromboxane controls the local vascular environment and is important in thromboregulation, which raises concern regarding the sequelae of unwanted inhibition of vascular COX-2, which could lead to both increased thrombogenicity (26,48) and increased atherosclerosis (49). This is an important point because nonselective COX inhibitors in general inhibit atherosclerosis in animal models (49). By blocking production of $PGI_{2\alpha}$, selective inhibition of COX-2 in vascular endothelium may enhance the actions of platelet TXA_2 (Fig. 23.2B).

Several lines of evidence support the notion that several of the COX-derived products are important "proinflammation" mediators: (a) PG synthesis is increased at sites of inflammation, (b) PG administration (e.g., intradermal injection) causes pathologic changes almost identical to those observed in inflammation, and (c) aspirin and other NSAIDs, molecules of differing chemical structure, share as a common action the ability to inhibit enzymes involved in PG biosynthesis. Increased biosynthesis of PG is an almost invariable consequence of tissue injury, whether physically-, chemically-, or immunologically-triggered.

A variety of inflammatory arthritides (e.g., RA, gout) are associated with increased levels of PGE_2 in the synovial fluid. Aspirin, one of the original (late 1800s) and most effective treatments for arthritis, is a potent inhibitor of PG biosynthesis (7). Aspirin successfully relieves the symptoms and signs of inflammation and causes a parallel decline in PG levels (7,8). Similar findings were demonstrated with various animal models of inflammation and arthritis, yet the mechanism of aspirin therapeutic agents has yet to be fully appreciated. PGs have pharmacologic actions that might differ from their endogenous roles; for example, local administration of PGE_2 causes many of the cardinal signs of inflammation. Injection of PGE_2 into human skin causes arteriolar dilatation and, as a result, redness and increased skin temperature. Moreover, PGE_2 causes fever when administered into the subarachnoid space and is one of the most pyretic substances known. By itself, PGE_2 does not produce pain or changes in vascular permeability and swelling, but does potentiate the effects of other autacoids such as histamine and serotonin. Although prostacyclin, thromboxane, PGD_2, and $PGF_{1\alpha}$ have all been identified in significant quantities at sites of inflammation, their precise role, namely spatial-temporal relationships, in mediating acute inflammation in humans is less clear. Prostacyclin, like PGE_2, causes marked vasodilatation and hyperalgesia (50). The actions of PGs on the acquired immune response are less well defined. In this context, PGE_2 inhibits the function of T and B lymphocytes and natural killer cell activity (Table 23.4). Recent evidence suggests

TABLE 23.4. *Major immunomodulatory actions of eicosanoids*

Product	Immunomodulatory effect
LTB_4	Stimulates phagocyte recruitment Inhibits immunoglobulin synthesis Inhibits helper cell (CD4) proliferation; induction of suppressor cell (CD8) proliferation Enhances NK cell activity Enhances monocyte cytokine production
LXA_4, LXB_4, and LX/ATL analogues	"Stop" neutrophil and eosinophil trafficking and functional responses Stimulate nonphlogistic recruitment of monocytes Block dendritic cell migration Stimulate the uptake and clearance by macrophages of apoptotic PMNs Regulate growth factors and angiogenesis via VEGF Block IL-12 production and regulates cytokine production Block T-cell cytokine release and signaling Up-regulate transcriptional corepressor NAB1
PGE_2	Inhibition of T- and B-lymphocyte activation Inhibition of NK cell activity

For original recent reports see references 102, 108, 126, and 128–130; for historical perspective and overviews of prostanoids and leukotrienes see references 5–9.

IL, interleukin; LT, leukotriene; LX, lipoxin; NK, natural killer; PMN, polymorphonuclear cell; PG, prostaglandin; VEGF, vascular endothelial growth factor.

that COX-2-derived products can also play a role in resolution or endogenous antiinflammation/wound healing (Fig. 23.3B). In this regard, PGE_2 and LXA_4 serve as key mediators (51–53). Also, it is important to note that neutrophils can induce COX-2 and switch its eicosanoid product profile (54).

Similar Reaction Mechanisms for Cyclooxygenases and Lipoxygenases

Both classes of enzymes, COX and LO, recognize the 1,4 cis-pentadiene structure present in polyunsaturated fatty acids. In the case of arachidonic acid, both enzymes abstract, in a stereospecific fashion, a methylenic hydrogen to insert molecular oxygen (the positional specificity of the hydrogen abstraction directs the insertion of molecular oxygen) (Fig. 23.4). Each enzyme transforms arachidonate to an unstable intermediate (COX generates PGG_2, and LO generates a hydroperoxyeicosatetraenoic acid) that is further transformed by specific enzymes to bioactive products. PGG/H synthase (also known as COX) abstracts the pro-S hydrogen at carbon 13 to stereospecifically insert oxygen at carbon 11, generating a putative 11-hydroperoxy-containing intermediate (39) (Fig. 23.4). The bis-oxygenase activity of this enzyme inserts oxygen at carbon 15 to generate the endoperoxide intermediate PGG_2, which is reduced at the carbon 15 hydroperoxy to PGH_2 that gives rise to individual PGs, TXs, or prostacyclin depending on the specific enzymes present in the cell type of origin (Fig. 23.2). Figure 23.2 also notes the hallmark bioactivity of each COX product next to their structure. The actions evoked by these compounds are highly stereoselective, which is a general theme in this area that is reflected in the recently cloned and identified receptors.

LIPOXYGENASES AND THEIR PRODUCTS: LEUKOTRIENES AND LIPOXINS

Three major types of LOs are observed in human tissues (i.e., 5-, 12-, and 15-LO), all of which are cloned (reviewed in references 55 and 56). The general reaction mechanisms of individual LOs are similar (Figs. 23.4–23.6). 5-LO, for

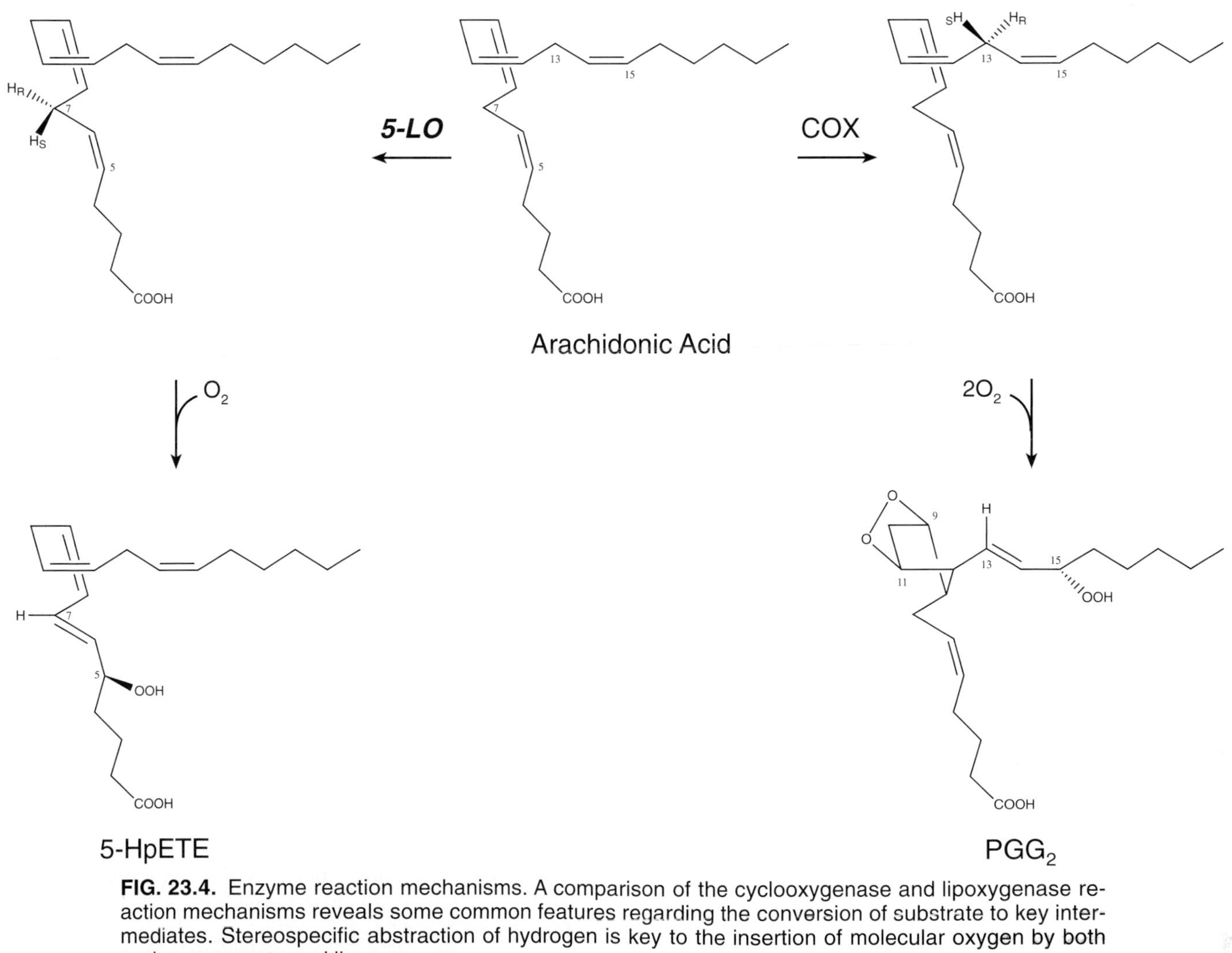

FIG. 23.4. Enzyme reaction mechanisms. A comparison of the cyclooxygenase and lipoxygenase reaction mechanisms reveals some common features regarding the conversion of substrate to key intermediates. Stereospecific abstraction of hydrogen is key to the insertion of molecular oxygen by both cyclooxygenases and lipoxygenases.

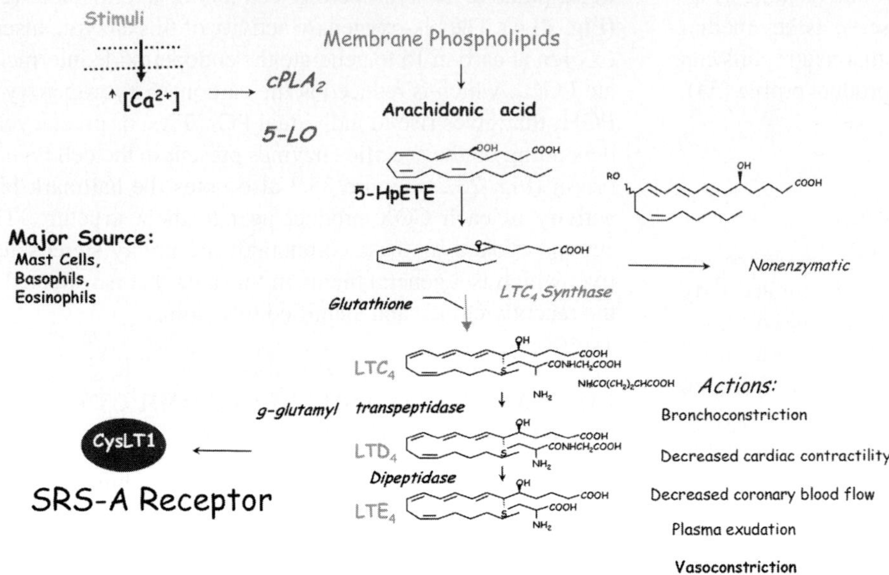

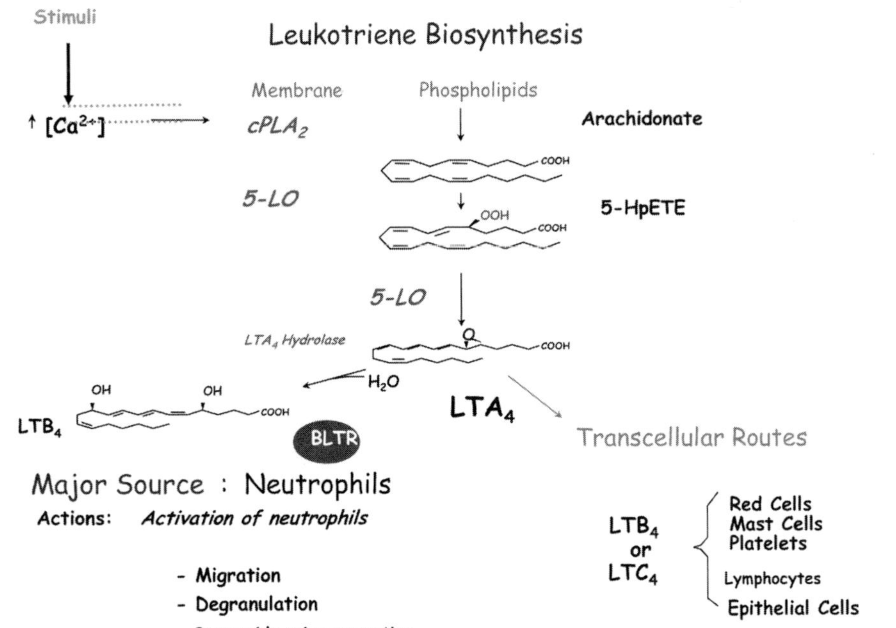

FIG. 23.5. Leukotriene biosynthesis. **A:** Synthesis of leukotrienes C4, D4, and E4 (peptido-leukotrienes) and their actions. **B:** Synthesis of leukotrienes B4. *BLTR,* LTB4 receptor; *CysLT1,* peptido-leukotriene receptor.

example, abstracts hydrogen at the 7-pro S position to insert molecular oxygen at carbon 5 of arachidonic acid. The product of this reaction contains a conjugated double bond and a hydroperoxy group at carbon 5 in the S configuration. 12-LO abstracts at 10-pro S and 15-LO at 13-pro S (Table 23.5). Thus, each enzyme generates a hydroperoxyeicosatetraenoic acid that carries a hydroperoxy group that is predominately in the S configuration at the LO-dictated carbon [i.e., 5(S)HPETE, 12(S)HPETE, and 15(S)HPETE]. Most LOs are responsible for insertion of oxygen in the S configuration. Recently, however, R LOs were reported (57), namely specific enzymes that insert oxygen in the R configuration. The function remains to be determined.

5-LO carries a second enzymatic activity and can abstract the 10-pro R hydrogen to yield the next key intermediate in LT biosynthesis (Fig. 23.5), namely, the 5(6)epoxide LTA_4 (55,58). Another important feature of the 5-LO is its requirement for several stimulatory cofactors (e.g., Ca^{+2}, ATP, FLAP). The structure of FLAP has been elucidated, and, upon cell activation, is translocated from the cytosol (Fig. 23.6) to its membrane association site and is thought to present arachidonic acid to 5-LO (23,59,60). Pharmacologic agents, which block both association of 5-LO with its membrane-bound activating protein (FLAP) and the utilization of substrate, inhibit LT production (61) (Figs. 23.5A and 23.6).

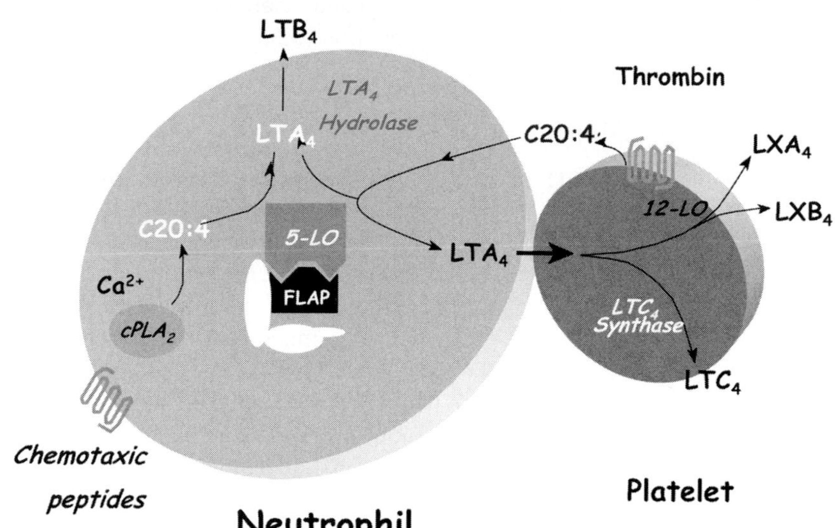

FIG. 23.6. Cell/cell interactions and transcellular biosynthesis of leukotrienes and lipoxins. Activated neutrophils generate leukotriene B_4 (LTB_4) from arachidonic acid-derived LTA_4 by the action of 5-lipoxygenase, but do not possess LTC_4-synthase activity. Platelets and endothelial cells, which themselves do not form LTC_4 from endogenous substrates, can generate LTC_4 in abundance from neutrophil-derived LTA_4. Platelets also generate lipoxins from leukocyte-derived LTA_4.

TABLE 23.5. *General features of key eicosanoid enzymes*

Enzyme	MW/Deduced primary structure	Hydrogen elimination	Primary product/function	Remarks
Cyclooxygenase (PGG/H synthase) *bis*-oxygenase	341 amino acids Integral membrane (endoplasmic reticulum and nuclear membrane)	13-pro S	PGG_2	Heme requirement; serine residue acetylated by ASA[a] platelet/ endothelial
COX-1 COX-2	Constitutive "Inducible isozyme"—except in vascular endothelial cells, where *in vivo* expression is upregulated by shear and flow forces[b]	13-pro S	PGG_2	
COX-3 P COXs				Acetaminophen sensitive[c]
5-lipoxygenase	MW 77,839 673 amino acids Cytosol to plasma membrane translocation	7-pro S 10-pro R	5-HPETE LTA_4	Leukocytes Three stimulatory factors (Ca^{2+}, ATP, FLAP)
12-lipoxygenase	MW 72,000	10-pro S	12-HPETE	Platelets
15-lipoxygenase	MW 73,000	13-pro S	15-HPETE	Lung Eosinophils
FLAP	MW 18,000		Associates with 5-LO	Leukocytes
LTA_4 hydrolase	MW 68,000–70,000		LTB_4	Ubiquitous distribution

For recent lipoxygenase reviews, see references 18, 55, 57, and 132.

[a]Acetylation of cyclooxygenases by aspirin causes a loss of PGG_2 generating activity because it places a bulky group in the protein which interferes with arachidonic acid (substrate conversion): an example of irreversible inhibition of prostaglandin formation and switch to lipoxygenation in the case of COX-2 (see references 39 and 131).

[b]In endothelial cells of vasculature, COX-2 appears to be up-regulated by physiologic flow and shear forces to produce PGI_2 (31).

[c]For COX-3 and related new isoforms of COX (designated f-COX). However, their function and sensitivity to NSAIDs remains to be established (see text for further details (30).

ASA, acetylsalicylic acid; FLAP, 5-lipoxygenase-activating protein; HPETE, hydroperoxyeicosatetraenoic acid; LO, lipoxygenase; LT, leukotriene; MW, molecular weight; PG, prostaglandin.

Leukotriene Biosynthesis and Cell Sources

Leukotrienes were elucidated in the mid-1970s and were so named because they were isolated from leukocytes and contain a conjugated triene structure (three conjugated double bonds) (6,7). The subscript numeral in leukotriene nomenclature refers to the number of double bonds in the precursor molecule. Leukotrienes of the 4 series are derived from arachidonic acid (eicosatetraenoic acid), which has four double bonds, whereas leukotrienes of the 5 series are generated from eicosapentaenoic acid (from fish oil), which contains five double bonds (62). Leukotrienes are formed from arachidonic acid by the initial action of the enzyme 5-LO (Fig. 23.5). This enzyme catalyzes two sequential reactions: (a) the insertion of molecular oxygen at the carbon 5 position of arachidonic acid (counting from the carboxylic acid end as one) to form 5-hydroperoxyeicosatetraenoic acid (5-HPETE) and (b) the subsequent transformation of 5-HPETE to an epoxide denoted LTA_4. LTA_4 is also a relatively short-lived molecule (with a half-life of seconds in the absence of stabilizing factors) that is rapidly transformed in a cell-specific manner, a situation analogous to the transformation of PGH_2 in PG biosynthesis.

The epoxide LTA_4 can be hydrated enzymatically to LTB_4 by LTA_4 hydrolase (Fig. 23.5A) (e.g., in neutrophils) or conjugated with glutathione to form LTC_4 (e.g., in mast cells and eosinophils) by LTC_4 synthetase, a glutathione-S-transferase. LTC_4 can be converted in turn to LTD_4 and LTE_4 by the successive elimination of glutamyl and glycine residues (Fig. 23.5B). These transformations are associated with relative loss of contractile activity (LTC_4 << LTE_4). The mixture of peptido-containing leukotrienes (LTC_4, LTD_4, and LTE_4), formerly known as slow-reacting substance of anaphylaxis (SRS-A) (7,62), is generated by mast cells following antigenic challenge and IgE receptor–mediated signal transduction (6,63).

5-Lipoxygenase

5-LO is a dual-function enzyme generating both 5(S)-HPETE and a subsequent epoxide (LTA_4) (Figs. 23.5 and 23.6) that is central to LT biosynthesis (Table 23.5 and Fig. 23.7). Within PMNs, LTA_4 is converted to the chemoattractant LTB_4, whereas when generated within eosinophils, mast cells, or macrophages, it is precursor to peptido-LTs (LTC_4, LTD_4, LTE_4). 5-LO (−/−) mice were prepared (64), and natural mutation noted in the promoter for 5-LO, which might have implications for anti-LT-based therapies (65). 5-LO of PMNs appears unique among LOs in that, upon cell activation, this LO translocates and interacts with a membrane-associated protein (18 kd) that brings about full activity of the 5-LO complex. This protein, termed FLAP (Fig. 23.6 and Table 23.5), is conserved across species at sites believed to interact with both 5-LO and inhibitors. FLAP-deduced amino acid sequences and hydropathy analyses suggest this is a transmembrane protein (59,66), as illustrated in Fig. 23.6. FLAP was targeted for development of novel 5-LO inhibitors, and several useful compounds were achieved by the Merck group (reviewed in references 6 and 61). To date, only a few 5-LO inhibitors are marketed in the United States (e.g., zileuton).

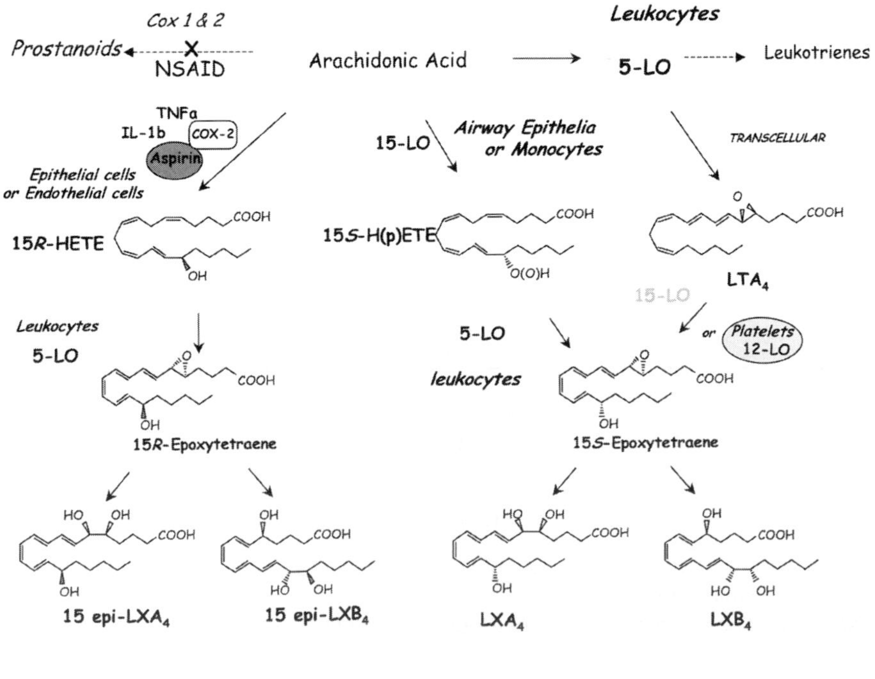

FIG. 23.7. Lipoxin and aspirin-triggered 15-epi-LX biosynthesis. *TNF-α,* tumor necrosis factor-α; *IL-1β,* interleukin-1β.

Actions of Leukotrienes

Figure 23.5 also lists the major actions of LT relevant to the immune response (1,62). LTB_4 is a potent activator of human neutrophils, whereas LTC_4, LTD_4, and LTE_4 display strikingly different biologic actions, causing, for example, smooth muscle contraction in a variety of tissues (6). These compounds are potent constrictors of bronchial smooth muscle. Their actions are rapid in onset and last for hours. Inhalation of LTC_4 or LTD_4 by healthy volunteers results in prolonged bronchoconstriction, and both LTC_4 and LTD_4 are vasoconstrictors. Nevertheless, systemic administration of LTC_4, LTD_4, and LTE_4 causes hypotension from (a) reduced myocardial contractility and coronary blood flow and (b) loss of plasma to the extravascular space as a consequence of increased vascular permeability. Because these compounds are released along with histamine following antigenic challenge of mast cells, eosinophils, or basophils, it is likely that they represent major inflammatory mediators derived from these cells (6).

Leukotrienes in Inflammation

Leukotrienes are important mediators of acute inflammation, including acute hypersensitivity. LTB_4 is a potent activator of neutrophil functional responses (i.e., generation of oxygen free radicals and release of lysosomal enzymes), and is an important early signal that mediates the migration of neutrophils to sites of inflammation (neutrophil chemotaxis; Fig. 23.5B). In health, approximately 50% of neutrophils circulate freely in blood, whereas approximately 50% are thought to crawl (stick and roll) along the endothelial surface lining of blood vessel walls (67). In inflammatory states, circulating neutrophils adhere to the endothelial cell layer, pass through the cells of the vessel wall (diapedesis), and migrate to the site of inflammation where they attack and ingest foreign antigen. This latter process of phagocytosis results in the formation of a phagosome, which fuses with neutrophil lysosomes to form phagolysosomes. Ingested particles are then destroyed within this organelle by proteases, hydrolases, and reactive oxygen species, with relative protection of host tissues (45–47). In addition, activated neutrophils generate and release more eicosanoids. LTB_4, through its interaction with two neutrophil cell surface receptors, BLT_1 and BLT_2 (68,69), is a potent stimulus for neutrophil adhesion, diapedesis, migration, the generation of reactive oxygen species, and lysosomal enzyme release (47).

Administration of LTB_4 *in vivo* is associated with increased neutrophil margination along vessel walls and migration to the extracellular space. LTB_4 is not believed to affect vascular tone directly, and induces plasma exudation via neutrophil-dependent mechanisms (70). Combined exposure to LTB_4 and PGE_2, a mild inducer of plasma exudation when given alone, results in a profound increase in vascular permeability (71). Therefore, in certain settings PGs and leukotrienes can act synergistically to promote inflammation. LTB_4 does not directly induce pain, but lowers the threshold for other stimuli. Leukotriene-deficient mice exhibit reduced collagen-induced arthritis (72) and LTB_4 receptor (termed BLTR) antagonists (69) have clear impact in disease models (61). Because these receptor antagonists were developed by classical pharmacology and medicinal chemistry, the cloning of these receptors will now open the way for more selective interventions and perhaps elucidation of a role for LTC_4 and LTD_4 in RA (68,69,73).

The peptido-containing leukotrienes (LTC_4, LTD_4, and LTE_4) have been identified in several experimental models of inflammation, and may be particularly important in the pathogenesis of hypersensitivity disorders such as asthma (74–76). Asthmatic subjects appear to be hypersensitive to these eicosanoids. In addition to their effects on vascular tone, LTC_4 and LTD_4 increase vascular permeability and increase the leakage of plasma and macromolecules from the intravascular space. Unlike LTB_4, leukotrienes C_4 and D_4 do not appear to directly affect human neutrophil functional responses and do not directly alter the pain threshold after topical administration. Also of interest, antileukotriene therapy, namely the LTC_4, LTD_4 receptor antagonist Singulair® (Merck, West Point, PA, U.S.A.), was introduced in the clinic for treatment of asthma; however, steroid treatment appears to be superior in recent clinical trials (77).

Leukotrienes are also important regulators of both cellular and humoral immunity. Table 23.4 summarizes some of the major effects of these compounds on the immune system. It should be noted, however, that the majority of these actions have been identified *in vitro* or in experimental models, and their clinical relevance remains a subject of interest.

Biosynthesis and Cell Sources of Lipoxins

Lipoxins are characterized structurally by the presence of four conjugated double bonds. These confer a characteristic appearance on ultraviolet spectroscopy, which is the hallmark of the compounds in this series and different from that seen with leukotrienes (78). Of interest, there appears to be an inverse relationship between the amount of LX, compared to LT formed *in vitro*, which suggests the potential for counterregulatory interactions between these two series of LO products. The sequential oxygenation of arachidonic acid at the carbon 15 and then carbon 5 position by 15- and 5-LO, respectively, results in the formation of lipoxins (*lipox*ygenase *in*teraction products) (62). These novel eicosanoids differ markedly from the leukotrienes in both their structure and biologic actions (Figs. 23.6 and 23.7). Dual oxygenation produces an epoxide intermediate denoted as 5,6-epoxytetraene, which is rapidly converted to

TABLE 23.6. *Leukotriene and lipoxin formation in humans*

- Asthma
- Aspirin-sensitive asthmatics (134)
- Angioplasty-induced plaque rupture (intraluminal generation) (136)
- Bone marrow generation
- Alterations in both LT and LX biosynthesis (defect in LX generation in chronic myeloid leukemia) (92)
- Glomerulonephritis (84,133)
- Sarcoidosis (135)
- Pneumonia
- Periodontal disease (137,138)
- Nasal polyps (139)
- Rheumatoid arthritis (140)

LT, leukotriene; LX, lipoxin.

either LXA_4 or LXB_4 by epoxide hydrolases. Also, LX formation can be achieved by oxygenation of leukocyte-derived LTA_4 by platelet LO through cell/cell interaction (78) (Figs. 23.6 and 23.7).

Lipoxins in Inflammation

Lipoxins are the more recently identified of the eicosanoids, yet it is already apparent that they have important actions on a number of inflammatory cells. Recent findings indicate that LXs emerge as specialized mediators of resolution (79,80). LXA_4 inhibits neutrophil chemotaxis and adhesion *in vitro*. The administration of LXs or their stable analogs *in vivo* does not provoke neutrophil adhesion to endothelial cells or neutrophil migration to the extracellular space. Instead, LXA_4 "stops" neutrophil migration (13,81,82). These compounds possess antiinflammatory or counterregulatory roles in many experimental animal models (79,83). In addition to their actions on human neutrophils, both LXA_4 and LXB_4 recruit eosinophils *in vivo,* and LXA_4 and aspirin-triggered lipoxin (ATL) analogue block dendritic cell migration, suggesting that they may regulate other facets of the immune response (Tables 23.2, 23.6, and 23.7). LXA_4 is a partial agonist on the vascular smooth muscle LTD_4 receptor (84,85). Along these lines, LXA_4 attenuates the actions of LTC_4 and LTD_4 on bronchial smooth muscle and the renal microcirculation, suggesting that these compounds may serve as nature's endogenous leukotriene antagonists as well as act at their own recognition sites, namely LX receptors (69).

There is compelling evidence indicating that the LXs may be important LO-derived lipid mediators involved in both acute inflammation and the control of cellular immunity (1,17). LXs, as well as LTs, are present in bronchoalveolar lavage samples from patients with sarcoidosis and pneumonia (Table 23.6). The possibility that LXs represent endogenous modulators of LT responses and pro-resolving mediators in inflammation is an area of active research in my laboratory. Specifically, we elucidated a novel mechanism of action for aspirin that involves the biosynthetic production of epimers of LX (Fig. 23.7). When aspirin is exposed to inflamed tissues or those in which COX-2 is up-regulated (86), acetylation by aspirin gives rise to novel 15-epimer LXs that carry potent antiinflammatory actions. Stable analogues of these native LXs, which resist rapid inactivation and are receptor mimetics, illuminate a new path to understanding the endogenous mechanisms of antiinflammation (reviewed in references

TABLE 23.7. *Molecular properties of enzymes in eicosanoid biosynthesis*

Enzyme	Protein size (no. of amino acids)[a]	Prosthetic group	Gene size (kb)	Exon no.	Putative *cis*-elements of promoter region	Chromosomal location
COX-1 (PGHS-I)	598 [576][b]	Heme	~22	11	Sp1, AP-2, GATA-1	9
COX-2 (PGHS-II)	603 [587][b]	Heme	>8.3	10	TATA, CRE, NFκB, Sp1, AP-2	1
5-LO	673	Fe	>82	14	Sp1, AP-2, NFκkB	10
12-LO	662	Fe	~17	14	Sp1, AP-2, GRE	17
15-LO	661	Fe	—	—	—	17
FLAP	160	—	>31	5	TATA, AP-2, GRE	13
LTA_4 hydrolase	610	Zn	>35	19	XRE, AP-2	12
LTC_4 synthase	149	—	~2.5	5	Sp1, AP-1, AP-2	5

[a]The number of amino acids in the polypeptide chain, excluding the initial methionine. Values within square braces represent processed proteins after removal of signal peptides.

[b]The native enzyme is glycosylated, which causes an increase in molecular weight in sodium dodecyl sulfate-polyacrylamide gel electrophoresis. Results are for human enzymes and are from the cited references.

COX, cyclooxygenase; FLAP, 5-lipoxygenase-activating protein; LO, lipoxygenase; LT, leukotriene; NFκB, nuclear factor κB.

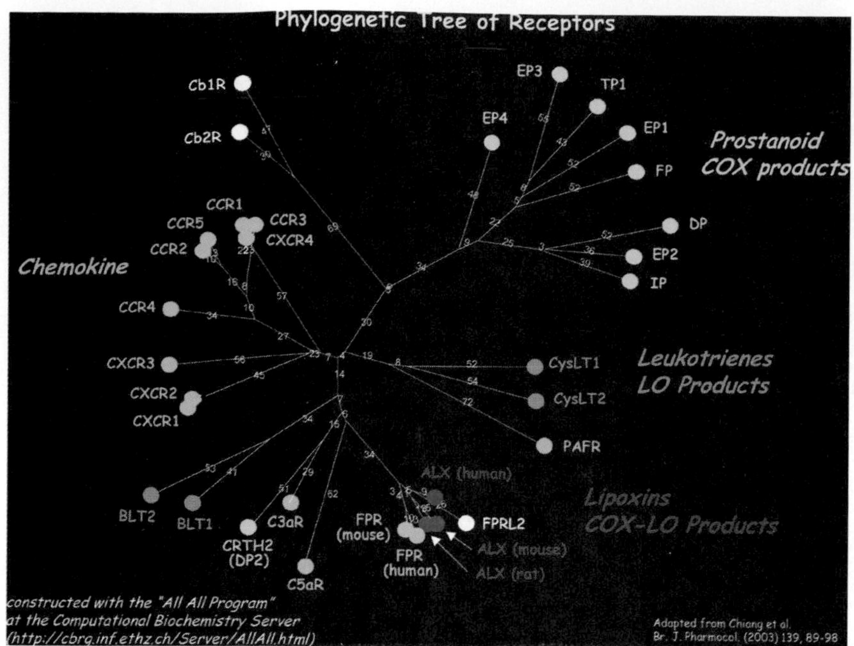

FIG. 23.8. Phylogenetic tree of G protein–coupled receptors (GPCRs) for eicosanoids and chemokines. The phylogenetic branches for prostaglandin, leukotriene, and lipoxin receptors indicate that receptors for linear eicosanoids, such as lipoxins and leukotrienes, are distinct from those of cyclic prostanoid receptors and that both classes are related to GPCRs for chemokines, yet structurally and functionally distinct. The numbers denote phylogenetic branches. For further details, see the website *cbrg.inf.ethz.ch/Server/AllAll.html* to construct the GPCR phylogenetic tree in the "All All Program."

1, 14, and 71). Several of these new ATL and LX analogues are topically and orally active and at least two orders of magnitude more potent than aspirin (83,87,88). Because they also regulate the chemokine-cytokine axis and enhance resolution of inflammation (reviewed in references 1 and 72), they represent a novel approach to controlling leukocyte traffic and inflammation by mechanisms that differ from both traditional antiinflammatory agents and other current eicosanoid-directed approaches (Figs. 23.6–23.8).

CELL/CELL INTERACTIONS FOR TRANSCELLULAR EICOSANOID BIOSYNTHESIS AND CELL/CELL COMMUNICATION

Acute inflammation is characterized by the local accumulation of inflammatory cells at the site of injury where they function in juxtaposition with, and often while adherent to, resident endothelial, epithelial, mesenchymal, and other inflammatory cells (Fig. 23.6). Arachidonic acid and other fatty acid–derived LO and COX products can be donated from one cell type to another so that different cell types cooperate with each other (i.e., pooling their enzymatic machinery) to generate eicosanoids and novel bioactive lipid mediators. In this way, cell types that on their own may not be able to generate a particular class of eicosanoid (e.g., cells that lack an LO) can generate eicosanoids from intermediates generated in other cells if they have the enzymes to convert the intermediate to a biologically active product (89–91). Figure 23.6 illustrates these events in the platelet/neutrophil interaction. In this example, neither neutrophils nor platelets alone can generate LTC_4, because neutrophils do not have LTC_4 synthetase and platelets do not possess a 5-LO activity. Nevertheless, when these different cell types interact, LTC_4 is formed in abundance because platelets can convert neutrophil-derived LTA_4 to LTC_4. Similarly, LTC_4 can be generated by endothelial cells from neutrophil-derived LTA_4.

LXs are also formed during platelet/neutrophil interaction (78,92). Platelets alone do not generate LX (Figs. 23.6 and 23.7). In contrast, when platelets and neutrophils interact (Fig. 23.9A), platelets can form LX from neutrophil-derived intermediates (93). Thus, the process of cell/cell interaction not only expands the array of eicosanoids that can be generated at sites of inflammation, but also amplifies the quantity of eicosanoids produced. These events are also subject to alterations following drug intervention within these pathways (Fig. 23.9B). Aspirin has a dramatic impact on cell/cell interactions and can lead to the biosynthesis of novel lipid mediators such as 15-epi-lipoxins (Fig. 23.7). The impact of NSAID and anti-LT therapies on transcellular eicosanoid biosynthesis remains to be fully appreciated.

REGULATION OF AUTACOIDS BY RAPID TRANSFORMATION AND INACTIVATION

In general, eicosanoids are rapidly generated, exert their actions, and then are further transformed. LTC_4 is metabolized to LTD_4 by γ-glutamyl transpeptidase (94). In many tissues, LTD_4 is a potent product, while its metabolite LTE_4

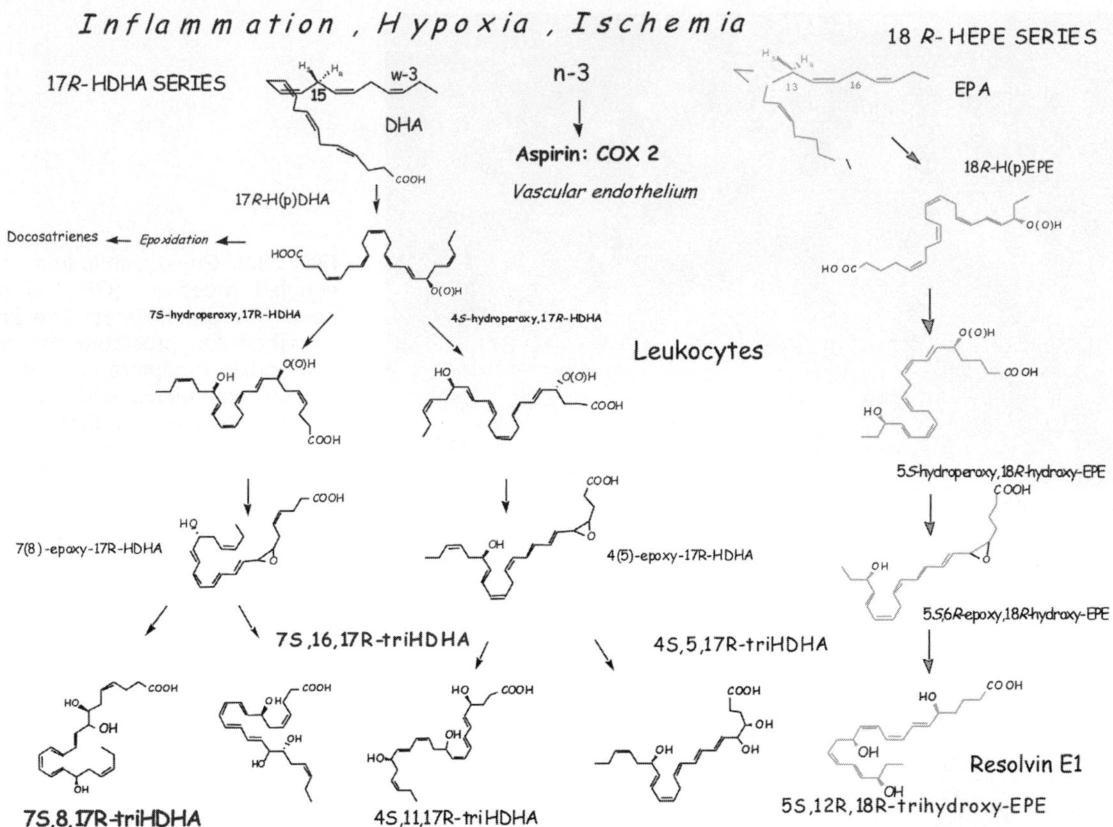

FIG. 23.9. Resolvin biosynthesis from ω-3 eicosapentanoic acid (EPA) and docosahexanoic acid (DHA). DHA is transformed by actylated COX-2 to form 17*R*-H(p)DHA or 17*R*-hydroperoxydocosahexaenoic acid. This intermediate is rapidly transformed by human leukocytes to produce two hydroperoxy-containing intermediates, the 7*S*-hydroperoxy and 4*S*-hydroperoxy intermediates from 17*R*-HDHA. Both intermediates are independently converted to epoxide-containing intermediates that open to four respective DHA-derived resolvins that each contain trihydroxy-containing structures. Eicosapentaenoic acid on the right is also transformed by acetylated COX-2 in vascular endothelium to produce 18*R*-hydroperoxy-eicosapentaenoic acid [18*R*(p)EPE] that is converted to a 5,6-epoxide and then open to resolvin E1, a trihydroxy EPA-derived product. These compounds have each been shown to be potent inhibitors of leukocyte infiltration (10,11) and are the first examples of potent bioactive products with increased biologic potency from their respective ω-3 precursors. See references 11 and 143 for further details.

generated by cysteinyl glycinase is generally regarded as an inactive component of SRS-A (6). LTB_4 is further metabolized by ω-oxidation by a P450-like enzyme found in neutrophils. LTB_4 is successively metabolized at the carbon 20 position to generate an inactive carbon 20-COOH-containing metabolite in neutrophils. Recently, LTB_4 was shown to undergo dehydrogenation in the kidney to give novel 12-oxo-metabolites (68). PGs are rapidly inactivated, as are LXs (95), which regulates their duration of action (14). In most cases, the metabolite does not activate the specific G protein-coupled receptor (GPCR) to transmit appropriate intracellular signals (69).

MOLECULAR ASPECTS OF EICOSANOID ENZYMES

All of the key enzymes in the formation of PG, TX, LT, LX, and epoxyeicosatetranoic acids (EETs) are cloned and sequenced, and for some of them, the complete gene structure and its promoter have been characterized (Table 23.7). This section briefly highlights advances in the understanding of the expression, regulation, and mechanism of the key enzymes.

Prostaglandin Endoperoxide Synthases

COX or PG endoperoxide synthase, the well-known target of NSAIDs (see Chapter 31), exists in two isoforms (Fig. 23.3) and possibly a third isoform, COX-3 (29,37,51), that are similar in terms of overall amino acid homology (~60%), catalytic properties, and substrate specificity (39).

COX-1 is currently regarded as a constitutive enzyme, required for basal formation of PGs, whereas COX-2 can be induced by a variety of agents such as cytokines, growth factors, and tumor promoters (96). Glucocorticoids can reverse induction of COX-2. COX-1 is expressed in gastric mucosa, and the gastric lesions frequently accompanying use of NSAIDs are believed to result from reduced formation of cytoprotective PGs. Recent advances in the understanding of these two enzymes has been reviewed (16,27, 97). COX-1 and COX-2 exhibit different profiles of inhibition when tested *in vitro* against a wide range of NSAIDs. The possibility of finding a selective COX-2 inhibitor with all the beneficial analgesic and antipyretic properties of classical NSAIDs such as aspirin, but without their negative side effects, has focused attention on this area of eicosanoid research (98,99). Both Searle (now together with Pharmacia, Pfizer, and Upjohn) and Merck introduced COX-2 selective inhibitors that at present are useful in the treatment of RA (Chapter 31). A current focus for more selective inhibitors is directed toward the specific PG synthases that convert PGH_2 to individual prostanoids (100) (Figs. 23.2 and 23.3).

Enzymes in Leukotriene Biosynthesis

The critical enzymes in the leukotriene cascade are purified, cloned, and sequenced. Computer-assisted sequence comparisons have identified segments conserved among isoenzymes and established unexpected relationships among proteins with a low degree of overall homology. Several conserved segments, including six histidines, have been identified among LO, and a so-called Src homology 3 (SH3) motif is present in the primary structure of 5-LO. Another striking example is the discovery of a zinc binding motif in LTA_4 hydrolase, similar to those present in certain zinc metalloproteases and aminopeptidases. As a result, LTA_4 hydrolase was found to contain one mole of zinc per mole of protein and to exhibit a previously unknown peptide cleaving activity (58,101). In addition, significant sequence similarities are present between LTC_4 synthase and FLAP, both of which are membrane proteins of similar molecular mass (63). 15-LO and its promoter are cloned, and recent studies provide clear evidence for its role in LX generation *in vivo* in glomerulonephritis (84) and in host defense mechanisms (102).

Gene Structures and Promoters of Enzymes in Eicosanoid Biosynthesis

Several genes and corresponding promoters are characterized (Table 23.7). With regard to COX (EC 1.14.99.1), COX-1 and COX-2 genes are divided into 11 and 10 exons, respectively. In agreement with the presumed functional dichotomy between COX isozymes, the genes are located on different chromosomes and the promoters exhibit distinct features (96). The promoter of human COX-1 lacks a canonical TATA box but instead is rich in GC, typical of a so-called housekeeping gene. In contrast, the COX-2 promoter contains a TATA box and several potential regulatory elements, including CRE, nuclear factor κB, nuclear factor IL-6 (C/EBPβ), MEF-2, Sp1, and AP2 sites.

The gene for human 5-LO (E.C. 1.13.11.34) spans more than 82 kb of DNA, consists of 14 exons, and is located on chromosome 10. As for COX-1, the promoter region lacks a TATA or CCAT box but contains multiple GC boxes (potential Sp1 sites) typical for housekeeping genes, which is of interest because 5-LO appears to be expressed exclusively in bone marrow–derived cells and displays natural mutations that apparently can alter transcription factor binding (65). The FLAP gene spans more than 31 kb on chromosome 13 and is divided into 5 exons. Its 5′-flanking region contains a TATA box and a possible GRE and AP-2 binding site. The gene for LTA_4 hydrolase is also large (>35 kb) and contains 19 exons, the smallest of which consists of only 24 bp. Surprisingly, components of the zinc binding motif are split between exons 10 and 11. The gene is located on chromosome 12, and the 5′-flanking region contains two XRE. Detailed promoter analysis is required to gain a better understanding of constitutive, induced, and cell type–specific expression of these enzymes.

EICOSANOID RECEPTORS

Many eicosanoids act via cell surface GPCRs that have been cloned in recent years. The PGs interact with specific receptors denoted in Fig. 23.2 (i.e., EP_{1-4}, DP, etc.) that transduce their signals. The classification of prostanoid receptors and their subtypes has been introduced (103). More recently, the LT and LX receptors (69) and their structure-function relationships for therapeutic intervention (reviewed in references 104 and 105) have been described. Results from receptor-deficient mice (reviewed in references 25 and 105) demonstrate the importance of prostanoids in inflammation. Of interest, most prostanoid receptor antagonists/mimetics were developed before the receptors were cloned (106), and some, such as misoprostal, are still used clinically in the treatment of RA (Chapter 31). It will be of interest to follow the development of novel therapeutics with the cloned receptors available (104).

The LXA_4 receptor (ALXR) was the first of the LO product receptors identified as an orphan GPCR (69) that proved distinct for the prostanoid receptors (107). The ALXR also interacts with stable LX and ATL analogues and appears to represent a novel antiinflammatory receptor that signals "stop" in the course of an inflammatory response (83). Its overexpression in transgenic mouse results in reduced inflammation (108; reviewed in reference 69). Also, both the LTB_4 (68) and $cysLT_1$ (73) receptors (denoted BLT_1 and $cysLT_1$) were identified as acting via orphan GPCR, as is the case with their respective second lower-affinity forms BLT_2 and $cysLT_2$ (69) (Fig. 23.8). Their elucidation will not only complement studies on signaling mechanisms, but will also facilitate identification of tissue display patterns and potential alternative functional receptors during disease that should yield insights into treatment or new functional roles for receptors and their ligands.

Surprisingly, indomethacin, a widely used NSAID, was recently found to activate a specific GPCR termed CRTH2 (chemoattractant receptor-homologous molecular expressed on T_H2 cells). Indomethacin, at submicromolar concentrations, stimulates Ca^{2+} mobilization via this receptor in its recombinant form when expressed in K562 cells, and also stimulates chemotaxis of T_H2 cells, eosinophils, and basophils via this GPCR. Other NSAIDs, including aspirin, sulindac, or diclofenac, do not appear to activate this GPCR. These exciting results (109) opened many new approaches for understanding the actions of NSAIDs and may provide a molecular basis for some of indomethacin's unwanted effects. It is noteworthy that LTB_4 and certain prostanoids can also act at intracellular sites via interaction with the peroxisome proliferator–activated receptor (PPAR) (41,110,111). In view of the nuclear localization of the COX and 5-LO systems (39,55,112), it is possible that eicosanoids could have nuclear functions like their cousins, the steroids, and act as transcription factor regulators (41). However, a systematic search for natural ligands of PPAR-α revealed only the high degree of flexibility of the PPAR systems as receptors for lipid ligands (111). In view of the antiinflammatory actions of ATL and LX and new methods for structure-based drug design, the presence of cell surface sites as well as potential intracellular sites of action for lipid mediators such as eicosanoids and resolvins provides many new avenues for rheumatologists to harness unwanted consequences of inflammation in a highly selective manner.

MULTIPLE NEW TARGETS FOR ANTIINFLAMMATORY AND PRORESOLVING THERAPIES

As illustrated in Figs. 23.3 and 23.6, there are many sites or targets along eicosanoid biosynthetic pathways at which to direct novel antiinflammatory therapies. A selective inhibitor of $cPLA_2$ would have the advantage of inhibiting the formation of PGs, leukotrienes, LX, and PAF (113). However, potential beneficial actions of eicosanoids in resolution and wound healing might be lost (Fig. 23.3). Corticosteroids are potent antiinflammatory compounds effective in the treatment of a wide variety of inflammatory and hypersensitivity states (see Chapter 34). In certain settings, corticosteroids can block PLA_2 activity *in vitro* and inhibit eicosanoid synthesis. Whether the antiinflammatory actions of corticosteroids are related to their ability to block PLA_2 activity *in vivo* is unclear, because corticosteroids can also inhibit a range of other functional responses by immune cells, including lymphocytes, monocytes, and natural killer cells. The generation of annexin-derived peptides, also known earlier as lipocortin 1 (114), that were recently found to act via specific GPCRs, as well as the recently discovered ALX receptor, open many new therapeutic possibilities (115).

There are a large number of relatively specific and potent inhibitors of COX activity available (e.g., aspirin, indomethacin, and ibuprofen) (Fig. 23.1). Their efficacy as antiinflammatory agents has been well demonstrated, and the resolution of inflammation is paralleled by a decline in tissue PG levels from COX-1 and an increase in PGE_2 from COX-2 that may play a different functional role in wound healing (53) and cell trafficking in resolution (116). It should be remembered, however, that PGs are intimately involved in many physiologic functions, such as fluid and electrolyte homeostasis and the control of vascular tone and tissue perfusion. For example, PGE_2 has natriuretic and diuretic properties, whereas PGE_2 and PGI_2 are vasodilators that appear to play an important role in the preservation of renal blood flow during renal ischemia. During the course of inflammation, PG and LTB_4 are temporally generated before LXA_4 in the murine air pouch, and PGE stimulates expression of 15-LO in human PMNs (116). Of particular interest, both PGE and PGD_2 stimulate 15-LO type I expression in a cyclic adenosine monophosphate–dependent fashion in human PMNs. PGE_2 appears to have a cytoprotective role in the upper gastrointestinal tract (117). Thus, COX inhibitors, while being effective antiinflammatory drugs, may also interfere with these homeostatic mechanisms and cause salt and water retention or gastrointestinal ulceration, exacerbate renal ischemia, and precipitate acute renal failure; hence the search for selective COX-1 and COX-2 inhibitors (98,118). Along these lines, LX and ATL stable analogues have an additive inhibitory action with glucocorticoids (114,119).

Several 5-LO inhibitors have reached clinical trials, and this continues to be an area of active research (120). Similarly, research is currently ongoing to synthesize drugs that selectively inhibit the various synthase enzymes, which are involved in the generation of selective individual eicosanoids or which antagonize the actions of specific eicosanoids with cells by blocking their interaction with cell surface receptors on target tissues. Also, the specific PG reductases are targets for more selective agents. The development of such agents will not only allow more specific, and hopefully more effective, antiinflammatory drug regimens, but will also enable a more complete dissection of the roles of individual eicosanoids in the pathophysiology of acute inflammation and hypersensitivity.

A nutritional approach to the manipulation of inflammation has been to modify the intake and content of dietary lipids using fish oils. The biochemical basis for this approach lies in the finding that in many settings LT derived from eicosapentaenoic acid (the 5 series) are less potent than those derived from arachidonic acid (the 4 series). The replacement of arachidonic acid at membrane storage sites in phospholipid by dietary fish oil–derived eicosapentaenoic acid results in a decrease in the agonist-induced formation of series 4 leukotrienes and can alter product formation by generating the less active 5 series leukotrienes (19,121). Investigators using this dietary approach have reported success in the treatment of arthritis and SLE. This is an important area of active research (63).

Novel Antiinflammatory Signals and Pathways: Resolvins and Docosatrienes

Over the past 25 years, numerous studies have reported that dietary supplementation with ω-3 polyunsaturated fatty acids (ω-3 PUFA) has beneficial effects in disease. Recent reviews discuss potential antithrombotic, immunoregulatory, and antiinflammatory responses relevant in arteriosclerosis, arthritis, and asthma, as well as antitumor and antimetastatic effects (122). The possible preventative or therapeutic actions of ω-3 PUFA supplementation in infant nutrition, cardiovascular diseases, and mental health led an international workshop to call for recommended dietary intakes (122), and data from one large trial that evaluated the benefits of aspirin with or without ω-3 PUFA supplementation for patients surviving myocardial infarction found a significant decrease in death in the group taking the supplement (123).

Fish oils or ω-3 PUFAs per se have been proposed to act by several possible mechanisms (122). None of the proposed explanations are widely accepted, largely because of the suprapharmacologic amounts (milligram to microgram range of ω-3 PUFAs) that are required *in vitro* to achieve the supposed beneficial effects. Because compelling molecular evidence has been lacking, and in view of beneficial profiles attributed to dietary ω-3 PUFAs and those of aspirin in a variety of diseases, we sought evidence for possible new lipid-derived signals that could explain the epidemiologic findings in humans.

Inflammatory exudates formed in murine dorsal pouches treated with ω-3 PUFAs and acetylsalicylic acid (ASA) generate several novel compounds (10), including 18*R*-hydroxy-eicosapentaenoic acid (18*R*-HEPE) and several trihydroxy-containing compounds derived from the ω-3 fish oil eicosapentaenoic acid (EPA) (C20:5) used as a ω-3 PUFA prototype. Human cells also generate these new 18R and 15R series of compounds from EPA that we termed resolvins (11), which carry intriguing bioactivities. When human endothelial cells expressing COX-2 are pulsed with EPA and treated with ASA, they generate 18*R*-HEPE or a mixture of 18*R*-HEPE and 15*R*-HEPE. A role for COX-2 in this biosynthetic pathway was confirmed with recombinant human COX-2, in which acetylation by ASA dramatically increased the production of both 18*R*-HEPE and 15*R*-HEPE, findings that could be of clinical significance (10).

When engaged in phagocytosis, activated human PMNs process the intermediates derived from acetylated recombinant COX-2 to produce two series of trihydroxy-containing compounds; one series carries an 18*R* position hydroxyl group, and the other series a hydroxyl group in the 15*R* position, which is related to 15-epi-LX_5. Trout macrophages and human leukocytes can indeed convert endogenous EPA to 15S-containing LX, also denoted as 5-series LX_5 (124). Briefly, we found that human PMNs take up and convert 18*R*-HEPE via 5-lipoxygenation to insert molecular oxygen and, in subsequent steps, form 5-hydro(peroxy)-18*R*-DiH(p)EPE and a more labile intermediate 5(6)epoxide that gives rise to 5,12,18*R*-triHEPE. In a similar biosynthetic pathway, 15*R*-HEPE released by endothelial cells is converted by activated PMNs via 5-lipoxygenation to a 5 series LXA_5 analogue that also retains the C15 *R* or epi configuration, namely 15-epi-LXA_5 (10). The stereochemistry of compounds in this pathway is different from those of the LO-driven pathways that give predominantly C15 S containing LX_5 structures (so-called 5 series of five double bonds) as with endogenous sources of EPA in trout macrophages (124). The chirality of the precursor with ASA-COX-2, predominantly *R*, is retained when converted by human PMNs to 15-epi-LXA_5 (10).

The newly described 18*R* series members might serve as dampers for inflammatory responses because 18*R*-HEPE exhibits some inhibitory activity and its product 5,12,18*R*-triHEPE potently inhibits PMN transmigration and infiltration (10). These results raise the question of whether arachidonate is the sole substrate for COX-2 in physiologic setting in human tissues or whether EPA or other PUFAs are important as well (10). Despite the many reports of possible beneficial impact of ω-3 PUFAs and EPA in humans (122,123), oxygenation by COX-2 to generate bioactive compounds, as referenced herein, has not been addressed. In fish leukocytes and platelets, both EPA (C20:5) and arachidonic acid are mobilized and converted to both 5 series and 4 series eicosanoids (including PG, LT, and LX) with roughly equal abundance (124). Given the gram amounts of ω-3 PUFAs taken as dietary supplements by humans (122,123) and the large area of the vasculature that can express COX-2 (vascular "hot spots" during local inflammation and under physiologic flow conditions *in vivo*), the conversion of EPA and docosahexaenoic acid (DHA) by vascular endothelial cells and neighboring cells could represent a significant *in vivo* source of these eicosanoids (Fig. 23.9). Indeed, studies by Garcia-Cardena et al. (31) indicate that shear force on endothelial cells up-regulates the expression of COX-2, which appears to be a major source of prostacyclin *in vivo* (32). Inhibition of vascular COX by COX-2-selected inhibitors appears to be responsible for increased thrombogenicity observed in some studies in individuals taking therapeutic doses of selective COX-2 inhibitors. It follows, then, that low-dose aspirin therapy and acetylation of vascular COX-2 provides a source of production of epimeric forms of oxygenated arachidonic acid such as 15*R*-HETE from arachidonic acid as well as the novel 17*R* and 18*R* products derived from DHA and EPA, respectively (Fig. 23.9). This previously unappreciated source of EPA and DHA utilization by vascular endothelial cells *in vivo* to produce novel products such as the resolvins and docosatrienes may explain in part some of the beneficial action of dietary supplementation of ω-3 PUFAs observed in many epidemiologic and clinical studies (123).

Inappropriate control of inflammation and its resolution is now recognized to contribute to many diseases. Aspirin as well as other NSAIDs that affect these signaling systems (Fig. 23.1) are in wide use, yet these agents are not without unwanted side effects, particularly in the kidney and stomach. The discovery of the second isoform of COX (reviewed in reference 27) sparked a large-scale search for safer aspirin-like drugs, namely COX-2 inhibitors, that would bypass the unwanted side effects of aspirin. Results reviewed here indicate that LX, their aspirin-triggered epimers (ATL), and broader arrays of aspirin-triggered lipid mediators derived from ω-3 PUFAs reveal previously unappreciated endogenous antiinflammation and proresolution signaling mechanisms that could offer new treatment approaches. The finding that LX counters inflammatory events led to a more general concept, namely that aspirin-triggered lipid mediators could serve as local mediators of antiinflammation or endogenous agonists that favor resolution of inflammation. Additional support for this notion that LXs are protective and that ATLs share this property (10,125) comes from the finding that LXA_4 stimulates macrophages to clear apoptotic PMNs (126) and regulates expression of cytokines and metalloproteases via LXA_4 receptors (127). These signaling pathways add a new dimension to the well-established use of low-dose ASA as a specific COX-1 inhibitor in platelets, namely, triggering of COX-2-generated protective products, which underscores the importance of transcellular biosynthetic signaling pathways.

CONCLUSION

Substantial progress was achieved with respect to the development of selective COX-1 and COX-2 inhibitors, LT receptor antagonists, cloning of enzymes and receptors, and new drugs entering the clinical arena. Also, the roles of transcellular eicosanoid biosynthesis in the formation of LT, LX, and other novel products, such as the resolvins and docosatrienes, are being elucidated. New bioactions for eicosanoids and the ω-3-derived resolvins were identified that give further insight to their important roles in cell signaling. The therapeutic uses of targeted, selective enzyme inhibitors (i.e., PG synthases, LTA_4 hydrolase, etc.) and receptor antagonists, as well as specific receptor agonists (i.e., ATL and LX stable analogues), are currently being evaluated. They represent important tools in unraveling the roles of eicosanoids and the contributions of novel lipid mediators in leukocyte and immune function. The role of cell-cell contact and adhesion in the generation of transcellular-derived products is being evaluated in the context of resolution of inflammation, and the potential intracellular actions of eicosanoids and lipid mediators continue to be intriguing areas for further research and development. Importantly, the spatial-temporal relationships and the topography that functionally links eicosanoid and lipid mediator production to subcellular addresses and intracellular signaling pathways await further study. These loci and signaling routes require molecular definition in order to appreciate the events key in the progression of arthritis and to stage appropriate targeted and more selective therapeutics for this and related diseases.

ACKNOWLEDGMENTS

This work was supported in part by Grants GM38765 and DK50305 (to C.N.S.) from the National Institutes of Health. I thank M. Halm Small for expert assistance in the preparation of this chapter and J. Bell for help with graphic illustrations.

REFERENCES

1. Serhan CN. Endogenous chemical mediators in anti-inflammation and pro-resolution. *Curr Med Chem* 2002;1:177–192.
2. Roman RJ, Alonso-Galicia M. P-450 eicosanoids: a novel signaling pathway regulating renal function. *News Physiol Sci* 1999;14:238.
3. Omura T. Forty years of cytochrome P450. *Biochem Biophys Res Commun* 1999;266:690–698.
4. Node K, Huo Y, Ruan X, et al. Anti-inflammatory properties of cytochrome P450 epoxygenase-derived eicosanoids. *Science* 1999;285: 1276–1279.
5. Bergström S. The prostaglandins: from the laboratory to the clinic. In: *Les Prix Nobel: Nobel Prizes, presentations, biographies and lectures*. Stockholm: Almqvist & Wiksell, 1982:129–148. Also available at *www.nobel.se*.
6. Holgate S, Dahlén S-E, eds. *SRS-A to leukotrienes: the dawning of a new treatment*. Oxford, UK: Blackwell Science, 1997.
7. Samuelsson B. From studies of biochemical mechanisms to novel biological mediators: prostaglandin endoperoxides, thromboxanes and leukotrienes. In: *Les Prix Nobel: Nobel Prizes, presentations, biographies and lectures*. Stockholm: Almqvist & Wiksell, 1982:153–174. Also available at *www.nobel.se*.
8. Vane JR. Adventures and excursions in bioassay: the stepping stones to prostacyclin. In: *Les Prix Nobel: Nobel Prizes, presentations, biographies and lectures*. Stockholm: Almqvist & Wiksell, 1982:181–206. Also available at *www.nobel.se*.
9. The Nobel Foundation. Elias James Corey: Prize for masterly development of organic synthesis, 1990 (press release). *www.nobel.se/chemistry/laureates/1990/press.html*.
10. Serhan CN, Clish CB, Brannon J, et al. Novel functional sets of lipid-derived mediators with antiinflammatory actions generated from omega-3 fatty acids via cyclooxygenase 2-nonsteroidal antiinflammatory drugs and transcellular processing. *J Exp Med* 2000;192:1197–1204.
11. Serhan CN, Hong S, Gronert K, et al. Resolvins: a family of bioactive products of omega-3 fatty acid transformation circuits initiated by aspirin treatment that counter pro-inflammation signals. *J Exp Med* 2002;196:1025–1037.
12. Hong S, Gronert K, Devchand P, et al. Novel docosatrienes and 17S-resolvins generated from docosahexaenoic acid in murine brain, human blood and glial cells: autacoids in anti-inflammation. *J Biol Chem* 2003;278:14677–14687.
13. Serhan CN, Maddox JF, Petasis NA, et al. Design of lipoxin A_4 stable analogs that block transmigration and adhesion of human neutrophils. *Biochemistry* 1995;34:14609–14615.
14. Clish CB, O'Brien JA, Gronert K, et al. Local and systemic delivery of a stable aspirin-triggered lipoxin prevents neutrophil recruitment *in vivo*. *Proc Natl Acad Sci U S A* 1999;96:8247–8252.
15. Serhan CN. Lipoxins and aspirin-triggered 15-epi-lipoxins. In: Gallin JI, Snyderman R, eds. *Inflammation: basic principles and clinical correlates*. Philadelphia: Lippincott Williams & Wilkins, 1999:373–385.
16. Needleman P, Isakson PC. The discovery and function of COX-2. *J Rheumatol* 1997;24(suppl 49):6–8.
17. McMahon B, Mitchell S, Brady HR, et al. Lipoxins: revelations on resolution. *Trends Pharmacol Sci* 2001;22:391–395.

18. Dennis EA. Phospholipase A_2 in eicosanoid generation. *Am J Respir Crit Care Med* 2000;161(suppl):32–35.
19. De Caterina R, Endres S, Kristensen SD, et al., eds. *n-3 Fatty acids and vascular disease.* London: Springer-Verlag, 1993.
20. Takasaki J, Kawauchi Y, Masuho Y. Synergistic effect of type II phospholipase A_2 and platelet-activating factor on Mac-1 surface expression and exocytosis of gelatinase granules in human neutrophils: evidence for the 5-lipoxygenase-dependent mechanism. *J Immunol* 1998;160:5066–5072.
21. Herschman HR. Prostaglandin synthase 2. *Biochim Biophys Acta* 1996;1299:125–140.
22. Tada K, Murakami M, Kambe T, et al. Induction of cyclooxygenase-2 by secretory phospholipases A_2 in nerve growth factor-stimulated rat serosal mast cells is facilitated by interaction with fibroblasts and mediated by a mechanism independent of their enzymatic functions. *J Immunol* 1998;161:5008–5015.
23. Bonventre JV, Huang Z, Taheri MR, et al. Reduced fertility and postischaemic brain injury in mice deficient in cytosolic phospholipase A_2. *Nature* 1997;390:622–625.
24. Uozumi N, Kume K, Nagase T, et al. Role of cytosolic phospholipase A2 in allergic response and parturition. *Nature* 1997;390:618–622.
25. Austin SC, Funk CD. Insight into prostaglandin, leukotriene, and other eicosanoid functions using mice with targeted gene disruptions. *Prostaglandins Other Lipid Mediat* 1999;58:231–252.
26. Marcus AJ, Broekman MJ, Pinsky DJ. COX inhibitors and thromboregulation. *N Engl J Med* 2002;347:1025–1026.
27. Herschman HR. Recent progress in the cellular and molecular biology of prostaglandin synthesis. *Trends Cardiovasc Med* 1998;8:145–150.
28. Vane JR, Botting RM, eds. *Therapeutic roles of selective COX-2 inhibitors.* London: William Harvey Press, 2001.
29. Willoughby DA, Moore AR, Colville-Nash PR. COX-1, COX-2, and COX-3 and the future treatment of chronic inflammatory disease. *Lancet* 2000;355:646–648.
30. Chandrasekharan NV, Dai H, Roos KLT, et al. COX-3, a cyclooxygenase-1 variant inhibited by acetaminophen and other analgesic/antipyretic drugs: cloning, structure, and expression. *Proc Natl Acad Sci U S A* 2002;99:13926–13931.
31. Garcia Cardena G, Comander J, Anderson KR, et al. Biomechanical activation of vascular endothelium as a determinant of its functional phenotype. *Proc Natl Acad Sci U S A* 2001;98:4478–4485.
32. Cheng Y, Austin SC, Rocea B, et al. Role of prostacyclin in the cardiovascular response to thromboxane A_2. *Science* 2002;296:539–541.
33. Serhan CN, Levy B. Success of prostaglandin E_2 in structure function is a challenge for structure-based therapeutics. *Proc Natl Acad Sci U S A* 2003;100:8609–8611.
34. Trebino CE, Stock JL, Gibbons CP. Impaired inflammatory and pain responses in mice lacking an inducible prostaglandin E synthase. *Proc Natl Acad Sci U S A* 2003;100:9044–9049.
35. Gilroy DW, Colville-Nash PR, Willis D, et al. Inducible cyclooxygenase may have anti-inflammatory properties. *Nat Med* 1999;5:698–701.
36. Willoughby DA, Moore AR, Colville-Nash PR. COX-1, COX-2, and COX-3 and the future treatment of chronic inflammatory disease. *Lancet* 2000;355:646–648.
37. Simmons DL, Botting RM, Robertson PM, et al. Induction of an acetaminophen-sensitive cyclooxygenase with reduced sensitivity to nonsteroid antiinflammatory drugs. *Proc Natl Acad Sci U S A* 1999;96:3275–3280.
38. Schwab JM, Schlusener HJ, Meyermann R, et al. COX-3 the enzyme and the concept: steps toward highly specialized pathways and precision therapeutics. *Prostaglandins Leukot Essent Fatty Acids* 2003;69:339–343.
39. van der Donk WA, Tsai A-L, Kulmacz RJ. The cyclooxygenase reaction mechanism. *Biochemistry* 2002;41:15451–15458.
40. Schievella AR, Regier MK, Smith WL, et al. Calcium-mediated translocation of cytosolic phospholipase A_2 to the nuclear envelope and endoplasmic reticulum. *J Biol Chem* 1995;270:30749–30754.
41. Serhan CN. Signalling the fat controller. *Nature* 1996;384:23–24.
42. Morham SG, Langenbach R, Loftin CD, et al. Prostaglandin synthase 2 gene disruption causes severe renal pathology in the mouse. *Cell* 1995;83:473–482.
43. Langenbach R, Morham SG, Tiano HF, et al. Prostaglandin synthase 1 gene disruption in mice reduces arachidonic acid-induced inflammation and indomethacin-induced gastric ulceration. *Cell* 1995;83:483–492.
44. Warner TD, Mitchell JA. Cyclooxygenase-3 (COX-3): filling in the gaps toward a COX continuum? *Proc Natl Acad Sci U S A* 2002;99:13371–13373.
45. Weissmann G. Aspirin. *Sci Am* 1991;264:84–90.
46. Cronstein BN, Montesinos MC, Weissmann G. Sites of action for future therapy: an adenosine-dependent mechanism by which aspirin retains its antiinflammatory activity in cyclooxygenase-2 and NFκB knockout mice. *Osteoarthritis Cartilage* 1999;7:361–363.
47. Pillinger MH, Abramson SB. The neutrophil in rheumatoid arthritis. *Rheumatic Dis Clin North Am* 1995;21:691–714.
48. FitzGerald GA. Parsing an enigma: the pharmacodynamics of aspirin resistance. *Lancet* 2003;361:542–544.
49. Linton MF, Fazio S. Cyclooxygenase-2 and atherosclerosis. *Curr Opin Lipidol* 2002;13:497–504.
50. Murata T, Ushikubi F, Matsuoka T, et al. Altered pain perception and inflammatory response in mice lacking prostacyclin receptor. *Nature* 1997;388:678–682.
51. Gilroy DW, Colville-Nash PR, Willis D, et al. Inducible cyclooxygenase may have anti-inflammatory properties. *Nat Med* 1999;5:698–701.
52. Jones MK, Wang H, Peskar BM, et al. Inhibition of angiogenesis by nonsteroidal anti-inflammatory drugs: insight into mechanisms and implications for cancer growth and ulcer healing. *Nat Med* 1999;5:1418–1423.
53. Bandeira-Melo C, Serra MF, Diaz BL, et al. Cyclooxygenase-2-derived prostaglandin E_2 and lipoxin A_4 accelerate resolution of allergic edema in *Angiostrongylus costaricensis*–infected rats: relationship with concurrent eosinophilia. *J Immunol* 2000;164:1029–1036.
54. Pouliot M, Gilbert C, Borgeat P, et al. Expression and activity of prostaglandin endoperoxide synthase-2 in agonist-activated human neutrophils. *FASEB J* 1998;12:1109–1123.
55. Haeggström JZ, Serhan CN. Update on arachidonic acid cascade: leukotrienes and lipoxins in disease models. In: Serhan CN, Ward PA, eds. *Molecular and cellular basis of inflammation.* Totowa, NJ: Humana Press, 1999:51–92.
56. Rowley AF, Kühn H, Schewe T, eds. *Eicosanoids and related compounds in plants and animals.* London: Portland Press, 1998.
57. Brash AR. Lipoxygenases: occurrence, functions, catalysis, and acquisition of substrate. *J Biol Chem* 1999;274:23679–23682.
58. Thunnissen MMGM, Nordlund P, Haeggström J. Crystal structure of human leukotriene A_4 hydrolase, a bifunctional enzyme in inflammation. *Nat Struct Biol* 2001;8:131–135.
59. Byrum RS, Goulet JL, Griffiths RJ, et al. Role of the 5-lipoxygenase-activating protein (FLAP) in murine acute inflammatory responses. *J Exp Med* 1997;185:1065–1075.
60. Surette ME, Palmantier R, Gosselin J, et al. Lipopolysaccharides prime whole human blood and isolated neutrophils for the increased synthesis of 5-lipoxygenase products by enhancing arachidonic acid availability: involvement of the CD14 antigen. *J Exp Med* 1993;178:1347–1355.
61. Showell HJ, Cooper K. Inhibitors and antagonists of cyclooxygenase, 5-lipoxygenase, and platelet activating factor. In: Gallin JI, Snyderman R, eds. *Inflammation: basic principles and clinical correlates.* Philadelphia: Lippincott Williams & Wilkins, 1999:1177–1193.
62. Samuelsson B, Dahlén SE, Lindgren JÅ, et al. Leukotrienes and lipoxins: structures, biosynthesis, and biological effects. *Science* 1987;237:1171–1176.
63. Penrose JF, Austen KF, Lam BK. Leukotrienes: biosynthetic pathways, release, and receptor-mediated actions with relevance to disease states. In: Gallin JI, Snyderman R, eds. *Inflammation: basic principles and clinical correlates.* Philadelphia: Lippincott Williams & Wilkins, 1999:361–372.
64. Chen XS, Sheller JR, Johnson EN, et al. Role of leukotrienes revealed by targeted disruption of the 5-lipoxygenase gene. *Nature* 1994;372:179–182.
65. In KH, Asano K, Beier D, et al. Naturally occurring mutations in the human 5-lipoxygenase gene promoter that modify transcription factor binding and reporter gene transcription. *J Clin Invest* 1997;99:1130–1137.
66. Mancini JA, Vickers PJ, O'Neill GP, et al. Altered sensitivity of aspirin-acetylated prostaglandin G/H synthase-2 inhibition by nonsteroidal anti-inflammatory drugs. *Mol Pharmacol* 1997;51:52–60.
67. Cotran RS, Kumar V, Collins T, eds. *Robbins pathologic basis of disease.* Philadelphia: WB Saunders, 1999.
68. Yokomizo T, Izumi T, Chang K, et al. A G-protein-coupled receptor for leukotriene B_4 that mediates chemotaxis. *Nature* 1997;387:620–624.

69. Brink C, Dahlén S-E, Drazen J, et al. International Union of Pharmacology XXXVII. Nomenclature for leukotriene and lipoxin receptors. *Pharmacol Rev* 2003;55:195–227.
70. Chiang N, Gronert K, Clish CB, et al. Leukotriene B_4 receptor transgenic mice reveal novel protective roles for lipoxins and aspirin-triggered lipoxins in reperfusion. *J Clin Invest* 1999;104:309–316.
71. Takano T, Clish CB, Gronert K, et al. Neutrophil-mediated changes in vascular permeability are inhibited by topical application of aspirin-triggered 15-epi-lipoxin A_4 and novel lipoxin B_4 stable analogues. *J Clin Invest* 1998;101:819–826.
72. Griffiths RJ, Smith MA, Roach ML, et al. Collagen-induced arthritis is reduced in 5-lipoxygenase-activating protein-deficient mice. *J Exp Med* 1997;185:1123–1129.
73. Lynch KR, O'Neill GP, Liu Q, et al. Characterization of the human cysteinyl leukotriene $CysLT_1$ receptor. *Nature* 1999;399:789.
74. Drazen JM, Israel E, O'Byrne PM. Treatment of asthma with drugs modifying the leukotriene pathway. *N Engl J Med* 1999;340:197–206.
75. Noonan MJ, Chervinsky P, Brandon M, et al. Montelukast, a potent leukotriene receptor antagonist, causes dose-related improvements in chronic asthma. *Eur Respir J* 1998;11:1232–1239.
76. Leff JA, Busse WW, Pearlman D, et al. Montelukast, a leukotriene-receptor antagonist, for the treatment of mild asthma and exercise-induced bronchoconstriction. *N Engl J Med* 1998;339:147–152.
77. Ducharme FM. Anti-leukotrienes as add-on therapy to inhaled glucocorticoids in patients with asthma: systematic review of current evidence. *BMJ* 2002;324:1545–1551.
78. Serhan CN, Sheppard KA. Lipoxin formation during human neutrophil-platelet interactions. Evidence for the transformation of leukotriene A_4 by platelet 12-lipoxygenase *in vitro*. *J Clin Invest* 1990;85:772–780.
79. Goh J, Godson C, Brady HR, et al. Lipoxins: pro-resolution lipid mediators in intestinal inflammation. *Gastroenterology* 2003;124:1043–1054.
80. Serhan CN, Chiang N. Lipid-derived mediators in endogenous anti-inflammation and resolution: lipoxins and aspirin-triggered 15-epi-lipoxins. *Sci World J* 2002;2:169–204.
81. Colgan SP, Serhan CN, Parkos CA, et al. Lipoxin A_4 modulates transmigration of human neutrophils across intestinal epithelial monolayers. *J Clin Invest* 1993;92:75–82.
82. Lee TH, Lympany P, Crea AE, et al. Inhibition of leukotriene B_4-induced neutrophil migration by lipoxin A_4: structure-function relationships. *Biochem Biophys Res Commun* 1991;180:1416–1421.
83. Takano T, Fiore S, Maddox JF, et al. Aspirin-triggered 15-epi-lipoxin A_4 and LXA_4 stable analogs are potent inhibitors of acute inflammation: Evidence for anti-inflammatory receptors. *J Exp Med* 1997;185:1693–1704.
84. Munger KA, Montero A, Fukunaga M, et al. Transfection of rat kidney with human 15-lipoxygenase suppresses inflammation and preserves function in experimental glomerulonephritis. *Proc Natl Acad Sci U S A* 1999;96:13375–13380.
85. Badr KF, DeBoer DK, Schwartzberg M, et al. Lipoxin A_4 antagonizes cellular and in vivo actions of leukotriene D_4 in rat glomerular mesangial cells: evidence for competition at a common receptor. *Proc Natl Acad Sci U S A* 1989;86:3438–3442.
86. Topper JN, Cai J, Falb D, et al. Identification of vascular endothelial genes differentially responsive to fluid mechanical stimuli: cyclooxygenase-2, manganese superoxide dismutase, and endothelial cell nitric oxide synthase are selectively up-regulated by steady laminar shear stress. *Proc Natl Acad Sci U S A* 1996;93:10417–10422.
87. Schottelius AJ, Giesen C, Asadullah K, et al. An aspirin-triggered lipoxin A_4 stable analog displays a unique topical anti-inflammatory profile. *J Immunol* 2002;169:7063–7070.
88. Gewirtz AT, Collier-Hyams LS, Young AN, et al. Lipoxin A_4 analogs attenuate induction of intestinal epithelial proinflammatory gene expression and reduce the severity of dextran sodium sulfate-induced colitis. *J Immunol* 2002;168:5260–5267.
89. Maclouf J, Folco G, Patrono C. Eicosanoids and iso-eicosanoids: constitutive, inducible and transcellular biosynthesis in vascular disease. *Thromb Haemost* 1998;79:691–705.
90. Marcus AJ. Platelets: their role in hemostasis, thrombosis, and inflammation. In: Gallin JI, Snyderman R, eds. *Inflammation: basic principles and clinical correlates.* Philadelphia: Lippincott Williams & Wilkins, 1999:77–95.
91. Doré M. Platelet-leukocyte interactions. *Am Heart J* 1998;135(suppl):146–151.
92. Stenke L, Reizenstein P, Lindgren JA. Leukotrienes and lipoxins—new potential performers in the regulation of human myelopoiesis. *Leuk Res* 1994;18:727–732.
93. Levy BD, Gronert K, Clish C, et al. Leukotriene and lipoxin biosynthesis. In: Laychock S, Rubin RP, eds. *Lipid second messengers.* Boca Raton, FL: CRC Press, 1999:83–111.
94. Habib GM, Shi Z-Z, Cuevas AA, et al. Leukotriene D_4 and cysteinyl-bis-glycine metabolism in membrane-bound dipeptidase-deficient mice. *Proc Natl Acad Sci U S A* 1998;95:4859–4863.
95. Clish CB, Levy BD, Chiang N, et al. Oxidoreductases in lipoxin A_4 metabolic inactivation. *J Biol Chem* 2000;275:25372–25380.
96. Yamamoto S, Yamamoto K, Kurobe H, et al. Transcriptional regulation of fatty acid cyclooxygenases-1 and -2. *Int J Tissue React* 1998;20:17–22.
97. Vane JR, Bakhle YS, Botting RM. Cyclooxygenases 1 and 2. *Annu Rev Pharmacol Toxicol* 1998;38:97–120.
98. Tan L, Chen C-y, Larsen RD, et al. An efficient asymmetric synthesis of a potent COX-2 inhibitor L-784,512. *Tetrahedron Lett* 1998;39:3961–3964.
99. Kalgutkar AS, Crews BC, Rowlinson SW, et al. Aspirin-like molecules that covalently inactivate cyclooxygenase-2. *Science* 1998;280:1268–1272.
100. Claveau D, Sirinyan M, Guay J, et al. Microsomal prostaglandin E synthase-1 is a major terminal synthase that is selectively up-regulated during cyclooxygenase-2-dependent prostaglandin E_2 production in the rat adjuvant-induced arthritis model. *J Immunol* 2003;170:4738–4744.
101. Rudberg PC, Tholander F, Thunnissen MMGM, et al. Leukotriene A_4 hydrolase: selective abrogation of leukotriene B_4 formation by mutation of aspartic acid 375. *Proc Natl Acad Sci U S A* 2002;99:4215–4220.
102. Aliberti J, Hieny S, Reis e Sousa C, et al. Lipoxin-mediated inhibition of IL-12 production by DCs: a mechanism for regulation of microbial immunity. *Nat Immunol* 2002;3:76–82.
103. Coleman RA, Smith WL, Narumiya S. International Union of Pharmacology classification of prostanoid receptors: properties, distribution, and structure of the receptors and their subtypes. *Pharmacol Rev* 1994;46:205–229.
104. Breyer MD. Prostaglandin receptors in the kidney: a new route for intervention? *Exp Nephrol* 1998;6:180–188.
105. Narumiya S, Sugimoto Y, Ushikubi F. Prostanoid receptors: structures, properties, and functions. *Physiol Rev* 1999;79:1193–1226.
106. Armstrong RA. Platelet prostanoid receptors. *Pharmacol Ther* 1996;72:171–191.
107. Toh H, Ichikawa A, Narumiya S. Molecular evolution of receptors for eicosanoids. *FEBS Lett* 1995;361:17–21.
108. Devchand PR, Arita M, Hong S, et al. Human ALX receptor regulates neutrophil recruitment in transgenic mice: roles in inflammation and host-defense. *FASEB J* 2003;17:652–659.
109. Hirai H, Tanaka K, Takano S, et al. Cutting edge: agonistic effect of indomethacin on a prostaglandin D_2 receptor, CRTH2. *J Immunol* 2002;168:981–985.
110. Devchand PR, Keller H, Peters JM, et al. The PPARα—leukotriene B_4 pathway to inflammation control. *Nature* 1996;384:39–43.
111. Wright HM, Clish CB, Mikami T, et al. A synthetic antagonist for the peroxisome proliferator-activated receptor γ inhibits adipocyte differentiation. *J Biol Chem* 2000;275:1873–1877.
112. Brock TG, Paine R III, Peters-Golden M. Localization of 5-lipoxygenase to the nucleus of unstimulated rat basophilic leukemia cells. *J Biol Chem* 1994;269:22059–22066.
113. Nagase T, Uozumi N, Ishii S, et al. Acute lung injury by sepsis and acid aspiration: a key role for cytosolic phospholipase A_2. *Nat Immunol* 2000;1:13–15.
114. Perretti M, Croxtall JD, Wheeler SK, et al. Mobilizing lipocortin 1 in adherent human leukocytes downregulates their transmigration. *Nat Med* 1996;22:1259–1262.
115. Perretti M, Chiang N, La M, et al. Endogenous lipid- and peptide-derived anti-inflammatory pathways generated with glucocorticoid and aspirin treatment activate the lipoxin A(4) receptor. *Nat Med* 2002;8:1296–1302.
116. Levy BD, Clish CB, Schmidt B, et al. Lipid mediator class switching during acute inflammation: signals in resolution. *Nat Immunol* 2001;2:612–619.
117. Wallace JL, Fiorucci S. A magic bullet for mucosal protection . . . and aspirin is the trigger! *Trends Pharmacol Sci* 2003;24:323–326.

118. Hawkey CJ. COX-2 inhibitors. *Lancet* 1999;353:307–314.
119. Filep JG, Zouki C, Petasis NA, et al. Anti-inflammatory actions of lipoxin A_4 stable analogs are demonstrable in human whole blood: modulation of leukocyte adhesion molecules and inhibition of neutrophil-endothelial interactions. *Blood* 1999;94:4132–4142.
120. Brooks CDW, Stewart AO, Kolasa T, et al. Design of inhibitors of leukotriene biosynthesis and their therapeutic potential. *Pure Appl Chem* 1998;70:271–274.
121. von Schacky C. ω-3 fatty acids in primary and secondary prevention of coronary artery disease. In: De Caterina R, Endres S, Kristensen SD, et al., eds. *n-3 Fatty acids and vascular disease*. London: Springer-Verlag, 1993:159–166.
122. Simopoulos AP, Leaf A, Salem N Jr. Workshop on the essentiality of and recommended dietary intakes for omega-6 and omega-3 fatty acids. *J Am Coll Nutr* 1999;18:487–489.
123. GISSI-Prevenzione Investigators. Dietary supplementation with n-3 polyunsaturated fatty acids and vitamin E after myocardial infarction: results of the GISSI-Prevenzione trial. Gruppo Italiano per lo Studio della Sopravvivenza nell'Infarto miocardico. *Lancet* 1999; 354:447–455.
124. Hill DJ, Griffiths DH, Rowley AF. Trout thrombocytes contain 12- but not 5-lipoxygenase activity. *Biochim Biophys Acta* 1999;1437:63–70.
125. Serhan CN, Chiang N. Lipid-derived mediators in endogenous antiinflammation and resolution: lipoxins and aspirin-triggered 15-epi-lipoxins. *Sci World* 2001. Accessed on-line at *www.thescientificworld.com*.
126. Godson C, Mitchell S, Harvey K, et al. Cutting edge: Lipoxins rapidly stimulate nonphlogistic phagocytosis of apoptotic neutrophils by monocyte-derived macrophages. *J Immunol* 2000;164:1663–1667.
127. Sodin-Semrl S, Taddeo B, Tseng D, et al. Lipoxin A_4 inhibits IL-1 beta-induced IL-6, IL-8, and matrix metalloproteinase-3 production in human synovial fibroblasts and enhances synthesis of tissue inhibitors of metalloproteinases. *J Immunol* 2000;164:2660–2666.
128. Fierro IM, Kutok JL, Serhan CN. Novel lipid mediator regulators of endothelial cell proliferation and migration: Aspirin-triggered-15*R*-lipoxin A_4 and lipoxin A_4. *J Pharmacol Exp Ther* 2002;300:385–392.
129. Levy BD, De Sanctis GT, Devchand PR, et al. Multi-pronged inhibition of airway hyper-responsiveness and inflammation by lipoxin A_4. *Nat Med* 2002;8:1018–1023.
130. Qiu F-H, Devchand PR, Wada K, et al. Aspirin-triggered lipoxin A_4 and lipoxin A_4 up-regulate transcriptional corepressor NAB1 in human neutrophils. *FASEB J* 2001;15:2736–2738.
131. Xiao G, Tsai A-L, Palmer G, et al. Analysis of hydroperoxide-induced tyrosyl radicals and lipoxygenase activity in aspirin-treated human prostaglandin H synthase-2. *Biochemistry* 1997;36:1836–1845.
132. Garg R, Kurup A, Mekapati SB, et al. Cyclooxygenase (COX) inhibitors: a comparative QSAR study. *Chem Rev* 2003;103:703–731.
133. Brady HR, Papayianni A, Serhan CN. Leukocyte adhesion promotes biosynthesis of lipoxygenase products by transcellular routes. *Kidney Int Suppl* 1994;45(suppl):90–97.
134. Levy BD, Bertram S, Tai HH, et al. Agonist-induced lipoxin A_4 generation: detection by a novel lipoxin A_4-ELISA. *Lipids* 1993;28: 1047–1053.
135. Lee TH, Crea AE, Gant V, et al. Identification of lipoxin A_4 and its relationship to the sulfidopeptide leukotrienes C_4, D_4, and E_4 in the bronchoalveolar lavage fluids obtained from patients with selected pulmonary diseases. *Am Rev Respir Dis* 1990;141:1453–1458.
136. Brezinski DA, Nesto RW, Serhan CN. Angioplasty triggers intracoronary leukotrienes and lipoxin A_4. Impact of aspirin therapy. *Circulation* 1992;86:56–63.
137. Pouliot M, Clish CB, Petasis NA, et al. Lipoxin A_4 analogues inhibit leukocyte recruitment to *Porphyromonas gingivalis*: a role for cyclooxygenase-2 and lipoxins in periodontal disease. *Biochemistry* 2000; 39:4761–4768.
138. Van Dyke TE, Serhan CN. Resolution of inflammation: a new paradigm for the pathogenesis of periodontal diseases. *J Dent Res* 2003: 82–90.
139. Edenius C, Kumlin M, Björk T, et al. Lipoxin formation in human nasal polyps and bronchial tissue. *FEBS Lett* 1990;272:25–28.
140. Thomas E, Leroux JL, Blotman F, et al. Conversion of endogenous arachidonic acid to 5,15-diHETE and lipoxins by polymorphonuclear cells from patients with rheumatoid arthritis. *Inflamm Res* 1995;44:121–124.
141. Capdevila J, Yadagiri P, Manna S, et al. Absolute configuration of the hydroxyeicosatetraenoic acids (HETEs) formed during catalytic oxygenation of arachidonic acid by microsomal cytochrome P-450. *Biochem Biophys Res Commun* 1986;141:1007–1011.
142. Roberts LJ II, Morrow JD. Products of the isoprostane pathway: unique bioactive compounds and markers of lipid peroxidation. *Cell Mol Life Sci* 2002;59:808–820.
143. Serhan CN, Oliw E. Unorthodox routes to prostanoid formation: new twists in cyclooxygenase-initiated pathways. *J Clin Invest* 2001:107: 1481–1489.

CHAPTER 24

Nitric Oxide and Related Compounds

Jim C. Oates and Gary S. Gilkeson

Nitric oxide (NO) is a short-lived, soluble intercellular messenger involved in neurotransmission, vascular dilatation, and antitumor and antimicrobial activity (1–4). The recognized effects of NO and its metabolites in cellular processes are ever increasing. The importance of NO in biology was perhaps best indicated by the recent awarding of the Nobel Prize to a trio of investigators who first described the biologic effects of NO. This chapter focuses on the effects of NO in inflammation, because this aspect of its function is most pertinent to the rheumatic diseases. Due to its host of effects in many clinical situations, production of NO cannot be classified as either solely harmful or beneficial (Table 24.1). In many inflammatory states, including autoimmune and infectious diseases, NO is overproduced in these patients compared with controls. Overproduction of NO is not specific for any disease state (Table 24.2). In some of these diseases, NO appears to be mediating tissue damage; in others it may be limiting the inflammatory response (1). Thus, each clinical state and inflammatory condition must be considered individually with regard to the role of NO in disease pathogenesis. This chapter reviews the biochemistry of NO production and metabolism, including discussion of the bioactive metabolites of NO referred to as reactive nitrogen species (RNS). The important cellular effects of NO will be reviewed. Finally, the evidence for a role for NO in various rheumatic diseases will be presented.

TABLE 24.1. *Pro- and antiinflammatory properties of nitric oxide*

- Proinflammatory properties
  - Induces cellular apoptosis, releasing autoantigens in apoptotic blebs
  - Induces cellular necrosis
  - Induces vasodilatation and vascular leakiness
  - Forms peroxynitrite that alters protein function (through nitration)
    - Induces cyclooxygenase-2
    - Induces thromboxane synthase
    - Inhibits prostacyclin synthase
    - Inhibits catalase
  - Contributes to oxidative stress
- Antiinflammatory properties
  - Induces apoptosis of infiltrating inflammatory and collagen-producing cells
  - Inhibits apoptosis of specific cells
  - Inhibits platelet aggregation and leukocyte adhesion
  - Inhibits expression of adhesion molecules

TABLE 24.2. *Rheumatic diseases in which nitric oxide is implicated in the pathogenesis*

	Human data	Animal models
Rheumatoid arthritis	Yes	Yes
Systemic lupus erythematosus	Yes	Yes
Lupus-related vasculitis	No	Yes
Scleroderma	Yes	Yes
Osteoarthritis	Yes	Yes
Giant-cell arteritis	Yes	No
Kawasaki disease	Yes	Yes
Behçet disease	Yes	No
Henoch-Schönlein purpura	Yes	No

BIOCHEMISTRY OF NITRIC OXIDE PRODUCTION

NO is produced via the oxidation of the amino acid arginine (Fig. 24.1) mediated by nitric oxide synthases (NOS) (1–4). The products of this reaction are NO and citrulline. NO is generated by at least three different forms of NOS: endothelial NOS (eNOS), neuronal NOS (nNOS), and inducible NOS (iNOS) (5). The genes that produce these synthases are, by convention, referred to as NOS1 for the protein nNOS, NOS2 for iNOS, and NOS3 for eNOS (1). eNOS and nNOS are constitutive enzymes that produce low levels of NO (picomolar amounts), are calcium dependent, and

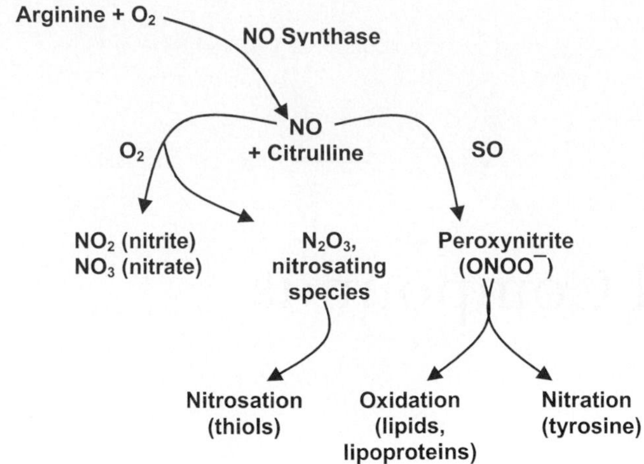

FIG. 24.1. Biochemistry of nitric oxide (NO) production. Arginine is converted to NO + citrulline via NO synthases. NO is then metabolized through different pathways, yielding a variety of biologic effects. *SO,* superoxide; *N_2O_3*, dinitrogen trioxide.

produce NO for only a short duration (1–5). The terms *constitutive* and *inducible* are relative, in that eNOS can be induced by certain stimuli and iNOS is constitutive in some cells (1). All forms of NOS require reduced nicotinamide adenine dinucleotide phosphate (NADPH) and tetrahydrobiopterin as cofactors. In the endothelium, NO is a smooth muscle relaxant and inhibits platelet binding and aggregation (6–8). Low-level production of NO by endothelial cells is, for the most part, considered antiinflammatory, due to its ability to relax smooth muscle, resulting in vasodilatation, while also blocking platelet aggregation and neutrophil adhesion (6–8). In the nervous system, NO produced by neuronal NOS serves as a neurotransmitter and appears to play a role in transmitting pain in animal models of inflammation and hyperalgesia and in inducing fever in response to lipopolysaccharide (LPS) *in vivo* (9–12). nNOS is overexpressed in stroke, Alzheimer disease, human immunodeficiency virus–related dementia, and Parkinson disease, but the role of nNOS in these diseases is not clear (13). In animal models of asthma, nNOS appears to reduce airway hyperresponsiveness in response to methacholine (14,15). The effect of neuronal NO production on inflammation, if any, is unclear (2). The end result of NO expression in inflammation (whether it is protective or deleterious) may depend on the quantity of NO produced in response to the inflammatory stimulus and the accompanying oxidative stress that would lead to pathogenic peroxynitrite ($ONOO^-$) production, as described below (16). For example, in one model of *Escherichia coli* meningitis, nNOS overexpression appeared to enhance the inflammatory response and subsequent brain injury (17).

The inducible form of nitric oxide synthase (iNOS) is capable of producing large quantities of NO (nanomolar to micromolar amounts) in response to immune stimuli and is found in (among other cells) hepatocytes, mesangial cells, lymphocytes, and macrophages (1,2). A variety of immune stimuli induce NO production, including LPS, interleukin-1β (IL-1β), interferon-γ (IFN-γ), IFN-α, and tumor necrosis factor-α (TNF-α) (1,5,18–22). Once activated, iNOS produces NO for an extended period (1,3,5).

The signaling pathways for induced NO production are at least partially known. One of the key convergence points for NO production is at the level of nuclear factor κB (NFκB) (1,5,23). NFκB is found in the cytoplasm linked with a protein-designated inhibitor of NFκB (IκB). Stimuli of NO production (i.e., LPS) leads to phosphorylation of IκB, which leads to uncoupling of IκB from NFκB. NFκB is then able to enter the nucleus and bind to the promoter region of a number of proinflammatory genes, including NOS2. The binding of NFκB to the NOS2 promoter region is required for enhanced NOS2-mediated production of NO (1,5,23). In macrophages, NO production also requires the interaction of CD40 and CD40 ligand (CD40L) (24). Although the role of NFκB in NOS2 transcriptional regulation is well described, a number of other transcription factors are being investigated as regulators of NOS2 transcription. Consensus sequences for binding of several transcription factors to the promoter region of human NOS2 have been described, including IFN-γ regulatory factor-1 (IRF-1), IFN-stimulated response element (ISRE), γ activation site (GAS), activator protein-1 (AP-1), CCAAT/enhancer-binding protein β (C/EBPβ) (25), and signal transducer and activator of transcription 1 α (STAT1-α), while an octamer factor-binding site has been described in the murine NOS2 promoter (26).

IMMUNE FACTORS IMPLICATED IN NITRIC OXIDE PRODUCTION

A number of inflammatory mediators that are known to be overproduced in inflammatory states are capable of inducing NO production (1,18–20,27). IFN-γ is a potent stimulus for NO production, especially when combined with other inflammatory factors (20). In strains of mice predisposed to developing a lupuslike disease (e.g., NZB/NZW or MRL/lpr mice), T cells at sites of tissue inflammation such as the glomerulus overproduced IFN-γ, and exogenous IFN-γ accelerated lupus renal disease (28,29). Mice treated with soluble IFN-γ receptor or an anti-IFN-γ monoclonal antibody had reduced disease (30,31). Similar to murine lupus, SLE patients exhibit increased expression of IFN-γ messenger RNA (mRNA) in peripheral blood mononuclear cells (PBMCs) (32,33). PBMCs obtained from lupus patients, however, produced reduced amounts of IFN-γ in a separate study (34). A recent study indicates that searching for expression of helper T cell subset 1 (T_H1) cytokines in PBMCs may not be as fruitful as looking at surrogate markers of T_H1 cytokine expression in tissue sites. Both IFN-γ and IL-2 mRNA are seen in increased amounts in the urine sediment of lupus patients with active nephritis compared with those in remission and those without nephritis (35). Another cytokine that stimulates murine NO production is IL-1β. IL-1β mRNA is overexpressed in lupus mice; levels are increased in the renal cortex, particularly in nephritic mice (34,36). IL-1β is also overproduced in patients with rheumatoid arthritis (RA) and in the rheumatoid synovium (37).

TNF-α is a potent stimulus for NO production in mice (22). Although the role of TNF-α in lupus is unclear (38–44), it is a key mediator of inflammation in RA (45). TNF-α activity was reduced in the PBMCs of lupus patients (43), but elevated levels of TNF-α antigen were found in glomerular mesangial cells (44). Localized production of TNF-α may result in elevated iNOS expression and renal damage in patients with lupus nephritis. The local presence of TNF-α in rheumatoid synovium may stimulate the enhanced NO production that occurs in the rheumatoid joint (45).

In contrast to their effect on NO production in murine macrophages, neither IFN-γ, TNF-α, IL-1β, nor IL-12, alone or in combination, induced NO production by normal human macrophages (46). A number of studies have demonstrated, however, that human macrophages can produce NO in certain disease states (47–49). Whether cytokines or other stimuli induce NO in these diseases is unclear; it is conceivable that an as yet undefined mediator stimulates macrophage NO production in humans. A potential mediator of enhanced NO production in humans is IFN-α. When IFN-α is used therapeutically in patients with hepatitis C, a small percentage of patients receiving IFN-α develop autoimmunity (50). Some hepatitis C patients treated with IFN-α developed elevated levels of serum NO, compared with untreated hepatitis C patients (51). IFN-α given *in vitro* stimulated NO production by PBMCs from normal individuals (51). Thus, IFN-α is a potential inducer of iNOS in humans.

CELLULAR EFFECTS OF NITRIC OXIDE AND REACTIVE NITROGEN SPECIES

Depending on the environment in which NO is released, the metabolism of NO varies significantly. The major pathways for NO metabolism are summarized in graphic form in Figs. 24.1 and 24.2. NO itself can act as a ligand for hemoproteins. In the case of guanylate cyclase, this results in activation of the enzyme. In an aqueous environment, NO can react with oxygen to form nitrogen dioxide, a potent oxidant that can react with anions of phenol or thiols. Nitrogen dioxide can form a dimer with itself [dinitrogen tetroxide (N_2O_4)] or combine with oxygen to form N_2O_3 (dinitrogen trioxide) (52). N_2O_4 can hydrolyze to form one nitrate ion (NO_3^-) and one nitrite ion (NO_2^-), whereas N_2O_3 is rapidly converted to NO_2^- in the absence of substrate. Both NO_3^- and NO_2^- (collectively called NO_X) can be measured in the serum or urine as stable oxidative products of NO. N_2O_4, N_2O_3, and NO itself are nitrosating agents (although *in vivo*, N_2O_3 appears to be the primary actor) and can easily react with thiols to form *S*-nitrosothiols (52). These compounds are biologically relevant because they serve to prolong the half-life of NO. These modified thiols can transport NO much farther from its origin than possible by mere diffusion. Thus, in biologic systems, the predominant products of NO and oxygen are likely NO_2^- and *S*-nitrosothiols (16). *S*-nitrosothiols can be measured in the serum or plasma along with NO_3^- and NO_2^-.

Whether superoxide (SO) is present when NO is formed has a profound effect on the metabolic fate of NO. When present in equimolar amounts, NO and SO combine to form peroxynitrite ($ONOO^-$), an important oxidizer and pathogenic mediator (16) (Figs. 24.1 and 24.2). Recently, it has been shown that iNOS, under certain conditions, can produce both NO and SO (53,54), Thus, iNOS alone can produce $ONOO^-$. However, $ONOO^-$ can also be produced when NO- and SO-producing cells are in close proximity (16). Peroxynitrite can be further metabolized to nitrate and a hydroxyl radical. Hydroxyl radicals are highly reactive and toxic to cells (53). $ONOO^-$ can react with a number of biologic molecules, including proteins, nucleic acids, and lipids. The most intensely studied biologic effect of peroxynitrite is the nitration of amino acids, primarily tyrosines and cysteines (53–56). This amino acid nitration can affect the function of proteins by either increasing activity (as in the case of thromboxane synthase) or decreasing activity (prostacyclin synthase and catalase) (57–62). Alternatively, $ONOO^-$ can serve as an enzyme substrate and increase activity in this fashion (as in the case of cyclooxygenase 2) (63). Because $ONOO^-$, like NO, has a short half-life, it cannot be directly measured. However, it can be indirectly measured as 3-nitrotyrosine in proteins that are formed as the result of the reaction between tyrosine and $ONOO^-$ (64). It should be noted that the leukocyte peroxidases myeloperoxidase and eosinophil peroxidase may also play a role in tyrosine nitration (65).

Peroxynitrite can react with lipoproteins and lipids alone. Interaction of peroxynitrite with lipids results in their oxidation, the most intensely studied example being low-density lipoprotein (LDL) (53). In contrast, NO inhibits the oxidation of LDL (53). Peroxynitrite can also oxidize lipids to form isoprostanes (66). Isoprostanes are biologically active, including functioning as an agonist for eicosanoid receptors (67–69). Thus, the indirect effects of NO via NO-derived RNS and the biochemical modifications they induce may be responsible for many of the biologic effects previously attributed to NO alone (53,54).

NO alone can have direct effects on cellular function through a number of different mechanisms. NO can bind to the heme group of cyclic guanylate cyclase, thereby activating the enzyme and resulting in increased levels of cyclic guanosine monophosphate (70). In the vascular endothelium, this results in smooth muscle relaxation. In addition, NO can also interact with the heme moieties of other proteins, including cytochrome P450, leading to reversible inhibition of the enzyme (4). NO can bind to nonheme irons, including those in aconitase and other proteins in the mitochondrial respiratory chain. Binding of NO to these iron-containing enzymes blocks the respiratory chain (1,2,4).

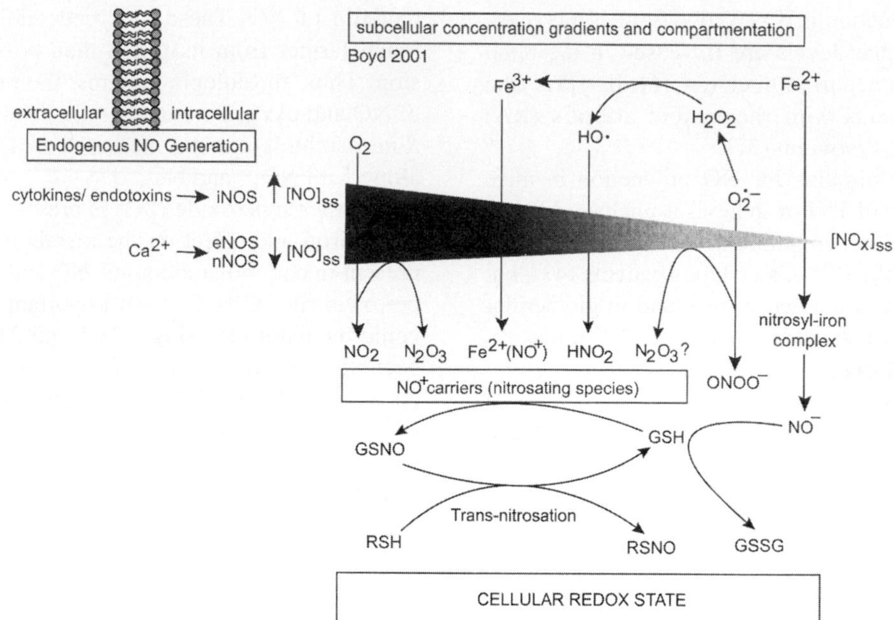

FIG. 24.2. Role of cellular microenvironment in nitric oxide (NO) chemistry. NO, synthesized by NO synthase either endogenous or exogenous to the cell, reaches a steady state, $[NO]_{ss}$, that is highly dependent on the relationship to the NO source and the cellular microenvironment. NO diffuses across cellular compartments in a concentration gradient in the cell. Reactions (redox or additive) occur with metals and oxygen-containing compounds in the local microenvironment that are also in a gradient. These reactions result in a number of nitrogen-containing compounds that are also in steady state $[NO_X]_{ss}$. Under physiologic conditions, NO^+ carriers contribute to nitrosation reactions with sulfhydryl (thiol) groups such as those with reduced glutathione (GSH) to form GSNO. These species can participate in transnitrosation reactions, whereby nitrosated thiols can transfer NO^+ from GSNO to another protein nitrosothiol (RSNO) or the reverse. GSH, under higher oxidant stress, can be oxidized to form GSSG; thus, the ratio of GSH/GSSG is a good index of redox potential in a cell. This ratio can be shifted by carriers of either NO^+ or NO^- depending on the redox state of the microenvironment. *GSNO,* S-nitrosoglutathione; *GSSG,* oxidized glutathione; *NOS,* NO synthase (e, endothelial; n, neuronal; i, inducible); *$[NO_X]_{ss}$,* steady state concentration of NO-related species; *RSH,* free or protein thiols; *RSNO,* S-nitrosothiols (free or protein). Reprinted from Boyd CS, Cadenas E. Nitric oxide and cell signaling pathways in mitochondrial-dependent apoptosis. *Biol Chem* 2002;383:411–23, with permission.

NO may also influence posttranslational modification of proteins, including inducing adenosine diphosphate (ADP) ribosylation. ADP ribosylation of actin may inhibit polymerization, adhesion, and migration of neutrophils (4).

NITRIC OXIDE AND APOPTOSIS

NO also plays an important role in apoptosis. Depending on the cell type and the presence of other factors locally released, NO can enhance apoptosis of some cells while inhibiting apoptosis of other cells. The potential for NO to induce apoptosis via mitochondrial-dependent mechanisms is highly dependent on cellular redox state and the relative concentration of NO in the mitochondria. At higher concentrations (<1 μM), NO can oxidize ubiquinol, leading to the generation of SO. At lower concentrations of NO (either as itself or as an *S*-nitrosothiol), the SO formed from mitochondrial respiratory activity tends to be converted by SO dismutase to hydrogen peroxide. At higher concentrations of NO, combination of SO and NO to form $ONOO^-$ is favored. $ONOO^-$ irreversibly damages mitochondrial adenosine triphosphate synthase, leading to release of cytochrome *c* and subsequent activation of caspase 9, which then promotes apoptosis. NO generation for these reactions can occur at the mitochondrial membrane or from extramitochondrial sources (71).

Cells that are sensitive to NO-induced apoptosis include fibroblasts, macrophages, pancreatic islet cells, smooth muscle cells, chondrocytes, and osteoblasts (70,72–75). Recently, mitochondrial NOS (mtNOS), nNOS with posttranslational modifications, has been identified and described (76) and may be an autocrine source of NO that induces apoptosis in cells such as thymocytes (77).

NO can induce cell death via multiple mechanisms, including activation of p53, and release of cytochrome *c* from mitochondria with subsequent activation of caspases (78). NO-induced apoptosis can occur when NO is produced by neighboring cells [such as thymic dendritic cells when presented with autoantigens (79)] or within the cell undergoing apoptosis, as described above (77).

NO also induces apoptosis by posttranslational modification of signal transduction proteins. For instance, although NO can activate all three mitogen-activated protein kinase (MAPK) pathways (ERK1/2, JNK, and p38), NO can shift the balance from ERK1/2 activation to JNK/p38 activation, which favors apoptosis. As with many processes involving NO, the degree of activation of each MAPK depends on the cellular environment in which NO is produced, the cell type, and the presence of ongoing proapoptotic stimuli (71).

NO, however, is not solely proapoptotic. It can block apoptosis by a variety of mechanisms, including *S*-nitrosylation of specific caspases, thereby inhibiting the more terminal portions of the apoptosis cascade (80–84). This antiapoptotic mechanism of NO appears most prevalent in hepatocytes (81). NO has also been demonstrated to interfere with Fas-mediated apoptosis (73,74,85). Although NO reduces apoptosis of murine B cells by increasing levels of Bcl-2, it appears to induce apoptosis in mesangial cells by decreasing Bcl-2 expression (86,87). Apoptosis of a Burkitt lymphoma cell line exposed to Epstein-Barr virus was inhibited by NO, suggesting a parallel inhibitory effect of NO on apoptosis of human and murine B cells (88).

Direct toxic effects of NO in areas of local release, such as the glomerulus, may be pathogenic in SLE. Recent studies indicate a key role for NO and SO production in induction of apoptosis of mesangial cells (73,74,85). Furthermore, apoptosis of mesangial cells appears to be a mechanism for the resolution of glomerular hypertrophy in induced glomerulonephritis models (89). NO also affects the production of extracellular matrix by mesangial cells, thereby modulating fibrosis (90). Thus, NO may have dual actions locally within the kidney. It may directly induce tissue damage, yet at the same time be a mediator of disease healing by inducing mesangial cell and macrophage apoptosis. Whether NO induces apoptosis in mesangial cells depends, as described above, on the overall reactive oxygen and nitrogen stress in mesangial cells at the time of exposure to NO (91).

An unusual but apparent key to the fate of a cell in an inflammatory setting is the inflammatory mediators being produced by the cell itself. Mesangial cells exposed to exogenous NO undergo apoptosis; however, if the mesangial cell is itself producing NO, it is protected from apoptosis (73,74). Products of the cyclooxygenase pathway and reactive oxygen species are also intricately involved with NO in the control of apoptosis in mesangial cells (92). One mechanism by which NO induces apoptosis is through induction of the enzyme poly (ADP-ribose) polymerase (PARP). Induction of PARP depletes the cell of NAD, interfering with key cellular processes and resulting in apoptosis (53).

In summary, NO has a host of cellular and molecular effects. These effects are not only due to NO, but are also a result of other RNS formed by the redox microenvironment at the site of NO production or distribution. Undoubtedly, a number of other important effects of NO remain to be clarified. Given this number of biologic effects of NO, it is perhaps not surprising that NO has been implicated in a number of disease processes. Most data and research into NO effects in rheumatology are centered on NO overproduction in inflammation. Underproduction of NO may be implicated in diseases in which vascular endothelial dysfunction is predominant, such as in Raynaud phenomenon and pulmonary hypertension. $ONOO^-$ actually inhibits NO production by eNOS via posttranslational modifications and promotes SO by the same modified enzyme (93). Thus, initial overproduction of NO by iNOS could lead to decreased endothelial production of NO by modified eNOS (93). Data implicating the role of NO *in vivo* in rheumatic and inflammatory diseases are discussed in the following sections.

ROLE OF INDUCED NITRIC OXIDE PRODUCTION IN IMMUNE DEFENSE

Mice genetically deficient in NOS2, or in whom NO production is blocked pharmacologically, are highly susceptible to specific infections, particularly intracellular infections like *Mycobacterium tuberculosis, Listeria monocytogenes,* and malaria (1). In contrast, mice that are not challenged with infections, but maintained in a normal laboratory environment, do not appear to be more susceptible to infection (1). Obviously, mice housed in animal facilities are not challenged with the wide range of pathogens they would face in the wild. Thus, NO appears important in normal immune function against certain pathogens, but NO-deficient mice are not totally defenseless against infection.

The role of NO in human disease was at one time questioned, due to the inability in the laboratory to stimulate human macrophages to produce NO using immune stimuli that are effective in rodent models (46). Subsequently, as shown below, production of NO above that of controls in a variety of human diseases has been documented. The inability to induce NO production in human macrophages appears to be explained by not using the proper immune stimuli rather than the inability of human cells to produce NO, because iNOS protein and mRNA can be isolated from inflammatory tissues in a number of autoimmune diseases as discussed below.

The role of induced NO production in human malaria has been of particular interest and may provide insight into NO production in rheumatic diseases. Studies of patients with malaria revealed that the severity of disease, especially central nervous system malaria, was inversely correlated with serum measures of NO production (serum NO_X) (48). Thus, in patients with high levels of serum NO_X, cerebral malaria was less common and less severe. These studies were performed primarily in Western Africa (48). Applicability of these findings to other geographic regions or ethnic populations is not clear. Subsequently, polymorphisms in the NOS2 gene promoter region have been identified. Two of these polymorphisms were reported to be linked with disease severity in West African patients with malaria (94,95).

These data suggest that the ability to respond to malaria infection with heightened NO production may be at least partially genetically determined. One of the NOS2 promoter polymorphisms was found primarily in Africa and was associated with increased NO production from isolated cells when compared to cells with the wild-type promoter (96). Thus, there may be phenotypes of NO production, with some individuals being high producers and others low producers. These phenotypes likely affect the ability to eliminate certain infections and might also affect the outcome of autoimmune responses (97).

NITRIC OXIDE IN ANIMAL MODELS OF INFLAMMATORY DISEASE

In MRL/MpJ-Fas^{lpr} (MRL-lpr) mice, a murine model of lupus, elevated levels of NO_X are present in the serum and urine prior to the onset of clinical disease, which is manifested by glomerulonephritis, vasculitis, and arthritis (98). Increased iNOS protein expression was present in the spleens and kidneys of these mice. Peritoneal macrophages exhibited increased spontaneous and induced iNOS expression and NO production compared with those from normal strains of mice (98). Nitrosylated hemoglobin increased with age in MRL-lpr mice, but not normal mice (99). Increased nitrosylated nonheme proteins were detected in diseased kidneys of MRL-lpr mice using electron paramagnetic imaging (99). When NO production was blocked in these mice using the arginine analog *N*-monomethyl arginine (NMMA), the clinical and pathologic disease in the mice was significantly diminished, demonstrating the importance of NO in autoimmunity and tissue damage in this disease model (98). A subsequent report demonstrated that NO production in MRL-lpr mice was IL-12 dependent (18). Linomide, another inhibitor of NO production, also prevented nephritis in MRL-lpr mice (100). Inhibition of NO, even after onset of disease, decreased renal disease severity in MRL-lpr mice, as well as another lupus-prone strain, NZB/NZW mice (101). Subsequently, aminoguanidine, a specific inhibitor of iNOS, was demonstrated to decrease renal disease severity in NZB/NZW mice. Another iNOS-specific inhibitor (L-NIL) abrogated disease in MRL-lpr mice, indicating a key role for induced NO production in renal disease in these mice (102,103).

In a rat glomerulonephritis model, NO production was localized to glomerular mesangial cells and infiltrating macrophages, supporting the hypothesis that NO is produced locally in immune-complex glomerulonephritis (104). Several other animal models of human diseases manifest enhanced NO production, including immune complex alveolitis, inflammatory bowel disease, experimental allergic encephalomyelitis (EAE), nonobese diabetic mice, and collagen-induced arthritis (1). In almost all instances, NO production was demonstrated locally at the site of tissue damage. Blocking NO production by NO inhibitors prevented disease in most models, indicating a critical role of NO in disease pathogenesis (1). Depending on the animal model and timing of treatment, however, blocking NO production may either worsen or improve disease (e.g., EAE). Cattell et al. have demonstrated that in certain induced models of acute proliferative glomerulonephritis, disease expression may be enhanced by blocking NO production (105). Thus, it is clear that NO is overproduced in a number of models of human inflammatory diseases. Blocking NO production is beneficial in most models of inflammatory disease but is deleterious in some, depending on the timing and method of treatment. There is no clear predictive model that will differentiate diseases in which blocking NO is harmful versus protective.

Understanding the role of induced NO in autoimmune disease was further complicated by studies of NOS2 knockout mice. When the NOS2 knockout gene was bred onto the MRL-lpr lupus background, there was no effect on renal disease or arthritis (106). Evidence of vasculitis was decreased in the NOS2 knockout mice compared with wild-type controls. In a model of autoantibody-mediated arthritis, histologic sections of joints from NOS2 knockout mice showed no reduction in the local inflammatory response, but cartilage degradation was less severe in the knockout mice when compared with the wild-type controls (107). The reason for the disparate results obtained with pharmacologic blockade of NO production versus genetic knockout of induced production remains unclear. Certainly, the immune system is notable for its alternative pathways that may become more activated with a congenital NOS2 defect versus pharmacologic blockade at or just prior to disease onset (108). The genetic knockout studies do indicate, however, that NO production is not required for disease onset or progression. Despite these findings, NO inhibition is still a viable therapeutic strategy in inflammatory diseases.

NITRIC OXIDE IN HUMAN DISEASE

The importance of NO in human rheumatic diseases is emerging through recent studies. Although it has been difficult to demonstrate NO production by either unstimulated or stimulated normal human PBMCs, increased iNOS expression and NO production can be detected in many human inflammatory and autoimmune diseases (35–37) (Table 24.2). The postulated mechanisms through which NO is pathogenic in various inflammatory diseases are discussed in the sections below and are briefly outlined in Fig. 24.3.

Rheumatoid Arthritis

In RA, increased iNOS expression was demonstrated in synoviocytes, and increased NO_X levels were present in synovial fluid (47). Serum NO_X levels from RA subjects and controls were assayed after all subjects were given a strict NO_X-free diet on an inpatient basis. RA subjects had significantly higher baseline serum NO_X levels than controls. The number of active joints in the RA patients correlated with

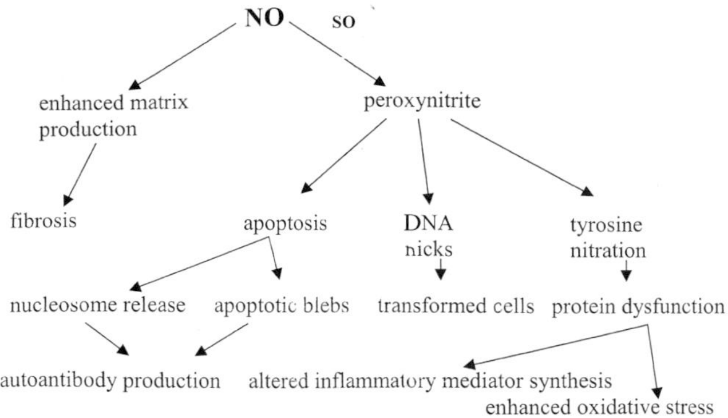

FIG. 24.3. Mechanisms of nitric oxide (NO)-mediated tissue damage in autoimmunity. NO can mediate tissue damage by enhancing matrix production, inducing apoptosis, transforming cells, or altering protein function through nitration. These NO effects can be direct actions of NO or through related nitrogen species (that form as NO interacts with the local redox state) such as peroxynitrite ($ONOO^-$). *SO*, superoxide.

iNOS expression by PBMCs. In addition, PBMCs from RA patients cultured for 5 days with either LPS, IFNγ, or both expressed iNOS, whereas those from controls did not (47). In a recent report, NO production in RA patients was shown to decrease in patients successfully treated with an anti-TNF-α monoclonal antibody (109). The decrease in iNOS expression by PBMCs correlated with the improvement in clinical disease activity. One mechanism by which NO is toxic in RA is through induction of chondrocyte apoptosis. As seen in other cell types, NO may only induce apoptosis of chondrocytes in the presence of reactive oxygen species (110). iNOS expression may also induce apoptosis of local osteoblasts, resulting in osteoporosis (111). Thus, NO is overproduced in RA, produced locally in the rheumatoid joint, correlated with disease activity, and decreased following successful treatment. There have been no trials of specific NO inhibitors in RA to determine if inhibiting NO production in humans is therapeutically effective, as has been shown in animal models of arthritis.

Systemic Lupus Erythematosus

Production of NO in lupus has been evaluated in several studies using a variety of measures of NO production. Lupus patients exhale increased levels of NO, suggesting increased NO production in this disease (112). Most exhaled NO is produced locally in the lungs, so these findings may not be generalizable to systemic NO production (112). In a retrospective analysis, sera from SLE patients had increased levels of NO metabolites (NO_X) when compared with healthy controls, and enhanced iNOS expression was demonstrated in dermal endothelial cells in patients with active disease (49). There was a correlation between the SLE Disease Activity Index (SLEDAI) scores overall, anti-DNA activity, and serum NO_X levels. A subsequent prospective study of patients with SLE followed over time found higher urinary NO_X levels in lupus patients compared with controls; however, no correlation with disease activity was found (113).

An additional retrospective analysis of the relationship between serum NO_X levels and disease activity in patients with lupus followed over time, however, revealed a correlation between NO production and disease activity both overall and in individual patients (114) (Fig. 24.4). In this study, patients were evaluated at baseline, during flare-ups, and after resolution of flare-ups. Lupus activity was determined by the SLEDAI; serum NO_X levels were measured in blood drawn at the time of the clinic visit. Lupus patients had significantly higher mean serum NO_X levels at baseline than controls. Serum NO_X levels correlated with SLEDAI scores in individual patients followed over time. Serum NO_X levels paralleled disease activity in the majority of the patients studied (Fig. 24.4). Proteinuria and SLEDAI renal activity scores also correlated with serum NO_X levels (114). There was no correlation between serum NO_X levels and creatinine. Thus, the correlation of renal disease markers and serum NO_X was not merely a reflection of poor renal clearance of NO_X. Serum NO_X and anti-DNA antibody titers correlated similarly with SLEDAI scores, and both were more closely associated with disease activity than complement measures. Serum NO_X and anti-DNA antibody titers did not correlate with each other, suggesting that these may be independent markers of disease activity. More recently, plasma nitrite, soluble thrombomodulin, and vascular cell adhesion molecule-1 levels were demonstrated to be higher in SLE patients, particularly those with renal involvement, than controls and had significant associations with disease activity in those with SLE (115). In the above studies, NO was overproduced in lupus patients versus controls; the reason for the conflicting results regarding correlation with disease activity is not clear.

A concern with many published studies using measurements of serum NO metabolites is that neither the patients or controls were on a low NO_X diet nor were tobacco use or medications controlled. Because diet, medications, and tobacco can affect both urinary and serum NO_X levels, these factors almost certainly affected the results obtained (47, 113,114). Despite these concerns, current published data support the hypothesis that lupus patients produce higher levels of NO than controls and that patients with active disease produce more NO than those with inactive disease.

An additional footprint of NO production is the nitration of tyrosine by peroxynitrite to form 3-nitrotyrosine (3NT). Proteins containing 3NT can be detected by immunoassay, and such assays have been used previously to measure NO production in other human diseases (58,116). Because nitration of tyrosines is mostly irreversible, the level of 3NT in serum proteins reflects the amount of NO produced over time and thus is somewhat analogous to the measure of glycosylated hemoglobin in diabetes.

Using a dot blot assay to assess levels of 3NT, 3NT-containing proteins were measured in the serum of lupus

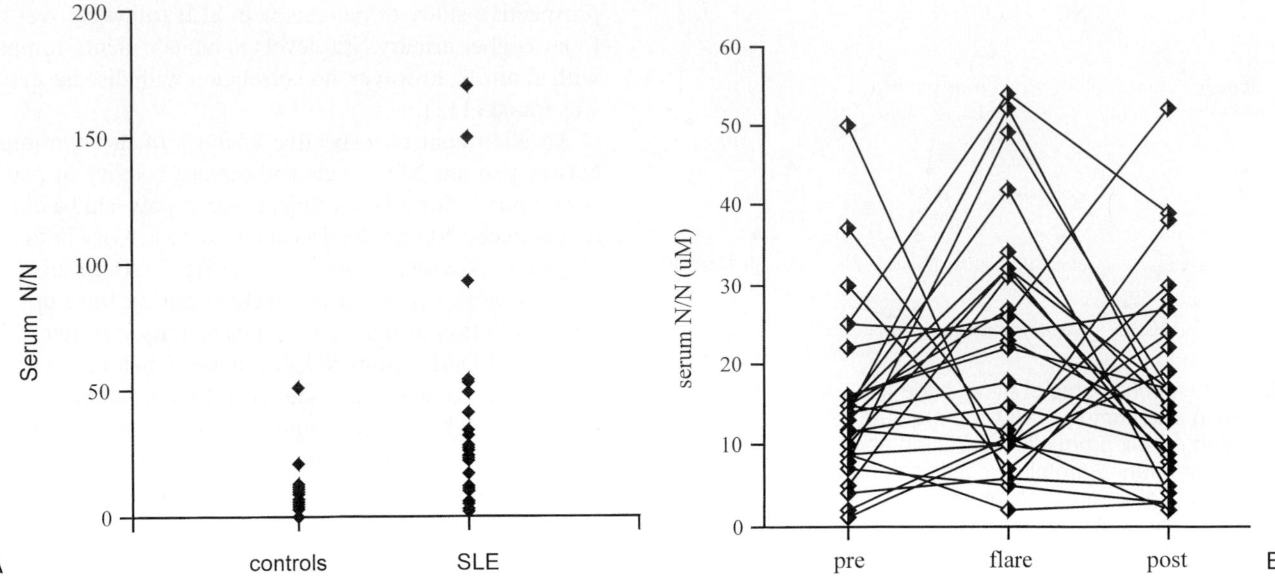

FIG. 24.4. A: Serum NO_x levels of systemic lupus erythematosus (SLE) patients versus controls. **B:** Serum NO_x levels before, during, and after a flare-up of disease [increase in SLE disease activity index (SLEDAI) score of 5] in patients with SLE. Neither patients nor controls were on a low-nitrate/nitrite (N/N) diet.

subjects and controls. A significant difference between serum 3NT in lupus patients versus controls was found (117). These results provide further confirmation that lupus patients overproduce NO when compared with controls. Furthermore, serum 3NT levels correlated with SLEDAI scores (Fig. 24.5). Banked sera from lupus patients were tested to compare SLE patients with SLEDAI scores of 0 versus SLE patients with SLEDAI scores greater than 1. Patients with higher SLEDAI scores had significantly higher serum 3NT levels.

FIG. 24.5. Serum nitrotyrosine (3NT) levels versus SLE disease activity index (SLEDAI) score in 16 patients with SLE. The correlation between serum 3NT levels and SLEDAI scores was $p = 0.002$.

When the patients were analyzed based on ethnic origin, the serum 3NT levels for African-American lupus patients were significantly greater than serum 3NT levels of white SLE patients (117). Some of the difference observed may reflect higher disease activity in the African-American patients. Serum 3NT levels were significantly higher in the African-American lupus patients compared with the African-American controls. These data suggest that there may be a difference in NO production both at baseline (controls) and with immune stimulation (lupus disease activity) between African Americans and whites. Differences in disease activity, however, could also be playing a role in these differences in NO production in lupus patients. A recent report found that African Americans are more resistant to NO-mediated vasodilatation than whites, perhaps providing a rationale for increased baseline secretion of NO by African Americans to maintain vascular relaxation and normal blood pressure (118). A more recent study reported that circulating endothelial cells were increased in SLE subjects in a manner that correlated with disease activity. Furthermore, these cells had an activated phenotype as measured by staining for 3NT (119).

Recent studies of iNOS expression in human kidney diseases are relevant to this review (120–122). In these studies, iNOS expression was demonstrated in the renal tissue of lupus patients. INOS expression, however, was found only in patients with class III (focal proliferative glomerulonephritis) and class IV [diffuse proliferative glomerulonephritis

(DPGN)] but not in all patients with class III or IV disease. It is likely that timing of the biopsy, concurrent therapy, and degree of disease activity and chronicity affected expression of iNOS in individual kidneys. For instance, both prednisone and mycophenolate mofetil are known to reduce iNOS expression (123–125). In one study, iNOS expression also was associated with apoptosis of mesangial cells, primarily in DPGN, suggesting another mechanism by which iNOS expression is pathogenic in lupus nephritis (122). INOS activity may also lead to fibrosis when L-arginine substrate is plentiful, because lupus-prone mice fed a higher L-arginine diet had greater mortality and renal fibrosis despite similar IgG and double-stranded DNA antibody deposition in the kidney (126).

One of the initial insults that may lead to lupus disease activity is UV exposure to the skin. For many lupus patients, this is the first manifestation of their SLE phenotype. In SLE and cutaneous LE subjects exposed to UVB light, iNOS expression in the epidermis was delayed but was markedly prolonged when compared with UVB-exposed control skin (127). This phenomenon occurs more frequently in SLE than in photosensitive annular erythematous lesions in subjects with Sjögren syndrome (128).

Increased iNOS expression in SLE may be due to enhanced local production of helper T cell subset 1 (T_H1) cytokines and other inflammatory mediators in tissues in which immune complex deposition and subsequent complement activation occurs. In a study from Hong Kong, serum IL-18 levels were increased in SLE subjects with renal disease when compared to controls, and these levels correlated with systemic measures of NO production (129). However, iNOS expression may also be affected by polymorphisms in the promoter region of NOS2 that increase transcription of NOS2 in the presence of inflammatory stimuli, such as those present in proliferative glomerular lesions in lupus. Recently, two such polymorphisms have been studied in lupus patients from eastern North Carolina and South Carolina. Among African-American women, both occurred more frequently in SLE subjects than race- and sex-matched controls (97). This association was not found when one of the NOS2 promoter polymorphisms was studied in a population of SLE subjects and controls from southern Spain (130).

Mechanisms of Nitric Oxide Production and Disease Modulation in Systemic Lupus Erythematosus

Modulation of Apoptosis

One mechanism by which NO may be important in the pathogenesis of lupus is by inducing apoptosis and release of nuclear material through membrane blebbing (131). As demonstrated in previous studies, NO increased murine thymocyte (72) and macrophage (70) apoptosis and thus increased nucleosomal constituents in the extracellular milieu. SLE patients have elevated percentages of PBMC apoptosis compared with healthy controls (132). Nuclear antigens released by enhanced apoptosis may play a role in the pathogenesis of disease by driving autoimmune responses (133). Supporting this hypothesis is a recent study demonstrating that lupus patients had increased apoptosis of monocytes during disease activity when compared to lupus patients with no activity and to healthy controls (134). If NO is increased during periods of disease activity, NO may lead to increased PBMC apoptosis or enhanced sensitivity to apoptosis induced by other factors (i.e., TNF-α). Other pathogenic mechanisms for NO are discussed in further detail in other parts of this chapter.

Nitric Oxide and Estrogen

Cytokines are not the only factors that may affect NO production in rheumatic diseases. For example, lupus is much more common in women than men (135). Obvious candidates for these differences are the immune effects of estrogen. Estrogen in a number of recent studies in mice and humans has been demonstrated to have significant effects on NO production (136–141). Several other immune effects are also modulated by estrogen; for example, B-cell and T-cell function is enhanced in women compared with men (135). Almost all immune cells express estrogen receptors, including macrophages, mesangial cells, and endothelial cells (135). Recent reports indicate that estrogens have variable effects on NO production, although the overall result in humans and animals is to enhance NO production (136–141). Estrogen replacement of postmenopausal women increases serum NO_X levels, likely due to enhanced NO production by eNOS (139). Enhanced endothelial NO production may account for the decrease in atherosclerosis in women due to the vasodilatory effects of NO (142). Estrogen also appears to modulate iNOS activity. Two studies found that estrogen inhibited the production of NO in IFN-γ-stimulated macrophage-like cells (136,140); a second study found no effect of physiologic levels of 17-β estradiol on induced iNOS expression in a murine macrophage cell line (143). A third study found increased iNOS expression in LPS-stimulated alveolar macrophages from rats treated with physiologic amounts of estrogen, whereas pharmacologic levels of estrogen inhibited iNOS expression (144).

The current literature supports NO as an important immune modulator that is overproduced in SLE. Activated macrophages are key pathogenic cells in human and murine lupus, especially in lupus nephritis; production of NO is part of this activated phenotype. The link between NO and disease activity, as well as the role of NO in disease pathogenesis in lupus, remains unclear.

Vasculitis

As noted above in the studies of MRL/lpr mice, either pharmacologic or genetic blockade of NO production led to a decrease in the incidence and severity of vasculitis in these mice (95). The role of NO in human vasculitis is less clear, but recent studies support the notion that NO is pathogenic in several types of vasculitis. A study by Weyand and colleagues demonstrated the presence of iNOS-producing macrophages within the vessel wall of patients with temporal arteritis at the site of tissue destruction (145). Borkowski et al. determined that 3NT staining in giant cell arteritis was restricted to the endothelial cells of newly formed microcapillaries and was isolated to the media in a manner that correlated with NOS3 expression, suggesting that $ONOO^-$ formation was from eNOS-derived NO and focal reactive oxygen species production (146). Similarly, in an experimental model of Kawasaki disease, iNOS and 3NT staining were enhanced in perivascular macrophages and coronary arterioles in clinically affected animals (147). In humans with Kawasaki disease, serum NO_X levels were increased compared with controls. This increase was reversed with intravenous immunoglobulin therapy (148). In Wegener granulomatosis, 3NT staining can be found in infiltrating inflammatory cells in the renal interstitium in association with iNOS staining (149). Serum nitrite levels were also higher in patients with active Behçet disease compared to those with inactive disease or to controls (150,151). Those with ocular disease had higher levels than those without ocular disease (150), and aqueous humor nitrite levels were higher in patients with ocular disease than in controls (152). Similarly, serum nitrite levels were increased in Henoch-Schönlein purpura subjects in a manner that correlated with disease activity (153). Bell and colleagues also found evidence for increased NO production in systemic vasculitides by measuring forearm endothelium-dependent vasodilator responses (154). These findings suggest that NO and its more reactive oxidative products may also play a critical role in tissue destruction in human vasculitides.

Scleroderma

Several studies have reported systemic measurements of NO in systemic sclerosis (SSc) (155–157). Serum NO_X levels were elevated in SSc subjects compared with controls in one study. Supernatants from stimulated SSc PBMCs contained more NO_X than controls. Urine isoprostanes were elevated in SSc subjects, suggesting an increased level of oxidative stress, perhaps mediated by peroxynitrite (66,158). Exhaled NO has also been used as a measure of systemic NO production in SSc, as in SLE. However, because NO has an extremely short half-life, exhaled NO may more accurately reflect pulmonary alveolar, interstitial, and vascular sources, as discussed previously (156). Those SSc subjects with interstitial lung disease exhibited the highest exhaled NO levels, suggesting that inflammatory pulmonary disease and iNOS activity in the alveoli or interstitium was the source of the NO. Those with SSc, but without pulmonary hypertension, had higher levels than controls (156). However, those with pulmonary hypertension, but no interstitial lung disease, had lower levels than controls, suggesting that local endothelial dysfunction caused reduced eNOS-derived pulmonary vascular NO production (159). The above data suggest that systemic NO production is elevated in SSc but that focal production of NO, perhaps by eNOS, is reduced in the pulmonary vascular endothelium of subjects with pulmonary hypertension. These data also suggest that among SSc subjects, systemic production of NO, presumably by infiltrating mononuclear and PBMC iNOS, is elevated.

The stimulus leading to overproduction of collagen by SSc fibroblasts is unknown. However, recent evidence points to NO as a potential mediator. In affected SSc skin, iNOS expression is increased among infiltrating mononuclear cells, endothelial cells, and fibroblasts (155). When these fibroblasts were isolated, iNOS protein was overexpressed compared with control fibroblasts (155). Data obtained from experiments in wound healing also point to NO as a mediator of collagen production. Experimental models of wound healing demonstrated increased NO production locally, perhaps by infiltrating macrophages (160,161). Among diabetics, in whom wound healing is impaired, local NO production in wounds was reduced compared with controls (162). Cultured wound fibroblasts produced abnormally large amounts of NO, and blockade of NO production impaired collagen synthesis (163). Similarly, NOS-deficient mice have impaired wound healing and collagen production that can be corrected with topical administration of an NOS2 complementary DNA–containing adenoviral vector (164). Because both wound fibroblasts and SSc fibroblasts express a heightened extracellular matrix synthesis phenotype, NO could play a role in mediating collagen synthesis in both.

The role of NO in SSc lung disease is also of potential interest and importance. In one study, lung biopsies from subjects with idiopathic pulmonary fibrosis revealed elevated levels of nitrotyrosine in airway epithelium, alveolar epithelium, macrophages, and neutrophils (165). Some subjects exhibited staining in vascular endothelium, smooth muscle cells, and lymphocytes. Staining for iNOS was increased in macrophages, neutrophils, and alveolar and airway epithelium with occasional expression in lymphocytes, vascular endothelial cells, and smooth muscle cells of both airways and vessels (165). Among SSc patients with active alveolitis (determined by the presence of increased polymorphonuclear cells on bronchoalveolar lavage), exhaled NO levels were significantly higher than controls or SSc patients with interstitial lung disease and no signs of active alveolitis (166).

eNOS expression, however, was reduced among subjects with pulmonary hypertension secondary to pulmonary fibrosis. Expression was present but reduced among those subjects with early or intermediate stage pulmonary fibrosis (165). In a second study, reductions in eNOS expression in the vascular endothelium in subjects with pulmonary hypertension was inversely correlated with the severity of lesions and with the level of pulmonary vascular resistance (167). Whether increased iNOS-derived peroxynitrite production is responsible for this reduced eNOS expression is unclear. However, peroxynitrite can reduce eNOS activity without reducing the protein concentration (93). In the tight-skin mouse model of SSc, loss of alternative endothelium-dependent vasodilation may lead to a compensatory upregulation of NO production. This, in turn, could lead to NO-mediated endothelial toxicity (168). These data begin to reconcile seemingly conflicting results in the literature regarding systemic measures of NO production in SSc. They do so by suggesting that early iNOS-dependent fibroblast, PBMC, and infiltrating mononuclear cell peroxynitrite production may lead to reduced eNOS-dependent NO production, which then can lead to enhanced vasoreactivity and thrombosis.

Osteoarthritis

Recent evidence supports a key role for NO in the pathogenesis of osteoarthritis (169,170). Several laboratories have demonstrated that NO is produced by chondrocytes (171–173). Similar to macrophages, NO production by chondrocytes depends on stimulation by immune factors. Factors that induce NO production in chondrocytes include LPS, IL-1β, TNF-α, IL-17, and IL-18 (172–175). Mechanical loading also induces NO production by cultured chondrocytes and meniscus explants (176–178). The ability of chondrocytes to produce NO appears to decrease with age (179,180). However, NO itself may not be the toxin of interest. It appears that NO contributes to chondrocyte damage only in the presence of concurrent production of reactive oxygen species (110).

In animal models of induced osteoarthritis, inhibition of NO by pharmacologic or genetic methods led to decreased development of arthritis (95,181,182). Blocking NO production did not affect inflammatory cell influx, but did block degradation of proteoglycan (183). More relevant to osteoarthritis, a recent study reported the effect of giving an iNOS-specific inhibitor (L-NIL) to a dog model of osteoarthritis (178,184). In this model, the anterior cruciate ligament is cut, leading to development of accelerated osteoarthritis in the operated knee when compared with the contralateral, control knee. When these dogs were treated with L-NIL, there was significantly less inflammation, cartilage loss, and osteophyte development than in dogs not receiving L-NIL (184). L-NIL treatment also resulted in reduced IL-1β and matrix metalloproteinases (collagenase-1 and stromelysin-1) production, suggesting a mechanism for this effect (178).

Supporting these *in vivo* data, NO inhibited matrix production by cultured chondrocytes, likely as a result of increased metalloproteinase production (185–187). NO may also directly increase degradation of matrix proteins (187). Furthermore, NO may induce apoptosis of chondrocytes (75). Together these NO-mediated effects would lead to loss of matrix and chondrocyte death, hallmark features of osteoarthritis.

In studies of patients with osteoarthritis, serum and joint fluid levels of NO_X were elevated (188). These findings suggest that NO is produced during the development of osteoarthritis and that blocking NO production might be of potential benefit in treating this disease (171,184).

SUMMARY

NO has many biologic effects and functions. As such, it has been implicated as being pathogenic in several diseases. Overproduction of NO has been demonstrated in a number of rheumatic diseases. Blocking NO production has been therapeutically successful in many animal models of rheumatic diseases, including SLE, RA, SSc, vasculitis, and osteoarthritis. These data suggest that overproduction of NO is pathogenic in these diseases. Due to its multiple functions, appropriate concern should be exercised in approaching human disease with NO inhibitors due to potential side effects. Undoubtedly, however, we will soon see therapeutic trials directed at inhibiting NO production in rheumatic diseases.

ACKNOWLEDGMENTS

This work was supported by grants from the Arthritis Foundation, Atlanta, GA; a University Research Committee grant from the Medical University of South Carolina; Grants K08AR002193, AI047469, AR045476, and AR04745 from the National Institutes of Health, Bethesda, MD; and Career Development and Merit Review grants from the Medical Research Service, Ralph H. Johnson VAMC, Charleston, SC.

REFERENCES

1. Nathan C. Inducible nitric oxide synthase: what difference does it make? *J Clin Invest* 1997;100:2417–2423.
2. Lowenstein CJ, Dinerman JL, Snyder SH. Nitric oxide: a physiologic messenger. *Ann Intern Med* 1994;120:227–237.
3. Lincoln J, Hoyle CHV, Burnstock G. *Nitric oxide in health and disease.* New York, NY: Cambridge University Press, 1997.
4. Clancy RM, Amin AR, Abramson SB. The role of nitric oxide in inflammation and immunity. *Arthritis Rheum* 1998;41:1141–1151.
5. Nathan C, Xie QW. Regulation of biosynthesis of nitric oxide. *J Biol Chem* 1994;269:13725–13728.
6. Sase K, Michel T. Expression of constitutive endothelial nitric oxide synthase in human blood platelets. *Life Sci* 1995;57:2049–2055.
7. Lopez-Farre A, Sanchez de Miguel L, Caramelo C, et al. Role of nitric oxide in autocrine control of growth and apoptosis of endothelial cells. *Am J Physiol* 1997;272:H760–H768.
8. Dhaunsi GS, Matthews C, Kaur K, et al. NO increases protein tyrosine phosphatase activity in smooth muscle cells: relationship to antimitogenesis. *Am J Physiol* 1997;272:H1342–H1349.
9. Osborne MG, Coderre TJ. Effects of intrathecal administration of nitric oxide synthase inhibitors on carrageenan-induced thermal hyperalgesia. *Br J Pharmacol* 1999;126:1840–1846.
10. Coutinho SV, Gebhart GF. A role for spinal nitric oxide in mediating visceral hyperalgesia in the rat. *Gastroenterology* 1999;116:1399–1408.
11. Tao YX, Johns RA. Activation and up-regulation of spinal cord nitric oxide receptor, soluble guanylate cyclase, after formalin injection into the rat hind paw. *Neuroscience* 2002;112:439–446.
12. Kozak W, Kozak A. Genetic models in applied physiology: selected contribution: differential role of nitric oxide synthase isoforms in

fever of different etiologies: studies using Nos gene-deficient mice. *J Appl Physiol* 2003;94:2534–2544.

13. Salerno L, Sorrenti V, Di Giacomo C, et al. Progress in the development of selective nitric oxide synthase (NOS) inhibitors. *Curr Pharm Des* 2002;8:177–200.
14. De Sanctis GT, MacLean JA, Hamada K, et al. Contribution of nitric oxide synthases 1, 2, and 3 to airway hyperresponsiveness and inflammation in a murine model of asthma. *J Exp Med* 1999;189:1621–1630.
15. Tulic MK, Wale JL, Holt PG, et al. Differential effects of nitric oxide synthase inhibitors in an *in vivo* allergic rat model. *Eur Respir J* 2000; 15:870–877.
16. Miranda KM, Espey MG, Jourd'heuil D, et al. The chemical biology of nitric oxide. In: Ignarro LJ, ed. *Nitric oxide biology and pathobiology.* New York: Academic, 2000:41–55.
17. Park WS, Chang YS, Lee M. 7-Nitroindazole, but not aminoguanidine, attenuates the acute inflammatory responses and brain injury during the early phase of *Escherichia coli* meningitis in the newborn piglet. *Biol Neonate* 2001;80:53–59.
18. Huang FP, Feng GJ, Lindop G, et al. The role of interleukin 12 and nitric oxide in the development of spontaneous autoimmune disease in MRL:MP-lpr:lpr mice. *J Exp Med* 1996;183:1447–1459.
19. Busse R, Mulsch A. Induction of nitric oxide synthase by cytokines in vascular smooth muscle cells. *FEBS Lett* 1990;275:87–90.
20. Mozaffarian N, Berman JW, Casadevall A. Immune complexes increase nitric oxide production by interferon-gamma-stimulated murine macrophage-like J774.16 cells. *J Leukoc Biol* 1995;57:657–662.
21. Taylor-Robinson AW, Liew FY, Severn A, et al. Regulation of the immune response by nitric oxide differentially produced by T helper type 1 and T helper type 2 cells. *Eur J Immunol* 1994;24:980–984.
22. Jiang H, Stewart CA, Tan SY, et al. Transfection of L929 cells with complement subcomponent C1q B-chain antisense cDNA inhibits tumor necrosis factor-alpha binding to mediate cytotoxicity and nitric oxide generation. *Cell Immunol* 1996;167:293–301.
23. Jiang C, Ting AT, Seed B. PPAR-gamma agonists inhibit production of monocyte inflammatory cytokines. *Nature* 1998;391:82–86.
24. Grewal IS, Flavell RA. The role of CD40 ligand in costimulation and T-cell activation. *Immunol Rev* 1996;153:85–106.
25. Pahan K, Jana M, Liu X, et al. Gemfibrozil, a lipid-lowering drug, inhibits the induction of nitric-oxide synthase in human astrocytes. *J Biol Chem* 2002;277:45984–45991.
26. Kleinert H, Boissel JP, Schwarz PM, et al. Regulation of the expression of nitric oxide synthase isoforms. In: Ignarro LJ, ed. *Nitric oxide biology and pathobiology.* New York: Academic, 2000:105–128.
27. Vodovotz Y, Geiser AG, Chesler L, et al. Spontaneously increased production of nitric oxide and aberrant expression of the inducible nitric oxide synthase *in vivo* in the transforming growth factor beta 1 null mouse. *J Exp Med* 1996;183:2337–2342.
28. Balomenos D, Rumold R, Theofilopoulos AN. Interferon-gamma is required for lupus-like disease and lymphoaccumulation in MRL-lpr mice. *J Clin Invest* 1998;101:364–371.
29. Schwarting A, Wada T, Kinoshita K, et al. IFN-gamma receptor signaling is essential for the initiation, acceleration, and destruction of autoimmune kidney disease in MRL-Fas(lpr) mice. *J Immunol* 1998; 161:494–503.
30. Ozmen L, Roman D, Fountoulakis M, et al. Experimental therapy of systemic lupus erythematosus: the treatment of NZB/W mice with mouse soluble interferon-gamma receptor inhibits the onset of glomerulonephritis. *Eur J Immunol* 1995;25:6–12.
31. Jacob CO, van der Meide PH, McDevitt HO. *In vivo* treatment of (NZB X NZW)F1 lupus-like nephritis with monoclonal antibody to gamma interferon. *J Exp Med* 1987;166:798–803.
32. Linker-Israeli M. Cytokine abnormalities in human lupus. *Clin Immunol Immunopathol* 1992;63:10–12.
33. al-Janadi M, al-Balla S, al-Dalaan A, et al. Cytokine profile in systemic lupus erythematosus, rheumatoid arthritis, and other rheumatic diseases. *J Clin Immunol* 1993;13:58–67.
34. Hagiwara E, Gourley MF, Lee S, et al. Disease severity in patients with systemic lupus erythematosus correlates with an increased ratio of interleukin-10:interferon-gamma-secreting cells in the peripheral blood. *Arthritis Rheum* 1996;39:379–385.
35. Chan RW, Tam LS, Li EK, et al. Inflammatory cytokine gene expression in the urinary sediment of patients with lupus nephritis. *Arthritis Rheum* 2003;48:1326–1331.
36. Boswell JM, Yui MA, Burt DW, et al. Increased tumor necrosis factor and IL-1 beta gene expression in the kidneys of mice with lupus nephritis. *J Immunol* 1988;141:3050–3054.
37. Gabay C, Arend WP. Treatment of rheumatoid arthritis with IL-1 inhibitors. *Springer Semin Immunopathol* 1998;20:229–246.
38. Jacob CO, McDevitt HO. Tumour necrosis factor-alpha in murine autoimmune "lupus" nephritis. *Nature* 1988;331:356–358.
39. Brennan DC, Yui MA, Wuthrich RP, et al. Tumor necrosis factor and IL-1 in New Zealand Black/White mice. Enhanced gene expression and acceleration of renal injury. *J Immunol* 1989;143:3470–3475.
40. Gordon C, Ranges GE, Greenspan JS, et al. Chronic therapy with recombinant tumor necrosis factor-alpha in autoimmune NZB/NZW F1 mice. *Clin Immunol Immunopathol* 1989;52:421–434.
41. Tomita Y, Hashimoto S, Yamagami K, et al. Restriction fragment length polymorphism (RFLP) analysis in the TNF genes of patients with systemic lupus erythematosus (SLE). *Clin Exp Rheumatol* 1993; 11:533–536.
42. Wilson AG, Gordon C, di Giovine FS, et al. A genetic association between systemic lupus erythematosus and tumor necrosis factor alpha. *Eur J Immunol* 1994;24:191–195.
43. Mitamura K, Kang H, Tomita Y, et al. Impaired tumour necrosis factor-alpha (TNF-alpha) production and abnormal B cell response to TNF-alpha in patients with systemic lupus erythematosus (SLE). *Clin Exp Immunol* 1991;85:386–391.
44. Malide D, Russo P, Bendayan M. Presence of tumor necrosis factor alpha and interleukin-6 in renal mesangial cells of lupus nephritis patients. *Hum Pathol* 1995;26:558–564.
45. Feldmann M, Charles P, Taylor P, et al. Biological insights from clinical trials with anti-TNF therapy. *Springer Semin Immunopathol* 1998; 20:211–228.
46. Weinberg JB, Misukonis MA, Shami PJ, et al. Human mononuclear phagocyte inducible nitric oxide synthase (iNOS): analysis of iNOS mRNA, iNOS protein, biopterin, and nitric oxide production by blood monocytes and peritoneal macrophages. *Blood* 1995;86:1184–1195.
47. St Clair EW, Wilkinson WE, Lang T, et al. Increased expression of blood mononuclear cell nitric oxide synthase type 2 in rheumatoid arthritis patients. *J Exp Med* 1996;184:1173–1178.
48. Anstey NM, Weinberg JB, Hassanali MY, et al. Nitric oxide in Tanzanian children with malaria: inverse relationship between malaria severity and nitric oxide production/nitric oxide synthase type 2 expression. *J Exp Med* 1996;184:557–567.
49. Belmont HM, Levartovsky D, Goel A, et al. Increased nitric oxide production accompanied by the up-regulation of inducible nitric oxide synthase in vascular endothelium from patients with systemic lupus erythematosus. *Arthritis Rheum* 1997;40:1810–1816.
50. Morris LF, Lemak NA, Arnett FC Jr, et al. Systemic lupus erythematosus diagnosed during interferon alfa therapy. *South Med J* 1996;89: 810–814.
51. Sharara AI, Perkins DJ, Misukonis MA, et al. Interferon (IFN)-alpha activation of human blood mononuclear cells *in vitro* and *in vivo* for nitric oxide synthase (NOS) type 2 mRNA and protein expression: possible relationship of induced NOS2 to the anti-hepatitis C effects of IFN-alpha *in vivo*. *J Exp Med* 1997;186:1495–1502.
52. Fukuto JM, Cho JY, Switzer CH. The chemical properties of nitric oxide and related nitrogen oxides. In: Ignarro LJ, ed. *Nitric oxide biology and pathobiology.* New York: Academic, 2000:23–40.
53. Patel RP, McAndrew J, Sellak H, et al. Biological aspects of reactive nitrogen species. *Biochim Biophys Acta* 1999;1411:385–400.
54. Sampson JB, Rosen H, Beckman JS. Peroxynitrite-dependent tyrosine nitration catalyzed by superoxide dismutase, myeloperoxidase, and horseradish peroxidase. *Methods Enzymol* 1996;269:210–218.
55. Beckman JS, Chen J, Ischiropoulos H, et al. Oxidative chemistry of peroxynitrite. *Methods Enzymol* 1994;233:229–240.
56. Khan J, Brennan DM, Bradley N, et al. 3-Nitrotyrosine in the proteins of human plasma determined by an ELISA method. *Biochem J* 1998; 330:795–801.
57. Privalle CT, Keng T, Gilkeson GS, et al. The role of nitric oxide and peroxynitrite in the pathogenesis of spontaneous murine autoimmune disease. In: Stamler J, Gross SS, Moncada S, eds. The biology of nitric oxide. New York: Elsevier, 1996.
58. MacMillan-Crow LA, Crow JP, Kerby JD, et al. Nitration and inactivation of manganese superoxide dismutase in chronic rejection of human renal allografts. *Proc Natl Acad Sci U S A* 1996;93:11853–11858.

59. Zou M, Martin C, Ullrich V. Tyrosine nitration as a mechanism of selective inactivation of prostacyclin synthase by peroxynitrite. *Biol Chem* 1997;378:707–713.
60. Zou MH, Yesilkaya A, Ullrich V. Peroxynitrite inactivates prostacyclin synthase by heme-thiolate-catalyzed tyrosine nitration. *Drug Metab Rev* 1999;31:343–349.
61. Ischiropoulos H. Biological tyrosine nitration—a pathophysiological function of nitric oxide and reactive oxygen species. *Arch Biochem Biophys* 1998;356:1–11.
62. Gow AJ, Duran D, Malcolm S, et al. Effects of peroxynitrite-induced protein modifications on tyrosine phosphorylation and degradation. *FEBS Lett* 1996;385:63–66.
63. Landino LM, Crews BC, Timmons MD, et al. Peroxynitrite, the coupling product of nitric oxide and superoxide, activates prostaglandin biosynthesis. *Proc Natl Acad Sci U S A* 1996;93:15069–15074.
64. Hensley K, Williamson KS, Floyd RA. Measurement of 3-nitrotyrosine and 5-nitro-gamma-tocopherol by high-performance liquid chromatography with electrochemical detection. *Free Radic Biol Med* 2000; 28:520–528.
65. Brennan ML, Wu W, Fu X, et al. A tale of two controversies: defining both the role of peroxidases in nitrotyrosine formation *in vivo* using eosinophil peroxidase and myeloperoxidase-deficient mice, and the nature of peroxidase-generated reactive nitrogen species. *J Biol Chem* 2002;277:17415–17427.
66. Moore KP, Darley-Usmar V, Morrow J, et al. Formation of F2-isoprostanes during oxidation of human low-density lipoprotein and plasma by peroxynitrite. *Circ Res* 1995;77:335–341.
67. Fukunaga M, Makita N, Roberts LJd, et al. Evidence for the existence of F2-isoprostane receptors on rat vascular smooth muscle cells. *Am J Physiol* 1993;264:C1619–C1624.
68. Morrow JD, Minton TA, Roberts LJd. The F2-isoprostane, 8-epi-prostaglandin F2 alpha, a potent agonist of the vascular thromboxane/endoperoxide receptor, is a platelet thromboxane/endoperoxide receptor antagonist. *Prostaglandins* 1992;44:155–163.
69. Morrow JD, Awad JA, Wu A, et al. Nonenzymatic free radical-catalyzed generation of thromboxane-like compounds (isothromboxanes) *in vivo*. *J Biol Chem* 1996;271:23185–23190.
70. Messmer UK, Lapetina EG, Brune B. Nitric oxide-induced apoptosis in RAW 264.7 macrophages is antagonized by protein kinase C– and protein kinase A–activating compounds. *Mol Pharmacol* 1995;47: 757–765.
71. Boyd CS, Cadenas E. Nitric oxide and cell signaling pathways in mitochondrial-dependent apoptosis. *Biol Chem* 2002;383:411–423.
72. Fehsel K, Kroncke KD, Meyer KL, et al. Nitric oxide induces apoptosis in mouse thymocytes. *J Immunol* 1995;155:2858–2865.
73. Muhl H, Sandau K, Brune B, et al. Nitric oxide donors induce apoptosis in glomerular mesangial cells, epithelial cells and endothelial cells. *Eur J Pharmacol* 1996;317:137–149.
74. Sandau K, Pfeilschifter J, Brune B. The balance between nitric oxide and superoxide determines apoptotic and necrotic death of rat mesangial cells. *J Immunol* 1997;158:4938–4946.
75. Blanco FJ, Ochs RL, Schwarz H, et al. Chondrocyte apoptosis induced by nitric oxide. *Am J Pathol* 1995;146:75–85.
76. Elfering SL, Sarkela TM, Giulivi C. Biochemistry of mitochondrial nitric-oxide synthase. *J Biol Chem* 2002;277:38079–38086.
77. Bustamante J, Bersier G, Romero M, et al. Nitric oxide production and mitochondrial dysfunction during rat thymocyte apoptosis. *Arch Biochem Biophys* 2000;376:239–247.
78. Ramachandran A, Levonen AL, Brookes PS, et al. Mitochondria, nitric oxide, and cardiovascular dysfunction. *Free Radic Biol Med* 2002; 33:1465–1474.
79. Aiello S, Noris M, Piccinini G, et al. Thymic dendritic cells express inducible nitric oxide synthase and generate nitric oxide in response to self- and alloantigens. *J Immunol* 2000;164:4649–4658.
80. Mohr S, Zech B, Lapetina EG, et al. Inhibition of caspase-3 by S-nitrosation and oxidation caused by nitric oxide. *Biochem Biophys Res Commun* 1997;238:387–391.
81. Kim YM, Talanian RV, Billiar TR. Nitric oxide inhibits apoptosis by preventing increases in caspase-3-like activity via two distinct mechanisms. *J Biol Chem* 1997;272:31138–31148.
82. Kim PK, Kwon YG, Chung HT, et al. Regulation of caspases by nitric oxide. *Ann NY Acad Sci* 2002;962:42–52.
83. Li J, Billiar TR, Talanian RV, et al. Nitric oxide reversibly inhibits seven members of the caspase family via S-nitrosylation. *Biochem Biophys Res Commun* 1997;240:419–424.
84. Leist M, Volbracht C, Kuhnle S, et al. Caspase-mediated apoptosis in neuronal excitotoxicity triggered by nitric oxide. *Mol Med* 1997; 3:750–764.
85. Nitsch DD, Ghilardi N, Muhl H, et al. Apoptosis and expression of inducible nitric oxide synthase are mutually exclusive in renal mesangial cells. *Am J Pathol* 1997;150:889–900.
86. Genaro AM, Hortelano S, Alvarez A, et al. Splenic B lymphocyte programmed cell death is prevented by nitric oxide release through mechanisms involving sustained Bcl-2 levels. *J Clin Invest* 1995; 95:1884–1890.
87. Messmer UK, Reed UK, Brune B. Bcl-2 protects macrophages from nitric oxide-induced apoptosis. *J Biol Chem* 1996;271:20192–20197.
88. Mannick JB, Asano K, Izumi K, et al. Nitric oxide produced by human B lymphocytes inhibits apoptosis and Epstein-Barr virus reactivation. *Cell* 1994;79:1137–1146.
89. Baker AJ, Mooney A, Hughes J, et al. Mesangial cell apoptosis: the major mechanism for resolution of glomerular hypercellularity in experimental mesangial proliferative nephritis. *J Clin Invest* 1994; 94:2105–2116.
90. Trachtman H, Futterweit S, Singhal P. Nitric oxide modulates the synthesis of extracellular matrix proteins in cultured rat mesangial cells. *Biochem Biophys Res Commun* 1995;207:120–125.
91. Brune B. Nitric oxide and apoptosis in mesangial cells. *Kidney Int* 2002;61:786–789.
92. von Knethen A, Brune B. Cyclooxygenase-2: an essential regulator of NO-mediated apoptosis. *FASEB J* 1997;11:887–895.
93. Sheehy AM, Burson MA, Black SM. Nitric oxide exposure inhibits endothelial NOS activity but not gene expression: a role for superoxide. *Am J Physiol* 1998;274:L833–L841.
94. Burgner D, Xu W, Rockett K, et al. Inducible nitric oxide synthase polymorphism and fatal cerebral malaria. *Lancet* 1998;352:1193–1194.
95. Kun JF, Mordmuller B, Lell B, et al. Polymorphism in promoter region of inducible nitric oxide synthase gene and protection against malaria. *Lancet* 1998;351:265–266.
96. Kun JF, Mordmuller B, Perkins DJ, et al. Nitric oxide synthase 2 (G-954C), increased nitric oxide production, and protection against malaria. *J Infect Dis* 2001;184:330–336.
97. Oates JC, Levesque MC, Hobbs MR, et al. Nitric oxide synthase 2 promoter polymorphisms and systemic lupus erythematosus in African-Americans. *J Rheumatol* 2003;30:60–67.
98. Weinberg JB, Granger DL, Pisetsky DS, et al. The role of nitric oxide in the pathogenesis of spontaneous murine autoimmune disease: increased nitric oxide production and nitric oxide synthase expression in MRL-lpr/lpr mice, and reduction of spontaneous glomerulonephritis and arthritis by orally administered NG-monomethyl-L- arginine. *J Exp Med* 1994;179:651–660.
99. Weinberg JB, Gilkeson GS, Mason RP, et al. Nitrosylation of blood hemoglobin and renal nonheme proteins in autoimmune MRL-lpr/lpr mice. *Free Radic Biol Med* 1998;24:191–196.
100. Hortelano S, Diazguerra MJM, Gonzalezgarcia A, et al. Linomide administration to mice attenuates the induction of nitric oxide synthase elicited by lipopolysaccharide-activated macrophages and prevents nephritis in Mrl/Mp-lpr/lpr mice. *J Immunol* 1997;158:1402–1408.
101. Oates JC, Ruiz P, Alexander A, et al. Effect of late modulation of nitric oxide production on murine lupus. *Clin Immunol Immunopathol* 1997;83:86–92.
102. Reilly CM, Farrelly LW, Viti D, et al. Modulation of renal disease in MRL/lpr mice by pharmacologic inhibition of inducible nitric oxide synthase. *Kidney Int* 2002;61:839–846.
103. Yang CW, Yu CC, Ko YC, et al. Aminoguanidine reduces glomerular inducible nitric oxide synthase (iNOS) and transforming growth factor-beta 1 (TGF-beta1) mRNA expression and diminishes glomerulosclerosis in NZB/W F1 mice. *Clin Exp Immunol* 1998;113:258–264.
104. Jansen A, Cook T, Taylor GM, et al. Induction of nitric oxide synthase in rat immune complex glomerulonephritis. *Kidney Int* 1994; 45:1215–1219.
105. Cattell V, Cook HT, Ebrahim H, et al. Anti-GBM glomerulonephritis in mice lacking nitric oxide synthase type 2. *Kidney Int* 1998;53: 932–936.
106. Gilkeson GS, Mudgett JS, Seldin MF, et al. Clinical and serologic manifestations of autoimmune disease in MRL-lpr/lpr mice lacking nitric oxide synthase type 2. *J Exp Med* 1997;186:365–373.

107. Kato H, Nishida K, Yoshida A, et al. Effect of NOS2 gene deficiency on the development of autoantibody mediated arthritis and subsequent articular cartilage degeneration. *J Rheumatol* 2003;30:247–255.
108. Steinman L. Some misconceptions about understanding autoimmunity through experiments with knockouts. *J Exp Med* 1997;185: 2039–2041.
109. Perkins DJ, St Clair EW, Misukonis MA, et al. Reduction of NOS2 overexpression in rheumatoid arthritis patients treated with anti-tumor necrosis factor alpha monoclonal antibody (cA2). *Arthritis Rheum* 1998;41:2205–2210.
110. Del Carlo M Jr, Loeser RF. Nitric oxide-mediated chondrocyte cell death requires the generation of additional reactive oxygen species. *Arthritis Rheum* 2002;46:394–403.
111. Armour KJ, Armour KE, van't Hof RJ, et al. Activation of the inducible nitric oxide synthase pathway contributes to inflammation-induced osteoporosis by suppressing bone formation and causing osteoblast apoptosis. *Arthritis Rheum* 2001;44:2790–2796.
112. Rolla G, Brussino L, Bertero MT, et al. Increased nitric oxide in exhaled air of patients with systemic lupus erythematosus. *J Rheumatol* 1997;24:1066–1071.
113. Gonzalezcrespo MR, Navarro JA, Arenas J, et al. Prospective study of serum and urinary nitrate levels in patients with systemic lupus erythematosus. *Br J Rheumatol* 1998;37:972–977.
114. Gilkeson G, Cannon C, Oates J, et al. Correlation of serum measures of nitric oxide production with lupus disease activity. *J Rheumatol* 1999;26:318–324.
115. Ho CY, Wong CK, Li EK, et al. Elevated plasma concentrations of nitric oxide, soluble thrombomodulin and soluble vascular cell adhesion molecule-1 in patients with systemic lupus erythematosus. *Rheumatology (Oxford)* 2003;42:117–122.
116. Granger DL, Miller WC, Hibbs JB. Methods of analyzing nitric oxide production in the immune response. In: Feelisch M, Stamler JS, eds. *Methods in nitric oxide research.* New York: John Wiley & Sons, 1996.
117. Oates JC, Christensen EF, Reilly CM, et al. Prospective measure of serum 3-nitrotyrosine levels in systemic lupus erythematosus: correlation with disease activity. *Proc Assoc Am Physicians* 1999;111: 611–621.
118. Cardillo C, Kilcoyne CM, Cannon RO 3rd, et al. Racial differences in nitric oxide-mediated vasodilator response to mental stress in the forearm circulation. *Hypertension* 1998;31:1235–1239.
119. Clancy R, Marder G, Martin V, et al. Circulating activated endothelial cells in systemic lupus erythematosus: further evidence for diffuse vasculopathy. *Arthritis Rheum* 2001;44:1203–1208.
120. Kashem A, Endoh M, Yano N, et al. Expression of inducible-NOS in human glomerulonephritis: the possible source is infiltrating monocytes/macrophages. *Kidney Int* 1996;50:392–399.
121. Furusu A, Miyazaki M, Abe K, et al. Expression of endothelial and inducible nitric oxide synthase in human glomerulonephritis. *Kidney Int* 1998;53:1760–1768.
122. Wang JS, Tseng HH, Shih DF, et al. Expression of inducible nitric oxide synthase and apoptosis in human lupus nephritis. *Nephron* 1997;77:404–411.
123. Yu CC, Yang CW, Wu MS, et al. Mycophenolate mofetil reduces renal cortical inducible nitric oxide synthase mRNA expression and diminishes glomerulosclerosis in MRL/lpr mice. *J Lab Clin Med* 2001;138:69–77.
124. Tapia E, Franco M, Sanchez-Lozada LG, et al. Mycophenolate mofetil prevents arteriolopathy and renal injury in subtotal ablation despite persistent hypertension. *Kidney Int* 2003;63:994–1002.
125. Lui SL, Tsang R, Wong D, et al. Effect of mycophenolate mofetil on severity of nephritis and nitric oxide production in lupus-prone MRL/lpr mice. *Lupus* 2002;11:411–418.
126. Peters H, Border WA, Ruckert M, et al. l-Arginine supplementation accelerates renal fibrosis and shortens life span in experimental lupus nephritis. *Kidney Int* 2003;63:1382–1392.
127. Kuhn A, Fehsel K, Lehmann P, et al. Aberrant timing in epidermal expression of inducible nitric oxide synthase after UV irradiation in cutaneous lupus erythematosus. *J Invest Dermatol* 1998;111: 149–153.
128. Tsukazaki N, Watanabe M, Shimizu K, et al. Photoprovocation test and immunohistochemical analysis of inducible nitric oxide synthase expression in patients with Sjögren's syndrome associated with photosensitivity. *Br J Dermatol* 2002;147:1102–1108.
129. Wong CK, Ho CY, Li EK, et al. Elevated production of interleukin-18 is associated with renal disease in patients with systemic lupus erythematosus. *Clin Exp Immunol* 2002;130:345–351.
130. Lopez-Nevot MA, Ramal L, Jimenez-Alonso J, et al. The inducible nitric oxide synthase promoter polymorphism does not confer susceptibility to systemic lupus erythematosus. *Rheumatology (Oxford)* 2003;42:113–116.
131. Lorenz HM, Grunke M, Hieronymus T, et al. *In vitro* apoptosis and expression of apoptosis-related molecules in lymphocytes from patients with systemic lupus erythematosus and other autoimmune diseases. *Arthritis Rheum* 1997;40:306–317.
132. Emlen W, Niebur J, Kadera R. Accelerated *in vitro* apoptosis of lymphocytes from patients with systemic lupus erythematosus. *J Immunol* 1994;152:3685–3692.
133. Elkon KB. Apoptosis in SLE—too little or too much? *Clin Exp Rheumatol* 1994;12:553–559.
134. Richardson BC, Yung RL, Johnson KJ, et al. Monocyte apoptosis in patients with active lupus. *Arthritis Rheum* 1996;39:1432–1434.
135. Steinberg AD, Melez KA, Raveche ES, et al. Approach to the study of the role of sex hormones in autoimmunity. *Arthritis Rheum* 1979; 22:1170–1176.
136. Hayashi T, Yamada K, Esaki T, et al. Effect of estrogen on isoforms of nitric oxide synthase: possible mechanism of anti-atherosclerotic effect of estrogen. *Gerontology* 1997;43:24–34.
137. Best PJ, Berger PB, Miller VM, et al. The effect of estrogen replacement therapy on plasma nitric oxide and endothelin-1 levels in postmenopausal women. *Ann Intern Med* 1998;128:285–288.
138. Lang U, Baker RS, Clark KE. Estrogen-induced increases in coronary blood flow are antagonized by inhibitors of nitric oxide synthesis. Eur J Obstet Gynecol Reprod Biol 1997;74:229–235.
139. Binko J, Majewski H. 17 Beta-estradiol reduces vasoconstriction in endothelium-denuded rat aortas through inducible NOS. *Am J Physiol* 1998;274:H853–H859.
140. Hayashi T, Yamada K, Esaki T, et al. Physiological concentrations of 17beta-estradiol inhibit the synthesis of nitric oxide synthase in macrophages via a receptor-mediated system. *J Cardiovasc Pharmacol* 1998;31:292–298.
141. Chao TC, Van Alten PJ, Walter RJ. Steroid sex hormones and macrophage function: modulation of reactive oxygen intermediates and nitrite release. *Am J Reprod Immunol* 1994;32:43–52.
142. Hayashi T, Fukuto JM, Ignarro LJ, et al. Gender differences in atherosclerosis: possible role of nitric oxide. *J Cardiovasc Pharmacol* 1995;26:792–802.
143. Woodfork KA, Schuller KC, Huffman LJ. Cytokine and nitric oxide release by J774A.1 macrophages is not regulated by estradiol. *Life Sci* 2001;69:2287–2294.
144. Devaux Y, Seguin C, Grosjean S, et al. Lipopolysaccharide-induced increase of prostaglandin E-2 is mediated by inducible nitric oxide synthase activation of the constitutive cyclooxygenase and induction of membrane-associated prostaglandin E synthase. *J Immunol* 2001; 167:3962–3971.
145. Weyand CM, Wagner AD, Bjornsson J, et al. Correlation of the topographical arrangement and the functional pattern of tissue-infiltrating macrophages in giant cell arteritis. *J Clin Invest* 1996;98:1642–1649.
146. Borkowski A, Younge BR, Szweda L, et al. Reactive nitrogen intermediates in giant cell arteritis: selective nitration of neocapillaries. *Am J Pathol* 2002;161:115–123.
147. Adewuya O, Irie Y, Bian K, et al. Mechanism of vasculitis and aneurysms in Kawasaki disease: role of nitric oxide. *Nitric Oxide* 2003;8:15–25.
148. Wang CL, Wu YT, Lee CJ, et al. Decreased nitric oxide production after intravenous immunoglobulin treatment in patients with Kawasaki disease. *J Pediatr* 2002;141:560–565.
149. Heeringa P, Bijl M, de Jager-Krikken A, et al. Renal expression of endothelial and inducible nitric oxide synthase, and formation of peroxynitrite-modified proteins and reactive oxygen species in Wegener's granulomatosis. *J Pathol* 2001;193:224–232.
150. Er H, Evereklioglu C, Cumurcu T, et al. Serum homocysteine level is increased and correlated with endothelin-1 and nitric oxide in Behçet's disease. *Br J Ophthalmol* 2002;86:653–657.
151. Evereklioglu C, Turkoz Y, Er H, et al. Increased nitric oxide production in patients with Behçet's disease: is it a new activity marker? *J Am Acad Dermatol* 2002;46:50–54.

152. Yilmaz G, Sizmaz S, Yilmaz ED, et al. Aqueous humor nitric oxide levels in patients with Behçet disease. *Retina* 2002;22:330–335.
153. Soylemezoglu O, Ozkaya O, Erbas D, et al. Nitric oxide in Henoch-Schonlein purpura. *Scand J Rheumatol* 2002;31:271–274.
154. Bruce IN, Harris CM, Nugent A, et al. Enhanced endothelium-dependent vasodilator responses in patients with systemic vasculitis. *Scand J Rheumatol* 1997;26:318–324.
155. Yamamoto T, Katayama I, Nishioka K. Nitric oxide production and inducible nitric oxide synthase expression in systemic sclerosis. *J Rheumatol* 1998;25:314–317.
156. Kharitonov SA, Cailes JB, Black CM, et al. Decreased nitric oxide in the exhaled air of patients with systemic sclerosis with pulmonary hypertension. *Thorax* 1997;52:1051–1055.
157. Yamamoto T, Sawada Y, Katayama I, et al. Increased production of nitric oxide stimulated by interleukin-1-beta in peripheral blood mononuclear cells in patients with systemic sclerosis. *Br J Rheumatol* 1998; 37:1123–1125.
158. Stein CM, Tanner SB, Awad JA, et al. Evidence of free radical-mediated injury (isoprostane overproduction) in scleroderma. *Arthritis Rheum* 1996;39:1146–1150.
159. Rolla G, Colagrande P, Scappaticci E, et al. Exhaled nitric oxide in systemic sclerosis: relationships with lung involvement and pulmonary hypertension. *J Rheumatol* 2000;27:1693–1698.
160. Schaffer MR, Tantry U, Gross SS, et al. Nitric oxide regulates wound healing. *J Surg Res* 1996;63:237–240.
161. Schaffer MR, Tantry U, van Wesep RA, et al. Nitric oxide metabolism in wounds. *J Surg Res* 1997;71:25–31.
162. Schaffer MR, Tantry U, Efron PA, et al. Diabetes-impaired healing and reduced wound nitric oxide synthesis: a possible pathophysiologic correlation. *Surgery* 1997;121:513–519.
163. Schaffer MR, Efron PA, Thornton FJ, et al. Nitric oxide, an autocrine regulator of wound fibroblast synthetic function. *J Immunol* 1997; 158:2375–2381.
164. Yamasaki K, Edington HD, McClosky C, et al. Reversal of impaired wound repair in iNOS-deficient mice by topical adenoviral-mediated iNOS gene transfer. *J Clin Invest* 1998;101:967–971.
165. Saleh D, Barnes PJ, Giaid A. Increased production of the potent oxidant peroxynitrite in the lungs of patients with idiopathic pulmonary fibrosis. *Am J Respir Crit Care Med* 1997;155:1763–1769.
166. Paredi P, Kharitonov SA, Loukides S, et al. Exhaled nitric oxide is increased in active fibrosing alveolitis. *Chest* 1999;115:1352–1356.
167. Giaid A, Saleh D. Reduced expression of endothelial nitric oxide synthase in the lungs of patients with pulmonary hypertension. *N Engl J Med* 1995;333:214–221.
168. Marie I, Beny JL. Endothelial dysfunction in murine model of systemic sclerosis: tight-skin mice 1. *J Invest Dermatol* 2002;119:1379–1387.
169. Evans CH, Stefanovic-Racic M, Lancaster J. Nitric oxide and its role in orthopaedic disease. *Clin Orthop* 1995:275–294.
170. Lotz M. The role of nitric oxide in articular cartilage damage. *Rheum Dis Clin North Am* 1999;25:269–282.
171. Maier R, Bilbe G, Rediske J, et al. Inducible nitric oxide synthase from human articular chondrocytes: cDNA cloning and analysis of mRNA expression. *Biochim Biophys Acta* 1994;1208:145–150.
172. Stadler J, Stefanovic-Racic M, Billiar TR, et al. Articular chondrocytes synthesize nitric oxide in response to cytokines and lipopolysaccharide. *J Immunol* 1991;147:3915–3920.
173. Palmer RM, Hickery MS, Charles IG, et al. Induction of nitric oxide synthase in human chondrocytes. *Biochem Biophys Res Commun* 1993;193:398–405.
174. Shalom-Barak T, Quach J, Lotz M. Interleukin-17-induced gene expression in articular chondrocytes is associated with activation of mitogen-activated protein kinases and NF-kappaB. *J Biol Chem* 1998;273:27467–27473.
175. Olee T, Hashimoto S, Quach J, et al. IL-18 is produced by articular chondrocytes and induces proinflammatory and catabolic responses. *J Immunol* 1999;162:1096–1100.
176. Fink C, Fermor B, Weinberg JB, et al. The effect of dynamic mechanical compression on nitric oxide production in the meniscus. *Osteoarthritis Cartilage* 2001;9:481–487.
177. Fermor B, Weinberg JB, Pisetsky DS, et al. The effects of static and intermittent compression on nitric oxide production in articular cartilage explants. *J Orthop Res* 2001;19:729–737.
178. Pelletier JP, Lascau-Coman V, Jovanovic D, et al. Selective inhibition of inducible nitric oxide synthase in experimental osteoarthritis is associated with reduction in tissue levels of catabolic factors. *J Rheumatol* 1999;26:2002–2014.
179. Das P, Schurman DJ, Smith RL. Nitric oxide and G proteins mediate the response of bovine articular chondrocytes to fluid-induced shear. *J Orthop Res* 1997;15:87–93.
180. Rediske JJ, Koehne CF, Zhang B, et al. The inducible production of nitric oxide by articular cell types. *Osteoarthritis Cartilage* 1994; 2:199–206.
181. Stefanovic-Racic M, Meyers K, Meschter C, et al. Comparison of the nitric oxide synthase inhibitors methylarginine and aminoguanidine as prophylactic and therapeutic agents in rat adjuvant arthritis. *J Rheumatol* 1995;22:1922–1928.
182. McCartney-Francis NL, Song X, Mizel DE, et al. Selective inhibition of inducible nitric oxide synthase exacerbates erosive joint disease. *J Immunol* 2001;166:2734–2740.
183. van de Loo FA, Arntz OJ, van Enckevort FH, et al. Reduced cartilage proteoglycan loss during zymosan-induced gonarthritis in NOS2-deficient mice and in anti-interleukin-1-treated wild-type mice with unabated joint inflammation. *Arthritis Rheum* 1998;41: 634–646.
184. Pelletier J, Jovanovic D, Fernandes JC, et al. Reduction in the structural changes of experimental osteoarthritis by a nitric oxide inhibitor. *Osteoarthritis Cartilage* 1999;7:416–418.
185. Clancy RM, Abramson SB, Kohne C, et al. Nitric oxide attenuates cellular hexose monophosphate shunt response to oxidants in articular chondrocytes and acts to promote oxidant injury. *J Cell Physiol* 1997;172:183–191.
186. Frenkel SR, Clancy RM, Ricci JL, et al. Effects of nitric oxide on chondrocyte migration, adhesion, and cytoskeletal assembly. *Arthritis Rheum* 1996;39:1905–1912.
187. Clancy RM, Rediske J, Tang X, et al. Outside-in signaling in the chondrocyte. Nitric oxide disrupts fibronectin-induced assembly of a subplasmalemmal actin/rho A/focal adhesion kinase signaling complex. *J Clin Invest* 1997;100:1789–1796.
188. Farrell AJ, Blake DR, Palmer RM, et al. Increased concentrations of nitrite in synovial fluid and serum samples suggest increased nitric oxide synthesis in rheumatic diseases. *Ann Rheum Dis* 1992;51: 1219–1222.

CHAPTER 25

Characteristics of Immune Complexes and Principles of Immune Complex Diseases

Robert P. Kimberly

Autoantibody production and the formation of antigen–antibody complexes are characteristic of many autoimmune diseases. These immune complexes may deposit directly from the circulation in tissues and vessel walls or form *in situ* within target tissues, leading to inflammation, tissue damage, and ultimately, to disease manifestations. Immune complexes also may interact with circulating cells and trigger proinflammatory cell programs. Whereas the recognized technical limitations in quantitating circulating immune complexes in clinical specimens may diminish the clinical utility of immune complex measurements, such difficulties do not diminish the biologic significance of immune complexes. Indeed, immune complexes play a central role in targeting antigen for processing and presentation, in addition to their potential role in disease pathogenesis emphasized by their association with a variety of clinical manifestations, including glomerulonephritis, arthritis, vasculitis, and pleuropericarditis.

Traditionally, activation of the complement cascade with the generation of chemotaxins and activators of inflammatory cells had been accepted as the primary pathophysiologic role of immune complexes in disease. Although complement activation clearly plays an important role in inflammation, evidence in both animal and human models also points toward a central role for immunoglobulin receptors in the development of inflammation and immune complex disease (1–4). This role is underscored by the recent recognition that C-reactive protein (CRP)-containing complexes, known to activate complement, use immunoglobulin receptors as their primary binding and activation receptors (5,6). Thus, immune complexes containing constituents of both the innate and adaptive immune systems share common effector pathways. These observations, coupled with studies of antigen presentation (7,8), B-lymphocyte physiology (9–12), and natural killer (NK) cell function (13,14), provide a broad biologic context for immune complexes, with a focus on several critical issues:

1. What determines the balance between proinflammatory receptor-mediated triggering of phagocytes and antiinflammatory receptor-mediated uptake and removal?
2. What role do immune complexes containing antibody or CRP play in the amplification of antigen presentation?
3. What role do immune complexes play in the regulation of B-cell function and antibody formation?
4. What role do immune complexes play in the modulation of NK function and survival?

To approach each of these questions, it is necessary to understand the physical and biologic properties of immune complexes, the characteristics of the receptors for both immunoglobulins (Fc receptors) and complement cleavage products with which they interact, and the nature of the cell types displaying these receptors. Formation of immune complexes per se is part of the normal immune response. Thus, the development of clinical disease reflects the persistent and excessive production of immune complexes that interact with the properties of the targeted tissues. This process is influenced by genetic variants in receptor structure (1,2,15) and, perhaps, by genetically-determined differences in the production of cytokines, which influence receptor function (16–19). The interplay between these host characteristics and both the qualitative and quantitative aspects of the humoral immune response plays an essential role in the development of immune complex–mediated disease.

PROPERTIES OF IMMUNE COMPLEXES

With the recognition that opsonins of both the innate and adaptive immune systems form complexes with target antigens and share some common effector mechanisms, the term immune complexes could be applied to CRP–target, C1q–target, serum amyloid protein–target, and mannose binding lectin–target complexes, just as it is applied classically to antibody–antigen complexes. Each of these opsonin–target systems plays a role in host defense and may provide important insights into the pathogenesis of immunologic disease (20–23). However, antibody–antigen immune complexes have received the most attention and are the focus of this chapter.

Antibody–antigen complexes vary in their potential to initiate an inflammatory response and induce tissue injury. This variation reflects the physical and chemical properties of the component antigens and their corresponding antibodies, as well as the properties of the combined antibody–antigen complex (Table 25.1). Antigens may differ in molecular size and in the number of antigenic determinants or epitopes per molecule. Larger antigens with multiple epitopes favor the formation of large complexes that promote rapid receptor-mediated clearance from the circulation, whereas smaller antigens are less effective in promoting rapid clearance. The distribution of charge on antigen influences the interaction of antigen with other molecules and tissues. For example, positively-charged antigens can interact with negatively-charged tissues, such as glomerular basement membrane, and facilitate deposition of antigen and antigen–antibody complexes (24). Such a mechanism can contribute to local immune complex formation and to the apparent tissue tropism of immune complexes in some diseases. Other characteristics of antigens also play an important role in determining the properties of antibody–antigen complexes. Glycoprotein antigens interact with lectinlike molecules, and when galactose residues are available for recognition, galactose receptors on hepatocytes can mediate the uptake of small immune complexes (25). Similarly, antigens containing nucleic acids, whether by size, charge, or specialized uptake mechanisms, may endow immune complexes with unique properties (26).

The characteristics of the corresponding antibodies also are essential in determining the overall properties of the immune complex. Immunoglobulin G (IgG), the most common constituent of immune complexes among the five classes of human immunoglobulins (IgG, IgM, IgA, IgE, and IgD), can bind antigen bivalently. If the bound epitopes reside on the same antigen molecule, the resultant monogamous bivalent interaction does not cross-link antigens into a lattice framework. In contrast, if the epitopes bound reside on different antigen molecules, antibody binding cross-links antigens into a larger network of molecules. This lattice formation is strongly influenced by many factors: the valence, distribution, and diversity of epitopes on the antigens; the valence and affinity of the antibodies (IgM and IgA typically have a valence greater than 2); the molar ratio of antigen to antibody; and the absolute concentrations of antigen and antibody. The biologic properties of the resultant immune complex reflect this lattice formation, modified by the intrinsic properties of the constituent antigens and antibodies.

TABLE 25.1. *Factors affecting properties of immune complexes*

Characteristics of the antigen
Physical size
Epitope density and distribution
Electrostatic charge and its distribution
Capacity for direct interaction with tissues
Concentration, Ab/Ag molar ratio
Characteristics of the antibody
Class and subclass
Capacity for complement fixation
Binding avidity
Electrostatic charge and its distribution
Concentration, Ab/Ag molar ratio

Ab/Ag, antibody/antigen

IMMUNOGLOBULIN G SUBCLASSES

IgG has four subclasses, each with distinct physicochemical properties that reflect differences in both primary amino acid sequence and in glycosylation of the subclass-specific heavy chains (27). The IgG subclasses differ significantly in the structure of the hinge region, which participates in the binding of both the early complement component C1q to IgG and IgG to Fcγ receptors. Not surprisingly, therefore, the subclasses differ both in complement activation and Fcγ receptor binding. Although tertiary structures of IgG are important for these interactions, a sequence motif in residues 318 to 322 of IgG heavy chain appears to be important for C1q binding (28). Residues 234 to 237 appear to be critical for Fcγ receptor binding, although different Fcγ receptors may be sensitive to different residues within this region (29) and to the state of heavy-chain glycosylation (30). The genes encoding IgG heavy chains, located on human chromosome 14q32 (see *genome.ucsc.edu*), have allelic variants known as Gm allotypes. Available data suggest that allotypic variations in the primary amino acid sequence of heavy chain does not affect complement fixation or receptor binding, but some studies suggest that Gm allotypes may be related to basal IgG concentration (31).

Although IgG1 is the most common immunoglobulin in serum and IgG2 is the second most common, the IgG subclass composition of immune complexes may vary depending on the nature of the inciting antigen as well as the cytokine milieu at the time of antigen presentation. Both IgG1 and IgG3 are directed primarily against protein antigens, predominate in many types of immune complexes, and activate complement efficiently (32,33). IgG2 is typically produced in response to polysaccharide antigens and may predominate in some autoantibody responses, such as anti-C1q (34). IgG2 does not activate the complement cascade well. IgG4, also a poor activator of complement, is an uncommon constituent of immune complexes. Thus, the nature of the IgG subclass in an immune complex can influence both the biologic properties of the immune complex *in vivo* and the ability to detect the immune complex in certain immune complex assays.

COMPLEMENT COMPONENTS AND COMPONENT DEFICIENCIES

Homozygous deficiencies in the early components of the complement cascade (C1q, C1r, C1s, C4, C2, and C3) are associated with a systemic lupus erythematosus (SLE)-like immune complex disease (see Chapter 21). Although these homozygous deficiencies are rare, heterozygous deficiency of C4 is much more common, and patients with SLE have an increased prevalence of C4A null alleles (35–38). Interpretation of the significance of this increased prevalence, especially in white patients, is complicated by the strong linkage disequilibrium of C4A null alleles with human leukocyte antigen DR3 (HLA-DR3) and the ancestral 8.1 major histocompatibility complex (MHC) haplotype. This raises the possibility of other, as yet unidentified, genes in an extended disease-associated haplotype. Nonetheless, the association of the C4A null allele with SLE in other ethnic populations, in the absence of an HLA-DR3 association, supports a pathophysiologic role. The mechanism for an association with C4A null, but not with C4B null, is not established. There is remarkable genomic variation in structure and C4 gene copy number (39–41), and the two gene products do have different properties. The C4A gene product is more efficient at forming amide links with amino groups, whereas the C4B gene product is more efficient at forming ester links with hydroxyl groups. Perhaps this difference influences the efficiency of immune complex solubilization and opsonization. Thus, a deficiency in the early components of the classic pathway of complement activation may lead to significant differences in the physical and biologic properties of the immune complexes and in their interaction with complement and Fcγ receptors.

CELL RECEPTORS FOR IMMUNE COMPLEXES

Complement Receptors

Complement receptors include those for intact C1q and those for proteolytic fragments of complement components. The cell-surface C1q binding protein, C1qRP, a 126,000-kd molecule expressed on phagocytes, enhances phagocytosis and may participate in the handling of C1q-opsonized immune complexes. Interestingly, several ligands, including C1q and mannose-binding lectin, can bind C1qRP, and C1q may have more than one cell surface–binding protein (42–44). This general theme parallels the interplay between antibody, CRP, and receptors for antibody (FcγR).

Cleavage of complement components leads to the potent anaphylatoxins, C3a and C5a, which bind to distinct receptors belonging to the seven transmembrane-spanning, serpentine receptor family (45,46). These receptors, found on myeloid cells as well as T cells and glomerular mesangial cells, activate proinflammatory cell programs, including enhanced adhesion and mediator release (47). Mice, genetically engineered to lack the C5a receptor, show marked reduction of inflammation in several models of immune complex–induced disease (48).

Cleavage of complement components also generates opsonic fragments of C3, and four structurally-distinct receptors can bind these fragments of C3 (Table 25.2).

TABLE 25.2. *Receptors for complement-derived opsonins*

Receptor	Molecular family	Molecular structure	Cell distribution	Ligand	Functions
CR1 (CD35)	RCA	90–280 kd; four alleles with variable number of SCRs	Erythrocytes Neutrophils Mononuclear phagocytes Mesangial phagocytes B lymphocytes T lymphocytes	C3b, C4b iC3b	Immune adherence Cofactor activity Enhanced phagocytosis Modulation of degranulation
CR2 (CD21)	RCA	145 kd	B lymphocytes Dendritic cells	iC3b C3dg EBV	B-cell activation Antigen localization Viral infection
CR3 (CD11b/18)	β_2 integrin	Two chains: α_M and β_2	Neutrophils	iC3b	Adhesion events (various ligands)
			Mononuclear phagocytes	C3dg Other proteins	Immune complex binding Enhanced phagocytosis
CR4 (CD11c/18)	β_2 integrin	Two chains: α_X and β_2	Neutrophils	iC3b	Adhesion events (various ligands)
			Mononuclear phagocytes	C3dg Other proteins	Immune complex binding Enhanced phagocytosis

SCR, short consensus repeat; RCA, regulaters of complement activation.

Complement receptors type 1 and 2 (CR1 and CR2) belong to the RCA (regulators of complement activation) family of molecules (49,50) (see Chapter 21). As members of the RCA family, CR1 and CR2 share common structural features—a 60– to 70–amino acid repeating substructure called the short consensus repeat (SCR) and groups of SCRs forming a long homologous repeat (LHR). CR1 (CD35) has four codominantly expressed alleles of different molecular size reflecting different numbers of component LHRs, the significance of which is not established (51). CR1 also has several polymorphic sites that may influence ligand binding (52). Distinct, albeit homologous, SCR sequences and different numbers of both SCRs and LHRs distinguish the structure of CR1 from that of CR2 (CD21). The tissue distribution of CR1 and CR2 also are substantially different. CR1 is widely distributed (erythrocytes, neutrophils, mononuclear phagocytes, mesangial cells, B cells, and some T cells), whereas CR2 is expressed only on B cells. CR1 preferentially binds C3b and C4b, the cleavage products of C3 and C4, and to a lesser degree, iC3b, the cleavage product of C3b. CR1 mediates binding of immune complexes to erythrocytes, participates in the handling of immune complexes, and has cofactor activity for C3b degradation. CR2 binds C3dg, a degradation product of iC3b, and does not participate in immune complex clearance. However, CR2 is important in modulating B-cell function and is a receptor for Epstein-Barr virus.

CR3 and CR4 are members of the family of β_2 integrins, and each comprises a unique α chain and a common β chain (designated $\beta2$) (53). Both CR3 and CR4 bind the C3 degradation products iC3b and C3dg and are found on fixed-tissue macrophages, mononuclear phagocytes, and polymorphonuclear leukocytes. These receptors likely play a role in immune complex uptake and destruction after cleavage of the immune complex–bound C3 to iC3b and C3dg by erythrocyte CR1. Unlike many complement component deficiencies that are associated with SLE-like immune complex disease, deficiencies of these β_2 integrin receptors are not associated with immune complex deposition. The clinical phenotype of β_2 deficiency (leukocyte adhesion deficiency type 1) involves loss of leukocyte adhesive properties, a decrease in phagocytic capacity, and severe impairment of host defenses against bacterial infections (54).

Receptors for Immunoglobulin G

Immune complexes containing IgG engage Fcγ receptors, which mediate internalization by fixed tissue macrophages (55). Depending on the target cell type, Fcγ receptor cross-linking also can stimulate cytokine synthesis, degranulation, release of inflammatory mediators and vasoactive amines, and antibody-directed cytolytic killing. In cells of lymphoid lineage, Fcγ receptor ligation can initiate cytokine synthesis and antibody-directed cytolytic killing, as well as regulation of cell activation and survival. Unlike CR1 through CR4, which bind complement cleavage products, Fcγ receptors bind native ligand. The affinity of this binding interaction varies substantially among different Fcγ receptors, with some receptors requiring multimeric ligand for effective engagement. Like many other receptors in the immune system, clustering or cross-linking of Fcγ receptors is essential for signal transduction.

Three highly homologous families of Fcγ receptor genes are classically recognized: *FCGR1*, *FCGR2*, and *FCGR3* (Table 25.3). In humans, all members of these families are encoded by distinct genes on human chromosome 1 and share the structural motif of immunoglobulin-like disulfide-linked extracellular domains common to the immunoglobulin supergene family (56–58). Although these receptors have similar primary sequences comprising their extracellular domains, they are not identical and have distinct ligand-binding properties. Even greater diversity in the structure of the transmembrane and cytoplasmic domains provides the basis for the range of functions that these receptors can elicit. Receptor isoforms, generated through alternative splicing, provide an additional dimension of variation in a variety of cell types. Interestingly, the completion of the human genome project has facilitated the discovery of a new family of Fc receptor homologues, the function of which is the subject of intense investigation (59–61).

FcγRIa (CD64), the receptor protein encoded by the *FCGR1A* gene, has three immunoglobulin-like disulfide-linked extracellular domains and is unique among all Fcγ receptors in its high affinity for monomeric IgG. It is constitutively expressed on monocytes and macrophages, may be expressed on a subset of dendritic cells (62), and can be induced in polymorphonuclear leukocytes by interferon-γ or granulocyte colony-stimulating factor. The *FCGR1* gene family contains three highly homologous genes, which encode distinct isoforms of FcγRI. Although spliced isoforms of the B gene product, for example, encode for a putative lower affinity receptor with two extracellular immunoglobulin-like domains, the biologic significance and distribution of these other putative, alternative *FCGR1* gene family products are not yet established (63).

The *FCGR2* gene family comprises low-affinity receptors that interact most effectively with multivalent immune complexes, multivalent IgG-opsonized particles, and IgG bound to the surface of the cell. FcγRII is expressed by platelets, myeloid cells, and lymphoid cells, including B lymphocytes. Like the *FCGR1* family of genes, the *FCGR2* family contains three distinct, yet highly homologous, genes (*FCGR2A*, *FCGR2B*, and *FCGR2C*), each of which gives rise to at least one expressed protein product. Alternative splicing of *FCGR2A* and *FCGR2B* results in expression of six different FcγRII isoforms. The extracellular and cytoplasmic domains of FcγRII family members exhibit significant differences. The cytoplasmic domain of FcγRIIa has an immunoreceptor tyrosine activation motif (ITAM), which serves as a docking site for src homology 2 (SH2)-containing cytoplasmic tyrosine kinases and adaptor mole-

TABLE 25.3. *Human Fcγ receptors*

Receptor family	Member genes	Molecular structure	Cell distribution	Ligand affinity	Functions
FcγRI (CD64)	A	70 kd 3 extracellular (EC) domains γ Chain	Mononuclear phagocytes Neutrophils (IFN-γ) Dendritic cells Mesangial cells	10^8–10^9 M^{-1}	Cell activation Phagocytosis, secretion, ADCC, gene activation Antigen processing
	B	? Protein	?		
	C	? Protein	?		
FcγRII (CD32)	A	45–50 kd 2 EC domains ITAM in cytoplasmic domain	Neutrophils Mononuclear phagocytes Platelets Eosinophils	<10^7 M^{-1}	Cell activation Phagocytosis, secretion, ADCC, gene activation
	B	45–50 kd 2 EC domains ITIM in cytoplasmic domain	B lymphocytes Neutrophils Mononuclear phagocytes		Cell inhibition
	C	45–50 kd 2 EC domains ITAM in cytoplasmic domain	NK cells		Cell activation
FcγRIII (CD16)	A	60–65 kd 2 EC domains γ Chain (or ζ in NK)	NK cells Mononuclear phagocytes Mesangial phagocytes Mast cells	~10^7 M^{-1}	Cell activation Phagocytosis, secretion, ADCC, gene activation
	B	60–80 kd 2 EC domains Heavily glycosylated GPI membrane ancho	Neutrophils Eosinophils	<10^7 M^{-1}	Cell activation

ADCC, antibody-dependent cellular cytotoxicity; ITAM, immunoreceptor tyrosine activation motif; ITIM, immunoreceptor tyrosine inhibition motif.

cules (Fig. 25.1). In contrast, FcγRIIb has an immunoreceptor tyrosine inhibition motif that can recruit the protein tyrosine phosphatases, SHP, SHIP and PTP1C (10–12). Additionally, two allelic forms of FcγRIIa have nonsynonymous single nucleotide polymorphisms that encode for single amino acid sequence differences in the extracellular domains. These polymorphisms significantly alter the binding of human IgG2, and to a lesser extent, of human IgG3 (64–66). FcγRIIa alleles are expressed codominantly on polymorphonuclear leukocytes, mononuclear phagocytes, and platelets. FcγRIIc may be uniquely expressed on natural killer (NK) cells. FcγRIIIa binds ligand with intermediate affinity and is expressed on human mononuclear phagocytes, mesangial cells, and NK cells. Like FcγRIa, FcγRIIIa associates with a homodimer of the γ chain, a member of the γ, ζ, η family of signal transduction molecules (67). In NK cells, FcγRIIIa also may associate with the ζ chain (13,14). These accessory chains, which contain ITAMs, also are found in association with the high-affinity receptor for IgE (FcεRI) and the T-cell receptor for antigen. Similar signal-transducing chains, Igα and Igβ, are expressed in association with the B-cell antigen receptor (67). FcγRIIIb, a low-affinity receptor, is expressed exclusively on neutrophils and eosinophils and is unique among human Fcγ receptors in the absence of a transmembrane domain and in the use of a glycosylphosphatidylinositol moiety to mediate attachment to the plasma membrane. FcγRIIIb has two predominant allelic forms, neutrophil antigen 1 (NA1) and NA2, which reflect genomically encoded nonsynonymous single nucleotide polymorphisms (SNPs) that change several amino acids in the expressed protein and influence the receptor's functional capacity (68,69). A third uncommon allele (SH) has no recognized biologic significance as yet.

Functional Properties of Complement and Fc Receptors

Several distinct functional properties characterize complement and Fcγ receptors. Whereas CR1 exerts an immediate effect on immune complex processing through its cofactor activity for C3b cleavage and immune complex solubilization, CR3 and CR4 on phagocytic cells are unable to internalize ligand without priming of the cell through other pathways. Fcγ receptors do not require such activation but are able to provide the necessary signals to capacitate complement receptors. Both complement and Fcγ

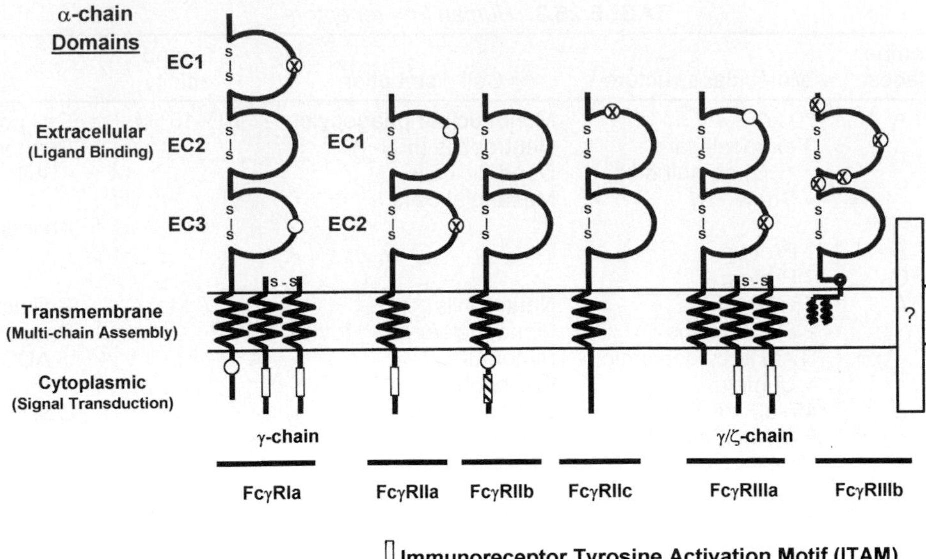

FIG. 25.1. Themes in Fcγ receptor (FcγR) structure and function. FcγRs are members of the immunoglobulin supergene family and have an α chain with two or three disulfide-linked immunoglobulin-like domains in the extracellular portion of the molecule, which is responsible for ligand binding. Except for the glycosylphosphatidylinositol-linked FcγRIIIb, all FcγRs have a transmembrane region. Some receptor forms associate with accessory chains, including the γ chain of the high-affinity FcγRI, ζ chain, and the β chain of the high-affinity FcγRI. The cytoplasmic regions of the α or accessory chains contain the immunoregulatory tyrosine activation motif (*ITAM*), which is essential for signal transduction. Signal transduction by the glycosylphosphatidylinositol-linked FcγRIIIb also involves tyrosine phosphorylation.

receptors can be activated—an event that may enhance quantitative capacity or engage new functional capabilities. As with many other immune system receptors, both complement and Fcγ receptors require clustering of at least two receptors on the same cell to initiate intracellular signaling. This requirement for clustering prevents circulating monomeric IgG or complement components from stimulating effector cells in the absence of opsonized antigen or opsonized target cells.

Increasing evidence suggests that individual Fcγ receptor forms may engage at least some distinct intracellular signaling elements. Nonetheless, general themes in signal transduction include rapid tyrosine phosphorylation of intracellular proteins, fluxes in intracellular calcium, increased phosphoinositide turnover, and membrane lipid remodeling (54–57). These events lead to effector functions, such as phagocytosis; release of inflammatory mediators, including prostaglandins, leukotrienes, and hydrolytic enzymes; synthesis and release of cytokines [e.g., interleukin-6 (IL-6), IL-8, and tumor necrosis factor-alpha (TNF-α)]; antibody dependent cellular cytotoxicity (ADCC); and activation of the oxidative burst. Multiple signaling pathways are certainly activated by a single receptor species, which in turn leads to multiple effector functions. Cross-linking of multiple receptor types, such as FcγRIII and FcγRII on neutrophils, leads to functional responses that are significantly greater than those initiated by either receptor form alone (70). Interaction between receptor types is especially important, given the presence of both complement and IgG in most immune complexes.

IMMUNE COMPLEX PROCESSING AND PATHOPHYSIOLOGY

Immune Adherence Reaction

In 1953, Nelson (71) described the immune adherence reaction, mediated by the binding of C3b fragments to CR1 on erythrocytes. Three decades later, Hebert et al. (72) demonstrated that complement-fixing immune complexes formed *ex vivo* and injected into primates became bound to erythrocytes through CR1. Immune complexes formed experimentally *in vivo* from free antibody and free antigen in the circulation also bind to erythrocytes in a complement-dependent manner (73). These observations, amplified by additional experiments in both humans and nonhuman primates (74–77), indicated that, in primates, complement-fixing circulating immune complexes interact with erythrocytes that express the majority of the available complement receptors in the circulation.

CR1-mediated binding of immune complexes to erythrocytes probably serves several potential roles (78–80). First, the erythrocyte likely serves to bind complement-opsonized immune complexes, partition them to the circulation, and decrease the probability of their deposition in tissues (81,82). Second, the erythrocyte acts as an immune complex "shuttle," facilitating immune complex presentation to, and uptake by, the fixed-tissue mononuclear phagocyte system, primarily in liver and spleen. Third, by providing CR1, which is a cofactor for the cleavage of immune complex–bound C3b to iC3b and C3dg, the erythrocyte accelerates complement-mediated immune complex solubilization into smaller, nonpathogenic complexes (83). Most probably, cleavage of erythrocyte CR1 by a cell surface metalloproteinase on the macrophage releases the immune complex from the erythrocyte. Other complement receptors on the macrophages of the mononuclear phagocyte system can bind to C3 degradation products, which may lead to complement-mediated recognition of the immune complex and uptake by phagocytes. Thus, complement and complement receptors play an important role in immune complex removal.

Role of Fcγ Receptors in the Handling of Model Immune Complexes

Work in several experimental animals has demonstrated the rapid removal of model immune complexes from the circulation by the mononuclear phagocyte system. Although the precise mechanisms of clearance depend on the properties of the complexes, uptake of large lattice complexes can proceed in the absence of complement and is mediated predominantly by the Kupffer cells of the liver (reviewed in reference 84). Nonetheless, debate about the relative roles of complement-mediated and Fcγ receptor–mediated mechanisms continues, driven in part by the different properties of model immune complexes used in these studies.

In addressing these differences, studies involving infusions of antireceptor monoclonal antibodies in chimpanzees (85,86) have provided important insights into the relationship between immune clearance of IgG-opsonized erythrocytes and soluble model immune complexes used by some investigators. These observations include recognition that (a) complement-mediated solubilization of complexes occurs *in vivo,* with resultant change in their clearance characteristics; (b) complement plays an important role in early, rapid uptake, whereas slower uptake, mostly in the spleen, is predominantly Fcγ receptor mediated; and (c) Fcγ receptors participate in hepatic as well as splenic handling of complexes, as evidenced by the role of Fcγ receptors in retention of immune complexes by the liver after initial complement-dependent binding.

With these insights and with the understanding that change in clearance kinetics due to altered solubilization involves mechanisms distinct from changes in clearance kinetics due to altered receptor-mediated uptake of immune complexes by phagocytes, observations with various model immune complexes, which initially may appear contradictory, are easily reconciled. For example, data using soluble aggregated IgG support the observation of decreased Fcγ receptor–mediated splenic clearance in SLE (87), whereas studies with tetanus toxoid antigen–antitetanus antibody and hepatitis B surface antigen–antibody complexes indicate an accelerated early phase of clearance in SLE (88). However, inferences about receptor function, made in studies with soluble immune complexes in hypocomplementemic SLE patients with low erythrocyte CR1 numbers, are confounded by concurrent changes in the efficiency of solubilization.

Accelerated early clearance may be due to poor solubilization of large immune complexes, which are then more rapidly cleared. In contrast, heat-aggregated IgG fixes less complement and is less susceptible to solubilization because of the nature of aggregation. Its clearance is more sensitive to Fcγ receptor–specific dysfunction. Indeed, erythrocytes opsonized with low levels of IgG anti-Rh(D) fix very little complement, and "solubilization" does not occur. Their clearance is a sensitive probe of Fcγ receptor–specific dysfunction.

Based on studies in chimpanzees, the following predictions for patients with immune complex disease can be made: normal to accelerated early clearance of immune complexes (depending on immune complex size, the degree of hypocomplementemia, and any altered solubilization), increased hepatic release of immune complexes due to Fcγ receptor dysfunction, and delayed Fcγ receptor–mediated splenic uptake. These predictions have been substantiated with soluble hepatitis B surface antigen–antibody complexes in studies extending over 60 minutes (74). Thus, studies with soluble immune complexes, coupled with observations using heat-aggregated IgG (87,88) and IgG-opsonized erythrocytes (89,90), clearly indicate that Fcγ receptor–specific dysfunction occurs in SLE, a prototypic immune complex disease, and contributes to abnormal immune complex handling in both the liver and the spleen.

EXPERIMENTAL MODELS OF IMMUNE COMPLEX DISEASE

Numerous studies in animal models have suggested that clearance of immune complexes by the mononuclear phagocyte system is an important determinant of immune complex deposition in tissues (reviewed in reference 84). In these studies, saturation of the mononuclear phagocyte system promoted deposition of infused complexes, whereas activation of these cells reduced deposition in the glomerulus. Similarly, in animal models characterized by endogenous immune complex formation, altered clearance of immune complexes occurs in conjunction with tissue deposition (91,92). Such studies have established several basic principles—the occurrence of mononuclear phagocyte system dysfunction, the importance of the test probe in assessing function, and the role of timing of the assessment relative to the disease state. These principles may also be important for the handling of antibody-opsonized nucleosomes and apoptotic material.

Models of Acute Immune Complex–Mediated Inflammation

The reverse passive Arthus reaction, in which antigen is injected intravenously and antibody is injected intradermally, has been used as one model of immune complex disease. The classic understanding of this model includes local formation of immune complexes with binding and activation of complement followed by generation of chemotactic peptides, neutrophil chemotaxis, neutrophil activation, and release of inflammatory mediators. Although complement depletion studies have supported a role for complement, other studies provide direct evidence for a pivotal role for Fcγ receptors. Using the reverse passive Arthus reaction, Hogarth et al. (93) studied the effects of soluble Fcγ receptor, which blocks Fcγ-receptor engagement by immune complexes, and demonstrated a marked reduction in inflammation. Additional experiments using *FCGR3*-deficient and FcγRI + FcγRIII–deficient mice have shown marked reduction in edema, hemorrhage, and neutrophil infiltration in homozygous knockout mice, and these observations strongly support the role of Fcγ receptors in mediating the inflammation characteristic of this immune complex disease model (3,4). Mast cells (94), neutrophils, macrophages (95), and dendritic cells, all of which express at least some FcγR, no doubt play pivotal roles in the inflammatory response.

Not surprisingly, the biology of immune complex–mediated disease is more intricate than a response mediated by a single receptor. Whereas the cutaneous reverse passive Arthus reaction appears to be initiated primarily by FcγRIII, immune complex peritonitis is mostly dependent on FcγRI (96). Coexpression of inhibitory receptors represents an important modulating factor, and receptors for chemotactic fragments of complement also play an important role (48). Interaction between and interdependence of different receptor systems is a common theme (97). Furthermore, models of spontaneous immune complex disease suggest that in addition to IgG and its receptors (98), CRP, C1q, and serum amyloid precursor also may play important roles (20–22).

ACQUIRED ABNORMALITIES IN IMMUNE COMPLEX HANDLING IN HUMAN IMMUNE COMPLEX DISEASE

Fc receptor–specific clearance by the mononuclear phagocyte system, measured with IgG-opsonized erythrocytes, is decreased in SLE (89,90) and other autoimmune diseases (99,100). This defect is not a fixed property, but rather a dynamic deficit that correlates with disease activity (90,101). This correlation has emphasized the possible role of altered Fcγ receptor function in disease pathogenesis, a view variably supported by studies of infused soluble model immune complexes. Experiments in nonhuman primates, using soluble complexes, IgG-opsonized erythrocytes, and antireceptor monoclonal antibody infusions, suggest a framework in which immune complex disease patients may have normal to accelerated early uptake of complexes, depending on the degree of hypocomplementemia, and altered solubilization, increased release of immune complexes from hepatic Kupffer cells due to Fcγ receptor dysfunction, and delayed Fcγ receptor–mediated splenic uptake. In this framework, studies with soluble immune complexes (74,77,88), heat-aggregated IgG (87), and IgG-opsonized erythrocytes (89,90) clearly indicate that Fcγ receptor–specific dysfunction occurs in SLE and contributes to abnormal immune complex handling in both the liver and the spleen.

Fcγ receptor dysfunction is not the only acquired mechanism for abnormal immune complex handling in immune complex disease. Hypocomplementemia may affect the kinetics and efficiency of immune complex opsonization and solubilization by complement, and some evidence suggests that complement receptor function also may be abnormal (102,103). Furthermore, SLE provides a striking example in which the number of CR1 molecules on erythrocytes may be reduced (103,104). Although an inherited expression polymorphism for CR1 density on erythrocytes has been demonstrated (105), the low levels of CR1 on erythrocytes in SLE are most probably acquired (106,107) and reflect an alteration in CR1 after binding of immune complexes and uptake by phagocytes in the liver. Indeed, repeated administration of antigen to immunized primates leads to *in vivo* immune complex formation and subsequent reduction in erythrocyte CR1 number. *In vitro* data indicate that the binding capacity of erythrocytes for immune complexes through CR1 correlates with the density of CR1 expression (108,109). Because complexes that are not bound to erythrocytes may be more easily deposited in the microvasculature of the lung and kidneys (110,111), the potential for altered CR1 expression to contribute to disease pathogenesis is clear.

Other mechanisms also play a role in immune complex handling. Exogenously-administered, soluble FcγRII can reduce the binding of immune complexes to Fcγ receptors (93). Soluble Fcγ receptor, secreted as an alternatively spliced product of FcγRIIa or derived from the proteolytic cleavage of FcγRIIIb on neutrophils, is present in normal sera (112–114). Levels of soluble FcγRIIIb increase during inflammation, which might impair the ability of immune complexes containing IgG to bind cell surface Fcγ receptors. Soluble Fcγ receptors might also alter the ability of complexes to activate complement and form the C3b required for solubilization and complement receptor interaction. The biologic significance of these soluble molecules is poorly understood, but along with antireceptor autoantibodies that have been described in patients with autoimmune immune complex disease (115,116), they represent areas for potential further insight and understanding of immune complex pathophysiology.

INHERITED FACTORS INFLUENCING IMMUNE COMPLEX HANDLING

Structural polymorphisms of CR1 do not appear to be primarily responsible for the reduction of CR1 on erythrocytes in SLE patients, but several allelic polymorphisms of CR1 have clear differences in functional capacity (52). Heritable differences in complement-dependent mechanisms are important in immune complex pathophysiology; both homozygous deficiencies of early complement components and heterozygous deficiencies of C4A are associated with an immune complex diathesis.

The allelic polymorphisms in immunoglobulin heavy chains (Gm allotypes) do not appear to alter complement fixation or Fcγ receptor binding, but there are several known SNPs in the coding regions of Fcγ receptor genes that alter the amino acid residue encoded. Known as non-synonymous SNPs, because they change coding sequence, these alleles have distinct functional capacities (Fig. 25.2). The two alleles of FcγRIIa, which were originally identified by their differential ability to bind murine IgG1, differ substantially in their binding capacity for human IgG2 (1). The allotype with histidine, rather than an arginine, in position 131 (FcγRIIa-H131) in the second extracellular domain, binds human IgG2 much more strongly than the allotype with arginine (FcγRIIa-R131). FcγRIIa-H131 is the only Fcγ receptor that binds IgG2 well, and it is under-represented in SLE patients, especially those with nephritis (1). Similarly, FcγRIIIa has two functional alleles that differ in their ability to bind human IgG1 and IgG3 (2). The allotype with valine in position 176 in extracellular domain two binds IgG1 nearly tenfold more avidly than the allotype with phenylalanine, and, like FcγRIIa-H131, it is under-represented in SLE patients. Association studies suggest that both genes may contribute to lupus severity, and the apparent predominant effect of FcγRIIIa may reflect the predominance of IgG1 and IgG3 among lupus autoantibodies. In contrast, SNPs in the neutrophil FcγRIIIb result in two major alleles (NA1 and NA2), which differ quantitatively in their capacity to activate neutrophils despite equivalent ligand binding and density of receptor expression (68,69), but which do not seem to be associated with SLE.

The most extreme model for the role of Fcγ receptors in human disease would be a naturally-occurring knockout (i.e., the null phenotype for one or more receptors) (117–120). Fcγ-receptor deficiency is rare, and no individuals lacking FcγRII have been described. Several individuals lacking FcγRIa appear to have a normal phenotype. *FCGR3B* deficiency in mothers is associated with neonatal neutropenia, but the reports of association with SLE may reflect disequilibrium with *FCGR2B* (119–122).

MECHANISMS OF TISSUE LOCALIZATION AND INJURY

Based on current knowledge of immune complex components, relevant cell surface receptors, and the status of the

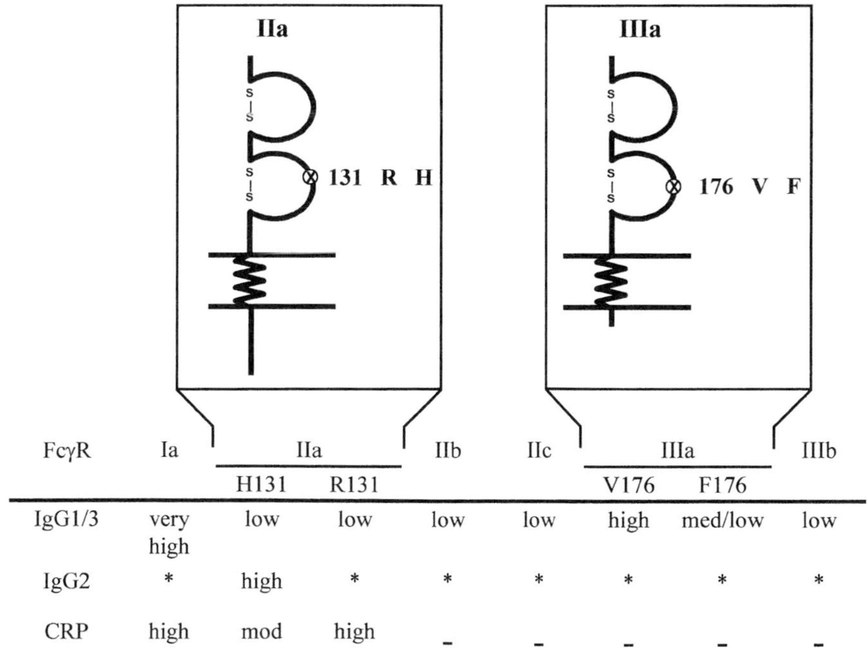

FcγR	Ia	IIa H131	IIa R131	IIb	IIc	IIIa V176	IIIa F176	IIIb
IgG1/3	very high	low	low	low	low	high	med/low	low
IgG2	*	high	*	*	*	*	*	*
CRP	high	mod	high	–	–	–	–	–

FIG. 25.2. Allelic polymorphisms of human Fcγ receptors (FcγRs). Several allelic systems in human FcγRs have been studied. The FcγRIIa polymorphism markedly affects the ability to bind human immunoglobulin G2 (IgG2), whereas the FcγRIIIa polymorphism affects IgG1 and IgG3 binding. The FcγRIIIb polymorphism does not affect ligand binding but does affect quantitative effector function through a mechanism that remains to be determined.

TABLE 25.4. *Factors affecting immune complex deposition*

Process	Mechanism
Rate of immune complex formation	Antibody synthesis Antigen synthesis and release
Rate of immune complex removal and degradation	Efficiency of complement fixation Erythrocyte CR1 level Immune complex solubilization Receptor-mediated immune complex uptake
Local tissue characteristics	Blood flow and pressure Basement membrane exposure Natural vs. injury-induced fenestrations Vascular permeability
Potential for directly targeted deposition	Tissue tropism for Ag, Ab, or complexes (e.g., charge-mediated *in situ* formation) Specific reactivity by Ab

Ab, antibody; Ag, antigen.

mononuclear phagocyte system, it is clear that many factors contribute to the level of circulating immune complexes and to the likelihood of abnormal tissue deposition (Table 25.4). The balance between production and removal is pivotal, and in the setting of chronic immune complex formation, a subtle shift in this balance that permits the persistence of even small amounts of phlogistic complexes may favor their gradual accumulation, especially in tissues that subserve filtering functions, with subsequent development of inflammation and tissue injury. Many different tissues can be sites for immune complex deposits (Table 25.5), and the individual properties of these target tissues are important in determining the processes involved in such deposition. For example, the architecture of the glomerular capillary loop is designed for rapid filtration. The glomerular capillary wall serves as a size and charge barrier to circulating macromolecules that have open access to the glomerular basement membrane through the fenestrated cytoplasmic extensions of endothelial cells (123–125). Thus, in addition to deposition through physical trapping, fixed negative charges in both the subendothelial and subepithelial regions of the glomerular capillary wall can contribute to immune complex accumulation through charge-directed deposition of circulating complexes or through charge-directed deposition of free antigen followed by *in situ* formation of complexes (126). Local *in situ* formation also can occur when antigen binds to glomerular basement membrane or becomes trapped in the glomerular mesangial matrix. Both direct deposition and local immune complex formation lead to a typically irregular, "lumpy-bumpy" pattern of deposits. In contrast, exposure of the glomerular basement membrane and its antigenic epitopes permits specifically reactive antibodies to bind in a typically smooth, uniform fashion, as found in Goodpasture syndrome.

TABLE 25.5. *Examples of tissue sites for immune complex deposition*

Organ system	Tissue structure
Cardiovascular system	Vascular basement membrane
Central nervous system	Choroid plexus
Endocrine system	Thyroid follicles, basement membrane
Kidney	Renal glomeruli, tubular basement membranes
Musculoskeletal system	Articular cartilage, synovial interstitial space
Pulmonary system	Alveolar walls
Skin	Dermal–epidermal junction

Subsequent persistence of immune complex deposits in the glomerulus depends on the initial properties of the complexes and their ability to rearrange into even larger complexes and eventually into immune precipitates recognized as electron-dense deposits (127). Immune complexes that cannot undergo rearrangement do not persist in the subendothelial space of the glomerulus for significant periods. Subepithelial deposits most commonly reflect local immune complex formation, at least in experimental models (128). The mesangium, which contains FcγRIIIa-bearing cells of mononuclear phagocyte lineage (129), also can accumulate immune deposits. The properties of these deposits may vary because they can include both positively- and negatively-charged antibodies.

Although other tissues, like the choroid plexus, share some structural features with the renal glomerulus, most tissues have properties that are quite distinct. Most vascular endothelium is not fenestrated and does not expose the underlying basement membrane to circulating immune complexes. Thus, in immune complex–mediated vasculitis, factors that include local hemodynamics (blood flow and pressures), preexistent injury with disruption of endothelial integrity, and the state of vascular permeability likely all contribute to the pathologic process. Inflammatory cell activation may contribute directly to deposition through accelerated endothelial cell injury and enhanced vascular permeability. This activation may proceed in part as a result of immune complex–initiated receptor engagement (130,131).

The possibility that immune complexes engage Fcγ receptors on circulating cells and initiate an inflammatory cell program might seem at odds with the concept that receptor-mediated uptake of immune complexes is protective for the host. It seems likely that receptor ligation on the fixed tissue macrophage in liver and spleen elicits a different set of cell programs than does ligation of receptors on mobile neutrophils and mononuclear phagocytes. Whether this is due to cell type, state of differentiation, or repertoire of receptors expressed remains to be established.

METHODS FOR DETECTION OF IMMUNE COMPLEXES

Because the antigen in any given circulating immune complex is usually not known, strategies for the detection of immune complexes must take advantage of the antigen-nonspecific properties of complexes. These include physical properties of size and solubility and biologic properties of complement fixation, preferential rheumatoid factor or protein A binding, and platelet aggregation (Table 25.6). Each approach relies on different properties of immune complexes, and given the potential variability in immune complex characteristics, variability among different assays based on these approaches is not uncommon. The variability in immune complex characteristics also underscores the difficulty in developing a suitable standard for comparing results from different assays, even within a single laboratory. These limitations, combined with the ability of nonspecifically-aggregated immunoglobulin (e.g., due to freezing/thawing) to yield false-positive results, have restricted the quantitative value of immune complex assays. Nonetheless, they have been used in a wide variety of immune complex diseases (132–134).

Only a small percentage of immune complexes precipitate in the cold, making cryoprecipitation an insensitive assay. Polyethylene glycol (PEG), 3.5% to 4.0%, also has been used to precipitate complexes, because immunoglobulin aggregates are less soluble in PEG than is monomeric immunoglobulin. PEG precipitates can be detected in up to 70% of immune complex disease patients, but as with cryoprecipitation, the results are not completely specific (135). Consequently, substantial effort has been devoted to developing sensitive and more specific assays based on characteristic biologic properties of immune complexes.

Aggregation of immunoglobulin promotes the binding of C1q, which can be measured directly. In the fluid-phase C1q-binding assay, purified and labeled C1q is added to the given serum specimen, and then immune complex bound C1q is precipitated with PEG (136). In the solid-phase C1q binding assay, C1q is adsorbed to the walls of the reaction well. The serum specimen is incubated in the well to allow immune complex binding to the adsorbed C1q, and then, after washing away nonbound proteins, the bound immune complexes are detected with a labeled antiimmunoglobulin (137). Both assays report positive binding in more than half of SLE patients.

Because many immune complexes activate the complement cascade *in vivo,* C3b and additional cleavage products may be covalently bound to the complexes. The presence of C3b, iC3b, or C3dg can be used as the basis for separation and detection of complement-fixing immune complexes. The general principles of separation, by means of covalently bound complement components and detection by antiimmunoglobulin reagents, have been used in a range of different assays. Strategies for the initial capture of im-

TABLE 25.6. *Common immune complex assays*

Assay	Detection principles	Comments
Physical		
PEG precipitation	Differential solubility: ICs less soluble in PEG than other serum proteins	Relatively crude; may be used as a separation step in other assays
Cryoprecipitation	Relative insolubility of some ICs at low temperatures	Sample handling important; many ICs soluble at low temperature
Complement component dependent		
Fluid-phase C1q binding	Binding of radiolabeled C1q to ICs	More sensitive to large complexes
Solid-phase C1q binding	Binding of ICs to immobilized C1q	
Raji cell binding	Binding of ICs containing iC3b or C3dg to CR2 on Raji cells	More sensitive to large complexes; requires complement fixation and cleavage to iC3b/C3dg
Conglutinin binding	Binding of ICs containing C3b to immobilized bovine conglutinin	More sensitive to large complexes; requires complement fixation and degradation to iC3b
Immunoglobulin dependent		
Monoclonal rheumatoid factor binding	Competition between IC and IgG for binding	Preferential detection of large complexes; rheumatoid factor can confound results
Staphylococcal protein A binding	Preferential binding of IgG aggregates in ICs, to protein A	Less bias toward large complexes; can be used to characterize IgG subclass within ICs

IC, immune complex; Ig, immunoglobulin; PEG, polyethylene glycol.

mune complexes have included immobilized complement-binding proteins, complement-binding monoclonal antibodies, and complement-binding cell surface receptors. For example, bovine conglutinin binds iC3b with high affinity (138). Immune complexes containing iC3b can bind to conglutinin and be separated from total serum immunoglobulin. The immunoglobulin in the complexes can then be quantitated by appropriately labeled antiimmunoglobulin reagents. The Raji cell–binding assay uses a parallel strategy with cell receptors (139). Raji cells are lymphoblastoid B-cell lines that express CR2 and bind C3dg-containing immune complexes. After separation from total serum, these bound complexes also are quantitated by antiimmunoglobulin reagents. Not surprisingly, each assay has some unique characteristics. The conglutinin assay, which depends on the presence of iC3b, cannot detect complexes that have only C3b and C3dg bound to immunoglobulin. Similarly, the Raji assay, requiring the use of intact lymphoblastoid cells, can be confounded by antilymphocyte antibodies that react directly through their antigen-binding domains with the Raji cells and lead to false-positive results (140). Raji cells also express a low-affinity FcγRIIb, which does not contribute substantially to immune complex binding.

Several assays have exploited complement-independent properties of immune complexes. Rheumatoid factors bind to the Fc portion of IgG, a binding that is more efficient for aggregated or immune complexed IgG than for monomeric IgG and that does not require the presence of complement components (141). Similarly, immobilized staphylococcal protein A binds to the Fc portion of IgG, with the multivalent binding of aggregated or complexed IgG exhibiting a significant competitive advantage over monomeric binding (142). Combinations of washing and competitive removal of the human monomeric IgG favor the exclusive binding of immune complexes in the test sample, which can be quantitated by labeled anti-IgG reagents. As expected from the principles of these assays, detection of larger complexes is more efficient than that of smaller complexes, and especially in the rheumatoid factor–binding assay, hypergammaglobulinemia can lead to false-positive results.

Because immune complexes vary in their properties, and different assays take advantage of different properties of these immune complexes, one might anticipate that the results of immune complex assays would show some variation (143,144). In general, larger lattice immune complexes are detected more readily by all assays, and results with techniques using similar principles are more highly correlated than are those using different principles. Specimen handling can be important, and the opportunity for erythrocyte CR1-mediated cleavage of C3b *in vitro* after phlebotomy can affect results (145). Much of this variability in sensitivity, specificity, and absolute levels can be anticipated from fundamental principles. Although diminishing the utility of immune complex assays in clinical diagnosis and management, these results do not diminish the importance of immune complexes in the disease process.

Immune Complexes in Rheumatic Diseases

Many rheumatic, infectious, and neoplastic diseases have been associated with the presence of circulating immune complexes (Table 25.7). Whereas the presence of immune complexes per se provides evidence for the activation of the humoral immune system, reflecting either an appropriate or a pathologic disease process, immune complexes assessed by antigen-nonspecific assays do not provide support for a specific diagnosis. Nonetheless, one might intuitively anticipate a correlation between the level of immune complexes and clinical disease activity for any given disease. This relationship has been explored in SLE and other diseases associated with immune complexes, but the results are in conflict, with some studies demonstrating a good correlation and others failing to find such a relationship. Methodologic issues in quantitative measurements of immune complexes and in quantitative assessment of disease activity have no doubt contributed to this variability. It also is important to recognize that not all circulating complexes have the same pathogenic properties, that individual host factors (including genetic variants of cell surface receptors) may alter the pathogenic potential of any given set of complexes, and that other mechanisms, including *in situ* com-

TABLE 25.7. *Diseases with positive tests for immune complexes*

Rheumatic and connective tissue diseases
Rheumatoid arthritis
Juvenile rheumatoid arthritis
Systemic lupus erythematosus
Sjögren syndrome
Mixed connective tissue disease
Progressive systemic sclerosis
Vasculitis syndromes
Cryoglobulinemia (hepatitis C)
Henoch-Schönlein purpura
Polyarteritis nodosa
Wegener granulomatosis
Hypocomplementemic urticarial vasculitis
Seronegative spondyloarthropathies
Infectious diseases
Bacterial infections
Acute (e.g., endocarditis, meningococcemia, gonococcemia, streptococcal infection)
Chronic (e.g., endocarditis, syphilis, recurrent otitis media, persistent bronchitis associated with cystic fibrosis)
Viral infections
Hepatitis B, hepatitis C, cytomegalovirus
Parasitic diseases
Toxoplasmosis, schistosomiasis, malaria
Neoplastic diseases
Lymphoproliferative disorders
Solid tumors (colonic, bronchogenic, and renal cell carcinomas)
Idiopathic diseases
Glomerulonephritis
Inflammatory bowel disease

plex formation, may contribute to tissue injury and disease activity. Thus, despite the intuitive appeal, it is not surprising that the correlation between immune complex levels and disease activity is variable.

Several lines of investigation suggest a new way of approaching immune complex disease and identifying risk factors for disease activity and severity. Certainly, the association of SLE with early complement component deficiencies and with the C4A null-phenotype is consistent with an important role for complement in effective immune complex processing and removal. The associations of FcγR allotypes with SLE provide non-MHC genetic risk factors, which may be most important in the context of nephritis. One can also anticipate functionally significant polymorphisms in cytokine genes that influence receptor function. Taken together with a profile of the genetic polymorphisms of the host, immune complex measurement with immunochemical characterization and with immunoglobulin class and IgG subclass identification may provide a risk index that can anticipate disease severity and help guide therapeutic decisions.

REFERENCES

1. Salmon JE, Millard S, Schacter L, et al. FcγRIIA alleles are heritable risk factors for lupus nephritis in African Americans. *J Clin Invest* 1996;97:1348–1354.
2. Wu J, Edberg JC, Redecha PB, et al. A novel polymorphism of FcγRIIIa (CD16) alters receptor function and predisposes to autoimmune disease. *J Clin Invest* 1997;100:1059–1070.
3. Hazenbos WL, Gesser JE, Hofhuis FMA, et al. Impaired IgG-dependent anaphylaxis and Arthus reaction in FcγRIII (CD16) deficient mice. *Immunity* 1996;5:181–188.
4. Sylvestre DL, Ravetch JV. Fc receptors initiate the Arthus reaction: redefining the inflammatory cascade. *Science* 1994;265:1095–1098.
5. Marnell LL, Mold C, Volzer MA, et al. C-reactive protein binds to FcγRI in transfected COS cells. *J Immunol* 1995;155:2185–2193.
6. Bharadwaj D, Stein MP, Volzer M, et al. C-reactive protein binds to FcγRIIA-transfected COS cells. *J Exp Med* 1999;190:585–590.
7. Amigorena S, Salamero J, Davoust J, et al. Tyrosine-containing motif that transduces cell activation signals also determines internalization and antigen presentation via type III receptors for IgG. *Nature* 1992; 358:337–341.
8. Haberman AM, Shlomchik MJ. Reassessing the function of immune-complex retention by follicular dendritic cells. *Nat Rev Immunol* 2003;3:757–763.
9. D'Ambrosio D, Hippen KL, Minskoff SA, et al. Recruitment and activation of PTP1C in negative regulation of antigen receptor signaling by FcγRIIB1. *Science* 1995;268:263–264.
10. Coggeshall KM. Regulation of signal transduction by the Fc gamma receptor family members and their involvement in autoimmunity. *Curr Dir Autoimmunity* 2002;5;1–29.
11. Vely F, Olivero S, Olcese L, et al. Differential association of phosphatases with hematopoietic co-receptors bearing immunoreceptor tyrosine-based inhibition motifs. *Eur J Immunol* 1997;27:1994–2000.
12. Daeron M. Fc receptor biology. *Annu Rev Immunol* 1997;15:203–234.
13. O'Shea JJ, Weisman AM, Kennedy IC, et al. Engagement of the natural killer cell IgG receptor results in tyrosine phosphorylation of the z chain. *Proc Natl Acad Sci U S A* 1991;88:350–354.
14. Ortaldo JR, Mason AT, O'Shea JJ. Receptor-induced death in human natural killer cells: involvement of CD16. *J Exp Med* 1995;181: 339–344.
15. Stein MP, Edberg JC, Kimberly RP, et al. C-reactive protein binding to FcγRIIa on human monocytes and neutrophils is allele specific. *J Clin Invest* 2000;105:369–376.
16. Jacob CO, Fronek Z, Lewis GD, et al. Heritable major histocompatibility complex class II–associated differences in production of tumor necrosis factor α: relevance to genetic predisposition to systemic lupus erythematosus. *Proc Natl Acad Sci U S A* 1990;87:1233–1237.
17. Gibson AW, Edberg JC, Wu J, et al. Novel single nucleotide polymorphisms in the distal IL-10 promoter affect IL-10 production and enhance the risk of systemic lupus erythematosus. *J Immunol* 2001;166: 3915–3922.
18. Eskdale J, Gallagher G, Verweij CL, et al. Interleukin 10 secretion in relation to human IL-10 locus haplotypes. *Proc Natl Acad Sci U S A* 1998;95:9465–9470.
19. Haukim N, Bidwell JL, Smith AJ, et al. Cytokine gene polymorphism in human disease: on-line databases, supplement 2. *Genes Immun* 2002;3:313–330.
20. Burlingame RW, Volzer MA, Harris J, et al. The effect of acute phase proteins on clearance of chromatin from the circulation of normal mice. *J Immunol* 1996;156:4783–4788.
21. Botto M, Dell'Agnola C, Bygrave AE, et al. Homozygous C1q deficiency causes glomerulonephritis associated with multiple apoptotic bodies. *Nat Genet* 1998;19:56–59.
22. Bickerstaff MC, Botto M, Hutchinson WL, et al. Serum amyloid P component controls chromatin degradation and prevents antinuclear autoimmunity. *Nat Med* 1999;5:694–697.
23. Garred P, Madsen HO, Halberg P, et al. Mannose-binding lectin polymorphisms and susceptibility to infection in systemic lupus erythematosus. *Arthritis Rheum* 1999;42:2145–2152.
24. Gauthier VJ, Mannik M, Striker GE. Effect of cationized antibodies in preformed immune complexes on deposition and persistence in renal glomeruli. *J Exp Med* 1982;156:766–777.
25. Finbloom DS, Magilavy DB, Harford JB, et al. The influence of antigen on immune complex behavior in mice. *J Clin Invest* 1981;68:214–244.
26. Emlen W, Mannik M. Clearance of circulating DNA-anti-DNA immune complexes in mice. *J Exp Med* 1982;155:1210–1215.
27. Jefferis R. Molecular structure of human IgG subclasses. In: Shakib F, ed. *The human IgG subclasses*. Oxford: Pergamon, 1990:15–30.
28. Duncan AR, Winter G. The binding site for C1q on IgG. *Nature* 1988; 332:738–740.
29. Duncan AR, Woof JM, Partridge LJ, et al. Localization of the binding site for the human high-affinity Fc receptor for IgG. *Nature* 1988; 332:563–564.
30. Krapp S, Mimura Y, Jefferis R, et al. Structural analysis of human IgG-Fc glycoforms reveals a correlation between glycosylation and structural integrity. *J Mol Biol* 2003;325:979–989.
31. Sarvas H, Vesterinen P, Makela O. Serum IgG2 concentration is associated with Gm-allotypes of IgG2 but not with the R131H polymorphism of human Fc-gamma receptor type IIa. *J Clin Immunol* 2002;22:92–97.
32. Rubin RL, Tang FL, Chan EKL, et al. IgG subclasses of autoantibodies in systemic lupus erythematosus, Sjögren's syndrome and drug-induced autoimmunity. *J Immunol* 1986;137:2528–2534.
33. Winkler TH, Henschel TA, Kalies I, et al. Constant isotype pattern of anti-dsDNA antibodies in patients with systemic lupus erythematosus. *Clin Exp Immunol* 1988;72:434–439.
34. Prada AE, Strife CF. IgG subclass restriction of autoantibody to solid-phase C1q in membranoproliferative and lupus nephritis. *Clin Immunol Immunopathol* 1992;63:84–88.
35. Moulds JM, Krych M, Holers VM, et al. Genetics of the complement system and rheumatic disease. *Rheum Dis Clin* 1992;18:893–914.
36. Dunckley H, Gatenby PA, Hawkins B, et al. Deficiency of C4A is a genetic determinant of systemic lupus erythematosus in three ethnic groups. *J Immunogenet* 1987;14:209–218.
37. Fan Q, Uring-Lambert B, Weill B, et al. Complement component C4 deficiencies and gene alterations in patients with systemic lupus erythematosus. *Eur J Immunogenet* 1993;20:11–21.
38. Welch TR, Brickman C, Bishof N, et al. The phenotype of SLE associated with complete deficiency of complement isotype C4a. *J Clin Immunol* 1998;18:48–51.
39. Dawkins R, Leelayuwat C, Gaudieri S, et al. Genomics of the major histocompatibility complex: haplotypes, duplication, retroviruses and disease. *Immunol Rev* 1999;167:275–304.
40. Yu CY. Molecular genetics of the human MHC complement gene cluster. *Exp Clin Immunogenet* 1998;15:213–230.
41. Chung EK, Yang Y, Rupert KL, et al. Determining the one, two, three or four long and short loci of human complement C4 in a major

histocompatibility complex haplotype encoding C4A or C4B proteins. *Am J Hum Genet.* 2002;71:810–822.
42. Nepomuceno RR, Ruiz S, Park M, et al. C1qRP is a heavily O-glycosylated cell surface protein involved in the regulation of phagocytic activity. *J Immunol* 1999;162:3583–3589.
43. Nicholson-Weller A, Klickstein LB. C1q-binding proteins and C1q receptors. *Curr Opin Immunol* 1999;11:42–46.
44. Ghebrehiwet B, Peerschke EI. Structure and function of gC1q-R: a multiligand binding cellular protein. *Immunobiology* 1998;199:225–238.
45. Gerard C, Gerard NP. C5a anaphylatoxin and its seven transmembrane-segment receptor. *Annu Rev Immunol* 1994;12:775–808.
46. Crass T, Ames RS, Sarau HM, et al. Chimeric receptors of the human C3a receptor and C5a receptor (CD88). *J Biol Chem* 1999;274:8367–8370.
47. Nataf S, Davoust N, Ames RS, et al. Human T cells express the C5a receptor and are chemoattracted to C5a. *J Immunol* 1999;162:4018–4023.
48. Höpken UE, Lu B, Gerard NP, Gerard C. Impaired inflammatory responses in the reverse Arthus reaction through genetic deletion of the C5a receptor. *J Exp Med* 1997;186:749–756.
49. Ahearn JM, Fearon DT. Structure and function of the complement receptors, CR1 (CD35) and CR2 (CD21). *Adv Immunol* 1989;46:183–219.
50. Krych M, Atkinson JP, Holers VM. Complement receptors. *Curr Opin Immunol* 1992;4:8–13.
51. Dykman TR, Hatch JA, Atkinson JP. Polymorphism of the human C3b/C4b receptors: identification of third allele and analysis of receptor phenotypes in families and patients with systemic lupus. *J Exp Med* 1989;159:691–703.
52. Birmingham DJ, Chen W, Liang G, et al. A CR1 polymorphism associated with constitutive erythrocyte CR1 levels affects binding to C4b but not C3b. *Immunology* 2003;108:531–538.
53. Kishimoto TK, Larson RS, Corbi AL, et al. The leukocyte integrins. *Adv Immunol* 1989;46:149–182.
54. Etzioni A. Adhesion molecule deficiencies and their clinical significance. *Cell Adhes Commun* 1994;2:257–260.
55. Kimberly RP, Salmon JE, Edberg JC. Receptors for immunoglobulin G: molecular diversity and implications for disease. *Arthritis Rheum* 1995;38:306–314.
56. Hogarth PM. Fc receptors are major mediators of antibody based inflammation in autoimmunity. *Curr Opin Immunol* 2002;14:798–802.
57. Dijstelbloem HM, van de Winkel JGJ, Kallenberg CG. Inflammation in autoimmunity: receptors for IgG revisited. *Trends Immunol* 2001; 22:510–516.
58. Ravetch JV, Bolland S. IgG Fc receptors. *Annu Rev Immunol* 2001; 19:275–290.
59. Davis RS, Wang YH, Kubagawa H, et al. Identification of a family of Fc receptor homologs with preferential B cell expression. *Proc Natl Acad Sci U S A* 2001,98:9772–9777.
60. Hatzivassiliou G, Miller I, Takizawa J, et at. IRTA1 and IRTA2, novel immunoglobulin superfamily receptors expressed in B cells and involved in chromosome 1q21 abnormalities in B cell malignancy. *Immunity* 2001;14:277–289.
61. Ehrhardt GRA, Davis RS, Hsu JT, et al. The inhibitory potential of Fc receptor homolog 4 on memory B cells. *Proc Natl Acad Sci U S A* 2003;100:13489–13494.
62. Fanger NA, Voigtlaender D, Liu C, et al. Characterization of expression, cytokine regulation, and effector function of the high affinity IgG receptor Fc gamma RI (CD64) expressed on human blood dendritic cells. *J Immunol* 1997;158:3090–3098.
63. Porges AJ, Redecha PB, Doebele R, et al. Novel Fcγ receptor I gene products in human mononuclear cells. *J Clin Invest* 1992;90:2102–2109.
64. Warmerdam PAM, van de Winkel JGJ, Vlug A, et al. A single amino acid in the second Ig-like domain of the human Fcγ receptor II is critical in human IgG2 binding. *J Immunol* 1991;147:1338–1343.
65. Salmon JE, Edberg JC, Brogle NL, et al. Allelic polymorphisms of human Fcγ receptor IIA and Fcγ receptor IIIB: independent mechanisms for differences in human phagocyte function. *J Clin Invest* 1992;89:1274–1281.
66. Parren P, Warmerdam PAM, Boeiji LCM, et al. On the interaction of IgG subclasses with the low affinity FcγRIIA (CD32) on human monocytes, neutrophils and platelets: analysis of a functional polymorphism to human IgG2. *J Clin Invest* 1992;90:1537–1546.
67. Keegan AD, Paul WE. Multi-chain immune recognition receptors: similarities in structure and signaling pathways. *Immunol Today* 1992; 13:63–68.
68. Salmon JE, Edberg JC, Kimberly RP. Fcγ receptor III on human neutrophils: allelic variants have functionally distinct capacities. *Clin Invest* 1990;85:1287–1295.
69. Salmon JE, Millard SS, Brogle N, Kimberly RP. Fcγ receptor IIIb enhances FcγRIIa function in an oxidant-dependent and allele-sensitive manner. *J Clin Invest* 1995;95:2877–2885.
70. Edberg JC, Salmon JE, Kimberly RP. Functional capacity of Fcγ receptor III (CD16) on human neutrophils. *Immunol Res* 1992;11: 239–251.
71. Nelson RA. The immune adherence phenomenon: an immunologically specific reaction between micro-organisms and erythrocytes leading to enhanced phagocytosis. *Science* 1953;118:733–737.
72. Cornacoff JB, Hebert LA, Smead WL. Primate erythrocyte-immune complex-clearing mechanism. *J Clin Invest* 1983;71:236–247.
73. Edberg JC, Kujala GA, Taylor RP. Rapid immune adherence reactivity of nascent, soluble antibody/DNA immune complexes in the circulation. *J Immunol* 1987;139:1240–1244.
74. Madi N, Steiger G, Estreicher J, et al. Immune adherence and clearance of hepatitis B surface Ag/Ab complexes is abnormal in patients with systemic lupus erythematosus. *Clin Exp Immunol* 1991;85:373–378.
75. Schifferli JA, Ng YC, Estreicher J, et al. The clearance of tetanus/anti-tetanus toxoid immune complexes from the circulation of humans: complement- and erythrocyte complement receptor 1–dependent mechanisms. *J Immunol* 1988;140:899–904.
76. Schifferli JA, Ng YC, Paccaud J-P, et al. The role of hypocomplementaemia and low erythrocyte complement receptor type 1 numbers in determining abnormal immune complex clearance in humans. *Clin Exp Immunol* 1989;75:329–335.
77. Davies KA, Hird V, Stewart S, et al. A study of *in vivo* immune complex formation and clearance in man. *J Immunol* 1990;144:4613–4620.
78. Hebert LA, Cosio FG. The erythrocyte-immune complex-glomerulonephritis connection in man. *Kidney Int* 1987;31:877–885.
79. Schifferli JA, Ng YC, Peters DK. The role of complement and its receptor in the elimination of immune complexes. *N Engl J Med* 1986; 315:488–495.
80. Davies KA, Chapman PT, Norsworthy PJ, et al. Clearance pathways of soluble immune complexes in the pig: insights into the adaptive nature of antigen clearance in humans. *J Immunol* 1995;155:5760–5768.
81. Hebert L. The clearance of immune complexes from the circulation of man and other primates. *Am J Kidney Dis* 1991;17:352–361.
82. Schifferli JA, Taylor RP. Physiological and pathological aspects of circulating immune complexes. *Kidney Int* 1989;35:993–1003.
83. Medof ME. Complement-dependent maintenance of immune complex solubility. In: Rother K, Till GO, eds. *The complement system.* Berlin: Springer-Verlag, 1988:418–437.
84. Mannik M. Pathophysiology of circulating immune complexes. *Arthritis Rheum* 1982;25:783–787.
85. Clarkson S, Kimberly R, Valinsky J, et al. Blockade of clearance of immune complexes by an anti-FcγR monoclonal antibody. *J Exp Med* 1986;164:474–489.
86. Kimberly R, Edberg J, Merriam L, et al. The *in vivo* handling of soluble complement fixing Ab/dsDNA complexes in chimpanzees. *J Clin Invest* 1989;84:962–970.
87. Lobatto S, Daha MR, Breedveld FC, et al. Abnormal clearance of soluble aggregates of human immunoglobulin G in patients with systemic lupus erythematosus. *Clin Exp Immunol* 1988;72:55–59.
88. Davies KA, Peters AM, Beynon HCL, et al. Immune complex processing in systemic lupus erythematosus: *in vivo* imaging and clearance studies. *J Clin Invest* 1992;90:2075–2083.
89. Parris TM, Kimberly RP, Inman RD, et al. Defective Fc receptor mediated mononuclear phagocyte function in lupus nephritis. *Ann Intern Med* 1982;97:526–532.
90. Kimberly RP, Parris TM, Inman RD, et al. Dynamics of mononuclear phagocyte system FcγR function in SLE: relation to disease activity and circulating immune complexes. *Clin Exp Immunol* 1983;51:261–268.
91. Hoffsten PE, Swerdlin JA, Bartell M, et al. Reticuloendothelial and mesangial function in murine immune complex glomerulonephritis. *Kidney Int* 1979;15:144–159.

92. Pappas MG, Nussenzweig RS, Nussenzweig V, et al. Complement-mediated defect in clearance and sequestration of sensitized, autologous erythrocytes in rodent malaria. *J Exp Med* 1981;67:183–192.
93. Ierino FL, Powell MS, McKenzie IFC, et al. Recombinant soluble human FcγRII: production, characterization and inhibition of the Arthus reaction. *J Exp Med* 1994;178:1617–1628.
94. Zhang Y, Ramos BF, Jakschik BA. Augmentation of reverse Arthus reaction by mast cells in mice. *J Clin Invest* 1991;88:841–846.
95. Marsh CB, Gadek JE, Kindt GC, et al. Monocyte Fcγ receptor cross-linking induces IL-8 production. *J Immunol* 1995;155:3161–3167.
96. Heller T, Gessner JE, Schmidt RE, et al. Fc receptor type I for IgG on macrophages and complement mediate the inflammatory response in immune complex peritonitis. *J Immunol* 1999;162:5657–5661.
97. Baumann U, Kohl J, Tschernig T, et al. A codominant role of FcRI/III and C5aR in the reverse Arthus reaction. *J Immunol* 2000;164:1065–1070.
98. Clynes R, Dumitru C, Ravetch JV. Uncoupling of immune complex formation and kidney damage in autoimmune glomerulonephritis. *Science* 1998;279:1052–1054.
99. Hamburger MI, Moutsopoulos HM, Lawley TJ, Frank MM. Sjögren's syndrome: a defect in reticuloendothelial system Fc-receptor-specific clearance. *Ann Intern Med* 1979;91:534–538.
100. Gordon PA, Davis P, Russel AS, et al. Splenic reticuloendothelial function in patients with active rheumatoid arthritis. *J Rheumatol* 1981;8:490–493.
101. Hamburger MI, Lawley TJ, Kimberly RP, et al. A serial study of reticuloendothelial system Fc receptor functional activity in systemic lupus erythematosus. *Arthritis Rheum* 1982;25:48–54.
102. Kimberly RP, Meryhew NL, Runquist OA. Mononuclear phagocyte function in SLE I: bipartite Fc- and complement-dependent dysfunction. *J Immunol* 1986;137:91–96.
103. Miyakawa Y, Yamada A, Kosaka K, et al. Defective immune adherence receptor (C3b) on erythrocytes from patients with systemic lupus erythematosus. *Lancet* 1981;2:493–497.
104. Ross GC, Yount WJ, Walport MJ, et al. Disease-associated loss of erythrocyte complement receptors (CR1, C3b receptors) in patients with systemic lupus erythematosus and other diseases involving autoantibodies and/or complement activation. *J Immunol* 1985;135:2005–2014.
105. Wilson JG, Wong WW, Schur PH, Fearon DT. Mode of inheritance of decreased C3b receptors on erythrocytes of patients with systemic lupus erythematosus. *N Engl J Med* 1982;307:981–986.
106. Walport MJ, Ross GD, Mackworth-Young C, et al. Family studies of erythrocyte complement type 1 levels: reduced levels in patients with SLE are acquired, not inherited. *Clin Exp Immunol* 1985;59:547–554.
107. Walport M, Ng YC, Lachmann PJ. Erythrocytes transfused into patients with SLE and haemolytic anaemia lose complement receptor type 1 from their cell surface. *Clin Exp Immunol* 1987;69:501–507.
108. Chevalier J, Kazatchkine MD. Distribution in clusters of complement receptor type one (CR1) on human erythrocytes. *J Immunol* 1989;142:2031–2036.
109. Horgan C, Taylor RP. Studies on the kinetics of binding of complement-fixing dsDNA/anti-DNA immune complexes to the red blood cells of normal individuals and patients with systemic lupus erythematosus. *Arthritis Rheum* 1987;27:320–329.
110. Waxman FJ, Hebert LA, Cornacoff JB, et al. Complement depletion accelerates the clearance of immune complexes from the circulation of primates. *J Clin Invest* 1984;74:1329–1340.
111. Waxman FJ, Hebert LA, Cosio FG, et al. Differential binding of immunoglobulin A and immunoglobulin G1 immune complexes to primate erythrocytes *in vivo*: immunoglobulin A immune complexes bind less well to erythrocytes and are preferentially deposited in glomeruli. *J Clin Invest* 1986;77:82–89.
112. Astier A, de la Salle H, de la Salle C, et al. Human epidermal Langerhans cells secrete a soluble receptor for IgG (FcγRII/CD32) that inhibits the binding of immune complexes to FcγR+ cells. *J Immunol* 1994;152:201–212.
113. Huizinga TWJ, De Haas M, Kleijer M, et al. Soluble Fcγ receptor III in human plasma originates from release by neutrophils. *J Clin Invest* 1990;86:416–423.
114. de Haas M, Kleijer M, Minchinton RM, et al. Soluble FcγRIIIa is present in plasma and is derived from natural killer cells. *J Immunol* 1994;152:900–907.
115. Boros P, Muryoi T, Spiera H, et al. Autoantibodies directed against different classes of FcγR are found in sera of autoimmune patients. *J Immunol* 1993;150:2018–2024.
116. Boros P, Odin JA, Chen J, et al. Specificity and class distribution of FcγR-specific autoantibodies in patients with autoimmune disease. *J Immunol* 1993;152:302–306.
117. Ceuppens JL, Baroja ML, van Vaeck F, et al. A defect in the membrane expression of high affinity 72 kD Fc receptors on phagocytic cells in four healthy subjects. *J Clin Invest* 1988;82: 571–578.
118. Edberg JC, Salmon JE, Whitlow M, et al. Preferential expression of human FcγRIIIPMN (CD16) in paroxysmal nocturnal hemoglobinuria. *J Clin Invest* 1991;87:58–67.
119. Huizinga TWJ, Kuijpers RWAM, Kleijer M, et al. Maternal genomic neutrophil FcRIII deficiency leading to neonatal isoimmune neutropenia. *Blood* 1990;76:1927–1932.
120. Fromont P, Bettaieb A, Skouri H, et al. Frequency of the polymorphonuclear neutrophil FcγRIII deficiency in the French population and its involvement in the development of neonatal alloimmune neutropenia. *Blood* 1992;79:2131–2134.
121. Clark MR, Lui L, Clarkson SB, et al. An abnormality of the gene that encodes neutrophil Fc receptor III in a patient with systemic lupus erythematosus. *J Clin Invest* 1990;86:341–346.
122. Enenkel B, Jung D, Frey J. Molecular basis of IgG Fc receptor III defect in a patient with systemic lupus erythematosus. *Eur J Immunol* 1991;21:659–663.
123. Gauthier VJ, Mannik M. A small proportion of cationic antibodies in immune complexes is sufficient to mediate their deposition in glomeruli. *J Immunol* 1990;145:3348–3352.
124. Gauthier VJ, Striker GE, Mannik M. Glomerular localization of preformed immune complexes prepared with anionic antibodies or with cationic antigens. *Lab Invest* 1984;50:636–644.
125. Gallo GR, Caulin-Glaser T, Lamm ME. Charge of circulating immune complexes as a factor in glomerular basement membrane localization in mice. *J Clin Invest* 1981;76:1305–1313.
126. Couser WG, Salant DJ. *In situ* immune complex formation and glomerular injury. *Kidney Int* 1980;17:1–13.
127. Mannik M, Agodoa LYC, David KA. Rearrangement of immune complexes in glomeruli leads to persistence and development of electron dense deposits. *J Exp Med* 1983;157:1516–1528.
128. Couser WG. Mechanisms of glomerular injury in immune complex disease. *Kidney Int* 1985;28:569–583.
129. Radeke HH, Gessner JE, Uciechowski P, et al. Intrinsic human glomerular mesangial cells can express receptors for IgG complexes (hFcγRIII-A) and the associated FcγRI γ chain. *J Immunol* 1994;153:1281–1287.
130. Hundt M, Zielinska-Skowronek M, Schmidt RE. Fcγ receptor activation of neutrophils in cryoglobulin-induced leukocytoclastic vasculitis. *Arthritis Rheum* 1993;36:974–982.
131. Porges AJ, Redecha PB, Kimberly WT, et al. Anti-neutrophil cytoplasmic antibodies engage and activate human neutrophils via FcγRIIA. *J Immunol* 1994;153:1271–1280.
132. Kimberly RP. Immune complexes in rheumatic diseases. *Rheum Dis Clin North Am* 1987:13:583–596.
133. McDougal JS, McDuffie FC. Immune complexes in man: detection and clinical significance. *Adv Clin Chem* 1985;24:1–60.
134. Theofilopoulos AN. Evaluation and clinical significance of circulating immune complexes. *Prog Clin Immunol* 1980;4:63–106.
135. Inman RD. Immune complexes in SLE. *Clin Rheum Dis* 1982;8:49–62.
136. Nydegger UE, Lambert PH, Gerber H, et al. Circulating immune complexes in the serum in systemic lupus erythematosus and in carriers of hepatitis B antigen: quantitation by binding to radiolabelled C1q. *J Clin Invest* 1974;54:297–309.
137. Hay FC, Niveham LJ, Roitt IM. Routine assay for the detection of known immunoglobulin class using solid phase C1q. *Clin Exp Immunol* 1976;24:396–400.
138. Eisenberg RA, Theofilopoulos AN, Dixon FJ. Use of bovine conglutinin for the assay of immune complexes. *J Immunol* 1977;118:1428–1434.
139. Theofilopoulos AN, Dixon FJ. Immune complexes in human diseases. *Am J Pathol* 1980;100:529–594.

140. Anderson CL, Stillman WS. Raji cell assay for immune complexes: evidence for detection of Raji-directed immunoglobulin G antibody in sera from patients with systemic lupus erythematosus. *J Clin Invest* 1980;66:353–360.
141. Gabriel A, Agnello V. Detection of immune complexes: the use of radioimmunoassays with C1q and monoclonal rheumatoid factor. *J Clin Invest* 1977;59:990–1001.
142. Inman RD, Redecha PB, Knechtle SJ, et al. Identification of bacterial antigens in circulating immune complexes of infective endocarditis. *J Clin Invest* 1982;70:271–280.
143. Lambert PH, Dixon FJ, Zubler RH, et al. A WHO collaborative study for the evaluation of eighteen methods for detecting immune complexes in serum. *J Clin Lab Immunol* 1978;1:1–15.
144. McDougal JS, Hubbard M, Strobel PL, et al. Comparison of five assays for immune complexes in the rheumatic diseases: performance characteristics of the assays. *J Lab Clin Med* 1982;100:705–719.
145. Taylor RP, Horgan C, Hooper M, et al. Dynamics of interaction between complement-fixing antibody/dsDNA immune complexes and erythrocytes: *in vitro* studies and potential general applications to clinical immune complex testing. *J Clin Invest* 1985;75:102–111.

CHAPTER 26

Apoptosis and Autoimmunity

John D. Mountz and Tong Zhou

Apoptosis is a physiologic process that mediates the death of selected cells. In contrast to necrosis, which is the result of strong nonspecific or toxic cell injury, apoptosis is initiated by specific ligand/receptor interactions, is tightly coupled to the phagocytosis of the cells that are undergoing apoptosis, and is an active process that requires energy. The morphology of the cell undergoes characteristic changes during apoptosis. The early stages of apoptosis are associated with a reduction in the volume of the cell and its nucleus (1–3). Subsequent alterations in the plasma membrane, including blebbing, precede nuclear condensation and fragmentation (Fig. 26.1). One of the distinctive features of apoptotic cell

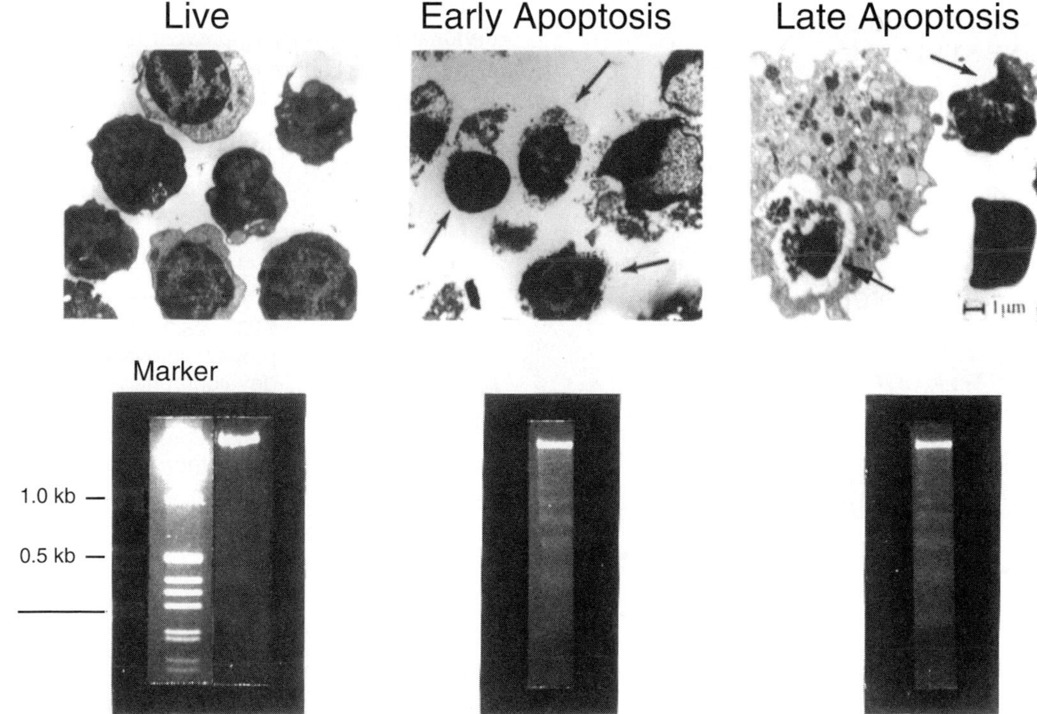

FIG. 26.1. Nuclear condensation, DNA fragmentation, and engulfment of cells during apoptosis. Anti-Fas-treated murine thymocytes were sorted into live, early apoptotic, and late apoptotic cells according to 7-AAD and Annexin V staining, and then further analyzed for characteristics of apoptosis using electron microscopy (×4,200) and agarose gel analysis to detect DNA fragmentation using ethidium bromide staining. Early apoptosis is characterized by nuclear condensation, cell shrinkage (*arrows*), and DNA cleavage. Late apoptotic cells were engulfed by a macrophage (*arrows*) and extensive DNA cleavage to small fragments of less than 200 bp (bottom panels).

death is the degradation of chromosomal DNA by endonucleases into oligomers consisting of multiples of 180 base pairs. This pattern of degradation results in the "ladder" of DNA on gel analysis that is often used as an assay for apoptosis. Apoptosis culminates in fragmentation of cells cultured *in vitro*, whereas the process of apoptosis *in vivo* leads to the rapid clearance of the apoptotic cells before they have undergone fragmentation. Although the clearance of apoptotic cells has been overlooked previously as a contributing factor in autoimmune disease processes, there is now evidence to suggest that engulfment of apoptotic cells may be defective in systemic lupus erythematosus (SLE) (4–6). Several macrophage receptors, including the receptors for phosphatidylserine, thrombospondin (including CD36 and the V_3 integrins), and glycoproteins that have lost terminal sialic acid residues, recognize their respective ligands on cells undergoing apoptosis (7). In lymphocytes, an asymmetric distribution of phospholipids across the plasma membrane is maintained in live cells by an adenosine triphosphate (ATP)-dependent translocase, which specifically transports aminophospholipids from the outer to the inner leaflet of the bilayer. During apoptosis, this enzyme is down-regulated, and a lipid flipsite, termed the scramblase, is activated. Together, these events lead to the appearance of phosphatidylserine, which is recognized by macrophages, on the cell surface of the apoptotic lymphocytes (8,9).

FUNCTION OF APOPTOSIS IN THE IMMUNE SYSTEM

Apoptosis is responsible for the efficient removal of thymocytes and B cells that express inappropriate receptors, including thymocytes that either do not rearrange the T-cell receptor or fail to undergo appropriate positive or negative selection and B cells that do not rearrange immunoglobulin genes normally (Fig. 26.2). Thus, apoptosis plays a key role in shaping the T- and B-cell repertoire (10). In young humans or mice, only approximately 2% of progenitor T cells or B cells develop fully; the other 98% are eliminated by apoptosis during cell development. Thus, apoptosis is responsible for eliminating a majority number of thymocytes, together with an equivalent proportion of B cells. Although most thymocytes undergo apoptosis, they are susceptible to apoptosis for only a brief period, spanning 3 days, that occurs during the early stages of their development. Because the process of apoptosis occurs rapidly, taking only 1 hour to complete, only 1% of thymocytes can be visualized as undergoing apoptosis on analysis of the thymus. Notably, these apoptotic cells are resident within macrophages (11).

Apoptosis also is involved in the removal of immune cells after they have undergone activation and proliferation during a normal immune response, through a process called activation-induced cell death (AICD) (12–16) (Fig. 26.2). This process efficiently removes inflammatory cells that produce proinflammatory cytokines and likely plays a key role in down-regulating the immune response. Thus, defects in AICD, even if minor, could potentially be a contributing factor in chronic autoimmune rheumatic diseases.

Apoptosis also plays an important role in the removal of damaged or senescent immune cells (17–19). Selective deletion of senescent T cells throughout the life of an individual is necessary to prevent the ongoing accumulation of these cells. Failure to clear these cells may affect the immune response and it is therefore of interest that a decline in some aspects of apoptosis function, including the expression and function of Fas, is apparent in T cells obtained

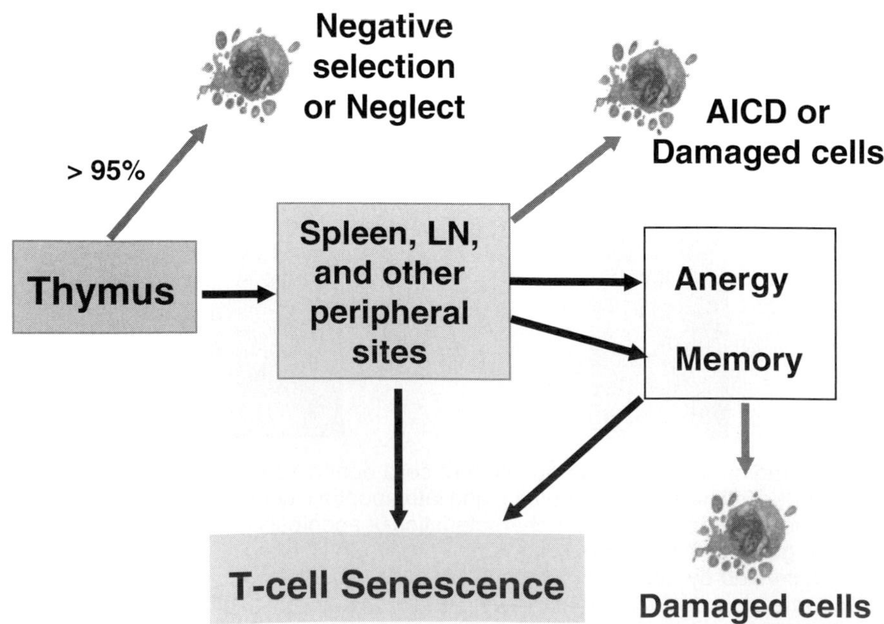

FIG. 26.2. Apoptosis is critical for proper removal of T cells at all stages of development. Apoptosis is responsible for the efficient removal of thymocytes that express inappropriate receptors that either do not rearrange the T-cell receptor or fail to undergo appropriate positive or negative selection. Apoptosis also is involved in the removal of T cells after they have undergone activation and proliferation during a normal immune response, in a process called activation-induced cell death (AICD). This process efficiently removes inflammatory cells producing proinflammatory cytokines and likely plays a key role in down-regulating the immune response. Apoptosis also plays an important role in the removal of damaged or senescent immune cells. Selective deletion of senescent T cells throughout life is necessary to prevent their accumulation.

from aged mice (17). Defective apoptosis, and resulting accumulation of senescent T and B cells, may contribute to late-age predisposition to autoimmune disease and age-associated increases in autoantibody production.

In summary, apoptosis is critical for the appropriate removal of immune cells at all stages of their development. Defects at any one of several points in the complex apoptotic pathways that underlie the removal of inflammatory cells could give rise to a prolonged or autoimmune inflammatory reaction, resulting in a chronic rheumatic disease.

TUMOR NECROSIS FACTOR LIGAND RECEPTOR SUPERFAMILY

The members of the tumor necrosis factor (TNF) receptor superfamily are involved intimately in the regulation of the proliferation and death of immune cells and are of particular interest in relation to their role in immunobiology and the pathogenesis of autoimmune disease (20). The number of receptors, and their corresponding ligands, that are recognized as members of the TNF receptor superfamily has increased rapidly, and the biologic functions of these molecules are now being revealed (Table 26.1). Therapeutic strategies that target members of the TNF receptor superfamily are being used for the treatment of autoimmune disease.

Structurally, the members of the TNF receptor and ligand superfamily share several common features (Fig. 26.3). All members of the receptor family are type I transmembrane proteins with conserved cysteine-rich repeats and a certain degree of homology in the extracellular domain. A subgroup of receptor family members contain a conserved cytoplasmic "death domain," which is responsible for transducing an apoptosis signal. All members of the ligand family are type II transmembrane proteins, which can be expressed in both a membrane-bound and a secreted form. The oligomerization of the receptor as a consequence of interaction with its ligand is required to deliver a functional signal. An immune cell may express either the receptor or ligand alone or express paired receptors and ligands on the cell surface simultaneously. Therefore, the interaction between the receptor and ligand in immune cells can be associated with both autocrine and paracrine responses.

Death Domain Receptors and Autoimmunity

The immunologic functions of most members of the TNF receptor and ligand family have been identified. All of the receptors with an apoptosis-inducing function are involved in the down-modulation of the immune response. One of the most important functions of the death receptors is to mediate the AICD of immune cells. AICD is a highly regulated event that involves several apoptosis signaling molecules, including Fas and the TNF receptor, which are expressed on different cell types, including B cells, T cells, and macrophages (21). The identification of mutations of the murine *fas* and *fas* ligand (*fasL*) genes over a decade ago indicated that the products of these genes are a pair of receptor/ligand molecules that are specialized to carry out the function of apoptosis (22,23). Moreover, the identification of mutated *fas* and *fasL* genes in the autoimmune *lpr/lpr* and *gld/gld* strains of

TABLE 26.1. *Summary of the major TNF ligand-receptor superfamily members that are associated with autoimmune disease*

Ligand	Receptor	Functions and connection with autoimmune disease
TNF-α		Increase in human RA patients
		TNFα transgenic mice develop arthritis spontaneously
	TNFR1 (CD120a)	Promotes apoptosis but also inflammatory response
	TNFR2 (CD120b)	Promotes apoptosis but also inflammatory response
FasL (CD95L, or CD178)		Mutation leads to generalized autoimmune disease in *gld* mice
	Fas (CD95)	Mutation leads to generalized autoimmune disease in *lpr* mice
TRAIL (Apo-2L)		Blockade leads to CIA and EAE
		Upregulation Inhibited the development of CIA
	TRAIL-R1 (DR4)	Induction leads to apoptosis or activation of NFκB and JNK pathways
	TRAIL-R2 (DR5)	Induction leads to apoptosis or activation of NFκB and JNK pathways
	TRAIL-R3 (DcR1)	Does not have a death domain and mainly inhibit apoptosis
	TRAIL-R4 (DcR2)	Has only a partial death domain and does not induce apoptosis
	DcR3	Can bind to FasL and prevent the FasL-mediated apoptosis
TWEAK		Induces apoptosis and costimulation of T cells
	DR3 (TWEAK-R, WSL-1, TRAMP, LARD)	Deficiency leads to abnormal thymocyte negative selection
Unidentified	DR6	Deficiency leads to increased T-cell proliferation and altered Th1 and Th2 response
BAFF (Blys, THANK, TALL-1, zTNF4)		Supports the survival and proliferation of activated B cells
		Blys transgenic mice develop lupus-like autoimmune disease
	TACI	Inhibits B cell activation
	BAFF-R	Deficiency lead to B-cell maturation defects
	BCMA	Does not appear to be crucial for B cell activation

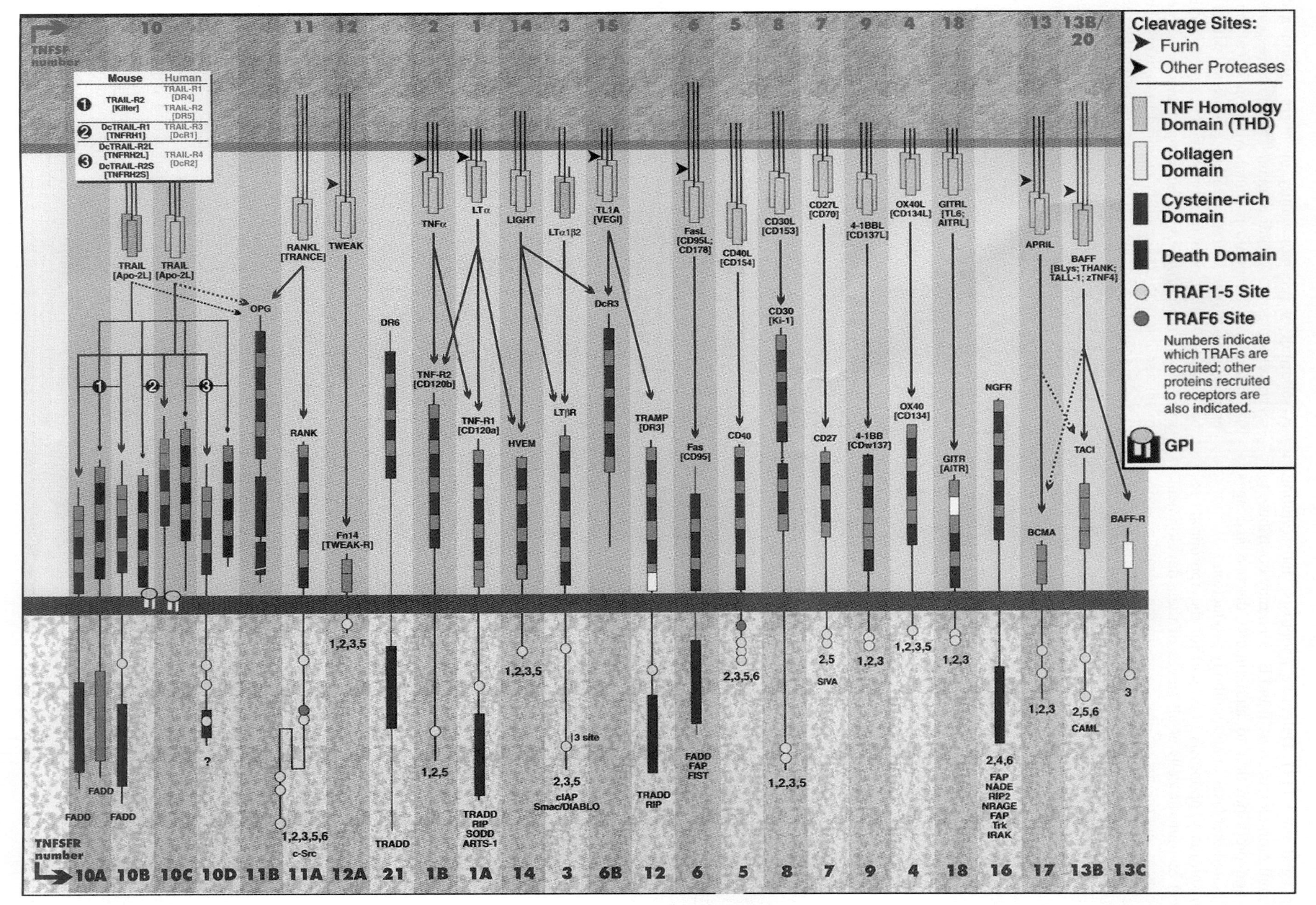

TNFSF number
10
11
12
2
1
14
3
15
6
5
8
7
9
4
18
13
13B/20
Mouse
Human
TRAIL-R2 [Killer]
TRAIL-R1 [DR4]
TRAIL-R2 [DR5]
DcTRAIL-R1 [TNFRH1]
TRAIL-R3 [DcR1]
DcTRAIL-R2L [TNFRH2L]
DcTRAIL-R2S [TNFRH2S]
TRAIL-R4 [DcR2]
TRAIL [Apo-2L]
TRAIL [Apo-2L]
OPG
RANKL [TRANCE]
RANK
TWEAK
Fn14 [TWEAK-R]
DR6
TNFα
TNF-R2 [CD120b]
LTα
TNF-R1 [CD120a]
LIGHT
HVEM
LTα1β2
LTβR
TL1A [VEGI]
DcR3
TRAMP [DR3]
FasL [CD95L; CD178]
Fas [CD95]
CD40L [CD154]
CD40
CD30L [CD153]
CD30 [Ki-1]
CD27L [CD70]
CD27
4-1BBL [CD137L]
4-1BB [CDw137]
OX40L [CD134L]
OX40 [CD134]
GITRL [TL6; AITRL]
GITR [AITR]
NGFR
APRIL
BCMA
BAFF [BLys; THANK; TALL-1; zTNF4]
TACI
BAFF-R
Cleavage Sites:
Furin
Other Proteases
TNF Homology Domain (THD)
Collagen Domain
Cysteine-rich Domain
Death Domain
TRAF1-5 Site
TRAF6 Site
Numbers indicate which TRAFs are recruited; other proteins recruited to receptors are also indicated.
GPI
FADD
FADD
FADD
?
1,2,3,5,6
c-Src
1,2,3,5
TRADD
1,2,5
TRADD
RIP
SODD
ARTS-1
1,2,3,5
3 site
2,3,5
cIAP
Smac/DIABLO
TRADD
RIP
FADD
FAP
FIST
2,3,5,6
1,2,3,5
2,5
SIVA
1,2,3
1,2,3,5
1,2,3
2,4,6
FAP
NADE
RIP2
NRAGE
FAP
Trk
IRAK
1,2,3
2,5,6
CAML
3
TNFSFR number
10A
10B
10C
10D
11B
11A
12A
21
1B
1A
14
3
6B
12
6
5
8
7
9
4
18
16
17
13B
13C

mice, respectively, provided the first evidence that autoimmune disease could result from defective apoptosis of immune cells (24,25). A major function of Fas-mediated apoptosis is in the AICD of T cells, which is critical for maintenance of peripheral T-cell tolerance. On activation, T cells express increased levels of both Fas and Fas ligand, which enables apoptosis to occur in an autocrine fashion (21,26). Studies using a T-cell receptor transgenic mouse model have demonstrated that failure of Fas-mediated apoptosis results in increased production of self-reactive T cells in the periphery (27) and decreased clonal deletion of superantigen-stimulated T cells (28). Other biologic functions of Fas-mediated apoptosis include (a) a role in the immunosurveillance function of cytotoxic T cells and natural killer (NK) cells, both of which express high levels of Fas ligand and mediate apoptosis of virally infected host cells; and (b) a role in immunoprivilege, in which expression of Fas ligand by "immunoprivileged" tissues and organs prevents attack by T cells and other inflammatory cells (21).

Defective apoptosis or reduction in the levels of apoptosis of autoimmune T cells may lead to the development of autoimmune disease, and it was therefore logical to assume that manipulation of the expression of Fas might be an effective therapeutic strategy. The feasibility of this approach has been limited to date, however, by the severe liver toxicity associated with administration of both soluble Fas ligand and agonistic anti-Fas antibodies (29,30). Strategies to avoid toxicity have included the local delivery of the *fasL* gene (31) and the development of monoclonal antibodies that target Fas and induce effects on inflammatory cells selectively, thereby bypassing the associated potential for liver toxicity (32,33).

Both TNF receptor 1 (TNFR1) and TNFR2 are involved in AICD of T cells through their interaction with TNF-α (20). Greatly accelerated lymphadenopathy and autoimmune disease in Fas and TNFRI double-deficient mice suggests that TNFR1 can serve as an alternative pathway to Fas in the induction of activation-induced cell death of T cells (34). TNFR2 has been shown to induce the proliferation of submaximally-activated naive cells, but apoptosis late in the activation process (35,36). Teh et al. (37) showed that $CD8^+$ T cells are resistant to AICD if they do not express TNFR2. A recent study by Elzey et al. (38) demonstrated that $TNFR2^{-/-}$ T cells did not undergo apoptosis when placed in the eyes of normal mice, whereas normal and $TNFR1^{-/-}$ T cells underwent apoptosis. *In vitro,* TNF enhanced the Fas-mediated apoptosis of unactivated T cells through decreased intracellular levels of Fas-associated death domain-like interleukin-1β (IL-1β)-converting enzyme (FLICE) inhibitory protein (FLIP) and increased production of the proapoptotic molecule Bax. This effect was mediated through the TNFR2 receptor.

The Tumor Necrosis Factor-Related Apoptosis-Inducing Ligand and Its Receptors

The TNF-related apoptosis-inducing ligand (TRAIL), another member of the TNF superfamily (39), has an apoptosis-inducing activity that is equivalent to that of TNF-α and Fas ligand. TRAIL has been of particular interest in the development of therapeutics because it differs from TNF-α and Fas ligand in that it induces apoptosis of tumor cells preferentially, with little or no effect on normal cells (40). At least five receptors for TRAIL have been identified, two of which, DR4 (TRAIL-R1) and DR5 (TRAIL-R2), are capable of transducing an apoptosis signal (41–43), whereas the other three [TRAIL-R3, -R4, and osteoprotegerim (OPG)] serve as decoy receptors to block TRAIL-mediated apoptosis (44–46). All five receptors for TRAIL share significant homology in their extracellular ligand–binding domain.

Recent studies indicate that defective TRAIL-mediated apoptosis has the potential to contribute to the development of autoimmune disease. Blockade of TRAIL-mediated apoptosis with the soluble receptor DR5 (47,48) has been shown to significantly increase the susceptibility of mice to collagen-induced arthritis and experimental allergic encephalitis. DR5 is of great interest because it is selectively expressed by abnormally-proliferating pathogenic cells. Selective targeting of DR5 may induce apoptosis of autoimmune cells.

A role for TRAIL-mediated apoptosis in AICD of T cells has been proposed (49,50), and the newly identified DR3

FIG. 26.3. The tumor necrosis factor (TNF) superfamily of ligands and receptors. The identified members of the TNF receptor superfamily (TNFSFR), as indicated in Table 26.1, include Fas, TNF receptor 1 (TNFR1) and TNFR2; cytoplasmic avian leukosis–sarcoma virus receptor (CAR)-1; death receptor (DR)3, DR4, DR5, and DR6; lymphotoxin (LT)βR; CD40; CD30; CD27; CDw137; OX40; glucocorticoid-induced TNF receptor (GITR); nerve growth factor receptor (NGFR); B-cell maturation antigen (BCMA); transmembrane activator and calcium modulator cyclophilin ligand interactor (TACI); and B cell–activating factor receptor (BAFFR). The decoy receptor (DCR)1/TRAIL receptor without an intracellular domain (TRID) does not have a death domain but binds to TNFR apoptosis inducing ligand (TRAIL). The extracellular region of these receptors carries two to six repeats of a cystine-rich subdomain that have approximately 25% homology. For example, Fas has three cystine-rich subdomains and TNFR1 has four such subdomains. The intracytoplasmic death domain is shown by the rectangular box, and the different TRAF sites are shown by different color-coated circles. (Modified and adapted from the ALEXIS Immunology catalog, with permission of the ALEXIS Platform, San Diego, CA).

(51) and DR6 (52) death receptors are likely to be involved in the regulation of the T-cell response. DR3 knockout mice exhibit abnormal negative selection in the thymus (53), and DR6 knockout mice exhibit an increased T-cell proliferative response and an imbalance in the helper T cell subset 1 (T_H1) and T_H2 responses (54).

Many receptors in the TNF receptor superfamily exhibit more than one function, in that they are able to induce apoptosis, but also can act as costimulatory molecules. For example, although TNFR1 and TNFR2 are capable of inducing cell death, they also can act to promote an inflammatory response. Previous studies have demonstrated that TNF receptor $p55^{-/-}p75^{-/-}$ double knockout mice are resistant to the development of experimental autoimmune myasthenia gravis induced by acetylcholine receptor immunizations (55) and MOG(35–55)-induced experimental autoimmune encephalomyelitis (EAE) (56). Similarly, the lymphotoxin-β receptor is capable of inducing cell death (57) but is also important for lymphoid organ development (58). In addition, a recently identified DR3 ligand can induce apoptosis of tumor cells and act as a costimulator of T cells.

In contrast to the death receptors, the survival receptors of the TNF receptor superfamily function as costimulatory molecules to stimulate activation and proliferation of immune cells. Despite the absence of the death domain, such molecules also may serve dual roles. For example, CD30 may serve as a pro-apoptosis receptor mediating cell death during thymic negative selection (59). Similarly, the interaction between CD27 and CD27L promotes both T-cell proliferation and the generation of cytotoxic T cell responses (60,61).

The interaction between the survival molecules CD40 and CD40L is required for T-dependent B-cell responses and for the immunoglobulin isotype switch. Thus, blockade of CD40/CD40L is under evaluation as a therapy for SLE and other autoimmune diseases (62,63). The newly identified herpes viral entry mediator interacts with its ligand, LIGHT, to costimulate T-cell proliferation in an autocrine fashion (64–66), and T cells expressing transgenic LIGHT exhibit hyperproliferation (67).

Taken together, these recent observations indicate the importance of individual death and survival receptors in the regulation of the immune response. They also emphasize the necessity for a full understanding of the molecular mechanisms in play because many of these molecules appear to have the capacity to mediate differential signaling and profoundly different outcomes depending on cell context. Given this caveat, these receptor/ligand interactions are excellent potential therapeutic targets for the treatment of autoimmune disease.

B Lymphocyte Stimulator and Its Receptor

B-lymphocyte stimulator (BLyS), a new member of the TNF superfamily, is also known as TALL-1 (TNF and apoptosis ligand-related leukocyte-expressed ligand 1), BAFF (B-cell activating factor belonging to the TNF family), THANK (TNF homologue that activates apoptosis, nuclear factor αB, and c-Jun NH_2-terminal kinase), and zTNF4 (68–72). BLyS is produced in both membrane-bound and secreted forms primarily by the cells of the myeloid lineage (73). In BLyS knockout mice, the numbers of mature B cells are decreased dramatically, marginal zone and follicular B cells are absent, and B-cell maturation is blocked at a transitional stage between the T1 and T2 types of immature B cells (74), indicating that BLyS is a crucial survival factor for B-cell development and maturation. BLyS also is essential for the effective induction of the antigen-specific antibody response. Treatment of immunized mice *in vivo* with a soluble BLyS receptor (TACI) inhibits the antibody response to both T-dependent and T-independent antigens and prevents the formation of the germinal centers (75). Moreover, exogenous BLyS augments B-cell proliferation induced by anti–immunoglobulin M (anti-IgM) *in vitro*, and treatment of mice with BLyS *in vivo* results in B-cell hyperplasia and elevated serum levels of immunoglobulins (68). These results suggest that BLyS supports the survival and proliferation of activated B cells.

At least three receptors for BLyS, known as transmembrane activator and calcium modulator cyclophilin ligand interactor (TACI), B cell maturation antigen (BCMA), and BAFF-R, have been identified. All three BLyS receptors are expressed primarily on cells of the B-cell lineage (72,75–79). Although BLyS binds to all three receptors with a similar affinity, the contribution of each receptor to B-cell function is quite different, as demonstrated by the results generated using receptor knockout mice. TACI knockout mice exhibit higher numbers of B cells and enhanced B-cell reactivity compared with wild-type mice (80,81). Thus, TACI most likely functions to inhibit B-cell activation and contributes to the maintenance of immunologic homeostasis. The BCMA-deficient mice that have been generated do not show significant defects in B-cell development or maturation, suggesting that it is unlikely that BCMA plays a crucial role in B-cell activation (82). BAFF-R, however, appears to be absolutely essential for the biologic function of BLyS. A/WySnJ mice, in which the *BAFF-R* locus is disrupted, exhibit a B-cell maturation deficiency (83). Notably, this phenotype is similar to that of BLyS-deficient mice.

BLyS and its receptors play a crucial role in B-cell development and survival. Defective expression of BlyS (74) and its principal receptor, BAFF-R (83), results in profound B-cell deficiency, whereas overexpression of BLyS leads to the development of a lupuslike autoimmune disease (84, 85). The BLyS transgenic mice develop a lupuslike autoimmune disease in which 100% of the mice are positive for circulating autoantibodies. The pattern of specificity of the autoantibodies is similar to that seen in SLE and includes rheumatoid factor, anti–double-stranded DNA (anti-dsDNA) antibodies, and anti–nuclear protein antibodies. All of the mice develop glomerulonephritis with aging, characterized by deposition of immune complexes in the kidney. Similarly, hyperimmunoglobulinemia occurs in all of the BLyS transgenic mice. Severe hyperplasia of the secondary lymphoid organs with marked accumulation of B cells and expansion of B-cell populations in the spleen and lymph nodes is notable (84,85). Thus, early and persistent overexpression of BLyS may result in loss of B-cell tolerance, autoantibody production, and the development of systemic autoimmune disease.

Regulation of Apoptosis Signaling

Functionally, the members of the TNF receptor superfamily can deliver signals leading to either apoptosis or proliferation and survival. The differentiation of function between cell death and proliferation depends on the type of cell and its functional status. The receptors of the superfamily share signal transduction pathways, with the apoptosis signal transduction being mediated through the Fas-associated death domain (FADD)/caspase 8 cascade, and the stimulatory signal transduction being mediated primarily by TNF receptor–associated factors and the nuclear factor κB (NFκB) pathway. The balanced expression of the death receptors and the survival receptors on immune cells and their appropriate signaling maintains the homeostasis of the immune system. Flexibility in the regulation of this homeostasis is provided by the dual function of some of the receptors. The intracellular segments of both DR4 and DR5 contain a death domain, and can transduce an apoptosis signal through a FADD- and caspase 8–dependent pathway (86); in addition, both of these receptors also can activate an NFκB and JNK pathway (41,87,88).

The family of *Bcl-2*-related proteins also function as regulators of apoptosis (Fig. 26.4). These molecules share homology at four conserved Bcl-2 homology (BH1–4) domain regions, which control the ability of these proteins to dimerize and affect apoptosis. The conserved domains BH1, BH2, and BH3 participate in the formation of various dimer pairs as well as the regulation of cell death (89). The Bcl-2 family includes the death antagonists Bcl-2, Bcl-X_L, Mcl-1, and A1, as well as the proapoptotic molecules Bax, Bcl-X_s, Bak, Bik, Bid, Bim, and Bad (90,91). The overall ratio of the death agonists to antagonists determines the susceptibility to a death stimulus. Bcl-X_L, Bcl-2, and Bax

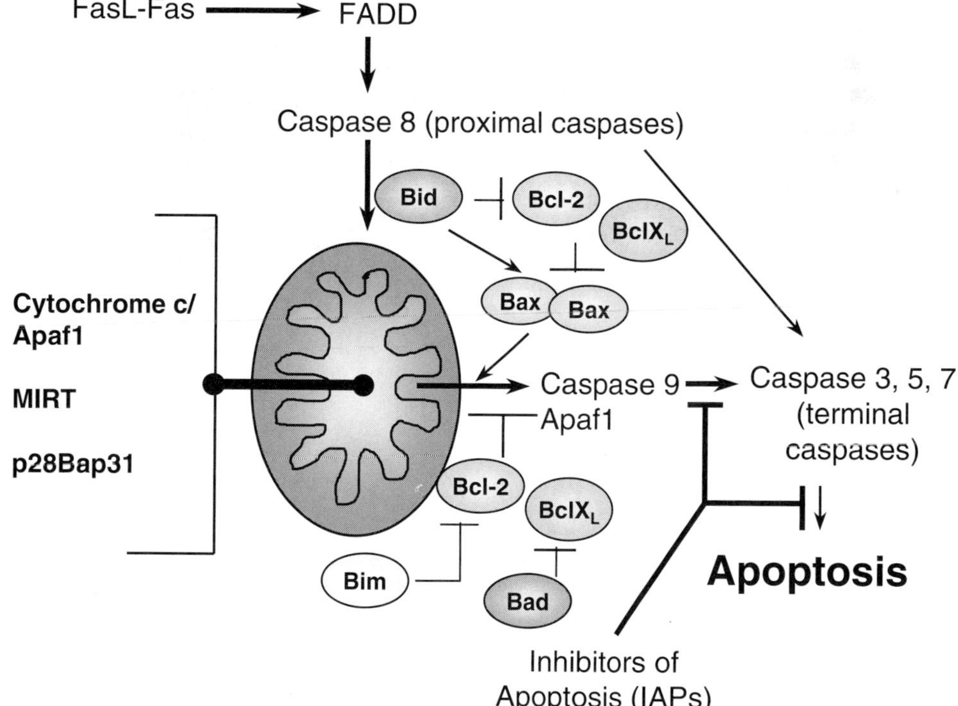

FIG. 26.4. Members of the Bcl-2 family of proteins: protein/protein interactions among Bcl-2 family members regulate apoptosis function. Activated caspase 8 is regulated by Bcl-2 family members and mitochondrial signaling. Active caspase 8 directly activates BH-3 interacting death domain (BID). *Bax* can form homodimers or heterodimers with either Bcl-2 or Bcl-X_L. Formation of Bax homodimers promotes cell death, whereas Bax heterodimerization with either Bcl-2 or Bcl-X_L blocks cell death. Bad, a proapoptotic Bcl-2 family member, heterodimerizes with Bcl-2 and Bcl-X_L and promotes cell death. Bid can be directly activated by Fas to promote cell death. It has been suggested that members of the Bcl-2 family play a role in mitochondrial ion channel formation and promote the release of cytochrome c from mitochondria. *FADD,* Fas-associated death domain protein.

also can form ion-conductive pores in artificial membranes. Bcl-2 and Bcl-X_L display a reciprocal pattern of expression during lymphocyte development.

Bid and Bad possess the minimal death domain BH3, and the phosphorylation of Bad at Ser112, Ser136, and Ser155 residue connects proximal survival signals to the Bcl-2 family. In contrast, the dephosphorylated (active) form of Bad binds to prosurvival Bcl-2 family members in the mitochondria. The binding of Bad to prosurvival Bcl-2 proteins is followed by the oligomerization of the proapoptotic Bcl-2 proteins Bax and Bak, which results in mitochondrial dysfunction, cytochrome *c* release, caspase activation, and apoptotic death (92,93).

T-cell apoptosis is associated with sequential activation of the caspases, which cleave after Asp residues, beginning with caspase 8 (Fig. 26.4). Caspases are expressed constitutively in most cells, residing in the cytosol as a single-chain proenzyme. These are activated to fully functional proteases by an initial proteolytic cleavage that divides the chain into large and small caspase subunits and a second cleavage that removes the N-terminal domain (prodomain). Inefficient activation of caspase 8 results in direct activation of Bid, a proapoptotic member of the Bcl-2 family, and the C-terminal fragment of Bid acts on mitochondria, triggering cytochrome *c* release (94–96). The released cytochrome *c* binds to apoptotic protease activating factor-1 (Apaf-1), which self-associates and binds to and activates caspase 9 (97). This is associated with a decrease in inner mitochondria membrane potential corresponding to the opening of the inner membrane permeability transition (PT) pore complex and loss of the ability to take up certain dyes (98). In immune cells in which this mitochondrial amplification loop is important, antiapoptotic Bcl-2 family members can suppress Fas-induced apoptosis (99). Bcl-2 and Bcl-X_L act to prevent cytochrome *c* release and thus interfere with this pathway.

Activated caspase 9 and 8 then act on the terminal caspases 3, 5, and 7 that are activated immediately before cell death (100). Strong signaling through the Fas receptor can lead directly to high levels of activated caspase 8 activity and immediate activation of terminal caspases 3, 6, and 7, resulting in the death of the cell (101–105).

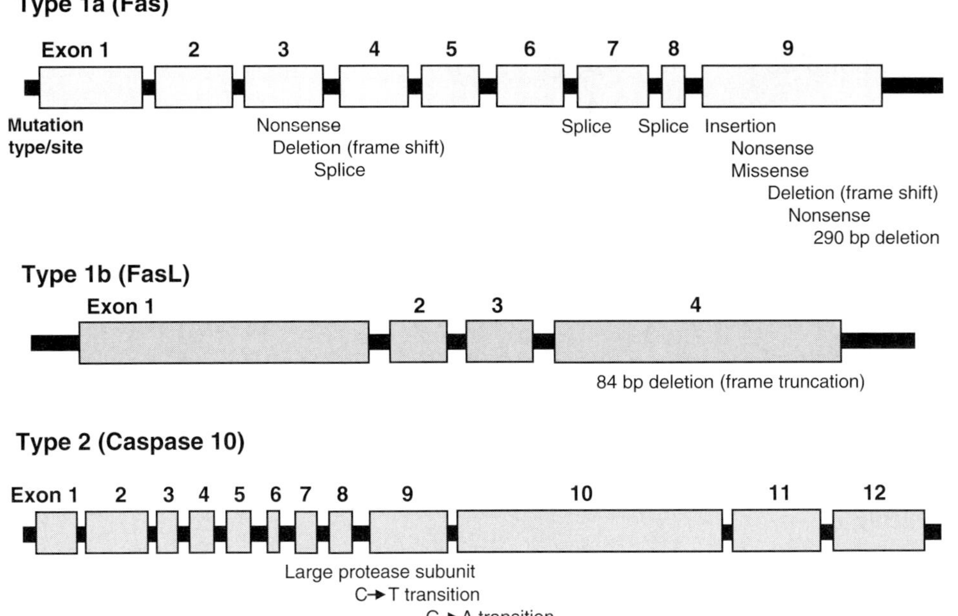

FIG. 26.5. Mutations of Fas-mediated apoptosis genes that have been identified to date in patients with autoimmune lymphoproliferative syndrome (ALPS) and systemic lupus erythematosus (SLE). The localization and type of mutations in patients are depicted below the exon drawing. **Top**: Distinct *Fas* mutations have been identified in patients with ALPS type IA that involve both the extracellular domain (ED) as well as the death domain (DD). Shown is the genomic organization of *Fas* with nine exons, including a transmembrane exon (exon 6) and a death domain, which is entirely encoded within exon 9. All of the mutations to date are single-nucleotide changes, except for a 290-bp homozygous deletion in exon 9 found in a severely affected daughter of related parents in a French study (217). **Center:** A patient with a mutation of Fas ligand is referred to as having ALPS type 1-B. The Fas ligand gene in this patient contained a 28–amino acid deletion within exon 4. **Bottom**: Caspase 10 mutation in two kindreds with ALPS type II. The first patient carries a C-to-T transition predicted to replace a leucine with phenylalanine in the p17 large subunit of the protease. The second patient carries a G-to-A transition predicted to replace a valine with an isoleucine, seven amino acids downstream of the QACQG active site in the p17 large subunit of the Caspase 10 gene (117).

The inhibitor of apoptosis (*IAP*) gene products play an evolutionarily conserved role in regulating programmed cell death in diverse species ranging from insects to humans. Human XIAP, cIAP1, and cIAP2 directly inhibit caspase 3, 6, and 7 (106–109). The IAPs also can block cytochrome *c*–induced activation of pro–caspase 9 and inhibit Fas-mediated apoptosis (105). The murine homologue of the human X-linked IAP, called miap, has been mapped to the X chromosome (110). We previously (111) showed that XIAP was up-regulated by TNF-α in rheumatoid arthritis synovial fibroblasts (RASF), and this up-regulation was inhibited using a dominant negative form of the inhibitor of nuclear factor κB (IκB) plus TNF-α. XIAP is an inhibitor of apoptosis after TNF-α signaling because transfection of primary RASF with an XIAP antisense adenovirus promoted apoptosis of RASF. Therefore, XIAP is a TNF-α-inducible specific inhibitor of apoptosis in RASF. This and other modulators of the TNF receptor or the Fas apoptosis pathway may be therapeutically beneficial in facilitating apoptosis of synovial tissue in patients with RA.

Autoimmune Lymphoproliferative Syndrome

More than 30 years ago, Canale and Smith, as well as others, reported a condition characterized by nonmalignant lymphadenopathy associated with autoimmune features in children (112). In humans, autoimmune lymphoproliferative syndrome (ALPS) is defined by functional analysis of lymphocyte sensitivity to Fas-induced apoptosis *in vitro*. The ALPS condition is characterized by splenomegaly or lymphadenopathy, autoimmune manifestations, hypergammaglobulinemia and $CD4^{-}CD8^{-}$ T cells in blood. T cells from ALPS patients can exhibit a complete deficiency in *Fas* (ALPS 0) due to genetic mutations of both Fas alleles. Other patients exhibit a partial Fas-induced apoptosis defect associated with normal or slightly reduced Fas expression due to an intrinsic Fas defect (ALPS type IA) (113–115) (Fig. 26.5) or a defect in the Fas signaling pathway (ALPS type II). Different mutation in caspase 10 have been shown to cause ALPS syndrome in two patients (ALPS type II) (116). ALPS not associated with a Fas-induced apoptosis defect can be due to a Fas ligand deficiency (ALPS type IB). We have identified one patient with ALPS type IB who has a mutation of *FasL* and lymphoproliferative disease and also exhibits an AICD defect of peripheral blood mononuclear cells (PBMCs) (117). In ALPS III, lymphocytes of patients exhibit a normal Fas/FasL pathway despite a typical ALPS phenotype, and no molecular basis has yet been established. Interestingly, although the type IA ALPS patients studied and one of their parents all are heterozygous for a mutation of *Fas,* the parents do not develop ALPS. Mice that are heterozygous for mutations of *Fas* (*lpr*/+) or *Fas* ligand (*gld*/+) do not develop lymphoproliferative disease. The mutant Fas molecules produced in the heterozygous mice act as dominant negatives and prevent functional trimer formation (117).

APOPTOSIS AND AUTOIMMUNE DISEASE

Based on experiments in *lpr* and *gld* mice that develop systemic autoimmune disease, the authors first proposed that humans with autoimmune disease may exhibit defects in apoptosis or AICD (118). In contrast to the studies of patients with ALPS syndrome, most studies of patients with SLE have indicated higher levels of apoptosis and AICD of PBMCs than found in controls. Accelerated *in vitro* apoptosis of PBMCs from patients with SLE was first reported by Emlen et al. (119), who found a 2.3-fold higher level of spontaneous apoptosis of lymphocytes from patients with SLE compared with normal controls. Other investigators then reported that PBMCs from patients with SLE exhibit higher levels of apoptosis after AICD (120) than controls. In contrast, short-term established T-cell lines from patients with SLE exhibit lower levels of anti-CD3-mediated AICD, which could be blocked in both control and SLE T cells by an IgG anti-*Fas* antibody (121). The analysis of activation pathways in SLE must take into account not only the differences between *in vitro* and *in vivo* environments, but also the mechanisms of activation of T cells. Different subpopulations of T cells may be more or less susceptible to AICD. The greater susceptibility to anti-CD3-induced apoptosis of $CD28^{+}$ T cells in patients with SLE than controls is consistent with loss of the peripheral T cells that express high levels of CD28 that is seen in patients with SLE (122). T cells from patients with SLE express increased levels of functional *Fas* ligand after anti-CD3 signaling (123,124). These types of experiments are normally performed by using T-cell receptor signaling of T cells from patients with SLE and normal controls, and testing these T cells using a chromium 51–labeled *Fas*-expressing target cell. There is an important distinction between membrane-bound Fas ligand, as determined by functional assays, and soluble Fas ligand, as can be measured in sera, in that soluble Fas ligand is an inhibitor of Fas-mediated apoptosis (125).

Although the Fas death domain family of molecules is the primary pathway for elimination of inflammatory cells, defects in these death domain molecules are observed only rarely in patients with SLE. Expression of the apoptotic ligands TRAIL, TNF-like weak inducer of apoptosis (TWEAK), and Fas ligand have been reported to mediate the autologous monocyte death induced by lupus T cells. This cytotoxicity is associated with increased expression of these molecules on activated T cells, rather than with an increased susceptibility of lupus monocytes to apoptosis induced by these ligands (126). Despite reported differences in apoptosis pathway molecules in SLE, defects in clonal deletion and tolerance induction have been difficult to analyze in humans with SLE. First, in contrast to experiments using TCR transgenic mice, self-reactive T cells in humans cannot be identified. Autoreactive T cells are only a small fraction of the activated T-cell population and have been made readily visible for the first time only through the use of TCR transgenic mice. Second, tolerance experiments such as introduction of a self-reactive T-cell or neonatal tolerance cannot be conducted in humans. Experimental studies of human PBMCs must resort to the analysis of the total population of T cells that express multiple specificities. Therefore, it has not been possible to determine whether there is a defect in AICD of a minor population of T cells with autoreactive specificities. The future direction and challenges in this area are to obtain T cells from patients with autoimmune diseases in which the autoreactive specificity is known, such as myelin basic protein–autoreactive T cells in patients with multiple sclerosis. This approach may now be feasible in that the class I or class II major histocompatibility complex (MHC) molecule tetramer system may be used to identify such T cells (127). Analysis of defective or normal AICD of these T cells should help clarify whether there is an AICD defect in autoreactive T cells in humans with autoimmune disease.

BLyS and Human Autoimmune Disease

High levels of BLyS have been found in serum samples from patients with SLE and rheumatoid arthritis (RA). The levels of BLyS in the sera of patients with SLE are significantly higher than those of healthy controls (128). The levels of BLyS also are elevated in the sera of patients with RA, with the levels of BLyS being even higher in the synovial fluid (129,130). The levels of BLyS in the sera of normal controls were approximately 5 ng/mL or less, whereas the levels in more than 30% of the SLE patients were greater than 10 ng/mL, with more than 10% of the patients having levels greater than 20 ng/mL. In a few patients, the BLyS levels were as high as 100 ng/mL. The data generated thus far suggest that higher serum levels of BLyS are associated with higher titers of anti-dsDNA and anti-Sm antibodies (128). Other investigators have examined the levels of BLyS in the sera of 195 patients with SLE, RA, and other rheumatic diseases, and found that 21% of these patients had significantly high levels of BLyS, and that high levels of BLyS correlated with high levels of IgG, anti-dsDNA antibody, and rheumatoid factors (131). More recently, we measured the serum levels of BLyS in 49 patients with primary's Sjögren's syndrome (SS), an autoimmune disease in which patients exhibit high levels of B-cell activation and autoantibody production. The serum levels of BLyS in patients with SS were significantly higher than those of healthy controls. Importantly, the high BLyS levels in the patients with SS patients correlated well with the titer of anti-SSA antibody, an autoantibody characteristic of SS, and with rheumatoid factor (132). The results of these studies are promising in that they suggest a link between levels of circulating BLyS and autoimmune disease. The results of further analysis of the correlation with disease activity will be of great interest.

Soluble Fas Is Correlated with Organ Damage

We have isolated chromosomal DNA for the human *fas* gene and characterized the intron/exon organization as well as the promoter region (133). A naturally-occurring, soluble, alternatively spliced form of human Fas that is capable of binding to Fas ligand and inhibiting apoptosis was then identified (134,135). Soluble Fas is normally present at serum levels of 0.2 to 2.0 ng/mL, and despite original controversy (136,137), is now known to be elevated in the sera of patients with SLE (138–143). Soluble Fas may play a role in both immune regulation and the regulation of FasL-mediated tissue damage in SLE (144). Levels of soluble Fas were quantitated in 39 patients with varying degrees of disease activity and disease severity over a period of 4 years (277 visits). Healthy age- and sex-matched volunteers served as controls. The Systemic Lupus Erythematosus Disease Activity Index (SLEDAI) scores of disease activity were measured, as were the Systemic Lupus International Collaborating Clinics/American College of Rheumatology (SLICC/ACR) scores of accumulative organ damage. The levels of autoantibodies and complement in the sera were determined and liver and kidney function tests performed. Levels of soluble Fas were elevated in the sera of patients with SLE (0.60 ng/mL) compared with controls (0.26 ng/mL). The levels of soluble Fas were found to correlate with the SLICC/ACR damage index, but not with the SLEDAI. In addition, soluble Fas levels correlated strongly with liver and renal function tests, including measurement of serum albumin, serum aspartate aminotransferase (AST), serum creatinine, and creatinine clearance, but did not correlate with inflammatory activity, as assessed by the erythrocyte sedimentation rate and serum levels of acute-phase reactants. These results corroborate the theory that serum levels of soluble Fas are elevated in patients with SLE. Because the levels of soluble Fas in the serum correlate with indices of organ damage but not with disease activity, we suggest that soluble Fas might be a marker of organ damage in SLE. We propose that, in patients with SLE, soluble Fas is produced primarily at sites of organ damage to counter the adverse effects of Fas ligand expression. These results are consistent with previous reports that increased levels of soluble Fas are associated with liver disease.

Bcl-2 and Interleukin-10

Many (145–147), but not all (148), investigators have reported high levels of Bcl-2 protein in circulating T cells or in PBMCs from patients with SLE. IL-10 has been shown to promote AICD in SLE patients, and it appears that the elevated spontaneous cell death *in vitro* results from *in vitro* T-cell activation and induction of IL-10 and Fas ligand (149). A genetic linkage has been reported between *IL-10* and *Bcl-2* genotypes and susceptibility to SLE (150). Short, tandem repeat sequences (microsatellites) within the noncoding region of these genes have been identified and used as genetic markers. This information has been used to examine a large Mexican-American cohort of 128 SLE patients and 223 ethnically matched controls (150). The DNA was analyzed using fluorescent-labeled primers and semiautomatic genotyping. The results of this study revealed a synergistic effect between susceptible alleles of *Bcl-2* and *IL-10* in determination of disease susceptibility, with inheritance of two alleles together increasing the odds of developing SLE by more than 40-fold (150). This is the first time a combination of two distinct genes that regulate apoptosis has been found to predispose humans to an autoimmune disease (151).

Decreased Clearance of Apoptotic Cells and Production of Autoantigens

More severe SLE disease is associated with a polymorphism of FcγRIII (CD16) (152), which alters the function of this receptor and predisposes to autoimmune disease. Patients with this polymorphism have more severe disease, as well as a greater level of NK cell activation and more rapid induction of AICD. There is a strong association of lupus nephritis with this low-binding Fc receptor phenotype. Despite a clear role for FcγRIII and decreased clearance of immune complexes, a clear relationship between Fc receptors and phagocytosis of apoptotic cells has yet to be established. The adherence of leukocytes to cells undergoing apoptosis has been reported to be dependent on $\alpha_{\nu}\beta_3$ (CD51/CD61, vitronectin receptor), CD36 (thrombospondin receptor), macrophage class A scavenger receptor, phosphatidyl serine translocated to the outer leaflet of apoptotic membranes, and CD14 (LPS-binding protein) (7). Defects in these clearance mechanisms have not yet been reported in patients with SLE; however, *in vitro* phagocytosis of autologous apoptotic cells in culture with PBMCs has been found to be defective in patients with SLE (5,6,153).

A high number of apoptotic cells or fragments of apoptotic cells in patients with SLE could be due to increased apoptosis. High levels of circulating apoptotic PBMCs and autoantigens resulting from abnormally increased apoptosis have been observed by many investigators in patients with SLE (4,5,154–156). Apoptotic cells among PBMCs from patients with SLE have been analyzed by annexin-V-FITC staining and flow cytometry and compared with the results generated using normal controls. No correlation was found between the percentage of apoptotic cells and either the Systemic Lupus Activity Measure (SLAM) score or therapy. It is possible, however, that the persistently circulating apoptotic waste may encounter inflammatory removal pathways and serve as an immunogen for the induction of autoreactive lymphocytes and as an antigen in immune complex formation (Fig. 26.6).

Apoptosis in the PBMCs of patients with SLE is associated with the generation of novel autoantigens. *In vivo*, the nucleosomes that are generated during apoptosis may lead to the production of antinucleosomal antibodies (4,5,155). In addition, protein fragments are generated during apoptosis through the activation of caspases. The cell surface blebbing of apoptotic cells constitutes a potentially autoantigenic particle in SLE (157). Apoptosis is associated with translocation of the phosphatidyl serine from the inner membrane leaflet to the outer membrane leaflet. Phosphatidyl serine is a potent procoagulant, and also can lead to generation of antiphospholipid antibodies (157–159). Different apoptotic stimuli, including Fas ligation, gamma radiation, and ultraviolet light irradiation, but not anti-CD3 ligation, lead to the generation of several distinct serine phosphorylated proteins (160–163). This protein phosphorylation precedes, or is coincident, with the induction of DNA fragmentation related to apoptosis. More than 75% of patients with SLE who produce antinuclear antibodies also produce antibodies to these novel phosphorylated proteins (164). A 72-kd signal recognition particle (SRP) protein is cleaved to a 66-kd amino-terminal fragment by caspase 3 and is an autoantigen in some patients with SLE (164). Therefore, proteins that are newly phosphorylated during apoptosis may be targets for autoantibody production in patients with SLE.

Treatment of Autoimmune Disease in Mice by Targeting Apoptosis Pathways

Human studies using direct signaling of apoptosis receptors have not been undertaken, to date, due to the risk of induction of apoptosis of normal cells. Mouse models of autoimmune disease have been used to develop and evaluate strategies that target apoptosis as a therapy for autoimmune disease.

Antigen presenting cells (APCs) play an important role in both the initiation of the T-cell response and the induction of T-cell tolerance. Many proposed treatments of autoimmune disease target the interaction between the APCs and T cells by modification of autoantigen processing by APCs and blockade of costimulation. Although autocrine suicide of the T cells is a major function of Fas-mediated apoptosis of T cells, the capacity of Fas ligand to mediate immune privilege function indicates that apoptosis of T cells also can occur in a paracrine fashion. Thus, the apoptosis-inducing capability of APCs may represent an essential component in the regulation of the immune response and might play a critical role in the induction and maintenance of T-cell tolerance. It is well established that a full T-cell activation response requires that the T cells receive two signals from APCs: one generated by the interaction between the TCR and the antigen complexed with the MHC molecules of APCs and the second one generated by pairs of costimulatory molecules on T cells and APCs. In the absence of costimulation, T cells become anergic, a mechanism by which T-cell tolerance is achieved. We propose that in the presence of an apoptosis-inducing molecule such as Fas ligand on APCs, the T cells are depleted. Because T cells interact directly with APCs during immune

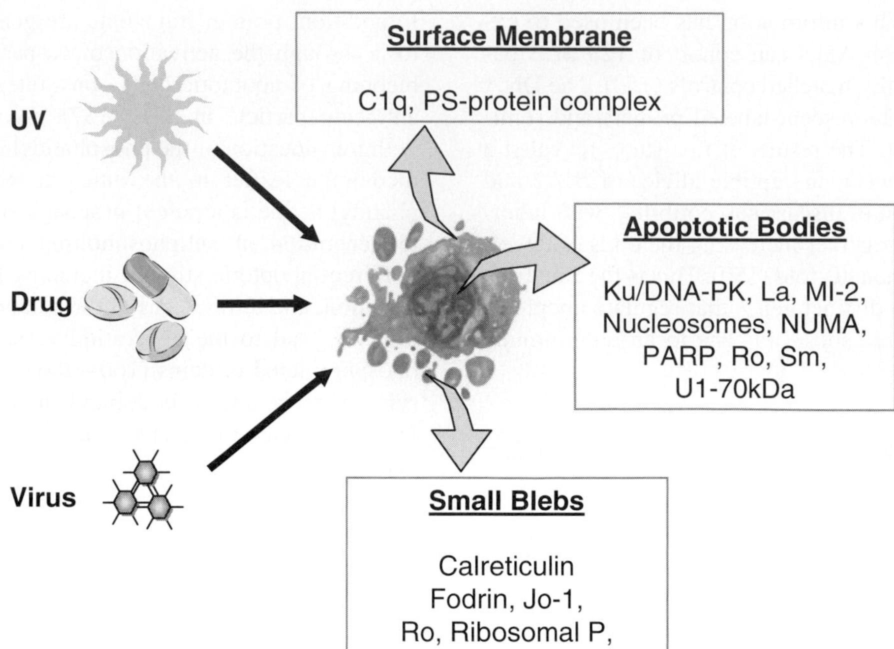

FIG. 26.6. Reduced clearance of antigen–antibody complexes in systemic lupus erythematosus (SLE). Different environmental stimuli or toxins including ultraviolet (UV) light, drugs, or viruses can induce apoptosis of cells and release previously sequestered antigens or newly generated antigens that are derived from (a) small blebs of plasma membrane that include endoplasmic reticulum and cytoskeletal components; (b) apoptotic bodies, including nucleoli; and (c) several autoantigens that become modified (e.g., by cleavage) during apoptosis. Apoptosis is associated with translocation of the phosphatidyl serine from the inner membrane leaflet to the outer membrane leaflet. Phosphatidyl serine is a potent procoagulant, and can lead to generation of antiphospholipid antibodies. When the normal clearance of apoptotic cells somehow is disturbed, such modified antigens might become exposed to the immune system. Failure to clear these antigens in an efficient manner might then lead to autoimmunization and the production of autoantibodies.

responses, Fas ligand–expressing APCs would only induce apoptosis in the responding activated T cells. Consequently, T-cell tolerance induced by this mechanism should be antigen specific. To test this hypothesis, the researchers examined whether allogeneic APCs that express Fas ligand are capable of inducing T-cell tolerance that is specific for the alloantigen being presented by APCs (165,166). Using H-2D^b/HY TCR transgenic mice, the researchers examined the extent and timing of antigen-specific clonal deletion of T cells by Fas ligand–expressing APCs. The Fas ligand–expressing APCs induced a rapid and much more efficient clonal deletion of antigen-specific T cells than that observed when AICD was induced (166). In animal models of autoimmune disease, the administration of Fas ligand–expressing APCs has been found to be effective in the treatment of several T cell–mediated autoimmune diseases, including post-murine cytomegalovirus (MCMV) infection–induced sialadenitis in *gld* mice (166), post-mycoplasma infection–induced arthritis in *gld* mice (167), and the collagen II–induced arthritis (CIA) of DBA/1j mice (168). In a parallel approach, we were able to deliver TRAIL *in vivo* using collagen II–pulsed dendritic cells (DCs) that had been transfected with a novel adenovirus system that was engineered to exhibit inducible TRAIL under the control of the doxycycline-inducible tetracycline response element. CIA-susceptible DBA/1j mice that were treated with these engineered DCs exhibited a significantly lower incidence of arthritis and infiltration of T cells in the joint than control-treated animals (169).

Development of a Novel Agonistic Monoclonal Antibody for DR5

To evaluate the therapeutic potential of targeting the death receptor for TRAIL, an agonistic monoclonal antibody (TRA-8) against human DR5 has been developed by us and others (170,171). The rationale for using an anti-DR5 antibody for the treatment of autoimmune disease is based on the observed and potential limitations of soluble TRAIL ligand-based therapy:

1. TRAIL has many receptors, including the death receptors, DR4 and DR5, and decoy receptors, DcR1, DcR1, and OPG. Thus, the ability of TRAIL to induce apoptosis can be reduced by the presence of the decoy receptors. In addition, ligation of a decoy receptor might

cause untoward side effects (e.g., ligation of OPG might cause osteoporosis).

2. The heterotypic cross-linking of both DR4 and DR5 might result in apoptosis of normal cells, with the major concern being hepatocellular toxicity (172).
3. In preclinical trials in animals, recombinant soluble TRAIL has exhibited an extremely short half-life *in vivo,* and its therapeutic application might be limited by its pharmacokinetics.

Unlike Fas, DR5 is not expressed by naïve T cells and B cells of normal individuals, and both activated T cells and B cells may express increased levels of DR5. Moreover, the apoptosis-inducing function of DR5 is restricted to a small portion of activated cells and is associated with fully activated blast cells, suggesting that the action of DR5 in AICD is more selective than that of Fas. It is possible that DR5 may be used to selectively target abnormal B cells because B lymphoma cells, Epstein-Barr virus–transformed B cells, and myeloma cells express high levels of DR5. Importantly, our preliminary data indicate that peripheral B cells from patients with SLE may express higher levels of DR5 than normal controls and are more susceptible to anti-DR5-induced apoptosis. In a human peripheral blood lymphocyte (PBL)/severe combined immune deficient (SCID) mouse chimeric model, anti-DR5 was found to exhibit a potent anti–T cell effect *in vivo.* Our studies of animal models of autoimmune disease indicate that TRAIL/DR5-mediated AICD can act as an alternative pathway to the AICD mediated by Fas in that T cells and B cells isolated from Fas-deficient *lpr/lpr* and Fas ligand–deficient *gld/gld* mice are highly susceptible to TRAIL-mediated apoptosis. The inoculation of host animals with a recombinant adenoviral vector encoding TRAIL (Ad/TRAIL) was found to significantly inhibit the graft versus host disease that is induced by *lpr/lpr* T cells. Treatment of *gld/gld* mice with the Ad/TRAIL was found to inhibit the development of lymphadenopathy and production of autoantibody, whereas the total numbers of circulating B cells and normal T cells were not affected. A similar effect was also observed in NZB/W F1 mice. Treatment with Ad/TRAIL, but not control vector, resulted in a time-dependent decrease in the serum levels of anti-dsDNA antibody (Liu et al., unpublished observation). Taken together, these results suggest that TRAIL might selectively induce apoptosis of those abnormal T cells and B cells that are highly proliferative and producing autoantibody. The data also support the concept that targeting of the DR5 death receptor may be a safe and effective therapy for autoimmune disease.

Prospects for Therapeutic Targeting of BLyS in Autoimmune Disease

We have recently demonstrated significant elevations of BLyS in the patients with SLE. The BLyS isolated from the sera of SLE patients had the same molecular weight as the natural soluble form and was able to stimulate B cell activation *in vitro.* Increased BLyS in SLE patients was partially associated with higher levels of anti-dsDNA of the IgG, IgM, and IgA classes, but not associated with disease activity. Our results suggest that BLyS may be a useful marker for early activation of an autoimmune diathesis and likely plays a critical role in triggering activation of self-Ag-driven autoimmune B cells in human SLE (128).

The considerable body of evidence implicating BLyS in the induction of B-cell autoimmunity has stimulated the testing of therapeutic strategies in many animal models of autoimmune disease and, not unsurprisingly, these have proven effective. A soluble form of the BLyS receptor, TACI-Fc, was first used for the treatment of lupus in the NZB/W F1 and MRL-*lpr/lpr* mouse models of this disease. Although only a modest reduction was achieved in the serum levels of anti-dsDNA antibody, the development of autoimmune nephritis was inhibited significantly, and survival was greatly enhanced (72). Administration of an Ad/TACI-Fc construct resulted in the achievement of serum levels of TACI-Fc as high as 300 μg/mL at 1 week after injection, with these levels being maintained for at least 3 months (Zhou et al., unpublished observation). The administration of Ad/TACI-Fc revealed the striking effect of TACI-Fc on B-cell autoimmunity. Treatment of young B6-*lpr/lpr* mice with Ad/TACI-Fc significantly inhibited age-associated increases in autoantibody production. In addition, treatment of older B6-*lpr/lpr* mice with Ad/TACI-Fc significantly inhibited ongoing autoimmune B-cell responses and reduced the levels of anti-dsDNA and rheumatoid factor of all immunoglobulin classes. The long-term follow-up of the Ad/TACI-Fc-treated B6-*lpr/lpr* mice indicates that none of these mice has developed immune complex deposition in the kidney to date. Furthermore, administration of TACI-Fc ameliorated the severity of CIA. Production of anticollagen antibody was inhibited, and interestingly, the collagen-specific T-cell response was almost completely abolished by TACI-Fc (173). These observations suggest that the anticollagen T-cell response might be driven in a B cell–dependent fashion and that inhibition of the B-cell autoimmune response to collagen by TACI-Fc is sufficient to eliminate both autoimmune T cells and B cells. In general, however, our results indicate that TACI-Fc treatment appeared to be more effective in B cell–dependent autoimmune diseases, such as SLE and arthritis, and less effective in T cell–dependent autoimmune diseases, such as the experimental autoimmune encephalitis model of multiple sclerosis and the nonobese diabetes (NOD) murine autoimmune model of diabetes (Zhou et al., unpublished observation). The data obtained thus far using animal models provide a rational basis for the use of BLyS antagonists in the treatment of patients with SLE. Our preliminary results indicate that *in vitro* treatment of the activated B cells of SLE patients with either TACI-Fc or a BLyS neutralizing monoclonal antibody inhibits production of anti-dsDNA and rheumatoid factor autoantibodies.

In addition to the targeting of BLyS with soluble forms of the BLyS receptors or BLyS neutralizing antibodies, the specific targeting of cell surface BLyS receptors with monoclonal antibodies might improve the selectivity and efficacy of the therapy. Our recent study indicates that the three BLyS receptors are differentially expressed during B-cell activation. BAFF-R is a default receptor for BLyS, which is involved in normal B-cell development and maturation. Although activated B cells are more susceptible to the blockade of BLyS, the dose and timing of the treatment must be carefully adjusted to minimize the effect on normal B cells. TACI is likely expressed by activated B cells and antibody-producing B cells, and importantly, serves as a negative regulator of B-cell activation. Thus, the targeting of TACI with an agonistic monoclonal antibody might selectively bind to activated cells and plasma cells and deliver a signal that inhibits B-cell activation and antibody production. BCMA also is expressed by activated B cells as well as plasma cells. Although the biologic function of BCMA is still unclear, it likely can serve as a marker for abnormal B cells, such as autoantibody-producing cells, B-cell lymphomas, and B-cell leukemias. Thus, anti-BCMA antibodies, armed with cytotoxic drugs or radioisotopes, might help to selectively eliminate pathogenic B cells.

Rheumatoid Arthritis and Apoptosis

Initial investigations of apoptosis in rheumatoid synovium indicated that apoptotic cells were confined to the synovial lining layer and that infiltrating T cells expressed high levels of Bcl-2 and were resistant to Fas-mediated apoptosis (91,174–177). In other studies, either lower expression of Bcl-2 in the synovial fluid T cells, or no significant difference in Bcl-2 expression in synovial tissue T cells of patients with RA compared with those of osteoarthritis (OA) and reactive arthritis has been reported (178,179). The levels of soluble Fas, which is capable of binding Fas ligand and inhibiting Fas-mediated apoptosis, are elevated in the synovial fluid of patients with RA (142,180). Other investigators have reported higher expression of Fas ligand and higher expression of Fas on activated T cells in RA synovium, together with a high sensitivity to apoptosis (181–185). Most studies, therefore, support the concept that T cells in the synovium of patients with RA are activated and, correspondingly, express increased levels of Fas and Fas ligand, and tend to undergo Fas-mediated apoptosis. The question remains, however, as to whether this up-regulation of apoptosis is sufficient to effectively eliminate the T cells that promote the inflammatory disease.

It has been reported that the synovial fibroblasts that undergo hyperplasia in patients with RA have several defects in Fas and Fas ligand expression, apoptosis function, and the expression of other apoptosis molecules, such as p53 (176,186). Analysis of fresh synovial tissue sections from patients with RA reveals higher apoptosis of the type A (macrophage-like) synovial lining cells with little apoptosis of type B (fibroblast-like) synovial cells. Synovial fibroblasts have been demonstrated to be sensitive to apoptosis in a human T-cell leukemia virus type 1 (HTLV-1) *tax* transgenic mouse model when high levels of anti-Fas antibody were injected intraarticularly (33). These and similar experiments were conducted using anti-Fas monoclonal antibody, including RK-8 and HFE-7A (187), which can cross-link Fas and induce apoptosis in some strains of mice without causing significant liver toxicity. Transfection of human Fas ligand into RA synovial fibroblasts that were transplanted into SCID mice also resulted in the induction of apoptosis (31,188). Similar results were obtained when an anti-Fas monoclonal antibody was used to induce apoptosis of human RA tissue engrafted into SCID mice (189). TNF-α has been shown to either inhibit (185) or facilitate (190) Fas signaling in human RA synovial fibroblasts. To date, the studies indicate that Fas apoptosis signaling may be defective in human synovial fibroblasts and that this signaling can be modulated by other cytokines, such as TNF-α and transforming growth factor-β, that are present in abundance in the joint tissue (191).

The authors have developed a novel antihuman DR5 antibody that can induce apoptosis of RA synovial fibroblasts (192). Synovial fibroblast cells isolated from patients with RA, but not those isolated from patients with OA, expressed high levels of DR5 similar to most malignantly transformed tissues and cells. In contrast, the expression of other death receptors, such as DR4, did not differ between RA and OA synovial cells. DR5-mediated apoptosis was highly selective for the RA synovial cells, because primary RA synovial cells but not OA synovial cells were susceptible to anti-DR5-mediated apoptosis. In contrast, there was no difference in Fas-mediated apoptosis between the two types of synovial cells. *In vitro* treatment of RA synovial cells with anti-DR5 strongly inhibited the production of matrix metalloproteinases induced by proinflammatory cytokines. In a human RA synovial cell xenograft model, treatment with anti-DR5 effectively inhibited hyperproliferation of RA synovial cells and completely prevented the bone erosion and cartilage destruction induced by RA synovial cells. These results indicate that increased DR5 expression and susceptibility to DR5-mediated apoptosis are characteristic of the proliferating synovial cells in RA and suggest that specific targeting of DR5 on RA synovial cells with an agonistic anti-DR5 antibody may be a potential therapy for RA.

Signaling Pathways of Apoptosis in Rheumatoid Arthritis Synovial Cells

The signaling pathway for Fas in synovial fibroblasts has not been studied extensively, but several observations indicate that Fas signaling is down-regulated. Fas apoptosis has been shown by one investigator to involve the Jun kinase and the AP-1 pathways, as well as ceramide signaling (193). Other investigators have reported that the Jun kinase path-

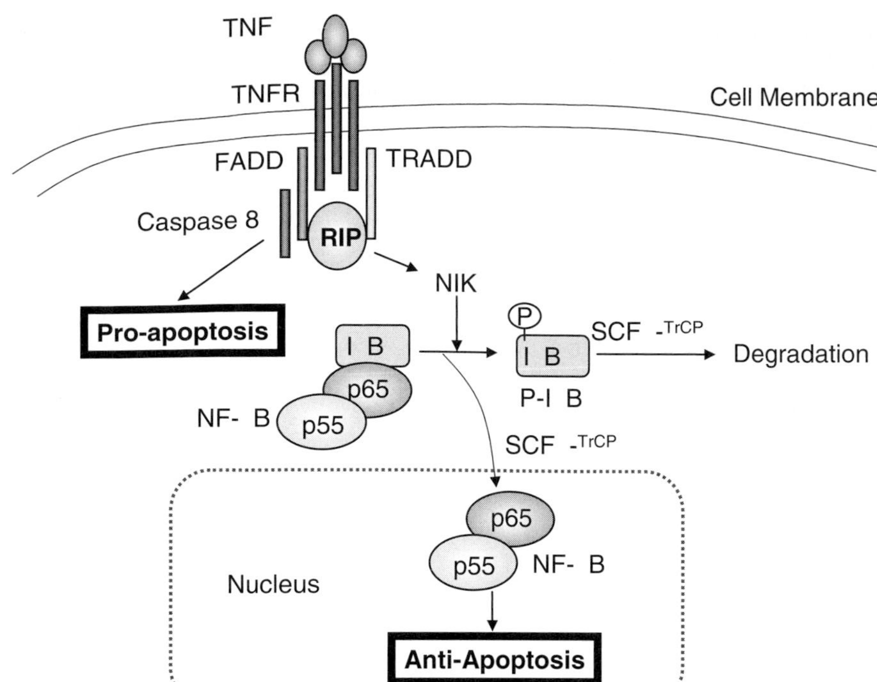

FIG. 26.7. Nuclear factor κB (NFκB) nuclear translocation. Signaling through tumor necrosis factor receptor 1 (TNFR1) activates the death-inducing signal complex (DISC), and also activates a second pathway leading to activation of NFκB-inducing kinase (NIK). NIK phosphorylates and activates IκB kinase, which, in turn, phosphorylates the inhibitor of NFκB protein (IκB). This results in disassociation of the IκB α and β chains from NFκB. IκB α and β are degraded in the proteosome, and NFκB is then translocated to the nucleus, resulting in the induction of antiapoptosis molecules, such as inhibitors of apoptosis (IAPs). *RIP,* receptor interacting protein; *FADD,* Fas-associated death domain protein.

way is a critical mitogen activated protein kinase (MAPK) pathway for IL-1-induced collagenase gene expression in synoviocytes and in arthritis, suggesting that Jun K is an important potential therapeutic target for RA (194). Another pathway of growth regulation in RA synovial fibroblasts involves TNF receptor signaling (Fig. 26.7). TNF receptor signaling can activate a potent antiinflammatory pathway by NFκB nuclear translocation (195–197). Studies in the streptococcal cell wall (SCW) model of arthritis in rats have indicated that introduction of a mutant form of inhibitor κBa (IκBa), which prevents nuclear translocation of NFκB, resulted in enhanced synovial apoptosis (198). A similar mutant form of IκB also has been used in human RA synovial cell lines to block nuclear translocation of NFκB in response to TNF-α (199,200). This leads to unopposed activity of the proapoptotic pathway and significant apoptosis of human RA synovial cells. Further understanding of regulation of Fas and TNF receptor apoptosis pathways in RA synovial fibroblasts should lead to insights into mechanisms for inducing apoptosis of these cells and inhibiting the synovial hyperplasia characteristic of RA. An important pathway of apoptosis resistance for some synovial cells appears to be expression of mutant p53 (176,186). It was hypothesized that free radical production associated with the highly oxidative environment present in the inflammatory synovium may lead to mutations of the p53 tumor suppressor gene (201). More recently, Yao et al. (202) demonstrated that overexpression of p53 resulted in significant apoptosis of human and rabbit synovial cells in culture. Furthermore, intraarticular injection of an Ad-p53 vector resulted in a significant reduction in the leukocytic infiltrate and extensive and rapid induction of synovial apoptosis in the rabbit knee without affecting cartilage metabolism. Thus, p53 may be a critical regulator of fibroblast-like synovial cell proliferation, apoptosis, and invasiveness. Abnormalities of p53 function might contribute to synovial lining expansion and joint destruction in RA.

Current Therapy for Rheumatoid Arthritis and Apoptosis

Most current therapies used for RA have been shown to induce apoptosis (187,203,204). Chloroquine inhibits growth of human umbilical vein endothelial cells by induction of apoptosis (205). This is associated with upregulation of Bcl-X without any change in Bcl-2. The folate antagonist methotrexate is used extensively to treat RA, as well as other chronic inflammatory diseases. It exerts an antiproliferative effect by inhibition of dihydrofolate reductase and other folate-dependent enzymes. Methotrexate has been found to induce apoptosis of T cells efficiently at a concentration of 0.1 to 10 mmol, in a cell cycle–dependent fashion independent of Fas and Fas ligand. *In vitro* activation of PBMCs from patients with arthritis after injection of methotrexate revealed an increased propensity toward apoptosis (206). Phototherapy, which is useful in the treatment of certain autoimmune diseases, may exert its effects by direct induction of the Fas-mediated apoptosis system (207), and by Fas-independent apoptosis systems (208). Soluble TNF-RII (Etanercept®) can inhibit the later stages of inflammatory disease of RA (209–213). In contrast, we and others have previously shown that TNF-α can inhibit development of autoimmune disease, and that TNFR1 knockout mice crossed with *lpr/lpr* mice develop an accelerated autoimmune disease (214,215). These apparently conflicting results obtained with TNF may be attributable to the dual signaling pathway of the TNF receptor. One pathway involves a proapoptotic mechanism and acts through TRADD, followed by FADD, and then caspase 8, as shown earlier for Fas. However, this pathway appears to be blocked in RA synovial cells. The second pathway, a proinflammatory pathway, is mediated primarily by nuclear translocation of NFκB, which induces transcription of proinflammatory cytokines as well as transcription of antiapoptosis molecules such as IAP. Sulfasalazine, which is widely used for RA, as well as for inflammatory bowel disease, can induce apoptosis of neutrophils *in vitro* (216). Neutrophil apoptosis can be blocked by specific inhibitors, including a tyrosine kinase inhibitor, protein kinase A inhibitors, and antioxidants. These results suggest that phosphorylation involving tyrosine kinases and protein kinase A, as well as generation of reactive oxygen species, is involved in sulfasalazine-mediated neutrophil apoptosis. Taken together, these results indicate that the achievement of a better understanding of the apoptosis pathways and their interplay under different physiologic conditions, together with the development of more specific and effective strategies for the manipulation of these pathways, is likely to be beneficial in the development of more effective therapies for rheumatic diseases.

CONCLUSION

In 1992, the first mutation of the gene that causes systemic autoimmune disease in mice was identified: the *lpr* gene, which is a mutation of the *fas* gene. Autoimmune *lpr* mice exhibit a defect in the AICD of their T cells and B cells *in vivo.* This leads to the failure of proper clearance and removal of immune cells and defective down-modulation of immune responses. Such observations kindled speculation that defects in apoptosis, including defects in Fas, Fas ligand, and Fas apoptosis signaling, might play a role in defective down-modulation of the hyperimmune response observed in human autoimmune diseases. Over the past 10 years, many scientists have analyzed different proapoptotic genes, such as *Fas, FasL, Bcl-X,* and the caspases, as well as antiapoptosis genes, including defects in the *Fas* and *FasL, Bcl-2,* and caspase inhibitors. Potential genetic defects have been analyzed at the RNA, protein, and functional levels in humans with autoimmune disease. Somewhat surprisingly, most studies indicate that there is excessive apoptosis of PBMCs in autoimmune disease, suggesting that human autoimmune disease is not due to defective apoptosis of immune cells. Other studies indicate, however, that specific cell populations may be more resistant to apoptosis, such as RA synovial fibroblasts that exhibit reduced apoptosis and perhaps contribute to the observed synovial hyperplasia in this disease. There also is increasing evidence to indicate that antigens exposed during excessive apoptosis, or the release of subcellular components from apoptotic cells, can lead to autoimmunization, autoantibody production, and induction of the inflammatory response. Moreover, defective engulfment and clearance of apoptotic immune cells may contribute to the *in vivo* release of previously sequestered antigens and the production of autoantibodies. Finally, defective apoptosis may lead to defective elimination of tissue damaged in response to genetic or environmental factors, such as the hyperproliferative cells of the rheumatoid synovium, resulting in an accumulation of dysfunctional cells.

REFERENCES

1. Cohen JJ, Duke RC, Fadok VA, et al. Apoptosis and programmed cell death in immunity. *Annu Rev Immunol* 1992;10:267–293.
2. Duke RC, Chervenak R, Cohen JJ. Endogenous endonuclease-induced DNA fragmentation: an early event in cell-mediated cytolysis. *Proc Natl Acad Sci U S A* 1983;80:6361–6365.
3. Wyllie AH. Glucocorticoid-induced thymocyte apoptosis is associated with endogenous endonuclease activation. *Nature* 1980;284:555–556.
4. Dieude M, Senecal JL, Rauch J, et al. Association of autoantibodies to nuclear lamin B1 with thromboprotection in systemic lupus erythematosus: lack of evidence for a direct role of lamin B1 in apoptotic blebs. *Arthritis Rheum* 2002;46:2695–2707.
5. Herrmann M, Voll RE, Zoller OM, et al. Impaired phagocytosis of apoptotic cell material by monocyte-derived macrophages from patients with systemic lupus erythematosus. *Arthritis Rheum* 1998;41: 1241–1250.
6. Kalden JR. Defective phagocytosis of apoptotic cells: possible explanation for the induction of autoantibodies in SLE. *Lupus* 1997;6:326–327.
7. Savill J. Apoptosis in resolution of inflammation. *J Leukoc Biol* 1997; 61:375–380.
8. Verhoven B, Krahling S, Schlegel RA, et al. Regulation of phosphatidylserine exposure and phagocytosis of apoptotic T lymphocytes. *Cell Death Differ* 1999;6:262–270.
9. Bratton DL, Fadok VA, Richter DA, et al. Appearance of phosphatidylserine on apoptotic cells requires calcium-mediated nonspecific flip-flop and is enhanced by loss of the aminophospholipid translocase. *J Biol Chem* 1997;272:26159–26165.
10. Golstein P, Ojcius DM, Young JD. Cell death mechanisms and the immune system. *Immunol Rev* 1991;121:29–65.
11. Surh CD, Sprent J. T-cell apoptosis detected in situ during positive and negative selection in the thymus. *Nature* 1994;372:100–103.
12. Dhein J, Walczak H, Baumler C, et al. Autocrine T-cell suicide mediated by APO-1/(Fas/CD95). *Nature* 1995;373:438–441.
13. Alderson MR, Tough TW, Davis-Smith T, et al. Fas ligand mediates activation-induced cell death in human T lymphocytes. *J Exp Med* 1995;181:71–77.
14. Green DR, Scott DW. Activation-induced apoptosis in lymphocytes. *Curr Opin Immunol* 1994;6:476–487.
15. Ju ST, Panka DJ, Cui H, et al. Fas(CD95)/FasL interactions required for programmed cell death after T-cell activation. *Nature* 1995;373: 444–448.
16. Brunner T, Mogil RJ, LaFace D, et al. Cell-autonomous Fas (CD95)/ Fas-ligand interaction mediates activation-induced apoptosis in T-cell hybridomas. *Nature* 1995;373:441–444.
17. Zhou T, Edwards CK 3rd, Mountz JD. Prevention of age-related T cell apoptosis defect in CD2-fas-transgenic mice. *J Exp Med* 1995;182: 129–137.
18. Thoman ML, Ernst DN, Hobbs MV, et al. T cell differentiation and functional maturation in aging mice. *Adv Exp Med Biol* 1993;330: 93–106.
19. Trainor KJ, Wigmore DJ, Chrysostomou A, et al. Mutation frequency in human lymphocytes increases with age. *Mech Ageing Dev* 1984;27: 83–86.
20. Chan KF, Siegel MR, Lenardo JM. Signaling by the TNF receptor superfamily and T cell homeostasis. *Immunity* 2000;13:419–422.

21. Nagata S. Apoptosis by death factor. *Cell* 1997;88:355–365.
22. Itoh N, Yonehara S, Ishii A, et al. The polypeptide encoded by the cDNA for human cell surface antigen Fas can mediate apoptosis. *Cell* 1991;66:233–243.
23. Suda T, Takahashi T, Golstein P, et al. Molecular cloning and expression of the Fas ligand, a novel member of the tumor necrosis factor family. *Cell* 1993;75:1169–1178.
24. Watanabe-Fukunaga R, Brannan CI, Copeland NG, et al. Lymphoproliferation disorder in mice explained by defects in Fas antigen that mediates apoptosis. *Nature* 1992;356:314–317.
25. Takahashi T, Tanaka M, Brannan CI, et al. Generalized lymphoproliferative disease in mice, caused by a point mutation in the Fas ligand. *Cell* 1994;76:969–976.
26. Nagata S, Golstein P. The Fas death factor. *Science* 1995;267:1449–1456.
27. Zhou T, Bluethmann H, Eldridge J, et al. Abnormal thymocyte development and production of autoreactive T cells in T cell receptor transgenic autoimmune mice. *J Immunol* 1991;147:466–474.
28. Zhou T, Bluethmann H, Zhang J, et al. Defective maintenance of T cell tolerance to a superantigen in MRL-lpr/lpr mice. *J Exp Med* 1992;176:1063–1072.
29. Ogasawara J, Watanabe-Fukunaga R, Adachi M, et al. Lethal effect of the anti-Fas antibody in mice. *Nature* 1993;364:806–809.
30. Tanaka M, Suda T, Yatomi T, et al. Lethal effect of recombinant human Fas ligand in mice pretreated with *Propionibacterium acnes. J Immunol* 1997;158:2303–2309.
31. Zhang H, Yang Y, Horton JL, et al. Amelioration of collagen-induced arthritis by CD95 (Apo-1/Fas)-ligand gene transfer. *J Clin Invest* 1997;100:1951–1957.
32. Ichikawa K, Yoshida-Kato H, Ohtsuki M, et al. A novel murine anti-human Fas mAb which mitigates lymphadenopathy without hepatotoxicity. *Int Immunol* 2000;12:555–562.
33. Fujisawa K, Asahara H, Okamoto K, et al. Therapeutic effect of the anti-Fas antibody on arthritis in HTLV-1 tax transgenic mice. *J Clin Invest* 1996;98:271–278.
34. Zhou T, Cheng J, Yang P, et al. Inhibition of Nur77/Nurr1 leads to inefficient clonal deletion of self-reactive T cells. *J Exp Med* 1996;183:1879–1892.
35. Kim EY, Teh HS. TNF type 2 receptor (p75) lowers the threshold of T cell activation. *J Immunol* 2001;167:6812–6820.
36. Grell M, Becke FM, Wajant H, et al. TNF receptor type 2 mediates thymocyte proliferation independently of TNF receptor type 1. *Eur J Immunol* 1998;28:257–263.
37. Teh HS, Seebaran A, Teh SJ. TNF receptor 2-deficient CD8 T cells are resistant to Fas/Fas ligand-induced cell death. *J Immunol* 2000;165:4814–4821.
38. Elzey BD, Griffith TS, Herndon JM, et al. Regulation of Fas ligand-induced apoptosis by TNF. *J Immunol* 2001;167:3049–3056.
39. Wiley SR, Schooley K, Smolak PJ, et al. Identification and characterization of a new member of the TNF family that induces apoptosis. *Immunity* 1995;3:673–682.
40. Gura T. How TRAIL kills cancer cells, but not normal cells. *Science* 1997;277:768.
41. Chaudhary PM, Eby M, Jasmin A, et al. Death receptor 5, a new member of the TNFR family, and DR4 induce FADD- dependent apoptosis and activate the NF-kappaB pathway. *Immunity* 1997;7:821–830.
42. Walczak H, Degli-Esposti MA, Johnson RS, et al. TRAIL-R2: a novel apoptosis-mediating receptor for TRAIL. *EMBO J* 1997;16:5386–5397.
43. Schneider P, Thome M, Burns K, et al. TRAIL receptors 1 (DR4) and 2 (DR5) signal FADD-dependent apoptosis and activate NF-kappaB. *Immunity* 1997;7:831–836.
44. Degli-Esposti MA, Dougall WC, Smolak PJ, et al. The novel receptor TRAIL-R4 induces NF-kappaB and protects against TRAIL-mediated apoptosis, yet retains an incomplete death domain. *Immunity* 1997;7:813–820.
45. Degli-Esposti MA, Smolak PJ, Walczak H, et al. Cloning and characterization of TRAIL-R3, a novel member of the emerging TRAIL receptor family. *J Exp Med* 1997;186:1165–1170.
46. Emery JG, McDonnell P, Burke MB, et al. Osteoprotegerin is a receptor for the cytotoxic ligand TRAIL. *J Biol Chem* 1998;273:14363–14367.
47. Hilliard B, Wilmen A, Seidel C, et al. Roles of TNF-related apoptosis-inducing ligand in experimental autoimmune encephalomyelitis. *J Immunol* 2001;166:1314–1319.
48. Song K, Chen Y, Goke R, et al. Tumor necrosis factor-related apoptosis-inducing ligand (TRAIL) is an inhibitor of autoimmune inflammation and cell cycle progression. *J Exp Med* 2000;191:1095–1104.
49. Miura Y, Misawa N, Maeda N, et al. Critical contribution of tumor necrosis factor–related apoptosis-inducing ligand (TRAIL) to apoptosis of human CD4$^+$ T cells in HIV-1-infected hu-PBL-NOD-SCID mice. *J Exp Med* 2001;193:651–660.
50. Martinez-Lorenzo MJ, Alava MA, Gamen S, et al. Involvement of APO2 ligand/TRAIL in activation-induced death of Jurkat and human peripheral blood T cells. *Eur J Immunol* 1998;28:2714–2725.
51. Chinnaiyan AM, O'Rourke K, Yu GL, et al. Signal transduction by DR3, a death domain-containing receptor related to TNFR-1 and CD95. *Science* 1996;274:990–992.
52. Pan G, Bauer JH, Haridas V, et al. Identification and functional characterization of DR6, a novel death domain-containing TNF receptor. *FEBS Lett* 1998;431:351–356.
53. Wang EC, Thern A, Denzel A, ET AL. DR3 regulates negative selection during thymocyte development. *Mol Cell Biol* 2001;21:3451–3461.
54. Liu J, Na S, Glasebrook A, et al. Enhanced CD4$^+$ T cell proliferation and Th2 cytokine production in DR6- deficient mice. *Immunity* 2001;15:23–34.
55. Goluszko E, Deng C, Poussin MA, et al. Tumor necrosis factor receptor p55 and p75 deficiency protects mice from developing experimental autoimmune myasthenia gravis. *J Neuroimmunol* 2002;122:85–93.
56. Suvannavejh GC, Lee HO, Padilla J, et al. Divergent roles for p55 and p75 tumor necrosis factor receptors in the pathogenesis of MOG(35–55)-induced experimental autoimmune encephalomyelitis. *Cell Immunol* 2000;205:24–33.
57. Rooney IA, Butrovich KD, Glass AA, et al. The lymphotoxin-beta receptor is necessary and sufficient for LIGHT-mediated apoptosis of tumor cells. *J Biol Chem* 2000;275:14307–14315.
58. Ettinger R, Browning JL, Michie SA, et al. Disrupted splenic architecture, but normal lymph node development in mice expressing a soluble lymphotoxin-beta receptor-IgG1 fusion protein. *Proc Natl Acad Sci U S A* 1996;93:13102–13107.
59. Amakawa R, Hakem A, Kundig TM, et al. Impaired negative selection of T cells in Hodgkin's disease antigen CD30-deficient mice. *Cell* 1996;84:551–562.
60. Hendriks J, Gravestein LA, Tesselaar K, et al. CD27 is required for generation and long-term maintenance of T cell immunity. *Nat Immunol* 2000;1:433–440.
61. Yang FC, Agematsu K, Nakazawa T, et al. CD27/CD70 interaction directly induces natural killer cell killing activity. *Immunology* 1996;88:289–293.
62. Durie FH, Foy TM, Noelle RJ. The role of CD40 and its ligand (gp39) in peripheral and central tolerance and its contribution to autoimmune disease. *Res Immunol* 1994;145:200–205; discussion 244–249.
63. Grewal IS, Flavell RA. CD40 and CD154 in cell-mediated immunity. *Annu Rev Immunol* 1998;16:111–135.
64. Harrop JA, McDonnell PC, Brigham-Burke M, et al. Herpesvirus entry mediator ligand (HVEM-L), a novel ligand for HVEM/TR2, stimulates proliferation of T cells and inhibits HT29 cell growth. *J Biol Chem* 1998;273:27548–27556.
65. Mauri DN, Ebner R, Montgomery RI, et al. LIGHT, a new member of the TNF superfamily, and lymphotoxin alpha are ligands for herpesvirus entry mediator. *Immunity* 1998;8:21–30.
66. Tamada K, Shimozaki K, Chapoval AI, et al. LIGHT, a TNF-like molecule, costimulates T cell proliferation and is required for dendritic cell-mediated allogeneic T cell response. *J Immunol* 2000;164:4105–4110.
67. Shaikh RB, Santee S, Granger SW, et al. Constitutive expression of LIGHT on T cells leads to lymphocyte activation, inflammation, and tissue destruction. *J Immunol* 2001;167:6330–6337.
68. Moore PA, Belvedere O, Orr A, et al. BLyS: member of the tumor necrosis factor family and B lymphocyte stimulator. *Science* 1999;285:260–263.
69. Shu HB, Hu WH, Johnson H. TALL-1 is a novel member of the TNF family that is down-regulated by mitogens. *J Leukoc Biol* 1999;65:680–683.
70. Schneider P, MacKay F, Steiner V, et al. BAFF, a novel ligand of the tumor necrosis factor family, stimulates B cell growth. *J Exp Med* 1999;189:1747–1756.
71. Mukhopadhyay A, Ni J, Zhai Y, et al. Identification and characterization of a novel cytokine, THANK, a TNF homologue that activates

apoptosis, nuclear factor-kappaB, and c-Jun NH2-terminal kinase. *J Biol Chem* 1999;274:15978–15981.

72. Gross JA, Johnston J, Mudri S, et al. TACI and BCMA are receptors for a TNF homologue implicated in B-cell autoimmune disease. *Nature* 2000;404:995–999.
73. Nardelli B, Belvedere O, Roschke V, et al. Synthesis and release of B-lymphocyte stimulator from myeloid cells. *Blood* 2001;97:198–204.
74. Schiemann B, Gommerman JL, Vora K, et al. An essential role for BAFF in the normal development of B cells through a BCMA-independent pathway. *Science* 2001;293:2111–2114.
75. Yan M, Marsters SA, Grewal IS, et al. Identification of a receptor for BLyS demonstrates a crucial role in humoral immunity. *Nat Immunol* 2000;1:37–41.
76. Yu G, Boone T, Delaney J, et al. APRIL and TALL-I and receptors BCMA and TACI: system for regulating humoral immunity. *Nat Immunol* 2000;1:252–256.
77. Yan M, Brady JR, Chan B, et al. Identification of a novel receptor for B lymphocyte stimulator that is mutated in a mouse strain with severe B cell deficiency. *Curr Biol* 2001;11:1547–1552.
78. Wu Y, Bressette D, Carrell JA, et al. Tumor necrosis factor (TNF) receptor superfamily member TACI is a high affinity receptor for TNF family members APRIL and BLyS. *J Biol Chem* 2000;275:35478–35485.
79. Marsters SA, Yan M, Pitti RM, et al. Interaction of the TNF homologues BLyS and APRIL with the TNF receptor homologues BCMA and TACI. *Curr Biol* 2000;10:785–788.
80. von Bulow GU, van Deursen JM, Bram RJ. Regulation of the T-independent humoral response by TACI. *Immunity* 2001;14:573–582.
81. Yan M, Wang H, Chan B, et al. Activation and accumulation of B cells in TACI-deficient mice. *Nat Immunol* 2001;2:638–643.
82. Xu S, Lam KP. B-cell maturation protein, which binds the tumor necrosis factor family members BAFF and APRIL, is dispensable for humoral immune responses. *Mol Cell Biol* 2001;21:4067–4074.
83. Thompson JS, Bixler SA, Qian F, et al. BAFF-R, a newly identified TNF receptor that specifically interacts with BAFF. *Science* 2001;293:2108–2111.
84. Khare SD, Sarosi I, Xia XZ, et al. Severe B cell hyperplasia and autoimmune disease in TALL-1 transgenic mice. *Proc Natl Acad Sci U S A* 2000;97:3370–3375.
85. Mackay F, Woodcock SA, Lawton P, et al. Mice transgenic for BAFF develop lymphocytic disorders along with autoimmune manifestations. *J Exp Med* 1999;190:1697–1710.
86. Kuang AA, Diehl GE, Zhang J, et al. FADD is required for DR4- and DR5-mediated apoptosis: lack of TRAIL-induced apoptosis in FADD-deficient mouse embryonic fibroblasts. *J Biol Chem* 2000;275:25065–25068.
87. Muhlenbeck F, Haas E, Schwenzer R, et al. TRAIL/Apo2L activates c-Jun NH2-terminal kinase (JNK) via caspase-dependent and caspase-independent pathways. *J Biol Chem* 1998;273:33091–33098.
88. Jeremias I, Debatin KM. TRAIL induces apoptosis and activation of NFkappaB. *Eur Cytokine Netw* 1998;9:687–688.
89. Chao DT, Korsmeyer SJ. BCL-2 family: regulators of cell death. *Annu Rev Immunol* 1998;16:395–419.
90. Strasser A, Puthalakath H, Bouillet P, et al. The role of bim, a proapoptotic BH3-only member of the Bcl-2 family in cell-death control. *Ann NY Acad Sci* 2000;917:541–548.
91. Mountz JD, Zhang HG. Regulation of apoptosis of synovial fibroblasts. *Curr Dir Autoimmun* 2001;3:216–239.
92. Wei MC, Zong WX, Cheng EH, et al. Proapoptotic BAX and BAK: a requisite gateway to mitochondrial dysfunction and death. *Science* 2001;292:727–730.
93. Cheng EH, Wei MC, Weiler S, et al. BCL-2, BCL-X(L) sequester BH3 domain-only molecules preventing BAX- and BAK-mediated mitochondrial apoptosis. *Mol Cell* 2001;8:705–711.
94. Green DR. Apoptotic pathways: the roads to ruin. *Cell* 1998;94:695–698.
95. Li H, Zhu H, Xu CJ, et al. Cleavage of BID by caspase 8 mediates the mitochondrial damage in the Fas pathway of apoptosis. *Cell* 1998;94:491–501.
96. Luo X, Budihardjo I, Zou H, et al. Bid, a Bcl2 interacting protein, mediates cytochrome c release from mitochondria in response to activation of cell surface death receptors. *Cell* 1998;94:481–490.
97. Zou H, Li Y, Liu X, et al. An APAF-1 cytochrome c multimeric complex is a functional apoptosome that activates procaspase-9. *J Biol Chem* 1999;274:11549–11556.
98. Green DR, Reed JC. Mitochondria and apoptosis. *Science* 1998;281:1300–1312
99. Hu Y, Benedict MA, Wu D, et al. Bcl-XL interacts with Apaf-1 and inhibits Apaf-1-dependent caspase-9 activation. *Proc Natl Acad Sci U S A* 1998;95:4386–4391.
100. Medema JP, Scaffidi C, Krammer PH, et al. Bcl-xL acts downstream of caspase-8 activation by the CD95 death-inducing signaling complex. *J Biol Chem* 1998;273:3388–3393.
101. Juo P, Kuo CJ, Yuan J, et al. Essential requirement for caspase-8/FLICE in the initiation of the Fas-induced apoptotic cascade. *Curr Biol* 1998;8:1001–1008.
102. Varfolomeev EE, Schuchmann M, Luria V, et al. Targeted disruption of the mouse Caspase 8 gene ablates cell death induction by the TNF receptors, Fas/Apo1, and DR3 and is lethal prenatally. *Immunity* 1998;9:267–276.
103. Peter ME, Kischkel FC, Scheuerpflug CG, et al. Resistance of cultured peripheral T cells towards activation-induced cell death involves a lack of recruitment of FLICE (MACH/caspase 8) to the CD95 death-inducing signaling complex. *Eur J Immunol* 1997;27:1207–1212.
104. Kennedy NJ, Budd RC. Phosphorylation of FADD/MORT1 and Fas by kinases that associate with the membrane-proximal cytoplasmic domain of Fas. *J Immunol* 1998;160:4881–4888.
105. Scaffidi C, Fulda S, Srinivasan A, et al. Two CD95 (APO-1/Fas) signaling pathways. *EMBO J* 1998;17:1675–1687.
106. Takahashi R, Deveraux Q, Tamm I, et al. A single BIR domain of XIAP sufficient for inhibiting caspases. *J Biol Chem* 1998;273:7787–7790.
107. Deveraux QL, Roy N, Stennicke HR, et al. IAPs block apoptotic events induced by caspase-8 and cytochrome c by direct inhibition of distinct caspases. *EMBO J* 1998;17:2215–2223.
108. Suzuki A, Tsutomi Y, Akahane K, et al. Resistance to Fas-mediated apoptosis: activation of caspase 3 is regulated by cell cycle regulator p21WAF1 and IAP gene family ILP. *Oncogene* 1998;17:931–939.
109. Duckett CS, Li F, Wang Y, et al. Human IAP-like protein regulates programmed cell death downstream of Bcl-xL and cytochrome c. *Mol Cell Biol* 1998;18:608–615.
110. Farahani R, Fong WG, Korneluk RG, et al. Genomic organization and primary characterization of miap-3: the murine homologue of human X-linked IAP. *Genomics* 1997;42:514–518.
111. Zhang HG, Huang N, Liu D, et al. Gene therapy that inhibits nuclear translocation of nuclear factor kappaB results in tumor necrosis factor alpha–induced apoptosis of human synovial fibroblasts. *Arthritis Rheum* 2000;43:1094–1105.
112. Wu J, Wilson J, He J, et al. Fas ligand mutation in a patient with systemic lupus erythematosus and lymphoproliferative disease. *J Clin Invest* 1996;98:1107–1113.
113. Fisher GH, Rosenberg FJ, Straus SE, et al. Dominant interfering Fas gene mutations impair apoptosis in a human autoimmune lymphoproliferative syndrome. *Cell* 1995;81:935–946.
114. Sneller MC, Wang J, Dale JK, et al. Clinical, immunologic, and genetic features of an autoimmune lymphoproliferative syndrome associated with abnormal lymphocyte apoptosis. *Blood* 1997;89:1341–1348.
115. Drappa J, Vaishnaw AK, Sullivan KE, et al. Fas gene mutations in the Canale-Smith syndrome, an inherited lymphoproliferative disorder associated with autoimmunity. *N Engl J Med* 1996;335:1643–1649.
116. Jackson CE, Puck JM. Autoimmune lymphoproliferative syndrome, a disorder of apoptosis. *Curr Opin Pediatr* 1999;11:521–527.
117. Wang J, Zheng L, Lobito A, et al. Inherited human caspase 10 mutations underlie defective lymphocyte and dendritic cell apoptosis in autoimmune lymphoproliferative syndrome type II. *Cell* 1999;98:47–58.
118. Mountz JD, Wu J, Cheng J, et al. Autoimmune disease. A problem of defective apoptosis. *Arthritis Rheum* 1994;37:1415–1420.
119. Emlen W, Niebur J, Kadera R. Accelerated *in vitro* apoptosis of lymphocytes from patients with systemic lupus erythematosus. *J Immunol* 1994;152:3685–3692.
120. Mysler E, Bini P, Drappa J, et al. The apoptosis-1/Fas protein in human systemic lupus erythematosus. *J Clin Invest* 1994;93:1029–1034.
121. Kovacs B, Vassilopoulos D, Vogelgesang SA, et al. Defective CD3-mediated cell death in activated T cells from patients with systemic lupus erythematosus: role of decreased intracellular TNF-alpha. *Clin Immunol Immunopathol* 1996;81:293–302.
122. Kaneko H, Saito K, Hashimoto H, et al. Preferential elimination of $CD28^{+}$ T cells in systemic lupus erythematosus (SLE) and the relation with activation-induced apoptosis. *Clin Exp Immunol* 1996;106:218–229.

123. Kovacs B, Liossis SN, Dennis GJ, et al. Increased expression of functional Fas-ligand in activated T cells from patients with systemic lupus erythematosus. *Autoimmunity* 1997;25:213–221.
124. Sakata K, Sakata A, Vela-Roch N, et al. Fas (CD95)-transduced signal preferentially stimulates lupus peripheral T lymphocytes. *Eur J Immunol* 1998;28:2648–2660.
125. Tanaka M, Itai T, Adachi M, et al. Downregulation of Fas ligand by shedding. *Nat Med* 1998;4:31–36.
126. Kaplan MJ, Lewis EE, Shelden EA, et al. The apoptotic ligands TRAIL, TWEAK, and Fas ligand mediate monocyte death induced by autologous lupus T cells. *J Immunol* 2002;169:6020–6029.
127. Altman JD, Moss PA, Goulder PJ, et al. Phenotypic analysis of antigen-specific T lymphocytes. *Science* 1996;274:94–96.
128. Zhang J, Roschke V, Baker KP, et al. Cutting edge: a role for B lymphocyte stimulator in systemic lupus erythematosus. *J Immunol* 2001;166:6–10.
129. Zhou T, Zhang J, Carter R, et al. BLyS and B cell autoimmunity. *Curr Dir Autoimmun* 2003;6:21–37.
130. Tan SM, Xu D, Roschke V, et al. Local production of B lymphocyte stimulator protein and APRIL in arthritic joints of patients with inflammatory arthritis. *Arthritis Rheum* 2003;48:982–992.
131. Cheema GS, Roschke V, Hilbert DM, et al. Elevated serum B lymphocyte stimulator levels in patients with systemic immune-based rheumatic diseases. *Arthritis Rheum* 2001;44:1313–1319.
132. Mariette X, Roux S, Zhang J, et al. The level of BLyS (BAFF) correlates with the titre of autoantibodies in human Sjögren's syndrome. *Ann Rheum Dis* 2003;62:168–171.
133. Cheng J, Liu C, Koopman WJ, et al. Characterization of human Fas gene. Exon/intron organization and promoter region. *J Immunol* 1995;154:1239–1245.
134. Cheng J, Zhou T, Liu C, et al. Protection from Fas-mediated apoptosis by a soluble form of the Fas molecule. *Science* 1994;263:1759–1762.
135. Liu C, Cheng J, Mountz JD. Differential expression of human Fas mRNA species upon peripheral blood mononuclear cell activation. *Biochem J* 1995;310(part 3):957–963.
136. Knipping E, Krammer PH, Onel KB, et al. Levels of soluble Fas/APO-1/CD95 in systemic lupus erythematosus and juvenile rheumatoid arthritis. *Arthritis Rheum* 1995;38:1735–1737.
137. Goel N, Ulrich DT, St Clair EW, et al. Lack of correlation between serum soluble Fas/APO-1 levels and autoimmune disease. *Arthritis Rheum* 1995;38:1738–1743.
138. Tokano Y, Miyake S, Kayagaki N, et al. Soluble Fas molecule in the serum of patients with systemic lupus erythematosus. *J Clin Immunol* 1996;16:261–265.
139. Jodo S, Kobayashi S, Kayagaki N, et al. Serum levels of soluble Fas/APO-1 (CD95) and its molecular structure in patients with systemic lupus erythematosus (SLE) and other autoimmune diseases. *Clin Exp Immunol* 1997;107:89–95.
140. Nozawa K, Kayagaki N, Tokano Y, et al. Soluble Fas (APO-1, CD95) and soluble Fas ligand in rheumatic diseases. *Arthritis Rheum* 1997; 40:1126–1129.
141. Rose LM, Latchman DS, Isenberg DA. Elevated soluble fas production in SLE correlates with HLA status not with disease activity. *Lupus* 1997;6:717–722.
142. Bijl M, van Lopik T, Limburg PC, et al. Do elevated levels of serum-soluble fas contribute to the persistence of activated lymphocytes in systemic lupus erythematosus? *J Autoimmun* 1998;11: 457–463.
143. Kovacs B, Szentendrei T, Bednarek JM, et al. Persistent expression of a soluble form of Fas/APO1 in continuously activated T cells from a patient with SLE. *Clin Exp Rheumatol* 1997;15:19–23.
144. Al-Maini MH, Mountz JD, Al-Mohri HA, et al. Serum levels of soluble Fas correlate with indices of organ damage in systemic lupus erythematosus. *Lupus* 2000;9:132–139.
145. Aringer M, Wintersberger W, Steiner CW, et al. High levels of bcl-2 protein in circulating T lymphocytes, but not B lymphocytes, of patients with systemic lupus erythematosus. *Arthritis Rheum* 1994;37: 1423–1430.
146. Ohsako S, Hara M, Harigai M, et al. Expression and function of Fas antigen and bcl-2 in human systemic lupus erythematosus lymphocytes. *Clin Immunol Immunopathol* 1994;73:109–114.
147. Komaki S, Kohno M, Matsuura N, et al. The polymorphic 43Thr bcl-2 protein confers relative resistance to autoimmunity: an analytical evaluation. *Hum Genet* 1998;103:435–440.
148. Rose LM, Latchman DS, Isenberg DA. Bcl-2 expression is unaltered in unfractionated peripheral blood mononuclear cells in patients with systemic lupus erythematosus. *Br J Rheumatol* 1995;34:316–320.
149. Georgescu L, Vakkalanka RK, Elkon KB, et al. Interleukin-10 promotes activation-induced cell death of SLE lymphocytes mediated by Fas ligand. *J Clin Invest* 1997;100:2622–2633.
150. Mehrian R, Quismorio FP Jr, Strassmann G, et al. Synergistic effect between IL-10 and bcl-2 genotypes in determining susceptibility to systemic lupus erythematosus. *Arthritis Rheum* 1998;41:596–602.
151. Singh RR, Hahn BH, Tsao BP, et al. Evidence for multiple mechanisms of polyclonal T cell activation in murine lupus. *J Clin Invest* 1998;102:1841–1849.
152. Wu J, Edberg JC, Redecha PB, et al. A novel polymorphism of FcgammaRIIIa (CD16) alters receptor function and predisposes to autoimmune disease. *J Clin Invest* 1997;100:1059–1070.
153. Perniok A, Wedekind F, Herrmann M, et al. High levels of circulating early apoptic peripheral blood mononuclear cells in systemic lupus erythematosus. *Lupus* 1998;7:113–118.
154. Stollar BD, Stephenson F. Apoptosis and nucleosomes. *Lupus* 2002; 11:787–789.
155. Licht R, van Bruggen MC, Oppers-Walgreen B, et al. Plasma levels of nucleosomes and nucleosome-autoantibody complexes in murine lupus: effects of disease progression and lipopolysaccharide administration. *Arthritis Rheum* 2001;44:1320–1330.
156. Courtney PA, Crockard AD, Williamson K, et al. Increased apoptotic peripheral blood neutrophils in systemic lupus erythematosus: relations with disease activity, antibodies to double stranded DNA, and neutropenia. *Ann Rheum Dis* 1999;58:309–314.
157. Casciola-Rosen L, Rosen A, Petri M, et al. Surface blebs on apoptotic cells are sites of enhanced procoagulant activity: implications for coagulation events and antigenic spread in systemic lupus erythematosus. *Proc Natl Acad Sci U S A* 1996;93:1624–1629.
158. Gaipl US, Beyer TD, Baumann I, et al. Exposure of anionic phospholipids serves as anti-inflammatory and immunosuppressive signal—implications for antiphospholipid syndrome and systemic lupus erythematosus. *Immunobiology* 2003;207:73–81.
159. Manfredi AA, Rovere P, Galati G, et al. Apoptotic cell clearance in systemic lupus erythematosus. I. Opsonization by antiphospholipid antibodies. *Arthritis Rheum* 1998;41:205–214.
160. Kamachi M, Le TM, Kim SJ, et al. Human autoimmune sera as molecular probes for the identification of an autoantigen kinase signaling pathway. *J Exp Med* 2002;196:1213–1225.
161. Utz PJ, Hottelet M, Schur PH, et al. Proteins phosphorylated during stress-induced apoptosis are common targets for autoantibody production in patients with systemic lupus erythematosus. *J Exp Med* 1997;185:843–854.
162. Utz PJ, Hottelet M, van Venrooij WJ, et al. Association of phosphorylated serine/arginine (SR) splicing factors with the U1-small ribonucleoprotein (snRNP) autoantigen complex accompanies apoptotic cell death. *J Exp Med* 1998;187:547–560.
163. Overzet K, Gensler TJ, Kim SJ, et al. Small nucleolar RNP scleroderma autoantigens associate with phosphorylated serine/arginine splicing factors during apoptosis. *Arthritis Rheum* 2000;43:1327–1336.
164. Utz PJ, Hottelet M, Le TM, et al. The 72-kd component of signal recognition particle is cleaved during apoptosis. *J Biol Chem* 1998; 273:35362–35370.
165. Zhang HG, Liu D, Heike Y, et al. Induction of specific T-cell tolerance by adenovirus-transfected, Fas ligand-producing antigen presenting cells. *Nat Biotechnol* 1998;16:1045–1049.
166. Zhang HG, Su X, Liu D, et al. Induction of specific T cell tolerance by Fas ligand-expressing antigen- presenting cells. *J Immunol* 1999; 162:1423–1430.
167. Hsu HC, Zhang HG, Song GG, et al. Defective Fas ligand-mediated apoptosis predisposes to development of a chronic erosive arthritis subsequent to *Mycoplasma pulmonis* infection. *Arthritis Rheum* 2001; 44:2146–2159.
168. Zhang HG, Yang P, Xie J, et al. Depletion of collagen II-reactive T cells and blocking of B cell activation prevents collagen II-induced arthritis in DBA/1j mice. *J Immunol* 2002;168:4164–4172.
169. Liu Z, Xu X, Hsu H-C, et al. CII-DC-AdTRAIL cell gene therapy inhibits infiltration of CII-reactive T cells and CII-induced arthritis. *J Clin Invest* 2003;112(9):1332–1341.
170. Ichikawa K, Liu W, Zhao L, et al. Tumoricidal activity of a novel anti-human DR5 monoclonal antibody without hepatocyte cytotoxicity. *Nat Med* 2001;7:954–960.

171. Odoux C, Albers A, Amoscato AA, et al. TRAIL, FasL and a blocking anti-DR5 antibody augment paclitaxel-induced apoptosis in human non-small-cell lung cancer. *Int J Cancer* 2002;97:458–465.
172. Jo M, Kim TH, Seol DW, et al. Apoptosis induced in normal human hepatocytes by tumor necrosis factor- related apoptosis-inducing ligand. *Nat Med* 2000;6:564–567.
173. Wang H, Marsters SA, Baker T, et al. TACI-ligand interactions are required for T cell activation and collagen-induced arthritis in mice. *Nat Immunol* 2001;2:632–637.
174. Firestein GS, Yeo M, Zvaifler NJ. Apoptosis in rheumatoid arthritis synovium. *J Clin Invest* 1995;96:1631–1638.
175. Perlman H, Liu H, Georganas C, et al. Differential expression pattern of the antiapoptotic proteins, Bcl-2 and FLIP, in experimental arthritis. *Arthritis Rheum* 2001;44:2899–2908.
176. Chou CT, Yang JS, Lee MR. Apoptosis in rheumatoid arthritis—expression of Fas, Fas-L, p53, and Bcl-2 in rheumatoid synovial tissues. *J Pathol* 2001;193:110–116.
177. Sioud M, Mellbye O, Forre O. Analysis of the NF-kappa B p65 subunit, Fas antigen, Fas ligand and Bcl-2-related proteins in the synovium of RA and polyarticular JRA. *Clin Exp Rheumatol* 1998;16:125–134.
178. Zdichavsky M, Schorpp C, Nickels A, et al. Analysis of bcl-2^+ lymphocyte subpopulations in inflammatory synovial infiltrates by a double-immunostaining technique. *Rheumatol Int* 1996;16:151–157.
179. Isomaki P, Soderstrom KO, Punnonen J, et al. Expression of bcl-2 in rheumatoid arthritis. *Br J Rheumatol* 1996;35:611–619.
180. Hasunuma T, Kayagaki N, Asahara H, et al. Accumulation of soluble Fas in inflamed joints of patients with rheumatoid arthritis. *Arthritis Rheum* 1997;40:80–86.
181. Asahara H, Hasumuna T, Kobata T, et al. Expression of Fas antigen and Fas ligand in the rheumatoid synovial tissue. *Clin Immunol Immunopathol* 1996;81:27–34.
182. Hashimoto H, Tanaka M, Suda T, et al. Soluble Fas ligand in the joints of patients with rheumatoid arthritis and osteoarthritis. *Arthritis Rheum* 1998;41:657–662.
183. Wang M, Keino H, Matsumoto I, et al. A single cell analysis of Fas ligand positive T cells in rheumatoid synovial fluid. *J Rheumatol* 2000;27:311–318.
184. Roessner K, Wolfe J, Shi C, et al. High expression of Fas ligand by synovial fluid-derived gamma delta T cells in Lyme arthritis. *J Immunol* 2003;170:2702–2710.
185. Wakisaka S, Suzuki N, Takeba Y, et al. Modulation by proinflammatory cytokines of Fas/Fas ligand-mediated apoptotic cell death of synovial cells in patients with rheumatoid arthritis (RA). *Clin Exp Immunol* 1998;114:119–128.
186. Firestein GS, Nguyen K, Aupperle KR, et al. Apoptosis in rheumatoid arthritis: p53 overexpression in rheumatoid arthritis synovium. *Am J Pathol* 1996;149:2143–2151.
187. Matsuno H, Yudoh K, Nakazawa F, et al. Antirheumatic effects of humanized anti-Fas monoclonal antibody in human rheumatoid arthritis/SCID mouse chimera. *J Rheumatol* 2002;29:1609–1614.
188. Okamoto K, Asahara H, Kobayashi T, et al. Induction of apoptosis in the rheumatoid synovium by Fas ligand gene transfer. *Gene Ther* 1998;5:331–338.
189. Sakai K, Matsuno H, Morita I, et al. Potential withdrawal of rheumatoid synovium by the induction of apoptosis using a novel *in vivo* model of rheumatoid arthritis. *Arthritis Rheum* 1998;41:1251–1257.
190. Kobayashi T, Okamoto K, Kobata T, et al. Tumor necrosis factor alpha regulation of the FAS-mediated apoptosis-signaling pathway in synovial cells. *Arthritis Rheum* 1999;42:519–526.
191. Kawakami A, Eguchi K, Matsuoka N, et al. Inhibition of Fas antigen-mediated apoptosis of rheumatoid synovial cells in vitro by transforming growth factor beta 1. *Arthritis Rheum* 1996;39:1267–1276.
192. Ichikawa K, Liu W, Fleck M, et al. TRAIL-R2 (DR5) mediates apoptosis of synovial fibroblasts in rheumatoid arthritis. *J Immunol* 2003; 171:1061–1069.
193. Okamoto K, Fujisawa K, Hasunuma T, et al. Selective activation of the JNK/AP-1 pathway in Fas-mediated apoptosis of rheumatoid arthritis synoviocytes. *Arthritis Rheum* 1997;40:919–926.
194. Han Z, Boyle DL, Chang L, et al. c-Jun N-terminal kinase is required for metalloproteinase expression and joint destruction in inflammatory arthritis. *J Clin Invest* 2001;108:73–81.
195. Lacey D, Sampey A, Mitchell R, et al. Control of fibroblast-like synoviocyte proliferation by macrophage migration inhibitory factor. *Arthritis Rheum* 2003;48:103–109.
196. Youn J, Kim HY, Park JH, et al. Regulation of TNF-alpha-mediated hyperplasia through TNF receptors, TRAFs, and NF-kappaB in synoviocytes obtained from patients with rheumatoid arthritis. *Immunol Lett* 2002;83:85–93.
197. Tomita T, Takano H, Tomita N, et al. Transcription factor decoy for NFkappaB inhibits cytokine and adhesion molecule expressions in synovial cells derived from rheumatoid arthritis. *Rheumatology (Oxford)* 2000;39:749–757.
198. Miagkov AV, Kovalenko DV, Brown CE, et al. NF-kappaB activation provides the potential link between inflammation and hyperplasia in the arthritic joint. *Proc Natl Acad Sci U S A* 1998;95: 13859–13864.
199. Makarov SS. NF-kappa B in rheumatoid arthritis: a pivotal regulator of inflammation, hyperplasia, and tissue destruction. *Arthritis Res* 2001;3:200–206.
200. Aupperle KR, Bennett BL, Boyle DL, et al. NF-kappa B regulation by I kappa B kinase in primary fibroblast-like synoviocytes. *J Immunol* 1999;163:427–433.
201. Aupperle KR, Boyle DL, Hendrix M, et al. Regulation of synoviocyte proliferation, apoptosis, and invasion by the p53 tumor suppressor gene. *Am J Pathol* 1998;152:1091–1098.
202. Yao Q, Wang S, Glorioso JC, et al. Gene transfer of p53 to arthritic joints stimulates synovial apoptosis and inhibits inflammation. *Mol Ther* 2001;3:901–910.
203. Herman S, Zurgil N, Langevitz P, et al. The induction of apoptosis by methotrexate in activated lymphocytes as indicated by fluorescence hyperpolarization: a possible model for predicting methotrexate therapy for rheumatoid arthritis patients. *Cell Struct Funct* 2003;28: 113–122.
204. Maciejewski JP, Risitano AM, Sloand EM, et al. A pilot study of the recombinant soluble human tumour necrosis factor receptor (p75)-Fc fusion protein in patients with myelodysplastic syndrome. *Br J Haematol* 2002;117:119–126.
205. Potvin F, Petitclerc E, Marceau F, et al. Mechanisms of action of antimalarials in inflammation: induction of apoptosis in human endothelial cells. *J Immunol* 1997;158:1872–1879.
206. Genestier L, Paillot R, Fournel S, et al. Immunosuppressive properties of methotrexate: apoptosis and clonal deletion of activated peripheral T cells. *J Clin Invest* 1998;102:322–328.
207. Morita A, Werfel T, Stege H, et al. Evidence that singlet oxygen-induced human T helper cell apoptosis is the basic mechanism of ultraviolet-A radiation phototherapy. *J Exp Med* 1997;186:1763–1768.
208. Ratkay LG, Chowdhary RK, Iamaroon A, et al. Amelioration of antigen-induced arthritis in rabbits by induction of apoptosis of inflammatory cells with local application of transdermal photodynamic therapy. *Arthritis Rheum* 1998;41:525–534.
209. Elliott MJ, Maini RN, Feldmann M, et al. Randomised double-blind comparison of chimeric monoclonal antibody to tumour necrosis factor alpha (cA2) versus placebo in rheumatoid arthritis. *Lancet* 1994; 344:1105–1110.
210. Murray KM, Dahl SL. Recombinant human tumor necrosis factor receptor (p75) Fc fusion protein (TNFR:Fc) in rheumatoid arthritis. *Ann Pharmacother* 1997;31:1335–1338.
211. Su X, Zhou T, Yang P, et al. Reduction of arthritis and pneumonitis in motheaten mice by soluble tumor necrosis factor receptor. *Arthritis Rheum* 1998;41:139–149.
212. Weinblatt ME, Kremer JM, Bankhurst AD, et al. A trial of etanercept, a recombinant tumor necrosis factor receptor:Fc fusion protein, in patients with rheumatoid arthritis receiving methotrexate. *N Engl J Med* 1999;340:253–239.
213. Moreland LW, Cohen SB, Baumgartner SW, et al. Long-term safety and efficacy of etanercept in patients with rheumatoid arthritis. *J Rheumatol* 2001;28:1238–1244.
214. Jacob CO, Hwang F, Lewis GD, et al. Tumor necrosis factor alpha in murine systemic lupus erythematosus disease models: implications for genetic predisposition and immune regulation. *Cytokine* 1991;3: 551–561.
215. Zhou T, Edwards CK 3rd, Yang P, et al. Greatly accelerated lymphadenopathy and autoimmune disease in lpr mice lacking tumor necrosis factor receptor I. *J Immunol* 1996;156:2661–2665.
216. Akahoshi T, Namai R, Sekiyama N, et al. Rapid induction of neutrophil apoptosis by sulfasalazine: implications of reactive oxygen species in the apoptotic process. *J Leukoc Biol* 1997;62:817–826.

CHAPTER 27

Structure, Function, and Genetics of the Human Leukocyte Antigen Complex in Rheumatic Disease

Jane A. Buckner and Gerald T. Nepom

The major histocompatibility complex (MHC) is a 3.6-Mb region located on the short arm of chromosome 6 (6p21.3) that contains over 200 genes, of which greater than 40% are involved in immune function (1). Among these genes are the human leukocyte antigen (HLA) class I and II molecules that are encoded in the class I and class II regions of the MHC, respectively. Other, related "nonclassical" HLA molecules involved in the signaling of innate immune responses are found in the class I region, and molecules involved in antigen processing are encoded in the class II region. The class III region contains a group of non-HLA genes, many of which participate in immune function. The HLA genes encoded by the MHC play a central role in the development and function of the adaptive immune response and are highly polymorphic. The polymorphic nature of these genes leads to the development of a diverse and unique immune response among individuals. Additionally, these genes play a role in the development of human disease, including transplant rejection, immune deficiencies, and autoimmunity. Understanding the molecular structure and the function of HLA molecules has enhanced our understanding of the complexity of the genetic heterogeneity found in the MHC and of the subsequent impact on the function of the immune system.

STRUCTURE AND FUNCTION OF HLA MOLECULES

The HLA class I and II molecules are membrane-bound proteins expressed on the cell surface that bind peptides. When expressed on the surface of various cell types, the complex of HLA molecule and peptide can then act as a ligand for the T-cell receptor (TCR) expressed on T lymphocytes. The structure of HLA molecules allows binding of peptides by the formation of a groove on a solvent-exposed surface. The groove is defined by a β-pleated sheet flanked by two α helixes (Fig. 27.1). Both class I and class II molecules conform to this design, but achieve it through different mechanisms. The amino acid residues that form the

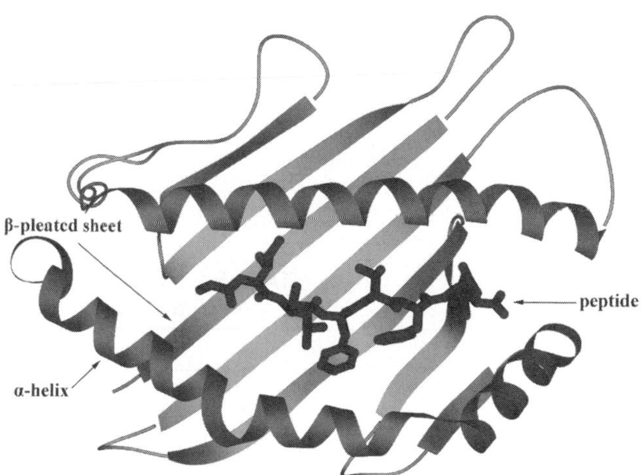

FIG. 27.1. Molecular model of the peptide-binding groove of a human leukocyte antigen molecule. The groove is defined by a β-pleated sheet flanked by two α helices, and peptides bind within the groove. [Derived from a major histocompatibility complex class I crystal structure, In: Stewart-Jones GB, McMichael AJ, Bell J. et at. A structural basis for immunodominant human T cell receptor recognition. *Nat Immunol* 2003;4:657, with permission].

groove determine the characteristics of the peptides that can bind within the groove. In the case of class I and class II molecules, for any allele a large number of peptides may bind within the binding groove if they conform to the same binding motif. These motifs are influenced by the size, charge, and hydrophobic properties of the pockets formed by the amino acids surrounding the binding groove. Binding motifs for many HLA molecules have been determined experimentally or through modeling, and these binding motifs can be used to predict which peptides will bind to specific HLA alleles (*syfpeithi.bmi-heidelberg. com/scripts/ MHCServer.dll/home.htm*; *www.imtech.res.in/ raghava/ propred*). An example of one such motif is shown in Table 27.1. The binding of peptides to HLA class I and II molecules leads to the availability of an array of HLA molecules bound to many different peptides on the cell surface. These are available to the T cell, and if the interaction between the TCR and HLA–peptide complex (trimolecular complex) is of sufficient strength, T-cell activation is initiated. Crystalographic structures have demonstrated that the interaction of TCR with class I or II molecules is characterized by the interaction of the variable regions of the TCR α and β chains (CDR1, CDR2, and CDR3) with residues from both the most polymorphic regions of the MHC molecule itself and the peptide bound in the groove (Fig. 27.2). The interaction of T cells with the HLA–peptide complex is important both during thymic development and later in the peripheral immune system. Within the thymus, a developing T cell expresses a unique TCR on its surface during maturation. In order for the T cell to proceed in development, its unique TCR must be able to interact with the HLA molecules present in the cortical epithelium. Those that bind with an adequate affinity to an expressed HLA molecule continue to mature, while those that cannot do so die of neglect (positive selection). Once past the cortical epithelium, thymocytes must then pass another test within the medullary region of the thymus. At this step, the T cell interacts with HLA molecules containing an array of self peptides. If the interaction of the TCR with HLA expressing self is too strong (high affinity for self), the cell is deleted (negative selection). Thus, any T cells that reach maturity must be able to interact with one of the HLA molecules expressed by the individual and must not be highly reactive to self. In this way, the HLA molecules determine the repertoire or complexity of an individual's T-cell responses. In the periphery, HLA molecules then display an array of peptides, both derived from self and foreign proteins, allowing the T cells to identify and respond to nonself challenges such as infections and tumors. These functions have been fine tuned within the HLA system by a division of labor between the class I and class II molecules. HLA class I molecules present peptides predominantly derived from intracellular proteins to $CD8^+$ cytotoxic T cells and class II molecules present peptides derived from extracellular proteins to $CD4^+$ helper T cells.

HLA CLASS I GENES AND MOLECULES

The class I molecule is a heterodimer composed of the polymorphic α chain, which includes an intracytoplasmic, transmembrane, and extracellular region, noncovalently complexed with the nonpolymorphic light chain, called β_2-microglobulin. The crystallographic structure of this portion of an HLA class I molecule is depicted in Fig. 27.3A (2). The α chain of class I is encoded by the HLA-A, B, and C transplantation antigens found in the class I region; these are also referred to as the class Ia molecules (3,4). β_2-microglobulin is encoded outside the MHC on chromosome 15. Genes that encode the α chain of class I are highly polymorphic. Currently, more than 250 alleles have been identified at the HLA-A locus, more than

TABLE 27.1. *of preferred peptide-binding motifs for selected DR alleles using the single letter amino acid code*

	Peptide anchor positions			
DRB1 allele:	1	4	6	9
*0101	F, Y, L, V, I, W	L, M, A	S, A, G	L, A, V, I
*0301	F, V, I, M, Y, L	D, E, A	K, R, H, E, Q	Y, L, F
*0401	Y, F, W, M, V, L	(*NOT* R, K)	T, S, N, Q, V	(*NOT* D, E)
*0402	V, I, L, M	(*NOT* D, E)	T, S, N, Q	(*NOT* D, E)
*1101	W, F, Y	M, L, V	R, K	
*1501	L, V, I	F, Y, I	I, L, V, M, F	

Examples of preferred peptide-binding motifs for selected DR alleles using the single-letter amino acid code. Anchor positions 1, 4, 6, and 9 represent sites within the antigen-binding groove of DR molecules that accommodate specific peptide side-chain amino acids. Peptides that contain these side-chain residues at each corresponding position have favorable binding properties, accounting for the allele-specific selection of particular peptide antigens.

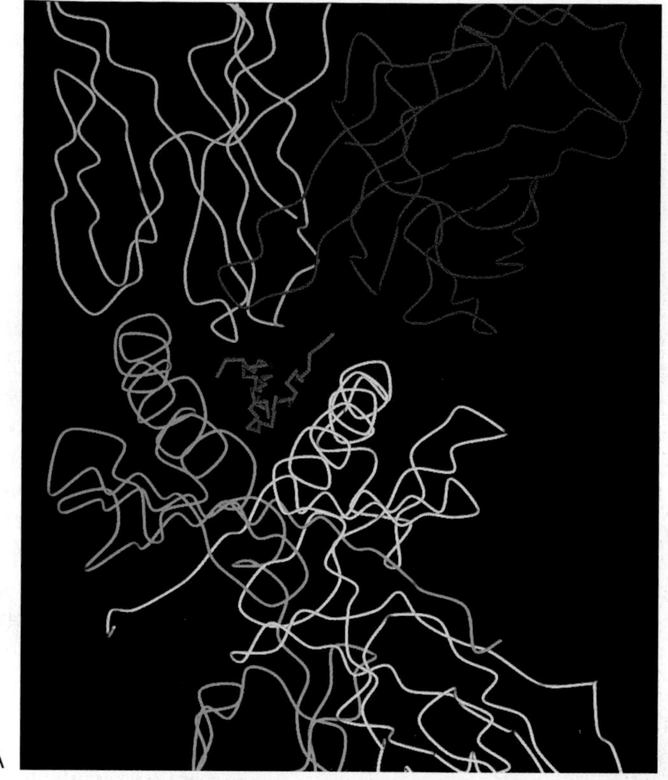

A

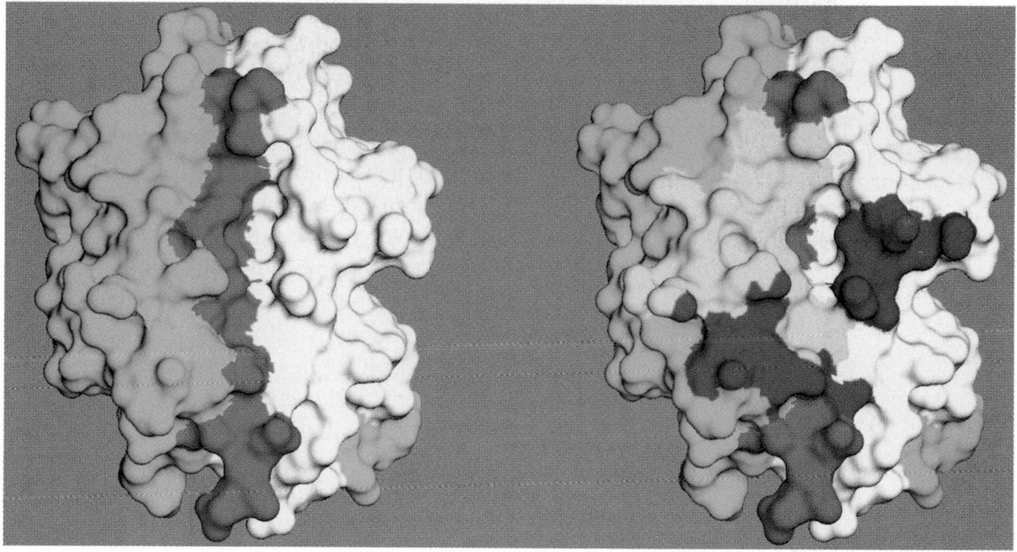

B

FIG. 27.2. The trimolecular complex. **A:** Demonstrates the backbone structures of the trimolecular complex. The T-cell receptor is on top, with the α chain in light blue and the β chain in red. The major histocompatibility complex (MHC) class II molecule is on the bottom, with the α chain in yellow and β chain in green. The peptide is shown in violet. (From Reinherz et al. *Science* 1999;286:1913, with permission.) **B:** The molecular surface of the MHC class II molecule with peptide is shown on the left. As in **A**, the α chain is yellow, the β chain is green, and the peptide is shown in violet. The image on the right shows the areas that contact the T-cell receptor (TCR), with the TCR-α chain contacts shown in dark blue and the TCR-β chain in light blue. Reinherz EL, Tank, Tang L, et al. The crystal structure of a T cell receptor in complex with peptide and MHC class II. *Science* 1999;286(S446)1913–1921.

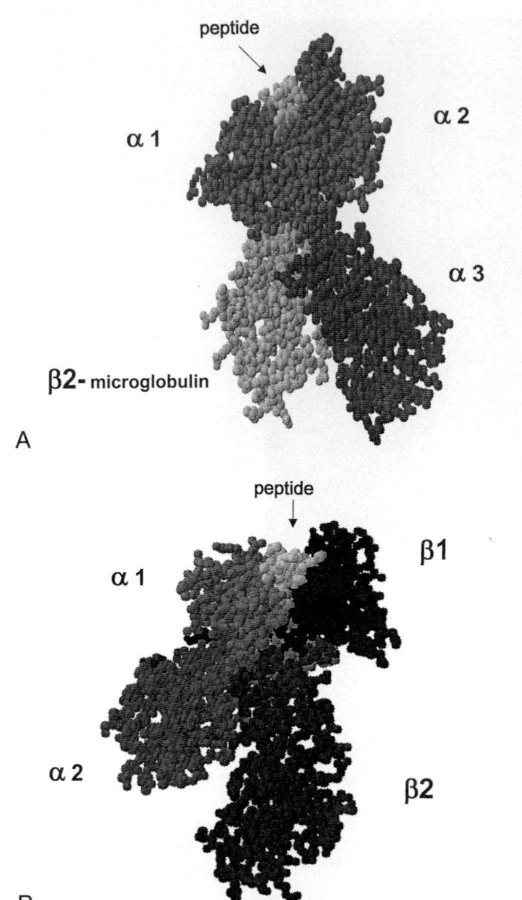

FIG. 27.3. A: Side view of a three-dimensional model of the class I molecule human leukocyte antigen A2 complexed with a peptide from influenza. The antigen-binding groove is pointing up and is occupied by peptide. **B:** Side view of a three-dimensional model of the class II molecule DRB1*0301 binding the class I–associated invariant chain peptide (CLIP). The peptide is in the antigen-binding groove, which is pointing up. The domains are homologous to those of the class I molecule in Fig. 27.4A.

500 at HLA-B, and more than 100 at HLA-C. The sequences of these genes and others in the MHC locus can be found online at *anthonynolan.org.uk* (5). The extracellular region of the α chain is divided into three domains: the α1, α2, and α3. The α1 and α2 domains form the antigen-binding groove, the sides of which are formed by two α helices, the base of which is a β-pleated sheet, as described above. The ends of the peptide binding groove are closed, limiting the size of the peptide that can be bound to no more than eight to ten amino acid residues in length. The α chain's extreme polymorphism is found predominantly within the α1 and α2 domains. These polymorphisms dictate the unique structural characteristics of the groove, conferring most of the variation in antigen-binding preferences among different alleles (6–8). The membrane-proximal α3 domain is relatively nonpolymorphic, it associates with β_2-microglobulin, which does not have a transmembrane or intracellular component (2,4), and with non-HLA molecules on the cell surface, such as CD8 (9).

CLASS I SYNTHESIS AND PEPTIDE BINDING

Class I molecules bind peptides derived from the endogenous antigen processing pathway. This pathway is specialized to deal with antigens synthesized within the cytosol, such as viral proteins in infected cells Fig. 27.4A (10–14). Newly synthesized class I α chains initially bind to a chaperone protein, calnexin in the endoplasmic reticulum (ER) (15,16). Once the α chain becomes associated with β_2-microglobulin, the class I complex is released from calnexin and binds calreticulin. The incompletely folded class I α chain/β_2-microglobulin heterodimer together with calreticulin bind the components of the peptide-loading complex. The order of events is not yet clear, but the mature loading complex includes calreticulin, class I α chain, β_2-microglobulin and tapasin which couples to the transporter associated with antigen processing (TAP)-1 portion of the TAP transporter (17,18) and ERP27, which is bound to tapasin via a disulfide bond (19). This interaction allows the newly synthesized class I molecule to sample and bind the peptides transported into the ER via the TAP transporter.

The peptides available for binding to class I in the ER are derived from cytosolic proteins. These proteins are degraded by proteasomes, a multiprotein complex with proteolytic activity. The character of the peptides produced by proteosomal cleavage is influenced by the state of the cell. Resting cells have a "conventional" proteosome, whereas cells that are exposed to interferon-γ (IFN-γ) at the site of an injury or inflammation synthesize three proteosome subunits, large multifunction proteosome 2 (LMP2), LMP7, and multicatalytic endopeptidase complex subunit-1 (MECL-1). These subunits replace the constitutively-expressed proteosome subunits (20). This appears to alter the specificity of polypeptide cleavage, generating peptides with carboxy-terminal residues that are preferred for association with both TAP and class I molecules. The TAP-1 and TAP-2 gene products form a heterodimer that crosses the membrane of the ER and transports the antigenic peptides into the lumen of the ER (21). When a suitable peptide is bound, the class I–peptide complex is stabilized, allowing it to leave the ER and traffic through the Golgi and post-Golgi compartments to the cell surface. Here, it is displayed and available to be recognized by appropriate $CD8^+$ T cells, signaling them to kill the virally-infected cell. Nearly all cells express HLA class I molecules constitutively, allowing this system to be active in nonimmune as well as in immune cells, which serves to protect nearly all cell types that can be infected with viruses. Exposure to interferons induces, even in cells outside the immune system, increased expression of a number of molecules making up this antigen-processing machinery, including class I α chain, β_2-microglobulin, LMP2, LMP7, and TAP-1 and 2, among others. In this way, any cell that may be infected with a virus has the capability of

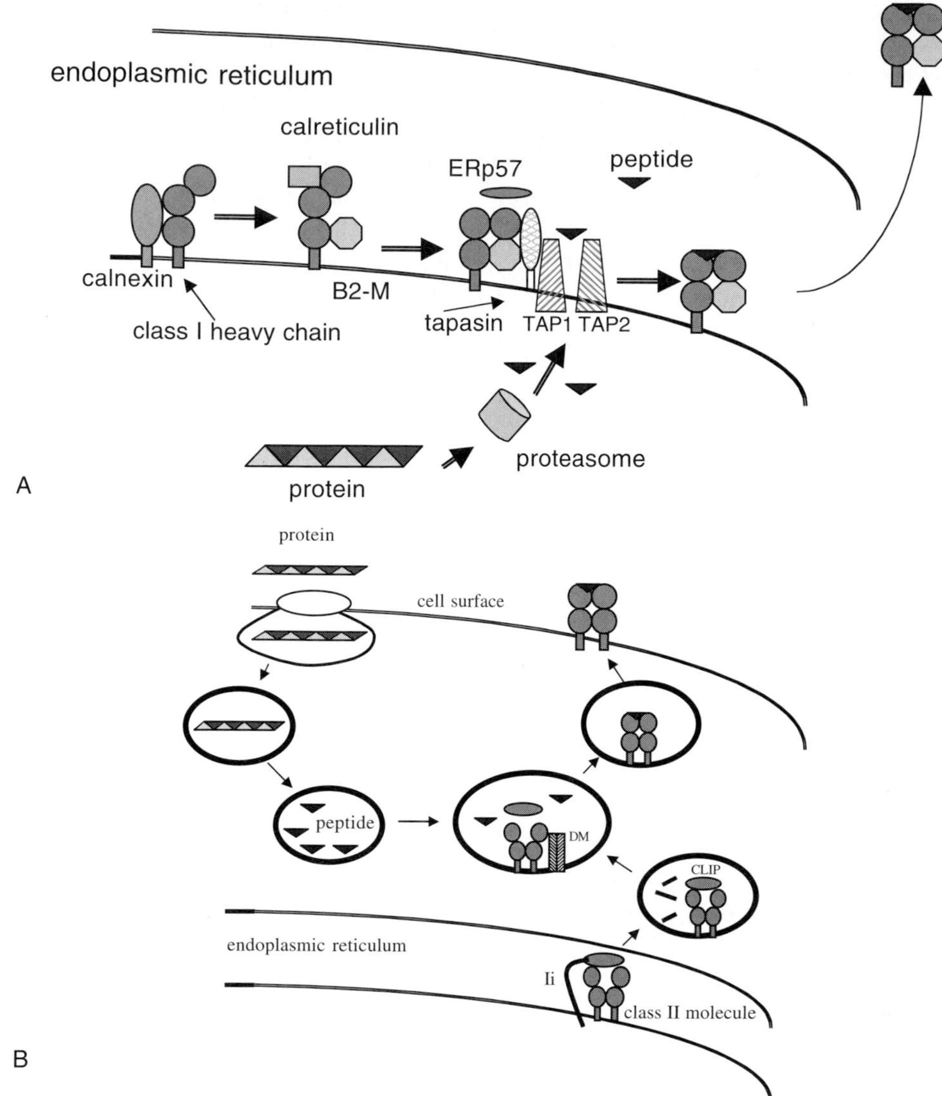

FIG. 27.4. Antigen processing pathways. **A:** Schematic representation of the endogenous antigen-processing pathway. Proteins from the cytosol (such as viral proteins) are degraded by proteasomes into peptides that are transported into the endoplasmic reticulum (ER) by TAP transporters. Within the ER, the chaperone molecules calnexin, calreticulin, and Erp57 assist in stabilizing and bringing together the class I heavy chain, β_2-microglobulin, and peptide forming the mature class I molecule, which is then transported to the cell surface via the Golgi and post-Golgi compartments. **B:** The endogenous antigen-processing pathway allows extracellular proteins to be taken up by the cell and processed into peptides within the acidic endocytic compartments. The class II α and β chains assemble in the ER with invariant chain (Ii), whose fragment class I–associated invariant chain peptide (CLIP) protects the antigen-binding groove from peptides present in the ER. After assembly, the class II–Ii complex exits the ER and traffics to the acidic vesicles, where enzymes, including cathepsins, cleave Ii until only CLIP remains in the antigen-binding groove. In a compartment known as the MIIC, human leukocyte antigen DM heterodimers then catalyze the exchange of CLIP for antigenic peptides. The fully-formed complex is then transported to the cell surface.

presenting class I/viral peptide complexes on its surface, marking it for elimination by cytotoxic T cells.

HLA CLASS II GENES AND MOLECULES

The HLA class II molecules are encoded within the HLA class II gene complex, which lies at the centromeric end of the MHC, and includes multiple gene loci, including the HLA-DP, DQ, and DR subregions (22). Class II molecules have a more restricted tissue distribution than class Ia molecules, being expressed primarily on cells of the immune system, including dendritic cells, macrophages, B cells, and activated T cells (23). However, expression of class II molecules can be induced in many other cell types following stimulation by cytokines such as IFN-γ or other agents (24). The crystal structure of class II molecules is homologous to that of class I antigens (25–27) (Fig. 27.3B). However, both the 34-kd α chain and a 29-kd β chain are encoded in the MHC, and both chains are anchored in the cell membrane and, like class Ia molecules, display tremendous polymorphism. More than 200 alleles are known at the DRB1 locus, 8 to 20 each at the DRB3, DRB4, and DRB5 loci, 20 at DQA1, more than 40 at DQB1, 17 at DPA1, and more than 80 at DPB1.

Both the α and β chains of class II consist of an intracellular portion, transmembrane portion, and extracellular portion that is subdivided into two domains. The α2 and β2 domains are membrane proximal and can be considered homologous to the α3 and β_2-microglobulin portions of the class I molecule. Part of the β2 domain interacts with CD4 molecules on the surface of T cells during an immune response. The α1 and β1 domains form the class II antigen-binding groove, homologous to the class I α1 and α2 domains, respectively. In class II antigens, however, the ends of the groove are open, allowing binding of peptides of varying lengths, up to 20 or more amino acid residues (28,29). The β1 domain contains most of the extreme polymorphism found in class II molecules, although the α chain does contribute some polymorphism in DP and DQ antigens. Polymorphism in class II β chains is concentrated in three hypervariable regions. In DR molecules, these occur in the regions from amino acids 9 through 13, 26 through 37, and 67 through 74. Variation among different DRβ amino acid sequences can be thought of as a matrix, with a "mix and match" pattern of hypervariable regions forming different alleles.

The gene organization of the class II region is complex. Each class II subregion, HLA-DP, DQ, and DR, contains a functional α chain gene as well as at least one functional β chain gene, along with a variable number of pseudogenes (30). For example, DP heterodimers are composed of an α chain encoded by the DPA1 locus and a β chain encoded by the DPB1 locus. DPA2 and DPB2 are pseudogenes and do not express a gene product. Similarly, DQA1 and DQB1 encode α and β chains, respectively, which dimerize to form the mature DQ antigen, whereas DQA2 and DQB2 are not expressed. Both the α and the β chains of DP and DQ antigens are polymorphic. This provides an additional level of variation, because, in some cases, an α chain encoded on one chromosome can dimerize not only with its cis-encoded β chain, but also with the β chain encoded on the other chromosome (31).

The DR subregion is even more complex. A single DR α chain, with limited polymorphism, is encoded by the DRA locus and can dimerize with β chains encoded by several different loci. Mature DR heterodimers formed by products of the DRA and DRB1 loci represent the class II antigen normally most abundant on the cell surface. However, that same α chain can also dimerize with a β chain encoded by the DRB3, DRB4, or DRB5 loci to form a second expressed DR molecule on some haplotypes. For example, in the DR3 haplotype, two mature DR molecules are expressed: one made up of the DR α chain and a β chain encoded by the DRB1 gene, and the other made up of the DR α chain and a β chain encoded by the DRB3 gene. A DR4 haplotype will express one DR molecule encoded by the DRA and DRB1 genes, and a second DR molecule encoded by the DRA and DRB4 genes. Some haplotypes, such as DR1 or DR8, express only one DR molecule, which is encoded by DRA and DRB1 genes. The number of pseudogenes also varies among different haplotypes.

Another level of polymorphism lies in the upstream promoters of class II genes. A limited number of polymorphisms in these regulatory regions have been shown to be functionally active and may result in different levels of constitutive or inducible class II expression, potentially altering the threshold for immune activation (32–35). The physiologic relevance of this category of polymorphism remains to be clarified.

Class II Synthesis and Peptide Binding

In contrast to the endogenous peptides that are bound by class I molecules, class II molecules largely bind peptides that originate from extracellular proteins. These peptides are made available to the class II molecule via the exogenous antigen-processing pathway (36–40) (Fig. 27.4B). This pathway involves extracellular antigens, such as bacteria or their products, which are internalized from the extracellular milieu through processes such as endocytosis by macrophages or facilitated receptor-mediated endocytosis by B cells. Once taken up by the cell, the antigenic protein enters vesicles known as endosomes, which become progressively more acidic as they move toward the center of the cell. Low pH activates acid proteases present within the vesicles to degrade antigenic proteins. In particular, cysteine proteases called cathepsins play a primary role in this pathway, especially cathepsins S and L.

Like class I molecules, HLA class II molecules are translocated into the ER as part of their synthetic pathway. Unlike class I molecules, however, class II molecules are destined to bind peptides that are processed and available in endocytic vesicles, not peptides present in the ER. Thus, the class II antigen-binding groove must be protected from binding peptides until the proper compartment is reached. This is accomplished by assembling the class II α and β chains with a third protein, encoded outside the MHC on chromosome 5, called the invariant chain (Ii) (36,37). The invariant chain noncovalently binds to the class II α and β chains, with part of it blocking the antigen-binding groove and preventing other peptides from binding there prematurely. A trimer of Ii chains with their associated class II α/β chains assembles into a nine-chain complex in the ER, which is then released from the ER and directed by the Ii to an appropriate acidic endosomal compartment where peptide is encountered. Proteases found in these compartments, such as cathepsins, progressively cleave portions of the invariant chain until only a fragment known as CLIP (class II–associated invariant chain peptide) remains bound to the antigen-binding groove of the class II α/β heterodimer, still preventing antigenic peptides from binding.

The exchange of CLIP for an appropriate antigenic peptide occurs in a late endosomal compartment known as MIIC (MHC class II compartment). This process is aided by an additional nonclassical HLA molecule known as HLA-DM. The α/β DM dimer remains intracellular and is abundant in MIIC vesicles. DM molecules appear to bind and stabilize classical class II dimers and catalyze the removal of CLIP from the antigen-binding groove to allow the binding of other antigenic peptides available in the compartment (41). In addition, DM has a peptide "editing" function, by which it can catalyze the release not only of CLIP, but also of antigenic peptides that have bound poorly in the groove, facilitating the binding of peptides with higher avidity and promoting the formation of stable HLA–peptide complexes (42,43). When stabilized by such peptides, the HLA–peptide complex moves to the cell surface, where it is available for recognition by $CD4^+$ T cells of appropriate specificity.

OTHER HLA GENES IN THE MHC

Both the class I and class II gene regions contain nonclassical HLA genes (Fig. 27.5). In the class I region, the HLA-E, F, and G genes are designated as class Ib genes. The HLA-E, F, and G genes encode molecules with a more limited tissue distribution and much less polymorphism (3,44,45). HLA-E regulates natural killer (NK) cells through its interaction with CD94/NKG2 receptors (44,45). It is expressed in all tissues that express classical class I, but unlike class I, it binds only one peptide, a conserved leader sequence peptide from class Ia molecules. HLA-G molecules have a more restricted expression profile and bind a restricted class of nonamers with specific amino acids at several positions. The function of HLA-G is not yet known; it binds to CD8 (46,47), but T cells restricted to HLA-G have not been identified, and soluble HLA-G has been reported to regulate T-cell function (48,49). HLA-G tetramers also bind Ig-like transcripts 2 (ILT2) and ILT4, and can protect NK targets from lysis likely through the NK receptor (KIR) 2DL4 (50,51). The high expression of HLA-G in the placenta suggests a role in immune tolerance (45,52,53). HLA-F is also expressed in the placenta, but its function has yet to be determined (54).

Other class I–like genes found in the class I region include HLA-HFE (formerly called HLA-H), MICA, and MICB. The HFE gene product is homologous to class I molecules and is also associated with β_2-microglobulin, but does not appear to bind peptides. Mutations in this gene are strongly associated with hereditary hemochromatosis, suggesting that HFE plays a role in iron metabolism (44,55). MICA and MICB share less than 30% homology with HLA class I molecules, do not associate with β_2-microglobulin, and display a fairly high degree of polymorphism. They are expressed primarily on thymic cortical epithelium and gastrointestinal epithelium in a stress-inducible manner. A receptor for both MICA and MICB, NKG2D, has been identified on NK cells, CD8αβ T cells, γδ T cells, and activated macrophages (56). Binding of MICA or MICB to NKG2D augments cytotoxic responses to some antigens (57,58).

In addition to DR, DQ, and DP, two nonclassical class II molecules, HLA-DM and HLA-DO, are found in the class II region. They differ from DR, DQ, and DP antigens by being expressed intracellularly in endosomal and lysosomal compartments and by being relatively nonpolymorphic (59–62). HLA-DM is a heterodimer encoded by the DMA and DMB genes. The three-dimensional crystal structure of DM reveals a structure homologous to classical class II molecules, except that the antigen-binding groove is almost completely closed (59). As described above, HLA-DM contributes to antigen processing by catalyzing the exchange of invariant chain peptides for antigenic peptides in class II molecules (60,63) HLA-DO also is a heterodimer, composed of a DN α chain encoded by the DNA gene and a DO β chain encoded by DOB. Its tissue distribution is more restricted, being expressed in B cells and thymic epithelium, and it appears to be a modulator of DM function (61–64).

NON-HLA GENES IN THE MHC

Interspersed within the MHC are a number of non-HLA genes (22,30,65). The low-molecular-weight peptides (LMP) and TAP genes, located in the class II region, participate in antigen processing and presentation by HLA class I mole-

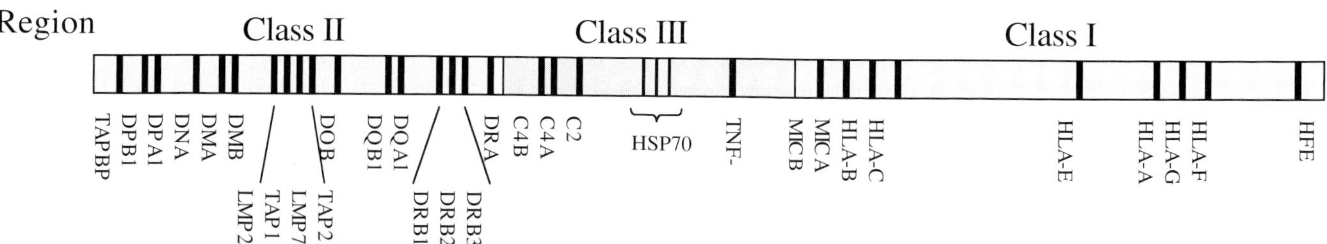

FIG. 27.5. Schematic map of the major histocompatibility complex.

cules (as described above). LMP2 and LMP7 are components of the proteasome, a large multiprotein complex with protease activity that degrades proteins and generates antigenic peptides for the class I processing pathway (66). TAP-1 and TAP-2 genes (for transporters associated with antigen processing) lie near the LMP genes and encode two proteins that form a heterodimer responsible for transporting cytosolic antigens into the endoplasmic reticulum, where they can be processed and bind class I molecules (67,68). Tapasin, whose gene lies centromeric to the DP genes, links immature class I molecules to the TAP-1 transporter.

A number of other expressed genes lie in the class III region of the MHC. These include the complement components C2, C4, and properdin factor B and the cytokines tumor necrosis factor-α (TNF-α) and lymphotoxin (also called TNF-β) (30,69). Heat-shock proteins (such as hsp70) are encoded in the same region (70), as is the enzyme 21-hydoxylase, important in steroid synthesis (71).

HLA TYPING METHODS AND NOMENCLATURE

Historically, HLA nomenclature has been complicated and frequently altered, making it difficult for the nonspecialist to keep up to date. These changes reflected the evolving understanding of the genetic organization and polymorphisms within the HLA region, limited largely by HLA typing methodology. Current nomenclature fortunately is based on a detailed genetic understanding of the region and is thus logical and consistent, albeit sometimes cumbersome.

Initial identification of HLA polymorphisms relied on serologically-based typing. Sera from multiparous women often contain antibodies against paternal HLA antigens to which the women were exposed during pregnancies. International workshops compared, standardized, and named serologic reactivities for the most common HLA-A, B, C, DR, and DQ types. The international workshops also standardized sets of homozygous typing cells (HTCs), lymphocytes from individuals homozygous at a particular class II locus, which were used in mixed lymphocyte response assays, a form of cellular typing. The precision of HLA analysis is much greater when examined at the DNA sequence level, as compared with the types defined by serologic and cellular methods. Thus, these serologic and cellular methods have been superseded by typing systems based on DNA sequences (72–74). Two methods are most commonly used; both are based on the polymerase chain reaction. One approach involves amplifying alleles at a particular locus by using primers hybridizing to conserved regions of all alleles, or a family of alleles, at that locus. The amplified product is then tested for hybridization with a series of labeled short sequence–specific oligonucleotide probes, each of which matches a sequence unique to a single allele. Often, there is not a single sequence stretch not shared by another allele, but rather a particular combination of polymorphic regions makes that allele unique, requiring interpretation of a pattern of hybridizations with multiple probes to determine the allele represented. A second approach, sequence-specific priming, amplifies DNA by using primers that hybridize to unique sequences of alleles where available, such that only that allele will amplify (75). Direct nucleotide sequencing provides a definitive alternative to these two methods and is now used routinely in some institutions.

These DNA-based techniques allow accurate and rapid identification of specific alleles; current nomenclature reflects this precision (76). Thus, an allele is named first by its locus (e.g., DRB1), followed by an asterisk and its allele number. The first two digits of this number refer to the family group of which the allele is a member (e.g., 04), and the second two digits signify the specific allele based on its sequence (e.g., 01). Thus, DRB1*0401 represents a single, specific nucleotide sequence, and DRB1*0404 represents a related but unique allele that is also in the DR4 family (in this example, the two alleles vary by three nucleotide substitutions). Occasionally, a fifth digit is added, such as in DRB1*11011 and DRB1*11012, indicating that a silent nucleotide sequence difference is present and does not alter the amino acid sequence of the alleles. This method of nomenclature describes alleles at an individual locus. In the case of DQ or DP, in which both the α and β chain genes are polymorphic, alleles at both loci must be specified to identify a mature molecule (e.g., DQA1*0101/DQB1*0501).

Because HLA genes are expressed codominantly, a single individual expresses two haplotypes, one inherited from the mother and one from the father. The alleles on a haplotype are essentially always inherited together in families, because loci in the HLA region are tightly linked. For example, one haplotype might be A*0101, B*0801, Cw*0201, DRA, DRB1*0301, DRB3*0101, DQA1*0101, DQB1*0201, DPA1*0101, DPB1*0401. Among populations, however, specific alleles may be found in combination with a variety of alleles at other loci. Over evolutionary time, one would expect that these alleles would randomly associate in all combinations. However, in some cases, particular haplotypic combinations occur with much greater frequency than expected by chance alone, suggesting that genetic or selection mechanisms may favor particular linkages. This phenomenon is termed linkage disequilibrium. A common example among the white population is the A*0101, B*0801, DR*0301 haplotype, which is intriguingly found to be increased in a number of autoimmune diseases.

HLA ASSOCIATIONS WITH DISEASE

The association of certain HLA specificities with rheumatic diseases was first described in the 1970s. The earliest, and still statistically the strongest, association noted was that of HLA-B27 with ankylosing spondylitis (AS) (77,78). The first class II–associated disease described was rheumatoid arthritis (RA), which was reported to be associated with DR4 (79,80). Since then, dozens of autoimmune diseases have been associated with a variety of both class I and class II HLA antigens (81). In general, these associations share a number of features. None is absolute: not all individuals with the disease have the associated allele, most individuals carrying that allele do not have disease, and even unaffected first-degree relatives may share the allele. Furthermore, the disease-associated gene is identical in patients and normal subjects. Thus, disease-associated HLA alleles confer disease susceptibility, or an increased risk, but are not absolute markers for any particular disease. A number of factors influence the strength of HLA genetic associations and can lead to seeming contradictions among different studies, emphasizing the need to be cautious in clinical applications of genetic analysis.

First, the population being studied is important. Different ethnic groups can vary dramatically in the background frequency of a particular allele. For example, the prevalence of HLA-B27 ranges from near zero in some African black populations (82) to approximately 50% among the Haida Indians of Canada (83). The frequency of AS seems to vary accordingly, being common in populations with a high prevalence of B27. It becomes obvious then that the control group with which the patient population is being compared must be ethnically similar to make a meaningful comparison.

Second, HLA-typing methods must be taken into account. Many early studies were performed by using serologic typing; however, most typing sera identify families of closely related specificities rather than individual alleles. If a disease is associated with a single allele or a subset of alleles within a family, then results of studies using such reagents will be diluted by inclusion of other nonassociated alleles within that specificity. DNA-based methods identifying individual alleles, however, should result in more accurate association statistics.

Improper statistical methods, too, can skew results. Population studies comparing the frequency of a particular HLA antigen in the control versus patient populations allow a statistical association to be established. Normally, an association is said to be statistically significant if the p value is less than 0.05, which indicates that the odds are less than 1 in 20 that the association has been found by chance alone. When one is investigating the possible association of a disease with hundreds of HLA alleles, it becomes likely that some associations will show up spuriously. To correct for this, the p value must be multiplied by the number of tests performed. For example, if one tests for 10 different DR alleles and finds an association with one at a p value of 0.006, then the corrected p value is 0.06, no longer statistically significant. If, however, one is trying to confirm a previous association, for example, the association of DRB1*0401 with RA, then one is essentially testing for a single allele, and correction of the p value is not necessary. True associations should be robust enough to remain reproducible and significant after proper statistical manipulation.

Finally, linkage disequilibrium is an important feature of HLA disease associations to be considered. As described earlier, usually the entire MHC is inherited as a block of genes, and within a population, certain alleles at different loci will frequently be inherited together. Thus, if a disease is found to be associated, for example, with DR3 (DRB1*0301) in whites, the alleles linked to this DR type will also likely be statistically associated with the disease, including DQA1*0101, DQB1*0201, HLA-B*0801, and HLA-A*0101. It can be difficult to pinpoint which allele is actually responsible for conferring disease risk. Furthermore, it is possible that another linked gene on the haplotype is the critical gene, such as a TNF-α allele. Usually this can be resolved, but it may take comprehensive studies in a number of different populations to unravel.

Despite these considerations, a number of rheumatic diseases have been convincingly associated with specific HLA alleles. Table 27.2 lists a number of these associations, along with their approximate strength of correlation, represented by relative risk (RR). This indicates the risk for a person to develop disease if the associated allele is present

TABLE 27.2. *HLA associations with rheumatic diseases*

Disease	Specificity	Allele	Approximate RR
Ankylosing spondylitis	B27		80–90
Reactive arthritis	B27		40
Psoriatic arthritis	B27		10
Behçet disease	B51	B*5101	3
Rheumatoid arthritis	DR4	DRB1*0401, *0404	6
Seropositive JRA	DR4	DRB1*0401, *0404	7
Pauciarticular JRA	A2		2–4
	DR5	DRB1*1101, *1104	3–7
	DR8	DRB1*0801	4–8
	DPw2.1	DPB1*0201	3–6
SLE	DR3		3–6
	DR2		2
Sjögren syndrome	DR3		6

Associations between human leukocyte antigen (HLA) alleles and susceptibility to some rheumatic diseases and their approximate relative risks (RR). Alleles in addition to those listed may also be associated.

compared with the risk for someone who does not have the allele, as calculated by the following formula: RR = (no. of patients having the allele × no. of controls not having the allele)/(no. of patients not having the allele × no. of controls having the allele).

HLA and Rheumatoid Arthritis

The association of RA with DR4 was first noted more than 20 years ago (79,80) and since then has been the most intensively studied HLA association among the rheumatic diseases, providing a good example of the complexities involved. DNA-based HLA-typing methods clarified that the association was with particular DR4-positive alleles (DRB1*0401, *0404, *0405, and *0408) and not with other DR4-positive alleles, such as *0402 and *0407 (84–87). Certain non-DR4 alleles also were found to be associated, such as DR1, although more weakly than DR4. Often, an association with DR1 was recognized only after removing all DR4-positive individuals from both patient and control groups, indicating that, among whites, DR1 accounts for most DR4-negative patients (84,87,88). Overall, the *0401 allele is the allele most strongly associated with RA.

When Gregersen et al. (89) sequenced individual DR4 alleles, they noted that all the alleles associated with RA share a very similar stretch of amino acid sequence, from amino acid 70 to 74 in the third hypervariable region of the DRB1 molecule (QKRAA in the *0401 allele, or QRRAA in the *0404 and *0101 alleles). From these observations emerged the shared epitope (SE) hypothesis, which suggests that the risk for RA is conferred by the structural element encoded by this small sequence stretch on susceptibility alleles, even though other polymorphic regions of the molecule can be quite different (89) (Fig. 27.6). Investigation of other ethnic populations in which DR4 alleles are uncommon reinforced this concept. For example, among several Native-American populations with a high prevalence of RA, an allele called DRB1*1402 is associated with disease (90,91). Its sequence is highly divergent from that of the DR4 genes, except for an exact match in the SE region. Similarly, the Spanish population has a relatively low prevalence of DR4 alleles; instead, DRB1*1001, which contains a variation of the SE (RRRAA), is most highly associated with RA in Spain (92). Among the Israeli Jewish population, the most common DR4 allele is DRB1*0402, which does not contain the SE, and in that population, DR1 and DRB1*1001 alleles are most highly associated with RA (93,94). In Japanese populations, RA is strongly associated with DRB1*0405, a DR4-positive allele that also contains the SE (95,96).

Not all patients in any study will have an SE allele. In some groups, such as American blacks, fewer than half of RA patients may possess an SE-positive allele, reflecting the relatively low background frequency of these alleles in that population (97). In the Hispanic population of the United States, there is no increase in SE alleles (98). Clearly, the SE is neither necessary nor sufficient for disease expression. Either a different mechanism accounts for disease in these individuals, or other genetic and environmental factors have contributed enough risk to push the individual over the threshold of disease expression.

Another area of complexity involves the clinical manifestations of RA. RA encompasses a spectrum of disease severity, from relatively mild articular disease to severe destructive arthritis accompanied by systemic features. Some studies investigating the HLA status of RA patients seen in primary care settings have found a prevalence of DR4 or SE-positive alleles lower than those previously reported when patients attended tertiary care centers, suggesting that these alleles contribute to disease severity as well as susceptibility (99). Indeed, many groups have reported an increased frequency of the SE, particularly when found on a DR4-positive allele, among patients with more erosive disease, as determined radiographically (100–102), as well as with serum rheumatoid factor (RF) positivity (100). In contrast, DR1 seems to be more frequent in patients with milder disease (96,103).

Furthermore, gene dosage contributes to disease manifestations as well, with a double dose of SE-positive alleles increasing risk for a severe disease course. Several studies have reported that the combination of DRB1*0401/ *0404 alleles confers a higher relative risk for disease compared with other genotypes (103–106). For example, one study reported a fourfold increased risk for disease among individuals carrying a single copy of the SE as compared with

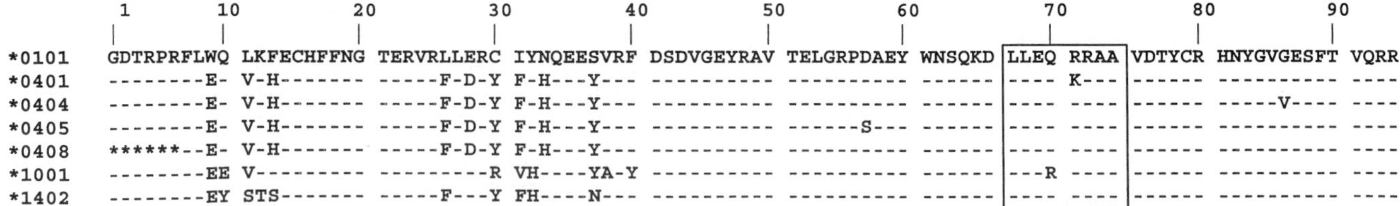

FIG. 27.6. The amino acid sequences of HLA-DRB1 alleles conferring susceptibility to rheumatoid arthritis (RA) are aligned. The "shared epitope" region, from amino acids 67 to 74, is boxed to highlight the residues characteristic of RA-associated alleles.

those without the SE. The risk for disease increased to eightfold among individuals with two SE-positive alleles, and jumped to 26-fold among those with the *0401/*0404 combination (103). Weyand et al. (107,108) developed a hierarchy of disease manifestations based on HLA genotypes. They suggested that, among RA patients, those carrying no SE-positive alleles were likely to have mild, RF-negative, nonerosive disease. The presence of an SE-positive, but DR4-negative, allele slightly increased the risk of more severe disease, whereas a single dose of an SE-positive, DR4-positive allele further increased the likelihood of RF-positive, erosive disease. Two doses of SE-positive alleles enhanced the risk for extraarticular disease: if one of the two were DR4 positive, nodular disease was most likely, whereas if both alleles were DR4-positive (such as *0401/*0404), the risk for major organ involvement increased. In their hierarchy, the *0401/*0401 homozygous combination presented the highest risk for vasculitis. Finally, Felty syndrome, a rare variant of RA that exhibits neutropenia and splenomegaly in addition to arthritis, has one of the strongest associations with DR4-positive susceptibility alleles, approaching 100% in some reports (109).

The possibility that other polymorphic genes in the MHC, particularly within the DRB1*01 and DRB1*04 haplotypes, may contribute to the MHC association with RA has been examined in several ways. A candidate gene approach has been taken for several genes, including other classical HLA genes, such as DQ and DP, as well as DM, TNF-α (110,111), hsp70 (112), and TAP genes (113). Although not all of these have been studied definitively, it is fair to say that, to date, no associations with particular alleles at any of these loci have been reproducibly reported that could not be accounted for by linkage with DR susceptibility genes. However, genome-wide linkage studies have been facilitated by the completion of the human genome and have been undertaken in RA. When family studies were conducted by Jawaheer et al., several regions of the MHC were linked with RA. The greatest linkage was seen at the DRB1 locus, mainly due to the DRB1*0401 and *0404 alleles. However, significant association was found in the region of TNF and a region flanking DRB1, as well a weaker signal in the class I region (114,115). These findings suggest that the role of the genes in the MHC may be more complex than an isolated association with DRB1 (116,117). Overall, it is clear that RA is strongly associated with the presence of the SE, particularly in DR4 alleles. It also is clear that the specific allele involved and the number of susceptibility alleles present are related to clinical manifestations of disease. The functional basis for this association is under intense investigation. In the meantime, the question of clinical utility for HLA typing arises. Is knowledge of HLA genotype useful for screening a population, for making a diagnosis in an individual patient, or for predicting disease course or guiding therapeutic decisions? One can address the first questions by calculating risk estimates for particular genes in a population, based on their background frequency in that population. For example, assuming that the prevalence of RA in North American whites is 1% and knowing the frequency of DR4 alleles in both normal individuals and RA patients in that population, one can conclude that the risk for developing RA in an individual who is positive for the DRB1*0401 allele is approximately 1 in 35 (118). Alternatively, this means that 97% of such individuals will not develop RA. The highest risk, that conferred by the presence of the *0401/*0404 genotype, reaches only 1 in 7. Clearly, then, HLA genotyping is not useful for general population screening or for diagnosis in an individual patient.

Conversely, once a diagnosis of RA is made, knowing the patient's genotype may be helpful in predicting disease course. The association studies discussed earlier that correlate disease severity with the presence and number of specific alleles have been augmented with recent prospective studies of this issue. Wagner et al. (119) followed up recently-diagnosed RA patients for a median of 2 years and reported that patients with an SE-positive, DR4-positive allele had a significantly increased risk for developing erosive disease (RR = 13.75). An independent, prospective study reported a similar result (RR = 13.5) for development of erosions after 1 year in the presence of either an SE allele or rheumatoid factor (105).

Furthermore, an additional study suggests that HLA genotyping may be helpful in guiding therapeutic decisions (120). In this report, several treatment protocols varying in aggressiveness were compared. The results indicated that patients carrying an SE-positive, DR4-positive allele required the most aggressive approach (in this case, the combination of methotrexate, hydroxychloroquine, and sulfasalazine) for a successful outcome, whereas patients without such an allele responded equally well to any of the treatment regimens. Additionally, individuals carrying two doses of the SE seemed to do even more poorly with the less aggressive treatments. An additional study conducted in the Netherlands also demonstrated more aggressive disease in SE-positive individuals, as defined by Sharp scores, and an improved response with more aggressive early therapy (121). These results suggest that RA patients carrying one, and especially two, SE-positive alleles may warrant earlier and more aggressive treatment to control disease and prevent erosions. The availability of more treatment options, including the newer biologic agents, makes the question of which individuals would benefit from earlier, more aggressive treatments more acute. Prospective studies are needed to clarify this issue, but it is likely that HLA markers will provide helpful information in this setting. Current technologic advances should make clinical DNA-based HLA typing feasible and available in the near future.

Other HLA-Associated Diseases

RA represents a disease in which the HLA association has been pinpointed to a small portion of the DRB1 molecule (i.e., the SE region). In contrast, AS illustrates a disease associated with a specificity, HLA-B27, present on a family of related alleles. It also is the best known of the relatively few HLA class I–associated diseases. Studies of this condition have reported a 90% to 95% prevalence of the B27 specificity in some white AS populations, making it one of the strongest HLA associations known (122,123). As with DR4 antigens, DNA sequencing revealed that the B27 specificity includes multiple alleles, at least 25 at latest count (B*2701, *2702, etc.). Several alleles, including B*2702, *2704, and *2705, have been well established as disease associated, with *2705 the predominant allele among North American whites. Most of the remaining alleles also have been at least anecdotally reported to be associated with disease, with the probable exceptions of B*2706 and *2709, suggesting that disease risk is due to a common feature shared by many of these alleles (124). One characteristic feature of HLA-B27 molecules is their unique preference for positively-charged peptides, particularly peptides carrying an arginine in the second position, leading some investigators to hypothesize that the interaction of the molecule with a particular arthritogenic peptide is responsible for disease development (124,125).

Elegant studies in animal models have provided the strongest direct evidence to date that HLA-B27 itself, rather than a linked gene, is responsible for disease. Transgenic rats were generated, in which an introduced HLA-B27 gene was expressed on all cells in the animals. Strikingly, most of these rats manifested pathology remarkably similar to that seen in human spondyloarthropathies. Furthermore, rats raised in a germ-free environment were partially protected from disease, implicating an interaction between genetic predisposition and microorganisms in the environment in disease expression (126). Similarly, expression of HLA-B27/h β_2-microglobulin in mice leads to spontaneous arthritis in mice (127); interestingly, this also occurs in mice, which express only the HLA-B27 gene without β_2-microglobulin (128). These animal models provide an unusual opportunity to uncover the molecular mechanisms involved in disease development.

Other diseases show a complex but reproducible association with alleles at multiple HLA loci. One example is pauciarticular juvenile rheumatoid arthritis (JRA), where DRB1*11 and *08 have been shown to confer increased risk for disease (129,130) and DRB1*08 has been shown to predict more persistent and severe disease (131). Certain heterozygous combinations of these alleles may increase risk synergistically (e.g., *1101/*0801). Individuals who possess the DP allele DPB1*0201 in addition to a DR susceptibility gene have an even higher risk for disease (132–135). In addition, a class I allele, HLA-A*0201, also has been associated with this form of JRA, implicating alleles at three different HLA loci in susceptibility to this condition (136). In some cases, HLA alleles may be associated with particular autoantibody production. For example, in systemic lupus erythematosus (SLE), the reported association of DR3 and DR2 specificities is generally stronger with the presence of anti-SSA (Ro) and anti-SSB (La) antibodies than with clinical disease itself (137–140). Furthermore, in primary Sjögren syndrome, an intriguing association has been reported between high levels of these same autoantibodies and the heterozygous combination of DR3, DQ2, DR2, and DQ1 haplotypes (more recently identified as the genotype DRB1*0301/*1501 in white patients) (141–143). This raises the possibility that, at least in some cases, HLA susceptibility genes direct the production of particular autoantibodies, which in turn are directly involved in the pathogenesis of disease.

Mechanistic Hypotheses to Explain HLA Associations with Disease

Clearly, genes found in the MHC locus are important in the development of autoimmunity. Among these genes, the most strongly associated with disease are the classical HLA molecules. The genes associated with autoimmunity vary with the disease, and it is likely that the underlying pathogenic mechanisms are heterogeneous. In cases where a class I or II allele is linked to disease, the pathogenic mechanism is likely due to an aspect of the immunologic function of these molecules, either in the development or activation of T cells, and thus hypotheses explaining the aberrant immune responses leading to HLA-associated autoimmunity should incorporate this function. As discussed earlier, the primary role of the extensive polymorphism within HLA molecules relates to their ability to bind a wide variety of antigenic peptides and present them to T lymphocytes. This suggests several potential mechanisms by which allelic polymorphisms may contribute to autoimmunity either by the presentation of unique self peptides, or enhanced development or propagation of pathogenic T cells. Four potential mechanistic models are described here.

HLA allelic differences tend toward a preference for particular peptides for binding and antigen presentation in two pivotal steps in the immune response: guiding T-cell development in the thymus and triggering an immune response in the periphery. One hypothesis to explain HLA-linked autoimmune disease suggests that the critical HLA alleles exert their effect during T-cell selection, which takes place in the fetal thymus. It is there that T cells expressing T-cell receptors with high affinity for their HLA/self peptide ligand are negatively selected, or deleted, whereas those with moderate affinity are positively selected. This process fulfills the need for developing a broad T-cell repertoire capable of responding to the myriad pathogenic antigens that the individual will see in his or her lifetime, while preventing damaging responses to the individual's own tissues. T cells specific for a particular autoantigen may be selected depending on the particular HLA allele, resulting in mature T cells that are capable, under the right conditions, of inappropriately recognizing and responding to self antigens.

The second model predicts that a critical recognition event between HLA-expressing antigen-presenting cells

(APCs) and mature T cells occurs in the peripheral immune system. There, the unique peptide-binding properties of the disease-associated HLA allele determine binding and presentation of a specific peptide that is related to the target tissue, such as the joint. This self peptide may be presented in the periphery, but not in the thymus, in scenarios where the APC is altered, or a "nonprofessional" APC, such as a synovial cell, is induced to express HLA and bind a unique set of peptides, which can activate pathogenic T cells.

A third theory is that of molecular mimicry. In this case, the T cell recognizes a self antigen as a structural mimic of a pathogen antigen, such as a peptide derived from a critical polymorphic portion of the HLA molecule itself (e.g., the SE region). By virtue of cross-reactivity, an antigenic mimic may successfully bypass normal tolerance mechanisms. Homologous amino acid sequence stretches between disease-associated HLA molecules and viral or bacterial proteins have been noted in support of this hypothesis, such as a portion of an Epstein-Barr virus glycoprotein that resembles the SE region (144). In this setting the polymorphic portion of the HLA molecule, with homology to a foreign peptide, would act as a peptide itself, being processed and then presented on another, intact HLA molecule.

A fourth possibility is that the threshold for activation of autoreactive T cells may be reached more readily by the HLA alleles that confer risk for autoimmunity. This could be achieved by increased levels of expression of the HLA molecule on the cell surface, or the predominance of a specific self peptide among those peptides presented on the cell surface. Alternatively, T cells may interact directly with polymorphic regions of HLA molecules, and that interaction may enhance the signal received by the T cell and may be relatively peptide-independent (145).

These models provide a mechanistic hypothesis that may explain the association between specific HLA alleles and particular autoimmune diseases. Numerous immunologic events underlie the development, maturation, and activation of an antigen-specific immune response, and the critical structural role of HLA molecules guides the outcome at each step. Combinations of these and possibly other models may be necessary to explain fully the HLA association with autoimmune disease. It also is important to remember that HLA contributes only part of the predisposition to these diseases, and other genetic, infectious, environmental, and developmental factors undoubtedly must work in concert to push an individual over the threshold of disease expression.

ACKNOWLEDGMENTS

We thank Matt Warren for his help with preparation of this manuscript and Eric Swanson for producing the molecular models used in the figures for this text. This chapter has been revised from the previous edition of this textbook with the permission of Barbara Nepom.

REFERENCES

1. Complete sequence and gene map of a human major histocompatibility complex. The MHC sequencing consortium. *Nature* 1999;401:921–923.
2. Bjorkman PJ, Saper MA, Samraoui B, et al. Structure of the human class I histocompatibility antigen, HLA-A2. *Nature* 1987;329:506–512.
3. Geraghty DE. Structure of the HLA class I region and expression of its resident genes. *Curr Opin Immunol* 1993;5:3–7.
4. Bjorkman P, Parham P. Structure, function, and diversity of class I major histocompatibility complex molecules. *Ann Rev Biochem* 1990;59:253–288.
5. Robinson J, Waller MJ, Parham P. et al. IMGT/HLA and IMGT/MHC: sequence databases for the study of the major histompatibility complex. *Nucleic Acids Research* 2003;31:311–314
6. Garrett TP, Saper MA, Bjorkman PJ, et al. Specificity pockets for the side chains of peptide antigens in HLA-Aw68. *Nature* 1989;342:692–696.
7. Madden DR. The three-dimensional structure of peptide-MHC complexes. *Annu Rev Immunol* 1995;13:587–622.
8. Bjorkman PJ, Saper MA, Samraoui B, et al. The foreign antigen binding site and T cell recognition regions of class I histocompatibility antigens. *Nature* 1987;329:512–518.
9. Gao MH, Walz M, Kavathas PB. Post-transcriptional regulation associated with control of human CD8A expression of CD4+ T cells. *Immunogenetics* 1996;45:130–135.
10. Van Kaer L. Major histocompatibility complex class I–restricted antigen processing and presentation. *Tissue Antigens* 2002;60:1–9.
11. Bijlmakers MJ, Pleogh HL. Putting together an MHC class I molecule. *Curr Opin Immunol* 1993;5:21–26.
12. Maffei A, Papadopoulos K, Harris PE. MHC class I antigen processing pathways. *Hum Immunol* 1997;54:91–103.
13. van Endert PM. Genes regulating MHC class I processing of antigen. *Curr Opin Immunol* 1999;11:82–88.
14. Pamer E, Cresswell P. Mechanisms of MHC class I–restricted antigen processing. *Ann Rev Immunol* 1998;16:323–358.
15. Vassilakos A, Cohen-Doyle MF, Peterson PA, et al. The molecular chaperone calnexin facilitates folding and assembly of class I histocompatibility molecules. *EMBO J* 1996;15:1495–1506.
16. Tector M, Salter RD. Calnexin influences folding of human class I histocompatibility proteins but not their assembly with beta 2-microglobulin. *J Biol Chem* 1995;270:19638–19642.
17. Ortmann B, Copeman J, Lehner PJ, et al. A critical role for tapasin in the assembly and function of multimeric MHC class I-TAP complexes. *Science* 1997;277:1306–1309.
18. Sadasivan B, Lehner PJ, Ortmann B, et al. Roles for calreticulin and a novel glycoprotein, tapasin, in the interaction of MHC class I molecules with TAP. *Immunity* 1996;5:103–114.
19. Dick TP, Bangia N, Peaper DR, et al. Disulfide bond isomerization and the assembly of MHC class I-peptide complexes. *Immunity* 2002;16:87–98.
20. Rock KL, Goldberg AL. Degradation of cell proteins and the generation of MHC class I-presented peptides. *Annu Rev Immunol* 1999;17:739–779.
21. Powis SJ. Major histocompatibility complex class I molecules interact with both subunits of the transporter associated with antigen processing, TAP1 and TAP2. *Eur J Immunol* 1997;27:2744–2747.
22. Ragoussis J, Monaco A, Mockridge I, et al. Cloning of the HLA class II region in yeast artificial chromosomes. *Proc Natl Acad Sci U S A* 1991;88:3753–3757.
23. Kappes D, Strominger JL. Human class II major histocompatibility complex genes and proteins. *Ann Rev Biochem* 1988;57:991–1028.
24. Skoskiewicz MJ, Colvin RB, Schneeberger EE, et al. Widespread and selective induction of major histocompatibility complex-determined antigens *in vivo* by gamma interferon. *J Exp Med* 1985;162:1645–1664.
25. Brown JH, Jardetzky TS, Gorga JC, et al. Three-dimensional structure of the human class II histocompatibility antigen HLA-DR1. *Nature* 1993;364:33–39.
26. Stern LJ, Brown JH, Jardetzky TS, et al. Crystal structure of the human class II MHC protein HLA-DR1 complexed with an influenza virus peptide. *Nature* 1994;368:215–221.
27. Dessen A, Lawrence CM, Cupo S, et al. X-ray crystal structure of HLA-DR4 (DRA1*0101, DRB1*0401) complexed with a peptide from human collagen II. *Immunity* 1997;7:473–481.

28. Chicz RM, Urban RG, Lane WS, et al. Predominant naturally processed peptides bound to HLA-DR1 are derived from MHC-related molecules and are heterogeneous in size. *Nature* 1992;358:764–768.
29. Kirschmann DA, Duffin KL, Smith CE, et al. Naturally processed peptides from rheumatoid arthritis associated and non-associated HLA-DR alleles. *J Immunol* 1995;155:5655–5662.
30. Carroll MC, Katzman P, Alicot EM, et al. Linkage map of the human major histocompatibility complex including the tumor necrosis factor genes. *Proc Natl Acad Sci U S A* 1987;84:8535–8539.
31. Kwok WW, Schwarz D, Nepom BS, et al. HLA-DQ molecules form a-b heterodimers of mixed allotype. *J Immunol* 1988;141:3123–3127.
32. Andersen LC, Beaty JS, Nettles JW, et al. Allelic polymorphism in transcriptional regulatory regions of HLA-DQB genes. *J Exp Med* 1991;173:181–192.
33. Perfetto C, Zacheis M, McDaid D, et al. Polymorphism in the promoter region of HLA-DRB genes. *Hum Immunol* 1993;36:27–33.
34. Singal DP, Qiu X, D'Souza M, et al. Polymorphism in the upstream regulatory regions of HLA-DRB genes. *Immunogenetics* 1993;37:143–147.
35. Louis P, Vincent R, Cavadore P, et al. Differential transcriptional activities of HLA-DR genes in the various haplotypes. *J Immunol* 1994; 153:5059–5067.
36. Cresswell P. Chemistry and functional role of the invariant chain. *Curr Opin Immunol* 1992;4:87–92.
37. Bertolino P, Rabourdin-Combe C. The MHC class II-associated invariant chain: a molecule with multiple roles in MHC class II biosynthesis and antigen presentation to CD4+ T cells. *Crit Rev Immunol* 1996;16:359–379.
38. Harding CV. Class II antigen processing: analysis of compartments and functions. *Crit Rev Immunol* 1996;16:13–29.
39. Watts C. Capture and processing of exogenous antigens for presentation on MHC molecules. *Annu Rev Immunol* 1997;15:821–850.
40. Pieters J. MHC class II restricted antigen presentation. *Curr Opin Immunol* 1997;9:89–96.
41. Green JM, Pierce SK. Class II antigen processing compartments and the function of HLA-DM. *Int Rev Immunol* 1996;13:209–219.
42. Vogt AB, Kropshofer H, Hammerling GJ. How HLA-DM affects the peptide repertoire bound to HLA-DR molecules. *Hum Immunol* 1997; 54:170–179.
43. Arndt SO, Vogt AB, Hammerling GJ, et al. Selection of the MHC class II-associated peptide repertoire by HLA-DM. *Immunol Res* 1997;16: 261–272.
44. Braud VM, Allan DS, McMichael AJ. Functions of nonclassical MHC and non-MHC-encoded class I molecules. *Curr Opin Immunol* 1999; 11:100–108.
45. O'Callaghan CA, Bell JI. Structure and function of the human MHC class Ib molecules HLA-E, HLA-F and HLA-G. *Immunol Rev* 1998; 163:129–138.
46. Fournel S, Aguerre-Girr M, Huc X, et al. Cutting edge: soluble HLA-G1 triggers CD95/CD95 ligand-mediated apoptosis in activated CD8+ cells by interacting with CD8. *J Immunol* 2000;164:6100–6104.
47. Sanders SK, Giblin PA, Kavathas P. Cell-cell adhesion mediated by CD8 and human histocompatibility leukocyte antigen G, a nonclassical major histocompatibility complex class 1 molecule on cytotrophoblasts. *J Exp Med* 1991;174:737–740.
48. Le Gal FA, Riteau B, Sedlik C, et al. HLA-G-mediated inhibition of antigen-specific cytotoxic T lymphocytes. *Int Immunol* 1999;11: 1351–1356.
49. Bainbridge DR, Ellis SA, Sargent IL. HLA-G suppresses proliferation of CD4 (+) T-lymphocytes. *J Reprod Immunol* 2000;48:17–26.
50. Rajagopalan S, Long EO. A human histocompatibility leukocyte antigen (HLA)-G-specific receptor expressed on all natural killer cells. *J Exp Med* 1999;189:1093–1100.
51. Ponte M, Cantoni C, Biassoni R, et al. Inhibitory receptors sensing HLA-G1 molecules in pregnancy: decidua-associated natural killer cells express LIR-1 and CD94/NKG2A and acquire p49, an HLA-G1-specific receptor. *Proc Natl Acad Sci U S A* 1999;96:5674–5679.
52. Le Bouteiller P, Blaschitz A. The functionality of HLA-G is emerging. *Immunol Rev* 1999;167:233–244.
53. Carosella ED, Dausset J, Rouas-Freiss N. Immunotolerant functions of HLA-G. *Cell Mol Life Sci* 1999;55:327–333.
54. Ishitani A, Sageshima N, Lee N, et al. Protein expression and peptide binding suggest unique and interacting functional roles for HLA-E, F, and G in maternal-placental immune recognition. *J Immunol* 2003; 171:1376–1384.
55. Feder JN, Gnirke A, Thomas W, et al. A novel MHC class I-like gene is mutated in patients with hereditary haemochromatosis [see comments]. *Nat Genet* 1996;13:399–408.
56. Wu J, Song Y, Bakker AB, Bauer S, et al. An activating immunoreceptor complex formed by NKG2D and DAP10. *Science* 1999;285:730–732.
57. Groh V, Rhinehart R, Randolph-Habecker J, et al. Costimulation of CD8alphabeta T cells by NKG2D via engagement by MIC induced on virus-infected cells. *Nat Immunol* 2001;2:255–260.
58. Das H, Groh V, Kuijl C, et al. MICA engagement by human Vgamma2Vdelta2 T cells enhances their antigen-dependent effector function. *Immunity* 2001;15:83–93.
59. Mosyak L, Zaller DM, Wiley DC. The structure of HLA-DM, the peptide exchange catalyst that loads antigen onto class II MHC molecules during antigen presentation. *Immunity* 1998;9:377–383.
60. Busch R, Mellins ED. Developing and shedding inhibitions: how the MHC class II molecules reach maturity. *Curr Opin Immunol* 1996;8: 51–58.
61. Jensen PE. Antigen processing: HLA-DO—a hitchhiking inhibitor of HLA-DM. *Curr Biol* 8:R128–R131.
62. Denzin, LK, Sant'Angelo DB, Hammond C, et al. Negative regulation by HLA-DO of MHC class II-restricted antigen processing. *Science* 1997;278:106–109.
63. Vogt AB, Kropshofer H. HLA-DM—an endosomal and lysosomal chaperone for the immune system. *Trends Biochem Sci* 1999;24: 150–154.
64. Kropshofer H, Vogt AB, Thery C, et al. A role for HLA-DO as a co-chaperone of HLA-DM in peptide loading of MHC class II molecules. *EMBO J* 1998;17:2971–2981.
65. Kelly A, Trowsdale J. Novel genes in the human major histocompatibility complex class II region. *Int Arch Allergy Immunol* 1994;103: 11–15.
66. Martinez CK, Monaco JJ. Homology of proteasome subunits to a major histocompatibility complex-linked LMP gene. *Nature* 1991; 353:664–667.
67. Monaco JJ. Genes in the MHC that may affect antigen processing. *Curr Opin Immunol* 1992;4:70–73.
68. Trowsdale J, Hanson I, Mockridge I, et al. Sequences encoded in the class II region of the MHC related to the "ABC" superfamily of transporters. *Nature* 1990;348:741–744.
69. Carroll MC, Campbell RD, Bentley DR, et al. A molecular map of the human major histocompatibility complex class III region linking complement genes C4, C2, and factor B. *Nature* 1984;307:237–241.
70. Sargent CA, Dunham I, Trowsdale J, et al. Human major histocompatibility complex contains genes for the major heat shock protein HSP70. *Proc Natl Acad Sci U S A* 1989;86:1968–1972.
71. Carroll MC, Campbell RD, Porter RR. The mapping of 21-hydroxylase genes adjacent to complement C4 genes in HLA, the major histocompatibility complex in man. *Proc Natl Acad Sci U S A* 1985;82:521–525.
72. Scharf SJ, Griffith RL, Erlich HA. Rapid typing of DNA sequence polymorphism at the HLA-DRB1 locus using the polymerase chain reaction and nonradioactive oligonucleotide probes. *Hum Immunol* 1991;30:190–201.
73. Erlich H, Bugawan T, Begovich AB, et al. HLA-DR, DQ, and DP typing using PCR amplification and immobilized probes. *Eur J Immunogen* 1991;18:33–55.
74. Hui KM, Bidwell JL. eds. *Handbook of HLA typing techniques.* Boca Raton: CRC Press, 1993.
75. Erlich HA, Opelz G, Hansen J. HLA DNA typing and transplantation. *Immunity* 2001;14:347–356.
76. Marsh SG, Albert ED, Bodmer WF, et al. Nomenclature for factors of the HLA system, 2002. *Tissue Antigens* 2002;60:407–464.
77. Brewerton DA, Hart FD, Nicholls A, et al. Ankylosing spondylitis and HLA-A27. *Lancet* 1973;1:904–907.
78. Schlosstein T, Terasaki PI, Bluestone R, et al. High association of an HLA antigen, w27, with ankylosing spondylitis. *N Engl J Med* 1973; 288:704–706.
79. McMichael SJ, Sasazuki T, McDevitt HO, et al. Increased frequency of HLA-Cw3 and HLA-Dw4 in rheumatoid arthritis. *Arthritis Rheum* 1977;20:1037–1042.
80. Stastny P. Association of the B-cell alloantigen DRw4 with rheumatoid arthritis. *N Engl J Med* 1978;298:869–871.
81. Tiwari J, Terasaki P. *HLA and disease associations.* New York: Springer-Verlag 1985:1–472.

82. Vartdal F, Johansen BH, Friede T, et al. The peptide binding motif of the disease associated HLA-DQ (alpha 1* 0501, beta 1* 0201) molecule. *Eur J Immunol* 1996;26:2764–2772.
83. Gofton JP. Epidemiology, tissue type antigens and Bechterew's syndrome (ankylosing spondylitis) in various ethnical populations. *Scand J Rheumatol* 1980;32(suppl):166–168.
84. Nepom GT, Byers P, Seyfried C, et al. HLA genes associated with rheumatoid arthritis. *Arthritis Rheum* 1989;32:15–21.
85. Ronningen KA, Spurkland A, Egeland T, et al. Rheumatoid arthritis may be primarily associated with HLA-DR4 molecules sharing a particular sequence at residues 67–74. *Tissue Antigens* 1990;36:235–240.
86. Wordsworth B, Lanchbury JSS, Sakkas LI, et al. HLA-DR4 subtype frequencies in rheumatoid arthritis indicate that DRB1 is the major susceptibility locus within the HLA class II region. *Proc Natl Acad Sci U S A* 1989;86:10049–10053.
87. Wallin J, Hillert J, Olerup O, et al. Association of rheumatoid arthritis with a dominant DR1/Dw4/Dw14 sequence motif, but not with T cell receptor b chain gene alleles or haplotypes. *Arthritis Rheum* 1991;34:1416–1424.
88. Thomsen M, Morling N, Snorrason E, et al. HLA-Dw4 and rheumatoid arthritis. *Tissue Antigens* 1979;13:56–60.
89. Gregersen PK, Silver J, Winchester RJ. The shared epitope hypothesis: an approach to understanding the molecular genetics of susceptibility to rheumatoid arthritis. *Arthritis Rheum* 1987;30:1205– 1213.
90. Willkens RF, Nepom GT, Marks CR, et al. The association of HLA-Dw16 with rheumatoid arthritis in Yakima Indians: further evidence for the "shared epitope" hypothesis. *Arthritis Rheum* 1991;34:43–47.
91. Nelson JL, Boyer G, Templin D, et al. HLA antigens in Tlingit Indians with rheumatoid arthritis. *Tissue Antigens* 1992;40:57–63.
92. Yelamos J, Garcia-Lozano JR, Moreno I, et al. Association of HLA-DR4-Dw15 (DRB1*0405) and DR10 with rheumatoid arthritis in a Spanish population. *Arthritis Rheum* 1993;36:811–814.
93. Schiff B, Mizrachi Y, Orgad S, et al. Association of HLA-Aw31 and HLA-DR1 with adult rheumatoid arthritis. *Ann Rheum Dis* 1982;41: 403–404.
94. Gao X, Gazit E, Livneh A, et al. Rheumatoid arthritis in Israeli Jews: shared sequences in the third hypervariable region of DRB1 alleles are associated with susceptibility. *J Rheumatol* 1991;18:801–803.
95. Takeuchi F, Nakano K, Matsuta K, et al. Positive and negative association of HLA-DR genotypes with Japanese rheumatoid arthritis. *Clin Exp Rheum* 1996;14:17–22.
96. Wakitani S, Murata N, Toda Y, et al. The relationship between HLA-DRB1 alleles and disease subsets of rheumatoid arthritis in Japanese. *Br J Rheumatol* 1997;36:630–636.
97. McDaniel DO, Alarcon GS, Pratt PW, et al. Most African-American patients with rheumatoid arthritis do not have the rheumatoid antigenic determinant (epitope). *Ann Intern Med* 1995;123:181–187.
98. Del Rincon I, Battafarano DF, Arroyo RA, et al. Ethnic variation in the clinical manifestations of rheumatoid arthritis: role of HLA-DRB1 alleles. *Arthritis Rheum* 2003;49:200–208.
99. Thomson W, Pepper L, Payton A, et al. Absence of an association between HLA-DRB1*04 and rheumatoid arthritis in newly diagnosed cases from the community. *Ann Rheum Dis* 1993;52:539–541.
100. Young A, Jaraquemada D, Awad J, et al. Association of HLA-DR4/Dw4 and DR2/Dw2 with radiologic changes in a prospective study of patients with rheumatoid arthritis. *Arthritis Rheum* 1984;27: 20–25.
101. Olsen NJ, Callahan LF, Brooks RH, et al. Associations of HLA-DR4 with rheumatoid factor and radiographic severity in rheumatoid arthritis. *Am J Med* 1988;84:257–264.
102. Wagner U, Kaltenhauser S, Pierer M, et al. Prospective analysis of the impact of HLA-DR and -DQ on joint destruction in recent-onset rheumatoid arthritis. *Rheumatology (Oxford)* 2003;42:553–562.
103. MacGregor A, Ollier W, Thomson W, et al. HLA-DRB1*0401/0404 genotype and rheumatoid arthritis: Increased association in men, young age at onset, and disease severity. *J Rheumatol* 1995;22:1032–1036.
104. Nepom GT, Seyfried CE, Holbeck SL, et al. Identification of HLA-Dw14 genes in DR4[+] rheumatoid arthritis. *Lancet* 1986;2:1002–1005.
105. Gough A, Faint J, Salmon M, et al. Genetic typing of patients with inflammatory arthritis at presentation can be used to predict outcome. *Arthritis Rheum* 1994;37:1166–1170.
106. Wordsworth P, Pile KD, Buckley JD, et al. HLA heterozygosity contributes to susceptibility to rheumatoid arthritis. *Am J Hum Genet* 1992;51:585–591.
107. Weyand CM, McCarthy TG, Goronzy JJ. Correlation between disease phenotype and genetic heterogeneity in rheumatoid arthritis. *J Clin Invest* 1995;95:2120–2126.
108. Weyand CM, Xie C, Goronzy JJ. Homozygosity for the HLA-DRB1 allele selects for extra-articular manifestations in rheumatoid arthritis. *J Clin Invest* 1992;89:2033–2039.
109. Campion G, Maddison PJ, Goulding N, et al. The Felty syndrome: a case-matched study of clinical manifestations and outcome, serologic features, and immunogenetic associations. *Medicine* 1990;69:69–80.
110. Newton J, Brown MA, Milicic A, et al. The effect of HLA-DR on susceptibility to rheumatoid arthritis is influenced by the associated lymphotoxin alpha-tumor necrosis factor haplotype. *Arthritis Rheum* 2003;48:90–96.
111. Low AS, Gonzalez-Gay MA, Akil M, et al. TNF +489 polymorphism does not contribute to susceptibility to rheumatoid arthritis. *Clin Exp Rheumatol* 2002;20:829–832.
112. Jenkins SC, March RE, Campbell RD, et al. A novel variant of the MHC-linked hsp70, hsp70-hom, is associated with rheumatoid arthritis. *Tissue Antigens* 2000;56:38–44.
113. Vejbaesya S, Luangtrakool P, Luangtrakool K, et al. Analysis of TAP and HLA-DM polymorphism in thai rheumatoid arthritis. *Hum Immunol* 2000;61:309–313.
114. Jawaheer D, Li W, Graham RR, et al. Dissecting the genetic complexity of the association between human leukocyte antigens and rheumatoid arthritis. *Am J Hum Genet* 2002;71:585–594.
115. Gregersen PK. Teasing apart the complex genetics of human autoimmunity: lessons from rheumatoid arthritis. *Clin Immunol* 2003; 107:1–9.
116. Cornélis F, Faure S, Martinez M, et al. New susceptibility locus for rheumatoid arthritis suggested by a genome-wide linkage study. *Proc Natl Acad Sci U S A* 1998;95:10746–10750.
117. Gregersen PK. The North American Rheumatoid Arthritis Consortium—bringing genetic analysis to bear on disease susceptibility, severity, and outcome. *Arthritis Care Res* 1998;11:1–2.
118. Nepom GT, Nepom BS. *Prediction of susceptibility to rheumatoid arthritis by human leukocyte antigen genotyping.* In: Nepom GT, ed. Rheumatic disease clinics of North America. Philadelphia: WB Saunders 1991:825–842.
119. Wagner U, Kaltenhauser S, Sauer H, et al. HLA markers and prediction of clinical course and outcome in rheumatoid arthritis. *Arthritis Rheum* 1997;40:341–351.
120. O'Dell JR, Nepom BS, Haire C, et al. HLA-DRB1 typing in rheumatoid arthritis: predicting response to specific treatments. *Ann Rheum Dis* 1998;57:209–213.
121. Lard LR, Boers M, Verhoeven A, et al. Early and aggressive treatment of rheumatoid arthritis patients affects the association of HLA class II antigens with progression of joint damage. *Arthritis Rheum* 2002;46:899–905.
122. Gonzalez S, Martinez-Borra J, Lopez-Larrea C. Immunogenetics, HLA-B27 and spondyloarthropathies. *Curr Opin Rheumatol* 1999; 11:257–264.
123. Al-Khonizy W, Reveille JD. The immunogenetics of the seronegative spondyloarthropathies. *Baillieres Clin Rheumatol* 1998;12:567–589.
124. Lamas JR, Paradela A, Roncal F, et al. Modulation at multiple anchor positions of the peptide specificity of HLA-B27 subtypes differentially associated with ankylosing spondylitis. *Arthritis Rheum* 1999; 42:1975–1985.
125. Parham P. B27 polymorphism and peptide repertoire. *Clin Rheumatol* 1996;15(suppl):72–73.
126. Taurog JD, Maika SD, Satumtira N, et al. Inflammatory disease in HLA-B27 transgenic rats. *Immunol Rev* 1999;169:209–223.
127. Khare SD, Hansen J, Luthra HS, et al. HLA-B27 heavy chains contribute to spontaneous inflammatory disease in B27/human beta2-microglobulin (beta2m) double transgenic mice with disrupted mouse beta2m. *J Clin Invest* 1996;98:2746–2755.
128. Khare SD, Luthra HS, David CS. Spontaneous inflammatory arthritis in HLA-B27 transgenic mice lacking beta 2-microglobulin: a model of human spondyloarthropathies. *J Exp Med* 1995;182:1153–1158.
129. Thomson W, Barrett JH, Donn R, et al. Juvenile idiopathic arthritis classified by the ILAR criteria: HLA associations in UK patients. *Rheumatology (Oxford)* 2002;41:1183–1189.

130. Zeggini E, Donn RP, Ollier WE, et al. Evidence for linkage of HLA loci in juvenile idiopathic oligoarthritis: independent effects of HLA-A and HLA-DRB1. *Arthritis Rheum* 2002;46:2716–2720.
131. Flato B, Lien G, Smerdel A, et al. Prognostic factors in juvenile rheumatoid arthritis: a case-control study revealing early predictors and outcome after 14.9 years. *J Rheumatol* 2003;30:386–393.
132. Nepom B. *The immunogenetics of juvenile rheumatoid arthritis.* In Athreya B, ed. Rheumatic disease clinics of North America. Philadelphia: WB Saunders 1991:825–842.
133. Nepom BS, Glass DN. Juvenile rheumatoid arthritis and HLA: report of the Park City III Workshop. *J Rheumatol* 1992;19:70–74.
134. Grom AA, Giannini EH, Glass DN. Juvenile rheumatoid arthritis and the trimolecular complex (HLA, T cell receptor, and antigen). Differences from rheumatoid arthritis. *Arthritis Rheum* 1994;37:601–607.
135. Albert ED, Scholz S. Juvenile arthritis: genetic update. *Baillieres Clin Rheumatol* 1998;12:209–218.
136. Zeggini E, Donn RP, Ollier WE, and Thomson, W. Evidence for linkage of HLA loci in juvenile idiopathic oligoarthritis: independent effects of HLA-A and HLA-DRB1 *Arthritis Rheum* 2002;46:2716–2720,
137. Harley JB, Moser KL, Gaffney PM, et al. The genetics of human systemic lupus erythematosus. *Curr Opin Immunol* 1998;10:690–696.
138. Tan FK, Arnett FC. The genetics of lupus. *Curr Opin Rheumatol* 1998;10:399–408.
139. Schur PH. Genetics of systemic lupus erythematosus. *Lupus* 1995;4: 425–437.
140. Galeazzi M, Sebastiani GD, Morozzi G, et al. HLA class II DNA typing in a large series of European patients with systemic lupus erythematosus: correlations with clinical and autoantibody subsets. *Medicine (Baltimore)* 2002;81:169–178.
141. Harley JB, Reichlin M, Arnett FC, et al. Gene interaction at HLA-DQ enhances autoantibody production in primary Sjögren's syndrome. *Science* 1986;232:1145–1147.
142. Guggenbuhl P, Jean S, Jego P, et al. Primary Sjögren's syndrome: role of the HLA-DRB1*0301-*1501 heterozygotes. *J Rheumatol* 1998;25:900–905.
143. Gottenberg JE, Busson M, Loiseau P, et al. In primary Sjögren's syndrome, HLA class II is associated exclusively with autoantibody production and spreading of the autoimmune response. *Arthritis Rheum* 2003;48:2240–2245.
144. Roudier J, Rhodes G, Petersen J, et al. Hypothesis: the Epstein-Barr virus glycoprotein gp110, a molecular link between HLA DR4, HLA DR1, and rheumatoid arthritis. *Scand J Immunol* 1988;27: 367–371.
145. Gebe JA, Novak EJ, Kwok WW, et al. T cell selection and differential activation on structurally related HLA-DR4 ligands. *J Immunol* 2001;167:3250–3256.

CHAPTER 28

Genetic Basis of Rheumatic Disease

John B. Harley and Amr H. Sawalha

The enormous complexity of biologic systems renders the understanding of disease states very difficult. In many situations the critical abnormalities that initiate these processes are not known. The basic understanding of the etiology of disease has a profound and practical influence on the development of treatment and preventive strategies.

Etiology derives from two sources: genetics and environment. The genetic differences between individuals in a species lead to structural differences. These in turn change the probability that a genetic difference will "cause" or explain the etiology of the observed phenotype of interest, for our purposes, a rheumatic disease. Often genetic causes interact with or require other genes or environmental factors to be fully expressed.

This chapter explores how rapidly improving modern genetic strategies and newly available genomic resources are being used to discover the genetic components of the etiology of rheumatic disorders. The environmental component of etiology for individual disorders is discussed in chapters elsewhere in this text.

The available conceptual and technical methods provide not only the opportunity for discovery, but also set the limits for what is possible to discover. Genetic discovery in human diseases now relies heavily on improved DNA technology, more incisive applied mathematical methods, and better infrastructure describing and accessing the human genome. Each of these areas is in the throes of fundamental and very rapidly paradigm-shifting changes. Cumulatively, they are making previously impenetrable problems in the rheumatic diseases accessible to genetic solution. Indeed, the new boundaries of what might be possible are not well defined. Disappointment, through failure to meet current expectations, seems inevitable, as do unexpected successes through brilliant and paradigm-challenging experiments.

This is an exciting time to work in human genetics, with the high drama of enormous effort and human enterprise pursuing the unfulfilled promise and hope offered by a rapidly changing discipline. Consequently, subsequent volumes of this text are likely to describe the genetic components of most rheumatic diseases with the kind of detail that is well beyond our present understanding.

In the previous era of human genetics, only two decades ago, the underlying genetics were understood by inferring genotypes from phenotypes. A phenotype is an observed characteristic (or set of characteristics) in an individual, whereas a genotype is the heritable property responsible for that phenotype. Today, a genotype is the actual DNA sequence itself, and when the DNA is different among the typed individuals, the genotype becomes a description of the DNA variation. The previous generation of geneticists would find polymorphic differences in proteins or body appearance or capabilities (e.g., tongue rolling), and then infer probabilities for the possible genotypes at each locus. This would then be used to explain the observed marker phenotype. The phenotype of interest was evaluated relative to these genotypic probabilities.

For example, the first genetic linkage in humans was published in 1935, when Penrose showed that red hair color was linked to blood type A and B using affected pairs of siblings (1). The genotypic difference for red hair is complicated, but he relied only on the inference obtained from the presence or absence of the phenotypes. The ABO blood type phenotype sufficiently limits the possible genotypes that may be present at this second locus, and thereby provides the analytic capability to discover linkage. Relative to previous generations of rheumatic disease geneticists, we now enjoy the enormous advantage of directly determining genotypes at the nucleic acid sequence level of DNA (or RNA). This profoundly simplifying advance has greatly increased our ability to identify genetic relationships.

Of course, the genomic infrastructural resources being made available are also extremely important. Genetic maps containing sequenced genes, microsatellites, single nucleotide polymorphisms (SNPs), and disease linkages are rapidly becoming more and more dense. Indeed, in early 2003 it was announced that the sequence of the human genome was complete. Those trying to use the currently available human genome sequence might disagree; however, the remaining ambiguities, gaps, and errors are being addressed and progressively eliminated.

Advances in applied mathematics have been as important for genetic progress as have advances in DNA manipulation, computer technology, and genomics. These methods further increase experimental productivity and make otherwise inaccessible genetic effects discoverable. Indeed, experimental design is dictated by the analytic methods available.

There are two standard strategies now used for disease-associated gene identification. The first is to test candidate genes for association. Here, a statistically-significant relationship is usually sought between a phenotype and an allele (also called a polymorphism) at a single locus. Rheumatic disease investigators have been exploring candidate genes for association for many decades. The many histocompatibility [human leukocyte antigen (HLA)] associations now known for the inflammatory disorders are among the best known examples of genetic association. In the next few years, the putative candidate gene associations are expected to substantially increase as the capacity to evaluate the entire genome for genetic association with a particular disease becomes a practical possibility.

The second strategy for disease-associated gene identification begins with genetic linkage. Once linkage has been established, efforts are made to confine the area of interest to the smallest genomic region possible. The region is then explored for candidate genes containing the polymorphisms responsible for the observed genetic linkage. This approach ultimately employs genetic association, but uses linkage to increase the prior probability of there being genetic association in a candidate region of the genome.

SEGREGATION

How does one tell if a particular phenotype represents a genetic problem amenable to solution? There are a few general rules. Identifying a genetic model explaining the mode of inheritance is powerful and virtually assures that there will be a successful outcome in the effort to find the responsible genes. The lower the genetic concordance between identical twins, the less likely that a genetic explanation for the phenotype will be found. A high identical twin concordance also helps, but may also be explained by a shared environment.

The distribution of diseases in the population varies according to the mechanisms by which they are generated. Some disorders appear to occur in families following the known rules of inheritance. These reflect the source of DNA as somatic DNA (Mendelian), sex-linked (X chromosome), patrilineal (Y chromosome), and matrilineal (mitochondrial DNA). Indeed, DNA is the repository for genetic information. Its variations, also called polymorphisms or alleles, at a gene (here meaning a locus) change the risk for a phenotype. The word *gene* is ambiguous, which leads to confusion. *Gene* is sometimes used to mean an allele and in other contexts is used to mean a locus. The ambiguity has historical roots, since the word *gene* preceded both the more specific use and meaning of allele and locus.

There are, for example, families whose members have a risk for calcium pyrophosphate deposition disease and the accompanying arthritis of pseudogout transmitted in an autosomal-dominant pattern of inheritance. Some disorders appear to be associated with the DNA of the mitochondria and are inherited only through the maternal lineage. Myopathies, such as myoclonic epilepsy with ragged red fibers, are examples of this form of inheritance.

Other diseases appear to have more complicated genetics. Although they appear to have a genetic component, the mechanism of inheritance responsible for the observed relationships is not apparent. Indeed, for many of the more common rheumatic disorders, such as rheumatoid arthritis (RA), systemic lupus erythematosus (SLE), osteoarthritis, and osteoporosis, it is widely suspected that many different genes are making variable contributions toward each of these phenotypes. These are commonly referred to as complex genetic disorders.

The effort to understand the pattern of disease phenotype inheritance is called segregation analysis. Knowing the pattern of disease inheritance is important. This can help determine which approach is more likely to be successful in finding the genes responsible.

Some diseases segregate as if they have a "founder effect." This means that the disease phenotype should theoretically be able to be traced to a single DNA variation in a single progenitor individual (Fig. 28.1). A founder effect means that the affected individuals share an original affected ancestor whose critical piece of DNA, which causes the disorder, is shared among subsequent progeny affecteds. The process of establishing and identifying the responsible DNA variation in the presence of a founder effect is different and, in some ways, simpler than in situations where no founder effect is present. Huntington chorea is perhaps the most classic example. Virtually all of the thousands of individuals at risk for Huntington chorea appear to be the descendant of a single individual (2). Hemochromatosis, by virtue of being concentrated in one ethnic group where an HLA association had been identified, had long been suspected to have a founder effect (3). This prediction was used to great advantage in the successful effort to identify the responsible gene.

Neils Risch developed a useful measure now commonly applied to the segregation analysis of complex diseases. The rate of phenotype concordance between a proband and his or her relatives versus the phenotype occurrence in the general population is used to assess the apparent capacity of a particular study to reveal underlying genetic effects (4). The rate of concordance of siblings of the proband divided by the rate of disease in the general population is such a

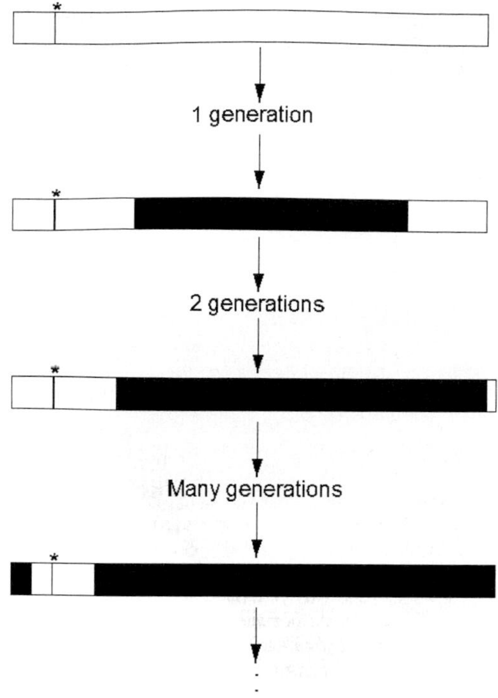

FIG. 28.1. Individual founder chromosome. A founder effect classically begins with the mutation of a single chromosome (*). Crossovers replace the chromosomal DNA from the founder (*white*) with DNA not from the founder chromosome (*black*) in affected individuals of subsequent generations. Crossovers continue to reduce the size of the region from the founder. Although subsequent affected individuals share the mutation (*) conferring risk for the phenotype and the surrounding DNA, the size of this shared founder DNA region varies among affected progeny. In addition, other founder DNA (*white*) will tend to be randomly distributed across the chromosome and will be present, on average, as a function of the number of generations and of the population structure (inbreeding).

measure and is referred to as the λs. The higher the λs, the greater the potential genetic contribution to the phenotype. Although one does not know in advance how complicated the genetics may be, this provides a general benchmark for how difficult the genetic answers may be to find. In addition, when the rate of concordance decreases by more than 3 for each degree of relationship, the genetics of the phenotype are predicted to be complex (4).

GENOTYPING

Genomic DNA is usually used at two levels: first, to establish genetic linkage by using genotypic markers, and second, to identify the responsible gene by testing for association. The latter finds the genotypes responsible for the observed phenotype from the evaluation of candidate genes. Candidate gene polymorphisms are often directly evaluated, and surprisingly, often positive results are found without any evidence for linkage having been previously collected. Identifying the genes and understanding their biology is the great challenge. If association studies will be eventually performed, directly evaluating promising candidate genes has the potential to greatly accelerate progress.

There are two types of genetic markers now ordinarily used for genotyping: microsatellites and SNPs (Fig. 28.2). Microsatellites are also called variable number tandem repeats because a sequence of two, three, or four nucleotides is repeated a variable number of times. The polymorphism or allele for that marker is based on the number of times the short sequence is repeated. There are estimated to be more than 50,000 microsatellites in the human genome.

Polymorphisms are usually identified after expansion using the polymerase chain reaction (Fig. 28.3). This requires the preparation of primers complementary to the DNA sequence flanking the variably repeated element and geometric expansion of the DNA through repetitious primer extension and DNA denaturation. The procedure has been

Panel A

Microsatellite Marker

Chromosome A (TCA is repeated three times):

AAG TTC <u>TCA TCA TCA</u> TAG GAT CTC

Chromosome B (TCA is repeated four times):

AAG TTC <u>TCA TCA TCA TCA</u> TAG GAT CTC

Panel B

Single Nucleotide Polymorphism (SNP) at FcγRIIA, H131R

Chromosome A:

lys phe ser *his* leu asp pro

AAA TTC TCC CAT TTG GAT CCC

Chromosome B:

AAA TTC TCC CGT TTG GAT CCC

lys phe ser *arg* leu asp pro

FIG. 28.2. Microsatellites and single nucleotide polymorphisms (SNPs). **A:** Polymorphic microsatellite compares a pair of alleles found on two individual's chromosomes, one with three repeats of the trinucleotide sequence and the other with four repeats. **B:** The single nucleotide polymorphism difference found at nucleotide position 394 of the FcγRIIA nucleotide sequence on chromosome 1q23.1. This polymorphism leads to a change within the amino acid at position 131 [histidine is changed to arginine (H131R)], which changes the affinity of IgG2 for this Fc receptor.

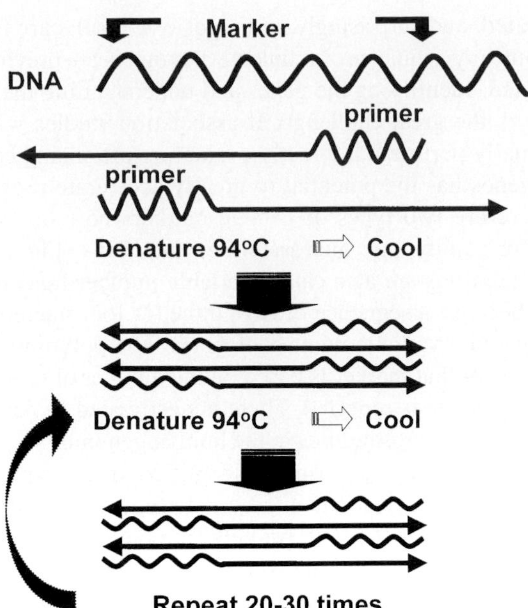

FIG. 28.3. The polymerase chain reaction geometrically expands specific DNA. Complementary oligonucleotide DNA primers locate the 3′ end of the DNA to be expanded. The intervening DNA is replicated. With each elevation of temperature (to 94°C) the DNA is denatured, allowing the primers to again locate the 3′ end of the target DNA for another round of DNA synthesis when the temperature is reduced. Repeating this cycle progressively produces larger and larger quantities of the target DNA sequence.

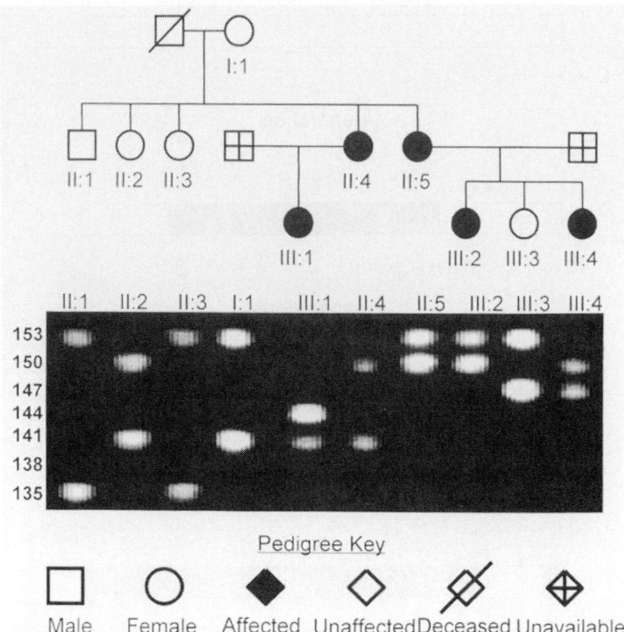

FIG. 28.4. Genotyping a pedigree multiplex for systemic lupus erythematosus. **Top:** A three-generation African-American pedigree is presented. A horizontal line connects spouses. The progeny of a mating divide horizontal lines with vertical lines. **Bottom:** The pedigree drawing has been redrawn so that the genotyping results at D12S1042 are given in the image from the polyacrylamide gel electrophoresis presented below. The alleles vary by the number of three-base repeats present (135 to 153 indicates the number of nucleotide bases in the DNA fragment). The larger alleles move relatively more slowly in the electric field and are therefore higher in the gel.

semiautomated, making possible the collection of thousands of genotypes a day (Fig. 28.4).

Single nucleotide polymorphisms are expected to supplant the microsatellites because there are so many more of them and their rate of mutation is so much lower. There is a relatively common SNP every 500 or fewer bases of the human genome, leading to the expectation that there would be on the order of 7,000,000 SNPs with which to perform human genetic analyses. In addition, DNA chip technologies evaluate tens or hundreds of thousands of these polymorphisms simultaneously and rapidly. The SNP Consortium has, to date, described 1.8 million SNPs. Many laboratories around the world joined this effort to identify SNPs and to provide them to a public database. This has been an extraordinary example of the power of cooperating through the Internet. The reader is invited to go to *snp.cshl.org/* and look up their favorite gene, locus, or chromosome location.

A current controversy focuses on how useful SNPs will prove to be. The mutation rate is not linear along the chromosome. Therefore, situations are expected in which the more recent and subpopulation variable SNPs would be the most useful for this approach, but they are generally less prevalent than the evolutionarily older SNPs. A recent study preliminarily reported to have failed to locate the well-known genetic defect for sickle cell anemia using this approach (5). Nevertheless, there is much hope that well-characterized SNPs, along with a detailed and accurate map of their location, will help solve a number of presently intractable problems. A central role for the SNPs in locating genetic effects is anticipated, but some work remains in order to understand their capabilities and to build the resources and databases needed to best exploit this promising approach.

Discovery of genetic effects by directly testing genes is intrinsically inefficient. There are on the order of 25,000 human genes, and an unknown number of polymorphisms. Any present effort to find disease genes in this way is bound to be incomplete with existing technology. On the other hand, the technical capacity to evaluate more than 100,000 SNPs routinely from a single individual should be available as this text is going to press. Such capability will revolutionize genetic analysis.

CROSSOVERS

Of course, the goal is to find the disease-associated genes and then to explain their role in pathophysiology of the phe-

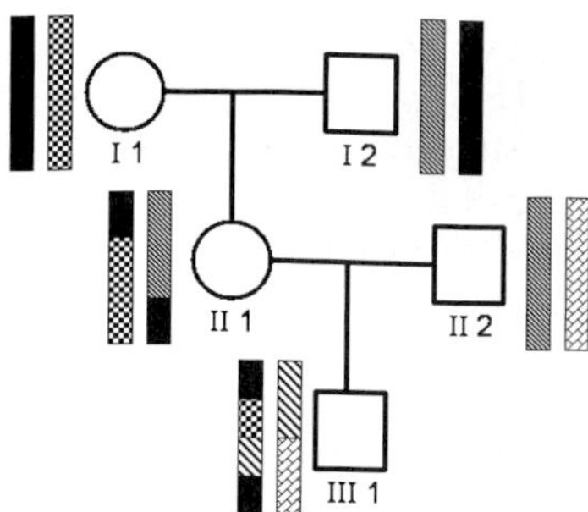

FIG. 28.5. Crossover. One chromosome is depicted for each of three founders (I1, I2, and II2) in a three-generation pedigree. The chromosomes of the progeny become mosaic constructions of the founders, as indicated.

notype. Finding the genes is made possible by the 37 crossovers (usually one or more per somatic chromosome) that occur every meiosis (the process by which the haploid DNA is generated for the egg and sperm) (Fig. 28.5). The haploid chromosomal DNA of the gamete then becomes a mosaic construction of the diploid chromosomal DNA from the parent. In each generation, the DNA is shuffled a little, since in the entire human genome there are about 37 crossovers, by definition one on average every 100 centiMorgans. Slowly, over the generations, each DNA base pair is randomized with its neighbors and provides the measure of genetic distance used in linkage and association studies to identify regions containing genes that cause observed effects.

LINKAGE AND ASSOCIATION

A phenotype being linked to a genetic marker usually means that a statistically-unexpected relationship is found between either the presence or absence of the phenotype in the family and the sharing of alleles at the marker locus within families. In contrast, most tests of allelic association evaluate relationships between the phenotype in members of a population (i.e., between families) and the particular alleles at a given marker. Thinking of this from another perspective, the tests for linkage usually rely on crossovers within pedigrees and are tests for involvement of a locus; they do not identify particular alleles. On the other hand, allelic association does identify a particular allele and also relies on crossovers within a population (i.e., between pedigrees).

The more crossovers there are between affecteds, the smaller the average piece of DNA that can be statistically related to genetic risk (Figs. 28.1 and 28.5). Most strong linkage effects are detected over 20 to 30 megabases of DNA, whereas tests of association usually operate over 0.1 megabases or less. There are some exceptions to this, such as the HLA region, in which genetic association effects are detected over 3.5 megabases. The region of the genome over which association can be detected is said to be in linkage disequilibrium.

Some populations have a much lower number of crossovers between affecteds. For example, in selected isolated populations, an association may be detected over a greater genomic distance. Also, when populations with different haplotype frequencies have been recently admixed, then association may be found over relatively large genetic distances. Such effects are predicted to be present in African-Americans.

Consequently, linkage is ordinarily used to identify genetic effects in a region, whereas association is usually used to narrow such a region. Indeed, association is sometimes used to find the disease gene itself. Associations of HLA-B27 with ankylosing spondylitis, HLA-DR4 with RA, and FcγRIIA alleles (histidine vs. arginine at amino acid 131) with lupus nephritis in African-Americans are but a few of the hundreds of genetic associations that have been found in the rheumatic diseases (6).

ASCERTAINMENT

Appropriate study designs greatly improve the prospect of a successful outcome of a genetic project, as they do in all science. What can be discovered is usually dictated by the study design, and study designs begin with the enrollment of the first subject. A critical question is how to collect the pedigrees and pedigree materials. The data collection, methods of analysis, and possible results are dramatically different when cohorts of cases and controls are collected, as opposed to, for example, multiplex, multigenerational pedigrees.

FOUNDERS AND ISOLATED POPULATIONS

Case-control designs are appropriate for some situations, particularly isolated populations and within populations with a founder effect for the phenotype of interest. Isolated populations offer special opportunities. The genetic variation in such groups is different from that in the general population. Usually, the number of possible genetic explanations is fewer, and hence, often easier to find. By evaluating three benign cholestatic jaundice patients (a known autosomal-recessive disorder) and their parents at 256 markers, Houwen and colleagues established a linkage on chromosome 18 (7). This is also the strategy used in the comprehensive genetic evaluation of the Icelandic population, which has recently become a commercial enterprise and is the focus of much discussion and controversy (8).

Tan et al. (10) and Arnett et al. (9) also used the isolated population strategy to study scleroderma in the Choctaw Indians. They showed two separate genomic regions, one containing the fibrillin gene and the other containing the HLA genes, to be genetic risk factors in these patients. The hope, of course, is that these same genes will be important in scleroderma patients from the general population. But, even if they are not, the genes responsible for the observed effects are still likely to be important in helping understand the pathogenesis of the disorder. Opportunities presented by isolated populations should not be ignored.

A founder effect, as mentioned previously, is the presence of a phenotype due to a common ancestral mutation. The founder is the first to pass the genotype to his or her offspring. The founder need not have the phenotype, only the mutation, and then only in his or her germline. An increased risk for the phenotype can be traced back through the generations (if the records existed) to the founder. How much of the neighboring genome is in linkage disequilibrium with the genotype conferring disease risk depends on how many generations ago the founder introduced the genotype. The more distant in the past, the smaller the region over which linkage disequilibrium will exist (Fig. 28.1). When founder effects are present, the gene can often be discovered by association studies, as was done for hemochromatosis (11).

TRANSMISSION DISEQUILIBRIUM

A popular technique for assessing association is the transmission disequilibrium test (TDT) (12). In its simplest form, the affected and either one of the parents is considered a unit, a case, and a matched control unit (Fig. 28.6), but only when that parent is heterozygous and the inheritance pattern is unambiguous. The test evaluates the distortion in the ratio of allele transmission to allele nontransmission from parent to progeny. The TDT is not susceptible to artifacts arising from population stratification because the control (which here is the nontransmitted allele) comes from the same parent as the case (the transmitted allele) and, hence, is taken from the same population.

AFFECTED SIBLING PAIRS

In situations where there is strong evidence for a genetic effect, but the mode of inheritance is not known, affected sibling pairs have been collected. Although there are many variations on the strategy for ascertaining affected sibling pairs, the most straightforward is the collection of the affected sibling pairs and their parents. At markers where both parents are heterozygous for different alleles, the test for linkage is based on the expected sharing of no alleles (0) and of two alleles (2) at a marker locus (Fig. 28.7). Given that a marker locus is fully linked to the disease gene, a concordant affected sibling pair would be expected to share no alleles 0% of the time and 2 alleles 100% of the time. The extent to which the sibling pairs differ from these expected values measures the probability of linkage at the locus.

Usually hundreds, if not thousands, of sibling pairs are needed to establish linkage in situations where the genetics are complex and the genetic effects at any given locus are thought to be relatively small. An often unstated assumption in the application of this method is that no other process is operating to select for or against particular alleles. For example, if an allele at the marker locus is recessive lethal, then no affected would be found who is homozygous for this allele at this locus. The distribution of allele sharing

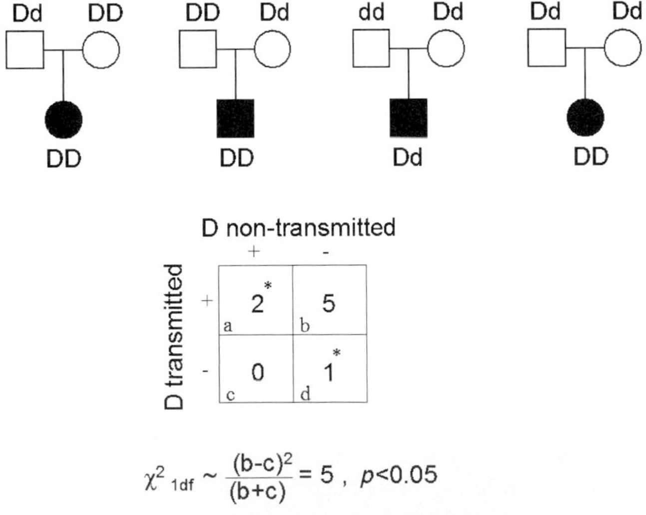

FIG. 28.6. The transmission disequilibrium test. Four pedigrees are shown in which the "D" and "d" alleles are shown for each pedigree member. In the first pedigree the parent-progeny unit from the father shows that D is transmitted and d is not transmitted. These are tallied, much like they are in the classic case with matched control design. Here $X^2 \sim [(b - c)^2/(b + c)] = 5$, which with one degree of freedom leads to $p < 0.05$. The odds ratio = b/c. Note the homozygous parents (either DD or dd) do not contribute. df, degree of freedom.

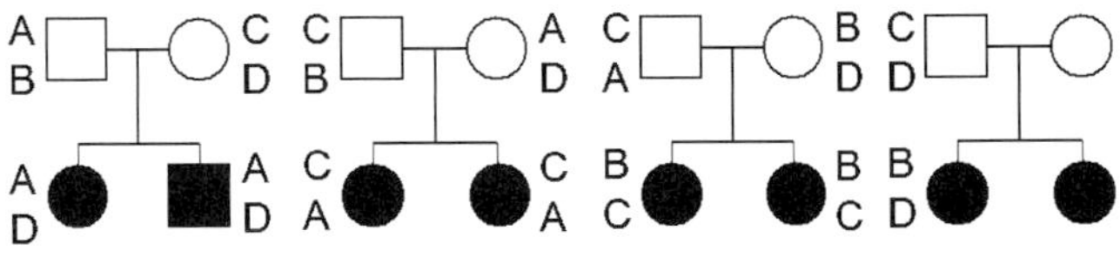

X= # sharing 2 alleles IBD= 4
Y= # sharing 0 alleles IBD= 0

$$\chi^2_{1df} = \Sigma \frac{(X-Y)^2}{(X+Y)} = 4, \ p<0.05$$

FIG. 28.7. Affected sibling pairs. The most informative situation is when both parents are differently heterozygous, which is the case for each pedigree presented. Here, all affected pairs share two alleles, providing some support for linkage ($p < 0.05$). To determine if there is genetic association, the allele frequencies of the cases are usually compared with controls. IBD, identical by descent; df, degree of freedom.

would be distorted from the expected for a reason other than linkage.

There are, of course, many variations of the affected sibling pair method presented above. One variation is the inclusion of unaffected siblings and other relative pairs. Another is using a quantitative, rather than qualitative, trait. Yet another is including only the siblings with the most extreme phenotype on a scale of measurement. A recent variation to this method is to evaluate genetic interactions as well as other possible covariates. All of the above-mentioned extensions increase the power to detect linkage and are, therefore, of great interest to geneticists. Several other mathematical accommodations and advances have been made, and many useful software programs are available but are beyond the scope of this discussion. However, the reader should be aware that many good choices are available once affected sibling pairs and their relatives have been ascertained.

EXTENDED MULTIPLEX PEDIGREES

Ascertainment of large pedigrees with several affecteds is very powerful. Clearly, the larger the pedigree is, the greater the potential to find several affecteds. This is the classic ascertainment strategy for simple or single-gene disorders when the segregation analysis supports an autosomal-dominant, autosomal-recessive, or X-linked mode of inheritance.

The classic method of analyzing these data is based on the work of Newton Morton, developed almost a half century ago (13). The likelihood ratio of the odds for linkage divided by the odds of no linkage is calculated by estimating the odds for linkage as a function of the recombination fraction (Fig. 28.8). The recombination fraction is a measure of distance from the marker in a single generation. The maximum evidence for linkage over the recombination interval of 0 to 0.5 is usually reported as the logarithm of the odds (LOD) score or the log of the likelihood ratio. For example, LOD scores of greater than 4 support linkage of specific regions of the genome in two hereditary forms of pseudogout (14,15). As the distance from the marker increases, the likelihood that there has been a crossover increases. A recombination fraction of 0.5 by this method is the equivalent of no linkage. Any recombination fraction less than this and convincingly present is consistent with linkage. Of course, small recombination fractions

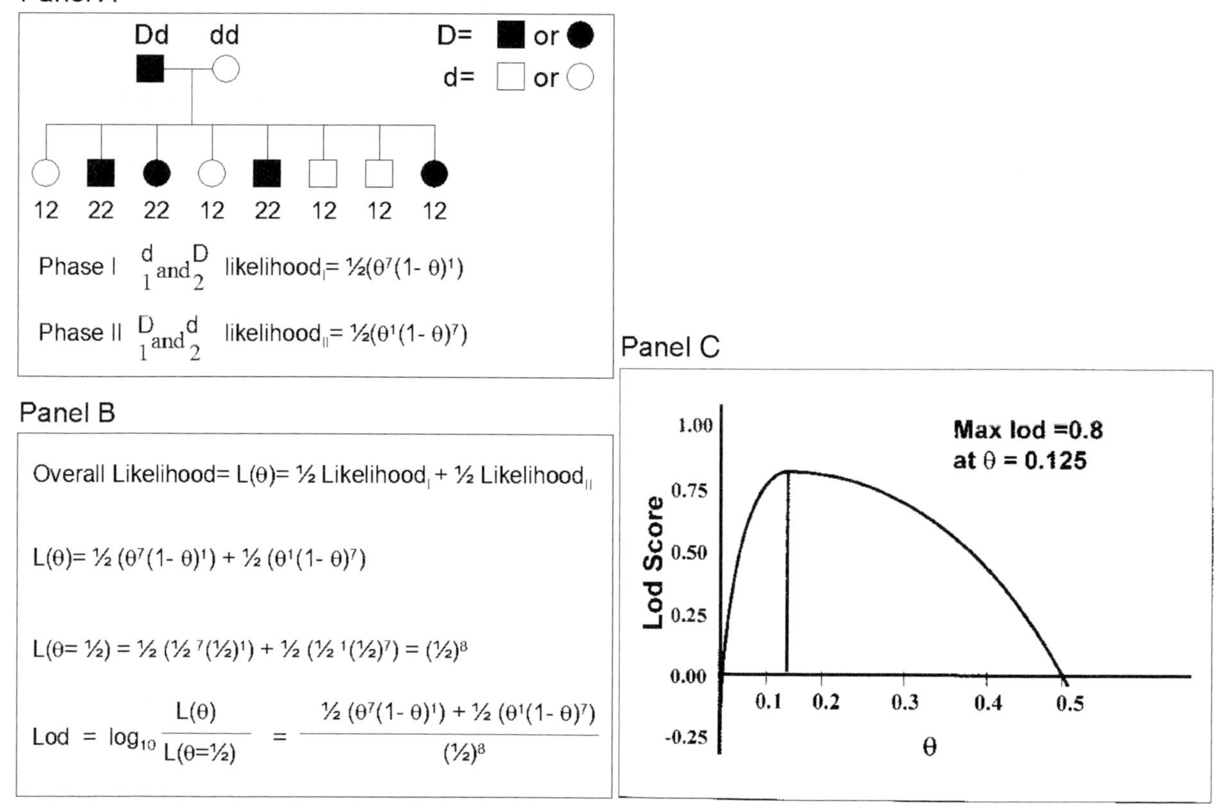

FIG. 28.8. Maximum likelihood ratio test for linkage. Consider a two-generation pedigree **(A)** when the phenotype is known to segregate as an autosomal dominant disorder. **B:** The LOD [$\log_{10}$ (likelihood of linkage/likelihood of no linkage)] as a function of the recombination fraction (θ). **C:** The plot of the LOD score as a function of θ. The maximum LOD score (0.8) is at θ = 0.125, some genetic distance from the marker.

produce the strongest evidence for linkage. A 1% recombination fraction is equivalent to 1 centiMorgan and is approximately 1 megabase of DNA.

As might be evident from this discussion, for the classic method of linkage by the likelihood ratio test, any error in pedigree relationship or genotyping will appear as an error in the estimate of the recombination fraction. The procedure maximzes the likelihood across the range of penetrance values possible and across genetic heterogeneity. This allows for refinement of the inheritance mechanism and increased power to detect linkage. Penetrance is the probability of having the phenotype, given the genotype. For example, the penetrance for a strict autosomal-dominant disorder is 100% for an individual heterozygous or homozygous for the responsible allele. Genetic heterogeneity is a measure of the proportion of the pedigrees linked at the locus of interest. Finally, with consideration of the genotypic data at neighboring loci simultaneously, LOD scores can be calculated at each interesting position using a specified model of inheritance. These multipoint LOD scores are the current standard for this kind of genetic analysis.

In recent years, other algorithms have been developed for extended multiplex pedigrees. Of these, the inheritance distribution pattern approach, based on the work of Leonid Kruglyak and colleagues, is widely used (16). This and other relative pair methods have been extended from the affected sibling pair approach to accommodate extended pedigrees.

GENOME SCAN FOR LINKAGE

Genome-wide scans are being conducted for most of the major disease problems thought to have a genetic component. This means that the entire collection of pedigrees, whether sibling pairs or multiplex families, is genotyped for markers at roughly equal spacing throughout the human genome, usually 120 to 400 microsatellites. This approach has led to evidence for additional genes (beyond HLA-B27) for the development of ankylosing spondylitis and is now being applied to many rheumatic disease problems with a genetic component (17).

SIGNIFICANT LOD SCORES AND *p* VALUES

The issue of deciding what level of significance is meaningful is not simple. Indeed, entire scientific disciplines have been organized around this issue. The critical decision is made when a linkage or association is sufficiently significant to imply or even identify a gene. Thankfully, there are some general rules to follow. First, one should know whether an important finding has been confirmed, since this greatly increases the confidence that a finding is correct. Confirmation by repetition is also a basic tenet of the scientific method. However, failure of other investigators to confirm a finding does not necessarily mean that a finding is not correct. This depends greatly on the context of both the original study and its replicate. In genetic situations where segregation analysis has established a simple genetic mechanism, failure to confirm a linkage usually means that there is a second gene in the pedigree or population being evaluated. In genetically complex diseases, pedigree collections are unintentionally enriched for some linkages and depleted for others, due to random variation in the population. Different genes will then be detected as a result of selecting different samples from the different populations. Thus, positive confirmation, rather than negative, is the most convincing, although there are many examples of initially convincing linkages that are now thought to have been false-positive linkage signals.

Most researchers express the significance of their results as either a probability (*p* value) or a likelihood (LOD score). The *p* value is the probability that the observation will occur by chance. The LOD score, as explained above, is the $\log_{10}$ of the likelihood that the marker is linked to a disease gene divided by the likelihood that the marker is not linked. LOD scores of greater than about 3.3 are estimated to be found by chance only once in every 20 genome scans using marker data that are not linked to a disease gene (18). Therefore, an LOD of about 3.3 is widely accepted as a threshold for significance in a genome scan, especially in complex genetics diseases. At times the expression of a *p* value as an LOD score is desired. This can be done by assuming a normal distribution, then determining the Z corresponding to the respective *p* value, and approximating $\chi^2 = \sim Z^2$ and LOD = $\sim(\chi^2 / 4.6)$. Using this method, the LOD of 3.3 is approximately equivalent to $p < 0.00002$.

CANDIDATE GENES

There are three important sources for candidate genes, or genes that have the potential to explain the known biology of the disease in question. First, work with the biology of the phenotype may raise the suspicion that a particular gene is related. This can be the result of brilliant thinking, as in the example of apolipoprotein E and Alzheimer disease (19). It can also be the result of a complete accident, as in the relationship of *HLA-B27* with ankylosing spondylitis. The latter association was found because ankylosing spondylitis patients were selected as controls for an inquiry into an association of gout with HLA (20). Second, linkage results may restrict the genes being considered to a relatively small region of the genome. Genes in this region are considered as candidates in an order of prior probability chosen by the investigator. Third, linkages or genes found in other species, usually from the mouse, may specifically suggest genomic regions or specific genes in humans.

This discussion would not be complete without addressing this third source in more detail. Mouse genetics in particular has played a substantial role in the discovery of genes important in human disease. Our capacity to manipulate the genetic composition of the mouse far exceeds what can be done in humans and is an approach proven to greatly accelerate progress.

Murine knockouts are animals with a dysfunctional gene at a particular locus. Transgenic mice have a gene or set of genes installed from another DNA source (e.g., human gene). Breeding programs manipulate genetic composition. Although these experiments often fail to produce the expected result, they offer profoundly important insights into the biology of the system being explored.

A few simple examples will serve to illustrate what is now possible. First, a transgenic mouse is available containing much of the human DNA for the variable regions of the immunoglobulin locus (21). These animals are presumed to have an enhanced capacity to imitate the human immune response. Second, a human transgenic rat has begun to suggest a role for the HLA-B27 allele in the inflammatory response (22). Third, breeding experiments have shown that the MRL *lpr/lpr* mouse defect is in the *fas* gene, which is responsible for lupus nephritis in this mouse. A large body of literature on apoptosis and autoimmunity has been spawned from this observation (23).

Ward Wakeland and his colleagues have been isolating the genes disposing to lupus in the NZM mouse [a fixed interstrain cross from the classic (NZB × NZW)F1 model of lupus]. They have evidence for at least eight genes (24,25). Some of these genetic effects are very close to one another, whereas others are on separate chromosomes. Even genes operating to suppress disease are suggested. The mouse offers the prospect of identifying these genes quickly, but gene identification even in the mouse can be problematic. The murine SLE locus *sle1* has been found to have at least four distinct components, located very close to one another on mouse chromosome 1 (26). Distinguishing the causative gene from among these haplotypes composed of multiple polymorphisms in neighboring, ancestrally-duplicated genes (i.e., *sle1*) presents a daunting level of complexity. The situation is much more complicated in humans, which should give pause to anyone who thinks that genetic solutions will rapidly follow the advancing technology.

Mouse genetics offers another advantage. Mouse genes and human genes are syntenic, meaning that the gene order on the chromosomes in the two species is similar. In humans and mice, they are astonishingly similar (over 95% identical). When a linkage is found in the mouse, it is likely to be in the same relative position in humans. This is a strategy for exploring candidate linkages that has been successfully applied. Once a gene is known in the mouse, the homologue can be directly explored in humans.

THE STATUS QUO

The methods used throughout this chapter have been used to identify rheumatic disease genes. With the phenotype as the bait, the new technologies and resources are aggressively being applied to go fishing for the linkages and genes that will explain etiology.

Familial Mediterranean Fever

Familial Mediterranean fever (FMF) is an autosomal-recessive autoimmune disease characterized by recurrent episodes of fever, serositis, arthritis, and skin rash. Pras et al. mapped the gene causing FMF to the short arm of chromosome 16 (27). Subsequently, the gene (*MEFV*) was cloned by two independent groups in 1997 (28,29). *MEFV,* predominantly expressed on myeloid cells, encodes for a 781–amino acid protein, pyrin or marenostrin, and appears to be up-regulated during myeloid differentiation (30). The *MEFV* gene has 10 exons. At least 29 mutations have been reported, mostly involving exons 10 and 2. The most common mutations are M694V, V726A, M694I, and M680I on exon 10 and E148Q on exon 2 (31). About 22% to 67% of the patients evaluated have the M694A mutation and 7% to 35% have V726A. M694A means that the DNA code has changed from the codon for methionone to the codon for alanine at amino acid position 694 of the pyrin protein molecule. Other mutations have been reported on exons 1, 3, 5, and 9. The severity of the disease and the risk for amyloidosis appear to vary among these different mutations. The homozygous state for the M964V mutation is indeed associated with a more severe disease and higher risk for amyloidosis (32,33). More recently, it has been shown that male sex, coupled with articular manifestations, is associated with a fourfold increase in the risk for amyloidosis among patients who are homozygous for the M964V mutation (34).

Pyrin consists of four functional subunits, which in order are the PYRIN domain (N-terminal), the B-box zinc-finger domain, a coiled-coil domain, and the B30.2 domain (C-terminal). The PYRIN domain is shared by a family of related proteins involved in apoptosis and inflammation (35). Interaction among these various PYRIN domain–containing proteins appears to be mediated via the PYRIN domain. In most FMF patients, the relevant mutations involve the C-terminal part of the molecule; thus, a full functional PYRIN domain is usually retained. In a recent study, macrophages from mice expressing a truncated pyrin molecule, yet retaining the PYRIN domain, produce elevated levels of interleukin (IL)-1β (36). In addition, macrophages derived from pyrin-truncated mice demonstrate impaired apoptosis (36).

Rheumatoid Arthritis

The familial clustering of RA (λs = 5), and a higher concordance in monozygotic twins compared to dizygotic twins support the role of genetic factors in the development of RA. The most consistent genetic association reported is with the HLA class II locus. Indeed, association with several HLA-DRB1 alleles has been confirmed, including the association with *HLA-DRB1*0401* and *HLA-DRB1*0404* (37,38). Other confirmed HLA associations include *HLA-DRB1 *0101, *0102, *0405, *0408, *1001,* and **1402*. The association between HLA-DRB1 alleles and disease severity and the presence of extraarticular manifestations has also been reported. In one study, all patients with nodular disease carried the genotype *HLA-DRB1*04/04* (39). *HLA-DRB1*0401* is associated with a higher frequency of bronchiectasis in RA patients (40).

Genome-wide scans performed in affected sibling pair families have confirmed a linkage on chromosome 6p21–23 (41–43). Other reported linkages include 1p36, Xq27 (44), 6q22(42), and 4q22–24 (43). Additional non-HLA genetic associations have also been reported. A linkage to the corticotropin-releasing hormone gene at chromosome 8q13 has been reported and replicated in a second group of RA sibling pair families, but the effect was not sufficient to be considered an established linkage (45). Similarly, linkage to chromosome 17q22 has been confirmed in affected sibling pair analysis (46). In addition, numerous other non-HLA associations have been reported and replicated, including insulin-dependent diabetes mellitus susceptibility locus *IDDM5* (47,48) and tumor necrosis factor (TNF) polymorphisms (49–52).

Osteoarthritis

A genetic component is clearly involved in susceptibility to developing osteoarthritis (OA), as suggested by twin studies, sibling risk, and familial aggregation. The disease has a $\lambda s = 2.32$ in a study of severe OA requiring joint replacement (53). Some suspect that the role of genetics in the development of OA is more important in women than in men (54). In addition, the locus-specific genetic susceptibility varies by articular location of the OA. Several linkages have been suggested by sibling pair analysis and by the rare OA pedigrees, including effects on chromosomes 2q, 4q, 6, 7p, 11q, 16p, and Xcen. Replicated linkage effects include chromosomes 2q and 4q (55). The effect on 4q12–21.2 produced a LOD = 3.9 in female sibling pairs with hip disease (56). In a fine mapping study of the chromosome 6 effect, the susceptibility locus was mapped between 70.5 and 81.9 centiMorgans from the 6p telomere in sibling pairs concordant for total hip replacement (57). Interestingly, stratification analysis suggested that this effect is completely accounted for by female total hip replacement families (maximum LOD = 4.6 at the marker D6S1573) (57). A recent genome-wide linkage analysis for hand OA revealed evidence for convincing linkages on chromosome 4q, 3p, and 2p (58). The maximum LOD score on chromosome 2 coincides with a gene encoding a noncollagenous cartilage extracellular matrix protein, matrilin-3. Further analysis revealed a novel missense mutation in the matrilin-3 encoding gene, *MATN3,* that was responsible for the observed linkage effect (58).

Several genetic association studies reported association between OA and polymorphisms in the type II collagen gene *COL2A1,* which constitutes a major protein in articular cartilage (59–61). The *COL2A1* gene is located on chromosome 12q12–13.1, very close to the vitamin D receptor (*VDR*) gene. The association between OA and the *VDR* gene has been repeatedly reported as well (62–65). In one study, the *COL2A1* gene was associated with joint narrowing and the *VDR* gene with osteophyte formation, both in patients with knee OA (66).

Osteoporosis

Osteoporosis is a major health problem that results in significant morbidity and mortality. Several environmental factors are clearly involved in the development of osteoporosis; however, the role of genetics is also central. This is supported by twin studies and familial aggregation. The disease is characterized by loss of bone mass, as identified by bone mineral density (BMD) studies. Quantitative trait loci (QTL) are chromosomal regions that contain genes regulating quantitative traits. A QTL approach has been used to identify genes or effects that regulate bone mineral density. Several genome-wide linkage studies have been performed to identify loci that are linked to bone mineral density. Evidence for established linkage, as defined by an LOD $\geq$ 3.3, has been reported on chromosomes 1p36 (67,68), 1q21 (69), and 11q12–13 (70). Other loci with evidence of suggested linkage include 2p23 (67), 4q33 (67), 2p21 (71), 5q33–35 (69), 6p11–12 (69), 7p22 (72), 12q24 (72), 13q33–34 (72), and 10q26 (72). Among the numerous linkages reported, only 1p36, 4q, and 13q have been replicated (67,68,72).

The effect on 11q12–13 is linked to rare bone diseases, including osteoporosis-pseudoglioma and high bone mass syndrome. Finer mapping and sequencing of this locus identified the gene responsible for this effect to be low-density lipoprotein receptor–related protein 5 (*LRP5*). Activating mutations in this gene are responsible for high bone mass syndrome, while on the other hand, inactivating mutations cause osteoporosis-pseudoglioma (73). A number of candidate genes have been studied in relation to BMD. Associations have been reported for *VDR* (74), collagen type I gene (*COL1A1*) (75,76), estrogen receptor gene (*ESR1*) (77,78), and parathyroid hormone receptor gene (*PTHR1*) (79).

Ankylosing Spondylitis

Ankylosing spondylitis is a potentially disabling disease with a major genetic component, suggested initially by familial aggregation. This was confirmed by the discovery of the strong association between the disease and *HLA-B27*, now confirmed well over 100 times. However, twin studies indicate that other genetic components are also involved, since the concordance rate in HLA-B27-positive dizygotic twins is lower than that in monozygotic twins (23% vs. 63%) (80).

Other HLA genes reportedly involved in the susceptibility to ankylosing spondylitis are *HLA-B60* (81) and *HLA-DRB1* (82). Non-HLA genes identified by the candidate gene approach reveal a potential association with TNF-α (83–85), IL-1 receptor antagonist (*IL-1ra*) (86,87), and cytochrome P450 2D6 (*CYP2D6*) gene polymorphisms (88,89). Genome-wide linkage studies have shown a significant effect on chromosome 16q (LOD = 4.7) (90). This effect on 16q exceeds the threshold for established linkage and has been confirmed (90,91). Other chromosomal effects suggested by genome-wide scans include loci on chromosomes 1p, 2q, 6p, 9q, 10q, and 19q (90).

Psoriatic Arthritis

About 15% to 30% of patients with psoriasis will develop psoriatic arthritis. Both psoriasis and, hence, psoriatic arthritis appear to have excessive paternal transmission (92). This means that progeny are more likely to develop psoriasis or psoriatic arthritis if the father has psoriasis or psoriatic arthritis. A strong association was repeatedly reported between psoriatic arthritis and *HLA-Cw*0602* (93). This HLA allele is also a recognized susceptibility locus for psoriasis and is, indeed, associated with earlier onset of the disease (94). MICA-A9 triplet repeat polymorphism, corresponding to the *MICA-002* allele, is associated with susceptibility to psoriatic arthritis, independent of the genetic effect of the nearby *HLA-Cw*0602* (95). The reported association with TNF-α polymorphisms has been inconsistent and, perhaps, explained by linkage disequilibrium with *HLA-Cw*0602*.

A recent genome-wide linkage study identified a susceptibility locus for psoriatic arthritis on chromosome 16q. When conditioned on paternal transmission, this effect gave an LOD score = 4.19, which exceeds the threshold for established linkage (96). In addition, an effect on chromosome 17q has been separately reported for both psoriasis and psoriatic arthritis (97,98).

Calcium Pyrophosphate Deposition Disease

The deposition of calcium-containing crystals within the articular cartilage induces an arthritis known as pseudogout. Calcium pyrophosphate crystal deposition increases with age and is associated with elevated pyrophosphate in the joints (99). Although mostly sporadic, rare forms of familial pseudogout with autosomal-dominant inheritance have been observed. Those have been linked to susceptibility loci at chromosome 8q (*CCAL1*) (100) and 5p (*CCAL2*) (101,102). It was recently described that families with the *CCAL2* effect have mutations in the human homologue of the mouse progressive ankylosis gene (*ANKH*) (103,104), which has previously been shown to be involved in pyrophosphate regulation and joint calcification.

Paget's Disease

Islands of increased bone turnover, resulting in disorganized bone growth, is characteristic of Paget's disease. This common disease often segregates in an autosomal-dominant manner with incomplete penetrance, although it has substantial genetic heterogeneity (105). Linkage studies identified a disease susceptibility gene on chromosome 6p21.3 (*PDB1*) (106) and 18q21–22 (*PDB2*) (107,108). The effect on chromosome 18q21–22 has been previously linked to a rare bone dysplastic disease, known as familial expansile osteolysis (109). However, unlike the case in familial expansile osteolysis, mutations in the receptor activator of the nuclear factor κB gene (*RANK*) mapped to the *PDB2* region (110) are not observed in classic Paget's disease (111). Interestingly, evidence of an osteosarcoma tumor suppressor gene (on chromosome 18q region) linked to Paget's disease has been reported (112). This might provide an explanation for the higher frequency of osteosarcoma in Paget's disease patients. Additional susceptibility loci for Paget's disease have been reported on chromosome 5q35-qter (*PDB3*) and 5q31 (*PDB4*) (113–115).

Systemic Lupus Erythematosus

SLE is a complex disease of controversial etiology. Both environmental and genetic factors contribute to its pathogenesis. Evidence for genetic contribution comes from twin studies and familial aggregation (λs = 10–20) (116–119). The known associated genetic polymorphisms and the linkages reported using genome-wide scans of multiplex pedigrees and affected sibling pair families further support a genetic component.

Studies of histocompatibility molecules have been performed in various SLE populations (120–132). The *DR2* and *DR3* alleles at HLA-DR have the most consistent association with SLE. As is true for all human histocompatibility associations, the pathophysiology and mechanistic details that explain this association are not known.

SLE is also associated with polymorphisms of at least *FcγRIIA* (133,134) and *FcγRIIIA* (135,136), and perhaps other Fc receptor genes. In both cases, the allele that binds immunoglobulin G (IgG) subtypes with lower affinity is associated with increased risk for SLE. These alleles are thought to have decreased capacity to clear immune complexes composed of the specific low-affinity IgG subtypes. These genes are neighbors on the human genome at chromosome 1q22–24, in a region also known to have genetic linkage with SLE. These two Fc receptors are separated by only 20 kb of genomic DNA and are in linkage disequilibrium.

Recently, alleles of *PDCD-1*, a T-lymphocyte transcription factor, have been implicated as being responsible for the linkage at 2q37 (137), first found in Nordic pedigrees multiplex for SLE. Further confirmation of this result is widely anticipated.

Several other genes are thought to increase susceptibility to the development of SLE without producing consistently convincing evidence of genetic association. These include polymorphisms involving *IL-10,* FAS (138,139) and FASL (140), the mannose-binding lectin genes (141–143), *Bcl-2* (144), *CTLA4* (145), the T-cell receptors (146), prolactin (147), *TNF-α* (148,149), and TNF receptors (150).

Genome-wide linkage studies in pedigrees multiplex for SLE have revealed some potentially important genetic polymorphisms. At least five linkages have been established and confirmed, including those at 1q23, 2q37, 4p16, 6p21, and 16q13, along with many others that have not yet produced such convincing results (151). Of these linkages, convincing associations potentially explaining them are found at *FcγRIIIA* (1q23) (152), *PDCD-1* (2q37) (137), and HLA-DR (6q21) (153). Many other genetic effects (>15) have been established and await confirmation (151). Progress in the human genome project and improved methods of analysis are anticipated to provide much more rapid progress toward a more complete genetic understanding than has been possible in the past.

Sjögren's Syndrome

Primary Sjögren's syndrome is a complicated polygenic disorder with many genes predicted to be interacting with environmental factors. Several HLA class II genes, in particular *HLA-DRB1*, *DRB3*, *DQA1*, and *DQB1*, have been associated with Sjögren's syndrome and the production of anti-Ro and anti-La autoantibodies (154). Using DNA methodologies, confirmed alleles include *HLA-DRB1*0301, -DRB1*1501, -DQA1*0103, -DQA1*0501, -DQB1*0201,* and *-DQB1*0601* (Fig. 28.9).

Numerous non-HLA genetic associations have been described, including polymorphisms of *IL-10* (155), *IL-1Ra* (156), *IL-6* (157), *Ro52* (158), *TAP2* (159), *GSTM1* (160), *MBL* (161,162), and FAS genes (163). However, confirmation is generally lacking with the non-HLA associations that have been reported for primary Sjögren's syndrome.

Hemochromatosis

Hemochromatosis is a common inherited disorder with an autosomal-recessive pattern of inheritance. The disease is characterized by iron overload and manifested by liver cirrhosis, symmetric OA, skin discoloration, cardiomyopathy, hypogonadism, diabetes, weakness, and lethargy. An environmental component is thought to have a major role in hemochromatosis because of alcohol abuse.

Epidemiologic data for hemochromatosis suggest a founder effect. There is a relatively high prevalence of affecteds among Northern Europeans, and the estimated gene frequency has been found to be over 10%, with 0.5% of the population being homozygous. For more than two decades, an association of HLA-A3 within Northern Europeans with hemochromatosis has been known (164). This means that the gene responsible for hemochromatosis tends to be found in haplotypes containing *HLA-A3*, or alternatively, that *HLA-A3* and the hemochromatosis gene are in linkage disequilibrium in people with Northern European ancestors. Consequently, a direct approach was taken seeking to

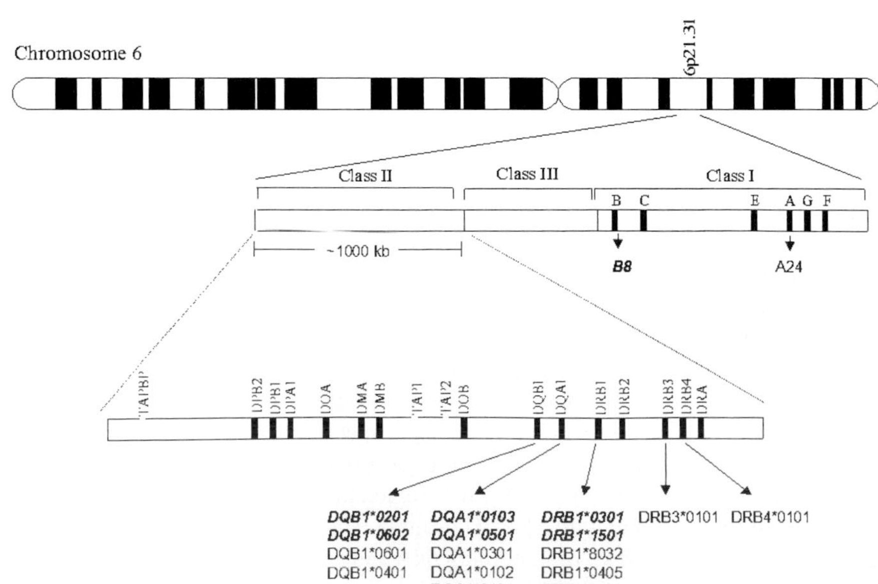

FIG. 28.9. The human leukocyte antigen (HLA) region on the short arm of chromosome 6 showing the HLA alleles associated with Sjögren's syndrome. Confirmed associations are in italics. Modified with permision from Sawalha et al. (154).

identify an increase in association between disease and genetic markers while moving farther away from *HLA-A3*.

This effort was a spectacular success and has identified the hereditary hemochromatosis gene, now designated *HFE*, which appears to be mutated in most hemochromatosis patients (165). The postulated founder effect is supported by a single amino acid coding change in the *HFE* gene, resulting in tyrosine being substituted for cysteine at amino acid position 282 (C282Y). The vast majority of hemochromatosis patients (>90%) are associated with being homozygous for C282Y (166). In addition, other mutations of *HFE* have been described, including H63D and S65C (167). The S65C mutation is associated with mild iron overload in individuals who are also heterozygous for the C282Y or the H63D mutations (168,169). Contrary to the initial impression, only a minority of the C282Y homozygotes develop clinical features of hemochromatosis (170). Indeed, in one study the penetrance of the C282Y homozygous genotype has been estimated to be 1% (171), providing more evidence consistent with the involvement of environmental or other genetic factors in the susceptibility to hemochromatosis and being more than 10-fold lower than estimates of the penetrance that had been made only a few years ago, before the knowledge of the specific mutation involved had been applied in population-based studies. New evidence for the involvement of other genes, including various iron absorption and metabolism genes, is therefore not unexpected (170).

Defining the genotype that confers risk provides a new perspective from which to evaluate related phenotypes. For example, nine pedigrees with juvenile hemochromatosis have been studied by a genome scan. A maximum LOD score of 5.16 was found on chromosome 1q (at D1S2344) (172). The affecteds in these pedigrees, having a younger age of onset (second and third decades of life) as well as showing no linkage to the region on chromosome 6p containing *HFE*, establish juvenile hemochromatosis (type 2) as a distinct phenotype and, therefore, presumably a distinct pathogenesis. Type 3 hemochromatosis is caused by a mutation in a transferrin receptor gene (*TFR2*) and is an autosomal-recessive disease (173–175). Types 4 and 5 are both autosomal dominant and are caused by mutations in the *ferroprotein 1* gene, which encodes for an intestinal iron transport molecule, and the *H-ferritin* gene, which encodes for the H subunit of the ferritin molecule (176–180).

Summary

This section is entitled "The Status Quo," which is misleading because of rapid progress in the genetic characterization of disease. New technologies promise to accelerate further the pace of discovery; indeed, the new genetic approaches discussed in the early part of the chapter promise to revolutionize our conception of how these diseases occur. The challenge is to understand more than the gene, to identify it, and then to place the gene in its pathophysiologic context so that the mechanism of disease is fully explained and understood. In some situations this has occurred quickly (e.g., familial Mediterranean fever or hemochromatosis). In others, many decades have passed finding us still waiting for the critical insight that explains the essential role of the allele in the disease process (e.g., ankylosing spondylitis and *HLA-B27*). To be more than curiosities or only diagnostic tests, the genetic advances must be accompanied by a deeper understanding of the biology of these illnesses.

THE FUTURE

As in other disciplines, situations in which the genetic model is known and the pedigree material is sufficient are likely to yield genes that contribute to the observed phenotype. Knowing the genetic solution is perhaps the easier part of the answer. We hope that explaining the genetics will lead to a solution to the more difficult problem of understanding the biology of the disease phenotypes.

In the more common disorders, where the genetic mechanisms are not known, genetic progress is more likely to be episodic and difficult. We are likely to repeat the experience of psychiatric and affective disorders where the difficulty of confirming alleged linkages threatens the entire effort of identifying genes.

For type 1 diabetes, approximately 2,000 pedigrees are available, and consequently, a variety of effects have been identified (181). These results would have been convincing, save for the failed effort to confirm their presence in a large American consortium (182). Although the differences have generated much speculation, the reasons for the discrepancies are, even now, not completely known. Understanding these issues is important for everyone interested in the genetics of complex diseases, particularly because type 1 diabetes has commanded many more resources than have been dedicated to any of the complex genetic rheumatic diseases.

No doubt, our progress in explaining the genetics of rheumatic diseases will repeat at least part of the history of affective disorders and diabetes. The major lesson would appear to be that important progress in the genetic characterization is now possible, even for complex disorders. On the other hand, we should not be lulled into complacency or false security. Rather, some genetic rheumatic disease problems are likely to be virtually intractable, even given the incredible technologic advances in progress. Nevertheless, as long as research continues genes will be identified, as a result of incredible persistence, almost unbelievable luck, or both. We can then focus on the biology of the identified genes.

There are only about 25,000 human genes. One day we will have the capacity to assess inexpensively all of them in a large number of individuals simultaneously and to efficiently evaluate all of the data thereby produced. Finding the responsible genes may then be less difficult than it is today.

But even when such an incredible capacity is commonly available, understanding the biology of the genes will remain a significant impediment requiring a profound understanding and insight. Actually, we are not helped much by finding the gene if our conceptual framework for it remains outside the context of its biologic action. Consequently, several decades will be required to understand the biology of many of the genetic effects now being discovered. One only needs to consider a few examples. HLA-B27 has been powerfully associated with ankylosing spondylitis and known for more than 30 years (20). Yet we do not understand the biology at a sufficiently fundamental level to appreciate why the association of HLA-B27 with ankylosing spondylitis exists. The molecular basis for sickle cell anemia has been known for an even longer time, but only now are we beginning to develop therapies capable of influencing the level of normal hemoglobin in these patients. Thus, finding genes in many situations is now possible, but not easy. Once done, however, the much more difficult task of explaining the biology will provide a daunting challenge for many years, and perhaps generations to come.

ACKNOWLEDGMENTS

We appreciate the support of the National Institutes of Health (Grants AI42460, AR12253, AI24717, RR15577, AI31584, AR01005, AR048940, and AR049084) and the U.S. Department of Veterans Affairs for our work.

REFERENCES

1. Penrose LS. The detection of autosomal linkage in data which consist of pairs of brothers and sisters of unspecified parentage. *Ann Eugen* 1935;6:133–138.
2. Almquist E, Andrew S, Theilmann J, et al. Geographical distribution of haplotypes in Swedish families with Hunington's disease. *Hum Genet* 1994;94:124–128.
3. Simon M, Bourel M, Fauchet R, et al. Association of HLA-A3 and HLA-B14 antigens with idiopathic haemochromatosis. *Gut* 1976;17: 332–334.
4. Risch N. Linkage strategies for genetically complex traits. I. Multilocus models. *Am J Hum Genet* 1990;46:222–8.
5. Pennisi E. A closer look at SNPs suggest difficulties. *Science* 1998; 281:1787–1789.
6. Salmon JE, Millard S, Schachter LA, et al. Fc gamma RIIA alleles are heritable risk factors for lupus nephritis in African-Americans. *J Clin Invest* 1996;97:1348–1354.
7. Houwen RHJ, Baharloo S, Blankenship K, et al. Genome screening by searching for shared segments: mapping a gene for benign recurrent intrahepatic cholestasis. *Nat Genet* 1994;8:380–386.
8. Stefansson K. Health care and privacy. An interview with Kari Stefansson, founder and CEO of decode Genetics in Reykjavik, Iceland. *EMBO Rep* 2001;2:964–967.
9. Arnett FC, Howard RF, Tan F, et al. Increased prevalence of systemic sclerosis in a native American tribe in Oklahoma: association with an Amerindian HLA haplotype. *Arthritis Rheum* 1996;39:1362–1370.
10. Tan FK, Stivers DN, Foster MW, et al. Association of microsatellite markers near the fibrillin gene on human chromosome 15q with scleroderma in a native American population. *Arthritis Rheum* 1998;41: 1729–1737.
11. Feder IN, Gnirke A, Thomas W, et al. A novel MHC class I–like gene is mutated in patients with hereditary haemochromatosis. *Nat Genet* 1996;13:399–408.
12. Spielman RS, McGinnis RE, Ewens WJ. Transmission test for linkage disequilibrium: the insulin gene region and insulin-dependent diabetes mellitus (IDDM). *Am J Hum Genet* 1993;52:506–516.
13. Morton NE. Sequential tests for the detection of linkage. *Am J Hum Genet* 1955;7:277–318.
14. Baldwin CT, Farrer LA, Adair R, et al. Anderson L. Linkage of early-onset osteoarthritis and chondrocalcinosis to human chromosome 8q. *Am J Hum Genet* 1995;56:692–697.
15. Hughes AE, McGibbon, Woodward E, et al. Localisation of a gene for chondrocalcinosis to chromosome 5p. *Hum Mol Genet* 1995;4: 1225–1228.
16. Krugylak L, Daly MJ, Reeve-Daly MP, et al. Parametric and nonparametric linkage analysis: a unified multipoint approach. *Am J Hum Genet* 1996;58:1347–1363.
17. Brown MA, Pile KD, Kennedy LG, et al. A genome-wide screen for susceptibility loci in ankylosing spondylitis. *Arthritis Rheum* 1998;41: 588–595.
18. Kruglyak L. Thresholds and sample sizes. *Nat Genet* 1996;14:132–133.
19. Corder EH, Saunders AM, Strittmatter WJ, et al. Gene dose of apolipoprotein E type 4 allele and the risk of Alzheimer's disease in late onset families. *Science* 1993;261:921–923.
20. Brewerton DA, Hart FD, Nicholls A, et al. Ankylosing spondylitis and HL-A27. *Lancet* 1973;1:904–907.
21. Fishwild DM, O'Donnell SL, Bengoechea T, et al. High-avidity human IgG kappa monoclonal antibodies from a novel strain of minilocus transgenic mice. *Nat Biotechnol* 1996;14:845–851.
22. Khare SD, Bull MJ, Hanson J, et al. Spontaneous inflammatory disease in HLA-B27 transgenic mice is independent of MHC class II molecules: a direct role for B27 heavy chains and not B27-derived peptides. *J Immunol* 1998;160:101–106.
23. Watanabe-Fukunaga R, Brannan CI, Copeland NG, et al. Lymphoproliferation disorder in mice explained by defects in Fas antigen that mediates apoptosis. *Nature* 1992;26:314–317.
24. Morel L, Wakeland EK. Susceptibility to lupus nephritis in the NZB/W model system. *Curr Opin Immunol* 1998;10:718–725.
25. Mohan C, Morel L, Yang P, et al. Genetic dissection of lupus pathogenesis: a recipe for nephrophilic autoantibodies. *J Clin Invest* 1999; 103:1685–1695.
26. Morel L, Blenman KR, Croker BP, et al. The major murine systemic lupus erythematosus susceptibility locus, Sle1, is a cluster of functionally related genes. *Proc Natl Acad Sci U S A* 2001;98:1787–1792.
27. Pras E, Aksentijevich I, Gruberg L, et al. Mapping of a gene causing familial Mediterranean fever to the short arm of chromosome 16. *N Engl J Med* 1992;326:1509–1513.
28. The French FMF Consortium. A candidate gene for familial Mediterranean fever. *Nat Genet* 1997;17:25–31.
29. The International FMF Consortium. Ancient missense mutations in a new member of the RoRet gene family are likely to cause familial Mediterranean fever. *Cell* 1997;90:797–807.
30. Centola M, Wood G, Frucht DM, et al. The gene for familial Mediterranean fever, MEFV, is expressed in early leukocyte development and is regulated in response to inflammatory mediators. *Blood* 2000;95: 3223–3231.
31. Hull KM, Shoham N, Chae JJ, et al. The expanding spectrum of systemic autoinflammatory disorders and their rheumatic manifestations. *Curr Opin Rheumatol* 2003;15:61–69.
32. Livneh A, Langevitz P, Shinar Y, et al. MEFV mutation analysis in patients suffering from amyloidosis of familial Mediterranean fever. *Amyloid* 1999;6:1–6.
33. Shohat M, Magal N, Shohat T, et al. Phenotype-genotype correlation in familial Mediterranean fever: evidence for an association between Met694Val and amyloidosis. *Eur J Hum Genet* 1999;7:287–292.
34. Gershoni-Baruch R, Brik R, Lidar M, et al. Male sex coupled with articular manifestations cause a 4-fold increase in susceptibility to amyloidosis in patients with familial Mediterranean fever homozygous for the M694V-MEFV mutation. *J Rheumatol* 2003;30:308–312.
35. Kastner DL, O'Shea JJ. A fever gene comes in from the cold. An editorial summarizing recent findings on the PYRIN family of proteins. *Nat Genet* 2001;29:241–242.
36. Chae JJ, Komarow HD, Cheng J, et al. Targeted disruption of pyrin, the FMF protein, causes heightened sensitivity to endotoxin and a defect in macrophage apoptosis. *Mol Cell* 2003;11:591–604.
37. Stastny P. Association of the B-cell alloantigen DRw4 with rheumatoid arthritis. *N Engl J Med* 1978;298:869–871.

38. Nepom GT, Seyfried CE, Holbeck SL, et al. Identification of HLA-Dw14 genes in DR4+ rheumatoid arthritis. *Lancet* 1986;1002–1005.
39. Weyand CM, Hicok KC, Conn DL, et al. The influence of HLA-DRB1 genes on disease severity in rheumatoid arthritis. *Ann Intern Med* 1992;117:801–806.
40. Toussirot E, Despaux J, Wendling D. Increased frequency of HLA-DRB1 *0401 in patients with RA and bronchiectasis. *Ann Rheum Dis* 2000;59:1002–1003.
41. Cornelis F, Faure S, Martinez M, et al. New susceptibility locus for rheumatoid arthritis suggested by a genome-wide linkage study. *Proc Natl Acad Sci U S A* 1998;95:10746–10750.
42. MacKay K, Eyre S, Myerscough A, et al. Whole-genome linkage analysis of rheumatoid arthritis susceptibility loci in 252 affected sibling pairs in the United Kingdom. *Arthritis Rheum* 2002;46:632–639.
43. Jawaheer D, Seldin MF, Amos CI, et al. A genomewide screen in multiplex rheumatoid arthritis families suggests genetic overlap with other autoimmune diseases. *Am J Hum Genet* 2001;68:927–936.
44. Shiozawa S, Hayashi S, Tsukamoto Y, et al. Identification of the gene loci that predispose to rheumatoid arthritis. *Int Immunol* 1998;10: 1891–1895.
45. Fife MS, Fisher SA, John S, et al. Multipoint linkage analysis of a candidate gene locus in rheumatoid arthritis demonstrates significant evidence of linkage and association with the corticotropin-releasing hormone genomic region. *Arthritis Rheum* 2000;43:1673–1678.
46. Barton A, Eyre S, Myerscough A, et al. High resolution linkage and association mapping identifies a novel rheumatoid arthritis susceptibility locus homologous to one linked to two rat models of inflammatory arthritis. *Hum Mol Genet* 2001;10:1901–1906.
47. Myerscough A, John S, Barrett JH, et al. Linkage of rheumatoid arthritis to insulin-dependent diabetes mellitus loci. *Arthritis Rheum* 2000; 43:2771–2775.
48. Cheng SF, Lum RF, Peden E, et al. Additional support for an autoimmune susceptibility gene(s) at 6q24–27. *Arthritis Rheum* 2001;44 (suppl):104.
49. Van Krugten MV, Huizinga TW, Kaijzel EL, et al. Association of the TNF +489 polymorphism with susceptibility and radiographic damage in rheumatoid arthritis. *Genes Immun* 1999;1:91–96.
50. Castro F, Acevedo E, Ciusani E, et al. Tumor necrosis factor microsatellites and HLA-DRB1*, HLA-DQA1*, and HLA-DQB1* alleles in Peruvian patients with rheumatoid arthritis. *Ann Rheum Dis* 2001;60: 791–795.
51. Waldron-Lynch F, Adams C, Amos C, et al. Tumor necrosis factor 5′ promoter single nucleotide polymorphisms influence susceptibility to rheumatoid arthritis (RA) in immunogenetically defined multiplex RA families. *Genes Immun* 2001;2:82–87.
52. Meyer JM, Han J, Moxley G. Tumor necrosis factor markers show sex-influenced association with rheumatoid arthritis. *Arthritis Rheum* 2001;44:286–295.
53. Chitnavis J, Sinsheimer JS, Clipsham K. Genetic influences in end-stage osteoarthritis: sibling risks of hip and knee replacement for idiopathic osteoarthritis. *J Bone Joint Surg Br* 1997;79:660–664.
54. Kaprio J, Kujala UM, Peltonen L, et al. Genetic liability to osteoarthritis may be greater in women than men. *BMJ* 1996;313:232.
55. Loughlin J. Genetic epidemiology of primary osteoarthritis. *Curr Opin Rheumatol* 2001;13:111–116.
56. Loughlin J, Mustafa Z, Irven C, et al. Stratification analysis of an osteoarthritis genome screen: suggestive linkage to chromosomes 4, 6 and 16. *Am J Hum Genet* 1999;65:1795–1798.
57. Loughlin J, Mustafa Z, Dowling B, et al. Finer linkage mapping of a primary hip osteoarthritis susceptibility locus on chromosome 6. *Eur J Hum Genet* 2002;10:562–568.
58. Stefánsson SE, Jónsson H, Ingvarsson T, et al. Genomewide scan for hand osteoarthritis: a novel mutation in matrilin-3. *Am J Hum Genet* 2003;72:1448–1459.
59. Hull R, Pope FM. Osteoarthritis and cartilage collagen genes. *Lancet* 1989;1:1337–1338.
60. Meulenbelt I, Bijkerk C, De Wildt SCM, et al. Haplotype analysis of three polymorphisms of the COL2A1 gene and associations with generalized radiologic osteoarthritis. *Ann Hum Genet* 1999;63:393–400.
61. Loughlin J, Irven C, Athanasou N, et al. Differential allelic expression of the type II collagen gene (COL2A1) in osteoarthritic cartilage. *Am J Hum Genet* 1995;56:1186–1193.
62. Keen RW, Hart DJ, Lanchbury JS, et al. Association of early osteoarthritis of the knee with a TaqI polymorphism of the vitamin D receptor gene. *Arthritis Rheum* 1997;40:1444–1449.
63. Uitterlinden AG, Burger H, Huang Q, et al. Vitamin D receptor genotype is associated with radiographic osteoarthritis at the knee. *J Clin Invest* 1997;100:259–263.
64. Jones G, White C, Sambrook P, et al. Allelic variation in the vitamin D receptor, lifestyle factors and lumbar spinal degenerative disease. *Ann Rheum Dis* 1998;57:94–99.
65. Videman T, Leppävuori J, Kaprio J, et al. Intragenic polymorphisms of the vitamin D receptor gene associated with intervertebral disc degeneration. *Spine* 1998;23:2477–2485.
66. Uitterlinden AG, Burger H, van Duijn CM, et al. Adjacent genes, for COL2A1 and the vitamin D receptor, are associated with separate features of radiographic osteoarthritis of the knee. *Arthritis Rheum* 2000;43:1456–1464.
67. Devoto M, Shimoya K, Caminis J, et al. First-stage autosomal genome screen in extended pedigrees suggests genes predisposing to low bone mineral density on chromosomes 1p, 2p and 4q. *Eur J Hum Genet* 1998;6:151–157.
68. Karasik D, Myers RH, Hannan MT, et al. Mapping of quantitative ultrasound of the calcaneus bone to chromosome 1 by genome-wide linkage analysis. *Osteoporos Int* 2002;70:457–462.
69. Koller DL, Econs MJ, Morin PA, et al. Genome screen for QTLs contributing to normal variation in bone mineral density and osteoporosis. *J Clin Endocrinol Metab* 2000;85:3116–3120.
70. Koller DL, Rodriguez LA, Christian JC, et al. Linkage of a QTL contributing to normal variation in bone mineral density to chromosome 11q12–13. *J Bone Miner Res* 1999;13:1903–1908.
71. Niu T, Chen C, Cordell H, et al. A genome-wide scan for loci linked to forearm bone mineral density. *Hum Genet* 1999;104:226–233.
72. Deng HW, Xu FH, Huang QY, et al. A whole-gemone linkage scan suggests several genomic regions potentially containing quantitative trait loci for osteoporosis. *J Clin Endocrinol Metab* 2002;87:5151–5159.
73. Ralston SH. Genetic control of susceptibility to osteoporosis. *J Clin Endocrinol Metab* 2002;87:2460–2466.
74. Morrison NA, Qi JC, Tokita A, et al. Prediction of bone density from vitamin D receptor alleles. *Nature* 1994;367:284–287.
75. Grant SF, Reid DM, Blake G, et al. Reduced bone density and osteoporosis associated with a polymorphic Sp1 binding site in the collagen type I [alpha] 1 gene. *Nat Genet* 1996;14:203–205.
76. Garnero P, Borel O, Grant SF, et al. Collagen I [alpha]1 Sp1 polymorphism, bone mass, and bone turnover in healthy French premenopausal women: the OFELY study. *J Bone Miner Res* 1998;13:813–817.
77. Sano M, Inoue S, Hosoi T, et al. Association of estrogen receptor dinucleotide repeat polymorphism with osteroporosis. *Biochem Biophys Res Commun* 1995;217:378–383.
78. Kobayashi S, Inoue S, Hosoi T, et al. Association of bone mineral density with polymorphism of the estrogen receptor gene. *J Bone Miner Res* 1996;11:306–311.
79. Duncan EL, Brown MA, Sinsheimer J, et al. Suggestive linkage of the parathyroid receptor type 1 to osteoporosis. *J Bone Miner Res* 1999; 14:1993–1999.
80. Brown MA, Kennedy LG, MacGregor AJ, et al. Susceptibility to ankylosing spondylitis in twins: the role of genes, HLA, and the environment. *Arthritis Rheum* 1997;40:1823–1828.
81. Robinson WP, van der LS, Khan MA, et al. HLA-Bw60 increases susceptibility to ankylosing spondylitis in HLA-B27+ patients. *Arthritis Rheum* 1989;32:1135–1141.
82. Brown MA, Kennedy LG, Darke C, et al. The effect of HLA-DR genes on susceptibility to and severity of ankylosing spondylitis. *Arthritis Rheum* 1998;41:460–465.
83. Hohler T, Schaper T, Schneider PM, et al. Association of different tumor necrosis factor alpha promoter allele frequencies with ankylosing spondylitis in HLA-B27 positive individuals. *Arthritis Rheum* 1998;41:1489–1492.
84. McGarry F, Walker R, Sturrock R, et al. The −308.1 polymorphism in the promoter region of the tumor necrosis factor gene is associated with ankylosing spondylitis independent of HLA-B27. *J Rheumatol* 1999;26:1110–1116.
85. Milicic A, Lindheimer F, Laval S, et al. Interethnic studies of TNF polymorphisms confirm the likely presence of a second MHC susceptibility locus in ankylosing spondylitis. *Genes Immun* 2000;1:418–422.
86. McGarry F, Neilly J, Anderson N, et al. A polymorphism within the interleukin 1 receptor antagonist (IL-1Ra) gene is associated with ankylosing spondylitis. *Rheumatology* 2001;40:1359–1364.

87. van der Paardt M, Crusius JB, Garcia-Gonzalez MA, et al. Interleukin-1beta and interleukin-1 receptor antagonist gene polymorphisms in ankylosing spondylitis. *Rheumatology* 2002;41:1419–1423.
88. Beyeler C, Armstrong M, Bird HA, et al. Relationship between genotype for the cytochrome P450 CYP2D6 and susceptibility to ankylosing spondylitis and rheumatoid arthritis. *Ann Rheum Dis* 1996;55: 66–68.
89. Brown MA, Edwards S, Hoyle E, et al. Polymorphisms of the CYP2D6 gene increase susceptibility to ankylosing spondylitis. *Hum Mol Genet* 2000;9:1563–1566.
90. Laval SH, Timms A, Edwards S, et al. Whole-genome screening in ankylosing spondylitis: evidence of non-MHC genetic-susceptibility loci. *Am J Hum Genet* 2001;68:918–926.
91. Brown MA, Pile KD, Kennedy LG, et al. A genome-wide screen for susceptibility loci in ankylosing spondylitis. *Arthritis Rheum* 1998; 41:588–595.
92. Rahman P, Gladman DD, Schentag CT, et al. Excessive paternal transmission in psoriatic arthritis. *Arthritis Rheum* 1999;42:1228–1231.
93. Höhler T, Märker-Hermann E. Psoriatic. Arthritis: clinical aspects, genetics, and the role of T cells. *Curr Opin Rheumatol* 2001;13: 273–279.
94. Al-Heresh AM, Proctor J, Jones SM, et al. Tumor necrosis factor-alpha polymorphism and the HLA-Cw*0602 allele in psoriatic arthritis. *Rheumatology* 2002;41:525–530.
95. Gonzalez S, Martinez-Borra J, Torre-Alonso JC, et al. The MICA-A9 triplet repeat polymorphism in the transmembrane region confers additional susceptibility to the development of psoriatic arthritis and is independent of the association of Cw*0602 in psoriasis. *Arthritis Rheum* 1999;42:1010–1016.
96. Karason A, Gudjonsson JE, Upmanyu R, et al. A susceptibility gene for psoriatic arthritis maps to chromosome 16q: evidence for imprinting. *Am J Hum Genet* 2003;72:125–131.
97. Tomfohrde J, Silverman A, Barnes R, et al. Gene for familial psoriasis susceptibility mapped to the distal end of human chromosome 17q. *Science* 1994;264:1141–1145.
98. Samuelsson L, Enlund F, Torinsson A, et al. A genome-wide search for genes predisposing to familial psoriasis by using a stratification approach. *Hum Genet* 1999;105:523–529.
99. Halverson PB, Derfus BA. Calcium crystal-induced inflammation. *Curr Opin Rheum* 2001;13:221–224.
100. Baldwin CT, Farrer LA, Adair R, et al. Linkage of early-onset osteoarthritis and chondrocalcinosis to human chromosome 8q. *Am J Hum Genet* 1995;56:692–697.
101. Hughes AE, McGibbon D, Woodward E, et al. Localization of a gene for chondrocalcinosis to chromosome 5p. *Hum Mol Genet* 1995;4: 1225–1228.
102. Andrew LJ, Brancolini V, de la Pena LS, et al. Refinement of the chromosome 5p locus for familial calcium pyrophosphate dehydrate deposition disease. *Am J Hum Genet* 1999;64:136–145.
103. Pendleton A, Johnson MD, Hughes A, et al. Mutations in ANKH cause chondrocalcinosis. *Am J Hum Genet* 2002;71:933–940.
104. Williams CJ, Zhang Y, Timms A, et al. Autosomal dominant familial calcium pyrophosphate dehydrate deposition disease is caused by mutation in the transmembrane protein ANKH. *Am J Hum Genet* 2002;71:985–991.
105. Nance MA, Nuttall FQ, Econs MJ, et al. Heterogeneity in Paget disease of the bone. *Am J Hum Genet* 2000;92:303–307.
106. Tilyard MW, Gardner RJ, Milligan L, et al. A probable linkage between familial Paget's disease and the HLA loci. *Aust N Z J Med* 1982;12:498–500.
107. Cody JD, Singer FR, Roodman GD, et al. Genetic linkage of Paget disease of the bone to chromosome 18q. *Am J Hum Genet* 1997;61: 1117–1122.
108. Haslam SI, Van Hul W, Morales-Piga A. Paget's disease of bone: evidence for a susceptibility locus on chromosome 18q and for genetic heterogeneity. *J Bone Miner Res* 1998;13:911–917.
109. Hughes AE, Shearman AM, Weber JL, et al. Genetic linkage of familial expansile osteolysis to chromosome 18q. *Hum Mol Genet* 1994;3:359–361.
110. Hughes AE, Ralston SH, Marken J, et al. Mutations in TNFRSF11A, affecting the signal peptide of RANK, cause familial expansile osteolysis. *Nat Genet* 2000;24:45–48.
111. Kormas N, Kennerson M, Hooper A, et al. Does the TNFRSFIIA insertion mutation occur in familial Paget's disease of bone in Australia? *Bone Suppl* 2000;27:25.
112. Nellissery MJ, Padalecki SS, Brkanac Z, et al. Evidence for a novel osteosarcoma tumor-suppressor gene in the chromosome 18 region genetically linked with Paget disease of bone. *Am J Hum Genet* 1998;63:817–824.
113. Laurin N, Brown JP, Lemainque A, et al. Paget disease of bone: mapping of two loci at 5q35-qter and 5q31. *Am J Hum Genet* 2001;69: 528–543.
114. Hocking LJ, Herbert CA, Nicholls RK, et al. Genomewide search in familial Paget disease of bone shows evidence of genetic heterogeneity with candidate loci on chromosomes 2q36, 10p13, and 5q35. *Am J Hum Genet* 2001;69:1055–1061.
115. Laurin N, Brown JP, Morissette J, et al. Recurrent mutation of the gene encoding sequestosome 1 (SQSTM1/p62) in Paget disease of bone. *Am J Hum Genet* 2002;70:1582–1588.
116. Hochberg MC. The application of genetic epidemiology to systemic lupus erythematosus. *J Rheumatol* 1987;14:867–869.
117. Sestak AL, Shaver TS, Moser KL, et al. Familial aggregation of lupus and autoimmunity in an unusual multiplex pedigree. *J Rheumatol* 1999;26:1495–1499.
118. Vyse TJ, Todd JA. Genetic analysis of autoimmune disease. *Cell* 1996;85:311–318.
119. Deapen D, Escalante A, Weinrib L, et al. A revised estimate of twin concordance in systemic lupus erythematosus. *Arthritis Rheum* 1992; 35:311–318.
120. Ahearn JM, Provost TT, Dorsch Ca, et al. Interrelationships of HLA-DR, MB, and MT phenotypes, autoantibody expression, and clinical features in systemic lupus erythematosus. *Arthritis Rheum* 1982;25:1031–1040.
121. Celada A, Barras C, Benzonana G, et al. Increased frequency of HLA-DRw3 in systemic lupus erythematosus. *Tissue Antigens* 1980; 15:283–288.
122. Gladman KK, Urowitz MB, Darlinkton GA. Disease expression and class II HLA antigens in systemic lupus erythematosus. *Lupus* 1999; 8:466–470.
123. Hashimoto H, Tsuda H, Matsumoto T, et al. HLA antigens associated with systemic lupus erythematosus in Japan. *J Rheumatol* 1985; 12:919–923.
124. Kachru RB, Sequeira W, Mittal KK, et al. A significant increase of HLA-DR3 and DR2 in systemic lupus erythematosus among blacks. *J Rheumatol* 1984;11:471–474.
125. Kawai T, Katoh K, Tani K, et al. HLA antigens in Japanese patients with central nervous system lupus. *Tissue Antigens* 1990;35:45–46.
126. Mehra NK, Pande I, Taneja V, et al. Major histocompatibility complex genes and susceptibility to systemic lupus erythematosus in northern India. *Lupus* 1993;2:313–314.
127. Reinertsen JL, Klippel JH, Johnson AH, et al. B-lymphocyte alloantigens associated with systemic lupus erythematosus. *N Engl J Med* 1978;299:515–518.
128. Reinharz D, Tiercy JM, Mach B, et al. Absence of DRw15/3 and DRw15/7 heterozygotes in Caucasian patients with systemic lupus erythematosus. *Tissue Antigens* 1991;37:10–15.
129. Reveille JD, Barger BO, Hodge TW. HLA-DR2-DRB1 allele frequencies in DR2-positive black Americans with and without systemic lupus erythematosus. *Tissue Antigens* 1991;38:178–180.
130. Scherak O, Smolen JS, Mayr WR. HLA-DRw3 and systemic lupus erythematosus. *Arthritis Rheum* 1980;23:954–957.
131. So AK, Fielder AH, Warner CA, et al. DNA polymorphism of major histocompatibility complex class II and class III genes in systemic lupus erythematosus. *Tissue Antigens* 1990;35:144–147.
132. Yen JH, Chen CJ, Tsai WC, et al. HLA-DMA and HLA-DMB genotyping in patients with systemic lupus erythematosus. *J Rheumatol* 1999;26:1930–1933.
133. Duits AJ, Bootsma H, Derksen RH, et al. Skewed distribution of IgG Fc receptor IIa (CD32) polymorphism is associated with renal disease in systemic lupus erythematosus patients. *Arthritis Rheum* 1995; 39:1832–1836.
134. Salmon JE, Millard S, Schachter LA, et al. Fc gamma RIIA alleles are heritable risk factors for lupus nephritis in African Americans. *J Clin Invest* 1996;97:1348–1354.

135. Wu J, Edberg JC, Redecha PB, et al. A novel polymorphism of Fc gamma RIIIa (CD16) alters receptor function and predisposes to autoimmune disease. *J Clin Invest* 1997;100:1059–1070.
136. Salmon JE, Ng S, Yoo DH, et al. Altered distribution of Fc gamma receptor IIIA alleles in a cohort of Korean patients with lupus nephritis. *Arthritis Rheum* 1999;42:818–819.
137. Prokunina L, Castillejo-Lopez C, Oberg F, et al. A regulatory polymorphism in PDCD1 is associated with susceptibility to systemic lupus erythematosus in humans. *Nat Genet* 2002;32:666–669.
138. Horiuchi T, Nishizaka H, Yasunaga S, et al. Association of Fas/APO-1 gene polymorphism with systemic lupus erythematosus in Japanese. *Rheumatology* 1999;38:516–520.
139. Lee YH, Kim YR, Ji JD, et al. Fas promoter −670 polymorphism is associated with development of anti-RNP antibodies in systemic lupus erythematosus. *J Rheumatol* 2001;28:2008–2011.
140. Wu J, Wilson J, He J, et al. Fas ligand mutation in a patient with systemic lupus erythematosus and lymphoproliferative disease. *J Clin Invest* 1996;98:1107–1113.
141. Garred P, Madsen HO, Halberg P, et al. Mannose-binding lectin polymorphisms and susceptibility to infection in systemic lupus erythematosus. *Arthritis Rheum* 1999;42:2145–2152.
142. Davies EJ, Teh LS, Ordi-Ros J, et al. A dysfunctional allele of the mannose binding protein gene associates with systemic lupus erythematosus in a Spanish population. *J Rheumatol* 1997;24:485–488.
143. Sullivan KE, Wooten C, Goldman D, et al. Mannose-binding protein polymorphism in black patients with systemic lupus erythematosus. *Arthritis Rheum* 1996;39:2046–2051.
144. Mehrian R, Quismorio FP, Strassmann G, et al. Synergistic effect between IL-10 and bcl-2 genotypes in determining susceptibility to systemic lupus erythematosus. *Arthritis Rheum* 1998;41:596–602.
145. Ahmed S, Ihara K, Kanemitsu S, et al. Association of CTLA-4 but not CD28 gene polymorphisms with systemic lupus erythematosus in the Japanese population. *Rheumatology* 2001;40:662–667.
146. Tebib JG, Alcocer-Varela J, Alarcon-Segovia D, et al. Association between a T cell receptor restriction fragment length polymorphism and systemic lupus erythematosus. *J Clin Invest* 1990;86:1961–1967.
147. Stevens A, Ray D, Alansari A, et al. Characterization of a prolactin gene polymorphism and its associations with systemic lupus erythematosus. *Arthritis Rheum* 2001;44:2358–2366.
148. Wilson AG, Gordon C, diGiovine FS, et al. A genetic association between systemic lupus erythematosus and tumor necrosis factor alpha. *Eur J Immunol* 1994;24:191–195.
149. Zuniga J, Vargas-Alarcon G, Hernandez-Pacheco G, et al. Tumor necrosis factor-alpha promoter polymorphisms in Mexican patients with systemic lupus erythematosus (SLE). *Genes Immun* 2001;2:363–366.
150. Komata T, Tsuchiya N, Matsushita M, et al. Association of tumor necrosis factor receptor 2 (TNFR2) polymorphism with susceptibility to systemic lupus erythematosus. *Tissue Antigens* 1999;53:527–533.
151. Kelly JA, Moser KL, Harley JB. The genetics of systemic lupus erythematosus: putting the pieces together. *Genes Immun* 2002;3(suppl 1):71–85.
152. Edberg JC, Langefeld CD, Wu J, et al. Genetic linkage and association of Fcγ receptor IIIA (CDE16A) on chromosome 1q23 with human systemic lupus erythematosus. *Arthritis Rheum* 2002;46:2132–2140.
153. Graham RR, Ortmann WA, Langefeld CD, et al. Visualizing human leukocyte antigen class II risk haplotypes in human systemic lupus erythematosus. *Am J Hum Genet* 2002;71:543–553.
154. Sawalha AH, Potts R, Schmid WR, et al. The genetics of primary Sjögren's syndrome. *Curr Rheumatol Rep* 2003;5:324–332.
155. Hulkkonen J, Pertovaara M, Antonen J, et al. Genetic association between interleukin-10 promotor region polymorphisms and primary syndrome. *Arthritis Rheum* 2001;44:176–179.
156. Perrier S, Coussediere C, Dubost JJ, et al. IL-1 receptor antagonist (IL-1RA) gene polymorphism in Sjögren's syndrome and rheumatoid arthritis. *Clin Immunol Immunopathol* 1998;87:309–313.
157. Hulkkonen J, Pertovaara M, Antonen J, et al. Elevated interleukin-6 plasma levels are regulated by the promoter region polymorphism of the IL6 gene in primary Sjögren's syndrome and correlate with the clinical manifestations of the disease. *J Rheumatol* 2001;40:656–661.
158. Nakken B, Jonsson R, Bolstad AI. Polymorphisms of the Ro52 gene associated with anti-Ro 52kd autoantibodies in patients with primary Sjögren's syndrome. *Arthritis Rheum* 2001;44:638–646.
159. Kumigai S, Kanagawa S, Morinobu A, et al. Association of a new allele of the TAP2 gene, TAP2*Bky2 (Val577), with susceptibility to Sjögren's syndrome. *Arthritis Rheum* 1997;40:1685–1692.
160. Morinobu A, Kanagawa S, Koshiba M, et al. Association of the glutathione S-transferase M1 homozygous null genotype with susceptibility to Sjögren's syndrome in Japanese individuals. *Arthritis Rheum* 1999;42:2612–2615.
161. Wang ZY, Morinobu A, Kanagawa S, et al. Polymorphisms of the mannose binding lectin gene in patients with Sjögren's syndrome. *Ann Rheum Dis* 2001;60:483–486.
162. Tsutsumi A, Sasaki K, Wakamiya N, et al. Mannose-binding lectin gene: polymorphisms in Japanese patients with systemic lupus erythematosus, rheumatoid arthritis and Sjögren's syndrome. *Genes Immun* 2001;2:99–104.
163. Bolstad AI, Wargelius A, Nakken B, et al: Fas and Fas Ligand gene polymorphisms in primary Sjögren's syndrome. *J Rheumatol* 2000; 27:2397–2405.
164. Simon M, Bourel M, Fauchet R, et al. Association of HLA-A3 and HLA-BI4 antigens with idiopathic haemochromatosis. *Gut* 1976;17: 332–334.
165. Feder JN, Gnirke A, Thomas W, et al. A novel MHC class I–like gene is mutated in patients with hereditary hemochromatosis. *Nat Genet* 1996;13:399–408.
166. Mura C, Raguenes O, Ferec C. HFE mutations analysis in 711 hemochromatosis probands: evidence for S65C implication in mild form of hemochromatosis. *Blood* 1999;93:2502–2505.
167. Pointon JJ, Wallace D, Merryweather-Clarke AT, et al. Uncommon mutations and polymorphisms in the hemochromatosis gene. *Genet Test* 2000;4:151–161.
168. Mura C, Raguenes O, Ferec C. HFE mutation analysis in 711 hemochromatosis probands: evidence for S65C implication in mild form of haemochromatosis. *Blood* 1999;93:2502–2505.
169. Wallace DF, Walker AP, Pietrangelo A, et al. Frequency of the S65C mutation of HFE and iron overload in 309 subjects heterozygous for C282Y. *J Hepatol* 2002;36:474–479.
170. Bomford A. Genetics of haemochromatosis. *Lancet* 2002;360:1673–1681.
171. Beutler E, Felitti VJ, Koziol JA, et al. Penetrance of 845G A (C282Y) HFE hereditary hemochromatosis mutation in the USA. *Lancet* 2002; 359:211–218.
172. Roetto A, Totaro A, Cazzola M, et al. Juvenile hemochromatosis locus maps to chromosome lq. *Am J Hum Genet* 1999;64:1388–1393.
173. Camaschella C, Roetto A, Cali A, et al. The gene TFR2 is mutated in a new type of haemochromatosis mapping to 7q22. *Nat Genet* 2000; 25:14–15.
174. Roetto A, Totaro A, Piperno A, et al. New mutations inactivating transferrin receptor 2 in hemochromatosis type 3. *Blood* 2001;97: 2555–2560.
175. Mattman A, Huntsman D, Lockitch G, et al. Transferrin receptor 2 (TfR2) and HFE mutational analysis in non-C282Y iron overload: identification of a novel TfR2 mutation. *Blood* 2002;100:1075–1077.
176. Njajou OT, Vaessen N, Joosse M, et al. A mutation in SLC11A3 is associated with autosomal dominant hemochromatosis. *Nat Genet* 2001;28:213–214.
177. Montosi G, Donovan A, Totaro A, et al. Autosomal dominant hemochromatosis is associated with a mutation in the ferroportin (SLC11A3) gene. *J Clin Invest* 2001;108:619–623.
178. Devalia V, Carter K, Walker AP, et al. Autosomal dominant reticuloendothelial iron overload associated with a three base pair deletion in the Ferroportin 1 gene (SLC11A3). *Blood* 2002;100:695–697.
179. Wallace DF, Pederson P, Dixon JL, et al. Novel mutation in ferroportin 1 is associated with autosomal dominant hemochromatosis. *Blood* 2002;100:692–694.
180. Kato J, Fujikawa K, Kanda M, et al. A Mutation in the iron-responsive element of H ferritin mRNA, causing autosomal dominant iron overload. *Am J Hum Genet* 2001;69:191–117.
181. Todd JA, Farrall M. Panning for gold: Genome-wide scanning for linkage in type 1 diabetes. *Hum Mol Genet* 1996;5:1443–1448.
182. Concannon P, Gogolin-Ewens KJ, Hinds DA, et al. A second generation screen of the human genome for susceptibility to insulin-dependent diabetes mellitus. *Nat Genet* 1998;19:292–296.

CHAPTER 29

Arthritis and Autoimmunity in Animals

Philip L. Cohen and Anita P. Kuan

Animal models of rheumatic diseases have provided insights into the pathogenesis and treatment of human illnesses for decades. It is the purpose of this chapter to review the principal animal models of arthritis and autoimmunity. It is not intended to be comprehensive or exhaustive, but rather to serve as an overview and guide to further reading.

ADVANTAGES AND LIMITATIONS OF ANIMAL MODELS

Animal models have many attractions to investigators, among them accessibility of tissues to pathologic examination, the genetic homogeneity of inbred rodent strains, and the ability to test therapeutic interventions. No perfect animal model of human disease exists, and rodents in particular have important physiologic and biochemical differences from humans. Nevertheless, animal models of arthritis and autoimmunity have led to important information about disease mechanisms and treatment.

Why Use an Animal Model?

The chief reasons to investigate disease in animals are ethical, practical, and genetic. Animals can be subjected to experiments that could not be contemplated in humans (e.g., experimental surgery, breeding, and drug treatment) and can be sacrificed to obtain tissue. Furthermore, many animals are small, have compressed life spans, and can be maintained under rigid experimental conditions. Most animals used as disease models are highly inbred, so that their genomes are identical, or nearly so. Mice have come to be, by far, the most widely used experimental animals, and for good reason. The mouse genome is sequenced, reagents exist for thousands of mouse genes and proteins, and technology is widely available to add, alter, or remove genes. Many knockout and transgenic mice are commercially available and allow rapid investigation of the influence of specific genes. Mice have a rapid generation time (21-day gestation period, 6 weeks to adulthood) and can be maintained on defined diets. Rats are still in use for certain models and have advantages inherent in their larger size. Yet less is known about their genetics, and reagents are more limited. Rabbits have been used in several models of experimental arthritis and have been favored recently in gene therapy experiments, because their relatively large joints make it easier to transfer vectors, to aspirate fluid, and to assess pathology (1).

Heterogeneity of Disease in Inbred Animals—Relevant to Human Disease?

Inbred rodents are housed under identical environmental conditions, usually in specific pathogen-free colonies. It may come as a surprise that, despite genetic and environmental identity between individual animals, there is considerable individual variation. Titers of autoantibodies can vary considerably, along with the degree and even the incidence of pathology. What can account for this variability? In some cases, there may be influences of birth order or placental position, but it is likely that the differences between individuals reflect the fundamental biologic complexity of higher organisms and the numerous stochastic events present in development. In particular, the immune system may be especially influenced by random processes, such as those involved in the generation of the receptors on T and B cells and in the selection of immune repertoires.

That even genetically-identical mice reared under controlled conditions display significant animal-to-animal differences is important in considering mechanisms of human diseases. For humans, disparity in phenotype between identical twins has been ascribed to different environmental influences. Although exogenous influences are undoubtedly important, it is also possible that variations in disease phenotype or expression parallel the animal situation, namely that nongenetic, nonenvironmental factors may be important in the precise disease encountered in individual patients.

Important Differences between Humans, Rodents, and Lagomorphs

Although the human and mouse genomes show over 90% homology, interspecies differences can be important in interpreting animal model findings. Laboratory mouse strains may not be representative of the species as a whole, having been derived from strains of Japanese mouse fanciers introduced early in the twentieth century to North America (2). Laboratory mouse strains are more closely related to each other than to wild mice. Both laboratory and wild strains have deleted large segments of their T-cell receptor V genes (3), and many have deficiencies in complement components (4).

In general, life is accelerated in mice compared with humans. Mice have a life span of 2 to 3 years, depending on strain (5). Unlike humans, they have an estrous cycle and give rise to 10 or more offspring from a single mating. Mice have a body temperature of 37°C, yet a normal adult heart rate of over 200 beats per minute (6). Their skin structure differs significantly from humans, whereas joint anatomy is similar (7). Drug doses, adjusted for body weight, can vary widely (e.g., effective cyclophosphamide doses in mice need to be much greater than human doses) (8). The composition of mouse blood is remarkably similar to that of humans, and blood chemistry values differ only slightly (7). Mice (unlike rabbits) have four immunoglobulin G (IgG) subclasses, analogous to human subclasses. Immunoglobulin metabolism is significantly faster in mice, and IgG levels are about 40% of humans (9). Unlike humans, mice are born before full establishment of the T-cell repertoire; consequently, neonatal thymectomy results in profound T-cell deficiency (10). In humans and many other mammals, T-cell development is nearly complete at birth. Responsiveness to corticosteroids differs markedly in rodents compared with humans. Administration of glucocorticoids causes profound thymic involution in adult mice with marked depletion of immature T lymphocytes (11). Human T cells, both mature and immature, are more resistant to glucocorticoid treatment.

Inducible versus Spontaneous Models of Disease

Animal models can either be induced by experimental manipulation or can occur spontaneously. Inducible models have the powerful advantage of a known inciting agent that can be given in precise quantities and at any time, and measured and tracked accurately during disease. For example, arthritis can be induced by giving highly purified collagen to appropriate mouse strains. Arthritogenic epitopes can be deduced and regulatory pathways can be elucidated by readministration of antigenic fragments or specific lymphocytes. The disadvantage of inducible models is the relevance of the artificial disease to spontaneous human illness. With rare exceptions, the causes of rheumatic diseases remain unknown.

Spontaneous models of autoimmune disease depend on the genetic constitution of animal strains. For single gene mutations, transgenes, and knockouts, inferences can be straightforward. For many important models, for example the New Zealand black/New Zealand white (NZB × NZW) model of lupus, the genes responsible are many and their interactions are complex (12). Relevance to human disease is always an issue. Inducible models often reveal important genetic susceptibility loci; conversely, spontaneous models are often influenced by environmental factors. This can be troublesome in comparing results from one colony to another, particularly if there are differences in microbial flora and in prevalence of enzootics.

Knockouts and Transgenes

Transgenic animals (usually mice) are produced by microinjection of genes into the male pronucleus of fertilized eggs (Fig. 29.1). Founder mice are derived and can be back-

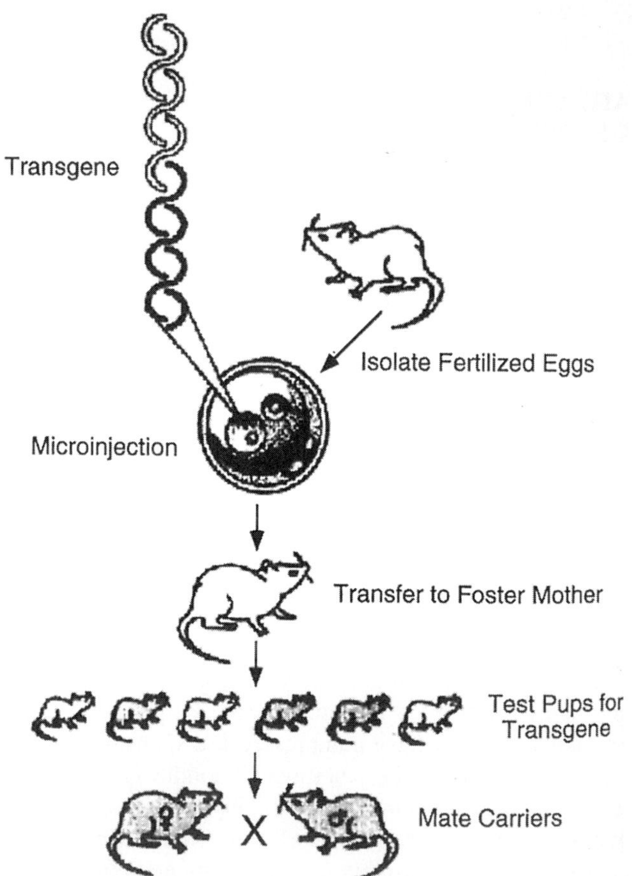

FIG. 29.1. Generation of transgenic mice. The gene to be introduced is isolated and microinjected into fertilized eggs. These one-cell mouse embryos are transferred to a foster mother and brought to term. Pups that carry the transgene become founder animals. Their heterozygous offspring are mated to generated homozygous transgenic animals.

crossed to any genetic background. Although conventional transgenic mice express randomly integrated genes in all tissues, it is possible to generate animals that express specific genes by using tissue-specific promoters (e.g., an insulin promoter can be used to achieve pancreatic beta cell–specific expression). Transgenes have been widely used to achieve generalized or tissue-specific expression of genes. Here, important considerations are the site of gene insertion (random for conventional transgenes, with the possibility of interactions with unknown genes); and the gene copy number, which can be quite variable. For example, spondylitic disease in rats is critically dependent on high numbers of human leukocyte antigen (HLA)-B27 gene copies.

It is now possible to insert transgenes selectively into relevant genetic loci (knock-ins), providing a further important manipulation to create interesting models of disease (13). For example, immunoglobulin heavy-chain genes can be inserted directly into the heavy-chain locus and can function as if they were normal endogenous genes, undergoing class switching and somatic mutation.

Targeted mutagenesis (knockout technology) depends on homologous recombination to localize DNA constructs so as to insert nonfunctional genes to cripple specific genes (Fig. 29.2). This powerful technique in effect introduces recessive nonfunctional mutations of genes. It can be combined with transgenic or transgenic knock-in technology to replace normal genes with engineered genes. Conditional knockouts allow the selective expression of genes in target tissues (13).

Custom-produced mice lacking one or more genes have proved especially invaluable in understanding the contributions of specific genes to disease pathogenesis. Such studies have led to a large number of artificial disease states, some intended and some unintended. It should be remembered that the phenotype of knockout mice reflects the absence of a gene product from the time of conception. This may lead to a different outcome than the deletion of a gene product in a mature animal. For example, the deletion of CD4 in mature animals using antibodies *in vivo* is quite different from knocking out the CD4 gene, which removes the gene from the earliest stages of development.

Animal Models: The Problem of Controls

Much animal experimentation takes the form of addressing the mechanism of disease in a genetic phenotype (often complex) and comparing with normal control animals. In some cases—for example, single-gene models like Fas deficiency or knockout strains,—inbred animals with a wild-type allele at the locus in question can be used as a control.

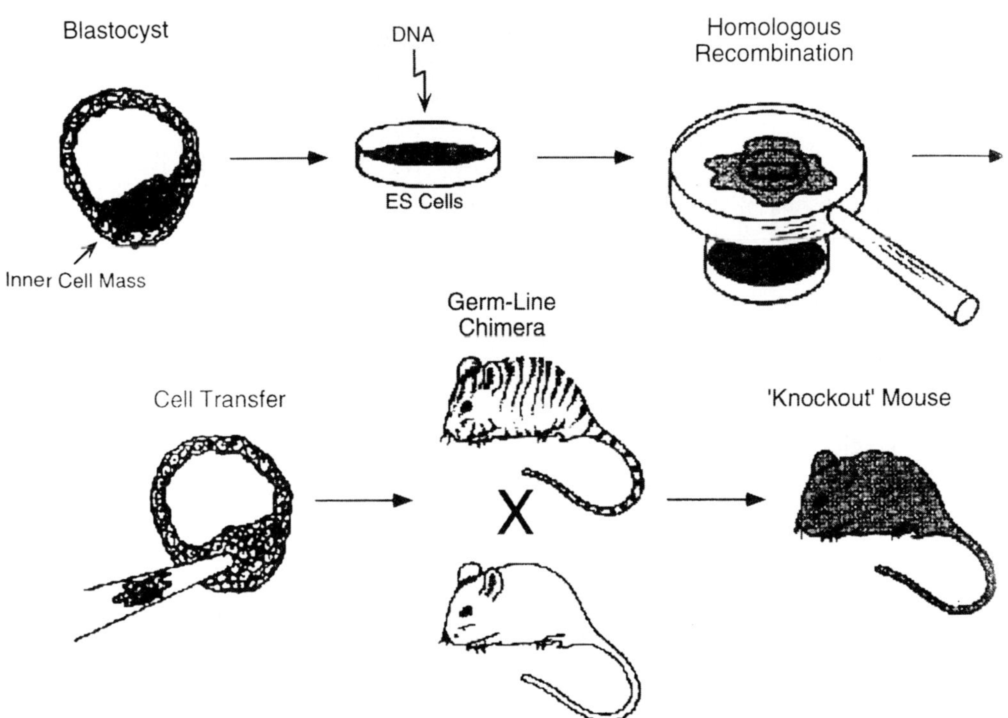

FIG. 29.2. Generation of knockout mice by targeted mutagenesis. Embryonic stem (ES) cells are isolated from the inner cell mass of a 3.5-day-old blastocyst embryo. They are grown *in vitro* like other cell lines. A DNA construct containing a mutated mouse gene is transferred into the ES cells. ES cells are selected in which the incoming DNA is recombined with homologous chromosomal sequences to create a mutation in the target gene. These cells are transferred into a recipient blastocyst, and germ line chimeras are generated. These chimeras are the founders of mouse lines that carry the selected mutation.

Day 39
1+ hind paws

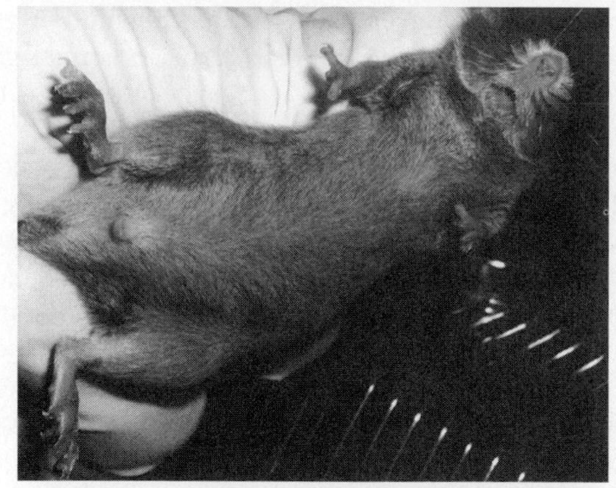
A

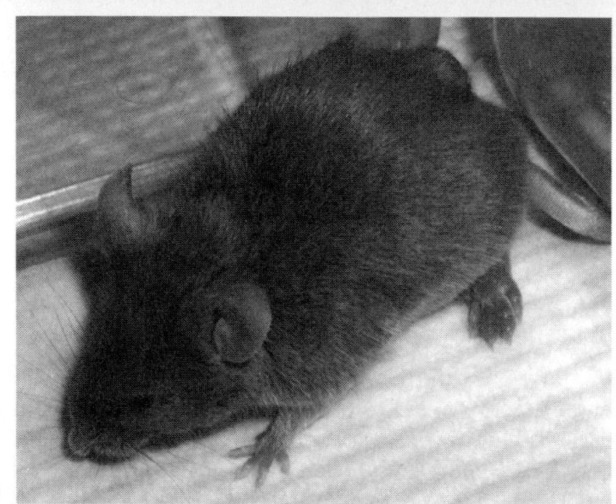
B

Day 45
3+ hind paws
1+ front paws

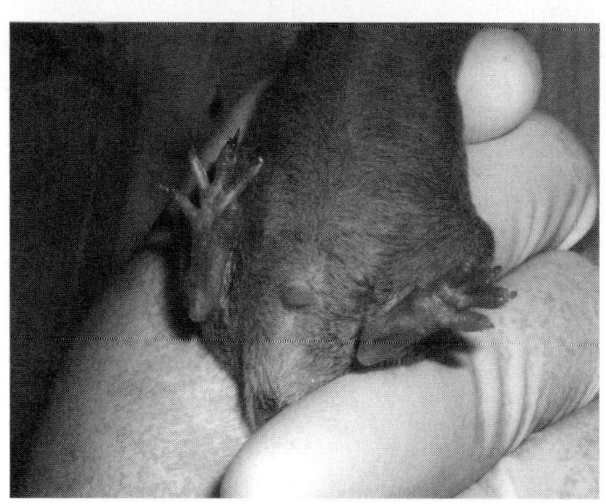
C

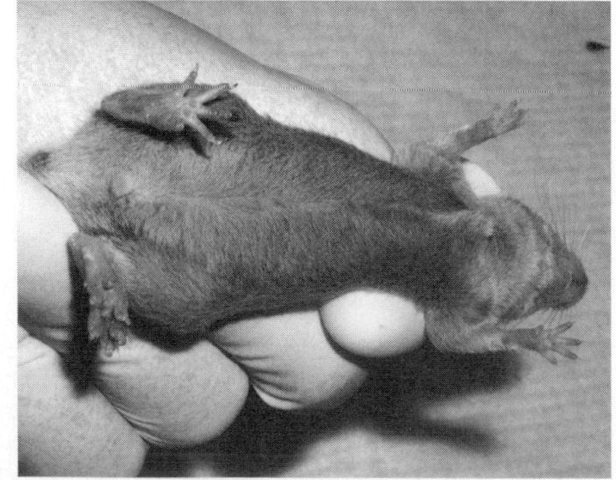
D

FIG. 29.3. Paw erythema and swelling are visible in these DBA/1 mice suffering from collagen-induced arthritis. "Days" are from initial injection of chicken collagen type II. Panels A and B show two views of a mouse at day 39. Panels C and D depict another mouse at day 15. Scoring is as indicated in the text. (Courtesy of Dr. Michael A. Maldonado, University of Pennsylvania.)

But, in other cases, there is no obvious control beyond selecting a "normal" strain; for example, much of the NZB and NZB/NZW literature relies on comparisons with BALB/c, selected presumably because it's major histocompatibility complex (MHC) is identical with NZB. In many experiments, C57BL/6 (B6) is considered a normal strain. The approach can be treacherous, in light of the many known abnormalities even in normal strains. Some, but comparatively few, investigators have used multiple strains for comparison with the autoimmune strain.

A newer problem concerns the widespread use of knockout mice as disease models. Invariably, embryonic stem cells from 129/Sv mice are used to generate the gene-deleted strain. Good experimental practice would require extensive backcrossing to a well-studied nonautoimmune genetic background, generally B6, but this is time consuming and expensive. Unfortunately, it is clear that the 129/Sv strain contains background genes that enhance the autoimmune phenotype (14). Although 129/Sv based knockouts remain of great value in autoimmunity studies, the complex influence of their background must be considered until mice are fully backcrossed onto other backgrounds.

Quantitation of Disease in Animal Models

Although there is no general agreement on this important issue, arthritis in animals is generally scored clinically using a scale assigning 0 to 3 points per paw. An unaffected joint is scored 0, mild swelling and erythema 1, moderate swelling and erythema 2, and severe swelling, erythema, or ankylosis 3; thus, the total score ranges from 0 to 12. Figure 29.3 shows an example of the scoring of arthritis in mice suffering from collagen-induced arthritis. For all such assessments, it is imperative that animals be scored blindly and by the same observer to minimize bias. Weight loss is an important clinical parameter that is sometimes neglected. Important information can be obtained using plain radiographs, and more recently, magnetic resonance imaging (MRI) has been used for clinical assessment. Histopathologic examination is of great value. Blood studies are of limited value in assessing arthritis activity: whole blood chemiluminescence reflects the degree of oxidative burst from neutrophils and has been advocated as a measure of total body inflammation (15). Sedimentation rate and C-reactive protein are not helpful in rodents, but measurement of serum amyloid protein is helpful in quantitating inflammation early in arthritis models (16).

Assessing murine systemic lupus erythematosus (SLE) is accomplished by measuring anti-DNA, antichromatin, and other antinuclear antibodies, either using conventional serology (usually enzyme-linked immunosorbent assay) or by a single-cell assay (usually enzyme-linked immunospot assay). Renal function is measured by creatinine or urea nitrogen testing, along with dipstick estimation of proteinuria and examination of kidneys by light and immunofluorescence microscopy after sacrifice. The degree of lymphadenopathy in lpr or gld mice can be assessed by weighing lymph nodes or counting total lymphoid cells. Survival is an important end point for many studies. An excellent practical reference gives important details for induction and measurement of experimental arthritis and SLE (17).

ANIMAL MODELS FOR TRANSPLANTATION OF HUMAN TISSUE

Mice with deficient immune systems have been useful as vehicles to study explanted human tissue. Severe combined immunodeficient (SCID) mice, genetically lacking a key recombinase needed for rearrangement of T- and B-cell genes, will accept human xenografts. Human immune progenitor cells have been used to reconstitute functional immune systems that will generate humoral and cellular responses to antigenic stimuli (18). Blood cells from patients with lupus and scleroderma have been observed to produce autoantibodies when transferred to SCID mice, but disease manifestations generally do not occur (19,20). Human synovium, transplanted under the skin or kidney capsule, shows persistent inflammation and has been used as an *in vivo* model of rheumatoid arthritis (RA) (21). Similarly, temporal artery fragments transferred into SCID mice have been used to study the role of cytokines in this illness (22).

ANIMAL MODELS OF INFLAMMATORY RHEUMATIC DISEASES

Collagen Arthritis

Collagen arthritis, inducible in rats, mice, and primates, has been studied as an arthritis model since the 1970s and is the most widely used animal model of arthritis (23). It has gained acceptance because of its reproducibility in diverse strains, its rapidity of onset, and its pathologic similarity to RA despite the uncertain link between anticollagen immunity and the human disease (24). Collagen-induced arthritis (CIA) results after injection of xenogeneic (usually bovine) collagen type II (CII) in adjuvant (25). Its course is chronically progressive, but a relapsing-remitting disease can be induced by immunization with murine CII (26).

After collagen immunization, susceptible animals (such as DBA/1 and B10RIII mice) develop articular fibrin deposition followed by pannus formation, marginal erosion of cartilage and subchondral bone, and joint destruction. An initial influx of neutrophils is followed by the arrival of macrophages, antibody-producing B cells, and $CD4^+$, $\alpha\beta$ T-cell receptor $(TCR)^+$ T lymphocytes (27). Pathology can be adoptively transferred using T cells, and to an extent, also by infusion of affected mouse serum containing antibodies to collagen. Despite many years of study, the relative contributions of T and B lymphocytes to disease are still controversial. Arthritis even develops (to a limited degree) in DBA/1 mice lacking T and B lymphocytes (Rag-1 knockouts), establishing an important role for innate immunity in pathogenesis (28).

The immune response to collagen is a potent cellular and humoral response, requiring costimulatory molecules such as B7–1, B7–2, CD28, CTLA4, CD40, and CD40L (23). CIA requires an intact complement system, because the full disease does not occur in the absence of complement components C5, C3, or factor B (29,30). During active arthritis, there is up-regulation in the joint of protooncogenes such as c-*fos*/AP-1, apoptosis-related molecules such as Fas, and adhesion molecules such as intercellular adhesion molecule-1 (31,32). Prostaglandins, leukotrienes such as LTB4, and oxidation products also appear to contribute significantly to the disease process (33). Production of chemokines, such as macrophage inhibitory protein-1α (MIP-1α), and proinflammatory cytokines, including tumor necrosis factor (TNF)-α, interleukin (IL)-1, and IL-6, also increase markedly during the active stages of the disease, and neutralizing TNF-α and IL-1 is effective in ameliorating arthritis, bone erosion, and joint inflammation (34). However, there may be different roles for TNF-α and IL-1 in the pathogenesis of CIA. TNF-α is important at the onset of arthritis but less so in later stages, whereas IL-1 plays a pivotal role at both early and late stages of disease (35). Mice overexpressing IL-1 receptor antagonist (IL-1Ra) have a significant reduction in the incidence and severity of CIA, whereas mice lacking IL-1Ra have a significantly earlier onset of CIA, with increased disease severity. The administration of a soluble fragment of the chain of the IL-15 receptor into susceptible DBA/1 mice also profoundly suppresses the development of CIA, as does systemic IL-4 (36,37). Granulocyte-macrophage colony-stimulating factor (GM-CSF) also is required for full expression of CIA (38). Levels of IL-2 and its receptor are elevated during active CIA, and IL-2 exacerbates disease if administered after its onset. Interestingly, IL-2 suppresses illness if given before onset of the disease or at its very beginning, apparently through stimulation of interferon-γ (IFN-γ) (39). In this regard, IFN-γ and IL-12 both play dual roles in CIA, that is, actively promoting arthritis during the induction phase and stimulating antiinflammatory mechanisms during the recovery phase (40,41). Sera from IFN-$\gamma R^{-/-}$ mice, which exhibit decreased incidence and severity of CIA, have lower levels of CII-specific IgG. This indicates that IFN-γ exacerbates CIA by affecting the levels of CII-specific IgG antibody, as well as by the imbalance of helper T cell subset 1 and 2 (T_H1/T_H2) cells (42). Anti-IL-12 also prevents the development and progression of CIA in IFN-$\gamma R^{-/-}$ mice.

Contrasting with the prominent expression of proinflammatory mediators, expression of antiinflammatory cytokines, such as IL-4 and IL-10, is minimal during the active stages of the disease, although IL-4 and IL-10 increase during the later stages.

The genetic aspects of CIA have been of special interest for many years. Non-MHC genes play an important role, with four principal quantitative trait loci identified in both rat and mouse (43). MHC genes are of key importance in CIA susceptibility. H-2^q and H-2^r MHC haplotypes, found in the susceptible DBA/1 (H-2^q) and B10.RIII (H-2^r) strains, are the most susceptible. Susceptibility to CIA in H-2^q mice maps to the class II-Aβ chain. CIA susceptibility in H-2^r strains is confined to certain species of type II collagen (porcine, bovine, deer). CIA-resistant haplotypes are H-2s, d, b, j, v, k, u, and p. However, B10.PL (H-2^u) and B.10M (H-2^f) show a low incidence of CIA when immunized with human CII.

Because of the strong linkage of RA to certain HLA haplotypes and the evidence that autoimmunity to CII may play a role in some cases of RA-like polyarthritis, considerable research has been devoted to the study of HLA in CIA using transgenic mice expressing human DQ and DR molecules (44). Mice with deleted endogenous class II genes but transgenic for the RA-associated genes, human HLA-DQA1*0301, DQB1*0302 (DQ8), are susceptible to severe CIA, whereas HLA-DQ6 transgenic mice are resistant. Double transgenic (DQ/DR) mice show contrasting effects. DQ8/DR2 mice exhibit significant decreases in disease incidence, whereas the DQ8/DR3 mice are susceptible to CIA. DQ8/DR2 mice show a T_H2 cytokine profile, whereas DQ8/DR3 mice show a T_H1 profile, indicating that DRB1 polymorphism can modulate both T_H1/T_H2 responses and CIA in mice. HLA-DR1 and HLA-DR4 transgenic mice immunized with either human or bovine CII also develop arthritis. The data indicate that both DQ and DR molecules can present CII, resulting in the development of arthritis. Recently, a regulatory and protective influence of CD8-bearing T cells has been reported in mice transgenic for RA MHC genes (45)

Sex and hormonal influences on CIA in mice have also been demonstrated (46). In DBA/1 and B10.RIII mice, males show a higher incidence of CIA and a more severe disease than do females, unlike RA in humans. This sex difference has been related to polymorphic genes on the X chromosome that suppress autoimmune responses rather than augmentation by Y chromosome–linked genes. Like RA, however, pregnancy delays the onset and causes clinical remission of CIA, which then flares up in the postpartum period. The protection afforded by pregnancy may result from elevated estrogen levels. Consistent with that view are the observations that treatment with estradiol and estriol or the estrogen metabolite 2-methoxyestradiol suppresses CIA. Moreover, administration of dihydroepiandrosterone, a weak androgen precursor of gonadal steroids, before CII immunization in DBA/1 male and female mice delays the onset and decreases the severity of disease, and decreases IgG anticollagen antibody levels. CIA development is also augmented by the pineal hormone melatonin, which most likely is secondary to stimulation of T-cell sensitization to collagen.

A Model for Relapsing Polychondritis

As indicated above, HLA-DQ8αβ (DQA1*0301/DQB*0302) transgenic mice with deletion of endogenous class II genes respond strongly to CII, developing severe arthritis, whereas DQ6αβ transgenic mice (DQA1*0103/DQB1*0601) are nonresponsive to CII. CII-immunized double transgenic DQ6αβ/8αβ ($A\beta^0$) mice, expressing both the α and β chains of DQ6 and DQ8 molecules, develop severe experimental polychondritis, exhibiting both polyarthritis and auricular chondritis (47). The clinical, serologic, and histologic manifestations of this experimental polychondritis resemble human relapsing polychondritis. The susceptibility of DQ6αβ/8αβ transgenic mice compared with resistance in the parental strains suggests that expression of both the DQ6αβ and DQ8αβ transgenes is important in susceptibility to experimental polychondritis.

K/B×N Mice: an Important New Model of Rheumatoid Arthritis

The serendipitous observation of severe erosive arthritis in mice with a transgenic TCR has led to important insights into disease mechanisms. The KRN TCR recognizes a peptide of bovine RNase in the context of $I\text{-}A^k$. The KRN TCR transgenic mouse was crossed with various mouse strains initially to introduce a restriction element for positive selection of the KRN TCR. The fortuitous breeding of the KRN mouse on the B6 background to the nonobese diabetic (NOD) mouse resulted in unexpected severe joint inflammation (48). Beginning at 1 month of age these K/B×N mice develop an arthritis characterized by symmetric joint disease with pannus formation and destructive bone and cartilage destruction of predominantly distal joints (48). K/B×N mice have elevated proinflammatory cytokine expression, hypergammaglobulinemia, and limited autoantibody production. However, K/B×N mice do not develop detectable rheumatoid factor. The disease is 100% penetrant and, remarkably, can be rapidly transferred by serum to normal strains. This latter property is a powerful aspect of this model, as investigators have exploited the multitude of mutant and knockout strains to address the cellular and molecular requirements for disease development in the adoptive host. In this model, autoantibody to the ubiquitous intracellular enzyme glucose-6-phosphate isomerase (GPI) is responsible for the development of arthritis. Just how this occurs is still under investigation, but it is clear that GPI is present in synovial tissue and that immune complexes of GPI and autoantibody are deposited *in situ*. Neutrophils, the alternative complement pathway, IL-1 signaling, and FcRs are required for paw swelling in this model. In contrast, complement component 4 (C4) and the complement receptors 1 and 2 are not required, suggesting K/B×N serum-induced RA is independent of the classical complement pathway (49).

How does the TCR transgene lead to autoimmunity? The KRN TCR has dual specificity, so that it binds not only an RNase-derived peptide, but also a peptide from GPI in the context of $I\text{-}A^{g7}$ (50,51). GPI is recognized as an autoantigen by both T and B cells, both of which are required for disease. Presumably, endogenous self peptide serves as an autoantigen, generating a potent cellular and humoral response. It is noteworthy that, despite the wide expression of GPI, autoimmunity is limited to the joint, probably due to unique aspects of its physiology and lymphatic drainage (52).

Studies using cell lineage knockout mice have shown that both T and B cells are required for disease initiation in the K/B×N model (53), and B cells secreting pathogenic antibodies are required to maintain the disease state. Despite the key role of anti-GPI in this model, the consensus is that such antibodies are not important in RA pathogenesis (54). Yet the demonstration that autoantibodies to an intracellular protein can so readily be generated via cross-reactive T cells and cause such profound disease has important implications for RA pathogenesis and has revived thinking about immune complexes in RA.

Proteoglycan-Induced Arthritis

Similar to type II collagen, proteoglycans are major structural components of the extracellular matrix of articular cartilage. Proteoglycan (PG)-induced arthritis is generated by intraperitoneal injection of cartilage PGs (human fetal cartilage PG digested with chondroitinase-ABC) in complete Freund's adjuvant (CFA) into a susceptible strain of mice (BALB/c), followed by injections of PG in incomplete Freund's adjuvant (IFA) 1 and 4 weeks later (55). Clinical features of the disease develop in 100% of animals, and include joint swelling and erythema that appear 9 to 12 days after the third injection and become maximal by 7 to 8 weeks. Later, a progressive chronic polyarthritis develops, characterized by destruction of cartilage and bone, osteophyte formation, and ankylosis of joints. Along with peripheral inflammatory joint disease, these animals develop perivertebral inflammation with erosion of the intervertebral discs and ankylosis of the spine. This model differs from other models of arthritis in its prominent axial involvement (56). Proteoglycans aggrecan and versican are the principal antigens in this model and share significant B- and T-cell epitope homology. Both proteoglycans are present in the intervertebral disc and hyaline cartilage of the sacroiliac joint, as well as in entheses. Whereas aggrecan is most concentrated in the nucleus of the intervertebral disc and in articular cartilages and end plates, versican is generally absent from these tissues, except in the sacroiliac joint, but is concentrated in ligaments and the annulus. Immunity to aggrecan results in anterior chamber eye inflammation and sacroiliitis.

The development of inflammatory joint disease depends on the expression of cell-mediated and humoral immunity to the antigen used for immunization (fetal human or canine cartilage PG) and to mouse cartilage PG. The role of antigen-specific lymphocytes in the induction of arthritis has been established by the ability to transfer disease to naive recipients using sensitized B and T lymphocytes (57).

Pristane-Induced Arthritis

In susceptible mice, such as DBA/1 and BALB/c, destructive arthritis is induced by two intraperitoneal injections, 50 days apart, of pristane (2,6,10,4-tetramethylpentadecane).

Unlike other arthritis models, the onset of murine, pristane-induced arthritis is delayed, and progression of disease extends for 100 to 200 days. Histologically, the arthritis is characterized by polymorphonuclear cell infiltration, synoviocyte hyperplasia, cartilage erosion, and the formation of pannus (58). B-cell activation and proliferation is suggested by the development of hypergammaglobulinemia and the appearance of antibodies to multiple targets, including 65-kd heat shock protein (hsp65), IgG, collagen types I and II, histones, single-stranded DNA (ssDNA), and other lupus-related antigens (59). A lupuslike syndrome is inducible using a slightly different protocol.

$CD4^+$ T-cell effector mechanisms appear to be pathogenically more important than antibody-dependent mechanisms, particularly T-cell responses to hsp65 (60). Preimmunization of mice with mycobacterial hsp65, but not the mammalian homologue hsp58, prevents the disease, as in several other experimental arthritis models (61). Protected mice exhibit elevated immune responses to hsp65, and disease protection is associated with the production of T_H2 cytokines.

Antigen-Induced Arthritis

Chronic arthritis induced by intraarticular injection of antigen into previously immunized animals has been used to study the mechanisms responsible for the maintenance of chronic inflammation. Experimental antigen-induced arthritis has been produced by systemic immunization with antigen in CFA followed by intraarticular injection of the same antigen (62,63). Antigens, such as fibrin, ovalbumin, bovine serum albumin, ferritin, and horseradish peroxidase, have been used. Rats, mice, and rabbits are susceptible to antigen-induced arthritis. This model is particularly useful if a monoarticular inflammatory arthritis is desired.

A few hours after intraarticular injection of the antigen, severe, acute joint swelling and exudation develops. The swelling usually decreases over 2 weeks, and about one third of the animals show synovial thickening lasting for 8 to 24 weeks. Invasive pannus and cartilage erosions develop after 4 to 6 weeks. The acute synovitis represents an Arthus reaction dependent on high titers of precipitating IgG antibodies and is characterized by infiltration with large numbers of polymorphonuclear lymphocytes, hemorrhagic change, vascular thrombosis, and tissue necrosis. As the arthritis progresses, synovial infiltration by macrophages ensues. Massive hyperplasia of synovial stromal connective tissue cells and increased numbers of lymphocytes and plasma cells are additional features. The lymphocytes congregate in structures resembling the lymphoid follicles commonly noted in the synovia of patients with RA. Plasma cells in the inflamed synovial membranes synthesize immunoglobulins directed against the inducing antigen. Chronicity of antigen-induced arthritis is suspected to be due in part to retained antigen in the joint, acting as a stimulus for prolonged local antibody synthesis and providing a source of complement-fixing antigen–antibody complexes. In addition, cell-mediated immunity also appears to be an important mechanism. Animals with antigen-induced arthritis exhibit flare-ups when challenged with intravenous injection of very small amounts of antigen. These flare-ups are due to local hypersensitivity, which is dependent, in part, on T lymphocytes that are retained in the joint.

Streptococcal–Cell Wall Arthritis

A single intraperitoneal injection of an aqueous suspension of cell wall peptidoglycan-polysaccharide fragments from group A streptococci induces severe erosive arthritis (64). An acute, thymic-independent, complement-dependent phase develops within 24 hours, in association with the deposition of cell wall fragments in the peripheral joints. The acute arthritis is characterized by high levels of proinflammatory TNF-α, IL-1, and chemokine production, and intense leukocyte infiltration. Although this system has been widely used as a model of RA, rats develop significant axial disease and do not generate rheumatoid factor. It might also be regarded as a model of reactive arthritis, because it is provoked by bacterial products.

This primary acute arthritic phase is followed by a chronic, secondary, thymic-dependent phase, which begins about 14 days after injection and is characterized by a fluctuating course. In affected joints, this chronic phase is associated with intense macrophage and T-lymphocyte infiltration, synovial hyperplasia, marginal and subchondral bone erosion, and cartilage destruction. The production of high levels of proinflammatory cytokines, growth factors, metalloproteinases, cyclooxygenase-2, and nitric oxide is also characteristic (65). Transforming growth factor (TGF)-β_1 appears to serve to inhibit the progression of inflammation and joint destruction (66). The kallikrein-kinin system is important for inflammation in this model (67), and arthritis can be blocked by treatment of rats with bradykinin receptor antagonists (68).

Intraarticular injection of streptococcal cell walls (SCWs) followed by intravenous challenge (reactivation) also results in destructive, lymphocyte-dependent monoarticular arthritis in rats and mice. Anti-IL-4, but not anti-IL-10 or anti-IFN-γ, is effective in lowering joint swelling in the reactivation model of SCW-induced arthritic rats, suggesting that T_H2 effector mechanisms, to some extent, may be operative in the reactivation model of arthritis. Alternatively, IL-4 may play a role in the development of T_H1-related inflammation. As in the systemic model, TNF-α plays a major role in the development of joint swelling, whereas IL-1 is dominant in mediating cartilage destruction and inflammatory cell influx in mice. As in RA patients, the transcription factor nuclear factor κB (NFκB) is activated in the synovia of rats with reactivation SCW-induced arthritis (69). *In vivo* suppression of NFκB in the synovia of rats with SCW- and pristane-induced arthritis, by either proteasomal inhibitors or intraarticular adenoviral gene transfer of the superrepressor inhibitor of κBa (IκBa), profoundly enhances apoptosis. Activation of

NFκB protects synovial cells against apoptosis and thus provides a potential link between inflammation and synovial hyperplasia. Intraarticular administration of NFκB decoys not only prevents the recurrence of SCW arthritis in treated joints but, in addition, reduces the severity of arthritis in untreated joints (69).

Susceptibility to streptococcal cell wall arthritis varies substantially among inbred rat strains. Lewis (LEW) rats (Rt1l) are the most widely studied susceptible strain, whereas F344 rats (RT1lv1), and to a lesser extent Buffalo (BUF) rats (RT1b), are the most widely studied resistant strains. The wide variation in susceptibility among inbred strains suggests that two or more genes regulate disease susceptibility.

Adjuvant-Induced Arthritis

Adjuvant-induced arthritis develops clinically about 10 to 14 days after susceptible rats, such as DA or LEW, are injected intradermally at the base of the tail with CFA (heat-killed *Mycobacterium tuberculosis* in IFA). Induction of the autoimmune disease, however, is not limited to *M. tuberculosis* in IFA; other bacterial types can be used, although the arthritogenicity varies. The type of oil, the dose, and the route of injection are also variable. Several inbred rat strains, such as BUF, F344, and Wistar-Kyoto (WKY), are noted for their relative resistance to antigen-induced arthritis (70).

Clinically, the disease is characterized by swelling and progressive destruction of peripheral joints. Histologically, the joints show granulocyte infiltration in the joint space, synovial hyperplasia and pannus formation, and mononuclear cell infiltration. The disease progresses rapidly over several weeks in what appears to be a monophasic process with marginal and subchondral periarticular bone erosion, cartilage loss, and periosteal new bone formation. Although the joint pathology of rat antigen-induced arthritis has clinical and histologic similarities to human RA, the development of periostitis and bony ankylosis, and most of the extraarticular manifestations, are more reminiscent of reactive arthritis or the spondyloarthropathies.

The role of heat shock proteins has been the subject of extensive investigation in this disease (71). This interest derives from the observation that mycobacterial hsp65, particularly amino acids 180 to 188, is a major antigenic target of the pathogenic T cells that develop in LEW rats (72). Following adjuvant injection, both antibodies and T-cell responses to hsp65 and the 180 to 188 epitope are detected by day 14, but there is no relationship between anti-hsp65 antibody titers and disease severity. However, one can transfer disease to naive recipient LEW rats with the hsp65 reactive T cells.

Pretreatment of animals with hsp65 protects animals from the development of active disease (73). There appears to be a spreading of tolerance to other arthritogenic epitopes within the inflamed joint (74).

Infectious Agents and Arthritis

Mycoplasma-*Induced Arthritis*

Autoimmune disease, including arthritis, may be triggered by infectious agents. *Mycoplasma* species are gram-negative microorganisms lacking rigid cell walls and may play a role in the genesis of arthritis. Whether mycoplasmas induce or perpetuate inflammatory joint diseases such as RA remains unclear. Experimental models of *Mycoplasma*-induced arthritis exist, some using mycoplasmas known to cause disease in humans.

Mycoplasma arthritidis causes chronic proliferative arthritis in mice and severe septic arthritis in rats (75,76). In mice, susceptibility to *M. arthritidis*–induced arthritis is associated with particular MHC haplotypes. In contrast, in rats, non-MHC genes determine susceptibility. *M. arthritidis* produces a soluble superantigen (SAg) that has been shown to regulate cytokine responses and to activate T lymphocytes in certain mouse strains following *in vivo* administration (75). Studying *M. arthritidis*–induced disease may thus serve as a model to investigate potential roles of SAgs in arthritis.

*Lyme Arthritis (*Borrelia burgdorferi*–Associated Arthritis)*

Injection of live *Borrelia burgdorferi* spirochetes into LEW rats induces Lyme disease, with an acute exudative polyarthritis, tendonitis, and bursitis by day 30. Lyme arthritis in mice is also strain dependent, with many mouse strains resistant to Lyme arthritis. A strong immune response to *B. burgdorferi* infection protects against Lyme arthritis because disease can be induced in the immunocompromised SCID mouse. Studies with various inbred mouse strains suggest disease susceptibility correlates with a T_H1 response, whereas a T_H2 response is associated with resistance to disease, and T cells are directly responsible for mediating inflammatory lesions (77). However, recent studies have demonstrated that T_H1 cells are not absolutely required for disease development (78–80). Passive administration of the OspA outer surface protein of *B. burgdorferi* can protect against infection and subsequent Lyme arthritis, leading to the development of the Lyme vaccine (81). MHC haplotype does not appear important in disease susceptibility, but the presence of the adhesion molecule decorin is essential for infection, because the organism expresses decorin-binding proteins (82,83).

HLA-B27 Transgenic Animals: Models for the Spondyloarthropathies

HLA-B27 is a major histocompatibility complex class I allele strongly associated with susceptibility to spondyloarthropathies. The risk for developing disease linked to HLA-B27 is the highest observed for any of the MHC-associated inflammatory disorders.

HLA-B27 alleles are normally noncovalently bound to β_2-microglobulin (β_2m) and associate with β_2m-presenting peptides for recognition by cytotoxic T lymphocytes (CTLs). Transgenic animal models confirm a role for HLA-B27 in pathogenesis, although the mechanism of action remains unclear. One long-standing hypothesis has been that HLA-B27 is an allele with abnormal characteristics related to the same residues that determine its peptide specificity. Its binding specificity thus results in the presentation of arthritogenic peptides that become targets of autoreactive CTLs. However, as yet no arthritic peptides have been found.

HLA-B27 Transgenic Rats

Transgenic rats expressing multiple copies of human HLA-B27 spontaneously develop inflammatory disease involving the gastrointestinal tract, peripheral and vertebral joints, male genital tract, skin, nails, and heart (84). Interestingly, the level of expression of functional human class I MHC molecules on the surface of lymphocytes correlates with susceptibility to disease. Adoptive transfer studies have confirmed a role for T cells in disease pathogenesis (85), arguing against the classical arthritogenic peptide model of disease. An environmental trigger appears to be necessary because transgenic rats housed in germ-free environments have reduced inflammatory disease.

HLA-B27 Transgenic Mice

HLA-B27 transgenic mice deficient in β_2m (B27/β_2m$^{-/-}$) do not express the HLA-B27 transgene on the cell surface. These mice develop nail changes, hair loss, and swelling in paws, which leads to ankylosis (86), whereas HLA-B27 transgenic mice with wild-type β_2m remain healthy. Environmental triggers also appear necessary in this model, because transgenic mice housed in a specific pathogen-free environment are unaffected. B27β_2m$^{-/-}$ mice containing the class II MHC knockout gene Aβ° have no H2-A or H2-E molecules. These mice still develop spontaneous disease (86); thus, the class II MHC molecule does not play a major role in B27/β_2m$^{-/-}$ inflammation. Mice expressing a hybrid B27 molecule with the peptide binding domain $\alpha1\alpha2$ of B27 and the $\alpha3$ domain from a H2-K^d mouse spontaneously develop arthritis and nail disease (87), indicating that the HLA-B27 may be acting as an antigen-presenting molecule. Further support for this hypothesis lies in the observation that HLA-B27 can form aberrant disulfide-linked homodimers that appear to retain their functional conformation and are able to bind peptide (88).

Tumor Necrosis Factor-α Transgenic Mice

Proinflammatory cytokines play a major role in chronic inflammatory diseases such as RA (89). Cytokines appear to drive the proliferation of synovial cells *in vitro* (90,91). Transgenic mice carrying a human TNF (hTNF) gene, modified at the 3′ end for enhanced translational efficiency and stabilization of mRNA, constitutively express TNF-α in the thymus, lung, spleen, kidney, brain, liver, gut, and joint tissues (92). At 3 to 4 weeks of age, swelling of the ankles and impairment of movement is evident, as is hyperplasia of the synovial membrane and polymorphonuclear and lymphocytic inflammatory infiltrates of the synovial space. This pathology is inherited with a 100% frequency in transgenic progeny. Treatment of these arthritic mice with anti-hTNF antibody completely prevents development of disease (92), confirming the role of TNF in the pathogenesis of the arthritis. Additionally, treatment with the antiinflammatory cytokines IL-4, IL-10, or IL-13 administered by gene therapy can decrease mRNA levels of both endogenous and transgenic cytokines, although only IL-4 demonstrated a slight attenuation of arthritis development (93).

Human T-Cell Leukemia Virus Type 1 Transgenic Mice

Human T cell leukemia virus type 1 (HTLV-1) is a known causative agent of adult T-cell leukemia. HTLV-1 infections can also cause autoimmune phenomena, including Sjögren syndrome and arthritis in a minority of infected individuals (94). The virus encodes a transcription transactivator, Tax, in the *p*X region. Mice transgenic for the HTLV-I *env-p*X region spontaneously develop a chronic inflammatory polyarthropathy (95,96). As early as 4 weeks of age, arthritis develops in multiple joints, and by 3 months 60% of mice are affected. Histopathology is similar to human RA, with marked synovial and periarticular inflammation. Autoimmunity is also observed, with antibodies to IgG, type II collagen, and HSP. The incidence of arthritis differs greatly among different background strains, ranging from 64% in BALB/c (H-2^d) to 0% to 2% in C57BL/6 (H-2^b) mice (97). Studies of congenic mouse strains transgenic for the HTLV-1 transgene show that the H-2 locus is not a major determinant of disease, and some background genes specific to BALB/c mice contribute to disease prevalence.

Tax is a nuclear phosphoprotein that transactivates the transcription of HTLV-1 and a variety of cellular genes, including IL-2, IL-2Rβ chain, c-*fos,* and TGF-β. It promotes nuclear translocation of NFκB and precursor proteins. Transgenic mice expressing the *tax* gene develop an RA-like inflammatory arthropathy similar to HTLV-1 transgenic mice, suggesting that the *tax* gene itself is arthritogenic (98).

ANIMAL MODELS OF SYSTEMIC SCLEROSIS

Genetically-Transmitted Models of Systemic Sclerosis

Tight Skin Mouse Model

The tight skin 1 (tsk1) mouse model is a spontaneous, dominant-negative mutation resulting from a duplication in the fibrillin-1 gene (99), resulting in abnormal fibrillin-1 protein and autoantibodies to fibrillin-1. Homozygous mice die *in utero* 8 to 10 days after gestation. In contrast, in heterozygous mice, disease starts at 1 to 2 weeks of age with a thickening and tightness of skin that is firmly bound to subcutaneous and deep muscular tissues (100). By 8 months of age, animals develop antinuclear antibody (ANA) titers (101). Biochemical and molecular abnormalities, as well as cutaneous and visceral changes, including greatly distended lungs histologically resembling human emphysema with little fibrosis and cardiac enlargement, closely resemble systemic scleroderma (SS) patients (102). Fibrillin-1 is a structural glycoprotein of connective tissue microfibrils that are present throughout the body. Fibrillin-1 transgenic mice expressing the tsk-1 mutated fibrillin-1 gene develop permanent cutaneous hyperplasia and produce antitopoisomerase I and antifibrillin-1 antibodies (103). Antibodies to fibrillin-1 have been found in SS patients of various ethnic groups, including Japanese and Native Americans (104,105). Additionally, in a population of Native Americans with the highest prevalence of SS known, there exists a strong association between a chromosomal region containing the fibrillin-1 gene and disease (105). Despite these findings, it is still unclear whether a defect in the fibrillin-1 gene is responsible for the development of disease in patients with SS.

The tight skin 2 (tsk2) mutant appeared in offspring of a 101/H mouse after ethylnitrosurea administration (106, 107). Tsk2 is inherited as an autosomal-dominant trait. Homozygous embryos die *in utero.* At 2 to 3 weeks of age, heterozygous tsk2 mice develop increased collagen deposition in the skin, similar to tsk1 and human scleroderma (106, 107). In contrast to tsk1, where the cellular immune system does not appear to be involved in the development of disease, infiltration by mononuclear cells is found in the lower dermis of tsk2 mice (107).

Avian Scleroderma

University of California, Davis (UCD) 200/206 chickens develop a spontaneous inherited scleroderma-like disease beginning 1 to 2 weeks after hatching. Disease appears to be inherited as an autosomal-recessive trait, with incomplete penetrance (108). Unlike other scleroderma models, UCD chickens display all three of the key signs of disease: endothelial lesions, inflammation, and collagen accumulation. They develop vascular occlusion, severe perivascular lymphocyte infiltration of skin and viscera, fibrosis of skin and internal organs, ANAs, anticardiolipin antibodies, antiendothelial cell antibodies, rheumatoid factors, anti-CII antibodies, and distal polyarthritis (108). Disease is significantly more fulminant in chickens than humans, with a 40% mortality rate and a large percentage of older chickens developing glomerulonephritis (109). Despite these differences from human disease, studies comparing skin lesion biopsies of UCD 200/206 chickens and human SS patients have demonstrated that endothelial cells are the primary target of autoimmune attack (110). Endothelial cells are the first cells to undergo apoptosis in the skin of UCD 200/206 chickens, apparently induced by antiendothelial antibodies (110).

Induced Models of Systemic Sclerosis

Bleomycin-Induced Fibrosis

Bleomycin is a glycopeptide antibiotic isolated from *Streptomyces verticillus* that inhibits DNA metabolism and is used as an antineoplastic agent. Parenteral administration of bleomycin induces a scleroderma-like disease in mice (111,112). Bleomycin administration results in cutaneous fibrosis, mononuclear cell infiltration of lung parenchyma, and accumulation of fibroblasts, leading to the development of pulmonary fibrosis in mice (111,112). Myofibroblasts have characteristics of fibroblasts and smooth muscle cells. They appear during wound healing and in fibrotic processes such as scleroderma. Studies showing increased smooth muscle actin expression by fibroblast cells from bleomycin-treated animals suggest that these cells are transdifferentiated into myofibroblasts (113). Additionally, peripheral blood mononuclear cells from bleomycin-treated mice release soluble factors, which may induce increased fibroblast differentiation (114). Pulmonary fibrosis results, at least in part, from an imbalance between oxidants and antioxidants (115). Oxygen free radicals are important initiators of tissue damage (116). Bleomycin is thought to bind to DNA and Fe^{2+}, forming a complex that induces production of reactive oxygen species (ROS), such as superoxide and hydroxyl radicals (117,118). Superoxide dismutases (SOD) catalyze the dismutation of O_2^- to H_2O_2. Yamamoto et al. have shown SOD inhibition of bleomycin-induced dermal sclerosis in mice (114), supporting the role of ROS in sclerosis. These studies suggest that SOD may have a therapeutic effect in SS.

Transforming Growth Factor-β–Induced Fibrosis

TGF-β is a known chemoattractant for fibroblasts (119) and increases their *in vitro* production of collagen and fibronectin (120,121). TGF-β can modify the extracellular matrix (ECM) by regulating proteins such as plasminogen activator and procollagenase (122–124). Thus, continuous elevated TGF-β levels induce deposition of the ECM that may lead to fibrosis.

Subcutaneous injection of TGF-β in newborn mice causes granulation tissue formation with subsequent abundant transient fibrosis (125). Injection of TGF-β into adult mice causes less tissue reaction. The induction of fibrosis seen in this model is reversible and transient; however, injection of TGF-β in combination with basic fibroblast growth factor (bFGF) produces more pronounced fibrotic change and prolonged, irreversible disease. *In vitro* studies showing increased mRNA levels of connective tissue growth factor (CTGF) in fibroblasts indicate activation by TGF-β. Based on studies using a combination of TGF-β, CTGF, and bFGF, it appears that TGF-β induces or initiates skin fibrosis while bFGF or CTGF are required to maintain this process (125).

Sclerodermatous Graft-Versus-Host Disease

The murine sclerodermatous graft-versus-host disease (Scl GVH) model of scleroderma is a particularly good model for a subset of SS patients that develop a rapidly progressive early cutaneous scleroderma. In this model, recipient mice transplanted with bone marrow and spleen cells from mice differing only in minor histocompatibility loci develop lung fibrosis and skin thickening. Pathology in Scl GVH mice is associated with an initial cutaneous inflammation consisting of monocytes/macrophages and T cells. Although T cells are critical in the initiation of immune reactions in the skin, characterization of the murine Scl GVH model shows that the predominant cells infiltrating the lungs and skin during early time points of disease when skin thickening is first apparent are macrophages, similar to patients with early progressive scleroderma (126). These macrophages express markers of activation and antigen presentation (127). Additionally, there is increased TGF-β mRNA expression and up-regulation of collagen mRNA and protein synthesis, leading to subsequent skin thickening and lung fibrosis (128).

Antibodies to TGF-β_1 prevent the infiltration of mononuclear cells into the skin and subsequent skin thickening and fibrosis (129). This suggests that monocyte activation by T cells may be the initiating event in scleroderma and Scl GVH. These monocytes infiltrate the skin and produce TGF-β_1 (129), which then causes collagen up-regulation, leading to fibrosis. As inflammatory immune cells induce matrix synthesis in scleroderma skin lesions and chemokines are involved in migration and recruitment of inflammatory cells, it is of interest that up-regulation of TGF-β_1 and monocyte chemotactic protein-1, MIP-1α, and RANTES (regulated upon activation normal T cell expressed and secreted) chemokine mRNA are associated with early time points in murine Scl GVH (127). These studies suggest different possible points for treatment in early scleroderma, that is, chemokine production, T-cell and monocyte/macrophage activation and homing to skin, and direct inhibition of TGF-β_1.

ANIMAL MODELS OF SYSTEMIC LUPUS

Animal strains developing lupus have proved to be among the most durable and successful disease models. Lupus in a mouse is usually defined by SLE-like autoantibodies (anti-DNA, antihistone, and others), together with immune-mediated kidney disease. Mice do not generally develop many of the important clinical features of SLE (serositis, discoid lesions, or other skin diseases in general), frank arthritis, or overt central nervous system disease (this is difficult to evaluate in mice). Their disease is relentlessly progressive and does not show the waxing/waning course typical of SLE. Mouse SLE is also much more amenable to therapeutic intervention by dietary manipulation, drugs, or even starvation. Despite these important differences, mouse lupus models have become widely accepted.

Inducible Models of SLE

Chronic Graft-Versus-Host Disease

Chronic GVH disease induced by infusion of class II MHC–reactive T cells into normal mice leads to the rapid (within 3 weeks) induction of antinuclear and antierythrocyte autoantibodies, together with immune-mediated renal disease and hemolytic anemia. Expression of disease is dependent on the nature of the MHC barrier between graft and host (I-A vs. I-E), and antibody production requires cell/cell interactions between alloreactive (graft) T cells and host B cells (130,131). Anti-DNA transgenes expressed in the host can become activated during experimental disease, allowing studies of tolerance in defined B-cell populations (132,133). The appeal of GVH as a model of SLE is its induction in normal animals, particularly B6, and the availability of many congenic strains to allow testing of the effects of other genes and exploration of mechanisms of lupuslike autoimmunity.

Pristane-Induced Lupus

The intraperitoneal injection of the aliphatic hydrocarbon pristane is followed by a lupuslike autoimmune disease characterized by autoantibodies to DNA and diverse nuclear antigens and by progressive glomerulonephritis (134). The injected oil elicits a chronic peritonitis with intense macrophage activation and cytokine production, with a key role identified for IL-6 and IL-10. Although there is a genetic influence on the spectrum of autoantibodies elicited, all immunocompetent mouse strains tested are susceptible (135). $CD4^+$ T lymphocytes are required for development of the autoimmune disease.

Blys Transgenic Mice

Blys, also known as APRIL, THANK, and zTNF4, is a key regulator of B-cell differentiation. Mice overexpressing this molecule develop a lupuslike disease with accompanying hyperactivation of B cells (136). Because Blys has been implicated in human SLE, this model may be of clinical importance.

Drug-Induced Lupus

Inducing lupus with the drugs commonly observed to cause human drug-induced lupus is difficult. Administration of procainamide or its metabolites directly to mice results in little autoimmunity; the variable degree of ANA production seen occurs only after many months of treatment. Intrathymic injection of procainamide hydroxylamine, however, causes a lupuslike syndrome. The mechanism appears to be disruption of positive thymic selection, with failure to establish tolerance to low-affinity selecting self antigens (137,138). Another model of drug-induced lupus is the adoptive transfer into mice of 5-azacytidine or procainamide-treated CD4 T cells. These inhibitors of DNA methylation induce overexpression of lymphocyte function–associated antigen-1 and secretion of T_H2 cytokines, and may lead to lysis of syngeneic macrophages with subsequent self-immunization (139).

Autoimmunity Due to Heavy Metals

Exposure to mercury, gold, and other heavy metals leads to autoimmunity in several strains of mice (140). Autoantibodies to nucleolar antigens have been particularly well studied in mercury-induced autoimmunity, susceptibility to which shows a marked dependence on MHC haplotype (141). T lymphocytes are required for expression of disease, which can be adoptively transferred via T cells (142). Mice given sufficient amounts of mercury develop membranous glomerulonephritis, with deposition of antibody and complement.

Genetically Transmitted Models of SLE

NZB and NZB Hybrid Mice

NZB mice were bred for other purposes and were serendipitously found to develop spontaneous autoimmune hemolytic anemia, antibodies to T cells, and ssDNA, along with increased levels of IgM and a high incidence of B-cell lymphoma. Remarkably, the offspring of crosses to NZW and SWR mice develop a much more severe autoimmune disease with many features of systemic lupus, notably immune complex renal disease and antibodies to single- and double-stranded DNA (dsDNA). Females have more rapid and severe disease, apparently due to the influence of female hormones, because disease severity can be modified by hormonal manipulations. The genetic basis of lupus susceptibility in NZB/NZW mice has been intensively studied and is quite complex. NZB contributes at least two genes, one tentatively identified as Ifi 202, an interferon-inducible gene (143). NZW's contribution is the result of three gene complexes, termed Sle 1, 2, and 3. The Sle 1 locus is composed of several genes (SLe 1a, b, c, and d) with complex interactions, and regulated by additional suppressor genes (144). SLe 1 is believed to be responsible for breaching of B-cell tolerance, whereas SLe 2 and 3 cause amplification of this lesion, decreased apoptosis, and T-cell hyperproliferation. The epigenetic interactions between these loci provide an important framework to think about the interactions that must be occurring among the multiple genes for human SLE susceptibility.

NZB/NZW F1 mice have been used for innumerable drug studies, genetic experiments, and other experimental manipulations. The responsiveness of their renal disease to alkylating agents has led to the use of cyclophosphamide in humans (145), and the T-cell dependence of their disease has been important in leading to clinical trials of antibodies to T cells, CD40L, and CTLA4 in human disease (146–149).

MRL, MRL/lpr Mice, and Fas and Fas Ligand Deficiency

MRL mice inherit a complex genetic background, which is expressed as a mild progressive autoimmune disease, with antinuclear antibodies and modest renal disease. When a hypofunctional CD95 mutation (Fas) is present on the MRL genetic background, a fulminant autoimmune disease occurs, with progressive immune complex renal disease, vasculitis, and early death (150). Because CD95 is a principal receptor-mediating apoptosis, the accelerating effect of lpr on autoimmunity is believed to be mostly due to aberrant T- and B-cell tolerance, probably in the periphery rather than in the developing thymus or fetal liver (151). MRL/lpr mice spontaneously develop anti-ssDNA and anti-dsDNA antibodies, IgG rheumatoid factor, cryoglobulinemia, and antibodies to Sm (152). Concurrently, they show massive enlargement of lymph nodes and, to a lesser extent, of spleen, mostly due to vastly increased numbers of anergic T lymphocytes that lack both CD4 and CD8 yet express numerous activation markers and some B-cell surface antigens. When the lpr mutation is bred onto other genetic backgrounds, a variable degree of mild autoimmunity results. For example, in the widely studied B6/lpr mice (convenient to use because of the many mutations, congenic strains, and transgenes/knockouts on B6), antibodies to DNA and chromatin develop at about 4 months of age, with little overt pathology beyond the massive lymphoproliferation (153). Gld is a point mutation in Fas ligand; mice homozygous for this defect develop a disease nearly identical to that of lpr mice (154).

Although MRL/lpr mice are far from an ideal model of SLE (the Fas gene is normal in human SLE and there is modest and variable lymphoid hyperplasia), the serologic similarities to the human illness and the rapidity of onset of disease have attracted many investigators to use these mice for therapeutic studies. The extensive diffuse lymphoproliferation affects the salivary and lacrimal glands, leading some investigators to use these animals as models of Sjögren syndrome (155). A rare human disorder termed autoimmune lymphoproliferative syndrome (or Canale-Smith syndrome) is caused by defects in expression or signaling through Fas (156). Inheritance is usually codominant. These individuals develop massive lymphoproliferation similar to lpr mice, primarily due to the accumulation of $CD4^{-}CD8^{-}$ T cells. Some individuals have been reported to develop lupuslike autoimmunity, yet most individuals have autoimmunity to erythrocytes and platelets.

BXSB Mice

This unique model has generated a substantial literature, despite ignorance of the mechanism whereby a Y chromosome–encoded gene (Yaa) induces a lupuslike disease in male offspring of mice with a poorly understood genetic propensity to develop autoimmunity (157). In adoptive transfer experiments, it has been shown that expression of Yaa in B cells is critically important for autoimmunity. It is of interest that BXSB × NZW mice develop an apparent antiphospholipid syndrome with coronary thrombosis, together with the appearance of antibodies to β_2 glycoprotein I (158). A delay in development in marginal zone B lymphocytes in BXSB mice has recently been recognized (159).

Anti-DNA Transgenes and Autoimmunity

An important new tool in understanding B-cell tolerance in autoimmunity comes from imposition of transgenes encoding antinuclear antibodies. Several heavy-chain genes have been studied intensively, notably 2–12, which encodes anti-Sm binding antibodies when paired with most light chains (160), and 3H9, which binds DNA when paired with most κ chains and with all λ chains (161). Anti-DNA producing B cells can thus be tracked in transgenic animals using antibodies to λ1. In normal mice, autoantibody-producing B cells are deleted or inactivated, or their specificity is altered by receptor editing (162,163). The 3H9 model has recently been modified by site-directed insertion of the heavy chain, so that it is in its normal position within the Ig gene locus and subject to class switching and normal Ig gene regulation (164).

Lupuslike Autoimmunity Due to Impaired Apoptotic Clearance

It has been proposed that the exposure during apoptosis of nuclear antigens may lead to self-immunization and autoimmunity. Several mouse models in which clearance of apoptotic cells is impaired have lent support to this hypothesis. Coincident with demonstrable apoptotic debris in their kidneys, mice deficient in C1q develop progressive autoimmunity and renal disease, similar to humans with this deficiency (165). Serum amyloid protein (SAP) binds to chromatin and is important in the catabolism of this molecule. SAP knockout mice develop antichromatin and anti-DNA antibodies, apparently due to the persistence of immunogenic chromatin (166). In this regard, DNase I–deficient mice also develop anti-DNA autoimmunity, probably due to the abnormal persistence of DNA derived from senescent cells when animals are lacking this enzyme (165). Finally, mice deficient in the membrane tyrosine kinase mer develop a lupuslike autoimmune disease with antibodies to DNA, chromatin, and phospholipids (167). The autoimmunity in mer-deficient mice is at least partially due to their impaired clearance of apoptotic cells, because mer binds to a protein (GAS-6) that in turn binds to exposed phosphatidylserine residues on apoptotic cells. Mer is also a key regulator of the production of inflammatory cytokines by macrophages that have ingested particles; autoimmunity in mer knockout mice is also probably due to the proinflammatory cytokines elaborated by the macrophages that have engulfed apoptotic cells.

Lupus Disease Due to Enhanced T-Cell Activation

T cells are regarded as important in the generation of autoantibodies in spontaneous lupus models and in human SLE. A number of models of mouse SLE have been described in recent years in mice in which T-cell activation is increased through deletion of regulatory pathways, or through imposition of transgenes controlling T-cell activation. These are summarized in Table 29.1.

TABLE 29.1. *Systemic lupus erythematosus models from increased T-cell activation*

Gene Defect	Mechanism	Reference
$p21^{-/-}$	↓ cyclin dependent kinase	186
$Gadd45a^{-/-}$	↑ T-cell proliferation	187
$E2F2^{-/-}$	↑ T-cell proliferation	188
$IEX\text{-}1^{-/-}$	↓ T-cell apoptosis	189
$Cbl\text{-}b^{-/-}$	↑ TCR signal transduction	190
$G2A^{-/-}$	Hyperresponsive T cells	191
CD45 inhibitory $wedge^{-/-}$	↑ TCR signal transduction	192
IFN-γ tg on keratin promoter	↑ T-cell activation	193
CD40L tg in epidermis	↑ T-cell activation	194

IFN, interferon; TCR, T-cell receptor; tg, transgene.

MODELS OF SYSTEMIC VASCULITIS

Palmerston North Mice

These mice develop a lupuslike progressive autoimmune disease (168). Accompanying this syndrome is a vasculitis affecting veins and arteries with abundant perivascular inflammation. The cells responsible for this process are $CD4^+$ T cells (169).

Interleukin-1 Infusion and Interleukin-1 Receptor Antagonist Knockout Mice

The administration to mice of IL-1 has been reported to cause intravascular inflammation (170), and a syndrome of severe spontaneous vasculitis occurs in mice lacking IL-1Ra (171). These animals develop neutrophilic vasculitis with $CD4^+$ cell infiltration, most prominently at the branch points of large arteries. The development of attenuated disease in heterozygotes implies that IL-1Ra must be present in sufficient quantities in normal individuals to prevent vessel inflammation. These studies were performed with IL-1Ra deficiency bred onto an outbred MF1 genetic background. When IL-1Ra deficiency (achieved through a gene knockout from another group) is bred onto a BALB/c, but not a C57BL/6, background, vasculitis is not seen but severe inflammatory erosive arthritis develops, emphasizing again the role of background genes in modulating pathology (172).

MODELS OF SJÖGREN'S DISEASE

Thymectomy at 3 days of age leads to a Sjögren syndrome–like infiltration of salivary and lacrimal glands in the NFS mouse (173). The disease is dependent on T lymphocytes and involves autoimmunity to the cytoskeletal protein fodrin (174). Another model is the HTLV tax transgenic mouse (175), discussed earlier. In addition, MRL/lpr and NOD mice (176) have been used as a model of Sjögren's disease.

ANTIPHOSPHOLIPID SYNDROME

Spontaneous thromboses and antiphospholipid antibodies have been reported in the BXSB × NZW mouse, and fetal wastage associated with these autoantibodies has also been observed in MRL/lpr mice. Recently, investigators have used passive transfer of human antiphospholipid syndrome sera to pregnant normal mice to induce fetal demise (177). Using this model, a key role for the complement system has been deduced in this process (Fig. 29.4). The C3 convertase inhibitor complement receptor 1–related gene/protein y (Crry)-Ig blocks fetal loss and growth retardation in mice. As another assay of the biologic activity of antiphospholipid autoantibodies, investigators have used the acceleration by autoantibodies of *in vivo* clotting in the ligated rat vena cava and in other traumatic models in which clotting is promoted (178).

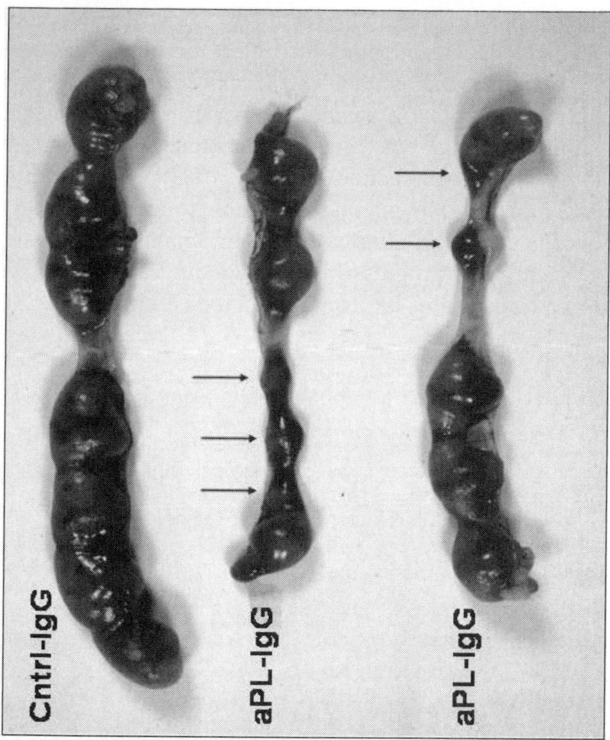

FIG. 29.4. Fetal resorption in mice treated with antiphospholipid antibodies. A uterus containing multiple normal mouse fetuses from a pregnant mouse given normal human immunoglobulin G (IgG) is shown on the left. To the right are uteri from two mice given IgG from a patient with antiphospholipid antibodies. Arrows indicate fetuses that have been resorbed. (Courtesy of Dr. Jane Salmon, Hospital for Special Surgery, New York.)

MODELS OF AUTOIMMUNE MYOSITIS

Several inducible models of polymyositis have been described (179). Infection with certain strains of coxsackie B virus leads to autoimmune muscle inflammation and progressive myopathy (180). T cells are required for muscle injury (181,182), as is active infection. Myositis can also be induced by immunizing SJL mice with rabbit myosin MB fraction, and disease can be ameliorated by administration of intravenous IgG (183).

Spontaneous muscle inflammation occurs in NOD mice overexpressing the β chain of IFN-γ, apparently through the effects of cytokine imbalance on NOD background genes (184). Conditional up-regulation in muscle of class I MHC genes has been reported to induce inflammatory myositis with antibodies to transfer RNA synthetases (185).

CONCLUSIONS

Animal models have been useful for many years in understanding basic inflammatory mechanisms and in designing treatments useful for humans. It is doubtful that many of the important developments in current antirheumatic therapy (e.g., TNF blockade and use of alkylating agents) could have been developed without widely accepted and well-characterized animal models. Molecular genetics has greatly increased the potential of models by permitting precise alteration or elimination of candidate genes in disease, by making possible dissection of illness due to multiple interacting genes, and by making it possible to assess the role of known genes on autoimmune and inflammatory processes. Continued rapid progress in understanding and treating inflammatory diseases is a certainty in the coming years.

REFERENCES

1. Kim, SH, Lechman ER, Kim S, et al. *Ex vivo* gene delivery of IL-1Ra and soluble TNF receptor confers a distal synergistic therapeutic effect in antigen-induced arthritis. *Mol Ther* 2002;6:591–600.
2. Crow JF. C. C. Little, cancer and inbred mice. *Genetics* 2002;161:1357–1361.
3. Jouvin-Marche E, Trede NS, Bandeira A, et al. Different large deletions of T cell receptor V beta genes in natural populations of mice. *Eur J Immunol* 1989;19:1921–1926.
4. Crawford K, Alper CA. Genetics of the complement system. *Rev Immunogenet* 2000;2:323–338.
5. Harman D. The aging process. *Proc Natl Acad Sci U S A* 1981;78:7124–7128.
6. Mazel JA, El-Sherif N, Buyon J, et al. Electrocardiographic abnormalities in a murine model injected with IgG from mothers of children with congenital heart block. *Circulation* 1999;99:1914–1918.
7. Green, EL, ed. *Biology of the laboratory mouse,* 2nd ed. New York: Mcgraw-Hill, 1966.
8. Waer, M, Van Damme B, Leenaerts P, et al. Treatment of murine lupus nephritis with cyclophosphamide or total lymphoid irradiation. *Kidney Int* 1988;34:678–682.
9. Israel EJ, Wilsker DF, Hayes KC, et al. Increased clearance of IgG in mice that lack beta 2-microglobulin: possible protective role of FcRn. *Immunology* 1996;89:573–578.
10. Miller JF. The thymus. Yesterday, today, and tomorrow. *Lancet* 1967;2:1299–1302.
11. O'Malley BW. Mechanisms of action of steroid hormones. *N Engl J Med* 1971;284:370–377.
12. Wakeland EK, Liu K, Graham RR, et al. Delineating the genetic basis of systemic lupus erythematosus. *Immunity* 2001;15:397–408.
13. Perkins AS. Functional genomics in the mouse. *Funct Integr Genomics* 2002;2:81 91.
14. Mitchell, DA, Pickering MC, Warren J, et al. C1q deficiency and autoimmunity: the effects of genetic background on disease expression. *J Immunol* 2002;168:2538–2543.
15. Miesel R, Dietrich A, Ulbrich N, et al. Assessment of collagen type II induced arthritis in mice by whole blood chemiluminescence. *Autoimmunity* 1994;19:153–159.
16. Bliven ML, Wooley PH, Pepys MB, et al. Murine type II collagen arthritis. Association of an acute-phase response with clinical course. *Arthritis Rheum* 1986;29:1131–1138.
17. Animal models for autoimmune and inflammatory disease. In: JC Coligan, ed. *Current protocols in immunology.* New York: John Wiley & Sons, 2003: Units 15.14, 15.15, 15.10, 15.20.
18. Vallet, V, Cherpillod J, Waridel F, et al. Fate and functions of human adult lymphoid cells in immunodeficient mice. *Histol Histopathol* 2003;18:309–322.
19. Ashany D, Hines J, Gharavi A, et al. Analysis of autoantibody production in SCID-systemic lupus erythematosus (SLE) chimeras. *Clin Exp Immunol* 1992;88:84–90.
20. Kraling BM, Juhasz I, Freundlich B, et al. Transplantation of systemic sclerosis (SSc) skin grafts into severe combined immunodeficient mice: increased presence of SSc leukocytes in SSc skin grafts and autoantibody production following autologous leukocyte transfer. *Pathobiology* 1996;64:99–114.
21. Rendt KE, Barry TS, Jones DM, et al. Engraftment of human synovium into severe combined immune deficient mice. Migration of human peripheral blood T cells to engrafted human synovium and to mouse lymph nodes. *J Immunol* 1993;151:7324–7336.
22. Brack A, Rittner HL, Younge BR, et al. Glucocorticoid-mediated repression of cytokine gene transcription in human arteritis-SCID chimeras. *J Clin Invest* 1997;99:2842–2850.
23. Luross JA, Williams NA. The genetic and immunopathological processes underlying collagen-induced arthritis. *Immunology* 2001;103:407–416.
24. Kraetsch HG, Unger C, Wernhoff P, et al. Cartilage-specific autoimmunity in rheumatoid arthritis: characterization of a triple helical B cell epitope in the integrin-binding-domain of collagen type II. *Eur J Immunol* 2001;31:1666–1673.
25. Stuart JM, Townes AS, Kang AH. Collagen autoimmune arthritis. *Annu Rev Immunol* 1984;2:199–218.
26. Malfait AM, Williams RO, Malik AS, et al. Chronic relapsing homologous collagen-induced arthritis in DBA/1 mice as a model for testing disease-modifying and remission-inducing therapies. *Arthritis Rheum* 2001;44:1215–1224.
27. Myers LK, Rosloniec EF, Cremer MA, et al. Collagen-induced arthritis, an animal model of autoimmunity. *Life Sci* 1997;61:1861–1878.
28. Plows D, Kontogeorgos G, Kollias G. Mice lacking mature T and B lymphocytes develop arthritic lesions after immunization with type II collagen. *J Immunol* 1999;162:1018–1023.
29. Wang Y, Kristan J, Hao L, et al. A role for complement in antibody-mediated inflammation: C5-deficient DBA/1 mice are resistant to collagen-induced arthritis. *J Immunol* 2000;164:4340–4347.
30. Hietala MA, Jonsson IM, Tarkowski A, et al. Complement deficiency ameliorates collagen-induced arthritis in mice. *J Immunol* 2002;169:454–459.
31. Shiozawa S, Shimizu K, Tanaka K, et al. Studies on the contribution of c-fos/AP-1 to arthritic joint destruction. *J Clin Invest* 1997;99:1210–1216.
32. Zhang HD, Yang YP, Horton JL, et al. Amelioration of collagen-induced arthritis by CD95 (APO-1/FAS)-ligand gene transfer. *J Clin Invest* 1997;100:1951–1957.
33. Griffiths, RJ, Smith MA, Roach ML, et al. Collagen-induced arthritis is reduced in 5-lipoxygenase-activating protein-deficient mice. *J Exp Med* 1997;185:1123–1129.
34. Saijo S, Asano M, Horai R, et al. Suppression of autoimmune arthritis in interleukin-1-deficient mice in which T cell activation is impaired due to low levels of CD40 ligand and OX40 expression on T cells. *Arthritis Rheum* 2002;46:533–544.
35. Joosten LA, Helsen MM, van de Loo FA, et al. Anticytokine treatment of established type II collagen-induced arthritis in DBA/1 mice. A comparative study using anti-TNF alpha, anti-IL-1 alpha/beta, and IL-1Ra. *Arthritis Rheum* 1996;39:797–809.
36. Ruchatz H, Leung BP, Wei XQ, et al. Soluble IL-15 receptor alpha-chain administration prevents murine collagen-induced arthritis: a role for IL-15 in development of antigen-induced immunopathology. *J Immunol* 1998;160:5654–5660.
37. Joosten LA, Lubberts E, Helsen MM, et al. Protection against cartilage and bone destruction by systemic interleukin-4 treatment in established murine type II collagen-induced arthritis. *Arthritis Res* 1999;1:81–91.
38. Campbell, IK, Bendele A, Smith DA, et al. Granulocyte-macrophage colony stimulating factor exacerbates collagen induced arthritis in mice. *Ann Rheum Dis* 1997;56:364–368.
39. Thornton, S, Boivin GP, Kim KN, et al. Heterogeneous effects of IL-2 on collagen-induced arthritis. *J Immunol* 2000;165:1557–1563.
40. Vermeire K, Heremans H, Vandeputte M, et al. Accelerated collagen-induced arthritis in IFN-gamma receptor-deficient mice. *J Immunol* 1997;158:5507–5513.
41. Matthys P, Vermeire K, Mitera T, et al. Anti-IL-12 antibody prevents the development and progression of collagen-induced arthritis in IFN-gamma receptor-deficient mice. *Eur J Immunol* 1998;28:2143–2151.
42. Kageyama Y, Koide Y, Yoshida A, et al. Reduced susceptibility to collagen-induced arthritis in mice deficient in IFN-gamma receptor. *J Immunol* 1998;161:1542–1548.
43. Yang HT, Jirholt J, Svensson L, et al. Identification of genes controlling collagen-induced arthritis in mice: striking homology with susceptibility loci previously identified in the rat. *J Immunol* 1999;163:2916–2921.
44. Taneja V, David CS. HLA class II transgenic mice as models of human diseases. *Immunol Rev* 1999;169:67–79.

45. Taneja V, Taneja N, Paisansinsup T, et al. CD4 and CD8 T cells in susceptibility/protection to collagen-induced arthritis in HLA-DQ8-transgenic mice: implications for rheumatoid arthritis. *J Immunol* 2002;168:5867–5875.
46. Wilder RL. Hormones and autoimmunity: animal models of arthritis. *Baillieres Clin Rheumatol* 1996;10:259–271.
47. Bradley DS, Das P, Griffiths MM, et al. HLA-DQ6/8 double transgenic mice develop auricular chondritis following type II collagen immunization: a model for human relapsing polychondritis. *J Immunol* 1998;161:5046–5053.
48. Kouskoff V, Korganow AS, Duchatelle V, et al. Organ-specific disease provoked by systemic autoimmunity. *Cell* 1996;87:811–822.
49. Solomon S, Kolb C, Mohanty S, et al. Transmission of antibody-induced arthritis is independent of complement component 4 (C4) and the complement receptors 1 and 2 (CD21/35). *Eur J Immunol* 2002; 32:644–651.
50. Basu, D, Horvath S, Matsumoto I, et al. Molecular basis for recognition of an arthritic peptide and a foreign epitope on distinct MHC molecules by a single TCR. *J Immunol* 2000;164:5788–5796.
51. Matsumoto, I, Staub A, Benoist C, et al. Arthritis provoked by linked T and B cell recognition of a glycolytic enzyme. *Science* 1999;286: 1732–1735.
52. Mandik-Nayak L, Wipke BT, Shih FF, et al. Despite ubiquitous autoantigen expression, arthritogenic autoantibody response initiates in the local lymph node. *Proc Natl Acad Sci U S A* 2002;99:14368–14373.
53. Korganow AS, Ji H, Mangialaio S, et al. From systemic T cell self-reactivity to organ-specific autoimmune disease via immunoglobulins. *Immunity* 1999;10:451–461.
54. Matsumoto I, Lee DM, Goldbach-Mansky R, et al. Low prevalence of antibodies to glucose-6-phosphate isomerase in patients with rheumatoid arthritis and a spectrum of other chronic autoimmune disorders. *Arthritis Rheum* 2003;48:944–954.
55. Glant TT, Mikecz K, Arzoumanian A, et al. Proteoglycan-induced arthritis in BALB/c mice. Clinical features and histopathology. *Arthritis Rheum* 1987;30:201–212.
56. Zhang Y, Shi S, Ciurli C, et al. Animal models of ankylosing spondylitis. *Curr Rheumatol Rep* 2002;4:507–512.
57. Mikecz K, Glant TT, Buzas E, et al. Proteoglycan-induced polyarthritis and spondylitis adoptively transferred to naive (nonimmunized) BALB/c mice. *Arthritis Rheum* 1990;33:866–876.
58. Hopkins SJ, Freemont AJ, Jayson MI. Pristane-induced arthritis in Balb/c mice. I. Clinical and histological features of the arthropathy. *Rheumatol Int* 1984;5:21–28.
59. Barker RN, Easterfield AJ, Allen RF, et al. B- and T-cell autoantigens in pristane-induced arthritis. *Immunology* 1996;89:189–194.
60. Levitt, NG, Fernandez-Madrid F, Wooley PH. Pristane induced arthritis in mice. IV. Immunotherapy with monoclonal antibodies directed against lymphocyte subsets. *J Rheumatol* 1992;19:1342–1347.
61. Thompson SJ, Francis JN, Siew LK, et al. An immunodominant epitope from mycobacterial 65-kDa heat shock protein protects against pristane-induced arthritis. *J Immunol* 1998;160:4628–4634.
62. Magilavy DB. Animal models of chronic inflammatory arthritis. *Clin Orthop* 1990;259:38–45.
63. Wooley PH. Animal models of rheumatoid arthritis. *Curr Opin Rheumatol* 1991;3:407–420.
64. Cromartie WJ, Craddock JG, Schwab JH, et al. Arthritis in rats after systemic injection of streptococcal cells or cell walls. *J Exp Med* 1977;146:1585–1602.
65. Houri JM, O'Sullivan FX. Animal models in rheumatoid arthritis. *Curr Opin Rheumatol* 1995;7:201–205.
66. Brandes ME, Allen JB, Ogawa Y, et al. Transforming growth factor beta 1 suppresses acute and chronic arthritis in experimental animals. *J Clin Invest* 1991;87:1108–1113.
67. Blais C Jr, Couture R, Drapeau G, et al. Involvement of endogenous kinins in the pathogenesis of peptidoglycan-induced arthritis in the Lewis rat. *Arthritis Rheum* 1997;40:1327–1333.
68. Uknis AB, DeLa Cadena RA, Janardham R, et al. Bradykinin receptor antagonists type 2 attenuate the inflammatory changes in peptidoglycan-induced acute arthritis in the Lewis rat. *Inflamm Res* 2001;50:149–155.
69. Miagkov AV, Kovalenko DV, Brown CE, et al. NF-kappaB activation provides the potential link between inflammation and hyperplasia in the arthritic joint. *Proc Natl Acad Sci U S A* 1998;95:13859–13864.
70. Waksman BH. Immune regulation in adjuvant disease and other arthritis models: relevance to pathogenesis of chronic arthritis. *Scand J Immunol* 2002;56:12–34.
71. Brahn E. Animal models of rheumatoid arthritis. Clues to etiology and treatment. *Clin Orthop* 1991;253:42–53.
72. van Eden, W, Thole JER, van der Zee R, et al. Cloning of the mycobacterial epitope recognized by T lymphocytes in adjuvant arthritis. *Nature* 1988;331:171–173.
73. Wendling U, Paul L, van der Zee R, et al. A conserved mycobacterial heat shock protein (hsp) 70 sequence prevents adjuvant arthritis upon nasal administration and induces IL-10-producing T cells that cross-react with the mammalian self-hsp70 homologue. *J Immunol* 2000; 164:2711–2717.
74. van Eden W, van der Zee R, Taams LS, et al. Heat-shock protein T-cell epitopes trigger a spreading regulatory control in a diversified arthritogenic T-cell response. *Immunol Rev* 1998;164:169–174.
75. Cole BC, Ward JR, Jones RS, et al. Chronic proliferative arthritis of mice induced by *Mycoplasma arthritidis*. I. Induction of disease and histopathological characteristics. *Infect Immun* 1971;4:344–355.
76. Washburn LR, Ramsay JR. Experimental induction of arthritis in LEW rats and antibody response to four *Mycoplasma arthritidis* strains. *Vet Microbiol* 1989;21:41–55.
77. McKisic MD, Redmond WL, Barthold SW. Cutting edge: T cell-mediated pathology in murine Lyme borreliosis. *J Immunol* 2000;164: 6096–6099.
78. Brown CR, Reiner SL. Experimental lyme arthritis in the absence of interleukin-4 or gamma interferon. *Infect Immun* 1999;67:3329–3333.
79. Potter MR, Noben-Trauth N, Weis JH, et al. Interleukin-4 (IL-4) and IL-13 signaling pathways do not regulate *Borrelia burgdorferi*–induced arthritis in mice: IgG1 is not required for host control of tissue spirochetes. *Infect Immun* 2000;68:5603–5609.
80. Glickstein L, Edelstein M, Dong JZ. Gamma interferon is not required for arthritis resistance in the murine Lyme disease model. *Infect Immun* 2001;69:3737–3743.
81. Fikrig E, Barthold SW, Kantor FS, et al. Protection of mice against the Lyme disease agent by immunizing with recombinant OspA. *Science* 1990;250:553–556.
82. Brown CR, Reiner SL. Genes outside the major histocompatibility complex control resistance and susceptibility to experimental Lyme arthritis. *Med Microbiol Immunol (Berl)* 2000;189:85–90.
83. Brown EL, Wooten RM, Johnson BJ, et al. Resistance to Lyme disease in decorin-deficient mice. *J Clin Invest* 2001;107:845–852.
84. Hammer RE, Maika SD, Richardson JA, et al. Spontaneous inflammatory disease in transgenic rats expressing HLA-B27 and human beta 2m: an animal model of HLA-B27-associated human disorders. *Cell* 1990;63:1099–1112.
85. Breban M, Fernandez-Sueiro JL, Richardson JA, et al. T cells, but not thymic exposure to HLA-B27, are required for the inflammatory disease of HLA-B27 transgenic rats. *J Immunol* 1996;156:794–803.
86. Khare, SD, Luthra HS, David CS. Spontaneous inflammatory arthritis in HLA-B27 transgenic mice lacking beta 2-microglobulin: a model of human spondyloarthropathies. *J Exp Med* 1995;182:1153–1158.
87. Khare SD, Lee S, Bull MJ, et al. Peptide binding alpha1alpha2 domain of HLA-B27 contributes to the disease pathogenesis in transgenic mice. *Hum Immunol* 1999;60:116–126.
88. Allen RL, O'Callaghan CA, McMichael AJ, et al. Cutting edge: HLA-B27 can form a novel beta 2-microglobulin-free heavy chain homodimer structure. *J Immunol* 1999;162:5045–5048.
89. Arend WP, Dayer JM. Inhibition of the production and effects of interleukin-1 and tumor necrosis factor alpha in rheumatoid arthritis. *Arthritis Rheum* 1995;38:151–160.
90. Butler DM, Piccoli DS, Hart PH, et al. Stimulation of human synovial fibroblast DNA synthesis by recombinant human cytokines. *J Rheumatol* 1988;15:1463–1470.
91. Gitter BD, Labus JM, Lees SL, et al. Characteristics of human synovial fibroblast activation by IL-1 beta and TNF alpha. *Immunology* 1989;66:196–200.
92. Keffer J, Probert L, Cazlaris H, et al. Transgenic mice expressing human tumour necrosis factor: a predictive genetic model of arthritis. *EMBO J* 1991;10:4025–4031.
93. Bessis N, Chiocchia G, Kollias G, et al. Modulation of proinflammatory cytokine production in tumour necrosis factor-alpha (TNF-alpha)-transgenic mice by treatment with cells engineered to secrete IL-4, IL-10 or IL-13. *Clin Exp Immunol* 1998;111:391–396.

94. Uchiyama T. Human T cell leukemia virus type I (HTLV-I) and human diseases. *Annu Rev Immunol* 1997;15:15–37.
95. Nerenberg MI. An HTLV-I transgenic mouse model: role of the tax gene in pathogenesis in multiple organ systems. *Curr Top Microbiol Immunol* 1990;160:121–128.
96. Iwakura Y, Tosu M, Yoshida E, et al. Induction of inflammatory arthropathy resembling rheumatoid arthritis in mice transgenic for HTLV-I. *Science* 1991;253:1026–1028.
97. Iwakura Y, Saijo S, Kioka Y, et al. Autoimmunity induction by human T cell leukemia virus type 1 in transgenic mice that develop chronic inflammatory arthropathy resembling rheumatoid arthritis in humans. *J Immunol* 1995;155:1588–1598.
98. Habu K, Nakayama-Yamada J, Asano M, et al. The human T cell leukemia virus type I-tax gene is responsible for the development of both inflammatory polyarthropathy resembling rheumatoid arthritis and noninflammatory ankylotic arthropathy in transgenic mice. *J Immunol* 1999;162:2956–2963.
99. Siracusa LD, McGrath R, Ma Q, et al. A tandem duplication within the fibrillin 1 gene is associated with the mouse tight skin mutation. *Genome Res* 1996;6:300–313.
100. Green MD, Sweet HO, Bunker LE. Tight-skin, a new mutation of the mouse causing excessive growth of connective tissue and skeleton. *Am J Pathol* 1976;892:493–512.
101. Tsuji-Yamada J, Nakazawa M, Takahashi K, et al. Effect of IL-12 encoding plasmid administration on tight-skin mouse. *Biochem Biophys Res Commun* 2001;280:707–712.
102. Jimenez SA, Millan A, Bashey RI. Scleroderma-like alterations in collagen metabolism occurring in the TSK (tight skin) mouse. *Arthritis Rheum* 1984;27:180–185.
103. Saito S, Nishimura H, Phelps RG, et al. Induction of skin fibrosis in mice expressing a mutated fibrillin-1 gene. *Mol Med* 2000;6:825–836.
104. Arnett FC, Bias WB, Reveille JD. Genetic studies in Sjögren's syndrome and systemic lupus erythematosus. *J Autoimmun* 1989;2:403–413.
105. Tan FK, Arnett FC, Antohi S, et al. Autoantibodies to the extracellular matrix microfibrillar protein, fibrillin-1, in patients with scleroderma and other connective tissue diseases. *J Immunol* 1999;163: 1066–1072.
106. Peters J, Ball ST. Tight skin-2 (Tsk-2). *Mouse News Lett* 1986;74: 91–92.
107. Christner PJ, Peters J, Hawkins D, et al. The tight skin 2 mouse. An animal model of scleroderma displaying cutaneous fibrosis and mononuclear cell infiltration. *Arthritis Rheum* 1995;38:1791–1798.
108. Gershwin ME, Abplanalp H, Castles JJ, et al. Characterization of a spontaneous disease of white leghorn chickens resembling progressive systemic sclerosis. *J Exp Med* 1981;153:1640–1659.
109. Gershwin ME, Abplanalp H, Castles JJ, et al. Characterization of a spontaneous disease of white leghorn chickens resembling progressive systemic sclerosis (scleroderma). *J Exp Med* 1981;153:1640–1659.
110. Sgonc R, Gruschwitz MS, Dietrich H, et al. Endothelial cell apoptosis is a primary pathogenetic event underlying skin lesions in avian and human scleroderma. *J Clin Invest* 1996;98:785–792.
111. Ichihashi M, Shinkai H, Takei M, et al. Analysis of the mechanism of bleomycin-induced cutaneous fibrosis in mice. *J Antibiot (Tokyo)* 1973;26:238–242.
112. Adamson IY, Bowden DH. The pathogenesis of bleomycin-induced pulmonary fibrosis in mice. *Am J Pathol* 1974;77:185–197.
113. Yamamoto T, Katayama I, Nishioka K. Fibroblast proliferation by bleomycin stimulated peripheral blood mononuclear cell factors. *J Rheumatol* 1999;26:609–615.
114. Yamamoto, T, Takagawa S, Katayama I, et al. Effect of superoxide dismutase on bleomycin-induced dermal sclerosis: implications for the treatment of systemic sclerosis. *J Invest Dermatol* 1999;113:843–847.
115. Strausz, J, Muller-Quernheim J, Steppling H, et al. Oxygen radical production by alveolar inflammatory cells in idiopathic pulmonary fibrosis. *Am Rev Respir Dis* 1990;141:124–128.
116. McCord JM. Oxygen-derived free radicals in postischemic tissue injury. *N Engl J Med* 1985;312:159–163.
117. Hay, J, Shahzeidi S, Laurent G. Mechanisms of bleomycin-induced lung damage. *Arch Toxicol* 1991;65:81–94.
118. Sugiura Y. Production of free radicals from phenol and tocopherol by bleomycin-iron(II) complex. *Biochem Biophys Res Commun* 1979; 87:649–653.
119. Postlethwaite AE, Keski-Oja J, Moses HL, et al. Stimulation of the chemotactic migration of human fibroblasts by transforming growth factor beta. *J Exp Med* 1987;165:251–256.
120. Raghow R, Postlethwaite AE, Keski-Oja J, et al. Transforming growth factor-beta increases steady state levels of type I procollagen and fibronectin messenger RNAs posttranscriptionally in cultured human dermal fibroblasts. *J Clin Invest* 1987;79:1285–1288.
121. Varga J, Rosenbloom J, Jimenez SA. Transforming growth factor beta (TGF beta) causes a persistent increase in steady-state amounts of type I and type III collagen and fibronectin mRNAs in normal human dermal fibroblasts. *Biochem J* 1987;247:597–604.
122. Laiho M, Saksela O, Keski-Oja J. Transforming growth factor-beta induction of type-1 plasminogen activator inhibitor. Pericellular deposition and sensitivity to exogenous urokinase. *J Biol Chem* 1987; 262:17467–17474.
123. Laiho M, Saksela O, Andreasen PA, et al. Enhanced production and extracellular deposition of the endothelial-type plasminogen activator inhibitor in cultured human lung fibroblasts by transforming growth factor-beta. *J Cell Biol* 1986;103:2403–2410.
124. Edwards DR, Murphy G, Reynolds JJ, et al. Transforming growth factor beta modulates the expression of collagenase and metalloproteinase inhibitor. *EMBO J* 1987;6:1899–1904.
125. Shinozaki M, Kawara S, Hayashi N, et al. Induction of subcutaneous tissue fibrosis in newborn mice by transforming growth factor beta-simultaneous application with basic fibroblast growth factor causes persistent fibrosis. *Biochem Biophys Res Commun* 1997;237:292–296.
126. Kraling BM, Maul GG, Jimenez SA. Mononuclear cellular infiltrates in clinically involved skin from patients with systemic sclerosis of recent onset predominantly consist of monocytes/macrophages. *Pathobiology* 1995;63:48–56.
127. Zhang Y, McCormick LL, Desai SR, et al. Murine sclerodermatous graft-versus-host disease, a model for human scleroderma: cutaneous cytokines, chemokines, and immune cell activation. *J Immunol* 2002; 168:3088–3098.
128. Jaffee BD, Claman HN. Chronic graft-versus-host disease (GVHD) as a model for scleroderma. I. Description of model systems. *Cell Immunol* 1983;77:1–12.
129. McCormick LL, Zhang Y, Tootell E, et al. Anti-TGF-beta treatment prevents skin and lung fibrosis in murine sclerodermatous graft-versus-host disease: a model for human scleroderma. *J Immunol* 1999;163:5693–5699.
130. Bradley DS, Jennette JC, Cohen PL, et al. Chronic graft versus host disease-associated autoimmune manifestations are independently regulated by different MHC class II loci. *J Immunol* 1994;152:1960–1969.
131. Morris SC, Cheek RL, Cohen PL, et al. Allotype-specific immunoregulation of autoantibody production by host B cells in chronic graft-versus host disease. *J Immunol* 1990;144:916–922.
132. Sekiguchi DR, Eisenberg RA, Weigert M. Secondary heavy chain rearrangement: a mechanism for generating anti-double-stranded DNA B cells. *J Exp Med* 2003;197:27–39.
133. Van Rappard-Van der Veen FM, Kiesel U, Poels L, et al. Further evidence against random polyclonal antibody formation in mice with lupus-like graft-vs-host disease. *J Immunol* 1984;132:1814–1820.
134. Satoh M, Kumar A, Kanwar YS, et al. Anti-nuclear antibody production and immune-complex glomerulonephritis in BALB/c mice treated with pristane. *Proc Natl Acad Sci U S A* 1995;92:10934–10938.
135. Satoh, M, Richards HB, Shaheen VM, et al. Widespread susceptibility among inbred mouse strains to the induction of lupus autoantibodies by pristane. *Clin Exp Immunol* 2000;121:399–405.
136. Dorner T, Putterman C. B cells, BAFF/zTNF4, TACI, and systemic lupus erythematosus. *Arthritis Res* 2001;3:197–199.
137. Rubin RL, Kretz-Rommel A. A nondeletional mechanism for central T-cell tolerance. *Crit Rev Immunol* 2001;21:29–40.
138. Kretz-Rommel A, Rubin RL. Disruption of positive selection of thymocytes causes autoimmunity. *Nat Med* 2000;6:298–305.

139. Yung RL, Quddus J, Chrisp CE, et al. Mechanism of drug-induced lupus. I. Cloned Th2 cells modified with DNA methylation inhibitors *in vitro* cause autoimmunity *in vivo*. *J Immunol* 1995;154:3025–3035.
140. Bagenstose LM, Salgame P, Monestier M. Murine mercury-induced autoimmunity: a model of chemically related autoimmunity in humans. *Immunol Res* 1999;20:67–78.
141. Hultman P, Enestrom S, Pollard KM, et al. Anti-fibrillarin autoantibodies in mercury-treated mice. *Clin Exp Immunol* 1989;78:470–477.
142. Pelletier L, Pasquier R, Rossert J, et al. Autoreactive T cells in mercury-induced autoimmunity. *J Immunol* 1988;140:750–754.
143. Rozzo SJ, Allard JD, Choubey D, et al. Evidence for an interferon-inducible gene, Ifi202, in the susceptibility to systemic lupus. *Immunity* 2001;15:435–443.
144. Morel L, Blenman KR, Croker BP, et al. The major murine systemic lupus erythematosus susceptibility locus, Sle1, is a cluster of functionally related genes. *Proc Natl Acad Sci U S A* 2001;98:1787–1792.
145. Steinberg AD, Krieg AM, Gourley MF, et al. Theoreticcal and experimental approaches to generalized autoimmunity. *Immunol Rev* 1990;118:129–163.
146. Wofsy D. The role of Lyt-2+ T cells in the regulation of autoimmunity in murine lupus. *J Autoimmun* 1988;1:207–217.
147. Connolly K, Roubinian JR, Wofsy D. Development of murine lupus in CD4-depleted NZB/NZW mice: sustained inhibition of residual CD4+ T cells is required to suppress autoimmunity. *J Immunol* 1992;149:3083–3088.
148. Daikh DI, Wofsy D. Cutting edge: reversal of murine lupus nephritis with CTLA4Ig and cyclophosphamide. *J Immunol* 2001;166:2913–2916.
149. Kalled SL, Cutler AH, Datta SK, et al. Anti-CD40 ligand antibody treatment of SNF1 mice with established nephritis: preservation of kidney function. *J Immunol* 1998;160:2158–2165.
150. Cohen PL, Eisenberg RA. Lpr and gld: single gene models of systemic autoimmunity and lymphoproliferative disease. *Annu Rev Immunol* 1991;9:243–269.
151. Singer GG, Abbas AK. The Fas antigen is involved in peripheral but not thymic deletion of T lymphocytes in T cell receptor transgenic mice. *Immunity* 1994;1:365–371.
152. Theofilopoulos AN, McConahey PJ, Izui S, et al. A comparative immunologic analysis of several murine strains with autoimmune manifestations. *Clin Immunol Immunopathol* 1980;15:258–278.
153. Izui S, Kelley VE, Masuda K, et al. Induction of various autoantibodies by mutant gene lpr in several strains of mice. *J Immunol* 1984;133:227–233.
154. Lynch DH, Watson JL, Alderson MR, et al. The mouse Fas-ligand gene is mutated in gld mice and is part of a TNF family gene cluster. *Immunity* 1994;1:131–136.
155. Jabs DA, Lee B, Prendergast RA. Role of T cells in the pathogenesis of autoimmune lacrimal disease in MRL/Mp-lpr/lpr mice. *Curr Eye Res* 1997;16:909–916.
156. Fleisher TA, Puck JM, Strober W, et al. The autoimmune lymphoproliferative syndrome. A disorder of human lymphocyte apoptosis. *Clin Rev Allergy Immunol* 2001;20:109–120.
157. Fossati L, Sobel ES, Iwamoto M, et al. The Yaa gene-mediated acceleration of murine lupus: Yaa− T cells from non-autoimmune mice collaborate with Yaa+ B cells to produce lupus autoantibodies *in vivo*. *Eur J Immunol* 1995;25:3412–3417.
158. Matsuura E, Kobayashi K, Kasahara J, et al. Anti-beta 2-glycoprotein I autoantibodies and atherosclerosis. *Int Rev Immunol* 2002;21:51–66.
159. Amano H, Amano E, Moll T, et al. The Yaa mutation promoting murine lupus causes defective development of marginal zone B cells. *J Immunol* 2003;170:2293–2301.
160. Retter MW, Cohen PL, Eisenberg RA, et al. Both Sm and DNA are selecting antigens in the anti-Sm B cell response in autoimmune MRL/lpr mice. *J Immunol* 1996;156:1296–1306.
161. Ibrahim SM, Weigert M, Basu C, et al. Light chain contribution to specificity in anti-DNA antibodies. *J Immunol* 1995;155:3223–3233.
162. Chen C, Nagy Z, Radic MZ, et al. The site and stage of anti-DNA B-cell deletion. *Nature* 1995;373:252–255.
163. Qian Y, Santiago C, Borrero M, et al. Lupus-specific antiribonucleoprotein B cell tolerance in nonautoimmune mice is maintained by differentiation to B-1 and governed by B cell receptor signaling thresholds. *J Immunol* 2001;166:2412–2419.
164. Chen C, Nagy Z, Prak EL, et al. Immunoglobulin heavy chain gene replacement: a mechanism of receptor editing. *Immunity* 1995;3:747–755.
165. Walport MJ. Lupus, DNase and defective disposal of cellular debris. *Nat Genet* 2000;25:135–136.
166. Paul E, Carroll MC. SAP-less chromatin triggers systemic lupus erythematosus. *Nat Med* 1999;5:607–608.
167. Cohen PL, Caricchio R, Abraham V, et al. Delayed apoptotic cell clearance and lupus-like autoimmunity in mice lacking the c-mer membrane tyrosine kinase. *J Exp Med* 2002;196:135–140.
168. Walker SE, Gray RH, Fulton M, et al. Palmerston North mice, a new animal model of systemic lupus erythematosus. *J Lab Clin Med* 1978;92:932–945.
169. Luzina IG, Knitzer RH, Atamas SP, et al. Vasculitis in the Palmerston North mouse model of lupus: phenotype and cytokine production profile of infiltrating cells. *Arthritis Rheum* 1999;42:561–568.
170. Rhodin J, Thomas T, Bryant M, et al. Animal model of vascular inflammation. *J Submicrosc Cytol Pathol* 1999;31:305–311.
171. Nicklin MJ, Hughes DE, Barton JL, et al. Arterial inflammation in mice lacking the interleukin 1 receptor antagonist gene. *J Exp Med* 2000;191:303–312.
172. Horai R, Saijo S, Tanioka H, et al. Development of chronic inflammatory arthropathy resembling rheumatoid arthritis in interleukin 1 receptor antagonist-deficient mice. *J Exp Med* 2000;191:313–320.
173. Haneji N, Hamano H, Yanagi K, et al. A new animal model for primary Sjögren's syndrome in NFS/sld mutant mice. *J Immunol* 1994;153:2769–2777.
174. Haneji N, Nakamura T, Takio K, et al. Identification of alpha-fodrin as a candidate autoantigen in primary Sjögren's syndrome. *Science* 1997;276:604–607.
175. Green, JE, Hinrich SH, Vogel J, et al. Exocrinopathy resembling Sjögren's syndrome in HTLV-1 tax transgenic mice. *Nature* 1989;341:72–74.
176. Cha S, Peck AB, Humphreys-Beher MG. Progress in understanding autoimmune exocrinopathy using the non-obese diabetic mouse: an update. *Crit Rev Oral Biol Med* 2002;13:5–16.
177. Holers VM, Girardi G, Mo L, et al. Complement C3 activation is required for antiphospholipid antibody-induced fetal loss. *J Exp Med* 2002;195:211–220.
178. Pierangeli SS, Gharavi AE, Harris EN. Experimental thrombosis and antiphospholipid antibodies: new insights. J Autoimmun 2000;15:241–247.
179. Nagaraju K, Plotz PH. Animal models of myositis. *Rheum Dis Clin North Am* 2002;28:917–933.
180. Ytterberg SR. Coxsackievirus B 1 induced murine polymyositis: acute infection with active virus is required for myositis. *J Rheumatol* 1987;14:12–18.
181. Ytterberg SR, Mahowald ML, Messner RP. Coxsackievirus B 1-induced polymyositis: lack of disease expression in nu/nu mice. *J Clin Invest* 1987;80:499–506.
182. Ytterberg SR, Mahowald ML, Messner RP. T cells are required for coxsackievirus B1 induced murine polymyositis. *J Rheumatol* 1988;15:475–478.
183. Wada J, Shintani N, Kikutani K, et al. Intravenous immunoglobulin prevents experimental autoimmune myositis in SJL mice by reducing anti-myosin antibody and by blocking complement deposition. *Clin Exp Immunol* 2001;124:282–289.
184. Serreze DV, Pierce MA, Post CM, et al. Paralytic autoimmune myositis develops in nonobese diabetic mice made Th1 cytokine-deficient by expression of an IFN-gamma receptor beta-chain transgene. *J Immunol* 2003;170:2742–2749.
185. Nagaraju K, Raben N, Loeffler L, et al. Conditional up-regulation of MHC class I in skeletal muscle leads to self-sustaining autoimmune myositis and myositis-specific autoantibodies. *Proc Natl Acad Sci U S A* 2000;97:9209–9214.
186. Balomenos D, Martin-Caballero J, Garcia MI, et al. The cell cycle inhibitor p21 controls T-cell proliferation and sex-linked lupus development. *Nat Med* 2000;6:171–176.

187. Salvador JM, Hollander MC, Nguyen AT, et al. Mice lacking the p53-effector gene Gadd45a develop a lupus-like syndrome. *Immunity* 2002;16:499–508.
188. Murga M, Fernandez-Capetillo O, Field SJ, et al. Mutation of E2F2 in mice causes enhanced T lymphocyte proliferation, leading to the development of autoimmunity. *Immunity* 2001;15:959–970.
189. Zhang Y, Schlossman SF, Edwards RA, et al. Impaired apoptosis, extended duration of immune responses, and a lupus-like autoimmune disease in IEX-1-transgenic mice. *Proc Natl Acad Sci U S A* 2002;99:878–883.
190. Bachmaier K, Krawczyk C, Kozieradzki I, et al. Negative regulation of lymphocyte activation and autoimmunity by the molecular adaptor Cbl-b. *Nature* 2000;403:211–216.
191. Le LQ, Kabarowski JH, Weng Z, et al. Mice lacking the orphan G protein-coupled receptor G2A develop a late-onset autoimmune syndrome. *Immunity* 2001;14:561–571.
192. Majeti R, Xu Z, Parslow TG, et al. An inactivating point mutation in the inhibitory wedge of CD45 causes lymphoproliferation and autoimmunity. *Cell* 2000;103:1059–1070.
193. Seery JP, Carroll JM, Cattell V, et al. Antinuclear autoantibodies and lupus nephritis in transgenic mice expressing interferon gamma in the epidermis. *J Exp Med* 1997;186:1451–1459.
194. Mehling A, Loser K, Varga G, et al. Overexpression of CD40 ligand in murine epidermis results in chronic skin inflammation and systemic autoimmunity. *J Exp Med* 2001;194:615–628.

CHAPTER 30

Infectious Agents in Chronic Rheumatic Diseases

Robert D. Inman and Andras Perl

The potential infectious origins of arthritis and autoimmunity have attracted both basic and clinical researchers throughout the twentieth century (1). The isolation of anthrax bacillus by Robert Koch at the end of the nineteenth century ushered in an era in which new organisms were isolated from a wide variety of diseases, and it was assumed that chronic arthritis would yield to the same kind of systematic study as pneumonia and meningitis. The early literature, however, is plagued by confusion and inconsistency in terminology, and this delayed a definitive distinction between septic arthritis and noninfected arthritis. The early reports of Schueller described a large number of patients in whom synovial fluid (SF) yielded recovery of unusual bacilli, but control patients were not examined and attention to aseptic technique was not stressed (2). The early twentieth century saw the theory of focal infection become dominant in the etiology of arthritis. It was presumed that organisms such as streptococci lurked in hidden sites of the body, such as the teeth or the tonsils, and that by disseminating to joints they could initiate and perpetuate chronic inflammation (3). Although this theory lacked any controlled experimental data to support it, and indeed, led to a vast number of tonsillectomies and high colonic enemas, some of the current concepts of persisting microbial antigens in chronic arthritis bear a relationship to these early concepts of pathogenesis.

The advent of molecular biology brought a new set of more sensitive techniques to the analysis of arthritis, but methods such as the polymerase chain reaction (PCR) have brought with them a new set of unanswered questions regarding the specificity of such results. Indeed, as will be discussed below, the immunologic footprint of a putative arthritogenic pathogen is often taken as compelling evidence of causality. Whether it is lingering evidence of recent microbes, implicated on a positive PCR test result, or the persistence of serum antibodies or antigen-specific T-cell responses, all such results must be interpreted cautiously in light of the prevalence of the pathogen in the control population from whom the case is drawn. Rigorous proof of a causal role for such microbial suspects is proving to be a more complex issue than Koch might have imagined at the end of the nineteenth century.

This chapter focuses on microbes as inciting or perpetuating factors in the pathogenesis of connective tissue disease (CTD). Known infections causing rheumatic disease in humans are used to illustrate the various microbe/host interactions that could lead to CTD, and the evidence for specific microbial involvement in each CTD is reviewed with emphasis on recent studies and controversial areas. Earlier work was discussed and referenced in previous editions of this book (1). Several reviews have addressed various aspects of this topic (4–9).

MICROBE/HOST INTERACTION

The clinical and immunologic sequelae to infection are as varied as the range of pathogens and the hosts they infect. Increasingly, the biochemical events that reflect the host/microbe interaction at the cellular level are being understood. The attachment and invasion of bacteria represent an interplay between invasion-related proteins of the bacteria, and surface receptors on host target cells. Analysis of these events has refined the concept of virulence of an organism from one that is a fixed property of a bacteria, like the Gram stain, to a dynamic concept that reflects both bacterial and host factors. Similarly, the B-cell and T-cell immune responses to viral and bacterial infections are shedding new light on antigenic recognition, cell signaling pathways in activation, and immunologic memory. Thus, the pathways from antecedent infection to subsequent arthritis are becoming defined. Local persistence of the intact pathogen may prove elusive to define at first, as was the case for *Borrelia burgdorferi* in Lyme arthritis. Local persistence of bacterial antigens is exemplified by post-*Yersinia* reactive arthritis (ReA), and perhaps, in a broader range of the spondyloarthropathies (SpAs). Deposition of circulating immune complexes, as in bacterial endocarditis, may result in a chronic synovitis that remains culture negative. Generation of arthritogenic toxins may occur as a sequela to infection with *Clostridium difficile*, or in the course of toxic shock syndrome. Antecedent infection may initiate an autoimmune attack on articular structures if the foreign antigens exhibit immunologic cross-reactivity with normal host tissues. Such molecular mimicry is reflected in the relationship between M protein of group A streptococcus and cardiac myosin. The example of acute rheumatic fever has significantly influenced theories of microbial pathogenesis (see Chapter 79).

Yet, even molecular mimicry, a cornerstone of this line of investigation, has come under rigorous scrutiny (10). The central notion of that theory is that if microbial antigens share elements recognized as antigenic by the immune system, then the stage is set for an activation of otherwise quiescent autoreactive T cells and B cells. Yet, it is evident that sequence homology between self and microbial proteins may be a relatively common event in biology, and that there is a degree of degeneracy in the binding of peptides to both major histocompatibility complex (MHC) molecules on antigen-presenting cells (APCs) and to T-cell receptors on responding T cells. Thus, rigorous proof of molecular mimicry in the pathogenesis of human arthritis and autoimmunity has proved elusive. But infection may provide the stimulus for breaking tolerance to self antigens through several nonspecific mechanisms unrelated to mimicry. Tissue damage and local necrosis of cells may uncover cryptic epitopes of self antigens. Reactivation of resting autoreactive T cells may occur in this manner (11). Inappropriate activation may occur secondary to up-regulation of MHC molecules and costimulatory molecules on APCs. Alternatively, nonspecific T-cell activation can occur as the result of the elaboration of bacterial proteins known as superantigens.

Conventional Antigens Versus Superantigens

It is now well established that T lymphocytes can recognize two different types of antigens: conventional antigens and superantigens. Conventional antigens require uptake and processing by specialized APCs. These antigens are processed into peptides and presented in a groove formed by polymorphic α and β chains of MHC class II molecules on the surface of APCs. T cells recognize this peptide–MHC complex mainly through the third hypervariable region of the T-cell receptor, consisting of variable/joining (VJ) and variable/diversity (VD) J segments of the T-cell receptor α and β chains, respectively (12). By contrast, superantigens are defined by their capacity to activate nearly all T cells expressing a particular T-cell receptor Vβ domain (13). Superantigens do not require processing because they can bind directly to MHC class II molecules (14) and can stimulate T cells when added to fixed APCs (15). Two main categories of superantigens have been described. Bacterial toxins, such as the enterotoxins or exotoxins of staphylococci, streptococci, mycoplasmas (16,17), and *Yersinia enterocolitica*, have been implicated in food poisoning, toxic shock syndrome, and potentially, in arthritis (18). Prototypical viral superantigens are encoded by mouse mammary tumor virus (MMTV)-related endogenous retroviruses (19). Such "self superantigens" lead to the clonal elimination, mainly in the thymus, of those T cells that express Vβ products reactive with superantigen (20). Since superantigen-reactive T cells promote infection of B cells by exogenous MMTV, intrathymic elimination of these autoreactive T cells confers significant protection against homologous MMTV infection and transmission (21). By analogy, endogenous retrovirus-encoded superantigens may also influence autoreactivity and susceptibility to retroviral infections in human (22). Skewing of the T-cell receptor Vβ repertoire, potentially reflecting a superantigen effect, in SF of patients with rheumatoid arthritis (RA) (23,24) and in peripheral blood of patients with Kawasaki disease has been reported (25). Another study found no evidence for superantigen effect in patients with Kawasaki disease (26). To date, no superantigen definitively mediating autoimmune disease in humans has been identified.

Human Endogenous Retroviruses and Molecular Mimicry

Human Endogenous Retroviruses: Associations with Molecular Mimicry and Genetic Susceptibility

The human genome contains a complex variety of endogenous retroviruses (ERVs) that may make up as much as 5% of human DNA (27,28). Whereas exogenous retroviruses are infectious, with a replication cycle that requires integration of proviral DNA into host cell DNA, ERVs are transmitted genetically in a classic mendelian fashion through the germ line as proviral DNA. As an example, human T-cell lymphotropic virus–related endogenous sequence-1 (HRES-1) is a defective provirus that may have entered the genome at the developmental stage of Old World primates (29).

Involvement of ERV in autoimmunity was initially proposed by studies of the New Zealand mouse model of systemic lupus erythematosus (SLE), based on finding ERV-encoded envelop glycoprotein antigen in immune complexes deposited in the kidney of diseased animals (30). A pathogenic role of retroviral elements has been further implicated by the discovery of (a) cross-reactive antibodies to gag proteins of human retroviruses in patients with autoimmune disease (31–33), and (b) autoimmune syndromes in patients infected by human retroviruses (34).

Striking amino acid homologies between certain nonhuman retroviral gag proteins (glycoprotein antigens forming the protein core of retroviral particles) and human autoantigens, U1 small nuclear ribonucleoprotein (snRNP) (35), topoisomerase I (36), and La (37) have suggested the possibility that the natural targets of cross-reactive antibodies of autoimmune patients may correspond to ERVs (Table 30.1). While the function of human ERVs (HERVs) is generally unknown, ERVs, which are expressed on the protein level, are likely targets of cross-reactivity for virally-induced immune responses (38). Such cross-reactivity (i.e., molecular mimicry between self antigens and viral proteins) has been proposed as a trigger of autoimmunity (39–41). Along this line, antibodies to the env protein of ERV-3 were reported in patients with SLE, with the highest prevalence in mothers of babies with complete heart block (42). Antibodies to a recombinant HERV-E 4–1 gag p30 protein were also reported in SLE patients (43). There are at least 85 copies of HERV-E/4–1 per haploid genome scattered on 12 different chromosomes (44). All isolates of HERV-E are either truncated or contain multiple stop codons in their open reading frames, thus rendering them incapable of encoding proteins (45). The recombinant antigen was generated by correcting several stop codons in a genomic 4–1 sequence (43). Existence of a native 4–1 gag p30 protein has not yet been reported. Therefore, the antigen responsible for triggering of these autoantibodies remains to be determined.

Interestingly, transcription of HERV-E, previously termed 4–1 (45,46), is also increased in patients with SLE (47). HERV-E *gag*-specific RNA is detectable in peripheral blood mononuclear cells of healthy donors (48). Thus, the amount, precise sequence, and chromosomal origin of lupus-specific HERV-E transcripts require further studies. HERV-E RNA was also noted in normal skin and keratinocyte cell lines (49). Transcription of ERV family members HERV-K, HERV-L, and ERV-9 was increased in ultraviolet B–irradiated skin and skin biopsy samples of lupus patients (49). Transcriptional inactivation of ERV is often associated with host-directed methylation of CpG islands in the ERV promoters (50). 5-azacytidine (5-AZA), a demethylating agent, was found to enhance expression of type C ERV in the mouse (51,42). 5-AZA was also described to enhance expression of HERV-E (4–1) RNA in normal lymphocytes (47). This mechanism is particularly interesting with regard to induction of T-cell autoreactivity by 5-AZA (53) and impaired DNA methylation in T cells of patients with SLE (54). Demethylation of DNA plays an important role in toxicity of hydralazine and other lupus-inducing drugs (54).The *gag* gene of HERV-E and human leukocyte antigen (HLA) class I antigen E share a 97 nucleotide region of 91% homology (55). Interestingly, 48% of Japanese lupus patients have antibody to HERV-E *gag*, which is thought to interfere with HLA-E-restricted CD8 T-cell responses (56).

HRES-1 is a human T-cell lymphotropic virus–related human endogenous retrovirus that encodes a 28-kd nuclear autoantigen. HRES-1 antibodies are detectable in up to half of the patients with SLE and overlap syndromes (57–61). HRES-1/p28 contains cross-reactive antigenic epitopes with human T-cell leukemia virus type 1 (HTLV-1) gagp24 and the 70-kd component of U1 snRNP (58). The retroviral *gag*-related region of the 70Kd U1 snRNP–derived protein shares three consecutive highly charged amino acids—Arg-Arg-Glu (RRE), an additional Arg, and functionally similar Arg/Lys residues—with HRES-1/p28 that represent cross-reactive epitopes between the two proteins (58). Interestingly, the RRE triplet is repeated three times in the 70Kd protein at residues 248 to 250, 418 to 420, and 477 to 479, respectively (GenEmbl accession number X04654). This suggests that recognition of the retroviral domain may lead to epitope spreading through binding to RRE triplets within the 70K protein. It is well known that highly charged

TABLE 30.1. *Molecular mimicry between viral proteins and autoantigens*

Autoantigen	Prevalence[a]	Viral protein	Virus	References
70k/U1 snRNP	30%	*gag*	MoMLV, HRES-1	334,335
HRES-1	21%–52%	*gag*p24	HTLV-I	335–338
Sm B/B′	30%	*gag*p24	HIV-1	339
C/U1 snRNP	30%	ICP4	HHV-1	340
Sm D	36%	EBNA-1	EBV	341
Sm B/B′	25%–40%	EBNA-1	EBV	342
La	15%	*gag*	FSV	343
p542	10%–50%	EBNA-1	EBV	344
Topoisomerase I	20%[b]	*gag*	MoMLV	345
HERV-E	48.3%	*gag*p30	MoMLV	43
ERV-3	32%	*env*	MoMLV	42

[a]Prevalence of antibodies in patients with systemic lupus erythematosus.

[b]Prevalence of antibodies in patients with scleroderma.

EBNA-1, Epstein-Barr nuclear antigen 1; EBV, Epstein-Barr virus; HHV-1, human herpes virus type 1; HIV-1, human immunodeficiency virus type 1; HRES-1, human T-cell lymphotropic virus-related endogenous sequence 1; HTLV-1, human T-lymphotropic virus type 1; ICP4, infected cell protein 4; MoMLV, moloney murine leukemia virus.

polypeptides can elicit high-titer antibodies (62). Therefore, the presence of charged amino acids in the mimicking epitopes may have important implications in triggering cross-reactive antibodies of high affinity. Autoantigenicity of ERVs may be a key factor in molecular mimicry (i.e., retargeting of an immune response raised by an exogenous retrovirus toward self proteins).

Polymorphic alleles have been identified in the long terminal repeat promoter region of the HRES-1 element, and a differential segregation of these alleles was noted in patients with SLE (63,64). Diminished frequency of genotype I alleles was associated with production of antibodies to HRES-1/p28 in patients with SLE (65,66). HRES-1 is a single-copy endogenous retroviral element that was mapped to chromosome 1 at band q42 (67) (see *gdbwww.gdb.org*). Mapping of this ERS-encoded lupus autoantigen to 1q42 identified this chromosomal location as a potential lupus susceptibility site (63), which was also suggested by independent screening studies based on segregation of polymorphic microsatellite markers (68–70). The notion that autoantigenicity of ERVs, such as HRES-1, is involved in the pathogenesis of autoimmunity could explain both the familial aggregation of autoimmune diseases and the detection of antiretroviral antibodies.

Regulation of Apoptosis by Viruses

Viral infections may have a role in dysregulation of apoptosis or programmed cell death (PCD) in SLE. Many viruses have evolved genes that can selectively inhibit or stimulate PCD. The suicide of an infected cell by internal activation of apoptosis or the killing of an infected cell by a cytotoxic T lymphocyte or natural killer (NK) cell may be viewed as a defense mechanism of the host to prevent viral propagation. In the early stages of infection, viral inhibitors of apoptosis allow for more extensive production of progeny. At later stages, viral inducers of apoptosis facilitate spread of progeny to uninfected cells (64).

Apoptosis, or PCD, represents a physiologic mechanism for elimination of potentially autoreactive lymphocytes during development (71) (see Chapter 26). Excess cells after completion of an immune response are also eliminated by apoptosis (72). Defects in signaling though the Fas pathway may contribute to autoimmunity in *lpr* and *gld* mice (73). Although mutations of the Fas receptor (FasR) or Fas ligand (FasL) have been associated with lupuslike autoimmune syndromes in mice with *lpr* or *gld* backgrounds, respectively (73), and FasR defects have been documented in a rare form of lymphoproliferative disease (autoimmune lymphoproliferation syndrome) in humans (74,75), Fas-mediated signaling appears to be intact in patients with SLE (76). Defective CD3-mediated cell death in lupus patients, possibly related to decreased intracellular synthesis of tumor necrosis factor-α (TNF-α), has been linked to persistence of autoreactive cells (77). Nevertheless, apoptosis appears to be accelerated in peripheral blood lymphocytes of lupus patients (78), and could be a mechanism responsible for chronic lymphopenia and compartmentalized release of nuclear autoantigens in patients with SLE (79). Dysregulation of apoptosis might be an important mechanism of viral-induced disease pathogenesis in systemic rheumatic diseases.

HUMAN MODELS FOR INFECTION IN THE CONNECTIVE TISSUE DISEASES

Animal models of chronic infection causing immunologically-mediated disease are discussed in Chapter 29. Several other known infections causing rheumatic disease in humans are also useful as models, some for articular, and others for systemic, CTD.

Viral Infection–Induced Arthritis Syndromes

Viral infections often lead to inflammatory syndromes in which arthralgias or arthritis may represent a major manifestation (Table 30.2). Most cases of viral arthritis, such as rubella or parvovirus B19, are short term and self-limited as a result of an efficient elimination of the organism by the immune system. Chronic arthropathies have been associated with persistent or latent viral infections, virus-induced autoimmunity, polyclonal B-cell activation, and immunodeficiency resulting in opportunistic infections, largely due to an inability of the immune system to eliminate the pathogen. This latter group of viruses include human immunodeficiency virus 1 (HIV-1), human T-cell lymphotropic virus type 1, and hepatitis C virus (HCV).

Virus-Induced Transient Arthritis Syndromes

Parvovirus B19

Parvovirus B19 is one of the most frequent causes of viral arthritis (20). Joint manifestations are temporally associated with production of anti-B19 immunoglobulin M (IgM) antibodies. Although involvement of B19 has been repeatedly raised in classic RA, large surveys failed to demonstrate an association between erosive RA and parvovirus B19 (80).

Rubella Virus

Rubella is known to cause mild and self-limited arthralgias and acute arthritis (81). Chronic arthropathy was reported in 1% to 4% of postpartum female recipients of the RA27/3 vaccine strain (82). Other studies found no increase of chronic arthritis in women receiving the RA27/3 rubella vaccine (83). Moreover, no rubella virus has been recovered from peripheral blood lymphocytes of persons with chronic arthropathy following rubella infection or vacci-

TABLE 30.2. *Virus-induced arthritis syndromes*

Virus	Arthritis frequency	Arthritis Type	Duration	Erosion	Other	References
Parvovirus B19	Children: 5%–10% Adults: 50%–70% Female:male = 2:1	Polyarticular, small and large joints, symmetric	2–8 wk, rarely chronic	No	Anemia Leukopenia Thrombopenia Vasculitis Autoantibodies	80,346
Rubella	10%–30%	Multiple small joints	5–10 days	No	Vaccine strain RA27/3 may induce arthritis	81,347
VZV	<1%	Monoarthritis	1–7 days	No	Life-long latency	98
EBV	1%–5%	Poly- or monoarthritis	1–12 wk	No	Autoantibodies	95
HBV	10%–25%	Symmetric, migratory	1–3 wk	No	Vasculitis	347
HCV	10%–50%	Polyarticular, symmetric	Chronic	No	Vasculitis Sjögren's disease Autoantibodies	42
HTLV-1	<1%	Oligoarthritis, large joints	Chronic	Yes	Sjögren's disease Polymyositis Autoantibodies CD4$^+$ T-cell expansion	107
HIV-1	10%–50%	Painful joint syndrome	1–2 days	No	Promotion of CD8$^+$ T cell–mediated autoimmunity	111
		Reiter syndrome	Chronic	Yes		
		Psoriatic arthritis	Chronic	Yes		
Alphaviruses	>50%	Symmetric, small joints	1 wk to months	No	Fever Myalgia Encephalitis	88
Adenovirus	Rare	Small and large joints	Transient or chronic	No	Pharyngitis	92,93
Coxsackie	Rare	Symmetric, small and large joints	Acute or chronic	No	Myocarditis Serositis Pleurodynia	94
Pogosta	8% Female:male > 1	Small joints of hand and foot	Acute and chronic	Yes	Rash Fever	89,90,348

EBV, Epstein-Barr virus (human herpesvirus 4); HBV, hepatitis B virus; HCV, hepatitis C virus; HIV-1, human immunodeficiency virus type 1; HTLV-1, human T cell lymphotropic virus type 1; VZV, varicella-zoster virus.

nation (84). Therefore, continued vaccination of rubella-susceptible females to reduce the risk for congenital malformations seems warranted.

Alphaviruses

These are arthropod-borne viruses, which include the chikungunya, o'nyong-nyong, Mayaro, Sindbis, Okelbo, Barmah Forest (BF), and Ross River (RR) viruses. Similar to the rubella virus, they belong to the Togavirus family, which contains a positive-strand RNA genome. The viruses are spread by mosquitoes in endemic areas of Australia (Sindbis, BF, and RR), South America (Mayaro), Northern Europe (Okelbo), and Asia and sub-Saharan Africa (chikungunya). They can cause an acute infectious illness with skin rash, fever, arthritis, myalgia, or encephalitis. RR virus is the etiologic agent of the best-studied epidemic polyarthritis (EPA) affecting up to 7,800 Australians annually (85). Persistent infections are believed to be responsible for chronic arthritis. CD4$^+$ T cells dominate in mononuclear synovial effusions of EPA patients, in contrast to CD8$^+$T cell infiltrates in skin rashes of RR virus-infected patients who made early and complete recoveries (86,87). EPA involves the small joints of the hand and often causes tendonitis. Symptoms may persist for months. The diagnosis is made by demonstrating IgM antibodies to RR virus (88). Pogosta disease is caused by an arbo A type alphavirus closely related to Sindbis. It is endemic in Finland, Sweden, and the Karelian region of Russia. Chronic inflammatory arthritis leading to bony erosion (89) of small joints of the hands has been documented 2.5 years after initial infection with Pogosta virus (90). Pogosta virus infection is confirmed by detection of viral RNA and IgM and IgG antibodies (90).

Adenoviruses

These viruses are a common cause of acute respiratory infections. Symmetric polyarthritis of small and large joints may occur within a week of respiratory symptoms (91). Recurrent chronic oligoarthritis due to adenovirus infection was rarely reported (92,93).

Coxsackieviruses

They belong to the Enterovirus group of viruses. More than 90% of coxsackievirus infections are asymptomatic or manifest in undifferentiated febrile illness. Spectrum and severity of disease manifestations vary with age, gender, and immune status of the host (94). Coxsackievirus arthritis, usually caused by group B virus, occurs with fever, serositis, pleurodynia, and rash. The arthritis is usually symmetric and polyarticular, involving both small and large joints.

Herpesviruses

After initial infection, viruses of the Herpesviridae family persist in the host with life-long latency. Therefore, several of these viruses have been considered as etiologic agents in autoimmune diseases, such as SLE, RA, or Sjögren syndrome. Epstein-Barr virus (EBV) infection causes arthralgias lasting for up to 4 months in 2% of patients with mononucleosis (95). Recently, EBV-positive lymphomas were described in methotrexate-treated RA patients (96,97). Interestingly, remission of lymphomas was noted after discontinuation of methotrexate (96). Herpes simplex virus type 1 (HSV-1) arthritis rarely lasts longer than two weeks. Varicella-zoster virus can cause monarthritis, mostly in the knee, as a rare complication of chickenpox (98). Cytomegalovirus (CMV) may be responsible for scleroderma-like changes in patients with chronic graft-versus-host disease (99). These patients carry CD13 autoantibodies that bind to skin and mucous membranes. CMV incorporates the human CD13 protein into its viral envelope, which may be responsible for generation of autoantibodies.

Hepatitis B Virus

Hepatitis B virus (HBV) can cause arthralgias and arthritis early after infection. Arthritis resolves in 2 to 6 weeks with the onset of jaundice. HBV also has been associated with polyarteritis nodosa and cryoglobulinemia.

Virus-Induced Chronic Rheumatic Diseases

Hepatitis C Virus

HCV has a wide pathogenic potential that is not limited to diseases of the liver (100). Despite high-titer antibody levels, greater than 80% of infected individuals become chronic virus carriers. Cryoglobulinemia is detectable in up to 40% to 50% of HCV-infected patients (101). Identification of HCV as the causal agent of most (>90%) type II or essential mixed cryoglobulinemias (EMCs) has been a major breakthrough in rheumatology during the past decade (102). Type II cryoglobulins are immune complexes composed of a monoclonal IgM/kappa rheumatoid factor (RF) and polyclonal IgG. The clinical syndrome of EMC is an immune complex vasculitis characterized by purpura, arthralgias, inflammatory arthritis, peripheral neuropathy, and glomerulonephritis (103). IgM/kappa-bearing B cells are clonally expanded in the peripheral blood of EMC patients (104). Infection by HCV may be directly responsible for the clonal expansion of B cells (105), which may lead to development of B-cell non-Hodgkin's lymphomas (100). HCV infection is associated with the production of autoantibodies. Up to 75% of the patients have high-titer RF, presumably produced by HCV-infected and clonally expanded B lymphocytes. Moreover, 50% or more of the patients have anti–smooth muscle antibodies. Low-titer antinuclear antibodies (ANAs) and anticardiolipin antibodies were noted in 10% to 30% of HCV-infected patients. Approximately 5% of patients may develop Sjögren syndrome, SLE, autoimmune thyroiditis, or scleroderma (106). Erosive/rheumatoid arthritis and polymyositis/dermatomyositis have been rarely documented (100).

Human T-Cell Lymphotropic Virus Type 1

Infection by human T-cell lymphotropic virus type 1 has been associated with adult T-cell leukemia (ATL), mycosis fungoides/Sézary syndrome, human T-cell lymphotropic virus type 1–associated myelopathy/tropic spastic paraparesis, human T-cell lymphotropic virus type 1–associated arthritis (HAA), polymyositis, and Sjögren syndrome (107). Despite high rates of infection in endemic areas where 30% or more of the population may be infected, relatively few (<1%) of infected individuals show disease manifestations attributable to human T-cell lymphotropic virus type 1. The lifetime risk for developing a human T-cell lymphotropic virus type 1–associated disorder is less than 5%. Polymyositis, Sjögren syndrome, and inflammatory arthritis may occur in the absence of leukemia. These complications are characterized by infiltration of the skeletal muscle, salivary glands, or synovium with human T-cell lymphotropic virus type 1–infected T lymphocytes. HAA is characterized by erosive symmetric polyarthritis, most often involving the hands. The patients may have RF or ANAs and usually satisfy the diagnostic criteria for RA (48). Arthroscopic studies revealed proliferative synovitis in HAA (108). T cells infiltrating the joint have indented cerebriform nuclei similar to those seen in ATL. The prevalence of RA is increased in the human T-cell lymphotropic virus type 1–infected population (0.56%) compared with the uninfected population of Japan (0.31%) (107). Thus, the relatively low disease frequency in virus-infected individuals strongly advocates for the role of factors other than human T-cell lymphotropic virus type 1 in the development of RA. Transgenic mice carrying the *tax* transactivator gene of human T-cell lymphotropic virus type 1 develop Sjögren syndrome and rheumatoid-like arthritis, suggesting a pathogenic role for the p40/tax protein (107). Human T-cell lymphotropic virus type 1 was also shown to induce polymyositis, arthritis, and uveitis in rhesus macaque monkeys (109), thus establishing a primate model of viral arthritis.

Human Immunodeficiency Virus Type 1

During the course of HIV-1 infection, three major phases can be distinguished. Within a few weeks after infection, extensive viremia occurs, giving rise to an acute mononucleosis-like syndrome. A second, and relatively latent, period represents an ongoing fierce battle between virus replication and replenishing of the $CD4^+$ T cell reservoirs. On average, 10 years following infection, diminished $CD4^+$ T cell function gives rise to opportunistic infections, lymphomagenesis, and autoimmune phenomena at the final stages of disease. Polyclonal B-cell activation and production of autoantibodies have been attributed to a shift from helper T cell subset 1 (T_H1) to T_H2 type predominance. Rheumatic diseases most commonly noted in patients with acquired immunodeficiency syndrome (AIDS) include ReA, psoriatic arthritis, spondylarthropathies, and diffuse infiltrative lymphocytosis syndrome. Interestingly, all of these syndromes have been associated with relative expansion of $CD8^+$ T cells, thus suggesting that HIV-1 infection accelerates HLA class I–restricted $CD8^+$ T cell-mediated autoreactivity (110). In turn, SLE, RA, and polymyositis, which are thought to be mediated by $CD4^+$ T cells, remit in some patients following infection by HIV-1 (111).

Other Infection-Related Arthropathies

Rheumatic fever is the generally accepted model for rheumatic disease due to a cross-reactive immune response to local host antigen and a component of a microbial agent (112). In recent years, its incidence is again increasing, and more cases with arthritis alone ("reactive") are being seen. Local presence of the microbe is not necessary. Following a group A streptococcal infection in the pharynx, the host antibody response to a streptococcal antigen cross-reacts with a host antigen present in the heart, resulting in local inflammation (carditis). The cycle is repeated or intensified with recurrent infections. A cross-reactive host antigen has been demonstrated in the heart and in joint tissues such as synovium. This model, also known as molecular mimicry, thus postulates a host antigen in joint tissues cross-reactive with a microbial antigen and is an attractive hypothesis for articular CTD. Substantial direct evidence exists for the model, but little for streptococcal infection as a causative agent in RA or juvenile rheumatoid arthritis (JRA) (1).

Lyme disease is perhaps the best microbial model for RA, combining three important factors: local infection, host immune response, and possibly, a local cross-reactive host antigen. The disease has a variety of acute and chronic manifestations, including proliferative arthritis. It is caused by infection with a group of diverse spirochetes called *Borrelia burgdorferi* sensu lato (113–115). Clinical manifestations may depend at least in part on the precise microbial species involved, and to further complicate investigation, mixed infections can occur (115). Antigen-specific immune responses have been demonstrated in blood, cerebrospinal fluid, and the joint (116), where the microbe has been shown to persist using culture and PCR (115), and may be accompanied by persistent IgM antibody responses. In Lyme neurologic disease, the spirochete and neuronal cells were found to share a cross-reactive antigen. The microorganism can also alter immune responses in various less antigen-specific ways, and chronicity may result from progressively increasing T-cell responses to persistent microbial antigens. Both antigen-specific and nonspecific mechanisms seem to be important in the pathogenesis of Lyme disease, but microbial persistence may be most critical for chronicity (1). The benefits of research on pathogenesis are nowhere more evident than in Lyme disease, where antibiotic treatment is curative (particularly during the early stages of the disease), and prevention by vaccination has now become possible (114).

Taken together, the data from these human models and from the animal models discussed in Chapter 29 support a pathogenic role both for microbial persistence with ongoing antigen-specific immune responses, and for less specific up-regulation of the immune response by microbial antigens, perhaps acting as superantigens, leading to immunodysregulation. Thus, all three factors in Table 30.3 could be important: a microbial infection, possibly in joint tissues, could induce local inflammation either by specific immune responses to the microbial antigen, an inflammation-altered host antigen, or a cross-reactive host antigen present locally; or less antigen-specific mechanisms could induce immunodysregulation. Local persistence of one or more of these processes then provides the perpetuating stimulus for recurrent or chronic arthritis, perhaps with microbial reinfections as an additional stimulus for exacerbations.

Many variations of this basic theme have been constructed to account for specific features of particular diseases. One is the bacterial debris hypothesis, in which endogenous gut bacteria provide microbial host antigen, and various immune complexes are formed by specific antibody, alteration of host IgG, and the induction of RF (117). Formation of such complexes locally in joints results in articular CTD, whereas circulating complexes lead to systemic CTD. This mechanism could account for rheumatic disease after intestinal bypass surgery or inflammatory bowel disease. Alternatively, endogenous or exogenous microbial antigens may cross-react with host antigens, which

TABLE 30.3. *Current hypotheses for a microbial role in articular CTD*

Sequence: general microbial hypothesis
Local microbial replication (bacteria, mycoplasma, or virus)
Microbe-specific immune response and/or nonspecific immunodysregulation
Local antigen(s): microbial, cross-reactive, and/or altered host
Local inflammation
Early arthritis
Persistent local antigen(s): microbial, cross-reactive, and/or altered host
Persistent local inflammation
Recurrent/chronic arthritis
Alternative sequence: bacterial debris hypothesis
Endogenous gastrointestinal bacterial antigens
Microbe-specific immune response
Nonspecific immune response: rheumatoid factor
Immune complex formation: local or systemic
Recurrent or chronic arthritis
Alternative sequence: cross-tolerance hypothesis
Endogenous or exogenous microbial infection
Microbe-specific immune response
Cross-reactive host antigen: HLA-B27, or other
Local inflammation
Recurrent or chronic arthritis

CTD, connective tissue disease; HLA, human leukocyte antigen.

may be MHC determined (118) (Table 30.2). Infection could also be involved in a variety of other mechanisms, including antiidiotype antibodies and cellular oncogene activation (119,120).

Systemic Connective Tissue Disease

Hepatitis B Vasculitis

Hepatitis B vasculitis probably results from the immune response to persistent systemic virus replication, with circulating immune complex formation and deposition (1). The clearance of such complexes may be impaired by defective Kupffer cell function due to viral damage and overload. Composition, size, complement fixing ability, and timing of the complexes are factors affecting potential pathogenicity. *In situ* immune complex formation may also occur, and factors in addition to the humoral immune response are probably involved. For instance, at the subcellular level, host genetic control of virus and virus component production apparently leads to vast excess of circulating hepatitis B surface antigen. The enhanced immunogenicity of the hepatitis B core antigen may reflect its ability to directly induce B-cell antibody production. Still, unrecognized virus strain variations or an abnormal cellular immune response might also be involved. Thus, hepatitis B infection can be viewed as the cause of a subset of necrotizing vasculitis, but only in concert with other equally critical host factors. An extraordinarily broad spectrum of immunopathology can occur during hepatitis B infections, ranging from often fatal vasculitis to acute arthritis, to both acute and chronic asymptomatic infections.

Hepatitis C Virus and Cryoglobulinemia

Cryoglobulins are immunoglobulins that spontaneously precipitate in the blood or serum, usually on cooling below 25°C. Type I cryoglobulins consist of monoclonal immunoglobulins, which cryoprecipitate by self-association through the Fc portion of the molecule. Mixed-type II cryoglobulins contain a monoclonal RF that cryoprecipitates after binding monoclonal or polyclonal IgGs. Mixed-type III cryoglobulins contain polyclonal RF, usually IgM or IgG, that binds polyclonal IgGs (121). The resulting circulating immune complexes cause a clinical syndrome of vascular purpura, arthritis/arthralgia, glomerulonephritis, and peripheral neuropathy (122). Mixed cryoglobulins have long been associated with chronic hepatitis (123). Since the recent documentation that HCV infection is responsible for about 90% of the cases of non-A, non-B hepatitis, a pathogenic role of HCV in mixed cryoglobulins has been actively investigated. Using a combination of enzyme-linked immunosorbent assay (ELISA) and recombinant protein-based immunoblot assays for antibody detection and reverse transcriptase–mediated PCR for demonstration of HCV RNA, it appears that 50% to 90% of patients with mixed cryoglobulins are infected with HCV. Cryoglobulins were cleared from the sera of 13 of 20 patients treated with interferon-α for 6 to 12 months with relief of associated symptoms. A direct role of HCV in pathogenesis of mixed cryoglobulins has been further substantiated by a 20- to 100-fold concentration of HCV RNA in the cryoprecipitate (124). By contrast, the concentration of anti-HCV antibodies was not higher in cryoprecipitates than in the whole serum or in cryoprecipitate-deprived supernatants in patients with mixed cryoglobulins (125).

If the virion is a key factor in cryoprecipitability of virion antigen–immunoglobulin complexes, one would anticipate higher concentration of antibody in the cryoglobulin. However, this is not fully understood at present. Moreover, HCV productively infects peripheral blood lymphocytes, and thus it could be involved in transformation and clonal expansion of RF-producing B lymphocytes (126,127). These results suggest that HCV may be the causative agent in more than half of the "essential" mixed cryoglobulins cases. In addition, as discussed in Chapter 128, persistent HCV infection has been associated with a number of syndromes: RA-like arthritis, glomerulonephritis, Sjögren syndrome, and other rheumatic diseases (128).

Retroviruses and Rheumatic Diseases

Retroviruses are distinguished by their ability to transcribe their RNA genome into DNA by reverse transcription (see Chapter 129). The resulting double-stranded DNA is integrated into the host cell nuclear DNA. Host cell enzymes will subsequently transcribe the integrated DNA back to RNA, which can then be translated into viral proteins and form the genetic material for newly assembled virions. This unusual life cycle, associated with a long-term latency without any virion production from integrated proviral DNA, has made detection of retroviral infection very difficult. Infectious human retroviruses have been divided into three major groups: lentiviruses, including HIV-1 and HIV-2; HTLV-1 and HTLV-2; and the spumaretroviruses (129). By contrast, endogenous retroviruses reflect an inability of the integrated provirus to produce infectious virions and represent a permanent integration into the germline DNA, as discussed previously.

AIDS is causally associated with infection by HIV-1 and HIV-2. *In vivo*, these viruses preferentially grow in macrophages/monocyte lineage cells in various organs or in T cells. Patients diagnosed with AIDS exhibit qualitative and quantitative defects in CD4 T lymphocytes, causing impaired cell-mediated immunity, subsequent opportunistic infections, and a high incidence of non-Hodgkin lymphomas and Kaposi sarcoma (130). Patients with AIDS can exhibit symptoms of autoimmune disorders, such as SLE and Sjögren syndrome. It has been proposed that autoimmune mechanisms are involved in the pathogenesis of AIDS (131). Thus, AIDS is another potential model for systemic, as well as articular, CTD.

Considering the pathogenesis of AIDS as a model for systemic CTD, a variety of mechanisms may be applicable. HIV binds to the T-cell CD4 receptor (132), thereby infecting this helper/inducer subset, and preferentially, either interferes with its function or actually kills it. In AIDS, the cellular immune functions are profoundly impaired because of the loss of $CD4^+$ T cells. Low numbers of $CD4^+$ T cells, as well as a low percentage of $CD4^+$ T cells relative to $CD8^+$ T cells, are seen in all AIDS patients. The profound immune deficiency can largely be explained by the central role of the $CD4^+$ T cell in the immune system—providing help to B cells for antibody synthesis, interacting with monocytes for delayed-type hypersensitivity, participating in the generation of cytotoxic T cells and NK cells, and producing a variety of cytokines. Immune dysregulation observed in individuals infected with HIV during progression toward AIDS has been accounted for by a shift from a T_H1-type response to a T_H2-like cytokine profile (133). A T_H1-type response is defined by strong cell-mediated immune reactivities with normal or increased levels of interleukin-2 (IL-2), IL-12, and interferon-γ (IFN-γ). A predominance of T_H2 responses is characterized by increased B-cell reactivity (hypergammaglobulinemia, autoantibody production) accompanied by an increase in IL-4, IL-5, IL-6, IL-10, or IL-13. It has been proposed that the T-cell death in AIDS is mediated by an increased rate of apoptosis or PCD (134). Interestingly, T_H1-type cytokines protect against apoptosis, whereas T_H2 cytokines increase PCD. HIV may use several mechanisms to deplete $CD4^+$ T cells at the later stages of disease. HIV induces oxidative stress (135,136) and enhances surface expression of FasL, resulting in acceleration of signaling through the Fas apoptosis pathway (137). In addition, cleavage of bcl-2 by HIV protease may expose the cell to a variety of apoptotic signals (138).

A variety of autoimmune laboratory phenomena are associated with HIV infection. Polyclonal hypergammaglobulinemia is commonly seen, with all immunoglobulin isotypes elevated to a degree that increases with the clinical course of infection. In patients with AIDS, ANAs are primarily directed against nucleosomes and histones, whereas anti-double-stranded DNA antibody titers are not different from those in healthy donors (139).

A variety of autoantibodies have been reported in AIDS. Nineteen sera from 151 patients with AIDS or AIDS-related complex (ARC) had low-titer positive ANA, but this is a higher frequency than reported in several subsequent studies. RF was found in 2 of 36 patients with ARC and 23 of 141 patients with AIDS, but none was positive by sheep cell agglutination. Anticardiolipin antibodies (ACLAs) were reported in 76% of HIV-infected individuals; in another study, ACLAs of the IgG class were present in 48% of intravenous drug users, 38% of homosexuals, and 14% of heterosexuals infected with HIV. ACLAs were not increased in HIV-negative sexual partners of HIV-infected patients and were not associated with thrombocytopenia, pneumonia due to *Pneumocystis carinii*, disease progression, or clinical stage. There appears to be no strong association between ACLAs and thrombotic episodes, in contrast to the case in patients with SLE (1).

Cytopenias are a common finding in the HIV-infected population. Thrombocytopenia, anemia, and neutropenia may all have their origins in autoantibody formation against the respective cellular substrates. Autoantibodies against platelets and neutrophils occur early in HIV infection, and their prevalence is correlated with disease progression, but they are associated with cytopenia only in a limited number of patients. Antilymphocyte antibodies have been observed with varying prevalence and may play a role in the lymphocytopenia of HIV infection. Reactivity of these antibodies is directed primarily against T cells. Recently, autoantibodies against denatured collagen were detected in all homosexual AIDS patients tested, in 60% of HIV-positive homosexuals, and in 22% or less of HIV-positive transfusion recipients and hemophiliacs. These antibodies reacted preferentially with types I and III collagen after heat denaturation. The significance of these autoantibodies is uncertain, but they may play a role in some of the clinical manifestations of AIDS (1).

A variety of clinical rheumatic syndromes have been associated with HIV infection (1). Several reports have described a sicca complex occurring in AIDS patients, in which parotid gland biopsy revealed lymphocytic infiltration and myoepithelial lesions characteristic of primary Sjögren syndrome. Unlike primary Sjögren syndrome, RF and anti-Ro or anti-La antibodies are not seen. Male predominance and diffuse lymphadenopathy also suggest the AIDS sicca complex rather than primary Sjögren syndrome. Another study described 17 patients with a diffuse infiltrative lymphocytic disorder resembling Sjögren syndrome (140). All patients had bilateral parotid enlargement, and xerostomia or xerophthalmia was present in most. There was a $CD8^+$ lymphocytosis present in the salivary gland biopsy samples as well as in peripheral blood. HLA-DR5 was most frequent in African-American patients. Despite lymphocytic infiltration of the lymph nodes, salivary gland, and gastrointestinal (GI) tract, opportunistic infections were rare and none of the patients has died with AIDS. Autoantibodies were generally absent. The syndrome appears to be an immunogenetically defined alteration in the immune response to HIV (140).

Polymyositis can be the first clinical manifestation of impending AIDS. Inflammatory infiltrates may or may not be present in the myopathy seen in these patients. *In situ* hybridization with the *tat* gene of HIV has demonstrated numerous infected cells in the inflammatory infiltrate in the muscle. A report of myositis coexisting with toxoplasma infection highlights the importance of excluding cofactors such as other infection in AIDS patients. Muscle disease may also be simulated by fibromyalgia, which has been reported in patients with HIV infection (1).

A summary of 14 cases of vasculitis with HIV infection highlighted the importance of angiocentric immunoproliferative disorders, including benign lymphocytic angiitis, lymphomatoid granulomatosis, and angiocentric lymphoma (141). This spectrum of disorders may all present with the clinical picture of systemic necrotizing vasculitis. Lymphoproliferation of T cells with angiocentric predisposition may be the underlying mechanism, although immune complex deposition or infectious cofactors remain possibilities.

There has been increasing awareness of the spectrum of inflammatory joint disease occurring in HIV infection, including septic arthritis, HIV-associated arthropathy, psoriatic arthritis, and ReA (1). Infections accounting for septic arthritis tend to be atypical organisms such as *Cryptococcus neoformans* or *Sporothrix schenckii*, although staphylococcal septic bursitis was recently reported. It is important to note that HIV and another pathogen may coexist in the joint, as was the case for a patient infected with *Histoplasma capsulatum*. The concept that HIV may be playing a primary pathogenic role in the arthropathy is supported by recovery of the virus from SF and tissue (142–144). "Primary" HIV arthropathy appears to present two clinical syndromes (144,145). One pattern is severe arthralgias involving primarily the lower extremity, with noninflammatory SF. There is no HLA-B27 association, and the syndrome is generally of short duration and responsive to NSAIDs. The second pattern is an asymmetric lower extremity polyarthritis, without extraarticular features of ReA or an HLA-B27 association.

Psoriatic arthritis has been reported in patients with HIV infection, although there is no consensus regarding the prevalence of this overlap. The course of psoriasis was followed in 13 patients from a population of more than 1,000 HIV-positive individuals; 4 with mild psoriasis demonstrated severe exacerbations as AIDS developed. Both the skin and joint inflammation can be very difficult to control in these patients. An asymmetric polyarthritis occurred in 33% of 18 men with HIV-associated psoriasis and correlated with the presence of HLA-B27. Extensive overlap between psoriatic arthritis and ReA was noted, and no excess of HLAs previously associated with psoriatic arthritis was seen (1).

The interface of ReA and HIV infection was highlighted previously. The arthritis had a defined microbial antecedent infection in only 3 of 13 patients with ReA and AIDS; 9 were HLA-B27 positive. ReA and AIDS appeared simultaneously in 4 patients, and in the others, AIDS either preceded or followed ReA. Two patients developed Kaposi's sarcoma and fulminant AIDS after receiving methotrexate therapy, emphasizing the need for caution in the use of immunosuppressive therapy in ReA. These patients may have no clinical manifestation of AIDS preceding ReA, and recognized bacterial triggering events may be absent. An HIV-related ReA not associated with HLA-B27 was reported in Zimbabwean patients. Most patients had clinical manifestations of AIDS coexisting with the ReA. In black Zimbabweans, there is a low prevalence of HLA-B27 (gene prevalence 0.68) and a low frequency of B27-associated SpAs (1).

The coexistence of AIDS and ReA has suggested several possibilities for the immunopathogenic basis for the overlap. The altered immune status in AIDS, with relatively increased cytotoxic T cells, may increase the likelihood of an abnormal immune response to bacterial infections, resulting in ReA. This is of interest because HLA-B27, being a class I HLA, is thought to play a critical role in the interaction of $CD8^+$ T cells with APCs. It is also apparent that severe ReA can occur in patients with virtually no circulating $CD4^+$ T cells, which may carry an important message about the cellular basis of inflammation in this disease. Nevertheless, the aberrant immune response to bacterial infection that results in ReA has not yet been characterized, so this proposed pathogenesis remains speculative. This also applies to a second explanation for the HIV/ReA association; the immunodeficient state of AIDS predisposes to infection by an arthritogenic organism. Recurrent GI infections are indeed common in AIDS patients, so this has some support from clinical observations. A third possibility is that activation of the immune system during acute ReA may contribute to reactivation of latent HIV infection. Currently, there is an incomplete understanding of the mechanism for latent HIV infection becoming activated, so this is difficult to prove. Finally, the overlap may represent an epidemiologic coincidence. It may be that there is a parallel increase in frequency of infections by both HIV and arthritogenic organisms in this patient population because of sexual habits. The resolution of these possibilities will require combined clinical laboratory studies, but likely will provide important insights into the immunopathogenesis of both AIDS and ReA. The impression from a prospective study is that rheumatic symptoms occur predominantly in patients with advanced HIV infection (146). Thus, the development of arthritis in such patients may constitute a poor prognostic sign, although continued late follow-up of such cohorts will be needed to resolve this issue.

Another human retrovirus, HTLV-1, has been recognized as the etiologic agent of adult T cell leukemia/lymphoma (147) and has been associated with tropical spastic paraparesis (146), mycosis fungoides (148–150), and a variety of autoimmune syndromes, including rheumatoid-like arthritis (151) and polymyositis (152,153). Sjögren syndrome has been observed in patients with tropical paraparesis (154) and intravenous drug abusers (155) frequently infected with HTLV-1 or HTLV-2 (156). The seroprevalence of HTLV-1 antibodies was significantly increased among patients with Behçet disease in southern Japan (32.1% vs. 12.3% in controls; $p < 0.01$), an area in which HTLV-1 is endemic (157). HTLV-1-associated inflammatory arthropathy (HAAP) appears to be a particularly interesting natural model for a retroviral involvement in rheumatic diseases. HTLV-1 proviral DNA and expression of the p40/*tax* transactivator gene was demonstrated in synovial tissue and cultured nonlymphoid synovial cells in two patients with HAAP (158). Moreover, HTLV-1-infected synovial cells displayed an increased rate of proliferation and production of proinflammatory lymphokines, including IL-1, IL-6, and granulocyte-monocyte colony-stimulating factor (GM-CSF).

The capability of HTLV-1 to infect synovial cells was independently demonstrated by coculture of synovial cells from biopsy tissue of HTLV-1-negative RA patients with HTLV-1 producing T-cell lines *in vitro*. Likewise, production of proinflammatory GM-CSF by synovial cells was augmented after infection with HTLV-1 (159). Transfection of synovial cells with the p40/*tax* gene of HTLV-1 increased proliferation and cytokine production of synovial cells (160). Another pathway by which HTLV-1 p40/*tax* may induce rheumatic disease is a direct stimulatory effect on expression of autoantigens. Expression of two potentially novel autoantigens (molecular weight 44 kd and 46 kd), detected by sera of progressive systemic sclerosis patients, were induced by p40/*tax* of HTLV (161). Because none of these patients was infected by HTLV-1, a protein functionally similar to p40/*tax* may be involved in eliciting autoantigen expression and a subsequent autoantibody response in a subset of autoimmune patients. Moreover, HTLV-1 p40/*tax* increases apoptosis (162), which can lead to autoantigen release, a hallmark of patients with SLE. A key role of the p40/*tax* gene in HTLV-1-associated autoimmune syndromes was further substantiated by development of HTLV-1 *tax* gene–carrying transgenic mice. These mice exhibit Sjögren syndrome accompanied by lymphocytic infiltration of the salivary glands (163) and chronic arthritis resembling RA (164). The RA-like picture in these mice is characterized by synovial and periarticular inflammation, synovial proliferation, and erosive changes in the joints (165). In HIV- and HTLV-associated diseases, immunologic aberrations result in a multisystem disease with a number of similarities to SLE and other autoimmune syndromes. There are almost certainly as yet undiscovered retroviruses in humans; these might affect different immunologically active cell subsets. Thus, the profound immunodysregulation elicited by human retroviral infections is a fascinating model for CTD.

EVIDENCE IMPLICATING INFECTIOUS AGENTS IN CONNECTIVE TISSUE DISEASE

Many attempts at implicating different classes of microorganisms in most rheumatic syndromes have been made over the past 70 years. With a few exceptions, promising early findings have generally not been substantiated subsequently. Earlier enthusiasm was discussed in detail and referenced in previous editions (1). More recent efforts and controversial areas are discussed subsequently.

Articular Connective Tissue Disease

Rheumatoid Arthritis

Extensive microbial studies with an imposing array of methods have been conducted over the years, in part because of the ready availability of specimens from this common disease (6–8,117,118,165–168). The enthusiasm for studying different classes of microbes was driven mostly by available methodology, thus the chronologic sequence from bacteria to mycoplasma to viruses. Earlier attempts at implicating bacteria and mycoplasma in RA did not yield consistent or reproducible results (1). Interest in bacteria and their constituents, however, has increased sharply in the past 15 years because of their increasingly well-documented role in both animal models and human disease, including Lyme disease and reactive and enteropathic arthritis; because of the identification of the causative bacterium in other nonrheumatic diseases such as Whipple disease (169) and bacillary angiomatosis-peliosis (170); and because of the potential importance of bacterial superantigens.

Studies of bowel bacterial flora in RA have continued, particularly on *Clostridium perfringens* and *Proteus mirabilis.* RA patients had more frequent carriage of clostridia, which decreased after sulfasalazine treatment, although this did not correlate with the antirheumatic effect of the medication. Higher carriage rates were associated with nonsteroidal antiinflammatory drug (NSAID) treatment both in RA and degenerative joint disease (DJD). The studies to date do not support a pathogenetic role for clostridia in RA (1). Nonetheless, these data, together with other studies showing small intestinal bacterial overgrowth (171) and abnormal bacterial cellular fatty acid levels in early RA (172), indicate that further study of this area is warranted.

Studies of humoral immune responses in RA have shown higher levels of *Klebsiella*-, *Streptococcus*-, and particularly *Proteus*-specific antibodies. The latter may be related to disease activity, particularly to C-reactive protein levels.

Antibody levels did decrease in patients with RA responding to a vegetarian diet. Higher proteus antibodies were found in several European countries (173), but were related to disease activity. Molecular mimicry could be involved in the increased *Proteus* antibodies, but apart from the serologic studies, there has been little evidence to support a pathogenetic role for *Proteus* in RA (1).

Specific synovial cellular responses to *Chlamydia* and *Salmonella,* as well as other microbial antigens, have been reported in RA, although peripheral blood cellular and humoral immune responses to these microbes were not increased. Several trials of antibiotic treatment for RA have shown modest benefit with minocycline, but this may be due to an effect on the inflammatory process rather than the antibacterial activity of the drug (1).

The possible role of heat shock proteins (HSPs) as cross-reactive antigens has been an interesting area of investigation in RA. Their widespread prevalence and high degree of conservation and homology across species from bacteria to humans make HSPs attractive candidates for cross-reactive immune responses leading to autoimmunity. HSPs increase in cells stressed by heat and other factors; they are classified by size and other characteristics, including function. Early studies, principally involving mycobacterial HSPs, suggested a role in RA. Elevated antibodies to mycobacterial 65-kd HSP were found; SF and cellular responses were also increased. *In vitro*, mycobacterial antigens stimulated RA mononuclear or synovial cells to destroy cartilage and to proliferate and form pannus. Certain HLA-DR phenotypes influenced immune responses to mycobacterial antigens, and RFs shared cross-reactivity with various microbial proteins (1,174). Subsequent studies were less impressive: synovial HSP levels were similar in RA and controls, and GI mucosal HSP expression was not related to disease activity or treatment. HSPs induced synovial cells to suppress cartilage formation; cellular responses to HSP were involved in joint destruction in both RA and JRA. SF cells had high responses to HSPs, associated with HLA-DR4-Dw15. Other studies did not find increased synovial cellular responses to HSPs and other bacterial antigens, or increased humoral immune responses to HSPs in RA (1). However, a study in long-standing RA again indicated that both IgG and IgM responses to HSP were increased. The responses did not seem to be related to HLA-DR phenotypes but did correlate with radiographic severity, and with RF. High responses were also found in mixed CTD and SLE. The investigators concluded that the HSP responses were probably autoantibodies, and possibly directed against articular HSPs exposed as a result of chronic joint inflammation. In any case, it seems clear that these HSP antibodies were markers for more severe RA (175). In summary, the pathogenetic role of both cellular and humoral immune responses to HSPs in RA remains unclear.

The most exciting area of recent investigation has been the application of PCR to detection of bacterial DNA in patients with rheumatoid and other chronic inflammatory arthritides. The PCR method has many pitfalls, but also shows great promise as a rapid and very sensitive method of diagnosis (176). Several recent studies have applied broad-range PCR tests that amplify 16s ribosomal RNA (rRNA) genes in clinical specimens. These genes contain regions conserved in all bacteria, which thus allow detection of any bacteria present without knowing the exact species. There are also variable fragments within the 16s rRNA regions that are also amplified and allow exact identification of the species. One study examined peripheral blood, SF, and synovial tissue from 20 patients with undifferentiated arthritis, along with other positive and negative control groups. Eight patients tested positive by 16s rRNA PCR, but further analysis to identify the species showed ambiguous sequences in all. Subsequent cloning studies in four patients showed multiple bacterial species: pseudomonas in all four, along with one or more *Mycobacteria, Neisseria,* and other species present (177). The detection of multiple species in single specimens suggests contamination even though stringent precautions were taken to prevent it in both this and subsequent studies. The latter used the same type of PCR method to examine SF from patients with RA, JRA, undifferentiated oligoarthritis, ReA, and other rheumatic diseases. Approximately half of the patients in each group (26 of 57) tested positive. Best-fit analysis of the PCR product showed six were *Bacillus,* probably due to airborne contamination. Of the remaining 21 positive results, *Chlamydia, Yersinia,* opportunistic pathogens including *Pseudomonas*, major pathogens including *Haemophilus influenzae* and *H. pasteurella,* as well as unidentifiable species were found. In this study, multiple species were not found in individual patients, but multiple different species were found among the group, including recognizable contaminants. The authors conclude that this kingdom-specific PCR technique is controversial and that further studies should clarify the significance of these provocative findings (178).

Studies to detect *Mycobacterium tuberculosis* in RA have continued to yield conflicting positive and negative results (1). PCR has also been applied here, both for clinical testing in suspected mycobacterial infections (179) and in patients with RA (180). The investigators used mycobacterial genus-specific PCR on SF or tissue from 40 patients with RA, 21 with undifferentiated arthritis, and other groups as positive and negative controls. Mycobacterial species were detected in three patients with RA and two from other negative control groups, which the authors interpreted as probably not substantiating a pathogenetic role for mycobacteria in RA (180). Although stringent precautions were taken, the study indicates the propensity of PCR to produce false-positive results despite the precautions.

Interest in mycoplasmas continues; they also express stress proteins and appear to function as superantigens in animal models (66,67). Previous efforts to identify mycoplasmas in RA have also been conflicting (1), but a recent study used a highly sensitive and specific forensic PCR method on 28 patients with RA. Fifteen tested positive compared with 3 of 32 controls. Most species were identified as *Mycoplasma penetrans* or *M. pneumoniae*, but 36% had several *Mycoplasma* species identified. The investigators suggested that this was evidence of systemic *Mycoplasma* infections in RA, but after reviewing other studies of *Mycoplasma* in RA, including some using PCR, they concluded that the actual role of *Mycoplasma* is uncertain (181). The use of PCR has clearly opened a new era of investigation into the role of bacteria and mycoplasma in RA, but the diversity of species identified in studies to date suggests either that multiple different environmental triggers may lead to chronic arthritis, or that technical refinements are needed in PCR methodology to increase specificity and reduce false-positive results.

Interest in viral candidates is also increasing, fueled by new technology. Earlier studies, both published and unpublished, were conflicting but, on balance, predominantly negative (1). The most credible current candidates continue to be parvovirus B19, rubella, retroviruses, and herpesviruses, including EBV and CMV, with others being less likely candidates (1,4,182,183). Increased synovial cellular immune responses suggested that mumps and adenovirus might be involved in RA (184), but no evidence for adenovirus, mumps, or measles was found in other studies (1,185).

Earlier studies of CMV in RA provided conflicting results. Studies using PCR found evidence of CMV in both synovial membrane and fluid and in blood, but they need to be interpreted with caution because CMV is such a common latent infection (1). Expansion of $CD4^{+}CD28^{-}$ T cells in RA was found to be associated with prior CMV infection, and so is probably not significant in the pathogenesis of RA (186). No increased prevalence of CMV antibodies was found in 52 RA patients with Felty syndrome, 15 of whom had large granular lymphocytosis (187). In sum, studies to date do not show any clear role for CMV in RA. Direct evidence for involvement of HSV and other herpesviruses was not found, including using PCR for HSV-1, HSV-2, and human herpesvirus type 6 (HHV-6). Fc-binding proteins of these viruses had been suggested as the stimulus for RF production in RA (1).

Regarding retroviruses, the manifestations of HTLV-1 infection include both oligoarthritis and polyarthritis, as discussed in the previous section and Chapter 129. HTLV-1 antibody studies in RA itself yielded conflicting results, but immunohistochemical evidence of HTLV-1 antigens was found in RA synovial tissues. An HTLV-1-infected SF cell line from an HTLV-1 arthritis patient secreted large amounts of cytokines. Retrovirus-like particles were seen in RA SFs, but other studies with a variety of methods, including PCR, failed to incriminate human retroviruses or other lentiviruses in RA (1). The *tax* gene of HTLV-1 alone, in transgenic mice, can elicit Sjögren syndrome (163) and chronic arthritis resembling RA (164). Therefore, recent data showing threefold increased prevalence of HTLV-1 *tax* antibodies and DNA in peripheral blood of patients with RA as compared with healthy blood donors are intriguing (188). No other gene of HTLV-1 was noted in these patients; thus, a viral origin of this *tax* sequence is unresolved. Multiple endogenous retrovirus transcripts have also been noted in RA, osteoarthritis, and normal synovial tissues (189). As discussed earlier, multiple endogenous retrovirus sequences are normally present in the genome of all humans, but aberrant expression could result in a variety of disease processes, including autoimmunity. Indeed, the L1 retrotransposon appears to be considerably overexpressed in RA synovial fibroblasts (190). This finding may be related to DNA hypomethylation in RA. Another study using PCR found evidence of an infectious retrovirus, provisionally termed HRV-5, in RA. Proviral DNA was found in almost half of the RA synovial tissue samples tested, but also in similar or greater frequency in reactive and psoriatic arthritis, and in osteoarthritis, as well as in RA and SLE blood samples. HRV-5 has not previously been associated with any human disease, nor has its human origin been confirmed (191). In sum, studies to date have not clearly implicated any retrovirus, endogenous or infectious, in the pathogenesis of RA.

Parvoviruses are small DNA viruses that can cause disease in many vertebrate species. The B19 strain causes erythema infectiosum, a rubella-like illness occurring mostly in children and often accompanied, particularly in adults, by a usually self-limited polyarthritis. RF is occasionally present, and the arthritis sometimes becomes chronic, both in adults and children (183,192). Studies of B19 antibody prevalence and viral persistence using PCR did not seem to indicate a pathogenetic role in adult RA (192–196). However, later studies also using serology and PCR did find evidence of B19 infection in patients with RA (197,198), and with arthritis of unknown origin (199). Antibodies to B19 may also cross-react as autoantibodies (200). B19 infection was also implicated in vasculitis (201), but not in that seen in essential mixed cryoglobulinemia (202). In contrast, other recent serologic studies found only a 2.7% (4 of 147) prevalence of recent B19 infection in patients with early inflammatory polyarthritis followed up for 3 years to ascertain their outcome. Three of the four patients appeared to have RA. The investigators concluded that B19 infection could only be causative for a very small proportion of RA, if any (203). Follow-up of 54 patients with recent B19 infection for a mean of 5 years found none with chronic inflammatory disease (204). A PCR study showed a higher prevalence of B19 DNA in synovial tissue from traumatic joint disease than from JRA (205). Taken together, it seems unlikely that parvovirus B19 causes very many cases of RA, or itself results in chronic arthritis.

EBV is a DNA herpesvirus that causes infectious mononucleosis and has been linked etiologically to Burkitt lymphoma and nasopharyngeal carcinoma. It also occasionally causes acute arthritis (206). EBV causes a persistent infection in B lymphocytes both *in vivo*, where proliferation is usually checked by T cells, and *in vitro*, where it is not. It is also a polyclonal B-cell activator. EBV was initially implicated in RA 30 years ago by the presence of anti-EBV antibodies in sera, and subsequent studies have continued to show elevated antibodies to various EBV antigens in RA. Antibodies to EBV-encoded antigens may cross-react with proteins present in host tissues; thus, molecular mimicry may be a mechanism for any role EBV might have in RA. The second line of evidence regarding EBV was that RA blood lymphocytes behaved differently *in vitro*, in particular, transforming into lymphoblastoid cell lines more readily than controls. This appears to be due to abnormal RA T-cell function *in vitro*, which may also be reflected *in vivo* (1,207). Higher EBV-induced *in vitro* immunoglobulin production was found in lymphocytes from patients with more severe RA (208).

Interestingly, EBV-associated lymphoproliferative disease in a patient with RA reversed when methotrexate was discontinued (209). Earlier studies, including some with PCR, did not show increased EBV antigen or DNA in RA tissues, including synovium, compared with controls (1). A higher prevalence of EBV DNA and RNA transcripts was found in RA synovial tissue and fluid, and in blood using PCR and immunohistochemistry (210–213). Recently, a close to tenfold elevation of EBV viral load was documented in peripheral blood mononuclear cells of 84 patients with RA compared to 69 normal controls and 22 patients with rheumatic conditions other than RA (214). An EBV-infected fibroblast cell line was propagated from RA synovial tissue (215). Higher EBV antibody responses continue to be found in RA sera compared with controls (211,213). Further evidence was presented to support the importance of molecular mimicry with an enhanced immune response in RA to the "shared epitope" (QKRAA) found in the host HLA-DRB 1*0401 or *0404 alleles and in the EBV glycoprotein 110 (gp110). This study showed that the epitope is also present in several bacterial species besides *Escherichia coli,* and is recognized by RA patients (215). RA synovial lymphocytes were also shown to recognize EBV antigens, particularly the transactivating proteins (216). Overall, the role of EBV in RA is unclear. It does not seem to be a primary etiologic agent, but may be a cofactor involved in defective immunoregulation or molecular mimicry. However, the abnormalities in EBV handling demonstrated in so many studies over the past 30 years could also be a consequence of immune dysregulation (207). Thus, EBV seems unlikely to be a prime cause of RA, but further studies are needed to determine its role in the disease (1).

Rubella has also been a perennial etiologic candidate in RA for 30 years, and controversial for most of that time. The various positive and negative studies have been summarized in previous editions (1). Rubella has been isolated from RA patients—apparently rubella-specific immune responses have been found, both systemically and locally in the joint—but negative results were obtained in other studies. As summarized above, epidemiologic studies seem to show that chronic arthritis, including RA, is rare following rubella vaccination. Peripheral blood and SF from 54 early RA patients was negative using a PCR sensitive enough to detect five rubella genome copies. One of 46 patients with other arthropathies, mostly ReA, was positive for rubella. Similar low rates of positivity in the RA and control populations were found for measles and mumps as well (185). In other studies of a possible link between rubella and autoimmunity, the interactions of the ribonucleoprotein complexes Ro and La, calreticulin, and the virus were explored (217,218), but no definite mechanisms established. Thus, at present, the balance of evidence for any role of rubella in RA seems to be negative.

Both humoral and cellular immune responses to other viruses have been examined in RA. Antibodies in serum and SF to herpes, measles, and other viruses were generally normal, including in siblings discordant for RA. B cells secreting antibody to various viruses were rarely found in blood and never in synovial tissue. Immunofluorescence revealed elevated measles-specific antibodies in RA sera, but neither this nor elevation of any virus antibody other than EBV has generally been found. RA SF lymphocytes differed from blood lymphocytes in being unable to support HSV replication, apparently due to a cell-to-cell interaction, perhaps mediated by interferon (1).

With regard to cellular responses in RA, earlier studies of blood lymphocytes had not shown virus-specific changes, but synovial lymphocytes may respond specifically, although often to several viruses (168). The local immune response continues to be a promising subject for investigation. In parallel with these generally inconclusive attempts at implicating specific viruses by different methods, several immunologic and other approaches have been used in an attempt to identify an antigen unique to rheumatoid synovial cells, whether or not of microbial origin. These attempts have yielded negative results to date (1). A cluster of 10 patients with RA developing after recombinant hepatitis B vaccination was described. The mechanism was thought to involve MHC class II–mediated T-cell activation in individuals with HLA class II genes expressing the rheumatoid "shared epitope." Certain hepatitis B vaccine peptides could be predicted to bind to the MHC class II molecules, thus triggering T-cell proliferation and activation, leading in some cases to persistent arthritis (219).

In JRA, models for microbial involvement are similar to those in the adult disease. Attempts at implicating specific antigens both in JRA and in other childhood rheumatic diseases were generally negative. Increased serum antibodies to bacterial peptidoglycan and inflammation of the gut were found in JRA and juvenile ankylosing spondylitis (AS). Disease exacerbation in JRA was associated with preceding viral infections, but serum antiviral antibodies were similar to controls. Interferon was not found in JRA sera, but *in vitro* production was similar or increased compared with controls. In contrast to adult RA, both blood and joint lymphocytes from JRA supported HSV growth normally (1).

Earlier studies of rubella in JRA were also conflicting (1,61). Claims of rubella isolation have not been confirmed. Other studies in JRA have provided some data implicating peptidoglycan, influenza A and other viruses, but not retroviruses or rubella (1). EBV infection seemed to trigger adult-onset Still's disease in an elderly woman (220); remission of JRA following varicella infection was also reported (221).

In summary, no firm evidence implicates specific microbial agents in RA or JRA at present. Persistence in RA joint tissues has not been convincingly shown for any microbe, although some of the candidate viruses, such as parvovirus B19 and rubella, could still act as initial triggers for RA. The evidence implicating other microbial agents, such as bacterial HSPs and EBV, suggests a mechanism involving molecular mimicry or cross-reactive antigens, or perhaps less antigen-specific activation of the immune system. Clearly, the most promising avenue of current investigation is the application of PCR to detection of microbial agents, particularly bacteria, in RA tissues. Another exciting area is the shared epitope in host HLA-DR molecules and various microbial agents such as EBV, with the potential to generate chronic synovitis via molecular mimicry. However, these and other studies directly or indirectly implicating other microbes all require confirmation.

Seronegative Spondyloarthropathies

The seronegative SpAs refer to a group of diseases that share several common features: (a) association with HLA-B27; (b) asymmetric oligoarthritis; (c) axial involvement, particularly of the sacroiliac joints; (d) enthesitis; and (e) characteristic extraarticular features, including acute anterior uveitis (222). The role of infection as a triggering factor is implicated with varying degrees of certainty among the subcategories: probable in ReA, possible in AS, and unresolved in psoriatic arthritis and enteropathic arthritis. The very definition of ReA—a sterile synovitis following an extraarticular infection—clearly implicates infection in its inclusion criteria. The SpAs and ReA, in particular, continue to occupy the conceptual ground somewhere between septic arthritis and the autoimmune rheumatic diseases such as RA.

There have been attempts to bring more order into the nomenclature of the SpAs (223–226). The historical approach has been established in the literature, but in the case of Reiter syndrome, the term has largely been abandoned because of its imprecise definition and because of the the role of Reiter himself in Nazi Germany during the second World War. The etiologic classification has the most intrinsic appeal and has fueled the search for definitive links between particular pathogens and ReA. Many of these studies represent guilt by association, in that the demonstration of a particular immune response profile by serology or cellular responses comes to define the identity of the causative pathogen even when there is no direct demonstration of the organism or its antigens in synovial tissues or fluid. However, the predictive power of a diagnostic test critically depends on the prevalence of positives in the healthy population at large (227).What constitutes the appropriate control group for these studies has not been consistently defined or applied. The mechanistic approach to classification of the SpAs awaits a better understanding of the molecular and cellular mechanisms underlying the chronic inflammation, but advances in clinical and experimental ReA hold the promise for this in the near future. Recent studies in ReA and undifferentiated oligoarthritis indicate that about 50% of such cases can be attributed to a specific pathogen by a combination of culture and serology, the predominant organisms being *Salmonella, Yersinia,* and *Chlamydia* (228). Species-specific analysis of serologic response to pathogens may further enhance this detection rate (229).

Studies on the epidemiology of ReA have shed new light on the frequency of this complication of enteric infections. A prospective study of the incidence of inflammatory joint disease in Sweden found that the annual incidence of ReA (28 per 100,000 population) exceeded that of RA (24 per 100,000 population), emphasizing the importance of ReA in the overall burden of rheumatic diseases (230). Studies on both sporadic (231) and outbreak (232) *Salmonella typhimurium* infections have further substantiated the role of *Salmonella* in triggering ReA. The frequency of this event has generally been in the range of 10% (233), but a recent study of 91 individuals exposed to food-borne *Salmonella enteritidis* reported that 17 developed ReA, so this may occur more frequently than previously thought (234). In a population-based study, it was determined that ReA is common after *Campylobacter* infections, with an annual incidence of 4.3 per 100,000 (235). These incidence figures are no doubt strongly influenced by the population under study. ReA appears to be more prevalent in Alaskan Eskimo populations (236), whereas the incidence of ReA after a *Salmonella* outbreak appears to be lower in children than adults (237).

One observation that may indirectly implicate microbial antigens of gut origin is the coexistence of inflammation in the GI tract and the joint. This relates both to postdysenteric ReA as well as to the arthritis associated with inflammatory bowel disease. It would appear that inflammatory lesions in the gut occur in 68% of patients with SpA, including patients with classical AS and no history of GI symptomatology (238–240). There is a correlation between the resolution of GI and joint inflammation, and this relationship may reflect altered bowel permeability and repeated microbial antigenemia as a mechanism, but this awaits formal proof. The range of pathogens may be broader than those classically linked to SpA (*Yersinia, Salmonella, Shigella, Chlamydia*), but often these organisms are not associated with the common clinical features summarized above.

More sophisticated techniques, such as PCR, may broaden the definition of the arthritogenic pathogens even further. Poststreptococcal ReA continues to attract the attention of investigators (241) and is the most common of arthritogenic bacteria beyond the gram-negative pathogens listed. Poststreptococcal arthritis in children is a potential predecessor of rheumatic heart disease, although the relationship with acute rheumatic fever is not clearly defined (242). A recent report of six adult patients with poststreptococcal ReA highlighted the important contribution of this entity in the differential diagnosis of acute polyarthritis (243). Another discriminating feature between poststreptococcal ReA and the more common forms is its association with HLA-DR alleles (DRB1*01) rather than with HLA-B27, suggesting that the cellular basis for the inflammation in the two syndromes may differ fundamentally (244). Other microbial triggers that have been implicated in association with arthritis recently have included bacille Calmette-Guérin (BCG) (245,246), HBV vaccination (247), Lyme vaccination (248), enterotoxigenic *E. coli* (249), and a broad range of parasites (250).

Studies have attempted to define the relative contribution of different pathogens to the general picture of ReA. However, the lack of universally agreed-upon classification criteria continues to pose problems for population studies of incidence and prevalence. In an urban sexually transmitted disease (STD) clinic, it was observed that 4.1% of patients with genital infection or inflammation had objective ReA, and chlamydial or nongonococcal STD syndromes accounted for 88% of these cases (251). In a recent population-based study to assess the relative contribution of different organisms to new-onset arthritis, *Campylobacter* predominated, with lesser roles ascribed to *Chlamydia trachomatis, B. burgdorferi, Chlamydia pneumoniae,* and parvovirus B19 (252).

One of the messages from these population-based surveys is that the prevalence of unclassified SpA and its natural history and prognosis remains an important unresolved area.

The SpAs represent an interplay of environmental and genetic factors. Recent population studies have begun to unravel new aspects of this dynamic interaction. In a study of twins with AS, it was concluded that genetic factors accounted for 97% of the determining influence, suggesting that an environmental trigger for the disease is likely to be ubiquitous and may contribute little to the population variance (253). When one includes the broader spectrum of the SpAs and the interplay between infection and genetics, the picture may be very different. In a large study addressing the prevalence of SpA in HLA-B27-positive and -negative blood donors, there was a prevalence of 13.6% among B27-positive individuals and 0.7% in the B27-negative population (254). The relative risk for developing SpA in B27-positive subjects was calculated as 20.7. Taking into account the frequency of B27 in the population studied, it was concluded that the SpAs have a prevalence of 1.9%, making this group of arthropathies among the most common rheumatic diseases. Other genetically-defined modulators of immune response, particularly those impacting host innate immunity, are attractive candidates for non-MHC genes that may contribute to disease susceptibility. Mannose-binding lectin was examined but did not differentiate ReA patients from controls (255). On the other hand, enhanced gene expression of host defense scavenger receptors was demonstrated in both ReA and RA patients (256). This continues to be an area of active investigation.

Clinical studies have provided a more complete picture of the manifestations and the clinical course of ReA. Thomson et al. (257) reported on a large cohort of *Salmonella* ReA patients at a 5-year follow-up interval after the initial infection. In 9 of the 27 patients, the arthritis resolved within 4 months of onset. Eighteen patients continued to have symptoms 5 years after onset, and in four of these the symptoms were severe enough to force a change of work. At the 5-year point, 37% had objective changes in the joints. These important long-term sequelae have rendered the issue of antibiotic therapy an important area for study. A 3-month, double-blind, randomized, placebo-controlled study found no benefit of ciprofloxacin treatment in patients with ReA and undifferentiated oligoarthritis (258). In subgroup analysis, ciprofloxacin was better than placebo in *Chamydia*-induced ReA but not in *Salmonella*- or *Yersinia*-induced ReA. This general impression was borne out in a report that lymecycline decreased the duration of acute arthritis in *Chlamydia*-induced ReA but not in other ReA (259). Of 17 patients followed for 10 years in this study, 1 patient had AS, 3 had radiographic sacroiliitis, and 3 had radiographic changes in peripheral joints, but long-term lymecycline treatment did not change the natural history of the disease. A 3-month trial of doxycycline for chronic SpA was no better than placebo for subsequent pain or functional status, but few patients had a causative organism identified (260). At present, the consensus that *Chlamydia*-induced ReA alone may be responsive to antibiotic treatment raises the interesting question that the pathogenesis of acute and chronic ReA induced by this organism may be very different from the enteric pathogens, but the critical differences at the cellular level have not been defined.

The most direct causal proof for microbes in ReA derives from demonstration of microbial antigens in the joint. The case for persisting intraarticular pathogens is strongest for *Chlamydia,* and several investigators have detected *Chlamydia* DNA or RNA by PCR in joints of patients with postchlamydial ReA. In an experimental model, it has been shown that synoviocyte-packaged *Chlamydia* can induce a chronic aseptic arthritis, and that the synoviocyte can serve as an important reservoir of microbial antigens within the joint tissues long after the organism can be cultured from the joint (261). There is some evidence that these persisting organisms in the joints are metabolically altered, and may have entered a quiescent phase that renders them more resistant to antibiotic treatment. This has been shown for *Chlamydia pneumoniae* (262), which, in terms of viability and metabolic activity, has been shown to have characteristics comparable to *C. trachomatis*. There is however a lower prevalence of *C. pneumoniae* DNA compared with *C. trachomatis* DNA in synovial tissues (263). But the significance of such findings for pathogenesis of joint disease remains an ongoing discussion (264). *Chlamydia* nucleic acids have been found in the synovium of some asymptomatic patients (265). On the other hand, bacterial DNA or RNA from a wide spectrum of bacteria, including species not previously associated with ReA, have been demonstrated in chronic arthritis patients in reports from Latin America (266,267), England (268), and the United States (269). DNA from a number of different strains of bacteria has been detected in the same joint in some patients. Thus, although the application of PCR technology has heightened the sensitivity of this quest, it has raised important questions about the specificity of the results. In addition to PCR analysis, gas chromatography–mass spectrometry has been applied to search for bacterial components in joint tissues (270). Using this technique, investigators have demonstrated that a bacterial component, muramic acid, is detected in synovial tissues from a few patients with advanced RA or OA. Once again, enhanced sensitivity has complicated the analysis of specificity (271). These different approaches to "microbe hunting" in the joints are summarized in Table 30.4. It is evident that positive results are not confined to the ReA category.

It is unresolved how these organisms gain access to the joints, but leukocytes that have internalized these pathogens may display altered migratory patterns that would accentuate homing to the joints (272). Those studies support the notion of a viable organism present, at least transiently, in the early stages of the synovitis. It is speculated that this may reflect defective killing of the organism, either by failure to internalize the pathogen or to effectively initiate intracellular killing. The cellular response to chlamydial infection has been studied by microarray techniques, and 18 genes appeared to be selectively up-regulated following infection with *C. trachomatis* (273). Infection of synoviocytes with *Chlamydia* induces IL-6 production (274) and HLA class I expression (275). The latter appears to be mediated by induction of interferon-β (IFN-β), which in turn stimulates synthesis of ISFG3γ, a transcription factor participating in the regulation of the HLA-1 gene. This host/microbial interaction has proved a fertile ground for exploring noncanonical roles for HLA-27, the latter being raised in part because of the sustained difficulty in using conventional structure and function for a mechanistic hypothesis of how B27 contributes to disease. Using transfected U937 cell lines, it has been observed that B27-positive cells kill *Salmonella* less efficiently than control cells (276), and that lipopolysaccharide (LPS) stimulation of these transfected cells suggests that HLA-B27 enhances nuclear factor κB activation and TNF-α secretion (277). In contrast, some investigators have found that HLA-B27 expression neither alters infection nor replication of *C. trachomatis* in cell lines (278). An alternative approach to studying transfected cell lines has been to analyze host/microbial interactions in the context of synoviocytes harvested from HLA-B27-positive patients (279). Using this approach, it was observed that HLA did not play a direct role either in internalization of *S. typhimurium*, or in the kinetics of intracellular killing of these organisms. In some patients, there was a paradoxic response to IFN-γ, which may provide a clue to aberrant handling of pathogens in the joint, but this is unresolved at present.

Indirect evidence implicating microbes in SpA has depended largely on the immunologic footprint left behind by the culprit, as reflected in the humoral or cellular immune response of the host. Serologic studies continue to contribute to this body of evidence. In the case of *Chlamydia*, the high prevalence of antichlamydial antibodies in the normal population (280) has led investigators to seek an antibody profile with sufficient sensitivity and specificity to be of diagnostic value. It has been proposed that IgG and IgA antibodies against major outer membrance protein (MOMP)-derived peptides and pgp3 may be useful in the diagnosis of *Chlamydia*-induced ReA (281). On the other hand, ReA may reflect a failure of host response to the infection. The male predominance of ReA may be related to a deficient humoral immune response to *Chlamydia*, secondarily leading to systemic dissemination of the organism (282). There has been continued interest in the possible role of *Klebsiella* in SpA. ELISA analysis earlier indicated that there was an increase

TABLE 30.4. *Detection of microbes in joint tissues by different methods*

	RA	ReA	AS	OA	Septic arthritis
Culture	–	–	–	–	+
EM	–	+[a]	ND	ND	+
IF/IHC	–	+[b]	ND	ND	+
PCR	+[c]/–[d]	+[a]	+[e]/–[f]	+[a]	+
GC-MS	+[d]	+[g]	ND	+[d]	+

Culture, EM, IF, and IHC are used for detecting intact organisms or their antigenic fragments; PCR for their nucleic acids; and GC-MS for their cell wall components.

[a]*Chlamydia* only.
[b]*Chlamydia, Salmonella*, and *Yersinia*.
[c]Pan-bacterial PCR.
[d]Reference 270.
[e]In juvenile AS patients.
[f]Nested PCR.
[g]Detection of muramic acid.

AS, ankylosing spondylitis; EM, electron microscopy; GC-MS, gas chromatography–mass spectroscopy; IF/IHC, immunofluorescence/immunohistochemistry; ND, not done; OA, osteoarthritis; PCR, polymerase chain reaction; RA, rheumatoid arthritis; ReA, reactive arthritis.

in serum IgG against particular capsular polysaccharides of *Klebsiella pneumoniae* in patients with AS. Underlying gut inflammation has been demonstrated in patients with SpA even in the absence of GI symptoms, and one study observed a correlation between gut inflammation and increased IgA antibodies to *Klebsiella* in patients with axial, but not peripheral, AS (283). Recent approaches to the specificity of this antibody response have addressed LPS, capsular polysaccharides, and bacterial HSPs (284–287). These findings are consistent with the notion of occult inflammation in the gut and altered bowel permeability, but provide a note of caution indicating the importance of including a range of control bacterial antigens in serologic studies of AS before ascribing a causal role to the gut microbes. A recent study of familial AS examined both humoral and cellular immune responses against *Klebsiella pneumoniae*. Although confirming that increased serum antibodies against *Klebsiella* are common, there was no specificity of this immune response for AS, arguing against a direct pathogenic role for this organism (288).

In acute anterior uveitis (AAU), a disease with an independent association with HLA-B27, there have been inconsistent results regarding anti-*Klebsiella* antibody profiles. One study observed higher IgA antibodies against *Klebsiella* in B27-negative patients with AAU (289). Patients with AAU have been shown to demonstrate increased frequency of antibodies to *Yersinia enterocolitica* compared with controls (290), and there is a significant cross-reactivity of anti-*Yersinia* antibodies with *Salmonella*, suggesting that different gram-negative bacteria may initiate overlapping immune responses in the initiation of the disease. All such data must be viewed in the context of the level of antibodies in the local control population, and in some countries this may be a significant background effect (291). A parallel approach to serologic testing has been to examine markers of host defense against these pathogens. It has been observed that patients with ReA have increased serum and SF levels of LPS binding protein, which may be an important intermediary factor in the generation of protective or deleterious cytokines such as TNF-α.

Analysis of cellular immune responses has continued to shed light both on potential triggering pathogens as well as on effector mechanisms. Isolation of T-cell clones from SF of patients with post-*Yersinia* ReA identified the triggering antigens to be proteins secreted by the organism, including a phosphatase, YopH, and determined that the clones utilized a limited set of T-cell receptor variable region gene segments (292). Using a similar approach for post-*Chlamydia* ReA, it has been observed that two antigens were immunodominant: the 57-kd HSP and the 18-kd histone-like protein Hc1 (293). Mapping the epitope in Hc1 using synthetic peptides identified a peptide containing a sequence motif compatible with binding to HLA-DR1, the restricting element for the T-cell clones. There has been an extensive body of evidence to support the notion of local generation of SF T cells specific for the triggering bacterium. A recent study addressed the corresponding T-cell reactivity in peripheral blood (294). In 24 of 87 patients with a bacteria-specific T-cell proliferative response in SF, there was a corresponding peripheral blood response to the same bacterium. The longitudinal profile of SF T-cell reactivity was studied in 28 patients with ReA (295). At different time points the same bacterium was always recognized in arthritis triggered by *Chlamydia, Shigella,* and *B. burgdorferi*, with a significant degree of variation in the magnitude of the proliferative response. Only the *Yersinia*-specific responses changed specificity, suggesting that the proliferative response to *Yersinia* is nonspecific in some patients. An analysis of the specificity of $CD4^+$ T-cell clones for *Yersinia* peptides was reported (296). Using overlapping synthetic peptides from *Yersinia* 60-kd HSP (hsp60), the specificity of the clones identified a core epitope that was presented in an MHC promiscuous manner, and this epitope was almost identical with the B27-restricted epitope of *Yersinia* hsp60. Analysis of $CR4^+$ T-cell responses to *Chlamydia trachomatis* revealed that in patients with ReA there were abundant blood and SF T cells specific for the 60-kd cysteine-rich outer membrane protein of *C. trachomatis*, and that this epitope was presented by HLA-DRB1*0401 (297). Expression libraries have also been used to provide a more comprehensive analysis of chlamydial antigenic recognition by $CD4^+$ T cells (S46), and flow cytometry may provide a method to quantitate the number of antigen-specific T cells against the triggering pathogen in ReA (298).

Analysis of T-cell subsets with respect to cytokine profiles is an additional method for studying the link between infection and ReA. Exposure to different pathogens can stimulate at least two patterns of cytokine production by $CD4^+$ T cells (T_H1 and T_H2). It has been long held that T_H1 cells mediate a protective role against intracellular pathogens. Thus, it would seem appropriate that these cells would be central in clinical complications of such infections. In a study of 11 patients with ReA, it was observed that stimulation of SF mononuclear cells resulted in secretion of low amounts of IFN-γ and TNF-α but high amounts of IL-10 (299). IL-10 was responsible for suppression of IFN-γ and TNF-α as judged by the effect of adding IL-10 or anti-IL-10 to the cells. The suppression of T_H1-like cytokines is likely mediated through suppression of IL-12 synthesis. In the synovial tissues of these patients, a higher number of cells were positive for the T_H2 cytokine IL-4, compared with the number of IFN-γ-secreting cells. This IL-10/IL-12 balance, resulting in a predominance of T_H2 cytokines, may contribute to the persistence of bacteria in the joint. In comparison with RA, SF levels of TNF-α in ReA are lower, despite comparable levels of IL-2 receptor, again implicating a relative deficiency of protective, antimicrobial cytokines in the local environment (300). The source of these cytokines may not only be the infiltrating immunoreactive mononuclear cells, but also the resident synoviocytes. When human synoviocytes are infected with *Chlamydia trachomatis in vitro*, there is generation of IL-6, transforming growth factor-β (TGF-β), and GM-CSF (301). The cells respond to IFN-γ with secretion of TNF-α, so this represents another contributory population of cells in the joint, in addition to B cells and T cells. Whether these cytokine profiles are primarily genetically defined is an important unanswered question (302). The non-B27 genes that are contributing to disease susceptibility in SpA patients have not been characterized adequately for a definitive answer. The TNF dependence of chronic inflammation in the spine draws indirect support from the dramatic changes that follow the institution of anti-TNF therapies in these patients. Yet the effect of a cytokine in the setting of infection can be helpful or harmful, depending on the window of time under observation. In studies of murine experimental *Yersinia*-induced arthritis, it has been observed that TNF-α is deleterious for the host in the acute phase of the infection, because there is a TNF-mediated apoptosis of $CD4^+$ cells (303). However, in the chronic phase of the disease, TNF-α is helpful for host defense, because TNF-mediated production of nitric oxide plays a critical role in clearance of the pathogen (304). It is recognized that reactivation of tuberculosis can occur following the institution of anti-TNF therapy in SpA patients, but experience to date has not unmasked quiescent pathogens in the treated patients in this population. Clearly vigilance is warranted as long-term experience with these agents grows.

The strong association of HLA-B27 with SpA has indirectly implicated microbial antigen–specific, MHC class I–restricted $CD8^+$ cytotoxic T lymphocytes (CTLs) as playing a role in the pathogenesis of these diseases. It is important to note in this context that $CD8^+$ T cells in SF may express NK cell receptors (305). Such cells reflect a high degree of heterogeneity in the expression of NK cell receptors, which may modulate their cytotoxicity and contribute to disease pathogenesis as a result. The fact that certain subtypes of HLA-B27 are more strongly associated with SpA than others has implicated T-cell specificities in a more precise fashion (306,307). The HLA-B*2709 subtype, although differing by a single amino acid (His116→Asp116) from the strongly AS-associated subtype B27*2705, is not found in AS patients. It has been shown that $CD8^+$ T cells can distinguish between these two B27 subtypes when presenting the same epitope derived from EBV LMP-2, suggesting that the subtypes may differ in presenting an arthritogenic peptide derived from microbial sources (308) A recent approach using peptide binding has addressed what might differentiate HLA-B*2704 (associated with SpA) from HLA-B*2706 (not associated with SpA). The main structural feature of peptides differentially bound to B*2704 was the presence of C-terminal Tyr or Arg together with a strong preference for aliphatic/aromatic P3 residues. This provides a distinctive profile of B*2704 and B*2706 binding that correlates with their differential association with SpA. An analysis of the specificity of T-cell clones demonstrated that target cells pulsed with *Yersinia* hsp60, but not with other *Yersinia* proteins, were successfully lysed by the CTLs, and that this killing was restricted by B27 (309). It was also observed that a single nonamer, 321 to 329, derived from *Yersinia* hsp60 was the dominant epitope in this recognition event. In another approach to this interaction, it was shown that T cells themselves can be infected with *Yersinia*, and that infected CTLs have a reduced lytic capacity against syngeneic and allogeneic infected target cells, implicating a breakdown in immune surveillance that could occur by this mechanism during the course of gram-negative bacterial infection (310). Using a computer-generated algorithm that incorporated HLA-B27 binding motifs and proteosome-generated motifs, an approach to identifying immunodominant peptides from *C. trachomatis* has been undertaken (311). Nine peptides so identified proved to be stimulatory for $CD8^+$ T cells, and many of these same peptides were recognized by $CD8^+$ T cells derived from patients with ReA. Peptide binding to these T cells was also demonstrated by tetramer staining. This may prove to be a valuable approach to identifying key peptides from arthritogenic pathogens.

Whether these microbial peptides share functional homology with self proteins, such as B27 itself, has remained unresolved. There is some supportive evidence for this notion of molecular mimicry in SpA (312,313), but the theory leaves important questions unanswered. For example, the target organ specificity of AS remains unexplained, as does the apparent frequency of homologous sequences, even among bacteria not commonly thought to be arthritogenic on clinical grounds. An immunodominant epitope from the *S. typhimurium* GroEL molecule was recognized by $CD8^+$ CTLs after natural infection in mice (314), and these CTLs cross-reacted with peptides derived from mouse hsp60. This provided a model that might link bacterial immunity with autoimmunity, although several aspects of this relationship remain unexplained (315). A dodecamer derived from the intracytoplasmic tail of HLA-B27 was found to be a natural ligand for disease-associated subtypes (B*2702, B*2704, B*2705) but not for non-disease-associated subtypes (B*2706, B*2709). This peptide showed striking homology with a region of the DNA primase from *Chlamydia trachomatis*. This indicated that some mimicry exists between B27-derived and chlamydial peptides that might relate to cross-reactivity of immune responses against microbial and endogenous antigens (316). In a study addressing CTL recognition of B27, it was observed in an animal model that prior expansion of an immune response against HLA-B27 results in a reduced threshold for generating a primary anti-*Chlamydia* CTL response (317). A subsequent study applied this system in B27-transgenic animals (318). Such animals are tolerant of immunization with B27 DNA, but if splenocytes from these animals are exposed to *Chlamydia in vitro*, then autoreactive CTLs with specificity for B27 are generated. The autoreactive epitope of HLA-B27 involves the lysine residue at position 70 in a critical way. This indicates a dynamic interrelationship between the pathogen and host B27 that may have important implications for the pathogenesis of ReA. These interactions might result in a break in self-tolerance, or perhaps an impaired clearance of the organism on the basis of impaired recognition of the organism as non-self.

Systemic Connective Tissue Disease

Systemic Lupus Erythematosus

Interest in the role of microbes in SLE, particularly viruses, has declined, both because of their secondary role in New Zealand mouse disease and because of many negative studies over the past 20 years (1). Earlier anaplasma and mycoplasma isolations from SLE patients have not been confirmed. Regarding viruses, the tubuloreticular structures found by electron microscopy in many SLE patients are not thought to be viral, but rather secondary to elevated IFN, levels frequently observed in sera from patients with active SLE. This initially suggested an antiviral response, but elevated levels were also found in other CTDs, and the IFN is an unusual acid-labile or leukocyte-derived type. Antibodies to IFN have been found in SLE, and may also be deposited in the kidney. Both IFN and the inclusions are also found in patients with AIDS. Interferons are a heterogeneous group of substances, including various kinds of viral- and immune-induced compounds, which can alter many cellular, including lymphocyte, functions. It is not clear whether the elevated levels in CTD are a cause or a result of lymphocyte dysfunction, but it seems more likely they are a direct result of lymphocyte activation rather than of viral infection. Various other electron microscopic inclusions have been seen in SLE tissues, but none is convincingly viral (1).

Retroviruses were initially implicated in the autoimmune disease of New Zealand mice, but it now appears that any viral pathogenetic role is secondary. Earlier studies in SLE, principally using immunofluorescence and radioimmunoassays with antiviral antisera, suggested that retrovirus expression was enhanced and that virus-related antigens were present in renal glomeruli. Specificity was difficult to prove, however, especially because these viruses acquire envelopes as they bud from host cells, incorporating and adsorbing components from both the cell and the culture medium. Thus, the antiviral reagents used invariably contained nonviral reactivities that often persisted even after extensive absorption. Antibody binding to the carbohydrate moiety of viral glycoproteins was shown to be one source of false-positive reactions (1).

Many other studies have not shown increased retrovirus expression in SLE. Some showed no difference between patients with SLE and normal individuals, including analysis of the retrovirus-like particles in placentas, their immunohistologic reactivity with viral antisera, and serum antibodies to retroviruses using cytotoxicity or viral enzyme inhibition. One study did show baboon endogenous virus enzyme inhibition by 20% of SLE sera, but most studies showed no evidence of viral expression. Thus, a pathogenetic role for any of the subhuman retroviruses studied in the past seems unlikely.

More recent studies have applied HTLV-1 reagents to the study of SLE. An increased prevalence of high IgM anti-HTLV-1 antibodies was found using enzyme immunoassay and protein immunoblotting. In contrast, IgG antibodies to HTLV-1 were not elevated in this or in other studies. Apparent antibody reactivity with both HTLV-1 and HIV antigens was found in SLE sera. Another study showed reactivity of unspecified autoimmune disease sera with murine retrovirus proteins using immunoblotting. Antibodies to HTLV-2 have not been found in SLE sera. Neither HTLV-1 or -2 nor HIV proviral sequences were found in SLE peripheral blood leukocytes, but protooncogene expression was increased in both SLE and other autoimmune diseases. Antibody reactivities to endogenous retroviruses are increased in both SLE and other autoimmune diseases, however (31,78,319). The latter probably reflects generalized lymphocyte activation, which can occur with retrovirus infection. Recent studies emphasize the interpretative difficulties caused by the wide reactivity of antibodies to HIV p24 gag protein, including demonstration of a significant cross-reaction with the Sm antigen. This suggests that molecular mimicry may be involved, but does not indicate which antigen, viral or cellular, was recognized first. It is clear that occasional SLE patients have been infected with HTLV-1, but this seems to occur at the same rate as the general population, and its effect on the course of the disease is unclear. Thus, the studies to date fail to implicate HTLV-1 in SLE but rather, as in multiple sclerosis, suggest the possibility that a related retrovirus might be involved. Considering the recent isolation of the human retroviruses, their tropism for T cells and synoviocytes (78,320), and their ability to cause immunoregulatory disturbances in both humans and animals, these viruses remain major etiologic candidates for SLE.

Other viruses, viral antigens, and viral genomes that have not been found as frequently, or at all, in SLE tissues include myxoviruses such as measles and influenza, papoviruses, and, recently, hepatitis B antigen in renal biopsies. Measuring specific antibody levels has not provided any clues either. Serum antibody levels, particularly against measles and rubella, are often increased in patients with SLE compared with controls, but this seems to be part of the general overproduction of antibodies so characteristic of the disease. As in the retrovirus studies, a major problem with these virus antibody tests is that they may also measure antibodies to nonviral antigens (medium, cellular components), which may also be increased in SLE.

There is an increased prevalence in SLE of antibodies to EBV early antigen, and, in a recent study, to the EB nuclear antigens EBNA-2 and EBNA-3, but not to synthetic peptides derived from EBNA-1. Two thirds of SLE patients had IgG antibodies to HSV-1, and one third to varicella-zoster virus. None had IgM antibodies, but controls were not included. Mothers of babies with congenital heart block, who may have SLE, had a slightly increased prevalence of CMV antibodies, but not of EBV capsid antibodies, compared with normal controls. Based on a PCR-based detection of viral DNA, prevalence of EBV infection may be increased among young patients with SLE (74). However, a recent epidemiologic study found no association between self-reported history of infectious mononucleosis and SLE risk. Further analysis provided little evidence of an increasing risk with older age at occurrence of mononucleosis (as a marker of late EBV infection) compared with people who reported no history of mononucleosis (75). The prevalence of hepatitis B antibody was increased in SLE, but not in RA, JRA, polymyalgia rheumatica, temporal arteritis, or other CTDs; this was not found in another study (1).

The response to immunization with both bacterial and viral antigens often seems to be blunted in patients with SLE, both *in vivo* and *in vitro*. The nature of the defect is not clear, but theoretically might reflect prior commitment to other antigens. The finding of antibodies to polynucleotides following viral illness was suggested as a possible mechanism for their occurrence in SLE and other CTDs. Cellular reactivity to viral antigens was generally reduced in SLE, probably owing to a generalized functional lymphocyte defect rather than to a failure of specific immune recognition (1).

The La (SS-B), Ro (SS-A), and Sm autoantibodies found in SLE and other CTDs recognize protein antigens in intracellular ribonucleoprotein particles, including snRNPs. The La antigen, in particular, appears to play a role in the functions of cellular messenger RNA (mRNA), but also binds to viral mRNAs, including EBV, adenovirus, vesicular stomatitis viruses, and, in a recent study, CMV. As noted previously, cross-reactivity was found between Sm and HIV p24; similar findings were also reported in Sjögren syndrome, as discussed below. Antibodies to native DNA in SLE sera inhibited adenovirus DNA synthesis *in vitro*. Thus, these autoantibodies react with cellular components that may also be involved in replication of several other viruses (1). U1 snRNP was shown to influence the formation of HIV-1 env mRNA that is regulated by rev of HIV-1 (321). Moreover, HTLV-1 p40/*tax* was found to influence the expression of novel autoantigens (151), raising the possibility that a viral infection may lead to autoantigenicity of self proteins. Whether viruses are actually involved in induction of specific autoantibodies is unknown, but a study indicates a possible mechanism by which viruses could trigger autoimmune abnormalities. Transgenic mice expressing the cell membrane–associated glycoprotein of vesicular stomatitis virus (VSV-G) are tolerant to this virus-derived self antigen. Autoantibodies to VSV-G cannot be induced by immunization with recombinant VSV-G but are triggered by infection with wild-type VSV. These results indicate that helper T-cell tolerance can be broken by viral infection, possibly through presentation of cryptic antigenic epitopes (322).

Earlier studies of antilymphocyte and other autoantibodies in family members of SLE patients, human contacts of canine SLE, and canine contacts of human SLE suggested possible horizontal transmission of an infectious agent. Subsequent studies comparing microbial antibody titers in SLE and examining households with canine SLE have not supported this idea. The origin of the autoantibodies is also heterogeneous; they can result from viral infection, but they may simply reflect disordered immunoregulation in SLE. More recent studies add parvovirus B19 to the infections known to induce anti-DNA or antilymphocyte antibodies transiently and, again, suggest anti-DNA antibodies can be induced by contact with SLE blood specimens. Whether viruses are actually involved in induction of any of these autoantibodies in SLE is unknown, but these studies indicate a possible mechanism by which viruses could trigger autoimmune abnormalities (1).

Despite the lack of evidence implicating infectious agents, it is still likely that SLE requires an initiating event, probably environmental, and possibly infectious. In the setting of genetically-determined perturbations of the immune system, an infectious trigger might be a trivial event clinically. Once triggered, the immunologic abnormalities might be self-perpetuating so that the persistent infection and foreign antigens, as found in hepatitis B vasculitis, might not be needed in SLE. Current evidence does not firmly implicate any specific microbial agent, but, on a theoretic basis, the human retroviruses are particularly attractive candidates. The data actually implicating them may reflect molecular mimicry and thus do not necessarily indicate a pathogenic role for infection.

Polymyositis and Dermatomyositis

The possible role of *Toxoplasma gondii* and picornaviruses continues to be investigated. Approximately 15% of patients with polymyositis have high serum *Toxoplasma* antibody levels, many with specific IgM antibodies, suggesting current or recent infection. Isolation attempts have been negative, however, and the clinical response to specific antimicrobial treatment equivocal. Immunofluorescence has occasionally demonstrated the microorganism in muscle. The etiologic role of toxoplasmosis remains to be established, because latent infection is common and could be secondarily activated by the myositis (1).

Various inclusions, possibly viral, have been found in myositis using the electron microscope; the most convincing are the crystalline picornavirus-like arrays. One study found these inclusions could be digested with amylase, however, suggesting they were in fact glycogen. Virus isolation attempts and antibody studies have generally not been revealing, but in some patients have implicated coxsackieviruses, which belong to the Picornaviridae family. More recent studies, particularly in juvenile dermatomyositis, have shown a higher prevalence of coxsackie B virus antibodies, and the presence of viral RNA in muscle. Another type of picornavirus, echoviruses, can cause a polymyositis-like clinical picture in hypogammaglobulinemia. The myositis-specific Jo-1 and other autoantibody specificities inhibited different aminoacyl-tRNA synthetases, cellular enzymes that can be involved in the replication of RNA viruses like picornaviruses and that also share sequences with EBV proteins. Clinically, autoantibodies to these enzymes were linked to interstitial lung disease. This work is analogous to that discussed previously showing that La and other autoantibodies in SLE recognize cellular nucleic acid proteins that can be involved in viral replication. Another point in favor of a role for coxsackieviruses is the excellent model of myositis in mice caused by the B1 virus.

Influenza virus occasionally causes a severe acute myositis, but may also cause a syndrome called benign acute childhood myositis, which may be a mild form of polymyositis. Inflammatory myopathy has occurred as a manifestation of both AIDS and HTLV-1 infection, but this association has also been disputed. Polymyositis has also been associated rarely with hepatitis B and BCG vaccination. Viruses have also been implicated occasionally in other forms of inflammatory muscle disease, but a recent study of mumps in inclusion body myositis yielded negative results. Polymyositis has occurred as an early manifestation of AIDS and HTLV-1 infection (152,153).

That such a variety of infectious agents has been implicated, but so rarely and in such a variety of myopathies, suggests again that the infectious triggers may be different in different patients. The underlying mechanisms may also be different, varying from direct invasion of muscle to various immunoregulatory disturbances. To date, *Toxoplasma*, coxsackieviruses, influenza virus, and perhaps the retroviruses have been implicated in myositis, but only in some cases.

Other Connective Tissue Diseases

Necrotizing vasculitis without evidence of hepatitis B infection presumably has other causes, possibly also infectious. Some adults presented with serous otitis media and episcleritis, a picture suggesting infection, but virus antibody studies have been inconclusive. *Streptococcus*, rubella vaccination, cytomegalovirus, and trichinosis have been implicated rarely in systemic vasculitis, but in most non–hepatitis B cases no agent can be identified. Herpes simplex and HTLV-1 have been implicated in cutaneous vasculitis, as has varicella-zoster in central nervous system vasculitis. Recent studies added EBV and HIV to the list. The purported efficacy of sulfamethoxazole-trimethoprim in some patients with Wegener granulomatosis suggested an infectious cause.

Infantile polyarteritis is the most severe form of Kawasaki disease, also called the mucocutaneous lymph node syndrome. It has become a major epidemic disease in Japan. Many cases appear to be linked to previous respiratory illnesses, but no specific agents have been identified. Various causes have been proposed, including rickettsia, rug shampoo mobilizing house dust mites, a variant strain *Propionibacterium acnes* spread by mites, a feline virus transmitted by fleas, and retroviruses. The latter were implicated by transient viral reverse transcriptase production from cultured blood mononuclear cells, which was also transmitted transiently to an established T-cell line. Rare, virus-like structures were also found in circulating mononuclear cells, but antibodies to HTLV-1 or -2, HIV, or simian immunodeficiency virus were not found. More recent etiologic studies continued to implicate environmental factors (possibly arthropod-borne and *P. acnes*) and added EBV, but removed, at least for now, retroviruses. Although not implicated in Kawasaki disease itself, streptococci were linked to a related syndrome, childhood polyarteritis nodosa. Involvement of a superantigen in Kawasaki disease remains controversial (25,26).

An infectious cause, particularly viral, has long been suspected in Behçet disease. Most studies have been negative, but several have suggested a possible viral role. As observed in RA synovial lymphocytes, HSV replication was impaired in blood lymphocytes from Behçet patients, and chromosomal abnormalities were frequent. Nucleic acid hybridization suggested that the herpes genome persists in lymphocytes, and blood mononuclear responses to both herpes and varicella-zoster were diminished. As in SLE, IFN levels were also increased in Behçet sera. Thus, herpesviruses may be candidate agents in this disease (1). Recent studies implicated hypersensitivity to streptococcal but not yersinial antigens. Prevalence of antibodies to HTLV-1 is increased in patients with Behçet syndrome in Japan (157).

In Henoch-Schönlein vasculitis preceding upper respiratory infections were frequently observed, but specific agents were not implicated. In polymyalgia rheumatica and giant cell arteritis, no evidence was found to implicate hepatitis B infection, but possible horizontal transmission between spouses was reported. EBV was not implicated in a recent study. The possible role of infection in fibromyalgia was reviewed, and studies regarding EBV were negative.

Goodpasture syndrome may follow influenza rarely. Viruslike structures have been found with the electron microscope, but no further evidence for an infectious etiology has been observed. In children, a variety of antigens may be involved in glomerulonephritis. Streptococcal infection has long been recognized as one of these, although the exact mechanism is still obscure (1).

In Sjögren syndrome, earlier studies implicated CMV, but recent interest has centered on EBV and retroviruses.

The possible role of EBV is controversial (323). The main evidence has been more frequent detection of EBV DNA in salivary gland tissue and blood using *in situ* hybridization and amplification with PCR. EBV DNA has been found in some studies, but not in others. An increased prevalence of antibodies to various EBV antigens has also been found in some studies, but not in another. Impaired *in vivo* regulation of EBV may be involved in these abnormalities, similar to that found earlier in RA. The evidence implicating retroviruses in Sjögren syndrome includes the similar clinical picture seen in some AIDS patients, the increased prevalence of serum antibodies to the HIV-1 group-specific protein, and the electron microscopic finding of retrovirus-like particles in cell cultures inoculated with Sjögren salivary tissue (324,325). HHV-6, the cause of exanthema subitum, has also been implicated in Sjögren syndrome, on the basis of a higher prevalence of antibody, but this was not confirmed with more sensitive methods in a later study (326). HHV-6 has also been associated with lymphoproliferative disease, and viral DNA was detected in lymphoma tissue from one patient with Sjögren syndrome (327). Recent studies suggest that EBV association does not lead to an increased occurrence of malignant lymphoma (328). Overall, in Sjögren syndrome the evidence implicating retroviruses and EBV is suggestive, but CMV and HHV-6 are also potential etiologic candidates.

In scleroderma, little evidence for a microbial etiology has been found, but a marker antibody in the disease was found to have a potential cross-reactivity to a retroviral protein, based on sequence similarities. In mixed CTD, two patients had HTLV-1 antibody, but most did not; patients with polymyositis were also negative. CMV and other viruses have been associated occasionally with both autoimmune hemolytic anemia and idiopathic thrombocytopenia. In the latter disease, some evidence of hepatitis B and other viral antigens has been found. Herpesviruses were implicated in a syndrome of arthralgias with acute urinary retention. Evidence for a chronic paramyxovirus infection has been found in Paget disease, and, more recently, in osteopetrosis as well.

In summary, although Sjögren syndrome is currently an active area of study, the rarity of most of these CTD syndromes is a major impediment to investigating their possible infectious etiologies.

Hepatitis B Syndromes

The spectrum of immunologic responses to hepatitis B infection is broad, ranging from the asymptomatic persistent virus carrier, through the acute arthritis-hepatitis syndrome, to fatal necrotizing vasculitis (1). Two other immunologically-mediated diseases have been associated with hepatitis B infection: membranous glomerulonephritis and EMC. The former has been associated with hepatitis B infection predominantly in childhood, where it appears to be the single most common cause of this form of glomerulonephritis. Hepatitis is often present, but may be subclinical or overshadowed by the renal disease. Considerable evidence has been found for an immune complex pathogenesis, but the viral antigens involved are still unclear. Treatment with IFN-α may offer some benefit in chronic hepatitis B infection.

The association of essential mixed cryoglobulinemia with hepatitis B infection has been more controversial. Initially, most patients were reported to have hepatitis B infection, but this finding was not confirmed subsequently. Nevertheless, it seemed clear that hepatitis B infection, chronic liver disease, and cryoglobulinemia were associated, and that many of the clinical manifestations of the latter were due to immune complex–mediated vasculitis. As discussed in a previous section, more recent studies have clearly incriminated hepatitis C as the prime cause of essential mixed cryoglobulinemia.

Reverse transcriptase activity was demonstrated in cultured T-cell lines, and antibodies capable of immunoprecipitating HTLV-1 proteins were noted in sera of a subset of patients with essential mixed cryoglobulinemia patients. The patients showing evidence for retroviral involvement were not infected with HTLV-1 (329), HCV, or HBV, and possessed no antibodies to HRES-1. These findings raise the possibility that an HTLV-related retrovirus may be involved in these patients.

Hepatitis B infection in humans continues to be unique because of the wide spectrum of associated immunologic disease. Hepatitis A can also be accompanied by arthralgias and rash acutely, and by arthritis, cutaneous vasculitis, and cryoglobulinemia with relapsing infection. Much has yet to be learned about both the viral and host factors involved in the pathogenesis of all hepatitis virus infections.

CONCLUSION

With the advent of molecular biology techniques, the genetic basis of human disease is increasingly being defined. The molecular basis of disease susceptibility in MHC class II–related diseases, such as RA, and MHC class I–related diseases, such as ReA, has brought MHC to the center stage of much current research in the rheumatic diseases. But in another interesting parallel between the rheumatologist and the microbiologist, genetic susceptibility is now an area of great interest in infectious diseases. Studies concerning the HLA alleles of South American Indians have identified limited HLA polymorphism, likely reflecting the smaller founder populations that colonized America from Asia 11,000 to 40,000 years ago (330,331). The nucleotide sequences of HLA-B alleles from these tribes differ from white, Oriental, and other populations. This indicates that the HLA-B locus can evolve rapidly in isolated populations. It is argued that the selective pressure on these populations was imposed by pathogen diversity. Indeed, it has been argued that infectious disease is the driving force behind MHC polymorphism in general (332). One supportive observation derives from the study of Hill and associates (333), who studied HLA alleles in children with severe malarial anemia or cerebral malaria. Out of 45 class I alleles studied, HLA-Bw53 was significantly reduced in frequency in the severely ill children. The notion that HLA-Bw53 is a protective allele against malaria is further supported by its geographic distribution; although rare elsewhere in the world, HLA-Bw53 reaches a frequency as high as 25% in malarial regions of Africa. The geographic aspects of host/pathogen interaction illustrated by these studies raise important questions about global frequencies of HLA-associated rheumatic diseases. A central example is the distribution of HLA-B27 in various parts of the world. It is recognized that the incidence of SpAs is closely related to the frequency of HLA-B27 in the regional population. The gene frequency varies widely from virtual absence in parts of the sub-Sahara to high frequencies in certain Indian tribes on the west coast of Canada. If infectious diseases are the key determinants in patterns of HLA polymorphism, the nature of the microbial factors selecting for or against HLA-B27 in different environments may hold a clue to the agents playing a role in B27-related SpAs.

It is noteworthy that the genetic mechanisms used by human hosts to respond to various pathogenic antigens are similar to microbial strategies to establish a niche in the host population and to maximize the basic reproductive rate. This illustrates a remarkably symmetric converging arms race between the pathogen and host. Both the microbe and the host immune response use gene conversion in an adaptive response to the interaction. Selection by the pathogens determines population susceptibility by driving MHC allelic polymorphisms, and host population herd immunity drives allelic polymorphism of dominant surface antigens of pathogens. If some of the rheumatic diseases reflect an interplay of pathogen and host susceptibility as discussed earlier in various categories of CTD, then the genetic analysis of both parties in this scenario should bring us closer to defining the microbial etiology of these diseases.

REFERENCES

1. Phillips PE, Inman RD, Christian CL. Infectious agents in chronic rheumatic disease. In: McCarty DJ, Koopman WJ, eds. *Arthritis and allied conditions,* 9th to 12th eds. Philadelphia: Lea & Febiger, 9th ed., 1979:320–328; 10th ed., 1985:431–449; 11th ed., 1989:482–504; 12th ed., 1993:541–564; 14th ed., 2001:635–654.
2. Hughes RA. The microbiology of chronic inflammatory arthritis: an historical review. *Br J Rheumatol* 1994;33:361–369.
3. Murray GR. Discussion on focal sepsis as a factor in disease. *Ap R Soc Med* 1926;1:1–26.
4. Behar SM, Porcelli SA. Mechanisms of autoimmune disease induction. *Arthritis Rheum* 1995;38:458–476.
5. Espinosa L, Goldenberg DL, Arnett FC, et al., eds. *Infections in the rheumatic diseases: a comprehensive review of microbial relations to rheumatic disorders.* Orlando, FL: Grune & Stratton, 1988.
6. Tan PLJ, Skinner MA. The microbial cause of RA: time to dump Koch's postulates. *J Rheumatol* 1992;19:1170–1172.
7. Burmester GR, Solback W. Hit and run, hit and hide or permanent hit: why it is premature to dump Koch's postulates in rheumatic diseases. *J Rheumatol* 1992;19.1173–1174.
8. Inman RD. The role of infection in chronic arthritis. *J Rheumatol* 1992;19(suppl 33):98–104.
9. Perl A. Mechanisms of viral pathogenesis in rheumatic disease. *Ann Rheum Dis* 1999;58:454–461.
10. Albert LJ, Inman RD. Molecular mimicry and autoimmunity. *N Engl J Med* 1999;341:2068–2074.
11. Horwitz MS, Bradley LM, Halbertson J, et al. Diabetes induced by Coxsackie virus: initiation by bystander damage and not molecular mimicry. *Nat Med* 1998;4:781–785.
12. Germain RN. MHC-dependent antigen processing and peptide presentation: providing ligands for T lymphocyte activation. *Cell* 1994;76: 287–299.
13. Kappler J, Kotzin B, Herron LR, et al. V-beta-specific stimulation of human T cells by staphylococcal toxins. *Science* 1989;244:811–813.
14. Fleischer B, Schrezemeier H. T cell stimulation by staphylococcal enterotoxins: clonally variable response and requirement for major histocompatibility complex class II molecules on accessory or target cells. *J Exp Med* 1988;167:1697–1705.
15. Fraser JD. High-affinity binding of staphylococcal enterotoxin A and B to HLA-DR. *Nature* 1989;339:221–223.
16. Fleischer B, Schrezemeier H. T cell stimulation by staphylococcal enterotoxins: clonally variable response and requirement for major histocompatibility complex class II molecules on accessory or target cells. *J Exp Med* 1988;167:1697–1705.
17. Marrack P, Kappler J. The staphylococcal enterotoxins and their relatives. *Science* 1990;248:705–711.
18. Stuart PM, Woodward JG. *Yersinia enterocolitica* produces superantigenic activity. *J Immunol* 1992;148:225–233.
19. Huber BT. Mls-genes and self-superantigens. *Trends Genet* 1992;8: 399–402.
20. Webb SR, Gascoigne NRJ. T-cell activation by superantigen. *Curr Opin Immunol* 1994;6:467–475.
21. Held W, Waanders GA, Shakov AN, et al. Superantigen-induced immune stimulation amplifies mouse mammary tumor virus infection and allows virus transmission. *Cell* 1993;74:529–540.
22. Kotzin BL, Leung DY, Kappler J, et al. Superantigens and their potential role in human disease. *Adv Immunol* 1993;54:99–166.
23. Paliard X, West SG, Lafferty JA, et al. Evidence for the effects of a superantigen in RA. *Science* 1991;253:325–329.
24. Uematsu Y, Wege H, Straus A, et al. The T-cell receptor repertoire in the synovial fluid of a patient with RA is polyclonal. *Proc Natl Acad Sci U S A* 1991;88:8534–8538.
25. Abe J, Kotzin BL, Jujo K, et al. Selective expansion of T cells expressing T-cell receptor variable regions V-beta 2 and V-beta 8 in Kawasaki disease. *Proc Natl Acad Sci U S A* 1992;89:4006–4070.
26. Pietra BA, De Inocencio J, Giannini EH, et al. TCR V beta family repertoire and T cell activation markers in Kawasaki disease. *J Immunol* 1994;153:1881–1888.
27. Krieg AM, Gourley MF, Perl A. Endogenous retroviruses: potential etiologic agents in autoimmunity. *FASEB J* 1992;6:2537–2544.
28. Perl A, Banki K. Human endogenous retroviral elements and autoimmunity: data and concepts. *Trends Microbiol* 1993;1:153–156.
29. Perl A, Rosenblatt JD, Chen IS, et al. Detection and cloning of new HTLV-related endogenous sequences in man. *Nucleic Acids Res* 1989; 17:6841–6854.
30. Izui S, McConahey PJ, Theophilopoulos AN, et al. Association of circulating retroviral gp70-anti-gp70 immune complexes with murine SLE. *J Exp Med* 1979;149:1099–1116.
31. Phillips PE, Johnston SL, Runge LA, et al. High IgM antibody to human T-cell leukemia virus type I in SLE. *J Clin Immunol* 1986;6: 234–241.
32. Talal N, Dauphinee MJ, Dang H, et al. Detection of serum antibodies to retroviral proteins in patients with primary Sjögren's syndrome (autoimmune exocrinopathy). *Arthritis Rheum* 1990;33:774–781.
33. Banki K, Maceda J, Hurley E, et al. Human T-cell lymphotropic virus (HTLV)-related endogenous sequence, HRES-1, encodes a 28-kDa protein: a possible autoantigen for HTLV-I gag-reactive autoantibodies. *Proc Natl Acad Sci U S A* 1992;89:1939–1943.
34. Via CS, Shearer GM. Autoimmunity and the acquired immune deficiency syndrome. *Curr Opin Immunol* 1989;1:753–756.
35. Query CC, Keene JD. A human autoimmune protein associated with U1 RNA contains a region of homology that is cross-reactive with retroviral p30gag antigen. *Cell* 1987;51:211–220.

36. Maul GG, Jimenez SA, Riggs E, et al. Determination of an epitope of the diffuse systemic sclerosis marker antigen DNA topoisomerase I: sequence similarity with retroviral p30 gag protein suggests a possible cause for autoimmunity in systemic sclerosis. *Proc Natl Acad Sci U S A* 1989;86:8492–8496.
37. Kohsaka H, Yamamoto K, Fujii H, et al. Fine epitope mapping of the human SS-B/La protein. Identification of a distinct autoepitope homologous to a viral gag polyprotein. *J Clin Invest* 1990;85:1566–1574.
38. Perl A. Role of endogenous retroviruses in autoimmune diseases [Review]. *Rheum Dis Clin North Am* 2003;29:123–143.
39. Oldstone MBA. Molecular mimicry and autoimmune disease. *Cell* 1987;50:819–820.
40. Perl A, Banki K. Molecular mimicry, altered apoptosis, and immunomodulation as mechanisms of viral pathogenesis in systemic lupus erythematosus. In: Kammer GM, Tsokos GC, eds. *Lupus: molecular and cellular pathogenesis.* Totowa, NJ: Humana Press, 1999:43–64.
41. Perl A. Mechanisms of viral pathogenesis in rheumatic diseases. *Ann Rheum Dis* 1999;58:454–461.
42. Li J-M, Fan WS, Horsfall AC, et al. The expression of human endogenous retrovirus-3 in fetal cardiac tissue and antibodies in congenital heart block. *Clin Exp Immunol* 1996;104:388–393.
43. Hishikawa T, Ogasawara H, Kaneko H, et al. Detection of antibodies to a recombinant gag protein derived from human endogenous retrovirus clone 4–1 in autoimmune diseases. *Viral Immunol* 1997;10:137–147.
44. Tristem M. Identification and characterization of novel human endogenous retrovirus families by phyligenetic screening of human genome mapping project database. *J Virol* 2000;74:3715–3730.
45. Wilkinson DA, Mager DL, Leong J-AC. Endogenous human retroviruses. In: Levy JA, ed. *The retroviridae.* New York: Plenum, 1994: 465–535.
46. Repaske R, Steele PE, O'Neill RR, et al. Nucleotide sequence of a full-length human endogenous retroviral segment. *J Virol* 1985;54:764–772.
47. Ogasawara H, Naito T, Kaneko H, et al. Quantitative analysis of messenger RNA of human endogenous retrovirus in systemic lupus erythematosus. *J Rheumatol* 2001;28:533–538.
48. Medstrand P, Lindeskog M, Blomberg J. Expression of human endogenous retroviral sequences in peripheral blood mononuclear cells of healthy individuals. *J Gen Virol* 1992;73:2463–2466.
49. Hohenadl C, Germaier H, Walchner M, et al. Transcriptional activation of endogenous retroviral sequences in human epidermal keratinocytes by UVB irradiation. *J Invest Dermatol* 1999;113:587–594.
50. Coffin JM, Hughes SH, Varmus HE. Retrotransposons, endogenous retroviruses, and the evolution of retroelements. In: Coffin JM, Hughes SH, Varmus HE, eds. *Retroviruses.* Cold Spring Harbor, NY: Cold Spring Harbor Laboratory Press, 1997:343–435.
51. Groudine M, Eisenman R, Weintraub H. Chromatin structure of endogenous retroviral genes and activation by an inhibitor of DNA methylation. *Nature* 1985;292:311–317.
52. Hsiao WL, Gattoni-Celli S, Weinstein IB. Effects of 5-azacytidine on expression of endogenous retrovirus-related sequences in C3H 10T1/2 cells. *J Virol* 1986;57:1119–1126.
53. Richardson BC, Strahler JR, Pivirotto TS, et al. Phenotypic and functional similarities between 5-azacytidine-treated T cells and a T-cell subset in patients with active systemic lupus erythematosus. *Arthritis Rheum* 1992;35:647–662.
54. Richardson B, Scheinbart L, Strahler J, et al. Evidence for impaired T cell DNA methylation in systemic lupus erythematosus and rheumatoid arthritis. *Arthritis Rheum* 1990;33:1665–1673.
55. Ogasawara H, Kaneko H, Hishikawa T, et al. Molecular mimicry between human endogenous retrovirus clone 4–1 and HLA class I antigen with reference to the pathogenesis of systemic lupus erythematosus. *Rheumatology* 1999;38:1163–1164.
56. Hishikawa T, Ogasawara H, Kaneko H, et al. Detection of antibodies to a recombinant gag protein derived from human endogenous retrovirus clone 4–1 in autoimmune diseases. *Viral Immunol* 1997;10:137–147.
57. Mueller-Lantzsch N, Sauter M, Weiskircher A, et al. Human endogenous retroviral element K10 (HERV-K10) encodes a full-length gag homologous 73-kDa protein and a functional protease. *AIDS Res Hum Retroviruses* 1993;9:343–350.
58. Perl A, Colombo E, Dai H, et al. Antibody reactivity to the HRES-1 endogenous retroviral element identifies a subset in patients with systemic lupus erythematosus and overlap syndromes: correlation with antinuclear antibodies and HLA class II alleles. *Arthritis Rheum* 1995; 38:1660–1671.
59. Brookes SM, Pandolfino YA, Mitchell TJ, et al. The immune response to and expression of cross-reactive retroviral gag sequences in autoimmune disease. *Br J Rheumatol* 1992;31:735–742.
60. Bengtsson A, Blomberg J, Nived O, et al. Selective antibody reactivity with peptides from human endogenous retroviruses and nonviral poly(amino acids) in patients with systemic lupus erythematosus. *Arthritis Rheum* 1996;39:1654–1663.
61. Li J, Fan AC, Horsfall C, et al. The expression of human endogenous retrovirus-3 in fetal cardiac tissue and antibodies in congenital heart block. *Clin Exp Immunol* 1996;104;388–393.
62. Sela M. Antigenicity: some molecular aspects. *Science* 1969;166: 1365–1374.
63. Magistrelli C, Banki K, Ferrante P, et al. Mapping and cloning of polymorphic genotypes of the HRES-1 LTR. *Arthritis Rheum* 1994;37 (suppl):316.
64. Perl A, Banki K. Molecular mimicry, altered apoptosis, and immunomodulation as mechanisms of viral pathogenesis in systemic lupus erythematosus. In: Kammer GM, Tsokos GC, eds. *Lupus molecular and cellular pathogenesis.* Totowa, NJ: Humana Press, 1999, pp 43–64.
65. Magistrelli C, Samoilova E, Agarwal RK, et al. Polymorphic genotypes of the HRES-1 human endogenous locus are associated with its autoantigenicity in SLE. *Arthritis Rheum* 1998;41(suppl): 282.
66. Magistrelli C, Samoilova E, Agarwal RK, et al. Polymorphic genotypes of the HRES-1 human endogenous retrovirus locus correlate with systemic lupus erythematosus and autoreactivity. *Immunogenetics* 1999;49:829–834.
67. Perl A, Isaacs CM, Eddy RL, et al. The human T-cell leukemia virus-related endogenous sequence (HRES1) is located on chromosomes 1 at Q42. *Genomics* 1991;11:1172–1173.
68. Tsao BP, Cantor RM, Kalunian KC, et al. Evidence for linkage of a candidate chromosome 1 region to human systemic lupus erythematosus. *J Clin Invest* 1997;99:725–731.
69. Gaffney PM, Kearns GM, Shark KB, et al. A genome-wide search for susceptibility genes in human systemic lupus erythematosus sib-pair families. *Proc Natl Acad Sci U S A* 1998;95:14875–14879.
70. Moser KL, Neas BR, Salmon JE, et al. Genome scan of human systemic lupus erythematosus: evidence for linkage on chromosome 1q in African-American pedigrees. *Proc Natl Acad Sci U S A* 1998;95: 14869–14874.
71. Cohen JJ, Duke RC, Fadok VA, et al. Apoptosis and programmed cell death in immunity. *Annu Rev Immunol* 1992;10:267–293.
72. Thompson CB. Apoptosis in the pathogenesis and treatment of disease. *Science* 1995;267:1456–1462.
73. Nagata S, Golstein P. The Fas death factor. *Science* 1995;267:1449–1456.
74. Fisher GH, Rosenberg FJ, Straus SE, et al. Dominant interfering Fas gene mutations impair apoptosis in a human autoimmune lymphoproliferative syndrome. *Cell* 1995;81:935–946.
75. Drappa J, Vaishnaw AK, Sullivan KE, et al. Fas gene mutations in the Canale-Smith syndrome, and inherited lymphoproliferative disorder associated with autoimmunity. *N Engl J Med* 1996;335:1643–1649.
76. Mysler E, Pini P, Drappa J, et al. The apoptosis-1/fas protein in human systemic lupus erythematosus. *J Clin Invest* 1994;93:1029–1034.
77. Kovacs B, Vassilopoulas D, Vogelgesang SA, et al. Defective CD3-mediated cell death in activated T cells from patients with systemic lupus erythematosus: role of decreased intracellular TN-alpha. *Clin Immunol Immunopathol* 1996;81:293–302.
78. Emlen W, Niebur JA, Kadera R. Accelerated *in vitro* apoptosis of lymphocytes from patients with systemic lupus erythematosus. *J Immunol* 1994;152:3685–3692.
79. Casciola-Rosen LA, Anhalt G, Rosen A. Autoantigens targeted in systemic lupus erythematosus are clustered in two populations of surface structures on apoptotic keratinocytes. *J Exp Med* 1994;179:1317–1330.
80. Naides SJ. Rheumatic manifestations of parvovirus B19 infection. [Review]. *Rheum Dis Clin North Am* 1998;24:375–401.
81. Phillips PE. Viral arthritis. *Curr Opin Rheumatol* 1997;9:337–344.
82. Tingle AJ, Mitchell LA, Grace M, et al. Randomised double-blind placebo-controlled study on adverse effects of rubella immunisation in seronegative women. *Lancet* 1997;349:1277–1281.

83. Ray P, Black S, Shinefield H, et al. Risk of chronic arthropathy among women after rubella vaccination. Vaccine Safety Datalink Team [see comments]. *JAMA* 1997;278:551–556.
84. Frenkel LM, Nielsen K, Garakian A, et al. A search for persistent rubella virus infection in persons with chronic symptoms after rubella and rubella immunization and in patients with juvenile rheumatoid arthritis. *Clin Infect Dis* 1996;22:287–294.
85. Flexman JP, Smith DW, Mackenzie JS, et al. A comparison of the diseases caused by Ross River virus and Barmah Forest virus. *Med J Aust* 1998;169:159–163.
86. Fraser JR, Becker GJ. Mononuclear cell types in chronic synovial effusions of Ross River virus disease. *Aust N Z J Med* 1984;14:505–506.
87. Fraser JR, Ratnamohan VM, Dowling JP, et al. The exanthem of Ross River virus infection: histology location of virus antigen and nature of inflammatory infiltrate. *J Clin Pathol* 1983;36:1256–1263.
88. Fraser JR. Epidemic polyarthritis and Ross River virus disease. *Clin Rheum Dis* 1986;12:369–388.
89. Luukkainen R, Laine M, Nirhamo J. Chronic arthritis after Sindbis-related (Pogosta) virus infection. *Scand J Rheumatol* 2000;29:399–400.
90. Laine M, Luukkainen R, Jalava J, et al. Prolonged arthritis associated with sindbis-related (Pogosta) virus infection. *Rheumatology* 2000; 39:1272–1274.
91. Panush RS. Adenovirus arthritis. *Arthritis Rheum* 1974;17:534–536.
92. Rahal JJ, Millian SJ, Noriega ER. Coxsackie and adenovirus infection. Association with acute febrile and juvenile rheumatoid arthritis. *JAMA* 1976;235:2496–2501.
93. Fraser KJ, Clarris BJ, Muirden KD, et al. A persistent adenovirus type 1 infection in synovial tissue from an immunodeficient patient with chronic, rheumatoid-like polyarthritis. *Arthritis Rheum* 1985; 28:455–458.
94. Modlin JF. Coxsackieviruses, echoviruses, and newer enteroviruses. In: Mandell GL, Bennett JE, Dolin R, eds. *Principles and practice of infectious diseases.* New York: Churchill Livingstone, 1995:1620–1636.
95. Ray CG, Gall EP, Minnich LL, et al. Acute polyarthritis associated with active Epstein-Barr virus infection. *JAMA* 1982;248:2990–2993.
96. Le Goff P, Chicault P, Saraux A, et al. Lymphoma with regression after methotrexate withdrawal in a patient with rheumatoid arthritis. Role for the Epstein-Barr virus. *Rev Rhum* 1998;65:283–286.
97. Natkunam Y, Elenitoba-Johnson KS, Kingma DW, et al. Epstein-Barr virus strain type and latent membrane protein 1 gene deletions in lymphomas in patients with rheumatic diseases. *Arthritis Rheum* 1997;40:1152–1156.
98. Stebbings S, Highton J, Croxson MC, et al. Chickenpox monoarthritis: demonstration of varicella-zoster virus in joint fluid by polymerase chain reaction. *Br J Rheumatol* 1998;37:311–313.
99. Naucler CS, Larsson S, Moller E. A novel mechanism for virus-induced autoimmunity in humans [Review]. *Immunol Rev* 1996;152: 175–192.
100. Ferri C, La Civita L, Longombardo G, et al. Mixed cryoglobulinaemia: a cross-road between autoimmune and lymphoproliferative disorders. *Lupus* 1998;7:275–279.
101. Akriviadis EA, Xanthakis I, Navrozidou C, et al. Prevalence of cryoglobulinemia in chronic hepatitis C virus infection and response to treatment with interferon-alpha. *J Clin Gastroenterol* 1997;25: 612–618.
102. Ferri C, Greco F, Longombardo G, et al. Association between hepatitis C virus and mixed cryoglobulinemia. *Clin Exp Rheumatol* 1991; 9:621–624.
103. Gorevic PD, Kassab HJ, Levo Y, et al. Mixed cryoglobulinemia: clinical aspects and long-term follow-up of 40 patients. *Am J Med* 1980; 69:287–308.
104. Perl A, Gorevic PD, Ryan DH, et al. Clonal B cell expansions in patients with essential mixed cryoglobulinaemia. *Clin Exp Immunol* 1989;76:54–60.
105. Ferri C, Monti M, La Civita L, et al. Infection of peripheral blood mononuclear cells by hepatitis C virus in mixed cryoglobulinemia. *Blood* 1993;82:3701–3704.
106. Jackson JM, Callen JP. Scarring alopecia and sclerodermatous changes of the scalp in a patient with hepatitis C infection. *J Am Acad Dermatol* 1998;39:824–826.
107. Nishioka K. HTLV-I arthropathy and Sjögren syndrome [Review]. *J Acquir Immune Defic Syndr Hum Retrovirol* 1996;13(suppl 1): 57 62.
108. Guerin B, Arfi S, Numeric P, et al. Polyarthritis in HTLV-1-infected patients. A review of 17 cases. *Rev Rhum* 1995;62:21–28.
109. Beilke MA, Traina-Dorge V, England JD, et al. Polymyositis, arthritis, and uveitis in a macaque experimentally infected with human T lymphotropic virus type I. *Arth Rheum* 1996;39:610–615.
110. Weitzul S, Duvic M. HIV-related psoriasis and Reiter's syndrome [Review]. *Semin Cutan Med Surg* 1997;16:213–218.
111. Espinoza LR, Cuellar ML. Retrovirus-associated rheumatic syndromes. In: Koopman WJ, ed. *Arthritis and allied conditions.* Baltimore: Williams & Wilkins, 1998:2361–2374.
112. Gibofsky A, Zabriskie JB. Rheumatic fever and poststreptococcal reactive arthritis. *Curr Opin Rheumatol* 1995;7:299–305.
113. Steere AC. Lyme disease. *N Engl J Med* 1989;321:586–596.
114. Evans J. Lyme disease. *Curr Opin Rheumatol* 1999;11:281–288.
115. van der Heijden IM, Wilbrink B, Rijpkema SGT, et al. Detection of *Borrelia burgdorferi* sensu stricto by reverse line blot in the joints of Dutch patients with Lyme arthritis. *Arthritis Rheum* 1999;42:1473–1480.
116. Fendler C, Wu P, Eggens U, et al. Longitudinal investigation of bacterium-specific synovial lymphocyte proliferation in reactive arthritis and Lyme arthritis. *Br J Rheumatol* 1998;37:784–788.
117. Bennett JC. The infectious etiology of RA: new considerations. *Arthritis Rheum* 1978;21:531–538.
118. Young CR, Ebringer A, Archer JR. Immune response inversion after hyper-immunization: possible mechanism in the pathogenesis of HLA-linked diseases. *Ann Rheum Dis* 1978;31:152–158.
119. Plotz PH. Autoantibodies are anti-idiotype antibodies to anti-viral antibodies. *Lancet* 1983;1:824–826.
120. Williams RC, Sibbet WL, Husby G. Oncogenes, viruses, or rheumogenes? *Am J Med* 1986;80:1011–1016.
121. Brouet JC, Clauvel JP, Danon F, et al. Biologic and clinical significance of cryoglobulins. *Am J Med* 1974;57:775–788.
122. Gorevic PD, Kassab HJ, Levo Y, et al. Mixed cryoglobulinemia: clinical aspects and long-term follow-up of 40 patients. *Am J Med* 1980; 69:287–308.
123. Levo Y, Gorevic PD, Hanna MD, et al. Liver involvement in the syndrome of mixed cryoglobulinemia. *Ann Intern Med* 1977;87:287–292.
124. Agnello V, Chung RT, Kaplan LM. A role for hepatitis C virus infection type II cryoglobulinemia. *N Engl J Med* 1992;327:1490–1495.
125. Cacoub P, Fabiani FL, Musset L, et al. Mixed cryoglobulinemia and hepatitis C virus. *Am J Med* 1994;96:124–132.
126. Ferri C, Monti M, La Civita L, et al. Infection of peripheral blood mononuclear cells by hepatitis C virus in mixed cryoglobulinemia. *Blood* 1993;82:3701–3704.
127. Perl A, Gorevic PD, Ryan DH, et al. Clonal B cell expansions in patients with essential mixed cryoglobulinemia. *Clin Exp Immunol* 1989;76:54–60.
128. Buskila D, Shnaider A, Neumann L, et al. Musculoskeletal manifestations and autoantibody profile in 90 hepatitis C virus infected Israeli patients. *Semin Arthritis Rheum* 1998;28:107–113.
129. Coffin JM. Genetic diversity and evolution of retroviruses. *Curr Top Microbiol Immunol* 1992;176:143–164.
130. Pantaleo G, Graziosi C, Fauci AS. The immunopathogenesis of human immunodeficiency virus infection. *N Engl J Med* 1993;328: 327–335.
131. Weiss RA. How does HIV cause AIDS? *Science* 1993;260:1273–1279.
132. McDougal JS, Kennedy MS, Sligh JM, et al. Binding of HTLV-III/LAV to T4+ T cells by a complex of the 100K viral protein and the T4 molecule. *Science* 1986;231:382–385.
133. Clerici M, Shearer GM. The Th1–Th2 hypothesis of HIV infection: new insights. *Immunol Today* 1994;15:575–581.
134. Meyaard L, Otto SA, Jonker RR, et al. Programmed death of T cells in HIV infection. *Science* 1992;257:217–219.
135. Pan H, Griep AE. Temporarily distinct patterns of p53-dependent and p53-independent apoptosis during mouse lens development. *Genes Dev* 1995;9:2157–2169.
136. Ehret A, Westendorp MO, Herr I, et al. Resistance of chimpanzee T cell to human immunodeficiency virus type I tat-enhanced oxidative stress and apoptosis. *J Virol* 1996;70:6502–6507.
137. Westendorp MO, Frank R, Ochsenbauer C, et al. Sensitization of T cells to CD95-mediated apoptosis by HIV-1 tat and gp120. *Nature* 1995;375:497–500.

138. Strack PR, Frey MW, Rizzo CJ, et al. Apoptosis mediated by HIV protease is preceded by cleavage of bcl-2. *Proc Natl Acad Sci U S A* 1996;93:9571–9576.
139. Viard J, Chabre H, Bach J. Autoantibodies to nucleosomes in HIV-1-infected patients. *J AIDS* 1994;7:1286–1293.
140. Itescu S, Brancato LJ, Buxbaum J, et al. A diffuse infiltrative CD8 lymphocytosis syndrome in HIV infection: a host immune response associated with HLA-DR5. *Ann Intern Med* 1990;112:3–10.
141. Calbrese LH, Estes M, Yen-Lieberman B, et al. Systemic vasculitis in association with HIV infection. *Arthritis Rheum* 1989;32:569–576.
142. Withrington RH, Cornes C, Harris JRW, et al. Isolation of HIV from synovial fluid of a patient with reactive arthritis. *BMJ* 1987;294:484.
143. Forster SM, Seifert MH, Keat AC, et al. Inflammatory joint disease and HIV infection. *BMJ* 1988;296:1625–1627.
144. Berman A, Espinoza LR, Diaz JD, et al. Rheumatic manifestations of HIV infection. *Am J Med* 1988;85:59–64.
145. Rynes RI, Goldenberg DL, DiGiacomo R, et al. AIDS-associated arthritis. *Am J Med* 1988;84:810–816.
146. Calabrese LH, Kelley DM, Myers A, et al. Rheumatic symptoms and HIV infection. *Arthritis Rheum* 1991;34:257–263.
147. Poiesz BJ, Ruscetti FW, Gazdar AF, et al. Detection and isolation of type C retrovirus particles from fresh and cultured lymphocytes of a patient with cutaneous T cell lymphoma. *Proc Natl Acad Sci U S A* 1980;77:7415–7419.
148. Gesain A, Barin F, Vernant JC, et al. Antibodies to human T-lymphotropic virus type-I in patients with tropical spastic paraparesis. *Lancet* 1985;2:407–410.
149. Hall WW, Liu CR, Schneewind O, et al. Deleted HTLV-I provirus in blood and cutaneous lesions of patients with mycosis fungoides. *Science* 1991;253:317–320.
150. Zucker-Franklin D, Coutavas EE, Rush MG, et al. Detection of human T-lymphotropic virus-like particles in cultures of peripheral blood lymphocytes from patients with mycosis fungoides. *Proc Natl Acad Sci U S A* 1991;88:7630–7634.
151. Nishioka K, Maruyama I, Sato K, et al. Chronic inflammatory arthropathy associated with HTLV-I. *Lancet* 1989;1:141.
152. Wiley CA, Nerenberg M, Cros D, et al. HTLV-I polymyositis in patients also infected with the human immunodeficiency virus. *N Engl J Med* 1989;320:292–995.
153. Masson C, Chauna MP, Hen D, et al. Myelopathy, polymyositis, and systemic manifestations associated with HTLV-I virus. *Rev Neurol* 1989;145:838–841.
154. Vernant JC, Maurs L, Gesain A. Endemic tropical spastic paraparesis associated human T-lymphotropic virus type I: a clinical and seroepidemiologic study of 25 cases. *Ann Neurol* 1987;21:123–130.
155. Smith FB, Rajdeo H, Panesar N, et al. Benign lymphoepithelial lesion of the parotid gland in intravenous drug users. *Arch Pathol Lab Med* 1988;112:742–745.
156. Robert-Guroff M, Weiss SH, Giron JA, et al. Prevalence of antibodies to HTLV-I, -II, and -III in intravenous drug abusers from and AIDS epidemic region. *JAMA* 1986;225:3133–3137.
157. Igakura T, Kawahigashi Y, Kanazawa H, et al. HTLV-I and Behçet's disease. *J Rheumatol* 1993;20:2175–2176.
158. Kitajima I, Yamamoto K, Sato K, et al. Detection of human T cell lymphotropic virus type I proviral DNA and its gene expression in synovial cells in chronic inflammatory arthropathy. *J Clin Invest* 1991;88:1315–1322.
159. Sakai M, Eguchi K, Terada K, et al. Infection of human synovial cells by human T cell lymphotropic virus type I. *J Clin Invest* 1993;92:1957–1966.
160. Nakajima T, Aono H, Hasunuma T, et al. Overgrowth of human synovial cells driven by the human T cell leukemia virus type I *tax* gene. *J Clin Invest* 1993;92:186–193.
161. Banki K, Ablonczy E, Nakamura M, et al. Effect of p40*tax* transactivator of human T cell lymphotropic virus type I on expression of autoantigens. *AIDS Res Hum Retroviruses* 1994;10:303–308.
162. Yamada T, Yamaoka S, Goto T, et al. The human T-cell leukemia virus type I tax protein induces apoptosis which is blocked by the bcl-2 protein. *J Virol* 1994;68:3374–3379.
163. Green JE, Hinrichs SH, Vogel J, et al. Exocrinopathy resembling Sjögren's syndrome in HTLV-I *tax* transgenic mice. *Nature* 1989;341:72–74.
164. Iwakura Y, Tosu M, Yoshida E, et al. Induction of inflammatory arthropathy resembling rheumatoid arthritis in mice transgenic for HTLV-I. *Science* 1991;253:1026–1028.
165. Ebringer A, Shiples M, eds. Pathogenesis of ankylosing spondylitis and RA. *Br J Rheumatol* 1988;27(suppl 2):1–176.
166. Venables PJW. Infection and RA. *Curr Opin Rheumatol* 1989;1:15–20.
167. Rodriguez MA, Williams RC. Infection and rheumatic diseases. *Clin Exp Rheumatol* 1989;7:91–97.
168. Phillips PE. How do bacteria cause chronic arthritis? *J Rheumatol* 1989;16:1017–1019.
169. Relman DA, Schmidt TM, MacDermott RP, et al. Identification of the uncultured bacillus of Whipple's disease. *N Engl J Med* 1992;237:293–301.
170. Tappero JW, Mohle-Boetani J, Koehler JE, et al. The epidemiology of bacillary angiomatosis and bacillary peliosis. *JAMA* 1993;269:770–775.
171. Henrickson AEK, Blomquist L, Nord C-E, et al. Small intestinal bacterial overgrowth in patients with RA. *Ann Rheum Dis* 1993;52:503–510.
172. Eerola E, Mottonen T, Hannonen P, et al. Intestinal flora in early RA. *Br J Rheumatol* 1994;33:1030–1038.
173. Rashid T, Darlington G, Kjeldsen-Kragh J, et al. Proteus IgG antibodies and C-reactive protein in English, Norwegian and Spanish patients with rheumatoid arthritis. *Clin Rheumatol* 1999;18:190–195.
174. Schultz DR, Arnold PI. Heat shock (stress) proteins and autoimmunity in rheumatic diseases. *Semin Arthritis Rheum* 1993;22:357–374.
175. Hayem G, DeBandt M, Palazzo E, et al. Anti-heat shock protein 70 kDa and 90 kDa antibodies in serum of patients with rheumatoid arthritis. *Ann Rheum Dis* 1999;58:291–296.
176. Louie JS, Liebling MR. The polymerase chain reaction in infectious and post-infectious arthritis: a review. *Rheum Dis Clin North Am* 1998;24:227–236.
177. Wilbrink B, van der Heijden IM, Schouls LM, et al. Detection of bacterial DNA in joint samples from patients with undifferentiated arthritis and reactive arthritis, using polymerase chain reaction with universal 16S ribosomal RNA primers. *Arthritis Rheum* 1998;41:535–543. (Correspondence: Steinman CR, Wilbrink B, et al. *Arthritis Rheum* 1998;41:2276–2279.)
178. Wilkinson NZ, Kingsley GH, Jones HW, et al. The detection of DNA from a range of bacterial species in the joints of patients with a variety of arthritides using a nested, broad-range polymerase chain reaction. *Rheumatology* 1999;38:260–266.
179. Harrington JT. The evolving role of direct amplification tests in diagnosing osteoarticular infections caused by mycobacteria and fungi. *Curr Opin Rheumatol* 1999;11:289–292.
180. van der Heijden IM, Wilbrink B, Schouls LM, et al. Detection of mycobacteria in joint samples from patients with arthritis using a genus-specific polymerase chain reaction and sequence analysis. *Rheumatology* 1999;38:547–553.
181. Haier J, Nasaralla M, Franco AR, et al. Detection of mycoplasmal infections in blood of patients with rheumatoid arthritis. *Rheumatology* 1999;38:504–509.
182. Naides SJ. Viral infection including HIV. *Curr Opin Rheumatol* 1993;5:468–474.
183. Naides SJ. Viral arthritis including HIV. *Curr Opin Rheumatol* 1995;7:337–342.
184. Ford DK, Stein HB, Schulzer M. Persistent synovial lymphocyte responses to mumps and adenovirus antigens. *J Rheumatol* 1988;15:1717–1719.
185. Zhang D, Nikkari S, Vainiopaa R, et al. Detection of rubella, mumps, and measles virus genomic RNA in cells from synovial fluid and peripheral blood in early rheumatoid arthritis. *J Rheumatol* 1997;24:1260–1265.
186. Hooper M, Kallas EG, Coffin D, et al. Cytomegalovirus seropositivity is associated with the expansion of $CD4^{+}CD28^{-}$ and $CD8^{+}CD28^{-}$ T cells in rheumatoid arthritis. *J Rheumatol* 1999;256:1452–1457.
187. Nelson PN, Pinto-Basto G, Shipp A, et al. No serological evidence to implicate a role for cytomegalovirus infection in the aetiology of Felty's syndrome. *Br J Rheumatol* 1998;37:1256–1257.
188. Zucker-Franklin D, Pankcake BA, Brown WH. Prevalene of HLTV-I Tax in a subset of patients with rheumatoid arthritis. *Clin Exp Rheumatol* 2002;20:161–169.
189. Nakagawa K, Brusic V, McColl G, et al. Direct evidence for the expression of multiple endogenous retroviruses in the synovial compartment in rheumatoid arthritis. *Arthritis Rheum* 1997;40:627–638.
190. Neidbart M, Rethage J, Kuchen S, et al. Retrotransposable L1 elements expressed in rheumatoid arthritis synovial tissue: association

with genomic DNA hypomethylation and influence on gene expression. *Arthritis Rheum* 2000;43:2634–2647.
191. Griffiths DJ, Cooke SP, Herve C, et al. Detection of human retrovirus 5 in patients with arthritis and systemic lupus erythematosus. *Arthritis Rheum* 1999;42:448–454.
192. Naides SJ. Rheumatic manifestations of parvovirus B19 infection. *Rheum Dis Clin North Am* 1998;24:375–401.
193. Nikkari S, Luukkainen R, Möttönen T, et al. Does parvovirus B19 have a role in RA? *Ann Rheum Dis* 1994;53:106–111.
194. Hajeer AH, MacGregor AJ, Rigby AS, et al. Influence of previous exposure to human parvovirus B19 infection in explaining susceptibility to RA: an analysis of disease discordant twin pairs. *Ann Rheum Dis* 1994;53:137–139.
195. Cassinotti P, Bas S, Siegl G, et al. Association between human parvovirus B19 infection and arthritis. *Ann Rheum Dis* 1995;54:498–500.
196. Nikkari S, Roivainen A, Hannonen P, et al. Persistence of parvovirus B19 in synovial fluid and bone marrow. *Ann Rheum Dis* 1995;54:597–600.
197. Takahashi Y, Murai C, Shibata S, et al. Human parvovirus B19 as a causative agent for rheumatoid arthritis. *Proc Natl Acad Sci U S A* 1998;95:8227–8232.
198. Murai C, Munakata Y, Takahashi Y, et al. Rheumatoid arthritis after human parvovirus B19 infection. *Ann Rheum Dis* 1999;58:130–132.
199. Cassinotti P, Siegel C, Michel B, et al. Presence and significance of human parvovirus B19 DNA in synovial membranes and bone marrow from patients with arthritis of unknown origin. *J Med Microbiol* 1998;56:199–204.
200. Lunardi C, Tiso M, Borgato L, et al. Chronic parvovirus B19 infection induces the production of anti-virus antibodies with autoantigen binding properties. *Eur J Immunol* 1998;28:936–948.
201. Cooper CL, Choudhri SH. Leukocytoclastic vasculitis secondary to parvovirus B19 infection. *Clin Infect Dis* 1998;26:849, 989.
202. Cacoub P, Boukli N, Hausfater P, et al. Parvovirus B19 infection, hepatitis C virus infection, and mixed cryoglobulinemia. *Ann Rheum Dis* 1998;57:422–424.
203. Harrison B, Silman A, Barrett E, et al. Low frequency of recent parvovirus infection in a population-based cohort of patients with early inflammatory polyarthritis. *Ann Rheum Dis* 1998;57:375–377.
204. Speyer I, Breedveld FC, Dijkmans BAC. Human parvovirus B19 infection is not followed by inflammatory joint disease during long term follow-up. A retrospective study of 54 patients. *Clin Exp Rheum* 1998;16:576–578.
205. Soderlund M, Von Essen R, Haapasaari J, et al. Persistence of parvovirus B19 DNA in synovial membranes of young patients with and without chronic arthropathy. *Lancet* 1997;349:1063–1065.
206. McCarty DJ, Csuka ME. Polysynovitis associated with acute Epstein-Barr virus infection. *J Rheumatol* 1998;25:2039–2040
207. Fox RI, Luppi M, Pisa P, et al. Potential role of EBV in Sjögren's syndrome and RA. *J Rheumatol* 1992;19(suppl 32):18–24.
208. Jokinen EI, Möttönen, Hannonen PJ, et al. Prediction of severe RA using EBV. *Br J Rheumatol* 1994;33:917–922.
209. Lioté F, Pertuiset é, Cochand-Priollet B, et al. Methotrexate related B lymphoproliferative disease in a patient with RA. Role of EBV infection. *J Rheumatol* 1995;22:1174–1178.
210. Zhang L, Nikkari S, Shurnik M, et al. Detection of herpesviruses by PCR in lymphocytes from patients with RA. *Arthritis Rheum* 1993;36:1080–1086.
211. Saal JG, Krimmel M, Steidle M, et al. Synovial Epstein-Barr virus infection increases the risk of rheumatoid arthritis in individuals with the shared HLA-DR4 epitope. *Arthritis Rheum* 1999;42:1485–1496.
212. Takei MK, Mitamura K, Fujiwara S, et al. Detection of Epstein-Barr virus-encoded small RNA 1 and latent membrane protein 1 in synovial lining cells from rheumatoid arthritis patients. *Int Immunol* 1997;9:739–743.
213. Blaschke S, Schwarz G, Moneke D, et al. Epstein-Barr virus infection in peripheral blood mononuclear cells, synovial fluid cells, and synovial membranes of patients with rheumatoid arthritis. *J Rheumatol* 2000;27:866–873.
214. Balandraud N, Meynard JB, Auger I, et al. Epstein-Barr virus load in the peripheral blood of patients with rheumatoid arthritis: accurate quantification using real-time polymerase chain reaction. *Arthritis Rheum* 2003;48:1223–1228.
215. Koide J, Takada K, Sugiura M, et al. Spontaneous establishment of an Epstein-Barr virus–infected fibroblast line from the synovial tissue of a rheumatoid arthritis patient. *J Virol* 1997;71:2478–2481.
216. La Cava A, Nelson JL, Ollier WER, et al. Genetic bias in immune responses to a cassette shared by different microorganisms in patients with rheumatoid arthritis. *J Clin Invest* 1997;100:658–663.
217. Pogue GP, Hofmann J, Duncan R, et al. Autoantigens interact with cis-acting elements of rubella virus RNA. *J Virol* 1996;70:6269–6277.
218. Cheng S-T, Nguyen TQ, Yang Y-S, et al. Calreticulin binds hYRNA and the 52-kDa polypeptide component of the Ra/SS-A ribonucleoprotein autoantigen. *J Immunol* 1996;156:4484–4491.
219. Pope JE, Stevens A, Howson W, et al. The development of rheumatoid arthritis after recombinant hepatitis B vaccination. *J Rheumatol* 1998;25:1687–1693.
220. Schifter T, Lewinski UH. Adult onset of Still's disease associated with Epstein-Barr virus infection in a 66-year-old woman. *Scand J Rheumatol* 1998;27:458–460.
221. Saulsbury FT. Remission of juvenile rheumatoid arthritis with varicella infection. *J Rheumatol* 1999;26:1606–1608.
222. Khan MA. Update on spondyloarthropathies. *Ann Intern Med* 2002; 136:896–907.
223. Inman RD. Classification criteria for reactive arthritis. *J Rheumatol* 1999;26:1219–1221.
224. Pacheco-Tena C, Burgos-Vargas R, Vazquez-Mellado J, et al. A proposal for the classification of patients to enter clinical and experimental studies on reactive arthritis. *J Rheumatol* 1999;26:1338–1347.
225. Sieper J, Braun J. Problems and advances in the diagnosis of reactive arthritis. *J Rheumatol* 1999;26:1124–1222.
226. Braun J, Kingsley G, van der Heijde D, et al. On the difficulties of establishing a consensus on the definition of and diagnostic criteria for reactive arthritis. *J Rheum* 2000;27:185–192
227. Sieper J, Rudwaleit M, et al. Diagnosing reactive arthritis. *Arthritis Rheum* 2002;46:319–327.
228. Fendler C, Laitko S, Sorensen H, et al. Frequency of triggering bacteria in patients with reactive arthritis and undifferentiated oligoarthritis and the relative importance of the tests used for diagnosis. *Ann Rheum Dis* 2001;60:337–343.
229. Nikkari S, Puolakkainen M, Narvanen A, et al. Use of a peptide based enzyme immunoassay in diagnosis of *Chlamydia trachomatis* triggered reactive arthritis. *J Rheumatol* 2001;28:2487–2493.
230. Soderlin MK, Borjesson O, Kautiainen H, et al. Annual incidence of inflammatory joint diseases in a population-based study in southern Sweden. *Ann Rheum Dis* 2002;61:911–915.
231. Buxton JA, Fyfe M, Berger S, et al. Reactive arthritis and other sequelae following sporadic *Salmonella typhimurium* infection in British Columbia, Canada—a case control study. *J Rheumatol* 2002;29:2154–2158.
232. Hannu T, Mattila L, Siitonen A, et al. Reactive arthritis following an outbreak of *Salmonella typhimurium* phage type 193 infection. *Ann Rheum Dis* 2002;61:264–266.
233. Hannu T, Mattila L, Siitonen A, et al. Reactive arthritis following an outbreak of *Salmonella typhimurium* phage type 193 infection. *Ann Rheum Dis* 2002;61:264–266.
234. Locht H, Molbak K, Krogfelt KA. High frequency of reactive arthritis symptoms after an outbreak of *Salmonella* enteritidis. *J Rheumatol* 2002:29:767–771.
235. Hannu T, Mattila L, Rautelin H, et al. Campylobacter-triggered reactive arthritis: a population-based study. *Rheumatology* 2002;41:312–318.
236. Boyer GS, Templin DW, Bowler A, et al. Spondyloarthropathy in the community: clinical syndromes and disease manifestations in Alaskan Eskimo populations. *J Rheumatol* 1999;26:1537–1544.
237. Rudwaleit M, Richter S, Braun J, et al. Low incidence of reactive arthritis in children following a salmonella outbreak. *Ann Rheum Dis* 2001;60:1055–1057.
238. Mielants H, Veys EM, Cuvelier C, et al. The evolution of spondyloarthropathies in relation to gut histology. III. Relation between gut and joint. *J Rheumatol* 1995;22:2279–2284.
239. Mielants H, Veys EM, Cuvelier C, et al. The evolution of spondyloarthropathies in relation to gut histology. II. Histological aspects. *J Rheumatol* 1995;22:2273–2278.

240. Mielants H, Veys EM, De Vos M, et al. The evolution of spondyloarthropathies in relation to gut histology. I. Clinical aspects. *J Rheumatol* 1995;22:2266–2272.
241. Birdi N, Hosking M, Clulow MK, et al. Acute rheumatic fever and poststreptococcal reactive arthritis: diagnostic and treatment practices of pediatric subspecialists, *J Rheumatol* 2001;28:1681–1688.
242. Moon RY, Greene MG, Rehe GT, et al. Poststreptococcal reactive arthritis in children: a potential predecessor of rheumatic heart disease. *J Rheumatol* 1995;22:529–532.
243. Aviles RJ, Ramakrishna G, Mohr DN, et al. Poststreptococcal reactive arthritis in adults: a case series. *Mayo Clin Proc* 2000;75:144–147.
244. Shulman ST, Ayoub EM. Poststreptococcal reactive arthritis. *Curr Opin Rheumatol* 2002;14:562–565.
245. Schwartzenberg JM, Smith DD, Lindsley HB. BCG-associated arthropathy mimicking undifferentiated spondyloarthropathy. *J Rheumatol* 1999;26:933–935.
246. Mas AJ, Romera M, Valverde-Garcia JM. Articular manifestations after the administration of intravesical BCG. *J Bone Spine* 2002; 69:92–93.
247. Maillefert JF, Sibilia J, Toussirot E, et al. Rheumatic disorders developed after hepatitis B vaccination. *Rheumatology* 1999;38:978–983.
248. Rose Cd, Fawcett PT, Gibney KM. Arthritis following recombinant outer surface protein A vaccination for Lyme disease. *J Rheumatol* 2001;28:2555–2557.
249. Locht H, Krogfelt KA. Comparison of rheumatological and gastrointestinal symptoms after infection with *Campylobacter jejuni/coli* and enterotoxigenic *Escherichia coli. Ann Rheum Dis* 2002:61:448–452.
250. Peng SL. Rheumatic manifestations of parasitic diseases. *Semin Arthritis Rheum* 2002;31:228–247.
251. Rich E, Hook EW 3rd, Alarcon GS, et al. Reactive arthritis in patients attending an urban sexually transmitted diseases clinic. *Arthritis Rheum* 1996;39:1172–1177.
252. Soderlin MK, Kautiainen H, Puolakkainen M, et al. Infection preceding early arthritis in southern Sweden: a prospective population-based study. *J Rheumatol* 2003;30:459–464.
253. Brown MA, Kennedy GL, MacGregor AJ, et al. Susceptibility to ankylosing spondylitis in twins—the role of genes, HLA, and environment. *Arthritis Rheum* 1997;40:1823–1828.
254. Braun J, Bollow M, Remlinger G, et al. Prevalence of spondyloarthropathies in HLA-B27 positive and negative blood donors. *Arthritis Rheum* 1998;41:58–67.
255. Locht H, Christiansen M, Laursen I. Reactive arthritis and serum levels of mannose binding lectin—lack of association. *Clin Exp Immunol* 2003;131:169–173.
256. Seta N, Granfors K, Sahly H, et al. Expression of host defense scavenger receptors in spondyloarthropathy. *Arthritis Rheum* 2001;44: 931–939.
257. Thomson GT, DeRubeis DA, Hodge MA, et al. Post-salmonella reactive arthritis: late sequelae in a point source cohort. *Am J Med* 1995; 38:618–627.
258. Sieper J, Fendler C, Laitko S, et al. No benefit of long-term ciprofloxacin treatment in patients with reactive arthritis and undifferentiated oligoarthritis: a three-month, multicente, double-blind, randomized, placebo-controlled study. *Arthritis Rheum* 42:1386–1396.
259. Laasila K, Lassonen L, Leirisalo-Repo M. Antibiotic treatment and long term prognosis of reactive arthritis. *Ann Rheum Dis* 2003;62: 655–658.
260. Smieja M, MacPherson DW, Kean W, et al. Randomised, blinded, placebo-controlled trial of doxycycline in chronic seronegative arthritis. *Ann Rheum Dis* 2001;60:1088–1094.
261. Inman RD, Chiu B. Synoviocyte-packaged *Chlamydia trachomatis* induces a chronic aseptic arthritis. *J Clin Invest* 1998;102:1776–1782.
262. Gerard HC, Schumacher HR, El-Gabalawy H, et al. *Chlamydia pneumoniae* present in the human synovium are viable and metabolically active. *Microb Pathog* 2000;29:17–24.
263. Schumacher HR, Gerard HC, Arayssi TK, et al. Lower prevalence of *Chlamydia pneumoniae* DNA compared with *Chlamydia trachomatis* DNA in synovial tissue of arthritis patients. *Arthritis Rheum* 1999;42:1889–1893.
264. Sigal LH. Synovial fluid polymerase chain reaction detection of pathogens—what does it really mean? *Arthritis Rheum* 2001;44: 2463–2485.
265. Schumacher HR, Arayssi T, Crane M, et al. *Chlamydia trachomatis* nucleic acids can be found in the synovium of some asymptomatic subjects. *Arthritis Rheum* 1999;42:1281–1284.
266. Cuchacovich R, Japa S, Huang WQ, et al. Detection of bacterial DNA in Latin American patients with reactive arthritis by polymerase chain reaction and sequencing analysis. *J Rheumatol* 2002: 29:1426–1429.
267. Pacheco-Tena P, De La Barrerra A, Lopez-Vidal Y, et al. Bacterial DNA in synovial fluid cells of patients with juvenile onset spondyloarthropathies. *Rheumatology* 2001;40:920–927.
268. Cox CJ, Kempsell KE, Gaston JS. Investigation of infectious agents associated with arthritis by reverse transcription of PCR of bacterial rRNA. *Arthritis Res Ther* 2002:1:1–8.
269. Gerard HC, Wang Z, Wang GF, et al. Chromosomal DNA from a variety of bacterial species is present in synovial tissue from patients with various forms of arthritis. *Arthritis Rheum* 2001;44:1689–1697.
270. Chen T, Rimpilainen M, Luukkainen R, et al. Bacterial components in the synovial tissue of patients with advanced rheumatoid arthritis or osteoarthritis: analysis with gas chromatography-mass spectrometry and pan-bacterial polymerase chain reaction. *Arthritis Rheum* 2003;49:328–334.
271. Zhang X, Pacheco-Tena C, Inman RD. Microbe hunting in the joints. *Arthritis Rheum* 2003;49:479–482.
272. Wuorela M, Tohka S, Granfors K, et al. Monocytes that have ingested *Yersinia enterocolitica* serotype 0:3 acquire capacity to bind to nonstimulated vascular endothelial cells via P-selectin. *Infect Immun* 1999;67:726–732.
273. Hess S, Rheinheimer C, Tidow F, et al. The reprogrammed host: *Chlamydia trachomatis*–induced upregulation of glycoprotein 130 cytokines, transcription factors and antiapoptotic genes. *Arthritis Rheum* 2001;44:2392–2401.
274. Hanada H, Ikeda-DantsujiY, Naito M, et al. Infection of human fibroblast-like synovial cells with *Chlamydia trachomatis* results in persistent infection and IL-6 production. *Microb Pathog* 2003;34: 57–63.
275. Rodel J, Vogelsang H, Prager K, et al. Role of IFN-stimulated gene factor 3γ and β-interferon in HLA class I enhancement in synovial fibroblasts upon infection with *Chlamydia trachomatis. Infect Immun* 2002;70:6140–6146.
276. Ekman P, Saarinen M, He Q, et al. HLA-B27-transfected and HLA-A2-transfected human monocytic U937 cells differ in their production of cytokines. *Infect Immun* 2002;70:1609–1614.
277. Pentinned MA, Holmberg CI, Sistonen L, et al. HLA-B27 modulates NFκB activation in human monocytic cells exposed to lipopolysaccharide. *Arthritis Rheum* 2002;46:2172–2180.
278. Young JL, Smith L, Matyszak MK, et al. HLA-B27 expression does not modulate intracellular *Chlamydia trachomatis* infection of cell lines. *Infect Immun* 2001;69:6670–6675.
279. Payne U, Inman RD. Determinants of synoviocyte clearance of arthritogenic bacteria. *J Rheumatol* 2003:30:1291–1297.
280. Erlacher L, Wintersberger W, Menschik M, et al. Reactive arthritis: urogenital swab culture is the only useful diagnostic method for detection of the arthritogenic infection in extra-articularly asymptomatic patients with undifferentiated oligoarthritis. *Br J Rheumatol* 1995;34:838–842.
281. Bas S, Genevay S, Schenkel MC, et al. Importance of species-specific antigens in the serodiagnosis of *Chlamydia trachomatis* reactive arthritis. *Rheumatology* 2002;41:1017–1020.
282. Bas S, Scieux C, Vischer TL. Male sex predominance in *Chlamydia trachomatis* sexually acquired reactive arthritis: are women more protected by anti-chlamydia antibodies? *Ann Rheum Dis* 2001;60: 605–611.
283. Maki-Ikola O, Leirisalo-Repo M, Turunen U, et al. Association of gut inflammation with increased serum IgA class *Klebsiella* antibody concentrations in patients with axial ankylosing spondylitis: implications for different aetiopathogenetic mechanisms for axial and peripheral AS. *Ann Rheum Dis* 1997;56:180–183.
284. Ahmadi K, Wilson C, Tiwana H, et al. Antibodies to *Klebsiella pneumoniae* lipopolysaccharide in patients with ankylosing spondylitis. *Br J Rheum* 1998;37:1299–1302.
285. Maki-Ikola O, Nissila M, Lehtinen K, et al. IgA class serum antibodies against three different *Klebsiella* serotypes in ankylosing spondylitis. *Br J Rheumatol* 1998:37:1299–1302.

286. Sahly H, Podschun R, Kekow J, et al. Humoral immune response to *Klebsiella* capsular polysaccharides in HLA-B27-positive patients with acute anterior uveitis and ankylosing spondylitis. *Autoimmunity* 1998;28:209–215.
287. Cancino-Diaz ME, Perez-Salazar JE, Dominguez-Lopez L, et al. Antibody responses to *Klebsiella pneumoniae* 60kD protein in familial and sporadic ankylosing spondylitis: role of HLA-B27 and characterization as a GroEl-like protein. *J Rheumatol* 1998;25:1756–1764.
288. Stone MA, Payne U, Lapp V, et al. *Klebsiella* is not the dominant microbial trigger in familial ankylosing spondylitis. *Arthritis Rheum* 2001;44(suppl):346.
289. Sprenkels SH, Uksila J, Vainiopaa R, et al. IgA antibodies in HLA-B27 associated acute anterior uveitis and ankylosing spondylitis. *Clin Rheumatol* 1996;15:52–56.
290. Careless DJ, Chiu B, Rabinovitch T, et al. Immunogenetic and microbial factors in acute anterior uveitis. *J Rheumatol* 1997;24:102–108.
291. Maki-Ikola O, Heesemann J, Toivanen A, et al. High frequency of *Yersinia* antibodies in healthy populations in Finland and Germany. *Rheumatol Int* 1997;16:227–229.
292. Lahesmaa R, Soderberg C, Bliska J, et al. Pathogen antigen-and superantigen-reactive synovial fluid T cells in reactive arthritis. *J Infect Dis* 1995;172:1290–1297.
293. Gaston JS, Deane KH, Jecock RM, et al. Identification of 2 *Chlamydia trachomatis* antigens recognized by synovial fluid T cells from patients with *Chlamydia*-induced reactive arthritis. *J Rheumatol* 1996;23:130–136.
294. Fendler C, Braun J, Eggens U, et al. Bacteria-specific lymphocyte proliferation in peripheral blood in reactive arthritis and related diseases. *Br J Rheumatol* 1998;37:520–524.
295. Fendler C, Wu P, Eggens U, et al. Longitudinal investigation of bacterium-specific synovial lymphocyte proliferation in reactive arthritis and Lyme arthritis. *Br J Rheumatol* 1998;37:784–788.
296. Mertz AK, Wu P, Stuniolo T, et al. Multispecific $CD4^+$ T cell response to a single 12-mer epitope od the immunodominant heat shock protein 69 of *Yersinia enterocolitica* in *Yersinia*-triggered reactive arthritis. *J Immunol* 2000;164;1529–1537.
297. Goodall JC, Beacock-Sharp H, Deane KH, et al. Recognition of the 60kD cysteine-rich outer membrane protein OMP2 by $CD4^+$ T cells from humans infected with *Chlamydia trachomatis. Clin Exp Immunol* 2001;136:488–493.
298. Thiel A, Wu P, Lauster R, et al. Analysis of the antigen-specific T cell response in reactive arthritis by flow cytometry. *Arthritis Rheum* 2000;43:2834–2842.
299. Yin Z, Braun J, Neure L, et al. Crucial role of interleukin-10/interleukin-12 balance in the regulation of the type 2 T helper cytokine response in reactive arthritis. *Arthritis Rheum* 1997;40:1788–1797.
300. Steiner G, Studnicka-Benke A, Witzmann G, et al. Soluble receptors for tumor necrosis factor and interleukin-2 in serum and synovial fluid of patients with rheumatoid arthritis, reactive arthritis, and osteoarthritis. *J Rheumatol* 1885;22:406–412.
301. Rodel J, Straube E, Lungerhausen W, et al. Secretion of cytokines by human synoviocytes during *in vitro* infection with *Chlamydia trachomatis. J Rheumatol* 1998;24:2161–2168.
302. Stone MA, Inman RD. The genetics of cytokines in ankylosing spondylitis. *J Rheumatol* 2001;28:1288–1293.
303. Zhao YX, Lajoie G, Zhang H, et al. Tumor necrosis factor p55-receptor-deficient mice respond to acute *Yersinia enterocolitica* infection with less apoptosis and more effective host resistance. *Infect Immun* 2000;68:1243–1251.
304. Zhao YX, Zhang H, Chiu B, et al. Tumor necrosis factor receptor p55 controls the severity of arthritis in experimental *Yersinia enterocolitica* infection. *Arthritis Rheum* 1999;42:1662–1672.
305. Dulphy N, Rabian C, Douay C, et al. Functional modulation of expanded $CD8^+$ synovial fluid T cells—NK cell receptor expression in HLA-B27-associated reactive arthritis. *Int Immunol* 2002;14:471–479.
306. Ren EC, Koh Wh, Sim D, et al. Possible protective role of HLA-B*2706 for ankylosing spondylitis. *Tissue Antigens* 1997;49:67–69.
307. D'Amato M, Fiorillo MT, Carcassi C, et al. Relevance of residue 116 of HLA-B27 in determining susceptibility to ankylosing spondylitis. *Eur J Immunol* 1995;25:3199–3201.
308. Fiorillo MT, Greco G, Maragno M, et al. The naturally occurring polymorphism Asp116 → HiS116, differentiating the ankylosing spondylitis-associated HLA-B*2705 from the non-associated HLA-B*2709 subtype, influences peptide-specific CD8 T cell recognition. *Eur J Immunol* 1998;28:2508–2516.
309. Ugrinovic S, Mertz A, Wu P, et al. A single nonamer from the *Yersinia* 60-kDa heat shock protein is the target of HLA-B27-restricted CTL response in *Yersinia*-induced arthritis. *J Immunol* 1997;159:5715–5723.
310. Ackermann B, Staege MS, Reske-Kunz AB, et al. Enterobacteria-infected T cells as antigen-presenting cells for cytotoxic CD8 T cells: a contribution to the self-limitation of cellular immune reactions in reactive arthritis? *J Infect Dis* 1997;175:1121–1127.
311. Kuon W, Holzhutter HG, Appel H, et al. Identification of HLA-B27-restricted peptides from the *Chlamydia trachomatis* proteome with possible relevance to HLA- B27-associated diseases. *J Immunol* 2001;167:4738–4746.
312. Lopez-Larrea C, Gonzalez S, Martinez-Borra J. The role of HLA-B27 polymorphism and molecular mimicry in spondyloarthropathy. *Mol Med Today* 1998;4:540–549.
313. Williams RC, Tsuchiya N, Husby G. Molecular mimicry, ankylosing spondylitis and reactive arthritis. *Scand J Rheumatol* 1992;21:105–108.
314. Lo WF, Woods AS, DeCloux A, et al. Molecular mimicry mediated by MHC class Ib molecules after infection with gram-negative pathogens. *Nat Med* 2000;6:215–218.
315. Albert LJ, Inman RD. Gram-negative pathogens and molecular mimicry: is there a case for mistaken identity? *Trends Microbiol* 2000;8: 446–447.
316. Ramos M, Alvarez I, Sesma L, et al. Molecular mimicry of HLA-B27-derived peptide ligand of arthritis-linked subtypes with chlamydial proteins. *J Biol Chem* 2002:277:37573–37581.
317. Popov I, Dela Cruz CS, Barber BH, et al. The effect of an anti-B27 immune response on CTL recognition of *Chlamydia. J Immunol* 2001;167:3375–3382.
318. Popov I, Dela Cruz CS, Barber BH, et al. Breakdown of CTL tolerance to self HLA-B*2705 induced by exposure to *Chlamydia trachomatis. J Immunol* 2002;169:4033–4038
319. Banki K, Colombo E, Sia F, et al. Oligodendrocyte-specific expression and autoantigenicity of transaldolase in multiple sclerosis. *J Exp Med* 1994;180:1649–1663.
320. Banki K, Tatum AH, Sciubba JJ, et al. Correlation of autoantigenicity with expression of a human endogenous retroviral element, HRES-1. *Arthritis Rheum* 1993;36(suppl):44.
321. Lu X, Heimer J, Rekosh D, et al. U1 small nuclear RNA plays a direct role in the formation of a rev-regulated human immunodeficiency virus env mRNA that remains unspliced. *Proc Natl Acad Sci U S A* 1990;87:7598–7602.
322. Zinkernagel RM, Cooper S, Chambers J, et al. Virus-induced autoantibody response to a transgenic viral antigen. *Nature* 1990;345: 68–71.
323. Fox RI. Sjögren's syndrome. Pathogenesis and new approaches to therapy. *Adv Exp Med Biol* 1998;438:891–902.
324. Kordossis T, Paikos S, Aroni K, et al. Prevalence of Sjögren's-like syndrome in a cohort of HIV-1-positive patients descriptive pathology and immunopathology. *Br J Rheumatol* 1998;37:691–695.
325. Williams FM, Cohen PR, Jumshyd J, et al. Prevalence of the diffuse lymphocytosis syndrome among patients with human immunodeficiency virus type-1-positive patients. *Arthritis Rheum* 1998;41:863–868.
326. Ranger-Rogez S, Vidal E, Labrousse F, et al. Large-scale study suggests no direct link between human herpesvirus-6 and primary Sjögren's syndrome. *J Med Virol* 1995;47:198–203.
327. Fox RI, Luppi M, Kang HI, et al. Detection of high levels of human herpes virus-6DNA in a lymphoma of a patient with Sjögren's syndrome. *J Rheumatol* 1993;20:764–765.
328. Hirose Y, Sugai S, Masaki Y, et al. Epstein-Barr virus study in malignant lymphoma in Sjögren's syndrome. *Int J Hematol* 1999;69:174–179.
329. Perl A, Gorevic PD, Condemi JJ, et al. Antibodies to retroviral proteins and reverse transcriptase activity in patients with essential cryoglobulinemia. *Arthritis Rheum* 1991;34:1313–1318.
330. Watkins DI, McAdam SN, Liu X, et al. New recombinant HLA-B alleles in a tribe of South America Amerindians indicate rapid evolution of MHC class I loci. *Nature* 1992;357:329–332.
331. Belich MP, Madrigal JA, Hildebrand WH, et al. Unusual HLA-B alleles in two tribes of Brazilian Indians. *Nature* 1992;357:326–329.

332. Howard JC. Disease and evolution. *Nature* 1991;352:565–567.
333. Hill AS, Allsopp CEM, Kwatkowski D, et al. Common West African HLA antigens are associated with protection from severe malaria. *Nature* 1991;352:595–600.
334. Query CC, Keene JD. A human autoimmune protein associated with U1 RNA contains a region of homology that is cross-reactive with retroviral $p30^{gag}$ antigen. *Cell* 1987;51:211–220.
335. Perl A, Colombo E, Dai H, et al. Antibody reactivity to the HRES-1 endogenous retroviral element identifies a subset of patients with systemic lupus erythematosus and overlap syndromes: correlation with antinuclear antibodies and HLA class II alleles. *Arthritis Rheum* 1995;38:1660–1671.
336. Banki K, Maceda J, Hurley E, et al. Human T-cell lymphotropic virus (HTLV)-related endogenous sequence, HRES-1, encodes a 28-kDa protein: a possible autoantigen for HTLV-I gag-reactive autoantibodies. *Proc Natl Acad Sci U S A* 1992;89:1939–1943.
337. Brookes SM, Pandolfino YA, Mitchell TJ, et al. The immune response to and expression of cross-reactive retroviral gag sequences in autoimmune disease. *Br J Rheumatol* 1992;31:735–742.
338. Bengtsson A, Blomberg J, Nived O, et al. Selective antibody reactivity with peptides from human endogenous retroviruses and nonviral poly(amino acids) in patients with systemic lupus erythematosus. *Arthritis Rheum* 1996;39:1654–1663.
339. Talal N, Garry RF, Schur PH, et al. A conserved idiotype and antibodies to retroviral proteins in systemic lupus erythematosus. *J Clin Invest* 1990;85:1866–1871.
340. Misaki Y, Yamamoto K, Yanagi K, et al. B cell epitope on the U1 snRNP-C autoantigen contains a sequence similar to that of the herpes simplex virus protein. *Eur J Immunol* 1993;23:1064–1071.
341. Sabbatini A, Bombardieri S, Migliorini P. Autoantibodies form patients with systemic lupus erythematosus bind a shared sequence of SmD and Epstein-Barr virus–encoded nuclear antigen EBNA I. *Eur J Immunol* 1993;23:1146–1152.
342. James JJ, Kaufman KM, Farris AD, et al. An increased prevalence of Epstein-Barr virus infection in young patients suggests a possible etiology for systemic lupus erythematosus. *J Clin Invest* 1997;100: 3019–3026.
343. Kohsaka H, Yamamoto K, Fujii H, et al. Fine epitope mapping of the human SS-B/La protein. Identification of a distinct autoepitope homologous to a viral gag polyprotein. *J Clin Invest* 1990;85:1566–1574.
344. Vaughan JH, Nguyen M-D, Valbracht JR, et al. Epstein-Barr virus–induced autoimmune responses II. Immunoglobulin G autoantibodies to mimicking and nonmimicking epitopes. Presence in autoimmune disease. *J Clin Invest* 1995;95:1316–1327.
345. Maul GG, Jimenez SA, Riggs E, et al. Determination of an epitope of the diffuse systemic sclerosis marker antigen DNA topoisomerase I: sequence similarity with retroviral p30 gag protein suggests a possible cause for autoimmunity in systemic sclerosis. *Proc Natl Acad Sci U S A* 1989;86:8492–8496.
346. Lunardi C, Tiso M, Borgato L, et al. Chronic parvovirus B19 infection induces the production of anti-virus antibodies with autoantigen binding properties. *Eur J Immunol* 1998;28:936–948.
347. Inman RD, Perl A, Phillips PE. Infectious agents in chronic rheumatic diseases. In: Koopman WJ, ed. *Arthritis and allied conditions. A textbook of rheumatology.* Philadelphia: Lea & Febiger, 1997:585–608.
348. Brummer-Korvenkontio M, Vapalahti O, Kuusisto P, et al. Epidemiology of Sindbis virus infections in Finland 1981–96: possible factors explaining a peculiar disease pattern. *Epidemiol Infect* 2002; 129:335–345.

SECTION III

Therapeutic Approaches in the Rheumatic Diseases

CHAPTER 31

Nonsteroidal Anti-Inflammatory Drugs

John S. Sundy

The nonsteroidal antiinflammatory drugs (NSAIDs) are a diverse group of compounds that includes salicylates, nonselective cyclooxygenase (COX) inhibitors, and the newer class of selective COX-2 inhibitors. NSAIDs are among the most widely used class of medications in the United States. They are effective across a wide spectrum of disorders that includes fever, inflammation, mild to moderate pain, and the prevention of cardiovascular syndromes. NSAIDs have a critical role in the management of numerous rheumatologic disorders. Their use is likely to grow as a result of emerging applications such as the prevention of some forms of cancer and Alzheimer disease.

The medicinal use of NSAIDs dates back several millennia to the use of willow bark to treat musculoskeletal pain (1). The active ingredient of willow bark, salicin, was extracted in 1828, and later obtained in crystalline form (1,2). Subsequently, sodium salicylate and aspirin were synthesized in 1875 and 1899, respectively (1,3). The first nonaspirin NSAID, phenylbutazone, was approved by the U.S. Food and Drug Administration (FDA) in 1949, followed by indomethacin in 1963 (4). Numerous other NSAIDs followed for the next 30 years. The most recent significant advance has been the introduction of the selective COX-2 inhibitors—celecoxib, rofecoxib, and valdecoxib—beginning in 1999 (5).

The NSAIDs are a mainstay in the pharmacologic armamentarium of rheumatologists. For treatment of mild to moderate musculoskeletal pain and osteoarthritis (OA), the NSAIDs are generally considered the pharmacologic treatment of choice (6–8). In contrast, NSAIDs have assumed an adjunctive position in the management of immune-mediated inflammatory diseases such as rheumatoid arthritis (RA), owing to the early use of immunomodulating therapy for these conditions.

Despite the prevalent use of NSAIDs, drug-related adverse events are a primary concern for clinicians. The high prevalence of NSAID-induced peptic ulcer disease (PUD) provided the impetus for the recent development of the new class of highly selective COX-2 inhibitor. Ongoing concerns relate to exacerbation of hypertension and congestive heart failure (CHF) and impairment of renal function in some patients using NSAIDs. The therapeutic benefits and widespread use of NSAIDs requires that physicians of all specialties, especially rheumatologists, be well versed in

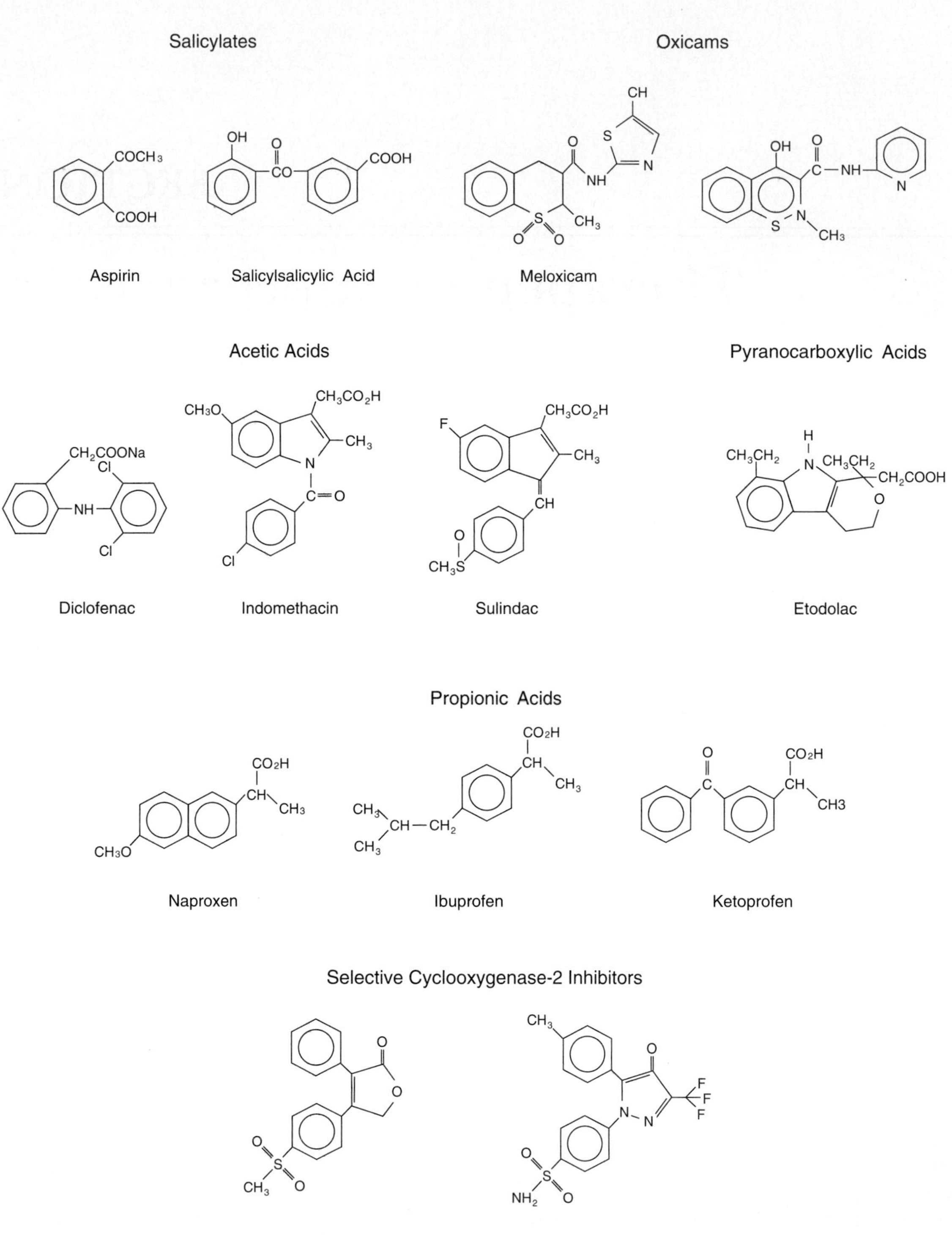

FIG. 31.1. Chemical structures of selected salicylates, nonselective nonsteroidal antiinflammatory drugs, and selective cyclooxygenase-2 inhibitors.

the appropriate prescribing and monitoring of patients taking NSAIDs. The efficacy of NSAIDs in specific rheumatologic disorders is discussed in detail throughout this text. This chapter will review the biochemical and pharmacologic rationale for the use of NSAIDs, and will review the strategies for anticipating and preventing adverse events of therapy.

CHEMISTRY

The NSAIDs may be divided into three major classes: aspirin and salicylates, nonselective NSAIDs, and selective COX-2 inhibitors (Fig. 31.1, Table 31.1). The prototype salicylate, aspirin, is the salicylic ester of acetic acid. Chemically, there are two classes of salicylates: esters of salicylic acid (e.g., salsalate), and salicylate esters of organic acids (e.g., acetylsalicylic acid or aspirin). Other compounds in clinical use include the salicylic acid salts (e.g., choline salicylate). A more clinically relevant classification scheme groups salicylates into acetylated (aspirin) and nonacetylated salicylates (all other salicylates in clinical use).

Among the nonselective NSAIDs are several subclasses grouped by chemical structure (Table 31.2). Despite the tradition of grouping nonselective NSAIDs by chemical structure, the designation carries no important significance for efficacy or safety. The third class of NSAIDs is the selective COX-2 inhibitors, which have negligible inhibition of COX-1 at therapeutic tissue concentrations (5).

Mechanism of Action

Despite the use of NSAIDs dating back to the early history of medicine, their mechanism of action was not identified until 1971 (9). The primary mechanism of action of NSAIDs is the inhibition of COX, a synthetic enzyme for prostaglandins (PGs). NSAIDs also have other potential mechanisms of action that may contribute to their clinical effectiveness.

Reduction of Prostaglandin Synthesis

The synthetic pathway for PG is reviewed in detail in Chapter 23. Briefly, arachidonic acid, the precursor to PGs, is produced in cells by cleavage of membrane phospholipids by phospholipase A. Cyclooxygenase and lipoxygenase convert arachidonic acid into PGs and leukotrienes, respectively (Fig. 31.2). PGG_2 and PGH_2 are the products of COX, and are subsequently converted to a variety of prostanoids by tissue-specific isomerases (5). For example, PGH_2 is converted to thromboxane A_2 in platelets.

Through the independent work of several laboratories, two isoforms of COX, designated COX-1 and COX-2, have been identified (10–15). COX-1 and COX-2 are associated with membranes in the endoplasmic reticulum and cell nucleus (16). As a generalization, COX-1 is constitutively expressed in most cell types and produces PGs important in normal tissue homeostasis, such as the maintenance of gastrointestinal mucosa and regulation of platelet function (17,18). COX-2 is induced in response to a variety of proinflammatory mediators, growth factors, and tumor promoters (13,14). This dichotomy is somewhat oversimplified because COX-2 is constitutively expressed in the kidney and the central nervous system, and COX-1 expression has also been shown to be regulated in some sites (19–22).

The inhibition of COX enzyme activity is the primary mechanism of action of NSAIDs as a class. Both isoforms of COX are inhibited by aspirin and NSAIDs. Aspirin is unique in that it irreversibly inhibits both isoforms of COX by acetylating a serine moiety (serine 530 of COX-1 and serine 516 of COX-2) (23,24). Two mechanisms of COX inhibition by nonselective NSAIDs have been identified. First, NSAIDs can mediate time-independent inhibition of COX that is dependent on drug concentration. Second, some NSAIDs (e.g., indomethacin and flurbiprofen) have the additional feature of inducing time-dependent structural changes in the active site of COX that may lead to near-irreversible inhibition of enzyme activity (25). The clinical significance of these distinct inhibitory mechanisms has not been investigated.

Aspirin and the nonselective NSAIDs inhibit both isoforms of COX with varying ratios of effect on COX-1 and COX-2. The fundamental hypothesis that derived from the discovery of COX-1 and COX-2 was that the therapeutic benefits of NSAIDs resulted from COX-2 inhibition, whereas the adverse events associated with NSAIDs resulted from COX-1 inhibition. Highly selective COX-2 inhibitors were developed with the objective of ameliorating the harmful effects associated with traditional NSAIDs. This objective has been partially achieved; however, COX-2 inhibitors possess many of the adverse renal effects observed with nonselective NSAIDs (see later section on Adverse Events Associated with NSAIDs).

Other Potential Mechanisms of Action

Many NSAIDs possess pharmacologic properties distinct from COX inhibition. The salicylates, with the exception of aspirin, have minimal inhibitory action on COX. Yet, salicylates demonstrate significant antiinflammatory activity and inhibit the production of PG synthesis in cell culture and in whole animals (26,27). The mechanism of PG inhibition by salicylates probably relates to suppressing the expression of COX itself, rather than inhibiting its function (26).

Other pharmacologic properties of NSAIDs include the inhibition of transcription factors, cell growth factors, and molecules that regulate apoptosis. At supratherapeutic concentrations, sodium salicylate inhibits the gene transcription regulator nuclear factor κB, which may, in part, contribute to reduced expression of chemokines and nitric oxide, and reduced tumor necrosis factor–induced signaling activity (28–31). COX-2 selective and nonselective

TABLE 31.1. *Characteristics of currently approved nonsteroidal antiinflammatory drugs (NSAIDs)*

Drug (trade names)	Indications and uses	Formulations	Daily dose	Metabolism	Half-life	Other considerations
Salicylates						
Aspirin	Arthralgia, dental pain, dysmenorrhea, fever, headache, JRA, migraine, mild pain, myalgia, OA, RA, prevention and treatment cardiovascular thrombosis	Numerous	Variable, depending on indication; maximum (adults) 2.4–5.4 g/day in 4 or more divided doses	Hepatic and renal	Acetylsalicylic acid 15–30 min; salicylate 2–30 h	Dose in children body weight <25 kg is 60–90 mg/kg/day. Serum salicylate levels may need to be monitored at higher doses.
Choline magnesium trisalicylate (Trilisate)	Fever, JRA, mild-moderate pain, OA, RA	Solution Tablets	3 g/day in divided doses	Hepatic and renal	Low dose 2–3 h; high dose 15–30 h	Dose in children <37 kg is 50 mg/kg/day. Serum salicylate levels may need to be monitored at higher doses.
Salsalate (Disalsid)	Mild moderate pain OA, RA	Capsules Tablets	2–4 g daily divided dose	Hepatic and renal	1 h	Serum salicylate levels may need to be monitored at higher doses.
Nonselective NSAIDs						
Naproxen (Naprosen, Anaprox)	Ankylosing spondylitis, arthralgia, bursitis, dental pain, dysmenorrhea, fever, gout arthritis, headache, JRA, mild-moderate pain, myalgia, OA, RA, tendinitis	Tablet Extended-release tablet Suspension	500–1,000 mg b.i.d.	Hepatic and renal	10–20 h	Dosage in children age >2 yr 10–15 mg/kg/day in 2 divided doses. Naproxen may falsely elevate urinary 17 ketosteroid concentrations and interfere with 5-hydroxyindoleacetic acid determination. Discontinue 72 h before testing.
Flurbiprofen (Ansaid)	Arthralgia, mild-moderate pain, miosis inhibition, myalgia, OA, RA	Tablets Ophthalmic solution	50–100 mg b.i.d.–t.i.d.; maximum 300 mg/day	Hepatic	3–9 h	
Diclofenac (Voltaren, Arthrotec)	Actinic keratoses, allergic conjunctivitis, ankylosing spondylitis, arthralgia, corneal ulcer, dysmenorrhea, headache, keratoconjunctivitis, migraine, mild-moderate pain, myalgia, OA, postoperative ocular inflammation, RA	Tablets Tablets (combination with misoprostol) Ophthalmic solution Topical solution	50–100 mg b.i.d.; maximum 225 mg/day	Hepatic	1–2 h	Cholestyramine reduced bioavailability of diclofenac. Diclofenac/misoprostol combination contraindicated in pregnancy because of abortifacient effect of misoprostol.
Sulindac (Clinoril)	Ankylosing spondylitis, arthralgia, bursitis, gouty arthritis, moderate pain, OA, RA, tendinitis	Tablets	150–200 mg b.i.d.	Hepatic	8–16 h	Nonindicated use in JRA 2–4 mg/kg/day suggested.

Oxaprozin (Daypro)	Moderate pain, OA, RA	Tablets	600–1200 mg qd	Hepatic	36–92 h	Non-indicated use in JRA of 10–20 mg/kg/day reported
Diflunisal (Dolobid)	Mild-moderate pain, OA, RA	Tablets	500–1,000 mg b.i.d.	Hepatic	8–12 h 68–138 h in severe renal disease	50% increase in acetaminophen plasma concentratrion following administration of diflunisal. Diflunisal is a salicylic acid derivative, association with Reye syndrome not known. Avoid in children. Diflunisal may falsely elevate serum salicylate levels.
Piroxicam (Feldene)	Arthralgia, headache, moderate pain, myalgia, OA, RA	Capsule	20 mg q.d.	Hepatic with enterohepatic recirculation	50 h	Particular caution in high-risk individuals. Plasma concentrations decreased by 20% when administered with aspirin.
Indomethacin (Indocin)	Ankylosing spondylitis, arthralgia, bursitis, gouty arthritis, moderate pain, myalgia, OA, patent ductus arteriosus, RA, severe pain, tendinitis	Capsules Extended-release capsules Suspension Suppositories Parenteral	25–50 mg t.i.d.–q.i.d.	Hepatic Some enterohepatic recirculation	Biphasic: 1 h initial; 2.6–11.2 h in second phase Prolonged half-life in neonates and premature neonates	Increased serum aminoglycoside concentrations in neonates; monitor aminoglycoside levels closely in all patients. Indomethacin augments the hypothalamic-pituitary-adrenal axis response to dexamethasone. Possible false normal results in patients with depressed response.
Ibuprofen (Motrin)	Arthralgia, dental pain, dysmenorrhea, fever, headache, JRA, migraine, mild-moderate pain, myalgia, OA, RA	Numerous	Adults: 400–800 mg t.i.d.–q.i.d. Children: 5–10 mg/kg	Hepatic	2–4 h	Safety demonstrated in children 6 mo of age and older.
Fenoprofen (Nalfon)	Arthralgia, mild-moderate pain, myalgia, OA, RA	Tablets Capsules	300–600 mg t.i.d.–q.i.d.; maximum 3,200 mg/day	Hepatic Enterohepatic recirculation	2.5–3.0 h	Aspirin can decrease fenoprofen plasma concentrations by 50% and reduce half-life. Phenobarbital can decrease plasma concentrations of fenoprofen. Monitor barbiturate levels after initiation or withdrawal of fenoprofen. Elevated free and total triiodithyronine plasma concentrations by some methods
Etodolac (Lodine)	Arthralgia, bone pain, dental pain, mild pain, moderate pain, myalgia, OA, RA	Tablets Extended-release tablets	600–1,200 mg daily	Hepatic	6–7 h	

Continued

TABLE 31.1. *Continued*

Drug (trade names)	Indications and uses	Formulations	Daily dose	Metabolism	Half-life	Other considerations
Ketoprofen (Orudis)	Arthralgia, dental pain, dysmenorrhea, fever, headache, mild-moderate pain, myalgia, OA, RA	Capsules Extended-release capsules Tablets	75 mg t.i.d. or 50 mg q.i.d.	Hepatic	1.1–4 h	Increased plasma concentration of ketoprofen when administered with probenecid.
Ketorolac (Toradol)	Allergic conjunctivitis, arthralgia, moderate pain, myalgia, ocular pain, ocular pruritus, photophobia, post-operative ocular inflammation	Tablets Parenteral (i.m. or i.v.) Ophthalmic solution	30 mg i.m./i.v. every 6 h; maximum 120 mg/day; do not use longer than 5 days 10 mg p.o. every 4–6 h; maximum of 40 mg daily for 5 days	Hepatic	Biphasic; terminal phase 4–6 h	Elimination half-life of ketorolac is doubled during administration with probenecid. Concomitant use should be avoided. Parenteral ketorolac can enhance the muscle relaxant effect of non-depolarizing skeletal muscle relaxants. Caution with concomitant use.
Meclofenamate, mefenamic acid (Ponstel)	Arthralgia, dysmenorrhea, mild-moderate pain, OA, RA	Capsule	50–100 mg t.i.d.–q.i.d.; maximum 400 mg/day Mefenamic acid: 250 mg every 6 h for 7 days; maximum 1,250 mg/day	Hepatic	2 h	Mefenamic acid may cause false-positive test result for urinary bile.
Meloxicam (Mobic)	OA	Tablets	7.5–15 mg q.d.	Hepatic	15–30 h	Cholestyramine may increase clearance meloxicam. No platelet inhibition at indicated doses.

Nabumetone (Relafen)	Moderate pain, OA, RA	Tablets	1,000 mg q.d.; maximum dose of 2,000 mg q.d.	Hepatic	24 h	
Tolmetin (Tolectin)	Arthralgia, JRA, moderate pain, myalgia, OA, RA	Tablets Capsules	400 mg t.i.d.–q.i.d.; maximum dose 2,000 mg/day	Hepatic	Biphasic: initial 1–2 h; terminal 5 h	Dosage in children age 2 yr and above 5–7 mg/kg/dose p.o. every 6–8 h. False-positive reaction for proteinuria on acid precipitation test; no effect on urine dipstick test for protein.
Selective COX-2 inhibitors						
Celecoxib (Celebrex)	Bone pain, dental pain, dysmenorrhea, FAP, headache, moderate-severe pain, OA, RA	Capsules	100–200 mg b.i.d.; 400 mg b.i.d. in FAP	Hepatic	11 h	Reduce dose 50% in setting of moderate liver dysfunction. Fluconazole inhibits celecoxib metabolism in the liver. Use lowest celecoxib dose with concomitant fluconazole.
Rofecoxib (Vioxx)	Bone pain, dental pain, dysmenorrhea, headache, mild-moderate pain, OA, RA	Tablet Suspension	12.5–25 mg q.d.; 50 mg q.d. for 5 days for pain	Hepatic	17 h	
Valdecoxib (Bextra)	Dysmenorrhea, OA, RA	Tablet	10 mg q.d.; 20 mg q.d. as needed for dysmenorrhea	Hepatic	8–11 h	

b.i.d., twice daily; FAP, familial adenomatous polyposis; i.m., intramuscularly; i.v., intravenously; JRA, juvenile rheumatoid arthritis; OA, osteoarthritis; p.o., by mouth; q.d., daily; RA, rheumatoid arthritis; t.i.d., three times daily.

TABLE 31.2. *Chemical classification of nonselective nonsteroidal antiinflammatory drugs (NSAIDs)*

Chemical class	Associated NSAIDs
Acetic acids	Diclofenac, indomethacin, sulindac, tolmetin
Fenamates	Meclofenamate, mefenamic acid
Napthylalkanones	Nabumetone
Oxicams	Meloxicam, piroxicam
Propionic acids	Enoprofen, flurbiprofen, ibuprofen, ketoprofen, naproxen, oxaprozin
Pyranocarboxylic acid	Etodolac
Pyrrolizine carboxylic acid	Ketorolac

NSAIDs have also been shown to inhibit angiogenesis through inhibition of mitogen-activated protein kinase (ERK2) in endothelial cells (32). Finally, when COX-2 is acetylated by aspirin, it acquires the ability to synthesize 15-hydroxyeicosatetraenoic acid, which is metabolized by 5-lipoxygenase to yield the antiinflammatory eicosanoid 15-epi-lipoxin A4 (33–35). This may contribute to the antiinflammatory actions of aspirin.

PHARMACODYNAMICS

Antiinflammatory Effect

PGs directly or indirectly mediate many of the manifestations of inflammation. The antiinflammatory properties of NSAIDs correlate with their ability to inhibit PG synthesis. The ability to inhibit COX is one method for assessing antiinflammatory activity. *In vitro* whole blood assays of COX-1 and COX-2 inhibition are used as a surrogate marker of antiinflammatory effectiveness and as a method for assessing the relative selectivity of an agent for COX-1 versus COX-2. An *in vivo* method for assessing the antiinflammatory effectiveness of NSAIDs is the administration of proinflammatory irritants, such as carrageenin, into the hind paw of rats. Other models include the induction of adjuvant arthritis, which results from administration of mycobacteria and oil into rat paws. Effective NSAIDs diminish the swelling and inflammatory infiltrates within the affected paw. Most compounds must demonstrate antiinflammatory effects in numerous *in vitro* and *in vivo* models to be considered for clinical development as an NSAID.

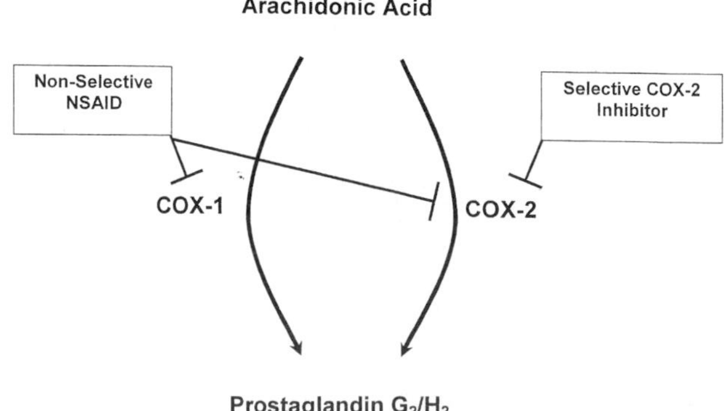

FIG. 31.2. Prostaglandin synthesis pathway with sites of nonsteroidal antiinflammatory drug inhibition.

Analgesic Effect

One of the primary uses of NSAIDs is to relieve pain. The NSAIDs were originally thought to influence pain sensation strictly in the peripheral nervous system, but recent data indicate that both peripheral and central pain pathways are inhibited. Three types of pain are recognized: physiologic pain, inflammatory pain, and neuropathic pain (36). Physiologic pain is characterized by a high threshold for stimulation, transient symptoms, and well-localized sensation. Inflammatory pain is characterized by heightened sensitivity of normal pain stimuli in response to tissue inflammation or injury. Neuropathic pain results from injury to neurons in the periphery or in the spinal cord and is characterized by hyperalgesia to noxious stimuli, allodynia, and spontaneous onset of pain symptoms. PGs are hypothesized to play a role in the induction of all three types of pain, and may act in both the peripheral and central nervous system.

Inflammation or injury in peripheral tissues leads to local up-regulation of PGs and other inflammatory mediators. This coincides with markedly increased expression of COX-2 by local tissue cells and infiltrating inflammatory cells (37). Evidence indicating that PGs induce hyperalgesia at peripheral sites of inflammation includes the induction of hyperalgesia by local injection of PGE_2 and reduction in the pain response by administration of neutralizing monoclonal antibodies to PGE_2. Therefore, an important aspect of the analgesic properties of NSAIDs relates to inhibition of tissue PG production in sites of inflammation or injury.

PGs produced in the central nervous system (CNS) also regulate pain symptoms. Both COX-1 and COX-2 are expressed in the CNS (38,39). COX-2 is expressed constitutively in the CNS, and is also up-regulated by peripheral inflammatory stimuli. Both constitutive and induced

COX-2 expression is inhibited by systemic glucocorticoids (38,40). COX-2 is the predominant isoform expressed in the rat spinal cord (41,42), whereas COX-1, but not COX-2, is expressed in nociceptive neurons in the dorsal root ganglion (43). During systemic inflammatory stimulation, COX-1, but not COX-2, is stably expressed in dorsal root ganglia, whereas COX-2 is markedly up-regulated within the spinal cord.

Receptors for PGs are widely expressed in neuronal cells of the CNS. The EP3 receptor for PGE_2 is expressed in ascending nociceptive pathways of the pontine parabrachial nucleus (44) and in thalamic nuclei (45) of rats. EP3 expression has also been detected in interleukin-1 (IL-1)-responsive neurons of nociceptive pathways in the preoptic area of the brain (46). Interestingly, COX-2 and EP3 expression colocalized to specific elements of the rat spinal cord that are associated with pain transmission (42). The expression of COX in association with receptors for PGs provides strong evidence for a role for PGE-induced hyperalgesia within the CNS (36).

Together these data demonstrate that PGs are important in regulating nociception in both the peripheral and CNS. The analgesic properties of NSAIDs most likely result from central and peripheral inhibition of PG production. Although comparative trials of the analgesic efficacy of NSAIDs have not been systematically studied, it is possible that variation in the analgesic effectiveness of NSAIDs may relate to differences in penetration of the drug into the CNS.

Antipyretic Effect

NSAIDs are effective at reducing fever in humans. Most evidence indicates that the febrile response is mediated through the production of PGE_2 in the CNS (47). Evidence supporting this includes the detection of increased levels of PGE_2 in the hypothalamus and the third ventricle during fever. Furthermore, deletion of the PGE_2 receptor EP3 in mice abrogates the febrile response to pyrogens such as IL-1β and lipopolysaccharide (48). The production of PGE_2 in the hypothalamus leads to the release of cyclic adenosine monophosphate, which functions as a neurotransmitter for neurons in the thermoregulatory center.

COX-2 is the primary source of PGE_2 that leads to a febrile response. Mice deficient in COX-1 exhibit normal febrile responses to intraperitoneal administration of lipopolysaccharide or IL-1β (49), whereas COX-2-deficient mice do not develop fever in response to these stimuli (49). The highly selective COX-2 inhibitor rofecoxib reduced naturally-occurring fever in humans (50). These data indicate that NSAIDs reduce fever by inhibiting COX-2 activity in the CNS. The mechanism by which acetaminophen reduces fever despite negligible COX-2 inhibitory activity *in vitro* remains unresolved. Some evidence suggests that acetaminophen is modified by oxidation in the CNS to gain COX inhibitory activity. Evidence for a third isoform of COX expressed in the CNS has also been presented (51).

Antiplatelet Effect

Among the benefits of NSAIDs, the role of low-dose aspirin in inhibiting platelet function has perhaps had the most significant impact on public health (52). Aspirin, but not the nonacetylated salicylates, irreversibly inhibit COX-1 in platelets, resulting in the inability to produce thromboxane A_2 in response to platelet activation (24). After exposure to aspirin, platelets are incapable of thromboxane production for the remainder of their circulating life span. As a result, the bleeding time of individuals treated with aspirin is prolonged for about 3 days after discontinuation of aspirin.

The nonselective NSAIDs inhibit COX reversibly. The effect of nonselective NSAIDs on platelet function depends on the drug's avidity for COX-1 and its half-life. Some NSAIDs, such as naproxen, have significant platelet-inhibiting function that lasts for several hours after dosing. Selective COX-2 inhibitors have no effect on platelet function because COX-2 is not expressed in platelets.

Other Effects

NSAIDs also have other unique pharmacodynamic properties. A reduction in uterine PG levels induces closure of the ductus arteriosis shortly after birth. Indomethacin is used to induce closure of a patent ductus arteriosis in infants. The uterine cramping of primary dysmenorrhea is also mediated by PG production. The pain associated with uterine cramping represents an inflammatory pain process associated with spasm of the uterine musculature. NSAIDs are uniquely effective in treating the pain of primary dysmenorrhea (53–55).

A role for NSAIDs in the chemoprevention of malignancy and Alzheimer disease has been the focus of much recent research (56,57). The rationale for this work is the observation that COX-2 expression is up-regulated in some tumors and the amyloid plaques of Alzheimer disease.

Interest in chemoprevention of cancer using NSAIDs originated with the observation that sulindac-induced polyp regression in patients with established familial adenomatous polyposis (FAP) (58). A subsequent randomized trial demonstrated that both sulindac and celecoxib caused regression of polyps in established FAP (59). Numerous epidemiologic studies have demonstrated that aspirin and nonselective NSAID use is associated with reduced risk for nonfamilial colon polyps and colon cancer (60–71). Two recent randomized controlled trials have shown that low-dose aspirin reduces the risk for recurrent colon polyps in patients with a prior history of benign adenomas or carcinoma of the colon (72,73). Although these findings are intriguing, endoscopic surveillance remains the method of choice for the prevention of colon cancer (74).

Alzheimer disease is associated with inflammatory responses in regions of the brain affected by plaque formation. In addition, COX-induced oxidation influences glutamate signaling pathways in the brain that may damage neurons (75,76). Several observational studies have suggested a reduced risk for Alzheimer dementia in patients taking NSAIDs (57). Regular use of NSAIDs by participants in the Rotterdam Study, a prospective cohort study, had a significantly lower risk [relative risk (RR) 0.20; 95% confidence interval (CI), 0.05–0.83] for developing dementia during follow-up (77). However, a randomized controlled trial of rofecoxib, naproxen, or placebo in patients with mild-to-moderate Alzheimer disease showed no benefit in slowing the progression of dementia (78). Additional studies are needed before definitive conclusions can be drawn on the effect of NSAIDs on Alzheimer disease.

ADVERSE EVENTS ASSOCIATED WITH NSAIDS

Comparative studies have shown that the efficacy of NSAIDs for most rheumatologic disorders is similar regardless of the particular drug used. Therefore, preventing and anticipating adverse events is a primary consideration when NSAIDs are prescribed. About one third of patients using NSAIDs will develop a persistent drug-related adverse event, leading 10% to discontinue treatment (79). NSAID use also increases the risk for hospitalization and death. Over-the-counter availability of NSAIDs and inadequate assessment of risk factors for NSAID toxicity by physicians are factors that may contribute to the number of drug-related adverse events (80). The spectrum of drug toxicities associated with NSAIDs is shown in Table 31.3 and reviewed in this section.

Gastrointestinal Toxicity

Gastrointestinal toxicity is perhaps the most important adverse event related to NSAIDs. Much of the history of NSAIDs has been driven by efforts to reduce gastrointestinal toxicity. Aspirin was developed as a solution to the high rate of gastrointestinal intolerance to sodium salicylate (1,3). By the 1930s there was evidence that aspirin caused gastric ulceration (81). The advent of nonaspirin NSAIDs was driven, in part, by efforts to identify a better tolerated alternative to aspirin (82). However, the NSAIDs were also demonstrated to cause substantial gastrointestinal injury (83–85). The discovery of the mechanism of action of NSAIDs (9) and the identification of two isoforms of COX (10–15) led to renewed efforts to improve the gastrointestinal safety of NSAIDs through the development of COX-2 inhibitors.

Epidemiology

Several gastrointestinal adverse events are associated with NSAIDs. The most common is dyspepsia. However, the most important is gastroduodenal ulceration. The epidemiology of NSAID-induced gastroduodenal ulcer has been well established (reviewed in reference 79). Serious gastrointestinal complications occurred in 0.7% of OA patients who took an NSAID for 1 year (86). The incidence was 1.3% to 1.5% annually among patients with RA (86,87). Low-dose aspirin used for prophylaxis of cardiovascular events has also been associated with a twofold increased risk for bleeding peptic ulcer (88). Mortality associated with NSAID-induced gastrointestinal toxicity is estimated to be 0.22% per year, or over 16,500 NSAID-related deaths annually (79,86).

TABLE 31.3. *Drug toxicities associated with nonsteroidal antiinflammatory drugs (NSAIDs)*

Gastrointestinal
Gastroduodenal ulcer
Dyspepsia
Lower gastrointestinal tract (ulcer, stricture, hemorrhage)
Hepatic toxicity (elevated liver enzymes, hepatic failure)
Renal
Peripheral edema
Acute reduction in renal function
Hyperkalemia
Interstitial nephritis with nephrotic syndrome
Renal papillary necrosis
Analgesic nephropathy
Cardiovascular
Exacerbation of hypertension
Exacerbation of congestive heart failure
Acute coronary syndromes (?)
Allergic, Pseudoallergic and Immunologic
NSAID-induced rhinitis and asthma
NSAID-induced urticaria and angioedema
Anaphylaxis
Cutaneous reactions
Hypersensitivity pneumonitis
Aseptic meningitis
Other
Salicylate toxicity
Reye syndrome

Mechanisms

The mechanisms by which NSAIDs cause gastrointestinal injury include both local and systemic effects (89). Local injury occurs as a result of the direct toxic effects of NSAIDs on mucosal cells. Aspirin and most NSAIDs are weak acids that remain in their nonionized form in the acidic environment of the stomach. As such, NSAIDs readily diffuse through the gastric mucous layer into the relatively neutral environment adjacent to epithelial cells. There, aspirin and NSAIDs become ionized, releasing hydrogen ions that injure the epithelium and increase mucosal permeability. The primary systemic effect of NSAIDs is inhibition of COX-1, which is necessary for the production of PGs important in maintaining the integrity of the gastric mucosa. The systemic effects of NSAIDs on mucosal PG production in the gastrointestinal tract are thought to be the most important factor leading to ulcer formation (79).

Risk Factors

Risk factors for NSAID-induced gastrointestinal ulcers relate predominantly to comorbid medical conditions. In fact, prior symptoms of dyspepsia were reported by only 19% to 41% of patients using NSAIDs who presented with serious gastroduodenal ulcer (90,91). The risk for severe gastrointestinal complications is associated with advancing age, prior history of peptic ulcer, concomitant corticosteroid use, high doses of NSAIDs, concomitant anticoagulation, and severe systemic illness (79,92) (Table 31.4, Fig. 31.3). Other possible risk factors include *Helicobacter pylori* infection, smoking, and alcohol use. These data demonstrate that dyspepsia is not a sensitive indicator of gastrointestinal complications from NSAIDs. Instead, risk factors for gastrointestinal toxicity should be assessed before NSAIDs are prescribed, even for short-term use.

Two types of risk factors for gastrointestinal toxicity have been defined in patients using NSAIDs: baseline risk and NSAID-attributable risk (93). Baseline risk is attributable to preexisting factors such as advanced age, prior PUD, or *H. pylori* infection. NSAID-attributable risk is that which exists in those patients without other ulcer risk factors. Although the incidence of gastrointestinal toxicity may be highest in those with high baseline risk (e.g., multiple ulcer risk factors), strategies used to reduce the risk for ulcers may be most effective in those patients who have only NSAID-attributable risk.

Prevention Strategies

Several strategies have been shown to reduce the incidence of gastrointestinal injury in patients using NSAIDs. When evaluating clinical trials of interventions to protect against NSAID-induced ulcers, it is important to draw a distinction between reduction in symptomatic ulcers and reduction in surrogate markers of ulcers such as superficial gastric erosions or ulcers detected by endoscopy. The most clinically-relevant outcome is reduction in painful ulcers, and ulcer complications such as perforation, bleeding, and obstruction. However, given the low frequency of these events in patients using NSAIDs, few studies have been performed that have sufficient power to detect a reduction in clinically-important ulcers. A summary of clinical trials of strategies to reduce NSAID-induced ulcers is summarized in the next section (Table 31.5).

TABLE 31.4. *Risk factors for severe nonsteroidal antiinflammatory drug (NSAID)-induced gastrointestinal ulcer*

Established risk factors
Advanced age
History of ulcer
Concomitant use of corticosteroids
Higher doses of NSAIDs, including use of more than one NSAID
Concomitant administration of anticoagulants
Serious systemic disorder
Possible risk factors
Concomitant infection with *Helicobacter pylori*
Cigarette smoking
Consumption of alcohol

From Wolfe MM, Lichtenstein DR, Singh G. Gastrointestinal toxicity of nonsteroidal antiinflammatory drugs. *N Engl J Med* 1999;340:1888–1899, with permission.

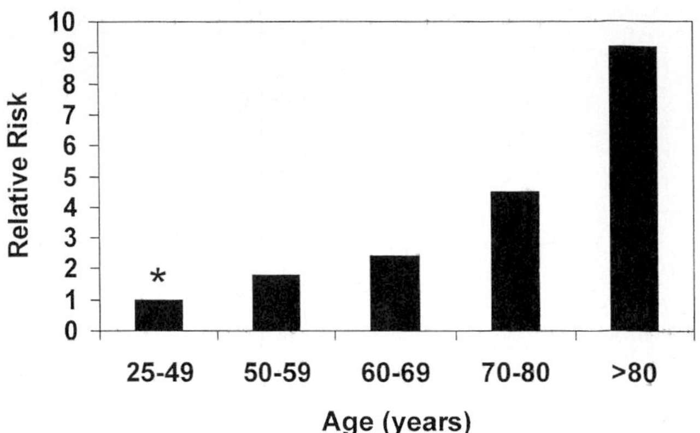

FIG. 31.3. Risk of nonsteroidal antiinflammatory drug–induced upper gastrointestinal bleeding increases with age. The relative risk for bleeding increases from 1.8 for individuals age 50 to 80 years to 9.2 for individuals older than 80 years. (Asterisk signifies individuals 25–49 years of age as a reference group) (92).

The following interventions have been shown to reduce endoscopic or symptomatic ulcers in patients taking NSAIDs:

1. *Misoprostol.* Misoprostol is an oral PGE_1 analogue that is approved for the prevention of NSAID-induced gastric ulcers. Its pharmacologic actions may be mediated by a cytoprotective effect on gastric mucosa and by inhibition of acid secretion from parietal cells. Coadministration of misoprostol with NSAIDs reduced endoscopic ulcers by 71% and symptomatic ulcers by 51% (87,94). Disadvantages of misoprostol include a high incidence (27%) of diarrhea and other gastrointestinal symptoms that often leads to discontinuation of treatment; especially at the most effective dosage of 800 μg/day (94). The requirement for dosing twice to four times daily may also lead to poor compliance.
2. *Proton pump inhibitors.* Proton pump inhibitors (PPIs) bind to the H^+/K^+ adenosine triphosphatase pump on the surface of parietal epithelial cells and inhibit secretion of hydrogen ions into the gastric lumen. PPIs are indicated for the treatment of gastric and duodenal ulcers. When used in combination with NSAIDs, PPIs reduce the risk for endoscopic gastroduodenal ulcers by 77%. PPIs are well tolerated and significantly reduce dyspepsia symptoms

TABLE 31.5. *Effectiveness and tolerability of strategies to reduce NSAID-induced gastrointestinal ulcer risk*

Intervention	Reduction in endoscopic ulcers	Reduction in clinically important ulcers	Tolerability of intervention	Source
Misoprostol vs. placebo	Gastric: RR = 0.26 (95% CI: 0.17–0.39) Duodenal: RR = 0.47 (95% CI: 0.33–0.69) Combined: RR = 0.29 (95% CI: 0.21–0.39)	Symptomatic and complicated ulcer: OR = 0.431 (95% CI 0.276–0.672; $p < 0.001$) Complicated ulcer: OR = 0.487 (95% CI 0.268–0.886; $p = 0.021$)	Excess dropout in misoprostol group due to gastrointestinal adverse events	87,94
High-dose H_2 antagonist vs. placebo	Gastric: RR = 0.44 (95% CI: 0.26–0.74) Duodenal: RR = 0.26 (95% CI: 0.11–0.65) Combined: RR = 0.41 (95% CI: 0.26–0.63)	No data	No excess dropouts Reduced abdominal pain treatment group	94
Proton pump inhibitor vs. placebo	Gastric: RR = 0.40 (95% CI: 0.32–0.51) Duodenal: RR = 0.19 (95% CI: 0.09–0.37) Combined: RR = 0.23 (95% CI: 0.18–0.31)	No data	No excess dropouts Significant reduction in dyspepsia	
Selective COX-2 inhibitor vs. nonselective NSAID	N/A	Symptomatic and complicated ulcer: CLASS (celecoxib): OR = 0.66 (95% CI 0.45–0.98; $p = 0.04$) VIGOR (rofecoxib): OR = 0.50 (95% CI 0.3–0.6; $p < 0.001$) Complicated ulcer: CLASS (celecoxib) OR = 0.77 (95% CI 0.41–1.46; $p = 0.45$) VIGOR (rofecoxib) OR = 0.40 (95% CI 0.3–0.6; $p = 0.005$)	No excess dropouts	94,96, 97,276

CI, confidence interval; COX-2, cyclooxygenase-2; H_2, histamine receptor-2; OR, odds ratio; RR, relative risk.

in patients taking NSAIDs (94). No trials have assessed the effectiveness of PPIs in preventing clinically significant NSAID-induced ulcers. However, among patients with a history of gastrointestinal bleeding and *H. pylori* infection, a PPI reduced the risk for rebleeding more effectively than eradication of *H. pylori* (4.4% vs. 19%) (95). These data provide circumstantial evidence that PPIs reduce the risk for clinically important ulcers.

3. *High-dose histamine (H_2) receptor antagonists.* H_2 antagonists reduce gastric acid secretion and accelerate the healing of peptic ulcers. When administered at standard doses, H_2 antagonists prevented endoscopically-detected duodenal, but not gastric ulcers in subjects taking NSAIDs. Double-dose H_2 antagonists reduced both gastric and duodenal ulcers by 56% and 74%, respectively (94). H_2 antagonists are well tolerated and may reduce the severity of dyspepsia symptoms associated with NSAID use.

4. *Highly selective COX-2 inhibitors.* The use of COX-2 inhibitors to minimize ulcer risk is an alternate strategy to combinations of drugs used in conjunction with nonselective NSAIDs. The rationale for using COX-2 inhibitors to prevent gastroduodenal ulcers was previously described. Pooled analysis of several endoscopic studies in subjects using celecoxib or rofecoxib demonstrated a 76% reduction in gastroduodenal ulcer risk compared with nonselective NSAIDs (94). Furthermore, two large randomized controlled trials have shown that both celecoxib (CLASS trial) and rofecoxib (VIGOR trial) reduce the risk for symptomatic gastroduodenal ulcers when compared with nonselective NSAIDs (96,97).

There exists ongoing controversy regarding the interpretation of the results of both trials. In the CLASS study, the predefined primary end point of a reduction in complicated ulcers was not achieved, whereas the secondary end point of reduction in complicated and symptomatic ulcers was achieved. Factors that may have contributed to this outcome include the inclusion in the CLASS trial of patients using low-dose aspirin. The VIGOR trial achieved its primary end point of reduction in complicated and symptomatic ulcers. However, the overall rate of serious adverse events was similar in both treatment arms, owing to a greater incidence of cardiovascular events in the rofecoxib group. Hypotheses that may explain these findings are discussed below in the section on cardiovascular adverse events.

Each of the strategies described above shows substantial evidence of effectiveness in preventing NSAID-induced ulcer. The only agents shown to reduce the risk for clinically-important ulcers are misoprostol, celecoxib, and rofecoxib. Given the high rate of gastrointestinal symptoms and the frequent dosing interval required with misoprostol, the COX-2 inhibitors have emerged as the preferred method for avoiding gastroduodenal ulcers in patients using NSAIDs. Regardless, all patients initiating therapy with NSAIDs who have one or more risk factors for gastroduodenal ulcer are candidates for treatment with one of the strategies above for reducing ulcer risk. Ongoing studies will answer important remaining questions regarding the cardiovascular safety of COX-2 inhibitors, the impact of daily low-dose aspirin on the gastrointestinal safety of COX-2 inhibitors, and the relative gastrointestinal safety of COX-2 inhibitors versus nonselective NSAIDs administered with a PPI.

Role of Helicobacter pylori *Infection*

Infection with *H. pylori* represents the primary overall risk factor for peptic ulcer disease in the general population. The possibility that *H. pylori* and NSAIDs interact to influence the risk for NSAID-induced ulcer has been the focus of several clinical trials (98). Most studies have shown that *H. pylori* does not increase the risk for endoscopic or clinical ulcer formation in NSAID users (99–104), whereas three studies indicated that eradication of *H. pylori* reduces the risk for recurrent ulcer (105–107). Studies investigating the effect of *H. pylori* infection on ulcer healing have yielded mixed results (108–111). Two studies showed no effect (110,111), and two studies showed the counterintuitive observation that *H. pylori* infection enhanced ulcer healing (108,109). Several case control studies indicate an increased risk for ulcer bleeding in patients with *H. pylori* infection who take NSAIDs (98). However, two prospective randomized trials demonstrate no benefit of *H. pylori* eradication in preventing recurrent bleeding in patients taking NSAIDs (95,112). The conflicting results regarding the importance of *H. pylori* in NSAID-induced ulcer require further studies. At present, screening for *H. pylori* infection in patients initiating NSAID therapy is not indicated (98). However, patients diagnosed with ulcer, regardless of their use of NSAIDs, should be screened for *H. pylori* and treated if infection is detected.

Dyspepsia

Dyspepsia comprises a number of gastrointestinal symptoms that are common in users and nonusers of NSAIDs (113,114). Its pathophysiologic mechanism is not well understood. Dyspepsia symptoms occurred at a rate of 69 to 85 events per 100 patient-years of therapy in a pooled analysis of comparative clinical trials of rofecoxib and nonselective NSAIDs (115). Dyspepsia is also a primary reason for discontinuation of NSAID therapy. The percentage of patients in the VIGOR and CLASS trials who discontinued treatment due to dyspepsia and related gastrointestinal symptoms (excluding ulcers) was as follows: naproxen 4.9%, rofecoxib 3.5%, celecoxib 8.7%, and diclofenac/ibuprofen 10.7% (96,97). It is likely that the discontinuation rate is higher outside of a clinical trial setting. The clinician is challenged by the finding that dyspepsia symptoms correlate with gastroduodenal ulcers in just 50% of patients, and up to 40% of patients with gastroduodenal ulcer have no prior symptoms of dyspepsia (116,117). Both H_2 receptor antagonists (118–121) and PPIs (108,109) reduce the incidence of dyspepsia in patients taking NSAIDs. However, Singh and colleagues have shown that asymptomatic patients taking standard doses of H_2 receptor antagonists had a higher rate of ulcer complications than those not using these medications (91). It is possible that H_2 receptor antagonists masked symptoms of dyspepsia but did not protect against the development of clinically-important ulcers (79). Patients who develop dyspepsia while on NSAIDs should be treated with a PPI rather than an H_2 receptor antagonist in order to diminish dyspepsia symptoms, and potentially reduce the risk for ulcer formation. Gastroduodenal ulcer should be ruled out in patients who do not have prompt resolution of dyspepsia symptoms, because ulcer may be present in about 50% (116).

Lower Gastrointestinal Tract Adverse Events

Lower gastrointestinal tract complications of NSAIDs include stricture, ulceration, and hemorrhage of the small bowel or colon (122–131). Estimates of the annual rate of lower tract complications range from 0.9% to 4% per year (130–132). Recent prospective data indicate that COX-2 inhibitors may be less likely to cause complicated lower gastrointestinal tract adverse events (132).

Hepatic Toxicity

The spectrum of NSAID-induced hepatic toxicity ranges from elevated liver transaminases to fulminant liver failure (133). Severe liver injury due to NSAIDs is rare, resulting in 2.2 hospitalizations per 100,000 population annually (134,135). Hepatocellular injury, characterized by elevated transaminases, is the most common form of NSAID-induced liver toxicity (133). Laboratory abnormalities usually resolve within several days to weeks if the NSAID is discontinued. Small elevations in transaminases of less than three times the upper limit of normal do not require discontinuation of NSAIDs unless they are associated with clinical signs of liver injury, reduced serum albumin levels, or prolonged prothrombin time which indicates impaired liver synthetic function. Cholestatic injury or mixed hepatocellular/cholestatic injury has also been described. Sulindac is one of the most common causes of NSAID-induced liver toxicity, and typically induces cholestatic or mixed liver injury (133,136). Aspirin causes predictable dose-related hepatocellular toxicity. Manifestations usually occur when blood levels are 25 mg/dL or higher (133). The nonacetylated salicylates may induce non-dose-related idiosyncratic toxicity. Several NSAIDs have been associated with a greater than acceptable risk for fulminant hepatic failure and have been removed from the market; they include, benoxaprofen, ibufenac, and cinchophen (133).

Renal Toxicity

Up to 5% of patients taking NSAIDs will develop a clinically-apparent renal adverse event (137). The most common manifestation is peripheral edema (138). Other toxicities include acute reduction in renal function, hyperkalemia, interstitial nephritis, and papillary necrosis (139). Renal adverse events are almost always reversible when detected early (140). Both nonselective and selective COX-2 inhibitors seem to have similar effects on the kidney (141).

COX-1 and COX-2 are expressed in discrete locations in the human kidney (19,142) and produce PGs important in regulating sodium and water reabsorption (20,143–145). COX-1 is expressed in the collecting duct, interstitial cells, the endothelium, and vascular smooth muscle cells. COX-2 is expressed in endothelial cells and vascular smooth muscle cells, as well as in podocytes of the glomerulus. Furthermore, COX-2 expression could be detected in macula densa cells of human kidney tissue obtained from patients with hyperreninemia (146). The constitutive and regulated expression of COX in the kidney illustrates the important role of local PG production in regulating normal and "stressed" kidney function. Decreased production of PGs is the primary mechanism underlying most NSAID-related renal adverse events (140).

Edema

NSAID-induced edema occurs in 1% to 5% of patients (137,147,148), and results from increased sodium reabsorption due to decreased PGE_2 production (149,150). Edema is usually reversible and mild, associated with 1 to 2 kg of weight gain (137). Onset is most pronounced during the first several days of NSAID use and may improve after renal handling of sodium returns toward baseline (151,152). Edema does not necessarily correlate with increased mean blood pressure. Some patients may develop severe edema that can progress to CHF (153). Risk factors for peripheral edema include CHF, diuretic use, cirrhosis, diabetes mellitus, renal insufficiency, and older age (138). NSAIDs may be continued in patients with mild edema in the absence of increased blood pressure, reduced renal function, or exacerbation of underlying disease such as CHF. However, patients require frequent and careful monitoring to detect onset of hypertension or the development of electrolyte or renal function abnormalities. In this setting, clinicians must determine whether the clinical benefits of NSAID therapy offset the risks.

Acute Reduction in Renal Function

Renal function is unaffected by NSAIDs in normal, healthy individuals. However, NSAIDs may cause rapid loss of renal function when given to patients with effective intravascular volume depletion or impaired organ perfusion. The mechanism of toxicity is inhibition of PG-mediated vasodilation, which results in renal ischemia. Patients at risk for acute loss in renal function include those with CHF, poor underlying renal function, cirrhosis, diabetes mellitus, advanced age, and dehydration due to diuretics or underlying medical conditions (140,154–160). Acute renal failure is more commonly associated with higher doses of NSAIDs, as well as NSAIDs with longer half-lives (161). Patients with risk factors for acute reduction in renal function should be reevaluated soon after initiating NSAIDs for signs of edema, weight gain, impaired renal function, or hyperkalemia. Acute reduction in renal function is reversible and usually resolves within several days if detected early (140). Renal failure may require dialysis if not detected early (158).

Hyperkalemia

NSAIDs may induce hyperkalemia by inhibiting PG-stimulated renin release in the kidney (140). Reduced renin leads to reduced aldosterone production and subsequent reduction in potassium excretion (140). Risk factors for NSAID-induced hyperkalemia are use of angiotensin-converting enzyme inhibitors, potassium-sparing diuretics, and potassium supplements (140,162–165). Underlying medical conditions that may contribute to hyperkalemia include heart failure, renal insufficiency, multiple myeloma, and diabetes mellitus (166–169). Discontinuation of NSAIDs corrects the hyperkalemia. However, NSAID-induced hyperkalemia has been reported to present with renal failure, quadriparesis, and fatal arrhythmia (162,163,170–173).

Interstitial Nephritis with Nephrotic Syndrome

A rare complication of NSAID use is interstitial nephritis, usually in association with nephrotic syndrome. Onset may range from 2 weeks to 18 months from initiation of NSAIDs (174). The syndrome is unique in that eosinophilia and urine eosinophils are usually not present. Patients usually present with clinical manifestations of nephrotic syndrome. The urine sediment demonstrates microscopic hematuria and tubular epithelial cell casts (140). There are no known risk factors, and the pathophysiologic mechanism is unknown. Renal biopsy demonstrates a unique pattern of interstitial nephritis with minimal change glomerulonephritis (175,176). Proteinuria often resolves with discontinuation of the NSAID. The benefit of corticosteroid treatment for interstitial nephritis has not been definitively shown (157,175). A trial of corticosteroids is recommended if proteinuria has not begun to resolve within 2 weeks of stopping NSAIDs (140).

Renal Papillary Necrosis

Acute renal papillary necrosis is a rare and irreversible form of NSAID-induced toxicity (177–179). The usual clinical scenario involves high doses of NSAIDs in a setting of severe dehydration. The clinical presentation may be minimally symptomatic or may mimic passage of a renal stone (140). The mechanism of injury is ischemic necrosis of the distal nephron caused by loss of PG-dependent vasodilation secondary to high local concentrations of NSAIDs. Affected individuals have difficulty forming a maximally concentrated urine (140).

Chronic renal papillary necrosis is the pathologic description of the clinical entity analgesic nephropathy (180, 181). Long-term, daily use of drug combinations containing two or more analgesics plus caffeine or codeine is associated with analgesic nephropathy (182). The analgesic combination most commonly associated with nephropathy is aspirin and phenacetin. The latter, a prodrug that is metabolized to acetaminophen, is no longer available in most countries. Other analgesic combinations associated with analgesic nephropathy include aspirin and acetaminophen, and aspirin or acetaminophen in conjunction with the pyrazolone class of analgesic drugs (not available in the United States) (183). There is no indication that acetaminophen or NSAIDs used as single agents cause analgesic nephropathy.

The clinical presentation of analgesic nephropathy is usually limited to polyuria and, occasionally, episodes of microscopic or gross hematuria during sloughing of necrosed renal papillae. As analgesic nephropathy progresses, the clinical manifestations are the nonspecific findings of renal failure (182). Women are affected more often than men. Patients may present with end-stage renal disease as the initial manifestation of analgesic nephropathy. Computed tomography of the abdomen usually demonstrates small kidneys with a “bumpy” contour, and calcifications of the renal papillae (184,185). Discontinuation of analgesic medications may arrest the progression to renal failure if detected early. Urologic malignancy, usually transitional cell carcinoma, may be a late complication in up to 8% of individuals with analgesic nephropathy (186–188).

Cardiovascular Adverse Reactions

Hypertension

Meta-analyses of numerous clinical trials performed prior to the advent of COX-2 inhibitors have shown that NSAIDs induce small elevations in blood pressure. Pope and colleagues compiled data from 54 clinical trials and determined that mean blood pressure was increased in NSAID users (189). Normotensive subjects had a mean increase in blood pressure of 1.1 mm Hg, whereas hypertensive subjects had an increase of 3.3 mm Hg. Similarly, Johnson and colleagues pooled data from 50 clinical trials and determined that mean blood pressure increased by 5 mm Hg in patients taking NSAIDs (190). The hypertensive effect was must pronounced in subjects with preexisting hypertension. Certain NSAIDs were more commonly associated with elevated blood pressure. Both meta-analyses found that naproxen and indomethacin had the greatest effect, whereas sulindac and aspirin were not significantly different from placebo. Although mean changes in blood pressure were low in the total cohort, some patients experienced large increases in blood pressure while taking NSAIDs.

COX-2 inhibitors have also been shown to have effects on blood pressure that are similar to nonselective NSAIDs. Trials of celecoxib and rofecoxib demonstrated increases in blood pressure (<3 mmHg systolic; <1 mmHg diastolic) that were not statistically significant (191). In a pooled analysis of clinical trials of rofecoxib in patients with OA or RA, the incidence of investigator-defined hypertension was related to daily dose: 12.5 mg, 2.8%; 25 mg, 4.0%; and 50 mg, 8.2% (192). In long-term gastrointestinal safety studies, the incidences of investigator-defined hypertension was 9.7% (rofecoxib 50 mg daily, twice the recommended daily dose) and 5.5% (naproxen 500 mg twice daily) (96). The incidences of investigator-defined hypertension in celecoxib long-term gastrointestinal safety studies were 2.0% (celecoxib 400 mg twice daily, twice the recommended daily dose), 2.0% (diclofenac 75 mg twice daily), and 3.1% (ibuprofen 800 mg three times daily) (97). The conclusion from these results is that the incidence of hypertension in patients taking COX-2 inhibitors is similar to that in patients taking nonselective NSAIDs.

In general, NSAIDs cause small mean increases in blood pressure. However, a small subset of patients may experience clinically significant increases in blood pressure that require intervention—either discontinuation of NSAIDs or intensified antihypertensive therapy. Risk factors for NSAID-induced hypertension include older age and preexisting hypertension (189). In fact, NSAID use is a predictor of hypertension in elderly patients (193). Furthermore, a prospective analysis of elderly patients demonstrated a 70% increased risk for initiating antihypertensive medications in NSAID users versus nonusers (194). All patients initiating long-term NSAID therapy should be monitored for increased blood pressure. Particular caution should be taken in those with preexisting hypertension and older patients.

Congestive Heart Failure

NSAIDs have been associated with CHF in several studies (195–202). Among elderly patients with known heart disease, NSAID use was associated with a 10-fold increased risk for hospital admission for a first episode of CHF, suggesting that NSAIDs may induce CHF (200,201). However, a large 7-year prospective cohort study by Feenstra and colleagues demonstrated that NSAID use did not cause new-onset CHF, but was highly associated with relapse of CHF (202) (Fig. 31.4). Among patients who filled one or more prescriptions for NSAIDs, the risk for incident heart failure was not significantly elevated (RR 1.2; 95% CI 0.8–1.8). However, after a first episode of CHF, patients had a 10-fold increased risk for recurrence (RR 9.9; 95% CI 1.7–57.0) when prescribed NSAIDs. This observation is consistent with the observed risk for fluid retention and elevated blood pressure in patients with reduced left ventricular function who use NSAIDs. Risk factors for exacerbation of CHF by NSAIDs include higher daily dose and the use of NSAIDs with longer half-lives (201). It is estimated that up to 19% of hospital admissions for CHF may be attributable to NSAIDs (201). NSAIDs should be avoided in patients with heart failure. Close monitoring of fluid status, blood pressure, and renal function is mandatory in any patient with a history of heart disease who is taking an NSAID.

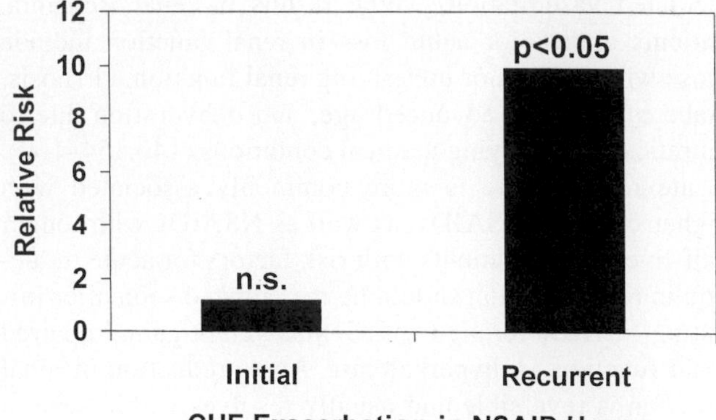

FIG. 31.4. Relative risk for exacerbation of congestive heart failure (CHF) in older patients using nonsteroidal antiinflammatory drugs (NSAIDs) (202). Patients without prior heart failure experienced no increased risk for CHF associated with NSAID use. Patients with a prior history of heart failure had a 10-fold increased risk for CHF exacerbation associated with NSAID use.

Myocardial Infarction and Stroke

The importance of low-dose aspirin in the prevention and management of acute coronary syndromes and stroke is well documented (203). A somewhat paradoxic concern relates to a potential association between selective COX-2 inhibitors and increased risk for myocardial infarction (204). Subjects receiving rofecoxib in the VIGOR trial experienced a higher risk for vascular events than those taking naproxen (20 versus 4 myocardial infarctions per 2,699 person-years of follow-up) (96). No increase in vascular events was observed in a metanalysis of randomized trials of rofecoxib (205). Similarly, celecoxib was not associated with an increased risk for vascular events in comparison with diclofenac or ibuprofen in the CLASS trial (97). Plausible hypotheses proposed to explain this observation include the known antiplatelet effects of naproxen relative to rofecoxib (206,207). Alternatively, selective COX-2 inhibition reduces prostacyclin production by endothelial cells, which normally prevents platelet aggregation and causes vasodilation. Prostacyclin inhibition in the absence of inhibition of thromboxane through COX-1 inhibition (which induces platelet aggregation) could potentially establish a prothrombotic state that might increase the risk for vascular events (208,209). Additional studies are needed to determine whether COX-2 inhibitors are associated with increased risk for vascular events.

Allergic and Pseudoallergic Reactions to NSAIDs

NSAIDs cause a variety of allergic, pseudoallergic, and immunologic reactions (210,211) (Table 31.3). NSAID-induced rhinitis and asthma (NIRA) is classically characterized by asthma, rhinitis or nasal polyps, and "aspirin sensitivity" (Samter triad). Chronic sinusitis has also been determined to be part of the syndrome of NIRA. Invariably, patients with NIRA have preexisting airway disease that often presents as persistent sinusitis or nasal polyps following a respiratory infection (210,211). Onset usually occurs in adulthood, and women are affected slightly more commonly than men. Symptoms often progress from isolated rhinitis or sinusitis to also include asthma. Exposure to aspirin or an NSAID may result in increased nasal congestion, rhinorrhea, or wheezing within 15 minutes to an hour (210). Symptoms may resolve within an hour or persist for a day or more. NIRA has been reported in 5% to 40% of patients with asthma, depending on the method used to assess sensitivity to NSAIDs (210,212,213).

The mechanism underlying AERS is not well established. The leading hypothesis is that inhibition of COX-1 reduces levels of PGE_2, which normally inhibits the production of leukotrienes by 5-lipoxygenase. Loss of 5-lipoxygenase inhibition leads to excessive production of leukotrienes, resulting in increased airway inflammation and bronchial responsiveness (214). Evidence supporting this hypothesis includes the finding of increased levels of urinary leukotrienes in aspirin-sensitive asthmatics compared with asthmatics who are not sensitive (215). Further evidence includes the ability of leukotriene-inhibiting drugs, such as montelukast, to reduce symptoms of asthma in patients with aspirin-sensitive disease (216,217). Because the presumed mechanism of action is not through the development of a specific immune response to the drug, symptoms may occur after the first dose of an NSAID.

There are important implications of NIRA in rheumatology practice. Physicians should be cautious about prescribing NSAIDs for patients with a history of nasal polyps, chronic sinusitis, or asthma. However, less than 10% of patients with asthma in the absence of nasal polyps will have increased symptoms when taking NSAIDs (210). Therefore, patients with asthma should not automatically be excluded from using NSAIDs. Definitive diagnosis of NIRA requires a provocative aspirin challenge, usually performed by an allergist.

Strategies that potentially enable use of aspirin or NSAIDs in patients with NIRA include (a) aspirin desensitization (218), (b) use of a selective COX-2 inhibitor (219–223), and (c) coadministration of a leukotriene inhibitor (216,217). Aspirin desensitization is usually performed by an allergist experienced in the management of patients undergoing provocative oral drug challenges. Progressive doses of aspirin are administered orally until a full dose (325 mg) is tolerated. About two thirds of patients are able to tolerate NSAIDs after 1 year of treatment (218). The patient may continue to use aspirin or another NSAID without concern for NIRA as long as a daily dose is administered. Interruption in aspirin or NSAID dosing for more than 24 hours requires that the desensitization procedure be repeated.

NSAID-induced urticaria/angioedema occurs in individuals with preexisting chronic urticaria or angioedema. Patients with idiopathic urticaria or angioedema may experience an exacerbation of symptoms after administration of an NSAID (224,225). Inhibition of COX-1 is thought to be the primary mechanism underlying increased urticaria or angioedema. Symptoms may occur after the first dose of the NSAID. The diagnosis may be confirmed by oral NSAID challenge. There are no *in vitro* tests or skin tests to confirm the presence of NSAID-induced urticaria or angioedema. About one third of patients with inactive urticaria symptoms have cross-reactivity to multiple NSAIDs, whereas two thirds of patients with active hives will be cross-reactive to multiple NSAIDs. Management strategies include (a) NSAID avoidance, (b) coadministration of an antihistamine or leukotriene antagonist (226–228), (c) a trial of an alternate NSAID, or (d) use of a selective COX-2 inhibitor (229–232). Desensitization is not effective in alleviating NSAID-induced urticaria or angioedema.

Angioedema and urticaria induced by NSAIDs may occur in patients with no preexisting history of chronic urticaria. Usually patients are sensitive to a single NSAID. The presumed mechanism is the induction of immunoglobulin E (IgE) antibody to the drug or a drug metabolite (210). As a result, symptoms do not occur after the first administration of the NSAID. Readministration of the NSAID after an acute episode of urticaria or angioedema could result in anaphylaxis. The appropriate management strategy is avoidance of the suspect drug and selection of an alternate NSAID when needed. Rarely, patients without a history of chronic urticaria or angioedema may develop urticaria or angioedema in response to multiple NSAIDs. Many of these patients ultimately develop chronic urticaria and would be classified as having NSAID-induced urticaria or angioedema as described above (233). Anaphylaxis may also occur after repeat use of a particular NSAID. The mechanism is presumed to be IgE mediated. Among patients presenting to emergency rooms with anaphylaxis in response to medications, half were sensitive to NSAIDs (234).

A variety of other allergic, pseudoallergic, and immunologic adverse events are associated with NSAIDs (211).

Cutaneous reactions associated with NSAIDs include maculopapular eruptions, fixed drug eruptions, erythema multiforme, Stevens-Johnson syndrome, leukocytoclastic vasculitis, pseudoporphyria, and photosensitivity responses (235–238). Aseptic meningitis has been associated with several NSAIDs (239,240). Hypersensitivity pneumonitis has rarely been associated with NSAIDs (241).

Salicylate Toxicity

Overdose of salicylates results in a characteristic syndrome of salicylate toxicity. Acute toxicity results from ingestion of more than 150 mg/kg of sodium salicylate. Lethal toxicity may occur after ingestion of more than 500 mg/kg. Clinical manifestations include mixed respiratory alkalosis and metabolic acidosis, altered mental status, hypernatremia, hypokalemia, dehydration, fever, and hyper- or hypoglycemia. Serum salicylate levels may be used to estimate the severity of intoxication (242). Treatment of acute salicylate overdose includes induction of emesis in conscious patients, gastric lavage, administration of activated charcoal, and supportive therapy.

Chronic salicylate toxicity, or salicylism, results from prolonged high doses of salicylates (242). Generally, the clinical manifestations are associated with administration of 100 mg/kg/day for 2 or more days. Factors that may lead to chronic intoxication include dehydration or concomitant use of bismuth compounds that contain salicylates. Symptoms include hearing loss, tinnitus, dizziness, confusion, tachycardia, nausea, and vomiting. Hyperventilation, mixed respiratory acidosis and metabolic acidosis, and hypoglycemia may also be present. Measurement of the serum salicylate level is not helpful in assessing the severity of chronic intoxication. Mild intoxication is treated by discontinuing salicylates. More severe toxicity is treated with supportive care and measures described above for acute intoxication.

Reye Syndrome

Reye syndrome is characterized by acute onset of fatty liver and encephalopathy in children less than 15 years of age (243). Typically, the syndrome is preceded by a viral infection such as chicken pox or influenza. Use of aspirin has been linked to Reye syndrome in several case-control studies (244,245). Clinical manifestations include persistent vomiting and stupor that progresses to seizures and coma. Laboratory findings may include elevated serum transaminases, prolonged prothrombin time, elevated serum ammonia, metabolic acidosis, and hypoglycemia. Jaundice is typically absent. Treatment is with infusions of fresh frozen plasma and glucose. The mortality rate exceeds 50%. Reye syndrome is rare, perhaps owing to the nearly universal avoidance of aspirin in children (246).

DRUG INTERACTIONS

Drug-drug interactions may occur among the entire class of NSAIDs, or may be unique to a particular NSAID (247, 248). Known interactions include the displacement of drugs from serum proteins, altered clearance or metabolism of drugs, and altered pharmacologic activity of drugs (e.g., antihypertensives) (248). Most drug-drug interactions involving NSAIDs are clinically insignificant in most patients. However, the marked variation of individual responses to drugs can lead to significant toxicity due to interactions.

One of the most common drug-drug interactions involving NSAIDs is blunting of the effect of antihypertensives. As a class, NSAIDs elevate mean blood pressure by 5 mm Hg in patients with controlled hypertension (189). This effect was most pronounced in patients treated with angiotensin-converting enzyme inhibitors, β blockers, or calcium channel blockers. NSAIDs also blunt the effects of diuretics (249). The risk for hyperkalemia is also increased in patients taking NSAIDs and angiotensin-converting enzyme inhibitors (162). The mechanism underlying these interactions is related to the inhibition of renal PG production by NSAIDs.

NSAIDs may increase serum levels of methotrexate by interfering with the function of a renal tubular anion transporter (250). The interaction of NSAIDs with methotrexate is most important in patients receiving high-dose methotrexate as chemotherapy, in which severe hematologic and gastrointestinal toxicity has been reported. Combinations of low-dose methotrexate and NSAIDs are routinely used in rheumatology practice. The systemic clearance of methotrexate was shown to be significantly reduced by NSAIDs in some studies (251,252), but not in others (253). All studies demonstrated significant variability between individuals in the effect of NSAIDs on methotrexate clearance. Patients taking methotrexate and NSAIDs should be carefully monitored for signs of methotrexate toxicity, especially in the setting of renal insufficiency.

NSAIDs interfere with excretion of lithium, which may lead to increased serum lithium concentrations (254). The effects occur within 5 to 7 days of initiating or discontinuing NSAIDs. Usually, the effect is not clinically important, but lithium toxicity in the setting of NSAID use has been reported (255). Patients should be monitored for lithium toxicity or decreased effectiveness of lithium when NSAIDs are initiated or withdrawn, respectively.

Patients taking NSAIDs may also frequently be taking low-dose aspirin for its antiplatelet effects. Because NSAIDs and aspirin bind to similar regions of COX-1, Catella-Lawson and colleagues hypothesized that certain NSAIDs may potentially inhibit the antiplatelet effect of aspirin (152). Their studies confirmed that ibuprofen administered prior to aspirin inhibited the antiplatelet effect of aspirin. Diclofenac, acetaminophen, and the COX-2 inhibitor rofecoxib did not inhibit the antiplatelet effect of aspirin. It is not yet known if ibuprofen negates the clinical benefits of daily low-dose aspirin, but use of this drug in patients taking low-dose aspirin for cardioprotection is not advised.

Other important drug interactions involving NSAIDs relate to the additive effects of shared toxicities. For instance, both NSAIDs and oral bisphosphonates are associated with increased risk for gastric ulcers. One study demonstrated that women taking alendronate and naproxen were more likely to develop endoscopically-detected gastric ulcers than women taking either agent alone (256). Similarly, combined use of NSAIDs with agents that impair renal function may lead to additive toxicity. An example is the increased risk for elevated serum creatinine and potassium in patients taking cyclosporine A and NSAIDs (257,258). Caution should be observed when combining NSAIDs with other nephrotoxic agents such as aminoglycosides, ganciclovir, cisplatin, and amphotericin B. Finally, NSAIDs can displace warfarin from plasma proteins, causing prolongation of the prothrombin time. The combination of impaired platelet function and gastrointestinal toxicity associated with nonselective NSAIDs and anticoagulation with warfarin is thought to lead to a significant increase in the incidence of bleeding gastroduodenal ulcers (79). With the availability of selective COX-2 inhibitors that have reduced ulcer risk and no effect on platelet function, aspirin and nonselective NSAIDs should be avoided in patients taking warfarin.

Inhibition of enzymes important in NSAID metabolism may lead to impaired clearance. Many NSAIDs (ibuprofen, celecoxib, diclofenac, flurbiprofen, meloxicam, and indomethacin) are metabolized by the 2C9 isozyme of cytochrome P450 (259–262). Drugs that inhibit 2C9 function may cause reduced rates of NSAID metabolism. Examples include fluconazole, metabolites of leflunomide, and voriconazole. The clinical significance of these interactions has not been studied. Many of the cytochrome P450 isozyme genes are polymorphic, and the importance of these polymorphisms with regard to drug toxicity is an area of intense research in the field of pharmacogenetics.

Salicylates may interact with other drugs as a result of high-protein binding (247). Warfarin is displaced from plasma proteins by salicylates. Other drugs that may be displaced from plasma proteins by salicylates are sulfonylureas, valproic acid, phenytoin, sulfonamides, and penicillins. The clinical significance of these interactions is usually related to high doses of salicylates.

PRACTICAL CONSIDERATIONS IN THE DOSING AND ADMINISTRATION OF NSAIDS

Drug Selection and Toxicity Monitoring

Among large groups of patients, most NSAIDs show similar levels of efficacy in disorders such as OA or RA. Therefore, considerations in the selection of NSAIDs may be focused on issues such as avoidance of adverse events. Therapy should be initiated with low doses that are titrated upward as needed, especially in the elderly and those with risk factors for adverse events such as hypertension and heart disease. Individual variability in clinical responsiveness to NSAIDs may be marked. Therefore, if the desired clinical response has not been achieved after 2 to 4 weeks of therapy, it is reasonable to switch to another NSAID. Some patients may try three to four NSAIDs before identifying a treatment that is effective and well tolerated.

A plan for monitoring potential drug toxicity should be implemented for each patient starting an NSAID. Patients should be advised to seek medical attention if persistent symptoms of dyspepsia or edema develop. Hypertensive patients should monitor their blood pressure frequently during the first several weeks of therapy and advised to report even modest increases. The elderly and patients with a history of heart disease or liver disease should be reevaluated after 2 to 6 weeks of therapy. Appropriate monitoring may include measurement of blood pressure, assessment of edema, and laboratory evaluation for signs of impaired renal function or hyperkalemia. Guidelines from the American College of Rheumatology recommend monitoring complete blood count, and possibly serum creatinine, aspartate aminotransferase (AST), and alanine aminotransferase (ALT) at least yearly (263). More frequent laboratory monitoring may be indicated in the elderly. Patients taking concomitant angiotensin-converting enzyme inhibitors or diuretics are recommended to have serum creatinine monitored weekly for 3 weeks upon initiating NSAID therapy.

Use in Children

NSAIDs are generally well tolerated in children; however, a limited number of systematic studies of efficacy and pharmacokinetics have been performed (264). Prolonged clearance of NSAIDs may be observed in neonates as a result of relatively lower glomerular filtration rates and immature hepatic cytochrome P450 system (265). The weight-adjusted elimination half-lives of NSAIDs in children are similar to those on adults (266). The gastrointestinal and renal safety profile of NSAIDs may be superior to that of adults, based on a small number of studies (264,265). However, severe and irreversible renal failure has been reported in neonates who received indomethacin to induce closure of a patent ductus arteriosus (267). Preliminary results of clinical trials using COX-2 inhibitors in children indicate that these drugs are well tolerated, although celecoxib was more rapidly cleared in children compared with adults (268,269).

Fertility, Pregnancy, and Lactation

PGs are involved in the implantation of embryos into the endometrium, and animal studies have shown that some

NSAIDs may reduce the number of successfully implanted embryos. However, there are no data to indicate that NSAIDs affect fertility in humans. NSAIDs cross the placenta, and tissue levels in the fetus are comparable with those in the mother. Limited studies with aspirin, naproxen, and ibuprofen do not indicate that these NSAIDs have teratogenic effects (270–272). Use of NSAIDs during the third trimester of pregnancy has been associated with premature closure of the ductus arteriosus or neonatal pulmonary hypertension (273). NSAIDs may also be associated with oligohydramnios, renal insufficiency in the fetus, maternal or fetal hemorrhage, and delayed onset and duration of labor (139,273). In general, NSAIDs are not recommended during pregnancy. An exception to this is the use of low-dose aspirin in the management of pregnant women with antiphospholipid antibody syndrome, a history of placental insufficiency, or risk factors for preeclampsia (273). NSAIDs are excreted into breast milk in many cases. Accordingly, use of NSAIDs in nursing mothers is not recommended.

FUTURE DIRECTIONS

The history of NSAIDs continues to be written with advances that improve the efficacy and safety of this important drug class. During the next 2 to 3 years several new COX-2 inhibitors will be introduced. Ongoing safety studies and cost-benefit analyses will better establish the most appropriate use of COX-2 inhibitors and nonselective NSAIDs (274). An emerging class of nitric oxide–releasing NSAIDs may offer a new strategy for added drug safety (275,276). Finally, it is hoped that the emerging field of pharmacogenetics will provide the tools to understand the mechanism behind the marked individual variability in both the clinical responses and adverse effects associated with NSAIDs.

REFERENCES

1. Jones R. Nonsteroidal anti-inflammatory drug prescribing: past, present, and future. *Am J Med* 2001;110(suppl 1A):4–7.
2. Leroux H. *J Chim Med* 1830;6:341.
3. Sneader W. The discovery of aspirin: a reappraisal. *BMJ* 2000;321 (7276):1591–1594.
4. Vieson K. Overview; Nonsteroidal antiinflammatory drugs. In: *Clinical pharmacology.* Vol. 2003. Gold Standard Multimedia, 2000.
5. FitzGerald GA, Patrono C. The coxibs, selective inhibitors of cyclooxygenase-2. *N Engl J Med* 2001;345:433–442.
6. Simon L, Lipman A, Jacox A, et al. *Guideline for the management of arthritis pain in osteoarthritis, rheumatoid arthritis, and juvenile chronic arthritis.* Glenview, IL: American Pain Society, 2002 (APS Clinical Practice Guidelines Series, No. 2).
7. American College of Rheumatology Subcommittee on Osteoarthritis Guidelines. Recommendations for the medical management of osteoarthritis of the hip and knee: 2000 update. *Arthritis Rheum* 2000; 43:1905–1915.
8. The management of persistent pain in older persons. *J Am Geriatr Soc* 2002;50(suppl):205–224.
9. Vane JR. Inhibition of prostaglandin synthesis as a mechanism of action for aspirin-like drugs. *Nat New Biol* 1971;231:232–235.
10. Pash JM, Bailey JM. Inhibition by corticosteroids of epidermal growth factor-induced recovery of cyclooxygenase after aspirin inactivation. *FASEB J* 1988;2:2613–2618.
11. Sebaldt RJ, Sheller JR, Oates JA, et al. Inhibition of eicosanoid biosynthesis by glucocorticoids in humans. *Proc Natl Acad Sci U S A* 1990;87:6974–6978.
12. Masferrer JL, Zweifel BS, Seibert K, et al. Selective regulation of cellular cyclooxygenase by dexamethasone and endotoxin in mice. *J Clin Invest* 1990;86:1375–1379.
13. Xie WL, Chipman JG, Robertson DL, et al. Expression of a mitogen-responsive gene encoding prostaglandin synthase is regulated by mRNA splicing. *Proc Natl Acad Sci U S A* 1991;88:2692–2696.
14. Kujubu DA, Herschman HR. Dexamethasone inhibits mitogen induction of the TIS10 prostaglandin synthase/cyclooxygenase gene. *J Biol Chem* 1992;267:7991–7994.
15. O'Banion MK, Winn VD, Young DA. cDNA cloning and functional activity of a glucocorticoid-regulated inflammatory cyclooxygenase. *Proc Natl Acad Sci U S A* 1992;89:4888–4892.
16. Toh H, Yokoyama C, Tanabe T, et al. Molecular evolution of cyclooxygenase and lipoxygenase. *Prostaglandins* 1992;44:291–315.
17. Morita I, Schindler M, Regier MK, et al. Different intracellular locations for prostaglandin endoperoxide H synthase-1 and -2. *J Biol Chem* 1995;270:10902–10908.
18. Smith WL. Prostanoid biosynthesis and mechanisms of action. *Am J Physiol* 1992;263(2 part 2):F181–F191.
19. Komhoff M, Grone HJ, Klein T, et al. Localization of cyclooxygenase-1 and -2 in adult and fetal human kidney: implication for renal function. *Am J Physiol* 1997;272(4 part 2):F460–F468.
20. Harris RC, McKanna JA, Akai Y, et al. Cyclooxygenase-2 is associated with the macula densa of rat kidney and increases with salt restriction. *J Clin Invest* 1994;94:2504–2510.
21. Rocca B, Spain LM, Pure E, et al. Distinct roles of prostaglandin H synthases 1 and 2 in T-cell development. *J Clin Invest* 1999;103:1469–1477.
22. Smith CJ, Morrow JD, Roberts LJ 2nd, et al. Induction of prostaglandin endoperoxide synthase-1 (COX-1) in a human promonocytic cell line by treatment with the differentiating agent TPA. *Adv Exp Med Biol* 1997;400A:99–106.
23. Loll PJ, Picot D, Garavito RM. The structural basis of aspirin activity inferred from the crystal structure of inactivated prostaglandin H2 synthase. *Nat Struct Biol* 1995;2:637–643.
24. Roth GJ, Majerus PW. The mechanism of the effect of aspirin on human platelets. I. Acetylation of a particulate fraction protein. *J Clin Invest* 1975;56:624–632.
25. Wu KK. Biochemical pharmacology of nonsteroidal anti-inflammatory drugs. *Biochem Pharmacol* 1998;55:543–547.
26. Wu KK, Sanduja R, Tsai AL, et al. Aspirin inhibits interleukin 1-induced prostaglandin H synthase expression in cultured endothelial cells. *Proc Natl Acad Sci U S A* 1991;88:2384–2387.
27. Weissmann G. Prostaglandins as modulators rather than mediators of inflammation. *J Lipid Mediat* 1993;6:275–286.
28. Kopp E, Ghosh S. Inhibition of NF-kappa B by sodium salicylate and aspirin. *Science* 1994;265:956–959.
29. Gautam SC, Pindolia KR, Noth CJ, et al. Chemokine gene expression in bone marrow stromal cells: downregulation with sodium salicylate. *Blood* 1995;86:2541–2550.
30. Farivar RS, Brecher P. Salicylate is a transcriptional inhibitor of the inducible nitric oxide synthase in cultured cardiac fibroblasts. *J Biol Chem* 1996;271:31585–31592.
31. Schwenger P, Skolnik EY, Vilcek J. Inhibition of tumor necrosis factor-induced p42/p44 mitogen-activated protein kinase activation by sodium salicylate. *J Biol Chem* 1996;271:8089–8094.
32. Jones MK, Wang H, Peskar BM, et al. Inhibition of angiogenesis by nonsteroidal anti-inflammatory drugs: insight into mechanisms and implications for cancer growth and ulcer healing. *Nat Med* 1999;5:1418–1423.
33. Lecomte M, Laneuville O, Ji C, et al. Acetylation of human prostaglandin endoperoxide synthase-2 (cyclooxygenase-2) by aspirin. *J Biol Chem* 1994;269:13207–13215.
34. Claria J, Serhan CN. Aspirin triggers previously undescribed bioactive eicosanoids by human endothelial cell-leukocyte interactions. *Proc Natl Acad Sci U S A* 1995;92:9475–9479.
35. Serhan CN, Takano T, Maddox JF. Aspirin-triggered 15-epi-lipoxin A4 and stable analogs on lipoxin A4 are potent inhibitors of acute inflammation. Receptors and pathways. *Adv Exp Med Biol* 1999;447: 133–149.

36. Ito S, Okuda-Ashitaka E, Minami T. Central and peripheral roles of prostaglandins in pain and their interactions with novel neuropeptides nociceptin and nocistatin. *Neurosci Res* 2001;41:299–332.
37. Seibert K, Zhang Y, Leahy K, et al. Pharmacological and biochemical demonstration of the role of cyclooxygenase 2 in inflammation and pain. *Proc Natl Acad Sci U S A* 1994;91:12013–12017.
38. Yamagata K, Andreasson KI, Kaufmann WE, et al. Expression of a mitogen-inducible cyclooxygenase in brain neurons: regulation by synaptic activity and glucocorticoids. *Neuron* 1993;11:371–386.
39. Breder CD, Smith WL, Raz A, et al. Distribution and characterization of cyclooxygenase immunoreactivity in the ovine brain. *J Comp Neurol* 1992;322:409–438.
40. Breder CD, Saper CB. Expression of inducible cyclooxygenase mRNA in the mouse brain after systemic administration of bacterial lipopolysaccharide. *Brain Res* 1996;713:64–69.
41. Beiche F, Scheuerer S, Brune K, et al. Up-regulation of cyclooxygenase-2 mRNA in the rat spinal cord following peripheral inflammation. *FEBS Lett* 1996;390:165–169.
42. Beiche F, Klein T, Nusing R, et al. Localization of cyclooxygenase-2 and prostaglandin E_2 receptor EP3 in the rat lumbar spinal cord. *J Neuroimmunol* 1998;89:26–34.
43. Chopra B, Giblett S, Little JG, et al. Cyclooxygenase-1 is a marker for a subpopulation of putative nociceptive neurons in rat dorsal root ganglia. *Eur J Neurosci* 2000;12:911–920.
44. Engblom D, Ek M, Hallbeck M, et al. Distribution of prostaglandin EP(3) and EP(4) receptor mRNA in the rat parabrachial nucleus. *Neurosci Lett* 2000;281:163–166.
45. Nakamura K, Kaneko T, Yamashita Y, et al. Immunohistochemical localization of prostaglandin EP3 receptor in the rat nervous system. *J Comp Neurol* 2000;421:543–569.
46. Ek M, Arias C, Sawchenko P, et al. Distribution of the EP3 prostaglandin E(2) receptor subtype in the rat brain: relationship to sites of interleukin-1-induced cellular responsiveness. *J Comp Neurol* 2000; 428:5–20.
47. Coceani F, Akarsu ES. Prostaglandin E_2 in the pathogenesis of fever. An update. *Ann NY Acad Sci* 1998;856:76–82.
48. Ushikubi F, Segi E, Sugimoto Y, et al. Impaired febrile response in mice lacking the prostaglandin E receptor subtype EP3. *Nature* 1998;395:281–284.
49. Li S, Wang Y, Matsumura K, et al. The febrile response to lipopolysaccharide is blocked in cyclooxygenase-2(−/−), but not in cyclooxygenase-1(−/−) mice. *Brain Res* 1999;825:86–94.
50. Schwartz JI, Chan CC, Mukhopadhyay S, et al. Cyclooxygenase-2 inhibition by rofecoxib reverses naturally occurring fever in humans. *Clin Pharmacol Ther* 1999;65:653–660.
51. Chandrasekharan NV, Dai H, Roos KL, et al. COX-3, a cyclooxygenase-1 variant inhibited by acetaminophen and other analgesic/antipyretic drugs: cloning, structure, and expression. *Proc Natl Acad Sci U S A* 2002;99:13926–13931.
52. Awtry EH, Loscalzo J. Aspirin. *Circulation* 2000;101:1206–1218.
53. Owen PR. Prostaglandin synthetase inhibitors in the treatment of primary dysmenorrhea. Outcome trials reviewed. *Am J Obstet Gynecol* 1984;148:96–103.
54. Morrison BW, Daniels SE, Kotey P, et al. Rofecoxib, a specific cyclooxygenase-2 inhibitor, in primary dysmenorrhea: a randomized controlled trial. *Obstet Gynecol* 1999;94:504–508.
55. Daniels SE, Talwalker S, Torri S, et al. Valdecoxib, a cyclooxygenase-2-specific inhibitor, is effective in treating primary dysmenorrhea. *Obstet Gynecol* 2002;100:350–358.
56. Subbaramaiah K, Dannenberg AJ. Cyclooxygenase 2: a molecular target for cancer prevention and treatment. *Trends Pharmacol Sci* 2003;24:96–102.
57. Aisen PS. Evaluation of selective COX-2 inhibitors for the treatment of Alzheimer's disease. *J Pain Symptom Manage* 2002;23(suppl):35–40.
58. Waddell WR, Loughry RW. Sulindac for polyposis of the colon. *J Surg Oncol* 1983;24:83–87.
59. Steinbach G, Lynch PM, Phillips RK, et al. The effect of celecoxib, a cyclooxygenase-2 inhibitor, in familial adenomatous polyposis. *N Engl J Med* 2000;342:1946–1952.
60. Giovannucci E, Egan KM, Hunter DJ, et al. Aspirin and the risk of colorectal cancer in women. *N Engl J Med* 1995;333:609–614.
61. Giovannucci E, Rimm EB, Stampfer MJ, et al. Aspirin use and the risk for colorectal cancer and adenoma in male health professionals. *Ann Intern Med* 1994;121:241–246.
62. Greenberg ER, Baron JA, Freeman DH Jr, et al. Reduced risk of large-bowel adenomas among aspirin users. The Polyp Prevention Study Group. *J Natl Cancer Inst* 1993;85:912–916.
63. Peleg, II, Maibach HT, Brown SH, et al. Aspirin and nonsteroidal anti-inflammatory drug use and the risk of subsequent colorectal cancer. *Arch Intern Med* 1994;154:394–399.
64. Thun MJ, Namboodiri MM, Calle EE, et al. Aspirin use and risk of fatal cancer. *Cancer Res* 1993;53:1322–1327.
65. Thun MJ, Namboodiri MM, Heath CW Jr. Aspirin use and reduced risk of fatal colon cancer. *N Engl J Med* 1991;325:1593–1596.
66. Collet JP, Sharpe C, Belzile E, et al. Colorectal cancer prevention by non-steroidal anti-inflammatory drugs: effects of dosage and timing. *Br J Cancer* 1999;81:62–68.
67. Logan RF, Little J, Hawtin PG, et al. Effect of aspirin and non-steroidal anti-inflammatory drugs on colorectal adenomas: case-control study of subjects participating in the Nottingham faecal occult blood screening programme. *BMJ* 1993;307:285–289.
68. Muscat JE, Stellman SD, Wynder EL. Nonsteroidal antiinflammatory drugs and colorectal cancer. *Cancer* 1994;74:1847–1854.
69. Peleg, II, Lubin MF, Cotsonis GA, et al. Long-term use of nonsteroidal antiinflammatory drugs and other chemopreventors and risk of subsequent colorectal neoplasia. *Dig Dis Sci* 1996;41:1319–1326.
70. Reeves MJ, Newcomb PA, Trentham-Dietz A, et al. Nonsteroidal anti-inflammatory drug use and protection against colorectal cancer in women. *Cancer Epidemiol Biomarkers Prev* 1996;5:955–960.
71. Smalley W, Ray WA, Daugherty J, et al. Use of nonsteroidal anti-inflammatory drugs and incidence of colorectal cancer: a population-based study. *Arch Intern Med* 1999;159:161–166.
72. Sandler RS, Halabi S, Baron JA, et al. A randomized trial of aspirin to prevent colorectal adenomas in patients with previous colorectal cancer. *N Engl J Med* 2003;348:883–890.
73. Baron JA, Cole BF, Sandler RS, et al. A randomized trial of aspirin to prevent colorectal adenomas. *N Engl J Med* 2003;348:891–899.
74. Imperiale TF. Aspirin and the prevention of colorectal cancer. *N Engl J Med* 2003;348:879–880.
75. McGeer PL, McGeer EG. The inflammatory response system of brain: implications for therapy of Alzheimer and other neurodegenerative diseases. *Brain Res Brain Res Rev* 1995;21:195–218.
76. Breitner JC. Inflammatory processes and antiinflammatory drugs in Alzheimer's disease: a current appraisal. *Neurobiol Aging* 1996;17: 789–794.
77. in t' Veld BA, Ruitenberg A, Hofman A, et al. Nonsteroidal antiinflammatory drugs and the risk of Alzheimer's disease. *N Engl J Med* 2001; 345:1515–1521.
78. Aisen PS, Schafer KA, Grundman M, et al. Effects of rofecoxib or naproxen vs placebo on Alzheimer disease progression: a randomized controlled trial. *JAMA* 2003;289:2819–2826.
79. Wolfe MM, Lichtenstein DR, Singh G. Gastrointestinal toxicity of nonsteroidal antiinflammatory drugs. *N Engl J Med* 1999;340:1888–1899.
80. Tamblyn R, Berkson L, Dauphinee WD, et al. Unnecessary prescribing of NSAIDs and the management of NSAID-related gastropathy in medical practice. *Ann Intern Med* 1997;127:429–438.
81. Douthwaite AH, Lintott GAM. Gastroscopic observation of effect of aspirin and certain other substances on stomach. *Lancet* 1938;2:1222–1225.
82. Bjorkman D. Commentary: Gastrointestinal safety of coxibs and outcomes studies: what's the verdict? *J Pain Symptom Manage* 2002;23 (suppl):11–14.
83. Sun DC, Roth SH, Mitchell CS, et al. Upper gastrointestinal disease in rheumatoid arthritis. *Am J Dig Dis* 1974;19:405–410.
84. Levy M. Aspirin use in patients with major upper gastrointestinal bleeding and peptic-ulcer disease. A report from the Boston Collaborative Drug Surveillance Program, Boston University Medical Center. *N Engl J Med* 1974;290:1158–1162.
85. Silvoso GR, Ivey KJ, Butt JH, et al. Incidence of gastric lesions in patients with rheumatic disease on chronic aspirin therapy. *Ann Intern Med* 1979;91:517–520.
86. Singh G, Triadafilopoulos G. Epidemiology of NSAID induced gastrointestinal complications. *J Rheumatol* 1999;26(suppl 56):18–24.

87. Silverstein FE, Graham DY, Senior JR, et al. Misoprostol reduces serious gastrointestinal complications in patients with rheumatoid arthritis receiving nonsteroidal anti-inflammatory drugs. A randomized, double-blind, placebo-controlled trial. *Ann Intern Med* 1995; 123:241–249.
88. Weil J, Colin-Jones D, Langman M, et al. Prophylactic aspirin and risk of peptic ulcer bleeding. BMJ 1995;310:827–830.
89. Schoen RT, Vender RJ. Mechanisms of nonsteroidal anti-inflammatory drug-induced gastric damage. *Am J Med* 1989;86:449–458.
90. Armstrong CP, Blower AL. Non-steroidal anti-inflammatory drugs and life threatening complications of peptic ulceration. *Gut* 1987;28: 527–532.
91. Singh G, Ramey DR, Morfeld D, et al. Gastrointestinal tract complications of nonsteroidal anti-inflammatory drug treatment in rheumatoid arthritis. A prospective observational cohort study. *Arch Intern Med* 1996;156:1530–1536.
92. Hernandez-Diaz S, Rodriguez LA. Association between nonsteroidal anti-inflammatory drugs and upper gastrointestinal tract bleeding/perforation: an overview of epidemiologic studies published in the 1990s. *Arch Intern Med* 2000;160:2093–2099.
93. MacDonald TM. Epidemiology and pharmacoeconomic implications of non-steroidal anti-inflammatory drug-associated gastrointestinal toxicity. *Rheumatology (Oxford)* 2000;39(suppl 2):13–20; discussion 57–59.
94. Rostom A, Dube C, Wells G, et al. Prevention of NSAID-induced gastroduodenal ulcers. *Cochrane Database Syst Rev* 2002: CD002296.
95. Chan FK, Chung SC, Suen BY, et al. Preventing recurrent upper gastrointestinal bleeding in patients with *Helicobacter pylori* infection who are taking low-dose aspirin or naproxen. *N Engl J Med* 2001;344:967–973.
96. Bombardier C, Laine L, Reicin A, et al. Comparison of upper gastrointestinal toxicity of rofecoxib and naproxen in patients with rheumatoid arthritis. VIGOR Study Group. *N Engl J Med* 2000; 343:1520–1528.
97. Silverstein FE, Faich G, Goldstein JL, et al. Gastrointestinal toxicity with celecoxib vs nonsteroidal anti-inflammatory drugs for osteoarthritis and rheumatoid arthritis: the CLASS study: A randomized controlled trial. Celecoxib Long-term Arthritis Safety Study. *JAMA* 2000;284:1247–1255.
98. Laine L. Review article: The effect of *Helicobacter pylori* infection on nonsteroidal anti-inflammatory drug-induced upper gastrointestinal tract injury. *Aliment Pharmacol Ther* 2002;16(suppl 1):34–39.
99. Laine L, Cominelli F, Sloane R, et al. Interaction of NSAIDs and *Helicobacter pylori* on gastrointestinal injury and prostaglandin production: a controlled double-blind trial. *Aliment Pharmacol Ther* 1995;9:127–135.
100. Thillainayagam AV, Tabaqchali S, Warrington SJ, et al. Interrelationships between *Helicobacter pylori* infection, nonsteroidal antiinflammatory drugs and gastroduodenal disease. A prospective study in healthy volunteers. *Dig Dis Sci* 1994;39:1085–1089.
101. Kim JG, Graham DY. *Helicobacter pylori* infection and development of gastric or duodenal ulcer in arthritic patients receiving chronic NSAID therapy. The Misoprostol Study Group. *Am J Gastroenterol* 1994;89:203–207.
102. Goggin PM, Collins DA, Jazrawi RP, et al. Prevalence of *Helicobacter pylori* infection and its effect on symptoms and non-steroidal anti-inflammatory drug induced gastrointestinal damage in patients with rheumatoid arthritis. *Gut* 1993;34:1677–1680.
103. Lanza FL, Evans DG, Graham DY. Effect of *Helicobacter pylori* infection on the severity of gastroduodenal mucosal injury after the acute administration of naproxen or aspirin to normal volunteers. *Am J Gastroenterol* 1991;86:735–737.
104. Bannwarth B, Dorval E, Caekaert A, et al. Influence of *Helicobacter pylori* eradication therapy on the occurrence of gastrointestinal events in patients treated with conventional nonsteroidal antiinflammatory drugs combined with omeprazole. *J Rheumatol* 2002;29: 1975–1980.
105. Taha AS, Dahill S, Morran C, et al. Neutrophils, *Helicobacter pylori*, and nonsteroidal anti-inflammatory drug ulcers. *Gastroenterology* 1999;116:254–258.
106. Chan FK, Sung JJ, Chung SC, et al. Randomised trial of eradication of *Helicobacter pylori* before non-steroidal anti-inflammatory drug therapy to prevent peptic ulcers. *Lancet* 1997;350:975–979.
107. Labenz J, Blum AL, Bolten WW, et al. Primary prevention of diclofenac associated ulcers and dyspepsia by omeprazole or triple therapy in *Helicobacter pylori* positive patients: a randomised, double blind, placebo controlled, clinical trial. *Gut* 2002;51:329–335.
108. Yeomans ND, Tulassay Z, Juhasz L, et al. A comparison of omeprazole with ranitidine for ulcers associated with nonsteroidal antiinflammatory drugs. Acid Suppression Trial: Ranitidine versus Omeprazole for NSAID-associated Ulcer Treatment (ASTRONAUT) Study Group. *N Engl J Med* 1998;338:719–726.
109. Hawkey CJ, Karrasch JA, Szczepanski L, et al. Omeprazole compared with misoprostol for ulcers associated with nonsteroidal antiinflammatory drugs. Omeprazole versus Misoprostol for NSAID-induced Ulcer Management (OMNIUM) Study Group. *N Engl J Med* 1998;338: 727–734.
110. Hawkey CJ, Tulassay Z, Szczepanski L, et al. Randomised controlled trial of *Helicobacter pylori* eradication in patients on non-steroidal anti-inflammatory drugs; HELP NSAIDs study. *Helicobacter* Eradication for Lesion Prevention. *Lancet* 1998;352:1016–1021.
111. Agrawal NM, Campbell DR, Safdi MA, et al. Superiority of lansoprazole vs ranitidine in healing nonsteroidal anti-inflammatory drug-associated gastric ulcers: results of a double-blind, randomized, multicenter study. NSAID-Associated Gastric Ulcer Study Group. *Arch Intern Med* 2000;160:1455–1461.
112. Chan FK, Sung JJ, Suen R, et al. Does eradication of *Helicobacter pylori* impair healing of nonsteroidal anti-inflammatory drug associated bleeding peptic ulcers? A prospective randomized study. *Aliment Pharmacol Ther* 1998;12:1201–1205.
113. Talley NJ, Zinsmeister AR, Schleck CD, et al. Smoking, alcohol, and analgesics in dyspepsia and among dyspepsia subgroups: lack of an association in a community. *Gut* 1994;35:619–624.
114. Talley NJ, Evans JM, Fleming KC, et al. Nonsteroidal antiinflammatory drugs and dyspepsia in the elderly. *Dig Dis Sci* 1995;40: 1345–1350.
115. Watson DJ, Harper SE, Zhao PL, et al. Gastrointestinal tolerability of the selective cyclooxygenase-2 (COX-2) inhibitor rofecoxib compared with nonselective COX-1 and COX-2 inhibitors in osteoarthritis. *Arch Intern Med* 2000;160:2998–3003.
116. Larkai EN, Smith JL, Lidsky MD, et al. Gastroduodenal mucosa and dyspeptic symptoms in arthritic patients during chronic nonsteroidal anti-inflammatory drug use. *Am J Gastroenterol* 1987;82: 1153–1158.
117. Pounder R. Silent peptic ulceration: deadly silence or golden silence? *Gastroenterology* 1989;96(part 2; suppl):626–631.
118. Bijlsma JW. Treatment of NSAID-induced gastrointestinal lesions with cimetidine: an international multicentre collaborative study. *Aliment Pharmacol Ther* 1988;2(suppl 1):85–95.
119. Lanza FL, Aspinall RL, Swabb EA, et al. Double-blind, placebo-controlled endoscopic comparison of the mucosal protective effects of misoprostol versus cimetidine on tolmetin-induced mucosal injury to the stomach and duodenum. *Gastroenterology* 1988;95:289–294.
120. Saunders JH, Oliver RJ, Higson DL. Dyspepsia: incidence of a non-ulcer disease in a controlled trial of ranitidine in general practice. *BMJ (Clin Res)* 1986;292:665–668.
121. Van Groenendael JH, Markusse HM, Dijkmans BA, et al. The effect of ranitidine on NSAID related dyspeptic symptoms with and without peptic ulcer disease of patients with rheumatoid arthritis and osteoarthritis. *Clin Rheumatol* 1996;15:450–456.
122. Matsuhashi N, Yamada A, Hiraishi M, et al. Multiple strictures of the small intestine after long-term nonsteroidal anti-inflammatory drug therapy. *Am J Gastroenterol* 1992;87:1183–1186.
123. Hershfield NB. Endoscopic demonstration of non-steroidal anti-inflammatory drug-induced small intestinal strictures. *Gastrointest Endosc* 1992;38:388–390.
124. Saw KC, Quick CR, Higgins AF. Ileocaecal perforation and bleeding—are non-steroidal anti-inflammatory drugs (NSAIDs) responsible? [comment]. *J R Soc Med* 1990;83:114–115.
125. Lang J, Price AB, Levi AJ, et al. Diaphragm disease: pathology of disease of the small intestine induced by non-steroidal anti-inflammatory drugs. *J Clin Pathol* 1988;41:516–526.
126. Bjarnason I, Price AB, Zanelli G, et al. Clinicopathological features of nonsteroidal antiinflammatory drug-induced small intestinal strictures. *Gastroenterology* 1988;94:1070–1074.
127. Sukumar L. Recurrent small bowel obstruction associated with piroxicam. *Br J Surg* 1987;74:186.

128. Fang WF, Broughton A, Jacobson ED. Indomethacin-induced intestinal inflammation. *Am J Dig Dis* 1977;22:749–760.
129. Sturges HF, Krone CL. Ulceration and stricture of the jejunum in a patient on long-term indomethacin therapy. *Am J Gastroenterol* 1973;59:162–169.
130. Bjorkman D. Nonsteroidal anti-inflammatory drug-associated toxicity of the liver, lower gastrointestinal tract, and esophagus. *Am J Med* 1998;105(suppl):17–21.
131. Kessler WF, Shires GT 3rd, Fahey TJ 3rd. Surgical complications of nonsteroidal antiinflammatory drug-induced small bowel ulceration. *J Am Coll Surg* 1997;185:250–254.
132. Laine L, Connors LG, Reicin A, et al. Serious lower gastrointestinal clinical events with nonselective NSAID or coxib use. *Gastroenterology* 2003;124:288–292.
133. Tolman KG. Hepatotoxicity of non-narcotic analgesics. *Am J Med* 1998;105(suppl):13–19.
134. Fry SW, Seeff LB. Hepatotoxicity of analgesics and anti-inflammatory agents. *Gastroenterol Clin North Am* 1995;24:875–905.
135. Carson JL, Strom BL, Duff A, et al. Safety of nonsteroidal antiinflammatory drugs with respect to acute liver disease. *Arch Intern Med* 1993;153:1331–1336.
136. Tarazi EM, Harter JG, Zimmerman HJ, et al. Sulindac-associated hepatic injury: analysis of 91 cases reported to the Food and Drug Administration. *Gastroenterology* 1993;104:569–574.
137. Whelton A, Hamilton CW. Nonsteroidal anti-inflammatory drugs: effects on kidney function. *J Clin Pharmacol* 1991;31:588–598.
138. Harris RC Jr. Cyclooxygenase-2 inhibition and renal physiology. *Am J Cardiol* 2002;89:10D–17D.
139. Henrich WL, Agodoa LE, Barrett B, et al. Analgesics and the kidney: summary and recommendations to the Scientific Advisory Board of the National Kidney Foundation from an Ad Hoc Committee of the National Kidney Foundation. *Am J Kidney Dis* 1996;27:162–165.
140. Whelton A. Nephrotoxicity of nonsteroidal anti-inflammatory drugs: physiologic foundations and clinical implications. *Am J Med* 1999;106(suppl):13–24.
141. Swan SK, Rudy DW, Lasseter KC, et al. Effect of cyclooxygenase-2 inhibition on renal function in elderly persons receiving a low-salt diet. A randomized, controlled trial. *Ann Intern Med* 2000;133:1–9.
142. Smith WL, Bell TG. Immunohistochemical localization of the prostaglandin-forming cyclooxygenase in renal cortex. *Am J Physiol* 1978;235:F451–F457.
143. Yang T, Singh I, Pham H, et al. Regulation of cyclooxygenase expression in the kidney by dietary salt intake. *Am J Physiol* 1998;274:F481–F489.
144. Ichihara A, Imig JD, Inscho EW, et al. Cyclooxygenase-2 participates in tubular flow-dependent afferent arteriolar tone: interaction with neuronal NOS. *Am J Physiol* 1998;275:F605–F612.
145. Harding P, Sigmon DH, Alfie ME, et al. Cyclooxygenase-2 mediates increased renal renin content induced by low-sodium diet. *Hypertension* 1997;29:297–302.
146. Komhoff M, Jeck ND, Seyberth HW, et al. Cyclooxygenase-2 expression is associated with the renal macula densa of patients with Bartter-like syndrome. *Kidney Int* 2000;58:2420–2424.
147. Whelton A, Maurath CJ, Verburg KM, et al. Renal safety and tolerability of celecoxib, a novel cyclooxygenase-2 inhibitor. *Am J Ther* 2000;7:159–175.
148. Gertz BJ, Krupa D, Bolognese JA, et al. A comparison of adverse renovascular experiences among osteoarthritis patients treated with rofecoxib and comparator non-selective non-steroidal anti-inflammatory agents. *Curr Med Res Opin* 2002;18:82–91.
149. Brater DC. Effects of nonsteroidal anti-inflammatory drugs on renal function: focus on cyclooxygenase-2-selective inhibition. *Am J Med* 1999;107(suppl):65–70; discussion 70–71.
150. Whelton A. Renal and related cardiovascular effects of conventional and COX-2-specific NSAIDs and non-NSAID analgesics. *Am J Ther* 2000;7:63–74.
151. Schwartz JI, Vandormael K, Malice MP, et al. Comparison of rofecoxib, celecoxib, and naproxen on renal function in elderly subjects receiving a normal-salt diet. *Clin Pharmacol Ther* 2002;72:50–61.
152. Catella-Lawson F, McAdam B, Morrison BW, et al. Effects of specific inhibition of cyclooxygenase-2 on sodium balance, hemodynamics, and vasoactive eicosanoids. *J Pharmacol Exp Ther* 1999;289:735–741.
153. Epstein M. Renal prostaglandins and the control of renal function in liver disease. *Am J Med* 1986;80:46–55.
154. Oates JA, FitzGerald GA, Branch RA, et al. Clinical implications of prostaglandin and thromboxane A2 formation (1). *N Engl J Med* 1988;319:689–698.
155. Walshe JJ, Venuto RC. Acute oliguric renal failure induced by indomethacin: possible mechanism. *Ann Intern Med* 1979;91:47–49.
156. Arisz L, Donker AJ, Brentjens JR, et al. The effect of indomethacin on proteinuria and kidney function in the nephrotic syndrome. *Acta Med Scand* 1976;199:121–125.
157. Kleinknecht C, Broyer M, Gubler MC, et al. Irreversible renal failure after indomethacin in steroid-resistant nephrosis. *N Engl J Med* 1980;302:691.
158. Blackshear JL, Napier JS, Davidman M, et al. Renal complications of nonsteroidal antiinflammatory drugs: identification and monitoring of those at risk. *Semin Arthritis Rheum* 1985;14:163–175.
159. Favre L, Glasson P, Vallotton MB. Reversible acute renal failure from combined triamterene and indomethacin: a study in healthy subjects. *Ann Intern Med* 1982;96:317–320.
160. McCarthy JT, Torres VE, Romero JC, et al. Acute intrinsic renal failure induced by indomethacin: role of prostaglandin synthetase inhibition. *Mayo Clin Proc* 1982;57:289–296.
161. Henry D, Page J, Whyte I, et al. Consumption of non-steroidal anti-inflammatory drugs and the development of functional renal impairment in elderly subjects. Results of a case-control study. *Br J Clin Pharmacol* 1997;44:85–90.
162. Hay E, Derazon H, Bukish N, et al. Fatal hyperkalemia related to combined therapy with a COX-2 inhibitor, ACE inhibitor and potassium rich diet. *J Emerg Med* 2002;22:349–352.
163. Jolobe OM. Nephrotoxicity in the elderly due to co-prescription of ACE inhibitors and NSAIDs. *J R Soc Med* 2001;94:657–658.
164. Akbarpour F, Afrasiabi A, Vaziri ND. Severe hyperkalemia caused by indomethacin and potassium supplementation. *South Med J* 1985;78:756–767.
165. Mor R, Pitlik S, Rosenfeld JB. Indomethacin- and moduretic-induced hyperkalemia. *Isr J Med Sci* 1983;19:535–537.
166. Galler M, Folkert VW, Schlondorff D. Reversible acute renal insufficiency and hyperkalemia following indomethacin therapy. *JAMA* 1981;246:154–155.
167. Nicholls MG, Espiner EA. Indomethacin-induced azotaemia and hyperkalaemia: a case study. *N Z Med J* 1981;94:377–379.
168. Findling JW, Beckstrom D, Rawsthorne L, et al. Indomethacin-induced hyperkalemia in three patients with gouty arthritis. *JAMA* 1980;244:1127–1128.
169. Paladini G, Tonazzi C. Indomethacin-induced hyperkalemia and renal failure in multiple myeloma. *Acta Haematol* 1982;68:256–260.
170. Kelley M, Bastani B. Ketorolac-induced acute renal failure and hyperkalemia. *Clin Nephrol* 1995;44:276–277.
171. Patel P, Mandal B, Greenway MW. Hyperkalaemic quadriparesis secondary to chronic diclofenac treatment. *Postgrad Med J* 2001;77:50–51.
172. Apostolou T, Sotsiou F, Yfanti G, et al. Acute renal failure induced by nimesulide in a patient suffering from temporal arteritis. *Nephrol Dial Transplant* 1997;12:1493–1496.
173. Pal B, Hutchinson A, Bhattacharya A, et al. Cardiac arrest due to severe hyperkalaemia in patient taking nabumetone and low salt diet. *BMJ* 1995;311:1486–1487.
174. Abraham PA, Keane WF. Glomerular and interstitial disease induced by nonsteroidal anti-inflammatory drugs. *Am J Nephrol* 1984;4:1–6.
175. Bender WL, Whelton A, Beschorner WE, et al. Interstitial nephritis, proteinuria, and renal failure caused by nonsteroidal anti-inflammatory drugs. Immunologic characterization of the inflammatory infiltrate. *Am J Med* 1984;76:1006–1012.
176. Levin ML. Patterns of tubulo-interstitial damage associated with nonsteroidal antiinflammatory drugs. *Semin Nephrol* 1988;8:55–61.

177. Husserl FE, Lange RK, Kantrow CM Jr. Renal papillary necrosis and pyelonephritis accompanying fenoprofen therapy. *JAMA* 1979;242: 1896–1898.
178. Shah GM, Muhalwas KK, Winer RL. Renal papillary necrosis due to ibuprofen. *Arthritis Rheum* 1981;24:1208–1210.
179. Morales A, Steyn J. Papillary necrosis following phenylbutazone ingestion. *Arch Surg* 1971;103:420–421.
180. Murray TG, Goldberg M. Analgesic-associated nephropathy in the U.S.A.: epidemiologic, clinical and pathogenetic features. *Kidney Int* 1978;13:64–71.
181. Nanra RS, Stuart-Taylor J, de Leon AH, et al. Analgesic nephropathy: etiology, clinical syndrome, and clinicopathologic correlations in Australia. *Kidney Int* 1978;13:79–92.
182. De Broe ME, Elseviers MM. Analgesic nephropathy. *N Engl J Med* 1998;338:446–452.
183. Elseviers MM, De Broe ME. A long-term prospective controlled study of analgesic abuse in Belgium. *Kidney Int* 1995;48:1912–1919.
184. Elseviers MM, De Schepper A, Corthouts R, et al. High diagnostic performance of CT scan for analgesic nephropathy in patients with incipient to severe renal failure. *Kidney Int* 1995;48:1316–1323.
185. Elseviers MM, Waller I, Nenoy D, et al. Evaluation of diagnostic criteria for analgesic nephropathy in patients with end-stage renal failure: results of the ANNE study. Analgesic Nephropathy Network of Europe. *Nephrol Dial Transplant* 1995;10:808–814.
186. Piper JM, Tonascia J, Matanoski GM. Heavy phenacetin use and bladder cancer in women aged 20 to 49 years. *N Engl J Med* 1985; 313:292–295.
187. Blohme I, Johansson S. Renal pelvic neoplasms and atypical urothelium in patients with end-stage analgesic nephropathy. *Kidney Int* 1981;20:671–675.
188. McCredie M, Stewart JH, Carter JJ, et al. Phenacetin and papillary necrosis: independent risk factors for renal pelvic cancer. *Kidney Int* 1986;30:81–84.
189. Johnson AG, Nguyen TV, Day RO. Do nonsteroidal anti-inflammatory drugs affect blood pressure? A meta-analysis. *Ann Intern Med* 1994; 121:289–300.
190. Pope JE, Anderson JJ, Felson DT. A meta-analysis of the effects of nonsteroidal anti-inflammatory drugs on blood pressure. *Arch Intern Med* 1993;153:477–484.
191. Komers R, Anderson S, Epstein M. Renal and cardiovascular effects of selective cyclooxygenase-2 inhibitors. *Am J Kidney Dis* 2001;38: 1145–1157.
192. Vioxx. Prescribing information, Merck, Inc.
193. Johnson AG, Simons LA, Simons J, et al. Non-steroidal anti-inflammatory drugs and hypertension in the elderly: a community-based cross-sectional study. *Br J Clin Pharmacol* 1993;35:455–459.
194. Gurwitz JH, Avorn J, Bohn RL, et al. Initiation of antihypertensive treatment during nonsteroidal anti-inflammatory drug therapy. *JAMA* 1994;272:781–786.
195. Schooley RT, Wagley PF, Lietman PS. Edema associated with ibuprofen therapy. *JAMA* 1977;237:1716–1717.
196. Tashima CK, Rose M. Letter: Pulmonary edema and salicylates. *Ann Intern Med* 1974;81:274–275.
197. Nevins M, Berque S, Corwin N, et al. Phenylbutazone and pulmonary oedema. *Lancet* 1969;2:1358.
198. Van den Ouweland FA, Gribnau FW, Meyboom RH. Congestive heart failure due to nonsteroidal anti-inflammatory drugs in the elderly. *Age Ageing* 1988;17:8–16.
199. Feenstra J, Grobbee DE, Mosterd A, et al. Adverse cardiovascular effects of NSAIDs in patients with congestive heart failure. *Drug Saf* 1997;17:166–180.
200. Heerdink ER, Leufkens HG, Herings RM, et al. NSAIDs associated with increased risk of congestive heart failure in elderly patients taking diuretics. *Arch Intern Med* 1998;158:1108–1112.
201. Page J, Henry D. Consumption of NSAIDs and the development of congestive heart failure in elderly patients: an underrecognized public health problem. *Arch Intern Med* 2000;160:777–784.
202. Feenstra J, Heerdink ER, Grobbee DE, et al. Association of nonsteroidal anti-inflammatory drugs with first occurrence of heart failure and with relapsing heart failure: the Rotterdam Study. *Arch Intern Med* 2002;162:265–270.
203. Collaborative meta-analysis of randomised trials of antiplatelet therapy for prevention of death, myocardial infarction, and stroke in high risk patients. *BMJ* 2002;324:71–86.
204. Baigent C, Patrono C. Selective cyclooxygenase 2 inhibitors, aspirin, and cardiovascular disease: a reappraisal. *Arthritis Rheum* 2003;48: 12–20.
205. Konstam MA, Weir MR, Reicin A, et al. Cardiovascular thrombotic events in controlled, clinical trials of rofecoxib. *Circulation* 2001; 104:2280–2288.
206. Van Hecken A, Schwartz JI, Depre M, et al. Comparative inhibitory activity of rofecoxib, meloxicam, diclofenac, ibuprofen, and naproxen on COX-2 versus COX-1 in healthy volunteers. *J Clin Pharmacol* 2000;40:1109–1120.
207. Watson DJ, Rhodes T, Cai B, et al. Lower risk of thromboembolic cardiovascular events with naproxen among patients with rheumatoid arthritis. *Arch Intern Med* 2002;162:1105–1110.
208. FitzGerald GA, Cheng Y, Austin S. COX-2 inhibitors and the cardiovascular system. *Clin Exp Rheumatol* 2001;19(suppl 25): 31–36.
209. Cheng Y, Austin SC, Rocca B, et al. Role of prostacyclin in the cardiovascular response to thromboxane A2. *Science* 2002;296:539–541.
210. Namazy JA, Simon RA. Sensitivity to nonsteroidal anti-inflammatory drugs. *Ann Allergy Asthma Immunol* 2002;89:542–550; quiz 550, 605.
211. Stevenson DD, Sanchez-Borges M, Szczeklik A. Classification of allergic and pseudoallergic reactions to drugs that inhibit cyclooxygenase enzymes. *Ann Allergy Asthma Immunol* 2001;87:177–180.
212. McDonald JR, Mathison DA, Stevenson DD. Aspirin intolerance in asthma. Detection by oral challenge. *J Allergy Clin Immunol* 1972;50:198–207.
213. Giraldo B, Blumenthal MN, Spink WW. Aspirin intolerance and asthma. A clinical and immunological study. *Ann Intern Med* 1969; 71:479–496.
214. Arm JP, O'Hickey SP, Spur BW, et al. Airway responsiveness to histamine and leukotriene E4 in subjects with aspirin-induced asthma. *Am Rev Respir Dis* 1989;140:148–153.
215. Christie PE, Tagari P, Ford-Hutchinson AW, et al. Urinary leukotriene E4 concentrations increase after aspirin challenge in aspirin-sensitive asthmatic subjects. *Am Rev Respir Dis* 1991;143:1025–1029.
216. Mastalerz L, Gawlewicz-Mroczka A, Nizankowska E, et al. Protection against exercise-induced bronchoconstriction by montelukast in aspirin-sensitive and aspirin-tolerant patients with asthma. *Clin Exp Allergy* 2002;32:1360–1365.
217. Dahlen SE, Malmstrom K, Nizankowska E, et al. Improvement of aspirin-intolerant asthma by montelukast, a leukotriene antagonist: a randomized, double-blind, placebo-controlled trial. *Am J Respir Crit Care Med* 2002;165:9–14.
218. Stevenson DD. Aspirin desensitization in patients with AERD. *Clin Rev Allergy Immunol* 2003;24:159–168.
219. Gyllfors P, Bochenek G, Overholt J, et al. Biochemical and clinical evidence that aspirin-intolerant asthmatic subjects tolerate the cyclooxygenase 2-selective analgetic drug celecoxib. *J Allergy Clin Immunol* 2003;111:1116–1121.
220. Woessner KM, Simon RA, Stevenson DD. The safety of celecoxib in patients with aspirin-sensitive asthma. *Arthritis Rheum* 2002;46: 2201–2206.
221. Martin-Garcia C, Hinojosa M, Berges P, et al. Safety of a cyclooxygenase-2 inhibitor in patients with aspirin-sensitive asthma. *Chest* 2002;121:1812–1817.
222. Szczeklik A, Nizankowska E, Bochenek G, et al. Safety of a specific COX-2 inhibitor in aspirin-induced asthma. *Clin Exp Allergy* 2001; 31:219–225.
223. Marks F, Harrell K, Fischer R. Successful use of cyclooxygenase-2 inhibitor in a patient with aspirin-induced asthma. *South Med J* 2001; 94:256–257.
224. Moore-Robinson M, Warin RP. Effect of salicylates in urticaria. *BMJ* 1967;4:262–264.
225. Sanchez-Borges M, Capriles-Hulett A, Caballero-Fonseca F. NSAID-induced urticaria and angioedema: a reappraisal of its clinical management. *Am J Clin Dermatol* 2002;3:599–607.

226. Perez C, Sanchez-Borges M, Capriles E. Pretreatment with montelukast blocks NSAID-induced urticaria and angioedema. *J Allergy Clin Immunol* 2001;108:1060–1061.
227. Pacor ML, Di Lorenzo G, Corrocher R. Efficacy of leukotriene receptor antagonist in chronic urticaria. A double-blind, placebo-controlled comparison of treatment with montelukast and cetirizine in patients with chronic urticaria with intolerance to food additive and/or acetylsalicylic acid. *Clin Exp Allergy* 2001;31:1607–1614.
228. Asero R. Leukotriene receptor antagonists may prevent NSAID-induced exacerbations in patients with chronic urticaria. *Ann Allergy Asthma Immunol* 2000;85:156–157.
229. Quiralte J, Saenz de San Pedro B, Florido JJ. Safety of selective cyclooxygenase-2 inhibitor rofecoxib in patients with NSAID-induced cutaneous reactions. *Ann Allergy Asthma Immunol* 2002;89: 63–66.
230. Pacor ML, Di Lorenzo G, Biasi D, et al. Safety of rofecoxib in subjects with a history of adverse cutaneous reactions to aspirin and/or non-steroidal anti-inflammatory drugs. *Clin Exp Allergy* 2002;32: 397–400.
231. Nettis E, Di PR, Ferrannini A, et al. Tolerability of rofecoxib in patients with cutaneous adverse reactions to nonsteroidal anti-inflammatory drugs. *Ann Allergy Asthma Immunol* 2002;88:331–334.
232. Sanchez Borges M, Capriles-Hulett A, Caballero-Fonseca F, et al. Tolerability to new COX-2 inhibitors in NSAID-sensitive patients with cutaneous reactions. *Ann Allergy Asthma Immunol* 2001;87: 201–204.
233. Asero R. Intolerance to nonsteroidal anti-inflammatory drugs might precede by years the onset of chronic urticaria. *J Allergy Clin Immunol* 2003;111:1095–1098.
234. Kemp SF, Lockey RF, Wolf BL, et al. Anaphylaxis. A review of 266 cases. *Arch Intern Med* 1995;155:1749–1754.
235. Davidson KA, Ringpfeil F, Lee JB. Ibuprofen-induced bullous leukocytoclastic vasculitis. *Cutis* 2001;67:303–307.
236. De Silva B, Banney L, Uttley W, et al. Pseudoporphyria and nonsteroidal antiinflammatory agents in children with juvenile idiopathic arthritis. *Pediatr Dermatol* 2000;17:480–483.
237. Cutaneous reactions to analgesic-antipyretics and nonsteroidal anti-inflammatory drugs. Analysis of reports to the spontaneous reporting system of the Gruppo Italiano Studi Epidemiologici in Dermatologia. *Dermatology* 1993;186:164–169.
238. Moore DE. Drug-induced cutaneous photosensitivity: incidence, mechanism, prevention and management. *Drug Saf* 2002;25:345–372.
239. Greenberg GN. Recurrent sulindac-induced aseptic meningitis in a patient tolerant to other nonsteroidal anti-inflammatory drugs. *South Med J* 1988;81:1463–1464.
240. Marinac JS. Drug- and chemical-induced aseptic meningitis: a review of the literature. *Ann Pharmacother* 1992;26:813–822.
241. Goodwin SD, Glenny RW. Nonsteroidal anti-inflammatory drug-associated pulmonary infiltrates with eosinophilia. Review of the literature and Food and Drug Administration Adverse Drug Reaction reports. *Arch Intern Med* 1992;152:1521–1524.
242. Yip L, Dart RC, Gabow PA. Concepts and controversies in salicylate toxicity. *Emerg Med Clin North Am* 1994;12:351–364.
243. Glasgow JF, Middleton B. Reye syndrome—insights on causation and prognosis. *Arch Dis Child* 2001;85:351–353.
244. Forsyth BW, Horwitz RI, Acampora D, et al. New epidemiologic evidence confirming that bias does not explain the aspirin/Reye's syndrome association. *JAMA* 1989;261:2517–2524.
245. Hall SM. Reye's syndrome and aspirin: a review. *Br J Clin Pract Suppl* 1990;70:4–11.
246. Belay ED, Bresee JS, Holman RC, et al. Reye's syndrome in the United States from 1981 through 1997. *N Engl J Med* 1999;340: 1377–1382.
247. Roberts LJ 2nd, Morrow JD. Analgesic-antipyretic and anti-inflammatory agents and drugs employed in the treatment of gout. In: Hardman JG, Limbird LE, eds. *Pharmacological basis of therapeutics,* 9th ed. New York: McGraw-Hill, 2001:687–731.
248. Brater DC. Drug-drug and drug-disease interactions with nonsteroidal anti-inflammatory drugs. *Am J Med* 1986;80:62–77.
249. Watkins J, Abbott EC, Hensby CN, et al. Attenuation of hypotensive effect of propranolol and thiazide diuretics by indomethacin. *BMJ* 1980;281:702–705.
250. Uwai Y, Saito H, Inui K. Interaction between methotrexate and nonsteroidal anti-inflammatory drugs in organic anion transporter. *Eur J Pharmacol* 2000;409:31–36.
251. Kremer JM, Hamilton RA. The effects of nonsteroidal antiinflammatory drugs on methotrexate (MTX) pharmacokinetics: impairment of renal clearance of MTX at weekly maintenance doses but not at 7.5 mg. *J Rheumatol* 1995;22:2072–2077.
252. Tracy TS, Krohn K, Jones DR, et al. The effects of a salicylate, ibuprofen, and naproxen on the disposition of methotrexate in patients with rheumatoid arthritis. *Eur J Clin Pharmacol* 1992;42: 121–125.
253. Iqbal MP, Baig JA, Ali AA, et al. The effects of non-steroidal anti-inflammatory drugs on the disposition of methotrexate in patients with rheumatoid arthritis. *Biopharm Drug Dispos* 1998;19:163–167.
254. Verbeeck RK. Pharmacokinetic drug interactions with nonsteroidal anti-inflammatory drugs. *Clin Pharmacokinet* 1990;19:44–66.
255. Ragheb M. The clinical significance of lithium-nonsteroidal anti-inflammatory drug interactions. *J Clin Psychopharmacol* 1990;10: 350–354.
256. Graham DY, Malaty HM. Alendronate and naproxen are synergistic for development of gastric ulcers. *Arch Intern Med* 2001;161: 107–110.
257. Kovarik JM, Mueller EA, Gerbeau C, et al. Cyclosporine and nonsteroidal antiinflammatory drugs: exploring potential drug interactions and their implications for the treatment of rheumatoid arthritis. *J Clin Pharmacol* 1997;37:336–343.
258. Tugwell P, Ludwin D, Gent M, et al. Interaction between cyclosporin A and nonsteroidal antiinflammatory drugs. *J Rheumatol* 1997;24: 1122–1125.
259. Davies NM, McLachlan AJ, Day RO, et al. Clinical pharmacokinetics and pharmacodynamics of celecoxib: a selective cyclo-oxygenase-2 inhibitor. *Clin Pharmacokinet* 2000;38:225–242.
260. Klose TS, Ibeanu GC, Ghanayem BI, et al. Identification of residues 286 and 289 as critical for conferring substrate specificity of human CYP2C9 for diclofenac and ibuprofen. *Arch Biochem Biophys* 1998; 357:240–248.
261. Yamazaki H, Inoue K, Chiba K, et al. Comparative studies on the catalytic roles of cytochrome P450 2C9 and its Cys- and Leu-variants in the oxidation of warfarin, flurbiprofen, and diclofenac by human liver microsomes. *Biochem Pharmacol* 1998;56:243–251.
262. Chesne C, Guyomard C, Guillouzo A, et al. Metabolism of meloxicam in human liver involves cytochromes P4502C9 and 3A4. *Xenobiotica* 1998;28:1–13.
263. Guidelines for monitoring drug therapy in rheumatoid arthritis. American College of Rheumatology Ad Hoc Committee on Clinical Guidelines. *Arthritis Rheum* 1996;39:723–731.
264. Hollingworth P. The use of non-steroidal anti-inflammatory drugs in paediatric rheumatic diseases. *Br J Rheumatol* 1993;32:73–77.
265. Berde CB, Sethna NF. Analgesics for the treatment of pain in children. *N Engl J Med* 2002;347:1094–1103.
266. Olkkola KT, Maunuksela EL. The pharmacokinetics of postoperative intravenous ketorolac tromethamine in children. *Br J Clin Pharmacol* 1991;31:182–184.
267. Cuzzolin L, Dal Cere M, Fanos V. NSAID-induced nephrotoxicity from the fetus to the child. *Drug Saf* 2001;24:9–18.
268. Pickering AE, Bridge HS, Nolan J, et al. Double-blind, placebo-controlled analgesic study of ibuprofen or rofecoxib in combination with paracetamol for tonsillectomy in children. *Br J Anaesth* 2002; 88:72–77.
269. Stempak D, Gammon J, Klein J, et al. Single-dose and steady-state pharmacokinetics of celecoxib in children. *Clin Pharmacol Ther* 2002;72:490–497.
270. Briggs GG, Freeman RK, Yaffe SJ. *Drugs in pregnancy and lactation: a reference guide to fetal and neonatal risk,* 6th ed. Philadelphia: Lippincott Williams & Wilkins, 2002.
271. Werler MM, Mitchell AA, Shapiro S. The relation of aspirin use during the first trimester of pregnancy to congenital cardiac defects. *N Engl J Med* 1989;321:1639–1642.

272. Collins E, Turner G. Letter: Salicylates and pregnancy. *Lancet* 1973; 2:1494.
273. Niebyl JR. Drugs in pregnancy and lactation. In: Gabbe SG, Niebyl JR, Simpson JL, eds. *Obstetrics: normal and problem pregnancies,* 4th ed. New York: Churchill Livingstone, 2002:221–50.
274. Laine L. Gastrointestinal safety of coxibs and outcomes studies: what's the verdict? *J Pain Symptom Manage* 2002;23(suppl):5–10; discussion 11–14.
275. Holm L, Phillipson M, Perry MA. NO-flurbiprofen maintains duodenal blood flow, enhances mucus secretion contributing to lower mucosal injury. *Am J Physiol Gastrointest Liver Physiol* 2002;283: G1090–G1097.
276. Wallace JL, Reuter B, Cicala C, et al. Novel nonsteroidal anti-inflammatory drug derivatives with markedly reduced ulcerogenic properties in the rat. *Gastroenterology* 1994;107:173–179.

CHAPTER 32

Methotrexate and Leflunomide: Use in the Treatment of Rheumatoid Arthritis and Other Rheumatic Disorders

Sergio M.A. Toloza and Graciela S. Alarcón

Patients with rheumatoid arthritis (RA) who are expected to have a poor outcome should be treated aggressively early in the disease course to prevent joint destruction. RA not only produces significant physical impairment and pain, but it also results in decreased life expectancy, comorbidities, and economic losses (1). Although methotrexate (MTX) may not prevent disease progression in patients with established disease, it may do so if patients are treated before joint damage ensues (2). Despite the availability of new drugs (e.g., leflunomide) and biologic therapies [tumor necrosis factor (TNF) and interleukin-1 (IL-1) inhibitors], MTX remains the drug with which all other treatment modalities for RA are compared (3–8). It is likely that MTX will remain an important antirheumatic drug for the next several years.

METHOTREXATE

Historical Overview

Aminopterin, a folic acid analogue and precursor of MTX, was first used for the treatment of RA (and psoriatic arthritis) by Gubner et al. in 1951 (9). Of seven patients receiving this analogue, six improved significantly. This initial report did not stimulate the use of either aminopterin or MTX by rheumatologists because they had just begun using cortisone, a compound thought to "cure" RA. Enthusiasm for cortisone and its derivatives decreased precipitously as serious side effects resulting from their use became evident. Dermatologists, however, instigated the use of MTX and demonstrated its efficacy for the cutaneous and articular manifestations of psoriasis (10). It was not until the 1980s that randomized clinical trials for RA were conducted in the United States and Canada (11–15), and MTX was accepted as a second-line agent for the treatment of this disease (16,17). MTX is still the preferred disease-modifying antirheumatic drug (DMARD) used in the Americas (18–21). Although concerns exist about its long-term toxicity (22), it is fair to say that the long-term "side effects" of RA are likely worse than those related to the administration of MTX (23).

Structure and Pharmacology

MTX is an analogue of folic acid. As shown in Fig. 32.1, both compounds are structurally similar, sharing pteridinyl, *para*-aminobenzoyl, and glutamyl moieties. MTX absorption from the gastrointestinal tract is dose dependent and is not affected by food (24–28); peak serum levels are achieved within 1 to 2 hours. At doses between 5 and 25 mg, MTX is well absorbed, exhibiting a bioavailability of approximately 60%. At much higher doses, it is not so well absorbed and is metabolized by the intestinal flora and excreted. When administered subcutaneously or intramuscularly, MTX is completely absorbed, and peak serum levels are achieved within an hour (24). Approximately 50% of MTX is protein bound and competes with other albumin-bound compounds (28–36). The main catabolic product of MTX, 7-hydroxymethotrexate, is almost entirely protein bound. MTX competes with folates for active transport into cells and undergoes polyglutamylation, primarily in the liver; MTX-polyglutamates can be converted back to MTX by hydrolytic enzymes, but MTX-polyglutamates may remain in the intracellular compartment for extended periods (32,37). 7-OH MTX is also polyglutamylated, but this compound is a much less potent inhibitor of dihydrofolic acid reductase.

Folic Acid

Methotrexate

FIG. 32.1. Chemical structures of folic acid and methotrexate.

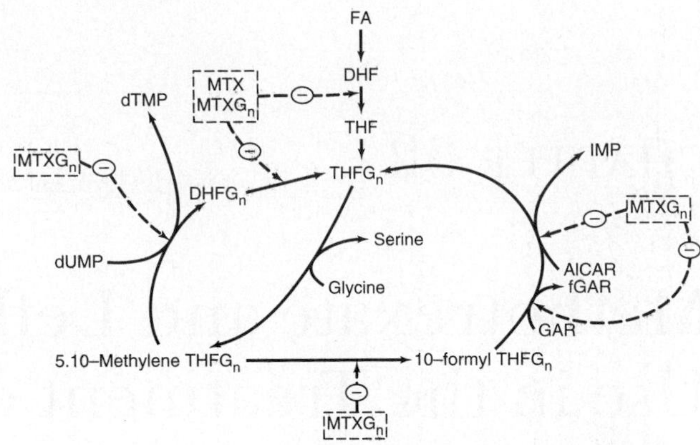

FIG. 32.2. Some folate-dependent metabolic pathways. *FA,* folic acid; *DHF, THF, DHFGn, THFGn,* dehydro- and tetrahydrofolic acid and their respective polyglutamates; *MTX, MTXGn,* methotrexate and methotrexate polyglutamates; *AICAR,* aminomidazole carboxymide riboside; *IMP, dUMP, dTMP,* inosine, desoxyuridine, and deoxythymidine monophosphates, respectively. (Modified from Baggott JE, Morgan SL, Ha T, et al. Antifolates in rheumatoid arthritis: a hypothetical mechanism of action. *Clin Exp Rheumatol* 1993;11(suppl):101–105, with permission.)

MTX is excreted primarily by the kidneys (80%) and, to a much lesser extent, by the biliary tract (10%–30%). Renal clearance of MTX occurs by glomerular filtration and tubular secretion and varies considerably among individuals. MTX toxicity depends, in large part, on the rate of clearance of the compound by the kidney, rather than on the peak dose achieved after its administration (38,39); thus, it should be used cautiously in patients with any degree of renal impairment. On the other hand, MTX should be avoided altogether in patients undergoing peritoneal dialysis as well as hemodialysis (unless high-flux hemodialysis membranes are used), because MTX is poorly dialyzable. Dialysis of any type has no effect in the clearance of MTX-polyglutamates (40).

Drug interactions with MTX occurs through several mechanisms (41,42), including interference with its absorption, distribution, and excretion (31,34,42,43). Additionally, use of MTX in conjunction with other antifolates such as trimethoprim-sulfamethoxazole may result in severe folate deficiency (44). Salicylates, as well as some absorbable antibiotics, are protein bound and may displace MTX, thereby enhancing its toxicity (29). Moreover, salicylates and nonsteroidal antiinflammatory drugs (NSAIDs) may potentiate the toxicity of MTX by altering its renal clearance. Fries et al. (45) have shown that patients receiving salicylates and MTX frequently exhibit increased (although generally within the normal range) serum transaminase levels and, therefore, this particular drug combination should be used with caution. Despite these considerations, patients generally tolerate the concomitant administration of MTX and an NSAID rather well (33,46–48); however, caution is indicated in the use of this combination in elderly patients, and as noted, particularly in patients with borderline renal function (38,39,49,50).

Mechanisms of Action and Biologic Effects

MTX, per se, can inhibit folic acid–dependent pathways by a number of mechanisms (Fig. 32.2). The one most commonly cited is inhibition of dihydrofolic acid reductase, preventing reduction of folic acid to dihydrofolic and tetrahydrofolic acid. The polyglutamyl derivatives of MTX are not only more potent inhibitors of this enzyme than MTX, but they also are inhibitors of several other enzymes in the folic acid pathway, including the so-called "distal enzymes." The antirheumatic properties of MTX appear to relate primarily to its effect on the distal rather than the proximal enzymes of the folic acid pathway. Among the distal enzymes, aminoimidazole-carboxamide-ribotide-transformylase (AICAR-*trans*-formylase) may be the most important (51). The distal enzymes thymidylate synthase and AICAR-transformylase are required for the synthesis of purines and pyrimidines (52,53).

Several lines of evidence suggest that inhibition of the proximal enzymes is not a prerequisite for the antirheumatic effect of MTX. Although the concomitant administration of MTX and folic acid, even at very large doses of the latter (54,55), does not affect the efficacy of MTX, this is not the case when the fully reduced compound folinic acid is concomitantly administered with MTX at moderate to high doses (56,57). Moreover, it has been shown that trimetrexate, a folic acid analogue that selectively inhibits dihydrofolic acid reductase, is not efficacious in animals with experimentally-induced arthritis, further supporting the notion that inhibition of this enzyme is not required for the antirheumatic properties of MTX (51).

Indirect evidence favoring AICAR-transformylase as the most important target of MTX has been provided by several groups of investigators. Cronstein et al. (58,59) have demonstrated that both MTX and AICAR (the substrate of AICAR-transformylate) induce release of adenosine, a potent antiinflammatory compound that inhibits neutrophil adherence to fibroblasts and endothelial cells. Addition of adenosine deaminase to the culture medium resulted in normalization of neutrophil adherence. Moreover, both MTX and adenosine inhibit leukocyte adhesion to postcapillary vessels, synthesis and release of leukotriene B_4, release of reactive oxygen metabolites, and production of tumor necrosis factor-α (TNF-α) (58,60–63), effects mediated by adenosine receptors on neutrophils (64,65). Adenosine also inhibits lymphocyte proliferation in response to mitogens; at the monocyte/macrophage level it inhibits production of TNF-α, IL-6, and IL-8, whereas it stimulates the production of a potent antiinflammatory cytokine, IL-10. Finally, adenosine also inhibits the release of some matrix metalloproteinases. These described effects are generally reversed by the administration of adenosine deaminase. Therefore, it is postulated that administration of MTX results in accumulation of AICAR and subsequent release of adenosine that interferes with the function of cellular elements critical to the inflammatory process in diseases such as RA. Unfortunately, there are no known folate analogues that selectively inhibit AICAR-transformylase without affecting other enzymes of the folate pathway; thus, it remains to be proven that this is the central inhibitory step accounting for the efficacy of MTX.

The biologic effects of MTX vary according to the dose. At high doses, it is a chemotherapeutic agent used for the treatment of choriocarcinoma and acute lymphocytic leukemia. In combination with other antineoplastic agents, it is used for the treatment of lymphomas and some solid tumors. At lower doses, it is an antirheumatic compound with antiinflammatory and immunosuppressive properties.

The effects of MTX on cytokines and other mediators of inflammation have been extensively studied (66–69). Segal (68) demonstrated decreased IL-1 activity, although IL-1 production was unaffected. Barrera et al. (70) showed decreased production of IL-1β by peripheral blood mononuclear cells from patients with active RA after the administration of a single dose of MTX; this effect was not observed in patients already receiving MTX. Although no relationship between serum levels of soluble IL-2 receptors and response to MTX in refractory RA (67) has been shown, decreased levels of IL-6 and soluble IL-2 receptors have been demonstrated in some patients after 12 weeks of therapy. Finally, Constantin et al. (71) have shown an increased expression of helper T cell subset 2 (T_H2) cytokine genes with corresponding decreases in expression of T_H1 cytokine genes in *ex vivo* peripheral blood mononuclear cells obtained from patients with RA being treated with MTX. Because proinflammatory cytokines are crucial for the expression of other molecules participating in the pathogenesis of RA (such as angiogenic factors, adhesion molecules, etc.), the reported *in vitro* effects of MTX are likely to be of importance in patients. MTX, after single or repeated doses, significantly decreases the production of leukotriene B_4 (72,73) and suppresses phospholipase A_2 activity (74,75). Thus, MTX decreases several mediators of inflammation, which likely explains the rapid clinical response observed in patients treated with this agent.

The immunosuppressive effects of MTX are less well established, and the literature must be examined carefully. In a number of reports, an effect of MTX on the immune system could not be demonstrated (14,15,76,77). Early *in vitro* experiments used culture media rich in folate (78) or tritiated thymidine to monitor DNA synthesis by treated cells (79). By using folate-depleted culture media and tritiated deoxyuridine to measure DNA synthesis, Hine et al. (80) demonstrated inhibition of lymphocyte proliferation by MTX. Inhibition was not observed when culture media with high folate content were used in the assays. Similar observations were reported by Olsen et al. (81,82). MTX has been shown to decrease levels of double-negative ($CD4^-$ and $CD8^-$) and γ/δ T cells in children with juvenile RA (83). More recently Genestier et al. (84) have demonstrated that MTX promotes apoptosis and clonal deletion of activated T cells in mixed lymphocyte reactions; these effects were not dependent on CD95 or its ligand. It was suggested that enhanced apoptosis of activated T cells might account for the immunosuppression observed in patients treated with low doses of MTX.

MTX affects the production of some autoantibodies, particularly rheumatoid factor (RF). Decreased serum levels of immunoglobulin (Ig) M (IgM) and IgA RF have been reported in patients with RA, regardless of clinical response, and peripheral blood mononuclear cells from MTX-treated patients with RA have been shown to produce less IgM RF than do cells from patients not treated with MTX (82).

The occurrence of opportunistic infections in patients treated with MTX also indicates an immunosuppressive effect of MTX. It can be argued that these are infrequent events and that affected patients are already immunocompromised by the underlying disease and by the use of corticosteroids. Nevertheless, infections have been reported in MTX-treated patients with RA, with some occurring in otherwise young and healthy individuals who have not received corticosteroids (85–112). In a group of nearly 80 MTX-treated patients with RA and a control group of approximately 150, a greater frequency of infections and antibiotic use was demonstrated in the MTX-treated patients (113). The majority of these infections were not life threatening, and it is possible that the increased use of antibiotics was influenced by knowledge that these patients were receiving MTX. In still another series (200 patients with RA from Mexico), MTX was found to be a risk factor for the occurrence of infections (114). Similar data have emerged from other reports (115).

Methotrexate in Rheumatoid Arthritis

Efficacy

As previously noted, MTX is currently an accepted therapeutic agent for RA. Four different, randomized, placebo-controlled clinical trials were conducted in the 1980s (11,

13–15). Subsequently, a metanalysis was published and served as the basis for a position paper by the American College of Physicians on the use of MTX and approval by the U.S. Food and Drug Administration (FDA) for its use in the treatment of RA (16,17,116).

The efficacy of MTX in improving several outcome measures in patients with RA has now been corroborated in many studies conducted around the world (3,19,21,117–131). As noted before, the efficacy of MTX may decrease substantially in patients consuming caffeine in large quantities (28). As with other DMARDs, the response to MTX occurs within weeks of initiation of the drug; likewise, discontinuation is usually followed by a flare-up of symptoms within a few weeks (132). It was initially thought that a favorable response to MTX was associated with the presence of human leukocyte antigen-DR2 (HLA-DR2) (15); such an assertion could not be validated in either our local Alabama patients (133) or in those participating in a multicenter study in the United States (134). More recently it has been postulated that genetic polymorphisms in the enzyme 5,10-methylenetetrahydrofolate reductase (MTHFR) may be associated with response to MTX (135).

The long-term efficacy of MTX in RA has been established by several investigators who followed up on treated patients over extended periods (22,119,121–123,126,128, 136). It also has been demonstrated indirectly by examining this drug's "survival curve" during several years of observation (128,136,137). At 5 years, MTX-treated patients with RA exhibited approximately a 50% probability of still taking MTX, as compared with 15% to 20% for other DMARDs such as gold salts and D-penicillamine (136). These data were generated before the use of folic acid supplementation, and it is entirely possible that continued MTX use could be even higher at the present time than previously reported; however, there are many more therapeutic options for patients with RA now than before, so it is possible that patients with incomplete responses are switched to other agents, and thus, "MTX survival" is no higher than previously reported. Discontinuation of MTX is primarily due to the occurrence and severity of adverse events rather than to lack of efficacy. Patients requiring higher doses are more likely to develop untoward side effects and discontinue the medication unless significant improvement occurs (138).

The efficacy of MTX in relation to other DMARDs is a matter of controversy and tends to reflect personal experience. MTX has been shown to be comparable with oral and parenteral gold salts (139,140) and azathioprine (141), but superior to hydroxychloroquine (142,143). It also has been shown to be comparable with leflunomide (144,145), but less potent than anti-TNF compounds, some of the newest antirheumatic products (146–150). When compared with other DMARDs in terms of its efficacy and toxicity, MTX has been found to be less toxic than parenteral gold salts and D-penicillamine, as toxic as sulfasalazine and oral gold salts, and more toxic than hydroxychloroquine. In short, among these drugs, MTX exhibits the best efficacy/toxicity ratio. It is uncertain whether MTX will remain the DMARD of choice in the United States over the next several years.

Prevention of disease progression of RA by MTX has not been definitely determined radiographically (3,140,151–157). Healing of erosions has been documented (158), but for the most part, disease progression continues, although at a lower rate than in patients treated with oral and parenteral gold salts, azathioprine, or NSAIDs according to some studies (3,159–161), and at the same rate according to others (162,163).

Further data supporting the view that MTX suppresses disease progression in RA comes from the leflunomide-MTX study, which demonstrated that patients treated with either of these two agents did not progress radiographically at the expected rate (estimated from the baseline erosion scores and disease duration) (164). On the other hand, all anti-TNF products compared with MTX have demonstrated some effect of MTX on disease progression, but not as substantial as that observed with either etanercept or infliximab (146,165). Finally, the data from Rich et al. (2) from our institution indicate that patients with RA who exhibited no evidence of joint destruction at the time of initiation of MTX were less likely to develop erosions than were those patients who began MTX with baseline evidence of joint destruction. This study, however, involved only a relatively small number of patients and awaits independent corroboration.

In summary, two arguments favor MTX over other DMARDs in terms of efficacy: (a) the survival curve of the drug, and (b) the (probably) slower rate of disease progression compared with other DMARDs (except anti-TNF products), as determined radiographically. Moreover, response to MTX occurs within weeks rather than months of drug initiation, an added reason to use it early in the course of the disease. It is not yet possible to determine definitively whether leflunomide (or anti-TNF therapy) exhibits a better efficacy/toxicity ratio than MTX. Thus, based on the available data, we favor the use of MTX as the first DMARD in patients with RA.

Toxicity

Adverse events encountered with MTX therapy are numerous and vary in severity from minor to fatal (21,22, 119,124,128,130,136,166–169). Predisposing factors to the occurrence of toxicity include (a) folate deficiency, (b) advanced age, (c) cumulative dose, (d) renal insufficiency, and (e) concomitant use of other antifolates (or other drugs such as NSAIDs). A C677T mutation in the MTHFR gene has been suggested to be a predisposing factor for liver toxicity as well as other MTX-associated untoward side effects (135, 170). From the therapeutic standpoint, the adverse events fall into four categories:

1. Events, such as stomatitis that can be alleviated by the administration of the fully oxidized form of folate
2. Events, such as moderate-to-severe bone marrow suppression that are reversed by the administration of the fully reduced form of folate (folinic acid)
3. True "idiosyncratic" or allergic reactions that may respond to the discontinuation of MTX (e.g., MTX-induced lung injury)
4. Events such as clinically-significant liver disease, as defined by the American College of Rheumatology (ACR) [advanced fibrosis, cirrhosis, or clinical evidence of hepatic failure, such as ascites or esophageal varices (171)] resulting from the intracellular accumulation of MTX-polyglutamates (172,173), and that do not predictably reverse with the administration of either the reduced or the oxidized form of folate or discontinuation of MTX

Table 32.1 summarizes the side effects reported with low doses of MTX in the treatment of RA.

TABLE 32.1. *Reported adverse events with low dose pulse methotrexate therapy*

Gastrointestinal tract	Oral ulcers
	Dyspepsia
	Abdominal pain
	Diarrhea
	Gastrointestinal bleeding
Hematopoietic system	Macrocytosis
	Cytopenias
Liver	Elevation of transaminases
	Fibrosis
	Cirrhosis
Lungs	Interstitial pneumonitis
	Diffuse interstitial fibrosis
Cardiovascular system	Atherogenesis (?)
Central nervous system	Headaches
	Dizziness
	Neurocognitive impairment
	Seizures
	Encephalopathy (?)
	Diabetes insipidus
	Dementia
	Optic neuropathy
Musculoskeletal system	Flare up of joint symptoms
	Osteopathy (?)
Skin and dane	Rash
	Alopecia
	Actinic keratosis
	Skin cancers (?)
	Dermatophytosis
Genitourinary tract	Erectile impotence
	Gynecomastia
	Peyrone disease
Reproductive system	Abortifacient/fetal death
	Chromosomal abnormalities
	Teratogenesis (aminopterine syndrome)
Infections and wound healing	Opportunistic and nonopportunistic infections
Neoplasia	Leukemia
	Lymphomas
	Lung cancer
Other	Nodulosis (cutaneous and visceral)
	Vasculitis

Adverse Events by Organ System

Gastrointestinal Tract

Gastrointestinal manifestations have been reported to occur in as many as 60% of MTX-treated patients with RA. Isolated or multiple painful ulcerations of the oral mucosa (or the gastrointestinal mucosa) occur and are exacerbated in temporal relation to the administration of the compound; they can be severe enough to preclude adequate nutritional intake. If concomitant thrombocytopenia occurs, there may be oozing of blood from these mucosal lesions. Dyspepsia, abdominal pain, and diarrhea also have been described (13–15,22,130,136,174). MTX may contribute to the occurrence of gastrointestinal bleeding in patients with underlying NSAID gastropathy and peptic ulcer disease (174). Most gastrointestinal manifestations can be mitigated by the concomitant administration of folic acid, a reduction in the weekly dose of MTX, or a change in route of administration (from oral to parenteral).

Hematopoietic System

The sustained administration of MTX results in folate deficiency and the occurrence of cytopenias of variable severity (37,44,99,103,104,110,174–199) and frequency (5%–25%). Overt hematologic toxicity is usually preceded by red blood cell (RBC) macrocytosis (200); however, some patients may have a dimorphic anemia owing to microscopic gastrointestinal blood loss, with the mean corpuscular volume (MCV) remaining within normal limits. In individuals with low intracellular folate stores, or in those concomitantly receiving another antifolate (44,201,202), clinically evident folate deficiency occurs more rapidly than in those not previously deficient. Severe preexisting folate depletion and the presence of other risk factors for MTX toxicity, particularly renal failure, are the most likely explanations for the reported occurrence of severe pancytopenia ensuing almost immediately after the initiation of MTX (181,183,189,196,197). A true allergic drug reaction to trimethoprim-sulfamethoxazole in patients developing *Pneumocystis carinii* pneumonia during the course of MTX treatment has been described (99,112). In these instances, however, MTX had been discontinued before the initiation of the second antifolate.

Severe cytopenias have been observed after a very small dose of MTX in patients with mild to moderate renal impairment or in those with end-stage renal disease undergoing dialysis (196–199). Another contributing factor to the occurrence of severe pancytopenia during the course of MTX therapy is the concomitant occurrence of a viral infection, particularly parvovirus B19, as illustrated by the case reported by Naides (203). Finally, dosing errors (daily rather than weekly) and accidental intake of MTX (by children) also have been reported as the cause of hematologic toxicity (177,195,204–206).

Liver

The occurrence of liver damage after prolonged administration of MTX for RA was a matter of serious concern to rheumatologists in the 1980s, based on previous experience with the drug in the treatment of psoriasis (172,207–220). Since then, it has become clear that clinically significant liver disease is less frequent than anticipated (168,207,211–213,215,221–224). Reasons for this apparent discrepancy include the method of administration (weekly in RA versus three times a week in patients with psoriasis) and, perhaps more important, the emphasis placed on alcohol abstinence when used in patients with RA. Drugs that may modulate the hepatotoxicity of MTX include NSAIDs and chloroquine (45,225). Whereas some NSAIDs may place a patient at greater risk for hepatotoxicity (45), chloroquine may actually exert some protection by decreasing the bioavailability of the drug (225). In fact, in the large database examined by Fries et al. (45), the combination of MTX and hydroxychloroquine resulted in the lowest levels of serum transaminases (with the highest levels observed in those patients taking combined aspirin and MTX, as already mentioned).

The incidence of clinically-significant liver disease in patients with RA treated with MTX is uncertain. Debate remains as to how to interpret histopathologically data obtained after MTX has been used, given the fact that patients with RA who have never been exposed to MTX may also have mild histopathologic abnormalities (226). The best estimate, derived from a survey of practicing members of the ACR, is of 1 case per 1,000 patients treated for 5 years (171). This figure is derived from practices serving predominantly Caucasian patients and uses only an approximate denominator. Higher incidences have been reported from tertiary care centers, but the effect of selection bias cannot be ignored. With nearly 2,000 patients treated at our institution over the past 20 years, we have yet to see a patient develop cirrhosis, and the same is true at other tertiary care facilities. Such cases have been reported in the literature or discussed among rheumatologists; some are, unfortunately, under consideration in courts of law (214,215,227).

Of note, whereas liver failure has resolved in a few patients after MTX discontinuation (228), some patients with MTX-induced liver injury have required transplantation (229). MTX liver concentrations measured serially over 3.5 years in a relatively small group of RA patients have not been found to be associated with either evidence of liver damage, drug efficacy, or toxicity (230). These data suggest that serum concentrations of MTX may not be useful predictors of liver damage in patients receiving this compound. It should be stressed that liver disease in MTX-treated RA patients does not uniformly imply that MTX is the culprit. Indeed, Bills et al. (231) reported a patient with RA and Felty syndrome who was treated with MTX and developed nodular regenerative hyperplasia of the liver, a condition described in association with Felty syndrome or RA alone. A patient with RA, heterozygous for α_1-antitrypsin deficiency (a known cause of cryptogenic cirrhosis), who developed end-stage liver disease after 8 years of MTX therapy has been reported (232). Thus, α_1-antitrypsin deficiency may well be another risk factor for liver disease in MTX-treated patients with RA. Finally, an elderly RA patient who was hepatitis B surface antigen positive, had antibodies to hepatitis B antigen, and was receiving MTX developed hepatic dysfunction. Upon MTX discontinuation, she developed fulminant and fatal hepatitis that proved to be due to a precore mutant virus. The researchers postulated that the discontinuation of MTX may have led to reactivation of the immune system and attack of the infected cells (233).

The survey of the ACR membership identified age, cumulative dose, and length of MTX treatment as risk factors predisposing to liver damage. When these risk factors were applied to an independent group of MTX-treated RA patients, they failed to identify a diabetic patient with significant liver disease (234). These investigators have thus suggested that diabetes be added to the list of risk factors for hepatotoxicity. From this study, as well as from careful analyses of laboratory data available from the manufacturers of MTX, it is evident that elevations of liver transaminases of any magnitude coupled with decreased serum albumin values (despite significant amelioration of RA disease activity) should not be dismissed, since they have been shown to be associated with the occurrence of clinically significant liver disease (171,219). The possibility that the concomitant administration of folic acid may in fact exert a hepatoprotective effect is suggested by the leflunomide versus MTX clinical trials data from the United States and Europe (144,145). The serum levels of liver transaminases in patients in the MTX arm were higher among the European patients who, by and large, did not receive folic acid supplementation, compared with patients in the United States, who almost all received this supplement (145,235).

Lung

Lung injury secondary to MTX continues to puzzle rheumatologists because it may occur at any time during treatment, even weeks after its discontinuation (37,169, 236–261). Risk factors predisposing to its occurrence have only recently been identified (262); they include increasing age, pleuropulmonary involvement due to RA, diabetes, and hypoalbuminemia (262). Although the majority of reported cases have occurred in patients with RA, lung injury also has been described in MTX-treated patients with asthma and primary biliary cirrhosis (247,248). Recently, a case of acute MTX lung injury was reported in a child with juvenile RA (263). Patients have either acute or subacute onset of cough, shortness of breath, and low-grade fever (264). On physical examination, they may appear ill with tachypnea and bibasilar rales; chest radiographs usually demonstrate bilateral interstitial parenchymal infiltrates, although pulmonary nodulosis also has been reported (265). Leukocytosis is quite common; blood and sputum cultures are negative, and commonly, there is some degree of hypoxemia (264). Serum concentrations of KL-6 (muciu-like high-molecular-weight glycoprotein) and surfactant protein D (both markers of pulmonary toxicity) have been reported elevated in two patients who developed MTX lung injury; a decrease in these markers paralleled these patients' clinical improvement (266). A transbronchial lung biopsy and bronchoalveolar lavage are generally required to rule out an opportunistic infectious process; it may be difficult to differentiate a patient with a disseminated infectious process from one with MTX lung injury (92,100,267), even after invasive studies are done (267). The presence of a lymphocytic alveolar infiltrate and peripheral eosinophilia should strongly favor the diagnosis of MTX lung injury (254); however, high-resolution computed tomography may reveal abnormalities in patients with normal chest radiographs but will not allow the distinction between an infectious process and MTX lung injury (268).

In mild cases of lung injury, symptoms may subside on discontinuation of MTX, but in more severe cases, parenteral corticosteroids and respiratory support may be needed. Some patients do die, often with a superimposed bacterial infection. In contrast to liver toxicity, no systematic efforts have been made to document the frequency of this complication. The available figures come from tertiary care centers and vary by ten-fold (0.7% to 7%). From the experience gathered at our institution, it appears (based on the number of cases observed and an estimated denominator) that the actual frequency of MTX-induced pulmonary injury is closer to 0.7% than to 7%. The multicenter, case-control study in which our institution participated (262) used the modified criteria of Searles and McKendry (254) to determine whether a purported case could be considered definite, probable, or neither (Table 32.2). Although in a few cases of MTX-induced pulmonary toxicity MTX has been successfully reintroduced (269), recurrences have been described in the multicenter study resulting in a fatal outcome in half the cases (264). Based on these data, we do not advocate the reintroduction of MTX once pulmonary toxicity has occurred (264).

TABLE 32.2. *Adverse pulmonary events to methotrexate: revised diagnostic criteria*

Major criteria
1. Hypersensitivity pneumonitis by histopathology (and without evidence of pathogenic organisms)
2. Radiologic evidence of pulmonary interstitial or alveolar infiltrates
3. Negative blood (if febrile) and initial sputum (if produced) cultures for pathogenic organisms
Minor criteria
1. Shortness of breath of less than 8 weeks
2. Nonproductive cough
3. O_2 saturation <90% at the time of initial evaluation on room air
4. DL_{CO} <70% of that predicted for age
5. White blood cell count <15,000 per mm^3

DL_{CO}, carbon monoxide diffusion capacity of the lungs.

From Alarcón GS, Kremer JM, et al. Risk factors for methotrexate-induced lung injury in patients with rheumatoid arthritis. A multicenter, case-control study. Methotrexate-Lung Study Group. *Ann Intern Med* 1997;127:356–364, with permission.

Cardiovascular System

Prolonged administration of MTX results in elevated blood levels of homocysteine, an amino acid known to induce atherosclerosis in experimental animals (270) and to be an independent risk factor for its occurrence in humans (271). Thus, there has been some concern regarding a possible increased frequency of coronary artery disease, a concern that has not been documented in the literature. In a cohort of patients (n = 152) followed up at our institution for a total of approximately 850 patient-years, excess deaths were not caused by heart disease or cerebrovascular accidents, but rather by infections (137). Recent data from the Wichita Arthritis Center in the United States (n = 1,240) do not support the occurrence of an excess number of deaths in MTX-treated RA patients, after adjusting for disease severity. To the contrary, patients on MTX had a mortality hazard ratio of 0.4 as compared with non-MTX users [(0.3 for cardiovascular (CV) mortality) (272)]. Accelerated CV disease thus remains a theoretic concern (273) that may be more likely to be validated in Europe than in the United States, because folic acid supplementation is not as commonly used there as it is in the United States (51,236,274).

Kidneys

MTX is not nephrotoxic, but renal impairment significantly increases the probability of MTX toxicity, particularly of the hematopoietic and gastrointestinal systems (275). Although MTX does not appear to produce renal insufficiency, a case report of a patient who apparently developed nephrotic syndrome secondary to MTX suggests that this compound is capable of rarely inducing renal injury (276). Corroboration is needed before nephrotic syndrome can be accepted as a complication, as opposed to a coincidental chance occurrence.

Central Nervous System

Manifestations of central nervous system toxicity vary in their severity and frequency, but for the most part are benign and fully reversible on drug discontinuation. However, dizziness, headaches, seizures, optic neuropathy, diabetes insipidus, and neurocognitive impairment have been reported (277–280). Leukoencephalopathy, temporally associated with the administration of MTX, has been reported in children receiving MTX intraventricularly for leukemia (281) and in adults receiving it intravenously for the treatment of soft tissue sarcomas without central nervous system metastasis (282), but not in patients with RA who receive much lower doses of MTX. A case of dementia also occurring in temporal association with the use of MTX has been reported (283), but it cannot be concluded that MTX caused it. Aminophylline has been shown to counteract the neurotoxicity of MTX (184).

Musculoskeletal System

As with gold salts and other DMARDs, a few MTX-treated patients with RA experience a postdose flare-up of their joint manifestations (284). In a few instances, these flare-ups are so severe and long lasting that patients are truly incapacitated for several days after the dose. These musculoskeletal symptoms are not influenced by the administration of either folic or folinic acid and may represent a true allergic reaction.

MTX in large doses can alter bone metabolism and is known to contribute to the occurrence of osteoporosis in patients receiving high doses as a chemotherapeutic agent (285,286). *In vitro* studies have shown, albeit inconsistently, that MTX interferes with osteoblast proliferation and differentiation (287,288). It is conceivable that with extended periods of treatment, MTX may lead to decreased bone formation and osteopenia, but this effect in the doses used for RA has not been demonstrated (289–292). The same is the case for children receiving MTX for the treatment of juvenile arthritis (293). A decrease in bone mineral density was observed among patients receiving MTX and corticosteroids, but not in those receiving MTX alone (294). Finally, there is a single case report of MTX osteopathy (microfractures) detected by technetium bone scan (295).

Skin

Rashes, usually mild and reversible, may occur early in treatment and likely represent allergic reactions to the drug. Cutaneous ulcerations over the knuckles and indurated, erythematosus papules consistent with a predominant hystiocytic inflammatory infiltrate in the dermis and distributed in the proximal aspect of the extremities have also been described in MTX-treated RA patients (296, 297). MTX may lead to worsening of actinic keratosis in patients being treated with topical 5-fluorouracil (298) as well as increased occurrence of dermatophytosis (299). Alopecia is rarely severe, but may be a disturbing side effect, particularly in women.

Genitourinary Tract

Erectile dysfunction has been described in patients treated with MTX (300). It usually subsides or improves after drug discontinuation or dose reduction. On questioning, some of these patients have been found to be using other agents (e.g., alcohol), with impotence occurring as a result of drug-drug synergism. Peyronie disease and gynecomastia also have been reported (301,302).

Reproductive System

Conception and pregnancy should be avoided during MTX therapy (303) because the drug may cause fetal death (abortifacient), chromosomal abnormalities, and birth defects (304–306). A washout period of at least 3 months is recommended. Unfortunately, many patients with RA may experience a flare-up within weeks of MTX discontinuation with conception not occurring. It should be stressed that men taking MTX also should discontinue the drug before impregnation, and possible conception, because MTX is accumulated intracellularly in both male and female reproductive cells.

A few pregnancies during treatment with MTX have been reported. Of 10 pregnancies, five terminated either by miscarriage or therapeutic abortion, and five proceeded to completion with no apparent ill effects in the newborns (304). A much different outcome, with the occurrence of multiple congenital abnormalities reminiscent of the fetal aminopterine syndrome, has been reported (307–309). Given that folate deficiency has been recognized as playing a major role in the occurrence of neural tube defects, and folate-enriched flour is now used in many countries to prevent their occurrence (310,311), it is not surprising that MTX use has been associated with birth defects. In short, MTX should be considered teratogenic, and sexually active women of childbearing age and men of any age should be counseled so that a reliable method of contraception is used.

Infections and Wound Healing

In addition to infections with uncommon organisms, an increase in the rate of infections has been observed during the perioperative period after major orthopedic procedures in patients who continue receiving the compound throughout the surgery (312). Perhala et al. (313), however, compared patients taking MTX with those not taking MTX and found no increase in the frequency of infections in the MTX group. In a study by Sany et al. (314), patients on MTX who discontinued the drug perioperatively were compared with those who continued it. Because no infections occurred in either group, the conclusion that there were no differences in the rate of infections in the two groups may not be valid.

A more definitive double-blind, case-control study involving patients randomized to MTX or placebo perioperatively was attempted in the United States but could not be completed (315). Data from two studies conducted in the United Kingdom clearly indicate that the rate of infection for elective orthopedic procedures (hand and wrist in one study and different procedures in the second) is comparable whether or not MTX is continued through the perioperative period (316,317). These two studies may change previous practice patterns that were based on empirically derived and incomplete data (312,315,318,319).

Neoplasia

MTX is a cocarcinogenic substance and may contribute to the risk for neoplasia. When MTX was first used for the treatment of psoriasis, there was concern regarding the possible increased risk for malignancies (320,321). Solid tumors, particularly lung cancer, were of particular concern (37,322). A higher than expected number of lung cancers (four cases) was observed in a cohort of 150 MTX-treated patients with RA followed up in Saskatoon, Canada (130), but all four patients were smokers at risk for the occurrence of lung cancer. In the cohort of patients followed up by our group since the early 1980s (about 850 patient-years of MTX exposure), the observed and expected number of malignancies were similar (137). Recently, melanomas have been reported in two RA patients who were treated with MTX, but a causal relationship could not be established (323).

The occurrence of lymphomas during MTX therapy has received increased attention over the past 12 years. A few years ago, these reports triggered a massive mailing from the drug's manufacturer to U.S. rheumatologists, advising them to discuss this possibility with patients.

The benefits of MTX treatment in RA generally exceed the risk for such occurrences (324). As with other malignancies (325), lymphoproliferative disorders have been reported to occur with increased frequency in patients with RA, and their occurrence in patients receiving MTX is, therefore, difficult to interpret (326–331). The possible role of MTX in the development of these malignancies is difficult to ignore, however, when some of the tumors regress after MTX discontinuation and without other therapeutic intervention (328). Cases of tumor regression have mostly involved Epstein-Barr virus (EBV)-related malignancies, some in unusual locations (93,328,332–342). A review article by Georgescu et al. (342) includes cases reported until 1996 and data from the cancer registries of several institutions. Additional cases have been published since then (343–347). We have observed three cases of lymphoma in about 2,000 MTX-treated RA patients; two of these lymphomas were EBV related; the other was a T cell–rich B-cell lymphoma. Three cases of lymphoma have been described in children receiving MTX for the treatment of juvenile RA (JRA) (348,349). Table 32.3 includes all published cases in adults and children, as well as the three unpublished cases from our institution.

Two additional studies deserve some comment, since in both studies an attempt was made at determining whether lymphomas in MTX-treated patients occur with frequency greater than expected. In the study by Dawson et al, 32 patients with lymphoma (23 in RA patients and 9 in Sjögren syndrome patients) were identified from the Arthritis Foundation membership of Washington State in the United States (350). The researchers concluded that lymphomas occurred more commonly than expected, but could not attribute this finding conclusively to the increase in MTX usage (350). In the French study by Mariette et al., 25 cases of lymphoma were identified over a 3-year period in MTX-treated RA patients. When compared with expected population figures, only Hodgkin lymphoma was felt to have occurred at a frequency greater than expected (351). The cases from these two studies have not been included in Table 32.3 because no sufficient detail about the cases is provided.

Miscellaneous

Nodulosis, generally peripheral, has been described during MTX treatment, but it has not been conclusively demonstrated to occur more frequently than in patients not treated with MTX. Indeed, nodules may regress in some patients treated with MTX (352–359). Nodules occur in crops, are rather small, and are distributed over the volar as well as the dorsal surface of the hands and feet. Because of their location, such nodules not only have a negative cosmetic effect but also impair hand function and the use of standard footwear. Some patients may elect to have these nodules removed; they tend to recur, however. Other patients may opt for discontinuing MTX, whereas others may prefer to leave the nodules alone and continue MTX, especially if they are experiencing significant clinical improvement. Colchicine has been successfully tried in some patients to reduce nodule size and prevent the occurrence of more nodules (360). Nodules have also been described along the tendon sheaths, such as the Achilles or the tibialis posterior (361); rupture of these tendons has been described (362).

Visceral nodulosis has been described in the lungs (265), the leptomeninges and brain (363), the heart (364–367), and the larynx (368). Although most cases of nodulosis have been reported in patients with RA, they may occur in patients with psoriatic arthritis and other rheumatic disorders (369,370).

Finally, leukocytoclastic vasculitis of variable severity, but generally not systemic, has been described in patients with RA treated with MTX (352,353,371–373) . Systemic vasculitis was reported in a patient with RA on discontinuation of MTX, suggesting instead that MTX may have been suppressing its clinical presentation (374). The occurrence of vasculitis as a consequence of MTX treatment is paradoxic because this drug currently is being used for the treatment of some chronic dermatoses that have a vasculitic

TABLE 32.3. *Lymphomas in patients receiving low-dose methotrexate for rheumatoid arthritis*

Author, year (reference)	Age (yr)	Gender	Disease duration (yr)	Rheumatoid factor	Sicca/other features	Months exposed to methotrexate/ weekly dose[a]	Tumor location	Cell type	EBV	Treatment	Outcome
Shiroky et al., 1991 (93)	83	F	23	Positive	No/No	84/10–15 mg p.o.	Diffuse lymphadenopathy	T cell	?	Spontaneous regression	Alive
Ellman et al., 1991 (338)	51	F	8	Positive	No/No	33/5–10 mg p.o.	Submandibular and intrathoracic lymphadenopathy	B cell	No	Chemotherapy	Alive
Kingsmore et al., 1992 (339)	44	M	7	?	No/No	29/? mg p.o.	Intraabdominal mass	B cell	?	Chemotherapy	Alive
	48	M	11	?	No/No	24/2.5–10 mg p.o.	Disseminated	B cell	?	Chemotherapy	Dead
Taillan et al., 1993 (340)	70	M	30	Positive	No/No	10/7.5–12.5 mg p.o.	Supraclavicular	B cell	?	Chemotherapy	Alive
Morris and Morris, 1993 (335)	72	M	20	Positive	?/No	11/7.5–15 mg p.o. and i.m.	Axilla	B cell	?	Chemotherapy	Alive
Kamel et al., 1993 (557)	86	F	18	Positive	No/No	36/7.5–10 mg p.o. and i.v.	Left thenar eminence	B cell	Yes	Spontaneous regression	Alive
Zimmer-Galler and Lie, 1994 (558)	64	F	?	Positive	No/Pulmonary interstitial fibrosis	16/7.5–10 mg p.o.	Choroidal → disseminated	B cell	?	None	Dead
Cobeta-Garcia et al., 1993 (559)	55	F	9	Positive	No/No	38/10 mg p.o.	Hepatosplemegaly, retroperitoneal adenopathy	T cell	?	Chemotherapy	Alive
Le Goff et al., 1994 (333)	47	F	23	Positive	Yes/No	33/7.5 mg p.o.	Left elbow and thigh	B cell	?	Chemotherapy	Alive
Lioté et al., 1995 (332)	57	F	24	Positive	No/No	60/10–15 mg p.o.	Diffuse lymphadenopathy	B cell	Yes	Spontaneous regression	Alive
Ferraccioli et al., 1995 (560)[b]	61	M	3	?	No/No	7/10 mg p.o.	Axilla	Reed-Sternberg	Yes	Chemotherapy and radiotherapy	Alive
Bachman, 1995 (561)	65	M	25	Positive	No/No	96/15 mg p.o.	Left inguinal	B cell	Yes	Spontaneous regression	Alive
	66	F	21	Positive	No/No	84/7.5–15 mg p.o.	Left ankle and hand, several feet joints	B cell	Yes	Spontaneous regression	Alive
Davies et al., 1995 (562)	?	?	21	?	No/?	?/?	?	NHL large cell B cell	No	Spontaneous regression	Alive
	?	?	20	?	No/?	?/?	?	B cell	No	Regression after chemotherapy	Alive
Stewart et al., 2001 (345)	55	M	16	?	History of CLL 9 years earlier	52/12.5 mg p.o.	Shoulder and axilla	B cell	No	Chemotherapy and rituximab	Alive
Baird et al., 2002 (344)	69	F	29	?	?/?	36/15 mg p.o.	Cervical adenopathy	B cell	No	Spontaneous regression	Alive
Lim and Bertouch, 2002, (343)	63	M	10	Positive	?/Splenomegaly	?/20 mg p.o. (plus cyclosporine)	Right gluteus muscle	B cell	No	Spontaneous regression	Alive
Jardine and Colls, 2002 (346)	80	F	> 4	?	?	78/7.5 mg p.o.	Hepatosplenomegaly, retroperitoneal lymphadenopathy	Hodgkin disease	?	None	Dead
Hirose et al., 2002 (347)	53	M	17	Positive	?/?	4/6 mg p.o	Chest wall	B cell	Yes	Chemotherapy	Dead
Alarcón and Heck, 1999	76	F	20	Positive	Yes/No	240/7.5–15 mg p.o.	Breast, lungs, mediastinum and CNS	B cell	No	None	Dead
	38	M	13	Positive	No/No	36	Meckel cave, CSF	B cell	No	Chemotherapy	Alive
Alarcón, 1999	56	F	20	Positive	No/No	120/15 mg p.o.	Intra/extrathecally (thoracic spine), bone marrow	T cell–rich B cell	No	Decompressive surgery	Dead

[a]An additional case of EBV-related lymphoma regressing after methotrexate discontinuation occurred in a patient with dermatomyositis and previous history of breast cancer.
[b]This patient had received azathioprine prior to methotrexate therapy. Cyclosporine was added to the regimen 2 months before tumor was discovered.
CLL, chronic lymphocytic leukemia; CNS, central nervous system; CSF, cerebrospinal fluid; EBV, Epstein-Barr virus; i.m., intramuscularly; i.v., intravenously; p.o., by mouth.

component, including ulceration in patients with rheumatoid vasculitis (375–377).

Monitoring

When MTX was first reintroduced into the rheumatologists' armamentarium in the early 1980s, monitoring followed the guidelines established years before by dermatologists for the treatment of psoriasis (212,213,378). In addition to laboratory testing to detect early hematologic and liver toxicity, dermatologists recommended performance of serial liver biopsies once the cumulative dose of MTX reached 1.5 g, and every 1.5 g thereafter. As early as 1989, however, rheumatologists questioned the validity of such an approach after comparing the risks of the liver biopsy procedure with the risk for developing clinically significant liver disease (379). It was thought that the risks (and cost) of the procedure did not justify the routine performance of liver biopsies either before or during the administration of MTX (207,211,379–382). Emerging evidence also indicated that the incidence of clinically significant liver disease secondary to MTX was much less than anticipated (211), hardly justifying the routine performance of liver biopsies. This sentiment was shared by patients as well (383).

Data obtained from a survey of the ACR membership provided an estimated frequency of clinically significant liver disease and identified possible risk factors (171). An ACR subcommittee was subsequently charged with the development of guidelines for monitoring treatment with MTX. This subcommittee reviewed and evaluated the literature, including unpublished laboratory data on file with the drug's manufacturer. It then developed a set of "suggested" guidelines for monitoring MTX therapy (384). These guidelines have received mixed reviews from the ACR membership (385–388), but have been found to have adequate sensitivity (80%) and specificity (82%) when the guidelines were applied to an existent cohort of MTX-treated patients with RA who had undergone liver biopsies according to the recommendations of their rheumatologists. This study, however, suggested that insulin-dependent diabetes mellitus be added as a risk factor for clinically significant liver disease (234). Recommended pretreatment laboratory evaluation includes a complete blood cell count (CBC) with differential, RBC indices, vitamin B_{12} and folate levels, a chemistry panel, and hepatitis serologies. Pretreatment liver biopsy was thought to be indicated only in patients previously exposed to hepatotoxic substances (e.g., history of alcohol use) or hepatic injury (e.g., hepatitis). Recently the ACR guidelines have been called into question, but this sentiment is not uniform among rheumatologists (389,390). Dermatologists, however, maintain a different view (382).

During MTX therapy, hematologic (CBC with platelet count and leukocyte differential), renal (creatinine), and liver (transaminases and albumin) laboratory tests are recommended every 6 to 8 weeks. Increased serum levels of transaminases or decreased serum albumin in a patient with otherwise well-controlled articular manifestations should alert the physician to the possible development of liver toxicity (171,210,232,391,392). If liver abnormalities persist despite discontinuation of other drugs (such as an NSAID known to be hepatotoxic), or reduction in the dose of MTX, a liver biopsy is indicated. If such a patient refuses to undergo a liver biopsy, MTX should be discontinued.

The ACR subcommittee recommended the use of the Roenigk system for grading liver biopsies (378): advanced fibrosis (III-B) and frank cirrhosis (IV) were deemed absolute contraindications to resumption of MTX, whereas mild portal inflammation and milder degrees of fibrosis (grades I, II, and III-A) were not. Other grading systems do not appear to offer an advantage over the Roenigk system and have not been adopted by the ACR (230,393). The indiscriminate use of liver biopsies was thought to have an unacceptable risk/benefit ratio because of the total number of biopsies needed to detect one single case of clinically significant liver disease and the cost of such a practice (171). Patients and physicians are not currently in favor of such an unselective approach (381,383,388). Based on the survey data, Bergquist et al. (394) were unable to demonstrate the cost effectiveness of performing routine liver biopsies within the first 5 years of MTX administration; at 10 years, they concluded that liver biopsies may be cost effective. Of interest, pediatric rheumatologists have adopted these ACR guidelines for children with JRA being treated with MTX (395).

Although not discussed in the guidelines, noninvasive imaging techniques may eventually permit accurate assessment of liver architecture and facilitate monitoring of patients in lieu of performing liver biopsies. These imaging techniques include high-resolution computed tomography (HRCT) (396,397), high-resolution ultrasonography, and single-photon emission computed tomography. Unfortunately, these techniques are thought to be more sensitive but less specific than biopsies and, at present, are not considered to be a substitute for them (396,397). Additionally, there is limited experience with these techniques, and their indiscriminate use will, by necessity, add to the already high overall cost of MTX treatment.

A survey of Canadian rheumatologists (398) indicated that only 17% performed routine liver biopsies after a given (but not specified) time, and 23% after a given (but not specified) cumulative dose. Pretreatment biopsies were performed by 62% of respondents when liver function test results were abnormal. Periodic (interval variable) laboratory tests were performed by 97% of the rheumatologists. Baseline chest radiographs and pulmonary function tests were performed only by a minority of respondents.

The ACR subcommittee did not address the monitoring of pulmonary parameters, including whether baseline chest radiographs and pulmonary function tests should be performed. Based on the multicenter case control study of

TABLE 32.4. *Recommendations for monitoring methotrexate therapy in rheumatoid arthritis*

Baseline
- CBC with differential and platelet count
- Vitamin B_{12} and folate levels
- Hepatitis B and C serologies
- Chest radiograph and pulmonary function tests[a]
- Pretreatment liver biopsy only if:
  - Prior excessive alcohol intake
  - Abnormal transaminases
  - Chronic hepatitis B and C infection

Follow-up (to be done at 6- to 8-week intervals)
- CBC with differential and platelet count
- Transaminases, albumin, creatinine
- Liver biopsy if:
  - 5 of 9 (or 6 of 12) transaminase determinations are abnormal (over 1 year), and do not subside with a decrease in the weekly dose of methotrexate, or discontinuation of NSAID, or
  - A decrease in serum albumin (in patients with well-controlled RA)

The following should be considered
- Age and cumulative dose predispose to liver toxicity, but pulmonary injury may occur at any time.
- Infections (and possibly lymphomas) need to be monitored.
- Other antifolates need to be administered with great caution.

From Kremer JM, Alarcón GS, Lightfoot RW Jr, et al. Methotrexate for rheumatoid arthritis. Suggested guidelines for monitoring liver toxicity. *Arthritis Rheum* 1994;37:316–328, with permission.

[a]If clinically indicated.

MTX lung injury, a chest radiograph appears reasonable in patients with suspected pulmonary involvement. In the absence of pulmonary symptoms, little justification exists for the routine periodic evaluation of pulmonary function tests, chest radiographs, or HRCTs during MTX therapy. Moreover, recent data suggest that in the large majority of MTX-treated RA patients, diverse pulmonary parameters (pulmonary function tests, HRCTs) remain unchanged over time (268). Table 32.4 summarizes the proposed guidelines for monitoring for MTX toxicity.

Wallace and Sherry (399) proposed that MTX toxicity can be avoided by determining the serum levels of MTX 1 and 24 hours after its administration and plotting the values in a nomogram they developed. As noted before, however, there is no relationship between hepatic tissue concentrations of MTX and liver damage, so it is unlikely that MTX serum concentrations will be useful in practice (230).

Folic Acid Versus Folinic Acid Supplementation

Folinic acid (or leucovorin), the fully reduced folate compound, has been used as the antidote for antifolates in cancer chemotherapy. Its administration during low-dose MTX therapy for RA decreases the occurrence of adverse toxic events. Unfortunately, it also decreases the efficacy of MTX, especially if used at high doses (45 mg/wk). The timing of the administration of both MTX and folinic acid is crucial in maintaining the antirheumatic effects of MTX (56,57,400–404). In contrast, folic acid supplementation, with doses as high as 27.5 mg/wk, does not abrogate the efficacy of MTX, but significantly reduces the occurrence of adverse toxic events, especially those that are clearly attributable to folate deficiency (e.g., alopecia, mucosal ulcerations, gastrointestinal symptoms, and cytopenias) (51, 54,274,405–410).

Data from a large randomized placebo-controlled trial suggest that folates (either folic or folinic acid) may also exert a hepatoprotective effect (411,412). In this 48-week study of over 400 RA patients, discontinuation of MTX occurred in 38% of placebo-treated, 17% of folic acid–supplemented, and 12% of folinic acid–supplemented patients. The main differences observed between the groups were in liver enzyme levels, which were higher in the placebo group than in the folate-supplemented patients; however, the beneficial effect of folate supplementation on other adverse events, considered to occur as a result of folate deficiency, was not observed in this study (411). A favorable effect of folic acid has also been reported in a small Japanese study (413). Even relatively small amounts of folic (or folinic) acid, such as that ingested with a folate-rich diet or with over-the-counter vitamin preparations, may suffice (55,414). Additional beneficial effects of folic acid supplementation relate to its possible role in the prevention of atherosclerosis (415) because its administration normalized the levels of homocysteine (412,416), as well as in the prevention of chromosomal abnormalities induced by MTX (306). The optimal ratio of MTX to folic acid has not yet been established, and the appropriate dose of folic acid to use in patients receiving high weekly doses of MTX has yet to be determined.

Despite convincing data favoring the routine use of folic acid supplementation (54,407,408,417,418), only about one third of Canadian rheumatologists followed this practice a few years ago (398). In Europe, the tendency has been toward decreasing the dose of MTX to minimize toxicity (419), rather than using folic acid supplementation (407,420,421).

This divergent practice became evident during the conduct of the European and U.S. trials of leflunomide versus MTX; most U.S. patients received folate supplementation, whereas most European patients did not (144,145). Whether the large randomized trial from the Netherlands will change this practice in Europe, remains to be determined (411,412).

It is unfortunate that information from privately owned patient drug education databases has been distributed to retailers warning patients to avoid taking folic acid concomitant with MTX. Our group has alerted the ACR, the FDA, and the rheumatology community regarding this misinformation in the hope that patients will be properly advised by their rheumatologists to disregard these recommendations (422). Additionally, the manufacturers still recommends withholding MTX for manifestations that are likely to resolve with folic acid supplementation.

Based on data alluded to previously, it is recommended that patients beginning MTX therapy be given folic acid concomitant with MTX to prevent untoward events that are clearly the result of folate deficiency, rather than waiting for RBC macrocytosis or overt toxicities to develop. Patients may start folic acid while their baseline laboratory or ancillary evaluation is being completed, and then proceed with the initiation of MTX while folic acid administration continues. However, it should be stressed that the administration of folic acid may precipitate or exacerbate the neurologic manifestations of vitamin B_{12} deficiency (423), which may be present in patients with RA (417).

Methotrexate in Juvenile Rheumatoid Arthritis

The use of MTX for the treatment of children with either systemic, pauciarticular, or polyarticular JRA has been a common practice over the past 14 years (48,424–429). Issues that should be addressed when dealing with children include the long-term safety of MTX (beyond 5 or 10 years), its effect on the reproductive system, and uncertainty about the frequency of serious adverse events (such as lung injury) observed in adults (424). Nevertheless, therapeutic inadequacy of other drugs and the weekly laboratory monitoring required for parenteral gold salt therapy have influenced pediatric rheumatologists toward an increased use of MTX in children with JRA. Jacobs has stated that he has not initiated gold salt treatment in children in the past several years, and he is not alone in this practice. MTX is now a standard antirheumatic drug in children with JRA, particularly in those with polyarticular, seropositive disease, who are more likely to develop joint destruction (430).

Children tolerate MTX quite well and, if properly supplemented with folic acid, tend not to experience gastrointestinal symptoms, alopecia, or cytopenias (431,432). One case of MTX lung injury (263) but no case of MTX-induced liver injury has been reported in children, but the cumulative experience in children is not as great as that in adults. Monitoring should be conducted by using the same guidelines as for adults because they seem to perform similarly (395). Parents need to be presented with balanced data concerning this drug's efficacy and toxicity profile, as well as the uncertainties concerning its long-term safety. Whether parents should be informed about the three cases of lymphoma reported in children taking MTX is a matter of clinical judgment. On the other hand, parents should be informed that MTX is the only DMARD that has been shown to improve the radiographic appearance of the carpal bones of children with JRA (433). In short, MTX offers some distinctive advantages over other DMARDs, not only in children with poly- and pauciarticular JRA, but also in those with the systemic febrile form of the disease (including its adult counterpart), as a steroid-sparing agent (434–436). Of course, like in adults, the availability of anti-TNF compounds and other biologic products may change the prescription patterns of MTX in children with juvenile arthritis (437).

Methotrexate in Other Arthropathies

MTX has been used for the treatment of patients with seronegative spondyloarthropathies, especially in patients with ankylosing spondylitis and significant peripheral arthritis, as well as for the treatment of chronic reactive arthritis (438). It also has been used successfully as a steroid-sparing agent in patients with inflammatory bowel disease and arthritis (439,440). Finally, MTX continues to be used for the treatment of psoriasis and psoriatic arthritis, with favorable results (10,129). Clinically-significant liver disease has been the major limiting factor in the use of this compound in patients with psoriasis. When alcohol ingestion is precluded and the total dose is given once weekly, however, there appears to be no greater risk for the occurrence of liver injury among patients with psoriasis than among those with RA. An additional concern regarding the use of MTX in psoriatic arthritis relates to its use in patients infected with the human immunodeficiency virus (HIV). These patients may experience worsening of skin manifestations while taking MTX for reasons that are not totally clear (441,442).

Methotrexate in Other Rheumatic and Nonrheumatic Disorders

Before MTX became widely used for the treatment of RA, it was used for the treatment of idiopathic inflammatory myopathy (either polymyositis or dermatomyositis) with impressive results (443). It was used primarily in patients who either did not respond to corticosteroids alone or who required sustained high doses of corticosteroids to control the inflammatory process. Doses are, for the most part, higher than those used in RA and are usually administered parenterally on a weekly basis. There have been no randomized, controlled trials of the use of MTX in polymyositis, dermatomyositis, or other systemic rheumatic disorders. In addition to polymyositis and dermatomyositis (443), MTX has been used in patients with scleroderma (444), Sjögren's syndrome (445), and systemic lupus erythematosus (SLE) (446–451) with or without renal or central nervous system involvement (452,453). Beneficial effects have been reported in both instances, but MTX has not replaced corticosteroids or other immunosuppressive agents, such as cyclophosphamide or azathioprine, for the treatment of patients with SLE.

MTX has been used by dermatologists for the treatment of some chronic dermatoses with a vasculitic component (RA included), usually at doses higher that those prescribed for patients with RA without vasculitis (376,377). Vasculitis, however, may occur *de novo* in patients with RA being treated with MTX, and its role in the treatment of vasculitis is then not clear. MTX also has been used in sarcoidosis, either limited to the skin or with organ system involvement (454–458) and in corticosteroid-dependent bronchial asthma (459). Although controversial because of its potential liver toxicity, MTX also has been used in some forms of liver disease, including primary biliary cirrhosis

(460) and idiopathic granulomatous hepatitis (461); in fact, and as noted before, fulminant viral hepatitis had been described in a patient receiving MTX, after its abrupt discontinuation (233).

MTX has been recommended as a steroid-sparing agent for the treatment of cutaneous polyarteritis nodosa, Behçet syndrome (375), Wegener granulomatosis (462), Takayasu arteritis, giant cell arteritis (and polymyalgia rheumatica) (463–465), and other forms of systemic vasculitis (466–468). Three randomized controlled trials using MTX, either instead of oral corticosteroids or in conjunction with them, have failed to show any beneficial effect from its administration (469–471). Use of MTX is justified primarily in the elderly, who are likely to experience significant deleterious effects from corticosteroids (e.g., osteoporosis, hypertension, diabetes, catabolic skin changes, and central nervous system toxicity).

Other Antifolates

A number of other folate antagonists exist, but their use in RA, other arthropathies, and other systemic rheumatic disorders is unlikely in the near future. Some of these antifolates have been tested in experimentally induced arthritis in animals (e.g., 10-deazaaminopterin and trimethotrexate 10-deazaadenosine) (472). Of them, 10-deazaaminopterin and 10-deazaadenosine have been tested in patients with RA. 10-deazaaminopterin but not 10-deazaadenosine appeared to be effective (473). However, whether 10-deazaaminopterin is less toxic than MTX (474,475) has not been determined to date.

Therapeutic Considerations

The oral route of administration of MTX is approved by the FDA. The high cost of the drug plus better tolerance of parenteral administration have been the primary reasons for switching from the oral to the parenteral route (7,476) which, in general, is though to be as effective as the oral route, although the contrary has been described (477). Some rheumatologists recommend the oral administration of the parenteral preparation in an effort to reduce treatment cost (478). Previously, weekly doses were generally divided into three doses, 12 hours apart. Many rheumatologists currently prescribe the entire dose either in one single intake or split into two doses for those patients taking more than 10 mg of MTX per week (24,479). Every-other-week dosing appears possible in patients doing well with the weekly dose, as recently shown by Pandya et al. (480). Intraarticular MTX has been used infrequently with variable success (481).

Understanding the pathogenesis of joint destruction in RA had prompted the initiation of MTX therapy (alone or in combination) earlier in the course of the disease, hoping to prevent the occurrence of destruction of articular and extraarticular structures. Some data support the notion that if MTX is given early, subsequent joint destruction may not occur (2). Of course, it can be argued that those patients who did not progress had spontaneous resolution of their arthritis, as had been reported for some individuals in cohorts of patients who fulfill criteria for the diagnosis of RA but who may not exhibit clinical evidence of the disease 5 years later (482). Such patients (reported rates vary between 10% and 20%), might be erroneously considered treatment successes if treated early, when in fact they have a self-limited form of the disease. The challenge for rheumatologists rests in their ability to identify early patients "destined" to have a progressive and destructive form of the disease and to treat them as early and aggressively as possible.

Whereas there has been significant progress in understanding the genetic basis for disease susceptibility and disease severity in RA, it is premature to recommend that all patients with new-onset polyarthritis be subjected to DNA analyses in search of the HLA-DRB1 alleles encoding the so-called "rheumatoid epitope" or other polymorphisms that, in conjunction with the rheumatoid epitope, may indicate a poor outcome (e.g., TNF-α polymorphisms), as described by Criswell et al. (483). Gough et al. (484) have shown that early polyarthritis in a significant proportion of patients who inherited the rheumatoid epitope evolved into a destructive arthropathy, but a significant proportion of healthy individuals and patients with a self-limited polyarthritis also exhibited the rheumatoid epitope. Moreover, the rheumatoid epitope has been found to be lacking in nearly two thirds of African-American patients with otherwise well-established and moderate-to-severe RA (485, 486). At this time, it would be erroneous to base treatment decisions solely on DNA analyses, even if such testing becomes commercially available at a reasonable cost.

McCarty et al. have proposed the use of multidrug therapy since the early 1980s for patients with RA (487,488). They initially used a combination of hydroxychloroquine, parenteral gold salts, azathioprine, and cyclophosphamide, but several patients developed malignant processes, which resulted in the replacement of cyclophosphamide with MTX, with excellent results (487,488).

Drugs tested in combination with MTX include oral gold (12), azathioprine (489,490), chloroquine, hydroxychloroquine (228,491–494), sulfasalazine (495–500), minocycline (493), cyclosporine (501–505), and leflunomide (506,507). The rationale behind the use of combination therapy comes from the oncology and infectious diseases experience—drugs may interfere with different mediators of inflammation and metabolic pathways and thus be synergistic. Ideally, each drug might be used at a reduced dose and be better tolerated, and the combination is more effective than either drug alone. For the most part, such data have not been generated for combination therapy in RA despite numerous trials, with the possible exception of cyclosporine. In the multicenter study by Tugwell et al. (501), patients with a partial response to MTX who were randomized to receive cyclosporine experienced additional improvement of their articular symptoms, which was not the case for those randomized to placebo. Moreover, patients initially randomized to placebo were administered cyclosporine, and they also improved significantly.

A promising combination therapy for RA is that proposed by O'Dell from the University of Nebraska (508). In this particular trial, patients received either MTX alone, MTX and sulfasalazine, or MTX, sulfasalazine, and hydroxychloroquine. Published data indicate that the triple DMARD combination is not only more effective than MTX or MTX plus sulfasalazine, but also is well tolerated. Long-term data suggest that this combination remains effective over time (509,510).

Finally, MTX has been used as the anchor drug in combination with biologic agents, including anti-CD4 and anti-TNF compounds (511). With the approval of TNF inhibitors, these agents are being used in combination with MTX in RA patients who are incomplete MTX responders.

Three recent studies have examined the combination of anti-TNF compounds and MTX (with etarnecept, the TEMPO trial; with adalimumab, Phase III trial; with infliximab, the ASPIRE trial) in patients with early, active RA (511a,511b,511c). These combinations (with anti-TNF compound) have clearly demonstrated a significant advantage in controlling disease activity, in avoiding functional decline and preventing structural damage over MTX alone (or MTX and placebo). For details of these trials, see chapter on combination therapy for RA. The long-term effects of this combination have yet to be determined.

Summary

MTX has become the most widely used DMARD for the treatment of RA in the Americas. The efficacy and toxicity of the compound are well known, and regimens capable of reducing its toxicity can be implemented. Concerns remain regarding its use, including the uncertainty about its long-term (beyond 5 or 10 years) possible hepatotoxic effect, the unpredictability of lung injury, and the possible occurrence of lymphomas. Proper knowledge of the pharmacokinetics of the drug, drug-drug interactions, and adequate clinical and laboratory monitoring are essential to assure maximal benefit and minimal toxicity from this compound.

Despite the advent of new therapies, MTX is likely to continue to be used as an anchor drug for the treatment of RA and other inflammatory arthropathies in years to come.

LEFLUNOMIDE

Leflunomide, a new immunomodulatory agent, was approved in 1998 by the FDA for the treatment of RA as an alternative agent to other DMARDs, such as MTX or sulfasalazine, if these agents proved to be ineffective or poorly tolerated.

Historical Overview

Leflunomide (HR486) was developed by Hoechst in the 1980s as a compound capable of preventing mitogen-stimulated lymphocyte proliferation. It was tested in different animal models, in which either inflammation or immunity needed to be suppressed (graft survival, adjuvant arthritis) and found to be effective (512).

Structure, Pharmacology, and Pharmacokinetics

Leflunomide, an isoxazol derivative, represents a novel immunoregulatory agent and a new generation of low-molecular-weight DMARD; it shares no structural relationship with existing immunomodulatory agents. Leflunomide [N-(4-trifluoromethylphenyl)-5-methylisoxazol-4-carboxamide] and its ring-open metabolite A77 1726 [3-cyano-3-hydroxy-N-(4-trifluoromethylphenyl)-croton-amide] have a molecular weight of 270 daltons.

Absorption of leflunomide from the intestinal tract is not interferred with by food; it is nearly 100% absorbed, with rapid nonenzymatic conversion to its active metabolite, malononitriloamide (A77 1726). This metabolite is nearly 100% protein bound (predominantly to albumin), and its levels are not influenced by age, gender, or body mass index. Because of its high protein-binding, the plasma half-life of A77 1726 is long (~15 days, range 5–40 days) (512). Leflunomide is metabolized and eliminated by the liver; due to its enterohepatic circulation, however, it can be easily and rapidly removed from the body with the administration of oral cholestyramine. Sixty percent to 70% of the drug is excreted in the urine as trifluoromethylaniline (TFMA)-oxanillic acid; a doubling of the free fraction of A77 1726 in patients ($n = 6$) receiving hemodialysis or peritoneal dialysis has been documented in single-dose studies (513).

Although leflunomide does not interact significantly with warfarin, oral contraceptives, oral hypoglycemic agents, or NSAIDs (514), it has been shown to increase the free fraction of diclofenac, ibuprofen, and tolbutamide at concentrations ranging from 13% to 50% of those achieved in the clinical setting. Leflunomide also inhibits CYP 450 2C9, which is responsible for the metabolism of many NSAIDs (513). However, the clinical significance of these properties is unknown. On the contrary, the concomitant administration of rifampin and leflunomide results in increases of the peak plasma levels of the latter; thus, this drug combination should be used cautiously (513).

Mechanisms of Action and Biologic Effects

Leflunomide inhibits the *de novo* pyrimidine ribonucleotide synthesis in activated lymphocytes during the G1 phase of their cell cycle; this inhibition occurs at the level of the enzyme dihydroorotate dehydrogenase (DHODH) and results in the inhibition of RNA and DNA synthesis with a significant decrease in the proliferation and differentiation of lymphocytes, particularly of T cells that are implicated in the pathogenesis of RA (512,515). This effect can be reversed with the addition of uridine (516). A77 1726 also inhibits several different tyrosine kinases in murine T cells; this effect does play an antiproliferative role in MRL/*lpr* mice (517), but it is not achieved in humans at the doses used for the treatment of RA (512).

Other important actions of leflunomide include the inhibition of membrane glycosylation, the inhibition of the expression of adhesion molecules on endothelial cells, the inhibition of chemokine expression (monocyte chemoattractant protein), the up-regulation of TGF-β1, an immunosuppressive cytokine, and the inhibition of cyclooxygenase-2 activity. The first two actions result from the inhibition of DHODH and represent a different mechanism of action than the arrest of the G1 phase of the cell cycle (512). Leflunomide also blocks the activation of nuclear factor κB, a transcription factor that regulates the expression of many of the genes that play critical role in immune and inflammatory responses, as has been shown in a bioassay using Jurkat human T cells treated with leflunomide (512,518); whether or not this action occurs *in vivo* in humans has yet to be determined.

Clinical Efficacy of Leflunomide in Rheumatoid Arthritis

The efficacy and safety of the long-term administration of leflunomide were assessed in an open-label study conducted in Croatia, Slovenia, and Yugoslavia in the early 1990s (519). The study involved 350 patients, with 255 completing 18 months of treatment with doses ranging from 5 to 25 mg per day. Leflunomide showed acceptable tolerability and clinical benefit.

Subsequently, Mladenovic et al. published the results of a randomized placebo-controlled dose-finding study also conducted in Eastern Europe and involving 402 patients. In this 24-week study, leflunomide improved all clinical variables in a dose-dependent manner; 55% for those on 10 mg/day and 60% for those on 25 mg/day. The response rate for the 5 mg/day dose was similar to that of placebo; it was felt that a dose of 20 mg/day would be associated with a maximal probability of success (164).

Using the information from these dose-finding studies, three randomized clinical trials were designed to determine the efficacy and toxicity of leflunomide for the treatment of RA as compared with placebo and other DMARDs. These three trials, United States 301 (US301), multinational 302 (MN302), and MN301, confirmed the efficacy and safety of leflunomide and were pivotal for its approval by the FDA in 1998 (144,145,520). The baseline characteristics of the patients who participated in these trials are shown in Table 32.5. Table 32.6 depicts the outcome data of these trials.

US301 (144) was a 52-week study that involved 482 RA patients. Patients were randomized to receive leflunomide (n = 182) 20 mg daily after an initial 3-day loading dose of 100 mg/day, MTX (n = 182) 7.5 mg per week, or placebo (n = 118). At week 9 of the study patients in the MTX arm were allowed to increase their dosage to 15 mg per week in the event of an inadequate therapeutic response (61% of the patients did so). US301 patients continued stable doses of prednisone (≤10 mg per day) and NSAIDs; they also received 1 to 2 mg of folic acid per day. The primary outcome measures in this study were a 20% improvement by ACR criteria (ACR20) and/or ACR success; the latter was defined as completing 52 weeks of initial therapy, with improvement of 20% or greater at end point. ACR response rates for improvement of 50% (ACR50) or greater and 70% (ACR70) or greater at 12 months were also determined.

In this study, the response rates of leflunomide and MTX were comparable but greater than with placebo for these four outcomes. Treatment with either active agent significantly improved the patient's quality of life as measured by the Health Assessment Questionnaire (HAQ), the Medical Outcomes Survey Short Form, and the Problem Elicitation Technique questionnaire (521–523). Analyses of the radiographic data demonstrated that both active compounds were superior to placebo in retarding disease progression (144).

MN302 (145) assessed the efficacy and safety of leflunomide as compared with MTX; this study differed from US301 in that there was no placebo group. MN302 was also important in demonstrating the long-term safety and

TABLE 32.5. *Baseline characteristics of rheumatoid arthritis patients in double-blind leflunomide studies*

Study	US301[a]			MN302[b]		MN301[c]		
Variable	Leflunomide (n = 182)	Methotrexate (n = 182)	Placebo (n = 118)	Leflunomide (n = 501)	Methotrexate (n = 498)	Leflunomide (n = 133)	Sulfasalazine (n = 133)	Placebo (n = 92)
Age (mean years)	54	53	55	59	58	58	59	59
% Women	73	75	70	71	71	76	69	75
Disease duration (mean years)	7	7	7	4	4	8	7	6
≤2 years (%)	39	40	33	44	43	38	42	45
>2 years (%)	61	60	67	56	47	62	59	55
Prior DMARD use (%)	56	60	56	66	67	60	49	47

[a]United States 301 (144).
[b]Multinational 302 (145).
[c]Multinational 301 (520).
DMARD, disease modifying antirheumatic drug.

TABLE 32.6. *American College of Rheumatology (ACR) response rates[a] in rheumatoid arthritis patients in double-blind leflunomide studies*

Study	Study type	Treatment duration (wk)	No. of patients: Leflunomide	No. of patients: Methotrexate (Sulfasalazine in MN301)[b]	No. of patients: Placebo	Outcome	Patients achieving outcome (%): Leflunomide	Patients achieving outcome (%): Methotrexate (Sulfasalazine in MN301)	Patients achieving outcome (%): Placebo	p
US301[c]	Placebo-controlled	52	182	182	118	ACR success	41	35	19	<0.001
						ACR20	52	46	26	<0.001
						ACR50	34	23	8	<0.001
						ACR70	20	9	4	<0.001
MN302[d]	Active-controlled	52	501	498	None	ACR20	51	65	NA[e]	<0.0001
						ACR50	31	44	NA	NA
						ACR70	10	16	NA	NA
MN301	Placebo-controlled	24	133	133	92	ACR20	55	56	29	0.0001[f]
						ACR50	33	30	14	0.002[f]

[a]Only ACR response rates are noted in table to facilitate comparison across trials.
[b]Multinational 301 (520).
[c]United States 301 (144).
[d]Multinational 302 (145).
[e]Not applicable.
[f]Leflunomide versus placebo.

efficacy of leflunomide. In this study, RA patients in the leflunomide group (n = 501) were dosed as in US301, but the daily dose could be reduced to 10 mg/day in case of an adverse event. Patients in the MTX group (n = 498) received 7.5 mg/wk until week 4; thereafter and up to week 12, this dosage could be increased to 15 mg. In this study the ACR20 response rate at 1 year was greater with MTX than with leflunomide; however, the difference between these rates was lost at 2 years. The rate of disease progression, as determined radiographically, was similar for both treatment groups. At 2 years, improvement in all clinical variables was maintained, but the rate of radiographic progression was smaller in the MTX-treated than in the leflunomide-treated patients. Folic acid supplementation was not mandated in MN302 and in fact occurred only in less than 10% of patients.

The last pivotal RA study, MN301 (520), compared the efficacy of leflunomide (n = 133) dosed as in US301 with that of sulfasalazine (n = 133) 0.5 g daily, titrated up to 2 g daily at week 4 and of placebo (n = 92). Similar ACR20 response rates were observed with leflunomide and sulfasalazine in this 24-week trial; however, response occurred sooner in the leflunomide-treated than in the sulfasalazine- or placebo-treated patients and was seen as early as 4 weeks. Furthermore, HAQ scores were significantly better in the leflunomide-treated patients than in those treated with placebo or sulfasalazine. Disease progression, as measured radiographically by the Larsen score, was significantly less pronounced in the leflunomide- and sulfasalazine-treated patients than in those treated with placebo. Patients (n = 230) who completed this study were given the option to be followed for 12 (n = 168) and 24 (n =146) months in double-blinded extension studies; patients in the placebo group were switched to sulfasalazine. At 1 year there were no statistically-significant differences between the two patient groups. The beneficial effects of leflunomide were maintained at 24 months, with leflunomide performing better that sulfasalazine in the global assessment scores, functional ability, ACR response rates, and in slowing the rate of disease progression as determined radiographically (524–526).

An open-label extension study of MN301 and MN302 was recently reported (527). In this study, a total of 214 patients (29 from MN301 and 185 from MN302) were enrolled and treated with leflunomide at the same daily maintenance dosage used in the original studies; however, patients were given the option to decrease the dose of leflunomide to 10 mg/day in case of an adverse event or to go back to 20 mg for lack of efficacy. The large majority of the patients, however, received 20 mg of leflunomide per day. Outcome measures included in this extension study were the same as in the original studies. The study was terminated when leflunomide became commercially available; by then, 163 patients (76%) had received leflunomide for a mean treatment duration of 4.6 years. Improvements in ACR20, 50, and 70 at year 4 or at study termination were 69%, 43%, and 20%, respectively. HAQ scores achieved at year 1 were maintained through year 4 or by the end point.

Adverse Events

In the context of the three pivotal trials described, patients receiving leflunomide experienced more adverse events than those receiving sulfasalazine but less than those receiving MTX. The most commonly reported adverse reactions associated with leflunomide in these trials were diarrhea, nausea, abdominal pain, elevations of the liver enzymes alanine aminotransferase (ALT) and aspartate aminotransferase

(AST), skin rashes, alopecia, and respiratory tract infections; most occurred in less than 20% of the patients. These data are depicted in Table 32.7.

The safety of leflunomide as compared with MTX was assessed in US301 and MN302. Patients on leflunomide tended to have more diarrhea, rash, and alopecia than those taking MTX, but the latter group developed more mouth ulcerations. The withdrawal rates for leflunomide due to adverse events were similar (22% in US301 and 20% in MN302); these rates were 10% and 15% for MTX. In US301, transaminase elevations were comparable in both treatment groups and were very uncommon (≤5%), whereas in MN302, the rate of significant liver enzyme elevations was approximately 5% in the leflunomide-treated patients but it was approximately 16% in MTX-treated subjects. The disparate transaminase results between these two trials have been interpreted as being possibly related to folate supplementation (common in US301, uncommon in MN302) (411), but whether or not that is the case remains to be determined.

No clinically-relevant changes in electrolytes or renal function have been reported in either US301 or MN302. Likewise, no hematologic adverse events were noted in US301; in contrast, leukopenia occurred at 1 year in 20 patients from MN302 treated with leflunomide, leading to 4 patients withdrawing from the trial. However, leukopenia was mild, ranging between 2,000 and 3,000 cells/mm^3. Eight additional patients experienced leukopenia during the second year of the study, and three were withdrawn from the study.

The safety of leflunomide as opposed to sulfasalazine was assessed in MN301. Withdrawals due to adverse events occurred in 14% of patients treated with leflunomide, 7% with placebo, and 19% with sulfasalazine. Common adverse reactions in this trial were diarrhea, nausea, alopecia, and skin rash, diarrhea and alopecia being more common in patients who received leflunomide than in those who received sulfasalazine. However, nausea was more common with sulfasalazine than with leflunomide. Hypertension in this study was observed in 6% of patients treated with leflunomide, 3% with placebo, and 4% with sulfasalazine, but drug-related hypertension occurred equally in both groups (2%). The frequency of ALT and AST elevations were similar with leflunomide and sulfasalazine; these elevations were 1.2 to 2.0 times above the upper normal limit. Like with US301 and MN302, no clinically-significant changes in electrolyte or renal function were seen with leflunomide in MN301. Clinically-relevant hematologic toxicities were not reported in this trial.

No new treatment-related adverse events occurred in patients from the MN301 and MN302 open-label extension study (527).

In clinical practice, most patients treated with leflunomide complain of gastrointestinal symptoms (nausea, diarrhea, abdominal pain) along with mild cutaneous manifestations (rash and pruritus). These manifestations usu-

TABLE 32.7. *Frequency of treatment-related adverse events in rheumatoid arthritis patients in double-blinded leflunomide studies*

Study	US301[a]			MN302[b]		MN301[c]		
Adverse event (%)	Leflunomide (n = 182)	Methotrexate (n = 182)	Placebo (n = 118)	Leflunomide (n = 501)	Methotrexate (n = 498)	Leflunomide (n = 133)	Sulfasalazine (n = 133)	Placebo (n = 92)
Gastrointestinal symptoms								
Diarrhea	34	20	17	18	7	12	6	4
Nausea	21	19	19	11	16	7	11	8
Dyspepsia	14	13	12	2	6	3	7	2
Abdominal pain	14	15	7	6	6	3	4	5
Abnormal ALT/AST[d]	15	12	3	5	16	2	4	0
Infections	57	60	48	5[e]	5[e]	1[f]	2[f]	3[f]
Allergic reactions	24	17	14	7[g]	5[g]	6[g]	7[g]	4[g]
Alopecia	10	6	1	17	10	6	4	2
Mouth ulcers	6	10	6	3	6	NA	NA	NA
Asthenia	6	3	NA	1	2	NA	NA	NA
Headache	12	14	NA	6	5	5	6	2
Hypertension								
All	11	3	5	NA	NA	2	2	1
New onset	2	2	0	NA	NA	NA	NA	NA

[a]United States 301 (144).
[b]Multinational 302 (145).
[c]Multinational 301 (520).
[d]Alanine-aminotransferase and aspartate-aminotransferase.
[e]Upper respiratory tract infections.
[f]All respiratory infections.
[g]MN302 and MN301 studies reported allergic reactions as rash.
NA, not available.

ally subside with reduction of the dose or discontinuation of the drug.

Liver Function Test Abnormalities and Hepatotoxicity

In clinical trials, 14% to 18% of patients had an elevation of ALT that was 1.2 to 2 times the upper limit of normal. Elevations greater than three times the upper limit of normal were seen in only 1.5% to 4.4% of the patients and were more frequent in patients receiving leflunomide than in those receiving placebo, but comparable with what occurred in those receiving either sulfasalazine or MTX. Liver enzyme abnormalities usually occurred within the first 6 months of treatment and were more frequent in patients with associated comorbidities. Acute liver injury did not occur in these trials (144,145,520).

In 2001, the European Medicines Evaluation Agency's (EMEA) scientific committee called attention to hepatotoxicity of variable degree occurring in leflunomide-treated RA patients (528). As noted in Table 32.8, the EMEA reported 296 cases of severe hepatic reactions in an estimated total drug exposure of 104,000 patient-years. Among these 296 cases, 232 patients presented with liver enzyme elevations, 129 had serious hepatic reactions, 2 had cirrhosis, and 15 presented with acute liver failure; 9 of these 15 patients died, but there were 6 additional deaths among the 129 patients. In all, leflunomide was implicated as the putative agent in 10 of the 15 deaths (528). Confounding factors present in the 129 patients with serious hepatic reactions included concomitant use of other hepatotoxic medications (n = 101, 78%) and associated comorbidities (previous history of alcohol abuse, liver failure, acute heart failure, severe pulmonary disease, or pancreatic carcinoma) (n = 33, 27%). Furthermore, over half of the patients with elevated liver enzymes were taking NSAIDs.

More recently, the FDA's Office of Drug Safety (ODS) (529) reported 102 cases of serious hepatic events since the approval of the drug until August 2002 in an estimated population exposure time of 90,266 to 166,172 person-years (529). As noted in Table 32.8, 54 cases of serious hepatic events were identified; 38 included cases of hepatitis and of jaundice and/or cholestasis. Acute liver injury occurred in the remaining 16; among them, 9 patients died, 8 from liver failure and 1 from concomitant interstitial lung disease. Only 1 patient underwent liver transplantation. The ODS staff concluded that the use of leflunomide constitutes a serious risk factor for acute liver injury and sided with the March 2002 Public Citizen Petition to the FDA requesting its removal from the market (530). Members of the FDA external advisory panel reviewed the same data, the data from all leflunomide clinical trials, and retrospective cohort data from three large national databases and reached a different conclusion, as did the ODS Director; the panel agreed with the ODS that serious life-threatening cases of hepatotoxicity had occurred in leflunomide-treated patients. However, the panel concluded that the evidence linking leflunomide with acute liver injury was inconclusive and confounded by the presence of comorbid conditions and the concomitant use of hepatotoxic drugs (529,530) and recommended not to remove leflunomide from the market.

Shortly after the EMEA (528) report, the ACR issued recommendations for monitoring patients receiving leflunomide, alone or in combination, for the occurrence of hepatotoxicity. These recommendations are shown in Tables 32.9 and 32.10. Of interest, only one of the cases of acute liver failure due to leflunomide has been published in standard rheumatology sources (531).

In summary, and in contrast with MTX, where elevations of liver enzymes occur over relatively long time periods and prior to the occurrence of fibrosis (and cirrhosis) (384),

TABLE 32.8. *Hepatic reactions reported in patients taking leflunomide*

Reporting agency variable	EMEA[a] n	FDA[b] n
All reactions	296	102
Serious reactions	129	54
Acute liver failure (ALF)	15	16
Fatal Outcome		
ALF	9	8
Other causes	6	1
All causes	15	9
Possibly leflunomide related	10	5
Time to reaction (mean days; range)	Variable (3–1,095)	135 (3–693)
Confounding factors (denominator)	129	54
Other hepatotoxic drugs (%)	78	74
Concomitant use of methotrexate and/or NSAIDs (%)	58	43
Comorbid conditions (%)	27	17

[a]European Medicines Evaluation Agency (528).
[b]Food and Drug Administration (529).
NSAIDs, nonsteroidal antiinflammatory drugs.

TABLE 32.9. *Leflunomide therapy monitoring in rheumatoid arthritis patients as per recommendations of the American College of Rheumatology*

Patients taking leflunomide as a single agent

Baseline
ALT and AST

First 6 months
ALT and AST monthly

Subsequently, if stable
ALT and AST every 2–3 months[a]

Patients taking leflunomide in combination with methotrexate

Baseline
ALT and AST

First 6 months of therapy
ALT and AST monthly

Subsequently, if stable
ALT and AST every 1–3 months[a]

Modified from Matteson E, Cush JJ. Reports of leflunomide hepatotoxicity in patients with rheumatoid arthritis. ACR Hotline. August 2001. *www.rheumatology.org/research/hotline/0801leflunomide.html,* with permission.

[a]More frequent monitoring if ALT/AST abnormalities occur (for further details refer to Table 32.10).

ALT, alanine aminotransferase; AST, aspartate aminotransferase.

acute liver failure, albeit quite infrequent, with leflunomide is unpredictable and thus should always be considered.

Infections

Infections were reported to occur in 1% to 5% of all patients in MN301 and MN302. They include upper and lower respiratory tract and urinary tract infections; they occurred at the same frequency in the leflunomide and MTX patient groups in MN302, but less frequently than in the sulfasalazine (and placebo) groups in MN301. In contrast, in US301, infections occurred in over 50% of leflunomide or MTX-treated patients and in nearly 50% of those treated with placebo. The most likely explanation for the tenfold infection rate discrepancy is that of reporting, which in US301 probably included, in addition to the above infections, others such as cutaneous, gynecologic, and other superficial infections. No opportunistic infections occurred in any of the three trials (144,145,520).

TABLE 32.10. *Leflunomide therapy monitoring in rheumatoid arthritis patients as per recommendations of the American College of Rheumatology*

In patients who develop:

- ALT or AST elevations greater than one times and less than two times above normal limits.
- Repeat testing as per Table 32.9, but no dose change is required.
- ALT or AST elevations two to three times above normal limits.
- A trial of dose reduction and repeat testing is warranted; drug should be discontinued if ALT or AST elevations greater than two times above normal limits persist.
- Persistently abnormal ALT/AST or elevations greater than three times above normal limits.
- Drug should be discontinued at once and cholestyramine elimination procedure instituted (as per Table 32.11).

Modified from Matteson E, Cush JJ. Reports of leflunomide hepatotoxicity in patients with rheumatoid arthritis. ACR Hotline. August 2001. *www.rheumatology.org/research/hotline/0801leflunomide.html,* with permission.

ALT, alanine aminotransferase; AST, aspartate aminotransferase.

Malignancies

In a 2-year study, male mice treated with leflunomide had an increased risk for lymphoma, whereas female mice had an increased incidence of bronchoalveolar adenomas and carcinomas (513). Lymphoproliferative disorders have been reported in patients from phase II and III trials, although not all of these few cases occurred in patients who received leflunomide (532). Long-term surveillance is needed to determine whether there is an increased risk for malignancy in leflunomide-treated patients.

Teratogenicity

Increased rates of congenital defects and fetal death have been shown in different animal species. Pregnancy outcomes of women treated with leflunomide early in their pregnancy are sparse, but fetal loss is expected (533). A registry of children born to women exposed to leflunomide during pregnancy has been established to monitor the possible teratogenic effects of the drug. This longitudinal cohort study is being conducted by the Organization of Teratology Information Services (OTIS) (534). As of July 9, 2003, 57 women have become pregnant while taking leflunomide; some elected to terminate their pregnancies, while others have delivered normal babies (KL Jones, personal communication, July 2003).

Rare Side Effects

Rare side effects have been reported in patients taking leflunomide alone or in combination with other DMARDs and include severe pancytopenia (535), vasculitis (536,537), anti–glomerular basement membrane antibody-mediated renal failure (538), reversible peripheral neuropathy (539), toxic epidermal necrolysis (540), and alopecia areata (541).

Leflunomide Use in Combination with Other Drugs

Combination of Leflunomide and Methotrexate

Weinblatt et al. have examined the combination of leflunomide and MTX in a 52-week study involving 30 patients with active RA despite treatment with MTX (average weekly dose of 17 mg for >6 months) (542,543). These patients received a two-day loading dose of leflunomide (100 mg/day) followed by 10 mg/day (could be increased to 20 mg/day if persistent disease activity was still present at 3 months); stable doses of prednisone (≤10 mg/day) and NSAIDs were allowed. Twenty-three patients completed 1 year of treatment; ACR20 response criteria was achieved by 53% of the patients. Two patients met ACR criteria for remission at 1 year. The combination treatment was well tolerated, and no significant negative drug interactions occurred.

In a subsequent 24-week study led by Kremer (507), 263 patients with persistent active RA despite stable MTX doses, were randomized to leflunomide or placebo. The percentage of patients on MTX and leflunomide who achieved ACR20 was approximately 46%, compared with 20% of those on MTX and placebo. Thirty-nine percent of the patients received 10 mg/day of leflunomide, and 55% received 20 mg; 6% received the drug every other day. The incidence of adverse events was quite high but comparable in the two groups (~90%); however, the reported adverse events were mild to moderate. Three patients (2%) were withdrawn from the trial due to persistently abnormal liver enzymes; this occurred in only two patients in the placebo group (1.5%).

Combination of Leflunomide and Infliximab

The safety and efficacy of the combination of leflunomide and infliximab has been assessed recently by Kiely et al. (544). In this 32-week study, 20 patients with active RA despite DMARD therapy were studied. At enrollment, DMARDs were stopped, prednisone was reduced to 7.5 mg/day (if taking it at higher dose) and NSAIDs were allowed to be continued. Four weeks after enrollment, patients received leflunomide 100 mg for 3 days followed by 20 mg daily (two patients were already taking 20 mg/day of leflunomide). At week 2, all patients were given infliximab 3 mg/kg, receiving further infusions at weeks 4, 8, 16, and 24.

Disease activity score at week 28 (DAS28) and ACR20, 50, and 70 or greater were assessed. Although 11 patients were withdrawn because of side effects, serious reactions occurred in only 4 patients and were all ascribed to infliximab. Eighty percent of the patients remaining on treatment by week 28 had achieved an ACR20 and 46% an ACR70 response.

Leflunomide in Other Rheumatic Diseases

Recent pilot studies have demonstrated the benefit of leflunomide for the treatment of patients with different rheumatic diseases, including SLE (545), Felty syndrome (546), psoriasis and psoriatic arthritis (547,548), Takayasu arteritis (549), antineutrophil cytoplasmic antibody–associated vasculitis (550,551), and adult-onset Still disease (552).

In an open-label study (545), 18 SLE women (15 of 18 fulfilling ACR criteria) with moderate disease activity as ascertained by the SLE Disease Activity Index (SLEDAI) score received the standard loading dose of leflunomide followed by 20 mg/day. In the subset of patients who fulfilled ACR criteria and completed the study (n = 12), there was a mean decrease in the SLEDAI score of 2.2; 8 of these 12 patients reported a subjective improvement. No major side effects were noted; diarrhea occurred in 7 patients (two stopped leflunomide) and rash occurred in 1 patient who also discontinued the medication (545). These data suggest that leflunomide may constitute an alternative therapeutic option for patients with SLE.

Dosage and Special Considerations

Given the half-life of leflunomide (15 days), an oral loading dose of 100 mg/day for 3 consecutive days is required to achieve a steady state. This loading dose is then followed by a daily maintenance dose of 20 mg.

Pediatric Population

Leflunomide is not recommended in children because it has not been studied in this patient population.

Elderly Population

Dose adjustment is not required in subjects over 65 years of age because there is no indication that age has an effect on the pharmacokinetics of the drug. However, caution is advised, especially in frail elderly individuals with associated comorbidities and borderline renal function.

Women of Childbearing Age

Sexually-active childbearing age women should be warned of the absolute contraindication of leflunomide intake during pregnancy; thus, pregnancy should be excluded and a safe method of contraception in place before leflunomide is prescribed to them. Women becoming pregnant while taking leflunomide should be administered cholestyramine to enhance the elimination of the drug. Table 32.11 describes this

TABLE 32.11. *Leflunomide elimination procedure*

Nonpregnancy and toxic or allergic reactions:
Cholestyramine: 4–8 g t.i.d. for 2–3 days
4 g t.i.d. for 1 day reduces leflunomide levels by about 50%; 5 days are considered adequate.
Pregnancy (planned or confirmed):
As above for a total of 11 days (consecutive or not), plus
Verification of plasma levels to <0.02 mg/L in two separate determinations at least 14 days apart.

Modified from Matteson E, Cush JJ. Reports of leflunomide hepatotoxicity in patients with rheumatoid arthritis. ACR Hotline. August 2001. *www.rheumatology.org/research/hotline/0801leflunomide.html,* with permission.

procedure in detail. The same procedure is indicated in women planning a pregnancy. Even if the washout is begun immediately after a woman notices a missed menstrual period, exposure to leflunomide during early organogenesis cannot be avoided; washouts beginning in the third week of pregnancy, however, do prevent the risk for microcephaly and mental retardation and should be instituted at once (533). Pregnancy outcome for the 160 women currently in the OTIS registry are not yet publicly available (RL Brent, personal communication, June 2003).

Levels of leflunomide metabolites in breast milk are unknown; lactation is thus not recommended if leflunomide is to be reinstituted immediately after delivery. For men taking leflunomide and wishing to father a child, the theoretical risk of a chromosomal abnormality or a point mutation is extremely small; the cholestyramine elimination procedure is not indicated for them.

End-stage Renal Disease and Dialysis

There is no clinical experience with the use of leflunomide in patients with mild-to-moderate renal impairment; as noted before, the free fraction of leflunomide is doubled in patients on hemodialysis or peritoneal dialysis. If leflunomide is used in patients with renal insufficiency, regardless of their dialysis status, close monitoring is indicated.

Hepatic Insufficiency

Leflunomide should be used with extreme caution (or not at all) in patients with preexisting and concomitant serious comorbidities, evidence of viral hepatitis (A, B, or C), liver insufficiency, history of alcohol abuse, and those receiving other potential hepatotoxic drugs.

Other Recommendations

The manufacturers of leflunomide do not recommend its use in patients with severe immunodeficiency, bone marrow dysplasia, or uncontrolled infections (513); cholestyramine should be administered to patients developing any serious toxic or allergic reaction as described in Table 32.11.

Guidelines

As noted, the ACR has issued guidelines to monitor leflunomide treatment (553). These guidelines are summarized in Tables 32.9 and 32.10.

Conclusions

Leflunomide is a DMARD that leads to suppression of T-cell proliferation with minimum effects on other cell types. The drug has proven to be efficacious for the treatment of RA, as evidenced clinically and radiographically in three large, double-blinded clinical trials. Leflunomide is generally well tolerated, with side effects ranging from mild to moderate gastrointestinal complaints, allergic reactions, alopecia, and liver enzyme elevation. In clinical trials the efficacy and safety of leflunomide have been comparable with sulfasalazine and MTX (554–556). Combination of the drug with MTX has resulted in additional benefit in patients with RA. The drug is contraindicated during (or before) pregnancy. Acute, unpredictable, and severe liver failure has been described rarely with the drug. At this point, the role of leflunomide in the management of RA remains to be determined.

REFERENCES

1. Yelin EH, Felts WR. A summary of the impact of musculoskeletal conditions in the United States. *Arthritis Rheum* 1990;33:750–755.
2. Rich E, Moreland LW, Alarcón GS. Paucity of radiographic progression in rheumatoid arthritis treated with methotrexate as the first disease-modifying anti-rheumatic drug. *J Rheumatol* 1999;26:259–261.
3. Bannwarth B, Labat L, Moride Y, et al. Methotrexate in rheumatoid arthritis. An update. *Drugs* 1994;47:25–50.
4. O'Dell JR. Methotrexate use in rheumatoid arthritis. *Rheum Dis Clin North Am* 1997;23:779–796.
5. Kremer JM. Safety, efficacy, and mortality in a long-term cohort of patients with rheumatoid arthritis taking methotrexate: followup after a mean of 13.3 years. *Arthritis Rheum* 1997;40:984–985.
6. Kremer JM. Historical overview of the treatment of rheumatoid arthritis with an emphasis on methotrexate. *J Rheumatol* 1996;23:34–37.
7. Kremer JM. Methotrexate and emerging therapies. *Rheum Dis Clin North Am* 1998;24:651–658.
8. Rau R, Schleusser B, Herborn G, et al. Longterm treatment of destructive rheumatoid arthritis with methotrexate. *J Rheumatol* 1997;24:1881–1889.
9. Gubner R, August S, Ginsberg V. Therapeutic suppression of tissue reactivity. II. Effect of aminopterin in rheumatoid arthritis and psoriasis. *Am J Med Sci* 1951;221:176–182.
10. Black RL, O'Brien WM, Van Scott EJ, et al. Methotrexate therapy in psoriatic arthritis. Double-blind study on 21 patients. *JAMA* 1964;189:743–747.
11. Williams HJ, Willkens RF, Samuelson COJ, et al. Comparison of low-dose oral pulse methotrexate and placebo in the treatment of rheumatoid arthritis. A controlled clinical trial. *Arthritis Rheum* 1985;28:721–730.
12. Williams HJ, Ward JR, Reading JC, et al. Comparison of auranofin, methotrexate, and the combination of both the treatment of rheumatoid arthritis. A controlled clinical trial. *Arthritis Rheum* 1992;35:259–269.
13. Thompson RN, Watts C, Edelman J, et al. A controlled two-centre trial of parenteral methotrexate therapy for refractory rheumatoid arthritis. *J Rheumatol* 1984;11:760–763.
14. Andersen PA, West SG, O'Dell JR, et al. Weekly pulse methotrexate in rheumatoid arthritis. Clinical and immunologic effects in a randomized, double-blind study. *Ann Intern Med* 1985;103:489–496.
15. Weinblatt ME, Coblyn JS, Fox DA, et al. Efficacy of low-dose methotrexate in rheumatoid arthritis. *N Engl J Med* 1985;312:818–822.
16. Tugwell P, Bennett K, Gent M. Methotrexate in rheumatoid arthritis. Indications, contraindications, efficacy, and safety. *Ann Intern Med* 1987;107:358–366.
17. Health and Public Policy Committee, American College of Physicians. Methotrexate in rheumatoid arthritis. *Ann Intern Med* 1987;107:418–419.
18. Alarcón GS. Methotrexate for the treatment of rheumatoid arthritis in the late 1990s. *Rheum Arthritis Idx Rev* 1999;1:4–5.
19. Carvallo AV, Wolff CF, Armas RM, et al. Artritis reumatoidea. Eficacia terapéutica del metotrexate y sus efectos hepatotóxicos. [Rheumatoid arthritis. Therapeutic efficacy of methotrexate and its hepatotoxic effects]. *Rev Med Chile* 1993;121:777–784.
20. Galindo-Rodríguez G, Avina-Zubieta JA, et al. Variations and trends in the prescription of initial second line therapy for patients with rheumatoid arthritis. *J Rheumatol* 1997;24:633–638.

21. Hanrahan PS, Scrivens GA, Russell AS. Prospective long-term follow-up of methotrexate therapy in rheumatoid arthritis: toxicity, efficacy and radiological progression. *Br J Rheumatol* 1989;28:147–153.
22. Furst DE, Erikson N, Clute L, et al. Adverse experience with methotrexate during 176 weeks of a longterm prospective trial in patients with rheumatoid arthritis. *J Rheumatol* 1990;17:1628–1635.
23. Pincus T, Callahan LF. The "side effects" of rheumatoid arthritis: joint destruction, disability and early mortality. *Br J Rheumatol* 1993;32: 28–37.
24. Jundt JW, Browne BA, Fiocco GP, et al. A comparison of low dose methotrexate bioavailability: oral solution, oral tablet, subcutaneous and intramuscular dosing. *J Rheumatol* 1993;20:1845–1849.
25. Teresi ME, Crom WR, Choi KE, et al. Methotrexate bioavailability after oral and intramuscular administration in children. *J Pediatrics* 1987;110:788–792.
26. Dupuis LL, Koren G, Silverman ED, et al. Influence of food on the bioavailability of oral methotrexate in children. *J Rheumatol* 1995; 22:1570–1573.
27. Kozloski GD, De Vito J, Kisicki JC, et al. The effect of food on the absorption of methotrexate sodium tablets in healthy volunteers. *Arthritis Rheum* 1992;35:761–764.
28. Nesher G, Mates M, Zevin S. Effect of caffeine consumption on efficacy of methotrexate in rheumatoid arthritis. *Arthritis Rheum* 2003; 48:571–572.
29. Stewart CF, Fleming RA, Germain BF, et al. Aspirin alters methotrexate disposition in rheumatoid arthritis patients. *Arthritis Rheum* 1991;34:1514–1520.
30. Bologna C, Anaya J-M, Bressolle F, et al. Correlation between methotrexate pharmacokinetic parameters, and clinical and biological status in rheumatoid arthritis patients. *Clin Exp Rheumatol* 1995;13:465–470.
31. Markham A, Faulds D. Methotrexate: a review of its pharmacodynamic and pharmacokinetic properties, and therapeutic efficacy in rheumatoid arthritis and other immunoregulatory disorders. *Clin Immunother* 1994;1:217–244.
32. Edelman J, Biggs DF, Jamali F, et al. Low-dose methotrexate kinetics in arthritis. *Clin Pharmacol Ther* 1984;35:382–386.
33. Rooney TW, Furst DE, Koehnke R, et al. Aspirin is not associated with more toxicity that other nonsteroidal antiinflammatory drugs in patients with rheumatoid arthritis treated with methotrexate. *J Rheumatol* 1993;20:1297–1302.
34. Jolivet J, Cowan KH, Curt GA, et al. The pharmacology and clinical use of methotrexate. *N Engl J Med* 1993;309:1094–1104.
35. Oguey D, Kolliker F, Gerber NJ, et al. Effect of food on the bioavailability of low-dose methotrexate in patients with rheumatoid arthritis. *Arthritis Rheum* 1992;35:611–614.
36. Hamilton RA, Kremer JM. Why intramuscular methotrexate may be more efficacious than oral dosing in patients with rheumatoid arthritis. *Br J Rheumatol* 1997;36:86–90.
37. Trenkwalder P, Eisenlohr H, Prechtel K, et al. Three cases of malignant neoplasm, pneumonitis, and pancytopenia during treatment with low-dose methotrexate. *Clin Invest* 1992;70:951–955.
38. Rheumatoid Arthritis Clinical Trial Archive Group. The effect of age and renal function on the efficacy and toxicity of methotrexate in rheumatoid arthritis. *J Rheumatol* 1995;22:218–223.
39. Bressolle F, Bologna C, Kinowski JM, et al. Effects of moderate renal insufficiency on pharmacokinetics of methotrexate in rheumatoid arthritis patients. *Ann Rheum Dis* 1998;57:110–113.
40. Wall SM, Johansen MJ, Molony DA, et al. Effective clearance of methotrexate using high-flux hemodialysis membranes. *Am J Kidney Dis* 1996;28:846–854.
41. Stewart CF, Evans WE. Drug-drug interactions with antirheumatic agents: review of selected clinically important interactions. *J Rheumatol* 1990;17:16–23.
42. Evans WE, Christensen ML. Drug interactions with methotrexate. *J Rheumatol* 1985;12:15–20.
43. Grosflam J, Weinblatt ME. Methotrexate: mechanism of action, pharmacokinetics, clinical indications, and toxicity. *Curr Opin Rheumatol* 1991;3:363–368.
44. Maricic M, Davis M, Gall EP. Megaloblastic pancytopenia in a patient receiving concurrent methotrexate and trimethoprim-sulfamethoxazole treatment. *Arthritis Rheum* 1986;29:133–135.
45. Fries JF, Singh G, Lenert L, et al. Aspirin, hydroxychloroquine, and hepatic enzyme abnormalities with methotrexate in rheumatoid arthritis. *Arthritis Rheum* 1990;33:1611–1619.
46. Anaya J-M, Fabre D, Bressolle F, et al. Effect of etodolac on methotrexate pharmacokinetics in patients with rheumatoid arthritis. *J Rheumatol* 1994;21:203–208.
47. Furst DE. Practical clinical pharmacology and drug interactions of low-dose methotrexate therapy in rheumatoid arthritis. *Br J Rheumatol* 1995;34:20–25.
48. Wallace CA, Smith AL, Sherry DD. Pilot investigation of naproxen/methotrexate interaction in patients with juvenile rheumatoid arthritis. *J Rheumatol* 1993;20:1764–1768.
49. Tett SE, Triggs EJ. Use of methotrexate in older patients. A risk-benefit assessment. *Drugs Aging* 1996;9:458–471.
50. Wolfe F, Cathey MA. The effect of age on methotrexate efficacy and toxicity. *J Rheumatol* 1991;18:973–979.
51. Baggott JE, Morgan SL, Ha T-S, et al. Antifolates in rheumatoid arthritis: a hypothetical mechanism of action. *Clin Exp Rheumatol* 1993;11(suppl):101–105.
52. Allegra CJ, Drake JC, Jolivet J, et al. Inhibition of phosphoribosylaminoimidazolecarboxamide transformylase by methotrexate and dihydrofolic acid polyglutamates. *Proc Natl Acad Sci U S A* 1985;82: 4881–4885.
53. Baggott JE, Vaughn WH, Hudson BB. Inhibition of 5-aminoimidazole-4-carboxamide ribotide transformylase, adenosine deaminase, and 5-adenylate deaminase by polyglutamates of methotrexate and oxidized folates and by 5′-aminoimidazole-4-carboxamide riboside and ribotide. *Biochem J* 1986;236:193–200.
54. Morgan SL, Baggott JE, Vaughn WH, et al. The effect of folic acid supplementation on the toxicity of low-dose methotrexate in patients with rheumatoid arthritis. *Arthritis Rheum* 1990;33:9–18.
55. Morgan SL, Baggott JE, Vaughn WH, et al. Supplementation with folic acid during methotrexate therapy for rheumatoid arthritis. A double-blind, placebo-controlled trial. *Ann Intern Med* 1994;121:833–841.
56. Joyce DA, Will RK, Hoffman DM, et al. Exacerbation of rheumatoid arthritis in patients treated with methotrexate after administration of folinic acid. *Ann Rheum Dis* 1991;50:913–914.
57. Tishler M, Caspi D, Fishel B, et al. The effects of leucovorin (folinic acid) on methotrexate therapy in rheumatoid arthritis patients. *Arthritis Rheum* 1988;31:906–908.
58. Cronstein BN, Eberle MA, Gruber HE, et al. Methotrexate inhibits neutrophil function by stimulating adenosine release from connective tissue cells. *Proc Natl Acad Sci U S A* 1991;88:2441–2445.
59. Cronstein BN. Leukocyte–endothelial interactions as a target for anti-inflammatory drugs: the mechanisms of action of colchicine and methotrexate. *Cliniguide Rheumatol* 1993;3:1–8.
60. Cronstein BN. The mechanism of action of methotrexate. *Rheum Dis Clin North Am* 1997;23:739–755.
61. Cronstein BN. Review: Molecular therapeutics: methotrexate and its mechanism of action. *Arthritis Rheum* 1996;39:1951–1960.
62. Cronstein BN, Naime D, Ostad E. The antiinflammatory mechanism of methotrexate. Increased adenosine release at inflamed sites diminishes leukocyte accumulation in an *in vivo* model of inflammation. *J Clin Invest* 1993;92:2675–2682.
63. Hausknecht RU. Methotrexate and misoprostol to terminate early pregnancy. *N Engl J Med* 1995;333:537–540.
64. Asako H, Wolf RE, Granger DN. Leukocyte adherence in rat mesenteric venules: effects of adenosine and methotrexate. *Gastroenterology* 1993;104:31–37.
65. Asako H, Kubes P, Baethge BA, et al. Colchicine and methotrexate reduce leukocyte adherence and emigration in rat mesenteric venules. *Inflammation* 1992;16:45–56.
66. Meyer FA, Yaron I, Mashiah V, et al. Methotrexate inhibits proliferation but not IL-1 stimulated secretory activities of cultured human synovial fibroblast. *J Rheumatol* 1993;20:238–242.
67. Polisson RP, Dooley MA, Dawson DV, et al. Interleukin-2 receptor levels in the sera of rheumatoid arthritis patients treated with methotrexate. *Arthritis Rheum* 1994;37:50–56.
68. Segal R, Mozes E, Yaron M, et al. The effects of methotrexate on the production and activity of interleukin-1. *Arthritis Rheum* 1989;32:370–377.
69. Wascher TC, Hermann J, Brezinschek R, et al. Serum levels of interleukin-6 and tumour-necrosis-factor-alpha are not correlated to disease activity in patients with rheumatoid arthritis after treatment with low-dose methotrexate. *Eur J Clin Invest* 1994;24:73–75.
70. Barrera P, Boerbooms AM, Demacker PN, et al. Circulating concentrations and production of cytokines and soluble receptors in rheumatoid arthritis patients: effects of a single dose methotrexate. *Br J Rheumatol* 1994;33:1017–1024.

71. Constantin A, Loubet-Lescoulie P, Lambert N, et al. Antiinflammatory and immunoregulatory action of methotrexate in the treatment of rheumatoid arthritis: evidence of increased interleukin-4 and interleukin-10 gene expression demonstrated *in vitro* by competitive reverse transcriptase-polymerase chain reaction. *Arthritis Rheum* 1998; 41:48–57.
72. Sperling RI, Coblyn JS, Larkin JK, et al. Inhibition of leukotriene B_4 synthesis in neutrophils from patients with rheumatoid arthritis by a single oral dose of methotrexate. *Arthritis Rheum* 1990;33:1149–1155.
73. Sperling RI, Benincaso AI, Anderson RJ, et al. Acute and chronic suppression of leukotriene B_4 synthesis *ex vivo* in neutrophils from patients with rheumatoid arthritis beginning treatment with methotrexate. *Arthritis Rheum* 1992;35:376–383.
74. Michaels RM, Chang ZL, Beezhold DH. Phospholipase A_2 activity in peripheral blood cells of rheumatoid arthritis patients treated with methotrexate: a preliminary study. *Clin Exp Rheumatol* 1994;12:643–648.
75. Michaels RM, Reading JC, Beezhold DH, et al. Serum phospholipase A_2 activity in patients with rheumatoid arthritis before and after treatment with methotrexate, auranofin, or combination of the two. *J Rheumatol* 1996;23:226–229.
76. Johnston CA, Russell AS, Kovithavongs T, et al. Measures of immunologic and inflammatory responses *in vitro* in rheumatoid patients treated with methotrexate. *J Rheumatol* 1986;13:294–296.
77. May KP, West SG, McDermott MT, et al. The effect of low-dose methotrexate on bone metabolism and histomorphometry in rats. *Arthritis Rheum* 1994;37:201–206.
78. Johnston C, Russell AS, Aaron S. The effect of *in vivo* and *in vitro* methotrexate on lymphocyte proliferation as measured by the uptake of tritiated thymidine and tritiated guanosine. *Clin Exp Rheumatol* 1988;6:391–393.
79. Alarcón GS, Everson MP, Krumdieck CL, et al. Activated lymphocytes in peripheral blood of patients with rheumatoid arthritis. *J Rheumatol* 1990;17:1712.
80. Hine RJ, Everson MP, Hardin JM, et al. Methotrexate therapy in rheumatoid arthritis patients diminishes lectin-induced mononuclear cell proliferation. *Rheumatol Int* 1990;10:165–169.
81. Olsen NJ, Murray LM. Antiproliferative effects of methotrexate on peripheral blood mononuclear cells. *Arthritis Rheum* 1989;32:378–385.
82. Olsen NJ, Callahan LF, Pincus T. Immunologic studies of rheumatoid arthritis patients treated with methotrexate. *Arthritis Rheum* 1987;30: 481–488.
83. Martini A. Association of methotrexate treatment with a decrease of double negative (CD4-CD8) and gamma/delta T cell levels in patients with juvenile rheumatoid arthritis. *J Rheumatol* 1993;20:1944–1948.
84. Genestier L, Paillot R, Fournel S, et al. Immunosuppressive properties of methotrexate: apoptosis and clonal deletion of activated peripheral T cells. *J Clin Invest* 1998;102:322–328.
85. Altz-Smith M, Kendall LG Jr, Stamm AM. Cryptococcosis associated with low-dose methotrexate for arthritis. *Am J Med* 1987;83:179–181.
86. Perruquet JL, Harrington TM, Davis DE. *Pneumocystis carinii* pneumonia following methotrexate therapy for rheumatoid arthritis. *Arthritis Rheum* 1983;26:1291–1292.
87. Salinier L, Jaureguilberry JP, Carloz E, et al. Methotrexate, prednisone: adverse reactions (serious), cytomegalovirus pneumonia. *Rev Intern Med* 1992;13(suppl 6):223.
88. Antonelli MA, Moreland LW, Brick JE. Herpes zoster in patients with rheumatoid arthritis treated with weekly, low-dose methotrexate. *Am J Med* 1991;90:295–298.
89. Cornelissen JJ, Bakker LJ, Van der Veen MJ, et al. *Nocardia asteroides* pneumonia complicating low dose methotrexate treatment of refractory rheumatoid arthritis. *Ann Rheum Dis* 1991;50:642–644.
90. Clerc D, Brousse C, Mariette X, et al. Cytomegalovirus pneumonia in a patient with rheumatoid arthritis treated with low dose methotrexate and prednisone. *Ann Rheum Dis* 1991;48:247–249.
91. Godeau B, Coutant-Perronne V, Le Thi Huong D, et al. *Pneumocystis carinii* pneumonia in the course of connective tissue disease: report of 34 cases. *J Rheumatol* 1994;21:246–251.
92. Law KF, Aranda CP, Smith RL, et al. Pulmonary cryptococcosis mimicking methotrexate pneumonitis. *J Rheumatol* 1993;20:872–873.
93. Shiroky JB, Frost A, Skeleton JD, et al. Complications of immunosuppression associated with weekly low dose methotrexate. *J Rheumatol* 1991;18:1172–1175.
94. Frieden TR, Bia FJ, Heald PW, et al. Cutaneous cryptococcosis in a patient with cutaneous T cell lymphoma receiving therapy with photopheresis and methotrexate. *Clin Infect Dis* 1993;17:776–778.
95. LeMense GP, Sahn SA. Opportunistic infection during treatment with low dose methotrexate. *Am J Respir Crit Care Med* 1994;150: 258–260.
96. Wollner AA, Mohle-Boetani J, Lambert RE, et al. *Pneumocystis carinii* pneumonia complicating low dose methotrexate treatment for rheumatoid arthritis. *Thorax* 1991;46:205–207.
97. Thomas E, Olive P, Mazyad H, et al. Cytomegalovirus-induced pneumonia in a rheumatoid arthritis patient treated with low dose methotrexate. *Clin Exp Rheumatol* 1997;15:583–584.
98. Stenger AA, Houtman PM, Bruyn GA, et al. *Pneumocystis carinii* pneumonia associated with low dose methotrexate treatment for rheumatoid arthritis. *Scand J Rheumatol* 1994;23:51–53.
99. Wyss E, Kuhn M, Luzi HP, et al. Fatal verlaufende *Pneumocystis-carinii*-pneumonie unter low-dose-methotrexat-und prednison-therapie wegen chronischer polyarthritis. [Fatal outcome of *Pneumocystis-carinii* pneumonia under low-dose methotrexate and prednisone therapy for chronic rheumatoid arthritis]. *Schweiz Rundsch Med Prax* 1994;83:449–452.
100. Aglas R, Rainer F, Hermann J, et al. Interstitial pneumonia due to cytomegalovirus following low-dose methotrexate treatment for rheumatoid arthritis. *Arthritis Rheum* 1995;38:291–292.
101. Ching DW. Severe, disseminated, life threatening herpes zoster infection in a patient with rheumatoid arthritis treated with methotrexate. *Ann Rheum Dis* 1995;54:155.
102. Roux N, Flipo RM, Cortet B, et al. *Pneumocystis carinii* pneumonia in rheumatoid arthritis patients treated with methotrexate. A report of two cases. *Rev Rheum* 1996;63:453–456.
103. Aspe de la Iglesia B, Sanchez-Burson J, Grana-Gil J, et al. Pancitopenia e infecciones oportunistas en artritis reumatoid tratada con metotrexato. [Pancytopenia and opportunistic infections in rheumatoid arthritis treated with methotrexate.] *Rev Clin Esp* 1990;187: 208–209.
104. Lang B, Riegel W, Peters T, et al. Low dose methotrexate therapy for rheumatoid arthritis complicated by pancytopenia and *Pneumocystis carinii* pneumonia. *J Rheumatol* 1991;18:1257–1259.
105. Lyon CC, Thompson D. Herpes zoster encephalomyelitis associated with low dose methotrexate for rheumatoid arthritis. *J Rheumatol* 1997;24:589–591.
106. Golden HE. Herpes zoster encephalomyelitis in a patient with rheumatoid arthritis treated with low dose methotrexate. *J Rheumatol* 1998;24:2487–2488.
107. McCambridge NM, Vogelgesang SA, Ockenhouse CF. *Listeria monocytogenes* infection in a patient treated with methotrexate for rheumatoid arthritis. *J Rheumatol* 1995;22:786–787.
108. O'Reilly S, Hartley P, Jeffers M, et al. Invasive pulmonary aspergillosis associated with low dose methotrexate therapy for rheumatoid arthritis: a case report of treatment with itraconazole. *Tubercle Lung Dis* 1994;75:153–155.
109. Flood DA, Chan CK, Pruzanski W. *Pneumocystis carinii* pneumonia associated with methotrexate therapy in rheumatoid arthritis. *J Rheumatol* 1991;18:1254–1256.
110. Kitsuwa S, Matsunaga K, Kawai M, et al. Pancytopenia and *Pneumocystis carinii* pneumonia associated with low dose methotrexate pulse therapy for rheumatoid arthritis—case report and review of literature. *Ryumachi* 1996;36:551–558.
111. Okuda Y, Oyama T, Oyama H, et al. *Pneumocystis carinii* pneumonia associated with low dose methotrexate treatment for malignant rheumatoid arthritis. *Ryumachi* 1995;35:699–704.
112. Chervrel G, Brantus JF, Sainte-Laudy J, et al. Allergic pancytopenia to trimethoprim-sulphamethoxazole for *Pneumocystis carinii* pneumonia following methotrexate treatment for rheumatoid arthritis. *Rheumatology* 1999;38:475–476.
113. Van der Veen MJ, van der Heide A, Kruize AA, et al. Infection rate and use of antibiotics in patients with rheumatoid arthritis treated with methotrexate. *Ann Rheum Dis* 1994;53:224–228.
114. Hernandez-Cruz B, Cardiel MH, Villa AR, et al. Development, recurrence, and severity of infections in Mexican patients with RA: a nested case-control study. *J Rheumatol* 1999;25:1900–1907.
115. Boerbooms AM, Kerstens PJ, van Loenhout JW, et al. Infections during low-dose methotrexate treatment in rheumatoid arthritis. *Semin Arthritis Rheum* 1995;24:411–421.

116. Paulus HE. FDA Arthritis Advisory Committee meeting: Methotrexate; guidelines for the clinical evaluation of antiinflammatory drugs; DMSO in scleroderma. *Arthritis Rheum* 1986;29:1289–1290.
117. Groff GD, Shenberger, Wilke WS, et al. Low dose oral methotrexate in rheumatoid arthritis: an uncontrolled trial and review of the literature. *Semin Arthritis Rheum* 1983;12:333–347.
118. Hoffmeister RT. Methotrexate therapy in rheumatoid arthritis: 15 years experience. *Am J Med* 1983;75:69–73.
119. Kremer JM, Lee JK. The safety and efficacy of the use of methotrexate in long-term therapy for rheumatoid arthritis. *Arthritis Rheum* 1986;29:822–831.
120. Weinblatt ME, Weissman BN, Holdsworth DE, et al. Long-term prospective study of methotrexate in the treatment of rheumatoid arthritis. 84-month update. *Arthritis Rheum* 1992;35:129–137.
121. Kremer JM, Lee JK. A long-term prospective study of the use of methotrexate in rheumatoid arthritis. Update after a mean of fifty-three months. *Arthritis Rheum* 1992;31:577–584.
122. Weinblatt ME, Trentham DE, Fraser PA, et al. Long-term prospective trial of low-dose methotrexate in rheumatoid arthritis. *Arthritis Rheum* 1988;31:167–175.
123. Kremer JM, Phelps CT. Long-term prospective study of the use of methotrexate in the treatment of rheumatoid arthritis. Update after a mean of 90 months. *Arthritis Rheum* 1992;35:138–145.
124. Drosos AA, Psychos D, Andonopoulos AP, et al. Methotrexate therapy in rheumatoid arthritis. A two year prospective follow-up. *Clin Rheumatol* 1990;9:333–341.
125. Willkens RF, Watson MA, Paxson CS. Low dose pulse methotrexate therapy in rheumatoid arthritis. *J Rheumatol* 1980;7:501–505.
126. Weinblatt ME, Maier AL. Longterm experience with low dose weekly methotrexate in rheumatoid arthritis. *J Rheumatol* 1990;17:33–38.
127. Weinblatt ME, Kaplan H, Germain BF, et al. Methotrexate in rheumatoid arthritis: effects on disease activity in multicenter prospective study. *J Rheumatol* 1991;18:334–338.
128. Buchbinder R, Hall S, Sambrook PN, et al. Methotrexate therapy in rheumatoid arthritis: a life table review of 587 patients treated in community practice. *J Rheumatol* 1993;20:639–644.
129. Abu-Shakra M, Gladman DD, Thorne JC, et al. Longterm methotrexate therapy in psoriatic arthritis: clinical and radiological outcome. *J Rheumatol* 1995;22:241–245.
130. McKendry RJ, Dale P. Adverse effects of low dose methotrexate therapy in rheumatoid arthritis. *J Rheumatol* 1993;20:1850–1856.
131. Nolla JM, Roig D, Lopez JA, et al. Metotrexato en la artritis reumatoidea. [Methotrexate in rheumatoid arthritis.] *Rev Esp Reumatol* 1988;15:49–53.
132. Kremer JM, Rynes RI, Bartholomew LE. Severe flare of rheumatoid arthritis after discontinuation of long-term methotrexate therapy. Double-blind study. *Am J Med* 1987;82:781–786.
133. Alarcón GS, Guyton JM, Acton RT, et al. DR2 positivity and response to methotrexate in rheumatoid arthritis. *Arthritis Rheum* 1986;29:151.
134. Alarcón GS, Billingsley LM, Clegg DO, et al. Lack of association between HLA-DR2 and clinical response to methotrexate in patients with rheumatoid arthritis. *Arthritis Rheum* 1987;30:218–220.
135. Urano W, Taniguchi A, Yamanaka H, et al. Polymorphisms in the methylenetetrahydrofolate reductase gene were associated with both the efficacy and the toxicity of methotrexate used for the treatment of rheumatoid arthritis, as evidenced by single locus and haplotype analyses. *Pharmacogenetics* 2002;12:183–190.
136. Alarcón GS, Tracy IC, Blackburn WD Jr. Methotrexate in rheumatoid arthritis. Toxic effects as the major factor in limiting long-term treatment. *Arthritis Rheum* 1989;32:671–676.
137. Alarcón GS, Tracy IC, Strand GM, et al. Survival and drug discontinuation analyses in a large cohort of methotrexate-treated rheumatoid arthritis patients. *Ann Rheum Dis* 1995;54:708–712.
138. Wilke WS, Mackenzie AH, Scherbel AL, et al. Toxicity from methotrexate may be dose related. *Arthritis Rheum* 1983;119–120.
139. Weinblatt ME, Kaplan H, Germain BF, et al. Low-dose methotrexate compared with auranofin in adult rheumatoid arthritis. A thirty-six-week, double-blind trial. *Arthritis Rheum* 1990;33:330–338.
140. López-Méndez A, Daniel WW, Reading JC, et al. Radiographic assessment of disease progression in rheumatoid arthritis patients enrolled in the Cooperative Systemic Studies of the Rheumatic Diseases Program randomized clinical trial of methotrexate, auranofin, or a combination of the two. *Arthritis Rheum* 1993;36:1364–1369.
141. Hamdy H, McKendry RJ, Mierins E, et al. Low-dose methotrexate compared with azathioprine in the treatment of rheumatoid arthritis. A twenty four-week controlled clinical trial. *Arthritis Rheum* 1987;30:361–367.
142. Felson DT, Anderson JJ, Meenan RF. The comparative efficacy and toxicity of second-line drugs in rheumatoid arthritis. Results of two metaanalyses. *Arthritis Rheum* 1990;33:1449–1461.
143. Hurst S, Kallan MJ, Wolfe FJ, et al. Methotrexate, hydroxychloroquine, and intramuscular gold in rheumatoid arthritis: relative area under the curve effectiveness and sequence effects. *J Rheumatol* 2002;29:1639–1645.
144. Strand V, Cohen S, Schiff M, et al. Treatment of active rheumatoid arthritis with leflunomide compared with placebo and methotrexate. *Arch Intern Med* 1999;159:2542–2550.
145. Emery P, Breedveld FC, Lemmel EM, et al. A comparison of the efficacy and safety of leflunomide and methotrexate for the treatment of rheumatoid arthritis. *Rheumatology* 2000;39:655–665.
146. Lipsky PE, van der Heijde DM, St Clair EW, et al. Infliximab and methotrexate in the treatment of rheumatoid arthritis. *N Engl J Med* 2000;343:1594–1602.
147. Bathon JM, Martin RW, Fleischmann RM, et al. A comparison of etanercept and methotrexate in patients with early rheumatoid arthritis. *N Engl J Med* 2000;343:1586–1593.
148. den Broeder AA, Joosten LA, Saxne T, et al. Long term anti-tumour necrosis factor alpha monotherapy in rheumatoid arthritis: effect on radiological course and prognostic value of markers of cartilage turnover and endothelial activation. *Ann Rheum Dis* 2002;61:311–318.
149. Weinblatt ME, Keystone EC, Furst DE, et al. Adalimumab, a fully human anti-tumor necrosis factor alpha monoclonal antibody, for the treatment of rheumatoid arthritis in patients taking concomitant methotrexate: the ARMADA trial. *Arthritis Rheum* 2003;48:35–45.
150. Cohen S, Hurd E, Cush J, et al. Treatment of rheumatoid arthritis with anakinra, a recombinant human interleukin-1 receptor antagonist, in combination with methotrexate: results of a twenty-four-week, multicenter, randomized, double-blind, placebo-controlled trial. *Arthritis Rheum* 2002;46:614–624.
151. Nordstrom DM, West SG, Andersen PA, et al. Pulse methotrexate therapy in rheumatoid arthritis. A controlled prospective roentgenographic study. *Ann Intern Med* 1987;107:797–801.
152. Jeurissen ME, Boerbooms AM, van de Putte LB, et al. Influence of methotrexate and azathioprine on radiologic progression in rheumatoid arthritis. A randomized, double-blind study. *Ann Intern Med* 1991;114:999–1004.
153. Rau R, Herborn G, Karger T, et al. Retardation of radiologic progression in rheumatoid arthritis with methotrexate therapy. A controlled study. *Arthritis Rheum* 1991;34:1236–1244.
154. Weinblatt ME, Polisson R, Blotner SD, et al. The effects of drug therapy on radiographic progression of rheumatoid arthritis. Results of a 36-week randomized trial comparing methotrexate and auranofin. *Arthritis Rheum* 1993;36:613–619.
155. Drosos AA, Karantanas AH, Psychos D, et al. Can treatment with methotrexate influence the radiological progression of rheumatoid arthritis? *Clin Rheumatol* 1990;9:342–345.
156. Sany J, Kaliski S, Couret M, et al. Radiologic progression during intramuscular methotrexate treatment of rheumatoid arthritis. *J Rheumatol* 1990;17:1636–1641.
157. Reykdal S, Steinsson K, Sigurjonsson K, et al. Methotrexate treatment of rheumatoid arthritis: Effects on radiological progression. *Scand J Rheumatol* 1989;18:221–226.
158. Wassenberg S, Rau R. Radiographic healing with sustained clinical remission in a patient with rheumatoid arthritis receiving methotrexate monotherapy. *Arthritis Rheum* 2002;46:2804–2807.
159. Alarcón GS, López-Méndez A, Walter J, et al. Radiographic evidence of disease progression in methotrexate treated and non-methotrexate disease modifying antirheumatic drug treated rheumatoid arthritis patients: a meta-analysis. *J Rheumatol* 1992;19:1868–1873.
160. Pincus T, Ferraccioli G, Sokka T, et al. Evidence from clinical trials and long-term observational studies that disease-modifying anti-rheumatic drugs slow radiographic progression in rheumatoid arthritis: updating a 1983 review. *Rheumatology* 2002;41:1346–1356.

161. Kerstens PJ, Boerbooms AM, Jeurissen ME, et al. Radiological and clinical results of longterm treatment of rheumatoid arthritis with methotrexate and azathioprine. *J Rheumatol* 2000;27:1148–1155.
162. Rau R, Herborn G, Menninger H, et al. Radiographic outcome after three years of patients with early erosive rheumatoid arthritis treated with intramuscular methotrexate or parenteral gold. Extension of a one-year double-blind study in 174 patients. Rheumatology 2002; 41:196–204.
163. Jones G, Halbert J, Crotty M, et al. The effect of treatment on radiological progression in rheumatoid arthritis: a systematic review of randomized placebo-controlled trials. *Rheumatology* 2003;42:6–13.
164. Mladenovic V, Domljan Z, Rozman B, et al. Safety and effectiveness of leflunomide in the treatment of patients with active rheumatoid arthritis. Results of a randomized, placebo-controlled, phase II study. *Arthritis Rheum* 1995;38:1595–1603.
165. Genovese MC, Bathon JM, Martin RW, et al. Etanercept versus methotrexate in patients with early rheumatoid arthritis: two-year radiographic and clinical outcomes. *Arthritis Rheum* 2002;46:1443–1450.
166. De La Mata J, Blanco FJ, Gomez-Reino JJ. Survival analysis of disease modifying antirheumatic drugs in Spanish rheumatoid arthritis patients. *Ann Rheum Dis* 1995;54:881–885.
167. Fries JF, Williams CA, Ramey D, et al. The relative toxicity of disease-modifying antirheumatic drugs. *Arthritis Rheum* 1993;36:297–306.
168. Nyfors A. Benefits and adverse drug experiences during long-term methotrexate treatment of 248 psoriatics. *Dan Med Bull* 1978;25: 208–211.
169. Sandoval DM, Alarcón GS, Morgan SL. Adverse events in methotrexate-treated rheumatoid arthritis patients. *Br J Rheumatol* 1995; 34:49–56.
170. van Ede AE, Laan RF, Blom HJ, et al. The C677T mutation in the methylenetetrahydrofolate reductase gene: a genetic risk factor for methotrexate-related elevation of liver enzymes in rheumatoid arthritis patients. *Arthritis Rheum* 2001;44:2525–2530.
171. Walker AM, Funch D, Dreyer NA, et al. Determinants of serious liver disease among patients receiving low-dose methotrexate for rheumatoid arthritis. *Arthritis Rheum* 1993;36:329–335.
172. Kremer JM, Galivan J, Streckfuss A, et al. Methotrexate metabolism analysis in blood and liver of rheumatoid arthritis patients. Association with hepatic folate deficiency and formation of polyglutamates. *Arthritis Rheum* 1986;29:832–835.
173. Kamen BA, Nylen PA, Camitta BM, et al. Methotrexate accumulation and folate depletion in cells as a possible mechanism of chronic toxicity to the drug. *Br J Haematol* 1981;49:355–360.
174. Gispen JG, Alarcón GS, Johnson JJ, et al. Toxicity to methotrexate in rheumatoid arthritis. *J Rheumatol* 1987;14:74–79.
175. Mackinnon SK, Starkebaum G, Willkens RF. Pancytopenia associated with low dose pulse methotrexate in the treatment of rheumatoid arthritis. *Semin Arthritis Rheum* 1985;15:119–126.
176. Basin KS, Escalante A, Beardmore TD. Severe pancytopenia in a patient taking low dose methotrexate and probenecid. *J Rheumatol* 1991;18:608–610.
177. Brown MA, Corrigan AB. Pancytopenia after accidental overdose of methotrexate. A complication of low-dose therapy for rheumatoid arthritis. *Med J Aust* 1991;155:493–494.
178. Al-Awadhi A, Dale P, McKendry RJ. Pancytopenia associated with low dose methotrexate therapy. A regional survey. *J Rheumatol* 1993; 20:1121–1124.
179. Casserly CM, Stange KC, Chren MM. Severe megaloblastic anemia in a patient receiving low-dose methotrexate for psoriasis. *J Am Acad Dermatol* 1993;29:477–480.
180. Akoun GM, Gauthier-Rahman S, Mayaud CM, et al. Leukocyte migration inhibition in methotrexate-induced pneumonitis. Evidence for an immunologic cell-mediated mechanism. *Chest* 1987;91:96–98.
181. Tanaka Y, Shiozawa K, Nishibayashi Y, et al. Methotrexate induced early onset pancytopenia in rheumatoid arthritis: Drug allergy? Idiosyncrasy? *J Rheumatol* 1992;19:1320–1321.
182. Berthelot J-M, Maugars Y, Prost A. Pancytopenia secondary to methotrexate therapy in rheumatoid arthritis: comment on the article by Gutierrez-Ureña et al. *Arthritis Rheum* 1997;40:193.
183. Berthelot JM, Maugars Y, Hamidou M, et al. Pancytopenia and severe cytopenia induced by low-dose methotrexate. Eight case-reports and a review of one hundred cases from the literautre (with twenty-four deaths). *Rev Rheum* 1995;62:477–486.
184. Bernini JC, Fort DW, Griener JC, et al. Aminophylline for methotrexate-induced neurotoxicity. *Lancet* 1995;345:544–547.
185. Bolla G, Disdier P, Harle JR, et al. Concurrent acute megaloblastic anaemia and pneumonitis: a severe side-effect of low-dose methotrexate therapy during rheumatoid arthritis. *Clin Rheumatol* 1993;12: 535–537.
186. Laroche F, Perrot S, Menkes CJ. Pancytopenies au cours de la polyarthrite rhumatoide traitée par methotrexate. [Pancytopenia in rheumatoid arthritis treated with methotrexate.] *Presse Med* 1996; 25:1144–1146.
187. Bruyn GA, Velthuysen E, Joosten P, et al. Pancytopenia related eosinophilia in rheumatoid arthritis: a specific methotrexate phenomenon? *J Rheumatol* 1995;22:1373–1376.
188. Franck H, Rau R, Herborn G. Thrombocytopenia in patients with rheumatoid arthritis on long-term treatment with low dose methotrexate. *Clin Rheumatol* 1996;15:266–270.
189. Gutierrez-Ureña S, Molina JF, García CO, et al. Pancytopenia secondary to methotrexate therapy in rheumatoid arthritis. *Arthritis Rheum* 1996;39:272–276.
190. Thevenet JP, Ristori JM, Cure H, et al. Pancytopenie au cours du traitement d'une polyarthrite rheumatoide par methotrexate après administration de trimethoprime-sulfamethoxazole. [Pancytopenia during treatment of rheumatoid arthritis with methotrexate after administration of trimethoprim-sulfamethoxazole.] *Presse Med* 1987; 16:1487.
191. Kevat SG, Hill WR, McCarthy PJ, Ahern MJ. Pancytopenia induced by low-dose methotrexate for rheumatoid arthritis. *Aust N Z J Med* 1988;18:697–700.
192. Maignen F, Guillot B, Pierron E, et al. L'intoxication aigue au methotrexate: à propos de 16 cas rapportes au Centre Anti-Poisons de Paris et revue de la litterature. [Acute methotrexate poisoning: apropos of 16 cases reported to the Paris Poison Control Center and review of the literature.] *Therapie* 1996;51:527–531.
193. Mayall B, Poggi G, Parkin JD. Neutropenia due to low-dose methotrexate therapy for psoriasis and rheumatoid arthritis may be fatal. *Med J Aust* 1991;155:480–484.
194. Noskov SM. Megaloblastic pancytopenia in a female patient with rheumatoid arthritis given methotrexate and amidopyrine simultaneously. [Megaloblasticheskaia pantsitopeniia u bol'noi revmatoidnym artritom pri odnovremennom primeneniem metotreksata i amidopirina.] *Ter Arkh* 1990;62:122–123.
195. Porawska W. Overdose of methotrexate with a fatal outcome in a patient with rheumatoid arthritis. [Przedawkowanie metotreksatu przyczyna zgonu chorej na reumatoidalne zapalenie stawow.] *Polskie Archi Med Wewnet* 1995;93:346–350.
196. Park GT, Jeon DW, Roh KH, et al. A case of pancytopenia secondary to low-dose pulse methotrexate therapy in a patient with rheumatoid arthritis and renal insufficiency. *Korean J Intern Med* 1999;14: 85–87.
197. Chatham WW, Morgan SL, Calvo F, et al. Renal failure, a risk factor for methotrexate toxicity. *Arthritis Rheum* 2000;43:1185–1186.
198. Calvo-Romero JM. Severe pancytopenia associated with low-dose methotrexate therapy for rheumatoid arthritis. *Ann Pharmacother* 2001;35:1575–1577.
199. Nakamura M, Sakemi T, Nagasawa K. Severe pancytopenia caused by a single administration of low dose methotrexate in a patient undergoing hemodialysis. *J Rheumatol* 1999;26:1424–1425.
200. Weinblatt ME, Fraser P. Elevated mean corpuscular volume as a predictor of hematologic toxicity due to methotrexate therapy. *Arthritis Rheum* 1989;32:1592–1596.
201. Groenendal H, Rampen FH. Methotrexate and trimethoprim-sulphamethoxazole—a potentially hazardous combination. *Clin Exp Dermatol* 1990;15:358–360.
202. Thomas MH, Gutterman LA. Methotrexate toxicity in a patient receiving trimethoprim-sulfamethoxazole. *J Rheumatol* 1986;13:440–441.
203. Naides SJ. Acute parvovirus B19-induced pancytopenia in the setting of methotrexate therapy for rheumatoid arthritis. *Arthritis Rheum* 1995;38:1023.
204. Myllykangas-Luosujarvi R, Aho K, Isomaki H. Death attributed to antirheumatic medication in a nationwide series of 1666 patients with rheumatoid arthritis who have died. *J Rheumatol* 1995;22: 2214–2217.

205. Lomaestro BM, Lesar TS, Hager TP. Errors in prescribing methotrexate. *JAMA* 1992;268:2031–2032.
206. Gibbon BN, Manthey DE. Pediatric case of accidental oral overdose of methotrexate. *Ann Emerg Med* 1999;34:98–100.
207. White-O'Keefe QE, Fye KH, Sack KD. Methotrexate and histologic abnormalities: a meta-analysis. *Am J Med* 1991;70:711–716.
208. Bjorkman DJ, Boschert M, Tolman KG, et al. The effect of long-term methotrexate therapy on hepatic fibrosis in rheumatoid arthritis. *Arthritis Rheum* 1993;36:1691–1696.
209. Aponte J, Petrelli M. Histopathologic findings in the liver of rheumatoid arthritis patients treated with long-term bolus methotrexate. *Arthritis Rheum* 1988;31:1457–1464.
210. Kremer JM, Lee RG, Tolman KG. Liver histology in rheumatoid arthritis patients receiving long-term methotrexate therapy. A prospective study with baseline and sequential biopsy samples. *Arthritis Rheum* 1989;32:121–127.
211. Bridges SL, Jr., Alarcón GS, Koopman WJ. Methotrexate-induced liver abnormalities in rheumatoid arthritis. *J Rheumatol* 1989;16: 1180–1183.
212. Robinson JK, Baughman RD, Auerbach R, et al. Methotrexate hepatotoxicity in psoriasis. Consideration of liver biopsies at regular intervals. *Arch Dermatol* 1980;116:413–415.
213. Dahl MG, Gregory MM, Scheuer PJ. Methotrexate hepatotoxicity in psoriasis—comparison of different dose regimens. *BMJ* 1972;1: 654–656.
214. Ahern MJ, Kevat S, Hill W, et al. Hepatic methotrexate content and progression of hepatic fibrosis: preliminary findings. *Ann Intern Med* 1991;50:477–480.
215. Phillips CA, Cera PJ, Mangan TF, et al. Clinical liver disease in patients with rheumatoid arthritis taking methotrexate. *J Rheumatol* 1992;19:229–233.
216. Boffa MJ, Chalmers RJ, Haboubi NY, et al. Sequential liver biopsies during long-term methotrexate treatment for psoriasis: a reappraisal. *Br J Dermatol* 1995;133:774–778.
217. Bjorkman DJ, Hammond EH, Lee RG, et al. Hepatic ultrastructure after methotrexate therapy for rheumatoid arthritis. *Arthritis Rheum* 1988;31:1465–1472.
218. Minocha A, Dean HA, Pittsley RA. Liver cirrhosis in rheumatoid arthritis patients treated with long-term methotrexate. *Vet Hum Toxicol* 1993;35:45–48.
219. Beyeler C, Reichen J, Thomann SR, et al. Quantitative liver function in patients with rheumatoid arthritis treated with low-dose methotrexate: a longitudinal study. *Br J Rheumatol* 1997;36:338–344.
220. Malatjalian DA, Ross JB, Willians CN, et al. Methotrexate hepatotoxicity in psoriatics: report of 104 patients from Nova Scotia, with analysis of risks from obesity, diabetes and alcohol consumption during long term follow-up. *Can J Gastroenterol* 1996;10:369 375.
221. Shergy WJ, Polisson RP, Caldwell DS, et al. Methotrexate-associated hepatotoxicity. retrospective analysis of 210 patients with rheumatoid arthritis. *Am J Med* 1988;85:711–774.
222. Zachariae H, Kragballe K, Sogaard H. Methotrexate induced liver cirrhosis. Studies including serial liver biopsies during continued treatment. *Br J Dermatol* 1980;102:407–512.
223. ter Borg EJ, Seldenrijk CA, Timmer R. Liver cirrhosis due to methotrexate in a patient with rheumatoid arthritis. *Neth J Med* 1996;49: 244–246.
224. West SG. Methotrexate hepatotoxicity. *Rheum Dis Clin North Am* 1997;23:883–915.
225. Seideman P, Albertioni F, Beck O, et al. Chloroquine reduces the bioavailability of methotrexate in patients with rheumatoid arthritis. A possible mechanism of reduced hepatotoxicity. *Arthritis Rheum* 1994;37:830–833.
226. Ros S, Juanola X, Condon E, et al. Light and electron microscopic analysis of liver biopsy samples from rheumatoid arthritis patients receiving long-term methotrexate therapy. *Scand J Rheumatol* 2002; 31:330–336.
227. Kujala GA, Shamma'a JM, Chang WL, et al. Hepatitis with bridging fibrosis and reversible hepatic insufficiency in a woman with rheumatoid arthritis taking methotrexate. *Arthritis Rheum* 1990;33: 1037–1041.
228. Clegg DO, Furst DE, Tolman KG, et al. Acute, reversible hepatic failure associated with methotrexate treatment of rheumatoid arthritis. *J Rheumatol* 1989;16:1123–1126.
229. Hakim NS, Kobienia B, Benedetti E, et al. Methotrexate-induced hepatic necrosis requiring liver transplantation in a patient with rheumatoid arthritis. *Int Surv* 1998;83:224–225.
230. Fathi NH, Mitros F, Hoffman J, et al. Longitudinal measurement of methotrexate liver concentrations does not correlate with liver damage, clinical efficacy, or toxicity during a 3.5 year double blind study in rheumatoid arthritis. *J Rheumatol* 2002;29:2092.
231. Bills LJ, Seibert D, Brick JE. Liver disease, erroneously attributed to methotrexate, in a patient with rheumatoid arthritis. *J Rheumatol* 1992;19:1963–1965.
232. Hilsden RJ, Urbanski SJ, Swain MG. End-stage liver disease developing with the use of methotrexate in heterozygous a1-antitrypsin deficiency. *Arthritis Rheum* 1995;38:1014–1018.
233. Ito S, Nakazono K, Murasawa A, et al. Development of fulminant hepatitis B (precore variant mutant type) after the discontinuation of low-dose methotrexate therapy in a rheumatoid arthritis patient. *Arthritis Rheum* 2001;44:339–342.
234. Erickson AR, Reddy V, Vogelgesang SA, et al. Usefulness of the American College of Rheumatology recommendations for liver biopsy in methotrexate-treated rheumatoid arthritis patients. *Arthritis Rheum* 1995;38:1115–1119.
235. Strand V, Morgan SL, Baggott JE, ET AL. Folic acid supplementation and methotrexate efficacy: comment on articles by Schiff, Emery et al, and others. *Arthritis Rheum* 2000;43:2615–2616.
236. Moreland LW, Fleischmann RM, for the Leflunomide RA Investigators Group, Strand V. Efficacy of leflunomide vs placebo vs methotrexate in early and late rheumatoid arthritis. *Arthritis Rheum* 1998; 41(suppl):155.
237. Elasser S, Dalquen P, Soler M, et al. Methotrexate-induced pneumonitis:appearance four weeks after discontinuation of treatment. *Am Rev Respir Dis* 1989;140:1089–1092.
238. Hand SH, Smith JK, Chaudhary BA. Methotrexate pneumonitis: a case report and summary of the literature. *J Med Assoc Ga* 1989; 78:625–628.
239. Barrera P, Van Ede A, Laan RF, et al. Methotrexate-related pulmonary complications in patients with rheumatoid arthritis: cluster of five cases in a period of three months. *Ann Rheum Dis* 1994;53: 479–480.
240. Carroll GJ, Thomas R, Phatouros CC, et al. Incidence, prevalence and possible risk factors for pneumonitis in patients with rheumatoid arthritis receiving methotrexate. *J Rheumatol* 1994;21:51–54.
241. Green L, Schattner A, Berkenstadt H. Severe reversible interstitial pneumonitis induced by low dose methotrexate: report of a case and review of the literature. *J Rheumatol* 1988;15:110–112.
242. Hilliquin P, Menkes CJ. Pneumopathies et traitement par le methotrexate dans la polyarthrite rheumatoide. [Lung diseases and treatment with methotrexate in rheumatoid arthritis.] *Rev Pneumol Clin* 1991;47:179–182.
243. Kaplan RL, Waite DH. Progressive interstitial lung disease from prolonged methotrexate therapy. *Arch Dermatol* 1978;114:1800–1802.
244. Van der Veen MJ, Dekker JJ, Dinant HJ, et al. Fatal pulmonary fibrosis complicating low dose methotrexate therapy for rheumatoid arthritis. *J Rheumatol* 1995;22:1766–1768.
245. Massin F, Coudert B, Marot JP, et al. La pneumopathie du methotrexate. [Pneumopathy caused by methotrexate.] *Rev Mal Respir* 1990;7: 5–15.
246. Scott DL, Greenwood A, Davies J, et al. Radiological progression in rheumatoid arthritis: do D-penicillamine and hydroxychloroquine have different effects? *Br J Rheumatol* 1990;29:126–127.
247. Sharma A, Provenzale D, McKusick A, et al. Interstitial pneumonitis after low-dose methotrexate therapy in primary biliary cirrhosis. *Gastroenterology* 1994;107:266–270.
248. Tsai JJ, Shin JF, Chen CH, et al. Methotrexate pneumonitis in bronchial asthma. *Intern Arch Allergy Immunol* 1993;100:287–290.
249. White DA, Rankin JA, Stover DE, et al. Methotrexate pneumonitis. Bronchoalveolar lavage findings suggest an immunologic disorder. *Am Rev Respir Dis* 1989;139:18–21.
250. Ridley MG, Wolfe CS, Mathews JA. Life threatening acute pneumonitis during low dose methotrexate treatment for rheumatoid arthritis: a case report and review of the literature. *Ann Rheum Dis* 1988;47: 784–788.
251. St.Clair EW, Rice JR, Snyderman R. Pneumonitis complicating low-dose methotrexate therapy in rheumatoid arthritis. *Arch Intern Med* 1985;145:2035–2038.

252. Cannon GW, Ward JR, Clegg DO, et al. Acute lung disease associated with low-dose pulse methotrexate therapy in patients with rheumatoid arthritis. *Arthritis Rheum* 1983;26:1269–1274.
253. Engelbrecht JA, Calhoon SL, Scherrer JJ. Methotrexate pneumonitis after low-dose therapy for rheumatoid arthritis. *Arthritis Rheum* 1983;26:1275–1278.
254. Searles G, McKendry RJ. Methotrexate pneumonitis in rheumatoid arthritis: potential risk factors. Four case reports and a review of the literature. *J Rheumatol* 1987;14:1164–1171.
255. Alarcón GS, Gispen JG, Koopman WJ. Severe reversible interstitial pneumonitis induced by low dose methotrexate. *J Rheumatol* 1989; 16:1007–1008.
256. Clarysse AM, Cathey WJ, Cartwright GE, et al. Pulmonary disease complicating intermittent therapy with methotrexate. *JAMA* 1969; 209:1861–1864.
257. Quadri F, Marone C. Schwere akute pneumopathie nach low-dose-methotrexate-therapi bei chronischer polyarthritis. [Acute pneumonitis after low dose methotrexate therapy for chronic polyarthritis.]. *Schweiz Med Wochenschr* 1989;119:1434–1436.
258. Carson CW, Cannon GW, Egger MJ, et al. Pulmonary disease during the treatment of rheumatoid arthritis with low dose pulse methotrexate. *Semin Arthritis Rheum* 1987;16:186–195.
259. Hargreaves MR, Mowat AG, Benson MK. Acute pneumonitis associated with low dose methotrexate treatment for rheumatoid arthritis: report of five cases and review of published reports. *Thorax* 1992; 47:628–633.
260. Sostman HD, Matthay RA, Putman CE, et al. Methotrexate-induced pneumonitis. *Medicine* 1976;55:371–388.
261. Golden MR, Katz RS, Balk RA, et al. The relationship of preexisting lung disease to the development of methotrexate pneumonitis in patients with rheumatoid arthritis. *J Rheumatol* 1995;22:1043–1047.
262. Alarcón GS, Kremer JM, Macaluso M, et al. Risk factors for methotrexate-induced lung injury in patients with rheumatoid arthritis. A multicenter, case-control study. Methotrexate-Lung Study Group. *Ann Intern Med* 1997;127:356–364.
263. Cron RQ, Sherry DD, Wallace CA. Methotrexate-induced hypersensitivity pneumonitis in a child with juvenile rheumatoid arthritis. *J Pediatr* 1998;132:901–902.
264. Kremer JM, Alarcón GS, Weinblatt ME, et al. Clinical, laboratory radiographic and histopathological features of methotrexate associated-lung injury in patients with rheumatoid arthritis: a multicenter study with literature review. *Arthritis Rheum* 1997;40:1829–1837.
265. Alarcón GS, Koopman WJ, McCarty MJ. Nonperipheral accelerated nodulosis in a methotrexate-treated rheumatoid arthritis patient. *Arthritis Rheum* 1993;36:132–133.
266. Miyata M, Sakuma F, Fukaya E, et al. Detection and monitoring of methotrexate-associated lung injury using serum markers KL-6 and SP-D in rheumatoid arthritis. *Intern Med* 2002;41:467–473.
267. Leduc D, De Vuyst P, Lheureux P, et al. Pneumonitis complicating low-dose methotrexate therapy for rheumatoid arthritis. Discrepancies between lung biopsy and bronchoalveolar lavage findings. *Chest* 1993;104:1620–1623.
268. Cleverly JR, Screaton NJ, Hiorns MP, et al. Drug-induced lung disease: high-resolution CT and histological findings. *Clin Radiol* 2002; 57:292–299.
269. Cook NJ, Carroll GJ. Successful reintroduction of methotrexate after pneumonitis in two patients with rheumatoid arthritis. *Ann Rheum Dis* 1992;51:272–274.
270. Morgan SL, Baggott JE, Refsum H, et al. Homocysteine levels in patients with rheumatoid arthritis treated with low-dose methotrexate. *Clin Pharmacol Ther* 1991;50:547–556.
271. Glueck CJ, Shaw P, Lang JE, et al. Evidence that homocysteine is an independent risk factor for atherosclerosis in hyperlipidemic patients. *Am J Cardiol* 1995;75:132–136.
272. Choi HK, Hernan MA, Seeger JD, et al. Methotrexate and mortality in patients with rheumatoid arthritis: a prospective study. *Lancet* 2002;359:1173–1171.
273. Landewe RB, van den Borne BE, Breedveld FC, et al. Methotrexate effects in patients with rheumatoid arthritis with cardiovascular comorbidity. *Lancet* 2000;355:1616–1617.
274. Morgan SL, Baggott JE, Alarcón GS. Methotrexate in rheumatoid arthritis. Folate supplementation should always be given. *Biodrugs* 1997;8:164–175.
275. Berthelot JM, Glemarec J, Chiffoleau A, et al. Traitements à faibles doses par le methotrexate dans la polyarthrite rheumatoide: facteurs de risque des complications graves. [Treatment with low dose methotrexate in rheumatoid arthritis: risk factors for severe complication.] *Therapie* 1997;52:111–116.
276. Jean G, Oueis E, Chazot C, et al. Nephrotic syndrome following initiation of methotrexate therapy for rheumatoid arthritis. *Clin Nephrol* 1998;50:198.
277. Wernick R, Smith DL. Central nervous system toxicity associated with weekly low-dose methotrexate treatment. *Arthritis Rheum* 1989; 32:770–775.
278. Thomas E, Leroux JL, Hellier JP, et al. Seizure and methotrexate therapy in rheumatoid arthritis. *J Rheumatol* 1993;20:1632.
279. Balachandran C, McCluskey PJ, Champion GD, et al. Methotrexate-induced optic neuropathy. *Clin Exp Ophthalmol* 2002;30:440–441.
280. Fernandez-Espartero MC, Rodriguez M, De La Mata J. Methotrexate-induced nephrogenic diabetes insipidus: first case report. *Rheumatology* 2002;41:233–234.
281. Worthley SG, McNeil JD. Leukoencephalopathy in a patient taking low dose oral methotrexate therapy for rheumatoid arthritis. *J Rheumatol* 1995;22:335–337.
282. Allen JC, Rosen G, Mehta BM, et al. Leukoencephalopathy following high-dose iv methotrexate chemotherapy with leucovorin rescue. *Cancer Tx Rep* 1980;64:1261–1273.
283. Pizzo PA, Bleyer WA, Poplack DG, et al. Reversible dementia temporally associated with intraventricular therapy with methotrexate in a child with acute myelogenous leukemia. *J Pediatr* 1976;88:131–133.
284. Halla JT, Hardin JG. Underrecognized postdosing reactions to methotrexate in patients with rheumatoid arthritis. *J Rheumatol* 1994;21: 1224–1226.
285. Schwartz AM, Leonidas JC. Methotrexate osteopathy. *Skel Radiol* 1984;11:13–16.
286. Nesbit M, Krivit W, Heyn R, et al. Acute and chronic effects of methotrexate on hepatic, pulmonary, and skeletal systems. *Cancer* 1976; 37:1048–1054.
287. Uehara R, Suzuki Y, Ichikawa Y. Methotrexate (MTX) inhibits osteoblastic differentiation in vitro: possible mechanism of MTX osteopathy. *J Rheumatol* 2001;28:251–256.
288. Minaur NJ, Jefferiss C, Bhalla AK, et al. Methotrexate in the treatment of rheumatoid arthritis. I. *In vitro* effects on cells of the osteoblast lineage. *Rheumatology* 2002;41:735–740.
289. Maenaut K, Westhovens R, Dequeker J. Methotrexate osteopathy, does it exist? *J Rheumatol* 1996;23:2156–2159.
290. Carbone LD, Kaeley G, McKown KM, et al. Effects of long-term administration of methotrexate on bone mineral density in rheumatoid arthritis. *Calcif Tissue Int* 1999;64:100–101.
291. Cranney AB, McKendry RJ, Wells GA, et al. The effect of low dose methotrexate on bone density. *J Rheumatol* 2001;28:2395–2399.
292. Minaur NJ, Kounali D, Vedi S, et al. Methotrexate in the treatment of rheumatoid arthritis. II. *In vivo* effects on bone mineral density. *Rheumatology* 2002;41:741–749.
293. Bianchi ML, Cimaz R, Galbiati E, et al. Bone mass change during methotrexate treatment in patients with juvenile rheumatoid arthritis. *Osteoporos Int* 1999;10:20–25.
294. Buckley LM, Leib ES, Cartularo KS, et al. Effect of low dose methotrexate on the bone mineral density of patients with rheumatoid arthritis. *J Rheumatol* 1997;24:1489–1494.
295. Stevens H, Jacobs JW, van Rijk PP, et al. Bone mass change during methotrexate treatment in patients with juvenile rheumatoid arthritis. *Clin Nucl Med* 2001;26:389–391.
296. Goerttler E, Kutzner H, Peter HH, et al. Methotrexate-induced papular eruption in patients with rheumatic diseases: a distinctive adverse cutaneous reaction produced by methotrexate in patients with collagen vascular diseases. *J Am Acad Dermatol* 1999;40:702–707.
297. Del Pozo J, Martinez W, Garcia-Silva J, et al. Cutaneous ulceration as a sign of methotrexate toxicity. *Eur J Dermatol* 2001;11:450–452.
298. Blackburn WD, Jr, Alarcón GS. Toxic response to topical fluorouracil in two rheumatoid arthritis patients receiving low-dose, weekly methotrexate. *Arthritis Rheum* 1990;33:303–304.
299. Bicer A, Tursen U, Cimen OB, et al. Prevalence of dermatophytosis in patients with rheumatoid arthritis. *Rheumatol Int* 2003;23:37–40.
300. Blackburn WD, Jr, Alarcón GS. Impotence in three rheumatoid arthritis patients treated with methotrexate. *Arthritis Rheum* 1989; 32:1341–1342.

301. Phelan MJ, Riley PL, Lynch MP. Methotrexate associated Peyronie's disease in the treatment of rheumatoid arthritis. *Br J Rheumatol* 1992;31:425–426.
302. Del Paine DW, Leek JC, Robbins DL. Gynecomastia associated with low dose methotrexate therapy. *Arthritis Rheum* 1980;26:691–692.
303. Ostensen M. Treatment with immunosuppressive and disease modifying drugs during pregnancy and lactation. *Am J Reprod Immunol* 1992;28:148–152.
304. Kozlowski RD, Steinbrunner JV, Mackenzie AH, et al. Outcome of first-trimester exposure to low-dose methotrexate in eight patients with rheumatic disease. *Am J Med* 1990;88:589–592.
305. Ross GT. Congenital anomalies among children born of mothers receiving chemotherapy for gestational trophoblastic neoplasma. *Cancer* 1976;37:1043–1047.
306. Shahin AA, Ismail MM, Saleh M, et al. Protective effect of folinic acid on low-dose methotrexate genotoxicity. *Z Rheumatol* 2001;60: 63–68.
307. Milunsky A, Graef JW, Gaynor MF Jr. Methotrexate-induced congenital malformations. *Pediatrics* 1968;72:790–795.
308. Buckley LM, Bullaboy CA, Leichtman L, et al. Multiple congenital anomalies associated with weekly low-dose methotrexate treatment of the mother. *Arthritis Rheum* 1997;40:971–973.
309. Krahenmann F, Ostensen M, Stallmach T, et al. *In utero* first trimester exposure to low-dose methotrexate with increased fetal nuchal translucency and associated malformations. *Prenat Diagn* 2002;22: 489–490.
310. Czeizel AE, Dudás I. Prevention of the first occurrence of neural-tube defects by periconceptional vitamin supplementation. *N Engl J Med* 1992;327:1832–1835.
311. Medical Research Council Vitamin SRG. Prevention of the first occurrence of neural-tube defects by periconceptional vitamin supplementation. *Lancet* 1991;338:131–137.
312. Bridges SL Jr, López-Méndez A, Han KH, et al. Should methotrexate be discontinued before elective orthopedic surgery in patients with rheumatoid arthritis? *J Rheumatol* 1991;18:984–988.
313. Perhala RS, Wilke WS, Clough JD, et al. Local infectious complications following large joint replacement in rheumatoid arthritis patients treated with methotrexate versus those not treated with methotrexate. *Arthritis Rheum* 1991;34:146–52.
314. Sany J, Anaya J-M, Canovas F, et al. Influence of methotrexate on the frequency of postoperative infectious complications in patients with rheumatoid arthritis. *J Rheumatol* 1993;20:1129–1132.
315. Alarcón GS, Moreland LW, Jaffe K, et al. Barriers encountered in the conduct of clinical studies: a case in point. Perioperatively discontinuation of methotrexate. *Controlled Clin Trials* 1995;16 (suppl):122.
316. Jain A, Witbreuk M, Ball C, et al. Influence of steroids and methotrexate on wound complications after elective rheumatoid hand and wrist surgery. *J Hand Surg* 2002;27:449–455.
317. Grennan DM, Gray J, Loudon J, et al. Methotrexate and early postoperative complications in patients with rheumatoid arthritis undergoing elective orthopaedic surgery. *Ann Rheum* 2001;60:214–217.
318. Sany J, Anaya J-M, Lussiez V, et al. Treatment of rheumatoid arthritis with methotrexate: a prospective open longterm study of 191 cases. *J Rheumatol* 1991;18:1323–1327.
319. Carpenter MT, West SG, Vogelgesang SA, et al. Postoperative joint infections in rheumatoid arthritis patients on methotrexate therapy. *Orthopedics* 1996;19:207–210.
320. Bailin PL, Tindall J, Roenigk HH Jr, et al. Is methotrexate therapy for psoriasis carcinogenic? A modified retrospective-prospective analysis. *JAMA* 1975;232:359–362.
321. Harris CC. Malignancy during methotrexate and steroid therapy for psoriasis. *Arch Dermatol* 1971;103:501–504.
322. Potter T, Hardwick N, Mulherin D. Multiple malignant melanomas in a patient with rheumatoid treated with methotrexate. *J Rheumatol* 1998;25:2282.
323. Jeannou J, Goupille P, Valat JP. Association of methotrexate, rheumatoid arthritis, and melanoma in 2 patients. *J Rheumatol* 1997;24: 1444–1445.
324. Thoburn R, Katz P. Lymphoproliferative disease in patients with autoimmune disease on low-dose methotrexate. *Am Coll Rheumatol Hotline* 1995;June:1.
325. Prior P. Cancer and rheumatoid arthritis: epidemiologic considerations. *Am J Med* 1985;78(suppl 1A):15–21.
326. Isomaki HA, Hakulinen T, Joutsenlahti U. Excess risk of lymphomas, leukemia and myeloma in patients with rheumatoid arthritis. *J Chronic Dis* 1978;31:691–696.
327. Moder KG, Tefferi A, Cohen MD, et al. Hematologic malignancies and the use of methotrexate in rheumatoid arthritis: a retrospective study. *Am J Med* 1995;99:276–281.
328. Pointud P, Prudat M, Peron J-M. Acute leukemia after low dose methotrexate therapy in a patient with rheumatoid arthritis. *J Rheumatol* 1993;20:1215–1216.
329. Ekstrom K, Hjalgrim H, Brandt L, et al. Risk of malignant lymphomas in patients with rheumatoid arthritis and in their first-degree relatives. *Arthritis Rheum* 2003;48:963–970.
330. Thomas E, Symmons DP, Brewster DH, et al. National study of cause-specific mortality in rheumatoid arthritis, juvenile chronic arthritis, and other rheumatic conditions: a 20 year followup study. *J Rheumatol* 2003;30:958–965.
331. Symmons DP, Ahern M, Bacon PA, et al. Lymphoproliferative malignancy in rheumatoid arthritis: a study of 20 cases. *Ann Rheum Dis* 1984;43:132–135.
332. Lioté F, Pertuiset E, Cochand-Priollet B, et al. Methotrexate related B lymphoproliferative disease in a patient with rheumatoid arthritis. Role of Epstein-Barr virus infection. *J Rheumatol* 1995;22:1174–1178.
333. Le Goff P, Koreichi A, Saraux A, et al. Lymphome au cours du traitement de la polyarthrite rhumatoide par le methotrexate a faible dose: un nouveau cas. [Lymphoma during treatment of rheumatoid arthritis with low-dose methotrexate: a new case.] *Rev Rhuma* 1994;61:357–358.
334. Marlier S, Chagnon A, Brocq O, et al. Lymphome sous methotrexate a faibles doses au cours d'une polyarthrite rheumatoide avec lymphopenie extrême. [Lymphoma induced by low-dose methotrexate in rheumatoid arthritis with severe lymphopenia.] *Ann Med Intern* 1995;146:206–208.
335. Morris CR, Morris AJ. Localized lymphoma in a patient with rheumatoid arthritis treated with parenteral methotrexate. *J Rheumatol* 1993;20:2172–2173.
336. Kleiman KS, Mahowald ML. Methotrexate and lymphoma a presentation of four cases and review of the literature. *J Clin Rheumatol* 1998;4:254–259.
337. Kamel OW, van de Rijn M, LeBrun DP, et al. Lymphoid neoplasms in patients with rheumatoid arthritis and dermatomyositis: frequency of Epstein-Barr virus and other features associated with immunosuppression. *Hum Pathol* 1994;25:638–643.
338. Ellman MH, Hurwitz H, Thomas C, et al. Lymphoma developing in a patient with rheumatoid arthritis taking low dose weekly methotrexate. *J Rheumatol* 1991;18:1741–1743.
339. Kingsmore SF, Hall BD, Allen NB, et al. Association of methotrexate, rheumatoid arthritis and lymphoma: Report of 2 cases and literature review. *J Rheumatol* 1992;19:1462–1465.
340. Taillan B, Garnier G, Castanet J, et al. Lymphoma developing in a patient with rheumatoid arthritis taking methotrexate. *Clin Rheumatol* 1993;12:93–94.
341. Usman AR, Yunus MB. Non-Hodgkin's lymphoma in patients with rheumatoid arthritis treated with low dose methotrexate. *J Rheumatol* 1996;23:1095–1098.
342. Georgescu L, Quinn GC, Schwartzman S, et al. Lymphoma in patients with rheumatoid arthritis: association with the disease state or methotrexate treatment. *Semin Arthritis Rheum* 1997;26:794–804.
343. Lim IG, Bertouch JV. Remission of lymphoma after drug withdrawal in rheumatoid arthritis. *Med J Aust* 2002;177:500–501.
344. Baird R, van Zyl-Smit RN, Dilke T, et al. Spontaneous remission of low-grade B-cell non-Hodgkin's lymphoma following withdrawal of methotrexate in a patient with rheumatoid arthritis: case report and review of the literature. *Br J Haematol* 2002;118:567–568.
345. Stewart M, Malkovska V, Krishnan J, et al. Lymphoma in a patient with rheumatoid arthritis receiving methotrexate treatment: successful treatment with rituximab. *Ann Rheum Dis* 2001;60:892–893.
346. Jardine DL, Colls BM. Hodgkin's disease following methotrexate therapy for rheumatoid arthritis. *N Z Med J* 2002;115:293–294.
347. Hirose Y, Masaki Y, Okada J, et al. Epstein-Barr virus–associated B-cell type non-Hodgkin's lymphoma with concurrent p53 protein expression in a rheumatoid arthritis patient treated with methotrexate. *Int J Hematol* 2002;75:412–415.
348. Padeh S, Sharon N, Schiby G, et al. Hodgkin's lymphoma in systemic onset juvenile rheumatoid arthritis after treatment with low dose methotrexate. *J Rheumatol* 1997;24:2035–2037.

349. Krugmann J, Sailer-Hock M, Muller T, et al. Epstein-Barr virus–associated Hodgkin's lymphoma and *Legionella pneumophila* infection complicating treatment of juvenile rheumatoid arthritis with methotrexate and cyclosporine A. *Hum Pathol* 2000;31:253–255.
350. Dawson TM, Starkebaum G, Wood BL, et al. Epstein-Barr virus, methotrexate, and lymphoma in patients with rheumatoid arthritis and primary Sjögren's syndrome: case series. *J Rheumatol* 2001;28: 47–53.
351. Mariette X, Caxals-Hatem D, Warszawki J, et al. Lymphomas in rheumatoid arthritis patients treated with methotrexate: a 3-year prospective study in France. *Blood* 2002;99:3909–3915.
352. Segal R, Caspi D, Tishler M, et al. Accelerated nodulosis and vasculitis during methotrexate therapy for rheumatoid arthritis. *Arthritis Rheum* 1988;31:1182–1185.
353. Jeurissen ME, Boerbooms AM, van de Putte LB. Eruption of nodulosis and vasculitis during methotrexate therapy for rheumatoid arthritis. *Clin Rheumatol* 1989;8:417–418.
354. Combe B, Didry C, Gutierrez M, et al. Accelerated nodulosis and systemic manifestations during methotrexate therapy for rheumatoid arthritis. *Eur J Med* 1993;2:153–156.
355. Falcini F, Taccetti G, Ernimi M, et al. Methotrexate-associated appearance and rapid progression of rheumatoid nodules in systemic-onset juvenile rheumatoid arthritis. *Arthritis Rheum* 1997;40:175–178.
356. Kerstens PJ, Boerbooms AM, Jeurissen ME, et al. Accelerated nodulosis during low dose methotrexate therapy for rheumatoid arthritis. An analysis of ten cases. *J Rheumatol* 1992;19:867–871.
357. Williams FM, Cohen PR, Arnett FC. Accelerated cutaneous nodulosis during methotrexate therapy in a patient with rheumatoid arthritis. *J Am Acad Dermatol* 1998;39:359–362.
358. Filosa G, Salaffi F, Bugatti L. Accelerated nodulosis during methotrexate therapy for refractory rheumatoid arthritis. A case report. *Adv Exp Med Biol* 1999;455:521–524.
359. Ahmed SS, Arnett FC, Smith CA, et al. The HLA-DRB1*0401 allele and the development of methotrexate-induced accelerated rheumatoid nodulosis: a follow-up study of 79 Caucasian patients with rheumatoid arthritis. *Medicine* 2001;80:271–278.
360. Abraham Z, Rosenbaum M, Rosner L. Colchicine therapy for low-dose-methotrexate-induced accelerated nodulosis in a rheumatoid arthritis patient. *J Dermatol* 1999;26:691–694.
361. Joosen H, Mellaerts B, Dereymaeker G, et al. Pulmonary nodule and aggressive tibialis posterior tenosynovitis in early rheumatoid arthritis. *Clin Rheumatol* 2000;19:392–395.
362. Patatanian E, Thompson DF. A review of methotrexate-induced accelerated nodulosis. *Pharmacotherapy* 2002;22:1157–1162.
363. Karam NE, Roger L, Hankins LL, et al. Rheumatoid nodulosis of the meninges. *J Rheumatol* 1994;21:1960–1963.
364. Raccaud O. Manifestations extra-articulaires de la polyarthrite rheumatoide lors d'un traitement de fond par methotrexate: à propos d'un cas de nodulose avec pericardite. [Extra-articular manifestations of rheumatoid arthritis at the time of basic methotrexate treatment: apropos of a case of nodulosis with pericarditis]. *Rev Med Suisse Rom* 1994;114:343–344.
365. Smith MD. Accelerated nodulosis, pleural effusion, and pericardial tamponade during methotrexate therapy. *J Rheumatol* 1995;22: 1439.
366. Bruyn GA, Essed CE, Houtman PM, et al. Fatal cardiac nodules in a patient with rheumatoid arthritis treated with low dose methotrexate. *J Rheumatol* 1993;20:912–914.
367. Abu-Shakra M, Nicol P, Urowitz MB. Accelerated nodulosis, pleural effusion, and pericardial tamponade during methotrexate therapy. *J Rheumatol* 1994;21:934–937.
368. Sorensen WT, Moller-Anderson K, Behrendt N. Rheumatoid nodules of the larynx. *J Laryngol Otol* 1998;112:573–574.
369. Nezondet-Chetaille AL, Brondino-Riquier R, Villani P, et al. Panniculitis in a patient on methotrexate for mixed connective tissue disease. *Joint Bone Spine* 2002;69:324–326.
370. Jang KA, Chio JH, Moon KC, et al. Methotrexate nodulosis. *J Dermatol* 1999;26:460–464.
371. Marks CR, Willkens RF, Wilske KR, et al. Small-vessel vasculitis and methotrexate. *Ann Intern Med* 1984;100:916.
372. Halevy S, Giryes H, Avinoach I, et al. Leukocytoclastic vasculitis induced by low-dose methotrexate: *in vitro* evidence for an immunologic mechanism. *J Euro Acad Dermatol Venereol* 1998;10:81–85.
373. Simonart T, Durez P, Margaux J, et al. Cutaneous necrotizing vasculitis after low dose methotrexate therapy for rheumatoid arthritis: a possible manifestation of methotrexate hypersensitivity. *Clin Rheumatol* 1997;16:623–625.
374. Rodriguez-Moreno J, del Blanco-Barnusell J, Castano-Moreno C, et al. Systemic rheumatoid vasculitis after discontinuation of methotrexate therapy. *J Rheumatol* 1992;19:178.
375. Jorizzo JL, White WL, Wise CM. Low-dose weekly methotrexate for unusual neutrophilic vascular reactions: cutaneous polyarteritis nodosa and Behçet's disease. *J Am Acad Dermatol* 1991;24:973–978.
376. Espinoza LR, Espinoza CG, Vasey FB, et al. Oral methotrexate therapy for chronic rheumatoid arthritis ulcerations. *J Am Acad Dermatol* 1986;15:508–512.
377. Williams HC, Pembroke AC. Methotrexate in the treatment of vasculitic cutaneous ulceration in rheumatoid arthritis. *J R Soc Med* 1989;82:763.
378. Roenigk HH Jr, Maibach HI, Auerbach R, et al. Methotrexate guidelines—revised. *J Am Acad Dermatol* 1982;6:145–155.
379. Cash JM, Swain M, Di Bisceglie M, et al. Massive intrahepatic hemorrhage following routine liver biopsy in a patient with rheumatoid arthritis treated with methotrexate. *J Rheumatol* 1992;19:1466–1468.
380. Weinblatt ME, Maier AL, Coblyn JS. Low dose leucovorin does not interfere with the efficacy of methotrexate in rheumatoid arthritis: an 8 week randomized placebo controlled trial. *J Rheumatol* 1993;20: 950–952.
381. Kremer JM. A debate: should patients with rheumatoid arthritis on methotrexate undergo liver biopsies? *Semin Arthritis Rheum* 1992; 21:376–386.
382. Dolan OM, Burrows D, Irvine A, et al. The value of a baseline liver biopsy prior to methotrexate treatment. *Br J Dermatol* 1994;131: 891–894.
383. Ferraz MB, Ciconelli RM, Vilar JM. Patient's preference regarding the option of performing unselective liver biopsy following methotrexate treatment in rheumatoid arthritis. *Clin Exp Rheumatol* 1994; 12:621–626.
384. Kremer JM, Alarcón GS, Lightfoot RW Jr, et al. Methotrexate for rheumatoid arthritis. Suggested guidelines for monitoring liver toxicity. *Arthritis Rheum* 1994;37:316–328.
385. Fries JF, Ramey DR, Singh G. Suggested guidelines for monitoring liver toxicity in rheumatoid arthritis patients treated with methotrexate: comment on the article by Kremer et al. *Arthritis Rheum* 1994; 37:1829–1834.
386. Newman ED, Harrington TM, Perruquet JL, et al. Creating a care-effective cost-effective strategy for methotrexate liver toxicity monitoring in rheumatoid arthritis: comment on the article by Kremer et al. *Arthritis Rheum* 1995;38:297–298.
387. Cash JM, Wilke WS. Guidelines for routine liver biopsy during methotrexate treatment. *Cleve Clin J Med* 1994;61:317–318.
388. Shiroky J. Liver biopsy in patients with rheumatoid arthritis taking methotrexate. *J Rheumatol* 1994;21:964–965.
389. Yazıcı Y, Erkan D, Paget SA. Monitoring methotrexate hepatic toxicity in rheumatoid arthritis: is it time to update the guidelines? *J Rheumatol* 2002;29:1586–1589.
390. Kremer JM. Not yet time to change the guidelines for monitoring methotrexate liver toxicity: they have served us well. *J Rheumatol* 2002;29:1590–1592.
391. Heathcote J. The significance of AST changes in patients with rheumatoid arthritis treated with methotrexate. *J Rheumatol* 1996;23:413–415.
392. Kremer JM, Kaye GI, Kaye NW, et al. Light and electron microscopic analysis of sequential liver biopsy samples for rheumatoid arthritis patients receiving long-term methotrexate therapy: followup over long treatment intervals and correlation with clinical and laboratory variables. *Arthritis Rheum* 1995;38:1194–1203.
393. Richard S, Guerret S, Gerard F, et al. Hepatic fibrosis in rheumatoid arthritis patients treated with methotrexate: application of a new semi-quantitative scoring system. *Rheumatology* 2000;39:50–54.
394. Bergquist SR, Felson DT, Prashker MJ, et al. The cost-effectiveness of liver biopsy in rheumatoid arthritis patients treated with methotrexate. *Arthritis Rheum* 1995;38:326–333.
395. Hashkes PJ, Balisteri WR, Bove KE, et al. The relationship of hepatotoxic risk factors and liver histology in methotrexate therapy for juvenile rheumatoid arthritis. *J Pediatr* 1999;134:47–52.
396. Arias JM, Morton KA, Albro JE, et al. Comparison of methods for identifying early methotrexate-induced hepatotoxicity in patients with rheumatoid arthritis. *J Nucl Med* 1993;34:1905–1909.

397. Verschuur AC, van Everdingern JJ, Cohen EB, et al. Liver biopsy versus ultrasound in methotrexate-treated psoriasis: a decision analysis. *Int J Dermatol* 1992;31:404–409.
398. Collins D, Bellamy N, Campbell J. A Canadian survey of current methotrexate prescribing practices in rheumatoid arthritis. *J Rheumatol* 1994;21:1220–1223.
399. Wallace CA, Bleyer WA, Sherry DD, et al. Toxicity and serum levels of methotrexate in children with juvenile rheumatoid arthritis. *Arthritis Rheum* 1989;32:677–681.
400. Shiroky JB, Neville C, Esdaile JM, et al. Low-dose methotrexate with leucovorin (folinic acid) in the management of rheumatoid arthritis. Results of a multicenter randomized, double-blinded, placebo-controlled trial. *Arthritis Rheum* 1993;36:795–803.
401. Hanrahan PS, Russell AS. Concurrent use of folinic acid and methotrexate in rheumatoid arthritis. *J Rheumatol* 1988;15:1078–1080.
402. Buckley LM, Vacek PM, Cooper SM. Administration of folinic acid after low dose methotrexate in patients with rheumatoid arthritis. *J Rheumatol* 1990;17:1158–1161.
403. Buckley LM. Reply: Folinic acid supplementation in patients with juvenile rheumatoid arthritis treated with methotrexate. *J Rheumatol* 1996;23:403–404.
404. Alarcón GS, Morgan SL. Folinic acid to prevent side effects of methotrexate in juvenile rheumatoid arthritis. *J Rheumatol* 1996;23:2184.
405. Gulko PS, Tracy IC, Baum SK, et al. Practice patterns in the use of supplemental folic acid in rheumatoid arthritis patients treated with methotrexate. *Rev Brasil Rheumatol* 1994;34:235–238.
406. Stewart KA, Mackenzie AH, Clough JD, et al. Folate supplementation in methotrexate-treated rheumatoid arthritis patients. *Semin Arthritis Rheum* 1991;20:332–338.
407. Morgan SL, Alarcón GS, Krumdieck CL. Folic acid supplementation during methotrexate therapy: it makes sense. *J Rheumatol* 1993;20:929–930.
408. Morgan SL, Baggott JE, Koopman WJ, et al. Folate supplementation and methotrexate. *Ann Rheum Dis* 1993;52:315–316.
409. Hunt RE, Phillips RM, Shergy WJ. Role of folic acid in limiting methotrexate related side effects. *Arthritis Rheum* 1987;30(suppl):253.
410. Griffith SM, Fisher J, Clarke S, et al. Do patients with rheumatoid arthritis established on methotrexate and folic acid 5 mg daily need to continue folic acid supplements long term? *Rheumatology* 2000;39:1102–1109.
411. van Ede AE, Laan RF, Rood MJ, et al. Effect of folic or folinic acid supplementation on the toxicity and efficacy of methotrexate in rheumatoid arthritis. A forty-eight week, multicenter, randomized, double-blind, placebo-controlled study. *Arthritis Rheum* 2001;44:1515–1524.
412. van Ede AE, Laan RF, Blom HJ, et al. Homocysteine and folate status in methotrexate-treated patients with rheumatoid arthritis. *Rheumatology* 2002;41:658–665.
413. Suzuki Y, Uchara R, Tajima C, et al. Elevation of serum hepatic aminotransferases during treatment of rheumatoid arthritis with low-dose methotrexate. Risk factors and response to folic acid. *Scand J Rheumatol* 1999;28:273–281.
414. Enderesen GK, Husby G. Folate supplementation during methotrexate treatment of patients with rheumatoid arthritis. An update and proposals for guidelines. *Scand J Rheumatol* 2001;30:129–134.
415. Morgan SL, Baggott JE, Lee JY, et al. Folic acid supplementation prevents deficient blood folate levels and hyperhomocysteinemia during longterm, low dose methotrexate therapy for rheumatoid arthritis: implications for cardiovascular disease prevention. *J Rheumatol* 1998;25:441–446.
416. Slot O. Changes in plasma homocysteine in arthritis patients starting treatment with low-dose methotrexate subsequently supplemented with folic acid. *Scand J Rheumatol* 2001;30:305–307.
417. Morgan SL, Baggott JE, Altz-Smith M. Folate status of rheumatoid arthritis patients receiving long-term, low-dose methotrexate therapy. *Arthritis Rheum* 1987;30:1348–1356.
418. Ortiz Z, Shea B, Súarez-Almazor M, et al. The efficacy of folic acid and folinic acid in reducing methotrexate gastrointestinal toxicity in rheumatoid arthritis. A metaanalysis of randomized controlled trials. *J Rheumatol* 1998;25:36–43.
419. Stenger AAME, Houtman PM, Bruyn GAW. Does folate supplementation make sense in patients with rheumatoid arthritis treated with methotrexate? *Ann Rheum Dis* 1992;51:1019–1020.
420. Jobanputra P, Hunter M, Clark D, et al. An audit of methotrexate and folic acid for rheumatoid arthritis. Experience from a teaching centre. *Br J Rheumatol* 1995;34:971–975.
421. Leeb BF. Should folate supplementation be routinely recommended for older patient receiving methotrexate? *Drugs Aging* 1994;5:319–322.
422. Morgan SL, Alarcón GS, Moreland LW. Improved methotrexate patient information. *Arthritis Rheum* 1995;38:874–875.
423. Pruthi RK, Tefferi A. Pernicious anemia revisited. *Mayo Clin Proc* 1994;69:144–150.
424. Graham LD, Myones BL, Rivas-Chacon RF, et al. Morbidity associated with long-term methotrexate therapy in juvenile rheumatoid arthritis. *J Pediatr* 1992;120:468–473.
425. Rose CD, Singsen BH, Eichenfield AH, et al. Safety and efficacy of methotrexate therapy for juvenile rheumatoid arthritis. *J Pediatr* 1990;117:653–659.
426. White P, Ansell BM. Methotrexate for juvenile rheumatoid arthritis. *N Engl J Med* 1992;326:1077–1078.
427. Giannini EH, Brewer EJ, Kuzmina N, et al. Methotrexate in resistant juvenile rheumatoid arthritis. Results of the U.S.A.–U.S.S.R. double-blind, placebo-controlled trial. *N Engl J Med* 1992;326:1043–1049.
428. Halle F, Prieur AM. Evaluation of methotrexate in the treatment of juvenile chronic arthritis according to the subtype. *Clin Exp Rheumatol* 1991;9:297–302.
429. Singsen BH, Goldbach-Mansky R. Methotrexate in the treatment of juvenile rheumatoid arthritis and other pediatric rheumatic and nonrheumatic disorders. *Rheum Dis Clin North Am* 1997;23:811–841.
430. Jacobs JC. Juvenile rheumatoid arthritis. In: *Pediatric rheumatology for the practitioner*, 2nd ed. New York: Springer-Verlag, 1992:231–359.
431. Morris PW, Bogle ML, Karkos J, et al. Folate supplementation in patients with juvenile rheumatoid arthritis being treated with methotrexate. *J Invest Med* 1995;43(suppl):36.
432. Ravelli A, Migliavacca D, Viola S, et al. Efficacy of folinic acid in reducing methotrexate toxicity in juvenile idiopathic arthritis. *Clin Exp Rheumatol* 1999;17:625–627.
433. Harel L, Wagner-Weiner L, Poznanski AK, et al. Effects of methotrexate on radiologic progression in juvenile rheumatoid arthritis. *Arthritis Rheum* 1993;36:1370–1374.
434. Aydintug AO, D'Cruz D, Cervera R, et al. Low dose methotrexate treatment in adult Still's disease. *J Rheumatol* 1992;19:431–435.
435. Kraus A, Alarcón-Segovia D. Fever in adult onset Still's disease. Response to methotrexate. *J Rheumatol* 1991;18:918–920.
436. Fautrel B, Borget C, Rozenberg S, et al. Corticosteroid sparing effect of low dose methotrexate treatment in adult Still's disease. *J Rheumatol* 1999;26:373–378.
437. Lovell DJ, Giannini EH, Jones OY, et al. Long-term efficacy and safety of etanercept in children with polyarticular-course juvenile rheumatoid arthritis: interim results from an ongoing multicenter, open label, extended-treatment trial. *Arthritis Rheum* 2003;48:218–226.
438. Creemers MC, Franssen JA, van de Putte LB, et al. Methotrexate in severe ankylosing spondylitis: an open study. *J Rheumatol* 1995;22:1104–1107.
439. Kozarek RA, Patterson DJ, Gelfand MD, et al. Methotrexate induces clinical and histologic remission in patients with refractory inflammatory bowel disease. *Ann Intern Med* 1989;110:353–356.
440. Feagan BG, Rochon J, Fedorak RN, et al. Methotrexate for the treatment of Crohn's disease. *N Engl J Med* 1995;332:292–297.
441. Winchester R, Bernstein DH, Fischer HD, et al. The co-occurrence of Reiter's syndrome and acquired immunodeficiency. *Ann Intern Med* 1987;106:19–26.
442. Masson C, Chennebault JM, Leclech C. Is HIV infection contraindication to the use of methotrexate in psoriatic arthritis? *J Rheumatol* 1995;22:2191.
443. Metzger AL, Bohan A, Goldberg LS, et al. Polymyositis and dermatomyositis: combined methotrexate and corticosteroid therapy. *Ann Intern Med* 1974;81:182–189.
444. van den Hoogen FH, Boerbooms AM, van de Putte LB. Methotrexate treatment in scleroderma. *Am J Med* 1989;87:116–117.
445. Skopouli FN, Jagiello P, Tsifetaki N, et al. Methotrexate in primary Sjögren's syndrome. *Clin Exp Rheumatol* 1996;14:555–558.
446. Davidson JR, Graziano FM, Rothenberg RJ. Methotrexate therapy for severe systemic lupus erythematosus. *Arthritis Rheum* 1987;30:1195–1196.

447. Rothenberg RJ, Graziano FM, Grandone JT, et al. The use of methotrexate in steroid-resistant systemic lupus erythematosus. *Arthritis Rheum* 1988;31:612–615.
448. Wilke WS, Krall PL, Scheetz RJ, et al. Methotrexate for systemic lupus erythematosus: a retrospective analysis of 17 unselected cases. *Clin Exp Rheumatol* 1991;9:581–588.
449. Asherson RA, Schatten S, Hughes GRV. Methotrexate in systemic lupus erythematosus. *J Rheumatol* 1997;24:610.
450. McCarty DH, Harman JG, Grassanovich JL, et al. Combination drug therapy of seropositive rheumatoid arthritis. *J Rheumatol* 1995;22:1636–1645.
451. Walz LeBlanc BA, Dagenais P, Urowitz MB, et al. Methotrexate in systemic lupus erythematosus. *J Rheumatol* 1994;21:836–838.
452. Ferraccioli GF, De Vita S, Bartoli E. Methotrexate benefits in patients with lupus with and without nephritis. *J Rheumatol* 1995;22:1442.
453. Gansauge S, Breitbart A, Rinaldi N, et al. Methotrexate in patients with moderate systemic lupus erythematosus (exclusion of renal and central nervous system disease). *Ann Rheum Dis* 1997;56:382–385.
454. Webster GF, Razsi LK, Sanchez M. Methotrexate therapy in cutaneous sarcoidosis. *Ann Intern Med* 1989;111:538–539.
455. Soriano FG, Caramelli P, Nitrini R, et al. Neurosarcoidosis: therapeutic success with methotrexate. *Postgrad Med J* 1990;66:142–143.
456. Toews GB, Lynch JPI. Methotrexate in sarcoidosis. *Am J Med Sci* 1990;300:33–36.
457. Lower EE, Baughman RP. The use of low dose methotrexate in refractory sarcoidosis. *Am J Med Sci* 1990;299:153–157.
458. Baughman RP, Lower EE. The effect of corticosteroid or methotrexate therapy on lung lymphocytes and macrophages in sarcoidosis. *Am Rev Respir Dis* 1990;142:1268–1271.
459. Mullarkey MF, Blumenstein BA, Andrade P, et al. Methotrexate in the treatment of corticosteroid-dependent asthma. *N Engl J Med* 1988;318:603–607.
460. Hoofnagle JH, Bergasa NV. Methotrexate therapy of primary biliary cirrhosis: promising but worrisome. *Gastroenterology* 1991;101:1440–1442.
461. Knox TA, Kaplan MM, Gelfand JA, et al. Methotrexate treatment of idiopathic granulomatous hepatitis. *Ann Intern Med* 1995;122:592–595.
462. de Groot K, Reinhold-Keller E, Tatsis E, et al. Therapy for the maintenance of remission in sixty-five patients with generalized Wegener's granulomatosis: methotrexate versus trimethoprim/sulfamethoxazole. *Arthritis Rheum* 1996;36:2052–2061.
463. Krall PL, Mazanec DJ, Wilke WS. Methotrexate for corticosteroid-resistant polymyalgia rheumatica and giant cell arteritis. *Cleve Clin J Med* 1989;56:253–257.
464. Hoffman GS, Leavitt RY, Kerr GS, et al. Treatment of glucocorticoid-resistant or relapsing Takayasu arteritis with methotrexate. *Arthritis Rheum* 1994;37:578–582.
465. Nesher G, Sonnenblick M. Steroid-sparing medications in temporal arteritis—report of three cases and review of 174 reported patients. *Clin Rheumatol* 1994;13:289–292.
466. Langford CA, Sneller MC, Hoffman GS. Methotrexate use in systemic vasculitis. *Rheum Dis Clin North Am* 1997;23:841–853.
467. Riente L, Taglione E, Berrettini S. Efficacy of methotrexate in Cogan's syndrome. *J Rheumatol* 1996;23:1830.
468. Wilke WS. Methotrexate use in miscellaneous inflammatory diseases. *Rheum Dis Clin North Am* 1997;23:855–883.
469. Spiera RF, Mitnick HJ, Kupersmith M, et al. A prospective, double-blind, randomized, placebo controlled trial of methotrexate in the treatment of giant cell arteritis (GCA). *Clin Exp Rheumatol* 2001;19:495–501.
470. Hoffman GS, Cid MC, Hellmann DB, et al. A multicenter, randomized, double-blind, placebo-controlled trial of adjuvant methotrexate treatment for giant cell arteritis. *Arthritis Rheum* 2002;46:1309–1318.
471. Jover JA, Hernandez-Garcia C, Morado JC, et al. Combined treatment of giant-cell arteritis with methotrexate and prednisone. A randomized, double-blind, placebo-controlled trial. *Ann Intern Med* 2001;134:106–114.
472. Baggott JE, Morgan SL, Freeberg LE, et al. Long-term treatment of the MRL/lpr mouse with methotrexate and 10-deazaaminopterin. *Agents Actions* 1992;35:104–111.
473. Cronstein BN, Chan ESL. The mechanisms of methotrexate's action in the treatment of inflammatory disease. In: Cronstein BN, Bertino JR, eds. *Methotrexate.* Basel: Birkhauser Verlag, 2000:65–82.
474. Alarcón GS, Castañeda O, Ferrandiz M, et al. Efficacy and safety of 10-deazaaminopterin in the treatment of rheumatoid arthritis. A one-year continuation, double-blind study. *Arthritis Rheum* 1992;35:1318–1321.
475. Alarcón GS, Castañeda O, Nair G, et al. 10-deazaaminopterin in the treatment of rheumatoid arthritis. *Ann Rheum Dis* 1992;51:600–603.
476. Michaels RM, Nashel DJ, Leonard A, et al. Weekly intravenous methotrexate in the treatment of rheumatoid arthritis. *Arthritis Rheum* 1982;25:339–341.
477. Rozin A, Schapira D, Balbir-Gurman A, et al. Relapse of rheumatoid arthritis after substitution of oral for parenteral administration of methotrexate. *Ann Rheum Dis* 2002;61:756–757.
478. Gertner E, Marshall PS. Oral administration of an easily prepared solution of injectable methotrexate diluted in water: a comparison of serum concentrations vs methotrexate tablets and clinical utility. *J Rheumatol* 1996;23:455–458.
479. Schnabel A, Herlyn K, Burchardi C, et al. Long-term tolerability of methotrexate at doses exceeding 15 mg per week in rheumatoid arthritis. *Rheumatol Int* 1996;15:195–200.
480. Pandya S, Aggarwal A, Misra R. Methotrexate twice weekly vs once weekly in rheumatoid arthritis: a pilot double-blind, controlled study. *Rheumatol Int* 2002;22:1–4.
481. Hall GH, Jones BJ, Head AC, et al. Intra-articular methotrexate. Clinical and laboratory study in rheumatoid and psoriatic arthritis. *Ann Rheum Dis* 1978;37:351–356.
482. Suárez-Almazor ME, Soskeine CL, Sanders LD, et al. Outcome in rheumatoid arthritis: a 1985 inception cohort study. *J Rheumatol* 1994;21:1438–1446.
483. Criswell LA, Mu H, Such CL, et al. Tumor necrosis factor (TNF) microsatellite polymorphism is associated with long-term RA outcomes. *Arthritis Rheum* 1997;40(suppl):330.
484. Gough A, Faint J, Salmon M, et al. Genetic typing of patients with inflammatory arthritis at presentation can be used to predict outcome. *Arthritis Rheum* 1994;37:1166–1170.
485. McDaniel DO, Alarcón GS, Pratt PW, et al. Most African-American patients with rheumatoid arthritis do not have the rheumatoid antigenic determinant (epitope). *Ann Intern Med* 1995;123:181–187.
486. Reveille JD, Alarcón GS, Fowler SE, et al. HLA-DRB1 genes and disease severity in rheumatoid arthritis. *Arthritis Rheum* 1996;39:1802–1807.
487. Csuka M, Carrera GF, McCarty DJ. Treatment of intractable rheumatoid arthritis with combined cyclophosphamide, azathioprine, and hydroxychloroquine. A follow up study. *JAMA* 1986;255:2315–2319.
488. McCarty DJ, Carrera GF. Intractable rheumatoid arthritis. Treatment with combined cyclophosphamide, azathioprine, and hydroxychloroquine. *JAMA* 1982;248:1718–1723.
489. Willkens RF, Urowitz MB, Stablein DM, et al. Comparison of azathioprine, methotrexate, and the combination of both in the treatment of rheumatoid arthritis. A controlled clinical trial. *Arthritis Rheum* 1992;35:849–856.
490. Jeurissen ME, Boerbooms AM, van de Putte LB, et al. Methotrexate versus azathioprine in the treatment of rheumatoid arthritis. A forty-eight-week randomized, double-blind trial. *Arthritis Rheum* 1991;34:961–972.
491. Trnavsky K, Gatterová J, Lindusková M, et al. Combination therapy with hydroxychloroquine and methotrexate in rheumatoid arthritis. *Z Rheumatol* 1993;52:292–296.
492. Ferraz MB, Pinheiro GR, Helfenstein M, et al. Combination therapy with methotrexate and chloroquine in rheumatoid arthritis. A multicenter randomized placebo-controlled trial. *Scand J Rheumatol* 1994;23:231–236.
493. Elkayam O, Yaron M, Zhukovsky G, et al. Toxicity profile of dual methotrexate combinations with gold, hydroxychloroquine, sulphasalazine and minocycline in rheumatoid arthritis patients. *Rheumatol Int* 1997;17:49–53.
494. Salaffi F, Carotti M, Cervini C. Combination therapy of cyclosporine a with methotrexate or hydroxychloroquine in refractory rheumatoid arthritis. *Scand J Rheumatol* 1996;25:16–23.
495. Haagsma CJ, van Riel PL, de Rooij DJ, et al. Combination of methotrexate and sulphasalazine vs methotrexate alone: a randomized open clinical trial in rheumatoid arthritis patients resistant to sulphasalazine therapy. *Br J Rheumatol* 1994;33:1049–1055.
496. Axtens RS, Morand EF, Littlejohn GO. Combination therapy with methotrexate and sulphasalazine in rheumatoid arthritis—tolerance of therapy. *Ann Rheum Dis* 1994;53:703.

497. Nisar M, Carlisle L, Amos RS. Methotrexate and sulphasalazine as combination therapy in rheumatoid arthritis. *Br J Rheumatol* 1994; 33:651–654.
498. Boers M, Verhoeven AC, Markusse HM, et al. Randomised comparison of combined step-down prednisolone, methotrexate and sulphasalazine with sulphasalazine alone in early rheumatoid arthritis. *Lancet* 1997;350:309–318.
499. Shiroky JB. Combination sulfasalazine and methotrexate in the management of rheumatoid arthritis. *J Rheumatol* 1996;23:72–74.
500. Haagsma CJ, Blom HJ, van Riel PL, et al. Influence of sulphasalazine, methotrexate, and the combination of both on plasma homocysteine concentrations in patients with rheumatoid arthritis. *Ann Rheum Dis* 1999;58:79–84.
501. Tugwell P, Pincus T, Yocum D, et al. Combination therapy with cyclosporine and methotrexate in severe rheumatoid arthritis. *N Engl J Med* 1995;333:137–141.
502. Schlesinger N, Huppert A, Hoch S. Cyclosporine and methotrexate for severe rheumatoid arthritis. *N Engl J Med* 1995;333:1567.
503. Stein CM, Pincus T, Yocum D, et al. Combination treatment of severe rheumatoid arthritis with cyclosporine and methotrexate for forty-eight weeks. An open-label extension study. *Arthritis Rheum* 1997; 40:1843–1851.
504. Giacomelli R, Cipriani P, Matucci Cerinic J, et al. Combination therapy with cyclosporine and methotrexate in patients with early rheumatoid arthritis soon inhibits TNFalpha production without decreasing TNFalpha in RNA levels. An *in vivo* and *in vitro* study. *Clin Exp Rheumatol* 2002;20:365–372.
505. Ferraccioli GF, Gremese E, Tomietto P, et al. Analysis of improvements, full responses, remission and toxicity in rheumatoid patients treated with step-up combination therapy (methotrexate, cyclosporin A, sulphasalazine) or monotherapy for three years. *Rheumatology* 2002;41:892–898.
506. Felson DT, Anderson JJ, Meenan RF. Use of short-term efficacy/toxicity tradeoffs to select second- line drugs in rheumatoid arthritis. A metaanalysis of published clinical trials. *Arthritis Rheum* 1992;35: 1117–1125.
507. Kremer JM, Genovese MC, Cannon GW, et al. Concomitant leflunomide therapy in patients with active rheumatoid arthritis despite stable doses of methotrexate. A randomized, double-blind, placebo-controlled trial. *Ann Intern Med* 2002;137:726–733.
508. O'Dell J, Haire C, Erikson N, et al. Triple DMARD therapy for rheumatoid arthritis: efficacy. *Arthritis Rheum* 1994;37(suppl):295.
509. O'Dell JR, Haire CE, Erikson N, et al. Treatment of rheumatoid arthritis with methotrexate alone, sulfasalazine and hydroxychloroquine, or a combination of all three medications. *N Engl J Med* 1996; 334:1287–1291.
510. O'Dell JR, Haire C, Erikson N, et al. Efficacy of triple DMARD therapy in patients with rheumatoid arthritis with suboptimal response to methotrexate. *J Rheumatol* 1996;44(suppl):72–74.
511. Weinblatt ME, Kremer JM, Bankhurst AD, et al. A trial of etanercept, a recombinant tumor necrosis factor receptor: Fc fusion protein, in patients with rheumatoid arthritis receiving methotrexate. *N Engl J Med* 1999;340:253–259.
511a. Klareskog L, van der Heijde D, de Jager JP, et al. Therapeutic effect of the combination of etarnecept and methotrexate compared with each treatment alone in patients with rheumatoid arthritis: double-blind randomised controlled trial. *Lancet* 2004;363:675–681.
511b. Keystone EC, Kavanaugh AF, Sharp JT, et al. Radiographic, clinical, and functional outcomes of treatment with adalimumab (a human anti-tumor necrosis factor monoclonal antibody) in patients with active rheumatoid arthritis receiving concomitant methotrexate therapy. *Arthritis Rheum* 2004;50:1400–1411.
511c. ASPIRE study Group. Largest-ever phase III early rheumatoid arthritis study shows REMICADE plus mehotrexate superior to standard of care. http://jnj.com/news/jnj_news/20030619_114821.htm. 2004
512. Fox RI, Herrmann ML, Frangou CG, et al. Short Analytical Review. Mechanism of action for leflunomide in rheumatoid arthritis. *Clin Immunol* 1999;93:198–208.
513. Aventis Pharmaceuticals. ARAVA prescribing information: Contraindications and warnings. April (*www.aventispharma-us.com/PIs/arava_TXT.html*), 2000.
514. Rozman B. Clinical pharmacokinetics of leflunomide. *Clin Pharmacokinet* 2002;41:421–430.
515. Breedveld FC, Dayer J-M. Leflunomide: mode of action in the treatment of rheumatoid arthritis. *Ann Rheum Dis* 2000;59:841–849.
516. Cherwinski HM, Byars N, Ballaron SJ, et al. Leflunomide interferes with pyrimidine nucleotide biosynthesis. *Inflamm Res* 1995;44:317–322.
517. Xu X, Blinder L, Shen J, et al. *In vivo* mechanism by which leflunomide controls lymphoproliferative and autoimmune disease in MRL/MpJ-lpr/lpr mice. *J Immunol* 1997;159:167–174.
518. Manna SK, Aggarwal BB. Immunosuppressive leflunomide metabolite (A77 1726) blocks TNF-dependent nuclear factor-kappa B activation and gene expression. *J Immunol* 1999;162:2095–2102.
519. Rozman B, Domljan Z, Popovic M, et al. Long term administration of leflunomide to patients with rheumatoid arthritis. *Arthritis Rheum* 1994;37(suppl):339.
520. Smolen JS, Kalden JR, Scott DL, et al. Efficacy and safety of leflunomide compared with placebo and sulphasalazine in active rheumatoid arthritis: a double-blind, randomised, multicentre trial. *Lancet* 1999;353:259–266.
521. Cohen S, Cannon GW, Schiff M, et al. Two-year, blinded, randomized, controlled trial of treatment of active rheumatoid arthritis with leflunomide compared with methotrexate. *Arthritis Rheum* 2001;44: 1984–1992.
522. Strand V, Tugwell P, Bombardier C, et al. Function and health-related quality of life. Results from a randomized controlled trial of leflunomide versus methotrexate or placebo in patients with active rheumatoid arthritis. *Arthritis Rheum* 1999;42:1870–1878.
523. Cohen S, Weaver A, Schiff M, et al., for the Leflunomide Study Group. Two-year treatment of active rheumatoid arthritis with leflunomide compared with placebo or methotrexate. *Arthritis Rheum* 1999;42 (suppl):271.
524. Scott DL, Smolen JS, Kalden JR, et al. Treatment of active rheumatoid arthritis with leflunomide: two year follow up of a double blind, placebo controlled trial versus sulfasalazine. *Ann Rheum Dis* 2001; 60:913–923.
525. Kalden JR, Scott DL, Smolen JS, et al. Improved functional ability in patients with rheumatoid arthritis—longterm treatment with leflunomide versus sulfasalazine. *J Rheumatol* 2001;28:1983–1991.
526. Larsen A, Kvien TK, Schattenkirchner M, et al. Slowing of disease progression in rheumatoid arthritis patients during long-term treatment with leflunomide or sulfasalazine. *Scand J Rheumatol* 2001;30: 135–142.
527. Kalden JR, Schattenkirchner M, Sörensen H, et al. The efficacy and safety of leflunomide in patients with active rheumatoid arthritis. A five-year followup study. *Arthritis Rheum* 2003;48:1513–1520.
528. The European Agency for the Evaluation of Medicinal Products. EMEA public statement on leflunomide (ARAVA)—severe and serious hepatic reactions. EMEA March 12 (Doc. Ref: EMEA/H/5611/01/en). 2001.
529. Arthritis Advisory Committee. Briefing information regarding ARAVA (leflunomide). Food and Drug Administration, March 5 (*www.fda.gov/ohrms/dockets/ac/03/briefing/3930b2.htm*), 2003. Aventis Pharmaceutical.
530. Moynihan R. FDA officials argue over safety of new arthritis drug. *BMJ* 2003;326:565.
531. Weinblatt ME, Dixon JA, Falchuk KR. Serious liver disease in a patient receiving methotrexate and leflunomide. *Arthritis Rheum* 2000; 43:2609–2613.
532. Kremer JM, Fox RI. Leflunomide. In: Koopman WJ, ed. *Arthritis and allied conditions. A textbook of rheumatology,* 14th ed. New York: Lippincott Williams & Wilkins, 2001:783–793.
533. Brent RL. Teratogen update: reproductive risks of leflunomide (Arava); a pyrimidine synthesis inhibitor: counseling women taking leflunomide before or during pregnancy and men taking leflunomide who are contemplating fathering a child. *Teratology* 2001;63:106–112.
534. Jones KL, Johnson DL, Chambers CD. Monitoring leflunomide (Arava) as a new potential teratogen. *Teratology* 2002;65: 200–202.
535. Auer J, Hinterreiter M, Allinger A, et al. Severe pancytopenia after leflunomide in rheumatoid arthritis. *Acta Med Aust* 2000;27:131–132.
536. Holm EA, Balslev E, Jemec GB. Vasculitis occurring during leflunomide therapy. *Dermatology* 2001;203:258–259.
537. Chan ATY, Bradlow A, McNally J. Leflunomide induced vasculitis—a dose-response relationship. *Rheumatology* 2003;42:492–493.

538. Bruyn GAW, Veenstra RP, Halma C, et al. Anti-glomerular basement membrane antibody-associated renal failure in a patient with leflunomide-treated rheumatoid arthritis. *Arthritis Rheum* 2003;48: 1164–1165.
539. Carulli MT, Davies UM. Peripheral neuropathy: an unwanted effect of leflunomide? *Rheumatology* 2002;41:952–953.
540. Soliotis F, Glover M, Jawad ASM. Severe skin reaction after leflunomide and etanercept in a patient with rheumatoid arthritis. *Ann Rheum Dis* 2002;61:850–851.
541. Gottenberg J-E, Venancie P-Y, Mariette X. Alopecia areata in a patient with rheumatoid arthritis treated with leflunomide. *J Rheumatol* 2002;29:1806–1807.
542. Mroczkowski PJ, Weinblatt ME, Kremer JM. Methotrexate and leflunomide combination therapy for patients with active rheumatoid arthritis. *Clin Exp Rheumatol* 1999;17(suppl):66–68.
543. Weinblatt ME, Kremer JM, Coblyn JS, et al. Pharmacokinetics, safety, and efficacy of combination treatment with methotrexate and leflunomide in patients with active rheumatoid arthritis. *Arthritis Rheum* 1999;42:1322–1328.
544. Kiely PDW, Johnson DM. Infliximab and leflunomide combination therapy in rheumatoid arthritis: an open-label study. *Rheumatology* 2002;41:631–637.
545. Remer CF, Weisman MH, Wallace DJ. Benefits of leflunomide in systemic lupus erythematosus: a pilot observational study. *Lupus* 2001;10:480–483.
546. Talip F, Walker N, Khan W, et al. Treatment of Felty's syndrome with leflunomide. *J Rheumatol* 2001;28:868–870.
547. Reich K, Hummel KM, Beckmann I, et al. Treatment of severe psoriasis and psoriatic arthritis with leflunomide. *Br J Dermatol* 2002; 146:335–336.
548. Cuchacovich M, Soto L. Leflunomide decreases joint erosions and induces reparative changes in a patient with psoriatic arthritis. *Ann Rheum Dis* 2002;61:942–943.
549. Haberhauer G, Kittl EM, Dunky A, et al. Beneficial effects of leflunomide in glucocorticoid-and methotrexate-resistant Takayasu's arteritis. *Clin Exp Rheumatol* 2001;19:477–478.
550. Cohen Tervaert JW, Stegeman CA, Kallenberg CG. Novel therapies for anti-neutrophil cytoplasmic antibody-associated vasculitis. *Curr Opin Nephrol Hypertens* 2001;10:211–217.
551. Gross WL. New concepts in treatment protocols for severe systemic vasculitis. *Curr Opin Rheumatol* 1999;11:41–46.
552. Pirildar T. Treatment of adult-onset Still's disease with leflunomide and chloroquine combination in two patients. *Clin Rheumatol* 2003;22:157.
553. Matteson E, Cush JJ. Reports of leflunomide hepatotoxicity in patients with rheumatoid arthritis. ACR Hotline. *www.rheumatology.org/research/hotline/0801leflunomide.html*, August, 2001.
554. Osiri M, Shea B, Robinson V, et al. Leflunomide for treating rheumatoid arthritis. *Cochrane Database Syst Rev* 2003;CD002047: Review.
555. Smolen JS, Emery P. Efficacy and safety of leflunomide in active rheumatoid arthritis. *Rheumatology* 2000;39:48–56.
556. Osiri M, Shea B, Robinson V, et al. Leflunomide for the treatment of rheumatoid arthritis: a systematic review and metaanalysis. *J Rheumatol* 2003;30:1182–1190.
557. Kamel OW, van de Rijn M, Weiss LM, et al. Brief report: Reversible lymphomas associated with Epstein-Barr virus occurring during methotrexate therapy for rheumatoid arthritis and dermatomyositis. *N Engl J Med* 1993;328:1317–1321.
558. Zimmer-Galler I, Lie JT. Choroidal infiltrates as the initial manifestation of lymphoma in rheumatoid arthritis after treatment with low-dose methotrexate. *Mayo Clin Proc* 1994;69:258–261.
559. Cobeta-Garcia JC, Ruiz-Jimeno MT, Fontova-Garrofe R. Non-Hodgkin's lymphoma rheumatoid arthritis and methotrexate. *J Rheumatol* 1993;20:200–202.
560. Ferraccioli GF, Casatta L, Bartoli E, et al. Epstein-Barr virus–associated Hodgkin's lymphoma in a rheumatoid arthritis patient treated with methotrexate and cyclosporin A. *Arthritis Rheum* 1995; 38:867–868.
561. Bachman TR, Sawitzke AD, Perkins SL, et al. Reversible lymphoma in rheumatoid arthritis patients treated with methotrexate: report of two cases. *Arthritis Rheum* 1996;39:325–329.
562. Davies JMS, Kremer JM, Furst DE, et al. Lymphomatous changes during methotrexate therapy. *Arthritis Rheum* 1995;38(suppl):204.

CHAPTER 33

Combination Drug Therapy

Michael J. Battistone and H. James Williams

Few areas in rheumatology have developed as rapidly within the past decade as has the use of combination therapy for rheumatoid arthritis (RA). In a broad sense, the concurrent use of multiple agents in RA is not new. For years, the model of the "therapeutic pyramid" has been taught and practiced, and patients have received combination treatment with nonsteroidal antiinflammatory drugs (NSAIDs) and low-dose corticosteroids while receiving second-line disease-modifying antirheumatic drugs (DMARDs), such as gold salts, hydroxychloroquine (HCQ), D-penicillamine (D-pen), methotrexate (MTX), sulfasalazine (SSZ), azathioprine (AZA), cyclosporine (CYA), or cytotoxic drugs. Combinations of DMARDs were first suggested for patients with refractory arthritis for whom "standard therapy" had failed (1–4), and initially, few studies were well controlled. In recent years, however, a large body of literature on the use of combination therapy in RA has emerged; much of the evidence supports implementing this approach early in the course of the disease.

We begin with a discussion of the scientific basis for DMARD combination therapy, drawing from examples with analogous diseases and experiences with animal models. The majority of this chapter is devoted to reviews of the most significant clinical reports and investigations of combinations of second-line agents in RA. We discuss both uncontrolled and controlled studies, organized with respect to number and type of drugs.

RATIONALE FOR COMBINATION THERAPY

As a general strategy, concurrent treatment with multiple drugs has been a standard approach to many conditions that bear some analogy to RA. Infectious diseases offer prime illustrations; the most successful regimens for serious infections such as human immunodeficiency virus, tuberculosis, and those caused by multidrug-resistant (MDR) bacteria are combination therapies. Treatments for neoplasia also are familiar examples, providing close parallel to the rheumatic diseases in the medications that are used, as well as in the method by which they are given. Indeed, combination therapy has become a recommended approach in treating many chronic conditions, including congestive heart failure (5,6), type 2 diabetes mellitus (7), most cases of hypertension (8), and severe asthma (9); combination therapy for rheumatic conditions is in harmony with this "climate change" in medical practice.

There are several potential advantages in combination therapy (10,11). It is possible that overall toxicity of combinations of DMARDs may be reduced compared with monotherapy, perhaps because combination regimens often feature lower doses of constituent drugs than are used in single-drug regimens. Some combinations may offer additional advantages; for example, when MTX and HCQ are used together, their toxicity may be muted even less than that of either drug alone (12). Several possible explanations for this have been proposed but not established (13,14). Two recent reviews address approaches for selecting combinations of agents for treating RA (15,16).

Another rationale for combining drugs to treat RA is the opportunity for synergy. In inflammatory arthritis, multiple and redundant pathways of the inflammatory cascades are activated; combination therapies use several agents to disrupt these pathways at multiple points. Until a central, "master switch" for controlling the inflammatory process is discovered and exploited, combination therapy seems to be the most effective and efficient method of treatment. This concept is further developed in an excellent review (17).

Finally, patients with RA who have not improved with monotherapy illustrate another theoretic advantage to combination therapy. "Resistant" RA may have immunologic parallels to MDR seen in oncologic diseases. In this setting, immunity to chemotherapeutic drugs is mediated by the adenosine triphosphate–dependent cell-membrane pump P-glycoprotein, which efficiently transports anticancer drugs out of cells, rendering them ineffective. An elegant hypothesis relating the mechanism of resistant RA to that of MDR infections has been proposed, providing a rationale for combination drug therapy based on molecular biology (18).

The experience of combination chemotherapy in RA patients who are treated for concurrent cancer also is enlightening. In two women with active erosive seropositive RA, acute myelogenous leukemia developed. The RA and the leukemia went into remission after treatment with cytosine arabinoside, daunorubicin hydrochloride, and m-AMSA (19). One patient remained in remission for both diseases after 8 months. The other woman had a recurrence of RA after 13 months, although the leukemia remained in remission. However, the RA was reportedly much less aggressive than it had been before the chemotherapy. Her rheumatoid factor levels had decreased with the initial chemotherapy and had become elevated again at the time of consolidation therapy. The rheumatoid factor decreased again with consolidation treatment, and has remained low even though the synovitis has returned.

Another woman with seropositive RA and immunoglobulin A deficiency subsequently developed features suggestive of an overlap connective tissue disease. A few years later, she developed symptoms of fever and weight loss, and was diagnosed with Hodgkin disease. The woman was treated with nitrogen mustard (later changed to cyclophosphamide because of myelosuppression), vincristine, procarbazine, and prednisone, and her RA and overlap connective tissue disease remitted (20). Severe RA, but not the other connective tissue disease symptoms, recurred after 3 years.

EXPERIENCE WITH ANIMAL MODELS

Combinations of DMARDs have been studied in both the collagen-induced arthritis (CIA) and adjuvant arthritis (AA) models. In the definitive review of animal experiments with combination therapy, Oliver and Brahn (21) observed that, as recently as 1996, surprisingly few investigations had been published. This continues to be the case.

In rats with CIA, combined treatment with relatively low doses of MTX and CYA resulted in suppression of the disease; interestingly, both agents were ineffective when used alone (22). In a later study with the same model, CYA was used in combination with AGM-1470, a potent inhibitor of angiogenesis. Although AGM-1470 demonstrated some efficacy when used as monotherapy (in both CIA and AA models), the addition of CYA increased the therapeutic response and did not increase toxicity (23). AGM-1470 also has been studied in combination with taxol, an antineoplastic drug, and with an anti-CD5 pan T-cell monoclonal antibody; in both cases, combined therapy was more effective in suppressing CIA activity than was single-agent treatment (24,25).

In rats with AA, therapy with CYA at the time of adjuvant immunization was shown to have a mixed effect; onset of arthritis was delayed, but severity was increased. Adding calcitriol, the active metabolite of vitamin D_3, to CYA at the time of immunization extended the disease-free interval even further, and also reduced the intensity of arthritis (26). This response is thought to be cytokine mediated, because earlier *in vitro* studies with calcitriol and CYA demonstrated synergistic inhibition of T-cell interleukin-2 (IL-2) (27). Finally, the rats that had been treated with CYA/calcitriol were less likely to develop hypercalcemia than were those treated with calcitriol alone, suggesting that some combination therapies may actually be less toxic than some monotherapies.

A more recent study, also involving rats with AA, evaluated the effects of treatment with an IL-1 receptor antagonist (IL-1ra) alone and in combination with MTX (28). With regard to paw swelling, treatment with the combination resulted in an 84% decrease, compared to a 47% decrease with MTX alone, and only a 6% decrease with IL-1ra monotherapy. Histologic evaluation of bone resorption demonstrated 97% inhibition for rats given the combination treatment, compared with 58% and 53% for MTX and IL-1ra monotherapy, respectively. The researchers concluded that the combination of IL-1ra and MTX conferred additive or synergistic benefit and encouraged clinical trials in humans with RA.

EARLY CLINICAL EXPERIENCES

Combination DMARD therapy has been used in practice much more extensively than has been reported in print. The earliest published experience was that of Sievers and Hurri (29), who described their experience with an antimalarial (usually chloroquine) and parenteral gold. They compared the course of 248 patients with RA who had received both drugs with 240 patients who had been treated with only the antimalarial, and observed more remissions and major improvements in the patients given the combination (43%) than in those who had taken only the antimalarial (36%). Despite these findings, fear of toxicity superseded fear of disease, and for almost 20 years, little attention was given to developing multidrug regimens.

The strategy of combination therapy was preserved by practicing rheumatologists, most notably Paul Young (Asheville, NC) and Arthur Scherbel (30). By the mid-1980s, this practice seemed fairly widespread: a survey of 92 Canadian and 77 Australian rheumatologists in 1986 revealed that combinations of antimalarials and parenteral gold were used by 31% of the Australians and 45% of the Canadians (31).

In little more than 10 years, combination therapy has gained essentially universal acceptance. In another survey involving 200 rheumatologists in the United States, 99% of the respondents reported using combination therapy in treating an estimated 24% of their patients. Furthermore,

39% endorsed the use of combination DMARDs as appropriate initial therapy (32). What developments led to such a significant shift in practice?

Initial Benchmarks

In 1982, McCarty and Carrera (3) described 17 patients with progressive, erosive, seropositive RA, refractory to standard therapy, who had been treated with a triple-drug regimen of cyclophosphamide (CTX), AZA, and HCQ. After a mean treatment course of 27 months, 5 patients enjoyed a complete remission, and radiographic evidence of recortication of erosions was observed in 9 patients. Although the results were encouraging, the researchers were careful to describe the regimen as experimental and did not recommend it for general use. In a follow-up report from the same group, the experience of 31 patients (including the original 17) was reviewed (2). Doses of CTX and AZA were adjusted to maintain a leukopenia of 2,500 cell to 4,000/mm^3 or until a "definite clinical response was noted." Maintenance dosages of HCQ were 100 to 400 mg/day (mean 210 mg/day), AZA 25 to 200 mg/day (mean 74 mg), and CYX 6 to 100 mg/day (mean 30 mg/day). Thirty patients improved during combination treatment. Sixteen patients achieved complete remission, seven others were in "near remission," and seven had a "partial response." Malignancies developed in four patients (erythroleukemia and colon, lung, and endometrial cancer), and three died. Other adverse effects included herpes zoster infections, pruritis, epigastric distress, and diarrhea (2,3). Many of these complications required discontinuation of the cytotoxic agents. Only six patients had no adverse effects. As important as these findings were, the greater impact came from the authors' willingness to present their data. These articles were the first turning point, making it acceptable to study and publish in this area.

Although there was new enthusiasm for combination therapy, investigations over the next decade produced mixed results in efficacy as well as toxicity, and most authorities found the accumulating data insufficient to provide clear recommendations for practice. Open, uncontrolled studies suggested greater efficacy for combinations of DMARDs, whereas randomized controlled trials generally failed to demonstrate a difference.

The second turning point came in 1995, when Tugwell et al. (33), writing for the Methotrexate-Cyclosporine Combination Study Group (MCCSG), reported the experience of a carefully selected population of patients who had only partial response to MTX, and who experienced clinically important benefit with the addition of CYA. Up to this time, most randomized controlled trials of two-DMARD combination therapy compared with monotherapy had failed to show any advantage for combination therapy (34); results of a meta-analysis suggested that a combination was not substantially more effective, but had greater toxicity (35). In 1994, Bensen et al. (36) reported the results of an open-label pilot study of 20 patients with partial response to MTX, and 20 patients with partial response to gold, who had improved with the addition of CYA, without significant adverse effects. These results were the impetus for the 1995 MCCSG study, a 6-month, randomized, double-blind trial in which 148 patients with a partial response to MTX, despite at least 3 months of therapy, were randomized to receive additional therapy with either CYA or placebo at initial dosages of 2.5 mg/kg of body weight per day, increased at regular intervals through the study by 0.5 mg/kg/day if active synovitis persisted. The primary outcome measure was the tender joint count, although there were statistically-significant differences between the treatment groups on all clinical measures. Adverse events were reported more often in the MTX/CYA group, but the researchers noted that the frequency and types of these side effects were similar to those seen in earlier studies of MTX and CYA as monotherapy.

Compared with earlier inconclusive work, the MCCSG study had a fundamental difference in design: a double arm used to compare the effect of two drugs in combination with the effect of only one of the constituent drugs used alone. Many previous investigations had used multiple-arm designs that included an evaluation of each drug as monotherapy. Because each group tended to improve somewhat, statistical power to detect significant differences between groups was hampered by regression to the mean, and well-designed projects often had negative results. The MCCSG approach, similar to that used in oncologic studies of combination chemotherapy, preserved statistical power and was able to demonstrate a significant result. Furthermore, these findings, easily generalized to clinical practice, introduced the concept of the "anchor drug." The anchor—in this case, MTX—serves to identify partial responders to monotherapy, and provides the foundation on which the combination regimen is constructed.

The findings of Tugwell's group illustrate the importance of study design. Discussions of how combination research ought to be conducted and interpreted were a prominent feature of the Chatham, Massachusetts, conference, convened in July 1995 (1 week before the MCCSG study was reported) to review the status and future of combination therapy in RA (37). Different strategies of data evaluation, including meta-analysis (38), use of longitudinal databases of unselected patients (39), cost-effectiveness and cost-utility comparisons (40), and area-under-the-curve analysis (41), have been reported and may further change the study of combination therapy. Today, most clinical studies of emerging RA treatments are designed as combination trials.

COMBINATIONS OF TWO DMARDS

Methotrexate and Sulfasalazine

In 1989, Shiroky et al. (42) published the report of four patients treated for a mean of 24 months. All were noted to have reduction in morning stiffness and number of involved joints, and in the three patients who had previously taken MTX, a reduction in MTX dose was possible. Concern for potential adverse reactions due to the combination of antifolate drugs without folate supplementation has been raised (43), but the significance has been disputed (44). Reviewing his experience on two occasions several years after his initial report, Shiroky (45,46) described the combination as "generally well tolerated." Moreover, flare-ups were observed after discontinuation of either MTX or SSZ in several patients.

In 1994, Nisar et al. (47) published their experience, in which 32 patients treated with MTX and SSZ were compared with 63 patients treated with MTX alone. In this study, toxicity was not increased in the combination group; however, there are few data to suggest that the combination provided added efficacy.

Later in 1994, Haagsma et al. (48) reported the combination of MTX and SSZ, studied in an open, randomized clinical trial of patients who had exhibited an inadequate response to SSZ monotherapy. Forty patients were randomly selected to receive either SSZ plus MTX or MTX alone. The mean decrement in Disease Activity Score (DAS) in the combination group was significantly greater than that seen in the MTX-only group, and there were no remarkable differences in toxicity. This report also examined the pharmacokinetics of MTX, finding no alteration when SSZ was given concomitantly (49). With a subset of 26 patients in this study, researchers found decreased production of interleukin-1β (IL-1β), IL-1ra, and circulating soluble receptors for tumor necrosis factor (TNF) (50).

In 1997, these investigators published a longer study with more subjects (51). One hundred five patients with early RA were randomized to receive SSZ, MTX, or both DMARDs, and were followed up by a single observer for 52 weeks. Outcome measures included the DAS, Ritchie articular index, swollen joint count, and erythrocyte sedimentation rate (ESR). Although trends favoring combination therapy were seen for each measure, there were no statistically significant differences in efficacy across groups (51). Also in 1997, Boers et al. (52) coordinated a multicenter, randomized controlled trial comparing SSZ (2 g/day) with a combination of SSZ plus MTX (7.5 mg/wk) and prednisolone (initially 60 mg/day, tapered in six weekly steps to 7.5 mg/day), in 155 patients with early RA. Over the course of the study, combination therapy was phased out; prednisone was discontinued after 28 weeks, and MTX was stopped after 40 weeks; SSZ was continued in all groups. Primary outcome measures included the pooled index (a weighted change score of five disease activity measures) and an assessment of radiographic damage. At 28 weeks, clinical improvements were significantly different, favoring the combined-therapy group; this was not sustained in subsequent weeks, after the discontinuation of steroid. Less radiographic damage, however, was noted in the combination group at 28, 56, and 80 weeks, statistically significant at all intervals. A more recent report demonstrates that the decrease in radiographic progression has persisted for 5 years after treatment in the study (53). These researchers also evaluated the cost effectiveness and cost-utility of early intervention in RA. In their analysis, the mean total costs per patient in the first 56 weeks of follow-up were $5,519 for combined treatment and $6,511 for treatment with SSZ alone (p = 0.37). They concluded that combined treatment was cost effective, giving greater efficacy at lower or equal cost (40).

Most recently, in 1999, Dougados et al. (54) reported the results of a randomized, controlled 52-week trial comparing SSZ and MTX as monotherapy, with these two DMARDs in combination. This project was similar in design to the work of Haagsma et al. in 1997, but included 205 participants, almost twice the number studied earlier (51). These patients, also DMARD naïve, were randomized to receive SSZ at dosages of 2,000 to 3,000 mg daily (n = 68); MTX, 7.5 to 15 mg/wk (n = 69); or the combination (n = 68). Outcome measures included the DAS and radiographic progression (modified Sharp score). Despite the greater statistical power, this study was unable to demonstrate significant differences in response, although adverse events, especially nausea, were observed more frequently in the combination group (91%) than in either monotherapy group (75% for both MTX and SSZ; p = 0.025). The results of this study also illustrate how improvement in all treatment groups results in regression to the mean and significantly dilutes statistical power.

Methotrexate and Antimalarials

In 1990, Schwarzer et al. (55) reported the results of an open study of 16 patients, each of whom had not responded to at least three DMARDs given as monotherapy. The patients were treated with HCQ (400 mg/day for 4 weeks, and then 200 mg/day thereafter) and cycling combination therapy, alternating monthly between SSZ 2 g/day and MTX 10 mg/wk. Improvements in a variety of measures were noted at 3 months, but at 12 months, only those measured by pain score (visual analogue) and ESR were sustained.

In 1993, Trnavsky et al. (56) published a randomized controlled study comparing the efficacy of MTX plus HCQ compared with HCQ alone. Twenty patients treated with MTX (7.5 mg/wk) and HCQ (200 mg daily) were compared with 20 who took only HCQ, by using six clinical variables, five laboratory tests, and one radiographic measure. In this study, improvements across all six clinical measures, in two laboratory tests, and in radiographic progression were observed in the combination group; responses in patients treated only with HCQ were limited to three of the clinical variables. Interestingly, statistical significance was demonstrated despite two treatment groups, differing from several trials that used a similar design to compare MTX with SSZ. This is most likely explained by the difference in efficacy between HCQ and SSZ; in contrast to patients treated with

SSZ, those who received HCQ, perhaps a less effective drug, did not improve to a degree that regression to the mean became significant, and statistical power was preserved.

Also in 1993, Clegg (57), writing for the HCQ/MTX study group, published an abstract describing the initial experience of a larger group of patients; detailed results after longer follow-up were presented in 1997 (58). In the first phase of the study, 141 patients were treated with HCQ (400 mg/day) and MTX (mean dosage, 9 mg/wk) during a 24-week, open-label phase. Then, responders (n = 121) were randomized into three groups: (a) HCQ with MTX as needed for disease exacerbation, (b) HCQ only, and (c) placebo with MTX as needed for flare-ups. In the second phase of the study, regimens that included maintenance HCQ delayed the onset of relapse ($p = 0.023$) and shortened the duration of flare-ups. Maintenance HCQ was well tolerated, and adverse events were equally distributed across treatment groups.

In 1994, Ferraz et al. (59) published a randomized controlled trial with 82 patients who received MTX (7.5 mg/wk) and either HCQ (250 mg/day) or placebo. Sixty-eight patients completed the study, and although all outcome measures improved significantly in both treatment groups, patients receiving the active combination had significantly lower joint counts, greater grip strength, and better functional ability at the conclusion of the study. Because mild adverse events were more frequently observed in the MTX plus HCQ group, the investigators concluded that this combination is slightly more efficacious and toxic than MTX plus placebo.

An explanation for the better performance of MTX plus HCQ has been provided by Carmichael et al. in 2002 (60). These investigators evaluated 10 healthy subjects to examine the bioavailability of MTX in the presence of HCQ and vice versa. In a randomized, crossover study, each subject received MTX and HCQ alone and in combination. The area under the concentration-time curve (AUC), was increased for MTX when taken with HCQ, whereas the AUC for HCQ was the same whether taken alone or with MTX. The maximum MTX concentration decreased, and the time to reach maximum MTX concentration was increased when MTX was taken with HCQ. These results suggest that the effect of HCQ on MTX metabolism may account for the increased potency and the sustained effects of MTX plus HCQ compared with monotherapy. The investigators also warned of the need for increased vigilance for MTX toxicity during combination therapy with HCQ.

Methotrexate and Gold

Few studies have focused on the combination of MTX and gold salts. In a 1988 abstract, Brawer (61) reported seven patients treated with parenteral gold, who relapsed after a mean duration of 4 years of successful therapy. MTX (mean dosage 11.5 mg/wk) was added to gold, with recapture of response, with an average follow-up of 19 months.

In 1990, Kantor et al. (62), writing for the Auranofin Cooperating Group, published an abstract describing 267 patients, previously untreated with DMARDs, who received auranofin and MTX as initial therapy. After a 6-month open study period, 89% of the patients had responded with at least a 50% reduction in total joint count, and a physician's global assessment of good or very good. One hundred seventy-four patients were randomized to another 6-month double-blind phase to either auranofin alone or to continued combination therapy. Benefits obtained during the initial phase were maintained in 74% of the combination patients and in 51% of the auranofin patients. Toxicity did not appear to be greatly increased on combination therapy.

In 1992, Williams et al. (63) reported the evaluation of 335 patients randomized to auranofin, MTX, or a combination of both in a 48-week, double-blind, placebo-controlled trial. Patients were allowed previous treatment with HCQ, but otherwise, had not been treated with second-line agents. No statistically-significant differences in clinical improvement outcomes were noted in the three groups. Withdrawals from the study were equal in the three groups, but the reasons for withdrawal varied. Withdrawals were more common in the combination group for adverse drug effects; however, this group had fewer withdrawals for lack of clinical response. A subsequent comparison of bony erosions in the three groups showed more erosions in patients receiving auranofin than in the other two groups; however, the progression of erosions in patients receiving a combination of MTX and auranofin was not different from the progression of erosions in patients receiving MTX alone (64).

Methotrexate and Azathioprine

In a 1987 abstract, Biro et al. (65) reported the course of 20 patients who had previously failed to improve with either MTX or AZA, who were then treated with the combination of the two drugs. The investigators noted improvements in several clinical and laboratory parameters and concluded that the combination was useful in resistant RA.

In 1992, Willkens et al. (66) presented the results of a 24-week, controlled, multicenter trial involving 212 patients randomized to one of three treatment groups: MTX alone, AZA alone, or the combination. One hundred fifty-eight patients completed the study, and there were significant differences between results from the primary and the intent-to-treat analyses. In the primary analysis, which included only patients who completed the study, the mean response was greater for AZA than for MTX, although the combination was the most powerful. In the intent-to-treat analysis, with withdrawals treated as therapy failures, there was no difference between MTX and combination therapy, although both of these groups were superior to AZA monotherapy.

Three years later, this group presented follow-up data, in which patients had been treated for 48 weeks, and included radiograph progression as an outcome measure (67). Of 209 patients who began this phase of the study, 110 remained in the group to which they had been randomized. Response rates were reported as 38% for combination therapy, 26% for AZA, and 45% for MTX ($p = 0.06$); interestingly, a trend toward decreased radiographic progression was seen in the MTX monotherapy group. The researchers concluded that the combination of MTX and AZA was not associated with greater toxicity than with either agent in single therapy, but this did not seem to provide greater benefit (68).

Finally, Blanco et al. (69) reported a series of 43 patients with RA refractory to MTX and who subsequently received MTX/AZA in combination. An acute febrile toxic reaction marked by fever, leukocytosis, and cutaneous leukocytoclastic vasculitis developed in four (9%) patients when AZA was added, resolving within days when the medications were discontinued. In two patients, rechallenge with the combination was associated with a new flare-up.

Methotrexate and Cyclosporine

As described earlier in this Chapter, the 1995 MCCSG study was important not only in that it demonstrated superior benefit for the combination of MTX and CYA, but also in that it highlighted an important point of study design. Tendency to improvement, likely with any therapy, causes regression to the mean, reducing statistical power and increasing the likelihood of type II error. In 1997, this group presented the results of the open-label extension of their initial report (70). In this phase of the investigation, 92 patients who had received MTX plus placebo during the initial 24 weeks were given MTX plus CYA; by the end of the extension period, most outcome measures in these patients were similar to those who had initially received combination therapy. In addition, the clinical improvements described in the combination group during the initial phase of the study were sustained during extension.

In 1996, Salaffi et al. (71) reported similar results from a smaller study, in which 14 patients with partial response to injectable MTX and 14 with partial response to HCQ received CYA in addition to their DMARD. Although patients in both groups improved, the combination of MTX plus CYA seemed slightly more efficacious and more toxic than HCQ plus CYA.

Success with the combination of MTX plus CYA over a longer period was reported in a letter by González-Gay et al. (72) in 1998, who followed up 11 patients for at least 3 years, without evidence of significant toxicity or loss of benefit.

More recently, a study from the Netherlands compared CYA in a dose of 2.5 to 5 mg/kg with the combination of CYA and MTX 7.5 to 15 mg/wk (73). The 120 RA patients were followed for 48 weeks. Withdrawals were similar in the two treatment groups but were more common for inefficacy on monotherapy and for adverse events on combination therapy. The patients on combination therapy had more improvement in clinical disease activity and had more slowing of radiographic progression.

Another recent report in 24 early RA patients demonstrated that the combination of MTX and CYA with prednisone lowered tumor necrosis factor (TNF) production without decreasing TNF messenger RNA expression to a greater degree than MTX and prednisone (74). The investigators suggested that this effect could be an explanation for the induction of immunosuppressive and therapeutic effects of the drug combination, although it could be a solitary effect of CYA. Consensus guidelines for the use of CYA in RA have been published, which include dosing recommendations for optimizing treatment, minimizing or avoiding adverse renal events, and managing CYA-associated hypertension (75). In these guidelines, the combination of MTX plus CYA is suggested for patients who exhibit only a partial response to CYA at the maximal tolerable dose of the drug.

Methotrexate and D-Penicillamine

A retrospective study of 16 patients treated with MTX and D-pen for periods ranging from 5 to 86 months was published in 1990 (76,77). These patients had demonstrated partial response to penicillamine monotherapy (mean dosage 750 mg/day), and MTX was added (mean dosage 10 mg/wk). Eight patients achieved complete remission, and no dropouts for drug toxicity were reported, although three patients were lost to follow-up and one patient died of undetermined cause.

Recently, successful treatment of MTX-induced nodulosis with D-pen has been reported (78). Three patients who experienced accelerated nodulosis after beginning MTX were treated with moderate dosages of D-pen (500 mg/day). This treatment was associated with regression of subcutaneous nodules in all patients, disappearance of vasculitic lesions in two cases, and resolution of pulmonary nodules in one patient.

Methotrexate and Leflunomide

Leflunomide (LEF) is the newest addition to the classical DMARD medications. It has been suggested that it has a high potential for success in combination therapy, particularly with MTX (79).

In 1999, Weinblatt et al. (80) published data describing the efficacy, safety, and pharmacokinetics of a combination of MTX and LEF in patients who had developed an unsatisfactory response to MTX alone. In this open-label study, 30 patients with active RA despite MTX (mean dosage 17 mg/wk) also were given LEF at dosages of 10 to 20 mg/ day. Sixteen (53%) patients met American College of Rheumatology 20% (ACR20) response criteria; two met ACR criteria for remission after 1 year. Seven patients withdrew—two voluntarily, three were withdrawn because of persistent liver enzyme elevations, and two withdrew because of lack of efficacy. Pharmacokinetic studies of both MTX and LEF did not detect any significant interactions.

An open-label study of 30 RA patients resistant to MTX who were subsequently given LEF was also reported in 1999 (81). Only 12 patients remained on the starting dosage of 10 mg/day LEF and 16 increased the dosage to 20 mg/day. Two patients decreased the dosage to 10 mg every other day because of toxicity, and 23 patients completed the 52-week trial. The patients improved overall, and two met the criteria for remission. The metabolism of each drug did not seem to be affected by the concomitant use of the other drug.

Recently, a double-blind, randomized controlled trial was reported where 263 RA patients who had persistent arthritis after at least 6 months of MTX therapy were randomized to have LEF or placebo added to their regimen (82). The patients on combination therapy had a significant improvement as measured by the ACR20 criteria compared with placebo (46% vs. 20%). Discontinuation rates and adverse events were similar in the two treatments groups. Appropriate liver enzyme and hematologic monitoring was recommended.

Sulfasalazine and Antimalarials

Other than the work by Schwarzer et al. described earlier (55), which used MTX and SSZ in cycling combination with HCQ, only one other study combining SSZ and antimalarials has been reported. In 1993, Faarvang et al. (83) reported a 6-month randomized controlled trial, in which 91 patients were randomized to receive SSZ, HCQ, or the combination of both. Sixty-two patients completed the study, and although the investigators reported better and faster response to the combination therapy, these differences were not statistically significant across the groups.

Sulfasalazine and Gold

In 1987, Dawes et al. (84) reported their 6-month open pilot study in which SSZ was added to the regimens of 25 patients who had had partial response to either gold or D-pen. Over the course of the study, 22 patients showed meaningful improvement in seven of eight clinical and laboratory outcome measures.

The following year, Farr et al. (85) reported the complementary study, in which 38 patients receiving established SSZ therapy were prescribed either gold (9 patients) or D-pen (29 patients). A favorable response was seen in 70% of the total group, although one third of the patients in both groups developed side effects requiring cessation of combination therapy.

Sulfasalazine and Cyclosporine

There is one study of CYA and SSZ reported in 1999 (86). The investigators studied the combination for 12 months in 45 patients with early active RA. The patients were evaluated by disease activity measures, which seemed to improve within 3 months. Seventy-eight percent of patients met European League Against Rheumatism (EULAR) response criteria at the end of the year. Seven patients did not complete the trial—five because of gastrointestinal side effects and two because of lack of response.

Sulfasalazine and Azathioprine

No significant studies have addressed the combination of SSZ and AZA, although two letters describing the treatment of patients with this regimen have been published (87,88).

Sulfasalazine and D-Penicillamine

In addition to the investigations by Dawes and Farr described earlier, Taggart et al. (89) performed an unblinded evaluation of 15 patients receiving SSZ and D-pen in comparison with 15 patients receiving SSZ alone. There was clinical improvement in both groups. The overall trend was for greater improvement in the combination group; however, differences between the groups achieved statistical significance in only two of the ten parameters evaluated. Adverse effects were slightly higher in the combination group.

In 1990, Scott and Huskisson (90) reported premature termination of a trial evaluating patients not adequately controlled with either D-pen or SSZ by itself who were randomized to receive an additional second-line agent or placebo. If the patients received SSZ originally, D-pen or placebo was added. If the patients originally received D-pen, SSZ or placebo was added. An interim analysis after the enrollment of 30 patients suggested that with the target population of 60 patients, demonstration of a significant difference between groups was unlikely.

Finally, in 1994, Borg et al. (91) reported two patients who developed signs and symptoms of drug-induced systemic lupus erythematosus while receiving combined therapy with SSZ and D-pen.

Antimalarials and Gold

In 1989, Scott et al. (92) published the results of a prospective study of the use of parenteral gold with either placebo or HCQ in 101 RA patients in a 12-month, parallel, double-blind, placebo-controlled trial. Eighteen withdrawals due to adverse effects occurred in the gold plus HCQ group versus 10 in the gold plus placebo group. Of 13 variables for clinical assessment, improvement in the gold plus HCQ group achieved statistical significance for overall disease activity index and C-reactive protein levels only at 12 months; however, there was an overall trend for approximately 20% to 25% greater improvement in patients receiving combination therapy.

In 1990, Luthra (93) presented an abstract describing 229 patients randomized to receive either auranofin, HCQ, or a combination of the two drugs for 24 weeks. No difference in clinical outcomes was identified in these groups, and the researchers concluded that "the evidence seems to suggest that combined therapy offers at best only marginal improvement over the two single therapies."

In 1993, Porter et al. (94) evaluated the benefit of adding HCQ versus placebo to the treatment of RA patients who had experienced a suboptimal response to injectable gold and found no efficacy or toxicity differences in the two groups.

Antimalarials and Cyclosporine

The 1996 study of Salaffi et al. (71), describing the efficacy and toxicity of this combination in 14 patients with partial response to HCQ, and comparing this with MTX plus CYA, was discussed earlier in this chapter.

In 1998, van den Borne et al. (95) published an investigation in which 88 patients with partial response to chloroquine were randomized to receive either placebo, CYA 1.25 mg/kg/day, or CYA 2.5 mg/kg/day. The primary outcome measures included the tender joint count for efficacy and the serum creatinine for toxicity. Both CYA groups experienced significant withdrawal rates for inefficacy or toxicity, and although the intent-to-treat analysis showed modest improvement in patients treated with CYA, this was accompanied by a statistically significant increase in serum creatinine.

Antimalarials and D-Penicillamine

The earliest report of this combination was published in 1982 by Martin et al. (96). This was a brief report of a 6-month open trial involving 45 patients. Although no outcome results or statistical analysis was presented, the investigators concluded that there was an advantage for combination therapy.

In 1984, Bunch et al. (97) published the results of a double-blind, placebo-controlled, 2-year study of 56 patients randomized to receive D-pen and HCQ in combination or either agent alone with the appropriate placebo. Combination therapy added no advantage over single-agent treatments, and D-pen alone appeared better than the combination. Although not statistically significant, side effects were more common in the D-pen-alone group than in the HCQ or D-pen plus HCQ groups.

In 1987, Gibson et al. (98) reported a 1-year, single-blind randomized study in which 72 patients were assigned to HCQ 250 mg/day, D-pen 750 mg/day, or the combination of both. All groups improved, and there were no significant differences in clinical response across the groups, although laboratory and radiologic measures favored the two groups receiving D-pen. Untoward drug effects were higher in patients on D-pen and were slightly increased in the combination group. Withdrawals for adverse events were higher in the combination group.

Gold and Cyclosporine

The 1994 open-label pilot study of Bensen et al. (36), which demonstrated efficacy for this combination in 20 patients with partial response to gold, was described briefly earlier in this chapter.

In 1996, Bendix and Bjelle (99) published a 6-month, randomized controlled trial in which 40 patients with decreasing response to parenteral gold were randomized to receive either CYA or placebo. Patients' global assessment was the only outcome measure significantly different between groups, favoring CYA over placebo. During the study, those treated with CYA had higher blood pressures and more evidence of renal insufficiency than those who received placebo, but these resolved by 6 months after completion of the project, and higher serum potassium levels were the only remaining differences between groups.

Gold and D-Penicillamine

In 1984, Bitter (4) reported clinical experience involving combination therapy with injectable gold and D-pen. Both agents were used alone, in combination, and with either levamisole or chlorambucil. The numbers of patients were small, with the largest groups containing only 12 subjects. No intergroup comparisons were reported, but the trend suggested a greater improvement in patients receiving combination therapies, with a concurrent increase in toxicity.

Gold and Cyclophosphamide

In 1998, Walters and Cawley (100) presented the results of a study evaluating methylprednisolone alone or combined with gold, intravenous CTX, or gold plus intravenous CTX. The numbers of patients were small (four or five in each group), and the patients and investigators were not blinded to the treatment course. There appeared to be no difference in patients receiving methylprednisolone alone compared with those receiving methylprednisolone and CTX. The two groups receiving gold had a greater improvement measured at 24 weeks than the groups not receiving gold. Adverse effects were not remarkably different in the treatment groups.

COMBINATIONS OF MULTIPLE DMARDS

Hydroxychloroquine, Azathioprine, and Cyclophosphamide

The benchmark contributions of McCarty, Csuka, and Carrera in the early and mid-1980s, which reported the use of multiple DMARDs in combination, have been described earlier in this chapter.

Hydroxychloroquine, Sulfasalazine, and Methotrexate

Of all the triple-DMARD combinations, this regimen has been the most extensively explored, primarily by the

Rheumatoid Arthritis Investigational Network (RAIN). In 1996, O'Dell et al. (101) published the results of a 2-year controlled study in which 102 patients with poor responses to at least one DMARD were randomized to receive MTX alone (7.5–17.5 mg/wk), a combination of SSZ (500 mg twice daily), and HCQ (200 mg twice daily), or all three drugs. In total, 50 patients had 50% improvement in composite symptoms of arthritis by 9 months, with benefit sustained at least 2 years without evidence of significant toxicity. These patients included 24 of 31 patients (77%) who had received the triple-drug combination, 12 of 36 patients (33%) treated with MTX alone, and 14 of 35 patients (40%) who had taken SSZ plus HCQ. Seven patients in the MTX-only group and three patients in both of the other two treatment groups were withdrawn due to drug toxicity.

In follow-up, O'Dell et al. (102), writing for the RAIN group, reported the open-label extension of their initial work, in which 28 patients who had not improved after treatment with either MTX alone (14 patients) or SSZ plus HCQ (14 patients) were given the combination of the three drugs. Both groups demonstrated significant statistical and clinical improvements across a range of clinical outcome measures.

The FIN-RA Co investigators, led by Mottonen, published a 2-year, multicenter trial comparing combination therapy with SSZ plus MTX plus HCQ plus prednisolone, with monotherapy in 199 patients (103). All patients randomized to monotherapy (n = 98) received SSZ initially, although 51 were switched to MTX over the course of the study. After 2 years, clinical response (ACR50) had been achieved in 71% and 58% of the combination and single-drug groups, respectively, with similar frequencies of adverse events.

In 1999, an interesting study was published by Calguneri et al. in which combination therapy with MTX plus SSZ plus HCQ was compared with each of these agents in monotherapy, as well as with MTX plus SSZ and MTX plus HCQ (104). Although improvements in clinical and laboratory parameters were seen in all groups, the triple-drug combination was more effective than any mono- or dual-drug regimen.

This approach was explored recently by the RAIN group in a 2-year study comparing 171 RA patients in three treatment groups: MTX plus HCQ, MTX plus SSZ, and the triple combination of MTX plus HCQ plus SSZ (105). MTX was given in a dosage of up to 17.5 mg/wk, SSZ in a dosage of up to 2 g/day, and HCQ in a dosage of up to 200 mg twice a day. The primary outcome measure was the percentage of patients in each group achieving an ACR20 response after 2 years. The triple combination was marginally superior to the combination of MTX plus HCQ (78% vs. 60%, $p = 0.05$) but clearly superior to the combination of MTX plus SSZ (78% vs. 49%, $p = 0.002$). The ACR50 showed similar results (55%, 40%, and 29%, respectively). All three combinations were well tolerated, with only 14 patients withdrawing for adverse effects.

A Finnish report examined radiographic evidence of cervical spine disease in 176 patients who had been treated either with monotherapy or a triple combination (106). Anterior atlantoaxial subluxation and atlantoaxial impaction were observed in patients who had received single-drug therapy (6.6% and 2.2%, respectively), but were not seen in the 85 patients on the combination regimen. This suggests that triple-combination therapy may retard the development of atlantoaxial disease.

Antimalarials, Methotrexate, and Cyclophosphamide

Recently, Keyszer et al. (107) reported the results of a matched-pair observational study in which 56 patients who had not responded to MTX were treated with the combination of MTX (15 mg/wk), HCQ (250 mg daily), and CTX (50 mg three times weekly). The primary end point, 50% improvement in swollen joint count, was required for continued participation in the treatment. Outcomes were compared with data collected in the same patients during the previous (unsuccessful) therapy with MTX, and with a matched-patient cohort that was given MTX monotherapy for the first time. In comparing single-subject data, combination therapy resulted in a significant decrease in the swollen joint count after 1 year, compared with the patients' prior experience with MTX monotherapy. In the matched-pair analysis, 13 (23%) patients in the combination group had a complete remission, compared with 26 (47%) patients in the MTX-only group. Toxicity was comparable in both groups, and the investigators concluded that this combination is "safe and beneficial" in patients for whom MTX monotherapy has been ineffective.

Several brief reports have described success with combinations of HCQ, MTX, and CTX (108–110).

Gold, Hydroxychloroquine, and Methotrexate

An open-label, 3-year study was conducted on patients with RA who were treated with injectable gold sodium thiomalate 50 mg/wk, HCQ 400 mg/day, and MTX 7.5 mg/wk (111). The dosage of HCQ and MTX was decreased to 200 mg/day and 5 mg/wk, respectively, and the gold injections were progressively increased in interval to every fourth week in the second and third year. Only 12 of the patients completed the study, but the researchers reported significant "amelioration" of clinical parameters in the first year that was maintained in the final 2 years; 10 of these patients did not demonstrate anatomic progression.

OTHER COMBINATIONS

In 1989, Langevitz et al. (112) published a brief report describing the successful treatment of intractable RA with MTX, AZA, and HCQ. In 1995, McCarty et al. (113) published a detailed analysis of his experience with combination DMARDs in 169 patients. Although various combinations were used in his cohort, the effectiveness of a triple-drug regimen of MTX and AZA, combined with an antimalarial, was investigated in depth. In reviewing the course of the entire cohort, the researchers found that combination therapy controlled joint inflammation in 167 patients; complete remission was reported in 43%.

Another step-up study was published in 2002 (114). There were three basic treatment groups for the 126 patients with RA. All three groups began as monotherapy with either MTX (group 1), CYA (group 2), or SSZ (group 3). After 6 months, patients who had not attained an ACR50 response in groups 1 and 2 were placed on MTX plus CYA. Those who still had not reached an ACR50 response at 12 months had SSZ added. Patients in group 3 remained on SSZ monotherapy for the duration of the study. After 18 months, the step-up approach led to about 90% of MTX and CYA patients reaching the ACR50 response compared with 24% of the SSZ monotherapy group. The step-up therapy resulted in slightly more adverse events.

In addition to the work already cited in this Chapter, several excellent reviews of combinations using two or more DMARDs have been published (115–124).

BLUEPRINTS OF THE NEW PYRAMIDS

In a 1989 editorial, Wilske and Healey (125), criticizing the traditional treatment pyramid on grounds that benefits are realized too slowly, proposed a "step-down bridge" approach, in which multiple DMARDs are initiated to control inflammation as quickly as possible, and then tapered as the activity of the disease permits. In this strategy, patients with RA are initially treated with prednisone 10 mg daily for 1 month. If synovitis is still present, combination therapy is recommended; this editorial suggested adding MTX, parenteral gold, oral gold, and HCQ to the daily dose of steroid. The regimen is then tapered sequentially, and drugs are discontinued one at a time until a maintenance medication is continued as monotherapy. The publication of this editorial prompted a reevaluation of the pyramid concept, and many leaders have expressed opinions as to whether this image ought to be remodeled, reformed, inverted, or abandoned (126–137).

In 1991, Wilke and Clough (138) suggested a similar approach, which they named graduated-step therapy. First, new patients with RA are stratified according to a disease activity index. Next, a specific treatment regimen, based on the severity of the disease, is used: the more severe the arthritis, the greater the number of DMARDs. Patients with mild disease receive HCQ and NSAIDS; for patients with moderate disease, a second DMARD is added (usually auranofin, SSZ, or MTX). Severe disease is treated with three DMARDs, adding parenteral gold, penicillamine, and AZA to the list of possible medications. In this method, patients are evaluated regularly, and a change in disease severity category may result in a change in therapy.

BIOLOGIC AGENTS IN COMBINATION THERAPY

The advent of effective biologic therapies for RA (see Chapters 39 and 40) has significantly broadened our therapeutic options, and the role of these agents in combination with traditional DMARDs and with other biologics is beginning to be explored. In 1995, Moreland et al. (139) published the results of a randomized controlled trial of 64 patients with RA refractory to MTX, who received either intravenous treatments with a chimeric anti-CD4 monoclonal antibody (cM-T412) or sham infusions, in combination with a stable dose of MTX. Despite significant peripheral T-cell depletion, this agent was neither clinically efficacious (using 50% improvement in swollen or tender joint counts) nor toxic. The early experience with combination therapy and biologic agents was also reviewed at the Chatham conference (140). In 2004, Klareskog et al. (142a) reported the Trial of Etanercept and Methotrexate with Radiographic Patient Outcomes (TEMPO), which compared etanercept (25 mg subcutaneously twice a week) combined with MTX (average dose 17 mg per week) to etanercept or MTX as monotherapy in 682 patients with RA. After 24 weeks, the combination therapy was significantly better than either monotherapy and the two single agents were similar in efficacy. After one year, the combination had less radiographic progression than either single agent although etanercept alone was superior to MTX alone. Adverse events were similar in all three treatment groups.

Etanercept

More promising were the results from the work of Weinblatt et al. (141), who investigated the efficacy of etanercept (a recombinant TNF receptor:FC fusion protein) in combination with MTX. In this study, 89 patients who had only partial response to MTX were randomized to receive either etanercept or placebo in combination with MTX. At 1 month, 56% of those who had received the active combination demonstrated an ACR20 response (the primary end point), compared with 20% who had received placebo; the difference at 6 months was even greater: 71% for those with active treatment compared with 27% in the comparison group. Statistically-significant differences also were found by using ACR50 and ACR70 response criteria at 6 months. Combination therapy also was associated with greater improvements in tender and swollen joint counts. Although localized reactions at the injection sites were common (42%), this was the only notable adverse event, and no patients were withdrawn from the study for this.

These results were confirmed by Bankhurst, who randomly assigned 30 RA patients on MTX to MTX plus placebo and 59 patients to MTX plus etanercept (142). After 24 weeks, 71% of the patients on the combination had achieved an ACR20 response as compared with 27% of the patients who continued MTX as monotherapy.

Infliximab

Treatment with infliximab, a chimeric monoclonal antibody against TNF, can lead to the formation of antibodies against infliximab. The development of these antibodies is associated with increased risk for infusion reactions and a reduced duration of response. The concomitant use of immunosuppressive therapy such as MTX or AZA reduces the antibody response, and it is recommended that infliximab be given as combination therapy with an immunosuppressive agent (143).

In 1998, Maini et al. (144) published an interesting study describing the use of infliximab in combination with MTX. One hundred one patients who had only a partial response to MTX were randomized across seven treatment categories. Six groups were given MTX (7.5 mg/wk) or placebo, plus an intravenous infusion of infliximab at 1, 3, or 10 mg/kg (weekly); the remaining group was given active MTX and placebo infusions. Approximately 60% of those who received either 3 or 10 mg/kg infusions achieved an ACR20 response, regardless of whether they received active or placebo MTX. At the lowest dose of infliximab, those who had been given active MTX had a prolonged response, compared with both the placebo/MTX and the placebo/infliximab groups. The researchers considered this to be evidence of apparent synergy, although this has been disputed (145).

Subsequently, these investigators conducted a double-blind, placebo-controlled trial in RA patients on MTX, using doses of infliximab of 3 mg/kg and 10 mg/kg and with infusions given either every 4 weeks or every 8 weeks (146). Four hundred twenty-eight patients were randomized to one of the four infliximab treatment groups or placebo. After 30 weeks of treatment, the infliximab plus MTX treatment groups all had greater clinical benefit than MTX as monotherapy, and the four infliximab groups were similar in ACR20 response. A subsequent 54-week follow-up on these patients demonstrated that radiographic evidence of RA progression was significantly decreased in the patients treated with infliximab and MTX (147).

A small study in which 28 patients on MTX (10 mg/wk) received a single blinded infusion of 5 mg/kg, 10 mg/kg, or 20 mg/kg infliximab or placebo has also been reported (148). Seventeen of the 21 patients receiving any dose of infliximab attained an ACR20 response, compared with only one of the seven patients on placebo. An open extension of the trial with infusions of 10 mg/kg at weeks 12, 20, and 28 showed that 53% of the patients maintained their response for 40 weeks.

There is one open-label study that examined the combination of infliximab and LEF in patients with RA (149). Twenty patients were followed for 32 weeks. Eleven patients withdrew for adverse events, commonly rash and pruritis. In those remaining on treatment, 80% attained an ACR20 response, with 46% also reaching an ACR70 response. Although the combination appears to be highly efficacious, its use may be limited by toxicity. In 2004, St. Clair et al. (149a) presented the findings of the Active-Controlled Study of Patients Receiving Infliximab for the Treatment of Rheumatoid Arthritis of Early Onset Study Group (ASPIRE). This trial studied 1049 patients with RA of less than three years duration who had not received MTX or TNF inhibitors. Patients were given MTX (up to 20 mg per week) and placebo or MTX and infliximab (3 mg/kg or 6 mg/kg) in the usual infliximab dosing schedule. At week 54, the patients receiving MTX and infliximab had more clinical improvement, less radiographic progression and greater physical function improvement than the patients on MTX and placebo. More infections, particularly pneumonia, were seen in the patients receiving infliximab.

Adalimumab

Adalimumab, a fully-human monoclonal antibody, is the newest TNF inhibitor. There is one randomized, double-blind, placebo-controlled 24-week study where adalimumab or placebo was added to MTX therapy in 271 RA patients (150). Three doses of adalimumab were evaluated: 20 mg, 40 mg, and 80 mg given subcutaneously every other week. All three doses of adalimumab with MTX achieved greater ACR20 response than MTX plus placebo (48%, 67%, and 65% vs. 15%, respectively.) The 40- and 80-mg doses of adalimumab reached ACR70 responses of 27% and 19%, respectively. Adverse events were similar in all treatment groups. In 2004, Keystone et al. (150a) reported that the addition of adulimumab to patients with an inadequate response to MTX resulted in greater improvement compared with the addition of placebo. Inadequate responders to MTX at doses of 12.5–25 mg/week were randomized to receive placebo or adulimumab 20 mg every other week or 40 mg every other week. The primary efficacy endpoint at 24 weeks (ACR 20) demonstrated significantly greater benefit with the addition of either dose of adulimumab. Primary endpoints at 52 weeks confirmed similar benefit in radiologic progression and physical function, in addition to sustained improvement in ACR 20 for both combinations compared to MTX alone. Adverse events were not increased in the patients on adulimumab.

Anakinra

Anakinra, an IL-1 receptor antagonist, has modest clinical benefit but does slow the progression of structural damage. A recent randomized, controlled trial examining the efficacy and safety of five doses of anikinra in combination with MTX was conducted in 419 patients with active RA despite MTX monotherapy (151). Patients were randomized to receive placebo, 0.04, 0.1, 0.4, 1.0, or 2.0 mg/kg of anakinra per day, in combination with their individual prestudy MTX dose. After 12 weeks of treatment, all anakinra plus MTX treatment groups had greater ACR responses than placebo plus MTX as monotherapy; similar findings were observed after 24 weeks, at study conclusion. Although anakinra was safe and well-tolerated, injection site reactions were common, and led to premature study withdrawal in 7% and 10% of those in the 1.0- and 2.0-mg/kg groups, respectively.

The combination of etanercept and anakinra in one small study and a larger controlled trial revealed an increase in serious infections, and the package insert for anakinra warns against this regimen until further studies demonstrate that it is safe (152,153).

CONCLUSION AND RECOMMENDATIONS

In recent years, combinations of two or more DMARDs have become established as mainstream treatments, and we have learned important lessons about study design and protocol development for evaluating combination therapy. Two-drug combination DMARD therapies appear effective in nonresponders or in partial responders to monotherapies. MTX seems to be the best anchor drug. Combinations of multiple DMARDs, especially triple therapy, may be more effective than two-drug combinations. The addition of newer biologic agents to traditional DMARDs holds future promise and the initial responses have been impressive, particularly in terms of halting structural damage. At least one combination (etanercept and anakinra) may be limited by safety concerns but more experience is needed with biologic or immunologic therapy and combinations of therapies.

The decision to use combination therapy as initial treatment is best left to the judgment of the individual physician, because there is good evidence that some patients will have a good response to monotherapy. We recommend combination DMARDs for those patients who have not responded (or only partially responded) to single-agent therapy, particularly with MTX. It is not yet possible to forecast which patients can be treated effectively with monotherapy, and which will require multiple agents, although the emerging field of pharmacogenomics may bring this to us soon. It may be that the next giant leap for RA treatment will come with the development of reliable, valid, and useful methods of predicting benefit or harm to individual patients when selecting from the broadening range of therapeutic options.

ACKNOWLEDGMENT

This work was supported by the Veterans Affairs Medical Research Program, the Western Institute for Biomedical Research, and the Nora Eccles Treadwell Foundation.

REFERENCES

1. Fowler PD, Dawes PT, Sheeran TP, et al. Combination therapy in rheumatoid arthritis: study design. *Br J Rheumatol* 1987;26:314–315.
2. Csuka ME, Carrera GF, McCarty DJ. Intractable rheumatoid arthritis: treatment with combined cyclophosphamide, azathioprine, and hydroxychloroquine: a follow-up study. *JAMA* 1986;255:2315–2319.
3. McCarty DJ, Carrera GF. Treatment of intractable rheumatoid arthritis with combined cyclophosphamide, azathioprine, and hydroxychloroquine. *JAMA* 1982;248:1718–1723.
4. Bitter T. Combined disease-modifying chemotherapy for intractable rheumatoid arthritis. *Clin Rheum Dis* 1984;10:417–428.
5. Consensus recommendations for the management of chronic heart failure. *Am J Cardiol* 1999;83:1A–38A.
6. Richards AM, Nicholls MG. Aldosterone antagonism in heart failure. *Lancet* 1999;354:789–790.
7. DeFronzo RA. Pharmacologic therapy for type 2 diabetes mellitus. *Ann Intern Med* 1999;131:281–303.
8. Chobanian AV, Bakris GL, Black HR, et al. The seventh report of the Joint National Committee on prevention, detection, evaluation, and treatment of high blood pressure. *JAMA* 2003;289:2560–2572.
9. National Asthma Education and Prevention Program. Expert panel report 2: guidelines for the diagnosis and management of asthma. NIH Publication No. 97-4051. Bethesda, MD: National Institutes of Health, 1997.
10. Pincus T, O'Dell JR, Kremer JM. Combination therapy with multiple disease-modifying antirheumatic drugs in rheumatoid arthritis: a preventive strategy. *Ann Intern Med* 1999;131:768–774.
11. Mottonen T, Hannonen P, Korpela M, et al. Delay to institution of therapy and induction of remission using single-drug or combination-disease-modifying antirheumatic drug therapy in early rheumatoid arthritis. *Arthritis Rheum* 2002;46:894–898.
12. Fries JF. Effectiveness and toxicity considerations in outcome directed therapy in rheumatoid arthritis. *J Rheumatol* 1996;23(suppl 44):102–106.
13. Fries JF, Singh G, Lenert L, et al. Aspirin, hydroxychloroquine, and hepatic enzyme abnormalities with methotrexate in rheumatoid arthritis. *Arthritis Rheum* 1990;33:1611–1619.
14. Seideman P, Albertioni F, Beck O, et al. Chloroquine reduces the bioavailability of methotrexate in patients with rheumatoid arthritis. A possible mechanism of reduced hepatotoxicity. *Arthritis Rheum* 1994;37:830–833.
15. Munster T, Furst D. Pharmacotherapeutic strategies for disease-modifying antirheumatic drug (DMARD) combinations to treat rheumatoid arthritis (RA). *Clin Exp Rheumatol* 1999:17(suppl 18):29–36.
16. Choy E. Panayi G. Mechanisms of action of second-line agents and choice of drugs in combination therapy. *Clin Exp Rheumatol* 1999; 17(suppl 18):20–28.
17. Harris ED Jr. The rationale for combination therapy of rheumatoid arthritis based on pathophysiology. *J Rheumatol* 1996;23(suppl 44): 2–4.
18. Salmon SE, Dalton WS. Relevance of multidrug resistance to rheumatoid arthritis: development of a new therapeutic hypothesis. *J Rheumatol* 1996;23(suppl 44):97–101.
19. Roubenoff R, Jones RJ, Karp JE, et al. Remission of rheumatoid arthritis with the successful treatment of acute myelogenous leukemia with cytosine arabinoside, daunorubicin, and m-AMSA. *Arthritis Rheum* 1987;30:1187–1190.
20. Cohen MG, Janssen B, Webb J. Response of rheumatoid arthritis to chemotherapy for Hodgkin's disease in a patient with IgA deficiency and overlap connective tissue disease. *Ann Rheum Dis* 1988;47:603–605.
21. Oliver SJ, Brahn E. Combination therapy in rheumatoid arthritis: the animal model perspective. *J Rheumatol* 1996;23(suppl 44):56–60.
22. Brahn E, Peacock DJ, Banquerigo ML. Suppression of collagen-induced arthritis by combination cyclosporin A and methotrexate therapy. *Arthritis Rheum* 1991;34:1282–1288.
23. Oliver SJ, Cheng TP, Banquerigo ML, et al. Suppression of collagen-induced arthritis by an angiogenesis inhibitor, AGM-1470, in combination with cyclosporin: reduction of vascular endothelial growth factor (VEGF). *Cell Immunol* 1995;166:196–206.
24. Peacock DJ, Banquerigo ML, Brahn E. An angiogenesis inhibitor in combination with anti-CD5 Mab suppresses established collagen-induced arthritis significantly more effectively than single agent therapy. *Arthritis Rheum* 1992;35(suppl):S140.
25. Oliver SJ, Banquerigo ML, Brahn E. Suppression of collagen induced arthritis using an angiogenesis inhibitor, AGM-1470, and a microtubule stabilizer, taxol. *Cell Immunol* 1994;157:291–299.
26. Boisser MC, Chiocchia G, Fournier C. Combination of cyclosporin A and calcitriol in the treatment of adjuvant arthritis. *J Rheumatol* 1992; 19:754–757.
27. Gepner P, Amor B, Fournier C. 1,25-Dihydroxyvitamin D_3 potentiates the in vitro inhibitor effects of cyclosporin A on T cells from rheumatoid arthritis patients. *Arthritis Rheum* 1989;32:31–36.

28. Bendele A, Sennello G, McAbee T, et al. Effects of interleukin 1 receptor antagonist alone and in combination with methotrexate in adjuvant arthritis rats. *J Rheumatol* 1999;26:1225–1229.
29. Seivers K, Hurri L. Combined therapy of rheumatoid arthritis with gold and chloroquine. I. evaluation of the therapeutic effect. *Acta Rheumatol Scand* 1963;9:48–55.
30. Ehrlich GE. Heroic treatment for nonmalignant disease. *JAMA* 1982; 248:1743–1744.
31. Bellamy N, Brooks PM. Current practice in antimalarial prescribing in rheumatoid arthritis. *J Rheumatol* 1986;13:551–555.
32. O'Dell J. Combination DMARD therapy for rheumatoid arthritis: apparent universal acceptance. *Arthritis Rheum* 1997;40(suppl):S50.
33. Tugwell P, Pincus T, Yocum D, et al. Combination therapy with cyclosporine and methotrexate in severe rheumatoid arthritis. *N Engl J Med* 1995;333:137–141.
34. Paulus HE. Protocol development for combination therapy with disease-modifying antirheumatic drugs. *Semin Arthritis Rheum* 1993;23(suppl 1):19–25.
35. Felson DT, Anderson JJ, Meenan RF. The efficacy and toxicity of combination therapy in rheumatoid arthritis (RA): a meta-analysis. *Arthritis Rheum* 1994;37:1487–1491.
36. Bensen W, Tugwell P, Roberts RM, et al. Combination therapy of cyclosporine with methotrexate and gold in rheumatoid arthritis (2 pilot studies). *J Rheumatol* 1994;21:2034–2038.
37. Wilske K, Yocum D. Rheumatoid arthritis: the status and future of combination therapy. *J Rheumatol* 1995;23(suppl 44):1–110.
38. Felson DT, Anderson JJ, Meenan RF. The comparative efficacy and toxicity of second-line drugs in rheumatoid arthritis: results of two meta-analyses. *Arthritis Rheum* 1990;33:1449–1461.
39. Pincus T. Limitations of randomized clinical trials to recognize possible advantages of combination therapies in rheumatic diseases. *Semin Arthritis Rheum* 1993;23(suppl 1):2–10.
40. Verhoeven AC, Bibo JC, Boers M, et al. Cost-effectiveness and cost-utility of combination therapy in early rheumatoid arthritis: randomized comparison of combined step-down prednisolone, methotrexate and sulphasalazine with sulphasalazine alone. *Br J Rheumatol* 1998; 37:1102–1109.
41. Pham B, Cranney A, Boers M, et al. Validity of area-under-the-curve analysis to summarize effect in rheumatoid arthritis clinical trials. *J Rheumatol* 1999;26:712–716.
42. Shiroky JB, Watts CS, Neville C. Combination methotrexate and sulfasalazine in the management of rheumatoid arthritis: case observations. *Arthritis Rheum* 1989;32:1160–1164.
43. Morgan SL, Baggott JE, Alarcón GS. Methotrexate and sulfasalazine combination therapy: is it worth the risk? *Arthritis Rheum* 1993;36: 281–282.
44. Shiroky JB. Unsubstantiated "risk" of antifolate toxicity with combination methotrexate and sulfasalazine therapy. *Arthritis Rheum* 1993; 36:1757.
45. Shiroky JB. Combination of sulphasalazine and methotrexate in the management of rheumatoid arthritis: view based on personal clinical experience. *Br J Rheumatol* 1995;34(suppl 2):109–112.
46. Shiroky JB. Combination sulfasalazine and methotrexate in the management of rheumatoid arthritis. *J Rheumatol* 1996;44(suppl): 69–71.
47. Nisar M, Carlisle L, Amos RS. Methotrexate and sulphasalazine as combination therapy in rheumatoid arthritis. *Br J Rheumatol* 1994;33: 651–654.
48. Haagsma CJ, van Riel PLCM, de Rooij DJRAM, et al. Combination of methotrexate and sulphasalazine vs. methotrexate alone: a randomized open clinical trial in rheumatoid arthritis patients resistant to sulphasalazine therapy. *Br J Rheumatol* 1994;33:1049–1055.
49. Haagsma CJ, Russel FGM, Vree TB, et al. Combination of methotrexate and sulphasalazine in patients with rheumatoid arthritis: pharmacokinetic analysis and relationship to clinical response. *Br J Clin Pharmacol* 1996;42:195–200.
50. Barrera P, Haagsma CJ, Boerbooms AMT, et al. Effect of methotrexate alone or in combination with sulphasalazine on the production and circulating concentrations of cytokines and their antagonists: longitudinal evaluation in patients with rheumatoid arthritis. *Br J Rheumatol* 1995;34:747–755.
51. Haagsma CJ, van Riel PLCM, de Jong AJL, et al. Combination of sulphasalazine and methotrexate versus the single components in early rheumatoid arthritis: a randomized, controlled, double-blind, 52 week clinical trial. *Br J Rheumatol* 1997;36:1082–1088.
52. Boers M, Verhoeven AC, Markusse HM, et al. Randomized comparison of combined step-down prednisolone, methotrexate and sulphasalazine with sulphasalazine alone in early rheumatoid arthritis. *Lancet* 1997;350:309–318.
53. Landewe RBM, Boers M, Verhoeven AC, et al. COBRA combination therapy in patients with early rheumatoid arthritis. Long-term structural benefits of a brief intervention. *Arthritis Rheum* 2002;46:347–356.
54. Dougados M, Combe B, Cantagrel A, et al. Combination therapy in early rheumatoid arthritis: a randomized, controlled, double blind 52 week clinical trial of sulphasalazine and methotrexate compared with the single components. *Ann Rheum Dis* 1999;58:220–225.
55. Schwarzer AC, Arnold MH, Kelly D, et al. The cycling of combination antirheumatic drug therapy in rheumatoid arthritis. *Br J Rheumatol* 1990;29:445–450.
56. Trnavsky K, Gatterova J, Linduskova M, et al. Combination therapy with hydroxychloroquine and methotrexate in rheumatoid arthritis. *Z Rheumatol* 1993;52:292–296.
57. Clegg DO. Combination hydroxychloroquine and methotrexate in the treatment of rheumatoid arthritis. *Arthritis Rheum* 1993; 36(suppl): S53.
58. Clegg DO, Dietz F, Duffy J, et al. Safety and efficacy of hydroxychloroquine as maintenance therapy for rheumatoid arthritis after combination therapy with methotrexate and hydroxychloroquine. *J Rheumatol* 1997; 24:1896–1902.
59. Ferraz MB, Pinheiro GRC, Helfenstein M, et al. Combination therapy with methotrexate and chloroquine in rheumatoid arthritis: a multicenter randomized placebo-controlled trial. *Scand J Rheumatol* 1994;23: 231–236.
60. Carmichael SJ, Beal J, Day RO, et al. Combination therapy with methotrexate and hydroxychloroquine for rheumatoid arthritis increases exposure to methotrexate. *J Rheumatol* 2002;29:2077–2083.
61. Brawer AE. The combined use of oral methotrexate and intramuscular gold in rheumatoid arthritis. *Arthritis Rheum* 1988;31:R10.
62. Kantor SM, Wallin BA, Grier CG, et al. Combination of auranofin and methotrexate as initial DMARD therapy in RA. *Arthritis Rheum* 1990;36(suppl):S60.
63. Williams HJ, Ward JR, Reading JC, et al. Comparison of auranofin, methotrexate, and the combination of both in the treatment of rheumatoid arthritis: a controlled clinical trial. *Arthritis Rheum* 1992;35: 259–269.
64. Lopez Mendez A, Daniel WW, Reading JC, et al. Radiographic assessment of disease progression in rheumatoid arthritis patients enrolled in the Cooperative Systematic Studies of the Rheumatic Diseases program randomized clinical trial of methotrexate, auranofin, or a combination of the two. *Arthritis Rheum* 1993;36:1364–1369.
65. Biro JA, Segal AM, Mackenzie AH, et al. The combination of methotrexate (MTX) and azathioprine (AZA) for resistant rheumatoid arthritis (RA). *Arthritis Rheum* 1987;30(suppl):S18.
66. Willkens RF, Urowitz MB, Stablein DM, et al. Comparison of azathioprine, methotrexate, and the combination of both in the treatment of rheumatoid arthritis: a controlled clinical trial. *Arthritis Rheum* 1992; 35:849–856.
67. Willkens RF, Sharp JT, Stablein D, et al. Comparison of azathioprine, methotrexate, and the combination of the two in the treatment of rheumatoid arthritis: a forty-eight-week controlled clinical trial with radiologic outcome assessment. *Arthritis Rheum* 1995;38:1799–1806.
68. Willkens RF, Stablein D. Combination treatment of rheumatoid arthritis using azathioprine and methotrexate: a 48 week controlled clinical trial. *J Rheumatol Suppl* 1996;23(suppl 44):64–68.
69. Blanco R, Martinez-Taboada VM, Gonzalez-Gay MA. Acute febrile toxic reaction in patients with refractory rheumatoid arthritis who are receiving combined therapy with methotrexate and azathioprine. *Arthritis Rheum* 1996;39:1016–1020.
70. Stein CM, Pincus T, Yocum D, et al. Combination treatment of severe rheumatoid arthritis with cyclosporine and methotrexate for forty-eight weeks: an open-label extension study. *Arthritis Rheum* 1997;40: 1843–1851.
71. Salaffi F, Carotti M, Cervini C. Combination therapy of cyclosporine A with methotrexate or hydroxychloroquine in refractory rheumatoid arthritis. *Scand J Rheumatol* 1996;25:16–23.
72. Gonzales-Gay MA, Blanco R, Garcia-Porrua C, et al. Long-term follow-up of patients receiving combined therapy with cyclosporine and methotrexate [Letter; comment]. *Arthritis Rheum* 1998;41:1703–1704.

73. Gerards AH, Landewe RB, Prins AP, et al. Cyclosporin A monotherapy versus cyclosporin A and methotrexate combination therapy in patients with early rheumatoid arthritis: a double blind randomized placebo controlled trial. *Ann Rheum Dis* 2003;62:291–296.
74. Giacomelli R, Cipriani P, Matucci CM, et al. Combination therapy with cyclosporine and methotrexate in patients with early rheumatoid arthritis soon inhibits TNF alpha production without decreasing TNF alpha mRNA levels. An *in vivo* and *in vitro* study. *Clin Exp Rheumatol* 2002;20:365–372.
75. Cush JJ, Tugwell P, Weinblatt M, et al. US consensus guidelines for the use of cyclosporin A in rheumatoid arthritis. *J Rheumatol* 1999; 26:1176–1186.
76. Williams HJ. Combination disease-modifying antirheumatic drug therapy in rheumatoid arthritis. In: van de Putte LBA, Furst DE, Williams HJ, et al., eds. *Therapy of systemic rheumatic disorders.* New York: Marcel Dekker, 1998:245–261.
77. Lee S, Solomon G. Combination D-penicillamine and methotrexate therapy: proposal for early and aggressive treatment for rheumatoid arthritis. *Bull Hosp Joint Dis Orthop Inst* 1990;50:160–168.
78. Dash S, Seibold JR, Tiku ML. Successful treatment of methotrexate induced nodulosis with D-penicillamine. *J Rheumatol* 1999;26:1396–1399.
79. Kremer JM. Methotrexate and leflunomide: biochemical basis for combination therapy in the treatment of rheumatoid arthritis. *Semin Arthritis Rheum* 1999;29:14–26.
80. Weinblatt ME, Kremer JM, Coblyn JS, et al. Pharmacokinetics, safety, and efficacy of combination treatment with methotrexate and leflunomide in patients with active rheumatoid arthritis. *Arthritis Rheum* 1999;42:1322–1328.
81. Mroczkowski PJ, Weinblatt ME, Kremer JM. Methotrexate and leflunomide combination therapy for patients with active rheumatoid arthritis. *Clin Exp Rheumatol* 1999;17(suppl 18):S66–68.
82. Kremer JM, Genovese MC, Cannon GW, et al. Concomitant leflunomide therapy in patients with active rheumatoid arthritis despite stable doses of methotrexate. A randomized, double-blind, placebo-controlled trial. *Ann Intern Med* 2002;137:726–733.
83. Faarvang KL, Egsmose C, Kryger P, et al. Hydroxychloroquine and sulphasalazine alone and in combination in rheumatoid arthritis: a randomized double blind trial. *Ann Rheum Dis* 1993;52:711–715.
84. Dawes PT, Sheeran TP, Fowler PD, et al. Improving the response to gold or D-penicillamine by addition of sulphasalazine: a pilot study in 25 patients with rheumatoid arthritis. *Clin Exp Rheumatol* 1987;5: 151–153.
85. Farr M, Kitas G, Bacon PA. Sulphasalazine in rheumatoid arthritis: combination therapy with D-penicillamine or sodium aurothiomalate. *Clin Rheumatol* 1988;7:242–248.
86. Rojkovich B, Hodinka L, Balint G, et al. Cyclosporin and sulfasalazine combination in the treatment of early rheumatoid arthritis. *Scand J Rheumatol* 1999;28:216–221.
87. Waterworth RF. The use of sulphasalazine and azathioprine in combination to treat rheumatoid arthritis. *Br J Rheumatol* 1989;28: 456.
88. Helliwell PS. Combination therapy with sulphasalazine and azathioprine [Letter]. *Br J Rheumatol* 1996;35:493–494.
89. Taggart AJ, Hill J, Astbury C, et al. Sulphasalazine alone or in combination with D-penicillamine in rheumatoid arthritis. *Br J Rheumatol* 1987;26:32–36.
90. Scott DL, Huskisson EC. Assessing combination therapy in rheumatoid arthritis: treatment with sulphasalazine and penicillamine. *Br J Rheumatol* 1990;29:313–314.
91. Borg AA, Davis MJ, Dawes PT, et al. Combination therapy for rheumatoid arthritis and drug-induced systemic lupus erythematosus. *Clin Rheumatol* 1994;13:522–524.
92. Scott DL, Dawes PT, Tunn E, et al. Combination therapy with gold and hydroxychloroquine in rheumatoid arthritis: a prospective, randomized, placebo-controlled study. *Br J Rheumatol* 1989;28:128–133.
93. Luthra HS, and The Midwest Cooperative Rheumatic Disease Study Group. Double-blind study comparing auranofin and hydroxychloroquine alone or in combination in rheumatoid arthritis. *Arthritis Rheum* 1990;33(suppl):S25.
94. Porter DR, Capell HA, Hunter J. Combination therapy in rheumatoid arthritis: no benefit of addition of hydroxychloroquine to patients with a suboptimal response to intramuscular gold therapy. *J Rheumatol* 1993;20:645–649.
95. van den Borne BEEM, Landewe RBM, Goei The HSG, et al. Combination therapy in recent onset rheumatoid arthritis: a randomized double blind trial of the addition of low dose cyclosporine to patients treated with low dose chloroquine. *J Rheumatol* 1998; 25:1493–1498.
96. Martin M, Dixon J, Hickling P, et al. A combination of D-penicillamine and hydroxychloroquine for the treatment of rheumatoid arthritis. *Ann Rheum Dis* 1982;41:208.
97. Bunch TW, O'Duffy JD, Tompkins RB, et al. Controlled trial of hydroxychloroquine and D-penicillamine singly and in combination in the treatment of rheumatoid arthritis. *Arthritis Rheum* 1984;27: 267–276.
98. Gibson T, Emery P, Armstrong RD, et al. Combined D-penicillamine and chloroquine treatment of rheumatoid arthritis: a comparative study. *Br J Rheumatol* 1987;26:279–284.
99. Bendix G, Bjelle A. Adding low-dose cyclosporin A to parenteral gold therapy in rheumatoid arthritis: a double-blind placebo-controlled study. *Br J Rheumatol* 1996;35:1142–1149.
100. Walters MT, Cawley M. Combined suppressive drug treatment in severe refractory rheumatoid disease: an analysis of the relative effects of parenteral methylprednisolone, cyclophosphamide, and sodium aurothiomalate. *Ann Rheum Dis* 1988;47:924–929.
101. O'Dell JR, Haire CE, Erikson N, et al. Treatment of rheumatoid arthritis with methotrexate alone, sulfasalazine and hydroxychloroquine, or a combination of all three medications. *N Engl J Med* 1996; 334:1287–1291.
102. O'Dell JR, Haire CE, Erikson N, et al. Efficacy of triple DMARD therapy in patients with RA with suboptimal response to methotrexate. *J Rheumatol Suppl* 1996;23(suppl 44):72–74.
103. Mottonen T, Hannonen P, Leirisalo-Repo M, et al. Comparison of combination therapy with single-drug therapy in early rheumatoid arthritis: a randomized trial. *Lancet* 1999;353:1568–1573.
104. Calguneri M, Pay S, Caliskaner Z, et al. Combination therapy versus monotherapy for the treatment of patients with rheumatoid arthritis. *Clin Exp Rheumatol* 1999;17:699–704.
105. O'Dell JR, Leff R, Paulsen G, et al. Treatment of rheumatoid arthritis with methotrexate and hydroxychloroquine, methotrexate and sulfasalazine, or a combination of the three medications. Results of a two-year, randomized, double-blind, placebo-controlled trial. *Arthritis Rheum* 2002;46:1164–1170.
106. Neva MH, Kauppi MJ, Kautiainen H, et al. Combination drug therapy retards the development of rheumatoid atlantoaxial subluxations. *Arthritis Rheum* 2000;43:2397–2401.
107. Keyszer G, Keysser C, Keysser M. Efficacy and safety of a combination of methotrexate, chloroquine, and cyclophosphamide in patients with refractory rheumatoid arthritis: results of an observational study with matched-pair analysis. *Clin Rheumatol* 1999;18:145–151.
108. Tiliakos NA. Low-dose cytotoxic drug combination therapy in intractable rheumatoid arthritis: two years later. *Arthritis Rheum* 1986;29(suppl):S79.
109. Butler D, Tiliakos N. Low-dose cytotoxic drug combination therapy in intractable rheumatoid arthritis [Abstract]. *Arthritis Rheum* 1985; 28(suppl):S15.
110. Tiliakos NA. Single-agent versus combination cytotoxic therapy: the case for combination therapy. In: Willkens RF, Dahl SL, eds. *Therapeutic controversies in the rheumatic diseases.* New York: Grune & Stratton, 1987:295–305.
111. Biasi D, Caramaschi P, Carletto A, et al. Combination therapy with hydroxychloroquine, gold sodium thiomalate and methotrexate in early rheumatoid arthritis. An open 3-year study. *Clin Rheumatol* 2000;19:505–507.
112. Langevitz P, Kaplinsky N, Ehrenfeld M, et al. Intractable RA—treatment with combined methotrexate, azathioprine and hydroxychloroquine. *Br J Rheumatol* 1989;28:271–272.
113. McCarty DJ, Harman JG, Grassanovich JL, et al. Combination drug therapy of seropositive rheumatoid arthritis. *J Rheumatol* 1995;22: 1636–1645.
114. Ferraccioli GF, Gremese E, Tomietto P, et al. Analysis of improvements, full responses, remission and toxicity in rheumatoid patients treated with step-up combination therapy (methotrexate, cyclosporin A, sulphasalazine) or monotherapy for three years. *Rheumatology* 2002;41:892–898.
115. Huskisson EC. Combination chemotherapy in rheumatoid arthritis. *Br J Rheumatol* 1987;26:243–244.

116. Paulus HE. Antimalarial agents compared with or in combination with other disease-modifying antirheumatic drugs. *Am J Med* 1988; 85(suppl 4A):45–52.
117. Jaffe IA. Combination therapy of rheumatoid arthritis: rationale and overview. *J Rheumatol* 1990;17(suppl 25):24–27.
118. Paulus HE. The use of combinations of disease-modifying antirheumatic agents in rheumatoid arthritis. *Arthritis Rheum* 1990;33: 113–120.
119. Boers M, Ramsden M. Longacting drug combinations in rheumatoid arthritis: a formal overview. *J Rheumatol* 1991;18:316–324.
120. Williams HJ. Combination second-line therapy for rheumatoid arthritis. *Br J Rheumatol* 1993;33:603–604.
121. Williams HJ. Overview of combination second-line or disease-modifying antirheumatic drug therapy in rheumatoid arthritis. *Br J Rheumatol* 1995;34(suppl 2):96–99.
122. O'Dell JR. Combination DMARD therapy for rheumatoid arthritis: a step closer to the goal. *Ann Rheum Dis* 1996;55:781–783.
123. Kremer JM. Methotrexate and emerging therapies. *Rheum Dis Clin North Am* 1998;24:651–658.
124. O'Dell JR. Triple therapy with methotrexate, sulfasalazine, and hydroxychloroquine in patients with rheumatoid arthritis. *Rheum Dis Clin North Am* 1998;24:465–477.
125. Wilske KR, Healey LA. Remodeling the pyramid: a concept whose time has come. *J Rheumatol* 1989;16:565–567.
126. Healey LA, Wilske KR. Reforming the pyramid: a plan for treating rheumatoid arthritis in the 1990s. *Rheum Dis Clin North Am* 1989; 15:615–619.
127. Hess EV, Luggen ME. Remodeling the pyramid: concept whose time has not yet come. *J Rheumatol* 1989;16:1175–1176.
128. Roth SH. Rethinking rheumatic disease therapy. *J Rheumatol* 1989; 16:1408–1409.
129. Malleson PN, Petty RE. Remodeling the pyramid: a pediatric prospective. *J Rheumatol* 1990;17:867–868.
130. Bensen WG, Bensen W, Adachi JD, et al. Remodeling the pyramid: the therapeutic target of rheumatoid arthritis. *J Rheumatol* 1990;17: 987–989.
131. Kantor TG. Order out of chaos: the primary mission of the pyramid. *J Rheumatol* 1990;17:1580–1581.
132. Pincus T, Callahan LF. Remodeling the pyramid or remodeling the paradigms concerning rheumatoid arthritis: lessons from Hodgkin's disease and coronary artery disease. *J Rheumatol* 1990;17:1582–1585.
133. McCarty DJ. Suppress rheumatoid inflammation early and leave the pyramid to the Egyptians. *J Rheumatol* 1990;17:115–118.
134. Klippel JH. Winning the battle, losing the war: another editorial about rheumatoid arthritis. *J Rheumatol* 1990;17:1118–1122.
135. Wilske KR. Inverting the therapeutic pyramid: observations and recommendations on new directions in rheumatoid arthritis therapy based on the author's experience. *Semin Arthritis Rheum* 1993; 23(suppl 1):11–18.
136. McCarty DJ. Personal experience in the treatment of seropositive rheumatoid arthritis with drugs used in combination. *Semin Arthritis Rheum* 1993;23(suppl 1):42–49.
137. Wilke WS, Sweeney TJ, Calabrese LH. Early, aggressive therapy for rheumatoid arthritis: concerns, descriptions, and estimate of outcome. *Semin Arthritis Rheum* 1993;23(suppl 1):26–41.
138. Wilke WS, Clough JD. Therapy for rheumatoid arthritis: combinations of disease-modifying drugs and new paradigms of treatment. *Semin Arthritis Rheum* 1991;21(suppl 1):21–34.
139. Moreland LW, Pratt PW, Mayes MD, et al. Double-blind placebo-controlled multicenter trial using chimeric monoclonal anti-CD4 antibody, cM-T412, in rheumatoid arthritis patients receiving concomitant methotrexate. *Arthritis Rheum* 1995;38:1581–1588.
140. Moreland LW. Initial experience combining methotrexate with biologic agents for treating rheumatoid arthritis. *J Rheumatol* 1996;23 (suppl 44):78–83.
141. Weinblatt ME, Kremer JM, Bankhurst AD, et al. A trial of etanercept, a recombinant tumor necrosis factor receptor: Fc fusion protein, in patients with rheumatoid arthritis receiving methotrexate. *N Engl J Med* 1999;340:253–259.
142. Bankhurst AD. Etanercept and methotrexate combination therapy. *Clin Exp Rheumatol* 1999;17(suppl 18):S69–72.
142a. Klareskog L, van der Heijde D, de Jager JP, et al. Therapeutic effect of the combination of etanercept and methotrexate compared with each treatment alone in patients with rheumatoid arthritis: double-blind randomized controlled trial. *Lancet* 2004;363:675–681.
143. Baert F, Norman M, Vermeire S, et al. Influence of immunogenicity on the long-term efficacy of infliximab in Crohn's disease. *N Engl J Med* 2003;348:601–608.
144. Maini RN, Breedveld FC, Kalden JR, et al. Therapeutic efficacy of multiple intravenous infusions of anti-tumor necrosis factor a monoclonal antibody combined with low-dose weekly methotrexate in rheumatoid arthritis. *Arthritis Rheum* 1998;41:1552–1563.
145. Rezaian MM. Do infliximab and methotrexate act synergistically in the treatment of rheumatoid arthritis? Comment on the article by Maini et al. [Letter and reply]. *Arthritis Rheum* 1999;42(suppl):1779–1781.
146. Maini R, St Clair EW, Breedveld F, et al. Infliximab (chimeric anti-tumour necrosis factor α monoclonal antibody) versus placebo in rheumatoid arthritis patients receiving concomitant methotrexate: a randomised phase III trial. *Lancet* 1999;354:1932–1939.
147. Lipsky PE, van der Heijde DM, St Clair EW, et al. Infliximab and methotrexate in the treatment of rheumatoid arthritis. *N Engl J Med* 2000;343:1594–1602.
148. Kavanaugh A, St Clair EW, McCune WJ, et al. Chimeric anti-tumor necrosis factor-α monoclonal antibody treatment of patients with rheumatoid arthritis receiving methotrexate therapy. *J Rheumatol* 2000;27:841–850.
149. Kiely PD, Johnson DM. Infliximab and leflunomide combination therapy in rheumatoid arthritis: an open-label study. *Rheumatology* 2002;41:631–637.
149a. St. Clair EW, van der Heijde DMFM, Smolen JS, et al. Combination of infliximab and methotrexate therapy for early rheumatoid arthritis. *Arthritis Rheum* 2004 (In Press).
150. Weinblatt ME, Keystone EC, Furst DE, et al. Adalimumab, a fully human anti-tumor necrosis factor alpha monoclonal antibody, for the treatment of rheumatoid arthritis in patients taking concomitant methotrexate: the ARMADA trial. *Arthritis Rheum* 2003;48: 35–45.
150a. Keystone EC, Kavanaugh AF, Sharp JT, et al. Radiographic, clinical, and functional outcomes of treatment with adalimumab (a human anti-tumor necrosis factor monoclonal antibody) in patients with active rheumatoid arthritis receiving concomitant methotrexate therapy. A randomized, placebo-controlled, 52-week trial. *Arthritis Rheum* 2004; 1400–1411.
151. Cohen S, Hurd E, Cush J, et al. Treatment of rheumatoid arthritis with anikinra, a recombinant human interleukin-1 receptor antagonist, in combination with methotrexate. *Arthritis Rheum* 2002;46: 614–624.
152. Schiff MH, Bulpitt K, Weaver AA, et al. Safety of combination therapy with anakinra and etanercept in patients with rheumatoid arthritis. *Arthritis Rheum* 2001;44(suppl):S79.
153. Genovese MC, Cohen S, Moreland L, et al. Combination therapy with etanercept and anakinra in the treatment of patients with rheumatoid arthritis who have been treated unsuccessfully with methotrexate. *Arthritis Rheum* 2004;50:1412–1419.

CHAPTER 34

Corticosteroids

Ioannis Tassiulas, Ronald L. Wilder, and Dimitrios T. Boumpas

Corticosteroids are one of the most controversial subjects in rheumatology. Their role in the pathogenesis of rheumatic diseases and their use in treatment of these diseases have been a source of continuous debate. Cortisone was first isolated from adrenal tissue in the 1930s by Mason et al. (1,2), but interest in corticosteroids soared when Hench et al. (3,4) described the dramatic antiinflammatory effects of cortisone in treating rheumatoid arthritis (RA). This surprising discovery resulted in a Nobel Prize in 1950. Enthusiasm for the pharmacologic use of corticosteroids in the treatment of inflammatory disease, however, was soon dampened by the recognition of the serious side effects that accompanied high-dose therapy. As a result of the controversy regarding the merits of corticosteroid therapy, many important issues were inadequately studied or ignored in subsequent years. For example, a widely held view was that corticosteroids were not important for normal *in vivo* regulation of inflammation, although they remain the most potent, naturally-occurring antiinflammatory agents known. Their antiinflammatory effects were considered a pharmacologic rather than a normal physiologic property. Moreover, the role of corticosteroids in systemic adaptive responses in reestablishing homeostasis and preserving physiologic integrity was not completely appreciated. These adaptive responses, collectively referred to as the "stress response," are now known to interconnect extensively with inflammatory and immune responses. A large body of molecular, cellular, and physiologic data regarding corticosteroids has been generated in the past 15 years, signaling intense interest in corticosteroids. These studies may ultimately delineate the role of corticosteroids in the pathogenesis of rheumatic and other inflammatory diseases as therapeutic options.

In this Chapter, we discuss the basic pharmacology of endogenous and synthetic corticosteroids, the molecular mechanisms of their action, and their antiinflammatory and immunosuppressive effects. Pharmacokinetics, drug interactions, and general principles of corticosteroid use, with an emphasis in the treatment of rheumatic diseases, are also presented. In addition, the adverse effects of corticosteroids and the corticosteroid resistance and withdrawal syndromes are reviewed.

PHYSIOLOGIC FUNCTIONS OF CORTICOSTEROIDS

The Hypothalamic-Pituitary-Adrenal Axis

The hypothalamic-pituitary-adrenal (HPA) axis regulates the adrenal secretion of corticosteroids (5). Corticotropin-releasing hormone (CRH), a 41–amino acid polypeptide synthesized in the hypothalamic paraventricular nucleus, stimulates the corticotrophic cells of the anterior pituitary to produce adrenocorticotropic hormone (ACTH). ACTH is synthesized as a precursor molecule, proopiomelanocortin, which consists of 290 amino acids and contains the sequence of α-melanocyte-stimulating hormone (α-MSH), β-lipotropic hormone, and β-endorphin. ACTH has a biologic half-life of 4 to 8 minutes, whereas synthetic ACTH (cosyntropin) has a longer half-life. A diurnal pattern of ACTH secretion exists, following the CRH pattern, with an increase in amplitude after 3 to 5 hours of sleep and reaching a maximum during the last few hours before awakening. The secretory pattern then declines progressively during the day and into the evening. The corresponding cortisol level is highest at the time of awakening, reaching its lowest point 1 to 2 hours after sleep begins. Corticosteroids secreted by the adrenal gland feedback suppress CRH and ACTH secretion and serve to limit the potential excessive fluctuation of the stress system. ACTH affects steroidogenesis acutely and chronically. Supraphysiologic levels of plasma ACTH cause adrenocortical hyperplasia and hypertrophy. Low levels of ACTH following corticosteroid administration result in decreased levels of all steroidogenic enzymes. Profound ACTH deficiency results in atrophy of the adrenal gland.

Cortisol, Adrenal Steroid Production, and Metabolism; synthetic Steroids

All steroid hormones produced by the adrenal cortex are derived from cholesterol and have a basic structure consisting of three cyclohexane rings and one cyclopendane ring (6,7) (Fig. 34.1). Six enzymatic reactions are involved in cortisol biosynthesis: the side chain cleavage enzyme P-450cytC converts cholesterol to pregnenolone in the inner mitochondrial membrane, which in turn is converted to progesterone by the enzyme 3β-hydroxysteroid dehydrogenase in the endoplasmic reticulum. Progesterone is initially converted to 17α-hydroxyprogesterone and finally to 11-deoxycortisol. Both these enzymatic reactions occur in the endoplasmic reticulum with the help of the enzymes P-450 C17 and P-450 C21, respectively. Finally, 11-deoxycortisol is converted to cortisol by P-450 C11 in the mitochondria. As cortisol is synthesized, it is rapidly secreted into the bloodstream, so there is little intraadrenal storage of this steroid. Once secreted, most of this cortisol (75%–80%) circulates in the plasma bound to transcortin, a specific corticosteroid-binding α_2-globulin. Secretion follows a circadian rhythm that achieves maximum plasma concentration between 8 and 10 p.m. In the context of stressful stimuli and HPA axis stimulation, these levels can increase to more than 60 μg/dL (8).

A number of synthetic corticosteroids have been developed. These compounds are more potent and possess fewer mineralocorticoid effects than cortisol. Regulatory mechanisms of synthetic corticosteroids with regard to binding to corticosteroid-binding globulin (CBG), tissue-specific metabolism, affinity for the corticosteroid receptors, and interaction with transcription factors may differ from those of endogenous corticosteroids (7). There is a need for synthetic corticosteroids with a safer side effect profile. Deflazacort, an oxazoline analogue of prednisolone, has a shorter plasma half-life and fewer mineralocorticoid effects (9–11). It is still debatable as to whether its adverse effects profile is superior to that of prednisone. Deflazacort is not currently approved for use in the United States. Budesonide is also a synthetic corticosteroid; it has high topical but low systemic corticosteroid activity, due to its rapid first-pass liver metabolism and inactivation. Thus, it is suitable only when topical antiinflammatory action is desired, such as in asthma (administered by inhalation), and in Crohn disease (administered as enemas) (12,13). Finally, the "dissociated" corticosteroids have potent activator protein-1 (AP-1) and nuclear factor κB (NFκB) transrepression activities (antiinflammatory) and weak transactivation properties that are likely responsible for the adverse effects of corticosteroids (14,15).

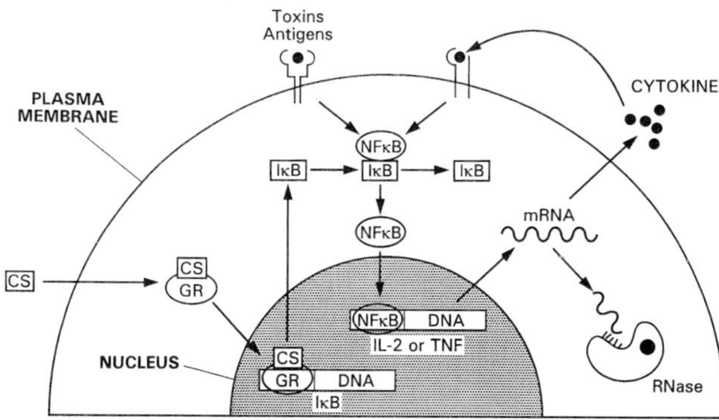

FIG. 34.1. Corticosteroid receptor antagonism of nuclear factor κB (NFκB). NFκB is an essential regulator of transcription for several genes involved in the immune and inflammatory response. Antigen, toxin, or cytokine [e.g., interleukin-2 (*IL-2*), tumor necrosis factor (*TNF*)] stimulation of cells leads to degradation of the inhibitor κB (IκB) and translocation of NFκB to the nucleus. The activated corticosteroid receptor (*GR*) either physically interacts with NFκB, preventing its binding to DNA, or binds to IκB. This dual inactivation provides a fail-proof mechanism. If any NFκB molecules escape the sequestration promoted by IκB, they are inactivated in the nucleus by associating with the GR. Corticosteroids also decrease the stability of messenger RNA. The combination of these effects leads to a dramatic decrease in cytokine production. Corticosteroids are unique among immunosuppressive agents because they inhibit both the production and action of cytokines.

MOLECULAR BIOLOGY OF CORTICOSTEROID ACTION

Corticosteroids exert most of their effects, including their antiinflammatory and immunosuppressive effects, primarily through interactions with specific, ubiquitously-expressed receptors (16). Corticosteroids circulate in the blood in either free form or in association CBG. The free form readily diffuses through the plasma membrane to bind the cytoplasmic glucocorticoid receptor (GR) (Fig. 34.1). GRs belong to the phylogenetically-conserved superfamily of nuclear "hormone receptors," which includes receptors for mineralocorticoids, androgens, progestins, estrogens, vitamin D, thyroid hormone, retinoic acid, and a growing number of so-called orphan receptors for which no specific ligand has yet been identified. In the hormone-bound state, these receptors specifically bind to and modulate the activity of target gene promoters and are, therefore, also known as ligand-dependent transcription factors.

Corticosteroids regulate gene expression by transcriptional, posttranscriptional, and posttranslational mechanisms (16). When inactive, GRs are part of a multiprotein complex that consists of the receptor, two molecules of 90-kd heat shock protein (hsp90), and one molecule each of hsp70 and hsp56, an immunophilin of the FK506- and rapamycin-binding class (17). Binding of a corticosteroid to its receptor triggers a conformational change, leading to its nuclear translocation and subsequent modulation of gene transcription (Fig. 34.1). GRs can stimulate transcription by binding to specific glucocorticoid response elements (GREs) in gene promoters, or can repress transcription by binding to negative GREs (18).

The molecular mechanisms underlying the antiinflammatory and immunosuppressive effects of corticosteroids have been investigated extensively. Two important mechanisms of action are inhibition of cytokine, chemokine, and adhesion molecule production and antagonism of the action of proinflammatory cytokines such as interleukin-1 (IL-1) and tumor necrosis factor (TNF). Inhibition of the transcription factors AP-1 and NFκB underlies both of these phenomena. Corticosteroids inhibit AP-1 and NFκB by a variety of mechanisms, depending on the cell type. One mechanism is by direct protein/protein interaction that leads to decreased transcriptional activity (19–24). Another important mechanism is the induction of IκBα transcription, an inhibitory molecule that tethers NFκB subunits in the cytoplasm (25,26). Recently, it has been shown that corticosteroids inhibit the Janus kinase signal transduction and activation of transcription (Jak-STAT) signaling pathway initiated by IL-2 and interferon-γ (IFN-γ) (27,28). This has important implications for the function of the innate immune system and the shaping of adaptive immune responses. Finally, corticosteroids can act posttranscriptionally and lead to either an increase or a decrease in messenger RNA (mRNA) stability of a number of cytokine genes (28,29).

One perceived paradoxic aspect of glucocorticoid (GC) biology is the rapidity with which the steroid is released after a stress event and the typically delayed cellular response that accompanies the actions of most steroids. Why are corticosteroids secreted so quickly, yet take hours or even days to exert a discernible response? A nongenomic action defines any action that does not directly influence gene expression initially, as do the classic steroid receptors, but rather drives more rapid effects such as the activation of signaling cascades. Corticosteroids occur naturally at high levels and often are used at high doses therapeutically; thus, nonspecific action at the membrane level must be considered. Steroids are highly lipophilic substances that tend to accumulate in lipid membranes. They might alter membrane fluidity and possibly influence the function of embedded proteins, such as ion channels or receptor proteins. However these phenomena are assumed to occur mainly at concentrations above 10 μ*M*, and there are many nongenomic CR effects that occur well below this concentration range (30,31).

Evidence for the existence of membrane steroid receptors comes from several types of observations. Electrophysiological studies demonstrated that membrane conductance can be modified within seconds of exposure to corticosteroids (32). A membrane corticosteroids receptor (CR) has been found in the brain of an amphibian, and it appears that it has similarities with opioid κ receptors (33). At the cellular level, high levels of dexamethasone have been reported to rapidly (in under 10 minutes) stabilize lysosomal membranes (34). A similar effect was detected after 24 hours, but this effect was sensitive to the GR antagonist RU486, whereas the rapid effect was insensitive to Ruy86. This indicates that a dual action occurs through classic and nonclassic receptors. Corticosteroids have also been shown to activate endothelial cell nitric oxide synthase in a nongenomic manner. This activity, which is mediated by phosphatidylinositol-3 kinase and Akt phosphorylation, leads to vasorelaxation, which may explain some of the acute cardioprotective and neuroprotective effects of corticosteroids (35,36). In contrast to these genomic effects in corticosteroids, nongenomic activities are observed at higher concentrations within seconds or minutes. Two types of specific and nonspecific nongenomic corticosteroid effects have been described. Specific, nongenomic corticosteroid effects occur within a few minutes and are considered to be mediated by steroid-selective membrane receptors (37). Nonspecific, nongenomic corticosteroid effects occur within seconds and appear to result from direct interactions with biologic membranes; these effects probably are of greatest clinical relevance when used in high-dose GC therapy (38).

ANTIINFLAMMATORY AND IMMUNOSUPPRESSIVE EFFECTS

Systemic inflammatory and immune-mediated diseases are the main clinical indications of exogenous corticosteroids. Corticosteroids are used to suppress inflammation and aberrant immune responses. There is growing evidence that endogenous corticosteroids play an important regulatory role in modulating immune responses that develop in response to venous stressors, such as infections. Corticosteroids initially help the development of adequate immune response against the invading pathogen, and later, after the infection has been confined, they act suppressively to restrain a potential deleterious "overshoot" of the same responses (39). Parameters such as serum levels and the timing of corticosteroid exposure relative to the initiation of stress determine their effects on the immune system. In general, higher corticosteroid levels are immunosuppressive, whereas lower physiologic levels may enhance immune responses (40). Endogenous corticosteroids (cortisol) appear to mediate both types of effects. Dexamethasone, a synthetic corticosteroid, mediates predominantly immunosuppressive effects; potential explanations for this include its inefficient binding to cortisol binding globulin, its longer half-life, its higher affinity for GRs, and absence of mineralocorticoid effects (41,42).

The clinically-detectable antiinflammatory effects of corticosteroids correlate with dose and duration of treatment. Corticosteroids inhibit vasodilation and vascular permeability, leading to decreased plasma exudation, erythema, and swelling. Corticosteroid inhibition on the up-regulation of inducible nitric oxide synthase by TNF-α, IL-1β and IFN-γ may contribute to this effect (43). Following corticosteroid administration, neutrophilic leukocytosis occurs, which peaks in 4 to 6 hours. At least two mechanisms mediate this phenomenon. First, there is an increased mobilization of the bone marrow reserve of neutrophil pool into the systemic circulation. Second, there is a decreased efflux of neutrophils from the circulation into sites of tissue inflammation. The mechanisms of changes in neutrophil trafficking in response to corticosteroid administration are not yet completely defined. Experimental models of inflammation suggest that corticosteroids impede granulocyte adherence to the vascular endothelium in response to inflammation (44) (Fig. 34.2). Thus, corticosteroids may alter adhesion molecules on the neutrophil or endothelial cell surfaces to interfere with the ability to traverse blood vessel walls to reach an inflammatory site. Support for this concept was initially provided by Cronstein et al., who demonstrated that corticosteroids suppressed neutrophil adhesion to endothelial cells by down-regulating the endothelial cell adhesion molecules E-selectin and intercellular adhesion molecule-1 (ICAM-1), which bind to specific ligands on neutrophils (45).

In contrast to peripheral neutrophilia, circulating levels of eosinophils, basophils, monocytes, and lymphocytes decrease upon even brief exposure to treatment corticosteroids (16,17). T cell numbers decrease more than B cells, and $CD4^+$ T cells decrease corticosteroid treatment more than $CD8^+$ T cells. Dexamethasone has been shown to down-regulate the lymphocyte adhesion molecules leukocyte function–associated antigen-1 (LFA-1) and to a lesser effect CD2 (46). These effects are mediated through the classic genomic action of corticosteroid receptors. There is evidence that non-genomic mechanisms are also involved in the regulation of cell adhesion events by corticosteroids. These changes in circulating cells are rapid (seconds to minutes) and involve cell membrane redistribution and modification of cellular adhesion molecule affinity and avidity status (44). Corticosteroids also have inhibitory effects on neutrophil function in a variety of *in vitro* assays evaluating phagocytosis and bactericidal ability; however, these effects occur at supraphysiologic and supratherapeutic drug concentrations. Granulocytes of patients receiving prednisolone or methylprednisolone have been observed to have normal phagocytic and bactericidal activity in other experiments (47). Although circulating neutrophil counts increase following corticosteroid administration, the number of circulating monocytes decrease within a few hours. From a functional standpoint, corticosteroids inhibit normal macrophage bactericidal and fungicidal activity *in vitro*, and monocytes from individuals receiving corticosteroids display diminished bactericidal ability as well.

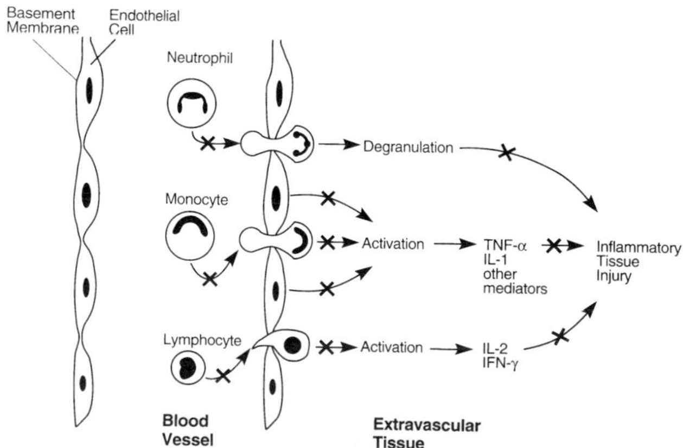

FIG. 34.2. Effects of corticosteroids on inflammatory cell recruitment and activation. Corticosteroids inhibit recruitment of leukocytes at inflammatory sites by blocking the adhesion of these cells to the endothelial cell wall. They also inhibit cellular activation and secretion of inflammatory mediators. Finally, they block the tissue effects of many cytokines and other inflammatory mediators.

Inhibition of synthesis or secretion of inflammatory mediators by different cells involved in the inflammatory response is central to the action of corticosteroids. Corticosteroids induce the transcription of lipocortin-1, a potent inhibitor of phospholipase A_2, which blocks eicosanoid generation and IL-1β-mediated (or lipopolysaccharide-mediated) cyclooxygenase-2 (COX-2) induction (48). Corticosteroids down-regulate the production of destructive tissue enzymes, such as collagenases. Inhibition of cytokine synthesis is another important antiinflammatory effect of corticosteroids. Synthesis of TNF-α, IL-1β, IL-2, IL-3, IL-6, IL-8, granulocyte-macrophage colony-stimulating factor, and IFN-γ is blocked by corticosteroids, whereas synthesis of the antiinflammatory cytokines TGF-β and IL-10 is either not affected, or is induced (49,50).

As stated previously, corticosteroids result in lymphopenia, which has been attributed to redirection of lymphocytes to bone marrow and spleen (51–53), but also to the skin and regional lymph nodes of inflammation sites. T-cell numbers decrease more than B cells, and CD4 T cells more than CD8 T cells (53). Corticosteroid-induced immunosuppression is mediated by inhibition of several stages of T-cell activation, including early tyrosine phosphorylation events (54), activation of Ca^{2+}/calmodulin-dependent protein kinase II (55), and calcineurin-dependent transactivating pathways (56). GCs inhibit IL-2 synthesis, which is critical for T-cell proliferative responses (57), and they inhibit signaling of this cytokine (58). Down-regulation of LFA-1, CD2, c-*myc*, and CD40 ligand, and induction of cyclic adenosine monophosphate (by inhibiting phosphodiesterase activity) further contribute to T-cell dysfunction (16). GCs also affect T-cell function indirectly by inhibiting the expression of major histocompatibility complex (MHC) class II and CD80 molecules on antigen-presenting cells.

B-cell function and immunoglobulin synthesis are relatively resistant to immunosuppressive GC effects. GCs also have important effects in shaping the developing immune responses because they favor deviation to helper T cell subset 2 (T_H2)-type cytokine formation by preferentially inhibiting IL-12 synthesis and sparing IL-4 and IL-10 (59,60). This effect might suggest that these agents are more potent in the treatment of diseases characterized by T_H1-type cytokine predominance, like rheumatoid arthritis

(RA). The ability of corticosteroids to induce apoptosis of double-positive thymocytes (60) and activated mature T cells (61) correlates with low cellular levels of *bcl*-2 and appears to have important implications for maintenance of central and possibly peripheral tolerance as well (60). Interestingly, T-cell receptor–mediated, activation-induced cell death and corticosteroid-mediated apoptosis are mutually antagonistic, an effect that may be partially due to downregulation of Fas ligand by corticosteroids (62). The degree to which corticosteroid-mediated apoptosis contributes to immunosuppression is not yet fully understood. Seki et al. demonstrated clinical resistance to corticosteroids in systemic lupus erythematosus (SLE) patients with decreased *in vitro* apoptosis of anti-CD3-activated peripheral blood mononuclear cells (63).

CELLULAR EFFECTS OF CORTICOSTEROIDS

Corticosteroids profoundly influence the function of a wide variety of organs and their component cells (Table 34.1). The effect of corticosteroids on a particular cell type depends on the concentration (physiologic or supraphysiologic) and type of corticosteroid (synthetic, naturally occurring, etc.), and varies with the receptor subtype to which the particular steroid binds. The outcome also varies with the phase of the cell cycle and stage of differentiation or activation of the cells. Some of this variation may possibly be attributable to differences in GR availability or affinity. In the case of immune cells, the effects also vary with timing and duration of exposure in relation to an antigenic or mitogenic stimulus, and in the case of both immune and nonimmune cells, also may be modulated by other hormonal or peptide regulators. For example, the absence of CBG in the eye may play a role in preventing immune responses at this site (64). In general, the transcriptional effects of corticosteroid on inflammation require supraphysiologic concentrations, similar to those obtained by high-dose daily or "pulse" corticosteroid therapy. Lower concentrations of corticosteroids are likely to involve posttranscriptional regulation of proinflammatory molecules.

TABLE 34.1. *Role of Endogenous Corticosteroids in Basal and Stress States*

Basal state
Maintenance of metabolic homeostasis
Blood glucose levels, liver glycogen content, excretion of water load, permissive effects on gluconeogenic and lipolytic activities of hormones
Maintenance of cardiovascular function
Adequate heart function and blood vessel tone, permissive effects on inotropic, chronotropic, and pressor activities of hormones
Maintenance of muscle work capacity
Maintenance of fetal lung surfactant
Stress states[a]
Adaptive changes in metabolic homeostasis
Increased blood glucose and liver glycogen content, insulin resistance, stimulation of ketogenesis, decreased growth factor action, decreased procollagen formation, suppression of fibroblast growth, decreased thyroid function and activation, gonadotropin suppression, and gonadal resistance to gonadotropins
Induction of enzymes increasing muscular metabolism
Induction of fetal lung surfactant
Detoxification of stress-induced toxic products, induction of glutamine synthetase, metallothionein, tyrosine aminotransferase, tryptophan oxygenase
Behavioral activation, euphoria, alertness
Immunosuppression, thymolysis, altered leukocyte traffic, antiinflammatory activity, suppression of inflammatory mediator production and effect (cytokines, prostanoids, kinins, serotonin, histamine, plasminogen activator, metalloproteinases)

[a]During stress state, negative feedback and tolerance mechanisms normally prevent prolonged hypersecretion of endogenous corticosteroids.

Modified from Laue L, Kawai S, Udelman R, et al. Glucocorticoid antagonists: pharmacological attributes of a prototype antiglucocorticoid (RU 486). In: Schleimer RP, Claman HN, Oronsky A, eds. *Anti-inflammatory steroid action: basic and clinical aspects.* San Diego: Academic, 1989:303–329, with permission.

Bone and Cartilage

Corticosteroids are involved in bone and calcium metabolism by a variety of mechanisms. The effects of corticosteroids in bone culture systems vary with concentration and time of exposure to the steroids. High concentrations of corticosteroids inhibit bone formation through direct inhibition of osteoblast replication and collagen and osteocalcin synthesis (65). This is partially attributable to inhibition of preosteoblast insulin-like growth factor-1 (IGF-1) production (66). Additionally, corticosteroids inhibit the bone synthesis of prostaglandin E_1 (PGE_1) and PGE_2, as well as vascular endothelial cell growth factor (VEGF), a major regulator of angiogenesis. Prostaglandins are potent stimulators of VEGF in osteoblasts. Both prostaglandins and VEGF play important roles in osteogenesis (67). Corticosteroids also directly suppress osteoclast function, but *in vivo,* this effect is usually obscured by the stimulatory effects of other factors such as parathyroid hormone (PTH) and IL-6 (68). During the first 6 months of corticosteroid therapy, bone is lost at a rapid rate, with reports of losses of up to 20% (Chapter 121). The use of greater than 7.5 mg/day of prednisone, or equivalent doses of other corticosteroids, appears to lead to clinically-significant bone loss in most individuals. A single daily dose of 2.5 mg of prednisone, however, can inhibit the nocturnal increase of osteocalcin, suggesting that even lower doses may have a deleterious effect (69). Corticosteroids decrease the renal absorption of calcium and phosphate, leading to hypercalciuria. They also interfere with the intestinal calcium absorption as a result of a direct effect on the duodenum and jejunum, which leads to a secondary increase in PTH (70). The influence of corticosteroids on chondrocytes is also dose- and time-dependent (71), the overall effect being stimulatory and increasing both glycosaminoglycan and DNA synthesis. Corticosteroids inhibit metalloproteinase production, although chondrocytes from patients with osteoarthritis (OA) have been seen to be hyporesponsive to corticosteroids (72).

Muscle

Corticosteroids may have a profound effect on muscle; the effects vary with dose and duration of treatment. High-dose corticosteroid therapy for more than 3 to 4 weeks is associated with selective skeletal muscle fiber atrophy, more prominent in type IIb glycolytic fibers, with relative sparing of type I fibers. Not only are different fiber types differentially affected, but different muscle groups also may be disproportionately involved (73). Certain muscle groups, such as those of the heart, those innervated by the cranial nerves, and those of respiration, have been viewed as generally resistant to GS-induced myopathy. Muscle atrophy is associated with negative nitrogen balance, resulting from decreased muscle protein synthesis, and increased nonlysosomally-mediated protein breakdown in association with antagonism of the antiproteolytic effect of insulin. Importantly, exercise antagonizes these myopathic effects (74).

Adipose Tissue

Corticosteroids also have biologic effects on adipose tissues that are similar to those on several other cell types. Adipose tissue and site specific effects include regulation of adipocyte differentiation from progenitor cells (75) and regulation of lipoprotein lipase activity. These effects appear to correlate with the level of CR expression, which also varies among different sites of adipose tissue. For example, receptor levels are higher in omental than in subcutaneous adipose tissues (76,77). These tissue-specific effects may determine the characteristic distribution of fat deposition that develops in settings of excess corticosteroids.

Pancreatic Cells

Corticosteroids enhance the response of pancreatic acinar cells to cholecystokinin by increasing the affinity of cholecystokinin for its receptors. They also reduce amylase secretion while increasing amylase activity, protein biosynthesis, steady-state mRNA levels, and gene transcription. Thus, although corticosteroids oppose several of the biologic effects of insulin and suppress insulin-stimulated metabolic responsiveness in many tissues, they are agonists of the effects of insulin on pancreatic amylase and cholecystokinin, and they enhance insulin secretion from β cells (78,79).

Liver

Amino acids are mobilized from multiple tissues in response to corticosteroids and reach the liver. They provide substrates for production of glucose and glycogen. In the liver, corticosteroids induce the transcription of several enzymes involved in gluconeogenesis and amino acid metabolism, including phosphoenolpyruvate carboxykinase (PEPCK), which controls the rate-limiting step in gluconeogenesis, glucose-6-phosphatase, and fructose-2,6-bisphosphatase (80). Corticosteroids regulate the transcription of PEPCK gene through two GR binding sites and two accessory factor binding sites. Corticosteroids also stimulate glycogen synthesis in the liver by activating glycogen synthase and inactivating glycogen phosphorylase.

Gastric Mucosa

The association between corticosteroids and peptic ulcer disease has been the subject of ongoing controversy for decades. In animal models, corticosteroids and ACTH delay but do not prevent ulcer healing. Prostaglandins, especially PGE_2, play an important cytoprotective role for the gastric mucosal epithelial cells. PGE_2 induces vasodilation, increases epithelial chloride secretion and vascular permeability, and promotes epithelial cell proliferation (81). Corticosteroids block arachidonic acid metabolism by inhibition of COX and phospholipase A_2 enzymes, which results in prostaglandin synthesis. COX has two isoforms: one that is constitutively expressed in most mammalian tissues (COX-1) and one that is induced (COX-2) and regulated by proinflammatory cytokines (i.e., IL-1, TNF-α). In the normal gastrointestinal tract, COX-1 expression is in abundance, whereas COX-2 is not expressed. A role for COX-2 in enhancing healing of peptic ulcers has been suggested based on animal studies (82). Several studies have demonstrated inhibition of COX-2 by corticosteroids *in vitro*. Also, it has been shown that corticosteroids suppress *in vivo* COX-2 transcription and enzyme activity. However, corticosteroids did not alter COX-1 mRNA or enzyme levels in murine peritoneal macrophages (83). IL-1 appears to have cytoprotective effects in the gastric mucosa; probable mechanisms include IL-1 production of PGE_2, as well as inhibition of acid secretion. IL-1 injections protect rats against gastric erosions secondary to aspirin, indomethacin, and ethanol (84). This IL-1-mediated cytoprotection may be impaired by corticosteroids. Corticosteroids alter the levels of lipid peroxidation products, nitric oxide levels, and the activity of antioxidant enzymes (85). All these effects may contribute to the development of gastropathy. Some studies suggest that corticosteroids released in response to stress protect gastric mucosa against stress-induced ulceration (86); this is mediated at least in part by maintaining gastric microcirculation.

In summary, there is no clear evidence that corticosteroids have clinically-significant effects on the gastric mucosa by themselves. However, the presence of comorbid conditions in patients or necessary medications with known deleterious effects on gastric mucosa, such as nonsteroidal antiinflammatory drugs (NSAIDs), could potentially accelerate peptic ulcer formation or inhibit their healing.

Central Nervous System

As in other systems, the effects of corticosteroids on cells of the central nervous system (CNS) vary with concentration and duration of exposure. High-dose, long-term corticosteroid exposure results in death of pyramidal cells in the Ammon horn portion of the hippocampus (87,88). Corticosteroids potentiate, whereas adrenalectomy protects against, neuronal loss associated with ischemia and exposure to excitatory neurotoxins. Basal levels of corticosteroids, however, protect against neuronal loss in the dentate gyrus of the hippocampus associated with adrenalectomy. This protection may be mediated through regulation of neuronal trophic factors, such as nerve growth factor. Corticosteroids also modify the functional activity of a variety of CNS cells. For example, corticosteroids regulate neuropeptide synthesis and secretion, neurotransmission, and neuronal cell membrane excitability (89). A major site of this effect appears to be through the regulation of prostaglandin signaling and the suppression of COX-2 induction (90). Additionally, corticosteroids lower the threshold for seizures, possibly by increasing the affinity and number of convulsant binding sites on the γ-aminobutyric acid (GABA)–benzodiazepine receptor complex (91). Corticosteroids also modulate other aspects of the GABA–benzodiazepine receptor complex, but their specific effects vary with concentration and different parts of the brain. The overall effect is to alter the sensitivity of a variety of neuronal cells to inhibition by GABA, which may amplify the effects of corticosteroids on synthesis and secretion of other neuronal products, as well as on complex functions such as cognition, mood, appetite, and other behavioral characteristics. Corticosteroids also modulate neurotransmitter systems, including the β-adrenergic–adenylate cyclase system in peripheral cells, such as lymphocytes, adipocytes, and muscle. In general, the effect is an enhancement of adenylate cyclase activity (92).

Neuroendocrine and Endocrine Systems

In addition to inhibition of hypothalamic CRH secretion and the pituitary release of ACTH, corticosteroids also affect the thyroid axis, growth, and gonadal axes (93). Excess corticosteroids inhibit the monodeiodination of thyroxine (T_4), resulting in decreased serum triiodothyronine (T_3) concentrations and increased reverse triiodothyronine (rT_3) concentrations (94). The GS-induced decreased production of T_3 in the periphery explains their utility in treating hyperthyroid storm. Excessive amounts of corticosteroid can also suppress thyroid-stimulating hormone (TSH) and decrease serum levels of total T_4 and total T_3. When corticosteroid therapy is withdrawn, serum TSH concentrations rebound to values in excess of pretreatment levels. Corticosteroid excess may play a role in the euthyroid sick syndrome (95).

Corticosteroids suppress growth and gonadal hormone synthesis and release. Pharmacologic amounts of corticosteroids inhibit growth; growth arrest is a hallmark of Cushing syndrome in children. With cortisol excess, the growth hormone response to growth hormone–releasing hormone is decreased, which results in a marked suppression of endogenous growth hormone (96).

CLINICAL PHARMACOLOGY OF CORTICOSTEROIDS

Structural Considerations and Potency

Corticosteroids (Fig. 34.3) are 21-carbon steroid molecules whose biologic activity requires the presence of a hydroxyl group at carbon 11 (C-11), a ketone oxygen at C-3, an unsaturated bond between C-4 and C-5, and a ketone oxygen at C-20. They also have a two-carbon chain at the 17 position and methyl groups at C-18 and C-19 (97). The principal, naturally-occurring plasma corticosteroid in humans is cortisol, or hydrocortisone. Figure 34.3 depicts some of the synthetic corticosteroids commonly used therapeutically. These synthetic agents were developed by modifying various sites on the cortisol molecule to enhance antiinflammatory and reduce mineralocorticoid activity. The 11-keto corticosteroids, cortisone and prednisone, must be converted *in vivo* to the 11-hydroxyl molecules (i.e., cortisol and prednisolone) to generate biologic activity. This conversion occurs primarily in the liver; therefore, they are only used systemically. Most of the corticosteroids are poorly soluble in water; conjugation of phosphate and hemisuccinate to C-21 increases solubility, resulting in formulations suitable for parenteral administration, such as methylprednisolone and cortisol. Corticosteroids intended for topical or local effects are 11-hydroxyl compounds with additional modifications at C-17 and C-21, which impede systemic absorption (e.g., triamcinolone acetonide). These modifications permit delivery of relatively large corticosteroid doses with reduced systemic effects. These compounds do not need bioconversion to generate biologic activity (97). The biologic effects of the various forms of corticosteroids traditionally are compared with respect to their GC and mineralocorticoid activity and their plasma half-life, as summarized in

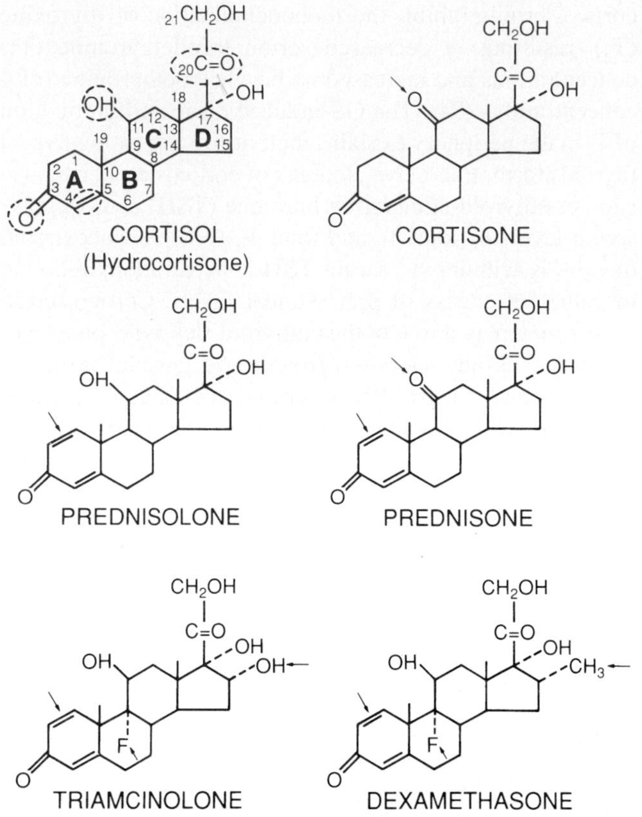

FIG. 34.3. Structure of commonly-used corticosteroids. The *arrows* indicate the structural differences between cortisol and each of the other compounds.

Table 34.2. In addition to dose and route of administration, absorption, metabolism, distribution, and elimination characteristics of these drugs influence the biologic effects. These corticosteroids may vary in different settings and patient subgroups.

Absorption, Metabolism, Distribution, and Elimination

Prednisone is the most commonly used corticosteroid in the United States. Prednisolone and methylprednisolone are alternatives, but they are more expensive.

Prednisone is 80% to 90% absorbed after oral administration, and absorption is not affected by food intake. Prednisone is biologically inactive and must be converted to prednisolone. This conversion, however, is rapid. Prednisone conversion is depressed in patients with severe liver disease (98), but it is doubtful that this factor is clinically significant (99). A large fraction of corticosteroids binds to serum proteins, and only their free fraction is biologically active. Of the two corticosteroid-binding proteins, transcortin (TC) binds to corticosteroids with high affinity and low capacity, whereas albumin binds with low affinity and high capacity. Because hydrocortisone and prednisone bind to both TC and albumin, their protein binding is concentration dependent and varies from 90% at lower doses to 60% at higher doses. In contrast, methylprednisolone and dexamethasone bind almost exclusively (99%) to albumin and, therefore, have concentration-independent protein-bound fractions (60%–70%). The difference in the plasma-free concentrations of dexamethasone and prednisone at standard oral doses may explain the better cerebrospinal fluid (CSF) penetration and better efficacy of the former in the preventive therapy of meningeal leukemia.

After oral administration, concentrations of prednisolone are only slightly lower than those after the same dose of intravenously administered prednisolone. Peak prednisolone concentrations are reached in 1 to 2 hours. These differences are not sufficient to recommend routine use of prednisolone in place of prednisone. Incomplete information is available on the *in vivo* distribution of corticosteroids. Prednisolone distributes well to most tissues, but there is little uptake in fat, brain, or CSF. About 60% of total pred-

TABLE 34.2. *Relative potencies of various corticosteroids*

Approximate equivalent	Plasma half-life (min)	Approximate relative potency: Glucocorticoid/mineralocorticoid	Doses (mg)
Short-acting			
Cortisol	100	1:1	20
Cortisone	100	1:1	25
Intermediate-acting			
Prednisolone	200	4:0–0.8	5
Methylprednisolone	200	5:0	4
Prednisone	200	4:0–0.8	5
Triamcinolone	200	5:0	4
Long-acting			
Dexamethasone	225	30:1	0.75
Mineralocorticoid			
Corticosterone		0.35:15	—
Fludrocortisone		10:125	—

Modified from Axelrod L. Side effects of glucocorticoid therapy. In: Schleimer RP, Claman HN, Oronsky A, eds. *Anti-inflammatory steroid action: basic and clinical aspects.* San Diego: Academic, 1989: 377–408, with permission.

nisolone uptake is in skeletal muscle (97). Cortisol and prednisolone are highly protein bound to two serum proteins: TC and albumin. As TC becomes saturated, free cortisol and prednisolone concentrations increase. Both free cortisol and prednisolone are eliminated more rapidly than protein-bound cortisol. By contrast, methylprednisolone and dexamethasone are minimally bound to TC, and elimination rates are constant (97); thus, the effects of these hormones are unaffected by changes in plasma protein levels. Corticosteroids are eliminated primarily by biotransformation to inactive compounds (100). Only a small fraction of the biologically-active parent compound is renally excreted. Principal transformations include reduction (in the liver and extrahepatic tissues) of the double bond between C-4 and C-5 and reduction (in the liver) of the ketone at C-3. Additionally, hepatic conjugation generates water-soluble sulfate esters of glucuronides, which are excreted through the urine. Neither biliary nor fecal excretion is of quantitative importance in humans. Certain disease states may alter corticosteroid metabolism. Severe liver disease and hypothyroidism impair elimination, whereas hyperthyroidism and renal disease accelerate elimination of corticosteroids. Disorders associated with hypoalbuminemia, such as nephrotic syndrome, may exhibit accelerated corticosteroid elimination. Disposition is apparently unimpaired in inflammatory bowel diseases (97).

Drug Interactions

Drugs that induce hepatic microsomal enzymes (especially CYP3A4), such as phenobarbital, phenytoin, rifampin, and carbamazepine, increase corticosteroid elimination. In contrast, ketokonazole, erythromycin, ethynylestradiol, and norethindrone inhibit CYP3A4 and can increase GC activity (101). Mifepristone (RU486), an antiprogestin drug marketed as an abortifacient, has potent anti-GC properties (at the level of GR) as well (102). Conversely, corticosteroids can also reduce the serum level of salicylates (103) and CYP3A4 substrates. Additionally, pulse GC can significantly potentiate the anticoagulant effect of warfarin, increasing the international normalized ratio 2 to 6 days after its administration in patients on oral anticoagulation therapy (104).

Biologic Response and Corticosteroid Resistance

The biologic effects of corticosteroids depend on their transport to cellular sites of action (Table 34.1). They enter cells by passive diffusion and, subsequently, bind cellular receptors. Although virtually all cells express corticosteroid receptors, lung, muscle, kidney, and small intestine tend to concentrate corticosteroids (i.e., tissue levels exceed plasma levels), whereas adipose tissue and brain do not (97). Corticosteroids have an immediate effect on cellular processes involving ion flux through specific ion channels (e.g., chloride). Effects requiring induction or inhibition of protein synthesis may require minutes to hours to appear. Different physiologic effects are often observed over time; thus, dose-response relationships are difficult to define.

In general, the biologic effects of corticosteroids depend on the total dose and cumulative duration of treatment. Immediate effects are noted in the CNS, the hypothalamic-pituitary-adrenal axis, and on electrolyte and glucose metabolism, whereas delayed responses are noted on adipose tissue and bone. Although high-dose and multidose daily administrations of corticosteroids are the most potent delivery schedules, the continuous exposure to supraphysiologic concentrations may be the most likely to produce adverse side effects. On the basis of these observations, the traditional goal of corticosteroid therapy has been to treat with the lowest possible effective dose and to minimize continuous exposure to supraphysiologic concentrations to decrease the risk for undesired side effects. In clinical practice, however, this objective is often difficult to achieve for several reasons, including patient and disease variability and imprecise measures of biologic effect. For example, it is widely appreciated that inflammation associated with SLE often requires substantially higher doses of corticosteroids to suppress disease activity than does RA (105). This apparent relative degree of "steroid resistance" has been suggested to reflect increased cortisol catabolism in patients with SLE compared with patients with RA. Steroid "resistance" has been the object of concern in a number of other conditions (106).

Clinical syndromes of corticosteroid resistance are due to generalized or tissue-specific defects of the GR transduction system. Generalized corticosteroid resistance is defined as hyposensitivity to cortisol in all tissues, including the hypothalamus and pituitary. Due to the impaired negative feedback, ACTH and cortisol levels are increased in this syndrome, compensating for the peripheral resistance. A point mutation in the GR hormone-binding domain has been identified as the cause of familial corticosteroid resistance in the first family reported with this condition (107). This mutation lowered the affinity (approximately three times) of the GR for its cognate hormone. Acquired generalized corticosteroid resistance has been observed in a subgroup of patients with acquired immunodeficiency syndrome (108). In these patients, the concomitantly elevated cortisol levels have not been sufficient to overcome the peripheral resistance, and symptoms of adrenal insufficiency have frequently been observed. The molecular mechanisms leading to this type of corticosteroid resistance are not known. Recently, Kino et al. reported that the *vpr* gene product of human immunodeficiency virus type 1 inhibits GR-mediated transactivation in HeLa cells (108,109). Tissue-specific corticosteroid resistance usually becomes clinically apparent because it is not compensated for by increased cortisol levels. This type of resistance may result in pathophysiologic (inflammatory) processes or may not allow corticosteroids to exert their physiologic (antiinflammatory effects) (110–113). Finally, corticosteroid resistance can also affect ACTH-producing cells; examples of "central" corticosteroid resistance include impaired negative feedback regulation and uninhibited ACTH production by pituitary adenomas (Cushing disease) and ectopic ACTH-secreting tumors (114,115).

ADVERSE EFFECTS OF CORTICOSTEROID TREATMENT

The discovery of the powerful antiinflammatory effects of corticosteroids in RA stimulated an enthusiastic exploration of their use as pharmacologic agents in a variety of diseases. One consequence of this historically-important finding was that the role of corticosteroids in normal physiology was neglected. For decades after their discovery, these unheralded antiinflammatory effects of the corticosteroids were thought to reflect unique pharmacologic properties that were distinct from their properties in usual physiologic contexts. The current view is that the physiologic and pharmacologic effects of corticosteroids are not distinct but reflect the same underlying biologic properties. It is now known that the effects of corticosteroids are on a continuum dependent on concentration, duration of exposure, and a multitude of cell and tissue variables. Moreover, the critical importance of corticosteroids in the regulation of adaptive responses has become better defined (116). In other words, corticosteroids are not simply powerful antiinflammatory "drugs"; rather, they are hormones with a multitude of important physiologic effects in the adaptation to stressful stimuli. One of these critical functions, as reviewed previously, is to suppress and restrain inflammatory and immune defense mechanisms and prevent overshoot that may result in self-injury and tissue destruction. In this sense, corticosteroids are adaptive and essential for survival.

As summarized in Table 34.1, many effects of corticosteroids facilitate the maintenance of physiologic homeostasis under resting or basal conditions. Other known effects of corticosteroids are observable in both the resting and the stress states, whereas some effects are most readily apparent in the stress state. The stress-related effects of corticosteroids mediate adaptive changes that facilitate the reestablishment, as opposed to the maintenance, of physiologic homeostasis (117). Therapeutic administration of corticosteroids may represent supplemental therapy if endogenous production of corticosteroids is "inadequate" to meet physiologic needs. When the dose for exogenously-administered corticosteroids exceeds physiologic needs, a syndrome of side effects develops that resembles Cushing syndrome [i.e., iatrogenic Cushing syndrome (Table 34.3)]. There are, however, differences between spontaneous and iatrogenic Cushing syndrome, in part because endogenous adrenal output of corticosteroids and androgens is suppressed in the iatrogenic disease but not in the spontaneous disease. These differences are summarized in Table 34.4. The extent to which manifestations of this iatrogenic syndrome develop depends on the total dose and cumulative duration of exposure to nonphysiologic concentrations.

TABLE 34.3. *Adverse effects of prolonged corticosteroid therapy*

Common
Hypertension
Negative balance of calcium and secondary hyperparathyroidism
Negative balance of nitrogen
Truncal obesity, moon facies, supraclavicular fat deposition, posterior cervical fat deposition (buffalo hump), mediastinal widening (lipomatosis), weight gain
Impaired wound healing; facial erythema; thin, fragile skin; violaceous striae; petechiae and ecchymoses
Acne
Suppression of growth in children
Secondary adrenal insufficiency secondary to hypothalamic-pituitary-adrenal axis suppression
Hyperglycemia, diabetes mellitus
Hyperlipoproteinemia; atherosclerosis
Sodium retention, hypokalemia
Increased risk for infection, neutrophilia, monocytopenia, lymphopenia, suppressed delayed-type hypersensitivity reactions
Myopathy
Osteoporosis, vertebral compression fractures
Osteonecrosis of femoral heads and other bones
Alterations in mood or behavior, such as euphoria, emotional lability, insomnia, depression; increased appetite
Uncommon
Metabolic alkalosis
Diabetic ketoacidosis; hyperosmolar, nonketotic diabetic coma
Peptic ulcer disease (usually gastric); gastric hemorrhage
"Silent" intestinal perforation
Increased intraocular pressure and glaucoma
Benign intracranial hypertension or pseudotumor cerebri
Spontaneous fractures
Psychosis
Rare
Sudden death with rapid administration of high-dose, pulse therapy
Cardiac valvular lesions in patients with systemic lupus erythematosus
Congestive heart failure in predisposed patients
Panniculitis (after withdrawal)
Hirsutism or virilism, impotence, secondary amenorrhea
Hepatomegaly due to fatty liver
Pancreatitis
Convulsions
Epidural lipomatosis
Exophthalmos
Allergy to synthetic corticosteroids resulting in urticaria, angioedema

Modified from Axelrod L. Side effects of glucocorticoid therapy. In: Schleimer RP, Claman HN, Oronsky A, eds. *Anti-inflammatory steroid action: basic and clinical aspects.* San Diego: Academic, 1989:377–408, with permission.

Both clinicians and patients should be aware that adverse effects of corticosteroid therapy are not uncommon, and some of them can be serious. Brief courses (i.e., up to 10 days) of high-dose corticosteroid therapy are probably well tolerated, and if adverse effects occur, such as Cushing

TABLE 34.4. *Iatrogenic versus spontaneous Cushing syndrome*

Features virtually unique to iatrogenic Cushing syndrome
Glaucoma
Posterior subcapsular cataracts
Osteonecrosis
Pseudotomor cerebri
Pancreatitis
Panniculitis
More common in spontaneous Cushing syndrome
Hypertension
Hirsutism, virilism
Striae, purpura, plethora
Altered menses
Impotence (men)
Shared clinical features
Centripetal obesity
Psychiatric symptoms
Poor wound healing
Osteoporosis
Glucose intolerance
Hypothalamic-pituitary-adrenal axis suppression

syndrome, glucose intolerance, and HPA axis suppression, they are rapidly reversible (118). More prolonged therapy, as is usually the case in most patients with systemic inflammatory diseases, invariably leads to complications. Some adverse effects (e.g., HPA axis suppression, glucose intolerance, osteonecrosis, cataracts) occur even with low-dose corticosteroids; others usually are associated with larger doses of corticosteroids (e.g., infection, psychosis, myopathy, and hyperlipidemia). Several of the side effects of particular importance to rheumatologic practice are reviewed here.

Bone Toxicity

GC-induced osteoporosis and osteonecrosis are frequent corticosteroid-induced adverse effects and contribute substantially to the morbidity associated with these agents (Chapter 121).

Osteoporosis

The main histologic findings in corticosteroid-induced osteoporosis are decreased bone formation rate, decreased thickness of trabeculae, and *in situ* bone death. Studies in a mouse model of corticosteroid-induced osteoporosis revealed an early (7 days after corticosteroid exposure) increase in osteoclast perimeter and bone resorption (119). Also, chronic corticosteroid exposure (27 days) led to decreases in bone turnover and bone formation, probably as a result of decreased osteoclastogenesis and osteoblastogenesis, respectively. Osteoblast function was further compromised as these cells underwent increased apoptosis (120). The augmented osteocyte apoptosis was proposed by the researchers as a potential mechanism for corticosteroid-induced osteonecrosis, because osteocytes are critical in sensing microdamage and regulating bone remodeling (120).

Corticosteroid-induced osteoporosis predominantly affects cancellous bone and the axial skeleton. Vertebral compression fractures secondary to bone loss are the most incapacitating sequelae of corticosteroid therapy. Rib and hip fractures are also common. The true incidence is uncertain, but may approach 30% to 90% (121–124). As expected, the incidence and severity of osteoporosis is closely related to the dose and duration of corticosteroid therapy. Dosages of prednisone of greater than 7.5 mg/day are considered significant, although some patients experience bone loss while taking smaller doses. Bone loss is greatest during the first 6 to 12 months of therapy and is most marked in trabecular bone. Some patients lose as much as 10% to 20% of their overall bone mass and even more in trabecular bone sites, particularly in the lumbar spine. Additional risk factors that accelerate bone loss or increase the risk for fracture include smoking, alcohol intake, sedentary lifestyle, a diet low in calcium and vitamin D, menopause, and, of course, the underlying disease process (125). Certain medications, such as thyroid hormone, anticonvulsants, cyclosporine, loop diuretics, lithium, and gonadotropin-releasing hormone agonists and antagonists, also increase bone loss. The risk for fracture is greatest in patients with the smallest initial bone masses and strength. Postmenopausal women are more sensitive to corticosteroid-induced osteoporosis than are premenopausal women, but at prednisone dosages equivalent to 7.5 mg/day or greater, bone loss develops in all patients. Corticosteroid doses should be kept as low as possible, and preventive measures should be used in all patients that require prolonged corticosteroid therapy.

Corticosteroids have important effects on bone through the indirect suppression of gonadal and adrenal androgen production and secretion. They inhibit intestinal calcium absorption and promote renal calcium excretion. This net calcium loss stimulates PTH secretion and promotes secondary hyperparathyroidism, which additionally contributes to bone loss. Plasma levels of PTH are increased in most patients taking high-dose corticosteroids. Osteoclast activity is increased, and osteoblast function is inhibited. The increased osteoclast activity is mainly the result of secondary hyperparathyroidism. Calcium and vitamin D supplementation can partially reverse these effects (123). Bone mineral density determination by dual-energy x-ray absorptiometry of the vertebral spine and hip is usually the first step in the evaluation of corticosteroid-induced osteopenia and osteoporosis (126). This technique appears to be the best method currently available for serial follow-up. Studies at 12-month intervals will usually identify patients with significant or continuing bone loss. Additional evaluation may include a 24-hour urine collection for calcium and creatinine, a serum measurement of intact PTH, and free testosterone level in men. The assessment of various biochemical markers of bone formation or bone resorption has not been established to have clinical utility in corticosteroid-induced bone loss.

Intensive efforts are ongoing to define appropriate measures to prevent and treat corticosteroid-induced osteopenia and osteoporosis. The best prevention is to minimize the dose and duration of exposure. Alternate-day therapy has not been shown to prevent bone loss (127). Pulse methylprednisolone therapy has not been adequately studied, although 1-g pulses of methylprednisolone given every other day for three doses transiently increase urinary excretion of calcium and hydroxyproline (128). Exercise (particularly weight bearing), smoking cessation, and minimizing alcohol consumption are recommended in appropriate situations. Daily elemental calcium intake should be at least 1,500 mg, and daily vitamin D intake 800 IU. Because most patients do not reach this level of intake through their diets, supplementation is advised. Supplementation of calcium and vitamin D have been shown to retard bone loss (129), but the long-term effect on preventing bone loss is not established. The assessment of dietary calcium intake should take into account the fact that typical servings of dairy products (e.g., a glass of milk or a serving of ice cream or yogurt) contain about 250 mg of calcium. Women treated with high-dose corticosteroids have low levels of estrone and androstenedione, and corticosteroid-treated, oophorectomized rats lose bone more rapidly than do corticosteroid-treated control rats. These observations could potentially support the use of estrogens (if there are no contraindications) in postmenopausal women and premenopausal women who become amenorrheic.

The best evidence regarding effective prevention and treatment of corticosteroid-induced osteoporosis exist for bisphosphonates, especially during initiation of corticosteroid therapy, when bone loss is the worse (130–132). Although there is some concern about the prolonged use of these agents in young individuals, due to their long-term retention in bones (133), this should not discourage physicians from prescribing them when clearly indicated in young patients. However, bisphosphonates should not be used in pregnancy or moderate-to-severe renal insufficiency. Discontinuation of the bisphosphonate should be considered when corticosteroid doses have been substantially tapered or there is stabilization of bone mineral density. Calcitonin has been recommended for corticosteroid-induced osteoporosis, but it may be less effective (134) than bisphosphonates. If the above measures fail, bone anabolic agents, such as low doses of slow-release sodium fluoride, could be used with caution (135). Other promising therapies for corticosteroid-induced osteoporosis have emerged. Specifically, daily subcutaneous injections of human PTH 1–34 in postmenopausal women, who also received hormone replacement therapy (HRT) and calcium supplementation, reversed corticosteroid-induced osteoporosis in the lumbar spine, whereas control therapy with HRT and calcium alone did not (136). Statins have also shown promise in treating corticosteroid-induced bone loss, since they appear to have bone anabolic activity (137–139). Finally, synthetic GC with dissociated transactivating and transrepressing activities have been proposed as potentially bone-sparing corticosteroid agents (140).

Osteonecrosis

Corticosteroids may induce infarctions of metadiaphyseal and epiphyseal bone (osteonecrosis). The likelihood of developing this complication is dependent on the dose and duration of exposure. No exposure is totally without risk because anecdotal observations have indicated that even short-term exposure (e.g., 7 days) may result in osteonecrosis in highly susceptible individuals. Although the mechanisms are not proven, several theories have been proposed. A vascular theory attributes the osteonecrosis to bone ischemia caused by corticosteroid-induced inhibition of angiogenesis in bone, secondary to suppressed VEGF production, promotes ischemia and possibly necrosis (141). A third hypothesis suggests that an ischemic bone collapse of the epiphysis is secondary to osteoporosis and the accumulation of unhealed trabecular microfractures. Finally, increased intraosseous pressure due to fat accumulation that leads to impaired sinusoidal blood flow within bone and to subsequent infarction (142) has been suggested as a cause of infarctions. The femoral heads and condyles, humoral heads, and tali seem to be most susceptible. Bilateral and polyarticular disease is common (143). In patients with SLE, osteonecrosis is common (occurs in about 12%) and is mostly likely to appear within 4 months of initiating high-dose oral therapy. Other factors such as anticardiolipin antibodies also may contribute to the risk for osteonecrosis in SLE patients (144). Osteonecrosis also occurs in other patient populations treated with high-dose corticosteroids, such as renal transplantation, leukemia and lymphoma, and Crohn disease. Intravenous pulse methylprednisolone therapy has been suggested to minimize the risk for osteonecrosis in patients with RA (145), but data are insufficient to support this conclusion. Clinicians should suspect osteonecrosis in the setting of new onset of joint pain, particularly in the hips in patients receiving high-dose corticosteroid treatment. Magnetic resonance imaging is particularly useful for diagnosis of early disease. For late disease, characteristic changes are observed on plain radiographs (142).

Myopathy

The development of myalgias and muscle weakness tends to parallel the development of other adverse effects of corticosteroids, particularly osteoporosis, but the development of myopathy is not strictly dose dependent. It is less common with dosages of prednisone of less than 30 mg/day and is an uncommon complication of alternate-day corticosteroid treatment. Myopathy may develop after only short exposure and may have an insidious or abrupt onset. It is usually most severe in the pelvic girdle, with lesser involvement of the shoulder girdle and distal muscles. Myalgias in the setting of high-dose corticosteroid treatment suggest the clinical diagnosis. Diagnosis is most difficult in SLE or polymyositis, in which an inflammatory myopathy may obscure the diagnosis. Elevated urine creatine in the presence of normal serum concentrations of muscle enzymes such as creatine kinase and aldolase is probably the best distinguishing feature, although this test has been questioned. Muscle biopsies show selective atrophy of type IIb fibers. Lactate dehydrogenase is normal, whereas glycogen synthase, β-hydroxyacyl-coenzyme A (CoA) dehydrogenase, and citric acid synthase are lower in patients with corticosteroid-induced myopathy compared with normal muscle (146). The myopathic changes are potentially reversible by decreasing corticosteroid dosage and increasing exercise (147).

Cardiovascular Effects

Hypertension, dyslipoproteinemias, atherosclerosis, and cardiac disease are more common in patients treated with long-term corticosteroids. Hypertension is partly due to the permissive effects of corticosteroids on the action of vasoactive substances (angiotensin II, catecholamines) on the vessel wall and myocardium that result in increased systemic vascular resistance and increased myocardial contractility (6,7). Inhibition of PGE_2 and the kallikrein system by corticosteroids also contributes to their adverse effects on blood pressure. The initiating event for the atherosclerotic lesion is generally believed to result from some form of intimal injury that serves as the nidus for the development of the atherosclerotic plaque. Corticosteroids, particularly with prednisone doses of more than 10 mg/day, antagonize insulin and contribute to hyperglycemia, hyperinsulinemia, hypercholesterolemia, and hypertriglyceridemia. Low-density lipoproteins and various apolipoproteins also may be elevated. All of these factors probably contribute to atherosclerotic plaque development (148). Data also have linked high-dose corticosteroid treatment of SLE with serious valvular pathology that may produce serious hemodynamic compromise requiring surgery. In contrast to classic Libman-Sacks verrucous vegetations, the valves are characterized by rigid thickening of the leaflets (149).

Infection

Corticosteroids predispose to infection and, at the same time, may mask clinical clues of infection as a result of their immunosuppressive and antiinflammatory effects. On the other hand, timely use of corticosteroids in *Pneumocystis carinii* pneumonia and *Haemophilus influenzae* meningitis improves the outcome probably because of reduction in the inflammatory response (150,151). In addition to the increased incidence of bacterial infections, corticosteroids can cause reactivation of latent tuberculosis or histoplasmosis and predispose to accelerated forms of infections due to herpes simplex virus.

Endogenous corticosteroids play a critical role in regulating normal host responses to infectious agents. Deficient corticosteroid production (e.g., hypoadrenalism, Addison disease) renders the host susceptible to severe and even life-threatening tissue injury secondary to the overwhelming effects of unrestrained and unchecked inflammation. Excess corticosteroid production (hyperadrenalism, Cushing syndrome), in contrast, leads to impaired host inflammatory and immune responses and an increased incidence and severity of infections. Infection was the reported cause of death in up to 50% of patients originally described with Cushing syndrome. Consistent with these observations, introduction of high-dose daily corticosteroids for treatment of rheumatic diseases was rapidly followed by reports documenting increased incidence and severity of infections (152,153). These observations have played a central role in the development of multiple alternative corticosteroid dosing schedules (Table 34.5). The risk for infection depends on the dose and duration of corticosteroid treatment. Daily administration of corticosteroids in doses approximating the normal basal physiologic production [i.e., 10 mg of cortisol (154) or about 2.5 mg of prednisone] does not impair normal protective host defenses, but doses in this range probably do partially restrain excessive activation of inflammatory mechanisms that may produce inappropriate self tissue injury. Daily corticosteroids equivalent to 10 mg of prednisone do not appreciably increase the incidence and severity of infection (154,155). Doses of prednisone approximating the range of corticosteroids produced during maximal stress responses (i.e., >100–300 mg of cortisol or 20–60 mg of prednisone) may have pronounced effects on host defense mechanisms, depending on the timing and duration

TABLE 34.5. *Alternatives to high-dose daily corticosteroid therapy*

Local
Topical
Intraarticular
Intrabursa
Peritendinous
Systemic
Physiologic, multiple low doses, oral, on as-needed schedule
Physiologic, single, daily a.m., oral, fixed or on as-needed schedule
Supraphysiologic, single a.m., alternate-day, oral
Physiologic, single a.m., alternate-day, oral
Intermittent, pulse or bolus therapy, i.v. or oral, many different dose (physiologic and supraphysiologic) and delivery schedules

I.V., intravenous.

of the corticosteroid treatment. Corticosteroid administration in multiple divided daily doses has maximal suppressive effects on host defense mechanisms. Daily morning doses have somewhat fewer inhibitory effects, and every-other-day dosing has even fewer effects. In fact, prednisone in doses of 40 to 120 mg every other day may not significantly increase the incidence and severity of infection.

The effects of suprapharmacologic pulse or bolus treatment in promoting infection are not completely defined. A single, suprapharmacologic bolus of corticosteroids does not increase the incidence of infection in normal volunteers, but repeated doses produce dramatic reduction in short- and long-term host defense mechanisms that could increase the risk for infection.

Total cumulative doses of greater than 700 mg are associated with progressively increased risk for infection (152). Continuous daily treatment for 30 days or more at a dosage of greater than 40 mg/day has a substantial effect on cell-mediated immune host defense mechanisms and markedly increases the risk for infection with facultative intracellular microbes. The primary risk is from organisms such as mycobacteria, fungi (e.g., *Cryptococcus neoformans,* occasionally *P. carinii*), and toxoplasmosis. Prophylaxis for *P. carinii* pneumonia should be considered in such patients. Moreover, although humoral defense mechanisms are less impaired, patients treated with corticosteroids with doses in this range develop more frequent and severe infections, particularly bacteremia, with acute pyrogenic organisms such as *Staphylococcus aureus,* group A streptococci, and *Escherichia coli.* This effect appears to be a consequence of the impaired influx of polymorphonuclear leukocytes to sites of infection. Therefore, signs and symptoms of infection, such as fever and malaise, are suppressed, and local symptoms and signs including redness, warmth, and exudates are usually diminished (153).

Except for herpes viruses, most types of viral infection are not a major problem during corticosteroid therapy. Patients treated with corticosteroids tolerate primary herpes infections less well. The incidence of herpes zoster is increased, but dissemination is uncommon. Purified protein derivative testing help identify patients exposed to tuberculosis who will be candidates for antituberculosis therapy before or during corticosteroid therapy. Immunizations with *H. influenzae* type B, tetanus toxoid, and pneumococcal vaccines should be considered in patients on chronic corticosteroid treatment. However, a trend toward lower protective antibody titers was noted for patients on immunosuppressive agents, perhaps suggesting that immunizations should best be administered before initiation of such therapy. Vaccinations for influenza, *Pneumococcus,* and tetanus are, therefore, recommended for such patients. In contrast, vaccinations with live attenuated viruses, such as oral polio, varicella, and measles/mumps/rubella (MMR), should be avoided in immunosuppressed patients because such vaccines may lead to disease (156). Notably, even contact with children vaccinated with the oral polio vaccine (but not MMR) is risky (156).

Chronic Suppression of the Hypothalamic-Pituitary-Adrenal Axis

Daily administration of corticosteroids at dosages above the normal basal equivalent of cortisol (~10 mg/day) (154) suppresses the HPA axis and may produce adrenocortical atrophy and potential secondary adrenal insufficiency. Daily, morning corticosteroid administration in the basal physiologic replacement range, alternate-day, and intermittent administration schedules do not significantly impair adrenocortical steroid output. However, suppression of the axis should be suspected in any patient treated daily with evening doses of corticosteroids, or doses above the physiologic replacement range. Patients treated with 20 to 30 mg of prednisone for as little as 5 days will develop HPA axis suppression, but function will rapidly return on discontinuing the corticosteroid administration. Longer duration and higher dose treatment produce more profound suppression (157). A major concern in such individuals is the development of acute adrenal insufficiency during general anesthesia and surgery, during major trauma, or in the setting of an acute infectious disease. Recovery of the hypothalamic-pituitary axis after discontinuation of corticosteroid therapy is more rapid than recovery of adrenocortical function. Although recovery of adrenocortical responses to stressful stimuli correlates with total dose and duration of corticosteroid therapy, it may require up to 12 months for function to return to precorticosteroid therapy levels. One should assume that all patients treated with daily corticosteroids at levels above the physiologic range for more than 1 month may have some degree of secondary adrenocortical insufficiency. Corticosteroid withdrawal should start by tapering the corticosteroid dose to physiologic levels (20 mg of hydrocortisone or 5 mg of prednisone in a single morning dose). Serum morning cortisol levels are measured, and only when they are more than 10 μg/dL can the maintenance dose be discontinued. However, these patients may still have abnormal cortisol responses to stress, and coverage should be given when necessary. Next, an acute ACTH test is performed (Table 34.6). If 30- or 60-minute cortisol serum levels, after subcutaneous injection of 250 mg of cosyntropin (synthetic $ACTH_{1-24}$), are more than 20 μg/mL, adrenal insufficiency is unlikely and stress corticosteroid supplementation is no longer necessary. However, exceptions can occur, and if there is any clinical suspicion of adrenal insufficiency (i.e., hypotension after surgery), corticosteroid coverage should be continued (158).

Central Nervous System

Mood changes occur in half the patients receiving corticosteroids (7). Depression is more common, but euphoria can also occur. Additionally, cognitive dysfunction and decreased duration of REM (rapid eye movement) sleep can be seen (7). Rarely, and especially with high corticosteroid doses, manic behavior, psychosis, or seizures can supervene during therapy, and need differentiation from primary

TABLE 34.6. *Assessment of adrenal function in patients treated with corticosteroids*

1. Withhold exogenous steroids for 24 hours.
2. Obtain plasma cortisol before ACTH administration.
3. Give cosyntropin (synthetic $ACTH_{1-24}$) 250 mg (25 units) as i.v. bolus or i.m. injection.
4. Obtain plasma cortisol 30 and 60 min after ACTH administration.
5. Performance of test in morning is customary, but not required.

Interpretation: normal response = plasma cortisol >18 mg/dL at 30 or 60 min after ACTH administration.

Traditional recommendations also specify an increment above baseline of 7 mg/dL at 30 min or 11 mg/dL at 60 min or a doubling of the baseline value at 60 min. These parameters are valid in normal, unstressed subjects, but are frequently misleading in ill patients with a normal hypothalamic-pituitary-adrenal axis, in whom stress may increase the baseline plasma cortisol level by an increase in endogenous ACTH levels.

ACTH, adrenocorticotropic hormone; i.m., intramuscular; i.v., intravenous.

Modified from Axelrod L. Side effects of glucocorticoid therapy. In: Schleimer RP, Claman HN, Oronsky A, eds. *Anti-inflammatory steroid action: basic and clinical aspects.* San Diego: Academic, 1989:377–408, with permission.

neuropsychiatric SLE (159,160). The distinction can be difficult, but the temporal relationship to increases in corticosteroid dose, along with lack of focal neurologic signs or CSF abnormalities, suggest the correct diagnosis. Discontinuation or reduction of corticosteroid therapy along with phenothiazine suffices to reverse corticosteroid-induced psychosis (160). Benign intracranial hypertension (pseudotumor cerebri) has been reported as a rare event during corticosteroid therapy.

Other Adverse Effects

Posterior subcapsular cataract formation is not uncommon with systemic, topical, or inhaled GC use; children may be more susceptible to this complication. Open-angle glaucoma may occur rapidly with topical ocular administration, but may take years before it occurs with systemic GC therapy. Glaucoma, in contrast to cataracts, often resolves with GC discontinuation (161). Hypersensitivity reactions and severe anaphylaxis to corticosteroids can rarely occur. Intravenous, intraarticular, soft tissue, and intradermal injections have been implicated, but association with topical and oral corticosteroid use also has been reported (162,163). Acne induced by pharmacologic doses of corticosteroids is a common complication (164). Common complications of topical corticosteroids applied to the face are rosacea and perioral dermatitis (165). Excessive hair growth in a hormonal-induced distribution characteristic of hirsutism may be noted alone or in conjunction with steroid acne. A telogen effluvium may infrequently occur 2 to 3 months after the initiation of high-dose corticosteroid treatment (166).

Corticosteroid Withdrawal Syndromes

Although addisonian crisis with nausea, vomiting, hypotension, fever, hypoglycemia, hyperkalemia, and hyponatremia is the most serious risk of corticosteroid-induced adrenal insufficiency, other corticosteroid withdrawal syndromes are commonly encountered. On decreasing corticosteroid doses, patients may develop a symptom complex, commonly called pseudorheumatism, characterized by diffuse aching in the muscles, bones, and joints; anorexia; nausea; weight loss; headache; and fever. Patients also may rapidly develop severe flare-ups of their underlying disease. These flare-ups may occur after reductions of high-dose, as well as low-dose, corticosteroid therapy, but are more common when dosage reductions within the physiologic range are made during therapy. Immediate flare-ups in clinical disease activity after abruptly stopping corticosteroids in patients with RA taking oral prednisolone at doses of 5 mg/day or less has been reported (167). Serum cortisol levels in these situations (i.e., disease flare-up while taking physiologic doses of cortisol-equivalent steroid) are confusing because they are frequently higher than "normal." Apparently, the antiinflammatory effects of cortisol are blunted. The development of corticosteroid withdrawal syndromes necessitates gradual corticosteroid dosage reduction, over a period of weeks to months, with frequent reassessment of the patient. Prolonged oral therapy with prednisone (2–5 mg) in the morning may be required to manage recurrent withdrawal symptoms.

Pregnancy

Corticosteroid therapy is generally considered safe during pregnancy and should not be withheld if life-threatening disease amenable to corticosteroid use develops. Most studies show no increased incidence of maternal, fetal, or neonatal deaths, toxemia, or uterine hemorrhage. Prednisone or prednisolone is the preferred corticosteroid because placental metabolism by 11β-dehydrogenase limits the exposure of the fetus to active corticosteroids. Only fluorinated corticosteroids (i.e., dexamethasone, betamethasone) can enter the fetal circulation in significant amounts, because they are only partially metabolized by the placental 11β-dehydrogenase. These are the agents of choice for incomplete heart block of neonatal lupus (168). In mice, corticosteroids have been associated with cleft palate, and studies have shown that corticosteroids are specifically involved in palatal morphogenesis (169). Mothers treated with corticosteroids during pregnancy may need stress corticosteroid doses in the peripartum period, especially when there is prolonged labor or delivery or if surgery is required (170). Careful monitoring of the babies for development of adrenal insufficiency is also recommended (170). Breast-feeding is generally safe, although it should probably be avoided if high therapeutic doses of corticosteroids are required. For patients receiving 20 mg/day or more of prednisone, avoiding breast-feeding during the first 3 to 4 hours after the dose should minimize the dose the infant receives (171).

ALTERNATIVE FORMS OF CORTICOSTEROID DOSING AND DELIVERY

Although highly effective in suppressing inflammation, long-term, high-dose (i.e., more than 0.6 to 1 mg/kg/day of prednisone), daily corticosteroid therapy is associated with an unacceptably high incidence of adverse effects. As a consequence, considerable effort has been devoted to developing alternative therapeutic routes and schedules to maximize effectiveness and minimize continuous exposure to supraphysiologic concentrations. Some of these approaches are listed in Table 34.5. Local therapy, when possible, is the safest route of administration. High doses of corticosteroids may be applied to the inflammatory site, so the risk for undesired side effects is minimized. Severe rheumatic disease manifestations, however, usually require systemic therapy.

Local Therapy

Topical corticosteroid therapy, because of the availability of a wide array of agents and vehicles, is an important method for delivering high doses of corticosteroids directly to an inflamed site, such as bronchial airways, the nasal mucosa, or skin. This approach generally avoids systemic side effects if low-potency corticosteroids are used for short periods. However, high-potency corticosteroids may produce systemic side effects, particularly in children (172). Topical therapy by the rheumatologist will be used most commonly in the treatment of discoid lupus. Subcutaneous atrophy and rosacea are common complications of topical therapy. Intraarticular injection of corticosteroids may be of great value in selected patients and clinical settings (see Chapter 35). Indications for intraarticular steroid injection include (a) to correct flexion deformities accompanying joint inflammation, (b) to control inflammation in one or more particularly troublesome joints in patients with polyarticular synovitis, (c) to control monoarticular or oligoarticular arthritis, and (d) to provide long-term control of joint or tendon sheath inflammation. Intraarticular injections should not be used for acute trauma, in the presence of infection, or in situations that may exacerbate a mechanical problem (e.g., tendon rupture). No long-term adverse effects of local corticosteroids on cartilage are usually apparent.

Low-Dose Daily Oral Therapy

Supraphysiologic daily therapy with prednisone dosages greater than 7.5 mg/day clearly have the most adverse effects. Single morning dosing is safer than single evening dosing, but the side effects of long-term exposure are still a major problem. Low-dose therapy in the physiologic range (<2.5–7.5 mg/day of prednisone) appears to be the safest route of daily corticosteroid treatment. Due to insufficient data, disagreement exists regarding the proper approach and effectiveness in specific clinical situations. Although a fixed, single, morning oral low dose of prednisone is most commonly used (e.g., 2–7.5 mg), as-needed daily dosing of prednisone (e.g., 0–7 mg) may be preferred by the patient and may be equally effective. Patients are often prescribed 11-mg prednisone tablets and instructed to take the medication as needed to achieve optimal relief of symptoms. Experience with this regimen in RA has indicated a high degree of patient acceptance and reduced overall prednisone doses compared with traditional fixed daily dosing schedules (173). As-needed self-dosing represents an attempt to match the dose of administered corticosteroids to disease activity and, in principle, to administer lower total cumulative doses over time compared with fixed-dose schedules. This approach is analogous to the method by which insulin is administered to patients with diabetes mellitus; that is, the amount of insulin administered is matched to the blood glucose level. Self-dosing appears to succeed in patients with RA because they are generally good self-assessors of disease activity. This may not be the case in other rheumatic diseases such as SLE or polymyositis. Whether this method of corticosteroid administration is safer than fixed-dose, daily administration is unclear.

Alternate-Day Therapy

Alternate-day therapy, as expected, is associated with fewer side effects than is high-dose daily therapy. The incidence of infections, myopathy, obesity, excessive appetite, growth inhibition in children, cushingoid facies, glucose intolerance, and suppression of the HPA axis is decreased. Bone loss and cataract occurrence are not decreased in this approach. Alternate-day therapy is generally not the first approach to treatment with corticosteroids. Patients are typically switched to an alternate-day regimen after disease is brought under control by a daily-dose regimen (16). The schedule for switching patients to an alternate-day therapy schedule is entirely empiric. Severity and nature of the underlying disease and the duration of daily corticosteroid therapy influence the time required to change to alternate-day treatment. However, symptoms on the "off" day are common and may hinder conversion. Adjunctive therapy with NSAIDs may be helpful, but physician support and encouragement are essential. In some conditions such as RA, "off" day symptoms are intolerable for the patient and preclude this approach.

High-Dose Pulse or Bolus Therapy

Pulse or bolus therapy is another dosing schedule that has received wide attention as an alternative approach to daily corticosteroid therapy (16,174–177). The intent of the approach is to maximize the antiinflammatory effects and to minimize side effects by confining exposure to high concentrations of corticosteroids to a very short time. The approach is controversial and elicits a wide spectrum of opinion, depending on the clinical condition, route, timing, dose, and type of corticosteroids. Much of the controversy revolves around long-term benefits of the therapy because outcome parameters vary in different studies. In general, high-dose, intravenous, pulse therapy (e.g., 1 g of methylprednisolone daily for 3 days) is a potent suppressant of a variety of inflammatory diseases over short periods (days to several weeks), but disease activity almost invariably recurs (178). Most physicians agree that the side effects are less common than those observed with the usual high-dose, daily therapeutic regimens. Controlled studies, which will define more accurately the value of this approach for various rheumatic conditions, are now appearing in the medical literature (176). In general, pulse therapy is initiated in patients with rapidly progressive, immunologically-mediated rheumatic conditions, such as severe lupus nephritis (176).

REFERENCES

1. Mason HL, Myers corticosteroid, Kendall EC. The chemistry of crystalline substances isolated from the suprarenal gland. *J Biol Chem* 1936;114:613–631.
2. Mason HL, Myers CS, Kendall EC. Chemical studies of the suprarenal cortex: the identification of a substance which processes the qualitative action of cortin. *J Biol Chem* 1936;116:267–276.
3. Hench PS, Kendall EC, Slocumb CH, et al. The effect of a hormone of the adrenal cortex (17-hydroxy-11-dehydrocorticosterone: compound E) and of pituitary adrenocorticotropic hormone on rheumatoid arthritis. *Proc Staff Meet Mayo Clin* 1949;24:181–197.
4. Hench PS, Kendall EC, Slocumb CH, et al. Effects of cortisone acetate and pituitary ACTH on rheumatoid arthritis, rheumatic fever and certain other conditions. *Arch Intern Med* 1950;85:545–666.
5. Chrousos GP. The hypothalamic-pituitary-adrenal axis and immune-mediated inflammation. *N Engl J Med* 1995;332:1351–1362.
6. Schimmer BP, Parker KL. Adrenocorticotropic hormone; adrenocortical steroids and their synthetic analogs; inhibitors of the synthesis and actions of adrenocortical hormones. In: Hardman JE, Limbird LE, Molinoff PB, et al., eds. *Goodman & Gilman's the pharmacological basis of therapeutics,* 9th ed. New York: McGraw-Hill, 1996:1459–1485.
7. Orth DN, Kovacs WJ. The adrenal cortex. In: Wilson JD, Foster DW, Kronenberg HM, et al., eds. *Williams textbook of endocrinology,* 9th ed. Philadelphia: WB Saunders, 1998:517–664.
8. Lamberts SWJ, Bruining HA, de Jong FH. Corticosteroid therapy in severe illness. *N Engl J Med* 1997;337:1285–1292.
9. Anonymous. Deflazacort—an alternative to prednisolone? *Drug Ther Bull* 1999;37:57–58.
10. Lipuner K, Casez JP, Horber FF, Jaeger P. Effects of deflazacort versus prednisone on bone mass, body composition, and lipid profile: a randomized, double blind study in kidney transplant patients. *J Clin Endocrinol Metab* 1998;83:3795–3802.
11. Barcelona JAS, Martin MC, Lopez VN, et al. An open comparison of the diabetogenic effect of deflazacort and prednisone at a dosage ratio of 1.5 mg:1 mg. *Eur J Clin Pharmacol* 1999;55:105–109.
12. Greenberg GR, Feagan BG, Martin F, et al. Oral budesonide for active Crohn's disease. *N Engl J Med* 1994;331:836–841.
13. Rutgeerts P, Lofberg R, Malchow H, et al. A comparison of budesonide with prednisolone for active Crohn's disease. *N Engl J Med* 1994;331: 842–845.
14. Vayssiere BM, Dupont S, Choquart A, et al. Synthetic glucocorticoids that dissociate transactivation and AP-1 transrepression exhibit anti-inflammatory activity *in vivo*. *Mol Endocrinol* 1997;11:1245–1255.
15. Van den Berghe W, Francesconi E, De Boscher K, et al. Dissociated glucocorticoids with antiinflammatory potential repress interleukin-6 gene expression by a nuclear factor-κB-dependent mechanism. *Mol Pharmacol* 1999;56:797–806.
16. Boumpas DT, Chrousos GP, Wilder RL, et al. Glucocorticoid therapy for immune-mediated diseases: basic and clinical correlates. *Ann Intern Med* 1993;119:1198–1208.
17. Boumpas DT, Paliogianni F, Anastassiou ED, et al. Glucocorticosteroid action on the immune system: molecular and cellular aspects. *Clin Exp Rheumatol* 1991;9:413–423.
18. Karin M. New twists in gene regulation by glucocorticoid receptor: is DNA binding dispensable? *Cell* 1998;93:487–490.
19. Diamond MI, Miner JN, Yoshinaga SK, et al. Transcription factor interactions: selectors of positive or negative regulation from a single DNA element. *Science* 1990;249:1266–1272.
20. De Boscher K, Schmitz ML, Van den Berghe W, et al. Glucocorticoid-mediated repression of nuclear factor-kappaB-dependent transcription involves direct interference with transactivation. *Proc Natl Acad Sci U S A* 1997;94:13504–13509.
21. Jonat C, Rahmsdorf HJ, Park KK. Antitumor promotion and anti-inflammation: down-modulation of AP-1 (Fos/Jun) activity by glucocorticoid hormone. *Cell* 1990;62:1189–1204.
22. Schule R, Rangarajan P, Kliewer S, et al. Functional antagonism between oncoprotein c-Jun and the glucocorticoid receptor. *Cell* 1990; 62:11217–11226.
23. Yang-Yen HF, Chambard JC, Sun YL, et al. Transcriptional interference between c-Jun and the glucocorticoid receptor: mutual inhibition of DNA binding due to direct protein-protein interaction. *Cell* 1990; 62:1205–1215.
24. Paliogianni F, Raptis A, Ahuja SS, et al. Negative transcriptional regulation of human interleukin 2 (IL-2) gene by glucocorticoids through interference with nuclear transcription factors AP-1 and NF-AT. *J Clin Invest* 1991;91:1481–1489.
25. Scheinman RI, Cogswell PC, Lofquist AK, et al. Role of transcriptional activation of IκBκ in mediation of immunosuppression by glucocorticoids. *Science* 1995;270:283–286.
26. Auphan N, DiDonato JA, Rosette C, et al. Immunosuppression by glucocorticoids: inhibition of NF-κB activity through induction of IκB synthesis. *Science* 1995;270:286–290.
27. Bianchi M, Meng C, Ivashkiv LB. Inhibition of IL-2-induced Jak-STAT signaling by glucocorticoids. *Proc Natl Acad Sci U S A* 2000;97:9573–9578.
28. Hu X, Li WP, Meng C, et al. Inhibition of IFN-γ signaling by glucocorticoids. *J Immunol* (in press).
29. Lee SW, Tsou AP, Chan H, et al. Glucocorticoids selectively inhibit the transcription of the interleukin-1β gene and decrease the stability of interleukin 1β mRNA. *Proc Natl Acad Sci U S A* 1988;85:1204–1208.
30. Boumpas DT, Anastassiou ED, Older SA, et al. Dexamethasone inhibits human interleukin 2 but not interleukin 2 receptor gene expression *in vitro* at the level of nuclear transcription. *J Clin Invest* 1991; 87:1739–1747.
31. Losel R, Wehling M. Nongenomic actions of steroid hormones. *Nature Rev Mol Cell Biol* 2003;4:46–56.
32. Borski RJ. Nongenomic membrane actions of glucocorticoids in vertebrates. *Trends Endocrinol Metab* 2000;11:427–436.
33. Orchinik M, Murray TF, Moore FL. A corticosteroid receptor in neuronal membranes. *Science* 1991;252:1828–1851.
34. Evans SJ, Murray TF, Moore FL. Partial purification and biochemical characterization of a membrane glucocorticoid receptor from an amphibian brain. *J Steroid Biochem Mol Biol* 2000;72:209–221.
35. Hinz B, Hirschelmann R. Rapid non-genomic feedback effects of CRF-induced ACTH secretion in rats. *Pharm Res* 2000;17:1273–1277.
36. Hafezi-Moghadam A, Simoncini T, Yang Z, et al. Acute cardiovascular protective effects of corticosteroids are mediated by non-transcriptional activation of endothelial nitric oxide synthase. *Nat Med* 2002;8:473–479.
37. Limbourg FP, Huang Z, Plumier JC, et al. Rapid nontranscriptional activation of endothelial nitric oxide synthase mediates increased cerebral blood flow and stroke protection by corticosteroids. *J Clin Invest* 2002;110:1729–1738.
38. Buttgereit F, Wehling M, Burmester GR. A new hypothesis of modular glucocorticoid actions: steroid treatment of rheumatic diseases revisited. *Arthritis Rheum* 1998;41:761–767.

39. Buttgereit F, Brand MD, Burmester GR. Equivalent doses and relative drug potencies for non-genomic glucocorticoid effects: a novel glucocorticoid hierarchy. *Biochem Pharmacol* 1999;58:363–368.
40. Sapolsky RM, Romero LM, Munck AU. How do glucocorticoids influence stress responses? Integrating permissive, suppressive, stimulatory, and preparative actions. *Endocrinol Rev* 2000;21:55–89.
41. Dhabhar FS, McEwen BS. Enhancing versus suppressive effects of stress hormones on skin immune function. *Proc Natl Acad Sci U S A* 1999;96:1059–1064.
42. Wilckens T, Derijk R. Glucocorticoids and immune functions: physiological relevance and potential of hormone dysfunction. *Trends Pharmacol Sci* 1995;16:193–197.
43. Wilckens T, Derijk R. Glucocorticoids and immune functions: unknown dimensions and new frontiers. *Immunol Today* 1997;18:418–424.
44. Geller DA, Nussler AK, DiSilvio M, et al. Cytokines, endotoxin, and glucocorticoids regulate the expression of inducible nitric oxide synthesis in hepatocytes. *Proc Natl Acad Sci U S A* 1993;90:522–526.
45. Pitzalis C, Pipitone N, Perretti M. Regulation of leukocyte-endothelial interactions by glucocorticoids. *Ann NY Acad Sci* 2002;966:108–118.
46. Cronstein BN, Kimmel SC, Levin RI, et al. A mechanism for the anti-inflammatory effects of corticosteroids: the glucocorticoid receptor regulates leukocyte adhesion to endothelial cells and expression of endothelial-leukocyte adhesion molecule 1 and intercellular adhesion molecule 1. *Proc Natl Acad Sci U S A* 1992;89:9991–9995.
47. Pitzalis C, Pipitone N, Bajocchi G, et al. Corticosteroids inhibit lymphocyte binding to endothelium and intercellular adhesion: an additional mechanism for their anti-inflammatory and immunosuppressive effect. *J Immunol* 1997;158:5007–5016.
48. Leonard JP, Silverstein RL. Corticosteroids and the hematopoietic system. In: Lin AN, Paget SA, eds. *Principles of corticosteroid therapy.* New York: Arnold, 2002:144–149.
49. O'Banion MK, Winn VD, Young DA. cDNA cloning and functional activity of a glucocorticoid-regulated inflammatory cyclooxygenase. *Proc Natl Acad Sci U S A* 1992;89:4888–4892.
50. Ayanlar Batuman O, Ferrero AP, Diaz A, et al. Regulation of transforming growth factor-β1 gene expression by glucocorticoids in normal human T lymphocytes. *J Clin Invest* 1991;88:1574–1580.
51. Visser J, van Boxel-Dezaire A, Methorst D, at al. Differential regulation of interleukin-10 (IL-10) and IL-12 by glucocorticoids *in vitro. Blood* 1998;91:4255–4264.
51. Fauci AS, Dale DC. The effect of hydrocortisone on the kinetics of normal human lymphocytes. *Blood* 1975;46:235–243.
52. Fauci AS. Mechanisms of corticosteroid action on lymphocyte subpopulations. Redistribution of circulating T and B lymphocytes to the bone marrow. *Immunology* 1975;28:669–680.
53. Ten Berge RJM, Sauerwein HP, Yong SL, et al. Administration of prednisolone *in vivo* affects the ratio of OKT4/OKT8 and the LDH-isoenzyme pattern of human T lymphocytes. *Clin Immunol Immunopathol* 1984;30:91–103.
54. Paliogianni F, Ahuja SS, Yamada H, et al. Glucocorticoids inhibit T cell proliferation by downregulating proliferative signals mediated through both T cell antigen and interleukin-2 receptors. *Arthritis Rheum* 1992;35(suppl):127.
55. Paliogianni F, Hama N, Balow JE, et al. Glucocorticoid-mediated regulation of protein phosphorylation in primary human T cells: evidence for induction of phosphatase activity. *J Immunol* 1995;155:1809–1817.
56. Paliogianni F, Boumpas DT. Glucocorticoids regulate calcineurin-dependent trans-activating pathways for interleukin-2 gene transcription in human T-lymphocytes. *Transplantation* 1995;59:1333–1339.
57. Vacca A, Martinotti S, Screpanti I, et al. Transcriptional regulation of the interleukin 2 gene by glucocorticoid hormones. Role of steroid receptor and antigen-responsive 5′-flanking sequences. *J Biol Chem* 1990:265:8075–8080.
58. Paliogianni F, Ahuja SS, Balow JP, et al. Novel mechanism for inhibition of human T cells by glucocorticoids (GC): GC modulate signal transduction through IL-2 receptor. *J Immunol* 1993;151:4081–4089.
59. Bischof F, Melms A. Glucocorticoids inhibit CD40 ligand expression of peripheral $CD4^+$ lymphocytes. *Cell Immunol* 1998;187:38–44.
60. Ashwell JD, Lu FWM, Vacchio MS. Glucocorticoids in T cell development and function. *Annu Rev Immunol* 2000;18:309–345.
61. Tuosto L, Cundari E, Montani MSG, et al. Analysis of susceptibility of mature human T lymphocytes to dexamethasone-induced apoptosis. *Eur J Immunol* 1994;24:1061–1065.
62. Yang Y, Mercep M, Ware CF, et al. Fas and activation-induced Fas ligand mediate apoptosis of T cell hybridomas: inhibition of Fas ligand expression by retinoic acid and glucocorticoids. *J Exp Med* 1995;181:1673–1682.
63. Seki M, Ushiyama C, Seta N, et al. Apoptosis of lymphocytes induced by glucocorticoids and relationship to therapeutic efficacy in patients with systemic lupus erythematosus. *Arthritis Rheum* 1998;41:823–830.
64. Knisely TL, Hosoi J, Nazareno R, et al. The presence of biologically significant concentrations of glucocorticoids but little or no cortisol binding globulin within aqueous humor: relevance to immune privilege in the anterior chamber of the eye. *Invest Ophthalmol Vis Sci* 1994;35:3711–3723.
65. Heinrichs AA, Bortell R, Rahman S, et al. Identification of multiple glucocorticoid receptor binding sites in the rat osteocalcin gene promoter. *Biochemistry* 1993;32:11436–11444.
66. McCarthy TL, Centrella M, Canalis E. Cortisol inhibits the synthesis of insulin-like growth factor-I in skeletal cells. *Endocrinology* 1990;126:1569–1575.
67. Harada S, Nagy JA, Sullivan KA, et al. Induction of vascular endothelial growth factor expression by prostaglandin E_2 and E_1 in osteoblasts. *J Clin Invest* 1994;93:2490–2496.
68. Defranco DJ, Lian JB, Glowacki J. Differential effects of glucocorticoid on recruitment and activity of osteoclasts induced by normal and osteocalcin-deficient bone implanted in rats. *Endocrinology* 1992;131:114–121.
69. Nielsen HK, Charles P, Mosekilde L. The effects of single oral doses of prednisone on the circadian rhythm of serum osteocalcin in normal subjects. *J Clin Endocrinol Metab* 1988;67:1025–1033.
70. Kimberg DV, Baerg RD, Gerson E. Effect of cortisone treatment on the active transport of calcium by the small intestine. *J Clin Invest* 1971;50:1309–1321.
71. Blondelon D, Adolphe M, Zizine L, et al. Evidence for glucocorticoid receptors in cultured rabbit articular chondrocytes. *FEBS Lett* 1980;117:195–199.
72. DiBattista JA, Martel-Pelletier J, Antakly T, et al. Reduced expression of glucocorticoid receptor levels in human osteoarthritic chondrocytes: role in the suppression of metalloprotease synthesis. *J Clin Endocrinol Metab* 1993;76:1128–1134.
73. Ferguson GT, Irvin CG, Cherniack RM. Effect of corticosteroids on respiratory muscle histopathology. *Am Rev Respir Dis* 1990;142:1047–1052.
74. Falduto MT, Young AP, Hickson RC. Exercise interrupts ongoing glucocorticoid-induced muscle atrophy and glutamine synthetase induction. *Am J Physiol* 1992;263:1157–1163.
75. Hauner H, Entenmann G, Wabitsch M, et al. Promoting effect of glucocorticoids on the differentiation of human adipocyte precursor cells cultured in a chemically defined medium. *J Clin Invest* 1989;84:1663–1670.
76. Fried SK, Russell CD, Grauso NL, et al. Lipoprotein lipase regulation by insulin and glucocorticoid in subcutaneous and omental adipose tissues of obese women and men. *J Clin Invest* 1993;92:2191–2198.
77. Pedersen SB, Jonler M, Richelsen B. Characterization of regional and gender differences in glucocorticoid receptors and lipoprotein lipase activity in human adipose tissue. *J Clin Endocrinol Metab* 1994;78:1354–1359.
78. Otsuki M, Okabayashi Y, Nakamura T, et al. Hydrocortisone treatment increases the sensitivity and responsiveness to cholecystokinin in rat pancreas. *Am J Physiol* 1989;257:364–370.
79. Logsdon CD. Glucocorticoids increase cholecystokinin receptors and amylase secretion in pancreatic acinar AR42J cells. *J Biol Chem* 1986;261:2096–2101.
80. Pilkis SJ, Granner DK. Molecular physiology of the regulation of hepatic gluconeogenesis and glycolysis. *Annu Rev Physiol* 1992;54:885–909.
81. Wolfe MM, Lichtenstein DR, Singh G. Gastrointestinal toxicity of nonsteroidal anti-inflammatory drugs. *N Engl J Med* 1999;24:1888–1899.
82. Stenson WF. COX-2 and wound healing in the stomach. *Gastroenterology* 1997;112:645–649.
83. Masferrer JL, Reddy ST, Zweifel BS, et al. Glucocorticoids regulate cyclooxygenase-2 but not cyclooxygenase-1 in peritoneal macrophage. *J Pharm Ther* 1994;270:1340–1344.

84. Robert A, Saperas E, Zhang W, et al. Gastric cytoprotection by intracisternal interleukin-1 beta in the rat. *Biochem Biophys Res Commun* 1991;174:1117–1124.
85. Bandyopadhyay U, et al. Dexamethasone makes the gastric mucosa susceptible to ulceration by inhibiting prostaglandin synthetase and peroxidase- two important gastroprotective enzymes. *Mol Cell Biochem* 1999;202:31–36.
86. Fileretova LP, Fileratov AA, Makar GB. Corticosterone increase inhibits stress-induced gastric erosions in rats. *Am J Physiol* 1998;6: 1024–1030.
87. McEwen BS. Protective and damaging effects of stress mediators. *N Engl J Med* 1998;338:171–179.
88. Sapolsky RM, Pulsinelli WA. Glucocorticoids potentiate ischemic injury to neurons: therapeutic implications. *Science* 1985;229:1397–1400.
89. Honkaniemi J, Pelto-Huikko M, Rechardt L, et al. Colocalization of peptide and glucocorticoid receptor immunoreactivities in rat central amygdaloid nucleus. *Neuroendocrinology* 1992;55:451–459.
90. Yamagata K, Andreasson KI, Kaufmann WE, et al. Expression of a mitogen-inducible cyclooxygenase in brain neurons: regulation by synaptic activity and glucocorticoids. *Neuron* 1993;11:371–386.
91. Schumacher M, McEwen BS. Steroid and barbiturate modulation of the GABAa receptor: possible mechanisms. *Mol Neurobiol* 1989;3: 275–304.
92. Davies AO. Steroid hormone-induced regulation of adrenergic receptors. In: Schleimer RP, Claman HN, Oronsky A, eds. *Anti-inflammatory steroid action: basic and clinical aspects.* San Diego: Academic, 1989:96–109.
93. Torpy DJ, Chrousos GP. The three-way interactions between the hypothalamic-pituitary-adrenal and gonadal axes and the immune system. *Baillieres Clin Rheumatol* 1996;10:181–198.
94. De Nayer P, Dozin B, Vandeput Y, et al. Altered interaction between triiodothyronine and its nuclear receptors in absence of cortisol: a proposed mechanism for increased thyrotropin secretion in corticosteroid deficiency states. *Eur J Clin Invest* 1987;17:106–110.
95. McIver B, Gorman CA. Euthyroid sick syndrome, an overview. *Thyroid* 1997;7:125–132.
96. Martinelli CE, Moreira AC. Relation between growth hormone and cortisol spontaneous secretion in children. *Clin Endocrinol* 1994;41: 117–121.
97. Szelzer SJ. General pharmacology of glucocorticoids. In: Schleimer RP, Claman HN, Oronsky A, eds. *Anti-inflammatory steroid action: basic and clinical aspects.* San Diego: Academic, 1989:353–376.
98. Powell LW, Axelsen E. Corticosteroids in liver disease: studies on the biological conversion of prednisone to prednisolone and plasma protein binding. *Gut* 1972;13:690–696.
99. Axelrod L. Glucocorticoid therapy. *Medicine (Baltimore)* 1976;55: 39–65.
100. Peterson RE, Wyngaarden JB, Guerra SL, et al. The physiological disposition and metabolic fate of hydrocortisone in man. *J Clin Invest* 1955;34:1779–1794.
101. Feldweg AM, Leddy JP. Drug interactions affecting the efficacy of corticosteroid therapy. A brief review with an illustrative case. *J Clin Rheumatol* 1999;5:143–150.
102. Spitz IM, Bardin CW. Mifepristone (RU 486)—a modulator of progestin and glucocorticoid action. *N Engl J Med* 1993;329:404–412.
103. Klinenberg JR, Miller F. Effect of corticosteroids on blood salicylate concentration. *JAMA* 1965;194:601–604.
104. Costedoat-Chalumeau N, Amoura Z, Aymard G, et al. Potentiation of vitamin K antagonists by high-dose intravenous methylprednisolone. *Ann Intern Med* 2000;132:631–635.
105. Chikanza LC, Panayi GS. The effects of hydrocortisone on *in vitro* lymphocyte proliferation and interleukin-2 and -4 production in corticosteroid sensitive and resistant subjects. *Eur J Clin Invest* 1993; 23:845–850.
106. Chrousos GP, Detera-Wadleigh SD, Karl M. Syndromes of glucocorticoid resistance. *Ann Intern Med* 1993;119:1113–1124.
107. Hurley DM, Accili D, Stratakis CA, et al. Point mutation causing a single amino acid substitution in the hormone binding domain of the glucocorticoid receptor in familial glucocorticoid resistance. *J Clin Invest* 1991;87:680–686.
108. Norbiato G, Bevilacqua M, Vago T, et al. Cortisol resistance in acquired immunodeficiency syndrome. *J Clin Endocrinol Metab* 1992; 74:608–613.
109. Kino T, Gragerov A, Kopp JB, et al. The HIV-1 virion associated protein Vpr is a coactivator of the human glucocorticoid receptor. *J Exp Med* 1999;189:51–62.
110. Kam JC, Szefler SJ, Surs W, et al. Combination IL-2 and IL-4 reduces glucocorticoid receptor-binding affinity and T cell responses to corticosteroids. *J Immunol* 1993;151:3460–3466.
111. Sher ER, Leung DY, Surs W, et al. Steroid-resistant asthma. Cellular mechanisms contributing to inadequate response to glucocorticoid therapy. *J Clin Invest* 1994;93:33–39.
112. Schlaghecke R, Kornely E, Wollenhaupt J, et al. Glucocorticoid receptors in rheumatoid arthritis. *Arthritis Rheum* 1992;35:740–744.
113. DiBattista JA, Martel-Pelletier J, Antakly T, et al. Reduced expression of glucocorticoid receptor levels in human osteoarthritic chondrocytes. Role in suppression of metalloprotease synthesis. *J Clin Endocrinol Metab* 1993;76:1128–1134.
114. Ray DW, Littlewood AC, Clark AJ, et. al. Human small cell lung cancer cell lines expressing the proopiomelanocortin gene have aberrant glucocorticoid receptor function. *J Clin Invest* 1994;93:1625–1630.
115. Karl M, Lamberts SWJ, Koper JW, et al. Cushing's disease preceded by generalized glucocorticoid resistance: clinical consequences of a novel, dominant-negative glucocorticoid receptor mutation. *Proc Assoc Am Physicians* 1996;108:296–307.
116. Wilder RL. Neuroendocrine-immune system interactions and autoimmunity. *Annu Rev Immunol* 1995;13:307–338.
117. Munck A, Guyre PM, Holbrook NJ. Physiological functions of glucocorticoids in stress and their relation to pharmacological actions. *Endocr Rev* 1984;5:25–44.
118. Baxter JD. Advances in glucocorticoid therapy. *Adv Intern Med* 2000;45:317–349.
119. Weinstein RS, Jilka RL, Parfitt AM, et al. Inhibition of osteoblastogenesis and promotion of apoptosis and osteocytes by glucocorticoids. Potential mechanisms of their deleterious effects on bone. *J Clin Invest* 1998;102:274–282.
120. Manolagas SC, Weinstein RS. New developments in the pathogenesis and treatment of steroid-induced osteoporosis. *J Bone Miner Res* 1999;14:1061–1066.
121. Lukert BP, Raisz LG. Glucocorticoid-induced osteoporosis: pathogenesis and management. *Ann Intern Med* 1990;112:352–364.
122. Reid IR. Steroid-induced osteoporosis. *Osteoporos Int* 1997;7(suppl 3):213–216.
123. Reid IR. Glucocorticoid effects on bone. *J Clin Endocrinol Metab* 1998;83:1860–1862
124. Zaqqa D, Jackson RD. Diagnosis and treatment of glucocorticoid-induced osteoporosis. *Cleve Clin J Med* 1999;66:221–230.
125. Kroger H, Honkanen R, Saarikoski S, et al. Decreased axial bone mineral density in perimenopausal women with rheumatoid arthritis: a population based study. *Ann Rheum Dis* 1994;53:18–23.
126. Zaqqa D, Jackson RD. Diagnosis and treatment of glucocorticoid-induced osteoporosis. *Cleve Clin J Med* 1999;66:221–230.
127. Gluck OS, Murphy WA, Hahn TJ, et al. Bone loss in adults receiving alternate day glucocorticoid therapy: a comparison with daily therapy. *Arthritis Rheum* 1981;24:892–898.
128. Bijlsma JW, Duursma SA, Bosch R, et al. Acute changes in calcium and bone metabolism during methylprednisolone pulse therapy in rheumatoid arthritis. *Br J Rheumatol* 1988;27:215–219.
129. Buckley LM, Leib ES, Cartularo KS, et al. Calcium and vitamin D_3 supplementation prevents bone loss in the spine secondary to low-dose corticosteroids in patients with rheumatoid arthritis: a randomized, double-blind, placebo-controlled trial. *Ann Intern Med* 1996;125:961–968.
130. Adachi JD, Bensen WG, Brown J, et al. Intermittent etidronate therapy to prevent corticosteroid induced osteoporosis. *N Engl J Med* 1997;337:382–387.
131. Saag KG, Emkey R, Schnitzer TJ, et al. Alendronate for the prevention and treatment of glucocorticoid-induced osteoporosis. Glucocorticoid-Induced Osteoporosis Study Group. *N Engl J Med* 1998;30:292–299.
132. Cohen S, Levy RM, Keller M, et al. Risedronate therapy prevents corticosteroid-induced bone loss. A twelve month, multicenter, randomized, double-blind, placebo-controlled, parallel-group study. *Arthritis Rheum* 1999;42:2309–2318.
133. Anonymous. Recommendations for the prevention and treatment of glucocorticoid-induced osteoporosis. American College of Rheumatology Task Force on Osteoporosis Guidelines. *Arthritis Rheum* 1996;39:1791–1801.

134. Healey JH, Paget SA, Williams-Russo P, et al. A randomized controlled trial of salmon calcitonin to prevent bone loss in corticosteroid-treated temporal arteritis and polymyalgia rheumatica. *Calcif Tissue Int* 1996;58:73–80.
135. Reid IR. Glucocorticoid osteoporosis-mechanisms and management. *Eur J Endocrinol* 1997;137:209–217.
136. Lane NE, Sanchez S, Modin GW, et al. Parathyroid hormone treatment can reverse corticosteroid-induced osteoporosis. Results of a randomized controlled clinical trial. *J Clin Invest* 1998;102:1627–1633.
137. Mundy G, Garett R, Harris S, et al. Stimulation of bone formation *in vitro* and in rodents by statins. *Science* 1999;286:1946–1949.
138. Meier CR, Schlienger RG, Kraenzlin ME, et al. HMG-CoA reductase inhibitors and the risk of fractures. *JAMA* 2000;283:3205–3210.
139. Wang PS, Solomon DH, Mogun H, et al. HMG-CoA reductase inhibitors and the risk of hip fractures in elderly patients. *JAMA* 2000; 283:3211–3216.
140. Manolagas SC, Weinstein RS. New developments in the pathogenesis and treatment of steroid-induced osteoporosis. *J Bone Miner Res* 1999;14:1061–1066.
141. Harada S, Nagy JA, Sullivan KA, et al. Induction of vascular endothelial growth factor expression by prostaglandin E_2 and E_1 in osteoblasts. *J Clin Invest* 1994;93:2490–2496.
142. Mankin HJ. Nontraumatic necrosis of bone (osteonecrosis). *N Engl J Med* 1992;326:1473–1479.
143. Zabinski SJ, Sculco TP, Dicarlo EF, et al. Osteonecrosis in the rheumatoid femoral head. *J Rheumatol* 1998;25:1674–1680.
144. Mok CC, Lau CS, Wong RW. Risk factors for avascular bone necrosis in systemic lupus erythematosus. *Br J Rheumatol* 1998;37:895–900.
145. Williams IA, Mitchell AD, Rothman W, et al. Survey of the long term incidence of osteonecrosis of the hip and adverse medical events in rheumatoid arthritis after high dose intravenous methylprednisolone. *Ann Rheum Dis* 1988;47:930–933.
146. Danneskiold-Samsoe B, Grimby G. The influence of prednisone on the muscle morphology and muscle enzymes in patients with rheumatoid arthritis. *Clin Sci* 1986;71:693–701.
147. LaPier TK. Glucocorticoid-induced muscle atrophy. The role of exercise in treatment and prevention. *J Cardiopulm Rehabil* 1997;17: 76–84.
148. Petri M, Perez-Gutthann S, Spence D, et al. Risk factors for coronary artery disease in patients with systemic lupus erythematosus. *Am J Med* 1992;93:513–519.
149. Galve E, Candell-Riera J, Pigrau C, et al. Prevalence, morphologic types, and evolution of cardiac valvular disease in systemic lupus erythematosus. *N Engl J Med* 1988;319:817–823.
150. Pareja JG, Garland R, Koziel H. Use of adjunctive corticosteroids in severe adult non-HIV pneumocystis carinii pneumonia. *Chest* 1998; 113:1215–1224.
151. McIntyre PB, Berkey CS, King SM, et al. Dexamethasone as adjunctive therapy in bacterial meningitis. A meta-analysis of randomized clinical trials since 1988. *JAMA* 1997;278:925–931.
152. Stuck AE, Minder CE, Frey FJ. Risk of infectious complications in patients taking glucocorticosteroids. *Rev Infect Dis* 1989;11:954–963.
153. Segal BH, Sneller MC. Infectious complications of immunosuppressive therapy in patients with rheumatic diseases. *Rheum Dis Clin North Am* 1997;23:219–237.
154. Esteban NV, Loughlin T, Yergey AL, et al. Daily cortisol production rate in man determined by stable isotope dilution/mass spectrometry. *J Clin Endocrinol Metab* 1991;72:39–45.
155. Caldwell JR, Furst DE. The efficacy and safety of low-dose corticosteroids for rheumatoid arthritis. *Semin Arthritis Rheum* 1991;21:1–11.
156. Singer NG, McCune J. Prevention of infectious complications in rheumatic disease patients: immunization, *Pneumocystis carinii* prophylaxis, and screening for latent infections. *Curr Opin Rheumatol* 1999;11:173–178.
157. Axelrod L. Glucocorticoid therapy. *Medicine (Baltimore)* 1976;55: 39–65.
158. Baxter JD. Advances in glucocorticoid therapy. *Adv Intern Med* 2000;45:317–349.
159. Wada K, Yamada N, Suzuki H, et al. Recurrent cases of corticosteroid-induced mood disorder: clinical characteristics and treatment. *J Clin Psychiatry* 2000;61:261–267.
160. Ling MHM, Perry PH, Tsuang MT. Psychiatric side effects of corticosteroid therapy. *Arch Gen Psychiatry* 1981;38:471–477.
161. Renfro L, Snow JS. Ocular effects of topical and systemic steroids. *Dermatol Clin* 1992;10:505–512.
162. Schonwald S. Methylprednisolone anaphylaxis *Am J Emerg Med* 1999;17:583–585.
163. Mace S, Vadas P, Pruzanski W. Anaphylactic shock induced by intraarticular injection of methylprednisolone acetate. *J Rheumatol* 1997; 24:1191–1194.
164. Monk B, Cunliffe WJ, Layton AM, et al. Acne induced by inhaled steroids. *Clin Exp Dermatol* 1993;18:148–150.
165. Omoto M, Sigiura H, Uehara M. Histopathologic features of recalcitrant erythema of the face in adult patients with atopic dermatitis. *J Dermatol* 1994;21:87–91.
166. Gallant C, Kenny P. Oral glucocorticoids and their complications: a review. *J Am Acad Dermatol* 1986;14:161–177.
167. Buchanan WW, Stephen LJ, Buchanan HM. Are "homeopathic" doses of oral corticosteroids effective in rheumatoid arthritis? *Clin Exp Rheumatol* 1988;6:281–284.
168. Saleeb S, Copel J, Friedman D, et al. Comparison of treatment with fluorinated glucocorticoids to the natural history of autoantibody-associated congenital heart block. Retrospective review of the research registry for neonatal lupus. *Arthritis Rheum* 1999;42:2335–2345.
169. Abbott BD, McNabb FM, Lau C. Glucocorticoid receptor expression during the development of the embryonic mouse secondary palate. *J Craniofac Genet Dev Biol* 1994;14:87–96.
170. Bermas BL, Hill JA. Effects of immunosuppressive drugs during pregnancy. *Arthritis Rheum* 1995;38:1722–1732.
171. Anderson PO. Corticosteroid use by breast-feeding mothers. *Clin Pharm* 1987;6:445.
172. Robertson DB, Maibach HI. Topical corticosteroids. In: Schleimer RP, Claman HN, Oronsky A, eds. *Anti-inflammatory steroid action: basic and clinical aspects.* San Diego: Academic, 1989:494–524.
173. Cash JM, Wilder RL. Refractory rheumatoid arthritis: therapeutic options. *Rheum Dis Clin North Am* 1995;21:1–18.
174. Cathcart ES, Idelson BA, Scheinberg MA, et al. Beneficial effects of methylprednisolone "pulse" therapy in diffuse proliferative lupus nephritis. *Lancet* 1976;1:163–166.
175. Kimberly RP, Lockshin MD, Sherman RL, et al. High dose intravenous methylprednisolone pulse therapy in systemic lupus erythematosus. *Am J Med* 1981;70:817–824.
176. Boumpas DT, Austin HAD, Vaughn EM, et al. Controlled trial of pulse methylprednisolone versus two regimens of pulse cyclophosphamide in severe lupus nephritis. *Lancet* 1992;340:741–745.
177. Gourley MF, Austin HA III, Scott D, et al. Methylprednisolone and cyclophosphamide, alone or in combination, in patients with lupus nephritis. *Ann Intern Med* 1996;125:549–557.
178. Kimberly RP. Glucocorticoids. *Curr Opin Rheumatol* 1994;6:273–280.
179. Laue L, Kawai S, Udelman R, et al. Glucocorticoid antagonists: pharmacological attributes of a prototype antiglucocorticoid (RU 486). In: Schleimer RP, Claman HN, Oronsky A, eds. *Anti-inflammatory steroid action: basic and clinical aspects.* San Diego: Academic, 1989:303–329.
180. Axelrod L. Side effects of glucocorticoid therapy. In: Schleimer RP, Claman HN, Oronsky A, eds. *Anti-inflammatory steroid action: basic and clinical aspects.* San Diego: Academic, 1989:377–408.

CHAPTER 35

Arthrocentesis Technique and Intraarticular Therapy

Gerald F. Moore

Arthrocentesis, removal of fluid from a joint cavity, has been a routine medical procedure since it was first described in the early 1950s (1). Analysis of joint fluid is required to make a diagnosis in conditions such as gout or to confirm the possibility of a septic joint. Analysis of joint fluid is described in detail in Chapter 4.

Intraarticular therapy, most commonly using a corticosteroid preparation, has been a valuable adjunct to the treatment of many types of arthritis. Early trials with cortisone were disappointing (1). One third of patients receiving a relatively small dose of hydrocortisone intraarticularly returned to pretreatment status within 1 week of the injection. Other trials with hydrocortisone (2) and later triamcinolone (3) demonstrated longer lasting effects. Therapeutic injection of a corticosteroid preparation or local anesthetic administration have been found to be effective treatments for soft tissue disease as well as for joint pathology.

ARTHROCENTESIS

Joint fluid has been examined since the time of Hippocrates. Rodnan's review (4) of several treatises on joints and joint fluid and the anatomy and physiology of the synovial membrane found in works by Hippocrates, Celsus, Galen, and Bichat, as well as Jean-Louis Margueron's description on the chemical analysis of synovium, are worth reading.

Joint aspiration is easily performed without major complications. One review of more than 100,000 injections in more than 4,000 patients found only 14 infections with coagulase-positive *Staphylococcus*—a rate of 1 in 286 patients (5). Another study reviewing 3,000 joint injections found no infectious complications (6).

In 1961, McCarty and Hollander (7) were the first to do a systematic analysis of synovial fluid in patients with gout. Uric acid crystals were identified in 15 (89%) of 18 specimens from patients with clinical diagnosis of gout. Incubation with uricase destroyed the crystals in 13 of 15 samples studied. Polarized light increased the rate of positive identification of uric acid crystals from 61% to 83%.

INDICATIONS

Arthrocentesis is required to fully evaluate a patient with a monarticular arthritis. Arthrocentesis also provides a route for the intraarticular injection of corticosteroids, radiopharmaceutical agents used to induce radiation synovectomy, or viscosupplementation with hyaluronan. Arthrocentesis may be used for the diagnosis and treatment of traumatic arthritis or intraarticular fractures. Pain from distention of the joint capsule by fluid accumulation (e.g., hemarthrosis or synovitis) can be relieved by removal of fluid via arthrocentesis. If more than one or two joints are involved, systemic therapy may be a more appropriate means of treatment.

Evaluation of Monarticular Arthritis

Arthrocentesis is the only definitive method to confirm the presence of an infectious agent in septic arthritis or crystals in gout or calcium pyrophosphate deposition disease. All patients with a monarticular arthritis should undergo joint aspiration when the diagnosis is not obvious from the history and physical examination. Examination of fluid also can help differentiate inflammatory from noninflammatory joint disease.

Injection of Therapeutic Agents

Intraarticular injections of corticosteroids are useful in the treatment of many local and systemic joint disorders.

Many conditions (other than trauma and infection) will respond at least temporarily with a decrease in swelling and other signs of inflammation. Corticosteroids should not be injected into infected joints in view of the risk for enhanced joint and bone destruction by responsible organisms.

McCarthy (8) listed indications for intraarticular corticosteroid injections: (a) to correct flexion deformities accompanying joint inflammation, (b) to control inflammation in one or more particularly troublesome joints in patients with polyarticular synovitis, (c) to control monarticular or oligoarticular arthritis, and (d) to provide longer-term control of joint or tendon sheath inflammation, essentially a medical synovectomy.

On occasion, injection of a local anesthetic such as lidocaine benefits the patient by immediately relieving pain. Relief of pain also indicates to the clinician that a corticosteroid preparation injected into the area might be helpful for longer-term control of symptoms. Saline lavage to reduce the inflammatory components of synovial fluid may be helpful in selected patients. Viscosupplementation by using hyaluronan preparations has recently been popularized as treatment for severe degenerative joint disease (Chapter 111) refractory to other measures.

Diagnosis and Treatment of Traumatic Arthritis

Occasionally, a patient does not remember a minor traumatic event necessitating joint aspiration to rule out septic or crystal-induced disease. The presence of significant amounts of blood in synovial fluid should suggest a traumatic event (either before or during arthrocentesis). Increased intraarticular pressure that decreases range of motion and causes pain in the joint may be reduced by removal of fluid.

Diagnosis of Intraarticular Fracture

Rarely an occult fracture may be suggested when fat globules are found mixed with intraarticular blood. This finding should prompt radiographic evaluation and orthopedic consultation and management, as appropriate.

Relief of Pain from Tense Effusion and Hemarthrosis

Fluid accumulates in response to an inflammatory condition or irritant such as blood. As the volume of fluid increases, the joint capsule becomes stretched, causing pain and discomfort. As fluid accumulates in the knee joint, the semimembranosus–gastrocnemius bursa distends and may develop into a popliteal cyst through a check-valve mechanism (9). Injection of corticosteroids into the joint space may help to decrease the production of synovial fluid and the pain associated with capsule distention.

Medical management was found to be superior to surgical treatment in one large review of more than 80 articles comparing needle aspiration with surgical drainage for septic joints (10). Seventy-five percent of the medically managed group responded favorably compared with 57% of the surgically-treated group. Surgical drainage should be used when medical management of the septic joint is unsuccessful or for joints, such as the hip, that technically are difficult to aspirate.

Obtaining Fluid for Gram Stain and Culture

One of the most important reasons for performing arthrocentesis is to rule out infection. Arthrocentesis provides easy access to joint fluid for Gram stain and culture. Repeated frequent joint aspirations (up to several times per day) may be necessary in septic arthritis to remove cellular debris and to speed healing.

RELATIVE CONTRAINDICATIONS TO ARTHROCENTESIS

There are no absolute contraindications to arthrocentesis. If septic arthritis is suspected, the joint should be aspirated to obtain fluid for Gram stain and culture, even when a relative contraindication is present. However, caution should be used in the following situations.

Overlying Cellulitis

Entering the joint space after the needle has passed through an infected area, such as a cellulitis, theoretically increases the risk for spread of infection into the joint cavity. The use of appropriate technique and avoidance of areas of obvious infection reduces the chance of transmitting infection into the joint space.

Bacteremia

Likewise, performing an arthrocentesis in a patient with documented bacteremia may spread infection into the joint. However, if the joint is suspected to be infected, it is still necessary to perform a diagnostic arthrocentesis for Gram stain and culture and to facilitate the removal of excessive fluid accumulation.

Bleeding Disorders

Patients with hemophilia, thrombocytopenia, or other coagulation disorders have the potential for intraarticular bleeding after insertion of the needle. Excessive movement of the needle tip while in the joint cavity should be avoided. Bleeding into the joint is infrequently seen and can usually be avoided by using the smallest-gauge needle that allows fluid to be easily aspirated or therapeutic injection performed (e.g., 22–25 gauge).

Prosthetic Joint

The presence of a prosthetic joint makes joint aspiration technically more difficult because of scarring from the surgical procedure and resulting change in anatomy. The prosthesis is a foreign body that increases the risk for infectious complications in the joint. Aspiration of the artificial joint should be avoided unless absolutely necessary for diagnosis. If there is any question of loosening of the prosthesis or underlying osteomyelitis, the patient should undergo orthopedic evaluation.

Failure of Previous Injections

A single joint should not be injected more than two to three times in 1 year (excluding viscosupplementation). Complications are more likely with more frequent injections. The lack of response to injections suggests the need for reevaluation of the treatment regimen and consideration of other intraarticular therapy, systemic therapy, or orthopedic intervention.

Uncooperative Patient

Arthrocentesis should not be performed on a patient who is unable to cooperate. Any unnecessary movement of the joint during aspiration can lead to damage of the cartilage or bleeding, which render interpretation of the joint fluid more difficult.

TECHNIQUE

Appropriate equipment should be readied (Table 35.1). Knowledge of the anatomy of the joint being aspirated is essential. The aspiration site is carefully chosen (usually extensor surfaces, except for the hip and ankle) to avoid contact with critical structures such as blood vessels and nerves.

TABLE 35.1. *Equipment needed*

Disposable gloves (do not need to be sterile)
Providone-iodine solution (or similar)
Alcohol wipes
Anesthetic: 1–2 mL lidocaine (1% without epinephrine) or ethyl chloride
Syringes and needles
One 3-mL syringe with 25-gauge needle for lidocaine (if used)
One 5-mL syringe with 18- to 22-gauge needle for administration of corticosteroid/lidocaine preparation (if used)
One (or more) 3- to 5-mL syringes with 18- to 25-gauge needles for obtaining fluid (size of syringe depends on volume of fluid expected, and size of needle depends on size of joint being aspirated)
Plastic bandage
Sterile container for culture and sensitivity
Test tube(s) with liquid anticoagulant for laboratory testing
Polarizing microscope with red filter, slides, and coverslips

Appropriate body fluid precautions are observed, including the use of disposable latex gloves. The site is cleansed appropriately with an iodophor (or similar) preparation. A sterile-field preparation is not necessary. In one small study, field preparations with a "swipe" with isopropyl alcohol or an "aseptic" technique using chlorhexidine demonstrated no difference in the incidence of positive cultures from needles used in either group (11). Local anesthesia is obtained with either an ethyl chloride spray or lidocaine injected subcutaneously. The needle is directed into the joint cavity (see later section on Technique for Specific Joints). Fluid should flow easily into the syringe.

If there is no fluid or very sluggish flow, several options should be considered:

1. No fluid is present.
2. Tissue is obstructing the lumen of the needle: try rotating the syringe and needle.
3. The needle is not actually in the joint cavity—pull back to the skin surface, and reinsert at a slightly different angle. Ultrasonographic guidance of the needle may be used when no fluid is obtained (12). Aspiration of a joint using ultrasound-guided aspiration (97% success rate) versus conventional technique (32% success) suggests that ultrasonography is a valuable adjunct for difficult aspirations (13).
4. No fluid is obtained because the patient has tensed muscles around the joint and obstructed synovial fluid flow. In this situation, keeping the needle still until the patient relaxes may allow synovial fluid to flow into the syringe.

If corticosteroids or other agents are to be injected, aspiration of synovial fluid prior to a corticosteroid injection will prolong the effectiveness of the treatment (14). After aspiration of fluid, the syringe should be removed from the needle while it is still in the joint space. The syringe containing the corticosteroid should be attached to the needle in the joint and an attempt to reaspirate fluid should be made to document that the needle remains in the joint space. If it is still in the joint space, corticosteroid can be safely injected. The injection should not require much pressure on the plunger. If significant pressure is required, the needle has left the joint space and should be reinserted properly.

A long-acting corticosteroid such as prednisolone or triamcinolone should be used for injection. The amount of corticosteroid administered is determined by the size of the joint injected. Because the knee is a large joint, a volume of 1 to 2 mL is appropriate (usually 40–80 mg of triamcinolone). Other joints may accommodate only 0.25 to 0.5 mL of a corticosteroid preparation.

Prolonged joint rest after injection for up to 3 weeks for upper extremity joints and 6 weeks for lower extremity joints has been recommended (8). A comparison of ordinary activity versus 24 hours of rest after corticosteroid injections of knees demonstrated that at 3 and 6 months, pain and stiffness assessments favored those patients treated with 24 hours of rest (15). A regimen of decreased activity for a few hours to days after injection is probably adequate.

COMPLICATIONS

Infections

If proper aseptic techniques for arthrocentesis are used, the risk for introducing infection into a joint is negligible. Most reports place the incidence at significantly less than 1% of all procedures (5,6). A review of the literature in 1989 identified 443 cases of reported postinjection bacterial arthritis (16). Predisposing factors for infection were diabetes mellitus, rheumatoid arthritis (RA), systemic steroid therapy, immunosuppressive therapy, and infection elsewhere in the body. Slightly fewer than half of the infections were due to staphylococcal species.

Iatrogenic infection can occur when a needle enters a joint through infected skin or subcutaneous tissue. This complication is estimated to occur in less than 1 in 10,000 arthrocenteses and may be increased by previous corticosteroid injection (17,18). A case report of *Staphylococcus aureus* infection of the wrist after injection of the carpal tunnel has been reported (19). Another report reviewing more than 3,000 periarticular and intraarticular injections noted no infections (6).

Bleeding

Significant bleeding after arthrocentesis is rare. It is best prevented by pressure over the puncture site after arthrocentesis. Arthrocentesis can safely be performed in patients with a bleeding diathesis or in patients taking anticoagulants if one is careful to avoid vessels and to use a small-gauge needle. Bleeding into a joint after arthrocentesis is usually self-limited and usually requires only observation. Treatment may rarely be required to reverse anticoagulation or to replace clotting factors.

Cartilage Injury

Injury to the cartilage by the needle is rare. Injury to cartilage can lead to focal degenerative change. This complication can be prevented by using the following techniques.

1. Aspirate as the joint space is entered to avoid going too deep.
2. Do not move the needle from side to side while in the joint.
3. Select a site and needle path that stays away from the cartilage.

Corticosteroid-Related Complications

Potential corticosteroid-related complications are listed in Table 35.2. When injected into soft tissues, fluorinated corticosteroids can cause significant atrophy of collagenous tissue and lead to ligament or tendon rupture or subcutaneous calcification (the atrophy may disappear in 2–3 years). Therefore, fluorinated corticosteroids are not recommended to be used for extraarticular injections. A crystal-induced arthritis (postinjection flare-up) sometimes occurs within hours of injection and can last for several days in up to 10% of patients (20).

TABLE 35.2. *Potential sequelae from intraarticular and periarticular corticosteroid injections*

Elevated serum glucose in diabetic patients
Erythema, warmth, diaphoresis of face and torso
Iatrogenic infection
Nerve damage (injection into nerve)
Pancreatitis
Posterior subcapsular cataracts
Postinjection flare
Radiologic changes
Charcot arthropathy
Osteonecrosis
Steroid arthropathy
Suppression of the hypothalamic/pituitary/adrenal axis
Tendon rupture
Tissue atrophy, fat necrosis, calcification
Uterine bleeding

Isolated reports of tendon rupture after soft tissue injections with corticosteroids have been documented after excessive administration of a corticosteroid preparation in one area or when the corticosteroid is injected directly into the tendon (21,22).

Three case reports illustrate other complications after corticosteroid arthrocentesis (19). In one patient, rupture of four digital flexor tendons developed after 29 corticosteroid injections. In another patient, a typical bowstring deformity involving the volar aspect of the hand at the metacarpophalangeal joint developed after 10 injections. The third case described flushing and warmth of the face and neck after intraarticular triamcinolone.

Side effects are not more common in children receiving intraarticular corticosteroid injections (23,24). Osteonecrosis was found in one injected hip but could not be shown to be attributable to the corticosteroid injection. Repeated joint injections in children probably do not increase the rate of radiographic deterioration of the joint.

Hormonal changes may occur secondary to intraarticular or soft tissue injections. Up to half of women in one series reported either delayed or early menstrual cycles (25). Rarely, patients receiving frequent intraarticular corticosteroid injections may demonstrate suppression of the hypothalamic-pituitary-adrenal axis (26). Plasma cortisol levels may be suppressed within hours of intraarticular injection, with the effect lasting for several days (27).

Significant elevation of the blood sugar may follow the intraarticular injection of corticosteroids. Type 1 diabetic patients should be warned to monitor their blood sugar levels closely for several days after injection.

Allergic and Local Reactions

Subcutaneous use of local anesthetics should be avoided in patients with known allergies. In these patients, local anesthesia may be obtained by ethyl chloride spray. Ethyl chloride works as a vapor coolant spray. Second-degree epidermolysis may occur if overzealous freezing of the skin occurs. An erythematous area may develop around the site and last for several days but will usually resolve without any significant long-term effects. Reports of flushing after intraarticular injections have been described (19,25) (Chapter 34). The incidence of postinjection flare-up, probably due to the ingestion of corticosteroid crystals by polymorphonuclear leukocytes, is low (2% of 100,000 injections in one series) (5).

Joint Instability

Instability of the joint may be seen with frequent joint injections (more than two per year per joint). Whether this results from a steroid or Charcot-like arthropathy or from progression of the underlying disease is unknown. In one large series of joint injections followed up for 10 years, repeatedly injected joints had less than a 1% incidence of joint instability (5). That number is probably close to the incidence of disease-related joint instability. The antiinflammatory effects of the corticosteroid preparation may potentiate the likelihood of developing joint instability.

Hypodermic Needle Separation

Two cases of hypodermic needle separation from the plastic hub during arthrocentesis have been reported (28). Removal of the separated needle from the soft tissue may require minor surgical exploration.

Dry Tap

Failure to obtain fluid may result from many factors (29). Most commonly, this is because no fluid is present. It may be difficult to determine whether fluid is present on physical examination, particularly in an obese patient. In the knee, the needle may enter the triangular fat pad on the medial aspect of the patellofemoral compartment. Chronically-inflamed synovium may undergo fat replacement (lipoma arborescens), making aspiration difficult. A medial plica in the knee may obstruct the lumen of the needle. Long-standing fluid with reabsorption over time can lead to development of a gelatinous material that is extremely difficult to aspirate.

TECHNIQUE FOR SPECIFIC JOINTS

The technique for each individual joint is described. Video examples of individual joint injections are available (30).

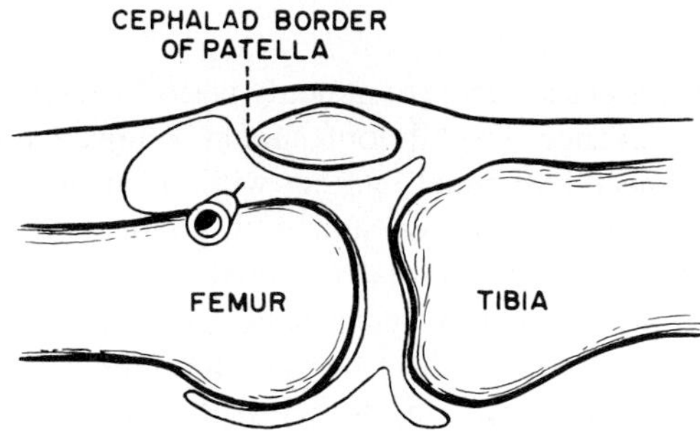

FIG. 35.1. Arthrocentesis of the right knee; lateral approach to the suprapatellar pouch.

Knee

The patient should be in the supine position with both legs extended as completely as possible. The knee to be aspirated should be completely exposed. A sheet or towel can be arranged around the knee to protect the patient's clothing. If the patient is unable to straighten the knee completely, a pillow should be placed beneath the knee to provide support.

The knee is usually aspirated through either a medial or lateral approach, although some prefer an anterior approach with the knee flexed at 90 degrees. Locate the patella, and ask the patient to relax so that the patella is freely movable. Injections are usually made at one of four positions (superior or inferior lateral and superior or inferior medial) in the palpable depression between the patella and femur.

Use a 22-gauge or larger needle (some prefer an 18- or 20-gauge needle) attached to a 3- to 5-mL syringe. After appropriate anesthesia is obtained, insert the needle into the space between the patella and femur parallel to the inferior border of the patella. Direct the needle toward the center of the patella. Insertion depth ranges from 2 cm in a normal, thin knee to more than 4 to 5 cm in grossly obese subjects, requiring the use of a 2.5-inch spinal needle. On entry into the synovial cavity, a small "give" may be felt. At that time, fluid should aspirate easily (Figs. 35.1 and 35.2).

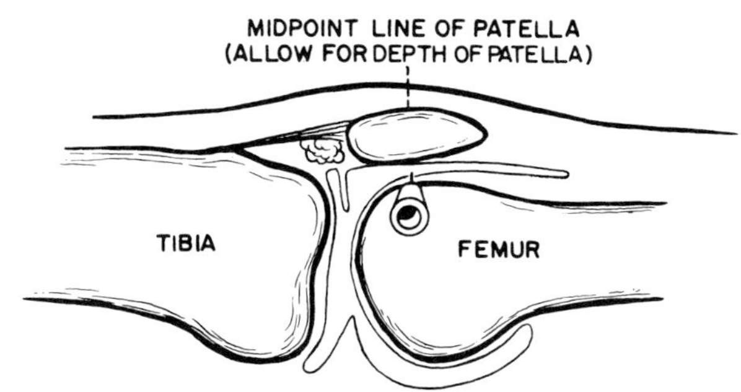

FIG. 35.2. Arthrocentesis of the right knee; medial approach under the patella.

Hip

Hip injections are most commonly performed under fluoroscopic guidance. The hip joint should be injected only by an experienced individual familiar with the anatomy of the joint. The patient is placed supine on a table with the hip extended and slightly internally rotated.

An 18- to 22-gauge spinal needle attached to a 10-mL syringe is typically used. In the anterior approach, a location approximately 2 to 3 cm below the anterior superior iliac spine and 2 to 3 cm lateral to the femoral artery can be used (Fig. 35.3).

After appropriate site preparation and administration of anesthetic, insert the needle under fluoroscopic guidance at a 60-degree angle in a posteromedial direction. Be careful to avoid the neurovascular bundle that lies medial to the injection site. Advance the needle until bone is encountered, and then withdraw slightly. After radiologic confirmation that the tip of the needle is in the vicinity of the joint capsule, aspiration or injection can be performed. Use a long-acting corticosteroid such as prednisolone or triamcinolone. Little pressure on the plunger of the syringe should be required.

Less commonly, a lateral approach is used: insert the needle anterior to the proximal tip of the greater trochanter and directed at a point midway between the symphysis pubis and the anterior superior iliac spine.

Ankle Joint

Ankle arthrocentesis is performed with the patient supine in a comfortable position. The foot should be in a neutral position with the heel resting on the table. Use an anterior approach. The area between the extensor hallucis longus and the tibialis anterior tendon should be identified near the medial malleolus (Fig. 35.4). A similar position and technique can be used for a subtalar approach (Fig. 35.5).

Use an 18- to 22-gauge needle attached to a 3- to 5-mL syringe. After preparing the site and administering the anesthetic, insert the needle parallel to the upper surface of the talus in the groove between the talus and tibia. At a depth of approximately 2 cm, the needle will enter the joint space. If present, fluid should be easily aspirated.

Metatarsophalangeal and Interphalangeal Joints of the Foot

Use a 25-gauge needle attached to a 1-mL syringe. After appropriate site preparation and administration of anesthetic, insert the needle perpendicular to the skin lateral to the extensor tendons, being careful to avoid the neurovascular bundle (Fig. 35.6). Because of the small size of these joints, careful probing of the area may be necessary to assure that the joint is entered appropriately. Insertion depth will be approximately 0.5 cm. Fluid is not usually easily aspirated.

When aspirating the first metatarsophalangeal joint to obtain fluid for crystals, use a medial approach. Because

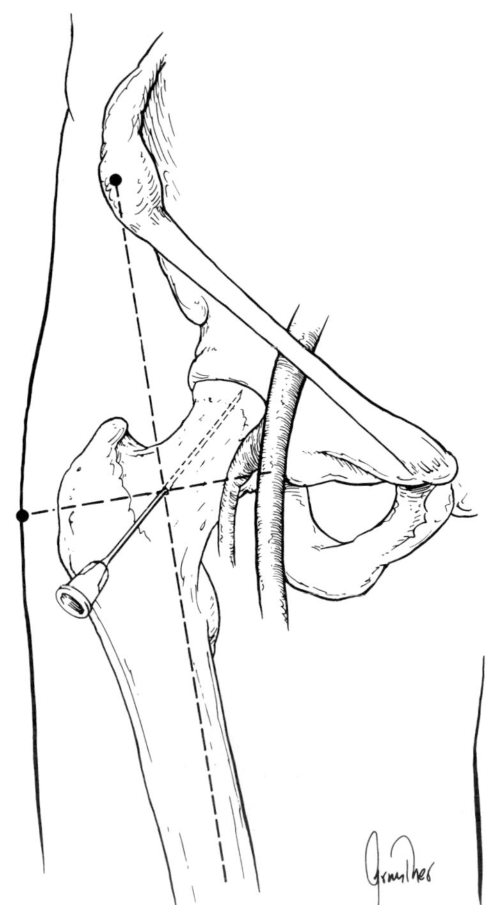

FIG. 35.3. Right hip.

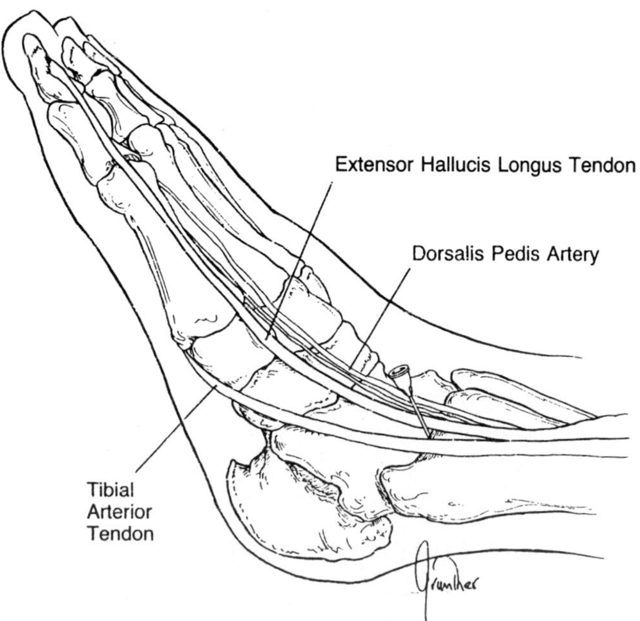

FIG. 35.4. Right ankle, anteromedial view.

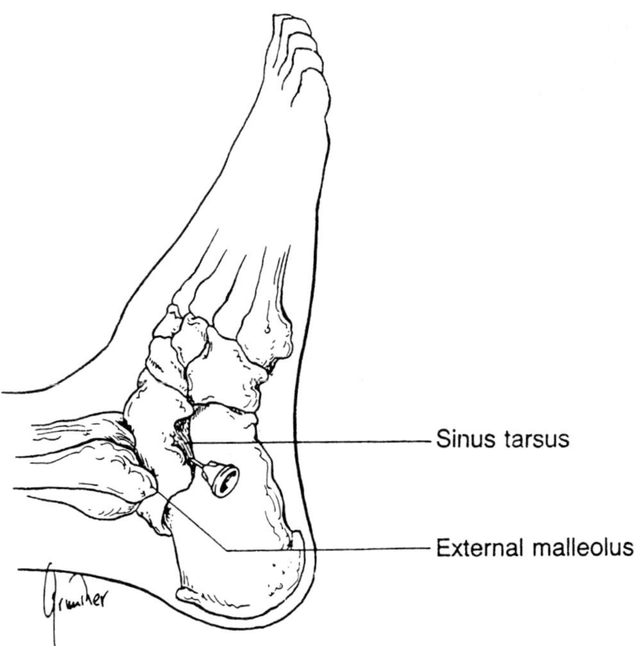

FIG. 35.5. Right subtalar joint, lateral view.

of possible severe discomfort for the patient, it may be appropriate to wait until acute inflammation begins to resolve. Crystals can usually be found between acute attacks of gout.

Shoulder

The patient is seated with the forearm flexed. Palpate the joint to determine the best place to aspirate. Any of three approaches for arthrocentesis of the shoulder can be used: anterior, lateral, or posterior. Anterior arthrocentesis is performed in the groove between the coracoid process and the humerus. Lateral injections are done inferior to the distal end of the acromion process. Posterior injections are done at the posterior tip of the acromion, aiming toward the coracoid process.

1. *Anterior approach.* The groove between the coracoid process and the humerus is identified. A 22-gauge or larger needle attached to a 3- to 5-mL syringe should be used. After appropriate site preparation and administration of anesthetic, insert the needle into the area just lateral and slightly inferior to the coracoid process (Fig. 35.7). The needle should be directed posteriorly. A small give may be felt when the joint capsule is entered. Insertion depth is approximately 2 cm in a normal-sized individual. Fluid should be easily aspirated if present.

2. *Lateral approach.* Palpate for the slight indentation just lateral to the distal acromion. Insert the needle horizontally in a medial and slightly posterior direction.

3. *Posterior approach.* Identify the posterior tip of the acromial process. Insert the needle medial to the head of the humerus in the general direction of the coracoid process.

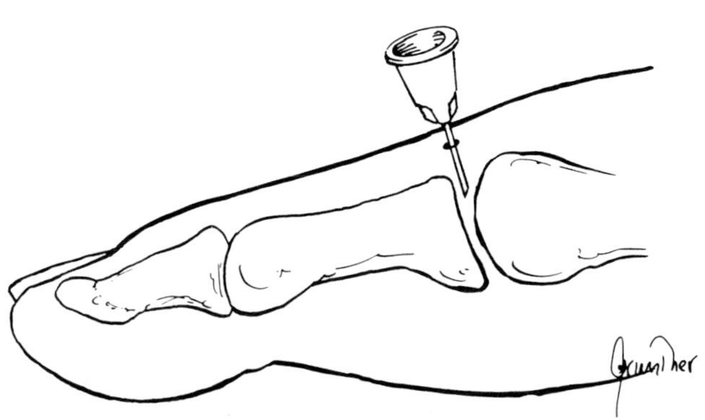

FIG. 35.6. Right first metatarsophalangeal joint, medial view.

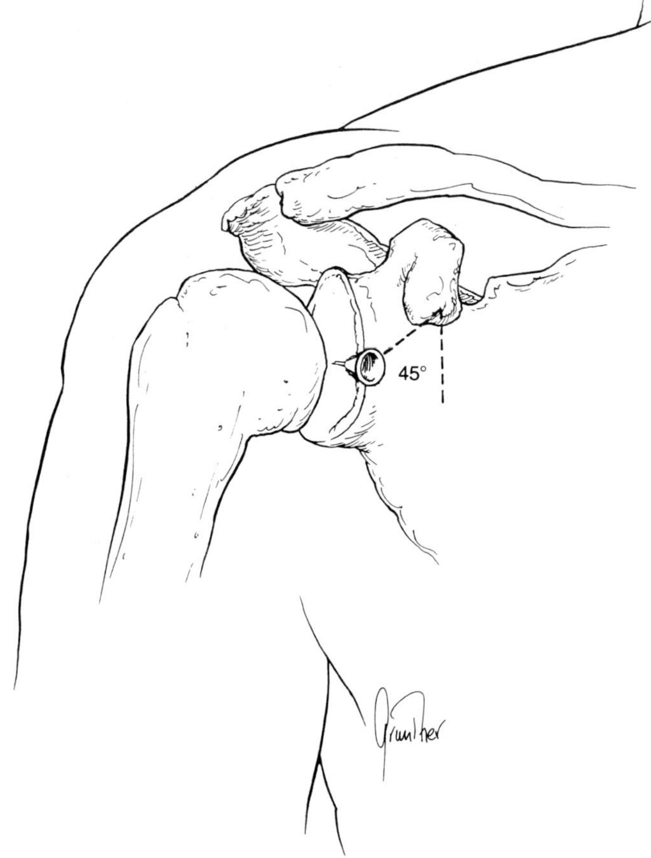

FIG. 35.7. Right shoulder.

Elbow

Arthrocentesis of the elbow is usually performed in the posterolateral area between the lateral epicondyle and the olecranon. The elbow should be partially flexed (~30–90 degrees), with the hand placed on the upper leg if sitting or on the abdomen if the patient is supine.

A 22-gauge or larger needle attached to a 3- to 5-mL syringe should be used. After appropriate site preparation

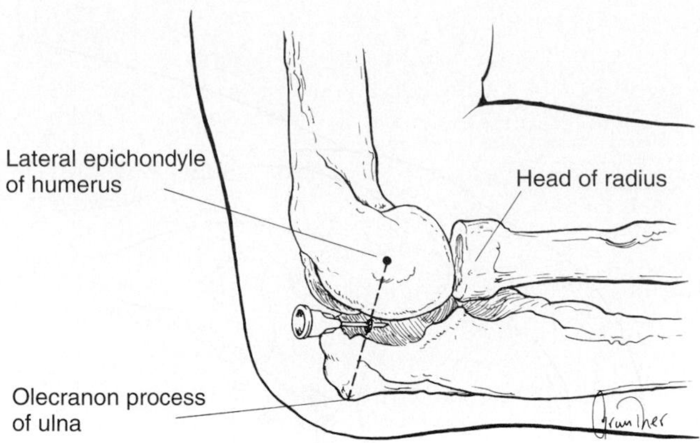

FIG. 35.8. Right elbow, lateral view.

and administration of anesthetic, insert the needle perpendicular to the skin in the area between the lateral epicondyle and the olecranon. The needle also may be positioned parallel to the radius and directed toward the hand (Fig. 35.8). The needle will need to be inserted approximately 1 cm in a normal-sized individual. Aspirate any fluid present. An alternative approach is to enter the joint posteriorly, inserting the needle superior to the olecranon and just lateral to the triceps tendon.

Wrist

Have the patient place the hand on a flat surface with the palm down. Place a small rolled-up towel beneath the wrist to flex the joint slightly. Arthrocentesis of the wrist is best performed on the dorsum of the wrist distal to the tip of the radius and to the ulnar side of the extensor tendon of the thumb. Alternatively, arthrocentesis may be performed distal to the ulnar styloid at the ulnar-carpal articulation (Fig. 35.9).

After appropriate site preparation and administration of anesthetic, insert the needle perpendicular to the skin directly over the radiocarpal joint between the extensor tendons of the thumb and the fingers (alternatively, the needle can be inserted distal to the ulnar styloid). The needle should be inserted approximately 1 cm before entering the joint. Fluid should be easily aspirated if present.

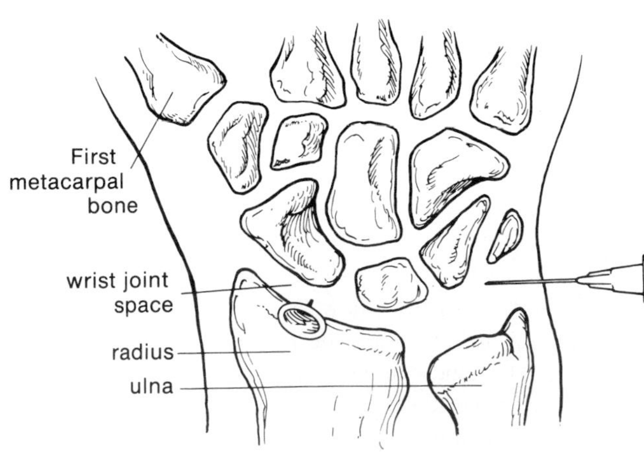

FIG. 35.9. Right wrist.

Metacarpophalangeal and Interphalangeal Joints of the Hand

Place the hand palmar side down on a table. The metacarpophalangeal joints of the hand are usually injected through a lateral approach, entering the joint space superior to the neurovascular bundle as it runs down the lateral aspect of the finger. By moving the finger and palpating the area, the joint line is usually easily identified.

For interphalangeal joint injections, an assistant can put pressure on the joint line opposite the intended insertion point to open up the joint. Enter the joint space superior to the neurovascular bundle on either side of the joint (Fig. 35.10).

A 25-gauge needle attached to a 1-mL syringe should be used. After appropriate site preparation and administration of anesthetic, insert the needle perpendicular to the joint space superior to the neurovascular bundle. Because of the small size of these joints, careful probing of the area may be necessary to ensure that the joint is entered appropriately. Insertion depth will be approximately 0.5 cm. Ordinarily fluid is not easily aspirated.

Temporomandibular Joint

The patient should be asked to open the mouth. The temporomandibular joint (TMJ) is best injected at a point approximately 2 cm in front of the tragus, just below the zygomatic arch. Care should be taken to avoid the temporal artery as well as the joint disc (Fig. 35.11).

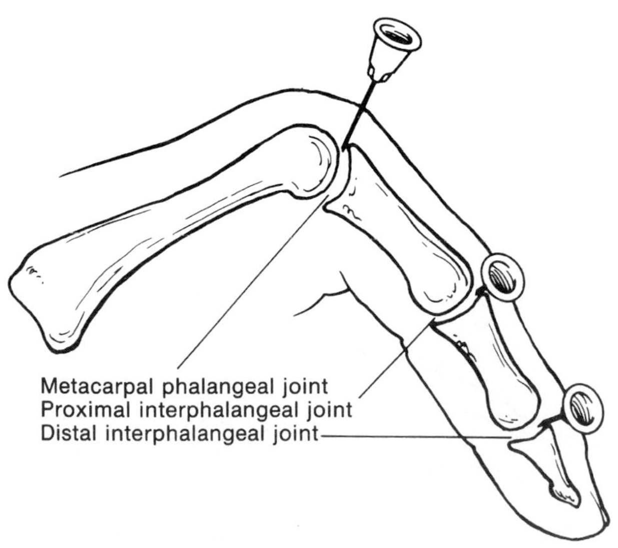

FIG. 35.10. Small joints of the hand.

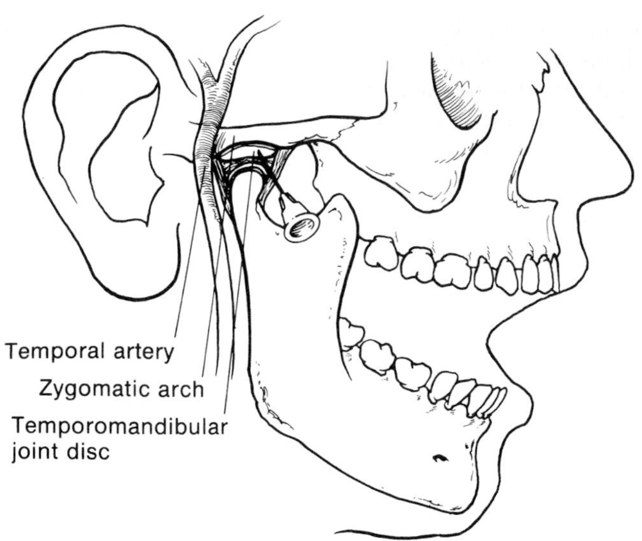

FIG. 35.11. Right temporomandibular joint.

INTRAARTICULAR THERAPY

Corticosteroids

The first report in the literature concerning the use of intraarticular corticosteroids was a personal communication by Thorn in 1950 on the use of 10 mg of hydrocortisone injected intraarticularly into the inflamed knee of a patient with RA (2). The knee improved significantly, but because of a generalized improvement thought to be due to a systemic effect, no further experiments were performed. During the next year, Hollander (2) subsequently injected seven knees of patients with RA with 25 mg of cortisone and found minimal benefit. Comparison of hydrocortisone with cortisone in 129 patients with 700 local injections demonstrated the superiority of hydrocortisone for intraarticular injections (2). The hypothesis was that hydrocortisone, one seventh less soluble than cortisone, resulted in a significant and durable "reservoir" of antiinflammatory compound in the joint.

Corticosteroids act through intracellular steroid receptors to control the rate of synthesis of messenger RNA and proteins (31) (reviewed in Chapter 34). Corticosteroids have effects on T and B cells and inhibit phospholipase A_2, with resultant decrease in the derivatives of arachidonic acid. They also may work by decreasing synthesis of the proteolytic enzyme stromelysin and the proinflammatory cytokine interleukin-1 (IL-1) in addition to reducing expression of the oncogenes c-*fos* and c-*myc*, which are important for the regulation of metalloproteinases and cytokine gene expression (31,32). In biopsy specimens of cartilage from the tibial plateaus of osteoarthritis (OA) patients who previously had received intraarticular injections with corticosteroids, metalloprotease activity was found to be normal compared with increased levels in controls not receiving the injections (33).

Neutrophil ingress into the joint is decreased by intravenous injection of 1 g of methylprednisolone, but egress from the joint is not effected (34). Magnetic resonance imaging with gadolinium performed before and after prednisolone sodium succinate was injected into the knees of six individuals with RA demonstrated reduced thickness of the synovium in two of six knees (35). Five of six patients improved clinically.

Efficacy in Osteoarthritis

Most studies in OA have found that intraarticular corticosteroids result in short-term benefit but are usually not any better than placebo after several months (reviewed in Chapter 111). A high placebo response to any injection is usually found in most studies. A review of seven controlled trials involving more than 300 OA patients treated with intraarticular steroids found that corticosteroid injections appear to be better than placebo in the first few weeks, but no long-term effect was found (31).

An early study of patients with OA receiving either placebo, hydrocortisone, saline, procaine, or lactic acid plus procaine did not demonstrate any differences between the modalities at a 6-week and 6-month follow-up (36). Significant improvement in the symptoms of OA was found in each group (varying from 78% to 92%). Intraarticular corticosteroid injection was found to be better than physiotherapy alone in 93 patients with adhesive capsulitis of the shoulder of less than 1 year's duration (37).

A controlled trial comparing methylprednisolone with saline given 8 weeks apart in the same joint demonstrated significant short-term benefit of the corticosteroid over the placebo. No clinical predictors of response were found (38). Another study of patients with OA of the knee treated with either triamcinolone or placebo demonstrated early benefit for the triamcinolone-treated subjects (78% response in the first week compared with 49% for the placebo) (39). At 6 weeks, the response rate was equal in the two groups (57% vs. 55%). Response to the injection was best predicted by the presence of joint effusion and aspiration of fluid at the time of injection.

Efficacy in Rheumatoid Arthritis

The long-term effectiveness of intraarticular corticosteroids in patients with RA is similar to that found in OA. In a 2-year follow-up study of patients with RA, 63 of 70 patients treated with corticosteroids did not have synovitis, whereas 28 of 59 patients not treated with corticosteroids had synovitis (19).

Most studies have recognized the benefit of using a longer-acting corticosteroid preparation such as triamcinolone. A randomized comparison of triamcinolone versus methylprednisolone in patients with RA revealed that at 6 months, three fourths of those treated with triamcinolone continued to have benefit compared with 58% of those treated with methylprednisolone (40).

An uncontrolled study of more than 100,000 injections in 4,000 patients over a 10-year period noted a 90% response rate to corticosteroid injection (5). A 7-year follow-up of some of those patients (100 patients with RA and 100 patients with OA) demonstrated that twice as many of the patients with OA still required injections to control their arthritis. One interesting side note: the investigators reported using corticosteroids 142 times in one joint without harm.

Efficacy in Capsulitis

The use of corticosteroids appears to be more efficient at increasing range of motion in patients with capsulitis when compared with distention of the capsule with both air and a local anesthetic (41).

Lavage

Joint lavage with saline has been used in situations in which corticosteroid injection is not thought to be appropriate. However, there are conflicting reports on the efficacy of lavage. There is some evidence that a lavage using 1 L of saline in patients with OA of the knee lasts longer than a routine corticosteroid injection (42). Pain relief with either lavage or corticosteroid injection is effective and twice as efficacious as placebo injection. Comparison of joint lavage (with or without corticosteroid) and nonsurgical synovectomy in another study found good to excellent results in one third of patients, regardless of the type of therapy (43). Similarly, a 1-L saline lavage was equal in effectiveness to diagnostic or therapeutic arthroscopy in patients with degenerative arthritis of the knee at 3-month follow-up (44). At 1-year follow-up, the knees treated with lavage were somewhat better than those knees having an arthroscopic procedure (58% vs. 44%). It should be noted that the cost of arthroscopy in this study was eight times the expense of saline lavage ($4,500 compared with $660 for lavage). A controlled trial of 180 patients randomized to arthroscopic débridement, arthroscopic lavage, or placebo failed to demonstrate a significant difference between any of the interventions (45).

Tidal irrigation may be less effective in the treatment of septic arthritis. A small study evaluated the benefit of tidal irrigation in 11 septic knees in 10 patients for whom treatment with repeated arthrocentesis failed (46). Only four of 11 responded to the tidal irrigation. Three of the nonresponders had a gram-negative infection.

VISCOSUPPLEMENTATION

Viscosupplementation was approved for use in the United States in 1997 as a medical device useful for treating refractory OA of the knee (Chapter 111). Hyaluronan (hyaluronic acid) is a long-chain polysaccharide made up of repeating disaccharide units of *N*-acetyl-glucosamine and glucuronic acid, which is produced by chondrocytes and synoviocytes (47). It is thought to have chondroprotective properties, resulting perhaps from its binding of inflammatory mediators and free radicals (48). Hyaluronan for medical use is extracted from umbilical cords, rooster comb, or bacterial cultures (48). Three to five weekly injections are usually recommended, depending on the preparation used. Before injection, synovial fluid should be removed from the joint so that the hyaluronan is not diluted.

Studies on the use of hyaluronan have not demonstrated a marked benefit of the treatment over conventional forms of therapy. However, in selected individuals with OA of the knee, hyaluronan may be appropriate therapy. A large controlled, randomized double-blind trial compared five weekly intraarticular injections of sodium hyaluronate (Hyalgan, Sanofi Pharmaceuticals, Inc., New York, NY, U.S.A.) with the nonsteroidal naproxen and with placebo in patients with OA of the knee (47). Reduction of pain with a 50-foot walk was found in all groups and persisted for the entire 6 months of the study. The only major complication was injection site discomfort in those receiving sodium hyaluronate. Other controlled studies of OA of the knee have not shown any benefit of hyaluronan over placebo (49–51). However, the subset of patients over 60 years of age with significant symptoms may be more likely to respond to intraarticular hyaluronan than to placebo.

At present, studies appear to show that hyaluronan may be as effective as NSAIDs in the treatment of OA of the knee (48). Patients for whom conservative therapy has failed and who are not candidates for orthopedic joint replacement may benefit from viscosupplementation. The high cost of the treatment may limit its usefulness.

RADIATION SYNOVECTOMY

Surgical synovectomy gives relief for 2 to 3 years but is technically difficult to do well and may result in loss of range of motion (52). As an alternative, radiopharmaceuticals such as yttrium 90, gold 198, erbium 169, rhenium 186, phosphorus 32, or dysprosium 165 administered into the joint cavity have been used as a method of nonsurgical synovectomy. Early concerns about leakage of the radiopharmaceuticals have been partially resolved by using agents such as dysprosium 165 that have short half-lives and decay primarily by beta emissions (52).

Radiation synovectomy may be more effective than older treatments such as intraarticular osmic acid. In patients with hemophilic arthropathy (53) and RA (54), radiation synovectomy with yttrium 90 or rhenium 186 may provide significant relief of symptoms when compared with osmic acid. Another study concluded that osmic acid might be better based on its longer duration of action and equal effectiveness compared with yttrium 90 (54). A review of the literature comparing the use of yttrium 90 synovectomy in

RA in comparison with placebo and intraarticular steroid failed to demonstrate a benefit for yttrium (55).

Surgical synovectomy is an effective form of therapy for patients in whom radiation synovectomy has failed (56). A report on the use of laser arthroscopic synovectomy in a limited number of patients suggests that patients with limited synovitis of the knee will respond well with reduced pain and swelling as well as a decrease in C-reactive protein. Patients with more active synovitis do not respond as well (57).

OTHER MEDICAL TREATMENTS

Many other substances have been injected intraarticularly, including osmic acid (53–56), morrhuate (58), superoxide dismutase (59), rifampin (60), and methotrexate (60, 61), as well as salicylates, phenylbutazone, and gold. Most of these treatments are not routinely used, because long-term benefits have not been demonstrated.

Osmic acid was first used for a chemical synovectomy in 1951. High fever and severe joint pain after injection limited its use until the addition of a corticosteroid was found to decrease the side effects. It has been used primarily in Europe, where reports of uncontrolled trials suggest that it may be as effective as radiation synovectomy. The material requires special handling, which limits its usefulness. Most reports in the literature on the use of osmic acid have been uncontrolled or unblinded (62–64). One controlled study comparing injections of osmic acid with triamcinolone in patients with RA of the knee noted decreased joint circumference and lowering of an inflammatory index with both treatments (65). No major side effects were noted.

REFERENCES

1. Hollander JL. The local effects of compound F (hydrocortisone) injected into joints. *Bull Rheum Dis* 1951;2:21–22.
2. Hollander JL, Brown EM Jr, Jessar RA, et al. Hydrocortisone and cortisone injected into arthritis joints. *JAMA* 1951;147:1629–1635.
3. McCarty DJ. Treatment of rheumatoid joint inflammation with triamcinolone hexacetonide. *Arthritis Rheum* 1972;15:157–173.
4. Rodnan GP, Benedek TG, Panetta WC. The early history of synovia (joint fluid). *Ann Intern Med* 1966;65:821–842.
5. Hollander JL, Jessar RA, Brown EM Jr. Intra-synovial corticosteroid therapy: a decade of use. *Bull Rheum Dis* 1961;XI:239–240.
6. Fitzgerald RH Jr. Intrasynovial injection of steroids. *Mayo Clin Proc* 1976;51:655–659.
7. McCarty DJ, Hollander JL. Identification of urate crystals in gouty synovial fluid. *Ann Intern Med* 1961;54:452–460.
8. McCarthy GM, McCarty DJ. Intrasynovial corticosteroid therapy. *Bull Rheum Dis* 1994;43:2–4.
9. Dixon Ast J, Graber J. *Local injection therapy in rheumatic diseases,* 3rd ed. Basel, Switzerland: Eular, 1989.
10. Broy SB, Schmid FR. A comparison of medical drainage (needle aspiration) and surgical drainage (arthrotomy or arthroscopy) in the initial treatment of infected joints. *Clin Rheum Dis* 1986;12:501–522.
11. Cawley PJ, Morris IM. A study to compare the efficacy of two methods of skin preparation prior to joint injection. *Br J Rheumatol* 1992; 31:847–848.
12. Koski JM. Ultrasound guided injections in rheumatology. *J Rheumatol* 2000;27:2131–2138.
13. Balint PV, Kane D, Hunter J, et al. Ultrasound guided versus conventional joint and soft tissue fluid aspiration in rheumatology practice: A pilot study. *J Rheumatol* 2002;29:2209–2213.
14. Weitoft T, Uddenfeldt P. Importance of synovial fluid aspiration when injecting intra-articular corticosteroids. *Ann Rheum Dis* 2000;59:233–235.
15. Chakravarty K, Pharoah PDP, Scott DGI. Intra-articular steroid therapy for knee synovitis: role of post injection rest. *Arthritis Rheum* 1992;35(suppl):200.
16. Von Essen R, Savolainen HA. Bacterial infection following intra-articular injection: a brief review. *Scand J Rheumatol* 1989;18:7–12.
17. Hasselbacher P. Arthrocentesis, synovial fluid analysis, and synovial biopsy. In: Klippel JH, Weyand CM, Wortman RL, et al., eds. *Primer on rheumatic diseases,* 11th ed. Atlanta: Arthritis Foundation, 1997: 98–104.
18. Östensson A, Geborek P. Septic arthritis as a non-surgical complication in rheumatoid arthritis: relation to disease severity and therapy. *Br J Rheumatol* 1991;30:35–38.
19. Gottlieb NL, Riskin WG. Complications of local corticosteroid injections. *JAMA* 1980;243:1547–1548.
20. Kahn CB, Hollander JL, Schumacher HR. Corticosteroid crystals in synovial fluid. *JAMA* 1970;211:807–809.
21. Schaffer TC. Joint and soft-tissue arthrocentesis. *Prim Care* 1993;20: 757–770.
22. Morgan J, McCarty DJ. Tendon ruptures in patients with systemic lupus erythematosus treated with corticosteroids. *Arthritis Rheum* 1974;17:1033–1036.
23. Sparling M, Malleson P, Wood B, et al. Radiographic followup of joints injected with triamcinolone hexacetonide for the management of childhood arthritis. *Arthritis Rheum* 1990;33:821–826.
24. Padeh S, Passwell JH. Intraarticular corticosteroid injection in the management of children with chronic arthritis. *Arthritis Rheum* 1998; 41:1210–1214.
25. Mens JMA, De Wolf AN, Berkhout BJ, et al. Disturbance of the menstrual pattern after local injection with triamcinolone acetonide. *Ann Rheum Dis* 1998;57:700.
26. Reid DM, Eastmond C, Rennie JAN. Hypothalamic-pituitary-adrenal axis suppression after repeated intra-articular steroid injections. *Ann Rheum Dis* 1986;45:87.
27. Bird HA, Ring EFJ, Bacon PA. A thermographic and clinical comparison of three intra-articular steroid preparations in rheumatoid arthritis. *Ann Rheum Dis* 1979;38:36–39.
28. Gottlieb NL. Hypodermic needle separation during arthrocentesis. *Arthritis Rheum* 1981;24:1593–1594.
29. Roberts WN, Hayes CW, Breitbach SA, et al. Dry taps and what to do about them: a pictorial essay on failed arthrocentesis of the knee. *Am J Med* 1996;100:461–464.
30. Moore GF. Arthrocentesis. In: Wigton RS, Tape TG, eds. *Mosby's primary care procedures.* CD-ROM series. St. Louis: CV Mosby, 1999.
31. Creamer P. Intra-articular corticosteroid injections in osteoarthritis: do they work and if so, how? *Ann Rheum Dis* 1997;56:634–636.
32. Anastassiades TP, Dwosh IL, Ford PM. Intra-articular steroid injections: a benefit or a hazard? *CMAJ* 1980;122:389–390.
33. Pelletier JP, Martel-Pelletier J, Cloutier JM, et al. Proteoglycan-degrading acid metalloprotease activity in human osteoarthritic cartilage, and the effect of intraarticular steroid injections. *Arthritis Rheum* 1987;30:541–548.
34. Youssef PP, Cormack J, Evill CA, et al. Neutrophil trafficking into inflamed joints in patients with rheumatoid arthritis, and the effects of methylprednisolone. *Arthritis Rheum* 1996;39:216–225.
35. Leitch R, Walker SE, Hillard AE. The rheumatoid knee before and after arthrocentesis and prednisolone injection: evaluation by Gd-enhanced MRI. *Clin Rheumatol* 1996;15:358–366.
36. Miller JH, White J, Norton TH. The value of intra-articular injections in osteoarthritis of the knee. *J Bone Joint Surg Br* 1958;40:636–643.
37. Carette S, Moffet H, Tardif J, et al. Intraarticular corticosteroids, supervised physiotherapy, or a combination of the two in the treatment of adhesive capsulitis of the shoulder: a placebo-controlled trial. *Arthritis Rheum* 2003;48:829–838.
38. Jones A, Doherty M. Intra-articular corticosteroids are effective in osteoarthritis but there are no clinical predictors of response. *Ann Rheum Dis* 1996;55:829–832.
39. Gaffney K, Ledingham J, Perry JD. Intra-articular triamcinolone hexacetonide in knee osteoarthritis: factors influencing the clinical response. *Ann Rheum Dis* 1995;54:379–381.

40. Jalava S, Saario R. Treatment of finger joints with local steroids. *Scand J Rheumatol* 1983;12:12–14.
41. Jacobs LGH, Barton MAJ, Wallace WA, et al. Intra-articular distension and steroids in the management of capsulitis of the shoulder. *BMJ* 1991;302:1498–1501.
42. Ravaud P, Moulinier L, Giraudeau B, et al. Effects of joint lavage and steroid injection in patients with osteoarthritis of the knee. *Arthritis Rheum* 1999;42:475–482.
43. Hilliquin P, Le Devic P, Menks C-J. Comparison of the efficacy of nonsurgical synovectomy (synoviorthesis) and joint lavage in knee osteoarthritis with effusions. *Rev Rheum* 1996;63:93–102.
44. Chang RW, Falconer J, Stulberg D, et al. A randomized, controlled trial of arthroscopic surgery versus closed-needle joint lavage for patients with osteoarthritis of the knee. *Arthritis Rheum* 1993;36:289–296.
45. Moseley JB, O'Malley K, Petersen NJ, et al. A controlled trial of arthroscopic surgery for osteoarthritis of the knee. *N Engl J Med* 2002; 347:81–88.
46. Ike RW. Tidal irrigation in septic arthritis of the knee: a potential alternative to surgical drainage. *J Rheumatol* 1993;20:2104–2111.
47. Altman RD, Moskowitz R, and the Hyalgan Study Group. Intraarticular sodium hyaluronate (Hyalgan) in the treatment of patients with osteoarthritis of the knee: a randomized clinical trial. *J Rheumatol* 1998;25:2203–2212.
48. George E. Intra-articular hyaluronan treatment for osteoarthritis. *Ann Rheum Dis* 1998;57:637–640.
49. Dahlberg L, Lohmander LS, Ryd L. Intraarticular injections of hyaluronan in patients with cartilage abnormalities and knee pain. *Arthritis Rheum* 1994;37:521–528.
50. Lohmander LS, Dalén N, Englund G, et al. Intra-articular hyaluronan injections in the treatment of osteoarthritis of the knee: a randomised, double blind, placebo controlled multicentre trial. *Ann Rheum Dis* 1996; 55:424–431.
51. Henderson EB, Smith EC, Pegley F, et al. Intra-articular injections of 750 kD hyaluronan in the treatment of osteoarthritis: a randomised single centre double-blind placebo-controlled trial of 91 patients demonstrating lack of efficacy. *Ann Rheum Dis* 1994;53:529–534.
52. Zuckerman JD, Sledge CB, Shortkroff S, et al. Treatment of rheumatoid arthritis using radiopharmaceuticals. *Nucl Med Biol* 1987;14: 211–218.
53. Molho P, Verrier P, Stieltjes N, et al. A retrospective study on chemical and radioactive synovectomy in severe haemophilia patients with recurrent haemarthrosis. *Haemophilia* 1999;5:115–123.
54. Sheppeard H, Aldin A, Ward DJ. Osmic acid versus yttrium-90 in rheumatoid synovitis of the knee. *Scand J Rheumatol* 1981;10:234–236.
55. Heuft-Dorenbosch LLJ, de Vet CW, van der Linder S. Yttrium radiosynoviorthesis in the treatment of knee arthritis in rheumatoid arthritis: a systemic review. *Ann Rheum Dis* 2000;59:583–586.
56. Combe B, Krause E, Sany J. Treatment of chronic knee synovitis with arthroscopic synovectomy after failure of intraarticular injection of radionuclide. *Arthritis Rheum* 1989;32:10–14.
57. Takagi T, Koshino T, Okamoto R. Arthroscopic synovectomy for rheumatoid arthritis using a holmium:YAG laser. *J Rheumatol* 2001;28: 1518–1522.
58. Menninger H, Reinhardt S, Söndgen W. Intra-articular treatment of rheumatoid knee-joint effusion with triamcinolone hexacetonide versus sodium morrhuate. *Scand J Rheumatol* 1994;23:249–254.
59. Mazieres B, Masquelier A-M, Capron M-H. A French controlled multicenter study of intraarticular orgotein versus intraarticular corticosteroids in the treatment of knee osteoarthritis: a one-year followup. *J Rheumatol* 1991;18(suppl 27):134–137.
60. Blyth T, Stirling A, Coote J, et al. Injection of the rheumatoid knee: does intra-articular methotrexate or rifampicin add to the benefits of triamcinolone hexacetonide? *Br J Rheumatol* 1998;37:770–772.
61. Dürk H, Kötter I, Saal JG. Intraarticular methotrexate (MTX) therapy in corticosteroid resistant monarthritis. *Arthritis Rheum* 1994;37 (suppl):252.
62. Hurri L, Sievers K, Oka M. Intra-articular osmic acid in rheumatoid arthritis. *Acta Rheum Scand* 1963;9:20–27.
63. Kajander A, Ruotsi A. The effect of intra-articular osmic acid on rheumatoid knee joint affections. *Ann Med Intern Fenn* 1967;57: 87–91.
64. Martio J, Isomäki H, Heikkola T, et al. The effect of intra-articular osmic acid in juvenile rheumatoid arthritis. *Scand J Rheumatol* 1972; 1:5–8.
65. Anttinen J, Oka M. Intra-articular triamcinolone hexacetonide and osmic acid in persistent synovitis of the knee. *Scand J Rheumatol* 1975;4:125–128.

CHAPTER 36

Hematopoietic Stem Cell Transplantation in Autoimmune Disease

Lynell W. Klassen

The relationship of autoimmune disease and histocompatible hematopoietic stem cells (HSCs) was first described in classic studies performed by Drs. Mortan and Denman and their associates (1,2). The ability to transfer autoimmune disease to normal animals by the infusion of HSCs opened a new arena for investigating the pathophysiology of autoimmunity, as well as the potential for applying such techniques in disease modification. At the same time, the use of clinical bone marrow transplantation, currently referred to as hematopoietic stem cell transplantation (HSCT), was also developed for malignant diseases. Recent years have seen a marked improvement in the techniques of HSCT. There has been a significant reduction in the morbidity of the procedure with improved therapeutic approaches for dealing with posttransplant complications and a clearer understanding of the mechanisms and timing of posttransplantation immune reconstitution. This large-scale experience with HSCT in malignant diseases, nonmalignant hematologic diseases, and certain metabolic diseases strengthened the association of the HSC with autoimmune disease. The observation that autoimmunity could be transferred from donors to recipients following HSCT (3–6), the reversal of autoimmune diseases in some recipients following HSCT (7–10), the autoimmune features of graft-versus-host disease (GVHD) following allogeneic transplantation (11–13), and the apparent induction of *de novo* autoimmune disease in some patients following HSCT (13) strengthened this relationship. Multiple investigators using various animal models of autoimmunity also demonstrated the ability to modify or cure disease manifestations with either allogeneic or autologous HSCT (14). All of these factors led to international efforts to investigate the use of HSC therapy for autoimmune diseases.

Although the concepts of HSCT are well known to hematologists and oncologists, the use of these techniques may be unfamiliar to many rheumatologists. The clear mortality and morbidity of these procedures, plus the potential for significant long-term complications, may make this therapeutic approach appear overly aggressive to many clinicians. This chapter reviews the rationale for using HSCT therapeutically in autoimmunity, outlines the general steps required in performing this procedure, discusses an approach to identify which patients would potentially benefit from such therapies, reviews the current status of this approach, and outlines the questions to be addressed in the future. Although the use of HSCT in autoimmune disease is still developmental, the current early approaches and clinical results predict it will remain an ongoing consideration for some patients with severe refractory autoimmune diseases.

STRATEGIES AND DEFINITIONS

Steps in Successful Hematopoietic Stem Cell Transplantation

Hematopoietic stem cell transplantation has been successfully used as a therapeutic modality in many different and diverse disease processes. Successful application of HSCT involves six steps (Table 36.1).

Step One

Patients must be identified with a sufficiently severe disease process so that the complications of HSCT warrant the application of a rather high-risk procedure. Issues of alternative experimental therapies, aggressive use of standard therapies, and relative costs must all be considered. It is important that all patients be advised of the appropriate (neither overstated nor understated) potential risk/benefit profile in HSCT.

TABLE 36.1. *Steps in successful hematopoietic stem cell transplantation (HSCT)*

Step number	Function
1	Identify significant autoimmune disease that is potentially curable by HSCT
2	Select the type of transplant to be used
3	Identify the source and mechanism of HSC collection, mobilization, processing, and preservation
4	Immunosuppress the recipient to alter autoimmune status and to allow growth of transplanted HSC
5	Transfer HSC
6	Deal with posttransplant complications

Step Two

The second decision is whether to use a source of stem cells taken from another individual (allogeneic transplantation) or to use the patient's own processed HSCs (autologous transplantation). A review of the relative advantages and disadvantages of the two very different transplantation techniques is outlined in Table 36.2.

Step Three

Once the type of transplantation has been identified, then a decision must be made regarding the source of the stem cells and the techniques to use in HSC collection and processing. In practice, stem cells are directly aspirated from the marrow cavity or are obtained by collecting peripheral blood progenitor cells (PBPCs) following apheresis of peripheral blood. The advantage of using a graft obtained from bone marrow tissue itself is the relatively high concentration of pleuripotent stem cells with a relatively low concentration of mature T cells. By comparison, PBPCs are diluted with many peripheral blood lymphocytes collected during the same apheresis.

TABLE 36.2. *Allogeneic versus autologous hematopoietic stem cell transplantation*

Allogeneic
Increased transplant-related mortality (15%–20%)
Increased posttransplant complications
Increased durability of disease remission
Increased cost of procedure
Significant incidence of acute and chronic graft-versus-host disease
Autologous
Lower transplant related mortality (<8%)
Rapid immune reconstitution
Increased disease relapse
Performed in appropriate outpatient setting

Although obtaining PBPCs is relatively easy, a variety of precollection treatments are usually given in order to stimulate (or "mobilize") the progenitor stem cells. For example, use of cyclophosphamide, granulocyte-colony-stimulating factor (GCSF), or both agents together, can increase the recovery of $CD34^+$ progenitor cells by a factor of 50 to 100 times. This mobilization phase significantly increases the number of HSCs retrieved and decreases the total amount of apheresis that must be performed. However, experience with using GCSF with other immunosuppressive agents indicates that some patients with autoimmune disease may experience a disease flare-up (15). For practical purposes, almost all autologous, and many allogeneic, HSCTs are currently performed using PBPCs. After obtaining the PBPC preparation, a decision must be made either to remove the contaminating mature lymphocytes (purged graft) or to leave the cell preparation intact (unpurged graft). The advantages of purged grafts are the greater chance of removing autoreactive cells prior to reinfusion (autologous) and a significant reduction in GVHD (allogeneic). The disadvantage is that purged grafts are more susceptible to rejection (or graft failure), which results in prolonged posttransplantation immunodeficiency and increased serious infections. A variety of techniques are available for removing a significant portion of the contaminating mature T cells, including use of monoclonal antibodies or physical cellular characteristics that differentiate T lymphocytes from progenitor stem cells. Alternatively, hematopoietic progenitor cells that are $CD34^+$ can be positively selected and concentrated. The apheresis technique itself removes most of the erythrocytes, and the resultant preparation has a hematocrit of around 3% to 5%. The HSC preparation (either processed or nonprocessed) then undergoes cryopreservation in dimethylsulfoxide using a controlled-rate freezer and is stored in nitrogen.

Step Four

The fourth step involves the preparation of the HSCT recipient with immunosuppressive agents to avoid transplanted stem cell rejection, eliminate any autoreactive lymphocytes, and produce marrow space for the growth of the transplanted progenitor cells. There are many different "conditioning" high-dose immunosuppressive protocols, but most utilize intensive cyclophosphamide therapy (200 mg/kg), cyclophosphamide plus total body irradiation, or a combination of cytotoxic agents such as cyclophosphamide plus busulfan. In addition, antithymocyte globulin (ATG) or other T-cell–directed antibodies may be given before or immediately after transplantation to reduce the number of host T cells and to induce enhanced immunosuppression. In general, intensifying the immunosuppressive and myelosuppressive properties of the conditioning regimen results in the potential for sustained disease control, but increases the immediate toxicity due to prolonged marrow aplasia, nonmarrow drug toxicities, and prolonged immune reconstitution. Decisions to use escalated immunosuppressive therapy enhance the potential for a positive clinical response, while also increasing the probability of transplant-related mortality and morbidity.

Step Five

Following treatment with the appropriate cytoreductive regimen, the HSC preparation is rapidly thawed by placing it in a 40°C water bath and infused intravenously as rapidly as tolerated without the removal of the cryoprotectant. Although the reinfusion is usually well tolerated, a significant portion of recipients will experience some nausea, abdominal cramping, flushing, transient hypertension, or dyspnea. In general, using PBPCs purged of lymphocytes results in fewer of these annoying but rarely life-threatening symptoms.

Step Six

A variety of posttransplantation complications must be successfully circumvented or managed. These include appropriate management of blood component support until the new bone marrow graft begins functioning and produces peripheral cells. The period of marrow aplasia is dependent on the type of immunosuppressive conditioning regimen, the type of stem cell transplant used (allogeneic vs. autologous), and the number of HSCs infused. The use of hematopoietic-colony-stimulating factors [GCSF or granulocyte-macrophage colony-stimulating factor (GM-CSF)] has significantly decreased the period of marrow aplasia and the subsequent immediate risk following bone marrow transplantation. With the use of growth factors, the period of marrow aplasia has been reduced from approximately 3 to 4 weeks to as little as 7 to 10 days. It is important to remember that HSC recipients are severely immunocompromised by the preparative regimen and thus are at risk for developing acute GVHD that can result from viable immunocompetent T lymphocytes present in platelet preparations. Therefore, all blood components must be irradiated before transfusion to eliminate viable, mature donor T cells and essentially remove the risk for acute GVHD.

Complications

Cytomegalovirus (CMV) can cause serious disease in both allogeneic and autologous graft recipients. Because CMV is transferable from healthy, seropositive blood donors by transfusion of any blood component containing leukocytes, all donors and recipients must be serotyped for CMV positivity in the early planning stages of transplantation. If a CMV-negative recipient receives a graft from a CMV-positive donor, then effective prophylaxis of CMV must be initiated. The use of prophylactic antibiotic and antifungal agents has now been standardized by most transplant centers. Although the specific types of antibiotics and the duration of therapy vary among the centers, it is clear that morbidity and mortality is decreased by standardized application of specific protocols for antimicrobial prophylaxis and treatment. Early rejection of allogeneic stem cells must be considered in all individuals, although it is unusual and is seen in fewer than 5% of transplant recipients. Less intensive immunosuppressive conditioning regimens have been associated with increased graft rejection when allogeneic HSCs are used.

A potentially devastating complication of HSCT is the development of acute GVHD. Requirements for the development of a classic graft-versus-host immune reaction include the transfer of immunocompetent donor lymphocytes with the capacity to divide in an immunocompromised recipient in the setting of antigenic differences between the donor and recipient tissue. Although the clinical course of acute GVHD is varied, it has been the direct cause of death in up to 10% of patients undergoing allogeneic HSCT and contributes to other posttransplantation complications by leading to an increased susceptibility to a variety of infections. While the classic acute GVHD is seen in the setting of an allogeneic transplantation, mild episodes of acute GVHD have been reported in patients undergoing autologous transplantation (13,16), suggesting that the pathophysiology of this process includes a loss of normal immunoregulatory influences that lead to an autoreactive state. The major target organs of acute GVHD are the skin, liver, and gastrointestinal tract.

Late complications attributable to HSCT are primarily dependent on whether an allogeneic or autologous graft was used. In the allogeneic setting, chronic GVHD is a significant complication that develops in approximately 50% of recipients (17). The clinical presentation of chronic GVHD has many characteristics in common with autoimmune disorders, such as scleroderma, systemic lupus erythematosus (SLE), induced autoimmune cytopenias, Sjögren's syndrome, and autoimmune hepatitis (12,13). The pathogenesis of chronic GVHD continues to evolve. However, it appears that damage to thymic tissue by cytotoxic immunosuppressive regimens may be one central contributing factor (17).

The induction of new autoimmune diseases that were not found in either the patient or the donor has been reported (13). These nontransmitted autoimmune diseases include hypothyroidism, hyperthyroidism, myasthenia gravis, and immune cytopenias. A variety of other autoimmune diseases have been described in case reports in the setting of allogeneic autologous stem cell transplantation. Although all of these posttransplantation autoimmune phenomena may well occur by different mechanisms, it is clear that allogeneic HSCT can result in the development of autoreactive clones, leading to pathogenic clonal B-cell expansion, the development of autoantibodies, and the development of autoimmune disease manifestations. Interestingly, a small number of autoimmune events have been reported following the use of autologous stem cell transplants (18,19).

There are other long-term complications of the intensely cytoreductive therapy used with either allo- or autotransplantation. Decreased reproductive capacity, cataracts, aseptic necrosis of bone, and secondary tumor development (usually lymphomas or leukemias) are all recognized long-term possibilities for recipients.

Types of Hematopoietic Stem Cell Transplantation

A variety of hematopoietic stem cell transplantations can be performed with the use of different donor and recipient combinations. The specific recipient-donor differences result in different posttransplantation complications and probably determine different outcomes in specific clinical diseases. The basis for these different approaches is determined by the antigenetic similarities on the surface membrane cell components that are coded for by the major histocompatibility complex (MHC). Transplantations are classified as follows:

Xenogeneic transplantation. Donor graft tissue comes from a species different from the recipient. There is no suggestion that xenogeneic HSCT will ever be used to treat clinical autoimmunity.

Allogeneic transplantation. Here the donor and recipient are the same species and have similar MHC transplantation antigens. The most common situation is to use human leukocyte antigen (HLA)-identical sibling donor cells. Because there are significant differences in the minor transplantation antigens, immune-based alloreactions can still occur.

Syngeneic transplantation. This type of transplantation involves the transfer of tissue between two genetically identical individuals (identical twins).

Autologous transplantation. The recipient's own HSCs are obtained, processed, stored, and reinfused following immunosuppression of the patient. Because there is no genetic difference between the "donor" and the "recipient," this is often referred to as an autologous marrow rescue. A major difficulty is the possibility that progenitor autoreactive clones will remain in the transfused stem cell preparation.

Unrelated versus related transplantation. The usual allogeneic transplants are between HLA-identical siblings. However, transplantation can be performed between donors and recipients who are MHC identical but unrelated. The chance for minor transplantation antigen differences is greater, leading to some increase in posttransplantation complications.

Unmatched or partially matched transplantation. Under certain circumstances, transplantation can occur between persons who are not completely MHC identical (related or nonrelated). Again, the increased degree of transplant antigen mismatch results in more complications.

RATIONALE FOR USE OF HEMATOPOIETIC STEM CELL TRANSPLANTATION IN AUTOIMMUNE DISEASES

Multiple factors provide a compelling rationale for considering HSCT in autoimmune diseases (Table 36.3). The current basic concepts of the pathogenesis of autoimmunity provide the underlying rationale for aggressive immunosuppressive therapy followed by the infusion of myeloprotective HSCs. The specific concepts of autoimmune dysregulation in a variety of rheumatologic disorders are discussed in detail in other portions of this text, and have been extensively reviewed elsewhere (14,20,21). In summary, it appears that autoimmune disease is the result of altered self, nonself discrimination with a loss of self tolerance, and the development of autoreactivity against self antigens. Available information from both animal and human studies suggests that T lymphocytes play a key role in the development and progression of specific autoimmune disease manifestations. In the context of a large body of information from murine models that suggests stem cells are involved in this process, the concept of an autoreactive progenitor cell has evolved (22). Although non-T-cell factors are certainly involved in the manifestation of many autoimmune processes, the interaction of both lymphoid and hematopoietic cells in early development provides a strong basic rationale for using lymphoablative techniques therapeutically.

For more than 20 years, preclinical studies using HSCT in animal models of autoimmunity have suggested efficacy in preventing, reversing, and even curing autoimmune manifestations. These specific experiments and the unique animal models relative to individual rheumatic diseases have

TABLE 36.3. *Rationale for use of hematopoietic stem cell transplantation (HSCT) in autoimmune diseases*

Immune pathogenesis of autoimmunity relative to the role of T cells, role of stem cells, and the concept of autoreactive progenitor cell
Preclinical studies using HSCT in animal models of autoimmunity
Transfer of autoimmune disease by donor cells into recipients undergoing HSCT for malignant diseases
Improvement or cure of coincidental autoimmunity in patients treated for another condition with HSCT
Long-term immune alterations following HSCT
Demonstration of increased therapeutic responses in autoimmune disease with increasing doses of immunosuppressive agents
Improvement of clinical response and decreasing toxicity with HSCT in malignant diseases
Common use of HSCT in immune mediated cytopenias

been discussed elsewhere in this text (see Chapter 29) and have been the subject of recent comprehensive reviews (14,20–22). The largest body of evidence uses spontaneous murine models of lupus, rodent models of adjuvant-induced inflammatory arthritis, models of multiple sclerosis in mice (experimental allergic encephalomyelitis), and models of diabetes using the spontaneous nonobese diabetic (NOD) mouse strains. Although the model systems vary, some general principles have evolved. In most model systems, early intervention with HSCT produces the most apparent and long-lasting disease remission (14). From studies of both NZW XB XSBF1 lupus-prone and NOD mice, the hypothesis developed that both the destruction of mature autoreactive lymphocytes and replacement with new HSCs are required for long-lasting disease modification (23). Other animal systems, such as the MRL/*lpr* mouse lupuslike model, suggest that relapses following HSCT are common, but often are associated with a reversal back to the recipient hematopoietic cell phenotype (24). The adjuvant arthritis model in rats surprisingly suggests that both autologous HSCs and allogeneic HSCs are effective in treating the inflammatory joint manifestations (25). Information using murine models of diabetes and lupus suggests that sublethal doses of radiation combined with infusion of allogeneic HSCs results in stable donor/recipient chimerism and disease suppression (26,27). These later observations raise the possibility of applying less intensive myelosuppressive techniques in HSCT for autoimmune disease.

Although the preclinical animal models have been central in understanding mechanistic issues, it is clear that their ability to predict clinical responses in patients often is limited. In human transplantation, it is well known that using patients with autoimmune disease as transplant donors can transfer the same disease manifestations to the recipient of an allogeneic transplantation (3–5). It appears that the transfer of either pathogenetic lymphocytes or so-called autoimmune progenitor cells will result in the development of autoreactive lymphoid clones from the donor that proliferate in the recipient and cause disease. The transfer of myasthenia gravis, diabetes, thyroiditis, autoimmune thrombocytopenic purpura, and celiac disease has been reported. In one patient undergoing allogeneic transplantation for acute myeloid leukemia, both the resolution of the recipient's own autoimmune process (pustular psoriasis) and the transfer of autoimmune thyroiditis from the donor sibling were noted (5). Although the transfer of an autoimmune disorder from the donor to the recipient has been clearly demonstrated, it should be emphasized that other reports have shown that recipients who have received unmanipulated marrow from HLA-identical donors affected either with SLE (28) or rheumatoid arthritis (RA) (29) have not experienced the development of those autoimmune diseases. Thus, the transfer of autoimmunity is neither predictable nor reproducible in humans. The transfer of an autoimmune disorder from a donor to a recipient strongly suggests the presence of human autoreactive progenitor cells that might, in turn, be successfully treated with normal HSC repopulation.

The most compelling rationale for the use of HSCT in autoimmune diseases is the well-described improvement or cure of coincidental autoimmunity seen in patients treated for another disease process. The specifics of these clinical observations have been detailed by other researchers (3,7, 8,30–33). In general, these observations suggest that both allogeneic and autologous HSCT can result in disease regression in RA, SLE, inflammatory bowel disease, and autoimmune cytopenias, as well as a variety of rare disorders such as Shulman syndrome, celiac disease, and others (9). Although the remission of autoimmunity appears to be more durable following allogeneic transplantation, recurrence of the original autoimmune disease has been described years after an apparent cure following allograft transplantation (34). Results of autologous transplantation are more varied with a few long-term remissions, but often rapid relapses are reported (35,36). All of these reports vary considerably in the patient disease status, duration of initial autoimmune process, use of T-cell depletion in the stem cell preparation, and initial immunosuppressive transplantation conditioning regimen. However, these results suggest that both long-lasting responses and treatment failures likely will be seen when a prospective approach to using HSCT in autoimmune disease is evaluated.

Support for the use of HSCT in autoimmune disease would be strengthened if mechanistic changes in immune status could be expected as a result of the transplantation procedure. It is clear that long-term immune alterations are seen in recipients following both allogeneic and autologous HSCT. Reconstitution of the immune system following both bone marrow and peripheral blood stem cell transplantations has been extensively reported (37–45). Although it has been suggested that reconstitution of the immune system in the setting of intensive lymphomyeloablation will result in redevelopment of ontogenesis and the resultant reacquisition of self-tolerance (3,14), it has also been demonstrated that T-cell reconstitution after HSCT follows a different and unique pattern (37). Effects of myeloablative therapy on both thymic and extrathymic function result in long-lasting absolute reduction in helper T cell ($CD4^+$) function. Although T-lymphocyte reconstitution occurs earlier following autologous repopulation, there is still a persistent depression in CD4 helper subsets that can last for years. In fact, high-dose chemotherapy itself has been shown to induce long-lasting loss of $CD4^+$ cells. Furthermore, selective differences in helper T cell subset 1 (T_H1) and T_H2 function have been suggested as a reason for long-lasting alloimmune suppression following stem cell transplantation (32). Thus, the presence of long-lasting immune dysregulation with a net effect of decreased $CD4^+$ function has encouraged the continued investigation of these approaches for controlling ongoing autoimmune diseases.

Observations suggesting a relationship between improved therapeutic response in autoimmune disease with increasing doses of immunosuppressive agents further support using HSCT as an adjunct therapy in high-dose immunosuppressive approaches (46–49). In this setting, infusion of the HSC is primarily viewed as a rescue process to decrease the complications of prolonged marrow aplasia. It is clear that high-dose immunosuppressive therapy itself can alter certain autoimmune processes without reinfusion of HSCs (50). Although such observations support the use of autologous HSCT as a rescue agent following intensive chemotherapy, the bulk of the experimental evidence suggests that the transfer or modulation of small numbers of lymphohematopoietic progenitor cells may directly contribute to clinical improvement.

The long history and standardized protocols now available for HSCT in malignancy strengthen the rationale for its use in autoimmune disease. There has been a clear improvement in clinical response and a decrease in toxicity in transplants used in the setting of malignancy. In addition, the rather routine use of HSCT in immune-mediated cytopenias, such as aplastic anemia and idiopathic thrombocytopenic purpura, have encouraged the application of this technology in other nonmalignant disease settings.

IDENTIFICATION OF CANDIDATES FOR HEMATOPOIETIC STEM CELL TRANSPLANTATION

The major issue in applying HSCT remains patient selection, both with reference to the specific disease groups considered and the development of clinical criteria for specific patient selection. Ideally, HSCT would be offered for the patients who were at high risk for progression to significant morbidity or mortality, have not or will not respond to effective conventional therapies, are rather early in their disease in order to minimize irreversible major organ damage, and have evidence that any existing structural tissue damage is reversible. Unfortunately, autoimmune diseases are notoriously unpredictable in their clinical course, and the ability to predict clear-cut prognostic factors early in a patient's disease is limited. It would be ideal to have clinical, genetic, or laboratory markers that could differentiate patients with poor prognoses. Although some patients with RA who have a DRb1 subtype marker (04–04) have a more destructive course, only recently have such genetic markers been used to identify patients who might have differential clinical responses to specific therapies (51). The dilemma remains that the best potential candidates for disease remission following HSCT are those with early disease, whereas the preferred candidates based on toxicity are those with advanced and far less reversible disease. As clearly demonstrated in the early experience with HSCT for malignancy, limiting patient selection to those with severe disease having few therapeutic options will result in an initial experience characterized by relatively high toxicity and low therapeutic responses. Fiscal considerations also become directly involved in patient selection. Although the initial costs of HSCT are high, a curative regimen could certainly be cost effective over the long term when compared with currently used multiple drug regimens and biologic therapies. To date, a careful cost analysis that would clearly define the fiscal advantages and disadvantages of HSCT in autoimmune disease has not been performed.

Several consensus reports regarding patient selection have been developed by rheumatologists and transplant physicians (52,53). It was recommended that HSCT should be considered in patients with specific rheumatic diseases only after demonstrating a failure to respond to conventional therapies, when there is evidence of severe life- and organ-threatening disease, and after two independent clinical specialists have evaluated the patient and determined that the quality of life could be improved following intensified immunologic manipulation. A group of specific potential rheumatic diseases have been identified (Table 36.4), and prospective randomized phase III trials for systemic sclerosis, multiple sclerosis, and RA have been proposed. A data registry has been established by the European Group for Bone Marrow Transplantation, the European League Against Rheumatism, and the International Bone Marrow Transplantation Registry for reporting patients who have been treated with HSCT for autoimmune diseases.

General principles for individual patient selection can be suggested based on results of these consensus conferences and by evaluating the increasing body of literature that details the specific responses of HSCT in human diseases. The following questions can be used to select individual patients for HSCT:

1. Does the patient have a definable rheumatic disease with a reasonable prediction of the future clinical course?
2. Is there evidence that the autoimmune disease is a significant threat to life or major organ function?

TABLE 36.4. *Consensus recommendation or rheumatic disease categories for HSCT*

Systemic sclerosis (scleroderma)
Systemic lupus erythematosus
Rheumatoid arthritis
Dermatomyositis
Necrotizing vasculitis
Antiphospholipid syndrome
Autoimmune pulmonary hypertension
Severe uncontrolled cryoglobulinemia

From Tyndall A, Gratwohl A. Blood and marrow stem cell transplants in auto-immune disease: a consensus report written on behalf of the European League against Rheumatism (EULAR) and the European Group for Blood and Marrow Transplantation (EBMT). *Bone Marrow Transplant* 1997; 19:643–645, with permission.

3. Has the patient failed appropriately aggressive conventional therapies?
4. Is there a reasonable suggestion from pathogenetic studies, preclinical models, or anecdotal clinical reports that the patient might respond to high-dose immunosuppressive therapy?
5. Does the patient lack serious major organ failure that would limit the application of aggressive immunosuppressive regimens or would significantly increase post-transplantation complications?
6. Has there been a realistic consideration of the financial issues?
7. Is there a clearly defined treatment protocol that has undergone prior ethical and investigative review?

It is obvious that the current situation of offering HSCT to high-risk patients will predict a worse overall clinical response to HSCT. However, until the specific toxicity of HSCT has been clearly defined in each autoimmune disease, the application of this intensive therapy in patients with early disease is premature.

EARLY APPROACHES AND RESULTS

By 2003, over 500 patients had been reported in the medical literature (21,53,54). These patients had been treated at multiple institutions with substantially different protocols, making overall interpretation of results and complications difficult. The largest group of patients have been treated for refractory multiple sclerosis. Systemic sclerosis and RA have been the most common rheumatic diseases treated. There have been around 50 patients with juvenile rheumatoid arthritis and SLE reported to the transplant registries. The remaining 15% of reports are from a variety of autoimmune neurologic, vasculitic, and rheumatic diseases. It is difficult to evaluate responses from such a heterogeneous group of patients treated under varying clinical protocols. However, summary reports from international databases suggest that around 70% of all patients undergoing HSCT have a clinically significant response, although relapses are seen in the majority of the cases (21,22,53,54). Procedure-related mortality associated with the stem cell mobilization phase is 1.5%, with an overall transplantation-related mortality rate of 8%. This treatment-related mortality is disease related, with a low incidence in RA (1.4%) and a higher rate in systemic sclerosis (10%–30%).

Although it is difficult to make statements about results in specific diseases because of the small number of patients, it appears that toxicity in systemic sclerosis is somewhat higher than in other rheumatic diseases. However, the response to HSCT has also been dramatic in some patients with this disease (54–56). The report by Fange and associates suggests that 70% of the patients had either major or partial responses. Of special interest is the rapid improvement seen in the skin scores. Multiple individual reports have detailed positive responses in applying HSCT to a wide variety of inflammatory conditions, including polychondritis, antiphospholipid syndrome, polyarteritis, and other disease processes (53,54). Although any analysis of early clinical reports is complicated by the fact that often only positive results are reported, the clinical experience suggests that a significant portion of patients with rheumatic disease will have disease remission or regression following HSCT. However, it is also apparent that the durability of the response is often limited and relapses occur frequently.

The concomitant report of three early studies using HSCT in the treatment of RA illustrates several important concepts for using this modality in other autoimmune diseases (56–58). A total of 16 patients were treated in three studies that had distinctive differences in design. A significant initial positive clinical response was seen in almost all patients. Many had highly resistant disease and had failed multiple disease-modifying regimens. Although some patients had an apparent significant and reasonably long-lasting response (9–20 months), others experienced either a partial response or had rather early relapses of their active synovitis. A large study reported by Moore and associates (59) continued and expanded these clinical observations. Thirty-three patients with severe RA received high-dose cyclophosphamide (200 mg/kg) followed by autologous stem cells that were either $CD34^+$ selected or unmanipulated. The overall 20% improvement by ACR criteria (ACR20) response rate was 70%, with an ACR70 response of around 40%. Unfortunately, virtually all patients relapsed with a median time to recurrence of around 6 months. There was no significant difference in response between the group that received T-cell depleted HSCs and those receiving unfractionated cells. Although significant differences existed in these specific protocols, several generalizations can be made. First, even long-standing refractory RA will respond to high-dose immunosuppression with autologous stem cell reconstitution. Second, disease remissions are often rather short-lived. Third, no clear advantage of *in vitro* manipulation of the PBPCs to remove lymphocytes was evident. Fourth, several patients with therapy-resistant RA had a suboptimal response to HSCT, but subsequently responded to standard disease-modifying agents. This suggests that HSCT may reset the disease to an earlier, more treatable phase (54). Fifth, it appears that changes will have to be made in either patient selection, the immunosuppressive regimen, or the manipulation of the HSC graft if a more significant clinical response following HSCT in RA is to occur.

One can view these early reports with either optimism or pessimism. Although sustained cure rates have not been uniformly obtained, these early results in autoimmune disease are positive when compared with the early history of HSCT in malignant diseases. It is reassuring that the early data suggest an overall transplant-related mortality rate of approximately 8% to 9%. This is somewhat higher than the widely accepted autotransplantation mortality risk for malignant diseases (<5%). However, this toxicity level is certainly appropriate given the early status of the clinical experience. In view of the well-established serious toxicity, continued emphasis should be placed on reducing the learning curve effect by applying this modality primarily in centers with established expertise in performing HSCT, evaluating the potential role of previous therapies on toxicity following HSCT, and looking specifically for increased organ toxicity in rheumatologic patients who undergo intensive immunosuppressive therapies.

TABLE 36.5. *Potential immunologic goals for use of hematopoietic stem cell transplantation in autoimmune diseases*

Destroy all autoreactive mature and progenitor cells and replace them with a normal immune system
Reduce the number of autoreactive cells to low levels, and allow for self-tolerance to be reestablished as the lymphoid population expands
Alter immunoregulatory circuits by the use of cytotoxic agents and reestablish more effective immune control mechanisms

QUESTIONS TO BE ADDRESSED AND FUTURE DIRECTIONS

After 20 years of preclinical animal studies and much anticipation, the application of HSCT to autoimmune disease is now a clinical reality. The use of HSCT for autoimmune disease will undoubtedly expand in the future. However, the status of our current experience and biologic knowledge raises obvious questions that must be addressed before these techniques will see widespread clinically use.

The first question is, which specific immunologic goal is to be achieved by the use of HSCT in autoimmune diseases (Table 36.5)? Although the approach, to date, has been empiric, current experience suggests that the choice of the cytoreductive regimen, the pretransplantation manipulation of the PBPCs, and the use of antirheumatic therapy posttransplantation may all result in the development of different immunologic responses following either allogeneic or autologous HSC reconstitution. The optimal goal would be to destroy all autoreactive mature and progenitor lymphoid cells and replace them with a normal nondiseased immune system. Because of the complex interaction of genetic, environmental, and pharmacologic factors in autoimmune disease expression, it is unlikely that such a goal can be reached unless allogeneic transplantation is used. At the present time, the toxicity and morbidity of an allogeneic transplant is unacceptable for most patients with autoimmune diseases. A more reasonable goal would be to reduce the number of autoreactive cells to very low levels and allow for the reestablishment of self-tolerance as the lymphoid populations reexpand. As mentioned above, there is some controversy as to whether the reconstitution of an immune system following autologous transplantation does indeed proceed by a process of "recapitulation of ontogenesis" resulting in a "new" immune system more amenable to therapeutic manipulation or whether the reconstituted immune system maintains the rheumatic disease phenotype.

Another goal is to alter immunoregulatory circuits primarily by using high-dose cytotoxic agents with or without radiation to reestablish more effective suppressive control of the immune system. This concept has been likened to a "resetting of the thermostat" (59). Research efforts to evaluate this possibility are concentrating on the role of T_H1/T_H2 cells in the expression and thus control of autoimmune disease manifestations. Although it is clear that high-dose cytotoxic agents or radiation produces long-lasting alterations in immunologic subsets, the relationship of these changes and the ability to predict exactly how HSCT will alter these control mechanism has not been established. Thus, our immune approach is still quite empiric. As better understanding of the immune control mechanisms in autoimmune disease and how HSCT alters these mechanisms is evident, more rational approaches to the selection of the specific techniques involved in HSCT can be made.

The second major question is, what are the clinical goals and expectations for the use of HSCT in autoimmune diseases? At present, the hope is to produce a cure or long-lasting remission by the use of this intensive therapy. The experience to date demonstrates that although the initial clinical response can be dramatic, it is usually not sustained. It is possible, however, that a partial response or a nondurable disease remission will allow a patient to again respond to standard disease-modifying therapies. The initial observations in RA suggest this may be a real possibility.

The third question is, can patients who will be highly refractory to standard therapy be identified early in their clinical course when HSCT would be expected to be more beneficial? Use of genetic markers in RA to predict response to therapy (51), the prospective application of disease activity index scores in SLE (59), the determination of functional assessment status (60,61), and the development of predictive cytokine profiles may all be useful in the future to identify patients for whom the application of HSCT would be reasonable.

The fourth question is, can the complications of allogeneic stem cell transplantation be reduced to the degree that application in autoimmune disease is acceptable? Although the immediate complications of allogeneic transplantation have remarkably improved during the past 20 years, an overall toxicity rate of 15% to 25% still limits its application in nonmalignant, nonlethal disease. New approaches using nonmyeloablative conditioning regimens may induce stable mixed chimeras that could produce significant immune alterations with fewer complications (27). The use of cord blood cells as a source of donor HSCs may also significantly decrease allogeneic transplantation complications if animal studies can be extrapolated to the clinical arena (62,63).

It is clear that HSCT procedures will continue to be used in selected patients with autoimmune diseases. The overall applicability of this approach in the clinical setting remains to be determined.

REFERENCES

1. Morton JI, Siegel BV. Transplantation of autoimmune potential. I. Development of antinuclear antibodies in H-2 histocompatible recipients of bone marrow from New Zealand Black mice. *Proc Natl Acad Sci U S A* 1974;71:2162–2165.
2. Denman AM, Russell AS, Denman EJ. Adoptive transfer of the diseases of New Zealand black mice to normal mouse strains. *Clin Exp Immunol* 1969;5:567–595.
3. Snowden JA, Brooks PM, Biggs JC. Haemopoietic stem cell transplantation for autoimmune diseases. *Br J Haematol* 1997;99:9–22.
4. Bargetzi MJ, Schonenberger A, Tichelli A, et al. Celiac disease transmitted by allogeneic non-T cell-depleted bone marrow transplantation. *Bone Marrow Transplant* 1997;20:607–609.
5. Kishimoto Y, Yamamoto Y, Ito T, et al. Transfer of autoimmune thyroiditis and resolution of palmoplantar pustular psoriasis following allogeneic bone marrow transplantation. *Bone Marrow Transplant* 1997;19:1041–1043.
6. Karthaus M, Gabrysiak T, Brabant G, et al. Immune thyroiditis after transplantation of allogeneic $CD34^+$ selected peripheral blood cells. *Bone Marrow Transplant* 1997;20:697–699.
7. Nelson JL, Torrez R, Louie FM, et al. Pre-existing autoimmune disease in patients with long-term survival after allogeneic bone marrow transplantation. *J Rheumatol Suppl* 1997;48:23–29.
8. Snowden JA, Kearney P, Kearney A, et al. Long-term outcome of autoimmune disease following allogeneic bone marrow transplantation. *Arthritis Rheum* 1998;41:453–459.
9. Cetkovsky P, Koza V, Cetkovska P, et al. Successful treatment of severe Shulman's syndrome by allogeneic bone marrow transplantation. *Bone Marrow Transplant* 1998;21:637–639.
10. Lopez-Cubero SO, Sullivan KM, McDonald GB. Course of Crohn's disease after allogeneic marrow transplantation. *Gastroenterology* 1998;114:433–440.
11. Klassen LW, Armitage JO, Warkentin PI. Bone marrow transplantation. In: Koepke JA, ed. *Practical laboratory hematology,* 1st ed. New York: Churchill Livingstone, 1991:547–571.
12. Rouquette-Gally AM, Boyeldieu D, Prost AC, et al. Autoimmunity after allogeneic bone marrow transplantation. A study of 53 long-term-surviving patients. *Transplantation* 1988;46:238–240.
13. Sherer Y, Shoenfeld Y. Autoimmune diseases and autoimmunity post-bone marrow transplantation. *Bone Marrow Transplant* 1998; 22:873–881.
14. von Bekkum DW. Experimental basis of hematopoietic stem cell transplantation for treatment of autoimmune diseases. *J Leukoc Biol* 2002;72:609–620.
15. Snowden JA, Biggs JC, Milliken ST, et al. A randomised, blinded, placebo-controlled, dose escalation study of the tolerability and efficacy of filgrastim for haemopoietic stem cell mobilisation in patients with severe active rheumatoid arthritis. *Bone Marrow Transplant* 1998;22: 1035–1041.
16. Hess AD, Fischer AC. Immune mechanisms in cyclosporine-induced syngeneic graft-versus-host disease. *Transplantation* 1989;48:895–900.
17. Ferrara JL, Deeg HJ. Graft-versus-host disease. *N Engl J Med* 1991; 324:667–674.
18. Fullerton SH, Woodley DT, Smoller BR, et al. Paraneoplastic pemphigus with autoantibody deposition in bronchial epithelium after autologous bone marrow transplantation. *JAMA* 1992;267:1500–1502.
19. Lambertenghi-Deliliers GL, Annaloro C, Della VA, et al. Multiple autoimmune events after autologous bone marrow transplantation. *Bone Marrow Transplant* 1997;19:745–747.
20. Ikehara S. Bone marrow transplantation for autoimmune diseases. *Acta Haematol* 1998;99:116–132.
21. Van Laar JM, Tyndall A. Intensive immunosuppression and stem-cell transplantation for patients with severe rheumatic autoimmune disease: a review. *Cancer Control* 2003;10:57–65.
22. Furst DE. Stem cell transplantation for autoimmune disease: progress and problems. *Curr Opin Rheumatol* 2002;14:220–224.
23. Ikehara S, Kawamura M, Takao F, et al. Organ-specific and systemic autoimmune diseases originate from defects in hematopoietic stem cells. *Proc Natl Acad Sci U S A* 1990;87:8341–8344.
24. Ishida T, Inaba M, Hisha H, et al. Requirement of donor-derived stromal cells in the bone marrow for successful allogeneic bone marrow transplantation. Complete prevention of recurrence of autoimmune diseases in MRL/MP-lpr/lpr mice by transplantation of bone marrow plus bones (stromal cells) from the same donor. *J Immunol* 1994;152: 3119–3127.
25. Knaan-Shanzer S, Houben P, Kinwel-Bohre EP, et al. Remission induction of adjuvant arthritis in rats by total body irradiation and autologous bone marrow transplantation. *Bone Marrow Transplant* 1991;8: 333–338.
26. Li H, Kaufman CL, Boggs SS, et al. Mixed allogeneic chimerism induced by a sublethal approach prevents autoimmune diabetes and reverses insulitis in nonobese diabetic (NOD) mice. *J Immunol* 1996; 156:380–388.
27. McSweeney PA, Storb R. Mixed chimerism: preclinical studies and clinical applications. *Biol Blood Marrow Transplant* 1999;5:192–203.
28. Sturfelt G, Lenhoff S, Sallerfors B, et al. Transplantation with allogeneic bone marrow from a donor with systemic lupus erythematosus (SLE): successful outcome in the recipient and induction of an SLE flare in the donor. *Ann Rheum Dis* 1996;55:638–641.
29. Snowden JA, Atkinson K, Kearney P, et al. Allogeneic bone marrow transplantation from a donor with severe active rheumatoid arthritis not resulting in adoptive transfer of disease to recipient. *Bone Marrow Transplant* 1997;20:71–73.
30. Marmont AM. Immune ablation with stem-cell rescue: a possible cure for systemic lupus erythematosus? *Lupus* 1993;2:151–156.
31. Tyndall A. Hematopoietic stem cell transplantation in rheumatic diseases other than systemic sclerosis and systemic lupus erythematosus. *J Rheumatol Suppl* 1997;48:94–97.
32. Marmont AM. Immune ablation followed by allogeneic or autologous bone marrow transplantation: a new treatment for severe autoimmune diseases? *Stem Cells* 1994;12:125–135.
33. Marmont AM. Stem cell transplantation for severe autoimmune diseases: progress and problems. *Haematologica* 1998;83:733–743.
34. McKendry RJ, Huebsch L, Leclair B. Progression of rheumatoid arthritis following bone marrow transplantation. A case report with a 13-year followup. *Arthritis Rheum* 1996;39:1246–1253.
35. Cooley HM, Snowden JA, Grigg AP, et al. Outcome of rheumatoid arthritis and psoriasis following autologous stem cell transplantation for hematologic malignancy. *Arthritis Rheum* 1997;40:1712–1715.
36. Euler HH, Marmont AM, Bacigalupo A, et al. Early recurrence or persistence of autoimmune diseases after unmanipulated autologous stem cell transplantation. *Blood* 1996;88:3621–3625.
37. Storek J, Witherspoon RP, Storb R. T cell reconstitution after bone marrow transplantation into adult patients does not resemble T cell development in early life. *Bone Marrow Transplant* 1995;16:413–425.
38. Cavenagh JD, Milne TM, Macey MG, et al. Thymic function in adults: evidence derived from immune recovery patterns following myeloablative chemotherapy and stem cell infusion. *Br J Haematol* 1997;97: 673–676.
39. Mall TN, Avigan D, Dupont B, et al. Immune reconstitution following T-cell depleted bone marrow transplantation: effect of age and post-transplant graft rejection prophylaxis. *Biol Blood Marrow Transplant* 1997;3:65–75.
40. Atkinson K. Reconstruction of the haemopoietic and immune systems after marrow transplantation. *Bone Marrow Transplant* 1990;5:209–226.
41. Witherspoon RP. Immunological reconstruction after allogeneic marrow, autologous marrow or autologous peripheral blood stem cell transplantation. In: Atkinson K, ed. *Clinical bone marrow transplantation.* Cambridge, MA: Cambridge University Press, 1994:62–72.
42. Roberts MM, To LB, Gillis D, et al. Immune reconstitution following peripheral blood stem cell transplantation, autologous bone marrow transplantation and allogeneic bone marrow transplantation. *Bone Marrow Transplant* 1993;12:469–475.

43. Olivieri A, Brunori M, Offidani M. A detailed study on immune recovery in 50 patients autotransplanted with blood progenitor cells. *Exp Hematol* 1996;24:1088.
44. Hakim FT, Cepeda R, Kaimei S, et al. Constraints on CD4 recovery postchemotherapy in adults: thymic insufficiency and apoptotic decline of expanded peripheral CD4 cells. *Blood* 1997;90:3789–3798.
45. Guillaume T, Rubinstein DB, Symann M. Immune reconstitution and immunotherapy after autologous hematopoietic stem cell transplantation. *Blood* 1998;92:1471–1490.
46. Wallace CA, Sherry DD. Trial of intravenous pulse cyclophosphamide and methylprednisolone in the treatment of severe systemic-onset juvenile rheumatoid arthritis. *Arthritis Rheum* 1997;40:1852–1855.
47. Reiner A, Gernsheimer T, Slichter SJ. Pulse cyclophosphamide therapy for refractory autoimmune thrombocytopenic purpura. *Blood* 1995;85:351–358.
48. Euler HH, Schroeder JO, Harten P, et al. Treatment-free remission in severe systemic lupus erythematosus following synchronization of plasmapheresis with subsequent pulse cyclophosphamide. *Arthritis Rheum* 1994;37:1784–1794.
49. Shaikov AV, Maximov AA, Speransky AI, et al. Repetitive use of pulse therapy with methylprednisolone and cyclophosphamide in addition to oral methotrexate in children with systemic juvenile rheumatoid arthritis—preliminary results of a longterm study. *J Rheumatol* 1992;19:612–616.
50. Brodsky RA, Petri M, Smith BD, et al. Immunoablative high-dose cyclophosphamide without stem-cell rescue for refractory, severe autoimmune disease. *Ann Intern Med* 1998;129:1031–1035.
51. O'Dell JR, Nepom BS, Haire C, et al. HLA-DRB1 typing in rheumatoid arthritis: predicting response to specific treatments. *Ann Rheum Dis* 1998;57:209–213.
52. Tyndall A, Gratwohl A. Blood and marrow stem cell transplants in auto-immune disease: a consensus report written on behalf of the European League against Rheumatism (EULAR) and the European Group for Blood and Marrow Transplantation (EBMT). *Bone Marrow Transplant* 1997;19:643–645.
53. Tyndall A, Passweg J, Gratwohl A. Haemopoietic stem cell transplantation in the treatment of severe autoimmune disease 2000. *Ann Rheum Dis* 2001;60:702–707.
54. Tyndall A, Koiket T. High dose immunoablative therapy with hematopoietic stem cell support in the treatment of severe autoimmune disease: current status and future direction. *Intens Med* 2002;41:608–612.
55. Farge D, Marollegu JD, Zohar S, et al. Autologous bone marrow transplantation in the treatment of refractory systemic sclerosis: early results from a French multicenter phase I-II study. *Br J Haematol* 2002;119:726–739.
56. Burt RK, Oyama Y, Traynor A, et al. Hematopoietic stem cell transplantation for systemic sclerosis with rapid improvement in skin scores: is neoangiogenesis occurring? *Bone Marrow Transplant* 2003;32(suppl):565–567.
57. Burt RK, Georganas C, Schroeder J, et al. Autologous hematopoietic stem cell transplantation in refractory rheumatoid arthritis: sustained response in two of four patients. *Arthritis Rheum* 1999;42:2281–2285.
58. Snowden JA, Biggs JC, Milliken ST, et al. A phase I/II dose escalation study of intensified cyclophosphamide and autologous blood stem cell rescue in severe, active rheumatoid arthritis. *Arthritis Rheum* 1999;42:2286–2292.
59. Moore J, Brooks P, Milliken S, et al. A pilot randomized trial comparing CD34-selected versus unmanipulated hemopoietic stem cell transplantation for severe refractory rheumatoid arthritis. *Arthritis Rheum* 2002;46:2301–2309.
60. Pincus T, Callahan LF. Taking mortality in rheumatoid arthritis seriously—predictive markers, socioeconomic status and comorbidity. *J Rheumatol* 1986;13:841–845.
61. Fries JF, Spitz P Kraines RG, et al. Measurement of patient outcome in arthritis. *Arthritis Rheum* 1980;23:137–145.
62. Ende N, Czarneski J, Raveche E. Effect of human cord blood transfer on survival and disease activity in MRL-lpr/lpr mice. *Clin Immunol Immunopathol* 1995;75:190–195.
63. Silberstein LE, Jefferies LC. Placental-blood banking—a new frontier in transfusion medicine. *N Engl J Med* 1996;335:199–201.

CHAPTER 37

Gene Therapy: Potential Applications in Arthritis

Ulf Müller-Ladner, Renate E. Gay, and Steffen Gay

About a decade ago, researchers were introducing the idea of gene transfer and gene therapy into the field of joint diseases. The challenges of gene therapy for arthritides, however, have not changed since the first experiments but technical advances such as new vector and model systems facilitated the rapid development of this young field. Because joints are difficult to target with the usual routes of application for drugs, including intravenous, intramuscular, and oral deliveries being of low efficacy, direct intraarticular application of vectors and *ex vivo* techniques, in which the target cells are transduced extraarticularly and reinjected into the joint (1), are the strategies most frequently used at present (2). During the development of gene therapy for arthritis, cytokines and cytokine inhibitors were the primary target genes (3), which paralleled the development of biologics for rheumatoid arthritis (RA). The use of animal models such as collagen-induced arthritis (CIA) also revealed that application of viral vectors into a joint showed (therapeutic) effects not only in nearby but in contralateral joints bearing the potential for a single joint-based treatment approach with systemic effects (3). Due to the increasing knowledge about cells that participate in the pathophysiologic process of arthritides, especially in RA, current target cells include synovial fibroblasts (SFs), macrophages, dendritic cells, lymphocytes, and chondrocytes (4–7). Future strategies will examine the potential of novel long-term expression vectors such as lentiviruses, the regulation (switch on/off) expression of genes, and the use of multipotent stem cells as vectors or target cells (5,8).

GOALS OF GENE THERAPY IN ARTHRITIS

For rheumatic diseases, and particularly in disabling arthritides including RA, gene therapy appears to be an attractive therapeutic strategy. On the other hand, one of the key difficulties in the design of gene therapy for such complex diseases is that the basic gene defects are not elucidated. Therefore, the approach required for gene therapy of the complex rheumatic diseases differs somewhat from the approaches developed for the treatment of mono- or oligogenetic diseases. Effective gene therapy for the treatment of the rheumatic diseases is, therefore, based on a two- or multistep approach: first, to evaluate the effects of gene transfer in cells involved in the pathogenic process of the disease, including the potential to reveal novel hitherto unknown pathways and interaction networks (9), and second, to transfer this knowledge in functional testing, including various animal and human model systems prior to application to patients suffering from the disease.

In addition, gene therapy for RA and other rheumatic diseases must address the issue that these diseases are systemic processes involving the "nonresident" immune system and frequently several target organs, of which some may show severe side effects. For example, adenoviruses are not only stable when circulating in the bloodstream, but intravenous administration of the present generation of adenovirus vectors delivers more than 90% of the virus to the liver, reducing substantially the titer of virus particles available for transduction of target cells in peripheral organs. In addition, the widespread distribution of the primary cellular receptor for adenoviruses currently precludes the targeting of disease-specific cell types and the comparison of disease-associated to nonassociated cells (10). Therefore, investigators are attempting to retarget adenovirus and to alter the normal tropism of the adenovirus vector to permit efficient targeted gene delivery to specific cell types (11,12). Another method for increasing adenovirus tropism for lymphocytes is the use of bispecific antibodies to bridge lymphocyte surface antigens to the adenovirus fiber knob (13,14). In addition, a goal of disease- or organ-specific gene therapy, such as targeting human chondrocytes in cartilage, is the ability to regulate gene expression by external "switches" that can be activated by addition or deletion of small molecule drugs or even by ultraviolet light. Using the latter, doses of up to 200 J/m^2 did not affect cell viability significantly, nor did it affect phenotypic appearance, rate of mitosis, or alteration in collagen messenger RNA (mRNA) synthesis (15).

In summary, the overall goals for a successful gene therapy of rheumatic diseases are selection of the appropriate target gene, a tissue or cell-specific delivery system, to avoid an immune response against the gene therapy vector or gene product, and the ability to regulate the gene transfer or the activation of the gene transcription by external stimuli.

TECHNIQUES AND STRATEGIES

In general, cells do not take up genes easily, which is mainly due to their size and polarity. Aside from viral vector systems that carry genes actively into the target cell, numerous nonviral strategies have been developed, including synthetic compounds, such as cationic liposomes and cationic polymers, which form a complex with DNA and fuse with the cell membrane prior to entry (16,17). A second problem is the sometimes intensive immune response to viral gene therapy vectors, especially to adenoviral vectors, which is frequently a significant limiting factor in the *in vivo* application of gene therapies (18,19). To overcome this problem, immunosuppressant drugs, anti-CD4 antibodies, and blocking costimulatory activity by cytotoxic T lymphocyte antigen-4 immunoglobulin (CTLA-4-Ig) (20–24) are used. Other strategies that specifically reduce immune reactions against adenoviruses include the pretreatment with adenovirus-infected antigen-presenting cells that express Fas ligand (25,26) and pretreatment with soluble tumor necrosis factor receptor (sTNFR) that neutralizes the large amounts of TNF-α produced by the immune system to attack the adenoviruses (27–30).

External modulation of the level of expression of gene therapy products can be achieved by the use of inducible promoters. Most of the current vector systems use a cytomegalovirus (CMV) promoter, because this viral promoter is active in a wide number of target cells to facilitate detectable transgene expression. When novel promoters are developed, at present the CMV promoter serves as the gold standard. In a recent CIA study, CMV-driven interleukin-1 receptor antagonist (IL-1Ra) synthesis resulted in high IL-1Ra levels and significant amelioration of arthritis; on the other hand, the C3-transactivator of transcription/HIV promoter (C3-Tat/HIV) showed an even better effect on inhibition of arthritis (31).

Another promoter system is the tetracycline system, which can be used as either an "on" or "off" switch system. These promoters require production of either the reverse tetracycline transactivator (rtTA) or the tetracycline transactivator (tTA), which, when activated by exogenously administered doxycycline, can bind to the tetracycline response element to induce or repress induction of the respective genes of interest (32–35). The attractive side of this system is the potential to initiate or stop the synthesis of the gene product of choice whenever needed, such as for flare-ups, given that the gene transfer itself is stable for an extended period of time (36). In a "TetON" setting, human primary SFs that were transduced with an IL-10 encoding AAV-tetON virus and injected into muscles of DBA1 mice, and application of doxycycline could sufficiently control IL-10 synthesis (37). Other studies have explored the potential of different ligands to regulate gene expression through the use of dimerizing agents to cross-link inactive domains in a chemical "two-hybrid" reaction using rapamycin-related compounds (38,39), or the insect hormone ecdysone, which, like progesterone, modifies the binding of a transcription factor to its cognate DNA sequence (40).

Adenoviruses

Replication-deficient adenoviruses are among the most widely used vector systems for gene therapy both *in vitro* and *in vivo*. The advantage of adenoviral vectors of serotypes 2 (Ad2) and 5 (Ad5), as compared with cationic liposomes and retroviral gene therapy, is mainly the high efficiency of introduction of a therapeutic gene into the target cells. This effect was used for one of the first gene therapy approaches about a decade ago, in which adenoviral vectors were used for gene transfer of β-galactosidase into synovial cells in the hind knees of New Zealand white rabbits, and efficient transduction of SFs and macrophages could be achieved for at least 8 weeks after infection (41). Of interest, adenovirus-based vectors can also be used to encode antisense gene segments as outlined below (42). After deletion of the E1 growth gene in first-generation adenoviruses developed for gene therapy, in the second generation of adenoviruses, deletion of the E2 and E4 genes was performed to achieve additional capacity for longer genes without exceeding the maximum packagable adenovirus genome length of 34 kb. In addition, the type of adenovirus may also play a significant role in efficacy of gene transfer, because neutralizing antibodies in synovial fluid from RA patients inhibited gene transfer, dependent on the type of adenovirus backbone used (43). Modification of the fiber coat proteins of the adenoviruses can also enhance efficiency of gene transfer (44).

In the third generation of adenoviruses, nearly all or all of the adenoviral genes are deleted, with the latter therefore named "gutless" (45–48), providing a maximum of 34 kb for therapeutic genes between the inverted terminal repeats (ITRs). Elimination of these sequences reduced immune reactions and expression in tissues that promote immune recognition (49). On the other hand, production of these gutless adenoviruses requires cotransduction with helper adenoviruses that carry the genes mandatory for adenoviral growth. Thus, helper adenoviruses that lack the

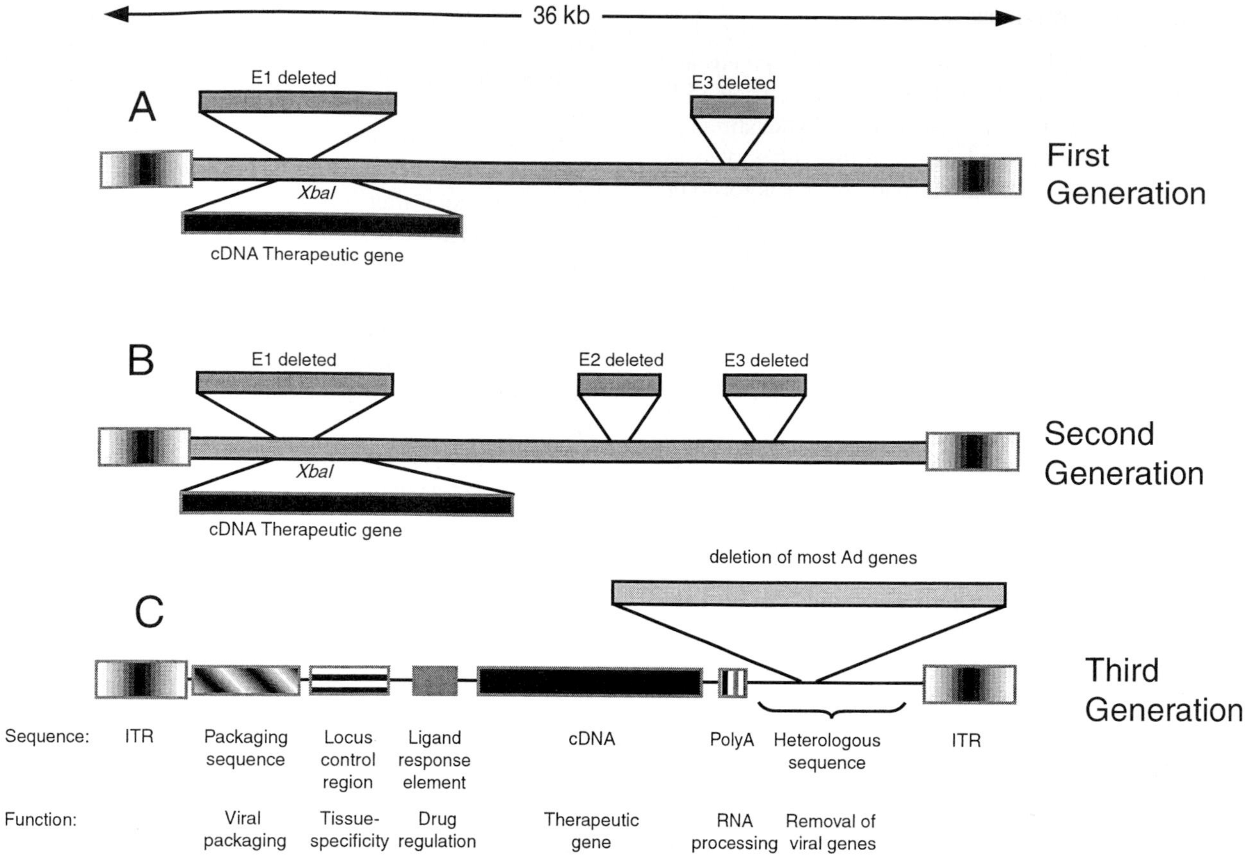

FIG. 37.1. Evolution of adenovirus gene therapy vectors using progressive deletion of adenovirus genes. **A:** The first-generation adenoviruses exhibited deletions of the E1 gene and the polylinker site. Thus, the capacity for insertion of therapeutic DNA was up to 8 kb. **B:** The second-generation adenovirus featured deletions of the E1, E3, and E4 genes. Thus, the capacity for insertion of therapeutic DNA was increased to 10 kb. **C:** The third-generation adenovirus exhibits deletion of all of the adenovirus genome and contains an adenoviral packaging sequence and inverted terminal repeats (*ITRs*). The indicated regulatory sequences are intended to confer tissue-specific, regulatable gene expression and the inability to synthesize natural viral gene products. This increases the capacity for insertion of therapeutic DNA to 34 kb and results in production of an adenovirus that is less antigenic due to deletion of the genes essential for adenovirus growth.

packaging signal need to be provided, and the absence of this signal prevents packaging of wild-type adenoviruses while facilitating packaging of the desired gene product. Figure 37.1. illustrates the evolution of adenovirus gene therapy vectors.

Adeno-Associated Viruses

An adeno-associated virus (AAV) bears a small, single-stranded genome of 4.6 kb and contains the AAV ITR and the AAV replication (*rep*) and capsid (*cap*) genes (50–52). To facilitate insertion of therapeutic genes, the *rep* and *cap* genes can be deleted and a therapeutic gene can be cloned between the AAV ITRs. AAVs also have the advantage of a low amount of foreign material introduced with the therapeutic gene. Owing to this advantage, the risk for inducing an immune response is low in combination with a gene product synthesis for up to 12 months (53). Of interest, AAV-dependent transgene expression appears to also be regulated by the local environment itself. Proinflammatory stimuli such as lipopolysaccharide (LPS) resulted in a higher and longer transgene expression in SFs than without this stimulus, and in LPS-induced arthritis in Sprague-Dawley rats, AAV-dependent IL-1Ra synthesis could even be reactivated after 3 months by a second application of LPS (54,55).

Owing to its small size, another advantage of AAV is its potential to transduce cells such as chondrocytes that are distant to the injection site or the vasculature. In cartilage organ cultures, AAVs could sufficiently transduce chondrocytes not only in the superficial layers of the cartilage but also in deeper layers (56), a property that may facilitate chondrocyte gene therapy in humans using an intraarticular injection approach. However, one of the remaining problems is to manufacture AAVs of high titer and high purity without contamination by wild-type AAVs.

Retroviruses and Lentiviruses

Retroviruses have also been developed extensively and used in a number of animal and human clinical trials (57–60). When produced as vectors, retroviruses do not stimulate synthesis of viral proteins and, because they integrate into the genome of the host cell, they provide the basis for long-term expression of the gene product of choice. Use of the retroviruses is limited, however, by the requirement for the target cell to divide to allow the virus to insert itself into the host DNA. This requirement carries with it the possibility of insertional mutagenesis. Similar to the adenovirus approaches, gene transfer using retroviruses also started about a decade ago and demonstrated that gene product (lacZ)-expressing cells were detectable in joints in bacterial cell wall–induced rat arthritis (61). One year later, using the Moloney murine leukemia virus (MMLV)-derived MFG vector, synthesis of IL-1Ra protein could be successfully achieved in joints of rabbits suffering from antigen-induced arthritis (62). Concomitant with the reduction of IL-1 in the joints, cartilage matrix metabolism and inhibition of matrix synthesis could also be down-regulated (62). Of interest, *ex vivo* gene transfer was equivalent to *in vivo* gene transfer with regard to transduction efficiency (59).

The "second generation" of retroviruses currently being investigated for treatment of arthritis are lentiviral vectors. Although the idea to be treated with an HIV-like virus most likely is not easy to understand for patients, *in vitro* and in animal models, using such constructs showed similar results as their predecessor "standard" retroviruses (63). Notably, long-term expression of gene products might also be achieved by using backbones of viruses that are known to cause remitting diseases such as herpesviruses, which was illustrated by the use of herpesviruses encoding IL-1Ra (64) or by preproenkephalin A precursor protein to inhibit arthritic symptoms in animal adjuvant arthritis (65).

Nonviral Vectors

Aside from direct injection of plasmid or naked DNA (66–69) and encapsulation of transduced cells into hollow fibers (70), the majority of nonviral vector systems are based on cationic liposomes that are designed to pass target cell membranes without the receptor mechanisms required for viral vector constructs. Because construction of liposomal carriers is easier than construction of viral vectors, numerous companies produce these systems for a variety of applications. However, due to their tumor-like properties, RA SFs are difficult to transduce with liposomal carriers, and efficacy of this transduction system still needs to be evaluated further for synovial macrophages. Commercially-available liposomes may also be used successfully to transduce chondrocytes, and have shown an efficiency of 41% for normal bovine chondrocytes, 21% for normal human chondrocytes, but only 8% for osteoarthritis chondrocytes (71).

Combination of viral vectors and liposomes increases the efficiency of gene transfer to chondrocytes without affecting the joint itself. An HVJ (hemagglutinating virus of Japan)-liposome suspension encoding for the SV40 large T antigen was injected into the knee joints of Lewis rats, and up to 30% of the cells were found to carry the SV40 antigen 3 weeks after injection (72). Double-stranded DNA can be transferred into the target cell using the HVJ-liposome technique. Using this method, nuclear factor κB (NFκB) decoy oligonucleotides could down-regulate the production of numerous molecules involved in pathophysiology of RA and particular joint destruction (73), including IL-1, IL-6, TNF-α, intracellular adhesion molecule (ICAM)-1, and collagenase-1, in RA SFs. This approach also illustrates the potential of gene transfer for proof-of-principle experiments targeting the signaling mechanisms operative in SFs (72,73).

Antisense Strategies

Although the idea to inhibit gene transcription and subsequent gene product synthesis by exposition of the target cell to antisense oligonucleotide constructs (ODN) is intriguing, only a few experimental settings have been successful. Among these, inhibition of key molecules of intracellular signaling and cellular proliferation revealed promising data. C-*myc* ODN down-regulated c-*myc* mRNA and protein expression, which resulted in the induction of apoptosis mediated by the caspase cascade (74). Similarly, c-*fos* and proliferating cell nuclear antigen ODN inhibited the stimulatory effects of IL-1 on SFs (75,76), and notch-1 ODN resulted in reduced proliferation of fibroblasts in combination with a lower response to TNF-α (77).

Proinflammatory pathways operative in human arthritis usually include the arachidonic acid–prostaglandin–cyclooxygenase cascade. Down-regulation of phospholipase A_2 and prostaglandin E_2 could be achieved by specific ODN (78). Antagonizing gene transcription of cyclooxygenase-2 following ODN by intraperitoneal injection into rats suffering from adjuvant arthritis showed amelioration of arthritic symptoms associated with lower levels of cyclooxygenase-2 (but not of cyclooxygenase-1) mRNA and protein (79).

Of interest, cartilage and matrix metabolism can also be modulated by antisense therapy. For example, treatment of injured ligaments with proteoglycan decorin antisense gene therapy resulted in larger collagen fibrils and improved mechanical parameters of the scarring process (80), and an antisense strategy against the hyaluronan receptor induced cartilage chondrolysis (81). Moreover, antisense ODN to urokinase-type plasminogen activator reduced proliferation of chondrocytes (82), and transfection with cathepsin B antisense reduced cathepsin B production by these cells by more than 75% (83).

Most intriguingly, antisense strategies were among the first to be transferred to human clinical trials. Patients with active RA were enrolled in a 6-month controlled trial and received a total of 13 anti-ICAM-1 antisense ODN infusions at a maximum of 2 mg/kg. This regimen was well tolerated and resulted in a maximum decrease of Paulus 50% criteria in 19% of the patients, although the overall efficacy was not significantly different from controls (84).

Ribozymes

Ribozymes are sequence-specific transcleaving ribozymes developed from self-cleaving RNA structures. In human T cell leukemia virus type 1 (HTLV-1)-associated arthropathy, a polyarticular arthritic disease similar to RA, hammerhead ribozymes targeted against the critical HTLV-1 *tax/rex* mRNA were used to inhibit synovial cell proliferation (85). Both *tax* mRNA expression as well as Tax protein synthesis were inhibited significantly followed by induction of apoptosis in ribozyme-treated SFs (85). Moreover, ribozymes against TNF-α showed not only an inhibitory effect on TNF-α synthesis but also on IL-6 production (86).

Ribozymes can also be designed against matrix-degrading enzymes such as stromelysin (87,88). In rabbit articular cartilage explants, ribozymes against stromelysin inhibited its expression after IL-1 stimulation but failed to protect cartilage from proteoglycan degradation (88). The cysteine proteinase cathepsin L cleaves, at least partially, collagen types I, II, IX, and XI, as well as certain proteoglycans, and is expressed by both synovial macrophages and SFs at sites of invasion into cartilage and bone. Transduction of RA SFs with cathepsin L ribozymes decreased the expression of cathepsin L mRNA up to 44%, and using an *in vitro* cartilage destruction assay, the release of sGAG decreased up to 60% (89). Table 37.1 summarizes the advantages and disadvantages of the different vector and gene transfer systems and techniques.

TABLE 37.1. *Gene transfer techniques and vectors*

	Advantage	Disadvantage
DNA-liposome	Simple No DNA size limitation Relatively low immunogenicity Versatility in conjugation to different targeting molecules Relatively safe	Low transduction inefficiency Requires preparation of large amount of highly pure DNA Requires large quantities of lipid carrier
Retrovirus	High-efficiency transduction, especially in replicating hematopoietic cells Long-term expression due to low immunogenicity plus integration into the genome Relatively large DNA fragment, up to 9 kb, can be inserted	Use restricted to dividing cells since this is required for integration and long-term expression Random integration can activate undesirable genes, such as protooncogenes Production of high titer retrovirus is limited due to necessity for a toxic replication-associated viral protein
Adenovirus	Growth characteristics and structural and nonstructural proteins are compatible with high-titer growth in cell lines Broad host range including different animals as well as humans Up to 8 kb of DNA can be inserted in E1/E3[a] deleted adenovirus Development of modified fiber holds promise for specific tropism Broad knowledge base of gene regulation provides potential for specific transgene transduction	Highly immunogenic Relatively short-term transient expression of gene
"Gutless" adenovirus	Insert up to 36 kb of DNA Low immunogenicity Long-term expression	Refinements required to produce "gutless" virus without contamination of E1 deleted helper virus Difficult to achieve high titers due to competition from helper virus
Adeno-associated virus (AAV)	Low immunogenicity Long-term expression No known pathogenic effect Broad host range Site specific integration on chromosome 19	Therapeutic gene limited in size to 4.8 kb Difficult to achieve high titer since growth requires adenovirus helper virus plus the requirement for *rep* and *cap* genes necessary for virus replication and packaging Hard to scale up growth for large quantity of viral production
Ribozymes/ Antisense	No limitation of target genes, low immunogenicity	Low-moderate efficacy, ribozymes difficult to synthesize

[a]E1/E3, deleted adenovirus is a second-generation adenovirus shown in Fig. 37.1.

APPLICATIONS AND TARGETS IN ANIMAL MODELS

Cytokines

Parallel to the wide application of cytokine inhibitors such as TNF-α and IL-1 antagonists in clinical rheumatology, numerous laboratories have evaluated the potential of overexpression of these joint-protective molecules by gene transfer. Inhibition of IL-1, which is mainly responsible for inflammation and cartilage degradation not only in RA but also in osteoarthritis, by soluble IL-1Ra (sIL-1Ra), has been among the first approaches in this emerging field (90–92). Encoded by a retrovirus, IL-1Ra was first introduced into lapine SFs in an *ex vivo* approach, and expression of gene product could be measured for up to 5 weeks (90). Rabbit knees, in which synovitis was induced by IL-1, could be protected from these proinflammatory and proliferative reactions by gene transfer of IL-1Ra (91), and in CIA, development of IL-1-triggered inflammation could be completely prevented when IL-1Ra-transduced cells were already producing IL-1Ra protein prior to IL-1 application (93). Interestingly, in bacterial cell wall arthritis, degradation of cartilage and bone could be attenuated but not completely inhibited (92), a finding that was similar in classic antigen-induced animal models as well as in the humanlike severe combined immunodeficient (SCID) mouse model for RA (94).

Notably, gene transfer into one joint sometimes showed so-called bystander effects, which in a human polyarticular setting might be desirable but is still not yet completely understood. The onset of CIA in "draining" ipsilateral joints in IL-1Ra retroviral gene transfer (93) could be ameliorated and disease activity of contralateral antigen-induced arthritis in IL-1Ra adenoviral-treated murine knee joints could be also attenuated (95). Current hypotheses to explain these bystander effects include transfer of mononuclear cells, dendritic cells, or parts of cells via the bloodstream (96).

In addition to RA, osteoarthritis (OA) has also been targeted using IL-1Ra gene transfer. *Ex vivo* gene transfer with IL-1Ra resulted in a marked reduction of lesions in experimental dog OA (58) and ameliorated various aspects of articular destruction in a rabbit OA model (57). The size of the joint does not appear to be a major limitation for this approach, because horses suffering from induced OA did show preservation of cartilage and overall mobility following adenoviral IL-1Ra gene transfer (97).

In contrast to the limited success of drug application of IL-4 to patients with different chronic inflammatory diseases, a large amount of data is addressing the effects of IL-4 in different forms of arthritis models. AAV-dependent gene therapy of CIA delayed the onset of arthritis and diminished the prevalence and intensity of the disease, and elevated IL-4 levels in murine serum could be measured from more than 4 months (98) up to more than 7 months (99). Independently from the type of gene transfer used, the beneficial influence of IL-4 is not limited to early CIA. Established CIA can also be efficiently ameliorated by overexpression of IL-4 (100–102), an effect that can be further optimized by gene transfer of the proapoptotic Fas ligand (103). Most interestingly, IL-4 gene therapy also significantly alters the destructive processes in arthritis models. Chondrocyte apoptosis and cartilage degradation could be inhibited by Ad5 IL-4 gene transduction into mice with CIA followed by reduction of cartilage breakdown and matrix metalloproteinase (MMP) synthesis, although some inflammatory reactions persisted (104). Similar beneficial effects could be observed with regard to inhibition of osteoclast formation, osteoprotegerin ligand synthesis, bone destruction (105), and vascularization (106). On the other hand, overexpression of IL-4 and its specific receptors revealed distinct molecular mechanisms modulated by this "antiinflammatory" helper T cell subset 2 (T_H2) cytokine, which challenge its "protective" role in inflammation (107).

Another key cytokine with inhibitory properties is IL-10. It is a pluripotent molecule that down-regulates proinflammatory cytokines such as IL-1, IL-2, IL-6, TNF-α, and interferon-γ, and is regarded as a potential therapeutic agent in inflammatory and allergic diseases. In murine CIA, even single administration of adenoviral gene transfer can inhibit the disease for an extended period of time (108), and CMV-based IL-10 gene transfer resulted in long-term down-regulation of proinflammatory T_H1 immune responses (109). Similar to IL-4, plasmid-encoded IL-10 gene transfer with macrophages as the target cells was also able to inhibit established CIA (110). At this point it needs to be stressed that animal models may reflect only part of the pathogenesis in RA. Here is an interesting example: although the transfer of IL-10 has been promising in the treatment of experimental arthritides, the application of IL-10 to patients with RA was not favorable. Other cytokines that were targeted by gene therapy were IL-12, showing modulation of the chemokine pattern in murine CIA (111), and IL-13, which was revealed to be a master switch for inflammation, chemokine production, vascularization, and severity of rat adjuvant arthritis (112).

One of the "dominant" proinflammatory cytokines on which research efforts are currently focused is TNF-α. TNF-α has properties similar to IL-1 and is produced by RA synovial macrophages, lymphocytes, endothelial cells, and some fibroblasts. TNF-α is arthritogenic in animals and contributes together with IL-1 to inflammatory pathways in human RA, partly by inducing IL-1 production. Other cytokines can modulate TNF-α expression, an effect that was also seen following gene transfer of interferon-β into immortalized fibroblasts in the CIA model (113). By analogy to IL-1, the natural antagonist of TNF-α is its shed soluble receptor, which is also present in RA synovium and maintains homeostasis by neutralizing the effects of TNF-α even under inflammatory conditions. Similar to the effects seen in human trials using etanercept, retroviral gene transfer of TNF receptor into splenocytes was able to inhibit arthritis in SCID mice (114), and AAV-based gene transfer of soluble TNF receptor into SFs could antagonize the proinflammatory stimulation with TNF-α (115). Of interest, presumably due to its pleiotropic nature, interference with TNF-dependent pathways can also result in unexpected effects. Intraarticular gene transfer of 55-KD TNF receptor type 1 was limited by an adenoviral synovitis that was resistant to TNF receptor overexpression (116), and an increased antibody response to collagen type II and TNF receptor itself can substantially antagonize the beneficial effects in CIA (117).

Signaling

Aberrant inter- and intracellular signaling belongs to the key pathophysiologic mechanisms in the development and perpetuation of arthritides, and numerous therapies target the interaction between cells or intracellular activation mechanisms. In this field, induction of apoptosis by adenovirus-based overexpression of Fas ligand in CIA belongs to the prototype models of gene therapy (118). Similar to current clinical trials, adenovirus-based inhibition of the interaction between antigen-presenting cells and lymphocytes by overexpression of the soluble CTLA-4Ig fusion protein were able to suppress established CIA, and secondary inflammatory parameters, such as anticollagen antibodies and interferon-γ production, were also found to be down-regulated (119). The effect of gene therapy was comparable with exogenous recombinant CTLA-4Ig, and this inhibitory effect lasted for up to 20 weeks (120); comparable long-term effects were required for successful gene transfer of transforming growth factor-β (TGF-β) to induce cartilage growth or to stimulate cartilage regeneration in orthopedic cartilage defect animal models (121).

Molecular research techniques in combination with different animal models have also revealed numerous novel aspects with regard to intra- and transcellular signaling and mechanisms of gene transcription. Transcription factors such as NFκB are activated by extracellular signals or cell/cell interactions that are converted into intracellular activation signals via receptor molecules located in the cell membrane. Activated transcription factors bind subsequently to their respective regulatory gene segments located mostly in the promoter region of their target genes and initiate or terminate gene transcription. Although used frequently in this context, NFκB is not an isolated transcription factor but the predominant member of a large family of dimeric transcription factors. NFκB is located in the cytoplasm and in quiescent cells, and a specific inhibitor (IκB) prevents the translocation of NFκB to the nucleus. Intraarticular injection of adenovirus-encoded inhibitor of NFκB kinase β (IKKβ) into normal Lewis rats resulted in initiation of arthritis, which not only indicated successful gene transfer but also proof of principle of the relevance of this signaling pathway for the development of arthritis in this model (122). Similar results were achieved when NFκB decoy oligonucleotides were used in an HVJ-liposome setting, which demonstrated that IL-1 and TNF-α production are also dependent on NFκB activity (123).

Inhibition of cellular growth is among the feasible targets for gene therapy of intracellular signaling pathways. The expression of cyclin-dependent kinase inhibitor p21(Cip1) is associated with growth-retardation of SFs *in vitro*, and in adjuvant arthritis, overexpression of this cell cyle inhibitor resulted in marked reduction of synovial proliferation and arthritis (124). Moreover, periarticular injection of adenovirus-encoded endogenous cytokine signaling repressor CIS3/SOCS3 also reduced the severity of CIA, potentially due to the inhibition of the IL-6-gp130-JAK-STAT3 signaling pathway (125).

Angiogenesis

To facilitate synovial activation and synovial inflammation, neoangiogenesis and long-term vascular proliferation are among the essential prerequisites for this process. Proangiogenic and proinflammatory stimuli and growth factors, including TNF-α, vascular endothelial cell growth factor (VEGF), their respective receptors fetal liver kinase-1 (flk-1) and fms-like tyrosine kinase (flt-1), and hypoxia-inducible factor-1α (HIF-1α) (126), contribute significantly to these mechanisms. Reduction of density of synovial vasculature, therefore, appears as an attractive goal for future gene therapeutic strategies. When mice suffering from CIA were challenged with a phage expressing RGD-containing cyclic peptide (RGD-4C) that binds to $\alpha_v\beta_3$ and $\alpha_v\beta_5$ vascular integrins, apoptosis of synovial vessels could be induced and subsequent inhibition of arthritis could be demonstrated (127).

Direct inhibition of vascular proliferation was achieved by lentiviral-based overexpression of the antiangiogenic factor endostatin in TNF-transgenic mice, which appeared to be predominantly due to the inhibition of janus kinase (JNK) (128). In CIA, retroviral gene transfer resulted in inhibition of pannus formation and cartilage erosion by overexpression of angiostatin (129). Because angiostatin has been proposed to be a useful inhibitor of angiogenesis in tumors driving metastasis in an inactive state, continuous delivery of this angiostatic molecule might be able to reduce synovial hyperplasia in human RA.

Similar to the strategy used in mouse testis, inhibition of VEGF-mediated angiogenesis in human arthritis might be achieved by antisense oligonucleotides targeting the VEGF receptors flk-1 and flt-1 (130). Interestingly, linking of inhibitory molecules, such as methotrexate to human serum albumin (HSA) (131), can be used to enhance antiangiogenic gene therapy. Adenoviral vectors encoding for urokinase plasminogen antagonist molecules fused to HSA could prolong the effect of urokinase plasminogen antagonist molecules–dependent inhibition of angiogenesis in CIA (132).

Adoptive Gene Transfer

The ability of T cells to migrate and accumulate at sites of inflammation, in general, and in arthritic joints, in particular, supports the idea that, aside from their common role as proinflammatory cells, they could serve as "intelligent" vectors for a targeted delivery of therapeutic gene products

(133–135). To test this idea, targeted adoptive cellular gene therapy, which combines retroviral transduction of target cells *ex vivo* and subsequent adoptive transfer of these cells into recipient animals by intravenous application, has been developed (136,137). Moreover, it has become clear that not only T cells can be used for the purpose of targeted adoptive cellular gene therapy, but also bone marrow-derived dendritic cells (DCs) (138,139), which also show a specific homing pattern (140). Efficient use of T cells and DCs as cellular vehicles for adoptive cellular gene therapy has been facilitated by the development of an MMLV-based bicistronic retroviral vector construct, termed pGCy, that allows for up to 60% transduction efficiency in T cells (134). An internal ribosome entry site enables the proportional expression of the gene of interest, and its YFP fluorescence can be used to analyze transduction efficiency and to sort successfully transduced cells by fluorescence-activated cell sorting. The construct has been examined when expressing several immune-modulating cytokines and cytokine inhibitors, including the IL-12 receptor antagonist IL-12p40, the T_H2 cytokine IL-4, and an anti-TNF scFv (antibody variable fragment single chain construct), and was tested in CIA with all three variants being capable to prevent CIA but not to ameliorate established disease (141–143).

Another variant of the retroviral vector described above encoding a firefly luciferase-GFP fusion protein was used for *in vivo* real-time bioluminescence imaging. This imaging technique illustrates the homing behavior of the vehicle cells *in vivo* by consecutive imaging of the same mice over a time period of several weeks after adoptive cell transfer. During the conversion of luciferin to oxyluciferin, which is catalyzed by luciferase released from the transferred cells, photons are emitted that penetrate the tissues and can be detected by a sensitive charge-coupled device camera. Representation of light signal intensity on a false color scale superimposed onto a gray scale body picture of the mice gives an image of the location of the transferred cells within the bodies of the mice (140,142,143).

The potential of this technique demonstrated that genetically-engineered T-cell hybridomas, primary T cells, and DCs can home to inflamed joints (143) and also demonstrated that YFP marker mRNA can be found in clinically uninflamed paws as early as 3 days after adoptive cell transfer and in inflamed joints as late as 55 days after transfer. Furthermore, the results showed that the initial homing of T-cell hybridomas to inflamed joints was independent of T-cell receptor (TCR) specificity, whereas the persistence of cells in the joints was not antigen dependent but chemokine mediated (142).

Matrix Metalloproteinases

Although belonging to the major theoretical approaches of joint protection, specifically targeting overexpression of inhibitors of MMPs by gene transfer is not presently reflected by an equivalent amount of experimental data. On the other hand, application of human tissue inhibitor of metalloproteinases-4 (TIMP-4) naked DNA by electroporation resulted in high TIMP-4 levels and significant amelioration of adjuvant arthritis (144). Of interest, the experiments also revealed some MMP-inhibitor-cytokine feedback loops, because TNFα and IL-1 were also down-regulated by TIMP-4 gene transfer (144). In murine gene therapy tumor models, TIMP-3 demonstrated to have anti-angiogenic and proapoptotic effects and could, therefore, also be used in the treatment of arthritis (145). On the other hand, disappointing results—at least with regard to inhibition of overall arthritic symptoms, sometimes even showing worsening of inflammation [e.g., following gene transfer of TIMP-1 (146)]—may have reduced the number of published data considerably. However, the most promising results were obtained by transferring TIMP-1 and TIMP-3 into SFs.

Ex Vivo Gene Transfer

One of the primary goals in the treatment of human RA is the inhibition of synovial activation and of joint destruction. Because SFs are one of the driving forces in this tissue, especially at the sites of invasion into the adjacent cartilage, various gene therapy strategies have been developed to interfere with long-term activation of rheumatoid SFs and to induce apoptosis in these cells. As outlined above, NFκB is one of the mediators for cellular activation, and inhibition of this nuclear transcription factor by adenoviral overexpression of its natural inhibitor IκB resulted in increased apoptosis of rheumatoid SFs. Interestingly, sole gene transfer was not effective, and TNF-α was required to initiate this process (147).

Inhibition of the cell cycle is another option for inhibition of uncontrolled cellular proliferation. Overexpression of the p16INK4a senescence gene not only could block efficiently synovial proliferation, but this mechanism appeared to be rather specific for RA (148). On the other hand, it is of interest that p16 appears induced at sites of cartilage invasion in the SCID mouse model of RA (149). Intracellular signaling kinases that are operative in human SFs or in other cells involved in joint destruction are also attractive targets for gene therapy approaches. Among them are *src* family tyrosine kinases that are involved in numerous intracellular signaling pathways in fibroblasts and osteoclasts. Adenovirus-mediated overexpression of the *csk* gene, which inhibits *src* kinases, not only reduced activity of *src* and slowed the growth rate of the fibroblasts, but it also showed an effect on proinflammatory IL-6 synthesis and on bone-resorbing activity of osteoclasts (150). Jun D is an antagonist of intracellular signaling protooncogene Ras-mediated RA SF transformation. Overexpression of jun D in RA SFs by transient transfection inhibited RA SF proliferation and down-regulated activator protein-1 (AP-1), thereby inhibiting the expression of cytokines IL-6 and IL-8 and of matrix-degrading MMPs (151).

Gene transfer to human synovial cells can be used to modulate the synthesis of proinflammatory molecules. Because IL-4 down-regulates a number of human cytokines similar to the situation in the animal models as outlined above, adenoviral vectors were used to overexpress IL-4 in human tissue and fibroblasts (152). Expression of the chemotactic cytokine IL-8 and the chemoattractant MCP-1 was reduced up to 60% and 88%, respectively, and a down-regulation of the synthesis of IL-1, TNF-α, and prostaglandin E_2 could also be found (152). Similarly, overexpression of inhibitory IL-13 following adenoviral gene transfer reduced IL-1 and TNF-α production by more than 80% (153).

Because the relative deficiency of IL-1Ra in comparison with IL-1 in the rheumatoid synovium contributes significantly to articular destruction (154), overexpression of this cartilage-protective molecule is most attractive for future *in vivo* human applications. Adenoviral gene transfer of IL-1Ra into SFs resulted in protection against IL-1-dependent production of proinflammatory mediators, such as IL-6, prostaglandin E_2, and nitric oxide. Successful gene transfer of protective cytokines, however, is not limited to SFs. Human chondrocytes transduced with the biologically-active IL-1Ra were resistant to IL-1-stimulated proteoglycan degradation and showed a down-regulation of nitric oxide and prostaglandin E_2 in cartilage culture (6,155).

The SCID Mouse Model

The SCID mouse model of RA was developed to simulate various aspects of a human joint (156) and offers the unique possibility of investigating human articular tissue under controlled conditions *in vivo*. In this model, complete human synovium or human SFs that have been obtained from RA, OA, and normal synovium by passaging *in vitro* are inserted into an inert gel sponge and coimplanted with a small block of fresh human cartilage under the kidney capsule or under the skin of SCID mice. Because the SCID mice cannot reject the implants, it is possible to study the interaction of synovial cells and the subsequent cartilage destruction in the absence of human inflammatory cells or associated factors (156–158), both as proof of principle as well as simulation of a preclinical gene therapy approach. This includes other approaches, such as the transfer of xenogeneic arthritis-inducing cells to study the effect of cytokines and growth factors (159). Figure 37.2 illustrates the potential of this model.

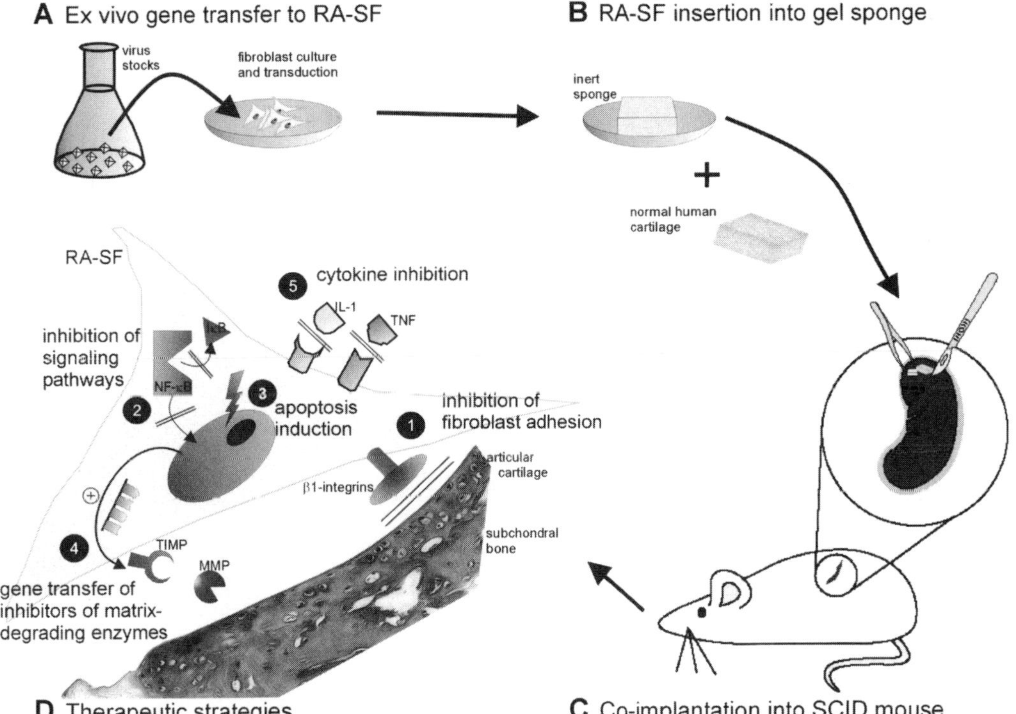

FIG. 37.2. The severe combined immunodeficiency (SCID) mouse model of rheumatoid arthritis (*RA*). **A:** Human synovial fibroblasts (*SF*) are isolated from RA, osteoarthritis (*OA*), and normal joint tissue specimens, purified by passaging *in vitro,* and transduced with retroviral or adenoviral constructs. **B:** Transduced fibroblasts are inserted into an inert gel sponge. **C:** The sponge and a small block of fresh normal human cartilage are coimplanted under the kidney capsule of SCID mice that do not reject the implants and, thus, allow undisturbed fibroblast/cartilage interaction in the absence of other components of the immune system. **D:** Currently, five strategies are used to antagonize the invasive and destructive behavior of RA SFs as shown in this figure: *1,* interference with RA SF adhesion to cartilage; *2,* inhibition of specific signaling pathways that are associated with the activation and destructive capacity of RA SF; *3,* induction of apoptosis to antagonize the RA SFs' extended lifespan; *4,* inactivation of matrix-degrading enzymes; and *5,* modulation of cytokine effects.

Targeting of cytokines was investigated as the first strategy in the SCID mouse model. Retroviral gene transfer of IL-1Ra and the binding soluble TNFp55 receptor into RA SFs were found to have little effect on RA SF invasiveness (94,160). In contrast, IL-1Ra gene transfer was highly chondroprotective, resulting in substantially less chondrocyte-mediated cartilage degradation. *In vitro* models of cartilage degradation showed that the intrinsic invasiveness of RA SFs is enhanced when exogenous IL-1 and TNF are added (161).

IL-10, which is known to have antiinflammatory properties, among other effects, and inhibits the production of IL-1 and TNF by synovial mononuclear cells (162), was also tested in the SCID mouse model. Retroviral transduction of RA SFs with murine and viral IL-10 significantly reduced cartilage invasion, while perichondrocytic cartilage degradation was not affected (160). Most intriguingly, complete inhibition of both cartilage invasion and perichondrocytic cartilage degradation by RA SFs could be observed when double gene transfer of IL-1Ra and IL-10 to RA SFs was performed (163). Figure 37.3 illustrates these effects. Moreover, molecular analysis revealed not only that the protective effects of this combination gene transfer were based on up-regulation of activin, but also revealed numerous links to pathways operative in the pathogenesis of RA (163).

Retroviral gene transfer of a dominant negative (dn) mutation variant of c-*raf* into RA SFs also resulted in reduced cartilage invasion. Of note, this blockade of the Ras-Raf-MAPK pathway by dn-c-*raf* did not abolish growth or induce apoptosis of RA SFs and, therefore, most likely is not sufficient to control the destructive capacity of RA SFs. However, when the cells were cotransfected with both dn-*raf* and dn-*myc*, the SFs became rapidly apoptotic (164). In another effort to enhance a physiologic joint-protective mechanism, tissue inhibitors of MMPs TIMP-1 and TIMP-3 were overexpressed in RA-SF by means of adenoviral gene transfer. Coimplantation of these cells with human cartilage into SCID mice led to a complete inhibition of cartilage destruction (165). Because TIMP-3 is also initiating the activation of TNF-α by TNF-α converting enzyme (TACE), the transfer of TIMP-3 to the rheumatoid synovium might inhibit both destruction and inflammation. Moreover, in an attempt to block the the plasminogen activator system, known to degrade different extracellular matrix components and to activate latent MMPs (166), adenoviral gene transfer of a cell surface–targeted plasmin inhibitor into RA SFs in the SCID mouse model resulted in a significant reduction of cartilage invasion (167). However, it was most notable that the inhibition of invasion of cartilage in the *in vivo* SCID mouse model was less significant than the inhibition of invasion in an *in vitro* model, indicating that *in vitro* models appear more limited for these studies than *in vivo* settings.

Based on the fact that local application of apoptosis-inducing anti-Fas (anti-CD95) antibodies can induce apoptosis in rheumatoid synovium, cells were transduced with the human Fas-ligand gene and applied to human synovium engrafted into SCID mice. The Fas ligand–transduced cells were able to induce apoptosis of synoviocytes and of mononuclear cells, illustrating the potential of gene therapy–based reduction of synovial growth (168). Fas-associated death domain protein (FADD), on the other hand, is one of the key mediators of apoptosis in synovial cells, and adenoviral FADD gene transfer into rheumatoid SFs resulted not only in apoptosis in cultured cells, but also increased apoptosis in synovium implanted into SCID mice (169). Interestingly, apoptosis was restricted to synovial cells and did not occur in chondrocytes.

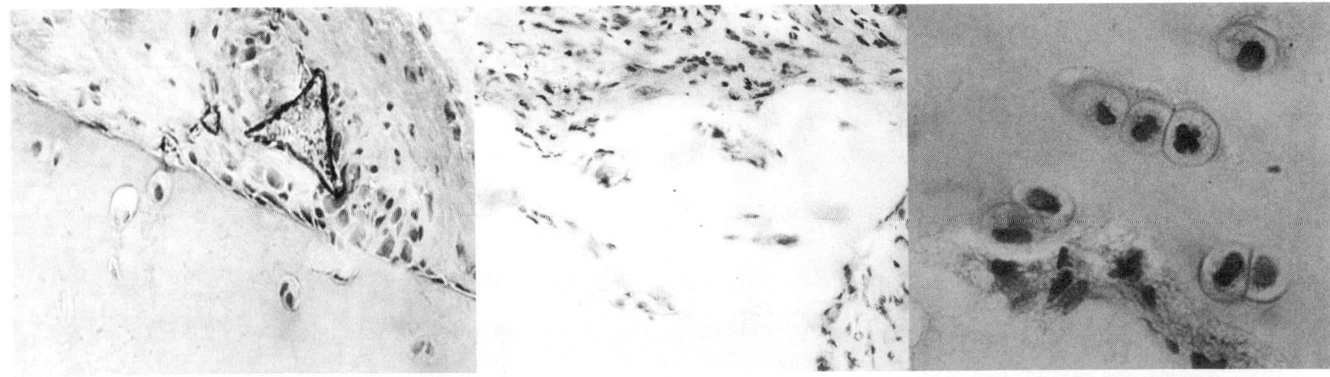

FIG. 37.3. Single and double retrovirus-based gene transfer of joint-protective molecules reveals different aspects of inhibition of cartilage degradation mediated by activated rheumatoid arthritis (RA) synovial fibroblasts (see Fig. 37.2.). **Left:** Overexpression of interleukin-1 receptor antagonist (IL-1ra) results in inhibition of perichondrocytic cartilage degradation but does not affect invasivity of RA synovial fibroblasts. **Middle:** Overexpression of IL-10 inhibits invasivity of the fibroblasts but leaves perichondrocytic cartilage degradation unaffected. **Right:** Double gene transfer of IL-1ra and IL-10 results in nearly complete inhibition of RA synovial fibroblast–driven cartilage destruction.

Human Gene Therapy

Because nature does not provide animal models that resemble human RA *in toto*, most animal models for RA facilitate only the evaluation of certain aspects of gene transfer approaches. Although successfully completed, this shortcoming includes gene therapy of transferred CIA arthritis into SCID mice (170) and gene therapy–dependent primate synovectomies by overexpression of herpes simplex virus thymidine kinase in combination with ganciclovir (171). On the other hand, the first human trials of gene therapy for RA were pioneered by Christopher Evans and Paul Robbins at the University of Pittsburgh in 1996 (172). These trials used a human IL-1Ra complementary DNA (cDNA) cloned into a retroviral vector, a derivative of MMLV. IL-1Ra was selected on the basis of its outstanding safety profile, its relevant biologic activity, its property as a naturally-occurring inhibitor of the biologic actions of IL-1, and the finding that recombinant protein can be administered at high doses without evidence of toxicity or adverse effects. The goals of these first human trials were designed to answer several questions, including (a) whether *ex vivo* transfer of human IL-1Ra gene into inflamed joints in humans would be successful and whether the transferred gene would be expressed intraarticularly in human joints; (b) whether a local biologic response to the transferred gene products occurs in the human joint; and (c) whether the procedure would be safe, feasible, and well tolerated. These first trials were performed by injection of metacarpophalangeal (MCP) joints that were removed shortly after intraarticular administration during the course of MTP joint replacement. This first clinical trial successfully demonstrated the feasibility of intraarticular gene transfer resulting in expression of a potentially therapeutic gene product, and subsequent clinical trials are planned or underway.

CONCLUSION

The intriguing variety of pathogenic pathways operative in RA as well as in other arthritides, which include activated T-cells, chemokines, proinflammatory cytokines, activated RA SFs, inter- and intracellular signaling pathways, and matrix-degrading enzymes, results in numerous challenges for the development of human gene therapy in these disease entities. Because no specific gene defect or "master switch" has been discovered so far, the complexity of the pathobiology may require an integrated approach targeting at least two pathways with avoiding major side effects. Therefore, elucidation and molecular analysis of *in vitro* and *in vivo* gene transfer experiments will be mandatory to be able to interfere with critical steps of the disease-specific pathways at distinct time points along the progression of the disease before a true gene therapy for the treatment of RA or OA might be approved. At present, we should consider gene transfer approaches to understand the functional relevance of key molecules in the destructive inflammatory process. In this regard, gene transfer experiments will not only help us to elucidate the functional role of novel gene sequences and molecules by analysis of the disease-specific mRNA/cDNA by applying a true "functional genomics" approach (173), but also to support the development of novel therapeutic targets.

ACKNOWLEDGMENTS

The work has been supported by the German Research Society (DFG No. Mu 1383/1–3 and 3–4) and the Swiss National Science Foundation (SNF 3200–64142.00).

REFERENCES

1. Bandara G, Robbins PD, Georgescu HI, et al. Gene transfer to synoviocytes: prospects for gene treatment of arthritis. *DNA Cell Biol* 1992;11:227–231.
2. Trucco M, Robbins PD, Thomson AW, et al. Gene therapy strategies to prevent autoimmune disorders. *Curr Gene Ther* 2002;2:341–354.
3. Van de Loo FA, van den Berg WB. Gene therapy for rheumatoid arthritis. Lessons from animal models, including studies on interleukin-4, interleukin-10, and interleukin-1 receptor antagonist as potential disease modulators. *Rheum Dis Clin North Am* 2002;28:127–149.
4. Bessis N, Doucet C, Cottard V, et al. Gene therapy for rheumatoid arthritis. *J Gene Med* 2002;4:581–591.
5. Pap T, Gay RE, Müller-Ladner U, et al. *Ex vivo* gene transfer in the years to come. *Arthritis Res* 2002;4:10–12.
6. Baragi VM, Renkiewicz RR, Jordan H, et al. Transplantation of transduced chondrocytes protects articular cartilage from interleukin 1-induced extracellular matrix degradation. *J Clin Invest* 1995;96: 2454–2460.
7. Doherty PJ, Zhang H, Manolopoulos V, et al. Adhesion of transplanted chondrocytes onto cartilage *in vitro* and *in vivo*. *J Rheumatol* 2000;27: 1725–1731.
8. Noel D, Djouad F, Jorgensen C. Regenerative medicine through mesenchymal stem cells for bone and cartilage repair. *Curr Opin Invest Drugs* 2002;3:1000–1004.
9. Neumann E, Kullmann F, Judex M, et al. Identification of differentially expressed genes in rheumatoid arthritis by a combination of cDNA array and RAP-PCR. *Arthritis Rheum* 2002;46:52–63.
10. Day CS, Kasemkijwattana C, Menetrey J, et al. Myoblast-mediated gene transfer to the joint. *J Orthop Res* 1997;15:894–903.
11. Bergelson JM, Cunningham JA, Droguett G, et al. Isolation of a common receptor for coxsackie B viruses and adenoviruses 2 and 5. *Science* 1997;275:1320–1323.
12. Wang X, Bergelson JM. Coxsackievirus and adenovirus receptor cytoplasmic and transmembrane domains are not essential for coxsackievirus and adenovirus infection. *J Virol* 1999;73:2559–2562.
13. Rogers BE, Douglas JT, Ahlem C, et al. Use of a novel cross-linking method to modify adenovirus tropism. *Gene Ther* 1997;4:1387–1392.
14. Wickham TJ, Segal DM, Roelvink PW, et al. Targeted adenovirus gene transfer to endothelial and smooth muscle cells by using bispecific antibodies. *J Virol* 1996;70:6831–6838.
15. Ulrich-Vinther M, Maloney MD, Goater JJ, et al. Light-activated gene transduction enhances adeno-associated virus vector mediated gene expression in human articular chondrocytes. *Arthritis Rheum* 2002;46: 2095–2104.
16. Zhang Y, Sekirov L, Saravolac E, et al. Stabilized plasmid-lipid particles for regional gene therapy: formulation and transfection properties. *Gene Ther* 1999;6:1438–1447.
17. Alton EW, Stern M, Farley R, et al. Cationic lipid-mediated CFTR gene transfer to the lungs and nose of patients with cystic fibrosis: a double-blind placebo-controlled trial. *Lancet* 1999;353:947–954.
18. Tripathy SK, Black HB, Goldwasser E, et al. Immune responses to transgene-encoded proteins limit the stability of gene expression after

injection of replication-defective adenovirus vectors. *Nat Med* 1996;2: 545–550.
19. van Ginkel FW, McGhee JR, Liu C, et al. Adenoviral gene delivery elicits distinct pulmonary-associated T helper cell responses to the vector and to its transgene. *J Immunol* 1997;159:685–693.
20. Vilquin JT, Guerette B, Kinoshita I, et al. FK506 immunosuppression to control the immune reactions triggered by first-generation adenovirus-mediated gene transfer. *Hum Gene Ther* 1995;6:1391–1401.
21. Kolls JK, Lei D, Odom G, et al. Use of transient CD4 lymphocyte depletion to prolong transgene expression of E1-deleted adenoviral vectors. *Hum Gene Ther* 1996;7:489–497.
22. Guerette B, Vilquin JT, Gingras M, et al. Prevention of immune reactions triggered by first-generation adenoviral vectors by monoclonal antibodies and CTLA4Ig. *Hum Gene Ther* 1996;7:1455–1463.
23. Schowalter DB, Meuse L, Wilson CB, et al. Constitutive expression of murine CTLA4Ig from a recombinant adenovirus vector results in prolonged transgene expression. *Gene Ther* 1997;4:853–860.
24. Sawchuk SJ, Boivin GP, Duwel LE, et al. Anti-T cell receptor monoclonal antibody prolongs transgene expression following adenovirus-mediated *in vivo* gene transfer to mouse synovium. *Hum Gene Ther* 1996;7:499–506.
25. Zhang HG, Bilbao G, Zhou T, et al. Fas ligand encoding a recombinant adenovirus vector for prolongation of transgene expression. *J Virol* 1998;72:2483–2490.
26. Zhang HG, Su X, Liu D, et al. Induction of specific T cell tolerance by Fas ligand-expressing antigen-presenting cells. *J Immunol* 1999;162: 1423–1430.
27. Kolls J, Peppel K, Silva M, et al. Prolonged and effective blockade of tumor necrosis factor activity through adenovirus-mediated gene transfer. *Proc Natl Acad Sci U S A* 1994;91:215–219.
28. Elkon KB, Liu CC, Gall JG, et al. Tumor necrosis factor alpha plays a central role in immune-mediated clearance of adenoviral vectors. *Proc Natl Acad Sci U S A* 1997;94:9814–9819.
29. Worgall S, Wolff G, Falck-Pedersen E, et al. Innate immune mechanisms dominate elimination of adenoviral vectors following *in vivo* administration. *Hum Gene Ther* 1997;8:37–44.
30. Zhang HG, Zhou T, Yang P, et al. Inhibition of tumor necrosis factor alpha decreases inflammation and prolongs adenovirus gene expression in lung and liver. *Hum Gene Ther* 1998;9:1875–1884.
31. Bakker AC, van de Loo FA, Joosten LA, et al. C3-Tat/HIV-regulated intraarticular human interleukin-1 receptor antagonist gene therapy results in efficient inhibition of collagen-induced arthritis superior to cytomegalovirus-regulated expression of the same transgene. *Arthritis Rheum* 2002;46:1661–1670.
32. Watusji T, Okamoto Y, Emi N, et al. Controlled gene expression with a reverse tetracycline-regulated retroviral vector (RTRV) system. *Biophys Res Commun* 1997;234:769–773.
33. Harding TC, Geddes BJ, Murphy D, et al. Switching transgene expression in the brain using an adenoviral tetracycline-regulatable system. *Nat Biotechnol* 1998;16:553–555.
34. Berens C, Schnappinger D, Hillen W. The role of the variable region in Tet repressor for inducibility by tetracycline. *J Biol Chem* 1997; 272:6936–6942.
35. Gossen M, Freundlieb S, Bender G, et al. Transcriptional activation by tetracyclines in mammalian cells. *Science* 1995;268:1766–1769.
36. Gould DJ, Berenstein M, Dreja H, et al. A novel doxycycline inducible autoregulatory plasmid which displays "on"/"off" regulation suited to gene therapy applications. *Gene Ther* 2000;7:2061–2070.
37. Apparailly F, Millet V, Noel D, et al. Tetracycline-inducible interleukin-10 gene transfer mediated by an adeno-associated virus:application to experimental arthritis. *Hum Gene Ther* 2002;13:1179–1188.
38. Ho SN, Biggar SR, Spencer DM, et al. Dimeric ligands define a role for transcriptional activation domains in reinitiation. *Nature* 1996; 382:822–826.
39. Rivera VM, Clackson T, Natesan S, et al. A humanized system for pharmacologic control of gene expression. *Nat Med* 1996;2:1028–1032.
40. No D, Yao TP, Evans RM. Ecdysone-inducible gene expression in mammalian cells and transgenic mice. *Proc Natl Acad Sci U S A* 1996;93:3346–3351.
41. Roessler BJ, Allen ED, Wilson JM, et al. Adenoviral-mediated gene transfer to rabbit synovium *in vivo*. *J Clin Invest* 1993;92:1085–1092.
42. Sidiropoulos P, Liu H, Mungre S, et al. Efficacy of adenoviral TNFα antisense is enhanced by macrophage specific promoter. *Gene Ther* 2001;8:223–231.
43. Goossens PH, Vogels R, Pieterman E, et al. The influence of synovial fluid on adenovirus-mediated gene transfer to the synovial tissue. *Arthritis Rheum* 2001;44:48–52.
44. Perlman H, Liu H, Georganas C, et al. Modifications in adenoviral coat fiber proteins and transcriptional regulatory sequences enhance transgene expression. *J Rheumatol* 2002;29:1593–1600.
45. Lieber A, He CY, Kirillova I, et al. Recombinant adenoviruses with large deletions generated by Cre-mediated excision exhibit different biological properties compared with first-generation vectors *in vitro* and *in vivo*. *J Virol* 1996;70:8944–8960.
46. Chen HH, Mack LM, Kelly R, et al. Persistence in muscle of an adenoviral vector that lacks all viral genes. *Proc Natl Acad Sci U S A* 1997; 94:1645–1650.
47. Clemens PR, Kochanek S, Sunada Y, et al. *In vivo* muscle gene transfer of full-length dystrophin with an adenoviral vector that lacks all viral genes. *Gene Ther* 1996;3:965–972.
48. Kochanek S, Clemens PR, Mitani K, et al. A new adenoviral vector: replacement of all viral coding sequences with 28 kb of DNA independently expressing both full-length dystrophin and beta-galactosidase. *Proc Natl Acad Sci U S A* 1996;93:5731–5736.
49. Nabel GJ. Development of optimized vectors for gene therapy. *Proc Natl Acad Sci U S A* 1999;96:324–326.
50. Fisher KJ, Jooss K, Alston J, et al. Recombinant adeno-associated virus for muscle directed gene therapy. *Nat Med* 1997;3:306–312.
51. Vincent KA, Piraino ST, Wadsworth SC. Analysis of recombinant adeno-associated virus packaging and requirements for rep and cap gene products. *J Virol* 1997;71:1897–1905.
52. Kaplitt MG, Leone P, Samulski RJ, et al. Long-term gene expression and phenotypic correction using adeno-associated virus vectors in the mammalian brain. *Nat Genet* 1994;8:148–154.
53. Koeberl DD, Bonham L, Halbert CL, et al. Persistent, therapeutically relevant levels of human granulocyte colony-stimulating factor in mice after systemic delivery of adeno-associated virus vectors. *Hum Gene Ther* 1999;10:2133–2140.
54. Pan RY, Xiao X, Chen SL, et al. Disease-inducible transgene expression from a recombinant adeno-associated virus vector in a rat arthritis model. *J Virol* 1999;73:3410–3417.
55. Pan RY, Chen SL, Xiao X, et al. Therapy and prevention of arthritis by recombinant adeno-associated virus vector with delivery of interleukin-1 receptor antagonist. *Arthritis Rheum* 2000;43:289–297.
56. Arai Y, Kubo T, Fushiki S, et al. Gene delivery to human chondrocytes by an adeno associated virus vector. *J Rheumatol* 2000;27: 979–982.
57. Fernandes J, Tardif G, Martel-Pelletier J, et al. *In vivo* transfer of interleukin-1 receptor antagonist gene in osteoarthritic rabbit knee joints: prevention of osteoarthritis progression. *Am J Pathol* 1999;154: 1159–1169.
58. Pelletier JP, Caron JP, Evans CH, et al. *In vivo* suppression of early experimental osteoarthritis by interleukin-1 receptor antagonist using gene therapy. *Arthritis Rheum* 1997;40:1012–1019.
59. Ghivizzani SC, Lechman ER, Tio C, et al. Direct retrovirus-mediated gene transfer to the synovium of the rabbit knee: implications for arthritis gene therapy. *Gene Ther* 1997;4:977–982.
60. Iyama S, Okamoto T, Sato T, et al. Treatment of murine collagen-induced arthritis by *ex vivo* extracellular superoxide dismutase gene transfer. *Arthritis Rheum* 2001;44:2160–2167.
61. Makarov SS, Olsen JC, Johnston WN, et al. Retrovirus mediated *in vivo* gene transfer to synovium in bacterial cell wall-induced arthritis in rats. *Gene Ther* 1995;2:424–428.
62. Otani K, Nita I, Macaulay W, et al. Suppression of antigen-induced arthritis in rabbits by *ex vivo* gene therapy. *J Immunol* 1996;156;3558–3562.
63. Gouze E, Pawliuk R, Pilapil C, et al. *In vivo* gene delivery to synovium by lentiviral vectors. *Mol Ther* 2002;5:397–404.
64. Oligino T, Ghivizzani S, Wolfe D, et al. Intra-articular delivery of a herpes simplex virus IL-1Ra gene vector reduces inflammation in a rabbit model of arthritis. *Gene Ther* 1999;6:1713–1720.
65. Braz J, Beaufour C, Coutaux A, et al. Therapeutic efficacy in experimental polyarthritis of viral-driven enkephalin overproduction in sensory neurons. *J Neurosci* 2001;21:7881–7888.
66. Song XY, Gu M, Jin WW, et al. Plasmid DNA encoding transforming growth factor-β1 suppresses chronic disease in a streptococcal cell wall-induced arthritis model. *J Clin Invest* 1998;101: 2615–2621.

67. Sant SM, Suarez TM, Moalli MR, et al. Molecular lysis of synovial lining cells by *in vivo* herpes simplex virus-thymidine kinase gene transfer. *Hum Gene Ther* 1998;9:2735–2743.
68. Dreja H, Annenkov A, Chernajovsky Y. Soluble complement receptor 1 (CD35) delivered by retrovirally infected syngeneic cells or by naked DNA injection prevents the progression of collagen-induced arthritis. *Arthritis Rheum* 2000;43:1698–1709.
69. Imagawa T, Watanabe S, Katakura S, et al. Gene transfer of a fibronectin peptide inhibits leukocyte recruitment and suppresses inflammation in mouse collagen-induced arthritis. *Arthritis Rheum* 2002;46: 1102–1108.
70. Bessis N, Honiger J, Damotte D, et al. Encapsulation in hollow fibres of xenogeneic cells engineered to secrete IL-4 or IL-13 ameliorates murine collagen-induced arthritis (CIA). *Clin Exp Immunol* 1999;117; 376–382.
71. Madry H, Trippel SB. Efficient lipid-mediated gene transfer to articular chondrocytes. *Gene Ther* 2000;7:286–291.
72. Tomita T, Hashimoto H, Tomita N, et al. *In vivo* direct gene transfer into articular cartilage by intraarticular injection mediated by HVJ (Sendai virus) and liposomes. *Arthritis Rheum* 1997;40:901–906.
73. Tomita T, Takano H, Tomita N, et al. Transcription factor decoy for NFκB inhibits cytokine and adhesion molecule expressions in synovial cells derived from rheumatoid arthritis. *Rheumatology* 2000;39: 749–757.
74. Hashiramoto A, Sano H, Maekawa T, et al. C-myc antisense oligodeoxynucleotides can induce apoptosis and downregulate Fas expression in rheumatoid synoviocytes. *Arthritis Rheum* 1999;42:954–962.
75. Morita Y, Kashihira N, Yamamura M, et al. Inhibition of rheumatoid synovial fibroblast proliferation by antisense oligonucleotides targeting proliferating cell nuclear antigen messenger RNA. *Arthritis Rheum* 1997;40:1292–1297.
76. Morita Y, Kashihira N, Yamamura M, et al. Antisense oligonucleotides targeting c-fos mRNA inhibit rheumatoid synovial fibroblast proliferation. *Ann Rheum Dis* 1998;57:122–124.
77. Nakazawa M, Ishii H, Aono H, et al. Role of notch-1 intracellular domain in activation of rheumatoid synoviocytes. *Arthritis Rheum* 2001;44:1545–1554.
78. Roshak A, Mochan E, Marshall LA. Suppression of human synovial fibroblast 85 kDa phospholipase A2 by antisense reduces interleukin-1β induced prostaglandin E_2. *J Rheumatol* 1996;23:420–427.
79. Yamada R, Sano H, Hla T, et al. Selective inhibition of cyclooxygenase-2 with antisense oligodeoxynucleotide restricts induction of rat adjuvant-induced arthritis. *Biochem Biophys Res Commun* 2000;269: 415–421.
80. Nakamura N, Hart DA, Boorman RS, et al. Decorin antisense gene therapy improves functional healing of early rabbit ligament scar with enhanced collagen fibrillogenesis *in vivo*. *J Orthop Res* 2000;18:517–523.
81. Chow G, Nietfeld JJ, Knudson CB, et al. Antisense inhibition of chondrocyte CD44 expression leading to cartilage chondrolysis. *Arthritis Rheum* 1998;41:1411–1419.
82. Fibbi G, Pucci M, Serni U, et al. Antisense targeting of the urokinase receptor blocks urokinase-dependent proliferation, chemoinvasion, and chemotaxis of human synovial cells and chondrocytes *in vitro*. *Proc Assoc Am Phys* 1998;110:340–350.
83. Zwicky R, Muntener K, Goldring MB, et al. Cathepsin B expression and down-regulation by gene silencing and antisense DNA in human chondrocytes. *Biochem J* 2002;367:209–217.
84. Maksymowych WP, Blackburn WD Jr, Tami JA, et al. A randomized, placebo controlled trial of an antisense oligodeoxynucleotide to intercellular adhesion molecule-1 in the treatment of severe rheumatoid arthritis. *J Rheumatol* 2002;29:447–453.
85. Kitajima I, Hanyu N, Kawahara K, et al. Ribozyme-based gene cleavage approach to chronic arthritis associated with human T cell leukemia virus type I: induction of apoptosis in synoviocytes by ablation of HTLV-I tax protein. *Arthritis Rheum* 1997;40:2118–2127.
86. Takahashi M, Funato Y, Suzuki Y, et al. Chemically modified ribozyme targeting TNF-α regulates TNF-α and IL-6 synthesis in synovial fibroblasts of patients with rheumatoid arthritis. *J Clin Immunol* 2002;22:228–236.
87. Flory CM, Pavco PA, Jarvis TC, et al. Nuclease-resistant ribozymes decrease stromelysin mRNA levels in rabbit synovium following exogenous delivery to the knee joint. *Proc Natl Acad Sci U S A* 1996;93: 754–758.
88. Jarvis TC, Bouhana KS, Lesch ME, et al. Ribozymes as tools for therapeutic target validation in arthritis. *J Immunol* 2000;165:493–498.
89. Schedel J, Seemayer CA, Neidhart M, et al. Targeting cathepsin L by specific ribozymes decreases cathepsin L protein synthesis and cartilage destruction in rheumatoid arthritis. *Gene Ther* (in press).
90. Bandara G, Mueller GM, Galea-Lauri J, et al. Intraarticular expression of biologically active interleukin 1-receptor antagonist protein by *ex vivo* gene transfer. *Proc Natl Acad Sci U S A* 1993;90:10764–10768.
91. Hung GL, Galea-Lauri J, Mueller GM, et al. Suppression of intra-articular responses to interleukin-1 by transfer of the interleukin-1 receptor antagonist gene to synovium. *Gene Ther* 1994;1:64–69.
92. Makarov SS, Olsen JC, Johnston WN, et al. Suppression of experimental arthritis by gene transfer of interleukin 1 receptor antagonist cDNA. *Proc Natl Acad Sci U S A* 1996;93:402–406.
93. Bakker AC, Joosten LA, Arntz OJ, et al. Prevention of murine collagen-induced arthritis in the knee and ipsilateral paw by local expression of human interleukin-1 receptor antagonist protein in the knee. *Arthritis Rheum* 1997;40:893–900.
94. Müller-Ladner U, Roberts CR, Franklin BN, et al. Human IL-1Ra gene transfer into human synovial fibroblasts is chondroprotective. *J Immunol* 1997;158:3492–3498.
95. Ghivizzani SC, Lechman ER, Kang R, et al. Direct adenovirus-mediated gene transfer of interleukin-1 and tumor necrosis factor α soluble receptors to rabbit knees with experimental arthritis has local and distal anti-arthritic effects. *Proc Natl Acad Sci U S A* 1998; 95:4613–4618.
96. Kim SH, Lechman ER, Kim S, et al. *Ex vivo* gene delivery of IL-1Ra and soluble TNF receptor confers a distal synergistic therapeutic effect in antigen-induced arthritis. *Mol Ther* 2002;6:591–600.
97. Frisbie DD, Ghivizzani SC, Robbins PD, et al. Treatment of experimental equine osteoarthritis by *in vivo* delivery of the equine interleukin-1 receptor antagonist gene. *Gene Ther* 2002;9:12–20.
98. Cottard V, Mulleman D, Bouille P, et al. Adeno-associated virus-mediated delivery of IL-4 prevents collagen-induced arthritis. *Gene Ther* 2000;7:1930–1939.
99. Watanabe S, Imagawa T, Boivin GP, et al. Adeno-associated virus mediates long-term gene transfer and delivery of chondroprotective IL-4 to murine synovium. *Mol Ther* 2000;2:147–152.
100. Boyle DL, Nguyen KH, Zhuang S, et al. Intra-articular IL-4 gene therapy in arthritis: anti-inflammatory effect and enhanced Th2 activity. *Gene Ther* 1999;6:1911–1918.
101. Kim SH, Evans CH, Kim S, et al. Gene therapy for established murine collagen-induced arthritis by local and systemic adenovirus-mediated delivery of interleukin-4. *Arthritis Res* 2000;2:293–302.
102. Bessis N, Cottard V, Saidenberg-Kermanach N, et al. Syngeneic fibroblasts transfected with a plasmid encoding interleukin-4 as non-viral vectors for anti-inflammatory gene therapy in collagen-induced arthritis. *J Gene Med* 2002;4:300–307.
103. Guery L, Batteux F, Bessis N, et al. Expression of Fas ligand improves the effect of IL-4 in collagen-induced arthritis. *Eur J Immunol* 2000;30:308–315.
104. Lubberts E, Joosten LA, van den Bersselaar L, et al. Adenoviral vector-mediated overexpression of IL-4 in the knee joint of mice with collagen-induced arthritis prevents cartilage destruction. *J Immunol* 1999;163:4546–4556.
105. Lubberts E, Joosten LA, Chabaud M, et al. IL-4 gene therapy for collagen arthritis suppresses synovial IL-17 and osteoprotegerin ligand and prevents bone erosion. *J Clin Invest* 2000;105:1697–1710.
106. Woods JM, Katschke KJ, Volin MV, et al. IL-4 adenoviral gene therapy reduces inflammation, proinflammatory cytokines, vascularization, and bony destruction in rat adjuvant-induced arthritis. *J Immunol* 2001;166: 1214–1222.
107. Chen Y, Rosloniec E, Goral MI, et al. Redirection of T cell effector function *in vivo* and enhanced collagen-induced arthritis mediated by an IL-2Rβ/IL-4Rα chimeric cytokine receptor transgene. *J Immunol* 2001;166:4163–4169.
108. Whalen JD, Lechman EL, Carlos CA, et al. Adenoviral transfer of the viral IL-10 gene particularly to mouse paws suppresses development of collagen-induced arthritis in both injected and uninjected paws. *J Immunol* 1999;162:3625–3632.
109. Miyata M, Sasajima T, Sato H, et al. Suppression of collagen-induced arthritis in mice utilizing plasmid DNA encoding interleukin-10. *J Rheumatol* 2000;27:1601–1605.

110. Fellowes R, Etheridge CJ, Coade S, et al. Amelioration of established collagen induced arthritis by systemic IL-10 gene delivery. *Gene Ther* 2000;7:967–977.
111. Parks E, Strieter RM, Lukacs NW, et al. Transient gene transfer of IL-12 regulates chemokine expression and disease severity in experimental arthritis. *J Immunol* 1998;160:4615–4619.
112. Woods JM, Amin MA, Katschke KJ Jr, et al. Interleukin-13 gene therapy reduces inflammation, vascularization and bony destruction in rat adjuvant-induced arthritis. *Hum Gene Ther* 2002;13: 381–393.
113. Triantaphyllopoulos KA, Williams RO, Tailor H, et al. Amelioration of collagen-induced arthritis and suppression of interferon-γ, interleukin-12, and tumor necrosis factor-α production by interferon-β gene therapy. *Arthritis Rheum* 1999;42:90–99.
114. Mageed RA, Adams G, Woodrow D, et al. Prevention of collagen-induced arthritis by gene delivery of soluble p75 tumour necrosis factor receptor. *Gene Ther* 1998;5:1584–1592.
115. Zhang HG, Xie J, Yang P, et al. Adeno-associated virus production of soluble tumor necrosis factor receptor neutralizes tumor necrosis factor α and reduces arthritis. *Hum Gene Ther* 2000;11:2431–2442.
116. Le CH, Nicolson AG, Morales A, Sewell KL. Suppression of collagen-induced arthritis through adenovirus-mediated transfer of a modified tumor necrosis factor α receptor gene. *Arthritis Rheum* 1997; 40:1662–1669.
117. Quattrochi E, Walmsley M, Browne K, et al. Paradoxical effects of adenovirus-mediated blockade of TNF activity in murine collagen-induced arthritis. *J Immunol* 1999;163:1000–1009
118. Zhang G, Yang Y, Horton JL, et al. Amelioration of collagen-induced arthritis by CD95 (Apo-1/Fas)-ligand gene transfer. *J Clin Invest* 1997;100:1951–1957.
119. Quattrochi E, Dallmann MJ, Feldmann M. Adenovirus-mediated gene transfer of CTLA-4Ig fusion protein in the suppression of experimental autoimmune arthritis. *Arthritis Rheum* 2000;53:1688–1697.
120. Ijima K, Murakami M, Okamoto H, et al. Successful gene therapy via intraarticular injection of adenovirus vector containing CTLA4IgG in a murine model of type II collagen-induced arthritis. *Hum Gene Ther* 2001;12:1063–1077.
121. Lee KH, Song SU, Hwang TS, et al. Regeneration of hyaline cartilage by cell-mediated gene therapy using transforming growth factor β1-producing fibroblasts. *Hum Gene Ther* 2001;12:1805–1813.
122. Tak PP, Gerlag DM, Aupperle KR, et al. Inhibitor of nuclear factor κB kinase β is a key regulator of synovial inflammation. *Arthritis Rheum* 2001;44:1897–1907.
123. Tomita T, Takeuchi E, Tomita N, et al. Suppressed severity of collagen-induced arthritis by *in vivo* transfection of nuclear factor κB decoy oligodeoxynucleotides as a gene therapy. *Arthritis Rheum* 1999;42: 2532–2542.
124. Nonomura Y, Kohsaka H, Nasu K, et al. Suppression of arthritis by forced expression of cyclin-dependent kinase inhibitor p21 (Cip1) gene into the joints. *Int Immunol* 2001;13:723–731.
125. Shouda T, Yoshida T, Hanada T, et al. Induction of the cytokine signal regulator SOCS3/CIS3 as a therapeutic strategy for treating inflammatory arthritis. *J Clin Invest* 2001;108:1781–1788.
126. Hollander AP, Corke KP, Freemont AJ, et al. Expression of hypoxia-inducible factor 1α by macrophages in the rheumatoid synovium: implications for targeting of therapeutic genes to the inflamed joint. *Arthritis Rheum* 2001;44:1540–1544.
127. Gerlag DM, Borges E, Tak PP, et al. Suppression of murine collagen-induced arthritis by targeted apoptosis of synovial neovasculature. *Arthritis Res* 2001;3:357–361.
128. Yin G, Liu W, An P, et al. Endostatin gene transfer inhibits joint angiogenesis and pannus formation in inflammatory arthritis. *Mol Ther* 2002;5:547–554.
129. Kim JH, Ho SH, Park EJ, et al. Angiostatin gene transfer as an effective treatment strategy in murine collagen-induced arthritis. *Arthritis Rheum* 2002;46:793–801.
130. Marchand GS, Noiseux N, Tanguay JF, et al. Blockade of *in vivo* VEGF-mediated angiogenesis by antisense gene therapy: role of Flk-1 and Flt-1 receptors. *Am Physiol Heart Circ Physiol* 2002;282: H194–H204.
131. Fiehn C, Müller-Ladner U, Stelzer EHK, et al. Albumin-based drug delivery as novel therapeutic approach for rheumatoid arthritis. *Arthritis Rheum* 2002;46(suppl):134.
132. Apparailly F, Bouquet C, Millet V, et al. Adenovirus-mediated gene transfer of urokinase plasminogen inhibitor inhibits angiogenesis in experimental arthritis. *Gene Ther* 2002;9:192–200.
133. Shaw MK, Lorens LB, Dhawan A, et al. Local delivery of interleukin 4 by retrovirus-transduced T lymphocytes ameliorates experimental autoimmune encephalomyelitis. *J Exp Med* 1997;185:1711–1714.
134. Costa GL, Benson JM, Seroogy CM, et al. Targeting rare populations of murine antigen-specific T lymphocytes by retroviral transduction for potential application in gene therapy for autoimmune disease. *J Immunol* 2000;164:3581–3590.
135. Annenkov A, Chernajovsky Y. Engineering mouse T lymphocytes specific to type II collagen by transduction with a chimeric receptor consisting of a single chain Fv and TCR zeta. *Gene Ther* 2000;7:714–722.
136. Tarner IH, Fathman CG. Gene therapy in autoimmune disease. *Curr Opin Immunol* 2001;13:676–682.
137. Slavin A, Tarner IH, Nakajima A, et al. Adoptive cellular gene therapy of autoimmune disease. *Autoimmun Rev* 2002;1:213–219.
138. Kim SH, Evans CH, Kim S, et al. Gene therapy for established murine collagen-induced arthritis by local and systemic adenovirus-mediated delivery of interleukin-4. *Arthritis Res* 2000;2:293–302.
139. Morita Y, Yang J, Gupta R, et al. Dendritic cells genetically engineered to express IL-4 inhibit murine collagen-induced arthritis. *J Clin Invest* 2001;107:1275–1284.
140. Tarner IH, Nakajima A, Staton TL, et al. Retroviral gene therapy of collagen-induced arthritis by local delivery of immunoregulatory molecules using antigen-specific T-cells and dendritic cells. *Arthritis Rheum* 2001;44(suppl):149.
141. Costa GL, Sandora MR, Nakajima A, et al. Adoptive immunotherapy of experimental autoimmune encephalomyelitis via T cell delivery of the IL-12 p40 subunit. *J Immunol* 2001;167:2379–2387.
142. Nakajima A, Seroogy CM, Sandora MR, et al. Antigen-specific T cell–mediated gene therapy in collagen-induced arthritis. *J Clin Invest* 2001;107;1293–1301.
143. Tarner IH, Nakajima A, Seroogy CM, et al. Retroviral gene therapy of collagen-induced arthritis by local delivery of IL-4. *Clin Immunol* 2002;105:304–314.
144. Celiker MY, Ramamurthy N, Xu JW, et al. Inhibition of adjuvant-induced arthritis by systemic tissue inhibitor of metalloproteinases-4 gene delivery. *Arthritis Rheum* 2002;46:3361–3368.
145. Ahonen M, Ala-Aho R, Baker AH, et al. Antitumor activity and bystander effect of adenovirally delivered tissue inhibitor of metalloproteinases-3. *Mol Ther* 2002;5:705–715.
146. Apparailly F, Noel D, Millet V, et al. Paradoxical effects of tissue inhibitor of metalloproteinases 1 gene transfer in collagen-induced arthritis. *Arthritis Rheum* 2001;44:1444–1454.
147. Zhang HG, Huang N, Liu D, et al. Gene therapy that inhibits nuclear translocation of nuclear factor κB results in tumor necrosis factor α-induced apoptosis of human synovial fibroblasts. *Arthritis Rheum* 2000;43:1094–1105.
148. Taniguchi K, Kohsaka H, Inoue N, et al. Induction of the p16INK4a senescence gene as a new therapeutic strategy for the treatment of rheumatoid arthritis. *Nat Med* 1999;5:760–767.
149. Künzler P, Kuchen S, Rihoskova V, et al. Induction of p16 at sites of cartilage invasion in the SCID mouse coimplantation model of rheumatoid arthritis. *Arthritis Rheum* 2003;48:2069–2073.
150. Takayanagi H, Juji T, Miyazaki T, et al. Suppression of arthritic bone destruction by adenovirus-mediated csk gene transfer to synoviocytes and osteoclasts. *J Clin Invest* 1999;104:137–146.
151. Wakisaka S, Suzuki N, Saito N, et al. Possible correction of abnormal rheumatoid arthritis synovial cell function by jun D transfection *in vivo*. *Arthritis Rheum* 1998;41:470–481.
152. Woods JM, Tokuhira M, Berry JC, et al. Interleukin-4 adenoviral gene therapy reduces production of inflammatory cytokines and prostaglandin E_2 by rheumatoid arthritis synovium *ex vivo*. *J Invest Med* 1999;47:285–292.
153. Woods JM, Katschke KJ Jr, Tokuhira M, et al. Reduction of inflammatory cytokines and prostaglandin E_2 by IL-13 gene therapy in rheumatoid arthritis synovium. *J Immunol* 2000;156:2755–2763.
154. Arend WP, Dayer J-P. Inhibition of the production and effects of interleukin-1 and tumor necrosis factor-α in rheumatoid arthritis. *Arthritis Rheum* 1995;38:151–160.
155. Attur MG, Dave MN, Leung MY, et al. Functional genomic analysis of type II IL-1β decoy receptor: potential for gene therapy in human arthritis and inflammation. *J Immunol* 2002;168:2001–2010.

156. Müller-Ladner U, Kriegsmann J, Franklin BN, et al. Synovial fibroblasts of patients with rheumatoid arthritis attach to and invade normal human cartilage when engrafted into SCID mice. *Am J Pathol* 1996;149:1607–1615.
157. Judex M, Neumann E, Fleck M, et al. "Inverse wrap": An improved implantation technique for virus-transduced synovial fibroblasts in the SCID mouse model for rheumatoid arthritis. *Mod Rheumatol* 2001:11;145–150.
158. Jorgensen C, Demoly P, Noel D, et al. Gene transfer to human rheumatoid synovial tissue engrafted in SCID mice. *J Rheumatol* 1997;24:2061–2062.
159. Chernajovsky Y, Adams G, Podhajcer OL, et al. Inhibition of transfer of collagen-induced arthritis into SCID mice by *ex vivo* infection of spleen cells with retroviruses expressing soluble tumor necrosis factor receptor. *Gene Ther* 1995;2:731–735.
160. Müller-Ladner U, Evans CH, Franklin BN, et al. Gene transfer of cytokine inhibitors into human synovial fibroblasts in the SCID mouse model. *Arthritis Rheum* 1999;42:490–497.
161. Neidhart M, Gay RE, Gay S. Anti-interleukin-1 and anti-CD44 interventions producing significant inhibition of cartilage destruction in an *in vitro* model of cartilage invasion by rheumatoid arthritis synovial fibroblasts. *Arthritis Rheum* 2000;43:1719–1728.
162. Isomaki P, Luukkainen R, Saario R, et al. Interleukin-10 functions as an antiinflammatory cytokine in rheumatoid synovium. *Arthritis Rheum* 1996;39:386–395.
163. Neumann E, Judex M, Kullmann F, et al. Inhibition of cartilage destruction by double gene transfer of IL-1Ra and IL-10 involves the activin pathway. *Gene Ther* 2002;9:1508–1519.
164. Nawrath M, Hummel KM, Pap T, et al. effect of dominant negative mutants of raf-1 and c-myc on rheumatoid arthritis synovial fibroblasts in the SCID mouse model. *Arthritis Rheum* 1998;41(suppl 9):95.
165. Van der Laan WH, Quax PHA, Seemayer CA, et al. Cartilage degradation and invasion by rheumatoid synovial fibroblasts is inhibited by gene transfer of TIMP-1 and TIMP-3. *Gene Ther* (in press).
166. Werb Z, Mainardi CL, Vater CA, et al. Endogenous activation of latent collagenase by rheumatoid synovial cells. Evidence for a role of plasminogen activator. *N Engl J Med* 1977;296:1017–1023.
167. Van der Laan WH, Pap T, Ronday HK, et al. Cartilage degradation and invasion by rheumatoid synovial fibroblasts is inhibited by gene transfer of a cell surface-targeted plasmin inhibitor. *Arthritis Rheum* 2000;43:1710–1718.
168. Okamoto K, Asahara H, Kobayashi T, et al. Induction of apoptosis in the rheumatoid synovium by Fas ligand gene transfer. *Gene Ther* 1998;5:331–338.
169. Kobayashi T, Okamoto K, Kobata T, et al. Novel gene therapy for rheumatoid arthritis by FADD gene transfer: induction of apoptosis of rheumatoid synoviocytes but not chondrocytes. *Gene Ther* 2000; 7:527–533.
170. Chernajovsky Y, Adams G, Triantaphyllopoulos K, et al. Pathogenic lymphoid cells engineered to express TGFβ1 ameliorate disease in a collagen-induced arthritis model. *Gene Ther* 1997:4:553–559.
171. Goossens PH, Schouten GJ, 't Hart BA, et al. Feasibility of adenovirus-mediated nonsurgical synovectomy in collagen-induced arthritis-affected rhesus monkeys. *Hum Gene Ther* 1999;10:1139–1149.
172. Evans CH, Robbins PD, Ghivizzani SC, et al. Clinical trial to assess the safety, feasibility, and efficacy of transferring a potentially anti-arthritic cytokine gene to human joints with rheumatoid arthritis. *Hum Gene Ther* 1996;7:1261–1280.
173. Müller-Ladner U, Distler O, Gay RE, et al. Genomics and rheumatology. Cutting Edge Reports 2001, *www.rheuma21st.com/archives/*

CHAPTER 38

Rehabilitation for Persons with Arthritis and Rheumatic Disorders

Vivian C. Shih and Rowland W. Chang

Arthritis is the leading cause of limitation of physical function in the United States. The Centers for Disease Control and Prevention (CDC) estimates that more than 7 million citizens are limited in their ability to dress, bathe, toilet, feed, groom, or transfer out of a bed or chair independently because of their arthritis (1). Arthritis has significant effects on the quality of life, both for the individual who experiences its painful symptoms and for the family members and caregivers of these sufferers. Compounding this, the nation bears significant medical and social costs for the treatment of the disease and its complications. Dunlop and colleagues estimate that the national economic burden due to arthritis was nearly \$125 billion in 1996 (expressed in 2000 dollars) (2).

Despite these sobering statistics, arthritis has been considered by many to be a minor medical disorder, described as a nuisance to most while severely limiting only a few. Arthritis has not assumed, in the public's eye or the media, the prominence of diseases such as breast cancer, which are more frightening and potentially fatal. The recent public health data outlining arthritis as the leading cause of functional limitation, physician visits, and missed workdays belie the notion that arthritis is a benign condition. Important goals of medical and rehabilitative care include effective ways to treat arthritis and reduce the pain, physical impairments, and functional limitations associated with the disease. Primary care physicians, rheumatologists, physiatrists, nurses, physical and occupational therapists, and surgeons all have the potential to contribute to care for arthritis patients with varying levels of needs and functional limitation. However, to date, integrated arthritis care has been elusive for most patients, because it requires ongoing coordination among a number of providers of different disciplines.

Rheumatology and rehabilitation have strong historical ties. Both disciplines' origins and early growth date back to the early 1900s. Because there were few medical treatments for arthritis during those times, rehabilitation was often all that was offered to a patient who had arthritis. Indeed, in many European hospitals, rheumatologists also often served as leaders of rehabilitation units, even until the 1980s.

Several factors have led to the relative isolation of these fields in recent years. On the rheumatology side, there has been a major scientific emphasis on the pathobiology—especially the immunology, biochemistry, and molecular biology—that explains many types of arthritis and rheumatic diseases. The vocabulary and conceptual frameworks of these sciences are different from those of rehabilitation science, which describe the pathoanatomy and pathophysiology of the joint as an organ, the understanding of which underpins much of the rehabilitation treatment of patients with arthritis. The major emphasis on pathoimmunology in rheumatology has led to the development of new biologic treatments for arthritis and other rheumatic diseases (see Chapters 39 and 40). Thus, it is understandable that recent and current generations of rheumatology trainees have been influenced less and less by the theoretical underpinnings of and experience with rehabilitation treatment, compared with those of medical treatment.

Similarly, in the middle and late 1900s the field of rehabilitation drifted away from patients with rheumatologic disorders because of its preoccupation with inpatient rehabilitation of patients with impairments from neurologic conditions and acute trauma, stroke and other brain injuries, spinal cord injuries, and amputations. It has only been in recent times that "musculoskeletal medicine" has become an attractive subspecialty for physiatrists, the medical specialists in physical medicine and rehabilitation.

Given these historical forces, why should a modern rheumatologist be interested in rehabilitation? The answer should be obvious to anyone who visits a typical rheumatology practice. Medical treatment cannot and will not address all the consequences of arthritis and rheumatic diseases that lead to functional limitation at least in the foreseeable future. Therefore, comprehensive care for persons with arthritis that aims to improve quality of life requires an interdisciplinary approach, using medications as well as appropriately-timed rehabilitation and surgical interventions. Perhaps a more compelling reason for rheumatologists to incorporate rehabilitation concepts into their patient management and to collaborate with rehabilitation providers is that the ideas and treatments associated with rehabilitation are likely to play an important role in public health strategies for the prevention and control of arthritis in our society.

This chapter describes a conceptual framework used by rehabilitation professionals that will allow readers to integrate their understanding of the pathophysiologic processes associated with arthritis with an understanding of joint pathology as well as the personal and societal consequences of joint and rheumatic disease. This framework helps guide the prescription of comprehensive medical and rehabilitative treatments, resulting in a holistic approach to arthritis care. A brief description of common rehabilitation strategies is presented along with their theoretical underpinnings. Finally, an evidence-based review of rehabilitation treatments for specific arthritis and rheumatic disease conditions is provided.

A CONCEPTUAL FRAMEWORK FOR INCORPORATING REHABILITATION INTO RHEUMATOLOGY PRACTICE

The challenge in choosing an appropriate integrative framework for rheumatology practitioners is related to the multiple perspectives one can take to understand and treat the problems presented by patients with arthritis and rheumatic disorders. We have the ability to intervene in inflammatory conditions at the cytokine and prostaglandin level, and we expect to be able to influence disease at the gene level in the not too distant future. These treatments are driven by viewing the patient from a molecular and cellular perspective. In contrast, viewing the patient's disorder from the joint or organ perspective, allows one to better understand the rationale for joint surgery and local exercise treatments for persons with arthritis. Similarly, considering the patient holistically allows one to assess and treat limitations of personal care (e.g., dressing, bathing, toileting, and grooming) and other physical function activities, such as ambulation. Rehabilitation treatments concentrate on enhancing outcomes at this level. Finally, taking the societal perspective on a patient's disorder allows one to consider both the patient's employment status and societal constraints on the ability of the patient to be productive. Thus, the appropriate conceptual framework that allows integration of medical, surgical, and rehabilitation treatment of arthritis and rheumatic disorders must necessarily be broad and comprehensive.

A conceptual framework that satisfies this breadth was promulgated by the World Health Organization (WHO) in the 1960s. Since then, this framework has been revised by several organizations and continues to undergo modification and refinement. One reason for the several revisions of the original WHO model is the ambiguity of the terms that were and are being used. We will present the framework proposed by the Institute of Medicine (IOM), which uses understandable terms and appropriately incorporates rehabilitation and modern molecular and cellular-based rheumatology practices (3).

An overview of the IOM framework is presented in the middle panel of Fig. 38.1, and rheumatologic examples of the major concepts are presented in Table 38.1. Understanding this framework might be facilitated by making some assumptions about causes and effect among the concepts of pathology, impairment, functional limitation, and disability, but one should recognize that, in reality, the relationships among these concepts are complex and certainly not linear.

Given this caveat, the framework begins with pathology, defined as "measurable cellular and tissue changes caused by disease, infection, trauma, congenital conditions, or other agents." This is the perspective that is taken by modern rheumatology, which has been greatly enhanced by successful laboratory-based research in recent times. Autoimmunity and inflammation are examples of pathologic concepts that are relevant in rheumatology.

Often, pathology leads to disruption at the organ level, classified as "impairment." The formal definition of impairment is "discrete loss and/or abnormality of mental, emotional, physiologic or anatomical structure or function." Most commonly the organ of interest in rheumatology is the joint, which is composed of articular and fibrocartilage, synovium, ligaments, tendons, bursae, muscles, and nerves. Thus, joint stiffness or instability, joint deformity, and joint pain are all examples of impairments common to persons with arthritis. Orthopedic surgery and exercise therapeutics address issues at this level.

Impairment can then lead to "functional limitation," defined as "restriction or lack of ability to perform an action or activity in the manner or within the range considered normal." Thus, limitations in ambulation, the ability to transfer from sitting to standing, or to dress, bathe, and toilet oneself are common examples of functional limitations traditionally addressed by rehabilitation professionals.

"Disability," then, is commonly a result of functional limitation. Disability is defined as "inability or limitation in performing socially defined activities and roles expected of individuals within a social and physical environment." Here is where the inability to gain employment or to be a housekeeper/caregiver in one's home as a social consequence of arthritis could be considered.

A comprehensive patient evaluation should evaluate and intervene at each of these levels. For example, the erythrocyte sedimentation rate or synovial fluid white cell count is

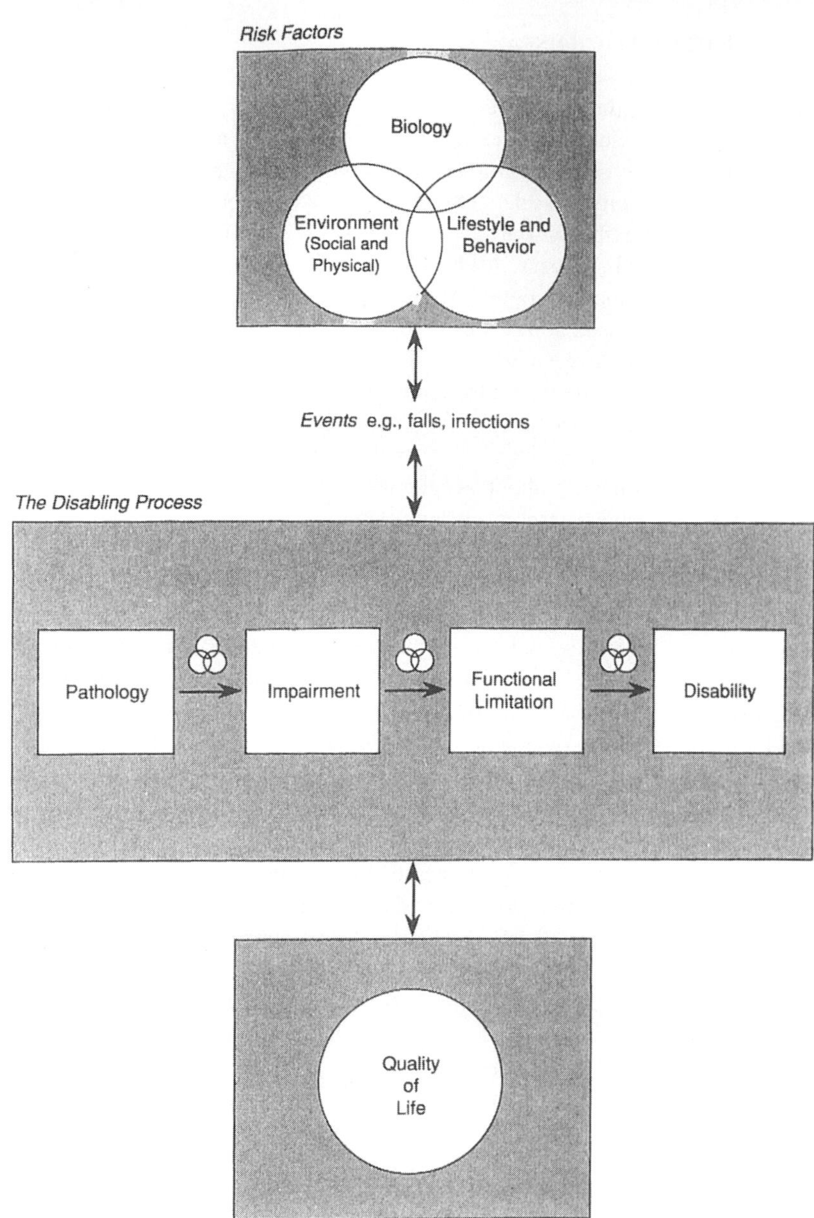

FIG. 38.1. Model of disability showing the interaction of the disabling process, quality of life, and risk factors. Three types of risk factors are included: biologic (e.g., Rh type); environmental [e.g., lead paint (physical environment) and access to care (social environment)]; and lifestyle and behavior (e.g., tobacco consumption). *Bidirectional arrows* indicate the potential for feedback. The potential for additional risk factors to affect the progression toward disability is shown between the stages of the model. The additional risk factors might include, depending on the stage of the model, diagnosis, treatment therapy, adequacy of rehabilitation, age of onset, financial resources, expectations, and environmental barriers. (From Pope AM, Tarlov AR, eds. *Disability in America: toward a national agenda for prevention.* Washington, DC: Institute of Medicine, National Academy Press, 1991, with permission.)

TABLE 38.1. *Definitions included in the Institute of Medicine's process of disablement and rheumatology examples*

Pathology	Impairment	Functional limitation	Disability
Interruption or interference of normal bodily processes or structures	Loss and/or abnormality of mental, emotional, physiologic, or anatomic structure or function: includes all losses or abnormalities, not just those attributable to active pathology; includes pain	Restriction or lack of ability to perform an action or activity in the manner or within the range considered normal that results from impairment	Inability or limitation in performing socially-defined activities and roles expected of individuals within a social and physical environment
Level of reference			
Cells and tissues	Organs and organ systems	Organism: action or activity performance	Society: task performance within the social and cultural context
Example			
Inflammation	Swelling, instability, pain	Restricted range of motion, limited walking, climbing	Cannot carry out groceries, can no longer jog
Denervated muscle due to trauma	Atrophy of muscle	Cannot pull with arm	Change of job, can no longer swim

Pathology, impairment, functional limitation determined by examination and testing. Disability is relational: functional limitation related to demands of tasks and roles.

Adapted from Pope AM, Tarlov AR, eds. *Disability in America: toward a national agenda for prevention.* Washington, DC: Institute of Medicine, National Academy Press, 1991, with permission.

used to assess the activity of the pathology in a patient with rheumatoid arthritis (RA). Joint examination and radiographic data define the joint impairments. Either self-report of how far the patient can walk without stopping or direct observation of gait would be one element of a functional limitation evaluation. Finally, asking how one is doing at work or at home would address disability status. Although time often limits the depth and breadth of a typical rheumatology evaluation, physiatrist consultation or direct referral to allied health professionals such as physical and occupational therapists, social workers, psychologists, and vocational counselors can provide more detailed information and intervention.

The application of this conceptual framework can be useful in solving complex problems presented by arthritis and rheumatic disease patients. For example, consider the patient with RA who complains of having more difficulty walking two blocks. This is a functional limitation complaint. One approach to this problem is to ask what impairments are contributing to this patient's functional limitation. Is it joint pain, swelling, deformity, or loss of joint motion? Or, is it muscle weakness or a lack of motor control? Once the relevant impairments are identified, one could ask, what disease processes are contributing to these impairments, and is there anything that can be done to modify these disease processes? If joint pain is the issue, is the pain due to active inflammation or is it due to an ongoing degenerative disease process? If muscle weakness is present, is it due to disuse atrophy or is there a myelopathy present due to cervical spine subluxation?

This conceptual framework is useful in directing treatment. Problems identified at the pathology level might be amenable to medical treatment. Problems identified at the impairment level can often be addressed by orthopedic surgery or rehabilitation strategies, even if medical treatment can modify the disease processes and pathologies that contribute to these impairments. Similarly, rehabilitation treatment to directly address functional limitations can be useful above and beyond what might be done to treat the impairments leading to these limitations. Finally, referrals to vocational counselors may be helpful to patients with disability concerns given the complexities of the assessments and potential solutions to securing a suitable job.

The ultimate utility of this conceptual framework is to provide more treatment opportunities that enhance the quality of life for persons with arthritis and rheumatic disease. As Fig. 38.1 depicts, quality of life is not just determined by pathology. All four elements of the disabling process should be addressed in order to maximize the patient's quality of life.

POTENTIAL REHABILITATION INTERVENTIONS: GENERAL CONCEPTS

Exercise and Physical Activity

Exercise is the rehabilitation strategy with the best theoretical rationale and has the most extensive evidence of efficacy in the literature related to patients with arthritis, musculoskeletal, and rheumatic conditions (4). It ameliorates many of the common impairments present by improving aerobic capacity, muscle strength, endurance, proprioception, and joint flexibility. Furthermore, exercise significantly reduces pain and stiffness. Additional benefits are decreased depression, reduced fatigue, resolution of sleep disturbances, and increased abilities to perform activities of daily living (ADLs) and level of independence (5–10).

In the past, physicians and other healthcare professionals have discouraged patients with arthritis and rheumatic disease from exercising or being physically active because of concerns about accelerated joint damage and pain. In the acute phases of inflammation, range of motion (ROM) and isotonic strengthening (continuous equal resistance) are believed to increase joint temperature and swelling, and potentially to accelerate joint deterioration. There is also concern about the deleterious effects of particular strengthening exercises on unstable joints. Unfortunately, the overemphasis on these theoretical negatives by healthcare providers has greatly overshadowed the important benefits of exercise and physical activity in arthritis. It is well known that those with arthritis have poorer muscle strength and endurance than the general population (5,11,12). Studies strongly indicate that aerobic and resistance exercises are significantly beneficial to patients with arthritis, including inflammatory arthritis, because they improve flexibility, strength, endurance, function, and cardiovascular fitness without aggravating the symptoms (5,6,9,13). For example, one study included subjects with RA and symptomatic weight-bearing joints in a 12-week graded aerobic exercise program. Significant improvements in aerobic capacity, overall physical activity, anxiety and depression, 50-foot walk time, grip strength, and flexibility were demonstrated and maintained after 1 year (5). A combined dance-based aerobic exercise and educational problem-solving, skills-building program improved quality of life measures and reduced 50-foot walk time (6,9). Yet another study of RA subjects indicated that a program of muscle strengthening exercises increased scores on physical fitness tests (13). In an extensive review of randomized control trials of dynamic exercise therapy for patients with RA, only six studies fulfilled the criteria of intensity levels greater than 60% maximal heart rate for at least 30 minutes, at least two sessions per week, and duration of greater than 6 weeks (14). Results indicate that dynamic exercise is effective for increasing muscle strength, physical capacity, and aerobic capacity without harmful increases in disease activity and pain.

In the Fitness Arthritis and Seniors Trial (FAST) for older adults with knee osteoarthritis (OA), the intervention groups (aerobic and resistance exercise participants) had modest improvements in measures of disability, physical performance, and pain compared with a health education–only cohort over a period of 18 months (15). Ettinger and colleagues found that benefits were seen in both sexes and in several subgroups: African Americans, obese patients, and persons over 70 years of age. Later on, Penninx and colleagues used the data from the FAST to assess whether the physical activity interventions could prevent the incidence of ADL disability (16). Again the intervention groups both had a significantly reduced 18-month incidence of ADL disability in older persons with knee OA compared with the health education–attention group. Interestingly, the individuals most compliant with the exercise program had the greatest reduction in risk for ADL disability. Another study by Baker and colleagues compared high-intensity home-based progressive strength training program to a nutrition education program (attention control) for adults age 55 and older with knee OA (17). The 4-month home program cohort had significantly decreased pain and improved self-reported physical function using the Western Ontario/McMaster Universities Osteoarthritis Index (WOMAC) and the Medical Outcomes Survey Short Form (SF-36) compared with the control cohort.

A specific exercise prescription that includes diagnosis, type of therapy, duration, intensity, frequency, precautions, and focus/goals should be offered to each individual patient (Table 38.2). An initial assessment of joint stability, effusions, and inflammation is critical so that potentially harmful exercises may be excluded. During acute joint inflammation, it is important not to overstretch periarticular tissues, because their reduced tensile strength may lead to tears and capsular ruptures. Isometric exercise is recommended during inflammation; it is used in conjunction with dynamic resistive and aerobic exercise programs once inflammation subsides. In isometric exercises, the length of the musculotendinous unit remains the same, unlike isotonic or isokinetic exercises, where the muscle length increases or decreases while muscle force or torque remain constant, respectively. Adequate warm-up prior to workouts and cool-down afterward with gentle stretching and light aerobics ensures safety and comfort.

Aquatic exercise is highly recommended for patients with high levels of pain or weakness. The warmth and buoyancy of a heated pool, typically above 85°F and ideally 90 to 93°F, provides an almost pain-free environment in which to exercise. Regular pool therapy has been demonstrated to improve strength and conditioning (18). Other aerobic exercise, such as low-impact aerobics, bicycling, and walking, are recommended to improve cardiovascular conditioning without increasing pain or inflammation (15).

TABLE 38.2. *Prescription: physical, occupational, or aquatic therapy*

Name: **Date:**
Diagnosis/indication:
Precautions: FWB, WBAT, PWB, NWB; no PROM; no deep heat; etc.
Frequency and duration: Sessions per week and number of weeks
Focus/goal: Increase balance, flexibility, strength, ADLs, ambulation, issue equipment/assistive devices, etc.
Modalities: Heat, cryotherapy, ultrasonography, TENS, etc.
Patient education: Home exercise program, joint protection techniques, energy-saving techniques, instruct on equipment
Physician Signature:

ADLs, activities of daily living; FWB, full weight bearing; NWB, non–weight bearing; PROM, passive range of motion; PWB, partial weight bearing; TENS, transcutaneous electrical nerve stimulation; WBAT, weight bearing as tolerated.

Patients with arthritis who have not previously exercised in a structured program and who have identified physical impairments (such as a joint contracture) will benefit from a referral to a physical therapist. This will best enable them to learn specifically which exercises are best for them and precisely how to perform them for the greatest benefit. The therapist may also review joint protection and energy conservation techniques along with providing necessary adaptive aids. A structured home exercise program will facilitate continued compliance and participation after the supervised therapy sessions are completed.

Patient compliance with exercise regimens is critical to the success of these interventions. Several strategies are proposed to improve patient compliance. These strategies include simplification of exercise regimens, setting of attainable goals, education about the importance of exercise, including social interaction, and regular follow-up and discussion of progress in exercise (19). Overall, patients with arthritis appear to be more compliant in supervised exercise classes than in home-based exercise programs (19).

The literature suggests that persons with arthritis are particularly inactive (20–22). This inactivity in patients with arthritis is associated with decreased function and increased medical costs (23). Investigators now distinguish between lifestyle physical activity (24,25), which includes participation in everyday activities (housework, occupational, leisure activities) and formal exercise, a subset of physical activity, which is "planned, structured, and repetitive, with the intent of improving or maintaining one or more facets of physical fitness or function" (26).

Much of the literature to date has focused on encouraging arthritis patients to participate in formal exercise programs, either at home or in the community. A review of randomized, controlled trials suggests that patients with arthritis, including RA and knee OA, who participate in exercise programs increase strength and functional status and decrease pain and fatigue without adversely affecting joint status (15,27–36). Exercise program participants also report improved self-efficacy (37) and quality of life (34). However, adherence rates vary between 50% and 75%, and long-term persistence has not been demonstrated in most cases (29,33,37–41).

Although formal exercise is commonly thought of as the way to meet physical activity goals, the energy expended in many everyday activities such as gardening and housekeeping is sufficient activity for some individuals with arthritis (42). For example, the recently revised Compendium of Physical Activities provides guidance about the amount of energy expended in the performance of everyday self-care, productive, and leisure activities, as well as exercise (42). Engaging in lifestyle physical activities has been shown to be as beneficial as formal exercise (24,25,43,44) in improving fitness and blood pressure and is more cost-effective than formal exercise programs (45) in the general population. Because adherence to exercise programs may be difficult, clinicians and public health professionals may wish to additionally promote everyday physical activities of moderate and high energy expenditure.

Current American College of Rheumatology (ACR) guidelines indicate that the goals of treatment for RA and knee OA are to decrease pain, prevent disability, and maintain joint integrity (particularly in RA) (46–48). The guidelines also suggest that medications should be used in conjunction with nonpharmacologic methods, such as education, physical activity, and psychological methods, although by far the lion's share of the guidelines are given over to medication use. In contrast, recent guidelines from the American Geriatric Society provide specific timing, intensity, and duration recommendations for stretching, strength, and aerobic exercise for OA (49).

Systemic and Local Joint Rest

Adequate systemic rest, including restorative sleep, is necessary for general health and imperative in the presence of chronic disease. General body rest is a known strategy to reduce systemic inflammation in RA. However, the known adverse effects of prolonged bed rest, including rapid reductions in strength and endurance, limit its use as a systemic therapy. During periods of acute inflammation, daily periods of intermittent rest breaks (30–60 minutes in duration) are typically recommended.

Resting splints and other orthotics are used to reduce pain and inflammation through strict immobilization of the joint (50,51). Numerous investigators have demonstrated the efficacy of splints in reducing pain (52). Although the duration of use to achieve pain reduction is not clear, most clinicians prescribe splint use throughout the day and night when inflammation is present and at night for several weeks once the inflammation has resolved. Patients are taught to self-manage splint use. Custom splints fabricated by occupational therapists or orthotists are expensive, but are often better tolerated than prefabricated splints.

Joint protection techniques can reduce repetitive joint loading and motion associated with increased pain in abnormal joints. Joint loading can be reduced through the modification of daily activities. For example, an individual with an impaired hip should carry heavy items in the ipsilateral hand or split the weight and carry half in each hand. Recreational activities should be low impact, such as swimming or bicycling. When standing at the sink, persons with back impairments should use a stool to elevate one leg. Individuals may also plan their kitchen so that frequently used items are at counter-height and easy-to-reach areas. The Arthritis Foundation provides outstanding practical literature on energy conservation and joint protection techniques for individuals with RA. Further patient-specific advice can be obtained with a referral to an occupational therapist.

Modalities

Superficial heat (hot packs, paraffin, wax baths, fluidotherapy, infrared radiation, and hydrotherapy) is used primarily to reduce pain and improve flexibility. Heat may reduce muscle guarding, increase blood flow, and increase the pain threshold of the sensory nerve. Heat increases extensibility of connective tissues, theoretically facilitating ROM therapies. However, the efficacy of superficial heat has not been clearly supported in clinical trials. Many patients report improvement in pain following heat treatments (53) despite the absence of substantiating literature (54). The daily use of heat does not appear to affect disease progression (55). In a recent review of seven randomized controlled trials by Robinson and colleagues, both moist heat and cryotherapy had no significant positive or negative effects on measurements of RA disease activity when compared with controls (56). However, because joint and skin temperatures elevate following superficial heat application, heat should be avoided during acute inflammatory flares. Deep heat (short-wave diathermy and ultrasonography) elevates joint, muscle, and connective tissue temperatures, but again, the current literature does not substantiate its use (57,58). General contraindications and precautions for therapeutic heat include acute inflammation, trauma, bleeding disorders, tissue insensitivity, inability to communicate pain, malignancy, edema, ischemia, and scar tissue (59).

Cold treatments (cold packs, ice massage, cold baths, and vapocoolant sprays) are used to reduce pain, swelling, and inflammation through slowing nerve conduction, decreasing muscle activity, releasing endorphins, or promoting vasoconstriction. Cold treatment is believed to reduce joint temperature by reducing skin temperature (60). The literature substantiating these effects is also limited.

Transcutaneous electrical nerve stimulation (TENS) theoretically reduces pain through stimulating large sensory fibers that overwhelm sensory receptors and block small pain fiber transmission to the spinal cord (61). It is reported to reduce pain in RA (62). The most common modes of TENS are high frequency, low frequency, and burst mode. High-frequency, with electrodes placed around the painful joint, uses a continuous train of 100-μsec pulses in a frequency of 70 to 100 Hz. Low-frequency uses wide 250-μsec pulses at a frequency of 1 to 3 Hz; electrodes are placed over motor points in the myotomes of muscles around the painful joint. In burst mode, current frequency is 70 Hz, delivered in small bursts at a rate of three per second. There is little evidence to support the use of one mode of TENS over the other in RA (63).

Orthotics and Assistive Devices

In addition to rendering local rest to painful and inflamed joints, splints and other orthotics are used to correct deformity and improve function by providing mechanical support for unstable joints and redirecting forces that are transmitted across joints during daily activities. For example, the use of soft heels has been shown to reduce lower extremity transmitted force during heel strike (64). Through shifting transmitted force, arch supports can reduce load transmitted to the medial compartment of the knee (64,65). The use of a cane in the hand opposite an impaired hip will reduce force transmitted to that hip by about 50% (66).

Psychological Therapies

Pain is a subjective experience, which cannot be directly measured or observed. The 1994 Task Force on Taxonomy of the International Association for the Study of Pain defined pain as "an unpleasant sensory and emotional experience associated with actual or potential tissue damage, or described in terms of such damage." Severity of disease is not a reliable marker for pain. The patient's perception of pain and subsequent functional limitation is influenced by much more than the physical changes at the tissue level. Thoughts and emotions contribute to the central descending control of peripheral nociception. Each individual's level of stress, anxiety, depression, and coping skills can greatly impact on perception of pain; treating those factors directly improves outcomes in arthritis and other chronic pain syndromes. Treatment of depression and mood disturbances is an important strategy in managing chronic pain.

One of the goals of psychological chronic pain therapy in general, and cognitive-behavioral therapies (CBTs) specifically, is to increase patients' self-efficacy skills. Self-efficacy has been defined as a person's belief in his or her own power to successfully manage a challenging situation. Self-efficacy training is a cornerstone to the rehabilitative management of arthritis patients. Even after controlling for disease severity, patient reports of high self-efficacy are significantly correlated with decreased pain and improved mood in persons with arthritis (67). There is evidence that patients who receive information about their disease fare better than those who are less knowledgeable (68). Monthly telephone calls from lay personnel even appear to improve pain (69). Stress management training, as one component of CBT, can reduce self-reported pain and improve coping strategies in persons with RA (70).

Biofeedback is also useful in the modulation of central control of pain, usually through electronic equipment that monitors a physiologic event and displays it to the therapist and patient. Relative to placebo or a no-treatment group, biofeedback group therapy appears to reduce pain and even joint inflammation in persons with RA (71). Finally, as discussed in the disease-specific sections that follow, treatment with antidepressants is useful to ameliorate common depressive symptoms as well as to provide direct analgesia.

Vocational Rehabilitation

Arthritis is the leading cause of work loss and second leading cause of payments for work disability in the United States (72). Work disability rates increase from about 25% of persons with less than 10 years of joint symptoms to nearly 90% of those with longer duration of disease (73). The greatest risk factors for work disability in those with arthritis appear to be advanced disease status, a physically demanding job, and older age (73).

Vocational rehabilitation services are useful to help retrain functionally-limited workers for jobs they can safely and effectively perform. Government-sponsored vocational rehabilitation services include assistance with job counseling and testing, job placement, assistance with resumes, interview skills training, and payments for job accommodations, training, educational programs, and travel. The Social Security Disability Insurance (SSDI) return to work program allows workers to retain their health benefits while transitioning to employment (74). When it appears that an individual with arthritis has impairments and functional limitations that ultimately preclude his ability to safely and effectively maintain employment, a disability application can be initiated. The Social Security Administration (SSA) defines disability as "the inability to engage in any substantial gainful activity by reason of any medically determinable physical or medical impairment which can be expected to result in death or which has lasted or can be expected to last for a continuous period of not less than 12 months" (75). The determination of disability is complex, not simply a result of a specific medical or physical impairment but a combination of physical, economic, social, and educational factors (76,77). Patients or physicians may initiate the process of disability by calling the SSA (1-800-772-1213). A specific history and physical examination is required in order to assess disease-specific disability criteria. The basics of the requisite examination are outlined in the medical evaluation form that is sent to the managing physician. The physician is required to document specifics about the history and physical examination but does not determine whether or not a patient receives disability. That determination is made at the SSA, minimizing potential conflicts between the physician and patient. Social, educational, and economic criteria are used in addition to those that are medically related in the determination of disability.

Although frank malingering is unusual, some patients may exaggerate their limitations in order to obtain disability benefits. This is particularly true in cases of worker's compensation, ongoing litigation, or other secondary-gain circumstances. Characteristics of persons with secondary gain include inconsistencies in their history and physical examination, excessive documentation of care, the use of multiple providers, anger, and symptom magnification. Symptom magnification, however, may be present in many other circumstances, such as in cases of depression and stress, and may not be indicative of malingering.

Alternative Medicine

Many patients today inquire about and participate in alternative treatments that include alternative medical systems, body work, mind-body interventions, and massage (78,79). In an outpatient telephone survey of six outpatient sites, approximately two thirds of the respondents had used complementary and alternative medicine therapies with only half discussing these with their physician (79). During patient visits, healthcare providers must ask if the patient is using alternative treatments in order to evaluate any potential harmful interactions. In alternative medical or healing systems, a model of the healing process includes remedies of different methods that may or may not be related to conventional Western practices. Examples of methods used for centuries in certain cultures include traditional Chinese, Ayurvedic (from India), and Native American medicine.

Body work encompasses the popular treatments of acupuncture, massage, craniosacral therapy, and structural integration (Rolfing) (78). These therapies are thought to improve the body by direct therapist-patient contact and manipulating the musculoskeletal system. Acupuncture involves the insertion of thin, noncutting, nonhollow needles into designated acupuncture points (or meridians) with manual manipulation or electrical current application (78, 80). Clinical studies supporting the use of acupuncture have been limited and are mostly case reports. However, a number of clinical trials have been performed demonstrating effectiveness in the treatment of musculoskeletal conditions (80). Christensen and colleagues report that acupuncture produces short-term improvement in pain and function for patients with severe knee OA as compared with a control cohort (81). This result is disputed in another trial using a placebo acupuncture group (82). In a randomized, controlled trial using relevant and irrelevant acupuncture cohorts compared with a nonsteroidal antiinflammatory control group, the individuals in the relevant acupuncture group had significantly greater pre- and posttreatment improvements in myofascial neck pain (83). In a review by Fargas-Babjak, the effectiveness of acupuncture for short- to long-term treatment of chronic pain was contradictory (84). Gaw and colleagues compared 40 patients with OA (hip, knee, cervical spine, fingers, or back) receiving either correct or incorrect acupuncture techniques (85). The treatment group had significantly decreased tenderness, pain, and increased physical activity levels.

Massage is thought to be generally safe and involves techniques that mobilize the skin and soft tissues (fascia, muscles) to relieve muscle spasms, pain, and stiffness. Patients usually find massage beneficial and pain relieving. Contraindications typically include applying pressure over areas of acute inflammation, skin infection, fracture, burns, venous thrombosis, and active cancerous tumors (86). In an extensive review by Furlan et al., massage was found to be superior to inert treatment, especially when combined with exercises and education (87). Massage was found to be inferior to manipulation. Finally, acupuncture massage was thought to be better than traditional Swedish massage.

Mind-body interventions include yoga, relaxation, and visualization. Yoga is an ancient technique originally from India that involves a combination of physical strength, flexibility, breathing techniques, meditation, and relaxation poses (78,88). In a randomized, controlled trial for individuals with hand OA, yoga at 60 minutes per week for 8 weeks has been found to increase activity and finger range of motion, as well as decrease tenderness (88). Pranayama yoga uses slow breathing techniques. Other studies on the benefits of yoga have focused on individuals with asthma, diabetes, hypertension, lipid profiles, and mood or vitality disorders (4). More studies are needed at this time, especially randomized, controlled trials with larger sample sizes, longer follow-up periods, and evaluation of long-term effects on musculoskeletal conditions. Relaxation is practiced to subjectively decrease arousal for conditions such as anxiety and stress. Visualization or guided imagery techniques produce psychological improvement through imagining a mental picture of what change is wanted and then producing it in the mind.

REHABILITATION STRATEGIES FOR OSTEOARTHRITIS AND OTHER NONINFLAMMATORY REGIONAL CONDITIONS

OA is a degenerative disorder of the joints, characterized by progressive loss of hyaline cartilage, overgrowth of subchondral bone, and atrophy and weakness of the periarticular muscles. It is an extraordinarily common disorder, perhaps affecting up to 40 million persons in the United States alone. OA may be responsible for over 10% of physician visits per year. The incidence of severe OA rises proportionately with increasing age and is a leading cause of impairment and functional limitations along with work disability in older adults (89). Studies have estimated that 70% of individuals over the age of 65 have radiographic evidence of OA. Both pharmacologic and nonpharmacologic treatments have been shown to be useful. Pharmacotherapy is aimed at reducing pain and inflammation when present. Rehabilitative techniques focus on exercise (to restore motion, strength, and endurance), superficial modalities, adaptive equipment and assistive devices, and education and counseling (90). Focusing of rehabilitation effects on regional body areas and active patient participation maximizes time utilization and goal orientation to decrease patient symptoms, increase function, and improve well-being.

Rehabilitation Interventions: General Concepts

Weight Loss

Obesity is a well-known risk factor for OA of the knee, but has not yet been established as a risk factor for hip OA.

Population studies report that obesity increases the risk for knee OA four to five times in individuals with body mass indexes (BMIs) of 30 to 35 (91). Framingham Study cohort data suggest that overweight individuals, particularly women, are more likely to develop knee OA (91). It has been demonstrated that obesity precedes OA and increases progression rates (91). Similarly, weight loss of even 12 pounds appears to reduce the incidence of symptomatic knee OA (92). In an 18-month randomized, single-blinded controlled trial of a combination of diet and exercise in obese, older adults with knee OA, the experimental group experienced the most positive effect on health-related quality of life not mediated by BMI or gender (93). Recent twin studies discovered a strong association between a high BMI and knee OA not mediated by genetic factors (94). Furthermore, the twins in the study did not have a greater prevalence of knee OA compared with the general population. In general, weight loss and exercise should be a standard recommendation of any arthritis treatment program.

Exercise

OA patients commonly incorrectly respond to their symptoms by limiting physical activity. The result is restricted joint ROM and disuse atrophy. This, in turn, promotes atrophy of cartilage and thinning of bone. Joint integrity is then further compromised, and pain ensues. Exercise is an extraordinarily promising avenue to reverse these physical impairments and functional limitations present in persons with OA. Often, it is difficult to exercise since the weight-bearing joints are affected, but exercise has been shown in numerous studies of patients with degenerative and inflammatory arthritis to reduce pain, assist in weight loss, and improve aerobic conditioning (5,95). Aquatic therapy is an option for individuals who need gravity relief and protection from fall injuries. Regular dynamic exercise is associated with increased blood flow and improved cartilage health, as well as increased ROM, strength, and periarticular muscle endurance. Exercise programs have been shown to improve flexibility, strength, endurance, function, cardiovascular fitness, and general health status without aggravation of arthritis symptoms or pathology (6,35,96). Dance-based aerobic exercise programs reduce pain and disability in persons with RA and OA (6). In contrast to previous recommendations against such exercise, aggressive muscle strengthening and endurance exercises improve strength, endurance, and function and reduce pain without significant exacerbation of disease (97,98). Cross-training techniques can prevent overuse injuries, decrease boredom, and, hopefully, increase patient participation.

Through amelioration of biomechanical and other periarticular soft tissue abnormalities, such as reversing a knee flexion contracture, exercise can substantially reduce pain. Tight, inflexible, and weak soft tissues are prone to injury and pain. Flexible, fatigue-resistant muscles function as more efficient shock absorbers, dampening the impact of force across the joint. Exercise protects joints by conditioning periarticular muscles to provide stability, strength, endurance, and power to avoid injury. However, caution should be used in strengthening quadriceps muscles in malaligned or lax knees due to the increased likelihood of tibiofemoral OA progression without correcting for these factors (99). Exercise-provided pain relief has been shown to be comparable with pharmacologic treatment and has the added benefits of improved physical functioning without medication-related side effects (100). Other potential gains of aerobic and strengthening activities include improved mood and stress reduction (100). Patient and physician-set goals should be attainable and may help improve adherence.

Modalities

Heat

The efficacy of heat modalities, either superficial or deep heat, in OA has not been proven. Ultrasonography, an example of deep heat, offered no additional benefits when used to facilitate standard physical therapy in the treatment of arthritic knee flexion contractures (57). Another example of deep heat is short-wave diathermy. Contraindications to the use of deep heat include the presence of reduced sensation, bleeding, severe inflammation, tumors, open or cavitary lesions, and fractures. Superficial heat such as moist or dry hot-packs applied for 15 to 30 minutes at a time are a common method for treating musculoskeletal disorders. Commonly, therapists will apply heat before stretching exercises to improve collagen elasticity, and then cold after exercises to decrease muscle soreness and pain (101). Heat is thought to reduce pain and muscle spasm and facilitate soft tissue stretching (52,102) by increasing blood flow to the skin and joint while diminishing joint stiffness (4).

Electrical Stimulation

The use of TENS in OA is controversial, with some studies indicating efficacy and others failing to demonstrate improvement compared with controls (i.e., mechanical massage, sham TENS, low-intensity TENS, electroacupuncture) (52,103). Most of the pain relief that did occur during the treatment sessions did not persist.

Cold

Cold therapy is useful in the initial treatment of painful acute musculoskeletal syndromes, such as spasm, soft tissue injury, and postoperative conditions. Again, application of cold to muscles is beneficial after strenuous exercise to decrease pain and muscle spasms (101). Its effect on joint temperature in OA has been debated (52).

Orthoses and Assistive Devices

The use of a cane or walking aid can decrease the joint compressive force generated by the ipsilateral hip abductor muscle contraction when used in the contralateral hand. Contralateral cane placement offers more load reduction than ipsilateral application. This load reduction is associated with pain relief in the affected joint (104). There are different types of canes available, such as the simple straight C-canes, functional grip canes, and quad canes. Tibial axial strain rates during walking, measured by percutaneous extensometers implanted 4 mm within the cortical bone, were significantly lowered by both ipsilateral and contralateral cane usage compared with no cane usage (105).

Patients with spine, hip, and knee OA frequently report that cushioned heel pads help reduce joint pain while walking (66). Foot orthotics, such as a total contact arch support with a medial wedge, can reduce knee pain in a patient with genu valgus and a pes planus deformity (64,65). Lateral-wedged insoles, at 5 to 10 degrees, can significantly decrease knee varus torque and associated pain in patients with medial compartment knee OA (106). An elastic knee sleeve used around an arthritic knee commonly reduces knee pain, despite the absence of demonstrable biomechanical reasons for this effect. It is thought that the sleeves may improve joint proprioception, warmth, or alter joint loading (104). Rigid knee orthoses are not well tolerated in patients with knee arthritis and instability or angular deformities. Obese individuals may not be able to don and keep a knee orthotic in proper position due to body habitus, and, thus, may need a restricting knee ankle-foot-orthosis, which is often not well tolerated. Medially taping the patella may help reduce anterior knee pain from patellofemoral syndrome, which is commonly associated with knee OA (107). This technique has been associated with superior pain relief when compared with lateral or neutral taping (107). Thus, orthotics and walking aids have the potential to provide pain relief and functional improvement when used in combination with other interventions, such as exercise and medications.

Psychological Therapies

Cognitive-Behavioral Therapies

CBTs are used to help patients understand how their thoughts, beliefs, expectations, and behaviors potentially impact their experience of pain. CBTs offer patients specific tools, such as distraction, imagery, pacing skills, and goal setting to give them control over their pain experience. Although there are clear benefits of CBT training with regard to improving pain as well as physical and psychological disability, these may tend to diminish over time without reinforcement. Involving a patient's family strengthens the social support system, which may help patients maintain gains for longer periods of time. Clinical research is needed to clarify which components of a CBT program are the most helpful, and how to match the timing of CBT with an individual patient's readiness to change (108). Coping skills training has been shown to reduce self-rated pain and psychological symptoms in persons will knee OA (109). The Arthritis Self-Management Program (ASMP), designed to improve coping skills through self-efficacy training, appears to reduce pain and arthritis-related physician visits (110). Telephone-based interventions that review educational information, medications, and problem-solving techniques have also been shown to reduce pain and improve function without substantially increasing costs (68).

Systemic Impairments and Limitations

Pain

A remarkable feature of OA is the lack of a strong correlation between symptoms and radiographic or clinical examination findings. Less than half of those with radiographic findings consistent with OA have corresponding symptoms. The specific factors that lead to painful OA are not clearly understood (90). In a large, prospective study of individuals with and without radiographic knee OA, psychological well-being and health status were important predictors of knee pain, independent of radiographic severity (111).

The synovial tissue and subchondral bone are thought to be less sensitive to pain than other articular structures. The development of osteophytes can cause pain through periosteal elevation. Bone cysts have the potential for causing pain, but there does not yet seem to be a radiographic correlation between the presence of bone cysts and pain (112). Increased growth in the subchondral cancellous bone can cause intraosseous venous engorgement and medullary hypertension, which have been shown to correlate with complaints of pain (113).

Extraarticular pain is a common phenomenon in OA. Bursae, tendons, entheses, and muscles are all supplied with nociceptors. Pain in or surrounding an arthritic joint may be only partially related, or even completely unrelated, to the articular pathology. Tendonitis, bursitis, and muscular strains and sprains are common impairments in persons with arthritic joints. Treatment of these conditions frequently ameliorates pain and functional limitations; the radiographic findings attributable to arthritis may have simply been incidental. Similarly, recent-onset biomechanical abnormalities around an arthritic joint, such as a knee flexion contracture, may convert a previously nonpainful, arthritic joint into a painful one. Reversing these impairments frequently alleviates pain, irrespective of the degree of radiographic joint abnormality. Treatment of pain symptoms in arthritis is always based on history and physical examination, not radiographic abnormalities.

Depression

Consistent with findings in many chronic diseases, persons with OA exhibit higher rates of depression than the general population. Overall, nearly 14% of persons with osteoarthritis report levels on the Arthritis Impact Measurement Scale (AIMS) consistent with probable depression. Depression rates are 17% in those with hip or knee OA and 23% in persons with neck involvement (114). Persons with arthritis (all types) have a significantly increased adjusted prevalence of past psychiatric disorders (affective, substance use, and anxiety) (115). Therefore, the management of OA should include screening for depression, which should also be addressed in the treatment plan.

Deconditioning

As noted elsewhere, physical deconditioning is common in OA and warrants treatment with exercise and physical therapy.

Hip Impairments and Limitations

The accurate diagnosis of hip region pain depends on a comprehensive history and careful musculoskeletal examination. The differential diagnosis includes articular hip pathology, bursitis and other soft tissue disorders, lumbar spine disease, abdominal tumors or infections involving the iliopsoas, referred pain from other joints such as the knee, and, occasionally, pelvic bony tumors or infection.

Osteoarthritic pain originating from the hip is insidious in onset, described as an aching discomfort in the groin, buttock, or lateral thigh, and exacerbated by weight-bearing activities and movement of the hip. Physical findings include hip flexion contracture (positive Thomas test); painful and limited passive/active ROM of the hip (particularly extension and internal rotation); weakness of hip musculature, especially the hip abductors (confirmed via positive Trendelenburg/single-leg stance test); leg length discrepancy; and, frequently, an antalgic gait with shortened stance and stride length, limited active hip flexion, lumbar spine hyperlordosis, and the characteristic abductor lurch gait. Patients with unilateral hip OA often compensate for the decreased hip motion by increasing pelvic mobility in the frontal and sagittal planes to decrease gait deviations and improve reduced walking speeds (116).

Therapeutic Interventions

The hip rehabilitation program is specific to the impairments identified. The prescription includes aerobic conditioning, muscle strengthening, ROM exercises, orthotics, functional training, ambulation aides, and education regarding proper body mechanics and energy conservation. Individuals with arthritis (all types) have exhibited decreased aerobic conditioning compared with age-matched normal subjects. Aerobic conditioning programs have resulted in improved aerobic capacity, 50-foot walk times, and scores for depression and anxiety in subjects with OA (5). In general, physical training programs should include 30 to 40 minutes of aerobic exercise (with warm-up and cool-down periods), maintaining a target heart rate or perceived exertion level, three to four times weekly. Aerobic conditioning programs should be of low impact, such as swimming or walking.

Strengthening exercises focus on the hip and lower back musculature, particularly the hip abductors and extensors. Active hip abductor strengthening exercises include side-lying leg lifts, prone "skateboard" abduction exercises, and standing abduction exercises. Weights to increase resistance are added according to patient tolerance. Hip extensors can be strengthened in supine or standing positions. Stretching exercises are exceedingly important, particularly in abduction and extension. Patients should lie prone daily for a few minutes to stretch hip flexors. Trunk strengthening and stretching exercises, shoe orthotics, and functional gait training are also important. Exercising in the pool is an efficient means of increasing strength, ROM, and endurance in a pain-free environment for those who fear falling and its related complications.

Educating the OA patient about energy conservation and joint protection completes the prescription. A referral to an occupational therapist will assist in evaluation of ADL performance and provision of necessary equipment along with the joint protection strategies (117). Understanding the hip joint as a simple lever system can direct the prescription of techniques to prevent abnormally high forces being distributed across the hip. For example, the loss of 1 pound of body weight translates to a 3-pound reduction in force distributed by the abductors. Use of a cane in the opposite hand acts to reduce the force generated by the abductors. Similarly, when reaching down to pick up an item, patients should support their weight on the contralateral hand (e.g., on a dresser) and lift with the ipsilateral hand. Heavy loads should be carried with two hands if possible, otherwise by the ipsilateral hand. These maneuvers tend to move the patient's center of mass toward the affected hip, thus reducing the need for the ipsilateral hip abductors to generate compressive and painful hip forces. Evaluation and issue of ambulation aides, such as canes, can be beneficial to decrease both the load throughout the joint and the pull of ipsilateral hip abductor muscles. Proper cane length is measured to the height of the patient's greater trochanter, allowing for approximately 20 degrees of elbow flexion. Adaptive equipment, including long-handled sponges, reachers, sock-donners, elevated toilet seats, grab bars, shower bench, and seat cushions may ease the performance of several functional tasks.

Knee Impairments and Limitations

The physical impairments common to individuals with knee OA include decreased aerobic capacity; muscle weakness, particularly of the hamstrings and quadriceps; decreased knee flexion and extension; gait disturbance; abnormal mechanical alignment with varus, valgus, and knee flexion deformities; other joint pathology such as OA of the hips, spine, or feet; and, potentially, neurologic disturbances, such as impaired sensation or proprioception.

The most common basic functional limitations in individuals with knee arthritis are difficulty walking for long distances or on uneven surfaces, climbing stairs, arising from low surfaces, kneeling, and performing lower extremity dressing. Knee stiffness after sitting for prolonged periods is common; this usually improves with warm-up stretches before moving. Patients often have difficulties performing more physically demanding tasks, such as housework, gardening, recreational sports, and carrying heavy objects.

Therapeutic Interventions

Rehabilitation goals include the improvement of physical symptoms, the correction of functional deficits, and improvement of quality of life. Referral to physical and occupational therapists will assist the patient in incorporating exercise and correct biomechanics. The challenge is motivating the individual to incorporate and integrate physical activity consistently into daily life in order to maintain gained benefits (118,119). In a prospective study, individually tailored physical therapy was shown to benefit those with severe OA of the knees, with improvements observed in strength, endurance, stair climbing, arising from a chair, pain, and walking ability (120). This section describes the common components of a rehabilitation prescription for knee OA.

Active-assisted and active ROM exercises are generally helpful. Because passive ROM exercise was reported to induce inflammation in canine knee joints with crystal-induced synovitis, vigorous passive stretching is usually not prescribed for patients with warm, swollen joints in the acute stage. Modalities applied beforehand, such as superficial or deep heat and cold, help patients tolerate the discomfort associated with ROM exercises.

Historically, the literature has suggested that high-resistance exercises increase strain on articular tissues and that certain types of exercise (particularly isotonic and isokinetic) are unsafe for individuals with arthritis or unstable joints. Consequently, initial muscle strengthening has traditionally been limited to isometric or isotonic programs with 1- to 2-pound weights. More recent studies seem to contradict this notion. In a rigorous, prospective, randomized trial, Fisher et al. (120) reported increased strength, endurance, and speed, with no adverse effects after a 16-week muscle-strengthening and endurance program in 15 subjects with advanced OA of the knee. In another 16-week randomized, controlled trial comparing dynamic versus isometric resistance training, both groups had improved functional ability and decreased knee pain compared with the control group (121).

In contrast to the traditional "open-chain" isotonic and isometric exercises, where the feet are not touching any surfaces, closed kinetic chain exercises are performed with the joint above (hip) and the joint below (ankle) "loaded." Standing and weight-shifting exercises that stress the various muscle groups around the knee are examples. These exercises are well tolerated by patients and may be quite beneficial in improving strength and reducing pain.

When a varus or valgus deformity is present, selected medial or lateral quadriceps strengthening exercises may be prescribed. Patients are taught to isolate and strengthen their medial or lateral quadriceps using electrical stimulation or surface electromyography for biofeedback. This treatment is commonly prescribed for patients with disproportionately weakened medial quadriceps and patellar subluxation.

Therapy to ameliorate functional limitations includes gait training and core strengthening, focusing on proper sequencing over both even and uneven surfaces; transfer training, particularly from low chairs, bathtubs, and cars; stair climbing; ADLs, focusing on lower extremity dressing and bathing with equipment; and instruction in energy conservation and proper body mechanics. Even though the therapy focus is on the knee and associated periarticular structures, attention must also be directed to pelvic and trunk stabilization and strengthening as part of the kinetic chain. Again, patient use of an ambulation aid, such as a cane in the contralateral hand, will help improve pain and function (117). For patients with balance deficits or disorders or severe knee disease bilaterally, a rolling or standard walker may be a better recommendation.

Foot orthotics are frequently prescribed, but have not been well studied in OA. For example, a medial sole wedge and total contact arch support may be appropriate for the patient with genu valgus and pronated feet. A heel lift may benefit a patient with a fixed knee contracture and apparent leg length discrepancy. Orthotics must be "broken in." Patients are instructed to alternate wearing them and not wearing them every 2 hours so that gradually they build up tolerance. Without this gradual introduction, back, knee, or foot pain as a consequence of the orthotic may be so severe that the patient will abandon the orthotic. Wearing shock-absorbing shoes with insoles is believed to benefit without supporting data (117). Knee orthotics may occasionally be prescribed for the purpose of correcting joint alignment, but rigid orthoses are poorly tolerated in individuals with varus or valgus deformities. Many patients report feeling increased knee stability when wearing an elastic bandage or gauntlet. Although these do not provide objective mechanical stability, the subjective improvement may justify its prescription.

Shoulder Impairments and Limitations

Osteoarthritis of the shoulder, although less common than hip and knee disease, can lead to significant functional limitation and disability, especially on the hand-dominant side. Pain and limitations from shoulder OA are usually a consequence of both articular disease and periarticular disease from overuse and chronic rotator cuff wear

TABLE 38.3. *Common causes of shoulder pain in shoulder osteoarthritis*

Glenohumeral synovitis
Swelling, warmth, and tenderness
Restricted active and passive ROM
Arm splinted in adduction and internal rotation
Glenohumeral degeneration
Muscle atrophy
Restricted ROM, particularly flexion, extension, abduction and minimal to no rotation
Radiographic evidence of cartilage and bone destruction
AC and SC joint degeneration
Shoulder arc painful, limited painful abduction
Tender joint, painful adduction with joint compression
Rotator cuff atrophy/tear/tendinitis
Impaired active abduction with better or full passive ROM
Painful active or restricted abduction, if acute night pain
Radiographs may reveal cephalad migration of humeral head
Arthrography reveals dye passed into bursae if cuff is torn
Impingement syndrome
"Catch" reported between 60 and 70 degrees is maximum at 100 to 120 degrees abduction
Pain with compression of subacrominal tissue occurs at 90 to 100 degrees flexion
Radiographic abnormalities are evident such as osteophytes and acrominal abnormalities
Subacromial/subdeltoid bursitis
Impaired and painful abduction and external rotation
Tenderness over superior lateral shoulder
Swelling, warmth, and erythema
Radiographs usually normal
Adhesive capsulitis
Diffuse pain and stiffness
Glenohumeral tenderness
Reduced passive and active ROM in all planes
Arthrogram may be abnormal with reduced joint volume

AC, acranioclavicular; ROM, range of motion; SC, sternoclavicular.

(Table 38.3). Often, the painful arthritic shoulder exhibits symptoms of multiple, intermingled diagnoses that are not easily separated into distinct clinical entities, such as impingement, rotator cuff injuries, adhesive capsulitis, and acromioclavicular joint injuries (see Chapter 106).

Shoulder dysfunction is primarily related to glenohumeral and acromioclavicular disease. However, the scapula and its associated movements should always be considered as well, since shoulder motion requires coordinated scapulohumeral movement. Other structures to consider in the kinetic chain are the back and lower limbs affecting shoulder movement. Sternoclavicular joint involvement only rarely causes functional limitation. In an attempt to limit shoulder pain of any cause, the patient splints the arm close to the body in adduction and internal rotation, resulting in capsular and ligamentous adhesions that limit range. Joint effusions limit both motion and strength, and occasional capsular ruptures can occur. Destruction of cartilage and subchondral bone causes pain and weakness as a result of reflex inhibition and biomechanical disadvantage. Weakness is exacerbated by muscle atrophy that accompanies disuse and inflammation. Glenohumeral synovitis often coexists with rotator cuff inflammation. Rotator cuff impairments, including tendonitis and tears, may cause profound functional limitations. Patients often report that associated pain is worse at night. Subdeltoid bursitis is a common comorbidity of glenohumeral arthritis and cuff tendonitis that further exacerbates pain and functional limitation. The end result is a patient with a painful shoulder, which cannot forward flex, abduct, or rotate. The patient may complain of difficulty performing functional tasks such as hair washing and styling, upper body dressing, orofacial hygiene, placing or retrieving items on shelves, and carrying heavy items.

Therapeutic Interventions for Acute-Phase Shoulder Impairments

An acutely inflamed or injured shoulder joint will benefit from local rest. The shoulder can be immobilized in an arm sling for 2 or 3 days until inflammation subsides. Prolonged rest is not advised in light of the muscle atrophy and adhesions associated with immobility. Gentle ROM exercises within pain-free arcs are important to minimize joint contractures during the acute inflammatory period. The critical amount of shoulder motion necessary for functional activities is 75 degrees of forward flexion, 75 degrees of abduction, 20 degrees of external rotation, and 45 degrees of internal rotation (9). Repetitive passive ROM probably causes some joint inflammation (122). The risk for joint contracture and muscle atrophy must be weighed against this potential disadvantage. Many clinicians, however, will prescribe gentle passive or active-assisted ROM in all planes of motion at least once daily. Ice application is particularly effective if used after therapy for 15 to 20 minutes. Isometric exercise is often painful during the acute stage of shoulder inflammation, so it is not routinely prescribed.

Therapeutic Interventions for Subacute and Chronic Phase Shoulder Impairments

At this point, the patient should benefit from a referral to physical therapy to learn and incorporate rehabilitation techniques that improve shoulder strength and ROM and prevent further impairments such as adhesive capsulitis. One of the main therapy goals is increasing glenohumeral movement and function with scapular control (123). Closed-chain axial proximal-to-distal kinetic chain exercises of shoulder-activating muscles coupled with scapular integrated patterns are used to achieve this goal. Active-assisted and active ROM exercises can be performed twice daily after analgesics or modalities have minimized pain and controlled inflammation. Movement exercises should focus on forward flexion, abduction, and internal and external rotation. At this early stage of rehabilitation, pendulum exercises are commonly prescribed (slow, progressive shoulder circumduction performed with the patient leaning forward on a chair or table with the arm dangling) and can be enhanced with light wrist weights.

Strengthening exercises, deferred through the acute phase, are then introduced, particularly isometric exercises, which are associated with the least amount of intraarticular pressure and joint stress (124). The patient is taught to contract the shoulder abductors, rotators, flexors, and extensors without limb movement. One set of contractions one or two times daily should be prescribed during the subacute phase. "Wall walking" is a simple, common active-assisted ROM and strengthening exercise used during this phase of recovery. The individual places his hand on the wall with his elbow extended and moves his arm along the wall in different directions.

When pain is resolved or the shoulder reaches maximal resolution of inflammation, the clinician should prescribe a comprehensive shoulder rehabilitation program. This program should address ROM, strength, endurance, functional task performance, adaptive equipment, and most importantly, education. Range-of-motion exercises should be prescribed as isolated active abduction, forward flexion, extension, both internal and external rotation, and full shoulder circles. It is imperative to understand the degree of articular damage before prescribing ROM or strengthening exercises. Aggressive stretching or vigorous isotonic strengthening exercises involving the shoulder should not be performed when there is significant joint destruction. Ultrasonography and other deep heat methods used prior to stretching maneuvers may enhance results.

When the joint space is relatively well preserved, strengthening exercise prescription should progress to more vigorous isometrics or isotonics. High-resistance, low-repetition isotonic exercises are probably not appropriate for arthritis patients because of the significant force distributed through the joints during these exercises (125). Light-weight repetitive exercises (using 1- to 2-pound cuff weights on the wrists), through a limited arc of motion, performed to the point of fatigue, are prescribed instead (125). This method of muscle strengthening probably produces comparable results without the consequent high levels of joint stress (126). Isokinetic exercises are not usually recommended for individuals with arthritis because of their associated high levels of joint stress. Isotonic exercise has been shown to be as effective as isokinetic exercise for muscle strengthening (127).

Endurance exercise should be prescribed to maximize overall health status, cardiovascular conditioning, and sense of well-being. Swimming is a particularly good endurance and strengthening activity for arthritis patients with shoulder impairments. Aerobic exercise should be performed at least three times weekly to obtain optimal cardiovascular results.

Functional limitations must be addressed. Adaptive equipment, such as dressing sticks or buttonhooks, will help the individual perform the simple ADLs that have been affected by shoulder immobility. In addition, compensatory techniques for achieving ADL performance can be learned from an occupational therapist. Environmental modifications, such as lowering the height of shelves and replacing doorknobs with levers can enhance independent function.

REHABILITATION STRATEGIES FOR RHEUMATOID ARTHRITIS AND OTHER INFLAMMATORY PERIPHERAL ARTHROPATHIES

Rheumatoid arthritis can be a devastating illness. The mortality of RA may be compared with that of diabetes (128). The typical outpatient with RA has a one-in-four chance of moderate-to-severe functional limitation. Nearly 50% of individuals who are employed at the time of diagnosis will find themselves out of the work force within 5 years due to joint destruction and deformity. Unfortunately, those with RA who do manage to continue working earn 50% to 75% less income compared with their age-matched controls (129). Rehabilitative therapies should be used early to help limit and prevent the severe physical impairments and functional limitations that occur from RA (130,131).

The cornerstones for the management of active RA are medications; joint immobilization to suppress synovitis locally; physical activity, including planned exercise to maintain joint motion, strength, and cardiovascular endurance; functional training, including the use of adaptive and assistive devices; education in joint protection, energy conservation, disease self-management; orthotics; environmental modification; and psychosocial, vocational, and avocational interventions. First and foremost, inflammation must be suppressed, because this is the cause of joint destruction and systemic deterioration. Once active inflammation is controlled, the rehabilitative measures described in the following sections will be most useful.

Systemic Impairments and Their Treatment

Fatigue

Fatigue is a complex perception arising from a combination of psychological, physiologic, and environmental factors. Fatigue is reported in about 90% of persons with RA (132). Pain, sleep disturbance, inactivity, and comorbidities contribute to the experience of fatigue. Muscle atrophy and deconditioning are also significant contributing factors. Similarly, the treatment of fatigue is therefore multifaceted, and includes control of inflammation, self-efficacy training, energy conservation technique instruction, measures to enhance restorative sleep, and regular physical activity and exercise (132).

Cardiorespiratory and Motor Deconditioning

Physical deconditioning is common in RA. Inflammation, reflex muscle inhibition from pain, neuropathies, myopathies, malnutrition, and disuse lead to muscle wasting.

RA cachexia reduces energy supply, limiting energy available for activity (133). Pain, depression, and fatigue limit motivation to be physically active. Recommended guidelines for physical activity in the general population are to accumulate 30 minutes of moderate-intensity physical activity [3.0–6.0 metabolic equivalents (METS)] on most days of the week (43). However, even low levels of physical activity impart significant benefits Thus, interventions tailored to move sedentary persons with arthritis out of the "sedentary" category stand to accrue physical activity benefits, even if they can only achieve less than the recommended levels of physical activity. Ideally, a physical activity program that enhances aerobic fitness should be incorporated into all treatment programs for RA. Recent evidence indicates that vigorous physical activity can lead to improved pain and functional outcomes for RA patients (14,134), and that improved outcomes of exercise programs are sustained after 1 year of follow-up (135). The bone mineral density of women with RA on low-dose prednisone can also be improved with regular exercise (32). Strength training has been shown to improve strength, disease activity, functional capacity, and bone mineral density in patients with early RA (136,137). New evidence continues to support the proposition that increasing physical activity behavior can be done without exacerbating RA (138). The challenge is helping sedentary patients change their behavior such that they can benefit from increased levels of physical activity (139).

Insomnia

Pain, morning stiffness, fatigue, limited daily activities, and other phenomena can lead to sleep disturbances in patients with RA. These are classified as dyssomnias (disorders of initiating or maintaining sleep, or of excessive sleepiness), parasomnias (sleepwalking, bruxism), sleep disorders associated with medical conditions (alcoholism, asthma, gastroesophageal reflux disease), and other unclassified disorders. Treatment is first aimed at the underlying cause. Education regarding good sleep hygiene principles (such as establishing regular nighttime rituals), behavioral therapies (stimulus control and relaxation training), and pharmacologic interventions (such as sedating tricyclic antidepressants) help facilitate restorative sleep (140).

Depression

Depression is a common comorbidity in patients with RA, a consequence of the complex psychosocial and physical manifestations of this chronic disease. Reported rates of depression in RA range from 10% to over 80%, with severe depression noted in approximately 20% (74,141,142).

Depression alone may be a significant predictor of functional limitation in RA, and must be approached as aggressively as any other impairment affecting function (143). The diagnosis of depression requires a thorough history, physical, and mental status examination augmented by the use of psychological tests. Referral to a psychologist or psychiatrist may be warranted to assist in diagnosis and treatment. A patient's initial complaints may be neurovegetative (e.g., poor appetite, impaired sleep, fatigue), and are easily confused with increased disease activity. Once diagnosed, major depression in RA appears to respond to aggressive treatment with antidepressants and psychotherapy; milder forms may also respond to antidepressants. Pain relief may accompany the pharmacologic, cognitive, and behavioral interventions used in treatment of depression since there are common underlying neurochemical mechanisms (71,141).

Regional and Anatomic Impairments and Functional Limitations

Ankle and Foot Impairments and Functional Limitations

The sequelae of ankle and foot pathology relate more to capsular malfunction than to bony destruction. Intertarsal, metatarsal, and phalangeal movement occur as a result of synovial proliferation with subsequent capsular weakening and ligamentous laxity. The forefoot initially undergoes changes at the metatarsal and proximal interphalangeal (PIP) joints. Loss of fat pads, abnormal long tendon forces, and involvement of the intrinsic and lumbrical muscles and toe flexors lead to toe abnormalities such as metatarsophalangeal hyperextension, PIP flexion deformities, and hammer toes. Hallux valgus results from a laterally directed force at the great toe, causing it to overlap the second. This results in a medial outpouching of the proximal first metatarsal head, pronation of the great toe phalanx, plantar migration of the abductor hallucis muscle, and asymmetric medial capsule weakening. Progressive skin irritation leads to callous and bunion formation. The development of hallux valgus is associated with spreading of the metatarsal ligaments, which increases vulnerability to pressure on interdigital nerves, particularly between the third and fourth metatarsal head, resulting in metatarsalgia. Ankle instability results from synovitis, capsular weakness, and tenosynovitis (particularly the Achilles and tibialis posterior tendons). Talocalcaneal valgus results in rotational and subluxing moments on the navicular head (also affected by tenosynovitis of the tibialis posterior muscle) and subtalar pronation. Because of this excessive pronation, the foot is less able to transform into the rigid structure necessary for proper push-off during ambulation. This makes the foot less capable of tolerating weight bearing and propulsion. These biomechanical abnormalities may lead to plantar fasciitis.

Tarsal tunnel syndrome, characterized by dysesthetic pain in the toes, sole, and heel, is not uncommon, resulting from tenosynovitis of the tibialis posterior, flexor digitorum longus, and flexor hallucis longus (90).

Therapeutic Interventions for Ankle and Foot Impairments

Orthotics and Shoe Management

The goals of orthotic and footwear prescriptions are relief of pain and normalization of limb biomechanics. Up to 90% of RA patients have foot involvement during the course of the disease, with 15% to 20% presenting with foot symptoms at disease onset. Well-designed orthotics can correct common calcaneal eversion and subtalar pronation. An ankle-foot orthosis (AFO) can be used to reduce pain and improve gait by immobilizing an ankle with chronic effusion and structural pathology.

Critical shoe structural components are those that potentially cause compression, specifically the toe box, heel counter, and vamp. A softer material is needed for shoe fabrication to accommodate abnormal foot anatomy. Shoes should have high and broad toe boxes, wide vamps, and nonconstraining heel counters to maximize inner shoe volumes and decrease metatarsal apposition. The sole of the shoe can be modified by the use of (a) a proximally placed metatarsal bar to relieve pressure on painful metatarsals, (b) a built-up lateral or medial undersurface to create a valgus or varus moment on the ankle, or (c) a rocker sole to alleviate metatarsal pressure, thus making the push-off phase of gait more comfortable and efficient (144).

Thermal Modalities

Superficial heat or cold applications penetrate the foot–ankle complex well. Thermal modalities with deeper penetration potential are used to improve connective tissue elasticity prior to stretching, and should be used cautiously in patients with acute inflammation, arterial disease, or sensory loss. Cold applications may be better tolerated if stroked or rubbed on, as opposed to continuous application. Patients should be cautioned about protecting the skin with a layer of cloth (such as a towel) before applying either thermal modality at home.

Exercise

Exercise prescription can be useful for reducing symptoms in the presence of foot and ankle impairments. The prescription should include (a) passive stretching of the Achilles and the peronei tendons, (b) active ROM exercises targeting the ankle and subtalar joints, (c) isometric exercises of the muscles of the anterior compartment, (d) concentric isotonic exercises of the posterior and anterior tibialis muscles from the elongated position, and (e) eccentric training of the gastroc-soleus complex and peronei muscles from the shortened position (90).

Knee Impairments and Functional Limitations

Knee synovitis leads to (a) increased nociceptive reflex associated with capsular distention, causing hamstring spasm and quadriceps inhibition; (b) deterioration of menisci, cruciate ligaments, and articular cartilage, resulting in knee instability, locking or catching sensations, and pain; (c) progressive synovial hypertrophy (pannus), which causes a physical impediment to motion that can progress to ankylosis; (d) posterior joint capsule, gastrocnemius, and semimembranosus tendon inflammation that may erode the bursa until it is confluent with the joint capsule, causing a Baker cyst; and (e) mechanical malalignment, such as genu varus, valgus, and flexion deformities.

Therapeutic Interventions for Knee Impairments

Acute Inflammatory Phase

1. *Orthotics.* Weight bearing should be minimized. A resting splint, such as a soft knee immobilizer, may be used to provide maximal extension and facilitate local joint rest. Pillows under the knee should be avoided when the orthotic is removed to minimize the risk for knee flexion contracture.
2. *Modalities.* Brief applications of cold modalities are best tolerated during acute inflammation. Frozen vegetable packages (which will provide natural thawing) are convenient. The use of superficial, moist heat can also provide patient comfort. Again, patients should be instructed to first place a towel or other piece of cloth on the skin to protect it from direct contact with the thermal modality.
3. *Exercise.* Quadriceps strength must be maintained through performance of isometric exercises (e.g., "quad sets"). Isotonic or isokinetic exercises are not recommended in the acute phase.

Subacute or Chronic Inflammatory Phase

Once the inflammatory process has been suppressed, the principles of specific joint rehabilitation for patients with RA resemble those of OA. Particular problems related to deformity and laxity are addressed below.

1. *Orthotics and assistive devices.* Chronic daytime use of knee orthoses is poorly tolerated by patients with long-standing arthritis. If a persistent knee flexion contracture occurs, a soft knee immobilizer or, in cases of hamstring tightness, an adjustable or spring-assisted knee extension orthosis may be worn at night.

If a valgus knee deformity exists, an ankle-foot orthotic may be prescribed to decrease the pronation moment at the subtalar joint. Additionally, building up the medial aspect of the foot creates a varus moment at the ankle and a varus moment at the knee. These are most successful in relieving pain if the medial knee compartment is relatively intact.

2. *Adaptive equipment.* Long-handled dressing equipment, such as a "sock-aid" or "reacher," will facilitate lower body dressing in the presence of a stiff knee. Elevated toilet seats and bath benches promote safety and independence in toileting and bathing.

3. *Assistive devices.* Canes, walkers, and crutches decrease the force on the knee during ambulation, and their use is encouraged.

4. *Thermal modalities.* In addition to the modalities listed for use in the acute phase, ultrasonography may be used when inflammation is not active and tissue stretching is desired. Transcutaneous nerve stimulation may be considered to assist with pain management for patients who are intolerant or refractory to oral analgesic agents. Topical capsaicin is a pharmacologic alternative for pain management.

5. *Exercise.* Generalized limb strengthening with a focus on the quadriceps should be performed through isotonic open-chain exercises, progressing to closed-chain concentric (muscle-shortening or -accelerating contraction) and eccentric (muscle-lengthening or -decelerating contraction) exercises. Stair-climbing exercises and inclined treadmill exercises may result in anterior knee pain syndromes and therefore should be avoided. Aquatic exercises facilitate aerobic training, but are not efficient in quadriceps-specific strengthening. For knee flexion contractures, slow hamstring stretching exercises are best tolerated, especially when preceded by superficial or deep heat.

6. *Energy conservation/joint protection.* Individuals may benefit from a referral to an occupational therapist to learn techniques for more efficient performance of ADLs, as well as strategies to conserve energy and minimize joint stress for their most important tasks. For example, repeated stair climbing (which greatly increases force on the knee) should be avoided; items can be safely stored in special baskets made for the stairs, and then transported upstairs in fewer trips (90).

Hip Impairments and Functional Limitations

The hip is involved in about 50% of individuals with RA. Articular cartilage loss occurs symmetrically, on both the femoral and acetabular surfaces, in contrast to the more focal deficits seen in OA. The femoral head may collapse, leading to bony ankylosis. Osteonecrosis of the femoral head may occur in patients after long-term corticosteroid treatment.

As the disease progresses, clinical symptoms become more pronounced, with increasing groin pain, joint stiffness, difficulty with ADLs, and antalgic gait development.

Therapeutic Interventions for Hip Impairments

1. *Orthotics and assistive devices.* Bracing of the hip joint is complicated by its proximal body position, difficulty with fitting supporting belts, and significant force generation across the joint. However, the use of ambulatory aids, such as a walker or cane, can provide considerable pain and biomechanical relief during gait. Patients with both upper and lower limb joint pathology may find platform walkers easier to use than standard walkers.

2. *Adaptive equipment.* Elevated toilet seats, bath chairs, safety rails, and raised seat cushions on chairs facilitate independent ADL performance for patients with hip disease by allowing for avoidance of painful hip positions during these activities. In addition, long-handled devices to assist with lower limb dressing and bathing compensate for limited hip motion and facilitate independence.

3. *Thermal modalities.* Superficial heat or cold may relieve the pain of superficial structures (such as trochanteric bursitis), but does not directly affect intrinsic joint pathology. In the absence of acute inflammation, ultrasonography may be used to facilitate soft tissue stretching around the joint.

4. *Exercise (acute stages).* Resting the joint with the patient in the prone position will help prevent hip flexion contractures. Alternatively, resting in the supine position with pillows under the buttocks to extend the hip without flexing the knee is recommended. Simple isometric contraction of hip musculature is also recommended to prevent disuse atrophy.

5. *Exercise (subacute and chronic stages).* Aquatic therapy is an excellent medium for isotonic and aerobic exercises. Hip extensors and the abductor muscles should be targeted. The use of stationary cycling, treadmill exercises, and progressive walking are recommended for gaining strength and endurance. Preexercise and postexercise stretching of the lower extremities is necessary.

Cervical Spine Impairments and Functional Limitations

Biomechanical disruption of the cervical spine is a result of elongation and destruction of the ligamentous supporting structures. Of particular importance is the excessive motion and subsequent subluxation of the occiput-atlas-axis complex (Table 38.4). The early recognition of atlantoaxial subluxation is critical. The normal atlantoaxial distance should be less than 3.5 mm, the lateral masses of the atlas-axis should be less than 2 mm apart, and the posterior atlanto-odontoid distance should be greater than 14 mm.

Therapeutic Interventions for Cervical Spine Impairments

1. *Orthotics.* Soft or semirigid cervical collars assist spinal muscles to relax and decrease spasms, but do not restrict motion. More aggressive immobilizing aids (occipital-cervical-thoracic orthoses) are indicated for patients with

TABLE 38.4. *Patterns of atlas-axial subluxation in rheumatoid arthritis*

Anterior: loss of integrity of the transverse and alar ligaments.
Posterior: principally because of erosion and fracture to bony elements creating a backward directional force.
Lateral: abnormal rotational forces theoretically created by both ligamentous and bony destruction.
Vertical: when the occipitoaxial and atlantoaxial joints erode to the point of significant joint space narrowing, the occiput-atlas-axis complex may collapse, resulting in upward migration of the odontoid.

mild subluxation without spinal cord impingement, and should be ordered with orthopedic consultation.

2. *Thermal modalities and traction.* The use of traction or manipulation in RA patients with neck pain is absolutely contraindicated, because occult ligamentous laxity may be present and may therefore threaten neurologic integrity. Superficial heat application or ultrasound modalities often provide welcome relief of the pain associated with tightly bound cervical muscles.

3. *Exercise.* Optimizing cervical ROM is best accomplished by regaining as much scapular and glenohumeral motion as possible. Physical therapists can apply soft tissue mobilization, deep friction rub, or gentle myofascial pain relief methods to assist in attaining this motion. Isometric exercises are performed by gently applying forward, backward, and lateral pressure with resistance from the hand. Isotonic exercise is not recommended.

4. *Energy conservation and joint protection.* Unloading the cervical spine can be accomplished by unweighting the loads carried by the upper limbs and using proper neck biomechanics. Suggested techniques are restricting the amount of weight lifted, lifting objects from a position close to the body, and keeping the neck in neutral positions when bending or performing overhead activities (90).

Wrist and Hand Impairments and Their Treatments

Swan Neck Deformity and Therapeutic Interventions

Swan neck deformity can occur as a result of two pathological processes. In the first process, metacarpophalangeal (MCP) joint synovitis alters the pull of the extensor tendons toward the palm, creating a flexion moment. This results in an unbalanced extensor moment on the PIP joint as the central slips of the extensor tendons become more taut. Subsequently, the distal interphalangeal (DIP) joints go passively into flexion. Alternatively, inflammation of the PIP joint that results in capsular expansion can cause asymmetric weakness on the volar aspect, creating a dorsally directed force on the extensor (lateral) tendon. This promotes an extension moment at the PIP joint and increased tension onto the centrally located flexor digitorum profundus (FDP) tendon, resulting in a DIP joint flexion moment (90).

Therapeutic interventions to reduce deformity include (a) digital massage, which may reduce edema and the risk of fibrous tissue development (but long-term efficacy evidence is lacking); (b) "ring splints," used principally over the PIP joint, are designed to create a flexion moment at the PIP joint, reversing the passive flexion moment at the DIP joint and offsetting MCP joint flexion deformity; and (c) stretching exercises that focus on elongation of intrinsic muscles, thus promoting MCP extension and PIP flexion (90,145,146). Heated paraffin may loosen soft tissue elements and provide transient analgesia before and after massage and stretching exercises.

Boutonniere Deformity and Therapeutic Interventions

Boutonniere deformity is caused by pathology at the PIP joint that results in PIP flexion, DIP extension, and MCP extension. Inflammation of the PIP joint causes joint expansion and overstretching of the joint capsule, which damages the extensor mechanism. This elongation and subsequent weakening of the extensor (central) tendons results in their lateral slippage, creating a flexion moment on the PIP. Concurrently, the two long lateral extensors inserting on the distal phalanx are displaced in a volar direction, creating an additional flexion moment at the PIP and a continual extension moment on the DIP.

Therapeutic interventions include (a) stretching exercises, which should encourage MCP flexion, PIP extension, and DIP flexion; (b) intrinsic muscle strengthening, which may provide some assistance with PIP extension and MCP flexion; and (c) use of orthotics, which should promote an extension moment at the PIP joint to create a DIP flexion moment or attempt to provide a DIP flexion moment with three points of pressure and reversal of PIP joint flexion. The latter is more difficult because the forcing of the DIP joint into flexion strongly inhibits the extensor mechanism, and PIP/MCP extension becomes limited (90,145,146). Again, heated paraffin may loosen soft tissue elements and provide transient analgesia before and after massage and stretching exercises.

Metacarpophalangeal Ulnar Deviation, Wrist Radial Deviation, and Therapeutic Interventions

Several factors are involved in the development of radial deviation of the wrist. First, wrist synovitis causes joint capsule weakness, with selective damage to the triangular fibrocartilage and disproportionate weakness on the ulnar side. Second, as inflammation increases and enzymatic destruction of intrinsic ligaments progresses, the proximal row carpal bones drift in a volar direction while the radius drifts dorsally. These processes, in addition to other deforming forces, cause an ulnar rotation of the proximal carpal bones, a radial rotation of the distal carpal bones, and a subsequent compensatory ulnar moment at the MCP joint—all adaptive mechanisms to realign the phalanx with the wrist. Digital ulnar deviation also occurs as a direct result of MCP synovitis, during which excessive capsular tension causes a volar shift of the superficial flexor tendons, resulting in an ulnar-directed force pull on the MCP and PIP joints.

Therapeutic interventions include the prescription of (a) resting splints, which may be useful in reducing pain and theoretically preventing progressive deformity by limiting ligamentous stretching and placing the joint at rest (this splint type is not intended to correct, but to prevent further deformity); (b) functional splints, which can be quite bulky, and difficult for patients to don themselves; (c) wrist/hand splints that focus on MCP radial return, which may improve hand function in some patients; and (d) carpal tunnel splints worn nightly, which are useful for patients who develop a compressive median neuropathy because of increased intracarpal canal pressures. Thumb pain/deformity commonly seen at the carpometacarpal (CMC) joint responds to semirigid orthotics that rest the joint but allow DIP and wrist/joint motion (90,145,146).

Joint protection is especially important for wrist/metacarpal pathology. Occupational therapy consults are appropriate for the provision of specific strengthening exercises, the design and fabrication of splints, and home, workplace, and task redesign (adaptive behavior) that encourages joint protection (90,145,146).

Intrinsic Muscle Tightness of the Hand and Therapeutic Interventions

Interossei, because of their unique insertion onto both the extensor mechanism dorsally and proximal phalanx volarly, create a flexion moment at the MCP joint and an extension moment at the PIP joint. Shortening of these muscle fibers occurs because of reflex spasms associated with juxtaposition to inflamed joint capsules, principally the MCP or PIP, resulting in a hand that has decreased functional grip and intrinsic hand weakness.

The focus of treatment for intrinsic tightness is on stretching shortened intrinsic muscles and other supportive connective tissues by providing MCP extension and PIP flexion. Prestretching use of paraffin and fluidotherapy may facilitate this process. Promoting functional skills that deemphasize MCP flexion/PIP extension may impede the process of intrinsic tightening. Such skills include the avoidance of habitual activities, such as sitting on the palms of the hands, or carrying drawstrings/purse strings or grocery bags with the palmar surface of the hand (90,145,146).

Work Disability Associated with Rheumatoid Arthritis

Work disability is a major problem for persons with RA. The prevalence rate ranges from 25% to 50% for persons in whom the disease has been present for up to 5 years, but skyrockets to 90% for persons with a 10-year history of RA (73,147). The most important risk factors for work disability are an aggressive disease process, physically demanding job, and older age (148).

Inadequate educational preparation, lack of family and co-worker support, coexistent depression, transportation difficulties, and other societal factors, as well as suboptimal employer disability management practices, all contribute to the degree of work disability. Disability in the performance of household chores is well documented in women with RA, negatively impacting self-esteem and family dynamics. Prevention and early intervention are the best methods to reduce disability, both inside and outside the home. Interventional strategies include patient and family vocational counseling, worksite modification, energy conservation strategies, employer counseling, and vocational retraining. Termination of employment may be the only option for some persons with severe RA. They may need assistance obtaining disability benefits through Social Security. Those who are likely to be disabled for at least 12 months and have contributed adequately to Social Security currently quality for SSDI. Those who have not contributed financially to Social Security but who have severe financial need are eligible for Social Security Insurance (SSI). Approval of benefits is based on medical disease criteria (such as radiographs and rheumatoid factor) or residual functional capacity when tests are inconclusive. Those persons who have received SSDI for 2 years are then eligible for Medicare benefits; those receiving SSI are immediately eligible for enrollment in the Medicaid program.

REHABILITATION STRATEGIES FOR SPONDYLOARTHROPATHIES

The spondyloarthropathies are a group of rheumatic diseases sharing various clinical, radiographic, and genetic features (149). This group of diseases includes ankylosing spondylitis (AS), Reiter syndrome, psoriatic arthritis, and arthritis of inflammatory bowel disease. A predictable pattern of AS emerges within the first 10 years of the disease. Fewer than 20% of patients with adult-onset AS deteriorate to a condition of significant functional limitation (150). In Reiter syndrome, disability usually occurs from arthritis of the foot and ankle, aggressive axial involvement, or blindness (149,151).

Rehabilitation Interventions: General Concepts

Exercise

Therapeutic exercise is a critically important component of treatment. A lifelong, individualized, well-instructed exercise program may help to maintain maximal ROM of the spine and costovertebral girdle joints, potentially preventing flexion contractures and loss of height. The exercise prescription should include ROM of the neck, shoulders, and hips; stretching of pectorals, paraspinal muscles, hip flexors, and hamstrings; deep breathing; and strengthening of back and hip extensors and abdominal muscles. If peripheral joint involvement is not significant, cardiovascular exercises with equipment (i.e., treadmill, stationary cycle) may improve endurance as well as lower body strength. Trunk and arm strengthening occurs with use of a cross-country ski machine (152). A recently published randomized controlled trial of home-based exercise confirmed exercise's efficacy for improving mobility in AS (153). Regular medical follow-up helps promote compliance. Before exercise, physical modalities such as heat, ice, massage, and TENS may be used to decrease pain and muscle spasm and to facilitate joint motion.

Physical fitness and sports activities assist in maintaining patient flexibility and strength, and patients should be encouraged to choose sports that promote good posture and back extension. In the early stages of spondylitis involving primarily low back pain, patients may be able to play basketball, volleyball, or tennis. In advanced disease processes, bicycling with upright handlebars or swimming may be more suitable. Swimming may require adaptation because of limited cervical motion (154). These activities, however, do not take the place of therapeutic exercise. Contact sports are not advised because of the risk for spinal fracture (90).

Other self-care measures are also appropriate for those with spinal arthropathies. Patients should be instructed in posture principles and the importance of recording key response variables, such as height and chest expansion.

Occupational and Physical Therapy

Occupational therapy is frequently prescribed for evaluation of and retraining in ADLs, as well as for work, avocational, or home adaptations. Assistive devices, such as reachers and long-handled tools, may be useful in compensating for decreased spinal motion during ADL performance, while wide-angled panoramic rearview or spot mirror placement may ease and improve visibility during driving.

In a study by Kraag and co-workers (155), a group of patients who received physiotherapy and disease-specific education for 4 months had greater improvement in fingertip-to-floor distance and function (measured by a modified Toronto ADL questionnaire for AS) than did control subjects. There were no significant changes in pain, spinal alignment, or Schober test results. Improvement in fingertip-to-floor distance was thought to be related to stretching of the hamstrings or muscles about the shoulder girdle, increased hip flexion, and compensation for the restricted movement by unaffected or mildly affected segments of the spine that responded to exercise. Fisher and co-workers (156) reported that cardiovascular fitness helped to maintain work capacity in patients with AS. Components of their regimen targeted improving spinal mobility and increasing cardiorespiratory fitness. A randomized controlled trial in 144 patients demonstrated that a program of group physical therapy was superior to home exercise in improving thoracolumbar mobility, fitness, and global effect on the health of AS patients. The program consisted of hydrotherapy, exercises, and sporting activities on a weekly basis for 3 hours per session (157).

Patient Education

Patient education is essential. Instruction in the natural history of the disease, the rationale for each treatment modality, and orientation to community resources should be offered to all patients. The Spondylitis Association of America, formerly the Ankylosing Spondylitis Association, is an excellent resource.

Spine Impairments

The ankylosed spine is frequently osteopenic and associated with ossification of spinal ligaments; therefore, the risk for fractures of the spine from even minor trauma is increased, especially in the cervical region (158). Because of the loss of ligamentous support, a fracture of an ankylosed spine is unstable. Spinal fractures should be considered in any patient with AS who experiences trauma. Unfortunately, plain film radiographs may not show the fracture. Tomography may be helpful, and radionuclide bone scan is particularly useful in patients with chronic pseudarthrosis (159).

The inflammatory process initiated by synovial tissue in the occipital-atlantoaxial articulation causes ligamentous laxity and bony destruction that can lead to upper cervical instability. Symptoms of atlantoaxial instability may vary from radiating pain in the occipital region caused by compression of the greater occipital nerve to radiating arm pain, hyperreflexia, and various degrees of sensory and motor loss in the limbs caused by compression of the spinal cord. Clinicians should base decisions about surgery on the presence of significant neurologic deficit, vertebral artery symptoms, and intractable pain, and not solely on the degree of subluxation seen radiographically. The latter does not correlate with the degree of neurologic impairment (160).

Cauda equina syndrome may begin late in the course of AS (159), even when the disease is inactive. The most frequent symptoms are cutaneous sensory loss in the lower lumbar and sacral dermatomes, disturbances in urinary and rectal sphincter function of lower motor neuron type, mild to moderate weakness in the lumbosacral myotomes, and pain in the rectum or lower limbs. This syndrome is associated with enlarged dural sleeves and arachnoid diverticula that erode the lamina of the lumbosacral spine. Radiographic evaluation by magnetic resonance imaging can establish the cauda equina diagnosis and exclude tumor as the cause of symptoms (161).

Therapeutic Interventions

Conservative treatment for upper cervical instability, which is satisfactory for controlling the symptoms of most patients, aims to relieve pain and discomfort, maintain or restore ROM and muscle strength, and help patients modify the ADLs that aggravate neck pain. Cervical collars, commonly used to relieve discomfort and protect the neck, are often prescribed to prevent sudden neck flexion and extension that could result in neurologic impairment or death (162). Hot and cold thermal modalities as well as TENS may relieve pain.

For fractures, nonoperative treatment with an emphasis on careful immobilization is often successful (163). Laminectomy is recommended for patients with progression of a neurologic lesion. Spinal fusion is recommended for fractures that cannot be externally stabilized (164).

Cardiopulmonary Involvement

Patients with AS rarely report respiratory symptoms or limitations. Despite diminished chest expansion secondary to costovertebral joint fusion, patients with AS have only minor restrictive changes with mildly reduced vital and total lung capacities on respiratory function tests (149). To compensate for the rigid chest wall, patients with AS rely on diaphragmatic movement in their respiratory function (156). Chest expansion exercises might be useful in preventing AS-related restrictive lung disease.

Aortic insufficiency and heart block are the most common cardiac complications associated with AS, resulting from inflammation of the aortic valve and root, as well as adjacent atrioventricular nodal tissue. Cardiac complications are more common in patients with long-standing disease (149).

Therapeutic Interventions

Patients should follow a therapeutic exercise program to maintain maximal ROM of the spine (costovertebral girdle joints), as well as a cardiovascular fitness program. Persons with AS who have aortic insufficiency or any other cardiac abnormalities should have an exercise tolerance test before starting a fitness program. Patients engaging in a modest amount of exercise regularly maintain a satisfactory work capacity despite restricted spinal and chest wall mobility (156). Restrictive lung disease may be further exacerbated when the patient is immobilized following trauma, surgery, or other medical illnesses, such that vigorous pulmonary therapy is indicated.

Heel Pain

Heel pain due to Achilles enthesopathy, Achilles bursitis, or plantar fasciitis frequently occurs in spondyloarthropathy (152). Inferior heel pain is most common and usually disappears spontaneously.

Therapeutic Interventions

Treatment includes heel pads, nonsteroidal antiinflammatory drugs, orthotics, and local injections of steroids. Injections into the Achilles tendon, however, should be avoided. Sulfasalazine may be prescribed for refractory heel pain.

Disability

Guillemin and co-workers (165) found that AS patients with peripheral joint involvement who were employed in physically-demanding occupations tended to have prolonged sick leaves, whereas long-term disability was more common when work demands involved exposure to cold conditions and prolonged standing activities. Employment in sedentary occupations and involvement in formal vocational rehabilitation programs was associated with a decreased incidence of long-term disability.

REHABILITATION STRATEGIES FOR INFLAMMATORY MYOPATHIES

Polymyositis (PM), dermatomyositis (DM), and inclusion body myositis (IBM) are acquired inflammatory myopathies. They are characterized by proximal and often symmetric muscle weakness of gradual onset. DM is accompanied by characteristic dermal changes, including a heliotrope rash on the eyelids and erythema over the knuckles (Gottron sign). IBM, first described in 1978, is characterized by marked quadriceps weakness and atrophy, involvement of distal muscles, minimal increase in serum muscle enzyme levels, and poor response to steroid treatment (166,167).

Associated functional limitations relate to weakness of the pelvic and shoulder girdles. Patients may have difficulty arising from a chair, going up stairs, getting in and out of the bathtub and car, lifting objects, dressing, combing their hair, and eating. Those with advanced disease have difficulty holding the head up and lifting the head off a pillow. Treatment programs for inflammatory myopathies require close follow-up and modification based on disease activity. Muscle strength and serum enzyme values should be monitored regularly during treatment. Of the two, muscle strength is the more important guide (168). The most critical clinical indicator for therapeutic monitoring is improved function, as reflected in the patient's ability to independently perform ADLs.

Rehabilitation Interventions

Modalities

Heat modalities may be used to treat myalgias. A cervical collar often proves helpful for a patient with weakness of the neck muscles.

Exercise, Rest, and Positioning

Bed rest with proper positioning is indicated in the acute phase. Passive ROM exercises should be performed during periods of severe inflammation and progress to active-assisted and active ROM exercises as disease activity decreases. Joint contractures can develop early and are particularly severe in children with DM, who need ongoing, careful ROM and stretching programs.

In the subacute phase, the rehabilitation program should include submaximal strengthening exercises and ambulatory and functional ADL performance. Exercises of the trunk and lower extremities against applied resistance, adjusted according to the strength of each muscle group, appear safe in the rehabilitation of PM and DM, without inducing a clinically-significant increase in the levels of serum muscle enzymes (168). An isometric program is useful for strengthening affected muscles in inactive or stable inflammatory muscle disease (169). The intensity of the exercise program should be monitored such that systemic fatigue is not encountered.

Orthotics, Assistive Devices, and Patient Education

Gradually progressive mobility training should be incorporated, including bed mobility, transfer skills, and ambulation with assistive devices. Patients who have marked quadriceps weakness may require a rigid ankle-foot orthotic in slight plantarflexion, which encourages knee extension during stance. Knee-ankle-foot orthoses can be used for severe limb weakness, but are often impractical for improving function because of their bulk and weight. The use of a motorized scooter or wheelchair should be considered for patients with progressive weakness who are no longer able to walk. These patients are candidates for motorized chairs because of their upper limb involvement, which prevents propelling a manual wheelchair. Patients may need adaptive equipment for dressing and reaching, as well as assistive devices in the bathroom. A mobile arm support (ball-bearing orthosis) allows a patient with weak proximal muscles to move more freely for ADLs and avocational and vocational activities. A common limitation in patients with proximal weakness is the inability to get up from a chair. Handrails and raised toilet seats assist independent function in the bathroom. Thick, firm seat cushions or increasing the height of a chair also facilitates independence with transfer activities. Seat-lift chairs that propel the patient from sit to stand are occasionally needed. Finally, patients should clearly understand the principles of energy conservation in order to maintain as much functional independence as possible.

Dysphagia Training

Dysphagia, reported in 12% to 38% of patients with PM and DM, predisposes the patient to aspiration (170). Although pharyngeal weakness usually responds to corticosteroid therapy, patients with dysphagia can benefit from a swallowing evaluation and retraining by a speech therapist to protect the airway and prevent aspiration pneumonia. The most common lung disease in PM and DM is pneumonia, generally due to aspiration (171).

CONCLUSION

This chapter has described a conceptual framework that includes medical, surgical, and rehabilitation management strategies; the theoretical underpinnings of rehabilitation interventions; and the empiric basis for appropriate rehabilitation treatment for specific joint and muscle diseases. Just as cell and molecular biologic research continues to offer the clinician and patient more therapeutic opportunities, rehabilitation research will undoubtedly also lead to innovative treatments that will capitalize on new discoveries related to the role of mechanics in the development and progression of many forms of arthritis, most notably OA. Although rehabilitation is often used in patients for whom medicine and surgery have failed, it is most likely that future strategies to prevent functional limitation and, indeed, to prevent the occurrence of some forms of OA will include exercises designed to maintain and improve the neurobiomechanical status of joints.

Finally, the future role of rehabilitation is also likely to include self-management programs. These programs are not traditionally offered in health-care settings, but in those that provide education that enables patients to engage in healthier lifestyles, and thus, improve their health status. The premier example of such a program for persons with arthritis is the Arthritis Foundation's Arthritis Self-Help Course. Physical activity and exercise will always be part of an arthritis self-management program; thus, rehabilitation researchers and practitioners will continue to be challenged to recommend simple but effective programs.

The likely result of these two trends will be to bring rehabilitation back into the mainstream of the care and prevention of arthritis and related disorders, thus reuniting the rehabilitation and rheumatology fields, as in times past.

REFERENCES

1. Centers for Disease Control and Prevention. Prevalence of Disabilities and Associated Health Conditions Among Adults—United States, 1999. *MMWR* 2001;50:120–125.
2. Dunlop DD, Manheim LM, Yelin EH, et al. The costs of arthritis. *Arthritis Rheum* 2003;49:101–113.
3. Pope A. *Disability in america: toward a national agenda for prevention.* Washington, DC: Institute of Medicine, National Academy Press, 1991.
4. Hanada EY. Efficacy of rehabilitative therapy in regional musculoskeletal conditions. *Best Pract Res Clin Rheumatol* 2003;17:151–166.
5. Minor MA, Hewett JE, Webel RR, et al. Efficacy of physical conditioning exercise in patients with rheumatoid arthritis and osteoarthritis. *Arthritis Rheum* 1989;32:1396–1405.
6. Perlman SG, Connell KJ, Clark A, et al. Dance-based aerobic exercise for rheumatoid arthritis. *Arthritis Care Res* 1990;3:29–35.
7. Nordemar R, Ekblom B, Zachrisson L, et al. Physical training in rheumatoid arthritis: a controlled long-term study. I. *Scand J Rheumatol* 1981;10:17–23.
8. Nordemar R. Physical training in rheumatoid arthritis: a controlled long-term study. II. Functional capacity and general attitudes. *Scand J Rheumatol* 1981;10:25–30.
9. Gerber LH. Exercise and arthritis. *Bull Rheum Dis* 1990;39:1–9.
10. Hicks JE. Exercise in patients with inflammatory arthritis and connective tissue disease. *Rheum Dis Clin North Am* 1990;16:845–870.
11. Clarke S, Burckhardt C, Bennett R. Exercise for prevention and treatment of illness. In: Goldberg L, Elliott D, eds. *Exercise for prevention and treatment of illness.* Philadelphia: FA Davis, 1994:83.
12. Basmajian J, Wolf S. *Therapeutic exercise,* 5th ed. Vol. 340. Baltimore: Williams & Wilkins, 1990.

13. Herbison GJ, Ditunno JF, Jaweed MM. Muscle atrophy in rheumatoid arthritis. *J Rheumatol* 1987;14(suppl 15):78–81.
14. Van Den Ende CH, Vliet Vlieland TP, Munneke M, et al. Dynamic exercise therapy for rheumatoid arthritis. *Cochrane Database Syst Rev* 2000;CD000322.
15. Ettinger WH Jr, Burns R, Messier SP, et al. A randomized trial comparing aerobic exercise and resistance exercise with a health education program in older adults with knee osteoarthritis. The Fitness Arthritis and Seniors Trial (FAST). *JAMA* 1997;277:25–31.
16. Penninx BW, Mesier SP, Rejeski J, et al. Physical exercise and the prevention of disability in activities of daily living in older persons with osteoarthritis. *Arch Intern Med* 2001;161:2309–2316.
17. Baker KR, Nelson ME, Felson DT, et al. The efficacy of home based progressive strength training in older adults with knee osteoarthritis: a randomized controlled trial. *J Rheumatol* 2001;28:1655–1665.
18. McNeal RL. Aquatic therapy for patients with rheumatic disease. *Rheum Dis Clin North Am* 1990;16:915–929.
19. Hoffman DF. Arthritis and exercise. *Prim Care* 1993;20:895–910.
20. Centers for Disease Control and Prevention. Prevalence of leisure-time physical activity among persons with arthritis and other rheumatic conditions—United States, 1990–1991. *MMWR* 1997;46:389–393.
21. Centers for Disease Control and Prevention. Monthly estimates of leisure-time physical inactivity—United States, 1994. *MMWR* 1997; 46:393–397.
22. Centers for Disease Control and Prevention. Prevalence and impact of chronic joint symptoms—seven states, 1996. *MMWR* 1998;47:345–351.
23. Wang G, Helmick CG, Macera C, et al. Inactivity-associated medical costs among US adults with arthritis. *Arthritis Rheum* 2001;45:439–445.
24. Dunn AL, Andersen RE, Jakicic JM. Lifestyle physical activity interventions. History, short- and long-term effects, and recommendations. *Am J Prev Med* 1988;15:398–412.
25. Dunn AL, Garcia ME, Marcus BH, et al. Six-month physical activity and fitness changes in Project Active, a randomized trial. *Med Exerc Sports Exerc* 1988;30:1076–1083.
26. DiPietro L. The epidemiology of physical activity and physical function in older people. *Med Sci Sports Exerc* 1996;28:596–600.
27. Minor MA. Exercise in the treatment of osteoarthritis. *Rheum Dis Clin North Am* 1999;25:397–415, viii.
28. Minor MA, Lane NE. Recreational exercise in arthritis. *Rheum Dis Clin North Am* 1996;22:563–577.
29. Baker KR, Nelson ME, Felson DT, et al. The efficacy of home based progressive strength training in older adults with knee osteoarthritis: a randomized controlled trial. *J Rheumatol* 2001;28:1655–1665.
30. Hakkinen A, Sokka T, Konaniemi A, et al. A randomized two-year study of the effects of dynamic strength training on muscle strength, disease activity, functional capacity, and bone mineral density in early rheumatoid arthritis. *Arthritis Rheum* 2001;44:515–522.
31. Ettinger WH, Burns R, Messier SP, et al. A randomized controlled trial comparing aerobic exercise and resistance exercise with a health education program in older adults with knee osteoarthritis. The Fitness Arthritis and Seniors Trial (FAST). *JAMA* 1997;277:25–31.
32. Westby MD, Wade JP, Rangno KK, et al. A randomized controlled trial to evaluate the effectiveness of an exercise program in women with rheumatoid arthritis taking low dose prednisone. *J Rheumatol* 2000;27:1674–1680.
33. O'Reilly SC, Muir KR, Doherty M. Effectiveness of home exercise on pain and disability from osteoarthritis of the knee: a randomized controlled trial. *Ann Rheum Dis* 1999;58:15–19.
34. Hopman-Rock M, Westhoff MH. The effects of a health educational and exercise program for older adults with osteoarthritis for the hip or knee. *J Rheumatol* 2000;27:1947–1954.
35. Kovar PA, Allegrante JP, MacKenzie CR, et al. Supervised fitness walking in patients with osteoarthritis of the knee. A randomized, controlled trial. *Ann Intern Med* 1992;116:529–534.
36. Neuberger GB, Press AN, Lindsley HB, et al. Effects of exercise on fatigue, aerobic fitness, and disease activity measures in persons with rheumatoid arthritis. *Res Nurs Health* 1997;20:195–204.
37. Bell MJ, Lineker SC, Wilkins AL, et al. A randomized controlled trial to evaluate the efficacy of community based physical therapy in the treatment of people with rheumatoid arthritis. *J Rheumatol* 1998;25: 231–237.
38. Deyle GD, Henderson NE, Matekel RL, et al. Effectiveness of manual physical therapy and exercise in osteoarthritis of the knee. *Ann Intern Med* 2000;132:173–181.
39. Moffet H, Noreau L, Parent E, et al. Feasibility of an 8-week dance-based exercise program and its effects on locomotor ability of persons with functional class III rheumatoid arthritis. *Arthritis Care Res* 2000; 13:100–111.
40. Rejeski WJ. Compliance to exercise therapy in older participants with knee osteoarthritis: implications for treating disability. *Med Sci Sports Exerc* 1997;29:977–985.
41. Thomas KS, Muir KR, Doherty M, et al. Home based exercise programme for knee pain and knee osteoarthritis: randomized controlled trial. *Br Med J* 2002;325:752.
42. Ainsworth BE, Haskell WL, Whitt MC, et al. Compendium of physical activities: an update of activity codes and MET intensities. *Med Sci Sports Exerc* 2000;32(suppl):498–516.
43. Pate RR, Pratt M, Blair SN, et al. Physical activity and public health: a recommendation from the Centers for Disease Control and Prevention and the American College of Sports Medicine. *JAMA* 1995;273:402–407.
44. Dunn AL, Marcus BH, Kampert JB, et al. Comparison of lifestyle and structured interventions to increase physical activity and cardiorespiratory fitness: a randomized trial. *JAMA* 1999;281:327–334.
45. Sevick MA, Dunn AL, Morrow MS, et al. Cost-effectiveness of lifestyle and structured exercise intervention in sedentary adults: results of Project Active. *Am J Prev Med* 2000;19:1–8.
46. Scottish Intercollegiate Guidelines Network (SIGN). *Management of early rheumatoid arthritis. A national clinical guideline.* Edinburgh, Scotland: SIGN: 2000:44.
47. American College of Rheumatology Subcommittee on Osteoarthritis Guidelines. Recommendations for the medical management of osteoarthritis of the hip and knee: 2000 update. *Arthritis Rheum* 2000;43: 1905–1925.
48. American College of Rheumatology Subcommittee on Rheumatoid Arthritis Guidelines. Guidelines for the management of Rheumatoid Arthritis: 2002 Update. *Arthritis Rheum* 2002;46:328–346.
49. American Geriatric Society. Exercise prescription for older adults with osteoarthritis pain: consensus practice recommendations. A supplement to the AGS Clinical Practice Guidelines on the management of chronic pain in older adults. *J Am Geriatr Soc* 2001;49:808–823.
50. Partridge R, Duthie J. Controlled trial of the effect of complete immobilization of the joints in rheumatoid arthritis. *Ann Rheum Dis* 1963; 22:91–99.
51. Gault S, Spyker J. Beneficial effect of immobilization of joints in rheumatoid arthritis and related arthritis: a splint study using sequential analysis. *Arthritis Rheum* 1969;12:34.
52. Nicholas JJ, Ziegler G. Cylinder splints: their use in the treatment of arthritis of the knee. *Arch Phys Med Rehabil* 1977;58:264–267.
53. Williams J, Harvey J, Tannebaum H. Use of superficial heat versus ice for rheumatoid arthritic shoulder: a pilot study. *Physiother Can* 1986; 38:8–13.
54. Green J, McKenna F, Redfern EJ, et al. Home exercises are as effective as outpatient hydrotherapy for osteoarthritis of the hip. *Br J Rheumatol* 1993;32:812–815.
55. Mainardi CL, Walter JM, Spiegel PK, et al. Rheumatoid arthritis: failure of daily heat therapy to affect its progression. *Arch Phys Med Rehabil* 1979;60:390–393.
56. Robinson V, Brosseau L, Casimiro L, et al. Thermotherapy for treating rheumatoid arthritis. *Cochrane Database Syst Rev* 2002:CD002826.
57. Falconer J, Hayes KW, Chang RW. Effect of ultrasound on mobility in osteoarthritis of the knee. A randomized clinical trial. *Arthritis Care Res* 1992;5:29–35.
58. Hashish I, Harvey W, Harris M. Anti-inflammatory effects of ultrasound therapy: evidence for a major placebo effect. *Br J Rheumatol* 1986;25:77–81.
59. Basford JR. Physical agents. *Rehabilitation medicine: principles and practice.* Philadelphia: Lippincott-Raven, 1998:483–503.
60. Oosterveld FG, Rasker JJ, Jacobs JW, et al. The effect of local heat and cold therapy on the intraarticular and skin surface temperature of the knee. *Arthritis Rheum* 1992;35:146–151.
61. Melzack R, Wall PD. Pain mechanisms: a new theory. *Science* 1965; 150:971–979.
62. Kumar VN, Redford JB. Transcutaneous nerve stimulation in rheumatoid arthritis. *Arch Phys Med Rehabil* 1982;63.595–596.

63. Hayes KW. Physical modalities. In: Wegener S, Belza B, Gall E, eds. *Clinical care in rheumatic diseases.* Atlanta: American College of Rheumatology, 1997:79–82.
64. Yasuda K, Sasaki T. The mechanics of treatment of the osteoarthritic knee with a wedged insole. *Clin Orthop* 1987;215:162–172.
65. Sasaki T, Yasuda K. Clinical evaluation of the treatment of osteoarthritic knees using a newly designed wedged insole. *Clin Orthop* 1987;22:181–187.
66. Voloshin A, Wosk J. Influence of artificial shock absorbers on human gait. *Clin Orthop* 1981;160:52–56.
67. Lefebvre JC, Keefe FJ, Affleck G, et al. The relationship of arthritis self-efficacy to daily pain, daily mood, and daily pain coping in rheumatoid arthritis patients. *Pain* 1999;80:425–435.
68. Weinberger M, Tierney WM, Booher P, et al. Can the provision of information to patients with osteoarthritis improve functional status? A randomized, controlled trial. *Arthritis Rheum* 1989;32:1577–1583.
69. Rene J, Weinberger M, Mazzuca SA, et al. Reduction of joint pain in patients with knee osteoarthritis who have received monthly telephone calls from lay personnel and whose medical treatment regimens have remained stable. *Arthritis Rheum* 1992;35:511–515.
70. Parker JC, Frank RG, Beck NC, et al. Pain management in rheumatoid arthritis patients. A cognitive-behavioral approach. *Arthritis Rheum* 1988;31:593–601.
71. Bradley LA. Psychosocial factors and arthritis. In: Schumacher HR, Klippel J, Koopman WK, eds. *Primer on rheumatic diseases.* Atlanta: Arthritis Foundation, 1993:319–322.
72. Yelin E. Arthritis. The cumulative impact of a common chronic condition. *Arthritis Rheum* 1992;35:489–497.
73. Yelin E, Henke C, Epstein W. The work dynamics of the person with rheumatoid arthritis. *Arthritis Rheum* 1987;30:507–512.
74. Katz PP, Yelin EH. Prevalence and correlates of depressive symptoms among persons with rheumatoid arthritis. *J Rheumatol* 1993;20:790–796.
75. Administration SS. Social Security Disability Benefits. Washington, DC: Social Security Administration, 1996.
76. Hadler NM. Medical ramifications of the federal regulation of the Social Security Disability Insurance program: Social Security and medicine. *Ann Intern Med* 1982;96:665–669.
77. Carey TS, Hadler NM. The role of the primary physician in disability determination for Social Security insurance and workers' compensation. *Ann Intern Med* 1986;104:706–710.
78. Shiflett SC. Complementary and alternative medicine. In: *Rehabilitation medicine: principles and practice.* Philadelphia: Lippincott-Raven, 1998:873–885.
79. Rao JK, Mihaliak K, Kroenke K, et al. Use of complementary therapies for arthritis among patients of rheumatologists. *Ann Intern Med* 1999;131:409–416.
80. Wright A, Sluka KA. Nonpharmacological treatments for musculoskeletal pain. *Clin J Pain* 2001;17:33–46.
81. Christensen BV, Juhl IU, Wilbek H, et al. Acupuncture treatment of knee arthrosis. A long-term study. *Ugeskr Laeger* 1993;155:4007–4011.
82. Takeda W, Wessel J. Acupuncture for the treatment of pain of osteoarthritic knees. *Arthritis Care Res* 1994;7:118–122.
83. Birch S, Jamison RN. Controlled trial of Japanese acupuncture for chronic myofascial neck pain: assessment of specific and nonspecific effects of treatment. *Clin J Pain* 1998;14:248–255.
84. Fargas-Babjak A. Acupuncture, transcutaneous electrical nerve stimulation, and laser therapy in chronic pain. *Clin J Pain* 2001;17(suppl):105–113.
85. Nicholas JJ. Physical modalities in rheumatological rehabilitation. *Arch Phys Med Rehabil* 1994;75:994–1001.
86. Brosseau L, Casimiro L, Milne S, et al. Deep transverse friction massage for treating tendinitis. *Cochrane Database Syst Rev* 2002: CD003528.
87. Furlan AD, Brosseau L, Imamura M, et al. Massage for low-back pain: a systematic review within the framework of the Cochrane Collaboration Back Review Group. *Spine* 2002;27:1896–1910.
88. Garfinkel MS, Schumacher HR Jr, Husain A, et al. Evaluation of a yoga based regimen for treatment of osteoarthritis of the hands. *J Rheumatol* 1994;21:2341–2343.
89. Centers for Disease Control and Prevention. Arthritis prevalence and activity limitations—United States. *MMWR* 1990;43:433–438.
90. Brander V, Oh T, Alpiner N. Rehabilitation of persons with arthritis. In: Grabois M, Garrison S, Hart K, eds. *Physical medicine and rehabilitation: the complete approach.* Malden, MA: Blackwell Scientific, 2000:1505–1533.
91. Felson DT, Anderson JJ, Naimark A, et al. Obesity and knee osteoarthritis. The Framingham Study. *Ann Intern Med* 1988;109:18–24.
92. Felson DT, Zhang Y, Anthony JM, et al. Weight loss reduces the risk for symptomatic knee osteoarthritis in women. The Framingham Study. *Ann Intern Med* 1992;116:535–539.
93. Rejeski WJ, Focht BC, Messier SP, et al. Obese, older adults with knee osteoarthritis: weight loss, exercise, and quality of life. *Health Psychol* 2002;21:419–426.
94. Manek NJ, Hart D, Spector TD, et al. The association of body mass index and osteoarthritis of the knee joint: an examination of genetic and environmental influences. *Arthritis Rheum* 2003;48:1024–1029.
95. Minor MA, Sanford MK. Physical interventions in the management of pain in arthritis: an overview for research and practice. *Arthritis Care Res* 1993;6:197–206.
96. Semble EL, Loeser RF, Wise CM. Therapeutic exercise for rheumatoid arthritis and osteoarthritis. *Semin Arthritis Rheum* 1990;20:32–40.
97. Fisher NM, Pendergast DR, Gresham GE, et al. Muscle rehabilitation: its effect on muscular and functional performance of patients with knee osteoarthritis. *Arch Phys Med Rehabil* 1991;72:367–374.
98. Ekdahl C, Broman G. Muscle strength, endurance, and aerobic capacity in rheumatoid arthritis: a comparative study with healthy subjects. *Ann Rheum Dis* 1992;51:35–40.
99. Sharma L, Dunlop DD, Cahue S, et al. Quadriceps strength and osteoarthritis progression in malaligned and lax knees [summary for patients in *Ann Intern Med* 2003;138(8):I1; PMID: 12693914]. *Ann Intern Med* 2003;138:613–619.
100. Bischoff HA, Roos EM. Effectiveness and safety of strengthening, aerobic, and coordination exercises for patients with osteoarthritis. *Curr Opin Rheumatol* 2003;15:141–144.
101. Puett DW, Griffin MR. Published trials of nonmedicinal and noninvasive therapies for hip and knee osteoarthritis. *Ann Intern Med* 1994;121:133–140.
102. Lehmann J, DeLateur B. Therapeutic heat. In: Lehmann JF, ed. *Therapeutic heat and cold.* Baltimore: Williams & Wilkins, 1982.
103. Reeve J, Menon D, Corabian P. Transcutaneous electrical nerve stimulation (TENS): a technology assessment. *Int J Technol Assess Health Care* 1996;12:299–324.
104. Buckwalter JA, Stanish WD, Rosier RN, et al. The increasing need for nonoperative treatment of patients with osteoarthritis. *Clin Orthop Rel Res* 2001;385:36–45.
105. Mendelson S, Milgrom C, Finestone A, et al. Effect of cane use on tibial strain and strain rates. *Am J Phys Med Rehabil* 1998;77:333–338.
106. Kerrigan DC, Lelas JL, Goggins J, et al. Effectiveness of a lateral-wedge insole on knee varus torque in patients with knee osteoarthritis. *Arch Phys Med Rehabil* 2002;83:889–893.
107. Cushnaghan J, McCarthy C, Dieppe P. Taping the patella medially: a new treatment for osteoarthritis of the knee joint? *BMJ* 1994;308:753–735.
108. Keefe FJ, Caldwell DS. Cognitive behavioral control of arthritis pain. *Med Clin North Am* 1997;81:277–290.
109. Keefe F, Caldwell DS, Williams D. Pain coping skills training in the management of osteoarthritis knee pain: a comparative study. *Behav Ther* 1990;21:49–62.
110. Lorig KR, Mazonson PD, Holman HR. Evidence suggesting that health education for self-management in patients with chronic arthritis has sustained health benefits while reducing health care costs. *Arthritis Rheum* 1993;36:439–446.
111. Davis MA, Ettinger WH, Neuhaus JM, et al. Correlates of knee pain among US adults with and without radiographic knee osteoarthritis. *J Rheumatol* 1992;19:1943–1949.
112. McCarthy C, Cushnaghan J, Dieppe P. Osteoarthritis. In: Wall PD, Melzack R, eds. *Textbook of pain.* Edinburgh: Churchill Livingstone, 1994:387–396.
113. Arnoldi CC, Djurhuus JC, Heerfordt J, et al. Intraosseous phlebography, intraosseous pressure measurements and 99mTC-polyphosphate scintigraphy in patients with various painful conditions in the hip and knee. *Acta Orthop Scand* 1980;51:19–28.
114. Dexter P, Brandt K. Distribution and predictors of depressive symptoms in osteoarthritis. *J Rheumatol* 1994;21:279–286.

115. Wells KB, Golding JM, Burnam MA. Affective, substance use, and anxiety disorders in persons with arthritis, diabetes, heart disease, high blood pressure, or chronic lung conditions. *Gen Hosp Psychiatry* 1989;11:320–327.
116. Watelain E, Dujardin F, Babier F, et al. Pelvic and lower limb compensatory actions of subjects in an early stage of hip osteoarthritis. *Arch Phys Med Rehabil* 2001;82:1705–1711.
117. Hochberg MC, Altman RD, Brandt KD, et al. Guidelines for the medical management of osteoarthritis. Part I. Osteoarthritis of the hip. American College of Rheumatology. *Arthritis Rheum* 1995;38:1535–1540.
118. Hochberg MC, Altman RD, Brandt KD, et al. Guidelines for the medical management of osteoarthritis. Part II. Osteoarthritis of the knee. American College of Rheumatology. *Arthritis Rheum* 1995;38:1541–1546.
119. van Baar M, Dekker J, Oostendorp RA, et al. Effectiveness of exercise program in patients with osteoarthritis of hip or knee: nine months follow-up. *Ann Rheum Dis* 2001;60:1123–1130.
120. Fisher NM, Gresham GE, Abrams M, et al. Quantitative effects of physical therapy on muscular and functional performance in subjects with osteoarthritis of the knees. *Arch Phys Med Rehabil* 1993;74:840–847.
121. Topp R, Woolley S, Hornyak J 3rd, et al. The effect of dynamic versus isometric resistance training on pain and functioning among adults with osteoarthritis of the knee. *Arch Phys Med Rehabil* 2002;83:1187–1195.
122. Agudelo CA, Schumacher HR, Phelps P. Effect of exercise on urate crystal-induced inflammation in canine joints. *Arthritis Rheum* 1972;15:609–616.
123. Kibler WB, McMullen J, Uhl T. Shoulder rehabilitation strategies, guidelines, and practice. *Orthop Clin North Am* 2001;32:527–538.
124. Jayson M, Dixon S. Intra-articular pressure in RA of the knee, part III: pressure changes during joint use. *Ann Rheum Dis* 1972;29:401.
125. DeLorme T, Watkins A. Techniques of progressive resistance exercise. *Arch Phys Med Rehabil* 1966;47:737.
126. DeLateur BJ, Lehmann JF, Fordyce WE. A test of the DeLorme axiom. *Arch Phys Med Rehabil* 1968;49:245–248.
127. DeLateur B, Lehmann JF, Warren CG, et al. Comparison of effectiveness of isokinetic and isotonic exercise in quadriceps strengthening. *Arch Phys Med Rehabil* 1972;53:60–64.
128. Spector TD. Rheumatoid arthritis. *Rheum Dis Clin North Am* 1990;16:513–537.
129. Pincus T, Callahan LF. Reassessment of twelve traditional paradigms concerning the diagnosis, prevalence, morbidity and mortality of rheumatoid arthritis. *Scand J Rheumatol Suppl* 1989;79:67–96.
130. Wilske KR, Healey LA. Remodeling the pyramid—a concept whose time has come. *J Rheumatol* 1989;16:565–567.
131. Alpiner N, Oh TH, Hinderer SR, et al. Rehabilitation in joint and connective tissue diseases. 1. Systemic diseases. *Arch Phys Med Rehabil* 1995;76(suppl):32–40.
132. Belza B. Fatigue. In: Wegner S, Belza B, Gall E, eds. *Clinical care in the rheumatic diseases.* Atlanta: American College of Rheumatology, 1996:117–120.
133. Roubenoff R. Exercise and inflammatory disease. *Arthritis Rheum* 2003;49:263–266.
134. van den Ende CH, Breedveld FC, le Cessie S, et al. Effect of intensive exercise on patients with active rheumatoid arthritis: a randomised clinical trial. *Ann Rheum Dis* 2000;59:615–621.
135. Lineker SC, Bell MJ, Wilkins AL, et al. Improvements following short term home based physical therapy are maintained at one year in people with moderate to severe rheumatoid arthritis. *J Rheumatol* 2001;28:165–168.
136. Hakkinen A, Sokka T, Konaniemi A, et al. A randomized two-year study of the effects of dynamic strength training on muscle strength, disease activity, functional capacity, and bone mineral density in early rheumatoid arthritis. *Arthritis Rheum* 2001;44:515–522.
137. Hakkinen A, Sokka T, Lietsalmi AM, et al. Effects of dynamic strength training on physical function, Valpar 9 work sample test, and working capacity in patients with recent-onset rheumatoid arthritis. *Arthritis Rheum* 2003;49:71–77.
138. Bearne LM, Scott DL, Hurley MV. Exercise can reverse quadriceps sensorimotor dysfunction that is associated with rheumatoid arthritis without exacerbating disease activity. *Rheumatology* 2002;41:157–166.
139. Gordon MM, Thomson EA, Madhok R, et al. Can intervention modify adverse lifestyle variables in a rheumatoid population? Results of a pilot study. *Ann Rheum Dis* 2002;61:66–69.
140. Wegener S. Sleep disturbance. In: Wegner S, Belza B, Gall E, eds. *Clinical care in the rheumatic diseases.* Atlanta: American College of Rheumatology, 1996:121–124.
141. Alarcon R, Glover S. Assessment and management of depression in rheumatoid arthritis. In: Biundo JM, ed. *Physical medicine and rehabilitation clinics of North America Joint disease.* Philadelphia: WB Saunders, 1994:837–858.
142. Frank RG, Beck NC, Parker JC, et al. Depression in rheumatoid arthritis. *J Rheumatol* 1988;15:920–925.
143. Beckham JC, D'Amico CJ, Rice JR, et al. Depression and level of functioning in patients with rheumatoid arthritis. *Can J Psychiatry* 1992;37:539–543.
144. Marlor J. Orthotic management of rheumatoid arthritis in the foot and ankle. In: *Rehabilitation of persons with rheumatoid arthritis.* Gaithersburg, MD: Aspen, 1996:109–117.
145. Robinson V, Brosseau L, Casimiro L, et al. Thermotherapy for treating rheumatoid arthritis. [Update of *Cochrane Database Syst Rev* 2002;1:CD002826; PMID: 11869637]. *Cochrane Database Syst Rev* 2002:CD002826.
146. Buljina AI, Taljanovic MS, Avdic DM, et al. Physical and exercise therapy for treatment of the rheumatoid hand. *Arthritis Rheum* 2001;45:392–397.
147. Reisine ST, Grady KE, Goodenow C, et al. Work disability among women with rheumatoid arthritis. The relative importance of disease, social, work, and family factors. *Arthritis Rheum* 1989;32:538–543.
148. Allaire SH, Anderson JJ, Meenan RF. Reducing work disability associated with rheumatoid arthritis: identification of additional risk factors and persons likely to benefit from intervention. *Arthritis Care Res* 1996;9:349–357.
149. Arnett FC. Seronegative spondylarthropathies. *Bull Rheum Dis* 1987;37:1–12.
150. Carette S, Graham D, Little H, et al. The natural disease course of ankylosing spondylitis. *Arthritis Rheum* 1983;26:186–190.
151. Fox R, Calin A, Gerber RC, et al. The chronicity of symptoms and disability in Reiter's syndrome. An analysis of 131 consecutive patients. *Ann Intern Med* 1979;91:190–193.
152. Amor B, Dougados M, Khan MA. Management of refractory ankylosing spondylitis and related spondyloarthropathies. *Rheum Dis Clin North Am* 1995;21:117–128.
153. Sweeney S, Taylor G, Calin A. The effect of a home based exercise intervention package on outcome in ankylosing spondylitis: a randomized controlled trial. *J Rheumatol* 2002;29:763–766.
154. Swezey R. *Straight talk on spondylitis,* 2nd ed. Sherman Oaks, CA: Spondylitis Association of America, 1992.
155. Kraag G, Stokes B, Groh J, et al. The effects of comprehensive home physiotherapy and supervision on patients with ankylosing spondylitis—a randomized controlled trial. *J Rheumatol* 1990;17:228–233.
156. Fisher LR, Cawley MI, Holgate ST. Relation between chest expansion, pulmonary function, and exercise tolerance in patients with ankylosing spondylitis. *Ann Rheum Dis* 1990;49:921–925.
157. Hidding A, van der Linden S, Boers M, et al. Is group physical therapy superior to individualized therapy in ankylosing spondylitis? A randomized controlled trial. *Arthritis Care Res* 1993;6:117–125.
158. Wade W, Saltzstein R, Maiman D. Spinal fractures complicating ankylosing spondylitis. *Arch Phys Med Rehabil* 1989;70:398–401.
159. Hunter T. The spinal complications of ankylosing spondylitis. *Semin Arthritis Rheum* 1989;19:172–182.
160. Fehring TK, Brooks AL. Upper cervical instability in rheumatoid arthritis. *Clin Orthop* 1987;221:137–148.
161. Ball G. Ankylosing spondylitis. In: McCarthy D, Koopman W, eds. *Arthritis and allied conditions: a textbook of rheumatology.* Philadelphia: Lea & Febiger, 1993:1051–1060.
162. Vanderschueren D, Decramer M, Van den Daele P, et al. Pulmonary function and maximal transrespiratory pressures in ankylosing spondylitis. *Ann Rheum Dis* 1989;48:632–635.
163. Haslock I. Ankylosing spondylitis. *Baillieres Clin Rheumatol* 1993;7:99–115.

164. Calin A, Elswood J. The outcome of 138 total hip replacements and 12 revisions in ankylosing spondylitis: high success rate after a mean followup of 7.5 years. *J Rheumatol* 1989;16:955–958.
165. Guillemin F, Briancon S, Pourel J, et al. Long-term disability and prolonged sick leaves as outcome measurements in ankylosing spondylitis. Possible predictive factors. *Arthritis Rheum* 1990;33:1001–1006.
166. Carpenter S, Karpati G, Heller I, et al. Inclusion body myositis: a distinct variety of idiopathic inflammatory myopathy. *Neurology* 1978;28:8–17.
167. Calabrese LH, Mitsumoto H, Chou SM. Inclusion body myositis presenting as treatment-resistant polymyositis. *Arthritis Rheum* 1987;30:397–403.
168. Escalante A, Miller L, Beardmore TD. Resistive exercise in the rehabilitation of polymyositis/dermatomyositis. *J Rheumatol* 1993;20:1340–1344.
169. Hicks JE, Miller F, Plotz P, et al. Isometric exercise increases strength and does not produce sustained creatinine phosphokinase increases in a patient with polymyositis. *J Rheumatol* 1993;20:1399–1401.
170. Benbassat J, Gefel D, Larholt K, et al. Prognostic factors in polymyositis/dermatomyositis. A computer-assisted analysis of ninety-two cases. *Arthritis Rheum* 1985;28:249–255.
171. Dickey BF, Myers AR. Pulmonary disease in polymyositis/dermatomyositis. *Semin Arthritis Rheum* 1984;14:60–76.

CHAPTER 39

Cytokine Inhibitors: Tumor Necrosis Factor and Interleukin-1

Uzma Haque and Joan M. Bathon

The development of inhibitors of the inflammatory cytokines tumor necrosis factor-α (TNF-α) and interleukin-1 (IL-1) has been heralded as one of the most important therapeutic advances in the treatment of rheumatoid arthritis (RA). From a conceptual viewpoint, they represent the first therapies for RA that evolved from an investigative "bench-to-bedside" approach. Studies with TNF inhibitors, in particular, provided proof of concept that inhibition of a single cytokine can markedly reduce the clinical expression of RA. From a practical viewpoint, they have proven to be efficacious not only in providing symptomatic relief but also in slowing structural damage to the joints. Although none of the current cytokine inhibitors has been shown to be dramatically superior to methotrexate (MTX) (the current gold standard treatment for RA), they provide highly effective alternative or adjunctive therapies for the patient who has had an inadequate response to, or cannot tolerate, MTX. This advantage, coupled with their scientific appeal and favorable efficacy and safety profiles, have led to the wide use of TNF inhibitors in RA, Crohn disease, and psoriatic arthritis, and investigations of their efficacy and safety in other chronic inflammatory conditions is also well advanced.

This chapter will focus on RA as a paradigm for examining TNF-α and IL-1 as targets for therapeutic intervention in chronic inflammatory states. Other conditions in which TNF and IL-1 inhibitors have been studied will be discussed briefly.

ROLE OF TUMOR NECROSIS FACTOR AND INTERLEUKIN-1 IN THE PATHOGENESIS OF RHEUMATOID ARTHRITIS

RA is an autoimmune disease characterized by intense inflammation that leads to joint destruction as well as extra-articular organ damage. Compared with normal synovium, the rheumatoid synovium is hypertrophic and highly vascularized, and exhibits increased numbers of macrophages and fibroblasts in the intimal lining, and lymphocytes, plasma cells and macrophages in the subintimal area (1). Destruction of articular cartilage and bone occurs, to a large degree, in areas contiguous to this hypertrophic synovium. In this milieu, molecules (both membrane and soluble) that are indicative of T-cell activation have been difficult to identify (2), and clinical trials targeted at the depletion or inhibition of activated T cells have demonstrated, for the most part, only modest clinical efficacy (3). In contrast, macrophage and fibroblast-derived cytokines are robustly expressed in rheumatoid synovium, including TNF-α, IL-1, IL-6, and granulocyte-macrophage colony-stimulating factor (GM-CSF) (2,4,5). These observations suggest that, although T cell–mediated, antigen-dependent processes are likely to be critical in the initiation of RA, chronic inflammation in the joint may be sustained to a large degree by innate immune responses involving macrophage- and fibroblast-derived cytokines (6).

In vitro studies have clarified the potent and overlapping biologic activities of TNF-α and IL-1. Both cytokines activate the transcription factor nuclear factor κB (NFκB), which in turn activates transcription of a set of proinflammatory genes, including adhesion molecules, IL-6, IL-8, GM-CSF, matrix metalloproteases, and prostanoids (7–11). These inflammatory mediators act in concert to promote bone and cartilage destruction as well as systemic cachexia. Furthermore, TNF-α and IL-1 amplify their own and each other's synthesis and, in combination, act synergistically to up-regulate a broad array of inflammatory pathways (12–15).

These *in vitro* data, which identified TNF-α and IL-1 as potential therapeutic targets for RA, were supported by data from animal models of arthritis. In the murine collagen-induced model of arthritis (CIA), expression of TNF-α and

IL-1 is abundantly up-regulated compared with unaffected controls (16–19). Inhibitors of TNF (soluble receptors or antibodies) prevent the onset or reduce the severity of established arthritis in this model (20–23), and mice deficient in soluble TNF receptor type I (p55) are resistant to the development of CIA (21). Furthermore, transgenic mice expressing human TNF-α develop a chronic symmetric erosive polyarthritis similar to human RA (24). Interestingly, another transgenic model in which only cell-associated, and not soluble, TNF-α is expressed also develop inflammatory polyarthritis (25,26).

Inhibitors of IL-1 [soluble receptor or IL-1 receptor antagonist (IL-1Ra)] administered by injection or by *ex vivo* gene transfer also ameliorate CIA and adjuvant- and antigen-induced arthritis in mice (27–31). Mice that are deficient in endogenous IL-1Ra, or are transgenic for human IL-1α, develop a chronic destructive inflammatory arthritis resembling human RA (32,33).

In rats with established CIA, combined treatment with polyethylene glycol (PEG)-ylated soluble TNF receptor and IL-1Ra was more effective than either cytokine inhibitor alone in alleviating the disease (34). Interestingly, treatment of transgenic TNF-α mice with IL-1Ra strongly ameliorated disease, suggesting that IL-1 is a downstream mediator of at least some of the effects of TNF (35). However, Niki et al. (33) demonstrated high levels of TNF-α messenger RNA (mRNA) in human IL-1α transgenic mice, confirming that IL-1 also induces TNF-α production *in vivo*. Some investigators have suggested that IL-1 and TNF-α have nonoverlapping biologic effects, such that IL-1 mediates cartilage and bone erosion, whereas TNF mediates joint inflammation (28,36). This hypothesis remains controversial, however, and it is likely that the *in vivo* actions of these cytokines are overlapping.

TUMOR NECROSIS FACTOR-α AND TUMOR NECROSIS FACTOR RECEPTORS

TNF-α, also known as cachectin, was originally named for its abilities to trigger necrosis of transplanted tumor cells and to induce wasting in chronic disease (37,38). TNF is produced primarily by macrophages and, to a lesser extent by T cells, and is a member of the TNF family of ligands and receptors (38). The polypeptide ligands are characterized by a common core sequence predicted to contain 10 β-sheet forming sequences and include TNF-α, lymphotoxin-α and -β, Fas ligand, CD40 ligand, and others (39) (Table 39.1). TNF-α is initially synthesized and expressed as a transmembrane molecule, but the extracellular portion is subsequently cleaved by TNF-α-converting enzyme (TACE) to release the soluble 17-kd molecule. Soluble TNF-α circulates as a homotrimer and, upon engagement of its cognate receptors, is believed to trigger a conformational change and dimerization or clustering of receptors (40).

TABLE 39.1. *Selected members of the tumor necrosis factor (TNF) ligand/receptor superfamily*

Ligands	Receptors
Lymphotoxin-α	TNF-R1 and -RII
TNF-α	TNF-RI and -RII
Lymphotoxin-β	LT-βR
OX40L	OX40
CD40L	CD40
Fas/Apo 1L	Fas/Apo 1
CD27L	CD27
CD30L	CD30
4-1BBL	4-1BB

For a complete list of TNF ligands and receptors, see reference 39.

There are two TNF receptors (TNF-R): the type I TNF-R (TNF-RI; p55 or p60; CD120a) and the type II TNF-R (TNF-RII; p75 or p80; CD120b) (40). There are two natural ligands for the TNF receptors: TNF-α and lymphotoxin-α. In contrast to the relatively restricted expression of TNF-α, TNF receptors are expressed by nearly every mammalian cell. Their ubiquitous expression and coupling to a variety of effector molecules explains the wide range of biologic activities of TNF-α. TNF-induced activation of the cysteine protease family of caspases leads to apoptotic cell death (41), whereas activation or enhanced synthesis of the transcription factors leads to induction of a wide array of protein and lipid inflammatory molecules (39,40). TNF signaling mechanisms have been reviewed in detail recently (39). The biologic activities of soluble TNF-α are thought to be mediated primarily through TNF-RI, whereas cell-associated TNF-α preferentially binds TNF-RII (42). Like TNF, the p55 and p75 TNF receptors can be cleaved from the cell surface by TACE (43). Soluble TNF receptors (sTNFRs) probably represent only a small fraction of total TNF receptors, but because they retain their ability to bind TNF-α, they may act as endogenous antagonists of circulating bioactive TNF-α (40).

INTERLEUKIN-1 AND INTERLEUKIN-1 RECEPTORS

The IL-1 superfamily consists of 10 closely related gene products. The four primary members are IL-1α, IL-1β, IL-1Ra, and IL-18. These molecules share considerable sequence homology and contain a β-pleated sheet structure (44). IL-1α and IL-β are agonists for the IL-1 receptor and are synthesized as 31-kd precursor molecules (pro-IL-1α and pro-IL-1β). Pro-IL-1α is retained intracellularly and can be cleaved by cysteine proteases called calpains to yield mature IL-1α, although pro-IL-1α is also biologically active (45). In contrast, pro-IL-1β requires proteolytic cleavage by the cysteine protease, caspase-1 (also known as IL-1β converting enzyme, or ICE), to yield the biologically-active mature 17-kd form of IL-1β (46,47). Mature IL-1β is secreted extracellularly and is believed to be responsible for the proinflammatory effects of IL-1. Another member of the IL-1 family is the IL-1Ra. Although originating from the same gene, there are multiple splice variants of IL-1Ra protein (48,49). The first to be described was the 22-kd secreted form of IL-1Ra. Secreted IL-1Ra (sIL-1Ra) is a pure receptor antagonist that binds IL-1R with an affinity comparable with that of IL-1β (50).

There are two immunoglobulin-like membrane-bound IL-1 receptors: type I (IL-1RI) and type II (IL-1RII). IL-1RI has a long cytoplasmic tail and is capable of intracellular signaling (51,52). Upon binding of IL-1β or IL-1α to IL-1RI, the recruitment of a second, structurally-distinct protein named the IL-1 receptor accessory protein (IL-1R AcP) is triggered (53,54). Assembly of this high-affinity receptor complex triggers subsequent transduction signaling. IL-1Ra lacks a binding domain for IL-1R AcP and, therefore, does not recruit this second chain to the receptor complex (55). IL-1-induced biologic responses require only 1% to 2% occupancy of IL-1RI, and extensive signal amplification further augments the biologic effects of IL-1 (50). In contrast to IL-1RI, IL-1RII has a short cytoplasmic tail and does not signal; it is likely to act as a decoy receptor for IL-1 (56). As with the TNF receptors, soluble forms of both IL-1RI and IL-1RII (sIL-1RI and sIL-1RII, respectively) are produced naturally and may act as endogenous antagonists of circulating bioactive IL-1β (57–59).

DEVELOPMENT OF TUMOR NECROSIS FACTOR AND INTERLEUKIN-1 ANTAGONISTS

Tumor Necrosis Factor Antagonists

The strategies for inhibiting TNF that have been most extensively studied to date are biologic, protein-based drugs, either monoclonal antibodies (MoAbs) directed against TNF or recombinant sTNFRs (Fig. 39.1). Both types of molecules will bind soluble TNF-α, effectively preventing the cytokine from engaging cell-associated TNF receptors and activating inflammatory pathways. The recombinant sTNFRs, but not anti-TNF MoAbs, will also bind lymphotoxin-α. TNF antagonists that are currently in clinical use or in development are listed in Table 39.2.

Recombinant sTNFRs have been engineered as fusion proteins in which the extracellular, ligand-binding portion of human TNF-RI or TNF-RII is coupled to a human immunoglobulin-like molecule. Even though cell-associated TNF-RI is thought to mediate the majority of the biologic effects of TNF *in vivo* (60), the native and engineered forms of both sTNF-RI and sTNF-RII all bind TNF with high affinity. These soluble receptor constructs consist entirely of human protein, but the linkage region between the receptor and the immunoglobulin molecule represents an unnatural sequence, and, therefore, has the potential for eliciting an antibody response.

Etanercept (sTNF-RII:Fc; Enbrel, Immunex Corp., Seattle, WA, U.S.A.), the only recombinant sTNFR currently approved by the U.S. Food and Drug Administration (FDA) for clinical use, is a dimeric construct in which two sTNF-RIIs (p75) are linked to the Fc portion of human IgG1 (60) (Fig. 39.1). Dimerization of the sTNF-RII results in a higher affinity for TNF-α (50- to 1,000-fold higher) than the monomeric receptor, and linkage to the Fc portion of human IgG1 prolongs its half-life (60). In RA patients, the serum half-life of etanercept is approximately 102 hours, and the drug is administered subcutaneously.

Conjugation with PEG is another mechanism for prolonging the half-life of receptors, and this strategy was used successfully to generate a monomeric construct of TNF-RI (PEG-p55sTNF-RI) (61). Soluble TNF-RI has also been dimerized by coupling to human IgG1-Fc, yielding the construct known as lenercept (p55sTNF-RI-Fc) (62,63). Neither of these constructs (PEG-p55sTNF-RI or p55sTNF-RI-Fc) have reached the stages of submission for FDA approval.

Two anti-TNF MoAbs have been approved by the FDA for clinical use (Table 39.2). Infliximab (Remicade, Centocor, Inc., Malvern, PA, U.S.A.) is a chimeric human/mouse anti-TNFα MoAb composed of the constant regions of human IgG1κ, coupled to the Fv region of a high-affinity neutralizing murine anti-human TNFα antibody (64) (Fig. 39.1). The antibody exhibits high affinity [association constant (K_a) 10^{10}/mol] for recombinant and natural human TNF-α, and neutralizes TNF-mediated cytotoxicity and other functions *in vitro* (64). The terminal half-life of infliximab is 8.0 to 9.5 days, and it is administered intravenously at approximately 8-week intervals following three loading doses.

Adalimumab (Humira, Abbott Laboratories, Abbott Park, Illinois) differs from infliximab in that its sequences are entirely human (Fig. 39.1). Generated by phase display technology with amino acid sequences only from the human germ line, it is indistinguishable in structure and function from natural human IgG1 (65). Adalimumab also has high specificity for TNFα [dissociation constant (K_d) = $6 \times 10^{-10} M$] and a terminal half-life comparable with that of human IgG1 (~2 weeks) (65) . It is administered subcutaneously. Other anti-TNF MoAbs that are not currently FDA approved for human use include CDP571, a humanized, complementarity determining region grafted MoAb (66), and CDP870, a PEGylated-linked Fab fragment (67).

Inhibition of TACE, which would prevent protease-mediated generation of soluble TNF-α (and soluble TNF receptors), is a third strategy to antagonize TNF and one that is currently under investigation (68,69).

Interleukin-1 Antagonists

Strategies for inhibition of IL-1 include the development of genetically-engineered, recombinant forms of IL-1Ra and

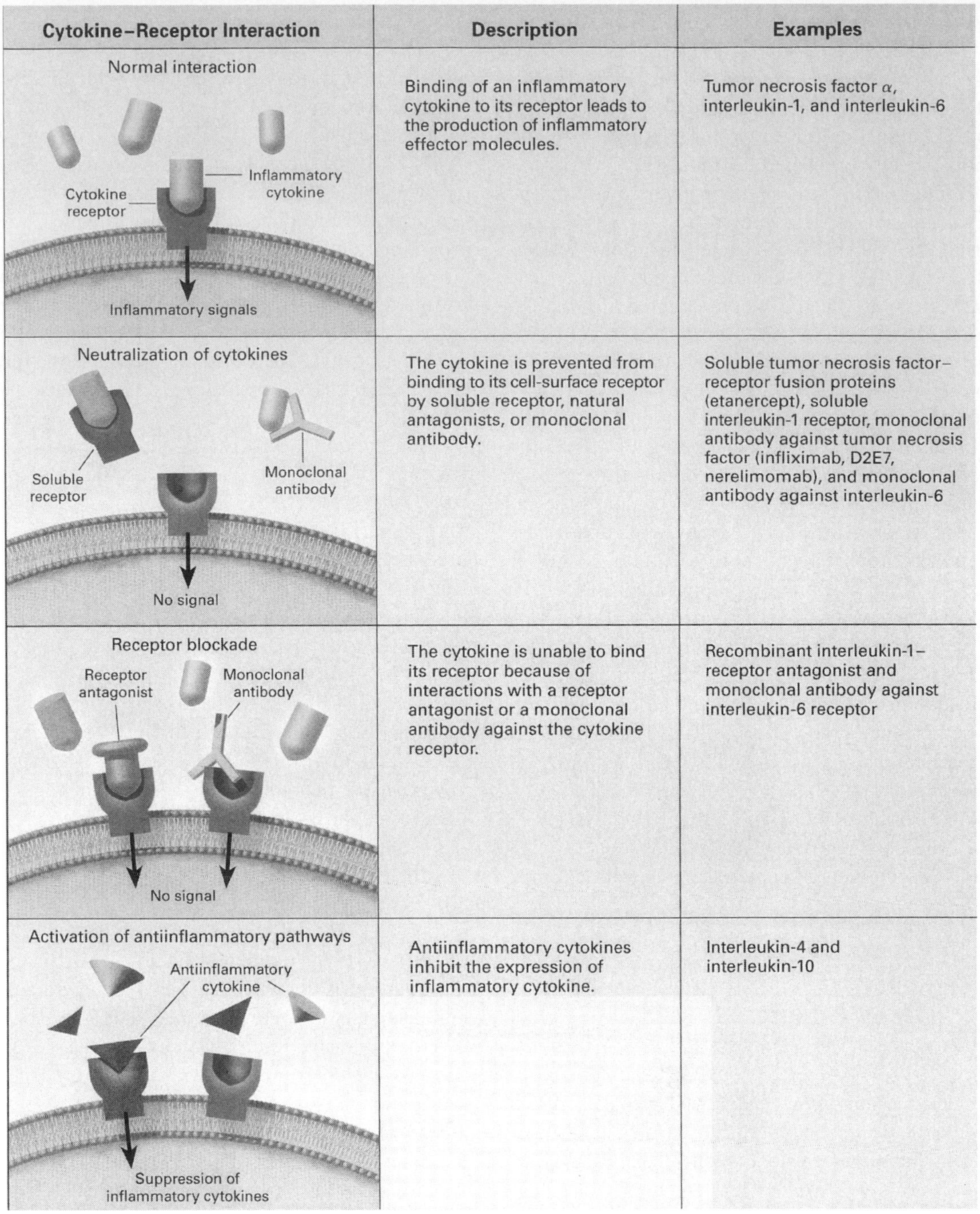

Cytokine–Receptor Interaction	Description	Examples
Normal interaction Inflammatory cytokine Cytokine receptor Inflammatory signals	Binding of an inflammatory cytokine to its receptor leads to the production of inflammatory effector molecules.	Tumor necrosis factor α, interleukin-1, and interleukin-6
Neutralization of cytokines Soluble receptor Monoclonal antibody No signal	The cytokine is prevented from binding to its cell-surface receptor by soluble receptor, natural antagonists, or monoclonal antibody.	Soluble tumor necrosis factor–receptor fusion proteins (etanercept), soluble interleukin-1 receptor, monoclonal antibody against tumor necrosis factor (infliximab, D2E7, nerelimomab), and monoclonal antibody against interleukin-6
Receptor blockade Receptor antagonist Monoclonal antibody No signal	The cytokine is unable to bind its receptor because of interactions with a receptor antagonist or a monoclonal antibody against the cytokine receptor.	Recombinant interleukin-1–receptor antagonist and monoclonal antibody against interleukin-6 receptor
Activation of antiinflammatory pathways Antiinflammatory cytokine Suppression of inflammatory cytokines	Antiinflammatory cytokines inhibit the expression of inflammatory cytokine.	Interleukin-4 and interleukin-10

FIG. 39.1. Cytokine/receptor interactions: descriptions and examples. (From Choi EH, Panayi GS. Cytokine pathways and joint inflammation in rheumatoid arthritis. *N Engl J Med* 2001;344:912, with permission.)

TABLE 39.2. *Tumor necrosis factor (TNF) inhibitors*

Generic name	Description	Target(s)	FDA approved	Refs.
Soluble TNF receptors				
Etanercept	sTNF-RII-Fc	TNF-α; lymphotoxin-α	Yes	86
Lenercept	sTNF-RI-Fc	TNF-α; lymphotoxin-α	No	62,194
NA	PEG-p55sTNF-RI	TNF-α; lymphotoxin-α	No	26
Anti-TNF monoclonal antibodies				
Infliximab	Mouse-human chimeric	TNF-α	Yes	64
Adalimumab	Human	TNF-α	Yes	65
CDP571	CDR grafted	TNF-α	No	66
CDP870	PEG-linked Fab	TNF-α	No	67

FDA, U.S. Food and Drug Administration; NA, not available.

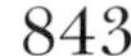

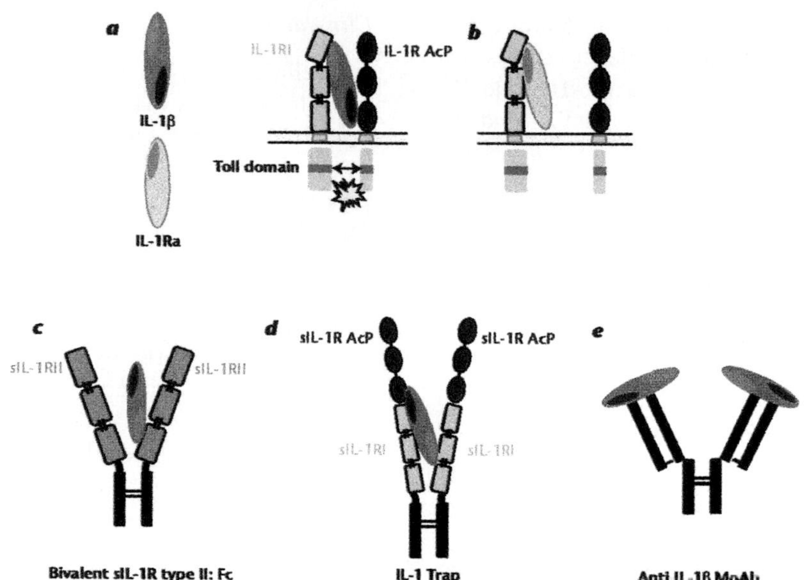

FIG. 39.2. Blocking interleukin-1 (IL-1) activity. **A:** The cytokine IL-1β has two different receptor binding sites (red and blue). The IL-1 receptor type I (IL-1RI) binds one site and the IL-1 receptor accessory protein (IL-1RAcP) engages the second site. The resulting complex activates the cell. The naturally-occurring IL-1 receptor antagonist (IL-1Ra) possesses only the type I receptor binding site. **B:** The antagonist occupies this receptor and prevents bona fide IL-1β from binding to cells. **C:** The soluble IL-1 receptor type II (sIL-1RII) is shown as a bivalent construction of the extracellular domains of the receptor; two identical chains are linked by the Fc segment of IgG1. **D:** The IL-1 trap contains the extracellular segment of both IL-1 receptor chains fused into a dimeric molecule using the complement domain of IgG1. The IL-1 trap allows high-affinity IL-1β binding similar to that on the cell surface. **E:** Monoclonal antibodies can bind and neutralize two IL-1β molecules. Cytokine traps may present some advantages over other cytokine-targeting agents. (From Greene GL. Setting the cytokine trap for autoimmunity. *Nat Med* 2003;9:20–22, with permission.)

soluble IL-1 receptors (Fig. 39.2, Table 39.3). Recombinant human IL-ra (rIL-1Ra; anakinra; Kineret, Amgen, Thousand Oaks, CA) is the only IL-1 antagonist approved by the FDA, and indications are currently limited to the treatment of adult RA. Anakinra differs from native nonglycosylated IL-1Ra only by the addition of an N-terminal methionine (70). Anakinra binds IL-1RI with an affinity equivalent to IL-1β (71), thereby preventing IL-1β from binding to cell-associated IL-1R1 (Fig. 39.2). Its terminal half-life is relatively short (4–6 hours) and, therefore, the drug must be administered daily by subcutaneous administration. *In vitro* data suggest that a 10- to 100-fold excess of IL-1Ra (relative to IL-1) is necessary to inhibit 50% of the biologic activity of IL-1 (72). Since only about 1% to 2% of IL-1RI need to be occupied to induce cell activation (52,73), a large excess of IL-1Ra (relative to IL-1) is theoretically needed to effectively block IL-1-induced inflammation. This potentially dose-limiting feature, coupled with its short-half life, may explain the relatively modest clinical efficacy of anakinra.

As with TNF, a second strategy for inhibition of IL-1 is through the development of sIL-1Rs. A recombinant sIL-1RI construct was developed and studied. Drevlow et al. (74) reported in patients with long-standing RA a marginal clinical benefit at the highest dose. This is likely due to the fact that sIL-1RI binds IL-1Ra more avidly than IL-1 and may, therefore, have a proinflammatory rather than an anti-inflammatory effect. Further clinical development of recombinant sIL-1RI was thus abandoned. Trials with recombinant sIL-1RII have been undertaken in animal models of arthritis (75). Human clinical trials are in progress at this time.

Recently, the development of the so-called IL-1 "trap" molecule has garnered considerable attention (76). The IL-1

TABLE 39.3. *Interleukin (IL)-1 inhibitors*

Name	Description	Target	Ref
Anakinra	IL-1 receptor antagonist (IL-1ra)	L-1-α and -β	70
sIL-1RI	Soluble IL-1 receptor type I	IL-1-α and -β	74
sIL-1RII	Soluble IL-1 receptor type II	IL-1-α and -β	75
IL-1 Trap	IL-1RI and IL-1RAcP fusion molecule	IL-1-α and -β	76

trap consists of two identical molecules covalently linked by disulfide bonds (Fig. 39.2). Each molecule consists of the two extracellular receptor sequences (IL-1RI and IL-1RAcP) necessary for high-affinity IL-1 binding and the Fc portion of human IgG1, arranged "in line" or sequentially. *In vitro,* the affinity constant of the IL-1 trap is approximately 1 to 2 p*M*, considerably higher than that of monomeric sIL-1RII (500 p*M*) or sIL-1RI (1–3 n*M*) (77). Furthermore, IL-1 trap exhibits a favorable terminal half-life in primates of 67 hours (76). This construct is now in clinical development and is discussed below.

MoAbs directed against IL-1α or IL-1β have not been evaluated in clinical trials to date, although these strategies have shown some promise in animal models of arthritis (78). Development of a small molecule inhibitor of ICE that would effectively limit the production of bioactive IL-1β is another strategy for IL-1 inhibition (79,80), and clinical trials have just begun with this approach.

CLINICAL TRIALS IN RHEUMATOID ARTHRITIS: EFFICACY OF CYTOKINE ANTAGONISTS

TNF and IL-1 antagonists have been studied extensively in clinical trials in RA (64,81–99). Both classes of inhibitors have clear efficacy in reducing symptomatology, slowing the progression of radiographically-evident joint damage, and down-regulating the inflammatory process. In addition, one or more of the TNF inhibitors have been demonstrated to reduce angiogenesis and leukocyte trafficking into joints, and to reverse the hematologic abnormalities that are typical of RA. The TNF antagonists are substantially more potent than IL-1Ra (Anakinra) but are also associated with a higher risk for infection and possibly other adverse events. These issues are discussed in detail below.

TNF Antagonists

The efficacy of each of the three approved TNF antagonists has been studied in patients with long-standing refractory RA in randomized, placebo-controlled trials, both as monotherapy and in combination with MTX (81–89,92, 93,98,99). Etanercept is the only TNF antagonist that has been studied as monotherapy in early disease (90), although clinical trials in early RA, in which infliximab or adalimumab is combined with MTX, are currently underway. The only direct comparison of efficacy and safety of a TNF antagonist to a nonbiologic disease-modifying antirheumatic drug (DMARD) was provided by the early RA trial with etanercept (90). The results of these various studies are summarized below.

Clinical Responses

In clinical trials of the TNF antagonists in long-standing refractory RA (81–89), the primary outcome was improvement in signs and symptoms of disease, as assessed by fulfillment of the American College of Rheumatology 20 (ACR20) (100) or Paulus 20 response criteria (101). The ACR20 and Paulus 20 responses are validated composite scores that contain physician, patient, and laboratory response elements (defined in Table 39.4) and are assessed as dichotomous variables. ACR50 and 70 scores are defined similarly by substituting a requirement for 50% and 70% improvement, respectively. The rank order of efficacy of the TNF antagonists cannot be discerned by the available clinical trials since there has been no head-to-head comparison of these agents. Comparison of ACR responses across clinical trials to discern relative efficacies is not valid because inclusion and exclusion criteria, duration of treatment, and statistical methods of analysis varied among the trials. Nonetheless, for the purposes of discussion, representative data from clinical trials with the various inhibitors are shown together in Tables 39.5 and 39.6 to provide an overview of the efficacy of these agents compared with their respective placebo-treated control populations. The data points selected and displayed in these tables represent ACR (or Paulus) responses to a dose of TNF antagonist used in each trial that most closely approximates the current FDA-approved starting dose, and represent the longest duration of randomized blinded treatment in each clinical trial cited (which corresponds in most cases, but not all, to the predefined primary outcome). In Table 39.5, ACR (or Paulus) responses are shown for each TNF antagonist as monotherapy compared with placebo, whereas Table 39.6 shows ACR responses to TNF antagonist in combination with MTX compared with MTX alone.

In the monotherapy trials shown in Table 39.5, all prior DMARDs were washed out for at least 4 weeks before the TNF antagonist (or placebo) was initiated. Despite varying

TABLE 39.4. *American College of Rheumatology (ACR) composite scores for assessing clinical responses in rheumatoid arthritis (100)*

ACR 20% Response
Must include both: (a) 20% improvement in tender joint count
(b) 20% improvement in swollen joint count.
And 20% improvement in three of five of the following criteria:
Patient pain assessment
Patient global assessment
Physician global assessment
Patient self-assessed disability
Acute phase reactant value (erythrocyte sedimentation rate or C-reactive protein)

ACR, American College of Rheumatology.

TABLE 39.5. *Placebo-controlled trials of cytokine inhibitors as montherapy in refractory rheumatoid arthritis*

	Response[a]					
	20%		50%		70%	
Clinical trial (ref)	Pl	Inh	Pl	Inh	Pl	Inh
TNF antagonists						
Infliximab (81)	8	79	8	58	NR	NR
Etanercept (87)	14	75	7	57	NR	NR
Etanercept (88)	11	59	5	40	1	15
Adalimumab (92)	19	46	8	22	2	12
IL-1 antagonist						
Anakinra (94)	27	43	NR	NR	NR	NR

Data are shown only for dose of cytokine inhibitors studied that most closely approximates the currently approved U.S. Food and Drug Administration starting dose, and for the longest time point evaluated in each trial, as follows: etanercept 16 mg/m^2 twice weekly at 3-month time point (87) or 25 mg twice weekly at 6-month time point (88); infliximab 10 mg/kg single dose at 1-month time point; adalimumab 40 mg twice monthly at 6-month time point; and anakinra 150 mg daily at 6-month time point.

[a]Percentage of subjects who met criteria for an ACR20/50/70 or Paulus 20/50/70 response criteria.

Inh, inhibitor; NR, not reported; Pl, placebo.

inclusion and exclusion criteria from trial to trial, the demographic characteristics of the enrolled subjects were remarkably similar across trials. Subjects were predominantly white women 50 to 60 years of age with disease duration of approximately 10 years and in whom disease had been poorly controlled on multiple, nonbiologic DMARDs. The majority of subjects were seropositive for rheumatoid factor and, at baseline, had a range of 28 to 35 tender joints and 20 to 25 swollen joints, and moderate-to-high elevation of C-reactive protein (CRP; range 3.6–6.7 mg/dL). As can be seen in Table 39.5, the ACR (or Paulus) response to each of TNF antagonists was robust and, in all cases, statistically superior to placebo at the dose represented. Clinical responses to the anti-TNF MoAbs have been observed to be rapid (days to weeks). Withdrawal of treatment with the TNF antagonists leads to a rapid rebound in clinical disease activity (86), indicating that inhibition of TNF is highly effective in suppressing the inflammatory process but is not curative.

In clinical trials in which combination treatment of TNF antagonist plus MTX was compared with MTX alone (Table 39.6), subjects were required to have been on a stable dose of MTX for at least 1 month prior to enrollment. Again, the subject populations studied were predominantly middle-aged, white women with long-standing, seropositive RA. Despite MTX, they exhibited moderate-to-marked disease activity at baseline (range of 24–35 tender joints and 17–23 swollen joints across the studies). The baseline levels of CRP were somewhat lower (range 2.0–3.1 mg/dL) than in the monotherapy trials, presumably due to a partial treatment effect from background MTX. ACR responses to each of the TNF antagonists (Table 39.6) were again observed to be quite robust, despite background MTX therapy, and nearly equivalent to those observed in the monotherapy

TABLE 39.6. *Placebo-controlled trials of cytokine inhibitors in combination with methotrexate (MTX) versus MTX alone in refractory rheumatoid arthritis*

	Percentage response[a]					
	20%		50%		70%	
Clinical trial (ref)	Pl	Inh	Pl	Inh	Pl	Inh
TNF antagonists						
Infliximab (84)	20	50	5	27	0	8
Etanercept (89)	27	71	3	39	0	15
Adalimumab (98)	15	67	8	55	5	27
IL-1 antagonist						
Anakinra (96)	23	42	4	24	0	10

Data are shown only for dose of cytokine inhibitors that most closely approximates the currently U.S. Food and Drug Administration recommended starting dose, and for the longest time point evaluated in each trial (24–30 weeks), as follows: infliximab 3 mg/kg every 8 weeks and median MTX dose of 15 mg/wk; etanercept 25 mg twice weekly and mean MTX dose of 18–19 mg/wk; adalimumab 40 mg twice monthly and mean MTX dose of 16–17 mg/wk; and anakinra 1 mg/kg daily and mean MTX dose of 16–18 mg/wk.

[a]Percentage of subjects who met criteria for an ACR20/50/70 response criteria.

Inh, inhibitor; Pl, placebo.

trials. All ACR responses to TNF antagonist plus MTX were statistically superior to MTX alone at the doses represented in Table 39.6. Recent data (unpublished) from another large trial have clearly demonstrated that the combination of TNF antagonist with MTX is markedly superior in efficacy compared to monotherapy with either agent. (See Chapters 32 and 33.)

TNF antagonists are also efficacious in children with polyarticular juvenile rheumatoid arthritis (JRA). In the largest study to date of a TNF inhibitor in children, Lovell et al. (102) reported superiority of etanercept to placebo in controlling the signs and symptoms of polyarticular JRA. Controlled trials of the anti-TNF MoAbs are currently in progress.

Structural Damage

The ACR response criteria measure improvements in signs and symptoms of RA. However, retardation of structural joint damage and prevention of disability are the ultimate goals of treatment of RA. Joint damage begins early, as evidenced radiographically by the appearance of articular erosions in the first year of disease in 40% of RA patients, and by the second year in 90% of patients (103, 104). Joint damage continues to accrue and accumulate throughout the course of the disease if left untreated or inadequately treated (103–106). These observations have prompted recommendations for the initiation of DMARDs early in disease (107). The ability of etanercept to slow radiographic progression was evaluated and compared with that of rapidly escalated MTX in a group of RA patients who had a mean duration of disease of only 1 year and who had never received MTX (90). Except for the short duration of disease, subjects were otherwise demographically similar to participants in prior RA trials and had very active disease (mean tender and swollen joint counts of 30 and 24, respectively; mean CRP range of 3.3–4.4 mg/dL). Radiographic damage was assessed by the modified Sharp score (103,108), a validated composite radiographic score of erosions and joint space narrowing in multiple joints of the hands, feet and wrists. The estimated mean annual rate of radiographic progression at the time of entry into the trial was 9 Sharp units/yr for both the etanercept and MTX groups; after 1 year of treatment with etanercept or MTX, the annual progression scores were only 1.00 and 1.59 Sharp units/yr, respectively. Furthermore, 72% of the etanercept group and 60% of the MTX group had no further erosions during the 12-month treatment period. These data confirmed the ability of a TNF antagonist as monotherapy to profoundly retard radiographically evident joint damage, and reaffirmed the capacity of MTX to do the same. In addition, the ACR20/50/70 responses in this early RA population in response to etanercept were very comparable with those seen in patients with advanced, refractory disease.

For patients who continue to develop radiographic joint damage despite treatment with MTX, the addition of a TNF antagonist can significantly reduce the rate of radiographic progression even late in the course of the disease. This was demonstrated by Lipsky et al. (85) in a combination trial comparing infliximab and MTX to MTX alone. In this study, 428 RA patients with a mean duration of disease of 10 years, mean tender and swollen joint counts at baseline of approximately 32 and 22, respectively, and mean baseline CRP of greater than or equal to 3.3 mg/dL despite treatment with MTX (mean dosage 16–17 mg/wk) were randomized to receive treatment with placebo or infliximab (one of four dosing schedules) while continuing MTX. After 1 year of treatment, the mean annual progression score in the MTX/placebo group was 7.0 Sharp units/yr, whereas the mean progression in the combined infliximab/ MTX groups was only 0.6 units/yr. The same trend was recently reported in a similarly designed trial with adalimumab wherein the MTX/placebo group progressed at 2.7 Sharp units/yr over 12 months compared with 0.1 Sharp units/yr in the adalimumab/MTX group (93). Thus, all three TNF antagonists are capable of profoundly slowing structural joint damage in RA.

Durability of Response

Antibodies directed against all three TNF antagonists have been observed to varying degrees, and this phenomenon may limit the half-life of the antagonist and thus the durability of the clinical response. In a study by Maini et al. (83), antibody responses to varying doses of infliximab, in the presence or absence of coadministered MTX, were evaluated. In general, the frequency of antichimeric antibodies was inversely proportional to the dose of infliximab but significantly suppressed in the presence of MTX. These data suggest that immunologic tolerance was induced at higher doses of infliximab, and tolerance was potentiated by the simultaneous administration of MTX.

Unpublished data presented to the FDA indicate that mean steady-state trough concentrations of adalimumab are also higher in the presence of MTX (5 and 8–9 μg/mL in the absence and presence of MTX, respectively), and there is higher apparent clearance of adalimumab in the presence of antiadalimumab antibodies (109). Nevertheless, the durability of clinical response to adalimumab as monotherapy does not appear to decline over 6 months (92). The prevalence of antietanercept antibodies reported in clinical trials is less than 10% (86–90), and no significant decay in the clinical response was observed during prolonged treatment with etanercept as monotherapy (90). Current FDA guidelines, therefore, advise the use of MTX with infliximab for the treatment of RA, whereas adalimumab and etanercept can be used as monotherapy or in combination with MTX (see later section on Current Indications for Tumor Necrosis Factor and Interleukin-1 Antagonists).

Interleukin-1 Antagonists

The efficacy of Anakinra has been evaluated in clinical trials of adult RA patients both as monotherapy and in combination with MTX (91,94–97). No studies in early RA have been conducted with anakinra.

The profile of adult RA subjects studied in the Anakinra trials was similar to that in the TNF studies (middle-aged white women with active disease), although the duration of disease tended to be lower in the Anakinra trials (4 years in the monotherapy trials and 6–9 years in the MTX combination trials) than the TNF antagonist trials. In general, the efficacy of Anakinra in relieving signs and symptoms of disease and in slowing radiographic progression is more modest than that of the TNF antagonists. For example, the ACR20 responses to Anakinra shown in Tables 39.5 and 39.6 were less than twofold higher than the corresponding placebo responses. In contrast, the ACR20 responses to the TNF antagonists ranged from 2.5- to 9.9-fold higher than their corresponding placebo responses. In contrast to the greater than 90% reduction in radiographic progression observed with the TNF antagonists alone or in combination with MTX, Anakinra treatment was associated with a 47% reduction in the rate of radiographic progression compared with placebo (95). It should be noted, however, that the radiographic scoring system used in the Anakinra trial was different from that used for the TNF antagonists.

No placebo-controlled data on the efficacy of Anakinra in juvenile RA are available yet. The efficacy of combining Anakinra with a TNF antagonist is currently under study in adult RA, although preliminary data from a small, open-label, pilot study suggested an unacceptably high rate of infection (see later section on Clinical Trials in Rheumatoid Arthritis: Safety of Cytokine Antagonists).

The relatively modest clinical responses of RA patients to anakinra may well be due to its short half-life. To more accurately assess the relative contribution of IL-1 to the inflammatory process in RA, clinical trials with a more stable and potent IL-1 antagonist will be necessary. The IL-1 trap molecule may provide such an opportunity because both *in vitro* and *in vivo* data confirm high (picomolar) affinity for IL-1, a slow off-rate from IL-1, and a prolonged terminal half-life (67 hours) (76). A phase I trial in RA patients suggested acceptable tolerability (110), but definitive conclusions about its efficacy and safety await large-scale phase II and III trials.

CLINICAL TRIALS IN RHEUMATOID ARTHRITIS: SAFETY OF CYTOKINE ANTAGONISTS

Tumor Necrosis Factor Antagonists

Etanercept, infliximab, and adalimumab were approved for RA by the FDA in 1998, 2000, and 2003, respectively. Safety data are available from controlled clinical trials for all three therapies, and postmarketing safety data for the first two. In controlled clinical trials in RA, the most common side effect was injection or infusion reactions. Overall, however, all three biologic agents were generally well tolerated, with no demonstrable major organ toxicities and no dose-limiting side effects. Based on the physiologic actions of these agents, however, there has been concern for the possibility of increased risk for infection and malignancy. Indeed, postmarketing data for etanercept and infliximab, and clinical trial data for adalimumab, have confirmed an apparent increased incidence of opportunistic infections in patients treated with these agents. No firm conclusions can be made as yet regarding the malignancy question. An additional concern is that these genetically-engineered proteins administered repeatedly over prolonged periods may elicit immune responses. These issues are addressed below.

Injection and Infusion Reactions

In placebo-controlled clinical trials for all three TNF antagonists, injection or infusion reactions were the most frequent and consistent side effect, although they rarely resulted in withdrawal of patients from the trials. Injection site reactions occur in 20% to 40% of patients treated with the subcutaneously-administered antagonists (etanercept and adalimumab) and consist of erythema and induration limited to the injection sites (86–90,92,93,98,99). Reactions occur early after initiation of treatment, are generally mild and self-limited, and usually resolve within the first month of treatment. The injection site reactions are limited to the skin and are not associated with other features of immediate hypersensitivity. No specific therapy is required, although antihistamines or topical corticosteroids may be helpful. Similarly, infusion reactions were the most common side effect of infliximab, manifested most frequently by headache and nausea, and less commonly by flushing or a reduction in blood pressure (64,81–85). The infusion reactions are transient and usually aborted by slowing the rate of infusion and, if needed, the addition of antihistamines or a bolus of corticosteroids. The frequency of infusion reactions does not increase over time of exposure to drug (85).

Infection

Multiple studies in humans and animals demonstrate the importance of TNF-α as a defense against infection by intracellular organisms. TNF is increased in the systemic circulation after administration of endotoxin or bacteria, and TNF and IL-1 are responsible for the physiologic alterations seen in septic shock (40). Indeed, in a human clinical trial of septic shock due to gram-positive organisms, treatment with etanercept was associated with increased mortality compared with treatment with placebo (111). Mice rendered deficient in TNF-α lack primary B-cell follicles and demonstrate impaired humoral immune responses to both T cell-dependent and T cell-independent antigens (112–114).

Granuloma formation is an important inflammatory host mechanism for containing the proliferation and spread of *Mycobacterium tuberculosis* (115). TNF-α plays a critical role, along with helper T cell subset 1 (T_H1) cytokines, in the initiation and maintenance of granulomas, presumably by mediating cell recruitment to the lung and activating mycobactericidal processes, such as inducible nitric oxide synthase (116). In animals infected with *M. tuberculosis*, neutralization of TNF inhibited macrophage recruitment and the development of well-differentiated granulomas, and resulted in mycobacterial proliferation and rapid animal death (117–120). Recently, it has been shown that lymphotoxin-α, the other cognate ligand of the TNF receptors, is also required for host defense against *M. tuberculosis* infections (121,122). Based on these data, it seemed plausible that chronic inhibition of TNF (or lymphotoxin-α) may predispose individuals to opportunistic infections.

In published placebo-controlled clinical trials of TNF antagonists in RA, no increase in the overall frequency of infections, or in the frequency of serious infections, was observed in patients treated with TNF antagonists compared with placebo (64,81–84,88,90,92,93,98,99). A trend toward more infection was observed, however, at the highest dose of infliximab (10 mg/kg) in the study by Maini et al. (84).

However, postmarketing surveillance data on the TNF antagonists from the FDA MedWatch program subsequently revealed a high number of reports of tuberculosis and other opportunistic infections (123–125). Estimated incidence rates of TNF inhibitor-associated tuberculosis in the United States in 2001 were 24 per 100,000 population for infliximab and 9 per 100,000 for etanercept, as compared with 6 per 100,000 for both the general U.S. population (126) and for nonbiologically-treated RA patients in the United States (127). Of note, MedWatch is a voluntary reporting system, and these calculated incidence rates were likely to be underestimates of the true incidence rates of tuberculosis in the infliximab- and etanercept-treated population during 2001. Importantly, over half of the patients with both etanercept- and infliximab-associated tuberculosis presented with miliary or extrapulmonary disease involving sites such as the meninges, pleura, peritoneum, muscle, spine, and joint (123,124). The majority of patients with infliximab- and etanercept-associated tuberculosis were also receiving other immunosuppressive agents, including MTX and prednisone. The median time to presentation of patients with infliximab-associated tuberculosis was only 3 months (range 1–12 months) after starting drug (123), suggesting that infection was due to reactivation of latent disease rather than to primary exposure. One new hypothesis for the apparent higher frequency and faster onset of tuberculosis in infliximab- compared with etanercept-treated patients is that TNF is more potently inhibited with the former agent. Support for this hypothesis (128) is derived from observations that (a) the half-life of infliximab is substantially longer than that of etanercept; (b) the off-rate of infliximab from TNF is considerably slower *in vitro* than that for etanercept; and (c) infliximab may induce lysis of bacteria-laden macrophages expressing transmembrane TNF while etanercept does not. Adalimumab also has a substantially longer half-life than etanercept, and 13 cases of tuberculosis were reported to the FDA in early phase I/II trials with this agent (129). Mandatory screening for latent tuberculosis in subsequent phase II/ III trials eliminated this problem.

Other opportunistic infections reported in patients treated with TNF antagonists include histoplasmosis, aspergillosis, coccidioidomycosis, listeriosis, *Pneumocystis carinii* pneumonia, cryptococcus infection, candidiasis, cytomegalovirus infection, sporothrix infection, and atypical mycobacteria infection (124,130,131). In addition, severe infections with common bacterial organisms such as *Staphylococcus aureus* have been reported both during the clinical trials and in postmarketing experience with all three TNF antagonists (124), although the rates of these infections compared with those in RA patients not receiving biologic therapy are unknown.

Pretreatment screening of patients for latent tuberculosis (and institution of antimicrobial therapy if positive) is strongly recommended prior to commencement of therapy with a TNF antagonist. Guidelines for assessing and treating latent tuberculosis have been published recently (126). In addition, vigilance for infections with common bacteria and other opportunistic organisms is indicated in patients treated with these agents, and all should be temporarily discontinued if an acute infection is present or suspected, keeping in mind the long half-life of the drugs.

Malignancy

The immune system has an important role in surveillance for malignancy, and TNF plays a role in initiating apoptosis of some types of tumor cells. Thus, an increased risk for malignancy is of theoretical concern with chronic TNF inhibition. Lymphomas, both Hodgkin and non-Hodgkin, have been a particular concern since their incidence is known to be increased in RA populations (132–136). The standardized incidence ratio (SIR) of lymphomas in RA patients in the prebiologic era compared with non-RA controls has been estimated at 2.4 to as high as 26 (132–136). Risk factors for the development of lymphoma in RA include duration and severity of disease, advanced age, exposure to immunosuppressive drugs (including cyclophosphamide and MTX), concomitant Sjögren's syndrome, and infection with Epstein-Barr virus (132,137–139). In a small number of RA patients, lymphomas have been observed to regress following discontinuation of immunosuppressive agent and without initiation of antilymphoma chemotherapy (140).

Given the complexity of risk factors for malignancies in RA and the limited experience with TNF antagonists to date, it has not been possible to ascertain with certainty whether this class of drug increases the risk for malignancies in general, or for lymphomas in particular, in RA patients. In RA clinical trials, no increase in the number or type of solid tumors was observed in patients treated with TNF antagonists (81–90,92,93,98,99) compared with placebo-treated controls. However, an apparent increase in the incidence of lymphomas was observed in clinical trials in patients treated with TNF antagonists when compared with matched non-RA controls from the National Cancer Institute's SEER (Surveillance, Epidemiology, and End Results) program data base, yielding a SIR ranging from 2.3 to 6.3 (129). Although this SIR range is elevated compared with non-RA controls, it is consistent with the SIR range previously reported for lymphomas in RA populations prior to the availability of biologics.

As in the prebiologic era, the majority (80%) of lymphomas reported in RA patients treated with TNF antagonists in both clinical trials and postmarketing data were of the non-Hodgkin type, and diffuse large B-cell and follicular lymphomas comprised the most common histologic subtypes (141). The median time to onset of lymphoma following initiation of anti-TNF therapy was short (8 weeks; range 2–52 weeks) in postmarketing series, whereas the time to onset in the clinical trials was longer (30–200 weeks). In the postmarketing series of 26 lymphomas, two regressed spontaneously following discontinuation of the TNF antagonist without antilymphoma chemotherapy.

In summary, incidence rates of solid tumors in RA patients are not increased by exposure to TNF antagonists. The incidence of lymphomas, particularly non-Hodgkin lymphomas, is increased in the RA population compared with matched controls. Available data to date do not suggest that TNF inhibition increases this risk for lymphoma. However, experience with the TNF antagonists is still relatively short (maximum exposure approximately 6 years in open-label extensions of clinical trials), and long-term observational studies with appropriate controls are needed to clarify this issue. Several patient registries have been established to monitor the long-term safety of these drugs.

Immunogenicity and Autoantibody Formation

Antibodies to all three TNF antagonists have been reported. Infliximab is a chimeric monoclonal antibody containing 25% mouse sequence with the potential for antimurine antibodies. Indeed, antiinfliximab antibodies do occur and can be suppressed effectively by concomitant administration of MTX. Infliximab has been administered as monotherapy for Crohn disease, and repeated dosing was associated with loss of efficacy; a 61% frequency of anti-infliximab antibodies has been noted (142,143).

Etanercept is composed entirely of human sequence, but neoepitopes could be generated at the joining region of TNF-RII to the immunoglobulin Fc region. In all published clinical trials to date, however, the incidence of antietanercept antibodies was routinely low (<10%), and the presence of antibodies had no apparent effect on efficacy (86–90).

Adalimumab contains 100% human sequence, but anti-adalimumab antibodies have been reported, albeit infrequently (109). In general, the presence of antibodies against TNF antagonists was not associated with an increased incidence of adverse events, although Crohn disease infusion reactions were more common in patients with antiinfliximab antibodies when infliximab was given as monotherapy (143).

Autoantibodies, particularly antinuclear (ANA) antibodies and anti–double-stranded DNA (anti-dsDNA) antibodies, have been reported in patients treated with TNF inhibitors. In clinical trials, 11% to 15% of etanercept-treated patients developed new positive ANA or anti-dsDNA antibodies (compared with 4% to 5% in placebo-treated controls) (86–90). None of these patients developed clinical signs or symptoms of systemic lupus erythematosus (SLE). However, a number of cases of SLE have been reported in postmarketing data in etanercept-treated individuals (144,145). In the infliximab trials, approximately 50% and 15% of infliximab-treated patients developed ANA and anti-dsDNA antibodies respectively, compared with approximately 20% and 0% of placebo-treated patients (64,81–85). Reports of SLE and lupuslike syndromes were rare and consisted mostly of cutaneous and pleuropericardial disease without the more serious renal or neurologic manifestations of lupus. Twelve percent of adalimumab-treated patients in controlled clinical trials developed ANA compared with 7% of placebo-treated patients, and one of these (out of a total of 2,334) developed a lupuslike syndrome that spontaneously resolved after discontinuation of adalimumab (109). It should be noted that the method of assessing anti-DNA antibodies varies between clinical trials and can yield widely different results (146). Furthermore, Charles et al. (146) demonstrated that even when antibodies occur with anti-TNF therapy, they are generally not pathogenic because of their isotype or other immunochemical properties.

Although issues of immunogenicity and autoantibody formation remain, continued efficacy and tolerability of both etanercept and infliximab in long-term trials provides increasingly stronger evidence to alleviate these concerns. Long-term data on adalimumab are not yet available.

Neurologic Events

Considerable evidence to date supports a role for TNF-α in the pathogenesis of autoimmune demyelinating disease. In experimental autoimmune encephalomyelitis (EAE), a murine model of multiple sclerosis (MS), treatment with TNF-α worsened, and treatment with anti-TNF antibody treatment ameliorated, disease activity (147, 148). In humans, the levels of TNF-α in the cerebrospinal fluid and sera of patients with MS correlated with disease activity (149), and TNF has been demonstrated at autopsy in active MS foci (150). However, in a randomized, placebo-controlled trial with lenercept (sTNF-RI-Fc) in 168 patients with MS (151), a significantly higher proportion of lenercept-treated, than placebo-treated, patients experienced disease exacerbations. There were no differences in the groups in any parameter measured by magnetic resonance imaging (MRI) of the brain (151). However, van Oosten et al. (152) reported an increase in the number of gadolinium-enhancing lesions observed in the brain MRIs of two MS patients following treatment with infliximab. Kassiotis et al. (153) showed that treatment of EAE mice with EAE with a TNF inhibitor is associated with prolongation of the life span of activated memory T cells.

In the RA and psoriatic arthritis clinical trials, no cases of new-onset demyelinating disease were reported with any of the TNF antagonists. However, Mohan et al. (154) surveyed the MedWatch postmarketing database and reported 20 patients, 18 treated with etanercept and 2 with infliximab, who developed new-onset neurologic signs and symptoms suggestive of a demyelinating process after receiving TNF antagonists. The most common presenting symptoms were paresthesias (13 of 20), visual disturbance due to optic neuritis (8 of 20), and confusion (5 of 20), and the less common were gait disturbance, apraxia, facial palsy and Guillain-Barré syndrome. Discontinuation of the TNF inhibitor led to partial or complete resolution of symptoms in some cases. A causal relationship of chronic TNF inhibition to the development of demyelinating disease remains unclear, however. The cases reported to date may represent spontaneous MS that develops at the rate of 3.2 cases per 100,000 persons per year (155). Robinson et al. (156) have raised doubt as to whether any of the TNF inhibitors are able to cross the blood-brain barrier. In the meantime, anti-TNF agents should not be used in patients with MS or other demyelinating diseases. In addition, patients treated with TNF inhibitors should be monitored for the development of new neurologic symptoms.

Congestive Heart Failure

As with MS, considerable evidence has accumulated to date pointing to a role for TNF-α in the pathogenesis of congestive heart failure (CHF), yet data from clinical trials in patients with CHF have suggested a detrimental, rather than therapeutic, effect of anti-TNF agents on CHF. TNF-α mRNA and protein are robustly expressed in the hearts of patients with myocarditis and end-stage CHF but not in normal hearts (157,158). TNF-α is a myocardial suppressant, as evidenced by its ability *ex vivo* to induce both immediate and delayed negative inotropic effects on myocardial contractility (159–161). In two different transgenic mouse models, cardiac-specific overexpression of TNF-α resulted in lethal myocarditis with cardiomyopathy and fatal ventricular arrhythmias (162–164), but could be prevented by administration of TNF antagonists (164,165).

A preliminary clinical trial of etanercept versus placebo in 47 patients with New York Heart Association (NYHA) class III to IV CHF provided encouraging results (166). Treatment with etanercept (5 or 12 mg/m^2) for 3 months resulted in a significant dose-dependent improvement in left ventricular function and remodeling, and a trend toward improved clinical parameters, compared with the placebo group. Subsequently, two large-scale placebo-controlled trials were undertaken, one with etanercept in NYHA class II to IV CHF patients, and one with infliximab in NYHA class III to IV CHF patients (167,168). However, both studies were terminated early—in the case of etanercept due to lack of efficacy, and in the case of infliximab due to an increase in CHF events and all-cause deaths in the infliximab-treated groups (167,168). Furthermore, in a review of postmarketing reports of CHF in etanercept and infliximab-treated patients, Kwon et al. (169) reported 38 patients with new-onset CHF, 19 of whom (50%) had no identifiable risk factors, and 10 of whom were younger than 50 years of age. Consequently, caution should be exercised in the use of TNF inhibitors in patients with CHF.

Other

No serious hematologic events occurred in controlled clinical trials of etanercept or infliximab in RA, JRA, or psoriatic arthritis. However, there have been rare case reports of pancytopenia, including aplastic anemia, in the postmarketing experience with both drugs. In animals, none of the TNF inhibitors has been associated with infertility or fetal loss. However, published data in humans are scarce (170). Postmarketing data with infliximab suggest that pregnant women exposed to the drug have fetal outcomes consistent with those expected in healthy women (171). All three TNF antagonists are currently classified by the FDA as category B (no evidence of risk) and are not recommended during pregnancy unless clearly needed.

INTERLEUKIN-1 ANTAGONISTS

In contrast to, and perhaps consistent with, its modest therapeutic efficacy in RA, Anakinra has proven to be remarkably safe in controlled clinical trials of the agent as monotherapy, in combination with MTX, and in combination with other nonbiologic DMARDs, for the treatment of RA (91,94–97). Injection site reactions were the most commonly observed adverse event in all of the published clinical trials. The frequency was dose related, occurring in 50%, 73%, and 81% of patients receiving Anakinra as monotherapy at doses of 30 mg, 75 mg, and 150 mg daily, respectively, compared with 25% of placebo-treated patients (94). At the FDA-approved dose of 100 mg daily in combination with other DMARDs, injection site reactions were reported at a frequency of 73% in Anakinra-treated, compared with 33% in placebo-treated, patients (97). As with the TNF inhibitors, the reactions consisted primarily of erythema and induration and usually resolved within the first month of treatment.

In the controlled clinical trials, as well as open-label extension studies, no increase in the occurrence of malignancies, either solid tumors or lymphomas, has been observed in anakinra-treated patients compared with placebo-treated patients, nor have the rates of malignancy exceeded those expected in the general population (91,94–97). In addition, no increase in the rate of overall infections was observed in clinical trials in patients treated with Anakinra, either alone or in combination with MTX, compared with controls (96). In a recently published large safety trial of 1,414 patients (97), a modest, but not statistically significant, increase in serious infections (requiring hospitalization or intravenous antibiotics) was observed in patients treated with Anakinra, in combination with one or more DMARDs compared with patients treated with DMARDs alone (2.1% vs. 0.4%, respectively; $p = 0.068$). This trial was designed to more closely approximate a clinical practice setting in that RA patients receiving one or more nonbiologic DMARDs and with comorbid illnesses, such as chronic cardiac and pulmonary diseases, were allowed to participate. Anakinra (or placebo) was added to existing therapy for 6 months. The majority of infections were pneumonias and cellulitis and appeared to be due to common bacterial pathogens. No risk factors for infection in Anakinra- vs. placebo-treated patients were identified in this study, although there was a trend toward a higher infection rate in asthma patients treated with Anakinra than in asthma patients treated with placebo. Importantly, no cases of tuberculosis or other opportunistic infections were reported in this trial or any other of the Anakinra clinical trials.

Combining Anakinra with a TNF inhibitor, however, appears to significantly increase the risk for serious infection. In a small open-label trial reported by Schiff et al. (172) in which anakinra (100 mg/day) was added to background treatment with etanercept (25 mg twice weekly) in 58 RA patients over 24 weeks, serious infections occurred in 4 patients (7%), and consisted of two cases each of pneumonia and cellulitis. No opportunistic infections were observed. Although there was no control group in this study, the rate of serious infection far exceeds that seen in clinical trials with either agent alone. A larger double-blind controlled trial comparing combination (etanercept/Anakinra) treatment with monotherapy has recently been published (172a). There was no synergistic or additive clinical benefit in efficacy, although serious infection occurred in 7% of the combination arm and in 0% in the monotherapy group (172a). Treatment with a combination of TNF and IL-1 antagonists is strongly discouraged.

Neutropenia was observed infrequently in the initial clinical trials with anakinra, but no cases of neutropenia or agranulocytosis were reported in the large safety trial (97). Antianakinra antibodies were observed infrequently in clinical trials (<1%), and were usually transient and rarely neutralizing.

CLINICAL TRIALS IN OTHER CHRONIC INFLAMMATORY DISEASES

Pathologic roles for TNF-α and IL-1 have been suggested for several other chronic inflammatory diseases (infectious and noninfectious, granulomatous and nongranulomatous). The only published clinical trials with Anakinra in diseases other than RA were those conducted in sepsis and acute graft-versus-host disease, and Anakinra proved ineffective for both conditions (173–175). The discussion below, therefore, focuses on clinical trials of TNF antagonists in non-RA conditions.

Inflammatory Bowel Disease

In patients with active and fistulizing Crohn's disease, two anti-TNF monoclonal antibodies have been demonstrated to be efficacious in placebo-controlled trials (143, 176–179). A single dose of infliximab (5 mg/kg, 10 mg/kg, or 20 mg/kg) was more effective in reducing disease activity at 4 weeks than placebo (65% response for the combined infliximab groups vs. 17% response in the placebo group, $p < 0.001$) (176). In subsequent trials (177,178), repeated administration of infliximab was effective in sustaining clinical response or remission, and safety profiles were similar to those seen in clinical trials of RA. As in the RA trials, the presence of antiinfliximab antibodies was associated with a shorter duration of action, and higher rate of infusion reactions, to infliximab when given as monotherapy, but antiinfliximab antibodies could be suppressed by concomitant immunosuppressive therapy (143) (e.g., MTX and azathioprine). A single dose of another anti-TNF MoAb, CDP571, was also found to be effective in a small placebo-controlled trial in Crohn disease, but repeated dosing had inconsistent effects (179).

Etanercept treatment of patients with Crohn disease, in contrast, was not associated with an improved clinical response compared with placebo when used at the recommended dosing schedule for RA (25 mg twice weekly) (180). Whether it would be efficacious at higher concentrations or with more frequent dosing remains unknown. Another soluble TNF receptor (p55TNFR; onercept) is under study in this disease (142). Currently, infliximab is the only TNF antagonist that is FDA approved for treatment of Crohn disease.

Psoriasis, Psoriatic Arthritis, and Ankylosing Spondylitis

Etanercept and infliximab have been demonstrated to have efficacy in the treatment of psoriasis, psoriatic arthritis, and ankylosing spondylitis (Chapters 63 and 64). Sixty patients with psoriatic arthritis were treated for 3 months with etanercept (25 mg subcutaneously twice weekly) or placebo in a phase II clinical trial (181). Study end points consisted of ACR20 and psoriatic arthritis response criteria (PsARC), as well as improvement in psoriatic skin lesions. At 3 months, 87% and 73% of etanercept-treated patients met PsARC and ACR response criteria, respectively, compared with 23% and 13% in the placebo group ($p < 0.001$ for comparisons for both end points). In addition, 21% of patients in the etanercept treatment group exhibited improvement in skin scores compared with 0% in the placebo arm ($p = 0.037$). Preliminary results from a phase III trial confirm these favorable clinical results and, in addition, suggest a disease-modifying effect of etanercept on the progression of radiographically-evident joint damage (182). Infliximab treatment at two doses (5 and 10 mg/kg) was also statistically significantly better than placebo in improving plaque-type psoriatic skin lesions (183); no published clinical trials of infliximab in psoriatic arthritis are available at the time of the writing of this chapter.

Results from several small placebo-controlled trials indicate that both etanercept and infliximab are efficacious in reducing clinical symptoms and radiologic signs of ankylosing spondylitis. In a trial of 40 patients treated with etanercept or placebo for 3 months (184), a statistically significant higher clinical response and greater improvement in spinal mobility were observed in the etanercept group compared with the placebo group ($p < 0.05$ for comparisons of both parameters). In another study of 70 patients with ankylosing spondylitis (185), 53% treated with infliximab for 12 weeks showed an improvement of 50% in a spondylitis activity index compared with 9% in the placebo group ($p < 0.0001$). Function and quality of life also improved to a greater degree in the infliximab group. Twenty of these patients underwent MRI evaluations of the spine (186). Using a novel MRI scoring system, active MRI lesion scores were observed to improve 40% to 60% in the infliximab group compared with 6% to 21% in the placebo group, and chronic MRI lesion scores improved 7% in the infliximab group and worsened by 35% in the placebo group. Van den Bosch et al. (187) also reported significantly greater improvement in physician and patient global assessments of disease activity in ankylosing spondylitis patients treated with infliximab compared with placebo. Several cases of disseminated tuberculosis and one case of allergic granulomatosis of the lung occurred in infliximab-treated patients in these trials.

Etanercept is the only TNF antagonist currently FDA approved for the treatment of psoriatic arthritis. Etanercept is approved for treatment of ankylosing spondylitis in the United States, and infliximab is approved in Europe.

Other Chronic Inflammatory Diseases

Dissolution of granulomas as a result of chronic TNF inhibition is detrimental in infectious granulomatous diseases such as tuberculosis but may be beneficial in noninfectious granulomatous states such as Wegener's granulomatosis, Behçet's disease, and sarcoidosis. An open-label safety trial of etanercept treatment in 20 patients with active Wegener's granulomatosis demonstrated a reduction in the mean Birmingham Vasculitis Activity Score from 3.6 at study entry to 0.6 at 6 months ($p < 0.001$) (188). Phase II/III trials of etanercept in Wegener's granulomatosis are currently underway. Etanercept treatment of patients with Behçet's disease was associated with a greater decrease in mucocutaneous manifestations than placebo treatment at 1 month (189). Several small case series of patients with uveitis treated with open-label etanercept and infliximab have yielded inconsistent results (190–192), and placebo-controlled trials have not yet been reported. Chronic inhibition of TNF-α has also been suggested as a rational therapeutic approach for sarcoidosis (193), but to date, no placebo-controlled clinical trials have been reported.

CURRENT INDICATIONS FOR TUMOR NECROSIS FACTOR AND INTERLEUKIN-1 ANTAGONISTS

Etanercept is currently FDA-approved for the treatment of both adults and children with moderately-to-severely active RA, and can be administered as monotherapy or in combination with MTX. Etanercept is also approved for the treatment of psoriatic arthritis and ankylosing spondylitis. The adult dose is 25 mg administered twice weekly by subcutaneous injection. The recommended dose for pediatric patients 4 to 17 years of age is 0.4 mg/kg (up to a maximum of 25 mg per dose) twice weekly.

Infliximab, in combination with MTX, is FDA approved for the treatment of adults with moderately to severely active RA. The recommended starting dose is 3 mg/kg administered intravenously at weeks 0, 2, and 6, followed by repeat administration every 8 weeks, and given in combination with MTX. If a clinical response is not observed, the dose of infliximab can be increased up to 10 mg/kg or the interval between doses can be shortened to 4–6 weeks. Infliximab is also indicated for the treatment of moderately to severely active or fistulizing Crohn's disease in patients who have had an inadequate response to conventional therapy. Infliximab is approved in Europe for treating ankylosing spondylitis.

Adalimumab is FDA approved for the treatment of adults with moderately-to-severely active RA who have had an inadequate response to one or more DMARDs. Adalimumab can be used alone or in combination with MTX or other DMARDs. The starting dose is 40 mg administered subcutaneously every other week, but the dosing interval can be reduced to weekly if an adequate clinical response is not observed.

Anakinra is FDA approved for treatment of adults with moderately-to-severely active RA who have failed one or more DMARDs. Anakinra can be used alone or in combination with MTX or other DMARDs. The dosage is 100 mg/day administered by subcutaneous injection.

For all four biologic therapies, caution is advised in the use of these agents in patients with a chronic infection or a history of recurrent infection. If a patient develops a serious infection while receiving a TNF or IL-1 inhibitor, the therapy should be discontinued until the infection has resolved. Pretreatment screening for latent tuberculosis is strongly recommended prior to use with a TNF inhibitor. The TNF inhibitors are relatively contraindicated in patients with congestive heart failure. All four therapies have an FDA category B designation (no evidence of risk) for pregnancy; they should be used during pregnancy only if clearly needed. Combinations of TNF and IL-1 inhibitors should not be used based on recent data showing no increased efficacy and increased toxity with the combination.

SUMMARY

In vitro and animal studies suggested that TNF and IL-1 are critical and proximal mediators of the inflammatory pathway in the rheumatoid joint. Proof-of-concept for this hypothesis has now been provided by a sizable number of clinical trials in RA. Not only do TNF and IL-1 inhibitors dramatically reduce markers of inflammation, but they also slow structural damage, and their efficacy appears to be as potent in early disease as in late disease. In human terms, these impressive results should translate in the long term to less disability and higher quality of life, for patients with RA and other chronic inflammatory diseases.

The robust responses to treatment with TNF inhibitors in RA, inflammatory bowel disease, and psoriasis are likely to be the tip of the iceberg. Any chronic (noninfectious) inflammatory disease in which the innate immune response predominates could be a potential target for anti-TNF therapy. The contribution of IL-1, independent of TNF-α, to the pathogenesis of chronic inflammatory states awaits full clarification pending the development of a more potent and durable IL-1 antagonist. The rebound in disease activity that occurs after cessation of anticytokine therapy indicates that the inflammatory cascade has been interrupted, but the underlying cause of the disease has not been addressed. Furthermore, the development or dissemination of opportunistic infections with chronic TNF inhibitors is a sobering reminder that endogenous TNF serves important homeostatic functions in host defense. Whether more potent IL-1 antagonists will be similarly associated with an increased risk for opportunistic infections remains to be determined.

REFERENCES

1. Choy EH, Panayi GS. Cytokine pathways and joint inflammation in rheumatoid arthritis. *N Engl J Med* 2001;344:907–916.
2. Firestein GS, Xu WD, Townsend K, et al. Cytokines in chronic inflammatory arthritis. 1. Failure to detect T-cell lymphokines (interleukin-2 and interleukin-3) and presence of macrophage colony-stimulating factor (CSF-1) and a novel mast-cell growth-factor in rheumatoid synovitis. *J Exp Med* 1988;168:1573–1586.
3. Moreland LW, Heck LW Jr, Koopman WJ. Biologic agents for treating rheumatoid arthritis. Concepts and progress. *Arthritis Rheum* 1997;40: 397–409.
4. Firestein GS, Alvaro-Gracia JM, Maki R, et al. Quantitative analysis of cytokine gene expression in rheumatoid arthritis. *J Immunol* 1990; 144:3347–3353.
5. Alvarogracia JM, Zvaifler NJ, Brown CB, et al. Cytokines in chronic inflammatory arthritis. 6. Analysis of the synovial-cells involved in granulocyte-macrophage colony-stimulating factor production and gene-expression in rheumatoid-arthritis and its regulation by IL-1 and tumor-necrosis-factor-alpha. *J Immunol* 1991;146:3365–3371.
6. Firestein GS, Zvaifler NJ. How important are T cells in chronic rheumatoid synovitis? *Arthritis Rheum* 1990;33:768–773.
7. Saklatvala J, Sarsfield SJ, Townsend Y. Pig interleukin 1. Purification of two immunologically different leukocyte proteins that cause cartilage resorption, lymphocyte activation, and fever. *J Exp Med* 1985; 162:1208–1222.
8. Dayer JM, Beutler B, Cerami A. Cachectin/tumor necrosis factor stimulates collagenase and prostaglandin E_2 production by human synovial cells and dermal fibroblasts. *J Exp Med* 1985;162:2163–2168.
9. Cavender D, Saegusa Y, Ziff M. Stimulation of endothelial cell binding of lymphocytes by tumor necrosis factor. *J Immunol* 1987;139: 1855–1860.
10. Gamble JR, Harlan JM, Klebanoff SJ, Vadas MA. Stimulation of the adherence of neutrophils to umbilical vein endothelium by human recombinant tumor necrosis factor. *Proc Natl Acad Sci U S A* 1985;82: 8667–8671.
11. Firestein GS. Rheumatoid synovitis and pannus. *Rheumatology,* 2nd edition. London: CV Mosby, 1999:13.1–13.24.
12. Dinarello CA, Cannon JG, Wolff SM, et al. Tumor-necrosis-factor (cachectin) is an endogenous pyrogen and induces production of interleukin-1. *J Exp Med* 1986;163:1433–1450.
13. Philip R, Epstein LB. tumor-necrosis-factor as immunomodulator and mediator of monocyte cytotoxicity induced by itself, gamma-interferon and interleukin-1. *Nature* 1986;323:86–89.
14. Ikejima T, Okusawa S, Ghezzi P, et al. Interleukin-1 induces tumor-necrosis-factor (TNF) in human peripheral-blood mononuclear-cells *in vitro* and a circulating TNF-like activity in rabbits. *J Infect Dis* 1990;162:215–223.
15. Dinarello CA, Ikejima T, Warner SJC, et al. Interleukin-1 induces interleukin-1. 1. Induction of circulating interleukin-1 in rabbits *in vivo* and in human mononuclear-cells *in vitro*. *J Immunol* 1987;139:1902–1910.
16. Marinova-Mutafchieva L, Williams RO, Mason LJ, et al. Dynamics of proinflammatory cytokine expression in the joints of mice with collagen-induced arthritis (CIA). *Clin Exp Immunol* 1997;107:507–512.
17. Mussener A, Litton MJ, Lindroos E, et al. Cytokine production in synovial tissue of mice with collagen-induced arthritis (CIA). *Clin Exp Immunol* 1997;107:485–493.
18. Stasiuk LM, Abehsira-Amar O, Fournier C. Collagen-induced arthritis in DBA/1 mice: cytokine gene activation following immunization with type II collagen. *Cell Immunol* 1996;173:269–275.
19. Thornton S, Duwel LE, Boivin GP, et al. Association of the course of collagen-induced arthritis with distinct patterns of cytokine and chemokine messenger RNA expression. *Arthritis Rheum* 1999;42: 1109–1118.
20. Williams RO, Feldmann M, Maini RN. Anti-tumor necrosis factor ameliorates joint disease in murine collagen-induced arthritis. *Proc Natl Acad Sci U S A* 1992;89:9784–9788.
21. Mori L, Iselin S, De Libero G, et al. Attenuation of collagen-induced arthritis in 55-kDa TNF receptor type 1 (TNFR1)-IgG1-treated and TNFR1-deficient mice. *J Immunol* 1996;157:3178–3182.
22. Thorbecke GJ, Shah R, Leu CH, et al. Involvement of endogenous tumor-necrosis-factor-alpha and transforming growth-factor-beta during induction of collagen type-II arthritis in mice. *Proc Natl Acad Sci U S A* 1992;89:7375–7379.
23. Piguet PF, Grau GE, Vesin C, et al. Evolution of collagen arthritis in mice is arrested by treatment with antitumor necrosis factor (TNF) antibody or a recombinant soluble TNF receptor. *Immunology* 1992; 77:510–514.
24. Keffer J, Probert L, Cazlaris H, et al. Transgenic mice expressing human tumour necrosis factor: a predictive genetic model of arthritis. *EMBO J* 1991;10:4025–4031.
25. Alexopoulou L, Pasparakis M, Kollias G. A murine transmembrane tumor necrosis factor (TNF) transgene induces arthritis by cooperative p55/p75 TNF receptor signaling. *Eur J Immunol* 1997;27:2588–2592.
26. Edwards CK, Chlipala ES, Dinarello CA, et al. Clinical and histopathologic characterization of arthritis in male and female tumor necrosis factor-alpha knockout [TNF-alpha(−/−)] and membrane-bound TNF-alpha transgenic [TNF-alpha (TgA86)] mice injected with *Mycoplasma pulmonis* of *Mycoplasma* arthritis. *Arthritis Rheum* 1999;42(suppl):120.

27. Bessis N, Guery L, Mantovani A, et al. The type II decoy receptor of IL-1 inhibits murine collagen-induced arthritis. *Eur J Immunol* 2000; 30:867–875.
28. Joosten LAB, Helsen MMA, Saxne T, et al. IL-1 alpha beta blockade prevents cartilage and bone destruction in murine type II collagen-induced arthritis, whereas TNF-alpha blockade only ameliorates joint inflammation. *J Immunol* 1999;163:5049–5055.
29. Bakker AC, Joosten LAB, Arntz OJ, et al. Prevention of murine collagen-induced arthritis in the knee and ipsilateral paw by local expression of human interleukin-1 receptor antagonist protein in the knee. *Arthritis Rheum* 1997;40:893–900.
30. Makarov SS, Olsen JC, Johnston WN, et al. Suppression of experimental arthritis by gene transfer of interleukin 1 receptor antagonist cDNA. *Proc Natl Acad Sci U S A* 1996;93:402–406.
31. Otani K, Nita I, Macaulay W, et al. Suppression of antigen-induced arthritis in rabbits by *ex vivo* gene therapy. *J Immunol* 1996;156: 3558–3562.
32. Horai R, Saijo S, Tanioka H, et al. Development of chronic inflammatory arthropathy resembling rheumatoid arthritis in interleukin 1 receptor antagonist-deficient mice. *J Exp Med* 2000;191:313–320.
33. Niki Y, Yamada H, Seki S, et al. Macrophage- and neutrophil-dominant arthritis in human IL-1 alpha transgenic mice. *J Clin Invest* 2001;107:1127–1135.
34. Bendele AM, Chlipala ES, Scherrer J, et al. Combination benefit of treatment with the cytokine inhibitors interleukin-1 receptor antagonist and PEGylated soluble tumor necrosis factor receptor type I in animal models of rheumatoid arthritis. *Arthritis Rheum* 2000;43: 2648–2659.
35. Probert L, Plows D, Kontogeorgos G, et al. The type-i interleukin-1 receptor acts in series with tumor-necrosis-factor (TNF) to induce arthritis in TNF-transgenic mice. *Eur J Immunol* 1995;25:1794–1797.
36. van den Berg WB. Uncoupling of inflammatory and destructive mechanisms in arthritis. *Semin Arthritis Rheum* 2001;30:7–16.
37. Carswell EA, Old LJ, Kassel RL, et al. An endotoxin-induced serum factor that causes necrosis of tumors. *Proc Natl Acad Sci U S A* 1975; 72:3666–3670.
38. Beutler B, Greenwald D, Hulmes JD, et al. Identity of tumour necrosis factor and the macrophage-secreted factor cachectin. *Nature* 1985; 316:552–554.
39. Wallach D, Varfolomeev EE, Malinin NL, et al. Tumor necrosis factor receptor and Fas signaling mechanisms. *Annu Rev Immunol* 1999;17: 331–367.
40. Bazzoni F, Beutler B. The tumor necrosis factor ligand and receptor families. *N Engl J Med* 1996;334:1717–1725.
41. Yonehara S, Ishii A, Yonehara M. A cell-killing monoclonal antibody (anti-Fas) to a cell surface antigen co-downregulated with the receptor of tumor necrosis factor. *J Exp Med* 1989;169:1747–1756.
42. Grell M, Douni E, Wajant H, et al. The transmembrane form of tumor-necrosis-factor is the prime activating ligand of the 80 kDa tumor-necrosis-factor receptor. *Cell* 1995;83:793–802.
43. Williams LM, Gibbons DL, Gearing A, et al. Paradoxical effects of a synthetic metalloproteinase inhibitor that blocks both p55 and p75 TNF receptor shedding and TNF alpha processing in RA synovial membrane cell cultures. *J Clin Invest* 1996;97:2833–2841.
44. Dinarello CA. Blocking interleukin-1 and tumor necrosis factor in disease. *Eur Cytokine Network* 1997;8:294–296.
45. Kobayashi Y, Yamamoto K, Saido T, et al. Identification of calcium-activated neutral protease as a processing enzyme of human interleukin-1-alpha. *Proc Natl Acad Sci U S A* 1990;87:5548–5552.
46. Black RA, Kronheim SR, Cantrell M, et al. Generation of biologically-active interleukin-1-beta by proteolytic cleavage of the inactive precursor. *J Biol Chem* 1988;263:9437–9442.
47. Wilson KP, Black JAF, Thomson JA, et al. Structure and mechanism of interleukin-1-beta converting-enzyme. *Nature* 1994;370:270–275.
48. Haskill S, Martin G, Van Le L, Morris J, et al. cDNA cloning of an intracellular form of the human interleukin 1 receptor antagonist associated with epithelium. *Proc Natl Acad Sci U S A* 1991;88:3681–3685.
49. Gabay C, Porter B, Fantuzzi G, et al. Mouse IL-1 receptor antagonist isoforms: complementary DNA cloning and protein expression of intracellular isoform and tissue distribution of secreted and intracellular IL-1 receptor antagonist *in vivo*. *J Immunol* 1997;159:5905–5913.
50. Arend WP. Interleukins and arthritis—IL-1 antagonism in inflammatory arthritis. *Lancet* 1993;341:155–156.
51. Sims JE, Gayle MA, Slack JL, et al. Interleukin 1 signaling occurs exclusively via the type I receptor. *Proc Natl Acad Sci U S A* 1993; 90:6155–6159.
52. Dower SK, Wignall JM, Schooley K, et al. Retention of ligand binding activity by the extracellular domain of the IL-1 receptor. *J Immunol* 1989;142:4314–4320.
53. Stahl N, Yancopoulos GD. The alphas, betas, and kinases of cytokine receptor complexes. *Cell* 1993;74:587–590.
54. Greenfeder SA, Nunes P, Kwee L, et al. Molecular-cloning and characterization of a 2nd subunit of the interleukin-1 receptor complex. *J Biol Chem* 1995;270:13757–13765.
55. Evans RJ, Bray J, Childs JD, et al. Mapping receptor binding sites in interleukin (IL)-1 receptor antagonist and IL-1 beta by site-directed mutagenesis. Identification of a single site in IL-1ra and two sites in IL-1 beta. *J Biol Chem* 1995;270:11477.
56. Colotta F, Re F, Muzio M, et al. Interleukin-1 type II receptor: a decoy target for IL-1 that is regulated by IL-4. *Science* 1993;261: 472–475.
57. Symons JA, Eastgate JA, Duff GW. Purification and characterization of a novel soluble receptor for interleukin 1. *J Exp Med* 1991;174: 1251–1254.
58. Arend WP, Malyak M, Smith MF Jr, et al. Binding of IL-1 alpha, IL-1 beta, and IL-1 receptor antagonist by soluble IL-1 receptors and levels of soluble IL-1 receptors in synovial fluids. *J Immunol* 1994;153: 4766–4774.
59. Giri JG, Wells J, Dower SK, et al. Elevated levels of shed type-II IL-1 receptor in sepsis—potential role for type-II receptor in regulation of IL-1 responses. *J Immunol* 1994;153:5802–5809.
60. Mohler KM, Torrance DS, Smith CA, et al. Soluble tumor necrosis factor (TNF) receptors are effective therapeutic agents in lethal endotoxemia and function simultaneously as both TNF carriers and TNF antagonists. *J Immunol* 1993;151:1548–1561.
61. Edwards CK. PEGylated recombinant human soluble tumour necrosis factor receptor type I (r-Hu-sTNF-RI): novel high affinity TNF receptor designed for chronic inflammatory diseases. *Ann Rheum Dis* 1999;58:73–81.
62. Lesslauer W, Tabuchi H, Gentz R, et al. Recombinant soluble tumor-necrosis-factor receptor proteins protect mice from lipopolysaccharide-induced lethality. *Eur J Immunol* 1991;21:2883–2886.
63. Kneer J, Leudin E, Lesslauer W, et al. An assessment of the effect of anti-drug antibody formation on the pharmacokinetics and pharmacodynamics of sTNFr55-IgG (Ro 45–2081-Lenercept [LEN]) (S.C.) in patients with rheumatoid arthritis (RA). *Arthritis Rheum* 1998;41 (suppl):58.
64. Elliott MJ, Maini RN, Feldmann M, et al. Treatment of rheumatoid arthritis with chimeric monoclonal antibodies to tumor necrosis factor alpha. *Arthritis Rheum* 1993;36:1681–1690.
65. van de Putte LBA, van Riel PLCM, den Broeder A, et al. A single dose placebo controlled phase 1 study of the fully human anti-TNF antibody D2E7 in patients with rheumatoid arthritis. *Arthritis Rheum* 1998;41(suppl):57.
66. Rankin EC, Choy EH, Kassimos D, et al. The therapeutic effects of an engineered human anti-tumour necrosis factor alpha antibody (CDP571) in rheumatoid arthritis. *Br J Rheumatol* 1995;34:334–342.
67. Choy EHS, Hazleman B, Smith M, et al. Efficacy of a novel PEGylated humanized anti-TNF fragment (CDP870) in patients with rheumatoid arthritis: a phase II double-blinded, randomized, dose-escalating trial. *Rheumatology* 2002;41:1133–1137.
68. Conway JG, Andrews RC, Beaudet B, et al. Inhibition of tumor necrosis factor-alpha (TNF-alpha) production and arthritis in the rat by GW3333, a dual inhibitor of TNF-alpha-converting enzyme and matrix metalloproteinases. *J Pharmacol Exp Ther* 2001;298:900–908.
69. Beck G, Bottomley G, Bradshaw D, et al. (E)-2(R)-[1(S)-(hydroxycarbamoyl)-4-phenyl-3-butenyl]-2′-isobutyl-2′-(methanesulfonyl)-4-methylvalerohydrazide (Ro 32–7315), a selective and orally active inhibitor of tumor necrosis factor-alpha convertase. *J Pharmacol Exp Ther* 2002;302:390–396.
70. Seckinger P, Klein-Nulend J, Alander C, et al. Natural and recombinant human IL-1 receptor antagonists block the effects of IL-1 on bone resorption and prostaglandin production. *J Immunol* 1990;145:4181–4184.

71. Hannum CH, Wilcox CJ, Arend WP, et al. Interleukin-1 receptor antagonist activity of a human interleukin-1 inhibitor. *Nature* 1990;343: 336–340.
72. Arend WP, Welgus HG, Thompson RC, et al. Biological properties of recombinant human monocyte-derived interleukin 1 receptor antagonist. *J Clin Invest* 1990;85:1694–1697.
73. Sims JE, Gayle MA, Slack JL, et al. Interleukin-1 signaling occurs exclusively via the type-I receptor. *Proc Natl Acad Sci U S A* 1993; 90:6155–6159.
74. Drevlow BE, Lovis R, Haag MA, et al. Recombinant human interleukin-1 receptor type I in the treatment of patients with active rheumatoid arthritis. *Arthritis Rheum* 1996;39:257–265.
75. Dawson J, Engelhardt P, Kastelic T, et al. Effects of soluble interleukin-1 type II receptor on rabbit antigen-induced arthritis: clinical, biochemical and histological assessment. *Rheumatology (Oxford)* 1999;38:401–406.
76. Economides AN, Carpenter LR, Rudge JS, et al. Cytokine traps: multi-component, high-affinity blockers of cytokine action. *Nat Med* 2003;9:47–52.
77. Dinarello CA. Biologic basis for interleukin-1 in disease. *Blood* 1996; 87:2095–2147.
78. vandenBerg WB, Joosten LAB, Helsen M, et al. Amelioration of established murine collagen-induced arthritis with anti-IL-1 treatment. *Clin Exp Immunol* 1994;95:237–243.
79. Ku G, Faust T, Lauffer LL, et al. Interleukin-1 beta converting enzyme inhibition blocks progression of type II collagen-induced arthritis in mice. *Cytokine* 1996;8:377–386.
80. Randle JCR, Harding MW, Ku G, et al. ICE/caspase-1 inhibitors as novel anti-inflammatory drugs. *Exp Opin Invest Drugs* 2001;10: 1207–1209.
81. Elliott MJ, Maini RN, Feldmann M, et al. Randomised double-blind comparison of chimeric monoclonal antibody to tumour necrosis factor alpha (cA2) versus placebo in rheumatoid arthritis. *Lancet* 1994; 344:1105–1110.
82. Elliott MJ, Maini RN, Feldmann M, et al. Repeated therapy with monoclonal antibody to tumour necrosis factor alpha (cA2) in patients with rheumatoid arthritis. *Lancet* 1994;344:1125–1127.
83. Maini RN, Breedveld FC, Kalden JR, et al. Therapeutic efficacy of multiple intravenous infusions of anti-tumor necrosis factor alpha monoclonal antibody combined with low-dose weekly methotrexate in rheumatoid arthritis. *Arthritis Rheum* 1998;41: 1552–1563.
84. Maini R, St Clair EW, Breedveld F, et al. Infliximab (chimeric anti-tumour necrosis factor alpha monoclonal antibody) versus placebo in rheumatoid arthritis patients receiving concomitant methotrexate: a randomised phase III trial. *Lancet* 1999;354:1932–1939.
85. Lipsky PE, van der Heijde DMFM, St Clair EW, et al. Infliximab and methotrexate in the treatment of rheumatoid arthritis. *N Engl J Med* 2000;343:1594–1602.
86. Moreland LW, Margolies G, Heck LW Jr, et al. Recombinant soluble tumor necrosis factor receptor (p80) fusion protein: toxicity and dose finding trial in refractory rheumatoid arthritis. *J Rheumatol* 1996;23: 1849–1855.
87. Moreland LW, Baumgartner SW, Schiff MH, et al. Treatment of rheumatoid arthritis with a recombinant human tumor necrosis factor receptor (p75)-Fc fusion protein. *N Engl J Med* 1997;337:141–147.
88. Moreland LW, Schiff MH, Baumgartner SW, et al. Etanercept therapy in rheumatoid arthritis. A randomized, controlled trial. *Ann Intern Med* 1999;130:478–486.
89. Weinblatt ME, Kremer JM, Bankhurst AD, et al. A trial of etanercept, a recombinant tumor necrosis factor receptor:Fc fusion protein, in patients with rheumatoid arthritis receiving methotrexate. *N Engl J Med* 1999;340:253–259.
90. Bathon JM, Martin RW, Fleischmann RM, et al. A comparison of etanercept and methotrexate in patients with early rheumatoid arthritis. *N Engl J Med* 2000;343:1586–1593.
91. Campion GV, Lebsack ME, Lookabaugh J, et al. Dose-range and dose-frequency study of recombinant human interleukin-1 receptor antagonist in patients with rheumatoid arthritis. The IL-1Ra Arthritis Study Group. *Arthritis Rheum* 1996;39:1092–1101.
92. van de Putte LB, Atkins C, Malaise M, et al. Adalimumab (D2E7) Monotherapy in the treatment of patients with severely active rheumatoid arthritis. *Arthritis Rheum* 2002;46(suppl 9):205.
93. Keystone E, Kavanaugh A, Sharp JT, et al. Adalimumab (D2E7), a fully human anti-TNF-alpha monoclonal antibody, inhibits the progression of structural joint damage in patients with active RA despite concomitant methotrexate therapy. *Arthritis Rheum* 2002;46(suppl 9):205.
94. Bresnihan B, Alvaro-Gracia JM, Cobby M, et al. Treatment of rheumatoid arthritis with recombinant human interleukin-1 receptor antagonist. *Arthritis Rheum* 1998;41:2196–2204.
95. Jiang Y, Genant HK, Watt I, et al. A multicenter, double-blind, dose-ranging, randomized, placebo-controlled study of recombinant human interleukin-1 receptor antagonist in patients with rheumatoid arthritis: radiologic progression and correlation of Genant and Larsen scores. *Arthritis Rheum* 2000;43:1001–1009.
96. Cohen S, Hurd E, Cush J, et al. Treatment of rheumatoid arthritis with anakinra, a recombinant human interleukin-1 receptor antagonist, in combination with methotrexate—results of a twenty-four-week, multicenter, randomized, double-blind, placebo-controlled trial. *Arthritis Rheum* 2002;46:614–624.
97. Fleischmann RM, Schechtman J, Bennett R, et al. Anakinra, a recombinant human interleukin-1 receptor antagonist (r-metHuIL-1ra), in patients with rheumatoid arthritis—a large, international, multicenter, placebo-controlled trial. *Arthritis Rheum* 2003;48:927–934.
98. Weinblatt ME, Keystone EC, Furst DE, et al. Adalimumab, a fully human anti-tumor necrosis factor alpha monoclonal antibody, for the treatment of rheumatoid arthritis in patients taking concomitant methotrexate: the ARMADA trial. *Arthritis Rheum* 2003;48: 35–45.
99. Furst D, Schiff M, Fleischmann RM, et al. Safety and efficacy of adalimumab (D2E7), a fully human anti-TNF-alpha monoclonal antibody, given in combination with standard anti-rheumatic therapy: safety trial of adalimumab in rheumatoid arthritis (STAR). *Arthritis Rheum* 2002;46(suppl 9):572.
100. Felson DT, Anderson JJ, Boers M, et al. The American College of Rheumatology preliminary core set of disease-activity measures for rheumatoid-arthritis clinical trials. *Arthritis Rheum* 1993;36:729–740.
101. Paulus HE, Egger MJ, Ward JR, et al. Analysis of improvement in individual rheumatoid-arthritis patients treated with disease-modifying antirheumatic drugs, based on the findings in patients treated with placebo. *Arthritis Rheum* 1990;33:477–484.
102. Lovell DJ, Giannini EH, Reiff A, et al. Etanercept in children with polyarticular juvenile rheumatoid arthritis. Pediatric Rheumatology Collaborative Study Group. *N Engl J Med* 2000;342:763–769.
103. van der Heijde DM, van Leeuwen MA, van Riel PL, et al. Biannual radiographic assessments of hands and feet in a three-year prospective followup of patients with early rheumatoid arthritis. *Arthritis Rheum* 1992;35:26–34.
104. Fuchs HA, Kaye JJ, Callahan LF, et al. Evidence of significant radiographic damage in rheumatoid arthritis within the first 2 years of disease. *J Rheumatol* 1989;16:585–591.
105. Plant MJ, Jones PW, Saklatvala J, et al. Patterns of radiological progression in early rheumatoid arthritis: results of an 8 year prospective study. *J Rheumatol* 1998;25:417–426.
106. Brook A, Corbett M. Radiographic changes in early rheumatoid disease. *Ann Rheum Dis* 1977;36:71–73.
107. Pincus T, Callahan LF. Remodeling the pyramid or remodeling the paradigms concerning rheumatoid arthritis—lessons from Hodgkin's disease and coronary artery disease. *J Rheumatol* 1990;17:1582–1585.
108. Sharp JT. Radiologic assessment as an outcome measure in rheumatoid arthritis. *Arthritis Rheum* 1989;32:221–229.
109. Adalimumab (Humira) package insert, 2003.
110. Guler H, Caldwell JR, Littlejohn T III, et al. A phase I, single dose escalation study of IL-1 trap in patients with rheumatoid arthritis. *Arthritis Rheum* 2001;44(suppl 9):370.
111. Fisher CJ Jr, Agosti JM, Opal SM, et al. Treatment of septic shock with the tumor necrosis factor receptor:Fc fusion protein. The Soluble TNF Receptor Sepsis Study Group. *N Engl J Med* 1996;334: 1697–1702.
112. Pasparakis M, Alexopoulou L, Episkopou V, et al. Immune and inflammatory responses in TNF alpha-deficient mice: a critical requirement for TNF alpha in the formation of primary B cell follicles, follicular dendritic cell networks and germinal centers, and in the maturation of the humoral immune response. *J Exp Med* 1996;184:1397–1411.

113. Rothe J, Lesslauer W, Lotscher H, et al. Mice lacking the tumour necrosis factor receptor 1 are resistant to TNF-mediated toxicity but highly susceptible to infection by *Listeria monocytogenes*. *Nature* 1993;364:798–802.
114. Erickson SL, Desauvage FJ, Kikly K, et al. Decreased sensitivity to tumor-necrosis-factor but normal T-cell development in TNF receptor-2-deficient mice. *Nature* 1994;372:560–563.
115. Chang J, Kaufmann SHE. Immune mechanisms of protection. In: Bloom BR, ed. *Tuberculosis: pathogenesis, protection, and control.* Washington, DC: 1994:389.
116. Gordon S, Keshav S, Stein M. BCG-induced granuloma-formation in murine tissues. *Immunobiology* 1994;191:369–377.
117. Kindler V, Sappino AP, Grau GE, et al. The inducing role of tumor necrosis factor in the development of bactericidal granulomas during BCG infection. *Cell* 1989;56:731–740.
118. Senaldi G, Yin S, Shaklee CL, et al. *Corynebacterium parvum*– and *Mycobacterium bovis* bacillus Calmette-Guerin–induced granuloma formation is inhibited in TNF receptor I (TNF-RI) knockout mice and by treatment with soluble TNF-RI. *J Immunol* 1996;157:5022–5026.
119. Bean AGD, Roach DR, Briscoe H, et al. Structural deficiencies in granuloma formation in TNF gene–targeted mice underlie the heightened susceptibility to aerosol *Mycobacterium tuberculosis* infection, which is not compensated for by lymphotoxin. *J Immunol* 1999;162:3504–3511.
120. Mohan VP, Scanga CA, Yu K, et al. Effects of tumor necrosis factor alpha on host immune response in chronic persistent tuberculosis: possible role for limiting pathology. *Infect Immun* 2001;69:1847–1855.
121. Bopst M, Garcia I, Guler R, et al. Differential effects of TNF and LT alpha in the host defense against M-bovis BCG. *Eur J Immunol* 2001;31:1935–1943.
122. Roach DR, Briscoe H, Saunders B, et al. Secreted lymphotoxin-alpha is essential for the control of an intracellular bacterial infection. *J Exp Med* 2001;193:239–246.
123. Keane J, Gershon S, Wise RP, et al. Tuberculosis associated with infliximab, a tumor necrosis factor alpha-neutralizing agent. *N Engl J Med* 2001;345:1098–1104.
124. Wallis WJ, Burge DJ, Holmdahl R, et al. Infection reports with etanercept (Enbrel) therapy. *Arthritis Rheum* 2001;44(suppl):154.
125. Manadan AM, Mohan AK, Cote TR, et al. Tuberculosis and etanercept treatment. *Arthritis Rheum* 2002;46(suppl):166.
126. Small PM, Fujiwara PI. Management of tuberculosis in the United States. *N Engl J Med* 2001;345:189–200.
127. Wolfe F, Rehman V, Lane NE, et al. Starting a disease modifying antirheumatic drug or a biologic agent in rheumatoid arthritis: standards of practice for RA treatment. *J Rheumatol* 2001;28:1704–1711.
128. Scallon B, Cai A, Solowski N, et al. Binding and functional comparisons of two types of tumor necrosis factor antagonists. *J Pharmacol Exp Ther* 2002;301:418–426.
129. U.S. Food and Drug Administration. Update on TNF-alpha blocking agents. 2003.
130. Slifman NR, Gershon SK, Lee JH, et al. *Listeria monocytogenes* infection as a complication of treatment with tumor necrosis factor alpha–neutralizing agents. *Arthritis Rheum* 2003;48:319–324.
131. Bergstrom L, Yocum D, Tesser J, et al. Coccidiomycosis (valley fever) occurring during infliximab therapy. *Arthritis Rheum* 2002; 46(suppl):169.
132. Kamel OW, Vanderijn M, Hanasono MM, et al. Immunosuppression-associated lymphoproliferative disorders in rheumatic patients. *Leuk Lymphoma* 1995;16:363–368.
133. Isomaki HA, Hakulinen T, Joutsenlahti U. Excess risk of lymphomas, leukemia and myeloma in patients with rheumatoid arthritis. *J Chronic Dis* 1978;31:691–696.
134. Gridley G, Mclaughlin JK, Ekbom A, et al. Incidence of cancer among patients with rheumatoid-arthritis. *J Natl Cancer Inst* 1993; 85:307–311.
135. Mellemkjaer L, Linet MS, Gridley G, et al. Rheumatoid arthritis and cancer risk. *Eur J Cancer* 1996;32A:1753–1757.
136. Thomas E, Brewster DH, Black RJ, et al. Risk of malignancy among patients with rheumatic conditions. *Int J Cancer* 2000;88:497–502.
137. Georgescu L, Quinn GC, Schwartzman S, et al. Lymphoma in patients with rheumatoid arthritis: association with the disease state or methotrexate treatment. *Semin Arthritis Rheum* 1997;26:794–804.
138. Kamel OW, Weiss LM, Vanderijn M, et al. Hodgkin's disease and lymphoproliferations resembling Hodgkin's disease in patients receiving long-term low-dose methotrexate therapy. *Am J Surg Pathol* 1996;20:1279–1287.
139. Baecklund E, Ekbom A, Sparen P, et al. Disease activity and risk of lymphoma in patients with rheumatoid arthritis: nested case-control study. *BMJ* 1998;317:180–181.
140. Salloum E, Cooper DL, Howe G, et al. Spontaneous regression of lymphoproliferative disorders in patients treated with methotrexate for rheumatoid arthritis and other rheumatic diseases. *J Clin Oncol* 1996;14:1943–1949.
141. Brown SL, Greene MH, Gershon SK, et al. Tumor necrosis factor antagonist therapy and lymphoma development: twenty-six cases reported to the Food and Drug Administration. *Arthritis Rheum* 2002;46:3151–3158.
142. Rutgeerts P, Lemmens L, Van Assche G, et al. Treatment of active Crohn's disease with onercept (recombinant human soluble p55 tumour necrosis factor receptor): results of a randomized, open-label, pilot study. *Aliment Pharmacol Ther* 2003;17:185–192.
143. Baert F, Noman M, Vermeire S, et al. Influence of immunogenicity on the long-term efficacy of infliximab in Crohn's disease. *N Engl J Med* 2003;348:601–608.
144. Shakoor N, Michalska M, Harris CA, et al. Drug-induced systemic lupus erythematosus associated with etanercept therapy. *Lancet* 2002; 359:579–580.
145. Mohan AK, Edwards ET, Cote TR, et al. Drug-induced systemic lupus erythematosus and TNF-alpha blockers. *Lancet* 2002;360: 646.
146. Charles PJ, Smeenk RJ, De Jong J, et al. Assessment of antibodies to double-stranded DNA induced in rheumatoid arthritis patients following treatment with infliximab, a monoclonal antibody to tumor necrosis factor alpha: findings in open-label and randomized placebo-controlled trials. *Arthritis Rheum* 2000;43:2383–2390.
147. Kuroda Y, Shimamoto Y. Human tumor necrosis factor-alpha augments experimental allergic encephalomyelitis in rats. *J Neuroimmunol* 1991;34:159–164.
148. Ruddle NH, Bergman CM, McGrath KM, et al. An antibody to lymphotoxin and tumor necrosis factor prevents transfer of experimental allergic encephalomyelitis. *J Exp Med* 1990;172:1193–1200.
149. Sharief MK, Hentges R. Association between tumor necrosis factor-alpha and disease progression in patients with multiple sclerosis. *N Engl J Med* 1991;325:467–472.
150. Hofman FM, Hinton DR, Johnson K, et al. Tumor necrosis factor identified in multiple sclerosis brain. *J Exp Med* 1989;170:607–612.
151. The Lenercept Multiple Sclerosis Study Group and the University of British Columbia MS/MRI Analysis Group. TNF neutralization in MS: results of a randomized, placebo-controlled multicenter study. *Neurology* 1999;53:457–465.
152. van Oosten BW, Barkhof F, Truyen L, et al. Increased MRI activity and immune activation in two multiple sclerosis patients treated with the monoclonal anti-tumor necrosis factor antibody cA2. *Neurology* 1996;47:1531–1534.
153. Kassiotis G, Kollias G. Uncoupling the proinflammatory from the immunosuppressive properties of tumor necrosis factor (TNF) at the p55 TNF receptor level: implications for pathogenesis and therapy of autoimmune demyelination. *J Exp Med* 2001;193:427–434.
154. Mohan N, Edwards ET, Cupps TR, et al. Demyelination occurring during anti-tumor necrosis factor alpha therapy for inflammatory arthritides. *Arthritis Rheum* 2001;44:2862–2869.
155. Jacobson DL, Gange SJ, Rose NR, et al. Epidemiology and estimated population burden of selected autoimmune diseases in the United States. *Clin Immunol Immunopathol* 1997;84:223–243.
156. Robinson WH, Genovese MC, Moreland LW. Demyelinating and neurologic events reported in association with tumor necrosis factor alpha antagonism: by what mechanisms could tumor necrosis factor alpha antagonists improve rheumatoid arthritis but exacerbate multiple sclerosis? *Arthritis Rheum* 2001;44:1977–1983.
157. Torre-Amione G, Kapadia S, Lee J, et al. Tumor necrosis factor-alpha and tumor necrosis factor receptors in the failing human heart. *Circulation* 1996;93:704–711.
158. Matsumori A, Yamada T, Suzuki H, et al. Increased circulating cytokines in patients with myocarditis and cardiomyopathy. *Br Heart J* 1994;72:561–566.

159. Heard SO, Perkins MW, Fink MP. Tumor necrosis factor-alpha causes myocardial depression in guinea pigs. *Crit Care Med* 1992; 20:523–527.
160. Pagani FD, Baker LS, Hsi C, et al. Left ventricular systolic and diastolic dysfunction after infusion of tumor necrosis factor-alpha in conscious dogs. *J Clin Invest* 1992;90:389–398.
161. Cain BS, Meldrum DR, Dinarello CA, et al. Tumor necrosis factor-alpha and interleukin-1beta synergistically depress human myocardial function. *Crit Care Med* 1999;27:1309–1318.
162. Kubota T, McTiernan CF, Frye CS, et al. Dilated cardiomyopathy in transgenic mice with cardiac-specific overexpression of tumor necrosis factor-alpha. *Circ Res* 1997;81:627–635.
163. Kadokami T, McTiernan CF, Kubota T, et al. Sex-related survival differences in murine cardiomyopathy are associated with differences in TNF-receptor expression. *J Clin Invest* 2000;106:589–597.
164. Li YY, Feng YQ, Kadokami T, et al. Myocardial extracellular matrix remodeling in transgenic mice overexpressing tumor necrosis factor alpha can be modulated by anti-tumor necrosis factor alpha therapy. *Proc Natl Acad Sci U S A* 2000;97:12746–12751.
165. Kubota T, Bounoutas GS, Miyagishima M, et al. Soluble tumor necrosis factor receptor abrogates myocardial inflammation but not hypertrophy in cytokine-induced cardiomyopathy. *Circulation* 2000; 101:2518–2525.
166. Bozkurt B, Torre Amione G, Warren MS, et al. Results of targeted anti-tumor necrosis factor therapy with etanercept (ENBREL) in patients with advanced heart failure. *Circulation* 2001;103:1044–1047.
167. Chung ES, Packer M, Lo KH, et al. Randomized, double-blind, placebo-controlled, pilot trial of infliximab, a chimeric monoclonal antibody tumor necrosis factor-α, in patients with moderate-to-severe heart failure: results of the Anti TNF Therapy Against Congestive Heart Failure (ATTACH) Trial. *Circulation* 2003;107:3133–3140.
168. Anker SD, Coats AJS. How to RECOVER from RENAISSANCE? The significance of the results of RECOVER, RENAISSANCE, RENEWAL and ATTACH. *Int J Cardiol* 2002;86:123–130.
169. Kwon HJ, Cote TR, Cuffe MS, et al. Case reports of heart failure after therapy with a tumor necrosis factor antagonist. *Ann Intern Med* 2003;138:807–811.
170. Sills ES, Perloe M, Tucker MJ, et al. Successful ovulation induction, conception, and normal delivery after chronic therapy with etanercept: a recombinant fusion anti-cytokine treatment for rheumatoid arthritis. *Am J Reprod Immunol* 2001;46:366–368.
171. Antoni C, Furst D, Manger B, et al. Outcome of pregnancy in women receiving Remicade (infliximab) for the treatment of Crohn's disease or rheumatoid arthritis. *Arthritis Rheum* 2001;44(suppl 9):152.
172. Schiff M, Bulpitt K, Weaver A, et al. Safety of combination therapy with anakinra and etanercept in patients with rheumatoid arthritis. *Arthritis Rheum* 2001;44(suppl 9):79.
172a. Genovese MC, Cohen S, Moreland C, et al. Combination therapy with etanercept and anakinra in the treatment of patients with arthritis who have been treated unsuccessfully with methotrexate. *Arthritis Rheum* 2004;50:1412–1419.
173. Antin JH, Weisdorf D, Neuberg D, et al. Interleukin-1 blockade does not prevent acute graft-versus-host disease: results of a randomized, double-blind, placebo-controlled trial of interleukin-1 receptor antagonist in allogeneic bone marrow transplantation. *Blood* 2002;100: 3479–3483.
174. Fisher CJ Jr, Dhainaut JF, Opal SM, et al. Recombinant human interleukin 1 receptor antagonist in the treatment of patients with sepsis syndrome. Results from a randomized, double-blind, placebo-controlled trial. Phase III rhIL-1ra Sepsis Syndrome Study Group. *JAMA* 1994;271:1836–1843.
175. Opal SM, Fisher CJ, Dhainaut JFA, et al. Confirmatory interleukin-1 receptor antagonist trial in severe sepsis: a phase III, randomized, double-blind, placebo-controlled, multicenter trial. *Crit Care Med* 1997;25:1115–1124.
176. Targan SR, Hanauer SB, van Deventer SJ, et al. A short-term study of chimeric monoclonal antibody cA2 to tumor necrosis factor alpha for Crohn's disease. Crohn's Disease cA2 Study Group. *N Engl J Med* 1997;337:1029–1035.
177. Rutgeerts P, D'Haens G, Targan S, et al. Efficacy and safety of retreatment with anti-tumor necrosis factor antibody (infliximab) to maintain remission in Crohn's disease. *Gastroenterology* 1999;117: 761–769.
178. Hanauer SB, Feagan BG, Lichtenstein GR, et al. Maintenance infliximab for Crohn's disease: the ACCENT I randomised trial. *Lancet* 2002;359:1541–1549.
179. Sandborn WJ, Feagan BG, Hanauer SB, et al. An engineered human antibody to TNF (CDP571) for active Crohn's disease: a randomized double-blind placebo-controlled trial. *Gastroenterology* 2001;120: 1330–1338.
180. Sandborn WJ, Hanauer SB, Katz S, et al. Etanercept for active Crohn's disease: a randomized, double-blind, placebo-controlled trial. *Gastroenterology* 2001;121:1088–1094.
181. Mease PJ, Goffe BS, Metz J, et al. Etanercept in the treatment of psoriatic arthritis and psoriasis: a randomised trial. *Lancet* 2000;356: 385–390.
182. Ory P, Sharp JT, Salonen D, et al. Etanercept (Enbrel) inhibits radiographic progression in patients with psoriatic arthritis. *Arthritis Rheum* 2002;46(suppl 9):196.
183. Chaudhari U, Romano P, Mulcahy LD, et al. Efficacy and safety of infliximab monotherapy for plaque-type psoriasis: a randomised trial. *Lancet* 2001;357:1842–1847.
184. Gorman JD, Sack KE, Davis JC. Treatment of ankylosing spondylitis by inhibition of tumor necrosis factor alpha. *N Engl J Med* 2002; 346:1349–1356.
185. Braun J, Brandt J, Listing J, et al. Treatment of active ankylosing spondylitis with infliximab: a randomised controlled multicentre trial. *Lancet* 2002;359:1187–1193.
186. Braun J, Baraliakos X, Golder W, et al. Magnetic resonance imaging examinations of the spine in patients with ankylosing spondylitis, before and after successful therapy with infliximab—evaluation of a new scoring system. *Arthritis Rheum* 2003;48:1126–1136.
187. Van den Bosch F, Kruithof E, Baeten D, et al. Randomised double-blind comparison of chimeric monoclonal antibody to tumor necrosis factor a (infliximab) versus placebo in active spondyloarthropathy. *Arthritis Rheum* 2001;44(suppl):153.
188. Stone JH, Uhlfelder ML, Hellmann DB, et al. Etanercept combined with conventional treatment in Wegener's granulomatosis: a six-month open-label trial to evaluate safety. *Arthritis Rheum* 2001;44:1149–1154.
189. Sfikakis PP. Behçet's disease: a new target for anti-tumor necrosis factor treatment. *Ann Rheum Dis* 2002;61(suppl 2):52–53.
190. El Shabrawi Y, Hermann J. Case series of selective anti-tumor necrosis factor a therapy using infliximab in patients with nonresponsive chronic HLA-B27-associated anterior uveitis: comment on the articles by Brandt et al. *Arthritis Rheum* 2002;46:2821–2822.
191. Sfikakis PP, Theodossiadis PG, Katsiari CG, et al. Effect of infliximab on sight-threatening panuveitis in Behçet's disease. *Lancet* 2001;358:295–296.
192. Foster CS, Tufail F, Waheed NK, et al. Efficacy of etanercept in preventing relapse of uveitis controlled by methotrexate. *Arch Ophthalmol* 2003;121:437–440.
193. Moller DR. Treatment of sarcoidosis—from a basic science point of view. *J Intern Med* 2003;253:31–40.
194. Kneer J, Leudin E, Lesslauer W, et al. An assessment of the effect of anti-drug antibody formation on the pharmacokinetics and pharmacodynamics of sTNFr55-IgG (Ro 45–2081-Lenercept [LEN]) (S.C.) in patients with rheumatoid arthritis (RA). *Arthritis Rheum* 1998;41 (suppl):58.

CHAPTER 40

Investigational Biologic Therapies for the Treatment of Rheumatic Diseases

Joseph Shanahan and Larry W. Moreland

New biologic agents have had tremendous impact on the treatment of rheumatic diseases, including rheumatoid arthritis (RA), psoriatic arthritis (PsA), and ankylosing spondylitis (AS). Advances in targeted therapies have suggested new possibilities for the treatment of other disorders, including systemic lupus erythematosus (SLE) and vasculitis. Biologic therapies targeting SLE and Wegener's granulomatosis are reviewed in more detail in Chapters 73 and 83, respectively. The testing of successful and unsuccessful treatment strategies has also shed new light on diseases pathology, particularly as novel agents modify ever more specific targets.

Biologic agents can be loosely categorized by the component of the autoimmune or inflammatory process that is targeted. For example, inhibitors of tumor necrosis factor-α (TNF-α) have been designed to block the activity of a proximal cytokine in the inflammatory cascade, thereby reducing downstream activities of numerous other inflammatory mediators, including cytokines, chemokines, and destructive enzymes. Other biologic agents, such as cytotoxic T-lymphocyte antigen-4 (CTLA-4) Ig or rituximab [anti-CD20 monoclonal antibody (MoAb) that targets B cells], target cells that play important roles in the pathogenesis and maintenance of autoimmune and inflammatory responses. Finally, some targets of drug development, such as matrix metalloproteinases (MMPs) or intracellular signaling molecules, are final common pathway molecules in the pathologic autoimmune and inflammatory cascades that characterize rheumatic diseases.

Powerful technologies, including recombinant DNA techniques and manufacturing of nonimmunogenic small molecules, MoAbs, soluble receptors, and cytokine traps, provide researchers with the tools they need to inhibit specific targets. Targets are typically identified from investigation of animal models of human disease and advances in understanding of human immunity. However, numerous targeted therapies have been ineffective in human disease. In most cases, failed therapy appears to be related to the redundancy inherent in the human immune system and inflammatory cascade. For instance, it is evident that TNF-α and interleukin-1 (IL-1) share many properties relevant to the pathology of RA, including stimulating release of IL-6, activating synovial macrophages and synovial fibroblasts, and inducing bone and joint destruction through various mediators. Described in Chapter 39, commercially-available inhibitors of both TNF and IL-1 reduce symptoms of RA disease activity and radiographic evidence of joint destruction in a significant proportion of, but not all, patients with RA. Due to concerns that RA pathology may be driven predominantly by either IL-1 or TNF-α, depending on the patient, a combination trial was performed using IL-1 receptor antagonist (anakinra) and a soluble TNF-α receptor (etanercept) (1). Although the combination appeared effective in this open-label pilot study, further trials have not been pursued due to an excessive number of infections. This experience provides an important lesson that the redundancy in human immune and inflammatory systems may be important to the maintenance of normal health.

As the field of biologic therapeutics continues to swiftly advance, the importance of biologic targets in maintaining human health must be considered as strongly as the role of these potential targets in promoting rheumatic disease. It will be important to maintain vigilance in both clinical trials and postmarketing surveillance for potential and unexpected toxicities and complications of altering immunity and inflammation with biologic agents. For example, the importance of TNF-α in developing and maintaining the integrity of inflammatory granulomas has been well described in several animal models of mycobacterial and other infections (2–7). Yet, in the clinical trials of soluble

TNF-α receptors and anti-TNF-α, only one case of reactivated latent tuberculosis was observed, and these agents were marketed with relatively modest concern for the potential of these infections (8). Fortunately, through careful postmarketing surveillance from manufacturers and investigation by the Center for Biologics Evaluation and Research at the U.S. Food and Drug Administration (FDA), the association between initiation of TNF-α-inhibiting therapy and reactivation of latent tuberculous infection was confirmed (9). Information on this association has now been disseminated so that clinical practice modifications can be instituted to protect at-risk patients.

This chapter will review emerging biologic therapies for the treatment of rheumatic disease. Review of each therapeutic target will include a brief explanation of the presumed mechanism of action as well as indicate the progression of the therapy in terms of clinical trials. For agents in which human exposure has been documented, a summary of efficacy and toxicity will be provided. In addition, we will also make brief mention of failed therapies.

CYTOKINES

The proinflammatory cytokines IL-1 and TNF-α have been successful targets of several new therapeutic agents in RA (see Chapter 39). Two anti-TNF-α MoAbs (infliximab and adalimumab) and a soluble TNF receptor (sTNFR)–Fc fusion molecule (etanercept) are approved for the treatment of RA. Etanercept has also been approved for use in the management of systemic-onset juvenile chronic arthritis, PsA, and AS. In addition, infliximab has been approved for Crohn disease. These TNF-α-inhibiting agents are also being evaluated for the treatment of Wegener's granulomatosis (10–12), and case reports suggest efficacy for TNF-α inhibition in giant cell arteritis (13), Behçet's disease (14–16), and adult-onset Still's disease (17–19). The only approved IL-1-inhibiting agent, Anakinra, is a recombinant IL-1ra product that has efficacy in the treatment of methotrexate-refractory RA. New therapeutic agents in development are designed to improve on existing agents through novel methods of inhibiting cytokine activity. These agents are primarily being studied for the treatment of RA.

Novel Methods of Inhibiting Tumor Necrosis Factor-α

Novel TNF inhibitors are presently in various stages of development. A soluble TNF receptor type I [polyethylene glycol (PEG)-sTNF-RI] reduces synovial expression of proinflammatory cytokines, including TNF-α, IL-2, interferon-γ (IFN-γ), and IL-17, and decreases synovitis in the adjuvant arthritis model of RA (20). Another product, CDP870 (PEG-ylated anti-TNF-α Fab′), consists of a PEG-ylated Fab′ fragment of an MoAb against TNF-α. CDP870, administered by intravenous infusion with a half-life of about 14 days, has been shown to reduce disease activity in phase II RA studies (21). A new recombinant soluble p55 receptor (TNF-RI) construct (onercept) may decrease Crohn's disease activity (22). An alternative approach to TNF blockade is the development of dominant negative TNF (DNTNF) inhibitors. These proteins, which do not bind to or signal through TNFR, sequester native TNF-α into inactive heterotrimers (Xencor Pharmaceuticals, *www.Xencor.com*). DNTNF is presently in the early stages of preclinical testing.

TNF-α exerts proinflammatory effects in two manners: through cell/cell interactions when bound to cell surfaces or as a soluble mediator after it is cleaved from cell surfaces. TNF-α converting enzyme (TACE), a transmembrane proteinase member of the ADAMT (a disintegrin and metalloprotease) family of proteases that cleaves surface-bound TNF-α to release soluble cytokine (23). Because TACE is overexpressed in rheumatoid synovium, it has been speculated that inhibiting release of soluble TNF-α may abrogate inflammation in diseases with significant TNF activity, such as RA (24). However, there are theoretic concerns that a compensatory increase in proinflammatory cell surface–bound cytokine might contravene the beneficial effects of TACE inhibition. In animal models, TACE inhibition reduces lipopolysaccharide (LPS)-induced serum TNF-α levels by up to 95%. The majority (>80%) of the unreleased cytokine is degraded within the cell, whereas the rest is expressed only transiently on the cell surface (25). Several TACE inhibitors are being investigated and have shown efficacy in controlling inflammatory arthritis in various animal models (25–29). Primarily, TACE inhibitors in development have been orally bioavailable metalloproteinases effective in limiting joint damage in animal models, while few some phase I human trials have been performed. However, some of the TACE inhibitors in development have broader inhibitory effects on MMPs in addition to TACE, which may enhance efficacy (30).

Targeting Interleukin-1 and Interleukin-18

IL-1 is a potent proinflammatory cytokine overexpressed by rheumatoid synovium that shares many biologic activities with TNF-α. The IL-1 family includes the membrane and soluble forms of IL-1 and several associated molecules. IL-1α is the membrane-bound form, which exerts biologic activity through intracellular signaling and cell-cell contact. IL-1β exists in a proform that is activated to its soluble form by a cysteine proteinase called IL-1 converting enzyme (ICE) that is also known as caspase 1 (31). IL-1α and IL-1β signal through a common receptor, IL-1 receptor type I (IL-1RI). However, IL-1 receptor accessory protein (IL-1RAcP) is a necessary component for IL-1β signaling (32,33). After binding to its receptor, IL-1 recruits IL-1RacP, which enhances the affinity of IL-1RI for IL-1. Two IL-1 family members down-regulate the proinflammatory effects of IL-1. First, the inhibitory molecule IL-1 receptor antagonist (IL-1Ra) competes with IL-1 for IL-1RI binding. In vivo concentrations of IL-1Ra must exceed IL-1 concentration by as much as 100-fold to achieve clinically relevant inhibition of IL-1 signaling. Anakinra, a recombinant IL-1Ra product administered daily by subcutaneous injection, significantly reduces disease activity in patients with methotrexate-refractory RA (34) (reviewed in Chapter 39). The second IL-1 regulatory mechanism is production of a decoy receptor, IL-1R type II (IL-1RII), which lacks a functional cytoplasmic tail, and, therefore, does not mediate signaling after binding IL-1 (35). IL-1RII, which may be present on cell surfaces or as a soluble molecule, binds IL-1β with high avidity, preventing interaction with IL-1RI.

Antagonizing IL-1 activity has proven to be an effective means of treating animal models of RA (36) and appears to be a particularly effective approach in reducing bone destruction in human RA (37). However, clinical improvement in symptoms and signs of inflammation in RA with Anakinra treatment has been relatively modest. Alternative approaches to inhibit IL-1 activity target each component of the IL-1 family (Fig. 40.1). A soluble, recombinant IL-1RII has shown preclinical efficacy and is presently in early phase clinical trials in RA. An IL-1 TRAP molecule, consisting of IL-1RI and IL-1RAcP, has entered phase II clinical trials in RA. Since IL-1 TRAP exhibits greater *in vitro* affinity for IL-1β than either IL-1Ra or the soluble ectodomains of IL-1RI and IL-1RII, it may be a more effective IL-1 antagonist than IL-1Ra (38). Another promising alternative for antagonizing IL-1 is ICE inhibition. Several ICE inhibitors are under development, but one agent, pralnacasan, has entered phase III clinical trials for RA. ICE inhibition is an attractive therapeutic option for two reasons. First, it prevents the release of active IL-1β and abrogates the attendant proinflammatory effects. Second, because ICE cleaves the proform of IL-18, the activity of this cytokine is also reduced.

IL-18 is a proinflammatory cytokine that up-regulates production of TNF-α, IFN-γ, granulocyte-macrophage colony-stimulating factor (GM-CSF), and nitric oxide (NO) in rheumatoid synovium (39). The relative impact of IL-18 on RA disease activity is unclear (40,41), but its activity may be potentiated by other cytokines such as IL-12 or IL-15, making it difficult to completely understand the importance of IL-18. Nevertheless, the potential exists that ICE inhibition exerts greater antiinflammatory potency than IL-1 blockade alone. However, other enzymes can cleave IL-1 and IL-18 proforms besides ICE. This enzymatic redundancy could mitigate the beneficial effects of ICE inhibition. Indeed, in animal models of sepsis, broad-spectrum caspase inhibitors reduced IL-1 expression, but left IL-18 levels unaffected (42).

Blocking IL-18 activity using both an anti-IL-18 MoAb and a recombinant form of IL-18 binding protein (IL-18bp) has been shown to effectively reduce inflammation in animal models of RA (43,44). IL-18bp is a naturally-occurring molecule that binds tightly to IL-18 at an approximately equimolar ratio (45). Administration of anti-IL-18 MoAb and IL-18bp to mice with collagen-induced arthritis (CIA) reduced clinical synovitis, and decreased synovial IL-1, TNF-α, and IFN-γ (43). However, IL-18bp did not attenuate disease activity in existing arthritis to the same degree as anti-IL-18.

Interleukin-6 Family

The IL-6 family of cytokines includes IL-6, IL-11, leukemia inhibitory factor (LIF), and oncostatin M. Although IL-6 exerts both proinflammatory and antiinflammatory effects, the presence of elevated IL-6 levels in RA synovial fluid and the increased IL-6 expression by RA synoviocytes suggests a pathogenic role for the IL-6 in inflammatory arthritis (46). The IL-6 cytokine family members are potential biologic targets for the treatment of RA and other rheumatic diseases.

IL-6 expression is up-regulated by TNF-α and IL-1 and exerts numerous proinflammatory effects, including enhanced expression of acute-phase reactants, T-cell proliferation, B-cell differentiation, osteoclast differentiation and activation, and enhanced leukocyte chemotaxis (46). Elevated concentrations of IL-6 and soluble IL-6 receptor (sIL-6R) are evident in rheumatoid synovium; however, the exact role of IL-6 in RA pathophysiology is unclear, primarily because IL-6 manifests antiinflammatory activities in certain model systems. For example, IL-6 reduces LPS-induced TNF-α and IL-1 release in cultured monocytes (47). However, in human RA, data suggest that IL-6 plays a primarily pathogenic role. IL-6 levels are elevated in RA synovial fluid and serum IL-6 levels correlate directly with radiographic joint damage and disease activity (48,49). Moreover, IL-6 levels decrease after successful treatment with disease-modifying antirheumatic agents (DMARDs), including TNF inhibitors in the treatment of AS (50).

IL-6-inhibiting therapy has been used in RA. An open-label trial of a murine anti-IL-6 MoAb has shown clinical improvement and reduction of serum C-reactive protein (CRP) levels in subjects with RA (51). A phase I/II study, in which a single intravenous dose of humanized soluble anti-IL-6 receptor MoAb (sIL-6R Ab) administered to subjects with active RA, has shown that CRP and erythrocyte sedimentation rates (ESRs) were normalized, and in the 5 mg/kg dose group, significantly more patients met American College of Rheumatology 20% improvement (ACR20) criteria than in the placebo group (52). Further phase II studies are underway.

IL-6 inhibition is under investigation for the treatment of other rheumatic diseases. For example, IL-6 inhibition with anti-IL-6R MoAb successfully reduced disease activity in a single patient with refractory, adult-onset Still's disease (53) and in two patients with refractory, systemic-onset, juvenile chronic arthritis (54). IL-6 may play a role in SLE disease activity based on the proinflammatory and B-cell proliferative effects of the cytokine. It has been suggested that the

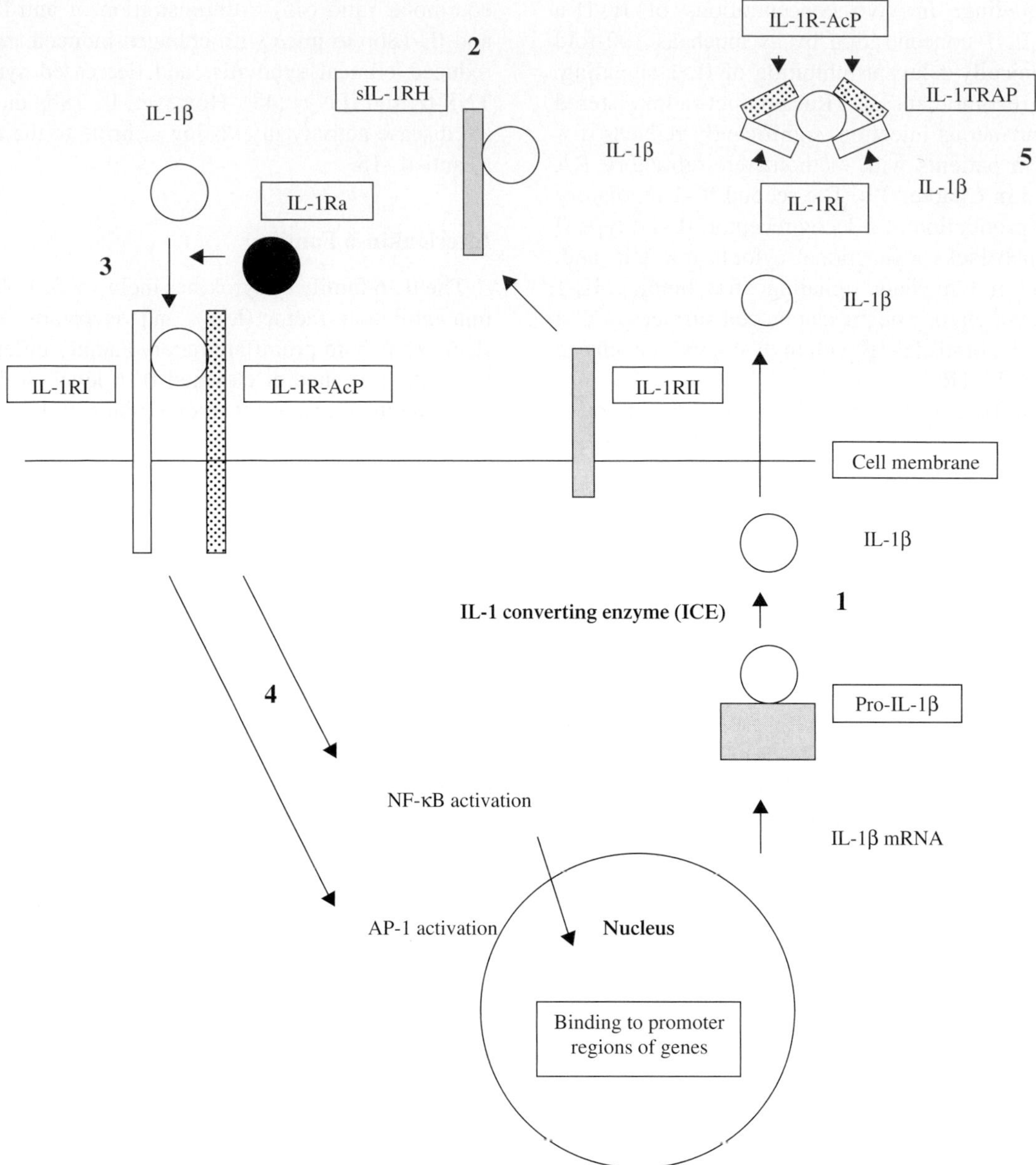

FIG. 40.1. Approaches to interleukin-1 (IL-1) inhibition. *1,* Inhibit production of mature IL-1β at the level of gene expression or by blocking IL-1 converting enzyme activity (pralnacasan); *2,* block extracellular IL-1β with using the decoy IL-1 receptor type II (sIL-1RII) or soluble IL-1 RI (IL-1TRAP); *3,* block the interaction of IL-1 with membrane-bound IL-1 type I receptor using IL-1ra (anakinra) or other synthetic molecule having similar properties; *4,* block the postreceptor effects of IL-1 by impeding nuclear factor κB or activator protein-1 activity. Adapted from Gabay C. IL = I inhibitors: novel agents in the treatment of rheumatoid arthritis. *Exp Opin Invest Drugs* 2000;9(1):115, with permission.

modest efficacy of anti-CD4 MoAb in SLE may be due in part to inhibition of cytokine release, particularly IL-6 production (55). In MRL *lpr/lpr* lupus-prone mice, IL-6-neutralizing antibodies that target IL-6R reduce glomerular damage and loss of renal function and lower anti–double-stranded DNA (anti-dsDNA) antibody titers (56). In addition, combination treatment with anti-CD4 and anti-IL-6 antibodies abrogated renal and serologic lupus activity in NZB/NZW mice (57).

IL-11 has potent antiinflammatory effects that include the inhibiting of degradative MMP expression and enhancing expression of tissue inhibitors of metalloproteinase (TIMPs), and decreasing proinflammatory cytokine production from activated macrophages via the inhibition of nuclear factor κB (NFκB) nuclear translocation (58). Systemic administration of IL-11 abrogated collagen-induced murine arthritis (59), and recombinant human IL-11 (rhIL-11) appeared to reduce Crohn's disease activity

(60). A clinical trial of rhIL-11 was conducted in RA; although tender joint counts were reduced in the highest dosing group, significant differences in ACR20 response were not observed (61). Further studies are needed to determine the efficacy of rh-IL-11 in RA.

Interleukin-17

The T cell–derived cytokine IL-17 has emerged as an important component of RA synovial and bone pathophysiology (62–64). IL-17 promotes articular cartilage degradation through increased MMP production and reduced TIMP expression (65,66) and by suppressing proteoglycan synthesis via NO production (67). Osteoclastogenesis and articular bone destruction is potentiated by IL-17 (63) through increased receptor activator of NF–κβ ligand (RANKL) expression (68). Some effects of IL-17 are independent of IL-1 (69), but synergy between IL-17, IL-1, and TNF-α in both synovitis and bone erosion is evident by studies in an *ex vivo* model using synovial and periarticular bone explants from patients with RA. In this *in vitro* system, the antagonism of IL-1 and IL-17 activity with sIL-1RII and s-IL-17R significantly enhanced the inflammatory effects of TNF inhibition with sTNFR (70). An IL-17 MoAb is also being studied in preclinical trials (71). IL-17 inhibition may be an attractive component of biologic combination therapy in RA, but such therapy may be limited by untoward effects on host T cell–mediated immunity (71).

Targeting T_H1-associated Inflammatory Cytokines: IL-12, IL-15, and IL-7

The cell-mediated immune response in RA is driven primarily by components of the helper T cell subset 1 (T_H1)-type immune response. T_H1-type responses, characterized chiefly by IL-2 and IFN-γ production, are dominated by T-cell activation and proliferation and proinflammatory cytokine expression. Polarization of the immune response toward the T_H1 phenotype is influenced by certain cytokines, including IL-12, IL-15, and IL-7, which are expressed by antigen-presenting cells such as dendritic cells and macrophages. In RA, each of these cytokines is expressed in the synovial lining layer (72–74). IL-12 is a potent inducer of T_H1 differentiation and IFN-γ production by T cells. The cytokine also suppresses the T_H2-type cytokines, such as IL-4, IL-5, and IL-10 (75). Importantly, IL-12 is part of a feedback loop including TNF-α and IFN-γ, in which each of these cytokines up-regulates the production of the other. This may be particularly important in RA, where high levels of TNF-α and IL-12 are detectable, but IFN-γ expression is modest. In murine CIA, anti-IL-12 MoAb treatment has had variable effects (76,77), but the efficacy of TNF-inhibiting treatment in ameliorating CIA was significantly enhanced when combined with anti-IL-12 MoAb (78). IL-12 also appears to play an important role in chronic inflammatory disorders, including Wegener's granulomatosis (79), and multiple sclerosis (MS) (80,81). Effective treatments for these diseases are often characterized by an ability to reduce IL-12 expression as part of their overall therapeutic effect. IL-12-inhibiting therapies, including MoAb against IL-12, have attenuated disease in animal models of MS. Human experience with biologic IL-12 inhibition is limited, but IL-12 appears to be a potential target for those diseases characterized by T_H1 immune responses. A phase I trial of a humanized anti-IL-12 MoAb in RA has been completed, but the results are not yet available.

IL-15 is a pleiotropic cytokine that stimulates T-cell activation and proliferation (82), promotes T-cell expression of TNF-α (83), and supports B cell and osteoclast maturation (84). IL-15 is evident in RA synovium and synovial fluid, and elevated IL-15 levels are detectable in SLE sera (85) and from myocytes of patients with inflammatory myopathy (86). IL-15 inhibition using soluble murine IL-15 receptor-α has been shown to decrease inflammatory synovitis in the murine CIA model (87). CRB-15, an IL-15-neutralizing biologic, is a fusion protein consisting of point-mutated IL-15 and human Fc Ig (88). Abrogation of clinical synovitis in a murine CIA model by CRB-15 correlated with a reduction in expression of proinflammatory cytokines. Initial release of phase I trial results of a humanized anti-IL-15 MoAb in RA reported 61% of patients treated with anti-IL-15 met ACR20 response criteria, whereas 39% and 26% met ACR50 and ACR70 criteria, respectively (press release, *www.genmab.com,* 2002).

IL-7 is an important growth factor for early T cells and plays a role in B-cell lymphopoiesis (89). Elevated serum IL-7 levels in patients with RA correlate with increased concentration of CRP (90). Fibroblast-like synoviocytes appear to be important producers of IL-7 (74). A key contribution of IL-7 is stimulation of TNF-α expression from macrophages and IL-6 and IL-1 expression from macrophages (91). Because IL-7 appears to support persistent T_H1 cytokine production by RA synovium and periarticular bone destruction, it is an attractive therapeutic target.

Macrophage Migration Inhibitory Factor

Macrophage migration inhibitory factor (MMIF) is a pleiotropic cytokine that is important to the development of both adaptive and innate immune responses (92). MMIF appears to influence innate immunity by controlling murine Toll-like receptor 4 (TLR4) expression (93), whereas effects on T-cell activation and proliferation by MMIF play a role in adaptive immune responses (94). Several researchers have shown excessive MMIF expression in RA synovial macrophages, fibroblast-like synoviocytes, and endothelial cells (92). In addition, administration of anti-MMIF to murine models of human disease results in abrogation of murine CIA and decreased vascularization of tumors. MMIF has several functions in RA inflammation. First, through down-regulation of the tumor suppressor protein p53, MMIF could contribute to the proliferation of fibroblast-like synoviocytes and neoangiogenesis that characterize the destructive rheumatoid pannus. Interestingly, studies have shown a potent glucocorticoid-antagonist effect for MMIF, particularly in terms of reversing glucocorticoid-induced suppression of TNF-α and IL-1 expression from activated macrophages (92). Small-molecule inhibitors of MMIF are in development for the treatment of RA and other inflammatory diseases.

Vasoactive Intestinal Peptide

Vasoactive intestinal peptide (VIP) is a pleiotropic neuropeptide produced by endocrine cells, neurons, and lymphocytes. VIP expression is increased in association with inflammation, and it appears to act as an endogenous antiinflammatory regulatory molecule (95). Signaling through a variety of receptors, VIP reduces expression of proinflammatory cytokines and mediators of tissue destruction, including TNF-α, IL-1, inducible nitric oxide synthetase, and MMPs. These effects result from at least two different mechanisms of action: inhibition of NFκB nuclear translocation and the up-regulation of antiinflammatory IL-10 expression. Exogenous administration of VIP to mice with CIA significantly reduced signs of synovitis, joint damage, and anti–collagen II autoantibodies (96). The tolerability and effectiveness of VIP as a therapy for human systemic inflammatory disease requires further study (97).

Altering the Balance of Inflammatory Subtypes via Cytokine Manipulation

Imbalance between T_H1- and T_H2-type immune responses has been considered an important component of rheumatic pathophysiology. RA and PSA are characterized by T_H1-type immune responses. The cytokine milieu in these diseases reflects excessive production of TNF-α and IL-12 and a relative paucity of IL-4 and IL-10. SLE is characterized by a T_H2-type immune response, with high levels of IL-10 expression and consequent maturation of autoreactive B cells and the attendant autoantibody production. Consequently, restoration of balance to immune responses is an attractive therapeutic goal for autoimmune disease. Systemic and intralesional administration of IL-10 has been effective in controlling psoriatic skin plaques (98–100), but systemic IL-10 did not benefit clinical measures of PsA (101). Recombinant human IL-10 also failed to show efficacy in clinical trials of RA treatment (102). IL-4 is a T_H2-type cytokine that acts to down-regulate T_H1-type proinflammatory cytokine expression. Recombinant human IL-4 (rhu IL–4) has been evaluated in RA and PsA with only modest clinical success. In a phase I trial in RA rhu IL–4, IL-4 therapy failed to result in clinical improvement, and further clinical development was halted. In an open-label trial of rhu IL-4 in psoriasis, histopathologic examination of lesional skin showed a clear shift toward T_H2 type inflammation, but only modest clinical benefits were observed (103). IL-11 is a pleiotropic T_H2-associated cytokine that is produced by articular chondrocytes and synoviocytes and that acts to reduce proinflammatory cytokine expression, NO production, and increase TIMP levels. As discussed previously, a phase I trial with rhIL-11 in RA has been completed.

IL-13 shares many of the antiinflammatory effects of IL-4, although its role in RA pathophysiology is controversial (104,105). However, overexpression of IL-13 delivered via adenoviral vector reduced synovitis and synovial TNF-α production in the rat adjuvant-induced arthritis model (106).

Targeting the pathogenic T_H2 cytokines in SLE is an attractive therapeutic biologic approach to this disease. Anti–IL–10 MoAb levels are elevated in SLE patients (107) and appear to correlate with disease activity (108,109). Furthermore, IL-10 delays onset of lupus-like disease in NZB/W mice (110). In an open label trial, six SLE patients with active disease received a murine anti-IL-10 MoAb (111). Improvements were noted in cutaneous and joint manifestations, and corticosteroid doses were lowered, but reactions to the murine antibody prevented retreatment. A humanized anti-IL-10 is expected to be used in future trials.

The interferons are a family of immunomodulatory cytokines categorized as type I (IFN-α and IFN-β) or type II (IFN-γ) interferons. As a predominant cytokine in T_H1-type immune responses, IFN-γ has broad proinflammatory effects. Down-regulating or inhibiting the function of this cytokine has been considered a target for the treatment of T_H1-mediated inflammatory disorders, and a phase I clinical trial in Crohn's disease suggested efficacy for an anti-IFN-γ MoAb (112). Type I interferons can promote T_H1 responses in certain situations, but manifest antiangiogenic, antiviral, and antiinflammatory effects in many contexts. IFN-α is an effective treatment for chronic hepatitis C infection, and eradication of viral infection appears to be an effective clinical intervention for hepatitis C–associated vasculitis and essential mixed cryoglobulinemia (113). Behçet's disease also responds to INF-α (114). In a randomized, controlled trial, 65% of INF-α-treated subjects achieved at least a partial remission in comparison with only 14% who received placebo (115). In contrast, anti-IFN-α MoAb is in development for the treatment of psoriasis, SLE, and Crohn's disease (Protein Design Labs, *www.pdl.com*). Clinical trials are awaited.

Since IFN-β down-regulates TNF-α and IL-1 production and up-regulates antiinflammatory cytokine expression and IL-1Ra levels, the interferon has been used to treat various inflammatory diseases. IFN-β is a highly effective treatment for relapsing-remitting MS. In preclinical studies of inflammatory arthritis, IFN-β abrogated joint damage and inflammation in murine CIA (116). In addition, IFN-β-deficient mice spontaneously develop severe osteopenia, suggesting that balance of this cytokine is important to the development of bone destruction in RA (117). In humans, IFN-β therapy was well tolerated, and improvement in RA activity was noted in an open-label study (118). Immunohistochemical analysis of synovial biopsies in these patients found a significant reduction in IL-1β, IL-6, and MMP-1 expression. Similar clinical benefits were observed in a small pilot study of six children with juvenile RA (118).

The myopathic lesions in inclusion body myositis (IBM) are characterized by cytotoxic T cells. The ability of IFN-β to counteract the immunostimulatory effects of IFN-γ, particularly the activation of cytotoxic T cells, suggests that this cytokine may be an effective therapy for IBM. In a placebo-controlled trial, 30 patients with IBM received weekly IFN-β (119). No differences in muscle strength between the groups were noted at 6 months in this pilot study; however, the treatment was generally well tolerated. A single case of refractory polymyositis treated successfully with IFN-β has been reported (120). Extended, placebo-controlled trials powered to assess efficacy are needed to determine the role of IFN-β in the treatment of RA and inflammatory muscle disease.

Placental Immunomodulator Ferritin

Pregnant women with RA and MS often experience remissions in disease activity during gestation. In RA, postpartum flare-ups of arthritis are observed frequently just weeks after delivery. It has been postulated that placental expression of immunosuppressive cytokines, including IL-10, serves to down-regulate the maternal immune response to the developing fetus. This phenomenon appears to be hormonally related. Indeed, in the murine CIA model, postpartum administration of estrogen can delay relapse of arthritis. During pregnancy a unique isoform of placental isoferritin (PLF), termed p43 PLF, is highly expressed in the placenta. The p43 component, called placental immunomodulator ferritin (PLIF), serves as an immunoregulatory cytokine. Recombinant PLIF inhibits T-cell proliferation in mixed lymphocyte reactions and human systems (121,122). In addition, administration of PLIF in murine zymogen-induced arthritis, and rat adjuvant-induced arthritis reduces synovitis, in part by up-regulating IL-10 production and by reducing IL-2 and TNF-α expression (122). Although direct evidence is lacking for PLIF as a mediator of pregnancy-induced RA remission, evidence suggests that pregnancy-associated remissions occur via mechanisms such as enhanced IL-10 production that could be due to PLIF activity. A recombinant PLIF molecule, C48, which consists of the active domain of PLIF, and has identical functions as PLIF in the aforementioned animal models, is a candidate therapy for RA.

Intracellular Signaling

Transcriptional Activation: Mitogen-Activated Protein Kinase and Nuclear Factor κB Pathways

The transcription of genes necessary to promote and maintain inflammatory and immune responses is mediated by the transcription factors NFκB and activating protein-1 (AP-1). Activity of these transcription factors is increased in diseases such as RA (123). Intracellular signaling cascades, in turn, regulate these transcription factors. NFκB, inactivated in the cytosol by a neutralizing binding molecule termed IκB, is activated by stimuli, including stress, endotoxin, and the inflammatory cytokines IL-1 and TNF-α, which disrupt IκB binding through the induction of IκB kinase (IKK) (124). IKK activation results in degradation of IκB permitting nuclear translocation of NFκB. The ensuing transcriptional activity leads to synthesis of IL-1, TNF-α, IL-8, cyclooxygenase-2 (COX-2), and IL-6 and promotion of inflammation (125). The antiinflammatory effects of some antirheumatic agents, including leflunomide, cyclosporine, and corticosteroids, have been attributed to inhibition of IKK activity and up-regulation of IκB expression (126, 127). Nuclear translocation of AP-1 results in the transcription of many of the same proinflammatory cytokines induced by NFκB, in addition to transcription of genes encoding matrix metalloproteinases and enzymes involved in the oxidative burst. AP-1 is a dimer of c-Fos and C-Jun, DNA-binding proteins for which transcriptional activity is up-regulated after phosphorylation by mitogen-activated protein kinase (MAPK) cascades. Three MAPK signaling cascades have been described: extracellular-regulated protein kinase (ERK), c-Jun N-terminal kinase (JNK), and p38 MAPK. JNK includes three kinases (JNK1, JNK2, and JNK3), while five p38 MAP kinases (α, β, β2, γ, and δ) have been described (128,129). p38α appears to be the most important kinase to be activated in inflammatory cells (128). JNK and p38 MAPK expression is up-regulated in RA, but not in osteoarthritis (OA) synovium (130), further supporting the notion that these signaling molecules may be important therapeutic targets for rheumatic diseases.

Antagonism and genetically-bred deficiency of JNK are associated with a partial defect in IL-1-induced AP-1 activity and reduced collagenase expression in murine models of inflammation (131,132). In adjuvant-induced arthritic rats, administration of a small molecule JNK inhibitor reduced paw swelling, and perhaps more importantly, almost completely inhibited radiographic joint damage, primarily via AP-1 blockade (133).

Small-molecule inhibitors of p38 MAPK have been shown to reduce LPS-induced TNF-α production, decrease mortality in endotoxin-induced shock, and abrogate synovitis in CIA and adjuvant-induced arthritis models (134–136). VX-745, an oral p38 MAPK inhibitor, has been tested in open-label and early-phase randomized, controlled trials in RA. After preclinical studies demonstrated efficacy in the murine CIA model (137), a dose escalation trial found favorable trends in ACR20 response and reduced tender and swollen joint counts and serum CRP levels (138). As with other p38 MAPK inhibitors, hepatotoxicity was a frequent side effect (128), as asymptomatic, reversible elevations in hepatic transaminases developed in 16% of treated subjects. A second-generation version of this agent is entering clinical trials.

Inhibitor of NFκB kinase β (IKKβ) has been identified as a key regulator of NFκB and should be considered a potential target for an antiinflammatory biologic agent (125). Rat adjuvant-induced arthritis activity was abrogated by intraarticular gene transfer of dominant negative IKKβ (125), whereas transfection of human RA fibroblast–like synoviocytes with adenoviral vectors encoding dominant negative IKK reduced NFκB activation and IL-6, IL-8, and intracellular adhesion molecule-1 (ICAM-1) expression (139). NFκB blockade inhibits TNF, IL-1, and IL-6 expression, while exerting little, if any, impact on IL-4, IL-10, IL-1Ra, and sTNFR production. The potential for restoring cytokine balance through NF-κB inhibition makes this approach an attractive option for the treatment of RA, PSA, and other inflammatory syndromes.

Efforts to inhibit NFκB activity have also included development of so-called dissociated steroids. These products retain transrepressive capabilities and inhibit AP-1 and NFκB activity while retaining transactivating effects. The goal for dissociated steroids is to retain antiinflammatory effects without causing side effects, such as osteoporosis, weight gain, and insulin resistance. An alternative method of inhibiting NFκB activity uses microcapsules of antisense oligomers to NFκB. Antisense oligomers to NFκB have reduced mortality and inhibited TNF-α expression in a rat model of endotoxic shock; moreover, antisense oligomers to NFκB decreased endotoxin-induced TNF-α, IL-1, and IL-6 expression in baboons (140). A variety of other NFκB inhibitors have shown efficacy in animal models of inflammation, including arthritis models (141–146).

JAK-STAT Pathway and Suppressors of Cytokine Signaling

Cytokines also promote transcription of proinflammatory genes by signaling through the JAK-STAT pathway. After binding to cognate receptors, cytokines activate a family of cytoplasmic kinases called Janus-activated kinases (JAK). Activated JAK kinases subsequently phosphorylate specific members of the family of signal transducers and activators of transcription (STAT), which dimerize, translocate to the nucleus, and initiate gene transcription. Knockout models have identified several STATs activated by various cytokines to transcribe critical genes for innate and acquired immune responses (147). JAK-STAT signaling is regulated by a variety of inhibitory cytoplasmic proteins, which act primarily to prevent prolonged and excessive activation of cell surface receptors. Direct inhibitory proteins, such as ubiquitin proteosome-dependent degradation of STAT proteins, and the protein inhibitor of activated STATs (PIAS) family of proteins, which bind directly to STAT dimers and impede DNA binding activity, are prominent among JAK-STAT inhibitors. In addition, STAT signaling induces the expression of regulatory molecules termed suppressors of cytokine signaling (SOCS). Members of the SOCS family down-regulate STAT-mediated gene transcription through interactions with JAK and STAT that antagonize the recruitment of STAT receptors. In murine models of inflammatory arthritis, SOCS-1 knockout mice suffered from more severe synovitis, whereas SOCS-1 overexpression reduced inflammation (148). Furthermore, periarticular injection of an adenovirus vector delivering SOCS-3/CIS3 reduced joint swelling and synovitis in both antigen-induced arthritis and CIA models (149). Targeting the JAK-STAT signaling pathway is a promising therapeutic alternative for the treatment of inflammatory diseases such as RA (150) .

Signal Transduction Targets in Systemic Lupus Erythematosus

Less is known of signal transduction pathways in SLE, although the effectiveness of glucocorticoids in reducing SLE disease activity is due in large part to disruption of NFκB and AP-1 signaling cascades. Lymphocyte activation and proliferation requires signal transduction via the intracellular Ras molecule. A novel Ras inhibitor, *S*-farnesylthiosalicylic acid (FTS), cleaves the membrane attachment site of Ras, releasing Ras into the cytosol, where it is degraded. Administration of FTS to MRL lpr/lpr lupus-prone mice reduces autoantibody levels, and decreases proteinuria, lymphadenopathy, spleen weight, and conconavalin A–induced lymphocyte proliferation (151).

T-CELL TARGETS

The crucial role of T cells in the pathogenesis and physiology of autoimmune diseases has been the target of numerous biologic therapies. However, T cell–depleting biologics, including MoAbs against CD4, CD5, and CD7, have shown limited efficacy in RA treatment. In addition, T cell–depleting therapy is complicated by prolonged lymphopenia and increased risk for infection. In contrast, nondepleting anti-CD4 MoAbs have shown some efficacy and less toxicity in the treatment of psoriasis (152) and RA (102). The effectiveness of nondepleting antibodies suggests that the therapeutic mechanism of these agents may include the induction of tolerance or suppressor cells. However, a phase II trial involving 155 subjects with active RA found no significant difference in ACR20 response between subjects treated with placebo (24%) and those receiving various doses of HuMax-CD4 (nondepleting anti-CD4 MoAb) (11%–29% met ACR20 criteria). Given these results, the ongoing phase III trial was closed to enrollment (press release, *www.genmab.com*). Studies of nondepleting OKTcdr4a are underway in PsA. A nondepleting anti-CD4 MoAb reduced lymphoproliferation and vasculitis in lupus-prone MRL/lpr mice, although survival was not prolonged in comparison with untreated mice (153). Further studies of anti-CD4 antibodies in SLE are required.

Anti-IL-2 Receptor Immunotoxins and Antibodies

Although biologic therapies directly targeting T cells have been generally disappointing, nonbiologic therapies that disrupt T-cell activities, such as cyclosporine, leflunomide, and mycophenolate, are effective in the treatment of a variety of autoimmune diseases. Therefore, alternative biologic approaches have targeted T-cell activation in order to replicate or improve on the immunomodulatory and anti-inflammatory effects of agents such as cyclosporine, which inhibits post–T-cell receptor (TCR) intracellular signaling in activated T cells, and sirolimus, an effective transplant rejection agent that inhibits post–IL-2 receptor intracellular signaling. Biologic agents that target the IL-2 receptor (anti-IL-2R, CD25) include denileukin diftitox (anti-IL-2 MoAb linked to diphtheria toxin, DAB486IL-2). After binding IL-2R, this compound is internalized, where it induces cell death. Denileukin diftitox reduces psoriatic plaque size (154), but only modest responses in RA have been reported (155). Another anti-IL2R product, daclizumab (humanized IgG1 MoAb against IL-2R), has been approved for the prevention of renal allograft rejection. This agent is presently being evaluated for preventing relapse in Wegener granulomatosis. Preclinical studies show that daclizumab abrogates collagen-induced arthritis in rhesus monkeys (156), so daclizumab may have efficacy in RA or PsA. Case reports describe rapid improvement in refractory plaque and pustular psoriasis and cyclosporine-sparing effects in psoriasis with basiliximab, another IL-2R MoAb developed for use in allograft rejection (157–159).

T-Cell Receptor and Vaccination Strategies

The TCR has been targeted directly with TCR peptide vaccination techniques and indirectly by administering anti–major histocompatibility complex (MHC) class II MoAbs. Although preclinical trials of these approaches were effective in reducing inflammatory arthritis, clinical studies in RA have resulted in only modest decreases in disease activity (102). Consensus peptides identified from V_H regions of murine anti-dsDNA antibodies have been used to vaccinate NZB/W lupus-prone mice. Vaccination reduces autoantibody levels, abrogates nephritis, and prolongs survival, in part through the induction of cytotoxic $CD8^+$ T cells, which appear to kill anti-dsDNA-producing B cells (160). Alternative strategies include vaccination with TNF-α, which has been shown to abrogate experimental murine cachexia and CIA (161). Further studies of vaccination strategies are under consideration in both RA and SLE.

Oral Tolerance

The induction of tolerance to specific antigens via repeated administration of low doses of antigen has been suggested as a possible therapy for autoimmune disease. Tolerance appears to be mediated by regulatory T cells that develop in gut-associated lymphoid tissue and then disperse to peripheral sites. On subsequent antigen exposure, these regulatory T cells down-regulate other T cells via a mechanism called bystander suppression (162). Although tolerance induction has been effective in abrogating disease activity in animal models of autoimmunity, including CIA and adjuvant-induced arthritis, trials in RA have failed to demonstrate efficacy. However, oral bovine collagen type I has been shown to modestly improve disease parameters in an open-label study in systemic sclerosis (163). It has been speculated that concomitant nonsteroidal antiinflammatory drug (NSAID) use in this study impaired the development of oral tolerance by depletion of the normal mucosal barrier of the gastrointestinal tract. A phase II trial is currently underway with modified enrollment criteria to minimize exposure to potential barriers for development of oral tolerance.

T-Cell Costimulatory Molecules

An exciting approach to inhibiting T-cell activation applies biologic therapies that interrupt T cell costimulatory signals. After TCR–CD4 or TCR–CD8 complexes recognize MHC-associated antigen, an essential "second signal" is required to activate T cells and B cells and to stimulate isotype switching (Fig. 40.2). There are multiple receptor-ligand pairs that can deliver a second signal that activates T cells (Table 40.1). In the absence of a second signal or if an inhibitory receptor-ligand pair provide a second signal, T-cell responsiveness is impaired and tolerance may develop. Biologic therapies that interfere with T-cell costimulatory signals have proven effective in preventing allograft rejection and treating several autoimmune and inflammatory diseases. It is important to note that multiple pairs of molecules can induce T-cell costimulation. This redundancy may prove to limit the effectiveness of biologic agents that inhibit the function of only one costimulatory pathway. On the contrary, many of these receptor-ligand pairs have additional functions. Therefore, depending on which receptor-ligand pair is targeted, inhibition of costimulatory molecules may lead to multiple antiinflammatory and immunomodulatory effects besides antagonizing T-cell activation, such as destabilizing the immune synapse, reducing immune cell chemotaxis, and impeding angiogenesis.

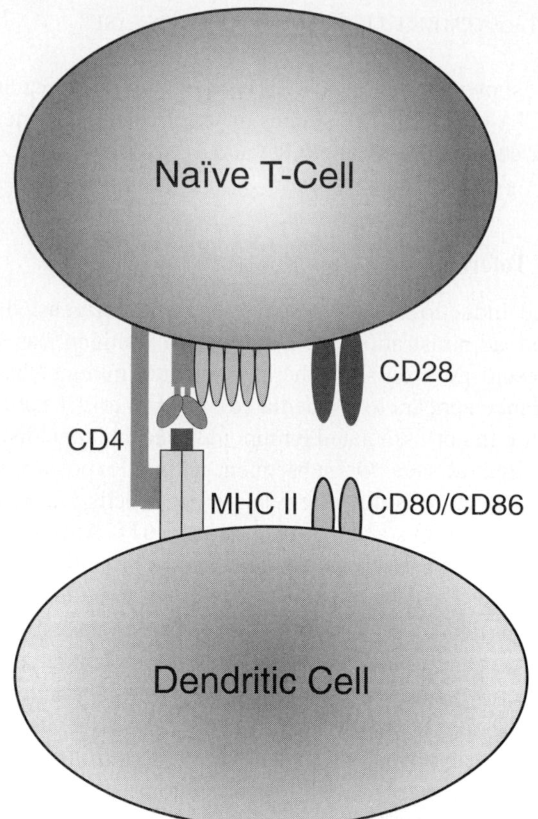

FIG. 40.2. T-cell costimulatory signaling. After ligation of the T-cell receptor with antigen processed by an antigen-presenting cell (APC), a second signal is transmitted by one of several T-cell surface molecules that interact with specific ligands on APC surfaces. In this figure, CD28 engages either B7–1 (CD80) or B7–2 (CD86) on the dendritic cell surface, which initiates an intracellular signaling cascade, resulting in T-cell activation, cytokine production, and proliferation. Reprinted from Sporki R, Perrin PJ. Continuation of memory T cells by a potential, thermocutic target for immunity? *Clinical Immunology* 2001;100:263–269, with permission.

CD28, B7–1 and B7–2, and CTLA4 Ig

The CD28 family includes receptor-ligand pairs that promote T cell activation through second-signal costimulation and induce tolerance through negative signaling (Table 40.2). CD28 is constitutively expressed on T-cell surfaces.

TABLE 40.2. *CD28 T-cell costimulatory family (CD28 and B7 families)*

Receptor	APC ligand	Outcome
CD28	B7.1 (CD80) B7.2 (CD86)	Increased cytokine production (e.g., IL-2) Enhanced proliferation Antiapoptotic signal
CTLA4 (CD152)	B7.1 (CD80) B7.2 (CD86)	"Off signal" Peripheral tolerance
ICOS	ByRP-1	Increased cytokine production (e.g., interferon-γ, IL-10)
PD1	PD-L1 PD-L2	"Off signal" Inhibition of proliferation

IL, interleukin.

Reprinted from Sporki R, Perrin PJ. Continuation of memory T cells by a potential, thermocutic target for immunity? *Clinical Immunology* 2001;100:263–269, with permission.

The B7 family of cell surface proteins [B7–1 (CD80) and B7–2 (CD86)], expressed on antigen-presenting cells and activated B cells, are the ligands for CD28. The primary effect of CD28-B7 interaction is to send a costimulatory signal to T cells in conjunction with TCR antigen recognition, which initiates T-cell activation. This costimulatory pathway is tightly regulated by the expression of cytotoxic T lymphocyte antigen 4 (CTLA-4, CD152) on activated T-cell surfaces, which binds to B7 molecules with greater affinity than CD28, thus inhibiting further T-cell activation. B7-CTLA-4 interaction sends negative signals to the T cell, resulting in tolerance instead of T-cell activation. Efforts to inhibit CD28 signaling include anti-B7 MoAbs, which have shown efficacy in preclinical allograft rejection studies and in chronic plaque psoriasis (164–166), and the development of CTLA-4Ig (abatacept), a soluble fusion protein composed of the extracellular domain of CTLA-4 and human Fc IgG1. In RA, abatacept has shown efficacy in patients with disease refractory to both methotrexate and TNF inhibitors. A phase II trial evaluated abatacept in 339 subjects with active RA on methotrexate (167). At 24 weeks, 60% of subjects treated with abatacept (10 mg/kg every other week) met ACR20 criteria in comparison with 35% in the placebo group. Also noted were significant improvement in quality of life measures (SF-36), and reductions in CRP and IL-6

TABLE 40.1. *T-cell costimulation: receptor-ligand pairs*

Family	T-cell surface receptor	Antigen-presenting cell ligand
Immunoglobulin superfamily	CD28	B7-1 B7-2
	ICOS	BRP-1
	CD2	CD58 (LFA-3)
Tumor necrosis factor (TNF)/TNF receptor superfamily	CD154 (CD40L)	CD40
	4-1BB	4-1BBL
	CD30	CD30L
	CD134	CD134L
	CD27	CD70
β_1 integrin	CD49d-CD26 (VLA-4)	VCAM-1, MadCAM-1, ICAM-4
β_2 integrin	CD11a/CD18	ICAM-1

ICAM, intercellular adhesion molecule; LFA, leukocyte-functional antigen; VCAM, vascular cell adhesion molecule; VLA, very late activation antigen.

levels. A second trial of low-dose CTLA4-Ig (2 mg/kg every other week) in subjects with active RA despite treatment with etanercept found trends toward clinical improvement in arthritis and quality of life in addition to reduced IL-6 levels (168). There were no significant toxicities noted in either study. Presently, two independent phase III studies of abatacept are underway in subjects with RA refractory to methotrexate and in subjects who have failed treatment with TNF inhibitors.

Abatacept is also being studied for use in SLE and psoriasis. Treatment of lupus-prone NZB/W mice with a murine CTLA4 construct prolonged survival and delayed the development of lupus features, including anti-dsDNA antibodies and nephritis (169,170). Preclinical studies of abatacept in BALB/c murine lupus models have shown reduced proteinuria and autoantibody levels in mice with early glomerulonephritis (171). However, no significant benefit was observed in the treatment of late disease. Wang and colleagues investigated combination treatment with abatacept and MoAb to CD40L (ligand for the costimulatory molecule CD40) in NZB/W mice with lupus (172). Combination therapy yielded significant improvement in survival and delays in proteinuria. Furthermore, a majority of mice responded to retreatment with the combination. However, unlike previous studies, monotherapy with either abatacept or anti-CD40L failed to alter disease course. Further studies aimed at understanding the pathophysiologic role of abatacept in the development and progression of SLE are needed. Administered to patients with refractory chronic plaque psoriasis, intravenous infusion of four doses of abatacept led to 50% reduction in psoriasis area and severity score (PASI) in almost half of subjects with refractory plaque psoriasis treated in an open-label study (173,174).

CD40 and CD40 Ligand

CD40 is expressed on numerous cell surfaces, including B cells, activated macrophages, dendritic cells, and endothelial cells whereas its cognate ligand, CD40L, is expressed on activated T cells. CD40L/CD40 interaction is required for B-cell maturation and germinal center formation (175). Therefore, biologic agents that interfere with CD40L activity have primarily been evaluated for treatment of SLE. However, disruption of CD40/CD40L interactions prevents murine CIA (176). In addition to the T-cell costimulatory effects of CD40/CD40L signaling, these findings suggest that blocking CD40L activity could be a useful RA therapy (177,178). Preclinical studies have shown that anti-CD40L MoAbs prevent or ameliorate nephritis in NZB/W and SNF1 mice (179,180).

Unfortunately, clinical trials of anti-CD40L antibody have been disappointing. In a phase II trial in SLE, IDEC-131, one of two anti-CD40L preparations that have been evaluated, failed to show significant differences in improvement of SLE disease activity as measured by SLEDAI scores between the treatment and placebo groups (181). Another anti-CD40L antibody, BG9588, was studied in an open-label, multidose trial in patients with proliferative lupus nephritis (182). The primary outcome measure for efficacy was 50% reduction in proteinuria without decline in renal function. The study was terminated before completion of enrollment due to thromboembolic events documented in this study and in concurrent studies of BG9588 in other clinical conditions. In the lupus nephritis study, two subjects suffered myocardial infarctions. At the time of termination, only 18 patients could be evaluated. Two subjects met criteria for improvement. In addition, hematuria resolved in all five subjects with hematuria at the screening visit. C3 concentrations increased, whereas anti-dsDNA antibody levels decreased, suggesting that the agent had a positive effect on lupus immunologic activity. Five subjects in the study underwent an extensive analysis of serum and peripheral blood mononuclear cells that showed treatment with anti-CD40L significantly reduced the number of IgG- and anti-dsDNA antibody-producing B cells (183). Importantly, these immunomodulatory effects persisted for several months after treatment. The thrombotic events observed in this study may be related to CD40L expression on activated platelets. However, thromboembolic complications have not been prominent in using other anti-CD40L antibodies. Because studies do suggest efficacy for anti-CD40L antibodies, more research into the role of CD40L in thrombosis and the effects of various therapeutic antibodies is required before further experimentation is attempted in humans.

CD11a/CD18 (Leukocyte Function–Associated Antigen-1) and the ICAM-1 Family

The cell surface protein CD11a/CD18 is a member of the β_2 integrin family. Expressed on neutrophils, macrophages, and lymphocytes, CD11a/CD18 binds to ICAM-1. CD11a/CD18 ligand binding activates T cells through costimulatory signals, enhances antigen-MHC recognition by the TCR via sealing the tight junction of the immune synapse, and facilitates T-cell extravasation into sites of inflammation (184–186). Although its importance as a T-cell costimulatory molecule may be modest compared with CD40L and B7–1/B7–2, inhibition of CD11a/CD18 binding may abrogate inflammatory processes by also impairing leukocyte chemotaxis. An MoAb against CD11a (efalizumab, humanized anti-CD11a-Ig) disrupts CD11a/CD18-ICAM-1 interaction. This agent significantly reduces PASI scores in patients with severe chronic plaque psoriasis (187,188). Phase II studies in PSA are underway. Although in preclinical studies efalizumab ameliorated murine CIA, a phase II trial observed no significant clinical improvement in RA patients treated with efalizumab (press release, *www.Xoma.com*). In NZB/W lupus-prone mice, anti-CD11a MoAb reduced anti-dsDNA antibody levels but had minimal effect on survival (189). In contrast, combination therapy with anti-CD11a and anti-ICAM-1 antibodies abrogated nephritis in a mouse model of graft-versus-host disease, which typically develops a lupuslike glomerulonephritis (190). Further preclinical investigation in SLE is needed, however, before efalizumab may be considered as part of combination biologic therapy.

The ICAM-1 family includes several members, so attempts to develop biologic inhibitors have had limited success. A murine anti-ICAM-1 MoAb (enlimomab, anti-ICAM-1 IgG2a) reduced disease activity in open-label studies in RA, but serum sickness reaction to murine Ig precluded further investigation of this agent (191–193). An antisense oligodeoxynucleotide to ICAM-1, which has been effective in Crohn's disease, has been studied in a double-blind, dose-finding study in active RA. Although the primary endpoint was not met, the drug was well tolerated, and further studies are anticipated (194).

Very Late Activation Antigen-4 (CD49d-CD26)

Very late activation antigen-4 (VLA-4; $\alpha_4\beta_1$ integrin) is expressed on leukocytes and binds both extracellular matrix proteins and cell surface adhesion molecules [vascular cell adhesion molecule (VCAM-1), ICAM-4, MadCAM01] (195). Like CD11a/CD18, VLA-4 plays an important role in recruiting lymphocytes and stabilizing the immune synapse. In addition, VLA-4 can function as a costimulatory molecule to activate T cells (196,197). Natalizumab, an anti-α_4 MoAb that blocks VLA-4 binding, reduces inflammatory plaque formation and clinical relapse in MS and reduces disease activity in Crohn's disease (198,199). In animal models of arthritis, antagonism of VLA-4 interaction with VCAM using soluble VCAM-1 anti–VCAM-1 and anti–VLAY antibodies abrogates synovitis, primarily through inhibition of VCAM-mediated chemotaxis of monocytes and T cells (200, 201). In the rat adjuvant arthritis model, monocytic chemotaxis to inflamed joints is mediated by α_4 integrin through a selectin-independent pathway (202). Thus, natalizumab has potential as a therapeutic agent for RA.

Leukocyte Function–Associated Antigen-3 and CD2

CD2 is a cell surface protein expressed on most T cells, although its expression is up-regulated on CD45RO$^+$ memory effector T cells. CD2 binding of its ligand, leukocyte function–associated antigen-3 (LFA-3; CD58), which is expressed on antigen-presenting cells, sends a costimulatory signal to activate T cells after antigen recognition by the TCR (203). CD2 signaling also up-regulates cytotoxic T cell activity (204). Alefacept, a soluble fusion protein composed of LFA-3 and human Fc Ig, engages CD2, preventing interaction with LFA-3 present on antigen-presenting cell surfaces. CD2 engagement by this fusion protein inhibits T-cell costimulation and induces apoptosis in memory effector (CD4$^+$ CD45RO$^+$ and CD8$^+$ CD45RO$^+$) T cells expressing CD2 (205). In chronic plaque psoriasis, alefacept significantly reduces PASI scores (206,207). The drug has been approved for use in psoriasis. A small open-label study of alefacept has been conducted in 11 subjects with active PsA (208). Six subjects (55%) met disease activity score (CRP-based) improvement criteria. In addition, synovial biopsies were performed before and after treatment in eight subjects. Alefacept responders had significantly greater reductions in CD4$^+$CD45RO$^+$ memory effector T cells in both serum and in the synovium and reduced CD68$^+$ macrophage numbers in the synovium. Similar reductions in memory effector T cells with sparing of CD45RA$^+$ naïve T cells, has been observed in clinical trials of chronic plaque psoriasis. The decrease in memory effector T cells appears to be a result of binding of the IgG1 portion of alefacept by Fcγ receptor III on natural killer cells, which mediate granzyme-induced apoptosis of the memory effector T cell.

CELL/CELL AND CELL/EXTRACELLULAR MATRIX INTERACTIONS

Cell/cell and cell/extracellular matrix (ECM) interactions are critical components of inflammatory and immune responses. Many proteins, including chemokines, chemokine receptors, integrins, and cell adhesion molecules, act in concert to mediate the effects of signaling from proinflammatory cytokines such as TNF-α and IL-1. Chemokines and their receptors are a large family of molecules integral to the development and maintenance of inflammation, particularly tissue trafficking of leukocytes. The integrins are a family of heterodimeric proteins responsible for cell/ECM interactions that support angiogenesis and mediate bone and cartilage destruction. Cell adhesion molecules (e.g., VCAM-1) mediate various inflammatory processes such as angiogenesis and leukocyte extravasation. All are potential targets for treatment of inflammatory diseases, including RA, PsA, MS, and inflammatory bowel disease. However, the clinical efficacy of biologic agents that target these molecules has been modest. Investigations suggest that redundancy in protein function and promiscuity of receptors will make it unlikely that blocking the function of a single protein or competitively binding a solitary receptor will be sufficient to significantly abrogate human disease.

Chemokines and Chemokine Receptors

Several groups have demonstrated that RA synovial fluid contains elevated levels of CC and CXC chemokines, and peripheral blood and synovial fluid cells express a variety of CCR chemokine receptors (reviewed in reference 209). The chemokines include both proinflammatory chemokines (multiple members of the CCL and CXCL families) and antiinflammatory chemokines such as the antiangiogenic factors CXCL9 and CXCL10. Various chemokine and chemokine receptor antagonists have been found to reduce synovitis in animal models of RA, but success in humans has been modest. Synovial biopsy studies have shown that increased synovial tissue IL-8 (CXCL-8) expression is associated with clinically-apparent synovitis (210). Unfortunately, placebo-controlled trials of a humanized anti-IL-8 (CXCL-8) MoAb did lead to significant improvement of RA or PsA disease activity, so further studies in these diseases have been abandoned (Abgenix website, *www.abgenix.com*). However, in a phase I study, an oral CCR1 antagonist significantly reduced synovial cellularity, T-cell infiltrate, and synovial macrophages, and trends toward clinical improvement were observed (211). A variety of chemokine antagonists and chemokine receptor blockers are in development for the treatment of RA, MS, psoriasis, and inflammatory bowel disease. The agents include MoAbs, truncated chemokines (functional receptor antagonists), soluble receptors, and chemokine toxins (reviewed in references 212 and 213). For example, Met-RANTES, a chemokine toxin consisting of the chemokine RANTES (regulated upon activation normal T cell expressed and secreted) and *Pseudomonas* toxin, which binds CCR5 and ablates cells expressing this receptor, has been shown to reduce synovitis in animal models (214,215).

$\alpha_v\beta$ Integrin

The integrins are a family of heterodimeric transmembrane proteins consisting of associated α and β subunits. Integrin-mediated cell/cell and cell/ECM interactions play important roles in angiogenesis and inflammation. The integrin $\alpha_v\beta_3$, has numerous ligands, including vitronectin, osteopontin, fibronectin, and fibrinogen, and interacts with multiple intracellular signaling molecules, such as paxillin and caspase 8 (reviewed in reference 216). It is highly expressed on the cell surfaces of differentiated osteoclasts and activated macrophages and endothelial cells. Given these characteristics, $\alpha_v\beta_3$ activity is likely an important mediator of inflammation, angiogenesis, and bone resorption in RA. Osteoclasts resorb bone in highly acidic resorption pits that are sealed off by a tight clear zone. $\alpha_v\beta_3$ expressed strongly at the clear zone mediates the attachment of the osteoclast to bone matrix, facilitating the development of resorption pits. Endothelial cells activated by TNF-α or growth factors express $\alpha_v\beta_3$, which mediates interaction between budding angiogenic sprouts and the surrounding ECM (217). The intense expression of $\alpha_v\beta_3$ in rheumatoid synovium suggests that the integrin may be important in the development of the tumorlike pannus that extends from inflammatory synovial tissue to erode into cartilage and periarticular bone (218,219). Various means of $\alpha_v\beta_1$ antagonism have been shown to reduce synovitis and inhibit periarticular bone destruction in animal models of RA (220,221). Vitaxin (Medi-522, Medimmune), an anti-$\alpha_v\beta_3$ MoAb, is presently in phase II trials for the treatment of RA. Vitaxin is unique because it targets a conformational epitope specifically formed by the association of α_v and β_3 integrins. By targeting a specific integrin association, the drug presumably avoids antagonizing the function of other integrins, thereby potentially reducing unwanted side effects.

CD44

CD44 is a polymorphic cell surface glycoprotein that exhibits a variety of cell-cell and cell-matrix functions, depending on differential splicing (reviewed in reference 222). CD44 and its principal ligand, hyaluronic acid, are highly expressed in the joints of patients with RA. CD44 appears to play an important role in endothelial adhesion of migrating inflammatory cells and in mediating destructive fibroblast/cartilage interactions. In murine CIA, neutralizing anti-CD44 antibodies that target conserved CD44 epitopes reduce synovial inflammation. Although CD44 is an attractive target for the treatment of human inflammatory arthritides, developing an agent that impairs only arthritogenic CD44 activity while avoiding antagonism of nonpathologic CD44 activities will be a difficult challenge.

Antagonizing Angiogenesis

Neovascularization entails a complex sequence of endothelial cell activation and proliferation, degradation and reformation of basement membrane, and proteolytic degradation of ECM. In RA, angiogenesis is driven by factors including fibroblast growth factor, vascular endothelial growth factor (VEGF), and transforming growth factor-β, all of which are strongly expressed in rheumatoid synovium (223). The necessary expression of growth factors, integrins, proteinases, and proliferative factors presents a multitude of potential targets to disrupt the process. As in many inflammatory actions, the efficacy of targeted therapy is limited by redundancy among various participating molecules. A number of small-molecule inhibitors of angiogenesis, including angiostatin, a fragment of fibrinogen, and endostatin, a collagen XVIII fragment, have been developed for the treatment of metastatic tumors. In experiments on the severe combined immunodeficient (SCID)-HuRAg murine model (human RA synovial tissue engrafted into SCID mice), endostatin has been shown to reduce synovial volume, inflammatory cell infiltrate, and number of vessels (224). VEGF, strongly expressed in RA synovium, where it is presumably induced by local tissue hypoxia and elevated TNF-α levels, appears to be an important mediator of angiogenesis in RA (223). A neutralizing soluble VEGF receptor 1:Fc chimeric protein (VEGFRI-Fc) has been shown to reduce endothelial proliferation in cultured human RA synovial tissue (225), and an anti-VEGF antibody abrogates murine CIA (226). In addition, small molecule inhibitors of VEGF receptor signaling tyrosine kinases and bevacizumab, a humanized anti-VEGF MoAb, which has shown efficacy in metastatic malignancy, are among the angiogenesis-blocking agents in development that may be candidates for RA therapy. Further study is necessary to determine the efficacy and safety of angiogenesis inhibitors in RA.

B CELLS

There has long been speculation regarding a primary role for humoral immunity and its effector cell, the B lymphocyte, in the pathogenesis of autoimmune disease. In disorders such as autoimmune thrombocytopenia and lupus nephritis, autoantibodies against platelets and dsDNA, respectively, promote platelet destruction and glomerular inflammation. However, conflicting evidence surrounding the pathogenicity of some autoantibodies, such as rheumatoid factor, and the inconsistent efficacy of antibody-reducing therapies, such as plasmapheresis, has directed research focus toward other inflammatory mononuclear cells, cytokines, and T cells as prime mediators of autoimmunity. Early reports of treating various autoimmune diseases with new biologic agents that selectively ablate B-cell subsets or reduce B-cell survival suggest efficacy in preclinical and clinical studies, fueling new interest in the role of the B cell in autoimmune pathophysiology.

Two biologic therapies that target B cells are currently under investigation for the treatment of a variety of autoimmune diseases: rituximab and anti–B lymphocyte stimulator (anti-BLyS) antibody. Rituximab (humanized anti-CD20 IgG1κ MoAb) depletes B cells expressing the CD20 cell surface antigen, which includes immature and mature naïve and memory B cells. Stable immunoglobulin levels are observed in humans treated with rituximab because plasma cells are spared. Rituximab ablates B cells through a combination of antibody- and complement-mediated cytotoxicity, in addition to activating apoptosis after cross-linking by FcR (227,228). B-lymphocyte stimulator (BLyS), also known as B-cell activating factor (BAFF), is a member of the TNF ligand superfamily. Expressed by monocytes, macrophages, and dendritic cells, BLyS exerts potent and necessary effects on B-cell maturation, differentiation, and survival (reviewed in reference 229). BLyS-deficient mice and transgenic mice overexpressing a BLyS-neutralizing TACI-Ig construct display marked reduction in mature B cell numbers, circulating immunoglobulin levels, and immunoglobulin responses to T cell–dependent and –independent antigens. BLyS binds to three receptors—BAFFR, TACI, and BCMA—although the BAFFR receptor appears most important for B-cell maturation effects of BLyS. In transgenic mice, BLyS overexpression results in polyclonal hypergammaglobulinemia and development of autoantibodies. Elevated serum BLyS levels are observed in human illness characterized by polyclonal hypergammaglobulinemia, including Sjögren's syndrome, SLE, RA, and human immunodeficiency virus infection (230–233). Although various means of inhibiting BLyS activity have been used to abrogate disease in experimental models of autoimmunity, a fully humanited anti-BLyS MoAb, antibody is currently being studied in phase I trials in SLE.

Rituximab (Anti-CD20)

Numerous case reports and small open-label trials suggest a role for rituximab in the treatment of various autoimmune disorders. In a study of rituximab treatment in refractory idiopathic thrombocytopenic purpura, over half of 25 subjects responded positively (234). In addition, case reports document improvement in refractory SLE-associated hemolytic anemia (235) and antineutrophil cytoplasmic antibody (c-ANCA)-positive Wegener's granulomatosis (236) after administration of rituximab. Preclinical studies with rituximab provide limited evidence for its use in autoimmune diseases such as RA. B cell–deficient mice are resistant to experimental autoimmune encephalitis, insulin-dependent diabetes (nonobese diabetic mice), and CIA (237,238). However, there are no active agents for animal models that are capable of mimicking the B-cell depletion induced in humans by rituximab, so extrapolation from animal models is based entirely on prevention of autoimmune disease in B cell–deficient mice. Nonetheless, formal investigation of rituximab for the treatment of RA and SLE has begun. Leandro and colleagues reported benefit in six subjects with refractory, active SLE treated with a 2-week regimen of rituximab (500 mg administered twice over 2 weeks) in combination with cyclophosphamide (750 mg twice) and high-dose steroids (239). C3 levels recovered in five patients with low values at entry, and improvement was observed in ESR, hemoglobin, and British Isles Assessment Group (BILAG) scores. Benefits appeared to be maintained for several months. In a phase I, dose escalation study of rituximab monotherapy in active, non-organ-threatening SLE, 16 subjects received increasing pulse doses of rituximab (240). No effect was observed in subjects at the low and mid-range doses, in which antichimeric antibodies developed. However, among 10 subjects who achieved good depletion of B-cell counts, a significant reduction from baseline was seen in Systemic Loupes Activity Measure (SLAM) score. Interestingly, anti-dsDNA levels declined in only one subject with prolonged B-cell depletion. Other investigators have observed similar outcome in an early-phase lupus study with rituximab (241). Phase II studies are now underway to examine the immunologic impact of rituximab and to determine the most effective dose.

Pilot studies of rituximab in various combinations with cyclophosphamide and glucocorticoids have suggested that such treatment can induce significant, long-lasting improvements in RA disease activity among refractory patients. Recurrence in some patients appears to coincide with recovery of B-cell counts and increasing rheumatoid factor titers (242). Edwards and colleagues reported impressive interim results of a phase II, placebo-controlled, randomized trial in subjects with methotrexate-refractory RA (243). In comparison with the placebo plus methotrexate group (33%), a significant percentage of subjects met ACR20 criteria in the three active treatment groups: rituximab alone (58%), rituximab plus methotrexate (84%), and rituximab plus cyclophosphamide (80%). Although the efficacy rate is striking, all subjects were treated with a tapering course of high-dose prednisone while receiving each of two 1,000-mg doses of rituximab two weeks apart. However, the intriguing reports of prolonged responses in the open-label studies bears careful long-term follow-up in this study.

B-Lymphocyte Stimulator

Various means of inhibiting BLyS activity in lupus-prone NZB/W mice and murine CIA have resulted in decreased autoantibody production and reduced tissue damage (244–246). Effective BLyS-inhibiting constructs have included TACI-Ig, BCMA-Ig, and BAFFR-Ig. In a phase I, dose-finding study in SLE, anti-BLyS MoAb (Lymphostat) or placebo was randomly given to 70 patients with SLE on standard therapies (press release, Human Genome Sciences, 2003). The agent was well tolerated, and significant reductions were observed in circulating $CD20^+$ B cells. BLyS may also be a useful target for the treatment of RA. Tan and colleagues found elevated levels of BLyS in the synovial fluid and BLyS expression on synovial monocytes in patients with RA, suggesting that local BLyS production might play a role in synovitis (247). Further studies in RA and other autoimmune diseases, including Sjögren syndrome, are under consideration.

Toleragens

Anti-dsDNA antibodies are specific markers for SLE and correlate with glomerulonephritis. In animal models, administration of anti-dsDNA antibodies can produce glomerular inflammation and proteinuria. Deposition of immune complexes of anti-dsDNA antibodies in the glomeruli leads to complement fixation and local tissue damage. LJP 394 was developed to treat lupus glomerulonephritis by reducing anti-dsDNA antibody levels and inducing tolerance in anti-dsDNA-producing B cells. The LJP 394 construct consists of four conjugated 20-mer dsDNA epitopes. In murine SLE-like disease, LJP 394 induces antigen-specific tolerance by cross-linking anti-dsDNA surface immunoglobulin, which initiates intracellular signaling cascades that ultimately lead to B-cell apoptosis or anergy (248). LJP 394 safely depletes anti-dsDNA antibody levels in humans by binding circulating anti-dsDNA into small, soluble complexes that do not appear to fix complement (249), although antibody levels returned after treatment was completed. In a phase III randomized, controlled trial in SLE patients with a history of previous SLE glomerulonephritis, but without active renal disease, intention-to-treat analysis found no difference between groups in the primary outcome, time to renal flare-up (250). However, in posthoc analysis of subjects with high-affinity anti-dsDNA antibodies for LJP 394, which made up 89% of the study population, a significant prolongation of time to renal flare-up and reduction in number of renal flare-ups were observed. Efficacy was also suggested in a small subset of subjects with baseline renal impairment (creatinine $\geq$1.5 mg/dL). However, intention-to-treat analysis of a subsequent phase III study that enrolled subjects with high-affinity antibodies failed to observe a significant difference in time to renal flare-up among 298 randomized subjects (press release, La Jolla Pharmaceuticals, *www.ljpc.com,* 2003). In this study, significant reductions in anti-dsDNA antibody titers and increases in C3 levels were seen. Further investigation is necessary to determine whether this agent will play a role in lupus management.

Another immunogen, LJP 1082, has been developed for treatment of antiphospholipid antibody syndrome. The epitopes represented on this immunogen consist of the first domain of β_2-glycoprotein-I, the target protein of many pathologic antiphospholipid antibodies. A phase I/II randomized, controlled trial in 20 subjects with antiphospholipid antibody syndrome observed a dose-dependent reduction in antibodies that bound the drug (press release, La Jolla Pharmaceuticals, *www.ljpc.com,* 2002). Further studies are underway to determine an appropriate dosing regimen and to evaluate efficacy in clinical parameters.

ACTIVATING APOPTOTIC PATHWAYS

Harnessing the body's own mechanism for eliminating autoreactive and otherwise abnormal cells has obvious appeal for the treatment of rheumatic diseases. Programmed cell death, termed apoptosis, represents a cascade of intracellular signaling and gene transcription that ultimately results in cell death characterized by inversion of the cell membrane. Apoptosis appears to be an efficient mechanism for the elimination of dying cells that limits the exposure of intracellular neoantigens to immune cells. The pathologic defect in the murine lupus model MRL lpr/lpr mouse is a defect in apoptosis that permits proliferation of autoreactive lymphocytes and the production of pathogenic autoantibodies. In human SLE, apoptosis appears normal, but defective clearance of apoptotic material may promote the activation of autoreactive lymphocytes (251–253). In RA, despite elevated expression of the apoptotic pathway receptor-ligand pair Fas/Fas ligand (FasL), fibroblast-like synoviocytes that form the invasive, tumorlike pannus appear resistant to apoptotic signaling (254). Given the relative deficit in apoptosis in RA and SLE, new biologic agents are being developed to target this pathway in order to enhance apoptosis in target cells. In preclinical studies, members of the TNF receptor family of proteins, including Fas and TRAIL receptors, have been shown to be potential targets for RA and SLE therapy. Several anti-Fas antibodies have been developed, although clinical utility has been limited by hepatotoxicity (255). One humanized anti-Fas MoAb has been shown to induce apoptosis in cultured cells transfected with FasL (256). Furthermore, this agent reduced inflammatory cell infiltrates and osteoclastogenesis in the SCID-huRAg model of RA (257). This anti-Fas MoAb initiates apoptosis only after cross-linking Fcγ receptor–positive cells. TRAIL is a TNF-like protein that stimulates activation-induced cell death in lymphocytes via signaling through any of several different receptors. Antibodies have been developed to the TRAIL receptors death receptor 4 and 5 with promising results evident in SLE animal models (Robert H. Carter, personal communication).

REDUCING INFLAMMATION-MEDIATED TISSUE DAMAGE AND END-ORGAN PATHOLOGY

Metalloproteinase Inhibitors

Destruction of the ECM characterizes both OA and inflammatory arthritis, such as RA and PsA. In the joint, ECM degradation is mediated by a family of zinc-containing endopeptidases called the MMPs. The MMPs are loosely grouped into gelatinases, stromelysins, and collagenases, based on their respective substrates. In health, MMPs are critical components of normal tissue remodeling, including wound healing, trophoblast implantation, and growth and development. In disease, MMP expression mediates spread of metastatic cancer and facilitates pathologic angiogenesis to support tumor growth. Excessive synovial and serum levels of MMPs are seen in RA and OA and appear to mediate both cartilage and bone damage (258). Natural MMP inhibitors include α_2-macroglobulin and the family of TIMPs; however, these enzymes appear to be underexpressed in RA and OA relative to high levels of MMPs (259–262). A host of MMP inhibitors have been developed for use in oncologic and rheumatic disease, including peptide and nonpeptide inhibitors, antisense constructs, and gene transfer of TIMPs (258,263–265). In animal models of both inflammatory arthritis and OA, MMP inhibitors have been shown to ameliorate joint destruction. Cevimastat (Trocade), a peptide inhibitor of three collagenases (MMP-1, MMP-8, and MMP-13) has been shown to be well tolerated in early phase studies in RA (266). However, radiographic disease progression was not halted in these RA patients, so drug development was discontinued in both RA and OA. Marimastat, another MMP inhibitor with a wide spectrum of activity, is in development for oncologic indications (267). Interestingly, its use has been associated with myalgia, stiffness, and occasionally an inflammatory arthritis.

Since MMP inhibitors will not affect the inflammatory component of RA, and may not have an immediate impact on pain and swelling in OA, proving efficacy with these agents will be difficult given the current available measures of disease activity. The most likely benefit of MMP inhibition, delay in progression or arrest of joint damage, may take years to detect in large-scale trials given the limited sensitivity of current imaging modalities. The future of MMP inhibitors will probably be a part of combination therapy in association with agents that can effectively reduce inflammation. In OA, it seems likely that timing of MMP inhibition will dictate the effectiveness of these agents. What remains to be determined is the optimal time to intervene with MMP inhibitors during the disease course of OA, although early treatment before extensive cartilage degradation occurs might permit natural cartilage repair mechanisms to reverse joint damage.

Inhibiting Nitric Oxide and Reactive Oxygen Intermediate Production

NO and reactive oxygen intermediates (ROI) are important mediators of inflammation through effects on gene transcription, direct cytotoxicity, and increased metalloproteinases expression. NO production is up-regulated in RA and OA joints by overexpression of inducible nitric oxide synthetase (iNOS) (268). NO is also involved in the tissue damage observed in SLE, Sjögren's syndrome, and vasculitis. NO is an important inducer of metalloproteinase expression, which appears to be a key mechanism of NO-induced joint damage in OA and RA. The ability to inhibit NO production has been considered an important mechanism of the purported antiinflammatory effects of tetracyclines in RA and OA. A variety of iNOS inhibitors have been developed for use in treatment of inflammatory disorders. These agents have included L-arginine derivatives that compete with arginine, a substrate for iNOS, at the active site, and metabolic inhibitors that act at either the active site or nearby residues. Preclinical models have not shown much success in ameliorating ongoing synovitis. A novel approach, to inhibit the homodimerization of iNOS, which is inactive as a monomer, includes the development of PPA250 (269). This agent has been shown to reduce NO production and ameliorate CIA arthritis in mice, even when administration was delayed until after the onset of arthritis.

NO is also a potent vasodilator that increases gastric blood flow and mucus formation, effects that counteract the deleterious impact of COX inhibition on the gut. As a result of these observations, a new class of NSAIDs is emerging: the COX-inhibiting NO donators. These agents are designed to deliver a COX inhibitor in addition to NO, with the goal of limiting COX-induced gastrointestinal toxicity. For one such COX-inhibiting NO donator, AZD3582, the primary metabolite of AZD3582 is naproxen. AZD3582 has recently completed phase II trials in the treatment of knee OA, which demonstrated beneficial effects on knee pain and good tolerability.

ROIs are generated in various forms of arthritis, including both OA and RA. In particular, the inflammatory process in RA contributes to superoxide anion production via direct release from osteoclasts, chondrocytes, neutrophils, activated macrophages, and synovial cells. Stimuli for ROI production include fragments of ECM, which activate synoviocytes and polymorphonuclear cells to release superoxide, and local ischemia-reperfusion cycles induced by tense effusions and mechanical use of the inflamed joint. Free radicals scavenge superoxide dismutase (SOD) enzymes under ordinary circumstances, a process that limits oxidative tissue damage. In RA, however, synovial tissue levels of SOD are depressed compared with normal tissue (270). Efforts to reduce ROI-mediated tissue damage have included the development of SOD products, including orgotein (bovine CuZnSOD) and SOD mimetics. In clinical trials in OA and RA, orgotein improved clinical measures of disease activity, including pain, swelling, stiffness, and function (271,272). Its wider use is limited by immune responses to its bovine extraction. A novel SOD mimetic, M40403, ameliorates CIA in a rat model of RA (273). This agent decreased bone and joint damage and histologic evidence of inflammation.

TARGETING COMPLEMENT

The wide-ranging inflammatory and immunomodulatory activities of the complement system play a variety of pathogenic roles in rheumatic disease, resulting in tissue damage in SLE, RA, and myositis. Complement activation is a critical component of both innate and acquired host defense. Therefore, biologic therapies designed to inhibit complement activity must be evaluated carefully for complications associated with impairment of opsonic and cytotoxic activities that protect the host from infection. Consequently, current therapies in development, such as the humanized anti-C5 MoAb (h5G1.1), target only a particular component of the complement cascade. In the case of h5G1.1, for example, only the formation of the membrane attack complex and production of C5a anaphylatoxin are impaired. H5G1.1 binds C5, preventing cleavage by C5 convertase. Preclinical studies have shown that inhibition of C5 activation by anti-C5 antibodies and C5a receptor antagonists reduces lupuslike disease in NZB/W lupus-prone mice (274), blocks antiphospholipid antibody–induced fetal loss in murine models (275), and limits synovitis in murine CIA (44,276, 277). Phase I/II human studies in RA, SLE, and dermatomyositis have been undertaken with h5G1.1 (278,279). Each study has shown good tolerability and suggested positive effects in reducing disease activity, particularly in terms of reducing inflammatory markers (press release, Alexion Pharmaceuticals, *www.alexionpharm.com*). However, further studies are necessary to quantify the magnitude of effect and to further assess toxicity. By inhibiting membrane attack complex formation, immune responses to *Neisseria* infection may be compromised; therefore, ongoing studies have carefully assessed disease risk for this organism. Alternative complement inhibitors soluble complement receptor type 1 (sCR1) and complement receptor 1–related gene protein y (Crry), which both target C3 convertase, have shown efficacy in animal models of inflammatory arthritis and antiphospholipid antibody syndrome (44,280–282), but are limited by high dosing requirements to achieve effect or less potency for inhibiting cytokine release than N5G1.1.

FC RECEPTORS

Fc receptors (FcRs) are expressed on many cells involved in inflammatory and immune responses, including macrophages, natural killer cells, and neutrophils. After binding to specific isotypes, FcR signaling promotes proinflammatory activities, including phagocytosis and antibody-dependent cell-mediated cytotoxicity (reviewed in reference 283). However, some FcRs function as regulatory molecules, such as the inhibitory FcγRIIb responsible for B-cell tolerance. Other FcRs regulate immune responses by influencing B-cell growth and immunoglobulin production. The critical role of FcγRs in mediating inflammation in SLE is evident in FcγR-deficient NZB/W mice, which are protected from developing glomerulonephritis (189). Furthermore, administration of soluble FcγRIII to NZB/W mice reduces anti-dsDNA antibody production and proteinuria and prolongs survival, possibly by competing with cell surface FcγRIII (284). The exact mechanism of action of soluble FcγRIII in this model is uncertain, but it has been speculated that immune complex deposition is altered, thereby reducing mesangial cell activation and production of inflammatory mediator ordinarily induced by large deposits of immune complexes. In contrast, transgenic mice overexpressing FcRγIIa develop rheumatoid-like erosive pannus and SLE-like glomerulonephritis (283). In RA, activated synovial macrophages express high levels of FcγRI (CD64), a high-affinity IgG1 receptor, in comparison with circulating macrophages (285). FcγRI is notable for its ability to efficiently endocytose bound antibodies. An immunotoxin created by conjugating anti-CD64 (FcγRI) to ricin A (CD64-RiA) is rapidly phagocytosed after binding to cell surface FcγRI, leading to rapid killing of RA synovial macrophages cultured with CD64-RiA. Treatment of RA synovial explants with CD64-RiA reduced TNF-α and IL-1 production and cartilage-degrading potential in the explants (285). Novel therapies targeting FcRs in SLE include TG19320, a synthetic molecule characterized by high-affinity binding to Fc immunoglobulin (286). Repeated treatment of the MRL lpr/lpr murine lupus model with TG19320 significantly prolonged survival, and delayed proteinuria. TG19320 presumably exerts beneficial effects by inhibiting IgG interaction with FcRs, which results in impaired immune complex deposition and smaller, more easily removable mesangial immune complexes. Given its tolerability in mice, molecules such as TG19320 are under consideration for treatment of human SLE.

TABLE 40.3. *Biologic agents no longer in development*

Biological target	Agent	Disease
T-cell depletion	Anti-CD7 MoAb	RA
	Anti-CD5 immunoconjugate	
	Anti-CD4	
	Primatised IgG, anti-CD4	
	Campath-1H	
T cells (nondepletion)	DAB486/389 IL-2	RA
	OKTcd4a MoAb	
	Primatised IgG1 anti-CD4 MoAb	
TNF-α	Lenercept (soluble p55TNF-R1-IgG1)	MS, RA
IL-4	Recombinant human IL-4	RA
IL-10	Recombinant human IL-10	RA, PSA
IL-11	Recombinant human IL-11	RA
Matrix metalloproteinases	Various MMP inhibitors: trocade, marimastat, batimistat, BAY 12–9566	RA, OA
E-selectin	Anti-E-selectin MoAb	Psoriasis
Chemokines	Anti-IL-8 MoAb	RA, psoriasis

IL, interleukin; MMP, matrix metalloproteinase; MoAb, monoclonal antibody; MS, multiple sclerosis; OA, osteoarthritis; PSA, psoriatic arthritis; RA, rheumatoid arthritis; TNF, tumor necrosis factor.

OSTEOCLAST DIFFERENTIATION

Bone destruction in RA is characterized radiographically by articular erosions. These erosions are formed primarily by differentiation and activation of bone-resorbing osteoclasts. Osteoclast progenitors are activated by the interaction of their receptor, RANK, with its ligand, RANKL. RANKL expression on T cells, osteoblasts, and fibroblasts is induced by TNF-α and IL-1. RANK/ RANKL interaction, in association with permissive levels of M-CSF, a necessary cofactor, induces osteoclast differentiation and activation. Uncontrolled osteoclast activation results in bone erosions, and probably periarticular osteopenia. A natural decoy receptor, osteoprotegerin (OPG), binds RANKL to prevent osteoclast activation; however, as with other antiinflammatory regulatory cytokines, synovial OPG levels are inadequate to control osteoclast differentiation and bone damage in patients with RA (287). A variety of osteoclast-targeted therapies, including OPG-Fc and bisphosphonates, have been shown to reduce or prevent bone erosions in animal models of arthritis, although significant improvements in synovial inflammation have not been observed. Treatment with OPG-Fc, a construct consisting of a truncated form of human OPG and IgG1 Fc, has been shown to reduce the number and size of bone erosions in the TNF-α-transgenic and CIA murine RA models and rats with adjuvant-induced arthritis (288–291). As an adjunct to antiinflammatory therapy, OPG may provide additional potency in preventing bone damage in RA (292).

CONCLUSION

The emergence of biologic therapies has had a striking positive impact on the treatment of rheumatic disease. However, currently-approved biologics are limited in terms of both efficacy and toxicity. Emerging therapies have also been limited by toxicity. Because many targets of biologics have important roles in normal tissue or immune homeostasis, the effects of blocking their activity can be unpredictable, if not detrimental. As a result, the clinical investigation of a number of treatments has been abandoned (Table 40.3). The use of biologic therapies has provided insight into various phenotypes among patients with the same disease classification. As research into novel biomarkers of disease activity and genetic investigation into disease etiology progress, reclassification of disease may permit more logical and informed use of targeted biologic therapy. For now, clinical investigation must proceed with caution, but agents that have or will be discarded due to failure to meet our present, unrefined standards of efficacy should not be forgotten. They may find a place in future therapeutic combinations. Advances in novel methods of targeted therapy, including antisense constructs, small molecule inhibitors, therapeutic vaccination, and gene therapy, may provide a more sophisticated approach to biologic therapy, thereby reducing toxicity and improving efficacy.

REFERENCES

1. Schiff M, Bulpitt K, Weaver A, et al. Safety of combination therapy with anakinra and etanercept in patients with rheumatoid arthritis. *Arthritis Rheum* 2001;44(suppl):79.
2. Bean A, Roach D, Briscoe H, et al. Structural deficiencies in granuloma formation in TNF gene-targeted mice underlie the heightened susceptibility to aerosol *Mycobacterium tuberculosis* infection, which is not compensated for by lymphotoxin. *J Immunol* 1999;162:3504–3511.
3. Ehlers S, Benini J, Kutsch S, et al. Fatal granuloma necrosis without exacerbated mycobacterial growth in tumor necrosis factor receptor p55 gene-deficient mice intravenously infected with *Mycobacterium avium. Infect Immun* 1999;67:3571–3579.
4. Kindler V, Sappino A, Grau G, et al. The inducing role of tumor necrosis factor in the development of bactericidal granulomas during BCG infection. *Cell* 1989;56:731–740.

5. Garcia I, Miyazaki Y, Marchal G, et al. High sensitivity of transgenic mice expressing soluble TNFR1 fusion protein to mycobacterial infections: synergistic action of TNF and IFN-gamma in the differentiation of protective granulomas. *Eur J Immunol* 1997;27:3182–3190.
6. Roach D, Bean A, Demangel C, et al. TNF regulates chemokine induction essential for cell recruitment, granuloma formation, and clearance of mycobacterial Infection. *J Immunol* 2002;168:4620–4627.
7. Senaldi G, Yin S, Shaklee C, et al. *Corynebacterium parvum*– and *Mycobacterium bovis* bacillus Calmette-Guerin–induced granuloma formation is inhibited in TNF receptor I (TNF-RI) knockout mice and by treatment with soluble TNF-RI. *J Immunol* 1996;157:5022–5026.
8. Maini R, St. Clair E, Breedveld F, et al. Infliximab versus placebo in rheumatoid arthritis patients receiving concomitant methotrexate: a randomised phase III trial. *Lancet* 1999;354:1932–1939.
9. Keane J, Gershon S, Wise RP, et al. Tuberculosis associated with infliximab, a tumor necrosis factor-α–neutralizing agent. *N Engl J Med* 2001;345:1098–1104.
10. Stone JH, Uhlfelder ML, Hellmann DB, et al. Etanercept combined with conventional treatment in Wegener's granulomatosis: a six-month open-label trial to evaluate safety. *Arthritis Rheum* 2001; 44:1149–1154.
11. The WGET Research Group. Design of the Wegener's Granulomatosis Etanercept Trial (WGET). *Controlled Clin Trials* 2002;23:450–468.
12. Booth AD, Jefferson HJ, Ayliffe W, et al. Safety and efficacy of TNFα blockade in relapsing vasculitis. *Ann Rheum Dis* 2002;61:559.
13. Cantini F, Niccoli L, Salvarani C, et al. Treatment of longstanding active giant cell arteritis with infliximab: report of four cases. *Arthritis Rheum* 2001;44:2933–2935.
14. Sfikakis PP. Behçet's disease: a new target for anti-tumour necrosis factor treatment. *Ann Rheum Dis* 2002;61:51–53.
15. Triolo G, Vadala M, Accardo-Palumbo A, et al. Anti-tumour necrosis factor monoclonal antibody treatment for ocular Behçet's disease. *Ann Rheum Dis* 2002;61:560–561.
16. Rozenbaum M, Rosner I, Portnoy E. Remission of Behçet's syndrome with TNFα blocking treatment. *Ann Rheum Dis* 2002;61:283–284.
17. Asherson RA, Pascoe L, Kraetsch HG, et al. Adult onset Still's disease: response to Enbrel. *Ann Rheum Dis* 2002;61:859–860.
18. Husni ME, Maier AL, Mease PJ, et al. Etanercept in the treatment of adult patients with Still's disease. *Arthritis Rheum* 2002;46:1171–1176.
19. Kraetsch HG, Antoni C, Kalden JR, et al. Successful treatment of a small cohort of patients with adult onset of Still's disease with infliximab: first experiences. *Ann Rheum Dis* 2001;60(suppl III):55–57.
20. Bush KA, Walker JS, Frazier J, et al. Effects of a PEGylated soluble TNF receptor type 1 (PEG sTNF-RI) on cytokine expression in adjuvant arthritis. *Scand J Rheumatol* 2002;31:198–204.
21. Choy EH, Hazleman B, Smith M, et al. Efficacy of a novel PEGylated humanized anti-TNF fragment (CDP870) in patients with rheumatoid arthritis: a phase II double-blinded, randomized, dose-escalating trial. *Rheumatology* 2002;41:1133–1137.
22. Rutgeerts P, Lemmens L, Van Assche G, et al. Treatment of active Crohn's disease with onercept (recombinant human soluble p55 tumour necrosis factor receptor): results of a randomized, open-label, pilot study. *Aliment Pharmacol Ther* 2003;17:185–192.
23. Black RA. Tumor necrosis factor-alpha converting enzyme. *Int J Biochem Cell Biol* 2002;34:1–5.
24. Ohta S, Harigai M, Tanaka M, et al. Tumor necrosis factor-alpha (TNF-alpha) converting enzyme contributes to production of TNF-alpha in synovial tissues from patients with rheumatoid arthritis. *J Rheum* 2001; 28:1756–1763.
25. Newton RC, Solomon KA, Covington MB, et al. Biology of TACE inhibition. *Ann Rheum Dis* 2001;60:25–32.
26. Beck G, Bottomley G, Bradshaw D, et al. (E)-2 (R)- (S)- (hydroxycarbamoyl)-4-phenyl-3-butenyl]-2′-isobutyl-2′- (methanesulfonyl)-4-methylvalerohydrazide (Ro 32–7315), a selective and orally active inhibitor of tumor necrosis factor-alpha convertase. *J Pharmacol Exp Ther* 2002;302:390–396.
27. Conway J, Andrews R, Beaudet B, et al. Inhibition of tumor necrosis factor-α (TNF-α) production and arthritis in the rat by GW3333, a dual inhibitor of TNF-α converting enzyme and matrix metalloproteinases. *J Pharmacol Exp Ther* 2001;298:900–908.
28. Doggrell S. TACE inhibition: a new approach to treating inflammation. *Exp Opin Invest Drugs* 2002;11:1003–1006.
29. Trifilieff A, Walker C, Keller T, et al. Pharmacological profile of PKF242–484 and PKF241–466, novel dual inhibitors of TNF-alpha converting enzyme and matrix metalloproteinases, in models of airway inflammation. *Br J Pharmacol* 2002;135:1655–1664.
30. Rabinowitz MH, Andrews RC, Becherer JD, et al. Design of selective and soluble inhibitors of tumor necrosis factor-alpha converting enzyme (TACE). *J Med Chem* 2001;44:4252–4567.
31. Dinarello CA. Interleukin-1 beta, interleukin-18, and the interleukin-1 beta converting enzyme. *Ann NY Acad Sci* 1998;856:1–11.
32. Greenfeder S, Nunes P, Kwee L, et al. Molecular cloning and characterization of a second subunit of the interleukin-1 receptor complex. *J Biol Chem* 1995;270:13757–13765.
33. Wesche H, Korherr C, Kracht M, et al. The interleukin-1 receptor accessory protein is essential for IL-1-induced activation of interleukin-1 receptor–associated kinase and stress-activated protein kinases. *J Biol Chem* 1998;272:7727–7731.
34. Cohen S, Hurd E, Cush J, et al. Treatment of rheumatoid arthritis with anakinra, a recombinant human interleukin-1 receptor antagonist, in combination with methotrexate: results of a twenty-four-week, multicenter, randomized, double-blind, placebo-controlled trial. *Arthritis Rheum* 2002;46:614–624.
35. Colotta F, Dower S, Sims J, et al. The type II decoy receptor: a novel regulatory pathway for interleukin 1. *Immunol Today* 1994;15:562–566.
36. van Den Berg W, Joosten L, Helsen M, et al. Amelioration of established murine collagen-induced arthritis with anti-IL-1 treatment. *Clin Exp Immunol* 1994;95:237–243.
37. Bresnihan B, Alvaro-Garcia J, Cobby M, et al. Treatment of rheumatoid arthritis with recombinant human interleukin-1 receptor antagonist. *Arthritis Rheum* 1998;41:2196–2204.
38. Economides A, Carpenter L, Rudge J, et al. Cytokine traps: multi-component, high-affinity blockers of cytokine action. *Nat Med* 2003; 9:47–52.
39. Gracie JA, Forsey RJ, Chan WL, et al. A proinflammatory role for IL-18 in rheumatoid arthritis. *J Clin Invest* 1999;104:1393–1401.
40. Bresnihan B, Roux-Lombard P, Murphy E, et al. Serum interleukin 18 and interleukin 18 binding protein in rheumatoid arthritis. *Ann Rheum Dis* 2002;61:726–729.
41. Joosten L, Radstake T, Lubberts E, et al. Association of interleukin-18 expression with enhanced levels of both interleukin-1β and tumor necrosis factor-α in knee synovial tissue of patients with rheumatoid arthritis. *Arthritis Rheum* 2003;48:339–347.
42. Oberholzer A, Harter L, Feilner A, et al. Differential effect of caspase inhibition on proinflammatory cytokine release in septic patients. *Shock* 2000;14:253–257.
43. Plater-Zyberk C, Joosten LA, Helsen MM, et al. Therapeutic effect of neutralizing endogenous IL-18 activity in the collagen-induced model of arthritis. *J Clin Invest* 2001;108:1825–1832.
44. Banda NK, Kraus D, Vondracek A, et al. Mechanisms of effects of complement inhibition in murine collagen-induced arthritis. *Arthritis Rheum* 2002;46:3065–3075.
45. Dinarello CA. Novel targets for interleukin 18 binding protein. *Ann Rheum Dis* 2001;60:18–24.
46. Wong P, Campbell I, Egan P, et al. The role of the interleukin-6 family of cytokines in inflammatory arthritis and bone turnover. *Arthritis Rheum* 2003;48:1177–1189.
47. Schindler R, Mancilla J, Endres S, et al. Correlations and interactions in the production of interleukin-6, IL-1, and tumor necrosis factor in human mononuclear cells. *Blood* 1980;75:40–47.
48. Dasgupta B, Corkill M, Kirkham B, et al. Serial estimation of interleukin-6 as a measure of systemic disease in rheumatoid arthritis. *J Rheumatol* 1992;19:22–25.
49. Kotake S, Sato K, Kim T, et al. Interleukin-6 and soluble interleukin-6 receptors in the synovial fluids from rheumatoid arthritis patients are responsible for osteoclast-like cell formation. *J Bone Miner Res* 1996;11:88–95.
50. Brandt J, Haibel H, Cornely D, et al. Successful treatment of active ankylosing spondylitis with the anti-tumor necrosis factor alpha monoclonal antibody infliximab. *Arthritis Rheum* 2000;43:1346–1352.
51. Wendling D, Racadot E, Wijdenes J. Treatment of severe rheumatoid arthritis by anti-interleukin-6 monoclonal antibody. *J Rheumatol* 1993;20:259–262.
52. Choy EH, Isenberg DA, Garrood T, et al. Therapeutic benefit of blocking interleukin-6 activity with an anti-interleukin-6 receptor monoclonal antibody in rheumatoid arthritis: a randomized, double-blind, placebo-controlled, dose-escalation trial. *Arthritis Rheum* 2002;46:3143–3150.

53. Iwamoto M, Nara H, Hirata D, et al. Humanized monoclonal anti-interleukin-6 receptor antibody for treatment of intractable adult-onset Still's disease. *Arthritis Rheum* 2002;46:3388–3389.
54. Yokota S, Miyamae T, Imigawa T, et al. Long-term therapeutic efficacy of humanized anti-IL-6-receptor antibody for systemic juvenile idiopathic arthritis. *Arthritis Rheum* 2002;46(suppl 9):479.
55. Brink I, Thiele B, Burmester GR, et al. Effects of anti-CD4 antibodies on the release of IL-6 and TNF-alpha in whole blood samples from patients with systemic lupus erythematosus. *Lupus* 1999; 8:723–730.
56. Kiberd BA. Interleukin-6 receptor blockage ameliorates murine lupus nephritis. *J Am Soc Nephrol* 1993;4:58–61.
57. Finck B, Chan B, Wofsy D. Interleukin 6 promotes murine lupus in NZB/NZW F1 mice. *J Clin Invest* 1994;94:585–591.
58. Trepecchio W, Wang L, Bozza M, et al. IL-11 regulates macrophage effector function through inhibition of nuclear factor-κB. *J Immunol* 1997;159:5661–5670.
59. Walmsely M, Butler D, Marinova-Mutafchieva L, et al. An anti-inflammatory role for interleukin-11 in established murine collagen-induced arthritis. *Immunology* 1998;95:31–37.
60. Sands B, Bank S, Sninsky C, et al. Safety and activity evaluation of rh-IL-11 in subjects with active Crohn's disease. *Gastroenterology* 1999;117:59–64.
61. Moreland LW, Gugliotti R, King K, et al. Results of a phase-I/II randomized, masked, placebo-controlled trial of recombinant human interleukin-11 in the treatment of subjects with active rheumatoid arthritis. *Arthritis Res* 2001;3:247–252.
62. Chabaud M, Durand JM, Buchs N, et al. Human interleukin-17: a T cell-derived proinflammatory cytokine produced by the rheumatoid synovium. *Arthritis Rheum* 1999;42:963–970.
63. Kotake S, Udagawa N, Takahashi N, et al. IL-17 in synovial fluids from patients with rheumatoid arthritis is a potent stimulator of osteoclastogenesis. *J Clin Invest* 1999;103:1345–1352.
64. Kehlen A, Thiele K, Riemann D, et al. Expression, modulation and signaling of IL-17 receptor in fibroblast-like synoviocytes of patients with rheumatoid arthritis. *Clin Exp Immunol* 2002;127:539–546.
65. Jovanovic DV, Martel-Pelletier J, Di Battista JA, et al. Stimulation of 92-kd gelatinase (matrix metalloproteinase 9) production by interleukin-17 in human monocyte/macrophages: a possible role in rheumatoid arthritis. *Arthritis Rheum* 2000;43:1134–1144.
66. Cai L, Yin JP, Starovasnik MA, et al. Pathways by which interleukin 17 induces articular cartilage breakdown *in vitro* and *in vivo*. *Cytokine* 2001;16:10–21.
67. Pacquelet S, Presle N, Boileau C, et al. Interleukin 17, a nitric oxide–producing cytokine with a peroxynitrite-independent inhibitory effect on proteoglycan synthesis. *J Rheumatol* 2002;29:2602–2610.
68. Lubberts E, van den Bersselaar L, Oppers-Walgreen B, et al. IL-17 promotes bone erosion in murine collagen-induced arthritis through loss of the receptor activator of NF-kappa B ligand/osteoprotegerin balance. *J Immunol* 2003;170:2655–2662.
69. Lubberts E, Joosten LA, Oppers B, et al. IL-1-independent role of IL-17 in synovial inflammation and joint destruction during collagen-induced arthritis. *J Immunol* 2001;167:1004–1013.
70. Chabaud M, Miossec P. The combination of tumor necrosis factor alpha blockade with interleukin-1 and interleukin-17 blockade is more effective for controlling synovial inflammation and bone resorption in an *ex vivo* model. *Arthritis Rheum* 2001;44:1293–1303.
71. Miossec P. Interleukin-17 in rheumatoid arthritis: if T cells were to contribute to inflammation and destruction through synergy. *Arthritis Rheum* 2003;48:594–601.
72. Sakkas LI, Johanson NA, Scanzello CR, et al. Interleukin-12 is expressed by infiltrating macrophages and synovial lining cells in rheumatoid arthritis and osteoarthritis. *Cell Immunol* 1998;188:105–110.
73. Morita Y, Yamamura M, Nishida K, et al. Expression of interleukin-12 in synovial tissue from patients with rheumatoid arthritis. *Arthritis Rheum* 1998;41:306–314.
74. Harada S, Yamamura M, Okamoto H, et al. Production of interleukin-7 and interleukin-15 by fibroblast-like synoviocytes from patients with rheumatoid arthritis. *Arthritis Rheum* 1999;42:1508–1516.
75. Hasko G, Szabo C. IL-12 as a therapeutic target for pharmacological modulation in immune-mediated and inflammatory diseases: regulation of T helper 1/T helper 2 responses. *Br J Pharmacol* 1999;127: 1295–1304.
76. Malfait A, Williams R, Malik A, et al. Chronic relapsing homologous collagen-induced arthritis in DBA/1 mice as a model for testing disease-modifying and remission-inducing therapies. *Arthritis Rheum* 2001;44:1215–1224.
77. Malfait AM, Butler DM, Presky DH, et al. Blockade of IL-12 during the induction of collagen-induced arthritis (CIA) markedly attenuates the severity of the arthritis. *Clin Exp Immunol* 1998;111:377–383.
78. Butler DM, Malfait AM, Maini RN, et al. Anti-IL-12 and anti-TNF antibodies synergistically suppress the progression of murine collagen-induced arthritis. *Eur J Immunol* 1999;29:2205–2212.
79. Lamprecht P, Kumanovics G, Mueller A, et al. Elevated monocytic IL-12 and TNF-alpha production in Wegener's granulomatosis is normalized by cyclophosphamide and corticosteroid therapy. *Clin Exp Immunol* 2002;128:181–186.
80. Ichikawa M, Koh CS, Inoue A, et al. Anti-IL-12 antibody prevents the development and progression of multiple sclerosis–like relapsing-remitting demyelinating disease in NOD mice induced with myelin oligodendrocyte glycoprotein peptide. *J Neuroimmunol* 2000;102: 56–66.
81. Brok HP, van Meurs M, Blezer E, et al. Prevention of experimental autoimmune encephalomyelitis in common marmosets using an anti-IL-12p40 monoclonal antibody. *J Immunol* 2002;169:6554–6563.
82. McInnes I, Mughales J, Field M, et al. The role of interleukin-15 in T cell migration and activation in rheumatoid arthritis. *Nat Med* 1996;2:175–182.
83. McInnes I, Leung B, Sturrock R, et al. Interleukin-15 mediates T cell-dependent regulation of tumor necrosis factor-a production in rheumatoid arthritis. *Nat Med* 1997;3:189–195.
84. Ogata Y, Kukita A, Kukita T, et al. A novel role of IL-15 in the development of osteoclasts: inability to replace its activity with IL-2. *J Immunol* 1999;162:2754–2760.
85. Aringer M, Stummvoll GH, Steiner G, et al. Serum interleukin-15 is elevated in systemic lupus erythematosus. *Rheumatology* 2001;40: 876–881.
86. Sugiura T, Harigai M, Kawaguchi Y, et al. Increased IL-15 production of muscle cells in polymyositis and dermatomyositis. *Int Immunol* 2002;14:917–924.
87. Ruchatz H, Leung BP, Wei XQ, et al. Soluble IL-15 receptor alpha-chain administration prevents murine collagen-induced arthritis: a role for IL-15 in development of antigen-induced immunopathology. *J Immunol* 1998;160:5654–5660.
88. Ferrari-Lacraz S, Neuberg M, Donskoy E, et al. A novel antagonist IL-15/Fc protein (CRB-15) shows therapeutic efficacy in an animal model of rheumatoid arthritis. *Arthritis Rheum* 2002;46(suppl 9):499.
89. Appasamy P. Biological and clinical implications of interleukin-7 and lymphopoiesis. *Cytokines Cell Mol Ther* 1999;5:25–39.
90. van Roon JA, Glaudemans KA, Bijlsma JW, et al. Interleukin 7 stimulates tumour necrosis factor alpha and Th1 cytokine production in joints of patients with rheumatoid arthritis. *Ann Rheum Dis* 2003;62: 113–119.
91. van Roon JAG, Glaudemans KAFM, Bijlsma JWJ, et al. Interleukin 7 stimulates tumour necrosis factor α and Th1 cytokine production in joints of patients with rheumatoid arthritis. *Ann Rheum Dis* 2003;62: 113–119.
92. Morand EF, Bucala R, Leech M. Macrophage migration inhibitory factor: an emerging therapeutic target in rheumatoid arthritis. *Arthritis Rheum* 2003;48:291–299.
93. Roger T, David J, Glauser M, et al. MIG regulates innate immune responses through modulation of toll-like receptor-4. *Nature* 2001;414: 920–924.
94. Bacher M, Metz C, Calandra T, et al. An essential regulatory role for macrophage migration inhibitory factor in T-cell activation. *Proc Natl Acad Sci U S A* 1996;93:7849–7854.
95. Delgado M, Abad C, Martinez C, et al. Vasoactive intestinal peptide in the immune system: potential therapeutic role in inflammatory and autoimmune diseases. *J Mol Med* 2002;80:16–24.
96. Delgado M, Abad C, Martinez C, et al. Vasoactive intestinal peptide prevents experimental arthritis by downregulating both autoimmune and inflammatory components of the disease. *Nat Med* 2001;7:563–568.
97. Firestein GS. VIP: a very important protein in arthritis. *Nat Med* 2001; 7:537–538.
98. Asadullah K, Sterry W, Stephanek K, et al. IL-10 is a key cytokine in psoriasis. Proof of principle by IL-10 therapy: a new therapeutic approach. *J Clin Invest* 1998;101:783–794.

99. Asadullah K, Docke WD, Ebeling M, et al. Interleukin 10 treatment of psoriasis: clinical results of a phase 2 trial. *Arch Dermatol* 1999; 135:187–192.
100. Asadullah K, Docke WD, Sabat RV, et al. The treatment of psoriasis with IL-10: rationale and review of the first clinical trials. *Exp Opin Invest Drugs* 2000;9:95–102.
101. McInnes IB, Illei GG, Danning CL, et al. IL-10 improves skin disease and modulates endothelial activation and leukocyte effector function in patients with psoriatic arthritis. *J Immunol* 2001;167: 4075–4082.
102. Moreland LW. Potential biologic agents for treating rheumatoid arthritis. *Rheum Dis Clin North Am* 2001;27:445–491.
103. Ghoreschi K, Thomas P, Breit S, et al. Interleukin-4 therapy of psoriasis induces Th2 responses and improves human autoimmune disease. *Nat Med* 2003;9:40–46.
104. Isomaki P, Luukkainen R, Toivanen P, et al. The presence of interleukin-13 in rheumatoid synovium and its antiinflammatory effects on synovial fluid macrophages from patients with rheumatoid arthritis. *Arthritis Rheum* 1996;39:1693–1702.
105. Woods JM, Haines GK, Shah MR, et al. Low-level production of interleukin-13 in synovial fluid and tissue from patients with arthritis. *Clin Immunol Immunopathol* 1997;85:210–220.
106. Woods JM, Amin MA, Katschke KJ Jr, et al. Interleukin-13 gene therapy reduces inflammation, vascularization, and bony destruction in rat adjuvant-induced arthritis. *Hum Gene Ther* 2002;13:381–393.
107. Houssiau F, Lefebvre C, Vanden Berge M, et al. Serum interleukin-10 titres in systemic lupus erythematosus reflect disease activity. *Lupus* 1995;4:393–395.
108. Park Y, Lee S, Kim D, et al. Elevated interleukin-10 levels correlated with disease activity in systemic lupus erythematosus. *Clin Exp Rheumatol* 1998;16:283–288.
109. Hagiwara E, Gourley M, Lee S, et al. Disease severity in patients with systemic lupus erythematosus correlates with an increased ratio of interleukin-10: interferon-γ-secreting cells in the peripheral blood. *Arthritis Rheum* 1996;39:379–385.
110. Ishida H, Muchamuel T, Sakaguchi S, et al. Continuous administration of anti-interleukin-10 antibodies delays the onset of autoimmunity in NZB/W F1 mice. *J Exp Med* 1994;179:305–310.
111. Llorente L, Richaud-Patin Y, Garcia-Padilla C, et al. Clinical and biologic effects of anti-interleukin-10 monoclonal antibody administration in systemic lupus erythematosus. *Arthritis Rheum* 2000;43: 1790–800.
112. Protein Design Labs Website. Protein design labs presents phase I/II clinical results with SMART anti-gamma interferon antibody in Crohn's disease. 2002.
113. Vassilopoulos D, Calabrese LH. Hepatitis C virus infection and vasculitis: implications of antiviral and immunosuppressive therapies. *Arthritis Rheum* 2002;46:585–597.
114. Zouboulis CC, Orfanos CE. Treatment of Adamantiades-Behçet disease with systemic interferon alpha. *Arch Dermatol* 1998;134:1010–1016.
115. Alpsoy E, Durusoy C, Yilmaz E, et al. Interferon alfa-2a in the treatment of Behçet disease: a randomized placebo-controlled and double-blind study. *Arch Dermatol* 2002;138:467–471.
116. Triantaphyllopoulos KA, Williams RO, Tailor H, et al. Amelioration of collagen-induced arthritis and suppression of interferon-gamma, interleukin-12, and tumor necrosis factor alpha production by interferon-beta gene therapy. *Arthritis Rheum* 1999;42:90–99.
117. Takayanagi H, Kim S, Matsuo K, et al. NRANKL maintains bone homeostasis through c-Fos-dependent induction of interferon-beta. *Nature* 2002;416:744–749.
118. van Holten J, Plater-Zyberk C, Tak PP. Interferon-β for treatment of rheumatoid arthritis? *Arthritis Res* 2002;4:346–352.
119. The Muscle Study G. Randomized pilot trial of betaINF1a (Avonex) in patients with inclusion body myositis. *Neurology* 2001;57:1566–1570.
120. Dressel A, Beuche W. Interferon beta-1a treatment of corticosteroid sensitive polymyositis. *J Neurol Neurosurg Psychiatry* 2002;72:676.
121. Moroz C, Traub L, Maymon R, et al. PLIF: a novel human ferritin subunit from placenta with immunosuppressive activity. *J Biol Chem* 2002;277:12901–12905.
122. Weinberger A, Halpern M, Zahalka MA, et al. Placental immunomodulator ferritin, a novel immunoregulator, suppresses experimental arthritis. *Arthritis Rheum* 2003;48:846–853.
123. Han Z, Boyle DL, Manning AM, et al. AP-1 and NF-kappaB regulation in rheumatoid arthritis and murine collagen-induced arthritis. *Autoimmunity* 1998;28:197–208.
124. Tak PP, Firestein GS. NF-kappaB: a key role in inflammatory diseases. *J Clin Invest* 2001;107:7–11.
125. Tak PP, Gerlag DM, Aupperle KR, et al. Inhibitor of nuclear factor kappaB kinase beta is a key regulator of synovial inflammation. *Arthritis Rheum* 2001;44:1897–1907.
126. Auphan N, DiDonato JA, Rosette C, et al. Immunosuppression by glucocorticoids: inhibition of NF-kappa B activity through induction of I kappa B synthesis. *Science* 1995;270:286–290.
127. Scheinman RI, Cogswell PC, Lofquist AK, et al. Role of transcriptional activation of I kappa B alpha in mediation of immunosuppression by glucocorticoids. *Science* 1995;270:283–286.
128. Herlaar E, Brown Z. p38 MAPK signaling cascades in inflammatory disease. *Mol Med Today* 1999;5:439–447.
129. Johnson GL, Lapadat R. Mitogen-activated protein kinase pathways mediated by ERK, JNK, and p38 protein kinases. *Science* 2002;298: 1911–1912.
130. Schett G, Tohidast-Akrad M, Smolen JS, et al. Activation, differential localization, and regulation of the stress-activated protein kinases, extracellular signal-regulated kinase, c-JUN N-terminal kinase, and p38 mitogen-activated protein kinase, in synovial tissue and cells in rheumatoid arthritis. *Arthritis Rheum* 2000;43:2501–2512.
131. Vincenti MP, Brinckerhoff CE. The potential of signal transduction inhibitors for the treatment of arthritis: is it all just JNK? *J Clin Invest* 2001;108:181–183.
132. Vincenti MP, Brinckerhoff CE. Transcriptional regulation of collagenase (MMP-1, MMP-13) genes in arthritis: integration of complex signaling pathways for the recruitment of gene-specific transcription factors. *Arthritis Res* 2002;4:157–164.
133. Han Z, Boyle DL, Chang L, et al. c-Jun N-terminal kinase is required for metalloproteinase expression and joint destruction in inflammatory arthritis. *J Clin Invest* 2001;108:73–81.
134. Badger AM, Cook MN, Lark MW, et al. SB 203580 inhibits p38 mitogen-activated protein kinase, nitric oxide production, and inducible nitric oxide synthase in bovine cartilage-derived chondrocytes. *J Immunol* 1998;161:467–473.
135. Jackson JR, Bolognese B, Hillegass L, et al. Pharmacological effects of SB 220025, a selective inhibitor of P38 mitogen-activated protein kinase, in angiogenesis and chronic inflammatory disease models. *J Pharmacol Exp Ther* 1998;284:687–692.
136. Kumar S, Votta BJ, Rieman DJ, et al. IL-1- and TNF-induced bone resorption is mediated by p38 mitogen activated protein kinase. *J Cell Physiol* 2001;187:294–303.
137. Haddad JJ. VX-745. Vertex Pharmaceuticals. *Curr Opin Invest Drugs* 2001;2:1070–1076.
138. Weisman M, Furst DE, Schiff M, et al. A double-blind, placebo-controlled trial of VX-745, an oral p38 mitogen activated protein kinase inhibitor, in patients with rheumatoid arthritis. Presented at the European League Against Rheumatism (EULAR) Meeting, 2002.
139. Aupperle K, Bennett B, Han Z, et al. NF-kappa B regulation by I kappa B kinase-2 in rheumatoid arthritis synoviocytes. *J Immunol* 2001;166:2705–2711.
140. Oettinger C, D'Souza M. Cell targeting by microencapsulated drug delivery, an improved method for cytokine inhibition. Presented at the Interscience Conference on Antimicrobrial Agents and Chemotherapy, 2002:B-956.
141. Aikawa Y, Yamamoto M, Yamamoto T, et al. An anti-rheumatic agent T-614 inhibits NF-kappaB activation in LPS- and TNF-alpha-stimulated THP-1 cells without interfering with IkappaBalpha degradation. *Inflamm Res* 2002;51:188–194.
142. Rioja I, Terencio MC, Ubeda A, et al. A new ditriazine inhibitor of NF-kappaB modulates chronic inflammation and angiogenesis. *Naunyn Schmiedebergs Arch Pharmacol* 2002;365:357–364.
143. Fitzpatrick LR, Wang J, Le T. Caffeic acid phenethyl ester, an inhibitor of nuclear factor-kappaB, attenuates bacterial peptidoglycan polysaccharide-induced colitis in rats. *J Pharmacol Exp Ther* 2001; 299:915–920.
144. Umezawa K, Ariga A, Matsumoto N. Naturally occurring and synthetic inhibitors of NF-kappaB functions. *Anticancer Drug Design* 2000;15:239–244.

145. Jeon KI, Jeong JY, Jue DM. Thiol-reactive metal compounds inhibit NF-kappa B activation by blocking I kappa B kinase. *J Immunol* 2000;164:5981–5989.
146. Anrather J, Csizmadia V, Brostjan C, et al. Inhibition of bovine endothelial cell activation *in vitro* by regulated expression of a transdominant inhibitor of NF-kappa B. *J Clin Invest* 1997;99:763–772.
147. Kisseleva T, Bhattacharya S, Braunstein J, et al. Signaling through the JAK/STAT pathway, recent advances and future challenges. *Gene* 2002;285:1–24.
148. Egan PJ, Lawlor KE, Alexander WS, et al. Suppressor of cytokine signaling-1 regulates acute inflammatory arthritis and T cell activation. *J Clin Invest* 2003;111:915–924.
149. Shouda T, Yoshida T, Hanada T, et al. Induction of the cytokine signal regulator SOCS3/CIS3 as a therapeutic strategy for treating inflammatory arthritis. *J Clin Invest* 2001;108:1781–1788.
150. Looney RJ, Boyd A, Totterman S, et al. Volumetric computerized tomography as a measurement of periprosthetic acetabular osteolysis and its correlation with wear. *Arthritis Res* 2002;4:59–63.
151. Katzav A, Kloog Y, Korczyn AD, et al. Treatment of MRL/lpr mice, a genetic autoimmune model, with the Ras inhibitor, farnesylthiosalicylate (FTS). *Clin Exp Immunol* 2001;126:570–577.
152. Gottlieb AB, Lebwohl M, Shirin S, et al. Anti-CD4 monoclonal antibody treatment of moderate to severe psoriasis vulgaris: results of a pilot, multicenter, multiple-dose, placebo-controlled study. *J Am Acad Dermatol* 2000;43:595–604.
153. Harper JM, Cook A. Beneficial effects of non-depleting anti-CD4 in MRL/Mp-lpr/lpr mice with active systemic lupus erythematosus and microscopic angiitis. *Autoimmunity* 2001;33:245–251.
154. Martin A, Gutierrez E, Muglia J, et al. A multicenter dose-escalation trial with denileukin diftitox (ONTAK, DAB (389)IL-2) in patients with severe psoriasis. *J Am Acad Dermatol* 2001;45:871–881.
155. Moreland LW, Sewell KL, Trentham DE, et al. Interleukin-2 diphtheria fusion protein (DAB486IL-2) in refractory rheumatoid arthritis. A double-blind, placebo-controlled trial with open-label extension. *Arthritis Rheum* 1995;38:1177–1186.
156. Brok HP, Tekoppele JM, Hakimi J, et al. Prophylactic and therapeutic effects of a humanized monoclonal antibody against the IL-2 receptor (DACLIZUMAB) on collagen-induced arthritis (CIA) in rhesus monkeys. *Clin Exp Immunol* 2001;124:134–141.
157. Bell HK, Parslew RA. Use of basiliximab as a cyclosporin-sparing agent in palmoplantar pustular psoriasis with myalgia as an adverse effect. *Br J Dermatol* 2002;147:606–607.
158. Owen CM, Harrison PV. Successful treatment of severe psoriasis with basiliximab, an interleukin-2 receptor monoclonal antibody. *Clin Exp Dermatol* 2000;25:195–197.
159. Salim A, Emerson RM, Dalziel KL. Successful treatment of severe generalized pustular psoriasis with basiliximab (interleukin-2 receptor blocker). *Br J Dermatol* 2000;143:1121–1122.
160. Hahn BH, Singh RR, Wong WK, et al. Treatment with a consensus peptide based on amino acid sequences in autoantibodies prevents T cell activation by autoantigens and delays disease onset in murine lupus. *Arthritis Rheum* 2001;44:432–441.
161. Dalum I, Butler DM, Jensen MR, et al. Therapeutic antibodies elicited by immunization against TNF-alpha. *Nat Biotechnol* 1999;17:666–669.
162. Weiner HL, Friedman A, Miller A, et al. Oral tolerance: immunologic mechanisms and treatment of animal and human organ-specific autoimmune diseases by oral administration of autoantigens. *Ann Rev Immunol* 1994;12:809–837.
163. McKown KM, Carbone LD, Bustillo J, et al. Induction of immune tolerance to human type I collagen in patients with systemic sclerosis by oral administration of bovine type I collagen. *Arthritis Rheum* 2000;43:1054–1061.
164. Gottlieb AB, Lebwohl M, Totoritis MC, et al. Clinical and histologic response to single-dose treatment of moderate to severe psoriasis with an anti-CD80 monoclonal antibody. *J Am Acad Dermatol* 2002;47:692–700.
165. Schopf RE. IDEC-114 (IDEC). *Curr Opin Invest Drugs* 2001;2:635–638.
166. Kirk AD, Tadaki DK, Celniker A, et al. Induction therapy with monoclonal antibodies specific for CD80 and CD86 delays the onset of acute renal allograft rejection in non-human primates. *Transplantation* 2001;72:377–384.
167. Kremer JR, Westhovens R, Leon R, et al. Treatment of rheumatoid arthritis by selective inhibition of T-cell activation with fusion protein CILA4Ig. *N Engl J Med* 2003;349:1907–1915.
168. Weinblatt M, Schiff M, Goldman M, et al. A pilot, multi-center, randomized, double-blind, placebo-controlled study of a co-stimulation blocker CTLA4-Ig (2 mg/kg) given monthly in combination with etanercept in active rheumatoid arthritis. *Arthritis Rheum* 2002;46 (suppl 9):204.
169. Mihara M, Tan I, Chuzhin Y, et al. CTLA4Ig inhibits T cell-dependent B-cell maturation in murine systemic lupus erythematosus. *J Clin Invest* 2000;106:91–101.
170. Finck BK, Linsley PS, Wofsy D. Treatment of murine lupus with CTLA4Ig. *Science* 1994;265:1225–1227.
171. Kitching AR, Huang XR, Ruth AJ, et al. Effects of CTLA4-Fc on glomerular injury in humorally-mediated glomerulonephritis in BALB/c mice. *Clin Exp Immunol* 2002;128:429–435.
172. Wang X, Huang W, Mihara M, et al. Mechanism of action of combined short-term CTLA4Ig and anti-CD40 ligand in murine systemic lupus erythematosus. *J Immunol* 2002;168:2046–2053.
173. Abrams JR, Lebwohl MG, Guzzo CA, et al. CTLA4Ig-mediated blockade of T-cell costimulation in patients with psoriasis vulgaris. *J Clin Invest* 1999;103:1243–1252.
174. Abrams JR, Kelley SL, Hayes E, et al. Blockade of T lymphocyte costimulation with cytotoxic T lymphocyte-associated antigen 4-immunoglobulin (CTLA4Ig) reverses the cellular pathology of psoriatic plaques, including the activation of keratinocytes, dendritic cells, and endothelial cells. *J Exp Med* 2000;192:681–694.
175. Clark LB, Foy TM, Noelle RJ. CD40 and its ligand. *Adv Immunol* 1996;63:43–78.
176. Durie FH, Fava RA, Foy TM, et al. Prevention of collagen-induced arthritis with an antibody to gp39, the ligand for CD40. *Science* 1993;261:1328–1330.
177. Foy TM, Durie FH, Noelle RJ. The expansive role of CD40 and its ligand, gp39, in immunity. *Semin Immunol* 1994;6:259–266.
178. Durie FH, Foy TM, Masters SR, et al. The role of CD40 in the regulation of humoral and cell-mediated immunity. *Immunol Today* 1994;15:406–411.
179. Mohan C, Shi Y, Laman JD, et al. Interaction between CD40 and its ligand gp39 in the development of murine lupus nephritis. *J Immunol* 1995;154:1470–1480.
180. Kalled SL, Cutler AH, Datta SK, et al. Anti-CD40 ligand antibody treatment of SNF1 mice with established nephritis: preservation of kidney function. *J Immunol* 1998;160:2158–2165.
181. Kalunian KC, Davis JC Jr, Merrill JT, et al. Treatment of systemic lupus erythematosus by inhibition of T cell costimulation with anti-CD154: a randomized, double-blind, placebo-controlled trial. *Arthritis Rheum* 2002;46:3251–3258.
182. Boumpas DT, Furie R, Manzi S, et al. A short course of BG9588 (anti-CD40 ligand antibody) improves serologic activity and decreases hematuria in patients with proliferative lupus glomerulonephritis. *Arthritis Rheum* 2003;48:719–727.
183. Huang W, Sinha J, Newman J, et al. The effect of anti-CD40 ligand antibody on B cells in human systemic lupus erythematosus. *Arthritis Rheum* 2002;46:1554–1562.
184. Van Seventer GA, Shimizu Y, Horgan KJ, et al. The LFA-1 ligand ICAM-1 provides an important costimulatory signal for T cell receptor-mediated activation of resting T cells. *J Immunol* 1990;144:4579–4586.
185. Dustin ML, Springer TA. T-cell receptor cross-linking transiently stimulates adhesiveness through LFA-1. *Nature* 1989;341:619–624.
186. Springer TA, Dustin ML, Kishimoto TK, et al. The lymphocyte function-associated LFA-1, CD2, and LFA-3 molecules: cell adhesion receptors of the immune system. *Ann Rev Immunol* 1987;5:223–252.
187. Papp K, Bissonnette R, Krueger JG, et al. The treatment of moderate to severe psoriasis with a new anti-CD11a monoclonal antibody. *J Am Acad Dermatol* 2001;45:665–674.
188. Gottlieb AB, Krueger JG, Wittkowski K, et al. Psoriasis as a model for T-cell-mediated disease: immunobiologic and clinical effects of treatment with multiple doses of efalizumab, an anti-CD11a antibody. *Arch Dermatol* 2002;138:591–600.
189. Connolly MK, Kitchens EA, Chan B, et al. Treatment of murine lupus with monoclonal antibodies to lymphocyte function-associated antigen-1: dose-dependent inhibition of autoantibody production and blockade of the immune response to therapy. *Clin Immunol Immunopathol* 1994;72:198–203.

190. Kootstra CJ, Van Der Giezen DM, Van Krieken JH, et al. Effective treatment of experimental lupus nephritis by combined administration of anti-CD11a and anti-CD54 antibodies. *Clin Exp Immunol* 1997;108:324–332.
191. Kavanaugh AF, Davis LS, Nichols LA, et al. Treatment of refractory rheumatoid arthritis with a monoclonal antibody to intercellular adhesion molecule 1. *Arthritis Rheum* 1994;37:992–999.
192. Kavanaugh AF, Davis LS, Jain RI, et al. A phase I/II open label study of the safety and efficacy of an anti-ICAM-1 (intercellular adhesion molecule-1; CD54) monoclonal antibody in early rheumatoid arthritis. *J Rheumatol* 1996;23:1338–1344.
193. Kavanaugh AF, Schulze-Koops H, Davis LS, et al. Repeat treatment of rheumatoid arthritis patients with a murine anti-intercellular adhesion molecule 1 monoclonal antibody. *Arthritis Rheum* 1997;40:849–853.
194. Maksymowych WP, Blackburn WD Jr, Tami JA, et al. A randomized, placebo controlled trial of an antisense oligodeoxynucleotide to intercellular adhesion molecule-1 in the treatment of severe rheumatoid arthritis. *J Rheumatol* 2002;29:447–453.
195. Hemler ME, Elices MJ, Parker C, et al. Structure of the integrin VLA-4 and its cell-cell and cell-matrix adhesion functions. *Immunol Rev* 1990;114:45–65.
196. Burkly LC, Jakubowski A, Newman BM, et al. Signaling by vascular cell adhesion molecule-1 (VCAM-1) through VLA-4 promotes CD3-dependent T cell proliferation. *Eur J Immunol* 1991;21:2871–2875.
197. Nojima Y, Humphries MJ, Mould AP, et al. VLA-4 mediates CD3-dependent CD4+ T cell activation via the CS1 alternatively spliced domain of fibronectin. *J Exp Med* 1990;172:1185–1192.
198. Ghosh S, Goldin E, Gordon FH, et al. Natalizumab for active Crohn's disease. *N Engl J Med* 2003;348:24–32.
199. Miller DH, Khan OA, Sheremata WA, et al. A controlled trial of natalizumab for relapsing multiple sclerosis. *N Engl J Med* 2003;348:15–23.
200. Kitani A, Nakashima N, Izumihara T, et al. Soluble VCAM-1 induces chemotaxis of Jurkat and synovial fluid T cells bearing high affinity very late antigen-4. *J Immunol* 1998;161:4931–4938.
201. Tokuhira M, Hosaka S, Volin MV, et al. Soluble vascular cell adhesion molecule 1 mediation of monocyte chemotaxis in rheumatoid arthritis. *Arthritis Rheum* 2000;43:1122–1133.
202. Birner U, Issekutz TB, Walter U, et al. The role of alpha (4) and LFA-1 integrins in selectin-independent monocyte and neutrophil migration to joints of rats with adjuvant arthritis. *Int Immunol* 2000; 12:141–150.
203. Brottier P, Boumsell L, Gelin C, et al. T cell activation via CD2 [T, gp50] molecules: accessory cells are required to trigger T cell activation via CD2-D66 plus CD2–9.6/T11 (1) epitopes. *J Immunol* 1985;135:1624–1631.
204. Danielian S, Fagard R, Alcover A, et al. The tyrosine kinase activity of p56lck is increased in human T cells activated via CD2. *Eur J Immunol* 1991;21:1967–1970.
205. Majeau GR, Meier W, Jimmo B, et al. Mechanism of lymphocyte function-associated molecule 3-Ig fusion proteins inhibition of T cell responses. Structure/function analysis *in vitro* and in human CD2 transgenic mice. *J Immunol* 1994;152:2753–2767.
206. Ellis CN, Krueger GG, and Alefacept Clinical Study G. Treatment of chronic plaque psoriasis by selective targeting of memory effector T lymphocytes. *N Engl J Med* 2001;345:248–255.
207. Krueger GG, Papp KA, Stough DB, et al. A randomized, double-blind, placebo-controlled phase III study evaluating efficacy and tolerability of 2 courses of alefacept in patients with chronic plaque psoriasis. *J Am Acad Dermatol*. 2002;47:821–833.
208. Kraan MC, van Kuijk AW, Dinant HJ, et al. Alefacept treatment in psoriatic arthritis: reduction of the effector T cell population in peripheral blood and synovial tissue is associated with improvement of clinical signs of arthritis. *Arthritis Rheum* 2002;46:2776–2784.
209. Godessart N, Kunkel SL. Chemokines in autoimmune disease. *Curr Opin Immunol* 2001;13:670–675.
210. Kraan MC, Patel DD, Haringman JJ, et al. The development of clinical signs of rheumatoid synovial inflammation is associated with increased synthesis of the chemokine CXCL8 (interleukin-8). *Arthritis Res* 2001;3:65–71.
211. Haringman JJ, Kraan MC, Smeets TJM, et al. Chemokine blockade and chronic inflammatory disease: proof of concept in patients with rheumatoid arthritis. *Arthritis Rheum* 2002;46(suppl):136.
212. Ajuebor MN, Swain MG, Perretti M. Chemokines as novel therapeutic targets in inflammatory diseases. *Biochem Pharmacol* 2002;63: 1191–1196.
213. D'Ambrosio D, Panina-Bordignon P, Sinigaglia F. Chemokine receptors in inflammation: an overview. *J Immunol Methods* 2003;273: 3–13.
214. Bruhl H, Cihak J, Stangassinger M, et al. Depletion of CCR5-expressing cells with bispecific antibodies and chemokine toxins: a new strategy in the treatment of chronic inflammatory diseases and HIV. *J Immunol* 2001;166:2420–2426.
215. Plater-Zyberk C, Hoogewerf AJ, Proudfoot AE, et al. Effect of a CC chemokine receptor antagonist on collagen induced arthritis in DBA/1 mice. *Immunol Lett* 1997;57:117–120.
216. Wilder RL. Integrin alpha V beta 3 as a target for treatment of rheumatoid arthritis and related rheumatic diseases. *Ann Rheum Dis* 2002;61:96–99.
217. Koch AE. The role of angiogenesis in rheumatoid arthritis: recent developments. *Ann Rheum Dis* 2000;59:65–71.
218. Johnson BA, Haines GK, Harlow LA, et al. Adhesion molecule expression in human synovial tissue. *Arthritis Rheum* 1993;36:137–146.
219. Walsh DA, Wade M, Mapp PI, et al. Focally regulated endothelial proliferation and cell death in human synovium. *Am J Pathol* 1998; 152:691–702.
220. Badger AM, Blake S, Kapadia R, et al. Disease-modifying activity of SB 273005, an orally active, nonpeptide alphavbeta3 (vitronectin receptor) antagonist, in rat adjuvant-induced arthritis. *Arthritis Rheum* 2001;44:128–137.
221. Gerlag DM, Borges E, Tak PP, et al. Suppression of murine collagen-induced arthritis by targeted apoptosis of synovial neovasculature. *Arthritis Res* 2001;3:357–361.
222. Naor D, Nedvetzki S. CD44 in rheumatoid arthritis. *Arthritis Res* 2003;5:105–115.
223. Brenchley PEC. Antagonising angiogenesis in rheumatoid arthritis. *Ann Rheum Dis* 2001;60(iii):71–74.
224. Matsuno H, Yudoh K, Uzuki M, et al. Treatment with the angiogenesis inhibitor endostatin: a novel therapy in rheumatoid arthritis. *J Rheumatol* 2002;29:890–895.
225. Sekimoto T, Hamada K, Oike Y, et al. Effect of direct angiogenesis inhibition in rheumatoid arthritis using a soluble vascular endothelial growth factor receptor 1 chimeric protein. *J Rheumatol* 2002;29: 240–245.
226. Sone H, Kawakami Y, Sakauchi M, et al. Neutralization of vascular endothelial growth factor prevents collagen-induced arthritis and ameliorates established disease in mice. *Biochem Biophys Res Commun* 2001;281:562–568.
227. Reff ME, Carner K, Chambers KS, et al. Depletion of B cells *in vivo* by a chimeric mouse human monoclonal antibody to CD20. *Blood* 1994;83:435–445.
228. Shan D, Ledbetter JA, Press OW. Signaling events involved in anti-CD20-induced apoptosis of malignant human B cells. *Cancer Immunol Immunother* 2000;48:673–683.
229. Stohl W. Systemic lupus erythematosus: a blissless disease of too much BLyS (B lymphocyte stimulator) protein. *Curr Opin Rheumatol* 2002;14:522–528.
230. Stohl W, Cheema GS, Briggs WS, et al. B lymphocyte stimulator protein-associated increase in circulating autoantibody levels may require CD4+ T cells: lessons from HIV-infected patients. *Clin Immunol* 2002;104:115–122.
231. Groom J, Kalled SL, Cutler AH, et al. Association of BAFF/BLyS overexpression and altered B cell differentiation with Sjögren's syndrome. *J Clin Invest* 2002;109:59–68.
232. Mariette X, Roux S, Zhang J, et al. The level of BLyS (BAFF) correlates with the titre of autoantibodies in human Sjögren's syndrome. *Ann Rheum Dis* 2003;62:168–171.
233. Cheema GS, Roschke V, Hilbert DM, et al. Elevated serum B lymphocyte stimulator levels in patients with systemic immune-based rheumatic diseases. *Arthritis Rheum* 2001;44:1313–1319.
234. Stasi R, Pagano A, Stipa E, et al. Rituximab chimeric anti-CD20 monoclonal antibody treatment for adults with chronic idiopathic thrombocytopenic purpura. *Blood* 2001;98:952–957.
235. Perrotta S, Locatelli F, La Manna A, et al. Anti-CD20 monoclonal antibody (Rituximab) for life-threatening autoimmune haemolytic anaemia in a patient with systemic lupus erythematosus. *Br J Haematol* 2002;116:465–467.

236. Specks U, Fervenza FC, McDonald TJ, et al. Response of Wegener's granulomatosis to anti-CD20 chimeric monoclonal antibody therapy. *Arthritis Rheum* 2001:44:2836–2840.
237. Noorchashm H, Noorchashm N, Kern J, et al. B-cells are required for the initiation of insulitis and sialitis in nonobese diabetic mice. *Diabetes* 1997;46:941–946.
238. Gausas J, Paterson PY, Day ED, et al. Intact B-cell activity is essential for complete expression of experimental allergic encephalomyelitis in Lewis rats. *Cell Immunol* 1982;72:360–366.
239. Leandro MJ, Edwards JC, Cambridge G, et al. An open study of B lymphocyte depletion in systemic lupus erythematosus. *Arthritis Rheum* 2002;46:2673–2677.
240. Anolik J, Campbell D, Felgar R, et al. B lymphocyte depletion in the treatment of systemic lupus erythematosus: a phase I/II trial of rituximab in SLE. *Arthritis Rheum* 2002;46(suppl 9):289.
241. Eisenberg R. Rituximab in lupus. *Arthritis Care Res* 2003;5:157–159.
242. Edwards JC, Cambridge G. Sustained improvement in rheumatoid arthritis following a protocol designed to deplete B lymphocytes. *Rheumatology* 2001;40:205–211.
243. Edwards JCW, Szczepanski L, Szechinski J, et al. Efficacy and safety of rituximab, a B-cell targeted chimeric monoclonal antibody: a randomized, placebo-controlled trial in patients with rheumatoid arthritis. *Arthritis Rheum* 2002;46(suppl):197.
244. Zhou T, Martin F, Liu W, et al. Adenoviral delivery of TACI-Fc reverses autoimmunity in mice [Abstract]. *Arthritis Rheum* 2001;44 (suppl 9):396.
245. Gross JA, Johnston J, Mudri S, et al. TACI and BCMA are receptors for a TNF homologue implicated in B-cell autoimmune disease. *Nature* 2000;404:995–999.
246. Gross JA, Dillon SR, Mudri S, et al. TACI-Ig neutralizes molecules critical for B cell development and autoimmune disease. Impaired B cell maturation in mice lacking BLyS. *Immunity* 2001; 15:289–302.
247. Tan SM, Xu D, Roschke V, et al. Local production of B lymphocyte stimulator protein and APRIL in arthritic joints of patients with inflammatory arthritis. *Arthritis Rheum* 2003;48:982–992.
248. Coutts SM, Plunkett ML, Iverson GM, et al. Pharmacological intervention in antibody mediated disease. *Lupus* 1996;5:158–159.
249. Furie RA, Cash JM, Cronin ME, et al. Treatment of systemic lupus erythematosus with LJP 394. *J Rheumatol* 2001;28:257–265.
250. Alarcon-Segovia D, Tumlin JA, Furie RA, et al. LJP 394 for the prevention of renal flare in patients with systemic lupus erythematosus: results from a randomized, double-blind, placebo-controlled study. *Arthritis Rheum* 2003;48:442–454.
251. Baumann I, Kolowos W, Voll RE, et al. Impaired uptake of apoptotic cells into tingible body macrophages in germinal centers of patients with systemic lupus erythematosus. *Arthritis Rheum* 2002;46:191–201.
252. Vaishnaw AK, Toubi E, Ohsako S, et al. The spectrum of apoptotic defects and clinical manifestations, including systemic lupus erythematosus, in humans with CD95 (Fas/APO-1) mutations. *Arthritis Rheum* 1999;42:1833–1842.
253. Herrmann M, Voll RE, Zoller OM, et al. Impaired phagocytosis of apoptotic cell material by monocyte-derived macrophages from patients with systemic lupus erythematosus. *Arthritis Rheum* 1998;41: 1241–1250.
254. Kurowska M, Rudnicka W, Kontny E, et al. Fibroblast-like synoviocytes from rheumatoid arthritis patients express functional IL-15 receptor complex: endogenous IL-15 in autocrine fashion enhances cell proliferation and expression of Bcl-x (L) and Bcl-2. *J Immunol* 2002;169:1760–1767.
255. Yonehara S. Death receptor Fas and autoimmune disease: from the original generation to therapeutic application of agonistic anti-Fas monoclonal antibody. *Cytokine Growth Factor Rev* 2002;13:393–402.
256. Matsuno H, Yudoh K, Nakazawa F, et al. Antirheumatic effects of humanized anti-Fas monoclonal antibody in human rheumatoid arthritis/SCID mouse chimera. *J Rheum* 2002;29:1609–1614.
257. Ogawa H, Nakayama J, Onozawa Y, et al. Anti-human Fas antibody suppresses osteoclastogenesis in rheumatoid arthritis through induction of T cell apoptosis. *Arthritis Rheum* 2002;46(suppl):210.
258. Close DR. Matrix metalloproteinase inhibitors in rheumatic diseases. *Ann Rheum Dis* 2001;60(iii):62–67.
259. Martel-Pelletier J, McCollum R, Fujimoto N, et al. Excess of metalloproteases over tissue inhibitor of metalloprotease may contribute to cartilage degradation in osteoarthritis and rheumatoid arthritis. *Lab Invest* 1994;70:807–15.
260. Dean DD, Martel-Pelletier J, Pelletier JP, et al. Evidence for metalloproteinase and metalloproteinase inhibitor imbalance in human osteoarthritic cartilage. *J Clin Invest* 1989;84:678–685.
261. Pelletier JP, Mineau F, Faure MP, et al. Imbalance between the mechanisms of activation and inhibition of metalloproteases in the early lesions of experimental osteoarthritis. *Arthritis Rheum* 1990; 33:1466–1476.
262. Yoshihara Y, Nakamura H, Obata K, et al. Matrix metalloproteinases and tissue inhibitors of metalloproteinases in synovial fluids from patients with rheumatoid arthritis or osteoarthritis. *Ann Rheum Dis* 2000;59:455–461.
263. Jackson C, Nguyen M, Arkell J, et al. Selective matrix metalloproteinase (MMP) inhibition in rheumatoid arthritis—targeting gelatinase A activation. *Inflamm Res* 2001;50:183–186.
264. Kafienah W, Al-Fayez F, Hollander AP, et al. Inhibition of cartilage degradation: a combined tissue engineering and gene therapy approach. *Arthritis Rheum* 2003;48:709–718.
265. Schett G, Hayer S, Tohidast-Akrad M, et al. Adenovirus-based overexpression of tissue inhibitor of metalloproteinases 1 reduces tissue damage in the joints of tumor necrosis factor alpha transgenic mice. *Arthritis Rheum* 2001;44:2888–2898.
266. Hemmings FJ, Farhan M, Rowland J, et al. Tolerability and pharmacokinetics of the collagenase-selective inhibitor trocade in patients with rheumatoid arthritis. *Rheumatology (Oxford)* 2001;40:537–543.
267. Nemunaitis J, Poole C, Primrose J, et al. Combined analysis of studies of the effects of the matrix metalloproteinase inhibitor marimastat on serum tumor markers in advanced cancer: selection of a biologically active and tolerable dose for longer-term studies. *Clin Cancer Res* 1998;4:1101–1109.
268. McInnes IB, Leung BP, Field M, et al. Production of nitric oxide in the synovial membrane of rheumatoid and osteoarthritis patients. *J Exp Med* 1996;184:1519–1524.
269. Ohtsuka M, Konno F, Honda H, et al. PPA250 [3- (2,4-difluorophenyl)-6-[2-[4- (1H-imidazol-1-ylmethyl) phenoxy]ethoxy]-2-phenylpyridine], a novel orally effective inhibitor of the dimerization of inducible nitric-oxide synthase, exhibits an anti-inflammatory effect in animal models of chronic arthritis. *J Pharmacol Exp Ther* 2002;303:52–57.
270. Marklund SL, Bjelle A, Elmqvist LG. Superoxide dismutase isoenzymes of the synovial fluid in rheumatoid arthritis and in reactive arthritides. *Ann Rheum Dis* 1986;45:847–851.
271. McIlwain H, Silverfield JC, Cheatum DE, et al. Intra-articular orgotein in osteoarthritis of the knee: a placebo-controlled efficacy, safety, and dosage comparison. *Am J Med* 1989;87:295–300.
272. Menander-Huber KB. Orgotein in the treatment of rheumatoid arthritis. *Eur J Rheumatol Inflamm* 1981;4:201–211.
273. Salvemini D, Mazzon E, Dugo L, et al. Amelioration of joint disease in a rat model of collagen-induced arthritis by M40403, a superoxide dismutase mimetic. *Arthritis Rheum* 2001;44:2909–2921.
274. Wang Y, Hu Q, Madri JA, et al. Amelioration of lupus-like autoimmune disease in NZB/WF1 mice after treatment with a blocking monoclonal antibody specific for complement component C5. *Proc Nat Acad Sci U S A* 1996;93:8563–8568.
275. Girardi G, Berman J, Spruce L, et al. A critical role for complement C5 in antiphospholipid antibody-induced pregnancy loss [Abstract]. *Arthritis Rheum* 2002;46(suppl):219.
276. Wang Y, Rollins SA, Madri JA, et al. Anti-C5 monoclonal antibody therapy prevents collagen-induced arthritis and ameliorates established disease. *Proc Nat Acad Sci U S A* 1995;92:8955–8959.
277. Woodruff TM, Strachan AJ, Dryburgh N, et al. Antiarthritic activity of an orally active C5a receptor antagonist against antigen-induced monarticular arthritis in the rat. *Arthritis Rheum* 2002;46:2476–2485.
278. Kaplan M. Eculizumab (Alexion). *Curr Opin Invest Drugs* 2002;3: 1017–1023.
279. Takada K, Bookbinder S, Furie R, et al. A pilot study of eculizumab in patients with dermatomyositis. *Arthritis Rheum* 2002;46(suppl): 489.
280. Holers VM, Girardi G, Mo L, et al. Complement C3 activation is required for antiphospholipid antibody-induced fetal loss. *J Exp Med* 2002;195:211–220.

281. Goodfellow RM, Williams AS, Levin JL, et al. Local therapy with soluble complement receptor 1 (sCR1) suppresses inflammation in rat mono-articular arthritis. *Clin Exp Immunol* 1997;110:45–52.
282. Goodfellow RM, Williams AS, Levin JL, et al. Soluble complement receptor one (sCR1) inhibits the development and progression of rat collagen-induced arthritis. *Clin Exp Immunol* 2000;119:210–216.
283. Hogarth PM. Fc receptors are major mediators of antibody based inflammation in autoimmunity. *Curr Opin Immunol* 2002;14:798–802.
284. Watanabe H, Sherris D, Gilkeson GS. Soluble CD16 in the treatment of murine lupus nephritis. *Clin Immunol Immunopathol* 1998;88:91–95.
285. Van Roon J, Van Vuuren A, Wijngaarden W, et al. Selective elimination of synovial inflammatory macrophages in rheumatoid arthritis by an Fc receptor I-directed immunotoxin. *Arthritis Rheum* 2003;48:1229–1238.
286. Marino M, Rossi M, Ruvo M, et al. Novel molecular targets for systemic lupus erythematosus. *Curr Drug Targets* 2002;3:223–228.
287. Haynes DR, Barg E, Crotti TN, et al. Osteoprotegerin expression in synovial tissue from patients with rheumatoid arthritis, spondyloarthropathies and osteoarthritis and normal controls. *Rheumatology* 2003;42:123–134.
288. Bolon B, Campagnuolo G, Feige U. Duration of bone protection by a single osteoprotegerin injection in rats with adjuvant-induced arthritis. *Cell Mol Life Sci* 2002;59:1569–1576.
289. Romas E, Sims NA, Hards DK, et al. Osteoprotegerin reduces osteoclast numbers and prevents bone erosion in collagen-induced arthritis. *Am J Pathol* 2002;161:1419–1427.
290. Campagnuolo G, Bolon B, Feige U. Kinetics of bone protection by recombinant osteoprotegerin therapy in Lewis rats with adjuvant arthritis. *Arthritis Rheum* 2002;46:1926–1936.
291. Redlich K, Hayer S, Maier A, et al. Tumor necrosis factor alpha-mediated joint destruction is inhibited by targeting osteoclasts with osteoprotegerin. *Arthritis Rheum* 2002;46:785–792.
292. Bolon B, Shalhoub V, Kostenuik PJ, et al. Osteoprotegerin, an endogenous antiosteoclast factor for protecting bone in rheumatoid arthritis. *Arthritis Rheum* 2002;46:3121–3135.

CHAPTER 41

Immunomodulatory Agents (Cyclosporine, Tacrolimus, Azathioprine, Cyclophosphamide, Mycophenolate Mofetil, and Chlorambucil)

Allen Dale Sawitzke and Grant W. Cannon

Immunomodulatory agents act through antiproliferative, immunoregulatory, and antiinflammatory mechanisms when they are used to treat rheumatic diseases. The precise mechanisms of action in rheumatic disease remain undefined and likely vary based on the disease process under consideration. This chapter will review two purine inhibitors, azathioprine (AZA) and mycophenolate mofetil; three calcineurin inhibitors, cyclosporine, tacrolimus (FK506), and sirolimus (rapamycin); and two alkylating agents, cyclophosphamide and chlorambucil. Antimetabolites (methotrexate) and antipyrimidines (leflunomide) are reviewed in Chapter 32.

Of these medications, only AZA and cyclosporine are currently approved by the U.S. Food and Drug Administration (FDA) for the treatment of a rheumatic disease. Nonetheless, well-designed clinical trials have demonstrated the other agents to be highly effective for specific situations. The lack of formal FDA approval requires the rheumatologist considering immunomodulatory drug therapy to carefully assess the potential risks and benefits and to completely discuss these factors with the patient before beginning treatment. Vigilant monitoring must be maintained once drug therapy is begun, because multiple potentially serious toxicities are also associated with use of these medications.

PURINE INHIBITION

Historical Overview

Synthesis of nucleic acids is critical to cellular division; hence, many medications have been developed that are modified purines or pyrimidines, including 6-mercaptopurine (6-MP), AZA, leflunomide, 5-fluorouracil, 2-chlorodeoxyadenosine, and allopurinol, among others (1). 6-MP was synthesized as a purine analogue for use in the treatment of malignancies. In the early 1960s, 6-MP was also reported to be effective in treating "autoimmune diseases" (2,3). Subsequent efforts were directed toward minimizing the rapid metabolism of 6-MP. AZA, or 6-[(1-methyl-4-nitro-imidazole-5-yl) thio] purine, was developed in response to this challenge (1,3) (Fig. 41.1A). Although AZA has some cytotoxic activity, its immunomodulatory properties are much more prominent at the doses usually used. AZA has been extensively used as an immunosuppressive agent for organ transplantation and for the treatment of autoimmune diseases, especially rheumatoid arthritis (RA) (4–8) and systemic lupus erythematosus (SLE) (4,5). Controlled trials have documented the effectiveness of AZA in RA (9–11), and long-term follow-up studies have confirmed continued clinical benefit (12–15). The role of AZA for treating SLE (16–24), polymyositis (25–28), and psoriatic arthritis (9, 13) remains controversial.

Mycophenolate mofetil also inhibits the *de novo* synthesis pathway of purine production. Its structure is shown in Fig. 41.1B. It is effective in organ transplantation (29–32) and is indicated for prevention of rejection of renal, hepatic, and cardiac transplants by the FDA. A case is now building for its use in SLE (33–35), and some interest in its use in polymyositis and RA has also been published (36–38).

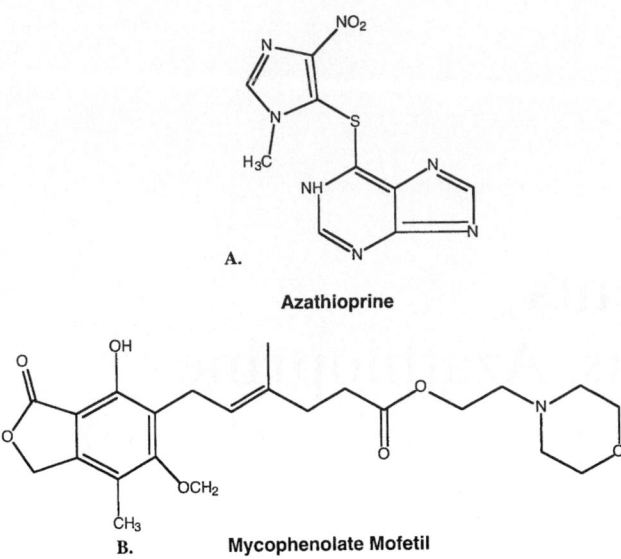

FIG. 41.1. Chemical structure of azathioprine (A) and mycophenolate mofetil (B).

Azathioprine

Pharmacology

Pharmacokinetics

AZA is well absorbed after oral administration. Approximately 30% of circulating AZA is protein bound, and 2% to 10% is excreted unchanged in the urine. In normal subjects, the plasma half-life of AZA is 3 hours (1). AZA itself is not an active compound, but is activated following nucleophilic attack, principally from glutathione, to form active 6-MP in the liver and erythrocytes (39,40) (Fig. 41.2). AZA metabolism is important because multiple metabolites of 6-MP have been identified, including the cytotoxic compounds 6-thioinosinic acid and its derivative, 6-thioguanylic acid (3). Genetic differences in metabolism change the expectations for adverse reactions as well as efficacy (41,42). Hypoxanthine phosphoribosyl transferase metabolizes 6-MP to 6-thioinosinic acid, which then suppresses several steps in the salvage synthesis of adenine and guanine by preventing interconversion of purine bases, especially inosinic and guanylic acid. Moreover, 6-thioinosinic acid acts as a feedback inhibitor of inosinic acid production, thereby inhibiting *de novo* biosynthesis of purine bases (40). 6-MP may also be incorporated into RNA and DNA as 6-thioguanine (6-TGN) (43), resulting in the cytotoxic effects of AZA at high doses. This may not be the principal action of the drug at the lower doses used to treat rheumatic diseases. AZA and 6-MP are ultimately metabolized to 6-thiouric acid by xanthine oxidase (XO) (40).

Allopurinol blocks XO, resulting in accumulation of selected metabolites. Although the pharmacokinetics of 6-MP are not significantly altered by allopurinol in all patients (44), the alteration of AZA metabolism by allopurinol is potentially life threatening if unrecognized. Hence, the simultaneous administration of AZA and allopurinol should be avoided. When AZA and allopurinol must be used concurrently, the dose of AZA must be reduced to 25% to 33% of the usual dose and close monitoring performed to avoid toxicity (40).

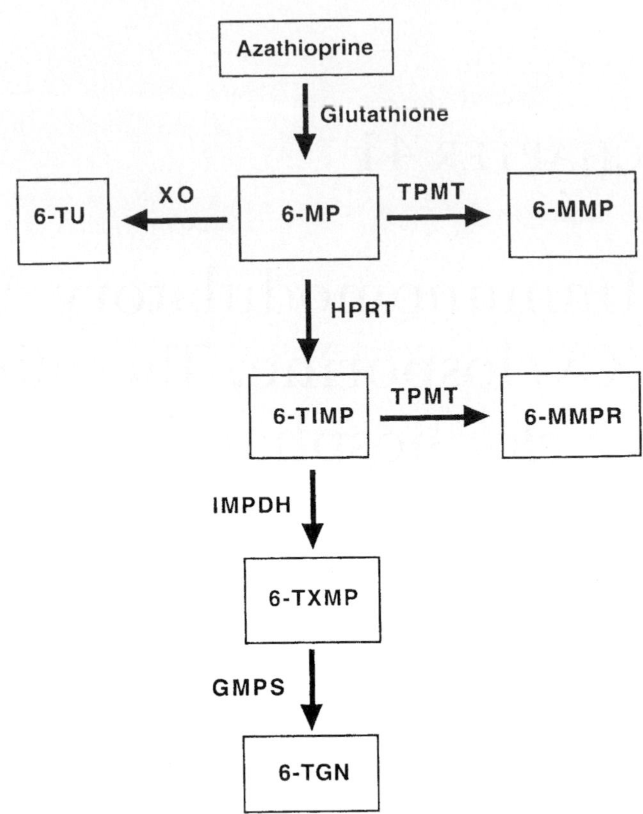

FIG. 41.2. Azathioprine and purine metabolic pathway. Azathioprine is readily converted through reaction with reactive thiols such as glutathione to 6-mercaptopurine. Thereafter, the relative enzyme activities determine the principal metabolites. Decreased TPMT activity results in more 6-TU and active metabolites such as 6-TGN, whereas inhibition of IMPDH (mycophenolate mofetil) results in more 6-TIMP, which inhibits *de novo* purine synthesis. HPRT, hypoxanthine phosphoribosyl transferase; IMPDH, inosine monophosphate dehydrogenase; 6-MP, 6-mercaptopurine; 6-TGN, 6-thioguanylic acid; 6-TIMP, 6-thioinosinic acid; TPMT, thiopurine methyltransferase; 6-TU, 6-thiouric acid; XO, xanthine oxidase.

Although hepatic metabolism is important, the effects of liver disease on AZA metabolism remain unpredictable. Some patients with liver disease have nearly normal AZA metabolism (45), whereas others, especially those with chronic liver disease, may be at higher risk for hematologic toxicity (46). The half-life of AZA may also increase in renal failure (47), although this effect is generally not clinically significant.

Role of Genetic Variation

A minority of Caucasians (0.3%) demonstrate little or no thiopurine methyltransferase (TPMT) activity in their erythrocytes, whereas another 10% have intermediate activities (48–50). Both of these groups of patients cannot as efficiently inactivate the AZA metabolites as homozygous high-activity patients (41), while increased levels of these same metabolites correlate with effectiveness in treating inflammatory bowel disease (51). Patients with low enzyme activity appear to have markedly increased levels of 6-TGN and hematologic adverse effects, as was highlighted by the case report of pancytopenia in a patient homozygous for TPMT deficiency (42). Concurrent administration of trimethoprim (52) or the use of angiotensin-converting enzyme inhibitors (53) may further increase the hematologic toxicity of AZA. How to best test patients for these effects remains under debate because ultimately it is the phenotype, not the genotype, that is most related to response to the medication (54,55). Proponents of genotype and of phenotype testing exist (51,56–58).

Proposed Mechanisms of Action

The mechanism of action of AZA in the treatment of rheumatic diseases is unclear, but both cytotoxic and immunosuppressive properties are likely involved. Lymphocytes are more dependent on the salvage pathway of purine synthesis than many other cells and are therefore more sensitive to AZA inhibition, as described above (59). In addition, AZA suppresses several immunologic functions *in vitro,* including natural killer cell activity (60), antibody production (61), antibody-dependent cellular cytotoxicity (60), and cellular immune responses (62). B cells are more affected than are T cells by AZA (63). Immunologic parameters (9) and cytokine levels (64,65) in patients receiving AZA are unaltered, although circulating AZA may interfere with interleukin-6 (IL-6) assays (64). AZA suppresses the production of autoantibodies in animal models of SLE (66) and has been reported to lower rheumatoid factor levels in RA patients (67,68), although this effect is not consistently seen (8,10,11,69,70). It is not clear whether this alteration of antibody levels is a primary or secondary drug effect (66,71).

Drug Monitoring

The recommended initial dose for AZA is 1 mg/kg/day, which may be increased to a maximum dose of 2.5 mg/kg/day in severe cases. Dose reductions should be considered for renal insufficiency and must be instituted if concurrent allopurinol is to be used (1). The application of genetic testing remains controversial because how to best apply the results to adjust management remains to be demonstrated. Recent changes to the "warnings" and "adverse reactions" sections of the product insert for AZA highlight an increasing role for TPMT genotyping. Complete blood counts, including platelet counts and differential, should be performed at initiation and at least every 2 weeks until stable and then every 1 to 3 months throughout therapy (72). The measurement of serum transaminase levels at baseline also seems appropriate (72), with repeated evaluation at every 3 to 6 months thereafter, although this was not recommended by the American College of Rheumatology (ACR) guidelines (72). Recommendations on its use in patients with hepatitis C virus infection are not available, but because both can adversely impact the liver, avoidance, if possible, seems appropriate. Clinical evaluation should include inquiries regarding gastrointestinal upset, stomatitis, skin rash, lymphadenopathy, and symptoms of infection.

Adverse Drug Effects

Adverse drug effects have been associated with AZA (Table 41.1). They prompt discontinuation of AZA in 19%

TABLE 41.1. *Adverse effects of azathioprine and mycophenolate mofetil*

Adverse effect	Azathioprine frequency	Mycophenolate frequency
Hematologic		
Leukopenia	+++[a]	++[a]
Thrombocytopenia	++[a]	+
Anemia	++[a]	++
Pure red cell aplasia	+	
Pancytopenia	+[a]	
Gastrointestinal		
Nausea/epigastric pain	+++[a]	++[a]
Stomatitis	++[a]	
Gastrointestinal hemorrhage	+[a]	
Gastric ulcer	+[a]	
Diarrhea	+[a]	+++[a]
Pancreatitis	+	
Hepatic		
Elevated liver enzymes	++[a]	+[a]
Cholestasis	+	
Fibrosis/cirrhosis	+	
Hypersensitivity hepatitis	+[a]	
Hepatic venoocclusive disease	+[a]	
Pulmonary		
Interstitial pneumonitis	+	
Diffuse alveolar damage	+	
Dermatologic		
Maculopapular rash	++[a]	
Generalized urticarial reactions	+[a]	
Reproductive		
Congenital deformities	+	
Chromosomal damage	+	
Miscellaneous		
Herpes zoster[a]	+[a]	+
Proteinuria[a]	+[a]	
Peripheral neuropathy	+	
Accelerated nodulosis[a]	+[a]	

[a]Reported during the treatment of rheumatic diseases.
+++, >10%; ++, <10% and >1%; +, <1%.

to 32% of patients (67,70,73,74). Patients experiencing mild toxicity often can continue their medication, because generally these events are rapidly reversible following dose reduction. Adverse events may be more frequent at higher doses (11,75). A survey of 546 patients found that a mean daily dose of 103 mg/day has a "surprisingly benign profile with relatively few serious therapeutic mishaps" (74). A retrospective review of 5,809 patients treated with disease-modifying antirheumatic disease (DMARD) therapy showed that patients remained on AZA longer than other DMARDs, with the exception of methotrexate, suggesting a good balance of efficacy and tolerability (76). Comparison with the newer DMARDs and biologic agents is not available.

Hematologic. Hematologic toxicity is a frequent complication of AZA therapy. Leukopenia (4,6,7,9,10,12,13, 68–70,73,75,77), thrombocytopenia (9,69,78), anemia (6, 13), pure red cell aplasia (77), and pancytopenia (14,79–81) have all been reported in RA patients, and severe leukopenia may predispose to serious infection (13). Lower activities of the enzymes of purine metabolism have been associated with increased toxicity (82,83), but these measurements remain complex. Specific rheumatic disease populations may have unique enzyme activities, because SLE patients appear to have lower TPMT activity (84). Attempts to identify patients at risk for serious complications by use of genetic markers have been reported (41,85,86). Interestingly, an increase in erythrocyte mean corpuscular volume (MCV) may be a readily available and simple marker related to *in vivo* 6-TGN levels that could be used to adjust therapy (87).

Gastrointestinal. Nausea, vomiting, and epigastric pain, sometimes accompanied by fever, are frequent complaints of patients receiving AZA (4,7,10,12,13,67,68,70,73–75,78). Symptoms commonly appear in the first week of therapy and reappear within hours of rechallenge. Less frequently, stomatitis (69), gastrointestinal hemorrhage (6), gastric ulcer (13), and diarrhea (69) occur. Pancreatitis has been seen during treatment of inflammatory bowel disease and renal transplantation with AZA (88–90).

Hepatic. Liver toxicity with AZA is rare (75,91–97). Mild elevations of aminotransferases are the most common finding in AZA-associated liver disease (75), but cirrhosis with fatal progressive liver failure during treatment with AZA has been reported (91). It is thought that the TGN is the principal hepatic toxin such that patients with homozygous low TPMT activity may be at highest risk. In some cases, hepatitis and abnormal liver enzymes have completely resolved following cessation of AZA (92). Some cases of fibrosis have not progressed on serial biopsies despite continued treatment with AZA (98,99). Other reported hepatic complications include cholestasis (92,93,95,96), a hypersensitivity hepatitis (94), and hepatic venoocclusive disease in an RA patient receiving AZA (97).

Pulmonary. Although pulmonary disease has rarely been reported during AZA treatment of rheumatic diseases, interstitial pneumonitis (100,101), diffuse alveolar damage (100), and respiratory failure (100) have occurred during its use in therapy of other disorders. Interestingly, bronchiolitis obliterans with organizing pneumonia (BOOP) has also reportedly been successfully treated with AZA (102).

Dermatologic. Maculopapular rashes, and less commonly generalized urticarial reactions, have been observed in most series of AZA therapy in RA (6,7,9,13,69,70,75,103). In some instances, skin reactions have prompted cessation of the drug, but more commonly, these side effects have not been serious. Psoriasis often improves in patients with psoriatic arthritis receiving AZA (7,9).

Reproductive. Although successful pregnancies have been reported in patients treated with AZA throughout pregnancy (104–106), the sexually active premenopausal female should practice adequate contraception. AZA and its metabolites cross the placenta (107), and significant neonatal complications and chromosomal damage have been observed in the offspring of patients receiving AZA during pregnancy (108–110). A report of nine pregnancies in six SLE patients treated with AZA during pregnancy (seven during the first trimester) reported three full-term good outcomes, two full-term small-for-date births, three preterm deliveries, and one miscarriage (106). In this study, pregnancy outcomes in SLE patients with previous immunosuppressive treatment were not different from pregnancy outcomes in other SLE patients without previous immunosuppressive treatment (106,111). Larger studies in transplant populations suggest that AZA is well tolerated in most pregnancies, resulting most often only in intrauterine growth retardation or premature delivery (112). AZA probably does not get into milk significantly, but may adversely effect immune benefits that would have been achieved through breast-feeding (113).

Malignancy. Prolonged AZA therapy has been associated with karyotypic abnormalities (12), and malignancies have occurred in RA patients during treatment with this drug (114–118). An epidemiologic study indicated that the prevalence of malignancies in nontransplant patients receiving AZA is increased compared with the expected rates (119). Complicating the evaluation of this study are reports of increased rates of malignancies in RA patients independent of cytotoxic antirheumatic therapy (118,120–124). Indeed, studies comparing the incidence of malignancies in patients with RA receiving AZA to those not so treated have not shown an increased risk for malignancy (118,120,121, 125–127). A study suggesting that AZA may increase malignancy rates in RA patients was complicated by the fact that many of these individuals also had received alkylating agents, which are known to induce malignancies (128). Although it remains controversial whether AZA increases the risk for malignancy in RA patients, the available data suggest that oncogenesis is not a major problem and that the risk with AZA, if any, is small. However, malignancies, especially squamous cell cancer of the skin, are clearly increased in renal transplant patients receiving AZA and corticosteroids (129). It has been speculated that some of these malignancies would have occurred independently of the immunosuppressive therapies (130). Studies in inflammatory bowel disease have not clearly shown an increase in cancer in patients treated with AZA (131,132).

Miscellaneous

Infections, particularly herpes zoster, may be increased in patients receiving AZA (9,13,70). Proteinuria (70), peripheral neuropathy (133), and accelerated nodulosis (134) have been observed in RA patients receiving AZA. Atrial fibrillation was reported during treatment of psoriasis with the drug (135). Hypersensitivity reactions characterized by fever, acute interstitial nephritis, and hepatitis also have been reported (94,136). The precise relationship of AZA to these uncommon events remains unknown.

Clinical Experience

Rheumatoid Arthritis

Dosages of AZA as used for the treatment of RA range from 1 to 4.8 mg/kg/day (13,14,137); however, the usual dosage is 1.25 to 2.5 mg/kg/day. Studies directly comparing 1.25 versus 2.5 mg/kg/day dosages have not demonstrated statistically significant differences in clinical outcomes, Although higher dosages may be more effective in controlling disease activity (11,75), adverse drug reactions are probably more common at the higher dosage (75). In a large multicenter trial evaluating the efficacy of AZA (1.25–1.5 mg/kg/day), 44% of patients experienced "important clinical improvement," defined as greater than 30% decrease in tender joints (73). Unlike the biologic agents, the slow onset of action by AZA necessitates a trial of at least 12 weeks to ensure an adequate opportunity for a clinical response. A recent Cochrane review suggested that "azathioprine appears to have a statistically significant benefit on the disease activity in joints of patients with RA" (138).

Evidence that AZA modifies the disease course of RA is lacking, and serial radiographs have demonstrated progression (13,67) or improvement (78) of bony erosions with AZA therapy. Although one study comparing gold salts and AZA indicated that fewer erosions developed during AZA therapy compared with gold salt therapy (70), analysis of radiographs in another prospective trial comparing methotrexate and AZA demonstrated significantly less radiologic progression in patients receiving methotrexate as compared with those receiving AZA (139,140).

Comparisons of AZA with D-penicillamine (67,69,73, 78), gold salts (68,70), cyclophosphamide (70), chloroquine (68), levamisole (78), and cyclosporine (141,142) have suggested that AZA is equally effective as these other agents. Comparisons of AZA and methotrexate in RA patients have produced conflicting results (143–147). A retrospective study and one prospective controlled trial comparing AZA and methotrexate found methotrexate to be superior to AZA (144). Three other prospective randomized trials, however, did not demonstrate a difference in efficacy between the two drugs (145–147). In one study, adverse drug effects were more frequent in the methotrexate group (146). In another study, the incidence of minor adverse effects was higher in RA patients receiving methotrexate compared with AZA, but the incidence of "major toxic reactions" was similar (148). Two other studies have suggested higher rates of adverse drug effects with AZA than methotrexate (144,147). Again, no data in comparison with modern biologic agents is available.

Systemic Lupus Erythematosus

AZA has been used to treat lupus nephritis (see Chapter 74), cutaneous lupus (24), and other manifestations of SLE (149,150). Results from long-term follow-up studies of lupus nephritis at the National Institutes of Health (NIH) have compared the efficacy of cytotoxic agents. These trials included patients randomized to receive AZA with prednisone (16,17,19–21,23). In general, these protocols have shown that cytotoxic drugs retard the progression of end-stage renal disease when compared with prednisone alone. The NIH results favor cyclophosphamide as the most effective agent, with AZA yielding an intermediate benefit (16). Other researchers have suggested that AZA is more effective than prednisone alone in SLE nephritis (18,22). The optimal role of AZA in the treatment of SLE remains difficult to define. It appears to be useful as a steroid-sparing agent, for management of arthritis and vasculitis, but rarely, if ever as the sole drug of choice for lupus nephritis (151, 152). It may be useful as a cyclophosphamide-sparing agent as well (153).

Autoimmune Hepatitis

Controlled and uncontrolled trials have shown AZA to be effective in treating autoimmune (lupoid) hepatitis whether associated with lupus or not (154–157). Most investigators now consider AZA with glucocorticoids to be the drugs of choice for treatment of patients with this disorder (158–160).

Inflammatory Muscle Disease

Uncontrolled series have reported improvement of inflammatory myopathies (see Chapter 75) treated with AZA (27,28). A small controlled trial evaluating AZA and prednisone versus prednisone alone in polymyositis patients showed no significant clinical difference after 3 months (25), but at 6 months the group receiving both AZA and prednisone experienced greater functional improvement and possibly a steroid-sparing effect (26). A retrospective study of 25 patients with polymyositis/dermatomyositis (PM/DM) demonstrated that 75% of patients had a good response to AZA (161). Combination oral methotrexate/AZA may benefit patients with treatment-resistant PM, including those who previously had inadequate responses to either methotrexate or AZA alone (162). A case of PM with associated BOOP reportedly responded to AZA (102). An uncontrolled study found that AZA may have a limited role in the treatment of inclusion body myositis (163).

Miscellaneous

Reiter's syndrome (see Chapter 65) has been treated with AZA with some success (164–166). A placebo-controlled trial in children with juvenile chronic arthritis (JCA) (see Chapter 63) demonstrated a trend toward greater clinical improvement in patients receiving AZA, but the difference was not statistically significant (167). Another study found that AZA was a useful drug in severe JCA, with acceptable side effects and noteworthy glucocorticoid-sparing effects (168). Uncontrolled studies have suggested improvement of psoriatic arthritis (169) (see Chapter 66) and psoriatic skin lesions with AZA (7,13). However, no controlled trial has yet verified this effect (170–172). Although alkylating agents appear to be the drug of choice for severe necrotizing vasculitis (173), AZA has been reported to be effective in some patients with Wegener's granulomatosis (174), Takayasu's arteritis (175,176), giant cell arteritis (177–180), and other necrotizing vasculitis syndromes (181).

Mycophenolate Mofetil

Pharmacology

Pharmacokinetics

Mycophenolate mofetil is a semisynthetic derivative of a fungal product that is rapidly absorbed and quickly converted by hydrolysis to the active agent mycophenolic acid (MPA). It has an oral bioavailability of 94% and is extensively protein bound, with an average half-life of 17.9 hours (182). It is inactivated by the liver and excreted into the gastrointestinal tract, where bacteria convert it to products that subsequently undergo an enterohepatic recirculation. Consequently, medications that affect enterohepatic circulation, including cholestyramine, may also affect mycophenolate mofetil levels. Excretion in the urine eliminates greater than 93% of the drug (182). Drug levels are increased by significant renal insufficiency.

The FDA has approved mycophenolate mofetil for the prevention of acute allograft rejection in renal, hepatic, and cardiac transplantation. Large trials have shown it to be superior to AZA for renal transplantation, with similar results in cardiac, pulmonary, and hepatic transplants. Descriptions of adverse drug reactions are almost exclusively from the transplantation literature.

Proposed Mechanism of Action

Through inhibition of inosine monophosphate dehydrogenase and the consequent increase in 6-thioinosinic acid (Fig. 41.2), MPA reversibly prevents the *de novo* synthesis of purines and hence of cell division. Because activated B and T cells are principally dependent on the *de novo* synthesis pathway to supply purines, they are much more affected by its blockade than are most somatic cells (182). This blockade prevents cell division, but also inhibits some specific cellular functions such as antibody formation by B cells. The blockade of immunoglobulin synthesis appears to be stronger than that observed with the use of AZA.

Adverse Drug Effects

Hematologic. Leukopenia is observed at a rate similar to that of AZA (Table 41.1), at 20% to 35% in patients treated for organ transplantation. Trials in RA have shown lymphopenia to be most common (183). Severe neutropenia is seen in only about 2% to 3% of patients. Anemia is observed in about 25% of patients, whereas thrombocytopenia is less common (10%) than observed with AZA (25%) (182).

Gastrointestinal. Diarrhea is common, occurring in up to 36% of patients, whereas dyspepsia and nausea are similar to the rates seen with AZA (182). Gastritis is also more frequent in treated patients than controls. All of these effects seem to be dose-related effects. The liver is not appreciably affected by low-dose mycophenolate mofetil, but in cardiac transplant studies using 3 g/day, transaminase elevations were seen in about 25% (182). Postmarketing surveillance has reported colitis and pancreatitis as well. Long-term safety studies in RA patients demonstrated diarrhea in 2.5%, nausea in 1.5%, and abdominal pain in 1.2% (183).

Pulmonary. Dyspnea and cough are reported to occur in 15% to 20% of patients treated with 2 to 3 g/day mycophenolate mofetil. It is unclear if these are dose related. Postmarketing reports include a fatal pulmonary fibrosis (182). An increase in pharyngitis may also be observed on 3 g/day.

Dermatologic. The skin is only rarely involved as a reaction to mycophenolate mofetil. Acne was the most common finding, occurring in about 10% of patients, a rate similar to other immunosuppressive medications. Rash is reported in 22% of cardiac transplant patients treated with 3 g/day mycophenolate mofetil.

Reproductive. Mycophenolate mofetil is characterized as category C by the FDA, because no adequate and well-controlled studies have been performed in pregnant women. Effective contraception is recommended before instituting medication and for at least 6 weeks after completing it. In rats, mycophenolate mofetil enters milk, but data are not available on human milk. Hence, breast-feeding is not advisable while taking mycophenolate mofetil.

Malignancy. Patients have developed lymphoma or lymphoproliferative disease following treatment with mycophenolate mofetil as well. However, the number of years of exposure remains small so that much needed long-term data are not available. Continued vigilance with interim assessments of lymphadenopathy and constitutional symptoms seems appropriate.

Infection. Infections have been more frequently reported, with rates up to 24% in the mycophenolate mofetil 3 g/day group, a rate similar to other immunosuppressive medications (182). The risk is also affected by concomitant steroid and cyclosporine use because most transplantation patients are concurrently taking these as well. Herpes simplex, herpes zoster, and tuberculosis have been reported. Serious postmarketing cases of endocarditis and meningitis have been reported (182).

Drug Monitoring

Most patients with rheumatic disease are treated with 1 to 2 g oral mycophenolate mofetil twice daily (37). Little is specifically prescribed for appropriate monitoring in rheumatic disease patients because the ACR guidance document for the treatment of RA did not include mycophenolate mofetil (72). It is prudent to follow CBC and transaminase levels at monthly intervals as well as checking for lymphadenopathy, fever, and chills clinically in these patients.

Clinical Experience

Rheumatoid Arthritis

Mycophenolate mofetil has been tested for use in RA (38), but limited data on efficacy have been published. In a randomized controlled trial of 217 patients, 1 g twice a day was superior to placebo in reducing the painful joint count and investigator global score ($p < 0.5$). Consequently, a 9-month trial comparing 178 patients in each of two groups, one given 1 g twice a day and the other 2 g twice a day orally was performed. Although only published in abstract form, the lower dose was better tolerated, and both dosages were minimally efficacious, showing ACR 20% improvement (ACR20) responses of 29.3% and 37.1%, respectively (184). Adverse events leading to discontinuation occurred in 15% and 25% of the two groups, respectively. The reported adverse events were primarily nausea, diarrhea, and dyspepsia. However, three deaths occurred in this trial that were thought to be unrelated to study medication. In a long-term safety study, only lymphopenia among blood tests was appreciably common, occurring in 20% of patients on at least one occasion (183). Subsequent trials in RA have not been reported, nor has a manuscript been published reporting these initial data.

Systemic Lupus Erythematosus

Experimental models of lupus nephritis (see Chapter 73) have shown that mycophenolate mofetil retards renal disease, and small series and case reports and abstracts highlight this medication's use for several manifestations of SLE (35,185,186) (see Chapter 74). A one-year randomized controlled trial examined the effects of mycophenolate mofetil in lupus nephritis (34). Patients with class IV nephritis were given either mycophenolate mofetil and steroids or cyclophosphamide for 6 months with steroids followed by AZA. Both groups had a reduction in proteinuria and stabilization of their serum creatinine. Long-term results are not available, but a trend toward loss of efficacy in the mycophenolate mofetil group has been suggested (35).

Case reports suggest that mycophenolate mofetil may be useful for treating cutaneous forms of SLE. In particular, subacute cutaneous lupus erythematosus (SCLE) may be responsive to mycophenolate mofetil (187). In summary, mycophenolate mofetil has been successful in treating some RA and SLE patients. Although it is reasonably well tolerated, its expense and lack of substantial long-term data limits its use at this time. Currently, it may be best thought of as an alternative to AZA for patients who cannot for one reason or another use AZA.

Miscellaneous

Efficacy of mycophenolate mofetil for the treatment of psoriatic arthritis, PM, and vasculitis has been reported (188).

Summary

AZA and mycophenolate mofetil are effective treatments for several rheumatic diseases. AZA may be helpful for patients with inflammatory polyarthritis, autoimmune hepatitis, SCLE and SLE, PM, or systemic vasculitis, whereas mycophenolate mofetil seems most useful for SCLE and SLE. The efficacy and toxicity of AZA in RA appear to be similar to that seen with other classical DMARDs, but its efficacy is likely less than that of the modern biologic agents. Head-to-head studies need be performed to clarify this issue. Regular monitoring for use of AZA, including genotyping of patients, is required to minimize potentially serious adverse drug events. The carcinogenicity of AZA is hotly debated and is still under active investigation, but the overall risk for rheumatic patients appears low. Less is known about the long-term consequences of mycophenolate mofetil use, but the initial results suggest that it offers some safety advantages over AZA, especially for the treatment of SLE.

CALCINEURIN INHIBITION

Historical Overview

Cyclosporine, tacrolimus (also known as FK506), and sirolimus (also known as rapamycin) (Fig. 41.3) have been critical in the development of successful organ transplantation. Preventing the rejection of allograft organs in transplant recipients through the immunosuppressive actions of these drugs has been a major advance and remains their principal

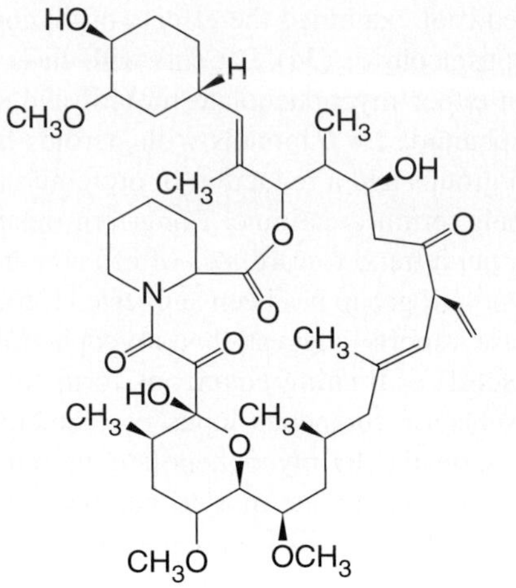

Tacrolimus

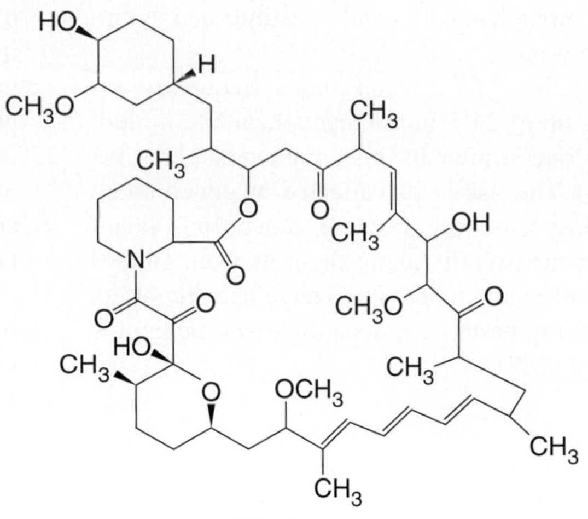

Sirolimus

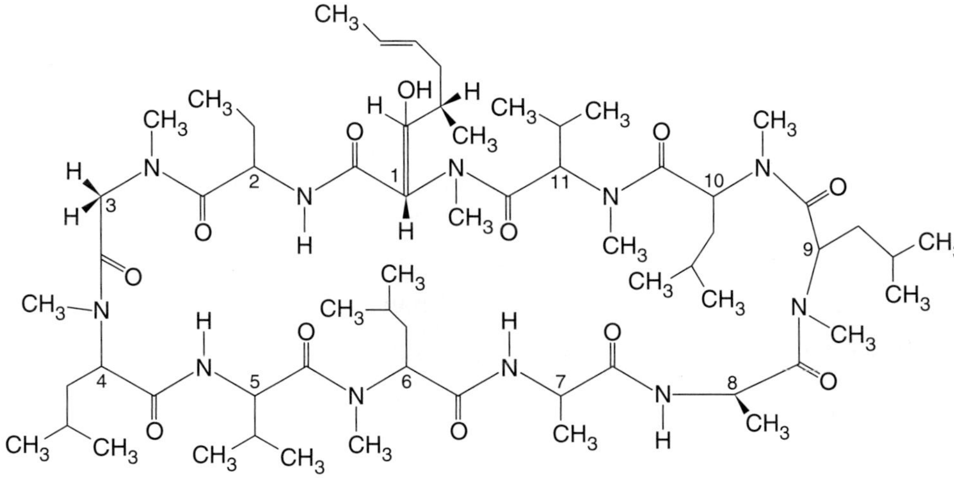

Cyclosporine

FIG. 41.3. Chemical structures of cyclosporine, tacrolimus, and sirolimus. (Modified from Sigal NH, Dumont FJ. Cyclosporin A, FK-506, and rapamycin: pharmacologic probes of lymphocyte signal transduction. *Annu Rev Immunol* 1992;10:519–560, with permission.)

use in clinical practice. Extensive experience during organ transplantation has provided useful information on the pharmacology, safety profile, mechanisms of action, and efficacy of these agents. Because of their immunosuppressive action, these drugs have also been evaluated in animal models and human rheumatic diseases.

Cyclosporine has an important, but limited, role in the treatment of rheumatic diseases. Both cyclosporine (189–196) and tacrolimus (197,198) have been demonstrated to be effective in the treatment of rheumatic diseases, and cyclosporine has been approved by the FDA for the treatment of RA (199). In addition to RA, cyclosporine has also been evaluated in patients with a variety of other rheumatic and autoimmune diseases to a much greater extent than either tacrolimus or sirolimus. Tacrolimus has been demonstrated to be effective in RA (197,198), but has limited clinical data on its use in other rheumatic diseases, and it has not been approved by the FDA for any indication other than prophylaxis against organ rejection (200). Sirolimus has demonstrated efficacy in animal models of arthritis (201), but human trials are not yet reported. As with tacrolimus, sirolimus in currently only approved by the FDA for prophylaxis against transplanted organ rejection (202).

In addition to their efficacy in organ transplantation management, all three drugs have the common features of being products from fungi, that operate on T cells to exert their effects, and to reduce T-cell cytokine production. Although the exact mechanism of action for each agent differs (each drug's mechanism is discussed below), their effects result from drug binding to a cytosolic protein, or immunophilin, specific for each agent (203) (see Fig. 41.4). The net result of these binding processes is to reduce T-cell cytokine secretion and T-cell proliferation. The differences and similarities in mechanism between the three agents produce common challenges and specific advantages and disadvantages. For example, each agent produces significant

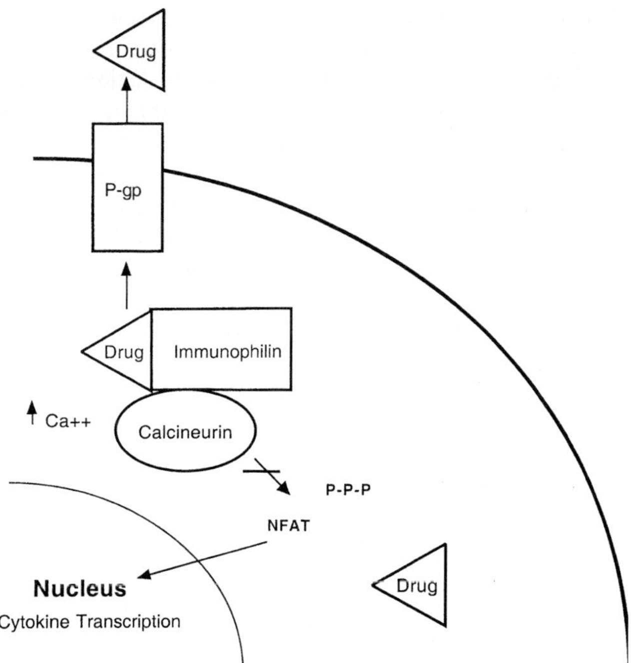

FIG. 41.4. Mechanism of calcineurin inhibitors. Medications of this family act by binding to an immunophilin specific for each drug. The drug–immunophilin complex then acts to bind and inactivate calcineurin (CyA and tacrolimus), resulting in failure to dephosphorylate NFAT, preventing its access to the nucleus to regulate transcription transcription. Sirolimus also binds to immunophilin to inhibit transcription although through another mechanism. P-glycoprotein acts to pump drug out of the cell. NFAT, nuclear factor of active T cells.

immunosuppression with associated risks for infection by impacting the common final pathways of T-cell cytokine expression, while at the same time each agent has different safety profiles on the basis of the drug's specific binding and other pharmacologic characteristics.

Cyclosporine

Pharmacology

Pharmacokinetics

Cyclosporine is a metabolite of the fungus *Beauveria nivea.* Two preparations of oral cyclosporine are produced commercially, Neoral (Novartis Pharmaceuticals, East Hanover, NJ, U.S.A.) (199), a microemulsion formulation, and Sandimmune (Novartis Pharmaceuticals) (204), an oil-based compound. The Neoral preparation immediately forms a microemulsion on exposure to an aqueous environment. Thus, cyclosporine in the Neoral preparation is generally more bioavailable than the cyclosporine in the Sandimmune preparation (205–207). Because of these differences in pharmacokinetics, Neoral and Sandimmune may not be used interchangeably without considerations to these pharmacokinetic differences and appropriate monitoring. Because the Neoral preparation is the FDA-approved compound for the treatment of RA, the pharmacokinetics of this agent will be discussed.

With oral administration, the absorption of cyclosporine is variable and incomplete (199). This variation in not only seen between individuals, but also within the same patient over time. Peak absorption occurs 1 to 2 hours after oral ingestion. The total area under the curve for oral administration ranges from 20% to 50% in renal transplant patients. Oral absorption is decreased with food. The volume of distribution for cyclosporine is 3 to 5 L/kg, with cyclosporine 90% protein bound. The elimination of cyclosporine from the blood is biphasic, with a terminal half-life of 8.4 hours (range 5–18 hours). Cyclosporine is metabolized by the cytochrome P450 3A enzyme system with over 25 metabolites, and it is eliminated primarily by biliary excretion. Little cyclosporine or its metabolites are excreted in the urine. In addition, mechanisms including the drug efflux pump, P-glycoprotein (P-gp), remove cyclosporine out of cells where it is inactive. Many medications, such as diltiazem, change the activity of this pump, resulting in changes in cyclosporine levels (208).

Potential Drug Interactions

Grapefruit and grapefruit juice affect the metabolism of cyclosporine (209,210). Multiple other agents may alter cyclosporine concentrations (199). For example, substances that inhibit the P450 3A enzyme system, such as several calcium channel blockers, some antifungal agents, erythromycin, clarithromycin (but not azithromycin), glucocorticoid, allopurinol, bromocriptine, danazol, metoclopramide, colchicine, and aminodarone, will increase cyclosporine (199). Several protease inhibitors are known to reduce P450 3A activity, but have not been formally studied with cyclosporine. Several drugs have been noted to decrease cyclosporine concentration, including nafcillin, rifampin, carbamazepine, phenobarbital, phenytoin, octreotide, ticlopidine, and orlistat. A serious interaction with St. John's Wort is reported, with marked reduction in cyclosporine blood levels and associated graft rejection in transplantation patients (211).

The coadministration of nonsteroidal antiinflammatory agents (NSAIDs) and cyclosporine should be given special attention. Both of these agents are known to have impact on renal physiology, and an additive decrease in renal function has been seen with the coadministration of naproxen and sulindac with cyclosporine (199). A study comparing the effects of adding either acetaminophen to indomethacin, ketoprofen, and sulindac to cyclosporine therapy did not detect a clinically significant change in renal function in RA patients treated with current NSAIDs and cyclosporine (212).

In addition to changes in cyclosporine level through drug interactions, cyclosporine has been noted to alter the metabolism of comedications. An increase in diclofenac blood levels has been observed in patients taking concurrent cyclosporine (199). This observation has been followed with a recommendation that diclofenac levels be reduced in patients receiving cyclosporine. The concurrent administration of cyclosporine with methotrexate has been noted to increase methotrexate levels without a concurrent change in the cyclosporine levels (199) and with no significant change in cyclosporine pharmacokinetics reported (213). Other interactions are reported with prednisolone, digoxin, and lovastatin, which have resulted in increased drug levels for these comedications (199).

Mechanism of Action

Cyclosporine acts on T cells by binding with a 17-kd protein, cyclophilin (203). Cyclophilin is a cytoplasmic binding protein referred to as an interphilin. By binding to cyclophilin (Fig. 41.4), cyclosporine forms a cyclophilin–cyclosporine complex, which inhibits the enzyme calcineurin. Calcineurin plays a key role in many T-cell regulatory functions involving regulatory proteins, signaling pathways, dynamic structural proteins, ion channels, and transcription regulation. This latter effect on transcription appears to be a critical component of cyclosporine's action (214). Multiple cytokine pathways are impacted, with a particularly important influence on interleukin-2 (IL-2) production and resultant T-cell activation (215). Other cytokine pathways involved include IL-3, IL-4, granulocyte-macrophage colony-stimulating factor (GM-CSF), tumor necrosis factor-α (TNF-α) (216), and interferon-γ (IFN-γ (215,217–220). The specifics of these interactions, which involve calcium dependent pathways and activation of specific nuclear transcription factors, are well described (203).

The observation that cyclosporine works through calcineurin inhibition provides the potential that the monitoring of calcineurin phosphatase activity may provide an additional avenue for monitoring cyclosporine therapy (203). If assays to evaluate the cyclosporine function can be developed, the potential exists to better target functional levels of the drug to the highest benefit to risk ratio. These hopes are somewhat limited by the challenges of inconsistent absorption of the oral drug, despite the development of the microemulsion preparation and other efforts to assure constant drug delivery.

Adverse Drug Effects

Renal. The renal adverse events of cyclosporine increase with dose and duration of therapy. Close monitoring of renal function (serum creatinine) and blood pressure are important because accurate measurement of renal function demonstrates a reduction in renal function in most patients receiving cyclosporine (221). In most cases, this renal impact is not clinically significant and is reversible on discontinuation of the drug. Although up to 50% of subjects in clinical trials developed an increase in creatinine, only 7% discontinued cyclosporine because of elevated creatinine (199). When an increase in creatinine is noted, this change most often occurs during the first 2 to 3 months of treatment and often remains stable as the drug in continued for the first year; however, an increase in creatinine may occur over time (222).

Irreversible renal damage is an uncommon but serious complication of cyclosporine therapy. Most information on this adverse event is reported in organ transplantation patients (223–225). The mechanism through which this renal injury develops has not been fully established, but may involve changes in renal blood flow, thromboxane, or endothelin levels (226). Pathologic findings on renal biopsy have included tubular vacuolization, tubular microcalcification, peritubular capillary congestion, arteriolopathy, and the striped form of interstitial fibrosis with tubular atrophy (199).

Hypertension is common during the treatment of RA with cyclosporine. The mechanism is not completely defined, but considered related to the renal effects of the drug. During clinical trials, hypertension was reported in up to 26% of patients and resulted in the discontinuation of therapy in approximately 5% of subjects (199,227). Because of the potential for hyperkalemia, concomitant therapy with potassium-sparing diuretics should be avoided (199,228,229).

Malignancy. Animal studies have suggested a trend for increased malignancies in rats and mice for lymphoma, hepatocellular carcinoma, and pancreatic islet cell adenomas. *In vitro* mutagenesis assays have been negative. During clinical observation in RA and organ transplant patients, the most common increase in malignancies has been non-Hodgkin's lymphoma and skin carcinoma. Although studies of RA patients have failed to show an increase in malignancies (230), an increased incidence of lymphoma and skin cancer has been observed in organ transplant recipients who have been treated with cyclosporine (199,231,232).

Reproductive. Cyclosporine should not be administered to pregnant women or nursing mothers. Cyclosporine has been shown to be toxic to the embryo and fetus in rat and rabbit models at high doses, but no clear evidence in animals models suggests teratogenicity. Limited experience during pregnancy has been reported, with most experience in organ transplantation patients, but good outcomes have been reported in many patients (233,234). Many complications were reported that may be related to the underlying medical conditions or drug effects. The complications include prematurity, low birth weight, preeclampsia, eclampsia, premature labor, abruptio placentae, oligohydramnios, Rh incompatibility, and fetoplacental dysfunction (199).

Other

Serious infections and infection characteristic of immunosuppression have been reported during treatment with cyclosporine (235). Elevation of hepatocellular enzymes and alkaline phosphatase, thrombocytopenia, and microangiopathic hemolytic anemia have been reported (199,236).

Dosing and Drug Monitoring

The initial dosage for RA patients is 2.5 mg/kg/day in two divided doses. If an insufficient clinical response is seen after 8 weeks and the drug is well tolerated, the dosage can be increased by 0.5 to 0.75 mg/kg/day. After 12 weeks the dosage can be increased again, but not to exceed a daily dose of 4 mg/kg. If no clinical benefit is seen after 16 weeks of therapy, cyclosporine should be discontinued (237).

Blood pressure should be monitored at baseline with at least two readings and a baseline creatinine measured. Blood pressure and creatinine should be measured at least every 2 weeks during the first 3 months and then monthly thereafter. These precautions should be repeated with a change in dose or significant change in comedication, which may alter cyclosporine pharmacokinetics such as changes in NSAIDs. If hypertension develops, the dose of cyclosporine should be reduced by 25% to 50%

Blood levels of cyclosporine can be measured and are frequently used in the management of patients with organ transplantation. In general, the monitoring of clinical response, blood pressure, and serum creatinine will be sufficient for management of RA patients and the measurement of cyclosporine blood levels is not routinely performed.

Clinical Experience

Rheumatoid Arthritis

Cyclosporine has been proven effective in RA as both monotherapy and in combination with other DMARDs. Multiple studies with cyclosporine as a single agent have shown efficacy greater than placebo (189–192,194,196, 238) and comparable efficacy to other DMARDs (239–241). These studies have included comparisons to AZA (239,240), D-penicillamine (241), methotrexate (242), leflunomide (242), levamisole (242), and gold (227,243). Efficacy has been demonstrated by improvement of the clinical features of RA and retardation of the progression of erosive disease on radiographs (196,244). A study comparing radiographic progression in RA patients treated with cyclosporine versus gold salts revealed no difference in radiographic progression (227,243). Cyclosporine has also been investigated in combination with other DMARDs, including methotrexate (222,245–247), chloroquine (248), hydroxychloroquine (249), and gold salts (250). These trials have demonstrated significant reduction in the signs and symptoms of RA during treatment using these combinations of DMARDs. However, although the use of the combination of methotrexate and cyclosporine in early RA patients provide more relief initially, the combination was not more efficacious than sulfasalazine alone over the long term (246). These data suggest that a "step up" approach would be a more effective use of these combinations. An attempt to "step down" from combination therapy of methotrexate and cyclosporine to monotherapy was associated with better clinical outcomes in patients assigned to methotrexate monotherapy (247).

Dose ranging studies have been performed and cyclosporine at 1.5 mg/kg/day has not been proven more effective than placebo (221), whereas dosages of over 2.5 mg/kg/day have consistently been efficacious (221). Even at 1.5 mg/kg/day, some renal impairment can be observed (221). Thus, there does not appear to be a cyclosporine dose that is effective in RA without some potential for significant renal impairment. The use of cyclosporine in combination with other DMARDs, although effective, does not appear to allow a lower dose of cyclosporine to be used.

In summary, cyclosporine is an efficacious treatment for RA and approved by the FDA for this indication. The decision to treat RA patients with cyclosporine requires the physician to balance the demonstrated efficacy of this drug with its potential toxicity. With the currently available options for the treatment of RA, cyclosporine is often reserved for patients who have failed traditional DMARDs or biologic agents. The current practice is to initiate treatment with the lowest effective dose followed by close monitoring for adverse events and dose adjustment if the cyclosporine is well tolerated with an increase in dose if required to achieve the desired clinical efficacy.

Topical Cyclosporine for Keratoconjunctivitis Sicca Syndrome

Recent evidence has demonstrated that inflammatory mechanisms are an important component of many dry eye conditions, including Sjögren's syndrome (251). In addition to treatment with artificial tears and lubricants, cyclosporine ophthalmic emulsion has recently been evaluated as a treatment option and has received FDA approval (252–254). The approved dose is one drop of the 0.05% cyclosporine ophthalmic emulsion twice daily. Clinical trials have demonstrated that treatment with two doses (0.05% and 0.1%) of topical cyclosporine is effective in increasing tear production measured by the Schirmer's test and clinical symptoms in patients with dry eye disease, including patients with Sjögren's syndrome (30%) (253). The most common adverse events reported were burning and stinging of the eyes during treatment. No systemic adverse events were noted. The majority of patients had no detectable systemic absorption.

Other Rheumatic Diseases

Current FDA-approved indications for cyclosporine include prophylaxis against organ transplant rejection, RA, and psoriasis. Several other immune-mediated inflammatory diseases have reportedly been responsive to treatment with cyclosporine. Before using cyclosporine for these unapproved indications, the physician and patient should completely evaluate the potential benefits and risks.

Although cyclosporine is approved for the treatment of psoriasis (199), it is not approved for psoriatic arthritis. It has been reported to be effective in uncontrolled trials of psoriatic arthritis, and clinical benefit was noted in the arthritis of patients with psoriatic arthritis included in studies for their psoriatic skin disease (255).

Open trials in patients with SLE have suggested improvement in SLE disease activity scores, antinuclear antibody levels, and steroid use (256–260). Although reductions in creatinine levels have been noted in SLE patients treated with cyclosporine, its use in patients with significant renal disease has been limited because of concern of its potential nephrotoxicity (261).

Case reports and case series have suggested efficacy for cyclosporine treatment of scleroderma (262–265), PM/DM (266–268), Behçet's syndrome (269,270), pyoderma gangrenosum (271–273), vasculitis (274,275), and JCA (276–279). In JCA patients, a particular role for cyclosporine has been suggested for treatment of the macrophage activation syndrome (280–282).

Tacrolimus

Pharmacology

Pharmacokinetics

Tacrolimus is a product of the fungus *Streptomyces tsukubaensis*. The absorption of tacrolimus after oral administration is incomplete and variable, with 20% to 25% bioavailability, and absorption is adversely impacted by food. Peak concentrations develop 1 to 3 hours after administration. The drug is 99% protein bound and well distributed throughout the body. It is metabolized by the cytochrome P450 system, leading to many drug-drug interactions that have also been reported with cyclosporine. Renal excretion is minimal.

Mechanism of Action

The mechanism of action for tacrolimus is similar to that for cyclosporine, except instead of binding to the interphilin cyclophilin, tacrolimus binds to the 12-kd interphilin FK binding protein (FKBP12) (203) (Fig. 41.4). The binding to FKBP12 and tacrolimus leads to a FKBP12–tacrolimus complex that inhibits the enzyme calcineurin in a similar manner to the cyclophilin–cyclosporine complex. Through this mechanism, tacrolimus has an influence on T-cell function and its cytokine products, similar to the actions of cyclosporine.

Adverse Drug Effects

The majority of information on the adverse events associated with tacrolimus have been established during the evaluation of this drug in organ transplant recipients. The safety issues observed during the treatment of rheumatic diseases are described in the clinical experience section (Table 41.2). Many of the adverse events with tacrolimus, particularly renal and hypertensive events, are similar to those seen with cyclosporine. However, the development of glucose intolerance and diabetes are unique adverse effects of tacrolimus.

Drug Monitoring

At the present time tacrolimus is not approved by the FDA for the treatment of rheumatic diseases; consequently, no recommended doses are available. In the double-blind study cited above, the researchers concluded that the optimal dosage for tacrolimus for the treatment of RA is probably between 1 and 3 mg/day (197). Monitoring guidelines and dosing have been developed for the use of this agent in organ transplant recipients. The data are not sufficient to

TABLE 41.2. *Adverse effects of cyclosporine and tacrolimus*

	Cyclosporine	Tacrolimus
Renal		
Renal insufficiency	++[a]	+++[a]
Hypertension	+++[a]	+++
Gastrointestinal		
Hepatotoxicity	++[a]	
Elevated liver enzymes		+++
Gastrointestinal upset	+++[a]	+++
Nausea	++[a]	+++[a]
Vomiting	++	+++
Diarrhea	++[a]	+++[a]
Constipation		+++
Anorexia		++
Oral ulcer	++[a]	
Hematologic		
Anemia		+++
Leukocytosis		+++
Thrombocytopenia	+	+++
Microangiopathic hemolytic anemia	+	
Metabolic		
Hyperkalemia	++	+++
Hyperglycemia		+++
Hyperuricemia		+
Hypomagnesemia		+++
Posttransplantation diabetes		+++
Neurologic		
Headaches	+++[a]	+++
Insomnia		+++
Seizures		
Encephalopathy		
Parethesia		+++
Tremor		+++
Reproductive	+	
Neonatal complication	+++	+++
Breast tenderness	+[a]	
Dermatologic		
Hypertrichosis	+	
Rash		+
Infections		
Bacterial infections	++[a]	+++
Herpes zoster	+[a]	+
Fungal infections	+[a]	
Potential for malignancies		
Lymphoma	+[a]	+
Skin	+	+
Other		
Gingival hyperplasia	+	+
Myocardial hypertrophy		+

[a]Reported during the treatment of rheumatic diseases.
+++, >10%; ++, <10% and >1%; +, <1%.

provide specific recommendations for this drug in the treatment of rheumatic diseases.

Clinical Experience

Published reports of clinical trials with tacrolimus in rheumatic diseases are limited in comparison with the larger experience with cyclosporine. An open-label study (198) and double-blind placebo-controlled trial (197) have reported the efficacy of tacrolimus in RA patients. In the open label study, 12 RA patients who had previously failed multiple DMARDs were treated with tacrolimus at 2 to 6 mg/day. Five patients did not complete the 6-month trial: three were withdrawn for gastrointestinal adverse events, one with chest pain, and one with neuropathic pain. All seven patients who were able to tolerate tacrolimus experienced an ACR20 response, and five patients met ACR50 response criteria.

The double-blind study involved comparison of three daily doses of tacrolimus (1, 3, or 5 mg) to placebo in 268 RA patients who were receiving concomitant weekly methotrexate (197). An ACR20 response was seen in 16% of placebo subjects and 29%, 34% and 50% of the tacrolimus-treated patients with increasing doses. Renal adverse events were also dose dependent. Discontinuation of tacrolimus was required if the serum creatinine increased to over 40% above baseline. The frequency of at least one elevated serum creatinine greater than 40% in the study was 7%, 9%, 19%, and 28% for patients treated with placebo and with 1, 3, and 5 mg tacrolimus daily, respectively. The rate of discontinuation for persistent elevated serum creatinine was 0%, 0%, 3% and 11%, respectively.

Sirolimus

Sirolimus, a metabolite of the fungus *Streptomyces hygroscopicus*, is an immunosuppressive agent given to prevent the rejection of organ transplants. Data in animal models suggest that sirolimus may also be an effective drug for the treatment of rheumatic diseases (201,283), but there are no clinical data to date in humans to support this hypothesis. Of interest, although the immunosuppressive effects of sirolimus are similar to those of cyclosporine and tacrolimus, the mechanism of action is different. Sirolimus binds to FKBP12, as does tacrolimus, but the sirolimus–FKBP12 complex has no impact on calcineurin (203). Rather, the complex binds to another protein, the mammalian target of rapamycin (mTOR), a key regulatory kinase. This complex inhibits the progression of T cells from the G_1 to S phase of the cell cycle, particularly IL-2-mediated T-cell proliferation. Because there is the potential for complimentary actions of sirolimus and cyclosporine, clinical trials of sirolimus in transplant recipients have studied the clinical efficacy of this drug when used in conjunction with cyclosporine and corticosteroids. Currently sirolimus is approved by the FDA for the prophylaxis of organ rejection in patients receiving renal transplants.

Summary

At the time of its initial investigation, cyclosporine was one of the few agents available for the treatment of RA. It offered an important alternative in patients with rheumatic diseases not responsive to other agents. The adverse events, particularly hypertension and renal impairment, and significant cost often limited its use to patients who had been refractory to less toxic and less expensive therapies. With the development of additional DMARDs for the treatment of RA and other rheumatic diseases, the role for cyclosporine has been under evaluation. The addition of these new therapies has reduced the number of RA patients who require cyclosporine therapy. Likewise, the impetus to fully investigate tacrolimus and sirolimus has also been diminished. Despite this overall move toward the use of other DMARDs, cyclosporine remains an important alternative for some patients with RA and other rheumatic diseases.

ALKYLATING AGENTS

Historical Overview

The biologic activity of alkylating agents was first recognized in the late 1800s (284). Nitrogen mustard was first used in the treatment of refractory RA in 1951 (285), and subsequently, cyclophosphamide and chlorambucil were more often used to treat rheumatic diseases. British and American investigators used cyclophosphamide predominantly, whereas chlorambucil was used extensively in France. Although clearly efficacious in several rheumatic diseases, the alkylating agents may produce significant short-term as well as long-term toxicity. Consequently, their role in rheumatic disease therapy remains under scrutiny.

Pharmacology

Pharmacokinetics

Cyclophosphamide is well absorbed after oral ingestion (1). It is an inactive compound that is activated in the liver by action of the cytochrome P450 mixed function oxidase system (1). Some metabolism may occur in the lung or kidney (284). It is first metabolized to 4-hydroxycyclophosphamide, which is in equilibrium steady state with aldophosphamide. Additional oxidation leads to formation of the inactive metabolites 4-ketocyclophosphamide and carboxy-phosphamide, as well as the active metabolites phosphoramide mustard and the toxin acrolein (1). The typical oral dosage is 1 to 2 mg/kg/day. Only 12% to 14% of the drug is bound to plasma proteins (286). Its plasma half-life is 2 to 10 hours, and less than 20% of the drug is excreted unchanged in the urine during the first 24 hours (284). Intravenous cyclophosphamide, often called "pulse cyclophosphamide," is typically given at a dose of 500 to 1,000 mg/m^2 at an interval of weekly to every 3 months, with monthly being the most common. When used intravenously, it undergoes metabolism similar to the oral form, since no significant differences in the levels of metabolites have been measured (287).

Drug interactions with cyclophosphamide appear to be rare, but enhanced cyclophosphamide toxicity during concurrent allopurinol therapy has been reported (288), perhaps secondary to inhibition of hepatic P450 enzymes (289). The activity of the inducible hepatic microsomal enzymes, and therefore the rate of cyclophosphamide metabolism, can be increased by prior exposure to various medications (284) including previous cyclophosphamide therapy (286). These interactions did not have a significant effect on the antineoplastic effects of cyclophosphamide in animal models (290–293). Steroids can inhibit cyclophosphamide metabolism (294), and in animal models, chloroquine has been shown to inhibit DNA repair enzymes, thereby increasing cyclophosphamide toxicity (295,296). However, most drug interactions with cyclophosphamide appear to have little clinical importance.

The pharmacokinetics of chlorambucil are not well defined (297,298). When used orally at dosages of 0.6 to 1.2 mg/kg/day, it is rapidly and almost completely absorbed, with peak plasma concentrations occurring 30 to 70 minutes after ingestion. The drug is extensively protein bound, principally by albumin (297,298). It is metabolized to phenylacetic acid mustard and other metabolites by the liver and exhibits a serum half-life of 1.5 to 1.7 hours (1). Twenty percent to 70% of labeled chlorambucil is excreted in the urine over the first 24 hours as various metabolites, with less than 1% being unchanged chlorambucil (299).

Proposed Mechanisms of Action

Cyclophosphamide and chlorambucil have demonstrated cytotoxic, immunosuppressive, and antiinflammatory properties. They are cytotoxic by virtue of alkylation of various cellular constituents, especially nucleic acids (300). Cyclophosphamide can alkylate even nondividing cellular DNA. The alkylation of guanine in DNA can lead to miscoding, destruction of the purine ring, and inhibition of DNA replication through DNA strand cross-linking (284). Some cell populations may be relatively protected from alkylating agents by having greater oxidative activity or a larger reservoir of protective thiol species (284). Cyclophosphamide can also phosphorylate compounds, which is not true of chlorambucil (301), but it is not clear if this relates to any clinical benefits or toxicities.

In vitro and *in vivo* studies in both animals and humans indicate that alkylating agents may alter immune function. Evaluation of cyclophosphamide *in vitro* is complicated because the compound is itself inactive; therefore, the effects of its active metabolites must be evaluated independently (302). The actions of alkylating agents on the immune system depend on the drug dose, the duration of therapy, and the temporal relationship of drug administration to an immune response. Depletion of lymphoid tissues (303–307), including both T cells and B cells (303,304,306–309) can occur following cyclophosphamide or chlorambucil therapy. Actively dividing cells are most effected by chlorambucil, and differential cytotoxicity for various lymphoid cell populations has been observed for cyclophosphamide (289,303,307,310–312). B cells more than T cells appear to be sensitive to cyclophosphamide (303,307,313). Low-dose cyclophosphamide therapy in children with minimal-change nephropathy is associated with a selective decrease in helper T-cell subsets, which normalize 6 to 12 months after completing pulse cyclophosphamide therapy (314). Cellular immune function can be either enhanced (315–320) or suppressed (304,321–325), depending on the experimental system examined. Enhancement of cellular immunity results from inhibition of suppressor function (319, 320) rather than from a direct enhancing property. Humoral immunity has generally been depressed (323,326–333), although rare examples of enhancement have been reported (334). Many immunologic parameters remain unaltered during cyclophosphamide treatment (335). Antiinflammatory effects of alkylating agents have also been documented (336).

In summary, alkylating agents appear to act principally through cytotoxic effects on the multitude of cell types involved in immune and inflammatory responses. The overall result appears to be both antiinflammatory and immunosuppressive, with decreases in cellular and humoral functions. Rarely, enhancement of the immune system may occur through selective inhibition of suppressor functions.

Adverse Drug Effects

Although alkylating agents are effective in the treatment of many rheumatic diseases, the adverse effects limit their long-term use (Table 41.3). Techniques to reduce toxicity without compromising efficacy have included dose reduction, the use of intermittent intravenous pulse therapy (337,338), and the addition of protective sulfhydryl molecules such as bladder infusions of *N*-acetyl cysteine (339) or oral or intravenous sodium 2-mercaptoethane sulfonate (MESNA) (340–342). Despite these innovations, alkylating agents still exhibit significant toxicities that must be considered in the risk/benefit assessment and reviewed with each patient before their use is considered. Long-term monitoring, even after discontinuation of the alkylating agent, is essential in order to minimize adverse effects in patients receiving these drugs.

TABLE 41.3. *Adverse effects of alkylating agents*

Adverse effect	Frequency
Hematologic	
Leukopenia	+++[a]
Thrombocytopenia	++[a]
Anemia	++[a]
Pancytopenia	+[a]
Eosinophilia	+[a,b]
Gastrointestinal	
Nausea/epigastric pain	+++[a]
Stomatitis	++[a]
Diarrhea	+[a]
Hepatotoxicity with cholestasis	+[a]
Infections	
Pneumonia	+[a]
Septic arthritis	+[a]
Sepsis	+[a]
Herpes zoster	++[a]
Urologic[c]	
Hemorrhagic cystitis	+++[a]
Carcinoma of the bladder	++[a]
Leiomyosarcoma	+
Pulmonary	
Pulmonary fibrosis	+
Pulmonary infiltrates	+[a]
Dermatologic	
Maculopapular rash	+[a]
Hair loss	+++[a]
Urticaria	+
Reproductive	
Male infertility	+++[a]
Ovarian failure	+++[a]
Teratogenicity	+[a]
Potential for malignancies	
Leukemia	++[a]
Lymphomas	++[a]
Solid tumors	+[a]
Chromosomal damage	+++[a]
Miscellaneous	
Impaired water excretion	+
Cardiotoxicity	+
Anaphylaxis	+
Acute oropharyngeal dysesthesias	+
Neuropathy	+[a]
Cutaneous vasculitis	+

[a]Reported during the treatment of rheumatic diseases.
[b]Reported only with chlorambucil.
[c]Reported only with cyclophosphamide.
+++, >10%; ++, <10% and >1%; +, <1%.

Hematologic

Hematologic complications are the most common adverse reactions, requiring either dose adjustment or drug discontinuation during treatment of rheumatic diseases with alkylating agents. Leukopenia (324,343–356), thrombocytopenia (343,344,347,355,357,358), anemia (including aplastic anemia) (344,350,351), pancytopenia (350,351, 359–361), and eosinophilia (344) have been reported. Leukopenia during cyclophosphamide treatment of RA is probably dose dependent (354). The hematologic abnormalities may persist for several months after the drug is stopped (343). Following pulse therapy with cyclophosphamide, blood leukocyte and platelet levels reach a nadir 8 to 12 days after dosing and return to normal in 2 to 3 weeks (362). The precise incidence of these complications is unclear because many investigators adjust the drug dose to maintain "mild leukopenia," generally in the range of 3,000 cells/mm^3 (356).

Deshayes et al. calculated the overall incidence of hematologic complications to be 20% during chlorambucil treatment, including leukopenia in 14%, thrombocytopenia in 8%, anemia in 5%, and pancytopenia in 3% (351). Others have reported the incidence of leukopenia to be as high as 50% (348). Thrombocytopenia and lymphopenia are more common in chlorambucil- than in cyclophosphamide-treated patients, and irreversible bone marrow failure may be also seen (360).

Gastrointestinal

Gastrointestinal upset (347,351–354,363–365), stomatitis (354,365,366), and diarrhea (354,357) are common complications during cyclophosphamide therapy. When given as a pulse, antiemetic therapy is typically required. Mild elevations of liver enzymes and slight impairment of hepatic metabolism are often seen in patients receiving high-dose cyclophosphamide therapy (366), and cholestasis has been reported (367). Additionally, patients with rheumatic diseases who developed hepatic necrosis during cyclophosphamide treatment have been reported (368). All these patients had been previously treated with AZA, and the researchers postulated that this might have predisposed them to develop hepatic injury during treatment with cyclophosphamide. It should be stressed that significant hepatic injury is uncommon. Gastrointestinal reactions are significantly less frequent with chlorambucil use, but nausea and emesis do occur.

Infectious

Significant infections can occur during treatment with alkylating agents (16,344,350,351,361,363,369,370), including pneumonia (346,363,369), septic arthritis (361), and septicemia (344,345,351,359,363,371). When *Pneumocystis carinii* pneumonia develops in patients with connective tissue diseases, these patients are most commonly being treated with both cyclophosphamide and prednisone (371). Herpes zoster frequently complicates treatment of rheumatic disease with cyclophosphamide (16,357,364, 365,372) or chlorambucil (344–347,350,355,356,359,361). The infections are often associated with leukopenia, but they may occur in the absence of peripheral blood abnormalities. A review by Bradley et al. did not find a correlation of infectious complications during cyclophosphamide treatment for vasculitis with leukopenia or concurrent corticosteroid therapy (370).

It is common to provide prophylactic treatment in patients treated with an oral alkylator to protect them from *Pneumocystis carinii* infection. Trimethoprim and sulfamethoxazole or dapsone are the usual recommendations (373–375). Concern over the use of sulfa drugs that may trigger flare-ups in SLE have limited this approach somewhat, and the use of pulse cyclophosphamide may have different prophylaxis requirements.

Urologic

Cyclophosphamide treatment may be complicated by hemorrhagic cystitis (16,331,332,335,346,347), chronic cystitis (376–378), carcinoma of the bladder (379–381), or leiomyosarcoma (382). These complications are probably caused by urinary excretion of the toxic metabolite acrolein (383). Efforts to reduce bladder exposure to this agent include the use of intravenous pulse therapy, abundant hydration, frequent voiding, and the use of agents with sulfhydryl groups to scavenge acrolein (384). The last is most commonly accomplished by coadministering MESNA at 20% of the cyclophosphamide dose, to be repeated at 3, 6, and 9 hours after infusion (385). One needs to be aware that serious allergy to the sulfhydryl component is relatively common. Pulse intravenous cyclophosphamide almost certainly lowers the risk for bladder toxicity as compared with daily oral cyclophosphamide (386).

Although hemorrhagic cystitis can occur in untreated necrotizing vasculitis (387), the occurrence of this complication in a patient receiving cyclophosphamide should prompt discontinuation of the drug. In a recent retrospective review of patients with Wegener's granulomatosis treated principally with oral cyclophosphamide, 50% developed nonglomerular hematuria. Of those with hematuria, 56% presented with microscopic hematuria and 44% had gross hematuria. Most patients did not have symptoms, and urinalysis was the most effective way to identify patients at risk for transitional cancer. Patients need be followed for many years even if their treatment had been stopped because 25% of patients developed hematuria after therapy was discontinued (388). Transitional cell cancer occurred in 5% of treated patients, a rate 31 times higher that the general population. Of note, none of the patients without a history of hematuria developed bladder cancer. The risk was 5% at 10 years after the first dose and 16% at 15 years. Urologic complications have not been reported with chlorambucil therapy. Thus, chlorambucil may offer an alternative therapy for patients whose course was complicated by urologic toxicity.

Pulmonary

Pulmonary fibrosis occurs in some patients receiving combination chemotherapy and has been attributed to both cyclophosphamide (389,390) and chlorambucil (391). However, pulmonary reactions during cyclophosphamide therapy are rare, and those reported in patients with rheumatic disease may have been due to infection or perhaps to the underlying rheumatic disease (353). The recent use of cyclophosphamide to treat active alveolitis in scleroderma adds support to this theory.

Dermatologic

Maculopapular rashes, severe enough to require discontinuing cyclophosphamide (364) or chlorambucil (344,346, 347,351,363), have been infrequently described. Alopecia (346,347,349,361,363,392), especially with cyclophosphamide, and urticaria (393) have also been observed.

Reproductive

Male infertility from alkylating agents results from either toxicity to the germinal epithelium in the seminiferous tubules (394–396) or to Leydig cell dysfunction (397, 398), which may be prolonged (394,395,398). It occurs in 50% to 60% of patients whether treated with pulse or oral therapy (394,399). Patients may become permanently sterile (398), but others have subsequently fathered normal children (400,401). Because recovery of fertility is variable, patients may wish to consider sperm banking before beginning treatment. One preliminary study suggests that administering exogenous testosterone prior to and during therapy with cyclophosphamide was protective of testicular function (399).

Ovarian failure and amenorrhea are well-documented complications of treatment with cyclophosphamide (352, 353,357,364,402) or chlorambucil (344,346,347,351). Ovarian fibrosis and follicular destruction often lead to permanent infertility. The rate of failure is closely related to the age of the woman, because increasing age portends a much higher risk (402). The use of pulse intravenous cyclophosphamide may produce less ovarian failure than daily oral treatment (403). Attempts to minimize ovarian toxicity have included giving pulse therapy at the time of the menses, inhibiting pituitary gonadotropins (403), and using oral contraceptives (398). To date, none of these has proven effective.

The teratogenic potential of cyclophosphamide and chlorambucil are not well defined, largely because most patients undergoing treatment with alkylating agents generally avoid pregnancies. However, chromosomal damage has been shown in RA patients receiving cyclophosphamide (404,405) and chlorambucil (404). The chromosomal damage may be less prominent with chlorambucil (406). Fetal abnormalities have been reported after treatment with oral and intravenous cyclophosphamide (407–411) and chlorambucil (412). Renal agenesis is the finding most often associated with chlorambucil use during pregnancy, whereas limb abnormalities are most common in cyclophosphamide (413). There have been reports of normal pregnancies after cyclophosphamide treatment as well (106,414,415).

Malignancy

The potential for induction of malignancies by alkylating agents is supported by reports of leukemia (117,343,350, 358,416–423), lymphoma (389,418,424,425), solid tumors (350,416,425), and chromosomal damage (405,406,426,427) in patients receiving these drugs. One case control and two cohort studies have evaluated the development of malignancies in RA patients receiving cyclophosphamide. A fourfold increase of solid tumors and a 16-fold increase in the incidence of lymphoreticular malignancy were observed in the patients who had received cyclophosphamide, compared with patients not receiving the drug (425). Another report of 39 RA patients receiving chlorambucil identified malignancies in 8 patients compared with only one malignancy in 30 control patients receiving AZA or 6-MP ($p < 0.03$) (426). A third study comparing 119 RA patients receiving cyclophosphamide to 119 matched controls, also found an increased risk of malignancy ($p < 0.01$), with the increased rate persisting over the entire 13 years of analysis (427).

Fewer data concerning induction of malignancy in patients given pulse intravenous cyclophosphamide are available. However, it appears to substantially reduce the incidence of hematopoietic-based tumors and to decrease the risk for bladder cancer.

Chlorambucil has been shown to be leukemogenic and seems to demonstrate a clear dose dependency to the relationship (301). It is thought that a course of less than 1 g is relatively safe in adults, but not so in children. Both solid and cutaneous tumors, as well as hematologic malignancies, have been reported in RA patients treated with chlorambucil (426). Similar problems have been observed in children treated for JCA (428). Thirty-eight deaths, including 15 malignancies (seven patients with lymphoma or leukemia), were reported in one series of 131 RA patients receiving chlorambucil between 1965 and 1973 (350). The prevalence of leukemia in 1,612 RA patients receiving chlorambucil was estimated at 0.74% (417).

The data strongly suggest that both cyclophosphamide and chlorambucil increase the risk for malignancy. This risk should be discussed with all patients before initiation of alkylating agents.

Miscellaneous

Rare complications reported with the use of cyclophosphamide include water retention (429), cardiac toxicity (362,430), anaphylaxis (431,432), acute oropharyngeal dysesthesias (433), neuropathy (434), and an acute hypersensitivity reaction (435). Although often used to treat severe vasculitis, cutaneous vasculitis resulting from cyclophosphamide therapy has been reported during the treatment of malignancy (436). Chlorambucil has been rarely associated with toxic epidermal necrolysis, pneumonitis (391,437), confusion, seizures, and drug fever.

Drug Monitoring

Both cyclophosphamide and chlorambucil require monitoring of CBCs and platelet counts every 1 to 2 weeks at the beginning of therapy and at least every 1 to 3 months throughout therapy (438). Patients receiving pulse intravenous cyclophosphamide should be monitored for leukopenia 8 to 12 days after treatment. They should also be instructed to maintain a high urine volume and frequent voiding and should be monitored for the development of cystitis using regular urinalyses. The ideal frequency for urinalysis is unknown, but it should probably be performed at least every 3 months while receiving cyclophosphamide. Urinalysis or urine cytologies should be continued every 6 to 12 months for years after discontinuation (438). Some recommend consideration of cystoscopy every 1 to 2 years (388). Measurement of liver function tests at baseline also seems appropriate, with repeated evaluation at 1 month and then every 3 to 6 months thereafter. Clinical evaluation should include inquiries regarding gastrointestinal upset, stomatitis, fever, hematuria, lymphadenopathy, and skin rash.

Clinical Experience

Cyclophosphamide and chlorambucil are approved by the FDA only for the treatment of malignancies. No alkylating agents are approved for the treatment of rheumatic disease. Some physicians have suggested that all patients with rheumatic disease receiving these cytotoxic agents should give informed consent before their administration. A thorough clinical evaluation should be conducted to ensure that the potential risks of this therapy are justified and minimized.

Rheumatoid Arthritis

Multiple uncontrolled (285,343,352,364) and controlled (354,357,365) trials have evaluated cyclophosphamide and chlorambucil therapy in RA patients. Clinical improvement, defined by diverse outcomes, occurred in 48% to 94% of patients (343). The daily dose of cyclophosphamide used in RA is generally 1 to 2 mg/kg. No difference in clinical benefit in patients treated with 75 mg/day versus 150 mg/day was shown (354), but a trend toward increased toxicity was observed in patients receiving the higher dose. Intravenous pulse cyclophosphamide alone in refractory RA did not result in significant clinical improvement (439,440).

Chlorambucil dosages range from 0.03 to 0.3 mg/kg/day, with the dose frequently adjusted to maintain mild leukopenia (343). Reduction in erythrocyte sedimentation rate (345,355,441) and rheumatoid factor (324,355,441), and healing of erosions (442) have been reported during the use of alkylating agent therapy. Because of their carcinogenicity, alkylating agents are rarely used to treat RA.

Systemic Lupus Erythematosus

Both cyclophosphamide (16,17,19,21,23,443,444) and chlorambucil (445) have been used to treat patients with SLE, especially those with glomerulonephritis (see Chapter 73). NIH studies have shown that progression to end-stage renal failure is reduced in patients receiving cytotoxic drugs in addition to corticosteroids as compared with patients receiving steroids alone (17,19,21,23,446,447). Pulse intravenous cyclophosphamide not only appears to be the most effective treatment for maintaining renal function, but also results in cost savings through prevention of dialysis and the reduced need for renal transplantation (448).

Pulse intravenous therapy has been used in a variety of dosages and schedules. Most regimens consist of intravenous cyclophosphamide (0.5–1.0 g/m^2) (443,444,449,450) given every 1 to 3 months with subsequent maintenance therapy (451), although weekly treatments at lower doses have also been advocated (452). Blood counts are obtained 8 to 12 days postinfusion to adjust subsequent doses in order to limit hematologic toxicity. A decrease in both B- and T-cell populations occurs, with B cells returning toward pretreatment levels more rapidly than T cells (443,444). In the early 1970s one report suggested that the use of cyclophosphamide without concurrent steroids in SLE was ineffective (353). More recently, a study compared pulse methylprednisolone to the combination of methylprednisolone and cyclophosphamide and to cyclophosphamide alone (385). The treatment groups induced renal remission in 29%, 85%, and 62%, respectively, clearly documenting the superiority of cyclophosphamide-containing regimens. Intermittent intravenous cyclophosphamide has also been used successfully in children with SLE nephritis; however, the long-term effects of this therapy in children are unknown (449). The use of plasmapheresis combined with pulse intravenous cyclophosphamide has been reported to be an especially effective treatment for severe SLE (453–455). For example, initial reports in 14 patients revealed that 8 of them were in "long-term stable remission" (456). However, long-term follow-up has highlighted an increased risk for mortality with this aggressive approach. A similarly aggressive approach using very high doses of cyclophosphamide as part of a conditioning regimen for subsequent autologous stem cell transplantation has recently been described for the treatment of SLE with some success (457). As a consequence of these early reports, other groups have tried higher than usual doses of cyclophosphamide in patients without subsequent stem cell transplantation. Encouraging results in patients with severe SLE have been noted (458).

Other manifestations of SLE, including autoimmune thrombocytopenia (459,460), aplastic anemia (461), vasculitis (462), transverse myelitis (463), neuropsychiatric lupus (464,465), massive pulmonary hemorrhage (466), interstitial pneumonitis (467), BOOP (468), pulmonary hypertension (469), and pneumatosis intestinalis (462), have also been successfully treated with pulse intravenous cyclophosphamide.

Vasculitis

Wegener's granulomatosis (see Chapter 84), a previously fatal disease, is suppressed predictably with cyclophosphamide. Long-term remissions are often obtained, and survival is clearly superior to that achieved with prednisone therapy alone (470). However, cyclophosphamide treatment failures have also been reported (174,471). Polyarteritis nodosa (181,472), Takayasu's arthritis (473) Churg-Strauss syndrome (176), systemic necrotizing vasculitis (173), and RA vasculitis (474) have all been effectively treated with cyclophosphamide, generally in combination with 0.5 to 1 mg/kg/day prednisone or equivalent corticosteroids.

The current question is whether the increased safety observed with intravenous pulse therapy should replace the traditional efficacy of oral cyclophosphamide for treatment of these disorders. One study partially addresses this by randomly assigning 50 patients with Wegener granulomatosis, all of whom were first treated with pulse therapy in combination with steroids, to continued oral or pulse maintenance therapy (475). Significantly fewer infectious complications occurred in the pulse intravenous group (40.7 vs. 69.6%), but more relapses of disease were seen than in the oral treatment group. Unfortunately, both groups had a higher mortality rate than expected, perhaps relating to the pulse induction. Of note, changing to oral therapy rescued patients who had failed pulse therapy, but none that failed oral therapy were successfully rescued by pulse therapy.

Systemic Sclerosis

Effective treatment of scleroderma with cyclophosphamide has been reported (405,476), but the use of cyclophosphamide for active scleroderma pulmonary disease is perhaps the most promising. Small pilot trials using oral or pulse therapy have shown beneficial effects on pulmonary disease progression (477–479), and an NIH-sponsored double-blind multicenter trial of oral cyclophosphamide versus placebo for the treatment of scleroderma pulmonary alveolitis is currently in progress. One small randomized controlled trial in patients with cryptogenic fibrosing alveolitis failed to show any benefit (480). Similarly, a 3-year placebo-controlled trial failed to show improvement using chlorambucil (481). Unfortunately, these trials have been small and lacking controls in some cases so that definitive recommendations are not yet possible.

Miscellaneous

Alkylating agents have been used to treat inflammatory muscle disease (353,482–487), as well as the interstitial lung disease associated with PM (488), essential mixed cryoglobulinemia (489), Behçet's syndrome (369,490,491), Goodpasture syndrome (492), Henoch-Schönlein purpura (493), and adult Still disease (494). Data are insufficient to predict results for any of these conditions. Cyclophosphamide has been used to treat JCA (495–498), and a very small pilot study has added pulse intravenous therapy to standard methotrexate (499). The researchers suggest that pulse intravenous cyclophosphamide added to methotrexate adds significantly to the treatment of severe cases of JCA.

Summary

Alkylating agents are often effective in suppressing disease activity in RA, SLE, systemic vasculitis, and (possibly) other rheumatic conditions. Toxic reactions, although common and often dose related, usually resolve after the drug is discontinued. The carcinogenicity of these agents is significant, and the risk continues for years after treatment has been discontinued, which dampens initial enthusiasm for their use in therapy of nonlethal diseases. Wegener granulomatosis, scleroderma lung disease, severe SLE (especially cerebritis and lupus nephritis), and aggressive necrotizing vasculitis represent diseases with such a grim prognosis that the potential benefit offered by alkylating agents justifies their continued use despite these risks. Efforts to improve safety may result in an enhanced applicability to rheumatic disease.

ACKNOWLEDGMENTS

This work was supported by the Vallois Egbert Foundation, Arthritis Foundation, and Veterans Affairs Medical Research.

REFERENCES

1. Chabner BA, Allegra CJ, Curt GA, et al. Antineoplastic agents. In: Hardman JG, Limbird LE, eds. *The pharmacological basis of therapeutics,* 9th ed. New York: McGraw-Hill, 1996:1233–1287.
2. Myles A. 6-Mercaptopurine (6MP) in the treatment of rheumatoid arthritis and related conditions. *Ann Rheum Dis* 1965;24:179–180.
3. Elion GB. Symposium on immunosuppressive drugs. Biochemistry and pharmacology of purine analogues. *Fed Proc* 1967;26:898–904.
4. Lorenzen I, Videbaek A. Treatment of connective tissue diseases with cytostatics. 6-mercaptopurine and azathioprine. *Ugeskr Laeger* 1965; 127:1531–1536.
5. Corley CC Jr, Lessner HE, Larsen WE. Azathioprine therapy of "autoimmune" diseases. *Am J Med* 1966;41:404–412.
6. Harris J, Jessop JD, Chaput de Saintonge DM. Further experience with azathioprine in rheumatoid arthritis. *BMJ* 1971;4:463–464.
7. Mason M, Currey HL, Barnes CG, et al. Azathioprine in rheumatoid arthritis. *BMJ* 1969;1:420–422.
8. Philips VK, Bergen W, Rothermich NO. Azathioprine therapy in twenty-five patients with rheumatoid arthritis. *Arthritis Rheum* 1967; 10:305.
9. Levy J, Paulus HE, Barnett EV, et al. A double-blind controlled evaluation of azathioprine treatment in rheumatoid arthritis and psoriatic arthritis. *BMJ* 1972;4:463–464.
10. Urowitz MB, Gordon DA, Smythe HA, et al. Azathioprine in rheumatoid arthritis. A double-blind, cross over study. *Arthritis Rheum* 1973; 16:411–418.
11. Urowitz MB, Hunter T, Bookman AAM. Azathioprine in rheumatoid arthritis: a double-blind study comparing full dose to half dose. *J Rheumatol* 1974;1:274–281.
12. Hunter T, Urowitz MB, Gordon DA, et al. Azathioprine in rheumatoid arthritis: a long-term follow-up study. *Arthritis Rheum* 1975;18: 15–20.
13. Pinals RS. Azathioprine in the treatment of chronic polyarthritis: longterm results and adverse effects in 25 patients. *J Rheumatol* 1976; 3:140–144.
14. DeSilva M, Hazleman BL. Long-term azathioprine in rheumatoid arthritis: a double-blind study. *Ann Rheum Dis* 1981;40:560–563.
15. Thompson PW, Kirwan JR, Barnes CG. Practical results of treatment with disease-modifying antirheumatoid drugs. *Br J Rheumatol* 1985; 24:167–175.
16. Austin HAD, Klippel JH, Balow JE, et al. Therapy of lupus nephritis. Controlled trial of prednisone and cytotoxic drugs. *N Engl J Med* 1986;314:614–619.
17. Steinberg AD, Decker JL. A double-blind controlled trial comparing cyclophosphamide, azathioprine and placebo in the treatment of lupus glomerulonephritis. *Arthritis Rheum* 1974;17:923–937.
18. Sztejnbok M, Stewart A, Diamond H, et al. Azathioprine in the treatment of systemic lupus erythematosus. A controlled study. *Arthritis Rheum* 1971;14:639–645.
19. Decker JL, Klippel JH, Plotz PH, et al. Cyclophosphamide or azathioprine in lupus glomerulonephritis. A controlled trial: results at 28 months. *Ann Intern Med* 1975;83:606–615.
20. Decker JL, Steinberg AD, Reinertsen JL, et al. NIH conference. Systemic lupus erythematosus: evolving concepts. *Ann Intern Med* 1979;91:587–604.
21. Dinant HJ, Decker JL, Klippel JH, et al. Alternative modes of cyclophosphamide and azathioprine therapy in lupus nephritis. *Ann Intern Med* 1982;96:728–736.
22. Cade R, Spooner G, Schlein E, et al. Comparison of azathioprine, prednisone, and heparin alone or combined in treating lupus nephritis. *Nephron* 1973;10:37–56.
23. Carette S, Klippel JH, Decker JL, et al. Controlled studies of oral immunosuppressive drugs in lupus nephritis. A long-term follow-up. *Ann Intern Med* 1983;99:1–8.
24. Tsokos GC, Caughman SW, Klippel JH. Successful treatment of generalized discoid skin lesions with azathioprine. Its use in a patient with systemic lupus erythematosus. *Arch Dermatol* 1985;121:1323–1325.
25. Bunch TW, Worthington JW, Combs JJ, et al. Azathioprine with prednisone for polymyositis. A controlled, clinical trial. *Ann Intern Med* 1980;92:365–369.
26. Bunch TW. Prednisone and azathioprine for polymyositis: long-term followup. *Arthritis Rheum* 1981;24:45–48.
27. Benson MD, Aldo MA. Azathioprine therapy in polymyositis. *Arch Intern Med* 1973;132:447–451.
28. McFarlin DE, Griggs RC. Treatment of inflammatory myopathics with azathioprine. *Trans Am Neurol Assoc* 1968;93:244–246.
29. Mycophenolate mofetil for the treatment of a first acute renal allograft rejection: three-year follow-up. The Mycophenolate Mofetil Acute Renal Rejection Study Group. *Transplantation* 2001;71:1091–1097.
30. Behrend M. Mycophenolate mofetil: suggested guidelines for use in kidney transplantation. *Biodrugs* 2001;15:37–53.
31. Di Maria L, Bertoni E, Rosati A, et al. Mycophenolate mofetil (MMF) in the treatment of chronic renal rejection. *Clin Nephrol* 2000;53: 33–34.
32. Mele TS, Halloran PF. The use of mycophenolate mofetil in transplant recipients. *Immunopharmacology* 2000;47:215–245.
33. Austin HA, Balow JE. Treatment of lupus nephritis. *Semin Nephrol* 2000;20:265–276.
34. Chan TM, Li FK, Tang CS, et al. Efficacy of mycophenolate mofetil in patients with diffuse proliferative lupus nephritis. Hong Kong-Guangzhou Nephrology Study Group. *N Engl J Med* 2000;343:1156–1162.
35. Mok CC, Lai KN. Mycophenolate mofetil in lupus glomerulonephritis. *Am J Kidney Dis* 2002;40:447–457.
36. Hachulla E. Dermatomyositis and polymyositis: clinical aspects and treatment. *Ann Med Interne (Paris)* 2001;152:455–464.
37. Schiff M. Emerging treatments for rheumatoid arthritis. *Am J Med* 1997;102(suppl):11–15.

38. Goldblum R. Therapy of rheumatoid arthritis with mycophenolate mofetil. *Clin Exp Rheumatol* 1993;11(suppl 8):117–119.
39. Clements PJ, Davis J. Cytotoxic drugs: their clinical application to the rheumatic diseases. *Semin Arthritis Rheum* 1986;15:231–254.
40. Bertino JR. Chemical action and pharmacology of methotrexate, azathioprine and cyclophosphamide in man. *Arthritis Rheum* 1973;16: 79–83.
41. Black AJ, McLeod HL, Capell HA, et al. Thiopurine methyltransferase genotype predicts therapy-limiting severe toxicity from azathioprine. *Ann Intern Med* 1998;129:716–718.
42. Leipold G, Schutz E, Haas JP, et al. Azathioprine-induced severe pancytopenia due to a homozygous two-point mutation of the thiopurine methyltransferase gene in a patient with juvenile HLA-B27-associated spondylarthritis. *Arthritis Rheum* 1997;40:1896–1898.
43. LePage GA. Incorporation of 6-thioguanine into nucleic acids. *Cancer Res* 1960;20:403–408.
44. Coffey JJ, White CA, Lesk AB, et al. Effect of allopurinol on the pharmacokinetics of 6-mercaptopurine (NSC 755) in cancer patients. *Cancer Res* 1972;32:1283–1289.
45. Bach JF, Dardenne M. Serum immunosuppressive activity of azathioprine in normal subjects and patients with liver diseases. *Proc R Soc Med* 1972;65:260–263.
46. Ware AJ, Luby JP, Hollinger B, et al. Etiology of liver disease in renal-transplant patients. *Ann Intern Med* 1979;91:364–371.
47. Maddocks JL. Clinical pharmacological observations on azathioprine in kidney transplant patients. *Clin Sci Mol Med* 1978;55:20P.
48. Corominas H, Domenech M, Gonzalez D, et al. Allelic variants of the thiopurine *S*-methyltransferase deficiency in patients with ulcerative colitis and in healthy controls. *Am J Gastroenterol* 2000;95:2313–2317.
49. Coulthard SA, Rabello C, Robson J, et al. A comparison of molecular and enzyme-based assays for the detection of thiopurine methyltransferase mutations. *Br J Haematol* 2000;110:599–604.
50. McLeod HL, Siva C. The thiopurine *S*-methyltransferase gene locus—implications for clinical pharmacogenomics. *Pharmacogenomics* 2002; 3:89–98.
51. Dubinsky MC, Yang H, Hassard PV, et al. 6-MP metabolite profiles provide a biochemical explanation for 6-MP resistance in patients with inflammatory bowel disease. *Gastroenterology* 2002;122:904–915.
52. Bailey RR. Leukopenia due to a trimethoprim-azathioprine interaction. *N Z Med J* 1984;97:739.
53. Gossmann J, Kachel HG, Schoeppe W, et al. Anemia in renal transplant recipients caused by concomitant therapy with azathioprine and angiotensin-converting enzyme inhibitors. *Transplantation* 1993;56: 585–589.
54. Ensom MH, Chang TK, Patel P. Pharmacogenetics: the therapeutic drug monitoring of the future? *Clin Pharmacokinet* 2001;40:783–802.
55. Schwartz JB. Pharmacogenetics: has it reached the clinic? *J Gend Specif Med* 2002;5:13–18.
56. Colombel JF, Ferrari N, Debuysere H, et al. Genotypic analysis of thiopurine *S*-methyltransferase in patients with Crohn's disease and severe myelosuppression during azathioprine therapy. *Gastroenterology* 2000;118:1025–1030.
57. Ansari A, Hassan C, Duley J, et al. Thiopurine methyltransferase activity and the use of azathioprine in inflammatory bowel disease. *Aliment Pharmacol Ther* 2002;16:1743–1750.
58. Schwab M, Schaffeler E, Marx C, et al. Azathioprine therapy and adverse drug reactions in patients with inflammatory bowel disease: impact of thiopurine *S*-methyltransferase polymorphism. *Pharmacogenetics* 2002;12:429–436.
59. Becher H, Weber M, Lohr GW. Purine nucleotide synthesis in normal and leukemic blood cells. *Klin Wochenschr* 1978;56:275–283.
60. Prince HE, Ettenger RB, Dorey FJ, et al. Azathioprine suppression of natural killer activity and antibody-dependent cellular cytotoxicity in renal transplant recipients. *Transplant Proc* 1984;16:1475–1477.
61. Diasio P. Immunomodulators: Immunosuppressives agents and Immunostimulants. In: Hardman JG, Limbird LE, eds. *The pharmacological basis of therapeutics,* 9th ed. New York: McGraw-Hill, 1996:1291.
62. Al-Safi SA, Maddocks JL. Strength of the human mixed lymphocyte reaction (MLR) and its suppression by azathioprine or 6-mercaptopurine. *Br J Clin Pharmacol* 1985;19:105–107.
63. Abdou NI, Zweiman B, Casella SR. Effects of azathioprine therapy on bone marrow-dependent and thymus-dependent cells in man. *Clin Exp Immunol* 1973;13:55–64.
64. Barrera P, Boerbooms AM, Janssen EM, et al. Circulating soluble tumor necrosis factor receptors, interleukin-2 receptors, tumor necrosis factor alpha, and interleukin-6 levels in rheumatoid arthritis. Longitudinal evaluation during methotrexate and azathioprine therapy. *Arthritis Rheum* 1993;36:1070–1079.
65. Crilly A, McInnes IB, Capell HA, et al. The effect of azathioprine on serum levels of interleukin 6 and soluble interleukin 2 receptor. *Scand J Rheumatol* 1994;23:87–91.
66. Hahn BH, Bagby MK, Hamilton TR, et al. Comparison of therapeutic and immunosuppressive effects of azathioprine, prednisolone and combined therapy in NZB-NZW mice. *Arthritis Rheum* 1973;16:163–170.
67. Berry H, Liyanage S, Durance R, et al. Trial comparing azathioprine and penicillamine in treatment of rheumatoid arthritis. *Ann Rheum Dis* 1976;35:542–543.
68. Dwosh IL, Stein HB, Urowitz MB, et al. Azathioprine in early rheumatoid arthritis. Comparison with gold and chloroquine. *Arthritis Rheum* 1977;20:685–692.
69. Berry H, Liyanage SP, Durance RA, et al. Azathioprine and penicillamine in treatment of rheumatoid arthritis: a controlled trial. *BMJ* 1976;1:1052–1054.
70. Currey HL, Harris J, Mason RM, et al. Comparison of azathioprine, cyclophosphamide, and gold in treatment of rheumatoid arthritis. *BMJ* 1974;3:763–766.
71. Gelfand MC, Steinberg AD, Nagle R, et al. Therapeutic studies in NZB-W mice. I. Synergy of azathioprine, cyclophosphamide and methylprednisolone in combination. *Arthritis Rheum* 1972;15:239–246.
72. Guidelines for the management of rheumatoid arthritis: 2002 Update. *Arthritis Rheum* 2002;46:328–346.
73. Paulus HE, Williams HJ, Ward JR, et al. Azathioprine versus D-penicillamine in rheumatoid arthritis patients who have been treated unsuccessfully with gold. *Arthritis Rheum* 1984;27:721–727.
74. Singh G, Fries JF, Spitz P, et al. Toxic effects of azathioprine in rheumatoid arthritis. A national post- marketing perspective. *Arthritis Rheum* 1989;32:837–843.
75. Woodland J, Chaput de Saintonge DM, Evans SJ, et al. Azathioprine in rheumatoid arthritis: double-blind study of full versus half doses versus placebo. *Ann Rheum Dis* 1981;40:355–359.
76. Wolfe F. The epidemiology of drug treatment failure in rheumatoid arthritis. *Baillieres Clin Rheumatol* 1995;9:619–632.
77. Old CW, Flannery EP, Grogan TM, et al. Azathioprine-induced pure red blood cell aplasia. *JAMA* 1978;240:552–554.
78. Halberg P, Bentzon MW, Crohn O, et al. Double-blind trial of levamisole, penicillamine and azathioprine in rheumatoid arthritis. Clinical, biochemical, radiological and scintigraphic studies. *Dan Med Bull* 1984;31:403–409.
79. Jeurissen ME, Boerbooms AM, van de Putte LB. Pancytopenia related to azathioprine in rheumatoid arthritis. *Ann Rheum Dis* 1988;47:503–505.
80. Nossent JC, Swaak AJ. Pancytopenia in systemic lupus erythematosus related to azathioprine. *J Intern Med* 1990;227:69–72.
81. Verhelst JA, Van den Enden E, Mathys R. Rapidly evolving azathioprine induced pancytopenia. *J Rheumatol* 1987;14:862.
82. Kerstens PJ, Stolk JN, De Abreu RA, et al. Azathioprine-related bone marrow toxicity and low activities of purine enzymes in patients with rheumatoid arthritis. *Arthritis Rheum* 1995;38:142–145.
83. Stolk JN, Boerbooms AM, De Abreu RA, et al. Azathioprine treatment and thiopurine metabolism in rheumatic diseases. Introduction and first results of investigation. *Adv Exp Med Biol* 1998;431:487–493.
84. Decaux G, Horsmans Y, Houssiau F, et al. High 6-thioguanine nucleotide levels and low thiopurine methyltransferase activity in patients with lupus erythematosus treated with azathioprine. *Am J Ther* 2001;8: 147–150.
85. Sebbag L, Boucher P, Davelu P, et al. Thiopurine *S*-methyltransferase gene polymorphism is predictive of azathioprine-induced myelosuppression in heart transplant recipients. *Transplantation* 2000;69:1524–1527.
86. Evans WE, Hon YY, Bomgaars L, et al. Preponderance of thiopurine *S*-methyltransferase deficiency and heterozygosity among patients intolerant to mercaptopurine or azathioprine. *J Clin Oncol* 2001;19: 2293–2301.
87. Decaux G, Prospert F, Horsmans Y, et al. Relationship between red cell mean corpuscular volume and 6-thioguanine nucleotides in patients treated with azathioprine. *J Lab Clin Med* 2000;135:256–262.

88. Guillaume P, Grandjean E, Male PJ. Azathioprine-associated acute pancreatitis in the course of chronic active hepatitis. *Dig Dis Sci* 1984;29:78–79.
89. Kawanishi H, Rudolph E, Bull FE. Azathioprine-induced acute pancreatitis. *N Engl J Med* 1973;289:357.
90. Taft PM, Jones AC, Collins GM, et al. Acute pancreatitis following renal allotransplantation. A lethal complication. *Am J Dig Dis* 1978; 23:541–544.
91. Zarday Z, Veith FJ, Gliedman ML, et al. Irreversible liver damage after azathioprine. *JAMA* 1972;222:690–691.
92. DePinho RA, Goldberg CS, Lefkowitch JH. Azathioprine and the liver. Evidence favoring idiosyncratic, mixed cholestatic-hepatocellular injury in humans. *Gastroenterology* 1984;86:162–165.
93. Jeurissen ME, Boerbooms AM, van de Putte LB, et al. Azathioprine induced fever, chills, rash, and hepatotoxicity in rheumatoid arthritis. *Ann Rheum Dis* 1990;49:25–27.
94. Meys E, Devogelaer JP, Geubel A, et al. Fever, hepatitis and acute interstitial nephritis in a patient with rheumatoid arthritis. Concurrent manifestations of azathioprine hypersensitivity. *J Rheumatol* 1992; 19:807–809.
95. Small P, Lichter M. Probable azathioprine hepatotoxicity: a case report. *Ann Allergy* 1989;62:518–520.
96. Sparberg M, Simon N, del Greco F. Intrahepatic cholestasis due to azathioprine. *Gastroenterology* 1969;57:439–441.
97. Lemley DE, DeLacy LM, Seeff LB, et al. Azathioprine induced hepatic veno-occlusive disease in rheumatoid arthritis. *Ann Rheum Dis* 1989;48:342–346.
98. Munro DD. Azathioprine in psoriasis. *Proc R Soc Med* 1973;66: 747–748.
99. DuVivier A, Munro DD, Verbov J. Treatment of psoriasis with azathioprine. *BMJ* 1974;1:49–51.
100. Bedrossian CW, Sussman J, Conklin RH, et al. Azathioprine-associated interstitial pneumonitis. *Am J Clin Pathol* 1984;82:148–154.
101. Carmichael DJ, Hamilton DV, Evans DB, et al. Interstitial pneumonitis secondary to azathioprine in a renal transplant patient. *Thorax* 1983;38:951–952.
102. Hsue YT, Paulus HE, Coulson WF. Bronchiolitis obliterans organizing pneumonia in polymyositis. A case report with longterm survival. *J Rheumatol* 1993;20:877–879.
103. Wijnands MJ, Perret CM, van Riel PL, et al. Generalized urticarial eruption during azathioprine treatment for rheumatoid arthritis. A case report and review of the literature. *Scand J Rheumatol* 1990; 19:167–169.
104. Sharon E, Jones J, Diamond H, et al. Pregnancy and azathioprine in systemic lupus erythematosus. *Am J Obstet Gynecol* 1974;118: 25–28.
105. Alstead EM, Ritchie JK, Lennard-Jones JE, et al. Safety of azathioprine in pregnancy in inflammatory bowel disease. *Gastroenterology* 1990;99:443–446.
106. Ramsey-Goldman R, Mientus JM, Kutzer JE, et al. Pregnancy outcome in women with systemic lupus erythematosus treated with immunosuppressive drugs. *J Rheumatol* 1993;20:1152–1157.
107. Saarikoski S, Seppala M. Immunosuppression during pregnancy: transmission of azathioprine and its metabolites from the mother to the fetus. *Am J Obstet Gynecol* 1973;115:1100–1106.
108. DeWitte DB, Buick MK, Cyran SE, et al. Neonatal pancytopenia and severe combined immunodeficiency associated with antenatal administration of azathioprine and prednisone. *J Pediatr* 1984;105: 625–628.
109. Cote CJ, Meuwissen HJ, Pickering RJ. Effects on the neonate of prednisone and azathioprine administered to the mother during pregnancy. *J Pediatr* 1974;85:324–328.
110. Leb DE, Weisskopf B, Kanovitz BS. Chromosome aberrations in the child of a kidney transplant recipient. *Arch Intern Med* 1971;128: 441–444.
111. Ramsey-Goldman R, Schilling E. Immunosuppressive drug use during pregnancy. *Rheum Dis Clin North Am* 1997;23:149–167.
112. Armenti VT, Ahlswede KM, Ahlswede BA, et al. National Transplantation Pregnancy Registry: analysis of outcome/risks of 394 pregnancies in kidney transplant recipients. *Transplant Proc* 1994; 26:2535.
113. Ostensen M, Husby G. Antirheumatic drug treatment during pregnancy and lactation. *Scand J Rheumatol* 1985;14:1–7.
114. Seidenfeld AM, Smythe HA, Ogryzlo MA, et al. Acute leukemia in rheumatoid arthritis treated with cytotoxic agents. *J Rheumatol* 1984; 11:586–587.
115. Tilson HH, Whisnant J. Pharmaco-epidemiology—drugs, arthritis, and neoplasms: industry contribution to the data. *Am J Med* 1985;78: 69–76.
116. Pitt PI, Sultan AH, Malone M, et al. Association between azathioprine therapy and lymphoma in rheumatoid disease. *J R Soc Med* 1987;80:428–429.
117. Vasquez S, Kavanaugh AF, Schneider NR, et al. Acute nonlymphocytic leukemia after treatment of systemic lupus erythematosus with immunosuppressive agents. *J Rheumatol* 1992;19:1625–1627.
118. Matteson EL, Hickey AR, Maguire L, et al. Occurrence of neoplasia in patients with rheumatoid arthritis enrolled in a DMARD Registry. Rheumatoid Arthritis Azathioprine Registry Steering Committee. *J Rheumatol* 1991;18:809–814.
119. Kinlen LJ, Sheil AG, Peto J, et al. Collaborative United Kingdom-Australasian study of cancer in patients treated with immunosuppressive drugs. *Br Med J* 1979;2:1461–1466.
120. Hazleman B. Incidence of neoplasms in patients with rheumatoid arthritis exposed to different treatment regimens. *Am J Med* 1985;78: 39–43.
121. Kinlen LJ. Incidence of cancer in rheumatoid arthritis and other disorders after immunosuppressive treatment. *Am J Med* 1985;78: 44–49.
122. Symmons DP, Ahern M, Bacon PA, et al. Lymphoproliferative malignancy in rheumatoid arthritis: a study of 20 cases. *Ann Rheum Dis* 1984;43:132–135.
123. Prior P, Symmons DP, Hawkins CF, et al. Cancer morbidity in rheumatoid arthritis. *Ann Rheum Dis* 1984;43:128–131.
124. Isomaki HA, Mutru O, Koota K. Death rate and causes of death in patients with rheumatoid arthritis. *Scand J Rheumatol* 1975;4:205–208.
125. Prior P. Cancer and rheumatoid arthritis: epidemiologic considerations. *Am J Med* 1985;78:15–21.
126. Symmons DP. Neoplasms of the immune system in rheumatoid arthritis. *Am J Med* 1985;78:22–28.
127. Silman AJ, Petrie J, Hazleman B, et al. Lymphoproliferative cancer and other malignancy in patients with rheumatoid arthritis treated with azathioprine: a 20 year follow up study. *Ann Rheum Dis* 1988; 47:988–992.
128. Lewis P, Hazleman BL, Hanka R, et al. Cause of death in patients with rheumatoid arthritis with particular reference to azathioprine. *Ann Rheum Dis* 1980;39:457–461.
129. Penn I, Halgrimson CG, Starzl TE. *De novo* malignant tumors in organ transplant recipients. *Transplant Proc* 1971;3:773–778.
130. Hoover R, Fraumeni JF Jr. Risk of cancer in renal-transplant recipients. *Lancet* 1973;2:55–57.
131. Fraser AG, Orchard TR, Robinson EM, et al. Long-term risk of malignancy after treatment of inflammatory bowel disease with azathioprine. *Aliment Pharmacol Ther* 2002;16:1225–1232.
132. van Hogezand RA, Eichhorn RF, Choudry A, et al. Malignancies in inflammatory bowel disease: fact or fiction? *Scand J Gastroenterol* 2002;(suppl 236)37:48–53.
133. Fathring MJG, Coxon AY, Sheaff PC. Polyneuritis associated with azathioprine sensitivity reaction. *BMJ* 1980;280:367.
134. Langevitz P, Maguire L, Urowitz M. Accelerated nodulosis during azathioprine therapy. *Arthritis Rheum* 1991;34:123–124.
135. Dodd HJ, Tatnall FM, Sarkany I. Fast atrial fibrillation induced by treatment of psoriasis with azathioprine. *BMJ* 1985;291:706.
136. Fields CL, Robinson JW, Roy TM, et al. Hypersensitivity reaction to azathioprine. *South Med J* 1998;91:471–474.
137. Kruger K, Schattenkirchner M. Comparison of cyclosporin A and azathioprine in the treatment of rheumatoid arthritis—results of a double-blind multicentre study. *Clin Rheumatol* 1994;13:248–255.
138. Suarez-Almazor ME, Spooner C, et al. Azathioprine for treating rheumatoid arthritis. *Cochrane Database Syst Rev* 2000:CD001461.
139. Jeurissen ME, Boerbooms AM, van de Putte LB, et al. Influence of methotrexate and azathioprine on radiologic progression in rheumatoid arthritis. A randomized, double-blind study. *Ann Intern Med* 1991;114:999–1004.
140. Kerstens PJ, Boerbooms AM, Jeurissen ME, et al. Radiological and clinical results of longterm treatment of rheumatoid arthritis with methotrexate and azathioprine. *J Rheumatol* 2000;27:1148–1155.

141. Kruger K. Use of cyclosporin A in chronic polyarthritis and other rheumatic diseases. *Z Rheumatol* 1995;54:89–95.
142. Ahern MJ, Harrison W, Hollingsworth P, et al. A randomised double-blind trial of cyclosporin and azathioprine in refractory rheumatoid arthritis. *Aust N Z J Med* 1991;21:844–849.
143. Sambrook PN, Champion GD, Browne CD, et al. Comparison of methotrexate with azathioprine or 6-mercaptopurine in refractory rheumatoid arthritis: a life-table analysis. *Br J Rheumatol* 1986;25:372–375.
144. Jeurissen ME, Boerbooms AM, van de Putte LB, et al. Methotrexate versus azathioprine in the treatment of rheumatoid arthritis. A forty-eight-week randomized, double-blind trial. *Arthritis Rheum* 1991;34:961–972.
145. Hamdy H, McKendry RJ, Mierins E, et al. Low-dose methotrexate compared with azathioprine in the treatment of rheumatoid arthritis. A twenty-four-week controlled clinical trial. *Arthritis Rheum* 1987;30:361–368.
146. Arnold MH, O'Callaghan J, McCredie M, et al. Comparative controlled trial of low-dose weekly methotrexate versus azathioprine in rheumatoid arthritis: 3-year prospective study. *Br J Rheumatol* 1990;29:120–125.
147. Wilkens RF, Urowitz MB, Strablein DM, et al. Comparison of azathioprine, methotrexate, and the combination of both in the treatment of rheumatoid arthritis. A controlled clinical trial. *Arthritis Rheum* 1993;36:1183–1184.
148. McKendry RJ, Cyr M. Toxicity of methotrexate compared with azathioprine in the treatment of rheumatoid arthritis. A case-control study of 131 patients. *Arch Intern Med* 1989;149:685–689.
149. Kaklamanis P, Vayopoulos G, Stamatelos G, et al. Chronic lupus peritonitis with ascites. *Ann Rheum Dis* 1991;50:176–177.
150. Callen JP, Spencer LV, Burruss JB, et al. Azathioprine. An effective, corticosteroid-sparing therapy for patients with recalcitrant cutaneous lupus erythematosus or with recalcitrant cutaneous leukocytoclastic vasculitis. *Arch Dermatol* 1991;127:515–522.
151. Contreras G, Roth D, Pardo V, et al. Lupus nephritis: a clinical review for practicing nephrologists. *Clin Nephrol* 2002;57:95–107.
152. Zimmerman R, Radhakrishnan J, Valeri A, et al. Advances in the treatment of lupus nephritis. *Annu Rev Med* 2001;52:63–78.
153. McCune J, Singer NG. Immunosuppressive drug treatment. *Curr Opin Rheumatol* 1997;9:191–199.
154. Rastogi H, Deodhar SD, Brown CH. Treatment of lupoid hepatitis with azathioprine. *Cleve Clin Q* 1967;34:97–104.
155. Heuckenkamp PU, Zollner N. On the effect of azathioprine on the course of 3 cases of lupoid hepatitis. *Verh Dtsch Ges Inn Med* 1968;74:897–901.
156. Krawitt EL. Autoimmune hepatitis: classification, heterogeneity, and treatment. *Am J Med* 1994;96(suppl):23–26.
157. Johnson PJ, McFarlane IG, Williams R. Azathioprine for long-term maintenance of remission in autoimmune hepatitis. *N Engl J Med* 1995;333:958–963.
158. Obermayer-Straub P, Strassburg CP, Manns MP. Autoimmune hepatitis. *J Hepatol* 2000;32(suppl 1):181–197.
159. Kanzler S, Lohr H, Gerken G, et al. Long-term management and prognosis of autoimmune hepatitis (AIH): a single center experience. *Z Gastroenterol* 2001;39:339–341, 344–348.
160. Gish RG, Mason A. Autoimmune liver disease. Current standards, future directions. *Clin Liver Dis* 2001;5:287–314.
161. Ramirez G, Asherson RA, Khamashta MA, et al. Adult-onset polymyositis-dermatomyositis: description of 25 patients with emphasis on treatment. *Semin Arthritis Rheum* 1990;20:114–120.
162. Villalba L, Hicks JE, Adams EM, et al. Treatment of refractory myositis: a randomized crossover study of two new cytotoxic regimens. *Arthritis Rheum* 1998;41:392–399.
163. Leff RL, Miller FW, Hicks J, et al. The treatment of inclusion body myositis: a retrospective review and a randomized, prospective trial of immunosuppressive therapy. *Medicine (Baltimore)* 1993;72:225–235.
164. Calin A. A placebo controlled, crossover study of azathioprine in Reiter's syndrome. *Ann Rheum Dis* 1986;45:653–655.
165. Creemers MC, van Riel PL, Franssen MJ, et al. Second-line treatment in seronegative spondylarthropathies. *Semin Arthritis Rheum* 1994;24:71–81.
166. Keat A, Rowe I. Reiter's syndrome and associated arthritides. *Rheum Dis Clin North Am* 1991;17:25–42.
167. Kvien TK, Hoyeraal HM, Sandstad B. Azathioprine versus placebo in patients with juvenile rheumatoid arthritis: a single center double blind comparative study. *J Rheumatol* 1986;13:118–123.
168. Savolainen HA, Kautiainen H, Isomaki H, et al. Azathioprine in patients with juvenile chronic arthritis: a longterm followup study. *J Rheumatol* 1997;24:2444–2450.
169. Goupille P, Soutif D, Valat JP. Treatment of psoriatic arthropathy. *Semin Arthritis Rheum* 1992;21:355–367.
170. Dutz JP, Ho VC. Immunosuppressive agents in dermatology. An update. *Dermatol Clin* 1998;16:235–251.
171. Hacker SM, Ramos-Caro FA, Ford MJ, et al. Azathioprine: a forgotten alternative for treatment of severe psoriasis. *Int J Dermatol* 1992;31:873–874.
172. Jones G, Crotty M, Brooks P. Psoriatic arthritis: a quantitative overview of therapeutic options. The Psoriatic Arthritis Meta-Analysis Study Group. *Br J Rheumatol* 1997;36:95–99.
173. Fauci AS, Katz P, Haynes BF, et al. Cyclophosphamide therapy of severe systemic necrotizing vasculitis. *N Engl J Med* 1979;301:235–238.
174. Brandwein S, Esdaile J, Danoff D, et al. Wegener's granulomatosis. Clinical features and outcome in 13 patients. *Arch Intern Med* 1983;143:476–479.
175. Hall S, Barr W, Lie JT, et al. Takayasu arteritis. A study of 32 North American patients. *Medicine (Baltimore)* 1985;64:89–99.
176. Lanham JG, Elkon KB, Pusey CD, et al. Systemic vasculitis with asthma and eosinophilia: a clinical approach to the Churg-Strauss syndrome. *Medicine (Baltimore)* 1984;63:65–81.
177. DeSilva M, Hazleman BL. Azathioprine in giant cell arteritis/polymyalgia rheumatica: a double- blind study. *Ann Rheum Dis* 1986;45:136–138.
178. Gross WL. New concepts in treatment protocols for severe systemic vasculitis. *Curr Opin Rheumatol* 1999;11:41–46.
179. Labbe P, Hardouin P. Epidemiology and optimal management of polymyalgia rheumatica. *Drugs Aging* 1998;13:109–118.
180. Eroglu Y, Duzovali O, Kavukcu S, et al. Combination of steroid with azathioprine in treatment of giant cell autoimmune hepatitis. *Turk J Pediatr* 1997;39:565–571.
181. Leib ES, Restivo C, Paulus HE. Immunosuppressive and corticosteroid therapy of polyarteritis nodosa. *Am J Med* 1979;67:941–947.
182. CellCept. *Physicians desk reference,* 57th ed. Vol. 1. 2003:2875–2883.
183. Schiff M, Leishman B. Long-term safety of CellCept (mycophenolate mofetil), a new therapy for rheumatoid arthritis. *Arthritis Rheum* 1998;41(suppl):155.
184. Schiff M, Stein G, Leishman B. CellCept (mycophenolate mofetil-MMF). A new treatment for RA: a 9-month randomized double-blind trial comparing 1g bid and 2g bid. *Arthritis Rheum* 1997;97(suppl):194.
185. Mok CC, Ho CT, Chan KW, et al. Outcome and prognostic indicators of diffuse proliferative lupus glomerulonephritis treated with sequential oral cyclophosphamide and azathioprine. *Arthritis Rheum* 2002;46:1003–1013.
186. Mok CC, Ho CT, Siu YP, et al. Treatment of diffuse proliferative lupus glomerulonephritis: a comparison of two cyclophosphamide-containing regimens. *Am J Kidney Dis* 2001;38:256–264.
187. Schanz S, Ulmer A, Rassner G, et al. Successful treatment of subacute cutaneous lupus erythematosus with mycophenolate mofetil. *Br J Dermatol* 2002;147:174–178.
188. Schneider C, Gold R, Schafers M, et al. Mycophenolate mofetil in the therapy of polymyositis associated with a polyautoimmune syndrome. *Muscle Nerve* 2002;25:286–288.
189. van Rijthoven AW, Dijkmans BA, Goei The HS, et al. Cyclosporin treatment for rheumatoid arthritis: a placebo controlled, double blind, multicentre study. *Ann Rheum Dis* 1986;45:726–731.
190. Dougados M, Amor B. Cyclosporin A in rheumatoid arthritis: preliminary clinical results of an open trial. *Arthritis Rheum* 1987;30:83–87.
191. Weinblatt ME, Coblyn JS, Fraser PA, et al. Cyclosporin A treatment of refractory rheumatoid arthritis. *Arthritis Rheum* 1987;30:11–17.
192. Dougados M, Awada H, Amor B. Cyclosporin in rheumatoid arthritis: a double blind, placebo controlled study in 52 patients. *Ann Rheum Dis* 1988;47:127–133.
193. Yocum DE, Klippel JH, Wilder RL, et al. Cyclosporin A in severe, treatment-refractory rheumatoid arthritis. A randomized study. *Ann Intern Med* 1988;109:863–869.

194. Tugwell P, Bombardier C, Gent M, et al. Low-dose cyclosporin versus placebo in patients with rheumatoid arthritis. *Lancet* 1990;335: 1051–1055.
195. Forre O, Group NAS. Cyclosporine as a disease modifier in rheumatoid arthritis [Abstract 198]. Presented at the 2nd Congress on Immunointervention in Autoimmune Diseases, Paris, France, 1991.
196. Forre O. Radiologic evidence of disease modification in rheumatoid arthritis patients treated with cyclosporine. Results of a 48-week multicenter study comparing low-dose cyclosporine with placebo. Norwegian Arthritis Study Group. *Arthritis Rheum* 1994;37:1506–1512.
197. Furst DE, Saag K, Fleischmann MR, et al. Efficacy of tacrolimus in rheumatoid arthritis patients who have been treated unsuccessfully with methotrexate: a six-month, double-blind, randomized, dose-ranging study. *Arthritis Rheum* 2002;46:2020–2028.
198. Gremillion RB, Posever JO, Manek N, et al. Tacrolimus (FK506) in the treatment of severe, refractory rheumatoid arthritis: initial experience in 12 patients. *J Rheumatol* 1999;26:2332–2336.
199. Cyclosporine Neoral. *Physicians desk reference.* 2002.
200. Tacrolimus. *Physicians desk reference.* 2003.
201. Carlson RP, Hartman DA, Tomchek LA, et al. Rapamycin, a potential disease-modifying antiarthritic drug. *J Pharmacol Exp Ther* 1993; 266:1125–38.
202. Sirolimus. *Physician's desk reference.* 2003.
203. Jorgensen KA, Koefoed-Nielsen PB, Karamperis N. Calcineurin phosphatase activity and immunosuppression. A review on the role of calcineurin phosphatase activity and the immunosuppressive effect of cyclosporin A and tacrolimus. *Scand J Immunol* 2003;57: 93–98.
204. Cyclosporine Sandimmune. *Physicians desk reference.* 2002.
205. Yocum DE, Allard S, Cohen SB, et al. Microemulsion formulation of cyclosporin (Sandimmun Neoral) vs Sandimmun: comparative safety, tolerability and efficacy in severe active rheumatoid arthritis. On behalf of the OLR 302 Study Group. *Rheumatology (Oxford)* 2000;39:156–164.
206. Sutherland DE, Gruessner RW, Dunn DL, et al. Lessons learned from more than 1,000 pancreas transplants at a single institution. *Ann Surg* 2001;233:463–501.
207. Anderson IF, Helve T, Hannonen P, et al. Conversion of patients with rheumatoid arthritis from the conventional to a microemulsion formulation of cyclosporine: a double blind comparison to screen for differences in safety, efficacy, and pharmacokinetics. *J Rheumatol* 1999;26:556–562.
208. Endo T, Kimura O, Sakata M. Effects of P-glycoprotein inhibitors on cadmium accumulation in cultured renal epithelial cells, LLC-PK1, and OK. *Toxicol Appl Pharmacol* 2002;185:166–171.
209. Yee GC, Stanley DL, Pessa LJ, et al. Effect of grapefruit juice on blood cyclosporin concentration. *Lancet* 1995;345:955–956.
210. Ioannides-Demos LL, Christophidis N, Ryan P, et al. Dosing implications of a clinical interaction between grapefruit juice and cyclosporine and metabolite concentrations in patients with autoimmune diseases. *J Rheumatol* 1997;24:49–54.
211. Ernst E. St John's Wort supplements endanger the success of organ transplantation. *Arch Surg* 2002;137:316–319.
212. Tugwell P, Ludwin D, Gent M, et al. Interaction between cyclosporin A and nonsteroidal antiinflammatory drugs. *J Rheumatol* 1997;24:1122–1125.
213. Baraldo M, Ferraccioli G, Pea F, et al. Cyclosporine A pharmacokinetics in rheumatoid arthritis patients after 6 months of methotrexate therapy. *Pharmacol Res* 1999;40:483–486.
214. Kronke M, Leonard WJ, Depper JM, et al. Cyclosporin A inhibits T-cell growth factor gene expression at the level of mRNA transcription. *Proc Natl Acad Sci U S A* 1984;81:5214–5218.
215. Sigal NH, Dumont FJ. Cyclosporin A, FK-506, and rapamycin: pharmacologic probes of lymphocyte signal transduction. *Annu Rev Immunol* 1992;10:519–560.
216. Giacomelli R, Cipriani P, Matucci Cerinic M, et al. Combination therapy with cyclosporine and methotrexate in patients with early rheumatoid arthritis soon inhibits TNFalpha production without decreasing TNFalpha mRNA levels. An *in vivo* and *in vitro* study. *Clin Exp Rheumatol* 2002;20:365–372.
217. Herold KC, Lancki DW, Moldwin RL, et al. Immunosuppressive effects of cyclosporin A on cloned T cells. *J Immunol* 1986;136:1315–1321.
218. Tocci MJ, Matkovich DA, Collier KA, et al. The immunosuppressant FK506 selectively inhibits expression of early T cell activation genes. *J Immunol* 1989;143:718–726.
219. Kim WU, Cho ML, Kim SI, et al. Divergent effect of cyclosporine on Th1/Th2 type cytokines in patients with severe, refractory rheumatoid arthritis. *J Rheumatol* 2000;27:324–331.
220. Ferraccioli G, Falleti E, De Vita S, et al. Circulating levels of interleukin 10 and other cytokines in rheumatoid arthritis treated with cyclosporin A or combination therapy. *J Rheumatol* 1998;25:1874–1879.
221. Altman RD, Schiff M, Kopp EJ. Cyclosporine A in rheumatoid arthritis: randomized, placebo controlled dose finding study. *J Rheumatol* 1999;26:2102–2109.
222. Stein CM, Pincus T, Yocum D, et al. Combination treatment of severe rheumatoid arthritis with cyclosporine and methotrexate for forty-eight weeks: an open-label extension study. The Methotrexate-Cyclosporine Combination Study Group. *Arthritis Rheum* 1997;40: 1843–1851.
223. Palestine AG, Austin HA 3rd, Balow JE, et al. Renal histopathologic alterations in patients treated with cyclosporine for uveitis. *N Engl J Med* 1986;314:1293–1298.
224. Olyaei AJ, de Mattos AM, Bennett WM. Nephrotoxicity of immunosuppressive drugs: new insight and preventive strategies. *Curr Opin Crit Care* 2001;7:384–389.
225. de Mattos AM, Olyaei AJ, Bennett WM. Nephrotoxicity of immunosuppressive drugs: long-term consequences and challenges for the future. *Am J Kidney Dis* 2000;35:333–346.
226. Prevot A, Semama DS, Tendron A, et al. Endothelin, angiotensin II and adenosine in acute cyclosporine A nephrotoxicity. *Pediatr Nephrol* 2000;14:927–934.
227. Kvien TK, Zeidler HK, Hannonen P, et al. Long term efficacy and safety of cyclosporin versus parenteral gold in early rheumatoid arthritis: a three year study of radiographic progression, renal function, and arterial hypertension. *Ann Rheum Dis* 2002;61:511–516.
228. Fleming DR, Ouseph R, Herrington J. Hyperkalemia associated with cyclosporine (CsA) use in bone marrow transplantation. *Bone Marrow Transplant* 1997;19:289–291.
229. Laine J, Holmberg C. Renal and adrenal mechanisms in cyclosporine-induced hyperkalaemia after renal transplantation. *Eur J Clin Invest* 1995;25:670–676.
230. van den Borne BE, Landewe RB, Houkes I, et al. No increased risk of malignancies and mortality in cyclosporin A-treated patients with rheumatoid arthritis. *Arthritis Rheum* 1998;41:1930–1937.
231. Krugmann J, Sailer-Hock M, Muller T, et al. Epstein-Barr virus–associated Hodgkin's lymphoma and *Legionella pneumophila* infection complicating treatment of juvenile rheumatoid arthritis with methotrexate and cyclosporine A. *Hum Pathol* 2000;31:253–255.
232. Zackheim HS. Cyclosporine-associated lymphoma. *J Am Acad Dermatol* 1999;40:1015–1016.
233. Hou S. Pregnancy in renal transplant recipients. *Adv Ren Replace Ther* 2003;10:40–47.
234. Airo P, Antonioli CM, Motta M, et al. The immune development in a child born to a cyclosporin A-treated woman with systemic lupus erythematosus/polymyositis. *Lupus* 2002;11:454–457.
235. Kim JH, Perfect JR. Infection and cyclosporine. *Rev Infect Dis* 1989; 11:677–690.
236. Wolyniec W, Debska-Slizien A, Chamienia A, et al. Cyclosporine A–related hemolytic uremic syndrome after living renal transplantation-case report. *Transplant Proc* 2002;34:569–571.
237. Cush JJ, Tugwell P, Weinblatt M, et al. US consensus guidelines for the use of cyclosporin A in rheumatoid arthritis. *J Rheumatol* 1999; 26:1176–1186.
238. Dougados M, Nguyen M, Duchesne L, et al. Evaluation of the usefulness of delayed-action preparations in the treatment of rheumatoid polyarthritis by analyzing the therapeutic maintenance dose. *Rev Rhum Mal Osteoartic* 1989;56:89–92.
239. Forre O, Bjerkhoel F, Salvesen CF, et al. An open, controlled, randomized comparison of cyclosporine and azathioprine in the treatment of rheumatoid arthritis: a preliminary report. *Arthritis Rheum* 1987;30:88–92.
240. Schattenkirchner M, Kruger K. Cyclosporin vs azathioprine in the treatment of rheumatoid arthritis—a controlled double-blind study [Abstract 198]. Presented at the 2nd Congress on Immunointervention in Autoimmune Diseases, Paris, France, 1991.

241. van Rijthoven AW, Dijkmans BA, The HS, et al. Comparison of cyclosporine and D-penicillamine for rheumatoid arthritis: a randomized, double blind, multicenter study. *J Rheumatol* 1991;18: 815–820.
242. Mitrovic D, Popovic M, Glisic B, et al. Cyclosporine in the treatment of autoimmune disorders: a 10-year experience. *Transplant Proc* 1998;30:4134.
243. Zeidler HK, Kvien TK, Hannonen P, et al. Progression of joint damage in early active severe rheumatoid arthritis during 18 months of treatment: comparison of low-dose cyclosporin and parenteral gold. *Br J Rheumatol* 1998;37:874–882.
244. Drosos AA, Voulgari PV, Katsaraki A, et al. Influence of cyclosporin A on radiological progression in early rheumatoid arthritis patients: a 42-month prospective study. *Rheumatol Int* 2000;19:113–118.
245. Tugwell P, Pincus T, Yocum D, et al. Combination therapy with cyclosporine and methotrexate in severe rheumatoid arthritis. The Methotrexate-Cyclosporine Combination Study Group. *N Engl J Med* 1995;333:137–141.
246. Proudman SM, Conaghan PG, Richardson C, et al. Treatment of poor-prognosis early rheumatoid arthritis. A randomized study of treatment with methotrexate, cyclosporin A, and intraarticular corticosteroids compared with sulfasalazine alone. *Arthritis Rheum* 2000; 43:1809–1819.
247. Marchesoni A, Battafarano N, Arreghini M, et al. Step-down approach using either cyclosporin A or methotrexate as maintenance therapy in early rheumatoid arthritis. *Arthritis Rheum* 2002;47: 59–66.
248. van den Borne BE, Landewe RB, Goei The HS, et al. Combination therapy in recent onset rheumatoid arthritis: a randomized double blind trial of the addition of low dose cyclosporine to patients treated with low dose chloroquine. *J Rheumatol* 1998;25:1493–1498.
249. Salaffi F, Carotti M, Cervini C. Combination therapy of cyclosporine A with methotrexate or hydroxychloroquine in refractory rheumatoid arthritis. *Scand J Rheumatol* 1996;25:16–23.
250. Bendix G, Bjelle A. Adding low-dose cyclosporin A to parenteral gold therapy in rheumatoid arthritis: a double-blind placebo-controlled study. *Br J Rheumatol* 1996;35:1142–1149.
251. Stern ME, Beuerman RW, Fox RI, et al. The pathology of dry eye: the interaction between the ocular surface and lacrimal glands. *Cornea* 1998;17:584–589.
252. Small DS, Acheampong A, Reis B, et al. Blood concentrations of cyclosporin a during long-term treatment with cyclosporin a ophthalmic emulsions in patients with moderate to severe dry eye disease. *J Ocul Pharmacol Ther* 2002;18:411–418.
253. Sall K, Stevenson OD, Mundorf TK, et al. Two multicenter, randomized studies of the efficacy and safety of cyclosporine ophthalmic emulsion in moderate to severe dry eye disease. CsA Phase 3 Study Group. *Ophthalmology* 2000;107:631–639.
254. Restasis. *Physicians desk reference.* 2003.
255. Gupta AK, Matteson EL, Ellis CN, et al. Cyclosporine in the treatment of psoriatic arthritis. *Arch Dermatol* 1989;125:507–510.
256. Isenberg DA, Snaith ML, Morrow WJ, et al. Cyclosporin A for the treatment of systemic lupus erythematosus. *Int J Immunopharmacol* 1981;3:163–169.
257. Feutren G, Querin S, Noel LH, et al. Effects of cyclosporine in severe systemic lupus erythematosus. *J Pediatr* 1987;111:1063–1068.
258. Tokuda M, Kurata N, Mizoguchi A, et al. Effect of low-dose cyclosporin A on systemic lupus erythematosus disease activity. *Arthritis Rheum* 1994;37:551–558.
259. Manger K, Kalden JR, Manger B. Cyclosporin A in the treatment of systemic lupus erythematosus: results of an open clinical study. *Br J Rheumatol* 1996;35:669–675.
260. Caccavo D, Lagana B, Mitterhofer AP, et al. Long-term treatment of systemic lupus erythematosus with cyclosporin A. *Arthritis Rheum* 1997;40:27–35.
261. ter Borg EJ, Tegzess AM, Kallenberg CG. Unexpected severe reversible cyclosporine A–induced nephrotoxicity in a patient with systemic lupus erythematosus and tubulointerstitial renal disease. *Clin Nephrol* 1988;29:93–95.
262. Worle B, Hein R, Krieg T, et al. Cyclosporin in localized and systemic scleroderma—a clinical study. *Dermatologica* 1990;181:215–220.
263. Zachariae H, Halkier-Sorensen L, Heickendorff L, et al. Cyclosporin A treatment of systemic sclerosis. *Br J Dermatol* 1990;122:677–681.
264. Gisslinger H, Burghuber OC, Stacher G, et al. Efficacy of cyclosporin A in systemic sclerosis. *Clin Exp Rheumatol* 1991;9:383–390.
265. Clements PJ, Lachenbruch PA, Sterz M, et al. Cyclosporine in systemic sclerosis. Results of a forty-eight-week open safety study in ten patients. *Arthritis Rheum* 1993;36:75–83.
266. Casato M, Bonomo L, Caccavo D, et al. Clinical effects of cyclosporin in dermatomyositis. *Clin Exp Dermatol* 1990;15:121–123.
267. Correia O, Polonia J, Nunes JP, et al. Severe acute form of adult dermatomyositis treated with cyclosporine. *Int J Dermatol* 1992;31: 517–519.
268. Mehregan DR, Su WP. Cyclosporine treatment for dermatomyositis/ polymyositis. *Cutis* 1993;51:59–61.
269. Diaz-Llopis M, Cervera M, Meenezo J. Cyclosporin-A treatment of Behçet's disease-a long-term study. *Curr Eye Res* 1990;9(suppl): 17–23.
270. Masuda K, Nakajima A, Urayama A, et al. Double-masked trial of cyclosporin versus colchicine and long-term open study of cyclosporin in Behçet's disease. *Lancet* 1989;1:1093–1096.
271. Elgart G, Stover P, Larson K, et al. Treatment of pyoderma gangrenosum with cyclosporine: results in seven patients. *J Am Acad Dermatol* 1991;24:83–86.
272. Matis WL, Ellis CN, Griffiths CE, et al. Treatment of pyoderma gangrenosum with cyclosporine. *Arch Dermatol* 1992;128:1060–1064.
273. Soria C, Allegue F, Martin M, et al. Treatment of pyoderma gangrenosum with cyclosporin A. *Clin Exp Dermatol* 1991;16:392–394.
274. Haubitz M, Koch KM, Brunkhorst R. Cyclosporin for the prevention of disease reactivation in relapsing ANCA-associated vasculitis. *Nephrol Dial Transplant* 1998;13:2074–2076.
275. Ghez D, Westeel PF, Henry I, et al. Control of a relapse and induction of long-term remission of Wegener's granulomatosis by cyclosporine. *Am J Kidney Dis* 2002;40:E6.
276. Ostensen M, Hoyeraal HM, Kass E. Tolerance of cyclosporine A in children with refractory juvenile rheumatoid arthritis. *J Rheumatol* 1988;15:1536–1538.
277. Pistoia V, Buoncompagni A, Scribanis R, et al. Cyclosporin A in the treatment of juvenile chronic arthritis and childhood polymyositis-dermatomyositis. Results of a preliminary study. *Clin Exp Rheumatol* 1993;11:203–208.
278. Gattorno M, Buoncompagni A, Faraci M, et al. Early treatment of systemic onset juvenile chronic arthritis with low-dose cyclosporin A. *Clin Exp Rheumatol* 1995;13:409–410.
279. Fautini F, Gerloui V, Gattinara M, et al. Long term therapy of severe unresponsive cases of juvenile chronic arthritis (JCA) with cyclosporin (CS): a seven year experience. *Arthritis Rheum* 1994;37 (suppl):277.
280. Ravelli A, De Benedetti F, Viola S, et al. Macrophage activation syndrome in systemic juvenile rheumatoid arthritis successfully treated with cyclosporine. *J Pediatr* 1996;128:275–278.
281. Prieur AM, Stephan JL. Macrophage activation syndrome in rheumatic diseases in children. *Rev Rhum Ed Fr* 1994;61:447–451.
282. Mouy R, Stephan JL, Pillet P, et al. Efficacy of cyclosporine A in the treatment of macrophage activation syndrome in juvenile arthritis: report of five cases. *J Pediatr* 1996;129:750–754.
283. Carlson RP, Hartman DA, Ochalski SJ, et al. Sirolimus (rapamycin, Rapamune) and combination therapy with cyclosporin A in the rat developing adjuvant arthritis model: correlation with blood levels and the effects of different oral formulations. *Inflamm Res* 1998;47: 339–344.
284. Kovarsky J. Clinical pharmacology and toxicology of cyclophosphamide: emphasis on use in rheumatic diseases. *Semin Arthritis Rheum* 1983;12:359–372.
285. Diaz CJ, Garcia EL, Mechante A. Treatment of rheumatoid arthritis with nitrogen mustard. Preliminary report. *JAMA* 1951;147:1418–1419.
286. Bagley CM Jr, Bostick FW, DeVita VT Jr. Clinical pharmacology of cyclophosphamide. *Cancer Res* 1973;33:226–233.
287. Moore MJ, Hardy RW, Thiessen JJ, et al. Rapid development of enhanced clearance after high-dose cyclophosphamide. *Clin Pharmacol Ther* 1988;44:622–628.
288. Allopurinol and cytotoxic drugs. Interaction in relation to bone marrow depression. Boston Collaborative Drug Surveillance Program. *JAMA* 1974;227:1036–1040.

289. Vesell ES, Passananti GT, Greene FE. Impairment of drug metabolism in man by allopurinol and nortriptyline. *N Engl J Med* 1970; 283:1484–1488.
290. Alberts DS, van Daalen Wetters T. The effect of phenobarbital on cyclophosphamide antitumor activity. *Cancer Res* 1976;36:2785–2789.
291. Hart LG, Adamson RH. Effect of microsomal enzyme modifiers on toxicity and therapeutic activity of cyclophosphamide in mice. *Arch Intern Pharmacodyn Ther* 1969;180:391–401.
292. Field RB, Gang M, Kline I, et al. The effect of phenobarbital or 2-diethylaminoethyl-2,2-diphenylvalerate on the activation of cyclophosphamide *in vivo*. *J Pharmacol Exp Ther* 1972;180:475–483.
293. Sladek NE. Therapeutic efficacy of cyclophosphamide as a function of its metabolism. *Cancer Res* 1972;32:535–542.
294. Hayakawa T, Kanai N, Yamada R, et al. Effect of steroid hormone on activation of Endoxan (cyclophosphamide). *Biochem Pharmacol* 1969;18:129–135.
295. Kovacs K, Steinberg AD. Cyclophosphamide. Drug interactions and bone marrow transplantation. *Transplantation* 1972;13:316–321.
296. Gaudin D, Yielding KL. Response of a "resistant" plasmacytoma to alkylating agents and x-ray in combination with the "excision" repair inhibitors caffeine and chloroquine. *Proc Soc Exp Biol Med* 1969; 131:1413–1416.
297. McLean A, Newell D, Baker G. The metabolism of chlorambucil. *Biochem Pharmacol* 1976;25:2331–2335.
298. Hartvig P, Simonsson B, Oberg G, et al. Inter- and intraindividual differences in oral chlorambucil pharmacokinetics. *Eur J Clin Pharmacol* 1988;35:551–554.
299. Alberts DS, Chang SY, Chen HS, et al. Pharmacokinetics and metabolism of chlorambucil in man: a preliminary report. *Cancer Treat Rev* 1979;6(suppl):9–17.
300. Kawabata TT, Chapman MY, Kim DH, et al. Mechanisms of *in vitro* immunosuppression by hepatocyte-generated cyclophosphamide metabolites and 4-hydroperoxycyclophosphamide. *Biochem Pharmacol* 1990;40:927–935.
301. Steinberg AD. Chlorambucil in the treatment of patients with immune-mediated rheumatic diseases. *Arthritis Rheum* 1993;36:325–328.
302. Shand FL, Howard JG. Induction *in vitro* of reversible immunosuppression and inhibition of B cell receptor regeneration by defined metabolites of cyclophosphamide. *Eur J Immunol* 1979;9:17–21.
303. Turk JL, Poulter LW. Selective depletion of lymphoid tissue by cyclophosphamide. *Clin Exp Immunol* 1972;10:285–296.
304. Turk JL, Poulter LW. Effects of cyclophosphamide on lymphoid tissues labelled with 5-iodo-2-deoxyuridine- 125 I and 51 Cr. *Int Arch Allergy Appl Immunol* 1972;43:620–629.
305. Clements PJ, Yu DT, Levy J, et al. Effects of cyclophosphamide on B- and T-lymphocytes in rheumatoid arthritis. *Arthritis Rheum* 1974;17:347–353.
306. Hurd ER, Giuliano VJ. The effect of cyclophosphamide on B and T lymphocytes in patients with connective tissue diseases. *Arthritis Rheum* 1975;18:67–75.
307. Stockman GD, Heim LR, South MA, et al. Differential effects of cyclophosphamide on the B and T cell compartments of adult mice. *J Immunol* 1973;110:277–282.
308. Girard D, Aloisi RM, Bliven ML, et al. Cyclophosphamide and 15(S)-15 methyl PGE1 correct the T/B lymphocyte ratios of NZB/NZW mice. *Agents Actions* 1990;29:333–341.
309. Dale DC, Fauci AS, Wolff SM. The effect of cyclophosphamide on leukocyte kinetics and susceptibility to infection in patients with Wegener's granulomatosis. *Arthritis Rheum* 1973;16:657–664.
310. Ozer H, Cowens JW, Colvin M, et al. *In vitro* effects of 4-hydroperoxycyclophosphamide on human immunoregulatory T subset function. I. Selective effects on lymphocyte function in T-B cell collaboration. *J Exp Med* 1982;155:276–290.
311. Kaufmann SH, Hahn H, Diamantstein T. Relative susceptibilities of T cell subsets involved in delayed-type hypersensitivity to sheep red blood cells to the *in vitro* action of 4- hydroperoxycyclophosphamide. *J Immunol* 1980;125:1104–1108.
312. Diamantstein T, Willinger E, Reiman J. T-suppressor cells sensitive to cyclophosphamide and to its *in vitro* active derivative 4-hydroperoxycyclophosphamide control the mitogenic response of murine splenic B cells to dextran sulfate. A direct proof for different sensitivities of lymphocyte subsets to cyclophosphamide. *J Exp Med* 1979; 150:1571–1576.
313. Takeno M, Suzuki N, Nagafuchi H, et al. Selective suppression of resting B cell function in patients with systemic lupus erythematosus treated with cyclophosphamide. *Clin Exp Rheumatol* 1993;11:263–270.
314. Feehally J, Beattie TJ, Brenchley PE, et al. Modulation of cellular immune function by cyclophosphamide in children with minimal-change nephropathy. *N Engl J Med* 1984;310:415–420.
315. Maguire HC Jr, Ettore VL. Enhancement of dinitrochlorobenzene (DNCB) contact sensitization by cyclophosphamide in the guinea pig. *J Invest Dermatol* 1967;48:39–43.
316. Turk JL, Parker D, Poulter LW. Functional aspects of the selective depletion of lymphoid tissue by cyclophosphamide. *Immunology* 1972;23:493–501.
317. Lagrange PH, Mackaness GB, Miller TE. Potentiation of T-cell-mediated immunity by selective suppression of antibody formation with cyclophosphamide. *J Exp Med* 1974;139:1529–1539.
318. Kerckhaert JA, Hofhuis FM, Willers JM. Influence of cyclophosphamide on delayed hypersensitivity and acquired cellular resistance to Listeria monocytogenes in the mouse. *Immunology* 1977;32:1027–1032.
319. Ferguson RM, Simmons RL. Differential cyclophosphamide sensitivity of suppressor and cytotoxic cell precursors. *Transplantation* 1978;25:36–38.
320. Rollinghoff M, Starzinski-Powitz A, Pfizenmaier K, et al. Cyclophosphamide-sensitive T lymphocytes suppress the *in vivo* generation of antigen-specific cytotoxic T lymphocytes. *J Exp Med* 1977; 145:455–459.
321. Maguire HC Jr. Specific acquired immune unresponsiveness to contact allergens with cyclophosphamide in the mouse. *Int Arch Allergy Appl Immunol* 1976;50:651–658.
322. Owens AH Jr, Santos GW. The effect of cytotoxic drugs on graft-versus-host disease in mice. *Transplantation* 1971;11:378–382.
323. Steinberg AD, Daley GG, Talal N. Tolerance to polyinosinic-polycytidylic acid in NZB-NZW mice. *Science* 1970;167:870–871.
324. Bontoux D, Kahan A, Brouilhet H, et al. Effect and mode of action of chlorambucil in rheumatoid disease. Value of the lymphoblastic transformation test. *Rev Rhum Mal Osteoartic* 1971;38:759–764.
325. Berenbaum MD, Brown IN. Prolongation of homograft survival in mice with single doses of cyclophosphamide. *Nature* 1963;200:84.
326. Stevenson HC, Fauci AS. Activation of human B lymphocytes. XII. Differential effects of *in vitro* cyclophosphamide on human lymphocyte subpopulations involved in B-cell activation. *Immunology* 1980; 39:391–397.
327. Santos GW, Owens AH Jr. 19S and 17S antibody production in the cyclophosphamide- or methotrexate-treated rat. *Nature* 1966;209: 622–624.
328. Kahn MF, De Seze S. The immunosuppressive agents in rheumatology. Indications, results and problems of long-term surveillance. *Ann Med Interne (Paris)* 1974;125:497–506.
329. Alepa FP, Zvaifler NJ, Sliwinski AJ. Immunologic effects of cyclophosphamide treatment in rheumatoid arthritis. *Arthritis Rheum* 1970;13:754–760.
330. Aisenberg AC. Immunosuppression by alkylating agents—tolerance induction. *Transplant Proc* 1973;5:1221–1226.
331. Kawaguchi S. Studies on the induction of immunological paralysis to bovine gamma-globulin in adult mice. II. The effect of cyclophosphamide. *Immunology* 1970;19:291–299.
332. Many A, Schwartz RS. On the mechanism of immunological tolerance in cyclophosphamide-treated mice. *Clin Exp Immunol* 1970;6: 87–99.
333. Turk JL, Parker D. Further studies on B-lymphocyte suppression in delayed hypersensitivity, indicating a possible mechanism for Jones-Mote hypersensitivity. *Immunology* 1973;24:751–758.
334. Duclos H, Galanaud P, Devinsky O, et al. Enhancing effect of low dose cyclophosphamide treatment on the *in vitro* antibody response. *Eur J Immunol* 1977;7:679–684.
335. Curtis JE, Sharp JT, Lidsky MD, et al. Immune response of patients with rheumatoid arthritis during cyclophosphamide treatment. *Arthritis Rheum* 1973;16:34–42.
336. Hersh EM, Wong VG, Freireich EJ. Inhibition of the local inflammatory response in man by antimetabolites. *Blood* 1966;27:38–48.
337. Balow JE, Austin HAd, Muenz LR, et al. Effect of treatment on the evolution of renal abnormalities in lupus nephritis. *N Engl J Med* 1984;311:491–495.

338. Sawitzky A, Rai KR, Glidewell O, et al. Comparison of daily versus intermittent chlorambucil and prednisone therapy in the treatment of patients with chronic lymphocytic leukemia. *Blood* 1977:50:1049–1059.
339. Parsons CL. Bladder surface glycosaminoglycan: efficient mechanism of environmental adaptation. *Urology* 1986;27:9–14.
340. Bryant BM, Jarman M, Ford HT, et al. Prevention of isophosphamide-induced urothelial toxicity with 2-mercaptoethane sulphonate sodium (mesnum) in patients with advanced carcinoma. *Lancet* 1980;2:657–659.
341. Ehrlich RM, Freedman A, Goldsobel AB, et al. The use of sodium 2-mercaptoethane sulfonate to prevent cyclophosphamide cystitis. *J Urol* 1984;131:960–962.
342. Hows JM, Mehta A, Ward L, et al. Comparison of mesna with forced diuresis to prevent cyclophosphamide induced haemorrhagic cystitis in marrow transplantation: a prospective randomised study. *Br J Cancer* 1984;50:753–756.
343. Cannon GW, Jackson CG, Samuelson CO Jr, et al. Chlorambucil therapy in rheumatoid arthritis: clinical experience in 28 patients and literature review. *Semin Arthritis Rheum* 1985;15:106–118.
344. Renier JC, Deshayes P, Houdent G, et al. Le traitement de la polyarthrite rhumatoide par le chlorambucil. Etude de 113 observations. *Arch Med Ouest* 1971;1:47–58.
345. Vignon G, Bied JC. Comparison of various immunosuppressive agents in the treatment of rheumatoid polyarthritis. 41 personal cases. *Rev Rhum Mal Osteoartic* 1971;38:785–795.
346. Cayla J, Rondier J. Treatment of 67 rheumatoid polyarthritis cases with chlorambucil. *Rev Rhum Mal Osteoartic* 1971;38:765–770.
347. Arlet J, Mole J, Debrock J. Our experience of chronic rheumatic polyarthritis therapy with immunosuppressive agents. Apropos of 41 cases. *Rev Rhum Mal Osteoartic* 1971;38:771–774.
348. Krel AA, Trifonov Iu I, Bolotin EV, et al. Cytopenic syndrome in rheumatoid arthritis patients treated with leukeran and azathioprine. *Sov Med* 1979;9:68–72.
349. Sauvezie B, Rampon S, Bussiere JL, et al. Value of the lymphoblastic transformation test with tritiated thymidine incorporation in the surveillance of immunosuppressive treatments in rheumatology. *Rev Rhum Mal Osteoartic* 1972;39:609–616.
350. Renier JC, Bregeon C, Bonnette C, et al. Evolution of patients with rheumatoid arthritis treated with immunosuppressive agents between 1965 and 1973. *Rev Rhum Mal Osteoartic* 1978;45:453–461.
351. Deshayes P, Renier JC, Bregeon C, et al. Side-effects and complications of immunosuppressive therapy in rheumatoid arthritis. *Rev Rhum Mal Osteoartic* 1971;38:797–806.
352. Fosdick WM, Parsons JL, Hill DF. Long-term cyclophosphamide therapy in rheumatoid arthritis. *Arthritis Rheum* 1968;11:151–161.
353. Fries JF, Sharp GC, McDevitt HO, et al. Cyclophosphamide therapy in systemic lupus erythematosus and polymyositis. *Arthritis Rheum* 1973;16:154–162.
354. Williams HJ, Reading JC, Ward JR, et al. Comparison of high and low dose cyclophosphamide therapy in rheumatoid arthritis. *Arthritis Rheum* 1980;23:521–527.
355. Seze Sd, Bedoiseau M, Debeyre N, et al. [Results of therapy of the immunodepressive type in 40 patients with severe rheumatoid polyarthritis]. *Semin Hop* 1967;43:3084–3091.
356. Amor B, Herson D, Cherot A, et al. Follow-up study of patients with rheumatoid arthritis over a period of more than 10 years (1966–1978): analysis of disease progression and treatment in 100 cases (author's translation). *Ann Med Interne* 1981;132:168–173.
357. Townes AS, Sowa JM, Shulman LE. Controlled trial of cyclophosphamide in rheumatoid arthritis. *Arthritis Rheum* 1976;19:563–573.
358. Aymard JP, Lederlin P, Witz F, et al. Acute leukemia following prolonged chlorambucil treatment of non-neoplastic disease—a study of two cases and literature review. *Acta Clin Belg* 1938;38:228–235.
359. Kahn MF, Bedoiseau M, Six B, et al. Chlorambucil in rheumatoid polyarthritis. *Rev Rhum Mal Osteoartic* 1971;38:741–748.
360. Rudd P, Fries JF, Epstein WV. Irreversible bone marrow failure with chlorambucil. *J Rheumatol* 1975;2:421–429.
361. Thorpe P. Rheumatoid arthritis treated with chlorambucil: a five-year follow-up. *Med J Aust* 1976;2:197–199.
362. Mullins GM, Colvin M. Intensive cyclophosphamide (NSC-26271) therapy for solid tumors. *Cancer Chemother Rep* 1975;59:411–419.
363. Renier JC, Bregeon C, Bonnette C. Results of immunosuppressive therapy in 78 patients with rheumatoid polyarthritis, treated for at least 4 years. *Rev Rhum Mal Osteoartic* 1975;42:399–407.
364. Smyth CJ, Bartholomew BA, Mills DM, et al. Cyclophosphamide therapy for rheumatoid arthritis. *Arch Intern Med* 1975;135:789–793.
365. A controlled trial of cyclophosphamide in rheumatoid arthritis. *N Engl J Med* 1970;283:883–889.
366. Honjo I, Suou T, Hirayama C. Hepatotoxicity of cyclophosphamide in man: pharmacokinetic analysis. *Res Commun Chem Pathol Pharmacol* 1988;61:149–165.
367. Bacon AM, Rosenberg SA. Cyclophosphamide hepatotoxicity in a patient with systemic lupus erythematosus. *Ann Intern Med* 1982; 97:62–63.
368. Shaunak S, Munro JM, Weinbren K, et al. Cyclophosphamide-induced liver necrosis: a possible interaction with azathioprine. *Q J Med* 1988;67:309–317.
369. O'Duffy JD, Robertson DM, Goldstein NP. Chlorambucil in the treatment of uveitis and meningoencephalitis of Behçet's disease. *Am J Med* 1984;76:75–84.
370. Bradley JD, Brandt KD, Katz BP. Infectious complications of cyclophosphamide treatment for vasculitis. *Arthritis Rheum* 1989;32: 45–53.
371. Kattwinkel N, Cook L, Agnello V. Overwhelming fatal infection in a young woman after intravenous cyclophosphamide therapy for lupus nephritis. *J Rheumatol* 1991;18:79–81.
372. Kahl LE. Herpes zoster infections in systemic lupus erythematosus: risk factors and outcome. *J Rheumatol* 1994;21:84–86.
373. Fishman JA. Prevention of infection caused by *Pneumocystis carinii* in transplant recipients. *Clin Infect Dis* 2001;33:1397–1405.
374. Hughes WT. Comparison of dosages, intervals, and drugs in the prevention of *Pneumocystis carinii* pneumonia. *Antimicrob Agents Chemother* 1988;32:623–625.
375. Omdal R, Husby G, Koldingsnes W. Intravenous and oral cyclophosphamide pulse therapy in rheumatic diseases: side effects and complications. *Clin Exp Rheumatol* 1993;11:283–288.
376. Schein PS, Winokur SH. Immunosuppressive and cytotoxic chemotherapy: long-term complications. *Ann Intern Med* 1975;82: 84–95.
377. Marsh FP, Vince FP, Pollock DJ, et al. Cyclophosphamide necrosis of bladder causing calcification, contracture and reflux; treated by colocystoplasty. *Br J Urol* 1971;43:324–332.
378. Johnson WW, Meadows DC. Urinary-bladder fibrosis and telangiectasia associated with long-term cyclophosphamide therapy. *N Engl J Med* 1971;284:290–294.
379. Fairchild WV, Spence CR, Solomon HD, et al. The incidence of bladder cancer after cyclophosphamide therapy. *J Urol* 1979;122:163–164.
380. Pearson RM, Soloway MS. Does cyclophosphamide induce bladder cancer? *Urology* 1978;11:437–447.
381. Wall RL, Clausen KP. Carcinoma of the urinary bladder in patients receiving cyclophosphamide. *N Engl J Med* 1975;293:271–273.
382. Thrasher JB, Miller GJ, Wettlaufer JN. Bladder leiomyosarcoma following cyclophosphamide therapy for lupus nephritis. *J Urol* 1990; 143:119–121.
383. deVries CR, Freiha FS. Hemorrhagic cystitis: a review. *J Urol* 1990; 143:1–9.
384. Scheef W, Klein HO, Brock N, et al. Controlled clinical studies with an antidote against the urotoxicity of oxazaphosphorines: preliminary results. *Cancer Treat Rep* 1979;63:501–505.
385. Gourley MF, Austin HA 3rd, Scott D, et al. Methylprednisolone and cyclophosphamide, alone or in combination, in patients with lupus nephritis. A randomized, controlled trial. *Ann Intern Med* 1996;125: 549–557.
386. De Vita S, Neri R, Bombardieri S. Cyclophosphamide pulses in the treatment of rheumatic diseases: an update. *Clin Exp Rheumatol* 1991;9:179–193.
387. Block JA. Hemorrhagic cystitis complicating untreated necrotizing vasculitis. *Arthritis Rheum* 1993;36:857–859.
388. Talar-Williams C, Hijazi YM, Walther MM, et al. Cyclophosphamide-induced cystitis and bladder cancer in patients with Wegener granulomatosis. *Ann Intern Med* 1996;124:477–484.
389. Spector JI, Zimbler H, Ross JS. Early-onset cyclophosphamide-induced interstitial pneumonitis. *JAMA* 1979;242:2852–2854.
390. Stentoft J. Progressive pulmonary fibrosis complicating cyclophosphamide therapy. *Acta Med Scand* 1987;221:403–407.
391. Carr ME Jr. Chlorambucil induced pulmonary fibrosis: report of a case and review. *Va Med* 1986;113:677–680.

392. Thorpe P, Hassal J, York J. Cytotoxic therapy in rheumatoid disease. *Med J Aust* 1971;2:796–798.
393. Lakin JD, Cahill RA. Generalized urticaria to cyclophosphamide: type I hypersensitivity to an immunosuppressive agent. *J Allergy Clin Immunol* 1976;58:160–171.
394. Fairley KF, Barrie JU, Johnson W. Sterility and testicular atrophy related to cyclophosphamide therapy. *Lancet* 1972;1:568–569.
395. Kumar R, Biggart JD, McEvoy J, et al. Cyclophosphamide and reproductive function. *Lancet* 1972;1:1212–1214.
396. Miller DG. Alkylating agents and human spermatogenesis. *JAMA* 1971;217:1662–1665.
397. Jacobson RJ, Sagel J, Distiller LA, et al. Leydig cell dysfunction in male patients with Hodgkin's disease receiving chemotherapy. *Clin Res* 1978;3437A:26.
398. Chapman RM, Sutcliffe SB, Rees LH, et al. Cyclical combination chemotherapy and gonadal function. Retrospective study in males. *Lancet* 1979;1:285–289.
399. Masala A, Faedda R, Alagna S, et al. Use of testosterone to prevent cyclophosphamide-induced azoospermia. *Ann Intern Med* 1997;126: 292–295.
400. Hinkes E, Plotkin D. Reversible drug-induced sterility in a patient with acute leukemia. *JAMA* 1973;223:1490–1491.
401. Blake DA, Heller RH, Hsu SH, et al. Return of fertility in a patient with cyclophosphamide-induced azoospermia. *Johns Hopkins Med J* 1976;139:20–22.
402. Boumpas DT, Austin HAd, Vaughan EM, et al. Risk for sustained amenorrhea in patients with systemic lupus erythematosus receiving intermittent pulse cyclophosphamide therapy. *Ann Intern Med* 1993; 119:366–369.
403. Klippel JH. Cyclophosphamide:ovarian and other toxicities. *Lupus* 1995;4:1–2.
404. Palmer RG, Dore CJ, Denman AM. Cyclophosphamide induces more chromosome damage than chlorambucil in patients with connective tissue diseases. *Q J Med* 1986;59:395–400.
405. Tolchin SF, Winkelstein A, Rodnan GP, et al. Chromosome abnormalities from cyclophosphamide therapy in rheumatoid arthritis and progressive systemic sclerosis (scleroderma). *Arthritis Rheum* 1974; 17:375–382.
406. Palmer RG, Dore CJ, Denman AM. Chlorambucil-induced chromosome damage to human lymphocytes is dose-dependent and cumulative. *Lancet* 1984;1:246–249.
407. Greenberg LH, Tanaka KR. Congenital anomalies probably induced by cyclophosphamide. *JAMA* 1964;188:423–426.
408. Sokal JE, Lessmann EM. Effects of cancer chemotherapeutic agents on the human fetus. *JAMA* 1960;172:1765–1777.
409. Toledo TM, Harper RC, Moser RH. Fetal effects during cyclophosphamide and irradiation therapy. *Ann Intern Med* 1971;74:87–91.
410. Gilchrist DM, Friedman JM. Teratogenesis and IV cyclophosphamide [Letter]. *J Rheumatol* 1989;16:1008–1009.
411. Kirshon B, Wasserstrum N, Willis R, et al. Teratogenic effects of first-trimester cyclophosphamide therapy. *Obstet Gynecol* 1988;72: 462–464.
412. Shotton D, Monie IW. Possible teratogenic effect of chlorambucil on a human fetus. *JAMA* 193;186:74–75.
413. Bermas BL, Hill JA. Effects of immunosuppressive drugs during pregnancy. *Arthritis Rheum* 1995;38:1722–1732.
414. Langevitz P, Klein L, Pras M, et al. The effect of cyclophosphamide pulses on fertility in patients with lupus nephritis. *Am J Reprod Immunol* 1992;28:157–158.
415. Blatt J, Mulvihill JJ, Ziegler JL, et al. Pregnancy outcome following cancer chemotherapy. *Am J Med* 1980;69:828–832.
416. Menkes CJ, Levy JP, Weill B, et al. [Acute leukemia with megakaryoblasts. Incidence following immunosuppressive treatment of rheumatoid polyarthritis]. *Nouv Presse Med* 1975;4:2869–2871.
417. Kahn MF, Arlet J, Bloch-Michel H, et al. Acute leukaemias after treatment using cytotoxic agents for rheumatological purpose. 19 cases among 2006 patients (author's translation). *Nouv Presse Med* 1979;8: 1393–1397.
418. Zittoun R, Debre P, Gardais J, et al. Small intestine lymphosarcoma after treatment of rheumatoid arthritis with chlorambucil. *Nouv Presse Med* 1972;1:2477–2479.
419. Prieur AM, Balafrej M, Griscelli C, et al. Results and long-term risks of immuno-suppressive treatment in chronic juvenile arthritis. Apropos of 40 cases. *Rev Rhum Mal Osteoartic* 1979;46:85–90.
420. Dumont J, Thiery JP, Mazabraud A, et al. Acute myeloid leukemia following non-Hodgkin's lymphoma: danger of prolonged use of chlorambucil as maintenance therapy. *Nouv Rev Fr Hematol* 1980; 22:391–404.
421. Berk PD, Goldberg JD, Silverstein MN, et al. Increased incidence of acute leukemia in polycythemia vera associated with chlorambucil therapy. *N Engl J Med* 1981;304:441–447.
422. Aymard JP, Frustin J, Witz F, et al. Acute leukaemia after prolonged chlorambucil treatment for non-malignant disease: report of a new case and literature survey. *Acta Haematol* 1980;63:283–285.
423. Fiere D, Felman P, Vu Van H, et al. Leucemies aigues myeloids après administration de chlorambucil. Deux observations. *Nouv Presse Med* 1978;7:156.
424. Chaplin H Jr. Lymphoma in primary chronic cold hemagglutinin disease treated with chlorambucil. *Arch Intern Med* 1982;142:2119–2123.
425. Baltus JA, Boersma JW, Hartman AP, et al. The occurrence of malignancies in patients with rheumatoid arthritis treated with cyclophosphamide: a controlled retrospective follow-up. *Ann Rheum Dis* 1983; 42:368–373.
426. Patapanian H, Graham S, Sambrook PN, et al. The oncogenicity of chlorambucil in rheumatoid arthritis. *Br J Rheumatol* 1988;27: 44–47.
427. Baker GL, Kahl LE, Zee BC, et al. Malignancy following treatment of rheumatoid arthritis with cyclophosphamide. Long-term case-control follow-up study. *Am J Med* 1987;83:1–9.
428. Kauppi MJ, Savolainen HA, Anttila VJ, et al. Increased risk of leukaemia in patients with juvenile chronic arthritis treated with chlorambucil. *Acta Paediatr* 1996;85:248–250.
429. DeFronzo RA, Braine H, Colvin M, et al. Water intoxication in man after cyclophosphamide therapy. Time course and relation to drug activation. *Ann Intern Med* 1973;78:861–869.
430. Herman EH, Mhatre RM, Waravdekar VS, et al. Comparison of the cardiovascular actions of NSC-109,724 (ifosfamide) and cyclophosphamide. *Toxicol Appl Pharmacol* 1972;23:178–190.
431. Karchmer RK, Hansen VL. Possible anaphylactic reaction to intravenous cyclophosphamide. Report of a case. *JAMA* 1977;237: 475.
432. Jones JB, Purdy CY, Bailey RT Jr. Cyclophosphamide anaphylaxis. *DICP* 1989;23:88–89.
433. Arena PJ. Oropharyngeal sensation associated with rapid intravenous administration of cyclophosphamide (NSC-26271). *Cancer Chemother Rep* 1972;56:779–780.
434. Sigal LH. Chronic inflammatory polyneuropathy complicating SLE: successful treatment with monthly oral pulse cyclophosphamide. *J Rheumatol* 1989;16:1518–1519.
435. Knysak DJ, McLean JA, Solomon WR, et al. Immediate hypersensitivity reaction to cyclophosphamide. *Arthritis Rheum* 1994;37:1101–1104.
436. Green RM, Schapel GJ, Sage RE. Cutaneous vasculitis due to cyclophosphamide therapy for chronic lymphocytic leukemia. *Aust N Z J Med* 1989;19:55–57.
437. Godard P, Marty JP, Michel FB. Interstitial pneumonia and chlorambucil. *Chest* 1979;76:471–473.
438. American College of Rheumatology Ad Hoc Committee on Clinical Guidelines. Guidelines for monitoring drug therapy in rheumatoid arthritis. *Arthritis Rheum* 1996;39:723–731.
439. Arnold MH, Janssen B, Schrieber L, et al. Prospective pilot study of intravenous pulse cyclophosphamide therapy for refractory rheumatoid arthritis. *Arthritis Rheum* 1989;32:933–934.
440. Horslev-Petersen K, Beyer JM, Helin P. Intermittent cyclophosphamide in refractory rheumatoid arthritis. *BMJ* 1983;287:711–712.
441. Renier JC, Deshayes P, Besson J, et al. Treatment of rheumatoid polyarthritis by chlorambucil. Apropos of 48 cases. *Presse Med* 1967;75: 2527–2530.
442. Iannuzzi L, Dawson N, Zein N, et al. Does drug therapy slow radiographic deterioration in rheumatoid arthritis? *N Engl J Med* 1983; 309:1023–1028.
443. McCune WJ, Golbus J, Zeldes W, et al. Clinical and immunologic effects of monthly administration of intravenous cyclophosphamide in severe systemic lupus erythematosus. *N Engl J Med* 1988;318:1423–1431.
444. McCune WJ, Fox D. Intravenous cyclophosphamide therapy of severe SLE. *Rheum Dis Clin North Am* 1989;15:455–477.

445. Snaith ML, Holt JM, Oliver DO, et al. Treatment of patients with systemic lupus erythematosus including nephritis with chlorambucil. *BMJ* 1973;2:197–201.
446. Balow JE, Austin HAd, Tsokos GC, et al. NIH conference. Lupus nephritis. *Ann Intern Med* 1987;106:79–94.
447. Steinberg AD, Steinberg SC. Long-term preservation of renal function in patients with lupus nephritis receiving treatment that includes cyclophosphamide versus those treated with prednisone only. *Arthritis Rheum* 1991;34:945–950.
448. McInnes PM, Schuttinga J, Sanslone WR, et al. The economic impact of treatment of severe lupus nephritis with prednisone and intravenous cyclophosphamide. *Arthritis Rheum* 1994;37:1000–1006.
449. Lehman TJ, Sherry DD, Wagner-Weiner L, et al. Intermittent intravenous cyclophosphamide therapy for lupus nephritis. *J Pediatr* 1989;114:1055–1060.
450. Bertoni M, Brugnolo F, Bertoni E, et al. Long term efficacy of high-dose intravenous methylprednisolone pulses in active lupus nephritis. A 21-month prospective study. *Scand J Rheumatol* 1994;23: 82–86.
451. Boumpas DT, Austin HAd, Vaughn EM, et al. Controlled trial of pulse methylprednisolone versus two regimens of pulse cyclophosphamide in severe lupus nephritis. *Lancet* 1992;340:741–745.
452. Houssiau FA, D'Cruz DP, Haga HJ, et al. Short course of weekly low-dose intravenous pulse cyclophosphamide in the treatment of lupus nephritis: a preliminary study. *Lupus* 1991;1:31–35.
453. Schroeder JO, Euler HH, Loffler H. Synchronization of plasmapheresis and pulse cyclophosphamide in severe systemic lupus erythematosus. *Ann Intern Med* 1987;107:344–346.
454. Dau PC, Callahan J, Parker R, et al. Immunologic effects of plasmapheresis synchronized with pulse cyclophosphamide in systemic lupus erythematosus. *J Rheumatol* 1991;18:270–276.
455. Barr WG, Hubbell EA, Robinson JA. Plasmapheresis and pulse cyclophosphamide in systemic lupus erythematosus. *Ann Intern Med* 1988;108:152–153.
456. Euler HH, Guillevin L. Plasmapheresis and subsequent pulse cyclophosphamide in severe systemic lupus erythematosus. An interim report of the Lupus Plasmapheresis Study Group. *Ann Med Interne* 1994;145:296–302.
457. Brunner M, Greinix HT, Redlich K, et al. Autologous blood stem cell transplantation in refractory systemic lupus erythematosus with severe pulmonary impairment: a case report. *Arthritis Rheum* 2002;46: 1580–1584.
458. Stewart M, Petri M. Lupus nephritis outcomes: health maintenance organizations compared to non-health maintenance organizations. *J Rheumatol* 2000;27:900–902.
459. Boumpas DT, Barez S, Klippel JH, et al. Intermittent cyclophosphamide for the treatment of autoimmune thrombocytopenia in systemic lupus erythematosus. *Ann Intern Med* 1990;112:674–677.
460. Roach BA, Hutchinson GJ. Treatment of refractory, systemic lupus erythematosus-associated thrombocytopenia with intermittent low-dose intravenous cyclophosphamide. *Arthritis Rheum* 1993;36:682–684.
461. Winkler A, Jackson RW, Kay DS, et al. High-dose intravenous cyclophosphamide treatment of systemic lupus erythematosus-associated aplastic anemia. *Arthritis Rheum* 1988;31:693–694.
462. Laing TJ. Gastrointestinal vasculitis and pneumatosis intestinalis due to systemic lupus erythematosus: successful treatment with pulse intravenous cyclophosphamide. *Am J Med* 1988;85:555–558.
463. Barile L, Lavalle C. Transverse myelitis in systemic lupus erythematosus—the effect of IV pulse methylprednisolone and cyclophosphamide. *J Rheumatol* 1992;19:370–372.
464. Boumpas DT, Yamada H, Patronas NJ, et al. Pulse cyclophosphamide for severe neuropsychiatric lupus. *Q J Med* 1991;81:975–984.
465. Stojanovich L, Stojanovich R, Kostich V, et al. Neuropsychiatric lupus favourable response to low dose i.v. cyclophosphamide and prednisolone (pilot study). *Lupus* 2003;12:3–7.
466. Fukuda M, Kamiyama Y, Kawahara K, et al. The favourable effect of cyclophosphamide pulse therapy in the treatment of massive pulmonary haemorrhage in systemic lupus erythematosus. *Eur J Pediatr* 1994;153:167–170.
467. Eiser AR, Shanies HM. Treatment of lupus interstitial lung disease with intravenous cyclophosphamide. *Arthritis Rheum* 1994;37:428–431.
468. Godeau B, Cormier C, Menkes CJ. Bronchiolitis obliterans in systemic lupus erythematosus: beneficial effect of intravenous cyclophosphamide. *Ann Rheum Dis* 1991;50:956–958.
469. Groen H, Bootsma H, Postma DS, et al. Primary pulmonary hypertension in a patient with systemic lupus erythematosus: partial improvement with cyclophosphamide. *J Rheumatol* 1993;20:1055–1057.
470. Fauci AS, Haynes BF, Katz P, et al. Wegener's granulomatosis: prospective clinical and therapeutic experience with 85 patients for 21 years. *Ann Intern Med* 1983;98:76–85.
471. Weiner SR, Paulus SR. Treatment of Wegener's granulomatosis with cyclophosphamide. Outcome analysis. *Arthritis Rheum Suppl* 1983; 26:65.
472. Fort JG, Abruzzo JL. Reversal of progressive necrotizing vasculitis with intravenous pulse cyclophosphamide and methylprednisolone. *Arthritis Rheum* 1988;31:1194–1198.
473. Shelhamer JH, Volkman DJ, Parrillo JE, et al. Takayasu's arteritis and its therapy. *Ann Intern Med* 1985;103:121–126.
474. Scott DG, Bacon PA. Intravenous cyclophosphamide plus methylprednisolone in treatment of systemic rheumatoid vasculitis. *Am J Med* 1984;76:377–384.
475. Guillevin L, Cordier JF, Lhote F, et al. A prospective, multicenter, randomized trial comparing steroids and pulse cyclophosphamide versus steroids and oral cyclophosphamide in the treatment of generalized Wegener's granulomatosis. *Arthritis Rheum* 1997;40:2187–2198.
476. Dau PC, Kahaleh MB, Sagebiel RW. Plasmapheresis and immunosuppressive drug therapy in scleroderma. *Arthritis Rheum* 1981;24: 1128–1136.
477. Silver RM, Warrick JH, Kinsella MB, et al. Cyclophosphamide and low-dose prednisone therapy in patients with systemic sclerosis (scleroderma) with interstitial lung disease. *J Rheumatol* 1993;20: 838–844.
478. Akesson A, Scheja A, Lundin A, et al. Improved pulmonary function in systemic sclerosis after treatment with cyclophosphamide [Comments]. *Arthritis Rheum* 1994;37:729–735.
479. Varai G, Earle L, Jimenez SA, et al. A pilot study of intermittent intravenous cyclophosphamide for the treatment of systemic sclerosis associated lung disease. *J Rheumatol* 1998;25:1325–1329.
480. Johnson MA, Kwan S, Snell NJ, et al. Randomised controlled trial comparing prednisolone alone with cyclophosphamide and low dose prednisolone in combination in cryptogenic fibrosing alveolitis. *Thorax* 1989;44:280–288.
481. Furst DE, Clements PJ, Hillis S, et al. Immunosuppression with chlorambucil, versus placebo, for scleroderma. Results of a three-year, parallel, randomized, double-blind study. *Arthritis Rheum* 1989; 32:584–593.
482. Kono DH, Klashman DJ, Gilbert RC. Successful IV pulse cyclophosphamide in refractory PM in 3 patients with SLE. *J Rheumatol* 1990; 17:982–983.
483. Bombardieri S, Hughes GR, Neri R, et al. Cyclophosphamide in severe polymyositis. *Lancet* 1989;1:1138–1139.
484. Cronin ME, Miller FW, Hicks JE, et al. The failure of intravenous cyclophosphamide therapy in refractory idiopathic inflammatory myopathy. *J Rheumatol* 1989;16:1225–1228.
485. El-Ghobarey A, Balint G, de Ceulaer K, et al. Dermatomyositis: observations on the use of immunosuppressive therapy and review of literature. Cairo–Glasgow study group. *Postgrad Med J* 1978;54: 516–527.
486. Hirano F, Tanaka H, Nomura Y, et al. Successful treatment of refractory polymyositis with pulse intravenous cyclophosphamide and low-dose weekly oral methotrexate therapy. *Intern Med* 1993;32: 749–752.
487. Sinoway PA, Callen JP. Chlorambucil. An effective corticosteroid-sparing agent for patients with recalcitrant dermatomyositis. *Arthritis Rheum* 1993;36:319–324.
488. al-Janadi M, Smith CD, Karsh J. Cyclophosphamide treatment of interstitial pulmonary fibrosis in polymyositis/dermatomyositis. *J Rheumatol* 1989;16:1592–1596.
489. Geltner D, Kohn RW, Gorevic P, et al. The effect of combination therapy (steroids, immunosuppressives, and plasmapheresis) on 5 mixed cryoglobulinemia patients with renal, neurologic, and vascular involvement. *Arthritis Rheum* 1981;24:1121–1127.

490. Mishima S, Masuda K, Izawa Y, et al. The eighth Frederick H. Verhoeff Lecture, presented by Saiichi Mishima, MD. Behçet's disease in Japan: ophthalmologic aspects. *Trans Am Ophthalmol Soc* 1979; 77:225–279.
491. Tabbara KF. Chlorambucil in Behçet's disease. A reappraisal. *Ophthalmology* 1983;90:906–908.
492. Erickson SB, Kurtz SB, Donadio JV Jr, et al. Use of combined plasmapheresis and immunosuppression in the treatment of Goodpasture's syndrome. *Mayo Clin Proc* 1979;54:714–720.
493. Grupe WE, Heymann W. Cytotoxic drugs in steroid-resistant renal disease. Alkylating and antimetabolic agents in the treatment of nephrotic syndrome, lupus nephritis, chronic glomerulonephritis, and purpura nephritis in children. *Am J Dis Child* 1966;112:448–458.
494. Sato M, Takeda A, Honzu H, et al. Adult Still's disease with Sjögren's syndrome successfully treated with intravenous pulse methylprednisolone and oral cyclophosphamide. *Intern Med* 1993; 32:730–732.
495. Buriot D, Prieur AM, Lebranchu Y, et al. [Acute leukemia in 3 children with chronic juvenile arthritis treated with chlorambucil]. *Arch Fr Pediatr* 1979;36:592–598.
496. Skoglund RR, Schanberger JE, Kaplan JM. Cyclophosphamide therapy for severe juvenile rheumatoid arthritis. *Am J Dis Child* 1971; 121:531–533.
497. Lehman TV, McCurdy D, Bernstein B, et al. Intravenous bolus cyclophosphamide (IV-C) therapy of lupus nephritis in childhood. *Arthritis Rheum* 1986;29(suppl):92.
498. Shaikov AV, Maximov AA, Speransky AI, et al. Repetitive use of pulse therapy with methylprednisolone and cyclophosphamide in addition to oral methotrexate in children with systemic juvenile rheumatoid arthritis—preliminary results of a longterm study. *J Rheumatol* 1992;19:612–616.
499. Wallace CA, Sherry DD. Trial of intravenous pulse cyclophosphamide and methylprednisolone in the treatment of severe systemic-onset juvenile rheumatoid arthritis. *Arthritis Rheum* 1997;40:1852–1855.

CHAPTER 42

Traditional Disease-Modifying Antirheumatic Drugs: Gold Compounds, D-Penicillamine, Sulfasalazine, and Antimalarials

W. Winn Chatham

With the goal of managing symptoms, improving function, and potentially arresting disease progression, experience with a number of drugs used to manage rheumatic diseases has developed over the past century. The utility of many traditional disease-modifying anti-rheumatic drugs (DMARDs) for treatment of rheumatoid arthritis (RA) was discovered either by happenstance or through efforts to use known properties of a compound to address purported triggers or pathophysiologic mechanisms underlying the disease. Increased knowledge of the immunologic events and inflammatory mediators underlying rheumatic disease has provided insight into potential mechanisms of DMARD efficacy, but much still remains to be learned with regard to why certain DMARDs are efficacious. Although the advent of biologic agents and pharmaceutical compounds that target established disease mechanisms will likely relegate use of traditional DMARDs to a passing era, an understanding of their use and toxicities remains important for current practice. This chapter discusses traditional DMARDs, emphasizing known biologic effects, optimal dosing and administration, known toxicities, and appropriate monitoring during their prescribed use. Methotrexate, leflunomide, cyclosporine, and azathioprine are covered in separate chapters.

GOLD COMPOUNDS

Dating back to the nineteenth century, gold salts were used for the treatment of infectious diseases, including tuberculosis. The purported antiseptic effects of gold salts prompted their use in a variety of infectious disorders with rheumatic manifestations (1). The benefits of aurothioglucose in the management of articular symptoms in patients with endocarditis and rheumatic fever were reported by Lande in 1927 (1). Based on these experiences and the hypothesis that rheumatoid joint inflammation might be a manifestation of infection with mycobacteria, gold salts were subsequently used for the treatment of RA and shown to be beneficial (2). Although a link between mycobacterial infection and RA remains to be established, the clinical experiences with gold compounds over the ensuing six decades resulted in widespread acceptance of the utility of gold in the management of RA and chronic synovitis associated with other diseases. Due to a relatively less favorable toxicity profile, the use of gold salts as a first-line DMARD for the treatment of RA has by and large been supplanted by use of weekly methotrexate and biologic reagents targeting cytokines implicated in the pathogenesis of RA and other chronic inflammatory arthritides. Gold salts are nonetheless highly effective and remain a therapeutic option for selected patients with chronic synovitis.

Chemistry

Elemental gold has multiple oxidation states (0, I, II, III, IV, and V), which result in a complex coordination chemistry. The most common oxidation states are I (Au^{+}) and III (Au^{+++}). These oxidized species form coordination bonds with ligands containing atoms with lone pairs of electrons that function as electron donors to the positively charged gold ions. The biochemistry and biologic activity of gold compounds is dependent on the number and types of ligands coordinated to gold, the coordination geometry (stereochemistry) around the gold, and the thermodynamic stability of the resulting compound. Metallic or colloidal gold (gold 0) is not biologically active, and simple salts of monovalent aurous gold such as gold chloride are not stable (3).

Gold preparations used in clinical practice consist of monovalent gold I (Au^+) complexed to organic molecules via a sulfur moiety (Fig. 42.1). Complexes consisting of gold in other oxidation states have unacceptable toxicity (gold III) or have not been studied. The gold thiolate compounds, such as gold sodium thiomalate (GST) and aurothioglucose, are hydrophilic and exist primarily as hexameric polymers, with two sulfur moieties in linear geometric coordination with each gold atom (Fig. 42.2). In aqueous solutions, both GST and aurothioglucose readily interact with other thiols, which can displace the drugs' thiolate ligands (3). This reactivity of gold compounds with thiols likely accounts for the biologic effects of gold salts.

Auranofin is a triethylphosphine gold compound that differs from the other compounds in that it is primarily a monomer with greater solubility in lipids. Unlike the other gold preparations, a significant percentage of auranofin can be absorbed following oral ingestion. Auranofin is capable of participating in phosphine transfer reactions, but the biologic significance of such reactions is unknown. The reactivity of auranofin with sulfhydryl groups is much weaker than that of the other gold compounds (3). Because reactivity with sulfhydryl groups may be responsible for much of the biologic activity of gold preparations, this may account for the clinical observation that auranofin is often less efficacious than aurothioglucose or GST in the management of rheumatoid synovitis.

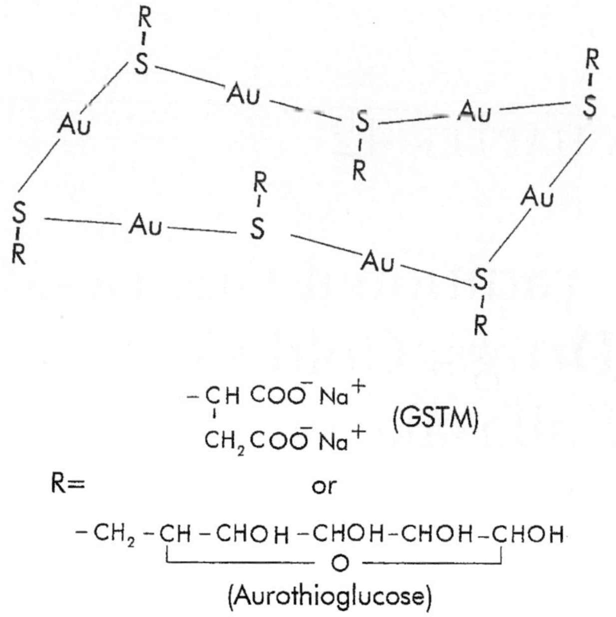

R= $-CH(COO^-Na^+)CH_2COO^-Na^+$ (GSTM) or $-CH_2-CH-CHOH-CHOH-CHOH-CHOH$ (ring O) (Aurothioglucose)

FIG. 42.2. Bonding of gold ions to sulfur atoms with formation of gold sodium thiomalate or aurothioglucose hexamers in aqueous solution.

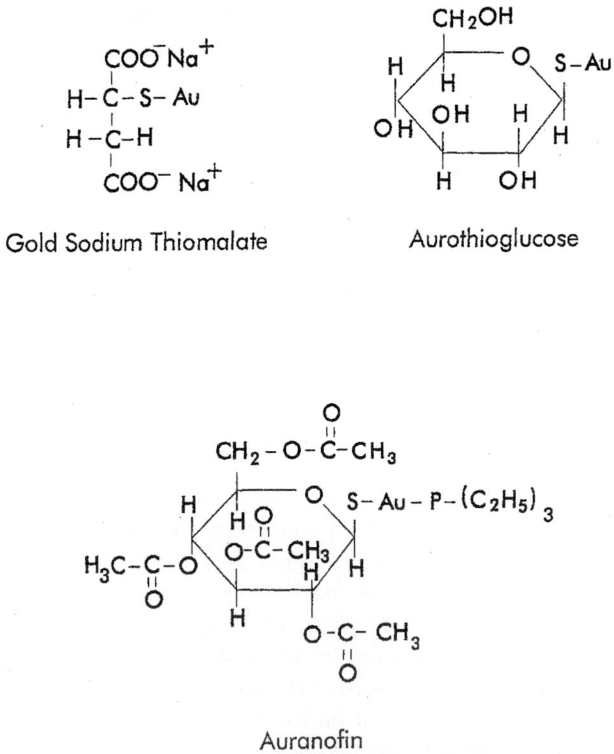

Gold Sodium Thiomalate

Aurothioglucose

Auranofin

FIG. 42.1. Chemical structures of commonly used gold preparations.

Biologic Effects

Although a primary mechanism underlying the clinical efficacy of gold salts has never been established, alterations in disease activity observed during treatment of RA with gold may be attributable, in part, to drug-induced alterations of protein function and alterations in cellular immunity. Although the capability of gold compounds to interact with protein sulfhydryl groups or disulfides can be readily demonstrated *in vitro,* the extent to which such interactions occur *in vivo* and mediate the biologic effects of therapeutic gold preparations is unknown.

In patients with RA, a decrease in the number of circulating $CD5^+$ B cells occurs following treatment with gold compounds (4). Treatment with GST results in decreased serum levels of circulating immune complexes, rheumatoid factor, and total levels of immunoglobulin. Whether these changes are primarily due to direct effects of gold compounds on B-cell function or the function of T cells responsible for inducing B-cell activation has not been delineated. The predominant attenuation in serum levels of immunoglobulin G1 (IgG1), IgG2, and IgG3 and absence in attenuation in levels of the helper T cell subset 2 (T_H2)-dependent IgG4 and IgE subclasses observed in the setting of gold treatment suggests that the effect of gold on immunoglobulin levels is mediated by attenuation in T_H1 responses (5).

Direct effects on B cells may nonetheless occur because auranofin and GST have been shown to inhibit IgM production by normal donor-derived B cells (6).

Gold compounds may interfere with antigen presentation by altering major histocompatibility complex (MHC)–peptide complexes (7,8). GST suppresses the differentiation of peripheral blood–derived dendritic cells and impairs dendritic cell production of IL-12 (9). These effects are consistent with the known inhibitory effects of auranofin and GST on transformation of lymphocytes in human mixed lymphocyte cultures and in response to a variety of mitogens *in vitro* (10,11). Despite the observed inhibitory effect on *in vitro* lymphocyte mitogenic responses, treatment of RA patients with GST has been shown to restore impaired mitogenic responses (12,13). Some of the observed changes in lymphocyte function noted in response to treatment with gold compounds may be due in part to the inhibitory effects of these compounds on monocyte and macrophage function. In rat models of adjuvant arthritis, GST alters the suppressive effects of splenic monocytes on mitogenic responses. The observed effects of gold compounds on dendritic cell function and monocyte-derived cytokines may furthermore account for the apparent skewing of T cells toward a T_H2 phenotype during treatment with gold (14).

Gold compounds may alter the influx of phagocytic cells into inflamed tissues via effects on synovial endothelial cells. In one study, treatment with parenteral gold compounds attenuated expression of the leukocyte adhesion ligand endothelium leukocyte adhesion molecule-1 (E-selectin) on synovial endothelial cells (15). Inhibitory effects of GST on synovial angiogenesis and synovial fibroblast proliferation have also been demonstrated and may contribute significantly to the efficacy of gold compounds in suppressing rheumatoid synovitis (16). Gold compounds also inhibit monocyte chemotaxis and attenuate the production of both monocyte chemotactic factor-1 (MCP-1) and interleukin-8 (IL-8) by cultured synoviocytes (17). These *in vitro* findings correlate well with synovial biopsy studies in which the numbers of monocytes in the synovial lining layer are markedly decreased within several weeks of GST treatment (18).

Production of IL-1β and other monocyte and macrophage products, including angiogenic factors and vascular endothelial growth factor (VEGF) required for synovial proliferation, is also markedly attenuated in the presence of gold or other thiol-containing compounds (19,20). The demonstrated inhibitory effects of some gold preparations on IκB kinase (IKK) as well as the binding of nuclear factor κB (NFκB) transcription factor to DNA may account for observed attenuation of cytokine-triggered monocyte/macrophage products (21). Such effects may account for the broad array of monocyte/macrophage cytokines and tumor necrosis factor-α (TNF-α)-dependent responses observed to be attenuated during gold therapy.

Neutrophil functions are also inhibited in the presence of gold compounds. Both GST and auranofin exert noncompetitive inhibitory effects on phospholipase C, a membrane-associated enzyme mediating neutrophil signal transduction (22). Variable effects on neutrophil chemotactic responses have been described (23,24). Gold compounds may also impair neutrophil phagocytic responses, since skin window techniques have demonstrated impaired phagocytic cell uptake of colloidal carbon particles in patients treated with GST (25). Neutrophil production of halogenated oxidants such as hypochlorous acid (HOCl) that promote protease activity is inhibited in the presence of GST or auranofin; thiol-containing gold compounds are also effective scavengers of HOCl (26).

Inhibition of yet other enzymes may contribute to the biologic activity of gold preparations. The activity of guinea pig peritoneal macrophage enzymes such as β-glucuronidase and acid phosphatase are inhibited by GST, and activity of these same enzymes in human synovial fluid as well as synovial cathepsins are also inhibited by GST (27,28). Both GST and auranofin have inhibitory effects on trypsinlike enzymes known to activate metalloproteases (28). Inhibition of both prostaglandin E_2 (PGE_2) synthesis and activity of the first component of complement (C1) in serum and synovial fluid has been observed in the presence of therapeutic concentrations of GST (29–31).

Clinical Efficacy and Therapeutic Uses

Rheumatoid Arthritis

The efficacy of gold compounds in the treatment of RA was first reported by Forestier, who noted benefit in over two thirds of 550 patients treated with gold salts (2). Double-blind studies of 1 to 5 years duration later confirmed the efficacy of GST in the treatment of RA (32). In the Empire Rheumatism study, improvement in the treated group was maintained for 1 year after the last injection, but lost at the end of 2 years (33). In these and subsequent studies with injectable gold preparations as well as auranofin, improvement in symptoms as assessed by functional capacity, number of joints involved, grip strength, and analgesic use has been well documented (34–36).

In addition to improvement in joint disease, treatment with gold compounds is associated with improvement in clinical laboratory parameters associated with disease activity. Serum rheumatoid factor titer, erythrocyte sedimentation rate (ESR), C-reactive protein (CRP) levels, fibrinogen levels, circulating immune complexes, and levels of gammaglobulin all have been shown to decrease significantly during treatment with gold compounds (37–39).

Progression of joint space narrowing and osseous erosions is diminished during treatment with GST, with the effect on erosion progression comparable with what is observed among patients taking methotrexate (40). Attenuation in these radiographic parameters of disease progression correlates with improvement in other clinical parameters of disease activity, such as joint swelling and tenderness.

Treatment with auranofin may also reduce progression of osseous erosions in patients with RA, but evidence in favor of such an effect was based on comparing longitudinal roentgenographic studies of the hands and wrists with studies in a placebo group drawn from a previous study (41). Longitudinal studies of erosion progression during chrysotherapy indicate that although erosions may progress during the initial 6 months of therapy, regression, and even healing, of erosions (demonstrated roentgenographically by erosion cortication) may occur after 6 to 18 months of treatment (42).

Little data have been published with regard to the effects of gold compounds on extraarticular manifestations of RA. In one controlled 6-month study, treatment with GST reduced the number of subcutaneous nodules (43). The extent to which chrysotherapy impacts on less frequently occurring extraarticular features such as serositis and vasculitis is not known. Gold compounds have been used with some success in the management of Felty's syndrome (44,45).

Although the frequency with which gold compounds induce remissions in RA has been difficult to determine accurately, complete remissions of disease activity have been reported in several studies (46–48). Reported remissions most commonly occurred when disease was present less than a year and when chrysotherapy extended beyond 18 to 36 months. Unfortunately, significant numbers of patients with RA will continue to have manifestations of active disease despite 4 to 6 months of weekly chrysotherapy or, after initially responding to gold therapy, develop recrudescence of disease activity despite continued treatment (49,50). For patients who respond well to parenteral chrysotherapy but subsequently develop increased disease activity during less frequently administered maintenance therapy, a return to weekly treatment was shown to be beneficial (51). Similarly, patients who achieve a clinical remission on chrysotherapy but then develop recrudescence of their disease following discontinuation of gold frequently respond favorably to a second course of gold (52).

Due to lack of initial response or subsequent escape from the initial beneficial effects of chrysotherapy and the significant numbers of patients who must discontinue treatment because of toxicity, only a minority of patients remain on gold treatment beyond 3 to 5 years (49,50). This likely accounts for results of some long-term (5-year) outcome assessments, which suggest that chrysotherapy does not significantly improve functional status and overall symptoms (53).

Juvenile Arthritis and Spondyloarthropathies

Parenteral gold compounds have been used with success in selected patients with juvenile arthritis (54). Trials to assess the efficacy of auranofin in juvenile arthritis yielded disappointing results with regard to efficacy (55,56). In patients with psoriatic arthritis or other spondyloarthropathies, both parenteral gold compounds and auranofin are effective in the management of peripheral joint synovitis (57–60). However, despite improvement in synovitis, gold therapy has not been shown to prevent progression of erosions in psoriatic arthritis (60). Toxicities associated with the use of gold salts in these disorders are comparable with those observed in patients with RA; there is no firm evidence to indicate that use of gold salts either improves or exacerbates psoriatic skin lesions.

Administration and Pharmacokinetics

With the exception of auranofin, all gold preparations are formulated for parenteral administration. The preparations traditionally used most commonly in the United States were GST and aurothioglucose. GST is dissolved in an aqueous solution that may be given intramuscularly; aurothioglucose is emulsified in sesame oil formulated for intramuscular administration. Conventionally, treatment with GST or aurothioglucose is initiated with a test dosage of 10 mg and 25 mg given 1 week apart, then weekly administration of 25 to 50 mg thereafter until the full therapeutic effect is achieved or toxicity develops. The recommended weekly dose for children with juvenile arthritis is 0.5 to 1.0 mg/kg aurothioglucose or GST (61,62). Although weekly doses in excess of 50 mg GST or aurothioglucose have been used in adults during the initial 4 to 6 months of chrysotherapy, such regimens result in significantly greater toxicity, but with little improvement in clinical response compared with conventional lower dose schedules (63,64).

Once a cumulative dose of 1,000 mg in adults or 15 mg/kg in children has been administered, and the desired clinical response has been achieved, the frequency of parenteral gold administration may be decreased to every 2 weeks or every 4 weeks. Alternatively, for patients who exhibit a suboptimal response after a 1,000-mg cumulative dose, increasing the weekly dose in 10- to 25-mg increments may result in further improvement (65,66). To avoid undue toxicity, it is generally recommended that the weekly dose in adults not exceed 100 mg.

In patients receiving GST or aurothioglucose, intravascular gold is predominantly (>90%) bound to plasma proteins such as albumin, complement, and immunoglobulins (67,68). Binding to cellular membranes and erythrocyte proteins accounts for the remainder of intravascular gold (69). In smokers, erythrocyte levels of elemental gold are elevated, presumably due to formation of gold complexes with cyanide and thiocyanate, which readily enter erythrocytes (70,71). Serum levels of elemental gold peak at approximately 700 μg/dL approximately 2 hours following a 50-mg test dose of GST (67,72). At 7 days, levels decrease to approximately 300 μg/dL (72). Peak levels for aurothioglucose are somewhat less, but trough levels at 7 days are comparable with those that occur with GST. After 2 months of weekly treatment with 50 mg of either preparation, serum levels of elemental gold remain fairly steady at 300 to 400 μg/dL; serum levels average about 25% of this concentration in patients receiving monthly injections (67,72). Following parenteral administration, gold diffuses rapidly into synovial fluid, with steady-state levels approximating 50% of serum levels (73).

Gold is distributed widely throughout the body. Greater than 85% of retained gold is stored in the bone marrow, liver, skin, and cortical bone (74). Tissue levels of gold are highest in organs composed of reticuloendothelial cells. Reported levels of gold in lymph nodes of patients receiving aurothioglucose approach 300 μg of elemental gold per gram of tissue wet weight; levels in the liver, spleen, kidney, and bone marrow range from 75 to 150 μg/g wet weight (75). Within cells, gold localizes predominantly to cell and organelle membranes (76). Localization of gold in synovial tissue during chrysotherapy may vary with disease activity and cellularity of the synovium, but measured levels of gold in synovium are lower than those found in the aforementioned tissues (77). Even smaller amounts of gold (<5 μg/g) accumulate in cartilage (74). In addition to synovial fluid, gold also diffuses into other body fluids during chrysotherapy, including breast milk and bile. However, measured concentrations of gold in these body fluids are much lower than concomitant serum concentrations.

During chrysotherapy with parenteral gold preparations, excretion of gold is primarily through the urine (two thirds) and feces (one third) (67,78). It is estimated that 40% of the daily excreted gold (urinary plus fecal) is derived from the most recently administered dose, with the remainder derived from previously administered doses (78). Urinary and fecal excretion studies with ^{195}Au-sodium thiomalate confirm that during weekly parenteral administration of GST, approximately 60% of each dose is retained in the body (78).

Effective dosing for auranofin in adults with RA or psoriatic arthritis may be as low as 1 mg daily, but the optimal dose appears to be 3 mg twice daily. Up to 9 mg daily may prove more effective in some patients, but dosing at this level is likely to be limited by gastrointestinal intolerance. The few studies in which auranofin was used in children indicate that dosages of 0.1 to 0.2 mg/kg/day were effective and well tolerated (79). In patients taking auranofin daily, serum levels of elemental gold gradually increase over a 3-month period (80,81). For patients taking 6 mg daily, the levels plateau at approximately 70 μg/dL; a 1-mg change in the daily dose usually will result in a 10 μg/dL change in the steady-state serum level (82). During treatment with auranofin, significant leukocyte uptake occurs, with up to 50% of the intravascular gold residing in the cellular fraction (83).

Absorption and excretion of auranofin is dose related. Virtually no auranofin is absorbed when the dose is less than 2 mg daily, whereas 25% to 30% of the administered dose is absorbed and retained when the daily dose is 6 mg (84). Less than 5% of gold ingested in auranofin appears in the urine, which probably accounts for the 21-day blood half-life of auranofin (84,85).

Toxicity and Side Effects

During the course of treatment with parenteral gold compounds, about 33% of patients experience adverse reactions (Table 42.1). Although the majority of these reactions are relatively mild and may require only temporary withholding of, or adjustments in, the dose of gold, severe mucocutaneous, bone marrow, or renal toxicity may require cessation of therapy. Less than 50% of patients treated with parenteral gold compounds remain on gold after 5 years, with approximately 60% of treatment terminations attributable to toxicity (50). Significantly fewer patients taking auranofin discontinue therapy because of toxic reactions (35,86).

Mucocutaneous Reactions

Dermatitis and stomatitis are the most frequent complications experienced, accounting for up to 75% of reported side effects (87). Cutaneous problems associated with chrysotherapy are highly variable with regard to appearance, severity, distribution, and duration. Reactions range from mild pruritus, seen commonly, to exfoliative dermatitis or toxic epidermal necrolysis, which are infrequent. Skin rashes associated with gold therapy may mimic other skin conditions such as psoriasis, pityriasis rosea, or lichen planus in both their gross and histologic appearance. However, in many patients gold-related skin lesions are difficult to classify into known dermatologic entities. Mucocutaneous may occur in the absence of other findings but are often accompanied by eosinophilia or mild proteinuria.

TABLE 42.1. *Toxicity of gold compounds*

Mucocutaneous
Oral ulcers
Pruritus
Erythematous rashes
Lichen planus
Exfoliative dermatitis
Renal
Proteinuria
Microscopic hematuria
Bone marrow
Leukopenia
Thrombocytopenia
Aplastic anemia
Gastrointestinal
Diarrhea
Enterocolitis
Cholestasis
Pulmonary
Acute pneumonitis
Interstitial pneumonitis
Neurologic
Sensory-motor polyneuropathy
Ocular or cutaneous chrysiasis
Nitritoid reactions
Postinjection arthralgia/myalgia

Contamination of gold salt preparations with nickel has been implicated as the possible cause of nonspecific skin rashes in patients with demonstrated *in vitro* lymphocyte proliferative responses to this metal (88). Several studies indicate that immunogenetic factors contribute to the development of mucocutaneous reactions to gold, and biooxidation of administered gold(I) compounds is likely required for sensitization (89–92).

The occurrence of oral ulcers or erythematous rashes during treatment with gold compounds usually does not mandate permanent discontinuance of chrysotherapy. Most mucocutaneous reactions can be managed successfully by withholding gold, treating oral lesions with topical anesthetic or corticosteroid gels, and managing pruritus symptoms with an antihistamine. More severe cutaneous reactions may require use of topical steroids and emollients; the use of systemic corticosteroids is of unproven utility. In the presence of bullous eruptions, exfoliative dermatitis, or lichen planus, chrysotherapy should not be reinstituted. In the absence of these more severe reactions, once the oral or cutaneous lesions have resolved, gold compounds can be reinstituted, albeit at a lower dose. If mucocutaneous symptoms do not recur, small increments in the weekly dose can be undertaken at 3- to 4-week intervals.

Chrysiasis

Chrysiasis, a gray-blue pigmentation of the skin that may occur in association with protracted parenteral chrysotherapy, is of little clinical significance. The mechanisms underlying development of chrysiasis are unknown, and the total dose of gold administered or concentration of gold in the skin does not appear to correlate with development of this relatively rare complication (93,94). Ocular chrysiasis, or deposition of gold salts in the cornea or (less frequently) the lens, is detectable with slit-lamp examination in virtually all patients who have received in excess of 1 g of parenteral gold compounds. These identified deposits are also of limited, if any, clinical significance.

Proteinuria

Proteinuria is the second most common side effect observed during chrysotherapy. Proteinuria occurs in approximately 10% of patients treated with gold compounds. The typical histologic lesions seen in renal biopsies of patients with gold-induced proteinuria are mesangial deposits of immune complexes in association with basement membrane deposits typically seen in classic idiopathic membranous glomerulonephritis (95). Although nephrotic syndrome and renal failure may occur in rare instances, proteinuria induced by gold compounds is usually mild and, when recognized early, typically resolves following discontinuation of gold therapy (96,97). In some patients treated with gold compounds, microscopic hematuria without evidence of renal insufficiency has been observed in the absence of other identifiable causes (98). In one study, proximal tubular damage manifested by elevated excretion of *N*-acetyl glucosaminidase was reported to occur more frequently than microalbuminuria during the induction phase of parenteral gold therapy (99).

Bone Marrow Toxicity

Toxicity to hematopoietic cells in the bone marrow constitutes the most serious adverse effect associated with the use of gold compounds. Gold may induce granulocytopenia, anemia, thrombocytopenia, or any combination of these entities. Severe, life-threatening leukopenia may develop at any time during treatment with parenteral or oral gold compounds, as may thrombocytopenia, which occurs in 1% to 3% of patients receiving gold compounds (100, 101). The prevalence of aplastic anemia is less than 0.5%, but development of this complication is ominous, with mortality rates reported to be as high as 60% (102). Management of severe leukopenia or marrow aplasia induced by gold is supportive, with judicious use of red cell or platelet transfusions for severe anemia or thrombocytopenia, respectively. Use of recombinant granulocyte-stimulating factor (GSF) may hasten marrow recovery in patients with severe neutropenia.

Eosinophilia occurs during chrysotherapy in 5% to 40% of patients (depending on the population reported and case definition) and may occur in the presence or absence of other manifestations of gold toxicity (103). Immunoglobulin deficiency affecting one or more isotypes has been reported to occur during treatment with gold compounds; hypogammaglobulinemia did not correlate with duration of therapy and was reversible following discontinuation of gold (104).

Nitritoid Reactions

Nitritoid reactions are vasomotor responses to injection of GST that induce symptoms of flushing, nausea, vomiting, sweating, or dizziness. The associated peripheral vasodilatation is usually well-tolerated but, in elderly patients with arteriosclerotic vascular disease, may result in stroke or myocardial infarction (105). Other transient symptoms reported to occur after administration of GST include arthralgias, myalgias, fatigue, and malaise (106). These symptom complexes are rarely seen following administration of aurothioglucose; classic nitritoid reactions have been reported with use of auranofin (107).

Other Organ Toxicity

Less frequently encountered complications of gold therapy involve the lung parenchyma, gastrointestinal tract, and peripheral nervous system. Gold compounds may induce an acute pulmonary syndrome of cough, fever, progressive dyspnea, and roentgenographic findings of diffuse infiltrates with patchy consolidation (108,109). The pulmonary syndrome typically resolves quickly upon withdrawal of gold treatment and institution of corticosteroids. Treatment with gold compounds may also be associated with insidious development of interstitial lung disease with impaired gas exchange. However, similar pulmonary function abnormalities occur in patients with untreated RA, and it may be difficult to determine whether observed changes in lung function are due to chrysotherapy or the underlying disease process. Distinguishing features that implicate gold-induced pulmonary disease rather than rheumatoid lung disease as the cause of lung abnormalities include the presence of skin rash, eosinophilia, lymphocytosis in bronchoalveolar lavage fluids, alveolar opacities on chest computed tomography (CT) scan, absent or low titer of rheumatoid factor titer, and absence of cutaneous nodules (110). In the setting of progressive lung function abnormalities, particularly if the rheumatoid disease is otherwise in remission, discontinuation of gold compounds may be advisable.

Enterocolitis is a potentially serious complication reported in patients receiving parenteral gold compounds. Presenting signs and symptoms may include nausea, vomiting, abdominal pain, and bloody or nonbloody diarrhea (111,112). Colonoscopic evaluation typically reveals mucosal edema and ulceration, but in some instances the enteritis may be limited to the ileum. Aggressive treatment is warranted because significant mortality occurs unless gold treatment is stopped and appropriate treatment with bowel decompression and antibiotics instituted. Corticosteroids are also frequently used in the management of gold-induced enterocolitis, but the efficacy of this intervention is uncertain (112). Mild, transient, dose-related lower gastrointestinal symptoms are associated with the use of auranofin. Change in stool consistency and frequency with or without abdominal cramping are among the most frequent side effects reported with the use of oral gold, but frank enterocolitis has not been reported with the use of auranofin (86). Biliary stasis is another uncommon side effect of chrysotherapy which may present as jaundice, pruritus, anorexia, or hepatomegaly; laboratory findings include elevated serum transaminase and alkaline phosphatase levels (113,114).

Although neurologic side effects of chrysotherapy are infrequent; the most commonly reported neurologic complication is polyneuropathy (115). A mixed, predominantly distal sensory motor neuropathy, as well as an acute polyneuropathy of the Guillain-Barré type, have been reported. Rarer complications attributed to gold compounds include encephalopathy and myopathy.

Therapeutic Considerations and Monitoring

Patient Selection

Clinical studies comparing GST with methotrexate for treatment of RA indicate that GST and methotrexate have comparable efficacy with respect to improvement in tender or swollen joints, ESR, CRP, and erosion scores, although methotrexate appears to be much better tolerated (116–119). One study comparing GST to methotrexate in patients with early erosive RA found that a greater percentage of patients achieved clinical remission when treated with GST (120). However, due to ease of administration, more rapid improvement in joint symptoms, and favorable tolerability, weekly administration of methotrexate has supplanted gold compounds as the initial DMARD prescribed for the majority of patients with active RA. The incorporation of specific TNF-α-inhibiting biologic therapies (etanercept, adalimumab, and infliximab) into treatment programs for RA and spondyloarthropathies has furthermore decreased the use of gold preparations. Gold preparations may nonetheless still be a useful option for management of RA or spondyloarthropathy-associated synovitis in selected patients with comorbidities related to liver disorders, significant preexisting lung disease, renal impairment, or significant infection risk that precludes use of other DMARDs or TNF inhibitors.

Cutaneous disorders, including psoriasis, are not contraindications to treatment with gold compounds, because there is no definitive evidence that chrysotherapy exacerbates preexisting skin diseases. Gold compounds have been used successfully in patients with preexisting leukopenia due to Felty's syndrome. Although there is little evidence implicating significant risk to the fetus or nursing infants of mothers treated with gold compounds, the safety of gold compounds in these settings has not been established. Accordingly, it remains common practice to avoid treating pregnant or nursing women with gold compounds. Alternatives to gold therapy should be considered for patients with preexisting proteinuria.

Gold compounds have been used in combination with other DMARDs (Chapter 33). In studies examining the effect of gold compounds in combination with methotrexate, hydroxychloroquine (HCQ), and cyclosporine, the tolerability and toxicity for the combination regimens are comparable to what is observed when the respective agents are used alone (121–124). However, outcomes of patients with established RA treated with methotrexate in combination with oral or parenteral gold are not significantly improved relative to patients treated with methotrexate alone (122,125).

Cost

The costs associated with parenteral chrysotherapy are significant. The present (2003) average retail cost for a 500-mg vial of GST or aurothioglucose ranges from \$140 to \$160. When laboratory charges for assessments of blood counts and urinalyses and costs for either visits to the physician's office or from a home health nurse for parenteral administration are added, the yearly cost of initiating and maintaining parenteral chrysotherapy may exceed \$2,500. Retail pharmacy costs for a 3-mg twice daily course of auranofin range from \$65 to \$80 a month; when the laboratory monitoring costs are added, the yearly cost for treatment with auranofin is approximately $1,500.

Toxicity Monitoring

Assessment of a complete blood count (CBC) is prudent prior to each dose of parenteral gold compound. The manufacturer's package insert recommends monthly blood counts for patients on stable doses of auranofin, with more frequent assessments following initiation of, or increments in, the dose of auranofin. Development of significant leukopenia (<3,500/mm^3), thrombocytopenia (<100,000/mm^3), or a persistent downward trend in the platelet count or hematocrit should prompt cessation of chrysotherapy. In the absence of other identifiable causes for observed cytopenias, treatment with gold compounds should not be reinstituted. Although gold compounds may be used in patients with preexisting leukopenia due to Felty's syndrome, exacerbation of leukopenia in this setting may require bone marrow evaluation to rule out toxic effects of gold on leukocyte precursors in the marrow.

A urinalysis should be performed at least monthly during treatment with gold to monitor for development of proteinuria. Proteinuria during chrysotherapy is frequently transient, responding to temporary withholding of gold; most patients can resume treatment at lower doses without recurrence of proteinuria. Gold is usually not reinstituted in patients who develop nephrotic range proteinuria (>1 g protein excreted per 24 hours). Although many patients with this degree of proteinuria improve spontaneously over several months following cessation of chrysotherapy, treatment with corticosteroids may be required to effect recovery of glomerular integrity. The prognosis for recovery of patients developing gold-induced nephrotic syndrome is good, with over 70% of patients recovering fully. Progression or persistence of proteinuria following withdrawal of gold should prompt evaluation to rule out other factors such as amyloidosis, glomerular toxicity induced by other drugs, or nephrosclerosis.

PENICILLAMINE AND BUCILLAMINE

Penicillamine was first identified by Abraham and colleagues in acid hydrolysates of penicillin (126). The compound was later identified in the urine of patients with liver disease receiving penicillin for intercurrent infections (127). The avidity of penicillamine for metal ions such as Pb^{2+} and Cu^{2+} prompted its use as a chelating agent in patients with lead poisoning and Wilson's disease. The observed reactivity of penicillamine with disulfide bonds to form mixed disulfides rendered the compound useful in preventing formation of cysteine calculi in patients with cystinuria (128). The potential effectiveness of penicillamine in disrupting disulfide bonds in IgM rheumatoid factors provided the initial rationale for its use in RA (129). Although significant dissociation of circulating rheumatoid factors has not been observed to occur in patients treated with penicillamine, improvement in synovitis and other disease manifestations was documented during clinical trials with the drug in the 1960s and early 1970s. Penicillamine has also been used in the treatment of primary biliary cirrhosis, chronic active hepatitis, and scleroderma, but the efficacy of the drug in these disorders remains to be established by controlled clinical trials.

Chemistry

Penicillamine is a sulfhydryl analogue of cysteine, containing two methyl groups on the β carbon (Fig. 42.3). Penicillamine may be prepared synthetically or purified from hydrolysates of natural penicillin. The compound may occur as a D- or L-isomer, but the synthesized D-isomer is the only compound available for clinical use. Similar to gold preparations used clinically, D-penicillamine has a sulfhydryl moiety capable of binding divalent metal cations or interacting with sulfhydryl residues on proteins. Penicillamine may also form thiazolidines with pyridoxal phosphate (vitamin B_6) or the aldehyde cross-links of type I collagen. Bucillamine is a recently synthesized analogue of penicillamine. The presence of two free sulfhydryl groups distinguishes it structurally and functionally from penicillamine (Fig. 42.3).

Biologic Effects

The sulfhydryl moiety of D-penicillamine is highly reactive. Accordingly, penicillamine shares many of the biologic effects noted for thiol-containing gold compounds. Penicillamine is a potent scavenger of HOCl and has inhibitory effects on the catalytic activity of myeloperoxidase (130). Attenuation of the activity of leukocyte proteases may occur as a consequence of either these antioxidant effects or the metal chelating properties of the drug. Sulfhydryl reactivity also may induce displacement of sulfhydryl-containing cytokines such as IL-1β from their protective binding sites on serum proteins (α_2-macroglobulin), rendering the cytokines potentially more susceptible to proteolytic inactivation (131). Chelation of zinc likely accounts for the observed inhibition of collagenase or stromelysin activity in the presence of penicillamine *in vitro*, but whether penicillamine is capable of inhibiting these enzymes *in vivo* has not been established.

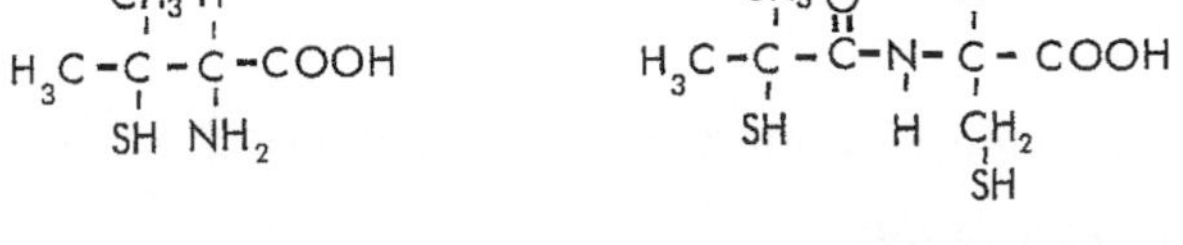

D-Penicillamine: $H_3C-C(CH_3)(SH)-C(H)(NH_2)-COOH$

Bucillamine: $H_3C-C(CH_3)(SH)-C(=O)-N(H)-C(H)(CH_2SH)-COOH$

FIG. 42.3. Chemical structures of D-penicillamine and bucillamine.

Penicillamine appears to modulate function of T- and B-cell lymphocytes. *In vitro* responsiveness of cultured human helper T cells to mitogens is suppressed in the presence of penicillamine (132); however, *ex vivo* studies to assess the function of lymphocytes obtained from patients with RA treated with penicillamine have yielded mixed results (133,134). In a small series of patients with scleroderma, treatment with penicillamine resulted in decreased numbers of circulating T cells with $CD4^+$ (helper/inducer) and $CD26^+$ (helper cells for B-cell differentiation) phenotypes (135). Indirect evidence that penicillamine alters T-cell regulatory function *in vivo* stems from the greater than expected number of autoimmune disorders such as pemphigus and myasthenia gravis observed in patients treated with penicillamine. Penicillamine may also modulate B-cell function, because spontaneous synthesis of IgM rheumatoid factors by cells derived from patients with RA is diminished following treatment with D-penicillamine.

Other biologic effects of penicillamine relate to the binding of penicillamine to thiazolidine residues on collagen chains. Penicillamine binds aldehyde moieties formed when lysyl residues are oxidized in a reaction catalyzed by lysyl oxidase. As a consequence, condensation of the aldehyde residues to form Schiff bases with formation of collagen cross-links characteristic of mature collagen is impaired. Despite this effect on maturation of collagen, use of penicillamine in doses employed for the treatment of RA does not appear to impair wound healing, and evidence of attenuation of fibrosis in disorders such as scleroderma has been inconclusive.

Bucillamine has biologic effects similar to penicillamine, but the presence of two, rather than one, sulfhydryl moieties appears to confer additional immunomodulatory attributes to this drug. Comparable inhibition of mitogen-induced T-cell proliferation and IL-2 production is observed in the presence of penicillamine and bucillamine (136). However, the inhibitory effect of penicillamine requires the presence of cupric ion and associated generation of hydrogen peroxide, whereas the inhibitory effect of bucillamine does not (137,138). Although penicillamine and bucillamine may indirectly inhibit B-cell activation via their inhibitory effects on T-cell activation, bucillamine also has been shown to have direct inhibitory effects on IgM production by cultured B cells (139). Similar to observed effects of GST on synovial production of VEGF, production of this angiogenic factor is inhibited in the presence of bucillamine (140). In studies of explanted RA synovial fibroblasts, bucillamine has been shown to inhibit synovial cell proliferation and production of IL-1β, an effect not observed in the presence of D-penicillamine (141).

Clinical Efficacy and Therapeutic Uses

In controlled clinical trials, penicillamine has been demonstrated to be as effective as gold and azathioprine in managing symptoms of RA (142–144). Because the dose must be increased gradually, clinical responses may not become apparent for several months after institution of therapy. In addition to improving fatigue and joint symptoms, an increase in hemoglobin and a decrease in both the serum rheumatoid factor titer and ESR have been shown to gradually occur (145). With prolonged administration, significant reductions in levels of serum and synovial fluid immune complexes also occur (146). Despite the clinical improvement reported in patients who are able to tolerate therapeutic doses of penicillamine, progression of radiographic erosions has not been shown to be altered in most clinical trials (147–149).

Case reports published over the years have suggested that penicillamine may be of benefit in patients with extraarticular manifestations of RA such as vasculitis (150), rheumatoid nodulosis (151,152), Felty's syndrome (153), amyloidosis (154), and rheumatoid lung disease (155). In one study of sequential lung function tests in patients with RA, the serial decline in diffusion capacity corrected for lung volume was significantly less for patients treated with penicillamine compared with patients not on therapy or treated with gold, chloroquine, or methotrexate (156). Among patients with initial volume-corrected diffusion capacity (DLCO) less than 80% of the predicted value, diffusion capacity improved for patients treated with penicillamine, suggesting that the drug may favorably affect disease-related changes in lung function.

Penicillamine also has demonstrated efficacy in the management of juvenile arthritis (157,158). However, unlike gold compounds, penicillamine does not appear to be useful in the management of psoriatic arthritis or the peripheral joint symptoms associated with other spondyloarthropathies (159). Due to a number of anecdotal reports attesting to the efficacy of penicillamine in the treatment of systemic sclerosis, controlled clinical trials have been instituted to determine its efficacy in this disorder (160). In one recent study comparing the efficacy of high-dose (750–1,000 mg/day) and low-dose (125 mg every other day) D-penicillamine in patients with scleroderma, no significant differences in skin thickness scores, incidence of scleroderma renal crisis, or mortality were noted between the two groups after 2 years of treatment (161).

Administration and Pharmacokinetics

Treatment with penicillamine is usually initiated with an oral daily dose of 250 mg. The daily dose is gradually increased in 125- to 250-mg increments every 8 to 10 weeks until the desired clinical response is achieved. Most therapeutic responses in adults require a dose of 500 to 750 mg daily. If the desired clinical effect has not been achieved after 6 months of treatment with this dose, gradual increases in the dose of up to 1,000 mg daily may benefit some patients (162,163). To avoid toxicity, it is generally recommended that increasing the daily dose above 500 mg be undertaken in 125-mg increments at timed intervals (162,163). For patients who have achieved the desired clinical response, there is evidence that responses can be maintained with discontinuous (1 week per month) therapy (164).

Penicillamine is rapidly absorbed following oral ingestion. Because chelation of penicillamine by dietary metals (particularly iron) or oxidation of penicillamine by other dietary constituents to form disulfides can significantly impair absorption, it is recommended that the drug be taken at least 1 hour before or 2 hours after meals (165). In patients receiving daily penicillamine, peak plasma concentrations approaching 60 μ*M* occur within 1.5 to 3 hours following ingestion; for patients ingesting daily doses of 500 to 750 mg, mean serum levels range from 15 to 35 μ*M* (165,166). Over two thirds of penicillamine in plasma exists either as penicillamine disulfide or as mixed disulfides with either free cysteine or (predominantly) cysteine residues on serum proteins such as albumin and ceruloplasmin. Levels of penicillamine-albumin disulfide measured in the synovial fluids of some patients with RA ranged from 50% to 84% of concomitant serum levels (167).

Penicillamine is eliminated primarily via the urinary tract as penicillamine disulfide, cysteine-penicillamine, homocysteine-penicillamine, or *S*-methyl-D-penicillamine (166). Studies with radiolabeled D-penicillamine indicate that the drug is rapidly eliminated via the kidneys, with 80% of urinary excretion occurring within 10 hours. Animal studies indicate that penicillamine is rapidly eliminated from the liver and kidneys, but is cleared slowly from collagen- and elastin-rich tissues such as skin and bone. Due to extensive protein binding in these tissues, excretion of drug and its metabolites persists for weeks or months following cessation of therapy.

TABLE 42.2. *Toxicity of D-penicillamine*

Mucocutaneous
Oral ulcers
Erythematous, maculopapular, or urticarial rashes
Lichen planus
Alopecia/dermatitis (zinc deficiency)
Penicillamine dermatopathy[a]
Elastosis perforans serpiginosa[a]
Cutis laxa[a]
Renal
Proteinuria
Microscopic hematuria
Rapidly progressive glomerulonephritis
Bone marrow
Thrombocytopenia
Leukopenia
Red cell aplasia
Aplastic anemia
Gastrointestinal
Hepatitis
Cholestasis
Pulmonary
Acute pneumonitis
Acute alveolar hemorrhage
Obliterative bronchiolitis
Hypogeusia
Pyridoxine deficiency
Breast hypertrophy
Autoimmune disorders
Pemphigoid/pemphigus
Myasthenia gravis
Lupus erythematosus
Polymyositis

[a]Seen primarily with protracted, high-dose therapy for Wilson's disease or cystinuria.

Toxicity and Side Effects

Similar to the side effects observed in patients treated with gold compounds, mucocutaneous, hematologic, and renal toxicity are often a limiting factors when using penicillamine in the treatment of RA (Table 42.2). Although most side effects are observed during the initial year or two of therapy, experience with dosing regimens indicates that early toxic reactions can be minimized by starting with low doses of drug and increasing the dose slowly in small increments. Major toxic reactions are less likely to occur after 18 months of treatment and attainment of a stable dose.

Dermatopathy

Cutaneous reactions are the most common side effects experienced during treatment with penicillamine. Erythematous, maculopapular, or urticarial rashes accompanied by pruritus or fever can appear during the first weeks of therapy, and likely reflect an acute sensitivity syndrome to the drug (168). Self-limited dryness and scaling of facial skin that is inconsequential may occur during the first few months of therapy. With prolonged use of penicillamine, the development of scaly erythematous lesions around skin folds in association with alopecia may indicate zinc deficiency occurring as a consequence of zinc chelation (169). Aphthous oral or genital ulcers may occur during treatment with penicillamine, particularly following dose increments. Lichen planus affecting the buccal mucosa or skin is rarely seen in patients with RA taking penicillamine, but occurs more commonly in patients with primary biliary cirrhosis treated with penicillamine (170). The occurrence of oral ulcers or stomatitis with vesicular or plaquelike erosive skin lesions may be indicative of an evolving pemphigoid reaction, mandating prompt cessation of penicillamine. Cutaneous lesions associated with other penicillamine-induced autoimmune diseases are discussed later.

Protracted treatment with high doses of penicillamine may result in cutaneous abnormalities occurring as a consequence of the drug's effects on maturation of collagen and elastin. These disorders have been seen primarily in patients with Wilson's disease or cystinuria taking daily doses of penicillamine in excess of 2 g or who have undergone greater than 5 to 6 years of uninterrupted treatment with penicillamine (168). Thinning and friability of the skin over bony prominences or sites subject to pressure, often accompanied by painless bleeding or ecchymosis, are characteristic features of penicillamine dermatopathy (168). Direct effects of penicillamine on elastin or localized deficiency of copper required for normal synthesis of elastin may result in elastosis perforans serpiginosa (171,172). Premature aging and wrinkling of the skin and findings of cutis laxa have been reported in women treated 10 years or longer with penicillamine (173).

Bone Marrow Toxicity

Penicillamine can effect all components of the bone marrow, but most commonly affects levels of circulating platelets. Decreases in the platelet count are often gradual, and usually resolve spontaneously or with diminution in the dose of penicillamine. However, thrombocytopenia or leukopenia may develop precipitously at any dose or at any time during treatment with penicillamine. Leukopenia occurs much less frequently during treatment with penicillamine than with gold compounds, but aplastic anemia may occur. Pure red cell aplasia during treatment of RA with penicillamine has also been reported (174).

Glomerulopathy

Proteinuria occurs in 10% to 20% of patients treated with penicillamine, and may progress to nephrotic syndrome if therapy is continued. Minimal changes are seen on light microscopy, but electron microscopic analysis of glomeruli from affected patients frequently reveals glomerular basement membrane deposits (175,176). Microscopic hematuria during treatment with penicillamine is often a benign occurrence not requiring discontinuance of therapy (177). However, rapidly progressive glomerulonephritis has been reported in patients with RA taking penicillamine, and careful inspection of the urinary sediment and monitoring of renal function is warranted in any patient developing hematuria or proteinuria (178,179).

Autoimmune Syndromes

In patients with RA, therapy with penicillamine is associated with a greater than expected occurrence of a variety of autoimmune syndromes (Table 42.2). A characteristic feature of these observed syndromes is tissue injury mediated by direct effects of autoantibodies. Interference with the normal homeostatic role of rheumatoid factor or antiidiotype antibodies during penicillamine therapy may result in excessive production and accumulation of autoantibodies (129,180).

Elevated titers of antibodies to striated muscle occur in up to 20% of patients with RA treated with penicillamine (181). Although the majority of these patients remain free of neuromuscular symptoms, a small percentage may develop antibodies to the acetylcholine receptor and myasthenia gravis. The clinical presentation of myasthenia gravis in patients receiving penicillamine is similar to that noted for patients with idiopathic myasthenia (181–183). Polymyositis occurring in the setting of penicillamine therapy may have clinical and serologic features identical to idiopathic polymyositis, including the presence of Jo-1 antibody and complications of heart block (184–186).

Although rarely occurring in penicillamine-treated Wilson's disease, pemphigus vulgaris and pemphigoid occur with higher frequency in patients with RA treated with penicillamine (168). Serum antibody specific for epidermal intracellular antigen has been demonstrated in these patients; presenting features may include stomatitis, gingivitis, bullae, plaques with vesicles, or scaly erosive lesions (168). Lupus-like syndromes and elevated titers of antinuclear antibodies occur with a greater than expected frequency in patients with RA or Wilson's disease treated with penicillamine. Erythematous skin rashes, nephritis, serositis, fever, and arthritis are reported presenting features (187).

Other Complications

Pulmonary complications of penicillamine therapy are relatively uncommon. Acute pulmonary hemorrhage may be seen in association with glomerulonephritis. Although this observed symptom complex resembles Goodpasture's syndrome, circulating antibodies to glomerular basement membrane are typically absent, and renal histology reveals granular rather than linear basement membrane deposits (188). Other reported pulmonary complications include development of diffuse infiltrates or irreversible airway obstruction with histologic findings of obliterative bronchiolitis (189–192).

Hypogeusia is commonly encountered during treatment with penicillamine. Blunting or loss of taste is usually transient, resolving in several months despite continuance of drug. Other, much less common side effects of penicillamine treatment include hepatotoxicity (193), cholestatic hepatitis (194), and benign breast hypertrophy (195,196). Due to the thiazolidine-forming properties of the drug, prolonged treatment with penicillamine may result in pyridoxine deficiency, particularly among patients with marginal nutritional status.

Therapeutic Considerations and Monitoring

Patient Selection

Due to the high prevalence of side effects, tolerability problems with long-term use, lack of a significant impact on prevention of structural damage in RA, and newer therapies with a much more favorable risk/benefit profile, penicillamine is now seldom used as a DMARD for treatment of RA. Prior to the advent of TNF-α-inhibiting biologic agents, penicillamine had some role in the treatment of patients with RA unable to use methotrexate and who had either failed to respond to or experienced unacceptable toxicity during chrysotherapy. Some clinicians have reported penicillamine to be useful in managing patients with severe pulmonary or cutaneous rheumatoid nodules, including accelerated nodule formation associated with use of methotrexate (152). Despite a lack of compelling data indicating efficacy in systemic sclerosis, penicillamine is still used in some centers as a treatment modality for selected patients with systemic sclerosis. Penicillamine should not be prescribed for patients who are pregnant, nursing infants, or for patients with significant preexisting proteinuria.

Toxicity Monitoring

Patients taking penicillamine require careful surveillance for mucocutaneous complications, with management of oral or cutaneous lesions depending on the severity and timing of the lesions. Mild rashes and pruritus during the first few weeks of therapy are common and frequently transient, requiring only symptomatic treatment with antihistamines and no adjustment in the dose of penicillamine. Oral ulcers or erythematous rashes occurring later in the course of therapy may be managed successfully by withholding penicillamine, then resuming treatment at a lower dose. Bullous or ulcerative cutaneous lesions occurring early or late during therapy, with or without stomatitis and gingivitis, may be indicative of evolving pemphigus or pemphigoid reaction, mandating permanent discontinuance of penicillamine. Confirmation of these lesions by skin biopsy may assist in management, because they may respond favorably to a brief course of systemic corticosteroids. Cutaneous lesions occurring in association with penicillamine-induced lupus syndromes will often resolve following discontinuation of the drug.

Aplastic anemia may occur at any time during treatment with penicillamine. A decrease in the platelet count below 100,000/mm^3 or the development of significant leukopenia (<3,000/mm^3) may portend development of aplastic anemia, and treatment should be discontinued immediately in this setting. For patients on stable doses of penicillamine, blood counts should be checked monthly, with more frequent assessments for several months following initiation of therapy or dose increments. Provided there is no concomitant decline in the peripheral leukocyte count and the platelet count does not fall below 100,000/mm^3, mild thrombocytopenia can usually be managed by a decrement in the daily dose of penicillamine. In patients who develop aplastic anemia during treatment with penicillamine, several weeks may be required for complete recovery of the bone marrow.

Patients receiving penicillamine should also have a complete urinalysis monthly concomitant with hematologic studies. Proteinuria during treatment with penicillamine is frequently transient, responding to temporary withholding of penicillamine; most patients can resume treatment at lower doses of drug without recurrence of proteinuria. Penicillamine is usually not reinstituted in patients who develop nephrotic range proteinuria (>1 g protein excreted per 24 hours).

Cost

The retail pharmacy cost for 100 125-mg tablets of D-penicillamine ranges from \$60 to \$80. The pharmacy and laboratory costs associated with initiating penicillamine at a dose of 250 mg per day with 125-mg increments in the dose every 8 weeks to a stable daily maintenance dose of 625 mg over a total treatment period of 1 year approximates \$2,100. These figures do not include costs associated with evaluation and the management of side effects often associated with penicillamine treatment.

SULFASALAZINE

Based on the premise that infection underlies development of RA, sulfasalazine (formerly referred to as salicylazosulfapyridin) was developed and synthesized as an antirheumatic agent in the late 1930s. Initial studies by Svartz, a collaborating developer of the drug, indicated favorable responses in patients with RA and ankylosing spondylitis treated with salicylazosulfapyridin (197). Due in part to later studies demonstrating only marginal efficacy of sulfasalazine in RA, its use as a DMARD for RA was overshadowed by chrysotherapy and more recently methotrexate. Studies demonstrating efficacy in the treatment of ulcerative colitis renewed interest in the use of sulfasalazine during the 1970s and 1980s as an antirheumatic agent for spondyloarthropathies as well as RA (198). Sulfasalazine gained even greater use in the 1990s incorporated into a DMARD combination regimen (see Chapter 33) with methotrexate and HCQ, demonstrated to be very effective in managing RA (199).

Chemistry and Biologic Effects

Sulfasalazine is an acid-soluble conjugate molecule consisting of a salicylate and sulfapyridine adjoined by an azo bond (Fig. 42.4). Following ingestion, the azo bond is re-

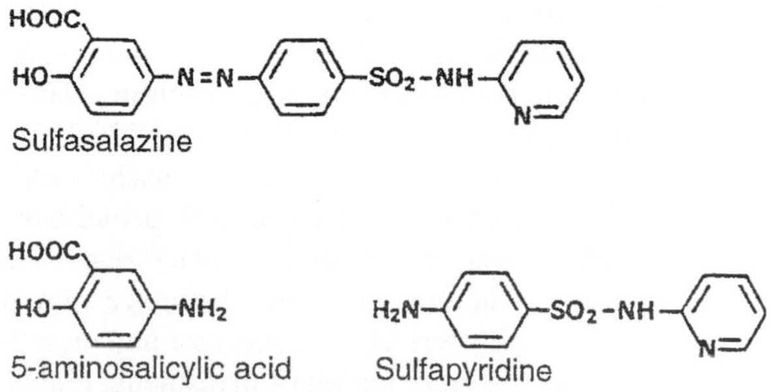

Sulfasalazine

5-aminosalicylic acid

Sulfapyridine

FIG. 42.4. Chemical structure of sulfasalazine.

duced and cleaved by bacterial organisms in the gut to yield 5-aminosalicylate and sulfapyridine.

The extent to which 5-amino salicylate and sulfapyridine contribute to the therapeutic efficacy of sulfasalazine has not been established. The liberated salicylate moiety is absorbed to a limited extent and has recognized antiinflammatory and oxidant-scavenging effects (200). Although it is speculated that sulfapyridine is responsible for much of the therapeutic efficacy of sulfasalazine, *in vitro* and *ex vivo* studies of cell function have provided conflicting data with regard to antiinflammatory or immunomodulatory effects of sulfasalazine and its principal metabolites. In *ex vivo* studies of neutrophils derived from RA subjects taking sulfasalazine, no significant effects of the drug on neutrophil chemotaxis or superoxide generation are observed (201). Sulfasalazine has been shown to attenuate neutrophil phagocytic responses and mononuclear cell mitogenic responses *in vitro*; however, these effects have not been demonstrated in the presence of salicylate or sulfapyridine (202). Moreover, at clinically relevant concentrations, sulfasalazine has been shown to accelerate apoptosis of neutrophils *in vitro,* but accelerated apoptosis has not been confirmed in the presence of 5-aminosalicylic acid (5-ASA) or sulfapyridine (203). In contrast, both sulfasalazine and sulfapyridine have been shown to impair intracellular signaling during neutrophil activation, attenuating intracellular calcium flux, generation of diacylglycerol, and production of inositol phosphates required for neutrophil effector responses (204).

More recent work has suggested that the antiinflammatory effects of sulfasalazine may be mediated by inhibition of aminoimidazole-carboxamide-ribotide (AICAR)-transformylase and accumulation of AICAR, an inhibitor of adenosine deaminase. The attendant increased release of adenosine from endothelial cells and occupancy of adenosine (A2) receptors on phagocytic cells may, therefore, result in attenuation of adhesion functions and transmigration of neutrophils and monocytes into inflamed tissues (205,206).

Significant decreases in IgA and IgM levels and IgM rheumatoid factor levels predictably occur during the course of treatment with sulfasalazine, with hypogammaglobulinemia occurring in up to 10% of patients treated with sulfasalazine (207–209). The mechanism for hypoglobulinemia is likely multifactorial, because sulfasalazine appears to affect the function of multiple cell types impacting immunoglobulin secretion. *In vitro* studies have documented suppression of IgM and IgG production by B cells in the presence of pharmacologic concentrations of sulfasalazine, sulfapyridine, and 5-ASA but not other metabolites (210). Attenuation in T-helper responses may be impacted during treatment. Sulfasalazine has been shown to accelerate apoptosis in T cells, but this effect was not observed in the presence of equal molar concentrations of 5-ASA or sulfapyridine (211,212). Other *in vitro* studies have shown suppression of IKKs by sulfasalazine in T-lymphocyte cell lines resulting in suppression of NFκB activation and associated T-cell responses (213). Finally, sulfasalazine may have global inhibitory effects on lymphocyte proliferation, since the intact molecule has been shown to be a potent inhibitor of the x(c)-plasma membrane cysteine transporter required for cellular uptake of cysteine, an essential nutrient for lymphoid cells (214).

The observed effects on immunoglobulin levels and acquired immunity may be indirect due to the effects of sulfasalazine on liberation of cytokines from monocytes and the associated activation and lineage commitment of T cells. Treatment with sulfasalazine *in vivo* or *in vitro* is associated with attenuated release of IL-12 and interferon-γ (IFN-γ) from murine peritoneal macrophages, resulting in the attenuation of T_H1 T-cell responses (215). Such findings in the murine model are consistent with reductions in IL-1 and TNF observed in patients with RA treated with sulfasalazine (216). Whether treatment with sulfasalazine promotes T_H2 over T_H1 responses in humans has not been confirmed, but such a scenario would be consistent with the demonstrated efficacy of sulfasalazine in RA and the seronegative spondyloarthropathies.

Clinical Efficacy and Therapeutic Use

Rheumatoid Arthritis

The clinical efficacy of sulfasalazine in RA has been established in randomized, placebo-controlled trials, with greatest efficacy noted in patients with relatively early RA (217–220). Although significant drop-out rates due to gastrointestinal intolerance have been observed in published trials, treatment with sulfasalazine over a sustained time period in one study was associated with a trend toward fewer erosions (220,221). In a 2-year study comparing the efficacy of sulfasalazine with HCQ, sulfasalazine was associated with significantly less radiologic manifestations of disease progression (222). In studies comparing treatment responses to sulfasalazine with other traditional DMARDs, sulfasalazine is shown to be comparable in efficacy to intramuscular gold, D-penicillamine and leflunomide (223–226). A metanalysis of clinical responses to traditional DMARDs has suggested that sulfasalazine and methotrexate may be of comparable efficacy in RA (227). However, a more recent study study comparing responses to sulfasalazine versus methotrexate found significantly higher response and remission rates in the methotrexate-treated group (228). Sulfasalazine has been reported to improve neutrophil counts and attenuate neutrophil-bound IgG in a patient with Felty's syndrome (229).

Several reports examining the use of sulfasalazine combined with methotrexate (see Chapter 33) in the treatment of RA have demonstrated the combination regimen to be reasonably well tolerated (230,231). Although improved efficacy of combined sulfasalazine and methotrexate treatment compared to treatment with either DMARD alone could not be demonstrated in one controlled study (232), several studies have demonstrated treatment with the combination of methotrexate, sulfasalazine, and HCQ to be superior in efficacy to treatment with the respective single-agent therapies (233–235).

Spondyloarthropathies

Efficacy of sulfasalazine has also been established in placebo-controlled studies of patients with spondyloarthropathies. In short (3-month) and longer duration (3-year) studies of patients with ankylosing spondylitis, sulfasalazine was shown to be superior to placebo in reducing signs and symptoms of peripheral arthritis; significant effects on the preservation of spinal mobility in these studies were not observed (236–238). However, other reports have indicated improvement in chest expansion following treatment with sulfasalazine (239,240).

In placebo-controlled studies of patients with psoriatic arthritis, significant improvements in peripheral joint swelling and pain are noted during treatment with sulfasalazine (241–243). The therapeutic dosages of sulfasalazine used in these studies were 2.0 g/day; exacerbations of psoriatic skin lesions were not observed. In several open studies, clinical responses to sulfasalazine in dosages ranging from 2.0 to 4.0 g/day have been observed in patients with Reiter syndrome and reactive, pauciarticular arthritis (244,245). Two placebo-controlled studies, including the Veterans Administration Cooperative trial, have confirmed at least some efficacy of sulfasalazine in the treatment of reactive arthritis (246,247). As observed for patients with ankylosing spondylitis treated with sulfasalazine, significant beneficial effects on axial symptoms has not been observed in the studies of patients with psoriatic arthritis or reactive arthritis treated with sulfasalazine (248).

Juvenile Inflammatory Arthritis

Favorable responses to sulfasalazine have been reported in children with juvenile inflammatory arthritis, and the drug has been reasonably well tolerated in children with inflammatory bowel disease (249). In a randomized, double-blind, placebo-controlled study from the Netherlands (Dutch Juvenile Arthritis Study Group), significant improvement in clinical as well as laboratory outcome measures were noted in children with oligoarticular and polyarticular juvenile chronic arthritis treated with 50 mg/kg/day sulfasalazine in doses of up to 2,000 mg daily (250). However, significant withdrawals from treatment (29%) due to gastrointestinal complaints or neutropenia were noted in the Dutch study.

Uveitis and Cutaneous Disorders

In an open, prospective study, sulfasalazine was reported to decrease the number of ocular flare-ups in patients with established recurrent acute anterior uveitis over a 1-year period relative to the year antedating treatment (251). Several collections of case reports indicate that sulfasalazine may be effective in patients with recalcitrant or severe atrophie blanche (252,253). Consistent with the known efficacy of sulfapyridine in the treatment of dermatitis herpetiformis, sulfasalazine is of reported efficacy in patients with this condition unable to tolerate dapsone (254). Several open pilot trials have also shown favorable responses in patients with discoid lupus unable to use antimalarials or thalidomide (255,256).

Administration and Pharmacokinetics

Treatment with sulfasalazine is best initiated incrementally to minimize intolerance. The usual starting dose is 500 mg twice daily, followed by increments of 500 mg/day at weekly intervals until the therapeutic dose of 2.0 to 3.0 g daily is attained. For the majority of patients, pushing the dose beyond 3.0 g daily does not afford additional benefit and may increase the likelihood of toxicity or intolerance.

Over 80% of ingested sulfasalazine remains intact and unabsorbed, passing into the colon, where the azo bond is reduced and cleaved by colonic bacteria to 5-ASA and sulfapyridine (257). Treatment with broad-spectrum antibiotics resulting in alteration of gut flora may, therefore, reduce sulfapyridine and 5-ASA bioavailability. Although most of the sulfapyridine is absorbed, 70% to 80% of the 5-ASA remains in the colon unabsorbed (258). Plasma levels of sulfapyridine peak 4 to 6 hours following ingestion of sulfasalazine, with subsequent metabolism in the liver by *N*-aceylation and ring hydroxylation followed by glucuronidation and biliary excretion. Absorbed 5-aminosalicylate is acetylated and excreted in the urine. Considerable individual variation exists in the rate of sulfapyridine metabolism; clinical efficacy has not been shown to correlate with sulfapyridine levels, but adverse events have been reported to occur more commonly among individuals with a slow acetylator phenotype (259–261).

Toxicity and Side Effects

Although most adverse reactions attributed to sulfasalazine (summarized in Table 42.3) are benign and reversible, just under one third of patients in reported clinical studies eventually discontinue sulfasalazine due to adverse effects of the drug. The majority of side effects appear to be dose-related and may occur more commonly in individuals with slow acetylator phenotype (262). However, acetylator phenotype may not be predictive of toxicity (263). Idiosyncratic reactions, including agranulocytosis and cutaneous or pulmonary hypersensitivity reactions are less predictable but usually occur early during the course of treatment.

Constitutional symptoms, including anorexia, headache, drowsiness, confusion, or malaise, typically manifest early during the course of treatment, are not uncommon with dos-

TABLE 42.3. *Toxicity of sulfasalazine*

Gastrointestinal
Nausea, vomiting
Anorexia
Abdominal pain, dyspepsia
Cutaneous
Photo-exanthem
Hypersensitivity reactions
Central nervous system
Headaches
Drowsiness
Confusion
Malaise
Hepatic
Elevated transaminase levels
Cholestasis
Hematologic
Macrocytosis
Megaloblastic anemia (corrected with folate)
Hemolysis with reticulocytosis
Leukopenia
Agranulocytosis
Methomoglobinemia
Hypersensitivity pneumonitis
Interstitial nephritis
Dysguesia
Male infertility [sperm dysfunction]
Drug-induced lupus

ing in excess of 4.0 g sulfasalazine daily, and may resolve with dose attenuation. Early macular or maculopapular skin rashes in sun-exposed skin that resolve with dose attenuation have also been reported (264,265). Skin reactions associated with urticaria, mouth ulcers, fever, or adenopathy should raise the suspicion of a hypersensitivity reaction and prompt discontinuation of the drug. Both Stevens-Johnson's syndrome and toxic epidermal necrolysis have been reported (266,267).

Hematologic

Sulfasalazine-induced neutropenia occurs in up to 4% of patients, most often occurring within the first several months of treatment (268,269). However, neutropenia may also occur much later, even several years following initiation of treatment. Although rare, agranulocytosis may occur during the first few months of treatment, and may require supportive care with antibiotics when accompanied by fever (270). Administration of granulocyte colony-stimulating factor may hasten recovery from sulfasalazine-induced agranulocytosis (271). Thrombocytopenia is a rarely reported complication of treatment with sulfasalazine (272). Macrocytosis may occur as a consequence of megaloblastic anemia arising from sulfasalazine-induced alterations in folate metabolism (273). However, the appearance of macrocytosis may also reflect reticulocytosis due to sulfasalazine-induced hemolysis, a condition that is usually dose related or associated with a slow acetylator phenotype (268).

Pulmonary

Hypersensitivity pneumonitis is the most frequent reported pulmonary complication of sulfasalazine treatment. Clinical features include cough, dyspnea, fever, and patchy infiltrates on chest radiographs, with most patients recovering completely following discontinuation of the medication (274–276). Fibrosing alveolitis and interstitial fibrosis have also been reported, although drug-induced effects may be difficult to distinguish from rheumatoid lung disease.

Gastrointestinal

Gastrointestinal intolerance to sulfasalazine is not uncommon, most commonly manifested by anorexia, nausea, and epigastric pain. Dose attenuation or use of enteric-coated preparations of the drug may render the drug more tolerable in patients who experience these side effects. Diarrhea and pancreatitis are rarely reported complications (277,278). Varying degrees of hepatotoxicity ranging from mild cholestasis to massive hepatic necrosis have been reported in the setting of treatment with sulfasalazine for inflammatory bowel disease or RA (279–281).

Renal

Renal toxicity associated with use of sulfasalazine is uncommon and rarely reported. However, recent reports of chronic interstitial nephritis developing in patients with inflammatory bowel disease treated with mesalamine (5-acetylsalicylate) emphasize that it may be prudent to periodically monitor serum creatinine levels in patients treated with sulfasalazine.

Reproductive

There is little reported evidence of teratogenicity or alterations in female fertility associated with use of sulfasalazine, but given the potential for alterations in folate absorption and metabolism, the current recommendations are to avoid treatment with the drug during pregnancy (282–284). Treatment with sulfasalazine is associated with infertility in men, inducing morphologic changes in and reduced motility of spermatozoa; abnormal penetration of ova has also been reported (285,286). Although the morphologic changes in spermatozoa may persist for months following discontinuation of sulfasalazine, the fertility changes in men are usually reversible.

Miscellaneous

Other miscellaneous reported side effects of sulfasalazine include seizures, tachycardia, Raynaud's, and dysgeusia, all of which resolved following dose attenuation or discontinuation of drug (287–290). Cyanosis unassociated with oxygen desaturation was reported in the original series of patients reported by Svartz, observed primarily in patients taking in excess of 4 g/day sulfasalazine (197). There are rare reports of sulfasalazine-induced lupus syndromes, including associated induction of anti-DNA antibodies (291,292).

Treatment Considerations and Monitoring

Patient Selection

Sulfasalazine is an effective DMARD for patients with RA, psoriatic arthritis, ankylosing spondylitis, or reactive arthritis who may not be suitable candidates for treatment with methotrexate or TNF-α inhibiting biologic therapy. It is still not uncommonly used and effective as a second or third agent in combination DMARD therapy with methotrexate (with or without HCQ) for management of RA. Given the salutary effects of the drug on enteric as well as joint inflammation, sulfasalazine may be particularly useful in patients with enteropathic arthritis associated with inflammatory bowel disease. Caution is required when using sulfasalazine in combination with azathioprine or 6-mercaptopurine (6-MP) due to drug interaction increasing levels of 6-MP (293).

Toxicity Monitoring

Since the uncommon but potentially life-threatening adverse effects on granulopoiesis most often occur early during the course of treatment, it is advisable to monitor blood counts at least monthly (or more frequently prior to the time of any dose escalation) during the first 3 to 6 months of treatment with sulfasalazine. Given the ongoing potential for drug-induced neutropenia or possible megaloblastic anemia at any time during the course of treatment, it is still recommended that blood counts be checked at 3-month intervals once a stable dose has been reached. Monitoring of liver function tests are advisable during the first few months of treatment to detect idiosyncratic effects on liver function. Given the reported occurrences of interstitial nephritis in patients treated with 5-aminosalicylate, monitoring of serum creatinine at 6-month intervals during the course of treatment is also now prudent.

Cost

The retail costs for a standard therapeutic dose of 1.0 g sulfasalazine twice daily is approximately $90 per month. Including laboratory cost for recommended blood count monitoring during the initial months of treatment and subsequent periodic monitoring of blood counts, creatinine, and liver function tests, the approximated yearly costs for treatment with sulfasalazine is $1,300.

ANTIMALARIALS: HYDROXYCHLOROQUINE, CHLOROQUINE, AND QUINACRINE

The beneficial effects of antimalarial drugs on manifestations of rheumatic disease were initially recognized in patients with discoid and systemic lupus erythematosus (SLE) during the early 1900s. Quinacrine, the first synthesized antimalarial, was later reported to be of benefit in patients with RA as well as SLE (294). Chloroquine and HCQ, developed as a consequence of efforts to synthesize antimalarial compounds that were better tolerated than quinacrine, were also observed to have beneficial effects in patients with RA and SLE. Although exact mechanisms of their efficacy for a given rheumatic disease manifestation have yet to be determined, HCQ and (to a much lesser extent) quinacrine and chloroquine are still commonly used in the management of SLE. Although gaining less favor as a first-line DMARD in the treatment of RA, HCQ is still not uncommonly used in combination DMARD regimens for treatment of RA. Antimalarials are also of reported benefit in the management of patients with other rheumatic diseases including psoriatic arthritis and sarcoidosis.

Chemistry and Biological Effects

HCQ and chloroquine are aromatic two-ringed 4-amino quinolone compounds; quinacrine has an additional aromatic ring with a methoxy group (Fig. 42.5). All three compounds are weak diprotic bases, a property that facilitates

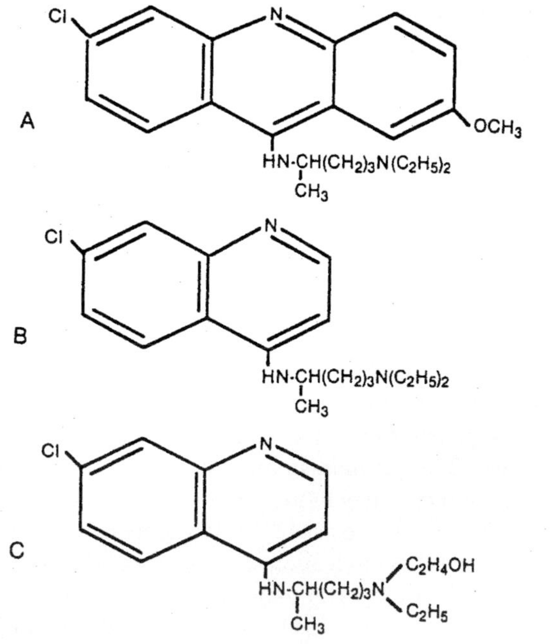

A: Quinacrine B: Chloroquine C: Hydroxychloroquine

FIG. 42.5. Chemical structures of antimalarials.

intracellular accumulation of the compounds in acidic organelles. At neutral pH of serum and interstitial fluids, antimalarials are uncharged and pass freely across cell membranes (295). Within the mildly acidic milieu of intracellular vesicles, the compounds become protonated and no longer freely diffuse across organelle membranes. The resulting partition gradient for uncharged drug may lead to over 100-fold excess concentration of drug within acidic vesicles (296). Increases in the pH of intracellular vesicles within malarial parasites resulting in impaired enzymatic breakdown of hemoglobin nutrients and impaired assembly and function of malarial proteins constitute proposed antiparasitic mechanisms of antimalarial efficacy.

The buffering effect of antimalarials and resulting pH changes within organelles has been readily demonstrated in phagocytic cells, and a relative increase in pH within the intracellular lysosomes of antigen-presenting cells constitutes the basis for a postulated mechanism of antimalarial efficacy in autoimmune disease (297–300). Efficient loading of antigen peptides onto MHC class II α and β chains requires displacement of the invariant chain (Ii) from the respective MHC chains, a reaction facilitated when hydrogen bonds mediating association of Ii with the MHC chains are disrupted by lowering of the ambient pH (299). Given the low affinity of autoantigen peptides for self MHC relative to that of nonself peptides, it has been postulated that antimalarial-induced increases in the pH of organelles involved in peptide loading may preferentially exclude loading of self peptides onto MHC chains, with the net result being attenuation in presentation autoantigens to T-cells and attendant autoimmune effector responses (300). Data from *in vitro* studies of lymphocyte function confirm that the impact of antimalarials on antigen-driven immune responses is likely mediated predominantly through effects on antigen processing and the accessory functions of monocytes (301). Effects on organelle acidification may furthermore account for observed inhibitory effects of antimalarials on signaling through toll-like receptors triggered by oligonucleotides (302).

Studies of lymphocyte proliferation in admixtures of mononuclear cells suggest that observed inhibitory effects of HCQ on proliferation of T cells or immunoglobulin secretion are also due to attenuation in secretion of monocyte cytokines (301,303). Observed effects of antimalarials on the production of oxidants and release of cytokines (IL-1β and TNF-α) by monocytes and macrophages vary with the activating ligand, the specific antimalarial used, and the effector response examined (303–305). Both HCQ and chloroquine have been shown to affect posttranslational modification of TNF-α, impairing the processing of membrane-bound pro-TNF to soluble mature protein (306). The observed inhibitory effects of HCQ on posttranslational processing of TNF-α are consistent with the observed inhibitory effects of the drug on posttranslational modification of other proteins, including gp120 required for assembly of HIV-1 in T-cells and monocytes (307,308).

Whether alterations in intracellular pH account for observed inhibitory effects of antimalarials on other phagocytic cell responses is uncertain. *In vitro* chemotactic responses of human neutrophils are impaired in the presence of HCQ and in animal models of inflammation, HCQ impairs neutrophil migration into inflamed tissues (309). Both HCQ and quinacrine attenuate arachidonic acid release and eicosanoid production induced by phorbol ester, suggesting that the drugs attenuate the activity of phospholipase A_2. HCQ, furthermore, impairs neutrophil production of superoxide, most likely through inhibitory effects on the liberation of inositol phosphates by membrane-associated phospholipases (310,311). Despite the observed inhibitory effects on neutrophil and monocyte function, antimalarial use has not been associated with an increased risk of or morbidity from infection.

Clinical Efficacy and Therapeutic Uses

Rheumatoid Arthritis and Juvenile Rheumatoid Arthritis

Controlled clinical trials have demonstrated efficacy of both chloroquine and HCQ in decreasing the number of tender and swollen joints as well as morning stiffness in patients with early or established RA (312–316). Similar improvements have been noted in children with JRA (317). However, the majority of controlled clinical trials have been of relatively short duration, and no studies to date have documented any effects of antimalarials on decreasing the incidence or progression of bone erosions in RA.

In a placebo-controlled study, HCQ has been shown to facilitate the tapering of glucocorticoids when used as a single DMARD (318). Similar steroid-sparing effects were noted in an open-label study adding HCQ as a second DMARD to patients with RA receiving methotrexate (319). Combination (see Chapter 33) of HCQ with other DMARDs, including azathioprine, sulfasalazine, penicillamine, and cyclophosphamide, have been reported. The triple therapy regimen of methotrexate, sulfasalazine, and HCQ has demonstrated benefits in patients with inadequate responses to methotrexate alone (199). The relative contributions of sulfasalazine and HCQ to the improved efficacy in studies using this combination are indeterminate, but a subsequent study found the combination of methotrexate and HCQ superior in efficacy to the combination of methotrexate and sulfasalazine (320). This efficacious regimen has not been associated with significant increases in bone marrow or liver toxicity, but gastrointestinal intolerance may limit compliance (321,322).

Systemic Lupus Erythematosus and Discoid Lupus

In controlled studies of patients with SLE, both chloroquine and HCQ have been shown to be efficacious in clearing or improving skin rashes, arthritis, pleuritic symptoms, and arthralgias (323–325). In these and other studies, chloroquine and HCQ also were shown to permit attenuation in the dose of administered corticosteroids (324–327). The benefits of maintaining patients with quiescent SLE on antimalarials was furthermore demonstrated in a drug withdrawal study in which patients maintained on HCQ were less likely to have flare-ups of disease (328). Although clinical trial data with quinacrine is limited, improvement in skin disease, arthralgias, and constitutional symptoms have been reported, and it has been the experience of some clinicians that the use of quinacrine in combination with HCQ may result in synergistic effects that improve disease activity (294,329,330). There are few controlled trials examining the efficacy of antimalarials in the treatment of discoid lupus; numerous published case series nonetheless document complete remissions or significant improvement in up to 90% of patients with discoid skin lesions treated with quinacrine, chloroquine, or HCQ (326,331–333). A majority of patients have been observed to relapse following discontinuation of treatment (324,326).

Antimalarials have been shown to have additional benefits in patients with SLE, including lowering of cholesterol levels and levels of low-density lipoproteins (334,335). Chloroquine as well as HCQ have known inhibitory effects on platelet aggregation with demonstrated efficacy in prevention of postoperative thrombosis (336–338); in a retrospective review, the frequency of thrombotic complications was observed to be lower in patients receiving antimalarials (339). HCQ may furthermore be of benefit in decreasing thrombotic complications among patients with antiphospholipid antibodies. Platelet activation, as measured by surface expression of glycoprotein IIb/IIIa induced by antiphospholipid antibodies and thrombin agonist receptor peptide, is abrogated in the presence of pharmacologic concentrations of HCQ (340). Furthermore, among patients with known antiphospholipid antibodies, use of HCQ was found to be more prevalent among patients with no known history of thrombosis relative to patients with a history of a documented thrombotic event (341).

Sjögren's Syndrome

Studies examining the efficacy of HCQ in Sjögren's syndrome have yielded conflicting results that are likely attributable in part to differences in entry criteria (342,343). In one controlled study of patients with active arthritis, skin rash, parotid swelling, elevated sedimentation rate, and hypergammaglobulinemia, treatment with HCQ resulted in significant improvement in the extraglandular manifestations as well as parotid swelling (342). In this same study, the appearance of monoclonal immunoglobulins was less frequent in the HCQ-treated group.

Other Rheumatic Conditions

In uncontrolled case series, decreases in the frequency and duration of symptoms of patients with palindromic rheumatism have been reported with administration of chloroquine (344,345). In children with dermatomyositis, significant decreases or resolution of skin rash has been reported in response to treatment with HCQ; myositis has not been reported to respond as well, although the prednisone dosages required to control muscle disease was lower following the addition of HCQ (346,347). In series of case reports, HCQ is reported to be of benefit in erosive osteoarthritis (348). In one controlled trial, HCQ was reported to be of benefit in decreasing joint flare-ups in patients with calcium pyrophosphate disease (349). In uncontrolled studies, patients with eosinophilic fasciitis failing to respond adequately to treatment with corticosteroids have responded favorably to HCQ (350). Patients with arthritis associated with hepatitis C may respond favorably to treatment with HCQ (351). Antimalarials have been used to prevent complications of graft-versus-host disease in patients who have undergone allogeneic bone marrow transplantation.

Administration and Pharmacokinetics

Recommended dosing of antimalarials is presently based on body weight, with the optimal therapeutic window for HCQ achieved using a daily dose of 6 to 7 mg/kg ideal body weight. Higher doses of antimalarials were administered during the early years of their use in treating rheumatic diseases, but the current dosing recommendations have evolved in efforts to improve tolerance and minimize ocular toxicity without compromising clinical efficacy. Loading doses of 600–800 mg/day administered for several weeks have been used with the goal of achieving a more rapid therapeutic effect, but there is little published data regarding the efficacy of this approach. The traditional dosages used for chloroquine are 3.5 to 4 mg/kg/day; quinacrine is usually prescribed in a dosage of 100 to 200 mg/day.

Although there is significant individual variation in fractional absorption, antimalarials are rapidly absorbed from the gastrointestinal tract and into the cellular compartments of the blood (295,352,353). Binding of the respective drugs to serum proteins is not extensive, averaging approximately 50% (354). Due to the weak diprotic base attribute, significant cellular concentration of antimalarials occurs in leukocytes, with *in vitro* studies demonstrating 20- to 100-fold intracellular concentration of the drugs within a 24-hour period (355). Antimalarials are deposited in tissues throughout the body, with intracellular binding particularly pronounced in pigmented tissues, including retinal cells and melanocytes (356).

Small amounts of HCQ and chloroquine may be excreted in the urine following initial dosing, but the drugs are slowly excreted with a serum half-life exceeding 45 days (357). Although a wide range of plasma levels are noted in patients with RA taking stable doses of 6 to 7 mg/kg/day HCQ, the average plasma level is reported to be approximately 0.9 μM, with whole blood concentrations averaging approximately 4 μM (357). Drug levels correlate poorly with efficacy, but an increased frequency of side effects has been reported among patients with elevated serum levels of HCQ and chloroquine (358,359). Antimalarials are oxidatively deaminated in the liver, with the desethylchloroquine or desethyl-HCQ excreted in the urine; the biologic or therapeutic effects of antimalarial metabolites are unknown (357).

Toxicity and Side Effects

Antimalarials are generally well tolerated, with an excellent safety profile. An extensive review and metanalysis of placebo-controlled clinical trials examining disease-modifying drugs used in RA found less toxicity related drug withdrawals among patients treated with antimalarials compared with other DMARDs (277). Commonly reported side effects after initiation of dosing of antimalarials, including nausea, abdominal bloating, diarrhea, headache, insomnia, and nervousness, are often dose dependent and frequently remit spontaneously. Cutaneous symptoms, including mild rashes or pruritis, as well as gastrointestinal intolerance, may improve with changing to alternative dosing preparations. Other reported side effects are summarized in Table 42.4; additional considerations with regard to ocular toxicity as well as some of the cutaneous and neuromuscular complications of antimalarials are discussed below.

Cutaneous Side Effects

Maculopapular rashes occur in up to 5% of patients taking antimalarials, usually recur with drug rechallenge, and are the most common side effect leading to discontinuation of treatment (324). Pigmentary changes in the skin are not uncommon, ranging from areas of relative hypopigmentation to areas of blue or black hyperpigmentation. Due to the increased deposition of antimalarials in melanin-containing cells, pigment changes are most commonly experienced in dark-skinned individuals but may occasionally occur in patients with light skin tone. Patients treated with quinacrine frequently develop a yellow skin discoloration, an effect reported to be attenuated by coadministration of β-carotene (294,324). Alopecia can occur as a consequence of antimalarial therapy, a complication that may be difficult to distinguish from alopecia occurring as a manifestation of lupus. Pruritis or a burning sensation in the skin exacerbated with bathing may limit use of antimalarials in some patients. Patients with psoriasis may experience exacerbations of psoriatic skin lesion dermatitis following administration of antimalarials, with some reports of exfoliative dermatitis.

Neuromuscular Complications

The majority of neurologic symptoms reported following initiation of antimalarials either abate spontaneously or resolve with dose attenuation. Uncommonly, a neuromuscular syndrome may evolve several months following initiation of antimalarial treatment that is associated with muscle weakness predominantly involving the proximal lower extremities (360,361). A vacuolar myopathy is the histologic feature found on muscle biopsy; creatine kinase levels are typically normal. Involvement of cardiac muscle may occur with presenting features of heart failure and atrioventricular conduction abnormalities (362,363).

TABLE 42.4. *Toxicity of antimalarials*

Cutaneous
Morbilliform or maculopapular rash
Exfoliative rash
Exacerbation of psoriasis
Increased skin pigmentation
Alopecia
Pruritis, burning sensations
Gastrointestinal
Anorexia
Nausea
Vomiting
Abdominal bloating/cramps
Diarrhea
Ocular
Corneal deposits with perceived halos
Impaired accommodation
Diplopia
Retinopathy
Pigment abnormalities
Scotomas
Impaired visual field or acuity
Neuromuscular
Headache
Insomnia
Mental irritability
Ototoxicity
Neural deafness
Tinnitus
Vestibular dysfunction
Psychosis
Neuromyopathy
Cardiac
Cardiomyopathy
Conduction abnormalities
Hematologic
Leukopenia
Agranulocytosis
Aplastic anemia

Ocular Toxicity

Antimalarial use may result in a variety of ocular effects, ranging from transient alterations in accommodation and benign corneal deposits to the more serious complications arising from retinal deposits. Transient blurring of vision or diplopia occurs not infrequently following initiation of therapy, usually resolves within 1 to 2 weeks, and usually does not require discontinuation of therapy. Corneal deposits may result in perception of halos around lights and are usually reversible following discontinuation of medication; commonly occurring in patients treated with chloroquine, symptomatic corneal deposits are reported to be much less frequent among patients treated with HCQ (364).

Retinal toxicity is a serious concern due to the potential for permanent visual loss. Relative to the initial experiences with chloroquine, retinopathy appears to occur less frequently among patients treated with HCQ, the majority of cases occurring when dosing exceeds 7 mg/kg/day (365–367). Physical manifestations of antimalarial retinopathy include pigment changes in the retina and clumping of retinal tissue, with occasional evolution of a concentric bull's eye lesion appearing on the macula. The findings of pigment changes on the retina (premaculopathy) often precede demonstrable or symptomatic visual loss and are usually reversible following discontinuation of the antimalarial. More advanced retinopathy may manifest as decreased visual acuity; ballooning of retinal pigmented epithelial cells may give rise to scotomas demonstrable on visual field testing (368). More advanced stages of retinopathy may persist or even progress despite discontinuation of drug (369,370). Despite these concerns, with the use of HCQ in lieu of chloroquine, avoidance of daily doses in excess of 7 mg/kg and regular ophthalmologic evaluations, visual loss can be prevented for the vast majority of patients (371).

Therapeutic Considerations and Toxicity Monitoring

Patient Selection

Given the demonstrated efficacy of antimalarials on cutaneous and articular manifestations, reported benefits on constitutional symptoms, and the favorable toxicity profile of HCQ, patients with SLE are likely to benefit from treatment with HCQ. Although the extent to which antimalarials prevent the development of lupus-related disease manifestations is not known, many clinicians favor initiation of HCQ as first-line therapy in patients presenting with signs and symptoms suggestive of SLE. HCQ is particularly useful as first-line therapy for patients with subacute cutaneous lupus or discoid lupus. For patients with skin manifestations of lupus not completely responsive to the usual doses of HCQ, the addition of quinacrine may be efficacious. HCQ may be the preferred choice of DMARD in patients presenting with palindromic rheumatism or for elderly patients presenting with mild RA who may have contraindications or intolerance to methotrexate. Addition of HCQ as a second DMARD is a reasonable option for patients not completely responding to methotrexate and unable to use or access biologic anti-TNF agents. Due to reported increases in blood levels and bioavailability of methotrexate following administration of HCQ (372), attention to frequent blood count monitoring is advised if this option is undertaken in patients with borderline renal function.

Toxicity Monitoring

Other than assessment for idiosyncratic hepatic or bone marrow toxicity during the first several months of treatment, treatment with antimalarials does not require regular monitoring of blood counts or liver chemistries. Regular monitoring for retinal toxicity is recommended. Guidelines have recently been issued by the American Academy of Ophthalmology regarding the timing and frequency of ocular examinations to monitor for development of antimalarial induced retinal toxicity (373):

1. All patients should undergo baseline examination of the retina through a dilated pupil and central visual field testing within the first year of treatment with HCQ.
2. For patients with normal baseline examination results, who are under the age of 60, who do not have significant renal disease, and who are taking less than 6.5 mg/kg/day of HCQ, no further ocular examination is required during the first 5 years of treatment with antimalarials.
3. For patients at higher risk (antimalarial treatment >5 years, HCQ dosing >6.5/mg/kg/day, high body fat, age >60, macular abnormalities on baseline examination, or renal impairment), yearly examinations are recommended.
4. More frequent ocular examinations (every 3–6 months) are warranted if possible retinopathy is suspected and the decision is to continue with antimalarial treatment.

There is still not uniform agreement with regard to the advisability of continuing treatment in low-risk individuals without an ocular examination during the first 5 years of treatment, and in the context of reported cases of retinal toxicity occurring early in the course of treatment, many clinicians continue to follow the 1996 American College of Rheumatology guidelines advocating a yearly ophthalmologic examination for patients receiving treatment with an antimalarial (374).

Cost

The retail cost for a month's treatment with 400 mg/day HCQ ranges from approximately $55 (generic preparation) to $80 (branded Plaquenil, Sanofi Pharmaceuticals, New York, NY, U.S.A.). Combined with costs for a yearly ophthalmologic examination, the approximate yearly costs for treatment with HCQ is $900. Quinacrine is available through compounding pharmacies at a cost of approximately $100/month for a daily dose of 100 mg.

MIZORIBINE

Mizoribine, also known as bredinin, is an imidazole nucleoside originally isolated from soil fungi (Fig. 42.6). Initially used as an antibiotic with fungal activity against *Candida albicans*, mizoribine was later noted to have immunosuppressive activity in animals of transplantation (375–377). Approved in Japan for use in renal transplantation, steroid-resistant nephrotic syndrome, and RA, mi-

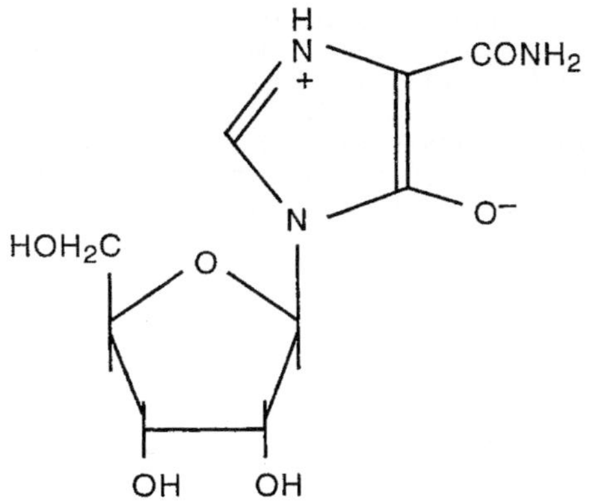

FIG. 42.6. Chemical structure of mizoribine.

zoribine is also being examined for efficacy in the management of lupus nephritis and multiple sclerosis.

Biologic Effects

Following oral administration, mizoribine is phosphorylated intracellularly by adenosine kinase to its active form, mizoribine 5′-monophosphate [MZ-5-P]. The activated compound selectively inhibits inosine monophosphate (IMP) dehydrogenase and guanosine monophosphate (GMP) synthetase, enzymes required for *de novo* synthesis of GMP from IMP. The resulting inhibition of guanine nucleotide synthesis has profound inhibitory effects on T-cell proliferation dependent on guanine nucleotide second messengers mediating the actions of T cell costimulatory factors (378). Mizoribine also inhibits the proliferation and function of immunoglobulin-secreting B cells, but through a different mechanism involving inhibition of cyclin A, a cell cycle regulatory protein critical to the progression of B cells from G1 phase to S phase (379). Decreased numbers of activated T cells and $CD5^+$ B cells in the peripheral blood of patients receiving mizoribine corroborate these effects *in vivo* (380).

Clinical Efficacy and Therapeutic Uses

In several studies of patients with RA treated for 16 to 48 weeks with mizoribine, improvements in morning stiffness, grip strength, and numbers of swollen and tender joints over baseline have been reported, with greater improvements noted in patients treated with higher dosages (300 mg/day vs. 150 mg/day) (381). However, no significant improvements in erythrocyte sedimentation rate were noted in these studies. In a double-blind study comparing mizoribine to placebo in patients with RA permitted to use nonsteroidal antiinflammatory drugs and low-dose corticosteroids, global assessments were improved in the mizoribine group, but no significant differences in morning stiffness, numbers of tender or swollen joints, grip strength, pain scales or activity of daily living scores between the two groups were observed (382). In another study comparing mizoribine to lobenzarit (another DMARD used in Japan for RA), radiographic progression was prevented in the mizoribine group (383). Improvements and steroid-sparing effects of mizoribine in cases of juvenile inflammatory arthritis have been reported (381). Favorable allograft survival rates have been reported for patients treated with mizoribine in combination with cyclosporine A (384).

Administration and Pharmacokinetics

Prescribed as a daily 150- to 300-mg dose, mizoribine is rapidly absorbed with maximum blood levels 90 minutes following ingestions. In animal models, complete elimination is noted within 24 hours, with 85% of the drug excreted in the urine (381,385).

Toxicity

Among patients with renal transplantation, nephrotic syndrome, lupus nephritis, and RA treated with mizoribine, minimal toxicity ascribed to the drug has been observed. The most common reported side effects have been transient gastrointestinal tract symptoms, with one case report of drug-induced pancreatitis (381). Significant hematologic toxicity has not been observed with mizoribine.

ACTARIT

Actarit (4-acetylaminophenylacetic acid) (Fig. 42.7) is a compound that was found to suppress inflammation in animal models of arthritis (386,387). Actarit was subsequently found to have beneficial immunomodulatory effects in humans and of benefit in patients with RA, for whom it has been used as a DMARD in Japan (388,389).

Biologic Effects and Efficacy

In cocultures of rheumatoid synovial cells, actarit suppresses synovial expression of matrix metalloproteinase 1 messenger RNA (mRNA) and cyclooxygenase-2 mRNA; actarit was also shown to attenuate spontaneous secretion of TNF-α and IL-1β and surface expression of CD44

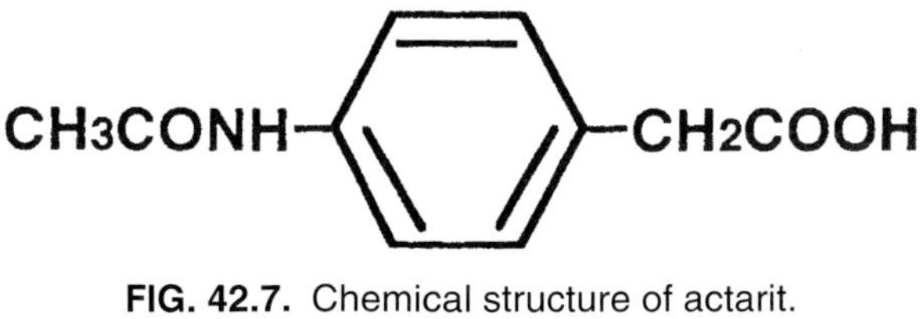

FIG. 42.7. Chemical structure of actarit.

and intercellular adhesion molecule-1 by the explanted cells (390). In experimental autoimmune encephalitis models, treatment with actarit suppresses infiltration of lymphocytes into the central nervous system; TNF-α and interferon-γ mRNA expression was attenuated and IL-10 mRNA up-regulated in the spleens of treated animals (391). In one clinical study of patients with RA not responding to gold therapy, addition of actarit was associated with significant improvement in numbers of painful and swollen joints, morning stiffness, and erythrocyte sedimentation rate (392).

LOBENZARIT

Lobenzarit (disodium 4-chloro-2,2′-iminodibenzoate) is an immunomodulating agent approved in Japan for the treatment of RA.

Biologic Effects and Efficacy

Lobenzarit has been shown to inhibit activated B cells. *In vitro* studies have shown that lobenzarit attenuates production of immunoglobulins, including anti-DNA antibodies and IgM rheumatoid factors, by peripheral B lymphocytes triggered by T cell–derived mitogens and staphylococcal proteins (393,394). The observed inhibition of IgM production was attributed to inhibitory effects of lobenzarit on cell cycle progression through the G1-S interphase required for terminal differentiation of activated B lymphocytes. In a double-blind controlled study of lobenzarit in patients with RA, lobenzarit was shown to be efficacious, improving a number of swollen joints (395). In an open clinical trial examining the effects of lobenzarit in patients with SLE, improvements in disease activity were noted, including resolution of leukopenia and decreases in the serum titers of antibodies to double-stranded DNA (396).

REFERENCES

1. Rodnan GP, Benedek TG. The early history of anti-rheumatic drugs. *Arthritis Rheum* 1970;13:145–165.
2. Forestier J. Rheumatoid arthritis and its treatment by gold salts. *J Lab Clin Med* 1935;20:837–840.
3. Sadler PJ. The comparative evaluation of the physical and chemical properties of gold compounds. *J Rheumatol* 1982;9(suppl 8):71–78.
4. Hassan J, Feighery C, Bresnihan B, et al. Effect of gold therapy on CD5+ B-cells and TCR gamma delta+ T-cells in patients with rheumatoid arthritis. *Rheumatol Int* 1991;11:175–178.
5. Kiely PD, Helbert MR, Miles J, Oliveira DB. Immunosuppressant effect of gold on IgG subclasses and IgE; evidence for sparing of Th2 responses. *Clin Exp Immunol* 2000;120:369–374.
6. Hirohata S, Nakanishi K, Yanagida T, et al. Synergistic inhibition of human B cell activation by gold sodium thiomalate and auranofin. *Clin Immunol* 1999;91:226–233.
7. Romagnoli P, Spinas GA, Sinigaglia F. Gold-specific T-cells in rheumatoid arthritis patients treated with gold. *J Clin Invest* 1992;89:254–256.
8. Griem P, Takahashi K, Kalbacher H, et al. The antirheumatic drug disodium aurothiomalate inhibits CD4+ T cell recognition of peptides containing two or more cysteine residues. *J Immunol* 1995;155:1575–1587.
9. Wang ZY, Morinobu A, Kawano S, et al. Gold sodium thiomalate suppresses the differentiation and function of human dendritic cells from peripheral blood monocytes. *Clin Exp Rheumatol* 2002;20:683–688.
10. Lies RB, Cardin C, Paulus HE. Inhibition by gold of human lymphocyte stimulation. *Ann Rheum Dis* 1977;36:216–218.
11. Waltz DT, DiMartino MJ, Griswold DE. Comparative pharmacologic and biologic effects of different gold compounds. *J Rheumatol* 1982; 9(suppl 8):54–60.
12. Lorber A, Jackson WH, Simon TM. Assessment of immune response during chrysotherapy. Comparison of gold sodium thiomalate vs. auranofin. *Scand J Rheumatol* 1981;10:129–137.
13. Lorber A, Simon TM, Leeb J, et al. Effect of chrysotherapy on parameters of immune response. J Rheumatol 1979;6(suppl 5):82–90.
14. Kim TS, Kang BY, Lee MH, et al. Inhibition of interleukin-12 production by auranofin, an anti-rheumatic gold compound, deviates CD4(+) T cells from the Th1 to the Th2 pathway. *Br J Pharmacol* 2001; 134:571–578.
15. Corkill MM, Kirkham BW, Haskard DO, et al. Gold treatment of rheumatoid arthritis decreases synovial expression of the endothelial leukocyte receptor ELAM-1. *J Rheumatol* 1991;18:1453–1460.
16. Matsubara T, Ziff M. Inhibition of human endothelial cell proliferation by gold compounds. *J Clin Invest* 1987;79:1440–1446.
17. Loetscher, Dewald B, Baggiolini M, et al. Monocyte chemoattractant protein 1 and interleukin 8 production by rheumatoid synoviocytes. Effects of anti-rheumatic drugs. *Cytokine* 1994;6:162–170.
18. Yanni G, Nabil M, Farahat MR, et al. Intramuscular gold decreases cytokine expression and macrophages in the rheumatoid synovial membrane. *Ann Rheum Dis* 1994;53:315–322.
19. Koch AE, Burrows JC, Polverini PJ, et al. Thiol-containing compounds inhibit the production of monocyte/macrophage derived angiogenic activity. *Agents Actions* 1991;34:350–357.
20. Nagashima M, Yoshino S, Aono H, et al. Inhibitory effects of anti-rheumatic drugs on vascular endothelial growth factor in cultured rheumatoid synovial cells. *Clin Exp Immunol* 1999;116:360–365.
21. Yang JP, Merin JP, Nakano T, et al. Inhibition of the DNA-binding activity of NF-kappa B by gold compounds *in vitro*. *FEBS Lett* 1995; 361:89–96.
22. Marki F, Stanton JL. Inhibition of phospholipase C by aurothiomalate and (triethylphosphine) gold complexes. *Arzneimittelforschung* 1992; 42:328–333.
23. Ho PPK, Young AL, Southard GL. Methyl ester of *N*-formylmethionyl-leucyl-phenylalanine. Chemotactic responses of human blood monocytes and inhibition of gold compounds. *Arthritis Rheum* 1978; 21:133–136.
24. Mowat AG. Neutrophil chemotaxis in rheumatoid arthritis. *Ann Rheum Dis* 1978;37:1–8.
25. Jessop JD, Vernon-Roberts B, Harris J. Effects of gold salts and prednisolone on inflammatory cells. *Ann Rheum Dis* 1973;32:294–300.
26. Cuperus RA, Muijsers AO, Wever R. Antiarthritic drugs containing thiol groups scavenge hypochlorite and inhibit its formation by myeloperoxidase from human leukocytes. A therapeutic mechanism of these drugs in rheumatoid arthritis? *Arthritis Rheum* 1985;28: 1228–1233.
27. Persellin RH, Ziff M. The effect of gold salts on lysosomal enzymes of the peritoneal macrophage. *Arthritis Rheum* 1966;9:57–65.
28. Paltemaa S. The inhibition of lysosomal enzymes by gold salts in human synovial fluid cells. *Acta Rheum Scand* 1968;14:161–168.
29. Schultz DR, Volanakis JE, Arnold PI, et al. Inactivation of C1 in rheumatoid synovial fluid, purified C1 and C1 esterase, by gold compounds. *Clin Exp Immunol* 1974;17:395–406.
30. Burge JJ, Fearson DT, Austen KF. Inhibition of the alternative pathway of complement by gold sodium thiomalate *in vitro*. *J Immunol* 1978;120:1625–1630.
31. Penneys NS, Ziboh V, Gottlieb NL, et al. Inhibition of prostaglandin synthesis and human epidermal enzymes by aurothiomalate *in vitro*: possible actions of gold in pemphigus. *J Invest Dermatol* 1974;63: 356–361.
32. Fraser TN. Gold therapy in rheumatoid arthritis. *Ann Rheum Dis* 1945;4:71–75.

33. Empire Rheumatism Council. Gold therapy in rheumatoid arthritis. Report of a multicenter controlled trial. *Ann Rheum Dis* 1961;20:315–334.
34. Sigler JW, Bluhm GB, Duncan H, et al. Gold salts in the treatment of rheumatoid arthritis: a double-blind study. *Ann Intern Med* 1974;80:21–26.
35. Ward JR, Williams HJ, Egger MJ, et al. Comparison of auranofin, gold sodium thiomalate, and placebo in the treatment of rheumatoid arthritis. *Arthritis Rheum* 1983;26:1303–1315.
36. Katz WA, Alexander S, Bland JH, et al. The efficacy and safety of auranofin compared to placebo in rheumatoid arthritis. *J Rheumatol* 1982;9(suppl 8):173–178.
37. Gottlieb NL, Kiem IM, Penneys NS, et al. The influence of chrysotherapy on serum proteins and immunoglobulin levels, rheumatoid factor, and antiepithelial antibody titers. *J Lab Clin Med* 1975;86:962–972.
38. Highton J, Panayi GS, Shephard P, et al. Fall in immune complex levels during gold treatment of rheumatoid arthritis. *Ann Rheum Dis* 1981;40:575–579.
39. Sharp JT, Lidsky MD, Duffy J. Clinical responses during gold therapy for rheumatoid arthritis: changes in synovitis, radiologically detectable erosive lesions, serum proteins, and serologic abnormalities. *Arthritis Rheum* 1982;25:540–549.
40. Rau R, Herborn G, Menninger H, et al. Radiographic outcome after three years of patients with early erosive rheumatoid arthritis treated with intramuscular methotrexate or parenteral gold. Extension of a one-year double-blind study in 174 patients. *Rheumatology (Oxford)* 2002;41:196–204.
41. Gofton JP, O'Brien W. Roentgenographic findings during auranofin treatment. *Am J Med* 1983;75(suppl):142–144.
42. Buckland-Wright JC, Clarke GS, Chikanza IC, Grahame R. Quantitative microfocal radiography detects changes in erosion area in patients with early rheumatoid arthritis treated with myochrysine. *J Rheumatol* 1993;20:243–247.
43. Huskisson EC, Gibson TJ, Balme HW. Trial comparing D-penicillamine and gold in rheumatoid arthritis. *Ann Rheum Dis* 1974;33:532–535.
44. Goldberg J, Pinals RS. Felty's syndrome. *Semin Arthritis Rheum* 1980;10:52–65.
45. Luthra HS, Conn DL, Ferguson RH. Felty's syndrome: response to parenteral gold. *J Rheumatol* 1981;8:902–909.
46. Adams CH, Cecil RL. Gold therapy in early rheumatoid arthritis. *Ann Intern Med* 1950;33:163–173.
47. Rothermich NO, Phillips VK, Bergen W. Chrysotherapy: a prospective study. *Arthritis Rheum* 1976;19:1321–1327.
48. Srinivasa NR, Miller BL, Paulus HE. Long-term chrysotherapy in rheumatoid arthritis. *Arthritis Rheum* 1979;22:105–110.
49. Sambrook TN, Browne CD, Champion GD, et al. Termination of treatment with gold sodium thiomalate in rheumatoid arthritis. *J Rheumatol* 1982;9:932–934.
50. Richter JA, Runge LA, Pinals RS, et al. Analysis of treatment terminations with gold and anti-malarial compounds in rheumatoid arthritis. *J Rheumatol* 1980;7:153–159.
51. Sagransky DM, Greenwald RA. Efficacy and toxicity of retreatment with gold salts: a retrospective review of 25 cases. *J Rheumatol* 1980;7:474–478.
52. Klinkhoff AV, Teufel A. The second course of gold. *J Rheumatol* 1995;22:1655–1656.
53. Epstein WV, Henk CJ, Yelin EH, et al. Effect of parenterally administered gold therapy on the course of adult rheumatoid arthritis. *Ann Intern Med* 1991;114:437–444.
54. Levinson JE. Gold salts in the rheumatic diseases. In: Moore TD, ed. *Arthritis in childhood.* Eightieth Ross conference in pediatric research. Columbus, OH: Ross Laboratories, 1981:120–124.
55. Giannini EH, Barron KS, Spencer CH, et al. Auranofin therapy for juvenile rheumatoid arthritis: results of the five year open label extension trial. *J Rheumatol* 1991;18:1240–1242.
56. Giannini EH, Cassidy JT, Brewer EJ, et al. Comparative efficacy and safety of advanced drug therapy in children with juvenile rheumatoid arthritis. *Semin Arthritis Rheum* 1993;23:34–46.
57. Dorwart BB, Gall EP, Schumacher HR, et al. Chrysotherapy in psoriatic arthritis. *Arthritis Rheum* 1978;21:513–515.
58. Richter MB, Kinsella P, Corbett M. Gold in psoriatic arthropathy. *Ann Rheum Dis* 1980;39:279–280.
59. Bruckle W, Dexel T, Grasedyck K, et al. Treatment of psoriatic arthritis with auranofin and gold sodium thiomalate. *Clin Rheumatol* 1994;13:209–216.
60. Mader R, Gladman DD, Long J, et al. Does injectable gold retard radiologic evidence of joint damage in psoriatic arthritis? *Clin Invest Med* 1995;18:139–143.
61. Hanson V. Dosage of gold salts in treatment of juvenile rheumatoid arthritis. *Arthritis Rheum* 1977;20(suppl 2):548.
62. Ansell BM. The management of juvenile chronic polyarthritis (Still's disease). *Practitioner* 1972;208:91–100.
63. Cats A. A multicenter controlled trial of the effects of different dosage of gold therapy, followed by maintenance dosage. *Agents Actions* 1976;6:355–363.
64. Furst D, Levine S, Srinivasa NR, et al. A double-blind trial of high versus conventional dosages of gold salts for rheumatoid arthritis. *Arthritis Rheum* 1977;20:1473–1480.
65. Rothermich NO, Phillips VK, Bergen W. Chrysotherapy: a prospective study. *Arthritis Rheum* 1976;19:1321–1327.
66. Smith RT, Peak WP, Kron KM. Increasing the effectiveness of gold therapy in rheumatoid arthritis. *JAMA* 1958;167:1197–1204.
67. Mascarhenas BR, Granda JL, Freyberg RH. Gold metabolism in patients with rheumatoid arthritis treated with gold compounds—reinvestigated. *Arthritis Rheum* 1972;15:391–402.
68. Lorber A, Bovy RA, Chang CC. Relationship between serum gold content and distribution to serum immunoglobulins and complement. *Nat New Biol* 1972;236:250.
69. Smith PM, Smith EM, Gottlieb NL. Gold distribution in whole blood during chrysotherapy. *J Lab Clin Med* 1973;82:930–937.
70. Graham GG, Haavisto TM, McNaught PJ, et al. The effect of smoking on the distribution of gold in blood. *J Rheumatol* 1982;9:527–531.
71. James DW, Ludvigsen NW, Cleland LG, et al. The influence of cigarette smoking on blood gold distribution during chrysotherapy. *J Rheumatol* 1982;9:532–535.
72. Gottlieb NL, Smith PM, Smith EM. Pharmacodynamics of ^{195}Au labeled aurothiomalate in blood. Correlation with course of rheumatoid arthritis, gold toxicity and gold excretion. *Arthritis Rheum* 1974;17:171–183.
73. Gerber RC, Paulus HE, Bluestone R. Kinetics of aurothiomalate in serum and synovial fluid. *Arthritis Rheum* 1972;15:625–629.
74. Gottlieb NL, Smith PM, Smith EM. Tissue gold concentrations in a rheumatoid arthritic receiving chrysotherapy. *Arthritis Rheum* 1972;15:16–20.
75. Grahame R, Billings R, Laurence M. Tissue gold levels after chrysotherapy. *Ann Rheum Dis* 1976;33:536–539.
76. Penneys NS, McCreary S, Gottlieb NL. Intracellular distribution of radiogold: localization to large granular membranes. *Arthritis Rheum* 1976;19:927–932.
77. Veron-Roberts B, Dore JL, Jessop JD, et al. Selective concentration and localization of gold in macrophages of synovial and other tissues during and after chrysotherapy in rheumatoid patients. *Ann Rheum Dis* 1976;35:477–486.
78. Gottlieb NL, Smith PM, Smith EM. Gold excretion correlated with clinical course during chrysotherapy in rheumatoid arthritis. *Arthritis Rheum* 1972;15:582–592.
79. Champion GD, Bieri D, Browne CD, et al. Auranofin in rheumatoid arthritis. *J Rheumatol* 1982;9(suppl 8):137–145.
80. Calin A, Saunders D, Bennett R, et al. Auranofin: one mg or 9 mg? The search for the appropriate dose. *J Rheumatol* 1982;9(suppl 8):146–148.
81. Giannini H, Brewer EJ Jr, Person PA. Auranofin in the treatment of juvenile rheumatoid arthritis. *J Pediatr* 1983;102:138–141.
82. Finkelstein AE, Roisman FR, Batista V. Oral chrysotherapy in rheumatoid arthritis: minimum effective dose. *J Rheumatol* 1980;7:160–168.
83. Walz DT, Griswold DE, DiMartino J, et al. Distribution of gold in blood following administration of auranofin. *J Rheumatol* 1979;6(suppl 5):56–60.
84. Blocka K, Furst DE, Landaw E, et al. Single-dose pharmacokinetics of auranofin in rheumatoid arthritis. *J Rheumatol* 1982;9(suppl 8):110–119.
85. Gottlieb NL. Comparative pharmacokinetics of parenteral and oral gold compounds. *J Rheumatol* 1982;9(suppl 8):99–109.
86. Blodgett RC, Heuer MA, Pietrusko RG. Auranofin: a unique oral chrysotherapeutic agent. *Semin Arthritis Rheum* 1984;13:255–273.

87. Penneys NS, Ackerman AB, Gottlieb NL. Gold dermatitis. *Arch Dermatol* 1974;109:372–376.
88. Choy EH, Gambling L, Best SL, et al. Nickel contamination of gold salts: link with gold-induced skin rash. *Br J Rheumatol* 1997;36:1054–1058.
89. Verwilghen J, Kingsley GH, Gambling L, Panayi GS. Activation of gold-reactive T lymphocytes in rheumatoid arthritis patients treated with gold. *Arthritis Rheum* 1992;35:1413–1418.
90. Pickl WF, Fischer GF, Fae I, et al. HLA-DR1-positive patients suffering from rheumatoid arthritis are at high risk for developing mucocutaneous side effects upon gold therapy. *Hum Immunol* 1993;38:127–131.
91. Rodriguez-Perez M, Gonzalez-Dominguez J, Mataran L, et al. Association of HLA-DR5 with mucocutaneous lesions in patients with rheumatoid arthritis receiving gold sodium thiomalate. *J Rheumatol* 1994;21:41–43.
92. Goldermann R, Schuppe HC, Gleichmann E, et al. Adverse immune reactions to gold in rheumatoid arthritis: lack of skin reactivity. *Acta Derm Venereol (Stockholm)* 1993;73:220–222.
93. Beckett VL, Doyle JA, Hadley GA, et al. Chrysiasis resulting from gold therapy in rheumatoid arthritis: identification of gold by x-ray microanalysis. *Mayo Clin Proc* 1982;57:773–777.
94. Jeffery DA, Biggs DF, Percy JS, et al. Quantitation of gold in skin in chrysiasis. *J Rheumatol* 1975;2:28–35.
95. Silverberg DS, Kidd EG, Shnitka TK. Gold nephropathy. A clinical and pathologic study. *Arthritis Rheum* 1970;13:812–825.
96. Vaamonde CA, Hunt FR. The nephrotic syndrome as a consequence of gold therapy. *Arthritis Rheum* 1970;13:826–834.
97. Davenport A, Maciver AG, Hall CL, et al. Do mesangial immune complex deposits affect the renal prognosis in membranous glomerulonephritis? *Clin Nephrol* 1994;41:271–276.
98. Korpela M, Mustonen J, Pasternack A, et al. Mesangial glomerulopathy in rheumatoid arthritis patients. *Nephron* 1991;59:46–50.
99. Wiland P, Szechinski J. *N*-acetyl-beta-D-glucosaminidase urinary excretion as an early indicator of kidney damage in rheumatoid arthritis patients starting on parenteral gold and Depo-Medrone/placebo injections. *Clin Rheumatol* 1999;18:106–113.
100. Deren B, Masi R, Weksler M. Gold-associated thrombocytopenia. *Arch Intern Med* 1974;134:1012–1015.
101. Stafford BT, Crosby WH. Late onset of gold-induced thrombocytopenia. *JAMA* 1978;239:50–51.
102. McCarty DJ, Brill JM, Harrop D. Aplastic anemia secondary to gold-salt therapy: report of a fatal case and a review of the literature. *JAMA* 1962;179:655–657.
103. Davis P, Hughes GRV. Significance of eosinophilia during gold therapy. *Arthritis Rheum* 1974;17:964–968.
104. Snowden N, Dietch DM, Teh LS, et al. Antibody deficiency associated with gold treatment: natural history and management in 22 patients. *Ann Rheum Dis* 1996;55:616–621.
105. Gottlieb NL, Brown HE Jr. Acute myocardial infarction following gold sodium thiomalate induced vasomotor (nitritoid) reaction. *Arthritis Rheum* 1977;20:1026–1028.
106. Halla JT, Hardin JG, Linn JE. Postinjection nonvasomotor reactions during chrysotherapy. *Arthritis Rheum* 1977;20:1188–1191.
107. Proudman SM, Cleland LG. Auranofin-induced vasomotor reaction. *Arthritis Rheum* 1992;35:1452–1454.
108. Winterbauer RH, Wilske KR, Wheelis RF. Diffuse pulmonary injury associated with gold treatment. *N Engl J Med* 1976;294:919–921.
109. Gould PW, McCormack PL, Palmer DG. Pulmonary damage associated with sodium aurothiomalate therapy. *J Rheumatol* 1977;4:252–260.
110. Tomioka R, King TE Jr. Gold-induced pulmonary disease: clinical features, outcome, and differentiation from rheumatoid lung disease. *Am J Respir Crit Care Med* 1997;155:1011–1020.
111. Stein HB, Urowitz MB. Gold-induced enterocolitis. *J Rheumatol* 1976;3:21–26.
112. Teodorescu V, Bauer J, Lichtiger S, et al. Gold-induced colitis: a case report and review of the literature. *Mt Sinai J Med* 1993;60:238–241.
113. Favreau M, Tannenbaum H, Lough J. Hepatic toxicity associated with gold therapy. *Ann Intern Med* 1977;87:717–719.
114. Howrie DL, Gartner JC Jr. Gold-induced hepatotoxicity: case report and review of the literature. *J Rheumatol* 1982;9:727–729.
115. Katrack SM, Pollock M, O'Brien CP, et al. Clinical and morphological features of gold neuropathy. *Brain* 1980;103:671–693.
116. Rau R, Herborn G, Karger T, et al. A double-blind comparison of parenteral methotrexate and parenteral gold in the treatment of early erosive rheumatoid arthritis: an interim report on 102 patients after 12 months. *Semin Arthritis Rheum* 1991;21(suppl 1):13–20.
117. Rau R, Herborn G, Karger T, et al. A double-blind randomized parallel trial of intramuscular methotrexate and gold sodium thiomalate in early erosive rheumatoid arthritis. *J Rheumatol* 1991;18:328–333.
118. Rau R, Herborn G, Menninger H, et al. Progression in early erosive rheumatoid arthritis: 12 month results from a randomized controlled trial comparing methotrexate and gold sodium thiomalate. *Br J Rheumatol* 1998;37:1220–1226.
119. Menninger H, Herborn G, Sander O, et al. A 36 month comparative trial of methotrexate and gold sodium thiomalate in the treatment of early active and erosive rheumatoid arthritis. *Br J Rheumatol* 1998;37:1060–1068.
120. Rau R, Herborn G, Menninger H, et al. Comparison of intramuscular methotrexate and gold sodium thiomalate in the treatment of early erosive rheumatoid arthritis: 12 month data of a double-blind parallel study of 174 patients. *Br J Rheumatol* 1997;36:345–352.
121. Porter DR, Capell HA, Hunter J. Combination therapy in rheumatoid arthritis—no benefit of addition of hydroxychloroquin to patients with a suboptimal response to intramuscular gold therapy. *J Rheumatol* 1993;20:645–649.
122. Rau R, Schleusser B, Herborn G, et al. Longterm combination therapy of refractory and destructive rheumatoid arthritis with methotrexate (MTX) and intramuscular gold or other disease modifying antirheumatic drugs compared to MTX monotherapy. *J Rheumatol* 1998;25:1485–1492.
123. Elkayam O, Yaron M, Zhukovsky G, et al. Toxicity profile of dual methotrexate combinations with gold, hydroxychloroquine, sulphasalazine and minocycline in rheumatoid arthritis patients. *Rheumatol Int* 1997;17:49–53.
124. Bendix G, Bjelle A. Adding low-dose cyclosporin A to parenteral gold therapy in rheumatoid arthritis: a double-blind placebo-controlled study. *Br J Rheumatol* 1996;35:1142–1149.
125. Williams HJ, Ward JR, Reading JC, et al. Comparison of auranofin, methotrexate, and the combination of both in the treatment of rheumatoid arthritis. *Arthritis Rheum* 1992;35:259–269.
126. Abraham EP, Chain E, Baker W, et al. Penicillamine: a characteristic degradation product of penicillin. *Nature* 1943;151:107.
127. Walshe JM. Disturbances of amino acid metabolism following liver injury. *Q J Med* 1953;22:483–505.
128. Crawhall JC, Scowen EF, Watts RWE. Effects of penicillamine on cystinuria. *BMJ* 1963;1:588–590.
129. Jaffe IA. Comparison of the effect of plasmapheresis and penicillamine on the level of circulating rheumatoid factor. *Ann Rheum Dis* 1963;22:71–76.
130. Cuperus RA, Muijsers AO, Wever R. Antiarthritic drugs containing thiol groups scavenge hypochlorite and inhibit its formation by myeloperoxidase from human leukocytes. A therapeutic mechanism of these drugs in rheumatoid arthritis? *Arthritis Rheum* 1985;28:1228–1233.
131. Teodorescu M, McAfee M, Skosey JI, et al. Covalent disulfide binding of IL-1β to α_2-macroglobulin: inhibition by D-penicillamine. *Mol Immunol* 1991;28:323–334.
132. Lipsky PE, Ziff M. Inhibition of human helper T cell function *in vitro* by D-penicillamine and $CuSO_4$. *J Clin Invest* 1980;65:1069–1076.
133. Zuckner J, Ramsey RH, Dorner RW, Gantner GE. D-penicillamine in rheumatoid arthritis. *Arthritis Rheum* 1970;13:131–138.
134. Brown-Galatola CH, Hall ND. Impaired suppressor cell activity due to surface sulphydryl oxidation in rheumatoid arthritis. *Br J Rheumatol* 1992;31:599–603.
135. Rosad M, Fiocco U, De Silvestro G, et al. Effect of D-penicillamine on the T cell phenotype in scleroderma. Comparison between treated and untreated patients. *Clin Exp Rheumatol* 1993;11:143–148.
136. Akamatsu T, Matsubara T, Saegusa Y, et al. Inhibition of mitogen-induced response of human peripheral blood mononuclear cells by bucillamine, a new antirheumatic sulfhydryl drug. *Rheumatol Int* 1994;13:197–201.
137. Hashimoto K, Lipsky PE. Immunosuppression by the disease modifying antirheumatic drug bucillamine: inhibition of human T lymphocyte function by bucillamine and its metabolites. *J Rheumatol* 1993;20:953–957.

138. Hirohata S, Lipsky PE. Regulation of B cell function by bucillamine, a novel disease modifying antirheumatic drug. *Clin Immunol Immunopathol* 1993;66:43–51.
139. Hirohata S, Lipsky PE. Comparative inhibitory effects of bucillamine and D-penicillamine on the function of human B cells and T cells. *Arthritis Rheum* 1994;37:942–950.
140. Nagashima M, Yoshino S, Aono H, et al. Inhibitory effects of antirheumatic drugs on vascular endothelial growth factor in cultured rheumatoid synovial cells. *Clin Exp Immunol* 1999;116:360–365.
141. Aono H, Hasunuma T, Fujisawa K, et al. Direct suppression of human synovial cell proliferation *in vitro* by salazosulfapyridine and bucillamine. *J Rheumatol* 1996;23:65–70.
142. Huskisson EC, Gibson TJ, Balme HW, et al. Trial comparing D-penicillamine in rheumatoid arthritis: preliminary report. *Ann Rheum Dis* 1974;33:532–535.
143. Berry H, Liyange R, Durance CG, et al. Trial comparing azathioprine and penicillamine in treatment of rheumatoid arthritis. *Ann Rheum Dis* 1976;35:542–543.
144. Dixon A St J, Davies J, Dormandy TL, et al. Synthetic D(-) penicillamine in rheumatoid arthritis. Double-blind controlled study of a high and a low dose regimen. *Ann Rheum Dis* 1975;34:416–421.
145. Jaffe IA. The effect of penicillamine on the laboratory parameters in rheumatoid arthritis. *Arthritis Rheum* 1965;8:1064–1079.
146. Jaffe IA. Penicillamine treatment of rheumatoid arthritis: effect on immune complexes. *Ann NY Acad Sci* 1975;256:330–337.
147. Wolfe F, Hawley DJ. Remission in rheumatoid arthritis. *J Rheumatol* 1985;12:245–252.
148. Pullar T, Hunter JA. Does second-line therapy affect the radiological progression of rheumatoid arthritis? *Ann Rheum Dis* 1984;43: 18–23.
149. Eberhardt K, Rydgren L, Fex E, et al. D-penicillamine in early rheumatoid arthritis: experience from a 2-year double blind placebo controlled. *Clin Exp Rheumatol* 1996;14:625–631.
150. Jaffe IA. Rheumatoid vasculitis report of a second case treated with penicillamine. *Arthritis Rheum* 1968;11:585–592.
151. Ginsberg MH, Genant HK, Yu TSF, et al. Rheumatoid nodulosis: an unusual variant of rheumatoid disease. *Arthritis Rheum* 1975;18: 49–58.
152. Dash S, Seibold JR, Tiku ML. Successful treatment of methotrexate induced nodulosis with D-penicillamine. *J Rheumatol* 1999;26:1396–1399.
153. Blau S, Meiselas L. Regression of splenomegaly with hematologic recovery in Felty's syndrome due to D-penicillamine. A case report. *Meadowbrook Hosp J* 1972;5:16.
154. Lake B, Andrews J. Rheumatoid arthritis with amyloidosis and malabsorption syndrome. Effect of D-penicillamine. *Am J Med* 1968;44: 105–115.
155. Lorber A. Penicillamine therapy for rheumatoid lung disease: effects of protein sulfhydryl groups. *Nature* 1966;210:1235–1237.
156. Haerdon J, Coolen L, Dequeker J. The effect of D-penicillamine on lung function parameters (diffusion capacity) in rheumatoid arthritis. *Clin Exp Rheumatol* 1993;11:509–513.
157. Ansell BM. Penicillamine, levamisole and cytotoxic drugs. In: Moore TD, ed. *Arthritis in childhood.* Eightieth Ross conference in pediatric research. Columbus, OH: Ross Laboratories, 1981:127–130.
158. Schairer H. Long-term follow-up of 285 cases of juvenile chronic polyarthritis treated with D-penicillamine or gold. In: *The care of rheumatic children.* EULAR bulletin. Monograph series no. 3:165. Basel, Switzerland: EULAR Publishers, 1978.
159. Bird HA, Dixon A St J. Failure of D-penicillamine to affect peripheral joint involvement in ankylosing spondylitis or HLA B-27 associated arthropathy. *Ann Rheum Dis* 1977;36:289.
160. Steen VD, Medsger TA Jr, Rodman GP. D-penicillamine therapy in progressive systemic sclerosis (scleroderma) a retrospective analysis. *Ann Intern Med* 1982;97:652–659.
161. Clements PJ, Furst DE, Wong WK, et al. High-dose versus low-dose D-penicillamine in early diffuse systemic sclerosis: analysis of a two-year, double-blind, randomized, controlled clinical trial. *Arthritis Rheum* 1999;42:1194–1203.
162. Jaffe IA. The technique of penicillamine administration in rheumatoid arthritis. *Arthritis Rheum* 1975;18:513–514.
163. Jaffe IA. D-penicillamine. *Bull Rheum Dis* 1978;28:948–952.
164. Doyle DV, Perrett D, Foster OJ, et al. The long-term use of D-penicillamine for treating rheumatoid arthritis: is continuous therapy necessary? *Br J Rheumatol* 1993;32:614–617.
165. Schnua A, Osman MA, Patel RB, et al. Influence of food on the bioavailability of penicillamine. *J Rheumatol* 1983;10:95–97.
166. Perrett D. The metabolism and pharmacology of D-penicillamine in man. *J Rheumatol* 1981;8(suppl 7):41–50.
167. Joyce DA, Day RO. D-penicillamine and D-penicillamine-protein disulfide in plasma and synovial fluid of patients with rheumatoid arthritis. *Br J Clin Pharmacol* 1990;30:511–517.
168. Sternlieb I, Fisher M, Scheinberg IH. Penicillamine-induced skin lesions. *J Rheumatol* 1981;8(suppl 7):149–154.
169. Klingberg WG, Prasad AS, Oberleas D. Zinc deficiency following penicillamine therapy. In: Prasad AS, ed. *Trace elements in human health and disease.* New York: Academic, 1976;1:51–65.
170. van de Staak WJBM, Cotton DWK, Jonckheer-Venneste MMH, et al. Lichenoid eruption following penicillamine. *Dermatologica* 1975; 150:372–374.
171. Pass F, Goldfischer S, Sternlieb I, et al. Elastosis perforans serpiginosa during penicillamine therapy for Wilson's disease. *Arch Dermatol* 1973;108:713–715.
172. Bardach H, Gebhart W, Niebauer G. "Lumpy-bumpy" elastic fibers in the skin and lungs of a patient with a penicillamine-induced elastosis perforans serpiginosa. *J Cutan Pathol* 1979;6:243–252.
173. Greer KS, Askew FC, Richardson DR. Skin lesions induced by penicillamine. Occurrence in a patient with hepatolenticular degeneration (Wilson's disease). *Arch Dermatol* 1976;112:1267–1269.
174. Tishler M, Kahn Y, Yaron M. Pure red cell aplasia caused by D-penicillamine treatment of rheumatoid arthritis. *Ann Rheum Dis* 1991;50:255–256.
175. Bacon PA, Tribe CR, Mackenzie JC, et al. Penicillamine nephropathy in rheumatoid arthritis. A clinical, pathological and immunological study. *Q J Med* 1976;45:661–684.
176. Dische FR, Swinson DR, Hamilton EBD, et al. Immunopathology of penicillamine induced glomerular disease. *J Rheumatol* 1976;3: 145–154.
177. Barraclough D, Cunningham TJ, Muirden KD. Microscopic hematuria in patients with rheumatoid arthritis on D-penicillamine. *Aust N Z J Med* 1981;11:706–708.
178. Almirall J, Alcorta I, Botey A, et al. Penicillamine-induced rapidly progressive glomerulonephritis in a patient with rheumatoid arthritis. *Am J Nephrol* 1993;13:286–288.
179. Macarron P, Garcia Crouzet J, Camus JP, et al. Lupus induced by D-penicillamine during the treatment of rheumatoid arthritis. *Ann Med Interne* 1974;125:71–80.
180. Macarron P, Garcia Diaz JE, Azofra JA, et al. D-penicillamine therapy associated with rapidly progressive glomerulonephritis. *Nephrol Dial Transplant* 1992:7:161–164.
181. Vardi P, Brik R, Barzilai D, et al. Frequent induction of insulin autoantibodies by D-penicillamine in patients with rheumatoid arthritis. *J Rheumatol* 1992;19:1527–1530.
182. Masters CL, Dawkins RL, Zilko PJ, et al. Penicillamine-associated myasthenia gravis, anti-acetylcholine receptor and antistriational antibodies. *Am J Med* 1977;63:689–694.
183. Dawkins RL, Garlepp MJ, McDonald BL, et al. Myasthenia gravis and D-penicillamine. *J Rheumatol* 1981;8(suppl 7):169–172.
184. Drosos AA, Christou L, Galanopoulou V, et al. D-penicillamine induced myasthenia gravis: clinical, serological and genetic findings. *Clin Exp Rheumatol* 1993;11:387–391.
185. Schrader PL, Peters HA, Dahl DS. Polymyositis and penicillamine. *Arch Neurol* 1972;27:456–457.
186. Jenkins EA, Hull RG, Thomas AL. D-penicillamine and polymyositis: the significance of the Jo-1 antibody. *Br J Rheumatol* 1993;32: 1109–1110.
187. Wright GD, Wilson C, Bell AL. D-penicillamine induced polymyositis causing complete heart block. *Clin Rheumatol* 1994;13:80–82.
188. Turner-Warwick M. Adverse reactions affecting the lung: possible association with D-penicillamine. *J Rheumatol* 1981;8(suppl 7)8: 166–168.
189. Eastmond CJ. Diffuse alveolitis as a complication of penicillamine treatment for rheumatoid arthritis. *BMJ* 1976;1:1506.
190. Petersen J. Moller I. Miliary pulmonary infiltrates and penicillamine. *Br J Radiol* 1978;51:915–916.

191. Geddes DM, Corrin B, Brewerton DA, et al. Progressive airway obliteration in adults and its association with rheumatoid disease. *Q J Med* 1977;46:427–444.
192. Lyle WH. D-penicillamine and fatal obliterative bronchiolitis. *BMJ* 1977;1:105.
193. Rosenbaum J, Katz WA, Schumacher HR. Hepatotoxicity associated with use of D-penicillamine in rheumatoid arthritis. *Ann Rheum Dis* 1980;39:152–154.
194. Jacobs JW, Van der Weide FR, Kruijsen MW. Fatal cholestatic hepatitis caused by D-penicillamine. *Br J Rheumatol* 1994;33:770–773.
195. Desai SN. Sudden gigantism of breasts: drug induced? *Br J Plast Surg* 1973;26:371–372.
196. Desautels JE. Breast gigantism due to D-penicillamine. *Can Assoc Radiol J* 1994;45:143–144.
197. Svartz N. Salazopyrin, a new sulfanilamide preparation. *Acta Med Scand* 1942;110:577.
198. McConkey B, Amos R, Durham S, et al. Sulphasalazine in rheumatoid arthritis. *BMJ* 1980;280:442.
199. O'Dell JR, Haire CE, Erikson N, et al. Treatment of rheumatoid arthritis with methotrexate alone, sulfasalazine and hydroxychloroquine, or a combination of all three medications. *N Engl J Med* 1996; 334:1287.
200. Williams J, Hallet M. Effect of sulphasalazine and its active metabolite, 5-aminosalicylic acid, on toxic oxygen metabolite production by neutrophils. *Gut* 1989;30:1581.
201. Storgaard M, Jensen MP, Stengaard-Pedersen K, et al. Effects of methotrexate, sulphasalazine and aurothiomalate on polymorphonuclear leucocytes in rheumatoid arthritis. *Scand J Rheumatol* 1996; 25:168–173.
202. Tsai CY, Wu TH, Yu CL, et al. The *in vitro* immunomodulatory effects of sulfasalazine on human polymorphonuclear leukocytes, mononuclear cells, and cultured glomerular mesangial cells. *Life Sci* 2000;67:1149–1161.
203. Akahoshi T, Namai R, Sekiyama N, et al. Rapid induction of neutrophil apoptosis by sulfasalazine: implications of reactive oxygen species in the apoptotic process. *J Leukoc Biol* 1997;62:817–826.
204. Carlin G, Djursater R, Smedegard G. Sulphasalazine inhibition of human granulocyte activation by inhibition of second messenger compounds. *Ann Rheum Dis* 1992;51:1230.
205. Gadangi P, Longaker M, Naime D, et al. The anti-inflammatory mechanism of sulfasalazine is related to adenosine release at inflamed sites. *J Immunol* 1996;156:1937–1941.
206. Morabito L, Montesinos MC, Schreibman DM, et al. Methotrexate and sulfasalazine promote adenosine release by a mechanism that requires ecto-5′-nucleotidase-mediated conversion of adenine nucleotides. *J Clin Invest* 1998;101:295–300.
207. Imai F, Suzuki R, Ishigashi T, et al. Effect of sulfasalazine on B cell hyperactivity in patients with rheumatoid arthritis. *J Rheumatol* 1994;21:612.
208. Symmons DPM, Salmon M, Farr M, et al. Sulfasalazine treatment and lymphocyte function in patients with rheumatoid arthritis. *J Rheumatol* 1988;15:575–579.
209. Nissila M, Lehtinen K, Leirisalo-Repo M. Sulfasalazine in the treatment of ankylosing spondylitis: a twenty-six week, placebo-controlled clinical trial. *Arthritis Rheum* 1988;31:1111–1116.
210. Hirohata S, Ohshima N, Yanagida T, et al. Regulation of human B cell function by sulfasalazine and its its metabolites. *Int Immunopharmacol* 2002;5:631–640.
211. Liptay S, Bachem M, Hacker G, et al. Inhibition of nuclear factor kappa B and induction of apoptosis in T-lymphocytes by sulfasalazine. *Br J Pharmacol* 1999;128:1361–1369.
212. Liptay S, Fulda S, Schanbacher M, et al. Molecular mechanisms of sulfasalazine-induced T cell apoptosis. *Br J Pharmacol* 2002;137: 608–620.
213. Weber CK, Liptay S, Wirth T, et al. Suppression of NF-kappaB activity by sulfasalazine is mediated by direct inhibition of IkappaB kinases alpha and beta. *Gastroenterology* 2000;119:1209–1218.
214. Gout PW, Buckley AR, Simms CR, et al. Sulfasalazine, a potent suppressor of lymphoma growth by inhibition of the x-cystine transporter: a new action for an old drug. *Leukemia* 2001;15:1633–1640.
215. Kang BY, Chung SW, Im SY, et al. Sulfasalazine prevents T-helper 1 immune response by suppressing interleukin-12 production in macrophages. *Immunology* 1999;98:98–103.
216. Danis VA, Franic GM, Rathjen DA, et al. Circulating cytokine levels in patients with rheumatoid arthritis: results of a double blind trial with sulphasalazine. *Ann Rheum Dis* 1992;51:945.
217. Pullar T, Hunter J, Capell H. Sulphasalazine in rheumatoid arthritis: a double blind comparison of sulphasalazine with placebo and sodium aurothiomalate. *BMJ* 1983;287:1102.
218. Australian Multicentre Clinic Trial Group. Sulphasalazine in early rheumatoid arthritis. *J Rheumatol* 1992;19:1672.
219. Pinals R, Kaplan S, Lawson J, et al. Sulphasalazine in rheumatoid arthritis: a double-blind placebo controlled trial. *Arthritis Rheum* 1986;29:1427.
220. Hannonen P, Mottonen T, Hakola M, et al. Sulphasalazine in early rheumatoid arthritis. *Arthritis Rheum* 1993;36:1501.
221. Mottonen T, Hannonen P, Leiroso-Repo M, et al. Comparison of combination therapy with single-drug therapy in early rheumatoid arthritis: a randomized trial. FIN-FACo trial group. *Lancet* 1999; 353:259–266.
222. Van der Heijde D, van Riel P, Nuver-Zwart E, et al. Sulphasalazine versus hydroxychloroquine in rheumatoid arthritis: 3-year follow-up. *Lancet* 1990;335:539.
223. Williams HJ, Ward JR, Dahl SL, et al. A controlled trial comparing sulfasalazine, gold sodium thiomalate, and placebo in rheumatoid arthritis. *Arthritis Rheum* 1988;31:702–713.
224. Neumann VC, Grindulis KA, Hbbal S, et al. Comparison between penicillamine and sulphasalazine in rheumatoid arthritis: Leeds-Birmingham trial. *BMJ* 1983;287:1099–1102.
225. Carroll GJ, Will RK, Breidahl PD, et al. Sulphasalazine versus penicillamine in the treatment of rheumatoid arthritis. *Rheumatol Int* 1989;8:251–255.
226. Smolen JS, Kalden JR, Scott DL, et al. Efficacy and safety of leflunomide compared with placebo and sulphasalazine in active rheumatoid arthritis: a double-blind, randomized, multi-centre trial. *Lancet* 1999;353:259–266.
227. Felson DT, Anderson JJ, Meenan RF. The comparative efficacy and toxicity of second-line drugs in rheumatoid arthritis: results of two meta-analyses. *Arthritis Rheum* 1990;33:1449–1461.
228. Svensson B, Ahlmen M, Forslind K. Treatment of early RA in clinical practice: a comparative study of two different DMARD/corticosteroid options. *Clin Exp Rheumatol* 2003;21:327–332.
229. Ishikawa K, Tsukada Y, Tamura S, et al. Salazosulfapridine-induced remission of Felty's syndrome along with significant reduction in neutrophil-bound immunoglobulin G. *J Rheumatol* 2003;30:404–406.
230. Haagsma CJ, van Riel PL, de Rooij DJ, et al. Combination of methotrexate and sulphasalazine vs methotrexate alone: a randomized open clinical trial in rheumatoid arthritis patients resistant to sulphasalazine therapy. *Br J Rheumatol* 1994;33:1049–1055.
231. Shiroky JB. Combination of sulphasalazine and methotrexate in the management of rheumatoid arthritis: view based on personal clinical experience. *Br J Rheumatol* 1995;34(suppl 2):109–112.
232. Dougados M, Combe B, et al. Combination therapy in early rheumatoid arthritis: a randomized, controlled, double blind 52 week clinical trial of sulphasalazine compared with the single components. *Ann Rheum Dis* 1999;58:220–225.
233. O'Dell JR, Haire CE. Treatment of rheumatoid arthritis with methotrexate alone, sulfasalazine and hydroxychloroquine, or a combination of all three medications. *N Engl J Med* 1996;334:1287–1291.
234. Mottonen T, Hannonen P, Leirisalo-Reppo M, et al. Comparison of combination therapy with single-drug therapy in early rheumatoid arthritis: a randomised trial. *Lancet* 1999;353:1568–1573.
235. Landewe RB, Boers M, Verhoeven AC, et al. COBRA combination therapy in patients with early rheumatoid arthritis: long-term structural benefits of a brief intervention. *Arthritis Rheum* 2002;46:347–356.
236. Clegg DO, Reda DJ, Weisman MH, et al. Comparison of sulfasalazine and placebo in the treatment of ankylosing spondylitis. *Arthritis Rheum* 1996;39:2004.
237. Kirwan J, Edwards A, Huitfeldt B, et al. The course of established ankylosing spondylitis and the effects of sulphasalazine over 3 years. *Br J Rheum* 1993;32:729.
238. Mielants H, Veys E. HLA-B27 related arthritis and bowel inflammation. Part 1. Sulfasalazine (Salazopyrin) in HLA-B27 related reactive arthritis. *J Rheumatol* 1985;12:287.
239. Feltelius N, Hallgren R. Sulphasalazine in ankylosing spondylitis. *Ann Rheum Dis* 1986;45:396–399.

240. Nissila M, Lehtinen K, Leirisalo-Repo M. Sulfasalazine in the treatment of ankylosing spondylitis: a twenty-six week, placebo-controlled clinical trial. *Arthritis Rheum* 1988;31:1111–1116.
241. Farr M, Kitas G, Waterhouse L, et al. Sulphasalazine in psoriatic arthritis: a double blind placebo-controlled study. *Br J Rheumatol* 1990;29:46.
242. Clegg DO, Reda DJ, Mejias E et al. Comparison of sulfasalazine and placebo in the treatment of psoriatic arthritis: a Department of Veterans Affairs Cooperative Study. *Arthritis Rheum* 1996;39:2013–2020.
243. Gupta AK, Grober JS, Hamilton TA, et al. Sulfasalazine therapy for psoriatic arthritis: a double blind, placebo controlled trial. *J Rheumatol* 1995;22:894.
244. Mielants H, Veys EM. HLA-B27 related arthritis and bowel inflammation. Part 1: sulfasalazine (salazopyrin) in HLA-B27 related reactive arthritis. *J Rheumatol* 1985;12:287–293.
245. Mielants H, Veys JM, Joos R, et al. Repeat ileocolonoscopy in reactive arthritis. *J Rheumatol* 1987;14:456–458.
246. Clegg DO, Reda DJ, Weisman MH, et al. Comparison of sulfasalazine and placebo in the treatment of reactive arthritis (Reiter's syndrome): a Department of Veterans Affairs Cooperative Study. *Arthritis Rheum* 1996;39:2021–2027.
247. Egsmose C, Hansen TM, Andersen LS, et al. Limited effect of sulphasalazine treatment in reactive arthritis: a randomized double blind placebo controlled trial. *Ann Rheum Dis* 1997;56:32–36.
248. Clegg DO, Reda DJ, Abdellatif M. Comparison of sulfasalazine and placebo for treatment of axial and peripheral articular manifestations of the seronegative spondyloarthropathies: a Department of Veterans Affairs Cooperative Study. *Arthritis Rheum* 1999;42: 2325–2329.
249. Grondin C, Malleson P, Petty R. Slow-acting antirheumatic drugs in chronic arthritis of childhood. *Semin Arthritis Rheum* 1988; 18:38.
250. van Rossum MA, Fiselier RJ, Franssen MJ, et al. Sulfasalazine in the treatment of juvenile chronic arthritis: a randomized. Double-blind, placebo-controlled, multicenter study: Dutch Juvenile Chronic Arthritis Group. *Arthritis Rheum* 1998;41:808–816.
251. Munoz-Fernandez S, Hidalgo V, Fernandez-Melon J, et al. Sulfasalazine reduces the number of flares of acute anterior uveitis over a one-year period. *J Rheumatol* 2003;30:1277–1279.
252. Gupta A, Goldfarb M, Voorhees J. The use of sulfasalazine in atrophie blanche. *Int J Dermatol* 1990;29:663–665.
253. Bisalbutra P, Kullavanijaya P. Sulfasalazine in atrophie blanche. *J Am Acad Dermatol* 1993;28:275–276.
254. Andreozzi R, Nuss D. Dermatitis herpetiformis: treatment with Azulfidine. *Cutis* 1974;13:366–370.
255. Artuz F, Lenk N, Deniz N, et al. Efficacy of sulfasalazine in discoid lupus erythematosus. *Int J Dermatol* 1996;35:746–748.
256. Delaporte E, Catteau N, Sabbagh N, et al. Treatment of discoid lupus erythematosus with sulfasalazine: 11 cases. *Ann Dermatol Venereol* 1997;124:151–156.
257. Schroder H, Campbell DES. Absorption, metabolism, and excretion of salicylazosulfapyridine in man. *Clin Pharmacol Ther* 1972;13: 539–551.
258. Klotz U, Maier KE. Pharmacology and pharmacokinetics of 5-aminosalicylic acid. *Dig Dis Sci* 1987;32(suppl):46–50.
259. Klotz U. Clinical pharmacokinetics of sulphasalazine: its metabolites, and other prodrugs of 5-aminosalicylic acid. *Clin Pharmacokinet* 1985;10:285–302.
260. Taggart AJ, McDermott BJ, Roberts SD. The effect of age and acetylator phenotype on the pharmacokinetics of sulfasalazine in patients with rheumatoid arthritis. *Clin Pharmacokinet* 1992;23: 311–320.
261. Das KM, Dubin R. Clinical pharmacokinetics of sulphasalazine. *Clin Pharmacokinet* 1976;1:406–425.
262. Tanaka E, Taniguchi A, Urano W, et al. Adverse effects of sulfasalazine in patients with rheumatoid arthritis are associated with diplotype configuration at the *N*-acetyltransferase 2 gene. *J Rheumatol* 2002;29:2492–2499.
263. Ricart E, Taylor WR, Loftus EV, et al. *N*-acetyltransferase 1 and 2 genotypes do not predict response or toxicity to treatment with mesalamine and sulphasalazine in patients with ulcerative colitis. *Am J Gastroenterol* 2002;97:1763–1768.
264. Taffet SL, Das KM. Sulfasalazine: adverse effects and desensitization. *Dig Dis Sci* 1983;28:833–842.
265. Scott DL, Dacre JE. Adverse reactions to sulfasalazine: the British experience. *J Rheumatol* 1988;15(suppl 16):17–21.
266. Rafouth R. Systemic granulomatous reaction to salicylazosulfapyridine in a patient with Crohn's disease. *Am J Dig Dis* 1974;19:465–469.
267. Maddocks JL, Slater DN. Toxic epidermal necrolysis, agranulocytosis, and erythroid hypoplasia associated with sulphasalazine. *J R Soc Med* 1980;73:587–588.
268. Das KM, Eastwood MA, McManus JA, et al. Adverse reactions during salicylazapyridine therapy and the relation with drug metabolism and acetylator phenotype. *N Engl J Med* 1973;289:491–495.
269. Capell HA, Pullar T, Hunter JA. Comparison of white blood cell dyscrasias during sulfasalazine therapy of rheumatoid arthritis and inflammatory bowel disease. *Drugs* 1986;32(suppl 1):44–48.
270. Deisu CL, Eckman E. Sulfasalazine associated agranulocytosis in Sweden 1972–1989: clinical features, and estimation of its incidence. *Eur J Clin Pharmacol* 1992;43:215–218.
271. Kuipers EJ, Vallenga E, de Wolf JT, et al. Sulfasalazine induced agranulocytosis treated with granulocyte-macrophage colony stimulating factor. *J Rheumatol* 1992;19:621–622.
272. Wijnands MJ, Allebes WA, Boerbooms AMT, et al. Thrombocytopenia due to aurothioglucose, sulphasalazine, and hydroxychloroquine. *Ann Rheum Dis* 1990;49:798–800.
273. Omer A, Mowat AG. Nature of anemia in rheumatoid arthritis: IX. Folate metabolism in patients with rheumatoid arthritis. *Ann Rheum Dis* 1968;27:414–424.
274. Averbuch M, Halpern Z, Hallak A, et al. Sulfasalazine pneumonitis. *Am J Gastroenterol* 1985;80:343–345.
275. Valcke Y, Pauwels R, Van Der Straeten M. Bronchoalveolar lavage in acute hypersensitivity pneumonitis caused by sulfasalazine. *Chest* 1987;92:572–573.
276. Jones GR, Malone DNS. Sulphasalazine induced lung disease. *Thorax* 1972;27:713–717.
277. Werlin S, Grand R. Bloody diarrhea: new complication of sulfasalazine. *J Pediatr* 1978;92:450–451.
278. Brazer SR, Medoff JR. Sulfonamide-induced pancreatitis. *Pancreas* 1988;3:583–586.
279. Haines JD Jr. Hepatotoxicity after treatment with sulfasalazine. *Postgrad Med J* 1986;79:193–198.
280. Mihas AA, Goldenberg DJ, Slaughlar RJ. Sulfasalazine toxic reactions: hepatitis, fever, and skin rash with hypocomplementemia and immune complexes. *JAMA* 1978;239:2590–2591.
281. Marinos G, Riley J, Painter DM, et al. Sulfasalazine-induced fulminant hepatic failure. *J Clin Gastroenterol* 1992;14:132–135.
282. Hoo JJ. Possible teratogenicity of sulfasalazine. *N Engl J Med* 1988; 318:1128.
283. Mogadam M, Dobbins WO III, Krelitz BI. The safety of corticosteroids and sulfasalazine in pregnancy associated with inflammatory bowel disease. *Gastroenterology* 1981;81:72–76.
284. Dhar J, Selhub J, Rosenberg IH. Azulfidine inhibition of folic acid absorption: confirmation of a specific saturable transport mechanism. *Gastroenterology* 1976;70:878A.
285. Toth A. Reversible toxic effect of salicylazosulfapyridine on semen quality. *Fertil Steril* 1979;31:538–540.
286. Riley SA. Sulfasalazine-induced abnormal sperm penetration. *Dig Dis Sci* 1988;33:1948.
287. Hill ME, Gordon C, Situnayake RD, et al. Sulfasalazine induced seizures and dysphasia. *J Rheumatol* 1994;21:748–749.
288. Neeman A, Berliner S, Shoenfeld Y, et al. Salazopyrine induced tachycardia [Letter]. *Biomedicine* 1980;33:1–2.
289. Reid J, Holt S, Housley E, et al. Raynaud's phenomenon induced by sulphasalazine. *Postgrad Med J* 1980;56:106–107.
290. Marcus RW. Sulfasalazine induced taste disturbances [Letter]. *J Rheumatol* 1991;18:634–635.
291. Chalmers I, Sitar D, Hunter T. A one-year, open, prospective study of sulfasalazine in the treatment of rheumatoid arthritis: adverse reactions in relation to laboratory variables, drug and metabolite serum levels and acetylator status. *J Rheumatol* 1990;17:764.
292. Caulier M, Dromer C, Andrieu V. Sulfasalazine induced lupus in rheumatoid arthritis. *J Rheumatol* 1994;21:750.
293. Lowry PW, Franklin CL, Weaver AL, et al. Leucopenia resulting from a drug interaction between azathioprine or 6-mercaptopurine and mesalamine, sulphasalazine, or balsalazide. *Gut* 2001;49:656–664.

294. Wallace D. Antimalarial agents and lupus. *Rheum Dis Clin North Am* 1994;20:243–263.
295. Krogstad DJ, Schlesinger PH. Acid-vesicle function, intracellular pathogens, and the action of chloroquine against *Plasmodium falciparum*. *N Engl J Med* 1987;317:542–549.
296. Homewood CA, Warhurst DC, Peters W, et al. Lysosomes pH and the antimalarial action of chloroquine. *Nature* 1972;235:50–52.
297. Ziegler HK, Unanue ER. Decrease in macrophage antigen catabolism caused by ammonia and chloroquine is associated with inhibition of antigen presentation to T cells. *Proc Natl Acad Sci U S A* 1982;79:175–178.
298. Unanue E. Antigen-presenting function of the macrophage. *Annu Rev Immunol* 1984;2:395–428.
299. Nowell J, Quaranta V. Chloroquine effects biosynthesis of Ia molecules by inhibiting dissociation of invariant (gamma) chains from α-β dimers in B cells. *J Exp Med* 1985;162:1371–1376.
300. Fox RI, Kang HI. Mechanism of action of antimalarial drugs: inhibition of antigen processing and presentation. *Lupus* 1993;2(suppl 1): 9–12.
301. Salmeron G, Lipsky PE. Immunosuppressive potential of antimalarials. *Am J Med* 1983;75:19–24.
302. Lee J, Chuang TH, Redecke V, et al. Molecular basis for the immunostimulatory activity of guanine nucleoside analogs: activation of Toll-like receptor 7. *Proc Natl Acad Sci USA* 2003;100(11):6646–6651.
303. Sperber K, Quraishi H, Kalb TH, et al. Selective regulation of cytokine secretion by hydroxychloroquine: inhibition of interleukin 1 alpha (IL-1-alpha) and IL-6 in human monocytes and T cells. *J Rheumatol* 1993;20:803–808.
304. Hurst NP, French JK, Bell AL, et al. Differential effects of mepacrine, chloroquine and hydroxychloroquine on superoxide anion generation, phospholipid methylation and arachidonic acid release by human blood monocytes. *Biochem Pharmacol* 1986;15; 35:3083–3089.
305. Bondeson J, Sundler R. Antimalarial drugs inhibit phospholipase A_2 activation and induction of interleukin 1beta and tumor necrosis factor alpha in macrophages: implications for their mode of action in rheumatoid arthritis. *Gen Pharmacol* 1998;30:357–366.
306. Jeong JY, Jue DM. Chloroquine inhibits processing of tumor necrosis factor in lipopolysaccharide-stimulated RAW 264.7 macrophages. *J Immunol* 1997;158:4901–4907.
307. Chiang G, Sassaroli M, Louie M, et al. Inhibition of HIV-1 replication by hydroxychloroquine: mechanism of action and comparison with zidovudine. *Clin Ther* 1996;18:1080–1092.
308. Sperber K, Kalb TH, Stecher VJ, et al. Inhibition of human immunodeficiency virus type 1 replication by hydroxychloroquine in T cells and monocytes. *AIDS Res Hum Retrovir* 1993;9:91–98.
309. Rhodes JM, McLaughlin JE, Brown DJ, et al. Inhibition of leucocyte motility and prevention of immune-complex experimental colitis by hydroxychloroquine. *Gut* 1982;23:181–187.
310. Hurst NP, French JK, Gorjatschko L, et al. Chloroquine and hydroxychloroquine inhibit multiple sites in metabolic pathways leading to neutrophil superoxide release. *J Rheumatol* 1988;15: 23–27.
311. Hurst NP, French JK, Gorjatschko L, et al. Studies on the mechanism of inhibition of chemotactic tripeptide stimulated human neutrophil polymorphonuclear leucocyte superoxide production by chloroquine and hydroxychloroquine. *Ann Rheum Dis* 1987;46: 750–756.
312. Cohen A, Calkins E. A controlled study of chloroquine as an antirheumatic agent. *Arthritis Rheum* 1958;1:297–308.
313. Freedman A, Steinberg VL. Chloroquine in rheumatoid arthritis: a double blindfold trial of treatment for one year. *Ann Rheum Dis* 1960;19:243–250.
314. Hamilton E, Scott J. Hydroxychloroquine in treatment of rheumatoid arthritis. *Arthritis Rheum* 1962;5:502–512.
315. Mainland D, Sutcliffe MI. Hydroxychloroquine in rheumatoid arthritis: a six-month, double blind trial. *Bull Rheum Dis* 1962;13:287–290.
316. HERA. A randomized trial of hydroxychloroquine in rheumatoid arthritis: the HERA study. *Am J Med* 1995;98:156–168.
317. Laaksonen L, Koskiadhde V, Juva K. Dosage of antimalarial drugs for children with juvenile RA. *Scand J Rheumatol* 1974;3:103–108.
318. Clark P, Casas E, Tugwell P, et al. Hydroxychloroquine compared with placebo in rheumatoid arthritis. *Ann Intern Med* 1993;119: 1067–1071.
319. Mottonen T, Hannonen P, Leirisalo-Repo M, et al. Comparison of combination therapy with single-drug therapy in early rheumatoid arthritis: a randomized trial. FIN-RACo trial group. *Lancet* 1999; 353:1568–1573.
320. O'Dell JR, Leff R, Paulsen G, et al. Treatment of rheumatoid arthritis with methotrexate and hydroxychloroquine, methotrexate and sulfasalazine, or a combination of the three medications: results of a two-year, randomized , double-blind, placebo-controlled trial. *Arthritis Rheum* 2002;46:1164–1170.
321. Furst DE. Update on clinical trials in the rheumatic diseases. *Curr Opin Rheumatol* 1998;10:123–128.
322. Avina-Zubieta JA, Galindo-Rodriguez G, Newman S, et al. Long-term effectiveness of antimalarial drugs in rheumatic diseases. *Ann Rheum Dis* 1998;57:582–587.
323. Ruzicka T, Sommerburg C, Goerz G, et al. Treatment of cutaneous lupus erythematosus with acitretin and hydroxychloroquine. *Br J Dermatol* 1992;127:513–518.
324. Dubois E. Antimalarials in the management of discoid and systemic lupus erythematosus. *Semin Arthritis Rheum* 1978;8:33–51.
325. Rudnicki R, Gresham G, Rothfeld N. The efficacy of antimalarials in systemic lupus erythematosus. *J Rheumatol* 1975;2:223–230.
326. Winkelman R, Merwin C, Brunsting L. Antimalarial therapy of systemic lupus. *Ann Intern Med* 1961;51:772–776.
327. Ziff M, Esserman P, McKwan C. Observations on the course and treatment of systemic lupus erythematosus. *Arthritis Rheum* 1958;1: 332–340.
328. Bykerk V, Sampalis J, Esdaile JM, et al. A randomized study of the effect of withdrawing hydroxychloroquine sulfate in systemic lupus erythematosus. *N Engl J Med* 1991;324:150–154.
329. Engel GL, Ramano J, Ferris EB. Effect of quinacrine (Atabrine) on the central nervous system. *Arch Neurol* 1947;58:337–350.
330. Tanenbaum L, Tuffanelli DL. Antimalarial agents: chloroquine, hydroxychloroquine and quinacrine. *Arch Dermatol* 1980;116:587–591.
331. O'Leary PA, Brunsting LA, Kierland RR. Quinacrine (Atabrine) hydrochloride in treatment of discoid lupus erythematosus. *Arch Dermatol Syph* 1953;67:633.
332. Rogers J, Finn OA. Synthetic antimalarial drugs in chronic discoid lupus erythematosus and light eruptions. *Arch Dermatol Syph* 1954; 70:61.
333. Kraak JH, van Ketel WG, Prakken JR, van Zwet WR. The value of hydroxychloroquine (Plaquenil) for the treatment of chronic discoid lupus erythematosus: a double-blind trial. *Dermatologica* 1965;130: 293.
334. Wallace JD, Metzger AL, Stecher VJ, et al. Cholesterol-lowering effect of hydroxychloroquine (Plaquenil) in rheumatoid disease patients: reversal of deleterious effects of steroids on lupus. *Am J Med* 1990;89:322.
335. Hodis HN, Quismorio FP Jr, Wickham E, et al. The lipid, lipoprotein and apolipoprotein effects of hydroxychloroquine in patients with SLE. *J Rheumatol* 1993;20:661.
336. Carter AE, Eban R, Perret RD. Prevention of post-operative deep venous thrombosis and pulmonary embolism. *BMJ* 1971;1:312–314.
337. Johnson R, Orth MC, Charnley J. Hydroxychloroquine in prophylaxis of pulmonary embolism following hip arthroplasty. *Clin Orthop* 1979;144:174–177.
338. Bertrand E, Cloitre B, Ticolat R, et al. Antiaggregation action of chloroquine. *Med Trop (Mars)* 1990;50:143–146.
339. Wallace DJ. Does hydroxychloroquine sulfate prevent clot formation in systemic lupus erythematosus? *Arthritis Rheum* 1987;30:1435–1436.
340. Espinola RG, Pierangeli SS, Ghara AE, et al. Hydroxychloroquine reverses platelet activation induced by human IgG antiphospholipid antibodies. *Thromb Haemost* 2002;87:518–522.
341. Erkan D, Yazici Y, Peterson MG, et al. A cross-sectional study of clinical thrombotic risk factors and preventive treatments in antiphospholipid syndrome. *Rheumatology* 2002;41:924–929.
342. Fox RI, Chan E, Benton L, et al. Treatment of primary Sjögren's syndrome with hydroxychloroquine. *Am J Med* 1988;85:62–67.

343. Kruize A, Hene R, Kallenberg C, et al. Hydroxychloroquine treatment for primary Sjögren's syndrome: a two-year double blind crossover trial. *Ann Rheum Dis* 1993;52:360.
344. Youssef W, Yan A, Russell A. Palindromic rheumatism: a response to chloroquine. *J Rheumatol* 1991;18:1.
345. Hannonen P, Mottonen T, Oka M. Treatment of palindromic rheumatism with chloroquine. *BMJ* 1987;294:1289.
346. Woo TY, Callen JP, Voorhees JJ, et al. Cutaneous lesions of dermatomyositis are improved by hydroxychloroquine. *J Am Acad Dermatol* 1984;10:592.
347. Olson NY, Lindsley CB. Adjunctive use of hydroxychloroquine childhood dermatomyositis. *J Rheumatol* 1989;16:12.
348. Bryant LR, DesRossier KF, Carpenter MT. Hydroxychloroquine in the treatment of erosive osteoarthritis. *J Rheumatol* 1995;22: 1527.
349. Rothschild BM. Prospective six-month double-blind trial of Plaquenil treatment of calcium pyrophosphate deposition disease (CPPD). *Arthritis Rheum* 1994;37(suppl 9):414.
350. Lakhanpal S, Ginsberg WW, Michet CJ, et al. Eosinophilic fasciitis: clinical spectrum and therapeutic response in 52 cases. *Semin Arthritis Rheum* 1988;17:221.
351. Lovy MR, Starkebaum G, Uberoi S. Hepatitis C infection presenting with rheumatic manifestations: a mimic of rheumatoid arthritis. *J Rheumatol* 1996;23:979.
352. Cutler DJ, MacIntyre AC, Tett SE. Pharmacokinetics and cellular uptake of 4-aminoquinolone antimalarials. *Agents Actions* 1988;24: 142–157.
353. Tett SE, Cutler DJ, Day RO. Bioavailability of hydroxychloroquine tablets assessed by deconvolution techniques. *J Pharm Sci* 1992; 81:55.
354. McLachlan AJ, Cutler DJ, Tett SE. Plasma protein binding of the enantiomers of hydroxychloroquine and metabolites. *Eur J Clin Pharmacol* 1993;44:481–484.
355. French J, Hurst N, O'Donnell M, et al. Uptake of chloroquine and hydroxychloroquine by human blood leukocytes *in vitro*: relation to cellular concentrations during antirheumatic therapy. *Ann Rheum Dis* 1992;46:42.
356. Wainer IW, Chen JC, Parenteau H, et al. Distribution of the enantiomers of hydroxychloroquine and its metabolites in ocular tissues of the rabbit after oral administration of racemic-hydroxychloroquine. *Chirality* 1994;6:347.
357. Miller DR, Khalil SKW, Nygard GA. Steady-state pharmacokinetics of hydroxychloroquine in rheumatoid arthritis patients. *Ann Pharmacother* 1991;25:1302–1305.
358. Miller D, Fiechtner J, Carpenter J, et al. Plasma hydroxychloroquine concentration and efficacy in rheumatoid arthritis. *Arthritis Rheum* 1987;30:567–571.
359. Frisk-Holmberg M, Bergkvist T, Domeij-Nyberg B, et al. Chloroquine serum concentration and side effects: evidence for dose-dependent kinetics. *Clin Pharmacol* 1979;25:345–350.
360. Whisnant J, Espinosa R, Kierland R, et al. Chloroquine neuromyopathy. *Mayo Clin Proc* 1963;23:502–510.
361. Estes ML, Ewing-Wilson D, Chou SM, et al. Chloroquine neuromyotoxicity: clinical and pathologic perspective. *Am J Med* 1987;82: 447.
362. Ratcliffe N. Diagnosis of chloroquine cardiomyopathy by endomyocardial biopsy. *N Engl J Med* 1987;316:191–204.
363. Veinot JP, Mai KT, Zarychanski R. Chloroquine related cardiac toxicity. *J Rheumatol* 1998;25:1221.
364. Finbloom DS, Silver K, Newsome DA, et al. Comparison of hydroxychloroquinie and chloroquine use and the development of retinal toxicity. *J Rheumatol* 1985;12:692–694.
365. Nylander U. Ocular damage in chloroquine retinopathy. *Ophthalmology (Copenh)* 1966;44:335–340.
366. Shearer R, Dubois E. Ocular changes induced by long-term hydroxychloroquine therapy. *Am J Ophthalmol* 1967;64:245–251.
367. Bernstein HN. Ocular safety of hydroxychloroquine. *Ann Ophthalmol* 1991;30:451–455.
368. Bernstein H, Ginsberg J. The pathology of chloroquine retinopathy. *Arch Ophthalmol* 1964;71:238–244.
369. Maurikakis M, Papazoglou S, Sfolalos PP, et al. Retinal toxicity in long-term hydroxychloroquine treatment. *Ann Rheum Dis* 1996;55: 187.
370. Brinkley J, Dubois E, Ryan S. Long-term course of chloroquine retinopathy after cessation of medication. *Am J Ophthalmol* 1979;88: 1–11.
371. Rynes RI, Bernstein HN. Ophthalmologic safety profile of antimalarials drugs. *Lupus* 1993;2(suppl 1):17.
372. Carmichael SJ, Beal J, Day RO, et al. Combination therapy with methotrexate and hydroxychloroquine for rheumatoid arthritis increases exposure to methotrexate. *J Rheumatol* 2002;29:2077–2083.
373. Marmor MF, Carr RE, Easterbrook M, et al. Recommendations on screening for chloroquine and hydroxychloroquine retinopathy. *Ophthalmology* 2002;109:1377–1382.
374. American College of Rheumatology Ad Hoc Committee on Clinical Guidelines. Guidleines for monitoring drug therapy in rheumatoid arthritis. *Arthritis Rheum* 1996;39:723–731.
375. Mizuno K, Tsujino M, Takada M, et al. Studies on bredinin. I. Isolation, characterization and biological properties. *J Antiobiot* 1974;27: 775–782.
376. Kamata K, Okubo M, Ishigamori E, et al. Immunosuppressive effect of bredinin on cell-mediated and humoral immune reactions in experimental animals. *Transplantation* 1983;35:144–149.
377. Yoshizawa M, Tsujino M, Mizuno K, et al. Immunosuppressive effect of mizoribine. II. Suppression of humoral and cellular immune response. *Clin Immunol* 1982;14:561–570.
378. Dayton JS, Turka LA, Thompson CB, et al. Comparison of the effects of mizoribine with those of azathioprine, 6-mercaptopurine, and mycophenolic acid on T cell lymphocyte proliferation and purine nucleotide metabolism. *Mol Pharmacol* 1992;41:671–676.
379. Hirohata S, Yanagida T. Inhibition of expression of cyclin A in human B cells by an immunosuppressant mizoribine. *J Immunol* 1995;155:5175–5183.
380. Nishioka K, Uchida S, Shiokawa Y. Effect of mizoribine on peripheral lymphocyte subsets in rheumatoid arthritis. *Clin Immunol* 1991; 23:904–912.
381. Takei S. Mizoribine in the treatment of rheumatoid arthritis and juvenile idiopathic arthritis. *Pediatr Int* 2002;44:205–209.
382. Shiokawa Y, Honma M, Schichikawa K, et al. Clinical evaluation of immunosuppressant, mizoribine, on rheumatoid arthritis. A double-blind placebo controlled study. *J Clin Exp Med* 1991;156: 811–831.
383. Shiokawa Y, Honma, Schichikawa K, et al. Clinical effectiveness of mizoribine in rheumatoid arthritis. A double-blind comparative study using lobenzarit sodium as a standard drug. *J Infect* 1991;11:375–396.
384. Marumo F, Okubo M, Yokota K, et al. A clinical study of renal transplant recipients receiving triple-drug therapy—cyclosporine A, mizoribine, and prednisolone. *Transplant Proc* 1988;20:406–409.
385. Murase J, Mizuno K, Kawai K, et al. Absorption, distribution, metabolism and excretion of bredinin in rats. *Pharmacometrics* 1978;15: 829–835.
386. Yoshida H, Fujisawa H, Abe C, et al. Effect of MS-932 (4-acetylaminophenylacetic acid) on articular lesions in MRL/I mice. *Int J Immunother* 1987;3:261–264.
387. Fujisawa H, Nishimura T, Motonaga A, et al. Effect of actarit on type II collagen-induced arthritis in mice. *Arzneim Forsch Drug Res* 1994;44:64–68.
388. Fujisawa H, Nishimura T, Inoue Y, et al. Antiinflammatory properties of the new antirheumatic agent 4-acetylaminophenylacetic acid. *Arzneim Forsch Drug Res* 1990;40:693–697.
389. Nakagawa Y, Ogawa T, Kobayashi M, et al. Immunopharmacological studies of 4-acetylaminophenylacetic acid. (MS-932). *Int J Immunother* 1990;6:131–140.
390. Takeba Y, Suzuki N, Wakisaka S, et al. Effects of actarit on synovial cell functions in patients with rheumatoid arthritis. *J Rheumatol* 1999;26:25–33.
391. Kawai K, Kobayashi Y, Hirayama M, et al. Suppressive effects of 4-acetylaminophenylacetic acid (actarit) on experimental autoimmune encephalomyelitis in rats. *Immunopharmacology* 1998;39: 127–138.
392. Sajurai T, Iso T, Inoue H, et al. [Effect of actarit combination therapy in patients with active rheumatoid arthritis resistant to gold agents] [Japanese] *Ryumachi* 2001;41:635–645.

393. Hirohata S, Shinohara S, Inoue T, et al. Regulation of B cell function by lobenzarit, a novel disease-modifying antirheumatic drug. *Arthritis Rheum* 1992;35:168–175.
394. Hirohata H. Regulation of *in vitro* anti-DNA antibody production by a novel disease modifying anti-rheumatic drug, Lobenzarit. *Clin Exp Rheumatol* 1992;10:357–363.
395. Shiokawa Y, Horiuchi Y, Mizushima Y, et al. A multicenter double-blind controlled study of lobenzarit, a novel immunomodulator, in rheumatoid arthritis. *J Rheumatol* 1984;11:615–623.
396. Hirohata S, Ohnishi K, Sagawa A. Treatment of systemic lupus erythematosus with lobenzarit: an open clinical trial. *Clin Exp Rheumatol* 1994;12:261–265.

CHAPTER 43

Tetracyclines and Alternative Therapies

Daniel O. Clegg and Christopher G. Jackson

The aim of this chapter is to provide an objective update on the use of tetracycline and tetracycline derivatives in the treatment of rheumatic diseases as well as to review a number of agents, often referred to as "complementary and alternative medicine (CAM)," most of which have not been evaluated in rigorous controlled trials.

TETRACYCLINES

Historical Overview

The tetracycline class of antibiotics was introduced in 1948 when the soil-resident fungi *Streptomyces aureofaciens* and *Streptomyces rimosus* were found to elaborate, respectively, chlortetracycline and oxytetracycline (1,2). The efficacy and tolerability of these compounds in the treatment of a large number of infectious processes soon became apparent, expanding the available antibacterial armamentarium that previously had consisted of penicillin, streptomycin, and the sulfonamides. The name *tetracycline* was derived from the fused four-benzene ring structure that is common to all members of this antibiotic class. Chemical alterations and substitutions on the side chains of the polycyclic core have produced a number of semisynthetic congeners that possess an essentially uniform spectrum of antimicrobial activity but a more convenient pharmacokinetic profile. The first of the semisynthetic derivatives, tetracycline, was released for clinical use in 1952, followed by doxycycline in 1966, and minocycline in 1972.

Interest in the tetracyclines for the treatment of musculoskeletal disorders originated with a report in 1948 that pleuropneumonia-like organisms, later known as mycoplasma, were capable of producing joint inflammation (3). Isolation of mycoplasma from the synovial fluid of patients with rheumatoid arthritis (RA) (4) coupled with the observation that mycoplasma species could inhibit the migration of leukocytes from RA patients (5) offered further support that mycoplasma might play a role in the etiopathogenesis of RA. The efficacy of the tetracyclines for mycoplasma-induced genitourinary tract infections quite logically led investigators to consider its potential as a therapy for RA. Although the early experience in RA was not encouraging, anecdotal use persisted with periodic reports of benefit that appeared predominantly in the lay press. More recently, interest in the tetracyclines was renewed when the semisynthetic derivatives minocycline and doxycycline were shown to have antiinflammatory and immunomodulatory properties apart from their antimicrobial activity. Minocycline, which has now been systematically investigated in the treatment of both early and established RA, will be discussed hereafter in much greater detail than doxycycline, for which only preliminary data exist.

Pharmacology

Minocycline is produced from tetracycline by substitutions at positions 6 and 7 of the polycyclic naphthacenecarboxamide core (Fig. 43.1). It is clinically available as a monohydrochloride, which is stable as a dry powder but quickly loses activity after being placed in solution. It is rapidly but incompletely absorbed from the gastrointestinal tract with maximal serum levels achieved at approximately 2 hours after oral ingestion (6,7). In contrast to the other tetracyclines, the absorption of minocycline is only slightly delayed and minimally diminished when taken with food. High intestinal drug levels occur with oral administration of the tetracyclines and produce a marked alteration in the normal enteric flora (8). The tetracyclines appear to pass through the inflamed synovium without difficulty and reach appreciable levels in the synovial fluid, even when admin-

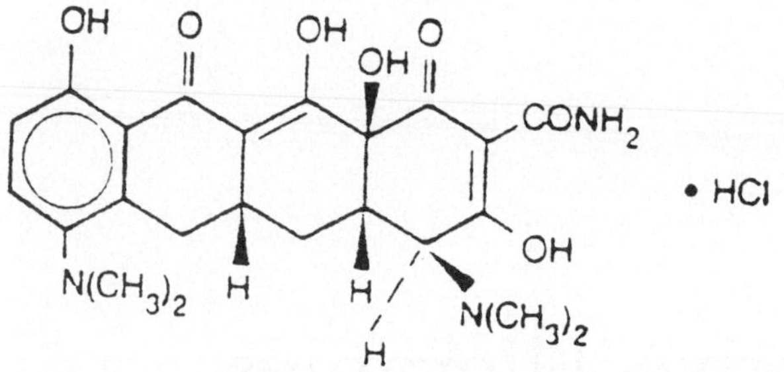

FIG. 43.1. Chemical structure of minocycline hydrochloride.

istered orally (9). Minocycline has a mean half-life of approximately 15 hours, which permits twice daily dosing in most treatment regimens. It is excreted in both the urine and the feces, but to a lesser extent than other tetracyclines because it is also extensively metabolized. Nonetheless, the presence of renal dysfunction causes significant prolongation of the serum half-life, which makes a dose reduction or the measurement of serum levels advisable, whereas no prolongation of the serum half-life is seen with hepatic failure (10). Minocycline undergoes enterohepatic recirculation and has a large volume of distribution because of significant fatty tissue stores, resulting in persistence of serum levels after treatment has been discontinued (11). The relationship between serum levels of minocycline and clinical efficacy and toxicity in the treatment of patients with rheumatic disease remains uncertain. A weak correlation between serum concentration and clinical response has been suggested, but no correlation of toxicity with serum levels is presently evident (12).

In comparison with minocycline, doxycycline (produced by substitutions at positions 5 and 6) has a similar serum half-life but slightly smaller volume of distribution. Doxycycline is unique among all the tetracyclines in having minimal urinary excretion so that neither serum levels nor half-life change in the setting of renal failure.

Mechanism of Action

No precise mechanism of action for the tetracycline derivatives in the treatment of rheumatic diseases is known; however, a number of potentially important effects have been described. For discussion purposes, these can be usefully classified as antibacterial, antiinflammatory, or immunomodulatory properties.

Antibacterial Properties

All tetracyclines, including minocycline, have a broad antimicrobial spectrum, with *in vitro* systems showing activity and clinical experience confirming efficacy in a wide array of infections caused by gram-negative and gram-positive organisms, including *Mycoplasma, Chlamydia,* and some mycobacterial strains (13). The antimicrobial action of the tetracyclines is primarily bacteriostatic and appears to involve inhibition of bacterial protein synthesis by binding to the 30S ribosomal subunit (14). Coliforms and gram-positive spore-forming bacteria residing within the gastrointestinal tract are particularly suppressed with persistent oral tetracycline use; however, no particular alteration in bowel flora is known to correlate with clinical efficacy. The significance and potential consequence of bacterial resistance that frequently emerges with prolonged tetracycline use, as used in current antirheumatic regimens, is unknown.

Antiinflammatory Properties

The antiinflammatory effects of tetracyclines appear to be independent of their antimicrobial activity, because chemically modified tetracycline derivatives that have no antibiotic effects exhibit antiinflammatory actions (15). In contrast to a relatively uniform spectrum of antimicrobial activity, disparate antiinflammatory effects have been observed for minocycline and doxycycline; however, the significance of these observed differences is unknown (16). Tetracyclines appear to affect a number of different inflammatory pathways by decreasing the synthesis of prostaglandins and leukotrienes through blockade of phospholipase A_2 (17–19), by modulating the production of nitric oxide and its active metabolites (20,21), and by acting as antioxidants (22,23). Tetracyclines also have been shown to inhibit the activity of host-derived collagenases and other matrix metalloproteinases (24–30). Interestingly, minocycline has been shown *in vivo* to inhibit collagenase in RA synovial tissue (31), whereas oral doxycycline has been shown to reduce collagenase and gelatinase activity in extracts of human OA cartilage (32). Compared with other antibiotics, the tetracyclines appear to be unique in this regard because similar anticollagenase activity is not seen with ampicillin, cloxacillin, or penicillin G (33). The mechanism by which metalloproteinase activity is affected remains unclear, but heavy metal ions are necessary for their structural integrity, and tetracycline-induced chelation of such ions may offer a possible explanation. Consistent with this idea is the observation that collagenase inhibition due to doxycycline *in vitro* can be reversed by the addition of calcium or zinc (33).

Immunomodulatory Properties

Several immunomodulatory actions have been attributed to the tetracyclines (34), including inhibition of protein synthesis in certain eukaryotic cells (35) and perturbation of a number of leukocyte functions, such as suppression of chemotaxis (36,37), depression of phagocytic activity (38), reduction of lymphocyte proliferation (39,40), and modulation of cytokine production (41–43). A reduction in delayed-type hypersensitivity is induced by tetracycline in mice bred in a germ-free environment, suggesting that the immunosuppressive effects of the tetracycline are independent of antimicrobial activity (44). No mechanism of action is known, but the potential importance of minocycline as a chelator of heavy metal ions is suggested by the observation that changes in intracellular calcium levels appear to correlate with altered lymphocyte transformation *in vitro* and with decreased joint inflammation in murine adjuvant and collagen arthritis *in vivo* (45).

Adverse Effects

The profile of adverse effects associated with tetracycline use in the treatment of infectious diseases is well established (46). However, information regarding the tolerability of the more long-term use required in antirheumatic regimens is much more limited. In general, minocycline in a dose of 200 mg daily has been well tolerated for sustained periods. As shown in Table 43.1, discontinuation rates for toxicity in the two largest minocycline trials were 6% and 12.5%, which both compare favorably with the average discontinuation rate of 15% associated with other second-line RA therapies (47). Specific adverse effects seen in these two trials are summarized in Table 43.2.

Autoimmune Syndromes

A number of autoimmune syndromes have been associated with minocycline use, including serum sickness (48, 49), polyarthritis (50–52), drug-induced systemic lupus erythematosus (SLE) (53–56), and vasculitis (57,58). Serologic abnormalities such as antinuclear antibodies and perinuclear antineutrophilic cytoplasmic antibodies (59) are not uncommon, although a relative absence of antihistone antibodies has been observed in drug-induced SLE due to tetracycline (60). In a reported series of 20 minocycline-induced lupus cases, polyarthritis was seen in all patients but renal disease in none (61), and all symptoms resolved within a mean of 15.7 weeks after discontinuation of therapy. Serum sickness most often appears within the first month of therapy, whereas other syndromes are usually seen with more prolonged use. Symptoms related to autoimmune syndromes generally resolve with cessation of tetracycline therapy (62).

TABLE 43.1. *Withdrawals due to toxicity with minocycline treatment in rheumatoid arthritis*

Study	Duration (wk)	Toxicity withdrawals
Kloppenburg et al. (89)	26	12.5%
MIRA (90)	48	6%

MIRA, monocycline in rheumatoid arthritis trial.

TABLE 43.2. *Adverse effects associated with minocycline treatment in rheumatoid arthritis*

Symptom	Kloppenburg	MIRA
Headache	2%	20%
Dizziness	40%	8%
Gastrointestinal	58%	24%
Skin	0%	5%

MIRA, monocycline in rheumatoid arthritis trial.

Central Nervous System

Headache and dizziness are experienced with minocycline to a degree much greater than that observed with other tetracycline derivatives. The dizziness is thought to be vestibular in origin, appears to be dose related, is probably more common in female patients, and seems to be reversible with drug discontinuation (63). Tetracycline in children has been associated with pseudotumor cerebri, but no etiology for headache in the adult population has been described. The frequency and severity of central nervous system symptoms have varied considerably in recent trials that used the same daily minocycline dose. These differences may be attributable to variations in the demographics of the study populations, particularly patient age.

Drug Interactions

As with other tetracyclines, minocycline should not be taken with dairy products, antacids, or iron supplements because of chelation that decreases absorption from the gastrointestinal tract.

Gastrointestinal

Nausea without emesis, presumably due to gastric irritation, is a common complaint, and it often subsides with continued therapy. Minocycline appears to produce less diarrhea than is seen with other tetracyclines, perhaps because of more complete gastrointestinal absorption. Increased hepatic transaminases as well as clinically evident hepatic dysfunction have been reported with minocycline and appear to occur predominantly in patients receiving larger doses (64–68). The potential for fatal hepatic injury exists, particularly with use in pregnancy (69).

Hematologic

The tetracyclines have been reported to cause abnormalities in the peripheral blood such as leukocytosis and lymphocyte atypia (70,71). This has been thought to be more likely to occur with prolonged therapy but was not a prominent occurrence in recent trials that used treatment durations of 6 and 12 months.

Hypersensitivity Reactions

A variety of cutaneous manifestations of hypersensitivity are known to occur with tetracycline administration, including morbilliform rashes, exfoliative dermatitis, photosensitivity, fixed drug eruptions, and erythema multiforme (72). More serious hypersensitivity reactions, including angioedema, anaphylaxis, and pneumonitis, have been reported but have not been demonstrated in published rheumatologic trials (73).

Pediatric

Tetracycline use in children and neonates is associated with a permanent brownish discoloration of the teeth. Its use should, therefore, be avoided in children under 8 years of age, as well as in pregnant women (74). Tetracycline deposition also occurs in fetal and adolescent skeletons and can result in significant retardation of bone growth in premature infants, which is reversible if treatment is not prolonged (75).

Renal

The tetracyclines are known to have an antianabolic effect, which may result in an increase in blood urea nitrogen and produce an exacerbation of preexisting renal dysfunction (76,77). Such effects are more common in malnourished individuals and seem to correlate with the degree of renal impairment and the severity of the malnourished state (78).

Skin

In addition to cutaneous manifestations of hypersensitivity, hyperpigmentation can occur with sustained use of minocycline (79–82).

Clinical Experience

Minocycline

As previously noted, the use of tetracycline derivatives in the treatment of RA originated with the hypothesis that an infectious agent, possibly mycoplasma, was important in the etiopathogenesis of the disease. Early reports by Brown et al. (83,84) and Sanchez (85) suggested clinical benefit associated with long-term tetracycline treatment. In 1971, Skinner et al. (86) reported a double-blind placebo-controlled study involving 30 RA patients treated for 1 year with tetracycline, 250 mg, or placebo daily. This dose of tetracycline was well tolerated, but no improvement of statistical significance was seen in the tetracycline-treated group as a whole or in any individual patient within that group. The researchers concluded that tetracycline did not appear to be beneficial therapy for RA, and formal interest in the use of the tetracyclines waned for a number of years.

The efficacy of tetracycline therapy in a number of apparently noninfectious inflammatory diseases, specifically periodontitis and acne vulgaris, coupled with persistent lay reports of tetracycline efficacy in RA, led to a 10-patient open trial reported by Breedveld and Trentham (87) in 1988. This 16-week dose-finding study involved a daily minocycline dose of 200 mg, escalated to a maximal dose of 400 mg daily if clinical disease activity persisted and no toxicity was evident. In contrast to tetracycline, which had been used in prior trials, minocycline produced significant vestibular side effects that resulted in the withdrawal of one patient and limited the dose in six others. All efficacy measures, including the number of swollen joints, Ritchie articular index, duration of morning stiffness, grip strength, erythrocyte sedimentation rate (ESR), and platelet count achieved statistical improvement by study completion when compared with pretreatment levels.

In 1992, Langevitz et al. (88) reported on 18 patients with more refractory RA treated for 48 weeks with minocycline 200 mg daily. At least two second-line agents had previously failed for all patients, who had active disease, as defined by clinical and laboratory measures. There were three withdrawals for lack of efficacy, two for adverse effects (dizziness and leukopenia), with one patient lost to follow-up. Three of the 12 patients completing the trial were judged to be in remission, with substantial and moderate improvement reported for the remaining 3 and 9 patients, respectively. Efficacy measures that achieved statistical significance included patient and physician global assessment, grip strength, and ESR.

The favorable experience of these two open trials led eventually to two large placebo-controlled minocycline trials, the first of which was conducted in the Netherlands, and the second in the United States.

Kloppenburg et al. (89) studied 80 patients with active RA equally randomized to treatment with either minocycline 200 mg daily or placebo over a period of 26 weeks. All patients had active inflammatory disease at study entry, with 89% being seropositive and 95% having erosive changes. All had been previously treated with at least one disease-modifying antirheumatic drug (DMARD), with 58 (69%) of the 80 study participants continuing on stable DMARD therapy during the study. There were five (12.5%) withdrawals from the minocycline group for toxicity that primarily manifested as gastrointestinal intolerance and dizziness. Efficacy measures that achieved statistical significance compared with placebo included morning stiffness ($p = 0.006$), functional capacity ($p = 0.002$), Ritchie articular index ($p = 0.002$), and number of swollen joints ($p = 0.008$). Additional evidence of minocycline efficacy was provided by a number of laboratory measures, including changes in the ESR, hemoglobin, platelet count, and C-reactive protein, which all achieved statistical significance (all p values <0.001).

The Minocycline in Rheumatoid Arthritis (MIRA) trial (90), conducted in the United States, also used a minocycline dosage of 200 mg/day but involved a larger study population (219 patients) and longer study duration (48 weeks). In contrast to the Kloppenburg trial, concomitant use of DMARDs was not permitted; however, the frequency of seropositivity (56%) and erosive disease (68%) was considerably lower, suggesting a study population with less aggressive disease. Clinical improvement became evident by 3 months, with joint swelling and joint tenderness achieving statistical significance ($p = 0.023$ and $p = 0.021$, respectively). Significant improvement also was observed in a number of laboratory parameters (the ESR, hematocrit, and platelet count all had p values of <0.001), consistent with the findings of the Kloppenburg study. No statistically significant difference in radiographic measures of disease progression was seen; however, a trend favoring minocycline treatment was suggested (91,92). Withdrawals for toxicity were less frequent (6%) than in the Kloppenburg trial, likely because the dose of minocycline could be adjusted downward if an adverse effect were suspected.

O'Dell et al. (93,94) evaluated minocycline versus placebo in early seropositive disease. Fifteen (65%) of the 23 patients treated with minocycline 200 mg daily achieved and maintained American College of Rheumatology 50% improvement (ACR50) responses by the conclusion of the 6-month blinded portion of the trial, compared with only 3 (13%) of the 23 placebo-treated patients. After a 4-year follow-up period in which first- and/or second-line therapy as well as steroids could be prescribed at the discretion of the treating physician, remissions were found to be more common and the need for second-line therapy less frequent in patients initially treated with minocycline compared with those initially treated with placebo. There were no withdrawals for dizziness or nausea, but three patients did withdraw because of hyperpigmentation, which improved after drug discontinuation.

More recently, O'Dell et al. (95) reported on a 2-year study of 60 RA patients with seropositive disease of less than 1 year's duration who were randomized to receive either minocycline 100 mg twice daily or hydroxychloroquine 200 mg twice daily. Eighteen of 30 patients (60%) receiving minocycline achieved and maintained ACR50 responses compared with 10 of 30 (33%) placebo-treated patients. Prednisone dosage at study completion was significantly lower in those receiving minocycline compared with hydroxychloroquine (0.81 mg/day vs. 3.21 mg/day), as was the patient's global assessment of disease activity.

Whether minocycline must be taken orally to be efficacious as an antirheumatic therapy is not known, because no clinical trial has used a parenteral or intraarticular route of administration. Interestingly, intraarticular injections of minocycline in an experimental model of synovitis in rabbits did not produce any benefit (96). The sclerosing property of the tetracyclines has been used with efficacy in the treatment of pleural and pericardial effusions, whereas a single report (97) has suggested that intrabursal tetracycline might be of benefit for olecranon bursitis in RA patients.

Doxycycline

Three placebo-controlled trials involving a total of 120 patients have investigated the efficacy of doxycycline in the treatment of RA (98–100). Although both oral and intravenous administration was well tolerated in general, no clinical suggestion of doxycycline benefit was suggested in any of the studies. A 3-month trial of doxycycline in chronic seronegative arthritis similarly failed to show improvement in pain or functional status compared with placebo (101). Preliminary studies using human OA cartilage as well as an animal model of OA have led to a large National Institute of Arthritis and Musculoskeletal and Skin Diseases (NIAMS)-sponsored trial of doxycycline in the prevention of knee OA, which is presently nearing completion (102–104).

ALTERNATIVE THERAPIES

History

Allopathic medical practice developed its roots in the nineteenth century as the burgeoning enthusiasm for scientific discovery was applied to the healing arts. Although it is doubtful that anyone would seriously challenge the advances that have come to the practice of medicine at the hand of rigorous scientific therapy, failure to meet or exceed the patient's perceived expectations often creates a frustrating gap between those expectations and reasonably attainable results. With ever-increasing frequency, patients are turning to complementary or alternative therapies in an effort to obtain an added measure of improvement. Physicians are similarly frustrated by the lack of evidence-based information to establish a foundation for the rational use of these therapies. In the past, studies attempting to demonstrate the efficacy of CAM have been fraught with serious flaws, including inadequacy of sample size, scientific design, statistical rigor, adequate or appropriate control groups, appropriate blinding and agent concealment, and recruitment bias. Of course, publication bias in the medical literature, even of trials that have been poorly developed and performed, is toward manuscripts that contain positive results. Consequently, due to a lack of scientifically credible information, both patients and health-care practitioners are often unable to develop appropriate therapeutic plans that include CAM. Adding to these concerns is the fact that currently, dietary supplements are more loosely regulated under the Dietary Supplement Health and Education Act 1994 (DSHEA) rather than the guidelines typically applied to pharmaceuticals by the Food and Drug Administration (FDA) which results in less rigorous regulation of the manufacturing, packaging and claims relating to efficacy and safety required for these substances. This less regulated environment can result in the arbitrary promotion or advocacy of dietary supplements and in unsubstantiated scientific claims or empiric utilization. In an effort that has encouraged rigorously designed scientific trials to address CAM efficacy, the National Institutes of Health established the Office of Alternative Medicine and, subsequently, the National Center for Complementary and Alternative Medicine (NCCAM). The stated mission of NCCAM is to "support rigorous research on complementary and alternative medicine, to train researchers in CAM, and to disseminate information to the public and professionals on which CAM modalities work, which do not, and why" (105). When the Office of Alternative Medicine was established in 1992, its budget was $2 million. The 2003 budget for NCCAM is $113.4 million (106).

Prevalence

Rheumatologic disorders may lend themselves to use of CAM due to the chronic nature of many of these illnesses (107) and to the circumstance that, in many cases, current "scientifically proven" treatments are only partially effective. A survey of CAM use by rheumatology patients (108) found that 63% of rheumatology patients had tried at least one CAM therapy for their rheumatologic condition. Over one half of the patients polled as part of this study were currently using CAM and only about one half of the patients identified had discussed CAM use with their physicians. Patients who reported they had OA and/or those who said they experienced chronic severe pain were more likely to be CAM users than other patients with rheumatologic diagnoses. When the investigators inquired about why patients did not disclose CAM use to their physicians, the most frequent response was that the physician did not ask. Few patients felt that that their treating physician would have disapproved of CAM usage as an adjunct to other prescribed antirheumatic therapies. Therefore, because of extensive CAM use and the underreporting of that usage, physicians should include a careful history of CAM exposure in order to anticipate the potential for both the salutary and adverse effects of these agents.

The reported reasons that patients expressed for adding CAM to their therapeutic approach to disease management are complex. Many patients who use CAM feel a sense of autonomy or empowerment in their choice to participate in the practice (107,109). Davidoff observed that "scientific medicine asserts that factors outside the patient, rather than within, are largely responsible for disease. Many alternative care systems, in contrast, are characterized by their intense conviction that the root cause, and, hence, the remedy for most illness lies deep within the patient, primarily in mind and spirit." Thus, patient autonomy and empowerment are often part of the perceived benefits of CAM. Although this can lead to a sense of control for the patient, it can also result in feelings of guilt or inadequacy when expected results are not obtained.

The ever more pervasive use of alternative therapies that has occurred over the past decade requires physicians to at least become familiar and even interested in their patients' CAM exposure. It is compelling to recognize that patient acceptance of CAM is increasing even though it is largely uncompensated by third-party payers. Although physicians should not feel threatened or defensive because of the growing use of CAM, to ignore its ubiquity as part of total patient care in rheumatology would be short-sighted. As Panush (110) stated, "This is reality. Deal with it. Discuss complementary and alternative therapies with patients."

Definition

Developing a consensus definition for CAMs is fraught with difficulty and controversy. Strongly held and defensible opinions are found among varied interests and factions. For the purposes of this chapter, CAM will be defined as therapies currently considered unconventional and thus not usually prescribed by allopathic physicians (108). It is important to remember that treatments once considered to be CAM can become important mainstream therapies. The discovery of the efficacy of digitalis glycosides in treating congestive heart failure (111) is an often stated example. In rheumatology, the use of gold salts in treating RA began from the observation that gold may have antituburculous properties under the assumption that both entities might have a common infectious cause (112).

Due, at least in part, to the lack of evidence-based information with which to make decisions, allopathic physicians can be perceived as having difficulty maintaining objectivity relating to issues of CAM therapy, possibly to the detriment of patient care. Alpert suggested consideration of the following five principles (113) when considering CAM in the practice setting:

1. Maintain an open-minded attitude about the potential new therapeutic interventions and include those commonly referred to as alternative.
2. Encourage carefully performed and appropriate controlled trials of these new therapies.
3. Do not ignore or ridicule the potential of the placebo effect to produce marked therapeutic benefit.
4. Do not accept all new therapies as efficacious on first acquaintance. Claims of therapeutic efficacy should be rationally examined and tested.
5. Avoid hubristic and arrogant attitudes toward alternative medical practices.

Recognition of and adherence to these principles will assist the treating physician in more completely understanding their patient's needs, as well as the patient's perception of underperformance of the prescribed regimen and whether patient expectations of prescribed therapy are realistic.

Placebo Effect

Efficacy in randomized controlled trials is defined as the difference between the effect of the active agent and effect seen in similar patients who receive placebo. The placebo effect can be profound and is likely a complex interaction among a number of factors including patient expectations, provider/patient interaction, the intensity of clinical monitoring, the frequency of patient encounters and so forth. Kaptchuk (114) suggests that alternative medicine may have an enhanced placebo effect. Potential reasons for such enhancement include:

1. Patient characteristics, including the requirement for personal involvement, and willingness to personally pay for agents used in alternative care.
2. Alternative practitioners may be more optimistic and enthusiastic as well as less constrained by objectivity, leading to "provider induced expectations" that have been shown to increase response (115).
3. Patients and physicians who use alternative medicines may find one another's beliefs more compatible and may potentially be less objective.
4. Diseases that lend themselves to treatment with alternative therapies are often more subjective and therefore more difficult to objectively assess in clinical trials.
5. The treatment and setting can effect response. Variables include the number of times per day an agent needs to be ingested or the need for a special device or regimen.

The allure of the patient being actively involved in the process of alternative medicine can add to the increased likelihood of placebo response. In some instances, one could argue that a placebo response could represent a legitimate outcome of patient management. This is especially true when the desired outcomes are relatively subjective, such as analgesia or improvement in stamina. The placebo effect has played a powerful role in determining the outcome of clinical trials in rheumatology. Results of some carefully designed trials in RA have been complicated by surprisingly high placebo effects (90,116). In addition to underscoring the importance of the placebo effect, these examples further validate the need for carefully controlled randomized clinical trials in order to objectively evaluate the efficacy of CAM agents. A number of reasons, including those detailed above suggest that the placebo response may play a role in trials with these agents. Future results from well-designed and carefully conducted trials will ultimately demonstrate whether these concerns are valid.

The objective of the subsections that follow is to summarize the most reliable published information currently available for CAM agents. Careful consideration was given to emphasize studies that were developed with prospective, controlled, and statistically sound design. At this time, such studies are relatively uncommon, at least partly due to the differences in regulatory requirements for CAM agents compared with FDA-regulated medications in the United States. The NCCAM is encouraging the development and implementation of trials that will assist in establishing the efficacy of many of these agents.

Glucosamine and Chondroitin Sulfate

Glucosamine

Glucosamine is a naturally-occurring amino-monosaccharide (Fig. 43.2) that is marketed in the United States as a dietary supplement. Glucosamine is extracted from shellfish, and persons with shellfish allergies should probably avoid exposure or should use with caution. Glucosamine has acceptance as a symptomatic slow-acting drug for OA (SYSADOA) in the treatment of OA in Europe (117). Glucosamine use for OA in the United States has been more controversial. In his books, Theodosakis (118,119) advocated use of glucosamine as part of a defined therapeutic approach in OA that, in addition to the supplements glucosamine and chondroitin, includes regular exercise, healthy diet and weight control, "traditional medications" as indicated, and a positive attitude.

In vivo, D-glucosamine is the hexosamine component of the glycosaminoglycans keratan sulfate and hyaluronic acid and thus likely plays an important role in cartilage metabolism. The mechanism of action of exogenously administered glucosamine has not been defined, but it has been suggested that *in vitro* addition of glucosamine to cultured human chondrocytes from osteoarthritic cartilage causes increased proteoglycan synthesis (120). At the present time, there is little *in vivo* evidence that orally administered glucosamine is incorporated into glycosaminoglycans and thus could be important in cartilage metabolism, although this theoretical mechanism of action has been proposed. A small study of glucosamine in dogs and humans demonstrated that glucosamine was well absorbed orally (121). Serum glucosamine levels following oral dosing are substantially less than levels following intravenous infusion, suggesting a first-pass effect in the liver that metabolizes glucosamine to carbon dioxide, water, and urea (122). Infusion of radio-labeled glucosamine in dogs demonstrates a rapid clearance from plasma (half-life 0.28 hours) and rapid incorporation into plasma proteins.

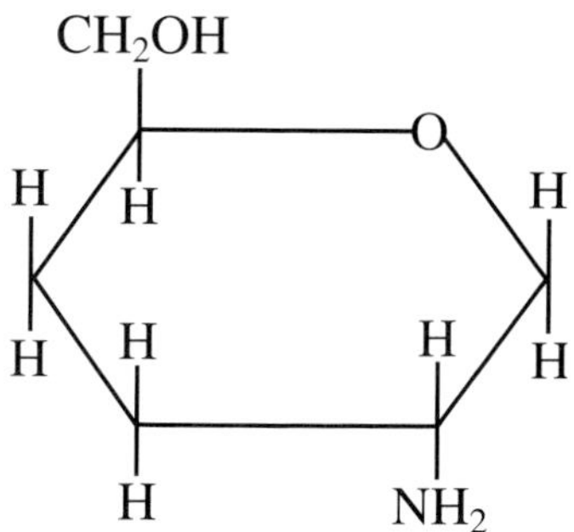

FIG. 43.2. Chemical structure of glucosamine.

Many of the controlled clinical trials with glucosamine in OA patients have been of marginal quality (123) due to insufficient sample size, lack of statistical rigor, potential for sponsor bias, inadequate concealment, and lack of intention-to-treat principles. After careful consideration, six studies were included in a systematic review (124–129). Each of these studies showed a positive effect, and the pooled effect size was deemed to be moderate. In general, studies with larger sample sizes tended to have smaller effect sizes.

Two other studies merit specific comment. Both of these recently published studies present data from patients who received long-term glucosamine therapy with the objective to evaluate symptomatic improvement and a change in the progressive loss of cartilage, and thus disease modification, using serially obtained standard anteroposterior, weight-bearing knee x-rays as the outcome measure.

The first study (130) reports 212 patients followed for 3 years on glucosamine 1,500 mg/day versus placebo. The study assessed change in medial compartment joint space width as determined on standing, weight-bearing anteroposterior knee radiographs as the primary outcome. The researchers reported that patients taking glucosamine experienced no loss in joint space, whereas placebo-treated patients continued to show progressive cartilage loss. Glucosamine-treated patients also experienced improved symptoms based on the total Western Ontario and McMaster's University OA Composite (WOMAC) index based on intent-to-treat statistical principles. In the second study (131), 202 patients received glucosamine 1,500 mg/day or placebo. Again, radiographic medial joint space narrowing as determined in the previously described study was the primary outcome measure. In this trial, patients taking glucosamine showed no progression of medial joint space narrowing, whereas placebo-treated patients experienced progressive narrowing. The study also reported a completer's analysis that demonstrated significant improvement in symptoms based on both the Lequesne and WOMAC indices. Substantial concerns have been raised about the validity of the radiographic outcome measure, which may be influenced by joint pain at the time the film was taken (132). Standardized radiographic protocols (133) will be necessary to demonstrate whether these agents are potentially disease modifying. However, the possibility of disease modification by glucosamine as determined by altering radiographic evidence of progressive joint space narrowing is an intriguing and important question.

The safety profile of glucosamine in published studies appears to be favorable. Few adverse events are reported and are generally minor, primarily consisting of gastrointestinal complaints including heartburn, diarrhea, constipation, epigastric pain, and nausea (134). One concern about the use of glucosamine is its potential to cause or worsen diabetes. In animal models, increased glucosamine levels in cells have been associated with insulin resistance (a major factor in the genesis of type 2 diabetes mellitus) and alterations in insulin production (135–137). Whether the doses commonly used in humans for the treatment of arthritis are sufficient to cause significant alterations in glucose homeostasis is unknown at this time.

Chondroitin

Chondroitin (Fig. 43.3) is a glycosaminoglycan that is a component of proteoglycans found in articular cartilage. Like glucosamine, chondroitin sulfate is recognized as a SYSADOA in Europe (117) and its use, although controversial in the United States, has been popularized in the lay press (118,119) as detailed in the glucosamine section above. Commercially available chondroitin is extracted from the cartilage of bovine trachea and is predominantly chondroitin 4 sulfate and chondroitin 6 sulfate. The pharmacokinetics of chondroitin are not clearly defined. Even though chondroitin is a large complex molecule, some degree of oral absorption has been demonstrated in humans. Determination of oral bioavailability has been attempted and is estimated to be in the range of 5% to 15% (138–140). It is further estimated that chondroitin serum levels at steady state are only 10%–20% higher than those seen following single dosing (140). Ronca and colleagues (141) have shown that orally administered chondroitin decreases granuloma formation in response to pellet, cotton, or sponge implants; ameliorates the inflammatory response in adjuvant arthritis; and

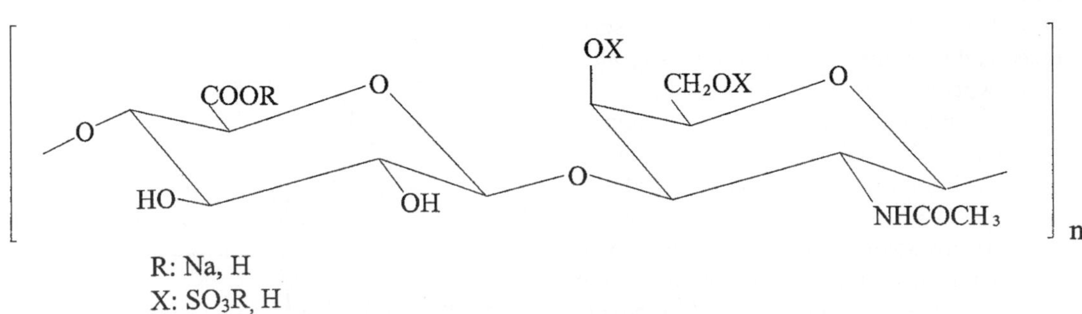

FIG. 43.3. Chemical structure of chondroitin.

diminishes lysosomal enzyme release in carrageenan-induced pleurisy. *In vitro,* addition of chondroitin sulfate to cultured human articular cartilage results in increased proteoglycans in the pericellular matrix and decreased collagenolytic activity. Injection of chondroitin into the rabbit knee resulted in increased hyaluronic acid production by synoviocytes (142).

A systematic review of clinical trials evaluating the efficacy of chondroitin in OA (123) identified nine trials that fulfilled inclusion criteria for the review (143– 151). In each instance, the outcome of the trial tended to be positive. One trial (144) demonstrated an effect size that was much larger than the other eight. Discounting that trial, pooled data from the remaining trials demonstrated a moderate to large effect size. As with glucosamine trials described above, the quality of these studies is hampered by faulty design, including a lack of intention-to-treat principles, industry sponsorship and inadequate allocation concealment. In general, studies with large numbers of patients and more rigorous design (146,150) tended to have lower treatment effect sizes.

Information about the safety of chondroitin is scant. The randomized controlled trials described above were of relatively short duration, and reported adverse events were minor and similar to placebo control groups (151). In fact, a meta-analysis found that the frequencies of side effects were consistently higher in the placebo groups when compared with the chondroitin groups (152). Overall, adverse events were uncommon. The most frequently reported side effects involved the gastrointestinal system and included epigastric distress, diarrhea, and constipation. Additionally, rashes, edema, alopecia, and extrasystoles were infrequently reported.

Combined Therapy with Glucosamine and Chondroitin

Published evidence evaluating the clinical efficacy of the combination of glucosamine and chondroitin is minimal. Clinical use of the drug combination is recommended in the lay literature (118,119). One animal study suggested that the combination of glucosamine/chondroitin/manganese resulted in increased glycosaminoglycan synthesis *in vivo* compared with either of the agents singly or with controls (153). Symptomatic and antiinflammatory improvement using glucosamine and chondroitin is reported in horses (154) and dogs (155). There are no published data suggesting that the safety profile of the combination would be any different from any of the agents ingested singly.

Omega-3 Fatty Acids

The efficacy of fish oils or flax seed oils containing ω-3 polyunsaturated fatty acids as dietary supplements has been most extensively studied in RA. These agents have been tested as complementary therapies in RA patients concurrently treated with nonsteroidal antiinflammatory drugs (NSAIDs) and DMARDs. In patients so treated, studies have demonstrated modest improvement in the number of tender joints (156–161) and in duration of morning stiffness (157,158). The minimum daily effective dose appears to be 3 g of eicosapentaenoic acid (EPA) or a metabolite, docosahexaenoic acid (DHA), and the minimum exposure for expected efficacy is at least 12 weeks. Studies do not demonstrate an advantage or rationale to recommend the use of one preparation over another. The mechanism of action has not been defined. It has been suggested that EPA and DHA may have antiinflammatory properties because they may act as substrates in leukotriene, prostaglandin, and thromboxane metabolism, leading to an antiinflammatory effect from altered eicosanoid metabolism in patients treated with fish oils (162).

S-adenosylmethionine

S-adenosylmethionine (SAMe) is a naturally occurring compound synthesized from L-methionine and adenosine triphosphate (ATP). SAMe plays a key role in transmethylation, transsulfuration, and aminopropylation (163). SAMe is marketed as a dietary supplement in the United States to promote joint health, mobility, and joint comfort (164). The mechanism of action for pain control is not known, and trials addressing the efficacy of SAMe are of variable quality. A meta-analysis was recently published that attempted to address the efficacy of SAMe relative to study quality, drug dosage and length of treatment (164). The authors identified 11 studies of sufficient quality to include in the analysis. In two studies, the comparator was placebo; in the remainder the comparator was an NSAID. This meta-analysis of clinical studies using SAMe indicated that SAMe had a comparable effect to NSAIDs in treating OA. The efficacy of SAMe over placebo was not clearly established. The authors' conclusions were additionally tempered because the trials were of relatively short duration and some studies used SAMe dosages higher than the recommended 800 mg/day for two weeks followed by 400 mg/day thereafter. Long-term efficacy of SAMe has not been addressed. Adverse events between SAMe and placebo were similar. SAMe was better tolerated than NSAIDs. SAMe is also promoted for the treatment of depression; no studies have been reported that monitor mood changes as an outcome of arthritis treatment.

Oral Collagen

Oral ingestion of undenatured type II bovine and chicken collagen has been studied in the treatment of RA. An early report of patients with long-standing RA (165) indicated efficacy and reported complete remission in four patients. However, the results of subsequent controlled trials were less encouraging (166–169). Orally induced immunologic tolerance is the most often suggested mechanism of action, and consistent with that theory, studies have suggested that maximal efficacy occurred at very low (20 μg/day) dosage forms (167). A trial designed to definitively demonstrate the efficacy of orally administered type II chicken collagen yielded negative results (unpublished data). Overall, if these treatments are effective, the salutary effect is small (169). Patients with allergies to chicken or eggs should take this agent with caution. No serious adverse events due to oral collagen were reported. In general, adverse events were similar in the placebo and active treatment arms, although one study showed increased liver enzymes compared with placebo (167).

Ginger

Ginger is a popular spice that is used in China as an antiinflammatory agent (170). As is common with herbal preparations, ginger is a complex mixture of constituents, including gingeroles, β-carotene, capsaicin, caffeic acid, and salicylate, but all in nonpharmacologic doses (171). Studies have shown that ginger may inhibit cyclooxygenase (172) and leukotriene synthesis (173), and reduce carrageenan-induced rat paw edema (174).

One study of 67 patients with OA of the hip or knee were randomized to one of three arms: ginger, ibuprofen, or placebo (175). The study had a 3-week crossover design and allowed for analgesic rescue with acetaminophen. The results indicated that ibuprofen was more effective than ginger and suggested that ginger was more effective than placebo based on assessment of pain on a visual analogue scale. The same trend was seen in acetaminophen consumption. Ibuprofen was more effective than ginger or placebo based on the Lequesne algofunctional index. Adverse events were minor; more episodes of dyspepsia were reported with ibuprofen. A second study compared ginger extract with placebo in 261 patients with OA of the knee using pain on standing as the primary outcome measure (171). The study design was blinded, randomized, and used intention-to-treat principles. The investigators reported improvement in knee pain on standing (p = 0.048). A secondary outcome measure that is well validated and widely used for assessing therapeutic response in patients with OA, the WOMAC index did not demonstrate improvement. The ginger extract was generally well tolerated, although mild gastrointestinal complaints, including eructation, dyspnea, and nausea, were noted (171). An accompanying editorial concluded that ginger should not be recommended for treatment of OA due to limited efficacy and lack of information about safety (176).

Devil's Claw (*Harpagophytum procumbens*)

Devil's claw is an herb native to South America and Namibia that is ingested as capsules or tea. Harpagoside is the active ingredient found in this herb. Therapy of low back pain has been evaluated in two studies (177,178). These studies suggested that there were more "pain-free" patients in the treated group. The initial primary outcome measures were not met. Adverse drug events were not specifically addressed, although one study suggested that this herb may interfere with ongoing warfarin therapy.

Willow Bark

White willow bark contains the salicylate salicin and is used in treating a number of musculoskeletal complaints. Ernest (179) reported a personal communication of a study in 78 patients with OA using willow bark extract (salicin 240 mg/day), who showed improvement based on the WOMAC pain index. Efficacy is felt to be similar to that of other salicylates, although it is difficult to obtain therapeutic salicylate doses because of the low concentration of salicin found in the herb. Concerns about its use in the pediatric population and the potential for inducing Reye syndrome have been raised. Like other salicylates, salicin can potentiate the effects of warfarin in patients and should be used cautiously in those patients.

Capsaicin

Capsaicin (trans-8-methyl-*N*-vanillyl-6-nonenamide) is extracted from the pepper *Capsicum frutescens.* Capsaicin is included as an effective option for topical therapy in the ACR management guidelines for OA (180) for the treatment of joint pain. Proposed mechanisms of actions include counterirritation of the skin and depletion of substance P in the small, superficial unmyelinated sensory neurons of the skin. McCarty found capsaicin effective in relieving articular hand pain in OA but not RA in a blinded, randomized controlled trial (181). Deal (182) demonstrated efficacy of topical capsaicin in knee pain of both OA and RA in a study with relatively small numbers. Blinding of capsaicin trials has been a challenging issue due to the unique burning sensation associated with the topical application of capsaicin. This reaction becomes less pronounced with prolonged usage. Application frequency in clinical trials was four times daily, and efficacy is typically seen in 5 to 7 days. Side effects reported with capsaicin have primarily been related to irritation of the skin where the agent is applied, which can be locally severe. Care must be taken to avoid contact with eyes or other tender tissues where exposure to capsaicin can result in serious burns.

Dimethyl Sulfoxide

Dimethyl sulfoxide (DMSO) is an industrial solvent that has been used in treating musculoskeletal conditions in animals for decades (183). After topical application, it readily penetrates soft tissues. DMSO rapidly produces a distinctive taste and odor on the breath following topical exposure. This physical property has made double-blind clinical trials assessing efficacy especially challenging. Some trials have used varying concentrations of DMSO (50%–95% in active study arm; 5%–10% in "placebo" arm) in an effort to maintain the blind effect (184). Early uncontrolled trials in treating both arthritis (185) and musculoskeletal injuries (186) demonstrated promising positive results. The results of randomized controlled clinical trials have been less consistent. Brown (187) reported excellent results in patients with acute musculoskeletal injuries who used high-dose compared with low-dose DMSO. However, a study of DMSO in treating epicondylitis or rotator cuff injuries showed no difference between 70% and 5% solutions (188). Likewise, a study of 100 patients with knee OA did not show a difference between DMSO and placebo (189). The mechanism of action of DMSO is not well understood. It is known to act as a scavenger of reactive oxygen metabolites and to stabilize lysosomal membranes, but how these findings translate to clinical utility has not been clarified. For more detailed information, the reader is referred to Trice and Pinals (183), who presented a comprehensive historical review of the use of DMSO in treating rheumatic conditions.

Chiropractic

The chiropractic was established in 1895 and is regulated through state licensure in all 50 United States, most European countries, Canada, and Australia. Currently there are over 50,000 chiropractors in the United States. Chiropractic services were first included in the payment structure of Medicare in the 1970s, and now most public and private payment plans cover chiropractic services. Few data are available that carefully evaluate the cost effectiveness of chiropractic care of musculoskeletal complaints, although a high degree of patient satisfaction and practitioner loyalty is seen among patients who use chiropractic services (190).

Most of the clinical research into musculoskeletal complaints addressed by the chiropractic has attempted to evaluate the treatment of low back and neck pain. Spinal manipulations are the procedures most commonly administered by chiropractors. These "adjustments" are generally accomplished manually, but perceived advantages among the various techniques are hotly contested among chiropractic practitioners. Physical therapy modalities such as temperature, therapeutic exercises, and general fitness recommendations are also commonly administered. Other forms of CAM, such as supplements, massage, and acupressure, are used by many chiropractors (191).

Studies indicate that musculoskeletal complaints comprise most chiropractic visits. Sixty percent have low back pain. Others include head, neck, and extremity pain. Over half of patients have chronic musculoskeletal complaints. Randomized clinical trials evaluating the efficacy of spinal manipulation in low back pain are difficult to design and to interpret, but tend clinically and statistically to favor manipulation, although the clinical advantage is not dramatic. A systematic review of many of these trials (192) concluded that the overall quality of the studies was low, but that spinal manipulation was likely to be an effective therapy for low back pain.

Homeopathy

Homeopathy was developed by German physician Samuel Christian Hahnemann in the latter part of the eighteenth century, at least partly in response to barbaric practices such as blood-letting, catharsis, and heavy metal administration that were widely used by the orthodox medical practitioners of the time. Because of the chronic nature of many of the rheumatic diseases and the relative inability to successfully manage them, patients turn to homeopathy as both alternative or complementary therapies to more fully address their complaints. There are two primary principles that underlie homeopathy. These are that signs and symptoms in a diseased individual can be cured with agents that would produce similar manifestations in a healthy individual and that serial dilutions of such remedies will maintain biologic activity if shaken or agitated between dilutions (193).

A meta-analysis of clinical trials addressing the efficacy of homeopathy has been published (194). Studies were identified for the analysis that addressed homeopathic approaches in RA, OA, and fibromyalgia. The meta-analysis concluded that the available homeopathic studies were suboptimal in a number of areas, including small sample size and marginal statistical design. The researchers concluded that there might have been an effect that could not be explained by placebo but that absolute superiority could not be demonstrated with the currently available data, and further study with rigorous design was necessary. Significant adverse events were not reported.

Use of homeopaths increased in the latter part of the twentieth century. It was estimated that there were over 5 million visits in the early 1990s (195). Patients who use homeopathy risk the inherent delay in instituting effective therapy. As more and more effective agents become available for treating rheumatic diseases, patients must be informed of that risk and encouraged not to abandon conventional approaches. Physicians must maintain an open dialogue, and evenly present therapeutic options based on the best available evidence-based information in an effort to optimize care of afflicted patients.

Acupuncture

Classically, acupuncture is an ancient Chinese practice believed to correct imbalances of flow of energies that are necessary for good health (Qi) through 12 primary channels or meridians and 8 "extraordinary" meridians. The practitioner assesses and seeks to identify the nature of the imbalance and then seeks to restore balance through manipulation of the appropriate acupuncture sites from among the approximately 360 sites along the meridians. Puncturing the skin with a long thin needle is the most common maneuver used by the practitioner. Heat, pressure, friction, suction, or electrical stimulation through the needles are also used (196).

Studies to address the efficacy of acupuncture are highly variable in quality. Blinding these trials is especially difficult because there may be some analgesic effect of sham acupuncture. Thomas (197) reports a study of 44 patients with OA of the cervical spine. Patients were randomly assigned to receive placebo, diazepam, sham acupuncture, and acupuncture. The results showed that acupuncture was more effective than placebo, but not more effective than diazepam or sham acupuncture in relieving pain. Berman reported a single blind study of acupuncture as adjunctive therapy of OA of the knee (198). The study included 58 patients on standard treatment with NSAIDs. The results of this 12-week trial showed significant improvement in self-reported pain and disability scores compared with the control group. Deluze and colleagues (199) reported a controlled trial of 70 patients with fibromyalgia using electroacupuncture versus sham superficial needling. Seven of eight of the outcome parameters showed improvement in the active group, and no significant improvement was seen in the sham group.

Although acupuncture may have a role in analgesia in the rheumatic diseases, data-driven evidence demonstrating efficacy through adequately designed clinical trials is still lacking. The trials that have been published to date have not had the statistical power to demonstrate differences if they exist. Additionally, the possibility that sham acupuncture may have analgesic propensity further complicates potential study designs (196). Common minor adverse events arising from acupuncture include rashes and bruising around the acupuncture site. Letters to journals have implicated hepatitis and human immunodeficiency virus infection (200,201). Use of licensed practitioners cognizant of the importance of sterile technique likely minimizes these problems.

SUMMARY

Open and controlled clinical trials have shown minocycline to be a well-tolerated and efficacious therapy for both early and established RA. Further study incorporating direct comparisons with other agents is needed to establish the proper place of minocycline in the management of RA and to elucidate its actual antirheumatic mechanism of action.

The role of CAM in the management of rheumatic diseases remains controversial and not surprisingly the content of this chapter will likely not be totally satisfactory to anyone. Those who believe the CAM has no place in the management of rheumatologic diseases are ignoring a large body of carefully constructed literature that demonstrates CAM as widely accepted, and to some degree almost universally practiced. Those who believe CAM to be mainstream will be disappointed that the researchers required agents and practices to have demonstrated efficacy and safety with some degree of scientific rigor in order to be included.

Because of extensive use, a working knowledge of CAM practices and agents is becoming ever more important in order for rheumatologists to provide comprehensive patient care. Studies indicate that patients will discuss CAM use if the physician inquires. A general lack of basic research to determine mechanisms of action followed by carefully designed adequately powered clinical trials will continue to hamper widespread acceptance of these agents in medical practice. Government regulations that permit the manufacture and distribution of CAM products under less stringent conditions than is currently required for pharmaceuticals will allow patient exposure to untested agents and will permit unsubstantiated claims that in the long run may not be in the patient's best interest.

CAM's increasing popularity and widespread use, combined with a dearth of evidence-based literature documenting either safety or efficacy, require that the patient and physician maintain an honest, open dialogue about all aspects of disease management. Studies suggest that patients will discuss CAM when queried. It is therefore incumbent on providers to have a working knowledge of the potential for efficacy, adverse events, and drug agent interactions with more conventional therapy in order to provide patients with recommendations best suited for their conditions. Ultimately, resolution of this quandary will require more careful regulation of CAM combined with thoughtfully designed studies that define its utility and safety.

REFERENCES

1. Duggar BM. Aureomycin: a new antibiotic. *Ann NY Acad Sci* 1948;51:175–342.
2. Bartz QR. Isolation and characterization of chloromycetin. *J Biol Chem* 1948;1172:445–450.
3. Dienes L, Ropes M, We S. The role of pleuropneumonia-like organisms in genitourinary and joint diseases. *N Engl J Med* 1948;238:509–515, 563–567.
4. Bartholomew L. Isolation and characterization of mycoplasma (PPLO) from patients with rheumatoid arthritis, systemic lupus erythematosus, and Reiter's syndrome. *Arthritis Rheum* 1965;8:376–388.
5. Williams M, Brostoff I, Roitt IM. Positive role of *Mycoplasma fermentans* in pathogenesis of rheumatoid arthritis. *Lancet* 1970;2:277–280.
6. Bernard B, Yin EJ, Simon HJ. Clinical pharmacologic studies with minocycline. *J Clin Pharmacol New Drugs* 1971;11:332–348.
7. Macdonald H, Kelly RG, Allen ES, et al. Pharmacokinetic studies on minocycline in man. *Clin Pharmacol Ther* 1973;14:852–861.
8. Hinton NA. The effect of oral tetracycline HCl and doxycycline on the intestinal flora. *Curr Ther Res* 1970;12:341–352.
9. Ehrlich GE. Concentrations of tetracycline and minocycline in joint effusions following oral administration. *Pa Med* 1972;75:47–49.
10. Devine LF, Johnson DP, Hagerman CR, et al. The effect of minocycline on meningococcal nasopharyngeal carrier state in naval personnel. *Am J Epidemiol* 1971;93:337–345.
11. Kunin CM, Finland M. Clinical pharmacology of the tetracycline antibiotics. *Arch Intern Med* 1959;104:1030–1050.

12. Kloppenburg M, Mattie H, Douwes N, et al. Minocycline in the treatment of rheumatoid arthritis: relationship of serum concentration to efficacy. *J Rheumatol* 1995;22:611–616.
13. Steigbigel NH, Reed CW, Finland M. Susceptibility of common pathogenic bacteria to seven tetracycline antibiotics in vitro. *Am J Med Sci* 1968;255:179–195.
14. Chopra I, Hawkey PM, Hinton M. Tetracyclines, molecular and clinical aspects. *J Antimicrob Chemother* 1992;29:245–277.
15. Golub LM, McNamara TF, D'Angelo G, et al. A nonantibacterial chemically modified tetracycline inhibits mammalian collagenase activity. *J Dent Res* 1987;66:1310–1314.
16. Sadowski T, Steinmeyer J. Minocycline inhibits the production of inducible nitric oxide synthase in articular chondrocytes. *J Rheumatol* 2001;28:336–340.
17. Pruzanski W, Greenwald R, Street I, et al. Inhibition of enzymatic activity of phospholipase A_2 by minocycline and doxycycline. *Biochem Pharmacol* 1992;44:1165–1170.
18. El Attar TMA, Lin HS, Schulz R. Effect of minocycline on prostaglandin formation in gingival fibroblasts. *J Periodontal Res* 1988;23:285–286.
19. Patel RN, Attur MG, Dave MN, et al. A novel mechanism of action of chemically modified tetracyclines: inhibition of COX-2-mediated prostaglandin E_2 production. *J Immunol* 1999;163:3459–3467.
20. Amin AR, Attur MG, Thakker GD, et al. A novel mechanism of action of tetracyclines: effects on nitric oxide synthases. *Proc Natl Acad Sci U S A* 1996;93:14014–14019.
21. Borderie D, Hernvann A, Hilliquin P, et al. Tetracyclines inhibit notrosothiol production by cytokine-stimulated osteoarthritis synovial cells. *Inflamm Res* 2001;50:409–414.
22. Van Barr H, Van De Kerkhof P, Mier P, et al. Tetracyclines are potent scavengers of the superoxide radical. *Br J Rheumatol* 1987;117:131–132.
23. Wasil M, Halliwell B, Moorhouse CP. Scavenging of hypochlorous acid by tetracycline, rifampicin and some other antibiotics: a possible antioxidant action of rifampicin and tetracycline. *Biochem Pharmacol* 1988;37:775–558.
24. Golub L, Ramamurthy N, McNamara T, et al. Tetracyclines inhibit tissue collagenase activity. *J Periodontal Res* 1984;19:651–655.
25. Golub L, Wolff M, Lee H. Further evidence that tetracyclines inhibit collagenase activity in human crevicular fluid and from other mammalian sources. *J Periodontal Res* 1985;20:12–13.
26. Golub LM. Reduction with tetracycline of excessive collagen degradation in periodontal and other diseases. *NY State Dent J* 1990;56: 24–26.
27. Golub L, Wolff M, Lee H. Further evidence that tetracyclines inhibit collagenase activity in human crevicular fluid and from other mammalian sources. *J Periodontal Res* 1985;20:12–13.
28. Greenwald RA. Treatment of destructive arthritic disorders with MMP inhibitors: potential role of tetracyclines. *Ann NY Acad Sci* 1994;732: 181–198.
29. Greenwald RA, Moak SA, Ramamurthy NS, et al. Tetracycline suppress matrix metalloproteinase activity in adjuvant arthritis and in combination with flurbiprofen ameliorate bone damage. *J Rheumatol* 1992; 19:927–938.
30. Greenwald RA, Moak SA, Golub LM. Low dose doxycycline inhibits pyridinolone excretion in selected patients with rheumatoid arthritis. *Ann NY Acad Sci* 1994;732:419–421.
31. Smith GN Jr, Yu LP Jr, Brandt KD, et al. Oral administration of doxycycline reduces collagenase and gelatinase activities in extracts of human osteoarthritis cartilage. *J Rheumatol* 1998;25:532–535.
32. Greenwald R, Golub L, Lavietes B. Tetracyclines inhibit human synovial collagenase *in vivo* and *in vitro*. *J Rheum* 1987;14:28–32.
33. Milwidsky A, Finci-Yeheskel Z, Mayer M. Direct inhibition of proteases and cervical plasminogen activator by antibiotics. *Am J Obstet Gynecol* 1992;166:606–612.
34. Yu LP, Smith GN, Hasty KA, et al. Doxycycline inhibits type XI collagenolytic activity of extracts from human osteoarthritic cartilage and of gelatinase. *J Rheum* 1991;18:1450–1452.
35. Kloppenburg M, Dijkmans BA, Verweij CL, et al. Inflammatory and immunological parameters of disease activity in rheumatoid arthritis patients treated with minocycline. *Immunopharmacology* 1996;31: 163–169.
36. Riesbeck K, Bredberg A, Forsgren A. Ciprofloxin does not inhibit mitochondrial functions but other antibiotics do. *Antimicrob Agents Chemother* 1990;34:167–169.
37. Martin R, Warr G, Couch R, et al. Effects of tetracycline on leukotaxis. *J Infect Dis* 1974;129:110–116.
38. Elewski BE, Lamb BAJ, Sams WMJ, et al. *In vivo* suppression of neutrophil chemotaxis by systemically and topically administered tetracycline. *J Am Acad Dermatol* 1983;8:807–812.
39. Forsgren A, Schmeling D, Quie P. Effect of tetracycline on the phagocytic function of human leukocytes. *J Infect Dis* 1974;130:412–415.
40. Thong Y, Ferrante A. Inhibition of mitogen-induced human lymphocyte proliferative responses by tetracycline analogues. *Clin Exp Immunol* 1979;35:443–446.
41. Ingham E, Turnbill L, Kearney J. The effects of minocycline and tetracycline on the mitotic response of human peripheral blood lymphocytes. *J Antimicrob Chemother* 1991;27:607–617.
42. Gearing AJH, Beckett P, Christodoulou M, et al. Processing of tumour necrosis factor-alpha precursor by metalloproteinases. *Nature* 1994; 370:555 557.
43. McGeehan GM, Becherer JD, Bast RC, et al. Regulation of tumour necrosis factor alpha by a metalloproteinase inhibitor. *Nature* 1994; 370:558–561.
44. Kloppenburg M, Brinkman BM, de Rooij-Dijk HH, et al. The tetracycline derivative minocycline differentially affects cytokine production by monocytes and T lymphocytes. *Antimicrob Agents Chemother* 1996;40:934–940.
45. MacDonald T, Carter P. Requirement for bacterial flora before mice generate cells capable of mediating the delayed hypersensitivity reaction to sheep red blood cells. *J Immunol* 1979;122:2624–2630.
46. Sewell KL, Breedveld F, Furrie E, et al. The effect of minocycline in rat models of inflammatory arthritis: correlation of arthritis suppression with enhanced T cell calcium flux. *Cell Immunol* 1996;167:195–204.
47. Neu HC. A symposium on the tetracyclines: a major appraisal. *Bull NY Acad Med* 1978;54:141–155.
48. Alarcon GS, Tracy IC, Strand GM, et al. Survival and drug discontinuation analyses in a large cohort of methotrexate-treated rheumatoid arthritis patients. *Ann Rheum Dis* 1995;54:708–712.
49. Levenson T, Masood D, Patterson R. Minocycline-induced serum sickness. *Allergy Asthma Proc* 1996;17:79–81.
50. Harel L, Amir J, Livni E, st al. Serum-sickness-like reaction associated with minocycline therapy in adolescents. *Ann Pharmacother* 1996;30:481–483.
51. Knights SE, Leandro MJ, Khamashta MA, et al. Minocycline-induced arthritis. *Clin Exp Rheumatol* 1998;16:587–590.
52. Gaffney K, Merry P. Antineutrophil cytoplasmic antibody-positive polyarthritis associated with minocycline therapy. *Br J Rheumatol* 1996;35:1327.
53. Byrne PAC, Williams BD, Pritchard MH. Minocycline-related lupus. *Br J Rheumatol* 1994;33:674–676.
54. McHugh NJ. Minocycline-induced lupus and autoimmune phenomena. *Lupus* 1999;8:417–418.
55. Angulo JM, Sigal LH, Espinoza LR. Coexistent minocycline-induced systemic lupus erythematosus and autoimmune hepatitis. *Semin Arthritis Rheum* 1998;28:187–192.
56. Angulo JM, Sigal LH, Espinoza LR. Minocycline induced lupus and autoimmune hepatitis. *J Rheumatol* 1999;26:1420–1421.
57. Schaffer JV, Davidson DM, NcNiff JM, et al. Perinuclear antineutrophilic cytoplasmic antibody-positive cutaneous polyarteritis nodosa associated with minocycline therapy for acne vulgaris. *J Am Acad Dermatol* 2001;44:198–206.
58. Schrodt BJ, Kuop-Shorten CL, Callen JP. Necrotizing vasculitis of the skin and uterine cervix associated with minocycline therapy for acne vulgaris. *South Med J* 1999;92:502–504.
59. Elkayam O, Yaron M, Caspi D. Minocycline induced arthritis associated with fever, livedo reticularis, and pANCA. *Ann Rheum Dis* 1996; 55:769–771.
60. Gordon MM, Porter D. Minocycline induced lupus:case series in the West of Scotland. *J Rheumatol* 2001;28:1004–1006.
61. Elkayam O, Yaron M, Caspi D. Minocycline-induced autoimmune syndromes: an overview. *Semin Arthritis Rheum* 1999;28:392–397.
62. Elkayam O, Levartovsky D, Brautbar C, et al. Clinical and immunological study of 7 patients with minocycline-induced autoimmune phenomena. *Am J Med* 1998:105:484–487.
63. Williams DN, Laughlin LW, Lee Y. Minocycline: possible vestibular side effects. *Lancet* 1974;2:744–746.
64. Lepper MH. Effect of large doses of aureomycin on human liver. *Arch Intern Med* 1951;88:271–283.

65. Burette A, Finet C, Prigogine T, et al. Acute hepatic injury associated with minocycline. *Arch Intern Med* 1984;144:1491–1492.
66. Malcolm A, Heap TR, Eckstein RP, et al. Minocycline-induced liver injury. *Am J Gastroenterol* 1996;91:1641–1643.
67. Matteson EL, Johnson BW, Maher JD. Arthralgias, myalgias, and autoimmune hepatitis with minocycline therapy. *J Rheumatol* 1998;25: 1653–1654.
68. Teitelbaum JE, Perez-Atayde AR, Cohen M, et al. Minocycline-related autoimmune hepatitis: case series and literature review. *Arch Pediatr Adolesc Med* 1998;1152:1132–1136.
69. Min DI, Burke PA, Lewis WD, et al. Acute hepatic failure associated with oral minocycline: a case report. *Pharmacotherapy* 1992;12: 68–71.
70. Erslev A. Hematopoietic depression induced by chloromycetin. *Blood* 1953;8:170–174.
71. Lupton JR, Figueroa P, Tamjidi P, et al. An infectious mononucleosis-like syndrome induced by minocycline; a third pattern of adverse drug reaction. *Cutis* 1999;64:91–96.
72. Morris WE. Photosensitivity due to tetracycline derivative. *JAMA* 1960;172:1155.
73. Guillon JM, Holy P, Autran B, et al. Minocycline-induced cell-mediated hypersensitivity pneumonitis. *Ann Intern Med* 1992;117:476–481.
74. Weyman J. Tetracyclines and teeth. *Practitioner* 1965;195:661–665.
75. Cohlan SQ, Bevelander G, Tiamsic T. Growth inhibition of prematures receiving tetracycline: clinical and laboratory investigation. *Am J Dis Child* 1963;105:453–461.
76. Walker RG, Thomson NM, Dowling JP, et al. Minocycline-induced acute interstitial nephritis. *BMJ* 1979;1:524.
77. Fabre J, Milek E, Kalfopoulos P. The kinetics of tetracycline in man: excretion, penetration in normal inflammatory tissues, behavior in renal insufficiency, and hemodialysis. *Schweiz Med Wochenschr* 1971;101:625–633.
78. Gabzuda GJ, Gocke TM, Jackson GG, et al. Some effects of antibiotics on nutrition in man including studies of the bacterial flora of the feces. *Arch Intern Med* 1958;101:476–513.
79. Angeloni VL, Salasche SJ, Ortiz R. Nail, skin, and scleral pigmentation induced by minocycline. *Cutis* 1987;40:229–234.
80. Fenske NA, Millns JL, Greer KE. Minocycline-induced pigmentation at sites of cutaneous inflammation. *JAMA* 1980;24:1103–1106.
81. Wasel NR, Schloss EH, Lin An. Minocycline-induced cutaneous pigmentation. *J Cutan Med Surg* 1998;3:105–108.
82. Eisen D, Hakim MD. Minocycline-induced pigmentation: incidence, prevention and management. *Drug Saf* 1998;431–440.
83. Brown TM, Bush S, Felts W. PPLO and their possible relation to articular disease. In: *American Rheumatism Association rheumatic diseases.* Philadelphia: WB Saunders, 1952:401.
84. Brown TM, Bush S, Felts W. Rheumatoid diseases and gout, long-term illnesses: management of the chronically ill patient. In: Wohl MG, ed. Long-Term Illness: Management of the Chronically Ill Patient. Philadelphia: WB Saunders, 1959:93–125.
85. Sanchez I. Tetracycline treatment in rheumatoid arthritis and other rheumatic diseases. *Braz Med* 1968;82:22–31.
86. Skinner M, Cathcart E, Mills J, et al. Tetracycline in the treatment of rheumatoid arthritis: a double-blind controlled study. *Arthritis Rheum* 1971;14:727–732.
87. Breedveld F, Trentham D. Suppression of collagen and adjuvant arthritis by a tetracycline. *Arthritis Rheum* 1988;31:R3.
88. Langevitz P, Bank I, Zemer D, et al. Treatment of resistant rheumatoid arthritis with minocycline: an open study. *J Rheumatol* 1992;19:1502–1504.
89. Kloppenburg M, Ferdinand C, Terwiel J, et al. Minocycline in active rheumatoid arthritis. *Arthritis Rheum* 1994;37:629–636.
90. Tilley BC, Alarcon GS, Heyse SP, et al. Minocycline in rheumatoid arthritis: a 48-week, double-blind, placebo-controlled trial. *Ann Intern Med* 1995;122:81–89.
91. Bluhm GB, Sharp JT, Tilley BC, et al. Radiographic results from the Minocycline in Rheumatoid Arthritis (MIRA) trial. *J Rheumatol* 1997; 24:1295–1302.
92. Alarcon GS, Bartolucci AA. Radiographic assessment of disease progression in rheumatoid arthritis patients treated with methotrexate or minocycline. *J Rheumatol* 2000; 27:530–534.
93. O'Dell JR, Haire CE, Palmer W, et al. Treatment of early rheumatoid arthritis with minocycline or placebo. *Arthritis Rheum* 19971;40:842–848.
94. O'Dell JR, Paulsen G, Haire CE, et al. Treatment of early seropositive rheumatoid arthritis with minocycline. *Arthritis Rheum* 1999;42: 1691–1695.
95. O'Dell JR, Blakely KW, Mallek JA, et al. Treatment of early seropositive rheumatoid arthritis: a two year, double-blind comparison of minocycline and hydroxychloroquine. *Arthritis Rheum* 2001;44: 2235–2241.
96. Weinberger A, Ben-gal T, Roizman P, et al. Intraarticular minocycline injection in experimental synovitis. *Clin Rheumatol* 1996;15: 290–294.
97. Hassell A, Fowler P, Dawes P. Intra-bursal tetracycline in the treatment of olecranon bursitis in patients with rheumatoid arthritis. *BJM* 1994;33:859–860.
98. St Clair EW, Wilkinson WE, Pisetsky DS, et al. The effects of intravenous doxycycline therapy for rheumatoid arthritis: a randomized, double-blind, placebo-controlled trial. *Arthritis Rheum* 2001;44: 1043–1047.
99. Van der Laan W, Molenaar E, Ronday K, et al. Lack of effect of doxycycline on disease activity and joint damage in patients with rheumatoid arthritis. A double blind, placebo controlled trial. *J Rheumatol* 2001;28:1967–1974.
100. Pillemer S, Gulko P, Ligier S, et al. Pilot clinical trial of intravenous doxycycline versus placebo for rheumatoid arthritis. *J Rheumatol* 2003;30:41–43.
101. Smieja M, MacPherson DW, Kean W, et al. Randomised, blinded, placebo controlled trial of doxycycline for chronic seronegative arthritis. *Ann Rheum Dis* 2001;60:1088–1094.
102. Yu LP Jr, Smith GN, Brandt, KD, et al. Reduction of the severity of canine ostoeoarthritis by prophylactic treatment with oral doxycycline. *Arthritis Rheum* 1992;35:1150–1159.
103. Yu LP Jr, Burr DB, Brandt KD, et al. Effects of oral doxycycline administration on histomorphometry and dynamics of subchondral bone in a canine model of osteoarthritis. *J Rheumatol* 1996;23:137–142.
104. Smith GN Jr, Yu LP Jr, Brandt KD, et al. Oral administration of doxycycline reduces collagenase and gelatinase activities in extracts of human osteoarthritis cartilage. *J Rheumatol* 1998;25:532–535.
105. NCCAM. About the National Center for Complementary and Alternative Medicine. 2003.
106. National Center for Complementary and Alternative Medicine. NCCAM funding: appropriations history.
107. Eisenberg DM, Davis RB, et al. Trends in alternative medicine use in the United States, 1990–1997: results of a follow-up national survey. *JAMA* 1998;280:1569–1575.
108. Rao JK, Mihaliak K, et al. Use of complementary therapies for arthritis among patients of rheumatologists. *Ann Intern Med* 1999;131: 409–416.
109. Davidoff F. Weighing the alternatives: lessons from the paradoxes of alternative medicine. *Ann Intern Med* 1998;129:1068–1070.
110. Panush RS. Shift happens: complementary and alternative medicine for rheumatologists. *J Rheumatol* 2002;29:656–658.
111. Whitfield AG. The William Withering bicentennial lecture. William Withering and "an account of the foxglove." *Q J Med* 1985;57:709–711.
112. Kean WF, Forestier F, et al. The history of gold therapy in rheumatoid disease. *Semin Arthritis Rheum* 1985;14:180–186.
113. Alpert JS. The relativity of alternative medicine. *Arch Intern Med* 1995;155:2385.
114. Kaptchuk TJ. The placebo effect in alternative medicine: can the performance of a healing ritual have clinical significance? *Ann Intern Med* 2002;136:817–825.
115. Crow R, Gage H, et al. The role of expectancies in the placebo effect and their use in the delivery of health care: a systematic review. *Health Technol Assess* 1999;3:1–96.
116. Williams HJ, Ward JR, et al. A controlled trial comparing sulfasalazine, gold sodium thiomalate, and placebo in rheumatoid arthritis. *Arthritis Rheum* 1988;31:702–713.
117. Pendleton A, Arden N, et al. EULAR recommendations for the management of knee osteoarthritis: report of a task force of the Standing Committee for International Clinical Studies Including Therapeutic Trials (ESCISIT). *Ann Rheum Dis* 2000;59:936–944.
118. Theodosakis J, Adderly B, et al. *The arthritis cure.* New York: St. Martin's, 1997.

119. Theodosakis J, Adderly B, et al. *Maximizing the arthritis cure.* New York: St. Martin's, 1998.
120. Bassleer C, Rovati L, et al. Stimulation of proteoglycan production by glucosamine sulfate in chondrocytes isolated from human osteoarthritic articular cartilage *in vitro. Osteoarthritis Cartilage* 1998;6: 427–434.
122. Deal CL, Moskowitz RW. Nutraceuticals as therapeutic agents in osteoarthritis. The role of glucosamine, chondroitin sulfate, and collagen hydrolysate. *Rheum Dis Clin North Am* 1999;25:379–395.
123. McAlindon TE, LaValley MP, et al. Glucosamine and chondroitin for treatment of osteoarthritis: a systematic quality assessment and meta-analysis. *JAMA* 2000;283:1469–1475.
124. Vajaradul Y. Double-blind clinical evaluation of intra-articular glucosamine in outpatients with gonarthrosis. *Clin Ther* 1981;3:336–343.
125. Reichelt A, Forster KK, et al. Efficacy and safety of intramuscular glucosamine sulfate in osteoarthritis of the knee. A randomised, placebo-controlled, double-blind study. *Arzneimittelforschung* 1994; 44:75–80.
126. Rovati L. The clinical profile of glucosamine sulfate as a selective symptom modifying drug in osteoarthritis: current data and perspectives. *Osteoarthritis Cartilage* 1997;5(suppl A):72.
127. Pujalte JM, Llavore EP, et al. Double-blind clinical evaluation of oral glucosamine sulphate in the basic treatment of osteoarthrosis. *Curr Med Res Opin* 1980;7:110–114.
128. Noack W, Fischer M, et al. Glucosamine sulfate in osteoarthritis of the knee. *Osteoarthritis Cartilage* 1994;2:51–59.
129. Houpt JB, McMillan R, et al. Effect of glucosamine hydrochloride in the treatment of pain of osteoarthritis of the knee. *J Rheumatol* 1999;26:2423–2430.
130. Reginster JY, Deroisy R, et al. Long-term effects of glucosamine sulphate on osteoarthritis progression: a randomised, placebo-controlled clinical trial. *Lancet* 2001;357:251–256.
131. Pavelka K, Gatterova J, et al. Glucosamine sulfate use and delay of progression of knee osteoarthritis: a 3-year, randomized, placebo-controlled, double-blind study. *Arch Intern Med* 2002;162:2113–2123.
131. Setnikar I, Giacchetti C, et al. Pharmacokinetics of glucosamine in the dog and in man. *Arzneimittelforschung* 1986;36:729–735.
132. Mazzuca SA, Brandt KD, et al. Knee pain reduces joint space width in conventional standing anteroposterior radiographs of osteoarthritic knees. *Arthritis Rheum* 2002;46:1223–1227.
133. Buckland-Wright JC, Wolfe F, et al. Substantial superiority of semiflexed (MTP) views in knee osteoarthritis: a comparative radiographic study, without fluoroscopy, of standing extended, semiflexed (MTP), and schuss views. *J Rheumatol* 1999;26:2664–2674.
134. Heyneman CA, Rhodes RS. Glucosamine for osteoarthritis: cure or conundrum? *Ann Pharmacother* 1998;32:602–603.
135. McClain DA, Crook ED. Hexosamines and insulin resistance. *Diabetes* 1996;45:1003–1009.
136. Rossetti L. Perspective: hexosamines and nutrient sensing. *Endocrinology* 2000;141:1922–1925.
137. Tang J, Neidigh JL, et al. Transgenic mice with increased hexosamine flux specifically targeted to beta-cells exhibit hyperinsulinemia and peripheral insulin resistance. *Diabetes* 2000;49:1492–1499.
138. Conte A, de Bernardi M, et al. Metabolic fate of exogenous chondroitin sulfate in man. *Arzneimittelforschung* 1991;41:768–772.
139. Conte A, Palmieri L, et al. Metabolic fate of partially depolymerized chondroitin sulfate administered to the rat. *Drugs Exp Clin Res* 1991;17:27–33.
140. Conte A, Volpi N, et al. Biochemical and pharmacokinetic aspects of oral treatment with chondroitin sulfate. *Arzneimittelforschung* 1995; 45:918–925.
141. Ronca F, Palmieri L, et al. Anti-inflammatory activity of chondroitin sulfate. *Osteoarthritis Cartilage* 1998;6(suppl A):14–21.
142. Nishikawa H, Mori I, et al. Influences of sulfated glycosaminoglycans on biosynthesis of hyaluronic acid in rabbit knee synovial membrane. *Arch Biochem Biophys* 1985;240:146–153.
143. Kerzberg EM, Roldan EJ, et al. Combination of glycosaminoglycans and acetylsalicylic acid in knee osteoarthrosis. *Scand J Rheumatol* 1987;16:377–380.
144. Rovetta G. Galactosaminoglycuronoglycan sulfate (matrix) in therapy of tibiofibular osteoarthritis of the knee. *Drugs Exp Clin Res* 1991;17:53–57.
145. L'Hirondel J. Double-blind clinical trial of oral chondroitin sulfate versus placebo for tibiofemoral osteoarthritis (125 patients). *Litera Rhumatol* 1992;14:77–84.
146. Mazieres B, Loyau G, et al. Chondroitin sulfate in the treatment of gonarthrosis and coxarthrosis. 5-months result of a multicenter double-blind controlled prospective study using placebo. *Rev Rhum Mal Osteoartic* 1992;59:466–472.
147. Pavelka K Jr, Sedlackova M, et al. Glycosaminoglycan polysulfuric acid (GAGPS) in osteoarthritis of the knee. *Osteoarthritis Cartilage* 1995;3:15–23.
148. Bourgeois P, Chales G, et al. Efficacy and tolerability of chondroitin sulfate 1200 mg/day vs chondroitin sulfate 3 × 400 mg/day vs placebo. *Osteoarthritis Cartilage* 1998;6(suppl A):25–30.
149. Bucsi L, Poor G. (1998). Efficacy and tolerability of oral chondroitin sulfate as a symptomatic slow-acting drug for osteoarthritis (SYSADOA) in the treatment of knee osteoarthritis. *Osteoarthritis Cartilage* 1998;6(suppl A):31–36.
150. Conrozier T. Anti-arthrosis treatments: efficacy and tolerance of chondroitin sulfates (CS 4&6). *Presse Med* 1998;27:1862–1865.
151. Uebelhart D, Thonar EJ, et al. Effects of oral chondroitin sulfate on the progression of knee osteoarthritis: a pilot study. *Osteoarthritis Cartilage* 1998;6(suppl A):39–46.
152. Leeb BF, Schweitzer H, et al. A metaanalysis of chondroitin sulfate in the treatment of osteoarthritis. *J Rheumatol* 2000;27:205–211.
153. Lippiello L, Woodward J, et al. *In vivo* chondroprotection and metabolic synergy of glucosamine and chondroitin sulfate. *Clin Orthop* 2000;381:229–240.
154. Hanson RR, Smolley LR, et al. Oral treatment with a glucosamine-chondroitin sulfate compound for degenerative joint disease in horses: 25 cases. *Equine Pract* 1997;19:16–20.
155. Canapp SO Jr, McLaughlin RM Jr, et al. Scintigraphic evaluation of dogs with acute synovitis after treatment with glucosamine hydrochloride and chondroitin sulfate. *Am J Vet Res* 1999;60:1552–1557.
156. Kremer JM, Jubiz W, et al. Fish-oil fatty acid supplementation in active rheumatoid arthritis. A double-blinded, controlled, crossover study. *Ann Intern Med* 1987;106:497–503.
157. Cleland LG, French JK, et al. Clinical and biochemical effects of dietary fish oil supplements in rheumatoid arthritis. *J Rheumatol* 1988;15:1471–1475.
158. Kremer JM, Lawrence DA, et al. Dietary fish oil and olive oil supplementation in patients with rheumatoid arthritis. Clinical and immunologic effects. *Arthritis Rheum* 1990;33:810–820.
159. van der Tempel H, Tulleken JE, et al. Effects of fish oil supplementation in rheumatoid arthritis. *Ann Rheum Dis* 1990;49:76–80.
160. Skoldstam L, Borjesson O, et al. Effect of six months of fish oil supplementation in stable rheumatoid arthritis. A double-blind, controlled study. *Scand J Rheumatol* 1992;21:178–185.
161. Kremer JM, Lawrence DA, et al. Effects of high-dose fish oil on rheumatoid arthritis after stopping nonsteroidal antiinflammatory drugs. Clinical and immune correlates. *Arthritis Rheum* 1995;38: 1107–1114.
162. Sperling RI. Dietary omega-3 fatty acids: effects on lipid mediators of inflammation and rheumatoid arthritis. *Rheum Dis Clin North Am* 1991;17:373–389.
163. Stramentinoli G. Pharmacologic aspects of *S*-adenosylmethionine. Pharmacokinetics and pharmacodynamics. *Am J Med* 1987;83: 35–42.
164. Soeken KL, Lee WL, et al. Safety and efficacy of *S*-adenosylmethionine (SAMe) for osteoarthritis. *J Fam Pract* 2002;51:425–430.
165. Trentham DE, Dynesius-Trentham RA, et al. Effects of oral administration of type II collagen on rheumatoid arthritis. *Science* 1993;261: 1727–1730.
166. Sieper J, Kary S, et al. Oral type II collagen treatment in early rheumatoid arthritis. A double-blind, placebo-controlled, randomized trial. *Arthritis Rheum* 1996;39:41–51.
167. Barnett ML, Kremer JM, et al. Treatment of rheumatoid arthritis with oral type II collagen. Results of a multicenter, double-blind, placebo-controlled trial. *Arthritis Rheum* 1998;41:290–297.
168. Cazzola M, Antivalle M, et al. Oral type II collagen in the treatment of rheumatoid arthritis. A six-month double blind placebo-controlled study. *Clin Exp Rheumatol* 2000;18:571–577.

169. Choy EH, Scott DL, et al. Control of rheumatoid arthritis by oral tolerance. *Arthritis Rheum* 2001;44:1993–1997.
170. Awang D. Ginger. *Can Pharm J* 1992;125:309–311.
171. Altman RD, Marcussen KC. Effects of a ginger extract on knee pain in patients with osteoarthritis. *Arthritis Rheum* 2001;44:2531–2538.
172. Mustafa T, Srivastava KC, et al. Drug development: report 9, pharmacology of ginger, *Zingiber officinale. J Drug Dev* 1993;6:25–89.
173. Kiuchi, F, Iwakami S, et al. Inhibition of prostaglandin and leukotriene biosynthesis by gingerols and diarylheptanoids. *Chem Pharm Bull (Tokyo)* 1992;40:387–391.
174. Mascolo N, Jain R, et al. Ethnopharmacologic investigation of ginger (*Zingiber officinale*). *J Ethnopharmacol* 1989;27:129–140.
175. Bliddal H, Rosetzsky A, et al. A randomized, placebo-controlled, cross-over study of ginger extracts and ibuprofen in osteoarthritis. *Osteoarthritis Cartilage* 2000;8:9–12.
176. Marcus DM, Suarez-Almazor ME. Is there a role for ginger in the treatment of osteoarthritis? *Arthritis Rheum* 2001;44:2461–2462.
177. Chrubasik S, Junck H, et al. Effectiveness of *Harpagophytum* extract WS 1531 in the treatment of exacerbation of low back pain: a randomized, placebo-controlled, double-blind study. *Eur J Anaesthesiol* 1999;16:118–129.
178. Chrubasik S, Zimpfer C, et al. Effectiveness of *Harpagophytum procumbens* in treatment of acute low back pain. *Phytomedicine* 1996;3:1–10.
179. Ernest E, Chrubasik S. Phyto-anti-inflammatories: a systematic review of randomized, placebo-controlled, double-blind trials. *Rheum Dis Clin North Am* 2000;26:13–27.
180. American College of Rheumatology Subcommittee on Osteoarthritis Guidelines. Recommendations for the medical management of osteoarthritis of the hip and knee: 2000 update. *Arthritis Rheum* 2000;43:1905–1915.
181. McCarthy GM, McCarty DJ. Effect of topical capsaicin in the therapy of painful osteoarthritis of the hands. *J Rheumatol* 1992;19:604–607.
182. Deal CL, Schnitzer TJ, et al. Treatment of arthritis with topical capsaicin: a double-blind trial. *Clin Ther* 1991;13:383–395.
183. Trice JM, Pinals RS. Dimethyl sulfoxide: a review of its use in the rheumatic disorders. *Semin Arthritis Rheum* 1985;15:45–60.
184. Williams HJ, Furst DE, et al. Double-blind, multicenter controlled trial comparing topical dimethyl sulfoxide and normal saline for treatment of hand ulcers in patients with systemic sclerosis. *Arthritis Rheum* 1985;28:308–314.
185. Steinberg A. The employment of dimethyl sulfoxide as an antiinflammatory agent and steroid-transporter in diversified clinical diseases. *Ann NY Acad Sci* 1967;141:532–550.
186. John H, Laudahn G. Clinical experiences with the topical application of DMSO in orthopedic diseases: evaluation of 4180 cases. *Ann NY Acad Sci* 1967;141:506–516.
187. Brown JH. Clinical experience with DMSO in acute musculoskeletal conditions comparing a noncontrolled series with a controlled double blind study. *Ann NY Acad Sci* 1967;141:496–505.
188. Percy EC, Carson JD. The use of DMSO in tennis elbow and rotator cuff tendonitis: a double-blind study. *Med Sci Sports Exerc* 1981;13:215–219.
189. Vuopala U, Vesterinen E, et al. The analgetic action of dimethyl sulfoxide (DMSO) ointment in arthrosis. A double blind study. *Acta Rheumatol Scand* 1971;17:57–60.
190. Fiechtner JJ, Brodeur RR. Manual and manipulation techniques for rheumatic disease. *Med Clin North Am* 2002;86:91–103.
191. Meeker WC, Haldeman S. Chiropractic: a profession at the crossroads of mainstream and alternative medicine. *Ann Intern Med* 2002;136:216–227.
192. Assendelft WJ, Koes BW, et al. The relationship between methodological quality and conclusions in reviews of spinal manipulation. *JAMA* 1995;274:1942–1948.
193. Jonas WB, Linde K, et al. Homeopathy and rheumatic disease. *Rheum Dis Clin North Am* 2000;26:117–123, x.
194. Linde K, Clausius N, et al. Are the clinical effects of homeopathy placebo effects? A meta-analysis of placebo-controlled trials. *Lancet* 1997;350:834–843.
195. Eisenberg DM, Kessler RC, et al. Unconventional medicine in the United States. Prevalence, costs, and patterns of use. *N Engl J Med* 1993;328:246–252.
196. Berman BM, Swyers JP, et al. The evidence for acupuncture as a treatment for rheumatologic conditions. *Rheum Dis Clin North Am* 2000;26:103–115, ix–x.
197. Thomas M, Eriksson SV, et al. A comparative study of diazepam and acupuncture in patients with osteoarthritis pain: a placebo controlled study. *Am J Chin Med* 1991;19:95–100.
198. Berman BM, Singh BB, et al. A randomized trial of acupuncture as an adjunctive therapy in osteoarthritis of the knee. *Rheumatology (Oxford)* 1999;38:346–354.
199. Deluze C, Bosia L, et al. Electroacupuncture in fibromyalgia: results of a controlled trial. *BMJ* 1992;305:1249–1252.
200. Cheng TO, Lee RJ, et al. Subacute bacterial endocarditis following ear acupuncture. *Int J Cardiol* 1985;8:97.
201. Vittecoq D, Mettetal JF, et al. Acute HIV infection after acupuncture treatments. *N Engl J Med* 1989;320:250–251.

CHAPTER 44

Mechanisms of Pain and Pain Modulation

Laurence A. Bradley

THE MULTIDIMENSIONAL NATURE OF PAIN

Pain is an "unpleasant sensory and emotional experience associated with actual or potential tissue damage, or described in terms of such damage" (1). Acute pain usually alerts an individual to the danger or presence of tissue damage, severity of the tissue damage, or the presence of an underlying disease process. In contrast, recurrent or chronic pain represents pain that persists despite appropriate medical care. Although recurrent and chronic pain may also signify the presence of disease (e.g., gastrointestinal reflux, rheumatoid arthritis) or central nervous system dysregulation (e.g., neuropathic pain), it frequently is only modestly correlated with either the presence of tissue damage (e.g., fibromyalgia) or severity of the damage (e.g., knee osteoarthritis) (2,3).

The above definition also conveys the subjective and multidimensional nature of pain. Health-care professionals tend to focus primarily on patients' verbal descriptions or behavioral displays of the location, frequency (as well as the intensity), and sensory (e.g., burning, aching) dimensions of pain because these data provide helpful information for medical decision making. However, it is equally important to attend to the cognitive and emotional dimensions of pain. That is, pain evokes various emotional responses and cognitions (e.g., expectations or beliefs) regarding the extent, severity, time course, and meaning of acute or recurrent pain episodes. These multiple dimensions of the pain experience, in conjunction with reflexive autonomic responses generated by pain, provide information about the individual's psychological status and they drive health-related behavior such as decisions to seek medical care or adherence with medical regimens (4,5).

It is important to note that pain-related cognitions and emotional responses are influenced by multiple factors, including the intensity and sensory dimensions of the pain, the individual's autonomic responses, history of illnesses and pain experiences, and cultural influences, as well as the responses of others to displays of verbal or motor pain behavior. Acute pain generally is associated with varying levels of anxiety. In contrast, chronic or recurrent pain that is not well controlled by pharmacologic or other therapies tends to be associated with depression or other negative emotional responses, especially among patients with poor coping resources. These negative emotional responses, in conjunction with negative, pain-related beliefs, may produce maladaptive behavioral responses (e.g., inappropriate medication usage, helplessness).

This chapter will describe the neural bases of pain and pain modulation. It begins with a discussion of the physiologic basis and neural representation of afferent nociceptive transmission. Special emphasis is devoted to the mechanisms underlying central sensitization given that increased spinal neural excitability contributes to many conditions characterized by chronic pain, including rheumatologic diseases. The chapter will then review descending neural pathways involved in pain modulation and the literature concerning abnormal pain inhibition in patients with rheumatologic diseases. The chapter will conclude with a review of quantitative sensory testing (QST) methods used in human studies of pain and pain modulation as well as new measures of cognitive and affective factors that may influence the pain responses of patients with rheumatologic diseases.

NEURAL MECHANISMS OF NOCICEPTION AND PAIN MODULATION

Ascending Nociceptive Pathways and Pain Processing

Nociceptors and Primary Afferents

The peripheral sensory fibers that innervate all body tissues respond to mechanical pressure as well as thermal (heat and cold), chemical, and metabolic (e.g., bradykinin, low pH) stimuli. These fibers include nociceptors that respond to noxious stimuli such as heat, cold, or mechanical pressure that are associated with potential or actual tissue damage. Signals from these nociceptors are transmitted by primary afferent fibers from peripheral tissues to the spinal cord and brain. These primary afferents have thinly myelinated (Aβ, Aδ) or unmyelinated (C) fibers that differ in function. Some A fiber afferents respond specifically to noxious mechanical stimuli, noxious thermal stimuli, or both. However, all A afferents are rapidly activated and transmit signals that tend to produce perceptions of relatively sharp pain that is referred to as "first pain." First pain, then, is particularly important in the avoidance of tissue-damaging stimuli that may threaten the integrity of the individual. In contrast, most C fiber afferents respond to noxious mechanical, thermal, and chemical stimuli. Some of the C fiber afferents do not respond to noxious stimuli unless they are sensitized by inflammatory agents. Nevertheless, all C fiber afferents are activated more slowly than the A afferents and tend to produce perceptions of aching or burning pain that is referred to as "second pain." Second pain tends to be more enduring and unpleasant than first pain and thus is highly relevant to pain associated with chronic medical conditions (6).

Spinothalamocortical Projections

The primary afferents ascend in a contralateral manner and enter the spinal cord through the medial division of the dorsal roots and terminate in lamina I and II of the superficial dorsal horn. Collaterals of these afferents also terminate in lamina V. The primary afferents activate secondary neurons within the dorsal horn through the release of several excitatory neurotransmitters (Fig. 44.1A,B). The main excitatory transmitter from the peripheral afferent fibers is glutamate, which acts on postsynaptic *N*-methyl-D-aspartate (NMDA) receptors of dorsal horn neurons. Other excitatory molecules include substance P and neurokinin A (NK), both of which act on postsynaptic NK receptors of the dorsal horn neurons as well as calcitonin gene-related peptide (CGRP), nerve growth factor, and dynorphin A (7). It should be noted that there are distinct types of neurons in lamina I and II that respond to specific stimuli within small receptive fields (e.g., in muscle or joint). The nociceptive-specific lamina I and II cells are dominated by A fiber input. The nociceptive neurons in lamina V respond to both noxious and nonnoxious mechanical stimuli. These neurons, termed wide dynamic range neurons, integrate afferent activity from all somatic tissues.

The signals generated by the secondary neurons within the dorsal horn are then transmitted to several brain regions via their axons, which travel in three primary ascending tracts that project to the thalamus and reticular formation. The spinothalamic tracts provide the major direct nociceptive input from the spinal cord to lateral, medial, and posterior thalamic nuclei (6). Direct spinothalamic tract projections to the ventral posterior lateral and ventral posterior inferior nucleus excite neurons with projections to the primary (S1) and secondary (S2) somatosensory cortices. These cortical regions are involved in discrimination of the intensity, spatial, and temporal aspects of pain as well as in the anticipation of painful stimuli (8). Spinothalamic tract projections to the posterior thalamic nuclei (i.e., pulvinar oralis, suprageniculate nucleus) excite neurons with projections to the insular cortex, which, because of its connections with the amygdala, prefrontal cortex, and cingulate cortex, is involved in affective, cognitive, and autonomic responses to nociception. One highly important function of the insular and prefrontal cortices may be the integration of nociceptive signals with memory to allow the individual to ascertain the meaning and potential threats associated with sources of painful stimuli (9).

Fibers in the anterior part of the anterolateral spinothalamic tract that originate in the contralateral posterior horns end in the gigantocellular part of the medulla and pons and in the lateral reticular nucleus. Fibers or collaterals from these areas terminate in the medial geniculate body, the posterior group, and the intralaminar nuclei of the thalamus (6). The intralaminar nuclei are an important group of medial thalamic nuclei that are considered to be a cranial extension of the brainstem reticular formation and have connections with both the prefrontal cortex and the cingulate cortex. The anterior cingulate cortex is an extensive area of the limbic cortex overlying the corpus collosum. It is especially important in pain processing because it is involved in the integration of cognition, affect, and response selection. In addition, descending connections of the anterior cingulate cortex to the medial thalamic nuclei and to the periaqueductal gray (PAG) in the brainstem suggest that this system may also be involved in the modulation of reflex responses to noxious stimuli.

Additional Nociceptive Pathways Involved in Pain Affect and Cognition

In addition to the classical spinothalamocortical pathways described above, several additional ascending nociceptive pathways recently have been mapped in animal studies that originate in the spinal cord and project to specific areas of the brainstem and then farther rostrally to various brain structures involved in emotional and cognitive processes (10). One pathway projects from the spinal dorsal horns to the dorsocaudal medulla (subnucleus reticularis dorsalis) and then to the ventromedian nucleus of the thalamus and the dorsolateral frontal lobes (11). Another ascending pathway projects from the spinal cord to the parabrachial nucleus (Pb) and then to the hypothalamus and amygdala (12). In addition, there are pathways that transmit nociceptive signals from the Pb to the (a) intralaminar thalamus and subsequently to the frontal cortices, and (b) central nucleus of the amygdala and on to the basal forebrain (13,14). It is likely that, in humans, these pathways

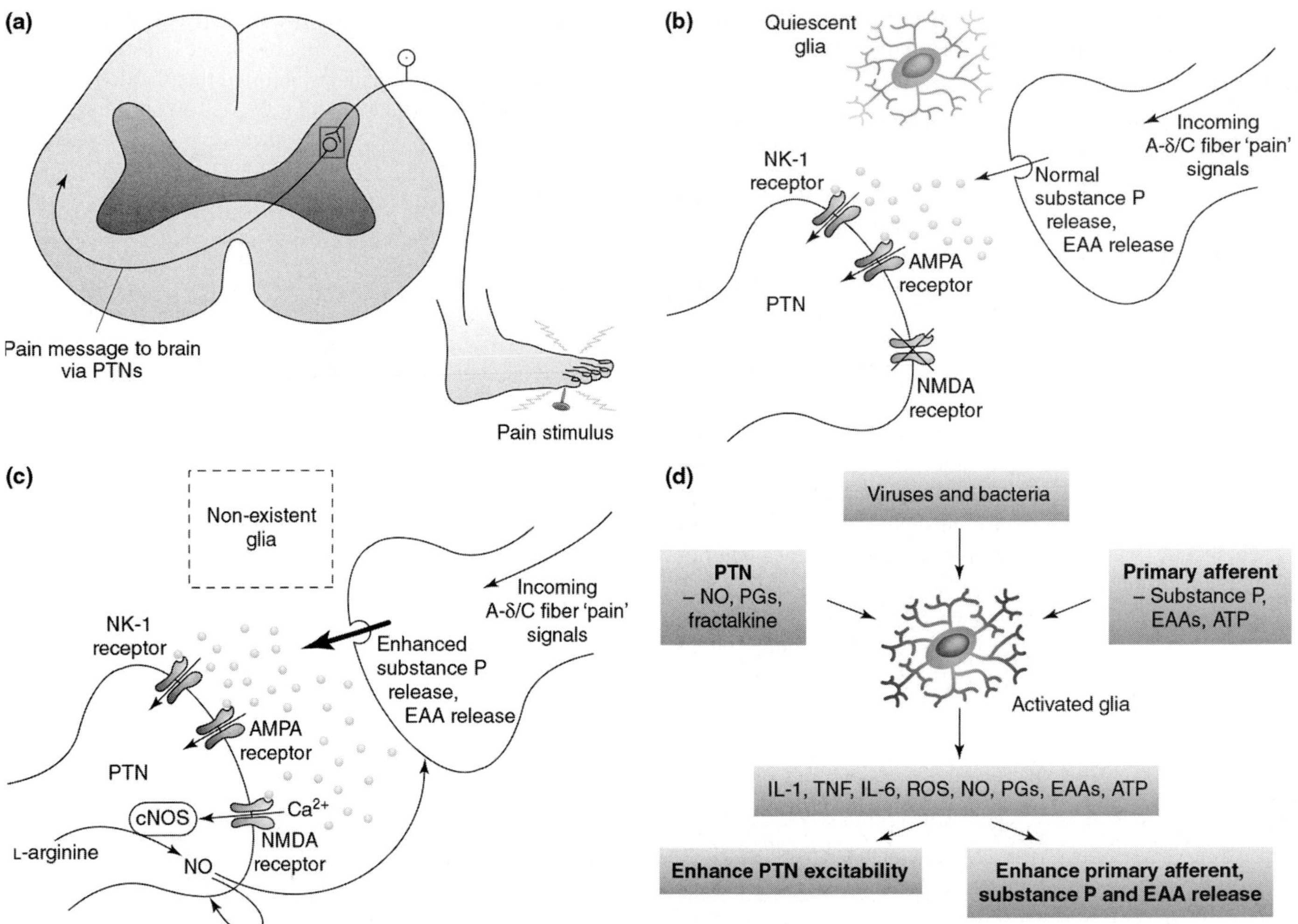

FIG. 44.1. A, B: Classic view of pain signaling. A noxious stimulus activates peripheral A-δ and C nerve fibers that transmit action potentials to their presynaptic terminals in the spinal dorsal horns. Substance P and excitatory amino acids (EAAs) are released that bind to and activate postsynaptic receptors [i.e., neurokinin (NK)-1, alpha-amino-3-hydroxy-5-methylisoxazole-4-proprionic acid (AMPA)] located on second-order pain transmission neurons (PTNs) that ascend to the brain carrying sensory input that may produce perceptions of pain. The *N*-methyl-D-aspartate (NMDA)-linked channels are inoperative because they are "plugged" by Mg^{2+} and the glia cells are not activated. **C:** Classic view of pathologic pain evoked by central sensitization. Intense or prolonged sensory input from A-δ and C afferents sufficiently depolarizes the dorsal horn neurons so that Mg^{2+} exits NMDA-linked ion channels. This is followed by an influx of extracellular Ca^{2+} and production of nitric oxide (NO), which diffuses out of the dorsal horn neurons. NO, in turn, promotes the exaggerated release of excitatory amino acids and substance P from presynaptic afferent terminals and causes the dorsal horn neurons to become hyperexcitable. Glia cell activation has not been considered relevant to central sensitization. **D:** Current view of pathologic pain. Glia cells are activated by release of viruses and bacteria as well as by release of NO, prostaglandins (PGs), fractalkine, substance P, adenosine triphosphate (ATP), and EAAs from primary afferents and PTNs. These glia cells release proinflammatory cytokines, NO, PGs, reactive oxygen species (ROS), ATP, EAAs such as glutamate, substance P, and calcitonin gene-related peptide (GGRP). These substances enhance depolarization of NMDA receptor sites in the dorsal horn and thus maintain or further drive pathological pain states. (Reproduced from Watkins LR, Milligan ED, Maier SF. Glial activation: a driving force for pathological pain. *Trends Neurosci* 2001;24:450–455, with permission.) *IL,* interleukin; *NOS,* nitric oxide synthase; *TNF,* tumor necrosis factor.

help mediate the interactions between pain and the cognitive and emotional responses observed in humans.

Representation of Nociceptive Transmission Associated with Pain Experience

Neuroimaging of pain-induced changes in functional brain activity dates back to 1976, when Ingvar and associates (15) showed that electrical stimulation of the fingers of eight healthy volunteers produced perceptions of mild pain and increased regional cerebral blood flow in the frontal cortex by 11% (Table 44.1). Most of the neuroimaging studies of healthy individuals performed from 1980 to 2000 in the 1990s focused primarily on the classical spinothalamocortical pathways described above. These studies consistently showed that phasic thermal nociceptive stimuli tend to increase functional activity in the contralateral hemisphere of several brain areas known to contribute to the experience of pain such as the S1, S2, thalamus, and insular and anterior cingulate cortices.

Recent studies have begun to examine very interesting issues such as the coding of changes in stimulus intensity, neural representations of individual differences in pain sensitivity, effects of experimental manipulations of pain-related affect, and brain activity associated with analgesic responses. With regard to coding of changes in stimulus intensity, Coghill and colleagues reported that the delivery of intensity-graded thermal stimuli (35° to 50°C) produce reliable increases in participants' ratings of pain intensity (20). More importantly, increases in stimulus intensity and perceived pain intensity show linear increases in functional activity within the (a) contralateral S1; (b) ipsilateral premotor area; and (c) contralateral and ipsilateral cerebellum, putamen, thalamus, insular cortex, anterior cingulate cortex, and S2 (Fig. 44.2). These findings suggest that, although specific brain regions tend to have particular roles in processing the sensory and cognitive-affective dimensions of pain, the processing of pain intensity tends to be distributed across multiple regions in both cerebral hemispheres. Intensity processing, then, is a critical component of the sensory, affective, and cognitive dimensions of the pain experience. In addition, the wide neural distribution of intensity processing may contribute to survival because it increases the likelihood that tissue damage can be detected even if extensive injury to the cerebral cortex occurs.

It is well-known that there are marked differences among individuals in their perceptions of the intensity of quantified stimuli in the laboratory. Coghill and colleagues (21)

TABLE 44.1. *Changes in regional cerebral blood flow (rCBF) in response to induction of experimental or clinical pain in healthy individuals*

Study	Subjects	Type of stimulation	rCBF changes
Ingvar et al. (15)	Healthy	Electrical	Frontal cortex
Jones et al. (16)	Healthy	Phasic thermal	Contralateral thalamus Contralateral lenticular nucleus Contralateral anterior cingulate cortex
Talbot et al. (17)	Healthy	Phasic thermal	Contralateral thalamus Contralateral anterior cingulate cortex Contralateral primary somatosensory cortex Contralateral secondary somatosensory cortex
Coghill et al. (18)	Healthy	Phasic thermal	Contralateral thalamus Contralateral insula Contralateral anterior cingulate cortex Contralateral primary somatosensory cortex Contralateral secondary somatosensory cortex
Casey et al. (19)	Healthy	Phasic thermal	Thalamus, bilateral Contralateral insula Contralateral anterior cingulate cortex Contralateral primary somatosensory cortex Contralateral secondary somatosensory cortex
Coghill et al. (20)	Healthy	Graded thermal	Cerebellum, bilateral Putamen, bilateral Thalamus, bilateral Insula, bilateral Anterior cingulate cortex, bilateral Secondary somatosensory cortex, bilateral Contralateral primary somatosensory cortex Contralateral supplementary motor area Ipsilateral ventral premotor area Ipsilateral prefrontal cortex

Adapted from Bradley LA, McKendree-Smith NL, Alberts KR, et al. Use of neuroimaging to understand abnormal pain sensitivity in fibromyalgia. *Curr Rheum Rep* 2000;2:141–148, with permission.

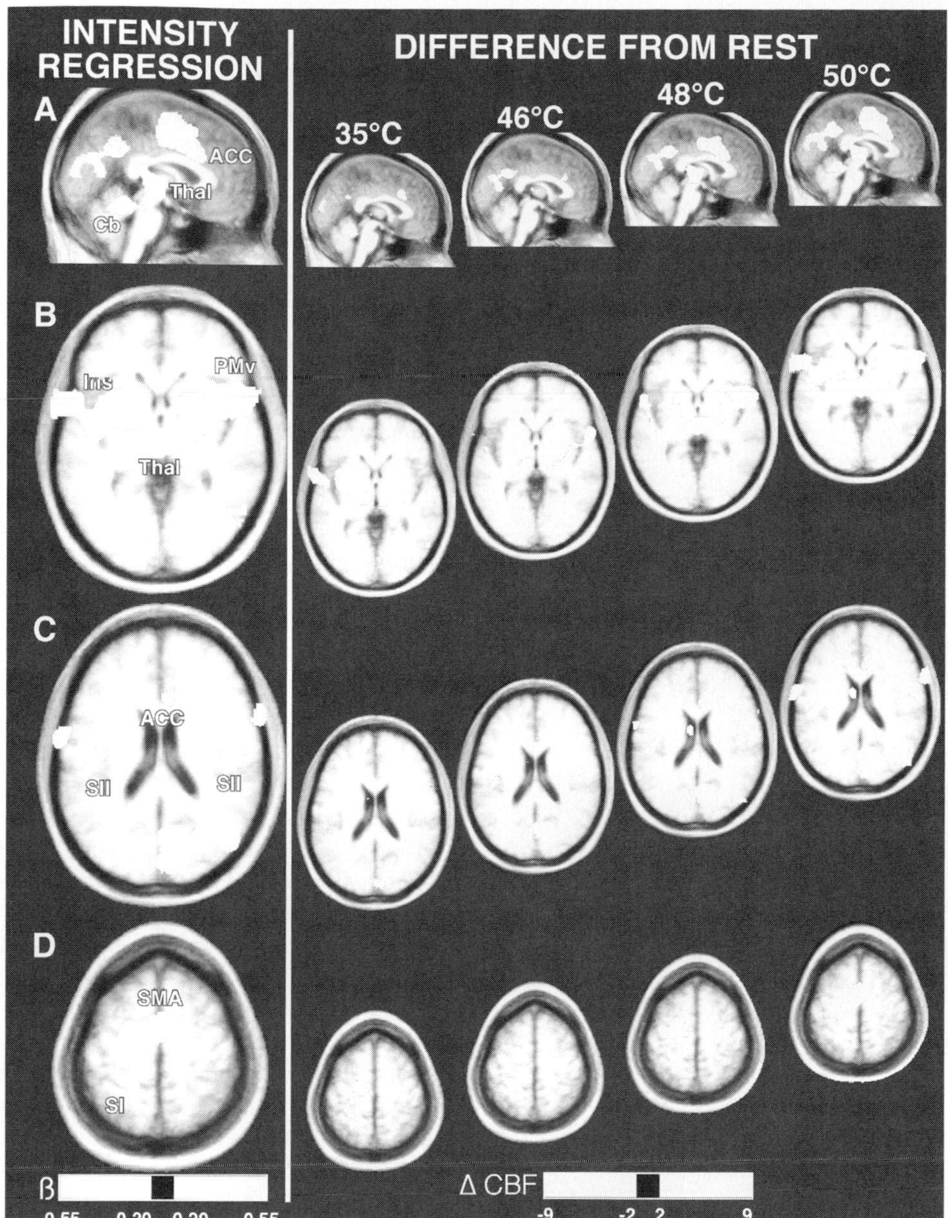

FIG. 44.2. Multiple regression analysis shows that activation within a wide array of brain areas is significantly related to stimulus intensity and subjects' perceptions of pain intensity (**left:** images are color coded such that red-yellow voxels are positively related to pain intensity, whereas blue-violet voxels are inversely related to pain intensity). Progressive increases in activation are evident within these areas as stimulus temperature increases [**right:** cerebral blood flow (CBF) difference between each temperature and rest]. *ACC,* anterior cingulate cortex; *Thal,* thalamus; *Cb,* cerebellum; *Ins,* insula; *PMv,* ventral premotor cortex; *SII,* secondary somatosensory cortex; *SI,* primary somatosensory cortex; *SMA,* supplementary motor area. (Reproduced from Coghill RC, Sang C, Maisog JM, Iadarola MJ. Pain intensity processing within the human brain: a bilateral, distributed mechanism. *J Neurophysiol* 1999;82:1934–1943, with permission.)

compared the changes in functional brain activity produced by a thermal stimulus of 49°C in healthy individuals who displayed relatively high levels of pain sensitivity [mean visual analogue scale (VAS) intensity rating = 7.4] or who showed relatively low levels of pain intensity (mean VAS intensity rating = 2.4). It was found that the high and low pain sensitivity groups did not differ with regard to activation changes in the thalamus, indicating that the group difference in intensity ratings was not due to variations in sensitivity of peripheral afferent or spinal mechanisms. However, the high pain sensitivity group displayed significantly greater levels of activation in the anterior cingulate cortex, prefrontal cortex, and S1 (Fig. 44.3). All of these brain regions are involved in intensity processing. Moreover, the anterior cingulate cortex and prefrontal cortex contribute to processing of affective and cognitive responses, attention, and memory (including memory of affective experiences). This finding validates the contribution of cognitive and emotional factors to individual differences in pain experience.

Several studies also have shown that the anterior cingulate cortex and insular cortex contribute to alterations in

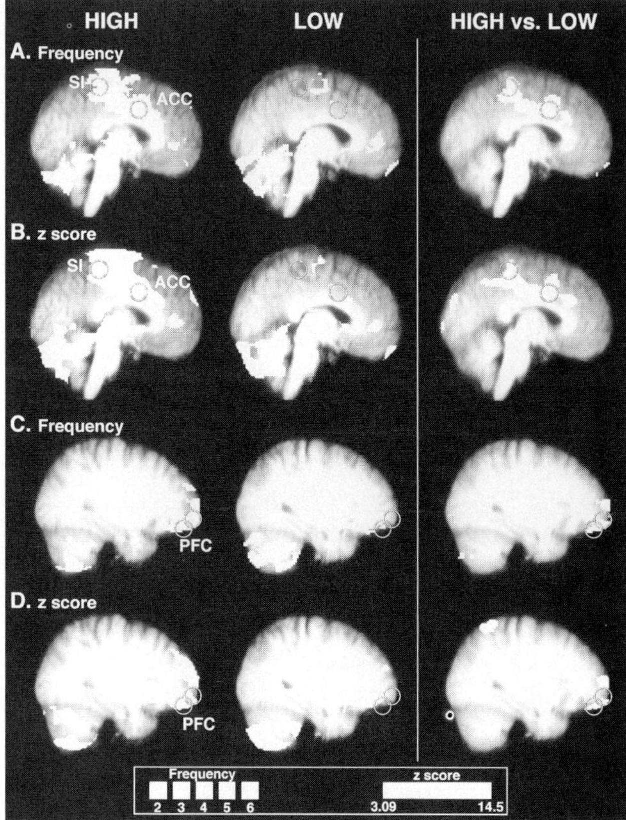

FIG. 44.3. Brain regions displaying different frequencies of activation between high- and low-sensitivity subgroups. Circles are centered on regions where the peak differences between groups were located. Colors in **A** and **C** correspond to the number of individuals displaying statistically significant activation at a given voxel (frequency), whereas colors in **B** and **D** correspond to the *z* score of the subgroup analysis. The most robust distinction in the frequency of activation between the high-sensitivity and low-sensitivity subgroups was located within a portion of the anterior cingulate cortex (ACC), where six of six of the highly sensitive subjects, but none of the insensitive subjects, displayed statistically significant activation. A large portion of the primary somatosensory cortex (SI) and spatially restricted regions of the ipsilateral (right) prefrontal cortex (PFC) also exhibited significantly more frequent activation in highly sensitive individuals than in insensitive individuals. (Reproduced from Coghill RC, McHaffie JG, Yen YF. Neural correlates of interindividual differences in the subjective experience of pain. *Proc Natl Acad Sci U S A* 2003;100:8538–8542, with permission.)

the affective dimension of pain that are not dependent on changes in stimulus intensity. For example, Rainville and colleagues (22) delivered hypnotic suggestions to healthy volunteers to increase or decrease the perceived unpleasantness of noxious, tonic heat stimuli without altering perceived stimulus intensity. They found that hypnotic suggestion of increased as well as decreased pain unpleasantness altered numerical ratings of this variable in the expected directions without changing ratings of pain intensity. Moreover, both types of hypnotic suggestion produced significant increases in activity of the anterior cingulate cortex, rostral insular cortex, and S1. There also was a significant correlation ($r = 0.42$) between hypnosis-induced changes in pain unpleasantness and increases in functional activity of the anterior cingulate cortex. Subsequent studies revealed that hypnotic suggestions of increased sensory intensity produce significant increases in ratings of both pain intensity and pain unpleasantness (23); however, altered pain intensity ratings are associated only with significant increases in activation of the S1 (24).

Compared with normal controls, patients with fibromyalgia show abnormal pain thresholds in response to low-intensity mechanical pressure and thermal stimuli (25,26). Gracely and colleagues (27) recently examined the neural correlates of this phenomenon using functional magnetic resonance imaging (fMRI). These investigators applied different levels of phasic pressure stimulation to the left thumbnail of patients with fibromyalgia (2.4 kg) and healthy controls (4.2 kg) for both groups to produce a mean rating of 11 on a 20-point scale of pain intensity. Neuroimaging of subjects' responses to stimulation revealed that, consistent with their verbal pain responses, both patients and controls exhibited significant increases in fMRI signal in the same brain regions (e.g., somatosensory cortices, insular cortex, putamen, cerebellum) in response to the stimulation. However, when the controls received pressure stimulation at the same low-intensity levels delivered to patients, they showed significant signal increases in only two brain regions; neither of these regions overlapped with those activated within the patient group. These findings suggest that enhanced pain perception in persons with fibromyalgia is associated with central augmentation of sensory input from the periphery.

Investigators have used neuroimaging to identify regions of enhanced brain activation that are associated with analgesic responses. For example, Petrovic and colleagues (28) reported that administration of both a μ-opioid agonist (remifentanil) and placebo in healthy individuals evoked reduced reports of pain intensity and activation of the rostral anterior cingulate cortex, a region that is rich in opiate receptors and receives input from cortical and limbic system regions. Placebo analgesia also evoked increased activation of the orbitofrontal cortex. In addition, there was covariation between activity in the rostral anterior cingulate cortex and the pons during both placebo and opioid analgesia. Therefore, the above findings suggest that cognitive input from higher order cortical regions may exert control over the analgesic systems of the brainstem during both placebo and opioid analgesia (29).

Zubieta and colleagues (30) recently used neuroimaging to examine the relationship between μ-opioid receptor-mediated neurotransmission and a common functional polymorphism of the cathechol-*O*-methyltransferase (COMT) gene. This gene codes the substitution of valine (val) by methionine (met) at codon 158 ($val^{158}met$) and is involved in metabolizing catecholamines. Thus, COMT helps modulate adrenergic/noradrenergic neurotransmission involved in pain modulation. Individuals with the val/val genotype have the highest activity of COMT, and those with the met/met genotype have the lowest activity of COMT, and heterozygous individuals (val/met) are intermediate.

With regard to the procedure, healthy subjects who were matched to one of the three COMT genotypes underwent neuroimaging during infusion of hypertonic saline in the masseter muscle that was titrated to levels that produced visual analogue ratings of pain intensity between 35 and 45 (of 100) units. These subjects also completed a standardized pain measure [McGill Pain Questionnaire (MPQ)] (31), which required them to choose quantified verbal descriptors (e.g., aching, miserable) to describe the sensory and affective dimensions of their subjective pain experience. It was found that, during the saline infusion, subjects with the met/met genotype, compared with the val/met subjects, showed lower μ-opioid system activation in the striatopallidal regions (nucleus accumbens, ventral pallidum, and subthalamic nucleus) and the amygdala. In addition, the val/val subjects, compared to those with the met/val genotype, displayed significantly higher μ-opioid system activation in the dorsal anterior cingulate, anterior thalamus, and cerebellar vermis. These findings were associated with group differences on two measures of pain. First, there was a linear correlation between genotype and sensory and affective MPQ scores in which the met/met subjects reported the highest levels of pain followed by the val/met and the val/val subjects, who reported the lowest levels of pain. Conversely, the volume of hypertonic saline required to produce pain was lowest in the met/met subjects, intermediate in the met/val subjects, and highest in the val/val subjects. These findings strongly suggest that the met/met genotype of COMT is associated with diminished μ-opioid system activation and enhanced pain responses in healthy persons. Additional studies are necessary to determine whether this genotype is also associated with disorders characterized by abnormalities in pain sensitivity or pain modulation.

Pathologic Pain

Tissue injury or infection evokes a local inflammatory response. This includes the production of eicosanoids (e.g., prostaglandins, bradykinin, lactic acid, super-oxide free radicals), as well as serotonin, histamine, and proinflammatory cytokines. These mediators, in turn, activate A and C afferent fiber endings (32). Under normal conditions, the blood-nerve barrier protects peripheral nerve fibers from eicosanoids and proinflammatory cytokines. However, induction of physical trauma or onset of autoimmune disease may damage myelin (33) or alter the blood-nerve barrier (34) and, thus, produce infiltration of immune cells, antibodies, and other immune products that may damage peripheral nerve fibers and produce pathologic pain conditions that are difficult to manage. For example, the widespread occlusion of peripheral nerve blood vessels associated with vasculitis disrupts the blood-nerve barrier and leads to edema and endoneurial immune cell migration. When this occurs, the peripheral nerve proteins P0 and P2, which are not normally encountered by macrophages, mast cells, or endothelial cells within the endoneurium, are responded to as nonself and generate an immune response (35). The ensuing release of proinflammatory cytokines, nitric oxide (NO), and reactive oxygen species (ROS) splits apart the layers of myelin surrounding the nerve. The myelin then becomes susceptible to degradation by the action of macrophages, and peripheral nerve structures such as ion channels and ion transporters are damaged by NO and ROS. The end result is peripheral nerve neuropathy and abnormal increases in nociceptive transmission that may lead to abnormal pain sensitivity. However, as described below, changes in spinal processing of the nociceptive input are also influenced by immune activation within the spinal cord and thus may contribute to abnormal pain sensitivity.

Central Sensitization

Prolonged or intense nociceptive input from peripheral afferents may produce a series of alterations in the function of spinal dorsal horn neurons that lead to hyperexcitability of these neurons and abnormal pain sensitivity. This phenomenon is referred to as central sensitization (Fig. 44.1C). Specifically, enhanced nociceptive input from peripheral afferents may sufficiently depolarize the dorsal horn neurons so that Mg^{2+} exits NMDA-linked ion channels. This is followed by an influx of extracellular Ca^{2+} and production of NO, which diffuses out of the dorsal horn neurons. NO, in turn, promotes the exaggerated release of excitatory amino acids and substance P from presynaptic afferent terminals and causes the dorsal horn neurons to become hyperexcitable (36). As a consequence, even low-intensity stimulation of the skin or deep muscle tissue will generate high levels of nociceptive input to the brain and displays of abnormal pain sensitivity or hyperalgesia. It is important to note that animal models of central sensitization have shown that central sensitization may be reversed if the initial source of nociceptive input is eliminated (36).

Recently, Watkins and colleagues (37) have provided evidence that dorsal horn glia cells also play a role in producing and maintaining abnormal pain sensitivity. Synapses within the central nervous system are encapsulated by glia cells that normally do not respond to nociceptive input from peripheral sites. However, following the initiation of central sensitization, spinal glia cells are activated by a wide array of factors that contribute to hyperalgesia such as immune activation within the spinal cord, substance P, excitatory amino acids, NO, and prostaglandins (Fig. 44.1D). Once activated, glia cells release several proinflammatory cytokines [e.g., tumor necrosis factor-α (TNF-α), interleukin-6 (IL-6), IL-1], substance P, NO, ROS, prostaglandins, excitatory amino acids, adenosine triphosphate, and fractalkine that, in turn, (a) further increase the release of excitatory amino acids and substance P from the Aδ and C afferents that synapse in the dorsal horn and (b) enhance the hyperexcitability of the dorsal horn neurons (37).

Activation of dorsal horn glia cells also may contribute to the perception of pain at sites distal to the source of nociceptive input. Milligan and her colleagues recently showed in rats that induction of a sciatic inflammatory neuropathy in one leg produces increased pain sensitivity to low-intensity pressure at the site of the neuropathy as well as at the same site in the contralateral leg (38). This mirror-image allodynia is reversed by intrathecal delivery of (a) fluorocitrate, a glial metabolic inhibitor; (b) CNI-1493, an inhibitor of p38 mitogen–activated kinases implicated in proinflammatory cytokine production and signaling; and (c) proinflammatory cytokine antagonists specific for IL-1, TNF-α, or IL-6.

Watkins and Maier (39) have suggested that cytokine-induced activation of spinal cord glia may contribute to the pain associated with inflammatory arthritis. No studies of animal models of arthritis have yet examined the role of spinal cord glial activation in abnormal pain responses. However, several studies that have used QST methods have produced evidence of abnormal pain sensitivity in humans with knee osteoarthritis (OA) and rheumatoid arthritis (RA) that is similar to the mirror-image allodynia described above. For example, Kosek and colleagues (40,41) assessed sensitivity to mechanical pressure in patients with unilateral hip OA prior to total joint replacement surgery and age-matched healthy controls. They found that the patients with hip OA, compared with controls, exhibited significantly lower pain thresholds in response to pressure stimulation at both the affected hip and the contralateral hip. Consistent with animal models of central sensitization, this mirror-image pain allodynia was eliminated after patients recovered from knee arthroplasty (Fig. 44.4). Similar findings indicative of central sensitization have been reported among patients with OA of the knee or lower extremities using hypertonic saline infusion of the tibialis muscle (42).

Animal models of central sensitization suggest that a prolonged period of nociceptive input may be necessary for abnormalities in pain processing to occur. Therefore, Leffler, Kosek, and their colleagues assessed pain sensitivity at inflamed and painful joints as well as in a pain-free area (e.g., thigh) in patients who had either a short (≤1 year) or long (>1 year) history of RA (43). The patients' responses were compared with those of healthy controls who were matched on age and site of stimulation. As expected, both groups of patients with RA, compared with controls, exhibited greater sensitivity to pressure at the painful and tender joint. However, only the patients with relatively long histories of RA showed greater sensitivity, compared with controls, to pressure stimulation of the pain-free area and to low-intensity thermal stimulation (i.e., cold threshold) of the painful and tender joint. These findings suggest that central sensitization in patients with RA may develop within 5 years after onset. However, it is necessary to attempt to replicate these observations in a prospective study of newly diagnosed patients.

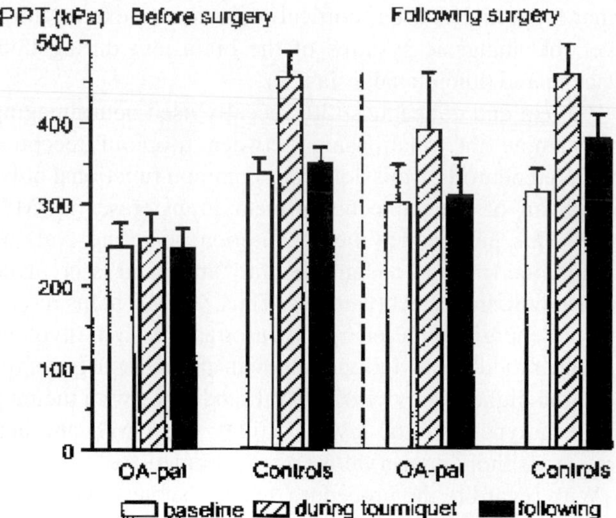

FIG. 44.4. Mean pressure pain thresholds (PPTs) (±SEM) in patients with knee osteoarthritis and healthy controls before and following surgery. Before surgery, patients, compared with controls, show significantly lower PPTs at baseline. In addition, only controls show statistically significant change in PPTs during ischemic counterstimulation. After withdrawal of ischemic counterstimulation, control subjects' PPTs return to baseline values. Following surgery, there is no difference in baseline PPTs between patients and controls. Ischemic counterstimulation produces significant increases in PPTs among both patients and controls. Also, PPTs decrease following withdrawal of ischemic counterstimulation. (Reproduced from Kosek E, Ordeberg G. Lack of pressure pain modulation by heterotopic noxious conditioning stimulation in patients with painful osteoarthritis before, but not following, surgical pain relief. *Pain* 2000;88:69–78, with permission.)

Cognitive and Affective Influences on Pain in Patients with Rheumatic Disease

A substantial amount of research has been devoted to associations between cognitive and affective factors and pain in patients with rheumatic disease and other rheumatologic disorders. This research has consistently shown that negative affective states and pain-related beliefs tend to increase reports of pain. For example, it has been found that a history of major depressive episode places patients with RA at risk for relatively high levels of pain and fatigue if the depressive episode is followed by persistent depressive symptoms (44,45). Similarly, anxiety about behaviors or events that are likely to evoke increased pain intensifies the pain and other somatic symptoms of patents with fibromyalgia (46). Conversely, self-management interventions designed to increase patients' perceptions of self-efficacy (i.e., perceived ability to perform actions that will increase symptom control) produce significantly greater improvements in pain and distress than credible attention/placebo interventions in patients with RA and OA (47,48).

Relatively little attention has been devoted to the effects of cognitive and affective factors on responses to experimental pain stimuli produced by QST in laboratory settings. Nevertheless, the few studies that have been performed have produced results similar to those described above. For example, Keefe and colleagues (49) found that patients with knee OA with high levels of self-efficacy for arthritis pain are less sensitive to thermal heat pain stimuli than those with low self-efficacy. Specifically, the patients with high self-efficacy display significantly higher pain threshold and pain tolerance levels than those with low self-efficacy. The high self-efficacy patients, compared to those with low self-efficacy, also rate the thermal stimuli as less unpleasant.

We recently compared MPQ pain affect ratings produced by patients with knee OA and age-matched healthy controls in response to phasic pressure of the left and right knee under two conditions (50) (Table 44.2). The first condition consisted of stimulation at touch threshold (1 kg). In the second condition, stimulation was calibrated to produce similar ratings of sensory pain intensity in both patients and controls. Both patients and controls underwent neuroimaging during the two stimulation conditions. We found that during painful stimulation, the patients produced significantly higher ratings of pain affect than controls, although there was no group difference in sensory pain intensity ratings. The patients, compared with controls, also reported significantly higher levels of catastrophizing (i.e., negative pain-related cognition) during painful stimulation and showed significantly greater increases from touch threshold to painful stimulation in activation of the anterior cingulate cortex. Moreover, additional analyses revealed that the group difference in catastrophizing mediated the difference in pain affect ratings between patients and controls.

TABLE 44.2. *Mean (±SEM) McGill Pain Questionnaire (MPQ) sensory and affective subscale scores of patients with knee osteoarthritis (OA) and healthy controls*

MPQ subscale	OA patients n = 11	Healthy controls n = 11	*p* value
Right knee			
Sensory	17.6 ± 2.0	15.17 ± 2.4	0.45
Affective	6.95 ± 1.9	1.76 ± 0.6	0.02
Left knee			
Sensory	18.3 ± 2.0	17.3 ± 2.5	0.76
Affective	7.0 ± 2.5	1.46 ± 0.7	0.003

Adapted from Bradley LA, BC, DeBerry JJ, et al. Lessons from fibromyalgia: generalized pain sensitivity in patients with knee osteoarthritis. In: Chadwick DJ, Goode J, ed. *Osteoarthritic joint pain (Novartis Foundation Symposium).* New York: Wiley, 2004, 258–276, with permission.

Patients with fibromyalgia are characterized by hypothalamis-pituitary-adrenal (HPA) axis dysregulation that may impair their ability to cope with environmental stressors (51). It is well-known that stressors evoke relatively low levels of cortisol release in patients with fibromyalgia (51). In addition, environmental stressors tend to increase circulating levels of IL-6 and TNF-α in healthy individuals (52). Thus, it is reasonable to predict that patients with fibromyalgia would report enhanced pain during exposure to stressors, and these enhanced pain responses may be mediated by alterations in production of cortisol or proinflammatory cytokines. Indeed, it has been found that fibromyalgia patients, compared with patients with knee OA, report significantly greater increases in their clinical pain following a 30-minute stress induction procedure (i.e., vivid recall of a personally relevant stressful event) (53). In addition, preliminary data from an ongoing study in our laboratory show that patients with fibromyalgia, compared with healthy controls, report significantly greater increases in subjective unpleasantness of thermal heat stimuli after only 4 minutes of vivid recall of personally relevant stressful events (Fig. 44.5). However, the patients do not differ from controls with regard to change in pain intensity ratings. We anticipate that as the study continues, we will be able to determine whether the group differences in stressor-evoked changes in pain unpleasantness are mediated by group differences in circulating levels of cortisol or proinflammatory cytokines.

Descending Antinociceptive Pathways and Pain Modulation

Melzack and Wall's original gate control theory posited that pain is produced by a dynamic neural system that includes both ascending nociceptive pathways from the periphery to the spinal cord and brain as well descending pathways that modulate nociceptive input (54). A large body of research generated by gate control theory has shown that the activity of several nerve pathways that originate in brainstem sites and descend to the spinal dorsal horns may inhibit transmission of nociceptive input to the brain, primarily through the release of serotonin, norepinephrine, opiates, and neurotensin. Indeed, the most recent revision of gate control theory posits that multiple environmental (e.g., noxious stimuli), biologic (e.g., genotype, function of the neuroendocrine axes and autonomic nervous system), cognitive (e.g., attention to sensory events), and

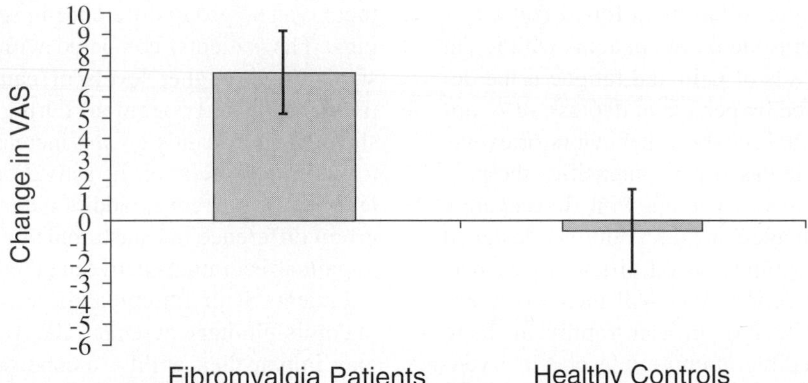

FIG. 44.5. Mean (±SEM) change scores on pain unpleasantness ratings of phasic thermal stimuli (range 45° to 49°C) in patients with fibromyalgia and healthy controls. Scores represent the difference between visual analogue scale (10 cm) pain unpleasantness rating produced after a 4-minute period of vividly imagining a personally relevant stressful event minus pain unpleasantness rating produced after a 4-minute period of vividly imagining a personally relevant, relatively neutral event. Patients with fibromyalgia produced significantly greater increases in pain unpleasantness ratings than healthy controls as a function of stressful imagery ($p = 0.01$). The order of presentation of the stimulus intensities as well as the stressful versus neutral imagery was counterbalanced across subjects to avoid bias.

affective (e.g., anxiety, depression) factors influence the transmission and inhibition of nociceptive input to the brain (55). These factors also influence the processing of nociceptive input in cortical and subcortical brain regions. Together, these complex interactions produce our perceptions of the sensory, intensity, and affective dimensions of pain and drive our behavioral expressions of pain (55).

The major anatomic components of the descending pain control system are the PAG, rostroventral medulla (RVM), dorsolateral and ventrolateral funiculi, cortical and limbic systems, and paraventricular nuclei of the hypothalamus. The PAG and the RVM play a major role in pain modulation because they are rich in opiate receptors. Indeed, it has been shown consistently that stimulation of the PAG reduces pain in both animals and humans (56,57). In addition, the PAG may be a key site for integration of pain and somatomotor adaptation through connections to stress response systems and other cortical and subcortical structures.

The PAG receives input from higher brain regions such as the frontal, cingulate, and insular cortex as well as the limbic system, septum, amygdala, and hypothalamus (58). The relay of input from the higher cortical areas to the PAG may mediate cognitive/affective modulation of pain perception (e.g., high self-efficacy, low catastrophizing). PAG neurons also project downward to the RVM and the locus ceruleus for relay to the spinal cord via noradrenergic pathways. Morphine and endogenous opioids produce antinociception and analgesia in descending modulatory circuits by activating μ-opioid receptors in these regions (59). This, in turn, activates pathways mediated by serotonin and norepinephrine in the RVM and locus ceruleus that descend to the spinal dorsal horn via projections in the dorsolateral funiculus and inhibit ascending nociceptive transmission (59). There also is a large projection from the ventrolateral part of the PAG to the nucleus raphe magnus of the RVM that is mediated by neurotensin, a tridecapeptide that contributes to activation of serotonergic descending modulatory pathways.

It should be noted that the RVM neurons that contribute to the activation of descending modulatory pathways to the spinal dorsal horn are termed OFF cells (60). However, the activity of these cells may be inhibited by other neurons within the RVM that are termed ON cells. Noradrenergic neurons that project to the RVM that stimulate α_1-receptor sites excite ON cells; however, descending noradrenergic neurons that stimulate α_2-receptor sites inhibit ON cell activity. Similarly, κ opiate receptor agonists within the RVM tend to antagonize μ receptor-mediated analgesia at this site.

The hypothalamus plays an important part in pain modulation due to its role in physiologic responses to stressors. Nociceptive stimuli may activate the ventrolateral PAG, which sends direct projections to the paraventricular nucleus of the hypothalamus (61). These projections terminate on the medial parvocellular nuclei that control neuroendocrine output by secretion of corticotropin-releasing hormone and arginine vasopressin, which subsequently activate pituitary-adrenal stress hormone production. Projections from the PAG also terminate in the magnocellular divisions of the paraventricular hypothalamus that stimulate vasopressin release from the posterior pituitary (62). There also is bidirectional communication between the hypothalamus and the PAG that is mediated by the activity of medial and lateral neurons that project directly to the PAG and medullary reticular formation.

The hypothalamus may contribute to analgesic responses through several descending pathways that inhibit ascending nociceptive transmission. These include a direct projection of the medial paraventricular nuclei of the thalamus to the dorsolateral funiculus as well as oxytocin- and vasopressin-containing neurons of the lateral hypothalamus that terminate in dorsal spinal lamina. In addition, some animal models of stress-induced analgesia suggest that pain inhibition is mediated by production of enkephalins in the adrenal medulla or β-endorphin in the pituitary (63). In contrast, impaired HPA axis function, in conjunction with persistent pain and psychological distress, may enhance the affective dimension of first pain produced by experimental stimuli. It was noted earlier that patients with fibromyalgia, compared with healthy controls, show greater stress-induced increases in pain unpleasantness ratings evoked by thermal heat stimuli. We also have made similar observations with patients with gastroesophageal reflux disease (GERD) and either high or low levels of anxiety in whom we evoked tonic visceral pain by a meal (i.e., pepperoni pizza and Coca-Cola) that reliably evokes increases in esophageal acid exposure (64). Following the meal, stressful tasks (e.g., performing complex timed, arithmetic problems) evoked significantly higher levels of painful reflux symptoms among patients with high levels of anxiety, compared to those with low anxiety levels, despite the fact that the patient groups did not differ in change in esophageal acid exposure. We subsequently examined the effects of a stress management procedure (i.e., progressive muscle relaxation training) and a credible attention/placebo on stress-induced changes in esophageal acid exposure and ratings of anxiety and painful reflux symptoms among GERD patients with high levels of anxiety (65). We found that relaxation training, compared to attention/placebo, produced significantly lower levels of stress-induced changes in painful reflux symptom ratings and in acid exposure.

Abnormal Pain Inhibition in Patients with Rheumatologic Disease

It was noted earlier that recent evidence from animal and human studies suggest that spinal and supraspinal events contribute to abnormal pain sensitivity in patients with rheumatic disease. There also is a small body of literature concerning central mechanisms that may contribute to abnormal pain inhibition in these patients. This literature has focused primarily on disease-related alterations in an endogenous analgesic system termed diffuse noxious inhibitory controls (DNIC). The typical laboratory study involving DNICs requires subjects to undergo a pain sensitivity task that requires them to rate the intensity of phasic, quantified, thermal, or mechanical pressure stimuli applied to the hand or arm. In one condition, the task is performed using standard laboratory procedures. In the second condition, however, the task is performed along with a counterirritation procedure, such as delivering a tonic pain stimulus (e.g., foot immersion in a hot water bath) to a different anatomic site. Among individuals with intact DNIC systems, the counterirritation procedure decreases the perceived intensity of the phasic stimuli. Animal models suggest that DNIC effects are mediated by supraspinal inhibition of wide dynamic range spinal neurons that receive input from both nociceptive and nonnociceptive primary afferents. The activity of spinal neurons that receive only nociceptive information from primary afferents is not influenced by DNIC (66,67).

A small number of studies have examined the extent to which DNIC effects are displayed among patients with rheumatologic conditions. Kosek and Ordeberg (40,41) reported that patients with unilateral hip OA, compared with controls, exhibited significantly lower pain thresholds in response to pressure stimulation at both the affected hip and the contralateral hip (Fig. 44.4). When the pressure pain threshold task was performed at the same time that ischemic stimulation was delivered to the arm, only the controls displayed a DNIC effect, (i.e., a significant increase in pressure pain threshold at the contralateral knee). Unlike the controls, the patients failed to show an increase in pain threshold at the unaffected, contralateral hip in response to ischemic counterstimulation. In addition, when the pressure pain threshold task was repeated in the absence of counterstimulation, the controls displayed a significant decrease in pain threshold while the patients showed no change on this measure. This provided reliable evidence that the DNIC effect shown by the controls was due to the counterstimulation, rather than task repetition. Kosek and Ordeberg then repeated the same procedures 5 months after the patients recovered from knee arthroplasty. There was no difference between patients and controls in pain threshold levels at the contralateral hip at baseline. Moreover, the abnormality in patients' pain modulation was reversed. That is, both the patients and controls displayed increased pain threshold levels at the contralateral hip in response to ischemic counterstimulation. Finally, both subject groups showed decreases in pain threshold levels when the task was repeated without counterstimulation. These findings strongly suggest that the abnormality in pain modulation displayed by the patients prior to arthroplasty was maintained by persistent nociceptive input from the affected knee and that cessation of nociceptive input allowed the patients' central pain inhibitory functions to return to normal.

In contrast to the results described above, efforts to document abnormalities in DNIC among patients with RA and fibromyalgia have produced negative or inconsistent results. It was noted earlier that Leffler, Kosek and their colleagues reported that, similar to their observations of patients with hip OA, patients with at least a 5-year history of RA exhibit greater pain sensitivity, compared with controls, to pressure stimulation of a pain-free area (43). However, when pain sensitivity was reassessed in conjunction with counterstimulation (i.e., hand and forearm immersion in a cold water bath), both the patients and controls showed significant decreases in pain sensitivity. Thus, DNIC-related pain modulation was preserved in the patients with RA. At present, the factors underlying the discrepant findings in patients with hip OA and RA are not known. It is possible, however, that differences between the patient groups in duration of disease, medication regimens, or counterstimulation procedures may underlie these findings.

With respect to fibromyalgia, Kosek and Hansson (68) initially reported that, unlike healthy controls, patients with this disorder did not display increases in pressure pain thresholds during counterstimulation with ischemic pressure, suggesting a dysfunction in systems subserving DNICs. Other investigators, however, have produced findings which suggest that several pain inhibition systems, including the system underlying DNIC, may function normally in patients with fibromyalgia. Staud and colleagues (69,70) showed that women with fibromyalgia, compared with healthy controls, report significantly higher levels of pain during exposure to phasic thermal heat or mechanical pressure stimuli as well as slower decay of pain perceptions after stimulation was terminated. This enhanced temporal summation of second pain is associated with hyperexcitability of spinal NMDA receptors induced by central sensitization (71). It has been found that administration of an NMDA antagonist (ketamine) (72) and fentanyl (73) reduces temporal summation of pain among patients with fibromyalgia and healthy controls. Staud and colleagues (74) also found that both healthy women and women with fibromyalgia show DNIC responses that are deficient compared with those of healthy men. This suggests that diminished DNIC effects on temporal summation of second pain may be gender specific, rather than a unique abnormality associated with fibromyalgia.

Nevertheless, there is evidence that exercise, which tends to activate endogenous opioid and adrenergic systems and diminish pain sensitivity in healthy persons, increases thermal pain sensitivity in patients with fibromyalgia (75). This may have important implications for exercise-based pain management programs for these patients. That is, patients with fibromyalgia may have difficulty in adherence with these programs due to the pain-enhancing effects of exercise. Indeed, Rooks and colleagues recently showed that in order to achieve positive results, it is necessary to gradually introduce fibromyalgia patients to exercise using 4 weeks of pool-based therapy before they engage in land-based therapy (76).

Preemptive Analgesia

Animal and human studies indicate that both peripheral inflammation and surgical trauma produce increased levels of cyclooxygenase-2 (COX-2) in the dorsal spinal cord that contribute to the synthesis of prostaglandins and subsequent development of central sensitization (77–79). Thus, enhanced spinal levels of COX-2 may also contribute to the abnormalities in pain modulation observed in patients with knee OA. These findings have generated interest in administering nonsteroidal antiinflammatory medications (NSAIDs) prior to and following total joint replacement procedures because these agents diminish inflammation associated with surgery, act in a synergistic fashion with opioids to enhance pain control, and may attenuate the development of central sensitization and hyperalgesia (80). However, nonselective NSAID therapy is potentially hazardous to patients because it is associated with enhanced bleeding during surgery (81).

Buvanendran and colleagues (79) recently reported the effects of administering the oral selective COX-2 inhibitor rofecoxib prior to and following knee arthroplasty in a sample of 70 patients. They compared the effects of a regimen of 50 mg of oral rofecoxib at 24 hours and at 1 to 2 hours before surgery, 50 mg daily for 5 days postoperatively, and 25 mg daily for another 8 days, versus matching placebo. It was found that preemptive analgesia with rofecoxib was superior to placebo with regard to (a) total epidural analgesic consumption and in-hospital opioid consumption; (b) pain intensity ratings during the hospital stay and 1 week after discharge; (c) postoperative vomiting; (d) knee flexion at discharge; and (e) time required in physical therapy to achieve effective joint range of motion. There was no group difference in intraoperative and postoperative surgical blood loss. Moreover, only the patients in the rofecoxib condition showed plasma and cerebrospinal fluid concentrations of COX-2 before the presurgical administration of spinal anesthetic. This finding suggests that the enhanced central levels of COX-2 prior to surgery helped mediate the superior pain control among patients in the rofecoxib condition.

Summary and Conclusions

The preceding discussion shows that a great deal of progress has been made in understanding the neural mechanisms that underlie pain and analgesia responses as well as the cognitive and affective factors that influence these responses. Human studies of pain sensitivity and pain modulation have been aided by the development of QST procedures that permit reliable measurement of individuals' responses to quantitative stimuli. In addition, neuroimaging procedures are beginning to produce valuable information concerning neural mechanisms underlying individual differences in pain sensitivity and the contribution of endogenous opioid activation systems involved in pain modulation.

The studies described above also have increased our understanding of centrally mediated factors that contribute to abnormal pain sensitivity or pain modulation in patients with rheumatologic diseases or disorders. There currently is reliable evidence that patients with knee or hip OA show abnormal pain sensitivity responses that may be produced by central sensitization. In addition, patients with hip OA display responses to DNIC procedures that suggest abnormalities in pain modulation systems. These abnormalities, however, are eliminated after total joint replacement surgery. In addition, postsurgical pain is reduced among these patients using preemptive analgesia with a selective COX-2 inhibitor.

There also is evidence of centrally mediated, abnormal pain sensitivity in patients with RA. Given the high levels of inflammation associated with RA, it is not surprising that patients with this disease would show abnormalities in pain processing consistent with central sensitization. In contrast to the literature on knee and hip OA, however, one study unexpectedly failed to find evidence of abnormal DNIC responses in patients with RA. It is possible that treatment of patients with biologic therapies that inhibit proinflammatory cytokines or factors associated with the specific QST or counterstimulation procedures used in this study may have contributed to the failure to observe abnormal pain modulation. Additional studies of pain modulation in patients with RA are necessary to resolve these issues.

Patients with fibromyalgia report pain in response to a wide array of low-intensity stimuli. Findings derived from studies involving neuroimaging and temporal summation procedures suggest that enhanced pain sensitivity in fibromyalgia may be mediated by central sensitization or other abnormalities that produce augmentation of sensory input. However, there is no consistent evidence that inflammation contributes to these abnormalities in central processing. Patients with fibromyalgia tend to show inhibited DNIC responses, although these are similar to the responses observed in healthy women. Nevertheless, patients with fibromyalgia do not show normal reductions in pain sensitivity following exercise. This suggests that fibromyalgia may be associated with abnormalities in endogenous opioid or adrenergic systems that diminish pain sensitivity in healthy persons. Nevertheless, additional work is needed to gain a better understanding of the central factors that contribute to the widespread pain and generalized pain sensitivity in patients with fibromyalgia. For example, Melzack (5) suggested that the spinal and supraspinal mechanisms involved in pain processing and pain modulation are influenced by genetic factors. It already has been shown that, compared with healthy women, a significantly greater proportion of patients with fibromyalgia are characterized by a functional polymorphism in the 5-HTT gene (82) (see Chapter 91). This polymorphism is associated with anxiety disorders and thus may contribute indirectly to abnormal pain responses. Additional progress in fibromyalgia research may be achieved through studies of functional polymorphisms in genes such as COMT that are associated with individual differences in pain sensitivity or pain modulation.

PAIN MEASUREMENT IN HUMAN STUDIES

This chapter has reviewed the neural mechanisms involved in pain and pain modulation as well as the progress we have made in understanding how centrally mediated alterations in these functions contribute to abnormal pain responses in patients with rheumatologic diseases or disorders. Given that many readers may not be familiar with many of the measurement procedures used in laboratory studies with humans, the final section of the chapter will briefly describe the major QST techniques used in human pain research as well as several standardized measures of cognitive and affective factors that are frequently used in these studies.

Quantitative Sensory Testing Procedures

Pain Threshold and Pain Tolerance

These probably are the most frequently used measures in studies of pain sensitivity in humans. Pain threshold represents the lowest stimulus intensity that first evokes an individual's report of pain. Pain tolerance represents the highest stimulus intensity or duration of stimulus exposure that an individual is willing to experience before he or she requests termination of the stimulus. Measurement of pain threshold or pain tolerance often involves administering a series of phasic stimuli or a tonic stimulus that increase in intensity at regular time intervals (e.g., 1 kg pressure per second). These are referred to as ascending method of limits procedures. It should be noted, however, that responses to these procedures may be highly influenced by psychological factors. For example, because individuals are instructed that stimulation will terminate when they report pain threshold or pain tolerance level, persons who are characterized by high levels of anxiety or fear of pain may prematurely report they have reached threshold or tolerance to avoid highly unpleasant sensory perceptions.

A sophisticated alternative to pain threshold measurement that decreases the influence of negative expectancies or other response biases involves the presentation of the phasic stimuli in a random sequence from two or more ascending "staircases" of stimuli. This random staircase procedure prevents the subject from correctly anticipating the intensity of the next stimulus he or she will experience. Therefore, the subject may attend more carefully to each stimulus in order to make accurate ratings. In addition, this method generally includes several measurements of pain threshold. These measurements are averaged to produce a more reliable measure of pain threshold. The random staircase procedure also may be used to evaluate pain tolerance, although the large number of stimulus presentations needed to achieve tolerance levels may reduce the feasibility of this procedure. It has been found that, among patients with fibromyalgia pain, the ascending method of limits does not evoke greater evidence of pain sensitivity than the random staircase procedure (83). Thus, the enhanced pain sensitivity displayed by these patients cannot be attributed primarily to response bias.

Magnitude Estimates of Pain Intensity and Unpleasantness

Measures of pain threshold or tolerance do not provide information concerning an individual's perception of the magnitude of intensity or unpleasantness evoked by stimuli of varying intensities. This information is necessary to examine the influence of environmental events (e.g., stressors) or treatment interventions (e.g., pharmacologic therapies) on individuals' pain perceptions. Magnitude estimate procedures are performed by presenting a series of phasic stimuli of different intensities, in random order. The subject rates the intensity or unpleasantness of each stimulus using a VAS or numerical category scale (0–100). The ratings produced for each pain dimension (intensity and unpleasantness) may then be transformed to power functions to assess the relationships between increases in stimulus intensity and changes in magnitude estimate. It should be noted, however, that it is necessary to instruct subjects concerning the difference between intensity and unpleasantness (e.g., intensity is like the volume on a radio; unpleasantness is the extent to which the music bothers you regardless of the volume). It also is necessary to provide subjects with the opportunity to practice rating stimuli on the dimensions of intensity and unpleasantness.

A good example of the use of magnitude estimates is a study of ethnic group differences on healthy individuals' perceptions of the intensity and unpleasantness of thermal stimuli (84). It was found that there was no difference between African Americans and whites in the power functions for pain intensity produced by thermal stimuli. However, the African Americans reported significantly higher levels of pain unpleasantness than did the whites in response to the same series of thermal stimuli. This relationship was especially pronounced at the lowest levels of stimulus intensity. The tendency of African Americans to report high levels of pain unpleasantness in response to relatively low-intensity stimulation may be relevant to the relationship between expectations of high levels of postsurgical pain among African-American patients with knee OA who are reluctant to undergo total joint replacement (85).

Temporal Summation

Brief, repetitive, thermal or pressure stimuli that are presented at noxious intensity levels with interstimulus intervals of less than 3 seconds produce a gradual and progressive increase in pain perception that is centrally rather than peripherally mediated. This phenomenon is associated with augmentation of input from C fiber nociceptors produced by hyperexcitability of spinal NMDA receptors. The usual temporal summation procedure requires subjects to rate the intensity of each stimulus using a 0 to 100 numerical scale, with 0 representing "no sensation," 20 representing "just painful," and "100" representing the "most intense pain imaginable." The procedure is terminated when subjects report a value of 100 or when a specified upper limit of stimuli have been presented. For subjects who terminate the procedure before the upper limit of stimuli have been presented, a value of 100 is assigned for all remaining stimulus presentations. Temporal summation typically occurs within the first several trials of the procedure. Thus, most investigators analyze their data in blocks of 5 to 10 stimulus presentations.

Another dimension of temporal summation is the amount of time required for cessation of pain reports after stimulation is terminated. Among healthy individuals, the perception of pain quickly dissipates after stimulation ends. However, one characteristic of abnormal temporal summation is slow decay of pain after repetitive stimulation ceases. As noted earlier in this chapter, Staud and colleagues found that patients with fibromyalgia, compared with controls, produce higher pain intensity ratings in response to repetitive thermal or mechanical pressure stimuli and they continue to report pain for longer time periods after stimulation ceases (69,70,73).

Diffuse Noxious Inhibitory Controls

The delivery of noxious stimulation may activate an endogenous analgesic system termed DNIC. The typical laboratory study involving DNICs requires subjects to undergo a pain sensitivity task that requires them to rate the intensity of phasic, quantified, thermal, or mechanical pressure stimuli applied to the hand or arm. In one condition, the task is performed using standard laboratory procedures. In the second condition, however, the task is performed along with a counterirritation procedure, such as delivering a tonic pain stimulus (e.g., foot immersion in a hot water bath) to a different anatomic site. Given that the counterirritation stimuli may be applied at any site, these stimuli are referred to as heterotopic noxious conditioning stimulation. Among individuals with intact DNIC systems, the counterirritation procedure decreases the perceived intensity of the phasic stimuli. Animal models suggest that DNIC effects are mediated by supraspinal inhibition of wide dynamic range spinal neurons that receive input from both nociceptive and nonnociceptive primary afferents. The activity of spinal neurons that receive only nociceptive information from primary afferents is not influenced by DNIC (66,67).

Measures of Cognitive and Affective Factors that Influence Pain Responses

Psychiatric Disorders

Psychiatric conditions, such as affective and anxiety disorders, may contribute to abnormal pain sensitivity due to their influence on brain structures involved in pain modulation (e.g., HPA axis, locus ceruleus) (86) and behavioral responses such as the use of maladaptive pain coping strategies (87,88). Two structured psychiatric interviews have been used extensively in studies of patients with persistent pain. Both of these interviews provide reliable and valid diagnoses based on the American Psychiatric Association's *Diagnostic and Statistical Manual of Mental Disorders,* 4th edition (DSM-IV) criteria. The first is the Diagnostic Interview Schedule (DIS) (89,90). The DIS is a highly structured interview that requires specialized training. However, training courses are offered twice each year at Washington University (DIS Training/Department of Psychiatry, 4940 Audobon Avenue, St. Louis, MO 63110). A computerized version of the DIS (CDIS-IV) also is available from Washington University. Nevertheless, potential users of the CDIS-IV should undergo training in order to best understand the structure of the DIS and to learn to respond appropriately to patients' questions regarding interview items.

The second psychiatric interview is the Structured Clinical Interview for DSM-IV (SCID) (91). The SCID was designed for use by experienced clinicians who may supplement the structured interview with (a) additional questions to clarify differential diagnosis, (b) challenges to inconsistencies in subjects' self-reports, or (c) ancillary information drawn from hospital records, family members, or other clinical staff. A detailed training manual and training videotapes are available to persons who wish to administer the SCID (91).

Self-Report Measures of Depression

Two of the most commonly used self-report measures of symptoms of depression are the Beck Depression Inventory (BDI) (92) and the Center for Epidemiological Studies–Depression Scale (CES-D) (93). Both measures are brief and easy to score and are characterized by high internal reliability. The BDI originally was developed to assess the cognitive components of depression. Nevertheless, it contains a large number of items concerning somatic symptoms that may artificially inflate the scores of patients with rheumatologic diseases (94). In contrast, the CES-D has relatively fewer items with somatic content. Therefore, the CES-D is more appropriate than the BDI for the evaluation of most patients (94).

Pain-Related Anxiety and Fear of Pain

The State-Trait Anxiety Inventory (STAI) and the Beck Anxiety Inventory (95,96) are the two most commonly used self-report measures in human pain research. Both of these questionnaires are brief and internally reliable. The STAI is particularly useful in laboratory studies because it includes one scale that evaluates symptoms of anxiety that the individual currently experiences (e.g., immediately before undergoing a pain sensitivity task) and another scale that evaluates symptoms of anxiety that the individual generally experiences across multiple situations.

There also are several relatively new standardized questionnaires that assess symptoms of anxiety or fear that are specific to the experience or avoidance of pain. The Pain Anxiety Symptoms Scale (PASS) (97) is the most frequently used measure of pain-related anxiety in the literature. This instrument includes 53 items that assess fear of pain in healthy persons and in patients with chronic pain across cognitive, behavioral, and physiological domains. The PASS consists of four subscales: Fear of Pain, Cognitive Anxiety, Somatic Anxiety, and Escape and Avoidance. The instrument is characterized by high internal reliability, and PASS scores are correlated with high scores on standardized measures of disability, self-reports of anxiety on a leg-raise exercise (98), and low scores on measures of lifting and carrying capacity (99). We also have found that high scores on the PASS among patients with fibromyalgia are associated with the tendency to report increases in pain and functional brain activity in the anterior cingulate cortex in response to low-intensity, nonnociceptive stimulation (100).

Catastrophizing

This construct is defined as an exaggerated negative orientation toward pain stimuli and pain experience (101). There are two standardized measures of catastrophizing. The first is the Pain Catastrophizing Scale (PCS) (102). The PCS includes three brief, internally reliable subscales that assess maladaptive cognitive and affective responses to pain: helplessness, magnification, and rumination. Helplessness refers to perceived difficulty in coping effectively with pain. Magnification represents a tendency to consistently anticipate that pain will produce highly negative consequences. Rumination reflects a high level of difficulty in distracting oneself from pain. A large number of studies have shown that high levels of catastrophizing are associated with self-reports of pain independently of affective disturbance and with poor psychosocial adjustment to persistent pain (101).

The second measure of catastrophizing is a subscale of the Coping Strategies Questionnaire described below. This subscale is identical to the helplessness subscale of the PCS.

Coping Strategies

Coping is considered to be a dynamic process that involves constantly changing cognitive and behavioral efforts to manage specific external or internal demands that are perceived to pose a threat to the well-being of the individual (103). The most frequently used measure of coping in pain research is the Coping Strategies Questionnaire (CSQ) (104). The CSQ includes seven internally reliable subscales: Diverting Attention, Reinterpreting Pain, Coping Self-Statements, Ignoring Pain, Praying or Hoping, Catastrophizing, and Increasing Activity. The CSQ also includes two additional scales that assess "perceived control over pain" and "perceived ability to control pain." The Catastrophizing subscale is consistently associated with self-reports of high levels of pain intensity or pain unpleasantness (50). However, findings concerning the correlates of the more adaptive

CSQ scales have been inconsistent. For example, there is evidence that a composite of Coping Self-Statements, Reinterpreting Pain, Ignoring Pain, Increasing Activity, and Diverting Attention is negatively associated with self-reports of disability (105). Nevertheless, there also are negative findings concerning this relationship (106).

Self-Efficacy

Self-efficacy represents the belief that one has the ability to successfully perform behaviors that are relevant to positive health status. Lorig and colleagues (107) developed and validated an arthritis self-efficacy scale that includes measures of self-efficacy for managing pain, disability, and other arthritis symptoms such as fatigue. Most research studies in the rheumatology literature have focused on self-efficacy for pain. These investigations have generally shown that high self-efficacy for pain is associated with improvement in self-management programs (108,109).

REFERENCES

1. IASP Subcommittee on Taxonomy. Pain terms: a list with definitions and notes on usage. *Pain* 1979;6:249–252.
2. Bradley LA, McKendree-Smith NL. Central nervous system mechanisms of pain in fibromyalgia and other musculoskeletal disorders: behavioral and psychologic treatment approaches. *Curr Opin Rheumatol* 2002;14:45–51.
3. Felson DT, Chaisson CE, Hill CL, et al. The association of bone marrow lesions with pain in knee osteoarthritis. *Ann Intern Med* 2001; 134:541–549.
4. Craig AD. Interoception: the sense of the physiological condition of the body. *Curr Opin Neurobiol* 2003;13:500–505.
5. Melzack R. From the gate to the neuromatrix. *Pain* 1999;6(suppl): 121–126.
6. Jones AKP. The contribution of functional imaging techniques to our understanding of rheumatic pain. *Rheum Dis Clin North Am* 1999;25: 123–152.
7. Pillemer SR, Bradley LA, Crofford LJ, et al. The neuroscience and endocrinology of fibromyalgia. *Arthritis Rheum* 1997;40:1928–1937.
8. Sawamoto N, Honda M, Okada T, et al. Expectation of pain enhances responses to nonpainful somatosensory stimulation in the anterior cingulate cortex and parietal operculum/posterior insula: an event-related functional magnetic resonance imaging study. *J Neurosci* 2000;20: 7438–7445.
9. Coghill RC, Sang CN, Maisog JM, et al. Pain intensity processing within the human brain: a bilateral distributed mechanism. *J Neurophysiol* 1999;82:1934–1943.
10. Rainville P. Brain mechanisms of pain affect and pain modulation. *Curr Opin Neurobiol* 2002;12:195–204.
11. Koyama T, Kato K, Mikami A. During pain-avoidance neurons in activated in the macaque anterior cingulate and caudate. *Neurosci Lett* 2000;283:17–20.
12. Bester H, Chapman V, Beeson JM, et al. Physiological properties of the lamina I spinoparabrachial neurons in the rat. *J Neurophysiol* 2000;83:2239–2259.
13. Desbos C, Villanueva L. The organization of lateral ventromedial thalamic connections in the rat: a link for the distribution of nociceptive signals to widespread cortical regions. *Neuroscience* 2001;102:885–898.
14. Bourgeais L, Guariau O, Bernard JF. Projections from the nociceptive area of the central nucleus of the amygdala to the forebrain: a PHA-L study in the rat. *Eur J Neurosci* 2001;14:229–255.
15. Ingvar DH, Rosen I, Elmquist D: Activation patterns induced in the dominant hemisphere by skin stimulation. In: Zimmerman Y, ed. *Sensory functions of the skin.* Oxford: Pergamon, 1976:549–559.
16. Jones AKP, Brown WD, Friston KJ, et al. Cortical and subcortical localization of response to pain in man using positron emission tomography. *Proc R Soc Lond B* 1991;244:39–44.
17. Talbot JD, Marrett S, Evans AC, et al. Multiple representations of pain in the human cerebral cortex. *Science* 1991;251:1355–1358.
18. Coghill RC, Talbot JD, Evans AC, et al. Distributed processing of pain and vibration by the human brain. *J Neurosci* 1994;14:4095–4108.
19. Casey KL, Minoshima S, Berger KL, et al. Positron emission tomographic analysis of cerebral structures activated specifically by repetitive noxious heat stimuli. *J Neurophysiol* 1994;71:802–807.
20. Coghill RC, Sang CN, Maisog JM, et al Pain intensity processing within the human brain: a bilateral, distributed mechanism. *J Neurophysiol* 1999;82:1934–1943.
21. Coghill RC, McHaffie JG, Yen YF. Neural correlates of interindividual differences in the subjective experience of pain. *Proc Natl Acad Sci U S A* 2003;100:8538–8542.
22. Rainville P, Duncan GH, Price DD, et al. Pain affect encoded in human anterior cingulate but not somatosensory cortex. *Science* 1997; 277:968–971.
23. Rainville P, Carrier B, Hofbauer RK, et al. Dissociation of sensory and affective dimensions of pain using hypnotic modulation. *Pain* 1999; 82:159–171.
24. Hofbauer RK, Rainville P, Duncan GH, et al. Cortical representation of the sensory dimension of pain. *J Neurophysiol* 2001;86:402–411.
25. Aaron LA, Bradley LA, Alarcón GS, et al. Psychiatric diagnoses are related to health care seeking behavior rather than illness in fibromyalgia. *Arthritis Rheum* 1996;39:436–445.
26. Gibson SJ, Littlejohn GO, Gorman MM, et al. Altered heat pain thresholds and cerebral event-related potentials following painful CO_2 laser stimulation in subjects with fibromyalgia syndrome. *Pain* 1994; 58:185–193.
27. Gracely RH, Petzke F, Wolf JM, et al. Functional magnetic resonance imaging evidence of augmented pain processing in fibromyalgia. *Arthritis Rheum* 2002;46:1333–1343.
28. Petrovic P, Kalso E, Petersson KM, et al. Placebo and opioid analgesia—imaging a shared neuronal network. *Science* 2002;295: 1737–1740.
29. Petrovic P, Ingvar M. Imaging cognitive modulation of pain processing. *Pain* 2002;95:1–5.
30. Zubieta JK, Heitzeg MM, Smith YR, et al. COMT val158met genotype affects mu-opioid neurotransmitter responses to a pain stressor. *Science* 2003;299:1240–1243.
31. Melzack R. The McGill Pain Questionnaire: major properties and scoring methods. *Pain* 1975;1:277–299.
32. Watkins LR, Maier SF. Beyond neurons: evidence that immune and glial cells contribute to pathological pain states. *Physiol Rev* 2002;82: 981–1011.
33. Smith KJ, Kapoor R, Felts PA. Demyelination: the role of reactive oxygen and nitrogen species. *Brain Pathol* 1999;9:69–92.
34. Greenacre S, Ridger V, Wilsoncroft P, et al. Peroxynitrite: a mediator of increased microvascular permeability? *Clin Exp Pharmacol Physiol* 1997;24:880–882.
35. Koski CL. Humoral mechanisms in immune neuropathies. *Neurol Clin* 1992;10:629–649.
36. Schaible H-G, Ebersberger A, von Banchet GS. Mechanisms of pain in arthritis. *Ann NY Acad Sci* 2001;966:343–354.
37. Watkins LR, Milligan ED, Maier SF. Glial activation: a driving force for pathological pain. *Trends Neurosci* 2001;24:450–455
38. Milligan ED, Twining C, Chacur M, et al. Spinal glia and proinflammatory cytokines mediate mirror-image neuropathic pain in rats. *J Neurosci* 2003;23:1026–1040.
39. Watkins LR, Maier SF. The pain of being sick: implications for brain-to-immune communication for understanding pain. *Ann Rev Psychol* 2000;51:29–57.
40. Kosek E, Ordeberg G. Lack of pressure pain modulation by heterotopic noxious conditioning stimulation in patients with painful osteoarthritis before, but not following, surgical pain relief. *Pain* 2000;88: 69–78.
41. Kosek E, Ordeberg G. Abnormalities of somatosensory perception in patients with painful osteoarthritis normalize following successful treatment. *Eur J Pain* 2000;4:229–238.
42. Bajaj P, Graven-Nielsen T, Arendt-Nielsen L. Osteoarthritis and its association with muscle hyperalgesia: an experimental, controlled study. *Pain* 2001;93:107–114.

43. Leffler AS, Kosek E, Lerndal T, et al. Somatosensory perception and function of diffuse noxious inhibitory controls (DNIC) in patients suffering from rheumatoid arthritis. *Eur J Pain* 2002;6:161–176.
44. Fifield J, Tennen H, Reisine S, et al. Depression and the long-term risk of pain, fatigue, and disability in patients with rheumatoid arthritis. *Arthritis Rheum* 1998;41:1851–1857.
45. Fifield J, McQuillan J, Tennen H, et al. History of affective disorder and the temporal trajectory of fatigue in rheumatoid arthritis. *Ann Behav Med* 2001;23:34–41.
46. Peters ML, Vlaeyen JW, van Drunen C. Do fibromyalgia patients display hypervigilance for innocuous somatosensory stimuli? Application of a body scanning reaction time paradigm. *Pain* 2000;86:283–292.
47. Bradley LA, Alberts KR. Psychological and behavioral approaches to pain management for patients with rheumatic disease. *Rheum Dis Clin North Am* 1999;25:215–232.
48. Bradley LA, McKendree-Smith NL, Cianfrini LR. Cognitive-behavioral therapy interventions for pain associated with chronic illnesses. *Semin Pain Med* 2004;1:38–45.
49. Keefe FJ, Lefebvre JC, Maixner W, et al. Self-efficacy for arthritis pain: relationship to perception of thermal laboratory pain stimuli. *Arthritis Care Res* 1997;10:177–184.
50. Bradley LA, BC, DeBerry JJ, et al. Lessons from fibromyalgia: generalized pain sensitivity in patients with knee osteoarthritis. In: Chadwick DJ, Goode J, ed. *Osteoarthritic joint pain (Novartis Foundation Symposium)*. New York: Wiley, 2004, 258–276.
51. Crofford LJ, Pillemer SR, Kalogeras KT, et al. Hypothalamic-pituitary-adrenal axis perturbations in patients with fibromyalgia. *Arthritis Rheum* 1994;37:1583–1592.
52. Goebel MU, Mills PJ, Irwin MR, et al. Interleukin-6 and tumor necrosis factor production. After acute psychological stress, exercise, and infused isoproterenol: differential effects and pathways. *Psychosom Med* 2000;62:591–598.
53. Davis MC, Zautra AJ, Reich JW. Vulnerability to stress among women in chronic pain from fibromyalgia and osteoarthritis. *Ann Behav Med* 2001;23:215–226.
54. Melzack R, Wall PD. Pain mechanisms: a new theory. *Science* 1965; 150:971–979.
55. Melzack R. Gate control theory: on the evolution of pain concepts. *Pain Forum* 1996;5:125–128.
56. Hosobuchi Y, Adams JE, Linchitz R. Pain relief by electrical stimulation of the central gray matter in humans and its reversal by naloxone. *Science* 1977;197:183–186.
57. Reynolds DV. Surgery in the rat during electrical analgesia induced by focal brain stimulation. *Science* 1969;164:444–445.
58. Mantyh PW. Forebrain projections to the periaqueductal gray in the monkey, with observations in the cat and rat. *J Compr Neurol* 1982; 206:146–158.
59. Yaksh TL. Pharmacology and mechanisms of opioid analgesic activity. *Acta Anaesthesiol Scand* 1997;41:94–111.
60. Fields HL, Heinricher MM, Mason P. Neurotransmitters in nociceptive modulatory circuits. *Ann Rev Neurosci* 1991;14:219–245.
61. Floyd NS, Keay KA, Arias CM, et al. Projections from the ventrolateral periaqueductal gray to endocrine regulatory subdivisions of the paraventricular nucleus of the hypothalamus in the rat. *Neurosci Lett* 1996;220:105–108.
62. Crofford LJ. Neuroendocrine abnormalities in fibromyalgia and related disorders. *Am J Med Sci* 1998;315:359–366.
63. Sternberg WF, Liebeskind JC. The analgesic response to stress: genetic and gender considerations. *Eur J Anaesthesiol Suppl* 1995;10: 14–17.
64. Bradley LA, Richter JE, Pulliam TJ, et al. The relationship between stress and symptoms of gastroesophageal reflux: the influence of psychological factors. *Am J Gastroenterol* 1993;88:11–19.
65. McDonald-Haile J, Bradley LA, Bailey MA, et al. Relaxation training reduces symptom reports and acid exposure in patients with gastroesophageal reflux disease. *Gastroenterology* 1994;107:61–69.
66. Le Bars D, Dickenson AH, Besson JM. Diffuse noxious inhibitory controls (DNIC). I. Effects on dorsal horn convergent neurones in the rat. *Pain* 1979;6:283–304.
67. Le Bars D, Dickenson AH, Besson JM. Diffuse noxious inhibitory controls (DNIC). II. Lack of effect on non-convergent neurones, supraspinal involvement and theoretical implications. *Pain* 1979;6: 305–327.
68. Kosek E, Hansson P. Modulatory influence on somatosensory perception from vibration and heterotopic noxious conditioning stimulation (HNCS) in fibromyalgia patients and healthy subjects. *Pain* 1997;70: 41–51.
69. Staud R Vierck CJ, Cannon RL, et al. Abnormal sensitization and temporal summation of second pain (wind-up) in patients with fibromyalgia syndrome. *Pain* 2001;91:165–175.
70. Staud R, Cannon RC, Mauderli AP, et al. Temporal summation of pain from mechanical stimulation of muscle tissue in normal controls and subjects with fibromyalgia syndrome. *Pain* 2003;102:87–95.
71. Price DD, Mao J, Frenk H, et al. The *N*-methyl-D-aspartate receptor antagonist dextromethorphan selectively reduces temporal summation of second pain in man. *Pain* 1994;59:165–174.
72. Graven-Nielsen T, Aspegren Kendall S, Henriksson KG, et al. Ketamine reduces muscle pain, temporal summation, and referred pain in fibromyalgia patients. *Pain* 2000;85:483–491.
73. Price DD, Staud R, Robinson ME, et al. Enhanced temporal summation of second pain and its central modulation in fibromyalgia patients. *Pain* 2002;99:49–59.
74. Staud R, Robinson ME, Vierck CJ, et al. Diffuse noxious inhibitory controls (DNIC) attenuate temporal summation of second pain in normal males but not in normal females or fibromyalgia patients. *Pain* 2003; 101:167–174.
75. Vierck CJ, Staud R, Price DD, et al. The effect of maximal exercise on temporal summation of second pain (windup) in patients with fibromyalgia syndrome. *J Pain* 2001;2:334–344.
76. Rooks DS, Silverman CB, Kantrowitz FG. The effects of progressive strength training and aerobic exercise on muscle strength and cardiovascular fitness in women with fibromyalgia: a pilot study. *Arthritis Rheum* 2002;47:22–28.
77. Seybold VS, Jia YP, Abrahams LG. Cyclo-oxygenase-2 contributes to central sensitization in rats with peripheral inflammation. *Pain* 2003; 105:47–55.
78. Woolf CJ, Chong MS. Preemptive analgesia—treating postoperative pain by preventing the establishment of central sensitization. *Anesth Analg* 1993;77:362–379.
79. Buvanendran A, Kroin JS, Tuman KJ, et al. Effects of perioperative administration of a selective cyclooxygenase 2 inhibitor on pain management and recovery of function after knee replacement: a randomized controlled trial. *JAMA* 2003;290:2411–2418.
80. Gordon SM, Brahim JS, Rowan J, et al. Peripheral prostanoid levels and nonsteroidal anti-inflammatory drug analgesia: replicate clinical trials in a tissue injury model. *Clin Pharmacol Ther* 2002;72:175–183.
81. Robinson CM, Christie J, Malcolm-Smith N. Nonsteroidal antiinflammatory drugs, perioperative blood loss, and transfusion requirements in elective hip arthroplasty. *J Arthroplasty* 1993;8:607–610.
82. Cohen H, Buskila D, Neumann L, et al. Confirmation of an association between fibromyalgia and serotonin transporter promoter region (5-HTTLPR) polymorphism, and relationship to anxiety-related personality traits. *Arthritis Rheum* 2002;46:845–847.
83. Petzke F, Clauw DJ, Ambrose K, et al. Increased pain sensitivity in fibromyalgia: effects of stimulus type and mode of presentation. *Pain* 2003;105:403–413.
84. Edwards RR, Fillingim RB. Ethnic differences in thermal pain responses. *Psychosom Med* 1999;61:346–354.
85. Ibrahim SA, Siminoff LA, Burant CJ, et al. Differences in expectations of outcome mediate African-American/white patient differences in "willingness" to consider joint replacement. *Arthritis Rheum* 2002; 46:2429–2435.
86. Clauw DJ, Chrousos GP. Chronic pain and fatigue syndromes: overlapping clinical and neuroendocrine features and potential pathogenic mechanisms. *Neuroimmunomodulation* 1997;4:134–153.
87. Vitaliano PP, Katon W, Maiuro RD, et al. Coping in chest pain patients with and without psychiatric disorders. *J Consult Clin Psychol* 1989; 57:338–343.
88. Bradley LA, Scarinci IC, Richter JE. Pain threshold levels and coping strategies among patients who have chest pain and normal coronary arteries. *Med Clin North Am* 1991;75:1189–1202.
89. Helzer JE, Robins LN. The Diagnostic Interview Schedule: its development, evaluation, and use. *Soc Psych Psychiatr Epidemiol* 1988;23: 6–16.
90. Robins LN, Helzer JE, Croughan J, et al. National Institute of Mental Health Diagnostic Interview Schedule. *Arch Gen Psych* 1981;38:381–389.

91. First MB, Spitzer RL, Gibbon M, et al. *User's guide for the Structured Clinical Interview for DSM-IV Axis I Disorders: SCID-I clinician version.* Washington, DC: American Psychiatric Press, 1997.
92. Beck AT, Ward CH, Mendelson M, et al. An inventory for measuring depression. *Arch Gen Psych* 1961;4:561–571.
93. Radloff L. The CES-D scale: a self-report depression scale for research in the general population. *J Appl Psychol Measure* 1977;1:385–401.
94. Bradley LA. Psychological dimensions of rheumatoid arthritis. In: Wolfe F, Pincus T, eds. *Rheumatoid arthritis: critical issues in etiology, assessment, prognosis, and therapy.* New York: Marcel Dekker, 1994:273–295.
95. Beck AT. *Beck Anxiety Inventory Manual.* San Antonio: Psychological Corporation, 1993.
96. Spielberger CD, Gorsuch RL, Lushene R. *The State-Trait Anxiety Inventory Manual.* Palo Alto, CA: Consulting Psychologists Press, 1970.
97. McCracken LM, Zayfert C, Gross RT. The Pain Anxiety Symptoms Scale: development and validation of a scale to measure fear of pain. *Pain* 1992;50:67–73.
98. McCracken LM, Spertus IL, Janeck AS, et al. Behavioral dimensions of adjustment in persons with chronic pain: pain-related anxiety and acceptance. *Pain* 1999;80:283–289.
99. Burns JW, Mullen JT, Higdon LJ, et al. Validity of the Pain Anxiety Symptoms Scale (PASS): prediction of physical capacity variables. *Pain* 2000;84:247–252.
100. Alberts KR, Bradley LA, Alarcón GS, et al. Anticipation of acute pain and high arousal feedback in women with fibromyalgia, high pain anxiety, and high negative affectivity evoke increased pain and anterior cingulated cortex activity without nociception. *Arthritis Rheum* 2000;43(suppl):173.
101. Sullivan MJL, Thorn B, Haythornthwaite JA, et al. Theoretical perspectives on the relation between catastrophizing and pain. *Clin J Pain* 2001;17:52–64.
102. Sullivan MJL, Bishop S, Pivik J. The Pain Catastrophizing Scale: development and validation. *Psychol Assess* 1995;7:524–532.
103. Burish TG, Bradley LA. Coping with chronic disease: definitions and issues. In: Burish TG, Bradley LA, eds. *Coping with chronic disease: research and applications.* New York: Academic, 1983:3–12.
104. Rosenstiel AK, Keefe FJ. The use of coping strategies in chronic low back pain patients: relationship to patient characteristics and current adjustment. *Pain* 1983;17:33–44.
105. Martin MY, Bradley LA, Alexander RW, et al. Coping strategies predict disability in fibromyalgia. *Pain* 1996;68:45–53.
106. Nicassio PM, Schoenfeld-Smith K, Radojevic V, et al. Pain coping mechanisms in fibromyalgia: relationship to pain and functional outcomes. *J Rheumatol* 1995;22:1552–1558.
107. Lorig K, Chastain RL, Ung E, et al. Development and evaluation of a scale to measure perceived self-efficacy in people with arthritis. *Arthritis Rheum* 1989;32:37–44.
108. Lorig K, Seleznick M, Lubeck D, et al. The beneficial outcomes of the arthritis self-management course are not adequately explained by behavior change. *Arthritis Rheum* 1989;32:91–95.
109. Lorig KR, Holman H. Self-management education: history, definition, outcomes, and mechanisms. *Ann Behav Med* 2003;26:1–7.

SECTION IV

Surgical Intervention in the Rheumatic Diseases

CHAPTER 45

Surgery of Arthritic Deformities of the Hand

Angela A. Wang and Andrew J. Weiland

The vast majority of hand surgery performed for arthritis deformities involves patients with osteoarthritis (OA) or rheumatoid arthritis (RA). Because the approaches to these two diseases are quite distinct, they are considered in separate sections.

RHEUMATOID ARTHRITIS

Rheumatoid arthritis is a chronic, systemic inflammatory disease involving the synovial lining of joints and tendons. All aspects of the joint, including both intraarticular and extraarticular structures, can be affected. Involvement in the hand is quite common, and patterns of involvement may vary. Synovial proliferation can both destroy articular cartilage and attenuate and invade the surrounding soft tissue–supporting structures, causing instability and secondary deformity; furthermore, the course of the disease can be highly variable. A recent article by Alderman et al. (1) highlighted a discrepancy in the perception of the effectiveness of RA hand surgery between hand surgeons and rheumatologists: rheumatologists viewed hand surgery as significantly less effective than did hand surgeons. There was not a clear reason for this discrepancy, however, this finding does underscore the need for close communication between the patient, the rheumatologist, the hand therapist, and the hand surgeon to provide optimal individualized treatment to the patient. Overall, hand surgery can have a very positive clinical effect, with decreased pain and improved dexterity and patient satisfaction (2).

Anatomy

The wrist area is composed of the distal radioulnar joint (DRUJ) and the radiocarpal joint. The DRUJ is the articulation of the distal radius with the distal ulna. The distal ulna is covered by the triangular fibrocartilage, which together with ulnocarpal and radioulnar ligaments, and the sheath of the extensor carpi ulnaris (ECU), comprise the triangular fibrocartilage complex (TFCC). The radiocarpal joint involves the articulation of the distal radius with mostly the scaphoid and lunate carpal bones.

The carpus includes the proximal carpal row (scaphoid, lunate, triquetrum, and pisiform) and the distal carpal row (trapezium, trapezoid, capitate, and hamate).

The distal carpal row articulates with the metacarpals through the carpometacarpal (CMC) joints, and the metacarpals articulate with the proximal phalanges through the metacarpophalangeal (MP) joints. The index, long, ring, and small digits have proximal interphalangeal (PIP) joints and distal interphalangeal (DIP) joints, whereas the thumb has only an interphalangeal (IP) articulation between the phalanges.

Nonoperative Treatment

The course of RA may be highly variable. Many patients are treated with medications such as corticosteroids, nonsteroidal antiinflammatory drugs (NSAIDs), immunosuppressive therapy, and the newer disease-modifying drugs, including biologic response modifiers. A more complete discussion of these medications can be found elsewhere in the text. This chapter focuses on surgical options.

Nonoperative treatments of RA hand problems include injections (of steroid and anesthetic), hand therapy, and splinting. These modalities are crucial in the early treatment of hand problems and may constitute definitive treatment. Mild inflammatory flare-ups in the hand and wrist often can be treated with an injection, followed by immobilization and gradual rehabilitation as inflammation subsides. Splinting of flexible deformities may allow the patient to carry on with activities of daily living and delay surgery until it becomes absolutely necessary.

Surgical Treatment

The goals of hand surgery in the RA patient are primarily pain relief, improvement of function, and the prevention of further damage to the hand and wrist. The benefits of cosmetic improvement and improved patient self-image, however, should not be overlooked. Often the deformity caused by the disease is more marked than the patient's symptoms. Indeed, RA patients may maintain a surprising level of function, given the external appearance of the hand. Therefore, surgical treatment is rendered based on the patient's complaints and severity of symptoms (3).

The overall medical condition of patients must be considered when planning hand surgery. RA is a systemic disease, affecting not only joints but also the cardiac, pulmonary, and renal systems. In addition to the routine preoperative medical evaluation, consideration should be given to specific medications associated with RA. Steroids may adversely affect the condition of the skin (it can be thinner and more fragile), but do not seem to cause increased wound infection (4). Methotrexate can affect liver function. Aspirin and other NSAIDs can affect platelet adhesion and exacerbate intraoperative bleeding and should be discontinued approximately 10 days before surgery.

It is common for patients with RA to have multiple joints involved with disease. Generally, large-joint surgery precedes correction of hand and finger deformities. However, patients frequently rely on their upper extremities when using walking aids, and stabilization of painful or unstable hand problems can facilitate rehabilitation for lower extremity surgery.

In the upper extremity, concomitant shoulder, elbow, wrist, and hand problems can exist. Usually, shoulder and elbow problems are addressed before hand and wrist problems to avoid hindering hand therapy with proximal areas of stiffness or pain. However, the patient should have a role in decision making, and those joints perceived to have the greatest disability, either functionally or with regard to pain, should be addressed first. In patients with bilateral involvement of the upper extremity, the surgeries should be staged, such that the patient is able to maintain one useful extremity while the other side is recovering and being rehabilitated (5).

Many upper extremity cases are preferably performed under regional anesthetic block (interscalene or axillary), but general anesthesia may be needed in cases of multiple procedures or iliac crest bone graft harvesting. The cervical spine should be examined preoperatively, and radiographs obtained, because potential cervical spine instability may influence the technique of anesthesia used. The temporomandibular joint may be involved with disease as well, potentially limiting the ability of the patient to open his or her mouth, which would again influence the choice of anesthesia technique (6).

The Wrist (Radiocarpal Joint): Soft Tissue

The wrist is the most frequently involved joint in the upper extremity in RA patients. Intraarticular synovial proliferation disrupts the wrist ligaments and causes rotatory instability of the scaphoid, eventually leading to palmar and ulnar subluxation of the carpus on the distal radius (Fig. 45.1).

Synovitis

Dorsal wrist tenosynovitis is usually painless (Fig. 45.2). However, the proliferative synovium may invade the substance of the tendon and can foreshadow extensor tendon rupture (7). Conservative therapy may consist of splinting and steroid injections, but excellent results and prophylaxis against tendon rupture are achieved with surgical tenosynovectomy. Each dorsal compartment is inspected, and the tenosynovium is carefully débrided (Fig. 45.3). Each tendon is inspected and repaired if frayed, or reconstructed if ruptured. A portion of the retinaculum may be transposed underneath the tendons to improve gliding. Intraarticular synovectomy can be performed at the same time, if indicated. Postoperatively, motion can and should begin immediately.

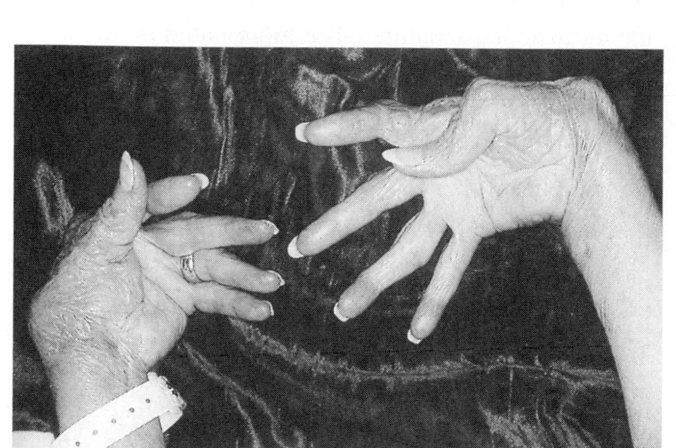

A

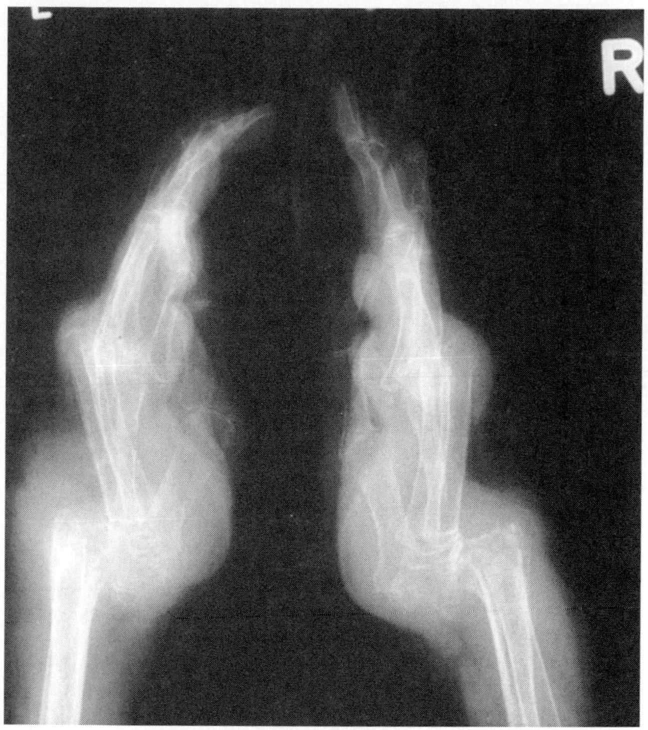

B

FIG. 45.1. **A:** Advanced deformities in the wrists of a patient with rheumatoid arthritis. Note the marked ulnar deviation at the wrist joints. **B:** Lateral wrist radiographs demonstrating severe palmar subluxation of the radiocarpal joint. Metacarpophalangeal joint subluxation also is seen in this patient.

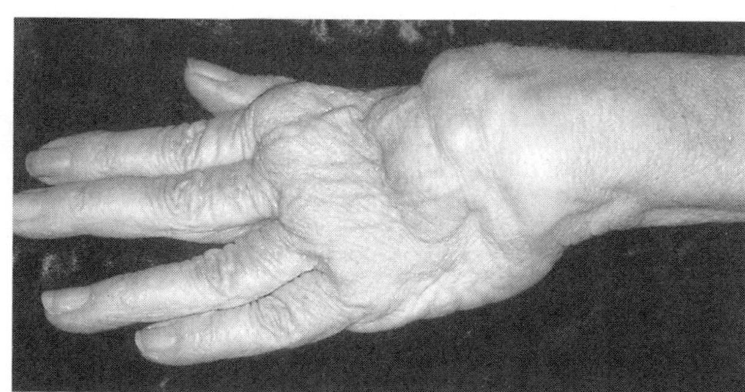

A

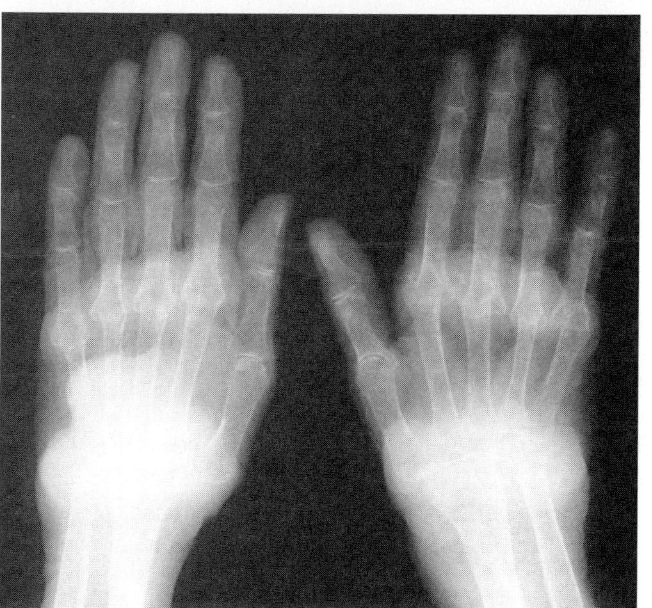

B

FIG. 45.2. **A:** A wrist with proliferative dorsal tenosynovitis. **B:** The dorsal wrist tenosynovitis has resulted in soft tissue swelling that can be detected on this posteroanterior radiograph.

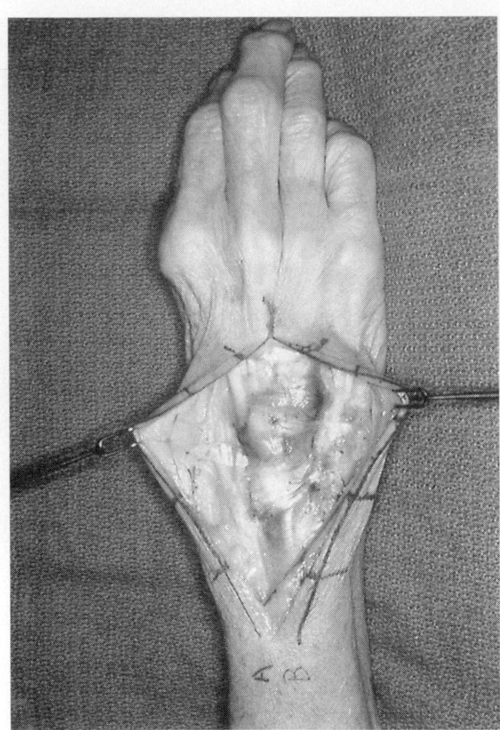

FIG. 45.3. An example of the longitudinal surgical approach to dorsal wrist tenosynovectomy. The inflamed tenosynovium can be seen bulging under the retinaculum.

Tendon Ruptures: Extensor

Extensor tendon ruptures around the wrist are commonly seen in RA patients. The ruptures are caused by a combination of synovial proliferation, which can penetrate the tendon, and attrition of the tendons passing over rough bony surfaces. Risk factors for rupture have been shown to include dorsal dislocation of the distal ulna, a radiographic scallop sign (erosion of the DRUJ), and tenosynovitis persisting for at least 6 months (8).

Clinically, loss of finger extension at the MP joint may be caused by extensor tendon rupture, but other causes should be ruled out. Differential diagnoses include ulnar subluxation of the tendon (disabling the extensor mechanism), dislocation of the MP joint, and posterior interosseous nerve compression (due to radiocapitellar synovitis). The examiner can determine continuity of the extensor tendon by testing the tenodesis effect. If the extensor tendon in question is intact, the tenodesis effect will be preserved: with passive wrist flexion, the fingers will extend.

In the wrist, the ulnar extensor tendons tend to be more frequently ruptured, with rupture of the small finger extensor tendon occurring most commonly. Isolated rupture of the small finger extensor may be a harbinger of more extensive tendon rupture if the inflammatory pathology is not addressed. As discussed previously, tendon rupture can be associated with attenuation of the tendon over a bony surface. On the ulnar side of the wrist, tendon rupture is usually due to dorsal subluxation of the distal ulna (caput ulnae syndrome; Fig. 45.4). Another extensor tendon rupture often seen is that of the extensor pollicis longus (EPL), which can rupture as it passes around the Lister tubercle on the distal radius. Integrity of the EPL can be tested by asking the patient to place the hand flat on a table and raise the thumb (if MP extension is not tested specifically, the examiner can be fooled into thinking the EPL is intact, because some patients can retain some thumb IP extension through the intrinsic musculature). The more radial digital extensor tendons are less frequently ruptured, and therefore, often remain available for reconstruction of other tendons.

Tendon ruptures may be repaired directly, but usually only if they are acute. More often, the tendon ends will have retracted, and direct repair will not be possible. Reconstruction can involve either tendon bridge grafting (from the palmaris longus or slips of the extensor digitorum communis) or tendon transfers. Fingers that have more than one extensor tendon are a good donor source for tendon transfers: the index finger possesses both the extensor digitorum communis (EDC) and the extensor indicis proprius, and the small finger has both the EDC and extensor digiti minimi. One of the tendons can be used for reconstruction, provided the other is intact. If several fingers are involved, the distal stumps can be secured in a side-to-side fashion and combined with a tendon transfer. If extensor tendon rupture is widespread and no extensor tendons remain for transfer, the flexor digitorum superficialis (FDS) tendons can be transferred dorsally to restore extension.

Generally results are better for single-tendon rupture than for multiple-tendon rupture. As discussed previously, the best therapeutic intervention is prevention, either by nonoperative measures to control inflammation, or by prophylactic tenosynovectomy, before tendon rupture occurs (9).

Postoperatively, the patients are immobilized for several weeks while the tendons heal. Hand therapists play a crucial

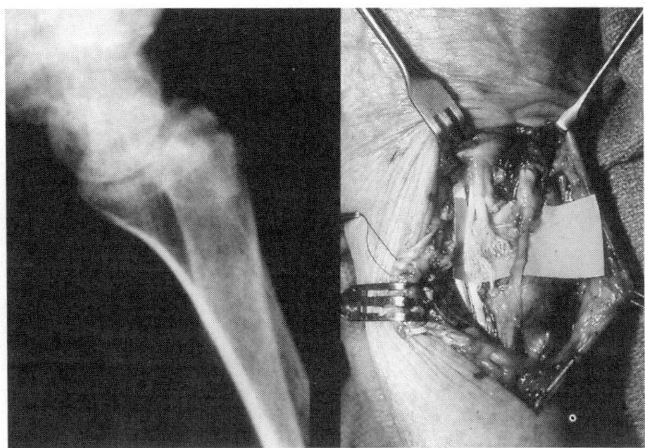

FIG. 45.4. Dorsal subluxation of the distal ulna (**left**), causing the corresponding tendon ruptures seen on the **right**.

role in postoperative management, providing custom splints and attentive regimens of controlled motion.

Tendon Ruptures: Flexor

Flexor tenosynovitis in the wrist and palm usually presents as decreased range of motion, but can also cause symptoms of median or ulnar nerve compression. In cases of nerve compression, early surgical decompression is warranted; routine carpal tunnel release is performed, and the carpal canal is explored as well, because synovium can act as a space-occupying lesion.

As in the dorsal wrist, some specific tendon ruptures can be attributed to a bony structure: the flexor pollicis longus (FPL) tendon may rupture as it passes over the rough prominence of the scaphoid (Mannerfelt lesion) or trapezium. Repair of the tendon also must address the underlying bone pathology, or it is likely that the patient will have a recurrence of the tendon rupture. Wrist flexor tendon repair is performed either primarily or by tendon grafting or transfer, as previously discussed.

The Wrist (Radiocarpal Joint): Bone

Wrist Arthroplasty

With severe articular destruction, surgical options become limited to wrist arthroplasty and arthrodesis. Arthroplasty is considered only if the patient has adequate bone stock and intact extensor tendons. Joint replacement options have included silicone and metal-on-plastic. Silicone implants have historically had difficulty with breakage, particularly at the distal stem–body interface. Total joint arthroplasties in the wrist may encounter problems similar to those seen in the hip and knee (loosening, dislocation, infection, and difficulty with revision), and have been associated with a relatively high complication rate (27%) (10). The greatest difficulty encountered with prosthetic placement, however, has been the problem of muscle imbalance across the wrist. Some of these difficulties are inherent in the patient population, which consists of severely involved, end-stage RA wrists with marked soft tissue and tendon imbalances (11). Wrist arthroplasty may be considered in a patient with bilateral disease: one wrist may undergo arthrodesis, with a contralateral arthroplasty to preserve wrist motion on one side.

Wrist Arthrodesis

Total wrist fusion provides excellent pain relief and stability in the RA wrist. Motion is, of course, sacrificed. Partial radiocarpal fusion may be considered in an effort to preserve some function; however, it should be remembered that stress will be transferred to adjacent joints. Wrist arthrodesis may be the procedure of choice in patients who have fixed carpal deformity, wrist instability, and poor bone stock or prior infection, or in heavy laborers (12). Several methods exist for wrist fusion, including plating and intermedullary rods, and bone grafting may be necessary. The optimal position for fusion has been debated, because slight wrist extension is used for most activities of daily living, with the exception of personal hygiene, in which the wrist is more often slightly flexed. Most investigators advocate fusion in a neutral position as a compromise. In patients with bilateral wrist disease, consideration may be given to arthrodesis in slightly different positions, or a unilateral wrist arthroplasty with contralateral wrist arthrodesis. Occasionally pseudoarthrosis (failure of fusion) may occur, but this may not be symptomatic, and no further treatment may be necessary.

The Distal Radioulnar Joint

The TFCC on the ulnar side of the wrist can be invaded by synovitis, causing destruction of the support of the DRUJ. The dorsal capsule of the ulna may become eroded as well, followed by dorsal subluxation of the distal ulna. This may in turn lead to tendon rupture, specifically rupture of the extensor tendons of the fourth and fifth fingers (Vaughan-Jackson sign; Fig. 45.5).

Synovial erosion of the DRUJ may be detected as a "scallop" sign at the area of the sigmoid notch on radiographs, and indicate impending extensor tendon rupture. Later in the disease process, degenerative changes and subluxation become obvious radiographically.

Initial treatment of inflammation of the DRUJ should consist of medical management, aided by splinting. Several procedures have been described to treat disorders of the DRUJ refractory to conservative treatment, including synovectomy, complete resection of the distal ulna, hemiresection with various soft tissue interpositions, and distal radioulnar fusion with proximal pseudoarthrosis (13). In the relatively low-demand rheumatoid population, a distal

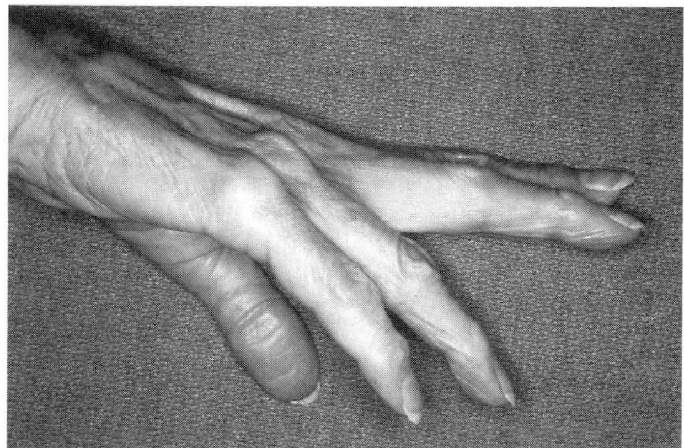

FIG. 45.5. Clinical appearance of a patient with rupture of the ring and small finger extensor tendons (Vaughn-Jackson lesion).

ulna resection (Darrach procedure) seems to provide good results. Attention is focused on avoiding subsequent instability of the distal ulnar stump, which can lead to painful or clicking forearm rotation, or extensor tendon rupture.

The Metacarpophalangeal Joint: Soft Tissue

The MP joint is a key joint for finger positioning and function, and is often affected in the RA hand. The classic deformity of ulnar drift is multifactorial, and involves ulnar deviation and palmar subluxation of the digit at the MP joint (Fig. 45.6). MP synovitis preferentially attenuates the radial sagittal band, causing loss of support of the dorsal, radial, and volar surfaces. In addition, RA involvement of the wrist causes supination of the carpus and palmar flexion of the scaphoid, which eventually leads to radial deviation of the metacarpals and compensatory ulnar deviation of the digits (14). Furthermore, ulnar drift can be accentuated by lateral pressure of the thumb on the fingers during pinching activities. Care should be taken when examining the MP joints to address concomitant problems with the digits, such as persistent finger deviation (e.g., boutonnière or swan-neck deformity), which can compromise the results of an otherwise satisfactory MP reconstruction. In addition, wrist pathology is usually addressed before MP reconstruction, because persistent wrist tendon imbalances can lead to recurrent MP deformity.

Synovitis

Mild involvement of the MP joints usually is seen as radial MP synovitis with slight extensor lag. These patients are usually managed medically, with occasional cortisone injections for discomfort, and splinting as needed. More extensive soft tissue deformity may be addressed with soft tissue rebalancing procedures (tendon centralization), along with synovectomy. This approach may be useful in a younger, higher-demand patient, in whom the function and longevity of silicone implants can be an issue.

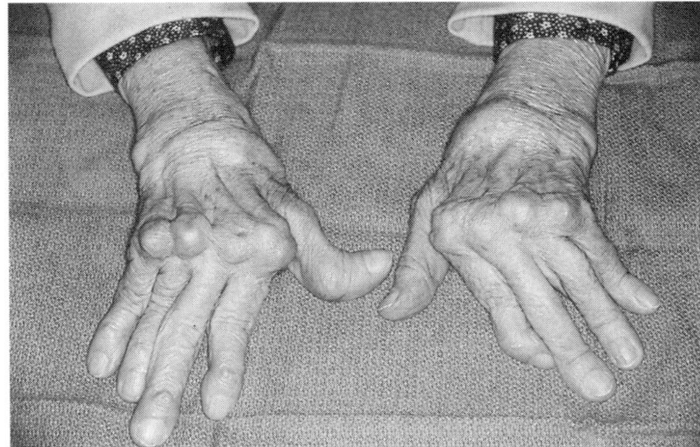

FIG. 45.6. A rheumatoid arthritis patient with involvement of the metacarpophalangeal joints. Note the severe ulnar drift of the fingers.

The Metacarpophalangeal Joint: Bone

Metacarpophalangeal Joint Arthroplasty

Severe MP destruction with fixed deformity may cause pain and loss of function. The treatment of choice is silicone implant arthroplasty (Fig. 45.7). The function of a silicone implant is to act as a spacer between the bones while early motion is started. The motion promotes development of a fibrous capsule around the joint. The implant is not fixed inside the bone, but rather pistons inside the medullary cavity, distributing the stresses on the implant over a wider area. This, in turn, decreases the potential for fracture of the implant with repeated bending over time. Postoperative therapy is essential, and the patients are placed in a dynamic splint with close attention to motion exercises.

The goal of MP arthroplasty surgery is not to regain a full range of motion of the MP joint, but to provide an arc of motion in a functional plane. Postoperatively, patients can expect to gain about 60 degrees of pain-free flexion with almost full extension, and grasp and pinch are improved as the fingers are centrally repositioned. Patients generally report a subjective functional improvement as well as great satisfaction with the improved appearance of the hand (15,16) (Fig. 45.8).

Complications can include implant fracture, which occurs mostly in the index and long fingers because of increased stresses on these fingers during pinch (Fig. 45.9). Reported rates of implant fracture have varied widely, rang-

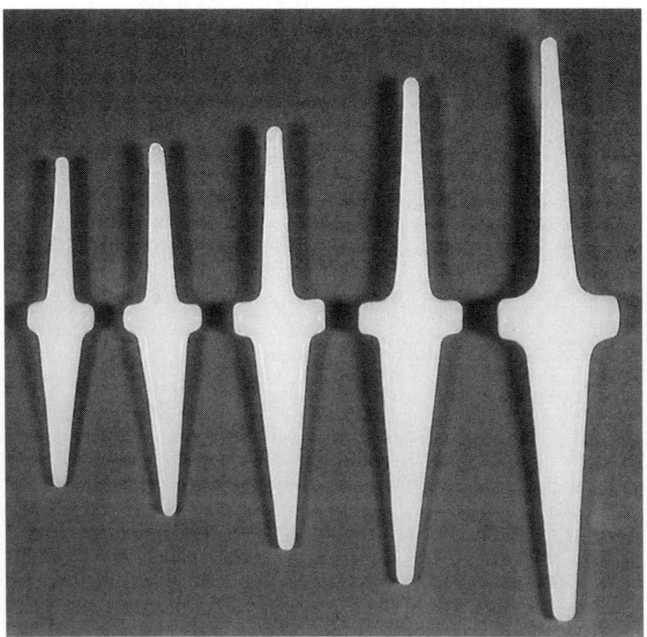

FIG. 45.7. Silicone implants for joint arthroplasty.

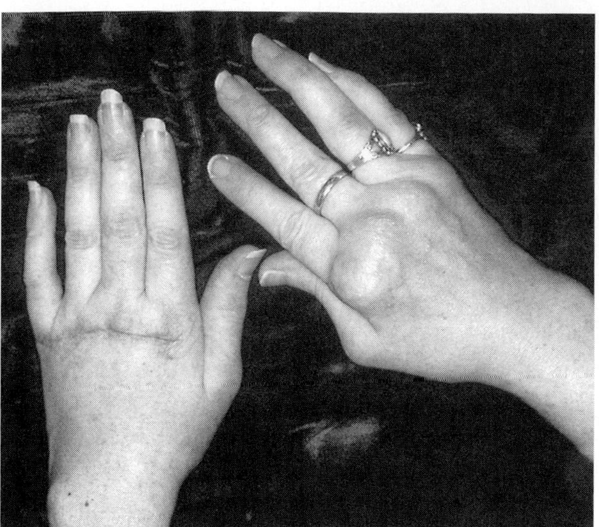

FIG. 45.8. Appearance of the left hand after metacarpophalangeal joint arthroplasty. The right (unoperated) hand is seen in comparison.

ing from 0 to 50%, however, good clinical results are usually maintained despite radiographic decline (17). Silicone particle disease is usually not a problem at the MP joint. Some more recently developed pyrolytic carbon joint implants may provide longer-lasting stability, as long as adequate bone stock exists to support the implant (18).

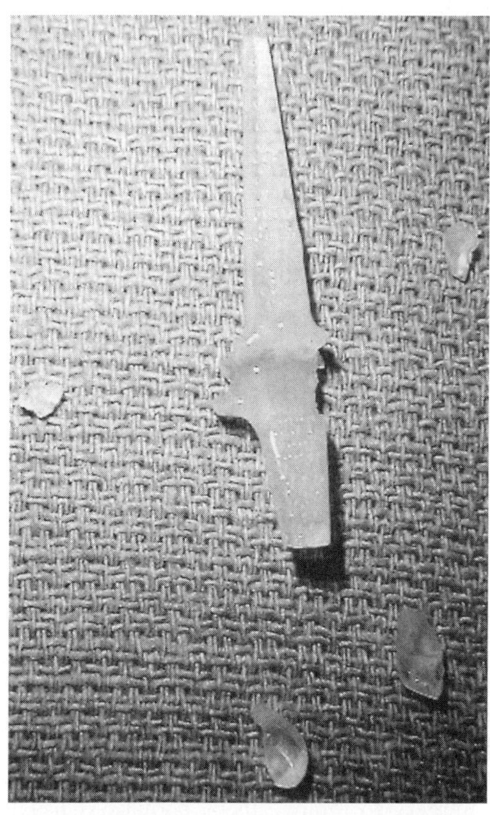

FIG. 45.9. A fractured silicone implant.

The Digits

Tenosynovitis

Digital flexor tenosynovitis can present with swelling, pain, stiffness, triggering, or flexor tendon rupture (Fig. 45.10). Early treatment may consist of steroid injection into the tendon sheath, but refractory inflammation should be treated with tenosynovectomy, especially because reconstruction after tendon rupture is more difficult and yields poor results (19). The entire flexor tendon should be explored, because tendon infiltration can be diffuse. The majority of the pulley system, particularly the A1 pulley, is usually preserved to minimize the risk of postoperative ulnar deviation. A single slip of the FDS tendon (usually ulnar) may be excised to decompress the flexor tendon sheath, if necessary (20). Range of motion should begin immediately postoperatively.

Boutonnière Deformity

Boutonnière deformity (flexion of the PIP joint with hyperextension at the DIP) is caused by PIP synovitis attenuation of the central slip and lateral bands. The lateral bands migrate volarly, becoming PIP flexors, and the joint may then "buttonhole" through the extensor apparatus (21). The deformity can range from mild to severe, depending on the suppleness of the joint and its ability to achieve passive correction. Nalebuff and Millender (22) have described stages of deformity that help to determine the appropriate treatment.

Stage I. Mild deformity and a slight extensor lag exists. PIP motion is good, and DIP joint may be slightly stiff. Treatment may consist of dynamic splinting, as well as PIP cortisone injection.

Stage II. Extensor lag of PIP measures greater than 30 to 40 degrees. Treatment may consist of soft tissue correction (shortening of the extensor mechanism), however, joint surfaces must be in good condition.

Stage III. Fixed flexion contracture and joint destruction. Joint may be repaired by PIP arthroplasty or arthrodesis. The DIP joint may be improved with a terminal extensor tendon release.

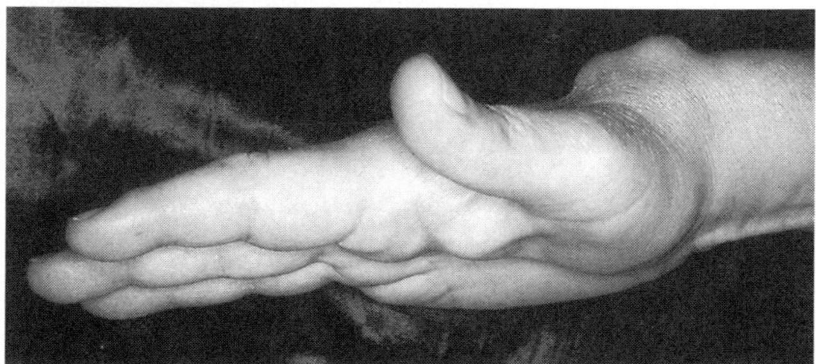

FIG. 45.10. A patient with flexor tenosynovitis of the index finger.

Swan-Neck Deformity

Swan-neck deformity (PIP hyperextension with DIP flexion) may be seen secondary to intrinsic imbalance, PIP volar plate attenuation, terminal extensor tendon rupture at the DIP joint, or FDS dysfunction (Fig. 45.11). Nalebuff (23) has categorized these based on level of severity.

Type I. Flexible PIP joint deformities may be treated with splinting (figure-of-eight splints). Surgery is aimed at eliminating DIP flexion (fusion) and limiting PIP hyperextension (flexor tenodesis, or retinacular ligament reconstruction).

Type II. These deformities have PIP joint mobility that is influenced by the position of the MP joints (which are subject to intrinsic muscle tightness). With MP extension, PIP flexion is limited (Bunnell intrinsic tightness test); with MP flexion, the intrinsics are relaxed, and more PIP flexion is possible. Flexible deformities can be treated with soft tissue reconstruction (e.g., intrinsic release), whereas fixed deformities must be treated with fusion or arthroplasty.

Type III. This deformity has PIP stiffness regardless of the MP position, and the joint is treated with either manipulation or lateral band release and PIP capsulotomy, followed by pinning in the flexed position.

Type IV. These deformities involve intraarticular joint destruction, and surgical treatment consists of salvage procedures, either arthrodesis or arthroplasty. Fusion may be considered in the index and long fingers, because a stable platform is essential for pinch, whereas arthroplasty may be considered in the ring and small fingers, since retention of flexion is preferable for grasping.

The Thumb

Classically, six types of thumb deformity have been described in RA (24–27):

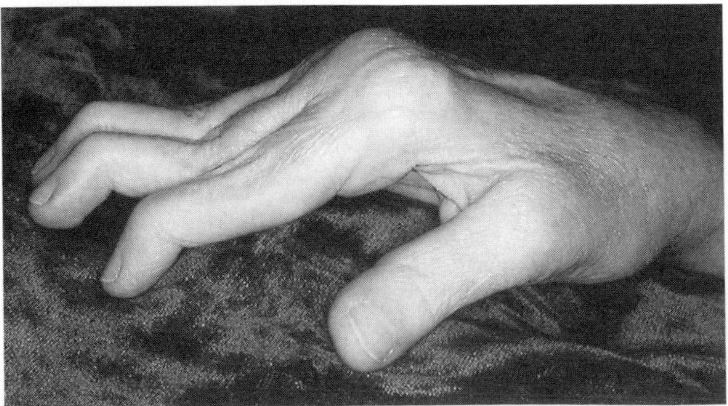

FIG. 45.11. Swan-neck deformities of the index, long, and ring fingers.

Type I: boutonnière deformity (MP flexion with IP hyperextension). This is the most commonly seen deformity of the thumb in RA patients and results from synovitis at the MP joint. The dorsal capsule is attenuated, leading to flexion at the MP joint with compensatory hyperextension at the IP joint. The deforming forces are accented with pinching and, over time, may become fixed. Early on, deformity in the extensor tissues can be reconstructed, whereas later stages require MP fusion.

Type II. This is similar to type I, but pathology includes the CMC joint. Treatment principles are similar to those described in types I and III.

Type III. Swan-neck deformity (MP hyperextension with IP flexion). This is the second most commonly seen deformity of the thumb in RA patients. In the swan-neck thumb, destruction begins at the CMC joint, leading to dorsoradial subluxation of the base of the first metacarpal. The first metacarpal then becomes adducted, and the MP joint is forced into hyperextension as compensation to allow the hand to grasp objects. Arthroplasty of the CMC joint may be necessary, but the pathology at the MP joint also must be addressed, either by capsulodesis of the MP joint or joint fusion. Implant arthroplasty of the CMC joint is generally not used in the rheumatoid population because of poor bone stock and weak capsular tissue.

Type IV: ulnar collateral ligament (UCL) laxity. This also is known as a gamekeeper's thumb, the etiology of which is weakening of the UCL at the MP joint from chronic synovitis. Synovectomy of the MP joint and reconstruction of the UCL may be performed, but if there are extensive articular changes, fusion may provide a better result.

Type V. This is uncommonly seen, and is similar to type III, but without CMC involvement. Treatment of the MP joint is all that is needed.

Type VI. This deformity is characterized by severe loss of bone and skeletal collapse (arthritis mutilans). The thumb becomes quite short and unstable. Treatment consists of fusion of the thumb, which should preferably take place before excessive bone loss occurs.

Rheumatoid Nodules

Rheumatoid nodules occur in the subcutaneous tissue and are seen in 20% to 30% of individuals with RA. They are associated with more aggressive, seropositive disease. The nodules are more common in the olecranon area and extensor surfaces. Occasionally, the nodules may become ulcerated or infected. Rheumatoid nodules may be excised if they become problematic to the patient (e.g., if they occur on resting skin surface or are tender).

Another type of nodulosis seems to involve only the hand (Fig. 45.12). These are rarely associated with systemic manifestations, and generally hand function is preserved. Surgery to remove these nodules is usually done for cosmesis (28).

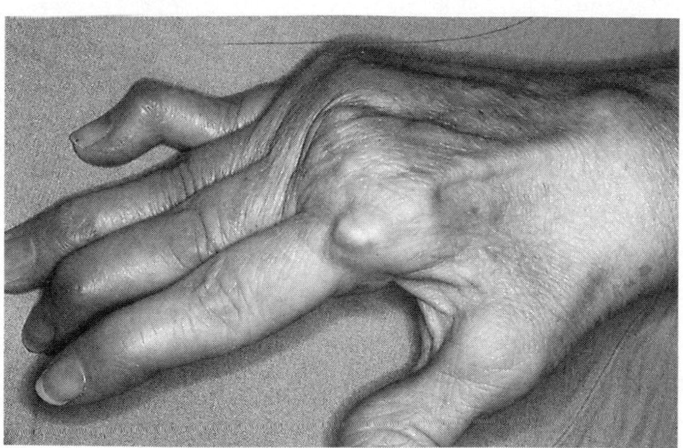

FIG. 45.12. A rheumatoid nodule is seen over the index metacarpophalangeal joint.

JUVENILE RHEUMATOID ARTHRITIS

Many of the reconstructive procedures discussed for the treatment of adult RA are not applicable in the child, because of the potential for growth arrest. Indeed, juvenile RA (JRA) is a different disease from adult RA. It is the most common connective tissue disease in childhood, and causes chronic synovial inflammation.

The articular effects of JRA are most commonly seen in the knees and wrists. In the wrist, the disease affects the ulnar side preferentially, with loss of wrist extension. Deformities of wrist flexion and ulnar deviation develop. In addition, patients may develop radial deviation at the MP joint (in contrast to adults with RA, who develop ulnar drift at the MP joint), and loss of finger flexion.

Radiographically, joint space narrowing may be seen, along with premature closure of epiphyses and periostitis. Later changes may include osteoporosis and bony erosions.

Occupational therapy should play an early role in patients with JRA. Range of motion exercises and a splinting program can help prevent contractures, which occur with growth. If surgery becomes necessary, special care must be directed to preserving the articular surfaces and the growth plate, and should preferably be delayed until skeletal maturity (29).

OSTEOARTHRITIS

Osteoarthritis is characterized by the degeneration of articular cartilage along with an attempt by the body to repair and remodel the cartilage. The cartilage first softens and fibrillates, followed by cracking and exposure of the subchondral bone. Eventually, the bone may become sclerotic and eburnated, with areas of bony cysts and spur formation. The term *primary OA* is given to the condition in which no underlying etiologic factor is present, and *secondary OA* is used when a previous factor can account for the changes (e.g., trauma, anatomic abnormality, or metabolic disease).

Primary OA in the hand characteristically involves the PIP and DIP joints of the fingers and the CMC and IP joints of the thumb. Patients commonly complain of joint pain and stiffness or deformity of the hand. Laboratory results are usually normal. Radiographic changes include narrowing of the joint space, sclerosis of the subchondral bone, subchondral cyst formation, and bony spurs (30).

Conservative treatment of OA of the hand and wrist includes patient education and therapy, splinting, NSAIDs, and intraarticular steroid injection (31,32). Patients should be educated as to the natural history of the disease and taught activity modification, depending on the severity of their symptoms. Generally, patients should be encouraged to exercise and maintain their range of motion as much as possible, with rest during symptomatic periods of flare-up. Therapeutic heat also may be used to increase blood flow and improve joint stiffness, but cold may be more helpful during acute flare-ups. Static splinting can immobilize the painful joint, particularly in the wrist or thumb, and still allow the patient to proceed with activities of daily living. NSAIDs can provide analgesia but do not alter the underlying course of the disease. They can also be associated with side effects, the most common of which is gastrointestinal irritation. A newer class of drugs, the cyclooxygenase-2 (COX-2) inhibitors, more specifically target the prostaglandins involved in inflammation without disturbing the effects of COX-1, which regulates the prostaglandins involved in gastrointestinal and platelet homeostasis. Finally, injection of intraarticular steroids into a specific joint may provide symptomatic relief and increased function. The addition of anesthetic to the steroid injection also can provide valuable information regarding the specificity of the diagnosis. Repeated injections are not indicated if the initial injection did not provide relief, and the need for frequent injections may alert the physician that more definitive treatment may be warranted.

Indications for surgery include intractable pain and limitation of function after conservative measures have been exhausted.

The Wrist

Pisotriquetral Joint

The pisiform is a sesamoid bone lying in the tendon of the flexor carpi ulnaris. It has a single articulation with the triquetrum, and OA of this joint can lead to ulnar-sided wrist pain in the region of the hypothenar eminence. The pain may be reproducible with direct pressure on the bone, passive side-to-side motion of the pisiform, and with extremes of palmar flexion and ulnar deviation. The diagnosis may be confirmed with an anesthetic injection directly into the pisotriquetral joint. The joint also may be viewed radiographically with the wrist in about 30 degrees of supination. Those patients with symptoms refractory to conservative treatment may undergo excision of the pisiform with good pain relief and minimal dysfunction (33).

Radiocarpal Arthroplasty

Arthroplasty of the radiocarpal joint has been used when it is desirable to maintain some range of motion in the wrist, for example, if other ispilateral upper extremity joints are severely arthritic, or if the contralateral wrist has already been fused. The most commonly used prosthesis is a cemented metal prosthesis.

Radiocarpal Arthrodesis

Arthrodesis of the wrist is an excellent, reliable treatment for correction of deformity, improvement of function, and pain relief in patients with degenerated radiocarpal joints. By correcting wrist alignment, providing stability, and eliminating painful motion, improvements in grip strength and overall function can be achieved. Many methods for arthrodesis have been described, and the more commonly used methods include plating (34) and intramedullary rods. The optimal position for fusion is neutral or slight extension.

The Distal Radioulnar Joint

Osteoarthritis at the DRUJ can be either primary or secondary to trauma, and can cause pain and occasionally extensor tendon ruptures (Fig. 45.13). Patients with symptomatic DRUJs have ulnar-sided wrist pain, along with some limitation of wrist and forearm range of motion, and decreased grip strength. Treatment of extensor tendon ruptures is generally the same as was described for rheumatoid patients, whereas treatment of the painful DRUJ is complex and controversial. Surgical options have included distal ulnar resection (Darrach procedure), distal ulnar recession, distal ulnar recession with hemiresection–interposition arthroplasty, and distal radioulnar arthrodesis with proximal ulnar pseudoarthrosis (Sauve-Kapandji procedure) (35). Generally speaking, the Darrach procedure is reserved for more elderly individuals with lower demands, whereas the reconstructive procedures may be considered in younger patients.

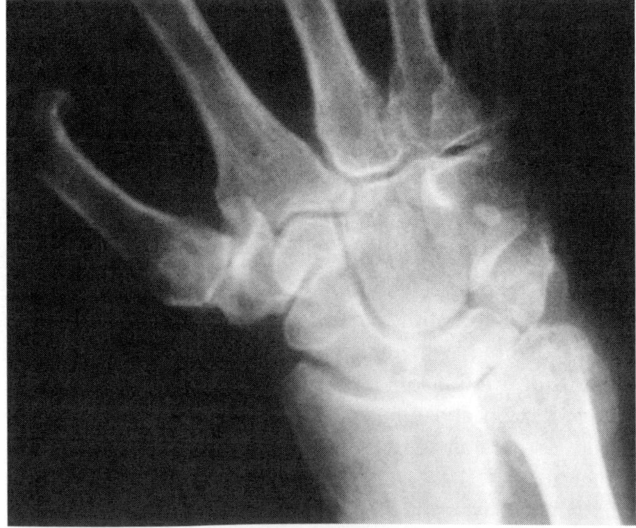

FIG. 45.13. Degenerative changes of the distal radioulnar joint.

The Metacarpophalangeal Joints

Primary osteoarthritic involvement of the MP joints of the fingers (except the thumb) is uncommon. Degenerative changes at the MP joint can result from trauma, infection, or RA, and certain systemic diseases may specifically affect the MP joint, for example, hemochromatosis and calcium pyrophosphate crystal deposition disease (36). Once marked degenerative changes have occurred, surgical options include fusion and arthroplasty. Fusion in digits other than the thumb is rarely indicated because of the resulting significant loss in finger function. The procedure for flexible silicone implant arthroplasty is similar to that described for RA in the preceding section. Newer pyrolytic carbon implants may also play a role in MP arthroplasty, given the sturdier bone stock and intact ligaments in patients with OA, as compared with RA (18).

The Digits

Proximal Interphalangeal Joints

Involvement of the PIP joint with OA is less common than involvement of the DIP, but may be more debilitating (Fig. 45.14). Advanced arthritis of the PIP joint can impair not only motion of the joint but also the functions of pinch (especially in the index and long fingers) and grasp (in the ulnar fingers) (37). The development of marginal osteophytes (Bouchard's nodes) can lead to progressive deformity of the fingers. The main surgical treatments available for the PIP are arthroplasty and arthrodesis. Each has benefits and drawbacks, and the choice depends partially on which finger is involved and the ultimate function desired by the patient (32).

Proximal Interphalangeal Joint Arthroplasty

Flexible silicone implants are available for PIP arthroplasty. Range of motion is partially preserved, with a flexion arc of 27 to 60 degrees reported (38). In addition, good pain relief is provided. However, problems have included periprosthetic bone resorption, limited lateral and rotational stability, and prosthetic fracture. Functional results have been seen to deteriorate with time, especially in young, active patients. Silicone interposition arthroplasty may be considered in the ulnar digits, where retention of flexibility is desired for maintenance of grasp (39).

New surface replacement arthroplasty prostheses have been developed (40). These prostheses are designed to minimize bony excision, preserve the collateral ligaments, and allow greater lateral stability. They have a greater need for

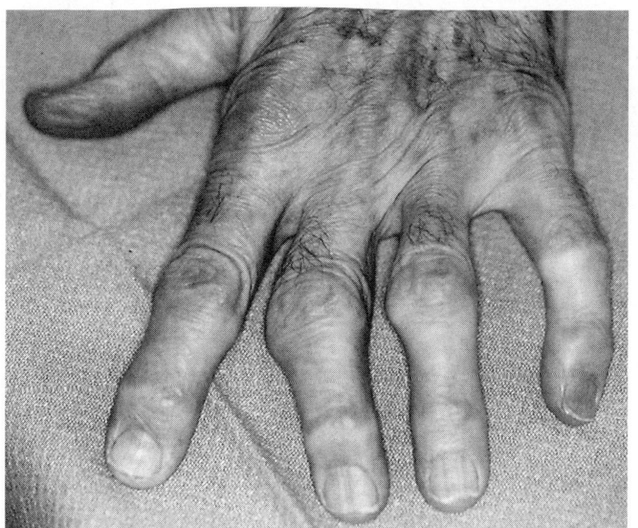

A

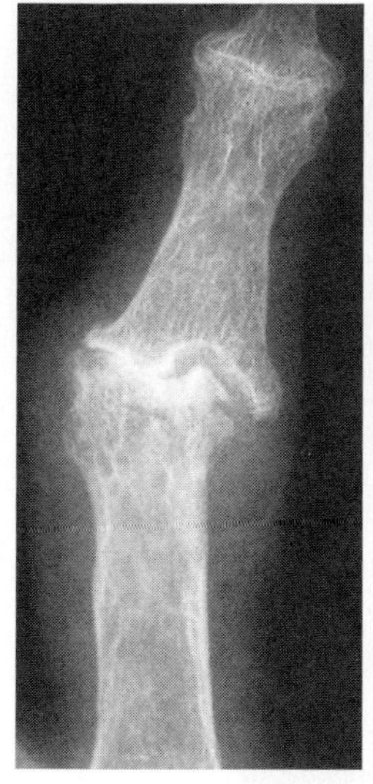

B

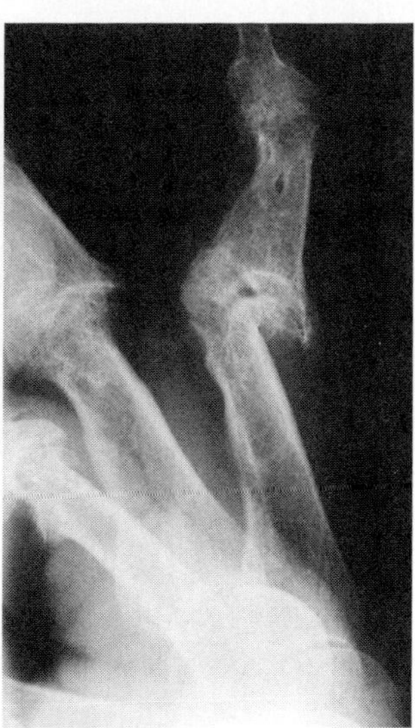

C

FIG. 45.14. A: Typical appearance of a hand with proximal interphalangeal (*PIP*) and distal interphalangeal (*DIP*) osteoarthritis. **B, C:** Posteroanterior and lateral radiographs of a PIP joint affected by osteoarthritis. There is severe joint destruction.

precision placement and alignment, as well as the addition of cement fixation. Pyrolytic carbon implants also exist for the PIP joint, but long-term results are still pending.

Proximal Interphalangeal Joint Arthrodesis

Arthrodesis provides pain relief and a durable, functional digit in the treatment of PIP arthritis. It is particularly useful in the radial digits, because a stable pain-free platform is essential for good lateral or key pinch function (38). Ideally, the patient should possess supple pain-free joints both proximal and distal to the joint in question, because arthrodesis will place increased stress across adjacent joints. The loss of mobility and cosmetic appearance of the finger is usually well tolerated by the patient. The position for fusion should be about 35 to 40 degrees of flexion for the index finger, increasing in a cascade of 5 degrees per finger, to about 55 degrees in the small finger. There should be no radial or ulnar deviation, and rotation should be neutral.

Methods of fixation are varied, including K-wires, tension-band techniques, screw fixation, and plating. Local or distal bone graft also may be used, and the finger is immobilized until the fusion has healed, usually about 6 to 8 weeks.

Distal Interphalangeal Joints

Involvement of the DIP joint with OA may be asymptomatic, deforming, or painful; furthermore, the radiologic appearance of the joint may not always correlate with the patient's symptoms (Fig. 45.15). Patients may develop hypertrophic osteophytes at the DIP joint, known as Heberden's nodes. Pain, along with deformity and instability, are the main indications for surgery.

Mucous Cysts

Osteoarthritis commonly occurs at the DIP joint. Occasionally a cyst may develop on the dorsum of the distal phalanx, usually to one side of the midline, in conjunction with the presence of an underlying osteophyte (Fig. 45.16). The

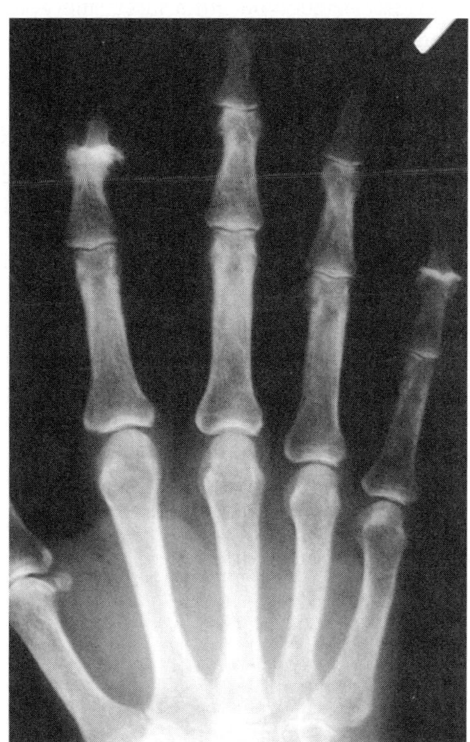

FIG. 45.15. Posteroanterior radiograph of distal interphalangeal osteoarthritis affecting the index and small fingers.

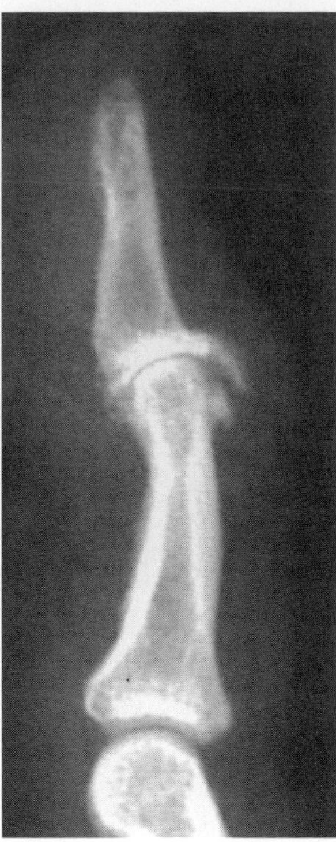

FIG. 45.16. Lateral radiograph of a distal interphalangeal joint demonstrating the dorsal bony spur typically associated with an overlying mucous cyst.

nail matrix may become involved, leading to indentation and grooving of the nail.

Mucous cysts can become quite large and compromise the overlying skin. If the cyst ruptures, there is a potential danger of infection. Aspiration of the cyst rarely eradicates it, but occasionally the cyst may spontaneously resolve. Definitive treatment usually consists of surgical excision of the cyst, along with débridement of the marginal osteophytes and excision of the cyst along with its stalk down to the joint. Sometimes, if the cyst is large, a skin graft or rotational flap may be needed to cover the deficit. Nail deformities should resolve after resection of the cyst and osteophytes, and recurrence is rare (41). If the articular cartilage is severely eroded and the patient has associated pain, consideration may be given to arthrodesis.

Distal Interphalangeal Joint Arthroplasty

Implant arthroplasty in the DIP joint may be performed if motion in the DIP joint must be preserved. This may be considered, for example, in a patient who has had previous PIP fusion. The results, however, are not as reliable as for fusion, and the main disadvantage is lack of stability (42).

Distal Interphalangeal Joint Arthrodesis

DIP joint arthrodesis is an excellent treatment for painful, deformed, or unstable joints. The joint is fused at approximately 0 degrees of flexion, in neutral radial and ulnar deviation. Slight supination may be added in the index and long fingers to aid pulp-to-pulp tip pinch with the thumb. Care is taken not to damage the germinal nail matrix, and supplemental bone graft may be used. Complications include infection, which is usually treated with oral antibiotics, and nonunion (43), but may not be symptomatic and may need no further treatment.

The Thumb

The Carpometacarpal Joint

The first CMC joint, or basal joint, is unique in possessing biconcave saddle-shaped articular surfaces that function as a universal joint. The two major axes of motion are flexion-extension and abduction-adduction. The exceptional mobility of the joint also makes it subject to large contact forces. Rotation, a primary component of thumb opposition, causes incongruity at the periphery of the joint, especially the palmar aspect; this is associated with wear of the palmar oblique or beak ligament. Factors associated with basal joint arthritis include gender (the condition commonly affects postmenopausal women), generalized ligamentous laxity, and a shallow joint surface (Fig. 45.17).

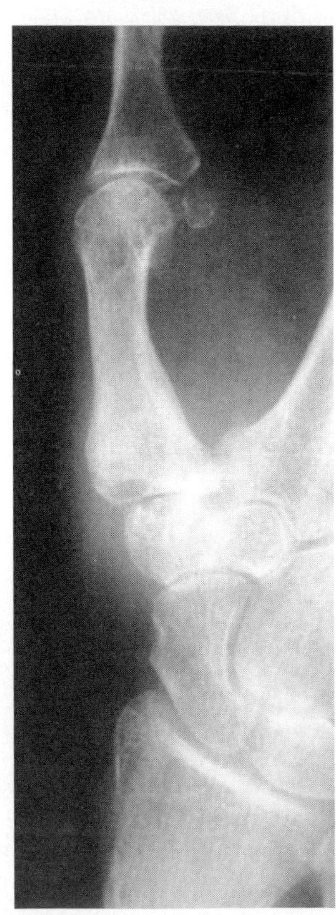

FIG. 45.17. Thumb carpometacarpal (*CMC*) arthrosis, demonstrating narrowing of the CMC joint space, and subchondral cyst formation (in the base of the thumb metacarpal).

The presenting symptoms are pain at the base of the thumb, especially with pinching activities. Progressive disease causes further loss of strength, increasing pain and crepitus, and decreased range of motion. Symptoms can be particularly marked, given the importance of prehensile grip in many activities of daily living. Pain at the base of the thumb due to OA should be distinguished from that of inflammation of the first dorsal compartment, or DeQuervain stenosing tenosynovitis. The Finklestein test (positive in DeQuervain syndrome) and the "grind test" (positive in CMC arthritis) may be useful in distinguishing between the two diseases.

Radiographically, progression of the disease has been characterized (44) (Table 45.1). In addition, a basal joint stress radiograph (PA radiograph of both hands taken with the lateral thumb tips pressed against each other) can provide an excellent pantrapezial joint view.

In evaluating a patient with basal joint disease, attention also must be directed to the MP joint. In advanced disease, dorsoradial subluxation of the base of the first metacarpal may develop, with a secondary compensatory deformity of hyperextension of the MP joint. The subluxation of the metacarpal bases results in adduction of the metacarpal, and loss of the first web space. The MP joint then becomes hyperextended (swan-neck deformity) to compensate for this loss, in an attempt to maintain the ability of the hand to accommodate large cylindrical objects (Fig. 45.18). Arthritic changes also may affect the MP joint; thus, any surgery of the CMC joint must also address abnormalities at the MP joint.

Several different options exist to address the first CMC joint; most provide good pain relief, with varying degrees of return of function.

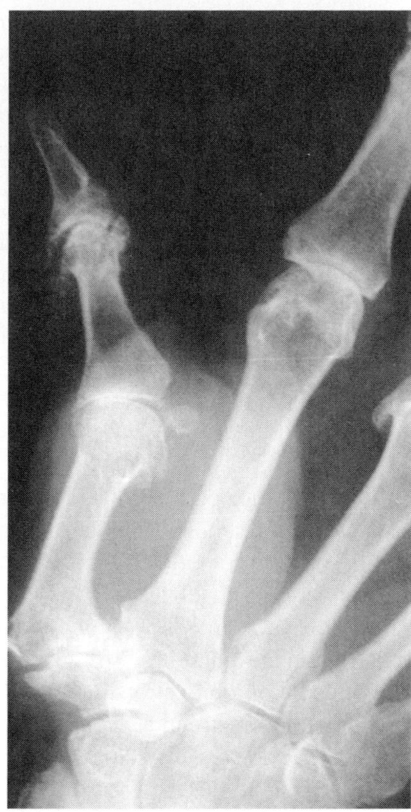

FIG. 45.18. Thumb carpometacarpal (*CMC*) arthrosis with involvement of the metacarpophalangeal (*MP*) joint. The MP joint typically hyperextends to compensate for the adduction deformity of the first metacarpal. The MCP joint also must be addressed at the time of CMC surgery.

Carpometacarpal Joint Arthroplasty

Excisional. Simple excision of the trapezium can alleviate pain and preserve thumb motion. Disadvantages include loss of thumb strength and stability.

Silicone. Many types of silicone implants exist, but all forms basically consist of a silicone spacer with an intramedullary portion extending into the thumb metacarpal. The major complication over time has been subluxation and instability of the prosthesis. Periprosthetic ligament reconstruction leads to greater stability of the implant, but also subjects it to greater forces across the basal joint, increasing the likelihood of prosthetic fragmentation. Silicone synovitis has been reported as a major problem, and overall, use of silicone implants is reserved for the very low-demand thumb (45,46).

Metal. These implants consist of a polyethylene cup, which is recessed into the trapezium, and a cemented cobalt chrome metacarpal component. Because of the large forces involved in the thumb and the small area of the implant–bone interface, loosening has been a problem over the long term.

Tendon Interposition. A portion of the trapezium or the complete trapezium is excised, and a spacer is fashioned out of donor fascia or tendon, usually the palmaris longus (if present), or a portion of the FCR, which is rolled up to resemble an "anchovy" (47,48). Theoretical problems include decreased pinch strength and thumb shortening.

TABLE 45.1. *Stages of carpometacarpal joint involvement in osteoarthritis*

Stage	Joint contour	Joint debris	Subluxation	ST joint
I	Normal/widened	None	None	Normal
II	Narrowed	<2 mm	None	Normal
III	Very narrow/gone	>2 mm	Present	Normal
IV	Obliterated	>2 mm	Present	Narrowed

Tendon Interposition with Ligament Reconstruction. To improve thumb function and prevent metacarpal subsidence, more recent efforts have focused on reconstruction of the palmar oblique ligament (49,50) (extends from the base of the thumb metacarpal to the base of the index metacarpal). This procedure reconstructs the palmar oblique ligament by using a portion or all of the FCR woven through a drill hole in the base of the metacarpal. The palmar oblique ligament is the primary stabilizer of the thumb in pronation in activities such as lateral pinch, and its reconstruction prevents "settling" of the thumb with time, generally resulting in better pinch strength than interposition arthroplasty alone.

Carpometacarpal Joint Arthrodesis

Fusion is primarily indicated for isolated degeneration of the CMC joint, and in the younger patient. Disadvantages include limitation of thumb motion, inability to flatten the hand, and transfer of stress to adjacent joints. However, patients seem to report little in the way of functional complaints (51,52). Fusion is sometimes difficult to accomplish even with prolonged immobilization; however, a fibrous union may be compatible with an acceptable result. Surgical techniques include K-wires and staples. The optimal position for fusion is 10 to 15 degrees of extension and 35 to 40 degrees of palmar abduction.

Thumb Metacarpophalangeal Joint Arthrodesis

Arthrodesis is a reliable method of treating the severely involved thumb MP joint, and is often performed in conjunction with arthroplasty of the first CMC joint. If there is significant degenerative arthritis, hyperextension greater than 25 to 30 degrees, or greater than 30 degrees of valgus laxity, consideration should be given to addressing the MP joint surgically (arthrodesis if the joint is degenerated; capsulodesis if the articular surfaces are good). Various methods exist to achieve arthrodesis (K-wires, screw), and the optimal position for fusion is 5 to 15 degrees of flexion, with slight pronation to aid pinch. Arthroplasty here is less successful because stability of the MP joint is crucial to overall function of the thumb.

Patients are generally very pleased with the results of MP fusion; given mobility of the CMC joint, function of the thumb is not significantly altered.

Interphalangeal Joint Arthrodesis

The thumb IP joint is affected by OA in a manner similar to that which was already discussed in the section on the digital DIP joint (Fig. 45.19). The treatment of thumb IP arthritis is also similar, with IP fusion having excellent results for pain relief and joint stability.

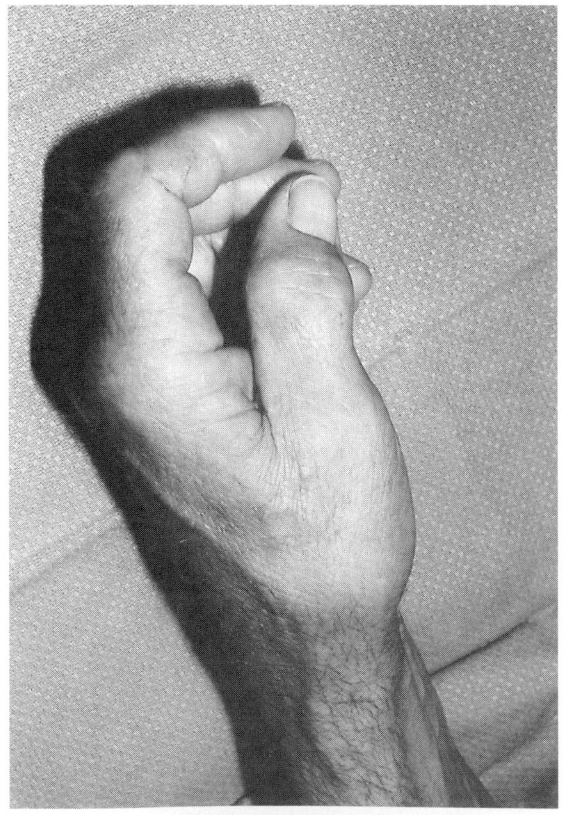

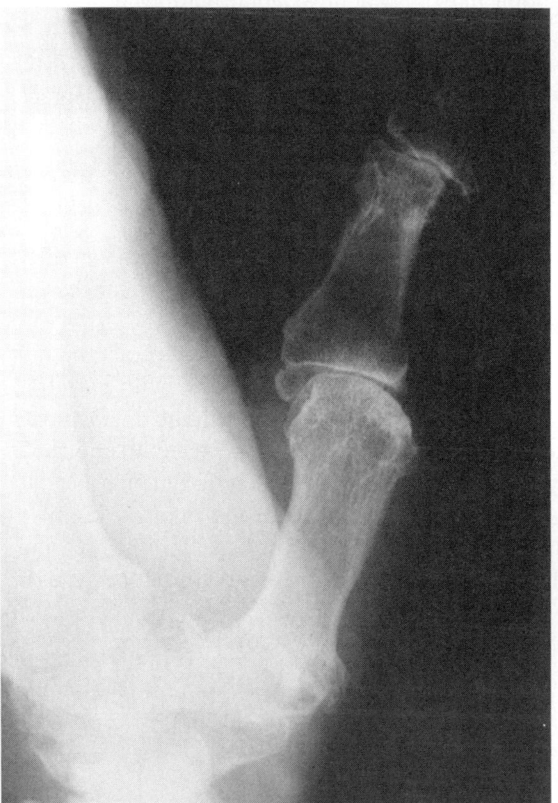

FIG. 45.19. A: Clinical appearance of thumb distal interphalangeal (*DIP*) osteoarthritis. **B:** Radiographic appearance of thumb DIP osteoarthritis. The DIP joint has subluxated laterally, probably due to repeated pinching forces against the index finger.

REFERENCES

1. Alderman AK, Chung KC, Kim HM, et al. Effectiveness of rheumatoid hand surgery: contrasting perceptions of hand surgeons and rheumatologists. *J Hand Surg* 2003;28:3–11.
2. Van Lankveld W, van't Pad Bosch R, van der Schaaf D, et al. Evaluating hand surgery in patients with rheumatoid arthritis: short-term effect on dexterity and pain and its relationship with patient satisfaction. *J Hand Surg* 2000;25;921–929.
3. Rosen A, Weiland AJ. Rheumatoid arthritis of the wrist and hand. *Rheum Dis Clin North Am* 1997;24:101–128.
4. Jain A, Witbreuk M, Ball C, et al. Influence of steroids and methotrexate in wound complications after elective rheumatoid hand and wrist surgery. *J Hand Surg* 2002;27A:449–455.
5. Blair WF. An approach to complex rheumatoid hand and wrist problems. *Hand Clin* 1996;12:615–628.
6. Mowat AG. Medical implications of orthopaedic surgery in rheumatic diseases. *Clin Rheum Dis* 1978;4:249–261.
7. Wilson RL, DeVito MC. Extensor tendon problems in rheumatoid arthritis. *Hand Clin* 1996;12:551–559.
8. Ryu J, Saito S, Honda T, et al. Risk factors and prophylactic tenosynovectomy for extensor tendon ruptures in the rheumatoid hand. *J Hand Surg* 1998;23:658–661.
9. Williamson SC, Feldon P. Extensor tendon ruptures in rheumatoid arthritis. *Hand Clin* 1995;11:449–459.
10. Gellman H, Hontas R, Brumfeld RH, et al. Total wrist arthroplasty in rheumatoid arthritis. *Clin Orthop* 1997;342:71–76.
11. Shapiro JS. The wrist in rheumatoid arthritis. *Hand Clin* 1996;12: 477–513.
12. Kobus RJ, Turner RH. Wrist arthrodesis for treatment of rheumatoid arthritis. *J Hand Surg* 1990;15:541–546.
13. Blank JE, Cassidy C. The distal radioulnar joint in rheumatoid arthritis. *Hand Clin* 1996;12:499–513.
14. Stirrat CR. Metacarpophalangeal joints in rheumatoid arthritis of the hand. *Hand Clin* 1996;12:515–529.
15. Gellman H, Stetson W, Brumfeld RH, et al. Silastic metacarpophalangeal joint arthroplasty in patients with rheumatoid arthritis. *Clin Orthop* 1997;342:16–21.
16. Kirschenbaum D, Schneider LH, Adams DC, et al. Arthroplasty of the metacarpophalangeal joints with use if silicone-rubber implants in patients who have rheumatoid arthritis. *J Bone Joint Surg Am* 1993;75: 3–12.
17. Schmidt K, Willburger RE, Meihlke RK, et al. Ten-year follow-up of silicone arthroplasty of the metacarpophalangeal joints in the rheumatoid hands. *Scan J Plast Reconstr Hand Surg* 1999;33:433–438.
18. Cook SD, Beckenbaugh RD, Redondo J, et al. Long-term follow-up of pyrolytic carbon metacarpophalangeal implants. *J Bone Joint Surg* 1999;81:635–648.
19. Ferlic DC. Rheumatoid flexor tenosynovitis and rupture. *Hand Clin* 1996;12:561–572.
20. Wheen DJ, Tonkin MA, Green J, et al. Long-term results following digital flexor tenosynovectomy in rheumatoid arthritis. *J Hand Surg* 1995;20:791–794.
21. Rizio L, Belsky MR. Finger deformities in rheumatoid arthritis. *Hand Clin* 1996;12:531–549.
22. Nalebuff EA, Millender LH. Surgical treatment of the boutonnière deformity in rheumatoid arthritis. *Orthop Clin North Am* 1975;6:753–763.
23. Nalebuff EA. The rheumatoid swan-neck deformity. *Hand Clin* 1989; 5:203–214.
24. Nalebuff EA. The rheumatoid thumb. *Rheum Dis Clin North Am* 1984; 10:589–595.
25. Stein AB, Terrano AL. The rheumatoid thumb. *Hand Clin* 1996;12: 541–549.
26. Terrano A, Millender L, Nalebuff E. Boutonnière rheumatoid thumb deformity. *J Hand Surg* 1990;15:999–1003.
27. Toledano B, Terrano A, Millender L. Reconstruction of the rheumatoid thumb. *Hand Clin* 1992;8:121–129.
28. Boland DM, Craig EV. Rheumatoid disease. *Hand Clin* 1989;5:359–371.
29. Simmons BP, Nutting JT, Bernstein RA. Juvenile rheumatoid arthritis. *Hand Clin* 1996;12:573–599.
30. Dray GJ, Jablon M. Clinical and radiologic features of primary osteoarthritis of the hand. *Hand Clin* 1987;3:351–367.
31. Docken WP. Clinical features and medical management of osteoarthritis at the hand and wrist. *Hand Clin* 1987;3:337–347.
32. Palmieri TJ, Grand FM, Hay EL, et al. Treatment of osteoarthritis in the hand and wrist: non-operative treatment. *Hand Clin* 1987;3:371–381.
33. Carroll RE, Coyle MP. Dysfunction of the pisotriquetral joint: treatment by excision of the pisiform. *J Hand Surg* 1985;10:703–707.
34. Leighton RK, Petrie D. Arthrodesis of the wrist. *Can J Surg* 1987;30: 115–116.
35. Minami A, Suzuki K, Suenaga N, et al. The Sauve-Kapandji procedure for osteoarthritis of the distal radioulnar Joint. *J Hand Surg* 1995;20:602–608.
36. Feldon P, Belsky MR. Degenerative diseases of the metacarpophalangeal joints. *Hand Clin* 1987;3:429–445.
37. Stern PJ, Ho S. Osteoarthritis of the proximal interphalangeal joint. *Hand Clin* 1987;3:405–412.
38. Pellegrini VD, Burton RI. Osteoarthritis of the proximal interphalangeal joint of the hand: arthroplasty or fusion? *J Hand Surg* 1990; 15:194–209.
39. Swanson AB. Implant resection arthroplasty of the proximal interphalangeal joint. *Ortho Clin North Am* 1974;4:1007–1029.
40. Linscheid RL, Murray PM, Vidal M-A, et al. Development of a surface replacement arthroplasty for proximal interphalangeal joints. *J Hand Surg* 1997;22:286–298.
41. Eaton RG, Dobranski AI, Little JW. Marginal osteophyte excision in treatment of mucous cysts. *J Bone Joint Surg Am* 1973;55:570–574.
42. Culver JE, Fleegler EJ, Osteoarthritis of the distal interphalangeal joint. *Hand Clin* 1987;3:385–404.
43. Burton RI, Margles SW, Lunseth PA. Small-joint arthrodesis in the hand. *J Hand Surg* 1986;11:678–682.
44. Eaton RG. Replacement of the trapezium for arthritis of the basal articulation: a new technique with stability by tenodesis. *J Bone Joint Surg Am* 1979;61:76–82.
45. Burton RI. Basal joint implant arthroplasty in osteoarthritis: indications, techniques, pitfalls, and problems. *Hand Clin* 1987;3:473–485.
46. Pellegrini VD, Burton RI. Surgical management of basal joint arthritis of the thumb. Part I. Long-term, results of silicone implant arthroplasty. *J Hand Surg* 1986;11:309–324.
47. Damen A, VanderLei B, Robinson PH. Carpometacarpal arthritis of the thumb. *J Hand Surg* 1996;21:807–812.
48. Froimson AI. Tendon interposition arthroplasty of the carpometacarpal joint of the thumb. *Hand Clin* 1987;3:489–503.
49. Burton RI, Pellegrini VD. Surgical management of basal joint arthritis of the thumb. Part II. Ligament reconstruction with tendon interposition arthroplasty. *J Hand Surg* 1986;11:324–332.
50. Tomaino MM, Pellegrini VD, Burton RI. Arthroplasty of the basal joint of the thumb. *J Bone Joint Surg Am* 1995;77:346–355.
51. Bamberger HB, Stern PJ, Kiefhaber TR, et al. Trapeziometacarpal joint arthrodesis: a functional evaluation. *J Hand Surg* 1992;17:605–611.
52. Chamay A, Paiget-Morerod F. Arthrodesis of the trapeziometacarpal joint. *J Hand Surg* 1994;19:489–497.

CHAPTER 46

Surgery of Shoulder Arthritis

D. Scott Devinney, Mark Frankle, Mark Mighell, and David Fisher

Surgical management of shoulder arthritis is evolving; minimally invasive surgery continues to play an important role for most arthritic conditions of the shoulder, including those in young or medically infirm patients. In shoulder arthroplasty, there have been many modifications to newer implants. Improving restoration of the anatomy by implants with varying offsets, an increased modular selection of implants, and different techniques of implant fixation has provided more reliable outcomes. The use of biologic resurfacing, with or without hemiarthroplasty, also has been tried in small numbers in younger patients. Additionally, the complex problem of patients with coexisting arthritis and irreparable cuff tears has been treated with a new semiconstrained reverse shoulder prosthesis that has provided encouraging results in terms of functional improvements and pain relief.

ANATOMY AND BIOMECHANICS

General Concepts

The shoulder is a complex joint that possesses the greatest degree of mobility of all the joints in the body. This mobility requires integrated motion of glenohumeral, scapulothoracic, acromioclavicular, and sternoclavicular joints, making it possible for the hand to move along the surface of a hypothetical sphere. The center of the sphere is located at the shoulder joint. Pathology affecting the shoulder girdle can impair the ability to place the hand along the surface of this sphere.

Radiographic studies of arm elevation have recorded a 2:1 ratio of glenohumeral to scapulothoracic motion when the humerus is elevated in the coronal plane. A similar analysis found a ratio of 5:4 after the first 30 degrees of elevation. These ratios are commonly accepted, and the motion termed humeroscapular or glenohumeral rhythm.

In elevation of the shoulder without rotator cuff pathology, the humeral head translates superiorly less than 2 to 3 mm. As the arm is elevated with the elbow extended, a maximum joint reactive force of 89% of body weight occurs at this 90 degree abduction angle. This decreases to 40% of body weight at 60 and 150 degrees of abduction. The addition of a 5-kg weight to the hand of this 90 degree abducted arm results in a joint reaction force that is 2.5 times body weight. Shear forces of the shoulder are highest between 30 and 60 degrees of abduction. The absence of a functional rotator cuff allows for increased translation with resultant increased shear forces (1–7). In the setting of total shoulder arthroplasty (TSA), lack of a functional rotator cuff contributes to glenoid stress through increased translation and is the primary reason for glenoid failure (termed rocking horse phenomenon).

In the nonpathologic shoulder, a balance of static and dynamic constraints acting across the joint achieves control of glenohumeral stability. The middle range of rotational joint stability is provided by the dynamic action of the rotator cuff and biceps through compression of the humeral head into the glenoid. The ligamentous structures function passively at the extreme positions of rotation, preventing excessive translation of the humeral head (Table 46.1). Tightening a portion of the capsule can increase translation of the humeral head during glenohumeral rotation. Translation occurs in the opposite direction of capsular tightening and can lead to instability and articular damage (capsulorrhaphy arthritis) and even impingement secondary to superior translation.

Another subset of patients presenting with lax capsuloligamentous complexes subluxate or dislocate in all directions with the shoulder at rest. This pathologic variant, called multidirectional instability, is typically seen in younger individuals and is not usually associated with arthritis.

The glenoid labrum not only reduces bearing stresses, but it also acts as an anchor for these capsuloligamentous structures, increasing the depth of the glenoid and facilitating the concavity compression mechanism as the humeral head is

TABLE 46.1. *Functions of ligamentous structures of the shoulder*

	Location	Insertion	Function
Superior glenohumeral ligament	Rotator interval (between supraspinatus and subscapularis)	Lesser tuberosity	Restraint to external rotation in adducted or slightly abducted arm; restraint to inferior translation in adducted arm; secondary restraint to posterior translation in adducted flexed and internally rotated shoulder
Coracohumeral ligament (two bands)	Coracoid base	Superior band: greater tuberosity/ anterior edge of supraspinatus Inferior band: lesser tuberosity/ superior border subscapularis	Restraint to inferior translation of adducted arm and to external rotation; secondary restraint to posterior instability with arm adducted, flexed, internally rotated
Middle glenohumeral ligament	Variable—anterior superior labrum, scapular neck, supraglenoid tubercle	Anterior to lesser tuberosity with subscapularis	Restraint to anterior translation with arm abducted 45 degrees; limits external rotation at 60 and 90 degrees of abduction
Inferior glenohumeral ligament	Anterior band from glenoid labrum at the 2 to 4 o'clock positions; posterior band from the 7 to 9 o'clock positions	Humeral head between subscapularis and triceps	Restraint to anterior translation in abducted externally rotated arm; restraint to posterior translation in abducted internally rotated arm

compressed in the glenoid during active elevation. Loss of the labrum, termed a Bankart lesion, can result in a 50% decrease in glenoid depth. Furthermore, the translational force required to dislocate the humeral head is 20% smaller after labrum excision. The additional stabilizing effect of intraarticular pressure is the result of a vacuum effect, which is present in a sealed joint compartment. This effect has been found to be minimal compared with the stabilizing actions of dynamic forces (rotator cuff) (1–5,8–16).

The heterogeneity of proximal humeral bony anatomy has had major implications for prosthetic design and development. Boileau and Walch first demonstrated the wide range of interpersonal variation in the inclination of the articular surface of the humerus relative to the orthopedic axis of the humerus. (The orthopaedic axis is the line that is formed when preparing the intramedullary canal of the humeral diaphysis for implantation of a straight stem.) This variation can be anywhere from 120 to 145 degrees. Furthermore, the amount of rotational angulation of the articular surface relative to the forearm (version) also has a large variation of 7 to 38 degrees. Finally, the articular surface can have variable translational offset from the center of the orthopedic axis, most commonly posterior and inferior up to 4 mm. The one constant relationship is the preservation of the amount of surface arc of articular cartilage on the humeral head of 140 degrees. These anatomic studies have produced several other biomechanical analyses that have evaluated the importance of restoration of the articular humeral anatomy with current prosthetic designs (17–20).

Glenohumeral positioning is of paramount importance in shoulder arthroplasty. Iannotti and Williams (21) have demonstrated that humeral articular malposition of 4 mm or less during prosthetic arthroplasty of the glenohumeral joint may lead to small alterations in humeral translations and range of motion. Williams and co-workers (22) have shown that inferior malposition of more than 4 mm can lead to increased subacromial contact, and offset of 8 mm in any direction results in significant decreases in passive range of motion. Therefore, if subacromial contact is to be minimized and glenohumeral motion maximized following shoulder replacement, anatomic reconstruction of the humeral head–humeral shaft offset to within 4 mm is desirable.

There are biomechanical and anatomic differences between second- and third-generation prosthetic shoulder joints. Pearl and Kurutz (18), using a three-dimensional cadaveric analysis, demonstrated that the variable geometry of the third-generation prosthetic systems allowed for significantly better replication of the three-dimensional position of the center of rotation and articulation point with preservation of the articular surface arc compared with the second-generation prosthetic systems. Current designs of modular implants have been investigated with a computer best-fit analysis. Results have shown that specific design features allow for improved biomechanical and anatomic measurements. Specifically, without prosthetic design features that allow for variations in inclination of the articular surface, stem-to-surface translational ability, and a selection of prosthetic head sizes of a specified anatomic thickness and corresponding radius of curvature allowing the surface arc to be 140 degrees, restoration of parameters would be possible only with a small number of current prosthetic designs.

Warner and co-workers (5) have compared hemiarthroplasty with use of a second-generation versus a third-generation design. Head-to-tuberosity height was greater than that on the contralateral normal side in patients who underwent hemiarthroplasty with a second-generation prosthesis. Moreover, these shoulders had a decreased radius of curvature of the articular surface and an increased lateral offset compared with these parameters in the uninvolved shoulder. In contrast, all radiographic parameters were reconstructed to 2 mm of normal (or less) in the patients who underwent hemiarthroplasty with a more adaptable design. However, there is no current evidence from any study that third-generation implants produce superior clinical outcomes. In fact, Friedman and co-workers (23) found no correlation between various radiographic measurements and functional score following TSA. They concluded that good surgical technique, including careful soft tissue balancing, appears to compensate for changes in the anatomic relationships among designs (6).

Pearl and co-workers have shown that a 4-mm offset between the articular surface and the intramedullary stem would be comparable with prosthetic designs that have multiple variable axes (such as translation inclination and rotation) in achieving anatomic restoration of vast numbers of humeri (18,19). These studies have influenced prosthetic manufacturers. There are many systems that provide a varying degree of flexibility when trying to reconstruct the articular surface relative to the intramedullary stem. Unfortunately, changes in clinical outcomes for TSA have yet to be demonstrated for these designs. The makers of one system have even abandoned using the stem to attach the articular surface. This resurfacing component has been used in some large shoulder replacements series in the United Kingdom but has yet to be used commonly in the United States. Concerns of reliable exposure to the glenoid, when glenoid resurfacing is indicated, continues to limit its use.

Glenohumeral Articulation

Evaluation of the normal shoulder articulation also has affected prosthetic design. Glenohumeral component mismatch (i.e., the difference in the radius of curvature between the humeral head and the glenoid) has important implications for joint loading, durability, and stability. Iannotti and Williams (21) have determined that there is a mismatch between the radius of curvature of the humeral head (which is more curved) and the radius of curvature of the glenoid (which is flatter). In the normal shoulder, the radius of curvature of the humeral head is no more than 2 to 3 mm smaller than that of the glenoid. Additionally, the normal glenoid is more constrained (has more depth) in the superoinferior direction than in the anteroposterior direction (9 mm vs. 5 mm). This allows the humeral head to translate on the glenoid with small changes in the contact forces of the head on the glenoid.

Glenohumeral mismatch is an important component of TSA. Walch and co-workers (24) have observed a significant linear relationship between mismatch and glenoid radiolucency scores, with lower scores associated with radial mismatches of more than 5.5 mm. This study represented an important step in establishing recommendations for the optimal amount of component mismatch. Prosthetic manufacturers now provide a limited mismatch between the articulation of the humeral head and the prosthetic glenoid radius of curvature.

The glenoid fossa is oriented in 7 degrees of retroversion relative to the scapula in 75% of individuals, with 5 degrees of superior tilt on average. The articular surface has a pear-shaped appearance, being wider in the inferior anteroposterior direction (29 mm vs. 23 mm). The average superoinferior dimension is 39 mm (6,17). In a study by Churchill and co-workers (17), 344 human scapular bones (172 matched pairs) were measured for glenoid height, width, inclination, and version. The sample consisted of 50 black men, 50 white men, 50 black women, and 22 white women, all of whom were 20 to 30 years of age at the time of death. Specifically, the glenoid version for black and white men measured 0.11 degrees and retroversion measured 2.87 degrees. The glenoid version for black and white women measured 0.30 degrees and retroversion measured 2.16 degrees. Relationships between glenoid size, inclination, and version are important to understand when a surgeon prepares to resurface the glenoid during TSA.

Bony lesions of the anterior or posterior glenoid rim decrease glenoid constraint. These lesions may result from an osseous Bankart lesion (bony Bankart), a displaced glenoid fracture, or wear of the glenoid rim related to recurrent instability. It is generally accepted that a fracture involving more than 25% of the glenoid surface should be repaired. Radiographic and intraoperative findings of the glenoid associated with arthritic changes include posterior glenoid erosion and central glenoid erosion associated with osteoarthritis (OA) and rheumatoid arthritis (RA). These changes are best viewed with the axillary radiograph or computed tomography (CT) scan and must be taken into account in any preoperative plan.

The amount of humeral head covered by the glenoid in the coronal plane (superoinferior) is 60% and in the axial plane (anteroposterior) plane is 46%. Overall, the glenoid covers 28% of the humeral articular cartilage at a given point of movement. This has led to the comparison of a golf ball resting on a tee, emphasizing the importance of the capsuloligamentous complex and rotator cuff musculature in providing stability. The Hill-Sachs lesion, an impression fracture of the articular surface caused by translation over the glenoid rim, has been reported in up to 80% of anterior dislocations, 25% of anterior subluxations, and almost 100% of cases of recurrent instability. With posterior instability, a reverse Hill-Sachs lesion results from impaction of the anterior articular surface when the humeral head dislocates over the posterior glenoid rim. When the lesion approaches 30% of the articular surface with associated instability, surgery is indicated (6).

Consideration of Muscle Forces

Primary movers of the shoulder include the deltoid, pectoralis major, latissimus dorsi, and teres major. These function in ways predictable to the line of their pull. Loss of deltoid function is disabling, has few surgical options, and commonly leads to a glenohumeral arthrodesis in the symptomatic patient.

The rotator cuff consists of the subscapularis, supraspinatus, infraspinatus, and teres minor muscles. The supraspinatus is active with glenohumeral elevation, and line of action is directed toward the glenoid providing compression. The infraspinatus and teres minor muscles function to externally rotate and extend the humerus. The infraspinatus also functions as a depressor of the humeral head and contributes to anterior and posterior stability. The subscapularis functions as an internal rotator of the humerus and a passive stabilizer to anterior subluxation and external rotation. Its lower fibers serve as a humeral head depressor. Together with the infraspinatus, the subscapularis provides a downward force on the humeral head resisting the shear forces of the deltoid during glenohumeral elevation. The coordinated function of the rotator cuff allows for rotation of the humerus on the glenoid while maintaining stability.

Ligamentous attachments are essential to stability of the shoulder. Ligamentocapsular release of contractures is required in the arthritic shoulder to obtain motion (Table 46.1). The coracoacromial arch consists of two bands. The coracoacromial ligament is considered more clinically important because it forms the roof above the supraspinatus, and variations in geometry and biomechanics have been found to be related to rotator cuff tears. Additionally, in the shoulder with a deficient rotator cuff, the coracoacromial ligament is important as a secondary restraint to prevent superior migration of the head. This restraint may provide a new fulcrum for the shoulder in the absence of rotator cuff function. Symptomatic arthritis of the glenohumeral joint in the setting of rotator cuff deficiency is characterized by chronic shoulder pain with superior or anterosuperior migration of the humeral head. It poses a complex problem for the orthopedic surgeon. Several theories have evolved, including localized RA, rapidly destructive arthritis of the shoulder, hemorrhagic shoulder of the elderly, Milwaukee shoulder syndrome/crystal-associated arthritis, and cuff tear arthropathy. Affected patients have massive rotator cuff tears, bone loss, and poor joint mechanics.

Blood Supply

The blood supply of the humeral head must be considered when evaluating patients with osteonecrosis, whether classified as primary or secondary to fracture. The ascending branch of the anterior humeral circumflex artery and its continuation as the arcuate artery are considered the main supply to the humeral head and articular surface (25, 26). Anastomosis has been shown between the anterior humeral circumflex, suprascapular, thoracodorsal, and posterior humeral circumflex arteries. The posteromedial vessels may provide perfusion of the humeral head in certain fractures, specifically a valgus impacted four-part fracture.

BIOMECHANICS OF FIXATION OF PROSTHESIS

The technique of TSA requires a method for securely and durably fixing the humeral component into the proximal part of the humerus. The complexities of the shape of the medullary canal include a substantial metaphyseal canal at the anatomic neck of the humerus where the proximal end of the prosthesis rests, a smaller canal in the diaphysis at the distal end of the prosthesis, and a taper between the two. Historically, this fixation has been accomplished by insertion of the component stem into unprepared bone, insertion of the component stem into a medullary canal that has been reamed to the stem diameter, or insertion of the component body into a medullary space that has been reamed and then broached. Traditionally, cement or use of a component with the capacity for tissue ingrowth has been used for fixation. Problems with these two types of fixation include the amount of bone loss that is associated with failure requiring revision surgery.

Sperling and co-workers (27) have alternately applied bone ingrowth on the undersurface of the head, and this has provided secure proximal fixation and the ability to exchange the prosthesis with minimal bone loss if revision is required. Because advantages exist for using a tissue ingrowth humeral component, a press-fitted component with ingrowth surfaces is currently used unless bone deficiencies prevent secure fixation without cement.

Another method of achieving this is a press-fit humeral component that has a tapered metaphyseal segment that provides fixation into the metaphyseal bone. This type of fixation also provides durability that is comparable with that reported for cemented components and superior to that reported for press-fit cylindrical components.

Traditional cemented glenoids have a keel, whereas newer designs provide for a pegged implant, and both of these are cemented into the glenoid vault. Connor used a photoelastic stress-freezing analysis to visualize and document the three-dimensional stress distribution patterns in a glenoid model for keeled and pegged component designs under physiologic loading conditions. He concluded that keeled components had higher glenoid surface contact stresses and higher volumetric stress shielding than did pegged components. In early pegged designs, the pegs were positioned too closely together. This resulted in the entire volume of the glenoid being removed with cavitary loss in revision surgery. At times, the anterior or posterior wall of the scapular neck was lost for reconstruction. Recent design changes in the peg positions represent attempts to deal with these difficulties. Wirth and co-workers have been able to demonstrate bone ingrowth into a polyethylene-pegged design (28).

Use of metal-backed glenoid components allows for bone ingrowth and provides stable fixation. However, problems have occurred either with overstuffing the soft tissue envelope or from polyethylene wear, which can provide metal wear particles leading to osteolysis. These findings have caused prosthetic manufacturers to offer an all-polyethylene component for cement and bone ingrowth fixation and a more limited role of metal backing as a means of component fixation.

In a study by Boileau and co-workers, 39 patients (40 shoulders; mean age 69 years) with primary OA were randomized to receive either a cemented all-polyethylene glenoid component or a cementless metal-backed component at the time of TSA. The presence of periprosthetic radiolucent lines was significantly greater with polyethylene than with metal-backed glenoids (85% vs. 25%). Of 20 radiolucent lines, 12 (60%) around polyethylene glenoids were present on immediate postoperative radiographs and 25% were progressive. No significant correlation was found between the presence of radiolucent lines around polyethylene glenoids and functional results. By contrast, periprosthetic radiolucent lines around metal-backed glenoids were rare but progressive when present. The incidence of loosening of metal-backed implants (4 cases, 20%) was significantly higher than that observed with polyethylene glenoids and was associated with component shift and severe osteolysis and increased pain. At a minimum of 3 years' follow-up, results of the study showed that the survival rate of cementless, metal-backed glenoid components is inferior to cemented all-polyethylene components; and the incidence of radiolucency at the glenoid–cement interface with all-polyethylene components is high and remains a concern. The high rate of loosening, because of the absence of ingrowth, the accelerated polyethylene wear, or both, led Boileau et al. to abandon the use of metal-backed glenoids (29).

ARTHRITIC CONDITIONS OF THE SHOULDER

Primary pathologic diseases treated by TSA have specific soft tissue problems that affect surgical approaches as well as prognostic outcomes (Tables 46.2 and 46.3).

Osteoarthritis

Primary OA is the most common arthritic process affecting the shoulder—up to 60% of patients undergoing TSA are diagnosed with primary OA. Men and women are affected equally, with the dominant arm involved twice as frequently as the nondominant arm. Classic radiographic findings of shoulder OA include osteophytes along the pos-

TABLE 46.2. *Pathology and surgical approaches of the most common conditions for which total shoulder arthroplasty is performed*

Disease	Surgical pathology	Surgical approach	Outcomes
Osteoarthritis	Intact rotator cuff, tight anterior structures, redundant posterior capsule, osteophytes inferior and medially on the humerus, posterior bone loss on the glenoid	Capsular release of anterior inferior capsule; avoid release of posterior capsule; modify retroversion to compensate for posterior glenoid wear; take down high side of glenoid to approach neutral version	Most reliable 95% good or excellent results, two thirds normal motion, loosening on glenoid side of 1% per year
Rheumatoid arthritis	Up to 60% associated rotator cuff tear or thinning, central erosion with synovitis at synovial folds; bony erosions at capsular junction	Very gentle with tissues; overall tissue quality will be poor; release capsule after synovectomy; may be unable to place glenoid with medial bone loss	Pain relief reliable; restoration of function less reliable; better if performed earlier in the disease progression prior to excessive tissue destruction
Posttraumatic arthritis	Complex scarring; malunited tuberosities produce chronic capsular contraction globally, and muscular imbalance can produce instability	Avoidance of tuberosity osteotomy; accept varus malalignment of neck shaft angle; reduce bulk of posterior malreduced greater tuberosity and then increase retroversion	If tuberosity osteotomy is required, only 50% chance of improvement; when no osteotomy is required, improvement in pain is reliable but no improvement in function
Osteonecrosis	The grade of the disease and the specific process will provide details of the anatomic changes; in general, the metaphyseal bone is brittle and sclerotic; often there are large cartilage flaps; bony deformity is uncommon	Preparation of the metaphyseal bone can produce fracture if careful broaching is not performed; hemiarthroplasty can be effective if the glenoid cartilage is normal	The most important factor is the grade of the disease; if little deformity, excellent outcomes are possible; patients with sickle cell disease have higher complication rates
Capsulorrhaphy arthritis	Capsular contracture anteriorly, bone loss posteriorly	Capsular release anteriorly more difficult than OA because multiple previous surgeries often make the intraoperative field scarred	80% good to excellent results; most patents are younger, so durability is a concern

TABLE 46.3. *History and radiographic findings of the most common conditions for which total shoulder arthroplasty is performed*

Type	History	Radiographic findings
Primary OA	Absence of major joint trauma, previous surgery, or other known causes of secondary OA joint disease	Joint space narrowing, sclerosis, periarticular osteophytes, posterior glenoid erosion, ± posterior subluxation of humeral head
Secondary OA	Evidence of major joint trauma or other known causes of secondary OA	Joint space narrowing, sclerosis, periarticular osteophytes, ± evidence of previous trauma
RA	Established RA diagnosis; muscle atrophy and weakness or bone on bone crepitus	Joint space narrowing, periarticular osteopenia, absence of osteophytes and sclerosis, periarticular erosions and medial glenoid erosion
Cuff tear arthropathy	Limited motion and function; weakness in elevation and rotation, diagnosis supported by previous rotator cuff tear	Superior displacement of humeral head (± collapse) with coracoacromial arch contact; secondary OA of the glenohumeral joint, ± erosion of greater tuberosity, ± contoured coracoacromial arch
Capsulorrhaphy arthropathy	Functionally restricted glenohumeral motion; previous repair for instability	Joint space narrowing, periarticular osteopenia, periarticular osteophytes, ± posterior glenoid erosion with posterior subluxation of humeral head
Osteonecrosis	Limited shoulder function, known risk factor	Sclerosis within humeral head, collapse of humeral head

OA, osteoarthritis; RA, rheumatoid arthritis.

terior and inferior portions of the humeral head with humeral head enlargement, joint space narrowing, subchondral sclerosis, and cysts (Fig. 46.1). Loose bodies within the joint, degeneration, and fibrosis of the rotator cuff muscles (especially subscapularis), along with anterior capsular contracture and posterior capsular distention are often noted at the time of surgery. The glenoid surface is eburnated with central and, more commonly, posterior erosion. The incidence of rotator cuff tears in patients with OA is less than 10%, although pain may be significant enough during muscle strength testing that a false-positive weakness may be noted. Clinically, patients complain of limited motion, impairment of activities of daily living, nocturnal pain, and activity-related pain. Radiographic studies should

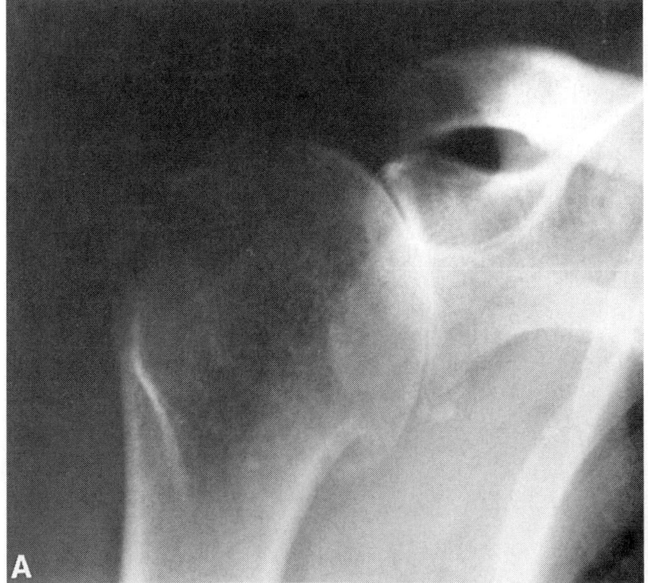

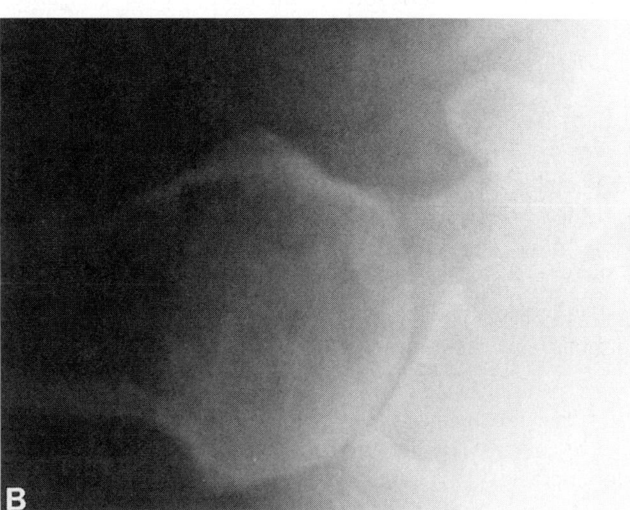

FIG. 46.1. Osteoarthritis. **A:** Nonspecific radiographic changes of osteoarthritis are seen in the shoulder, as in other joints. These include loss of the articular cartilage, subchondral sclerosis and cysts (especially in the superior central area, which is in contact with the glenoid with the arm elevated), and marginal osteophytes. Changes specific to the shoulder include the osteophytes on the inferior aspect of the humeral head and glenoid and enlargement and flattening of the humeral head. **B:** Posterior erosion of the glenoid with posterior subluxation of the humeral head is seen on the axial view in about one third of cases. It might relate to the etiology of the arthrosis and is important to consider technically during the surgery. There may be large osteochondral loose bodies inferiorly or anteriorly in the subscapularis recess or embedded in the soft tissues (not seen on these radiographs)

include true anteroposterior (AP) and axillary views. Osteophyte formation, bone loss, humeral head collapse, and elevation of the humerus with a compromised subacromial space should be reviewed on the AP view. The axillary or West Point view allows evaluation of posterior glenoid bone stock. A CT scan is also recommended when considering glenohumeral replacement to better assess the glenoid erosion.

The most common causes of secondary OA include trauma, instability, and previous surgeries. The association of joint instability and arthritis in the shoulder is not as clear as it is in other joints. In the classic case of a shoulder dislocation with a traumatic anterior labral injury (termed traumatic, unidirectional, Bankart surgery, or TUBS), nearly 20% of patients so affected will develop OA years later. Marx and associates studied patients with OA who had undergone hemiarthroplasty or TSA. The risk for developing severe arthrosis of the shoulder was found to be 10 to 20 times greater for individuals who had a previous dislocation of the shoulder (6,30,31). Individuals with multidirectional instability rarely develop OA, although following stabilization procedures, the incidence is higher (32–36).

Less commonly reported causes of secondary OA include infection, osteonecrosis, RA, and Paget disease. Metabolic conditions that have been associated with the development of arthritis include sickle cell disease, ochronosis, gout, and the epiphyseal dysplasias.

Rheumatoid Arthritis

RA is the second most common diagnosis for patients undergoing TSA and accounts for approximately 30% of patients undergoing this procedure. The entire shoulder girdle is susceptible to the destructive process seen in RA, with the acromioclavicular joint involved in up to two thirds of patients. Concomitant acromioclavicular and glenohumeral involvement occurs in 50% of patients, the extent of which varies among patients. Physical examination findings include decreased painful motion, weakness, and muscle atrophy and crepitation.

Typical radiographic features of the acromioclavicular joint include inferior joint line erosions. Radiographic findings of the glenohumeral joint vary depending on duration and severity of disease. Classic findings include osteopenia, juxtaarticular erosions, and concentric articular cartilage loss with humeral head collapse and centralization of the glenoid (Fig. 46.2).

Neer has described three types of glenohumeral RA based on radiographic appearance. The "dry type" is associated

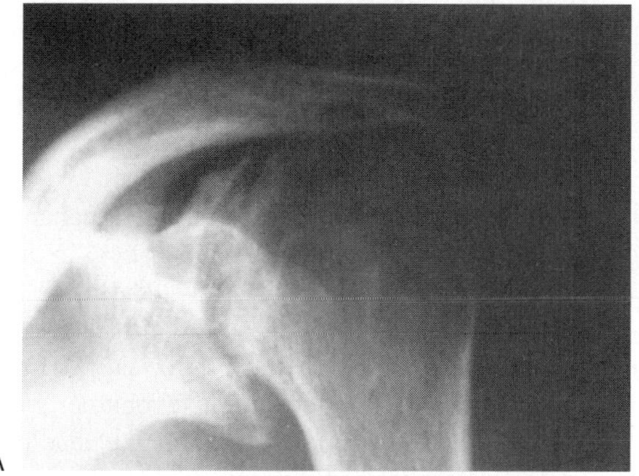
A

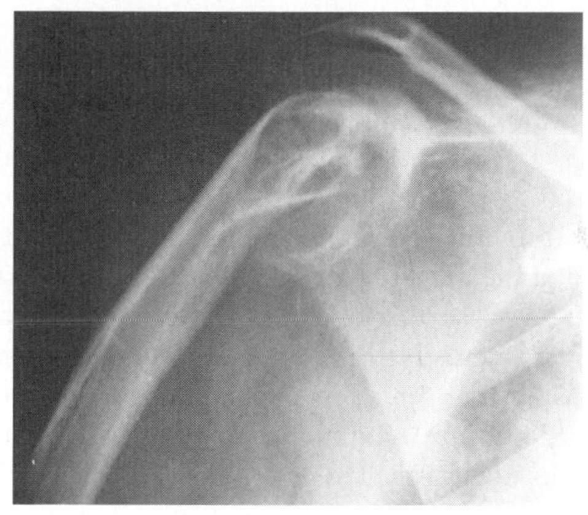
B

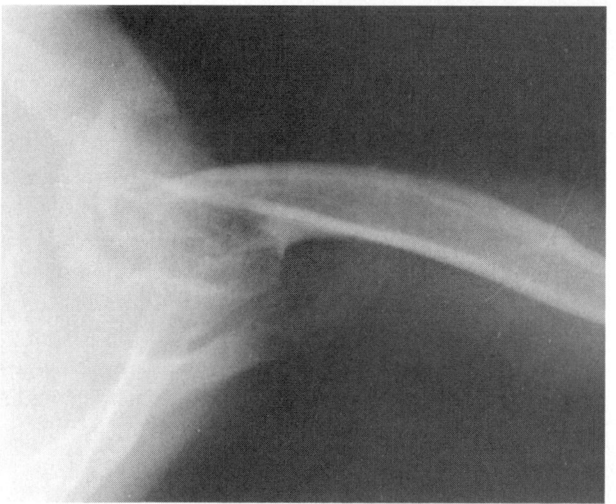
C

FIG. 46.2. Rheumatoid arthritis. **A:** Typical radiographic findings. There are osteopenia and joint destruction, with complete loss of the articular cartilage, erosion of the glenoid and humeral head, leading to medial migration of the humeral head into the glenoid and under the acromion. This is a moderately advanced stage, which seriously alters the biomechanics and, therefore, function of the shoulder. Further erosion of the glenoid can preclude the insertion of a glenoid component. If total shoulder replacement is likely to be required, it might be prudent to intervene before such severe changes and especially before the rotator cuff is destroyed. Anteroposterior **(B)** and axial views **(C)** of the shoulder of a 30-year-old patient with juvenile rheumatoid arthritis. There is virtually complete loss of the glenoid bone stock and the humeral head itself. The most important factor, however, is the destruction of the rotator cuff.

with joint space narrowing, subchondral cyst, erosions, and marginal osteophytes. Marginal erosions characterize the wet type, with the proximal humerus often acquiring a smooth pointed contour. The "wet and resorptive phases" are characterized by destruction of cartilage and bone with centralization and distortion of the glenohumeral joint. In the "wet type," a high incidence of rotator cuff rupture and early radiographic progression, which precedes glenoid damage, have been found. This type may require early synovectomy (37–42).

Full-thickness rotator cuff rupture occurs from 8% to 50% of patients and in approximately 30% of those undergoing TSA. If the rotator cuff is not torn, most patients exhibit thinning or attenuation with contracture of the cuff and capsule, leading to concentric glenohumeral erosion. With the presence of a large rotator cuff tear, imbalanced forces may result in superior translation of the humeral head. Progressive superior and medial glenoid wear then will ensue, often into the base of the coracoid. The long head of the biceps is typically ruptured in advanced disease.

The presence of a rotator cuff tear has been shown to adversely affect the overall functional score, range of motion, and glenoid component fixation in traditional TSA, prompting many surgeons to advocate earlier treatment prior to advanced bone and soft tissue destruction (6,40,43–46). CT scans are obtained during preoperative planning to assess osseous morphology in preparation for arthroplasty.

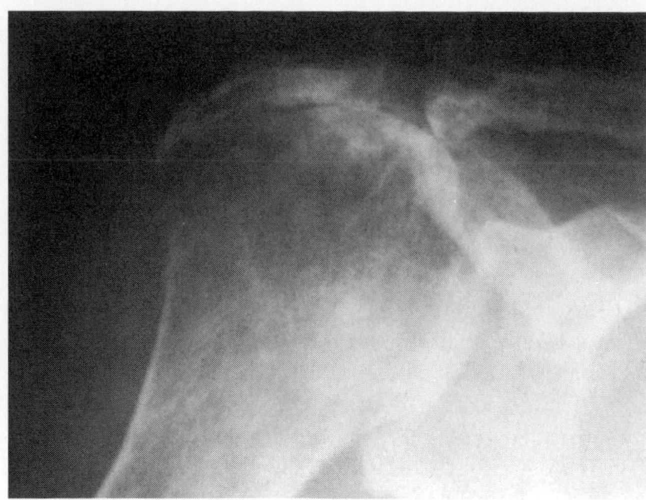

FIG. 46.3. Cuff tear arthropathy. With massive tears of the rotator cuff, the humeral head can subluxate superiorly and articulate with the undersurface of the acromion, which becomes concave. Erosions and sclerotic changes occur in the humeral head, the acromion, and the acromioclavicular joint. Arthritic changes include collapse of the humeral head. This condition is a most difficult treatment challenge.

Rotator Cuff Arthropathy

Rotator cuff arthropathy is a term that was first used by Neer and co-workers (47) in 1983 to describe glenohumeral arthritis in the setting of a chronic massive rotator cuff tear with associated instability and humeral head collapse. Superior migration of the humerus is characteristic and results in erosion of the caudal surface of the acromion and eburnation of the greater tuberosity (Fig. 46.3). Patients often are older women with shoulder symptoms of long duration. The dominant side is most commonly affected; however, bilateral involvement has been reported in up to 60% of cases. Symptoms include joint pain, loss of motion, and recurrent swelling of the shoulder. The pain typically interferes with sleep and intensifies with activity. Many patients report having received multiple steroid injections, but there is no proven correlation between these injections and progression of disease. Clinically, patients often exhibit atrophy of the supra- and infraspinatus fossa. A swollen fluid-filled appearance at the superficial shoulder may be present secondary to leakage of joint fluid into the glenohumeral bursa. Patients exhibit loss of both passive and active motion, rotator cuff weakness, and, often, credits. Attempts at active forward flexion or abduction result in superior elevation of the shoulder. Evidence of subluxation or dislocation anterosuperior is termed superior escape, resulting in a condition that is even more difficult to treat with conventional shoulder arthroplasty than with traditional rotator cuff arthropathy secondary to loss of the constraining effect of the coracoacromial arch.

Radiographic findings include loss of glenohumeral joint space, subarticular sclerosis, and collapse of proximal humeral articular surface with proximal migration of the humeral head, which erodes the undersurface of the acromion. Superior and medial erosion result in acetabularization of the glenoid and acromion with rounding of the greater tuberosity.

According to some researchers, mechanical and nutritional factors are believed to be critical in the pathogenesis of rotator cuff arthropathy (47). The force couple balance between the rotator cuff and deltoid are lost along with the compressive effect of the rotator cuff, resulting in instability and loss of concentric glenohumeral motion. A suspension bridge model, in which the leading edge of the detached rotator cuff tendon behaves biomechanically like a cable, has been used to explain the nonprogressive nature of some rotator cuff tears. This allows some patients who have a large or massive tear to maintain the transverse force couple and thus retain the ability to actively elevate the shoulder. The location of the "cable" or tendon attachment on the tuberosities results in either stable or unstable glenohumeral kinematics (6). The combination of glenohumeral instability due to the loss of primary and secondary stabilizers and loss of normal articular cartilage often results in the generation of calcium phosphate crystals. These crystal aggregates, which may originate from the damage to the articular cartilage or from the degenerative changes in the rotator cuff tendons, accelerate additional degenerative changes. Although arthropathy develops in only a small percentage of patients with rotator cuff tears, patients who are affected have massive rotator cuff tears, bone loss, and poor joint mechanics that pose great challenges for even the most experienced surgeon using traditional treatment methods. It is estimated that 50% of octogenarians will have a full-thickness rotator cuff tear. In the United States, 17 million persons suffer from a full-thickness rotator cuff tear. Neer and co-workers estimate that 4% of all patients with a full-thickness rotator cuff tear will develop rotator cuff arthropathy (47).

Postcapsulorrhaphy Arthritis

Neer and associates first described an arthropathy associated with patients who experienced recurrent dislocations and had undergone instability repair. These patients accounted for 10% of their patients undergoing TSA. This is one of the most common causes of arthritis in individuals under 50 years of age, with one report citing an average age of 38 years. The incidence of arthritis following some anterior procedures for glenohumeral instability has been reported in up to 80% of surgically treated shoulders. The condition is believed to result from excessive soft tissue tension, usually on the anterior aspect, with subluxation and subsequent glenoid erosion in the posterior direction. Although successful in approximately 95% of cases, the Putti-Platt procedure, in which the subscapularis and anterior capsule are shortened, has been associated with OA changes in up to 61% of patients by one researcher at a mean follow-up of 22 years (30,35,36). Secondary degenerative changes also have been reported after the Magnuson-Stack procedure, the Du Tot capsulorrhaphy, the Bristow procedure, and Bankart repairs.

Although less common, anterior subluxation can occur through a posterior tightening procedure. Care must be taken to balance capsular tension on all sides of the joint. Intraarticular placement of hardware or placement of bone graft in the face of instability can result in arthritis.

Evaluation of the degree of motion loss (especially passive motion) is required in surgical decision making as well as prognosis. Extensive soft tissue releases, anteroinferior capsulotomies, and subscapularis lengthening are required for severe loss of external rotation.

Shoulder arthroplasty for treatment of OA of the glenohumeral joint following instability surgery in this relatively young group of patients provides pain relief and improved motion but is associated with high rates of revision surgery and unsatisfactory results owing to component failure, instability, and pain secondary to glenoid arthritis (33,48). Estimated component survival is 97% (91%–100%) at 2 years, 86% (74%–99%) at 5 years, and 61% (42%–86%) at 10 years.

Osteonecrosis

Nontraumatic osteonecrosis of the humeral head results from vascular compromise to the region. The incidence of osteonecrosis in patients undergoing TSA is approximately 3%.

Patients typically present with shoulder pain that is worse with motion and night pain. In contrast to other arthropathies, pain at rest is not common. On physical examination, motion is decreased, with active motion commonly limited by pain. Eventual humeral head collapse and capsular contracture may occur.

The disease process is classified most commonly using the radiographic staging system of Cruess (Table 46.4). Magnetic resonance imaging (MRI) may first detect pathology before collapse is seen radiographically. Osteoporosis, osteosclerosis, and eventual subchondral collapse may be seen. In the end stage, the irregular humeral head destroys the glenoid articular cartilage, resulting in secondary degenerative joint disease (Fig. 46.4). Symptomatic progression has been reported in approximately 70% of patients. Either a hemiarthroplasty or TSA is indicated in patients with stage III, IV, or V osteonecrosis in whom nonsurgical management has failed. In patients with stage V disease, a TSA should be performed (6,25, 43,49–54).

Sickle Cell Disease

Radiographic evidence of humeral head osteonecrosis has been reported in 5.6% to 28% of patients with sickle cell disease, making sickle cell disease and other hemoglobinopathies some of the most common causes of osteonecrosis worldwide. Bilateral involvement has been reported in 44% to 71% of patients. One study described osteonecrosis of the humeral head as most problematic for sickle cell patients of all ages with hemoglobin S/S.

Patients with hemoglobin S/C and S/B+ thalassemia tended to develop osteonecrosis later in life. Many patients with abnormal examinations and normal radiographs may require MRI evaluation to confirm the diagnosis. Bone infarctions can develop and become secondarily infected, resulting in osteomyelitis and a septic joint and need to be considered by the clinician. Treatment for uncomplicated osteonecrosis is similar to that for osteonecrosis from other etiologies, although there have been reports of reversal of early osteonecrosis with bone marrow transplantation in younger patients. The mechanism of this remains unclear (55,56).

TABLE 46.4. *Stages of osteonecrosis*

Stage	Abnormality
I	Documented only by magnetic resonance imaging or bone scan
II	Localized or mottled sclerosis
III	Crescent sign present
IV	Collapse of humeral head subchondral bone
V	Degenerative changes both sides of joint

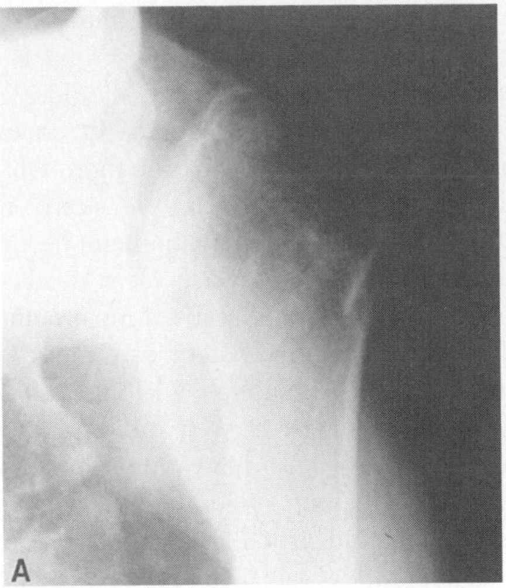

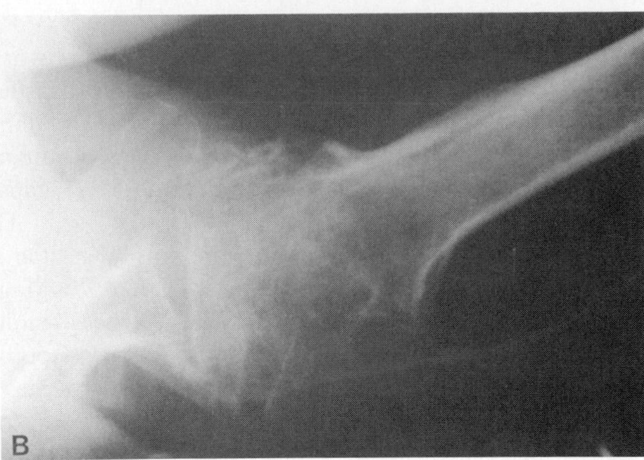

FIG. 46.4. A, B: Avascular necrosis. Avascular necrosis of the humeral head in a 60-year-old alcoholic. Changes include flattening of the humeral head and secondary osteoarthritis due to the longstanding history.

Posttraumatic Arthritis

Posttraumatic arthritis has many causes, the most common of which is proximal humeral malunion, nonunion, or osteonecrosis secondary to fracture. Proximal humeral malunion that has more than 2 mm of articular incongruity is considered a risk factor. In one series, posttraumatic osteonecrosis is more prevalent after displaced three- and four-part fractures. Reported rates range from 3% to 25% for three-part fractures and as high as 90% in four-part fractures. Less common causes of posttraumatic arthritis include chronic unreduced dislocations, recurrent dislocations, and glenoid malunion or nonunion. Posttraumatic arthritis accounts for approximately 13% of patients undergoing TSA. Patients typically have pain, stiffness, and loss of function. Other complicating factors include brachial plexus and axillary nerve injuries. An MRI may be required for the definitive diagnosis of posttraumatic osteonecrosis (6,44,51,52,57).

MANAGEMENT OF GLENOHUMERAL ARTHRITIS

Nonsurgical Treatment

The mainstay of nonsurgical treatment remains medical management with the use of nonsteroidal antiinflammatory drugs (NSAIDs). Nutritional supplementation with glucosamine and chondroitin sulfate also may provide symptomatic improvement in some patients. In patients with inflammatory arthritis (e.g., RA), oral steroids or other disease-modifying antirheumatic drugs may be used. Adjunctive use of steroids into affected joints, bursa, or tendon sheaths is useful in controlling acute inflammation in inflammatory arthropathies. The use of intraarticular injections in primary or secondary OA is less successful, and the use of these in both inflammatory and OA patients should be limited owing to the known deleterious effects on soft tissues and articular cartilage.

Physical therapy to maintain motion and strength is useful; however, in the case of advanced joint incongruity, symptoms may be worsened on attempts to regain motion. Isometric strengthening exercises may be more suitable in some patients secondary to joint inflammation and destruction.

Surgical Treatment

Arthroscopic Débridement/Synovectomy

In RA patients, five radiographic patterns have been identified and correlated with the optimal surgical treatment of the shoulder (40,42) (Table 46.5).

Arthroscopic synovectomy usually affords pain relief and improved range of motion in nonprogressive RA, and only pain relief for the erosive type. To achieve increases in motion in the erosive type, implant arthroplasty is often required. It is generally accepted that in the presence of destructive changes, arthroscopic synovectomy does not eliminate pain or restore motion.

The value of either arthroscopic or open joint débridement for degenerative arthritis of the shoulder is small, unless damage is confined to early changes. For instance, arthroscopic or open joint débridement may be efficacious if the humeral head remains spherical and centralized in the glenoid. In 61 patients, followed for a minimum of 2 years, Cameron and co-workers (58) evaluated the ability of arthroscopic débridement and capsular release to provide lasting pain relief and improved function. The patients had substantial and lasting reduction in pain and improvement in function. Patient satisfaction increased considerably, and

TABLE 46.5. *Radiographic patterns of shoulders seen in patients with rheumatoid arthritis*

Type of disease	Radiographic appearance	Treatment
Nonprogressive	Small erosions only, even after extended disease onset	Arthroscopic synovectomy
Arthrosis-like	Osteophytes, joint space narrowing, sclerosis of subchondral bone	Conservative
Erosive	Marginal lesions without collapse	Implant arthroplasty
Collapse	Coalescence of large subchondral cysts with collapse of subchondral trabeculae	Implant arthroplasty
Mutilating	Severe bone destruction and absorption, "cut off" appearance	Implant arthroplasty

53 indicated that they would have the surgery again. Notably, osteochondral lesions with an area greater than 20 mm^2 were associated with clinical failure and a return of pain. A good candidate was described as having a congruent, centered joint, little or no osteophyte formation, mild or no subchondral sclerosis or cyst formation, and an osteochondral lesion of less than 20 mm^2.

O'Driscoll has identified negative prognostic factors for arthroscopic débridement and capsular release, including pain in the midrange of motion, painful crepitus, and pain with glenohumeral compression during rotation. He concluded that the technique is useful for pain relief but is unreliable for improvement in motion. The majority of patients believe that it is worthwhile, so it may be indicated for patients in whom arthroplasty is neither appropriate nor desirable (6,59).

Bishop and co-workers (59) evaluated arthroscopic abrasion arthroplasty as a temporizing procedure for patients with glenohumeral arthritis. Twenty-seven shoulders in 26 patients were evaluated at a mean of 56 months postoperatively. In 8 cases, a congruous joint could not be created arthroscopically, and a TSA was performed. In the remaining cases, forward elevation improved from 107 to 131 degrees, external rotation with the arm at the side improved from 18 to 31 degrees, and the American Shoulder and Elbow Surgeons (ASES) shoulder score improved from 45 to 75 points. Most patients had a good or an excellent result, irrespective of age. Bishop concluded arthroscopic abrasion might be effective for delaying or obviating the need for shoulder replacement as long as strict selection criteria are met.

Resection Arthroplasty

Resection arthroplasty has limited indications. It has a potential use in severe septic arthritis with extensive glenohumeral osteomyelitis. A joint resection also results after the removal of infected or mechanically compromised implants. Poor function, weakness, instability, and unpredictable pain relief result. Maximum active abduction is rarely greater than 70 degrees (44,60).

Arthrodesis

Arthrodesis was once considered the most reliable form of treatment for advanced arthritic changes prior to arthroplasty. Today its indications are limited and include painful paralysis about the shoulder of both the deltoid and rotator cuff and persistent septic arthritis. Although pain relief is considered acceptable in approximately 75%, patients are not able to perform work at or above shoulder level. No single position of an arthrodesis allows for the performance of all activities of daily living (34,44,60). In our experience, and as reported by our European counterparts, a reverse TSA provides a much more functional outcome in cases of refractory instability and previous failed reconstructive procedures, provided there is a functional deltoid muscle and conventional arthroplasty is not possible. Conversion of a failed arthroplasty to an arthrodesis is always possible.

Soft Tissue Reconstructions

When surgically addressing postcapsulorrhaphy arthropathy, the degree of loss of external rotation and arthritic changes needs to be quantified. The type of capsulorrhaphy previously performed must be known when planning a revision procedure. Release of anterior structures, including the capsule, with subscapularis lengthening, is most commonly performed in the presence of mild arthritic changes and significant external rotation loss.

MacDonald and associates (61) have reported on subscapularis release with mild to severe arthritic changes present. Patients reported significant pain relief with an average increase of 27 degrees of external rotation. In patients who have undergone an anterior shoulder capsulorrhaphy with limitation of external rotation of 0 degrees at 6 months, some investigators recommend an anterior release at that time to prevent glenohumeral arthritis (6,56). Older patients and those with advanced symptomatic arthropathy require a prosthetic replacement. Even then, the operation will necessitate lengthening of the anterior structures.

Core Decompression

Results of core decompression for osteonecrosis are mixed, although there is evidence it is helpful in earlier stages of the disease. LaPorte and co-workers (62) reported on 63 shoulders with osteonecrosis of multiple etiologies with a 10-year follow-up evaluation. For stage I, core decompression was 94% successful. Stages II, III, and IV had success rates of 88%, 70%, and 14%, respectively. LaPorte et al. recommended core decompression for stages I to III and arthroplasty for stage IV and higher. Other researchers have reported poor results using core decompression for stage III, and its treatment remains controversial (52). Importantly, when performing core decompression, care must be taken to drill or ream lateral to the bicipital groove.

Interposition Arthroplasty

Resurfacing with fascia lata, capsule, or allograft sutured over a débrided glenoid and coupled with hemiarthroplasty has been described. Burkhead has reported on 13 patients followed for more than 2 years; 10 had an excellent result in terms of function and pain relief, and 2 had a satisfactory result (6).

Yamaguchi and co-workers (63) presented initial results associated with a novel nonprosthetic shoulder arthroplasty involving meniscal allograft interposition. The lateral meniscus was chosen for use as allograft tissue because of its established history for synovial-based healing, its structural characteristics, its wedge shape (to compensate for glenoid wear), and its durability. Seven consecutive patients who underwent interpositional arthroplasty were evaluated after a mean duration of follow-up of 24 months. Postoperatively, all patients were satisfied and reported minimal or no pain, and the average ASES score was 72 points. The technique was thought to be comparable with other interpositional techniques at the time of short-term follow-up while offering potential long-term advantages.

Conventional Arthroplasty

The primary indication for performing hemiarthroplasty or TSA is pain relief. It is indicated in the active patient with arthritic changes in which medical management has failed and simpler procedures are not indicated. In most studies, reliable pain relief has been reported following both hemiarthroplasty and TSA, with 71% to 100% of patients reporting mild to no pain. Contraindications for conventional shoulder arthroplasty include chronic infections, combined paralysis of deltoid and rotator cuff, and uncontrolled instability.

Improved motion and function are secondary goals of prosthetic replacement. Multiple studies have been reviewed, with elevation showing increases between 27 and 50 degrees and external rotation between 16 and 43 degrees (64–80). In general, preoperative active range of motion is typically less than half of normal, and patients can be expected to gain two thirds normal motion postoperatively. Some investigators believe that results correlate with the diagnostic category, with osteonecrosis and OA showing better functional gains than RA, cuff tear arthropathy, and posttraumatic arthritis. In reviewing subsets of osteonecrosis, inferior results can be expected in traumatic osteonecrosis as compared with steroid-induced disease. In one study, patients with steroid-induced osteonecrosis had an average of 75% of full forward elevation versus 50% in the trauma group. The presence of a rotator cuff tear has repeatedly been shown to directly correlate with poorer functional outcomes following shoulder arthroplasty.

In certain situations, implantation of the humeral component alone has been proposed, with the underlying reason being that the surface of the glenoid is judged to be in good condition with minimal deformity or incongruity. Accepted indications for humeral head replacement alone include osteonecrosis of the humeral head, recent four-part and head-splitting fractures of the proximal humerus, recent three-part fractures of the proximal humerus in older persons, malunions and nonunion of old proximal humeral fractures, insufficient glenoid bone stock to support a humeral component, and rotator cuff arthropathy. Patients in most series report slightly improved pain scores and satisfaction with glenoid resurfacing (6,43,81).

The reported incidence of radiolucent lines surrounding the glenoid component has been between 22% and 95% of patients. Incidences of clinical loosening or failure in short- to medium-term studies have been reported to be significantly lower. One recent report cited a long-term incidence of 44% of patients developing clinical loosening after presenting with lucency (80). The ability to safely implant the glenoid with an evaluation of glenoid bone stock must be taken into account. We prefer CT scans on all patients in addition to the axillary radiographic view to evaluate glenoid bone stock and version.

Results of solo humeral head replacement show that they tend to deteriorate at a faster rate than total shoulder replacements, even though glenoid radiolucencies often are present. Once posterior glenoid erosion occurs following a solo humeral head replacement, the success rate declines to 33% (6,43,82,83).

It has been found that more than 50% of a well-reviewed group of patients had pain, and 26% had been converted from hemiarthroplasty to TSA within 10 years of the index operation. Most patients with painful glenoid arthrosis after hemiarthrosis have marked pain relief and improvement in motion after revision to a TSA. This revision can be technically challenging because of the presence of scar tissue, muscle-tendon weakness, and bone loss (79,84).

Arthroplasty in the Rotator Cuff–Deficient Patient

The patient with an arthritic shoulder associated with a deficient rotator cuff represents a major problem. This can have many causes, including RA, cuff tear arthropathy, prior trauma, primary OA in the presence of a massive rotator cuff tear, and arthritis following a failed rotator cuff repair. Long-term efficacy of arthroscopic treatment is questionable in patients with advanced arthritis; arthrodesis is unacceptable to many patients, leaving arthroplasty as the only viable surgical option.

Glenoid resurfacing has been associated with a high degree of glenoid component loosening secondary to the rocking horse phenomenon caused by eccentric loading of the glenoid secondary to the deficient rotator cuff. Additionally, superior migration of the humeral head persists following TSA, placing the deltoid in a mechanically disadvantaged position and resulting in poor postoperative active elevation. Hemiarthroplasty has been proposed to prevent the rocking horse phenomenon. Use of large head prosthesis allows articulation with the glenoid and undersurface of the acromion. Pain relief has been acceptable, although active elevation has remained somewhat limited, rarely exceeding 120 degrees postoperatively. Hemiarthroplasty can be associated with a poor outcome if the acromiohumeral arch is damaged, either because of arthritis or because of previous surgery (extensive acromioplasty). Some investigators have proposed partial repair of the rotator cuff coupled with humeral arthroplasty and report satisfactory results at up to 7 years' follow-up. Other surgeons have used a bipolar design humeral arthroplasty with varying results, reporting good pain relief with limitation of glenohumeral mobility, which rarely exceeds 90 degrees (76, 85–90). Results of hemiarthroplasty for a rotator cuff–deficient shoulder from several authors are reported in Table 46.6.

Reverse design shoulder prosthesis places a cup within the proximal humerus and a hemisphere fixed to the glenoid. The prosthetic design relies on the deltoid to provide active elevation. Short- and mid-term results using reverse-design prostheses in the treatment of the cuff-deficient arthritic shoulder are encouraging. Schematically, reverse-design prostheses compared with hemiarthroplasty have a better chance of obtaining good function. Our European counterparts have demonstrated encouraging results using reverse-design prostheses with a lowered medialized center of rotation (Delta III, DePuy, Saint Priest France). Scapular notching has been consistently noted to varying degree and requires long-term evaluation (91–94). Recently, a reverse prosthesis (Encore, Austin, TX, U.S.A.) has been introduced in the United States with a more lateralized center of rotation and improved baseplate fixation and is currently under investigational study.

Historical Perspective of Constrained Prosthetic Design for the Rotator Cuff–Deficient Shoulder

Scales introduced constrained TSA in 1960 with the Stanmore Constrained prosthesis. This prosthesis mimicked a locked total hip design. In 1972, Kolbel introduced the first reverse prosthesis. The design incorporated a locking mechanism between the ball and socket. The ball was fixed by screw fixation via an outrigger to the scapula, whereas the socket was cemented into the humerus. The locking mechanism was designed to disengage prior to exposure of a force great enough to fracture the glenoid. Neer tried several versions of constrained shoulder; the Mark III was his final version. This prosthesis had a ball with a large diameter attached to a keel-shaped glenoid. The glenoid was cemented, and the humeral component rotated in a cemented stem. Glenoid fixation failure prompted him to abandon the use of a constrained device. In 1973, Kessel designed a reverse prosthesis with an uncemented glenoid. Kessel's glenoid had a large center screw for fixation with a cemented humerus. The joint had a snap-fit locking mechanism. In 1976, Reeves and Buechel changed the glenoid fixation by incorporating spikes for enhanced scapular attachment. In Buechel's design, the glenoid sphere articulated with a larger sphere that articulated with the cup on the humeral side.

Finally, in 1990, Grammont developed a semiconstrained reverse ball and socket. There was no locking mechanism between the components. The matched geometry between the humeral and the glenoid components provided stability owing to a deepened socket. This design diminished the

TABLE 46.6. *Reported results of shoulder hemiarthroplasty for treatment of glenohumeral arthritis with severe rotator cuff deficiency*

Authors	No. of procedures	Mean years of age (range)	Follow-up (yr)	No or mild postoperative pain	Pre-/postoperative active elevation (degrees)	Successful results
Arntz et al. (1993)	18	71 (54–84)	3 (2–10)	61%	66 (44–90)/112 (70–160)	Not reported
Williams and Rockwood (1996)	21	72 (59–80)	4 (2–7)	86%	70 (0–155)/120 (15–160)	86%
Field et al. (1997)	16	74 (62–83)	3 (2–5)	81%	60 (40–80)/100 (80–130)	63%
Zuckerman et al. (2000)	15	73 (65–81)	2 (1–5)	47%	69 (20–140)/86 (45–140)	Not reported
Sotelo and Cofield (2002)	33	69 (50–87)	5 (2–11)	73%	72 (30–150)/91 (40–165)	67%

force on the glenoid-prosthetic bone attachment. Furthermore, all previous reverse designs had a lateral offset of the humeral component relative to the glenoid surface. The lateral offset provided an improved fulcrum for deltoid function. The lateral offset also increased the torque of the resultant joint reactive force, which further stressed the glenoid–prosthetic bone attachment. This attachment site has proven to be the site of failure in previous designs. In addition to the medial offset, the deltoid is lengthened in response to an increased inferior offset. Thus, in the rotator cuff–deficient shoulder, the glenohumeral fulcrum could be stabilized via the ball-and-socket joint articulation. The deltoid can then be lengthened because of the increased inferior displacement. This increase in the length of the muscle can enhance deltoid function. Several hundred of these implants have been used in Europe since 1990, with 80% of patients reporting good to excellent results.

In 1997, we developed the Encore reverse shoulder prosthesis (RSP). The initial impetus to develop this was because of the inability to get the Grammont prosthesis to the United States. There was concern with the Grammont's medial encroachment. This medial encroachment was reported in 10% of patients at follow-up. Considering this as a possible source of mechanical failure, it was suggested that less medial offset could be an improvement. Other problems, such as unscrewing the glenosphere (glenoid ball) from the baseplate, suggested another source of design improvement. In accordance with the Kessel design, the Encore RSP improved the method of baseplate fixation to the glenoid by incorporating a large center screw. Additional transfixation screws also were implemented into the design. The glenosphere is attached to the baseplate with a Morse taper. The final modification made is the medial offset. The RSPs medial offset is more medial than previous designs but is 9 mm lateral to the Grammont. This was done to minimize medial encroachment. The improvement of glenoid fixation allows for a greater joint reactive force. The glenoid fixation also provides for a more anatomic reconstruction with the lateral offset. The increased inferior offset is similar to the Grammont. They both provide for improved deltoid efficiency. The greater inferior offset provides some improvement of strength, despite resultant loss of power from the poor rotator cuff musculature.

Reverse Total Shoulder Arthroplasty

Indications and Contraindications

A reverse shoulder prosthesis is indicated when a patient has failed all nonoperative treatments and continues to have functionally disabling pain and poor active shoulder elevation in conditions outlined in Table 46.7.

The RSP is contraindicated in patients with axillary nerve palsy; active infection; insufficient bone to seat the implant components; muscular, neurologic, or vascular deficiencies, which compromise the affected extremity; alcoholism or other addictions; or high levels of physical activity (e.g., competitive athletes, manual laborers).

TABLE 46.7. *Indications for a reverse shoulder prosthesis*

Arthritis and an irreparable, massive rotator cuff tear.
Massive, irreparable rotator cuff tear and coracoacromial arch deficiency resulting in anterosuperior escape.
Failed rotator cuff repair with secondary arthritis and superior humeral head migration.
Failed shoulder arthroplasty with an irreparable, massive rotator cuff tear, coracoacromial arch deficiency, or both.
A functional deltoid must be present in all cases.

Preoperative Planning

In primary cases, a detailed history, physical examination, and radiographs confirming shoulder arthritis and an irreparable rotator cuff tear must be present. In revision cases, previous operative notes can be helpful. Anterosuperior escape is more common in patients who have had previous shoulder surgery that involved releasing the coracoacromial ligament. The humeral head or humeral head prosthesis can be palpated underneath the skin and jumps forward with attempted arm elevation. A CT scan of the shoulder allows for proper evaluation of glenoid version and glenoid bone stock. An MRI is occasionally helpful in equivocal cases.

The humeral stem size may be templated from an AP radiograph. The stem is intended for cement fixation and comes in four sizes: 5, 6, 7, and 8 mm. The humeral polyethylene socket comes in three sizes: neutral, +4, and +8. The size is an intraoperative decision depending on soft tissue tension and proximal humeral bone loss. Generally, the neutral liner is used in primary cases. The baseplate central screw comes in two lengths: 25 and 30 mm. A depth gauge is used intraoperatively to determine the proper length. The glenoid head is 32 mm in diameter and comes in two neck lengths: neutral and −4 mm. Generally, the neutral head is used in primary cases. The −4 mm size may be used in very tight revision shoulders.

Operative Technique

General endotracheal anesthesia combined with an interscalene nerve block is preferable prior to positioning. The patient is placed in the upright beach-chair position, with the operative arm draped free. An extended deltopectoral approach is used. We prefer to free the deltoid muscle from the cephalic vein by ligating the lateral tributaries and leaving the vein medial with the pectoralis major muscle. Approximately two thirds of the pectoralis major tendon insertion is released.

Humeral Exposure. The deep spaces of the subdeltoid, subacromial, and subcoracoid are developed.

The remnant subscapularis tendon is released from the lesser tuberosity and proximal humerus. Externally rotating the arm places tension on the muscle and facilitates its release from bone. The shoulder is then atraumatically dislocated anteriorly with further gentle external rotation and extension. The humerus is often osteopenic and can be fractured if excessive force is used to dislocate the shoulder.

Humeral Neck Cut. A humeral neck cut is then made using a version osteotomy guide affixed onto the anterior humeral shaft. The alignment rod, screwed into the version guide, is placed parallel to the forearm, creating a preferred neck cut in 30 degrees of retroversion. Two holes are drilled through the guide with a 2-mm drill, and pins are tapped into the drill holes to secure the guide to the shaft. Hohmann retractors are placed medially around the proximal humerus to protect the axillary nerve. The neck cut is made with an oscillating saw followed by removal of the pins and the version guide.

Canal Preparation. A T-handled canal finder is used to sound the medullary canal, which is entered far lateral on the neck cut surface. Sequential hand reamers (6–10 mm) are used to open the canal until some resistance is met. The humerus is then broached beginning with a no. 6 broach. The broach handle's alignment rod is placed parallel to the forearm to maintain 30 degrees of humeral retroversion.

The broach handle is gently impacted with a mallet until the notch on the handle contacts the lateral humeral cortex. This countersinks the broach into the metaphysis of the proximal humerus. Generally, the final broach is equal to or smaller than the final diaphyseal reamer. Broach sizes are no. 6 to no. 10. The humeral stem implant comes in four sizes: 5, 6, 7, and 8 mm. The humeral stem is designed for cement implantation. To obtain a 2-mm cement mantle, the humeral stem implant should be two sizes smaller than the final broach.

Proximal Humerus Preparation. The nose of the metaphyseal reamer is placed inside the opening in the broach. The metaphysis is prepared using the power reamer; the lateral humeral cortex is protected with the surgeon's hand during metaphyseal reaming to prevent fracture. Reaming is performed incrementally with the small-, medium-, and large-sized reamers to prepare proximal bony support for the humeral polyethylene socket.

After removal of the metaphyseal reamer, a trial humeral socket is fitted into the broach. The humeral polyethylene socket comes in three sizes: neutral, +4, and +8. A burr may be used to remove excess bone from the medial margin of the broach such that the socket sits flush within the broach and on the prepared bony bed without impingement. The trial socket is then removed, leaving the broach in the humerus.

Glenoid Exposure. A glenoid retractor is placed on the posteroinferior rim of the glenoid to displace the humerus posteriorly. Extensive soft tissue releases may be necessary to gain optimal visualization and access to the glenoid. The coracohumeral ligament is released from the lateral coracoid to free the subscapularis and to visualize the lateral coracoid base. The glenohumeral ligaments, capsule, and labrum are released and excised from the glenoid beginning at the 12 o'clock position and ending at the 6 to 7 o'clock position. The axillary nerve is at risk for injury near the 5 to 6 o'clock position.

Glenoid Preparation. A centering hole is drilled in the glenoid and sequential reaming of the glenoid is performed beginning with the starter reamer and progressing up to the larger sized reamers. The glenoid reamers produce a bony surface congruent with the back of the glenoid baseplate implant. A 2.5-mm drill is then used to drill through the centering hole and exit out the anterior cortex of the scapula. The direction should be in line with the previous glenoid reamers so that the glenoid baseplate will sit flush with the bone. The central fixed angle 6.5-mm screw of the glenoid baseplate comes in 25-mm and 30-mm lengths.

Glenoid Baseplate Insertion. The appropriate glenoid baseplate implant is then screwed into the prepared glenoid using a hand-held ratchet screwdriver. Occasionally, a 6.5-mm tap is used to prepare the far cortex for central screw purchase. When fully seated, the baseplate is flush with the glenoid, and the scapula rotates when attempting to turn the screwdriver further.

A 2.5-mm drill is used to drill through the 4 holes in the periphery of the baseplate. Care is taken to stay within the cortices of the glenoid and scapula in two of the four drill holes to minimize stress risers from the peripheral screws. The drill may need to be angled slightly for this to occur. Depth gauge measurements are taken and appropriate length Encore self-tapping 3.5-mm cortical screws are inserted with a power screwdriver. Final seating of the screws is obtained with a hand-held screwdriver. The screw heads must be at or below the surface of the baseplate to prevent impingement when seating the glenoid head.

Glenoid Head Insertion. After all soft tissue and debris are circumferentially cleared from the baseplate, the glenoid head is placed over the Morse taper of the baseplate and impact with three to four firm taps with a mallet onto the black impactor. Often, the glenoid retractor must be removed to provide clearance for placement of the glenoid head onto the baseplate. A −4 mm glenoid head is available for special situations, such as revision surgery when the soft tissue envelope is extensively contracted.

Trial Reduction. The surface of the glenoid head is protected with the black plastic handle retractor. The proximal humerus is delineated anteriorly by pulling it laterally while extending and externally rotating the arm. The patient should be completely relaxed to facilitate reduction of the humeral socket onto the glenoid head.

The shoulder is reduced by pulling on the socket and proximal humerus laterally to clear it from the glenoid head while flexing and internally rotating the arm. A gentle but appreciable "clunk" should be experienced. If the shoulder reduces too easily, there is not enough tension present and the next size larger humeral socket should be tried. If the shoulder is not reducible, there may be soft tissue impingement, the patient is not relaxed, or occasionally not enough proximal humerus has been milled with the metaphyseal reamer. The ideal tension allows nearly full elevation in primary cases. In revision cases, elevation is dependent on many variables of altered native anatomy; however, 120 degrees of elevation is often achieved. With the arm at the side, externally rotate the shoulder to assess stability. If the socket dislocates off the glenoid head, there is not enough tension, thus necessitating a thicker socket, either +4 or +8. In most primary cases, a neutral liner suffices because some subscapularis is present, which, when repaired to the proximal humerus, limits excessive external rotation. In revision cases with proximal humerus bone loss, bone grafting, use of a thicker socket, or both achieves adequate soft tissue tension.

Cementing of the Humeral Stem. If the stability and motion are satisfactory, the shoulder is dislocated and the trial humeral components are removed. After clearing the humeral canal of debris, an appropriately sized cement restrictor is inserted into the humeral canal, 1.5 cm distal to the length of the humeral stem prosthesis.

The polyethylene humeral socket is placed via its Morse taper into the opening of the humeral stem implant in the correct orientation. The socket is impacted onto the stem with three to four firm taps onto the impactor with a mallet. Transosseous holes are drilled with a 2-mm drill into the proximal humerus for reattachment of any remaining subscapularis. No. 1 braided sutures are passed through the holes.

Cement, which should be in the doughy stage, is introduced into the humeral canal using a retrograde technique with a cement gun. The assembled humeral prosthesis is delivered into the humerus in the established 30 degrees of retroversion. Light taps may be used with the mallet onto the impactor placed on the socket to fully seat the prosthesis.

Final Reduction and Closure. Reduction of the humeral prosthesis onto the glenoid head is then performed. The arm is then placed in about 30 degrees abduction and slight external rotation. Any remaining subscapularis is reattached with the previously placed sutures in the proximal humerus. The shoulder is put through a final range of motion to assess a safe range for postoperative therapy. Routine closure is performed in layers. The arm is placed in a shoulder immobilizer.

Postoperative Rehabilitation. Generally, supine passive range of motion is instituted by a therapist the day after surgery. The usual parameter is 90 degrees elevation and 0 degrees external rotation. A shoulder immobilizer is maintained for 4 weeks while passive range of motion exercises are done. A sling is then worn for the next 4 weeks. During this time active assisted range of motion is done. Active range of motion is begun after 8 weeks. Resistive exercises are delayed until the remnant subscapularis tendon insertion has healed, usually at 12 weeks. In revision cases, it is not unusual to withhold therapy for a brief period.

Results

We have implanted 66 shoulders (20 men and 46 women; average age 69 years, range 34–86 years) with the reverse total shoulder replacement in two groups of patients at our institution. Follow-up has averaged 11 months (range 2–62 months). Group I patients (n = 27) are primary cases of an irreparable rotator cuff tear (IRCT) with glenohumeral arthritis or coracoacromial arch deficiency. Group II patients (n = 39) are revision cases of failed surgeries, including rotator cuff repair with secondary arthritis, hemiarthroplasty, or TSA who have an IRCT or coracoacromial arch deficiency.

Both groups had statistically significant ($p < 0.05$) improvements in postoperative outcome scores. Patients in group I, however, had more clinically relevant improvements in pain and function than did patients in group II. Patients in group I had improvements in total ASES from 35 to 68, ASES for pain from 18 to 38, and ASES for function from 16 to 30. Patients in group II had improvements in total ASES from 31 to 51, ASES for pain from 16 to 32, and ASES for function from 15 to 19. VAS for pain and function improved from 7 to 2 and from 2.5 to 6 in patients in group I, whereas it improved from 7 to 4 and from 2 to 4 in patients in group II. Positive responses on the SST improved from 1 to 5 in patients in group I and from 1 to 3 in patients in group II. Active forward elevation increased from 64 to 118 degrees in patients in group I, whereas it increased from 52 to 80 degrees in patients in group II. Complications occurred only in patients in group II and included component disassociation (n = 1), glenoid loosening (n = 1), recurrent instability (n = 2), and infection (n = 1).

GENERAL CONSIDERATION FOR SHOULDER ARTHROPLASTY

Conventional shoulder arthroplasty for patients with an irreparable rotator cuff tear and glenohumeral arthritis or coracoacromial arch deficiency provides adequate pain relief but not predictable function. Reverse TSA has yielded significant improvements in primary and revision cases. In primary cases, the RSP provides predictable improvements in pain and function with minimal complications. In revision cases, there has been a higher complication rate, and improvements in pain and function are less reliable. With proper patient selection, adherence to sound surgical technique and adequate postoperative protection, the reverse shoulder replacement can be beneficial in difficult shoulder conditions when no other surgical option is available. Long-term results are pending.

Conventional Total Shoulder Arthroplasty

The goal of arthroplasty is to improve the quality of life through relief of pain, improvement in function, or both. It is indicated when the goal cannot be met by medical management or simpler procedures. There appears to be a double standard for judging the results of replacement of the shoulder compared with the hip or knee. If a patient cannot reach high overhead after shoulder arthroplasty, many would say that the operation was not particularly successful—an opinion derived from the fact that such motion is important in the shoulder. What about expectations for hip or knee arthroplasty? If a normal range of motion were also important in those joints, would we be as satisfied? Consider those cultures where people sit with their legs crossed or folded beneath the body. Full range of motion would be considered just as important as pain relief for a satisfactory result. This is one reason why total knee replacement is considered not as successful in Japan as it is in North America. Finally, the technique of shoulder arthroplasty involves intricate soft tissue surgery. Although surface replacement provides pain relief, it is the soft tissue part of the operation that determines the functional outcome. It is certainly a more demanding procedure than is knee or hip joint replacement.

Preoperative Evaluation

Preoperative evaluation includes assessment of the patient's motivation and general health, history of previous injections, surgery or infection, use of corticosteroids, and functional limitations. Involvement of the other joints in the ipsilateral and contralateral upper extremities is determined. Requirements for walking aids as a result of lower extremity problems are relevant to the postoperative rehabilitation program. Finally, the spouse or other family member should learn the passive range of motion exercises needed during the first 6 weeks postoperatively. The physical examination should include determination of the soft tissue quality, muscle strength, and shoulder stability. Active and passive ranges of motion are recorded and include elevation in the functional plane (forward and slightly to the side), external rotation with the arm at the side and at 99 degrees of abduction, internal rotation at 90 degrees of abduction, and the highest vertebral segment that can be reached behind the back. The ability of the patient to perform most functional activities can be predicted from these measurements. These ranges of motion are recorded again preoperatively when the patient is under anesthesia.

Preoperative radiographs include AP views in full external and internal rotation as well as an axillary view. The AP views are obtained with the patient angled 30 to 45 degrees to the x-ray beam so that the scapula, and not the torso, is perpendicular to the beam. This shows the joint surface that cannot be assessed on typical AP views obtained in many radiology departments.

Contraindications

Shoulder arthroplasty is contraindicated by active infection or when neuromuscular control is impossible as a result of loss of either deltoid or rotator cuff muscle function. Lack of one or the other alone is not a contraindication.

Consideration of Other Joint Involvement

The shoulder links the hand to the body and position on the surface of a hypothetical sphere. The elbow permits the hand to reach places within the sphere. Arthritic involvement of an ipsilateral shoulder or elbow increases the demands on the other. Thus, replacement of one joint may obviate the need for replacing the other when both are damaged. A likely explanation for this is that elimination of pain in one of the joints eliminates its detrimental effects on the biomechanics and function of the other.

If both the elbow and shoulder joints definitely require placing, the one that is most painful or dysfunctional should be replaced first. Consideration is given to the expected outcome, expected rehabilitation, and whether any period of serious temporary disability is likely postoperatively. Technical considerations, such as the requirement of external shoulder rotation for positioning of the limb during elbow replacement surgery, also might influence the decision. Sequential replacement of both joints on the same day is possible technically, although the postoperative rehabilitation of one joint can at times interfere with that of the other.

Concomitant involvement of lower extremity joints is important also, especially if walking aids are required. Crutches cannot be used after total elbow replacement for 6 weeks, unless the triceps mechanism is left intact (it is usually detached in surgery). O'Driscoll has had experience with leaving it intact and has noticed a profound improvement in the postoperative recovery and rehabilitation period. Whether or not there will be a long-term difference in outcome is unclear. The surgery is far more difficult and takes longer than if the triceps mechanism is removed. It is possible only in cases of significant bone loss or destruction. Weight bearing is also undesirable immediately after total shoulder replacement. Thus, if surgery is also required on the lower extremity joint, it should be delayed for at least 3 months following replacement of either the shoulder or the elbow (95,96).

Postoperative Rehabilitation

This is more important to the eventual function of the shoulder than it is for arthroplasty of any other joint. There are three phases. During the first 6 weeks, the goal is to prevent the soft tissue repair from being stretched or avulsed. Active movements are not permitted, and extension is limited so that the elbow is kept anterior to the coronal plane (by placing folded sheets behind the elbow and by wearing a special shoulder immobilizer while lying in bed). Equally important is the prevention of stiffness. Passive range of motion exercises begins the day after operation. This is to maintain the elevation and external rotation that were regained at the time of surgery. Initially, internal rotation is not encouraged so that the anterosuperior soft tissue repair in the rotator cuff interval is not stretched. This would predispose to anterosuperior glenohumeral joint subluxation during active elevation. A member of the patient's family can do these passive exercises.

From 6 weeks to 3 months (second phase), full active exercises are added, and passive stretching is vigorously pursued. Finally, 3 months postoperatively (third phase), a full strengthening program is commenced. Neer has popularized the notion of "limited goals" applying to patients in whom the goals of surgery cannot be met (e.g., irreparable massive cuff tear) or who are incapable of participating in the full rehabilitation program. These patients are given a modified rehabilitation program from the start. They often obtain pain relief but little or no functional improvement (43,77).

Complications in Conventional Total Shoulder Arthroplasty

In a meta-analysis reviewing complications (Table 46.8), the order of frequency of major complications for unconstrained implants are glenoid loosening, subluxation or dislocation, and rotator cuff tearing. Humeral loosening, infection, and nerve injury were much less common. Glenoid arthritis, rotator cuff insufficiency, and glenohumeral instability are the most common complications reported with the use of a hemiarthroplasty. Constrained implants historically have higher rates of complications and are now infrequently used. However, there has been a resurgence in their use in Europe with the Grammont Delta III prosthesis and in the United States with the Encore RSP, which is currently undergoing an investigational study by the Food and Drug Administration for its use in rotator cuff arthropathy.

Expected Results

There have been numerous reports of the successful use of shoulder arthroplasty for glenohumeral OA. Historically, the most commonly used shoulder arthroplasty has been the Neer design. Neer himself reported an 86% excellent or satisfactory result in TSA patients.

Torchia and associates (80) recently analyzed the long-term results at the Mayo Clinic using the Neer prosthesis for TSA. They determined the probability of prosthesis survival as 93% at 10 years and 87% after 15 years. The patient's age, sex, preoperative diagnosis, condition of the rotator cuff, and preoperative range of motion did not affect the probability of prosthesis survival. The most common cause of failure was glenoid loosening (4%). At an average follow-up of 12.2 years, excellent pain relief was reported in 83% of patients. Range of motion was significantly improved. Functional gains were directly related to the condition of the rotator cuff. Humeral loosening was not associated with pain but was seen more frequently with press-fit fixation. At an average radiographic follow-up of 9.6 years, there were no signs of loosening of cement-fixed prostheses; however, the study group was small. In contrast, the press-fit group had a 49% incidence of radiographic loosening. Clinically, there was no pain associated with the loosening. The Neer prosthesis used was a smooth-surfaced design; therefore, it is recommended that if press-fit fixation is used, a tissue ingrowth stem should be implanted. Other authors have reported the survivorship of the Neer unconstrained TSA at 94.4% at 5 years and 71% at 11 years, with the incidence of component revision reported to be between 0% and 13%.

Goldberg and Smith evaluated the function of 124 shoulders with primary degenerative joint disease by patient self-assessment with the Simple Shoulder Test before and sequentially after standardized TSA technique. Patients reported that they could perform 3.8 ± 0.3 (SEM) of the 12 Simple Shoulder Test functions before surgery. The total number of performable functions was consistent at different

TABLE 46.8. *Complications of total shoulder arthroplasty*

Complications	Unconstrained (%)	Constrained (%)	Hemiarthroplasty (%)
Glenoid loosening	4.7 (0–36)	11.8 (0–25)	0
Humeral loosening	0.4 (0–6.9)	1.0 (0–7.7)	0
Subluxation	0.9 (0–12.5)	0	0
Dislocation	2.7 (0–18.2)	9.4 (6–16.7)	1.7 (2–6.6)
Rotator cuff tear	2.2 (0–16.6)	0	2.7 (2–11.5)
Infection	0.5 (0–3.9)	2.9 (0–15.4)	0
Nerve injury	0.5 (0–2)	0	0.4 (0–2)

follow-up intervals: 8.0 ± 0.4 at 6 months, 9.5 ± 0.4 at 1 year, 10.0 ± 0.3 at 2 years, 9.2 ± 0.4 at 3 years, 9.6 ± 0.4 at 4 years, and 10.0 ± 0.4 at 5 years. The investigators concluded that TSA provides substantial and durable improvement in shoulder function (70).

In another study, Matsen and co-workers looked at additional preoperative considerations to a successful outcome. One hundred thirty-four shoulders having TSA for degenerative glenohumeral joint disease had an average follow-up of 3.4 ± 1.8 years. The Short Form-36 (SF-36) comfort score improved from 39 to 61 ($p < 0.0001$). The overall well being of the patient before surgery was strongly correlated with the quality of the outcome from TSA for degenerative glenohumeral joint disease (76).

Boorman and Kopjar studied 91 patients and compared their responses to the eight quantitative domains of the SF-36 before surgery and at 30 to 60 months after surgery. These preoperative and postoperative scores were compared with data from age-matched and gender-matched controls. Although the improvements were significant and similar to the postoperative scores reported for total hip arthroplasty and coronary bypass procedures, the scores did not reach those of the general population (97).

Literature comparing hemiarthroplasty and TSA seems to favor the former when arthritis and cuff deficiency coexist and the later in OA and RA when the rotator cuff is intact. Some studies have attempted to compare hemiarthroplasty with TSA. Boyd and co-workers found a similar but unmatched series comparison that at 44 months follow-up hemiarthroplasty and TSA produced similar results in terms of functional improvement. Pain relief, range of motion, and patient satisfaction were better with TSA than with hemiarthroplasty in the rheumatoid population. Progressive glenoid loosening was found in 12% of total shoulder arthroplasties, but no correlation with pain relief or range of motion was noted (82).

Gartsman and co-workers randomized 51 shoulders into hemiarthroplasty or TSA groups to compare pain and functional outcome. Specific criteria for inclusion in the study were OA, intact rotator cuff, and concentric glenoid. Results demonstrated that TSA provided superior pain relief and equal results for elevation and external rotation versus hemiarthroplasty (81).

Jensen and Rockwood reported on 117 shoulders with OA, 25% of which had an irreparable rotator cuff tear. At 58-month follow-up, they found no difference in motion, pain relief, and ability to perform activities of daily living in patients treated with hemiarthroplasty and TSA.

In summary, unconstrained TSA provides pain relief in 90% to 95% of patients. Motion for a patient with primary OA undergoing TSA approximates two thirds of normal. The same is true for patients with proximal humeral osteonecrosis and secondary glenoid arthritis. RA affects soft tissues and bone to a greater extent and typically results in motion that is between one half and two thirds normal. The rheumatoid patient requires earlier intervention with synovectomy or arthroplasty performed prior to rotator cuff compromise. Glenoid bone stock should be carefully assessed with axillary radiographs and CT scan. In old trauma and revision surgery, extensive scarring and contracture can further compromise motion after surgery. In these cases, soft tissue releases must be performed with lengthening of tendons.

Glenoid erosion, humeral head subluxation, and a severe preoperative loss of passive motion of the shoulder have significant effects on outcome, whereas a repairable full-thickness tear of the rotator cuff isolated to the supraspinatus tendon did not affect outcome. On the basis of these data, we recommend the use of a glenoid component in shoulders with glenoid erosion and in the presence of a small, repairable tear of the supraspinatus tendon when there is coexistent glenoid arthritis. Humeral head subluxation consistently results in a less-favorable outcome regardless of whether a hemiarthroplasty or a TSA is performed. This anatomic factor must be considered in preoperative surgical planning and counseling. Return to active motion depends on the surgeon and postoperative management. Our experience with the Encore RSP as well as the European experience with the Grammont reverse TSA has resulted in predictable pain relief and improved function in the patient with rotator cuff deficiency when compared with conventional hemiarthroplasty in short-term comparison for rotator cuff arthropathy. Long-term results are needed in this most difficult patient population.

REFERENCES

1. Harryman DT 2nd, Sidles JA, Clark JM, et al. Translation of the humeral head on the glenoid with passive glenohumeral motion. *J Bone Joint Surg Am* 1990;72:1334–1343.
2. Karduna AR, Williams GR, Williams JL, et al. Kinematics of the glenohumeral joint: influences of muscle forces, ligamentous constraints, and articular geometry. *J Orthop Res* 1996;14:986–993.
3. Kumar VP, Balsubramaniamk P. The role of atmospheric pressure in stabilizing the shoulder: an experimental study. *J Bone Joint Surg Br* 1985;67:719–721.
4. McMahon PJ, Debski RE, Thompson WO, et al. Shoulder muscle forces and tendon excursions during glenohumeral abduction in the scapular plane. *J Shoulder Elbow Surg* 1995;4:199–208.
5. Novotny JE, Nichols CE, Beynnon BD. Normal kinematics of the unconstrained glenohumeral joint under coupled moment loads. *J Shoulder Elbow Surg* 1998;7:629–639.
6. Norris TR. *Orthopaedic knowledge update: shoulder and elbow,* 2nd ed. American Academy of Orthopaedic Surgeons, Rosemont, IL, 2002.
7. Young DC, Rockwood CA Jr. Complications of a failed Bristow procedure and their management. *J Bone Joint Surg Am* 1991;73:969–981.
8. Arwert HJ, deGroot J, Van Woensel WW, et al. Electromyography of shoulder muscles in relation to force direction. *J Shoulder Elbow Surg* 1997;6:360–370.
9. Lazarus MD, Sidles JA, Harryman DT 2nd, et al. Effect of a chondral-labral defect on glenoid concavity and glenohumeral stability: a cadaveric model. *J Bone Joint Surg Am* 1996;78:94–102.
10. Lee SB, Kim KJ, O'Driscoll SW, et al. Dynamic glenohumeral stability provided by the byte rotator cuff muscles in the mid-range and end-range of motion: a study in cadavera. *J Bone Joint Surg Am* 2000;82:849–857.

11. O'Brien SJ, Neves MC, Arnoczky SP, et al. The anatomy and histology of the inferior glenohumeral ligamentous complex of the shoulder. *Am J Sports Med* 1990;18:449–456.
12. Pagnani MJ, Deng XH, Warren RF, et al. Role of the long head of the biceps brachii in glenohumeral stability: a biomechanical study in cadavera. *J Shoulder Elbow Surg* 1996;5:255–262.
13. Soslowsky LJ, Malicky DM, Blasier RB. Active and passive factors in inferior glenohumeral stabilization: a biomechanical model. *J Shoulder Elbow Surg* 1997;6:371–379.
14. Steinbeck J, Liljenqvist U, Jerosch J. The anatomy of the glenohumeral ligamentous complex and its contribution to anterior shoulder stability. *J Shoulder Elbow Surg* 1998;7:122–126.
15. Warner JJ, Deng XH, Warren RF, et al. Static capsuloligamentous restraints to superior-inferior translation of the glenohumeral joint. *Am J Sports Med* 1992;20:675–685.
16. Boileau P, Walch G. The three-dimensional geometry of the proximal humerus: implications for surgical technique and prosthetic design. *J Bone Bone Joint Surg Br* 1997;79:857–865.
16. Yamaguchi K, Riew KD, Galatz LM, et al. Biceps activity during shoulder motion: an an electromyographic analysis. *Clin Orthop* 1997; 336:122–129.
17. Churchill RS, Brems JJ, Kotschi H, et al. Glenoid size, inclination, and version: an anatomic study. *J Shoulder Elbow Surg* 2001;10:327–332.
18. Pearl ML, Kurutz S. Geometric analysis of commonly used prosthetic systems for proximal humeral replacement. *J Bone Joint Surg Am* 1999;81:660–671.
19. Pearl ML, Volk AG. Coronal plane geometry of the proximal humerus relevant to prosthetic arthroplasty. *J Shoulder Elbow Surg* 1996;5: 320–326.
20. Robertson DD, Yuan J, Bigliani LU, et al. Three-dimensional analysis of the proximal part of the humerus: relevance relevance to arthroplasty. *J Bone Joint Surg Am* 2000;82:1594–1602.
21. Iannotti JP, Williams GR. Total shoulder arthroplasty: factors influencing prosthetic design. *Orthop Clin North Am* 1998;29:377–391.
22. Williams GR Jr, Wong KL, Pepe MD, et al. The effect of articular malposition after total shoulder arthroplasty on glenohumeral translations, range of motion, and subacromial impingement. *J Shoulder Elbow Surg* 2001;10:399–409.
23. Friedman RJ, Hawthorne KB, Genez BM. The use of computerized tomography in the measurement of glenoid version. *J Bone Joint Surg Am* 1992;74:1032–1037.
24. Walch G, Edwards TB, Boulahia A, et al. The influence of glenohumeral prosthetic mismatch on glenoid radiolucent lines: results of a multicenter study. *J Bone Joint Surg Am* 2002;84A:2186–2191.
25. Cushner MA, Friedman RJ. Osteonecrosis of the humeral head. *J Am Acad Orthop Surg* 1997;5:339–346.
26. Gerber C, Schneeberger AG, Vinh TS. The arterial vascularization of the humeral head: an anatomical study. *J Bone Joint Surg Am* 1990;72: 1486–1494.
27. Sperling JW, Cofield RH, O'Driscoll SW, et al. Radiographic assessment of ingrowth total shoulder arthroplasty. *J Shoulder Elbow Surg* 2000;9:507–513.
28. Wirth MA, Korvick DL, Basamania CJ, et al. Radiologic, mechanical, and histologic evaluation of 2 glenoid prosthesis designs in a canine model. Radiologic, mechanical, and histologic evaluation of 2 glenoid prosthesis designs in a canine model. *J Shoulder Elbow Surg* 2001; 10:140–148.
29. Boileau P, Avidor C, Krishnan SG, et al. Cemented polyethylene versus uncemented metal-backed glenoid components in total shoulder arthroplasty: a prospective, double-blind, randomized study. *J Shoulder Elbow Surg* 2002;11:351–359.
30. Brems JJ. Arthritis of dislocation. *Orthop Clin North Am* 1998;29: 453–466.
31. Marx RG, McCarty EC, Montemurno TD, et al. Development of arthrosis following dislocation of the shoulder: a case-control study. *J Shoulder Elbow Surg* 2002;11:1–5.
32. Banas MP, Dalldorf PG, Sebastianelli WJ, et al. Long-term follow-up of the modified Bristow procedure. *Am J Sports Med* 1993;21:666–671.
33. Bigliani LU, Weinstein DM, Glasgow MT, et al. Glenohumeral arthroplasty for arthritis after instability surgery. *J Shoulder Elbow Surg* 1995;4:87–94.
34. Hawkins RJ, Neer CS 2nd. A functional analysis of shoulder fusions. *Clin Orthop* 1987;223:65–76.
35. Hawkins RJ, Angelo RL. Glenohumeral osteoarthrosis: a late complication of the Putti-Platt repair. *J Bone Joint Surg Am* 1990;72:1193–1197.
36. van der Zwaag HM, Brand R, Obermann WR, et al. Glenohumeral osteoarthrosis after Putti-Platt repair. *J Shoulder Elbow Surg* 1999;8: 252–258.
37. Cuomo F, Greller MJ, Zuckerman JD. The rheumatoid shoulder. *Rheum Dis Clin North Am* 1998;24:67–82.
38. Lehtinen JT, Belt EA, Lyback CO, et al. Subacromial space in the rheumatoid shoulder: a radiographic 15-year follow-up study of 148 shoulders. *J Shoulder Elbow Surg* 2000;9:183–187.
39. Matthews LS, LaBudde JK. Arthroscopic treatment of synovial diseases of the shoulder. *Orthop Clin North Am* 1993;24:101–109.
40. Neer CS 2nd. Glenohumeral arthroplasty. In: Neer CS, ed. *Shoulder reconstruction*. Philadelphia: WB Saunders, 1990:143–172.
41. Rozing PM, Brand R: Rotator cuff repair during shoulder arthroplasty in rheumatoid arthritis. *J Arthroplasty* 1998;13:311–319.
42. Wakitani S, Imoto K, Saito M, et al. Evaluation of surgeries for rheumatoid shoulder based on the destruction pattern. *J Rheumatol* 1999; 26:41–46.
43. Cofield RH. Degenerative and arthritic problems of the glenohumeral joint. In: Rockwood CA, Matsen F, eds. *The shoulder.* Philadelphia: WB Saunders, 1990:678–749.
44. Crosby LA, Arroyo JS, Bigliani L, et al. *Total shoulder arthroplasty,* 1st ed. American Academy of Orthopaedic Surgeons, Rosemont, IL, 2000.
45. Figgie HE 3rd, Inglis AE, Goldberg VM, et al. An analysis of factors affecting the long-term results of total shoulder arthroplasty in inflammatory arthritis. *J Arthroplasty* 1988;3:123–130.
46. Friedman RJ, Thornhill TS, Thomas WH, et al. Non-constrained total shoulder replacement in patients who have rheumatoid arthritis and class-IV function. *J Bone Joint Surg Am* 1989;71:494–498.
47. Neer CS 2nd, Craig EV, Fukuda H. Cuff T-tear arthropathy. *J Bone Joint Surg Am* 1983;65:1232–1244.
48. Sperling JW, Antuna SA, Sanchez-Sotelo J, et al. Shoulder arthroplasty for arthritis after instability surgery. *J Bone Joint Surg Am* 2002; 84:1775–1781.
49. Basamania CJ, Jaramillo JC, Wirth MA, et al. Treatment of posttraumatic versus atraumatic avascular necrosis of the shoulder. 64th Annual Meeting of the Proceedings of the American Academy of Orthopaedic Surgeons, Rosemont, IL, 1997:51.
50. Gerber C, Hersche O, Berberat C. The clinical relevance of posttraumatic avascular necrosis of the humeral head. *J Shoulder Elbow Surg* 1998;7:586–590.
51. Hattrup SJ, Cofield RH. Osteonecrosis of the humeral head: relationship of disease stage, extent, and cause to natural history. *J Shoulder Elbow Surg* 1999;8:559–564.
52. L'Insalata JC, Pagnani MJ, Warren RF, et al. Humeral head osteonecrosis: clinical course and radiographic predictors of outcome. *J Shoulder Elbow Surg* 1996;5:355–361.
53. Mont MA, Maar DC, Urquhart MW, et al. Avascular necrosis of the humeral head treated by core decompression: a retrospective review. *J Bone Joint Surg Br* 1993;75:785–788.
54. Mont MA, Payman RK, LaPorte DM, et al. Atraumatic osteonecrosis of the humeral head. *J Rheumatol* 2000;27:1766–1773.
55. Hernigou P, Bernaudin F, Reinert P, et al. Bone-marrow transplantation in sickle-cell disease: effect on osteonecrosis: a case report with a four-year follow-up. *J Bone Joint Surg Am* 1997;79:1726–1730.
56. Milner PF, Kaus AP, Sebes JI, et al. Osteonecrosis of the humeral head in sickle cell disease. *Clin Orthop* 1993:289:136–143.
57. Wiater JM, Flatow EL. Posttraumatic arthritis. *Orthop Clin North Am* 2000;31:63–76
58. Cameron BD, Galatz LM, Ramsey ML, et al. Non-prosthetic management of grade IV osteochondral lesions of the glenohumeral joint. *J Shoulder Elbow Surg* 2002;11:25–32.
59. Bishop J, Nevaiser TJ, Nevaiser RJ. Arthroscopic abrasion arthroplasty for glenohumeral arthritis: analysis of outcome as a temporizing procedure. Paper presented at the AAOS Meeting, Dallas, TX, February 13–17, 2002.
60. Cofield RH. Shoulder arthrodesis and resection arthroplasty. *Instr Course Lect* 1985;34:268–277.
61. MacDonald PB, Hawkins RJ, Fowler PJ, et al. Release of the subscapularis for internal rotation contracture and pain after anterior repair for recurrent anterior dislocation of the shoulder. *J Bone Joint Surg Am* 1992;74:734–737.

62. LaPorte DM, Mont MA, Mohan V, et al. Osteonecrosis of the humeral head treated by core decompression. *Clin Orthop* 1998;355:254–260.
63. Yamaguchi K, Ball CM, Galatz LM, et al. Meniscal allograft interposition arthroplasty of the arthritic shoulder: early results and a review of the technique. Presented at ASES Specialty Day, Dallas, TX, February 16, 2002.
64. Amstutz HC, Sew Hoy AL, Clarke IC. UCLA anatomic total shoulder arthroplasty. *Clin Orthop* 1981;155:7–20.
65. Amstutz HC, Thomas BJ, Kabo JM, et al. The Dana total shoulder arthroplasty. *J Bone Joint Surg Am* 1988;70:1174–1182.
66. Barrett WP, Franklin JL, Jackins SE, et al. Total shoulder arthroplasty. *J Bone Joint Surg Am* 1987;69:865–872.
67. Cofield RH. Total shoulder arthroplasty with the Neer prosthesis. *J Bone Joint Surg Am* 1984;66:899–906.
68. Frich LH, Moller BN, Sneppen O. Shoulder arthroplasty with the Neer Mark-II prosthesis. *Arch Orthop Trauma Surg* 1988;107:110–113.
69. Godeneche A, Boileau P, Favard L, et al. Prosthetic replacement in the treatment of osteoarthritis of the shoulder: early results of 268 cases. *J Shoulder Elbow Surg* 2002;11:11–18.
70. Goldberg BA, Smith K, Jackins S, et al. The magnitude and durability of functional improvement after total shoulder arthroplasty for degenerative joint disease. *J Shoulder Elbow Surg* 2001;10:464–469.
71. Gristina AG, Romano RL, Kammire GC, et al. Total shoulder replacement. *Orthop Clin North Am* 1987;18:445–453.
72. Hawkins RJ, Bell RH, Jallay B. Total shoulder arthroplasty. *Clin Orthop* 1989;242:188–194.
73. Hawkins RJ, Greis PE, Bonutti PM. Treatment of symptomatic glenoid loosening following unconstrained shoulder arthroplasty. *Orthopedics* 1999;22:229–234.
74. Jensen KL, Rockwood CA Jr. Shoulder arthroplasty in recreational golfers. *J Shoulder Elbow Surg* 1998;7:362–367.
75. Jensen KL, Williams GR Jr, Russell IJ, et al. Rotator cuff tear arthropathy. *J Bone Joint Surg Am* 1999;5181:1312–1324.
76. Matsen FA 3rd, Antoniou J, Rozencwaig R, et al Correlates with comfort and function after total shoulder arthroplasty for degenerative joint disease. *J Shoulder Elbow Surg* 2000;9:465–469.
77. Neer CS 2nd, Watson KC, Stanton FJ. Recent experience in total shoulder replacement. *J Bone Joint Surg Am* 1982;64:319–337.
78. Sperling JW, Cofield RH, Rowland CM. Neer hemiarthroplasty and Neer total shoulder arthroplasty in patients fifty years old or less: long-term results. *J Bone Joint Surg Am* 1998;80:464–473.
79. Torchia ME, Cofield RH, Settergren CR. Total shoulder arthroplasty with the Neer prosthesis: long-term results. *J Shoulder Elbow Surg* 1997;6:495–505.
80. Wretenberg PF, Wallensten R. The Kessel total shoulder arthroplasty. A 13- to 16-year retrospective followup. *Clin Orthop* 1999;365:100–103.
81. Gartsman GM, Roddey TS, Hammerman SM. Shoulder arthroplasty with or without resurfacing of the glenoid in patients who have osteoarthritis. *J Bone Joint Surg Am* 2000;82:26–34.
82. Boyd AD Jr, Thomas WH, Scott RD, et al. Total shoulder arthroplasty versus hemiarthroplasty: indications for glenoid resurfacing. *J Arthroplasty* 1990;5:329–336.
83. Levine WN, Djurasovic M, Glasson JM, et al. Hemiarthroplasty for glenohumeral osteoarthritis: results correlated to degree of glenoid wear. *J Shoulder Elbow Surg* 1997;6:449–454.
84. Cofield RH, Edgerton BC. Total shoulder arthroplasty: complications and revision surgery. *Instr Course Lect* 1990;39:449–462.
85. Field LD, Dines DM, Zabinski SJ, et al. Hemiarthroplasty of the shoulder for rotator cuff arthropathy. *J Shoulder Elbow Surg* 1997;6:18–23.
86. Lee DH, Niemann KM. Bipolar shoulder arthroplasty. *Clin Orthop* 1994;30:97–107.
87. Nwakama AC, Cofield RH, Kavanagh BF, et al. Semiconstrained total shoulder arthroplasty for glenohumeral arthritis and massive rotator cuff tearing. *J Shoulder Elbow Surg* 2000;9:302–307.
88. Sanchez-Sotelo J, Cofield RH, Rowland CM. Shoulder hemiarthroplasty for glenohumeral arthritis associated with severe rotator cuff deficiency. *J Bone Joint Surg Am* 2001;83:1814–1822.
89. Yamaguchi K, Sher JS, Andersen WK, et al. Glenohumeral motion in patients with rotator cuff tears: a comparison of asymptomatic and symptomatic shoulders. *J Shoulder Elbow Surg* 2000;9:6–11.
90. Zuckerman JD, Scott AJ, Gallagher MA. Hemiarthroplasty for cuff tear arthropathy. *J Shoulder Elbow Surg* 2000;9:169–172.
91. Boulahia A, Edwards TB, Walch G, et al. Early results of a reverse design prosthesis in the treatment of arthritis of the shoulder in elderly patients with a large rotator cuff tear. *Orthopedics* 2002;25:129–133.
92. Grammont PM, Baulot E. Delta shoulder prosthesis for rotator cuff rupture. *Orthopaedics* 1993;16:65–68.
93. Rittmeister M, Kerschbaumer F. Grammont reverse total shoulder arthroplasty in patients with rheumatoid arthritis and nonreconstructible rotator cuff lesions. *J Shoulder Elbow Surg* 2001;10:17–22.
94. Valenti P, Boutens D, Nerot C. Delta 3 reversed prosthesis for osteoarthritis with massive rotator cuff tear: long term results (>5 years). *Shoulder Prostheses* 2000;253–259.
95. Friedman RJ, Ewald FC. Arthroplasty of the ipsilateral shoulder and elbow in patients who have rheumatoid arthritis. *J Bone Joint Surg Am* 1987;69:661–666.
96. Gill DR, Cofield RH, Morrey BF. Ipsilateral total shoulder and elbow arthroplasties in patients who have rheumatoid arthritis. *J Bone Joint Surg Am* 1999;81:1128–1137.
97. Boorman RS, Kopjar B, Fehringer E, et al The effect of total shoulder arthroplasty on self-assessed health status is comparable to that of total hip arthroplasty and coronary artery bypass grafting. *J Shoulder Elbow Surg* 2003;12:158–163.

CHAPTER 47

Surgical Management of Elbow Arthritis

Bradford O. Parsons and Michael Hausman

The surgical management of elbow arthritic conditions, including rheumatoid arthritis (RA), posttraumatic stiffness and arthrosis, and primary osteoarthritis (OA), has continued to expand and evolve. Elucidation of arthroscopic anatomy of the elbow has enabled arthroscopic techniques for contracture release, synovectomy, and débridement of the arthritic elbow to be used with increased frequency and wider application. Results of prosthetic replacement of the elbow have also continued to improve with increased understanding of pathologic and normal elbow anatomy and kinematics, especially with respect to instability patterns of the elbow. As a result of the expanding knowledge and advances in technique, a range of options for treating a patient with an arthritic elbow are now available.

ANATOMY, BIOMECHANICS, AND KINEMATICS

The primary function of the elbow is to position and stabilize the hand in space. As such, the elbow is critically important in activities of daily living as well as recreational and occupational activities. Although often felt to be a non-weight-bearing joint, the elbow does function as a load-bearing joint in the course of normal daily activity, and can bear forces up to three times body weight (1).

The elbow has been described as a trochoginglymoid joint that possesses 2 degrees of motion (flexion-extension and pronation-supination) through three articulations (the ulnohumeral, radiohumeral, and radioulnar joints). The ulnohumeral joint, originally felt to strictly act as a hinge joint, actually has a helical motion of the flexion axis. The center of the flexion-extension axis of the elbow is through the center of the arcs formed by the capitellum and the trochlear sulcus (2–4). The deviation from a strict uniaxial articulation at extremes of flexion and extension has caused some to term the elbow as a "loose hinge" joint (3–7). Rotation of the forearm relative to the arm occurs through the radiohumeral and radioulnar articulations, and is independent of elbow position (8).

The normal arc of flexion of the elbow is from 0 degrees or slightly hyperextended to 150 degrees, and arc of rotation averages around 75 degrees pronation to 85 degrees supination (1). Patients with posttraumatic stiffness, inflammatory arthritis, or OA can have substantial loss of motion from both extrinsic and intrinsic etiologies (9–12). Morrey et al. (13) have shown the functional flexion arc of motion to be from 30 to 130 degrees. Functional foreman rotation requires a total motion arc of 100 degrees, evenly divided between supination and pronation.

Elbow stability throughout the arcs of motion is maintained by an almost equal contribution from the osseous anatomy and soft tissue structures. The ulnohumeral articulation provides the majority of the static osseous constraint of the joint and along with the anterior band of the medial collateral ligament (MCL) and the lateral ulnar collateral ligament (LUCL) complex is a primary constraint to instability (14). The LUCL complex has been found to be integral in the prevention of posterolateral rotatory instability, which is a common instability pattern (15–17). Secondary constraints include the radiohumeral articulation, the common flexor and extensor tendon origins, and the anterior capsule. These primary and secondary restraints combine to make the elbow one of the most congruous and stable joints in the body.

Thorough knowledge of the functional anatomy and biomechanics of the normal elbow enables the clinician to better understand the pathologic processes and changes seen in the stiff, arthritic, or unstable elbow. Additionally, this knowledge has facilitated in the development and improvement of total elbow arthroplasty.

PATIENT EVALUATION

It is important to first take a detailed history and perform a thorough physical examination when evaluating a patient with elbow arthritis. The history should include onset and progression of symptoms. Attention should be directed to symptoms of instability, increasing stiffness, or neurologic changes in the arm, because each of these symptoms can affect the choice of treatment of the patient. History of prior surgical procedures of the elbow should be obtained. Patients may report locking or occasional episodes of sudden pain and swelling, possible hallmarks of loose bodies, or osteochondral lesions in the elbow.

The physical examination should attempt to differentiate between pain from neurologic, mechanical, inflammatory, and osteoarthritic causes. The examination should begin with inspection of the elbow for signs of effusion or synovitis, and the elbow is examined for tenderness. Range of motion, both active and passive, is assessed, and pain at the terminal points of flexion or extension is elicited. Terminal extension pain can be a sign of impingement of the olecranon into the fossa, whereas terminal flexion pain can be due to abutment of the coronoid in its humeral fossa.

As stated with the history, it is important to examine for signs of instability, especially in the patient with a history of RA or posttraumatic arthritis, or in patients who have undergone lateral elbow procedures. Valgus instability can be a sign of MCL insufficiency, and is best evaluated with the humerus externally rotated with a valgus stress applied to the elbow in approximately 30 degrees of flexion. Recently, the moving valgus stress test has been shown to be a valuable aid in diagnosing partial tears of the MCL (18). Varus stress is checked with the humerus in internal rotation. A more specific test for LUCL deficiency is the lateral pivot shift test (15). This is performed with the patient lying supine with the arm overhead and involves extending the elbow with an applied valgus axial stress while the forearm is supinated. The radial head subluxates posteriorly as the elbow is brought into extension, during which an awake patient may exhibit signs of apprehension.

A complete neurologic examination of the upper extremity is important because of the association of ulnar nerve entrapment with elbow arthritis. It is important to separate pain from neurologic, mechanical, inflammatory, and osteoarthritic causes.

Radiographic analysis using anteroposterior and lateral radiography is often sufficient to identify the majority of sources of pain in the elbow. Stress radiography may be helpful in confirming instability. Computed tomography (CT) scans can be helpful in localizing heterotopic ossification, osteophytes, or loose bodies, and reconstructions can help delineate subchondral bone destruction in patients with advanced rheumatoid disease. Magnetic resonance imaging (MRI) may be useful in diagnosing osteochondritis dessicans lesions, loose bodies, rice bodies, synovial lesions such as pigmental villonodular synovitis, or rupture of the collateral ligaments.

Elbow Instability

Elbow instability is a major cause of premature degenerative changes. The patient with an unstable elbow can present with a spectrum of complaints, from pain at extremes of elbow motion to recurrent subluxation or dislocation of the elbow. As stated previously, the MCL and LUCL are the two primary ligamentous stabilizers of the elbow. Instability can arise secondary to trauma, recurrent trauma (e.g., throwing), inflammatory disease, and iatrogenic causes (e.g., transection of the LUCL during the Kocher approach, or radial head resection).

The MCL can be damaged after traumatic dislocation of the elbow or radial head fracture, but most commonly is injured in the overhead throwing athlete who sustains gradual attenuation of the ligament due to high valgus loads (19, 20). Resection of the radial head, either during treatment of radial head fracture or in combination with synovectomy in patients with RA removes the secondary valgus restraint and may result in attenuation of the MCL and late valgus instability (21–23).

LUCL injury rarely occurs after excessive or repetitive isolated varus stress and is most commonly seen following elbow dislocation in the young, athletic population (24), or after iatrogenic injury during lateral elbow procedures performed via a Kocher approach (25,26). Injury to the LUCL has been shown to result in a posterolateral rotatory instability pattern (15,24,25).

Chronic laxity of the elbow alters the biomechanics of the joint. With valgus instability the medial olecranon can impinge on the medial wall of the olecranon fossa, resulting in synovitis and degenerative changes such as osteophytes and loose bodies (Fig. 47.1). Additional changes may be seen in the radiocapitellar joint due to abnormally high compressive forces across this joint in the elbow with a deficient MCL. Chronic posterolateral rotatory instability can result in progressive articular damage that occurs with each subluxation of the elbow.

Surgical Management

Reconstruction of the MCL or LUCL has been shown to provide symptomatic relief and can, in the case of throwing athletes with MCL insufficiency, allow a return to preinjury activity levels (25,27–30). The primary indication for ligament reconstruction is patients who have symptomatic ligamentous insufficiency and have failed nonoperative modalities, including rest and physical therapy. Additionally, stabilization of the elbow may help prevent later secondary arthritic changes in the elbow (28).

Reconstruction of the MCL is performed using autograft, most commonly palmaris tendon from the ipsilateral arm. The technique, originally presented by Jobe and associates (28), has been well described (Fig. 47.2). An additional method of MCL reconstruction using a "docking technique" has also been described (31).

Reconstruction of the LUCL using either tendon graft (24) or lateral triceps fascia (29) has been described. The original technique, as described by Nestor and O'Driscoll (24), uses a palmaris tendon graft, which is positioned through the ligament isometric points on the humerus and

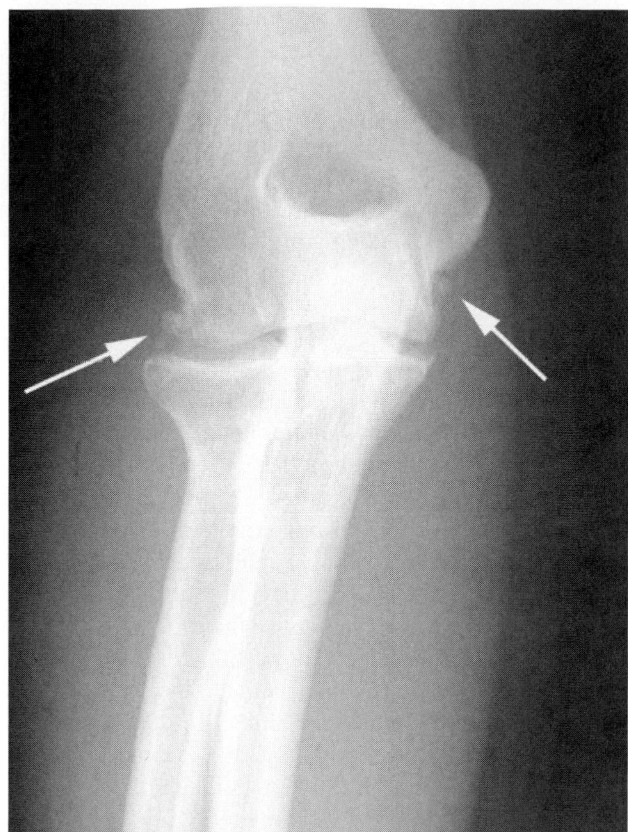

A

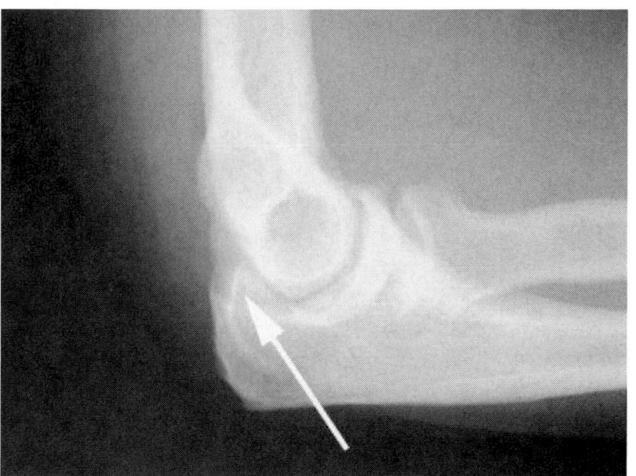

B

FIG. 47.1. Chronic valgus instability, due to attenuation or rupture of the medial collateral ligament (*MCL*) can result in characterisitic arthritic changes in the elbow. Anteroposterior **(A)** and lateral **(B)** elbow radiographs can show medial olecranon impingement, osteophytes, and loose bodies. Additionally, osteophytes can be seen along the lateral border of the radiocapitellar joint.

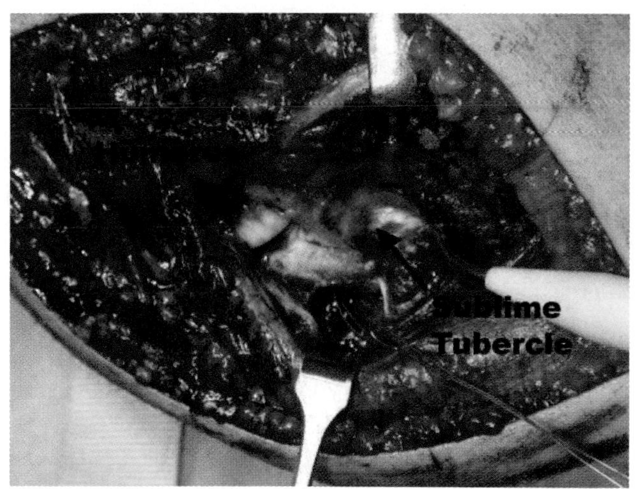

A

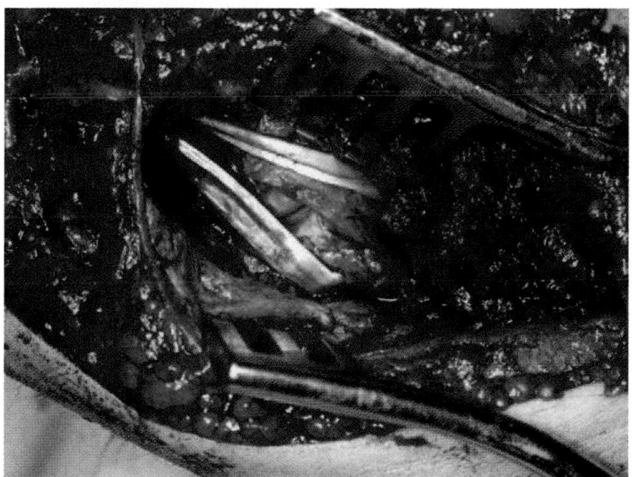

B

FIG. 47.2. Medial collateral ligament (MCL) reconstruction using palmaris graft as described by Jobe and colleagues (28). **A:** Intraoperative photo of a patient with absent medial collateral ligament after trauma. The anterior band of the MCL should travel from the medial epicondyle of the humerus to the sublime tubercle of the ulna. **B:** Palmaris tendon reconstruction of the MCL. (Reprinted from Parsons BO, Hausman M. Medial collateral and lateral ulnar collateral ligament reconstruction. In: Simonian PT, ed. *Techniques of sports medicine.* New York: Thieme, in press, with permission.)

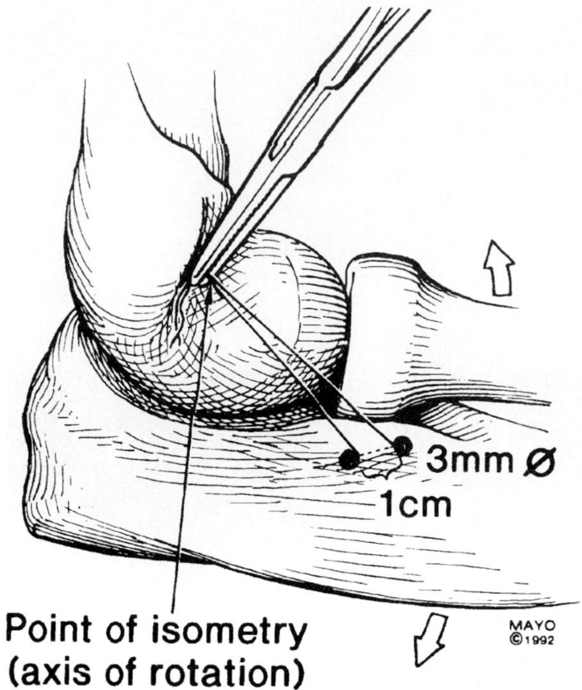

FIG. 47.3. The lateral ulnar collateral ligament (LUCL) can be reconstructed using a palmaris graft as described by Nestor and colleagues (24). The isometric origin of the LUCL on the lateral epicondyle is identified using suture passed through the ulnar tunnels deep to the supinator crest of the ulna, as shown. (Reprinted from Nestor BJ, O'Driscoll SW, Morrey BF. Ligamentous reconstruction for posterolateral rotatory instability of the elbow. *J Bone Joint Surg Am* 1992; 74:1235, with permission.)

ulna (Fig. 47.3). This can be technically challenging and is not uniformly successful, with some repairs having persistent posterolateral corner laxity in extension. A modified technique, described by DeLaMora and Hausman (29), using lateral triceps fascia, was developed because of the occasional failures of the anatomic, isometric reconstruction (Fig. 47.4). This procedure, although not isometric, yields a reconstruction that is taut in extension and does not inhibit flexion. This modification can be used alone or in combination with tendon autograft reconstruction.

Results

Ligamentous reconstruction on either the medial or lateral side of the elbow improves joint stability, thus improving symptomatic instability in most patients (24). Ligamentous repair using native tissue has not shown reliable results and probably has limited application in the adult patient (24,25,29,30). MCL reconstruction using a palmaris tendon graft has shown good results and enabled overhead throwing athletes to resume preinjury levels of sporting activity. Conway and associates (30) reported that 80% of 56 overhead throwing athletes had good or excellent results at an average follow-up of 6.3 years. Azar and associates (31) reported 79% successful outcomes in 59 patients after an average follow-up of 35.4 months. Series with long-term follow-up after LCL reconstruction with either the palmaris tendon autograft or lateral triceps fascia are not available, but series with short-term follow-up have shown reliable results with either procedure (24,29). Nestor and associates (24) reported that 10 of 11 patients remained stable after reconstruction using tendon graft at an average follow-up of 42 months.

The Stiff Elbow

As stated previously, the functional range of motion is from 30 to 130 degrees of flexion-extension, and a 100 degree arc of supination-pronation (13). Some patients, however, are intolerant of even mild contractures that allow a functional range of motion. Also, stiffness may cause pain by altering the normal kinetics of elbow motion, and abnormally load the joint surface. In general, extension loss is more common than loss of flexion, especially in the arthritic elbow. Elbow contractures can commonly occur following trauma to the elbow, and may also be seen in the arthritic elbow. In 200 patients with posttraumatic contracture, 38% had sustained fracture-dislocation of the elbow, 20% resulted from simple dislocations, and 30% were associated with fractures (32). Heterotopic ossification may be a cause of posttraumatic contracture, and can occur after burns, closed head injuries, and fracture-dislocation of the elbow (33–37). Synovitis associated with inflammatory arthritis also can result in contracture (38).

Classification

Elbow contractures are classified by the underlying pathology as extrinsic, intrinsic, or mixed (10). Extrinsic contractures arise in the muscles, ligaments, and most commonly the anterior or posterior capsules. Heterotopic ossification and scarred tissue from burns are other causes of extrinsic contractures. Intrinsic contractures are defined by intraarticular adhesions or intraarticular malunions. Osteophytes and loose bodies can also cause intrinsic contractures. Most patients present with extrinsic contractures, and those patients with intrinsic abnormalities often have secondary extrinsic pathology, yielding a mixed pattern.

Nonoperative Management

Most management of elbow contractures is nonoperative, especially those of recent onset or without "hard" end points of motion (which may herald bony impingement or heterotopic ossification). The principle of nonoperative treatment is to minimize inflammation while gradually increasing motion. Early range of motion exercises, stretching, and splinting are mainstays of nonoperative treatment.

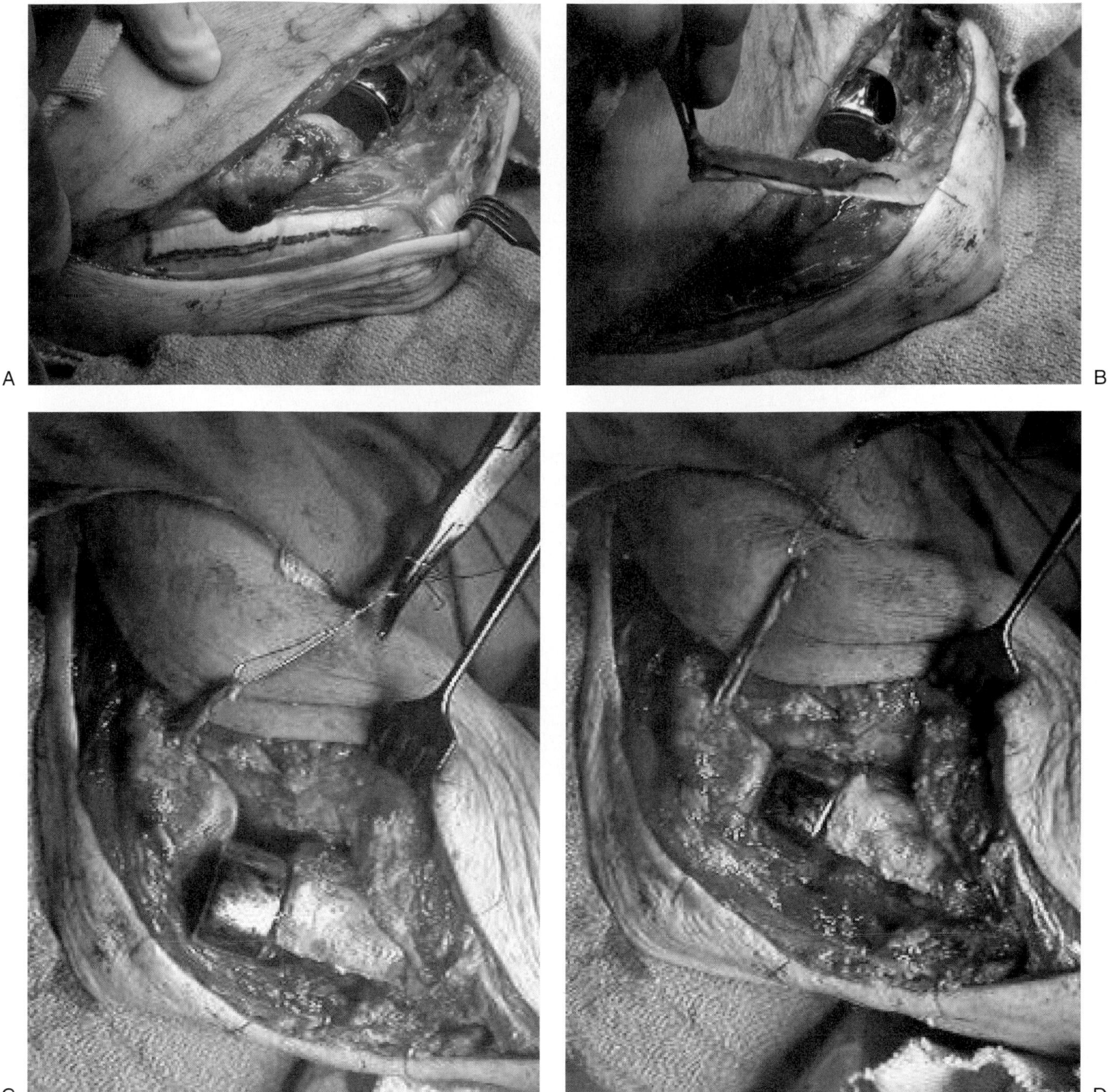

FIG. 47.4. Lateral triceps fascia reconstruction of the lateral ulnar collateral ligament (LUCL). An alternative to the use of tendon graft reconstruction of the LUCL is to use a strip of lateral triceps fascia **(A, B)**. **C, D:** After appropriate placement and tensioning of the fascial strip, stabilization of the radiocapitellar joint, especially in extension, is obtained. (Reprinted from Parsons BO, Hausman M. Medial collateral and lateral ulnar collateral ligament reconstruction. In: Simonian PT, ed. *Techniques of sports medicine.* New York: Thieme, in press, with permission.)

Patient-oriented static splints are used between periods of therapy, and nighttime splinting is used to position the elbow in the direction in which motion is most lacking (Fig. 47.5). Static splinting has been shown to yield an increase of motion (up to 43 degrees in some studies) in appropriately indicated patients (39–41).

Alternatively, dynamic splinting has been used, but is controversial because some feel it may cause increased inflammation and exacerbate the contracture. Manipulation under anaesthesia is also controversial and may result in an exuberant inflammatory response. Contractures that inhibit flexion greater then 90 degrees should not be manipulated

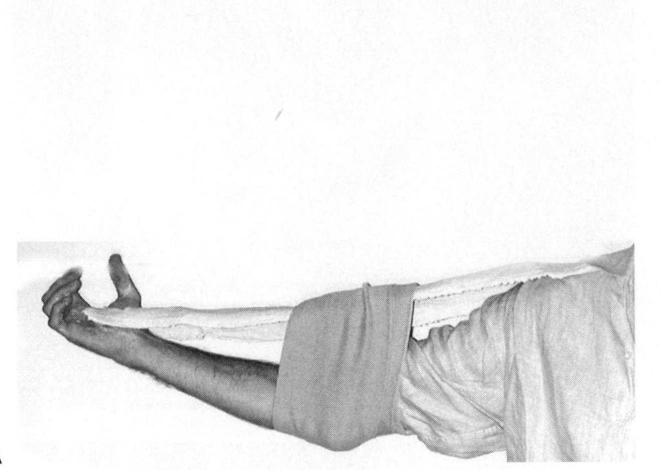
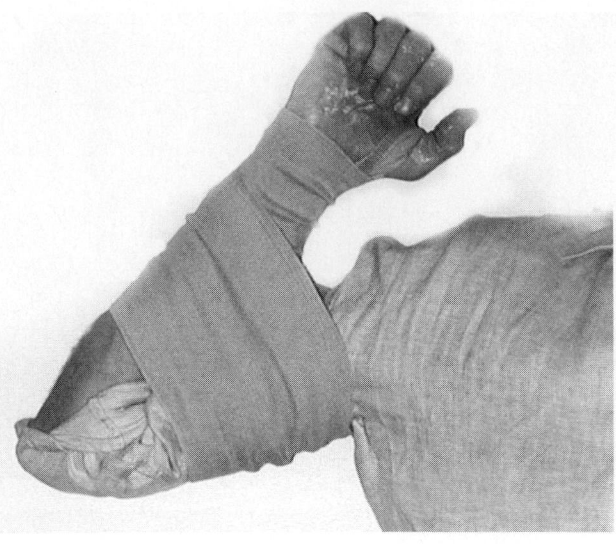

A B

FIG. 47.5. Static splinting for the treatment of contracture. **A:** A simple extension static splint can be made by using a splint constructed of either plaster or fiberglass that extends from the shoulder to the hand along with an Ace wrap around the elbow, as shown. **B:** A flexion static splint can be made from an Ace wrap placed taut around the forearm.

without examination and possible release of the ulnar nerve, because the nerve can be scarred in the cubital tunnel, and aggressive manipulation can result in a transient or permanent palsy (42,43).

Surgical Management

Surgical management is usually successful in restoring functional motion in those patients who have failed nonoperative treatment. Historically, the gold standard for extrinsic contracture management has been open capsular release, performed via a variety of surgical approaches (10,43–55). Regardless of approach, 95% of patients improve after release, and 80% regain a functional range of motion (56). Marti and associates (54) reported an average increase of 54 degrees of motion and 94% patient satisfaction after open release of 47 contracted elbows. Severe contractures with calcification of the collateral ligaments may necessitate release of the ligaments and reconstruction to maintain elbow stability (56). In these situations, hinged external fixators can maintain stability during postoperative range of motion until the ligament reconstructions heal (56).

Open techniques can also address intraarticular malunion or bony impingement at the time of contracture release. Resection of osteophytes on the olecranon or coronoid, as well as treatment of bony encroachment in their respective fossae, can be performed. Intrinsic contractures with significant joint destruction may require distraction and interposition arthroplasty to resolve the patient's symptoms of pain in conjunction with elbow stiffness. The techniques and success of these procedures will be discussed in later sections on management of the arthritic elbow.

Arthroscopic Management

Over the past decade more surgeons have been using arthroscopy to perform capsular release for extrinsic and intrinsic contractures. Arthroscopic techniques include procedures ranging from anterior capsular detachment, capsulotomy, to full capsulectomy. In addition, bony procedures involving reshaping of the coronoid, olecranon, and their fossae are possible. Reported complications of elbow arthroscopy have included transient and permanent nerve injuries, superficial and deep infection, persistent drainage from portal sites, and compartment syndrome (57–65). However, refinement in technique and instrumentation, along with improved knowledge of the three-dimensional anatomy of the elbow, have decreased neurologic complications, even while the complexity of arthroscopic elbow procedures has increased (42,56). Better understanding of the pathologic anatomy of the contracted elbow, specifically the decreased capacity of the capsule, has also enabled improved technique, including the use of retractors (rather then fluid distention), to protect neurologic structures during capsulectomy (42,66).

Arthroscopy offers the advantages of improved visualization of the elbow joint, decreased risk for infection, and less postoperative scarring that makes this technique an attractive alternative to traditional open procedures. In the hands of an experienced elbow arthroscopist familiar with the three-dimensional anatomy of the elbow, nearly all of the factors involved in both intrinsic and extrinsic contractures can be addressed, including the capsular, osseous, and articular pathology (65,67–69).

Indications for arthroscopic release are the same as for those of open capsular release. Arthroscopic release is contraindicated in the ankylosed elbow that prevents cannula entry and joint distention. An additional contraindication is the patient with a history of previous surgery that alters the normal anatomy of the neurovascular structures, such as ulnar nerve transposition. Such altered anatomy can increase the risk for injury to neurovascular structures (70,71).

Results of arthroscopic contracture release have been comparable with open techniques (57,72–76). Ball and associates (76) reported an increase of nearly 42 degrees in the arc of motion in 14 contracted elbows with a minimum of 1 year of follow-up. Kim and colleagues (75) obtained an average increase of 44 degrees of motion in 63 patients treated arthroscopically for posttraumatic or degenerative stiffness. They found that 92% of their patients had significant increase in motion after release. Similarly, Phillips and colleagues (72) reported an average increase of 41 degrees after release. Arthroscopy has now been shown to be a safe and reliable technique when properly performed in experienced hands, and current literature highlights the expanding role of arthroscopy in the treatment of the stiff elbow.

ETIOLOGY OF ELBOW ARTHRITIS

Elbow arthritis generally falls into one of three categories: inflammatory (most commonly RA or hemophilic), posttraumatic degenerative arthritis, and primary OA. RA frequently affects the elbow, can often be bilateral, and usually involves other joints. Posttraumatic arthritis can affect any age, whereas primary OA is most commonly seen in male heavy laborers.

Rheumatoid Arthritis

RA affects 1% to 2% of the general population (77,78) and involves the elbow joint in 20% to 50% of patients (79). Patients with RA of the elbow can have significant pain, loss of motion, and instability that limits function. Complaints of pain and loss of function are common in all stages of RA. Patients often have a persistent mild flexion contracture and synovitis in early stages of disease. With disease progression, joint destruction and instability can occur, with up to 25% of patients with advanced RA exhibiting signs and symptoms of instability (80).

The ulnohumeral joint is most commonly affected in early stages, but as the disease progresses, the remainder of the elbow can be involved. The spectrum of destruction that occurs in RA of the elbow is described by the Mayo classification, which stratifies radiographic signs of articular changes and bone destruction (81) (Fig. 47.6). Type I is

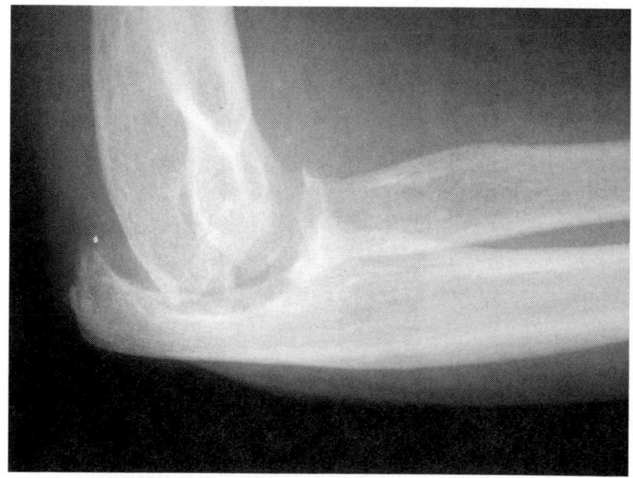

A

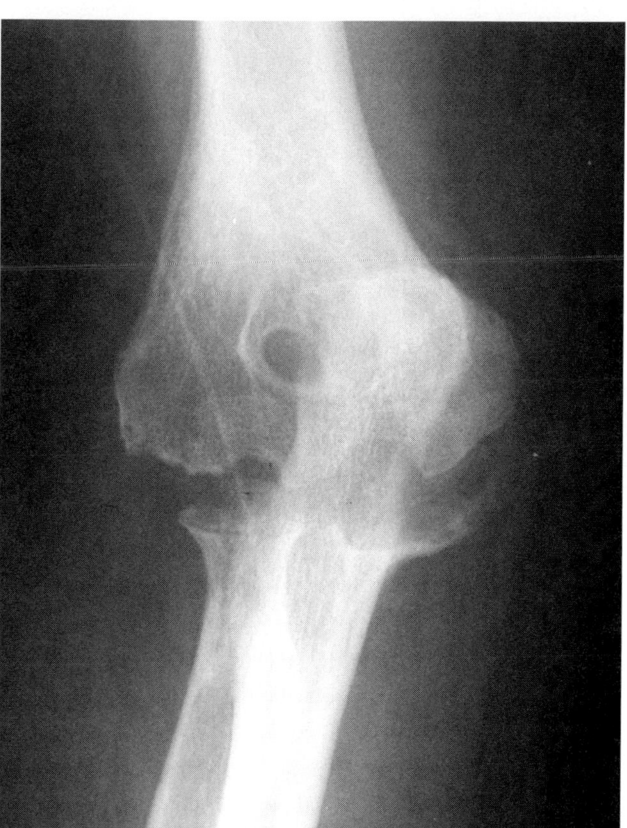

B

FIG. 47.6. Characteristic radiographs of Stage IIIb rheumatoid arthritis showing the bony resorption and loss of the normal contour of the articular surfaces.

defined by synovitis and pain without radiographic changes. Type II is characterized by loss of joint space but intact subchondral bone. Patients with type III elbows have alteration in the subchondral architecture of the elbow and are divided into types IIIa and IIIb, with the latter having loss of the normal contour of the articular surface. Type IV elbows have gross deformity and instability, sometimes termed a flail elbow. Type V was added to include patients with ankylosis of the elbow.

Posttraumatic Arthritis

Posttraumatic arthritis can affect patients of any age or sex. It is a common sequela of intraarticular comminuted fractures of the elbow. Stiffness is often the primary complaint, followed by pain. Treatment is tailored to the patient and is dependent on the age, occupation, degree of pathology, and evidence of stiffness or instability.

Primary Osteoarthritis

Unlike posttraumatic arthritis, OA has a consistent presentation. Most patients are men, involved in heavy labor, and around 50 years of age. This process is also seen in patients who were throwing athletes. It is rare in women. Patients often have a contracture at presentation, usually loss of terminal extension, and the primary complaint is often pain at the extremes of motion. Complaints of locking or clicking are also common, and may be signs of loose bodies.

Examination may reveal impingement at terminal flexion or extension, due to abutment of osteophytes. Pain throughout the arc of motion can be a sign of more extensive articular cartilage damage. Patients may also have symptoms of ulnar nerve neuropathy from impingement of osteophytes on the nerve. Radiographs (Fig. 47.7) and CT scans are used to reveal loss of joint space, loose bodies, and position of osteophytes. Osteophytes most commonly occur on the olecranon and coronoid, but as disease progresses, the radiocapitellar and radioulnar joint can also be involved.

NONSURGICAL MANAGEMENT

The mainstays of medical management involve decreasing inflammation, maintaining or improving joint motion, prevention of progression, and pain relief. Nonsteroidal antiinflammatory drugs (NSAIDs) are used in all three types of elbow arthritis. Medical treatment of RA is discussed elsewhere in this text. Acute flare-ups often respond to a short period of immobilization and NSAIDs. Long-term immobilization is contraindicated, however, because of the possibility of causing contracture.

In patients with an inflamed elbow with effusion or synovitis, aspiration and corticosteroid injections can be helpful in alleviating the symptoms of the acute episode. This is a temporary intervention in most cases, and an injection

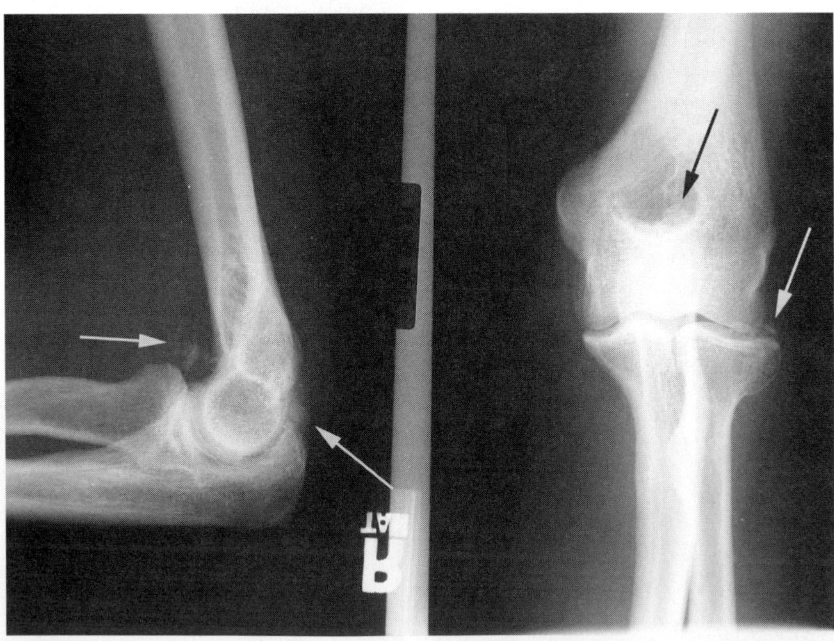

FIG. 47.7. Osteoarthritis of the elbow is most frequently seen in male laborers and overhead throwing athletes. Radiographs typically demonstrate olecranon and coronoid osteophytes and loss of joint space, but radiocapitellar osteopytes and loose bodies can also be observed.

may be repeated in a few months if symptoms were alleviated. In general, two to three injections of corticosteroid are the maximum number that should be administered.

Static splinting, as described in the section on instability, can be helpful in improving motion in the acutely contracted elbow. This should be done in conjunction with an active therapy program. Some have used braces to try to maintain articular congruency in the unstable elbow during activities of daily living. However, most braces end up limiting the patient's use of the extremity because they are cumbersome and difficult to maintain in the proper alignment and may actually increase varus or valgus stress on the elbow.

Patients with RA who have signs of acute synovitis may respond to chemical synovectomy. Synovectomy with agents such as gold 198, P-chromic phosphate, osmic acid, and yttrium 90 have been reported (82–85). However, concerns over articular cartilage damage or chromosomal mutation resulting in malignancy have limited the application of this technique.

SURGICAL MANAGEMENT

Surgical treatment should be considered in the patient who has failed to improve after a reasonable period of nonsurgical treatment. Options include débridement of arthritic changes, synovectomy of the inflamed elbow, capsular release of the stiff elbow (discussed previously), and arthroplasty. Arthroplasty options include interposition arthroplasty with or without joint distraction or prosthetic elbow arthroplasty. Arthroscopy has now been used with success, in lieu of open techniques, for all procedures with the exception of joint arthroplasty. Arthrodesis or resection arthroplasty is currently rarely indicated, usually only in a refractory septic elbow, because these procedures fail to restore functional use of the extremity (86–89). Treatment options are indicated based on patient disease progression, age, expectations and functional demands of the patient.

Open Débridement

Arthrotomy and débridement have been performed to remove loose bodies, excise osteophytes, and reshape intraarticular malunions. General indications include a painful elbow with evidence of terminal impingement due to osteophytes, associated contracture, or loose bodies that have failed nonsurgical treatment. These procedures are generally successful in the patient with early arthritic changes and loss of motion. Older patients (>60 years of age) with extensive arthritis may require replacement arthroplasty.

A variety of approaches have been used to perform débridement with or without contracture release, and most have shown good results (53,67,90–97). However, simply removing loose bodies without addressing the osteophytes or articular changes has been shown to yield inferior results (88). Most techniques involve reshaping of the olecranon tip and widening the fossa to relieve impingement, as in the Outerbridge-Kashiwagi (O-K) procedure (88,94–96) or ulnohumeral arthroplasty (98). Increasing understanding of pathoanatomy of the arthritic elbow has revealed that impingement may occur anteriorly, both in the coronoid fossa and between the radial head and the supracapitellar aspect of the distal humerus. Resection of coronoid osteophyte and reshaping of the coronoid fossa, as well as deepening of the supracapitellar area, can be performed. More extensive arthritic change, especially in the patient too young for prosthetic replacement, may be addressed by three-compartment (anterior ulnohumeral, posterior ulnohumeral, and radiocapitellar) débridement, as described by Tsuge and colleagues (53).

Long-term results are available for débridement. Oka (91) reported that 48 athletes and heavy laborers treated with débridement had pain relief and improved motion at an average follow-up of 60 months. All patients returned to their sport or occupation, and long-term results (>5 years) in 20 patients revealed mild recurrence of arthritic symptoms or radiographic changes. Minami and colleagues (96) reported that 55% of 44 elbows treated with the O-K procedure had no or mild pain after 10 years, whereas 90% had good relief in the early postoperative period (95). Morrey and colleagues report similar results (97). Similarly, Tsuge and Mizuseki (53) reported an average increase of motion of 34 degrees and good pain relief at a mean of 64 months of follow-up. Open débridement yields predictable improvement in pain and stiffness in the younger patient with elbow arthritis, but mild recurrence of symptoms can be expected at long-term follow-up.

Arthroscopic Débridement

As discussed in the section on arthroscopic capsular release, the use of arthroscopy for treatment of elbow pathology has exponentially increased in the past decade. This includes arthroscopic débridement of arthritic changes. Initially, arthroscopy was used for removal of loose bodies and reshaping of the olecranon and olecranon fossa (64, 65,68,99). As with treatment of contracture, advances have increased the capability of arthroscopic management of arthritic change. All three compartments are now accessible with arthroscopy using retractors, and visualization may be better than that of open techniques.

Few studies are available on the outcome of arthroscopic débridement, but all report results similar to the successes reported for the open procedures (64,65,67–69,100–102) (Fig. 47.8). Ogilvie and colleagues (68) reported a successful decrease in pain and increase in strength and motion in 21 patients who underwent arthroscopic débridement of posterior arthritis of the elbow. Similarly, Savoie and colleagues (69) reported an average increase of 81 degrees of

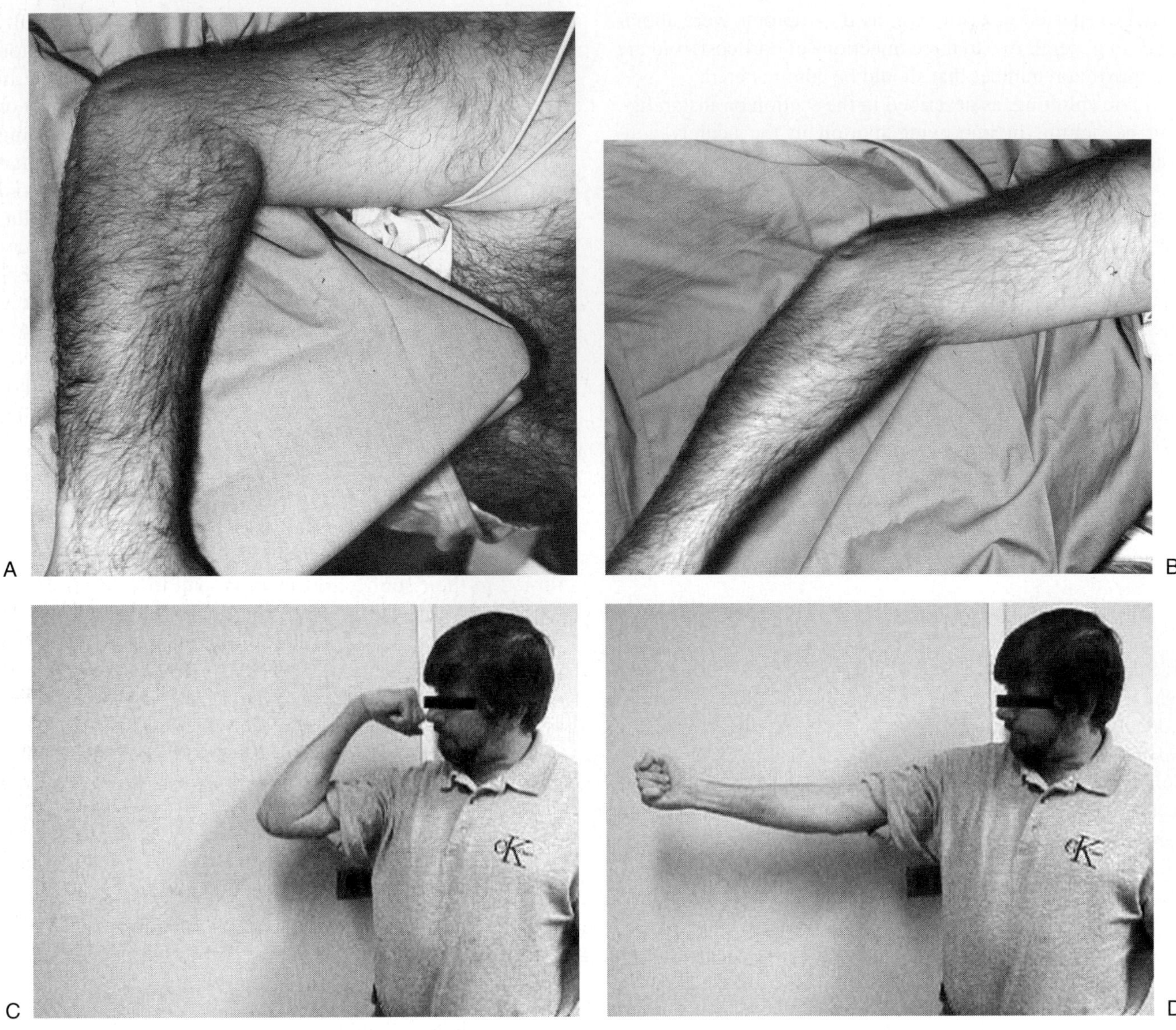

FIG. 47.8. Arthroscopic elbow contracture release. **A, B:** Preoperative flexion and extension in patient with early elbow arthritis with contracture. **C, D:** Postoperative range of motion following arthroscopic débridement and contracture release. Patient has a nearly full range of flexion and extension.

motion (49 degrees flexion, 32 degrees extension) and significant decrease in pain (based on analogue pain scores) in 24 patients. One prospective study (67) compared the results of the open O-K procedure with an arthroscopic variant. There was no difference in patient satisfaction between procedures, and there was a trend toward improved pain relief with arthroscopy. This study found that the O-K procedure resulted in significantly increased flexion (15 vs. 4 degrees, $p < 0.05$), although the researchers admitted to the fact that a more extensive capsular release and débridement was performed with the O-K procedure. Based on the previously presented data on arthroscopic versus open capsular release procedures, this deficit in motion should be overcome if a more extensive arthroscopic procedure addressing both the arthritic change and the restrictive capsule is performed.

Synovectomy With or Without Radial Head Excision

Synovectomy has been proven to be an effective treatment of inflammatory arthritis of the elbow. Open synovectomy is the gold standard and can be performed through a variety approaches (38). The goal of treatment is pain relief, not necessarily improvement in range of motion. In fact, less than a 90 degree arc of motion is a contraindication to synovectomy in some reports (103). Indications for synovectomy include the patient with painful synovitis without instability that has been refractory to nonoperative management. Most studies report better results when synovectomy is performed for early stages of the disease (Mayo I and II) (79,104–106). Some studies have found improved function and pain relief when synovectomy is performed, even in later stages of disease (79,103,107–109).

Historically, a lateral-based approach that also involves excision of the radial head, as first described by Smith-Peterson in 1943 (110), has most commonly been used. Numerous reports have described the successful improvement of motion and decrease in pain after routine excision of the radial head (79,104–107,111,112).

Recently, however, the need for radial head excision has been questioned. Biomechanical studies have shown an alteration of elbow kinematics after radial excision, and clinical studies have revealed the possibility of more rapid ulnohumeral degeneration and instability (21,22,113–115) (Fig. 47.9). Resection of the radial head removes a secondary valgus restraint, and in the MCL-deficient patient, or the rheumatoid patient with progressive attenuation of the MCL, results in progressive valgus instability. Additionally, some clinical studies have shown no difference in results with or without radial head excision (109,116). It would seem from a review of the literature that the main advantage of radial head excision is improved visualization of the joint via a lateral-based approach. However, if joint visualization can be achieved by arthroscopy, then a thorough synovectomy can be performed without removing the radial head. Our view is that radial excision should not be performed; rather, synovectomy and débridement of arthritic changes while maintaining lateral column length and secondary valgus restraint by leaving the radial head intact should be considered.

Most studies report initial relief of pain in 70% to 90% of patients after synovectomy with or without radial head excision in the short term (20,21,38,79,103–107,109,111, 112,114,116,117). However, the rate of recurrent synovitis after open synovectomy has ranged from 16% to 43% (79,106,107,114,118), and late (5–10 years) follow-up data reveal success rates in the 60% to 75% range (38,119). One study has shown an attrition rate of 2.6% per year (118). As opposed to pain relief, postoperative range of motion is less predictable, with results ranging from 55% to 80% in most series (38).

Arthroscopic Synovectomy

Arthroscopy offers many attractive advantages when performing a synovectomy of the elbow. The radial head does not need to be excised for visualization of the joint. Additionally, patients with a painful synovitis and contracture can have both problems addressed via arthroscopy. A complete synovectomy can be performed arthroscopically with protection of neurovascular structures using retractors. It

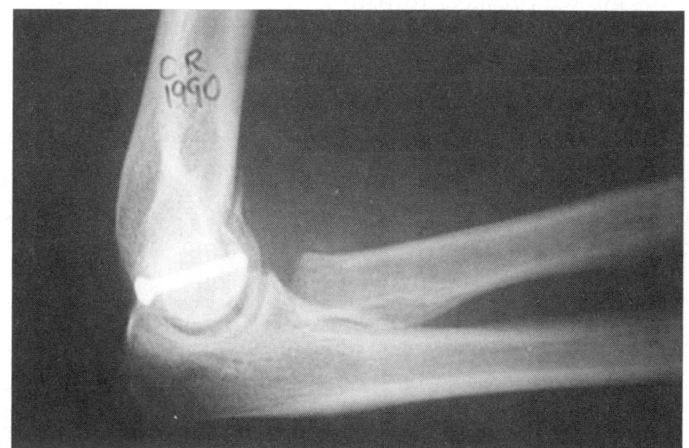

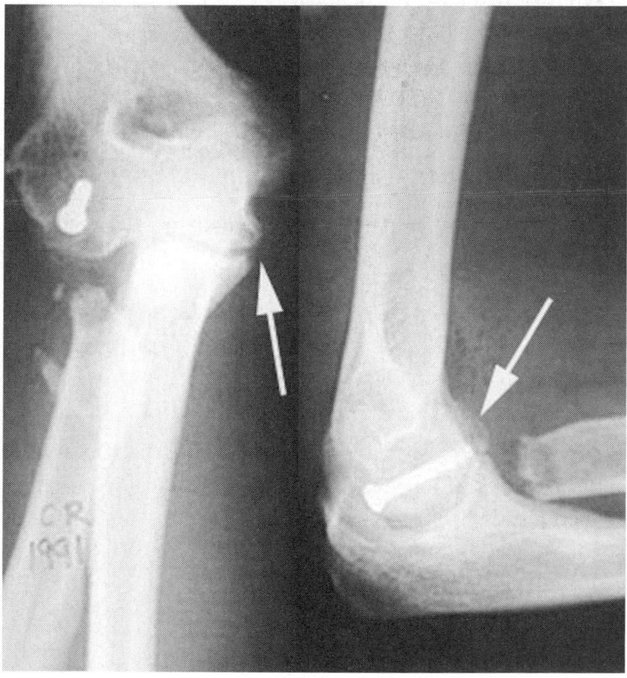

FIG. 47.9. Progressive arthritis following radial head excision. **A:** A postoperative lateral radiograph following capitellar open reduction and internal fixation and radial head excision. The elbow joint is congruent, with no evidence of arthrosis. **B:** Follow-up anteroposterior and lateral radiograph of the same elbow 1 year later. Note the osteophytes and changes along the coronoid and medial ulnohumeral joint (*arrows*). Excision of the radial head should be avoided because of potential acceleration of instability and arthritic changes of the elbow.

cannot be understated, however, that arthroscopic synovectomy and capsular release is a technically demanding procedure. Kelly and colleagues (42) found that the most significant risk factor for development of a nerve palsy following elbow arthroscopy was an underlying diagnosis of RA and contracture. This is likely due to the "thin and filmy capsule" and "altered osseous architecture" found in rheumatoid elbows, which obscure the normal, anatomic landmarks (42,60).

As with débridement of arthritis, there are only a few literature reports on the success of arthroscopic synovectomy (118,120,121). Horiuchi and colleagues (118) reported successful pain relief in 76% of elbows at 2-year follow-up. All the patients with early stage (type I or II) disease had resolution of pain. They did not see a significant improvement in range of motion, but did not perform a capsulectomy in any of the patients. Five of their 24 patients (24%) had recurrent synovitis at latest follow-up. Similar results were reported by Lee and Morrey (120) on 14 arthroscopic synovectomies. They had 93% of patients achieve a good or excellent subjective rating initially, which deteriorated to 57% good or excellent results at average follow-up of 42 months. Both studies had a few cases of transient neuropraxia, which resolved.

These results are comparable to those achieved with open techniques previously mentioned, but have the advantages of decreased morbidity and faster rehabilitation, and they are associated with a minimally invasive technique. The major advantage of arthroscopic synovectomy is preservation of the radial head, especially in patients who may ultimately develop elbow instability as a result of their underlying disease.

Distraction and Interposition Arthroplasty

Interposition arthroplasty is performed to resurface an arthritic elbow in an attempt to provide pain relief and either maintain or improve motion. Although primarily described for the treatment of the young patient (<60 years of age) with OA or posttraumatic arthritis, it is also applicable to the RA elbow. It can be performed in conjunction with capsular release prostectomy to treat patients with combined intrinsic and extrinsic contractures as well. In general, if less then half of the articular surface of the joint is covered with hyaline cartilage, interposition arthroplasty should be considered, with or without distraction (10) (Fig. 47.10).

The main indication for distraction interposition arthroplasty is to treat the arthritic stiff elbow with pain and loss of motion that is refractory to nonoperative treatment. The main contraindication is a patient with inadequate bone stock and untreatable instability as a result of bone loss, especially the lateral condyle and capitellum. It is also contraindicated in uncooperative patients who will not take care of the distraction device or follow postoperative protocol, patients with significant joint instability (unless a concomitant ligament reconstruction is performed), patients who need the elbow to function as a weight-bearing joint (i.e., crutch walkers, etc.), or patients with septic arthritis (93,122–124). Patients need to understand preoperatively the lower demands they may have to place on their elbow after this procedure.

Interposition arthroplasty involves removal of the articular surface and resurfacing with an interposition tissue, most commonly fascia lata, but a variety of tissues have been used, including skin, muscle, fat, fascia, allograft fascia, and so forth (10,12,93,122,125–128). A variety of approaches are available depending on the preference of the surgeon (10,122–124,127). As recommended in the section describing synovectomy, it is preferable to preserve the radial head to prevent late instability. Interposition arthroplasty is most commonly performed with distraction, obtained by using a hinged external fixator across the elbow joint. Three fixators are mainly used, the Dynamic Joint Distractor (Howmedica, Rutherford, NJ, U.S.A.) (10), the Compass Elbow Hinge (Smith and Nephew Richards, Memphis, TN, U.S.A.) (52), and the Orthofix Hinge (EBI). Distraction allows for range of motion without graft dislodgement, as well as maintaining articular congruency in the patient with a ligament reconstruction. The Compass Elbow Hinge and Orthofix Hinge can gradually stretch the contracted joint with a worm gear mechanism. Precise positioning of the axis of rotation is difficult but critical to success.

Results of distraction and interposition arthroplasty are best examined based on the underlying cause of arthritis. When used in the treatment of RA, most studies report improvement in motion and pain relief (129–132). Cheng and Morrey (132) found that 67% of patients had satisfactory relief of pain, and that instability, both before and after surgery, was associated with a poor outcome. Ruther and colleagues (130) reported 69% patient satisfaction, and 70% of patients had no or minimal activity restriction at 10 years of follow-up. Ljung and associates (131) reported similar results with respect to pain improvement, but felt that the long-term results (>10 years) were inferior to total elbow arthroplasty, especially in the patients with elbow instability.

When performed in patients with posttraumatic or OA elbows, arthroplasty yields results similar to those of RA patients. Cheng and Morrey found 69% of their patients were satisfied at average follow-up of 5 years (132). Kita (126) and Morrey (10,127) also found improvement in motion and pain relief after interposition arthroplasty. In general, functional motion is restored in more than 80% of patients.

Complications from this procedure can occur in up to 25% of patients, including pin tract infection, instability, ulnar nerve irritation, and bone resorption (10,93,123,124, 126–129,133). Clearly this is a technically demanding procedure that requires appropriate indications and should be performed in appropriate patients. However, when these criteria are met, it is possible to restore functional, often pain-free motion in the patient with elbow arthritis who is too young or too high demand for prosthetic replacement.

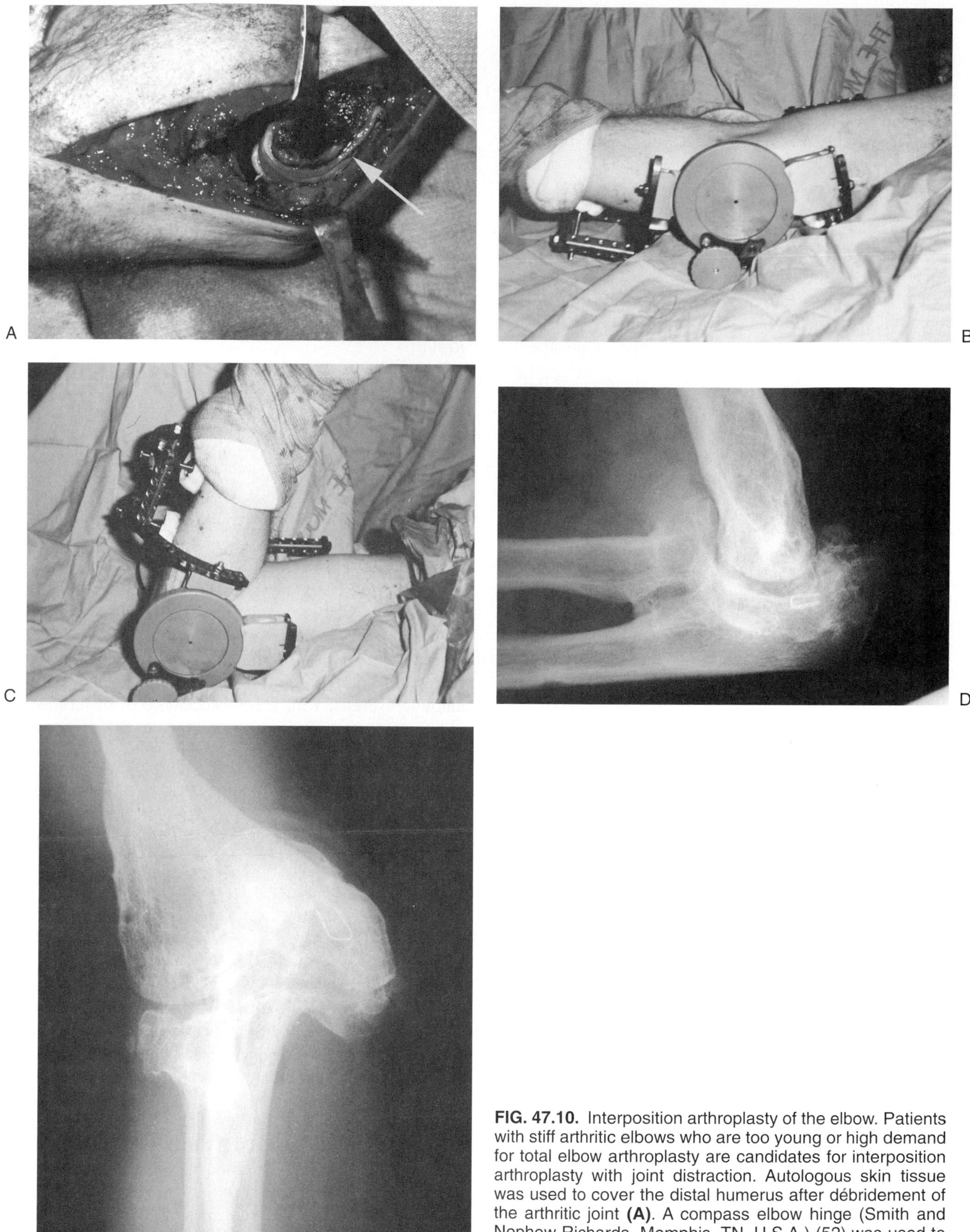

FIG. 47.10. Interposition arthroplasty of the elbow. Patients with stiff arthritic elbows who are too young or high demand for total elbow arthroplasty are candidates for interposition arthroplasty with joint distraction. Autologous skin tissue was used to cover the distal humerus after débridement of the arthritic joint **(A)**. A compass elbow hinge (Smith and Nephew Richards, Memphis, TN, U.S.A.) (52) was used to distract the joint and allow for a stable range of motion postoperatively **(B, C)**. Follow-up radiographs at 10 years are typical of the distorted anatomy, but a joint space is maintained **(C, D, E)**.

Total Elbow Arthoplasty

Total elbow arthroplasty continues to be a reliable procedure in patients with elbow arthritis for the relief of pain and loss of motion. Prosthetic design and increased knowledge of elbow biomechanics and kinematics has improved the results of elbow replacement compared with early prostheses (81,110,134–143). Conventional prostheses attempt to strike a balance between articular stability and excessive constraint. Articular stability is necessary to have a functional elbow that does not dislocate, but too much constraint applies excessive force to the bone–cement interface, possibly resulting in premature loosening. Total elbow prostheses are generally divided into two categories: unlinked (sometimes called "unconstrained") and linked ("semiconstrained"). Surgical approach is dependent on the type of prosthesis being implanted.

Unlinked prostheses rely on the capsuloligamentous tissues, muscles, and design of the implant to maintain articular congruency (144). Numerous unlinked prosthesis are currently available (131,135,137,141,143,145–152). The theoretical advantage of an unlinked prosthesis is decreased stress transfer to the bone–cement interface, thereby resulting in lower aseptic loosening rates (153). Depending on the design characteristics of the articular segment of the prosthesis, there is a variable amount of intrinsic constraint to an unlinked prosthesis. Regardless of design, unlinked prostheses require an intact MCL, LUCL, and possibly an intact radial head (154,155). As such, incorrect component placement can result in joint maltracking, excessive wear, and instability, which has been the major problem associated with unlinked prostheses (110,135–137,141–143,156).

The original linked prostheses were nearly fully constrained and as a result had unacceptable rates of aseptic loosening (157). O'Driscoll and colleagues (7) have found that a linked prosthesis that behaves as a "loose hinge" mimics the motion of a normal elbow. Newer prostheses using the loose hinge linked design have had similar loosening rates compared with unlinked designs (140,158–162). Linked designs allow for a broader indication of total elbow arthroplasty, including patients with instability, intraarticular fractures, as well as poor bone stock (163–171).

Indications

The most common indication for total elbow arthroplasty is a painful, stiff elbow as a result of RA. With improved results in many patients has come a broader indication to include patients with posttraumatic arthritis and primary OA. These patient populations have been found to have higher complication rates than the RA population, and careful consideration of patient demands, functional level, and age needs to occur prior to replacement. Replacement in the posttraumatic or OA elbow is generally reserved for the patient over 60 years of age, or those patients that have failed either débridement or interposition arthroplasty procedures (159). Recently, surgeons have begun using primary replacement in the management of intraarticular fractures, nonunions, and tumors (166–170,172,173).

Contraindications

Active septic arthritis is an absolute contraindication to elbow replacement. Relative contraindications include patients who have had a previous septic arthritis, patients with inadequate bone stock or muscle function, and patients with neuropathic joints. Additionally, patients with attenuated or dysfunctional collateral ligaments and elbow instability should not undergo an unlinked total elbow replacement.

Results

Numerous reports are available detailing the results of both unlinked and linked elbow replacements. In most series, 90% of patients obtain initial pain relief and a functional arc of motion after elbow replacement (147,174). Many studies have shown that functional improvement is reliably obtained after replacement (147,158,159,161,174,175).

The majority of studies examining the results of unlinked total elbows involve patients with RA. In these patients, most studies report a functional range of motion (as mentioned previously, flexion-extension of 30 to 130 degrees and forearm rotation arc of motion of 100 degrees) and greater than 80% relief of pain (137,147,150,174). The largest series of unlinked prostheses used in patients with RA reported excellent results using the capitellocondylar total elbow prosthesis, with a 1.5% incidence of dislocation or aseptic loosening after average follow-up of 6 years (137). Tanaka and associates (176) reported a 90% survival of an unlinked prosthesis used in 47 patients with RA. Average elbow function was substantially improved at late follow-up (11–16 years). However, other studies have shown the dislocation rate to range from 5% to 20% (87,137,145,148,152, 170). Aseptic loosening rates have ranged from 0 to 33%, with revision rates ranging between 0 and 36%, in studies with an average follow-up of at least 3 years (137,141,143, 145–148,174).

Functional improvement and pain relief with linked, semiconstrained total elbow replacement is similar to unlinked replacement in RA patients, with nearly 90% of patients regaining functional range of motion and pain relief (158). However, linked replacements generally have shown lower aseptic loosening rates than unlinked replacements in RA patients, with numerous studies reporting loosening rates lower than 10% (138,140,158). Gill and Morrey (158) reported the long-term (10–15 years) follow-up results of linked replacement in RA patients. Ninety-seven percent of patients were pain free at follow-up, and the average arc of motion was between 28 degrees of flexion and 131 degrees of extension. They concluded that the rate of survival at 10 years was 92%, with 86% excellent results. One study has compared the results of unlinked and linked prostheses

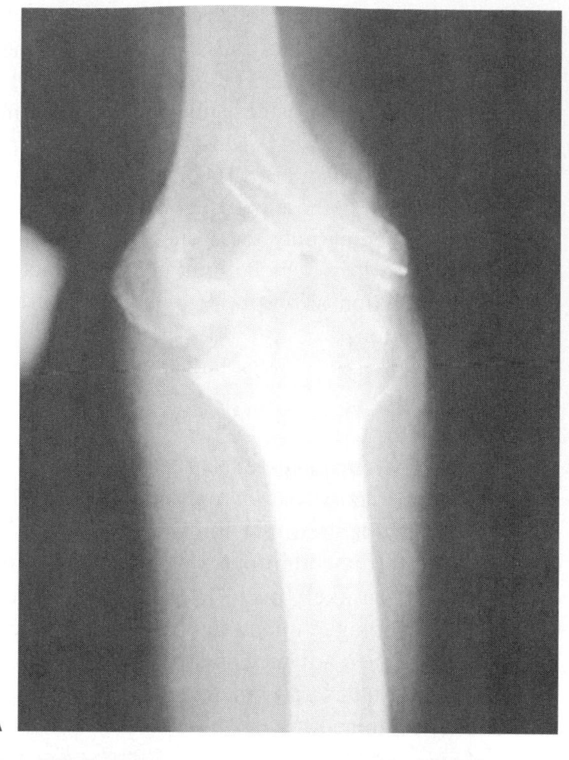

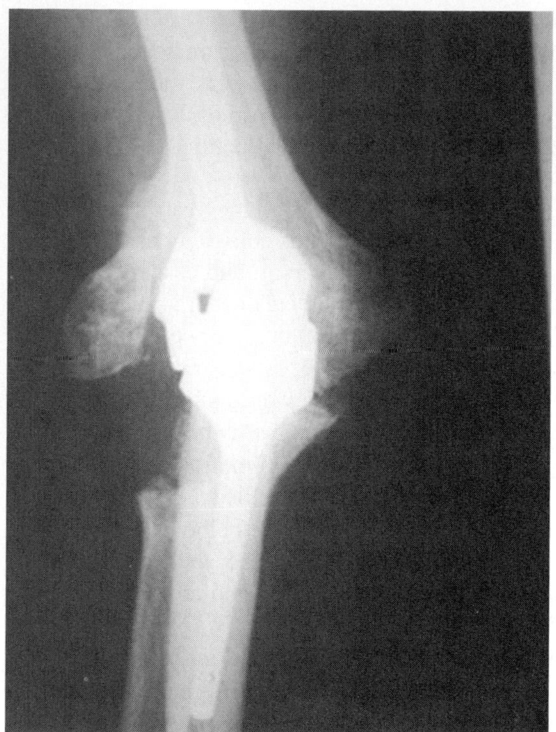

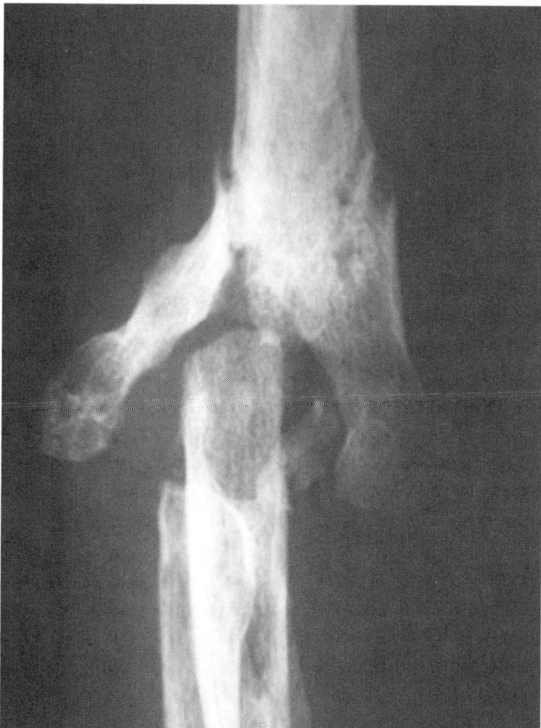

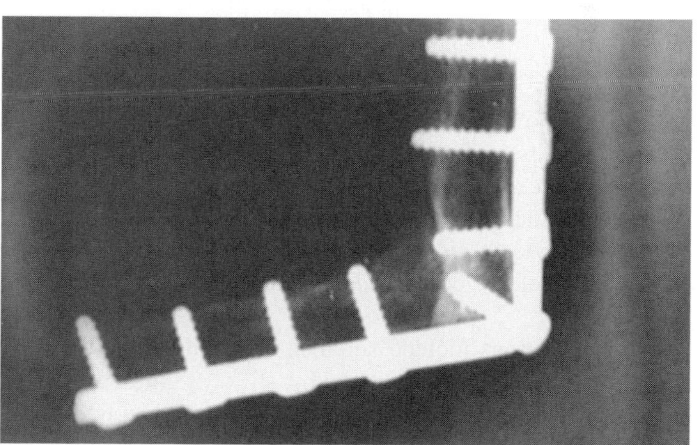

FIG. 47.11. A potentially devastating complication of total elbow arthroplaslty is an infected prosthesis. This patient had a total elbow arthroplasty placed for treatment of fracture nonunion with significant destruction of articular cartilage **(A)**. The implant became infected **(B)**, necessitating removal **(C)** and eventual arthrodesis of the elbow **(D)**, an unsatisfactory and nonfunctional outcome.

used to treat elbow arthritis of variable causes (162). In this study, 22 of 26 patients had RA. When matched for age at time of replacement, no difference was found between prosthetic design at minimum follow-up of 2 years with respect to loosening rates, patient satisfaction, or functional performance.

The results of linked replacement in the treatment of posttraumatic and OA elbows are not as consistent as in the RA population (140,159,160). Hildebrand and associates (159) reported the difference in results between 18 patients with RA versus 18 patients with noninflammatory etiologies at an average follow-up of 4 years after total elbow arthroplasty. The subjective functional score was significantly higher (90) for the RA group compared with the posttraumatic/traumatic group (78). No difference in motion was found between the two groups. Kraay and colleagues (140) found that the survival rate of semiconstrained elbows was significantly higher in the RA patients (3- and 5-year survival rates of 92% and 90%) compared with posttraumatic or other diagnoses (3- and 5-year survival rates of 73% and 53%). They found that the aseptic loosening rate was higher in the elbows with posttraumatic arthritis. Some of the differences between groups observed may be due to higher demands placed on the elbow by patients with posttraumatic or primary OA compared to patients with RA. In general, patients with RA have lower functional demands than the other category of patients, with the exception of patients using crutches for ambulation.

Complications

Infection remains the most difficult complication in total elbow arthoplasty. Infection rates range from 0 to 11% among reports of both unlinked and linked prostheses (137,139,140,143,145–148,158,174) (Fig. 47.11). One possible reason for the relatively high infection rate associated with total elbow arthroplasty may be the subcutaneous location of the elbow joint. Acute infections are managed with urgent surgical débridement and culture-directed intravenous antibiotics. Chronic infections often necessitate removal of the prosthesis and result in resection arthoplasty and a flail elbow or arthrodesis, both unsatisfactory options.

Other complications include subluxation or dislocation of unlinked prostheses, ulnar neuropathy, stiffness, intraoperative or postoperative periprosthetic fractures, and aseptic loosening and triceps insufficiency. Subluxed prostheses may initially be treated with an attempt at bracing or immobilization, but in general require conversion to a linked prosthesis if dislocation occurs after the acute perioperative period. Ulnar nerve symptoms are most often transient following operative neuropraxia. Fracture treatment is individualized to each case. Postoperative stiffness is best addressed acutely with therapy and static splinting (as described previously in the section on The Stiff Elbow).

Finally, a symptomatic, loose prosthesis with osteolysis is the most common cause of failed elbow replacement at late follow-up. Most often this is a result of polyethylene wear, but can be a result of prosthesis instability (in unlinked prostheses) (110,135–137,141–143,156) or rarely fracture of the linkage mechanism (158,160,171). Revision arthoplasty may be an option in these patients. However, failed prostheses due to loosening may result in an elbow with unreconstructable bone loss, which, similar to a septic prosthesis, results in resection arthroplasty or arthrodesis and a limb with poor traction.

SUMMARY

The surgical management of elbow arthritis has expanded dramatically in the previous decade. Numerous options are available to the surgeon treating patients with any of the arthritic conditions of the elbow. Continued advances will most likely occur in arthroscopic management of elbow pathology, including fracture treatment. Additionally, continued advances in prosthetic design are likely as the biomechanics and kinematics of elbow replacement are further examined.

REFERENCES

1. An KN, Morrey BF. Biomechanics of the elbow. In: Morrey BF, ed. *The elbow and its disorders.* Philadelphia: WB Saunders, 1985:43–61.
2. Ishizuki M. Functional anatomy of the elbow joint and three-dimensional quantitative motion analysis of the elbow joint. *Nippon Seikeigeka Gakkai Zasshi* 1979;53(8):989–996.
3. London JT. Kinematics of the elbow. *J Bone Joint Surg Am* 1981;63 (4):529–535.
4. Morrey BF, Chao EY. Passive motion of the elbow joint. *J Bone Joint Surg Am* 1976;58(4):501–508.
5. Chao EY, Morrey BF. Three-dimensional rotation of the elbow. *J Biomech* 1978;11(1–2):57–73.
6. Morrey BF, An KN. Functional anatomy of the ligaments of the elbow. *Clin Orthop* 1985;201:84–90.
7. O'Driscoll SW, et al. Kinematics of semi-constrained total elbow arthroplasty. *J Bone Joint Surg Br* 1992;74(2):297–299.
8. Hollister AM, Gellman H, Waters RL. The relationship of the interosseous membrane to the axis of rotation of the forearm. *Clin Orthop* 1994;298:272–276.
9. Cooney WP. Elbow arthroplasty: indications and implant selection. In: Morrey BF, ed. *The elbow and its disorders.* Philadelphia: WB Saunders, 1993:464.
10. Morrey BF. Post-traumatic contracture of the elbow. Operative treatment, including distraction arthroplasty. *J Bone Joint Surg Am* 1990: 72(4):601–618.
11. Morrey BF. Distraction arthroplasty. Clinical applications. *Clin Orthop* 1993;293:46–54.
12. Lee DH. Posttraumatic elbow arthritis and arthroplasty. *Orthop Clin North Am* 1999;30(1):141–162.
13. Morrey BF, Askew LJ, Chao EY. A biomechanical study of normal functional elbow motion. *J Bone Joint Surg Am* 1981;63(6):872–877.
14. O'Driscoll SW, et al. The unstable elbow. *Instr Course Lect* 2001;50: 89–102.
15. O'Driscoll SW, Bell DF, Morrey BF. Posterolateral rotatory instability of the elbow. *J Bone Joint Surg Am* 1991;73(3):440–446.
16. O'Driscoll SW, Horii E, Morrey BF, et al. Anatomy of the ulnar part of the lateral collateral ligament of the elbow. *Clin Anat* 1992;5:296–303.
17. O'Driscoll SW, et al. Elbow subluxation and dislocation. A spectrum of instability. *Clin Orthop* 1992;280:186–197.

18. Ball CM, Galatz LM, Yamaguchi K. Elbow instability: treatment strategies and emerging concepts. *Instr Course Lect* 2002;51:53–61.
19. Kuroda S, Sakamaki K. Ulnar collateral ligament tears of the elbow joint. *Clin Orthop* 1986;208:266–271.
20. Wilson FD, et al. Valgus extension overload in the pitching elbow. *Am J Sports Med* 1983;11(2):83–88.
21. Rymaszewski LA, et al. Long-term effects of excision of the radial head in rheumatoid arthritis. *J Bone Joint Surg Br* 1984;66(1):109–113.
22. Jensen SL, Olsen BS, Sojbjerg JO. Elbow joint kinematics after excision of the radial head. *J Shoulder Elbow Surg* 1999;8(3):238–241.
23. Morrey BF. Radial head fracture. In: Morrey BF, ed. *The elbow and its disorders.* Philadelphia: WB Saunders, 2000:341.
24. Nestor BJ, O'Driscoll SW, Morrey BF. Ligamentous reconstruction for posterolateral rotatory instability of the elbow. *J Bone Joint Surg Am* 1992;74(8):1235–1241.
25. Morrey BF, O'Driscoll SW. Lateral collateral ligament injury. In: Morrey BF, ed. *The elbow and its disorders.* Philadelphia: WB Saunders, 2000:556.
26. Morrey BF. Reoperation for failed tennis elbow surgery. *J Shoulder Elbow Surg* 1992;1:47.
27. Jobe FW, Elattrache NS. Diagnosis and treatment of ulnar collateral ligament injuries in athletes. In: Morrey BF, ed. *The elbow and its disorders.* Philadelphia: WB Saunders, 2000.
28. Jobe FW, Stark H, Lombardo SJ. Reconstruction of the ulnar collateral ligament in athletes. *J Bone Joint Surg Am* 1986;68(8):1158–1163.
29. DeLaMora SN, Hausman MR. A simple technique for lateral ulnar collateral ligament reconstruction using lateral triceps fascia. *Orthopedics* 2002;25(9):909.
30. Conway JE, et al. Medial instability of the elbow in throwing athletes. Treatment by repair or reconstruction of the ulnar collateral ligament. *J Bone Joint Surg Am* 1992;74(1):67–83.
31. Azar FM, et al. Operative treatment of ulnar collateral ligament injuries of the elbow in athletes. *Am J Sports Med* 2000;28(1):16–23.
32. Mohan K. Myositis ossificans traumatica of the elbow. *Int Surg* 1972; 57(6):475–478.
33. Engber WD, Reynen P. Post-burn heterotopic ossification at the elbow. *Iowa Orthop J* 1994;14:38–41.
34. Evans EB, Smith JR. Bone and joint changes following burns. *J Bone Joint Surg Am* 1966;48:643–669.
35. Garland DE, O'Hollaren RM. Fractures and dislocations about the elbow in the head-injured adult. *Clin Orthop* 1985;168:38–41.
36. Hastings H 2nd, Graham TJ. The classification and treatment of heterotopic ossification about the elbow and forearm. *Hand Clin* 1994; 10(3):417–437.
37. Seth MK, Khurana JK. Bony ankylosis of the elbow after burns. *J Bone Joint Surg Br* 1985;67(5):747–749.
38. Nestor BJ. Surgical treatment of the rheumatoid elbow. An overview. *Rheum Dis Clin North Am* 1998;24(1):83–99.
39. Bonutti PM, et al. Static progressive stretch to reestablish elbow range of motion. *Clin Orthop* 1994;303:128–134.
40. Green DP, McCoy H. Turnbuckle orthotic correction of elbow-flexion contractures after acute injuries. *J Bone Joint Surg Am* 1979;61(7): 1092–1095.
41. Gelinas JJ, et al. The effectiveness of turnbuckle splinting for elbow contractures. *J Bone Joint Surg Br* 2000;82(1):74–78.
42. Kelly EW, Morrey BF, O'Driscoll SW. Complications of elbow arthroscopy. *J Bone Joint Surg Am* 2001;83(1):25–34.
43. Wada T, et al. The medial approach for operative release of post-traumatic contracture of the elbow. *J Bone Joint Surg Br* 2000;82(1): 68–73.
44. Gates HS, Sullivan FL, Urbaniak JR. Anterior capsulectomy and continuous passive motion in the treatment of post-traumatic flexion contracture of the elbow: A prospective study. *J Bone Joint Surg Am* 1992; 74:1229–1234.
45. Boerboom AL, et al. Arthrolysis for post-traumatic stiffness of the elbow. *Int Orthop* 1993;17(6):346–349.
46. Cohen MS, Hastings H 2nd. Post-traumatic contracture of the elbow. Operative release using a lateral collateral ligament sparing approach. *J Bone Joint Surg Br* 1998;80(5):805–812.
47. Hepburn GR, Crivelli KJ. Use of the elbow Dynasplint for reduction of elbow flexion contractures: a case report. *J Orthop Sports Phys Ther* 1984;5:269–274.
48. Husband JB, Hastings H 2nd. The lateral approach for operative release of post-traumatic contracture of the elbow. *J Bone Joint Surg Am* 1990;72(9):1353–1358.
49. Mansat P, Morrey BF. The column procedure: a limited lateral approach for extrinsic contracture of the elbow. *J Bone Joint Surg Am* 1998;80(11):1603–1615.
50. Mih AD, Wolf FG. Surgical release of elbow-capsular contracture in pediatric patients. *J Pediatr Orthop* 1994;14(4):458–461.
51. Rymaszewski LA, Glass K, Parikh R. Post-traumatic elbow contracture treated by arthrolysis and continual passive motion under brachial plexus anaesthesia. *J Bone Joint Surg Br* 1996;76(30)(suppl):1996.
52. Hotchkiss RN, An KN, Weiland AJ, et al. Treatment of severe elbow contractures using the concepts of Ilizarov. *Trans AAOS* 1994;61:1994.
53. Tsuge K, Mizuseki T. Debridement arthroplasty for advanced primary osteoarthritis of the elbow. Results of a new technique used for 29 elbows. *J Bone Joint Surg Br* 1994;76(4):641–646.
54. Marti RK, et al. Progressive surgical release of a posttraumatic stiff elbow. Technique and outcome after 2–18 years in 46 patients. *Acta Orthop Scand* 2002;73(2):144–150.
55. Kraushaar BS, Nirschl RP, Cox W. A modified lateral approach for release of posttraumatic elbow flexion contracture. *J Shoulder Elbow Surg* 1999;8(5):476–480.
56. King GJ, Faber KJ. Posttraumatic elbow stiffness. *Orthop Clin North Am* 2000;31(1):129–143.
57. Jones GS, Savoie FH 3rd. Arthroscopic capsular release of flexion contractures (arthrofibrosis) of the elbow. *Arthroscopy* 1993;9(3):277–283.
58. Lynch GJ, et al. Neurovascular anatomy and elbow arthroscopy: inherent risks. *Arthroscopy* 1986;2(3):190–197.
59. Papilion JD, Neff RS, Shall LM. Compression neuropathy of the radial nerve as a complication of elbow arthroscopy: a case report and review of the literature. *Arthroscopy* 1988;4(4):284–286.
60. Ruch DS, Poehling GG. Anterior interosseous nerve injury following elbow arthroscopy. *Arthroscopy* 1997;13(6):756–758.
61. Rupp S, Tempelhof S. Arthroscopic surgery of the elbow. Therapeutic benefits and hazards. *Clin Orthop* 1995;313:140–145.
62. Schneider T, et al. Long-term results of elbow arthroscopy in 67 patients. *Acta Orthop Belg* 1994;60(4):378–383.
63. Thomas MA, Fast A, Shapiro D. Radial nerve damage as a complication of elbow arthroscopy. *Clin Orthop* 1987;215:130–131.
64. O'Driscoll SW, Morrey BF. Arthroscopy of the elbow. Diagnostic and therapeutic benefits and hazards. *J Bone Joint Surg Am* 1992;74(1): 84–94.
65. Redden JF, Stanley D. Arthroscopic fenestration of the olecranon fossa in the treatment of osteoarthritis of the elbow. *Arthroscopy* 1993; 9(1):14–16.
66. Gallay SH, Richards RR, O'Driscoll SW. Intraarticular capacity and compliance of stiff and normal elbows. *Arthroscopy* 1993;9(1):9–13.
67. Cohen AP, Redden JF, Stanley D. Treatment of osteoarthritis of the elbow: a comparison of open and arthroscopic debridement. *Arthroscopy* 2000;16(7):701–706.
68. Ogilvie-Harris DJ, Gordon R, MacKay M. Arthroscopic treatment for posterior impingement in degenerative arthritis of the elbow. *Arthroscopy* 1995;11(4):437–443.
69. Savoie FH 3rd, Nunley PD, Field LD. Arthroscopic management of the arthritic elbow: indications, technique, and results. *J Shoulder Elbow Surg* 1999;8(3):214–219.
70. Baker CL, Brooks AA. Arthroscopy of the elbow. *Clin Sports Med* 1996;15(2):261–281.
71. O'Driscoll SW. Arthroscopic treatment for osteoarthritis of the elbow. *Orthop Clin North Am* 1995;26(4):691–706.
72. Phillips BB, Strasburger S. Arthroscopic treatment of arthrofibrosis of the elbow joint. *Arthroscopy* 1998;14(1):38–44.
73. Byrd JW. Elbow arthroscopy for arthrofibrosis after type I radial head fractures. *Arthroscopy* 1994;10(2):162–165.
74. Timmerman LA, Andrews JR. Arthroscopic treatment of posttraumatic elbow pain and stiffness. *Am J Sports Med* 1994;22(2):230–235.
75. Kim SJ, Shin SJ. Arthroscopic treatment for limitation of motion of the elbow. *Clin Orthop* 2000;375:140–148.
76. Ball CM, et al. Arthroscopic treatment of post-traumatic elbow contracture. *J Shoulder Elbow Surg* 2002;11(6):624–629.
77. Wolfe AM, Kellgren JH, Masi AT. The epidemiology of rheumatoid arthritis: a review. II. Incidence and diagnostic criteria. *Bull Rheum Dis* 1968;19(3):524–529.

78. Wolfe AM. The epidemiology of rheumatoid arthritis: a review. I. Surveys. *Bull Rheum Dis* 1968;19(2):518–523.
79. Porter BB, Richardson C, Vainio K. Rheumatoid arthritis of the elbow: the results of synovectomy. *J Bone Joint Surg Br* 1974;56B (3):427–437.
80. Amis AA, et al. A functional study of the rheumatoid elbow. *Rheumatol Rehabil* 1982;21(3):151–157.
81. Morrey BF, Adams RA. Semiconstrained arthroplasty for the treatment of rheumatoid arthritis of the elbow. *J Bone Joint Surg Am* 1992;74(4):479–490.
82. Goldberg VM, Rashbaum R, Zika J. The role of osmic acid in the treatment of immune synovitis. *Arthritis Rheum* 1976;19(4):737–742.
83. Merchan EC, et al. Long term follow up of haemophilic arthropathy treated by Au-198 radiation synovectomy. *Int Orthop* 1993;17(2): 120–124.
84. Rivard GE, et al. Synoviorthesis with colloidal 32P chromic phosphate for the treatment of hemophilic arthropathy. *J Bone Joint Surg Am* 1994;76(4):482–488.
85. Stucki G, et al. Efficacy and safety of radiation synovectomy with yttrium-90: a retrospective long-term analysis of 164 applications in 82 patients. *Br J Rheumatol* 1993;32(5):383–386.
86. Coonrad RW. History of total elbow arthroplasty. In: Inglis AE, ed. *Upper extremity joint replacement.* St. Louis: CV Mosby, 1979:75.
87. Goldberg VM, et al. Total elbow arthroplasty. *J Bone Joint Surg Am* 1988;70(5):778–783.
88. Gutow AP, Wolfe SW. Infection following total elbow arthroplasty. *Hand Clin* 1994;10(3):521–529.
89. Morrey BF, Bryan RS. Infection after total elbow arthroplasty. *J Bone Joint Surg Am* 1983;65(3):330–338.
90. Oka Y, Ohta K, Saitoh I. Debridement arthroplasty for osteoarthritis of the elbow. *Clin Orthop* 1998;351:127–134.
91. Oka Y. Debridement arthroplasty for osteoarthrosis of the elbow: 50 patients followed mean 5 years. *Acta Orthop Scand* 2000;71(2): 185–190.
92. Forster MC, Clark DI, Lunn PG. Elbow osteoarthritis: prognostic indicators in ulnohumeral debridement—the Outerbridge-Kashiwagi procedure. *J Shoulder Elbow Surg* 2001;10(6):557–560.
93. Knight RA, Van Zandt IL. Arthroplasty of the elbow and end-result study. *J Bone Joint Surg Am* 1952;34:610–618.
94. Kashiwagi D. Osteoarthritis of the elbow joint. In: Kashiwagi D, ed. *Elbow joint.* Amsterdam: Elsevier Science, 1985:177–188.
95. Minami M, Ishii S. Outerbridge-Kashiwagi arthroplasty for osteoarthritis of the elbow joint. In: Kashiwagi D, ed. *Elbow joint.* Amsterdam: Elsevier Science, 1985:189–196.
96. Minami M, Kato S, Kashiwagi D. Outerbridge-Kashiwagi's method for arthroplasty of osteoarthritis of the elbow: 44 elbows followed for 8–16 years. *J Orthop Sci* 1996;1:11.
97. Morrey BF. Primary degenerative arthritis of the elbow. Treatment by ulnohumeral arthroplasty. *J Bone Joint Surg Br* 1992;74(3):409–413.
98. Morrey BF. Primary degenerative arthritis of the elbow: ulnohumeral arthroplasty. In: Morrey BF, ed. *The elbow and its disorders.* Philadelphia: WB Saunders, 2000:799.
99. Ward WG, Anderson TE. Elbow arthroscopy in a mostly athletic population. *J Hand Surg [Am]* 1993;18(2):220–224.
100. Boe S. Arthroscopy of the elbow. Diagnosis and extraction of loose bodies. *Acta Orthop Scand* 1986;57(1):52–53.
101. McGinty JB. Arthroscopic removal of loose bodies. *Orthop Clin North Am* 1982;13(2):313–328.
102. O'Driscoll SW. Elbow arthroscopy for loose bodies. *Orthopedics* 1992;15(7):855–859.
103. Linclau LA, Winia WP, Korst JK. Synovectomy of the elbow in rheumatoid arthritis. *Acta Orthop Scand* 1983;54(6):935–937.
104. Ferlic DC, et al. Elbow synovectomy in rheumatoid arthritis. Long-term results. *Clin Orthop* 1987;220:119–125.
105. Summers GD, Taylor AR, Webley M. Elbow synovectomy and excision of the radial head in rheumatoid arthritis: a short term palliative procedure. *J Rheumatol* 1988;15(4):566–569.
106. Vahvanen V, Eskola A, Peltonen J. Results of elbow synovectomy in rheumatoid arthritis. *Arch Orthop Trauma Surg* 1991;110(3):151–154.
107. Brumfield RH Jr, Resnick CT. Synovectomy of the elbow in rheumatoid arthritis. *J Bone Joint Surg Am* 1985;67(1):16–20.
108. Saito T, et al. Radical synovectomy with muscle release for the rheumatoid elbow. *Acta Orthop Scand* 1986;57(1):71–73.
109. Tulp NJ, Winia SP. Synovectomy of the elbow in rheumatoid arthritis. Long-term results. *J Bone Joint Surg Br* 1989;71(4):664–666.
110. Smith-Peterson MN, Aufranc OE, Larson CB. Useful surgical procedures for rheumatoid arthritis involving joints of the upper extremity. *Arch Surg* 1943;46:764–770.
111. Herold N, Schroder HA. Synovectomy and radial head excision in rheumatoid arthritis. 11 patients followed for 14 years. *Acta Orthop Scand* 1995;66(3):252–254.
112. Inglis AE, Ranawat CS, Straub LR. Synovectomy and debridement of the elbow in rheumatoid arthritis. *J Bone Joint Surg Am* 1971;53 (4):652–662.
113. Fuchs S, Chylarecki C. Do functional deficits result from radial head resection? *J Shoulder Elbow Surg* 1999;8(3):247–251.
114. Gendi NS, et al. Synovectomy of the elbow and radial head excision in rheumatoid arthritis. Predictive factors and long-term outcome. *J Bone Joint Surg Br* 1997;79(6):918–923.
115. Bakalim G. Fractures of radial head and their treatment. *Acta Orthop Scand* 1970;41(3):320–331.
116. Copeland SA, Taylor JG. Synovectomy of the elbow in rheumatoid arthritis: the place of excision of the head of the radius. *J Bone Joint Surg Br* 1979;61(1):69–73.
117. Lonner JH, Stuchin SA. Synovectomy, radial head excision, and anterior capsular release in stage III inflammatory arthritis of the elbow. *J Hand Surg [Am]* 1997;22(2):279–285.
118. Horiuchi K, et al. Arthroscopic synovectomy of the elbow in rheumatoid arthritis. *J Bone Joint Surg Am* 2002;84(3):342–347.
119. Woods DA, et al. Surgery for rheumatoid arthritis of the elbow: a comparison of radial-head excision and synovectomy with total elbow replacement. *J Shoulder Elbow Surg* 1999;8(4):291–295.
120. Lee BP, Morrey BF. Arthroscopic synovectomy of the elbow for rheumatoid arthritis. A prospective study. *J Bone Joint Surg Br* 1997;79 (5):770–772.
121. Ramsey ML. Elbow arthroscopy: basic setup and treatment of arthritis. *Instr Course Lect* 2002;51:69–72.
122. Froimson AI, Silva JE, Richey D. Cutis arthroplasty of the elbow joint. *J Bone Joint Surg Am* 1976;58(6):863–865.
123. Wright PE. Resection and anatomic elbow arthroplasty with and without interposition: indications and results. *AAOS Instr Course Lect* 1991;40:57.
124. Wright PE, Froimson AI, Stewart MJ. Reconstructive procedures of the elbow. In: Morrey BF, ed. *The elbow and its disorders.* Philadelphia: WB Saunders, 1993:611.
125. Ewald FC. Reconstruction of complex elbow problems. *AAOS Instr Course Lect* 1986;35:108.
126. Kita M. Arthroplasty of the elbow using J-K membrane: an analysis of 31 cases. *Acta Orthop Scand* 1977;48:450.
127. Morrey BF. Posttraumatic stiffness: distraction arthroplasty. *Orthopedics* 1992;15(7):863–869.
128. Shahriaree H, et al. Excisional arthroplasty of the elbow. *J Bone Joint Surg Am* 1979;61(6A):922–927.
129. Uuspaa V. Anatomical interposition arthroplasty with dermal graft. A study of 51 elbow arthroplasties on 48 rheumatoid patients. *Z Rheumatol* 1987;46(3):132–135.
130. Ruther W, Tillman K, Backenhohler G. Resection interposition arthroplasty of the elbow in rheumatoid arthritis. *J Orthop Rheum* 1992;5:31.
131. Ljung P, et al. Interposition arthroplasty of the elbow with rheumatoid arthritis. *J Shoulder Elbow Surg* 1996;5(2 part 1):81–85.
132. Cheng SL, Morrey BF. Treatment of the mobile, painful arthritic elbow by distraction interposition arthroplasty. *J Bone Joint Surg Br* 2000;82(2):233–238.
133. Wright PE, Froimson AI, Morrey BF. Interposition arthroplasty of the elbow. In: Morrey BF, ed. *The elbow and its disorders.* Philadelphia: WB Saunders, 2000:718.
134. Brumfield RH Jr, et al. Total elbow arthroplasty. *J Arthroplasty* 1990; 5(4):359–363.
135. Davis RF, et al. Nonconstrained total elbow arthroplasty. *Clin Orthop* 1982;171:156–160.
136. Dennis DA, et al. Capitello-condylar total elbow arthroplasty for rheumatoid arthritis. *J Arthroplasty* 1990;5(suppl):83–88.
137. Ewald FC, et al. Capitellocondylar total elbow replacement in rheumatoid arthritis. Long-term results. *J Bone Joint Surg Am* 1993;75 (4):498–507.

138. Gschwend N, Simmen BR, Matejovsky Z. Late complications in elbow arthroplasty. *J Shoulder Elbow Surg* 1996;5(2 part 1):86–96.
139. Gschwend N, Scheier NH, Baehler AR. Long-term results of the GSB III elbow arthroplasty. *J Bone Joint Surg Br* 1999;81(6):1005–1012.
140. Kraay MJ, et al. Primary semiconstrained total elbow arthroplasty. Survival analysis of 113 consecutive cases. *J Bone Joint Surg Br* 1994;76(4):636–640.
141. Kudo H, Iwano K, Nishino J. Total elbow arthroplasty with use of a nonconstrained humeral component inserted without cement in patients who have rheumatoid arthritis. *J Bone Joint Surg Am* 1999; 81(9):1268–1280.
142. Lyall HA, et al. Results of the Souter-Strathclyde total elbow arthroplasty in patients with rheumatoid arthritis. A preliminary report. *J Arthroplasty* 1994;9(3):279–284.
143. Poll RG, Rozing PM. Use of the Souter-Strathclyde total elbow prosthesis in patients who have rheumatoid arthritis. *J Bone Joint Surg Am* 1991;73(8):1227–1233.
144. King GJ, et al. *In vitro* stability of an unconstrained total elbow prosthesis. Influence of axial loading and joint flexion angle. *J Arthroplasty* 1993;8(3):291–298.
145. Kudo H, Iwano K, Watanabe S. Total replacement of the rheumatoid elbow with a hingeless prosthesis. *J Bone Joint Surg Am* 1980;62(2): 277–285.
146. Lowe LW, et al. The development of an unconstrained elbow arthroplasty. A clinical review. *J Bone Joint Surg Br* 1984;66(2):243–247.
147. Yanni ON, et al. The Roper-Tuke total elbow arthroplasty. 4- to 10-year results of an unconstrained prosthesis. *J Bone Joint Surg Br* 2000;82(5):705–710.
148. Weiland AJ, et al. Capitellocondylar total elbow replacement. A long-term follow-up study. *J Bone Joint Surg Am* 1989;71(2):217–222.
149. Ruth JT, Wilde AH. Capitellocondylar total elbow replacement. A long-term follow-up study. *J Bone Joint Surg Am* 1992;74(1):95–100.
150. Sorbie C, et al. The development of a surface arthroplasty for the elbow. *Clin Orthop* 1986;208:100–103.
151. Trail IA, Nuttall D, Stanley JK. Survivorship and radiological analysis of the standard Souter-Strathclyde total elbow arthroplasty. *J Bone Joint Surg Br* 1999;81(1):80–84.
152. King GJ, et al. Kinematic and stability of the Norway elbow. A cadaveric study. *Acta Orthop Scand* 1993;64(6):657–663.
153. Schneeberger AG, et al. Kinematics and laxity of the Souter-Strathclyde total elbow prosthesis. *J Shoulder Elbow Surg* 2000;9 (2):127–134.
154. Trepman E, Vella IM, Ewald FC. Radial head replacement in capitellocondylar total elbow arthroplasty. 2- to 6-year follow-up evaluation in rheumatoid arthritis. *J Arthroplasty* 1991;6(1):67–77.
155. Schemitsch EH, Ewald FC, Thornhill TS. Results of total elbow arthroplasty after excision of the radial head and synovectomy in patients who had rheumatoid arthritis. *J Bone Joint Surg Am* 1996;78 (10):1541–1547.
156. King GJ, et al. Motion and laxity of the capitellocondylar total elbow prosthesis. *J Bone Joint Surg Am* 1994;76(7):1000–1008.
157. Garrett JC, et al. Loosening associated with G.S.B. hinge total elbow replacement in patients with rheumatoid arthritis. *Clin Orthop* 1977; 127:170–174.
158. Gill DR, Morrey BF. The Coonrad-Morrey total elbow arthroplasty in patients who have rheumatoid arthritis. A ten to fifteen-year follow-up study. *J Bone Joint Surg Am* 1998;80(9):1327–1335.
159. Hildebrand KA, et al. Functional outcome of semiconstrained total elbow arthroplasty. *J Bone Joint Surg Am* 2000;82(10):1379–1386.
160. Schneeberger AG, Hertel R, Gerber C. Total elbow replacement with the GSB III prosthesis. *J Shoulder Elbow Surg* 2000;9(2):135–139.
161. Canovas F, Ledoux D, Bonnel F. Total elbow arthroplasty in rheumatoid arthritis: 20 GSBIII prostheses followed 2–5 years. *Acta Orthop Scand* 1999;70(6):564–568.
162. Wright TW, Wong AM, Jaffe R. Functional outcome comparison of semiconstrained and unconstrained total elbow arthroplasties. *J Shoulder Elbow Surg* 2000;9(6):524–531.
163. Yamaguchi K, Adams RA, Morrey BF. Infection after total elbow arthroplasty. *J Bone Joint Surg Am* 1998;80(4):481–491.
164. Mansat P, Morrey BF. Semiconstrained total elbow arthroplasty for ankylosed and stiff elbows. *J Bone Joint Surg Am* 2000;82(9):1260–1268.
165. Schneeberger AG, Adams R, Morrey BF. Semiconstrained total elbow replacement for the treatment of post-traumatic osteoarthrosis. *J Bone Joint Surg Am* 1997;79(8):1211–1222.
166. Cobb TK, Morrey BF. Total elbow arthroplasty as primary treatment for distal humeral fractures in elderly patients. *J Bone Joint Surg Am* 1997;79(6):826–832.
167. Sperling JW, Pritchard DJ, Morrey BF. Total elbow arthroplasty after resection of tumors at the elbow. *Clin Orthop* 1999;367:256–261.
168. Ramsey ML, Adams RA, Morrey BF. Instability of the elbow treated with semiconstrained total elbow arthroplasty. *J Bone Joint Surg Am* 1999;81(1):38–47.
169. Inglis AE, et al. Total elbow arthroplasty for flail and unstable elbows. *J Shoulder Elbow Surg* 1997;6(1):29–36.
170. Figgie MP, et al. Salvage of non-union of supracondylar fracture of the humerus by total elbow arthroplasty. *J Bone Joint Surg Am* 1989;71(7):1058–1065.
171. King GJ, Adams RA, Morrey BF. Total elbow arthroplasty: revision with use of a non-custom semiconstrained prosthesis. *J Bone Joint Surg Am* 1997;79(3):394–400.
172. Figgie HE 3rd, Inglis AE, Mow C. Total elbow arthroplasty in the face of significant bone stock or soft tissue losses. Preliminary results of custom-fit arthroplasty. *J Arthroplasty* 1986;1(2):71–81.
173. Morrey BF, Adams RA. Semiconstrained elbow replacement for distal humeral nonunion. *J Bone Joint Surg Br* 1995;77(1):67–72.
174. Rozing P. Souter-Strathclyde total elbow arthroplasty. *J Bone Joint Surg Br* 2000;82(8):1129–1134.
175. Dainton JN, Hutchins PM. A medium-term follow-up study of 44 Souter-Strathclyde elbow arthroplasties carried out for rheumatoid arthritis. *J Shoulder Elbow Surg* 2002;11(5):486–492.
176. Tanaka N, et al. Kudo total elbow arthroplasty in patients with rheumatoid arthritis: a long-term follow-up study. *J Bone Joint Surg Am* 2001;83(10):1506–1513.

CHAPTER 48

Correction of Arthritic Deformities of the Spine

Gregory J. Przybylski and James P. Hollowell

The inflammatory effects of various forms of arthritis on the cartilaginous and discoligamentous support structures of the spine result in the development of a wide-range of spinal instabilities and deformities. Although many deformities are asymptomatic, some result in significant pain, whereas others cause neurologic dysfunction, including spinal cord compression and myelopathy. Both the neurologic as well as structural consequences of arthritis on the spine must be considered together in formulating the appropriate treatment plan for patients with spinal deformities. Although correction of a deformity may represent one goal of treatment, this may not always be achievable. In fact, deformity correction may result in neurologic consequences that were not present preoperatively. On the other hand, treatment of myelopathy with spinal cord decompression may advance preexisting spinal instability, resulting in further progression of spinal deformity postoperatively. As a result, one must evaluate the interaction of treatments for spinal cord compression and spinal deformity in order to successfully manage patients with spinal consequences of arthritis. Because each form of arthritis has characteristic effects on the spine, the surgical management of spinal deformity will be examined individually in rheumatoid arthritis (RA), ankylosing spondylitis (AS), and osteoarthritis (OA).

RHEUMATOID ARTHRITIS

Most of the spinal manifestations of RA are observed in the craniocervical region. Although radiographic abnormalities of the cervical spine are observed in as many as half of patients with RA (1–3), many patients are not symptomatic. The incidence of cervical spine involvement has been associated with the severity of peripheral joint involvement (3,4). For example, only one third of patients with the least erosive forms developed cervical deformities, whereas nearly all with more erosive forms of RA developed cervical deformities in a study of 161 patients followed for a mean duration of 10 years (3). The most common abnormalities observed in decreasing order of frequency are atlantoaxial subluxation, cranial settling, and subaxial subluxation (3,5,6). Although Collins et al. (7) found that 61% of 113 patients with RA treated for joint disease had cervical spine abnormalities, including atlantoaxial subluxation, superior odontoid migration, or subaxial subluxation, only half had symptoms of their cervical disease. However, this does not imply that patients free of pain or neurologic dysfunction should not undergo radiographic evaluation and possibly surgery. In a 10-year study of 41 patients, Rana (8) observed progressive atlantoaxial subluxation in 27%. Boden and co-workers (9) followed 73 patients with RA over a mean period of 7.3 years, and found that 58% of these patients developed a neurologic deficit. In fact, rapid deterioration and death are known to occur. In a study of 241 patients with RA, Riise et al. observed an eight times greater mortality rate in those with atlantoaxial instability, despite adjustments for seropositivity, degree of erosiveness, and steroid use (10). Although the major indications for surgical treatment are pain and neurologic dysfunction, patients with severe deformity or canal compromise without pain or neurologic dysfunction may also benefit from surgery. In patients with good neurologic function preoperatively, the operative mortality rate is relatively low (3%) (5,8,11), and relief of pain and prevention of progressive neurologic dysfunction can be achieved (11). For example, approximately two thirds of patients had relief of occipital neuralgia and had improvement by at least one functional class 2 years postoperatively (12).

The initial radiographic assessment of the cervical spine should include lateral spine films with dynamic views in flexion and extension. Several measurements should be made on the images. The anterior atlantodental interval (ADI) is the distance between the posterior margin of the anterior arch of C1 and the anterior surface of the odontoid process (dens). Excessive enlargement of this distance in flexion implies ineffective restraint by the transverse ligament to prevent atlantoaxial instability. Whereas the normal anterior ADI is less than 3 mm in adults, studies in patients with RA have suggested that an anterior ADI exceeding 8 mm (8,13) represents instability that should be treated with a spinal arthrodesis. More recently, it has been appreciated that the posterior ADI may have more value in predicting neurologic compromise (7,9,14). The posterior ADI, measured as the distance between the posterior odontoid and the anterior margin of the posterior arch of C1, represents the spinal canal diameter and reflects the maximum space available for the spinal cord. However, measurements from magnetic resonance imaging (MRI) studies that include soft tissue abnormalities such as thickened ligaments or a pannus may demonstrate further canal narrowing compared with the posterior ADI. Boden and colleagues (9) demonstrated in long-term follow-up that a posterior ADI of less than 14 mm was 97% sensitive in predicting subsequent neurologic deterioration, whereas the anterior ADI did not correlate with paralysis. Moreover, Hamilton et al. found that 60% of patients with atlantoaxial compression on initial MRI treated nonoperatively deteriorated neurologically over a median of 1 year (15).

Additional measurements can be made on the neutral lateral cervical images to identify the presence of cranial settling and subaxial instability. Pathologic rostral displacement of the odontoid can be diagnosed if the tip of the odontoid extends more than 4.5 mm above a line connecting the hard palate to the occiput on a lateral radiograph (McGregor line). Other measures such as the Clark station, Redlund-Johnell value, and Ranawat index are also used to assess vertical settling and superior dental migration. These correlate well with the development of neurologic compromise, with a 94% sensitivity and 91% negative predictive value using any of these criteria (16). Finally, a subaxial subluxation is considered significant if it exceeds 20% of the vertebral body diameter or 4 mm (6). More recently, it has been demonstrated that the sagittal diameter of the canal correlates better with the subsequent development of neurologic compromise. Patients with canal diameters of less than 13 mm are at highest risk (9).

Although an MRI should be obtained in patients with neurologic deficits, it should also be considered in patients with superior migration of the odontoid, a posterior ADI less than 14 mm, or a subaxial canal diameter of less than 14 mm. Because the MRI identifies soft tissues, including the spinal cord and ligaments, the study allows a better assessment of the actual canal diameter. Dvorak et al. (17) demonstrated that more than 3 mm of pannus was present in two thirds of patients with atlantoaxial subluxation. It has been demonstrated that there is invariable cord compression in rheumatoid patients when the space available for the spinal cord is 13 mm or less (18). MRI is also used to detect the degree of superior migration of the odontoid and cord angulation. The cervicomedullary angle is determined by the angle of the cervical cord and the medulla. Measures less than 135 degrees are significant for cranial settling and have been shown to correlate with myelopathy (19). Functional MRI studies with flexion and extension images have also been used to reveal dynamic cord compression (20).

Anterior atlantoaxial subluxation is much more common than posterior displacement. The latter is usually related to erosion or fracture of the odontoid process. Atlantoaxial subluxation is potentiated by the axial orientation of the C1–2 facets, eventually developing as a result of ligamentous destruction and lack of bony constraint. Histopathologic analysis of patients undergoing transoral odontoid resection revealed ligamentous destruction and replacement of synovium with fibrous tissue (21). It was felt that the osseous erosion results from instability rather than acute inflammation. Progressive displacement is not directly correlated with the development of neurologic abnormalities (5). In some patients, the anterior ADI actually decreases with aging, likely related to cranial settling with descent of the arch of C1 toward the wider body of C2. However, this is not associated with improvement in the dimensions of the spinal canal.

Neurologic abnormalities do not usually develop with pure atlantoaxial subluxation until the anterior ADI becomes greater than 9 mm or the posterior ADI less than 14 mm (9,13). Because of joint stiffness and deformity, pain associated with movement, and the presence of muscle wasting, the early indicators of myelopathy including hyperreflexia, ankle clonus, and proprioceptive deficits may be masked. Consequently, the transition from seemingly normal spinal cord function to severe myelopathy can be relatively abrupt. In a prospective study, death could be attributed to atlantoaxial subluxation in 5% of the patients (8). Autopsies performed in 104 patients with RA demonstrated that atlantoaxial subluxation was the major cause of death in eight patients and a contributing factor in two. Seven of the deaths were sudden. The radiographic diagnosis of atlantoaxial subluxation had been made in two of these patients, and none of the patients had definite evidence of myelopathy prior to death (22). Because early physical findings may be subtle, one must rely on other symptoms of cord dysfunction such as a sense of limb heaviness, imbalance, or paresthesias in the trunk and limbs associated with movement of the head and neck. Unfortunately, once myelopathy becomes severe, recovery following surgical treatment may be less than adequate, and surgical mortality is dramatically increased (11,23). In fact, Casey et al. recommended prophylactic stabilization and arthrodesis before the onset of severe neurologic dysfunction, given the higher surgical morbidity and mortality in patients unable to ambulate preoperatively (24). Consequently, with radiographically demonstrable progression of atlantoaxial subluxation, it is prudent to perform a fusion before the displacement becomes sufficient to produce myelopathy.

Studies have demonstrated that the severity of preoperative neurologic deficit correlates with postsurgical neurologic recovery (11,23,25). Surgical results in patients with basilar invagination alone or with associated subluxation are much worse than in those with isolated atlantoaxial or subaxial subluxation (26). Boden et al. (9) has demonstrated that patients with a posterior ADI of less than 10 mm before surgery have a poor prognosis for recovery of motor function. Moreover, when associated with basilar invagination, significant neurologic recovery occurred only when the posterior ADI measured at least 13 mm preoperatively.

The most common indication for surgical treatment in atlantoaxial subluxation is occipital pain. Good relief of symptoms can be anticipated (11,27). Even an asymptomatic patient with an MRI revealing less than 13 mm of space available for the spinal cord or a cervicomedullary angle of less than 135 degrees should strongly be considered for atlantoaxial arthrodesis (1). Although isolated subluxation of C1 on C2 can be effectively treated by posterior C1–2 wiring and interlaminar fusion, pseudarthrosis rates are significantly increased in patients with RA compared with others having atlantoaxial instability. Although fusion rates with this technique can be further improved with postoperative immobilization in a halo device, newer techniques allow for atlantoaxial transarticular screw fixation, which permit better deformity correction as well as a higher fusion rate (28). Biomechanical studies have demonstrated that transarticular C1–2 screw fixation is an excellent alternative for stabilization of atlantoaxial subluxation. This procedure avoids the passage of sublaminar wires in a potentially narrowed canal (29–32). Another recent advance in spinal fixation involves pedicle fixation in the cervical spine (33). This technique can also be used in the absence of laminae that have been removed for decompression. Traditionally, placement of screws into the small pedicles of the cervical spine had been considered relatively hazardous. However, technologic advances in stereotactic computer image-guided intraoperative navigational systems have substantially improved the safety of cervical pedicle fixation as well as other fixation and decompression procedures of the spine (34,35). Extension of the fusion rostrally to the occiput or caudally to the subaxial spine may be necessary if fixation to the atlas or axis is inadequate. A variety of rigid devices are now available to provide reliable fixation of the cranium to the upper cervical spine (26,36,37) (Fig. 48.1). Because many of these patients have decreased bone

A

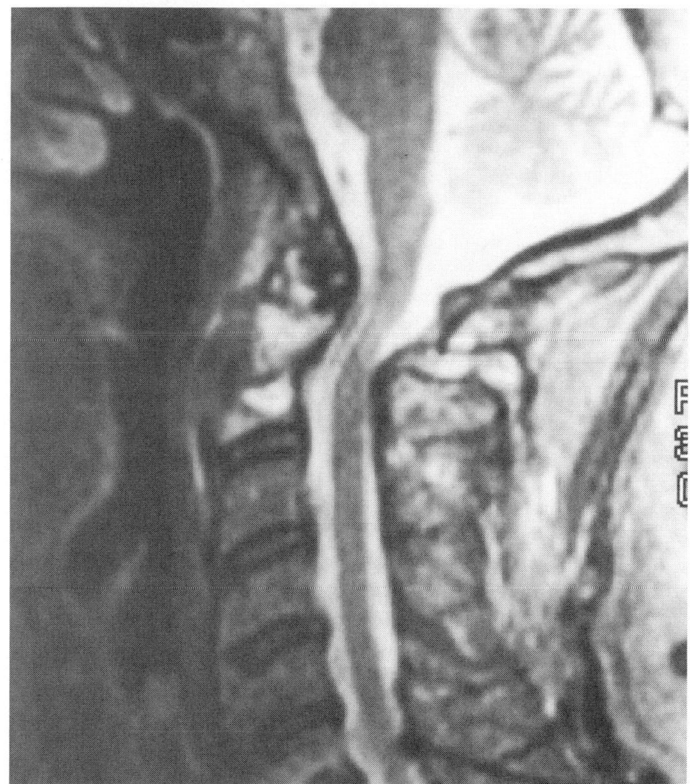

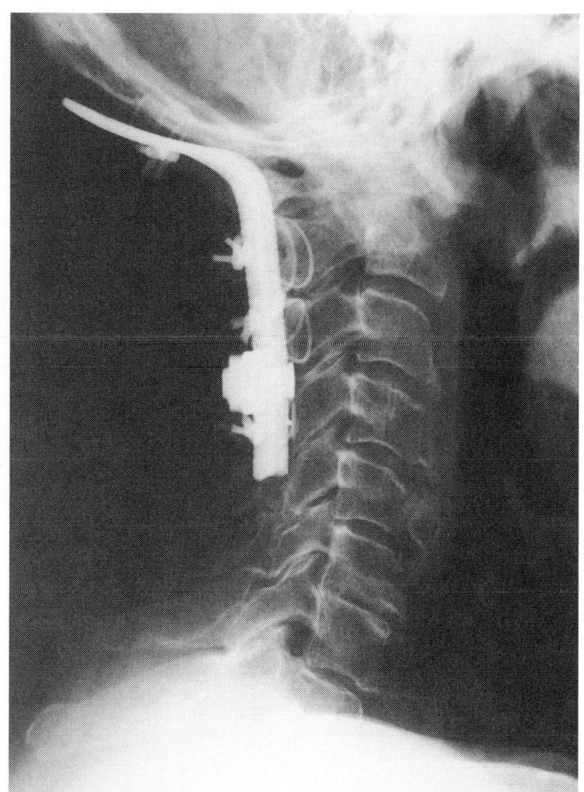

B

FIG. 48.1. A: T2-weighted sagittal magnetic resonance imaging (MRI) of the spine of a 60-year-old man with a 10-year history of rheumatoid arthritis, recently with increasing neck pain, quadriparesis, and difficulty swallowing. MRI reveals retrolisthesis of C1 on C2, and severe erosive destruction of the odontoid. Marked pannus nearly occludes the left vertebral artery and causes spinal cord compression. **B:** Lateral plain film obtained after anterior high retropharyngeal decompression and posterior stabilization with fusion. Device permits realignment and secure stabilization. The patient experienced significant reversal of symptoms.

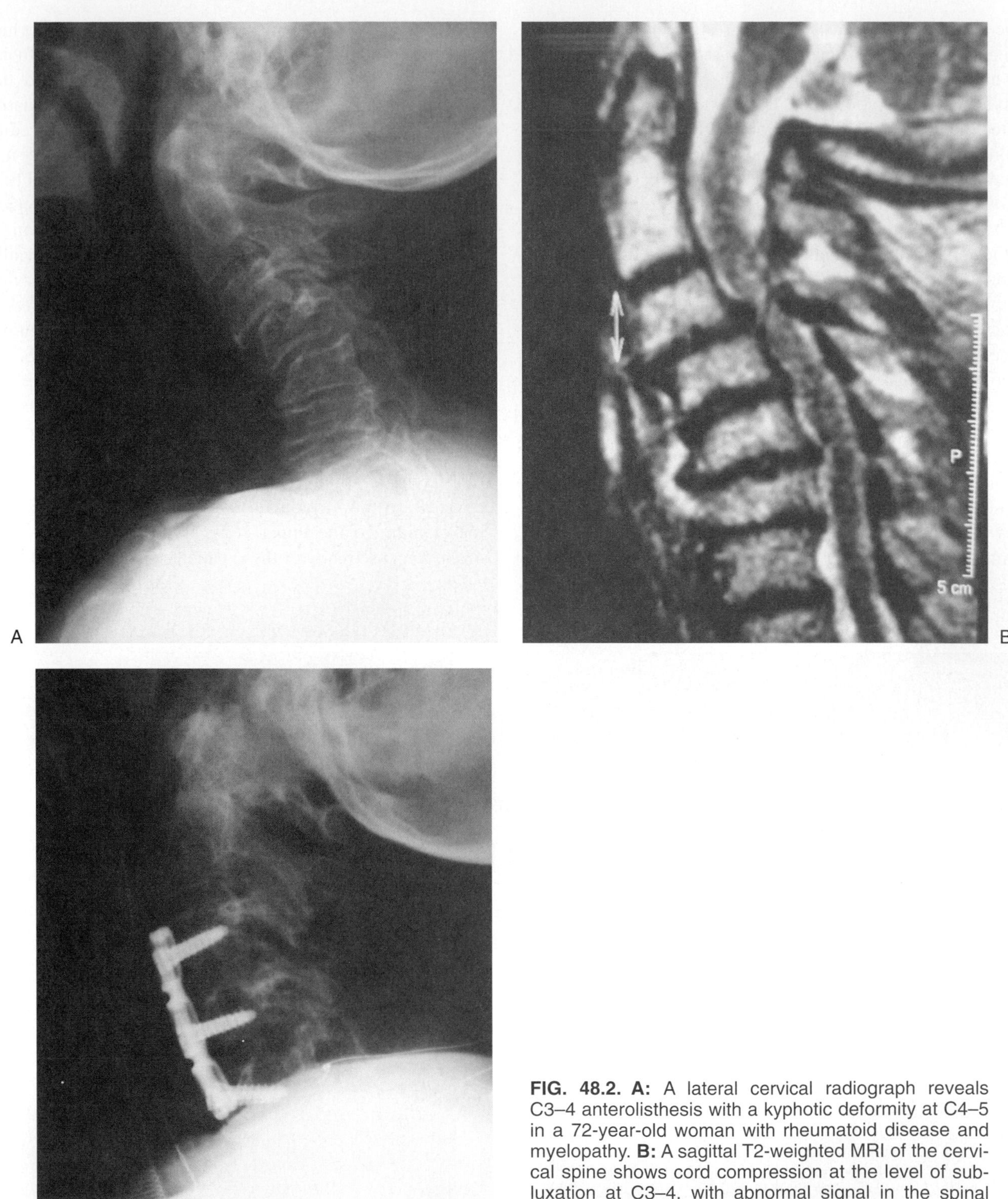

FIG. 48.2. A: A lateral cervical radiograph reveals C3–4 anterolisthesis with a kyphotic deformity at C4–5 in a 72-year-old woman with rheumatoid disease and myelopathy. **B:** A sagittal T2-weighted MRI of the cervical spine shows cord compression at the level of subluxation at C3–4, with abnormal signal in the spinal cord at the level of compression. **C:** A postoperative lateral cervical radiograph reveals correction of the subluxation and reduction of the deformity with anterior C3–5 arthrodesis and plate fixation.

mineral content, are taking corticosteroids, and are difficult to immobilize in an orthosis because of frailty and deformity, the incidence of pseudarthrosis is significantly greater when compared with the results following fusion for odontoid fracture, approximating 9% in a large series of patients (5,38).

The incidence of neurologic dysfunction is greater in patients with cranial settling. In addition to myelopathy, lower cranial nerve palsies may occur. When combined with atlantoaxial subluxation, myelopathy can develop with a smaller ADI than if atlantoaxial subluxation is an isolated finding. Because pain and neurologic dysfunction are related to cranial settling, a C1–2 fusion is inadequate and occipitocervical fusion is required to prevent further descent of the head and further neurologic compression (Fig. 48.1). Because retrodental rheumatoid inflammatory granulations may regress with immobilization, a posterior fusion can be sufficient for many patients (39,40). Persistent neurologic abnormalities may result from continued compression of the odontoid at the cervicomedullary junction, which may require a transoral approach for resection of the odontoid.

Finally, translational displacement may occur at subaxial levels. The indications for surgical treatment are severe axial pain, radicular pain, and myelopathy, or a combination of symptoms. As with atlantoaxial subluxation, detection of early myelopathy may be difficult. In patients undergoing operations for local pain or radiculopathy, a posterior approach for fusion, and foraminotomy when necessary, may be preferable to an anterior operation because stabilization is effective with less frequent complications. Patients with myelopathy may be placed in skeletal traction to evaluate whether a deformity is reducible. If the patient has a straight or lordotic spine, a posterior arthrodesis with plate or rod fixation can be performed. However, if the myelopathy persists or the patient has an uncorrected anterior deformity, an anterior approach for midsagittal decompression and interbody fusion is required (Fig. 48.2). In a small retrospective study of 40 patients with an average 21 years of symptoms, three fourths treated surgically had pain relief and the majority of nonambulators walked (41). Although the perioperative mortality rate was nearly 10%, the group of patients treated nonoperatively because of medical comorbidities had a nearly 50% mortality rate within 6 months.

It is also important to note that after successful atlantoaxial or craniocervical fusion, subaxial subluxation may occur (38,42) (Fig. 48.3). Of patients undergoing craniocervical fusion, 36% developed subaxial subluxation requiring surgery 2 to 3 years after the initial surgery. Of those undergoing atlantoaxial stabilization, only 5.5% developed subaxial subluxation requiring surgery an average of 9 years after the initial surgery (38). Clearly, patients should be followed closely after undergoing surgery, particularly after craniocervical fusions. Some surgeons recommend long segment stabilization in patients with progressive mutilating RA. Although all patients treated with spinal fusion stabilized or improved compared with those treated nonoperatively, subsequent deterioration of segments adjacent to the surgical fusion may limit persistent long-term improvement (43).

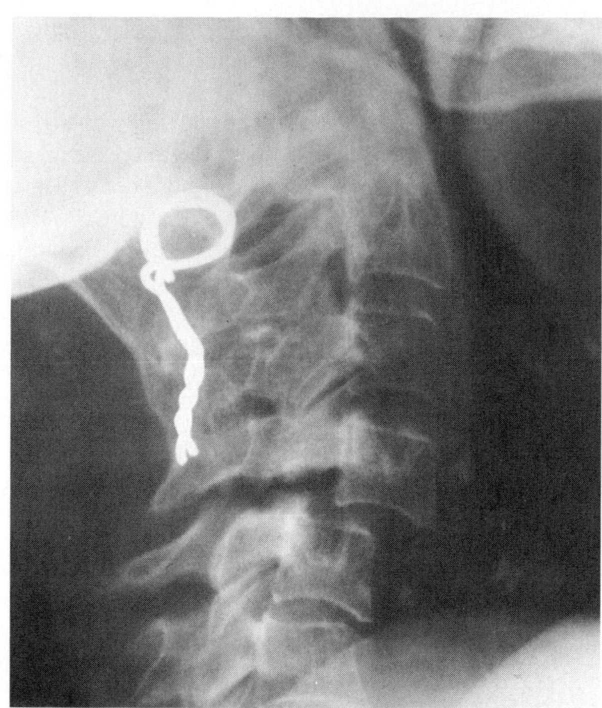

FIG. 48.3. This patient with rheumatoid arthritis had undergone fusion 3 years previously because of posterior displacement of C1 on C2 secondary to erosion and fracture of the odontoid. Although wiring and bone grafting had been limited to C1–2, the fusion has extended to the occiput and to C4. The patient had neck pain and early myelopathy, which were relieved by fusion.

Patients with associated secondary amyloidosis have a greater propensity to cervical instability. For example, three fourths of RA patients with secondary amyloidosis had subaxial subluxation, compared with less than one fourth without amyloidosis. Similarly, basilar invagination was seen in more than half and atlantoaxial subluxation was observed in 40%, nearly twice as often as in patients without amyloidosis. Laiho et al. concluded that patients with RA and secondary amyloidosis developed more severe spinal manifestations (44).

Lumbar spinal involvement can also be seen in RA, but is less commonly observed in mutilating forms of RA (45). In a series of 103 patients, Kawaguchi et al. found more than half with radiographic abnormalities and nearly half had low back pain. The latter was seen more often in patients with significant end-plate erosion. In addition, lumbar fractures were more commonly observed in RA patients treated with pulse steroid therapy (45). The bone mineral density as measured by dual-energy x-ray absorptiometry had a sensitivity of 82% and a negative predictive value of 90% among a cohort of RA patients (46). Criteria associated with compression factors included age, weight, inflammation, immobility, and steroid overuse. Among 205 patients with RA treated with steroids, 25% had vertebral deformities and 8% had clinically acute vertebral fractures compared with 13% having deformities and 1.5% having acute fractures in 205 RA patients not treated with steroids (47). DeNijs et al. reported that each 1-mg increase in daily dosage of steroid increased the risk for both deformity and clinically symptomatic acute vertebral fracture (47). Although management of acute fractures typically involved prolonged external bracing, percutaneous vertebral augmentation with polymethylmethacrylate has significantly improved the quality of life of many patients with osteoporotic compression fractures and may additionally reduce deformity (48).

ANKYLOSING SPONDYLITIS

Spinal deformity in ankylosing spondylitis may be related to the disease itself producing kyphosis, or to an acute traumatic event (1,49,50). Atlantoaxial subluxation was observed in 23% of 103 patients in one study (51). In patients with severe kyphotic deformity with functional impairment, an osteotomy and stabilization can provide substan-

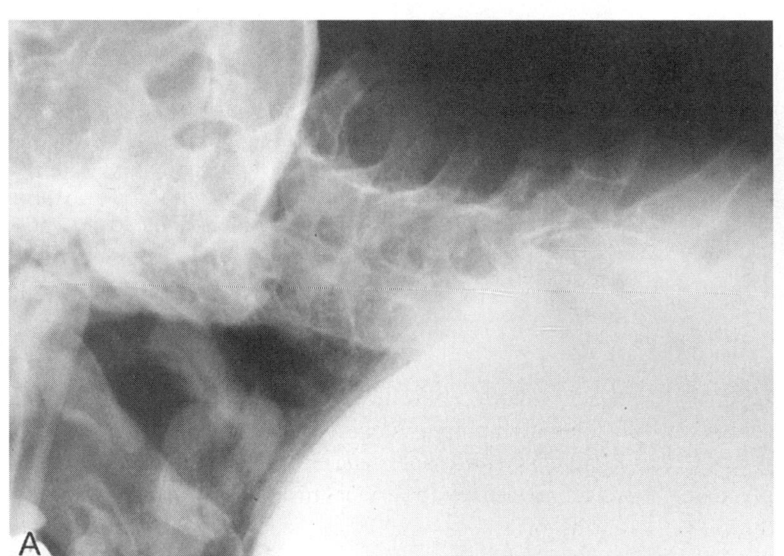

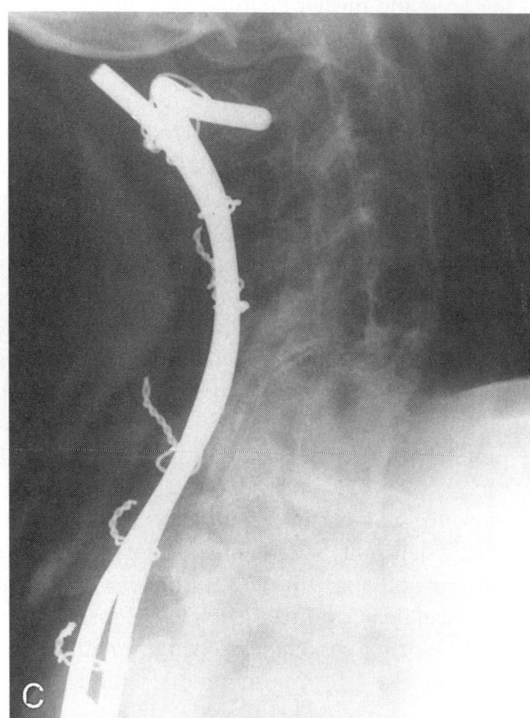

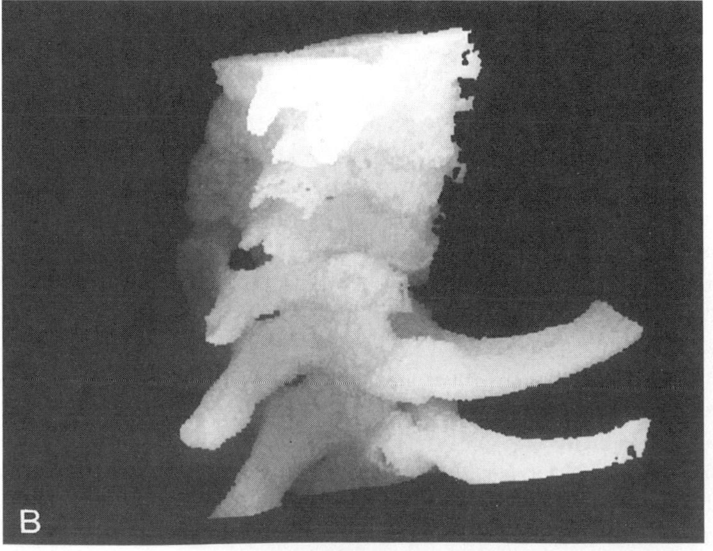

FIG. 48.4. A: Lateral cervical spine film in a patient with ankylosing spondylitis who developed immediate flexion rotation deformity after falling backward and striking his occiput on a table. A halo cast had been used without success and his chin eventually came to rest on the right clavicle. Because of difficulty eating, he lost 60 pounds in 12 weeks. Spine films and several computed tomography (CT) scans did not identify the area of injury. **B:** Three-dimensional CT scan demonstrated the fracture at C5–6. The patient was placed in 5 pounds of skeletal traction and reduction occurred suddenly 4 hours later. **C:** After Luque rods were wired to the spinous processes, the patient was turned and a bone graft was placed between the widely separated anterior portions of the C5 and C6 vertebral bodies.

tial correction (52). Although in most patients the kyphosis is most severe in the thoracic spine, it is safer and easier to do the osteotomy in the lumbar region where the canal is larger and the cauda equina more forgiving (53–55). In patients with a primary cervicothoracic kyphosis, an osteotomy should be performed at the cervicothoracic junction to maintain sagittal plane balance (54,56). Surgical techniques using one or more osteotomies are successful at achieving adequate deformity correction, permitting good forward vision and pain relief in patients with severe chin-on-chest deformity. Halm and co-workers (57) demonstrated excellent overall improvement of health status after deformity correction as assessed by the Modified Arthritis Impact Measurement Scales. Early techniques were unfortunately associated with a high rate of complications, including death and new neurologic deficits (54). More recent techniques have used safer types of reduction, better fixation, and intraoperative neurologic monitoring to substantially reduce these risks. However, clinical outcomes may not be related to the degree of deformity correction (52).

Fractures in patients with ankylosing spondylitis are frequently caused by relatively minor trauma, and might not be recognized until the advent of significant myelopathy (49,50,58,59). The mortality rate may be as high as 35% in patients with ankylosing spondylitis who sustain cervical fractures (60). Neurologic deficits occur in 57% to 75%, and associated spinal epidural hematomas are common (58,60). The mechanism of injury typically involves hyperextension (59). Because of the ligamentous ossification, fractures typically cause complete vertebral disruption, creating highly unstable injuries. The stiffness of the vertebral column above and below the fracture and the absence of any ligamentous connection across the fracture make it difficult to maintain alignment in an orthosis. Treatment by skeletal traction alone requires at least 4 to 6 weeks in bed and may be accompanied by significant risks such as delayed quadriparesis (49,58). Furthermore, if there is significant kyphotic deformity, application of skeletal traction becomes difficult. Direct axial traction across a cervical deformity can result in spinal angulation, cord compression, and paralysis. It is also difficult to safely place a halo vest or a Minerva cast.

Patients who are neurologically intact, without significant kyphotic deformity and with reasonable alignment of the vertebral column, can be treated in an orthosis (59). However, if there is neurologic deficit, substantial malalignment, or fracture in the presence of kyphosis, surgical treatment with fusion and posterior metallic fixation provides the best opportunity for neurologic recovery and early mobilization of the patient. Because ligamentous ossification interferes with facet and laminar fixation, an alternative way to achieve fixation is to secure metallic rods to the spinous processes by wires passed through holes in the base of the processes (61) (Fig. 48.4). If reconstruction of the spinal canal is required to remove bone anterior to the spinal cord, this can be done during the same operation after stabilization with posterior instrumentation has been accomplished.

Similar considerations apply to fractures in the thoracic portion of the vertebral column. Correction of kyphosis should be avoided, because this might be followed by increased neurologic deficit. If reconstruction of the spinal canal is not necessary, wiring of rods to the spinous processes may be sufficient in conjunction with onlay bone grafting for spinal fusion. Alternatively, segmental pedicle fixation in the thoracolumbar spine allows excellent internal stabilization. With neurologic deficit secondary to deformity of the spinal cord by bone anterior to it, a lateral extracavitary approach to the vertebral column allows reconstruction of the spinal canal and placement of posterior instrumentation through the same incision during the operation.

OSTEOARTHRITIS

Degenerative osteoarthritis typically effects the cervical and lumbar spine. In the cervical spine, the C5–6 and C6–7 levels are most commonly affected, whereas the L4–5 and L5–S1 levels are most commonly affected in the lumbar spine. Although most patients are asymptomatic, some develop radiculopathy that responds well to simple decompressive procedures. Even in patients who develop myelopathy, spinal deformity requiring treatment is much less common compared with RA patients.

Some patients develop cervical subaxial subluxation similar to that seen in RA patients (Fig. 48.5). Moreover, progressive disc degeneration in OA results in progressive cervical kyphosis, thereby limiting the utility of dorsal reconstructive operations. Even after anterior surgery, progressive kyphosis may continue. In nearly 100 patients undergoing one- or two-level corpectomies, progressive postoperative segmental kyphosis was observed. Most of the loss of lordosis occurred at the fused segments, with stabilization after 1 year (62). Consequently, internal fixation is frequently performed to limit the degree of postoperative kyphotic progression.

Two common types of thoracolumbar region deformity are encountered in OA. The most commonly observed subluxation is degenerative spondylolisthesis, which usually occurs at L4–5 in women. The vertical orientation of the articular processes at this level allows translational movement to occur with anterior displacement of L4 on L5. Neurogenic claudication can be produced by the consequent stenosis of the spinal canal. Usually in these patients the symptoms of pain associated with walking are much more prominent than the physical findings. Occasionally, however, radiculopathy is significant. A posterior approach for resection of lamina and the medial portions of the apophyseal joints can sufficiently enlarge the canal to relieve symptoms of claudication. Progression of displacement is not common unless a bilateral facetectomy has been done. Fusion is sometimes required for

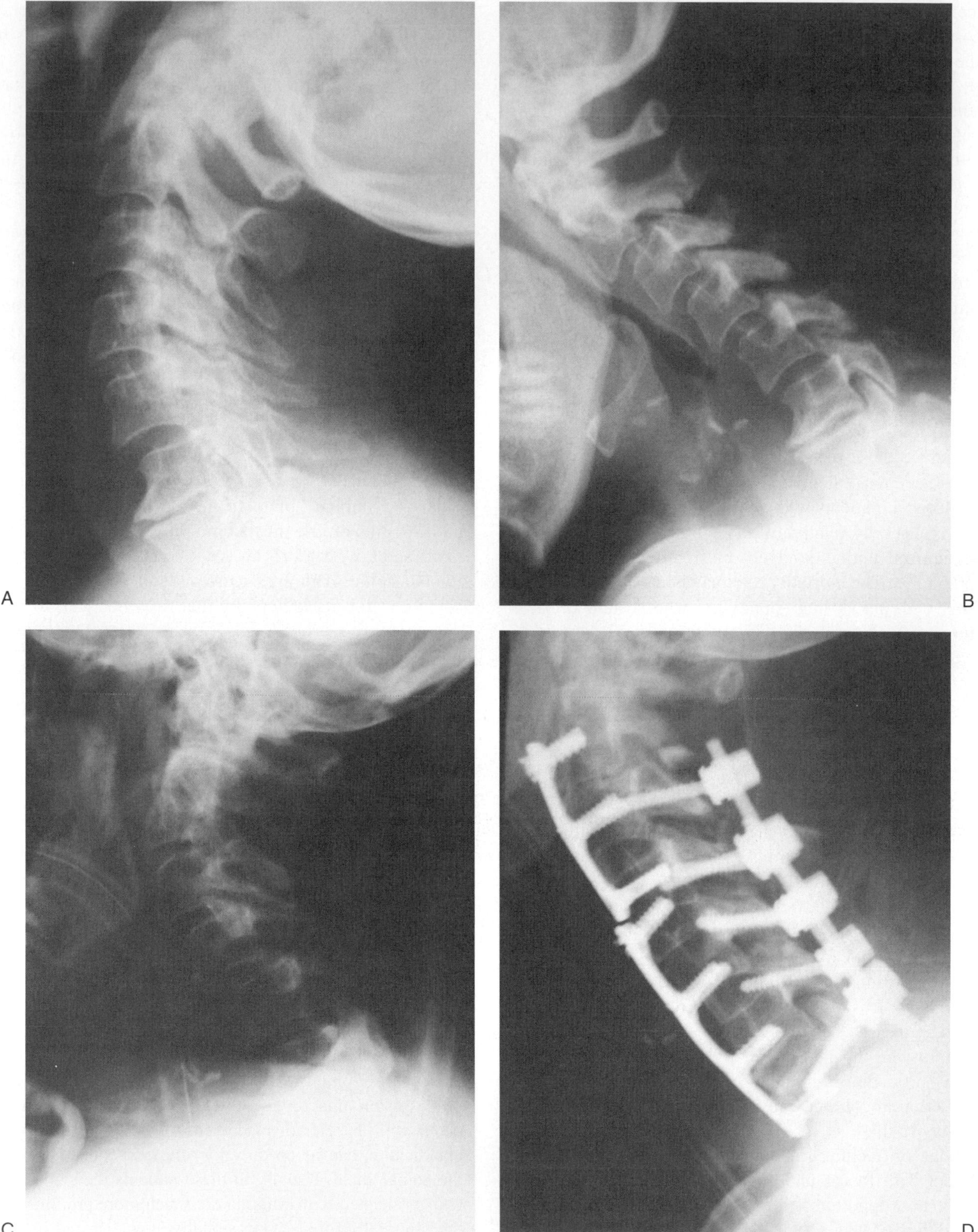

FIG. 48.5. A: A lateral cervical radiograph in extension reveals normal cervical alignment in this 62-year-old woman with OA and slowly progressive myelopathy. **B:** A lateral cervical radiograph in flexion reveals multilevel subaxial subluxation at C2–3, C3–4, and C4–5. **C:** A lateral cervical radiograph after posterior cervical laminectomy at C4–6 without stabilization reveals progressive subaxial deformity. **D:** A postoperative lateral cervical radiograph demonstrates reduction of the deformity with an anterior and posterior cervical arthrodesis from C2 to T1.

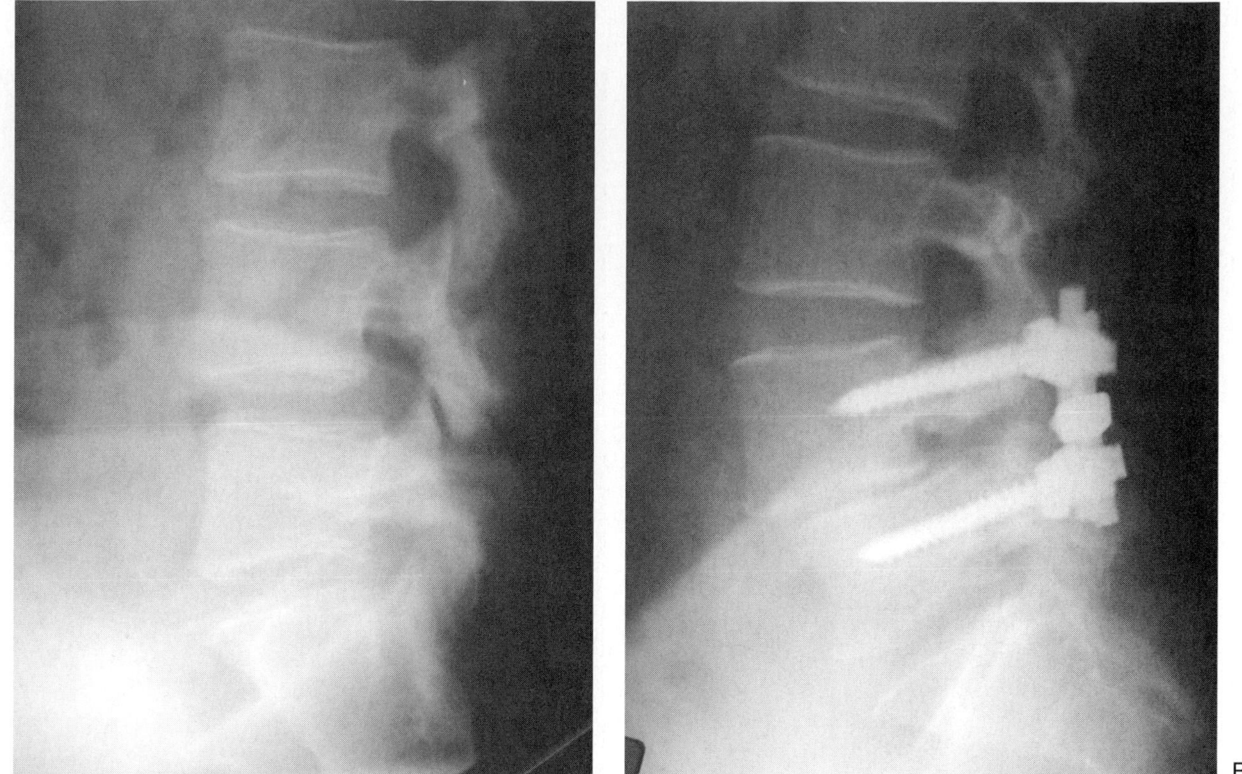

FIG. 48.6. A: A lateral lumbar radiograph in extension reveals a degenerative L4–5 spondylolisthesis with widening of the L4–5 facet joint in this 45-year-old man with mechanical back pain and an L5 radiculopathy. **B:** A postoperative lumbar radiograph demonstrates stabilization of the L4–5 segment with posterior pedicle screw fixation and posterolateral arthrodesis.

relief of back pain related to facet arthropathy or progressive instability (Fig. 48.6).

Less frequently, a progressive degenerative scoliosis develops (63,64). Pain is sometimes related to facet arthropathy, but is usually secondary to entrapment of the roots in the lateral recess of the spinal canal and in the stenotic root foramina on the concave side of the curve. Resection of sufficient bone to unroof the nerve roots may further destabilize the vertebral column with progression of deformity and recurrent symptoms (Fig. 48.7). Consequently, these pa-

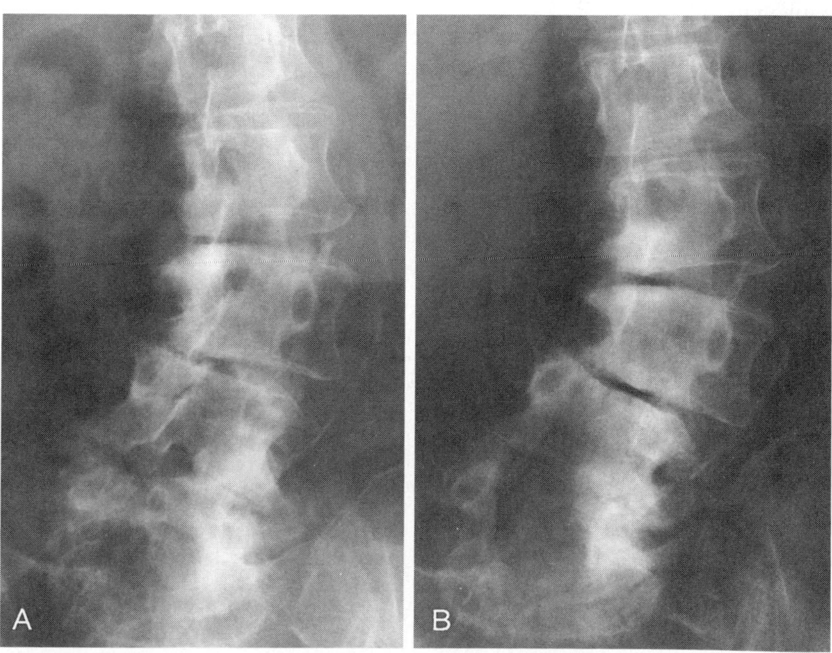

FIG. 48.7. A: Preoperative films from a patient with degenerative lumbar scoliosis and neurogenic claudication. The symptoms were relieved after a laminectomy from L2 to L5. **B:** This film was taken 2 years later. Back pain and a left L5 radiculopathy had developed. The scoliosis has become more pronounced, with approximation of L4 and L5 to the left iliac crest.

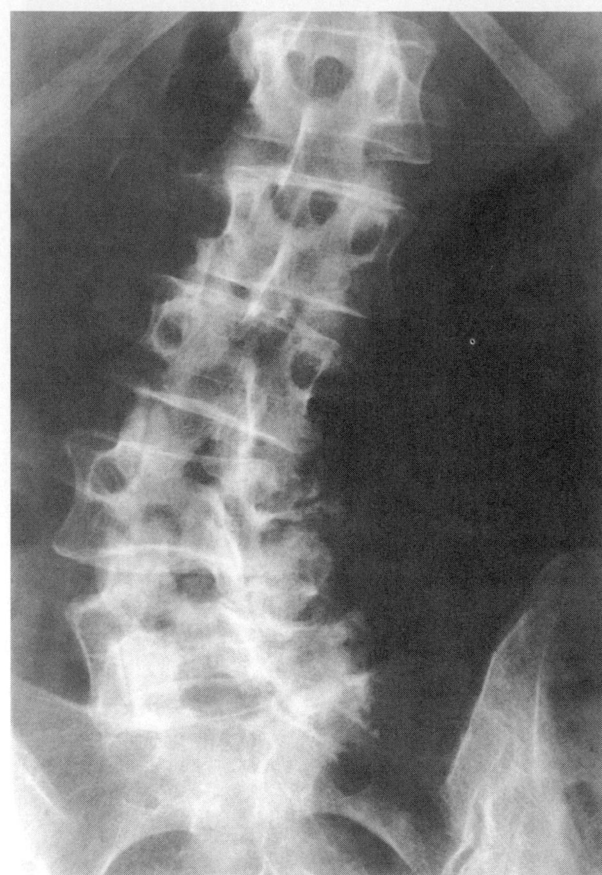

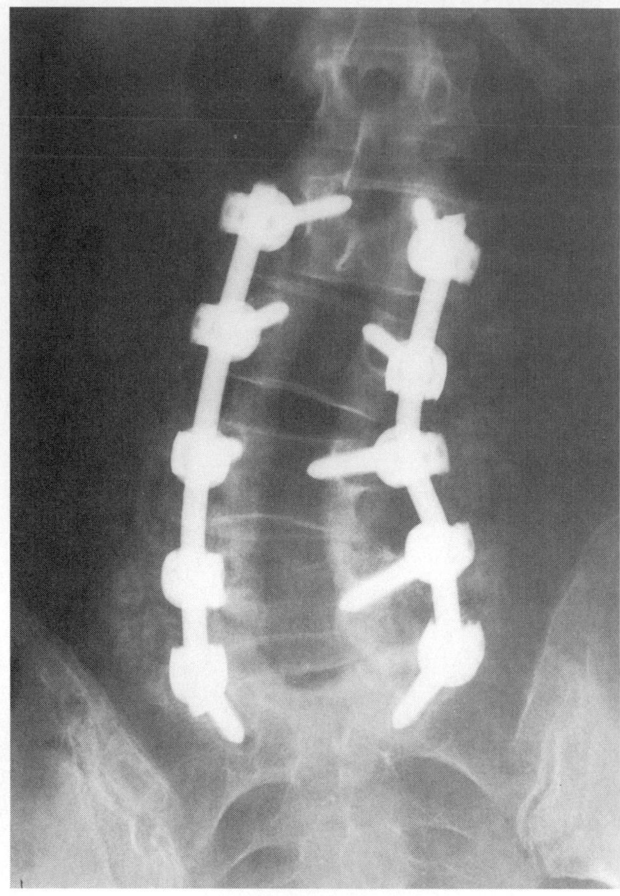

A B

FIG. 48.8. A: Lumbar spine films from a 58-year-old woman with progressive scoliosis and back and leg pain. **B:** The symptoms were relieved after laminectomy from L2 to the sacrum. Fixation was performed from L2 to the sacrum with pedicle screws aided by computer-guided intraoperative navigational system due to the small size and variable angles of the pedicles. The patient experienced near-complete relief of preoperative symptoms.

tients may require a spine stabilization and fusion as well as laminectomy. The addition of metallic instrumentation provides support against progression of the deformity until the fusion becomes solid (Fig. 48.8). Although pedicle fixation is often used, the accuracy and safety of screw placement can be improved with the utilization of stereotactic computer image-guided intraoperative navigational systems (34). However, correction of this type of deformity, a formidable procedure, is rarely, if ever, necessary.

REFERENCES

1. Reiter MF, Boden SD. Inflammatory disorders of the cervical spine. *Spine* 1998;23:2755–2766.
2. Gurley JP, Bell GR. The surgical management of patients with rheumatoid cervical spine disease. *Rheum Dis Clin North Am* 1997;23:317–332.
3. Fujiwara K, Owaki H, Fujimoto M, et al. A long-term follow-up of cervical lesions in rheumatoid arthritis. *J Spinal Disord* 2000;13:519–526.
4. Oda T, Fujiwara K, Yonenobu K, et al. Natural course of cervical spine lesions in rheumatoid arthritis. *Spine* 1995;20:1128–1135.
5. Pellicci PM, Ranawat CS, Tsairis P, et al. A prospective study of the progression of rheumatoid arthritis of the cervical spine. *J Bone Joint Surg Am* 1981;63:342–350.
6. Yonezawa T, Tsuji H, Matsui H, et al. Subaxial lesions in rheumatoid arthritis. Radiographic factors suggestive of lower cervical myelopathy. *Spine* 1995;20:208–215.
7. Collins DN, Barnes CL, FitzRandolph RL. Cervical spine instability in rheumatoid patients having total hip or knee arthroplasty. *Clin Orthop* 1991;Nov:127–135.
8. Rana NA. Natural history of atlanto-axial subluxation in rheumatoid arthritis. *Spine* 1989;14:1054–1056.
9. Boden SD, Dodge LD, Bohlman HH, et al. Rheumatoid arthritis of the cervical spine. A long-term analysis with predictors of paralysis and recovery. *J Bone Joint Surg Am* 1993;75A:1282–1297.
10. Riise T, Jacobsen BK, Gran JT. High mortality in patients with rheumatoid arthritis and atlantoaxial subluxation. *J Rheumatol* 2001;28:2425–2429.
11. Peppelman WC, Kraus DR, Donaldson WFd, et al. Cervical spine surgery in rheumatoid arthritis: improvement of neurologic deficit after cervical spine fusion. *Spine* 1993;18:2375–2379.
12. Van Asselt KM, Lems WF, Bongartz EB, et al. Outcome of cervical spine surgery in patients with rheumatoid arthritis. *Ann Rheum Dis* 2001;60:448–452.
13. Weissman BN, Aliabadi P, Weinfeld MS, et al. Prognostic features of atlantoaxial subluxation in rheumatoid arthritis patients. *Radiology* 1982;144:745–751.
14. Boden SD. Rheumatoid arthritis of the cervical spine. Surgical decision making based on predictors of paralysis and recovery. *Spine* 1994;19:2275–2280.
15. Hamilton JD, Johnston A, Madhok R, et al. Factors predictive of subsequent deterioration in rheumatoid cervical myelopathy. *Rheumatology* 2001;40:811–815.

16. Riew KD, Hillibrand AS, Palumbo MA, et al. Diagnosing basilar invagination in the rheumatoid patient. The reliability of radiographic criteria. *J Bone Joint Surg Am* 2001;83:194–200.
17. Dvorak J, Grob D, Baumgartner H, et al. Functional evaluation of the spinal cord by magnetic resonance imaging in patients with rheumatoid arthritis and instability of upper cervical spine. *Spine* 1989;14:1057–1064.
18. Kawaida H, Sakou T, Morizono Y, et al. Magnetic resonance imaging of upper cervical disorders in rheumatoid arthritis. *Spine* 1989;14:1144–1148.
19. Bundschuh C, Modic MT, Kearney F, et al. Rheumatoid arthritis of the cervical spine: surface-coil MR imaging. *AJR* 1988;151:181–187.
20. Roca A, Bernreuter WK, Alarcon GS. Functional magnetic resonance imaging should be included in the evaluation the cervical spine in patients with rheumatoid arthritis. *J Rheumatol* 1993;20:1485–1488.
21. O'Brien MF, Casey AT, Crockard A, et al. Histology of the craniocervical junction in chronic rheumatoid arthritis: a clinicopathological analysis of 33 operative cases. *Spine* 2002;27:2245–2254.
22. Mikulowski P, Wollheim FA, Rotmil P, et al. Sudden death in rheumatoid arthritis with atlanto-axial dislocation. *Acta Med Scand* 1975;198:445–451.
23. Casey AT, Crockard HA, Bland JM, et al. Surgery on the rheumatoid cervical spine for the non-ambulant myelopathic patient—too much, too late? [Comments]. *Lancet* 1996;347:1004–1007.
24. Casey AT, Crockard HA, Pringle J, et al. Rheumatoid arthritis of the cervical spine: current techniques for management. *Orthop Clin North Am* 2002;33:291–309.
25. Casey AT, Crockard HA, Bland JM, et al. Predictors of outcome in the quadriparetic nonambulatory myelopathic patient with rheumatoid arthritis: a prospective study of 55 surgically treated Ranawat class IIIb patients. *J Neurosurg* 1996;85:574–581.
26. Casey AT, Crockard HA, Stevens J. Vertical translocation. Part II. Outcomes after surgical treatment of rheumatoid cervical myelopathy. *J Neurosurg* 1997;87:863–869.
27. McRorie ER, McLoughlin P, Russell T, et al. Cervical spine surgery in patients with rheumatoid arthritis: an appraisal. *Ann Rheum Dis* 1996;55:99–104.
28. Grob D, Dvorak J, Panjabi MM, et al. The role of plate and screw fixation in occipitocervical fusion in rheumatoid arthritis. *Spine* 1994;19:2545–2551.
29. Stillerman CB, Wilson JA. Atlanto-axial stabilization with posterior transarticular screw fixation: technical description and report of 22 cases. *Neurosurgery* 1993;32:948–955.
30. Naderi S, Crawford NR, Song GS, et al. Biomechanical comparison of C1-C2 posterior fixations. Cable, graft, and screw combinations. *Spine* 1998;23:1946–1955; discussion 1955–1956.
31. Hurlbert RJ, Crawford NR, Choi WG, et al. A biomechanical evaluation of occipitocervical instrumentation: screw compared with wire fixation. *J Neurosurg* 1999;90:84–90.
32. Grob D, Crisco JJ III, Panjabi MM, et al. Biomechanical evaluation of four different posterior atlantoaxial fixation techniques. *Spine* 1992;17:480–490.
33. Abumi K, Kaneda K, Shono Y, et al. One-stage posterior decompression and reconstruction of the cervical spine by using pedicle screw fixation systems. *J Neurosurg* 1999;90:19–26.
34. Kalfas IH, Kormos DW, Murphy MA, et al. Application of frameless stereotaxy to pedicle screw fixation of the spine. *J Neurosurg* 1995;83:641–647.
35. Welch WC, Subach BR, Pollack IF, et al. Frameless stereotactic guidance for surgery of the upper cervical spine [see comments]. *Neurosurgery* 1997;40:958–963; discussion 963–964.
36. Heidecke V, Rainov NG, Burkert W. Occipito-cervical fusion with the cervical Cotrel-Dubousset rod system. *Acta Neurochir* 1998;140:969–976.
37. Vale FL, Oliver M, Cahill DW. Rigid occipitocervical fusion. *J Neurosurg* 1999;91:144–150.
38. Kraus DR, Peppelman WC, Agarwal AK, et al. Incidence of subaxial subluxation in patients with generalized rheumatoid arthritis who have had previous occipital cervical fusions. *Spine* 1991;16:S486–489.
39. Zygmunt S, Saveland H, Brattstrom H, et al. Reduction of rheumatoid periodontoid pannus following posterior occipito-cervical fusion visualised by magnetic resonance imaging. *Br J Neurosurg* 1988;2:315–320.
40. Grob D, Wursch R, Grauer W, et al. Atlantoaxial fusion and retrodental pannus in rheumatoid arthritis. *Spine* 1997;22:1580–1583; discussion 1584.
41. Falope ZF, Griffiths JD, Platt PN, et al. Cervical myelopathy and rheumatoid arthritis: a retrospective analysis of management. *Clin Rehabil* 2002;16:625–629.
42. Agarwal AK, Peppelman WC, Kraus DR, et al. Recurrence of cervical spine instability in rheumatoid arthritis following previous fusion: can disease progression be prevented by early surgery. *J Rheumatol* 1992;19:1364–1370.
43. Omura K, Hukuda S, Katsuura A, et al. Evaluation of posterior long fusion versus conservative treatment in the progressive rheumatoid cervical spine. *Spine* 2002;27:1336–1345.
44. Laiho K, Kaarela K, Kauppi M. Cervical spine disorders in patients with rheumatoid arthritis and amyloidosis. *Clin Rheumatol* 2002;21:227–230.
45. Kawaguchi Y, Matsuno H, Kanamori M, et al. Radiologic findings of the lumbar spine in patients with rheumatoid arthritis, and a review of pathologic mechanisms. *J Spinal Disord Tech* 2003;16:38–43.
46. Haugeberg G, Orstavik RE, Uhlig T, et al. Clinical decision rules in rheumatoid arthritis: do they identify patients at high risk for osteoporosis? Testing clinical criteria in a population based cohort of patients with rheumatoid arthritis recruited from the Oslo Rheumatoid Arthritis Register. *Ann Rheum Dis* 2002;61:1085–1089.
47. De Nijs RN, Jacobs JW, Bijlsma JW, et al. Prevalence of vertebral deformities and symptomatic vertebral fractures in corticosteroid treated patients with rheumatoid arthritis. *Rheumatology* 2001;40:1375–1383.
48. Garfin SR, Yuan HA, Reily MA. Kyphoplasty and vertebroplasty for treatment of painful osteoporotic compression fractures. *Spine* 2001;26:1511–1515.
49. Broom MJ, Raycroft JF. Complications of fractures of the cervical spine in ankylosing spondylitis. *Spine* 1988;13:763–766.
50. Fox MW, Onofrio BM, Kilgore JE. Neurological complications of ankylosing spondylitis. *J Neurosurg* 1993;78:871–878.
51. Ramos-Remus C, Gomez-Vargas A, Guzman-Guzman JL, et al. Frequency of atlantoaxial subluxation and neurologic involvement in patients with ankylosing spondylitis [Comments]. *J Rheumatol* 1995;22:2120–2125.
52. Kim KT, Suk KS, Cho YJ, et al. Clinical outcome results of pedicle subtraction osteotomy on ankylosing spondylitis with kyphotic deformity. *Spine* 2002;27:612–618.
53. van Royen BJ, Slot GH. Closing-wedge posterior osteotomy for ankylosing spondylitis. Partial corporectomy and transpedicular fixation in 22 cases. *J Bone Joint Surg Br* 1995;77:117–121.
54. Gerscovich EO, Greenspan A, Montesano PX. Treatment of kyphotic deformity in ankylosing spondylitis. *Orthopedics* 1994;17:335–342.
55. Thiranont N, Netrwichien P. Transpedicular cancellation closed wedge vertebral osteotomy for treatment of fixed flexion deformity of spine in ankylosing spondylitis. *Spine* 1993;18:2517–2522.
56. McMaster MJ. Osteotomy of the cervical spine in ankylosing spondylitis. *J Bone Joint Surg Br* 1997;79:197–203.
57. Halm H, Metz-Stavenhagen P, Zielke K. Results of surgical correction of kyphotic deformities of the spine in ankylosing spondylitis on the basis of the modified arthritis impact measurement scales. *Spine* 1995;20:1612–1619.
58. Graham B, Van Peteghem PK. Fractures of the spine in ankylosing spondylitis. Diagnosis, treatment, and complications. *Spine* 1989;14:803–807.
59. Hitchon PW, From AM, Brenton MD, et al. Fractures of the thoracolumbar spine complicating ankylosing spondylitis. *J Neurosurg* 2002;97:218–222.
60. Murray GC, Persellin RH. Cervical fracture complicating ankylosing spondylitis: a report of eight cases and review of the literature. *Am J Med* 1981;70:1033–1041.
61. Drummond DS, Keene JS. Spinous process segmental spinal instrumentation. *Orthopedics* 1988;11:1403–1410.
62. Rajshekhar V, Arunkumar MJ, Kumar SS. Changes in cervical spine curvature after uninstrumented one- and two-level corpectomy in patients with spondylotic myelopathy. *Neurosurgery* 2003;52:799–804; discussion 804–805.
63. Grubb SA, Lipscomb HJ, Coonrad RW. Degenerative adult onset scoliosis. *Spine* 1988;13:241–245.
64. Benner B, Ehni G. Degenerative lumbar scoliosis. *Spine* 1979;4:548–552.

CHAPTER 49

Correction of Arthritic Deformities of the Hip

Charles L. Nelson and Edward J. Stolarski

Arthritic hip deformities unresponsive to conservative management remain a common cause of significant morbidity. Pain and diminished function related to hip pathology often result in diminished physical and psychological well-being. Individuals with symptoms unresponsive to conservative treatment may benefit from surgical correction. Surgical correction in the form of total hip arthroplasty has been shown to decrease pain, improve function, and improve both the physical and psychological well-being of properly selected patients. Studies have demonstrated 90% survivorship at 20-year follow-up (1).

Surgical procedures other than total hip arthroplasty that may be appropriate for arthritic hip deformities include hemiarthroplasty, hip arthrodesis, femoral and acetabular osteotomies, hip arthroscopy, bone grafting or decompression procedures about the hip, hip débridement and/or synovectomy, and ablative hip procedures. Careful patient and procedural selection are critical to successful outcome.

EVALUATION OF ARTHRITIS DEFORMITIES OF THE HIP

Evaluation of arthritic hip deformities begins with a detailed history and physical examination. The history should clearly outline the character, location, and duration of symptoms. Whether the symptoms began insidiously or suddenly should be ascertained. Preceding trauma or surgery involving the hip must be clearly outlined. When the symptoms occur, associated activities and the chronicity of the symptoms are critical to the establishment of an appropriate differential diagnosis. The review of systems should note the presence of associated constitutional symptoms, other musculoskeletal complaints, or symptoms involving other organ symptoms. The history and examination should attempt to exclude referred pain, particularly from the lumbosacral spine, knee, abdomen, or retroperitoneum.

Patients with pain related to hip pathology typically will localize their pain to the groin region, sometimes with radiation into the anterior or medial thigh or to the knee. Hip pain as a rule does not radiate below the knee. Pain over the lateral aspect of the hip or the buttocks also may be secondary to hip pathology. However, if the pain is primarily buttock pain, particularly when associated with neurologic symptoms, or with radiation into the lateral or posterior thigh, the lumbosacral spine should be strongly considered as a potential source of the patient's symptoms. Arthritic pain is generally exacerbated by activity. Early in the course of arthritic conditions of the hip, pain is noted during the first couple of steps after arising from a seated position, resolving with continued ambulation.

On physical examination, patients with severe pain related to hip pathology often have a positive Trendelenburg sign. When asked to stand on the involved lower extremity alone, the patient is unable to maintain a level pelvis, and there is a drop of the contralateral pelvis. The sensitivity of the Trendelenburg sign may be increased by asking the patient to bring the uninvolved knee to the chest while in the standing position on the involved extremity. Examination of gait may demonstrate a limp. As in all significant lower extremity ailments, the gait may be antalgic with shortened stance phase.

Specific elements suggestive of hip pathology include an abductor lurch, or Trendelenburg gait. An abductor lurch is a natural response to decrease joint-reactive forces across the hip by centering body weight closer to the hip in stance phase and thereby decreasing hip pain. A Trendelenburg gait is secondary to hip abductor deficiency secondary to pain, or actual weakness in chronic conditions.

Determination of apparent and actual leg length discrepancy is critical during the evaluation of arthritic hip deformities, because certain surgical procedures may be associated with either shortening or lengthening of the limb. Accurate measurement of leg lengths in the absence of fixed unilateral hip contractures or fixed pelvic obliquity is possible by having the patient stand on wooden blocks of known thickness until the pelvis is level, with both hands on the iliac crest. True leg lengths refer to the distance between the anterior superior iliac spine and ipsilateral medial malleolus compared with the identical measurements for the contralateral limb. Apparent leg lengths are measured from a central single point such as the umbilicus to the medial malleolus on each side. Positioning of both limbs in identical position regarding flexion/extension, abduction/adduction, and internal/external rotation is critical for accuracy with both of these measurements. The hip and knee should be evaluated for contractures, which could affect the functional leg length after correction with surgery.

After examination of leg lengths and gait, palpation of bony and soft tissue structures of the hip and pelvis is performed. Areas of tenderness are noted. An inguinal hernia is an extrinsic source of groin pain, which may be palpated while asking the patient to cough. On occasion a synovial cyst emanating from an arthritic hip may be seen as an inguinal hernia. When a mass is palpated, the examiner should note the consistency, mobility, and size of the mass. Active and passive range of motion of both hips should be assessed. Any pain with hip motion should be noted.

Physical examination of the hip is incomplete without examination of the pelvis, lumbosacral spine, and lower extremities. Referred or radicular pain from the lumbosacral spine often manifests as hip pain. Sacroiliac pain also may be interpreted as hip pain. The FABER test involves flexion, abduction, and external rotation of the hip. Pain in the region of the sacroiliac joint with this maneuver may indicate sacroiliitis. Rarely knee pain may radiate to the proximal thigh or hip. Examination of the entire extremity is important before considering surgical intervention, because procedures on the hip may alter leg lengths, kinematics of gait, and joint biomechanics.

Neurovascular examination begins with assessment of the neurologic status of the extremity. Manual motor testing of the lower extremities allows identification of significant weakness, but is not accurate to detect subtle weakness due to the increased lower extremity strength of most patients compared with the upper extremity strength of the examiner. Sensory examination includes sensation to light touch, pinprick, or temperature, as well as proprioception. Patellar tendon and Achilles tendon reflexes should be evaluated, particularly when there is concern regarding spinal pathology. Vascular examination includes palpation of the femoral, popliteal, dorsalis pedis, and posterior tibial pulses. Concerns regarding the vascular status can be evaluated with an ankle brachial index (an index of the perfusion pressure at the brachium compared with the perfusion pressure at the ankle) in selected cases. In addition to palpation, swelling, edema, or skin changes suggestive of chronic venous insufficiency should be noted.

Pain related to an intraarticular hip condition will often be associated with diminished motion of the hip and with pain at the extremes of hip rotation or flexion. Active hip flexion against resistance with the ipsilateral knee extended will generally reproduce the patient's pain in intraarticular hip pathology. Tenderness over the greater trochanter may be present with intraarticular hip pathology, but should raise suspicion of trochanteric bursitis. Clicking, locking, snapping, or catching symptoms or signs in association with hip pain should alert the examining physician to the possibility of labral pathology, snapping iliopsoas tendon, snapping iliotibial band, or exostosis around the hip.

Patients with labral tears also may complain of symptoms of instability of the hip. Patients with an anterior labral tear may reproduce pain and clicking with extension, internal rotation, and adduction of the hip from a flexed, abducted, externally rotated position (2). Tears involving the posterior acetabular labrum generally lead to reproduction of symptoms with extension, abduction, and external rotation from a flexed, adducted, and internally rotated position (2). Unlike in the United States, where most acetabular labral tears involve the anterior labrum, in Japan, most of these tears appear to be posterior (2–5). Japanese investigators have noted pain with axial compression of the flexed hip as consistent with labral pathology in their population (5). Pain with internal rotation of the flexed hip was typically noted in patients with posterior labral tears in their experience as well.

Severe pain with short-arc range of motion, particularly in a febrile patient, should alert the examiner to the possibility of septic arthritis. Patients with inflammatory arthritis of the hip, avascular necrosis (AVN) with collapse, severe osteoarthritis (OA), or occult fracture also may be seen with severe pain in a limited range of motion.

Once septic arthritis is excluded, acute onset of significant hip pain requires careful evaluation to rule out AVN, transient osteoporosis, stress fracture, or occult fracture. Both AVN and transient osteoporosis initially appear with fairly good range of motion of the hip. Both usually occur with intraarticular hip pain manifesting as groin pain at the extremes of hip rotation or with active flexion of the hip against resistance. The history should evaluate risk factors for AVN, including trauma, systemic steroid intake, excessive ethanol intake, and history of systemic lupus erythematosus, sickle cell anemia, Gaucher disease, and conditions leading to a hypercoagulable state. Acute pain without abnormalities on plain radiographs, or with subtle osteopenia in a middle-aged man or third-trimester pregnant female, should lead to a strong suspicion of transient osteoporosis. Stress fracture may be secondary to overuse with normal bone or may be pathologic in patients with osteoporosis or osteomalacia (Fig. 49.1). Stress fracture should be strongly considered in athletic, amenorrheic women who have recently advanced the intensity of their workouts.

Increased femoral anteversion and improved comfort in abduction and internal rotation of the hip should alert the examiner to the possibility of acetabular dysplasia. Some patients with these symptoms will recall a prior treat-

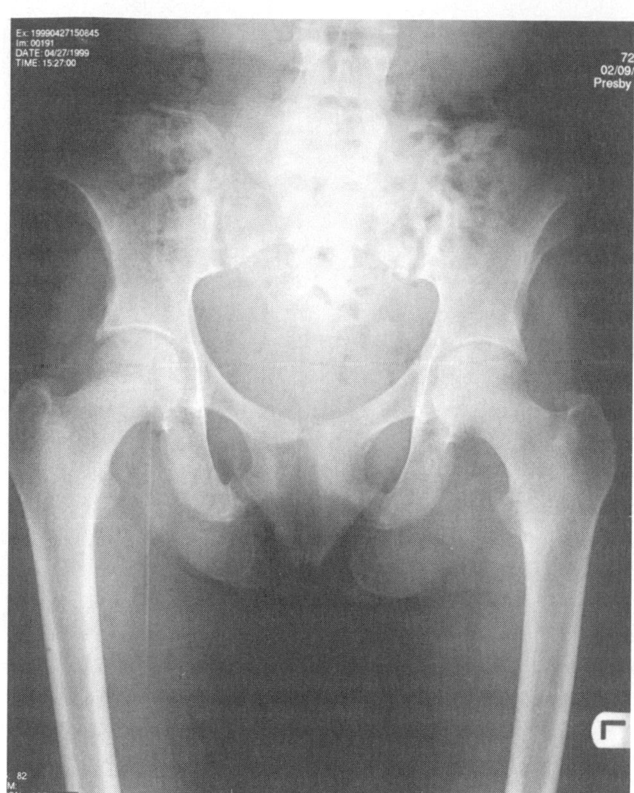

FIG. 49.1. Twenty-year-old woman with nutritional rickets secondary to a combination of insufficient sunlight and vitamin D intake. She complained of left hip pain with running or extensive walking. Radiographs demonstrate a stress fracture below the left lesser trochanter, as well as an asymptomatic stress fracture over the lateral aspect of the right proximal femur. Note the widening of the sacroiliac joints and symphysis pubis consistent with a diagnosis of osteomalacia.

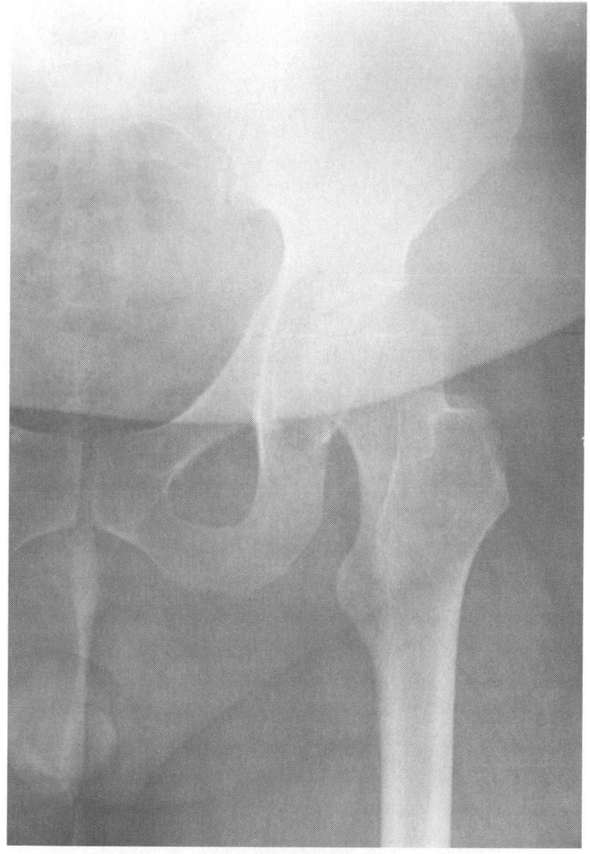

FIG. 49.2. Anteroposterior radiograph of the hip in a 44-year-old man with mild developmental dysplasia of the left hip. There is decreased lateral coverage with a diminished lateral center edge angle. There is excessive valgus angulation of the femoral neck.

ment or symptoms during childhood, but many will not. Increased femoral anteversion is suggested on physical examination when there is increased internal rotation of the hip and decreased external rotation in the prone patient with the knees flexed. Most patients with acetabular dysplasia have diminished anterior and lateral coverage. Standard radiographs demonstrate diminished coverage of the femoral head with a decreased lateral center edge angle (Fig. 49.2). In most cases, the inclination of the acetabular index angle (6) will be increased to greater than 10 degrees. A diminished anterior center edge angle may be appreciated on a weight-bearing lateral view of the acetabulum, the false-profile view (Fig. 49.3). The false-profile view (7) provides a tangential lateral view, allowing an accurate depiction of anterior acetabular coverage.

Laboratory evaluation is indicated for selected patients with a history of clinical or radiographic findings suggestive of inflammatory arthritis, Lyme disease, septic arthritis, osteoporosis, osteomalacia, or neoplasm. Complete blood count with differential, erythrocyte sedimentation rate, C-reactive protein, rheumatoid factor, antinuclear antibody, and Lyme titer may be helpful in evaluating infectious or inflammatory conditions. Alkaline phosphatase, serum protein electrophoresis, and urine protein electrophoresis may be helpful in evaluating for bony neoplasms involving the hip or pelvis. Alkaline phosphatase, blood urea nitrogen, creatinine, 25-hydroxyvitamin D_3, 1,25-dihydroxyvitamin D_3, and parathyroid hormone levels may be helpful in evaluating for metabolic bone disease.

Radiographic examination begins with plain radiographs in the anteroposterior pelvis view, the anteroposterior view of the involved hip in 15 degree internal rotation, and lateral view of the hip. A cross-table lateral view provides lateral views of both the acetabulum and proximal femur. The frog lateral view does not provide a lateral view of the acetabulum, but provides a better lateral view of the femoral head, allowing improved detection of subtle collapse or displacement in AVN or slipped capital femoral epiphysis. As noted earlier, the false-profile view is helpful when evaluating patients with acetabular dysplasia for deficient anterior coverage.

Computed tomography (CT) scans may be useful in the evaluation of some individuals with osteonecrosis, stress

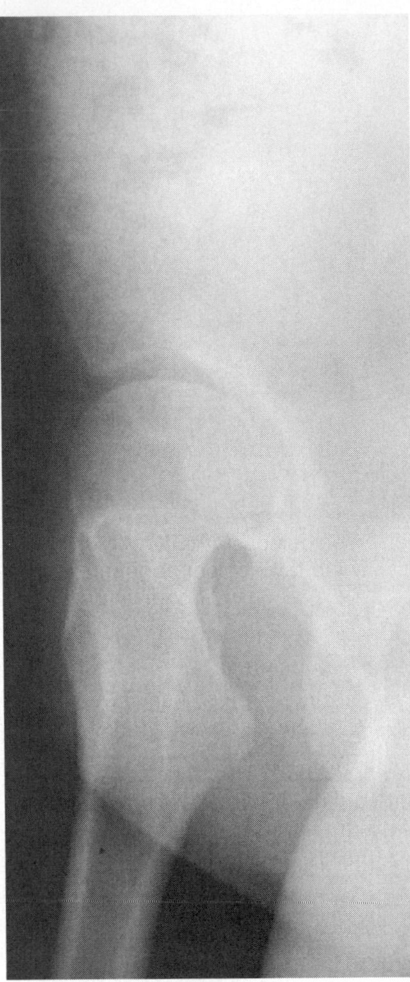

FIG. 49.3. False-profile radiograph of the acetabulum in a 20-year-old woman with unilateral acetabular dysplasia. Although this patient has deficient lateral coverage, the false-profile view demonstrates reasonable anterior coverage.

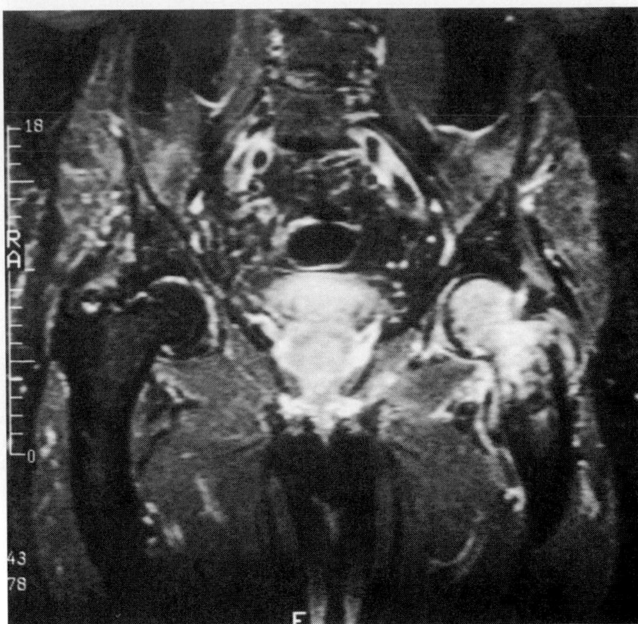

FIG. 49.4. Characteristic T2-weighted magnetic resonance image of a 62-year-old man with transient osteoporosis (bone marrow edema syndrome). Note the diffuse increased signal on T2-weighted imaging involving the entire head and extending to the intertrochanteric line, on the left side. Radiographs demonstrate unilateral decrease in bone mineral density.

fracture, and occult femoral neck fracture. CT scans also are valuable for preoperative planning for patients with acetabular dysplasia, particularly after prior hip surgery. Magnetic resonance imaging (MRI) and bone scintigraphy are valuable in the assessment of AVN, transient osteoporosis (Fig. 49.4), stress fracture, occult fracture, osteomyelitis, synovial disorders, loose bodies, and bony neoplasms. MRI also allows evaluation of soft tissue neoplasms. MR arthrography with intraarticular gadolinium is useful in detecting acetabular labral tears and is at this time considered the diagnostic modality of choice (8,9).

Urban et al. (10) demonstrated 90% sensitivity and 91% accuracy in evaluating acetabular labral tears. High-resolution MRI using special surface coils, without arthrography, has also been advocated for the detection of acetabular labral tears, but the accuracy is unknown (11).

Hip arthroscopy is valuable as both a diagnostic and therapeutic modality in the evaluation of arthritic hip conditions. Arthroscopy allows direct visualization, probing, and, at times, treatment of pathologic hip conditions.

ETIOLOGY

Severe end-stage arthritic deformities of the hip develop secondary to multiple causes. Despite multiple etiologies with characteristic findings early in the course of the disease, the final common pathway involves loss of articular cartilage with marked destructive changes involving the hip joint in end-stage disease. The inability of hip radiographs of patients with end-stage destruction of the hip to distinguish the etiology of the arthritic process has led to controversy regarding the etiology of OA in many cases.

The most common arthritic affliction of the hip is OA. As noted earlier, controversy exists as to the etiology of OA in many cases. The term *primary OA* refers to the development of OA without injury or known predisposing factor. In theory, breakdown of articular cartilage may be secondary to defective articular cartilage unable to withstand normal stress, or secondary to mechanical failure where normal articular cartilage fails secondary to abnormal mechanical loads. The mechanical theory of OA presumes that joints function properly within a narrow range of mechanical load (12,13). Abnormally low loads lead to atrophy, and abnormally high loads lead to cartilage destruction and OA (13).

Historically, most OA was believed to be idiopathic or primary (14) (Table 49.1). The prevailing opinion at this

TABLE 49.1. *Osteoarthritis of the hip in 124 patients*

Idiopathic coxarthrosis	58
Congenital hip disease	21
Adolescent cox vara	6
Legg-Calvé Perthes	2
Septic arthritis	2
Rheumatoid arthritis	2
Arthrokatadysis	2
Posttraumatic arthrosis	2
Trochanteric fracture	1
Acromegaly	1
Paget's disease	1
Osteonecrosis	1
Neurotrophic	1

Modified from Lloyd-Roberts GC. Osteoarthritis of the hip. *J Bone Joint Surg Br* 1955;37:8–47, with permission.

time is that most OA is secondary to a mechanical cause, often related to an unrecognized pediatric hip affliction. Stulberg et al. (15) identified the presence of developmental hip dysplasia, Legg-Calvé-Perthes disease, or slipped capital femoral epiphysis, in 79% of 125 patients with degenerative hip arthritis. Careful history, physical examination, and close scrutiny of radiographs will often provide insight into the etiology of OA in what were previously believed to be idiopathic cases.

Developmental hip dysplasia, the most common of the childhood hip disorders, refers to a spectrum of disorders of the hip with abnormal development of the acetabulum, and at times proximal femur, associated with deficient coverage of the femoral head. The mildest forms are associated with slight uncoverage of the femoral head without subluxation. Subluxation, typically accompanied by an oblique acetabular roof angle, occurs with more advanced dysplasia. Complete dislocation of the femoral head with or without development of a pseudoacetabulum is the most advanced form of hip dysplasia. Crowe (16) has classified acetabular dysplasia based on the degree of subluxation. Type I dysplasia is characterized by less than 50% femoral head subluxation, type II dysplasia by 50% to 75% subluxation, type III dysplasia by greater than 75% subluxation, and type IV dysplasia by complete dislocation (16).

Legg-Calvé-Perthes disease (17–19) is a poorly understood disorder of the hip, which typically is seen in a child between the ages of 4 and 8 years. The older the child the poorer the prognosis because the femoral head has less remodeling potential than in the younger child. Treatment during childhood is controversial, and many cases are managed with conservative treatment modalities. The major anatomic abnormality noted in adult patients with symptoms related to prior Legg-Calvé-Perthes disease is deformity of the femoral head with flattening and coxa magna. Unsuccessful containment of the femoral head during acetabular development can lead to abnormality in the development of the acetabulum as well. Secondary arthritic deformities of the hip are hypothesized to develop because of the mechanical consequences of the deformity. Resulting incongruity between the acetabulum and femoral head and joint subluxation or impingement with hinge abduction may lead to destruction of articular cartilage.

Slipped capital femoral epiphysis generally affects overweight adolescents or skeletally immature individuals with endocrine abnormalities such as hypothyroidism. The disorder is characterized by an epiphyseal fracture, typically with posterior displacement of the femoral head on the neck. Treatment during childhood generally involves pinning *in situ.* Some patients may develop chondrolysis or AVN, leading to subsequent joint destruction. Deformity of the proximal femur with impingement or incongruity also may lead to significant hip arthritis later in life.

Rare congenital conditions leading to significant arthritic hip involvement before or during adulthood include multiple epiphyseal dysplasia and spondyloepiphyseal dysplasia. Hip involvement in multiple epiphyseal dysplasia and spondyloepiphyseal dysplasia is indistinguishable from Legg-Calvé-Perthes disease, with the exception that the spine or other joints are involved with the latter two disorders, and the presentation is typically at an earlier age.

Posttraumatic arthritis of the hip is not uncommon. Traumatic conditions leading to arthritic deformities of the hip include acetabular fractures, femoral head fractures, hip dislocations, or fracture-dislocations of the hip with damage to the femoral head, acetabulum, or both. Acetabular fractures after prior surgical intervention are at significant risk for the development of heterotopic ossification, resulting in greater challenges during subsequent reconstruction (Fig. 49.5). Femoral neck fractures may be complicated by nonunion and AVN, leading to subsequent hip arthritis. The incidence of nonunion and AVN after femoral neck fracture varies according to the degree of displacement of the fracture (20). Barnes et al. (21) evaluated the results of 1,503 subcapital femur fractures. Displaced fractures were associated with nonunion after reduction and internal fixation in 33% of the patients. AVN with late segmental collapse in united fractures occurred in an additional 24% in female and 15% in male subjects. Asnis et al. (22) reported only a 4% nonunion rate with a 22% AVN rate in 141 consecutive patients with intracapsular femoral neck fractures after internal fixation with multiple cannulated screws within 2 days of injury. Patients in whom satisfactory reduction could not be obtained, who had preexisting arthritis, or in whom the fracture was present for more than 2 days were managed by hemiarthroplasty, and were not included in this study. Sixty-five percent of patients in the study had a displaced fracture. The mean age was 62 years.

Nontraumatic AVN of the hip is another hip condition often progressing to disabling arthritis of the hip (see Chapter 107). The etiology of AVN is poorly understood. AVN may result from direct cellular damage, intravascular occlusion, or extravascular compression (23). Direct cellular damage is usually from radiation therapy or chemotherapy. Obstruction of vascular outflow may lead to development of

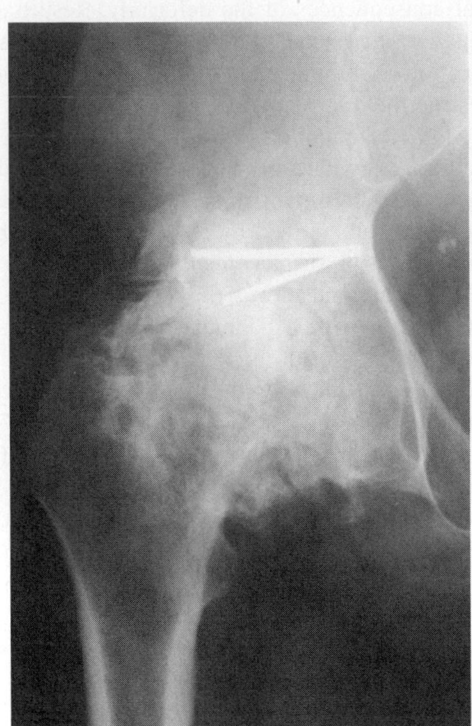

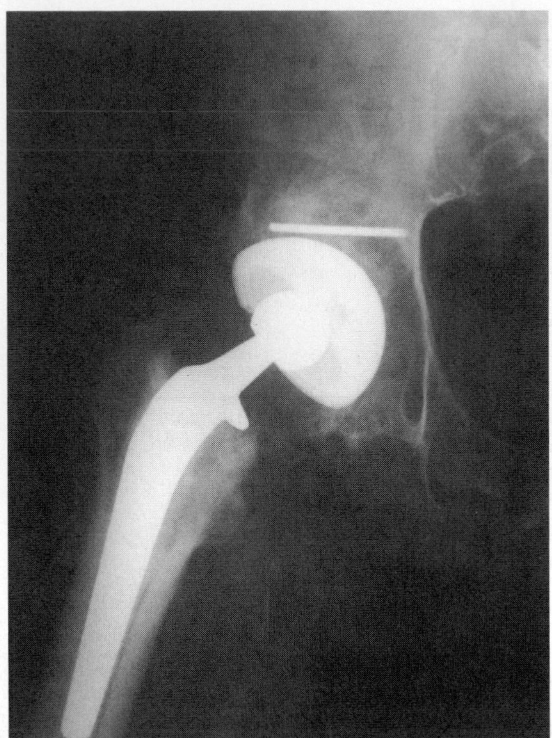

FIG. 49.5. Posttraumatic arthritis in a 57-year-old man with severe heterotopic ossification 25 years after an acetabular fracture treated surgically. **A:** Preoperative anteroposterior radiograph demonstrating severe posttraumatic arthritis with extensive heterotopic ossification. He has severe hip pain with severe limitation in hip motion. **B:** Postoperative anteroposterior radiograph after right hybrid total hip replacement with resection of heterotopic bone and postoperative radiation therapy for prophylaxis against the recurrence of heterotopic bone.

an intraosseous compartment syndrome in the femoral head. Ischemia, whether related to vascular occlusion involving inflow vessels or secondary to increased interosseous pressure, leads to osteocyte cell death. Regardless of the cause, AVN of the femoral head is characterized by death of the subchondral bone. Radiographs are initially normal. Progressive involvement leads to sclerosis or cyst formation involving the femoral head. Later subchondral or articular collapse occurs, resulting in joint incongruity and ultimately arthritic deterioration. Although there are cases of resolution of symptoms without collapse of the femoral head in patients with AVN managed conservatively, the majority of patients with symptoms secondary to AVN will progress to femoral head collapse and secondary OA of the hip without surgical intervention. Risk factors for nontraumatic AVN include alcoholism, systemic corticosteroid use, sickle cell anemia, systemic lupus erythematosus (independent of steroid use), Gaucher disease, irradiation, burns, familial lipid disorders, and hypercoagulable states (24–26).

Inflammatory conditions that may lead to arthritis hip deformities include rheumatoid arthritis (RA), juvenile RA, seronegative spondyloarthropathies, crystal-induced arthropathies, infections, and Lyme disease. RA is the most common inflammatory condition involving the hip. It is characterized by synovitis early in the course of the disease, followed by later cartilage and joint destruction. Radiographs generally demonstrate involvement of both hips with symmetric joint space narrowing, with or without cyst formation, and with significantly less osteophyte formation and subchondral sclerosis compared with OA (Fig. 49.6). Approximately 3% of individuals with severe arthritic hip deformities have RA. Combining all other forms of inflammatory arthritis makes up less than 1% of severe arthritic hip deformities requiring surgical intervention.

Seronegative spondyloarthropathies potentially involving the hip include ankylosing spondylitis, Reiter's syndrome, arthritis of inflammatory bowel disease, and psoriatic arthritis. In contrast to RA, these condition are more common in men than women. Ankylosing spondylitis is the most common of these conditions with regard to involvement of the hip. Although not diagnostic, a positive HLA-B27 antigen is found in the majority of patients with ankylosing spondylitis (25).

Septic arthritis of the hip occurs most commonly in children. Children are believed to be susceptible to hematogenous osteomyelitis and septic arthritis because of their unique metaphyseal blood supply. Septic arthritis is an uncommon source of adult hip pathology. Elderly and immunosuppressed adults, particularly after injury or with preexisting arthritis, appear to be at greatest risk in the adult

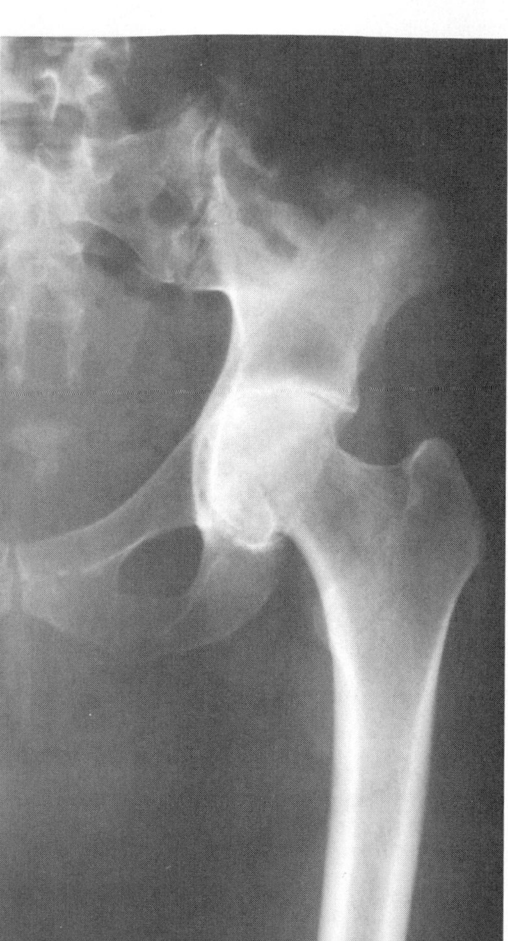

FIG. 49.6. Anteroposterior radiograph of the left hip in a 61-year-old woman with rheumatoid arthritis (RA) and severe involvement of both hips. The radiograph demonstrates characteristic findings of RA with symmetric (medial and superior) joint space narrowing, cyst formation, and absence of marked osteophyte formation or subchondral sclerosis.

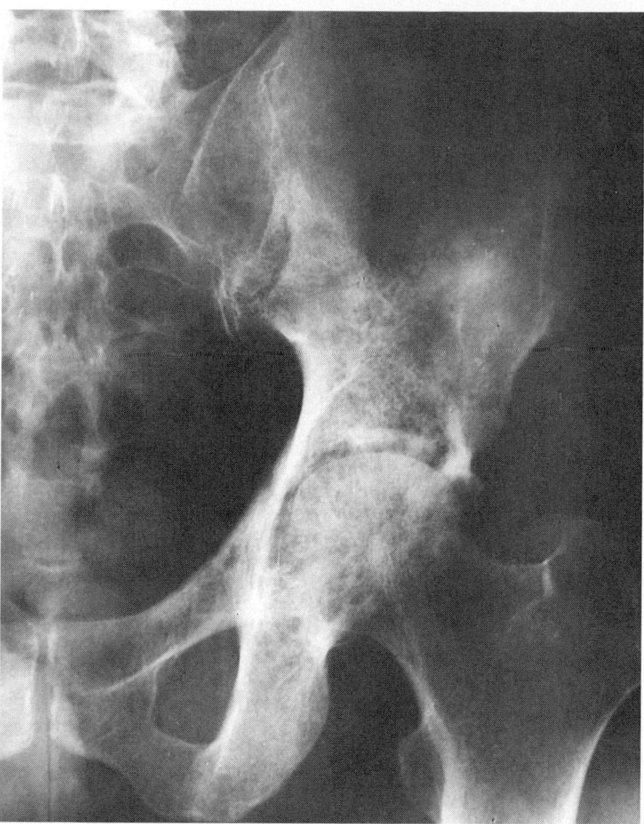

FIG. 49.7. Septic arthritis of the left hip. There is loss of the articular cartilage and subchondral bone of both the acetabulum and femoral head with cyst formation and radiolucencies of both sides of the joint and hemipelvis.

population (27). The patient may have sudden or insidious onset of constant hip pain, often associated with fever, chills, or sweats. On examination, the joint is irritable, and there is generally significant pain with any passive or active motion of the hip. Radiographs typically demonstrate arthritic changes or no abnormalities initially. Radiographs later often show complete loss of the joint space with cyst formation on both sides of the joint (Fig. 49.7) and periosteal reaction with associated osteomyelitis. If not diagnosed and treated promptly, the infection may lead to permanent joint destruction. When septic arthritis is considered in the differential diagnosis after history and physical examination, immediate blood culture, laboratory studies, and hip aspiration with Gram stain, aerobic and anaerobic incubation of synovial fluid, and synovial fluid cell count (and differential) and crystal analysis should be obtained. Empiric antibiotics are begun immediately after obtaining cultures. Treatment involves emergency irrigation and débridement of the hip. Hip arthrodesis, resection arthroplasty, and staged total hip arthroplasty are salvage options after significant arthritic deterioration or with chronic infections (26).

Benign and malignant primary neoplastic processes and secondary metastatic processes may lead to arthritic hip deformities as well (see Chapter 105). An exhaustive review of these disorders is beyond the scope of this chapter. All benign and malignant epiphyseal or metaphyseal bone tumors may affect the hip joint. Synovial disorders including synovial chondromatosis and pigmented vilonodular synovitis may occur initially as synovitis or loose bodies, later leading to hip arthritis. Benign tumorlike conditions such as Paget's disease and fibrous dysplasia often lead to severe deformity, particularly of the proximal femur, and may culminate in joint incongruity and secondary arthritic deformities.

Rare local and systemic disorders potentially leading to arthritic deformities of the hip include arthrokatadysis, hemophilia, hemochromatosis, and acromegaly. Arthrokatadysis or Otto pelvis refers to idiopathic protrusio acetabuli. Many inflammatory, infectious, metabolic, traumatic, and postsurgical conditions are recognized as predisposing factors for secondary protrusio acetabuli, but the pathogenesis of the idiopathic form is unknown. The disorder is often bilateral and is more common in female patients. Genetic

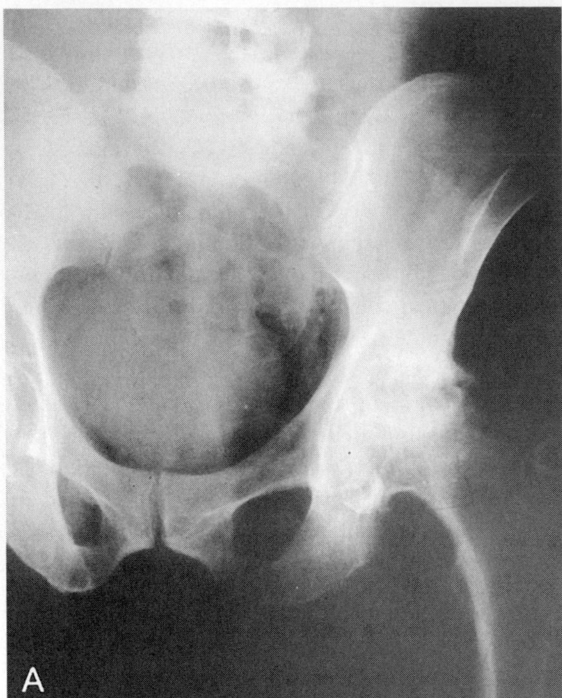

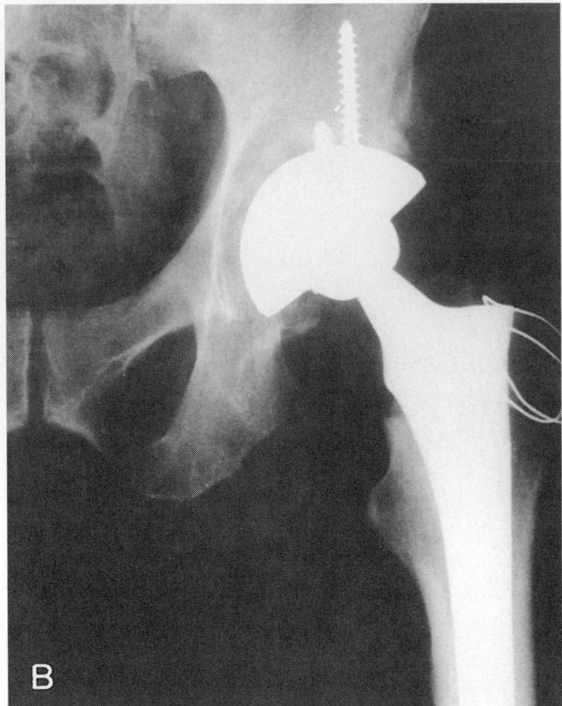

FIG. 49.8. Hemochromatosis with destruction of the left hip treated with a cementless total hip arthroplasty. **A:** This anteroposterior radiograph demonstrates destruction of the left hip secondary to hemochromatosis. **B:** Cementless total hip arthroplasty 3 years after surgery has restored painless function. No radiolucent lines are evident. There has been remodeling of the cut surface of the calcar femorale.

factors and abnormality of the triradiate cartilage have been proposed as etiologic factors (27–29). Protrusio acetabuli leads to a decreased range of motion, impingement, and secondary OA. Repeated hemarthroses secondary to hemophilia may lead to synovitis and secondary hip arthritis. Abnormal iron metabolism in hemochromatosis results in synovial deposition of iron with development of secondary hip OA (Fig. 49.8). Acromegaly, a disorder caused by abnormally high levels of growth hormone, can lead to arthritic hip deformities as well. Hypertrophy of both bone and cartilage may lead to early widening of joint spaces with subsequent narrowing and arthritic deformity resulting from joint incongruity or impingement.

SURGICAL PROCEDURES FOR THE ARTHRITIC HIP

Before planning surgical intervention for an arthritic hip deformity, nonsurgical management options should be considered. Nonsurgical management begins with patient education, activity modification, and consideration for use of an ambulatory aid (cane, crutches, walker). Weight loss is advisable in the overweight patient. Analgesics and nonsteroidal antiinflammatory drugs (NSAIDs) may help ameliorate pain. Antibiotics and cytotoxic medications may be appropriate for some infectious, immune-mediated, or neoplastic conditions unresponsive to analgesics and NSAIDs. These agents have significant potential side effects and are best administered by a rheumatologist or oncologist experienced in their use.

Surgical intervention is appropriate when conservative modalities fail to alleviate symptoms satisfactorily. The pathology present must be potentially amenable to the surgical procedure proposed. Proper informed consent is mandatory. The condition must be serious enough that the patient accepts the risks of surgery.

Whether a given surgical procedure should be considered depends on the age of the patient, the associated pain and functional disability, the expectations of the patient, the potential benefit of the procedure to the patient, and the surgical procedure proposed. Only minimally invasive or preventive reconstructive procedures are appropriate for young patients with mild arthritic involvement. Salvage or ablative procedures should be reserved for significant disability and pathology.

Hip Arthroscopy

Hip arthroscopy is a surgical procedure valuable for both diagnostic and therapeutic purposes. Although less invasive than arthrotomy, hip arthroscopy is associated with significant risks. The most common complication is a traction neuropraxia. The location of the hip and surrounding neurovascular structures is associated with the risk for direct neurovascular injury from arthroscopic instruments as well. Currently, therapeutic indications for hip arthroscopy include resection or repair of acetabular labral tears, synovial biopsy, synovectomy, removal of loose bodies, treatment of chondral injuries involving the hip, and irrigation and débridement in septic arthritis (30).

Decompression and Bone-Grafting Procedures

Core decompression and bone-grafting procedures of the hip are indicated primarily for the treatment of AVN in a precollapse stage before the development of arthritic deterioration. Core decompression involves creating a tract from the lateral aspect of the femur, above the level of the lesser trochanter, which extends into the necrotic bone in the femoral head. Advocates for core decompression alone, core decompression with cancellous bone grafting, core decompression with fibular strut allografting, and core decompression with vascularized fibular autografting all exist (31–34). The results have been varied in the literature, with some centers having good results with low complication rates, and others having poor results with high complication rates (31–35). There are no good randomized prospective studies demonstrating an advantage of one technique over another.

Pelvic Osteotomies

Pelvic osteotomies are indicated primarily for selected individuals with developmental hip dysplasia or Legg-Calvé-Perthes disease. Pelvic osteotomies may be categorized as either reconstructive or salvage osteotomies. Reconstructive osteotomies reorient existing acetabular articular cartilage to provide a more favorable mechanical environment for existing articular cartilage. The goal of these procedures is to prevent impending articular cartilage deterioration before the development of significant hip arthritis. Salvage osteotomies provide coverage without articular cartilage to create a more stable mechanical environment. These procedures are indicated for young patients with more significant arthritic involvement who are not good candidates for reconstructive osteotomies after advanced disease or incongruity, and are not good candidates for total hip arthroplasty because of age.

Reconstructive osteotomies of the pelvis include the Salter innominate osteotomy, the double innominate osteotomy, the triple innominate osteotomies of Steel or Tonnis, the Bernese periacetabular osteotomy, and the Wagner or dial spherical osteotomies (36–42). The Salter innominate osteotomy involves a single osteotomy of the innominate bone. Although significant rotation is often possible in the immature pelvis through the symphysis pubis and triradiate cartilage, this osteotomy does not allow sufficient correction in most skeletally mature patients. Rotation by the Salter innominate osteotomy also leads to lateralization of the acetabulum, increasing the hip joint–reactive forces. Double and triple innominate osteotomies allow improved rotation compared with the Salter innominate osteotomy, but rotation remains somewhat limited because of the soft tissue restraints. The spherical osteotomies are technically demanding and associated with a risk of intraarticular fracture and AVN of the acetabulum (42). Many surgeons now consider the Bernese periacetabular osteotomy (Fig. 49.9) the reconstructional acetabular osteotomy of choice for adult patients with acetabular dysplasia.

There appear to be several advantages of the Bernese periacetabular osteotomy (43). The acetabulum may be rotated independent of the strong sacrospinous and sacrotuberous ligaments. The acetabulum is an independent fragment and can be medialized to a normal position, allowing reduction of joint-reactive forces. Maintenance of an intact posterior column facilitates early rehabilitation without postoperative immobilization or bracing. The initial results after periacetabular osteotomy are encouraging for patients

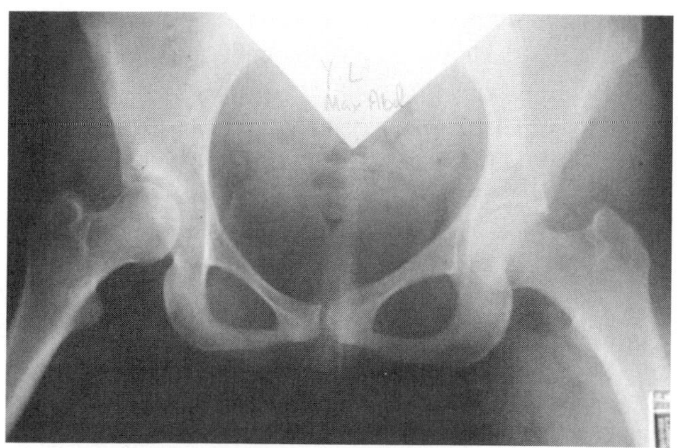

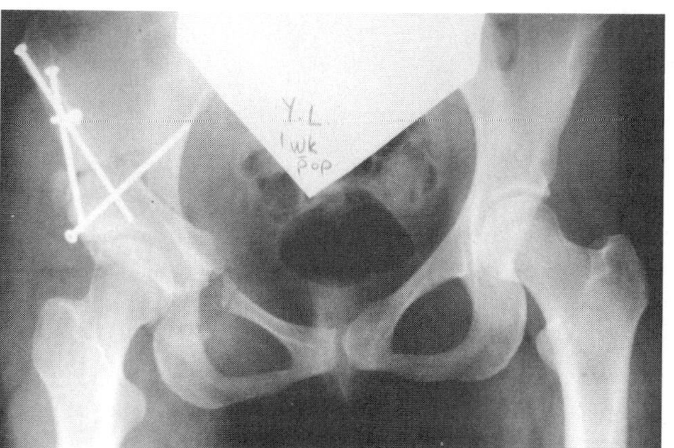

FIG. 49.9. This 20-year-old woman has developmental dysplasia of the hip. **A:** Maximal abduction anteroposterior radiograph of the pelvis demonstrating a congruous joint with improved lateral coverage in maximal abduction. **B:** Postoperative radiograph after Bernese periacetabular osteotomy.

with mild or moderate arthritis. However, intermediate and long-term results are not yet available. Trousdale et al. (43) reported the initial experience of 42 periacetabular osteotomies at a mean 4-year follow-up. Ninety-seven percent of patients with mild or moderate arthritis had a good or excellent result. Eighty-nine percent of individuals with significant arthritis had a poor result. The Bernese periacetabular osteotomy is technically difficult and associated with a high complication rate (43). The ideal candidate for periacetabular osteotomy is a young patient with hip dysplasia, but mild arthritis. The hip must be congruous. The patient should be more comfortable and have an improved radiographic appearance in abduction and internal rotation.

Pelvic salvage osteotomies include the Chiari osteotomy and the acetabular shelf procedure (44–48). Both procedures provide additional bone support superiorly at the lateral edge of the acetabulum. The Chiari osteotomy involves a transverse osteotomy at the level of the lateral bony margin of the acetabulum, extending into the greater sciatic notch. The acetabulum is displaced medially relative to the lateral aspect of the ilium. The ilium provides bony coverage over the hip capsule in the region of the uncovered femoral head. The results of the Chiari osteotomy in some series are surprisingly good, considering that the femoral head is not covered with articular cartilage. Hogh and Macnicol (49) reported 88% improvement in pain within the first year. Although the results deteriorated with time, four of the seven patients with 18-year follow-up had good function and mild pain. There are several variations of the acetabular shelf procedure (45–48,50) (Fig. 49.10). All of these procedures attempt to transfer hinged or free bone graft to cover the uncovered area of the femoral head overlying the hip capsule. Summers et al. (50) reviewed their experience with acetabular shelf osteotomies, noting 66% with good results at mean 16-year follow-up.

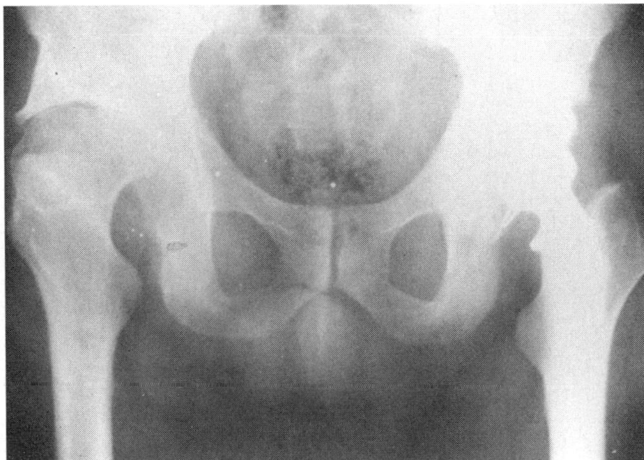

FIG. 49.10. Anteroposterior radiograph of the pelvis several years after a right acetabular shelf procedure. Note that the location of the acetabular shelf is at the same level as the subchondral bone of the acetabulum. There is a cemented total hip arthroplasty on the left side.

Proximal Femoral Osteotomies

Osteotomies of the proximal femur are indicated for selected patients with acetabular dysplasia, femoral neck nonunion, slipped capital femoral epiphysis, Legg-Calvé-Perthes disease, and AVN with femoral head collapse. Proper patient selection, preoperative planning, and precise technical correction is critical to successful outcome after proximal femoral osteotomies.

Proximal femoral varus osteotomy is indicated for acetabular dysplasia with coxa valga only when the clinical and radiographic appearance of the hip is improved with hip abduction. The patient should note improved comfort in abduction. The hip joint should be congruent with improved coverage of the femoral head in abduction. The acetabular index angle should ideally be less than 10 degrees (Fig. 49.11), or the varus intertrochanteric osteotomy should be combined with a pelvic osteotomy to restore a normal acetabular roof angle. The patient must have satisfactory range of abduction so that he or she is not left with an adduction contracture after the osteotomy. There is obligate extremity shortening and abductor weakness with varus intertrochanteric osteotomies of the femur. The patient should be aware of this before surgery. Preoperative planning is critical to successful outcome after any acetabular or femoral osteotomy. The addition of flexion, extension, or internal or external rotation to the osteotomy may be advantageous, based on the anatomy of the proximal femur and acetabulum. In planning a varus intertrochanteric osteotomy, we can estimate the optimal magnitude of correction based on the degree of hip abduction resulting in the optimal radiographic appearance and patient comfort. When planning a valgus intertrochanteric osteotomy, we can estimate the optimal magnitude of correction based on the degree of hip adduction resulting in the optimal radiography appearance and patient comfort. Technically, it is important to mark rotation before and after osteotomy to assure appropriate rotational correction. Preparing the channel for the blade plate before completing the osteotomy is advisable, because attempting to make the channel in a free proximal fragment is more difficult. Medial displacement of the distal fragment should be planned to restore the mechanical axis and align the femoral canal with the piriformis fossa.

Valgus intertrochanteric osteotomy may be indicated for some patients with congenital coxa vara, arthrokatadysis (Fig. 49.12), Legg-Calvé-Perthes disease with coxa magna, or hip dysplasia with a mushroom-cap deformity of the femoral head. Patients with the latter two conditions may have pain with abduction secondary to impingement and hinge abduction (42). Valgus intertrochanteric osteotomy is indicated when there is improvement in patient comfort and radiographic appearance with hip adduction. Valgus femoral osteotomy is occasionally accompanied by an ac-

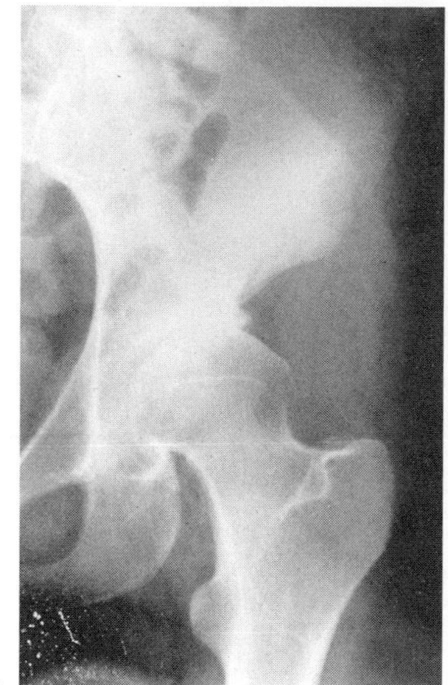

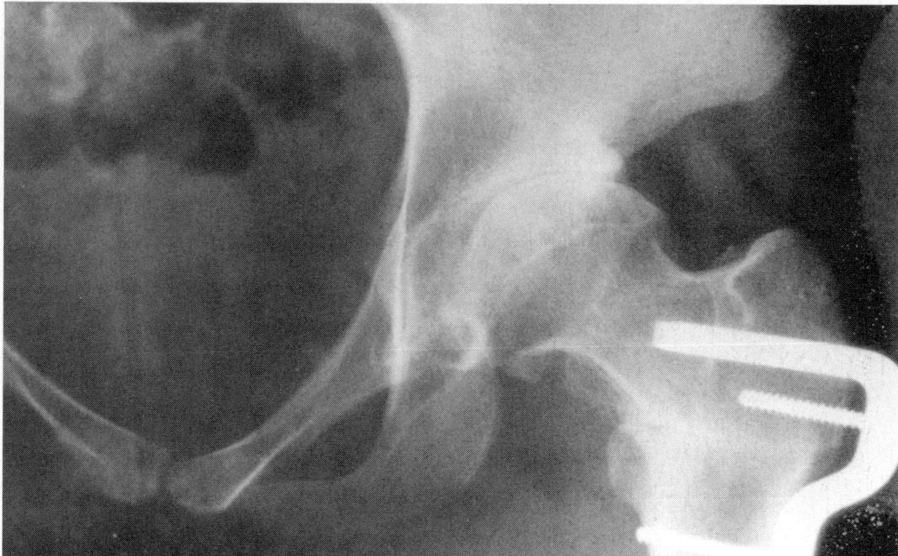

FIG. 49.11. Preoperative and postoperative radiographs of the left hip in a patient with osteoarthritis secondary to acetabular dysplasia. **A:** Anteroposterior radiograph demonstrating nearly complete obliteration of the superior joint space and an increased center edge angle of Wiberg, consistent with a diagnosis of acetabular dysplasia. Note that although the acetabulum has some lateral uncoverage, the acetabular index angle is horizontal. **B:** Anteroposterior radiograph of the left hip after varus intertrochanteric osteotomy, demonstrating some restoration of the superior joint space by rotating existing lateral femoral articular cartilage.

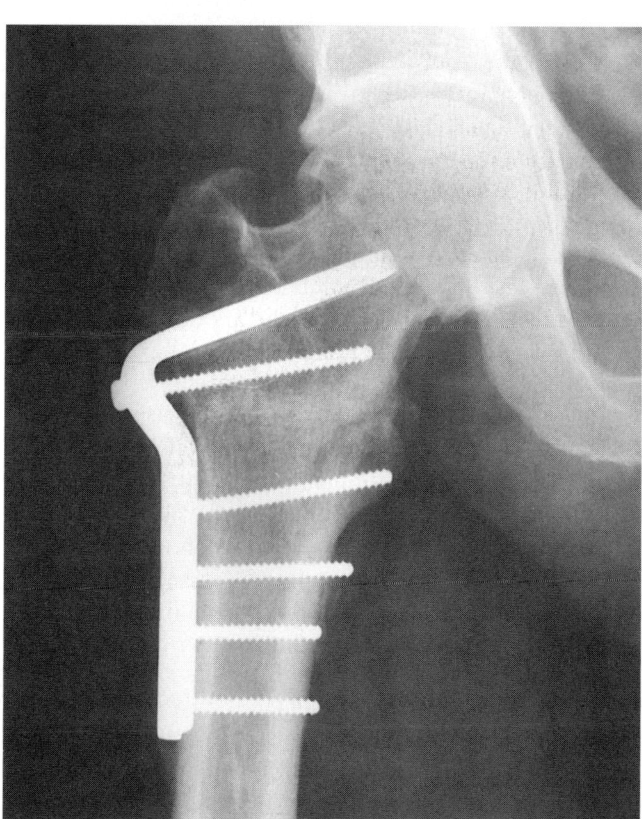

FIG. 49.12. Arthrokatadysis of the right hip in a 30-year-old man treated with valgus osteotomy. Early osteoarthritic alterations of the hip characterized by femoral head osteophytic formation and medial joint space narrowing secondary to the protrusion are evident on the anteroposterior radiograph. Two years after osteotomy, he had returned to manual labor.

etabular shelf procedure or a Chiari osteotomy to provide improved coverage of the femoral head.

Although satisfactory range of motion is generally a prerequisite to varus or valgus intertrochanteric osteotomy, there may be occasional indications for intertrochanteric osteotomies without satisfactory motion. After either surgical or spontaneous arthrodesis of the hip in a nonfunctional position, an intertrochanteric or subtrochanteric osteotomy allows proper alignment of the limb (Fig. 49.13). The result is a functional arthrodesis. Valgus osteotomies in the trochanteric region or at the base of the femoral neck also have been advocated to provide a more favorable biomechanical alignment to allow healing after nonunions of femoral neck fractures. Valgus or flexion osteotomies in the trochanteric region, or at the base of the femoral neck, may be considered for some patients with symptomatic healed displaced slipped capital femoral epiphysis (51).

The goal of proximal femoral osteotomy in the management of AVN is to rotate the area of articular collapse out from under the weight-bearing aspect of the hip joint. Most lesions are anterior and superior. Before considering any femoral osteotomy for AVN, the area of involvement must be assessed. Lesions with a combined arc of greater than 200 degrees on the anteroposterior and lateral radiographs are not amenable to standard intertrochanteric osteotomy of the proximal femur because of inability to rotate the lesion out of the weight-bearing aspect of the acetabulum (42). The osteotomy correction should be in the opposite direction, and of the same magnitude as the position (flexion, extension, abduction, adduction) where the area of involve-

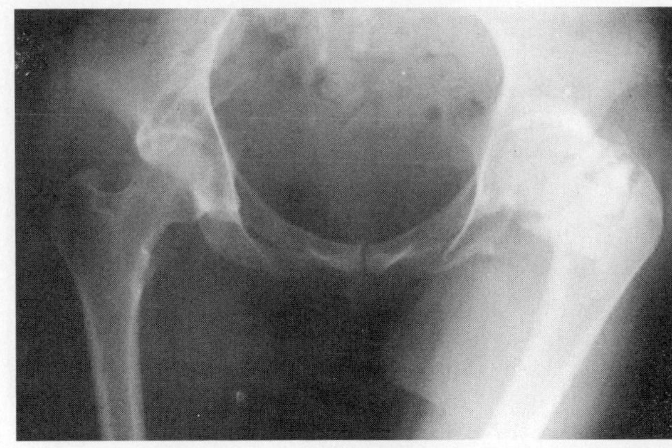
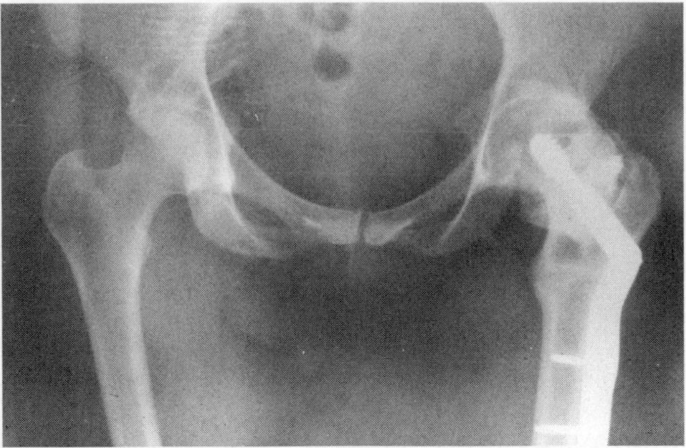

FIG. 49.13. Posttraumatic spontaneous arthrodesis of the hip in marked adduction, leading to marked disability. **A:** Anteroposterior radiograph of the pelvis, demonstrating posttraumatic adduction deformity with marked heterotopic ossification and functional arthrodesis. **B:** Anteroposterior radiograph of the pelvis after valgus intertrochanteric osteotomy.

ment has been transferred out of the weight-bearing region of the hip joint. Sugioka et al. (52) have reported success with a rotational intertrochanteric osteotomy in Japan. The excellent results reported by Sukioka et al. have not been successfully reproduced in North America.

Hip Arthrodesis

Hip arthrodesis (Fig. 49.14) is rarely performed at this time despite excellent long-term results with regard to pain relief and function. Once solid fusion of the hip occurs, pain relief is predictable. Hip arthrodesis is more durable than total hip arthroplasty; therefore, young patients are able to perform manual work successfully and engage in impact activities. Sponceller et al. (53) evaluated the results of 53 patients after hip arthrodesis at a mean 38-year follow-up (minimum 20 years). Seventy-eight percent were satisfied with their arthrodesis. Eighty-five percent of these patients worked outside of the home. Eighteen percent of the working patients performed heavy manual labor. Many patients participated in sporting activities.

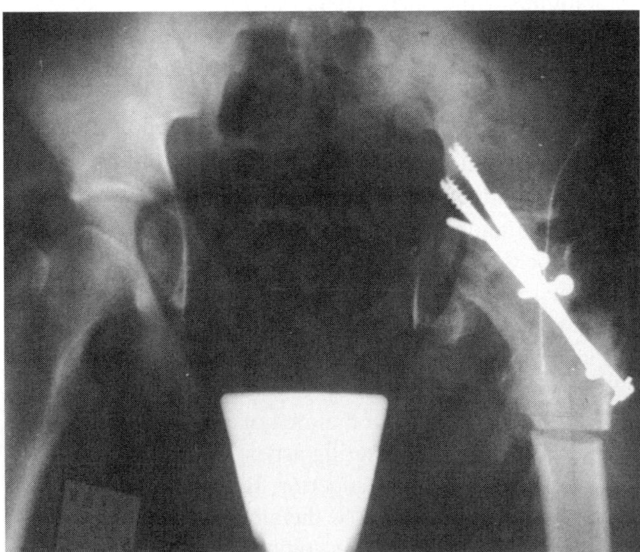

FIG. 49.14. Anteroposterior radiograph of the pelvis after hip arthrodesis with subtrochanteric osteotomy in a 300-pound 18-year-old man with end-stage avascular necrosis of the hip. Subtrochanteric osteotomy was performed to reduce the moment arm and improve the union rate of the arthrodesis in this large individual. The subtrochanteric osteotomy healed uneventfully with a spica cast, and allowed optimal positioning of the extremity.

There are several major reasons for the infrequency of hip arthrodesis today. These include the success of total hip arthroplasty, patients' preconceptions regarding the disability associated with arthrodesis, the technical difficulty of arthrodesis, the detrimental effect of arthrodesis on subsequent total hip replacement, and the deleterious effects of arthrodesis on the lower back, ipsilateral knee, and contralateral hip.

Callaghan et al. (54) evaluated the effects of hip arthrodesis on other joints. Sixty percent of patients developed significant ipsilateral knee pain at a mean of 23 years after hip arthrodesis. Chronic low back pain developed in 60% of patients at a mean of 25 years after hip arthrodesis. Twenty-five percent developed contralateral hip pain. All patients undergoing subsequent conversion to total hip arthroplasty due to low back pain noted relief of low back pain after hip replacement. Sponceller et al. (53) noted slightly lower rates of low back pain or ipsilateral knee pain at similar follow-up. Surgical arthrodesis of the hip compromises the results of total hip arthroplasty, particularly when the abductors are not preserved (55,56). Strathy and Fitzgerald (55) evaluated the results of 80 total hip arthroplasty procedures after either spontaneous or surgical hip arthrodesis. The investigators noted a high failure rate after conversion of surgical arthrodesis, especially if more than one attempt to achieve an arthrodesis was required. Among the 40 patients undergoing conversion of a surgically arthrodesed hip with minimum 9-year follow-up, there was a 20% rate of infection. An additional 30% of patients required revision for aseptic loosening or dislocation.

Total Hip Arthroplasty

The modern era of total hip replacement began with the introduction of low-friction arthroplasty by Sir John Charnley (57). Before the development of his low-friction design, Charnley noted early failures using a large-head press-fit stem with a Teflon acetabular component. During his first 4 years of performing total hip replacements from 1958 to 1962, his design evolved to the low-friction design consisting of a monoblock stainless-steel femoral component with a 22.25-mm diameter head articulating with a high-molecular-weight polyethylene acetabular component. Both components were fixed to the bone with polymethylmethacrylate bone cement.

Total hip arthroplasty resulted in such profound improvement in pain relief and function that many other procedures were essentially abandoned, except in younger patients. As the results and techniques improved, the indications expanded to include younger and more active patients. The use of total hip replacement in younger and more active patients, combined with occasional setbacks regarding implant design, has led to higher failure rates (58), sometimes with profound osteolysis, and associated bone loss (Fig. 49.15). The difficulty of salvaging these situations has resulted in pharmacologic, technical, and design modifications to prevent or lessen these problems.

Since the development of low-friction arthroplasty, advances and retreats have occurred regarding surgical technique, component design, and component fixation (59–62). Stainless steel has been replaced with titanium or cobalt-chromium in many designs. These superalloys have dramatically reduced the incidence of femoral stem fractures. Advances have been made with regard to cementing technique. First-generation cementing technique involved finger packing doughy cement into an unplugged femoral canal. Second-generation cement techniques involved the addition of pulsatile lavage of the femoral canal as well as retrograde injection of cement with a cement gun. The results after cemented femoral fixation with second-generation techniques are improved over those with first-generation technique in most series. Third- and fourth-generation cement techniques have evolved with the concepts of porosity reduction of cement, pressurization, surface modifications, and proximal and distal cement centralizers. Long-term results are not yet available to determine whether third- and fourth-generation techniques (Fig. 49.16) will be associated with improved outcome compared with second-generation techniques. Failures of cemented fixation, particularly in young active patients after first-generation cement technique, led to alternative methods of prosthetic fixation to bone.

The most popular methods of prosthetic fixation at this time include cementing both components, hybrid fixation with cement fixation of the femoral component and bone ingrowth into a porous-coated acetabular component (Fig. 49.17), and noncemented fixation with bone ingrowth into both femoral and acetabular components (Fig. 49.18). Hydroxyapatite has become increasingly popular as a means of enhancing bone ongrowth or ingrowth in noncemented applications. Many first-generation cementless femoral designs were associated with high failure rates, leading some

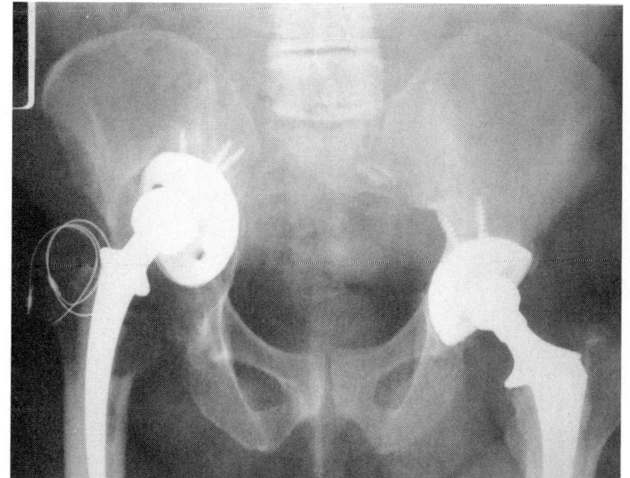

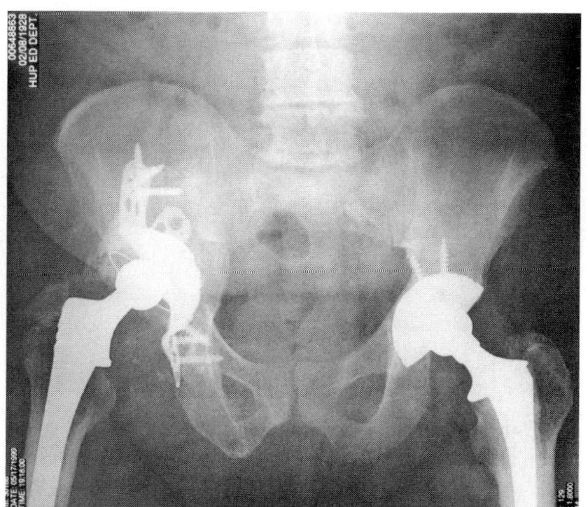

FIG. 49.15. This 71-year-old man had severe acetabular bone loss associated with a loose uncemented acetabular component 7.5 years after an acetabular revision. **A:** Preoperative anteroposterior view of the pelvis demonstrating the loose right acetabular component with severe bone loss. Review of prior radiographs demonstrated migration of the acetabular component with progressive bone loss. **B:** Anteroposterior radiograph of the pelvis 6 weeks after revision total hip arthroplasty with an acetabular reconstruction cage and allograft bone. Note that the femoral component was loose as well and required revision.

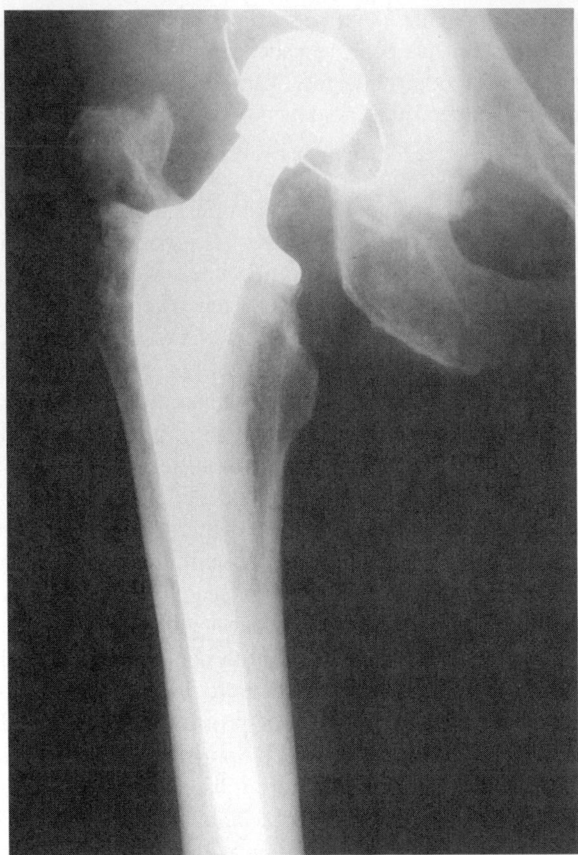

FIG. 49.16. Cemented total hip arthroplasty in a 70-year-old woman. Both the femoral and acetabular components were cemented using a fourth-generation cement technique. This anteroposterior radiograph was taken 45 years after surgery. The patient remains active without pain. There are no radiolucent lines in the bone–cement interface of either component. There has been a fracture of the posterior portion of the greater trochanter.

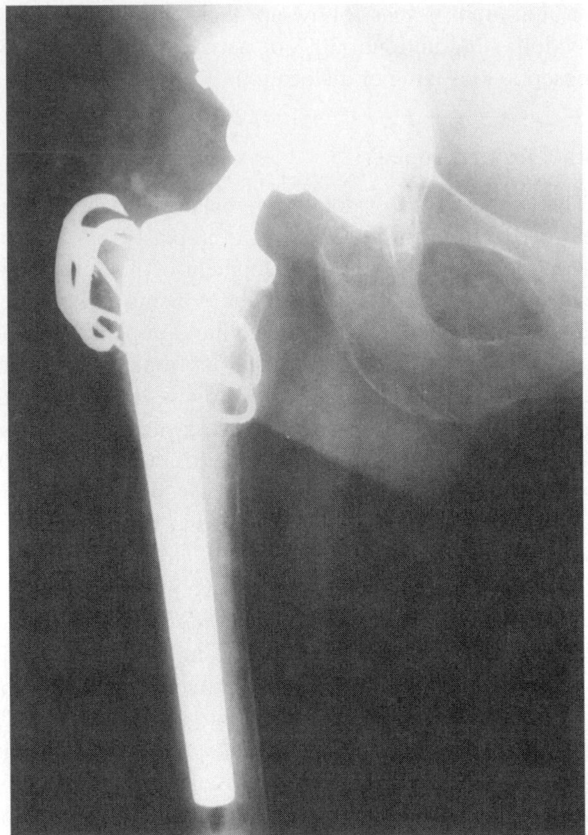

FIG. 49.17. Hybrid total arthroplasty of the right hip, characterized by a cemented femoral component and a cementless acetabular component in a 60-year-old woman with rheumatoid arthritis. The femoral cortices are thin because of severe osteoporosis. However, there were no radiolucent lines 4 years after surgery about either the cemented femoral component or the cementless acetabular component. A Dall-Miles cable grip and cables were used to reattach the greater trochanter at the time of the surgical procedure.

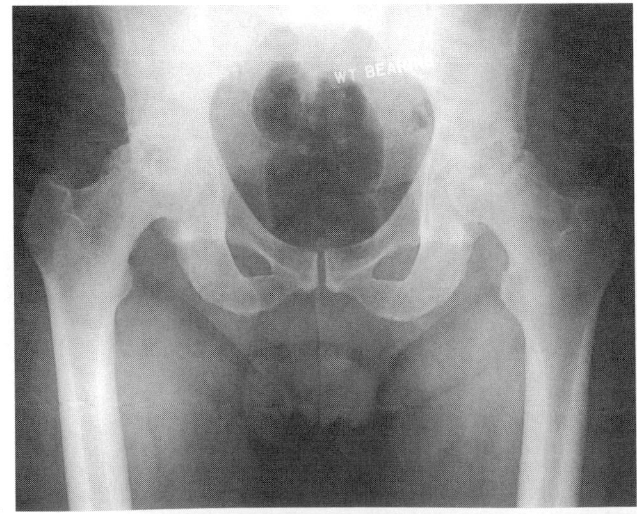

A

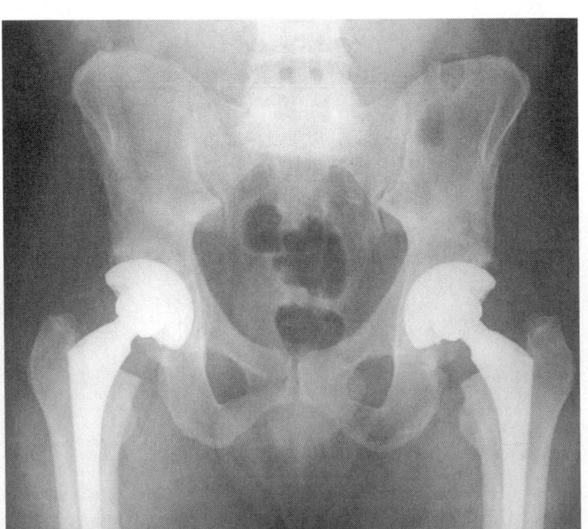

B

FIG. 49.18. This 54-year-old man had severe osteoarthritis of both hips. **A:** Preoperative anteroposterior radiograph of the pelvis demonstrating severe OA of both hips. **B:** Anteroposterior radiograph 6 months after bilateral uncemented total hip arthroplasties.

investigators to abandon noncemented femoral designs. Many early porous-coated acetabular designs, conversely, were associated with encouraging short- and intermediate-term results. These results, combined with improved cemented femoral results with second-generation and subsequent techniques, even in younger patients (63), led to increased interest in hybrid total hip replacement. Fully coated noncemented femoral components and certain circumferentially proximally coated tapered and hydroxyapatite-coated femoral designs have been associated with encouraging intermediate-term results, leading to interest in noncemented applications at many centers.

The standard articulating surface remains an ultra-high-molecular-weight acetabular liner against a polished cobalt-chrome head. However, there is increasing interest in ceramic against ultra-high-molecular-weight polyethylene articulations, ceramic-on-ceramic articulations, and metal-on-metal articulations using highly polished cobalt-chrome articulating surfaces. Although alternative bearings such as ceramic/ceramic or metal/metal have been championed by some investigators to decrease wear and improve longevity of total hip replacement, other investigators have attempted to improve the wear characteristics of polyethylene with cross-linking. A ceramic head articulating with a ceramic liner results in the least amount of wear debris and hopefully a longer-lasting implant. This is a promising alternative for the younger patient. The risk for fracture of the ceramic components is about 1 in 10,000, and must be taken into consideration. Ceramic fracture is a catostrophic failure and results in a difficult revision because of the debris (64). Another alternative is a ceramic head and highly cross-linked polyethylene articulation (65).

Modularity has resulted in positive and negative effects. Modularity allows customization of implant to anatomy (Fig. 49.19), combination of materials, decreased inventory, and the possibility of partial component exchange as opposed to revision. However, modularity also introduces the potential of dissociation, and fretting or wear at the junction between components.

Controversy continues with regard to the best mode and technique of fixation, implant design, and articulating surfaces. Excellent results are possible with a number of designs. The appropriate design is probably dependent on the patient's age, activity level, anatomy, goals, and associated medical conditions, as well as the skills of the surgeon.

Recently, less invasive surgical approaches have been advocated with proposed advantages including more rapid rehabilitation, less blood loss, improved cosmesis, and a more stable soft tissue envelop. Using specialized instruments, it is now possible to perform a total hip arthroplasty through a 5- to 10-cm incision. A two-incision approach with two 3-cm incisions is also being evaluated. Early results are showing a decreased hospital stay, early improved functional results, and earlier return to work (66,67). The

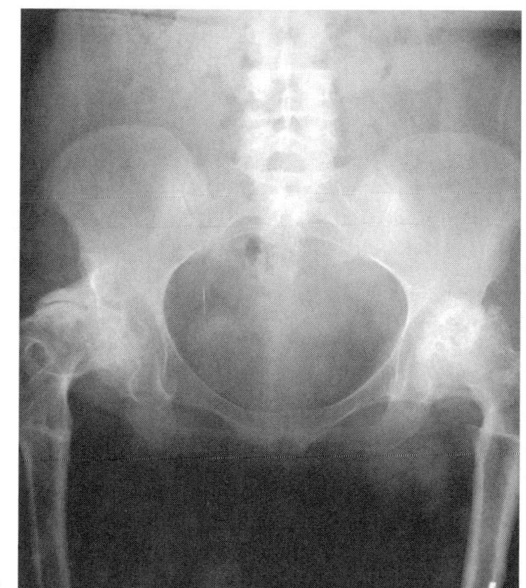

A

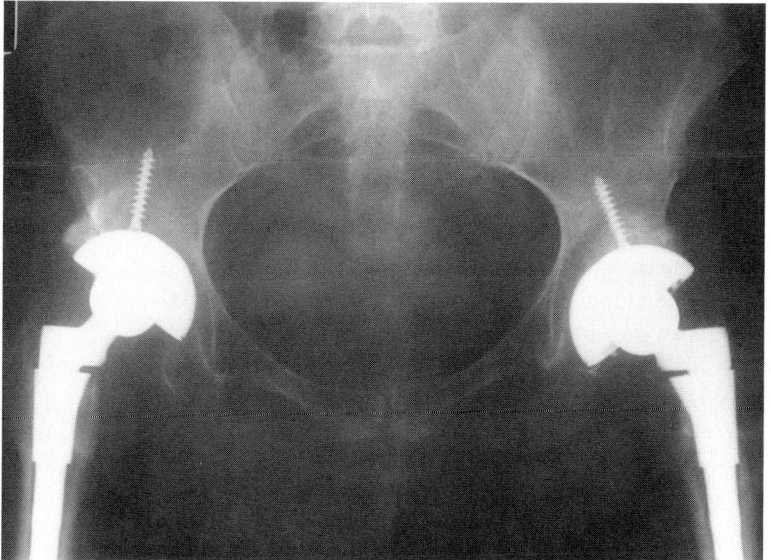

B

FIG. 49.19. This 52-year-old woman had severe osteoarthritis of both hips secondary to acetabular dysplasia. She underwent a right acetabular shelf procedure combined with a proximal femoral osteotomy 12 years before her initial evaluation and then a left proximal femoral osteotomy 8 years before evaluation. **A:** Preoperative anteroposterior view of the pelvis demonstrating severe arthritic involvement of both hips with alteration of her anatomy after prior surgical procedures. Standard nonmodular components are not compatible with the anatomy present without reosteotomizing the femur, or calcar replacement. **B:** Postoperative radiograph after bilateral uncemented total hip arthroplasty procedures with a modular prosthesis allowing adaptation to the postosteotomy deformity with restoration of normal femoral anteversion.

two-incision technique preserves the attachments of both the abductor muscles and short external rotator. This technique has been performed on an outpatient basis. Proponents of the two-incision technique claim significantly improved hip stability compared with traditional techniques minimizing the need for hip precautions to prevent dislocation following surgery.

Complications after total hip arthroplasty have been described in depth in the past. In his original article outlining his experience with low-friction arthroplasty, Charnley (57) listed his complications. Despite short follow-up, the complications described encompass most of the short-term and long-term complications recognized today. The short-term complications most commonly attributed to total hip arthroplasty today include wound drainage or dehiscence, wound hematoma, infection, deep venous thrombosis, pulmonary embolism, neurovascular injury, periprosthetic fracture, and heterotopic ossification. Bowel and bladder dysfunction may be related to postsurgical pain and postoperative narcotics. Infection and periprosthetic fracture also may occur as late complications. Aseptic loosening, osteolysis, and bone remodeling are long-term complications after hip replacement. Implant failure such as ceramic fracture or fracture of a metallic prosthesis is generally a late complication, but may occur at any time.

CONCLUSION

When conservative management fails, total hip arthroplasty and joint-preserving alternatives to hip replacement provide the orthopedic surgeon with an armamentarium to improve markedly the physical, psychological, and functional state of many patients with significant arthritic hip deformities. There are advantages and disadvantages of each of the procedures described for a particular patient and surgeon. The pathology, goals, and expectations of the patient, and the experience of the surgeon are critical before recommending surgical intervention for any patient. High patient satisfaction may be anticipated in most cases, provided the clinician uses sound clinical judgment, properly assesses patient's goals and expectations, and communicates realistic expectations to the patient. New implant technology may result in decreased wear debris and a longer period of time before need for revision. Improvements on surgical techniques and bone loss management allow improved outcomes when revision surgery becomes necessary. These improvements make total hip arthroplasty a more viable option for the younger patient with severe arthritic deformities.

REFERENCES

1. Schulte KR, Callaghan JJ, Kelley SS, et al. The outcome of Charnley total hip arthroplasty with cement after a minimum twenty-year follow-up: the results of one surgeon. *J Bone Joint Surg Am* 1993; 75:961–975.
2. Fitzgerald RH. Acetabular labral tears. *Clin Orthop* 1995;311:60–68.
3. McCarthy JC, Busconi B. The role of hip arthroscopy in the diagnosis and treatment of hip disease. *Can J Surg* 1995;38(suppl 1):13–17.
4. Fario LA, Glick JM, Sampson TG. Hip arthroscopy for acetabular labral tears. *Arthroscopy* 1999;15:132–137.
5. Hase T, Ueo T. Acetabular labral tear: arthroscopic diagnosis and treatment. *Arthroscopy* 1999;15:138–141.
6. Tonnis D. *Congenital dysplasia and dislocation of the hip in children and in adults.* Heidelberg: Springer, 1987.
7. Lequesne M, de Seze S. Le faux profil du bassin: nouvelle incidence radiographique pour Petude de la hanche: son utilité dans les dysplasies et les differentes coxopathies. *Rev Rhum Mal Osteoartic* 1961; 28:643.
8. Hofmann S, Tschauner C, Urban M, et al. Clinical and diagnostic imaging of the labrum in lesions of the hip joint. *Orthopade* 1998;27: 681–689.
9. Leunig M, Werlen S, Ungersbock A, et al. *J Bone Joint Surg Br* 1997;79:230–234.
10. Urban M, Hofmann S, Czerny C, et al. MRI arthrography in labrum lesions of the hip joint: method and diagnostic value. *Orthopade* 1998; 27:691–698.
11. Niitsu M, Mishima H, Itai Y. High resolution MR imaging of the hip using pelvic phased-array coil. *Nippon Acta Radiol* 1997;57:58–60.
12. Bombelli R, ed. *Structure and function in normal and abnormal hips: how to rescue mechanically jeopardized hips,* 3rd ed. Berlin: Springer-Verlag, 1993.
13. Pauwels F. *Biomechanics of the normal and disabled hip.* Heidelberg: Springer, 1976.
14. Lloyd-Roberts GC. Osteoarthritis of the hip. *J Bone Joint Surg Br* 1955;37:8–47.
15. Stulberg SD, Cordell LD, Harris WH, et al. Unrecognized childhood hip disease: a major cause of idiopathic osteoarthritis of the hip. In: Amstutz HC, ed. *The hip.* St. Louis: CV Mosby, 1975:212–228.
16. Crowe JF, Mani VJ, Ranawat CS. Total hip replacement in congenital dislocation and dysplasia of the hip. *J Bone Joint Surg Am* 1979;61: 15–23.
17. Legg AT. An obscure affection of the hip joint. *Boston Med Surg J* 1910;162:202.
18. Calve J. Sur une forme particuliere de coxalgie greffe, et sur des deformations caracteristiques de l'extreite superieure de femur. *Rev Chir* 1910;42:54.
19. Perthes G. Uber arthritis deformans juvenilis. *Dtsch Z Chir* 1910; 10:111.
20. Sevitt S. Avascular necrosis and revascularization of the femoral head after intracapsular fractures. *J Bone Joint Surg Br* 1964;46:270–296.
21. Barnes R, Brown JT, Garden RS, et al. Subcapital fractures of the femur: a prospective review. *J Bone Joint Surg Br* 1976;58:2–24.
22. Asnis SE, Wanek-Sgaglione L. Intracapsular fractures of the femoral neck: results of cannulated screw fixation. *J Bone Joint Surg Am* 1994; 76:1793–1803.
23. Aaron RK. Osteonecrosis: etiology, pathophysiology, and diagnosis. In: Callaghan JJ, Rosenberg AG, Rubash HE, eds. *The adult hip.* Philadelphia: Lippincott-Raven, 1998:451–466.
24. Steinberg DR, Steinberg ME. Osteonecrosis. In: Kelley WN, Harris ED, Ruddy S, et al., eds. *Textbook of rheumatology.* Philadelphia: WB Saunders, 1989:1749–1773.
25. Taurog JD. Genetics and immunology of the spondyloarthropathies. *Curr Opin Rheumatol* 1989;1:144–150.
26. Berman AT, Quartararo L. Septic arthritis, In: Callaghan JJ, Rosenberg AG, Rubash HE, eds. *The adult hip.* Philadelphia: Lippincott-Raven, 1998:575–591.
27. Hooper JC, Jones EW, Primary protrusio of the acetabulum. *J Bone Joint Surg Br* 1971;53:23–29.
28. Alexander C. The etiology of primary protrusio acetabuli. *Br J Radiol* 1965;38:567–580.
29. MacDonald D. Primary protrusio acetabuli: report of an affected family. *J Bone Joint Surg Br* 1971;53:30–36.
30. McCarthy JC, Day B, Busconi B. Hip arthroscopy: applications and technique. *J Acad Orthop Surg* 1995;3:115–122.
31. Fairbank AC, Bhatia D, Jinnah RH, et al. Long-term results of core decompression for ischaemic necrosis of the femoral head. *J Bone Joint Surg Br* 1995;77:42–49.
32. Steinberg ME. Core decompression of the femoral head for avascular necrosis: indications and results. *Can J Surg* 1995;38(suppl):18–24.

33. Buckley PD, Gearan PF, Petty RW. Structural bone-grafting for early atraumatic avascular necrosis of the femoral head, *J Bone Joint Surg Am* 1991;73:1357–1364.
34. Urbaniac J. Treatment of osteonecrosis of the femoral head with free vascularized fibular grafting. *J Bone Joint Surg Am* 1995;77:681–694.
35. Camp JF, Cowell CW. Core decompression of the femoral head for osteonecrosis. *J Bone Joint Surg Am* 1986;68:1313–1319.
36. Salter RB. Innominate osteotomy in the treatment of congenital dislocation and subluxation of the hip. *J Bone Joint Surg Br* 1961;43:518–539.
37. Sutherland DH, Greenfield R. Double innominate osteotomy. *J Bone Joint Surg Am* 1977;59:1082.
38. Steele HH. Triple osteotomy of the innominate bone. *J Bone Joint Surg Am* 1973;55:343.
39. Tonnis D. *Huftluxation und Hufttkopfnekose, Eine Sammel-statistik des Arbeitskieises fur Huftdysplasie Enke*. Stuttgart: Bucherei des Orthopoden Bd, 1978:581.
40. Eppright RH. Dial osteotomy of acetabulum in the treatment of dysplasia of the hip. *J Bone Joint Surg Am* 1975;57:1172.
41. Ganz R, Klaue K, Vinh TS, et al. A new periacetabular osteotomy for the treatment of hip dysplasias: technique and preliminary results. *Clin Orthop* 1988;232:26–36.
42. Millis MB, Murphy SB, Poss R. Osteotomies about the hip for prevention and treatment of osteoarthrosis. *Instr Course Lect* 1996;45:209–226.
43. Trousdale RT, Ekkernkamp A, Ganz R, et al. Periacetabular and intertrochanteric osteotomy for the treatment of osteoarthrosis in dysplastic hips. *J Bone Joint Surg Am* 1995;77:73–85.
44. Chiari K. Medial displacement osteotomy of the pelvis. *Clin Orthop* 1974;98:55–71.
45. Gill AB. Operation for old irreducible congenital dislocation of the hip. *J Bone Joint Surg Am* 1928;10:696–711.
46. Staheli LT. Slotted acetabular augmentation. *J Pediatr Orthop* 1981; 1:321–327.
47. Lowman CL. The double-leaf shelf operation for congenital dislocation of the hip. *J Bone Joint Surg Am* 1931;13:511–514.
48. Saito S, Takaoka K, Ono K. Tectoplasty for painful dislocation or subluxation of the hip: long-term evaluation of a new acetabuloplasty. *J Bone Joint Surg Br* 1986;68:55–60.
49. Hogh J, Macnicol MF. The Chiari pelvic osteotomy: a long-term review of clinical and radiographic results. *J Bone Joint Surg Br* 1987; 69:365–373.
50. Summers BN, Turner A, Wynn-Jones CH. The shelf operation in the management of late presentation of congenital hip dysplasia. *J Bone Joint Surg Br* 1988;70:63–68.
51. Schai PA, Exner GU, Hansch O. Prevention of secondary coxarthrosis in slipped capital femoral epiphysis: a long-term study after corrective intertrochanteric osteotomy. *J Pediatr Orthop* 1996;5:135–143.
52. Sugioka Y, Hotokebuchi T, Tsutsui H. Transtrochanteric anterior rotational osteotomy for idiopathic and steroid induced necrosis of the femoral head: indications and long-term results. *Clin Orthop* 1992; 277:111–120.
53. Sponceller PD, McBeath AA, Perpich M. Hip arthrodesis in young patients: a long-term follow-up study. *J Bone Joint Surg Am* 1984;66: 853–859.
54. Callaghan JJ, Brand RA, Pedersen DR. Hip arthrodesis. *J Bone Joint Surg Am* 1985;67:1328–1335.
55. Strathy GM, Fitzgerald RH. Total hip arthroplasty in the ankylosed hip: a ten year follow-up. *J Bone Joint Surg Am* 1988;70:963–966.
56. Brewster RC, Coventry MB, Johnson EW. Conversion of the arthrodesed hip to a total hip arthroplasty. *J Bone Joint Surg Am* 1975; 57:27–30.
57. Charnley J. Total hip replacement by low-friction arthroplasty. *Clin Orthop* 1970;72:7–21.
58. Chandler HP, Reineck FT, Wixson RL, et al. Total hip replacement in patients younger than 30 years old. *J Bone Joint Surg Am* 1981;63: 1426.
59. Law WA. Late results of vitallium-mold arthroplasty of the hip. *J Bone Joint Surg Am* 1962;44:1497.
60. McKee GK, Watson-Ferrar J. Replacement of the arthritic hip by the McKee-Ferrar prosthesis *J Bone Joint Surg Br* 1966;48:245–259.
61. Langenskiold A, Salenius P. Total hip replacement of the hip by the McKee-Ferrar prosthesis. *Clin Orthop* 1970;72:104–105.
62. Chapchal G, Muller W. Total hip replacement with the McKee prosthesis. *Clin Orthop* 1970;72:115–122.
63. Mulroy WF, Estok DM, Harris WH. Total hip arthroplasty with use of so-called second generation cementing techniques: a fifteen year average follow-up study. *J Bone Joint Surg Am* 1995;77:1845.
64. Allain J, Delcrin J, Migaud H, et al. Revision total hip arthroplasty performed after fracture of a ceramic femoral head. A multicenter survivorship study. *J Bone Joint Surg Am* 2003;85:825.
65. Urban JA, Garvin KL, Boese CK, et al. Ceramic-on-polyethylene bearing surfaces in total hip arthroplasty. Seventeen to twenty-one-year results. *J Bone Joint Surg Am* 2001;83(11):1688.
66. Berger RA. Mini-incisions: two for the price of one! Presented at Current Concepts in Joint Replacement–Winter 2001, Orlando, FL, December 13, 2001.
67. Rodrigo JJ. Interview on minimally invasive hip surgery. *Orthopedics* 2002;25(10):1016.

CHAPTER 50

Surgical Treatment of Knee Arthritis

K. David Moore and John M. Cuckler

Surgical intervention in the management of knee arthritis may be appropriate if medical and less invasive modalities fail to control pain, instability, or other symptoms related to the underlying arthritic condition. Selection of the appropriate intervention will depend on the age, activity status, and life expectancy of the patient, in addition to the precise underlying etiology of the arthritic problem. Knowledge of the relative risks and benefits of each surgical procedure will help the clinician managing the arthritic knee to appropriately refer a patient for surgical intervention.

Surgery for knee arthritis can range in complexity from simple arthroscopic débridement to total knee arthroplasty (TKA). Other procedures that may be appropriate for selected patients include synovectomy, osteotomy, unicompartmental replacement, and even arthrodesis. Cartilage implantation or transplantation procedures may also prove to be useful therapeutic options. A review of the relative indications and contraindications of these techniques and the documented risks and benefits for these procedures will help physicians managing patients with knee arthritis to participate in the decision-making process with both the patient and the consulting surgeon.

SURGICAL CONSIDERATIONS

The underlying etiology and pattern of knee arthritis should be considered when selecting possible surgical interventions for a specific patient. In general, arthritis of the knee (as with other joints) can be categorized as noninflammatory or inflammatory in etiology. Noninflammatory arthritis is by far the most common presentation of knee arthritis, and typically will occur as involvement of one or two of the three compartments of the knee. Osteoarthritis (OA) in the knee is typically seen with medial hemijoint involvement, although concurrent involvement of the patella femoral joint is common. Early diagnosis of OA of the knee is most easily made with a standing anteroposterior (AP) view of the knee (Figs. 50.1 and 50.2). Asymmetric loss of the medial hemijoint articular space will usually precede, by some years, the appearance of osteophytes, sclerosis, or other radiographic signs consistent with OA. In contrast, inflammatory arthritis of the knee typically occurs with a symmetric loss of the articular space in both the medial and

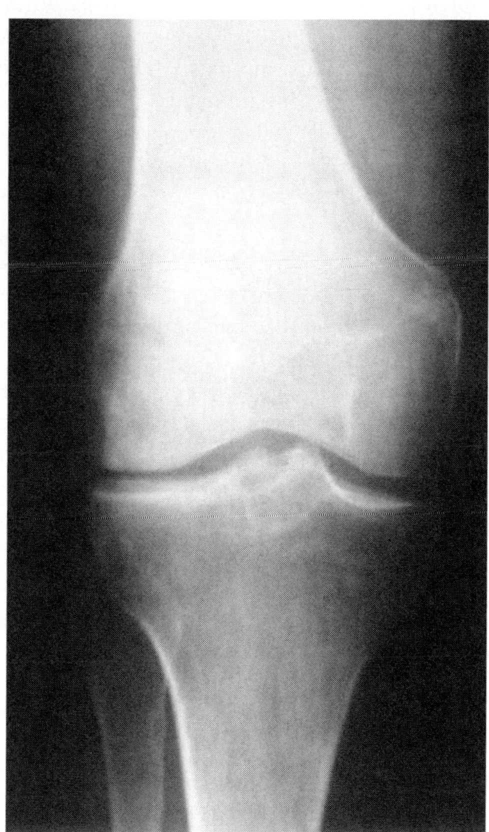

FIG. 50.1. Supine anteroposterior radiographs of the left knee of a 62-year-old man.

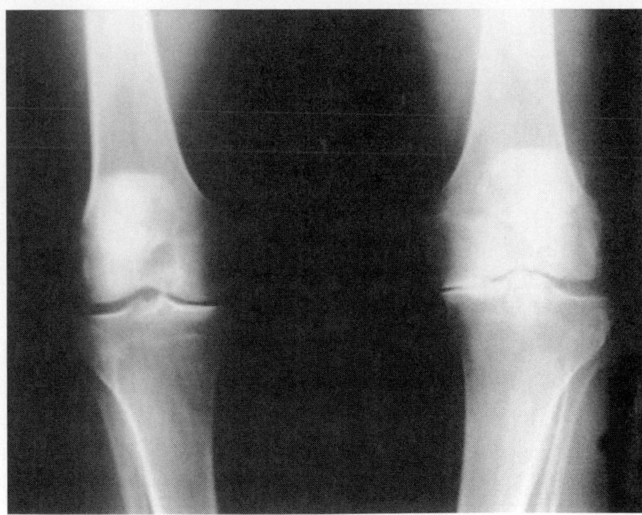

FIG. 50.2. Standing anteroposterior radiographs of the patient obtained the same day. Note the loss of medial articular space and the obvious varus alignment of the femorotibial axis, confirming the clinical diagnosis of osteoarthritis. This patient would have a low probability of lasting improvement from arthroscopic débridement.

lateral hemijoints when viewed on a standing AP view of the knee.

Noninflammatory arthritic conditions of the knee may be appropriate for surgical interventions such as arthroscopic débridement, cartilage auto- or allograft procedures, osteotomy, unicompartmental arthroplasty, TKA, or in rare cases, arthrodesis. In contrast, inflammatory arthritic syndromes are more amenable to surgical interventions such as synovectomy, total arthroplasty, or rarely, arthrodesis.

THE ROLE OF ARTHROSCOPY IN MANAGEMENT OF THE ARTHRITIC KNEE

The technique of arthroscopic surgery in the knee has advanced rapidly over the past 20 years (see Chapter 5). The procedure is now routinely performed as outpatient surgery, and rehabilitation is relatively rapid compared with previous open arthrotomy techniques. The procedures may be performed under local, regional, or general anesthetic, as dictated by the needs of the surgeon and the patient. The procedures generally take no longer than 1 hour and are not associated with significant blood loss.

The power of the arthroscope lies in its ability to provide an accurate diagnosis of the intraarticular structures within the knee joint. The accuracy of arthroscopy approaches 100% with regard to diagnosis of intraarticular pathology and has been shown to be more precise and sensitive than noninvasive magnetic resonance imaging (MRI) (1,2). In contrast, studies such as the MRI become less reliable with increasing age of the patient, because of the ambiguity inherently resulting from degenerative changes within the joint. Increasing age leads to loss of proteoglycan and consequently the water content in the cartilaginous structures of the joint, which can lead to equivocal interpretation of MRIs with regard to the existence of meniscal tears versus simple degeneration of structures (3,4).

The role of arthroscopy in the management of various forms of knee arthritis is still evolving. Unfortunately, the data available in the current literature are in general marred by the absence of prospective, randomized, and blinded assessment designs. Additionally, the characterization of the extent of intraarticular pathology and the precise nature of the intraarticular surgery are difficult to compare among published reports of these procedures. However, sufficient clinical data are beginning to accrue to guide the clinician in the use of this technology for patients with both inflammatory and noninflammatory arthritic disorders.

Arthroscopy for Osteoarthritis of the Knee

Judicious selection of patients is critical to successful outcome of arthroscopic treatment of patients with noninflammatory arthritis of the knee. Diagnostic arthroscopy may be of help in the OA knee in at least five situations: a painful swollen knee with normal radiographs and noninflammatory fluid; clinical and radiographic OA with pain out of proportion to radiographic findings and refractory to conventional medical therapy; chronic, stable (radiographic) OA with sudden, profound worsening of symptoms; OA with primarily "mechanical" symptoms; and OA with unexpected synovial fluid characteristics (5). However, it appears that the enthusiasm of the surgeon for débridement of articular cartilage or meniscal lesions must be tempered by careful preoperative evaluation.

It is unclear whether simple saline irrigation of the joint (which is a routine part of the arthroscopic procedure) may in and of itself produce significant clinical improvement. A study by Chang et al. (6) that randomly compared arthroscopic surgery with closed-needle joint lavage in patients with OA of the knee concluded that overall, there was no significant difference at 1 year after the procedure between those patients who had undergone the surgical procedure and those who had simply undergone irrigation of the joint. However, it was observed that patients with meniscal tears had a higher probability of improvement after arthroscopic surgery than did those patients with articular cartilage lesions who had undergone débridement. Merchan and Galindo (7) concluded in their prospective study of arthroscopic débridement of the arthritic knee versus nonoperative conservative treatment that surgically débrided patients had significant improvement compared with those patients conservatively managed. Their conclusions suggested that patients with a normal femorotibial mechanical axis with sudden onset of knee pain were the best candidates for arthroscopic débridement. This is similar to the conclusions of Baumgaertner et al. (8), who, in a retrospective review of patients with OA of the knee, found that symptoms of long duration, or more advanced arthritis as evidenced by loss of the normal valgus femorotibial alignment, were more likely to produce poor outcomes of arthroscopic débridement. The review by Rand (9) confirms the efficacy of débridement of degenerative meniscal tears in patients with degenerative arthritis of the knee as long as preoperative radiographs do not demonstrate subchondral sclerosis or osteophyte formation in the involved hemijoint. Other reported series confirm these results (10,11).

In contradistinction to the studies outlined above, Dervin et al. (12) prospectively studied 126 patients undergoing arthroscopic débridement for OA. They noted an overall success rate of only 44%. Only patients with medial joint line tenderness, a positive Steinmann test result for meniscal irritability, and the presence of an unstable meniscal tear at the time of arthroscopy had a sustained, clinically significant improvement. Most recently, Moseley et al. (13) called into question the efficacy of arthroscopy in OA. These researchers randomized 165 patients with knee OA to receive arthoscopic débridement, arthroscopic lavage, or placebo surgery. No differences in pain or function was noted in any of the three treatment groups compared with placebo.

Arthroscopic débridement of articular cartilage lesions is also controversial. Débridement of articular cartilage lesions seen in knee OA is variously referred to as "chondroplasty" or "abrasion chondroplasty," which is sometimes accompanied by simultaneous penetration of the subchondral bone, which is referred to as "subchondral drilling" or "subchondral picking" (14). These procedures in humans are performed to attempt to stimulate resurfacing of a denuded area of subchondral bone by fibrocartilage, although animal experiments have not consistently demonstrated success with these procedures (15). More recent attempts at resurfacing chondral injuries have used autogenous "plug grafts" of articular cartilage and subchondral bone from nonarticulating sections of the femoral condyles, a procedure known as "mosaicplasty" (16–18). Results at 2 to 3 years after transplantation appear to demonstrate viable hyaline cartilage according to anecdotal reports; the procedure is not indicated for OA or in patients over 50 years of age.

The functional long-term outcomes of arthroscopic procedures do not appear to provide consistent positive benefits to patients. In a retrospective study by Bert and Maschka (19), the 5-year outcomes of abrasion arthroplasty and débridement versus débridement alone in 126 patients with unicompartmental OA revealed that those patients who underwent arthroscopic débridement alone had a better outcome than did those who underwent an abrasion chondroplasty and arthroscopic débridement simultaneously. These researchers concluded that abrasion arthroplasty may not produce as good a result as simple arthroscopic débridement of degenerative lesions of both articular cartilage and menisci.

Other reports suggest that abrasion chondroplasty or subchondral bone penetration may be at best transient. Johnson has reported that although 75% of OA patients treated with abrasion arthroplasty reported initial "satisfactory" improvement, only 12% had no symptoms at 2-year follow-up (20). Friedman et al. reported on 73 patients treated with débridement and abrasion arthroplasty and at an average of 12 months after treatment, 60% were "improved," 34% were unchanged, and 6% were worse (21). Linschoten and Johnson have concluded that the outcome of arthroscopic débridement is directly related to the status of the articular cartilage at the time of surgery (22).

In summary, the "ideal" patient for an arthroscopic evaluation in noninflammatory knee arthritis is a patient with a near-normal femoral tibial alignment, without significant osteophyte formation or subchondral sclerosis. Patients with degenerative tears of menisci and resulting mechanical symptoms generally have better outcomes than do those with degenerative meniscal tears plus full-thickness lesions of the articular cartilage. It does not appear that abrasion arthroplasty offers significant long-term improvement in patients with knee OA.

Risks of Arthroscopic Surgery

Relative to other surgical procedures, the risks of arthroscopic surgery are minimal. They are primarily confined to the inherent risk of the anesthetic used. The risk for infection from the procedure has been estimated at less than 0.5% (23). As with surgical procedures in general, increased risk for infection appears to be related to length of the procedure, patient comorbid conditions such as diabetes, treatment with immunosuppressive medications, and the use of intraoperative intraarticular steroids at the conclusion of the procedure. The use of intraarticular long-acting corticosteroids at the end of an arthroscopic procedure is favored by some surgeons in an effort to minimize postoperative synovitis. Thrombophlebitis is a potential risk of arthroscopic procedures (24,25); the risk for deep vein thrombosis is quite low, but the risk is related to use of a tourniquet and age of the patient. Other possible complications include instrument breakage, hemarthrosis, and nerve injury; these are less common than deep vein thrombosis or infection (26,27).

Recovery from arthroscopic procedures is relatively fast, with most patients returning to their preoperative status within 2 weeks of the procedure. Most patients with knee OA who undergo arthroscopic débridement continue to require appropriate medical management.

SYNOVECTOMY OF THE KNEE

In clinical situations where inflammatory arthritis [e.g., rheumatoid arthritis (RA)] is unresponsive to medical therapy, synovectomy of the knee is often successful in decreasing swelling and pain. Indications for synovectomy are not clearly established, but generally the criteria of failure of appropriate medical management for a period of 6 to 12 months in the absence of significant radiographic changes may be accepted as an appropriate indication for consideration of synovectomy.

The advent of the arthroscope has led to resurgence in interest in synovectomy as a palliative procedure for inflammatory arthritis. Traditional open synovectomy has been associated with loss of motion in the knee joint. Multiple reports of the outcome of arthroscopic synovectomy appear to indicate that loss of motion is less a problem than is seen after open synovectomy, and that the outcome of arthroscopic synovectomy in palliation of inflammatory arthritis is equally effective.

A review by Doets et al. concluded that although arthroscopic synovectomy in patients with RA produced "fair or good" results in 50% of the cases, half of the 83 patients in this series had undergone total knee replacement at a mean interval of 4 years after synovectomy (28). These researchers concluded that early synovectomy did not prevent progression of the degenerative process in patients with RA. This conclusion is similar to that of McEwen, who concluded that open synovectomy in patients with RA of the knee did not slow the progression of the disease process (29). Matsui et al. have also reported gradual deterioration in clinical function among both patients who had undergone open synovectomy and those who had undergone arthroscopic synovectomy in RA of the knee (30). However, arthroscopic synovectomy was associated with less loss of motion and more rapid return of function than was open synovectomy.

Arthroscopic synovectomy appears to be a useful alternative to open synovectomy in the management of septic arthritis (31). Schoen et al. reported 80% success in using arthroscopic synovectomy in the management of refractory chronic Lyme arthritis of the knee among 16 patients followed up for 3 to 8 years (32).

The advantage of arthroscopic synovectomy therefore appears to be shorter hospitalization and more rapid rehabilitation with less risk of loss for motion than that associated with open synovectomy. Arthroscopic synovectomy in patients with RA may be associated with moderate blood loss. Generally, a suction drain is left in the joint for at least 24 hours. Most patients are hospitalized 24 to 48 hours after arthroscopic synovectomy. Early range of motion, with or without the use of continuous passive motion machines, is important to minimize the risk of loss of motion after this procedure. Although synovectomy may transiently reduce the swelling associated with inflammatory arthritis of the knee, it does not appear that synovectomy significantly alters the progression of degenerative changes in the articular cartilage of the joint (33–37).

OSTEOTOMY

Osteotomy of the knee is an option when noninflammatory OA involves a single weight-bearing compartment of the knee (38). Alternatives to osteotomy include unicompartmental replacement, TKA, and knee arthrodesis. Generally, osteotomy is preferred for young, active patients. Unicompartmental or total knee arthroplasty is reserved for elderly, low-demand patients. Arthrodesis is a salvage procedure, rarely used as a primary surgical intervention for the treatment of arthritic disorders of the knee.

Unilateral wear of a weight-bearing compartment of the knee invariably leads to deformity of the normal femorotibial axis. The normal anatomic valgus angulation between the femoral and tibial long axes is 6 degrees. Deviation from this alignment leads to increased stress on the medial or lateral compartment, thus accelerating the degenerative process and exacerbating the symptoms associated with the OA. McKellop et al. have demonstrated in cadaver knees that increased contact pressures in the medial or lateral hemijoint occur with varus or valgus deformity (39).

Osteotomy about the knee joint attempts to restore the valgus femorotibial axis of 6 degrees through a resection of either proximal tibial or distal femoral bone. Generally, varus deformities about the knee are treated with proximal tibial osteotomy, whereas valgus deformities of the knee are treated with distal femoral osteotomies. The technique of osteotomy must be designed to maintain a joint surface level with the ground at heel strike, while maintaining physiologic function of the collateral ligaments of the joint. These principles guide the surgeon in selecting the site of osteotomy for restoration of the anatomic axis of the joint.

Medial Degenerative Arthritis

Varus deformities of the knee are the result of loss of the articular space in the medial hemijoint. A standing, weight-bearing AP view of the knee will demonstrate loss of the medial articular space, and loss of the normal valgus femorotibial angle.

The ideal candidate for osteotomy of medial OA of the knee is the young, active patient without significant ligamentous laxity or patellofemoral arthritis. Osteotomy does not preclude subsequent total knee replacement, and therefore is an ideal procedure to provide pain relief and improve function for those patients not judged to be suitable candidates for arthroplasty. However, some researchers have reported suboptimal results of conversion of the previously osteotomized knee to a TKA because of subsequent technical difficulties (40,41).

The technique of proximal tibial osteotomy generally involves removal of a wedge of bone, tapered from the lateral cortex to the medial cortex. After removal of the wedge of bone, the osteotomy must be immobilized to allow bony healing. Immobilization can be accomplished with the use of a cylinder cast from the groin to the ankle, a knee brace, or internal or external fixation. The extremity is generally immobilized for approximately 6 weeks after surgery to achieve bony healing. Partial weight bearing on crutches is generally necessary for the first 6 postoperative weeks, followed by the use of a cane for 6 weeks.

The initial results of proximal tibial osteotomy for varus medial OA of the knee are quite good, but tend to decline with longer follow-up. Coventry et al. reported, in their follow-up of 87 proximal tibial osteotomies at a median length of follow-up of 10 years, 90% good or excellent results at 5 years and 65% good or excellent results at 10 years (42). Successful outcome was associated with a valgus femorotibial angle of 8 degrees or more and body weight less than 1.32 times the ideal weight. Insall et al. in 95 cases found good or excellent results in 85% at 5 years and 63% at 9 years of follow-up (43). Similarly, Yasuda et al. found 88% of patients with satisfactory results at 6-year follow-up and 63% satisfactory results at 10 years (44). Berman et al. reported a series of 39 high tibial osteotomies where 57% had a good result at 15-year follow-up, with better outcomes obtained in those patients under 60 years of age, with less than 12 degrees of preoperative angular deformity, arthrosis limited to the medial compartment, and preoperative motion of at least 90 degrees (45).

Surgical risks of osteotomy include intraarticular fracture, peroneal palsy, compartment syndrome, and delayed or nonunion. The risk for infection does not differ substantially from that in other open orthopedic procedures. Deep vein thrombosis is a risk and requires appropriate prophylaxis (46).

Recovery from tibial osteotomy may take 3 to 6 months, although improvement in knee function may be observed up to 1 year after osteotomy. Weidenhielm et al. have demonstrated equivalent improvement in knee pain and gait function in a comparison of patients undergoing high tibial osteotomy or prosthetic unicondylar replacement of the knee (47). However, Weale et al. reported better results with unicompartmental replacements versus high tibial osteotomy both in terms of pain control and survivorship at 12 to 17 years' follow-up (48).

No absolute physical limitations need be placed on a patient after tibial osteotomy. This is in contradistinction to the usual recommendations for avoidance of high-impact activity after TKA. Thus, the procedure is ideal for the young, active, or heavy patient with unicompartmental medial OA.

Lateral Degenerative Arthritis

Loss of the lateral articular space of the knee leads to progressive increase in valgus angulation of the femorotibial angle. Correction of this deformity with osteotomy generally is accomplished by removal of a wedge of bone from the distal femur. This allows restoration of the femorotibial angle to approximately 0 degrees, thus decreasing the contact stress in the degenerative lateral compartment.

The surgical technique involves removal of a medially based wedge in the supracondylar region of the distal femur. This requires internal fixation, usually with a blade plate device, to achieve bony union. The results of the less commonly performed distal femoral osteotomy for correction of valgus deformities are similar to those described earlier for proximal tibial osteotomy, with clinical improvement gradually declining over time. Selection of patients for distal femoral osteotomy should use clinical guidelines similar to those described for proximal tibial osteotomy.

UNICONDYLAR ARTHROPLASTY

In patients with unilateral OA of the knee, it is intuitively appealing to resurface only the involved portion of the joint. Although the unicondylar arthroplasty seeks to accomplish this, experience has shown that patient selection and surgical technique are critical to a successful outcome. The ideal candidate for unicondylar arthroplasty is a sedentary patient with a body weight of less than 180 pounds. Absence of symptomatic patellofemoral OA also is important for satisfactory postoperative function. The integrity of cruciate ligaments is controversial with regard to success of this technique (49). Relative contraindications to unicondylar arthroplasty include inflammatory arthritis, severe deformity or loss of motion in the knee, and high-activity expectations postoperatively. As with any arthroplasty, the presence of active or recent infection is an absolute contraindication.

Initial reports of unicondylar arthroplasties demonstrated poor outcomes, generally related to surgical technique, poor implant design, or improper patient selection (50–52). However, more recent studies have shown improvement in outcome. Scott et al. reported 85% survivorship among 100 consecutive unicompartmental arthroplasties with follow-up times of 8 to 12 years (53). Heck et al. reported 91% survivorship of almost 300 unicondylar arthroplasties at 10 years (54). In a prospective randomized study comparing the results of unicondylar versus total knee arthroplasty, Newman et al. demonstrated equivalent survivorship at 5-year follow-up, with better motion and less perioperative morbidity in the unicondylar group (55).

Unicondylar knee designs are particularly amenable to minimally invasive surgical techniques, which offer the potential advantages of decreased hospital stays and quicker recovery. However, there is currently a dearth of published information on the intermediate to long-term results of unicompartmental arthroplasty using minimally invasive techniques (56).

The risks of unicondylar arthroplasty are similar to those of TKA, although postoperative recovery from unicondylar arthroplasty tends to occur more rapidly. Conversion of a failed unicondylar arthroplasty to a TKA is potentially associated with technical difficulties, and the results of such conversions may not be so optimal as the results of primary TKA (57,58).

TOTAL KNEE ARTHROPLASTY

Total knee arthroplasty is the current treatment of choice for bi- or tricompartmental OA of the knee and inflammatory arthritis of the knee (Fig. 50.3). Indications for TKA

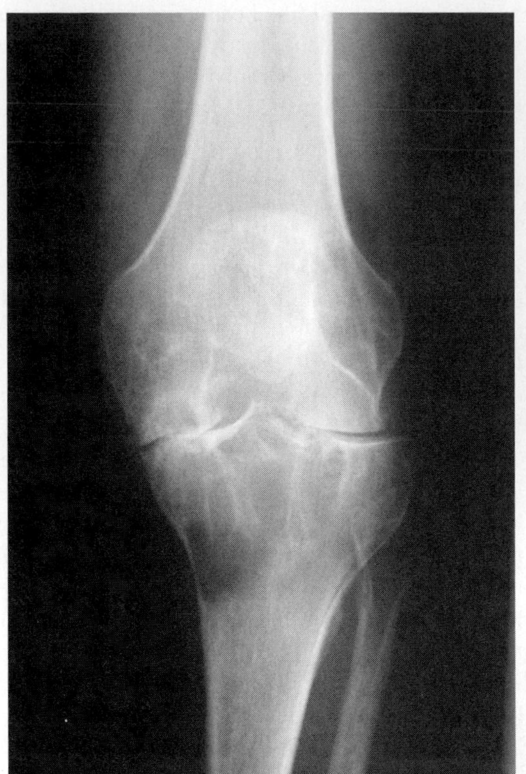
A

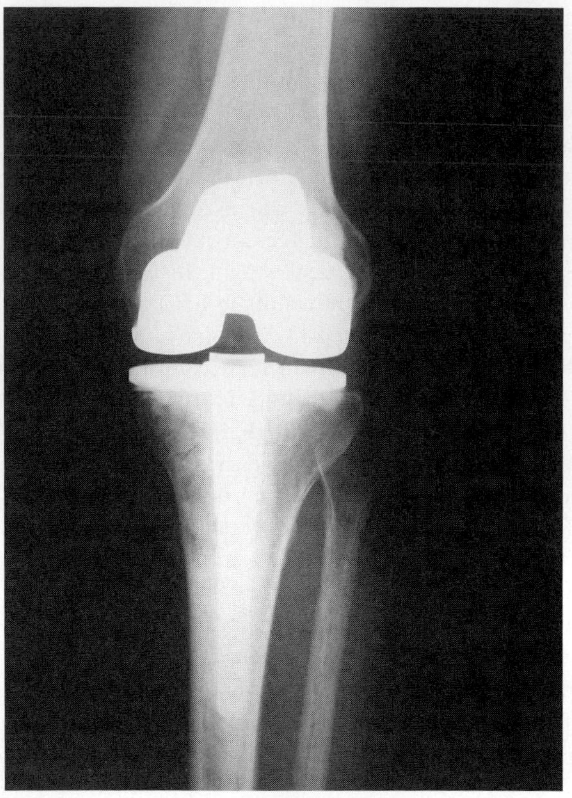
B

FIG. 50.3. A, B: Pre- and postoperative images of a 64-year-old patient with rheumatoid arthritis with large subchondral cysts. All three components have been fixed with polymethylmethacrylate bone cement, which appears as the irregular white material adjacent to the components. The larger cystic lesions were packed with cancellous bone graft. Ultra-high-molecular-weight polyethylene is the non-radiodense material between the femoral and tibial metal components, which provides the low-friction articular surface for the tibial prosthesis. To bypass areas weakened by cystic changes, a longer stem was used on the tibial component.

include pain refractory to medical management, or more rarely instability due to bone erosion and malalignment. However, the current limitations of the biomaterials used for a TKA define limits for application of this procedure. Polyethylene wear and bone loss due to osteolysis may eventually lead to loosening of the implant–bone interface. Additionally, potential complications such as early mechanical loosening due to prosthesis malposition or other factors, patellar subluxation, and even late hematogenous sepsis should temper the clinician's enthusiasm for this procedure if reasonable alternatives exist, such as osteotomy or unicompartmental arthroplasty.

Relative contraindications to TKA include high-activity expectations and long life expectancy. Absolute contraindications include the presence of active infection, including conditions that may produce nonhealing ulcers of the ipsilateral lower extremity, severe neurologic compromise of the limb, absent extensor mechanism, and prior arthrodesis.

Risks of TKA include infection (0.5%–2%), patellar subluxation, wound-healing complications, and deep vein thrombosis. Deep infection requires removal of the prosthesis to achieve control of the infection. Schoifet and Morrey have shown that simple débridement of the infected knee prosthesis followed by intravenous antibiotics failed to control the infection in 65% of patients, particularly in the elderly (59). Better results are accomplished by removal of the components, débridement of the joint, and placement of an antibiotic-loaded spacer. Prosthesis removal is generally followed by 4 to 6 weeks of intravenous antibiotic therapy. Reimplantation after infection has been successful in 90% of cases (60).

Patellar complications are the most frequent problem after TKA (61,62); the most common complication is lateral subluxation or dislocation of the patella, which is a result of both preoperative factors and intraoperative technical aspects of the reconstruction (63–65). On physical examination, the patella can be palpated lateral to the midlongitudinal axis of the femur when the knee is flexed; on active extension of the knee, sudden relocation to the midline is observed. Surprisingly, this subluxing patella is not usually painful, but rather produces a feeling of instability or insecurity. A dislocated patella severely compromises quadriceps strength and function. The solution to this complication requires soft tissue realignment procedures, or even revision of the TKA if component malalignment is the source of the subluxation.

Wound-healing complications are increased in patients with prior multiple surgeries about the knee, or systemic conditions such as diabetes or RA (66,67). To avoid sepsis, early intervention in the form of débridement and coverage with a local muscle or fasciocutaneous flap is necessary and generally quite successful (68).

Without appropriate prophylaxis, deep vein thrombosis may occur in up to 71% of patients, with associated pulmonary embolism in 22% (69). However, it appears that the majority of deep vein thrombosis occurs below the popliteal crease, which represents a low risk for embolization (70).

The prosthetic replacement may be implanted with either the use of polymethylmethacrylate bone cement, or the use of porous ingrowth from mechanical fixation of the components (71). The use of bone cement is the gold standard in TKA, and appears to be more consistently successful than cementless fixation of knee prostheses (72). The 10-year survivorship of TKA has been reported to be as high as 95%, with 15-year survivorship reported in excess of 90% (73–79). In contrast to the long-term results of total hip arthroplasty, TKA in the patient no more than 55 years of age also appears to be durable, with survivorship estimated at 99% at 10 years and 95% at 15 years (80,81).

PATELLOFEMORAL ARTHRITIS

Isolated OA of the patellofemoral joint is usually the result of patellar malalignment or trauma, such as hard falls or fractures of the patella. In the younger patient with OA of the patellofemoral joint, treatment usually consists of a physical therapy regimen designed to improve dynamic patellar tracking. On occasion, realignment procedures to restore normal patellar tracking are indicated. More advanced degrees of degeneration may benefit from débridement or anterior translocation of the tibial tubercle (Macquet procedure) in an effort to decrease patellofemoral contact stresses. Patellectomy has been advocated for advanced patellofemoral arthritis; however, the removal of the patella significantly weakens quadriceps function and can compromise the outcome of later TKA. In addition, abrasion of the quadriceps tendon on the anterior femoral condyles after patellectomy can also produce disabling pain (82).

Patellofemoral prosthetic arthroplasty is on occasion an appropriate option in the management of these patients. In performing the patellofemoral arthroplasty, the anterior femoral condyles are resurfaced along with the patella; the medial and lateral weight-bearing portions of the knee are untouched. Outcomes of patellofemoral arthroplasty are still evolving; one report indicates 88% good or excellent results in patients who were followed for 5.8 years (83).

OTHER SURGICAL ALTERNATIVES

Other alternatives in the surgical management of knee arthritis such as fusion, homologous cartilage implantation, and allograft resurfacing are occasionally appropriate for highly selected patients. A brief discussion of these alternatives is necessary to provide a comprehensive overview of the surgical management of the arthritic knee.

Cartilage Implantation

The elusive goal of biologic resurfacing of injured articular cartilage has led to intensive efforts to stimulate and repair both isolated and generalized articular defects in the knee. Transplanted heterologous or homologous chondrocytes, periosteum, and perichondrium have all been used in this effort, particularly in experimental animal models. Human experience is more limited, and therefore, such procedures should still be regarded as experimental, without proven long-term benefit.

Peterson et al. have published the most significant study to date of the efficacy of autologous chondrocyte implantation (84). Cultured autologous chondrocytes were implanted under a homologous patch of periosteum sewn over the articular defect. In their report, with 67-month follow-up, 58 patients with an average age of 26.4 years were treated for isolated articular cartilage defects of a single femoral condyle. Of the 58 patients, 53 demonstrated "good or excellent" results.

Patellar resurfacing for chondromalacia patella has been less successful, as have the limited number of tibial plateau implants (85). However, these initial reports are encouraging because repeated arthroscopic examinations and biopsy of the resurfaced areas demonstrated "hyaline-like" cartilage in 10 of 15 patient biopsy samples, with the remainder demonstrating "fibrous-hyaline" cartilage. Whether this procedure will in fact prevent subsequent OA remains to be proven.

Other approaches to biologic resurfacing, such as the use of carbon fiber implants show promising results, but await long-term follow-up and multicenter trials to confirm the initial results (86,87). Investigations of the utility of resorbable scaffolds impregnated with chondrocytes (88,89) and the use of cytokines and growth factors to attempt to stimulate cartilaginous healing are still in early clinical trials (90,91).

Allograft Resurfacing of the Arthritic Knee

Gross et al. have reported the use of fresh, small-fragment osteochondral allograft resurfacing of the knee, primarily after traumatic injuries resulting in secondary OA (92). In their series of 91 patients, 75% "success" at 5 years, 64% at 10 years, and 63% at up to 14 years of follow-up were observed. Unipolar grafts had better survival than bipolar (i.e., resurfacing of both femoral and tibial surfaces simultaneously), and younger patients had better outcomes than older (>60 years) patients. Correction of malalignment with the appropriate osteotomy at or before resurfacing was considered essential. Flynn et al. have reported similar success with the use of fresh-frozen osteoarticular allografts in the treatment of avascular necrosis of the knee, with 70% "satisfactory" results among 17 patients at a mean follow-up of 4.2 years (93).

Meniscal allografts also are currently being used clinically (94,95). The primary indication for this new and experimental technique appears to exist in the young athlete with irreparable damage to a meniscus, with or without concurrent anterior cruciate ligament injury and repair. The long-term survivorship of meniscal transplants is currently unknown, and their efficacy in preventing subsequent degenerative disease is unknown. Although experimental evidence in animals is encouraging (96), there is MRI and histologic evidence of an inflammatory response and degeneration at the meniscal–capsular junction in humans who have received meniscal transplants (97,98). A recent report of the outcome of meniscal transplantation in unicompartmental arthritis describes a 10% incidence of degenerative tears within an average of 21 months after surgery. This series is difficult to assess because of the high number of concomitant procedures such as osteotomy or cruciate reconstruction that accompanied the transplant; however, approximately 85% of cases were judged to be "good or excellent" at average 31-month follow-up (99). Further follow-up of these cases will be necessary to place this procedure in the proper clinical context.

Knee Fusion

Arthrodesis, or fusion of the knee joint, may be the treatment of choice for the young, active, or heavy patient with end-stage knee arthritis, or in those patients for whom there is a relative or absolute contraindication to arthroplasty (100). Knee fusion is reserved for those patients with unilateral disease, and also is appropriate as a salvage procedure for the infected arthroplasty for which appropriate treatment fails (101). Although some functional limitations obviously exist after knee fusion following failed TKA, the overall level of function and patient satisfaction is surprisingly high, even when compared with functioning primary TKAs (102).

When knee fusion is performed as a primary procedure, there is little shortening of the extremity, as compared with fusion after failed TKA, when shortening of 1.5 inches or more may result. Although no activity restrictions must be placed on the patient after fusion, some gait disability will be the inevitable result, leading to awkwardness in stair climbing and sitting, for example. Because of scarring of the extensor mechanism after knee arthrodesis, conversion of the fused knee back to a TKA should be discouraged (103,104).

CONCLUSIONS

Surgical intervention in the arthritic knee must always be tempered by an objective assessment of the relative risks and benefits for the procedures appropriate to a given patient. The young, active, or obese patient should resort to prosthetic arthroplasty only if all other surgical alternatives are inappropriate. Osteotomy about the knee for unicompartmental arthritis will generally be preferred for the patient under 50 years of age, with normal life expectancy and reasonable activity expectations. Arthroscopic débridement should be considered for those patients with mechanical symptoms and little or no loss of articular space as visualized on weight-bearing films.

Prosthetic TKA is the treatment of choice for patients older than 60 years with bicompartmental or tricompartmental arthritis. Inflammatory arthritis also is a relative indication for TKA, rather than partial replacement. However, overweight or very active patients older than age 50 may be considered for procedures such as osteotomy if appropriate. The prospect of wear and ultimate loosening of a prosthetic arthroplasty must be weighed against the potential need for replacement surgery if osteotomy fails to produce symptomatic relief.

Procedures to resurface articular cartilage injuries biologically must still be regarded as experimental, because no long-term evidence exists that these procedures will prevent the subsequent development of degenerative changes. These procedures should be confined to young individuals with limited hyaline cartilage lesions, as opposed to those with more advanced and diffuse degenerative disease. However, the tremendous promise and potential for the use of cytokines and growth factors to alter the response of cartilage to injury and subsequent degeneration may emerge as the ultimate treatment for the arthritic knee.

REFERENCES

1. Blackburn WD Jr, Bernrutter WK, Ronninger M, et al. Arthroscopic evaluation of knee articular cartilage: a comparison with plain radiographs and magnetic resonance imaging. *J Rheumatol* 1994;21:675–679.
2. Fischer SP, Fox JM, DelPizzo W, et al. Accuracy of diagnoses from magnetic resonance imaging of the knee: a multi-center analysis of one thousand and fourteen patients. *J Bone Joint Surg Am* 1991;73:2–10.
3. Ochi M, Sumen Y, Kanda T, et al. The diagnostic value and limitation of magnetic resonance imaging on chondral lesions in the knee joint. *Arthroscopy* 1994;10:17600–17683.
4. Boden SD, Davis DO, Dina TS, et al. A prospective and blinded investigation of magnetic resonance imaging of the knee: abnormal findings in asymptomatic subjects. *Clin Orthop* 1992;282:177–185.
5. Ike RW. The role of arthroscopy in the differential diagnosis of osteoarthritis of the knee. *Rheum Dis Clin North Am* 1993;19:673–696.
6. Chang RW, Falconer J, Stuelberg SD, et al. A randomized, controlled trial of arthroscopic surgery versus closed needle joint lavage for patients with osteoarthritis of the knee. *Arthritis Rheum* 1993;36:289–296.
7. Merchan EC, Galindo E. Arthroscope-guided surgery versus nonoperative treatment for limited degenerative osteoarthritis of the femorotibial joint in patients over 50 years of age: a prospective comparative study. *Arthroscopy* 1993;9:663–667.

8. Baumgaertner MR, Cannon WD Jr, Vittori JM, et al. Arthroscopic debridement of the arthritic knee. *Clin Orthop* 1990;253:197–202.
9. Rand JA. Arthroscopic management of degenerative meniscus tears in patients with degenerative arthritis. *Arthroscopy* 1985;1:253–258.
10. Aichroth PM, Patel DV, Moyes ST. A prospective review of arthroscopic debridement for degenerative joint disease of the knee. *Int Orthop* 1991;15:351–355.
11. Ogilvie-Harris DJ, Fitsialos DP. Arthroscopic management of the degenerative knee. *Arthroscopy* 1991;7:151–157.
12. Dervin GF, Stiell IG, Rody K, et al. Effect of arthroscopic debridement for osteoarthritis of the knee on health-related quality of life. *J Bone Joint Surg Am* 2003;85:10–19.
13. Moseley JB, O'Malley K, Petersen NJ, et al. A controlled trial of arthroscopic surgery for osteoarthritis of the knee. *N Engl J Med* 2002;347:81–88.
14. Johnson LL. Arthroscopic abrasion arthroplasty: historical and pathologic perspective: present status. *Arthroscopy* 1986;2:54–69.
15. Kim HK, Moran ME, Salter RB. The potential for regeneration of articular cartilage in defects created by chondral shaving and subchondral abrasion: an experimental investigation in rabbits. *J Bone Joint Surg Am* 1991;73:1301–1315.
16. Berlet GC, Mascia A, Miniaci A. Treatment of unstable osteochondritis dissecans lesions of the knee using autogenous osteochondral grafts (mosaicplasty). *Arthroscopy* 1999;15:312–316.
17. Kish G, Modis L, Hangody L. Osteochondral mosaicplasty for the treatment of focal chondral and osteochondral lesions of the knee and talus in the athlete: rationale, indications, techniques, and results. Clin Sports Med 1999;18:45–66.
18. Hangody L, Kish G, Karpati Z, et al. Arthroscopic autogenous osteochondral mosaicplasty for the treatment of femoral condylar articular defects: a preliminary report. *Knee Surg Sports Traumatol Arthrosc* 1997;5:262–267.
19. Bert JM, Maschka K. The arthroscopic treatment of unicompartmental gonarthrosis: a five-year follow-up study of abrasion arthroplasty plus arthroscopic debridement and arthroscopic debridement alone. *Arthroscopy* 1989;5:25–32.
20. Johnson LL. The sclerotic lesion: pathology and the clinical response to arthroscopic abrasion arthroplasty. In: Ewing JW, ed. *Articular cartilage and knee joint function: basic science and arthroscopy.* New York: Raven, 1990:319–333.
21. Friedman MJ, Berasi CC, Fox JM, et al. Preliminary results with abrasion arthroplasty in the osteoarthritic knee. *Clin Orthop* 1984;182: 200–205.
22. Linschoten NJ, Johnson CA. Arthroscopic debridement of knee joint arthritis: effect of advancing articular degeneration. *J South Orthop Assoc* 1997;6:25–36.
23. Armstrong RW, Bolding F, Joseph R. Septic arthritis following arthroscopy: clinical syndromes and analysis of risk factors. *Arthroscopy* 1992;8:213–223.
24. Poulsen KA, Borris LC, Lassen MR. Thromboembolic complications after arthroscopy of the knee. *Arthroscopy* 1993;9:570–573.
25. Savarese A, Lunghli E, Bundassi P, et al. Thromboembolic complications in arthroscopic surgery of the knee. *Ital J Orthop Traumatol* 1992;18:485–490.
26. Small NC. Complications in arthroscopic surgery of the knee and shoulder. *Orthopedics* 1993;16:985–988.
27. Kieser C. A review of the complications of arthroscopic knee surgery. *Arthroscopy* 1992;8:79–83.
28. Doets HC, Bierman BT, von Soesbergen RM. Synovectomy of the rheumatoid knee does not prevent deterioration. *Acta Orthop Scand* 1989;60:523–525.
29. McEwen C. The treatment of rheumatoid arthritis: report of results at the end of five years. *J Rheumatol* 1988;15:764–769.
30. Matsui N, Taneda Y, Ohta H, et al. Arthroscopic versus open synovectomy in the rheumatoid knee. *Int Orthop* 1989;13:17–20.
31. Jerosch J, Hoffstetter I, Schroder M, et al. Septic arthritis: arthroscopic management with local antibiotic treatment. *Acta Orthop Belg* 1995; 61:126–134.
32. Shoen RT, Aversa JM, Rahn DW, et al. Treatment of refractory chronic Lyme arthritis with arthroscopic synovectomy. *Arthritis Rheum* 1991; 34:1056–1060.
33. Paus AC, Dale K. Arthroscopic and radiographic examination of patients with juvenile rheumatoid arthritis before and after open synovectomy of the knee joint: a prospective study with a 5 year follow-up. *Ann Chir Gynaecol* 1993;82:55–61.
34. Smiley P, Wasilewski S. Arthroscopic synovectomy. *Arthroscopy* 1990;6:18–23.
35. Doets HC, Berman BT, von Soesbergen RM. Synovectomy of the rheumatoid knee does not prevent deterioration. *Acta Orthop Scand* 1989;60:523–525.
36. McEwen C. The treatment of rheumatoid arthritis: report of results at the end of five years. *J Rheumatol* 1988;15:764–769.
37. Canale ST, Dugdale M, Howard BC. Synovectomy of the knee in young patients with hemophilia. *South Med J* 1988;81:1480–1486.
38. Buckwalter JA, Lohmander S. Operative treatment of osteoarthrosis: current practice and future development. *J Bone Joint Surg Am* 1994; 76:1405–1418.
39. McKellop HA, Sigholm G, Redfern FC, et al. The effect of simulated fracture-angulations of the tibia on cartilage pressures in the knee joint. *J Bone Joint Surg Am* 1991;73:1382–1391.
40. Jackson M, Sarangi PP, Newman JH. Revision total knee arthroplasty: comparison of outcome following primary tibial osteotomy or unicompartmental arthroplasty. *J Arthroplasty* 1994;9:539–542.
41. Mont MA, Alexander N, Krackow KA, et al. Total knee arthroplasty after failed high tibial osteotomy. *Orthop Clin North Am* 1994;25: 515–525.
42. Coventry MB, Ilstrup DM, Wallrichs SL. Proximal tibial osteotomy: a critical long-term study of eighty-seven cases. *J Bone Joint Surg Am* 1993;75:196–201.
43. Insall JN, Joseph DM, Msika C. High tibial osteotomy for varus gonarthrosis: a long-term follow-up study. *J Bone Joint Surg Am* 1984;66:1040–1048.
44. Yasuda K, Majima T, Tsuchida T, et al. A ten- to 15-year follow-up observation of high tibial osteotomy in medial compartment osteoarthrosis. *Clin Orthop* 1992;282:186–195.
45. Berman AT, Bosacco SJ, Kirshner S, et al. Factors influencing long-term results in high tibial osteotomy. *Clin Orthop* 1991;272:192–198.
46. Turner RS, Griffiths H, Heatley FW. The incidence of deep-vein thrombosis after upper tibial osteotomy: a venographic study. *J Bone Joint Surg Br* 1993;75:942–944.
47. Weidenhielm L, Olsson E, Brostrom LA, et al. Improvement in gait one year after surgery for knee osteoarthrosis: a comparison between high tibial osteotomy and prosthetic replacement in a prospective randomized study. *Scand J Rehabil Med* 1993;25:25–31.
48. Weal AE, Newman JH. Unicompartmental arthroplasty and high tibial osteotomy for osteoarthrosis of the knee: a comparative study with a 12- to 17-year follow-up period. *Clin Orthop* 1994;302:134–137.
49. Kozinn SC, Scott R. Current concepts review: unicondylar knee arthroplasty. *J Bone Joint Surg Am* 1989;71:145–150.
50. Insall J, Aglietti P. A five to seven-year follow-up of unicondylar arthroplasty. *J Bone Joint Surg Am* 1980;62:1329–1337.
51. Laskin RS. Unicompartmental tibiofemoral resurfacing arthroplasty. *J Bone Joint Surg Am* 1978;60:182–185.
52. Marmor L. Unicompartmental knee arthroplasty: ten- to 13-year follow-up study. *Clin Orthop* 1988;226:14–20.
53. Scott RD, Cobb AG, McQueary FG, et al. Unicompartmental knee arthroplasty: eight- to 12-year follow-up evaluation with survivorship analysis. *Clin Orthop* 1991;271:96–100.
54. Heck DA, Marmor L, Gibson A, et al. Unicompartmental knee arthroplasty: a multicenter investigation with long-term follow-up evaluation. *Clin Orthop* 1993;286:154–159.
55. Newman JH, Ackyroyd CE, Shah NA. Unicompartmental or total knee replacement? Five year results of a prospective, randomized trial of 102 osteoarthritic knees with unicompartmental arthritis. *J Bone Joint Surg* 1998;80:862–865.
56. Romanowski MR, Repicci JA. Minimally invasive unicondylar arthroplasty: eight-year follow-up. *J Knee Surg* 2002;15:17–22
57. Padgett DE, Stern SH, Insall JN. Revision total knee arthroplasty for failed unicompartmental replacement. *J Bone Joint Surg* 1991;73: 186–190.
58. Lai CH, Rand JA. Revision of failed unicompartmental total knee arthroplasty. *Clin Orthop* 1993;287:193–201.
59. Schoifet S, Morrey B. Treatment of infection after total knee arthroplasty by debridement with retention of the components. *J Bone Joint Surg Am* 1990;72:1383–1390.
60. Windsor RE. Management of total knee arthroplasty infection. *Orthop Clin North Am* 1991;22:531–538.

61. Healy WL, Wasilewski SA, Takei R, et al. Patellofemoral complications following total knee arthroplasty: correlation with implant design and patient risk factors. *J Arthroplasty* 1995;10:197–201.
62. Brick GW, Scott RD. The patellofemoral component of total knee arthroplasty. *Clin Orthop* 1988;231:163–178.
63. Harrison MM, Cooke TD, Fischer SB, et al. Patterns of knee arthrosis and patellar subluxation. *Clin Orthop* 1994;309:56–63.
64. Rhoads D, Noble P, Reuben J, et al. The effect of femoral component position on patellar tracking after total knee arthroplasty. *Clin Orthop* 1990;260:43–51.
65. Rand JA. Patellar resurfacing in total knee arthroplasty. *Clin Orthop* 1990;260:110–117.
66. Ecker ML, Lotke PA. Postoperative care of the total knee patient. *Orthop Clin North Am* 1989;20:55–62.
67. Wong RY, Lotke PA, Ecker ML. Factors influencing wound healing after total knee arthroplasty. *Orthop Trans* 1986;10:497.
68. Greenberg B, LaRossa D, Lotke PA, et al. Salvage of jeopardized total-knee prosthesis: the role of the gastrocnemius muscle flap. *Plast Reconstr Surg* 1989;83:85–89.
69. Lynch J, Baker P, Polly R, et al. Mechanical measures in the prophylaxis of postoperative thromboembolism in total knee arthroplasty. *Clin Orthop* 1990;250:24–29.
70. Lotke PA, Ecker ML, Alavi A, et al. Indications for the treatment of deep venous thrombosis following total knee replacement. *J Bone Joint Surg Am* 1984;66:202–208.
71. Rand JA. Cement or cementless fixation in total knee arthroplasty? *Clin Orthop* 1991;273:52–62.
72. Rand JA, Ilstrup D. Survivorship analysis of total knee arthroplasty. *J Bone Joint Surg Am* 1991;73:397–409.
73. Malkani AL, Rand JA, Bryan RS, et al. Total knee arthroplasty with the Kinematic condylar prosthesis: a ten-year follow-up study. *J Bone Joint Surg Am* 1995;77:423–431.
74. Ritter MA, Herbst SA, Keating EM, et al. Long-term survival analysis of a posterior cruciate-retaining total condylar total knee arthroplasty. *Clin Orthop* 1994;309:136–145.
75. Ranawat CS, Flynn WF Jr, Deshmukh RG. Impact of modern technique on long-term results of total condylar knee arthroplasty. *Clin Orthop* 1994;309:131–135.
76. Ranawat CS, Flynn WF Jr, Saddler S, et al. Long-term results of the total condylar knee arthroplasty: a 15-year survivorship study. *Clin Orthop* 1993;286:94–102.
77. Stern SH, Insall JN. Posterior stabilized prosthesis: results after follow-up of nine to twelve years. *J Bone Joint Surg* 1992;74:980–986.
78. Schai PA, Thornhill TS, Scott RD. Total knee arthroplasty with the PFC system: results at a minimum of ten years and survivorship analysis. *J Bone Joint Surg Br* 1998;80:850–858.
79. Gill GS, Joshi AB, Mills DM. Total condylar knee arthroplasty: 16- to 21- year results. *Clin Orthop* 1999;367:210–215.
80. Duffy GP, Trousdale RT, Stuart MJ. Total knee arthroplasty in patients 55 years old or younger: 10- to 17-year results. *Clin Orthop* 1998; 356:22–27.
81. Gill GS, Chan KC, Mills DM. 5- to 18-year follow-up study of cemented total knee arthroplasty for patients 55 years old or younger. *J Arthroplasty* 1997;12:49–54.
82. Oberlander MA, Baker CL, Morgan BE. Patellofemoral arthrosis: the treatment options [Review]. *Am J Orthop* 1998;27:263–270.
83. Krajca-Radcliffe JB, Coker TP. Patellofemoral arthroplasty: a 2- to 18-year follow-up study. *Clin Orthop* 1996;330:143–151.
84. Peterson L, Minas T, Brittberg M, et al. Treatment of osteochondritis dissecans of the knee with autologous chondrocyte transplantation. *J Bone Joint Surg* 2003;85(suppl 2):17–24.
85. Brittberg M, Lindahl A, Nilsson A, et al. Treatment of deep cartilage defects in the knee with autologous chondrocyte transplantation. *N Engl J Med* 1994;331:889–895.
86. Muckle DS, Minns RJ. Biological response to woven carbon fibre pads in the knee: a clinical and experimental study. *J Bone Joint Surg Br* 1990;72:60–62.
87. Pongor P, Betts J, Muckle DS, et al. Woven carbon surface replacement in the knee: independent clinical review. *Biomaterials* 1992;13: 1070–1076.
88. Freed LE, Grande DA, Lingbin Z, et al. Joint resurfacing using allograft chondrocytes and synthetic biodegradable polymer scaffolds. *J Biomed Mater Res* 1994;28:891–899.
89. Hendrickson DA, Nixon AJ, Grande DA, et al. Chondrocyte-fibrin matrix transplants for resurfacing extensive articular cartilage defects. *J Orthop Res* 1994;12:485–497.
90. Hunziker EB, Rosenberg L. Induction of repair in partial thickness articular cartilage lesions by timed release of TGF-beta [Abstract]. *Trans Orthop Res Soc* 1994;19:236.
91. Trippel SB. Growth factor actions on articular cartilage [Review]. *J Rheumatol Suppl* 1995;43:129–132.
92. Beaver RJ, Mahomed M, Backstein D, et al. Fresh osteochondral allografts for post-traumatic defects in the knee: a survivorship analysis. *J Bone Joint Surg Am* 1992;74:105–110.
93. Flynn JM, Springfield DS, Mankin HJ. Osteoarticular allografts to treat distal femoral osteonecrosis. *Clin Orthop* 1994;303:38–43.
94. Veltri DM, Warren RF, Wickiewicz TL, et al. Current status of allograft meniscal transplantation. *Clin Orthop* 1994;303:44–55.
95. Garrett JC, Steensen RN, Steensen RN. Meniscal transplantation in the human knee: a preliminary report. *Arthroscopy* 1991;7:57–62.
96. Jackson DW, McDevitt CA, Simon TM, et al. Meniscal transplantation using fresh and cryopreserved allografts: an experimental study in goats. *Am J Sports Med* 1992;20:644–656.
97. Patten RM, Rolfe BA. MRI of meniscal allografts. *J Comput Assist Tomogr* 1995;19:243–246.
98. Rode SA, Seneviratne A, Suzuki K, et al. Histological analysis of human meniscal allografts: a preliminary report. *J Bone Joint Surg Am* 2000;82:1071–1087.
99. Cameron JC, Saha S. Meniscal allograft transplantation for unicompartmental arthritis of the knee. *Clin Orthop* 1997;337:164–171.
100. Cuckler JM, Rhoad RC. Alternatives to hip, knee, and ankle total joint arthroplasty [Review]. *Curr Opin Rheumatol* 1991;3:81–87.
101. Damron TA, McBeath AA. Arthrodesis following failed total knee arthroplasty: comprehensive review and meta-analysis of recent literature. *Orthopedics* 1994;18:361–368.
102. Benson ER, Resine ST, Lewis CG. Functional outcome of arthrodesis for failed total knee arthroplasty. *Orthopedics* 1998;21:875–879.
103. Cameron HU. Role of total knee replacement in failed knee fusions. *Can J Surg* 1987;30:25–27.
104. Holden DL, Jackson DW. Considerations in total knee arthroplasty following previous knee fusion. *Clin Orthop* 1987;227:223–228.

CHAPTER 51

Arthritis of the Foot and Ankle

Greg A. Horton and Charles L. Saltzman

Arthritic problems of the foot and ankle may result from posttraumatic, degenerative, or inflammatory processes. The basic principles of evaluation and management are similar for the variety of arthritic problems encountered. The primary focus of this chapter is on rheumatoid arthritis (RA), which may affect a variety of joints, resulting in disabling pain and deformity. The frequently encountered osteoarthritic (OA) problems involving the first metatarsophalangeal joint and the ankle joint also are addressed. Clinical evaluation and conservative foot care are discussed in detail. Surgical indications, operative principles and complications, as well as a number of specific operative procedures, also are outlined.

Whereas RA may affect any joint, foot and ankle involvement is frequent and many times heralds the onset of the disease process. Series documenting foot and ankle involvement in patients with RA reveal that nearly 90% of patients will develop foot symptoms over the course of their disease (1). The frequency and degree of foot and ankle problems are directly proportional to the disease duration (2–4). Forefoot involvement has been reported to occur more frequently and earlier in the disease course than hindfoot involvement. Symptomatic involvement of the midfoot is less common. Hindfoot involvement tends to occur later in the disease process. Although any of the hindfoot joints may be affected, talonavicular involvement is reported to be most common.

The mechanical stresses of weight bearing are responsible for the deformities that occur over time. In the forefoot, this consists of a valgus deformity of the great toe and lesser metatarsophalangeal subluxation or dislocation (Figs. 51.1 and 51.2). Hindfoot deformities frequently result in a planovalgus or flat-foot deformity. Hindfoot involvement typically results in valgus deformity. There is some controversy over the prevalence of posterior tibial tendon insufficiency in patients with RA (5). Although many patients demonstrate a planovalgus foot deformity of the hindfoot, it is unclear if this is secondary to subtalar joint instability, rupture of the spring ligament, or posterior tibial tendon dysfunction.

Primary OA problems also are common in the foot and ankle. The most frequent is OA of the first metatarsopha-

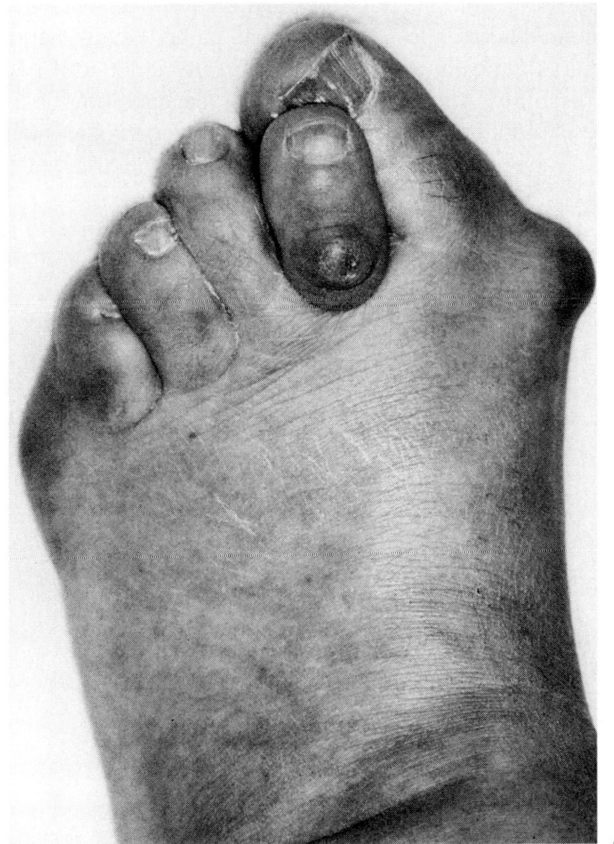

A

FIG. 51.1. A: The rheumatoid forefoot typically deforms in a characteristic pattern. Joint laxity allows the shoe to shape the forefoot into a "pied du rond" *Continued*

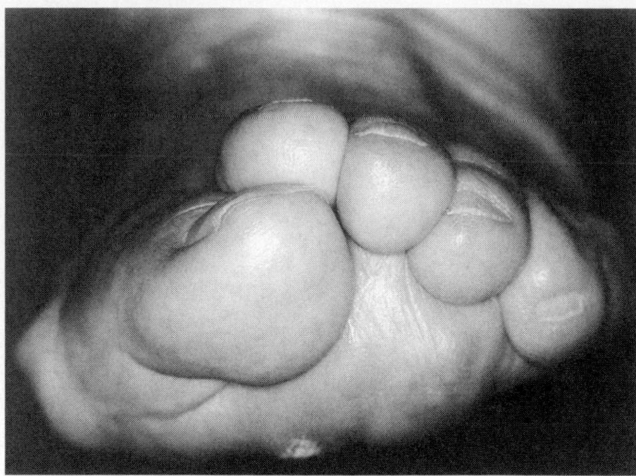

B

FIG. 51.1. *Continued* **(B)**. Hallux valgus and subluxation/deviation of the lesser metatarsophalangeal joints is common.

langeal joint or hallux rigidus. Hallux rigidus is a term used to describe a symptom complex that results in functional limitation of motion of the first metatarsophalangeal joint. This limitation of motion results from a reactive proliferation of bone along the dorsal aspect of the joint and is associated with painful limited motion. Hallux rigidus is a local arthritic process, typically without accompanying degeneration of other joints of the foot and ankle or appendicular skeleton. Although less common than hallux valgus, hallux rigidus is typically associated with greater amount of pain and disability. Although posttraumatic degeneration of the ankle is the most frequent cause of ankle arthritis, primary degenerative arthritis does occur. Frequently attributed to primary OA, chronic lateral ankle instability is another common cause of ankle arthropathy.

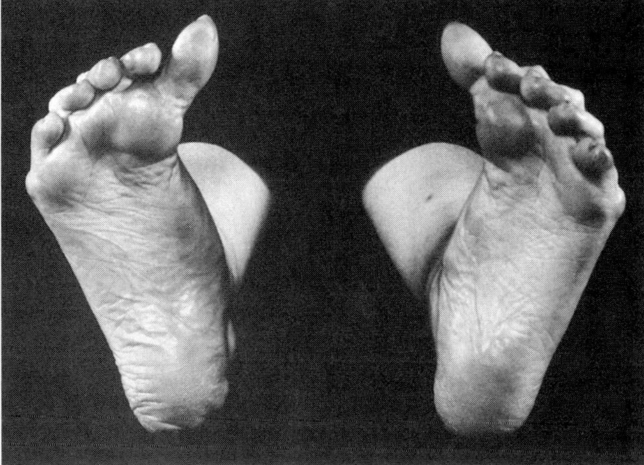

FIG. 51.2. With rheumatoid disease, the first metatarsophalangeal joint occasionally subluxates into a varus position, and the lesser toes follow. The medial buttress of the hallux is essential to control the lesser toes, and is the basis for improved forefoot surgical results with fusion of the first metatarsophalangeal joint.

CLINICAL EVALUATION

The clinical evaluation begins with a careful history in an attempt to identify the area of maximal pain and deformity. The overall activity level should be evaluated and correlated with the patient's goals and expectations. The history should elicit the chief complaint, be it pain from synovitis, shoe-wear difficulty, hammering of the toes, plantar callosities, or hindfoot deformity.

Physical examination of the foot and ankle should be performed in a systematic fashion and should include an observation of the patient's gait. All too often the examination is performed with the patient sitting, and essential findings related to deformity with weight bearing are missed. The physical examination should include an examination of the shoes. Wear patterns provide important information about deformity and areas of increased pressure. The height of the heel and volume of the toe box should be observed. Deformity and wear of the shoe should be carefully correlated with the patient's symptoms and foot alignment. Inspection of the foot should identify edema, skin integrity, and the presence of any skin lesions, nodules, or callosities (Fig. 51.3). The toes should be spread to allow inspection. Areas of synovial thickening are often grossly apparent and

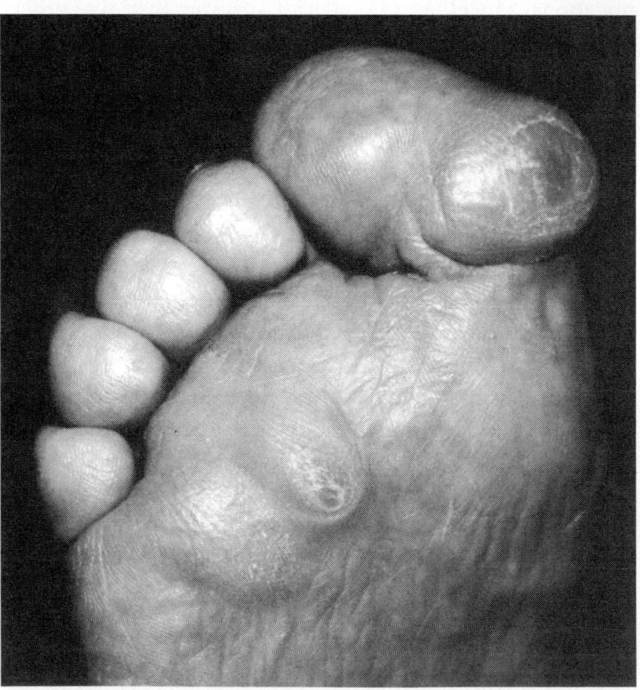

FIG. 51.3. Rheumatoid nodules often form in regions of high friction. The plantar-medial surface of the first interphalangeal joint is a common site and often secondary to a hallux valgus deformity. Surgical treatment usually involves realignment of the hallux and nodule excision.

may be associated with increased warmth. This is commonly seen in the dorsal aspect of the midfoot and forefoot as well as along the medial aspect of the hindfoot.

The metatarsophalangeal region is a common site of pathology in patients with RA. Dorsal subluxation or dislocation of the proximal phalanges typically occurs with hammering of the lesser toes. The plantar aspect of the forefoot should be carefully examined to identify areas of pain and increased pressure (Fig. 51.4).

The vascular status of the foot should be thoroughly evaluated. Capillary refill, skin temperature, and hair distribution may give some gross estimation of the vascular status of the foot. Posterior tibial and dorsalis pedis pulses should be palpated. Venous outflow of the foot should be estimated. RA patients can have vasculitic skin changes or distal phalangeal punctate lesions, presumably from immune complex deposition. Noninvasive vascular studies or formal vascular referral may be indicated if the vascular status is in question.

The neurologic status of the foot also is evaluated. It is not uncommon to find subtle neuropathy in patients with long-standing RA. Diabetes, often from long-term steroid use, may coexist and contribute to the potential for neuropathy. Synovitis along the medial aspect of the ankle may cause irritation of the tibial nerve in the region of the tarsal tunnel. Percussion of the nerve along its course may elicit tingling, which may be indicative of irritation or compression. Mononeuritis multiplex may occur with foot drop, and

A

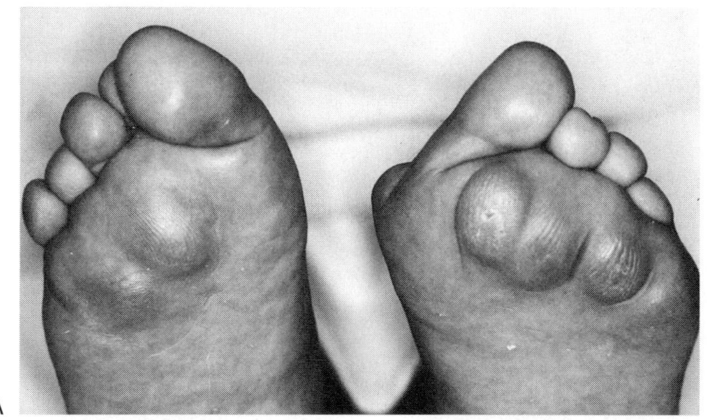

B

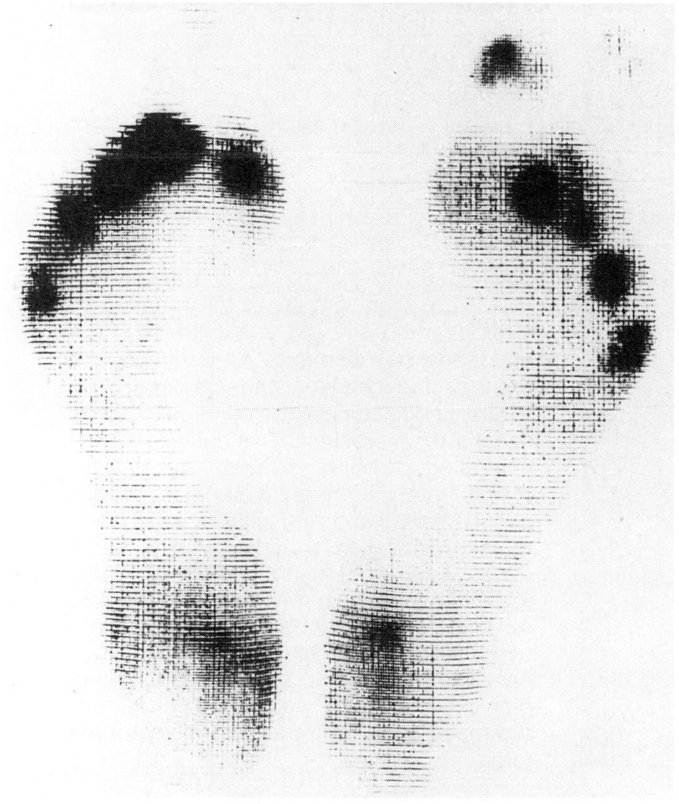

FIG. 51.4. Photograph **(A)** and Harris mat print **(B)** of a typical patient with rheumatoid forefoot deformities. The peak pressures under the central metatarsal heads can reach 20 times normal and are a source of considerable discomfort to patients. The goal of treatment is to reduce pressure on the metatarsal heads.

should be considered with focal peripheral nerve dysfunction. Motor function and muscle strength is evaluated. Range of motion of the ankle, subtalar, transverse tarsal, and metatarsophalangeal joints should be estimated. Restriction of motion, instability, pain, or crepitus should be noted.

Radiographic imaging is an important part of the evaluation of foot and ankle problems (Fig. 51.5). Routine standard projections include anteroposterior, lateral, and (internal) oblique views of the foot and an anterior mortise view of the ankle. For evaluation of deformity and surgical planning, patient weight-bearing radiographs are impera-

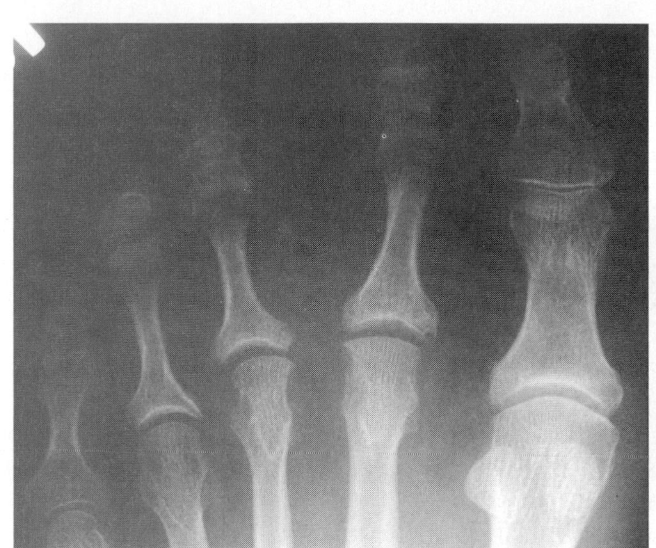
A

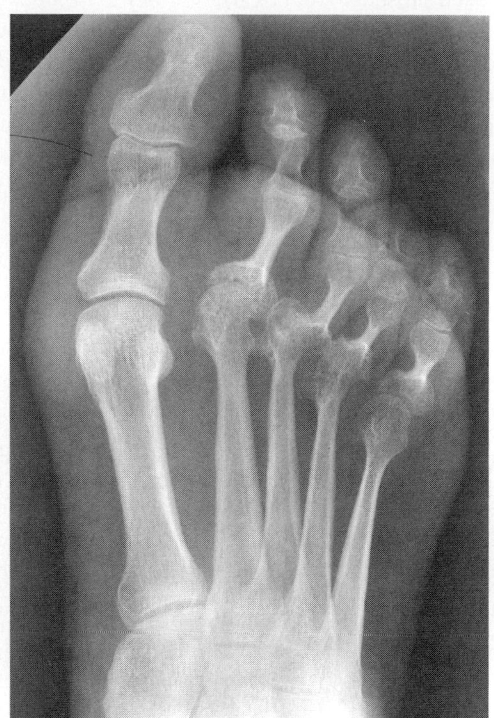
B

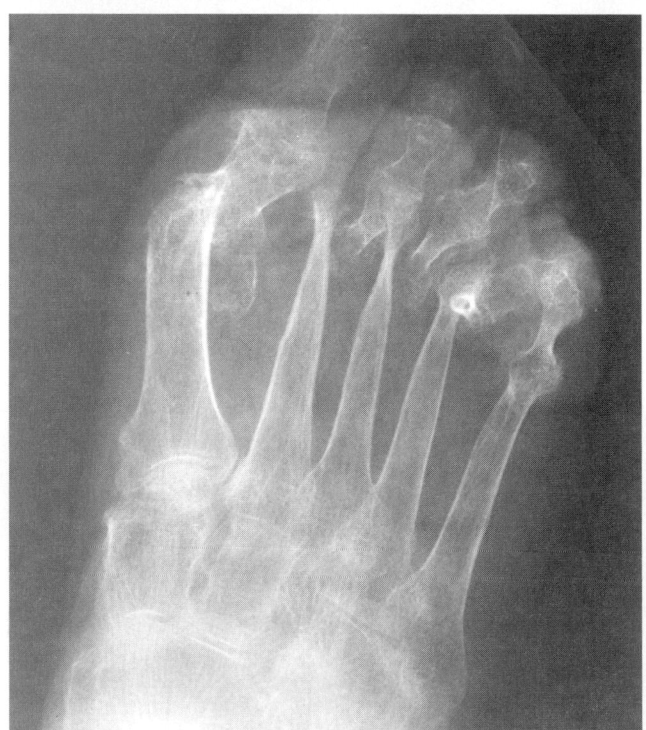
C

FIG. 51.5. Radiographs of the rheumatoid forefoot with early **(A)**, moderate **(B)**, and end-stage **(C)** changes. **A:** Early on, the radiographic changes can be subtle, revealing pauciarticular osteoporosis and a few marginal erosions. This patient had toe spreading, probably secondary to synovitis. Unfortunately, in the early stage of the disease, swelling and pain in this location is all too often mistaken for and surgically treated as an interdigital neuroma. **B:** Later the forefoot joints begin to subluxate. The central metatarsophalangeal joints are usually most affected. **C:** With severe erosive disease, the entire metatarsophalangeal region dislocates, with secondary penciling of the metatarsal neck and deformities of the toes.

tive; they give insight into the alignment and joint congruency of the foot and ankle, when it functions in physiologic loading.

CONSERVATIVE CARE

Nonoperative foot care and patient education are important aspects in the management of foot and ankle problems. Patients should be encouraged to wear shoes of proper size and avoid the temptation to sacrifice comfort for style. The shoe should be supportive and comfortable, allowing accommodation of a deformity, if present. Patients with RA often have dorsal dislocation of the metatarsophalangeal joints, hallux valgus, and hammering of the lesser toes. A shoe with an extra-depth toe box allows accommodation of this increased forefoot volume. If an orthotic device is to be worn inside the shoe, the volume occupied by the orthosis must be considered when sizing the shoe.

Many types of soft-soled wide shoes, including jogging shoes, are commercially available for men and women. A wide assortment of extra-depth shoes are now available off the shelf, and custom-made shoes are infrequently used because of their high cost, cosmetic concerns, and narrow indications. External modification of the shoe is used at times to alter the weight-bearing pattern during gait. An orthotic device may be added to provide cushion or alter the biomechanical configuration of the foot. Although it is not necessary to possess information on all types of shoe wear and orthoses, it is necessary to be able to communicate the goals with both the patient and the orthotist. Any shoe, shoe-wear modification, or orthosis must be evaluated by the prescribing physician to ensure that the fabrication is satisfactory and that the goals of the device are being met. A working relationship with a certified pedorthotist or orthotist is particularly helpful.

An orthosis is a device that is used to serve as an interface between the foot and the floor (shoe). A soft orthosis is most desirable for patients with RA and is used mainly to provide cushion and reduce friction. More rigid devices, or the combination of a rigid outershell with softer inner layers, may be used at times to try to correct the position of the foot. It is important to understand that no orthosis can be expected to correct a fixed deformity. More commonly, the interface between the floor and the foot is accommodated to fit the shape of the foot. Toe slings, sleeves, and corn pads (nonmedicated) are readily available and often extremely helpful.

For patients with hindfoot, midfoot, or ankle pain associated with instability or deformity, an orthotic device can be used that extends from the leg across the ankle to incorporate the foot. This is known as an ankle-foot orthosis (AFO). An AFO can be custom molded from hard plastic or leather and metal. The correct prescription for each patient depends on several factors, including quality of the skin, whether static correction is required, and whether unloading is necessary. Patients who require unloading of part of the foot or ankle to reduce pain will need circumferential bracing of the leg.

Because of concomitant hand and upper extremity involvement, many patients have difficulty donning and doffing a brace and are unable to perform routine nail care. Shoe and brace use are often simplified by applying Velcro strapping systems. Paring of plantar callosities is another important conservative measure. An intractable plantar keratosis is a hyperkeratotic skin lesion on the planter aspect of the foot and is the result of increased pressure, typically from the underlying deformity of the metatarsal heads. Trimming of the callus allows better evaluation of the underlying deformity and may also provide significant pain relief.

SURGICAL CONSIDERATIONS

Rheumatoid foot disorders may have a variable clinical course from patient to patient. It is important to estimate the natural history of each case and plot the current status in the course of the patient's RA. Acute inflammation may be associated with synovitis and joint erosions. This is best treated with medications in the rheumatologist's armamentarium. In the absence of deformity, surgery is rarely indicated for acute inflammatory problems. If nonsurgical measures, including immobilization, fail, a synovectomy may be considered. When soft tissue deformity occurs, surgical intervention may consist of synovectomy, capsular releases, and realignment procedures. For patients with long-standing RA, the problem is usually one of deformity due to either bony erosion or capsuloligamentous instability. The deformity may result in pain and difficulty with ambulation. Surgical intervention is appropriate at this stage and typically consists of arthroplasty or arthrodesis procedures.

Many surgeons prefer nonsteroidal antiinflammatory drugs (NSAIDs) to be discontinued before an operative procedure because of the potential for increased bleeding. Because of the theoretic risks for wound complications and infection, the use of methotrexate in the perioperative period has received some attention. A decrease in wound tensile strength has been demonstrated in animal studies. However, clinical studies have not supported the need to discontinue the use of methotrexate routinely in the perioperative period (6–9).

Although most forefoot and midfoot operative procedures can be performed under an ankle block, many hindfoot and ankle procedures require the use of regional or general anesthesia. For patients who require endotracheal intubation, lateral flexion and extension cervical spine radiographs should be obtained to rule out cervical spine instability. This is particularly important for RA patients with progressive extremity erosive disease because the severity of hand and foot involvement has been shown to correlate directly with cervical spine subluxation (10).

The extent of upper extremity involvement should be carefully evaluated when contemplating lower extremity reconstructive procedures because many patients require protected weight bearing postoperatively. Preoperative assessment by a physical therapist may be useful in the patient who is identified at risk for postoperative ambulatory difficulties. Platform crutches or walkers are helpful. Those with generalized polyarticular disease and poor hand, wrist, elbow, and shoulder function may require an electric wheelchair for several months after surgery. Advanced planning for the postoperative convalescence is enormously beneficial to patients and their families.

Frequently multiple areas of joint deterioration and deformity occur, potentially affecting the hip, knee, and foot. When no significant deformity is present, the most symptomatic area of pain should be addressed first. Often there is multilevel deformity. A valgus knee and ipsilateral planovalgus foot deformity in a patient with RA is a common example. There is debate among surgeons regarding which should be addressed first. It is our opinion that the knee should be corrected first. This allows some accommodation of the foot before performing a hindfoot arthrodesis and optimization of foot arthrodesis position.

Many patients have bilateral foot difficulties and request simultaneous surgical reconstruction of both feet. For all patients, but RA patients in particular, convalescence from bilateral surgical foot procedures of any significance can be exceedingly difficult. Except for relatively simple procedures such as hammer toe procedures, staged unilateral foot surgery is generally performed in the presence of bilateral disease.

The main complications after surgery on the foot and ankle include skin slough, infection, nonunion, and malunion. It is important to anticipate possible sources of complications because many times a complication can be minimized or resolved with early retention and treatment. The best preventive measures for wound infections are careful patient selection, meticulous soft tissue handling intraoperatively, and perioperative antibiotics. Despite the use of these measures, superficial and deep infections occasionally occur. Although superficial cellulitis and wound erythema can be treated with antibiotics, a deep infection necessitates operative débridement, usually with retention of internal fixation. This allows consolidation of the proposed arthrodesis site. Therapeutic or suppressive antibiotic therapy often is necessary, followed by hardware removal after consolidation.

Forefoot

Surgical reconstruction of RA forefoot deformities can be rewarding for both the patient and the surgeon. Pain relief and patient satisfaction are high, and ambulatory capacity is greatly enhanced for a properly performed forefoot reconstruction. The most frequent reasons that operative intervention of the forefoot is performed for RA are hammer toes and other painful lesser toe deformities, dislocation of the lesser metatarsophalangeal joints, and severe hallux valgus deformity (11,12). In earlier stages of foot involvement, isolated toe deformities or single metatarsophalangeal joint involvement may occur. Frequently, more severe and combined deformities occur. It is important to understand that a hallux valgus or bunion deformity in a patient with RA is distinctly different from the hallux valgus deformity frequently encountered in the middle-aged woman. If this is not understood, incorrect or insufficient surgical procedures may result in an unacceptably high recurrence rate.

Hammer toe deformities usually result in stiff and deformed toes. A flexion deformity at the distal interphalangeal joint, as well as extension at the metatarsophalangeal joint, may accompany flexion deformity at the proximal interphalangeal joint. Pain and callus may be present over the dorsum of the proximal interphalangeal joint, the tip of the toe, or beneath the metatarsal head. A hammer toe is repaired by excision of the distal portion of the proximal phalanx. For several weeks, the toe is stabilized with a K-wire, which is easily removed in the office. Weight bearing, as tolerated, in a postoperative shoe is allowed. Patients should be counseled that swelling of the toe might persist for several weeks postoperatively.

Synovitis of the lesser metatarsophalangeal joints may be associated with pain as well as capsular attenuation. Intra-articular corticosteroid injections can help quell an isolated metatarsophalangeal synovitis. Occasionally, a local synovectomy may be of benefit. More common is dislocation of

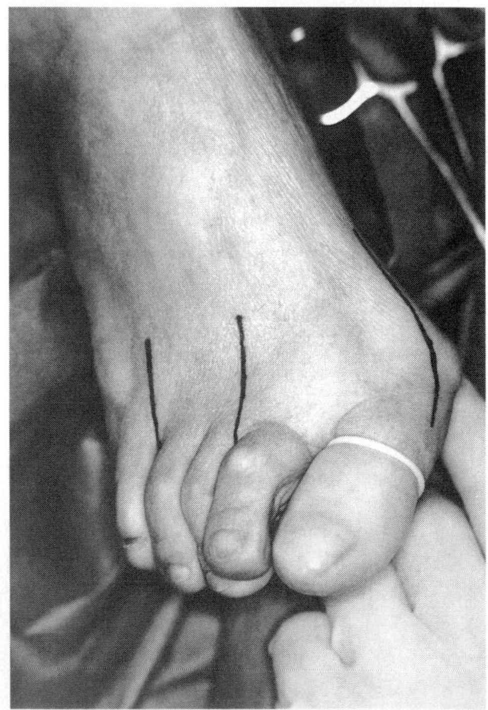

FIG. 51.6. Typical incisions required for a rheumatoid forefoot reconstruction. Because of the relatively large amount of dissection required, and the need for multiple incisions, this relatively immunosuppressed patient population is at relatively high risk for complications.

one or several of the lesser metatarsal heads. This is a dorsal dislocation with resultant plantar pressure from the uncovered metatarsal heads after distal migration of the plantar fat pad. Surgical correction of this consists of multiple metatarsal head removal at the level of the metatarsal neck, typically through dorsal incisions (Fig. 51.6). Concomitant hammer toe deformities are addressed with a formal hammer toe procedure or a closed osteoclasis of the toe deformity. The toes are stabilized with K-wires for several weeks; the wires are removed in the office. Some surgeons prefer simple hemiarthroplasty of the proximal interphalangeal joint as described earlier, whereas others recommend proximal interphalangeal joint fusion for the RA hammer toes after metatarsal head excision. Depending on the extent of the surgery and the intraoperative findings, some weight bearing, as tolerated in a postoperative shoe, may be allowed. Occasionally, ectopic bone may form about the end of the cut metatarsal, resulting in a recurrent plantar callus.

Advanced hallux valgus deformity in RA is most effectively treated with an arthrodesis of the metatarsophalangeal joint (13). The benefits of this procedure include stable alignment of the toe, pain relief, and improved stability of the medial side of the foot. The failure rate of implant arthroplasty of the first metatarsophalangeal joint makes this a less desirable choice in all but the most low-demand patients, or perhaps, in patients with a fused first interphalangeal joint. The hallux is positioned into about 10 to 15 degrees of valgus and about 5 to 10 degrees of dorsiflexion in relation to the floor. A variety of techniques for bone preparation and internal fixation have been advocated. Depending on the quality of the bone and fixation, the postoperative immobilization involves either a short-leg cast, a removable boot, or a postoperative shoe until satisfactory union occurs, usually by 10 to 12 weeks (Fig. 51.7).

Treatment of hallux rigidus in non-RA patients frequently involves an attempt to salvage the joint with a débridement or cheilectomy procedure (14). The dorsal proliferative bone is removed to allow an improvement of dorsiflexion and relieve the jamming phenomenon that occurs. Although the

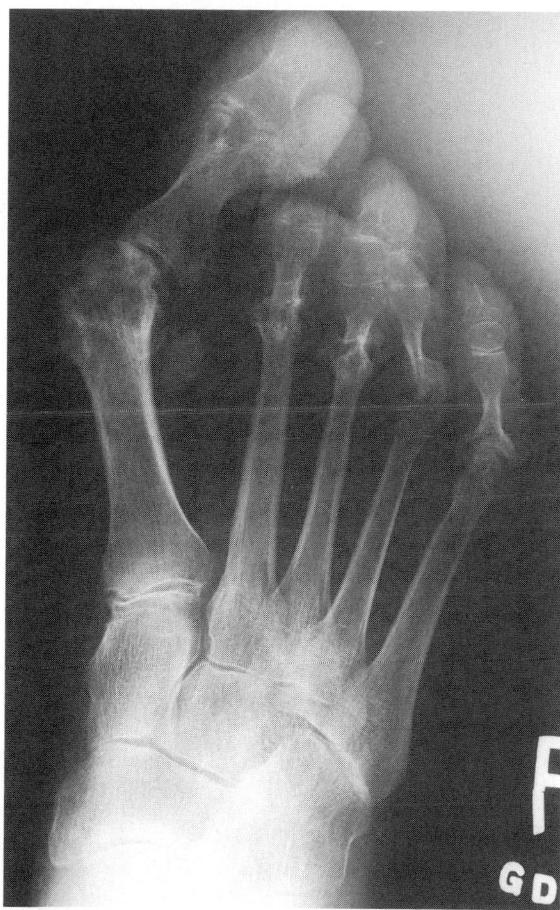

A

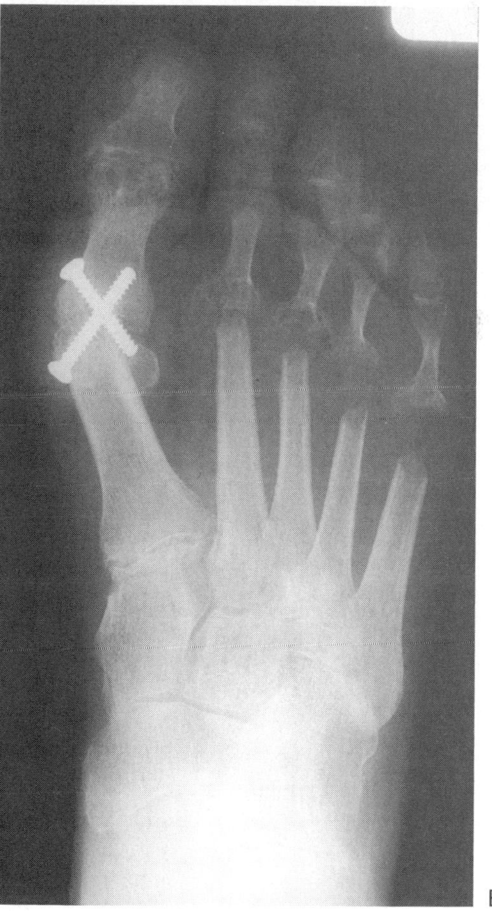

B

FIG. 51.7. Example of 57-year-old woman with a 15-year history of rheumatoid disease with severe metatarsalgia unresponsive to nonoperative means. **A:** Preoperative radiograph shows severe forefoot deformity. **B:** Surgery involved first metatarsophalangeal fusion, lesser metatarsal head resection, and resection/stabilization of the interphalangeal joints. She had an excellent clinical result and has requested the same procedure for her other foot.

underlying joint is not normal, patients typically have significant relief of pain. Further deterioration of the joint may occur over time. The treatment of advanced OA arthritis of the first metatarsophalangeal joint or salvage of a failed cheilectomy procedure is usually an arthrodesis procedure. In low-demand patients, a joint-resection arthroplasty or polymeric silicone (Silastic) replacement can be considered.

Hindfoot

Hindfoot surgical intervention typically consists of arthrodesis or fusion procedures. With laxity of the ligamentous supporting tissues of the subtalar or talonavicular joint, a collapse of the calcaneus into valgus may produce a severe flat-foot deformity and marked prominence of the talar head. Patients may complain of lateral pain secondary to impingement between the calcaneus and the tip of the fibula. If performed relatively early in the course of a significant flat-foot deformity, an isolated subtalar fusion may suffice (15). With longer established deformities and subluxation of the talonavicular joint, a triple arthrodesis (fusion of the talonavicular, calcaneocuboid, and subtalar joints) may be required (Fig. 51.8). The goal is a foot that is plantigrade or flat to the ground. Patients are kept non–weight bearing for a minimum of 6 weeks in a short-

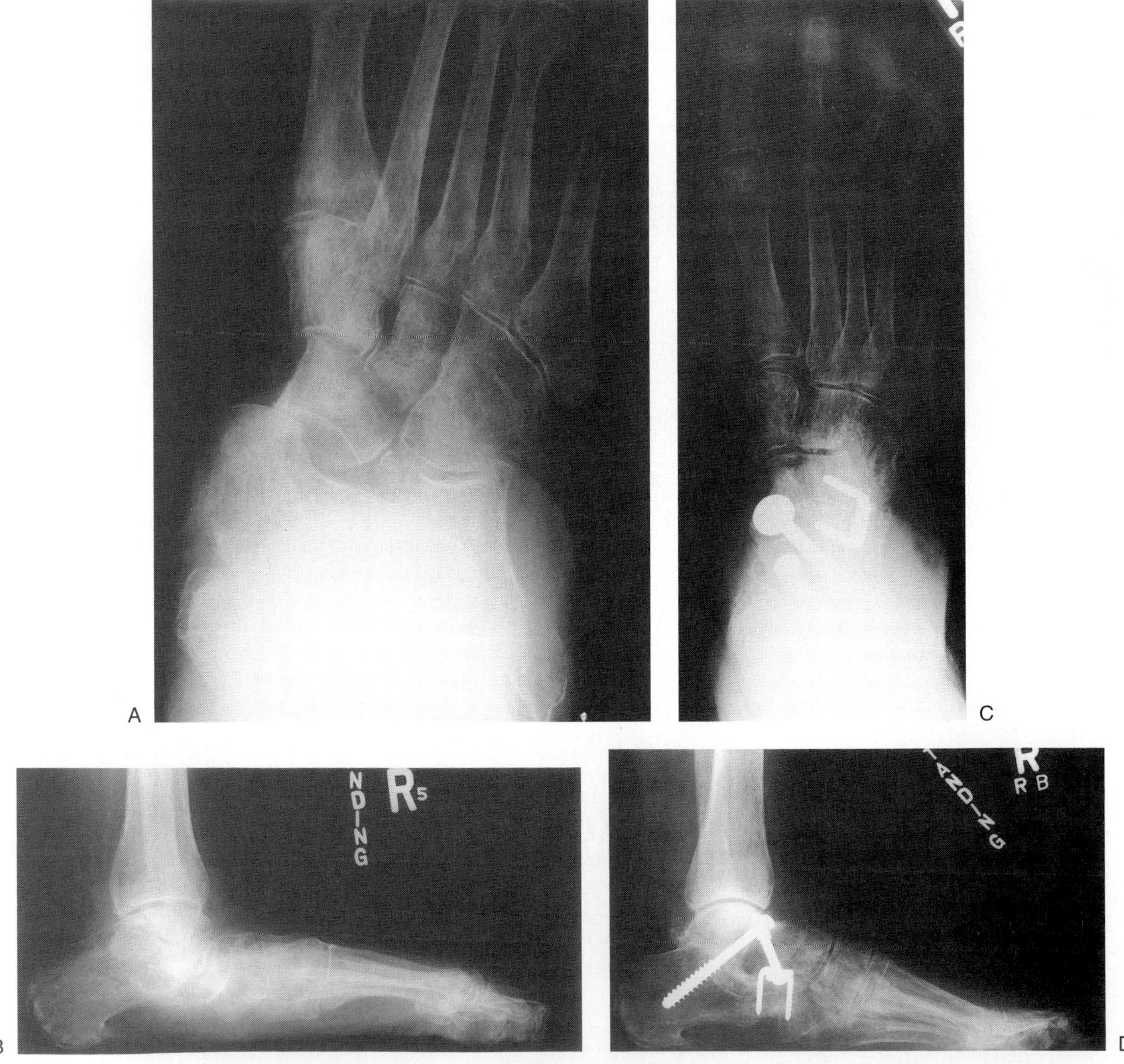

FIG. 51.8. A, B: Anteroposterior and lateral radiographs of a 72-year-old patient with unbraceable deformity of the hindfoot. In her custom brace, she developed recurrent ulceration along the medial aspect of the talar head. **C, D:** She was treated with a triple arthrodesis and became brace free.

leg cast followed by another 6 weeks of immobilization in an ambulatory cast.

Ankle

The optimal surgical treatment of end-stage ankle arthritis remains somewhat a matter of controversy, with some surgeons advocating fusion and others supporting the benefits of joint replacement. At present, most surgeons continue to perform ankle arthrodeses for ankle arthritis, but the tide of opinion is slowly changing toward the use of ankle arthroplasty. The complexities of all of the surgical considerations regarding whether to consider a joint replacement for a given patient, and if so, which design is optimal, are beyond the scope of this chapter. However, certain fundamental concepts are relevant.

Ankle fusion procedures are typically effective in relieving pain. A successful arthrodesis procedure may require 3 to 4 months of cast immobilization, of which the first half is non–weight bearing. Total convalescence time before most patients can walk comfortably averages 6 months, but for some patients, the swelling persists until a year or so after surgery. Approximately 5% to 10% of attempted fusions fail to fuse, and can require secondary surgeries to obtain satisfactory fusion. Fusion of the ankle eliminates substantial flexion/extension foot and ankle motion, and reduces some inversion/eversion motion. Over time, other joints are required to compensate for this loss of motion by increasing their natural range. The subtalar joint often deteriorates after ankle arthrodesis, and sometimes other hindfoot and midfoot joints are affected. This can require further surgery or prolonged use of bracing or ambulatory aids.

Similarly, ankle joint replacement carries its own intrinsic advantages and potential disadvantages. Historically, ankle joint replacement was associated with a high rate of wound complications and implant subsidence. With newer implant designs and improved surgical techniques, these problems have decreased, but have not been eliminated. The intrinsic advantage of a replacement is that, when successful, it maintains motion and reduces strain on adjacent joints. The primary disadvantage is that if it fails, salvage can be very challenging. With a wider variety of newer noncemented designs, salvage to another replacement after aseptic failure is possible, and can be considered an alternative to conversion to an ankle arthrodesis. Salvage after infection remains a major concern. Although most deep infections of ankle implants resolve with aggressive surgical débridement and appropriate antibiotics, not all do. The patient with a chronic, painful deep infection unresponsive to surgical and medical means may require a below-knee amputation to become functional again.

No consensus exists regarding the indications for ankle arthroplasty. In general, patients who are "ideal" are elderly or have low physical demands, with good bone stock and normal vascularity, and good hindfoot alignment. In particular, patients with bilateral ankle degenerative disease or those with ipsilateral hindfoot disease, especially after a triple arthrodesis, are good candidates because bilateral ankle fusions and pantalar fusion are extremely functionally limiting (Fig. 51.9). Contraindications include profound immunosuppression, neuromuscular imbalance, neuropathic (Charcot) joints, nonreconstructable hindfoot alignment, and talar avascular necrosis (for ingrowth talar components). Despite these relatively clear-cut indications and contraindications, most patients fall into a gray zone for decision making. We have no really firm concept of how young is too young, or what activities are allowed or prohibited. The RA patients are often good candidates because of other concomitant foot and ankle joint disease and low activity levels. Of concern, however, are patients receiving immunosuppressive drugs or those with low bone mineral density. As improved implant designs become available, and more options for revision ankle arthroplasty are possible, it

A

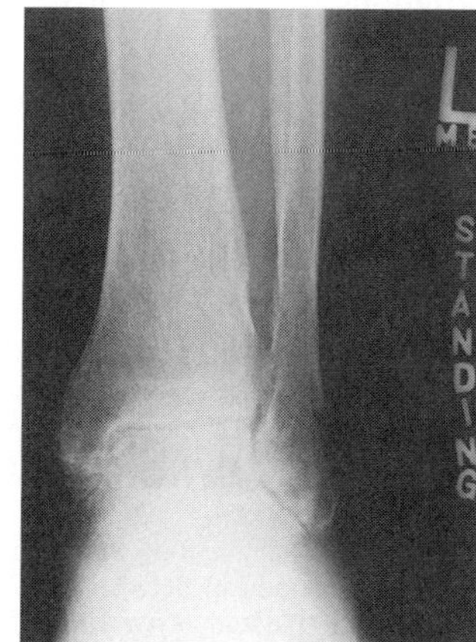

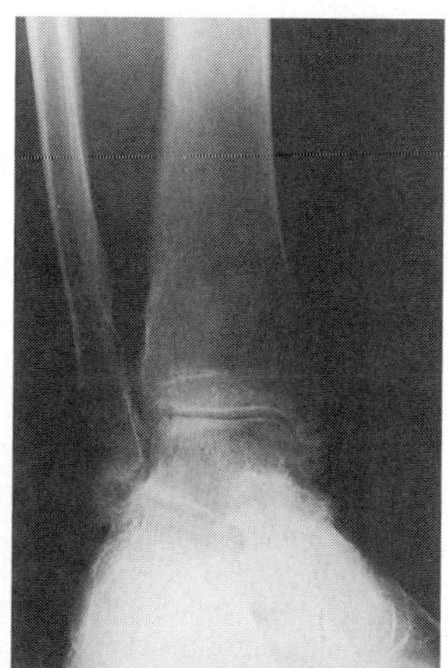

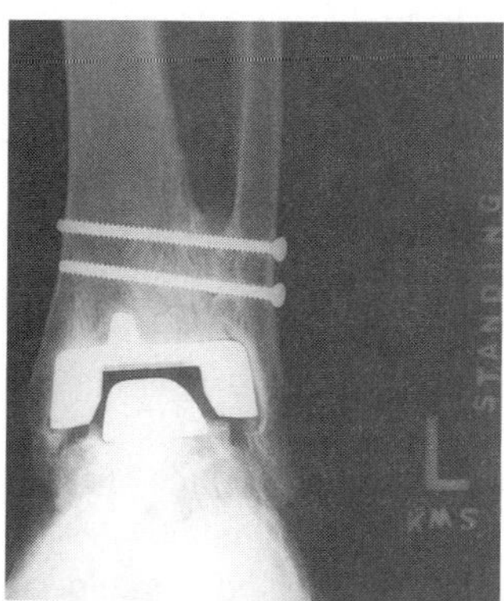

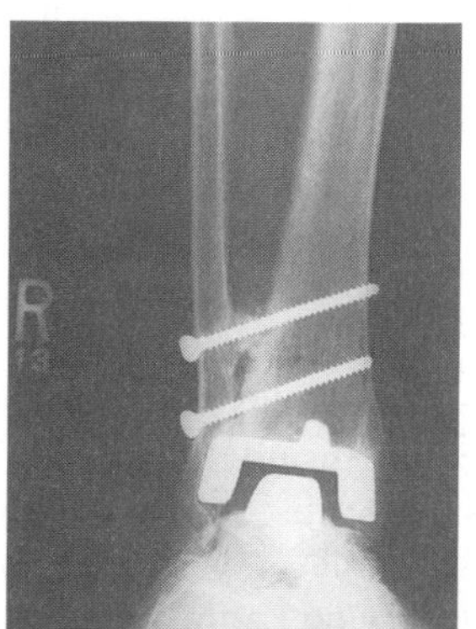

B

FIG. 51.9. Total ankle replacement can be considered for the rheumatoid arthritis patient, especially with bilateral involvement and ipsilateral hindfoot disease **(A)**. This patient had bilateral replacements performed with excellent clinical results **(B)**.

is likely that the average age of ankle replacement will decline, and the accepted activity level will increase.

CURRENT TRENDS

Treatment alternatives for ankle arthritis continue to gain interest and enthusiasm. Total ankle arthroplasty has continued to grow in popularity, gaining acceptance in mainstream orthopedic meetings and peer-reviewed publications. Some of this gain in popularity has been driven, in part, by the health-care consumer. As outcomes become better understood and more predictable, patients and doctors alike look to be part of this emerging technology.

Although a successful ankle arthrodesis predictably results in pain reduction, the long-term effects on adjacent joints is a concern. A recent long-term follow-up of isolated ankle fusions has highlighted this (16). While in general a satisfactory procedure, follow-up after two decades has shown an increase in peritalar arthritis. Increased stress in the adjacent joints of the foot following ankle arthrodesis results in accelerated wear and tear. Of interest is that no increased incidence in knee degeneration was observed in patients with an isolated ankle arthrodesis. Over time, an increase in activity limitation and pain was noted secondary to the degenerative changes in the subtalar and transverse tarsal region. The paradox is that those patients who are younger and more active are typically less well suited for ankle arthroplasty. The younger patient with posttraumatic arthrosis continues to be best suited for an ankle joint fusion.

Distraction arthroplasty represents a joint-sparing approach that may have a role in the algorithm of treatment alternatives. Joint distraction is a relatively new approach to ankle arthritis. By application of an external frame, the ankle joint is gradually mechanically separated. Distraction of 5 mm is maintained over a 3-month period with the use of the external frame. The patient is allowed to bear full weight while the frame is in place. The exact mechanism by which clinical and radiographic improvement are achieved is unclear. It has been suggested that by distracting the joint and relieving the mechanical stress, the residual articular cartilage may be able to mount some type of a reparative response. Long-term studies are lacking, but encouraging early results have been reported (17). A recent report has indicated that at 1 year following distraction, 70% of patients showed significant clinical improvement. Continued clinical improvement over time was reported as this cohort was followed for up to 5 years. Radiographic improvement has also been demonstrated with widening of the joint space over time. A potential advantage of this technique is that it does not disturb the native anatomic structures. This easily allows a subsequent reconstructive procedure whether it is an arthrodesis or an arthroplasty. Although the exact role of distraction arthroplasty has yet to be defined, continued scrutiny of the results will likely aid in establishing its place in the treatment algorithm.

Cartilage transplantation has been used effectively to treat isolated defects of the talus. This is typically used for larger osteochondritis dissecans lesions of the talar body. Current techniques include autologous osteochondral grafting, allogenic osteochondral grafting, and autologous chondroctye transplantation. Although useful for isolated talar dome lesions, autologous grafting has a number of limitations. Because of limited donor availability, the size of the lesion must be considered. In addition, it is difficult to address the tibial side of the joint with current surgical techniques. Diffuse articular involvement is not appropriate for autologous techniques. Once secondary bony changes occur, the role for any type of autologous grafting becomes questionable.

In an attempt to find an alternative to replacement arthroplasty and arthrodesis, a limited number of centers have explored the use of osteoarticular allogenic en bloc arthroplasty. The technique resects the diseased distal tibia and talar dome as a block. An osteoarticular shell matching the resection block is then obtained from a fresh cadaveric specimen. The graft is fashioned to fit in the defect and is held with screw fixation.

Complications of this procedure have included intraoperative fractures, graft collapse requiring revision, and reoperation for talofibular débridement. Because the talofibular articulation is not addressed with this technique, significant arthrosis in this region may be a relative contraindication. Follow-up at 21 months has demonstrated improvement in subjective scores of pain and function (18). Ankle range of motion was only modestly improved. The availability of fresh specimens will likely limit this technology to selected, typically academic, tertiary centers.

In summary, it is clear that no one treatment is appropriate for all patients with ankle arthritis. A number of factors, including age, weight, alignment, activity level, and underlying disease process, play a role in deciding the most appropriate treatment. The expectations of the patient and the experience of the orthopedic surgeon may also influence the treatment plan. Ankle arthrodesis remains a standard approach to treat end-stage ankle arthritis. Outcomes are generally satisfactory, although concerns regarding the eventual development of contiguous foot degenerative disease are genuine. Ankle arthroplasty is an alternative to fusion, and offers the potential for painless, preserved motion. However, concerns with salvage options remain, and the exact indications/contraindications for ankle joint replacement are not fully delineated.

REFERENCES

1. Michelson J, Easley M, Wigley FM, et al. Foot and ankle problems in rheumatoid arthritis. *Foot Ankle Int* 1994;15:608.
2. Spiegel TM, Spiegel JS. Rheumatoid arthritis in the foot and ankle: diagnosis, pathology and treatment: the relationship between foot and ankle deformity and disease duration in 50 patients. *Foot Ankle* 1982; 2:318.
3. Vainio K. Rheumatoid foot: clinical study with pathological and roentgenographical comments. *Ann Chir Gynaecol* 1956;45(suppl):1.

4. Vidigal E, Jacoby RK, Dixon AS, et al. Prospective study of the radiological changes in hands, feet and cervical spine in adult rheumatoid disease. *Ann Rheum Dis* 1983;42:613.
5. Michelson J, Easley M, Wigley FM, et al. Posterior tibial tendon dysfunction in rheumatoid arthritis. *Foot Ankle Int* 1995;16:157.
6. Bland KI, Palin WE, von Fraunhofor JA, et al. Experimental and clinical observations of the effects of cytotoxic chemotherapeutic drugs on wound healing. *Ann Surg* 1984;199:782–790.
7. Calnan J, Davies A. The effect of methotrexate on wound healing: an experimental study. *Br J Cancer* 1965;19:505.
8. Perhala RS, Wilke WS, Clough JD, et al. Local infectious complications following large joint replacement in rheumatoid arthritis patients treated with methotrexate versus those not treated with methotrexate. *Arthritis Rheum* 1991;34:146–152.
9. Sany J, Anaya JM, Canovas F, et al. Influence of methotrexate on the frequency of postoperative infectious complications in patients with rheumatoid arthritis. *J Rheumatol* 1993;20:1129–1132.
10. Rasker JJ, Cosh JA. Radiological study of cervical spine and hand in patients with rheumatoid arthritis of 15 years duration: an assessment of the effect of corticosteroid treatment. *Ann Rheum Dis* 1978;37:592.
11. Mann RA, Schakel ME II. Surgical correction of rheumatoid forefoot deformities. *Foot Ankle Int* 1995;16:1–6.
12. McGarvey SR, Johnson KA. Keller arthroplasty in combination with resection arthroplasty of lesser metatarsophalangeal joints in rheumatoid arthritis. *Foot Ankle Int* 1988;9:75–80.
13. Mann RA, Thompson FM. Arthrodesis of the first metatarsophalangeal joint for hallux valgus in rheumatoid arthritis. *J Bone Joint Surg Am* 1984;66:687–692.
14. Mann RA, Clanton TO. Hallux rigidus: treatment by cheilectomy. *J Bone Joint Surg Am* 1988;70:400–406.
15. Mann RA, Baumgarten M. Subtalar fusion for isolated subtalar disorders: preliminary report. *Clin Orthop* 1988;226:260–265.
16. Coester LM, Saltzman CL, Leupold J, et al. Long-term results following ankle arthrodesis for post-traumatic arthritis. *J Bone Joint Surg Am* 2001;83:219–228.
17. Marijnissen ACA, van Roermund PM, van Melkebeek J, et al. Clinical benefit of joint distraction in the treatment of ankle osteoarthritis. *Foot Ankle Clin North Am* 2003;8:335–346.
18. Tontz WL, Bugbee WD, Brage ME. Use of allografts in the management of ankle arthritis. *Foot Ankle Clin North Am* 2003;8:361–373.

SECTION V

Rheumatoid Arthritis

CHAPTER 52

Etiology and Pathogenesis of Rheumatoid Arthritis

David A. Fox

The etiology of rheumatoid arthritis (RA) is still unknown, despite important progress in understanding many aspects of its pathogenesis. Proposed causes for RA include (a) specific genetic polymorphisms or combinations of genetic factors; (b) pathogenic immune and inflammatory responses triggered by infectious agents; (c) autoimmunity directed against components of synovium and cartilage, mediated either by pathogenic autoantibodies or by autoreactive T cells; (d) disordered regulation of production of proinflammatory and tissue destructive cytokines; and (e) transformation of the cellular constituents of the synovial lining into autonomous, tissue-invasive cells.

The view that RA is a multifactorial process, requiring a combination of genetic, environmental, and immune-mediated factors, has gained wide acceptance. Understanding of how these components of the cause of RA interrelate remains incomplete, although insights into the biology of proinflammatory cytokines have highlighted the important roles of these mediators at all stages of the disease. It is possible that the multiple elements that lead to RA operate as "risk factors," with several possible combinations of predisposing factors capable of producing clinical disease through mechanisms and pathways that are at least partially distinct. Alternatively, evolution of clinical RA could require a specific sequence of events involving the immune system and the joints. One approach to framing this question is to consider two very different disease states, reactive arthritis and atherosclerosis. In reactive arthritis it seems clear that disease is initiated by an infectious organism, although the primary site of infection is not usually within the joint. In the setting of the correct genetic background, episodic or chronic arthritis may occur. Although we still have much to learn about the mechanisms for this sequence of events, the order of occurrence of the key elements in disease pathogenesis seems fairly clear. In atherosclerosis, on the other hand, a heterogeneous mixture of genetic and environmental factors combine in different ways to produce a tissue remodeling process with a typical anatomic distribution and functional consequences. No single risk factor is considered indispensable for disease. Does RA, like reactive arthritis, involve a prototypic sequential pathway of events operating on a specific genetic substrate? Or, does it, like atherosclerosis, target particular tissues but use a variety of mechanisms and predisposing factors to generate a unique lesion?

Another key unresolved question concerning RA is whether or not it fundamentally is an autoimmune disease. Immune mechanisms are prominent in RA synovium, but the nature and significance of specific antigenic targets remains controversial and confusing. Specific genetic polymorphisms of immune response molecules predispose to RA, but, as in other putatively autoimmune diseases, the mechanism of this effect remains unproven.

RA has both systemic and articular manifestations. Most work on understanding the etiology and pathogenesis of RA has focused on the joint, as will the preponderance of the discussion in this chapter. However, the prominent systemic manifestations of RA are only partly explained by events that can be observed in synovium and adjacent tissues. It remains possible that primary stages of this disease, especially immunologic aspects of its pathogenesis, may occur elsewhere (e.g., in the gastrointestinal tract or lymphoid organs), and then localize to the joint. The factors that could contribute to localizing a systemic, immune-mediated disease to diarthrodial joints are not clear, but may include the specialized structure of synovial tissue, its very rich blood supply, preferential expression of specific antigens in synovium or cartilage, and the unique combination of cell types that can interact in the inflamed joint (including a variety of cells of the immune system, synovial fibroblasts, and chondrocytes).

Any convincing, unifying explanation for the etiology and pathogenesis of RA must be consistent with a diversity of clinical and epidemiologic observations. These include the apparent absence of RA from the Old World until the past few hundred years, the typically symmetric and precisely mapped distribution of involvement among the axial and appendicular joints (which is far more striking than in other forms of joint inflammation), and the effects of gender and pregnancy on the incidence and course of RA.

It is convenient and useful to conceptualize RA as having distinct pathogenetic stages as it evolves from inflammation of joints to tissue destruction and deformity. However, recent findings have tended to blur the discreteness and significance of these stages. For example, it is now known that cartilage and bone erosion can begin early in the course of disease. On the other hand, the nature of the T-cell infiltrate is not demonstrably different in very late disease compared with relatively early disease. The existence of preclinical RA is supported by the finding that, in patients with early disease, clinically uninvolved joints can show characteristic histologic changes, and by the detection of characteristic autoantibodies before onset of clinical disease. The probable existence of several stages of pathogenetically significant but clinically undetectable RA, before the patient or physician is aware of illness, makes definition of the precise onset of RA (and of a possible etiology) particularly difficult. In view of all of the above considerations, and in light of the enormous morbidity and significant mortality of RA, the etiology of this disease can legitimately be viewed as one of the great unsolved mysteries of modern medicine.

GENETIC FACTORS IN RHEUMATOID ARTHRITIS

The existence of a genetic predisposition to RA is strongly supported by a frequency of concordance for RA in monozygotic twins that is much higher than in the general population, and also higher than in fraternal twins or other siblings. Although previous estimates for disease concordance in monozygotic twins ranged from 30% to 50%, more recent studies indicate that the true concordance is lower, between 12% and 15%, compared with 4% in fraternal twins and 1% or less in the general population (1–5). In a relatively isolated and homogeneous population (Iceland), it has been shown that RA patients were more closely related than sets of control subjects, consistent with descent from a small number of founders. Increased risk for RA was found in both first- and second-degree relatives (6). It may be more than simple coincidence that one of the first written descriptions of RA appears in a 1782 textbook authored by Jon Petursson, an Icelandic physician (7).

Association with Class II Major Histocompatibility Complex Alleles

It has been estimated that no more than one half of the genetic predisposition to RA resides in the major histocompatibility complex (MHC), with the remainder of genetic predisposition residing in other loci that are not yet conclusively defined, but that are the target of current investigation (1,5,8–11) (Table 52.1). Both case control studies and analysis of multicase families are being utilized; fortunately, RA typically displays fairly similar genotypic and phenotypic characteristics whether ascertained in family studies or as sporadic incident cases (5,12,13), with the possible exception of slightly greater association with HLA-DR4 in familial RA (13).

Several protein products encoded by genes of the MHC are responsible for presentation of peptide antigens to T lymphocytes. In general, class II MHC molecules (HLA-DR, DQ, and perhaps DP) present peptides to $CD4^+$ T cells, whereas class I MHC molecules (HLA-A, B, and C) present peptide antigens to $CD8^+$ T cells. In the 1970s, Stastny first reported a linkage of RA to the HLA-DR4 allele (14). In white patients with RA who have detectable rheumatoid factor, as many as 60% to 70% of individuals carry the DR4 allele, compared with 30% of controls (14–16). The existence of subtypes of HLA-DR4 confers additional complexity to this association, and it is the Dw4 and Dw14 molecules (subtypes of DR4 that are encoded by the DRB1*0401 and DRB1*0404 alleles) that are specifically associated with RA in whites. In Japanese individuals with RA, the specific association is with the Dw15 subtype of DR4 encoded by the DRB1*0405 allele (17). In certain

TABLE 52.1. *Gene loci proposed to affect susceptibility to rheumatoid arthritis and/or severity of rheumatoid arthritis*

Class II MHC
HLA-DR
HLA-DQ
HLA-DP
HLA-DM
Other MHC-linked genes (class III MHC)
TNF-α
C4
Heat shock protein 70
Hormone-related genes
Prolactin
Estrogen synthase
Estrogen receptor
Corticotropin releasing hormone
Non-MHC genes associated with immune and inflammatory responses
Lymphocyte-associated
T-cell receptor α
T-cell receptor δ
T-cell receptor β
Immunoglobulin G heavy chain
Immunoglobulin kappa light chain
FcγRIII-A
Stimulatory killer cell immunoglobulin-like receptor 2 (KIR2DS2)
Cytotoxic T-lymphocytic antigen 4 (CTLA4)
Cytokines/cytokine receptors
TNF receptor II
Chemokine receptor CCR5
IL-10
IL-1
IL-1 receptor antagonist
Macrophage migration inhibitory factor
IL-3
Other
Mannose binding lectin
Stromelysin 1 (matrix metalloproteinase 3)
Natural resistant-associated macrophage protein 1 (NRAMP1)

HLA, human leukocyte antigen; IL, interleukin; MHC, major histocompatibility complex; TNF, tumor necrosis factor.

Native American populations and in Israeli Jews, non-DR4 alleles (DR6 and DR1, respectively) are associated with risk for RA (18,19). Clarification of the probable molecular basis for these different genetic associations became clear once the amino acid sequence and three-dimensional structure of MHC molecules were obtained. Each DRB1 susceptibility allele carries the sequence QKRAA or QRRAA from amino acids 69 to 74 of the DR β chain, whereas DR alleles not associated with RA have different sequences in this region (in the amino acid single letter code Q indicates glutamine, K lysine, R arginine, and A alanine). This stretch of amino acids is positioned along the floor of the antigen binding groove of the DR molecule, such that it could contribute to the selection of specific peptides presented by DR molecules to $CD4^+$ T lymphocytes. This five–amino acid sequence has been termed the "shared epitope" (20).

Although the evidence for linkage of the shared epitope sequence to RA in many populations is strong, the mechanism by which it confers risk remains unknown, and several different alternatives are possible. The shared epitope is more clearly associated with seropositive RA (21) and with male patients who develop RA at a young age (22). Furthermore, other class II MHC genes have also been proposed to play a role in RA susceptibility (8,23–25), and in some populations HLA-DQ has been suggested to be even more important than HLA-DR (24), with homozygosity for DQ3 an especially strong predisposing genotype for RA (26). Whether DQ alleles confer risk for RA only because of linkage disequilibrium with HLA-DR, or whether they carry independent disease association remains controversial (27–30), and may depend on the specific ethnic group that is analyzed. HLA-DM functions during antigen trafficking and loading onto class II MHC dimers inside antigen-presenting cells. Initial studies suggested that associations of HLA-DM polymorphisms with RA were weak at best (8,31). A more recent study of a French RA cohort found an altered frequency of alleles at the HLA-DMA locus but not at HLA-DMB (32).

Roles of Other MHC Loci

A variety of genes not directly involved in antigen presentation are also located within the MHC locus. These non–class I or non–class II genes encode a heterogeneous group of proteins and are collectively termed class III MHC loci. Extensive haplotype analysis of multicase families suggests that at least two areas of the MHC outside the class II loci have genetic effects in RA (33). Polymorphisms associated with the tumor necrosis factor-α (TNF-α), complement component C4, and 70-kd heat shock protein (hsp70) genes have been linked to RA susceptibility (34–39).

In view of the important role of TNF-α in RA, with very high production of this cytokine in inflamed RA synovium, it will be important to clarify whether the linkages between susceptibility to RA and TNF locus microsatellite polymorphisms (5,34–36,40–43) can be correlated with functional effects on levels of TNF production. Linkage disequilibrium with HLA-DR may limit the extent of RA susceptibility that can be attributed to the TNF locus (44). Additional unknown genes telomeric to the TNF locus may be independent risk factors for RA (45,46). Two reports link a single nucleotide polymorphism in exon 6 of the TNF receptor II gene to familial RA in whites (47,48). This gene is located on chromosome 1, and the effects of the polymorphism on TNF receptor expression or function are not known.

C4 null alleles are more convincingly associated with systemic lupus erythematosus (SLE) than with other rheumatologic diseases. Nevertheless, some evidence links C4 locus polymorphisms with both risk for (37) and severity of (38) RA. The hsp70 gene cluster is positioned adjacent to complement genes found in the MHC complex. Three hsp70 proteins are encoded by MHC-linked genes. In one of these, hsp70-hom, a coding region polymorphism was linked to RA in one study (49).

The killer cell immunoglobulin-like receptor (KIR) gene family is expressed on cytotoxic lymphocytes. One study has shown that the KIR2DS2 receptor, which is thought to activate cytotoxic cell function, is found more frequently on the expanded subset of $CD4^+$ $CD28^-$ cells in patients with rheumatoid vasculitis, compared with RA or normal controls (50). This association may reflect a genetic polymorphism in the complex loci that control KIR expression, although direct demonstration of DNA polymorphisms at such loci in rheumatoid vasculitis are not yet available. Altered allele frequencies of the MHC class I gene HLA-C, a putative ligand for KIR2DS2, was found in the same group of rheumatoid vasculitis patients (50).

Hormonal Effects and the Genetics of Rheumatoid Arthritis

Important hormonal influences in RA are supported by several lines of evidence. RA is at least twice as common in women as in men. Onset of disease appears to be rare in pregnancy, whereas amelioration of preexisting RA can be observed. On the other hand, the postpartum period may carry an increased risk for onset of new RA (51). Evidence that exogenous estrogens can affect the incidence and severity of RA is controversial. Likewise, the effect of fecundity (with the suggestion that nulliparity carries increased risk for subsequent development of RA) requires confirmation. A marker in an intron of the estrogen synthase locus was shown to exhibit increased allele sharing in sibling pair analysis of RA patients (52). However, the functional significance of this polymorphism in the regulation of estrogen metabolism is not yet clear.

The prolactin gene is located close to the MHC complex on chromosome 6. In view of a reported association of RA with breast-feeding, which is a high prolactin state, a role for dysregulated production of prolactin and the prolactin gene locus in susceptibility to RA has been proposed (53). In women with RA, breast-feeding may be associated with a slightly greater risk of postpartum flare-up compared with postpartum RA patients who do not breast-feed (54). The hypothalamic-pituitary-adrenal axis regulates responses to inflammation. A genetic defect in corticotropin-releasing hormone (CRH) controls arthritis susceptibility in the rat, and has been postulated in human RA (55). In RA patients, a microsatellite linkage has been observed close to the CRH gene (56,57).

Recent work has discerned a novel connection between effects of pregnancy on the course of RA and products of the class II MHC gene locus. In analyzing the extent of maternofetal disparity for class II alleles, it was found that remission of RA during pregnancy was associated with extensive disparity of both DR and DQ alleles, whereas ongoing active RA tended to occur in women with a higher degree of maternofetal class II MHC identity (58). These findings may suggest that a reduction in the activity of RA during pregnancy may reflect specific immunologic events rather than general immunosuppressive effects of pregnancy.

Other Rheumatoid Arthritis Gene Loci

Preliminary evidence also implicates other gene loci associated with the immune response in susceptibility to RA. T-cell receptors (TCRs) for antigen are expressed as heterodimers, generally disulfide-linked, in association with the CD3 molecular complex on the T-cell surface. Most T cells express the $\alpha\beta$ receptor, and a minority express the $\gamma\delta$ receptor. There is no evidence for deletions in the TCR gene loci or inheritance of unique TCR genes in RA. However, some evidence suggests association of RA with various polymorphisms in the TCR gene regions, including the TCRA (α-chain) locus, the closely linked TCRD (δ-chain) locus, and possibly the TCRB (β-chain) locus (59). The largest study of TCR polymorphisms in these loci in RA identified a greater incidence, at the TCRAV8S1 locus, of the genotype II allele compared with the genotype I allele in RA patients, but did not find any association with polymorphisms in the TCRB region (60). No influence of HLA-DR alleles on the frequency of TCR allele polymorphisms was found in this study. The significance of this weak TCRA association and possible mechanisms by which it might influence disease pathogenesis remain unknown.

Immunoglobulin gene rearrangements generate the vast majority of the diversity expressed by both cell surface immunoglobulin and secreted antibodies. However, several polymorphisms, termed allotypes, exist in both immunoglobulin heavy and light chains. Associations of RA with specific IgG allotypes or with genetic polymorphisms linked to allotypes have been demonstrated (61). The functional importance of such polymorphisms in normal immune responses or in immune-mediated diseases such as RA remains unclear. In Czech but not British patients with RA who lacked the shared epitope, an altered frequency of a polymorphism was found in a heavy-chain gene that encodes a sequence frequently present in antibodies with rheumatoid factor activity (62). Immunoglobulin receptors expressed by inflammatory cells represent one pathway by which immune complexes can initiate inflammation in synovium. A functional polymorphism in the coding region of Fc γ receptor IIIA has been associated with both RA and SLE susceptibility and severity (63–65).

The chemokines are a large family of chemoattractant cytokines that play a crucial role in the influx of leukocytes into sites of inflammation, including inflamed joints in RA. Leukocyte subsets express several distinct chemokine receptors, with complex and overlapping binding specificity for individual chemokines. One recent report suggests that patients with RA have a different distribution of alleles of the chemokine receptor CCR5 compared with healthy controls or patients with SLE. None of the RA patients, compared with a small percentage of the other groups, were homozygous for a CCR5 allele that includes a 32–base pair genomic deletion, which renders this chemokine receptor nonfunctional and provides resistance to HIV-1 infection (66). Because memory T cells that infiltrate RA synovium express the CCR5 receptor, the implication is that a functional CCR5 receptor may be a necessary permissive factor for the development of RA. However, it has been found that CCR5 is not important in lymphocyte chemoattraction by RA synovial fluid (67).

Other cytokine and proinflammatory genes are potential candidate loci for RA susceptibility or resistance. The cytokine macrophage migration inhibitory factor (MIF) is a proinflammatory cytokine with allelic polymorphisms in the promotor region (68,69). A polymorphism associated with lower MIF expression is associated with lesser severity of RA (69). A single nucleotide polymorphism in the interleukin-3 (IL-3) promotor is associated with RA in Japanese subjects, but is apparently not associated with altered promotor function (70). Interferon-γ (IFN-γ) is the prototypic cytokine associated with helper T cell subset 1 (T_H1) immune responses that are believed to be dominant in RA and several other immune-mediated diseases. One case-control study found an association between an allelic polymorphism in the first intron of the IFN-γ gene and both incidence and severity of RA (71), but other investigators were unable to confirm these results (72,73). Stromelysin-1, also known as matrix metalloproteinase-3 (MMP-3), is one of the tissue-destructive enzymes present in RA pannus. An MMP-3 promotor allele was found to associate with rapid joint destruction in RA, but not risk for onset of RA (74).

The mannose-binding lectin (MBL) is an acute-phase response serum protein that is part of the innate immune response. A point mutation in the coding region and a promotor polymorphism that are associated with low MBL serum levels were each found to be genetic risk factors for onset of RA (75), and for RA severity (76). If confirmed, this could implicate ineffective innate responses to a microbial pathogen in the etiology of RA. The natural resistant-associated macrophage protein 1 (NRAMP1) appears to have a role in macrophage activation and cytokine synthesis. A coding region polymorphism in NRAMP1 was weakly linked to RA in one study (77), and a functional promotor polymorphism was associated with susceptibility to RA in shared epitope-negative patients, and with radiographically severe disease (78).

Various other chromosomal loci have been tentatively implicated as being associated with RA using gene mapping studies (79–81) (Table 52.1). However, genomewide linkage analyses have not yet been in agreement about which non-MHC loci are associated with RA (5,10,11,82). A metanalysis identified a region on chromosome 16 by pooling data from four studies, although none of the individual studies had linked this area to RA (11). Some of the loci identified in mapping studies are in the general neighborhood of genes associated with immune responses, and it is likely that well-controlled investigations of sufficient size will yield definitive identification of non-MHC RA-associated genes within the next few years (1). At this time, however, all genetic associations with RA other than at the class II MHC locus should be considered preliminary, with additional studies required to confirm their validity or functional significance. Furthermore, current knowledge suggests that no single genetic trait will prove to be either necessary or sufficient to lead to the development of RA (9). Genetic associations may exist for severity and extra-articular complications of RA that are distinct from genetic factors that affect the risk for developing RA.

Another approach to understanding gene expression in specific diseases makes use of emerging complementary DNA microarray technology and other sensitive methods to survey the levels of expression of a large number of genes in diseased tissue. These approaches, which are being introduced as an analytical tool in RA (83,84), are more likely to yield insights into levels of expression of genes involved in disease pathogenesis rather than inherited polymorphisms that govern disease susceptibility. Nevertheless, the importance of levels of expression of individual genes in inflammatory arthritis is highlighted by transgenic mice that overexpress TNF-α. In such mice, inflammatory, erosive arthritis is the major phenotypic abnormality (85).

ROLE OF INFECTION IN RHEUMATOID ARTHRITIS

Despite intensive efforts to identify an infectious organism, or class of organisms, as the cause of RA, convincing evidence for an infectious etiology of RA is not available. The strongest evidence for a role of infection in triggering RA is indirect and derives from historic and paleologic studies (86). Landré-Beauvais is generally credited with the first clear description of RA, in 1800, although Sydenham as early as 1676 and Petursson in 1782 also may have identified RA. The prevailing concept is that the RA cannot be conclusively identified in ancient human remains from the Old World, or as a distinct disorder in writings of Greek and Roman authors (87), although this view has recently been challenged (88). In contrast, other forms of arthritis such as ankylosing spondylitis (AS), osteoarthritis (OA), and gout are easily detectable from these eras. Hand deformities suggestive of RA have been recognized in European Renaissance art (88,89), although the reliability and significance of these observations remains in dispute. Some evidence for RA has been found in skeletal remains from ancient North America (87,88,90), and the Mexican physician Alonso Lopez de Hinejosos may have described RA as a second type of "gout" in 1578 (88). If RA first existed in the New World and then appeared in Europe only after arrival in the Americas of European settlers, this would be strong, but indirect, evidence for a critical, transmissible environmental agent. Although an infectious organism or group of organisms would be the most likely candidates for such an agent, other environmental factors are conceivable. For example, the prevalence of RA can be correlated with factors as diverse as dietary composition (91,92), smoking (93,94), and exposure to cats (95).

Specific Pathogens Suspected to Have a Role in Rheumatoid Arthritis

Attempts to implicate specific organisms in the etiology of RA date back to at least the 1920s. Table 52.2 lists some of the more prominent candidate organisms. Because the clinical onset of RA does not overtly cluster in space or time, it seems possible that a ubiquitous organism, perhaps presumed to be nonpathogenic, could trigger RA, given an appropriate mix of host factors, including genetic background. Alternatively, it is possible that infections that cause RA do cluster in space and time, but that the infectious event is subclinical, perhaps not initially located within joints, and followed by a highly variable latent period before expression of joint inflammation. The notion that infection, if important in RA, may not be directly present in the joints themselves, gains support from repeated failures to consistently document the presence of a unique organism in RA synovial tissue. Approaches used have included a wide range of culture techniques, immunologic analyses, *in situ* hybridization, and polymerase chain reaction strategies for amplification of nucleic acid sequences from classes of organisms. Unless microorganisms exist that are refractory to detection by all such techniques as are currently used, chronic, clinically established RA is not accompanied by direct infection of synovial tissue itself. This does not exclude infection as a transient mechanism for synovial injury and initiation of an immune-mediated pathogenetic cascade.

The rationale for consideration of the various organisms listed in Table 52.2 (and of others not listed) has varied according to the organism. For viruses, such as parvovirus, rubella, and the retrovirus human T cell leukemia virus type 1 (HTLV-1), clinical syndromes resembling RA are known to be caused by these organisms. However, for parvovirus and rubella virus, the arthritis, while fairly symmetric, inflammatory, and at times accompanied by serologic abnormalities (such as the presence of rheumatoid factor) (96), is not typically progressive or erosive. Detection of parvovirus DNA in RA synovium more than in OA (97) may reflect the far greater number of leukocytes present in RA synovial tissue. HTLV-1, on the other hand, can cause a chronic erosive arthropathy, but only in patients who can clearly be shown to have systemic and synovial infection with this retrovirus (98). Studies using mice transgenic for the HTLV-1 *tax* gene provide an interesting model for a direct role of retroviral gene products in orchestrating synovial inflammation and cartilage damage (99). In one study, 25 of 101 RA patients compared with 8% of healthy controls had detectable HTLV-1 tax sequences and antibodies to Tax in their peripheral blood. Only 1 RA patient was infected with HTLV-1 (100). In HTLV-1 endemic areas, association between HTLV-1 infection and RA is not evident (101). Could another retrovirus, not yet identified, be a cause of RA? In synovium, sequences corresponding to endogenous human retroviral components have been detected (102), but infectious retroviruses have not been isolated (103). Expression of endogenous retroviral sequences can be interpreted as a consequence of cell activation during an immune/inflammatory response.

TABLE 52.2. *Microbial organisms proposed as possible triggers for rheumatoid arthritis*

Bacterial
Gram positive cocci
Mycobacteria
Proteus
Escherichia coli
Mycoplasma
Viral
Epstein-Barr virus
Parvovirus
Retroviruses
Cytomegalovirus
Rubella
Human herpes virus 6

Serologic evidence has been proposed to implicate a variety of organisms in the etiology of RA, including Epstein-Barr virus (EBV) (104), parvovirus B19 (105), and *Proteus mirabilis* (106). However, interpretation of elevated antibody titers or an elevated percentage of positive titers is complicated, given the potential artifacts in such assays that can be caused by the presence of rheumatoid factor, other autoantibodies that may cross-react against microbial determinants, and dysregulated antibody responses that can accompany an autoimmune disease such as RA that has a significant systemic component. In order for serologic studies to provide convincing evidence for a microbial association, convincing longitudinal data will be needed in large numbers of patients, with stringent controls for antibody specificity and disease specificity. Therapeutic immunizations, such as the hepatitis B vaccine, have also been anecdotally linked to RA, but such a link is not supported by epidemiologic evidence (107).

EBV has received attention in connection with RA for several reasons. First, a primary target for EBV infection (apart from pharyngeal epithelium) is the B lymphocyte. Second, it has been observed that outgrowth of EBV-transformed B lymphoblastoid lines occurs more rapidly from peripheral blood samples of RA patients compared with controls, a phenomenon that is probably due to an elevated EBV DNA load (108). This likely occurs due to defective regulation of EBV-transformed B cells by T cells and monocytes, which occurs as a consequence of disease activity of RA rather than in connection with the etiology (109–111). A third connection between EBV and RA centers on the observation that synovial T lymphocytes from patients with RA can recognize and respond to EBV antigens (112). Such responses occur within expanded T-cell clonotypes that can be identified according to their TCRB variable gene usage. However, such T-cell responses to EBV antigens are not unique to synovial T cells, or to RA. A fourth link is the observation that bone marrow progenitor cells from RA patients are particularly effective in supporting transformation and outgrowth of B lymphoblasts infected with EBV (113). A fifth connection has been the observation that the shared epitope sequence contained within the RA susceptibility MHC class II alleles corresponds to an amino acid sequence within the EBV gp110 protein (114). This is one mechanism by which EBV could provoke autoreactivity. Expansion of a T-cell subset by an EBV superantigen could also trigger autoreactive T cells (115). Polyclonal activation of B lymphocytes by EBV could lead to production of autoantibodies. Nevertheless, most patients infected with EBV do not develop RA, some patients with RA have no evidence of EBV infection, and whether synovial tissue in RA is specifically infected by EBV remains controversial (116–119). Other autoimmune diseases, such as SLE (120), have been proposed as more likely to be etiologically connected with EBV.

The possible role of mycobacteria in RA arises from somewhat different lines of evidence. Adjuvant arthritis, one of the most interesting animal models of RA, is triggered by mycobacterial products and is mediated by T cell–dependent mechanisms (121). Evidence has been provided for cross-reactivity of cartilage components with mycobacterial antigens and for reactivity of synovial T cells from patients with RA to some of these antigens (122). Part of the response to mycobacteria in adjuvant arthritis is directed against heat shock proteins. In human disease, T-cell responses against heat shock proteins can be found both in RA and in other forms of joint inflammation (123). Whether these responses are triggered by microbial heat shock proteins or by human heat shock proteins released from dying cells in inflammatory lesions remains unsettled. Considerable sequence differences exist between microbial heat shock antigens and their human homologues. A distinct heat shock protein termed DNAj contains, in *Escherichia coli*, the QKRAA shared epitope sequence. Like the EBV antigen containing this sequence, immune responses to this region of *E. coli* DNAj are more readily observed in patients with RA than in other individuals (124). A link between *P. mirabilis* infection and RA has been proposed, based in part on immunologic cross-reactivity between *Proteus* antigen and both the shared epitope and components of articular cartilage (125,126).

An attempt to link mycoplasma with RA was based in part on the ability of mycoplasma superantigens to potently activate T lymphocytes and to exacerbate experimental arthritis in animal models (127). Tetracycline antibiotics, which can eradicate mycoplasma infections, have been used to treat RA. However, despite some efficacy of such antibiotics in RA, their antimicrobial specificity is broad, and tetracyclines can also function as MMP inhibitors. Recent intensive searches for mycoplasma in RA synovium have been unsuccessful.

Despite the frustrating lack of a clear connection between any microbial agent and the etiology of RA, it would be premature to abandon consideration of a central role for an infectious organism or class of organisms in this disease. The complex interplay between microorganisms and the immune system is by no means fully understood. A variety of potential indirect mechanisms for triggering of RA by microbes remains to be carefully examined. The capacity of RA synovium to retain bacterial products that may be deposited in immune system antigen-presenting cells due to extraarticular infection could be relevant to amplification or even initiation of disease (128). Overall, however, evidence for molecular mimicry between microorganisms and autoantigens as a cause for RA remains distinctly unconvincing (129).

ROLE OF AUTOANTIBODIES IN THE PATHOGENESIS OF RHEUMATOID ARTHRITIS

Although T lymphocytes greatly outnumber B lymphocytes in most RA synovial tissues, synovium is nevertheless an active site of B-cell differentiation. Plasma cells are present and synovial tissue is an antibody-producing organ in RA. Peripheral blood B lymphocytes in RA show evidence of oligoclonality (130,131), as well as elevated percentages of $CD5^+$ B cells (132), a subset associated with autoantibody production. B cells that have undergone receptor editing (a second round of immunoglobulin gene rearrangement that can occur in differentiated B cells) can accumulate in RA synovium and may be autoreactive (133–135). The B-cell population in RA synovium includes a $CD20^+$ $CD38^-$ subset that responds to activation stimuli with a high level of immunoglobulin production without cell proliferation (136). Cytokines that mediate B-cell chemotaxis (137) and differentiation into plasma cells (138) are found in RA synovial tissue or fluid.

The recombination activating genes (RAG) and terminal deoxynucleotidyl transferase (TdT) enzymes are expressed in RA synovium, consistent with *in situ,* active immunoglobulin gene rearrangement (139). The total synovial B cell pool likely includes both cells that matured *in situ*, as well as cells recruited to synovium after maturation elsewhere (139), potentially in other inflamed joints (140). These cells show a high rate of somatic mutation (141). Their survival may be enhanced through interactions with synovial fibroblasts (142), as well as with other immune system cells and mediators.

Rheumatoid factors are autoantibodies that recognize the Fc portion of IgG. The discovery of rheumatoid factor and its association with RA were milestones in the development of concepts of autoimmunity, and presence of elevated rheumatoid factor continues to be one of the American College of Rheumatology criteria for RA. Nevertheless, the role of rheumatoid factor, both in regulation of normal immune responses and in the pathogenesis of RA, remains incompletely understood. Rheumatoid factor is discussed in detail in Chapter 58, and some of the pieces of evidence for its importance in RA are summarized in Table 52.3. However, to date, no specific type of rheumatoid factor has been conclusively associated uniquely with RA, and a variety of other immune-mediated and infectious diseases that do not involve erosive joint damage can be characterized by high titers of circulating rheumatoid factor. A decline in the rheumatoid factor titer is not a consistently reliable early marker for response of RA to therapeutic intervention. Most importantly, a subset of patients with RA is seronegative (i.e., lacks elevations in rheumatoid factor). Although such patients overall tend to have milder disease, a subset of this seronegative group goes on to develop severe joint damage that is not otherwise distinguishable from patients with seropositive RA. In light of currently available evidence, a reasonable conclusion is that rheumatoid factor represents an important pathway for amplification of articular disease and development of extraarticular complications, but that it is not a required factor in the etiology or pathogenesis of RA.

Antinuclear antibodies of a variety of specificities can also be found in RA (Table 52.4), generally, but not exclusively, in patients with elevated titers of rheumatoid factor. Such antibodies do not currently have a unique role in disease pathogenesis, but may be additional markers for disease severity. Anticardiolipin antibodies may be found in RA, but are probably less frequently associated with thrombotic complications than in SLE. Antineutrophil cytoplasmic antibodies are found in some patients with RA, but are not necessarily a marker for vasculitic complications.

Anticollagen antibodies are of potential pathogenic interest given the important role of humoral responses to collagen, in conjunction with T-cell responses, in the rodent collagen arthritis model for RA (see Chapter 29). Arthritis can also be produced in mice by intravenous injection of large quantities of anticollagen antibodies, which lead to joint inflammation by a complement dependent pathway (143). Antibodies to both native and denatured type II collagen can be found in patients with RA (144–147), but are even more characteristic of relapsing polychondritis and are present in other rheumatologic disorders. Nonetheless, collagen epitopes targeted by anticollagen antibodies in RA differ from those found in other human diseases, but correspond to targets of pathogenic antibodies in murine collagen-induced arthritis (148). Whether such antibodies arise prior to or as a result of cartilage damage in RA is controversial (149,150). Antibodies to type IX collagen are more common in RA than in control subjects, but are detected in fewer than 50% of patients (151). Synovial tissue has been demonstrated to be a site of anticollagen antibody synthesis (152), and such antibodies are contained within immunoglobulins that can be eluted from articular cartilage (153). Antibodies to small proteoglycans can also be detected in RA (154), as can antibodies to cartilage oligomeric matrix protein (155).

A variety of antibodies directed against structures produced by keratinized epithelia have been found in sera from patients with RA (156–158). Included in this group are the antikeratin antibodies and antiperinuclear factor. The molecular targets of these antibodies overlap (158), and include filaggrin, vimentin (formerly termed the Sa antigen), and other peptides. It is now understood that such proteins become autoantigenic through deimination of arginine to citrulline, with citrulline being an essential component of the epitope recognized by these autoantibodies (160–163). Anti–citrulline-containing peptides (anti-CCPs) are up to 96% specific and 70% sensitive for RA (160), and may be detected very early in RA, even prior to onset of clinical symptoms. Such antibodies, like rheumatoid factors, are

TABLE 52.3. *Rheumatoid factor: evidence for a role in the pathogenesis of rheumatoid arthritis (RA)*

- Most patients with RA have elevated levels of rheumatoid factor.
- High titers of rheumatoid factor correlate with severe articular disease and with development of extraarticular manifestations.
- Preexisting elevations of rheumatoid factor predict subsequent development of RA.
- Rheumatoid factor production is prominent in RA synovial tissue, and such rheumatoid factors show evidence of antigen-driven affinity maturation.
- Rheumatoid factor can enhance formation of pathogenic immune complexes.
- B cells bearing surface rheumatoid factor can trap antigens contained in immune complexes and present them to primed T cells.

TABLE 52.4. *Antigenic targets of autoantibodies in rheumatoid arthritis*

Immune system molecules
IgG (RF)[a]
gp130 (cytokine receptor subunit)
Immunoglobulin heavy chain binding protein
Interleukin-1α
B7-H1
Connective tissue components
Type II collagen
Type IX collagen
Citrullinated peptides (e.g., citrullinated fibrin, filaggrin, vimentin)
Cartilage oligomeric matrix protein
Proteoglycan
Keratin
Intracellular antigens
Nuclear antigens (ANA)[a]
Neutrophil cytoplasmic antigens (ANCA)[a]
Glucose-6-phosphate isomerase (anti-GPI)[a]
Calpastatin
α-enolase
Calreticulin

[a]Antibody abbreviations in parentheses.

produced locally in RA synovium (164,165), where citrullinated fibrin may be their primary antigenic target (166, 167). Some patients who lack rheumatoid factor have detectable anti-CCP, which may be of diagnostic value (168). Like rheumatoid factor, anti-CCP predicts severe destructive disease when present in early RA (169–171).

Calpastatin is a natural inhibitor of calpains, a subset of cysteine proteinases. Antibodies to calpastatin have been identified in approximately 50% of patients with RA (172). It has been proposed that neutralizing antibodies to this proteinase inhibitor could promote overactivation of tissue-destructive cysteine proteinases in synovial tissue (172). Alternatively, because calpains degrade CCPs, overactivity of such proteins could also help to clear autoantigens in RA (162).

Autoantibodies to a soluble form of the gp130 signaling subunit that is part of the receptor for IL-6 and other cytokines were detected in 73% of RA patients and correlated with disease severity (173). Soluble gp130 is believed to regulate proinflammatory effects of IL-6 (173). Antibodies to B7-H1 (a cell surface molecule expressed on both T cells and antigen-presenting cells) have also been found in RA, and can coactivate T cells (174). Not all autoantibodies found in RA are pathogenic; high levels of autoantibodies to IL-1α are associated with a more favorable prognosis (175).

A new autoantibody specificity has recently been defined in RA as a result of experiments involving the K/BxN transgenic mouse (176). This animal produces high-titer autoantibodies against glucose-6-phosphate isomerase (GPI), an enzyme that is strongly expressed in synovial tissue (177), and arthritis is transferable by serum in this model (178). Joint inflammation in this system is dependent on neutrophils, Fc receptors, the alternative pathway of complement, and mast cells (179,180), and the synovial tissue contains more neutrophils than are found in RA synovium (176). Production of anti-GPI in these mice occurs primarily in lymph nodes that drain arthritic joints (181). Despite an initial report associating anti-GPI antibodies with human RA at high sensitivity and specificity (177), subsequent work showed that such antibodies are rarely found in RA and lack disease specificity (182). Antibodies to another glycolytic pathway enzyme, α-enolase, have also been reported in RA (183).

In addition to the presence of numerous autoantibodies, IgG in RA is abnormally galactosylated (184) due to reduced activity of galactosyl transferase in RA B cells (185). The reasons for this abnormality are not yet well defined, and it is not absolutely specific to RA. Although some undergalactosylated IgG molecules may be particularly good targets for rheumatoid factor binding, a clear link between galactosylation abnormalities of IgG and autoantibody contributions to pathogenesis of RA is not yet available.

Pathogenic autoantibodies, particularly rheumatoid factor (Table 52.3), probably do assume an important role in the pathogenesis of RA. Particular autoantibodies may be especially important in some extraarticular manifestations of RA, such as antineutrophil antibodies in Felty syndrome (186). Nevertheless, no single autoantibody appears to be indispensable for the development of RA. Furthermore, a condition not easily distinguished from RA has been reported as a frequent occurrence in patients with agammaglobulinemia (187). Although such patients can develop chronic infectious polyarthritis with organisms such as mycoplasma that may be difficult to culture, chronic joint infection is unlikely to explain every case of inflammatory polyarthritis in these patients. This suggests that joint inflammation typical of RA can develop in the complete absence of antibody responses, although such cases may show less erosive damage that is typical of RA (188). B cells may be important in RA as antigen-presenting and cytokine-secreting cells essential for maintaining integrity and erosive properties of synovial tissue (189), functions that are not due to autoantibody production. Recent encouraging therapeutic trials of B-cell depletion by monoclonal antibody infusions in RA support this concept (190).

CELLULAR IMMUNE MECHANISMS IN RHEUMATOID ARTHRITIS

T lymphocytes were not considered to have an important role in RA until it was demonstrated in the 1970s that the largest mononuclear cell population and the great majority of lymphocytes present in RA synovial tissue were T cells (191,192). Subsequently, the hypothesis that RA was similar to a delayed hypersensitivity reaction was proposed (193). Table 52.5 outlines the multiple and quite convincing lines of evidence that substantiate a central role for T cells in RA. T cells in synovium are concentrated in perivascular clusters, together with other leukocytes (Fig. 52.1), and are also scattered throughout less densely infiltrated portions of synovium. Most T cells in RA synovium are CD4$^+$, but the

TABLE 52.5. *Evidence for a central role for T cells in rheumatoid arthritis (RA)*

Large numbers of T cells and antigen-presenting cells are present in synovial tissue and fluid.
Synovial T cells express activation and memory makers.
T-cell subsets, and possibly clonal T cell populations, accumulate in RA joints in a nonrandom manner.
RA is associated with specific MHC class II alleles (DR and/or DQ).
T cells and specific clonal T-cell populations are central to the induction and regulation of several animal models of RA.
T cell–directed therapeutic interventions may be effective in RA, and are clearly effective in animal models.
T-cell cytokines, such as IFN-γ and IL-17, that are present in RA joints, mediate biologic effects highly relevant to the pathogenesis of joint inflammation and damage.
Cytokines that promote T-cell activation and T_H1 differentiation, such as IL-15 and IL-12, are present in RA synovium at physiologically significant concentrations.

IFN, interferon; IL, interleukin; MHC, major histocompatibility complex; T_H1, helper T cell subset 1.

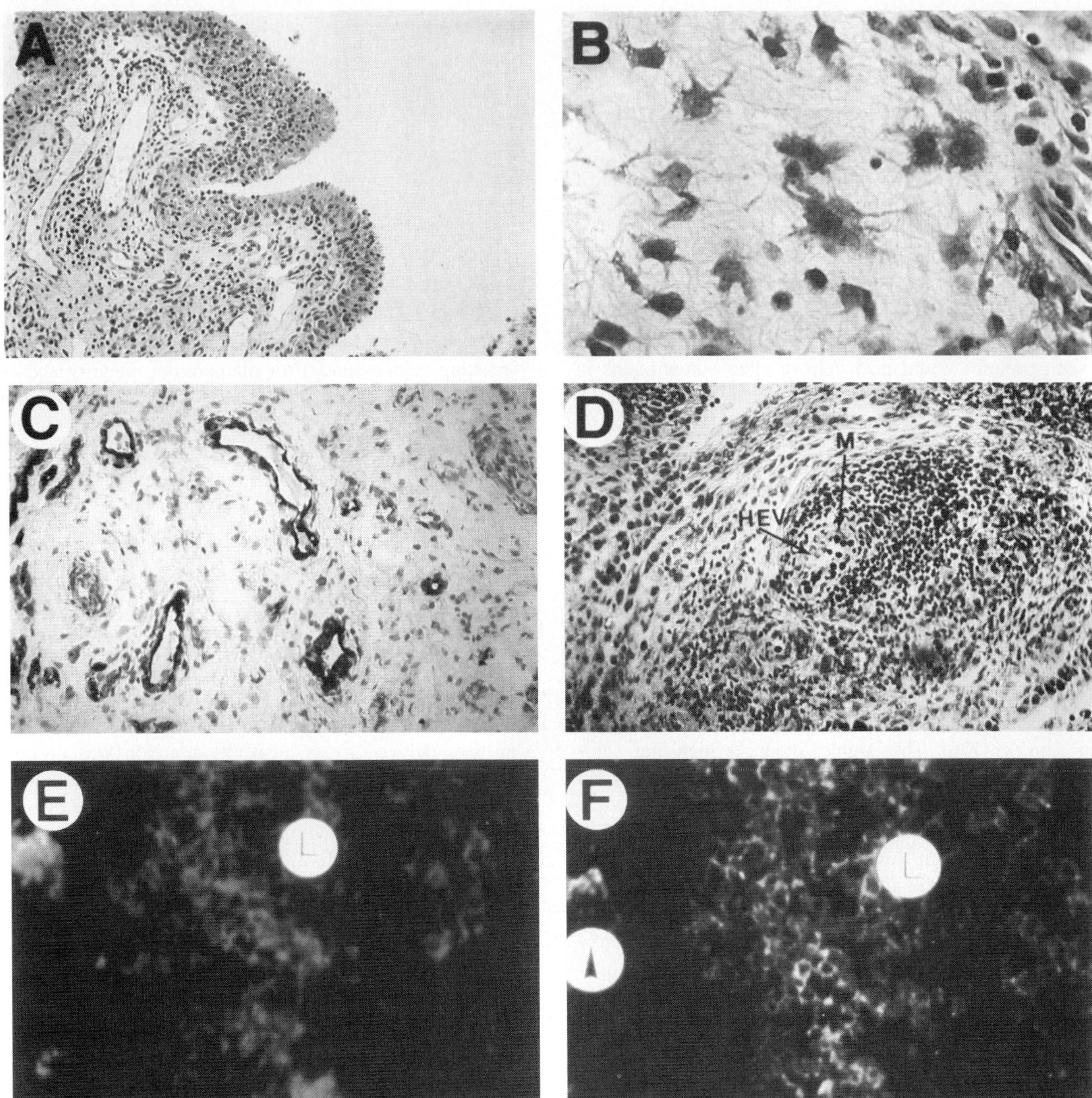

FIG. 52.1. Role of the cellular immune response in rheumatoid arthritis (RA) synovium. **A:** Low-power view of RA synovial tissue, illustrating hyperplasia of the synovial lining layer and infiltration of mononuclear cells. **B:** High-power view of RA synovium stained with anti-CD60, which identifies a variety of cell populations in this tissue. Cell/cell interactions between lymphocytes and antigen-presenting cells are visible in the center of the panel. **C**: Frozen section of RA synovial tissue, immunostained to identify vascular structures, including both thin-walled and thick-walled venules. **D:** Frozen section illustrating perivascular mononuclear cell aggregate around a high endothelial venule (*HEV*). Purified peripheral blood monocytes (*M*) have been overlaid onto this section and adhere to the luminal and cut surfaces of the HEV. **E, F:** Immunofluorescence photomicrographs of a perivascular mononuclear cell infiltrate stained with anti-CD3 **(F)**, which identifies nearly all mature T-lymphocytes, and with anti-CD60 **(E)**, which identifies most synovial T-lymphocytes and selected other cell populations. *L* indicates lymphoid aggregate and the arrow in **F** indicates a non–T cell that is CD60 positive. [Reprinted from references 403 **(A, B)**, 404 **(C, D)**, and 204 **(E, F)**, with permission.]

CD4:CD8 ratio is closer to 1:1 than is generally found in RA peripheral blood. Synovial tissue also contains multiple types of antigen-presenting cells (macrophages, dendritic cells, B lymphocytes, and even synovial fibroblasts), and these various cell types interact with T lymphocytes in synovial tissue (Figs. 52.1 and 52.2).

T-cell Subsets and Activation Pathways in Rheumatoid Arthritis

In RA, synovial T cells differ in several ways from peripheral blood T cells found in the same patients (194–203). Most cells in synovial tissue are memory cells, as classified by expression of distinct CD45 isoforms such as CD45RO (199–201). Synovial T cells also express surface structures indicative of prior activation (194–203), but their specific phenotype is puzzling, based on the sequence of expression of surface molecules known to occur with T-cell activation *in vitro*. For example, RA synovial T cells express CD69, a marker of very early T-cell activation (203), as well as class II MHC (194,195), which is a marker for later stages of T-cell activation. However, fewer cells express CD25, the high-affinity IL-2 receptor (204), which usually appears after expression of CD69 and before expression of class II MHC during T-cell activation. A subset of the $CD4^+$ $CD25^+$ cells in synovial fluid possesses regulatory function (205),

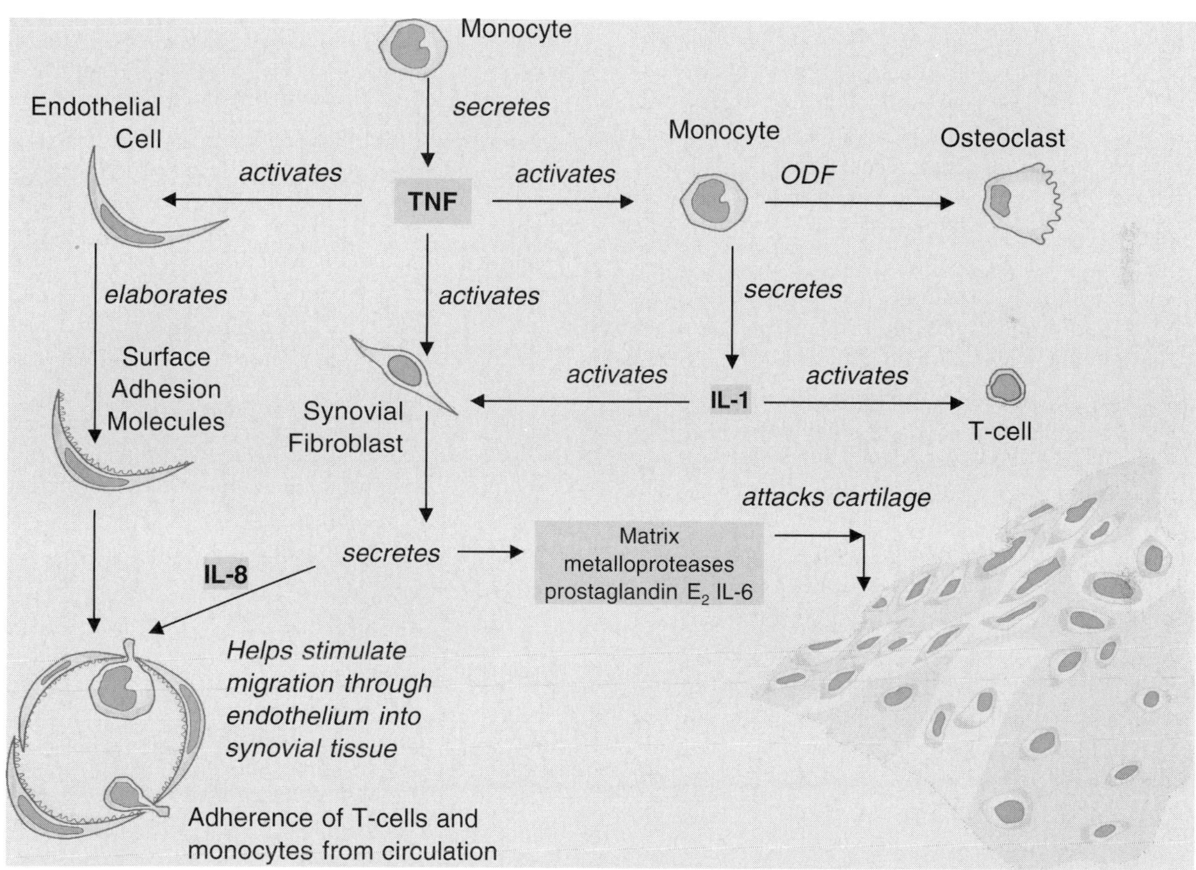

FIG. 52.2. Role of tumor necrosis factor (TNF) and other cytokines in intercellular communication and inflammation in rheumatoid arthritis (RA) synovium. Leukocytes, including T cells, monocytes, dendritic cells, and B cells, all enter synovium after adhering to activated endothelium in the synovial micovasculature. Some synovial macrophages differentiate into osteoclasts under the influence of osteoclast differentiation factor (ODF, also known as receptor activator of nuclear factor κB ligand). Interactions among the leukocyte populations include both cell-cell recognition events and cytokine activation of cell differentiation programs. Such interactions lead to activation, proliferation, and aggressive functional behavior of the synovial fibroblast, which is shown at the leading edge of destruction of articular cartilage and subchondral bone. Tumor necrosis factor (TNF) and other selected cytokines that regulate these processes are shown, with arrows indicating the cell populations that secrete these cytokines and selected cellular targets for cytokine actions. Important actions of TNF and interleukin-1 (IL-1) include up-regulation of cytokine, chemokine, prostaglandin, and protease production by synovial fibroblasts, monocytes and other cells; and induction of adhesion molecules on vascular endothelium. Leukocyte-endothelial adhesion is followed by ingress of leukocytes in the presence of chemokines (chemotactic cytokines) such as IL-8. Extracellular matrix components, not shown here, also regulate the distribution of inflammatory cells within subregions of synovium, release of cells from synovial tissue into synovial fluid, and activation of inflammatory cell subsets.

and their removal enhances disease severity in an animal model of RA (206).

T cells that express the γδ TCR dimer are a small minority of peripheral blood T cells, in contrast to the majority, which express the αβ dimer. The γδ cells are distinct with respect to antigen recognition and activation mechanisms (207–209). Some evidence indicates that this subset is overrepresented in RA synovial tissue and fluid (210–212). Because various animal models indicate that γδ T cells can either incite or regulate (213,214) immune-mediated disease, the precise role of these cells in RA is not yet certain.

T cells express a variety of costimulatory molecules that receive and transduce signals during the process of T-cell activation. One such molecule is CD28, which is normally expressed on almost all $CD4^+$ cells and a subset of $CD8^+$ cells. Ligands termed B7–1 and B7–2 (CD80 and CD86, respectively) are expressed on antigen-presenting cells and bind to CD28. Both CD28 and its ligands are expressed in RA synovial tissue (215,216). However, in some patients with RA, an expanded subset of unusual $CD4^+$ $CD28^-$ cells has been detected in peripheral blood and occasionally in the joint (217), possibly resulting from down-regulation of CD28 expression on T cells by TNF-α (218). These cells are autoreactive (217), resistant to apoptosis (219), and oligoclonal (219,220), and may rely primarily on costimulatory signals that engage surface molecules other than CD28, including receptors usually found on natural killer cells (221,222). Interpretation of this phenomenon is complex, because only a minority of RA patients show expansion of the $CD4^+$ $CD28^-$ subset, and the $CD4^+$ cells that do express CD28 may have increased cell surface density of CD28 during active disease (223).

Molecules other than CD28 that can deliver activating or coactivating signals to T cells include CD2, CD11a/CD18 (LFA-1), CD6, and CD60. These molecules are expressed on the great majority of T cells found in RA synovial fluid and tissue. With the exception of CD60, which is present on a minority of peripheral blood T cells in both normal individuals and patients with RA (204,224), all of these structures are also expressed on most circulating T cells. A role for these structures (and other structures) in T-cell activation is suggested by mitogenic effects of monoclonal antibodies against such molecules (204,224–226). Except for CD60, whose ligand is unknown, each of these molecules has well-characterized ligands that are expressed by various antigen-presenting cells, including cells in RA synovial tissue (227). Another molecule of significant importance in the interaction of T cells with antigen-presenting cells is the CD40 ligand (CD154), which appears on the cell surface early in the course of T-cell activation. This molecule binds to CD40, a cell membrane protein expressed by virtually all antigen-presenting cells, and activates a variety of functional programs in such cells, including expression of ligands for CD28. Both CD40 and its ligands are expressed by cells within RA synovium, and this molecular interaction may have an important role in the formation of germinal center–like structures in synovial tissue (228). Certain costimulatory ligands may be more abundant in inflamed joints than in other compartments. Thrombospondin-1 can costimulate T cells by cross-linking a distinct receptor on antigen-presenting cells (CD47) with a different receptor on T cells (CD36) (229). Vascular cell adhesion molecule 1 (VCAM-1, CD106) may promote activation and survival of both B and T cells in RA synovium, and may also mediate leukocyte-endothelial adhesion (230).

T cells are therefore not only present in abundance in RA synovial tissue, but also express surface structures that facilitate interactions with ligands on adjacent antigen-presenting cell populations. Nevertheless, several observations, summarized in Table 52.6, have led to an alternative viewpoint that T cells are not of great importance in the pathogenesis of RA (231). At present there is no agreement as to which, if any, antigenic targets for T cells are of importance in initiating or perpetuating RA. If self antigen cannot be shown to play an important role, the notion that RA is an autoimmune disease is difficult to sustain. Identification of pathogenic T cell clones has been difficult, and depletion of T cells has not proven thus far to be as useful a therapeutic strategy as cytokine blockade. In some assays, synovial T cells appear to be anergic (232,233). Until recently, the cytokines known to be abundant in RA synovium were not primarily of T-cell origin, and prototypic T-cell cytokines such as IL-2 were difficult to detect. More recently, however, discovery of additional cytokines, either produced by or acting upon T cells in RA synovium, has helped provide a clearer picture of how T-cell functions can be integrated logically into inflam-

TABLE 52.6. *Evidence against a central role for T cells in rheumatoid arthritis (RA)*

RA has not been proven to be an autoimmune disease.
T-cell responses to specific antigens have not been shown to trigger or perpetuate RA.
Demonstration of oligoclonal T cells in RA synovial tissue and fluid has been difficult, and different oligoclonal populations appear in different patients.
T cell–derived cytokines are less abundant in the joint than are cytokines produced by other cell types.
Erosion of cartilage and bone does not always correlate with inflammation, and may become independent of regulation by T cells, at least temporarily.
Depletion of T cells by monoclonal antibodies may not be therapeutic in RA.
Association of RA with the HLA-DR "shared epitope" is not consistently strong in all ethnic or racial groups.
RA may improve, concurrent with T-cell depletion in HIV infection, but exceptions to this pattern have been observed.
In some assays synovial T cells exhibit anergy.

HIV, human immunodeficiency virus; HLA, human leukocyte antigen.

matory and tissue destructive interactions that occur in synovial tissue.

Antigen Targets of Rheumatoid Arthritis T Cells

Various microbial antigens and autoantigens (Table 52.7) have been investigated as possible targets of T cell–directed responses in RA. The microbial antigens include both superantigens (which activate large families of T-cell clones sharing related but not identical Vβ sequences), and conventional peptide antigens, which are products of protein processing and are presented within the peptide binding cleft of MHC molecules. Because synovial tissue has many of the features of an activated lymphoid organ, it is likely that both primary and secondary immune responses to a variety of microorganisms encountered systemically will be reflected in T-cell specificities within synovial tissue. Bacterial antigens that are concentrated in lymphoid organs and that elicit T-cell responses in RA (234) can also be detected in RA synovial tissue (235). Many of these responses have no direct relationship to RA, but instead signify concurrent and essentially unrelated exposure to microbial agents (236). Enhanced synovial T-cell responses to multiple pathogens are consistent with migration to the joint of activated T cells with a variety of specificities (237). In other cases (such as responses to HTLV-1), T-cell activation by microorganisms occurs in syndromes that mimic RA, but similar responses do not generally occur in RA itself. Other responses may reflect cross-reactivity between microbial antigens and autoantigens. EBV contains a 110-kd glycoprotein, which contains the QKRAA shared epitope motif. Synovial T cells from patients with RA respond to EBV antigens, but this also is seen in spondyloarthropathies (112). The DNAj heat shock protein of *E. coli* also contains this sequence. T cells with specificity for the shared epitope sequence can be demonstrated in RA synovium (124), although the immunizing antigen that initially generated such T-cell responses is not clear.

A variety of interesting autoantigen targets have also been investigated (238–252), some only recently (Table 52.7). Some of these, such as type II collagen, gp39, cartilage link protein, and others, are arthritogenic in rodents. Posttranslational modifications of proteins, such as glycosylation, may be essential in the generation of immunogenic autoantigens (251). None of these responses has been found to associate uniformly with RA. Nonetheless, autoantigen T-cell targets that are expressed primarily or specifically in synovium and cartilage are credible candidates for amplification and perpetuation of destructive immune responses that localize to the joint, even though detectable antigen-specific T-cell populations are a small subset of synovial T cells (249). Some autoantigens, such as the molecular chaperone known as BiP (immunoglobulin binding protein), may elicit regulatory or antiinflammatory responses in both RA and animal models (253–255). Analysis of mutation frequencies at the hypoxanthine-guanine phosphoribosyl transferase (HPRT) locus in synovial and peripheral blood T cells in RA suggests that antigen-stimulated lymphocytes may recirculate from synovium back into the systemic pool, but that the primary location for activation is in the joint itself (256).

To date, attempts to treat RA by inducing tolerance to specific autoantigens has yielded an unimpressive level of clinical benefit (257–258). Although the relative importance of various antigenic targets for T cells in RA is not yet clear, substantial effort has been directed at analysis of the expressed T-cell repertoire in the joint, in the hopes of identifying pathogenic clones of lymphocytes (59). T-cell clones achieve diversity during development through combinatorial rearrangement of germ line gene segments, addition and deletion of nucleotides at the junctions of these segments, and variable pairing of receptor subunits, the α and β chains in most mature T cells. When T-cell clones are activated and expanded by encounter with antigen, the unique TCR sequences of clones can potentially be detected within heterogeneous T-cell populations. A variety of techniques have been used for this purpose, including Southern blot analysis, polymerase chain reaction (PCR) techniques, PCR followed by gel electrophoresis, and sequencing of large numbers of TCR gene segments. For analysis of RA synovial tissue or fluid T cells, control samples in various studies have included RA peripheral blood, normal peripheral blood, or

TABLE 52.7. *Proposed antigenic targets for T cells in rheumatoid arthritis*

Microbial Antigens	Autoantigens
Superantigens, such as staphylococcal toxins	Collagen (type II and other types)
Epstein-Barr virus antigens	gp39
Heat shock proteins	Cartilage link protein
Mycobacterial antigens	Cartilage proteoglycan
Parvovirus antigens	205-kd synovial fluid antigen
Peptidoglycan from gram-positive bacteria	Immunoglobulin binding protein (BiP)
	Heat shock proteins
	Class II MHC (shared epitope)
	IgG (Fc portion)
	RA33 (heterogeneous nuclear ribonucleoprotein A2)
	Filaggrin
	Glycosaminoglycans

lesional cells from other forms of arthritis. Numerous studies of the expressed T-cell repertoire in RA have been published, but the results do not yield a uniform or clear picture (59,259–273). Most of these studies have analyzed the αβ TCR, whereas fewer have examined the γδ chain usage. Selective expansion of various TCR V region genes has been observed in synovial tissue or synovial fluid T cells in numerous studies, and this is referred to as "skewing" or "bias" in TCR repertoire expression. However, the specific genes overexpressed are not consistent from study to study, and there is no clear correlation with stage of RA, early versus late. Oligoclonal $CD8^+$ T cells in synovial fluid may represent expanded clones that previously responded to systemic viral pathogens and subsequently migrated to the joint in a nonspecific manner (236). To this point, a clear link has not yet been established between expanded clonotypes and target antigens in the joint, nor is there convincing evidence for pathogenic clones in RA that are distinct from T cells found in other forms of arthritis, with the possible exception of circulating clonal populations in Felty syndrome. It should be emphasized that T cells in RA synovium are significantly heterogeneous, with quite sensitive techniques required to demonstrate expansion of clonal populations. It is not known whether the pattern of TCR expression in the joint is different from what would be observed in lymphoid organs of RA patients, and it is likely that some oligoclonal responses seen in the joint occur systemically, whereas others are more specific to the joint (274). Differences in clonal expansions from patient to patient, even among patients who share MHC alleles, suggest that ongoing inflammation in RA synovium may reflect responses to a variety of foreign or self antigens, which can be processed and presented to synovial T cells by any of several antigen-presenting cell populations in synovial tissue.

The Role of MHC Alleles in Rheumatoid Arthritis

Lack of certainty regarding the importance of antigen-specific T-cell responses in RA contributes to the difficulty in understanding precisely how the known MHC allele predisposition to RA contributes to disease pathogenesis. Surprisingly, despite the association of various MHC alleles with many systemic and articular diseases, in no case is the precise mechanism for disease predisposition firmly established. On first glance, presentation of an arthritogenic antigen to $CD4^+$ T cells by the class II shared epitope-containing alleles seems to be the most direct and plausible explanation, and some candidate peptides can bind to the shared epitope (275,276). Moreover, there is some evidence that in RA, relative to normal controls, alleles bearing the shared epitope are selectively overexpressed on the cell surface (277). Attempts to isolate unique, endogenous, arthritogenic peptides from MHC alleles that contain the shared epitope (admittedly, a technically daunting task) have as yet not been successful (278), However, an epitope of type II collagen that is arthritogenic in rodents can bind to both HLA-DR1 and DR4 (279), and other antigens may bind more strongly to class II molecules bearing the shared epitope compared with other HLA-DR molecules (280). In addition, peptides in which arginine is converted to citrulline bind more avidly to HLA-DRB1*0401 (281).

Some Caucasian patients with seropositive disease [perhaps as many as 27% (21)] do not have any MHC alleles that contain the shared epitope. In addition, two copies of the shared epitope may confer greater risk of disease, augmented disease severity, and greater incidence of extraarticular manifestations compared with one copy (282–285). If presentation of arthritogenic antigen were the mechanism for the shared epitope effect, the shared epitope should behave as a dominant rather than a codominant trait in view of the abundant expression of MHC molecules on antigen-presenting cells. Therefore, a variety of other potential explanations for association of the shared epitope with RA, some of which are listed in Table 52.8, need to be considered. It is even possible that, as in type I diabetes, absence of the disease-associated allele is protective, rather than presence of the disease-associated allele being pathogenic. Alternatively, some HLA-DR alleles may be protective against the development of RA, in both shared epitope positive and negative individuals, based on polymorphisms (e.g., DERAA) in the same region of HLA-DRB1 that contains the shared epitope (5,26,43,286,287). The same alleles may also reduce severity of RA (28). Mechanisms proposed

TABLE 52.8. *Possible mechanisms for the association of rheumatoid arthritis (RA) with class II major histocompatibility complex (MHC) polymorphisms*

Presentation of arthritogenic antigens to $CD4^+$ T cells by RA-associated class II alleles
Specific overexpression of class II alleles that bear the shared epitope, compared with their level of cell surface expression in normal controls without RA, leading to increased presentation of autoantigens to T cells
Linkage to other genes in or near the class II MHC locus
Altered T-cell selection in thymic development, leading to expanded populations of potentially arthritogenic T cells
Cross-reactivity between foreign antigen and the "shared epitope" (QKRAA or QRRAA)
Differences in surface expression and intracellular trafficking or stability of specific MHC alleles
Aberrant signaling through MHC alleles
"Holes" in the T-cell repertoire that lead to an inability to respond to an antigen that would otherwise protect against the development of RA
Absence of a particular set of T-cell receptors due to negative selection
Absence of MHC molecules capable of presenting a critical antigen to a particular set of T cell receptors
Lack of protective MHC alleles
Altered affinity of shared epitope alleles for chaperone proteins, causing altered pattern of antigen loading onto MHC molecules
Direct stimulation of T cells by the shared epitope on MHC molecules of antigen-presenting cells

for such protective effects include presentation of HLA-DR-derived peptides by HLA-DQ molecules (288,289), or distinct binding properties between chaperone heat shock proteins and specific HLA-DR molecules (290,291).

The MHC molecules also play an important role in shaping the T-cell repertoire during T-cell development in the thymus. In this process, negative and positive selection are controlled by MHC molecules along with antigenic peptides encountered during thymic development. Analysis of naive CD4+ peripheral blood T cells has led to the hypothesis that the shared epitope molds the expressed TCR repertoire in a unique manner. Furthermore, shared epitope–positive RA patients differ from HLA-matched normal individuals in the repertoire of their resting T cells, which is more restricted in RA patients that in controls (292,293). Whether such observations truly reflect unique features of intrathymic development, or are linked to T-cell responses related to disease, is not yet known. It has been proposed that this contracted T-cell repertoire represents premature senescence and distortion of both thymic output and homeostatic T-cell proliferation, and leads to overrepresentation of CD28− and autoreactive T cells (294). An aberrant pattern of expression of surface markers on circulating memory T cells in RA further supports the concept that T-cell differentiation is fundamentally abnormal in this disease (295).

Another possible relationship between the shared epitope and thymic T-cell development has been proposed. It is known that MHC sequences can be processed and presented to T cells by other MHC molecules. In view of the finding that synovial fluid T cells from patients with early RA can recognize peptides containing QKRAA (contained in several microbial antigens), it has been suggested that positive selection of T cells reactive with the shared epitope can occur in the thymus, producing lymphocytes that can later create an arthritogenic response after reacting to shared epitope sequences in microbial antigens (124). A different potential mechanism for the shared epitope effect springs from the observation that this sequence can alter intracellular trafficking of class II molecules, affecting loading or presentation of antigens as well as the extent of surface expression of MHC proteins (296). Such differences may reflect variations in stability of the complexes formed between various HLA-DR alleles and intracellular nonantigen class II ligands such as CLIP (class II associated invariant chain peptide) (280). It has been speculated that low stability of the association of 0404 and 0401 alleles with CLIP could facilitate loading and presentation of autoantigens by these shared epitope alleles. At this time, therefore, it is not possible to reach a conclusion regarding the mechanism by which MHC alleles predispose to RA or affect severity. However, a variety of distinct and provocative potential mechanisms have been proposed. The testing of these hypotheses may shed important light on the etiology and pathogenesis of RA. The close relationship of the shared epitope to RA is emphasized by a similar genetic association with a polyarthritis that resembles RA in another species, the dog (297).

THE ROLE OF CYTOKINES IN RHEUMATOID SYNOVITIS

Cytokines are peptide molecules that orchestrate and regulate immune and inflammatory responses. Most cytokines act in a paracrine manner, but numerous examples of autocrine and endocrine effects of cytokines are also available. Many cytokines have been detected in RA synovium and synovial fluid, some at very high levels (298). Animal studies, *in vitro* experiments, and, more recently, therapeutic trials in patients with RA all indicate that cytokines play a central role in joint inflammation and joint destruction in RA (see Chapters 19 and 54). Some of the more important cytokines present in RA synovium are listed in Table 52.9.

Roles of Tumor Necrosis Factor and Interleukin-1 in Rheumatoid Arthritis

Of special importance in RA are the proinflammatory cytokines TNF-α and IL-1β, which are produced primarily by cells of the monocyte/macrophage lineage (299–312). TNF-α can also be made by activated T cells. The high levels of TNF-α and IL-1β in RA synovium and the multiple biologic effects of these cytokines place them in a central role in the pathogenesis of joint inflammation and destruction. Biologic activities of these cytokines (see Chapter 19) include activation of a variety of cells of the immune system, acceleration of bone and cartilage breakdown (302–304,307,309) both by direct effects and through activation of synovial fibroblast (301,303), and a variety of systemic manifestations of chronic inflammatory disease (305). IL-1β probably plays a more important role in activation of matrix metalloprotease and prostaglandin release by synovial fibroblasts, whereas TNF-α is more important in induction of expression of adhesion molecules on synovial endothelium, as well as on synovial tissue cell subsets (313). TNF-α also up-regulates production of IL-1β (305), and both cytokines help to induce production of IL-6. It is likely that any stimulus capable of activating macrophages induces TNF release (314). Expression of adhesion molecules, such as selectins and their ligands, on synovial microvasculature results in rolling and eventual arrest of leukocytes traversing this circulatory bed (315). Leukocyte subsets are then acted on by the large family of chemotactic cytokines termed chemokines (IL-8 and many others), to facilitate migration through the microvascular wall into synovial tissue (315,316). At least a dozen chemokines are produced in RA synovium (316), probably stimulated to a great extent by TNF-α and IL-1β. These chemokines, such as IL-8 and monocyte chemotactic protein-1, have powerful proinflammatory and, in some cases, angiogenic effects (317–319).

TABLE 52.9. *Role of cytokines in rheumatoid arthritis synovium*

	Producing Cells		Target Cells		
Cytokine	T cells	Synovial Macrophages and/or Fibroblasts	T cells	Synovial Macrophages and/or Fibroblasts	Other
IFN-γ	+	−	−	+	−
IL-1β	+	++	+	++	Osteoclast
TNF-α	+	++	+	++	Endothelium
IL-6	+/−	+	+	−	Hepatocyte, chondrocyte
IL-8	+/−	+	+/−	−	Neutrophil
IL-10	+	++	+	+	−
IL-12	−	+	+	−	−
IL-15	−	+	+	−	−
IL-17	+	−	−	+	−
IL-18	−	+	+	+	−
RANKL	+	+	−	+	
MIF	+	++	+/−	+	

For production of cytokines, quantitative differences between cell types are indicated using arbitrary designations of −, +/−, +, and ++. Synovial B lymphocytes and dendritic cells are also sources of and targets for cytokines. RANKL (receptor activator of NFκB ligand, also known as osteoclast differentiation factor) stimulates a subset of synovial macrophages to differentiate into osteoclasts.

IFN-γ, interferon-γ; IL, interleukin; MIF, macrophage migration inhibitory factor; TNF-α, tumor necrosis factor-α.

Cytokine inhibitors or antagonists are also produced in RA synovial tissue (299). Large quantities of the IL-1 receptor antagonist are present, but a substantial excess of the antagonist is required to effectively neutralize the capacity of IL-1 to trigger signal transduction in target cells by receptor binding. Therefore, the concentration of IL-1 receptor antagonist is generally insufficient to overcome the actions of IL-1 (320,321). Soluble TNF receptors are released at sites of inflammation by shedding from the cell surface and have been documented in RA synovium (322). As with the IL-1 receptor antagonist, the levels of soluble TNF receptors seem to be generally insufficient to functionally neutralize the large quantities of TNF-α produced locally. However, therapeutic strategies that augment such endogenous attempts at cytokine homeostasis have great promise in the treatment of RA (see Chapter 39). TNF-α can be effectively neutralized, either with a monoclonal antibody or a genetically engineered soluble dimeric form of the p75 TNF receptor. TNF neutralization is effective in animal model systems and in cell culture assays, and has produced significant clinical responses in treatment of RA. Neutralization of IL-1 is also a logical approach to treatment of RA. Although IL-6 has both pro- and antiinflammatory capabilities, in RA the proinflammatory effects appear to dominate; thus, IL-6 may also be a valid therapeutic target (323).

Cytokine Production by T-cell Subsets in Rheumatoid Arthritis

Cytokines that regulate T-cell function or that are produced by T-cell subsets are often classified as T_H1, T_H2, or T_H3 (also termed type 1, type 2, and type 3). IFN-γ is a prototypic T_H1 cytokine, whereas IL-4 is a T_H2 cytokine and transforming growth factor-β (TGF-β) a T_H3 cytokine. T_H1 function is associated with delayed-type hypersensitivity and cytotoxic T-cell responses, whereas T_H2 function is paramount in allergic diseases and some parasitic infections. RA has been viewed as primarily a T_H1 disease (324–326). The myeloid dendritic cell subset that promotes T_H1 differentiation is present in RA synovial fluid (327). Levels of IFN-γ detectable in synovial tissue are low but functionally significant (328,329). T cells taken from synovial tissue or fluid can readily be stimulated to produce IFN-γ (330). T_H1 responses dominate whether RA T cells are activated by peptide antigen (331) or by monoclonal antibody to T-cell surface structures (332). The production of IFN-γ in RA is partly due to its synthesis by a T-cell subset that also bears natural killer cell markers (333). Biologic effects attributable at least in part to IFN-γ (such as strong class II MHC expression on a variety of cell types) are readily demonstrable in RA synovium, and other cytokines associated with activation of T_H1 responses, such as IL-12, are also present in synovial tissue (334). IL-15 and IL-18 probably synergize with IL-12 in supporting T_H1 differentiation, and both of these cytokines are readily detectable in RA synovium (335–337). IL-18 has broad proinflammatory effects that may include chemotactic (338) and angiogenic (339) activities. In contrast, IL-4 is rarely detected (340), and the capacity of synovial T cells to produce IL-4 is lower than their capacity to produce IFN-γ (341). Unexpectedly, individual synovial T cells can sometimes produce both T_H1 and T_H2 cytokines following *in vitro* stimulation (330). Rheumatoid nodules consistently show T_H1 dominance (342), but more data are needed regarding the T-cell cytokine phenotype of other extraarticular RA lesions.

IL-2 is barely detectable in RA synovial tissue or fluid (343,344), and a small minority of T cells express the high-affinity IL-2 receptor (204). These findings were viewed at one time as indicating dormancy of T cells in RA synovium, and perhaps only a limited role for T cells in chronic RA (231). However, it is now understood that other cytokines, especially IL-15, can have T-cell growth factor activity and can substitute for IL-2, even utilizing some of the subunits of the IL-2 receptor (345). The properties of RA synovial T cells can be mimicked by peripheral blood T cells activated by IL-15 or other cytokines more closely than by T cells activated through triggering of the antigen receptor (346). In addition, IL-15 can stimulate oligoclonal T-cell expansion (347) and induces expression of CD154, which is critical to T-cell interactions with non–T cells (348).

T lymphocytes can also release proinflammatory cytokines in RA. In addition to their minor contribution to TNF-α production, T cells in RA synovium make IL-17, which has direct effects on synovial fibroblasts, inducing production of proinflammatory mediators such as MMPs, prostaglandins, chemokines, nitric oxide, and IL-6 (349–353). IL-17 has multiple isoforms, which can also activate a variety of other cells in the joint (350). Synthesis of IL-17 can be induced by IL-15 (354), thus defining a fibroblast/T-cell cytokine axis, relatively independent of the monokines TNF and IL-1, that can also mediate joint destruction both in RA and in animal models (350,352,353, 355). T cells and other cells in RA also produce MIF. MIF activates macrophage cytokine synthesis, antagonizes glucocorticoids, and has multiple other proinflammatory effects (356,357).

The cytokine known as receptor activator of nuclear factor κB ligand (RANKL) or osteoclast differentiation factor (ODF) is critical to osteoclast formation and bone erosion in RA (358) (see Chapter 54). RANKL can be produced by activated T cells and by osteoblasts, and its osteoclastogenic effects are potentiated by TNF-α (359). The production of key cytokines by T cells in RA, including IFN-γ, IL-17, and RANKL (and some TNF-α), emphasizes the key role of these cells, together with synovial macrophages and fibroblasts, in the pathogenesis of the destruction of cartilage and bone that is typical of RA.

Immunoregulatory or antiinflammatory cytokines that are detectable in RA also may become useful as therapeutic agents. IL-10, previously classified as a T_H2 cytokine, is now viewed as capable of regulating a variety of T-cell responses, and IL-10 is produced within RA synovial tissue (360), but at inadequate levels to control T_H1 cells (361). IL-10-producing T cells are sometimes referred to as T_{R1} cells. Transforming growth factors are a family of cytokines that exist in both latent and active forms. Although TGF-β can have some immunosuppressant and antiinflammatory effects, its precise role in RA appears to be complex and to some degree pathogenic. Whether members of this cytokine family will be ultimately useful as therapeutic agents is unknown.

CELL/CELL INTERACTIONS IN RHEUMATOID ARTHRITIS

Cells in inflammatory lesions communicate both by molecular messengers such as cytokines and through direct cell/cell interactions, mediated by binding of receptors and reciprocal ligands on cell membranes in direct contact. Several types of cell/cell interactions are important in the development of rheumatoid synovitis, and some of these are listed in Table 52.10. For example, binding of circulating leukocytes to activated endothelium is an absolute prerequisite for development of a chronic inflammatory lesion. Such binding is mediated through a variety of specialized cell adhesion molecules (see Chapter 20) (362,363). The existence of distinct adhesion molecules expressed in the synovial microvasculature has been inferred (364), but not yet proven. It is likely that the precise combination of expressed selectins, integrins, and chemokines creates a unique milieu in inflamed synovium that regulates ingress of a combination of leukocyte populations. Use of specific chemokines/chemokine receptor pairs, as well as glycosylated adhesion ligands, defines T-cell subsets that preferentially migrate into and accumulate in synovial tissue (365–367).

T-cell responses in RA synovium are triggered by interaction of T cells with professional antigen-presenting cells, including dendritic cells, monocyte/macrophage cells, and B lymphocytes (368). Highly activated dendritic cells are present in both RA synovial tissue and fluid, and can be observed to interact with clustering T lymphocytes (369).

Although extensive infiltration of synovium by lymphocytes is typically found in RA and although the synovial histology is similar in large and small joints (370), RA patients can be classified into histologic subsets based on the characteristics of the cellular infiltrate. In about 50% of patients from whom synovial tissue is recovered at arthroplasty, the infiltrates are diffuse, lacking specific microstructures (371). In other patients, clusters of T and B cells are found, either as lymphoid aggregates or as true lymphoid follicles that contain germinal centers (371). These germinal centers contain follicular dendritic cells, and expression of key molecules associated with germinal center formation in lymphoid organs is specifically detected in this type of RA synovial tissue (371). $CD8^+$ T cells have an unexpectedly important role in supporting cytokine production and overall structural integrity of these ectopic germinal centers (372).

TABLE 52.10. *Cell-cell interactions in rheumatoid arthritis synovium*

Leukocyte-endothelial
T cell–dendritic cell
T cell–macrophage
Macrophage-fibroblast
T cell–fibroblast
B cell–fibroblast

It has also recently been found that synovial fibroblasts can interact directly with T cells, or with membranes of activated T cells, at least in cell culture systems (373–377). Such interactions can contribute both to activation of the T cell and the fibroblast, and likely occur *in vivo,* given the large numbers of these cell types present in RA synovium. T-cell activation and differentiation can also be triggered by cytokines found in RA synovium, without engagement of the T-cell antigen receptor, and such cytokine-activated T cells induce monocytes to produce TNF (346).

Macrophage/fibroblast interactions are mediated in large part by cytokines, but direct cell/cell communication undoubtedly occurs in RA synovial tissue, where these two synovial cell subsets are directly contiguous. An interesting interaction of the synovial fibroblasts with B lymphocytes has also been detected, in which fibroblasts can provide signals that promote survival and differentiation of B cells, protecting the B lymphocyte from apoptosis (378–380).

These cell/cell interactions and cytokine-related effects are likely to explain the unusual patterns of cell differentiation found in RA synovium. Particularly striking is the distinct, virtually unique phenotype of the RA synovial fibroblast (381,382). These fibroblasts exhibit many of the characteristics of transformed cells, including aggressive growth, the capacity to deeply invade adjacent tissues, and accumulation of mutations in tumor suppresser genes such as p53 (383, 384) (see Chapter 54). Whether abnormalities of the synovial fibroblasts are entirely secondary to chronic inflammation or whether they also reflect primary events involved in the etiology of RA is a critical issue for further investigation. The recent demonstration that mesenchymal precursor cells can circulate and migrate into joints by both systemic and local routes is prompting a reexamination of the role of synovial fibroblasts in the initiation of RA (385,386).

Interactions between extracellular matrix components (such as hyaluronan, fibronectin, laminin, and minor collagen types) and cell surface receptors specific for these molecules also regulate cell activation and migration in RA synovium (387–389). The repertoire of cell surface integrins, other adhesion molecules, and extracellular ligands expressed in synovium is unique in some respects, such as abundance of an alternatively spliced isoform of fibronectin (389), expression by synovial fibroblasts of splice variants of the CD44/hyaluronan receptor that are associated with tissue invasive properties (390), and expression of VCAM-1 on fibroblasts as well as endothelial cells (376,387).

ROLES OF THE INNATE AND ADAPTIVE IMMUNE RESPONSES IN RHEUMATOID ARTHRITIS

Innate immune responses can be viewed as components of host defense that do not require presensitization to specific antigen. For many years, attention was focused primarily on adaptive immune responses (autoantibodies and autoreactive T cells) as central to the pathogenesis and even etiology of RA. Innate immune mechanisms include not only pattern recognition receptors (Toll-like receptors and others), acute phase reactants, components of the complement cascade, phagocytic cells, and many cytokines, but also natural killer lymphocytes and even some polyreactive antibodies and T-cell effector functions. Innate immune responses precede and control the adaptive immune response, and are also engaged by the effector arms of adaptive immunity in ways that blur the boundary between these two systems.

Increasing attention is being focused on the role of innate immunity in RA (391,392). Relevant observations, some mentioned in earlier sections of this chapter, include the following:

1. Early stages of inflammatory arthritis involve cytokine-dependent synovial infiltration of myeloid and mesenchymal cells, changes in the bone marrow adjacent to inflamed joints, and possibly direct communication between adjacent bone marrow and synovium, all prior to influx of lymphocytes (391,393,394).
2. Toll-like receptors (TLRs) are expressed in RA synovium, with particularly strong expression of TLR-2, which is activated by various bacterial peptidoglycans and lipoproteins (395). The most important ligands of TLR-2 in RA synovium remain to be defined.
3. C-reactive protein (CRP) appears to directly activate complement in RA, and the levels of circulating CRP–complement fragment complexes correlate with clinical parameters (396,397).
4. Complement receptors are highly expressed on various cell types in RA synovium, complement components such as C3 are also synthesized locally (398), and various RA models are highly complement dependent (143, 179,399).
5. Genetic defects in mannose binding lectin have been associated with RA (75,76).
6. T cells can activate synovial fibroblasts without exposure to antigen (377), and cytokine-activated T cells are potent inducers of monocyte-macrophage activation (346).
7. A subset of natural killer cells that can produce IFN-γ is expanded in RA synovial fluid (400).

Inflammation and activation of innate immune pathways in RA could be promoted by local ongoing extravascular coagulation, which is triggered by tissue factor and leads to extensive fibrin deposition (401,402). Fibrinogen is converted to fibrin by thrombin, a serine protease that also exerts proinflammatory effects on endothelium through the protease activated receptor 1 (PAR-1), which is abundantly expressed in RA synovial tissue (401). Fibrin can activate synovial fibroblasts, and deiminated fibrin is a major target of autoantibodies in RA that are directed at citrullinated peptides (166,167).

CONCLUSION

Understanding of the etiology and pathogenesis of RA is evolving rapidly. Fundamental components of pathogenesis have been elucidated, and the value of these concepts is already evident in new forms of treatment for RA. The major issues regarding etiology, however, have remained unresolved. Attempts to explain RA using classic concepts of autoimmunity or response to microbial infection have been unsuccessful. Understanding this disease may require developing new conceptual models for how pathologic cell/cell interactions originate and cause tissue destruction. Such models will build on our growing understanding of the links between innate and adaptive immune responses, and the other pathways that produce tissue damage and inflammation. New therapeutic targets will likely be identified as the pathways that produce RA are more clearly defined.

REFERENCES

1. Seldin M, Amos C, Ward R, et al. The genetics revolution and the assault on rheumatoid arthritis. *Arthritis Rheum* 1999;42(6):1071–1079.
2. Aho K, Koskenvuo M, Tuominen J, et al. Occurrence of rheumatoid arthritis in a nationwide series of twins. *J Rheumatol* 1986;13:899–902.
3. Silman A, MacGregor A, Thompson W, et al. Twin concordance rates for rheumatoid arthritis: results from a nationwide study. *Br J Rheumatol* 1993;32:903–907.
4. Jarvinen P, Aho K. Twin studies in rheumatic diseases. *Arthritis Rheum* 1994;24:19–28.
5. Huizinga T. Genetics in rheumatoid arthritis. *Curr Rheum Rep* 2002; 4:195–200.
6. Grant S, Thorleifsson G, Frigge M, et al. The inheritance of rheumatoid arthritis in Iceland. *Arthritis Rheum* 2001;44(10):2247–2254.
7. Jonsson H, Helgason J. Rheumatoid arthritis in an Icelandic textbook from 1782. *Scand J Rheumatol* 1996;25:134–137.
8. Reveille J. The genetic contribution to the pathogenesis of rheumatoid arthritis. *Curr Opin Rheumatol* 1998;10:187–200.
9. Jirholt J, Lindqvist A, Holmdahl R. The genetics of rheumatoid arthritis and the need for animal models to find and understand the underlying genes. *Arthritis Res* 2001;3(Rev):87–97.
10. Jawaheer D, Seldin M, Amos C, et al. Screening the genome for rheumatoid arthritis susceptibility genes. *Arthritis Rheum* 2003;48(4): 906–916.
11. Fisher S, Lanchbury J, Lewis C. Meta-analysis of four rheumatoid arthritis genome-wide linkage studies: confirmation of a susceptibility locus on chromosome 16. *Arthritis Rheum* 2003;48(5):1200–1206.
12. Radstake T, Barrera P, Albers J, et al. Familial vs sporadic rheumatoid arthritis (RA). A prospective study in an early RA inception cohort. *Rheumatology* 2000;39:267–273.
13. Laivoranta-Nyman S, Mottonen T, Luukkainen R, et al. Immunogenetic differences between patients with familial and non-familial rheumatoid arthritis. *Ann Rheum Dis* 2000;59:173–177.
14. Stastny P. Association of the B-cell alloantigen DRw4 with rheumatoid arthritis. *N Engl J Med* 1978;298:869–871.
15. Nepom G, Byers P, Seyfried C, et al. HLA genes associated with rheumatoid arthritis: identification of susceptibility alleles using specific oligonucleotide probes. *Arthritis Rheum* 1989;32:15–21.
16. Wordsworth B, Lanchbury J, Sakkas L, et al. HLA-DR4 subtype frequencies in rheumatoid arthritis indicate that DRB1 is the major susceptibility locus within the HLA class II region. *Proc Natl Acad Sci U S A* 1989;86:10049–10053.
17. Takeuchi F, Matsuta K, Watanabe Y, et al. Susceptibility epitope on HLA-DR B chain for rheumatoid arthritis and the effect of the positivity on the clinical features. *J Immunogenet* 1989;16:475–483.
18. Templin D, Boyer G, Lanier A, et al. Rheumatoid arthritis in Tlingit Indians: clinical characterization and HLA associations. *J Rheumatol* 1994;21:1238–1244.
19. Gao X, Brautbar C, Gazit E, et al. A variant of HLA-DR4 determines susceptibility to rheumatoid arthritis in a subset of Israeli Jews. *Arthritis Rheum* 1991;34:547–551.
20. Gregersen P, Silver J, Winchester R. The shared epitope hypothesis: an approach to understanding the molecular genetics of susceptibility to rheumatoid arthritis. *Arthritis Rheum* 1987;30:1205–1213.
21. Fries J, Wolfe F, Apple R, et al. HLA-DRB1 genotype associations in 793 white patients from a rheumatoid arthritis inception cohort. *Arthritis Rheum* 2002;46(9):2320–2329.
22. del Rincon I, Battafarano D, Arroyo R, et al. Heterogeneity between men and women in the influence of the HLA-DRB1 shared epitope on the clinical expression of rheumatoid arthritis. *Arthritis Rheum* 2002; 46(6):1480–1488.
23. Singal D, Green D, Reid B, et al. HLA-D region genes and rheumatoid arthritis (RA): importance of DR and DQ genes in conferring susceptibility to rheumatoid arthritis. *Ann Rheum Dis* 1992;51:23–28.
24. Zanelli E, Krco C, Baisch J, et al. Immune response of HLA-DQ8 transgenic mice to peptides from the third hypervariable region of HLA-DRB1 correlates with predisposition to rheumatoid arthritis. *Proc Natl Acad Sci U S A* 1996;93:1814–1819.
25. Pascual M, Nieto A, Lopez-Nevot M, et al. Rheumatoid arthritis in southern Spain: toward elucidation of a unifying role of the HLA class II region in disease predisposition. *Arthritis Rheum* 2001;44(2):307–314.
26. Seidl C, Korbitzer J, Badenhoop K, et al. Protection against severe disease is conferred by DERRA-bearing HLA-DRB1 alleles among HLA-DQ3 and HLA-DQ5 positive rheumatoid arthritis patients. *Hum Immunol* 2001;62:523–529.
27. de Vries N, van Elderen C, Tijssen H, et al. No support for HLA-DQ encoded susceptibility in rheumatoid arthritis. *Arthritis Rheum* 1999; 42(8):1621–1627.
28. Wagner U, Kaltenhauser S, Pierer M, et al. Prospective analysis of the impact of HLA-DR and -DQ on joint destruction in recent-onset rheumatoid arthritis. *Rheumatology* 2003;42:553–562.
29. Zanelli E, Breedveld F, de Vries R. HLA class II association with rheumatoid arthritis: facts and interpretations. *Hum Immunol* 2000;61: 1254–1261.
30. Fugger L, Svejgaard A. Association of MHC and rheumatoid arthritis: HLA-DR4 and rheumatoid arthritis—studies in mice and men. *Arthritis Res* 2000;2(3):208–211.
31. Pinet V, Combe B, Avinens O, et al. Polymorphism of the HLA-DMA and DMB genes in rheumatoid arthritis. *Arthritis Rheum* 1997;40(5): 854–858.
32. Toussirot E, Sauvageot C, Chabod J, et al. The association of HLA-DM genes with rheumatoid arthritis in eastern France. *Hum Immunol* 2000;61:303–308.
33. Jawaheer D, Li W, Graham R, et al. Dissecting the genetic complexity of the association between human leukocyte antigens and rheumatoid arthritis. *Am J Hum Genet* 2002;71:585–594.
34. Mulcahy B, Waldron-Lynch F, McDermott M, et al. Genetic variability in the tumor necrosis factor-lymphotoxin region influences susceptibility to rheumatoid arthritis. *Am J Hum Genet* 1996;59:676–683.
35. Hajeer A, John S, Ollier W, et al. Tumor necrosis factor microsatellite haplotypes are different in male and female patients with rheumatoid arthritis. *J Rheumatol* 1997;24:217–219.
36. Mu H, Chen J, Jiang Y, et al. Tumor necrosis factor a microsatellite polymorphism is associated with rheumatoid arthritis severity through an interaction with the HLA-DRB1 shared epitope. *Arthritis Rheum* 1999;42(3):438–442.
37. Takeuchi F, Mimori A, Matsuta K, et al. Association of complement alleles C4AQO and C4B5 with rheumatoid arthritis in Japanese patients. *Arthritis Rheum* 1989;32:691–698.
38. Paimela L, Leirisalo-Repo M, Lokki M, et al. Prognostic significance of complement alleles Bf and C4 in early rheumatoid arthritis. *Clin Rheumatol* 1996;15:594–598.
39. Quadri S, Taneja V, Mehra N, et al. HSP70–1 promoter region alleles and susceptibility to rheumatoid arthritis. *Clin Exp Rheumatol* 1996; 14:183–185.
40. Newton J, Brown M, Milicic A, et al. The effect of HLA-DR on susceptibility to rheumatoid arthritis is influenced by the associated lymphotoxin A–tumor necrosis factor haplotype. *Arthritis Rheum* 2003;48(1):90–96.

41. Martinez A, Fernandez-Arquero M, Pascual-Salcedo D, et al. Primary association of tumor necrosis factor-region genetic markers with susceptibility to rheumatoid arthritis. *Arthritis Rheum* 2000;43(6):1366–1370.
42. Meyer J, Han J, Moxley G. Tumor necrosis factor markers show sex-influenced association with rheumatoid arthritis. *Arthritis Rheum* 2001; 44(2):286–295.
43. Tuokko J, Nejentsev S, Luukkainen R, et al. HLA haplotype analysis in Finnish patients with rheumatoid arthritis. *Arthritis Rheum* 2001; 44(2):315–322.
44. Yen J-H, Chen C-J, Tsai W-C, et al. Tumor necrosis factor microsatellite alleles in patients with rheumatoid arthritis in Taiwan. *Immunol Lett* 2002;81:177–182.
45. Zanelli E, Jones G, Pascual M, et al. The telomeric part of the HLA region predisposes to rheumatoid arthritis independently of the class II loci. *Hum Immunol* 2001;62:75–84.
46. Ota M, Katsuyama Y, Kimura A, et al. A second susceptibility gene for developing rheumatoid arthritis in the human MHC is localized within a 70-kb interval telomeric of the TNF genes in the HLA class III region. *Genomics* 2001;71:263–270.
47. Barton A, John S, Ollier W, et al. Association between rheumatoid arthritis and polymorphism of tumor necrosis factor receptor II, but not tumor necrosis factor receptor I, in Caucasians. *Arthritis Rheum* 2001;44(1):61–65.
48. Dieude P, Petit E, Cailleau-Moindrault S, et al. Association between tumor necrosis factor receptor II and familial, but not sporadic, rheumatoid arthritis. *Arthritis Rheum* 2002;46(8):2039–2044.
49. Jenkins S, March R, Campbell R, et al. A novel variant of the MHC-linked hsp70, hsp70-hom, is associated with rheumatoid arthritis. *Tissue Antigens* 2000;56:38–44.
50. Yen J-H, Moore B, Nakajima T, et al. Major histocompatibility complex class I–recognizing receptors are disease risk genes in rheumatoid arthritis. *J Exp Med* 2001;193(10):1159–1167.
51. Barrett J, Brennan P, Fiddler M, et al. Does rheumatoid arthritis remit during pregnancy and relapse postpartum? Results from a nationwide study in the United Kingdom performed prospectively from late pregnancy. *Arthritis Rheum* 1999;42(6):1219–1227.
52. John S, Myerscough A, Eyre S, et al. Linkage of a marker on intron D of the estrogen synthase locus to rheumatoid arthritis. *Arthritis Rheum* 1999;42(8):1617–1620.
53. Brennan P, Ollier W, Worthington J, et al. Are both genetic and reproductive associations with rheumatoid arthritis linked to prolactin? *Lancet* 1996;348:106–109.
54. Barrett J, Brennan P, Fiddler M, et al. Breast-feeding and postpartum relapse in women with rheumatoid and inflammatory arthritis. *Arthritis Rheum* 2000;43(5):1010–1015.
55. Straub R, Cutolo M. Involvement of the hypothalamic-pituitary-adrenal/gonadal axis and the peripheral nervous system in rheumatoid arthritis: viewpoint based on a systemic pathogenetic role. *Arthritis Rheum* 2001;44(3):493–507.
56. Fife M, Fisher S, John S, et al. Multipoint linkage analysis of a candidate gene locus in rheumatoid arthritis demonstrates significant evidence of linkage and association with the corticotropin-releasing hormone genomic region. *Arthritis Rheum* 2000;43(8):1673–1678.
57. Fife M, Steer S, Fisher S, et al. Association of familial and sporadic rheumatoid arthritis with a single corticotropin-releasing hormone genomic region (8q12.3) haplotype. *Arthritis Rheum* 2002;46(1):75–82.
58. Nelson J, Hughes K, Smith A, et al. Maternal-fetal disparity in HLA class II alloantigens and the pregnancy-induced amelioration of rheumatoid arthritis. *N Engl J Med* 1993;329:466–471.
59. Fox D, Singer N. T cell receptor rearrangements. In: Miossec P, van den Berg WB, Firestein GS, eds. *T cells in Arthritis (Progress in Inflammation Research).* Basel: Birkhauser, 1998:19–53.
60. Cornelis F, Hardwick L, Flipo R, et al. Association of rheumatoid arthritis with an amino acid allelic variation of the T cell receptor. *Arthritis Rheum* 1997;40(8):1387–1390.
61. Sherritt M, Tait B, Varney M, et al. Immunosusceptibility genes in rheumatoid arthritis. *Hum Immunol* 1996;51:32–40.
62. Vencovsky J, Zd'arsky E, Moyes S, et al. Polymorphism in the immunoglobulin VH gene V1–69 affects susceptibility to rheumatoid arthritis in subjects lacking the HLA-DRB1 shared epitope. *Rheumatology* 2002;41:401–410.
63. Nieto A, Caliz R, Pascual M, et al. Involvement of Fcγ receptor IIIA genotypes in susceptibility to rheumatoid arthritis. *Arthritis Rheum* 2000;43(4):735–739.
64. Morgan A, Keyte V, Babbage S, et al. FcγRIIIA-158V and rheumatoid arthritis: a confirmation study. *Rheumatology* 2003;42:528–533.
65. Morgan A, Griffiths B, Ponchel F, et al. Fcγ receptor type IIIA associated with rheumatoid arthritis in two distinct ethnic groups. *Arthritis Rheum* 2000;43(10):2328–2334.
66. Gomez-Reino J, Pablos J, Carreira P, et al. Association of rheumatoid arthritis with a functional chemokine receptor, CCR5. *Arthritis Rheum* 1999;42(5):989–992.
67. Santiago B, Galindo M, Rivero M, et al. The chemoattraction of lymphocytes by rheumatoid arthritis—synovial fluid is not dependent on the chemokine receptor CCR5. *Rheumatol Int* 2002;22(3):107–111.
68. Gregersen P, Bucala R. Macrophage migration inhibitory factor, MIF alleles, and the genetics of inflammatory disorders: incorporating disease outcome into the definition of phenotype. *Arthritis Rheum* 2003; 48(5):1171–1176.
69. Baugh J, Chitnis S, Donnelly S, et al. A functional promoter polymorphism in the macrophage migration inhibitory factor (MIF) gene associated with disease severity in rheumatoid arthritis. *Genes Immun* 2002;3:170–176.
70. Yamada R, Tanaka T, Unoki M, et al. Association between a single-nucleotide polymorphism in the promoter of the human interleukin-3 gene and rheumatoid arthritis in Japanese patients, and maximum-likelihood estimation of combinatorial effect that two genetic loci have on susceptibility to the disease. *Am J Hum Genet* 2001;68:674–685.
71. Khani-Hanjani A, Lacaille D, Hoar D. Association between dinucleotide repeat in non-coding region of interferon-gamma gene and susceptibility to, and severity of, rheumatoid arthritis. *Lancet* 2000; 356:820–825.
72. Vandenbroek K, Goris A, Billiau A, et al. Interferon gamma gene in rheumatoid arthritis. *Lancet* 2000;356(Corr):2191–2192.
73. Pokorny V, McLean L, McQueen F, et al. Interferon-gamma microsatellite and rheumatoid arthritis. *Lancet* 2001;358(9276):122–123.
74. Constantin A, Lauwers-Cances V, Navaux F, et al. Stromelysin 1 (matrix metalloproteinase 3) and HLA-DRB1 gene polymorphisms: association with severity and progression of rheumatoid arthritis in a prospective study. *Arthritis Rheum* 2002;46(7):1754–1762.
75. Ip W, Lau L, Chan S, et al. Mannose-binding lectin and rheumatoid arthritis in southern Chinese. *Arthritis Rheum* 2000;43(8):1679–1687.
76. Graudal N, Madsen H, Tarp U, et al. The association of variant mannose-binding lectin genotypes with radiographic outcome in rheumatoid arthritis. *Arthritis Rheum* 2000;43:515–521.
77. Singal D, Li J, Zhu Y, et al. NRAMP-1 gene polymorphisms in patients with rheumatoid arthritis. *Tissue Antigens* 2000;55:44–47.
78. Rodriguez M, Gonzalez-Escribano M, Aguilar F, et al. Association of NRAMP1 promoter gene polymorphism with the susceptibility and radiological severity of rheumatoid arthritis. *Tissue Antigens* 2002;59 (4):311–315.
79. Yamada R, Tanaka T, Ohnishi Y, et al. Identification of 142 single nucleotide polymorphisms in 41 candidate genes for rheumatoid arthritis in the Japanese population. *Hum Genet* 2000;106(3):293–297.
80. Jawaheer D, Seldin M, Amos C, et al. A genomewide screen in multiplex rheumatoid arthritis families suggests genetic overlap with other autoimmune diseases. *Am J Hum Genet* 2001;68:927–936.
81. Barton A, Eyre S, Myerscough A, et al. High resolution linkage and association mapping identifies a novel rheumatoid arthritis susceptibility locus homologous to one linked to two rat models of inflammatory arthritis. *Hum Mol Genet* 2001;10(18):1901–1906.
82. MacKay K, Eyre S, Myerscough A, et al. Whole-genome linkage analysis of rheumatoid arthritis susceptibility loci in 252 affected sibling pairs in the United Kingdom. *Arthritis Rheum* 2002;46(3):632–639.
83. Heller R, Schena M, Chai A, et al. Discovery and analysis of inflammatory disease-related genes using cDNA microarrays. *Proc Natl Acad Sci U S A* 1997;94:2150–2155.
84. Neumann E, Kullmann F, Judex M, et al. Identification of differentially expressed genes in rheumatoid arthritis by a combination of complementary DNA array and RNA arbitrarily primed-polymerase chain reaction. *Arthritis Rheum* 2002;46(1):52–63.
85. Keffer J, Probert L, Cazlaris H, et al. Transgenic mice expressing human tumor necrosis factor: a predictive genetic model of arthritis. *EMBO J* 1991;10:4025–4031.
86. Short C. The antiquity of rheumatoid arthritis. *Arthritis Rheum* 1974; 17:193–205.

87. Rothschild B. Rheumatoid arthritis at a time of passage. *J Rheumatol* 2001;28:245–250.
88. Aceves-Avila F, Medina F, Fraga A. The antiquity of rheumatoid arthritis: a reappraisal. *J Rheumatol* 2001;28:751–757.
89. Dequeker J. Arthritis in Flemish paintings (1400–1700). *BMJ* 1977; 1:1203–1205.
90. Rothschild B, Woods R, Rothschild C, et al. Geographic distribution of rheumatoid arthritis in ancient North America: implications for pathogenesis. *Semin Arthritis Rheum* 1992;22:181–187.
91. Grant W. The role of meat in the expression of rheumatoid arthritis. *Br J Nutr* 2000;84:589–595.
92. Cerhan J, Saag K, Merlino L, et al. Antioxidant micronutrients and risk of rheumatoid arthritis in a cohort of older women. *Am J Epidemiol* 2003;157(4):345–354.
93. Olsson A, Skogh T, Wingren G. Comorbidity and lifestyle, reproductive factors, and environmental exposures associated with rheumatoid arthritis. *Ann Rheum Dis* 2001;60:934–939.
94. Mattey D, Hutchinson D, Dawes P, et al. Smoking and disease severity in rheumatoid arthritis: association with polymorphism at the glutathione S-transferase M1 locus. *Arthritis Rheum* 2002;46(3):640–646.
95. Penglis P, Bond C, Humphreys I, et al. Genetic susceptibility and the link between cat exposure and rheumatoid arthritis. *Semin Arthritis Rheum* 2000;30(2):111–120.
96. Naides S, Field E. Transient rheumatoid factor positivity in acute human parvovirus B19 infection. *Arch Intern Med* 1988;148:2587–2589.
97. Takahashi Y, Murai C, Shibata S, et al. Human parvovirus B19 as a causative agent for rheumatoid arthritis. *Proc Natl Acad Sci U S A* 1998;95:8227–8232.
98. Sato M, Maruyama I, Maruyama Y, et al. Arthritis in patients infected with human T lymphotropic virus type I. *Arthritis Rheum* 1991;34 (6):714–721.
99. Iwakura Y, Tosu M, Yoshida E, et al. Induction of inflammatory arthropathy resembling rheumatoid arthritis in mice transgenic for HTLV-I. *Science* 1991;253:1026–1028.
100. Zucker-Franklin D, Pancake B, Brown W. Prevalence of HTLV-I tax in a subset of patients with rheumatoid arthritis. *Clin Exp Rheumatol* 2002;20:161–169.
101. Sebastian D, Nayiager S, York D, et al. Lack of association of human T cell lymphotrophic virus type 1 (HTLV-1) infection and rheumatoid arthritis in an endemic area. *Clin Rheumatol* 2003;22:30–32.
102. Neidhart M, Rethage J, Kuchen S, et al. Retrotransposable L1 elements expressed in rheumatoid arthritis synovial tissue. *Arthritis Rheum* 2000;43(12):2634–2647.
103. Seemayer C, Kolb S, Neidhart M, et al. Absence of inducible retroviruses from synovial fibroblasts and synovial fluid cells of patients with rheumatoid arthritis. *Arthritis Rheum* 2002;46(10):2811–2816.
104. Silverman S, Schumacher H. Antibodies to Epstein-Barr viral antigens in early rheumatoid arthritis. *Arthritis Rheum* 1981;24:1465–1468.
105. Hajeer A, MacGregor A, Rigby A, et al. Influence of previous exposure to human parvovirus B19 in explaining susceptibility of rheumatoid arthritis: an analysis of disease discordant twin pairs. *Ann Rheum Dis* 1994;53:137–139.
106. Ebringer A, Khalafpour S, Wilson C. Rheumatoid arthritis and *Proteus*: a possible aetiological association. *Rheum Int* 1989;9:223–228.
107. Sibilia J, Maillefert J. Vaccination and rheumatoid arthritis. *Ann Rheum Dis* 2002;61:575–576.
108. Balandraud N, Meynard J, Auger I, et al. Epstein-Barr virus load in the peripheral blood of patients with rheumatoid arthritis: accurate quantification using real-time polymerase chain reaction. *Arthritis Rheum* 2003;48(5):1223–1228.
109. Hasler F, Bluestein H, Zvaifler N, et al. Analysis of the defects responsible for the impaired regulation of EBV-induced B cell proliferation by rheumatoid arthritis lymphocytes. II. Role of monocytes and the increased sensitivity of rheumatoid arthritis lymphocytes to prostaglandin. *Eur J Immunol* 1983;131(2):768–772.
110. Ollier W. Rheumatoid arthritis and Epstein-Barr virus: a case of living with the enemy? *Ann Rheum Dis* 2000;59(7):497–499.
111. Toussirot E, Wendling D, Tiberghien P, et al. Decreased T cell precursor frequencies to Epstein-Barr virus glycoprotein gp110 in peripheral blood correlate with disease activity and severity in patients with rheumatoid arthritis. *Ann Rheum Dis* 2000;59:533–538.
112. Bonneville M, Scotet E, Peyrat M, et al. T cell reactivity to Epstein-Barr virus in rheumatoid arthritis. In: Miossec P, van den Berg WB, Firestein GS, eds. *T Cells in Arthritis (Progress in Inflammation Research)*. Basel: Birkhauser, 1998:149–167.
113. Hirohata S, Yanagida T, Nakamura H, et al. Bone marrow CD34+ progenitor cells from rheumatoid arthritis patients support spontaneous transformation of peripheral blood B cells from healthy individuals. *Rheumatol Int* 2000;19:153–159.
114. Roudier J, Petersen J, Rhodes G, et al. Susceptibility to rheumatoid arthritis maps to a T cell epitope shared by the HLA-Dw4 DR beta-1 chain and the Epstein-Barr virus glycoprotein gp110. *Proc Natl Acad Sci U S A* 1989;86:5104–5108.
115. Sutkowski N, Palkana T, Ciurli C, et al. An Epstein-Barr virus–associated superantigen. *J Exp Med* 1996;184:971–980.
116. Saal J, Krimmel M, Steidle M, et al. Synovial Epstein-Barr virus infection increases the risk of rheumatoid arthritis in individuals with the shared HLA-DR4 epitope. *Arthritis Rheum* 1999;42(7):1485–1496.
117. Edinger J, Bonneville M, Scotet E, et al. EBV gene expression not altered in rheumatoid synovia despite the presence of EBV antigen-specific T cell clones. *J Immunol* 1999;162:3694–3701.
118. Niedobitek G, Lisner R, Swoboda B, et al. Lack of evidence for an involvement of Epstein-Barr virus infection of synovial membranes in the pathogenesis of rheumatoid arthritis. *Arthritis Rheum* 2000; 43(1):151–154.
119. Takeda T, Mizugaki Y, Matsubara L, et al. Lytic Epstein-Barr virus infection in the synovial tissue of patients with rheumatoid arthritis. *Arthritis Rheum* 2000;43(6):1218–1225.
120. James J, Kaufman K, Farris A, et al. An increased prevalence of Epstein-Barr virus infection in young patients suggests a possible etiology for systemic lupus erythematosus. *J Clin Invest* 1997;100(12): 3019–3026.
121. Cohen I, Holoshitz J, van Eden W, et al. T lymphocyte clones illuminate pathogenesis and affect therapy of experimental arthritis. *Arthritis Rheum* 1985;28:841–845.
122. Holoshitz J, Klajman A, Drucker I, et al. T lymphocytes of rheumatoid arthritis patients show augmented reactivity to a fraction of mycobacteria cross-reactive with cartilage. *Lancet* 1986;2:305–309.
123. Gaston J, Life P, Bailey L, et al. *In vitro* responses to a 65-kilodalton mycobacterial protein by synovial T cells from inflammatory arthritis patients. *J Immunol* 1989;143:2494–2500.
124. Albani S, Keystone E, Nelson J, et al. Positive selection in autoimmunity: Abnormal immune responses to a bacterial dnaJ antigenic determinant in patients with early rheumatoid arthritis. *Nat Med* 1995;1(5):448–452.
125. Wilson C, Tiwana H, Ebringer A. Molecular mimicry between HLA-DR alleles associated with rheumatoid arthritis and *Proteus mirabilis* as the aetiological basis for autoimmunity. *Microbes Infect* 2000;2: 1489–1496.
126. Rashid T, Tiwana H, Wilson C, et al. Rheumatoid arthritis as an autoimmune disease caused by *Proteus* urinary tract infections: a proposal for a therapeutic protocol. *IMAJ* 2001;3:675–680.
127. Cole B, Griffiths M. Triggering and exacerbation of autoimmune arthritis by the mycoplasma arthritidis superantigen MAM. *Arthritis Rheum* 1993;36:990–994.
128. van der Heijden I, Wilbrink B, Tchetvcrikov I, et al. Presence of bacterial DNA and bacterial peptidoglycans in joints of patients with rheumatoid arthritis and other arthritides. *Arthritis Rheum* 2000;43 (3):593–598.
129. Albert L. Infection and rheumatoid arthritis: guilt by association? *J Rheumatol* 2000;22(3):564–566.
130. Fox D, Smith B. Evidence for oligoclonal B cell expansion in the peripheral blood of patients with rheumatoid arthritis. *Ann Rheum Dis* 1986;45:991–995.
131. McGee B, Small R, Singh R, et al. B lymphocyte clonal expansion in rheumatoid arthritis. *J Rheumatol* 1996;23:36–43.
132. Plater-Zyberk C, Maini R, Lam K, et al. A rheumatoid arthritis B cell subset expresses a phenotype similar to that in chronic lymphocytic leukemia. *Arthritis Rheum* 1985;28:971–976.
133. Meffre E, Davis E, Schiff C, et al. Circulating human B cells that express surrogate light chains and edited receptors. *Nat Immunol* 2000;1(3):207–213.
134. Itoh K, Meffre E, Albesiano E, et al. Immunoglobulin heavy chain variable region gene replacement as a mechanism for receptor revi-

sion in rheumatoid arthritis synovial tissue B lymphocytes. *J Exp Med* 2000;192(8):1151–1164.
135. Zhang Z, Wu X, Limbaugh B, et al. Expression of recombination-activating genes and terminal deoxynucleotidyl transferase and secondary rearrangement of immunoglobulin κ light chains in rheumatoid arthritis synovial tissue. *Arthritis Rheum* 2001;44(10): 2275–2284.
136. Reparon-Schuijt C, van Esch W, van Kooten C, et al. Presence of a population of CD20$^+$,CD38$^-$ B lymphocytes with defective proliferative responsiveness in the synovial compartment of patients with rheumatoid arthritis. *Arthritis Rheum* 2001;44(9):2029–2037.
137. Shi K, Hayashida K, Kaneko M, et al. Lymphoid chemokine B cell–attracting chemokine-1 (CXCL13) is expressed in germinal center of ectopic lymphoid follicles within the synovium of chronic arthritis patients. *J Immunol* 2001;166:650–655.
138. Tan S-M, Xu D, Roschke V, et al. Local production of B lymphocyte stimulator protein and APRIL in arthritic joints of patients with inflammatory arthritis. *Arthritis Rheum* 2003;48(4):982–992.
139. Magalhaes R, Stiehl P, Morawietz L, et al. Morphological and molecular pathology of the B cell response in synovitis of rheumatoid arthritis [Review]. *Virchows Arch* 2002;441(5):415–427.
140. Souto-Carneiro M, Krenn V, Hermann R, et al. IgVH genes from different anatomical regions, with different histopathological patterns, of a rheumatoid arthritis patient suggest cyclic re-entry of mature synovial B-cells in the hypermutation process. *Arthritis Res* 2000; 2(4):303–314.
141. Pyon H, Ha-Lee Y, Song G, et al. Analysis of Ig κ light chain gene variable regions expressed in the rheumatoid synovial B cells. *Scand J Rheumatol* 2001;53:503–509.
142. Reparon-Schuijt C, van Esch W, van Kooten C, et al. Regulation of synovial B cell survival in rheumatoid arthritis by vascular cell adhesion molecule 1 (CD106) expressed on fibroblast-like synoviocytes. *Arthritis Rheum* 2000;43(5):1115–1121.
143. Grant E, Picarella D, Burwell T, et al. Essential role for the C5a receptor in regulating the effector phase of synovial infiltration and joint destruction in experimental arthritis. *J Exp Med* 2002;196(11): 1461–1471.
144. Clague R, Moore L. IgG and IgM antibody to native type II collagen in rheumatoid arthritis serum and synovial fluid. Evidence for the presence of collagen-anti-collagen immune complexes in synovial fluid. *Arthritis Rheum* 1984;27:1370–1377.
145. Rowley M, Tait B, Mackay I, et al. Collagen antibodies in rheumatoid arthritis. Significance of antibodies to denatured collagen and their association with HLA-DR4. *Arthritis Rheum* 1986;29:174–184.
146. Watson W, Cremer M, Wooley P, et al. Assessment of the potential pathogenicity of type II collagen autoantibodies in patients with rheumatoid arthritis. *Arthritis Rheum* 1986;29:1316–1321.
147. Terato K, Shimozuru Y, Katayama K, et al. Specificity of antibodies to type II collagen in rheumatoid arthritis. *Arthritis Rheum* 1990;33: 1493–1500.
148. Burkhardt H, Koller T, Engstrojm A, et al. Epitope-specific recognition of type II collagen by rheumatoid arthritis antibodies is shared with recognition by antibodies that are arthritogenic in collagen-induced arthritis in the mouse. *Arthritis Rheum* 2002;46(9):2339–2348.
149. Mottonen T, Hannonen P, Oka M. Antibodies against native type II collagen do not precede the clinical onset of rheumatoid arthritis. *Arthritis Rheum* 1988;31:776–779.
150. Cook A, Rowley M, Mackay I, et al. Antibodies to type II collagen in early rheumatoid arthritis. *Arthritis Rheum* 1996;39(10):1720–1727.
151. Williams D. Autoantibodies in rheumatoid arthritis. In: Klippel JH, Dieppe PA, eds. Rheumatology. St. Louis: CV Mosby, 1998:section 5, 9.1–9.8.
152. Tarkowski A, Klareskog L, Carlsten H, et al. Secretion of antibodies to types I and II collagen by synovial tissue cells in patients with rheumatoid arthritis. *Arthritis Rheum* 1989;32:1087–1092.
153. Jasin H. Autoantibody specificities of immune complexes sequestered in articular cartilage of patients with rheumatoid arthritis and osteoarthritis. *Arthritis Rheum* 1985;28:241–248.
154. Polgar A, Falus A, Koo E, et al. Elevated levels of synovial fluid antibodies reactive with the small proteoglycans biglycan and decorin in patients with rheumatoid arthritis or other joint diseases. *Rheumatology* 2003;42:522–527.
155. Souto-Carneiro M, Burkhardt H, Muller E, et al. Human monoclonal rheumatoid synovial B lymphocyte hybridoma with a new disease-related specificity for cartilage oligomeric matrix protein. *J Immunol* 2001;166:4202–4208.
156. Janssens X, Veys E, Verbruggen G, et al. The diagnostic significance of the antiperinuclear factor for rheumatoid arthritis. *J Rheumatol* 1988;15:1346–1350.
157. Vincent C, Serre G, Lapeyre F, et al. High diagnostic value in rheumatoid arthritis of antibodies to the stratum corneum of rat oesophagus epithelium, so-called "anti-keratin antibodies." *Ann Rheum Dis* 1989; 48:712–722.
158. Simon M, Girbal E, Sebbag M, et al. The cytokeratin filament-aggregating protein filaggrin is the target of the so-called "antikeratin antibodies," autoantibodies specific for rheumatoid arthritis. *J Clin Invest* 1993;92:1387–1393.
159. Sebbag M, Simon M, Vincent C, et al. The cytokeratin filament-aggregating protein filaggrin is the target of the so-called "antikeratin antibodies," autoantibodies specific for rheumatoid arthritis. *J Clin Invest* 1993;92:1387–1393.
160. van Venrooij W, Pruijn G. Citrullination: a small change for a protein with great consequences for rheumatoid arthritis. *Arthritis Res* 2000; 2(4):249–251.
161. Menard H, Lapointe E, Rochdi M, et al. Insights into rheumatoid arthritis derived from the Sa immune system. *Arthritis Res* 2000;2 (6):429–432.
162. Zhou Z, Menard H. Autoantigenic posttranslational modifications of proteins: does it apply to rheumatoid arthritis? *Curr Opin Rheumatol* 2002;14:250–253.
163. Baeten D, Peene I, Union A, et al. Specific presence of intracellular citrullinated proteins in rheumatoid arthritis synovium. *Arthritis Rheum* 2001;44(10):2255–2262.
164. Masson-Bessiere C, Sebbag M, Durieux J-J, et al. In the rheumatoid pannus, anti-filaggrin autoantibodies are produced by local plasma cells and constitute a higher proportion of IgG than in synovial fluid and serum. *Clin Exp Immunol* 2000;119:544–552.
165. Reparon-Schuijt C, van Esch W, van Venrooij W, et al. Secretion of anti-citrulline-containing peptide antibody by B lymphocytes in rheumatoid arthritis. *Arthritis Rheum* 2001;44(1):41–47.
166. Schellekens G, de Jong B, van den Hoogen F. Citrulline is an essential constituent of antigenic determinants recognized by rheumatoid arthritis-specific autoantibodies. *J Clin Invest* 1998;101:273–281.
167. Masson-Bessiere C, Sebbag M, Girbal E, et al. The major synovial targets of the rheumatoid arthritis-specific antifilaggrin autoantibodies are deiminated forms of the α- and β-chains of fibrin. *J Immunol* 2001;166:4177–4184.
168. Goldbach-Mansky R, Lee J, McCoy A, et al. Rheumatoid arthritis associated autoantibodies in patients with synovitis of recent onset. *Arthritis Res* 2000;2(3):236–243.
169. Kroot E-J, de Jong B, van Leeuwen M, et al. The prognostic value of anti-cyclic citrullinated peptide antibody in patients with recent-onset rheumatoid arthritis. *Arthritis Rheum* 2000;43(8):1831–1835.
170. Meyer O, Labarre C, Dougados M, et al. Anticitrullinated protein/peptide antibody assays in early rheumatoid arthritis for predicting five year radiographic damage. *Ann Rheum Dis* 2003;62:120–126.
171. Vencovsky J, Machacek S, Sedova L, et al. Autoantibodies can be prognostic markers of an erosive disease in early rheumatoid arthritis. *Ann Rheum Dis* 2003;62:427–430.
172. Menard H, El-Amine M. The calpain-calpastatin system in rheumatoid arthritis. *Immunol Today* 1996;17:545–547.
173. Tanaka M, Kishimura M, Ozaki S, et al. Cloning of novel soluble gp130 and detection of its neutralizing autoantibodies in rheumatoid arthritis. *J Clin Invest* 2000;106(1):137–144.
174. Dong H, Strome S, Matteson E, et al. Costimulating aberrant T cell responses by B7-H1 autoantibodies in rheumatoid arthritis. *J Clin Invest* 2003;111(3):363–370.
175. Miossec P. Anti-interleukin 1a autoantibodies. *Ann Rheum Dis* 2002; 61:577–579.
176. Korganow A, Ji H, Mangialaio S, et al. From systemic T cell self-reactivity to organ-specific autoimmune disease via immunoglobulins. *Immunity* 1999;10:451–461.
177. Schaller M, Burton D, Ditzel H. Autoantibodies to GPI in rheumatoid arthritis: linkage between an animal model and human disease. *Nat Immunol* 2001;2(8):746–753.
178. Matsumoto I, Staub A, Benoist C, et al. Arthritis provoked by linked T and B cell recognition of a glycolytic enzyme. *Science* 1999;286: 1732–1735.

179. Ji H, Ohmura K, Mahmood U, et al. Arthritis critically dependent on innate immune system players. *Immunity* 2002;16:157–168.
180. Wipke B, Allen P. Essential role of neutrophils in the initiation and progression of a murine model of rheumatoid arthritis. *J Immunol* 2001;167:1601–1608.
181. Mandik-Nayak L, Wipke B, Shih F, et al. Despite ubiquitous autoantigen expression, arthritogenic autoantibody response initiates in the local lymph node. *Proc Natl Acad Sci U S A* 2002;99(22):14368–14373.
182. Matsumoto I, Lee D, Goldbach-Mansky R, et al. Low prevalence of antibodies to glucose-6-phosphate isomerase in patients with rheumatoid arthritis and a spectrum of other chronic autoimmune disorders. *Arthritis Rheum* 2003;48(4):944–954.
183. Saulot V, Vittecoq O, Charlionet R, et al. Presence of autoantibodies to the glycolytic enzyme α-enolase in sera from patients with early rheumatoid arthritis. *Arthritis Rheum* 2002;46(5):1196–1201.
184. Parekh R, Dwek R, Sutton B, et al. Association of rheumatoid arthritis and primary osteoarthritis with changes in the glycosylation pattern of total serum IgG. *Nature* 1985;316:452–457.
185. Axford J, Mackenzie L, Lydyard P, et al. Reduced B-cell galactosyltransferase activity in rheumatoid arthritis. *Lancet* 1987;2:1486–1488.
186. Ditzel H, Masaki Y, Nielsen H, et al. Cloning and expression of a novel human antibody-antigen pair associated with Felty's syndrome. *Proc Natl Acad Sci U S A* 2000;97(16):9234–9239.
187. Good R, Rotstein J, Mazzitello W. The simultaneous occurrence of rheumatoid arthritis and agammaglobulinemia. *J Clin Invest* 1957; 49:343–357.
188. Pipitone N, Jolliffe V, Cauli A, et al. Do B cells influence disease progression in chronic synovitis? Lessons from primary hypogammaglobulinaemia. *Rheumatology* 2000;39:1280–1285.
189. Takemura S, Klimiuk P, Braun A, et al. T cell activation in rheumatoid synovium is B cell dependent. *J Immunol* 2001;167:4710–4718.
190. De Vita S, Zaja F, Sacco S, et al. Efficacy of selective B cell blockade in the treatment of rheumatoid arthritis. *Arthritis Rheum* 2002;46(8): 2029–2033.
191. Van Boxel J, Paget S. Predominantly T cell infiltrate in rheumatoid synovial membranes. *N Engl J Med* 1975;293:517–520.
192. Bankhurst A, Husby G, Williams R. Predominance of T cells in the lymphocytic infiltrates of synovial tissues in rheumatoid arthritis. *Arthritis Rheum* 1976;19:555–562.
193. Janossy G, Panayi G, Duke O, et al. Rheumatoid arthritis: a disease of T lymphocyte/macrophage immunoregulation. *Lancet* 1981; 2:839–842.
194. Burmester G, Yu D, Irani A, et al. Ia$^+$ T cells in synovial fluid and tissues of patients with rheumatoid arthritis. *Arthritis Rheum* 1981;24: 1370–1376.
195. Fox R, Fong S, Sabharwal N, et al. Synovial fluid lymphocytes differ from peripheral blood lymphocytes in patients with rheumatoid arthritis. *J Immunol* 1982;128:351–354.
196. Hemler M, Glass D, Coblyn J, et al. Very late activation antigens on rheumatoid synovial fluid T lymphocytes. Association with stages of T cell activation. *J Clin Invest* 1986;78:696–702.
197. Tak P, Hintzen R, Teunissen J, et al. Expression of the activation antigen CD27 in rheumatoid arthritis. *Clin Immunol Immunopathol* 1996;80(2):129–138.
198. Veys E, Hermanns P, Verbruggen G, et al. Evaluation of T cell subsets with monoclonal antibodies in synovial fluid in rheumatoid arthritis. *J Rheumatol* 1982;9:821–826.
199. Emery P, Gentry K, Mackay I, et al. Deficiency of the suppressor inducer subset of T lymphocytes in rheumatoid arthritis. *Arthritis Rheum* 1987;30:849–856.
200. Morimoto C, Romain P, Fox D, et al. Abnormalities in CD4$^+$ T lymphocyte subsets in inflammatory rheumatic diseases. *Am J Med* 1988; 84:817–825.
201. Kohem C, Brezinschek R, Wisbey H, et al. Enrichment of differentiated CD45RB dim, CD27$^-$ memory T cells in the peripheral blood, synovial fluid, and synovial tissue of patients with rheumatoid arthritis. *Arthritis Rheum* 1996;39:844–854.
202. Mizokami A, Eguchi K, Kawakami A, et al. Increased population of high fluorescence 1F7 (CD26) antigen on T cells in synovial fluid of patients with rheumatoid arthritis. *J Rheumatol* 1996;23:2022–2026.
203. Isomaki P, Aversa G, Cocks B, et al. Increased expression of signaling lymphocytic activation molecule in patients with rheumatoid arthritis and its role in the regulation of cytokine production in rheumatoid synovium. *J Immunol* 1997;159:2986–2993.
204. Fox D, Millard J, Kan L, et al. Activation pathways of synovial T lymphocytes. Expression and function of the UM4D4/CDw60 antigen. *J Clin Invest* 1990;86:1124–1136.
205. Cao D, Malmstrom V, Baecher-Allan C, et al. Isolation and functional characterization of regulatory CD25^{bright}CD4$^+$ T cells from the target organ of patients with rheumatoid arthritis. *Eur J Immunol* 2003;33:215–223.
206. Morgan M, Sutmuller R, Witteveen H, et al. CD25$^+$ cell depletion hastens the onset of severe disease in collagen-induced arthritis. *Arthritis Rheum* 2003;48(5):1452–1460.
207. Holoshitz J, Vila L, Keroack B, et al. Dual antigenic recognition by cloned T cells. *J Clin Invest* 1992;89:308–314.
208. Tanaka Y, Morita C, Tanaka Y, et al. Natural and synthetic nonpeptide antigens recognized by human gamma delta T cells. *Nature* 1995;375:115–158.
209. Haftel H, Chang Y, Hinderer R, et al. Induction of the autoantigen proliferating cell nuclear antigen in T lymphocytes by a mycobacterial antigen. *J Clin Invest* 1994;94:1365–1372.
210. Lunardi C, Marguerie C, Walport M, et al. T γδ cells and their subsets in blood and synovial fluid from patients with rheumatoid arthritis. *Br J Rheumatol* 1992;31(8):527–530.
211. Bucht A, Soderstrom K, Hultman T, et al. T cell receptor diversity and activation markers in the V_d1 subset of rheumatoid synovial fluid and peripheral blood T lymphocytes. *Eur J Immunol* 1992;22(2): 567–574.
212. Meliconi R, Uguccioni M, D'Errico A, et al. T cell receptor γδ positive lymphocytes in synovial membrane. *Br J Rheumatol* 1992;31(1): 59–61.
213. Peterman G, Spencer C, Sperling A, et al. Role of γδ T cells in murine collagen-induced arthritis. *J Immunol* 1993;151(11):6546–6558.
214. Pelegri C, Kuhnlein P, Buchner E, et al. Depletion of γδ T cells does not prevent or ameliorate, but rather aggravates, rat adjuvant arthritis. *Arthritis Rheum* 1996;39(2):204–215.
215. Lui M, Kohsaka H, Sakurai H, et al. The presence of co-stimulatory molecules CD86 and CD28 in rheumatoid arthritis synovium. *Arthritis Rheum* 1996;39:110–114.
216. Sfikakis P, Zografou A, Viglis V, et al. CD28 expression on T cell subsets *in vivo* and CD28-mediated T cell response *in vitro* in patients with rheumatoid arthritis. *Arthritis Rheum* 1995;38:649–654.
217. Schmidt D, Goronzy J, Weyand C. CD4$^+$ CD7$^-$ CD28$^-$ T cells are expanded in rheumatoid arthritis and are characterized by autoreactivity. *J Clin Invest* 1996;97(9):2027–2037.
218. Bryl E, Vallejo A, Weyand C, et al. Down-regulation of CD28 expression by TNF-α. *J Immunol* 2001;167:3231–3238.
219. Vallejo A, Schirmer M, Weyand C, et al. Clonality and longevity of CD4$^+$ CD28^{null} T cells are associated with defects in apoptotic pathways. *J Immunol* 2000;165:6301–6307.
220. Wagner U, Pierer M, Kaltenhauser S, et al. Clonally expanded CD4$^+$CD28^{null} T cells in rheumatoid arthritis use distinct combinations of T cell receptor BV and BJ elements. *Eur J Immunol* 2003; 33:79–84.
221. Warrington K, Takemura S, Goronzy J, et al. CD4$^+$,CD28$^-$ T cells in rheumatoid arthritis patients combine features of the innate and adaptive immune systems. *Arthritis Rheum* 2001;44(1):13–20.
222. Namekawa T, Snyder M, Yen J-H, et al. Killer cell activating receptors function as costimulatory molecules on CD4$^+$CD28^{null} T cells clonally expanded in rheumatoid arthritis. *J Immunol* 2000; 165:1138–1145.
223. Salazar-Fontana L-I, Sanz E, Merida I, et al. Cell surface CD28 levels define four CD4$^+$ T cells subsets: abnormal expression in rheumatoid arthritis. *Clin Immunol* 2001;99(2):253–265.
224. Higgs J, Zeldes W, Kozarsky K, et al. A novel pathway of human T lymphocyte activation. Identification by a monoclonal antibody generated against a rheumatoid synovial T cell line. *J Immunol* 1988; 140:3758–3765.
225. Meuer S, Hussey R, Fabbi M, et al. An alternative pathway of T cell activation: a functional role for the 50 kd T11 sheep erythrocyte receptor protein. *Cell* 1984;36:897–906.
226. Bott C, Doshi J, Morimoto C, et al. Activation of human T cells through CD6; functional effects of a novel anti-CD6 monoclonal antibody and definition of four epitopes of the CD6 glycoprotein. *Int Immunol* 1993;5:783–792.

227. Levesque M, Heinly C, Whichard L, et al. Cytokine-regulated expression of activated leukocyte cell adhesion molecule (CD166) on monocyte-lineage cells and in rheumatoid arthritis synovium. *Arthritis Rheum* 1998;41:2221–2229.
228. Wagner U, Kurtin P, Wahner A, et al. The role of $CD8^+$ $CD40L^+$ T cells in the formation of germinal centers in rheumatoid synovitis. *J Immunol* 1998;161:6390–6397.
229. Vallejo A, Mugge L, Klimiuk P, et al. Central role of thrombospondin-1 in the activation and clonal expansion of inflammatory T cells. *J Immunol* 2000;164:2947–2954.
230. Carter R, Wicks I. Vascular cell adhesion molecule 1 (CD106): a multifaceted regulator of joint inflammation. *Arthritis Rheum* 2001; 44(5):985–994.
231. Firestein G, Zvaifler N. How important are T cells in chronic rheumatoid synovitis? *Arthritis Rheum* 1990;33:768–773.
232. Ponchel F, Wilson K, Ali M, et al. Rheumatoid arthritis synovial T cells regulate transcription of several genes associated with antigen-induced anergy. *J Clin Invest* 2001;107(4):519–528.
233. Corrigall V, Solau-Gervais E, Panayi G. Lack of CD80 expression by fibroblast-like synoviocytes leading to anergy in T lymphocytes. *Arthritis Rheum* 2000;43(7):1606–1615.
234. Schrijver I, Melief M, Markusse H, et al. Peptidoglycan from sterile human spleen induces T cell proliferation and inflammatory mediators in rheumatoid arthritis patients and healthy subjects. *Rheumatology* 2001;40:438–446.
235. Schrijver I, Melief M, Tak P, et al. Antigen-presenting cells containing bacterial peptidoglycan in synovial tissues of rheumatoid arthritis patients coexpress costimulatory molecules and cytokines. *Arthritis Rheum* 2000;43(10):2160–2168.
236. Fazou C, Yang H, McMichael A, et al. Epitope specificity of clonally expanded populations of $CD8^+$ T cells found within the joints of patients with inflammatory arthritis. *Arthritis Rheum* 2001;44(9):2038–2045.
237. Shadidi K, Aarvak T, Jeansson S, et al. T cell responses to viral, bacterial and protozoan antigens in rheumatoid inflammation. Selective migration of T cells to synovial tissue. *Rheumatology* 2001;40:1120–1125.
238. Cuesta I, Sud S, Song Z, et al. T cell receptor (V_b) bias in the response of rheumatoid arthritis synovial fluid T cells to connective tissue antigens. *Scand J Rheumatol* 1997;26(3):166–173.
239. Snowden N, Reynolds I, Morgan K, et al. T cell responses to human type II collagen in patients with rheumatoid arthritis and healthy controls. *Arthritis Rheum* 1997;40(7):1210–1218.
240. Londei M, Savill C, Verhoef A, et al. Persistence of collagen type II–specific T cell clones in the synovial membrane of a patient with rheumatoid arthritis. *Proc Natl Acad Sci U S A* 1989;86:636–640.
241. Verheijden G, Rijinders A, Bos E, et al. Human cartilage glycoprotein-39 as a candidate autoantigen in rheumatoid arthritis. *Arthritis Rheum* 1997;40:1115–1125.
242. Guerassimov A, Zhang Y, Banerjee S, et al. Cellular immunity to the G1 domain of cartilage proteoglycan aggrecan is enhanced in patients with rheumatoid arthritis but only after removal of keratan sulfate. *Arthritis Rheum* 1998;41(6):1019–1025.
243. Toyosaki T, Tsuruta Y, Yoshioka T, et al. Recognition of rheumatoid arthritis synovial antigen by $CD4^+$, $CD8^-$ T cell clones established from rheumatoid arthritis joints. *Arthritis Rheum* 1998;41(1): 92–100.
244. Cope A, Patel S, Hall F, et al. T cell responses to a human cartilage autoantigen in the context of rheumatoid arthritis-associated and nonassociated HLA-DR4 alleles. *Arthritis Rheum* 1999;42(7):1497–1507.
245. Blass S, Schumann F, Hain N, et al. p205 is a major target of autoreactive T cells in rheumatoid arthritis. *Arthritis Rheum* 1999;42(5): 971–980.
246. Fritsch R, Eselbock D, Skriner K, et al. Characterization of autoreactive T cells to the autoantigens heterogeneous nuclear ribonucleoprotein A2 (RA33) and filaggrin in patients with rheumatoid arthritis. *J Immunol* 2002;169:1068–1076.
247. Wang J, Roehrl M. Glycosaminoglycans are a potential cause of rheumatoid arthritis. *Proc Natl Acad Sci U S A* 2002;99(22):14362–14367.
248. Fang Q, Yan-Yang S, Cai W, et al. Cartilage-reactive T cells in rheumatoid synovium. *Int Immunol* 2000;12(5):659–669.
249. Kotzin B, Falta M, Crawford F, et al. Use of soluble peptide-DR4 tetramers to detect synovial T cells specific for cartilage antigens in patients with rheumatoid arthritis. *Proc Natl Acad Sci U S A* 2000; 97(1):291–296.
250. Tsark E, Wang W, Teng Y, et al. Differential MHC class II–mediated presentation of rheumatoid arthritis autoantigens by human dendritic cells and macrophages. *J Immunol* 2002;169(11):6625–6633.
251. Backlund J, Carlsen S, Hoger T, et al. Predominant selection of T cells specific for the glycosylated collagen type II epitope (263–270) in humanized transgenic mice and in rheumatoid arthritis. *Proc Natl Acad Sci U S A* 2002;99(15):9960–9965.
252. Baeten D, Boots A, Steenbakkers P, et al. Human cartilage gp-39^+, $CD16^+$ monocytes in peripheral blood and synovium. *Arthritis Rheum* 2000;43(6):1233–1243.
253. Corrigall V, Bodman-Smith M, Fife M, et al. The human endoplasmic reticulum molecular chaperone BiP is an autoantigen for rheumatoid arthritis and prevents the induction of experimental arthritis. *J Immunol* 2001;166:1492–1498.
254. Blab S, Union A, Raymackers J, et al. The stress protein BiP is overexpressed and is a major B and T cell target in rheumatoid arthritis. *Arthritis Rheum* 2001;44(4):761–771.
255. Bodman-Smith M, Corrigall V, Kemeny D, et al. BiP, a putative autoantigen in rheumatoid arthritis, stimulates IL-10-producing CD8-positive T cells from normal individuals. *Rheumatology* 2003;42: 637–644.
256. Cannons J, Karsch J, Birnboim H, et al. HRPT-mutant T cells in the peripheral blood and synovial tissue of patients with rheumatoid arthritis. *Arthritis Rheum* 1998;41(10):1772–1782.
257. Choy E, Scott D, Kingsley G, et al. Control of rheumatoid arthritis by oral tolerance. *Arthritis Rheum* 2001;44(9):1993–1997.
258. Kavanaugh A, Genovese M, Baughman J, et al. Allele and antigen-specific treatment of rheumatoid arthritis: A double-blind, placebo controlled phase 1 trial. *J Rheumatol* 2003;30:449–454.
259. Brennan F, Allard S, Londei M, et al. Heterogeneity of T cell receptor idiotypes in rheumatoid arthritis. *Clin Exp Rheumatol* 1988;73:417–423.
260. Gudmundsson S, Ronnelid J, Karlsson-Parra A, et al. T cell receptor V-gene usage in synovial fluid and synovial tissue from RA patients. *Scand J Rheumatol* 1992;36(5):681–688.
261. Williams W, Fang Q, Demarco D, et al. Restricted heterogeneity of T cell receptor transcripts in rheumatoid synovium. *J Clin Invest* 1992;90(2):326–333.
262. Jenkins R, Nikaein A, Zimmermann A, et al. T cell receptor V_b gene bias in rheumatoid arthritis. *J Clin Invest* 1993;92(6):2688–2701.
263. Struyk L, Kurnick J, Hawes G, et al. T cell receptor V-gene usage in synovial fluid lymphocytes of patients with chronic arthritis. *Hum Immunol* 1993;37(4):237–251.
264. Zagon G, Tumang J, Li Y, et al. Increased frequency of V_b17-positive T cells in patients with rheumatoid arthritis. *Arthritis Rheum* 1994; 37(10):1431–1440.
265. Alam A, Lule J, Coppin H, et al. T cell receptor variable region of the β-chain gene use in peripheral blood and multiple synovial membranes during rheumatoid arthritis. *Hum Immunol* 1995;42(4):331–339.
266. Fitzgerald J, Ricalton N, Meyer A, et al. Analysis of clonal $CD8^+$ T cell expansions in normal individuals and patients with rheumatoid arthritis. *J Immunol* 1995;154(7):3538–3547.
267. Huchenq A, Champagne E, Sevin J, et al. Abnormal T cell receptor V_b gene expression in the peripheral blood and synovial fluid of rheumatoid arthritis patients. *Clin Exp Rheumatol* 1995;13(1):29–36.
268. Melchers I, Peter H, Eibel H. The T and B cell repertoire of patients with rheumatoid arthritis. *Scand J Rheumatol Suppl* 1995;101:153–162.
269. Jenkins R, McGinnis D. T cell receptor V_b gene utilization in rheumatoid arthritis. *Ann NY Acad Sci* 1995;756:159–172.
270. Hingorani R, Monteiro J, Pergolizzi R, et al. CDR3 length restriction of T cell receptor β-chains in $CD8^+$ T cells of rheumatoid arthritis patients. *Ann NY Acad Sci* 1995;756:179–182.
271. Alam A, Lule J, Lambert N, et al. Use of T cell receptor V genes in synovial membrane in rheumatoid arthritis. *Ann NY Acad Sci* 1995; 756:199–200.
272. Gonzalez-Quintial R, Baccala R, Pope R, et al. Identification of clonally expanded T cells in rheumatoid arthritis using a sequence enrichment nuclease assay. *J Clin Invest* 1996;97(5):1335–1343.
273. Hingorani R, Monteiro J, Furie R, et al. Oligoclonality of V_b3 TCR chains in the $CD8^+$ T cell population of rheumatoid arthritis patients. *J Immunol* 1996;156(2):852–858.

274. Rittner H, Zettl A, Jendro M, et al. Multiple mechanisms support oligoclonal T cell expansion in rheumatoid synovitis. *Mol Med* 1997; 3(7):452–465.
275. Woulfe S, Bono C, Zacheis M, et al. Negatively charged residues interacting with the p4 pocket confer binding specificity to DRB1 * 0401. *Arthritis Rheum* 1995;38:1744–1753.
276. Hammer J, Gallazzi F, Bono E, et al. Peptide binding specificity of HLA-DR4 molecules: correlation with rheumatoid arthritis association. *J Exp Med* 1995;181:1847–1855.
277. Kerlan-Candon S, Louis-Plence P, Wiedemann A, et al. Specific overexpression of rheumatoid arthritis-associated HLA-DR alleles and presentation of low-affinity peptides. *Arthritis Rheum* 2001;44 (6):1281–1292.
278. Kirschman D, Duffin K, Smith C, et al. Naturally processed peptides from rheumatoid arthritis associated and non-associated HLA-DR alleles. *J Immunol* 1995;155:5655–5662.
279. Rosloniec E, Whittington K, Zaller D, et al. HLA-DR1 (DRB1*0101) and DR4 (DRB1*0401) use the same anchor residues for binding an immunodominant peptide derived from human type II collagen. *J Immunol* 2002;168:253–259.
280. Patil N, Pashine A, Belmares M, et al. Rheumatoid arthritis (RA)-associated HLA-DR alleles form less stable complexes with class II–associated invariant chain peptide than non-RA HLA-DR alleles. *J Immunol* 2001;167:7157–7168.
281. Hill J, Southwood S, Sette A, et al. The conversion of arginine to citrulline allows for a high-affinity peptide interaction with the rheumatoid arthritis–associated HLA-DRB1*0401 MHC class II molecule. *J Immunol* 2003;171:538–541.
282. Weyand C, Xie C, Goronzy J. Homozygosity for the HLA-DRB1 allele selects for extra-articular manifestations in rheumatoid arthritis. *J Clin Invest* 1992;89:2033–2039.
283. Weyand C, Hicok C, Conn D, et al. The influence of HLA-DRB1 genes on disease severity in rheumatoid arthritis. *Ann Intern Med* 1992;117:801–806.
284. Evans T, Han J, Singh R. The genotypic distribution of shared-epitope DRB1 alleles suggests a recessive mode of inheritance of the rheumatoid arthritis disease-susceptibility gene. *Arthritis Rheum* 1995;38:1754–1761.
285. Moreno I, Valenzuela A, Garcia A, et al. Association of the shared epitope with radiological severity of rheumatoid arthritis. *J Rheumatol* 1996;23:6–9.
286. de Vries N, Tijssen H, van Riel P, et al. Reshaping the shared epitope hypothesis: HLA-associated risk for rheumatoid arthritis is encoded by amino acid substitutions at positions 67–74 of the HLA-DRB1 molecule. *Arthritis Rheum* 2002;46(4):921–928.
287. Vos K, van der Horst-Bruinsma I, Hazes J, et al. Evidence for a protective role of the human leukocyte antigen class II region in early rheumatoid arthritis. *Rheumatology* 2001;40:133–139.
288. Snijders A, Elferink D, Geluk A, et al. An HLA-DRB1-derived peptide associated with protection against rheumatoid arthritis is naturally processed by human APCs. *J Immunol* 2001;166:4987–4993.
289. Taneja V, David C. Association of MHC and rheumatoid arthritis: regulatory role of HLA class II molecules in animal models of RA—studies on transgenic/knockout mice. *Arthritis Res* 2000;2(3):205–207.
290. Auger I, Lepecuchel L, Roudier J. Interaction between heat-shock protein 73 and HLA-DRB1 alleles associated or not with rheumatoid arthritis. *Arthritis Rheum* 2002;46(4):929–933.
291. Maier J, Haug M, Foll J, et al. Possible association of non-binding of HSP70 to HLA-DRB1 peptide sequences and protection from rheumatoid arthritis. *Immunogenetics* 2002;54:67–73.
292. Walser-Kuntz D, Weyand C, Weaver A, et al. Mechanisms underlying the formation of the T cell receptor repertoire in rheumatoid arthritis. *Immunity* 1995;2(6):597–605.
293. Wagner U, Koetz K, Weyand C, et al. Perturbation of the T cell repertoire in rheumatoid arthritis. *Proc Natl Acad Sci U S A* 1998;95: 14447–14452.
294. Koetz K, Bryl E, Spickschen K, et al. T cell homeostasis in patients with rheumatoid arthritis. *Proc Natl Acad Sci U S A* 2000;97(16): 9203–9208.
295. Ponchel F, Morgan A, Bingham S, et al. Dysregulated lymphocyte proliferation and differentiation in patients with rheumatoid arthritis. *Blood* 2002;100:4550–4556.
296. Auger I, Escola J, Gorvel J, et al. HLA-DR4 and HLA-DR10 motifs that carry susceptibility to rheumatoid arthritis bind 70-kD heat shock proteins. *Nat Med* 1996;2:306–310.
297. Ollier W, Kennedy L, Thomson W, et al. Dog MHC alleles containing the human RA shared epitope confer susceptibility to canine rheumatoid arthritis. *Immunogenetics* 2001;53(8):669–673.
298. Vervoordeldonk M, Tak P. Cytokines in rheumatoid arthritis. *Curr Rheum Rep* 2002;4:208–217.
299. Arend W, Dayer J. Cytokines and cytokine inhibitors or antagonists in rheumatoid arthritis. *Arthritis Rheum* 1990;33:305–315.
300. Brennan F, Maini R, Feldmann M. Cytokine expression in chronic inflammatory disease. *Br Med Bull* 1995;51:368–384.
301. Postlethwaite A, Lachman L, Kang A. Induction of fibroblast proliferation by interleukin-1 derived from human monocytic leukemia cells. *Arthritis Rheum* 1984;27:995–1001.
302. Tyler J. Articular cartilage cultured with catabolin (pig interleukin 1) synthesizes a decreased number of normal proteoglycan molecules. *Biochem J* 1985;227:869–878.
303. Dayer J, Beutler B, Cerami A. Cachectin/tumor necrosis factor stimulates collagenase and prostaglandin E_2 production by human synovial cells and dermal fibroblasts. *J Exp Med* 1985;162:2163–2168.
304. Dewhirst F, Stashenko P, Mole J, et al. Purification and partial sequence of human osteoclast-activating factor: Identify with interleukin 1β. *J Immunol* 1985;135:2562–2568.
305. Dinarello C, Cannon J, Wolff S, et al. Tumor necrosis factor (cachectin) is an endogenous pyrogen and induces production of interleukin 1. *J Exp Med* 1986;163:1433–1450.
306. Mochan E, Uhl J, Newton R. Interleukin 1 stimulation of synovial cell plasminogen activator production. *J Rheumatol* 1986;13:15–19.
307. Bertolini D, Nedwin G, Bringman T, et al. Stimulation of bone resorption and inhibition of bone formation *in vitro* by human tumor necrosis factor. *Nature* 1986;319:516–518.
308. Miossec P, Dinarello C, Ziff M. Interleukin-1 lymphocyte chemotactic activity in rheumatoid arthritis synovial fluid. *Arthritis Rheum* 1986;29:461–470.
309. Saklatvala J. Tumor necrosis factor-α stimulates resorption and inhibits synthesis of proteoglycan in cartilage. *Nature* 1986;322:547–549.
310. Strieter R, Kunkel S, Showell H, et al. Endothelial cell gene expression of a neutrophil chemotactic factor by TNF-α, LPS, and IL-1β. *Science* 1989;243:1467–1469.
311. Leirisalo-Repo M, Paimela L, Jaattela M, et al. Production of TNF by monocytes of patients with early rheumatoid arthritis is increased. *Scand J Rheumatol* 1995;24:366–371.
312. Paleolog E, Young S, Stark A, et al. Modulation of angiogenic vascular endothelial growth factor by tumor necrosis factor α and interleukin-1 in rheumatoid arthritis. *Arthritis Rheum* 1998;41:1258–1265.
313. Dayer J. The pivotal role of interleukin-1 in the clinical manifestations of rheumatoid arthritis. *Rheumatology* 2003;42(suppl 2):3–10.
314. Gracie J, Leung B, McInnes I. Novel pathways that regulate tumor necrosis factor-α production in rheumatoid arthritis. *Curr Opin Rheumatol* 2002;14:270–275.
315. Oppenheimer-Marks N, Lipsky P. Adhesion molecules in arthritis control of T cell migration into the synovium. In: Miossec P, van den Berg WB, Firestein GS, eds. *T cell in arthritis (progress in inflammation research).* Basel: Birkhauser, 1998:129–148.
316. Koch A, Kunkel S, Strieter R. Cytokines in rheumatoid arthritis. *J Invest Med* 1995;43:28–38.
317. Kraan M, Patel D, Haringman J, et al. The development of clinical signs of rheumatoid synovial inflammation is associated with increased synthesis of the chemokine CXCL8 (interleukin-8). *Arthritis Res* 2001;3(1):65–71.
318. Hayashida K, Nanki T, Girschick H, et al. Synovial stromal cells from rheumatoid arthritis patients attract monocytes by producing MCP-1 and IL-8. *Arthritis Res* 2001;3(2):118–126.
319. Szekanecz Z, Koch A. Chemokines and angiogenesis. *Curr Opin Rheumatol* 2001;13:202–208.
320. Firestein G, Boyle D, Yu C, et al. Synovial interleukin-1 receptor antagonist and interleukin-1 balance in rheumatoid arthritis. *Arthritis Rheum* 1994;37:644–652.
321. Arend W, Gabay C. Physiologic role of interleukin-1 receptor antagonist. *Arthritis Res* 2000;2(4):245–248.
322. Cope A, Aderka D, Doherty M, et al. Increased levels of soluble tumor necrosis factor receptors in the sera and synovial fluid of patients with rheumatic diseases. *Arthritis Rheum* 1992;35:1160–1169.

323. Wong P, Campbell I, Egan P, et al. The role of the interleukin-6 family of cytokines in inflammatory arthritis and bone turnover. *Arthritis Rheum* 2003;48(5):1177–1189.
324. Miossec P. The TH1/TH2 cytokine balance in arthritis. In: Miossec P, van den Berg WB, Firestein GS, eds. *T cells in arthritis (progress in inflammation research).* Basel: Birkhauser, 1998:93–109.
325. Bakakos P, Pickard C, Wong W, et al. Simultaneous analysis of T cell clonality and cytokine production in rheumatoid arthritis using three-colour flow cytometry. *Clin Exp Immunol* 2002;129:370–378.
326. Gerli R, Bistoni O, Russano A, et al. *In vivo* activated T cells in rheumatoid synovitis. Analysis of Th1- and Th2-type cytokine production at clonal level in different stages of disease. *Clin Exp Immunol* 2002;129:549–555.
327. Santiago-Schwarz F, Anand P, Liu S, et al. Dendritic cells (DCs) in rheumatoid arthritis (RA): progenitor cells and soluble factors contained in RA synovial fluid yield a subset of myeloid DCs that preferentially activate Th1 inflammatory-type responses. *J Immunol* 2001; 167(3):1758–1768.
328. Firestein G, Zvaifler N. Peripheral blood and synovial fluid monocyte activation in inflammatory arthritis: II. Low levels of synovial fluid and synovial tissue interferon suggest that γ-interferon is not the primary macrophage activating factor. *Arthritis Rheum* 1987;30: 864–871.
329. Canete J, Martinez S, Farres J. Differential Th1/Th2 cytokine patterns in chronic arthritis: interferon γ is highly expressed in synovium of rheumatoid arthritis compared with seronegative spondyloarthropathies. *Ann Rheum Dis* 2000;59:263–268.
330. Morita Y, Yamamura M, Kawashima M, et al. Flow cytometric single-cell analysis olf cytokine production by CD4⁺ T cells in synovial tissue and peripheral blood from patients with rheumatoid arthritis. *Arthritis Rheum* 1998;41(9):1669–1676.
331. Park S-H, Min D-J, Cho M-L, et al. Shift toward T helper 1 cytokines by type II collagen-reactive T cells in patients with rheumatoid arthritis. *Arthritis Rheum* 2001;44(3):561–569.
332. Wong W, Vakis S, Ayre K, et al. Rheumatoid arthritis T cells produce Th1 cytokines in response to stimulation with a novel trispecific antibody directed against CD2, CD3, and CD28. *Scand J Rheumatol* 2000;29:282–287.
333. Maeda T, Yamada H, Nagamine R, et al. Involvement of CD4⁺, CD57⁺ T cells in the disease activity of rheumatoid arthritis. *Arthritis Rheum* 2002;46(2):379–384.
334. Morita Y, Yamamura M, Nishida K. Expression of interleukin-12 in synovial tissue from patients with rheumatoid arthritis. *Arthritis Rheum* 1998;41(2):306–314.
335. McInnis I, Al-Mughales J, Field M, et al. The role of interleukin-15 in T cell migration and activation in rheumatoid arthritis. *Nat Med* 1996;2:175–182.
336. Gracie J, Forsey R, Chan W, et al. A pro-inflammatory role for interleukin-18 in rheumatoid arthritis. *J Clin Invest* 1999;104:1393–1401.
337. Yamamura M, Kawashima M, Taniai M, et al. Interferon-γ-inducing activity of interleukin-18 in the joint with rheumatoid arthritis. *Arthritis Rheum* 2001;44(2):275–285.
338. Komai-Koma M, Gracie J, Wei X, et al. Chemoattraction of human T cells by IL-18. *J Immunol* 2003;170:1084–1090.
339. Park C, Morel J, Amin M, et al. Evidence of IL-18 as a novel angiogenic mediator. *J Immunol* 2001;167:1644–1653.
340. Miossec P, Navillat M, Dupuy d'Angeac A, et al. Low levels of interleukin-4 and high levels of transforming growth factor beta in rheumatoid arthritis. *Arthritis Rheum* 1990;33:1180–1187.
341. Davis L, Cush J, Schulze-Koops H, et al. Rheumatoid synovial CD4⁺ T cells exhibit a reduced capacity to differentiate into IL-4 producing T-helper-2 effector cells. *Arthritis Res* 2001;3(1):54–64.
342. Hessian P, Highton J, Kean A, et al. Cytokine profile of the rheumatoid nodule suggests that it is a Th1 granuloma. *Arthritis Rheum* 2003;48(2):334–338.
343. Husby G, Williams R. Immunohistochemical studies of interleukin-2 and interferon-γ in rheumatoid arthritis. *Arthritis Rheum* 1985;28: 174–181.
344. Firestein G, Xu W, Townsend K, et al. Cytokines in chronic inflammatory arthritis: I. Failure to detect T cell lymphokines (interleukin 2 and interleukin 3) and presence of macrophage colony-stimulating factor (CSF-1) and a novel mast cell growth factor in rheumatoid synovitis. *J Exp Med* 1988;168:1573–1586.
345. Tagaya Y, Bamford R, DeFilippis A, et al. IL-15: a pleiotropic cytokine with diverse receptor/signalling pathways whose expression is controlled at multiple levels. *Immunity* 1996;4:329–336.
346. Brennan F, Hayes A, Ciesielski C, et al. Evidence that rheumatoid arthritis synovial T cells are similar to cytokine-activated T cells: Involvement of phosphatidylinositol 3-kinase and nuclear factor κB pathways in tumor necrosis factor a production in rheumatoid arthritis. *Arthritis Rheum* 2002;46(1):31–41.
347. Masuko-Hongo K, Kurokawa M, Kobata T, et al. Effect of IL15 on T cell clonality *in vitro* and in the synovial fluid of patients with rheumatoid arthritis. *Ann Rheum Dis* 2000;59:688–694.
348. Mottonen M, Isomaki P, Luukkainen R, et al. Interleukin-15 up-regulates the expression of CD154 on synovial fluid T cells. *Immunol* 2000;100:238–244.
349. Chabaud M, Fossiez F, Taupin J, et al. Enhancing effect of IL-17 on IL-1-induced IL-6 and leukemia inhibitory factor production by rheumatoid arthritis synoviocytes and its regulation by TH2 cytokines. *J Immunol* 1998;161:409–414.
350. Miossec P. Interleukin-17 in rheumatoid arthritis: if T cells were to contribute to inflammation and destruction through synergy. *Arthritis Rheum* 2003;48(2):594–601.
351. Kehlen A, Thiele K, Riemann D, et al. Expression, modulation and signalling of IL-17 receptor in fibroblast-like synoviocytes of patients with rheumatoid arthritis. *Clin Exp Immunol* 2002;127:539–546.
352. Chabaud M, Lubberts E, Joosten L, et al. IL-17 derived from juxta-articular bone and synovium contributes to joint degradation in rheumatoid arthritis. *Arthritis Res* 2001;3(3):168–177.
353. Chabaud M, Garnero P, Dayer J, et al. Contribution of interleukin 17 to synovium matrix destruction in rheumatoid arthritis. *Cytokine* 2000;12(7):1092–1099.
354. Ziolkowska M, Koc A, Luszczykiewicz G, et al. High levels of IL-17 in rheumatoid arthritis patients: IL-15 triggers *in vitro* IL-17 production via cyclosporin A–sensitive mechanism. *J Immunol* 2000;164: 2832–2838.
355. Bush K, Farmer K, Walker J, et al. Reduction of joint inflammation and bone erosion in rat adjuvant arthritis by treatment with interleukin-17 receptor IgG1 Fc fusion protein. *Arthritis Rheum* 2002;46 (3):802–805.
356. Morand E, Bucala R, Leech M. Macrophage migration inhibitory factor: an emerging therapeutic target in rheumatoid arthritis. *Arthritis Rheum* 2003;48(2):291–299.
357. Lacey D, Sampey A, Mitchell R, et al. Control of fibroblast-like synoviocyte proliferation by macrophage migration inhibitory factor. *Arthritis Rheum* 2003;48(1):103–109.
358. Gravallese E, Goldring S. Cellular mechanisms and the role of cytokines in bone erosions in rheumatoid arthritis. *Arthritis Rheum* 2000; 43(10):2143–2151.
359. Lam J, Takeshita S, Barker J, et al. TNF-α induces osteoclastogenesis by direct stimulation of macrophages exposed to permissive levels of RANK ligand. *J Clin Invest* 2000;106(12):1481–1488.
360. Katsikis P, Chu C, Brennan F, et al. Immunoregulatory role of interleukin 10 in rheumatoid arthritis. *J Exp Med* 1994;179:1517–1527.
361. Yudoh K, Matsuno H, Nakazawa F, et al. Reduced expression of the regulatory CD4⁺ T cell subset is related to Th1/Th2 balance and disease severity in rheumatoid arthritis. *Arthritis Rheum* 2000;43(3): 617–627.
362. Salmi M, Rajala P, Jalkanen S. Homing of mucosal leukocytes to joints: distinct endothelial ligands in synovium mediate leukocyte-subtype specific adhesion. *J Clin Invest* 1997;99(9):2165–2172.
363. Irjala H, Elima K, Johansson E, et al. The same endothelial receptor controls lymphocyte traffic both in vascular and lymphatic vessels. *Eur J Immunol* 2003;33:815–824.
364. Lee L, Buckley C, Blades M, et al. Identification of synovium-specific homing peptides by *in vivo* phage display selection. *Arthritis Rheum* 2002;46(8):2109–2120.
365. Nanki T, Hayashida K, El-Gabalawy H, et al. Stromal cell-derived factor-1-CXC chemokine receptor 4 interactions play a central role in CD4⁺ T cell accumulation in rheumatoid arthritis synovium. *J Immunol* 2000;165(11):6590–6598.
366. Homma T, Hosono O, Iwata S, et al. Recognition of cell surface GD3 by monoclonal antibody anti-6C2 in rheumatoid arthritis synovial fluid: expression on human T cells with transendothelial migratory activity. *Arthritis Rheum* 2001;44(2):296–306.

367. Nanki T, Imai T, Nagasaka K, et al. Migration of CX3CR1-positive T cells producing type 1 cytokines and cytotoxic molecules into the synovium of patients with rheumatoid arthritis. *Arthritis Rheum* 2002; 46(11):2878–2883.
368. Aarvak T, Natvig J. Cell-cell interactions in synovitis: antigen presenting cells and T cell interaction in rheumatoid arthritis. *Arthritis Res* 2001;3(1):13–17.
369. Tsai V, Zvaifler N. Dendritic cell–lymphocyte clusters that form spontaneously in rheumatoid arthritis synovial effusions differ from clusters formed in human mixed leukocyte reactions. *J Clin Invest* 1988;82:1731–1745.
370. Kraan M, Reece R, Smeets T, et al. Comparison of synovial tissues from the knee joints and the small joints of rheumatoid arthritis patients. *Arthritis Rheum* 2002;46(8):2034–2038.
371. Takemura S, Braun A, Crowson C, et al. Lymphoid neogenesis in rheumatoid synovitis. *J Immunol* 2001;167:1072–1080.
372. Kang Y, Zhang X, Wagner U, et al. CD8 T cells are required for the formation of ectopic germinal centers in rheumatoid synovitis. *J Exp Med* 2002;195(10):1325–1336.
373. Bornbara M, Webb D, Conrad P, et al. Cell contact between T cells and synovial fibroblasts causes induction of adhesion molecules and cytokines. *J Leukoc Biol* 1993;54:399–406.
374. Rezzonico R, Burger D, Dayer J. Direct contact between T lymphocytes and human dermal fibroblasts or synoviocytes down-regulates types I and III collagen production via cell-associated cytokines. *J Biol Chem* 1998;273(30):8720–8728.
375. Burger D, Rezzonico R, Li J, et al. Imbalance between interstitial collagenase and tissue inhibitor of metalloproteinases 1 in synoviocytes and fibroblasts upon direct contact with stimulated T lymphocytes. *Arthritis Rheum* 1998;41(10):1748–1759.
376. Tsai C, Diaz L, Singer N, et al. Human T lymphocytes respond to bacterial superantigens presented by cultured rheumatoid arthritis synoviocytes. *Arthritis Rheum* 1996;39:125–136.
377. Yamamura M, Gupta R, Morita Y, et al. Effector function of resting T cells: activation of synovial fibroblasts. *J Immunol* 2001;166: 2270–2275.
378. Dechanet J, Merville P, Durand I, et al. The ability of synoviocytes to support terminal differentiation of activated B cells may explain plasma cell accumulation in rheumatoid synovium. *J Clin Invest* 1995;95:456–463.
379. Edwards J, Leigh R, Cambridge G. Expression of molecules involved in B lymphocyte survival and differentiation by synovial fibroblasts. *Clin Exp Rheumatol* 1997;108:407–414.
380. Lindhout E, van Eijk M, van Pel M, et al. Fibroblast-like synoviocytes from rheumatoid arthritis patients have intrinsic properties of follicular dendritic cells. *J Immunol* 1999;162:5949–5956.
381. Firestein G. Invasive fibroblast-like synoviocytes in rheumatoid arthritis: passive responders or transformed aggressors? *Arthritis Rheum* 1996;39:1781–1790.
382. Pap T, Muller-Ladner U, Gay R, et al. Fibroblast biology: role of synovial fibroblasts in the pathogenesis of rheumatoid arthritis. *Arthritis Res* 2000;2(5):361–367.
383. Firestein G, Echeverri F, Yeo M, et al. Somatic mutations in the p53 tumor suppressor gene in rheumatoid arthritis synovium. *Proc Natl Acad Sci U S A* 1997;94:10895–10900.
384. Muller-Ladner U, Nishioka K. p53 in rheumatoid arthritis: friend or foe? *Arthritis Res* 2000;2(3):175–178.
385. Corr M, Zvaifler N. Mesenchymal precursor cells. *Ann Rheum Dis* 2002;61:3–5.
386. Jorgensen C, Noel D, Gross G. Could inflammatory arthritis be triggered by progenitor cells in the joints? *Ann Rheum Dis* 2002;61:6–9.
387. Liao H, Haynes B. Role of adhesion molecules in the pathogenesis of rheumatoid arthritis. *Rheum Dis Clin North Am* 1995;21(3):715–740.
388. Shang X, Lang B, Issekutz A. Adhesion molecule mechanisms mediating monocyte migration through synovial fibroblast and endothelium barriers: role for CD11/CD18, very late antigen-4 (CD49d/CD29), very late antigen-5 (CD49e/CD29), and vascular cell adhesion molecule-1 (CD106). *J Immunol* 1998;160(1):467–474.
389. Elices M, Tsai V, Strahl D, et al. Expression and functional significance of alternatively spliced CSI fibronectin in rheumatoid arthritis microvasculature. *J Clin Invest* 93:405–416.
390. Wibulswas A, Croft D, Pitsillides A, et al. Influence of epitopes CD44v3 and CD44v6 in the invasive behavior of fibroblast-like synoviocytes derived from rheumatoid arthritic joints. *Arthritis Rheum* 2002;46(8):2059–2064.
391. Arend W. The innate immune system in rheumatoid arthritis. *Arthritis Rheum* 2001;44(10):2224–2234.
392. Klinman D. Does activation of the innate immune system contribute to the development of rheumatoid arthritis? *Arthritis Rheum* 2003;48 (3):590–593.
393. Firestein G, Zvaifler N. How important are T cells in chronic rheumatoid synovitis? T cell-independent mechanisms from beginning to end. *Arthritis Rheum* 2002;46(2):298–308.
394. Marinova-Mutafchieva L, Williams R, Funa K, et al. Inflammation is preceded by tumor necrosis factor–dependent infiltration of mesenchymal cells in experimental arthritis. *Arthritis Rheum* 2002;46(2): 507–513.
395. Seibl R, Birchler T, Loeliger S, et al. Expression and regulation of toll-like receptor 2 in rheumatoid arthritis synovium. *Am J Pathol* 2003;162(4):1221–1227.
396. Molenaar E, Voskuyl A, Familian A, et al. Complement activation in patients with rheumatoid arthritis mediated in part by C-reactive protein. *Arthritis Rheum* 2001;44(5):997–1002.
397. Atkinson J. C-reactive protein: a rheumatologist's friend revisited. *Arthritis Rheum* 2001;44(5):995–996.
398. Neumann E, Barnum S, Tarner I, et al. Local production of complement proteins in rheumatoid arthritis synovium. *Arthritis Rheum* 2002;46(4):934–945.
399. Banda N, Kraus D, Vondracek A, et al. Mechanisms of effects of complement inhibition in murine collagen-induced arthritis. *Arthritis Rheum* 2002;46(11):3065–3075.
400. Dalbeth N, Callan M. A subset of natural killer cells is greatly expanded within inflamed joints. *Arthritis Rheum* 2002;46(7):1763–1772.
401. Busso N, Hamilton J. Extravascular coagulation and the plasminogen activator/plasmin system in rheumatoid arthritis. *Arthritis Rheum* 2002;46(9):2268–2279.
402. Busso N, Morard C, Salvi R, et al. Role of the tissue factor pathway in synovial inflammation. *Arthritis Rheum* 2003;48(3):651–659.
403. Carr K, Lowry T, Li L, et al. Expression of CD60 on multiple cell lineages in inflammatory synovitis. *Lab Invest* 1995;73:332–338.
404. Grober J, Bowen B, Ebling H, et al. Monocyte-endothelial adhesion in chronic rheumatoid arthritis. *In situ* detection of selectin and integrin-dependent interactions. *J Clin Invest* 1993;91:2609–2619.

CHAPTER 53

Pathology of Rheumatoid Arthritis and Associated Disorders

Laura P. Hale

Rheumatoid arthritis (RA) is a systemic disease that involves the diarthrodial joints and associated soft tissues, as well as multiple extraarticular tissue sites. The pathology of RA joint lesions historically has been limited to the study of synovium obtained at late stages of the disease during joint replacement surgery or at autopsy. Increased use of closed-needle synovial biopsies and arthroscopic surgical procedures during the past decade has increased our knowledge of histopathologic characteristics of synovial tissue in normal individuals and during the early stages of RA and associated disorders (1,2). Studies of extraarticular lesions in RA patients have clarified the pathogenesis of many of these RA-associated syndromes. Extraarticular lesions are also important clinically, because most of the excess mortality in patients with RA occurs in patients with severe extraarticular disease (3). This chapter reviews the histopathology of normal and RA synovium and extraarticular lesions of RA. Current knowledge regarding their immunopathogenetic mechanisms is also discussed.

HISTOLOGY OF NORMAL SYNOVIUM

Normal synovium consists of a synovial lining layer one to two cells thick facing the articular cavity and underlying loose connective tissue stroma containing scattered macrophages, fibroblasts, and vessels (Fig. 53.1) (see Chapters 7 and 12). Synovial lining cells lack a basement membrane; this allows rapid exchange of nutrients between blood and the synovial fluid. A layer of type VI collagen is located beneath the synovial lining cells. Type VI collagen has the ability to bind both to cells and to interstitial collagens, thus providing support for synovial lining cells and preventing lining cells from dislodging due to mechanical stress generated during joint movement (4). Capillaries are present within or immediately adjacent to the synovial lining layer, with small venules, arterioles, and lymphatics present in synovial connective tissue stroma (5).

Synovial lining cells are of two basic types, designated type A macrophage-like synoviocytes and type B fibroblast-like synoviocytes (see Chapter 12). Type A macrophage-like synoviocytes express macrophage lineage markers (e.g., CD14 and CD68) and are phagocytic, as demonstrated by the presence of multiple endocytotic vesicles. Type B fibroblast-like synoviocytes exhibit secretory features and an active Golgi apparatus, indicative of protein synthetic activity (6). The relative proportion of type A and B synoviocytes in normal synovium varies from place to place within samples and between samples (7).

The origin of type A macrophage-like synoviocytes was demonstrated by an elegant series of experiments using beige mice, a strain that carries a mutation resulting in giant granule formation within secondary lysosomes. Radiation chimeras of normal and beige mice receiving grafts of beige bone marrow contained giant granules in type A synoviocytes. These granules were neither seen in normal control tissue nor in type B synoviocytes of normal mice receiving beige bone marrow, definitively establishing that type A synoviocytes originate in the bone marrow (8,9).

Type B fibroblast-like synoviocytes have generally been considered to be mesenchymal cells, but their origin has not been definitively established. Direct comparison of the immunophenotypes of cultured fibroblast-like synoviocytes, dermal fibroblasts, and human umbilical vein endothelial cells using a panel of 84 monoclonal antibodies (MoAbs) and two lectins demonstrated that, although the immunophenotypes of all three cell types were highly concordant, none of the markers tested were specific for fibroblast-like synoviocytes (10). Endothelial cells can be distinguished from fibroblast-like synoviocytes by the

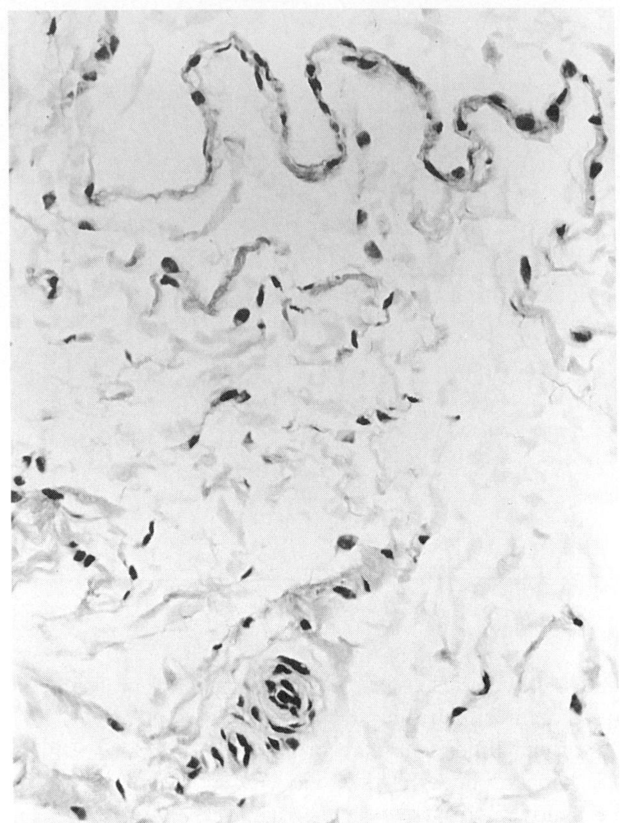

FIG. 53.1. Normal synovium from the metacarpophalangeal joint of a patient with acute traumatic tendon rupture. A single layer of synovial lining cells overlies loose connective tissue containing scattered fibroblasts, macrophages, and blood vessels (hematoxylin and eosin stain, original magnification ×320).

reactivity of endothelial cells with the *Ulex europus* lectin UEA-1, as well as MoAbs specific for von Willebrand factor and CD31 (10).

Type B fibroblast-like synoviocytes can be identified by their uridine diphosphoglucose dehydrogenase (UDPGD) activity, reflecting their ability to synthesize glycosaminoglycans including hyaluronan (11). Although the presence of prolyl 4-hydroxylase has been reported to be a marker for fibroblast-like synoviocytes, MoAbs specific for this enzyme also react with dermal fibroblasts and human umbilical vein endothelial cells (10). This finding is not surprising since prolyl 4-hydroxylase plays an important role in collagen synthesis, which occurs in endothelial cells as well as fibroblasts. No surface markers have been found that distinguish fibroblast-like synoviocytes from activated fibroblasts derived from other anatomic sites such as skin (10).

The extracellular matrix in normal synovium contains collagens, fibronectin, tenascin, and hyaluronan, as well as smaller quantities of other proteins and proteoglycans. Tenascin is present in a fine meshwork just below and extending into the synovial lining layer and in the walls of blood vessels in normal synovium (12,13). Hyaluronan surrounds the lining layer cells, but little is present in the deeper layers (14).

PATHOLOGIC CHANGES IN SYNOVIUM IN RHEUMATOID ARTHRITIS

The histopathologic appearance of synovium in RA is characterized by marked angiogenesis and influx of inflammatory leukocytes that lead to changes in tissue architecture and extracellular matrix composition and organization, as well as changes in the underlying cartilage and bone. RA synovium differs significantly from normal synovium in expression of cell surface adhesion molecules, proteinases, and proteinase inhibitors, as well as the array of cytokines expressed by components of the synovial microenvironment. The clinical symptoms of RA and subsequent joint destruction result from these pathologic changes.

Synovial Architecture in Rheumatoid Arthritis

The architectural changes seen in RA synovium include edema, hypertrophy and hyperplasia of synovial lining, proliferation of fibroblasts and blood vessels, deposition of fibrin, and increased villus formation. These manifestations, however, vary from tissue to tissue, as well as with disease stage.

Edema and fibrin deposition are among the earliest changes seen in RA synovial tissue (15,16). The presence of edema in synovial tissue specimens is demonstrated by the presence of spaces between collagen fibrils and around cellular structures (17). Extravascular fibrin is deposited most prominently in areas lining the synovial space, but also throughout the interstitium (16). Together, these changes are responsible for the early clinical signs of RA, such as swelling of affected joints.

Hypertrophy refers to an increase in the size of cells within an organ, whereas hyperplasia refers to an increase in the number of cells present. The synovial lining layer in inflamed joints is both hypertrophic and hyperplastic (Fig. 53.2), averaging three to seven cell layers in thickness as compared with the one to two cell layers seen in normal synovium. Synovial lining hyperplasia is accompanied by increased villus formation, which transforms the normally smooth synovial lining contour to one covered with delicate and bulbous villi (Fig. 53.3).

The simplest explanation for the increased synovial lining thickness in inflammatory synovium is an increased mitotic rate; however, the rarity of mitotic figures, low expression of antigens associated with cellular proliferation (18), and low rates of DNA synthesis (19,20) are more consistent with a slowly renewing population. Type A macrophage-like synoviocytes are derived through migration from the bone marrow, and synovial lining hyperplasia in RA therefore may result from increased recruitment of precursor cells from the bone marrow. Animal models demonstrate that synovial lining hyperplasia in acute experimentally induced arthritis

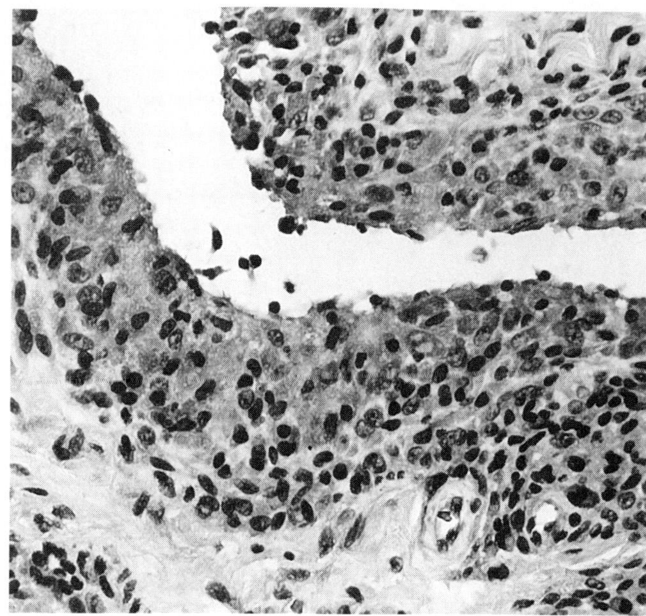

FIG. 53.2. Synovial lining hyperplasia in rheumatoid arthritis (hematoxylin and eosin stain, original magnification ×325).

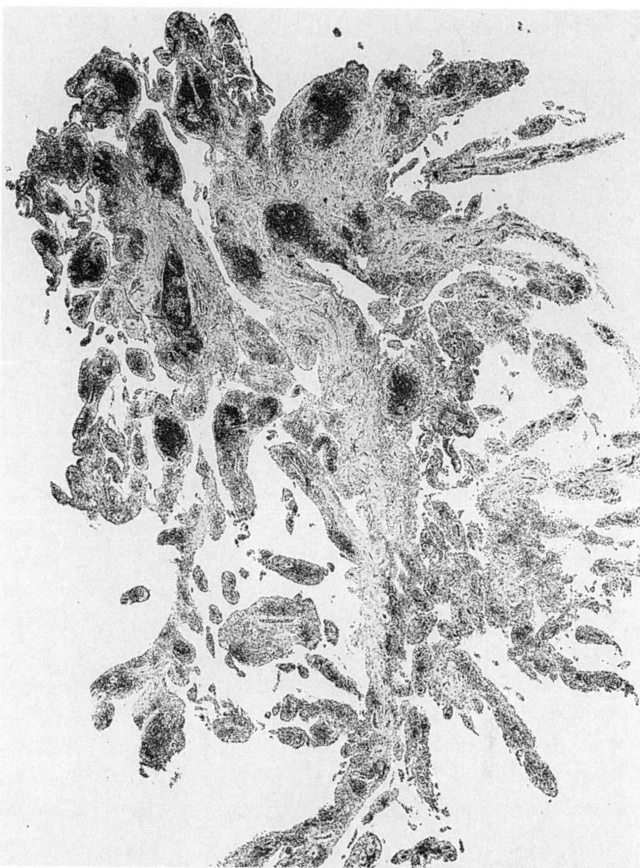

FIG. 53.3. Villous synovial hyperplasia in rheumatoid arthritis. Numerous frondlike projections and multiple nodular mononuclear inflammatory cell aggregates are present (hematoxylin and eosin stain, original magnification ×11.5).

is mainly due to the recruitment of bone marrow–derived mononuclear phagocytes (21) (see Chapter 30). Synovial biopsy samples from patients with early and advanced RA showed that increased macrophage infiltration correlates with expression of monocyte chemoattractant protein-1 (MCP-1) and macrophage inflammatory protein-1α (MIP-1α), chemokines that recruit macrophages (22). Clinical responses to disease-modifying antirheumatic drugs (DMARDs) are associated with a marked reduction in macrophages within the synovial lining layer, with less dramatic changes in the sublining layer (23). Defective cell death pathways have also been suggested to contribute to the synovial hyperplasia in RA. Synovial cells have been shown to be sensitive to apoptosis via the CD95 (Fas)/Fas ligand and tumor necrosis factor-α (TNF-α) pathways; however, the numbers of apoptotic cells observed in rheumatoid synovium are generally low (24,25). Induction of gene products that confer resistance to apoptosis has been documented in joints of patients with RA (24,25).

Some of the earliest cellular changes seen in RA synovium are endothelial swelling and transformation of blood vessels to those with high endothelial cells (high endothelial venules) (15), which provide a means for leukocytes to access synovium. Lymphocytes exit the blood through high endothelial venules to form perivascular infiltrates consisting of large numbers of $CD4^+$ T cells, smaller numbers of $CD8^+$ T cells, and B cells, surrounded by macrophages (Fig. 53.4). In addition to morphologic and functional changes in existing vessels, vascular proliferation is also present in RA. The extent of vascular proliferation and neovascularization depends on the balance between angiogenic and angiostatic mediators produced within rheumatoid synovium (26), as well as on the rate of cell death (27). Vascular endothelial growth factor (VEGF) is abundant in synovium, and is produced in response to tumor necrosis factor-β (TGF-β) and to a lesser extent interleukin-1 (IL-1). VEGF expression is also increased by hypoxia, which is physiologically present in the joint cavity (28). The proangiogenic growth factor angiopoietin-1 is also expressed in rheumatoid synovium in response to TNF-α (29). Gene therapy with the angiogenesis inhibitors angiostatin and endostatin or direct intrasynovial injection of endostatin inhibits development and severity of inflammatory arthritis in murine models (30–32). The fumagillin-derived angiogenesis inhibitor TNP-470 inhibits angiogenesis and synovial cell proliferation in human synovial tissues grafted into severe combined immunodeficient (SCID) mice (33). A soluble VEGF receptor 1 protein fused to the Fc portion of human immunoglobulin G1 (IgG1) inhibits *in vitro* growth of endothelial cells derived from synovium of patients with active RA (34). These promising experimental studies suggest the need for clinical studies to determine whether antiangiogenic therapies will prove beneficial in human patients with RA.

The architectural and cellular changes that occur in RA can be monitored by magnetic resonance imaging (MRI)

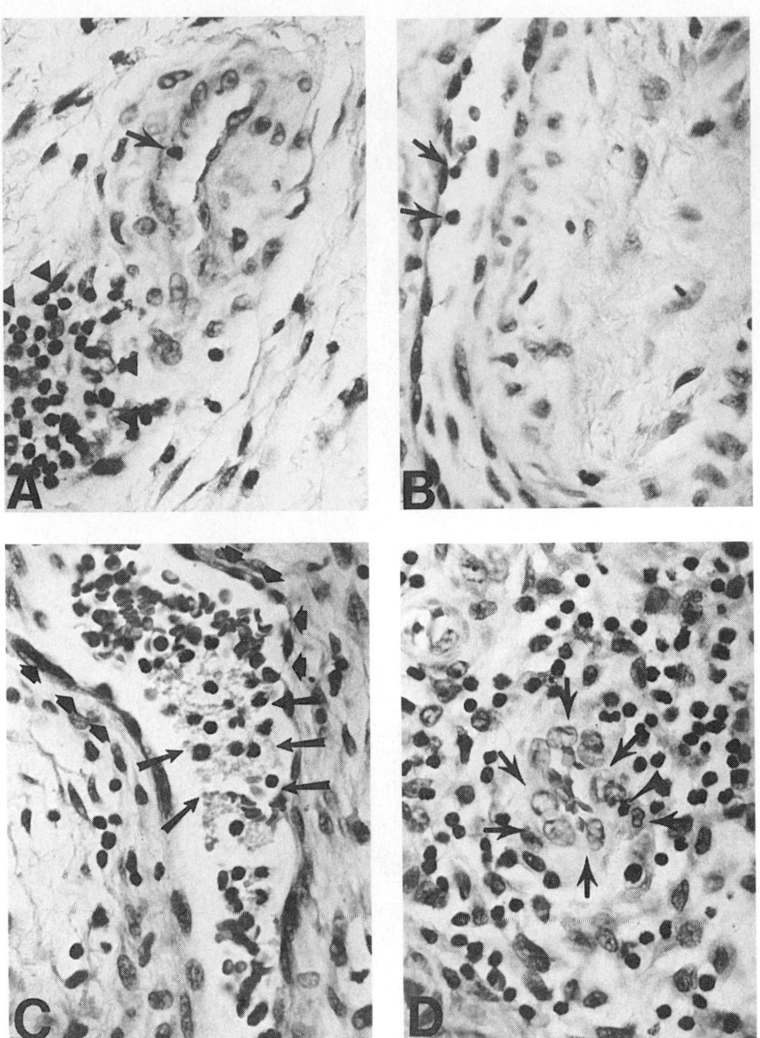

FIG. 53.4. Synovial vessels in rheumatoid arthritis. **A, B:** Mononuclear and polymorphonuclear leukocytes adherent to synovial vascular endothelium (*arrows*), as well as extravasating lymphocytes (*arrowheads*) **(A)**. **C:** Platelet aggregation in the lumen of a synovial vessel (*arrows*). **D:** High endothelial venule (*arrows*) with extravasating leukocytes around the vessel and one leukocyte (*arrowhead*) in the lumen bound to endothelium (hematoxylin and eosin stain, original magnification ×400).

and determination of synovial membrane volume. Recent studies have confirmed that measurement of synovial membrane volume provides an objective and noninvasive method to monitor disease activity and to predict progressive joint destruction in RA (35). Serial biopsies of knee or small joints can also be used to monitor changes in disease activity associated with DMARD therapy (36). Within the knee joint, biopsies taken from the suprapatellar pouch, medial gutter, and the cartilage–pannus junction provide representative samples for histology, immunohistology, and cytokine analysis (37).

Cell Composition of Synovium in Rheumatoid Arthritis

Cells enter the synovium via the circulation, then migrate through the synovial lining under the influence of chemotactic stimuli. Chemotactic cytokines, or chemokines, play an important role in this process (38). Chemokines bound to endothelial cell proteoglycans attract T cells and stimulate their integrin-mediated adhesion and extravasation into synovium (39). Adhesion molecules on various cell types within the synovial microenvironment may enhance, retard, or prevent the passage of these cells deeper into the synovium (see later section on the Role of Immune and Endothelial Cell Adhesion Molecules in the Pathogenesis of Rheumatoid Arthritis, and Chapter 20). Chemokines also may recruit endothelial cell precursors and thus drive the process of angiogenesis that is characteristic of inflammatory synovium (26).

RA synovium is characterized by the presence of diffuse (Fig. 53.5A) or nodular (Fig. 53.5B) mononuclear inflammatory cell infiltrates within synovial tissue. Tissues with nodular lymphoid aggregates (follicular synovitis) appear to be more frequently seen at arthroplasty; thus, the presence of focal lymphoid aggregates may represent a patient population at greater risk for joint destruction (40). Patients with follicular synovitis have increased serum TNF-α levels relative to RA patients with diffuse synovial infiltrates (41). Germinal centers present within synovium have been hypothesized to be sites for isotype switching and affinity maturation of the plasma cell precursors producing rheumatoid factors. This process requires follicular dendritic cells,

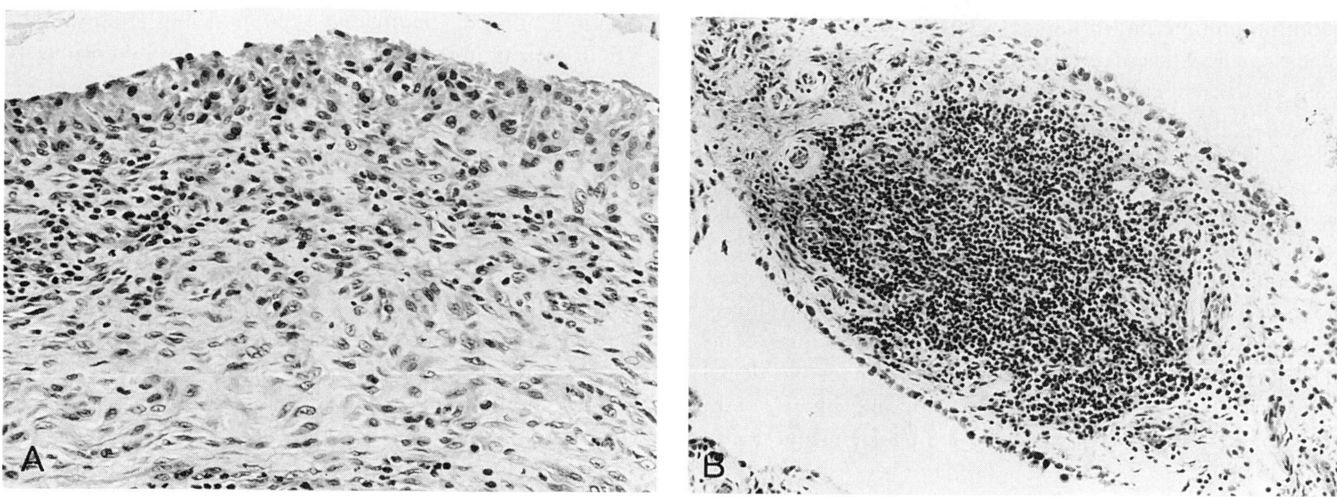

FIG. 53.5. Synovitis in rheumatoid arthritis. Diffuse **(A)** and nodular **(B)** mononuclear inflammatory cell infiltrates are present within rheumatoid arthritis synovium. [Hematoxylin and eosin stain; original magnifications ×250 **(A)** and ×170 **(B)**.]

which are present in tissues with follicular synovitis (42). Immature CD1a$^+$ dendritic cells appear to accumulate in RA synovium relative to mature CD83$^+$ dendritic cells, which may reflect differential expression of chemokines that govern the migration of these two dendritic cell subsets in and out of synovium (43).

The cellular infiltrate in RA synovium is composed primarily of small lymphocytes, macrophages, and plasma cells, despite the large proportion of synovial fluid cells that are polymorphonuclear leukocytes. Comparisons of the characteristics and the cellular subsets represented by the RA synovial infiltrate with those of similar cell types present in the peripheral blood and in the synovial fluid have been the subject of intense investigation over the past several decades. The predominant population of T cells present in RA synovium consists of cells with the surface phenotype of CD4$^+$, CD45RO^{hi+}, CD29^{hi+}, CD11a/CD18(LFA-1)$^{hi+}$, CD49d/CD29(VLA-4)$^{hi+}$, CD44^{hi+}, and CD7^{lo+}, a phenotype characteristic of memory T cells. These findings may reflect the enhanced ability of these cells to transmigrate through endothelium (44). However, several investigators have documented defective apoptosis of T cells in rheumatoid synovium, which could favor *in situ* expansion of autoreactive T cells (45,46). The majority of investigations have focused on T lymphocytes, since the genetic associations between class II major histocompatibility complex (MHC; HLA-DR) phenotype and RA suggest that presentation of antigen to effector T cells is involved in the pathogenesis of the disease (reviewed in reference 47). B cells are also relatively enriched in RA synovium. Immunoglobulin (e.g., rheumatoid factors) made by RA synovial B cells contributes to immune complex–mediated reactions locally.

In normal human immune responses, processed antigen binds to the groove of MHC molecules on antigen-presenting cells. The antigen-binding site of T-cell receptors expressed on the cell surface of the small percentage of lymphocytes recognizing that particular epitope then interact with the processed antigen, resulting in an antigen-specific response. Superantigens bind to common regions of T-cell receptors at a site distinct from the antigen recognition domain, which results in the activation of large numbers of T cells that express specific T-cell receptor Vβ (TCRBV) genes, bypassing the steps of antigen processing and recognition. An immune response initiated by antigen-specific proliferation of cells or by superantigen stimulation can result in skewing of the T-cell repertoire due to *in situ* expansion of cells expressing particular TCRBV genes (48–50). Thus, overrepresented TCRBV genes would suggest an antigen or superantigen-driven immune response such as an infectious agent might invoke.

The T-cell repertoire in RA is controversial, with conflicting results from studies examining the clonality and TCRBV usage by synovial T cells. Association with particular MHC class II types may bias the T-cell repertoire through positive or negative selection. Current data indicate that the T-cell receptor repertoire in RA synovial fluid is polyclonal, with enrichment of certain TCRBV sequences (51). Clonal populations of CD4$^+$ CD7$^-$ CD28$^-$ autoreactive T cells are frequently found in RA patients with extraarticular manifestations of RA (52,53). Extensive sequence analysis of T-cell clones isolated from RA synovium and blood at different time points suggests a dynamic T-cell receptor selection process, which is more consistent with an antigen-driven response to an as yet unidentified antigen (54). However, the mechanism resulting in TCRBV gene bias has not yet been definitively established.

Despite considerable evidence linking T cells to the initiation and maintenance of synovitis in RA (55), many disease manifestations cannot be adequately explained by T cell–mediated processes alone. Therefore, the role of nonimmunologic but inflammatory pathways in the pathogenesis of RA has also received attention. It is postulated that two distinct cellular pathways play a role in the pathogenesis of RA: a T cell–dependent pathway and a synovial cell–dependent pathway. In this latter pathway, interactions between resident synovial cells and extracellular matrix proteins or cytokines perpetuate synovial hyperplasia and progressive joint destruction (56).

Animal studies recently showed that mice lacking mast cells fail to develop inflammatory arthritis in response to arthritogenic serum (57). Human RA synovium demonstrates accumulations of mast cells that can be identified with histologic stains such as toluidine blue or with immunostains for tryptase or CD117 (c-*kit*) (Fig. 53.6). These mast cells are activated and have been shown to release proinflammatory cytokines and activated metalloproteinases at sites of cartilage destruction (58–60), suggesting that they contribute to the pathogenesis of RA. Among the cytokines produced by mast cells is TNF-α, a cytokine shown to be pivotal in driving ongoing joint inflammation in RA. Mast cells accumulate in situations with ongoing angiogenesis, and several mediators produced by mast cells themselves stimulate angiogenesis (61), one of the characteristic lesions in rheumatoid synovium. For example, the VEGF present in rheumatoid synovium is located primarily within mast cells (62). More research is needed to determine whether anti–mast cell therapies may prove beneficial to patients with RA (63).

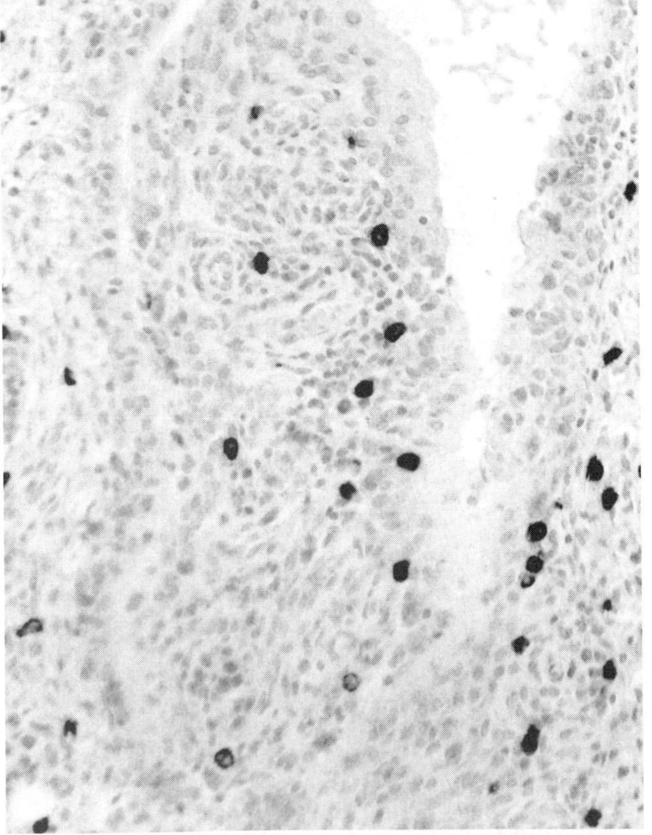

FIG. 53.6. Mast cells can be identified in rheumatoid arthritis synovium using CD117 (c-*kit*) immunostaining (dark color). Mast cells are typically located beneath the synovial lining layer, and are not present within lymphocyte clusters.

Changes in Periarticular Cartilage and Bone in Rheumatoid Arthritis

Morphologic studies of RA synovium and cartilage at various stages of disease progression have led to an understanding of the sequence of events leading to joint destruction in RA. The normal interface between synovium and cartilage, the marginal transitional fibroblastic zone, is a wedge-shaped tongue of fibroblast-like cells that extends from the synovium onto the cartilage surface (64). Blood vessels are particularly numerous in the area in which cartilage, bone, and synovium meet (65). In RA, synovial fibroblasts activated by interaction with cytokines and inflammatory cells undermine this interface (66–68). The invading cells form the pannus, a granulation tissue characterized by proliferation of blood vessels and influx of a variety of inflammatory cell types, that extends to cover the articular cartilage (Fig. 53.7). Pannus has been described as a tumorlike tissue, with invasive capability. Histopathologic studies of the cartilage–pannus junction in RA show penetration of the cartilage by blood vessels, mononuclear cells, and fibroblasts (69). Disruption of the synovial–cartilage interface and high expression of matrix metalloproteinases (MMPs) contributes to cartilage destruction. Later in the course of the disease, the cellular pannus is replaced by the fibrous pannus, a relatively avascular layer of fibroblast-like cells and collagen between the synovium and the cartilage surface (65,66). This layer may further contribute to cartilage degradation by interfering with its nutrient supply from the synovial fluid (69). Extension of the synovial inflammatory process into the capsular and periarticular tissues including menisci, with subsequent tissue destruction, leads to joint instability and the characteristic subluxations of joints.

Destruction of periarticular soft tissues can be attributed to direct release of proteolytic enzymes from pannus (70). Erosion of bone, however, occurs in areas contiguous to the pannus as well as in regions adjacent to bone marrow distant from the site of inflammation. Therefore, the bone erosions are not only due to the local effects of pannus, but also likely due to induction and differentiation of osteoclast precursors under the influence of proinflammatory cytokines.

Synovial and Cartilage Extracellular Matrix Changes in Rheumatoid Arthritis

The extracellular matrix in RA and other forms of synovitis shows changes in the relative amounts of collagens, fibronectin, tenascin, hyaluronan, and other proteins and proteoglycans normally present in synovium, as well as in their distribution within synovial tissue.

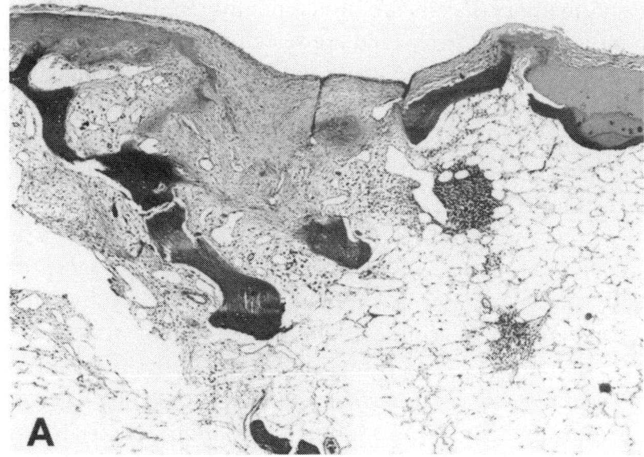

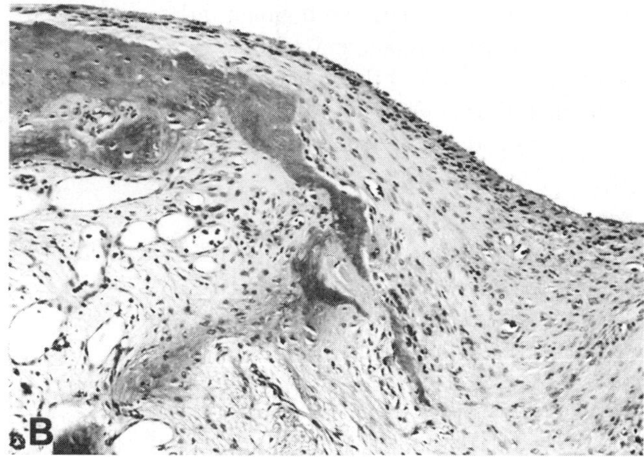

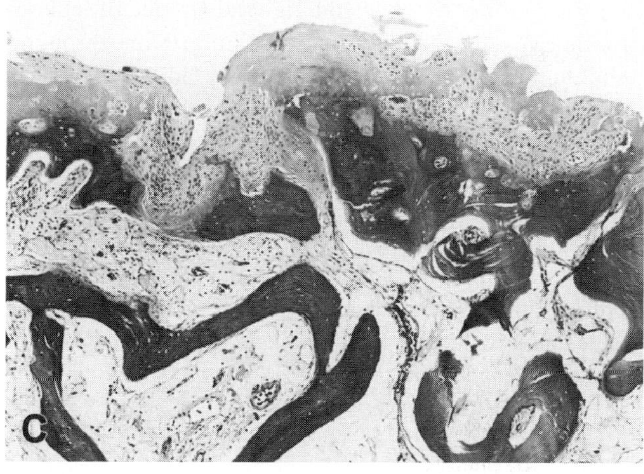

FIG. 53.7. Destruction of articular cartilage in rheumatoid arthritis. **A:** Articular surface of metacarpophalangeal joint demonstrating invasion and lysis of articular cartilage by pannus. Note penetration of pannus into the marrow space. **B:** Higher magnification of central portion of **A**, showing active granulation tissue pannus invading through cartilage into the underlying bone. **C:** Articular surface from the same patient showing undermining of articular cartilage by pannus in multiple locations. [Hematoxylin and eosin stain; original magnifications ×25 **(A)**, ×130 **(B)**, and ×52 **(C)**.]

Fibronectin is a major extracellular matrix component in synovium, which colocalizes with fibrin and collagen. Fibronectin plays a central role in cell/cell and cell/matrix interactions through ligation of cell surface integrins and may influence tissue organization by providing appropriate support for proliferation and differentiation of cells within tissue. Fibronectin is both derived from the plasma and synthesized *in situ* by synovial lining cells (71). It is prominently deposited at sites of synovial hyperplasia (71,72). Fibronectin has been documented on the surface of articular cartilage in RA, but not in joints with osteoarthritis (OA) or trauma (73). Fibronectin may provide a support for the extension of pannus over the cartilage surface, as well as the subsequent invasion of the cartilage by the pannus. Fibronectin fragments are found in synovial fluid (74,75) and are associated with immune complexes in RA (75).

Tenascin is normally found only in the synovial lining layer and perivascular areas. However, it is also found in lymphoid aggregates and in areas of fibrosis in inflammatory synovitis. Levels of tenascin messenger RNA (mRNA) and protein are increased in the synovial lining layer and perivascular areas of RA relative to those found in normal synovium (12,13). The cells expressing tenascin mRNA do not express CD14 and do not react with macrophage-specific monoclonal antibodies; thus, they are likely to be type B fibroblast-like synoviocytes (13). Expression of tenascin is also increased in articular cartilage of diseased joints (12). RA pannus contains high levels of tenascin in both the pericellular and adjacent interterritorial regions of the residual articular cartilage (12). Tenascin deposition correlates with intensity of inflammation, with no difference between OA and RA synovium. Increases in tenascin expression can be induced by IL-1 in synovial fibroblast cultures, suggesting a mechanism for the changes seen in inflammatory synovium (13). Tenascin can modify the binding of cells to fibronectin and interfere with T-cell activation through CD3, thus potentially influencing local inflammatory activity (13).

In contrast to its presence predominantly in the synovial lining layer in normal synovium, hyaluronan shows intense staining throughout RA synovium. Hyaluronan is most notably associated with blood vessels and areas of dense cellular infiltration in RA. The distribution of hyaluronan in OA varies according to the degree of inflammation (14).

In addition to changes in the distribution of extracellular matrix proteins present in normal synovium, inflammation is associated with deposition of additional proteins, including fibrin within RA synovium (16). The extravascular fibrin meshwork serves as a matrix onto which inflammatory and endothelial cells can migrate and adhere. The "rice bodies" frequently seen in synovial fluid are composed of aggregates of organizing fibrin. Ongoing deposition of extracellular matrix proteins and subsequent organization may eventually lead to joint fibrosis and ankylosis.

ROLE OF IMMUNE AND ENDOTHELIAL CELL ADHESION MOLECULES IN THE PATHOGENESIS OF RHEUMATOID ARTHRITIS

Extraordinary progress has been made recently in elucidating the earliest manifestations of inflammation in RA. Joint tissues reacting to an as yet unidentified injury respond with increased angiogenesis, formation of high endothelial venules, and increased expression of cellular adhesion molecules and inflammatory cytokines, thereby creating an environment that is proinflammatory and procoagulatory. A small subset of circulating T cells, B cells, and macrophages preferentially adhere to the abnormal endothelium, initiating and perpetuating the inflammatory process.

Adhesion molecules mediate interactions between (a) leukocytes and endothelium, (b) leukocytes and the extracellular matrix, (c) leukocytes and synoviocytes, and (d) leukocytes and other leukocytes. The number of lymphocytes migrating into a tissue is determined by adhesion molecules expressed on both lymphocytes and endothelium. Activated and memory T cells are preferentially recruited into sites of inflammation (76,77) and are selectively retained by binding to the extracellular matrix (76–78). Nonspecific T cells recruited to the joint may be activated by cytokines or following binding of their adhesion molecules to the extracellular matrix, because many ligands of adhesion molecules mediate costimulation of T-cell activation (79,80).

Four major families of adhesion molecules—the integrins, immunoglobulin superfamily, selectins, and proteoglycans (e.g., CD44)—are expressed in RA synovium (see Chapter 20). Rolling of blood-borne leukocytes along endothelial surfaces is primarily mediated by interactions of selectins with their carbohydrate ligands. Cleavage of selectins and subsequent induction of high-affinity forms of integrins and adhesion molecules from the immunoglobulin superfamily mediates the tight adherence of leukocytes to the vessel endothelium. Transmigration through the endothelial wall is then mediated by additional adhesion molecules, including CD106 and integrins. This discussion focuses on a few receptor/ligand pairs that are expressed or up-regulated in the RA synovial microenvironment and play important roles in cellular migration or activation.

CD54 (intercellular adhesion molecule-1, ICAM-1) is a 50-kd member of the immunoglobulin superfamily expressed on the luminal and lateral surfaces of endothelial cells and absent from the endothelial cell surface adjacent to the basement membrane (Fig. 53.8A). CD54 on endothelial

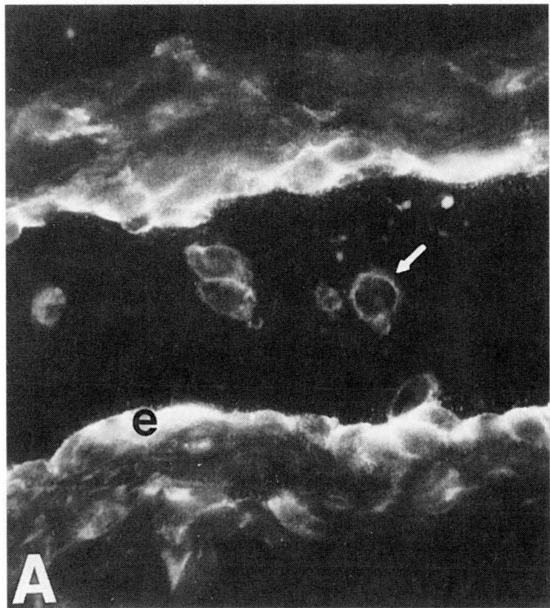

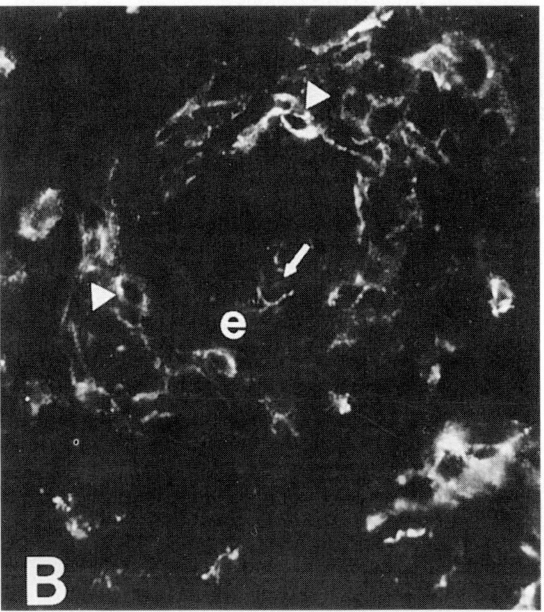

FIG. 53.8. Immunolocalization of the adhesion receptor/ligand pair CD54 [intercellular adhesion molecule-1 (ICAM-1)] **(A)** and CD11a/CD18 [leukocyte function–associated antigen-1 (LFA-1)] **(B)** in inflammatory synovium. **A:** Vessel endothelium (*e*) and intravascular mononuclear cells (*arrowhead*) are ICAM-1 positive. **B.** Note LFA-1-positive mononuclear cells adherent to vessel endothelium (*arrow*) and present in perivascular tissues (*arrowheads*). (Immunofluorescence, original magnification ×400.) (Reproduced from Hale LP, Martin ME, McCollum DE, et al. Immunohistologic analysis of the distribution of cell adhesion molecules within the inflammatory synovial microenvironment. *Arthritis Rheum* 1989;32:22–30, with permission.)

cells binds to leukocyte function antigen-1 (LFA-1, CD11a/CD18) on leukocytes during the process of leukocyte extravasation into synovium. Continued expression of LFA-1 on subintimal lymphocytes and macrophages (Fig. 53.8B) (81,82) directs the traffic of LFA-1-positive leukocytes from vascular endothelium to CD54-positive cells of the subintima and intima (82). The CD54/LFA-1–mediated binding of T cells to synovial fibroblasts is also reported to contribute to costimulation of T-cell activation and cytokine secretion by synovial fibroblasts (79,83). DMARD treatment leading to clinical response or remission is associated with decreased CD54 expression in synovial tissue of RA patients (84).

CD106 (vascular cell adhesion molecule-1, VCAM-1) is a 90- to 110-kd member of the immunoglobulin superfamily that mediates adhesion and subsequent transmigration of inflammatory cells through activated vascular endothelium or synovial fibroblasts (85). CD106 binds to very late antigen-4 (VLA-4, CD49d/CD29), an $\alpha_4\beta_1$ integrin found on lymphocytes, monocytes, and eosinophils but minimally on neutrophils (86). The VLA-4/CD106 pathway mediates recruitment of activated lymphocytes to inflamed synovium in RA. $\alpha_4\beta_7$ integrin also binds to CD106 and fibronectin, similar to VLA-4. Sixty-two percent of synovial membrane T cells express high-density $\alpha_4\beta_7$, in contrast to 4.7% of synovial fluid and 9.1% of peripheral blood leukocytes (PBLs). The expression of $\alpha_4\beta_7$ may thus provide a mechanism by which certain T cells adhere to rheumatoid synovium while others remain in synovial fluid (87).

The endothelial leukocyte adhesion molecule CD62E (ELAM-1, E selectin) is not detectable on the endothelium of normal synovial vessels; however, it is expressed on synovial venules and capillaries in areas close to the intima and the joint cavity in RA synovium. By binding to its sialyl-Lewis^X carbohydrate ligand on various proteins, CD62E plays a role in directing the migration of leukocytes into the inflamed synovial membrane (88).

Thus, the expression of CD54, CD106, and CD62E are important in directing migration of inflammatory cells into synovial tissue. β_1 integrins such as VLA-2 (CD49b/CD29, collagen receptor), VLA-4 and VLA-5 (CD49d/CD29 and CD49e/CD29, fibronectin receptors), and VLA-6 (CD49f/CD29, laminin receptor) on leukocytes then bind to their extracellular matrix ligands, favoring retention of inflammatory cells within the synovium. Binding of β_1 integrins to both fibronectin and laminin facilitates T-cell costimulation (89). Integrin engagement by extracellular matrix substrates has also been shown to regulate the proliferation, expression of MMPs, and invasion of synovial fibroblasts into cartilage (68,90).

Levels of the CD44 adhesion molecule, a principal ligand for hyaluronan as well as other extracellular matrix proteins, are markedly increased in RA and correlate with disease activity in inflammatory synovitis (77,91). CD44 has been implicated in leukocyte rolling on endothelium (92) as well as costimulation of T-cell activation (93,94). CD44 cross-linking and binding to hyaluronan was recently shown to markedly up-regulate CD106 expression and subsequent CD106-mediated cell adhesion as well as integrin-mediated binding of synovial cells to T cells (95). This enhanced adhesion may cause cellular activation, further contributing to inflammation. The interaction of synovial fibroblasts with cartilage has also been shown to be dependent on CD44, and antibodies to CD44 can markedly inhibit cartilage destruction (96).

ROLE OF CYTOKINES IN THE PATHOGENESIS OF RHEUMATOID ARTHRITIS

Cytokines are important regulators of inflammation in RA (97,98). Many studies have measured levels of cytokines in rheumatoid synovial tissues (reviewed in reference 99). Proinflammatory cytokines present in synovium include TNF-α, IL-1β, IL-6, granulocyte monocyte-colony stimulating factor (GM-CSF), monocyte-colony stimulating factor (M-CSF), and the chemokine IL-8. Antiinflammatory cytokines include IL-10, IL-11, and TGF-β. Receptor antagonists, including IL-1 receptor antagonist and soluble forms of the TNF receptor, are present in rheumatoid synovium. The level of inflammation within the rheumatoid joint is regulated by the balance of proinflammatory and antiinflammatory cytokines (99).

The discoveries that TNF-α is a major regulator of IL-1 production and that neutralization of TNF-α inhibits other proinflammatory cytokines have led to the concept that TNF-α is the dominant mediator of the cytokine cascade that causes the inflammation and joint destruction in RA (97). Fifty percent to 90% of cells in the synovial lining layer express TNF receptors, and thus may potentially respond to this cytokine (100). Three major mechanisms have been proposed for the effects of TNF-α blockade on joint pathology: deactivation of the proinflammatory cytokine cascade, interruption of cellular recruitment by effects on adhesion molecules or chemokines, and regulation of angiogenesis (97). Exciting progress has been made recently in treating RA patients with antagonists of TNF-α, including recombinant human TNF receptor p75 Fc fusion protein and chimeric monoclonal anti-TNF-α antibodies. Randomized, placebo-controlled multicenter clinical trials of these agents have confirmed their efficacy in decreasing inflammation and joint damage (reviewed in reference 99).

Histologic patterns of inflammation in RA correlate with tissue cytokine profiles. Synovial tissues with diffuse lymphoid infiltration typically have low-level transcription of interferon-γ (IFN-γ), IL-4, IL-1β, and TNF-α. IFN-γ is the predominant cytokine in synovial tissues with lymphoid follicles and germinal centers (follicular synovitis), which also have abundant IL-10 and virtually undetectable IL-4. Synovial tissues with granuloma formation (granulomatous synovitis) demonstrate high transcription of IFN-γ, IL-4, IL-1β, and TNF-α (101). Rheumatoid nodules have prominent expression of IL-1β and TNF-α, along with IFN-γ, IL-12, IL-18, IL-15, and IL-10 (102). Sequential biopsies

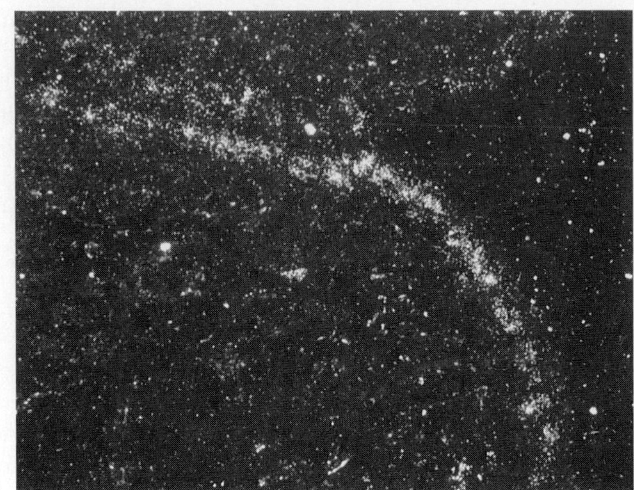

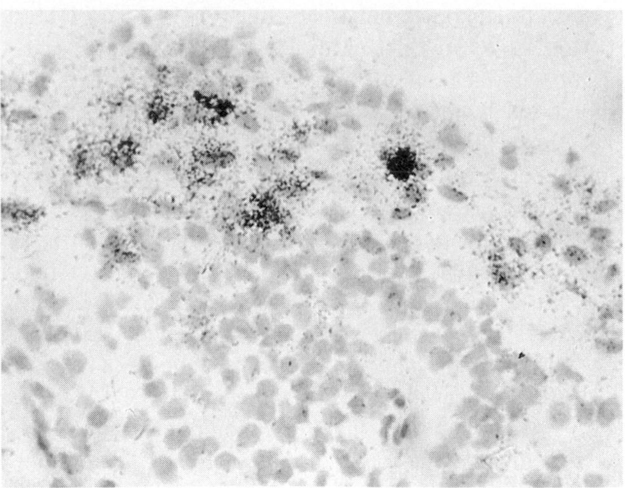

A B

FIG. 53.9. Matrix metalloproteinase 1 (collagenase) expression in rheumatoid synovium. **A:** Dark-field view shows production of collagenase by synovial lining cells. **B:** Bright-field view demonstrates expression of collagenase by synovial lining cells and by subintimal cells as well. (Courtesy of S. Spence McCachren.)

show that patients who have a clinical response or achieve remission with DMARD therapy have decreased TNF-α and IL-1β in synovial tissue following treatment (84).

ROLE OF METALLOPROTEINASES IN TISSUE INJURY IN RHEUMATOID ARTHRITIS

Degradation of the extracellular matrix is characteristic of RA and ultimately results in destruction of cartilage, ligaments, and bone. The proteolytic enzymes primarily responsible for this destruction are known as MMPs. MMPs are synthesized as proenzymes, then secreted and cleaved to active forms by proteolytic enzymes such as trypsin, plasmin, and tryptase. MMP-1 (tissue collagenase) degrades native triple helical collagen types I, II, III, VII, and X. MMP-2 (gelatinase/type IV collagenase) degrades denatured collagen as well as native collagen types IV, V, and VII. MMP-3 (stromelysin-1) has broad specificity, including proteoglycans, fibronectin, collagen types IV and IX, and laminin. MMP-3 also removes the amino-terminal propeptides from type I procollagen and can proteolytically activate MMP-1 (103). Together, these three MMPs can degrade the majority of extracellular matrix components. The action of MMPs is regulated by tissue inhibitors of metalloproteinases (TIMPs), which bind stoichiometrically (1:1) to MMPs to inhibit proteolytic activity of these enzymes *in vivo* (104).

Immunohistochemical studies of synovium demonstrate abundant MMP-1, MMP-3, and TIMP-1 within synovium even in early RA (105); however, because these proteins are secreted and may be adsorbed onto a variety of cell types, *in situ* hybridization studies are required to demonstrate which cells produce these proteins. *In situ* hybridization studies show definitively that synovial lining cells are the major site of MMPs and TIMP-1 production in both RA and OA (Fig. 53.9) (106). High expression of MMP-1 mRNA in the synovial lining layer soon after symptom onset identifies those patients who develop rapidly progressive erosive disease (107).

Tissue levels of metalloproteinases and metalloproteinase inhibitors are regulated by systemic and local cytokine concentrations. For example, IL-6 increases TIMP-1 expression, but does not induce metalloproteinase expression (108,109). IL-1β and TNF-α induce expression of MMP-1 and MMP-3, but not TIMP-1 (110). Corticosteroids inhibit expression of MMP-1, MMP-2, and TIMP-1 (111). MMP levels are higher in RA compared with OA; however, TIMP-1 levels are similar in these two diseases. This may account for the increased incidence of joint erosion in RA as compared with OA (111). Gene therapy to increase the expression of TIMP-1 and TIMP-3 markedly reduces the invasiveness of rheumatoid synovial fibroblasts in a SCID mouse model (112). Thus, therapies that increase expression of metalloproteinase inhibitors in the pannus may help to prevent joint destruction in RA.

An MMP-like activity termed aggrecanase has been identified in synovial and joint capsule tissue, where it is associated with pathologic degradation of cartilage (113, 114). Aggrecanase is also present in cartilage (115) and can be released from cartilage upon coculture with synoviocytes (114). Two aggrecanase genes have been identified: aggrecanase-1 (a disintegrin and metalloproteinase with thrombospondin motifs, ADAMTS-11) and aggrecanase-2 (ADAMTS-5) (116,117).

HISTOPATHOLOGY OF RHEUMATOID NODULES

Rheumatoid nodule formation is one of the most common extraarticular manifestations of RA and occurs in up to 50% of patients at some time during their disease course

(118). Rheumatoid nodules are most commonly found within subcutaneous tissue overlying the olecranon process of the ulna, and are less frequently found in tendons, tendon sheaths, and periarticular subcutaneous tissue, particularly in areas prone to pressure or trauma. Rheumatoid nodules have also been documented in nearly all tissues and organs (119), including heart and large vessels, cardiac valves, kidney, meninges and spinal cord (120,121), larynx (122,123), lung and pleura, synovium, and the orbit (124). MRI may be useful for diagnosis of extraarticular rheumatoid nodules (121,125,126); however, biopsy may still be required to rule out malignancy or infectious disease in some cases (127–129).

A typical excised rheumatoid nodule consists of firm, tan tissue. Sectioning reveals a soft yellow center surrounded by white to yellow fibrous tissue. Histologically, rheumatoid nodules consist of a central region of necrosis, with palisading histiocytes, fibroblasts, and a mixed inflammatory infiltrate (Fig. 53.10). The central core of a rheumatoid nodule contains fibrinoid necrotic material. The term *fibrinoid* refers to intensely eosinophilic fibrillar material with a similar appearance to fibrin in hematoxylin and eosin–stained sections. A variety of histochemical and immunohistochemical techniques have shown that the necrotic material may be composed of collagen, lipids, nucleoproteins, acid mucopolysaccharides, and serum proteins, including immunoglobulin, as well as fibrin (130,131). Cellular debris from necrotic macrophages or other cell types may also be present (132). Although the necrotic material is lipid rich, calcification rarely occurs.

The cells palisading around the central core have been determined to be elongated macrophages or histiocytes by immunohistochemical studies (132–134). The characteristic radial orientation occurs due to alignment of the elongated macrophages along collagen fibers. Adhesion molecules expressed by palisading cells are generally similar to those expressed by macrophages present within synovium (135, 136). Multinucleated giant cells with a macrophage surface phenotype (134) may be located adjacent to the palisaded layer. These giant cells have high expression of variants of the CD44 hyaluronate receptor containing exon v9, which is involved in the formation of syncytia by activated macrophages (137,138).

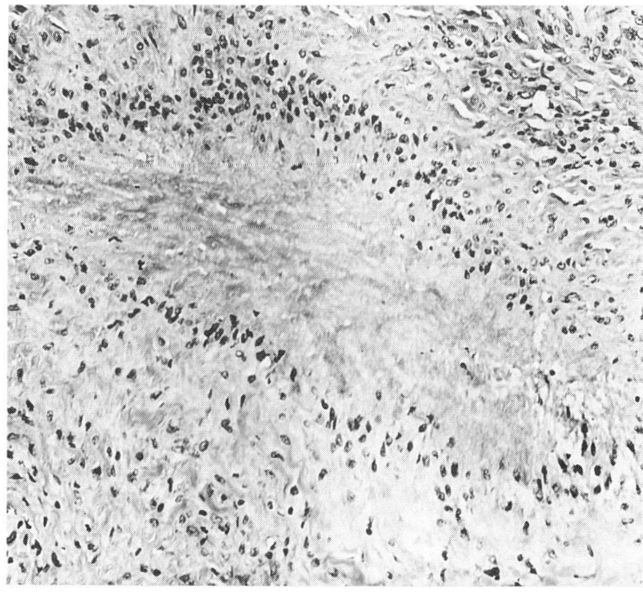

FIG. 53.10. Subcutaneous rheumatoid nodule from the olecranon bursa shows typical palisading borders and central fibrinoid necrosis (hematoxylin and eosin stain, original magnification ×170).

The third component of a rheumatoid nodule is granulation tissue, composed of a proliferation of fibroblasts and small vessels with a variable inflammatory infiltrate, which surrounds the palisaded layer. In long-established nodules this area may become sclerotic. Other diseases in which subcutaneous nodules are present include tuberculosis, necrobiosis lipoidica, granuloma annulare, erythema nodosum, tophaceous gout, and xanthoma tuberosum, as well as idiopathic nodulosis, also called subcutaneous granuloma annulare. Nodules resulting from most of these diseases can usually be distinguished from rheumatoid nodules histologically. Histochemical or immunohistochemical studies may be helpful in the diagnosis of difficult cases. For example, the necrotic material within nodules of idiopathic nodulosis is generally Alcian blue positive, whereas that within rheumatoid nodules is Alcian blue negative (139).

Rheumatoid nodules can also be diagnosed by fine-needle aspiration (FNA) as opposed to excisional biopsy. The FNA findings include all of the standard histologic features discussed above. Elongated macrophages with round to oval nuclei and well-defined borders may be abundant, in association with long strands of fibrin or collagen. Multinucleated giant cells may also be present. The background is markedly granular and necrotic. The main differential diagnosis of rheumatoid nodules in FNA biopsies includes mycobacterial or fungal infection and sarcoidosis (140).

Adults and children receiving methotrexate may experience accelerated nodulosis, with a characteristically abrupt onset beginning months to years after initiation of methotrexate therapy (141–143). An increase in number and size of rheumatoid nodules has also been reported during cyclosporine therapy for RA (144). Methotrexate-induced nodules may be larger and present in increased numbers; however, histologic examination does not permit a distinction between methotrexate-induced nodules and standard rheumatoid nodules (145). Methotrexate-induced nodules generally regress upon discontinuation of methotrexate therapy (141,142).

VASCULITIS SYNDROMES ASSOCIATED WITH RHEUMATOID ARTHRITIS

Vasculitis is a serious complication of RA usually occurring in seropositive patients with long-standing erosive nodular disease (146). Vasculitis, defined as inflammatory injury to blood vessels, is classified according to the anatomic site and size of vessel, the presence or absence of necrosis, and the clinical manifestations. Rheumatoid vasculitis may affect blood vessels of all sizes, although it usually affects small- and medium-sized arteries. Inflammation is generally greatest in the adventitia, but may be observed in all layers of the vessel wall. The inflammatory infiltrate is predominantly mononuclear, and consists mostly of lymphocytes. Neutrophils and plasma cells may also be present. The inflammation may be associated with intimal proliferation and thrombosis, with subsequent intimal fibrosis and recanalization. Healed vasculitic lesions involving arteries may be identified by the presence of fibrosis associated with prominent, sharply defined defects in the internal elastic lamina.

Patients with RA may demonstrate a necrotizing arteritis of small- and medium-sized arteries indistinguishable from polyarteritis nodosa. When multiple organs are affected, this form of vasculitis can be life threatening due to visceral infarction (147). Pulmonary hypertension is a rare complication of pulmonary vasculitis. Another clinical picture consists of involvement of venules by fibrinoid necrosis with neutrophils and nuclear debris (leukocytoclastic vasculitis), variable mononuclear infiltrate, and extravasation of erythrocytes. All of these lesions may coexist in a single patient at the same time or sequentially (148). Aortitis with and without aortic insufficiency has been reported as a rare, but serious, form of vasculitis associated with RA (149,150).

Clinical manifestations of RA vasculitis vary according to the size of vessel involved. Larger vessel vasculitis results in digital gangrene, gastrointestinal bleeding or stricture (151), nailfold infarcts, cutaneous ulcers, and internal organ involvement. Small vessel necrotizing vasculitis results in palpable purpura and systemic manifestations. In the absence of systemic vasculitis, cutaneous manifestations of RA include nailfold telangiectasia with thromboses, minute digital ulcers, digital petechiae, livedo reticularis, and digital pulp papules (Bywater lesions). Bywater lesions show histologic changes of leukocytoclastic vasculitis (152). Peripheral neuropathy and visceral infarction may result from vasculitic involvement of vessels supplying nerves and viscera. Lesions with clinicopathologic features of both leukocytoclastic vasculitis and early palisading granuloma have been described and proposed to be a link between vasculitis and rheumatoid nodules (153).

Immune complexes have been demonstrated in involved tissues of patients with active vasculitis, but not in patients with inactive disease (154). These studies combined with the presence of high levels of rheumatoid factor, cryoglobulins, and decreased circulating complement in patients with RA vasculitis (15) provide evidence that immune complex deposition and complement activation play a role in the pathogenesis of rheumatoid vasculitis. Antiendothelial antibodies may also play a role in the pathogenesis of rheumatoid vasculitis (155,156).

The diagnosis of RA vasculitis is most often made on clinical grounds, because typical ischemic ulcers or mononeuritis multiplex in the clinical setting of RA generally indicate the presence of vasculitis (15). Biopsy of a skin lesion, an affected nerve or other involved tissue generally has higher diagnostic yield than "blind" rectal biopsy (148). The presence of perivascular infiltrates at least three cell layers thick surrounding at least 50% of a vessel wall in muscle biopsy samples has been reported to be specific and to be more sensitive than the finding of fibrinoid necrosis in rheumatoid vasculitis (157). Levels of circulating cellular fibronectin have also been shown to be elevated in patients with rheumatoid vasculitis as compared to RA patients without vasculitis (158). Levels of circulating TNF-α and IL-6 are significantly higher in RA patients with vasculitis as compared to those without vasculitis, implicating the cytokine network in regulating cellular activation associated with microvascular damage (159).

PATHOLOGIC LESIONS OF THE LUNGS AND PLEURA IN RHEUMATOID ARTHRITIS

The reported prevalence of pulmonary involvement in RA has varied widely depending on the diagnostic methods and criteria used, with the highest reported percentages in autopsy series and the lowest in radiographic studies. Despite these variations, it is clear that pulmonary and pleural lesions are common in RA. Autopsy examination of a series of 30 patients with RA showed evidence of pleural inflammation in 22 patients (73%) (160). Five percent of a series of 180 unselected patients with RA demonstrated radiographic evidence of a pleural effusion (161). Types of pulmonary involvement seen in RA include chronic pleuritis with or without effusion, interstitial pneumonitis and fibrosis, bronchiolitis, intrapulmonary rheumatoid nodules with or without pneumoconiosis, and pulmonary vasculitis.

Pleuritis and Pleural Effusion in Rheumatoid Arthritis

The chronic pleuritis associated with RA may be extensive with formation of pleural adhesions. The majority of tissue samples for histologic examination are obtained by needle biopsy at the time of therapeutic or diagnostic thoracentesis. However, when required clinically, better morphology may be achieved using thoracoscopy (162). Diagnostic histologic features of RA pleura include elongated palisaded epithelioid macrophages replacing the mesothelial surface, scattered multinucleated giant cells, and underlying granulation tissue stroma (162,163). The surface layer may detach easily on needle biopsy, resulting in detached strips of epithelioid cells and "naked" stroma. Normal pleural structures such as mesothelial cells are characteristically not evident (162). This histologic appearance is most consistent with an "inside-out" rheumatoid nodule arranged linearly along the pleural surface, with its fibrinoid necrotic center open toward the pleural cavity.

A pleural effusion may accompany histologic evidence of pleuritis. The effusion may be unilateral despite the presence of systemic disease, and may be large enough to cause respiratory failure (163). The pleural fluid glucose level is characteristically low, with values below 20 to 30 mg/dL in 70% to 80% of patients (164). This very low glucose level is thought to be due to a defect in the transport of glucose across the inflamed pleura rather than due to the increased usage of glucose seen in malignant pleural effusions (165). The low fluid pH results from decreased diffusion of metabolites across the thickened and inflamed pleura (166). Pleural fluid lactate dehydrogenase is elevated, generally greater than 1,000 IU/L, indicative of an exudate. Pleural fluid hyaluronan levels are also elevated (167). Cholesterol crystals, when present, can be identified by polarization microscopy.

The cytologic picture of rheumatoid pleural effusion is considered to be pathognomonic (168) (Fig. 53.11). The classic cytologic triad consists of the presence of elongated spindle-shaped macrophages, multinucleated giant cells, and necrotic debris resulting from breakdown of macrophages and other cell types (132). The number of elongated macrophages seen in rheumatoid effusions varies. They are generally not abundant, and occasionally will not be observed in the specimen (168). They are up to 160 mm in length, with generally uniform thickness and pointed ends, and may occasionally be multinucleated. The multinucleated giant cells seen in RA effusions are also not numerous and may even be absent. They are round to oval and up to 150 mm in diameter, with 20 or more nuclei distributed randomly or in a horseshoe or flower petal arrangement. These giant cells have cytologic characteristics and immunohistologic phenotypes otherwise similar to those of the elongated macrophages. The necrotic material is variously described as granular, amorphous, "soft," and "fluffy," and may be so abundant as to dominate the smear. The color of this material varies from shades of light green to red, pink, or orange in Papanicolaou-stained smears, and is usually eosinophilic in hematoxylin and eosin–stained cell block preparations. The necrotic material present in RA effusions can be distinguished from fibrin by the dense, sharply demarcated, angulated, islandlike appearance in RA effusions as well as by strong but nonspecific reactivity of RA necrotic material with antiimmunoglobulin antisera (169). Fibrin generally has a more strandlike histologic appearance and is nonreactive with antiimmunoglobulin antisera.

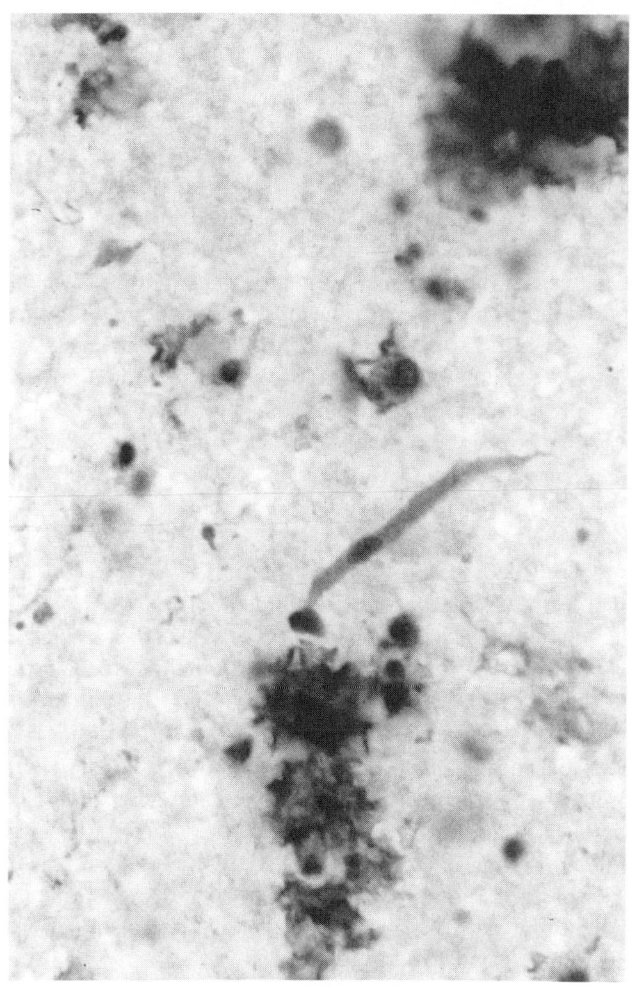

FIG. 53.11. Rheumatoid pleuritis. Elongated spindle-shaped macrophage is present in a background of amorphous granular material and inflammatory cells. Although not shown in this field, giant multinucleated macrophages are often seen (smear of pleural fluid, Papanicolaou stain).

Mesothelial cells are rarely observed in RA pleural effusions, most likely due to extensive involvement of the pleural surface (170). Cholesterol clefts, caused by the dissolution of cholesterol crystals during slide preparation, appear as trapezoid-shaped clear spaces in smears or as lancet-shaped empty spaces in paraffin-embedded material. These crystals are formed when cholesterol accumulates due to breakdown of cellular membranes of necrotic macrophages and other cell types in pleural effusions of long duration (168,170). The presence of cholesterol crystals is indicative of the chronicity of the effusion but is not specific for RA effusions.

The presence of the classic triad of elongated spindle-shaped macrophages, multinucleated giant cells, and necrotic debris in pleural fluid is diagnostic of RA. However, rheumatoid pleuritis may also be diagnosed with one or two of these cytologic features in the appropriate clinical setting. A high index of suspicion and acquaintance with its unique cytology are key to making this diagnosis (171).

Pulmonary Lesions in Rheumatoid Arthritis

Interstitial lung disease occurs in 10% to 50% of patients with RA (172–175). The majority of these patients have subclinical disease detectable on chest radiographs and pulmonary function testing. However, RA-associated pulmonary fibrosis can be progressive, may respond poorly to therapy, and has an overall poor prognosis (176). The form of interstitial lung disease most frequently seen in RA is called diffuse interstitial pulmonary fibrosis or usual interstitial pneumonitis. Atypical pulmonary infections (particularly due to mycobacteria, *Pneumocystis carinii,* or cytomegalovirus) and drug-induced interstitial disease must also be considered in the differential diagnosis (176).

The presence of rheumatoid nodules in lung tissue is specific for and diagnostic of RA-associated lung disease. Other histologic findings in RA pulmonary fibrosis (usual interstitial pneumonitis) are similar to those present in usual interstitial pneumonitis from other causes. Early lesions are characterized by prominent lymphoplasmacytic interstitial infiltrates and hyperplasia of type II alveolar cells. The intense inflammation occurring within the alveolar walls results in deposition of interstitial collagen, with progressive loss of alveolar capillaries due to fibrosis. The loss of capillaries stimulates medial hypertrophy in pulmonary arterioles and small arterioles, leading to pulmonary hypertension. As fibrosis progresses, pulmonary architecture is destroyed. The end-stage lesion is honeycombing, which may alternate with areas of active interstitial inflammation (177,178). The pathogenesis of RA pulmonary fibrosis is still unclear. Genetic factors including α1-protease inhibitor subtype, and altered host immunologic and tissue repair responses have been suggested as possible pathogenetic mechanisms (176). Direct immunofluorescence studies of lung tissue from patients with RA and pulmonary fibrosis show granular deposits of IgG and IgM in the septal capillaries, suggesting that the initial lung injury may result from immune complex deposition (179).

Other pulmonary manifestations of RA include bronchiolitis obliterans with or without organizing pneumonia, follicular bronchitis, and diffuse alveolar hemorrhage due to pulmonary capillaritis. Biopsy remains the gold standard for diagnosis of these disorders.

Caplan Syndrome

The syndrome of rheumatoid nodules with pneumoconiosis was first described by Caplan in 1953 as a characteristic lung disease of coal workers with RA (180). These patients had multiple discrete pulmonary nodules (0.5–5 cm) or masses of smaller nodules on chest radiographs. Histopathologically, nodules in Caplan syndrome have zones of necrotic material, primarily collagen, with adjacent reactive coal dust–laden macrophages, and a prominent lymphoplasmacytic infiltrate. As lesions mature, rings of coal dust are deposited in collagen scars. These nodules have been compared with standard rheumatoid nodules; however, the classic palisaded layers of macrophages are not generally observed (181). Twenty-five percent of patients with pneumoconiosis and RA have the pulmonary nodules of Caplan syndrome, an incidence of pulmonary involvement that is much greater than that in patients with RA alone (182). The therapy of these nodules is directed toward treatment of the underlying RA. Caplan syndrome has recently been expanded to include RA patients exposed to other dusts, including inhalable silica.

INVOLVEMENT OF THE HEART AND PERICARDIUM IN RHEUMATOID ARTHRITIS

The overall prevalence of cardiac abnormalities in autopsy studies of RA patients ranges from 30% to 50%; however, many of these patients do not experience clinical cardiac symptoms (183–185). Cardiac involvement in RA is primarily manifested by rheumatoid nodules, myocarditis or coronary artery vasculitis, and chronic pericarditis.

Cardiac rheumatoid nodules are histologically similar to those observed elsewhere and have been reported in all portions of the heart, including epicardium, myocardium, endocardium, and valve rings and cusps (149,186–191). Valvular or conduction disturbances may result from involvement of these structures by nodule formation, including embolization from affected valves (189). Rheumatoid nodules can also present as a cardiac mass lesion that results in severe heart failure (192). Myocarditis is common in autopsy studies of RA patients (186). The inflammatory infiltrate in RA myocarditis consists principally of plasma cells, lymphocytes, and histiocytes. Coronary arteritis is seen in about 20% of RA patients at autopsy (193). Severe and life-threatening clinical cardiac symptoms can result solely from RA-associated lesions (190–192).

Of patients with long-standing RA, 20% to 40% have evidence of pericardial involvement (194). This most commonly takes the form of fibrinous pericarditis, which may progress to fibrosis of the pericardium with adhesion formation. Rheumatoid nodules can also occur in the pericardium. When rheumatoid nodules are present in a linear array, the cytologic picture is identical to that observed in rheumatoid pleural effusions.

OCULAR LESIONS IN RHEUMATOID ARTHRITIS

The most common ocular manifestation of RA is keratoconjunctivitis sicca, which is present in 15% to 25% of patients (195,196). Patient symptoms include ocular redness, dryness, gritty or burning sensations, and photophobia. Slit-lamp examination reveals conjunctival injection, poor tear meniscus, and devitalized corneal epithelial cells. Biopsy samples from lacrimal glands demonstrate degeneration of lacrimal gland acini, with a mononuclear infiltrate consisting predominantly of lymphocytes and plasma cells present in and around the secretory ducts and acinar epithelium. Fibrosis of lacrimal glands may eventually result from chronic inflammation (197).

In addition to corneal changes resulting from keratoconjunctivitis sicca, RA patients may develop sterile central ulceration or peripheral ulcerative keratitis. Biopsies of conjunctival and corneal tissues in RA patients with sterile corneal ulceration show abundant mononuclear cell infiltrates consisting predominantly of activated lymphocytes and macrophages and expression of MHC class II (HLA-DR) antigens on conjunctival epithelial cells (198). Cytokines released by the infiltrating mononuclear cells may contribute to ulcer formation by inducing the production and release of proteolytic enzymes (199). Peripheral ulcerative keratitis can be associated with systemic vasculitis and aggressive immunosuppression may be required to prevent poor outcome (200).

Other ophthalmic manifestations of RA include episcleritis and scleritis (201). Episcleritis is classically sudden in onset, and self-limited but recurrent (202). In addition to episcleritis, episcleral nodules resembling rheumatoid nodules may develop in patients with RA (203). One of three patients with scleritis have RA, although this complication is present in less than 0.7% of all patients with RA (204). RA patients typically have the necrotizing form of scleritis. Scleromalacia perforans results when necrotizing scleritis thins the underlying sclera sufficiently to allow uveal prolapse (196). Rheumatoid necrotizing scleritis may be the first indication of clinically occult systemic vasculitis, and is associated with high mortality if not treated with systemic immunosuppressive therapy (201,202,204).

The most prominent histopathologic features of rheumatoid scleritis are vasculitis, scleral necrosis, and granulomatous inflammation surrounding the necrotic sclera in zones populated first by predominantly neutrophils and histiocytes, then by lymphocytes and plasma cells (205). Reactive proliferation of fibroblasts and blood vessels is typically not present (206).

Retinal vasculitis, demonstrated by diffuse leakage from the retinal capillaries during fluorescein angiography and cystoid macular edema, may occur in the absence of signs of vasculitis elsewhere in the body (207), and in the absence of clinical and ophthalmologic signs of retinal vessel inflammation (208).

LYMPHADENOPATHY IN RHEUMATOID ARTHRITIS

Lymphadenopathy is common in RA and may occur in 50% to 75% of patients (209,210). Lymph nodes frequently are examined via biopsy to exclude the presence of malignant lymphoma, which may be increased in RA patients (211). The histologic findings in RA lymph nodes are follicular hyperplasia with active germinal centers and polyclonal plasma cell infiltration in the interfollicular area (212–214). Proliferation of vascular endothelium and infiltration of the lymph node capsule and adjacent adipose tissue may also be observed. IL-6 production is particularly high in RA lymph nodes and may contribute significantly to the observed lymphadenopathy (213). RA lymph nodes may contain periodic acid-Schiff (PAS)-positive, Congo red–negative extracellular hyaline material, which in some cases may almost totally obliterate nodal architecture (215).

SPLEEN IN RHEUMATOID ARTHRITIS

Splenomegaly is common in RA patients, and patients with RA are at increased risk for spontaneous splenic rupture (216). However, the best known association of splenic involvement in RA is Felty syndrome, defined by the combination of RA, splenomegaly, and neutropenia. Felty syndrome occurs in less than 1% of RA patients (217). The splenomegaly of Felty syndrome varies from massive to subclinical, requiring radiographic studies for detection. Splenic enlargement occurs primarily due to expansion of the sinusoidal (red) pulp (218–220), and is indicated histologically by increased separation of arteries and trabeculae (218). Hyperplastic germinal centers are also generally present, and may be numerous (219). Granulocytes may be seen in T-cell areas of the spleen, despite the extremely low numbers of circulating granulocytes (219). Clusters of plasma cells may be seen prominently within the sinuses, often accompanied by immunoblasts (218,221). Patients with Felty syndrome are at increased risk for development of splenic abscess (216).

LIVER LESIONS ASSOCIATED WITH RHEUMATOID ARTHRITIS

Nodular regenerative hyperplasia is an uncommon disease of the liver that has been reported in association with RA, usually but not limited to patients with Felty syndrome (222–224). Nodular regenerative hyperplasia is defined pathologically by small nodules of regenerating hepatocytes distributed diffusely throughout the liver. Although grossly resembling micronodular cirrhosis, nodular regenerative hyperplasia is microscopically distinguished from cirrhosis by the lack of fibrous septa surrounding the nodules. Compressed reticulin fibers and atrophic hepatocytes are, however, seen at the periphery of the nodules. The pathogenesis of nodular regenerative hyperplasia has not been well defined, although hepatic arteritis has been postulated to play a role in the etiology of at least some cases (222). Most patients with nodular regenerative hyperplasia are asymptomatic. However, some patients may present with portal hypertension (splenomegaly, esophageal varices) and intrahepatic cholestasis (224).

MUSCLE LESIONS IN RHEUMATOID ARTHRITIS

Muscle involvement in RA most frequently occurs as a complication of RA vasculitis. Patients may present with muscle pain or proximal muscle weakness. Muscle enzymes may be elevated, with electromyographic evidence consistent with inflammatory myopathy (225). Muscle frequently is examined via biopsy simultaneously with nerve in patients undergoing evaluation for sensory or sensorimotor neuropathy. The results of muscle biopsy in these patients may show fibrosis, inflammatory infiltrates within muscle fibers, necrotizing vasculitis of perimysial medium-sized arteries, atrophy, or necrosis (226). In one series of 28 patients undergoing simultaneous nerve and muscle biopsy, vasculitis was present in 86% of muscle biopsy samples as compared with 64% of nerve biopsy samples (227).

DRUG-RELATED HISTOPATHOLOGIC CHANGES THAT FREQUENTLY OCCUR IN RHEUMATOID ARTHRITIS

The differential diagnosis of disease-related versus drug treatment–related changes in RA patients is often difficult due to the disease-associated histopathologic changes in multiple organs, and the resemblance of these changes to those caused by antirheumatic therapy (228). The organs most often affected by drug toxicity are the lung, liver, and kidney.

Antirheumatic agents implicated in pulmonary parenchymal disease include penicillamine, gold salts, methotrexate, aspirin and other nonsteroidal antiinflammatory drugs (NSAIDs), and rarely colchicine. The clinical syndromes associated with these drugs include hypersensitivity pneumonitis (methotrexate, gold, NSAIDs, penicillamine, sulfasalazine); chronic alveolitis/fibrosis (penicillamine, gold, NSAIDs, sulfasalazine); acute interstitial disease (sulfasalazine); pulmonary-renal syndrome similar to Goodpasture syndrome (penicillamine); bronchiolitis obliterans (penicillamine, gold); and noncardiogenic pulmonary edema (salicylates, NSAIDs, colchicine) (229,230). Therapy with TNF inhibitors is associated with an increased incidence of opportunistic infections, including tuberculosis and histoplasmosis (231,232).

Acute methotrexate-induced pulmonary toxicity may occur in 3% to 12% of methotrexate-treated patients (233–235). Clinical symptoms include fever, progressive dyspnea, and nonproductive cough, symptoms that also may be associated with infection. Consequently, bronchoalveolar lavage or lung biopsy may be required to rule out opportunistic infections such as *Pneumocystis carinii* pneumonia (236,237) or cryptococcosis (238). The histopathologic findings in methotrexate-induced pneumonitis include interstitial and sometimes alveolar infiltrates composed predominately of mononuclear cells, proliferation of type I and II pneumocytes, bronchiolitis, granulomatous inflammation, and infiltration by eosinophils, changes that are consistent with a drug hypersensitivity reaction. Methotrexate-induced pneumonitis generally regresses on discontinuation of methotrexate therapy (235). In severe cases, diffuse alveolar damage may be present (239). Open lung biopsy is generally used; however, transbronchial biopsy has been used successfully to diagnose methotrexate-induced pneumonitis (240). Although pulmonary fibrosis is a well-known complication of methotrexate treatment of malignancy, results of high-resolution computed tomography and serial pulmonary function tests in methotrexate-treated and control patients with RA do not support an association of low-dose methotrexate therapy with chronic interstitial lung disease (241).

Severe liver toxicity as a complication of methotrexate therapy is more common in patients with preexisting liver disease, alcohol abuse, diabetes mellitus, advanced age, and renal insufficiency. Methotrexate therapy may be relatively contraindicated in these patients. The weekly low-dose methotrexate regimen usually used in patients with RA has a low, but definite, risk for hepatic toxicity (242–245). The total cumulative dose, heavy alcohol consumption, and advanced age are important risk factors for development of severe liver disease (244,246). Liver biopsy is the gold standard for diagnosis of methotrexate-induced liver abnormalities. Histopathologic findings include hepatic fibrosis and cirrhosis. Both of these entities feature deposition of excess extracellular matrix material consisting predominantly of collagen; however, the hepatic architecture is relatively preserved in hepatic fibrosis, and the lesion is reversible. As fibrosis progresses to cirrhosis, the relationships between portal triads and central veins are distorted, nodules are present, and the lesion is generally irreversible. The degree and type of liver dysfunction associated with hepatic fibrosis is correlated with the location of the collagen deposition (periportal, pericentral, or perisinusoidal) and the resulting disturbance in blood flow (247). In an autopsy study of 188 patients with RA who died prior to the widespread use of methotrexate, serious fibrotic liver disease was rare in patients without an underlying cause of liver pathology (e.g., alcohol abuse or viral hepatitis) (248). This supports the current practice of limiting pretreatment liver biopsies to patients with suspected liver disease.

Hepatotoxicity resulting from therapy with gold salts is rare, dose related, and occurs after prolonged treatment. Gradual improvement of liver function generally follows discontinuation of the drug. Histopathologic examination of biopsy specimens shows submassive loss of hepatocytes, collapse of reticulin framework, and mixed cellular infiltrates consisting of lymphocytes, neutrophils, macrophages, and occasional eosinophils present in lobules and portal tracts. Macrophages contain dark granules, which can be identified as containing gold by electron probe microanalysis (249). The mechanism by which gold results in hepatic toxicity is not known. Lipogranulomas containing brown and black gold deposits may be seen in the liver of asymptomatic patients up to 10 years after cessation of gold therapy (250).

Renal toxicity resulting from penicillamine or parenteral gold therapy is most commonly manifested by proteinuria. Renal biopsy may be required if proteinuria persists after drug discontinuation, to rule out amyloidosis or other renal diseases. The most common histopathologic finding in gold or penicillamine nephropathy is membranous glomerulonephritis (251,252). Gold deposits may be identified within kidney tissue by histochemical stains or electron microscopy (251).

Ocular complications resulting from treatment of RA include deposition of gold particles, which do not affect vision, in the lens and posterior corneal stroma following treatment with gold salts (253), as well as the development of posterior subcapsular cataracts in patients treated with corticosteroids (196) .

DIFFERENTIAL HISTOPATHOLOGIC DIAGNOSIS OF CHRONIC SYNOVITIS

No histopathologic features exist that by themselves allow definitive diagnosis of the chronic active synovitis caused by RA from other forms of chronic synovitis (17). However certain histopathologic features that are characteristic of the synovitis of RA occur less frequently in other forms of synovitis. These include (a) moderate to marked proliferation of synovial cells often accompanied by palisading; (b) presence of non–foreign body type giant cells; (c) presence of lymphoid aggregates containing germinal centers; (d) moderate to marked infiltration of the sublining layer by plasma cells; (e) moderate to marked proliferation of granulation tissue; (f) fibrin deposition or fibrinoid necrosis; and (g) synovial accumulations of hemosiderin. A semiquantitative grading scale using these features has been developed that may allow synovial biopsy results from patients with RA to be distinguished from those with OA (254); however, use of this scale has not been widely adopted (2). A high percentage of synovial vessels with perivascular lymphocyte infiltrates may predict patients at high risk for erosive disease (255).

Osteoarthritis is characterized by gradual loss of extracellular matrix by the articular cartilage with resultant progressive joint erosion. The earliest changes are swelling of cartilage, followed by depletion of proteoglycan from the cartilage in the face of increased synthesis (256). The proteoglycans present in OA have altered biochemical properties, which may be attributed to proteolytic digestion of the hyaluronic acid–binding regions and the core protein of aggrecan, the principal large proteoglycan of cartilage. MMP-3 is produced by chondrocytes and synovial lining cells in the regions of cartilage breakdown and may be important in proteoglycan degradation (257). IL-1 produced by chondrocytes in OA cartilage induces degradation of the matrix. Prostaglandin derivatives, TNF-α, and TGF-β induce the synthesis of lytic enzymes by chondrocytes and also inhibit matrix synthesis (258).

Arthritis occurs in 5% to 7% of patients with psoriasis and may precede the appearance of skin lesions. Although clinical features may resemble RA, the presence of an asymmetric oligoarticular distribution, the presence of dactylitis, distal interphalangeal joint involvement, or the absence of rheumatoid factor suggest consideration of psoriatic arthritis. Careful physical examination should search for psoriatic skin lesions or nail dystrophic changes, including nail pits. The histologic findings in synovium from patients with psoriatic arthritis generally show a scant inflammatory infiltrate with slight synovial lining hyperplasia, changes similar to but milder than those seen in RA (17,259). Comparison of synovial membrane needle biopsy samples from patients with psoriatic arthritis and with RA, matched for disease duration, show that there is significantly less synovial lining hyperplasia in psoriatic arthritis, averaging three cell layers in depth (range 2–5), as compared with nine cell layers in RA (range 3–32) (260). Fewer tissue macrophages are present, and the number of vessels present in the subintimal layer of synovium is markedly increased in psoriatic arthritis. Numbers of B cells, T cells, and T-cell subsets are similar in RA and psoriatic arthritis, with similar expression of CD54 and CD106. CD62E expression is less intense in psoriatic arthritis as compared with RA (260). Because CD62E may mediate monocyte adherence, the lack of CD62E expression in psoriatic synovial membranes may explain the histopathologic findings of fewer macrophages and lack of lining layer hyperplasia as compared with RA.

Synovium from patients with systemic lupus erythematosus (SLE) most frequently exhibits synovial lining hyperplasia, scant inflammatory infiltrate, congestion and edema, fibrinoid necrosis and intimal fibrosis of synovial blood vessels, and fibrin deposition on the synovial surface (261). However, these findings are not specific for SLE.

Synovial tissue from patients with reactive arthropathy generally does not exhibit the villous hyperplasia, synovial lining hypertrophy, or focal lymphoid aggregates commonly seen in RA patients (262). Additional differences between RA and reactive arthritis include low to absent expression of HLA-DQ antigens by synovial vessels in reactive arthritis (262). Activated T lymphocytes in the synovial fluid in reactive arthritis are generally $CD8^+$, whereas the activated T cells in RA synovial fluid are predominately $CD4^+$ (263).

Synovial tissue from patients with spondyloarthropathy exhibits increased synovial vascularity microscopically and macroscopically compared with RA, with a tortuous vessel pattern. Numbers of T and B lymphocytes are decreased relative to rheumatoid synovium (264).

SYNDROMES ASSOCIATED WITH RHEUMATOID ARTHRITIS

Amyloidosis

Amyloidosis (see Chapter 93) is defined as a group of biochemically diverse conditions in which normally innocuous soluble proteins polymerize to form insoluble fibrils (265). The fibrils associate with proteoglycans and proteins derived from plasma or with extracellular matrix proteins to form amyloid deposits. These deposits occupy extracellular spaces in a variety of organs with resulting destruction of normal tissue architecture and function.

Amyloidosis associated with inflammation or reactive systemic amyloidosis occurs in 2% to 23% of patients with RA (266), rendering this one of the major causes of secondary amyloidosis (267,268). The major risk factor for amyloidosis in RA is continuously active disease (269). Cytokines produced by activated mononuclear phagocytes in RA enhance the expression of acute-phase serum amyloid A proteins, as well as the expression of proteolytic enzymes that convert these precursors to amyloid AA fibrils by proteolytic removal of a portion of the C-terminal domain (265).

The definitive histologic demonstration of amyloid involves the examination of tissue sections stained with Congo red stain using polarization microscopy. Amyloid deposits appear homogeneous, amorphous, and red when viewed under light microscopy. The amorphous appearance is deceiving, however, because amyloid deposits demonstrate birefringence under polarization microscopy even in the unstained state, indicating the presence of highly ordered structures. Congo red staining markedly enhances the birefringence of the amyloid deposits, resulting in strong apple-green birefringence. This characteristic staining pattern has been linked to the parallel arrangement of linear Congo red dye molecules along the axis of the amyloid fibril (270). Fibrin deposits, which may appear similar to amyloid deposits in hematoxylin and eosin–stained sections, as well as elastin fibers, are also Congophilic; however, they do not exhibit apple-green birefringence (271). Collagen fibrils are birefringent under polarized light. The collagen birefringence, however, is not enhanced by Congo red staining (272).

A variety of tissues have been commonly examined via biopsy for the diagnosis of amyloidosis, including the upper gastrointestinal tract, rectum, gingiva, conjunctiva, and kidney. Needle or aspiration biopsies of subcutaneous abdominal fat have gained favor due to the simplicity, increased safety and patient tolerance, and decreased cost compared with other biopsy sites (273,274). Aspirated material must contain not only fat droplets but also adipose tissue fragments visible to the eye in order to be useful for diagnosis. However, the sensitivity and diagnostic yield for gastrointestinal biopsies has remained consistently higher than that for abdominal fat biopsies (273,275).

Sjögren's Syndrome

Sjögren's syndrome (see Chapter 78) consists of the combination of keratoconjunctivitis sicca, xerostomia with or without salivary gland enlargement, and RA or one of the other connective tissue diseases. The diagnosis of Sjögren's syndrome is most frequently made by biopsy of minor salivary glands present in the lip. The characteristic histologic feature is the presence of a predominantly lymphocytic infiltrate in an otherwise normal salivary gland. Diagnostic criteria include the presence of at least four lobules of salivary gland, containing at least two foci of lymphocytes per 4 mm^2 area, with each focal aggregate composed of greater than 50 lymphocytes (Fig. 53.12). These lymphocytic aggregates should appear in nearly all glands present in the biopsy (276). Plasma cells and histiocytes may also be present.

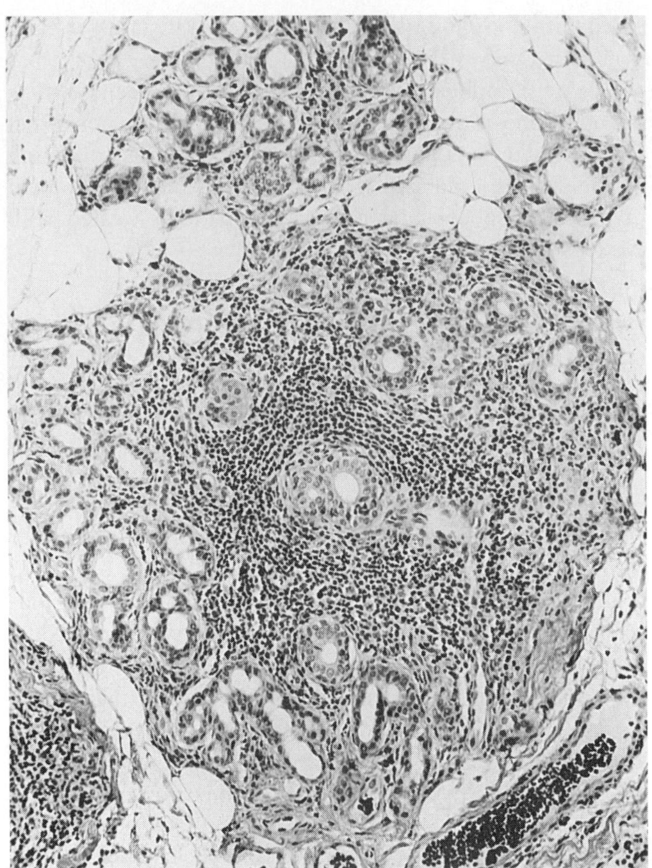

FIG. 53.12. Sjögren's syndrome, labial salivary gland. An intense lymphoplasmacytic infiltrate surrounds salivary ducts (hematoxylin and eosin stain, original magnification ×130).

In Sjögren's syndrome, the lung may be involved in a lymphoproliferative process similar to that seen in salivary and lacrimal glands, resulting in loss of mucous gland secretions within the trachea and chronic bronchitis (277). Lymphocytic interstitial pneumonitis may be present with prominent lymphocytic infiltrates in and around bronchioles (278).

Patients with Sjögren's syndrome may develop "pseudolymphomas," which demonstrate partial obliteration of lymph node architecture by a heterogeneous interfollicular infiltrate of macrophages, plasma cells, small lymphocytes, and immunoblasts. Monocytoid B cells may be present within the sinuses. These lymph nodes should be carefully evaluated immunohistochemically for focal areas of plasma cell clonality, which indicates evolution to malignant lymphoma, for which patients with Sjögren's syndrome are at increased risk (279).

SUMMARY

RA is a systemic disease with pathologic manifestations in many organs. The migration of leukocytes to synovium, followed by initiation of a complex cascade of pathologic immune-mediated events, results in cartilage, soft tissue, and bone destruction. The knowledge that is now available regarding the molecules and cytokines involved in tissue damage in RA is providing new prospects for treatment of this chronic and destructive disease.

REFERENCES

1. Bresnihan B, Tak PP, Emery P, et al. Synovial biopsy in arthritis research: five years of concerted European collaboration. *Ann Rheum Dis* 2000;59:506–510.
2. Katrib A, McNeil HP, Youssef PP. What can we learn from the synovium in early rheumatoid arthritis? *Inflamm Res* 2002;51:170–175.
3. Turesson C, O'Fallon WM, Crowson CS, et al. Occurrence of extra-articular disease manifestations is associated with excess mortality in a community based cohort of patients with rheumatoid arthritis. *J Rheumatol* 2002;29:62–67.
4. Okada Y, Naka K, Minamoto T, et al. Localization of type VI collagen in the lining cell layer of normal and rheumatoid synovium. *Lab Invest* 1990;63:647–656.
5. Wilkinson LS, Edwards JCW. Microvascular distribution in normal human synovium. *J Anat* 1989;167:129–136.
6. Zvaifler NJ, Firestein GS. Pannus and pannocytes: alternative models of joint destruction in rheumatoid arthritis. *Arthritis Rheum* 1994;37: 783–789.
7. Edwards JCW, Wilkinson LS, Pitsillides AA. Palisading cells of rheumatoid nodules: comparison with synovial intimal cells. *Ann Rheum Dis* 1993;52:801–805.
8. Edwards JCW, Willoughby DA. Demonstration of bone marrow-derived cells in synovial lining by means of giant intercellular granules as genetic markers. *Ann Rheum Dis* 1982;41:177–182.
9. Edwards JCW. The origin of the type A synovial lining cell. *Immunobiology* 1982;161:227–231.
10. Schwachula A, Riemann D, Kehlen A, et al. Characterization of the immunophenotype and functional properties of fibroblast-like synoviocytes in comparison to skin fibroblasts and umbilical vein endothelial cells. *Immunobiology* 1994;190:67–92.
11. Wilkinson LS, Pitsillides AA, Worral JG, et al. Light microscope characterisation of the fibroblast-like synovial lining cell. *Arthritis Rheum* 1992;35:1179–1184.
12. Salter DM. Tenascin is increased in cartilage and synovium from arthritic knees. *Br J Rheum* 1993;32:780–786.
13. McCachren SS, Lightner VA. Expression of human tenascin in synovitis and its regulation by interleukin-1. *Arthritis Rheum* 1992;35:1185–1196.
14. Worrall JG, Bayliss MT, Edwards JCW. Morphological localization of hyaluronan in normal and diseased synovium. *J Rheumatol* 1991;18: 1466–1472.
15. Vollertsen RS, Conn DL. Vasculitis associated with rheumatoid arthritis. *Rheum Clin North Am* 1990;16:445–461.
16. Weinberg JB, Pippen AMM, Greenberg CS. Extravascular fibrin formation and dissolution in synovial tissue of patients with osteoarthritis and rheumatoid arthritis. *Arthritis Rheum* 1991;34:996–1005.
17. Soren A. *Histodiagnosis and clinical correlation of rheumatoid and other synovitis.* Philadelphia: JB Lippincott, 1978.
18. Lalor PA, Mapp PI, Hall PA, Revell PA. Proliferative activity of cells in synovium as determined by a monoclonal antibody Ki-67. *Rheumatol Int* 1987;7:183–186.
19. Coulton LA, Henderson B, Bitensky L, et al. DNA synthesis in human rheumatoid and non-rheumatoid synovial lining. *Ann Rheum Dis* 1980; 39:241–247.
20. Coulton LA, Henderson B, Chayen J. The assessment of DNA-synthetic activity. *Histochemistry* 1981;72:91–99.
21. Dreher R. The origin of synovial type A cells during inflammation: an experimental approach. *Immunobiology* 1982;161:232–245.
22. Katrib A, Tak PP, Bertouch JV, et al. Expression of chemokines and matrix metalloproteinases in early rheumatoid arthritis. *Rheumatology* 2001;40:988–994.
23. Smith MD, Kraan MC, Slavotinek J, et al. Treatment-induced remission in rheumatoid arthritis patients is characterized by a reduction in macrophage content of synovial biopsies. *Rheumatology* 2001;40:367–374.
24. Wakisaka S, Suzuki N, Takeba, et al. Modulation by proinflammatory cytokines of Fas/Fas ligand-mediated apoptotic cell death of synovial cells in patients with rheumatoid arthritis (RA). *Clin Exp Immunol* 1998;114:119–128.
25. Sugiyama M, Tsukazaki T, Yonekura A, et al. Localisation of apoptosis and expression of apoptosis related proteins in the synovium of patients with rheumatoid arthritis. *Ann Rheum Dis* 1996;55:442–449.
26. Szekanecz Z, Koch AE. Chemokines and angiogenesis. *Curr Opin Rheumatol* 2001;13:202–208.
27. O'Donnell K, Harkes IC, Dougherty L, et al. Expression of the receptor tyrosine kinase Ax1 and its ligand Gas6 in rheumatoid arthritis: evidence for a novel endothelial cell survival pathway. *Am J Pathol* 1999;154:1171–1180.
28. Berse B, Hunt JA, Diegel RJ, et al. Hypoxia augments cytokine (transforming growth factor-beta (TGF-beta) and IL-1-induced vascular endothelial growth factor secretion by human synovial fibroblasts. *Clin Exp Immunol* 1999;115:176–182.
29. Gravallese EM, Pettit AR, Lee R, et al. Angiopoietin-1 is expressed in the synovium of patients with rheumatoid arthritis and is induced by tumour necrosis factor α. *Ann Rheum Dis* 2003;62:100–107.
30. Yin G, Liu W, An P, et al. Endostatin gene transfer inhibits joint angiogenesis and pannus formation in inflammatory arthritis. *Mol Ther* 2002;5:547–554.
31. Kim J-M, Ho S-H, Park E-J, et al. Angiostatin gene transfer as an effective treatment strategy in murine collagen-induced arthritis. *Arthritis Rheum* 2002;46:793–801.
32. Matsuno H, Yudoh K, Uzuki M, et al. Treatment with the angiogenesis inhibitor endostatin: a novel therapy in rheumatoid arthritis. *J Rheumatol* 2002;29:890–895.
33. Nagashima M, Tanaka H, Takahashi H, et al. Study of the mechanism involved in angiogenesis and synovial cell proliferation in human synovial tissues of patients with rheumatoid arthritis using SCID mice. *Lab Invest* 2002;82:981–988.
34. Sekimoto T, Hamada K, Oike Y, et al. Effect of direct angiogenesis inhibition in rheumatoid arthritis using a soluble vascular endothelial growth factor receptor 1 chimeric protein. *J Rheumatol* 2002;29:240–245.
35. Ostergaard M, Hansen M, Stoltenberg M, et al. Magnetic resonance imaging-determined synovial membrane volume as a marker of disease activity and a predictor of progressive joint destruction in the wrists of patients with rheumatoid arthritis. *Arthritis Rheum* 1999;42: 918–929.
36. Kraan MC, Reece RJ, Smeets TJM, et al. Comparison of synovial tissues from the knee joints and small joints of rheumatoid arthritis patients:implications for pathogenesis and evaluation of treatment. *Arthritis Rheum* 2002;46:2034–2038.
37. Kirkham B, Portek I, Lee CS, et al. Intraarticular variability of synovial membrane histology, immunohistology, and cytokine mRNA expression in patients with rheumatoid arthritis. *J Rheumatol* 1999;26: 777–784.
38. Szekanecz Z, Strieter RM, Kunkel SL, et al. Chemokines in rheumatoid arthritis. *Springer Semin Pathol* 1998;20:115–132.
39. Tanaka Y, Fujii K, Hubscher S, et al. Heparan sulfate proteoglycan on endothelium efficiently induces integrin-mediated T cell adhesion by immobilizing chemokines in patients with rheumatoid synovitis. *Arthritis Rheum* 1998;41:1365–1377.
40. Yanni G, Whelan A, Feighery C, et al. Morphometric analysis of synovial membrane blood vessels in rheumatoid arthritis: associations with the immunohistologic features, synovial fluid cytokine levels, and the clinical course. *J Rheumatol* 1993;20:634–638.
41. Klimiuk PA, Sierakowski S, Latosiewicz, et al. Serum cytokines in different histological variants of rheumatoid synovitis. *J Rheumatol* 2001;28:1211–1217.
42. Takemura S, Braun A, Crowson C, et al. Lymphoid neogenesis in rheumatoid synovitis. *J Immunol* 2001;167:1072–1080.
43. Page G, Lebecque S, Miossec P. Anatomic localization of immature and mature dendritic cells in an ectopic lymphoid organ: correlation with selective chemokine expression in rheumatoid synovium. *J Immunol* 2002;168:5333–5341.
44. Oppenheimer-Marks N, Davis LS, Lipsky PE. Transendothelial migration of T cells in chronic inflammation. *Clin Trends* 1994;2:58–64.
45. Salmon M, Scheel-Toellner D, Huissoon AP, et al. Inhibition of T cell apoptosis in the rheumatoid synovium. *J Clin Invest* 1997;99:439–446.
46. Schirmer M, Vallejo AN, Weyand CM, et al. Resistance to apoptosis and elevated expression of Bcl-2 in clonally expanded $CD4^{+}CD28^{-}$ T cells from rheumatoid arthritis patients. *J Immunol* 1998;161:1018–1025.
47. Jenkins JK, Hardy KJ, McMurray RW. The pathogenesis of rheumatoid arthritis: guide to therapy. *Am J Med Sci* 2002;323:171–180.

48. Firestein GS. Mechanisms of tissue destruction and cellular activation in rheumatoid arthritis. *Curr Opin Rheum* 1992;4:348–354.
49. Richardson BC. T cell receptor usage in rheumatic disease. *Clin Exp Rheum* 1992;10:271–283.
50. Pluschke G, Ginter A, Taube H, et al. Analysis of T cell receptor Vβ regions expressed by rheumatoid synovial T lymphocytes. *Immunobiology* 1993;188:330–339.
51. Goronzy JJ, Zettl A, Weuand CM. T cell receptor repertoire in rheumatoid arthritis. *Int Rev Immunol* 1998;17:339–363.
52. Martens PB, Goronzy JJ, Schaid D, et al. Expansion of unsual CD4+ T cells in severe rheumatoid arthritis. *Arthritis Rheum* 1997;40:1106–1114.
53. Schmidt D, Goronzy JJ, Weyand CM. CD4+ CD7− CD28− T cells are expanded in rheumatoid arthritis and are characterized by autoreactivity. *J Clin Invest* 1996;97:2027–2037.
54. Alam A, Lambert N, Lule J, et al. Persistence of dominant T cell clones in synovial tissues during rheumatoid arthritis. *J Immunol* 1996;156:3480–3485.
55. Weyand CM. New insights into the pathogenesis of rheumatoid arthritis. *Rheumatology* 2000;39:3–8.
56. Yamanishi Y, Firestein GS. Pathogenesis of rheumatoid arthritis: the role of synoviocytes. *Rheum Clin North Am* 2001;27:355–371.
57. Lee DM, Friend DS, Gurish MF, et al. Mast cells: a cellular link between autoantibodies and inflammatory arthritis. *Science* 2002;297:1689–1692.
58. Tetlow LC, Wooley DE. Mast cells, cytokines, and metalloproteinases at the rheumatoid lesion: dual immunolocalisation studies. *Ann Rheum Dis* 1995;54:896–903.
59. Wooley DE, Tetlow LC. Mast cell activation and its relation to proinflammatory cytokine production in the rheumatoid lesion. *Arthritis Res* 2000;2:65–74.
60. Kobayashi Y, Okunishi H. Mast cells as a target of theumatoid arthritis treatment. *Jpn J Pharmacol* 2002;90:7–11.
61. Hiromatsu Y, Toda S. Mast cells and angiogenesis. *Microscopy Res Tech* 2003;60:64–69.
62. Yamada T, Sawatsubashi M, Yakushiji H, et al. Localization of vascular endothelial growth factor in synovial membrane mast cells: examination with "multi-labeling subtraction immunostaining." *Virchows Arch* 1998;433:567–570.
63. Wooley DE. The mast cell in inflammatory arthritis. *N Engl J Med* 2003;348:1709–1710.
64. Allard SA, Muirden KD, Maini RN. Correlation of histopathologic features of pannus with patterns of tissue damage in different joints in rheumatoid arthritis. *Ann Rheum Dis* 1991;50:278–283.
65. Allard SA, Bayliss MT, Maini RN. The synovium-cartilage junction of the normal human knee: implications for joint destruction and repair. *Arthritis Rheum* 1990;33:1170–1179.
66. Shiozawa S, Shiozawa K, Fujita T. Morphologic observations in the early phase of the cartilage-pannus junction: light and electron microscopic studies of active cellular pannus. *Arthritis Rheum* 1983;26:472–478.
67. Scott BB, Weisbrot LM, Greenwood JD, et al. Rheumatoid arthritis synovial fibroblast and U937 macrophage/monocyte cell line interaction in cartilage degradation. *Arthritis Rheum* 1997;40:490–498.
68. Wang AZ, Wang JC, Fisher GW, et al. Interleukin-1 beta-stimulated invasion of articular cartilage by rheumatoid synovial fibroblasts is inhibited by antibodies to specific integrin receptors and by collagenase inhibitors. *Arthritis Rheum* 1997;40:1298–1307.
69. Kobayashi I, Ziff M. Electron microscopic studies of the cartilage-pannus junction in rheumatoid arthritis. *Arthritis Rheum* 1975;18:475–483.
70. Krane SM, Conca W, Stephenson ML, et al. Mechanisms of matrix degradation in rheumatoid arthritis. *Ann NY Acad Sci* 1990;580:340–354.
71. Waller HA, Butler MG, McClean JGB, et al. Localisation of fibronectin mRNA in the rheumatoid synovium by in situ hybridisation. *Ann Rheum Dis* 1992;51:735–740.
72. Cutolo M, Picasso M, Ponassi M, et al. Tenascin and fibronectin distribution in human normal and pathological synovium. *J Rheumatol* 1992;19:1439–1447.
73. Shiozawa K, Shiozawa S, Shimizu S, et al. Fibronectin on the surface of articular cartilage in rheumatoid arthritis. *Arthritis Rheum* 1984;27:615–622.
74. Clemmensen I, Andersen RB. Different molecular forms of fibronectin in rheumatoid synovial fluid. *Arthritis Rheum* 1984;25:25–31.
75. Griffiths AM, Herbert KE, Perret D, et al. Fragmented fibronectin and other synovial fluid proteins in chronic arthritis: their relation to immune complexes. *Clin Chim Acta* 1989;184:133–146.
76. Pitzalis C, Kingsley GH, Covelli M, et al. Selective migration of the human helper-inducer memory T cell subset: confirmation by *in vivo* cellular kinetic studies. *Eur J Immunol* 1991;21:369–376.
77. Brennan FR, Mikecz K, Glant TT, et al. CD44 expression by leucocytes in rheumatoid arthritis and modulation by specific antibody: implications for lymphocyte adhesion to endothelial cells and synoviocytes *in vitro. Scand J Immunol* 1997;45:213–220.
78. Lanchbury JS, Pitzalis C. Cellular immune mechanisms in rheumatoid arthritis and other inflammatory arthritides. *Curr Opin Immunol* 1993;5:918–924.
79. Van Seventer GA, Newman W, Shimizu Y, et al. Analysis of T cell stimulation by superantigen plus major histocompatibility complex class II molecules or by CD3 monoclonal antibody: costimulation by purified adhesion ligands VCAM-1, ICAM-1, but not ELAM-1. *J Exp Med* 1991;174:901–913.
80. Miyake S, Yagita H, Maruyama T, et al. β1 integrin-mediated interaction with extracellular matrix proteins regulates cytokine gene expression in synovial fluid cells of rheumatoid arthritis patients. *J Exp Med* 1993;177:863–868.
81. Hale LP, Martin ME, McCollum DE, et al. Immunohistologic analysis of the distribution of cell adhesion molecules within the inflammatory synovial microenvironment. *Arthritis Rheum* 1989;32:22–30.
82. Athanasou NA, Quinn J. Immunocytochemical analysis of human synovial lining cells: phenotypic relation to other marrow derived cells. *Ann Rheum Dis* 1991;50:311–315.
83. Nakatsuka K, Tanaka Y, Hubscher S, et al. Rheumatoid synovial fibroblasts are stimulated by cellular adhesion to T cells through lymphocyte function associated antigen-1/intercellular adhesion molecule-1. *J Rheumatol* 1997;24:458–464.
84. Smith MD, Slavotinek J, Au V, et al. Successful treatment of rheumatoid arthritis is associated with a reduction in synovial membrane cytokines and cell adhesion molecule expression. *Rheumatology* 2001;40:965–977.
85. Shang XZ, Lang BJ, Issekutz AC. Adhesion molecule mechanisms mediating monocyte migration through synovial fibroblast and endothelium barriers: role for CD11/CD18, very late antigen-4 (CD49d/CD29), very late antigen-5 (CD49e/CD29), and vascular cell adhesion molecule (CD106). *J Immunol* 1998;160:467–474.
86. Elices MJ, Osborn L, Takada Y, et al. VCAM-1 on activated endothelium interacts with the leukocyte integrin VLA-4 at a site distinct from the VLA-4/fibronectin binding site. *Cell* 1990;60:977–984.
87. Lazarovits AI, Karsh J. Differential expression in rheumatoid synovium and synovial fluid of α2β7 integrin: a novel receptor for fibronectin and vascular cell adhesion molecule-1. *J Immunol* 1993;151:6482–6489.
88. Veale DJ, Maple C. Cell adhesion molecules in rheumatoid arthritis. *Drugs Aging* 1996;9:87–92.
89. Shimizu Y, van Seventer GA, Horgan KJ, et al. Costimulation of proliferative responses of resting CD4+ T cells by the interaction of VLA-4 and VLA-5 with fibronectin or VLA-6 with laminin. *J Immunol* 1990;145:59–67.
90. Sarkissian M, Lafyatis R. Integrin engagement regulates proliferation and collagenase expression of rheumatoid synovial fibroblasts. *J Immunol* 1999;162:1772–1779.
91. Haynes BF, Hale LP, Patton KL, et al. Measurement of an adhesion molecule as an indicator of inflammatory disease activity: up-regulation of the receptor for hyaluronate (CD44) in rheumatoid arthritis. *Arthritis Rheum* 1991;34:1434–1443.
92. DeGrendele HC, Estess P, Siegelman MH. Requirement for CD44 in activated T cell extravasation into an inflammatory site. *Science* 1997;278:672–675.
93. Denning SM, Le PT, Singer KH, et al. Antibodies against the CD44 p80, lymphocyte homing receptor molecule augment human peripheral blood T cell activation. *J Immunol* 1990;144:7–15.
94. Shimizu Y, Van Seventer GA, Siriganian R, et al. Dual role of the CD44 molecule in T cell adhesion and activation. *J Immunol* 1989;143:2457–2463.
95. Fujii K, Tanaka Y, Hubscher S, et al. Cross-linking of CD44 on rheumatoid synovial cells up-regulates VCAM-1. *J Immunol* 1999;162:2391–2398.
96. Neidhart M, Gay RE, Gay S. Anti-interleukin 1 and anti-CD44 interventions producing significant inhibition of cartilage destruction in an

in vitro model of cartilage invasion by rheumatoid arthritis synovial fibroblasts. *Arthritis Rheum* 2000;43:1719–1728.

97. Feldmann M, Maini RN. Role of cytokines in the pathogenesis of rheumatoid arthritis. *Rheumatology* 1999;38:3–7.
98. Brennan FM, Maini RN, Feldmann M. Role of pro-inflammatory cytokines in rheumatoid arthritis. *Springer Semin Immunopathol* 1998;20:133–147.
99. Feldmann M, Maini RN. Anti-TNFα therapy of rheumatoid arthritis: what have we learned? *Annu Rev Immunol* 2001;19:163–196.
100. Alsalamah S, Winter K, Al-Ward R, et al. Distribution of TNF-alpha, TNF-R55, and TNF-R75 in the rheumatoid synovial membrane. *Scand J Immunol* 1999;49:278–285.
101. Klimiuk PA, Goronzy JJ, Bjoronsson J, et al. Tissue cytokine patterns distinguish variants of rheumatoid synovitis. *Am J Pathol* 1997;151: 1311–1319.
102. Hessian PA, Highton J, Kean A, et al. Cytokine profile of the rheumatoid nodule suggests that it is a Th1 granuloma. *Arthritis Rheum* 2003;48:334–338.
103. Firestein GS, Paine M. Stromelysin and tissue inhibitor of metalloproteinase (TIMP) gene expression in rheumatoid arthritis synovium. *Am J Pathol* 1992;140:1309–1314.
104. Iwata K, Yamashita K, Kodama S, et al. Significance of tissue inhibitor of metalloproteinases (TIMP) in synovial fluid of rheumatoid arthritis. *Matrix* 1992;1:332–333.
105. Katrib A, Tak PP, Bertouch JV, et al. Expression of chemokines and matrix metalloproteinases in early rheumatoid arthritis. *Rheumatology* 2001;40:988–994.
106. McCachren SS, Haynes BF, Niedel J. Localization of collagenase mRNA in rheumatoid arthritis synovium by *in situ* hybridization histochemistry. *J Clin Immunol* 1990;135:1055–1064.
107. Cunnane G, Fitzgerald O, Hummel KM, et al. Synovial tissue protease gene expression and joint erosions in early rheumatoid arthritis. *Arthritis Rheum* 2001;44:1744–1753.
108. Sato T, Ito A, Mori Y. Interleukin 6 enhances the production of tissue inhibitor of metalloproteinases (TIMP) but not that of matrix metalloproteinases by human fibroblasts. *Biochem Biophys Res Commun* 1990;170:824–829.
109. Lotz M, Guerne PA. Interleukin-6 induces the synthesis of tissue inhibitor of metalloproteinases-1/erythroid potentiating activity (TIMP-1/EPA). *J Biol Chem* 1991;266:2017–2020.
110. MacNaul KL, Chartrain N, Lark M, et al. Discoordinate expression of stromelysin, collagenase, and tissue inhibitor of metalloproteinases-1 in rheumatoid synovial fibroblasts: synergistic effects of interleukin-1 and tumor necrosis factor-α on stromelysin expression. *J Biol Chem* 1990;265:17238–17245.
111. Firestein GS, Paine MM, Littman BH. Gene expression (collagenase, tissue inhibitor of metalloproteinases, complement, and HLA-DR) in rheumatoid arthritis and osteoarthritis synovium. *Arthritis Rheum* 1991;34:1094–1105.
112. van der Laan WH, Quax PHA, Seemayer CA, et al. Cartilage degradation and invasion by rheumatoid synovial fibroblasts is inhibited by gene transfer of TIMP-1 and TIMP-3. *Gene Ther* 2003;10:234–242
113. Lark MW, Bayne EK, Flanagan J, et al. Aggrecan degradation in human cartilage. Evidence for both matrix metalloproteinase and aggrecanase activity in normal, osteoarthritic, and rheumatoid joints. *J Clin Invest* 1997;100:93–106.
114. Vankemmelbeke MN, Ilic MZ, Handley CJ, et al. Coincubation of bovine synovial or capsular tissue with cartilage generates a soluble "aggrecanase" activity. *Biochem Biophys Res Commun* 1999;255: 686–691.
115. Arner EC, Pratta MA, Trzaskos JM, et al. Generation and characterization of aggrecanase: a soluble, cartilage-derived aggrecan-degrading ability. *J Biol Chem* 1999;274:6594–6601.
116. Abbaszade I, Liu RQ, Yang F, et al. Cloning and characterization of ADAMTS11, an aggrecanase from the ADAMTS family. *J Biol Chem* 1999;274:23443–23450.
117. Tortorella MD, Burn TC, Pratta MA, et al. Purification and cloning of aggrecanase-1: a member of the ADAMTS family of proteins. *Science* 1999;284:1664–1666.
118. Moore CP, Willkens RF. The subcutaneous nodule: its significance in the diagnosis of rheumatic disease. *Semin Arthritis Rheum* 1977;7: 63–79.
119. Hurd ER. Extraarticular manifestations of rheumatoid arthritis. *Semin Arthritis Rheum* 1979;8:151–176.
120. Karam NE, Roger L, Hankins LL, et al. Rheumatoid nodulosis of the meninges. *J Rheumatol* 1994;21:1960–1963.
121. Sasaki S, Nakamura K, Oda H, et al. Thoracic myelopathy due to intraspinal rheumatoid nodules. *Scand J Rheumatol* 1997;26:227–228.
122. Friedman BA, Rice DH. Rheumatoid nodules of the larynx. *Arch Otolaryngol* 1975;101:361–363.
123. Woo P, Mendelsohn J, Humphrey D. Rheumatoid nodules of the larynx. *Otolaryngol Head Neck Surg* 1995;113:147–150.
124. Konishi T, Saida T, Nishitani H. Orbital apex syndrome caused by rheumatoid nodules. *J Neurol Neurosurg Psychiatry* 1986;49:460–462.
125. Starok M, Eilenberg SS, Resnick D. Rheumatoid nodules: MRI characteristics. *Clin Imaging* 1998;22:216–219.
126. El-Noueam KI, Giuliano V, Schweitzer ME, et al. Rheumatoid nodules: MR/pathological correlation. *J Comput Assist Tomogr* 1997;21: 796–799.
127. Adelman HM, Dupont EL, Flannery MT, et al. Case report: recurrent pneumothorax in a patient with rheumatoid arthritis. *Am J Med Sci* 1994;308:171–172.
128. Laloux L, Chevalier X, Maitre B, et al. Unusual onset of rheumatoid arthritis with diffuse pulmonary nodulosis: a diagnostic problem. *J Rheumatol* 1999;26:920–922.
129. Appleton MA, Ismail SM. Ulcerating rheumatoid nodule of the vulva. *J Clin Pathol* 1996;49:85–87.
130. Fukase M, Koizumi F, Wakaki K. Histopathologic analysis of sixteen subcutaneous nodules. *Acta Pathol Jpn* 1980;30:871–882.
131. Ziff M. The rheumatoid nodule. *Arthritis Rheum* 1990;33:761–767.
132. Nosanchuk JS, Naylor B. A unique cytologic picture in pleural fluid from patients with rheumatoid arthritis. *Am J Clin Pathol* 1968;50: 330–335.
133. Duke OL, Hobbs S, Panayi GS, et al. A combined immunohistological and histochemical analysis of lymphocyte and macrophage subpopulations in the rheumatoid nodule. *Clin Exp Immunol* 1984;56: 239–246.
134. Athanasou NA, Quinn J, Woods CG, et al. Immunohistology of rheumatoid nodules and rheumatoid synovium. *Ann Rheum Dis* 1988;47: 398–403.
135. Elewaut D, De Keyser F, De Wever N, et al. A comparative phenotypical analysis of rheumatoid nodules and rheumatoid synovium with special reference to adhesion molecules and activation markers. *Ann Rheum Dis* 1998;57:480–486.
136. Wikaningrum R, Highton J, Parker A, et al. Pathogenetic mechanisms in the rheumatoid nodule: comparison of proinflammatory cytokine production and cell adhesion molecule expression in rheumatoid nodules and synovial membranes from the same patient. *Arthritis Rheum* 1998;41:1783–1797.
137. Levesque ML, Radcliff G, Haynes BF. *In vitro* culture of human peripheral blood monocytes induces monocyte-hyaluronan binding and upregulates monocyte variant CD44 isoform expression. *J Immunol* 1996;156:1557–1565.
138. Hale LP, Haynes BF, McCachren SS. CD44 variants in human inflammatory synovitis. *J Clin Immunol* 1995;15:300–311.
139. Patterson JW. Rheumatoid nodule and subcutaneous granuloma annulare: a comparative histologic study. *Ann J Dermatopathol* 1988; 10:1–8.
140. Filho JS, Soares MF, Wal R, et al. Fine needle aspiration cytology of pulmonary rheumatoid nodule: case report and review of the major cytologic features. *Diagn Cytopathol* 2002;26:150–153.
141. Alarcon GS, Koopman WJ, McCarty MJ. Nonperipheral accelerated nodulosis in a methotrexate-treated rheumatoid arthritis patient. *Arthritis Rheum* 1993;36:132–133.
142. Williams FM, Cohen PR, Arnett FC. Accelerated cutaneous nodulosis during methotrexate therapy in a patient with rheumatoid arthritis. *J Am Acad Dermatol* 1998;39:359–362.
143. Falcini F, TaccettiG, Ermini M, et al. Methotrexate-associated appearance and rapid progression of rheumatoid nodules in systemic-onset juvenile rheumatoid arthritis. *Arthritis Rheum* 1997;40:175–178.
144. Spadaro A, Fiore D, Iagnocco A, et al. Rheumatoid nodules and cyclosporin A treatment. *Int J Clin Pharmacol Res* 1994;14:75–78.
145. DiFrancesco L, Miller F, Greenwald RA. Detailed immunohistologic evaluation of a methotrexate-induced nodule. *Arch Pathol Lab Med* 1994;118:1223–1225.
146. Danning CL, Illei GG, Boumpas DT. Vasculitis associated with primary rheumatologic diseases. *Curr Opin Rheumatol* 1998;10:58–65.

147. Babian M, Nasef S, Soloway G. Gastrointestinal infarction as a manifestation of rheumatoid vasculitis. *Am J Gastroenterol* 1998;93:119–120.
148. Scott DGI, Bacon PA, Tribe CR. Systemic rheumatoid vasculitis: a clinical and laboratory study of 50 cases. *Medicine* 1981;60:288–297.
149. Reimer KA, Rodgers RF, Oyasu R. Rheumatoid arthritis with rheumatoid heart disease and granulomatous aortitis. *JAMA* 1976;235:2510–2512.
150. Gravallese EM, Corson JM, Coblyn JS, et al. Rheumatoid aortitis: a rarely recognized but clinically significant entity. *Medicine* 1989;68:95–106.
151. Kuehne SE, Gauvin GP, Shortsleeve MJ. Small bowel stricture caused by rheumatoid vasculitis. *Radiology* 1992;184:215–216.
152. Craig SD, Jorizzo JL, White WL, et al. Cutaneous signs of rheumatic disease: acral purpuric papules in a patient with clinical rheumatoid arthritis. *Arthritis Rheum* 1994;37:957–959.
153. Smith ML, Jorizzo JL, Semble E, et al. Rheumatoid papules: lesions showing features of vasculitis and palisading granuloma. *J Am Acad Dermatol* 1989;20:348–352.
154. Conn DL, McDuffie FC, Dyck PJ. Immunopathologic study of sural nerves in rheumatoid arthritis. *Arthritis Rheum* 1972;15:135–143.
155. Van der Zee JM, Heurkens AHM, van der Voort EAM, et al. Characterization of anti-endothelial antibodies in patients with rheumatoid arthritis complicated by vasculitis. *Clin Exp Rheumatol* 1991;9:589–594.
156. Salih AM, Nixon NB, Dawes PT, et al. Soluble adhesion molecules and anti-endothelial cell antibodies in patients with rheumatoid arthritis complicated by peripheral neuropathy. *J Rheumatol* 1999;26:551–555.
157. Voskuyl AE, van Duinen SG, Zwinderman AH, et al. The diagnostic value of perivascular infiltrates in muscle biopsy specimens for the assessment of rheumatoid vasculitis. *Ann Rheum Dis* 1998;57:114–117.
158. Voskuyl AE, Emeis JJ, Hazes JM, et al. Levels of circulating cellular fibronectin are increased in patients with rheumatoid vasculitis. *Clin Exp Rheumatol* 1998;16:429–434.
159. Kuryliszyn-Moskel A. Cytokines and soluble CD4 and CD8 molecules in rheumatoid arthritis: relationships to systemic vasculitis and microvascular capillaroscopic abnormalities. *Clin Rheumatol* 1998;17:489–495.
160. Baggenstoss AH, Rosenberg EF. Visceral lesions associated with chronic infectious (rheumatoid) arthritis. *Arch Pathol* 1943;35:503–516.
161. Horler AR, Thompson M. The pleural and pulmonary complications of rheumatoid arthritis. *Ann Intern Med* 1959;51:1179–1203.
162. Aru A, Engel E, Francis D. Characteristic and specific histological findings in rheumatoid pleurisy. *Acta Path Microbiol Immunol Scand* 1986A;94:57–62.
163. Pritikin ND, Jensen WA, Yenokida GG, et al. Respiratory failure due to a massive rheumatoid pleural effusion. *J Rheumatol* 1990;17:673–675.
164. Tarn AC, Lapworth R. Biochemical analysis of pleural fluid: what should we measure? *Ann Clin Biochem* 2001;38:311–322.
165. Dodson WH, Hollingsworth JW. Pleural effusion in rheumatoid arthritis: impaired transport of glucose. *N Engl J Med* 1966;275:1337–1342.
166. Joseph J, Sahn SA. Connective tissue diseases and the pleura. *Chest* 1993;104:262–270.
167. Soderblom T, Pettersson T, Nyberg P, et al. High pleural fluid hyaluronan concentrations in rheumatoid arthritis. *Eur Respir J* 1999;13:519–522.
168. Naylor B. The pathognomonic cytologic picture of rheumatoid pleuritis: the 1989 Maurice Goldblatt cytology award lecture. *Acta Cytol* 1990;34:465–473.
169. Boddington MM, Spriggs AI, Morton JA, et al. Cytodiagnosis of rheumatoid pleural effusions. *J Clin Pathol* 1971;24:95–106.
170. Engel U, Aru A, Francis D. Rheumatoid pleurisy: specificity of cytologic findings. *Acta Path Microbiol Immunol Scand* 1986A;94:53–56.
171. Chou C-W, Chang S-C. Pleuritis as a presenting manifestation of rheumatoid arthritis:diagnostic clues in pleural fluid cytology. *Am J Med Sci* 2002;323:158–161.
172. Shiel WC Jr, Prete PF. Pleuropulmonary manifestations of rheumatoid arthritis. *Semin Arthritis Rheum* 1984;13:235–243.
173. Gilligan DM, O'Connor CM, Ward K, et al. Bronchoalveolar lavage in patients with mild and severe rheumatoid lung disease. *Thorax* 1990;45:591–596.
174. Suzuki A, Ohosone Y, Obana M, et al. Cause of death in 81 autopsied patients with rheumatoid arthritis. *J Rheumatol* 1994;21:33–36.
175. Gabbay E, Lake FR, Cameron D, et al. Interstitial lung disease in recent onset rheumatoid arthritis. *Am J Respir Crit Care Med* 1997;156:528–525.
176. Gochuico BR. Potential pathogenesis and clinical aspects of pulmonary fibrosis associated with rheumatoid arthritis. *Am J Med Sci* 2001;321:83–88.
177. Colby TV. Pathologic aspects of bronchiolitis obliterans organizing pneumonia. *Chest* 1992;102(suppl):38–43.
178. Sternberg SS, ed. *Diagnostic surgical pathology,* 3rd ed. Philadelphia: Lippincott Williams & Wilkins, 1999:1018.
179. Magro CM, Morrison C, Pope-Harman A, et al. Direct and indirect immunofluorescence as a diagnostic adjunct in the interpretation of nonneoplastic medical lung disease. *Am J Clin Pathol* 2003;119:279–289.
180. Caplan A. Certain unusual radiological appearances in the chest of coal miners suffering from rheumatoid arthritis. *Thorax* 1953;8:29–37.
181. Williams WJ. Caplan's syndrome. *Br J Clin Pract* 1991;45:285–288.
182. Shannon TM, Gale ME. Noncardiac manifestations of rheumatoid arthritis in the thorax. *J Thorac Imaging* 1992;7:19–29.
183. Goehrs HR, Baggenstoss AH, Slocumb CH. Cardiac lesions in rheumatoid arthritis. *Arthritis Rheum* 1960;3:298–308.
184. Mody GM, Stevens JE, Meyers OL. The heart in rheumatoid arthritis—a clinical and echocardiographic study. *Q J Med* 1987;65:921–928.
185. Bonfiglio T, Atwater EC. Heart disease in patients with seropositive rheumatoid arthritis: a controlled autopsy study and review. *Arch Intern Med* 1969;124:714–719.
186. Lebowitz WB. The heart in rheumatoid arthritis: a clinical and pathologic study of 62 cases. *Ann Intern Med* 1963;58:102–123.
187. Suriani RJ, Lansman S, Konstadt S. Intracardiac rheumatoid nodule presenting as a left atrial mass. *Am Heart J* 1994;127:463–465.
188. Webber MD, Selsky EJ, Roper PA. Identification of a mobile intracardiac rheumatoid nodule mimicking an atrial myxoma. *J Am Soc Echocardiogr* 1995;8:961–964.
189. Mounet FS, Soula P, Concina P, et al. A rare case of embolizing cardiac tumor: rheumatoid nodule of the mitral valve. *J Heart Valve Dis* 1997;6:77–78.
190. Chand EM, Freant LJ, Rubin JW. Aortic valve rheumatoid nodules producing clinical aortic regurgitation and a review of the literature. *Cardiovasc Pathol* 1999;8:333–338.
191. Shimaya K, Kurihashi A, Masago R, et al. Rheumatoid arthritis and simultaneous aortic, mitral, and tricuspid valve incompetence. *Int J Cardiol* 1999;71:181–183.
192. Abbas A, Byrd BF. Right-sided heart failure due to right ventricular cavity obliteration by rheumatoid nodules. *Am J Cardiol* 2000;86:711–712.
193. Morris PB, Inber MJ, Heinsimer JA, et al. Rheumatoid arthritis and coronary arteritis. *Am J Cardiol* 1986;57:689–690.
194. Cotran RS, Kumar V, Collins T. *Robbins pathologic basis of disease,* 6th ed. Philadelphia: WB Saunders, 1999:589.
195. Thompson M, Eadie S. Keratoconjunctivitis sicca and rheumatoid arthritis. *Ann Rheum Dis* 1956;15:21–25.
196. Reddy CV, Foster CS. Adult rheumatoid arthritis. In: Albert DM, Jakobiec FA, eds. *Principles and practice of ophthalmology.* Philadelphia: WB Saunders, 1994.
197. Sjögren H, Bloch KJ. Keratoconjunctivitis sicca and the Sjögren syndrome. *Surv Ophthalmol* 1971;16:145–159.
198. Michels ML, Cobo LM, Caldwell DS, et al. Rheumatoid arthritis and sterile corneal ulceration. *Arthritis Rheum* 1984;27:606–616.
199. Dayer J-M, Russell RGG, Krane SM. Collagenase production by rheumatoid synovial cells: stimulation by a human lymphocyte factor. *Science* 1977;195:181–183.
200. Squirrell DM, Winfield J, Amos RS. Peripheral ulcerative keratitis "corneal melt" and rheumatoid arthritis: a case series. *Rheumatology* 1999;38:1245–1248.
201. Hazleman BL. Rheumatic disorders of the eye and the various structures involved. *Br J Rheumatol* 1996;35:258–268.
202. Watson PG, Hayreh SS. Scleritis and episcleritis. *Br J Ophthalmol* 1976;60:163–191.

203. Verhoeff FH, King MJ. Scleromalacia perforans. *Arch Ophthalmol* 1938;20:1013–1035.
204. McGavin DDM, Williamson J, Forrester JV, et al. Episcleritis and scleritis: a study of their clinical manifestations and associations with rheumatoid arthritis. *Br J Ophthalmol* 1976;60:192–226.
205. Riono WP, Hidayat AA, Rao NA. Scleritis: a clinicopathologic study of 55 cases. *Ophthalmology* 1999;106:1328–1333.
206. Rao NA, Marak GE, Hidayat AA. Necrotizing scleritis: a clinicopathologic study of 41 cases. *Ophthalmology* 1985;92:1542–1549.
207. Matsuo T, Koyama T, Morimoto N, et al. Retinal vasculitis as a complication of rheumatoid arthritis. *Ophthalmologica* 1990;201:196–200.
208. Giordano N, D'Ettorre M, Biasi G, et al. Retinal vasculitis in rheumatoid arthritis: an angiographic study. *Clin Exp Rheumatol* 1990; 8:121–125.
209. Motulsky AG, Weinburg S, Saphir O, et al. Lymph nodes in rheumatoid arthritis. *Arch Intern Med* 1952;90:660–676.
210. Robertson MDJ, Dudley HF, White WF, et al. Rheumatoid lymphadenopathy. *Ann Rheum Dis* 1968;27:253–260.
211. Symmons DPM, Ahern M, Bacon PA, et al. Lymphoproliferative malignancy in rheumatoid arthritis: a study of 20 cases. *Ann Rheum Dis* 1984;43:132–135.
212. Kojima M, Hosomura Y, Itoh H, et al. Reactive proliferative lesions in lymph nodes from rheumatoid arthritis patients: a clinicopathological and immunohistological study. *Acta Pathol Jpn* 1990;40:249–254.
213. Numata Y, Matsuura Y, Onishi S, et al. Case report: interleukin-6 positive follicular hyperplasia in the lymph node of a patient with rheumatoid arthritis. *Am J Hematol* 1991;36:282–284.
214. Kondratowicz GM, Symmons DPM, Bacon PA, et al. Rheumatoid lymphadenopathy: a morphological and immunohistochemical study. *J Clin Pathol* 1990;40:106–113.
215. McCluggage WG, Bharucha H. Lymph node hyalinisation in rheumatoid arthritis and systemic sclerosis. *J Clin Pathol* 1994;47:138–142.
216. Fishman D, Isenberg DA. Splenic involvement in rheumatic diseases. *Semin Arthritis Rheum* 1997;27:141–155.
217. Rosenstein ED, Kramer N. Felty's and pseudo-Felty's syndromes. *Semin Arthritis Rheum* 1991;21:129–142.
218. Laszlo J, Jones R, Silberman HR, et al. Splenectomy for Felty's syndrome: clinicopathological study of 27 patients. *Arch Intern Med* 1978;138:597–602.
219. van Krieken JHJM, Breedveld FC, te Velde J. The spleen in Felty's syndrome: a histological, morphometrical, and immunohistochemical study. *Eur J Hematol* 1988;40:58–64.
220. Campbell DA, Corman LC, Williams RC Jr. Splenectomy as treatment for nonhealing soft tissue defect after total knee arthroplasty in a patient with Felty's syndrome. *J Rheumatol* 1992;19:1126–1129.
221. Barnes CG, Turnbull AL, Vernon-Roberts B. Felty's syndrome: a clinical and pathological survey of 21 patients and their response to treatment. *Ann Rheum Dis* 1971;30:359–374.
222. Young ID, Segura J, Ford PM, et al. The pathogenesis of nodular regenerative hyperplasia of the liver associated with rheumatoid vasculitis. *J Clin Gastroenterol* 1992;14:127–131.
223. Ruiz FP, Martinez FJO, Mendoza ACZ, et al. Nodular regenerative hyperplasia of the liver in rheumatic diseases: report of seven cases and review of the literature. *Semin Arthritis Rheum* 1991;21:47–54.
224. Goritsas C, Roussos A, Ferti A, et al. Nodular regenerative hyperplasia in a rheumatoid arthritis patient without Felty's syndrome. *J Clin Gastroenterol* 2002;35:363–364.
225. Kraus A, Palacios A, Munoz L. Muscular involvement in systemic rheumatoid vasculitis. *Br J Rheumatol* 1992;31:355–356.
226. Chang DJ, Paget SA. Neurologic complications of rheumatoid arthritis. *Rheum Clin North Am* 1993;19:955–973.
227. Puechal X, Said G, Job-Deslandre C, et al. Muscular involvement in systemic rheumatoid vasculitis. *Br J Rheumatol* 1993;32:766–767.
228. Cannon GW. Pulmonary complications of antirheumatic therapy. *Semin Arthritis Rheum* 1990;19:353–364.
229. Zitnik RJ, Cooper JAD Jr. Pulmonary disease due to antirheumatic agents. *Clin Chest Med* 1990;11:139–150.
230. Hamadeh MA, Atkinson J, Smith LJ. Sulfasalazine-induced pulmonary disease. *Chest* 1992;101:1033–1037.
231. Keane J, Gershon S, Wise RP, et al. Tuberculosis associated with infliximab, a tumor necrosis factor (alpha)-neutralizing agent. *N Engl J Med* 2001;345:1098–1104.
232. Lee J-H, Slifman NR, Gershon SK, et al. Life-threatening histoplasmosis complicating immunotherapy with tumor necrosis factor α antagonists infliximab and etanercept. *Arthritis Rheum* 2002;46:2565–2570.
233. Hargreaves MR, Mowat AG, Benson MK. Acute pneumonitis associated with low dose methotrexate treatment for rheumatoid arthritis: report of five cases and review of published reports. *Thorax* 1992; 47:628–633.
234. Carroll GJ, Thomas R, Phatouros CC, et al. Incidence, prevalence, and possible risk factors for pneumonitis in patients with rheumatoid arthritis receiving methotrexate. *J Rheumatol* 1994;21:51–54.
235. St. Clair EW, Rice JR, Snyderman R. Pneumonitis complicating low-dose methotrexate therapy in rheumatoid arthritis. *Arch Intern Med* 1985;145:2035–2038.
236. Lang B, Riegel W, Peters T, et al. Low dose methotrexate therapy for rheumatoid arthritis complicated by pancytopenia and *Pneumocystis carinii* pneumonia. *J Rheumatol* 1991;18:1257–1259.
237. Flood DA, Chan CK, Pruzanski W. *Pneumocystis carinii* pneumonia associated with methotrexate therapy in rheumatoid arthritis. *J Rheumatol* 1991;18:1254–1256.
238. Law KF, Aranda CP, Smith RL, et al. Pulmonary cryptococcosis mimicking methotrexate pneumonia. *J Rheumatol* 1993;20:872–873.
239. Carson CW, Cannon GW, Egger MJ, et al. Pulmonary disease during the treatment of rheumatoid arthritis with low dose pulse methotrexate. *Semin Arthritis Rheum* 1987;16:186–195.
240. Leduc D, De Vuyst P, Lheureux P, et al. Pneumonitis complicating low-dose methotrexate therapy for rheumatoid arthritis: discrepancies between lung biopsy and bronchoalveolar lavage findings. *Chest* 1993;104:1620–1623.
241. Dawson JK, Graham DR, Desmond J, et al. Investigation of the chronic pulmonary effects of low-dose oral methotrexate in patients with rheumatoid arthritis: a prospective study incorporating HRCT scanning and pulmonary function tests. *Rheumatology* 2002;41:262–267.
242. Shergy WJ, Polisson RP, Caldwell DS, et al. Methotrexate-associated hepatotoxicity: retrospective analysis of 210 patients with rheumatoid arthritis. *Am J Med* 1988;85:771–774.
243. Aponte J, Petrelli M. Histopathologic findings in the liver of rheumatoid arthritis patients treated with long-term bolus methotrexate. *Arthritis Rheum* 1988;31:1457–1464.
244. Walker AM, Funch D, Dreyer NA, et al. Determinants of serious liver disease among patients receiving low-dose methotrexate for rheumatoid arthritis. *Arthritis Rheum* 1993;36:329–335.
245. Phillips CA, Cera PJ, Mangan TF, et al. Clinical liver disease in patients with rheumatoid arthritis taking methotrexate. *J Rheumatol* 1992;19:229–233.
246. Whiting-O'Keefe QE, Fye KH, Sack KD. Methotrexate and hepatic abnormalities: a meta-analysis. *Am J Med* 1991;90:711–716.
247. Kremer JM, Koff R. A debate: should patients with rheumatoid arthritis on methotrexate undergo liver biopsies? *Semin Arthritis Rheum* 1992;21:376–386.
248. Ruderman EM, Crawford JM, Maier A, et al. Histologic liver abnormalities in an autopsy series of patients with rheumatoid arthritis. *Br J Rheumatol* 1997;36:210–213.
249. Fleischner GM, Morecki R, Hanaichi T, et al. Light- and electron-microscopical study of a case of gold salt-induced hepatotoxicity. *Hepatology* 1991;14:422–425.
250. Landas SK, Mitros FA, Furst DE, et al. Lipogranulomas and gold in the liver in rheumatoid arthritis. *Am J Surg Pathol* 1992;16:171–174.
251. Silverberg DS, Kidd EG, Shnitka TK, et al. Gold nephropathy: a clinical and pathologic study. *Arthritis Rheum* 1970;13:812–825.
252. Hall CL, Jawad S, Harrison PR, et al. Natural course of penicillamine nephropathy: a long-term study of 33 patients. *BMJ* 1988;296:1083–1086.
253. McCormick SA, DiBartolomeo AG, Raju VK, et al. Ocular chrysiasis. *Ophthalmology* 1985;92:1432–1435.
254. Koizumi F, Matsuno H, Wakaki K, et al. Synovitis in rheumatoid arthritis: scoring of characteristic histopathological features. *Pathol Int* 1999;49:298–304.
255. Fonseca JE, Canhao H, Resende C, et al. Histology of synovial tissue: value of semiquantitative analysis for the prediction of joint erosions in rheumatoid arthritis. *Clin Exp Rheumatol* 2000;18:559–564.

256. Kulka JP, Bocking D, Ropes MW, et al. Early joint lesions of rheumatoid arthritis: report of 8 cases with knee biopsies of lesions of less than one year's duration. *Arch Pathol* 1955;59:129–139.
257. Okada Y, Shinmei M, Tanaka O, et al. Location of matrix metalloproteinase 3 (stromelysin) in osteoarthritic cartilage and synovium. *Lab Invest* 1992;66:680–690.
258. Cotran RS, Kumar V, Collins T. *Robbins pathologic basis of disease,* 6th edition. Philadelphia: WB Saunders, 1999:1248–1251.
259. Cooper NS, Soren A, McEwen C, et al. Diagnostic specificity of synovial lesions. *Hum Pathol* 1981;12:314–328.
260. Veal D, Yanni G, Rogers S, et al. Reduced synovial membrane macrophage numbers, ELAM-1 expression, and lining layer hyperplasia in psoriatic arthritis as compared with rheumatoid arthritis. *Arthritis Rheum* 1993;36:893–900.
261. Natour J, Montezzo LC, Moura LA, et al. A study of synovial membrane of patients with systemic lupus erythematosus (SLE). *Clin Exp Rheum* 1991;9:221–225.
262. Barkley D, Allard S, Feldmann M, et al. Increased expression of HLA-DQ antigens by interstitial cells and endothelium in the synovial membrane of rheumatoid arthritis patients compared with reactive arthritis patients. *Arthritis Rheum* 1989;32:955–963.
263. Nordstrom DC. DNA synthesis in CD4- and CD8-positive cells in synovial fluid of patients with reactive and rheumatoid arthritis. *Rheumatol Int* 1989;8:269–272.
264. Baeten D, Demetter P, Cuvelier C, et al. Comparative study of synovial histology in rheumatoid arthritis, spondyloarthropathy, and osteoarthritis: influence of disease duration and activity. *Ann Rheum Dis* 2000;59:945–953.
265. Sipe JS. Amyloidosis. *Ann Rev Biochem* 1992;61:947–975.
266. Pai S, Helin H, Isomaki H. Frequency of amyloidosis in Estonian patients with rheumatoid arthritis. *Scand J Rheumatol* 1993;22:248–249.
267. Dhillon V, Woo P, Isenberg D. Amyloidosis in the rheumatic diseases. *Ann Rheum Dis* 1989;48:696–701.
268. Husby G. Amyloidosis. *Semin Arthritis Rheum* 1992;22:67–82.
269. Tiitinen S, Kaarela K, Helin H, et al. Amyloidosis—incidence and early risk factors in patients with rheumatoid arthritis. *Scand J Rheumatol* 1993;22:158–161.
270. Glenner GG, Page DL. Amyloid, amyloidosis, and amyloidogenesis. *Int Rev Exp Pathol* 1976;15:1–92.
271. Glenner GG, Eanes ED, Bladen HA, et al. β-pleated sheet fibrils: a comparison of native amyloid with synthetic protein fibrils. *J Histochem Cytochem* 1974;22:1141–1158.
272. Wolman M. Amyloid, its nature and molecular structure: comparison of a new toluidine blue polarized light method with traditional procedures. *Lab Invest* 1971;25:104–110.
273. Klemi PJ, Sorsa S, Happonen RP. Fine needle aspiration biopsy from subcutaneous fat: an easy method to diagnose secondary amyloidosis. *Scand J Rheumatol* 1987;16:429–421.
274. Breedveld FC, Markusse HM, MacFarlane JD. Subcutaneous fat biopsy in the diagnosis of amyloidosis secondary to chronic arthritis. *Clin Exp Rheumatol* 1989;7:407–410.
275. Kuroda T, Tanabe N, Sakatsume M, et al. Comparison of gastroduodenal, renal, and abdominal fat biopsies for diagnosing amyloidosis in rheumatoid arthritis. *Clin Rheumatol* 2002;21:123–128
276. Sternberg SS, ed. *Diagnostic surgical pathology,* 3rd ed. Philadelphia: Lippincott Williams & Wilkins, 1999:855–856.
277. Wells AU, du Bois RM. Bronchiolitis in association with connective tissue disorders. *Clin Chest Med* 1993;14:655–666.
278. Strimlan CV, Rosenow EC, Divertie MB, et al. Pulmonary manifestations of Sjögren's syndrome. *Chest* 1976;70:354–361.
279. Kassan SS, Thomas TL, Moutsopoulos HM, et al. Increased risk of lymphoma in sicca syndrome. *Ann Intern Med* 1978;89:888–892.

CHAPTER 54

Mechanisms of Tissue Damage in Rheumatoid Arthritis

Hugo E. Jasin

Rheumatoid arthritis (RA) is characterized by chronic inflammation involving connective tissues throughout the body, but particularly diarthrodial joints. When the duration and severity of the inflammatory process reach a certain threshold, irreversible tissue damage occurs. The relative inability of the body's repair mechanisms to orchestrate *restitutio ad integrum* of the affected joint tissues also influences the degree of functional disability of a given patient affected with the disease. In this chapter, the mechanisms that play a role in the mediation of the pathologic changes described in Chapter 53 are discussed, including synovitis, cartilage, and soft connective tissue damage, pannus formation, fibrosis, and bone resorption. It is likely that many, if not most, of the inflammatory mechanisms known to be operative in RA are similar to those present in other chronic inflammatory processes. Currently, detailed descriptions of many potentially pathogenic mechanisms are available, but these mechanisms have been studied in isolation and are derived from *in vitro* analysis of rheumatoid tissues and fluids and investigation of experimental animal models. At this stage of our knowledge, however, it is not possible to assemble the pieces of the puzzle so as to be able to weigh the relative importance of each mechanism, cell, enzyme, cytokine, and so forth in the process of tissue damage and repair. This is, in part, due to the lack of adequate models that mimic the conditions present in the rheumatoid joint, particularly when the element of time is considered. To describe adequately the multiple pathogenic mechanisms operative in the rheumatoid process, it is necessary to analyze events occurring in the synovial membrane, synovial fluid, and articular cartilage compartments.

SYNOVIAL MEMBRANE

It is reasonable to assume that the early pathogenic events in RA occur at the level of the synovial membrane. The reasons for the preferential homing of inflammatory cells to this particular type of connective tissue are not well understood. It has been adduced that the synovium may be selected because it is subjected to mechanical trauma, its capillary walls are fenestrated (1), and it differs from undifferentiated connective tissue by the presence of a lining layer composed of phagocytic macrophage-like type A cells and fibroblastic type B cells (see Chapter 12). It should be pointed out that rheumatoid inflammation involves only synovial joints, sparing synarthroses and amphiarthroses. Moreover, joint immobilization and local neurologic compromise, which ameliorate the intensity of inflammation, underscore the importance of mechanical factors in RA. Another mechanism that may explain the involvement of diarthrodial joints in immunologically driven diseases is indicated by the observation that animals with experimental arthritis treated with a monoclonal antibody against CD44, a hyaluronic acid receptor present in most activated cells, experience rapid resolution of inflammation (2,3). Other studies have shown that cross-linking the CD44 receptor in rheumatoid synovial cells up-regulates the expression of adhesion molecules on these cells (4,5). These studies suggest that high concentrations of hyaluronate may be responsible for the homing of inflammatory cells to the synovial membrane. It is also clear that many of the factors and cells (to be discussed later) that are present in synovial fluid and contribute to irreversible joint damage derive directly or indirectly from the inflamed synovium.

Several investigators have studied the pathologic features of early rheumatoid synovitis (<12 months' duration) in an attempt to gain insights into the pathogenesis of rheumatoid inflammation (6–11). The evidence at hand suggests that in early synovitis the common histologic features include (a) lining layer hyperplasia, (b) microvascular alterations including hyperemia, capillary proliferation, small vessel occlusion,

TABLE 54.1. *Features of early synovitis in rheumatoid arthritis*

Lining cell layer hyperplasia
Hyperemia
Capillary proliferation
Perivascular CD4+ lymphocyte infiltration
B-lymphocyte infiltration
Expression of MHC class II markers

MHC, major histocompatibility complex.

and endothelial cell swelling, (c) perivascular accumulation of CD4+ lymphocytes of variable intensity, (d) presence of B cells and plasma cells commensurate with the degree of clinical inflammation, and (e) expression of class II major histocompatibility complex (MHC) markers by synoviocytes and mononuclear cells, and (f) presence of collagenase and cathepsin messenger RNA in the intima and subintima (Table 54.1). As the disease progresses to its chronic stage, the well-known, albeit nonspecific, histologic features of rheumatoid synovitis develop.

LYMPHOCYTES

Multiple studies of the immunologic status of the rheumatoid synovium suggest that infiltrating lymphoid cells exhibit markers of activation, such as MHC determinants and adhesion molecules (12–17). Prima facie evidence of activation and maturation of the T cells include the preponderance of CD45RO+ "memory T cells," as well as recent evidence suggesting that the cytokine profile appears to be skewed towards the helper T cell subset 2 (T_H2) phenotype of lymphocytes (see Chapter 19). These infiltrating T cells presumably mediate the activation and maturation of antibody-forming B cells by direct contact signaling, in concert with synoviocytes with accessory cell function (18,19) and cytokines such as interleukin-2 (IL-2), IL-3, IL-4, and IL-10 (20).

The origin of the exuberant cellular infiltration within the synovial membrane and the mechanisms involved in its maintenance are still unresolved. Several lines of evidence suggest that circulating helper T lymphocytes are of pivotal importance in this process. Significant amelioration of inflammatory activity in RA has been observed following depletion of recirculating lymphocytes by thoracic duct drainage (21) and total lymphoid irradiation (22,23). Modulation of disease activity by treatment with cyclosporine A (24) and anecdotal reports of disease remission in patients with RA and concomitant acquired immune deficiency syndrome (AIDS) (25,26), in which there is depletion of CD4+ T cells, provide additional evidence for the importance of helper T-cell function in RA. However, others (27) have reported continuing inflammatory activity in patients with AIDS and low circulating CD4 cells as evidence that in the later stages of the disease, the process may become "lymphocyte independent" (28). The unimpressive therapeutic effects of treatment with monoclonal antibodies against CD4 T cells reinforces this view (17).

The increased susceptibility to RA in subjects with alleles of human leukocyte antigen (HLA)-DR exhibiting the QKRAA motif (29) and the influence of these HLA-DRB1 alleles on disease severity (30) have prompted many investigators to study the possible selective expansion of the T-cell receptor repertoire in blood and affected joints under the assumption that one particular "arthritogenic" peptide present in the groove of the HLA-DR4 molecule may stimulate the proliferation of T cells bearing a particular T-cell receptor configuration (31). These studies have yielded variable results, perhaps due to the heterogeneity of the patient populations used, the methodology used to select the T cells to be studied, and the phenomenon of "epitope spreading" (32). Although some researchers found selective expansion of some Vβ alleles in synovial lymphocytes not seen in the circulating cell population (32a–35), others failed to do so (36–40). It is likely, however, that the circulating T cells homing to the synovium may be selected because of prior activation outside the joint. Indeed, the numbers of T lymphocytes bearing activation markers and adhesion molecules (15,41), and the levels of soluble T-cell activation products such as IL-2 and IL-2 receptors (42,43) are increased in the blood of patients with active RA.

The mechanisms whereby these activated T cells home to the inflamed synovium are under study (44–46). Adhesion molecule synthesis and expression appear to be upregulated in the microvasculature of rheumatoid synovium (47–50) (Table 54.2), probably as a result of exposure of the endothelial cells to cytokines such as IL-1 and tumor necrosis factor-α (TNF-α) (20). With the data available thus far, it is not possible to pinpoint which of the several adhesion families of molecules known to be operative in inflammatory foci play a major role in rheumatoid synovitis. Recent evidence suggests that adherence to endothelial cells in rheumatoid synovium involves predominantly the vascular cell adhesion molecule-1 (VCAM-1) and endothelial leukocyte adhesion molecule-1 (ELAM-1) counter-receptors (51–53). It is likely, however, that the process of cell adhesion and migration into tissues develops as a cooperative interaction between several receptors and ligands (54,55). Interaction of these adhesion molecules with their respective receptors and counterreceptors expressed in circulating activated cells may result in the selective homing of cell subpopulations. Pertinent to the preferential accumulation of selective T-cell receptor specificities is the observation that memory T-helper lymphocytes expressing the CD45RO+ marker show increased ability both to bind to, and migrate into, inflamed tissues (56–59).

Although the T cells infiltrating the synovium express a wide array of activation markers (see Chapter 53), it is paradoxic that they appear to be relatively unresponsive to stimuli that normally induce proliferation. Moreover, many

TABLE 54.2. *Adhesion molecules detected in human rheumatoid synovial tissue*

Adhesion molecules	Present in synovium			
	Endothelium	Leukocytes	Lining cells	Fibroblasts
E-selectin	Yes[a]	No	No	No
L-selectin	No	Yes	Yes	No
P-selectin	Yes	No	No	No
ICAM-1	Yes[a]	Yes	Yes[a]	Yes
ICAM-2	Yes	No	No	No
ICAM-3	No	Yes	Yes	?
PECAM	Yes	Yes	Yes[a]	?
VCAM-1	Yes[a]	No	No	No
VLA-1–6	No	Yes	No	No
LFA 1	No	Yes[a]	No	No
MAC-1	No	Yes[a]	No	No
β_3 integrins	Yes[a]	No	Yes	No
HCAM (CD44)	Yes	Yes	Yes[a]	Yes[a]

[a]Increased expression of the adhesion molecule in rheumatoid as compared with osteoarthritic synovial tissue. (Reproduced with permission from Mickecz K, Brennan FR, Kim JH, Glant TT. The role of adhesion molecules in the development of autoimmune arthritis. *Scand J Rheumatol* 1995;24(suppl 101):99–106.)

studies suggest that synovial T cells synthesize relatively low levels of cytokines such as IL-2 and interferon-γ (IFN-γ) (60,61). Thus, the bulk of the proinflammatory cytokines and inhibitors secreted by the synovial cellular infiltrate probably originate from macrophages, fibroblast-like cells, and chondrocytes (see Chapters 11, 12, and 14). Recent studies have unraveled several mechanisms that may contribute to the seemingly abnormal behavior of the synovial T cells. Prolonged exposure of T-cell clones to TNF-α inhibited subsequent proliferative responses to antigen challenge, as well as production of IL-2, IL-10, and IFN-γ, and expression of the IL-2 receptor α chain. Of interest in this regard, treatment of patients with RA with anti-TNF monoclonal antibody restored the proliferative responses of blood lymphocytes to recall antigens (62). Transforming growth factor-β (TGF-β) has been shown to exert powerful inhibitory effects on T lymphocytes. In rheumatoid synovial fluid, it may account for a significant fraction of the antiproliferative effect on helper T cells (63,64). This factor also inhibits IL-1-induced lymphocyte proliferation (65). The important modulatory activity of TGF-β is underscored by studies in TGF-β knockout mice showing that these animals develop widespread visceral infiltration of mononuclear cells, resulting in generalized inflammatory disease (66). Another cytokine produced by synovial mononuclear cells, IL-10 (67–69) has been shown to be a major inhibitory factor of inflammatory responses by inhibition of T_H1 function (70) and IFN-γ production by synovial cells (67). IL-10 also mediates inhibition of accessory CD28/B7 receptor interactions, and it interferes with the antigen-presenting capacity of synovial macrophages (71). Prostaglandins also exert a modulatory effect on helper T cells. In the presence of prostaglandin E_2, T_H1 responses are suppressed and T_H0-like responses are shifted toward a T_H2-like pattern reflected in increased secretion of IL-4 and IL-5 (72). Similarly, nitric oxide (NO) inhibits secretion of IL-2 and IFN-γ by murine T cells without affecting production of IL-4 by T_H2 cells (73). The underlying defective T-cell responses have been recently identified as being the consequence of impaired signal transduction via the TCR/CD3 complex (74).

Circulating and synovial B lymphocytes also show evidence of activation in RA. In patients with active disease, circulating, activated B cells spontaneously secrete rheumatoid factor *in vitro* (75,76). This correlates with the degree of clinical inflammatory activity in individual patients (77,78), again suggesting that cell activation may originate in central lymphoid organs. Prima facie evidence of B-lymphocyte activation at the level of the synovial membrane is demonstrated histologically by the abundance of plasma cells in chronic RA (see Chapters 52 and 53), and by classic studies showing that the rheumatoid synovial cells synthesize and secrete large amounts of immunoglobulins (79,80), which in some cases may account for as much as 20% of all the immunoglobulins produced by the body (80). In the case of immunoglobulin-producing cells, it is well established that B lymphocytes programmed to secrete antibodies of selective specificities are enriched in rheumatoid synovium. Several studies have shown that rheumatoid synovial cells synthesize and secrete large amounts of rheumatoid factor in seropositive patients (81,82). Similarly, plasma cells in the synovial infiltrate have been shown to produce autoantibodies directed against collagen type II (83,84). It is likely that a significant proportion of the immune complexes found in synovium (85), synovial fluid (86), and cartilage (87,88) derive from locally synthesized autoantibodies. An additional interesting function for the synovial B cells in RA has also been reported (89). Based on synovial tissue transfer into severe combined immunodeficient (SCID) mouse chimeras and B-cell depletion studies, it was found that T-cell activation and cytokine secretion depended on the presence of B lymphocytes. Lymphoid follicles devoid of B cells failed to activate T lymphocytes.

NONLYMPHOCYTIC CELLS

A major cellular component of the inflamed rheumatoid synovial membrane includes the tissue macrophage and macrophage-like cells. These probably originate from bone marrow–derived, rapidly dividing precursors, and, as previously indicated for T and B lymphocytes, they circulate as monocytes, exhibiting evidence of activation (42,90,91). Blood monocytes from patients with RA spontaneously secrete greater amounts of prostaglandin E2, leukotriene B4, IL-1β (90), and angiotensin-converting enzyme (91) than their normal counterparts. Other studies suggest that they adhere to activated endothelial cells in inflamed rheumatoid synovium mainly by interacting with the P-selectin adhesion molecule (92). Cells with tissue macrophage characteristics constitute a major population in rheumatoid tissue. They are closely associated with T cells in relatively acellular, transitional, and lymphocyte-rich areas of synovium (93), suggesting that they may function as antigen-presenting cells (94). Additionally, they may contribute directly to the wide array of cytokines and chemokines (95–97) and indirectly to the proteolytic enzymes and arachidonate metabolites synthesized locally and secreted into the synovial cavity. A balanced review on the relative importance of the mononuclear phagocyte in the rheumatoid inflammatory process has been published (98).

Studies dealing with the characterization of synovial nonlymphocytic mononuclear cells have recognized two types of cells with dendritic appearance but with widely differing phenotypes (99–101). One population appears to be nonphagocytic, lacks Fcγ receptors and monocyte and fibroblast membrane markers, and expresses large amounts of HLA-DQ surface antigens (101). These cells have been shown to produce IL-1 (100), so they may be related to previously described dendritic cells in other tissues and blood (102), which are highly efficient antigen-presenting cells. Although there is evidence that the autoantibodies produced by rheumatoid synovial B lymphocytes and plasma cells exhibit features of an antigen-driven immune response (103), the identity of the cells responsible for antigen presentation within the synovial cell exudate remains unresolved (104).

A second population of cells with dendritic cell characteristics isolated from rheumatoid synovium appears to be of the fibroblast lineage (99,101). These cells divide rapidly *in vitro,* are devoid of phagocytic capacity, lack monocyte/macrophage markers, are HLA-DR$^+$/DQ$^-$, and produce IL-1. Their dendritic appearance results from exposure to prostaglandin E2, and activation of adenyl cyclase (105). These cells may be related to a pannus cell population that is also HLA-DR$^+$/DQ$^-$ (106), suggesting that they may play an important role in cartilage damage in RA. Recent evidence indicates that interaction of fibroblast-like synoviocytes with B lymphocytes induces increased survival and terminal differentiation of the latter cells resulting in increased antibody production (107). A related cell type with characteristics resembling "nurse cells" first described by Wekerle (108), believed to play an important role in T-cell maturation in mice, have been recently isolated from rheumatoid synovial membrane (109). These cells spontaneously produced large amounts of proinflammatory cytokines, and when in direct contact with B cells, they induced proliferation and immunoglobulin synthesis *in vitro*.

Another cell type that may play a role in the rheumatoid inflammatory process is the mast cell (see Chapter 17). These cells have been found in increased numbers in the rheumatoid synovium (110,111) and in areas of cartilage erosion (112). Their abundance correlates with the degree of clinical activity (110) and synovial cell infiltration (113). Synovial mast cells have been shown to be fully functional in that they are able to degranulate and secrete histamine in the presence of secretagogues or when their Fcε receptors are cross-linked with anti-IgE antibodies (114). Moreover, rheumatoid synovial fluids have been shown to contain increased levels of histamine (113,114) and tryptase (115) when compared with plasma. Although their role in joint inflammation has not been fully defined, activated mast cells can secrete a wide array of cytokines (116–119), including IL-3 and IL-4, TGF-β, granulocyte macrophage-colony stimulating factor (GM-CSF), and chemotactic factors (120), in addition to the traditional preformed products such as histamine, heparin, and tryptase. Recent studies indicate that mast cells acting through some of the above-mentioned cytokines, particularly IL-4 and TGF-β, may be involved in the process of fibrosis (121–123). The potential importance of mast cells in the generation of joint inflammation has been recently highlighted in a murine model of autoimmune arthritis in K/BxN mice (124). In this model, erosive arthritis results from an autoantibody response to a ubiquitous enzyme, glucose 6-phosphate isomerase. The arthritis appears to be solely dependent on the presence of the autoantibody since it can be generated passively in unrelated animals by transfer of serum from the K/BxN mice. However, mice lacking mast cells were resistant to the development of arthritis, and the susceptibility was restored after mast cell engraftment (124).

In summary, the inflammatory synovitis in RA is characterized by evidence of widespread activation of all cell types involved. Whether maintenance of a sustained inflammatory process depends on continuous migration of activated cells from the circulation, or the inflammatory synovitis becomes autonomous in the established disease is still an open question. It is clear, however, that the inflamed tissue is the main source of cells, cytokines, growth and inhibitory factors, chemokines, and lytic enzymes in pannus and synovial fluid that will determine the ultimate functional fate of the involved joint.

SYNOVIAL FLUID

Cells

The composition of the synovial fluid in RA is the end result of a complex influx and efflux of cells, cell fragments, and secreted molecules, which originate in blood, lymph, synovium, and cartilage. As in many other chronic inflammatory arthritides, the predominant cell is the polymorphonuclear neutrophil. There are multiple chemotactic factors in synovial membrane and fluid that result in the continuous influx of these cells into the synovial cavity. Polymorphonuclear neutrophils adhere to the activated synovial capillary endothelial cells by interacting with the previously mentioned adhesion molecules; they then migrate to the synovial cavity, where they accumulate and eventually die (perhaps by apoptosis) in a short period of time. Given the short life span of these cells, it has been calculated that approximately 1 billion cells may migrate into a large joint in a patient with active disease (125). Although *in vitro* studies suggest that polymorphonuclear neutrophils are rapidly phagocytosed early in apoptosis, recent observations indicate that inflammatory synovial fluids contain significant amounts of oligonucleosomal DNA complexes, a marker of apoptotic cell death (126). These nuclear products have been reported to stimulate lymphocyte proliferation and IgG synthesis (127). Morphologic studies have shown that synovial fluid polymorphonuclear neutrophils exhibit evidence of activation and degranulation, probably as a result of their encounter with immune complexes, cartilage fragments, proinflammatory complement components, chemokines, and so forth. The processes of activation, phagocytosis (regurgitation while feeding, reverse endocytosis), and *in situ* cell death contribute to the accumulation in synovial fluid of potentially noxious polymorphonuclear neutrophil products such as serine proteases, collagenase, oxygen radicals, arachidonate products, fibronectin, and so forth.

Synovial fluid lymphocytes in RA also show evidence of activation (128). As described for the synovial membrane T cells, the synovial fluid contains a disproportionate number of memory $CD4^+$ lymphocytes (129,130) exhibiting activation markers and adhesion molecules (129–133). In contrast to the synovial T-cell infiltrate, however, the synovial fluid is relatively rich in suppressor/cytotoxic $CD8^+$ cells (129–131). A third T-lymphocyte population described in rheumatoid synovial fluids has the $CD3^+$ $CD4^-$ $CD8^-$ and γ/δ T-cell receptor phenotype (131). Interestingly, clones generated from these cells were reactive to mycobacterial antigens (134). The role that $CD8^+$ and γ/δ cells may play in rheumatoid inflammation and tissue damage is unknown. It has been shown recently, however, that peripheral blood and synovial fluid T lymphocytes from patients with RA react against articular chondrocyte membrane antigens (135) and link proteins (136). Although the responding cells have not been characterized further, it is possible that T cell–mediated cytotoxicity may contribute to the destructive process in RA.

B lymphocytes constitute a small proportion of the synovial fluid cell exudate. These cells also show evidence of activation and spontaneous secretion of immunoglobulins (137). Moreover, they are enriched in rheumatoid factor–producing plasma cells when compared with B cells obtained from blood (76,138), therefore contributing to the generation of immune complexes in the synovial fluid.

Enzymes and Inhibitors

In addition to pannus, the composition of rheumatoid synovial fluid that constantly bathes the articular cartilage, intraarticular ligaments, and synovial membrane plays a pivotal role in the destructive process of the affected joints. In addition to the normal constituents, the inflammatory synovial fluid represents a complex mixture of components originating from blood, synovial membrane, and cartilage. Thus, it is particularly difficult to sort out the importance of the individual active factors present in the synovial fluid vis-à-vis the inflammatory manifestations and deleterious effects on the joint tissues.

Several types of proteolytic enzymes derived from synovial cells, synovial fluid exudate, and chondrocytes have been detected in rheumatoid joint fluid. Serine proteases from polymorphonuclear neutrophils, including elastase, cathepsin G, and proteinase 3, constitute a large fraction of the total enzyme content in rheumatoid synovial fluids (139,140). Except for a minority of fluids with very high cell counts, spontaneous proteolytic activity is usually not detectable in most specimens due to the presence of enzyme inhibitors in excess. The plasma-derived protein inhibitors α_1 protease inhibitor and α_2-macroglobulin form complexes with the neutral proteases in synovial fluid (141, 142), resulting in enzymatic inhibition. It is likely, however, that the neutral proteases are at least partially responsible for cartilage matrix proteoglycan degradation in RA. Neutrophil elastase has been detected at the sites of cartilage erosion in cartilage–pannus junctions (143,144). Although very few granulocytes are usually seen along the cartilage surface in inflammatory arthritides, the presence of immune complexes sequestered on the superficial layer of rheumatoid cartilage (87,88,145,146) suggests that these cells may attach to the surface and undergo a process akin to "frustrated phagocytosis" (147), forming a compartment between the cartilage and cell membrane that is impervious to the high-molecular-weight inhibitors present in synovial fluid. Moreover, other evidence suggests that a significant proportion of freshly collected cell-free rheumatoid synovial fluids are able to degrade cartilage proteoglycans when applied directly to frozen sections of tissue (148). This process appeared to be mediated by neutrophil elastase because the degrading activity was prevented by a specific inhibitor of this enzyme. Although elastase complexes to the above mentioned inhibitors, proteases bound to α_2-macroglobulin are unstable (149), and the α_2-macroglobulin–elastase complex has been found to retain activity against low-molecular-weight substrates (150), some proteins (151,152), and cartilage itself (153).

The polymorphonuclear neutrophil–derived metalloproteinases, collagenase (matrix metalloproteinase-8, MMP-8) and gelatinase (MMP-9) have also been implicated in the process of tissue damage (154). This type of enzymatic activity has been detected in rheumatoid synovial fluids even in the presence of the above-mentioned inhibitors and tissue inhibitor of metalloproteinase (TIMP) (155,156). Quantitative measurements of MMP in synovial fluids suggest that the most abundant enzyme types are MMP-1 (collagenase) and MMP-3 (stromelysin), derived from fibroblasts and chondrocytes (157).

The precise role that the proteases in synovial fluid play in the process of articular cartilage damage in RA has been difficult to assess due to the many factors that contribute to the modulation of their enzymatic activity. These enzymes are synthesized as inactive proenzymes or zymogens. They are probably activated *in vivo* by the action of other proteases, as shown in Fig. 54.1. Evidence has indicated that the plasminogen activator–plasmin system may be involved in protease activation (158–160). Additionally, other enzyme systems such as kallikrein (158), cathepsin B (158), and mast cell-derived tryptase (161), as well as oxygen radicals (162), have been shown to activate tissue metalloproteinases. Stromelysin itself is part of the activation network because it is able to activate matrix collagenase (163,164). Elucidation of the fine structure of MMP-2, one of the proteases that degrade collagen type IV has shown that proteolytic cleavage of the propeptide that normally shields the catalytic cleft uncovers this domain, allowing water molecules to enter the cleft and disrupt the coordination of a cysteine with Zn^{2+} ion (165). Once in the active form, metalloproteinases are irreversibly inhibited by locally synthesized TIMP. Clearly, the ability of active MMPs to mediate tissue destruction depends on the perturbation of the balance between enzyme and inhibitor production in the area undergoing degradation (166). In addition to their direct role in tissue destruction, the metalloproteinases have been indirectly implicated in the process of angiogenesis, both as promoters of the process and in the generation of peptides from various protein substrates with antiangiogenic properties (167). The role of synovial fluid cytokines in the modulation of synthesis of enzymes and inhibitors will be discussed below.

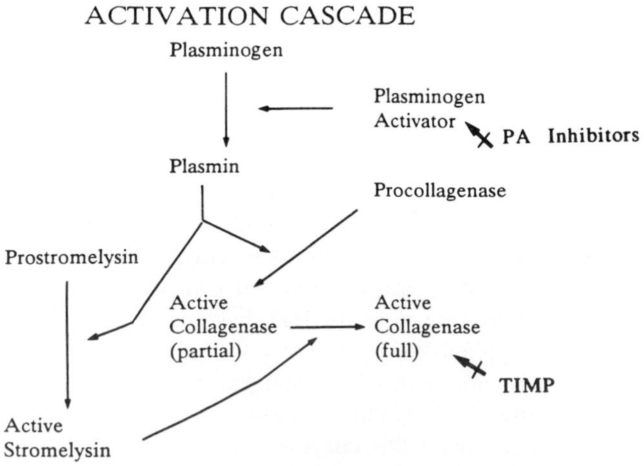

ACTIVATION CASCADE
Plasminogen
Plasminogen Activator
PA Inhibitors
Plasmin
Procollagenase
Prostromelysin
Active Collagenase (partial)
Active Collagenase (full)
TIMP
Active Stromelysin

FIG. 54.1. Probable events in the proteolytic cascade leading to activation of collagenase. *PA*, plasminogen activator; *TIMP*, tissue inhibitor of metalloproteinase.

Cytokines and Inhibitors

There is now clear evidence that the cytokines secreted by the inflamed synovium and chondrocytes in RA play a significant role in the process of tissue damage (168–170). As mentioned previously, it is paradoxic that in the face of evident T-cell activation in the synovial membrane cellular infiltrate, there is a relative lack of T lymphocyte–derived cytokines. The failure to detect their presence in the inflamed joint, however, does not necessarily mean that they do not play a role in the maintenance of local cellular responses such as T- and B-lymphocyte activation and differentiation. In an adoptive transfer model of antigen-induced arthritis, naive mice infused with T lymphocytes expressing the transgenic T-cell receptor specific for the intraarticularly injected antigen develop a chronic destructive synovitis. Only a minority of cells bearing the transgenic receptor were detected in areas of synovium affected with severe inflammation. Moreover, only rare cells expressed a message for IFN-γ or IL-2, whereas abundant expression of macrophage-derived cytokines was observed (170), indicating that in this T lymphocyte–dependent arthritis model, as in RA, a joint inflammatory response may develop in the face of low local expression of T cell–derived lymphokines.

Many studies are available concerning the detection of cytokines, cytokine inhibitors, and chemokines in rheumatoid synovial fluid, and their *in vitro* and *in vivo* effects on biologic phenomena pertinent to tissue destruction (171–214) (Table 54.3). However, the coexistence in synovial fluids of factors that may exert synergistic and opposing effects on cells, and the presence of inhibitors and soluble receptors, has made it difficult to delineate the relative importance that each may have in the process of tissue damage. For instance, IL-1 has been found in rheumatoid fluids (171,172), as well as its high-affinity receptor antagonist IL-1Ra (173). The latter molecule interferes with IL-1 binding to its receptor (174), so that effective inhibition of IL-1 activity can be achieved with 10- to 100-fold excess concentrations of IL-1Ra. In rheumatoid synovial fluids, IL-1Ra is found in 1.2- to 3.6-fold molar excess with respect to IL-1 (174). One of the best studied actions of IL-1 and TNF-α is the induction of *in vitro* chondrocyte-mediated cartilage explant resorption by a combination of a decrease in matrix macromolecular synthesis and an increase in secretion of proteases (154). However, whereas

TABLE 54.3. *Biologic effects of synovial fluid cytokines and other factors in rheumatoid arthritis*

Adhesion molecule expression	Chemotaxis	Macrophage activation	Lytic enzyme secretion	Matrix macromolecule synthesis	Angiogenesis	Fibrosis
IL-1↑[176]	IL-1↑[170]	IL-1↑[188]	IL-1↑[153]	IL-1↓[195]	TNF-α↑[199]	IL-1↑[208]
TNF-α↑[177]	TNF-α↑[180]	TNF-α↑[189]	TNF-α↑[191]	TNF-α↓[191]	IL-8↑[200]	TNF-α↑[208]
IFN-γ↑[178]	IL-8↑[181]	IFN-γ↑[190]	TGF-β↓[179]	IFN-γ↓[190]	FGF↑[201]	TGF-β↑[179]
TGF-β↑[179]	TGF-β↑[183]		FGF↑[192]	TGF-β↑[196]	TGF-β↑[202]	PGDF↑[203]
	MCP-1↑[184]		IL-4↓[193]	IGF-I↑[197]	PGDF↑[203]	FGF↑[209]
	MIP-1↑[185]		IL-10↑[194]	CTAP-III↑[198]	IGF-1↑[204]	IL-4↓[210]
	RANTES↑[186]		IL-8↑[182]	IL-10↓[194]	IFN-γ↓[205]	IL-10↑[194]
	PGDF↑[187]		IL-11↓[211]		PD-ECGF↑[206]	IFN-γ↓[212]
			OSM↑[213]		VEGF↑[207]	
			IL-18↑[214]			

Reference numbers are in superscript.

↑, Activation; ↓, inhibition. IL-1, interleukin-1; IL-4, interleukin-4; IL-8, interleukin-8; IL-10, interleukin-10; IL-11, interleukin-11; IL-18, interleukin-18; TNF-α, tumor necrosis factor-α; IFN-γ, interferon-γ; TGF-β, transforming growth factor-β; FGF, fibroblast growth factor; PGDF, platelet-derived growth factor; IGF-1, insulin-like growth factor-1; CTAP-III, connective tissue activating peptide-III; OSM, oncostatin M; PD-ECGF, platelet-derived endothelial cell growth factor; VEGF, vascular endothelial growth factor; MCP-1, monocyte chemoattractant peptide-1; MIP-1, macrophage inflammatory peptide-1.

incubation of cartilage explants with rheumatoid synovial fluids resulted in matrix depletion, which was variably inhibited by specific antisera to IL-1 or TNF-α, exposure of normal cartilage explants to the purified cytokines did not (175). This suggests that synergistic effects between cytokines may be operative *in vivo*. Recent evidence has suggested that TNF-α in particular plays a pivotal role in the rheumatoid inflammatory process (199). In transgenic mice that constitutively express the human TNF-α gene product, a spontaneous chronic arthritis characterized by synovitis, cartilage destruction, and bony erosions develops that is prevented by the administration of anti-TNF-α antibodies (215). This cytokine is present in rheumatoid serum, synovial tissues, and fluids (216,217), and its level correlates with disease severity (218). Additional evidence is provided by the efficacy of anti-TNF-α monoclonal antibodies or soluble TNF-α receptors in which administration of these agents to patients with active disease results in significant amelioration of inflammatory activity and arrest of structural damage (219,221) (see Chapter 39). Although there is compelling evidence that individual cytokines are important in the process of tissue damage, it is likely that their combined action and that of many additional factors contribute to the process (222).

One of the oldest cytokines, migration inhibitory factor (MIF), has recently been highlighted as playing a role in inflammatory arthritis (reviewed in reference 223). Elevated levels of MIF are present in rheumatoid synovial fluids in greater concentrations that in osteoarthritic synovial fluids. MIF is part and parcel of the cytokine network, in that it is partially responsible for the continuous secretion of TNF-α, and it stimulates prostaglandin secretion from RA fibroblasts, as well as up-regulates expression of metalloproteinases from the same cells, independently of IL-1 (224).

Antibodies, Immune Complexes, and Complement

Rheumatoid synovial fluids contain a variety of antibodies derived from blood and local synthesis. The synovial membrane plasma cells probably contribute a major portion of the autoantibodies found in the fluids (79,80). The presence of immune complexes containing IgM and IgG rheumatoid factors and collagen-anticollagen has been analyzed in several studies (225–227). Other specificities that may contribute to tissue damage include cytotoxic antibodies directed against chondrocyte membrane antigens (228–230). There is also evidence that immune complex–like material generated by oxygen radical–mediated covalent cross-linking of IgG (231) is present in rheumatoid synovial fluids (232). The oxidatively modified IgG reacts preferentially with rheumatoid factor (233), thus contributing to the immune complex burden present in the fluid.

Classic studies have shown that activation of the complement cascade takes place within the joint cavity, resulting in low levels of C3 (234) and in the generation of proinflammatory peptides such as C3a and C5a (235–237). C5a in particular is not only a potent chemotactic factor for neutrophils, but it is also able to activate and induce degranulation of these inflammatory cells (236), thus contributing part of the lytic enzymes and other deleterious factors found in synovial fluids. This process may be compounded by the fact that some of the complement components are also synthesized by the synovial cells (238).

C5a has also been shown to exacerbate inflammatory reactions by up-regulation of the activating Fcγ receptors (FcγRI and III) and down-regulating the inhibitory receptor FcγRII (239). These receptors have been under intense scrutiny recently as the main bridging structures mediating immune complex interaction with inflammatory cells in autoimmune diseases. In RA for instance, FcγR receptors in synovium and macrophages are highly expressed compared with controls resulting in much higher production of TNF-α and metalloproteinases after stimulation with immune complexes (240), leading to increased tissue destruction (241). Moreover, in parallel with studies undertaken in systemic lupus erythematosus, recent work suggests that certain FcγR genetic polymorphisms, particularly FcγRIII, may correlate with susceptibility (242) and severity (243) in RA.

Arachidonate Metabolites

The local synthesis of prostaglandins and leukotrienes in synovial fluids has been studied extensively (244) (see Chapter 23). Similar to the difficulty in defining the precise inflammatory role of the synovial fluid cytokine network, the role of prostaglandins is also unclear because both pro- (245) and antiinflammatory (245–248) activities have been reported. The latter results from interference with the stimulus-response coupling of inflammatory cells, and is associated with an increase in intracellular cyclic adenosine monophosphate (cAMP) levels (245). The difficulty in dissecting the biologic activities of these products is compounded by the fact that their secretion is regulated by cytokines (249,250). Other studies suggest that these compounds contribute to the modulation of the immune response by inhibiting IL-1 and TNF-α synthesis (251), IL-2 secretion (252), antigen-specific T-cell cytotoxicity (253), and natural killer cell activity (254). Prostaglandin E_2 has been shown to suppress T_H1-like responses and to shift T_H0-like responses toward a T_H2-like humoral pattern (255). This, in conjunction with IL-4 and IL-10, may explain why the synovial membrane T lymphocytes tend to exhibit such a phenotype. Some of the catabolic effects of IL-1, including stimulation of plasminogen activator and macrophage collagenase secretion, may be mediated by prostaglandin E_2 and increases in intracellular cAMP levels (256,257).

In contrast to the prostaglandins, the inflammatory role of the other family of arachidonate metabolites, the leukotrienes, appears to be well established (258). Inflammatory stimuli induce the release of arachidonic acid, the precursor of both prostaglandins and leukotrienes (259), activating the enzyme 5-lipoxygenase and its activating protein (260), and giving rise to the common precursor of the leukotriene family, leukotriene A_4. This product is synthesized by a variety of inflammatory cells of myeloid origin, such as neutrophils, eosinophils, monocyte/macrophages, mast cells, and B lymphocytes (259,261). Subsequently, this precursor molecule can be converted to other active metabolites by endothelial cells and platelets (261). The leukotrienes have a variety of proinflammatory activities, including the induction of neutrophil chemotaxis and aggregation (262), neutrophil adherence to endothelial cells (263), induction of neutrophil degranulation and lysosomal enzyme release (264), and mediation of pain (265), among others. Additionally, they play a role in the modulation of the immune response by increasing secretion of IL-1 (266), IL-2, and IFN-γ by T cells (267), and of IL-6 (268). Antiinflammatory effects also have been reported for one of the by-products of leukotriene metabolism (269), 15-hydroxy-eicosatetraenoic acid (15-HETE), which has been shown to inhibit leukotriene biosynthesis (270) and carrageenan-induced experimental arthritis (271). In patients with RA, serum and synovial fluid levels of leukotrienes are substantially higher than in patients with osteoarthritis (272,273), and synovial fluid leukotriene concentrations correlate with other parameters of inflammatory activity (274). Administration to patients with RA of a 5-lipoxygenase inhibitor in a placebo-controlled study showed partial amelioration of disease activity when compared with controls (275).

Oxygen Free Radicals

Activation of phagocytic cells within the inflamed joint gives rise to large amounts of highly reactive oxygen-derived products that in conjunction with cell peroxidases, free divalent metals, halide ions, and other substrates play a major role in defense mechanisms against infection and in the generation of tissue injury in acute and chronic inflammatory reactions (276–278). Several oxygen-derived free radicals have been implicated directly or indirectly in rheumatoid inflammation. In response to external stimuli, phagocytic cells trigger a respiratory burst that results in increased oxygen utilization, anaerobic glycolysis, and the generation of superoxide ion (O_2^-) and H_2O_2. Although superoxide does not diffuse well out of the cells, H_2O_2 does, and this powerful oxidant, together with superoxide produced extracellularly, has been shown to produce a variety of effects pertinent to the process of tissue injury. Production of oxygen-derived products by polymorphonuclear leukocytes develops in an explosive fashion and is short lived, whereas monocytes are able to release H_2O_2 for up to 7 days when appropriately stimulated (279,280). Table 54.4 shows some of the biologic effects mediated by oxygen free radicals within the inflamed joint. One of the best established effects of oxygen products is the mediation of depolymerization of synovial fluid hyaluronate (281,282). Abnormally short hyaluronate chains are a hallmark of inflammatory synovial fluids, and oxidative processes may provide an explanation for this observation (278) in the face of undetectable hyaluronidase activity in rheu-

TABLE 54.4. *Biologic effects of intraarticular oxidant molecules*

Depolymerization of hyaluronate
Protein cross-linking
Generation of aggregated IgG
Activation of metalloproteinases
Inactivation of protease inhibitors
Generation of noxious lipid peroxides
Generation of chemotactic prostanoids
DNA damage
Apoptosis

Ig, immunoglobulin.

matoid fluids. Although there is evidence that collagen and proteoglycans may be modified by *in vitro* oxidative attack, evidence for an *in vivo* effect of oxygen free radicals is lacking, except for the demonstration that polymorphonuclear leukocytes are able to covalently cross-link anticollagen antibodies bound to cartilage by a H_2O_2-myeloperoxidase-Cl^-–dependent mechanism (231). Chemical modification of other synovial fluid macromolecules pertinent to the process of tissue injury include activation of latent metalloproteinases (283), inactivation of α_1-protease inhibitor (284), and generation of potentially injurious oxidized lipoproteins (285,286), chemotactic prostanoids (287), and aggregated IgG (232, 233). The effect of oxidative attack on a variety of cells has also been proposed as one of the pathogenic mechanisms operative in inflammatory arthritis. Oxygen free radicals are able to damage nuclear DNA, thereby inducing mutations (288) and programmed cell death (289,290). Moreover, several studies have shown that these products can inhibit cellular metabolic activity, particularly cartilage macromolecular synthesis by chondrocytes (291).

One of the strongest oxidizing radicals potentially generated as a by-product of the respiratory burst is the hydroxyl radical (•OH). This reactive species has been postulated to be generated by H_2O_2 in the presence of ferrous ion (Haber-Weiss reaction) as follows: $Fe^{3+} + O_2^- \rightarrow Fe^{2+} + O_2$; $Fe^{2+} + H_2O_2 \rightarrow OH^- + \bullet OH$. Generation of hydroxyl radical by this reaction has been implicated in a variety of pathogenic processes in inflammation (276–278); however, using specific methodology for the detection of this radical, it has been difficult to show that phagocytes can indeed generate the hydroxyl radical (292,293). One appealing exception is the possible role of •OH in the severe exacerbation of rheumatoid inflammatory activity in patients given an intravenous infusion of iron-dextran for the treatment of iron deficiency (294). Careful studies have shown the presence of free catalytic iron in synovial fluids (295); therefore, this environment is probably conducive to the generation of this oxidant. Moreover, other reactions involving hypochlorous acid, superoxide, or NO have been shown to generate •OH independently of catalytic iron (292). The ischemia-reperfusion phenomenon (296) has been postulated to be operative in the rheumatoid joint as an additional source of oxygen free radicals. In this reaction, anoxia activates xanthine oxidase, which, as the oxygen tension increases, gives rise to superoxide ions as a by-product of oxidation of xanthine and hypoxanthine. Low oxygen tension is present in the inflamed joint (297), suggesting that this mechanism may be operative in RA (298). It is difficult to determine the importance of many of the observations described above because the majority of the *in vitro* studies dealing with the role of oxidative mechanisms in tissue injury fail to take into consideration the protective mechanisms present in serum and within cells (278). A wide variety of radical scavengers are present in normal serum, including proteins with free sulfhydryl groups, free amino acids (cysteine, methionine, tyrosine, alanine, and histidine), uric acid, ascorbate, α-tocopherol, and so forth. Enhanced production of oxygen free radicals has been proposed to explain the observed decrease of free sulfhydryl group concentration in rheumatoid sera (299); other studies have found increased antioxidant activity in serum and synovial fluids (300). Despite the well-known cytotoxic activity of oxygen products, even the cells that produce these radicals appear to be protected from their deleterious effects. Intracellular compounds containing sulfhydryl groups, the glutathione-glutathione reductase system in particular (301), and iron chelation by lactoferrin (302) and ferritin (303) contribute to limit oxidant-mediated injury within cells. These considerations have raised understandable interest in the therapeutic use of radical scavengers for the treatment of RA. Thus far, there is little evidence to show significant antiinflammatory effects by antioxidant preparations such as chemically modified superoxide dismutase (277).

Nitric Oxide

The discovery that NO synthesized by endothelial cells was essential for the regulation of blood pressure gave rise to a large number of studies implicating this gas in the maintenance of homeostasis, defense mechanisms against infection, and acute and chronic inflammatory processes (304–306). In addition to its physiologic role in the maintenance of vascular tone, NO has been shown to be a neurotransmitter, inhibit platelet aggregation, mediate penile erection, and, at least in animals, contribute to intracellular killing of parasites. NO is produced as a by-product of the oxidation of L-arginine to citrulline, catalyzed by a group of enzymes, the NO synthases. These belong to two major families: the constitutive forms (cNOS) responsible for continuous low level synthesis, particularly in endothelial cells and neurons, and the inducible forms (iNOS), synthesized within a few hours following cell stimulation with bacterial products such as endotoxin, or cytokines, particularly IL-1 and TNF-α. NO is produced in humans by a variety of cells, including endothelial cells, smooth muscle cells, platelets, neurons, chondrocytes (307), synovial cells (308), and polymorphonuclear cells (309).

As was the case with oxygen free radicals, NO and its derivatives exhibit both proinflammatory and antiinflammatory activities. The direct effects of NO in inflammatory foci are probably exerted at a short distance from its source, since its half-life in physiologic conditions is only a few seconds. However, nitrosylation products such as peroxinitrite, nitryl chloride (310), nitrogen dioxide ions (311), and *S*-nitrosothiols are more stable and may mediate some of the *in vivo* biologic effects attributed to NO. Peroxinitrites are generated by NO and the superoxide ion according to the following reaction: $\bullet O_2^- + \bullet NO^- \rightarrow ONOO^- + H^+$, which may decompose to yield the hydroxyl radical in the absence of iron as another possible pathway for tissue injury. This radical has been the focus of increased interest as a possible mediator of cytotoxicity (312,313). Another possible pathogenic pathway may involve the oxidation product of NO,

TABLE 54.5. *Biologic effects of nitric oxide pertinent to inflammatory arthritis*

Proinflammatory	Antiinflammatory
DNA damage	Inhibition of cell adhesion
Respiratory chain inactivation	Inhibition of superoxide ion production
Vascular damage	Inactivation of superoxide ion
Edema formation	Inhibition of IL-6 secretion
Stimulation of angiogenesis	Suppression of T-cell proliferation
Stimulation of metallo-proteinase activity	Suppression of Th1 cytokine production
Chondrocyte apoptosis	

IL, interleukin.

NO_2, which when reacting with hydrogen peroxide forms $NO_2^{\bullet}$, a highly active radical capable of nitrosylating and aggregating proteins (314). Table 54.5 summarizes some of the biologic effects of NO pertinent to tissue injury in RA. NO-mediated cytotoxicity may be due to its effects on DNA, which undergoes deamination (315) and other forms of chemical damage (316), and on the mitochondrial respiratory chain by inactivation of iron-sulfur-containing enzymes (317). Immune complex–mediated vascular damage with increased capillary permeability and edema formation has been shown to depend on NO production (318,319). Recent studies have shown that NO stimulates endothelial cell proliferation and migration, and that it mediates angiogenesis induced by substance P and prostaglandin E_2 (320). Complementary studies have shown that NO is also able to modulate leukocyte adhesion (321).

The dual capabilities of NO may be due to a dose effect; thus, low concentrations produced by cNOS may induce a given response, whereas higher levels due to cell activation and iNOS synthesis may induce an opposite response. For instance, induction of low levels of NO synthesis in chondrocytes stimulates prostaglandin production, whereas maximal stimulation of NO results in inhibition of prostaglandin synthesis (322). Other possible antiinflammatory effects include inhibition of neutrophil adhesion to endothelial cells (321), inhibition of superoxide production by neutrophils, and inhibition of IL-6 secretion by Kupffer cells (322). It has been deduced that the antiinflammatory properties of NO may depend on its ability to quench superoxide as discussed above.

NO has been shown to modulate several cellular immune mechanisms. In rodents, suppression of T-cell proliferation mediated by macrophage activation depends on NO production by these cells (323). NO also may be partially responsible for the low levels of T_H1-dependent cytokines, IL-2 and IFN-γ, synthesized by rheumatoid synovial T cells. Activated murine T_H1, but not T_H2, cell lines produced a large amount of NO, which also inhibited secretion of the above-mentioned cytokines (324). In humans, administration of IL-2 results in increased excretion of urinary nitrite, an indirect measure of enhanced NO production (325).

The observation that cytokine-stimulated chondrocytes release large amounts of NO (307) has prompted a series of studies on the biologic effects of this mediator on the process of cartilage degradation. Both the well-known IL-1-mediated inhibition of proteoglycan synthesis and increased metalloproteinase activity in chondrocytes were shown to be partially mediated by NO (326–328). Moreover, NO was found to mediate inhibition of IL-1 receptor antagonist (329), suggesting that this molecule may play an important role in cartilage damage in inflammatory arthritides. Cytokine-stimulated chondrocytes develop increased sensitivity to oxidant injury, which was demonstrated to depend on NO synthesis by these cells (330). In contrast, NO protected chondrocytes from cytotoxic attack by activated polymorphonuclear leukocytes (331).

Direct evidence derived from animal models and human disease is available to suggest that NO plays a role in the inflammatory process. Administration of an inhibitor of NO synthesis significantly reduced glomerulonephritis and arthritis in the MRL-*lpr/lpr* mouse (332) and synovial inflammation and tissue damage in animals with streptococcal cell wall–induced arthritis (333). A similar effect was observed in rats with adjuvant arthritis (334). Conversely, knockout mice lacking iNOS were able to mount joint inflammatory responses similar to those in the wild-type littermates (335,336). In patients with RA, nitrite concentrations in serum and synovial fluids were increased, suggesting increased NO synthesis *in vivo* (337). Along the same lines, an oxidative by-product of peroxinitrite, 3-nitrotyrosine, was also elevated in patients with advanced rheumatoid disease (338), and 3-nitrotyrosine-containing proteins have been found in abundance in rheumatoid synovia (339). It is apparent from these considerations that this area of inquiry is changing rapidly, and that delineation of the relative importance of NO in rheumatoid inflammation requires further work (340).

Kinins and Neuropeptides

The kallikrein-kininogen system has been implicated in the rheumatoid inflammatory process (341). Kallikrein itself, a serine protease present in plasma and tissues, mediates neutrophil chemotaxis (342), cell aggregation (343), and degranulation (344), and it is also able to activate latent collagenase (345). Acting on kininogen, it generates kinin peptides that can cause arteriolar dilatation, constriction of venules, increased capillary permeability, and elicitation of pain. Both kinins and kallikrein have been detected in rheumatoid synovial fluid (346,347), suggesting that they may play a proinflammatory role. As previously discussed, however, the synovial fluids also contain large amounts of the protease inhibitors α_1-antitrypsin and α_2-macroglobulin complexed to the active enzyme. A positive correlation between the synovial fluid levels of tissue kallikrein and the degree of joint pain and inflammation has been reported (348). It was postulated that as neutrophils degranulate within the joint cavity, kallikrein is released from lysosomes, where it can act on kininogen bound to the cell surface before it is inactivated by inhibitors. An inflammatory role for this system is supported by the finding that administration of a specific inhibitor of kallikrein to rats with streptococcal peptidoglycan–induced arthritis resulted in partial control of the inflammatory activity (349).

Stimulation of peripheral afferent nerves induces local inflammation as a result of the release of a family of biologically active peptides, the neurokinins. The main components of this group include substance P, calcitonin gene–related peptide, and vasoactive intestinal polypeptide (350). These neurotransmitters mediate a variety of inflammation-related phenomena, including vasodilatation, chemotaxis, and activation of neutrophils (351) and macrophages; mast cell degranulation; increased expression of endothelial adhesion molecules (352); and stimulation of IL-1 secretion (353) (Table 54.6). The evidence that they may play an inflammatory role in RA derives from studies showing increased levels of these neuropeptides, particularly substance P, in rheumatoid synovial fluids (354,355). Additionally, some studies have shown that the inflamed synovium itself appears to be depleted of these mediators (356,357), suggesting an active secretory process. On this basis, the topical application of capsaicin, a substance extracted from capsicum (hot pepper) that depletes nerve endings of substance P, has been used with positive results in patients with RA (358).

Proteolytic Fragments

The accumulation of inflammatory cells in rheumatoid synovial fluids and the activation of chondrocytes results in release of enzymes that are responsible for the generation of proteolytic fragments from plasma and connective tissue macromolecules. These fragments may have potent biologic activities, and may also serve as markers of disease severity or tissue damage (359,360).

A potentially important mediator of inflammation and tissue damage in the rheumatoid joint is fibronectin, a ubiquitous glycoprotein with multiple functions, particularly cell adhesion, which is present in plasma and all connective tissues. In the rheumatoid joint, fibronectin is found in large amounts in synovium, synovial fluid, and the cartilage–pannus junction (361). Proteolytic fragments that are generated by enzymes such as elastase, cathepsins, and collagenase and are present in synovial fluids (362) have been shown to have potent biologic effects (Table 54.7). Whereas intact fibronectin has chemotactic activity only for fibroblasts (363), fragments containing the cell-binding domain mediate monocyte/macrophage chemotaxis (364) and neutrophil degranulation (365), increase expression of matrix-degrading enzymes in chondrocytes (366), and depress proteoglycan synthesis in these cells (367). In rheumatoid synovial fluids, depletion of fibronectin-like material with gelatin inhibits fibroblast migration by 75% (362), suggesting that this molecule may have an important role in pannus formation. Fibronectin has several cell-binding domains with affinity for the cell surface adhesion molecules very late antigen-3 (VLA-3), VLA-4, and VLA-5. This property has been exploited by the use of synthetic cell adhesion inhibitory peptides to suppress ongoing streptococcal cell wall arthritis in rats (368).

TABLE 54.6. *Biologic activities of neurokinins*

Vasodilatation
Chemotaxis of neutrophils and macrophages
Neutrophil and macrophage activation
Neutrophil and macrophage degranulation
Mast cell degranulation
Stimulation of IL-1 secretion
Increased expression of adhesion molecules

IL, interleukin.

TABLE 54.7. *Biologic activities of fibronectin and its proteolytic fragments*

Fibroblast chemotaxis
Macrophage chemotaxis
Neutrophil degranulation
Increased expression of chondrocyte proteases
Depression of proteoglycan synthesis

Proteolytic fragments with biologic activity that are derived from other macromolecules may also contribute to the inflammatory process. Collagen fragments are of particular interest because they have multiple biologic activities, including chemotaxis for macrophages (369), macrophage activation (370), and secretion of IL-1 (371). Moreover, they have been detected in rheumatoid synovial fluids (372).

There is abundant evidence to indicate that the coagulation cascade also may participate in the rheumatoid inflammatory process (373). Histologic techniques have shown the presence of several components of the cascade in rheumatoid synovial tissue (374), including fibrin and plasmin-derived fibrin degradation products (375). The latter have been shown to mediate macrophage chemotaxis (376). Additionally, active enzyme components of the cascade such as plasmin and thrombin can induce cartilage matrix degradation (373,377).

The role of angiogenesis in the arthritic process is under active investigation in many laboratories (378). High serum levels of vascular endothelial growth factor (VEGF) are associated with early radiographic joint damage, and conversely, decreases in VEGF concentrations are seen in patients exhibiting clinical improvement (379). Similar results have been reported in studies dealing with another group of angiogenic factors, the angiopoietins (380). Of particular interest are the family of peptides derived from plasmin with potent antiangiogenic capacity (angiostatins). Several metalloproteinases active in the inflamed joint have been shown to generate both pro- and antiangiogenic molecules (177). In addition, peptides produced by chondrocytes and other cells such as TIMPs have been shown to exhibit antiangiogenic activity (381). There are no studies dealing with the properties of rheumatoid synovial fluids with regard to their putative pro- or antiangiogenic activities.

CARTILAGE AND PANNUS

Loss of joint function in RA is the result of irreversible damage to the articular cartilage as a direct consequence of the sustained chronic inflammatory process. The mechanisms operative in cartilage damage in RA are not completely understood. It is likely, however, that the inability of chondrocytes to maintain tissue integrity as a result of cell death and metabolic abnormalities induced by factors secreted by cells in inflamed synovium, invasive pannus, and synovial fluid play a major role in the process of cartilage destruction. Additionally, proteolytic enzymes and other factors from pannus cells and synovial fluid acting directly on the cartilage matrix also contribute to the destructive process. At the present time it is not possible to single out any of the factors listed in Table 54.8 as being mainly responsible for irreversible damage. It is likely that the concerted action of many of the factors listed in the table acting over a protracted period of time is responsible. Synthesis and degradation of cartilage macromolecules in normal adult tissue is probably a tightly regulated process, because the chemical composition of adult cartilage matrix remains fairly constant, changing only slowly with age. Thus, cartilage matrix degradation in pathologic conditions could result from a decrease in the rate of macromolecule synthesis, an increase in the rate of proteoglycan and collagen breakdown, or a combination of both. Matrix proteoglycans are highly susceptible to degradation by various proteolytic enzymes, such as cathepsins, elastase, and metalloproteinases. These macromolecules are the components most readily lost in pathologic conditions. Proteoglycans are also rapidly restored by chondrocytes, however, so that irreversible damage is thought to occur only when collagen fibers are degraded, because this structural component cannot be replaced in a manner that would maintain the integrity of this tissue. There is good evidence suggesting that active proteolytic enzymes may be responsible for degradation of the matrix proteoglycans. The collagen type II fiber appears to be relatively resistant to enzymatic attack, however, and the rheumatoid synovial fluids usually lack active collagenase due to the presence of excess inhibitors. Thus, it is likely that collagen degradation may be due to collagenase secreted by activated chondrocytes and fibroblastic pannus.

Chondrocyte Apoptosis and Cytotoxicity

Widespread chondrocyte death near the surface of the affected joint has been reported in pannus-free areas of rheumatoid cartilage (382). It is likely that several mechanisms may be operative to explain this observation. Studies have shown that IL-1-mediated induction of NO synthesis by chondrocytes may induce apoptosis (programmed cell death) (383). However, chondrocyte apoptosis occurred only if oxygen radical quenchers were added to the culture, suggesting that superoxide reduced the levels of biologically active NO. Conversely, stimulation of oxygen radical synthesis in the presence of iNOS induced cell necrosis (383). Because both oxidant species are probably produced by stimulated chondrocytes *in vivo,* it is difficult to ascertain the precise role of these mechanisms in cartilage cell death *in vivo.* Evidence of apoptosis has been demonstrated in rheumatoid synovial tissues (384,385) and cartilage (386), and its by-product, oligonucleosomal bodies, has been detected in rheumatoid synovial fluids (126).

As the extracellular matrix in cartilage is degraded by the inflammatory process, it is likely that chondrocytes are exposed to immunologic attack by cells and antibodies. Several studies have provided some evidence of lymphocyte-mediated chondrocyte cytotoxicity in RA. Chondrocytes obtained from rheumatoid cartilage express class I and II MHC antigens (387), as well as tissue-specific determinants (388). Moreover, rheumatoid T lymphocytes demonstrate a striking proliferative response when exposed to human chondrocytes (389). Several potential autoantigens have been identified (390–392), although their importance in the process of tissue damage has yet to be determined. Direct evidence of cell-mediated chondrocyte cytotoxicity has been more difficult to obtain (393), even though the rheumatoid synovium appears to be enriched for natural killer and cytotoxic T lymphocytes as evidenced by the presence of molecular markers specific for cytotoxic cells [e.g., granzyme A and perforin (394,395)]. Autoantibody-

TABLE 54.8. *Factors involved in cartilage damage in rheumatoid arthritis*

Cartilage	Synovial fluid	Pannus
Articular surface disruption	Lymphocytes	"Transformed" fibroblasts
Chondrocyte apoptosis	Neutrophils	Macrophages
Chondrocyte cytotoxicity	Active proteases	Endothelial cells
Inhibition of protein synthesis	Cytokines	Neutrophils
Increased synthesis of proteinases	Proinflammatory peptides	
Oxygen radicals and nitric oxide	Cytotoxic antibodies	
Immune complexes	Immune complexes	
Decreased synthesis of protease inhibitors	Neurokinins	
	Coagulation cascade	

mediated chondrocyte cytotoxicity may also play a role in cartilage damage in RA. Complement-dependent cytotoxic antibodies have been detected in rheumatoid sera (396,397) and synovial fluids (385). The specificities of most of the reactive antibodies have not been well characterized, but autoantibodies directed against collagen type II have been shown to contribute to chondrocyte killing (398). The chondrocytes in the superficial layer of cartilage appeared to be more susceptible to cytotoxicity (398), supporting the possible role of synovial fluid–derived antibodies in the widespread superficial cell death observed in electron microscopic studies (382).

Chondrocyte Activation

Histologic studies of rheumatoid cartilage have revealed areas of matrix depletion in the perilacunar area, indicating that macromolecular degradation takes place in areas adjacent to deep chondrocytes (399). The importance of this observation became apparent when it was first realized that chondrocytes had the capability to digest the surrounding matrix when appropriately stimulated (400). These observations coincided with characterization of cytokines and their effects on cellular events. It soon became apparent that proinflammatory cytokines, particularly IL-1 and TNF-α, were able to induce chondrocytes to secrete metalloproteinases such as collagenase and stromelysin (401,402), mediate cartilage resorption in organ culture (196,403), and inhibit matrix macromolecule synthesis (193,404), precisely the alterations conducive to irreversible cartilage damage. Several chondrocyte-derived enzymes have been implicated in the process of matrix degradation. In human cartilage, cytokines may exert their action predominantly by inhibiting protein synthesis rather than by stimulating matrix macromolecule degradation (405). There is no evidence to suggest digestion of the sugar chain moieties by active polysaccharidases, although a lysosomal hyaluronidase active in acid pH has been described (406). Much of the matrix proteoglycan degradation in arthritic cartilage occurs by protease attack on the protein core. Two main enzyme systems have been described: a metalloproteinase (stromelysin) activation cascade and the recently characterized aggrecanases (407–410). Cleavage of the protein core by these two systems takes place between the G1 and G2 interglobular domains of the peptide chain close to the hyaluronate binding site. Metalloproteinases attack the peptide chain between Asn341 and Phe342 (411), and aggrecanase cleaves it between Glu373 and Ala374 (412). The resulting neoepitopes have been shown to coexist and accumulate in inflammatory synovial fluids (413,414), but it is unclear at this point which of the two enzymatic processes is predominant in rheumatoid cartilage.

Irreversible cartilage damage is usually the consequence of collagen fiber degradation. Immunochemical studies have detected the presence of collagen type II α-chain fragments cleaved at the site, indicative of collagenase action (415), and this enzyme is present in damaged tissue, particularly at the cartilage–pannus junction (416,417). Electron microscopic studies have also shown evidence of widespread fiber damage (418), with a concomitant alteration of the normal biomechanical properties of the tissue. Although only collagenase is able to cleave the collagen fiber within the collagen fold, other proteinases such as elastase and stromelysin can degrade the nonhelical domain of the molecule (419), no doubt contributing to the destructive process. Following collagenase cleavage at the specific sites, the resulting fragments undergo denaturation at body temperature, becoming susceptible to further enzymatic attack by a variety of proteases.

Pannus

Although it is widely believed that cartilage resorption is almost always associated with the presence of invasive pannus in RA, this granulation tissue is not specific for the disease because other human and animal chronic arthritides also exhibit the presence of this invasive tissue. It is also likely that pannus invasion into the cartilage is a relatively late event, suggesting that this process represents a nonspecific phenomenon resulting from previous alterations of the articular cartilage by the inflammatory process. For instance, widespread chondrocyte death near the surface of the affected joint has been reported in pannus-free areas (382), and loss of matrix macromolecules around chondrocytes has been reported (399), lending some credence to the hypothesis that cartilage alteration may precede invasion by the pannus. Additionally, the surface of pannus-free cartilage shows the presence of embedded immune complexes in a large proportion of surgical specimens (87,88), which disappear as pannus invasion proceeds (420).

Recent evidence suggests that the articular cartilage surface may be the structure that sustains the earliest damage in inflammatory arthritis. This layer has been the subject of some controversy in the past. It has been argued that the surface differs from other cartilage deeper layers only in the spatial arrangement of the collagen fibers and the relative paucity of matrix proteoglycan (421). Using electron microscopic analysis, however, several investigators have observed a thin, irregular, granular electron-dense layer containing anionic charges (421). Other studies have shown that this layer appears to resist extraction with high ionic strength reagents, hyaluronidase, chondroitinase ABC, or keratinase, but is partially disrupted by collagenase and removed by trypsin. The normal articular surface does not support adhesion of inflammatory or connective tissue cells (422,423). Some studies have implicated fibronectin as a possible factor facilitating pannus invasion into cartilage in RA (424,425). Other studies have shown that the macromolecules present on the normal surface (426) may act as a possible barrier to cell adhesion in the intact cartilage and that these proteoglycans are exquisitely sensitive to attack by serine esterases in polymorphonuclear leukocytes (425).

Two of the small nonaggregating proteoglycans that appear to play a role in the prevention of cell adhesion to the cartilage surface are decorin and fibromodulin. In the case of fibromodulin, this molecule prevents fibroblast adhesion to the surface by masking the cell-binding domain (RGD) of fibronectin. Decorin appears to inhibit collagen-dependent cell binding (423). Another possible protective mechanism that may prevent cell adhesion to the surface is suggested by the capability of chondrocytes to secrete large quantities of nitric oxide, a powerful inhibitor of leukocyte adhesion (292). Thus, it is likely that invasion of pannus into the articular surface is preceded by damage to the surface by the inflammatory exudate in the synovial fluid, since incubation for 1 hour with as few as 100 neutrophils/mm^3 is sufficient to induce detectable damage to the surface, as revealed by the exposure of collagen type II epitopes that were previously covered by the macromolecules that form part of the articular surface (425). Damage to the articular surface of rheumatoid cartilage, as gauged by the availability of collagen type II epitopes to bind antibody, has been reported (427).

There is considerable controversy with regard to the cellular nature of the invasive pannus. Most studies agree that two histologic types are prevalent in RA: the inflammatory type containing macrophages, neutrophils, mast cells, and endothelial cells, and the fibroblastic transitional type (reviewed in reference 428). It has been hypothesized that the fibroblast-like cells may be derived from transformed chondrocytes with the capacity to synthesize cartilage matrix macromolecules. The latter type of pannus is mostly present in large joints, where juxtaarticular erosions are rare and progressive loss of cartilage is prevalent, whereas the invading inflammatory pannus is more common in small joints, where bony erosions are more frequent (428). The phenotype of the fibroblast-like cells in synovium and pannus has also been the focus of considerable attention (429). It has been deduced that these cells represent mesenchymal cells that under the influence of cytokines and other factors develop into a "transformed," aggressive phenotype, with enhanced proliferative activity, increased expression of oncogenes and adhesion molecules, and the capacity to secrete large quantities of cytokines and proteolytic enzymes (429–433). A body of evidence is accumulating that suggests that these cells may not only be the main mediators of cartilage and bone damage in RA, but that they become autonomous and independent of T-cell influences (429). This hypothesis is based on the following observations: (a) the relative dearth of T_H1-derived lymphokines and little evidence of T-lymphocyte activation in rheumatoid synovium and pannus; (b) the studies of MRL/l mice, which indicate the development of spontaneous arthritis with cartilage lesions induced by polyhedral cells similar to those described in the rheumatoid pannus and in the apparent absence of T lymphocytes (433); (c) studies of c-*fos* transgenic mice in which antigen-induced arthritis develops in the absence of T cells (434); and (d) the observation that rheumatoid synovium and human cartilage implanted in SCID mice develop a pannuslike appearance with focal cartilage erosions induced by fibroblast-like cells of human origin in the apparent absence of human or murine T cell influences (435). It is suggested, therefore, that the development of pannus may occur independently of T cell–driven inflammatory activity, and is perhaps initiated by a retrovirus infection, which is transported to the joint by monocyte precursors of type A synoviocytes and eventually lodges in chondrocytes (429). Alternatively, it is possible that the abnormal immune mechanisms undeniably operative in RA may be responsible for the initial transformation of mesenchymal cells into an autonomous phenotype.

BONE

It is likely that all the pathogenic mechanisms discussed earlier play a role in the development of bone resorption analogous to their role in cartilage damage. In parallel with the evidence suggesting that chondrocyte activation and inflammatory cells may mediate digestion of the surrounding matrix, there is evidence that both the osteoblast, a stromal cell, and the osteoclast, a hematopoietic cell, working in tandem (436), may be responsible for part of the resorptive activity taking place adjacent to the inflamed joint (437). In parallel with the process of chondrocyte activation, there is evidence to suggest that the osteoblast responds to the stimuli provided by proinflammatory cytokines and other factors to secrete proteases, modify the bone matrix, and facilitate osteoclast-mediated bone resorptive activity. Additionally, histologic studies have underscored the role of the pannus, which commonly invades the subchondral bone and generates juxtaarticular erosions, a radiologic hallmark of small joints in RA. Pertinent to this aspect of bone destruction is the observation that the activated fibroblasts induce osteoclastogenesis (438) and that inhibition of one of the systems involved in fibroblast and osteoclast activation, the cytoplasmic tyrosine kinases of the Src family, results in inhibition of bone resorption *in vitro* and in the adjuvant arthritis model in the rat (439).

Other recent studies, mostly in animal models, have further clarified the molecular mechanisms operative in bone remodeling and bony erosions in inflammatory arthritis. These studies have demonstrated the pivotal role of the TNF family molecule receptor activator of nuclear factor κB ligand (RANKL, or osteoprotegerin ligand) and its receptor RANK in osteoclast activation, bone remodeling, bony erosions, and osteoporosis (440). High levels of osteoprotegerin and RANKL are found in the serum of RA patients, which normalize after TNF-α treatment (441).

SUMMARY

It is readily apparent from the above considerations that the process of joint destruction in RA is the result of an extremely complex interaction of proinflammatory and modulatory activities working in concert for prolonged periods of time. It is usually customary to complete a review of this nature with a schematic drawing summarizing the researcher's bias. At this stage of our knowledge, the task would be futile, since it is not possible to assign the proper weight to any of the phenomena described. Moreover, it would be equally difficult to attempt to unravel the mechanisms of action of the many therapeutic agents used to control the disease, because for every steroidal or nonsteroidal antiinflammatory agent, disease-modifying agent, antimalarial, antibiotic, monoclonal antibody, cytokine inhibitor, and so forth, there are studies demonstrating that they can affect many of the *in vivo* and *in vitro* processes described in this chapter. It is therefore reasonable to conclude that the process of joint destruction in RA is probably the consequence of a sustained multipronged attack by cells and soluble factors originating in the inflamed synovium, synovial fluid, cartilage, and pannus. The success of anti-TNF-α therapy, however, suggests that some of the pathogenic factors may be at crucial sites in the complex web, resulting in chronic joint inflammation. It is obvious that interventions aimed at controlling these important nodes of such a complex tree may be successful, at least for the prevention of irreversible joint damage and loss of function. Truly effective control of the disease, and perhaps prevention, will only come with the identification of all the genetic and environmental factors responsible for the initiation of the inflammatory process.

REFERENCES

1. Schumacher HR. The microvasculature of the synovial membrane of the monkey: ultrastructural studies. *Arthritis Rheum* 1969;12:387–404.
2. Mikecz K, Brennan FR, Kim JH, Glant TT. Anti-CD44 treatment abrogates tissue oedema and leukocyte infiltration in murine arthritis. *Nat Med* 1995;1:558–563.
3. Mikecz K, Dennis K, Kim JH. Modulation of hyaluronan receptor (CD44) function *in vivo* in a murine model of rheumatoid arthritis. *Arthritis Rheum* 1999;42:659–668.
4. Fujii K, Tanaka Y, Hubscher S, et al. Cross-linking of CD44 on rheumatoid synovial cells upregulates VCAM-1. *J Immunol* 1999;162:2391–2398.
5. Siegelman MH, Stanescu D, Estes P. The CD44-initiated pathway of T-cell extravasation uses VLA-4 but not LFA-1 for firm adhesion. *J Clin Invest* 2000;105:683–691.
6. Kulka JP, Bocking D, Ropes MW, et al. Early joint lesions of rheumatoid arthritis. *Arch Pathol* 1955;59:129–150.
7. Schumacher HR, Kitridou RC. Synovitis of recent onset. A clinicopathologic study during the first months of disease. *Arthritis Rheum* 1972;15:465–485.
8. Soden M, Rooney M, Cullen A, et al. Immunohistologic features in the synovium obtained from clinically uninvolved knee joints of patients with rheumatoid arthritis. *Br J Rheumatol* 1989;28:287–292.
9. Schumacher HR, Bautista BB, Krauser RE, et al. Histological appearance of the synovium in early rheumatoid arthritis. *Semin Arthritis Rheum* 1994;23:3–10.
10. Zvaifler NJ, Boyle D, Firestein G. Early synovitis—synoviocytes and mononuclear cells. *Semin Arthritis Rheum* 1994;23:11–16.
11. Tak PP, Smeets TJM, Daha MR, et al. Analysis of the synovial infiltrate in early rheumatoid synovial tissue in relation to local disease activity. *Arthritis Rheum* 1997;38:34–42.
12. Lindblad S, Hedfors E. Intra-articular variation in synovitis. Local macroscopic and microscopic signs of inflammatory activity are significantly correlated. *Arthritis Rheum* 1985;28:977–986.
13. Duke O, Panayi GS, Poulter LW. An immunohistological analysis of lymphocyte subpopulations and their microenvironment in the synovial membranes of patients with rheumatoid arthritis using monoclonal antibodies. *Clin Exp Immunol* 1982;49:22–30.
14. Poulter LW, Duke O, Panayi GS, et al. Activated T lymphocytes of the synovial membrane in rheumatoid arthritis and other arthropathies. *Scand J Immunol* 1985;22:683–690.
15. Cush JJ, Lipsky PE. Phenotypic analysis of synovial tissue and peripheral blood lymphocytes isolated from patients with rheumatoid arthritis. *Arthritis Rheum* 1988;31:1230–1238.
16. Nakao H, Eguchi K, Kawakami A, et al. Phenotype characterization of lymphocytes infiltrating synovial tissue from patients with rheumatoid arthritis: analysis of lymphocytes isolated from minced synovial tissue by dual immunofluorescence staining. *J Rheumatol* 1990;17:142–148.
17. Fox DA. The role of T cells in the immunopathogenesis of rheumatoid arthritis. *Arthritis Rheum* 1997;40:598–609.
18. Lindhout E, van Eijk M, van Pel M, et al. Fibroblast-like synoviocytes from rheumatoid arthritis patients have intrinsic properties of follicular dendritic cells. *J Immunol* 1999;162:5949–5956.
19. Shimaoka Y, Attrep JF, Hirano T, et al. Nurse-like cells from bone marrow and synovium of patients with rheumatoid arthritis promote survival and enhance function of human B cells. *J Clin Invest* 1998;102:606–618.
20. Koch AE, Kunkel SL, Strieter RM. Cytokines in rheumatoid arthritis. *J Invest Med* 1995;43:28–38.
21. Paulus HE, Machleder EL, Levine S, et al. Lymphocyte involvement in rheumatoid arthritis: studies during thoracic duct drainage. *Arthritis Rheum* 1977;20:1249–1262.
22. Gaston JSH, Strober S, Solovera JJ, et al. Dissection of the mechanism of immune injury in rheumatoid arthritis, using total lymphoid irradiation. *Arthritis Rheum* 1988;31:21–30.
23. Trentham DE, Belli JA, Bloomer WD, et al. 2000-Centigray total lymphoid irradiation for refractory rheumatoid arthritis. *Arthritis Rheum* 1987;30:980–987.
24. Weinblatt ME, Coblyn JS, Frazer PA, et al. Cyclosporin A treatment of refractory rheumatoid arthritis. *Arthritis Rheum* 1987;30:11–17.
25. Jaffe IA. Rheumatoid arthritis and AIDS [Letter]. *J Rheumatol* 1989;16:845.
26. Amor B. Rheumatoid arthritis and AIDS [Reply]. *J Rheumatol* 1989;16:845.
27. Ornstein MH, Kerr LD, Spiera H. A reexamination of the relationship between active rheumatoid arthritis and the acquired immunodeficiency syndrome. *Arthritis Rheum* 1995;38:1701–1706.
28. Firestein GS. Invasive fibroblast-like synoviocytes in rheumatoid arthritis. Passive responders or transformed aggressors? *Arthritis Rheum* 1996;39:1781–1790.
29. Gregersen P, Silver J, Winchester RJ. The shared epitope hypothesis: an approach to understanding the molecular genetics of susceptibility to rheumatoid arthritis. *Arthritis Rheum* 1987;30:1205–1213.
30. Weyand CM, Xie C, Goronzy JJ. Homozygosity for the HLA-DRB1 allele selects for extra-articular manifestations in rheumatoid arthritis. *J Clin Invest* 1992;89:2033–2039.
31. Wedderburn LR. Tracking T cells in arthritis. *Rheumatology* 2000;39:458–462.
32. Steinman L. Escape from "Horror Autotoxicus": pathogenesis and treatment of autoimmune disease. *Cell* 1995;80:7–10.

32a. Stamenkovic IM, Stegagno M, Wright KA, et al. Clonal dominance among T-lymphocyte infiltrates in arthritis. *Proc Soc Natl Acad Sci U S A* 1988;85:1179–1183.

33. Pallard X, West SG, Lafferty JA, et al. Evidence for the effects of a superantigen in arthritis. *Science* 1991;253:325–329.
34. Howell MD, Diveley JP, Lundeen KA, et al. Limited T-cell receptor β-chain heterogeneity among IL-2 receptor-positive synovial T cells suggests a role for superantigen in rheumatoid arthritis. *Proc Soc Natl Acad Sci U S A* 1991;88:10921–10925.
35. Jenkins RN, Nikaein A, Zimmermann A, et al. T cell receptor Vβ gene bias in rheumatoid arthritis. *J Clin Invest* 1993;92:2688–2701.

36. Williams WV, Fang Q, Demarco D, et al. Restricted heterogeneity of T cell receptor transcripts in rheumatoid synovium. *J Clin Invest* 1992;90:326–333.
37. Sottini A, Imberti L, Gorla R, et al. Restricted expression of T cell receptor Vβ but not Vα genes in rheumatoid arthritis. *Eur J Immunol* 1991;21:461–466.
38. Gudmundsson S, Ronnelid J, Karlssoon-Parra A, et al. T-cell receptor V-gene usage in synovial fluid and synovial tissue from RA patients. *Scand J Immunol* 1992;36:681–688.
39. Goronzy JJ, Bartz-Bazzanella P, Hu W, et al. Dominant clonotypes in the repertoire of peripheral CD4+ T cells in rheumatoid arthritis. *J Clin Invest* 1994;94:2068–2076.
40. Struyk L, Hawes GE, Chatila MK, et al. Review: T cell receptors in rheumatoid arthritis. *Arthritis Rheum* 1995;38:577–589.
41. Smith MD, Roberts-Thompson PJ. Lymphocyte surface marker expression in rheumatic diseases: evidence for prior activation of lymphocytes *in vivo*. *Ann Rheum Dis* 1990;49:81–87.
42. Schulze-Koops H, Davis LA, Kavanaugh AF, et al. Elevated cytokine messenger RNA levels in the peripheral blood of patients with rheumatoid arthritis suggest different degrees of myeloid cell activation. *Arthritis Rheum* 1997;40:639–647.
43. Keystone EC, Snow KM, Bombardier C, et al. Elevated soluble interleukin-2 receptor levels in the sera and synovial fluids of patients with rheumatoid arthritis. *Arthritis Rheum* 1988;31:844–849.
44. Ziff M. Role of endothelium in chronic inflammatory synovitis. *Arthritis Rheum* 1991;34:1345–1352.
45. Paleolog EM. Angiogenesis: a critical process in the pathogenesis of RA-a role for VEGF? *Br J Rheumatol* 1996;35:917–920.
46. Walsh DA. Angiogenesis and arthritis. *Rheumatology* 1999;38:103–112.
47. Hale LP, Martin ME, McCollum DE, et al. Immunohistologic analysis of the distribution of cell adhesion molecules within the inflammatory synovial microenvironment. *Arthritis Rheum* 1989;32:22–30.
48. Koch AE, Burrows JC, Haines GK, et al. Immunolocalization of endothelial and leukocyte adhesion molecules in human rheumatoid and osteoarthritic synovial tissues. *Lab Invest* 1991;64:313–320.
49. Lazarovits AI, Karsh J. Differential expression in rheumatoid synovium and synovial fluid of $\alpha_4\beta_7$ integrin. *J Immunol* 1993;151:6482–6489.
50. Hamann A, Syrbe U. T-cell trafficking into sites of inflammation. *Rheumatology* 2000;39:696–699.
51. Postigo AA, Garcia-Vicuña R, Diaz-Gonzales F, et al. Increased binding of synovial T lymphocytes from rheumatoid arthritis to endothelial leukocyte adhesion molecule-1 (ELAM-1) and vascular cell adhesion molecule-1 (VCAM-1). *J Clin Invest* 1992;89:1445–1452.
52. Van Dinther-Janssen ACHM, Horst E, Koopman G, et al. The VLA4/VCAM-1 pathway is involved in lymphocyte adhesion to endothelium in rheumatoid arthritis. *J Immunol* 1991;147:4207–4210.
53. Morales-Ducret J, Wayner E, Elices MJ. α_4/β_1 integrin (VLA-4) ligands in arthritis. Vascular cell adhesion molecule-1 expression in synovium and on fibroblast-like synoviocytes. *J Immunol* 1992;149:1424–1431.
54. Springer TA. Traffic signals for lymphocyte recirculation and leukocyte emigration: the multistep paradigm. *Cell* 1994;76:301–314.
55. Mojcik CF, Shevach EM. Adhesion molecules. A rheumatologic perspective. *Arthritis Rheum* 1997;40:991–1004.
56. Shimizu Y, Shaw S, Graber N, et al. Activation-independent binding of human memory T cells to adhesion molecule ELAM-1. *Nature* 1991;349:799–802.
57. Pitzalis C, Kingsley GH, Haskard DO, et al. The preferential accumulation of helper-inducer T lymphocytes in inflammatory lesions: evidence for regulation by selective endothelial and homotypic adhesion. *Eur J Immunol* 1988;18:1397–1404.
58. Pitzalis C, Kingsley GH, Covelli M, et al. Selective migration of the human helper-inducer memory T cell subset: confirmation by *in vivo* cellular kinetic studies. *Eur J Immunol* 1991;21:369–376.
59. Pietschmann P, Cush JJ, Lipsky PE, et al. Identification of subsets of human T cells capable of enhanced transendothelial migration. *J Immunol* 1992;149:1170–1178.
60. Firestein GS, Zvaifler NJ. Peripheral blood and synovial fluid monocyte activation in inflammatory arthritis. II. Low levels of synovial fluid and synovial tissue interferon suggest that γ-interferon is not the primary macrophage activating factor. *Arthritis Rheum* 1987;30:864–871.
61. Firestein GS, Xu W-D, Townsend K, et al. Cytokines in chronic inflammatory arthritis. I. Failure to detect T cell lymphokines (interleukin 2 and interleukin 3) and presence of macrophage colony stimulating factor (CSF-1) and a novel mast cell growth factor in rheumatoid synovitis. *J Exp Med* 1988;168:1573–1586.
62. Cope AP, Londei M, Chu R, et al. Chronic exposure to tumor necrosis factor (TNF) *in vitro* impairs the activation of T cells through the T cell receptor/CD3 complex; reversal *in vivo* by anti-TNF antibodies in patients with rheumatoid arthritis. *J Clin Invest* 1994;94:749–760.
63. Lotz M, Kekow J, Carson D. Transforming growth factor-B and cellular immune responses in synovial fluids. *J Immunol* 1990;144:4189–4194.
64. Miossec P, Naviliat M, D'Angeac AD, et al. Low levels of interleukin-4 and high levels of transforming growth factor β in rheumatoid synovitis. *Arthritis Rheum* 1990;33:1180–1187.
65. Wahl SM, Allen JB, Wong HL, et al. Antagonistic and agonistic effects of transforming growth factor-β and IL-1 in rheumatoid arthritis. *J Immunol* 1990;145:2514–2519.
66. Shull MM, Ormsby I, Kier AB, et al. Targeted disruption of the mouth transforming growth factor-β1 gene results in multifocal inflammatory disease. *Nature* 1992;359:693–699.
67. Katsikis PD, Cong-Qiu C, Brennan FM, et al. Immunoregulatory role of interleukin 10 in rheumatoid arthritis. *J Exp Med* 1994;179:1517–1527.
68. Cush JJ, Splawski JB, Thomas R, et al. Elevated interleukin-10 levels in patients with rheumatoid arthritis. *Arthritis Rheum* 1995;38:96–104.
69. Brennan FM. Interleukin-10 and arthritis. *Rheumatology* 1999;38:293–297.
70. Howard M, O'Garra A, Ishida H, et al. Biological properties of interleukin 10. *J Clin Immunol* 1992;12:239–247.
71. Mottonen M, Isomaki P, Saario R, et al. Interleukin-10 inhibits the capacity of synovial macrophages to function as antigen-presenting cells. *Br J Rheumatol* 1998;37:1207–1214
72. Gold KN, Weyand CM, Goronzy JJ. Modulation of helper T cell function by prostaglandins. *Arthritis Rheum* 1994;37:925–933.
73. Taylor-Robinson AW, Liew FY, Severn A, et al. Regulation of the immune response by nitric oxide differentially produced by T helper type 1 and T helper type 2 cells. *Eur J Immunol* 1994;24:980–984.
74. Maurice MM, Lankester AC, Bezemer AZ, et al. Defective TCR-mediated signaling in synovial T cells in rheumatoid arthritis. *J Immunol* 1997;159:2973–2978.
75. Olsen N, Ziff M, Jasin HE. *In vitro* synthesis of immunoglobulins and IgM-rheumatoid factor by blood mononuclear cells of patients with rheumatoid arthritis. *Rheumatol Int* 1982;2:59–66.
76. Olsen N, Jasin HE. Synthesis of RF *in vitro*: implications for the pathogenesis of rheumatoid arthritis. *Semin Arthritis Rheum* 1985;15:146–156.
77. Olsen N, Ziff M, Jasin HE. Spontaneous synthesis of IgM rheumatoid factor by blood mononuclear cells from patients with rheumatoid arthritis: effect of treatment with gold salts or D-penicillamine. *J Rheumatol* 1984;11:17–21.
78. Boling EP, Ohishi T, Wahl SM, et al. Humoral immune function in severe, active rheumatoid arthritis. *Clin Immunol Immunopathol* 1987;43:185–194.
79. Smiley JD, Sachs C, Ziff M. *In vitro* synthesis of immunoglobulins by rheumatoid synovial membrane. *J Clin Invest* 1968;47:624–632.
80. Sliwinski AJ, Zvaifler NJ. *In vivo* synthesis of IgG by rheumatoid synovium. *J Lab Clin Med* 1970;76:304–310.
81. Wernick RM, Lipsky PE, Marban-Arcos E, et al. IgG and IgM rheumatoid factor synthesis in rheumatoid synovial membrane cell cultures. *Arthritis Rheum* 1985;28:742–752.
82. Natvig JB, Munthe E. Self-associating IgG rheumatoid factor represents a major response of plasma cells in rheumatoid inflammatory tissue. *Ann NY Acad Sci* 1975;256:88–95.
83. Mestecki J, Miller EJ. Presence of antibodies to cartilage-type collagen in rheumatoid synovial tissue. *Clin Exp Immunol* 1975;22:453–456.
84. Tarkowski A, Klareskog L, Carlsten H, et al. Secretion of antibodies to types I and II collagen by synovial tissue cells in patients with rheumatoid arthritis. *Arthritis Rheum* 1989;32:1087–1092.
85. Munthe E, Natvig JB. Characterization of IgG complexes in eluates from rheumatoid tissue. *Clin Exp Immunol* 1971;8:249–262.

86. Winchester RJ, Agnello V, Kunkel HG. Gamma globulin complexes in synovial fluids of patients with rheumatoid arthritis. *Clin Exp Immunol* 1970;6:689–706.
87. Cooke TD, Hurd E, Jasin HE, et al. The identification of immunoglobulins and complement in rheumatoid articular collagenous tissues. *Arthritis Rheum* 1975;18:541–551.
88. Jasin HE. Autoantibody specificities of immune complexes sequestered in articular cartilage of patients with rheumatoid arthritis and osteoarthritis. *Arthritis Rheum* 1985;28:241–248.
89. Takemura S, Klimiuk PA, Braun A et al. T cell activation in rheumatoid synovium is B cell dependent. *J Immunol* 2001;167:4710–4718.
90. Fuji I, Shingu M, Nobunaga M. Monocyte activation in early onset rheumatoid arthritis. *Ann Rheum Dis* 1990;49:497–503.
91. Goto M, Fujisawa M, Yamada A, et al. Spontaneous release of angiotensin converting enzyme and interleukin 1β in peripheral blood monocytes from patients with rheumatoid arthritis under a serum free condition. *Ann Rheum Dis* 1990;49:172–176.
92. Grober JS, Bowen BL, Ebling H, et al. Monocyte-endothelial adhesion in chronic rheumatoid arthritis. *In situ* detection of selectin and integrin-dependent interactions. *J Clin Invest* 1993;91:2609–2619.
93. Iguchi T, Kurosaka M, Ziff M. Immunoelectron microscopic study of HLA-DR and monocyte/macrophage staining cells in the rheumatoid synovial membrane. *Arthritis Rheum* 1986;29:600–613.
94. Barkley D, Allard S, Feldman M, et al. Increased expression of HLA-DQ antigens by interstitial cells and endothelium in the synovial membrane of rheumatoid arthritis patients compared with reactive arthritis patients. *Arthritis Rheum* 1989;32:955–963.
95. Poubelle PM, Damon M, Blotman F, Dayer J-M. Production of mononuclear cell factor by mononuclear phagocytes from rheumatoid synovial fluid. *J Rheumatol* 1985;12:412–417.
96. Firestein GS, Alvaro-Garcia JM, Maki R. Quantitative analysis of cytokine gene expression in rheumatoid arthritis. *J Immunol* 1990; 144:3347–3353.
97. Dayer J-M, de Rochemontieix B, Burrus B, et al. Human recombinant interleukin 1 stimulates collagenase and prostaglandin E_2 production by human synovial cells. *J Clin Invest* 1986;77:645–648.
98. Burmester GR, Stuhlmüller B, Keyszer G, et al. Mononuclear phagocytes and rheumatoid arthritis. *Arthritis Rheum* 1997;40:5–18.
99. Burmester GR, Dimitriu-Bona A, Waters SJ, et al. Identification of three major synovial lining cell populations by monoclonal antibodies directed to Ia antigens and antigens associated with monocytes/macrophages and fibroblasts. *Scand J Immunol* 1983;17:69–82.
100. Goto M, Sasano M, Yamanaka H, et al. Spontaneous production of an interleukin 1-like factor by cloned rheumatoid synovial cells in long-term culture. *J Clin Invest* 1987;80:786–796.
101. Burmester GR, Jahn B, Zacher J, et al. Differential expression of Ia antigens by rheumatoid synovial lining cells. *J Clin Invest* 1987; 80:595–604.
102. Steinman RM, Adams JC, Cohn ZA. Identification of a novel cell type in peripheral lymphoid organs of mice. I. Morphology, quantitation and tissue distribution. *J Exp Med* 1973;137:1142–1162.
103. Deftos M, Olee T, Carson DA, et al. Defining the genetic origins of three rheumatoid synovium-derived IgG rheumatoid factors. *J Clin Invest* 1994;93:2545–2553.
104. Geppert TD, Jasin HE. Antigen presentation in the rheumatoid joint [Editorial]. *J Rheumatol* 1991;18:309–311.
105. Baker DG, Dayer J-M, Roelke M, et al. Rheumatoid synovial cell morphologic changes induced by a mononuclear cell factor in culture. *Arthritis Rheum* 1983;26:8–14.
106. Klareskog L, Johnell O, Hulth A. Expression of HLA-DR and HLA-DQ antigens on cells within the cartilage-pannus junction in rheumatoid arthritis. *Rheumatol Int* 1984;4:11–15.
107. Dechanet J, Merville P, Durand I, et al. The ability of synoviocytes to support terminal differentiation of activated B cells may explain plasma cell accumulation in rheumatoid synovium. *J Clin Invest* 1995;95:456–463.
108. Wekerle H, Ketelsen UP, Ernst M. Thymic nurse cells. Lymphoepithelial cell complexes in murine thymuses: morphological and serological characterization. *J Exp Med* 1980;151:925–944
109. Takeuchi E, Tomita T, Toyosaki-Maeda T, et al. Establishment and characterization of nurse cell-like stromal cell lines from synovial tissues of patients with rheumatoid arthritis. *Arthritis Rheum* 1999; 42:221–228.
110. Crisp AJ, Chapman CM, Kirkham SE, et al. Articular mastocytosis in rheumatoid arthritis. *Arthritis Rheum* 1984;27:845–851.
111. Godfrey HP, Ilardi C, Engber W, et al. Quantitation of human synovial mast cells in rheumatoid arthritis and other rheumatic diseases. *Arthritis Rheum* 1984;27:852–856.
112. Bromley M, Fisher WD, Wooley DE. Mast cells at sites of cartilage erosion in the rheumatoid joint. *Ann Rheum Dis* 1984;43:76–79.
113. Malone DG, Irani A-M, Schwartz LB, et al. Mast cell numbers and histamine levels in synovial fluids from patients with diverse arthritides. *Arthritis Rheum* 1986;29:956–963.
114. Gruber B, Poznansky M, Boss E, et al. Characterization and functional studies of rheumatoid synovial mast cells: activation by secretagogues, anti-IgE, and a histamine-releasing lymphokine. *Arthritis Rheum* 1986;29:944–955.
115. Frewin DB, Cleland LG, Johnsson JR, et al. Histamine levels in human synovial fluid. *J Rheumatol* 1986;13:13–14.
116. Plaut M, Pierce JH, Watson CJ, et al. Mast cell lines produce lymphokines in response to cross-linkage of Fcε R1 or to calcium ionophores. *Nature* 1989;339:64–67.
117. Burd PR, Rogers HW, Gordon JR, et al. Interleukin 3-dependent and -independent mast cells stimulated with IgE and antigen express multiple cytokines. *J Exp Med* 1989;170:245–257.
118. Wodnar-Filipowicz A, Heusser CH, Moroni C. Production of the haemopoietic growth factor GM-CSF and interleukin-3 by mast cells in response to IgE receptor-mediated activation. *Nature* 1989;339: 150–152.
119. Gordon JR, Galli SJ. Mast cells as a source of both preformed and immunologically inducible TNFα-cachectin. *Nature* 1990;346:274–276.
120. Center DM. Identification of rat mast cell–derived chemoattractant factors for lymphocytes. *J Allergy Clin Immunol* 1983;71:29–35.
121. Postlethwaite AE, Holness MA, Katai H, et al. Human fibroblasts synthesize elevated levels of extracellular matrix in response to interleukin 4. *J Clin Invest* 1990;90:1479–1485.
122. Claman HN. Mast cells and fibrosis. *Rheum Dis Clin North Am* 1990;16:141–151.
123. Gruber BL, Kew RR, Jelaska A, et al. Human mast cells activate fibroblasts. Tryptase is a fibrogenic factor stimulating collagen messenger ribonucleic acid synthesis and fibroblast chemotaxis. *J Immunol* 1997;158:2310–2317.
124. Lee DM, Friend DS, Gurish MF, et al. Mast cells: a cellular link between autoantibodies and inflammatory arthritis. *Science* 2002;297: 1689–1692.
125. Hollingsworth JW, Siegel ER, Creasey WA. Granulocyte survival in synovial exudate of patients with rheumatoid arthritis and other inflammatory joint diseases. *Yale J Biol Med* 1967;39:289–297.
126. Rumore PM, Yu D, Steinman CR. Presence and pathophysiologic significance of apoptotically derived oligonucleosomal complexes in RA synovial fluid. *Arthritis Rheum* 1994;37(suppl):311.
127. Bell DA, Morrison B, Vandenbygaart P. Immunogenic DNA-related factors. Nucleosomes spontaneously released from normal murine lymphoid cells stimulate proliferation and immunoglobulin synthesis of normal mouse lymphocytes. *J Clin Invest* 1990;85:1487–1496.
128. Cush JJ, Lipsky PE. Cellular basis for joint inflammation. *Clin Orthop* 1991;265:9–22.
129. Fox RI, Fong S, Sabharwal N, et al. Synovial fluid lymphocytes differ from peripheral blood lymphocytes in patients with rheumatoid arthritis. *J Immunol* 1982;128:351–354.
130. Smith MD, Roberts-Thompson PJ. Lymphocyte surface marker expression in rheumatic diseases: evidence for prior activation of lymphocytes in vivo. *Ann Rheum Dis* 1990;49:81–87.
131. Reme T, Portier M, Frayssinoux F, et al. T cell receptor expression and activation of synovial lymphocyte subsets in patients with rheumatoid arthritis. Phenotyping of multiple synovial sites. *Arthritis Rheum* 1990; 33:485–492.
132. Hemler M, Glass D, Coblyn JS, et al. Very late activation antigens on rheumatoid synovial fluid T lymphocytes. Association with stages of T cell activation. *J Clin Invest* 1986;78:696–702.
133. Konttinen Y, Bergroth V, Nykanen P. Lymphocyte activation in rheumatoid arthritis synovial fluid *in vivo*. *Scand J Immunol* 1985; 22:503–507.
134. Holoshitz J, Koning F, Coligan J, et al. Isolation of $CD4^-$ $CD8^-$ mycobacteria-reactive T lymphocyte clones from rheumatoid arthritis synovial fluid. *Nature* 1989;339:226–229.

135. Alsalameh S, Mollenhauer J, Hain N, et al. Cellular immune response toward human articular chondrocytes. T cell reactivities against chondrocyte and fibroblast membranes in destructive joint diseases. *Arthritis Rheum* 1990;33:1477–1486.
136. Guerassimov A, Zhang Y, Banerjee S, et al. Autoimmunity to cartilage link protein in patients with rheumatoid arthritis and ankylosing spondylitis. *J Rheumatol* 1998;25:1480–1484.
137. Al-Balaghi S, Strom H, Moller E. High incidence of spontaneous Ig-producing lymphocytes in peripheral blood and synovial fluid of patients with active seropositive rheumatoid arthritis. *Scand J Immunol* 1982;16:69–76.
138. Vaughan JH, Chihara T, Moore TL, et al. Rheumatoid factor-producing cells detected by direct hemolytic plaque assay. *J Clin Invest* 1976;58:933–941.
139. Breedveld FC, Lafeber GJM, Siegert CEH, et al. Elastase and collagenase activities in synovial fluids of patients with arthritis. *J Rheumatol* 1987;14:1008–1012.
140. Gysen P, Malaise M, Gaspar S, et al. Measurement of proteoglycans, elastase, collagenase and protein in synovial fluid in inflammatory and degenerative arthropathies. *Clin Rheumatol* 1985;4:39–50.
141. Borth W, Dunky A, Kleesiek K. α2-Macroglobulin complexes as correlated with α1-proteinase inhibitor-elastase complexes in synovial fluids of rheumatoid arthritis patients. *Arthritis Rheum* 1986;29:319–325.
142. Kuramitsu K, Yoshida A. Plasma and synovial fluid levels of granulocytal elastase-α-1 protease inhibitor complex in patients with rheumatoid arthritis. *Rheumatol Int* 1990;10:51–56.
143. Menninger H, Putzier R, Mohr W, et al. Granulocyte elastase at the sites of cartilage erosion by rheumatoid synovial tissue. *Z Rheumatol* 1980;39:145–156.
144. Velbart M, Fehr K. Degradation *in vivo* of articular cartilage in rheumatoid arthritis and juvenile chronic arthritis by cathepsin G and elastase from polymorphonuclear leukocytes. *Rheumatol Int* 1987;7: 195–202.
145. Ishikawa H, Smiley JD, Ziff M. Electron microscopic demonstration of immunoglobulin deposition in rheumatoid cartilage. *Arthritis Rheum* 1975;18:563–576.
146. Ohno O, Cooke TD. Electron microscopic morphology of immunoglobulin aggregates and their interactions in rheumatoid articular collagenous tissues. *Arthritis Rheum* 1978;21:516–527.
147. Henson PM, Henson JE, Fittschen C, et al. Phagocytic cells: degranulation and secretion. In: Gallin JL, Goldstein IM, Snyderman R, eds. *Inflammation: basic principles and clinical correlates.* New York: Raven, 1988:363–390.
148. Larbre J-P, Moore AR, Da Silva JAP, et al. Direct degradation of articular cartilage by rheumatoid synovial fluid: contribution of proteolytic enzymes. *J Rheumatol* 1994;21:1796–1801.
149. Baumstark JS. Studies on the elastase serum protein interaction. II. On the digestion of human α2-macroglobulin, an elastase inhibitor by elastase. *Biochem Biophys Acta* 1970;207:318–330.
150. Barrett AJ, Starkey PM. The interaction of α_2-macroglobulin with proteinases. *Biochem J* 1973;133:709–724.
151. Harpel PC, Moresson MW. Degradation of human fibrinogen by plasma α_2-macroglobulin enzyme complexes. *J Clin Invest* 1973;52: 2175–2184.
152. Galdston M, Levytska V, Liener IE, et al. Degradation of tropoelastin and elastin substrates by human neutrophil elastase free and bound to α_2-macroglobulin in serum of the M and Z (pi) phenotypes for α_1-antitrypsin. *Am Rev Respir Dis* 1979;119:435–441.
153. Moore AR, Appelboam A, Kawabata K. Destruction of articular cartilage by alpha2 macroglobulin-elastase complexes: role in rheumatoid arthritis. *Ann Rheum Dis* 1999;58:109–113.
154. Murphy G, Hembry RM. Proteinases in rheumatoid arthritis. *J Rheumatol* 1992;19(suppl):61–64.
155. Harris ED Jr, DiBona DR, Krane SM. Collagenase in human synovial fluid. *J Clin Invest* 1969;48:2104–2113.
156. Cawston TE, Mercer E, de Silva M, et al. Metalloproteinases and collagenase inhibitors in rheumatoid synovial fluid. *Arthritis Rheum* 1984;27:285–290.
157. Clark IM, Powell LK, Ramsey S, et al. The measurement of collagenase, tissue inhibitor of metalloproteinases (TIMP), and collagenase-TIMP complex in synovial fluids from patients with osteoarthritis and rheumatoid arthritis. *Arthritis Rheum* 1993;36:372–379.
158. Eeckhout Y, Vaes G. Further studies on the activation of procollagenase, the latent precursor of bone collagenase: effects of lysosomal cathepsin B, plasmin and kallikrein and spontaneous activation. *Biochem J* 1977;166:21–31.
159. Werb Z, Mainardi C, Vater CA, et al. Endogenous activation of latent collagenase by rheumatoid synovial cells: evidence for a role of plasminogen activator. *N Engl J Med* 1977;296:1017–1023.
160. Nagase H, Enghild JJ, Suzuki K, et al. Stepwise activation mechanisms of the precursor of matrix metalloproteinase 3 (stromelysin) by proteinases and (4-aminophenyl)mercuric acetate. *Biochemistry* 1990;29:5783–5789.
161. Gruber BL, Marchese MJ, Suzuki K, et al. Synovial procollagenase activation by human mast cell tryptase dependence upon matrix metalloproteinase 3 activation. *J Clin Invest* 1989;84:1657–1662.
162. Weiss SJ, Peppin G, Ortiz X, et al. Oxidative autoxidation of latent collagenase by human neutrophils. *Science* 1985;227:747–749.
163. Murphy G, Cockett MI, Stephens PE, et al. Stromelysin is an activator of procollagenase. A study with natural and recombinant enzymes. *Biochem J* 1987;248:265–268.
164. Ito A, Nagase H. Evidence that rheumatoid synovial matrix metalloproteinase 3 is an endogenous activator of procollagenase. *Arch Biochem Biophys* 1988;267:211–216.
165. Morgunova E, Tuuttila A, Bergmann U, et al. Structure of human pro-matrix metalloproteinase-2: activation mechanism revealed. *Science* 1999;284:1667–1670.
166. Murphy G, Reynolds JJ. Extracellular matrix degradation. In: Royce PM, Steinman B, eds. *Connective tissue and its heritable disorders.* New York: Wiley-Liss, 1993:287–316.
167. Stetler-Stevenson WG. Matrix metalloproteinases in angiogenesis: a moving target for therapeutic intervention. *J Clin Invest* 1999;103: 1237–1241.
168. Arend WP. Cytokines and cellular interactions in inflammatory arthritis. *J Clin Invest* 2001;107:1081–1082.
169. La Cava A. Cytokines and autoimmune rheumatic diseases. *Int J Adv Rheumatol* 2003;1:10–19.
170. Devore-Carter D, Gay RM, Weaver CT, et al. New model of antigen-induced murine arthritis. *FASEB J* 1995;9:A786.
171. Miossec P, Dinarello CA, Ziff M. Interleukin 1 lymphocyte chemotactic activity in rheumatoid arthritis synovial fluid. *Arthritis Rheum* 1986;29:461–470.
172. Symons JA, McDowell TL, DiGiovine FS, et al. Interleukin 1 in rheumatoid arthritis: potentiation of immune responses within the joint. *Lymphokine Res* 1989;8:365–372.
173. Malyak M, Swaney RE, Arend WP. Levels of synovial fluid interleukin-1 receptor antagonist in rheumatoid arthritis and other arthropathies. *Arthritis Rheum* 1993;36:781–789.
174. Firestein GS, Boyle DL, Yu C, et al. Synovial interleukin-1 receptor antagonist and interleukin-1 balance in rheumatoid arthritis. *Arthritis Rheum* 1994;37:644–652.
175. Hollander AP, Atkins RM, Eastwood DM, et al. Human cartilage is degraded by rheumatoid arthritis synovial fluid but not by recombinant cytokines in vitro. *Clin Exp Immunol* 1991;83:52–57.
176. Mantovani A, Bussolini F, Dejana E. Cytokine regulation of endothelial cell function. *FASEB J* 1992;6:2591–2599.
177. Gamble JR, Harlan JM, Klebanoff SJ, et al. Stimulation of the adherence of neutrophils to umbilical vein endothelium by human recombinant tumor necrosis factor. *Proc Natl Acad Sci U S A* 1985;82: 8667–8681.
178. Yu C-L, Haskard D, Cavender D, et al. Human gamma interferon increases the binding of T lymphocytes to endothelial cells. *Clin Exp Immunol* 1985;62:554–560.
179. Border WA, Noble NA. Transforming growth factor β in tissue fibrosis. *N Engl J Med* 1994;331:1286–1292.
180. Ming WJ, Bersani L, Mantovani A. Tumour necrosis factor is chemotactic for monocytes and polymorphonuclear leucocytes. *J Immunol* 1987;138:1469–1474.
181. Koch AE, Kunkel SL, Burrows JC, et al. Synovial tissue macrophages as a source of the chemotactic cytokine IL-8. *J Immunol* 1991;147:2187–2195.
182. Matsukawa A, Yoshimura T, Maeda T, et al. Neutrophil accumulation and activation by homologous IL-8 in rabbits. IL-8 induces destruction of cartilage and production of IL-1 and IL-1 receptor antagonist *in vivo. J Immunol* 1995;154:5418–5425.
183. Fava RA, Olsen NJ, Postlethwaite AE, et al. Transforming growth factor β1 (TGF-β1) induced neutrophil recruitment to synovial tis-

sues: implications for TGF-β-driven synovial inflammation and hyperplasia. *J Exp Med* 1991;173:1121–1132.
184. Akahoshi T, Wada C, Endo H, et al. Expression of monocyte chemotactic and activating factor in rheumatoid arthritis. *Arthritis Rheum* 1993;36:762–771.
185. Koch AE, Kunkel SL, Harlow LA, et al. Macrophage inflammatory protein-1α: a novel chemotactic cytokine for macrophages in rheumatoid arthritis. *J Clin Invest* 1994;93:921–928.
186. Rathanaswami P, Hachicha M, Sadick M, et al. Expression of the cytokine RANTES in human rheumatoid synovial fibroblasts. *J Biol Chem* 1993;268:5834–5839.
187. Remmers EF, Sano H, Wilder RL. Platelet-derived growth factors and heparin-binding (fibroblast) growth factors in the synovial tissue pathology of rheumatoid arthritis. *Semin Arthritis Rheum* 1991;21: 191–199.
188. Kirkham B. Interleukin-1, immune activation pathways, and different mechanisms in osteoarthritis and rheumatoid arthritis. *Ann Rheum Dis* 1991;50:395–400.
189. Larsen CG, Zachariae C, Oppenheim JJ, et al. Production of monocyte chemotactic and activating factor (MCAF) by human dermal fibroblasts in response to interleukin 1 or tumour necrosis factor. *Biochem Biophys Res Commun* 1989;160:1403–1408.
190. Bonnem EM, Oldham RK. Gamma-interferon: physiology and speculation on its role in medicine. *J Biol Response Mod* 1987;6:275–301.
191. Saklatvala J. Tumour necrosis factor α stimulates resorption and inhibits synthesis of proteoglycan in cartilage. *Nature* 1986;322:547–549.
192. Phadke K. Fibroblast growth factor enhances the interleukin 1 mediated chondrocyte protease release. *Biochem Biophys Res Commun* 1987;142:448–453.
193. Shingu M, Miyauchi S, Nagai Y, et al. The role of IL-4 and IL-6 in IL-1-dependent cartilage matrix degradation. *Br J Rheumatol* 1995; 34:101–106.
194. Reitamo S, Remitz A, Tamai K, et al. Interleukin-10 modulates type I collagen and matrix metalloproteinase gene expression in cultured human skin fibroblasts. *J Clin Invest* 1994;94:2489–2492.
195. Tyler JA. Articular cartilage cultured with catabolin (interleukin 1) synthesizes a decreased number of normal proteoglycan molecules. *Biochem J* 1985;227:869–878.
196. Morales TI, Roberts AB. Transforming growth factor β regulates the metabolism of proteoglycans in bovine cartilage organ cultures. *J Biol Chem* 1988;263:12828–12831.
197. Trippel SB, Corvol MT, Dumontier MF, et al. Effect of somatomedin c/insulin-like growth factor 1 on cultured growth plate and articular chondrocytes. *Pediatr Res* 1989;25:76–82.
198. Castor CW, Smith EM, Hossler PA, et al. Detection of connective tissue activating peptide-III isoforms in synovium from osteoarthritis and rheumatoid arthritis patients: patterns of interaction with other synovial cytokines in cell culture. *Arthritis Rheum* 1992;35:783–793.
199. Brennan FM, Maini RN, Feldmann M. TNFα—a pivotal role in rheumatoid arthritis. *Br J Rheumatol* 1992;31:293–298.
200. Koch A, Polverini PJ, Kunkel SL, et al. Interleukin-8 as a macrophage-derived mediator of angiogenesis. *Science* 1992;258:1798–1801.
201. Montesano R, Vasalli J-D, Baird A, et al. Basic fibroblast growth factor induces angiogenesis *in vitro*. *Proc Natl Acad Sci U S A* 1986; 83:7297–7301.
202. Heimark RL, Twarzik DR, Schwatz SM. Inhibition of endothelial regeneration by type-beta transforming growth factor from platelets. *Science* 1986;233:1078–1080.
203. Grotendorst GR, Grotendorst CA, Gilman T. Production of growth factors at the site of tissue repair. *Prog Clin Biol Res* 1988;266: 47–54.
204. Rapolee DA, Mark D, Banda MJ, et al. Wound macrophages express TGF-α and other growth factors *in vivo*: analysis by mRNA typing. *Science* 1988;241:708–712.
205. Kovacs EJ, DiPietro LA. Fibrogenic cytokines and connective tissue production. *FASEB J* 1994;8:854–861.
206. Ishikawa F, Miyazono K, Hellman U, et al. Identification of angiogenic activity and the cloning and expression of platelet-derived endothelial cell growth factor. *Nature* 1989;338:557–561.
207. Koch AE, Harlow LA, Haines GK, et al. Vascular endothelial growth factor: a cytokine modulating endothelial function in rheumatoid arthritis. *J Immunol* 1994;152:4149–4156.
208. Thorton SC, Pot SB, Walsh BJ, et al. Interaction of immune and connective tissue cells: the effects of lymphokines and monokines on fibroblast growth. *J Leukocyte Biol* 1990;47:312–320.
209. Butler DM, Leizer T, Hamilton JA. Stimulation of human synovial fibroblast DNA synthesis by platelet-derived growth factor and fibroblast growth factor. *J Immunol* 1988;142:3098–3103.
210. Vannier E, Miller LC, Dinarello CA. Coordinated anti-inflammatory effects of interleukin-4: IL-4 suppresses IL-1 production but up-regulates gene expression and synthesis of interleukin-1 receptor antagonist. *Proc Natl Acad Sci U S A* 1992;89:4076–4080.
211. Hermann JA, Hall MA, Maini RN, et al. Important immunoregulatory role of interleukin-11 in the inflammatory process in rheumatoid arthritis. *Arthritis Rheum* 1998;41:1388–1397.
212. Goldring MB, Birkhead J, Sandell LJ, et al. Immune interferon suppresses levels of procollagen in mRNA and type II collagen synthesis in cultured human articular and costal chondrocytes. *J Biol Chem* 1986;261:9049–9056.
213. Cawston TE, Curry VA, Summers CA, et al. The role of oncostatin M in animal and human connective tissue collagen turnover and its localization within the rheumatoid joint. *Arthritis Rheum* 1998;41: 1760–1771.
214. Olee T, Hashimoto S, Quach J, et al. IL-18 is produced by articular chondrocytes and induces proinflammatory and catabolic responses. *J Immunol* 1999;162:1096–1100.
215. Keffer J, Probert L, Cazlaris H, et al. Transgenic mice expressing human tumour necrosis factor: a predictive genetic model of arthritis. *EMBO J* 1991;10:4025–4031.
216. Saxne T, Palladino MA Jr, Heinegard D, et al. Detection of tumor necrosis factor α but not tumor necrosis factor β in rheumatoid arthritis synovial fluid and serum. *Arthritis Rheum* 1988;31:1041–1045.
217. Chu CQ, Field M, Feldmann M, et al. Localization of tumor necrosis factor α in synovial tissues and at the cartilage-pannus junction in patients with rheumatoid arthritis. *Arthritis Rheum* 1991;34:1125–1132.
218. Manicoourt D-H, Triki R, Fukuda K, et al. Levels of circulating tumor necrosis factor α and interleukin-6 in patients with rheumatoid arthritis. *Arthritis Rheum* 1993;36:490–499.
219. Roubenoff R, Roubenoff RA, Cannon JG, et al. Rheumatoid cachexia: cytokine-driven hypermetabolism accompanying reduced body cell mass in chronic inflammation. *J Clin Invest* 1994;93:2379–2386.
220. Genovese MC, Bathon JM, Martin RW, et al. Etanercept versus methotrexate in patients with early rheumatoid arthritis. *Arthritis Rheum* 2002;46:1443–1450.
221. Lipsky PE, van der Heijde DMFM, St Clair EW, et al. Infliximab and methotrexate in the treatment of rheumatoid arthritis. *N Engl J Med* 2000;343:1594–1602.
222. Epstein FH. Cytokine pathways and joint inflammation in rheumatoid arthritis. *N Engl J Med* 2001;344:907–911.
223. Morand EF, Bucala R, Leech M. Macrophage migration inhibitory factor. An emerging therapeutic target in rheumatoid arthritis. *Arthritis Rheum* 2003;48:291–299.
224. Gregersen PK, Bucala R. Macrophage migration inhibitory factor, MIF alleles, and the genetics of inflammatory disorders: incorporating disease outcome in the definition of phenotype. *Arthritis Rheum* 2003;48:1171–1176.
225. Winchester RJ, Agnello V, Kunkel HG. Gamma globulin complexes in synovial fluids of patients with rheumatoid arthritis. *Clin Exp Immunol* 1970;6:689–706.
226. Menzel J, Steffen C, Kolarz G, et al. Demonstration of antibodies to collagen and of collagen-anticollagen immune complexes in rheumatoid arthritis synovial fluids. *Ann Rheum Dis* 1976;35:446–450.
227. Jasin HE. Autoantibody specificities of immune complexes sequestered in articular cartilage of patients with rheumatoid arthritis and osteoarthritis. *Arthritis Rheum* 1985;28:241–248.
228. Mollenhauer J, von der Mark K, Burmester G, et al. Serum antibodies against chondrocyte cell surface proteins in osteoarthritis and rheumatoid arthritis. *J Rheumatol* 1988;15:1811–1817.
229. Mettal D, Brune K, Mollenhauer J. Cytotoxic effects of rheumatoid arthritis sera on chondrocytes. *Biochim Biophys Acta* 1992;1138: 85–92.
230. Takagi T, Jasin HE. Interactions of synovial fluid immunoglobulins with chondrocytes. *Arthritis Rheum* 1992;35:1502–1509.

231. Jasin HE. Oxidative cross-linking of immune complexes by human polymorphonuclear leukocytes. *J Clin Invest* 1988;81:6–15.
232. Jasin HE. Oxidative modification of inflammatory synovial fluid immunoglobulin G. *Inflammation* 1993;17:167–181.
233. Lunec J, Griffiths HR, Brailsford S. Oxygen free radicals denature human IgG and increase its reactivity with rheumatoid factor antibody. *Scand J Rheumatol* 1988;75(suppl):140–147.
234. Pekin TJ, Zvaifler NJ. Hemolytic complement in synovial fluid. *J Clin Invest* 1964;43:1372–1382.
235. Elmgreen J, Hansen TM. Subnormal sensitivity of neutrophils to complement split-product C5a in rheumatoid arthritis: relation to complement catabolism and disease extent. *Ann Rheum Dis* 1985; 44:514–518.
236. Goldstein IM, Weissmann G. Generation of C5-derived lysosomal enzyme-releasing activity (C5a) by lysates of leukocyte lysosomes. *J Immunol* 1974;113:1583–1588.
237. Kitsis E, Weissmann G. The role of the neutrophil in rheumatoid arthritis. *Clin Orthop Rel Res* 1991;265:63–72.
238. Breitner S, Störkel S, Reichel W, et al. Complement components C1q, C1r/C1s, and C1INH in rheumatoid arthritis. *Arthritis Rheum* 1995;38:492–498.
239. Ravetch JV. A full complement of receptors in immune complex disease. *J Clin Invest* 2002;110:1759–1761.
240. Blom AB, Radstake TRDJ, Holthuysen AEM, et al. Increased expression of Fcγ receptors II and III on macrophages of rheumatoid arthritis patients results in higher production of tumor necrosis factor α and matrix metalloproteinase. *Arthritis Rheum* 2003;48:1002–1014.
241. Nabbe KCAM, Blom AB, Holthuysen AEM, et al. Coordinate expression of activating Fcγ receptors II and III and inhibiting Fcγ receptor type II in the determination of joint inflammation and cartilage destruction during immune complex-mediated arthritis. *Arthritis Rheum* 2003;48:255–265.
242. Nieto A, Cáliz R, Pascual M, et al. Involvement of Fcγ receptor IIIA genotypes in susceptibility to rheumatoid arthritis. *Arthritis Rheum* 2000;43:735–739.
243. Brun JG, Madland TM, Vedeler CA. Immunoglobulin G Fc-receptor IIA, IIIA, and IIIB polymorphisms related to disease severity in rheumatoid arthritis. *J Rheumatol* 2002;29:1135–1140.
244. Robinson DR, Dayer JM, Krane SM. Prostaglandins and their regulation in rheumatoid arthritis. *Ann NY Acad Sci* 1979;332:279–294.
245. Abramsom SH, Weissmann G. The mechanism of action of nonsteroidal antiinflammatory drugs. *Arthritis Rheum* 1989;32:1–9.
246. Zurier RB, Quagliatta F. Effect of prostaglandin E_1 on adjuvant arthritis. *Nature* 1971;234:304–305.
247. Weissmann G, Dukor P, Zurier RB. Effect of cyclic AMP on release of lysosomal enzymes from phagocytes. *Nature (New Biol)* 1971; 231:131–135.
248. Oppenheimer-Marks N, Kavanaugh AF, Lipsky PE. Inhibition of the transendothelial migration of human T lymphocytes by prostaglandin E_2. *J Immunol* 1994;152:5703–5713.
249. Fu J-Y, Masferrer JL, Seibert K, et al. The induction and suppression of prostaglandin H_2 synthase (cyclooxygenase) in human monocytes. *J Biol Chem* 1990;265:16737–16740.
250. Jones D, Carlton P, McIntyre T, et al. Molecular cloning of human prostaglandin endoperoxide synthase type 2 and demonstration of expression in response to cytokines. *J Biol Chem* 1993;268:9049–9054.
251. Scales WE, Chensue SW, Otterness I, et al. Regulation of monokine gene expression: prostaglandin E_2 suppresses tumor necrosis factor but not interleukin-1α or β mRNA and cell-associated activity. *J Leukoc Biol* 1989;45:416–421.
252. Anastassiou ED, Paliogianni F, Balow JP, et al. Prostaglandin E_2 and other cAMP-elevating agents modulate IL-2 and IL-2Rα gene expression at multiple levels. *J Immunol* 1992;148:2845–2852.
253. Ratcliffe LT, Lukey PT, Meyers OL, et al. Prostanoid modulation of synovial antigen-specific CD4+ T-cell cytotoxic function in rheumatoid arthritis. *Br J Rheumatol* 1995;34:113–120.
254. Linnemeyer PA, Pollack SB. Prostaglandin E_2-induced changes in the phenotype, morphology and lytic activity of IL-2 activated natural killer cells. *J Immunol* 1993;150:3747–3754.
255. Gold KN, Weyand CM, Goronzy JJ. Modulation of helper T cell function by prostaglandins. *Arthritis Rheum* 1994;37:925–933.
256. Mochan E, Uhl J, Newton R. Evidence that interleukin-1 induction of synovial cell plasminogen activator is mediated via prostaglandin E_2 and cAMP. *Arthritis Rheum* 1986;29:1078–1084.
257. Wahl LM, Mergenhagen SE. Regulation of monocyte/macrophage collagenase. *J Oral Pathol* 1988;17:452–455.
258. Henderson WR Jr. The role of leukotrienes in inflammation. *Ann Intern Med* 1994;121:684–697.
259. Clark MA, Ögü LE, Conway TM, et al. Cloning of a phospholipase A_2-activating protein. *Proc Natl Acad Sci U S A* 1991;88:5418–5422.
260. Jakobsson P-J, Odlander B, Steinhilber B, et al. Human B lymphocytes possess 5-lipoxygenase activity and convert arachidonic acid to leukotriene B_4. *Biochem Biophys Res Commun* 1991;178:302–308.
261. Claesson HE, Haeggström J. Human endothelial cells stimulate leukotriene synthesis and convert granulocyte released leukotriene A_4 into leukotrienes B_4, C_4, D_4 and E_4. *Eur J Biochem* 1988;173:93–100.
262. Palmer RM, Stepney RJ, Higgs GA, et al. Chemokinetic activities of arachidonic and lipoxygenase products on leukocytes of different species. *Prostaglandins* 1980;20:411–418.
263. Tonnesen MG. Neutrophil-endothelial cell interactions: mechanisms of neutrophil adherence to vascular endothelium. *J Invest Dermatol* 1989;93(suppl):53–58.
264. Sha'afi RI, Naccache PH, Molski TF, et al. Cellular regulatory role of leukotriene B4: its effect on cation homeostasis in rabbit neutrophils. *J Cell Physiol* 1981;108:401–408.
265. Levine JD, Lau W, Kwiat G, et al. Leukotriene B_4 produces hyperalgesia that is dependent on polymorphonuclear leukocytes. *Science* 1984;225:743–745.
266. Rola-Pleszczynski M, Bouvrette L, Gingras D, et al. Identification of interferon-gamma as the lymphokine that mediates leukotriene B_4-induced immunoregulation. *J Immunol* 1987;139:513–517.
267. Rola-Pleszczynski M, Chavaillaz PA, Lemaire I. Stimulation of interleukin 2 and interferon gamma production by leukotriene B_4 in human lymphocyte cultures. *Prostaglandins Leukot Med* 1986;23: 207–210.
268. Rola-Pleszczynski M, Stañkova J. Leukotriene B_4 enhances interleukin-6 (IL-6) production and IL-6 messenger RNA accumulation in human monocytes *in vitro*: transcriptional and posttranscriptional mechanisms. *Blood* 1992;80:1004–1011.
269. Serhan CN, Drazen JM. Antiinflammatory potential of lipoxygenase-derived eicosanoids: a molecular switch at 5 and 15 positions? *J Clin Invest* 1997;99:1147–1148.
270. Ternowitz T, Fogh K, Kragballe K. 15-Hydroxy-eicosatetraenoic acid (15-HETE) specifically inhibits LTB4-induced chemotaxis of polymorphonuclear leukocytes. *Skin Pharmacol* 1988;1:93–99.
271. Fogh K, Hansen ES, Herlin T, et al. 15-Hydroxy-eicosatetraenoic acid (15-HETE) inhibits carrageenan-induced experimental arthritis and reduces synovial fluid leukotriene B_4 (LTB_4). *Prostaglandins* 1989;37:213–228.
272. Davidson EM, Rae SA, Smith SM. Leukotriene B_4 a mediator of inflammation present in synovial fluid in rheumatoid arthritis. *Ann Rheum Dis* 1983;42:677–679.
273. Koshihara I, Isono T, Oda H, et al. Measurement of sulfidopeptide leukotrienes and their metabolism in human synovial fluid of patients with rheumatoid arthritis. *Prostaglandins Leukot Essent Fatty Acids* 1988;32:113–119.
274. Ahmadzadeh N, Shingu M, Nobunaga M, et al. Relationship between leukotriene B_4 and immunological parameters in rheumatoid synovial fluids. *Inflammation* 1991;15:497–503.
275. Weinblatt ME, Kremer JM, Coblyn JS, et al. Zileuton, a 5-lipoxygenase inhibitor in rheumatoid arthritis. *J Rheumatol* 1992;19:1537–1541.
276. Weiss SJ. Tissue destruction by neutrophils. *N Engl J Med* 1989;320: 365–376.
277. Greenwald RA. Oxygen radicals, inflammation, and arthritis: pathophysiological considerations and implications for treatment. *Semin Arthritis Rheum* 1991;20:219–240.
278. Miller RA, Britigan BE. The formation and biologic significance of phagocyte-derived oxidants. *J Invest Med* 1995;43:39–49.
279. Cohen MS, Mesler DE, Snipes RG, et al. 1,25-dihydroxyvitamin D_3 activates secretion of hydrogen peroxide by human monocytes. *J Immunol* 1986;136:1049–1053.
280. Jasin HE. Cross-linking of immune complexes by human mononuclear phagocytes. *Inflammation* 1987;11:117–129.
281. Greenwald RA, Moak SA. Degradation of hyaluronic acid by polymorphonuclear leukocytes. *Inflammation* 1986;10:15–30.
282. Uchiyama H, Dobashi Y, Phkouchi K, et al. Chemical changes involved in the oxidative reductive depolymerization of hyaluronic acid. *J Biol Chem* 1990;265:7753–7759.

283. Weiss SJ, Peppin G, Ortiz X, et al. Oxidative autoxidation of latent collagenase by human neutrophils. *Science* 1985;227:747–749.
284. Carp H, Janoff A. Potential mediator of inflammation: phagocyte derived oxidants suppress the elastase inhibitory capacity of alpha 1-proteinase inhibitor *in vitro*. *J Clin Invest* 1980;66:987–995.
285. Cathcart MK, McNally AK, Morel DW, et al. Superoxide anion participation in human monocyte-mediated oxidation of low-density lipoprotein and conversion of low-density lipoprotein to a cytotoxin. *J Immunol* 1989;142:1963–1969.
286. Winyard PG, Tatzber F, Esterbauer H, et al. Presence of foam cells containing oxidised low density lipoprotein in the synovial membrane from patients with rheumatoid arthritis. *Ann Rheum Dis* 1993; 52:677–680.
287. Perez HD, Weksler BB, Goldstein I. Generation of a chemotactic lipid from arachidonic acid by exposure to a superoxide generating system. *Inflammation* 1980;4:313–320.
288. Bashir S, Denman MA, Blake DR, et al. Oxidative DNA damage and cellular sensitivity to oxidative stress in human autoimmune diseases. *Ann Rheum Dis* 1993;52:659–666.
289. Carson DA, Seto S, Wasson DB, et al. DNA strand breaks, NAD metabolism, and programmed cell death. *Exp Cell Res* 1986;164:273–281.
290. Hildeman DA, Mitchell, Kappler J, et al. T cell apoptosis and reactive oxygen species. *J Clin Invest* 2003;111:575–581.
291. Bates EJ, Johnson CC, Lowther DA. Inhibition of proteoglycan synthesis by hydrogen peroxide in cultured bovine articular cartilage. *Biochim Biophys Acta* 1985;838:221–228.
292. Rosen GM, Pou S, Ramos CL, et al. Free radicals and phagocytic cells. *FASEB J* 1995;9:200–209.
293. Leeuwenburgh C, Rasmussen JE, Hsu FF, et al. Mass spectrometric quantification of markers for protein oxidation by tyrosyl radical, copper, and hydroxyl radical in low density lipoprotein isolated from human atherosclerotic plaques. *J Biol Chem* 1997;272:3520–3526.
294. Winyard PG, Chirico S, Blake DR. Mechanism of exacerbation of rheumatoid synovitis by total-dose iron infusion: in vivo demonstration of iron promoted oxidant stress. *Lancet* 1987;1:69–72.
295. Bettner GR, Chamulitrat W. The catalytic activity of iron in synovial fluid as monitored by the ascorbate free radical. *Free Radical Biol Med* 1990;8:55–56.
296. Downey JM. Free radicals: their involvement during long-term myocardial ischemia and reperfusion. *Ann Rev Phys* 1990;52:487–504.
297. Levick JR. Hypoxia and acidosis in chronic inflammatory arthritis: relation to vascular supply and dynamic effusion pressure. *J Rheumatol* 1989;17:579–581.
298. Blake DR, Unsworth J, Outhwaite JM, et al. Hypoxic reperfusion injury in the inflamed human joint. *Lancet* 1989;1:289–292.
299. Hall ND, Maslen CL, Blake DR. The oxidation of serum sulphydryl groups by hydrogen peroxide secreted by stimulated phagocytic cells in rheumatoid arthritis. *Rheumatol Int* 1984;4:35–38.
300. Gutteridge JMC. Antioxidant properties of the proteins ceruloplasmin, albumin, and transferrin: a study of their activity in serum and synovial fluid from patients with rheumatoid arthritis. *Biochim Biophys Acta* 1986;869:119–127.
301. Heffner JE, Repine JE. Pulmonary strategies of antioxidant defense. *Am Rev Respir Dis* 1989;140:531–554.
302. Britigan BE, Hassett DJ, Rosen GM, et al. Neutrophil degranulation inhibits potential hydroxyl radical formation: differential impact of myeloperoxidase and lactoferrin release on hydroxyl radical production by iron supplemented neutrophils assessed by spin trapping. *Biochem J* 1989;264:447–455.
303. Balla G, Jacob HS, Balla J, et al. Ferritin: a cytoprotective oxidant stratagem of endothelium. *J Biol Chem* 1992;267:18148–18153.
304. Moncada S, Higgs A. The L-arginine-nitric oxide pathway. *N Engl J Med* 1993;329:2002–2012.
305. Lowenstein CJ, Dinerman JL, Snyder SH. Nitric oxide: a physiologic messenger. *Ann Intern Med* 1994;120:227–237.
306. Lotz M. The role of nitric oxide in articular cartilage damage. *Rheum Dis Clin North Am* 1999;25:269–282.
307. Stadler J, Stefanovic-Racic M, Billiar TR, et al. Articular chondrocytes synthesize nitric oxide in response to cytokines and lipopolysaccharide. *J Immunol* 1991;147:3915–3920.
308. McInnes IB, Leung BP, Field M, et al. Production of nitric oxide in the synovial membrane of rheumatoid and osteoarthritic patients. *J Exp Med* 1996;184:1519–1524.
309. Wheeler MA, Smith SD, Garcia-Cerdeza G, et al. Bacterial infection induces nitric oxide synthase in human neutrophils. *J Clin Invest* 1997;99:110–116.
310. Eiserich JP, Cross CE, Jones AD, et al. Formation of nitrating and chlorinating species by reaction of nitrite with hypochlorous acid. *J Biol Chem* 1996;271:19199–19203.
311. Van der Vliet A, Eiserich JP, Halliwell B, et al. Formation of reactive nitrogen species during peroxidase-catalized oxidation of nitrate: a potential additional mechanism of nitric oxide-dependent toxicity. *J Biol Chem* 1997;272:7617–7620.
312. Beckman JS, Beckman TW, Chen J. Apparent hydroxyl radical production by peroxinitrite: implications for endothelial injury from nitric oxide and superoxide. *Proc Natl Acad Sci U S A* 1990;87: 1620–1624.
313. Lipton SA, Choi Y-B, Pan Z-H, et al. A redox-based mechanism for the neuroprotective and neurodestructive effects of nitric oxide and related nitroso-compounds. *Nature (London)* 1993;364:626–631.
314. Uesugi M, Hayashi T, Jasin HE. Covalent cross-linking of immune complexes by oxygen radicals and nitrite. *J Immunol* 1998;161: 1422–1427.
315. Wink DA, Kasprzak KS, Maragos CM, et al. DNA deaminating ability and genotoxicity of nitric oxide and its progenitors. *Science* 1992; 254:1001–1003.
316. Nguyen R, Brunson D, Crespi CL, et al. DNA damage mutation in human cells exposed to nitric oxide in vitro. *Proc Natl Acad Sci U S A* 1992;89:3030–3034.
317. Stadler J, Billiar TR, Curran RD, et al. Effect of exogenous and endogenous nitric oxide on mitochondrial respiration of rat hepatocytes. *Am J Physiol* 1991;260:C910–C916.
318. Mulligan MS, Heirel JM, Marletta MA, et al. Tissue injury caused by deposition of immune complexes is L-arginine dependent. *Proc Natl Acad Sci U S A* 1991;88:6338–6342.
319. Hughes SR, Williams TJ, Brain SD. Evidence that endogenous nitric oxide modulates oedema formation induced by substance P. *Eur J Pharmacol* 1990;191:481–484.
320. Ziche M, Morbidelli L, Masini S, et al. Nitric oxide mediates angiogenesis *in vivo* and endothelial cell growth and migration *in vitro* promoted by substance P. *J Clin Invest* 1994;94:2036–2044.
321. Kubes P, Suzuki M, Granger DM. Nitric oxide: an endogenous modulator of leukocyte adhesion. *Proc Natl Acad Sci U S A* 1991;88: 4651–4655.
322. Stadler J, Harbrecht BG, DiSilvio M, et al. Endogenous nitric oxide inhibits the synthesis of cyclooxygenase products and interleukin-6 by rat Kupffer cells. *J Leukoc Biol* 1993;53:165–172.
323. Hoffman RA, Langrher JM, Billiar TR, et al. Alloantigen-induced activation of rat splenocytes is regulated by the oxidative metabolism of L-arginine. *J Immunol* 1990;145:2220–2226.
324. Taylor-Robinson AW, Liew FY, Xu D, et al. Regulation of the immune response by nitric oxide differentially produced by T helper type 1 and T helper type 2 cells. *Eur J Immunol* 1994;24:980–984.
325. Hibbs JB, Westenfelder G, Taitor R, et al. Evidence for cytokine-inducible nitric oxide synthesis from L-arginine in patients receiving interleukin-2 therapy. *J Clin Invest* 1992;89:867–877.
326. Lin PP, Hughes CE, Clark JB, et al. Inhibitors of nitric oxide synthetase reverse the IL-1 induced inhibition of aggrecan biosynthesis but not its degradation. *Trans Orthop Res Soc* 1995;20:217.
327. Studer RK, Georgescu HI, Miller LA, et al. Inhibition of transforming growth factor β production by nitric oxide-treated chondrocytes. Implications for matrix synthesis. *Arthritis Rheum* 1999;42:248–257.
328. Murrell GAC, Jang D, Williams RJ. Nitric oxide activates metalloprotease enzymes articular cartilage. *Biochem Biophys Res Commun* 1995;206:15–21.
329. Pelletier J-P, Mineau F, Ranger P, et al. The synthesis of nitric oxide induced by IL-1 in human chondrocytes markedly reduced the synthesis of IL-1 receptor antagonist (IL-1ra): a possible role in osteoarthritic cartilage degradation. *Trans Orthop Res Soc* 1995;20: 352.
330. Abramson SB, Clancy R, Koehne C, et al. Nitric oxide mediates cytokine dependent susceptibility to oxidant injury in articular chondrocytes. *J Invest Med* 1995;43:246A.
331. Fujita I, Saura R, Matsubara T, et al. Inhibition of neutrophil-mediated chondrocyte cytotoxicity by nitric oxide generated by articular chondrocytes; a novel protective mechanism of cartilage degradation. *Trans Orthop Res Soc* 1994;19:472.

332. Weinberg JB, Granger DL, Pisetsky DS, et al. The role of nitric oxide in the pathogenesis of spontaneous autoimmune disease: increased nitric oxide production and nitric oxide synthase expression in MRL-lpr/lpr mice, and reduction of spontaneous glomerulonephritis and arthritis by orally administered N^G-monomethyl-L-arginine. *J Exp Med* 1994;179:651–660.
333. McCartney-Francis N, Allen JB, Mizel DE, et al. Suppression of arthritis by an inhibitor of nitric oxide synthase. *J Exp Med* 1993;178: 749–754.
334. Stefanovic-Racic M, Meyers K, Meschter C, et al. *N*-monomethyl arginine, an inhibitor of nitric oxide synthase, suppresses the development of adjuvant arthritis in rats. *Arthritis Rheum* 1994;37:1062–1069.
335. Brown CR, Reiner SL. Development of lyme arthritis in mice deficient in inducible nitric oxide synthase. *J Infect Dis* 1999;179:1573–1576.
336. Gilkerson GS, Mudgett JS, Seldin ME, et al. Clinical and serologic manifestations of autoimmune diseases in MRL-lpr/lpr mice lacking nitric oxide synthase type 2. *J Exp Med* 1997;186:365–373.
337. Farrell AJ, Blake DR, Palmer RMJ, et al. Increased concentrations of nitrite in synovial fluid and serum samples suggest increased nitric oxide synthesis in rheumatic diseases. *Ann Rheum Dis* 1992;51:1219–1222.
338. Kaur H, Halliwell B. Evidence for nitric oxide-mediated damage in chronic inflammation. Nitrotyrosine in serum and synovial fluid from rheumatoid patients. *FEBS Lett* 1994;350:9–12.
339. Sandhu JK, Robertson S, Birnboim HC, et al. Distribution of protein nitrotyrosine in synovial tissues of patients with rheumatoid arthritis and osteoarthritis. *J Rheumatol* 2003;30:1173–1181.
340. Clancy RM, Amin AR, Abramson SB. The role of nitric oxide in inflammation and immunity. *Arthritis Rheum* 1998;41:1141–1151.
341. Colman RW, Sartor RB, Adam AA, et al. The plasma kallikrein-kinin system in sepsis, inflammatory arthritis, and enterocolitis. *Clin Rev Allergy Immunol* 1998;16:365–384.
342. Schapira M, Despland E, Scott CF, et al. Purified plasma kallikrein aggregates human blood neutrophils. *J Clin Invest* 1982;69:1199–1202.
343. Kaplan AP, Kay AB, Austen KF. A prealbumin activator of prekallikrein. 3. Appearance of chemotactic activity for human neutrophils by the conversion of human prekallikrein to kallikrein. *J Exp Med* 1972;135:81–97.
344. Wachtfogel YT, Kucich U, James H, et al. Human plasma kallikrein releases neutrophil elastase during blood coagulation. *J Clin Invest* 1983;72:1672–1677.
345. Nagase H, Cawston TE, De Silva M, et al. Identification of plasma kallikrein as an activator of latent collagenase in rheumatoid synovial fluid. *Biochim Biophys Acta* 1982;702:133–142.
346. Melmon KL, Webster ME, Golfinger SE, et al. The presence of kinin in inflammatory synovial effusions from arthritides of varying etiologies. *Arthritis Rheum* 1967;10:13–20.
347. Selwyn B, Figueroa CD, Fink E, et al. A tissue kallikrein in the synovial fluid of patients with rheumatoid arthritis. *Ann Rheum Dis* 1989; 48:128–133.
348. Rahman MM, Lemon MJC, Elson CJ, et al. Proinflammatory role of tissue kallikrein in modulating pain in inflamed joints. *Br J Rheumatol* 1995;34:88–90.
349. Dela Cadena RA, Stadnicki A, Uknis AB, et al. Inhibition of plasma kallikrein prevents peptidoglycan-induced arthritis in the Lewis rat. *FASEB J* 1995;9:446–452.
350. Konttinen YT, Kemppinen P, Segerberg M, et al. Peripheral and spinal mechanisms in arthritis, with particular reference to treatment on inflammation and pain. *Arthritis Rheum* 1994;37:965–982.
351. Ohlen A, Thureson-Klein A, Lindbom L, et al. Substance P activates leukocytes and platelets in rabbit microvessels. *Blood Vessels* 1989; 26:84–94.
352. Smith CH, Barker JNWN, Morris RW, et al. Neuropeptides induce rapid expression of endothelial cell adhesion molecules and elicit granulocytic infiltration in human skin. *J Immunol* 1993;151:3274–3282.
353. Kimball ES, Persico FJ, Vaught JL. Substance P, neurokinin A, and neurokinin B, induce generation of IL-1-like activity in P338 D 1 cells. Possible relevance to arthritic disease. *J Immunol* 1988;141: 3564–3569.
354. Devillier P, Weill BJ, Menkes CJ, et al. Elevated levels of tachykinin-like immunoreactivity in joint fluids in patients with rheumatic inflammatory diseases. *N Engl J Med* 1986;314:1323.
355. Matucci-Cerinic M, Marabini S, Partsch G, et al. High levels of substance P in rheumatoid arthritis synovial fluid. Lack of substance P production by synoviocytes *in vitro*. *Clin Exp Rheumatol* 1991;9: 440–442.
356. Menkes CJ, Renoux M, Loussadi S, et al. Substance P levels in the synovium and synovial fluid from patients with rheumatoid arthritis and osteoarthritis. *J Rheumatol* 1993;20:714–717.
357. Mapp P, Kidd BL, Gibson SJ, et al. Substance P, calcitonin gene-related peptide, and C-flanking peptide of neuropeptide Y are present in normal synovium but depleted in patients with rheumatoid arthritis. *Neuroscience* 1990;37:143–153.
358. Deal CL, Schnitzer TJ, Lipstein E, et al. Treatment of arthritis with topical capsaicin: a double-blind trial. *Clin Ther* 1991;13:383–395.
359. Poole AR, Dieppe P. Biological markers in rheumatoid arthritis. *Semin Arthritis Rheum* 1994;23(suppl):17–31.
360. Maånsson B, Carey D, Alini M, et al. Cartilage and bone metabolism in rheumatoid arthritis. Differences between rapid and slow progression of disease identified by serum markers of cartilage metabolism. *J Clin Invest* 1995;95:1071–1077.
361. Carsons S, Lavietes BB, Diamond HS. Role of fibronectin in rheumatic diseases. In: Mosher DF, ed. *Fibronectin*. San Diego: Academic, 1989:327–361.
362. Carsons S, Lavietes BB, Diamond HS, et al. The immunoreactivity, ligand, and cell binding characteristics of rheumatoid synovial fluid fibronectin. *Arthritis Rheum* 1985;28:601–612.
363. Postlethwaite AE, Keski-Oja J, Balian G, et al. Induction of fibroblast chemotaxis by fibronectin. Localization of the chemotactic region to a 140,000-molecular weight non-gelatin-binding fragment. *J Exp Med* 1981;153:494–499.
364. Clark RAF, Wickner NE, Doherty DE, et al. Cryptic chemotactic activity of fibronectin for human monocytes resides in the 120kDa fibroblastic cell-binding fragment. *J Biol Chem* 1988;263:12115–12123.
365. Wachtfogel YT, Abrams W, Kucich U, et al. Fibronectin degradation products containing the cytoadhesive tetrapeptide stimulate human neutrophil degranulation. *J Clin Invest* 1988;81:1310–1316.
366. Homandberg GA, Meyers R, Williams J. Intraarticular injection of fibronectin fragments causes severe depletion of cartilage proteoglycans *in vivo*. *J Rheumatol* 1993;20:1378–1382.
367. Homandberg G, Xie DL, Bewsey K. Fibronectin samples depress proteoglycan synthesis and cause apparent irreversible cartilage damage *in vitro*. *Trans Orthop Res Soc* 1993;18:685.
368. Wahl SM, Allen JB, Hines KL, et al. Synthetic fibronectin peptides suppress arthritis in rats by interrupting leukocyte adhesion and recruitment. *J Clin Invest* 1994;94:655–662.
369. Postlethwaite AE, Kang AH. Collagen- and collagen-peptide-induced chemotaxis of human blood monocytes. *J Exp Med* 1976;143:1299–1307.
370. Hanauske-Abel HM, Poutz BF, Schorlemmer HU. Cartilage specific collagen activates macrophages and the alternative pathway of complement: evidence for an immunopathogenic concept of rheumatoid arthritis. *Ann Rheum Dis* 1982;41:168–176.
371. Goto M, Yoshinoya S, Miyamoto T, et al. Stimulation of interleukin-1α and interleukin-1β release from human monocytes by cyanogen bromide peptides of type II collagen. *Arthritis Rheum* 1988;31:1508–1514.
372. Cheung HS, Ryan LM, Kozin B, et al. Identification of collagen subtypes in synovial fluid sediments from arthritic patients. *Am J Med* 1980;68:73–79.
373. Furmaniak-Kazmierczak E, Cooke TDV, Manuel R, et al. Studies of thrombin-induced proteoglycan release in the degradation of human and bovine cartilage. *J Clin Invest* 1994;94:472–480.
374. Weinberg JB, Pippen AMM, Greenberg CS. Extravascular fibrin formation and dissolution in synovial tissue of patients with osteoarthritis and rheumatoid arthritis. *Arthritis Rheum* 1991;34:996–1005.
375. Jespersen J, Brommer EJP, Haverkate F, et al. Degradation products of fibrin and of fibrinogen in synovial fluid and in plasma of patients with rheumatoid arthritis. *Fibrinolysis* 1989;3:183–196.
376. Richardson DL, Pepper DS, Kay AB. Chemotaxis for human monocytes by fibrinogen-derived peptides. *Br J Haematol* 1976;32:507–513.
377. Busso N, Hamilton JA. Extravascular coagulation and the plasminogen activator/plasmin system in rheumatoid arthritis. *Arthritis Rheum* 2002;46:2268–2279.

378. Firestein GS. Starving the synovium: angiogenesis and inflammation in rheumatoid arthritis. *J Clin Invest* 1999;103:3–4.
379. Ballara S, Taylor PC, Reusch P, et al. Raised serum vascular endothelial growth factor levels are associated with destructive change in inflammatory arthritis. *Arthritis Rheum* 2001;44:2055–2064.
380. Fearon U, Griosios C, Fraser A, et al. Angiopoietins, growth factors, and vascular morphology in early arthritis. *J Rheumatol* 2003;30: 260–268.
381. Anand-Apte B, Pepper MS, Voest E, et al. Inhibition of angiogenesis by tissue inhibitor of of metalloproteinase-3. *Invest Ophthalmol Vis Sci* 1997;38:817–823.
382. Mitchell N, Shepard N. The ultrastructure of articular cartilage in rheumatoid arthritis: a preliminary report. *J Bone Joint Surg Am* 1970;52: 1405–1423.
383. Blanco FJ, Ochs RL, Schwarz H, et al. Chondrocyte apoptosis induced by nitric oxide. *Am J Pathol* 1995;146:75–85.
384. Nakajima T, Aono H, Hasunumat T, et al. Apoptosis and functional Fas antigen in rheumatoid arthritis synoviocytes. *Arthritis Rheum* 1995; 38:485–491.
385. Firestein GS, Yeo M, Zvaifler NJ. Apoptosis in rheumatoid arthritis synovium. *J Clin Invest* 1995;96:1631–1638.
386. Kim HA, Song YW. Apoptotic chondrocyte death in rheumatoid arthritis. *Arthritis Rheum* 1999;42:1528–1537.
387. Burmester GR, Menche D, Merryman P, et al. Application of monoclonal antibodies to the characterization of cells eluted from human articular cartilage. Expression of Ia antigen in certain diseases and identification of an 85-KD cell surface molecule accumulated in the pericellular matrix. *Arthritis Rheum* 1983;26:1187–1195.
388. Glant T, Mikecz K. Antigenic profiles of human, bovine and canine articular chondrocytes. Cell Tissue Res 1986;244:359–369.
389. Alsalameh S, Mollenhauer J, Hain N, et al. Cellular immune response toward human articular chondrocytes. T cell reactivities against chondrocyte and fibroblast membranes in destructive joint diseases. *Arthritis Rheum* 1990;33:1477–1486.
390. Steenbakkers PGA, Baeten D, Rovers E, et al. Localization of MHC class II/human cartilage glycoprotein-39 complexes in synovia of rheumatoid arthritis patients using complex-specific monoclonal antibodies. *J Immunol* 2003;170:5719–5727.
391. Verheijden GFM, Rijnders AWM, Bos E, et al. Human cartilage glycoprotein-39 as a candidate autoantigen in rheumatoid arthritis. *Arthritis Rheum* 1997;40:1115–1125.
392. Blass S, Schumann F, Hain NAK, et al. P205 is a major target of autoreactive T cells in rheumatoid arthritis. *Arthritis Rheum* 1999;42: 971–980
393. Yamaga KM, Bolen H, Kimura L, et al. Enhanced chondrocyte destruction by lymphokine-activated killer cells. Possible role in rheumatoid arthritis. *Arthritis Rheum* 1983;36:500–513.
394. Tak PP, Kummer JA, Hack CE, et al. Granzyme-positive cytotoxic cells are specifically increased in early rheumatoid synovial tissue. *Arthritis Rheum* 1994;37:1735–1743.
395. Müller-Ladner U, Kriegsmann J, Tschopp J, et al. Demonstration of granzyme A and perforin messenger RNA in the synovium of patients with rheumatoid arthritis. *Arthritis Rheum* 1995;38:477–484.
396. Mollenhauer J, von der Mark K, Burmester G, et al. Serum antibodies against chondrocyte cell surface proteins in osteoarthritis and rheumatoid arthritis. *J Rheumatol* 1988;15:1811–1817.
397. Mettal D, Brune K, Mollenhauer J. Cytotoxic effects of rheumatoid arthritis sera on chondrocytes. *Biochim Biophys Acta* 1992;1138:85–92.
398. Takagi T, Jasin HE. Interactions of synovial fluid immunoglobulins with chondrocytes. *Arthritis Rheum* 1992;35:1502–1509.
399. Mitchell N, Shepard N. Changes in proteoglycan and collagen in rheumatoid arthritis. *J Bone Joint Surg Am* 1978;60:349–354.
400. Jasin HE. Factors controlling articular cartilage degradation by activation of chondrocytes. In: Weissmann G, ed. *Advances in inflammation research.* Vol. 5. New York: Raven, 1983:87–105.
401. Lefevre V, Peeters-Joris C, Vaes G. Modulation by interleukin-1 and tumor necrosis factor α of production of collagenase, tissue inhibitor of metalloproteinases and collagen types in differentiated and dedifferentiated articular chondrocytes. *Biochim Biophys Acta* 1990;1052: 366–378.
402. Saklatvala J, Pilsworth LMC, Sarsfield SJ, et al. Pig catabolin is a form of interleukin 1; cartilage and bone resorb, fibroblasts make prostaglandin and collagenase, and thymocyte proliferation is augmented in response to one protein. *Biochem J* 1984;224:461–466.
403. Krakauer T, Oppenheim JJ, Jasin HE. Human interleukin 1 mediates cartilage matrix degradation. *Cell Immunol* 1985;91:92–99.
404. Tyler JA, Benton HP. Synthesis of type II collagen is decreased in cartilage cultured with interleukin-1 while the rate of extracellular degradation remains unchanged. *Coll Relat Res* 1988;8:393–405.
405. Hollander AP, Atkins RM, Eastwood DM, et al. Human cartilage is degraded by rheumatoid arthritis synovial fluid but not by recombinant cytokines in vitro. *Clin Exp Immunol* 1991;83:52–57.
406. Barrett AJ, Heath MF. Lysosomal enzymes. In: Dingle JT, ed. *Lysosomes, a laboratory handbook.* Amsterdam: North Holland, 1977:19–145.
407. Sandy JD, Flannery CR, Neame PJ, et al. The structure of aggrecan fragments in human synovial fluid: evidence for the involvement in osteoarthritis of a novel proteinase which cleaves glu 373-Ala 374 bond of the interglobular domain. *J Clin Invest* 1992;89:1512–1516.
408. Lohmander LS, Neame PJ, Sandy JD. The structure of aggrecan fragments in human synovial fluid. Evidence that aggrecanase mediates cartilage degradation in inflammatory joint disease, joint injury, and osteoarthritis. *Arthritis Rheum* 1993;36:1214–1222.
409. Arner EC. Aggrecanase-mediated cartilage degradation. *Curr Opin Pharm* 2002;2:322–329.
410. Tortorella MD, Burn TC, Pratta MA, et al. Purification and cloning of aggrecanase-1: a member of the ADAMTS family of proteins. *Science* 1999;284:1664–1666.
411. Fosang AJ, Neame PJ, Hardingham TE, et al. Cleavage of cartilage proteoglycan between G1 and G2 domains by stromelysin. *J Biol Chem* 1991;266:15579–15582.
412. Sandy JD, Neame PJ, Boynton RE, Flannery CR. Catabolism of aggrecan in cartilage explants: identification of a major cleavage site within the interglobular domain. *J Biol Chem* 1991;266:8683–8685.
413. Fosang AJ, Last K, Brown L, et al. Identification of metalloproteinase-derived aggrecan fragments with FFGVG N-terminal sequence in human synovial fluids. *Trans Orthop Res Soc* 1995;20:4.
414. Fosang AJ, Last K, Maciewicz RA. Aggrecan is degraded by matrix metalloproteinases in human arthritis. Evidence that matrix metalloproteinase and aggrecanase can be independent. *J Clin Invest* 1996; 98:2292–2299.
415. Dodge GR, Poole AR. Immunohistochemical detection and immunochemical analysis of type II collagen degradation in human normal, rheumatoid and osteoarthritic articular cartilage and in explants of bovine articular cartilage cultured with interleukin 1. *J Clin Invest* 1989;83:647–661.
416. Nguyen Q, Mort JS, Roughley PJ. Preferential mRNA expression of prostromelysin relative to procollagenase and *in situ* localization in human articular cartilage. *J Clin Invest* 1992;89:1189–1197.
417. Martel-Pelletier J, Clouthier J-M, Pelletier J-P. *In vivo* effects of antirheumatic drugs on neutral collagenolytic proteases in human rheumatoid arthritis cartilage and synovium. *J Rheumatol* 1988;15: 1198–1204.
418. Dodge GR, Pidoux I, Poole AR. The degradation of type II collagen in rheumatoid arthritis: an immunoelectron microscopic study. *Matrix* 1991;11:330–338.
419. Wu J-J, Lark M, Chun LE, et al. Sites of stromelysin cleavage in collagens type II, IX, X, and XI of cartilage. *J Biol Chem* 1991;266: 5625–5628.
420. Shiozawa S, Jasin HE, Ziff M. Absence of immunoglobulins in rheumatoid cartilage-pannus junctions. *Arthritis Rheum* 1980;23:816–821.
421. Jasin HE. The articular cartilage surface as a target organ [Editorial]. *Clin Exp Rheumatol* 1994;12:469–472.
422. Ugai K, Ziff M, Jasin HE. Interaction of polymorphonuclear leukocytes with immune complexes trapped in joint collagenous tissues. *Arthritis Rheum* 1979;22:353–364.
423. Noyori K, Jasin HE. Inhibition of human fibroblast adhesion by cartilage surface proteoglycans. *Arthritis Rheum* 1994;37:1656–1663.
424. Shiozawa S, Yoshihara R, Kuroki Y, et al. Pathogenic importance of fibronectin in the superficial region of articular cartilage as a local factor for the induction of pannus extension on rheumatoid articular cartilage. *Ann Rheum Dis* 1992;51:869–873.
425. Jasin HE, Taurog JD. Mechanisms of disruption of the articular cartilage surface in inflammation. Neutrophil elastase increases availability of collagen II epitopes for binding with antibodies on the surface of articular cartilage. *J Clin Invest* 1991;87:1531–1536.

426. Noyori K, Takagi T, Jasin HE. Characterization of the macromolecular components of the articular cartilage surface. *Rheumatol Int* 1998;18:71–77.
427. Noyori K, Koshino T, Takagi T, et al. Binding characteristics of anti-collagen type II antibody to the surface of diseased human cartilage as a probe for tissue damage. *J Rheumatol* 1994;21:293–296.
428. Allard SA, Muirden KD, Maini RN. Correlation of histopathological features of pannus with patterns of damage in different joints in rheumatoid arthritis. *Ann Rheum Dis* 1991;50:278–283.
429. Zvaifler NJ, Firestein GS. Pannus and pannocytes. Alternative models of joint destruction in rheumatoid arthritis. *Arthritis Rheum* 1994;37:783–789.
430. Fassbender HG. Histomorphological basis of articular cartilage destruction in rheumatoid arthritis. *Coll Rel Res* 1983;3:141–155.
431. Gay S, Gay RE, Koopman WJ. Molecular and cellular mechanisms of joint destruction in rheumatoid arthritis: two cellular mechanisms explain joint destruction? *Ann Rheum Dis* 1993;52(suppl):39–47.
432. Imamura F, Hiroyuki A, Hosunune T, et al. Monoclonal expansion of synoviocytes in rheumatoid arthritis. *Arthritis Rheum* 1998;41:1979–1986.
433. O'Sullivan FX, Fassbender HG, Gay S, et al. Etiopathogenesis of rheumatoid arthritis-like disease in MRL/l mice. I. The histomorphologic basis of joint destruction. *Arthritis Rheum* 1985;28:529–536.
434. Shiozawa S, Tanaka Y, Fujita T, et al. Destructive arthritis without lymphocyte infiltration in H2-c-*fos* transgenic mice. *J Immunol* 1992;148:3100–3104.
435. Geiler T, Kriegsmann J, Keyszer GM, et al. A new model for rheumatoid arthritis generated by engraftment of rheumatoid synovial tissue and normal human cartilage into SCID mice. *Arthritis Rheum* 1994;37:1664–1671.
436. Parfitt AM. The coupling of bone formation to bone resorption: a critical analysis of the concept and of its relevance to the pathogenesis of osteoporosis. *Metab Bone Dis Rel Res* 1982;4:1–6.
437. Manolagas SC, Gilka RL. Bone marrow, cytokines and bone remodeling. *N Engl J Med* 1995;332:305–311.
438. Takayanagi H, et al. A new mechanism of bone destruction in rheumatoid arthritis: synovial fibroblasts induce osteoclastogenesis. *Biochem Biophys Res Commun* 1997;240:279–286.
439. Takayanagi H, Juji T, Miyasaki T, et al. Suppression of arthritic bone destruction by adenovirus-mediated csk gene transfer to synoviocytes and osteoclasts. *J Clin Invest* 1999;104:137–146.
440. Nakashima T, Wada T, Penninger JM. RANKL and RANK as novel therapeutic targets for arthritis. *Curr Opin Rheumatol* 2003;15:280–287.
441. Ziolkowska M, Kurowska M, Radzikovska A, et al. High levels of osteoprotegerin and soluble receptor activator of nuclear factor kappa B ligand in serum of rheumatoid arthritis patients and their normalization after anti-tumor necrosis factor alpha treatment. *Arthritis Rheum* 2002;46:1744–1753.

CHAPTER 55

Rheumatoid Arthritis: The Clinical Picture

James R. O'Dell

Rheumatoid arthritis (RA) is a lifelong disease of unknown cause where no cures are available. Early and accurate diagnosis is critical for optimal outcomes but cannot be established by a single blood test or biopsy. Many effective therapies for RA are now available, but tests that would allow clinicians to select the best therapy for each individual patient remain to be elucidated. Therefore, the diagnosis of RA continues to require clinical skills and experience, whereas management puts a premium on the physician's ability to practice the art, as well as the science, of medicine.

RA is a systemic inflammatory disease with its primary manifestation in the synovium. The hallmark of the disease is a chronic, symmetric polyarthritis (synovitis) that typically affects the hands, wrists, and feet initially, and later may involve any joint lined by a synovial membrane, most frequently the knees, ankles, hips, elbows, and shoulders. Why RA has a particular predilection for the synovial joints has not been elucidated and remains one of the keys to pathogenesis. Although RA primarily involves the synovium, features of systemic disease are present in almost all patients and range in severity from fatigue, low-grade fevers, and mild to moderate anemias, to serositis (pleural or pericardial effusions) and severe multisystemic vasculitis. Fortunately, significant advances in therapy have recently occurred, but despite these advances, RA continues to result in substantial morbidity (1) for most patients and premature mortality in many (1–3).

EPIDEMIOLOGY

RA is a common illness affecting all racial groups worldwide, although it is seen more commonly in some populations than others (see Chapter 1). The prevalence in most cohorts averages approximately 1% (4,5), although some estimates are somewhat lower (6). The extremes of involvement include the Chippewa and Pima Amerindians in the United States, of whom over 5% have RA (7), and a population in rural western Nigeria where no affected persons were found (8). The more generally accepted prevalence rates have been derived from population samples, and the definition of what constitutes RA obviously greatly affects the estimates.

Incidence rates have been found to be less than (9), or the same as (10), several decades ago. A study in Minnesota found an incidence of 50 per 100,000 person-years in men and 98 per 100,000 person-years in women; the preponderance of women was marked in the younger age groups, but nearly equal for patients over 75 (5). The incidence of RA increases with age, with female excess in each age range found in most studies (5,9,11). There has been suggestion that not as many individuals are severely affected as in decades past (12). It is hoped that new and better treatments will continue to decrease the consequences of RA.

ESTABLISHING THE DIAGNOSIS

The importance of making an accurate diagnosis of RA as early as possible cannot be overemphasized. All modern treatment paradigms stress early, aggressive disease-modifying antirheumatic drug (DMARD) therapy (13,14); it is critical to ensure that effective treatments are begun when they have the maximum chance of making the biggest differences, while at the same time protecting patients who do not have RA from the potential toxicities of therapies. The diagnosis of RA is a clinical one, based almost exclusively on the history and physical examination. No single finding, either on examination or from laboratory testing, is pathognomonic for RA. Therefore, a set of seven criteria have been established for classification purposes (14) (Table 55.1), and although strictly speaking they were not developed for diagnostic purposes, they are widely used as such. The presence of four of seven criteria is required to establish the presence of RA for study purposes. These criteria include morning stiffness of at least 1-hour's duration

TABLE 55.1. *1987 American College of Rheumatology revised criteria for the classification of rheumatoid arthritis (traditional format)*

Criterion	Definition
Morning stiffness	Morning stiffness in and around the joints, lasting at least 1 hour before maximal improvement
Arthritis of three or more joint areas	At least three joint areas simultaneously with soft tissue swelling or joint fluid observed by a physician; the 14 possible areas are (right or left): PIP, MCP, wrist, elbow, knee, ankle, and MTP joints
Arthritis of hand joints	At least one area swollen in a wrist, MCP, or PIP joint
Symmetric arthritis	Simultaneous involvement of the same joint areas on both sides of the body (bilateral involvement of PIP, MCP, or MTP acceptable without perfect symmetry)
Rheumatoid nodules	Subcutaneous nodules over bony prominences or extensor surfaces, or in juxtaarticular regions, observed by a physician
Serum rheumatoid factor	Abnormal amount of serum rheumatoid factor by any method for which the result has been positive in <5% of control subjects
Radiographic changes	Erosions or unequivocal bony decalcification localized in or most marked adjacent to the involved joints (osteoarthritis changes excluded), typical of rheumatoid arthritis on posteroanterior hand and wrist radiographs

For classification purposes, a patient is said to have rheumatoid arthritis if four of seven criteria are satisfied. Criteria 1–4 must have been present for at least 6 weeks. Patients with two clinical diagnoses are not excluded.

MCP, metacarpophalangeal; MTP, metatarsophalangeal; PIP, proximal interphalangeal.

From Arnett FC, Edworth SM, Bloch DA, et al. The American Rheumatism Association 1987 revised criteria for the classification of rheumatoid arthritis. *Arthritis Rheum* 1988;31:315–324, with permission.

in and around the joints, simultaneous soft tissue swelling in three or more joint groups observed by the physician, involvement of the hands, symmetric involvement (i.e., same joint on right as on left side of body), rheumatoid nodules, serum rheumatoid factor (RF), and radiographic damage typical of RA on hand and wrist radiography (bone erosion). Importantly, in the case of the first four criteria, the patient must have had these present for a minimum of 6 weeks. This requirement is necessary since there are many other causes of symmetric polyarthritis (viral and others) that may mimic RA, but are of short duration. Unfortunately, this need to wait a minimum of 6 weeks for a definitive diagnosis can be frustrating for the patient and the physician and, worse, often results in significant delays in therapy.

A criticism of the 1987 American College of Rheumatology (ACR) criteria (15) is that relatively more importance is assigned to the hands than the feet; some investigators have shown that clinical involvement and radiographic damage in the feet may precede that seen in the hands and wrists (16). Despite these limitations, the classification criteria for RA are helpful guidelines to use when considering the diagnosis of RA.

Recently, antibodies to cyclic citrullinated peptide (CCP) have been shown to be very specific (17–21), although not very sensitive, for RA. Additionally, in some cases they are present years before the clinical diagnosis is made (19). If further studies corroborate these findings, anti-CCP antibodies may be useful in the early diagnosis of RA.

The diagnosis of RA should be considered in any patient with polyarticular inflammatory arthritis of greater than 6 weeks' duration, especially if the hands and feet are involved. As mentioned above, the history is critical in suggesting and then confirming the diagnosis. The patient response to the question "What is the worst time of day for your joints?" is often telling. Patients with inflammatory arthritis such as RA usually report significant morning stiffness (often greater than 1 hour), whereas patients with osteoarthritis (OA) and other mechanical syndromes are usually worse later in the day after activity. Additionally, significant fatigue may be present even in early RA. Early physical findings of disease include soft tissue joint swelling and joint tenderness to palpation. Joint distribution is critical in diagnosis. Initially, RA is often limited to the hands and feet. In the hands, it is the proximal interphalangeal (PIP) joints and metacarpophalangeal (MCP) joint that are most likely to be involved early. Figure 55-1 compares and contrasts the joints most commonly involved in the two most common kinds of arthritis: RA and OA. In the hand, the distal interphalangeal (DIP) joints are characteristically involved in OA (Heberden nodes) but seldom involved in RA, the PIPs may be involved with either, whereas MCP involvement is the rule in RA and seldom occurs in OA. The wrist is frequently involved in RA, whereas only the first CMC joint is commonly involved in OA. A remarkable feature of RA is the symmetry of involvement; interestingly, patients with prior cerebrovascular accidents may have sparing of the plegic side (22), suggesting that neural mechanisms are involved (23).

If synovial-based inflammation persists over time, permanent damage, including tendon, ligament, cartilage, and subchondral bone destruction, will occur, with resultant joint deformity and limited motion. Although inflammation and deformity are most often seen initially in the hands and

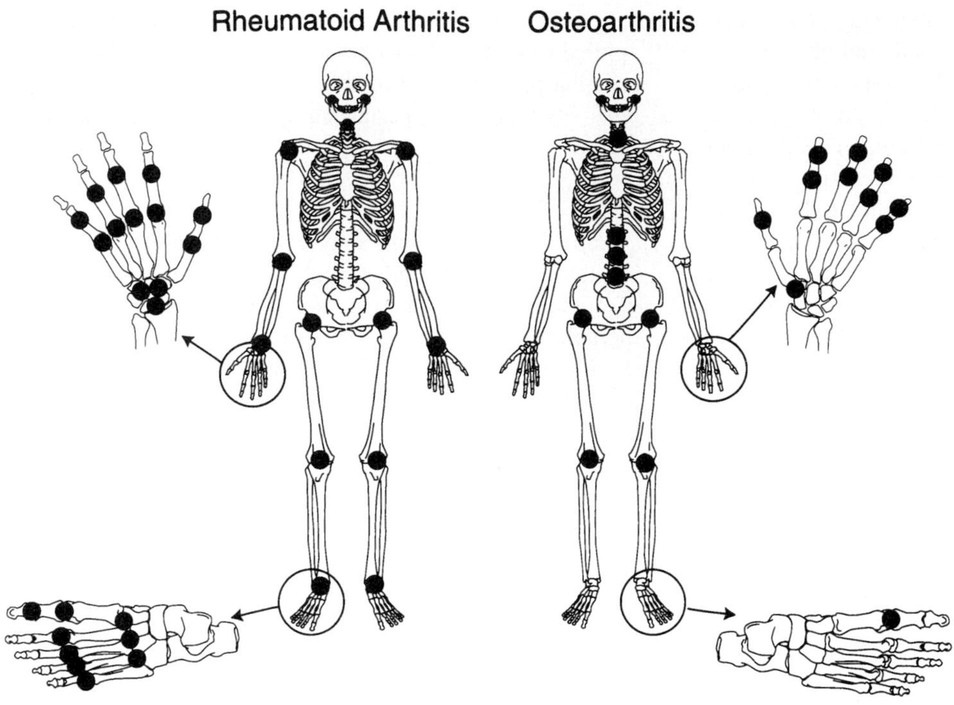

FIG. 55.1. The joint distribution of the two most common forms of arthritis—rheumatoid arthritis (*RA*) and osteoarthritis (*OA*)—are compared and contrasted. Joints involved in these arthritides are noted by the *black circles* over involved joint areas.

feet, later the disease often extends to larger joints, and involvement of the knees, hips, and shoulders accounts for significant morbidity, including work disability in a large percentage of patients.

A major difference in the pathophysiology of RA versus OA or mechanical joint problems is the presence of extensive synovial-based inflammation. The cardinal signs of inflammation were stated by Celsus: "*rubor et tumor cum calore et dolore*" ("redness and swelling with heat and pain"). And *functio laesa* (disturbed function) was later attributed to Galen. Joint tenderness, swelling, stiffness, and pain on motion are the features of inflammation experienced by the patient with RA (24).

GENDER AND HORMONAL INFLUENCES

The incidence of RA is two to three times greater in women (4,9). The greatest differences in incidence are in patients under age 50, an age at which RA is uncommon in men. Therefore, hormonal mechanisms are felt to play a part (25); somewhat paradoxically, the use of oral contraceptives and pregnancy are protective with respect to the development of RA, and 75% of pregnancies in patients with RA result in a significant decrease in symptoms (26). In the postpartum period, there is a relative increase in the incidence of RA, which suggests a "catch-up" phenomenon (27). In a similar fashion, oral contraceptives seem to be protective only during use (6). Breast-feeding appears to encourage the development of RA, perhaps, in part, by the actions of prolactin, a known proinflammatory cytokine (28). Finally, hormonal replacement therapy in women does not result in an increase in the activity of disease (29). Some have suggested that males with RA may have mild testosterone deficiencies (30) and replacement may result in some decrease in RA symptoms.

GENETICS

First-degree relatives of those with RA are at increased risk for developing the disease (31), with siblings of severely affected RA patients at highest risk (32). Monozygotic twins have a concordance rate of about 12% to 15%, whereas dizygotic twins have a rate about one fourth of this (33).

In populations of northern European descent, human leukocyte antigen (HLA)-DR4 is associated with both an increased incidence of RA (34) and with more severe disease (32). This is felt to be due primarily to a relevant shared DRB1 epitope found in certain subtypes of HLA-DR4, HLA-DR1, and HLA-Dw16 (see Chapter 27). Monozygosity for HLA-DR4 or this particular DRB1 epitope may predispose to seropositivity and more severe disease (35,36). Monozygotic twins who were homozygous for the DRB1 shared epitope had a fivefold increased risk of concordance for RA (37).

CLINICAL PICTURE

Stiffness

Morning stiffness is a hallmark of the inflammatory arthritides. Joint stiffness is a major symptom of most types of arthritis, and RA, in particular, is often accompanied by significant stiffness early in the day that may at times be disabling. Prolonged stiffness has been included in RA classification criteria (Fig. 55.1); when quantifying stiffness for clinical monitoring, it may be preferable to identify the length of time to maximal improvement (38). Other inflammatory conditions, such as systemic lupus erythematosus (SLE), ankylosing spondylitis, and polymyalgia rheumatica, are also accompanied by morning stiffness. The presence of morning stiffness may better discriminate a primary inflammatory process from other joint processes (39). Edema of the synovium and periarticular structures contributes to stiffness in RA by mechanically interfering with the usual motion of the joint. Stiffness is most pronounced after sleep, in part due to redistribution of interstitial fluid while sleeping. Although stiffness is usually most prominent around clinically involved joints, generalized morning stiffness, a feeling that all muscles have gelled or thickened, is also characteristic of RA.

On physical examination, stiffness is manifested by limitation of motion that may vary with the time of day, unlike that due to articular surface derangement or soft tissue contractures about the joint. A circadian rhythm is followed with patients unable to fully extend or flex the fingers in the early morning, but attaining best hand function and least pain and stiffness in mid-afternoon (40). Severe stiffness in the hands may improve with heat (41), but is most effectively relieved with active exercise (42).

Pain

Unfortunately, pain is a major problem for most patients with RA and is often what brings them to the physician's office. Pain is difficult to quantify, although its relief is a major end point used to measure the effectiveness of therapy (43,44) (Table 55.2). Pain thresholds among patients vary greatly with seemingly similar degrees of inflammation or joint damage as assessed by examination. RA patients as a group tend to minimize symptoms and often complain very little, even when obvious swelling and deformities are present. Joints with rapidly evolving effusions, as seen in early disease, or swollen joints with an applied load, may be extremely painful due to high intra-articular pressures that lead to excessive stresses on the extensively innervated, periarticular supporting structures.

TABLE 55.2. *American College of Rheumatology core set of disease activity measures for rheumatoid arthritis*

Disease activity measure
1. Tender joint count
2. Swollen joint count
3. Patient's assessment of pain
4. Patient's global assessment of disease activity
5. Physician's global assessment of disease activity
6. Patient's assessment of physical function
7. Acute-phase reactant value

For trial duration ≥1 year and agent being tested as a disease-modifying antirheumatic drug, also perform radiography or other imaging technique.

To meet improvement requirement, three of parameters 3 through 7 must improve by a specified amount.

Tenderness

Palpation of the joints may elicit tenderness, and counting the number of tender joints is also a major end point of clinical trials used to demonstrate the effectiveness of therapies (Table 55.2). Tenderness thresholds also vary significantly among patients and with the method of applying force used to elicit tenderness (45,46). The examiner should try to apply approximately the same pressure for each patient examined to standardize responses over time for each patient and between patients. Different observers will apply pressure at different sites and intensity and may arrive at varying conclusions about the same patient (47). The enlarged synovial membrane, periarticular ligaments, and supporting structures are the major pain-sensitive structures. Severe muscle tenderness should suggest another diagnosis such as fibromyalgia or a regional pain disorder. Bony prominences are generally tender, because periarticular structures are more superficial and therefore more sensitive to palpation at these sites.

A lateral squeeze of the MCP and metatarsophalangeal (MTP) joint row will detect tenderness in inflamed joints (48). Tenderness of three or all four of these joint groups is seen almost exclusively in patients with RA (49).

Pain on Motion

Pain on motion is often used as a surrogate for tenderness in joints that are difficult to palpate directly due to overlying muscle and other tissues; these include the cervical spine, shoulder, and hip (48). Pain on motion of the joint may be due to noninflammatory processes that also interfere with the joint's normal, almost frictionless, motion (50), including damage of cartilage and bone. Additionally, joint instability or subluxation may cause pain on motion.

Swelling

Joint swelling is a seminal finding for the diagnosis of RA, and is a major end point of therapeutic trials (Table 55.2). Swelling of a joint may result from proliferation of the synovial tissues, effusions, or from bony proliferation. In RA, the first two processes predominate, while bony proliferation around joints should suggest another type of process, such as OA. Early in the disease process there is an influx of inflammatory cells into the synovial membrane and concomitant angiogenesis, infiltration of chronic inflammatory (mononuclear) cells, proliferation of resident synovial cells, and resultant marked histologic changes—a joint lining membrane that is normally two cell layers thick changes to a thickened membrane that may be hundreds of cell layers thick, often having villous projections into the joint space. This soft tissue swelling is most evident in the small joints of the hands and feet: in the MCP and MTP joints, the outline of the base of the proximal phalanx may become indistinct, and in the PIP joints of the fingers, fusiform swelling is noted due to the anatomy of the synovial reflections (Fig. 55.2).

If synovial proliferation is abundant, a doughy texture may be felt due to the resultant soft tissue mass. Such synovial proliferation is commonly identified in the PIP, MCP, elbow, ankle, MTP, and knee joints, as well as in the flexor tendons of the fingers, the common extensor compartment of the dorsal wrist, and the extensor carpi ulnaris tendon sheath (Fig. 55.2). Swelling in the hip and shoulder joints may be difficult to ascertain on physical examination, unless it is severe (51).

Joint effusions also contribute to swelling. When the effusion is placed under increased pressure with joint flexion, the synovium may be forced between articular structures, and a portion becomes trapped and separated from the rest of the joint, forming what is called a Baker cyst. More fluid is forced into the structure, with subsequent loading of the distended joint, and a one-way valve effect may prevent the fluid from returning to the joint (52). Baker cysts were originally described in the knee, and although a similar phenomenon may be seen in most peripheral joints (53), they are most commonly recognized in the knee, where the larger the effusion, the more likely there will be a painful cyst (54). Dissection of a Baker cyst most often occurs in the posterior calf and often presents with only mild symptoms, such as a feeling of fullness. However, rupture of a Baker cyst at the knee often produces significant soft tissue swelling and pain in the calf that may resemble acute thrombophlebitis, often termed pseudothrombophlebitis syndrome (55), with extravasation of inflammatory joint contents along fascial planes as far as the ankle and dorsal foot (56). It is important to differentiate this syndrome from deep vein thrombosis, because anticoagulation of patients with a ruptured Baker cyst will result in increased bleeding into the calf and increased pain.

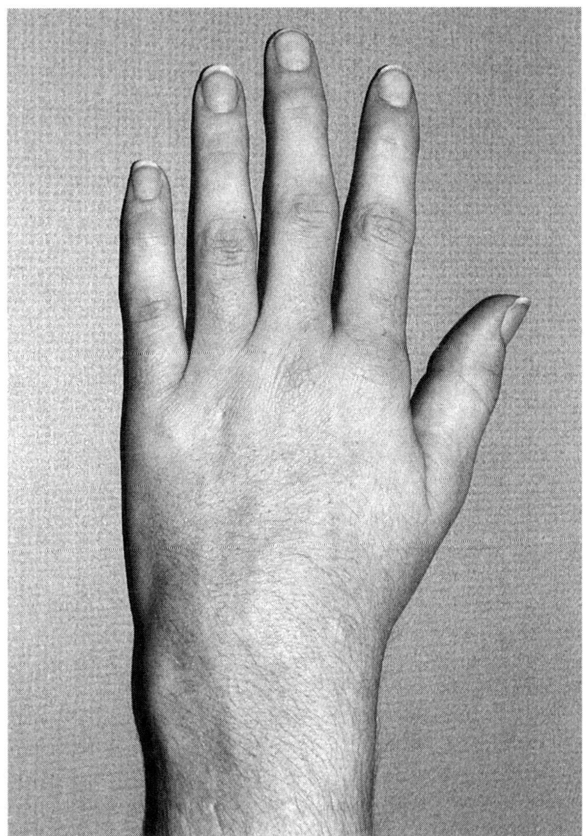

FIG. 55.2. Fusiform swelling and erythema about the proximal interphalangeal joints, most marked in the long finger. Swelling at the metacarpophalangeal joints has caused loss of definition of joint margins. The extensor carpi ulnaris tendon sheath (sixth dorsal compartment of the wrist) has synovial thickening and swelling.

Deformity

Joint deformities develop over time as articular and supporting structures are damaged by the inflammatory process. Joint effusions, which seem benign, particularly if the patient does not complain of symptoms, lead to stretching of tendons and ligaments and, if allowed to persist, will result in deformities and disability. The small joints of the hands and feet are particularly susceptible to this; greater than 10% of RA patients will develop deformity of the small joints of the hands within the first 2 years of disease (57), and at least one third develop such deformities over time (58). This phenomenon may result in the seemingly paradoxic situation in which deformities become more pronounced as the synovitis is controlled and the joint effusions resolve. Joint instability is seen if disruption of supporting structures has occurred. Loss of cartilage as a result of enzymatic and mechanical degradation, combined with stretching and weakening of the periarticular ligaments and their attachments, allows forces acting across the joints to deform them.

Unfortunately, once deformities develop they are permanent. Therefore, initiating treatment early to prevent this is crucial. All too often clinicians wait until obvious deformities are present before effective disease-modifying treatments are pursued.

Limitation of Motion

Limitation of motion occurs as a result of articular surface damage, joint and tendon sheath swelling, or alteration of joint-supporting structures. Effusions may limit joint motion because of pain or by causing sufficient tightness of the joint capsule to impede joint mobility. Fibrosis involving tendons and muscles may limit normal joint motion and result in flexion contractures. Joint deformities and subluxations invariably limit motion due to mechanical factors.

Effects of Rheumatoid Arthritis on Specific Joints

Fingers

Nonreducible flexion at the PIP joint with concomitant hyperextension of the DIP joint of the finger (boutonnière deformity, Fig. 55.3) occurs as a consequence of synovitis with stretching of, or rupture of, the PIP joint through the central extensor tendon with concomitant volar displacement of the lateral bands. When the lateral bands have subluxed far enough to pass the transverse axis of the joint, they become flexors of the PIP joint. Hyperextension of the DIP joint will occur as the tendons shorten with time. There may be a compensatory and reducible hyperextension at the MCP joint.

Hyperextension at the PIP joint with flexion of the DIP joint (swan-neck deformity, Fig. 55.4) may be initiated by (a) disruption of the extensor tendon at the DIP joint with secondary shortening of the central extensor tendon and hyperextension of the PIP joint, or (b) volar herniation of the PIP joint capsule due to weakening from chronic synovitis with subsequent tightening of the lateral bands and central extensor tendon (59). The lateral bands may become shortened over time and lie dorsally, limiting PIP flexion and ineffectively extending the DIP joint. Flexor tenosynovitis may also play a role by limiting the ability of the sublimis tendon to flex the PIP joint. Lupus has a particular predilection for the PIP joints and often produces reducible swan-neck deformities, whereas boutonnière deformities are almost never seen in lupus.

Intrinsic muscle (interossei, lumbricals) tightness may cause major declines in mobility of the fingers. This is evident on examination when the PIP joint cannot be flexed while the MCP joint is fully extended, but can be flexed if the MCP joint is in flexion (Bunnell test); primary PIP joint pathology would be evident with the MCP joint in either position. To assess this accurately, the phalanx must be aligned with the metacarpal, since the intrinsics on the ulnar side will be slack when ulnar deviation at the MCP joint exists, thus allowing more motion.

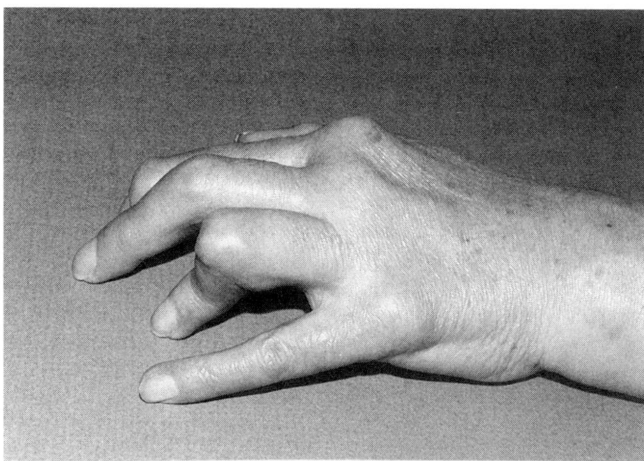

FIG. 55.3. A boutonnière deformity of the ring finger, flexion deformity of the long finger proximal interphalangeal joint, and mild swan-neck deformity of the index finger. Extensive synovitis at the metacarpophalangeal joints obscures the usual definition of joint margins.

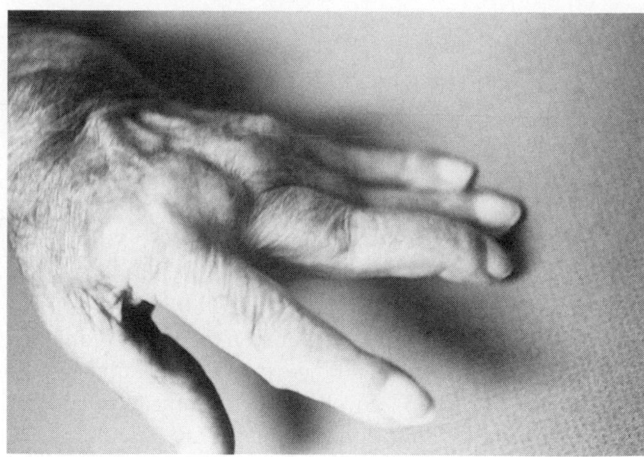

FIG. 55.4. Swan-neck deformities of long, ring, and little fingers, with concomitant subluxation of the metacarpophalangeal joints.

Flexor tenosynovitis of the fingers is common and portends a poor prognosis (16). Stiffness and crepitance along the tendon sheath with limitations of flexion (Fig. 55.5) and extension may follow. "Triggering" of the finger occurs when thickening or nodule formation of the tendon interacts with the concomitant tenosynovial proliferation, trapping the tendon (stenosing tenosynovitis). Tendon rupture

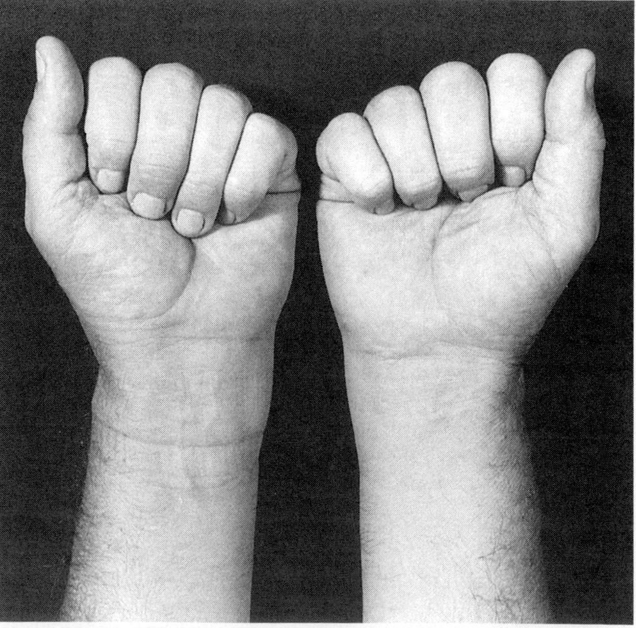

FIG. 55.5. Flexor tenosynovitis at the wrist and in the palm leading to decreased flexion of the fingers of the left hand.

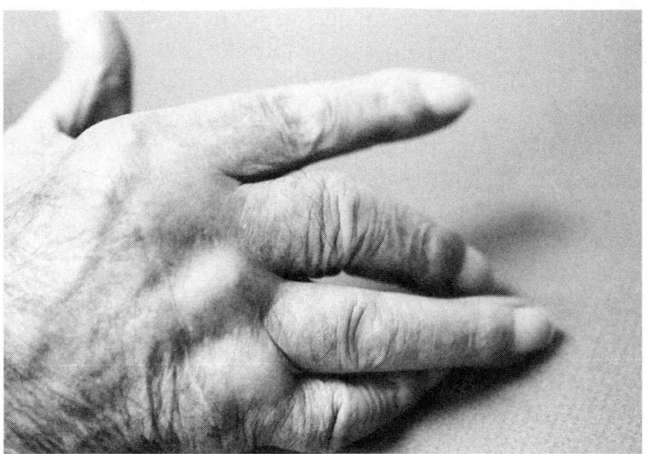

FIG. 55.6. Arthritis mutilans: the long proximal interphalangeal joint has been destroyed by rheumatoid arthritis. Deflection of the distal portion of the phalanx is due to the pull of gravity.

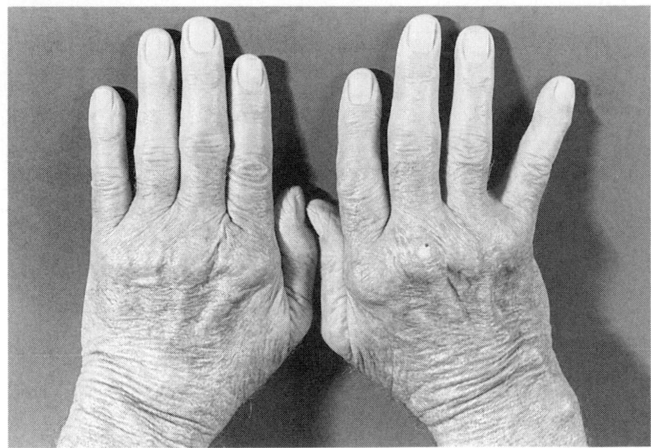

FIG. 55.7. Subcutaneous tissue atrophy, metacarpophalangeal joint proliferative synovitis with loss of joint definition, and mild proximal interphalangeal joint enlargement. There is slight volar subluxation of the metacarpophalangeal joints and mild ulnar deviation at the metacarpophalangeal joints of the right hand. Involvement of the dominant (right) hand is more pronounced.

may occur due to infiltrative synovitis in the digit or bony erosions that produce surfaces that cut the tendon at the wrist (especially the flexor pollicis longus).

Arthritis mutilans ("opera glass hands") results if destruction is severe and extensive, with dissolution of bone. In the small joints of the hands, the phalanges may shorten and the joints become grossly unstable. Pulling on the fingers during examination may lengthen the digit much like opening opera glasses, or the joint may bend in unusual directions merely under the pull of gravity (Fig. 55.6).

Metacarpophalangeal Joints

Two typical deformities may occur at the MCP joints that alter the alignment of the palmar skeletal arches and the stability of the fingers: volar subluxation of the fingers relative to the metacarpal bones and ulnar deviation (Fig. 55.7). Most cases of ulnar deviation are accompanied by counterpoised radial deviation of the wrist, roughly proportional to the degree of ulnar deviation of the fingers (60). Although RA is the most common cause of ulnar deviation, other arthritides, as well as certain neurologic deficiencies, may result in ulnar deviation as well.

The volar plate is firmer and more substantial than other portions of the MCP joint capsule and therefore effectively limits extension and dorsal movement at the joint. The greater relative strength of the flexor muscles, as compared with the extensors, causes volar migration of the proximal phalanx after synovial-based inflammation has weakened ligament and tendon insertions about the MCP joint capsule (61).

Ulnar deviation occurs after synovitis has led to stretching and attenuation of the volar plate and collateral ligaments, allowing dislocation of the flexor tendon volarward and ulnarward (62). The supporting structures of the extensor tendons also may become attenuated or destroyed by synovial distention and invasion, loosening the tendons so that they no longer ride centrally and dorsally over the metacarpal head, but move into the cleft between the MCP joints (58). If the extensor tendon subluxation is beyond the transverse axis of the MCP joint, the tendon will become a flexor at that joint, further limiting active extension of the fingers.

Wrists

The wrist is the site of multiple problems in patients with RA. Disruption of the radioulnar joint with dorsal subluxation of the ulna (caput ulna) and rotation of the carpus on the distal radius with an ulnarly translocated lunate are common (63). The combination of ulnar drift of the fingers and carpal rotation is known as a "zigzag" deformity (Fig. 55.8). Shortening of the carpal height (noted on radiographs), due in part to cartilage loss, is seen with rotational deformities.

Dorsal subluxation of the ulna often allows the ulnar styloid to be depressed volarly on examination much like depressing a piano key (piano key styloid). Subluxation may lead to rupture of the extensor tendons of the little, ring, and long fingers (Fig. 55.9), because the end of the distal ulna may be roughened secondary to erosion of bone and may abrade the tendons as they move back and forth during normal hand function, much like a rope being frayed while rubbing over a sharp rock. This process is especially likely to lead to tendon rupture if there is associated tenosynovitis.

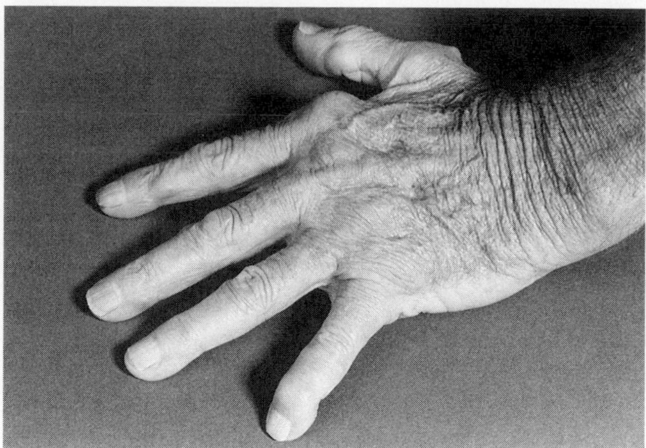

FIG. 55.8. "Zigzag" deformity with ulnar deviation of the fingers at the metacarpophalangeal joints and clockwise rotation of the carpus on distal radius.

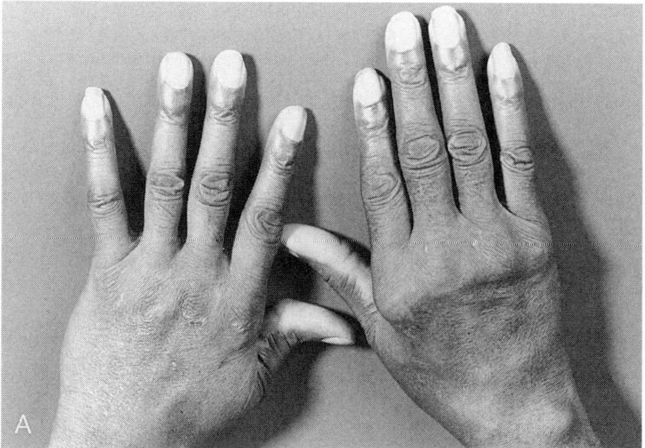

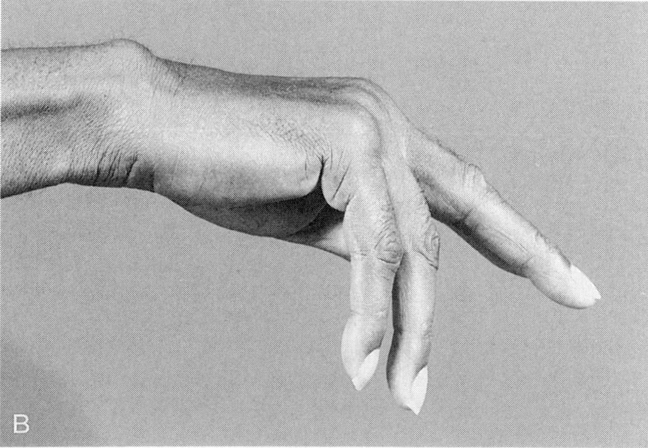

FIG. 55.9. A: More extensive involvement of the dominant (right) hand. Early volar subluxation of the metacarpophalangeal joints and a "doughy" synovitis are present. Subluxation of the right radioulnar joint with dorsal ulnar styloid subluxation is evident. **B:** A lateral view showing the dorsal subluxation of the ulnar styloid. The ability to extend the little and ring fingers fully has been lost due to rupture of the extensor tendons at the ulnar styloid.

Entrapment neuropathy may result from synovitis about the flexor tendons. Entrapment of the median nerve as it passes through the carpal tunnel (carpal tunnel syndrome) leads to decreased sensation on the palmar aspect of the thumb, index, and long fingers, and radial aspect of the ring finger, and later to weakness and atrophy of the muscles in the thenar eminence (Fig. 55.10). These symptoms are often most prominent at night and frequently awaken patients from sleep. Patients generally report pain, numbness, and tingling in the hand. This awakening from sleep may be one reason why patients do not always give a history of the classic cutaneous distribution. In RA patients, median nerve decompression should be considered before significant atrophy of the thenar eminence has occurred. Thenar atrophy can be evaluated by comparing the thenar mass to the contralateral side with the hands in the modified prayer position (Fig. 55.11). The mass of the thenar eminence of the dominant thumb is normally slightly larger.

Less commonly, entrapment of the ulnar nerve at the wrist causes decreased sensation over the little finger and the ulnar aspect of the ring finger and decreased interosseous muscle strength and mass.

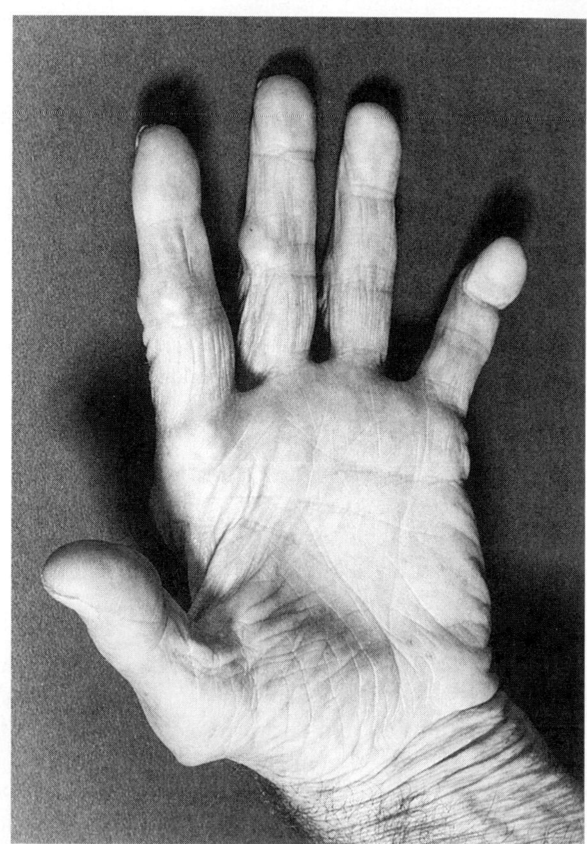

FIG. 55.10. Sequelae of carpal tunnel syndrome, with thenar eminence atrophy. Rheumatoid nodules are present at the index and long proximal interphalangeal joints. Traumatic disruption of the little finger distal interphalangeal joint has led to a swan-neck deformity.

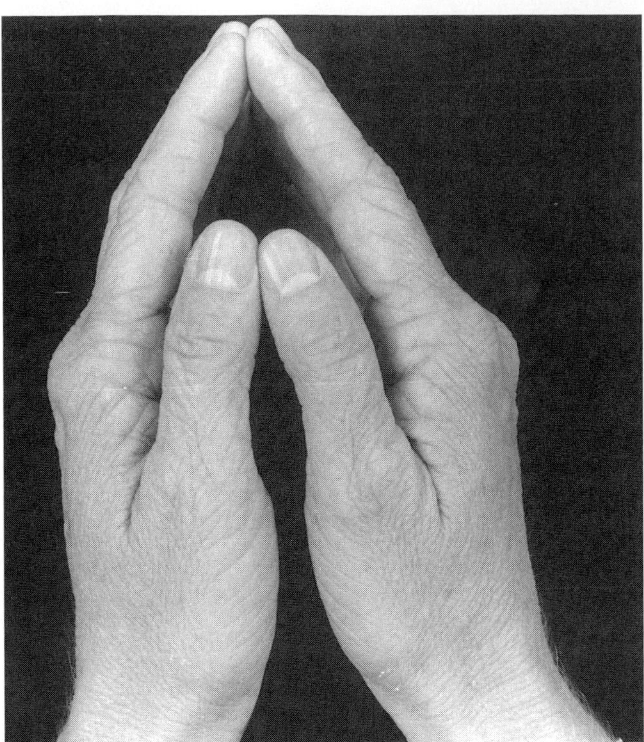

FIG. 55.11. This patient has early carpal tunnel syndrome. With the hands placed in a modified prayer position, the mass of the thenar eminence is compared. In a normal patient, the thenar eminence should be relatively equal, although usually somewhat larger on the dominant hand. In this right-handed patient, the thenar eminence is smaller on the right than the left, indicating early thenar atrophy.

Elbow

Elbow involvement is often detected by palpable synovial proliferation at the radiohumeral joint and frequently is accompanied by a flexion deformity. If synovitis or effusion is present in the elbow, complete extension will not occur; therefore, complete extension is an excellent sign that significant synovitis or effusion is not present. Olecranon bursal involvement is common, as are rheumatoid nodules in the bursa and along the extensor surface of the ulna.

Shoulders

The shoulders are frequently involved, manifested by tenderness, nocturnal pain, and limited motion. Nocturnal pain is particularly troubling; it is often difficult for patients with shoulder problems to find a comfortable position for sleep. Initially, swelling occurs anteriorly, but may be difficult to detect and is present on examination only in a minority of patients at any point in time (50). Rotator cuff degeneration secondary to synovitis may limit abduction and rotation. Superolateral migration of the humerus occurs with complete tears. Glenohumeral damage leads to pain both with motion and at rest, and typically leads to severely restricted motion. Acromioclavicular arthritis is not as frequent or as disabling.

Chest Wall

Chronic synovitis of the sternoclavicular and manubriosternal joints may lead to destruction and instability. The latter joint is rarely involved without extensive joint destruction elsewhere.

Feet and Ankles

Ankle joint involvement is seldom seen in the absence of midfoot or MTP involvement (64). The ankle does not often deform, because it is a mortice joint. Major structural changes occur in the midfoot and foot due to the combination of chronic synovitis and weight bearing. Posterior tibialis tendon involvement or rupture may lead to subtalar subluxation that results in eversion and migration of the talus laterally (65). Midfoot disease leads to loss of normal arch contour with flattening of the feet (Fig. 55.12).

MTP joint inflammation occurs in most patients, and is often one of the earliest disease manifestations. Due to the heavy loads they bear, the MTP joints become deformed over time. The great toe typically develops hallux valgus (bunion); subluxation of the phalanx at the MTP joint of the other toes (64) is predominantly dorsal (Fig. 55.13). The toes may exhibit compensatory flexion due to a fixed length of the flexor tendons, resulting in hammer toes (named because they resemble piano key hammers). When dorsal subluxation occurs, the soft tissue pad on the plantar surface of the metatarsal heads is displaced, allowing the metatarsal heads to protrude and become the primary weight-bearing surface; this is painful and calluses develop. This results in patients feeling that they are walking with pebbles in their shoes.

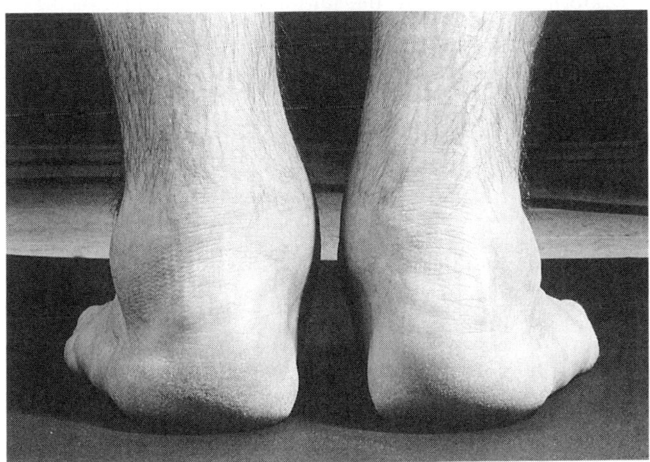

FIG. 55.12. Marked ankle and midfoot synovitis. There is also loss of definition of the arch and eversion at the subtalar joint.

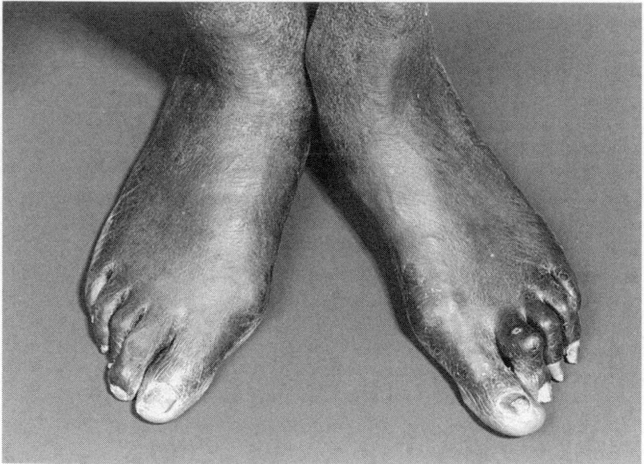

FIG. 55.13. Mild hallux valgus, with dorsal subluxation of the metatarsophalangeal joints and resultant "hammer toe" deformities of the second through fifth toes. Midfoot instability has led to eversion, with concomitant flattening of the feet.

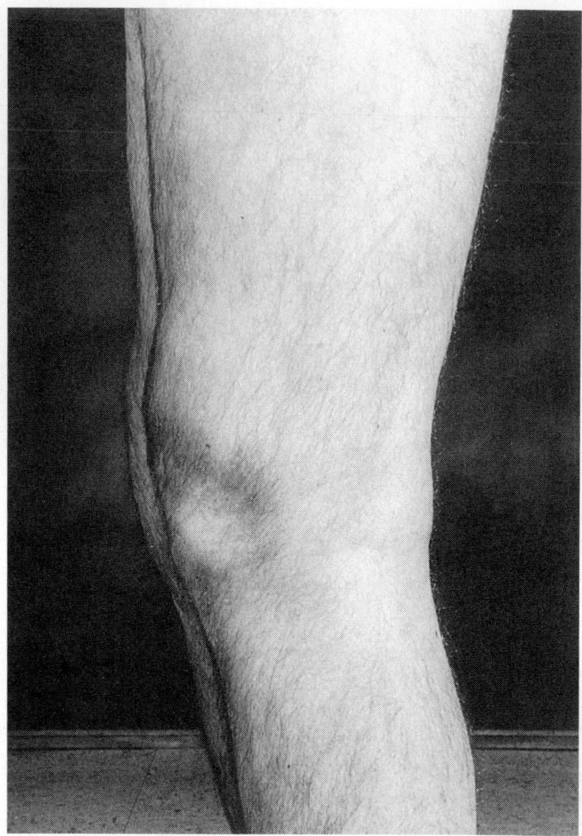

FIG. 55.14. Lateral view of a patient with rheumatoid arthritis affecting the knees. There is quadriceps atrophy, marked synovial proliferation with joint effusion in the suprapatellar pouch, and fullness in the popliteal space due to a small synovial (Baker) cyst.

Knees

The knees may develop large effusions and abundant proliferation of synovium (Fig. 55.14). Persistent effusions may lead to inhibition of quadriceps function by spinal reflexes with subsequent atrophy (66). Instability may develop after progressive loss of cartilage and weakening of ligaments; deformity may include genu valgus or varus and flexion deformities. With chronic effusions, the knee is more comfortable in the flexed position, and flexion deformities occur that greatly increase the work expended to walk. Baker cysts are common.

Hips

The hips are difficult to examine by direct inspection or palpation. However, limited motion or pain with internal or external rotation are the hallmarks of hip involvement. Patients with true hip joint pathology will have pain in the midgroin with rotation or with weight bearing. The Patrick maneuver (flexion, external rotation, and abduction) is abnormal in this situation. A flexion deformity may be demonstrable by flexing one hip of a supine patient while restricting pelvic motion by keeping the other hip in the neutral position on the examination table—if the hip cannot be maintained in the neutral position, a contracture is present. An abnormal gait with compensatory flexion at the ipsilateral knee usually results.

Cervical Spine

Neck pain on motion and occipital headache are common manifestations of cervical spine involvement, and occur in a majority of patients with persistent disease for more than 10 years (67). The atlantoaxial joint is a synovial-lined joint and is susceptible to the same proliferative synovitis and subsequent instability that are seen in the peripheral joints. Patients generally do fine when they are in control of their neck motion, but may experience problems when others try to flex their neck, as when attempting to obtain good flexion radiographs or helping the patient into a fetal position to perform a lumbar puncture. One should consider the possibility of significant C1–2 instability before a patient with RA undergoes surgical procedures in order to avoid compromise to the cervical cord or brainstem during intubation or as the patient is transferred while asleep. Patients with severe destruction in the hands (arthritis mutilans) are likely to have symptomatic cervical spine abnormalities, as are those patients taking significant amounts of corticosteroids for control of RA (68).

Neurologic involvement ranges from radicular pain to a variety of spinal cord lesions that may result in weakness (including quadriparesis), sphincter dysfunction, sensory deficits, and pathologic reflexes. Transient ischemic attacks (with fluctuations of blood pressure and alteration in breathing patterns) and cerebellar signs may reflect vertebral artery impingement from cervical subluxation or basilar artery impingement from upward migration of the dens. Radiculopathy is most common at the C2 root, although symptomatic subluxations may occur at any level.

Cricoarytenoid Joint

Because synovial tissue is present around the cricoarytenoid joint, involvement of this joint may occur in up to one fourth of RA patients (69). A fullness that is aggravated by speaking or swallowing is usually the initial symptom. Pain may be referred to the ear and typically is increased by swallowing. Hoarseness and inspiratory symptoms may develop. Severe involvement may produce enough restriction of joint motion to cause acute, life-threatening dyspnea, and emergent tracheotomy may be required (70).

Extraarticular Manifestations

Rarely, a patient will present with extraarticular manifestations (see Chapter 56) prior to the onset of arthritis. Extraarticular manifestations (Table 55.3) clearly demonstrate that RA is a systemic disease that can affect multiple organs through chronic inflammation. They occur almost exclusively in patients with RF, and their presence portends a poor prognosis (71). Some are more common in men [pleural involvement (72), vasculitis (73), and pericarditis (74)], but the proportion of men and women involved with other manifestations is similar to that of RA overall (71).

Rheumatoid nodules occur in approximately 25% of RA patients (75), but in less than 10% of patients in the first year of disease (76). They are most commonly found on extensor surfaces, sites of frequent mechanical irritation, or over joints. The olecranon process (Fig. 55.15), proximal ulna, back of the heels (Fig. 55.16), occiput, and ischial

TABLE 55.3. *Extraarticular manifestations of rheumatoid arthritis*

Heart	Pericarditis, premature atherosclerosis, vasculitis, valvular and valve ring nodules
Lung	Pleural effusions, interstitial lung disease, bronchiolitis obliterans, rheumatoid nodules, vasculitis
Skin	Nodules, fragility, vasculitis
Neurologic	Entrapment neuropathy, cervical myelopathy, mononeuritis multiplex (vasculitis), peripheral neuropathy
Hematopoietic	Anemia, thrombocytosis, lymphadenopathy, Felty's syndrome
Bone	Osteopenia
Eye	Keratoconjunctivitis sicca, episcleritis, scleritis, scleromalacia perforans, peripheral ulcerative keratopathy
Kidney	Amyloidosis, vasculitis

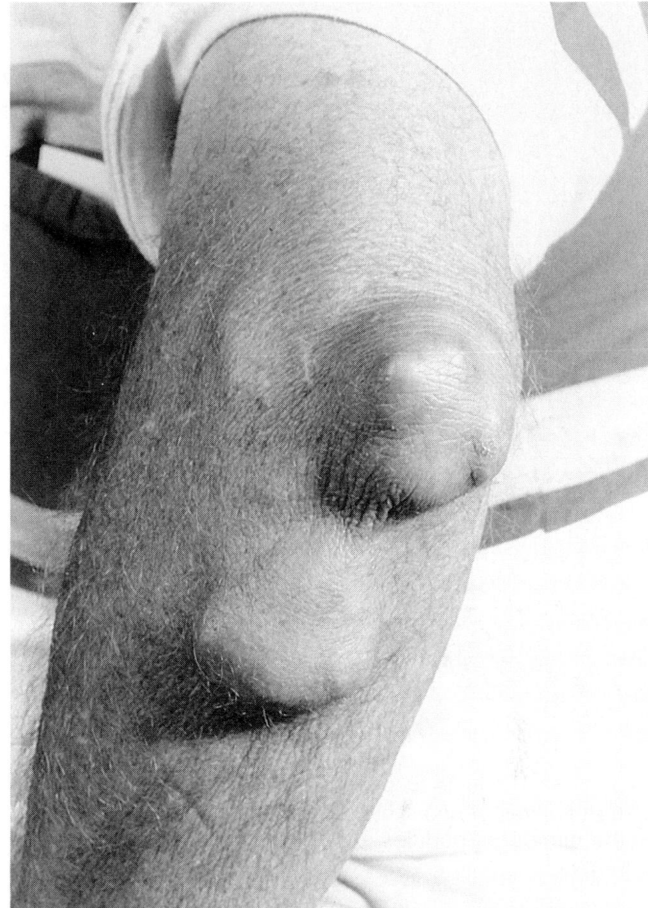

FIG. 55.15. Large rheumatoid nodules in the olecranon bursa and along the extensor surface of the proximal ulna; each mass is a collection of multiple smaller nodules. A small effusion is present in the olecranon bursa.

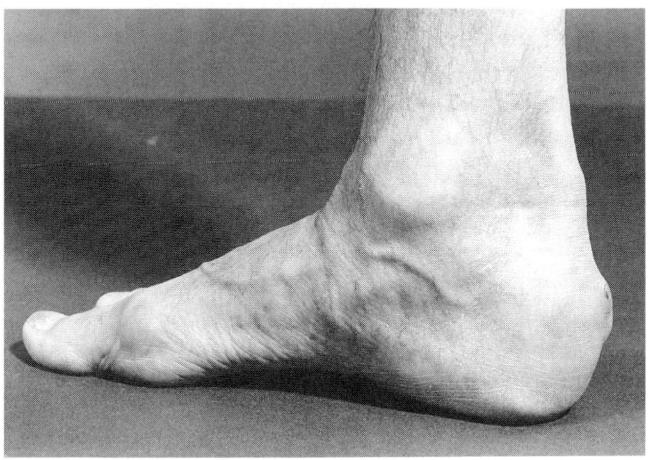

FIG. 55.16. Lateral view of rheumatoid nodules at the Achilles tendon insertion on the calcaneus and in the midportion of the tendon. Friction from shoewear has led to breakdown of the skin over the calcaneus.

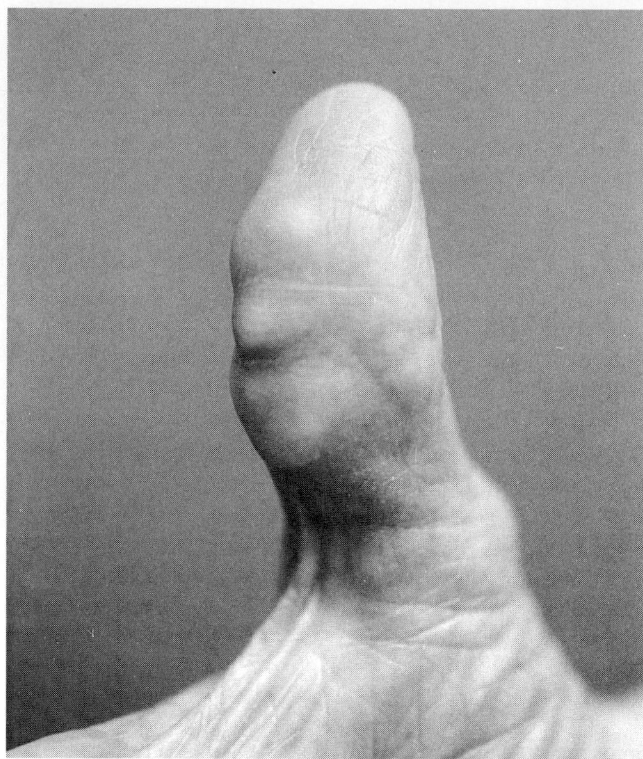

FIG. 55.17. Multiple small rheumatoid nodules in the thumb pad over sites of use. This patient experienced an increase in the number of nodules after the initiation of methotrexate therapy.

tuberosities are common periosteal sites for their development. They may also form in subcutaneous tissues of the finger (Fig. 55.17), toe and heel pads, tendons, and viscera. RF is almost invariably present, and if absent, other diagnoses, such as chronic tophaceous gout, should be entertained. There often is a discrepancy between the level of articular inflammation and the progression of nodule formation. Patients with rheumatoid nodulosis have a great number of nodules, usually subcutaneous, and may have little active synovitis (77). In a similar fashion, patients treated with methotrexate who have a good response of their articular inflammation may have a seemingly paradoxic rapid increase in the number of nodules (78,79).

IMAGING

Conventional Radiography

Radiographic evaluation of patients with RA may be performed initially to aid in diagnosis (15,80), but thereafter is used to assess the course of disease, response to therapy, and need for surgical intervention. The ability of therapeutic agents to slow the radiographic progression of RA has been considered the gold standard of efficacy and therefore is a key outcome measure in clinical trials (Table 55.2). Radiographic abnormalities of RA can be broadly divided into those due to acute inflammation and those due to articular and periarticular destruction.

Abnormalities seen in soft tissue suggest acute inflammation and include periarticular swelling, loss of definition of tissue planes (as around fat pads), and evidence of joint effusions. Osteopenia is commonly seen in the periarticular regions, as well as in the long bones of the hands and feet, and is due, in part, to the cumulative effects of inflammation over the course of disease (81). Bone mineral density of the lumbar spine assessed by dual-energy absorptiometry can decrease within the first few months of disease (82,83), and the decline is greater with more severe disease. Disease-modifying antirheumatic drugs (gold, methotrexate, biologicals) can have a significant sparing effect on metacarpal osteoporosis in RA, indicating that control of synovitis may prevent or reverse the osteopenia (84).

Radiographic changes that are irreversible include erosion of bone, joint space narrowing, ankylosis (rarely seen), and malalignment, although the latter may be somewhat dependent on the positioning of the joint by the technician for the radiograph. Radiographic erosions (Fig. 55.18) represent loss of cortical bone and take place initially at the margin of the joint [bare area (85)], where the synovium ap-

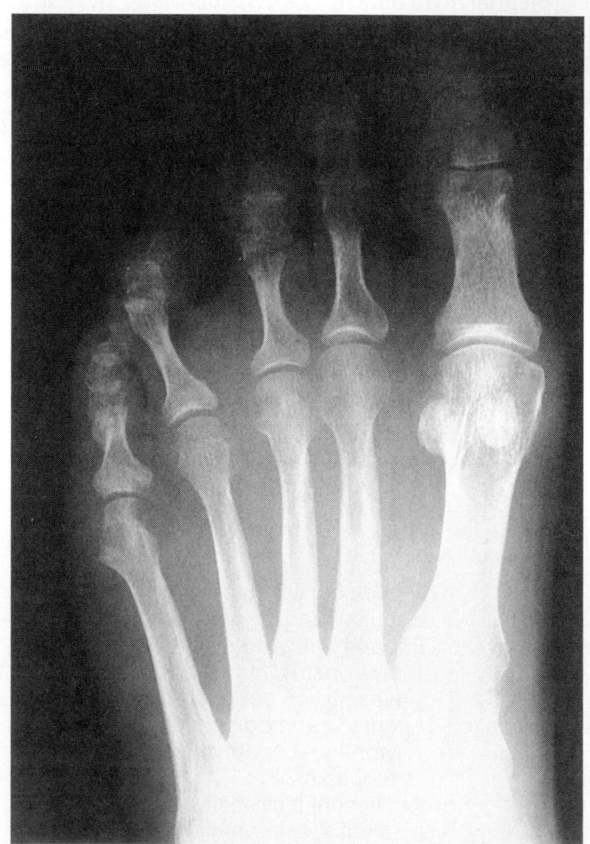

FIG. 55.18. Erosion of the medial and lateral margins of the fifth metatarsal head in a patient with recent-onset rheumatoid arthritis. There is no significant joint space narrowing.

proximates bone without intervening cartilage (Fig. 55.19). At other locations in the joint, the cartilage protects the subchondral bone from erosion, but is itself degraded, and damage is manifest as diffuse joint space narrowing; this is unlike the focal joint space narrowing that is commonly seen in OA (Fig. 55.20). Table 55.4 compares and contrasts the radiographic features of the two most common kinds of arthritis. Although diffuse joint space narrowing is commonly seen in other types of chronic inflammatory arthritis, in conjunction with marginal erosions and osteopenia, it is highly characteristic of RA. The small joints of the hands and feet commonly exhibit both erosion and joint space narrowing, whereas the knee and hip have a predominance of joint space narrowing (Fig. 55.21). This difference is due in part to the fact that the cartilage–pannus junction at these sites is different histopathologically, with an invasive pannus most common in the small joints and a metaplastic reaction at the articular surface more common in the large joints (86).

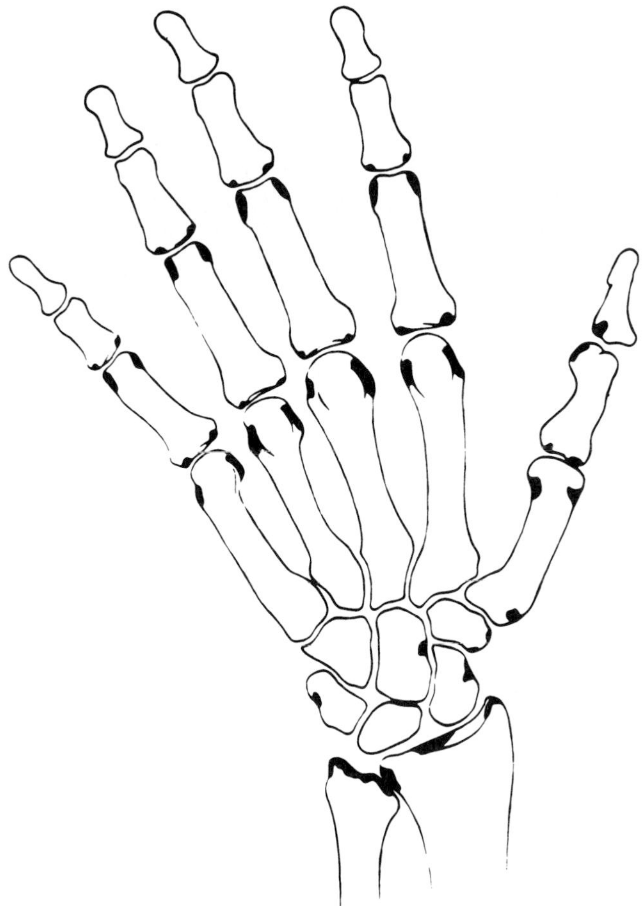

FIG. 55.19. "Bare areas" in the hand described by Martel et al. (85). These are intraarticular sites of bone not covered with cartilage and susceptible to direct attack by the rheumatoid synovial pannus. (From Martel W, Hayes JT, Duff IF. The pattern of bone erosion in the hand and wrist in rheumatoid arthritis. *Radiology* 1965;84:204–214, with permission.)

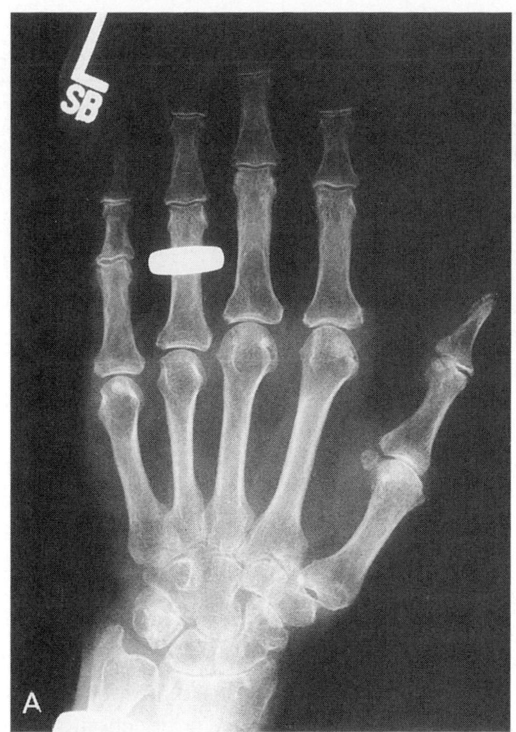

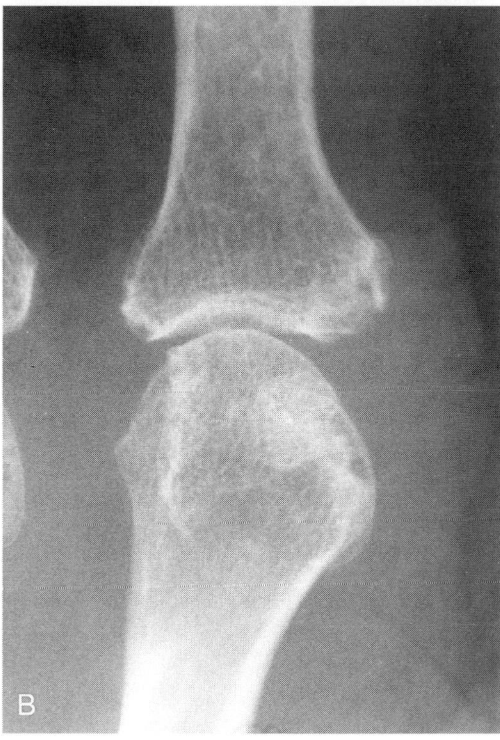

FIG. 55.20. A: Hand radiograph of a patient with rheumatoid arthritis. There is joint space narrowing in all metacarpophalangeal joints, as well as in the midcarpal and radiocarpal joints. Cystic changes have occurred in the proximal carpal row, and erosions are seen in the long and index metacarpophalangeal joints. **B:** Enlargement of the index metacarpophalangeal joint seen in **A** demonstrating diffuse joint space narrowing and erosions of bone on both sides of the joint on the medial and lateral aspects. The erosions have occurred within the joint at sites where there is no cartilage ("bare areas").

TABLE 55.4. *Contrasting radiographic features*

	Rheumatoid arthritis	Osteoarthritis
Sclerosis	±	++++
Osteophytes	±	++++
Osteopenia	+++	0
Symmetry	+++	+
Erosions	+++	0
Cysts	++	++
Narrowing	+++	+++

Radiographic evidence of damage (erosions) occurs in almost all patients with RA who are seropositive for RF and are followed for more than 5 years. In one notable study, 99% of RF-positive patients had erosions at follow-up (87). The initial changes may occur early in the course of disease, especially in the hands, where studies show erosions in 30% to 60% of patients in the first 2 years (88–90). Destructive changes of the hip, knee, ankle, shoulder, and elbow joints occur later than those in the hands (91). Damage in the hands and wrists may be more marked in the dominant hand and in the joints used most heavily (second MCP > fourth MCP), presumably a reflection of increased mechanical stress, as well as increased inflammation that may result from use (92,93).

Joint subluxation and dislocation are common (50), especially in the small joints of the hands and feet. MCP subluxation is generally seen with concomitant radiocarpal rotation (Fig. 55.22). MTP subluxation is common in the toes other than the great toe; the great toe more commonly develops hallux valgus, contributing to the deformities at the other MTP joints (Fig. 55.23).

Reparative bone changes (osteophytes) are unusual in active seropositive RA, but may occur if the disease is controlled. However, patients with seronegative (for RF) RA may have less osteopenia and may make new bone even in the presence of active inflammation (94). These differences are especially evident in the wrist (95), and are somewhat similar to those seen with adult Still disease (96). Erosive seronegative patients appear to have HLA-DR phenotypes similar to those of seropositive patients with erosive disease (97).

Bony ankylosis is becoming increasingly uncommon, but may occur when cartilage loss is extreme and joint surfaces

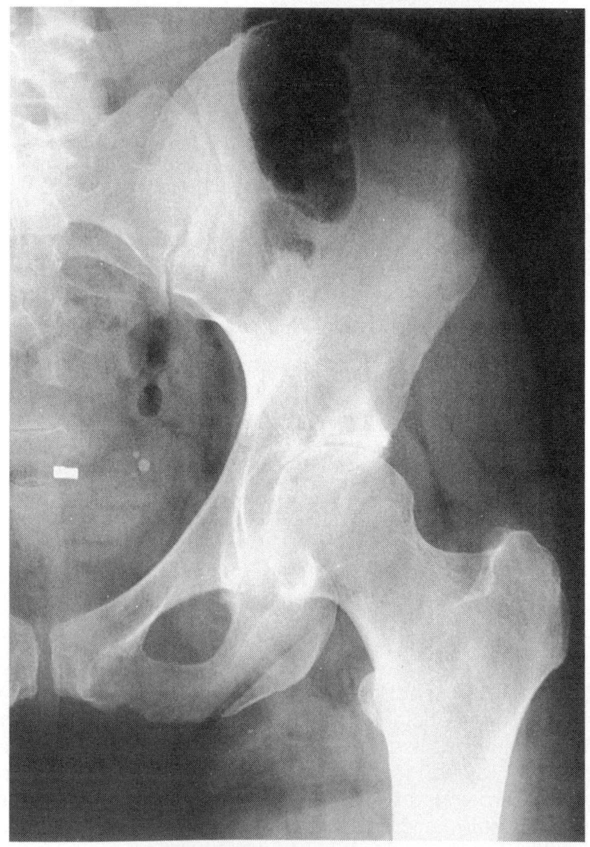

FIG. 55.21. Hip radiograph of a patient with RA. There is diffuse joint space narrowing, small cysts in the femoral head and acetabulum, and little reparative bony change.

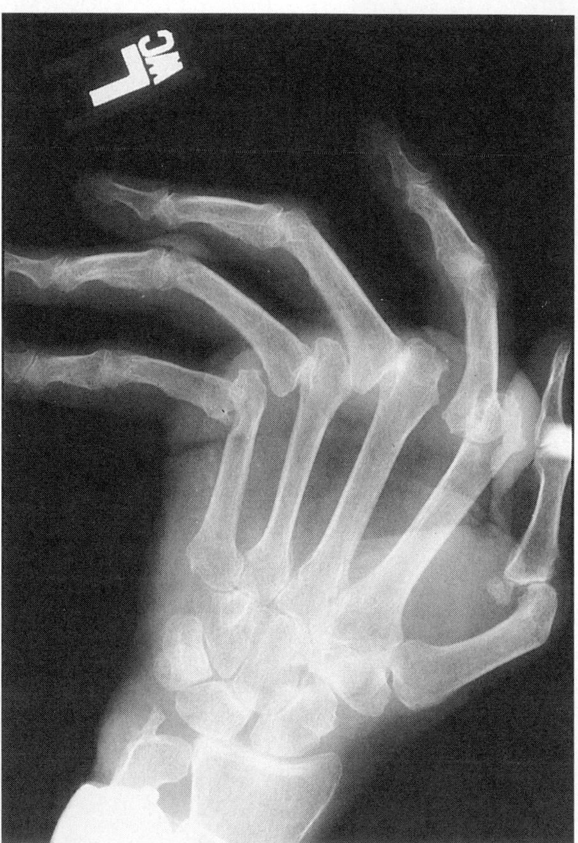

FIG. 55.22. Severe metacarpophalangeal joint subluxations in the volar and ulnar directions. There is concomitant clockwise rotation of the carpus on the distal radius ("zigzag" deformity). Erosions of the ulnar styloid and metacarpal heads are evident.

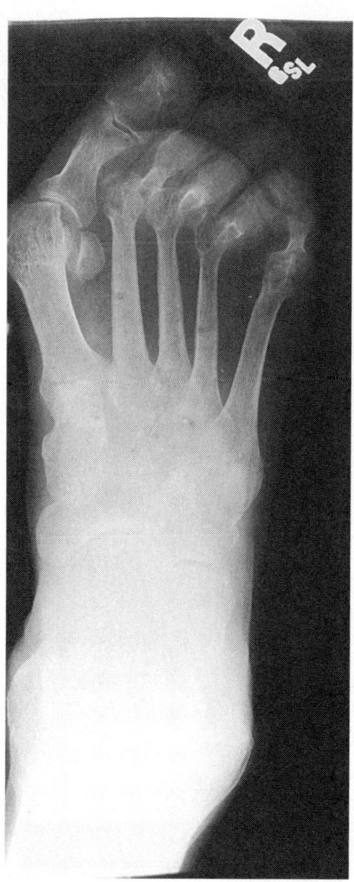

FIG. 55.23. Hallux valgus and dorsal subluxation of the toes at the remaining metatarsophalangeal joints.

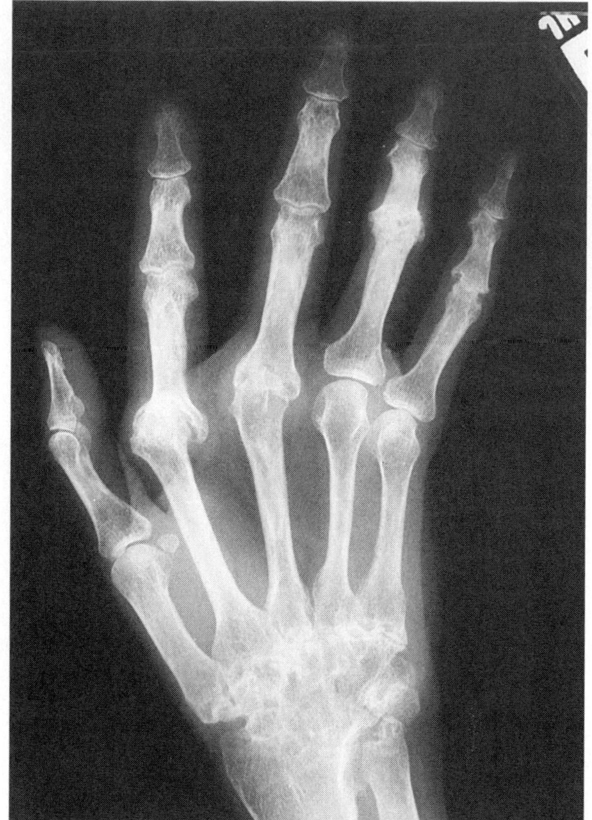

FIG. 55.24. Ankylosis of the carpal rows in a patient with long-standing RA. Erosions are prominent in the little finger proximal interphalangeal joint and about the distal ulna. Some repair is evident at the long and index metacarpophalangeal joints with osteophyte formation; the arthritis had been relatively quiescent in this patient for several years.

are juxtaposed, allowing fusion of the joint (Fig. 55.24). It is seen in the small joints of the hands, wrists, feet, and ankles; ankylosis of large joints is especially rare in RA. The prevalence of ankylosis increases with duration of disease, the presence of subcutaneous nodules, and disease activity (98–100).

Cervical spine radiographic abnormalities may include atlantoaxial (C1–2) subluxation, superior migration of the odontoid, subaxial arthritis, and collapse of the lateral masses of C1 from erosion at the facet joints.

Erosion of the odontoid (Fig. 55.25), accompanied by invasion and damage of the transverse ligament and alar ligaments (attachments from the odontoid process to the occipital condyles) by pannus, leads to instability. Atlantoaxial subluxation is often the initial abnormality (101) and is demonstrated by comparing lateral cervical spine films obtained in extension, when subluxation should be minimal, and in flexion, when the subluxation is maximal with protrusion of the odontoid into the neural canal (Fig. 55.26). Risk for myelopathy increases with progressive C1–2 subluxation, especially with superior migration of the odontoid (102); those with C1–2 subluxation over 10 mm are especially at risk. If erosion is severe, the odontoid may fracture

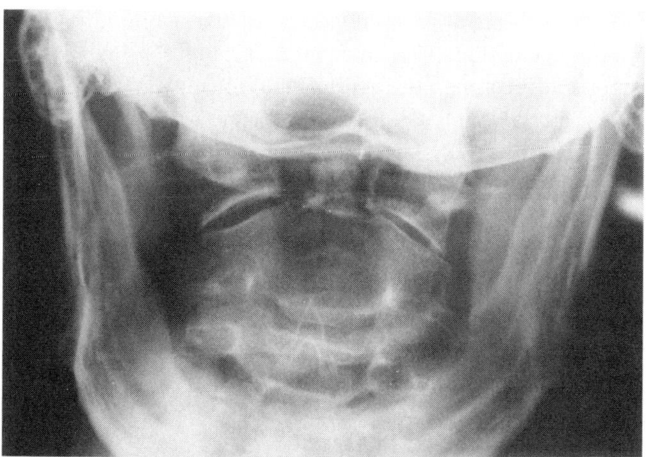

FIG. 55.25. Anteroposterior radiograph of the C1–2 articulation showing facet joint space narrowing on the patient's left (patient is facing the observer) and erosion at the base of the odontoid. Both findings are typical for rheumatoid arthritis.

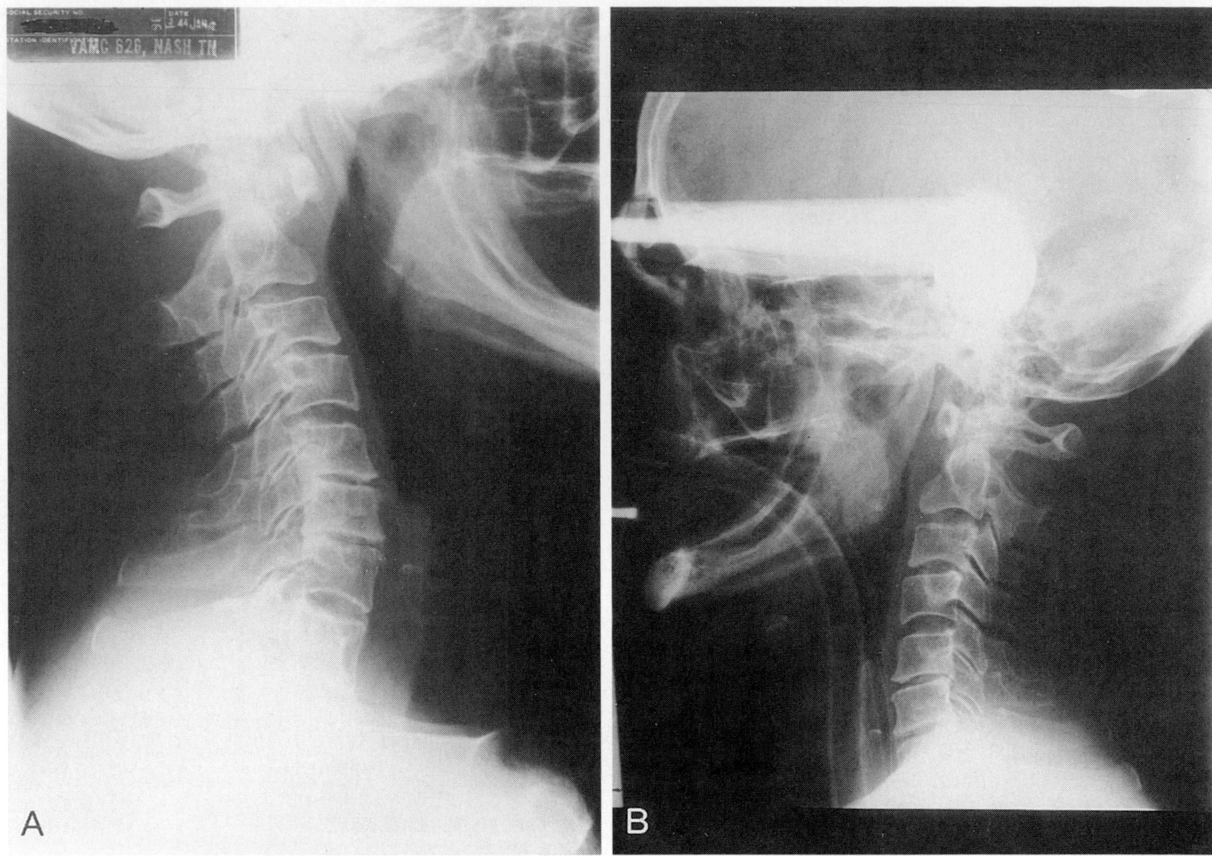

FIG. 55.26. **A:** Lateral flexion view of a rheumatoid arthritis patient with 12 mm of C1–2 anterior subluxation (distance between the odontoid peg and the C1 arch anterior to the peg). C5–6 and C6–7 disc space narrowing is also noted. **B:** The same patient as in **A** after cervical spine stabilization by a "halo," with reduction of the subluxation.

or even disappear, allowing posterior subluxation of C1–2 to occur.

Unilateral significant erosion at the C1–2 facet joints may allow rotatory instability (103) and bilateral C1–2 facet erosion may cause upward migration of the odontoid into the foramen magnum (104). When this "cranial settling" occurs, there is less room in the neural canal for movement between the odontoid (and its surrounding pannus) and the spinal cord (105) before compression and myelopathy occur. The odontoid may also impinge on the basilar artery or brainstem, with resultant vertebrobasilar insufficiency or damage to the medullary respiratory centers.

Subluxations below the C1–2 level may also occur, more commonly in those with C1–2 subluxation. The most common sites are C2–3 and C3–4 (Fig. 55.27). Subluxations greater than 3.5 mm with flexion are associated with an increased risk for myelopathy.

Scintigraphy

Articular inflammation may be documented by increased localization of radionuclide to the joint. Because this is a sensitive technique that may show abnormalities before synovitis is apparent on physical examination, and certainly before radiographic abnormalities occur, it is occasionally used to document the presence of an inflammatory arthropathy in patients with suggestive histories and normal examination results. Its major advantage is in simultaneously documenting the extent of inflammation in all joints with minimal radiation exposure. Joints that are persistently abnormal on scintigraphy are more likely to exhibit damage over time (106). Distinguishing rheumatoid inflammation from other causes (e.g., infection and mechanical abnormalities) may not be possible; therefore, the specificity of this imaging modality is limited. Scintigraphy is not recommended during the routine workup or monitoring of RA.

Magnetic Resonance Imaging and Ultrasonography

Studies in hands and wrists have documented the ability of magnetic resonance imaging (MRI) to detect inflammation in tendon sheaths, early abnormalities in carpal bones, and reduction in cartilage thickness prior to abnormalities

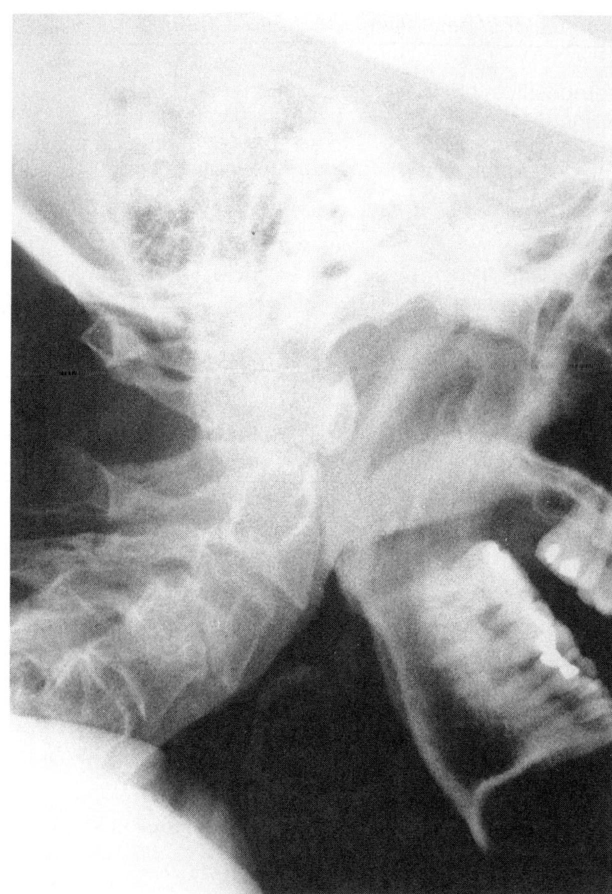

FIG. 55.27. A lateral radiograph of a rheumatoid arthritis patient experiencing severe upper extremity neurologic decline due to C2–3 and C3–4 anterior subluxations. The odontoid is not visible due to severe erosion.

appearing on conventional radiographs (107). Other studies have shown similar sensitivity for ultrasonography (US) of the small joints of the hands (107,108). However, the significance of erosions seen only on MRI or US is not known (i.e., do they progress to radiographically detectable lesions or do they heal spontaneously or with treatment?). MRI and US results are now appearing in some clinical trials and may provide an approach to monitoring progression that is both safe and more rapidly responsive to therapy. However, MRI is a very costly modality, and currently there is little use for MRI in the routine diagnosis or monitoring of patients with RA.

MRI of the cervical spinal cord, on the other hand, is superior to other modalities, and its use is routine in the evaluation of patients suspected of serious cervical spine disease. MRI may demonstrate impingement on the cervical cord by synovial pannus about the odontoid, impression of the medulla by upward migration of the odontoid, or impingement of the cervical cord by subaxial subluxations (Fig. 55.28).

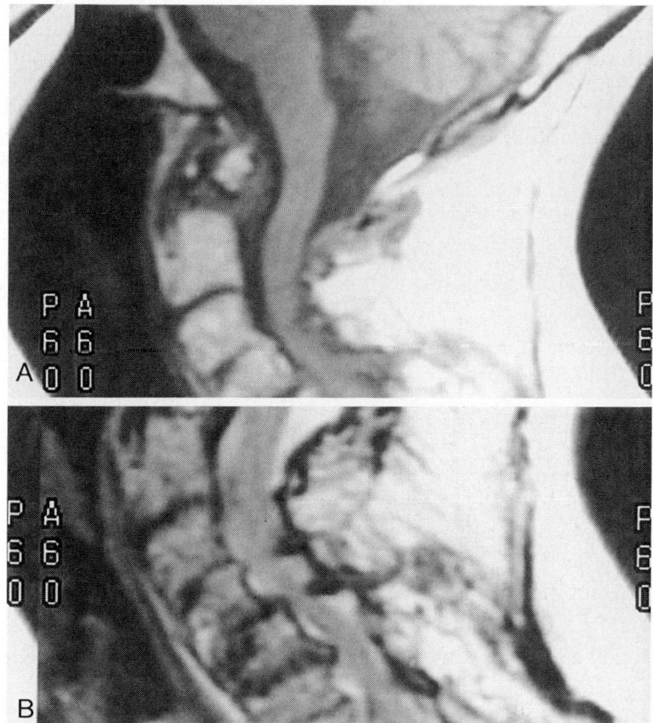

FIG. 55.28. A: T1-weighted magnetic resonance imaging (MRI) of the cervical spine of a patient with RA with a large pannus about the odontoid and fracture-dislocation of the odontoid from the body of C2. **B:** Same patient as in **A**, demonstrating extensive subluxation with impingement on the spinal canal at C3–4, C4–5, and C5–6.

LABORATORY MEASURES

Rheumatoid Factor

The term *rheumatoid factor* is unfortunate; it makes everyone immediately think of RA. RF (see Chapter 58) is not a diagnostic test; the presence of RF does not establish the diagnosis of RA, nor does its absence rule out the diagnosis. RF may be seen in many clinical settings other than RA. In most surveys of patients seen in a clinical setting, about three fourths of RA patients will have a positive RF test result. Various investigators have found that the presence of RF bears some relationship to the onset of RA. In one series, RF was present in about 33% of patients within 3 months of onset of disease, another 40% developed RF within the next 9 months, and the remainder who developed RF did so after the first 12 months of disease (12% were persistently seronegative in this report) (109). The presence of RF in high titers has been observed primarily in those with more severe disease, especially those with systemic vasculitis (71).

The mere presence of RF may confer susceptibility to RA. Family studies have shown that family members with RF have a higher relative risk for developing RA (Table 55.5). Population studies also show that the likelihood of

TABLE 55.5. *Presence of rheumatoid factor (RF) as a predictor of developing rheumatoid arthritis*

Studies of family members of patients with rheumatoid arthritis	
Walker et al. (236)	19 of 213 family members seropositive for RF by latex fixation test at baseline; 3 developed rheumatoid arthritis versus none of the seronegative patients
Silman (33)	24 of 370 family members seropositive for RF by ELISA at baseline; 4 seropositive, 10 seronegative at baseline developed rheumatoid arthritis (note: all but 2 developing rheumatoid arthritis had RF at follow-up)
Population studies	
del Puente (237)	
(prospective; Pima Amerindians)	2.6/1,000 incidence rate in those with RF <1:32, 16.6/1,000 incidence rate in those with RF >1:32; incidence rate increased with age and RF titers (48.3/1,000 incidence rate for RF >1:256)
Aho (110)	
(retrospective; 1972–1977 sample)	16 of 32 developing rheumatoid arthritis had a positive RF latex test result prior to developing rheumatoid arthritis
(prospective; 1978–1980 sample)	15 of 34 developing rheumatoid arthritis had a positive RF latex test result prior to developing rheumatoid arthritis

ELISA, enzyme-linked immunosorbent assay.

developing RA is much higher in individuals seropositive for RF (Table 55.5). Many individuals who develop RA, as many as half in some studies, may have been positive for RF for years before the onset of arthritis (110). However, because only a minority of people with RF will develop RA over time, its use as a prognostic or screening test is limited.

Many illnesses that induce chronic immune stimulation may lead to the presence of RF (see Chapter 58). Smoking has been shown to be associated with both a higher incidence of RF (111) and an increased risk for developing RA in males (112). The majority of studies have found that the presence of RF increases with age in the general population (113), although one study in a rheumatology referral clinic found no such trend (114). The predictive value of the test depends strongly on the pretest probability of having RA. Indeed, at least a 10% to 20% pretest probability of RA is required before the test is useful (114) (i.e., RF testing should not be performed as a diagnostic test in patients without inflammatory arthritis).

Acute-Phase Reactants

Systemic inflammation induces the production by the liver of a number of proteins, which are known as acute-phase reactants (see Chapters 22 and 57). These include fibrinogen, C-reactive protein (CRP), serum amyloid A protein, serum amyloid P protein, haptoglobin, ferritin, ceruloplasmin, and others. Clinical measurement of these proteins is largely restricted to CRP and evaluation of the erythrocyte sedimentation rate (ESR). Fibrinogen concentration, the major determinant of the ESR, takes 3 to 5 days to reach maximal levels after an acute stimulus and a comparable time to return to normal levels. In contrast, CRP levels increase rapidly after a stimulus (within hours) and decay within days after the stimulus resolves.

Sequential monitoring of either the ESR or CRP levels to assess the level of systemic inflammation in RA is reasonable, especially when physical signs may be hard to interpret (e.g., assessing swelling in an obese person, assessing swelling and tenderness in a patient with severely damaged joints, or assessing tenderness in a patient with a low pain threshold). The magnitude of elevation of the ESR over time (area under the curve) is strongly associated with radiographic erosions (115). Although the use of the ESR is more widespread, the CRP may more closely reflect current disease activity as assessed by other measures (116,117).

Anemia

An anemia of chronic disease is commonly seen in patients with RA, and the severity of this anemia correlates with disease activity. It is characterized by a low serum iron with normal iron stores and a blunted response to erythropoietin (118). The actions of cytokines commonly elaborated at sites of inflammation in RA, including interleukin-1 and tumor necrosis factor-α, impair iron metabolism and erythropoiesis in the marrow (119). In general, effective treatment of the disease will result in an improvement in the anemia, but many of the drugs used for treatment may also result in bone marrow depression.

Iron deficiency anemia may occur from blood losses during menses, phlebotomy, and gastrointestinal bleeding. A careful search for a gastrointestinal source is required when hematochezia (occult or frank) is present, because a sizable proportion of patients will have sources other than ulcerations caused by medication (120). However, patients with RA have a significantly reduced mortality risk from gastrointestinal malignancies (121), possibly due to chronic nonsteroidal antiinflammatory drug (NSAID) therapy.

Thrombocytosis

Platelet counts often parallel acute-phase reactants and are elevated in active RA, usually in association with other extraarticular manifestations (122); in these instances, platelet counts tend to be inversely correlated with the hematocrit.

Despite the elevated platelet levels, platelet survival may be decreased in active RA, with thrombocytosis representing marrow hyperresponsiveness to the decreased platelet survival (123).

Anti-CCP Antibodies

Antibodies directed against CCPs have been shown to be present in a significant percentage of patients (50%–70%) with established RA (18) and interestingly in one study were identified in approximately half of patients years before they developed symptoms of RA (19). The specificity of anti-CCP antibodies in published studies has been approximately 96% (17–21). Furthermore, anti-CCP antibodies predict erosive disease (18–21).

ASSESSING PATIENT STATUS

The status of an individual patient at any point in time should always be assessed relative to treatment goals. Specific treatment goals are well accepted and easy to understand in such conditions as hypertension, hyperlipidemia, or diabetes; however, in RA, goals are more difficult to quantify, but no less important. It is impossible to evaluate the effectiveness of treatment without a goal. With improving therapies (see Chapter 59), remission is becoming a more realistic, although still elusive, goal. No one single measure adequately describes the status of a patient with RA. Rather, combinations of abnormalities detected by laboratory testing, physical examination, radiographic examination, and assessment of pain and functional status are used. The ACR has recommended a core set of composite criteria (Table 55.2) for the evaluation of therapies in patients with RA (43). The components of this core set are excellent parameters to follow in individual patients in clinical practice, as well as in clinical research situations. A 20% improvement level has been set as the minimum required to show efficacy of a drug over placebo. This requires that both the tender and swollen joint counts be improved by this amount, and that three of the five parameters below the line show similar degrees of improvement. Increasingly, rheumatologists are not satisfied with this modest degree of improvement, and are adjusting therapies to achieve ACR50 or ACR70 responses (improvement of parameters by 50% and 70%, respectively).

Some measures, such as radiographs, joint deformity, and limitation of motion, are essentially measurements of joint damage. Other measures attempt to quantify the presence of inflammation and include joint tenderness and swelling, elevation of acute-phase reactants, and morning stiffness. Pain and decrements in function result from a combination of the effects of joint damage and inflammation.

For the short-term management of patients, parameters that assess acute inflammation are the most helpful, because most current medical interventions are aimed primarily at controlling the inflammatory response. Recording the joints that are swollen and tender at each patient encounter will document ongoing inflammation (24). Acute-phase reactants (ESR or CRP) may also be useful parameters to follow intermittently. Time-integrated ESR has been shown to be strongly correlated with radiographic progression (115). Joints that are persistently swollen over time, as opposed to those that are merely tender, are more likely to become damaged (124), which emphasizes the need to assess this parameter carefully. However, measures of inflammation may fluctuate widely over the course of disease, and do not necessarily worsen over time, despite long-term functional declines (109,125–128).

On the other hand, measures of damage (radiographs, limitation of joint motion) will generally worsen over time (128), and are correlated with a decline in functional status (127,129). Radiographs are included in the recommended evaluation for patients in studies if they are of a 1-year duration or longer. Examinations performed to establish disability primarily focus on measures of damage (130), because these are unlikely to improve.

FUNCTIONAL STATUS

Classification of functional status in RA has been according to the American Rheumatism Association (ARA) Functional Class Criteria (131), revised in 1991 by the ACR (132) (Table 55.6). It is a 4-point scale rating limitations in self-care and vocational and avocational activities, thus describing the global consequences of RA. It is a quick method for describing status, and allows grouping of patients for studies.

Functional status instruments are sensitive to change and may be preferable for monitoring outcomes in patient care and clinical research (132). Functional status questionnaires may allow numerical quantification of functional status and thus assess the combined effects of inflammation and

TABLE 55.6. *Revised criteria for classification of functional status in rheumatoid arthritis*

Class I	Completely able to perform usual activities of daily living (self-care, vocational, and avocational)
Class II	Able to perform usual self-care and vocational activities, but limited in avocational activities
Class III	Able to perform usual self-care activities, but limited in vocational and avocational activities
Class IV	Limited in ability to perform usual self-care, vocational, and avocational activities

Usual self-care activities include dressing, feeding, bathing, grooming, and toileting. Avocational (recreational and/or leisure) and vocational (work, school, homemaking) activities are patient desired and age and sex specific.

From Hochberg MC, Chane RW, Dwosh I, et al. The American College of Rheumatology 1991 revised criteria for the classification of global functional status in rheumatoid arthritis. *Arthritis Rheum* 1992;25:498–502, with permission.

Activities And Lifestyle Index

The questions below concern your daily activities. The few minutes you spend answering these questions can provide a more complete picture of how a medical condition may affect your life, adding to information from standard medical tests such as blood tests and X-rays. Please try to answer each question, even if you do not think it is related to you or any condition you may have. Please answer exactly as you think or feel, as there are no right and wrong answers.

Please check (✓) the **ONE** best answer for your abilities.

AT THIS MOMENT, are you able to:	**Without ANY Difficulty**	**With SOME Difficulty**	**With MUCH Difficulty**	**UNABLE To Do**
a. Dress yourself, including tying shoelaces and doing buttons?	____	____	____	____
b. Get in and out of bed?	____	____	____	____
c. Lift a full cup or glass to your mouth?	____	____	____	____
d. Walk outdoors on flat ground?	____	____	____	____
e. Wash and dry your entire body?	____	____	____	____
f. Bend down to pick up clothing from the floor?	____	____	____	____
g. Turn regular faucets on and off?	____	____	____	____
h. Get in and out of a car?	____	____	____	____

• **How Much Pain Have You Had Because Of Your Condition IN THE PAST WEEK?**

Place a mark on the line below to indicate how severe your pain has been:

NO PAIN |————————————————————| PAIN AS BAD AS IT COULD BE

FIG. 55.29. The difficulty scale (top) of the modified Stanford Health Assessment Questionnaire. This version is graded 0 to 3 (analogous to American College of Rheumatology functional class), with higher values given for increased difficulty. The visual analogue pain scale (bottom) is a 10-cm scale. Both instruments entail patient self-reporting and have been validated for use in rheumatoid arthritis. (From Callahan LF, Pincus T. A clue from a self-report questionnaire to distinguish rheumatoid arthritis from noninflammatory diffuse musculoskeletal pain: the P-VAS:D-ADL ratio. *Arthritis Rheum* 1990;33:1317–1322, with permission.)

damage. They are useful instruments for long-term outcome measurement, are standard in outcomes assessment research, and are part of the core set of evaluation criteria (Table 55.2). The Stanford Health Assessment Questionnaire (HAQ) (133), its modified version (mHAQ) (Fig. 55.29) (134), and the Arthritis Impact Measurement Scale (135) are the most commonly used instruments. These instruments have been translated into other languages, and culture-specific tasks have been incorporated to assess functional status optimally.

Routine assessment of the patient should also ascertain the level of patient pain and function by direct questioning. Quantification of pain may best be performed with a 10-cm visual analogue pain scale (Fig. 55.29), allowing patients to serve as their own control over time. It has been found that horizontal scales perform better than vertical ones, and some investigators prefer to have descriptions of pain severity during intervals of time, as opposed to a single point in time (44).

COURSE OF ILLNESS

Remission

Criteria for clinical remission include absence of fatigue, absence of joint pain by history, absence of synovial swelling, absence of joint tenderness, normal sedimentation rate, and morning stiffness of less than 15 minutes. The patient must meet five of these criteria to be classified as being in remission (136). The proportion of patients with resolution of polyarticular inflammatory arthritis over time depends on the method of ascertainment. In population studies, where few patients have RF or radiographic damage (and do not fulfill 1987 ACR classification criteria for RA), the majority of patients are in remission within 3 to 5 years (137,138). For patients seen in medical settings, however, only about 15% will achieve remission (139,140) or normal functional status a decade later (132).

Work Disability and Costs

Significant functional declines and work disability occur in RA patients (1). One study reported that three fourths of RA patients followed in rheumatology clinics changed jobs due to the illness and more than half became disabled within a decade (141). Another study showed that one fourth of RA patients are unable to work just 6.4 years after diagnosis and half are not able to work after 20 years (142). The loss of income over time is the greatest financial burden, far surpassing direct medical costs (143). Lifetime costs of RA are comparable with those for coronary artery disease or stroke (144). There are emerging data to show that early consistent use of DMARDs can improve long-term function outcomes (145–147) and one population based study has demonstrated a significant decrease in need for joint replacement surgery (148).

Self-reported functional status and the physical demands of work are the best predictors of disability (149). Lack of autonomy over the work schedule, the pace of work, and the nature of the job all increase the likelihood of becoming disabled (150). Social responsibilities at home reduce the likelihood of becoming disabled, whereas lack of a supportive household increases the likelihood (151).

FACTORS AFFECTING OUTCOME

Age of Onset and Gender

In patients under 50 years of age, women tend to have a worse prognosis with regard to persistence and severity of disease (152). Pregnancy may lead to a remission of RA, with return of the synovitis postpartum; HLA mismatches between mother and fetus may predict this favorable response during pregnancy (153). Replacement androgen therapy for males with low serum testosterone levels may improve clinical and laboratory parameters (154).

Benign RA of the aged (155) probably includes those with remitting, seronegative, symmetric synovitis with pitting edema (RS3PE) and polymyalgia rheumatica, as well as mild seronegative RA, and has a relatively good prognosis. However, older patients with seropositive RA appear to have immunogenetic profiles (156) and clinical courses similar to those of younger patients (157–159), and early aggressive therapy is especially important, because older patients typically have less reserve.

Smoking

Smoking appears to make RA worse (160) and may be a risk factor for developing RA (161–167). One study found that smokers are more likely to be seropositive, have nodules, and to have radiographic erosions (160). Evidence that smoking cessation can ameliorate disease has not yet been shown. RA patients have a significantly increased morbidity from cardiovascular disease, infections (particularly pulmonary infections), and osteoporosis. The potential role of smoking in exacerbating these issues may be significant (reviewed in references 168 and 169).

Type of Onset

RA may have an insidious onset over years or appear dramatically overnight, although in most patients the disease evolves over a period of a few months. Prognosis does not appear to depend on the mode of onset (170). With an abrupt onset, however, infection, systemic vasculitis, and RS3PE (171) also need to be considered. Those with malaise and weight loss at the onset of illness (172,173) have a less favorable functional outcome.

Education

The level of formal education, even after adjustment for economic status, has been found to be predictive of outcome in patients with RA, with poorer clinical status (174) and premature mortality (2) seen in those who did not finish high school. This may be a surrogate measure for other behavioral, cognitive, or psychological variables that influence one's abilities to cope with a chronic illness (175). Similar trends have been seen with other chronic diseases (176).

Joint Involvement

The joints involved in a cross-section of patients with well-established disease (median duration 10 years) attending a rheumatology clinic are listed in Table 55.7 (50); similar patterns of involvement have also been documented in RA patients participating in clinical trials (51). Other investigators have found more frequent involvement of the foot and ankle joints (177). Small joints are invariably involved, with MCP involvement most common. One series showed that joint groups not involved with inflammation (swelling and tenderness) over the first year of disease were unlikely to be involved over the course of the disease (178). Deformities may take years to develop, although in one group of RA patients hand deformities developed in 15% of patients within the first 2 years of disease (57). As expected, limitation of joint motion and deformity are more extensive in disabled RA patients compared with those still able to work (179).

Radiographic Damage

Damage as detectable by radiographs occurs within the first several years of disease in a majority of RA patients followed in rheumatology clinics (89,90,140,180). Clinical parameters that predict the development of destructive radiographic changes in the hands and wrists over time include persistently swollen joints (124,181–185); elevation

TABLE 55.7. *Percentage of rheumatoid arthritis patients with abnormalities in specific joints seen in an outpatient setting*

Joint	Swelling	Tenderness	Pain on Motion	Limitation of Motion	Deformity
Temporomandibular (TM)	3	17	9	21	—
Sternoclavicular (SC)	3	11	1	—	—
Acromioclavicular (AC)	0	22	3	—	—
Shoulder	0	21	52	43	4
Elbow	26	35	25	34	36
Wrist	66	55	58	71	35
Metacarpophalangeal (MCP) index[a]	82	51	24	34	31
Proximal interphalangeal (PIP) index[a]	36	40	23	35	24
Hip	—	5	19	18	1
Knee	33	38	34	11	11
Ankle	40	38	34	29	5
Subtalar	7	5	11	16	3
Tarsometatarsal	11	11	19	23	3
Metatarsophalangeal (MTP) great[a]	24	42	12	6	38

[a]Values for index MCP and PIP joints shown as representative joints of these rows of joints; values for great MTP joints shown as representative of this row of joints.

Adapted from Fuchs HA, Brooks RH, Callahan LF, et al. A simplified twenty-eight-joint quantitative articular index in rheumatoid arthritis. *Arthritis Rheum* 1989;32:531–537, with permission.

of acute-phase reactants (115,181–183,186,187); the presence of RF (181,182,184,188), which may be a surrogate for the presence of HLA-DR4 (35); the presence of HLA-DR4/Dw4 (189,190), DR1 (187), or DRB1*0401 (36); and flexor tendonitis of the fingers (16). Almost all hand and foot joints developing erosions over a 2-year study of newly diagnosed RA patients were persistently abnormal on scintigraphy (106).

Mortality

Mortality rates are increased at least twofold for RA patients and are related to disease severity (191). Up to one third of deaths may be directly attributable to the disease itself (2), with increases in the rates of cardiovascular and infectious causes seen as well (192).

Mortality is correlated with the arthritis itself, in that prognosis is worse in those with the greatest number of abnormal joints (2). Involvement of large joints portends a worse prognosis than synovitis restricted to hands and feet (175), but rarely occurs without concomitant involvement of the small joints. A recent study (193) has shown that methotrexate-treated patients have significantly decreased overall mortality risks (OD = 0.4) with a significantly decreased cardiovascular mortality risk (OD = 0.3).

DIFFERENTIAL DIAGNOSIS

When presented with a patient who has joint pain, the physician's first challenge is to discern if the problem is due to mechanical derangements, OA, or the presence of inflammation. Stiffness, swelling, tenderness, warmth, and pain with motion are hallmarks of active inflammation in the joint. The presence of severe morning stiffness is indicative of an inflammatory process; gelling of the joints for merely a few minutes in the morning and after rest is more consistent with OA and tendonitis.

The diagnosis of RA is most difficult in early disease or when relatively few joints are involved, and unfortunately, diagnosis is usually delayed several months after the onset of symptoms, limiting the initiation of early treatment. Reasons for the delay include asymmetric involvement, absence of RF, less severe disease at onset, and the tendency for symptoms to fluctuate early in the disease course (194). Distinguishing RA from other causes of chronic inflammatory arthritis or transient synovitis syndromes (e.g., postviral) is difficult early in the disease. Seropositivity for RF and fulfillment of the 1987 ACR criteria for classification of RA increase the likelihood of RA (195).

OTHER RHEUMATOLOGIC CAUSES OF INFLAMMATORY ARTHRITIS

Signs and symptoms of inflammatory arthritis may be associated with many other syndromes besides RA. A history directed at eliciting the associated features of other arthritides is essential; thus, the presence of photosensitivity or nephritis should suggest the possibility of SLE; the Raynaud phenomenon should bring to mind the possibility of systemic sclerosis or SLE, although about 1% of RA patients will have the Raynaud phenomenon; and conjunctivitis and dactylitis should suggest reactive arthritis. Systemic vasculitis, such as polyarteritis nodosa or Wegener granulomatosis, may be associated with disabling joint pain, although objective signs of arthritis are infrequent. Finally, hypothyroidism can produce rheumatic symptoms, and also is seen in increased association with RA (196,197).

Spondyloarthropathies

The spondyloarthropathies (reactive arthritis and some types of psoriatic arthritis; see Chapters 64 and 65) may appear similar to RA at presentation. In most cases, differences in the history or on physical examination will distinguish them from RA (Table 55.8). The nature of the joint inflammation is often different, with a great deal of inflammation found at the enthesis or site of tendon insertions (e.g., Achilles tendon insertion, plantar fascia, shafts of fingers or toes). Asymmetric oligoarthritis (less than four joints), usually of the weight-bearing joints, is common in these disorders with or without sacroiliac and spinal involvement. Recognizing the importance of a focused history, asking about conjunctivitis/iritis, urethritis, and mucocutaneous manifestations is key. Additionally, inflammatory symptoms of the axial skeleton would strongly suggest the diagnosis of one of the spondyloarthropathies.

Adult-Onset Still's Disease

Still's disease or systemic onset juvenile RA has systemic features as a major manifestation and therefore should be easy to separate from RA in most cases (see Chapter 61). Fever, rash, leukocytosis, lymphadenopathy, pleuropericarditis, sore throat, and hepatosplenomegaly (198) are common in addition to the arthritis. When adults are affected they are usually under 40 years of age and commonly present with fever of unknown origin (see Chapter 60). The characteristic evanescent, macular, salmon-colored rash usually appears on the torso and upper arms and may be brought out by mechanical stimulation of the skin (Köbner phenomenon). It is most evident at times of fever, which characteristically occurs in the evening, with resolution by the following morning. Hectic fever curves with two or more spikes per day are also common. Amyloidosis may develop after years of disease, more commonly in adult-onset disease (96).

In Still's disease, elevated ESR and leukocytosis are seen in over 90% of patients (199). Anemia, hypoalbuminemia, and abnormal liver function tests are seen in a majority of patients. Antinuclear antibodies (ANAs) and RF are present in less than 10% (200). Curiously, extreme elevation of ferritin (>1,000 ng/L) may be seen in a majority of patients; such elevations are not generally seen in other forms of inflammatory arthritis, suggesting a relative specificity of this finding (201). Ferritin levels may fluctuate with disease activity, as does the ESR (202).

Treatment is aimed at controlling the inflammatory process. An initial trial of salicylates is warranted, although most patients will eventually require corticosteroids for control of systemic symptoms (200). Second-line antiinflammatory drugs (gold, methotrexate) have been used successfully to control the synovitis, decrease the frequency of attacks, or to decrease the dose of steroids necessary for overall control.

Palindromic Rheumatism

Palindromic rheumatism is a remitting, recurring, nondestructive, inflammatory arthritis with recurrences over at least 6 months (203). The accompanying pain has been likened to that of gout, with maximum intensity within hours and pain severe enough to confine patients to bed. A palindrome is a word or a sentence that reads the same backward as it does forward. Therefore, the name *palin-*

TABLE 55.8. *Attributes on physical examination that help distinguish rheumatoid arthritis from spondyloarthropathy*

Rheumatoid arthritis	Spondyloarthropathy
Articular Involvement	
Symmetric	Asymmetric
Polyarthritis	Oligoarthritis
Prominent in hands	Mostly weight bearing joints
Fusiform swelling in fingers	Dactylitis ("sausage digits")
Rows of joints involved	Ray involvement (e.g., all joints of a particular digit)
Spinal instability (cervical)	Spinal ankylosis (all regions)
Extraarticular Involvement	
Rheumatoid nodules	Psoriasiform rash
Serositis (pleuropericarditis)	Mucositis (diarrhea, oral ulcers, urethritis, conjunctivitis)
Vasculitis, ischemic ulcers	No vasculitis
Nodules on valves	Aortitis, chronic aortic insufficiency
Acute valvular insufficiency	Heart block
Scleritis, ulcerative keratopathy, keratoconjunctivitis sicca	Uveitis
Splenomegaly, reactive adenopathy	
Periarticular osteoporosis	Reactive bone formation
	Inflammatory bowel disease

dromic rheumatism was coined to describe the rapid appearance and disappearance of the arthritis, because the attacks may last for hours or days (rarely greater than a week), with complete resolution between attacks. Each attack generally involves only a few joints, with the joints ultimately involved being similar to those involved in typical RA; the MCP, wrist, shoulder, knee, ankle, foot, and elbow are each affected in over 33% of reported patients (204).

Concomitant inflammation of tendons or paraarticular structures is seen in over 25% of patients (204). Subcutaneous nodules may appear with the arthritis attacks and resolve in less than a week. The ESR may be elevated during an attack, but should normalize between attacks. Radiographs do not show bony erosions or cartilage loss (by definition).

The disease will eventually evolve into typical RA over time in 25% to 50% of the patients (204–206). The presence of RF, female gender, and the involvement of PIP and wrist joints have been shown to be a risk factor for the development of RA in some (205), but not all, studies. Female patients with RF and early hand involvement were eight times more likely to develop RA than patients with only one of these features (205). Other laboratory analyses are not predictive of evolution into RA (ESR, ANA, synovial fluid analyses, complement) (204,207).

Treatment generally involves administration of NSAIDs for the acute inflammation with consideration of second-line antirheumatic drugs in patients with frequent recurrences. Hydroxychloroquine has been useful in decreasing the frequency and duration of attacks in patients with persistent palindromic rheumatism (206). If the patient evolves to RA then they should be treated as such.

Remitting Seronegative Symmetric Synovitis with Pitting Edema

A peculiar inflammatory arthritis affecting primarily the elderly (men more than women) designated RS3PE, has been described by McCarty and colleagues (208). It is characterized by abrupt onset of marked dorsal swelling of the hands with pitting edema, wrist synovitis, and flexor tendinitis of the fingers; similar swelling and synovitis may also be seen in the feet and ankles. Patients can often precisely pinpoint the time of onset. In general, the prognosis is excellent, although RS3PE occurring with an underlying malignancy as a paraneoplastic syndrome has been reported (209). Patients have, for the most part, responded dramatically to low-dose steroids (171,210); treatment with a combination of hydroxychloroquine and NSAIDs (208) has also yielded good results. RF is not present and radiographic joint destruction does not occur. Remission is the rule within a year, although one patient had arthritis for 3 years (208). Residual, mild, asymptomatic flexion contractures in the fingers and wrists are common. HLA-B7 has been present in a majority of cases (171,208). Hemiplegic individuals do not develop the synovitis on the plegic side, similar to joint involvement in RA (211). Finally, some have suggested overlap with polymyalgia rheumatica in some cases (210).

Polymyalgia Rheumatica

Polymyalgia rheumatica (see Chapter 85) generally presents with an abrupt onset of pain and stiffness in the shoulder and hip girdles of patients over 50 years of age. Fever, weight loss, and lethargy can occur and may be severe. Inflammatory arthritis of the shoulders and hips is suggested by bone scan (212,213), although swelling may be difficult to detect (clinical symptoms localize much more to the proximal musculature). The stiffness is often severe enough to awaken patients if they roll over in bed at night, and restriction of shoulder movement secondary to pain and soft tissue contracture is common. The stiffness and restricted mobility are exquisitely sensitive to treatment with low-dose prednisone, with 10 mg/day often sufficient to control the process. Relapse after discontinuing or reducing the corticosteroid dose is frequent, and up to half of the patients require treatment beyond 2 years (214–216).

Polymyalgia rheumatica may be seen alone as a symptom complex or be associated with giant cell arteritis (217); it may also be part of the spectrum of RA (218,219). An elevation of the ESR is usual, but RF is generally absent. An abnormal temporal artery biopsy differentiates giant cell arteritis from polymyalgia rheumatica, and should usually be obtained in the setting of a new headache, jaw claudication, sudden visual loss, significant weight loss, or extreme elevation of the ESR (>100 mm/h) (see Chapter 85). Persistent small joint synovitis of the hands and feet distinguishes RA from polymyalgia rheumatica, although morning stiffness may otherwise be identical. RA of acute onset with polymyalgia rheumatica symptoms in the elderly often has an excellent prognosis (155). Genetic predisposition is inferred by the presence of HLA-DR4 in polymyalgia rheumatica as observed in giant cell arteritis and RA (220), although the genetics of polymyalgia rheumatica may more closely resemble that associated with giant cell arteritis than RA (221).

Rhupus

About 1% to 2% of patients with SLE will have concurrent RA, which has been labeled by some as rhupus (222). The clinical manifestations include an erosive (by radiographs) polyarthritis typical of RA and cutaneous or renal features of SLE (223); serositis is common, but could be attributed to either RA or SLE. RF and ANA are typically present, and anti-Ro (SS-A) antibody is seen in about half the patients; hypocomplementemia is common, and anti-DNA is often present in patients with glomerulonephritis

(224). HLA typing shows an increase in both HLA-DR4 (as expected in RA) and HLA-DR3 (as expected in SLE) (224). Management directed at both features of rheumatoid and lupus may be necessary.

Importantly, the treatment of RA with sulfasalazine (225), and D-penicillamine (226) has been associated with drug-induced lupus. The presence of antinuclear antibodies, photosensitive rash, and serositis are the most common manifestations. The medication must be stopped and the associated inflammatory process treated; corticosteroids may be required.

VIRAL ARTHRITIS

Polyarthritis may be the presenting feature of viral infections. Clues pointing toward the etiologic agent may be evident in the history and examination. Fever and cutaneous manifestations may suggest that an infectious process is present.

Rubella

Rubella virus has been associated with a polyarthritis affecting primarily the MCP and PIP joints of the hands, wrists, knees, and ankles. The onset usually coincides with the exanthem, cervical adenopathy, and fever. The arthritis usually resolves within a few days or weeks, although it may persist for months. The wild virus is more likely to cause synovitis (227); *in vitro* studies show that the wild virus and vaccine strains associated with a high incidence of synovitis replicates and persists in fetal synovial cultures better than strains that are relatively nonarthritogenic (228). As in RA, young women are most susceptible, with about half of those infected with wild virus exhibiting arthritis and 14% experiencing arthritis after vaccination; recurrent arthritis of up to 18 months' duration was seen in 30% of those infected with wild virus (227). There are reports of chronic arthritis developing after rubella infection with both the wild virus and vaccine (229); intravenous gamma globulin has been variably effective in treatment, but more conventional treatment with NSAIDs is generally used. Except in these rare cases of chronic arthritis, proliferative synovitis as seen in RA does not occur.

Parvovirus

Human parvovirus B19 causes fifth disease in children and adults, bone marrow suppression (including aplastic crisis in those with hemolytic anemias), and hydrops fetalis (230). A macular rash (often with the appearance of a slapped cheek) and flulike symptoms may precede the arthritis (231). This may present as a symmetric polyarthritis with swelling and tenderness of the small joints of the hands, wrists, and knees, primarily in women and children. The onset of arthritis is often abrupt, with the patient suddenly being unable to get out of bed in the morning due to pain (232). The course is generally limited to less than 2 months, although a chronic arthropathy has been described that can fulfill criteria for seronegative RA with a relatively benign outcome (233).

Hepatitis B and C

Hepatitis B and C have been reported to cause polyarthritis that is sometimes accompanied by RF, but generally only lasts a few days to a few weeks. Both should be considered in the differential diagnosis of polyarthritis of short duration. Hepatitis C is also associated with RF, cryoglobulinemia, and a nondestructive arthritis (234), and has been reported to cause a chronic polyarthritis resembling RA. In some cases, the arthritis has responded dramatically to treatment of the underlying hepatitis C infection.

IMPORTANT CONDITIONS THAT OFTEN OCCUR WITH RHEUMATOID ARTHRITIS

Fibromyalgia

Fibromyalgia is a common problem and is often seen in patients with RA. In general, a patient with fibromyalgia is easy to distinguish from a patient with RA. However, when fibromyalgia occurs with RA, as it does in 10% to 20% of patients (235), it can confuse the clinical situation. The clinician should be on the lookout for this and not treat the aches and pains of fibromyalgia with increasing doses of DMARDs or steroids.

Osteoporosis

Patients of both sexes with RA have a significantly greater risk for osteoporosis. The reasons for this are multifactorial and include active RA, gender (most are women), treatment (especially steroids), and decreased activity. This risk should be recognized early, and all patients should be on calcium and vitamin D, especially if they are taking steroids, which decrease the gastrointestinal absorption of calcium. Bisphosphonates should be used aggressively in this patient population, particularly in patients on steroids.

CONCLUSION

The diagnosis and assessment of RA may be facilitated by laboratory and radiographic examinations. Ultimately, however, the diagnosis is primarily dependent on the clinical skills of the physician. Indeed, there are few areas left in medicine in which the physician, relying on experience, patience, and powers of observation, can make such a difference in the lives of patients. The early recognition of C1–2 subluxation, constrictive pericarditis, or systemic vasculitis may be life saving, and much morbidity can be avoided by prompt treatment of entrapment neuropathies and referral at the appropriate time to orthopedic surgeons skilled in joint replacement.

More importantly, the experienced rheumatologist can establish the diagnosis and initiate treatment early. With the growing realization that structural damage in RA is a cumulative result of joint inflammation, and that irreversible changes occur very early in the course, there is a clear consensus that early initiation of appropriate treatment is essential (see Chapter 59). Finally, to optimally manage patients with RA, since there is seldom, if ever, one correct medication for a given situation, the rheumatologist must be skilled in the art, as well as the science, of medicine.

ACKNOWLEDGMENTS

I thank Drs. Howard A. Fuchs and John S. Sergent for their contributions to this chapter.

REFERENCES

1. Scott DL, Symmons DPM, Coulton BL, et al. Long-term outcome of treating rheumatoid arthritis: results after 20 years. *Lancet* 1987;1: 1108–1111.
2. Pincus T, Brooks RH, Callahan LF. Prediction of long-term mortality in patients with rheumatoid arthritis according to simple questionnaire and joint count measures. *Ann Intern Med* 1994;120:26–34.
3. Wolfe F, Mitchell DM, Sibley JT, et al. The mortality of rheumatoid arthritis. *Arthritis Rheum* 1994;37:481–494.
4. Gabriel SE, Crowson CS, O'Fallon WM. The epidemiology of rheumatoid arthritis in Rochester, Minnesota, 1955–1985. *Arthritis Rheum* 1999;42:415–420.
5. Kellgren JH. Epidemiology of rheumatoid arthritis. *Arthritis Rheum* 1966;9:658–674.
6. Silman AJ, Hochberg MC. Rheumatoid arthritis. In: Silman AJ, Hochberg MC, eds. *Epidemiology of the rheumatic diseases.* Oxford: Oxford University Press, 1993:7–68.
7. del Puente A, Knowler WC, Pettitt DJ, et al. High incidence and prevalence of rheumatoid arthritis in Pima Indians. *Am J Epidemiol* 1989;129:1170–1187.
8. Silman AJ, Ollier W, Holligan S, et al. Absence of rheumatoid arthritis in a rural Nigerian population. *J Rheumatol* 1993;20:618–622.
9. Linos A, Worthington JW, O'Fallon WM, et al. The epidemiology of rheumatoid arthritis in Rochester, Minnesota: a study of incidence, prevalence and mortality. *Am J Epidemiol* 1980;111:87–98.
10. Chan KA, Felson DT, Yood RA, et al. Incidence of rheumatoid arthritis in central Massachusetts. *Arthritis Rheum* 1993;36:1691–1696.
11. Dugowson CE, Koepsell TD, Vooigt LF, et al. Rheumatoid arthritis in women—incidence rates in group health cooperative, Seattle, Washington, 1987–1989. *Arthritis Rheum* 1991;34:1502–1507.
12. Aho K, Tuomi T, Palosuo T, et al. Is seropositive rheumatoid arthritis becoming less severe? *Clin Exp Rheumatol* 1989;7:287–290.
13. American College of Rheumatology Subcommittee on Rheumatoid Arthritis Guidelines. 2002 Update: guidelines for the management of rheumatoid arthritis. *Arthritis Rheum* 2002;46:328–346.
14. O'Dell JR. Treating rheumatoid arthritis early: a window of opportunity. *Arthritis Rheum* 2002;46:283–285.
15. Arnett FC, Edworthy SM, Bloch DA, et al. The American Rheumatism Association 1987 revised criteria for the classification of rheumatoid arthritis. *Arthritis Rheum* 1988;31:315–324.
16. Mottonen TT. Prediction of erosiveness and rate of development of new erosions in early rheumatoid arthritis. *Ann Rheum Dis* 1988;47:648–653.
17. Goldbach-Mansky R, Lee J, McCoy A, et al. Rheumatoid arthritis associated autoantibodies in patients with synovitis of recent onset. *Arthritis Res* 2002;2(3):236–243.
18. Schellekens GA, Visser H, de Jong BA, et al. The diagnostic properties of rheumatoid arthritis antibodies recognizing a cyclic citrullinated peptide. *Arthritis Rheum* 2000;43(1):155–163.
19. Nielen MMJ, van Schaardenburg D, van de Stadt RJ, et al. Autoantibodies in serum of blood donors precede symptoms of rheumatoid arthritis (RA) by 1 to 6 years. *Arthritis Rheum* 2002;46(9)(suppl):370.
20. Jansen AL, van der Horst-Bruinsma I, van Schaardenburg D, et al. Rheumatoid factor and antibodies to cyclic citrullinated peptide differentiate rheumatoid arthritis from undifferentiated polyarthritis in patients with early arthritis. *J Rheumatol* 2002;29(10):2074–2076.
21. Vencovsky J, Machacek S, Sedova L, et al. Autoantibodies can be prognostic markers of an erosive disease in early rheumatoid arthritis. *Ann Rheum Dis* 2003;62(5):427–430.
22. Bland JH, Eddy WM. Hemiplegia and rheumatoid arthritis. *Arthritis Rheum* 1968;11:72–78.
23. Konttinen YT, Kemppinen P, Gegerberg M, et al. Peripheral and spinal neural mechanisms in arthritis, with particular reference to treatment of inflammation and pain. *Arthritis Rheum* 1994;37:965–982.
24. Fuchs HA, Anderson JJ. Joint assessment. In: Wolfe F, Pincus T, eds. *Rheumatoid arthritis: critical issues in etiology, assessment, prognosis and therapy.* New York: Marcel Dekker, 1994:151–165.
25. Wilder RL. Hormones, pregnancy, and autoimmune diseases. *Ann NY Acad Sci* 1998;840:45–50.
26. Nelson JL, Ostensen M. Pregnancy and rheumatoid arthritis. *Rheum Dis Clin North Am* 1997;23:195–212.
27. Silman A, Kay A, Brennan P. Timing of pregnancy in relation to the onset of rheumatoid arthritis. *Arthritis Rheum* 1992;35:152–155.
28. Brennan P, Silman A. Breast-feeding and the onset of rheumatoid arthritis. *Arthritis Rheum* 1994;37:808–813.
29. Van Vollenhoven RF, McGuire JL. Estrogen, progesterone, and testosterone: can they be used to treat autoimmune diseases? *Cleve Clin J Med* 1994;61:276–284.
30. Wilder RL. Adrenal and gonadal steroid hormone deficiency in the pathogenesis of rheumatoid arthritis. *J Rheumatol* 1996;44:10–12.
31. Silman AJ, Hennessy E, Ollier WER. Incidence of rheumatoid arthritis in a genetically predisposed population. *Br J Rheumatol* 1992;31:365–368.
32. Deighton CM, Roberts DF, Walker DJ. Effect of disease severity on rheumatoid arthritis concordance in same sexed siblings. *Ann Rheum Dis* 1992;51:943–945.
33. Silman AJ, MacGregor AJ, Thomson W, et al. Twin concordance rates for rheumatoid arthritis: results from a nationwide study. *Br J Rheumatol* 1993;32:903–907.
34. Stastny P. Association of the B-cell alloantigen DRw4 with rheumatoid arthritis. *N Engl J Med* 1978;298:869–871.
35. Olsen NJ, Callahan LF, Brooks RH, et al. Associations of HLA-DR4 with rheumatoid factor and radiographic severity in rheumatoid arthritis. *Am J Med* 1988;84:257–264.
36. Weyand CM, Hicok KC, Conn D, et al. The influence of HLA-DRB1 genes on disease severity in rheumatoid arthritis. *Ann Intern Med* 1992;117:801–806.
37. Jawaheer D, Thomson W, MacGregor AJ, et al. "Homozygosity" for the HLA-DR shared epitope contributes the highest risk for rheumatoid arthritis concordance in identical twins. *Arthritis Rheum* 1994; 37:681–686.
38. Hazes JM, Hayton R, Burt J, et al. Consistency of morning stiffness: an analysis of diary data. *Br J Rheumatol* 1994;33:562–565.
39. Hazes JMW, Hayton R, Silman AJ. A reevaluation of the symptom of morning stiffness. *J Rheumatol* 1993;20:1138–1142.
40. Bellamy N, Sothern RB, Campbell J, et al. Circadian rhythm in pain, stiffness and manual dexterity in rheumatoid arthritis: relation between discomfort and disability. *Ann Rheum Dis* 1991;50:243–248.
41. Bromley J, Unsworth A, Haslock I. Changes in stiffness following short-and long-term application of standard physiotherapeutic techniques. *Br J Rheumatol* 1994;33:555–561.
42. Dellhag B, Wollersjo I, Bjelle A. Effect of active hand exercise and wax bath treatment in rheumatoid arthritis patients. *Arthritis Care Res* 1992;5:87–92.
43. Felson DT, Anderson JJ, Boers M, et al. The American College of Rheumatology preliminary core set of disease activity measures for rheumatoid arthritis clinical trials. *Arthritis Rheum* 1993;36:729–740.
44. Buchanan WW, Tugwell P. Traditional assessments of articular diseases. *Clin Rheum Dis* 1983;9:515–529.

45. Klinkhoff AV, Bellamy N, Bombardier C, et al. An experiment in reducing interobserver variability of the examination of joint tenderness. *J Rheumatol* 1988;15:492–494.
46. Atkins CJ, Zielinski A, Klinkhoff AV, et al. An electronic method for measuring joint tenderness in rheumatoid arthritis. *Arthritis Rheum* 1992;35:407–410.
47. Hart LE, Tugwell P, Buchanan WW, et al. Grading of tenderness as a source of interrater error in the Ritchie articular index. *J Rheumatol* 1985;12:716–717.
48. Ritchie DM, Boyle JA, McInnes JM, et al. Clinical studies with an articular index for the assessment of joint tenderness in patients with rheumatoid arthritis. *Q J Med* 1968;37:393–406.
49. Rigby AS, Wood PHN. The lateral metacarpophalangeal/metatarsophalangeal squeeze: an alternative assignment criterion for rheumatoid arthritis. *Scand J Rheumatol* 1991;20:115–120.
50. Fuchs HA, Brooks RH, Callahan LF, et al. A simplified twenty-eight-joint quantitative articular index in rheumatoid arthritis. *Arthritis Rheum* 1989;32:531–537.
51. Fuchs HA, Pincus T. Reduced joint counts in controlled clinical trials in rheumatoid arthritis. *Arthritis Rheum* 1994;37:470–475.
52. Jayson MIV, Dixon ASJ. Valvular mechanisms in juxta-articular cysts. *Ann Rheum Dis* 1970;29:415–420.
53. Palmer DG. Synovial cysts in rheumatoid disease. *Ann Intern Med* 1969;70:61–68.
54. Szer IS, Klein-Gitelman M, Denardo BA, et al. Ultrasonography in the study of prevalence and clinical evolution of popliteal cysts in children with knee effusions. *J Rheumatol* 1992;19:458–462.
55. Katz RS, Zizic TM, Arnold WP, et al. The pseudothrombophlebitis syndrome. *Medicine* 1997;56:151–164.
56. Kraag G, Thevathasan EM, Gordon DA, et al. The hemorrhagic crescent sign of acute synovial rupture. *Ann Intern Med* 1976;85:477–478.
57. Eberhardt K, Johnson PM, Rydgren L. The occurrence and significance of hand deformities in early rheumatoid arthritis. *Br J Rheumatol* 1991;30:211–213.
58. Smith RJ, Kaplan EB. Rheumatoid deformities at the metacarpophalangeal joints of the fingers. *J Bone Joint Surg Am* 1967;49:31–47.
59. Dreyfus JN, Schnitzer TJ. Pathogenesis and differential diagnosis of the swan-neck deformity. *Semin Arthritis Rheum* 1983;13:200–211.
60. Read GO, Solomon L, Biddulph S. Relationship between finger and wrist deformities in rheumatoid arthritis. *Ann Rheum Dis* 1983;42:619–625.
61. Smith EM, Juvinall RC, Bender LF, et al. Flexor forces and rheumatoid metacarpophalangeal deformity. *JAMA* 1966;198:150–154.
62. Hakstian RW, Tubiana R. Ulnar deviation of the fingers; the role of joint structure and function. *J Bone Joint Surg* 1967;49:299–316.
63. DiBenedetto MR, Lubbers LM, Coleman CR. Relationship between radial inclination angle and ulnar deviation of the fingers. *J Hand Surg [Am]* 1991;16:36–39.
64. Vidigal E, Jacoby RK, Dixon ASJ, et al. The foot in chronic rheumatoid arthritis. *Ann Rheum Dis* 1975;34:292–297.
65. Anderson EG. The rheumatoid foot: a sideways look. *Ann Rheum Dis* 1990;49:851–857.
66. Jones DW, Jones DA, Newham DJ. Chronic knee effusion and aspiration: the effect on quadriceps inhibition. *Br J Rheumatol* 1987;26:370–374.
67. Komusi T, Munro T, Harth M. Radiologic review: the rheumatoid cervical spine. *Semin Arthritis Rheum* 1985;14:187–195.
68. Rasker JJ, Cosh JA. Radiological study of cervical spine and hand in patients with rheumatoid arthritis of 15 years' duration: an assessment of the effects of corticosteroid treatment. *Ann Rheum Dis* 1978;37:529–535.
69. Leicht MJ, Harrington TM, Davis DE. Cricoarytenoid arthritis: a cause of laryngeal obstruction. *Ann Emerg Med* 1987;16:885–888.
70. Lawry GV, Finerman ML, Hanaffee WN, et al. Laryngeal involvement in rheumatoid arthritis: a clinical, laryngoscopic and computerized tomographic study. *Arthritis Rheum* 1984;27:873–882.
71. Gordon DA, Stein JL, Broder I. The extra-articular features of rheumatoid arthritis: a systematic analysis of 127 cases. *Am J Med* 1973;54:445–452.
72. Walker WC, Wright V. Rheumatoid pleuritis. *Ann Rheum Dis* 1967;26:467–471.
73. Scott DGI, Bacon PA, Tribe CR. Systemic rheumatoid vasculitis: a clinical and laboratory study of 50 cases. *Medicine* 1981;60:288–297.
74. Hara KS, Ballard DJ, Ilstrup DM, et al. Rheumatoid pericarditis: clinical features and survival. *Medicine* 1990;69:81–91.
75. Kaye BR, Kaye RL, Bobrove A. Rheumatoid nodules: review of the spectrum of associated conditions and a proposal of a new classification, with a report of four seronegative cases. *Am J Med* 1984;76:279–292.
76. Symmons DPM, Barrett EM, Bankhead CR, et al. The incidence of rheumatoid arthritis in the United Kingdom: results from the Norfolk Arthritis Register. *Br J Rheumatol* 1994;33:735–739.
77. Ching DWT, Petrie JP, Klemp P, et al. Injection therapy of superficial rheumatoid nodules. *Br J Rheumatol* 1992;31:775–777.
78. Segal R, Caspi D, Tishler M, et al. Accelerated nodulosis and vasculitis during methotrexate therapy for rheumatoid arthritis. *Arthritis Rheum* 1988;31:1182–1185.
79. Fuchs HA. Rheumatoid vasculitis with worsening nodulosis. *J Rheumatol* 1990;17:123–124.
80. Renner WR, Weinstein AS. Early changes of rheumatoid arthritis in the hand and wrist. *Radiol Clin North Am* 1988;26:1186–1193.
81. Stashenko P, Dewhirst FE, Peros WJ, et al. Synergistic interactions between interleukin-1, tumor necrosis factor and lymphotoxin in bone resorption. *J Immunol* 1987;138:1464–1468.
82. Shenstone BD, Mahmoud A, Woodward R, et al. Longitudinal bone mineral density changes in early rheumatoid arthritis. *Br J Rheumatol* 1994;33:541–545.
83. Gough AKS, Lilley J, Eyre S, et al. Generalised bone loss in patients with early rheumatoid arthritis. *Lancet* 1994;344:23–27.
84. Kalla AA, Meyers OL, Chalton D, et al. Increased metacarpal bone mass following 18 months of slow-acting antirheumatic drugs for rheumatoid arthritis. *Br J Rheumatol* 1991;30:91–100.
85. Martel W, Hayes JT, Duff IF. The pattern of bone erosion in the hand and wrist in rheumatoid arthritis. *Radiology* 1965;84:204–214.
86. Allard SA, Muirden KD, Maini RN. Correlation of histopathological features of pannus with patterns of damage in different joints in rheumatoid arthritis. *Ann Rheum Dis* 1991;50:278–283.
87. Kaarela K, Luukkainen R, Koskimies S. How often is seropositive rheumatoid arthritis an erosive disease? A 17-year followup study. *J Rheumatol* 1993;20:1670–1673.
88. Brook A, Corbett M. Radiographic changes in early rheumatoid disease. *Ann Rheum Dis* 1977;36:71–73.
89. van der Heijde DMFM, van Leeuwen MA, van Riel PLCM, et al. Biannual radiographic assessments of hands and feet in a three-year prospective followup of patients with early rheumatoid arthritis. *Arthritis Rheum* 1992;35:26–34.
90. Van der Heijde DM. Joint erosions and patients with early rheumatoid arthritis. *Br J Rheumatol* 1995;34:74–78.
91. de Carvalho A, Graudal H, Jorgensen B. Radiologic evaluation of the progression of rheumatoid arthritis. *Acta Radiol Diagn* 1980;21:115–121.
92. Boonsaner K, Louthrenoo W, Meyer S, et al. Effect of dominancy on severity in rheumatoid arthritis. *Br J Rheumatol* 1992;31:77–80.
93. Owsianik WDJ, Kundi A, Whitehead JN, et al. Radiological articular involvement in the dominant hand in rheumatoid arthritis. *Ann Rheum Dis* 1980;39:508–510.
94. Burns TM, Calin A. The hand radiograph as a diagnostic discriminant between seropositive and seronegative "rheumatoid arthritis": a controlled study. *Ann Rheum Dis* 1983;42:605–612.
95. El-Khoury GY, Larson RK, Kathol MH, et al. Seronegative and seropositive rheumatoid arthritis: radiographic differences. *Radiology* 1988;168:517–520.
96. Cabane J, Michon A, Ziza J-M, et al. Comparison of long term evolution of adult onset and juvenile onset Still's disease, both followed up for more than 10 years. *Ann Rheum Dis* 1990;49:283–285.
97. Vehe RK, Nepom GT, Wilske KR, et al. Erosive rheumatoid factor negative and positive rheumatoid arthritis are immunogenetically similar. *J Rheumatol* 1994;21:194–196.
98. Kaye JJ, Callahan LF, Nance EP, et al. Bony ankylosis in rheumatoid arthritis: association with longer duration and greater severity of disease. *Invest Radiol* 1987;22:303–309.
99. Sharp JT, Lidsky MD, Collins LC, et al. Methods of scoring the progression of radiologic change in rheumatoid arthritis. *Arthritis Rheum* 1971;14:706–720.

100. Thould AK, Simon G. Assessment of radiologic changes in the hands and feet in rheumatoid arthritis. *Ann Rheum Dis* 1965;25:220–228.
101. Nakano KK, Schoene WC, Baker RA, et al. The cervical myelopathy associated with rheumatoid arthritis: analysis of 32 patients, with 2 postmortem cases. *Ann Neurol* 1978;3:144–151.
102. Weissman BW, Aliabadi P, Weinfield MS, et al. Prognostic features of atlantoaxial subluxation in rheumatoid arthritis patients. *Radiology* 1982;144:745–751.
103. Bogduk N, Major GAC, Carter J. Lateral subluxation of the atlas in rheumatoid arthritis: a case report and post-mortem study. *Ann Rheum Dis* 1984;43:341–346.
104. Santavirta S, Hopfner-Hallikainen D, Paukku P, et al. Atlantoaxial facet joint arthritis in the rheumatoid cervical spine. A panoramic zonography study. *J Rheumatol* 1988;15:217–223.
105. Kauppi M, Hakala M. Prevalence of cervical spine subluxations and dislocations in a community-based rheumatoid arthritis population. *Scand J Rheumatol* 1994;23:133–136.
106. Mottonen TT, Hannonen P, Toivanen J, et al. Value of joint scintigraphy in the prediction of erosiveness in early rheumatoid arthritis. *Ann Rheum Dis* 1988;47:183–189.
107. Peterfy CG. New developments in imaging in rheumatoid arthritis. *Curr Opin Rheumatol* 2003;15(3):288–295.
108. Weidekamm C, Koller M, Weber M, et al. Diagnostic value of high-resolution B-mode and Doppler sonography for imaging of hand and finger joints in rheumatoid arthritis. *Arthritis Rheum* 203;48(2): 325–333.
109. Jacoby RK, Jayson MIV, Cosh JA. Onset, early stages and prognosis of rheumatoid arthritis: a clinical study of 100 patients with 11-year followup. *BMJ* 1973;2:96–100.
110. Aho K, Heliovaara M, Maatela J, et al. Rheumatoid factors antedating clinical rheumatoid arthritis. *J Rheumatol* 1991;18:1282–1284.
111. Tuomi T, Heliovaara M, Palosuo T, et al. Smoking, lung function and rheumatoid factors. *Ann Rheum Dis* 1990;49:753–756.
112. Heliovaara M, Aho K, Aromaa A, et al. Smoking and risk of rheumatoid arthritis. *J Rheumatol* 1993;20:1830–1835.
113. Tuomi T, Aho K, Palosuo T, et al. Significance of rheumatoid factors in an eight-year longitudinal study on arthritis. *Rheumatol Int* 1988; 8:21–26.
114. Wolfe F, Cathey MA, Roberts FK. The latex test revisited: rheumatoid factor testing in 8267 rheumatic disease patients. *Arthritis Rheum* 1991;34:951–960.
115. Wolfe F, Sharp JT. Radiographic outcome of recent-onset rheumatoid arthritis: a 19-year study of radiographic progression. *Arthritis Rheum* 1998;41:1571–1582.
116. Walsh L, Davies P, McConkey B. Relationship between erythrocyte sedimentation rate and serum C-reactive protein in rheumatoid arthritis. *Ann Rheum Dis* 1979;38:362–363.
117. Thompson PW, Silman AJ, Kirwan JR, et al. Articular indices of joint inflammation in rheumatoid arthritis: correlation with the acute-phase response. *Arthritis Rheum* 1987;30:618–623.
118. Baer AN, Dessypris EN, Goldwasser E, et al. Blunted erythropoietin response to anaemia in rheumatoid arthritis. *Br J Haematol* 1987; 66:559–564.
119. Krantz SB. Pathogenesis and treatment of anemia of chronic disease. *Am J Med Sci* 1994;307:353–359.
120. Pye G, Ballantyne KC, Armitage NC, et al. Influence of non-steroidal anti-inflammatory drugs on the outcome of faecal occult blood tests in screening for colorectal cancer. *BMJ* 1987;294:1510–1511.
121. Gridley G, McLaughlin JK, Ekborn A, et al. Incidence of cancer among patients with RA. *J Natl Cancer Inst* 1993;85:307–311.
122. Hutchinson RM, Davis P, Jayson MIV. Thrombocytosis in rheumatoid arthritis. *Ann Rheum Dis* 1976;35:138–142.
123. Farr M, Scott DL, Constable TJ, et al. Thrombocytosis of active rheumatoid disease. *Ann Rheum Dis* 1983;42:545–549.
124. Scott DL, Dawes PT, Fowler PD, et al. Antirheumatic drugs and joint damage in rheumatoid arthritis. *Q J Med* 1985;54:49–59.
125. Pincus T, Brooks RH, Callahan LF. Joint count scores for tenderness and swelling are improved over 5 years, while scores for joint deformity and limited motion, as well as for radiographic and functional status, show disease progression in patients with rheumatoid arthritis. *Arthritis Rheum* 1994;37(suppl):40.
126. Mulherin D, FitzGerald O, Bresnihan B. An analysis of the discrepancy between the clinical and radiologic course in rheumatoid arthritis [Abstract]. *Arthritis Rheum* 1994;37(suppl):251.
127. Capell HA, Murphy EA, Hunter JA. Rheumatoid arthritis: workload and outcome over 10 years. *Q J Med* 1991;79:461–476.
128. Graudal HK, Graudal N, Jurik AG. On the course of seropositive rheumatoid arthritis during and after long-term gold therapy. *Scand J Rheumatol* 1994;23:223–230.
129. Pincus T, Callahan LF, Brooks RH, et al. Self-report questionnaire scores in rheumatoid arthritis compared with traditional physical, radiographic and laboratory measures. *Ann Intern Med* 1989;110: 259–266.
130. Engelberg AL. *Guides to the evaluation of permanent impairment*, 3rd ed. Chicago: American Medical Association, 1988.
131. Ropes MW, Bennett GA, Cobb S, et al. A 1958 revision of diagnostic criteria for rheumatoid arthritis. *Bull Rheum Dis* 1958;9:175–176.
132. Hochberg MC, Chang RW, Dwosh I, et al. The American College of Rheumatology 1991 revised criteria for the classification of global functional status in rheumatoid arthritis. *Arthritis Rheum* 1992;25: 498–502.
133. Fries JF, Spitz P, Kraines RG, et al. Measurement of patient outcome in arthritis. *Arthritis Rheum* 1980;23:137–145.
134. Pincus T, Summey JA, Soraci SAJ, et al. Assessment of patient satisfaction in activities of daily living using a modified Stanford Health Assessment Questionnaire. *Arthritis Rheum* 1983;26:1346–1353.
135. Meenan RF, Gertman PM, Mason JH. Measuring health status in arthritis: the Arthritis Impact Measurement scales. *Arthritis Rheum* 1980;23:146–152.
136. Pinals RS, Masi AT, Larsen RA, et al. Preliminary criteria for clinical remission in rheumatoid arthritis. *Arthritis Rheum* 1981;24:1308–1315.
137. O'Sullivan JB, Cathcart ES. The prevalence of rheumatoid arthritis: follow-up evaluation of the effect of criteria on rates in Sudbury, Massachusetts. *Ann Intern Med* 1972;76:573–577.
138. Mikkelsen WM, Dodge HJ, Duff IF, et al. Estimates of the prevalence of rheumatic diseases in the population of Tecumseh, Michigan, 1959–60. *J Chron Dis* 1967;20:351–369.
139. Wolfe F, Hawley DJ. Remission in rheumatoid arthritis. *J Rheumatol* 1985;12:245–252.
140. Eberhardt KB, Rydgren LC, Pettersson H, et al. Early rheumatoid arthritis—onset, course and outcome over 2 years. *Rheumatol Int* 1990;10:135–142.
141. Yelin E, Meenan R, Nevitt M, et al. Work disability in rheumatoid arthritis: effects of disease, social and work factors. *Ann Intern Med* 1980;93:551–556.
142. Wolfe F, Hawley DJ. The longterm outcomes of rheumatoid arthritis: work disability: a prospective 18 year study of 823 patients. *J Rheumatol* 1998;25:2108–2117.
143. Meenan RR, Yelin EH, Henke CJ, et al. The costs of rheumatoid arthritis: a patient oriented study of chronic disease costs. *Arthritis Rheum* 1978;21:827–833.
144. Stone C. The lifetime costs of rheumatoid arthritis. *J Rheumatol* 1984;11:819–827.
145. Fries JF, Williams CA, Morfeld D, et al. Reduction of long-term disability in patients with rheumatoid arthritis by disease-modifying antirheumatic drug-based treatment strategies. *Arthritis Rheum* 1996; 39:616–622.
146. Egsmose C, Lund B, Borg G, et al. Patients with rheumatoid arthritis benefit from early second-line therapy: 5-year follow-up of a prospective double-blind placebo-controlled study. *J Rheumatol* 1995;22:2208–2213.
147. Boers M, Verhoeven AC, Markusse HM, et al. Random comparison of combination step-down prednisolone, methotrexate and sulfasalazine with sulfasalazine alone in early rheumatoid arthritis. *Lancet* 1997;350:309–318.
148. Da Silva E, Doran MF, Crowson CS, et al. Declining use of orthopedic surgery in patients with rheumatoid arthritis? Results of a long-term, population-based assessment. *Arthritis Rheum* 2003;49 (2):216–220.
149. Eberhardt K, Larsson BM, Nived K. Early rheumatoid arthritis—some social, economical and psychological aspects. *Scand J Rheumatol* 1993;22:119–123.
150. Yelin E, Henke C, Epstein W. The work dynamics of the person with rheumatoid arthritis. *Arthritis Rheum* 1987;30:507–512.
151. Reisine ST, Grady KE, Goodenow C, et al. Work disability among women with rheumatoid arthritis: the relative importance of disease, social, work, and family factors. *Arthritis Rheum* 1989;32:538–543.

152. Masi AT, Maldonado-Cocco JA, Kaplan SB, et al. Prospective study of the early course of rheumatoid arthritis in young adults: comparison of patients with and without rheumatoid factor positivity at entry and identification of variables correlating with outcome. *Semin Arthritis Rheum* 1976;5:299–326.
153. Nelson JL, Hughes KA, Smith AG, et al. Maternal-fetal disparity in HLA class II alloantigens and the pregnancy-induced amelioration of rheumatoid arthritis. *N Engl J Med* 1993;329:466–471.
154. Cutolo M, Balleari E, Giusti M, et al. Androgen replacement therapy in male patients with rheumatoid arthritis. *Arthritis Rheum* 1991;34: 1–5.
155. Corrigan AB, Robinson RG, Terenty TR, et al. Benign rheumatoid arthritis of the aged. *BMJ* 1974;1:444–446.
156. Terkeltaub R, Decary R, Esdaile J. An immunogenetic study of older age onset rheumatoid arthritis. *J Rheumatol* 1984;11:147–152.
157. Kavanaugh AF. Rheumatoid arthritis in the elderly: is it a different disease? *Am J Med* 1997;103(suppl):40–48.
158. Pease CT, Bhakta BB, Devlin J, et al. Does the age of onset of rheumatoid arthritis influence phenotype? A prospective study of outcome and prognostic factors. *Rheumatology (Oxford)* 1999;38:228–234.
159. Lance NJ, Curran JJ. Late-onset, seropositive, erosive rheumatoid arthritis. *Semin Arthritis Rheum* 1993;23:177–182.
160. Saag KG, Cerhan JR, Kolluri S, et al. Cigarette smoking and rheumatoid arthritis severity. *Ann Rheum Dis* 1997;56:463–469.
161. Hazes JM, Dijkmans BA, Vandenbrouke JP, et al. Lifestyle and the risk of rheumatoid arthritis: cigarette smoking and alcohol consumption. *Ann Rheum Dis* 1990;49:980–982.
162. Vessey MP, Villard-Mackintosh L, Yeates D. Oral contraceptives, cigarette smoking and other factors in relation to arthritis. *Contraception* 1987;35:457–465.
163. Avila MH, Liang MH, Willett WC, et al. Reproductive factors, smoking, and the risk for rheumatoid arthritis. *Epidemiology* 1990;1:285–291.
164. Heliovaara M, Aho K, Aromaa A, et al. Smoking and risk of rheumatoid arthritis. *J Rheumatol* 1993;20:1830–1835.
165. Voigt LF, Koepsell TD, Nelson JL, et al. Smoking, obesity, alcohol consumption, and the risk of rheumatoid arthritis. *Epidemiology* 1994;5:525–532.
166. Silman AJ, Newman J, MacGregor AJ. Cigarette smoking increases the risk of rheumatoid arthritis: results from a nationwide study of disease-discordant twins. *Arthritis Rheum* 1996;39:732–735.
167. Uhlig T, Hagen KB, Kvien TK. Current tobacco smoking, formal education, and the risk of rheumatoid arthritis. *J Rheumatol* 1996; 26:47–54.
168. Deighton C. Smoke gets in your joints? *Ann Rheum Dis* 1997;56: 453–454.
169. Wilson K, Goldsmith CH. Does smoking cause rheumatoid arthritis? *J Rheumatol* 1999;26:1–3.
170. Luukkainen R, Isomaki H, Kajander A. Prognostic value of the type of onset of rheumatoid arthritis. *Ann Rheum Dis* 1983;42:274–275.
171. Russell EB, Hunter JB, Pearson L, et al. Remitting, seronegative, symmetrical synovitis with pitting edema—13 additional cases. *J Rheumatol* 1990;17:633–639.
172. Feigenbaum SL, Masi AT, Kaplan SB. Prognosis in rheumatoid arthritis: a longitudinal study of newly diagnosed younger adult patients. *Am J Med* 1979;66:377–384.
173. Fleming A, Crown JM, Corbett M. Prognostic value of early features in rheumatoid disease. *BMJ* 1976;1:1243–1245.
174. Callahan LF, Pincus T. Formal education level as a significant marker of clinical status in rheumatoid arthritis. *Arthritis Rheum* 1988;31:1346–1357.
175. Pincus T, Brooks RH, Callahan LF. Prediction of long-term mortality in patients with rheumatoid arthritis according to simple questionnaire and joint count measures. *Ann Intern Med* 1994;120:26–34.
176. Adler NE, Boyce WT, Chesney MA, et al. Socioeconomic inequalities in health: no easy solution. *JAMA* 1993;269:3140–3145.
177. Michelson J, Easley M, Wigley FM, et al. Foot and ankle problems in rheumatoid arthritis. *Foot Ankle Int* 1994;15:608–613.
178. Roberts WN, Daltroy LH, Anderson RJ. Stability of normal joint findings in persistent classic rheumatoid arthritis. *Arthritis Rheum* 1988;31:267–271.
179. Callahan LF, Bloch DA, Pincus T. Identification of work disability in rheumatoid arthritis: physical, radiographic and laboratory variables do not add explanatory power to demographic and functional variables. *J Clin Epidemiol* 1992;45:127–138.
180. Fuchs HA, Cow JJ, Callahan LF, et al. Evidence of significant radiographic damage in rheumatoid arthritis within the first 2 years of disease. *J Rheumatol* 1989;16:585–591.
181. van der Heijde DMFM, van Riel PLCM, van Leeuwen MA, et al. Prognostic factors for radiographic damage and physical disability in early rheumatoid arthritis. A prospective follow-up of 147 patients. *Br J Rheumatol* 1992;31:519–525.
182. Kaarela K. Prognostic factors and diagnostic criteria in early rheumatoid arthritis. *Scand J Rheumatol* 1991;57(suppl):1–54.
183. Dawes PT, Fowler PD, Clarke S, et al. Rheumatoid arthritis: treatment which controls the C-reactive protein and erythrocyte sedimentation rate reduces radiological progression. *Br J Rheumatol* 1986;25:44–49.
184. Young A, Corbett M, Winfield J, et al. A prognostic index for erosive changes in the hands, feet and cervical spine in early rheumatoid arthritis. *Br J Rheumatol* 1988;27:94–101.
185. Ingeman-Nielson M, Halskov O, Hanses TM, et al. Clinical synovitis and radiological lesions in rheumatoid arthritis. *Scand J Rheumatol* 1983;12:237–240.
186. Amos RS, Constable TJ, Crockson RA, et al. Rheumatoid arthritis: relation of serum C-reactive protein and erythrocyte sedimentation rates to radiographic changes. *BMJ* 1977;1:195–197.
187. Stockman A, Emery P, Doyle T, et al. Relationship of progression of radiographic changes in hands and wrists, clinical features and HLA-DR antigens in rheumatoid arthritis. *J Rheumatol* 1991;18:1001–1007.
188. Caruso I, Santandrea S, Puttini PS, et al. Clinical, laboratory and radiographic features in early rheumatoid arthritis. *J Rheumatol* 1990; 17:1263–1267.
189. Luukkainen R, Kaarela K, Isomaki H, et al. The prediction of radiological destruction during the early stage of rheumatoid arthritis. *Clin Exp Rheumatol* 1983;1:295–298.
190. Young A, Jarquemada D, Awad J, et al. Association of HLA-DR4/Dw4 and DR2/Dw2 with radiologic changes in a prospective study of patients with rheumatoid arthritis: preferential relationship with HLA-Dw rather than HLA-DR specificities. *Arthritis Rheum* 1984; 27:20–25.
191. Wolfe F, Mitchell DM, Sibley JT, et al. The mortality of rheumatoid arthritis. *Arthritis Rheum* 1994;37:481–494.
192. Pincus T, Callahan LF. Taking mortality in rheumatoid arthritis seriously-predictive markers, socioeconomic status and comorbidity [Editorial]. *J Rheumatol* 1987;14:240–251.
193. Choi HK, Hernan MA, Seeger JD, et al. Methotrexate and mortality in patients with rheumatoid arthritis: a prospective study. *Lancet* 2002;359:1173–1177.
194. Chan KA, Felson DT, Yood RA, et al. The lag time between onset of symptoms and diagnosis of rheumatoid arthritis. *Arthritis Rheum* 1994;37:814–820.
195. Wolfe F, Ross K, Hawley DJ, et al. The prognosis of rheumatoid arthritis and undifferentiated polyarthritis syndrome in the clinic: a study of 1141 patients. *J Rheumatol* 1993;20:2005–2009.
196. Andonopoulos AP, Siambi V, Makri M, et al. Thyroid function and immune profile in rheumatoid arthritis: a controlled study. *Clin Rheumatol* 1996;15:599–603.
197. Shiroky JB, Cohen M, Ballachey ML, et al. Thyroid dysfunction in rheumatoid arthritis: a controlled prospective study. *Ann Rheum Dis* 1993;52:454–456.
198. Bywaters EGL. Still's disease in the adult. *Ann Rheum Dis* 1974;30: 121–132.
199. Yamaguchi M, Ohta A, Tsunematsu T, et al. Preliminary criteria for classification of adult Still's disease. *J Rheumatol* 1992;19:424–430.
200. Ohta A, Yamaguchi M, Kaneoka H, et al. Adult Still's disease: review of 228 cases from the literature. *J Rheumatol* 1987;14:1139–1146.
201. Gonzalez-Hernandez T, Martin-Mola E, Fernandez-Zamorano A, et al. Serum ferritin can be useful for diagnosis in adult onset Still's disease. *J Rheumatol* 1989;16:412–413.
202. Schwarz-Eywill M, Heilig B, Bauer H, et al. Evaluation of serum ferritin as a marker for adult Still's disease activity. *Ann Rheum Dis* 1992;51:683–685.
203. Hench PS, Rosenberg EF. Palindromic rheumatism. *Arch Intern Med* 1944;73:293–321.
204. Guerne P-A, Weisman MH. Palindromic rheumatism: part of or apart from the spectrum of rheumatoid arthritis. *Am J Med* 1992;93:451–460.

205. Gonzalez-Lopez L, Gamez-Nava JI, Jhangri GS, et al. Prognostic factors for the development of rheumatoid arthritis and other connective tissue diseases in patients with palindromic rheumatism. *J Rheumatol* 1999;26:540–545.
206. Hannonen P, Mottonen T, Oka M. Palindromic rheumatism: a clinical survey of sixty patients. *Scand J Rheumatol* 1987;16:413–420.
207. Williams MH, Sheldon PJHS, Torrigiani G, et al. Palindromic rheumatism: clinical and immunological studies. *Ann Rheum Dis* 1971; 30:375–380.
208. McCarty DJ, O'Duffy JD, Pearson L, et al. Remitting seronegative symmetrical synovitis with pitting edema. RS3PE syndrome. *JAMA* 1985;254:2763–2767.
209. Sibilia J, Friess S, Schaeverbeke T, et al. Remitting seronegative symmetrical synovitis with pitting edema (RS3PE): a form of paraneoplastic polyarthritis? *J Rheumatol* 1999;26:115–120.
210. Cantini F, Salvarani C, Olivieri I, et al. Remitting seronegative symmetrical synovitis with pitting oedema (RS3PE) syndrome: a prospective follow-up and magnetic resonance imaging study. *Ann Rheum Dis* 1999;58:230–236.
211. Pariser KM, Canoso JJ. Remitting, seronegative (a)symmetrical synovitis with pitting edema—two cases of RS3PE. *J Rheumatol* 1991; 18:1260–1262.
212. O'Duffy JD, Hunder GG, Wahner HW. A follow-up study of polymyalgia rheumatica: evidence of chronic axial synovitis. *J Rheumatol* 1980;7:685–693.
213. Koski JM. Ultrasonographic evidence of synovitis in axial joints in patients with polymyalgia rheumatica. *Br J Rheumatol* 1992;31:201–203.
214. Behn AR, Perera T, Myles AB. Polymyalgia rheumatica and corticosteroids: how much for how long? Ann Rheum Dis 1983;42:374–378.
215. Ayoub WT, Franklin CM, Torretti D. Polymyalgia rheumatica: duration of therapy and long-term outcome. *Am J Med* 1985;79:309–315.
216. Kyle V, Hazelman BL. Stopping steroids in polymyalgia rheumatica and giant cell arteritis. *BMJ* 1990;300:344–345.
217. Hunder G. Immunogenetics and polymyalgia rheumatica. *Br J Rheumatol* 1990;29:321–324.
218. Healey LA. Polymyalgia rheumatica and seronegative rheumatoid arthritis may be the same entity. *J Rheumatol* 1992;19:270–272.
219. Robbins DL, White RH. Interrelationships between polymyalgia rheumatica and polyarthritis. *J Rheumatol* 1988;15:1323–1325.
220. Sakkas LI, Loqueman N, Panayi GS, et al. Immunogenetics of polymyalgia rheumatica. *Br J Rheumatol* 1990;29:331–334.
221. Weyand CM, Hunder NNH, Hicok KC, et al. HLA-DRB1 alleles in polymyalgia rheumatica, giant cell arteritis, and rheumatoid arthritis. Arthritis Rheum 1994;37:514–520.
222. Panush RS, Edwards NL, Longley S, et al. "Rhupus" syndrome. *Arch Intern Med* 1988;148:1633–1636.
223. Fischman AS, Abeles M, Zanetti M, et al. The coexistence of rheumatoid arthritis and systemic lupus erythematosus: a case report and review of the literature. *J Rheumatol* 1981;8:405–415.
224. Brand CA, Rowley VJ, Tait BD, et al. Coexistent rheumatoid arthritis and systemic lupus erythematosus: clinical, serological, and phenotypic features. *Ann Rheum Dis* 1992;51:173–176.
225. Siam AR, Hammoudeh M. Sulfasalazine induced systemic lupus erythematosus in a patient with rheumatoid arthritis. *J Rheumatol* 1993; 20:207.
226. Chalmers A, Thompson D, Stein HE, et al. Systemic lupus erythematosus during penicillamine therapy for rheumatoid arthritis. *Ann Intern Med* 1982;97:659–663.
227. Tingle AJ, Allen M, Petty RE, et al. Rubella-associated arthritis. I: Comparative study of joint manifestations associated with natural rubella infection and RA27/3 rubella immunization. *Ann Rheum Dis* 1986;45:110–114.
228. Miki NPH, Chantler JK. Differential ability of wild-type and vaccine strains of rubella virus to replicate and persist in human joint tissue. *Clin Exp Rheumatol* 1992;10:3–12.
229. Mitchell LA, Tingle AJ, Shukin R, et al. Chronic rubella vaccine-associated arthropathy. *Arch Intern Med* 1993;153:2268–2274.
230. Torok TJ. Parvovirus B19 and human disease. *Adv Intern Med* 1992;37:431–455.
231. White DG, Woolf AD, Mortimer PP, et al. Human parvovirus arthropathy. *Lancet* 1989;1:419–421.
232. Reid DM, Reid TMS, Brown T, et al. Human parvovirus-associated arthritis: a clinical and laboratory description. *Lancet* 1985;1:422–425.
233. Naides SJ, Scharosch LL, Foto F, et al. Rheumatologic manifestations of human parvovirus B19 infection in adults: initial two-year clinical experience. *Arthritis Rheum* 1990;33:1297–1309.
234. Rivera J, Garcia-Monforte A, Pineda A, et al. Arthritis in patients with chronic hepatitis C virus infection. *J Rheumatol* 1999;26:420–424.
235. Wolfe F, Cathey MA, Kleinheksel SM. Fibrositis (fibromyalgia) in rheumatoid arthritis. *J Rheumatol* 1984;11:814 818.
236. Walker DJ, Pound JD, Griffiths ID, et al. Rheumatoid factor tests in the diagnosis and prediction of rheumatoid arthritis. *Ann Rheum Dis* 1986;45:684–690.
237. Del Puente A, Knowler WC, Pettitt DJ, et al. The incidence of rheumatoid arthritis is predicted by rheumatoid factor titer in a longitudinal population study. *Arthritis Rheum* 1988;31:1239–1244.

CHAPTER 56

Extraarticular Manifestations of Rheumatoid Arthritis

Fraser N. Birrell and John D. Isaacs

Although the prevalence of rheumatoid arthritis (RA) may be declining (1), extraarticular disease (EAD) remains common, with nodules affecting 15% to 40% of Western (2,3) and 2% to 10% of Asian RA patients (4–6). Despite the perception that severe EA manifestations are becoming rarer in RA, 8% of a recent Swedish case series (7) developed severe EAD over a 10-year follow-up period. Longer-term data from the Mayo Clinic (since 1955; median 15-year follow-up) indicated that 38% of patients with RA (169 of 424) had nodules and that 15% of patients (63 of 424) with severe EAD had an increased risk for mortality (8). Thus, EAD remains common, is associated with severe RA, and is predictive of morbidity and mortality (9). Although treatment of RA is improving, EAD is likely determined by genetic predisposition and will therefore continue to be observed.

The pathogenesis of EAD in RA is not well understood. A recent cytokine profiling study has produced convincing evidence that the rheumatoid nodule is a helper T cell subset 1 (T_H1) granuloma (10). Furthermore, the finding of FcγRIIIa (CD16) expression at sites prone to EAD and on pallisading histiocytes within rheumatoid nodules (11) suggests a role for local tumor necrosis factor-α (TNF-α) and interleukin-1 (IL-1) production from infiltrating mononuclear cells, perhaps as a consequence of immune complex binding. Consistent with this hypothesis, a recent small case control study found the presence of antinuclear antibodies and rheumatoid nodules to be the only significant predictors of other extraarticular manifestations (12), suggesting humoral factors to be important.

Although long recognized as a systemic condition, the importance of inflammation in driving the atherosclerotic disease process has only recently become an area of research interest. This is of considerable interest to academicians as an elegant example of the convergence of ideas and value of interdisciplinary collaboration in addressing major causes of population morbidity and mortality. However, its relevance is equally great to the practicing rheumatologist, who must recognize that patients with long-standing RA are likely to die prematurely from atherosclerotic disease. Thus, other cardiovascular risk factors should be assessed and treated appropriately. Although observational, the recent finding of improved cardiovascular mortality rates in those treated with disease-modifying drugs such as methotrexate (13) further supports current strategies for aggressive control of inflammation.

SYSTEMIC FEATURES

The systemic features of RA can be divided into early and late manifestations. Early features include nodules, anorexia, and weight loss; less frequently, lymphadenopathy or fever can occur.

Rheumatoid Nodules

Nodules have a firm, rubbery consistency and characteristically occur subcutaneously on extensor surfaces over the elbows or other bony prominences (Fig. 56.1). However, they may occur in any organ or tissue layer. They must be distinguished from gouty tophi, xanthomata, and lipomata. Like other EA manifestations, rheumatoid nodules are strongly associated with seropositivity for rheumatoid factor, but other influences must operate, because the prevalence of nodules is at most half that of seropositivity. A recent study found that seropositivity, smoking, and human leukocyte antigen (HLA) DRB1*0401 were the only factors independently associated with nodules (14). The effect of treatment on nodules is not certain. Indeed, numerous case reports (15,16) and short series have suggested methotrexate therapy may be accompanied by the onset or worsening of

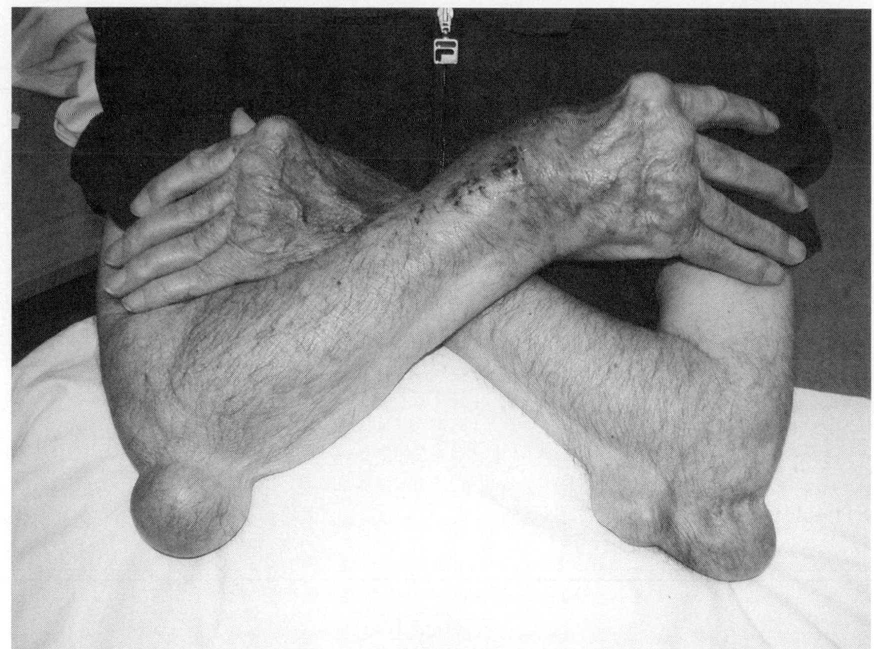

FIG. 56.1. Severe rheumatoid nodules over extensor surfaces of the arms of a patient with rheumatoid arthritis.

nodulosis. However, a recent review concluded that the evidence was poor for causality in the 58 reported cases (17). Case reports linking other drugs, including etanercept (18), to the development of nodules have also appeared.

Amyloidosis

An important late systemic manifestation of RA is secondary Amyloid A amyloidosis. Amyloid deposition occurs in many organs, including kidneys, intestines, liver, spleen, and heart. It is also a rare cause of carpal tunnel syndrome. Deposits form following persistent elevation of serum amyloid A, one of the acute-phase reactants. Diagnosis is confirmed by biopsy of involved tissue, typically a deep rectal or renal biopsy. Congo red stain reveals typical amorphous pink staining with apple-green birefringence under polarized light. The presence and extent of systemic amyloid deposition can be revealed using serum amyloid P component radiolabeled with iodine 131 or iodine 123 (19), although this technique is only available in highly specialized centers. Improved control of inflammation with more aggressive disease-modifying antirheumatic drug (DMARD) regimens and availability of anti-TNF therapies for refractory disease should reduce the incidence of amyloidosis. A recent study has demonstrated regression of amyloidosis following treatment with infliximab (20).

Vasculitis

The incidence of clinically evident systemic rheumatoid vasculitis is around 12.5 per million population per annum (21). It most commonly affects the skin: splinter hemorrhages, periungual infarcts, digital necrosis, or sharply demarcated, painful ulceration may all occur (Figs. 56.2 and 56.3). Isolated splinter hemorrhages are often found in patients with nodular disease without other vasculitic phenomena and do not require specific therapy. Vasculitis has been shown to be associated with high rheumatoid factor and antinuclear antibody (ANA) titers (22), male gender, erosions and other EAD (23). A more recent case control study concluded that the three clinical predictors of rheumatoid vasculitis were peripheral neuropathy, purpura/petechiae, and other EAD (24). In this study the only diagnostically useful laboratory markers were the presence of IgA rheumatoid factor and low C3 complement component. Cryoglobulins should be considered in the investigation of rheumatoid-associated vasculitis, particularly in the presence of Raynaud phenomenon or livedo reticularis.

Apart from the skin, rheumatoid vasculitis frequently affects the peripheral nerves, with either mononeuritis multiplex (in 10%) or a symmetric peripheral neuropathy (in 45%) (25), although reports of muscle (26), brain (27), aorta (28), and intraabdominal involvement (29) demonstrate that ischemia of any end organ, including large vessel disease, may also occur. A postmortem study showed that 30% of RA patients had systemic angiitis, irrespective of the cause of death (30).

Intriguingly, drug-induced vasculitis in RA patients has been reported in association with one of the drugs linked to nodulosis, etanercept (31–33), as well as infliximab (34) and leflunomide (35). This provides indirect evidence for multiple pathogenetic mechanisms in RA: a TNF-α-dependent

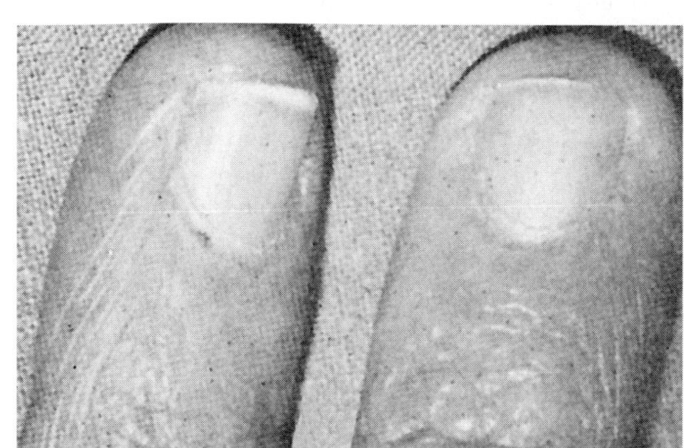

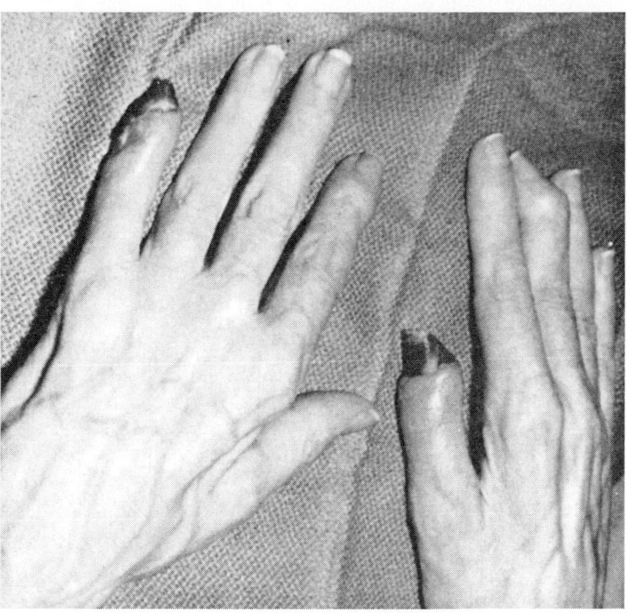

FIG. 56.2. Rheumatoid vasculitis. **A:** Patient with rheumatoid arthritis and systemic vasculitis showing periungual infacts. **B:** Same patient as in **A** with gangrene of the fingers as a result of digital vasculitis.

pathway, leading to synovitis and erosions, and an alternative pathway exacerbated by TNF-α blockade, contributing to EAD, including nodules and vasculitis. These reports also attest to the dual immunoregulatory roles of TNF-α, which can act in both pro- and antiinflammatory fashions (36).

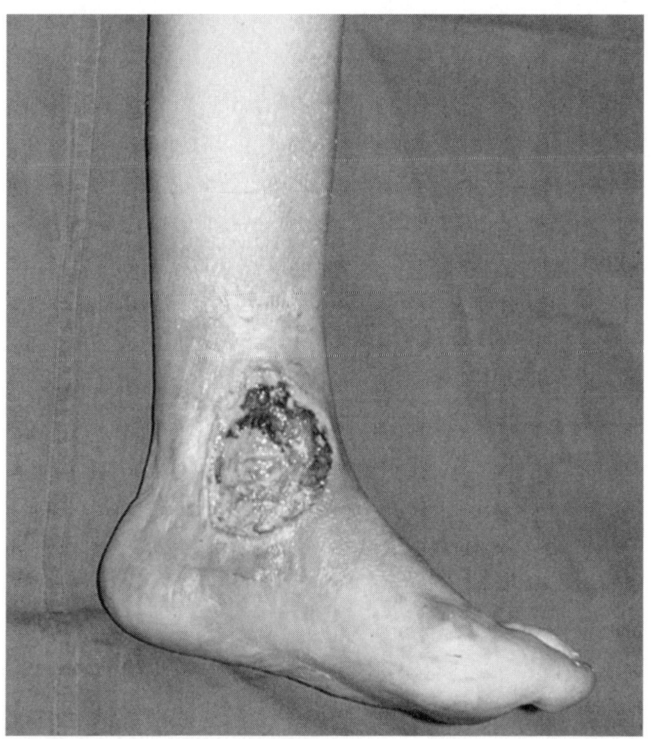

FIG. 56.3. Vasculitic leg ulcer in a patient with rheumatoid arthritis.

Hematologic

RA can affect any of the three main blood cell lineages: erythrocytes, leukocytes, and platelets.

Erythrocytes

Anemia is a common EA manifestation of RA. The prevalence depends on the duration, severity, and activity of the disease. In an early study, approximately 30% of patients with RA were observed to be anemic (37); however, because anemia correlates closely with disease activity, the prevalence depends on the patient population under study. There are several recognized patterns of anemia in RA (38):

1. Normocytic and normochromic; this is the most common pattern and strongly suggests the anemia of chronic disease (although this may also be microcytic and hypochromic). Typical laboratory findings include low serum iron levels and iron-binding capacity with a low or normal saturation. Ferritin levels are relatively high, and erythropoietin levels are low (39). The underlying mechanism is poor iron utilization from stores in the reticuloendothelial system. Increased production of proinflammatory cytokines in the bone marrow contributes to this ineffective erythropoiesis (40–43), and the anemia responds to effective medical therapy of RA. Some patients have been successfully treated with erythropoietin prior to collection of autologous blood for intraoperative replacement prior to joint replacement surgery (44,45).
2. Microcytic hypochromic, suggesting iron deficiency. In contrast to the anemia of chronic disease, serum iron levels are low, with a compensatory increase in iron binding

leading to low saturation. Erythropoietin levels are high. Low ferritin levels are strongly predictive of iron deficiency, but, as an acute-phase protein, normal or high levels can mask low iron stores in RA (39). The most common underlying cause is chronic blood loss as a result of long-term use of nonsteroidal antiinflammatory drugs (NSAIDs), although the increasing use of gastroprotective agents and cycooxygenase-2 inhibitors should reduce the incidence. Gastrointestinal malignancy must be considered in the approach to patients with chronic gastrointestinal blood loss.

3. Macrocytic, suggesting folate deficiency. The use of prophylactic folic acid in conjunction with methotrexate has reduced, but not entirely eliminated, the occurrence of macrocytic anemia. Dietary folate deficiency, alcohol consumption, or hypothyroidism should be considered if the patient is not taking methotrexate. Frank megaloblastosis is rare, and would suggest coexistent vitamin B_{12} deficiency from pernicious anemia.

4. Aplastic: usually associated with drugs, particularly gold, and reported with methotrexate and leflunomide, especially in combination with (46) or without infliximab (47). There are also reports of aplasia associated with viral infection in RA (48).

5. Hemolytic anemia has been reported (49), but is rare.

Different forms of anemia may coexist, particularly iron deficiency and the anemia of chronic disease (50).

Leukocytes

Leukocyte cell counts are normal in most RA patients, but approximately 1% of patients with RA develop leukopenia and splenomegaly. This triad, designated Felty syndrome, was described in 1924 in five patients (51). In addition, there may be variable reduction of other marrow lineages. Felty's syndrome generally occurs in the setting of severe arthritis, although synovitis may be inactive. There is an increased susceptibility to infections, particularly in association with ulceration of the lower extremities. Weight loss is common (52). Felty's syndrome is associated with high titers of rheumatoid factor and positivity for antinuclear antibodies, and patients are generally HLA-DR4 positive (53). It is rare in African-American patients (54). The mechanisms underlying neutropenia in Felty's syndrome have been elusive, but include increased destruction (55), increased margination (56), increased endocytosis of immune complexes (57), antineutrophil antibodies (58), decreased granulopoiesis (59), and immune-mediated bone marrow suppression (60,61). The management of Felty's syndrome is that of the underlying RA (62–66), although the potential association of most DMARDs with neutropenia can complicate monitoring (38). Granulocyte-macrophage colony-stimulating factor (GM-CSF) (67) and G-CSF (68) have been used for severe neutropenia, particularly in association with infection, but the occurrence of side effects, including flare-ups of arthritis and new leukocytoclastic vasculitis, is of concern. Recent results suggest that G-CSF should be administered at the lowest dose needed to elevate the neutrophil count above 1,000/μL (69). Flare-ups of arthritis with improvement in neutropenia have been observed in other settings (70) and argue for the importance of granulocytes in RA synovitis. Spontaneous remission in Felty syndrome has been observed, but is rare (71). Splenectomy improves the leukopenia, but the results are generally short lived, and splenectomy is best avoided unless a life-threatening situation exists (72).

A syndrome of clonal or polyclonal large granular lymphocyte (LGL) expansion associated with neutropenia and RA has been described (73,74); the clinical behavior can be either extremely benign or frankly malignant (38). These patients have associated splenomegaly and increased susceptibility to infections. In a typical population of patients with LGL expansion, about 26% of the patients had associated RA (75). Conversely, in a study of patients with presumed Felty syndrome, 19% had LGL expansion (76). In LGL leukemia, soluble Fas ligand appears to induce apoptosis of neutrophils (69). In contrast, recent evidence suggests that blockade of Fas signaling by soluble Fas may lead to apoptosis resistance of leukemic LGLs themselves (77).

Lymphopenia suggests coexistent pathology such as lupus overlap or human immunodeficiency virus infection, although drug-induced lymphopenia should also be considered (e.g., methotrexate) (78). Occasional cases of eosinophilia have been reported (79–81), associated with severe disease activity and EA features, but the significance is uncertain; a drug reaction should always be considered (82).

Platelets

Thrombocytosis is associated with active disease, as a manifestation of the acute-phase response. Complications from thrombocytosis are rare in RA (83). Thrombocytopenia is usually drug induced (84), but purpura is more commonly iatrogenic and related to corticosteroid use.

Immunodeficiency and Infection

The predisposition of patients with RA to infection has long been recognized (85); this includes susceptibility to atypical infections (86) and tumors associated with infection, such as Kaposi sarcoma (87), caused by Kaposi sarcoma–associated herpes virus infection (88). Immunodeficiency in RA is also manifested by susceptibility to tumors of the immune system such as myeloma and mucosal-associated lymphoid tissue lymphoma (38). Immunodeficiency probably reflects three contributing factors: immunosuppressive drugs; the effect of chronic disease, including malnutrition; and disease-specific factors. With regard to the latter, T cells from patients with RA are hypoproliferative and exhibit dysregulated signaling (89–92). The hypoproliferation is reversed by TNF-α blockade (93), and recent research has demonstrated that chronic exposure to TNF-α suppresses T-cell signaling, uncoupling T-cell receptor signal transduction pathways by impairing the assembly and stability of the T-cell receptor–

CD3 complex at the cell surface (94,95). Additionally, other abnormalities in RA suggest premature aging of the immune system. These include abnormal clonal expansions and a distorted T-cell repertoire consistent with dysregulated proliferation and maturation of lymphocytes (96–100).

Cardiovascular

Although the excess mortality associated with RA has been recognized for at least two decades (101), the appreciation of cardiovascular risk is more recent (102). This association is significant, however, within large population-based studies, such as the Nurses' Health Study (103), confirming that the relative risk for myocardial infarction in women with RA is twice that of women without RA; women who have RA for at least 10 years have three times the risk for myocardial infarction. The mechanisms involved are not well understood (104), but there are associations between C-reactive protein (CRP) levels and cardiovascular outcome for both acute coronary syndromes (105) and long-term risk for cardiovascular (106,107) and cerebrovascular disease (108,109), independent of lipid levels (110). In a Dutch study (111), the influence of CRP on progression of atherosclerosis, as assessed by ultrasonography, was as high as that associated with the traditional cardiovascular risk factors of elevated cholesterol, hypertension, and smoking. Intriguingly, use of a statin in high-risk individuals both reduces CRP levels (112) and the association of cardiovascular risk with inflammatory markers (113). These findings suggest that RA is one of a number of drivers of inflammation that lead to a nonspecific increase in vascular risk. Therapy should therefore be directed at both the underlying inflammation and other cardiovascular risk factors in patients with RA.

Other effects of RA on the heart are less important. Although investigations have indicated frequent minor abnormalities, clinical significance is rare (114). These include pericardial, myocardial, and endocardial disease.

Pericarditis

Autopsy studies reveal up to 30% of patients with RA have pericarditis, although an echocardiographic study has suggested the proportion affected may be as high as 50%. However, only 3% present with clinical symptoms (115). Small effusions may be detected incidentally (116) and do not require treatment, but clinicians should be alert to the possibility of pericardial tamponade and constrictive pericarditis (116–118), which require prompt intervention. Patients with pericardial disease have reduced survival compared with the general population, but have not been compared to other RA populations (116).

Myocarditis

Bonfiglio and Atwater (119), in an autopsy study of RA, observed that nonspecific myocardial inflammation occurred in 7 of 47 patients. These findings were confirmed by Cruickshank (120), Gowans (121), and others (115). Rheumatoid nodules of varying sizes may also occur, and these, or myocardial fibrosis, can lead to conduction abnormalities (119, 122,123). However, frank cardiac failure in RA patients is not likely to be a consequence of atherosclerotic disease.

Endocarditis

Baggenstross and Rosenberg (124) first described necrotizing granulomata similar to rheumatoid nodules in the aortic and mitral valves, which was confirmed by others (125). These may be asymptomatic or lead to valvular dysfunction (125–127).

Coronary Vasculitis

Vasculitis of the coronary vessels is rare and occurs in the setting of systemic vasculitis. It may be asymptomatic, but rare cases of associated myocardial infarction have been reported (128).

Respiratory

Lung involvement in RA is probably underrecognized. Pleural involvement is common (50% postmortem), but chest radiography is insensitive to early changes. An Italian study performed high-resolution computed tomography (HRCT) scans on 72 lifelong nonsmoking patients with RA without symptoms or signs of pulmonary disease and mean disease duration of 7 years (129). Abnormalities were found in 30% of the patients assessed via HRCT, compared with 10% assessed via plain radiography. These findings included irregular pleural margins (14%); septal/subpleural lines (18%) (both compatible with pulmonary fibrosis); ground-glass opacities (8%); pulmonary nodules (predominantly subpleural, 8%); bronchiectasis/bronchioloectasis (15.2%); and subpleural cysts (3%). No patient in this small, selected group had evidence of honeycombing fibrosis on HRCT.

The key clinical aspects of rheumatoid lung disease are interstitial disease and pleural effusion. For interstitial disease, excluding drug involvement is important, because methotrex ate, gold, and D-penicillamine can induce pneumonitis. The RA patient presenting with a pleural effusion can also present a diagnostic problem, and pleural aspiration is often required to distinguish between the exudates of a rheumatoid effusion (with rheumatoid factor positivity, a high lactate dehydrogenase level, and reduced glucose and complement levels), pleuritis associated with underlying infection (rheumatoid factor negative, normal complement), or a transudate from cardiac failure or nephrosis. With the decline of the mining industry, the syndrome of miners with pneumoconiosis developing massive multiple nodules with progressive massive fibrosis originally described by Caplan (130) is now uncommon.

The understanding of lung disease in RA has been hampered by confusing classifications with the use of terms not generally understood by nonspecialists. With respect to interstitial pneumonias, confusion has arisen about the relationship of the previous imprecise term *idiopathic pulmonary fibrosis* (IPF) to the new nomenclature *idiopathic interstitial pneumonias* (IIP) and *usual interstitial pneumonia* (UIP), based on defined histologic features. This is best viewed from the perspective of the severe UIP category, which has median survival of 3 years—UIP is a subset of IIP, itself a subset of IPF (131).

Although UIP is the predominant histologic subtype found with RA, it is not clear that these patients have the same prognosis as those with truly idiopathic UIP, although a prospective study of 29 patients with RA and HRCT-diagnosed alveolitis followed for 2 years found that 4 (14%) died from respiratory failure (132), suggesting a similarly poor prognosis as idiopathic UIP. In this cohort, one third progressed—the only independent predictor of progression was diffusion capacity, with a cut-off of less than 54% of predicted total lung carbon monoxide diffusion suggested as a threshold predicting progression (sensitivity 80%; specificity 93%).

Bronchiolitis obliterans with organized pneumonia has been described in RA patients, but is rare. The clinical features are not specific; histology reveals proliferative bronchiolitis in the airway and organizing pneumonia in the alveoli (133).

Renal

Currently, mesangial glomerulonephritis is the most frequent biopsy finding in RA patients presenting with renal disease (134), although drug-induced disease is common, secondary to both NSAIDs and DMARDs. Glomerulonephritis and interstitial renal disease are uncommon in the absence of vasculitis, although an early postmortem study of 132 patients found that 90% had nephrosclerosis, 14% systemic vasculitis, 11% amyloidosis, and 8% each had membranous or focal glomerular disease; 23% had evidence of renal impairment prior to death (135).

Gastrointestinal

Clinical involvement of the gastrointestinal tract in RA is unusual aside from the complications of therapy (see Chapter 55). Mild abnormalities in liver function tests are frequently seen, especially alkaline phosphatase, but these are usually transient, and pathology reveals minimal nonspecific changes, in the absence of coexistent liver pathology, such as infection or autoimmune hepatitis (136).

Other gut pathology is rare: an association of Crohn's disease with RA has been reported, but the low coincidence of the two disorders suggests this was a chance finding (137). Involvement of the mesenteric arteries with small bowel infarction is a rare complication of RA vasculitis (138).

Neurologic

Both peripheral and central neurologic consequences are observed in RA. Peripheral nervous system involvement in RA includes compression neuropathies: carpal tunnel syndrome, ulnar nerve entrapment at the elbow, and tarsal tunnel syndrome. There is no controlled evidence for treatment of these compression syndromes in RA. Conservative therapy with corticosteroid injection or splinting appears effective in the short term for idiopathic carpal tunnel syndrome (139), but surgery gives better long-term results (140).

Other peripheral manifestations are rarer and include sensory or sensorimotor peripheral neuropathy and mononeuritis multiplex as a consequence of vasculitis of the vasa nervorum. Autonomic neuropathy in RA has been reported, and subclinical forms may be more common than previously recognized (141), but the significance of this finding is unclear.

Cervical myelopathy from atlantoaxial subluxation or pannus is a further compressive phenomenon, similar to peripheral nerve syndromes. There is a high prevalence in patients with long-standing, severe disease. A Finnish series of 147 RA patients with amyloidosis showed atlantoaxial impaction in 52% and atlantoaxial subluxation in 40% (142). Instability may be detected with greater sensitivity by plain flexion-extension radiographs than by magnetic resonance imaging alone (143), suggesting that radiography should precede more sophisticated imaging. The latter is required to assess pannus volume and cord compression, however. The brain can be affected by systemic vasculitis, as mentioned above (27).

Psychiatric

Depression is common in RA, affecting 40% of patients in a recent case series (144). A Finnish study showed that female suicides are overrepresented in RA sufferers and that 50% had made a previous attempt, suggesting there is a window of opportunity for treatment (145). There is cross-sectional evidence that much of the effect of pain on cognition is mediated through depression (146). This is one example of progress toward a more holistic approach to the impact of RA, using a biopsychosocial model for assessment and treatment, which will require rigorous appraisal (147).

Bone

In addition to erosive disease, RA has more generalized effects on the skeleton. Bone density is decreased at both periarticular and distant skeletal sites and correlates with disease activity (148), leading to secondary osteoporosis in a proportion of patients.

A recently described cytokine system, including receptor activator of nuclear factor κB ligand (RANKL), its cellular receptor, receptor activator of nuclear factor κB (RANK), and the decoy receptor osteoprotegerin (OPG) has been implicated in this bone loss. Activated $CD4^+$ T cells and synovial fibroblasts derived from RA synovium express RANKL, which is an important factor in osteoclast formation, fusion, activation, and survival (149). Other proinflammatory mediators, including TNF-α, likely also contribute to osteoporosis in RA, which may be modulated by vitamin D (150). Vitamin D receptor genotype was shown to be predictive of severity of bone loss in women with RA (151). A recent study of monocytes from RA patients and controls confirmed increased osteoclast activity in RA, but did not demonstrate enhanced sensitivity to RANKL, 1,25 hydroxy vitamin D_3, or inflammatory cytokines (152).

Bone infection and avascular necrosis may also complicate RA. There is a paucity of controlled evidence for the factors predictive of avascular necrosis, but case reports and a small, uncontrolled, prospective study implicate steroids as the likely cause (153).

Eye

Eye involvement in RA is common, with keratoconjunctivitis sicca, or dry eyes (xerophthalmia), the most frequent complication. Secondary Sjögren syndrome is the usual cause, affecting up to one third of patients and often associated with a dry mouth (xerostomia), and vaginal dryness, leading to dyspareunia. The diagnosis is supported by a positive Schirmer test result, reduced salivary flow rate, and/or minor salivary gland biopsy results. The latter may reveal a lymphocytic infiltrate, with destruction of the glandular tissue. Drugs are another common cause of dry eyes in patients (154) and should always be considered, especially in patients over the age of 55 years (155). Treatment with artificial tears is usually appropriate; salivary substitutes are less commonly used by patients, who prefer to sip water regularly.

Episcleritis, inflammation of the layer superficial to the sclera, occurs in less than 1% of patients with RA and is a benign, self-limiting condition. It presents with focal dusky redness and irritation of the eye. There may be nodular or diffuse injection of the episcleral vessels. The diagnosis may be confirmed by blanching that occurs following the application of phenylephrine drops. Scleritis is a more aggressive process, characterized by an intensely painful inflammation of the sclera itself. The pattern may be diffuse or nodular but, unlike episcleritis, scleral necrosis and thinning may occur, revealing the blue-black underlying choroid and carrying a risk for perforation. By contrast, in scleromalacia perforans the thinning is often painless and the injection minimal. In severe cases, perforation of the sclera may still occur (Fig. 56.4).

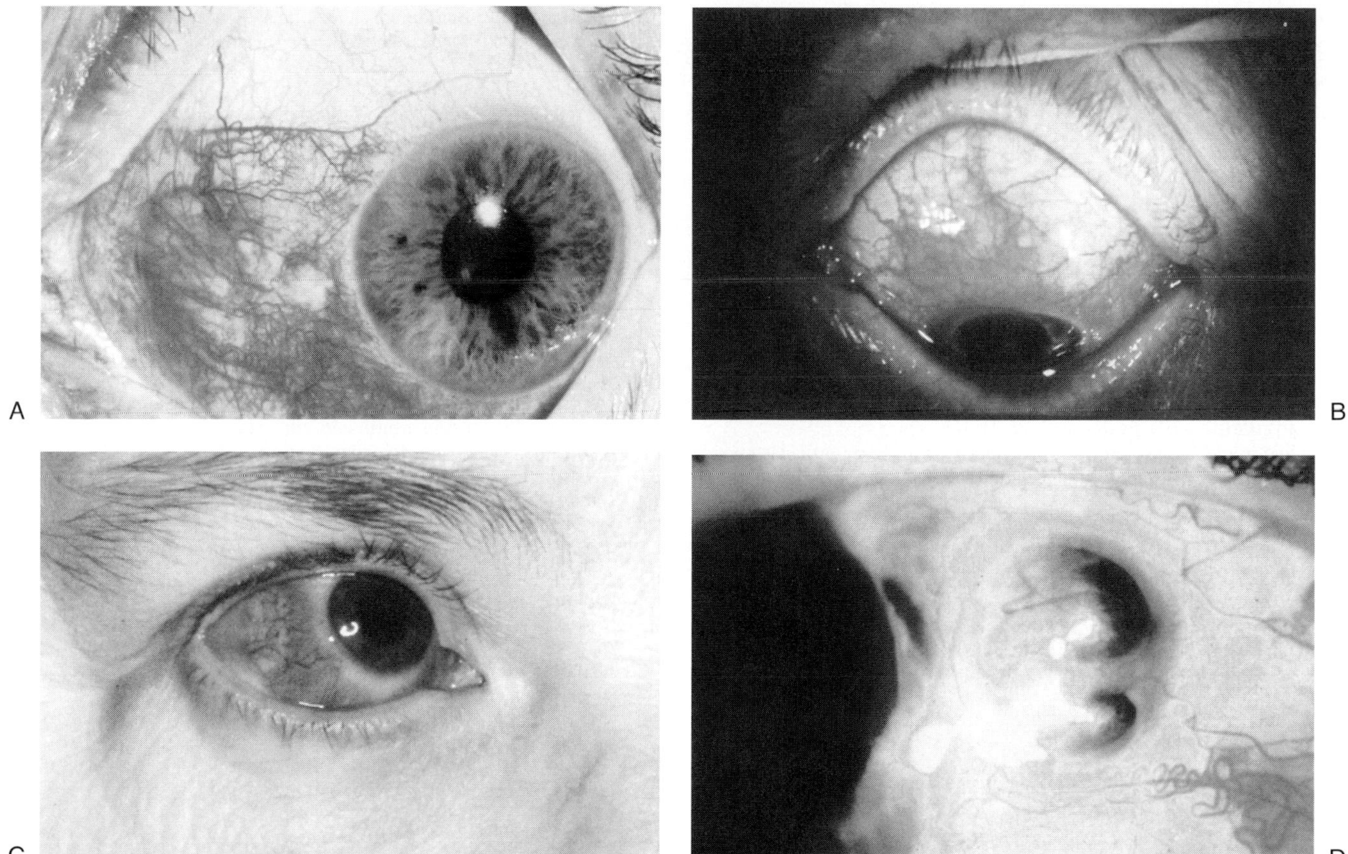

FIG. 56.4. A: Diffuse episcleritis. **B:** Nodular scleritis. **C:** Scleromalacia resulting from previous episodes of scleritis. **D:** Scleromalacia perforans. (From Conn DL. Rheumatoid neuropathy. In: Utsinger PD, Zvaifler NJ, Ehrlich GE, eds. *Rheumatoid arthritis.* Philadelphia: Lippincott, 1985:344, with permission.)

Other sites of inflammation within the eye include the central cornea, leading to painful acute necrotizing keratitis, and the peripheral cornea, where the insidious onset of peripheral ulcerative keratitis can lead to "corneal melt." Destructive processes involving the sclera and cornea are ophthalmologic emergencies.

As with other EA manifestations, rheumatoid eye disease may respond differently to disease-modifying treatment. A small retrospective case series showed a differential effect of anti-TNF-α therapy on eye disease associated with RA and other inflammatory disease: only 6 of 16 patients experienced eye improvement, and several developed deterioration or new eye problems, although all patients had improvement in arthritis (156). This further supports the role of multiple pathogenic mechanisms in this challenging disease.

SUMMARY

EAD remains prevalent in patients with severe RA. The mechanism remains unclear, but distinctive features of EAD include timing (such as the late onset of eye disease); serologic association with high rheumatoid factor titers and antinuclear factor positivity; and sometimes a paradoxic response to therapy. These features raise the possibility of a differing pathogenesis than synovial disease. Alternatively, they may demarcate a subset of RA patients with a different genetic predisposition in whom pathogenesis differs from those with less severe disease. Regardless of the etiology and pathogenesis, it remains essential for the practicing rheumatologist to remain aware of these potentially serious complications of RA occurring outside the joints and synovium.

REFERENCES

1. Symmons D, Turner G, Webb R, et al. The prevalence of rheumatoid arthritis in the United Kingdom. *Rheumatology* 2002;41:793–800.
2. Arnett FC, Edworthy SM, Bloch DA, et al. The American Rheumatism Association 1987 revised criteria for the classification of rheumatoid arthritis. *Arthritis Rheum* 1988;31:315–324.
3. Cimmino MA, Salvarani C, Macchioni P, et al. Extra-articular manifestations in 587 Italian patients with rheumatoid arthritis. *Rheumatol Int* 2000;19:213–217.
4. Mangat G. A comparative study of rheumatoid arthritis in Malaysian and British hospitals. *Br J Rheumatol* 1988;27(suppl):70–71.
5. Chopra A. The pattern of rheumatoid arthritis in the Indian population: a prospective study. *Br J Rheumatol* 1988;27:454–456.
6. Griffiths B, Situnayake RD, Clark B, et al. Racial origin and its effect on disease expression and HLA-DRB1 types in patients with rheumatoid arthritis: a matched cross-sectional study. *Rheumatology* 2000;39 (8):857–864.
7. Lindqvist E, Saxne T, Geborek P, et al. Ten year outcome in a cohort of patients with early rheumatoid arthritis: health status, disease process, and damage. *Ann Rheum Dis* 2002;61(12):1055–1059.
8. Turesson C, O'Fallon WM, Crowson CS, et al. Occurrence of extra-articular disease manifestations is associated with excess mortality in a community based cohort of patients with rheumatoid arthritis. *J Rheumatol* 2002;29(1):62–67.
9. Gabriel SE, Crowson CS, Kremers HM, et al. Survival in rheumatoid arthritis: a population-based analysis of trends over 40 years. *Arthritis Rheum* 2003;48(1):54–58.
10. Hessian PA, Highton J, Kean A, et al. Cytokine profile of the rheumatoid nodule suggests that it is a Th1 granuloma. *Arthritis Rheum* 2003; 48(2):334–338.
11. Edwards JCW, Blades S, Cambridge G. Restricted expression of Fc gammaRIII (CD16) in synovium and dermis: implications for tissue targeting in rheumatoid arthritis (RA). *Clin Exp Immunol* 1997;108:401.
12. Turesson C, Jacobsson L, Bergstrom U, et al. Predictors of extra-articular manifestations in rheumatoid arthritis. *Scand J Rheumatol* 2000;29(6):358–364.
13. Choi HK, Hernan MA, Seeger JD, et al. Methotrexate and mortality in patients with rheumatoid arthritis: a prospective study. *Lancet* 2002; 359(9313):1173–1177.
14. Mattey DL, Dawes PT, Fisher J, et al. Nodular disease in rheumatoid arthritis: association with cigarette smoking and HLA-DRB1/TNF gene interaction. *J Rheumatol* 2002;29(11):2313–2318.
15. Segal R, Caspi D, Tishler M, et al. Accelerated nodulosis and vasculitis during methotrexate therapy for rheumatoid arthritis. *Arthritis Rheum* 1988;31(9):1182–1185.
16. Jeurissen ME, Boerbooms AM, van de Putte LB. Eruption of nodulosis and vasculitis during methotrexate therapy for rheumatoid arthritis. *Clin Rheumatol* 1989;8(3):417–419.
17. Patatanian E, Thompson DF. A review of methotrexate-induced accelerated nodulosis [Review]. *Pharmacotherapy* 2002;22(9):1157–1162.
18. Kekow J, Welte T, Kellner U, et al. Development of rheumatoid nodules during anti-tumor necrosis factor alpha therapy with etanercept. *Arthritis Rheum* 2002;46(3):843–844.
19. Hawkins PN, Aprile C, Capri G, et al. Scintigraphic imaging and turnover studies with iodine-131 labelled serum amyloid P component in systemic amyloidosis. *Eur J Nucl Med* 1998;25(7):701–708.
20. Elkayam O, Hawkins PN, Lachmann H, et al. Rapid and complete resolution of proteinuria due to renal amyloidosis in a patient with rheumatoid arthritis treated with infliximab. *Arthritis Rheum* 2002; 46(10):2571–2573.
21. Watts RA, Carruthers DM, Symmons DP, et al. The incidence of rheumatoid vasculitis in the Norwich Health Authority. *Br J Rheumatol* 1994;33(9):832–833.
22. Quismorio FP, Beardmore T, Kaufman RL, et al. IgG rheumatoid factors and anti nuclear antibodies in rheumatoid vasculitis. *Clin Exp Immunol* 1983;52(2):333–340.
23. Voskuyl AE, Zwinderman AH, Westedt ML, et al. Factors associated with the development of vasculitis in rheumatoid arthritis: results of a case-control study. *Ann Rheum Dis* 1996;55(3):190–192.
24. Voskuyl AE, Hazes JM, Zwinderman AH, et al. Diagnostic strategy for the assessment of rheumatoid vasculitis. *Ann Rheum Dis* 2003;62 (5):407–413.
25. Voskuyl AE, Hazes JM, Zwinderman AH, et al. Diagnostic strategy for the assessment of rheumatoid vasculitis. *Ann Rheum Dis* 2003;62 (5):407–413.
26. Zwinderman AH, Voskuyl AE, Schelhaas DD, et al. Diagnostic strategies for the histological examination of muscle biopsy specimens for the assessment of vasculitis in rheumatoid arthritis. *Stat Med* 2000; 19(24):3433–3447.
27. Ando Y, Kai S, Uyama E, et al. Involvement of the central nervous system in rheumatoid arthritis: its clinical manifestations and analysis by magnetic resonance imaging. *Intern Med* 1995;34(3):188–191.
28. Gravallese EM, Corson JM, Coblyn JS, et al. Rheumatoid aortitis: a rarely recognized but clinically significant entity. *Medicine (Baltimore)* 1989;68(2):95–106.
29. Achkar AA, Stanson AW, Johnson CM, et al. Rheumatoid vasculitis manifesting as intra-abdominal hemorrhage. *Mayo Clin Proc* 1995;70 (6):565–569.
30. Suzuki A, Ohosone Y, Obana M, et al. Cause of death in 81 autopsied patients with rheumatoid arthritis. *J Rheumatol* 1994;21(1):33–36.
31. Galaria NA, Werth VP, Schumacher HR. Leukocytoclastic vasculitis due to etanercept. *J Rheumatol* 2000;27:2041–2044.
32. McCain ME, Quinet RJ, Davis WE. Etanercept and infliximab associated with cutaneous vasculitis. *Rheumatology* 2002;41:116–117.
33. Livermore PA, Murray KJ. Anti-tumour necrosis factor therapy associated with cutaneous vasculitis. *Rheumatology (Oxford)* 2002;41 (12):1450–1452.
34. McIlwain L, Carter JD, Bin-Sagheer S, et al. Hypersensitivity vasculitis with leukocytoclastic vasculitis secondary to infliximab. *J Clin Gastroenterol* 2003;36(5):411–413.
35. Chan ATY, Bradlow A, McNally J. Leflunomide induced vasculitis—a dose-response relationship. *Rheumatology* 2003;42(3):492–493.

36. Cope AP. Regulation of autoimmunity by proinflammatory cytokines. *Curr Opin Immunol* 1998;10(6):669–676.
37. Nilsson F. Anemia problems in rheumatoid arthritis. *Acta Med Scand* 1948;130(210):1–93.
38. Bowman SJ. Hematological manifestations of rheumatoid arthritis. *Scand J Rheumatol* 2002;31(5):251–259.
39. Mulherin D, Skelly M, Saunders A, et al. The diagnosis of iron deficiency in patients with rheumatoid arthritis and anemia: an algorithm using simple laboratory measures. *J Rheumatol* 1996;23:237–240.
40. Cavill I, Bentley D. Erythropoiesis in the anaemia of rheumatoid arthritis. *Br J Haematol* 1982;50:583–590.
41. Jongen-Lavrencic M, Peeters HR, Wognum A, et al. Elevated levels of inflammatory cytokines in bone marrow of patients with rheumatoid arthritis and anemia of chronic disease. *J Rheumatol* 1997;24:1504–1509.
42. Voulgari PV, Kolios G, Papadopoulos GK, et al. The role of cytokines in the pathogenesis of anemia of chronic disease in rheumatoid arthritis. *J Appl Biomater* 1999;92:153–160.
43. Vaiopoulos G, Boki K, Coulocheri S, et al. Hemoglobin levels correlate with serum soluble CD23 and TNF-Rs concentrations in patients with rheumatoid arthritis. *Haematologia* 1998;29:89–99.
44. Mercuriali F, Gualtieri G, Sinigaglia L, et al. Use of recombinant human erythropoietin to assist autologous blood donation by anemic rheumatoid arthritis patients undergoing major orthopedic surgery. *Transfusion* 1994;34:501–506.
45. Mercuriali F. Epoetin alfa for autologous blood donation in patients with rheumatoid arthritis and concomitant anemia. *Semin Hematol* 1997;33:18–20.
46. Infliximab/leflunomide/methotrexate: pancytopenia in an elderly patient (first report with infliximab): case report. *Reactions Weekly* 2003; 945:8.
47. Hill RL, Topliss DJ, Purcell PM. Pancytopenia associated with leflunomide and methotrexate. *Ann Pharmacother* 2003;37(1):149.
48. Kamper AM, Malbrain M, Zachee P, et al. Parvovirus infection causing red cell aplasia and leukopenia in rheumatoid arthritis. *Clin Rheumatol* 1994;13(1):129–131.
49. Maharaj D. Autoimmune haemolytic anaemia associated with rheumatoid arthritis and paroxysmal nocturnal haemoglobinuria. *Acta Haematol* 1986;75(4):241.
50. Das Gupta A, Abbi A. High serum transferrin receptor level in anemia of chronic disorders indicates coexistent iron deficiency. *Am J Hematol* 2003;72(3):158–161.
51. Felty AR. Chronic arthritis in the adult, associated with splenomegaly and leucopenia: a report of five cases of an unusual clinical syndrome. *Johns Hopkins Hosp Bull* 1924;35:16–20.
52. Campion G, Maddison PJ, Goulding N, et al. The Felty syndrome: a case-matched study of clinical manifestations and outcome, serologic features, and immunogenetic associations. *Medicine (Baltimore)* 1990; 69(2):69–80.
53. Lanchbury JS, Jaeger EE, Sansom DM, et al. Strong primary selection for the Dw4 subtype of DR4 accounts for the HLA-DQw7 association with Felty's syndrome. *Hum Immunol* 1991;32:56–64.
54. Termini TE, Biundo JJ, Ziff M. The rarity of Felty's syndrome in blacks. *Arthritis Rheum* 1979;22:999–1005.
55. Calabresi P, Edwards EA, Schilling RE. Fluorescent antiglobulin studies in leukopenic and related disorders. *J Clin Invest* 1959;38:2091–2106.
56. Vincent PC, Levi JA, Macqueen A. The mechanism of neutropenia in Felty's syndrome. *Br J Haematol* 1974;27:463–475.
57. Hurd ER, Andries M, Ziff M. Phagocytosis of immune complexes by polymorphonuclear leucocytes in patients with Felty's syndrome. *Clin Exp Immunol* 1977;28:413–425.
58. Starkebaum G, Arend W, Nardella F, et al. Characterization of immune complexes and immunoglobulin G antibodies reactive with neutrophils in the sera of patients with Felty's syndrome. *J Lab Clin Med* 1980;96:238–251.
59. Gupta RC, Robinson WA, Albrecht D. Granulopoietic activity in Felty's syndrome. *Ann Rheum Dis* 1975;34:156–161.
60. Starkebaum G, Singer J, Arend W. Humoral and cellular immune mechanisms of neutropenia in patients with Felty's syndrome. *Clin Exp Immunol* 1980;39:307–314.
61. Abdou N. Heterogeneity of bone marrow-directed immune mechanisms in the pathogenesis of neutropenia of Felty's syndrome. *Arthritis Rheum* 1983;26:947–953.
62. Luthra HS, Conn DL, Ferguson RH. Felty's syndrome: response to parenteral gold. *J Rheumatol* 1981;8:902–909.
63. Lakhanpal S, Luthra HS. D-penicillamine in Felty's syndrome. *J Rheumatol* 1985;12:703–706.
64. Ruderman M, Miller LM, Pinals RS. Clinical and serological observations on 27 patients with Felty's syndrome. *Arthritis Rheum* 1968;11: 377–384.
65. Fiechtner JJ, Miller DR, Starkebaum G. Reversal of neutropenia with methotrexate treatment in patients with Felty's syndrome. Correlation of response with neutrophil-reactive IgG. *Arthritis Rheum* 1989;32: 194–201.
66. Tan N, Grisanti MW, Grisanti JM. Oral methotrexate in the treatment of Felty's syndrome. *J Rheumatol* 1993;20:599–601.
67. Starkebaum G. Use of colony-stimulating factors in the treatment of neutropenia associated with collagen vascular disease. *Curr Opin Hematol* 1997;4:196–199.
68. Hellmich B, Schnabel A, Gross WL. Treatment of severe neutropenia due to Felty's syndrome or systemic lupus erythematosus with granulocyte colony stimulating. *Semin Arthritis Rheum* 1999;29:82–99.
69. Starkebaum G. Chronic neutropenia associated with autoimmune disease [Review]. *Semin Hematol* 2002;39(2):121–127.
70. Dillon AM, Luthra HS, Conn DL, et al. Parenteral gold therapy in the Felty syndrome. Experience with 20 patients. *Medicine* 1986;65:107–112.
71. Luthra HS, Hunder GG. Spontaneous remission of Felty's syndrome. *Arthritis Rheum* 1975;18:515–517.
72. Luthra HS. Felty's syndrome: a therapeutic dilemma? [Editorial]. *J Rheumatol* 1989;16:864–866.
73. Saway PA, Prasthofer EF, Barton JC. Prevalence of granular lymphocyte proliferation in patients with rheumatoid arthritis and neutropenia. *Am J Med* 1989;86:303–307.
74. Bowman SJ, Sivakumaran M, Snowden N, et al. The large granular lymphocyte syndrome with rheumatoid arthritis. Immunologenetic evidence for a broader description of Felty's syndrome. *Arthritis Rheum* 1994;37:1326–1330.
75. Dhodapkar MV, Li CY, Lust JA, et al. Clinical spectrum of clonal proliferations of T-large granular lymphocytes: a T-cell clonopathy of undetermined significance? *Blood* 1994;84:1620–1627.
76. Bowman SJ, Bhavnani M, Geddes GC, et al. Large granular lymphocyte expansions in patients with Felty's syndrome: analysis using anti-T cell receptor V beta-specific monoclonal antibodies. *Clin Exp Immunol* 1995;101:18–24.
77. Liu JH, Wei S, Lamy T, et al. Blockade of Fas-dependent apoptosis by soluble Fas in LGL leukemia. *Blood* 2002;100(4):1449–1453.
78. Roux N, Flipo RM, Cortet B, et al. *Pneumocystis carinii* pneumonia in rheumatoid arthritis patients treated with methotrexate. A report of two cases [Review]. *Rev Rhum Engl Ed* 1996;63(6):453–456.
79. Winchester RJ, Koffler D, Litwin SD, et al. Observations on the eosinophilia of certain patients with rheumatoid arthritis. *Arthritis Rheum* 1971;14:650–665.
80. Panush RS, Franco AE, Schur PH. Rheumatoid arthritis associated with eosinophilia. *Ann Intern Med* 1971;75:199–205.
81. Chaudhuri K, Dubey S, Zaphiropoulos G. Idiopathic hypereosinophilic syndrome in a patient with long-standing rheumatoid arthritis: a case report. *Rheumatology (Oxford)* 2002;41(3):349–3450.
82. Savolainen HA, Leirisalo-Repo M. Eosinophilia as a side-effect of methotrexate in patients with chronic arthritis. *Clin Rheumatol* 2001; 20(6):432–434.
83. Ehrenfeld M, Penchas S, Eliakim M. Thrombocytosis in rheumatoid arthritis. Recurrent arterial thromboembolism and death. *Ann Rheum Dis* 1977;36:579–581.
84. Grove ML, Hassell AB, Hay EM, et al. Adverse reactions to disease-modifying anti-rheumatic drugs in clinical practice. *Q J Med* 2001; 94(6):309–319.
85. Cohen C. Staphylococcal septicaemia with multiple pyoarthrosis complicating rheumatoid disease. *Gerontol Clin (Basel)* 1965;7(4):231–246.
86. Sepkowitz KA. Opportunistic infections in patients with and patients without acquired immunodeficiency syndrome [Review]. *Clin Infect Dis* 2002;34(8):1098–1107.
87. Louthrenoo W, Kasitanon N, Mahanuphab P, et al. Kaposi's sarcoma in rheumatic diseases. *Semin Arthritis Rheum* 2003;32(5):326–333.
88. Dedicoat M, Newton R. Review of the distribution of Kaposi's sarcoma-associated herpesvirus (KSHV) in Africa in relation to the incidence of Kaposi's sarcoma. *Br J Cancer* 2003;88(1):1–3.

89. Allen ME, Young SP, Michell RH, et al. Altered T lymphocyte signaling in rheumatoid arthritis. *Eur J Immunol* 1995;25(6):1547–1554.
90. Carruthers DM, Naylor WG, Allen ME, et al. Characterization of altered calcium signalling in T lymphocytes from patients with rheumatoid arthritis (RA). *Clin Exp Immunol* 1996;105(2):291–296.
91. Carruthers DM, Arrol HP, Bacon PA, et al. Dysregulated intracellular Ca^{2+} stores and Ca^{2+} signaling in synovial fluid T lymphocytes from patients with chronic inflammatory arthritis. *Arthritis Rheum* 2000; 43(6):1257–1265.
92. Ali M, Ponchel F, Wilson KE, et al. Rheumatoid arthritis synovial T cells regulate transcription of several genes associated with antigen-induced anergy. *J Clin Invest* 2001;107(4):519–528.
93. Cope AP, Londei M, Chu NR, et al. Chronic exposure to tumor necrosis factor (TNF) *in vitro* impairs the activation of T cells through the T cell receptor/CD3 complex; reversal *in vivo* by anti-TNF antibodies in patients with rheumatoid arthritis. *J Clin Invest* 1994;94(2):749–760.
94. Isomaki P, Panesar M, Annenkov A, et al. Prolonged exposure of T cells to TNF down-regulates TCR zeta and expression of the TCR/CD3 complex at the cell surface. *J Immunol* 2001 1;166(9):5495–5507.
95. Cope AP. Studies of T-cell activation in chronic inflammation. *Arthritis Res* 2002;4(3)(suppl):197–211.
96. Walser-Kuntz DR, Weyand CM, Fulbright JW, et al. HLA-DRB1 molecules and antigenic experience shape the repertoire of CD4 T cells. *Hum Immunol* 1995;44(4):203–209.
97. Schmidt D, Goronzy JJ, Weyand CM. $CD4^+$ $CD7^-$ $CD28^-$ T cells are expanded in rheumatoid arthritis and are characterized by autoreactivity. *J Clin Invest* 1996 1;97(9):2027–2037.
98. Martens PB, Goronzy JJ, Schaid D, et al. Expansion of unusual $CD4^+$ T cells in severe rheumatoid arthritis. *Arthritis Rheum* 1997;40(6):1106–1114.
99. Wagner UG, Koetz K, Weyand CM, et al. Perturbation of the T cell repertoire in rheumatoid arthritis. *Proc Natl Acad Sci U S A* 1998; 95(24):14447–14452.
100. Ponchel F, Morgan AW, Bingham SJ, et al. Dysregulated lymphocyte proliferation and differentiation in patients with rheumatoid arthritis. *Blood* 2002;100(13):4550–4556.
101. Mitchell D, Spitz P, Young D, et al. Survival, prognosis, and causes of death in rheumatoid arthritis. *Arthritis Rheum* 1986;29:706–714.
102. Wolfe F, Mitchell D, Sibley J, et al. The mortality of rheumatoid arthritis. *Arthritis Rheum* 1994;37:481–494.
103. Solomon DH, Karlson EW, Rimm EB, et al. Cardiovascular morbidity and mortality in women diagnosed with rheumatoid arthritis. *Circulation* 2003;107(9):1303–1307.
104. Goodson N. Coronary artery disease and rheumatoid arthritis. *Curr Opin Rheumatol* 2002;14(2):115–120.
105. Liuzzo G, Biasucci LM, Gallimore JR, et al. Prognostic value of C-reactive protein and plasma amyloid A protein in severe unstable angina. *N Engl J Med* 1994;331:417–424.
106. Thompson SG, Kienast J, Pyke SDM, et al. Hemostatic factors and the risk of myocardial infarction or sudden death in patients with angina pectoris. *N Engl J Med* 1995;332:635–641.
107. Ridker PM, Cushman M, Stampfer MJ, et al. Inflammation, aspirin, and the risk of cardiovascular disease in apparently healthy men. *N Engl J Med* 1997;336:973–979.
108. Rost NS, Wolf PA, Kase CS, et al. Plasma concentration of C-reactive protein and risk of ischemic stroke and transient ischemic attack: the Framingham study. *Stroke* 2001;32:2575–2579.
109. Curb JD, Abbott RD, Rodriguez BL, et al. C-reactive protein and the future risk of thromboembolic stroke in healthy men. *Circulation* 2003;107(15):2016–2020.
110. Ridker PM, Glynn RJ, Hennekens CH. C-reactive protein adds to the predictive value of total and HDL cholesterol in determining risk of first myocardial infarction. *Circulation* 1998;97:2007–2011.
111. van der Meer IM, de Maat MPM, Hak AE, et al. C-reactive protein predicts progression of atherosclerosis measured at various sites in the arterial tree: the Rotterdam Study. *Stroke* 2002;33(12):2750–2755.
112. Ridker PM, Rifai N, Pfeffer MA, et al. Long-term effects of pravastatin on plasma concentration of c-reactive protein. *Circulation* 1999; 100(3):230–235.
113. Ridker PM, Rifai N, Pfeffer MA, et al. Inflammation, pravastatin, and the risk of coronary events after myocardial infarction in patients with average cholesterol levels. *Circulation* 1998;98(9):839–844.
114. Kitas G, Banks MJ, Bacon PA. Cardiac involvement in rheumatoid disease [Review]. *Clin Med* 2001;1(1):18–21.
115. Maione S, Valentini G, Giunta A, et al. Cardiac involvement in rheumatoid arthritis: an echocardiographic study. *Cardiology* 1993;83: 234–239.
116. Wislowska M, Sypula S, Kowalik I. Echocardiographic findings and 24-h electrocardiographic Holter monitoring in patients with nodular and non-nodular rheumatoid arthritis. *Rheumatol Int* 1999;18:163–169.
117. Thould AK. Constrictive pericarditis in rheumatoid arthritis. *Ann Rheum Dis* 1986;45:89–94.
118. Thadani U, Iveson JM, Wright V. Cardiac tamponade, constrictive pericarditis and pericardial resection in rheumatoid arthritis. *Medicine* 1975;54:261–270.
119. Bonfiglio T, Atwater EC. Heart disease in patients with seropositive rheumatoid arthritis: a controlled autopsy study and review. *Arch Intern Med* 1969;124:714–719.
120. Cruickshank B. Heart lesions in rheumatoid arthritis. *J Pathol Bacteriol* 1958;76:223–240.
121. Gowans JDC. Complete heart block with Stokes-Adams syndrome due to rheumatoid heart disease. *N Engl J Med* 1960;262:1012–1014.
122. Bely M, Apathy A, Beke-Martos E. Cardiac changes in rheumatoid arthritis. *Acta Morphol Hung* 1992;40:1–4.
123. Badui E, Jiminez J, Saldivar C, et al. The heart and rheumatoid arthritis. Prospective study of 100 cases. *Arch Inst Cardiol Mex* 1987;57:159–167.
124. Baggenstross AH, Rosenberg EF. Cardiac lesions associated with chronic infectious arthritis. *Arch Intern Med* 1941;67:241–258.
125. Prakash R, Atassi A, Poske R, et al. Prevalence of pericardial effusion and mitral-valve involvement in patients with rheumatoid arthritis without cardiac symptoms. An echocardiographic evaluation. *N Engl J Med* 1973;289:597–600.
126. Cathcart ES, Spodick DH. Rheumatoid heart disease: a study of the incidence and nature of cardiac lesions in rheumatoid arthritis. *N Engl J Med* 1962;266:959–964.
127. Camilleri JP, Douglas-Jones AG, Pritchard MH. Rapidly progressive aortic valve incompetence in a patient with rheumatoid arthritis. *Br J Rheumatol* 1991;30:379–381.
128. Voyles WF, Searles RP, Bankhurst AD. Myocardial infarction caused by rheumatoid vasculitis. *Arthritis Rheum* 1980;23:860–863.
129. Carotti M, Salaffi F, Manganelli P, et al. [The subclinical involvement of the lung in rheumatoid arthritis: evaluation by high-resolution computed tomography]. *Reumatismo* 2001;53(4):280–288 (in Italian).
130. Caplan A. Certain unusual radiographic appearances in the chest of coal-miners suffering from rheumatoid arthritis. *Thorax* 1953;8: 29–37.
131. Ryu JH, Colby TV, Hartman TE. Idiopathic pulmonary fibrosis: current concepts. *Mayo Clin Proc* 1998;73(11):1085–1101.
132. Dawson JK, Fewins HE, Desmond J, et al. Predictors of progression of HRCT diagnosed fibrosing alveolitis in patients with rheumatoid arthritis. *Ann Rheum Dis* 2002;61(6):517–521.
133. Anaya JM, Diethelm L, Ortiz LA, et al. Pulmonary involvement in rheumatoid arthritis. *Semin Arthritis Rheum* 1995;24:242–254.
134. Korpela M, Mustonen J, Teppo AM, et al. Mesangial glomerulonephritis as an extra-articular manifestation of rheumatoid arthritis. *Br J Rheumatol* 1997;36(11):1189–1195.
135. Boers M, Croonen AM, Dijkmans BA, et al. Renal findings in rheumatoid arthritis: clinical aspects of 132 necropsies. *Ann Rheum Dis* 1987;46(9):658–663.
136. Kojima H, Uemura M, Sakurai S, et al. Clinical features of liver disturbance in rheumatoid diseases: clinicopathological study with special reference to the cause of liver disturbance. *J Gastroenterol* 2002;37(8):617–625.
137. Toussirot E, Wendling D. Crohn's disease associated with seropositive rheumatoid arthritis. *Clin Exp Rheumatol* 1997;15(3):307–311.
138. Mosley JG, Desai A, Gupta I. Mesenteric arteritis. *Gut* 1990;31(8): 956–957.
139. Marshall S, Tardif G, Ashworth N. Local corticosteroid injection for carpal tunnel syndrome [Review]. *Cochrane Database Syst Rev* 2002;(4):CD001554.

140. Gerritsen AA, de Vet HC, Scholten RJ, et al. Splinting vs surgery in the treatment of carpal tunnel syndrome: a randomized controlled trial. *JAMA* 2002;288(10):1245–1251.
141. Gozke E, Erdogan N, Akyuz G, et al. Sympathetic skin response and R-R interval variation in cases with rheumatoid arthritis. *Electromyogr Clin Neurophysiol* 2003;43(2):81–84.
142. Laiho K, Kaarela K, Kauppi M. Cervical spine disorders in patients with rheumatoid arthritis and amyloidosis. *Clin Rheumatol* 2002;21(3):227–230.
143. Laiho K, Soini I, Kautiainen H, et al. Can we rely on magnetic resonance imaging when evaluating unstable atlantoaxial subluxation? *Ann Rheum Dis* 2003;62(3):254–256.
144. Dickens C, Jackson J, Tomensen B, et al. Association of depression and rheumatoid arthritis. *Psychosomatics* 2003;44(3):209–215.
145. Timonen M, Viilo K, Hakko H, et al. Suicides in persons suffering from rheumatoid arthritis. *Rheumatology (Oxford)* 2003;42(2):287–291.
146. Brown SC, Glass JM, Park DC. The relationship of pain and depression to cognitive function in rheumatoid arthritis patients. *Pain* 2002;96(3):279–284.
147. Keefe FJ, Smith SJ, Buffington AL, et al. Recent advances and future directions in the biopsychosocial assessment and treatment of arthritis [Review]. *J Consult Clin Psychol* 2002;70(3):640–655.
148. Devlin J, Lilley J, Gough A, et al. Clinical associations of dual-energy X-ray absorptiometry measurement of hand bone mass in rheumatoid arthritis. *Br J Rheumatol* 1996;35(12):1256–1262.
149. Hofbauer LC, Heufelder AE. Role of receptor activator of nuclear factor-kappaB ligand and osteoprotegerin in bone cell biology. *J Mol Med* 2001;79(5–6):243–253.
150. Gravallese EM. Bone destruction in arthritis. *Ann Rheum Dis* 2002;61(2):84–86.
151. Gough A, Sambrook P, Devlin J, et al. Effect of vitamin D receptor gene alleles on bone loss in early rheumatoid arthritis. *J Rheumatol* 1998;25(5):864–868.
152. Hirayama T, Danks L, Sabokbar A, et al. Osteoclast formation and activity in the pathogenesis of osteoporosis in rheumatoid arthritis. *Rheumatology (Oxford)*. 2002;41(11):1232–1239.
153. van Vugt RM, Sijbrandij ES, Bijlsma JW. Magnetic resonance imaging of the femoral head to detect avascular necrosis in active rheumatoid arthritis treated with methylprednisolone pulse therapy. *Scand J Rheumatol* 1996;25(2):74–76.
154. Hay EM, Thomas E, Pal B, et al. Weak association between subjective symptoms or and objective testing for dry eyes and dry mouth: results from a population based study. *Ann Rheum Dis* 1998;57(1):20–24.
155. Schein OD, Hochberg MC, Munoz B, et al. Dry eye and dry mouth in the elderly: a population-based assessment. *Arch Intern Med* 1999;159(12):1359–1363.
156. Smith JR, Levinson RD, Holland GN, et al. Differential efficacy of tumor necrosis factor inhibition in the management of inflammatory eye disease and associated rheumatic disease. *Arthritis Rheum* 2001;45(3):252–257.

CHAPTER 57

Laboratory Findings in Rheumatoid Arthritis

W. Winn Chatham and Warren D. Blackburn, Jr.

A number of laboratory test results may be abnormal in patients with rheumatoid arthritis (RA), reflecting the systemic inflammatory nature of the disease. Whereas laboratory result abnormalities in RA are frequently nonspecific and observed in other inflammatory disorders, certain tests may be useful in diagnosis of the disease. Furthermore, some of the changes seen in RA may reflect disease activity and portend outcome. It must be remembered that there is no uniformly accepted gold standard to measure outcome in RA. Measures of outcome or disease activity have included functional parameters, radiographic analysis, and a variety of laboratory tests. Because RA is predominantly an articular disease, evidence of joint destruction has frequently been put forth as the outcome to measure. Unfortunately, plain radiographs and other imaging procedures such as magnetic resonance imaging (MRI) do not necessarily reflect the ongoing process, but rather reflect the cumulative effect of the disease. Moreover, it is not feasible to serially image all involved joints in RA. Functional outcome evaluations, although clearly of importance to the physician caring for the patient with RA, may reflect a number of factors other than ongoing disease activity. Certain laboratory tests may provide insight regarding the progression of the disease and, perhaps, response to therapy.

This chapter evaluates the laboratory findings in RA, focusing on their relationship to disease activity and the mechanisms, where understood, that account for these abnormalities.

HEMATOLOGIC ABNORMALITIES

Erythrocytes

Anemia is a common finding in patients with active RA, but in most patients hemoglobin levels are not less than 10 g/dL (1,2) (Table 57.1). Typically, the anemia is normocytic and either normochromic or hypochromic. Serum iron levels are usually low normal or decreased, but there is generally not a significant increase in iron binding capacity (3–6). Bone marrow examination typically reveals normal iron stores, unless there is another cause of iron loss. Even in those with decreased iron stores, the levels frequently do not correlate with the degree of anemia (7–11). Because transferrin behaves as an acute-phase protein, it is frequently elevated in patients with RA and does not necessarily reflect iron stores (12,13). Similarly, serum transferrin receptor levels have not been found to be predictive of iron deficiency in RA (14). At a molecular level, 5-aminolevulinate synthase activity is suppressed in marrow and in purified erythroblasts obtained from RA patients with anemia of chronic disease (15).

Although there may be other factors contributing to the anemia seen in patients with RA, the predominant cause is the so-called anemia of chronic disease (13). This anemia is principally due to underproduction of red blood cells (16). In response to the anemia, levels of erythropoietin increase in RA, but the increase is less than would be expected in normal individuals with the same degree of anemia (16,17). Correspondingly, healthy individuals with erythropoietin levels comparable with those present in patients with RA would be polycythemic. These observations indicate that the response to erythropoietin in RA is blunted.

The anemia of chronic disease appears to be attributable to interaction of inflammatory cytokines with the bone marrow. Evidence supporting this view comes from studies in both animals and patients with disease (18–24). Repetitive exogenous administration of interleukin-1 (IL-1) to mice induces anemia (18). *In vitro* studies of human bone marrow have also demonstrated that both blast-forming units–erythroid (BFU-E) and colony-forming units–erythroid (CFU-E) are inhibited by IL-1 (18,19). This inhibition is not direct, because removal of T cells blocks the inhibition of CFU-E (20).

TABLE 57.1. *Characteristics of anemia in rheumatoid arthritis*

RBC morphology	Normochromic or hypochromic
Serum iron	Usually low
TIBC	Normal
Transferrin	Elevated
Bone marrow iron	Usually normal
Erythropoietin	Increased
RBC life span	Normal or slightly decreased

RBC, red blood count; TIBC, total iron-binding capacity.

Supernatants obtained from cultures of IL-1-activated T cells also inhibit CFU-E (20), an effect neutralized by antibodies to interferon-γ (IFN-γ) (20). Incubation of bone marrow cultures with IFN-γ also inhibits red cell formation. Other inflammatory cytokines present in the serum of patients with RA may further contribute to the development of anemia. Tumor necrosis factor-α (TNF-α), when administered to animals and human subjects, also causes anemia and inhibits CFU-E in animal studies (22). *In vitro* studies of marrow from patients with RA and anemia of chronic disease have similarly demonstrated that TNF-α decreases erythroid colony-forming units, and anti-TNF antibodies increase them (25). As with IL-1, the effects of TNF-α on the bone marrow appear to be indirect and may be mediated by IFN-γ (24). Interestingly, IL-1, TNF-α, and transforming growth factor-β (TGF-β) have all been shown to inhibit production of erythropoietin by hepatoma cell lines. Not surprisingly, further studies have suggested that inhibition of erythropoiesis in RA is likely due to the synergistic effect of multiple cytokines on the bone marrow (reviewed in reference 13). Indeed, evaluations of patients with RA and anemia of chronic disease demonstrate a correlation between serum TNF-α and IL-6 measurements, and anemia (25,26) and elevated bone marrow production of both IL-6 and TNF-α (27). However, *in vitro* addition of IL-6 to marrow results in inconsistent effects on red cell production (26).

Additional evidence suggests that impairment of iron metabolism also occurs in RA patients with anemia. As noted earlier, serum iron levels are frequently low, despite the presence of adequate iron stores (3,4). In most cases, the anemia associated with active RA is not corrected by the administration of iron or other hematinics. Additionally, the observation that the anemia can be corrected by the administration of erythropoietin argues against the notion that a problem with iron metabolism is the principal determinant of the anemia (28).

In practice, correction of the anemia of chronic disease associated with RA can be accomplished with exogenous administration of erythropoietin. Unfortunately, improvement of disease symptoms is inconsistent with the erythropoietin-induced resolution of the anemia (28,29). Administration of erythropoietin, however, may be useful in patients who, for other reasons, are not tolerant of the degree of anemia sometimes seen in RA or for those undergoing surgery in whom transfusion requirements may be diminished by use of this treatment.

Leukocytes

Circulating white blood cell counts can vary widely in patients with RA. Patients with active disease frequently have elevated white counts. This appears to be largely attributable to molecules released during the inflammatory response. For example, in contrast to its effects on erythroid precursors, IL-1β does not inhibit colony-forming units–granulocyte macrophage (CFU-GM). In fact, IL-1β increases the production of both granulocyte-macrophage colony-stimulating factor (GM-CSF) and granulocyte colony-stimulating factor (G-CSF) (13). TNF-α has a similar effect and may increase CFU-GM (22). GM-CSF is present in the synovia of patients with RA (30).

Patients treated with corticosteroids may also have elevated white counts due to the factors discussed above and due to decreased margination, decreased emigration from the bloodstream, and increased marrow production (31–33).

White blood cell differential counts are usually normal, but may exhibit elevated numbers of granulocytes. Eosinophilia may occur in patients with severe disease or those with high-titer rheumatoid factor, and an apparent correlation has been observed with several extraarticular features, including vasculitis, subcutaneous nodules, and serositis (34,35).

Less frequently, white blood cell counts are decreased in RA. The triad of leukopenia, splenomegaly, and deforming arthritis was described by Felty (36) in 1924. Granulocytopenia accounts for most of the leukopenia, because monocyte and eosinophil counts are usually normal. The association of this syndrome with other extraarticular features of the disease—including vasculitis, weight loss, and anemia—has been well documented (37–41). Recurrent infections are sometimes seen, but typically only when neutrophil counts are dramatically reduced, typically less than $1{,}000/mm^3$ (39–42). Other factors that appear to increase the risk for infections in patients with Felty's syndrome include severe disability, skin ulcers, immunosuppressive therapy, and hypocomplementemia (39–42).

Studies of patients with RA and leukopenia suggest that multiple factors may contribute to the leukopenia. Not all patients have splenomegaly, and response to splenectomy is inconsistent (39–43). Indeed, even those patients who initially respond to splenectomy may have recurrence of their leukopenia. In some patients, the decrease in circulating leukocytes may simply be due to an increased marginated leukocyte population (44), and synovial fluid leukocyte counts can remain elevated in patients with peripheral neutropenia (45). Circulating neutrophils obtained from patients with RA exhibit detectable surface immunoglobulins (46–49). Although such findings may simply reflect binding of immunoglobulin complexes to surface Fc receptors, rather than antibodies directed against cell surface determinants (50), there is a correlation between levels of circulating immune complexes and neutropenia (51). Other factors potentially contributing to the neutropenia seen in these patients include suppression of bone marrow function by suppressor cells, suppressive cytokines, or decreased production of granulopoietic factors (52–59).

Subsequent to the observations reported by Felty, expansion of large granular lymphocytes (LGLs) in the bone marrow or peripheral blood has been noted in some patients with RA and neutropenia (60–66) (Table 57.2). In a large series of patients with RA, approximately 1.7% had neutropenia, approximately one third of whom had bone marrow evidence of LGL expansion (65). Between 20% and 30% of patients with expansion of LGLs have RA (65). The clinical presentation of LGLs in the setting of RA is variable. Patients with RA may develop expansion of LGLs in the absence of either splenomegaly or neutropenia. Other patients have a normal total white count because of the increased numbers of circulating lymphocytes, but are neutropenic. Initial reports suggested that patients with expansion of LGLs had more severe arthritis; however, later reports have indicated that disease severity can be quite variable (65–68). The LGLs are derived from either a natural killer lineage or from activated cytotoxic T cells and can be separated by cell surface phenotypic markers. In the latter case, analysis of T-cell receptors from these cells are consistent with an antigen-driven process (69). LGLs typically express CD2, CD8, CD16, and CD57 (65,66), or CD2, CD8, CD16, and CD56 (65,68). Occasionally, patients are found with expansion of LGLs expressing neither CD4 nor CD8 (68). Approximately half of the patients have evidence of clonal expansion of these cells, but frank leukemia is unusual in RA (68,70). Patients with RA and LGL expansion, as with patients with classic Felty's syndrome, are likely to be DR4 positive (66). The mechanism by which LGL expansion results in neutropenia has not been fully elucidated, but cells with the phenotypes seen in this syndrome may interfere with marrow production of neutrophils by either direct cellular cytotoxicity or through production of cytokines, which inhibit the marrow (71–73).

The functional status of granulocytes harvested from patients with RA is variable, and differing results are likely due to the relative state of activation of the cells and the milieu from which they are harvested (74–77). There is no convincing evidence for overall granulocyte dysfunction in RA. Cells exposed to certain cytokines, including TNF-α and IL-1, may respond more vigorously than control cells (78,79). However, activation of cells by complement cleavage fragments or 5-lipoxygenase products, as may occur in synovial fluid, may result in inhibition of responses to other activating ligands (80,81). In synovial fluid, other factors, including certain apolipoproteins, may also interfere with activation of neutrophils (82). Decreased functional activity of synovial fluid granulocytes related to microbicidal responses may partially explain why patients with RA are predisposed to develop septic arthritis.

TABLE 57.2. *Large granular lymphocytes in rheumatoid arthritis*

Source	NK cells or cytotoxic T cells
Cell markers	CD2, CD8, CD16, and CD57 or CD56
Total white cell count	Normal or decreased
Neutrophil counts	Frequently decreased
Clonal expansion	Frequently present
Leukemia	Unusual in rheumatoid arthritis

NK, natural killer.

Circulating total lymphocytes in patients with RA are usually normal. Lymphocyte surface markers have been cataloged in patients, and the numbers or percentages of cells bearing CD4 or CD8 are for the most part unchanged (83–86).

CD45 expression has been investigated on peripheral blood T cells in patients with RA (84,87,88). CD45RA expression delineates T cells that are considered naive, whereas CD45RO represents primed T cells. In contrast to synovial fluid, where there is increased expression of CD45RO (particularly in conjunction with expression of CD45RBdull), in peripheral blood there do not appear to be differences in cells expressing CD45RO (87,88).

Cells expressing the surface marker CD7 (one of the earliest markers in T-cell ontogeny) may be present in lower numbers in patients with RA. Cells phenotypically described as $CD7^-$ $CD4^+$ $CD45RA^-$, however, may be more prevalent. Of note, these cells have been shown *ex vivo* to provide considerable help to B cells in inducing immunoglobulin M (IgM) and, in particular, IgM rheumatoid factor synthesis, and may play a similar role *in vivo* (89).

T cells bearing CD57, a 110-kd glycoprotein expressed by natural killer cells and small granular lymphocytes, are increased in RA (90). The majority of these $CD3^+$ $CD57^+$ cells are also $CD8^+$ $CD45RA^+$. In peripheral blood, they predominantly express the αβ T-cell receptors and rarely are found to express CD16, CD28, or DR. In synovial fluid, phenotypically similar cells are more likely to express DR. The percentage of these cells in peripheral blood is correlated with disease duration, but their presence has not been correlated with sedimentation rate, C-reactive protein, levels of rheumatoid factor, or other measures of disease activity. It has been suggested that these cells exert a suppressive role in regulating synovial T cells.

Expression of the adhesion protein L selectin on $CD4^+$ T cells is also reported to be normal in RA (91). The IL-2 receptor may be present in lower numbers on T cells in RA (83,85,92,93). The clinical significance of such findings is not clear, however.

Based on the hypothesis that T cells may be pivotal in initiating RA, characteristics of the T-cell receptor have been investigated in peripheral blood, synovium, and synovial fluid of patients with the disease. The percentage of $CD3^+$ cells expressing the αβ T-cell receptor has been reported to be both increased and decreased in peripheral blood and synovial fluid when compared with healthy controls (94–96). Utilization of specific Vγ or Vδ chains does not appear to be different in patients with established disease compared with healthy controls (96). Using the polymerase chain reaction, at best a semiquantitative molecular technique, no clear pattern of Vβ usage had been established in cells from peripheral blood (97). A more direct evaluation using monoclonal antibodies to five β chains has indicated that Vβ gene product utilization by peripheral blood lymphocytes is not different between patients with seropositive RA and normal controls, with the exception of possible overexpression of Vβ17 (98). Vβ17 representation by peripheral T cells was more common in RA than in other inflammatory conditions. Similar findings have been noted in synovial fluid and synovium. There appears to be no consistent distribution of Vβ17 between $CD4^+$ or $CD8^+$ T cells, suggesting that the increased utilization occurs in both types of cells. Interestingly, expression of activation antigens such as the IL-2 receptor is more frequently found on Vβ17-positive T cells that also express CD4, a finding noted in synovial fluid even in instances where Vβ17 utilization was not increased (98). T cells expressing Vβ chains are responsive to superantigens, but it has not been established whether these cells are expanded by this mechanism or by antigen-specific mechanisms (99,100). Evaluation of Vα gene expression, also determined by utilization of monoclonal antibodies, has suggested that there may be oligoclonal expansion of T cells with apparent overexpression of cells utilizing Vα2 (101).

The number of B cells in peripheral blood of patients with RA is usually normal (102). Evidence of B-cell activation can be found in peripheral blood B cells with increased expression of CD21 (C3d receptor) (103). A subset of B cells expressing CD5 may be increased in RA (94, 104–106). CD5 is a pan–T-cell marker and also has been found on B cells in chronic lymphocytic leukemia, human immunodeficiency virus infection, and posttransplantation. *Ex vivo* stimulation of $CD5^+$ B cells leads to preferential production of a number of autoantibodies, including rheumatoid factor and antibodies recognizing single-stranded DNA (107,108). Overall, the number of $CD5^+$ B cells increases with age and appears to be genetically linked, because levels are correlated within families (108–110). In twins discordant for RA, the numbers of $CD5^+$ B cells were not different (109,110). In culture supernatants from $CD5^+$ B cells, apparent monomeric IgM can be detected on Western blots. The presence in peripheral blood of this low-molecular-weight (8S) IgM has been correlated with severity of disease and vasculitis (108). There does not appear to be a correlation between the number of $CD5^+$ B cells and the amount of 8S IgM, however.

Platelets

Platelet counts are frequently elevated in patients with RA, and this generally correlates with anemia, leukocytosis, and titer of rheumatoid factor (111). Platelets from patients with RA exhibit lower levels of serotonin and connective tissue–activating factor, but increased platelet-associated IgG (112,113).

ERYTHROCYTE SEDIMENTATION RATE

The most frequently used laboratory measure of inflammation or "disease activity" in RA is the erythrocyte sedimentation rate (ESR) (see also Chapter 22). The test reports the rate of sedimentation of red cells in anticoagulated blood [ethylenediaminetetraacetic acid (EDTA) or citrate] in a cylinder. Several methods have been developed to measure ESR, but the Westergren method has been adopted as the standard technique. Two milliliters of blood is collected into 0.5 mL of anticoagulant and placed in a 200-mm Westergren tube. The tube is placed upright on a stable surface and the zone of clearing in the column is measured and expressed in millimeters per hour. Measurement of the ESR is simple, inexpensive, and reproducible, but may be influenced by a variety of factors.

The predominant determinant of the ESR is aggregation or rouleaux formation of red cells (114). Erythrocytes are inherently attracted to each other by van der Waals forces. These forces are counterbalanced by repulsive forces due to the charged residues on surface molecules. In the normal situation, repulsive forces are in moderate excess and there is little aggregation. However, a third factor that modulates the degree of rouleaux formation is the media in which the cells are bathed (115). Molecules with an asymmetric charge distribution can essentially dissipate the repulsive charges and enhance rouleaux formation. Of the acute-phase proteins, fibrinogen, due to its asymmetry and concentration, has the greatest effect on the sedimentation rate (116,117). Fibrinogen levels do not peak for days or longer after the acute event, however, and may take even longer to return to normal after the event subsides (118). Other molecules, including α_2- and γ-globulins that are asymmetrically charged, although to a lesser extent than fibrinogen, may nonetheless influence sedimentation rates (119). Although γ-globulins have only a fraction of the effect on ESR that fibrinogen does, the remarkable elevation in ESR seen in patients with plasma cell dyscrasias is explained by the high levels of these antibody proteins (120,121).

To a lesser degree, ESR is influenced by erythrocyte size and shape. Alterations lead to interference with rouleaux formation and a paradoxic decrease in ESR, even when there are detectable increases in acute-phase proteins (122,123). Additionally, anemia may increase sedimentation rate, whereas polycythemia decreases ESR. Other factors, including certain drugs, may influence measurement of ESR. Heparin and intramuscular injection of certain compounds such as benzathine penicillin, for example, may increase the sedimentation rates, whereas sodium valproate may decrease the measurement (124,125). Estrogens and pregnancy increase the sedimentation rate (126–128). Older individuals and women tend to have higher ESR (129–132). Unfortunately, there is no simple or consistent means to adjust the sedimentation rates to account for these factors. Patients with cryoglobulins, whose blood is cooled prior to measuring the ESR, may have an artifactually decreased ESR, because fibrinogen may be incorporated into the precipitated cryoglobulin (133).

In broad terms, ESR does correlate with activity of disease in RA (134,135). Worsening disease is usually associated with an increase in ESR, and remission with normalization of this test. Those who have consistently elevated ESR are more likely to require total joint arthroplasty (136). At least 5% of patients with clinically active disease may have a normal ESR, however (137,138). Despite its simplicity, the ESR only indirectly measures the acute-phase response and, as noted earlier, may be altered by a number of factors. This might lead the unwary clinician to alter therapy based on incorrect assumptions.

C-REACTIVE PROTEIN AND OTHER ACUTE-PHASE PROTEINS

Acute-phase proteins are frequently elevated in patients with RA. These proteins are produced predominantly by the liver in response to certain cytokines, many of which are produced in excess in patients with RA. As discussed in Chapter 22, the extent and time course of responses of acute-phase proteins are quite diverse. Intuitively, one would expect that proteins that respond promptly with dramatic increases in levels would be the most useful for following disease activity. In contrast to proteins such as α_1-macroglobulin and C3, which generally only increase approximately 1.5-fold over baseline, C-reactive protein, serum amyloid A, serum amyloid P, and α_2-macroglobulin may increase several hundred– to even a thousand-fold. Fibrinogen, the major determinant of the ESR, may only increase about two- to fourfold above baseline levels. Moreover, serum amyloid A and C-reactive protein increase very rapidly, over hours, after the acute-phase response is initiated. They peak in 1 to 3 days and levels return rapidly back to baseline after the acute event has resolved (139, 140). Fibrinogen, on the other hand, may not reach peak levels until much later and may take another week to return to baseline (141). Metabolism of C-reactive protein does not appear to be altered in patients with RA, indicating that increases in C-reactive protein reflect enhanced production (142).

Although three proteins—C-reactive protein, serum amyloid A, and serum amyloid P—are markedly elevated in RA, only measurement of C-reactive protein is now broadly available. Sensitive enzyme-linked immunosorbent assays (ELISAs) that can detect C-reactive protein in normal individuals have become available. Studies evaluating C-reactive protein and disease activity date back nearly 30 years. In 1972, McConkey et al. (143) followed 187 patients with RA for 3 years and concluded that acute-phase proteins, particularly C-reactive protein, reflected exacerbations and remissions of this disease (143). C-reactive protein better reflected disease activity than either haptoglobin or the ESR. Mallya and colleagues (144) studied 99 patients with RA in a more quantitative manner. An evaluation of disease activity using an index consisting of morning stiffness, visual analogue scale, grip strength, articular index, hemoglobin levels, and ESR correlated with levels of C-reactive protein (144). In this study, it was noted that C-reactive protein was a better indicator of disease activity than ESR. C-reactive protein has also been shown to correlate with hand bone mineral density, grip strength, and disability (145).

C-reactive protein has also been correlated with radiographic evidence of disease progression. Larsen followed 200 patients with long-standing RA (146) and evaluated serial radiographs of the hand using a conventional scoring method (147). C-reactive protein levels correlated with both a defined erosion and damage score, and also correlated with progression of the erosion score. On the other hand, ESR did not correlate with either the damage or erosion score in individuals with disease duration of less than 10 years. Because C-reactive protein changes fairly rapidly in response to changes in the inflammatory response, serial measures of C-reactive protein may better reflect overall disease activity than a single reading. Van Leeuwen et al. (148) measured C-reactive protein every month for 2 years in 110 patients with newly diagnosed RA. They derived a score reflecting integration of C-reactive protein levels over time and compared it with radiographic progression of disease. Radiographic progression correlated with time-integrated C-reactive protein levels; the time-integrated C-reactive protein levels also predicted radiographic progression (149). Similar observations have been made using time-integrated ESR (150).

As patients with RA respond to therapeutic interventions, concomitant decreases in levels of C-reactive protein occur. Gold sodium thiomalate treatment in 50 patients resulted in significant decrements in IL-6, which paralleled decrements in C-reactive protein and ESR (151). Other studies have shown similar reduction in acute-phase proteins with other conventional disease-modifying antirheumatic drugs (DMARDs), including sulfasalazine, penicillamine, and methotrexate (152–155). CRP levels and ESR are also dramatically reduced in patients treated with TNF-α-blocking biologic reagents (156,157). Similarly, corticosteroids, administered as either an intraarticular injection or systemic treatment, also produce significant reductions in both C-reactive protein and ESR (158–161). In contrast, most studies suggest that nonsteroidal antiinflammatory drugs (NSAIDs) alone do not result in reduction of C-reactive protein in RA.

Alterations in C-reactive protein also appear to correlate with disease progression in patients treated with slow-acting drugs. Scott and colleagues (161) evaluated 43 patients with RA of less than 4 years' duration who were treated with either hydroxychloroquine or penicillamine and followed for 12 months. Both drugs resulted in equivalent decrements in disease activity as measured by an articular index and

C-reactive protein levels. Furthermore, radiographic progression of disease in each group was equivalent. In a series of 150 patients with RA treated with either dapsone, penicillamine, or gold, the groups could not be differentiated at 6 months regardless of the changes in sedimentation rate or C-reactive protein levels. There was no further radiographic progression over the next 6 months of observation in patients in whom there was normalization of C-reactive protein levels and ESR. In contrast, patients in whom C-reactive protein levels did not consistently normalize had significant radiographic progression (160). More recent studies have confirmed the findings that normalization or reduction of C-reactive protein significantly slows radiographic progression (162,163) and is associated with functional improvement as measured by the Health Assessment Questionnaire (163).

Measurement of levels of many other acute-phase proteins is either not routinely available to the clinician or has not been extensively evaluated. Levels of β_2-microglobulin, transferrin, ceruloplasmin, α_1-antiprotease, and antichymotrypsin are elevated in patients with RA (164–168). Preliminary studies have suggested that levels of serum amyloid A may parallel changes seen with C-reactive protein (169). Similarly, α_1-acid glycoprotein levels are elevated in the serum of patients with RA and generally correlate with disease activity. Levels of α_1-acid glycoprotein also have been shown to correlate better with C-reactive protein than with ESR (170) and also correlate with radiographic disease progression (171).

In summary, these observations indicate that certain acute-phase proteins such as C-reactive protein correlate with disease activity in patients with RA. Moreover, clinical responses to therapy may be predicted by decrements in C-reactive protein levels. Because patients differ considerably in terms of the specific joints involved and the number of joints involved, a systemic measure of disease activity may not reflect the course of an individual joint. Measurement of acute-phase proteins is most useful in evaluating individual responses because a patient with aggressive disease involving multiple small joints may have an acute-phase protein response that is less than that which occurs in a patient who has fewer, but larger, joints involved. Even with these measures, care must be taken in their clinical utilization. C-reactive protein and other acute-phase proteins are produced in response to certain cytokines and are at best surrogate markers of disease activity. It is certainly conceivable that there may be situations where C-reactive protein does not accurately reflect disease activity. For example, protease inhibitors might interfere with tissue injury and limit radiographic progression, without affecting cytokine and acute-phase protein responses.

CYTOKINES AND RELATED PROTEINS

A number of cytokines and related molecules, predominantly of macrophage or fibroblast origin, have been detected in either the serum, synovium, or synovial fluid of patients with RA (172). Many of these molecules play an important role in mediating the disease and may be responsible for regulating levels of proteases and other proteins that are directly responsible for the tissue injury and inflammation seen in RA. Measurement of these proteins may predict the course of the disease. Alternatively, since a number of cytokines are present and likely responsible for the full presentation of the disease, it may be that measurement of a single cytokine or, for that matter, a small battery of cytokines will not fully predict the course.

Early studies in RA frequently employed bioassays to measure certain cytokines. An advantage of these assays is that they measure biologically active material. Unfortunately, these assays are frequently cumbersome and time consuming, and drugs and other related molecules may interfere (173). As a result, they have not been extensively used. With the development of sensitive ELISA assays, some studies have been performed correlating disease activity with levels of specific molecules. In contrast to bioassays, these results may not reflect biologically active material and may not distinguish cytokine conjugated with a soluble receptor or an antagonist from the free form of the molecule.

TNF-α and IL-6 have been the subject of several studies in patients with RA. IL-6 and, to a lesser extent, TNF-α are responsible for inducing production of acute-phase proteins. Both of these cytokines also have deleterious effects on articular cartilage. In a study of 35 patients treated with corticosteroids, levels of TNF-α and IL-6 generally correlated with serum levels of hyaluronan, and therefore it was suggested that these levels may correlate with tissue injury (174). Not surprisingly, both TNF-α and IL-6 correlated with levels of ESR, C-reactive protein, and fibrinogen (174,175). In this study, however, 14% of the patients had no detectable levels of TNF-α in the serum, and approximately 50% had levels no different from those of normal controls (174). Similarly, in 10% of the patients there was no detectable IL-6, and approximately one third of the patients had levels that were no different from those of normal controls. In other studies, absence of detectable circulating levels of TNF-α was noted in up to 30% of patients (173, 176). Correlation of IL-6, but not TNF-α, with C-reactive protein and ESR has been noted in other studies (175,177). Interestingly, after treatment with methotrexate, the correlation between IL-6 and C-reactive protein was lost (177). Treatment of patients who have RA with methotrexate or azathioprine with clinical improvement resulted in decreases in levels of IL-6, but not TNF-α (173). Similarly, in a study examining the effects of the investigational drug tenidap, clinical improvement, and decreases in IL-6, C-reactive protein, and ESR were noted but no changes in TNF-α serum levels were noted (170). Levels of IL-6 have also been shown to decline after chrysotherapy (175). However, neither IL-6 nor TNF-α consistently correlate with clinical parameters of disease activity, including duration of disease, Ritchie articular index, duration of morning stiffness, erosion score, or number of tender joints (173). Moreover, TNF-α levels do not correlate with bone erosion scores (178). In one prognostic study, IL-6 was shown to correlate with disease activity and was a better clinical outcome marker than TNF-α (179).

Soluble TNF-receptor (sTNFR) can be detected in serum from patients with RA. sTNFR exists in both a 55- and 75-kd form, and may play a role in neutralizing the activity of TNF. Levels of both of these proteins are increased in RA. Levels of the 55-kd form have been observed to decrease with methotrexate therapy (173). sTNFR levels do not correlate with TNF-α levels or with clinical measures of disease activity (173).

IL-1β production by mononuclear cells from patients with RA is higher than controls. Of note, this increased production correlated with the increased resting energy expenditure seen in patients with RA (180). Based on this observation, IL-1β and TNF-α have been postulated to account for these findings and the overall decreased body mass seen in patients with rheumatoid cachexia. Measurement of IL-1β in sera of patients with RA is not a useful measure of disease activity, however, because it is infrequently detected in sera (169,176).

IL-10, a cytokine with both anti- and proinflammatory activity, is present in rheumatoid synovium. Increased levels of IL-10 have been found in synovial fluid and serum of patients with RA. However, IL-10 levels do not appear to correlate with standard measures of disease activity, including morning stiffness, global assessments, or joint counts (181). Furthermore, no correlations have been noted between IL-10 levels and laboratory measures of disease activity, including ESR, C-reactive protein, or with titers of rheumatoid factor.

A number of other cytokines have been detected in either serum or synovial fluid from patients with RA. Monocyte chemotactic factor has been found in synovial fluid (182–184). This molecule is chemotactic for monocytes and induces their activation. Leukemia inhibitory factor is produced by synovial cells and chondrocytes in response to a number of cytokines, including IL-1, IL-6, TGF-β, and TNF-α (185). It stimulates loss of proteoglycan from cartilage and induction of acute-phase proteins, and has been detected in synovial fluid. IgG2b-inducing activity has also been found in rheumatoid synovial fluid (186,187). This molecule is a T-cell replacing factor and induces IgG production. Other cytokines, including GM-CSF and TGF-β have also been detected in patients with RA, but data regarding measures of these cytokines in relation to disease activity and outcome are not yet available.

IL-2 receptors are expressed on activated T cells in response to IL-1. Activated T cells also release a truncated form of the α chain of the receptor, and these soluble receptors (sIL-2R) have been detected in serum and synovial fluid of patients with RA. Serum levels of the sIL-2R have been correlated with ESR (173,188), whereas synovial fluid levels of sIL-2R have been correlated with ESR and C-reactive protein. In some studies, levels of sIL-2R seem to correlate with both tender and swollen joint counts (188), whereas no correlation has been found in others (173,189). Levels of sIL-2R after therapy also have been variable (190–192) and have not been shown to be predictive of clinical outcomes in patients treated with either gold or sulfasalazine (189).

Intercellular adhesion molecule-1 (ICAM-1), is the counterreceptor for leukocyte function–associated antigen-1 (CD11a/CD18) and MAC-1 (CD11b/CD18). ICAM-1 is cleaved from the surface of expressing cells and has been measured in serum of patients with RA. Serum levels of ICAM-1 have been found to be higher than synovial fluid levels. There is a general correlation with joint score and ESR, but not C-reactive protein, morning stiffness, or global assessment of disease activity (193).

CONNECTIVE TISSUE PROTEINS

Considerable effort has been directed toward measuring components of cartilage or other connective tissue in serum, urine, or synovial fluid from patients with RA. To a large extent, these efforts have been hampered by the fact that many of the molecules studied are not limited to articular cartilage. Nonetheless, measurement of some of these molecules may have utility for clinical research and appears to be a fruitful area for further investigation.

Hyaluronic acid is synthesized by a variety of cellular elements, including synovial lining cells from patients with RA (194–197). Hyaluronate synthesis is increased by TNF-α and IL-1β. In general, hyaluronate levels are increased in the serum of patients with RA and parallel levels of acute-phase proteins and clinical measures of disease activity (198–202). Levels of hyaluronate are decreased when therapy with corticosteroids is instituted. Elevated levels of hyaluronate may predict the development of erosions in patients with very early RA (203), and may predict large rather than small joint damage (204).

Aggrecan levels also have been measured in the serum of patients with RA. Aggrecan consists of a core protein and attached proteoglycan side chains. It is retained in cartilage through its interaction with hyaluronic acid stabilized by link protein. Progressive proteolytic degradation of aggrecans occurs with the release of keratan- and chondroitin sulfate–rich proteoglycan fragments. Levels of aggrecan can be measured by immunoassays. High levels of fragments of proteoglycan are seen in synovial fluid of patients with RA. Individuals with high levels tend to have more destruction of involved joints (205,206). Levels of keratan sulfate, a sugar moiety from proteoglycan, are inversely correlated with measures of acute-phase proteins and IL-1β and TNF-α (207). It has been suggested, but not supported by experimental data, that this apparent paradox may be explained by a decrease in substrate related to the impaired synthesis of proteoglycan seen in the presence of inflammatory cytokines (208).

C-propeptide is a molecule that may reflect type II collagen synthesis. This protein is released from procollagen as collagen is incorporated into fibrils. Despite the fact that a number of inflammatory cytokines inhibit cartilage synthesis, C-propeptides levels have been noted to be increased in serum of patients with RA (209). Whether this represents compensatory collagen production in involved cartilage is not yet clear. The α chain of type II collagen has been detected in rheumatoid synovial fluids and serum. Levels in serum are not elevated above levels in normal individuals, however, suggesting that this may not be a useful measure in following the course of RA (208).

In some studies, an epitope has been detected in cartilage from patients with RA that is not usually found in normal cartilage, but is present on the largest aggrecan molecules of fetal cartilage (210). This epitope is found in increased levels in synovial fluid obtained from patients with RA, and levels are increased in association with increased synovial fluid leukocyte counts (211). Although it has been proposed as a marker for proteoglycan synthesis, it is not clear that this is the case. Serum levels are detectable in only half the patients with active RA (211).

High concentrations of a large-molecular-weight cartilage protein termed cartilage oligomeric protein are found in synovial fluid. This anionic pentameric molecule appears to be specific for cartilage. Serum levels are detectable in some patients with rapidly progressive erosive disease (212) and appear to be predictive of large joint damage in patients with RA (213,214).

Other molecules have been evaluated as possible measures of disease activity in RA. In many tissues other than skin, collagen is cross-linked through aldehydes derived from lysine and hydroxylysine. In cartilage, this cross-linker is predominantly in the hydroxylysyl form, pyridinoline, which is also present in bone. Both lysine and hydroxylysine forms are excreted by the kidney and can be detected in the urine by high-performance liquid chromatography (HPLC). Urinary levels in patients with RA are elevated and have been correlated with ESR, and more closely with C-reactive protein, as well as with pain and, inversely, with grip strength (215). The lysyl-pyridinoline form, called deoxypyridinoline, is the major collagen cross-linker in bone, and its levels are also increased in the urine of patients with RA (216). This has been only weakly correlated with ESR.

Measurement of pyridinoline and deoxypyrodinoline may be complicated by several factors. Patients taking corticosteroids may have further elevation of their urinary levels of these metabolites, despite clinical improvement, presumably related to increased bone resorption associated with glucocorticoid usage (216). Bisphosphonates, on the other hand, decrease levels of this cross-linker (217,218). Because measurement of collagen cross-links is performed on urine, there is concern about following levels in individuals with changing renal function. In patients with stable renal function, urinary levels of these cross-linkers have not been found to be correlated with creatinine clearance (219). Sulfasalazine interferes with detection of these cross-linkers when measured by HPLC (220).

Osteocalcin (bone Gla protein) is sometimes detectable in serum from patients with RA. This relatively small molecule is released from bone osteoblasts. Unfortunately, its serum half-life is quite short and several factors affect its measurement (221,222). Indeed, there is daily variability in its serum levels, with peaks at midday and nadirs at night. Conflicting results have been obtained from studies of patients with early RA or with established disease (223–227). Although the mean osteocalcin levels were no different in patients with RA compared with normal controls, patients with more severe disease radiographically had higher serum levels (228). In older patients with RA, levels were increased and correlated with ESR (229). Penicillamine and antimalarials increased serum osteocalcin levels, whereas acute-phase protein levels were decreased (224).

Bone sialoprotein is a phosphoprotein that constitutes about 12% of the noncollagenous bone proteins and has been implicated in bone mineralization. Synovial fluid levels of the molecule correlated with radiographic evidence of knee damage (228). There was no correlation between serum concentrations and the degree of joint damage, however.

Ultimately, cartilage destruction in RA is mediated by enzymatic degradation and in particular by a range of matrix metalloproteinases (MMPs). MMP-1 and MMP-3 are elevated in the synovial fluid and serum of patients with RA. Moreover, MMP-3 levels correlate with other inflammatory markers and decrease with therapy (230,231).

AUTOANTIBODIES OTHER THAN RHEUMATOID FACTOR

In addition to rheumatoid factor (see Chapter 58), a plethora of autoantibodies have been detected in sera obtained from patients with RA. Many are found in a minority of patients or have not been demonstrated to have any specific pathologic or clinical association, however. Cataloging each of these is beyond the scope of this chapter, which focuses on autoantibodies that either have been used in clinical practice or that appear to have some predictive or discriminatory value.

Antinuclear Antibodies

Antinuclear antibodies have been reported in up to 60% of patients with RA (232–234). The presence of these antibodies does not necessarily indicate that there are overlapping rheumatic features. The presence of antinuclear antibodies in the serum of patients with RA is associated with more severe articular disease and, in one study, with the presence of vasculitis (233). Patients with RA and neutropenia frequently have antinuclear antibodies of the IgE or IgD isotype (235,236). When patients with RA are studied, those who have features of Sjögren syndrome are more likely to have detectable antinuclear antibodies (234). Specific antinuclear antibodies are sometimes detectable in sera from patients with RA who do not have evidence of other rheumatic diseases. For example, Sm and double-stranded DNA (dsDNA) antibodies are found in about 2% and 3%, respectively, of RA sera, and antibodies to ribonucleoprotein have been found in 10% (237,238). Antibodies to Sjögren syndrome antigen-A (SS-A) and Sjögren syndrome antigen-B (SS-B) are often detected in RA sera, particularly in patients who have features of Sjögren syndrome (234, 238,239).

Anticyclic Citrullinated Peptide Antibodies

Antiperinuclear factor (APF), antikeratin antibodies (AKAs), and antibodies to Sa antigen are antibody systems described and analyzed over the past four decades that appeared to have sensitivity and perhaps specificity rivaling or exceeding that of rheumatoid factor. Despite their apparent specificity for RA, clinical use of these respective autoantibodies was limited due to exacting technical and substrate requirements required for performing the assays reliably. The more recent discovery that citrulline is an essential constituent of the antigenic determinant of APF, AKA, and anti-Sa has permitted the development of standardized substrates for more reliable detection of these antibodies (240–243). Referred to presently as anti–cyclic citrullinated peptide (anti-CCP) antibodies, a brief review of the characterization of the anti-CCP antibodies is useful to appreciate their significance in RA.

Antibodies directed against a perinuclear factor expressed in human buccal epithelial cells and reactive with keratohyalin granules were described to be frequently present in sera obtained from patients with RA (244). Depending on the serum dilution evaluated, APFs have been found in 70% to 90% of patients with RA (245,246). The specificity of these antibodies for RA may exceed 80% (245, 246). Correlations between the presence and titer of antiperinuclear antibodies and severity of disease have been inconsistent, and these antibodies do not appear to correlate with extraarticular features (246–248). Assays for antiperinuclear antibodies were problematic, because only a small percentage of human buccal mucosal cells have sufficient concentration of antigen to be useful, and cultured cells do not express a sufficient concentration of the antigen.

Antibodies directed against "keratin" occur in patients with RA (249–254). Initial studies using rat esophageal epithelium as the substrate demonstrated that sera from patients with RA frequently had antibodies that bound to the stratum corneum. These antibodies, which also react with the stratum corneum of human skin, are found in patients with more severe disease (253). In a large series of over 4,000 patients from several laboratories, antikeratin antibodies above a certain titer were rarely found in patients who did not have RA, and it was concluded that the presence of this antibody was the most specific serologic test for RA (249). In another study of 39 patients with RA, 26% had antikeratin antibodies in predisease serum samples (254). The patients with antikeratin antibodies, also had rheumatoid factor (RF) detected by the latex fixation test.

Based on the distribution of staining in these immunofluorescence studies, it was assumed that these antibodies bound to cytokeratins. Studies using purified proteins later demonstrated that these antibodies predominantly recognize filaggrin, an intermediate filament-associated protein that plays a role in aggregation of cytokeratin filaments during mammalian epidermal terminal differentiation (255). Sera from patients with RA react with the neutral and acidic isoforms of filaggrin. However, immunoabsorption with filaggrin did not completely abolish binding to the stratum corneum, leaving open the possibility that there may be other antigens partially responsible for reactivity. In one study of patients with RA, 75% had antibodies to filaggrin that correlated with the intensity of staining to rat esophageal stratum corneum, whereas in patients with other rheumatic diseases or healthy controls, only 11% and 3%, respectively, had evidence of antibodies to filaggrin (255). These antibodies have been detected in sera of patients with RF-negative erosive arthritis (256).

Subsequent colocalization studies indicated that antibodies to keratin-bound filaggrin localize with the perinuclear granules, and titers of "antikeratin" were found to correlate with antiperinuclear antibodies (257). These findings raised the issue of whether these systems were measuring identical or related antigens and studies comparing serum from RA patients for reactivity in both systems indicated a significant, but not complete, degree of overlap (256,258–260). Because the conversion of arginine residues in filaggrin to citrulline by peptidylarginine deaminase was known to be a posttranslational occurrence during cell differentiation, the role of citrulline in the epitope specificity of APF and AKA was examined (240). Affinity-purified RA sera–derived antibodies to citrulline-containing peptides were found to be reactive with filaggrin and positive in traditional immunofluorescence-based assays for APF and AKA (240). With confirmation of the citrulline moiety as the determinant on proteins recognized by APF and AKA (241), standardized CCP substrates that mimic conformational citrullinated filaggrin epitopes have been used to develop successive generation (CCP1, then CCP2) ELISAs that are now widely available for detection of anti-CCP.

Anti-Sa is another antibody that may be detected in sera of patients with early RA. This antibody recognizes posttranslationally modified vimentin, a cytoskeletal intermediate filament protein found in human spleen or placenta mesenchymal cells. Anti-Sa is present in about one third of patients with early RA (261,262) and ultimately in about one half. It occurs in about 30% of patients who are seronegative and in about one half of seropositive patients. It is rarely seen in patients who do not have RA. Recent studies indicate that antibodies in RA sera recognizing Sa have specificity for citrullinated vimentin, and anti-Sa are now considered part of the anti-CCP system (242).

The context in which anti-CCP antibodies likely develop in RA is of interest. Several isotypes of peptidylarginine deaminase (PAD) have been identified in RA synovium that induce citrullination of synovial proteins, and citrullinated proteins as well as local production of anti-CCP has been demonstrated in rheumatoid joints (263,264). The large numbers of neutrophils frequently present in rheumatoid joints may also comprise a potential source of PAD (265). The additional finding that citrullinated peptides have greater affinity for HLA DR4A (DRB1*0401 or *0404) antigen binding grooves relative to corresponding arginine containing peptides provides a linkage of citrullinated peptide–induced immune responses to the shared epitope hypothesis of RA pathogenesis (266).

The utility and role of anti-CCP in the early diagnosis and management of RA is still evolving. Given that the specificity of anti-CCP for RA is 95% to 98% and the sensitivity of CCP2 ELISA reagents for detecting anti-CCP in patients with early RA approximates 70%, anti-CCP may be useful in predicting which patients with early, undifferentiated synovitis are likely to develop RA (267). A recent study using stored sera found anti-CCP to be present 1 to 5 years before the onset of arthritis (268). The presence of anti-CCP appears to be a significant risk factor for predicting erosive disease, equaling or exceeding that of the presence of IgM rheumatoid factor (269,270).

Antibodies to Rheumatoid Arthritis Nuclear Antigens

Antigens that have been termed RA nuclear antigens (RANAs) are frequently recognized by sera obtained from patients with RA. Some of these antibodies have rheumatoid factor activity. These antibodies also react with synthetic peptides corresponding to segments of Epstein-Barr virus nuclear antigen 1 (EBNA-1) (271,272). The majority of seropositive patients with RA are positive for RANA. Antibodies are also found that recognize a 33-kd nuclear protein (RA33) identified as the A2 protein of the heterogeneous nuclear ribonucleoprotein (273). This antibody has been detected in approximately 35% of patients with RA. Antibodies to RA33 are detectable in seronegative patients with RA with greater frequency than in seropositive patients (273). Apart from mixed connective tissue disease, where the antibody may be detected in nearly two thirds of patients, it is rarely detected in other rheumatic diseases (274). The presence of antibodies to RA33 does not appear to correlate with other antibodies seen in RA, including rheumatoid factor, antiperinuclear antibodies, or antikeratin antibodies (274). The presence of antibodies to RA33 may correlate with evidence of more severe disease, as indicated by radiographic erosions and elevated ESR (274). Perhaps more interestingly, antibodies to RA33 may occur in the sera of patients with early RA, even prior to clinical onset (273). Although these antibodies are not present in all patients destined to develop RA, they rarely occur in sera from patients with other diseases.

Antineutrophil Cytoplasmic Antibodies

Antineutrophil cytoplasmic antibodies (ANCAs) are also detected in serum from patients with RA. ANCAs are present in roughly one third of patients with RA (275). Most of these antibodies are perinuclear ANCA (pANCA) (276–278). The pANCA is found more often in patients with long-standing or active disease, in patients with Felty syndrome (276,277,279,280), and in a group with RA and renal disease (281). Cytoplasmic ANCA (cANCA) appear to be infrequent in patients with RA. Antibodies directed against lactoferrin are found more often in sera from patients with RA than antibodies to myeloperoxidase (275,276,279,282). Antibodies to lactoferrin have been found more frequently in patients with rheumatoid vasculitis (275,283,284), but this has not been a uniform finding (276,285).

Antibodies to Collagen and Lamins

Anticollagen antibodies are of interest because of their potential as disease mediators. Indeed, antibodies to type II collagen have been found in sera, synovial fluid, and eluates from cartilage of patients with RA (286,287). B cells obtained from some rheumatoid synovium have been shown to produce anticollagen antibodies (288). Despite the considerable homology between type II collagen and the collagen-like region of complement component C1q, studies evaluating cross-reactivity between these two proteins have been negative (289). Overall, the prevalence of these antibodies varies widely, perhaps related to methodology or patient selection (290,291). However, studies attempting to correlate synovial fluid antibodies to type II collagen and cartilage damage as measured by release of glycosaminoglycans into the synovial fluid have not shown an association (292,293).

Antibodies to the intermediate filament proteins lamins are found in sera of patients with RA, as well as systemic lupus erythematosus and chronic active hepatitis (294–296). Antibodies from patients with RA are more likely to bind to the second coil of the central α-helical domain of the protein (296). In patients with RA who have detectable serum levels of these antibodies, there does not appear to be an association with liver disease, but the antibodies do occur in patients with milder, less erosive disease (295).

Antibodies to Cytokines and Other Functional Proteins

Several antibodies have been detected in sera of patients with RA that have the potential for modulating disease activity. Lipocortin 1 may have a role in mediating the antiinflammatory effects of glucocorticoids. In a series of patients with RA with high titers of antibodies to lipocortin 1, clinical and lymphopenic responses to glucocorticoids were found to be blunted (297). Antibodies have also been detected to IL-8 and TNF-α in sera of patients with RA (298,299). The antibodies to TNF-α appear to neutralize the function of this important cytokine (298). Antibodies to IL-8 correlate with measures of disease activity such as C-reactive protein (300). Occasional patients with RA have antibodies to clotting factors such as factor VIII (301, 302). These patients may have catastrophic hemorrhagic complications. Antibodies to soluble vascular cell adhesion molecule-1 have been detected in serum from some patients with RA with a peripheral neuropathy (303). Antibodies to pyruvate dehydrogenase (frequently detected in patients with primary biliary cirrhosis) are detected in approximately 10% of patients with RA and approximately 25% of those with Sjögren syndrome (304). Those with Sjögren syndrome are more likely to have elevated liver function tests and extraglandular features of the disease. Antibodies to insulin are detected in some patients with RA and appear to be related to prior therapy with penicillamine, because titers decrease after drug withdrawal (305).

CHOLESTEROL AND SERUM LIPIDS

As with many inflammatory disorders, changes in plasma lipids and lipoproteins occur in RA that, to some extent, reflect the acute-phase response. Total cholesterol levels are typically decreased (306). This is accounted for predominantly by decreases in high-density lipoprotein (HDL) and low-density lipoprotein (LDL) cholesterol (307). Very-low-density lipoprotein (VLDL) cholesterol is for the most part unchanged. HDL obtained from patients with RA or volunteers undergoing an experimentally induced acute-phase response is enriched with serum amyloid A (308,309). Serum amyloid A may substitute for apolipoprotein A-I in HDL, resulting in a particle that is denser and has a shorter half-life (308). This reduced A-I may be one factor leading to the increased atherosclerotic complications sometimes seen in patients with RA. Lipoprotein lipase activity and mass are diminished in sera of RA patients and the decrease correlates with acute-phase proteins such as C-reactive protein (310). This may also be associated with premature atherosclerosis by promoting macrophage lipid metabolism.

Triglyceride levels are decreased in patients with RA (311). Overall, fatty acid levels are normal, but there are decreases in linolenic and arachidonic acid with an increase in oleic acid levels (312,313).

OTHER SERUM COMPONENTS

Albumin levels typically are decreased in patients with RA and reflect decreased production, a finding typical of the acute-phase response (314–316). Studies of albumin metabolism have indicated that there is also increased metabolism, which generally correlates with disease activity (315). β_2-glycoprotein levels are also decreased in patients with RA (317).

Immunoglobulin levels in RA are either normal or increased (318,319). Levels of IgG and IgA are more likely to be increased, and increased levels can be noted in 15% to 20% of patients (318–320). Decreased galactosylation of serum IgG has also been described (321–326). Decreased B-cell galactosyl transferase activity may account for this finding (317). The IgG sugar moieties from patients with RA are more likely to terminate in *N*-acetylgalactosamine in lieu of galactose (323–325). These IgG molecules may aggregate more readily and function less efficiently (321,326). Overall, there is a modest correlation between the decreased IgG galactosylation and disease activity.

Cryoglobulins are occasionally detected in patients with RA and are usually associated with IgM rheumatoid factor activity (327). Immune complexes are detectable and correlate with extraarticular features and vasculitis (328). However, the variety of tests to measure immune complexes have not generally been found to be particularly useful in monitoring disease.

Total serum complement levels and levels of C3 and C4 are generally normal or slightly increased in RA (329,330). As evidenced by increased levels of C3d and C4d in the serum of untreated patients, there is increased metabolism of some of the early complement components (330). Levels of terminal complement components are frequently elevated (331). Occasional patients, representing up to 5% of those with RA, are hypocomplementemic (332). Hypocomplementemia usually occurs in patients with severe disease who seem predisposed to bacterial infections or in those with clinical evidence of systemic vasculitis (333, 334). Homozygous or heterozygous C2 deficiency has been reported in 1.4% of patients (335).

Except as noted earlier, routine chemistries are generally normal in patients with RA. Elevation of serum liver enzymes usually is modest and may not reflect abnormalities in the liver (336–339). Elevated levels of serum lactate dehydrogenase are likely neutrophil in origin, whereas 5-nucleotidase may be from synovium (336). An exception may be the modest elevations of alkaline phosphatase reported in about one third of patients (336). Bilirubin, serum glutamic-oxaloacetic transaminase, and glutamic-pyruvic transaminase levels are typically normal unless there is another hepatic insult (337–341). An evaluation of nearly 1,000 patients with RA uncovered either clinical or biochemical evidence of liver disease in only 0.7% (340). When liver biopsies are performed, changes, if present, are typically mild or nonspecific (341,342).

Although lean body mass is decreased in patients with RA, caloric intake generally approximates normal levels (180). Similarly, gastrointestinal absorption does not appear to be impaired. Decreased body mass, which, in its severe form, has been termed rheumatoid cachexia, has been correlated with increased resting metabolic rates and production of catabolic cytokines, particularly IL-1β and TNF-α (180). Preoperative nutritional support decreases the likelihood of complications in RA patients undergoing joint replacement (343).

Intake of a number of trace elements and vitamins, including vitamin E, folic acid, pyridoxine, magnesium, and zinc, is marginal in patients with RA (180). Interestingly, younger patients are more likely to have deficient intake than their older counterparts. Despite decreased intake, levels of these vitamins and minerals are normal in both older and younger patients. The decrease in folate intake may have clinical relevance, however, because folate supplementation appears to decrease the risk for methotrexate-induced side effects without altering efficacy (344,345).

In comparison with healthy controls, vitamin A and E levels are lower in RA (346). These vitamins have primary antioxidant capacity. Decreases in vitamin A levels are associated with decreased levels of retinol-binding protein, which is produced in the liver by a zinc-dependent enzyme. Decreased levels of retinol-binding protein are correlated with low zinc levels. Decrements in vitamin E levels are more frequently seen in individuals with seropositive disease.

Vitamin B_6 levels are normal or decreased in patients with RA. Vitamin B_6 is an important cofactor involved in protein and energy metabolism. Total vitamin B_6 includes pyridoxine, pyridoxal, pyridoxamine, and pyridoxal-5′-phosphate (PLP). PLP is the only form that is metabolically active, and it is formed from the other nonphosphorylated forms by a series of tightly controlled enzymatic steps. Levels of PLP in plasma are decreased in patients with RA, and the decrement has been inversely correlated with spontaneous production of TNF-α, but not IL-1β, by mononuclear cells cultured *ex vivo* as well as directly with other measures of disease activity, including ESR and pain on a visual analogue scale (347). In this same study, PLP levels in erythrocytes were noted to be normal. Exogenous administration of vitamin B_6 does not appear to be helpful (348).

In contrast to these findings, serum levels of copper are moderately increased (349,350). As might be expected, ceruloplasmin, an acute-phase protein, is elevated and accounts for the increased levels of serum copper (351). Selenium, another antioxidant, and some other trace metals, including aluminum, strontium, and chromium, are decreased, whereas levels of barium, cesium, tin, and molybdenum are elevated (352–356).

URINARY AND RENAL FINDINGS

Routine urinalysis in RA is generally normal. Protein detectable by dipstick analysis at greater than trace levels is observed in less than 10% of patients (135). Proteinuria, as noted by routine dipstick analysis, related to RA is most often associated with treatment or, rarely, with the development of amyloidosis. However, using more sensitive measures, proteinuria is detected in over one-half of patients with RA but in only 15% of controls, and only in a minority could the findings be related to drugs or vasculitis (357). The appearance of cellular elements is also unusual and should prompt a search for secondary causes. Patients with secondary Sjögren syndrome and vaginal dryness appear to be more susceptible to urinary tract infections and chronic pyuria (358).

Modest decreases (30%–40%) in creatinine clearance, which have not been clearly attributed to drug therapy, occur in patients with RA (359). In contrast, serum creatinine levels are slightly decreased, reflecting decreased body mass (360). Examination of tissue obtained from renal biopsies reveals infrequent or mild abnormalities. When abnormalities are noted, mesangial changes are most frequently seen (361). Immunofluorescence studies for immunoglobulin and complement are typically negative.

PLEURAL FLUIDS

Abnormalities of the pleura are common in RA. In autopsy studies, up to 70% of patients with RA had detectable pleural abnormalities (362); however, only about 5% have clinically detectable abnormalities (363,364). Patients with pleural effusions are usually older men with long-standing disease (364,365). Acute rheumatoid pleural effusions are usually exudative, but often have a normal pH and glucose. Chronic rheumatoid effusions are also typically exudative in character, with elevations of total protein and lactate dehydrogenase. Additionally, chronic effusions typically have a very low glucose level, which is thought to be due to thickening of the pleura and decreased diffusion of glucose into the pleural space (366,367). Increased production of lactic acid and decreased pleural fluid pH (often to pH 7.0) are observed in association with the low glucose.

Pleural fluid complement levels are usually depressed (368,369), but with elevated levels of terminal activation components and an increased ratio of C4d to C4 compared with that seen in malignant or tuberculous effusions (370). Rheumatoid factor levels are elevated, and there is evidence of local production (371). Rheumatoid pleural effusions are cellular, with the predominant components being neutrophils and monocytes. Frank empyemas are not rare. Pleural fluid cytology is somewhat distinctive, with findings of multinucleated giant cells, elongated macrophages, and a background of granular necrotic debris (372–374). In one series of 2,800 pleural fluid samples, 12 of 15 samples from patients with RA had these characteristic cytologic findings (375); however, they were found in none of the non-RA fluids. Others have noted similar findings in tuberculous pleural effusions (376). Hyaluronan levels in RA pleural effusions are elevated and similar to those seen with malignancies (377).

ELECTROPHYSIOLOGIC STUDIES

When present, abnormalities on electrophysiologic testing of patients with RA represent unusual extraarticular complications of the disease (378–380). Myopathic findings may be seen in those with complications due to drug therapy or in those who have overlap symptoms. The mild distal sensory neuropathy occasionally seen in RA may be detected as slowing during nerve conduction velocity testing. The less common mononeuritis multiplex seen as a manifestation of rheumatoid vasculitis can readily be detected with electrophysiologic studies. Other abnormalities may reflect compression neuropathies due to either synovium or mechanical deformity. In one study, 20% of patients with RA had electrophysiologic evidence of carpal tunnel syndrome (379). Abnormalities on either electromyograms or nerve conduction studies are sometimes seen in patients who have entrapment of the ulnar nerve at the elbow or tarsal tunnel syndrome. Patients with RA who have cervical spine involvement may have evidence of cervical radiculopathies or upper motor neuron findings in the lower vertebral segments (381). Cranial nerve abnormalities are sometimes present in those with vertical subluxation of the odontoid, including decreased sensation over the ophthalmic and maxillary divisions of cranial nerve V.

REFERENCES

1. Engstedt L, Strandberg O. Haematological data and clinical activity of the rheumatoid diseases. *Acta Med Scand* 1966;180:13.
2. Samson D, Haliday D, Gumpel JM. Role of ineffective erythropoiesis in the anaemia of rheumatoid arthritis. *Ann Rheum Dis* 1977;36:181–185.
3. Freireich EJ, Ross JF, Bayles TB, et al. Radioactive iron metabolism and erythrocyte survival studies of the mechanism of the anemia associated with rheumatoid arthritis. *J Clin Invest* 1957;36:1043–1058.
4. Ebaugh FG, Peterson RE, Rodnan GP. Symposium on rheumatic diseases: anemia of rheumatoid arthritis. *Med Clin North Am* 1955;39: 489–498.
5. Roberts FD, Hagedon AB, Slocumb CH. Evaluation of the anemia of rheumatoid arthritis. *Blood* 1963;21:470–478.
6. Johansson SV, Strandberg PO. Haem biosynthesis studied in patients with rheumatoid arthritis. *J Clin Pathol* 1972;25:159–162.
7. McCrea PC. Marrow iron examination in the diagnosis of iron deficiency in rheumatoid arthritis. *Ann Rheum Dis* 1958;17:89–96.
8. Alexander WRM, Richmond J, Roy LMH. Nature of anaemia in rheumatoid arthritis. III. Survival of transfused erythrocytes in patients with rheumatoid arthritis. *Ann Rheum Dis* 1956;15:12–20.
9. Brendstrup P. Serum copper, serum iron and total iron-binding capacity of serum in patients with chronic rheumatoid arthritis. *Acta Med Scand* 1953;146:384–392.
10. Jeffrey JR. Some observations on anemia in rheumatoid arthritis. *Blood* 1953;8:502–518.
11. Nilsson F. Anemia problems in rheumatoid arthritis. *Acta Med Scand* 1948;210(suppl):1–193.
12. Blake DR, Bacon PA. Serum ferritin and rheumatoid disease. *BMJ* 1981;282:1273–1274.
13. Krantz SB. Pathogenesis and treatment of the anemia of chronic disease. *Am J Med Sci* 1994;307:353–359.
14. Nielsen OJ, Andersen LS, Hansen NE, et al. Serum transferrin receptors levels in anaemic patients with rheumatoid arthritis. *Scand J Clin Lab Invest* 1994;54:75–82.
15. Houston T, Moore M, Porter D, et al. Abnormal haem biosynthesis in anaemia of rheumatoid arthritis. *Ann Rheum Dis* 1994;53:167–170.
16. Baer AN, Dessypris EN, Goldwasser E, et al. Blunted erythropoietin response to anaemia in rheumatoid arthritis. *Br J Haematol* 1987;66: 559–564.
17. Hochberg MC, Arnold CM, Hogans BB, et al. Serum immunoreactive erythropoietin in rheumatoid arthritis: impaired response to anemia. *Arthritis Rheum* 1988;31:1318–1321.
18. Maury CPJ, Andersson LC, Teppo AM, et al. Mechanism of the anaemia in rheumatoid arthritis: demonstration of raised interleukin 1b concentrations in anemic patients and of interleukin 1 mediated suppression of normal erythropoiesis and proliferation of human erythroleukemia (HEL) cells *in vitro*. *Ann Rheum Dis* 1988;47:972–978.
19. Eastgate JA, Symons JA, Wood NC. Correlation of plasma interleukin 1 levels with disease activity in rheumatoid arthritis. *Lancet* 1988;2:706–709.
20. Means RT, Dessypris EN, Krantz SB, et al. Inhibition of human erythroid colony-forming units by interleukin-1 is mediated by gamma interferon. *J Cell Physiol* 1992;150:59–64.
21. Teppo AM, Maury CJ. Radioimmunoassay of tumor necrosis factor in serum. *Clin Chem* 1987;33:2024–2027.
22. Blick M, Sherwin SA, Rosenblum M, et al. Phase I study of recombinant tumor necrosis factor in cancer patients. *Cancer Res* 1987;47: 2986–2989.
23. Means RT, Dessypris EN, Krantz SB, et al. Inhibition of human erythroid colony-forming units by tumor necrosis factor requires accessory cells. *J Clin Invest* 1990;86:538–541.
24. Means RT, Krantz SB. Inhibition of human erythroid colony-forming units by tumor necrosis factor requires beta interferon. *J Clin Invest* 1993;91:416–419.
25. Vreugdenhil G, Lowenberg B, Van Eijk HG, et al. Tumor necrosis factor alpha is associated with disease activity and the degree of anemia in rheumatoid arthritis. *Eur J Clin Invest* 1992;22:488–493.
26. Vreugdenhil G, Lowenberg B, van Eijk HG, et al. Anaemia of chronic disease in rheumatoid arthritis. Raised serum interleukin-6 levels and effects of IL-6 and anti-IL-6 on *in vitro* erythropoiesis. *Rheumatol Int* 1990;10:127–130.
27. Jongen-Lavrencic M, Peeters HR, Wognum A, et al. Elevated levels of inflammatory cytokines in bone marrow of patients with rheumatoid arthritis and anemia of chronic disease. *J Rheumatol* 1997;24:1504–1509.
28. Pincus T, Olsen NJ, Russell IJ. Multicenter study of recombinant human erythropoietin in correction of anemia in rheumatoid arthritis. *Am J Med* 1990;89:161–168.
29. Peeters HR, Jongen-Lavrencic M, Bakker CH, et al. Recombinant human erythropoietin improves health-related quality of life in patients with rheumatoid arthritis and anaemia of chronic disease: utility measures correlate strongly with disease activity measures. *Rheumatol Int* 1999;18:201–206.
30. Xu WD, Firestein GS, Taetle R, et al. Cytokines in chronic inflammatory arthritis II granulocyte-macrophage colony-stimulating factor in rheumatoid synovial effusions. *J Clin Invest* 1989;83:876–882.
31. Johnson NJ, Dodd K. Symposium on rheumatic diseases: juvenile rheumatoid arthritis. *Med Clin North Am* 1955;39:459–487.
32. Toumbis A, Franklin EC, McEwen R. Clinical and serological observations in patients with juvenile rheumatoid arthritis and their relatives. *J Pediatr* 1963;62:463–473.
33. Bishop CR, Athens JW, Boggs DR, et al. Leukokinetic studies. XIII, A non-steady state kinetic evaluation of the mechanism of cortisone-induced granulocytosis. *J Clin Invest* 1968;47:249–260.
34. Sylvester RA, Pinals RS. Eosinophilia in rheumatoid arthritis. *Ann Allergy* 1970;28:565–568.
35. Winchester RJ, Koffler D, Litwin SD. Observations on eosinophilia of certain patients with rheumatoid arthritis. *Arthritis Rheum* 1971;14: 650–665.
36. Felty AR. Chronic arthritis in the adult, associated with splenomegaly and leucopenia. *Johns Hopkins Hosp Bull* 1924;35:16–23.
37. Ruderman M, Miller LM, Pinals RS. Clinical and serologic observations on 27 patients with Felty's syndrome. *Arthritis Rheum* 1968;11: 377–382.
38. Sienknecht CW, Urowitz MD, Pruzanski W. Felty's syndrome. Clinical and serological analysis of 34 cases. *Ann Rheum Dis* 1977;36: 500–507.
39. Heyn J. Non-articular Felty's syndrome. *Scand J Rheumatol* 1982;11: 47–51.
40. Laszlo J, Jones R, Silberman HR. Splenectomy for Felty's syndrome: clinicopathological study of 27 patients. *Arch Intern Med* 1978;138: 597–602.
41. Riley SM, Aldrete JS. Role of splenectomy in Felty's syndrome. *Am J Surg* 1975;130:51–52.
42. Breedveld FC, Fibbe WE, Hermans J. Factors influencing the incidence of infections in Felty's syndrome. *Arch Intern Med* 1987;147: 915–920.

43. Logue GL, Huang AT, Shimm DS. Failure of splenectomy in Felty's syndrome. The role of antibodies supporting granulocyte lysis by lymphocytes. *N Engl J Med* 1981;304:580–583.
44. Vincent PC, Levi JA, MacQueen A, et al. The mechanism of neutropenia in Felty's syndrome. *Br J Haematol* 1974;27:463–475.
45. Hollingsworth JW, Siegal ER, Creasey WA. Granulocyte survival in synovial exudate of patients with rheumatoid arthritis and other inflammatory joint diseases. *Yale J Biol Med* 1967;39:289–296.
46. Wiik A, Munthe E. Complement-fixing granulocyte-specific antinuclear factors in neutropenic cases of rheumatoid arthritis. *Immunology* 1974;26:1127–1134.
47. Weisman M, Zvaifler NJ. Cryoimmunoglobulinemia in Felty's syndrome. *Arthritis Rheum* 1976;19:103–110.
48. Andreis M, Hurd ER, Lospalluto J. Comparison of the presence of immune complexes in Felty's syndrome and rheumatoid arthritis. *Arthritis Rheum* 1978;21:310–315.
49. Hurd ER, Chubick A, Jasin HE. Increased C1q binding immune complexes in Felty's syndrome. *Arthritis Rheum* 1979;22:697–702.
50. Goldschmeding R, Breedveld FC, Engel Freit CP. Lack of evidence for the presence of neutrophil autoantibodies in the serum of patients with Felty's syndrome. *Br J Haematol* 1988;68:37–40.
51. Logue G. Felty's syndrome: granulocyte-bound immunoglobulin G and splenectomy. *Ann Intern Med* 1976;85:437–442.
52. Greenberg PL, Schrier SL. Granulopoiesis in neutropenic disorders. *Blood* 1973;41:753–760.
53. Gupta R, Robinson WA, Albrecht C. Granulopoietic activity in Felty's syndrome. *Ann Rheum Dis* 1975;34:156–161.
54. Goldberg J, Pinals RS. Felty's syndrome. *Semin Arthritis Rheum* 1980;10:52–65.
55. Duckham DJ, Rhyne RL, Smith FE. Retardation of colony growth of *in vitro* bone marrow culture using sera from patients with Felty's syndrome, disseminated lupus erythematosus (SLE), rheumatoid arthritis, and other disease states. *Arthritis Rheum* 1975;18:323–333.
56. Goldberg LS, Bacon PA, Bucknall RC. Inhibition of human bone marrow–granulocyte precursors by serum from patients with Felty's syndrome. *J Rheumatol* 1980;7:275–278.
57. Abdou NI, NaPombejara C, Balentine L. Suppressor cell-mediated neutropenia in Felty's syndrome. *J Clin Invest* 1978;61:738–743.
58. Bagby GC Jr, Gabourel JD. Neutropenia in three patients with rheumatic disorders: suppression of granulopoiesis by control-sensitive thymus-dependent lymphocytes. *J Clin Invest* 1979;64:72–82.
59. Slavin S, Liang MH. Cell-mediated autoimmune granulocytopenia in a case of Felty's syndrome. *Ann Rheum Dis* 1980;39:399–402.
60. Cooper SM, Roessner K, Ferriss JA. Increase in OKM1$^+$ granular lymphocytes in patients with rheumatoid arthritis. *Arthritis Rheum* 1987;30:1089–1096.
61. Linch DC, Newland AC, Turnbull AL. Unusual T cell proliferations and neutropenia in rheumatoid arthritis: comparison with classical Felty's syndrome. *Scand J Haematol* 1984;33:342–350.
62. Wallis WJ, Loughran TP, Kadin ME. Polyarthritis and neutropenia associated with circulating large granular lymphocytes. *Ann Intern Med* 1985;103:357–362.
63. Loughran TP, Starkebaum G, Kidd P. Clonal proliferation of large granular lymphocytes in rheumatoid arthritis. *Arthritis Rheum* 1988; 31:31–36.
64. Semenzato G, Pandolfi F, Chisesi T. The lymphoproliferative disease of granular lymphocytes: a heterogeneous disorder ranging from indolent to aggressive conditions. *Cancer* 1987;60:2971–2987.
65. Saway PA, Prasthoper EF, Barton JC, et al. Prevalence of granular lymphocyte proliferation in patients with rheumatoid arthritis and neutropenia. *Am J Med* 1989;86:303–307.
66. Bowman SJ, Sivakumaran M, Snowden N. The large granular lymphocyte syndrome with rheumatoid arthritis. *Arthritis Rheum* 1994; 37:1326–1330.
67. Gonzales-Chambers R, Przepiorka D, Winkelstein A. Lymphocyte subsets associated with T cell receptor b-chain gene rearrangements in patients with rheumatoid arthritis and neutropenia. *Arthritis Rheum* 1992;35:516–520.
68. Dhodapkar MV, Li CY, Lust JA. Clinical spectrum of clonal proliferations of T-large granular lymphocytes: a T-cell clonopathy of undetermined significance? *Blood* 1994;84:1620–1627.
69. Bowman SJ, Hall MA, Panayi GS, et al. T cell receptor alpha-chain and beta-chain junctional region homology in clonal CD3$^+$, CD8$^+$ T lymphocyte expansions in Felty's syndrome. *Arthritis Rheum* 1997;40:615–623.
70. Meliconi R, Kingsley GH, Pitzalis C. Analysis of lymphocyte phenotype and T cell receptor genotype in Felty's syndrome. *J Rheumatol* 1992;19:1058–1064.
71. Pistoia V, Zupo S, Corcione A. Production and inhibition of haemopoiesis by NK cells: a model for immune-mediated haemopoietic suppression. *Clin Exp Rheumatol* 1989;7(suppl 3):91–94.
72. Hansson M, Kiessling R, Andersson B. Human fetal thymus and bone marrow contain target cells for natural killer cells. *Eur J Immunol* 1981;11:8–12.
73. Degliantoni G, Murphy M, Kobayashi M. Natural killer (NK) cell-derived hematopoietic colony-inhibiting activity and NK cytotoxic factor. Relationship with tumour necrosis factor and synergism with immune interferon. *J Exp Med* 1985;162:1512–1530.
74. Wenger ME, Bole GG. Nitroblue tetrazolium dye reduction by peripheral leukocytes from rheumatoid arthritis and systemic lupus erythematosus patients measured by a histochemical and spectrophotometric method. *J Lab Clin Med* 1973;82:513–521.
75. Mowat AG, Baum J. Chemotaxis of polymorphonuclear leukocytes from patients with rheumatoid arthritis. *J Clin Invest* 1971;50:2541–2549.
76. King SL, Parker J, Cooper R. Polymorphonuclear leukocyte function in rheumatoid arthritis. *Br J Rheumatol* 1986;25:26–33.
77. Ozaki Y, Ohashi T, Niwa Y. Oxygen radical production by neutrophils from patients with bacterial infection and rheumatoid arthritis. *Inflammation* 1986;10:119–130.
78. Test ST. Effect of tumor necrosis factor on the generation of chlorinated oxidants by adherent human neutrophils. *J Leukoc Biol* 1991; 50:131–139.
79. Nathan CF. Neutrophil activation on biological surfaces. Massive secretion of hydrogen peroxide in response to products of macrophages and lymphocytes. *J Clin Invest* 1987;80:1550–1560.
80. Chatham WW, Turkiewicz A, Blackburn WD. Determinants of neutrophil HOCL generation: ligand-dependent responses and the role of surface adhesion. *J Leukoc Biol* 1994;56:654–660.
81. Chatham WW, Blackburn WD. Fixation of C3 to IgG attenuates neutrophil HOCl generation and collagenase activation. *J Immunol* 1993; 151:949–958.
82. Blackburn WD, Dohlman JG, Pillion DJ, et al. Apolipoprotein A-I diminishes neutrophil activation. *J Lipid Res* 1991;32:1911–1918.
83. Ichikawa Y, Shimizu H, Yoshida M. Activation antigens expressed on T-cells of the peripheral blood in Sjögren's syndrome and rheumatoid arthritis. *Clin Exp Rheumatol* 1990;8:243–249.
84. Morimoto C, Romain PL, Fox DA. Abnormalities in CD4$^+$ T-lymphocyte subsets in inflammatory rheumatic diseases. *Am J Med* 1988;84: 817–825.
85. Cush JJ, Lipsky PE. Phenotypic analysis of synovial tissue and peripheral blood lymphocytes isolated from patients with rheumatoid arthritis. *Arthritis Rheum* 1988;31:1230–1238.
86. Ichikawa Y, Shimizu H, Takahasi M. Lymphocyte subsets of the peripheral blood in Sjögren's syndrome and rheumatoid arthritis. *Clin Exp Rheumatol* 1989;7:55–61.
87. Braun J, Grolms M, Sieper J. Three-colour flow cytometric examination of CD4/CD45 subsets reveals no differences in peripheral blood and synovial fluid between patients with reactive arthritis and rheumatoid arthritis. *Clin Exp Rheumatol* 1994;12:17–22.
88. Matthews N, Emery P, Pilling D. Subpopulations of primed T helper cells in rheumatoid arthritis. *Arthritis Rheum* 1993;36:603–607.
89. Lazarovits AI, White MJ, Karsh J. CD7$^-$ T cells in rheumatoid arthritis. *Arthritis Rheum* 1992;35:615–624.
90. d'Angeac AD, Monier S, Jorgensen S. Increased percentage of CD3$^+$, CD57$^+$ lymphocytes in patients with rheumatoid arthritis. Correlation with duration of disease. *Arthritis Rheum* 1993;36:608–612.
91. Tedder TF, Penta AC, Levine AB. Expression of the human leukocyte adhesion molecule, LAM-1. Identity with the TQ1 and Leu-8 differentiation antigens. *J Immunol* 1990;144:532–540.
92. Laffon A, Sanchez-Madrid F, Ortiz de Landaturi M. Very late activation antigen on synovial fluid T cells from patients with rheumatoid arthritis and other rheumatic diseases. *Arthritis Rheum* 1989;32:386–392.
93. Emery P, Wood N, Gentry K. High-affinity interleukin-2 receptors on blood lymphocytes are decreased during active rheumatoid arthritis. *Arthritis Rheum* 1988;31:1176–1181.
94. Taniguchi O, Miyajima H, Hirano T. The leu-1 B-cell subpopulation in patients with rheumatoid arthritis. *J Clin Immunol* 1987;7:441–448.

95. Brennan F, Plater-Zyberk C, Maini RN. Coordinate expansion of "fetal type" lymphocytes (TCR gamma delta+T and CD5+B) in rheumatoid arthritis and primary Sjögren's syndrome. *Clin Exp Immunol* 1989;77:175–178.
96. Lunardi C, Marquerie C, Walport MJ. Tgd cells and their subsets in blood and synovial fluid from patients with rheumatoid arthritis. *Br J Rheumatol* 1992;31:527–530.
97. Jenkins RN, Nikaein A, Zimmerman A. T cell receptor Vb gene bias in rheumatoid arthritis. *J Clin Invest* 1993;92:2688–2701.
98. Zagon G, Tumane JR, Li Y. Increased frequency of Vb17-positive T cells in patients with rheumatoid arthritis. *Arthritis Rheum* 1994; 37:1431–1440.
99. Friedman SM, Crow MK, Tumang JR. Characterization of human T cells reactive with the mycoplasma arthritidis-derived superantigen (MAM): generation of monoclonal antibody against Vb17, the T cell receptor gene product expressed by a large fraction of MAM-reactive human T cells. *J Exp Med* 1991;174:891–900.
100. Chothia C, Boswell DR, Lesk AM. The outline structure of the T-Cell α/β receptor. *EMBO J* 1988;7:3745–3755.
101. Bröker BM, Korthauer U, Heppt P. Biased T cell receptor V gene usage in rheumatoid arthritis. Oligoclonal expansion of T cells expressing Va2 genes in synovial fluid but not in peripheral blood. *Arthritis Rheum* 1993;36:1234–1243.
102. Holoshitz J, Koning F, Coligan JC. Isolation of CD4$^-$ CD8$^-$ mycobacteria-reactive T lymphocyte clones from rheumatoid arthritis synovial fluid. *Nature* 1989;339:226–229.
103. Hildebrandt S, von der Heydt I, von Wichert P. Expression of CD 21, CD 22, and the mouse erythrocyte receptor on peripheral B lymphocytes in rheumatoid arthritis. *Ann Rheum Dis* 1988;47:588–594.
104. Plater-Zyberk C, Maini RN, Lam K. A rheumatoid arthritis B cell subset expresses a phenotype similar to that in chronic lymphocytic leukemia. *Arthritis Rheum* 1985;28:971–976.
105. Youinou P, Mackenzie L, Katsikis P. The relationship between CD5-expressing B lymphocytes and serologic abnormalities in rheumatoid arthritis patients and their relatives. *Arthritis Rheum* 1990;33:339–348.
106. Kazbay K, Osterland CK. The frequency of leu 1+B cells in autoantibody positive and negative autoimmune diseases and in neonatal cord blood. *Clin Exp Rheumatol* 1990;8:231–235.
107. Taniguchi O, et al. The leu-1 B-cell subpopulation in patients with rheumatoid arthritis. *J Clin Immunol* 1987;7:441–448.
108. Xu H, Geddes R, Roberts-Thomson PJ. Low molecular weight IgM and CD5 B lymphocytes in rheumatoid arthritis. *Ann Rheum Dis* 1994;53:383–390.
109. Youinou P, Mackenzie L, Katsiku P. The relationship between CD5-expressing B lymphocytes and serologic abnormalities in rheumatoid arthritis and their relatives. *Arthritis Rheum* 1990;33:339–348.
110. Kipps TJ, Vaughan JH. Genetic influence on the levels of circulating CD5 B lymphocytes. *J Immunol* 1987;139:1060–1064.
111. Hutchinson RM, Davis P, Jayson MI. Thrombocytosis in rheumatoid arthritis. *Ann Rheum Dis* 1976;35:138–142.
112. Horn A, Avenarius HJ, Deicher H. Thrombocyte function and thrombocyte-associated immunoglobulins in patients with systemic lupus erythematosus and chronic polyarthritis. *Klin Wochenschr* 1990;68: 460–465.
113. Endresen GK. Evidence for activation of platelets in the synovial fluid from patients with rheumatoid arthritis. *Rheumatol Int* 1989;9: 19–24.
114. Bedell SE, Bush BT. Erythrocyte sedimentation rate. From folklore to facts. Am J Med 1985;78:1001–1009.
115. Pollack W. Some physicochemical aspects of hemagglutination. *Ann NY Acad Sci* 1965;127:892–895.
116. Talstad I, Haugen HF. The relationship between the erythrocyte sedimentation rate (ESR) and plasma proteins in clinical materials and models. *Scand J Clin Lab Invest* 1979;39:519–523.
117. Palmblad J, Karlsson CG, Levi L. The erythrocyte sedimentation rate and stress. *Acta Med Scand* 1979;205:517–520.
118. Glynn LE. Symposium on inflammation and role of fibrin in the rheumatic diseases. *Bull Rheum Dis* 1963;14:323–326.
119. Hardwicke H, Squire JR. The basis of the erythrocyte sedimentation rate. *Clin Sci* 1952;11:333–335.
120. Drivsholm A. Myelomatosis. *Acta Med Scand* 1964;176:509–524.
121. Ucci G, Riccardi A, Luoni R, et al. Presenting features of monoclonal gammopathies. An analysis of 684 newly diagnosed cases. Cooperative group for the study and treatment of multiple myeloma. *J Intern Med* 1993;234:165–173.
122. Lascari AD. The erythrocyte sedimentation rate. *Pediatr Clin North Am* 1972;19:1113–1121.
123. Lawrence C, Fabry ME. Erythrocyte sedimentation rate during steady state and painful crisis in sickle cell anemia. *Am J Med* 1986;81: 801–808.
124. Penchas S, Clay CM, Simpson MR. Heparin and ESR. *Arch Intern Med* 1978;138:1864–1865.
125. Hutchinson RM, Clay CM, Simpson MR, et al. Lowered erythrocyte-sedimentation rate with sodium valproate. *Lancet* 1978;2:1309.
126. Fahraeus R. The suspension stability of blood. *Physiol Rev* 1929;9: 241–274.
127. Fahraeus R. The suspension stability of the blood. *Acta Med Scand* 1921;55:1–228.
128. Burton JL. Effect of oral contraceptives on erythrocyte sedimentation rate in healthy young women. *BMJ* 1967;3:214–215.
129. Boyd RV, Hoffbrand BI. Erythrocyte sedimentation rate in elderly hospital in-patients. *BMJ* 1966;1:901–902.
130. Milne JS, Williamson J. The ESR in older people. *Gerontol Clin* 1972;14:36–42.
131. Miller A, Green M, Robinson D. Simple rule for calculating normal erythrocyte sedimentation rate. *BMJ* 1983;286:266.
132. Shearn MA, Kang IY. Effect of age and sex on the erythrocyte sedimentation rate. *J Rheumatol* 1986;13:297–298.
133. Haeney MR. Erroneous values for the total white cell count and ESR in patients with cryoglobulinemia. *J Clin Pathol* 1976;29:894–897.
134. Komatsubara Y, Hiramatsu S, Hongo J. Multi-variate analysis of serum protein in rheumatoid arthritis. *Scand J Rheumatol* 1976;5: 97–102.
135. Short CL, Dienes L, Bauer W. Rheumatoid arthritis: a comparative evaluation of commonly employed diagnostic tests. *JAMA* 1937;108: 2087–2091.
136. Wolfe F, Zwillich SH. The long-term outcomes of rheumatoid arthritis: a 23-year prospective, longitudinal study of total joint replacement and its predictors in 1,600 patients with rheumatoid arthritis. *Arthritis Rheum* 1998;41:1072–1982.
137. Dawson MH, Sia RHP, Boots RH. The differential diagnosis of rheumatoid and osteoarthritis: the sedimentation reaction and its value. *J Lab Clin Med* 1930;15:1065–1071.
138. Richardson AT. Routine clinical pathology in rheumatoid arthritis. *Proc R Soc Med Lond* 1957;50:466–469.
139. Kushner I, Broder ML, Karp D. Control of the acute phase response. Serum C-reactive protein kinetics after acute myocardial infarction. *J Clin Invest* 1978;61:235–242.
140. Tillett WS, Francis T. Serological reactions in pneumonia with a non-protein somatic fraction of pneumococcus. *J Exp Med* 1930;52:561–571.
141. Gitlin JD, Colten HR. Molecular biology of the acute phase plasma proteins. In: Pick E, Landy M, ed. *Lymphokines,* vol 14. San Diego: Academic, 1987:123–153.
142. Vigushin DM, Pepys MB, Hawkins PN. Metabolic and scintigraphic studies of radioiodinated human C-reactive protein in health and disease. *J Clin Invest* 1993;91:1351–1357.
143. McConkey B, Crockson RA, Crockson AP. The assessment of rheumatoid arthritis. A study based on measurements of the serum acute-phase reactants. *Q J Med* 1972;41:115–125.
144. Mallya RK, de Beer FC, Berry H, et al. Correlation of clinical parameters of disease activity in rheumatoid arthritis with serum concentrations of C-reactive protein and erythrocyte sedimentation rate. *J Rheumatol* 1982;9:224–228.
145. Devlin J, Lilley J, Gough A, et al. Clinical associations of dual-energy x-ray absorptiometry measurement of hand bone mass in rheumatoid arthritis. *Br J Rheumatol* 1996;35:1256–1262.
146. Larsen A. The relation of radiographic changes to serum acute-phase proteins and rheumatoid factor in 200 patients with rheumatoid arthritis. *Scand J Rheumatol* 1988;17:123–129.
147. Larsen A, Dale K, Eek M. Radiographic evaluation of rheumatoid arthritis and related conditions by standard reference films. *Acta Radiol Diagn* 1977;18:481–491.
148. van Leeuwen MA, van Rijswijk MH, van der Heijde DMFM, et al. The acute-phase response in relation to radiographic progression in early rheumatoid arthritis: a prospective study during the first three years of the disease. *Br J Rheumatol* 1993;32(suppl 3):9–13.

149. van Leuwen MA, van Rijswijk MH, Sluiter WJ, et al. Individual relationship between progression of radiological damage and the acute phase response in early rheumatoid arthritis. Towards development of a decision support system. *J Rheumatol* 1997;24:20–27.
150. Wolfe F, Sharp JT. Radiographic outcome of recent onset rheumatoid arthritis: a 19 year study of radiographic progression. *Arthritis Rheum* 1998;41:1571–1582.
151. Madhok R, Crilly A, Murphy E, et al. Gold therapy lowers serum interleukin 6 levels in rheumatoid arthritis. *J Rheumatol* 1993;20: 630–633.
152. Situnayake RD, McConkey B. Clinical and laboratory effects of prolonged therapy with sulfasalazine, gold or penicillamine: the effects of disease duration on treatment response. *J Rheumatol* 1990;17: 1268–1273.
153. McConkey B, Crockson RA, Crockson AP, et al. The effects of some anti-inflammatory drugs on the acute-phase proteins in rheumatoid arthritis. *Q J Med NS* 1973;42:785–791.
154. Scott DL, Dawes PT, Fowler PD, et al. Anti-rheumatic drugs and joint damage in rheumatoid arthritis. *Q J Med* 1985;54:49–59.
155. Herborn RR, Menninger G, Sangha O. Progression in early erosive rheumatoid arthritis. 12 months results from a randomized controlled trial comparing methotrexate and gold sodium thiomalate. *Br J Rheumatol* 1998;37:1220–1226.
156. Elliott MJ, Maini RN, Feldman M, et al. Repeated therapy with monoclonal antibody to tumour necrosis factor alpha (cA2) in patients with rheumatoid arthritis. *Lancet* 1994; 344(8930):1125–1127.
157. Kremer JM, Weinblatt ME, Bankhurst AD, et al. Etanercept added to background methotrexate therapy in patients with rheumatoid arthritis: continued observations. *Arthritis Rheum* 2003;48:1493–1499.
158. Taylor HG, Fowler PD, David MJ, et al. Intra-articular steroids: confounder of clinical trials. *Clin Rheumatol* 1991;10:38–42.
159. Luqmani RA, Sheeran TP, Winkles J, et al. Cytokines and the acute phase response in rheumatoid arthritis. *Br J Rheumatol* 1991;30 (suppl 2):6.
160. Dawes PT, Fowler PD, Clarke S, et al. Rheumatoid arthritis: treatment which controls the C-reactive protein and erythrocyte sedimentation rate reduces radiological progression. *Br J Rheumatol* 1986; 25:44–49.
161. Scott DL, Greenwood A, Davies J, et al. Radiological progression in rheumatoid arthritis: do D-penicillamine and hydroxychloroquine have different effects? *Br J Rheumatol* 1990;29:126–127.
162. Yamanaka MY, Higami H, Kashiwazaki S. Time lab between active joint inflammation and radiological progression in patients with early rheumatoid arthritis. *J Rheumatol* 1998;25:427–432.
163. Gough DJ, Huissoon A, Perkins P, et al. The acute phase and functions in early rheumatoid arthritis, C-reactive protein levels correlate with functional outcome. *J Rheumatol* 1997;24:9–13.
164. Walters MT, Stevenson FK, Goswami R, et al. Comparison of serum and synovial fluid concentrations of beta 2-microglobulin and C-reactive protein in relation to clinical disease activity and synovial inflammation in rheumatoid arthritis. *Ann Rheum Dis* 1989;48:905–911.
165. Denko CW, Gabriel P. Serum proteins—transferrin, ceruloplasmin, albumin, 1-antitrypsin—in rheumatic disorders. *J Rheumatol* 1979;6: 664–672.
166. Brackertz D, Hagmann J, Kueppers F. Proteinase inhibitors in rheumatoid arthritis. *Ann Rheum Dis* 1975;34:225–230.
167. Kosaka S, Tazawa M. Alpha-1-antichymotrypsin in rheumatoid arthritis. *Tohoku J Exp Med* 1976;119:369–375.
168. Swedlund HA, Hunder GG, Gleich GJ. Alpha-1-antitrypsin in serum and synovial fluid in rheumatoid arthritis. *Ann Rheum Dis* 1974;33: 162–164.
169. Littman BH, Drury CE, Zimmerer RO, et al. Rheumatoid arthritis treated with tenidap and piroxicam. Clinical associations with cytokine modulation by tenidap. *Arthritis Rheum* 1995;38:29–37.
170. Nakamura T, Board PG, Matsushita K. α_1-Acid glycoprotein expression in human leukocytes: possible correlation between α_1-acid glycoprotein and inflammatory cytokines in rheumatoid arthritis. *Inflammation* 1993;17:33–45.
171. Coste J, Spira A, Clerc D, et al. Prediction of articular destruction in rheumatoid arthritis: disease activity markers revisited. *J Rheumatol* 1997;24:28–34.
172. Chen E, Keystone EC, Fish EN. Restricted cytokine expression in rheumatoid arthritis. *Arthritis Rheum* 1993;36:901–910.
173. Barrera P, Boerbooms AM, Janssen EM. Circulating soluble tumor necrosis factor receptors, interleukin-2 receptors, tumor necrosis factor α, and interleukin-6 levels in rheumatoid arthritis. *Arthritis Rheum* 1993;36:1070–1079.
174. Manicourt D-H, Triki R, Fukuda K. Levels of circulating tumor necrosis factor a and interleukin-6 in patients with rheumatoid arthritis. *Arthritis Rheum* 1993;36:490–499.
175. Dasgupta B, Corkill M, Kirkham B. Serial estimation of interleukin 6 as a measure of systemic disease in rheumatoid arthritis. *J Rheumatol* 1992;19:22–25.
176. Danis VA, Frenic GM, Rathjen DA, et al. Circulating cytokine levels in patients with rheumatoid arthritis: results of a double-blind trial with sulphasalazine. *Ann Rheum Dis* 1992;51:946–950.
177. Wascher TC, Hermann J, Brezinschck R, et al. Serum levels of interleukin-6 and tumour-necrosis-factor-alpha are not correlated to disease activity in patients with rheumatoid arthritis after treatment with low-dose methotrexate. *Eur J Clin Invest* 1994;24:73–75.
178. Fong KY, Boey ML, Koh WN. Cytokine concentrations in the synovial fluid and plasma of rheumatoid arthritis patients: correlation with bony erosions. *Clin Exp Rheumatol* 1994;12:55–58.
179. Straub RH, Muller-Ladner U, Lichtinger T, et al. Decrease of interleukin 6 during the first 12 months is a prognostic marker for clinical outcome during 36 months treatment with disease-modifying anti-rheumatic agents. *Br J Rheumatol* 1997;36:1298–1303.
180. Roubenoff R, Roubenoff RA, Cannon JG. Rheumatoid cachexia: cytokine-driven hypermetabolism accompanying reduced body cell mass in chronic inflammation. *J Clin Invest* 1994; 93:2379–2386.
181. Cush JJ, Splawski JB, Thomas R. Elevated interleukin-10 levels in patients with rheumatoid arthritis. *Arthritis Rheum* 1995;38:96–104.
182. Akahoshi T, Weda C, Endo H. Expression of monocyte chemotactic and activating factor in rheumatoid arthritis. Regulation of its production in synovial cells by interleukin-1 and tumor necrosis factor. *Arthritis Rheum* 1993;36:762–771.
183. Villiger PM, Terkeltaub R. Production of monocyte chemoattractant protein-1 by inflamed synovial tissue and cultured synoviocytes. *J Immunol* 1992;149:722–727.
184. Harigai M, Hara U, Yoshimura T. Monocyte chemoattractant protein-1 (MCP-1) in inflammatory joint diseases and its involvement in the cytokine network of rheumatoid synovium. *Clin Immunol Immunopathol* 1993;69:83–91.
185. Campbell IK, Waring P, Noval U. Production of leukemia inhibitory factor by human articular chondrocytes and cartilage in response to interleukin-1 and tumor necrosis factor a. *Arthritis Rheum* 1993;36: 790–794.
186. Abedi-Valugerdi M, Ridderstad A, Strom H. Relationship between IgG2b-inducing activity in rheumatoid arthritis synovial fluid and other well-known cytokines and inflammatory mediators. *Arthritis Rheum* 1991;34:1461–1465.
187. Ridderstad A, Abedi-Valugerdi MA, Strom H. Selective presence of IgG2b inducting factor in synovial fluid of patients with rheumatoid arthritis. *Cytokine* 1993;5:589–594.
188. Wolf RE, Brelsford WG, Hall VC. Cytokines and soluble interleukin 2 receptors in rheumatoid arthritis. *J Rheumatol* 1992;19:524–528.
189. Merkel PA, Dooley MA, Dawson DV, et al. Interleukin 2 receptor levels in sera of patients treated with sulfasalazine, parenteral gold or placebo. *J Rheumatol* 1996;23:1856–1861.
190. Campes DH, Horwitz DA, Quismoro FP. Serum levels of interleukin-2 receptor and activity of rheumatic diseases characterized by immune system activation. *Arthritis Rheum* 1988;31:1358–1364.
191. Wood NC, Symons JA, Duff GW. Serum interleukin-2 receptor in rheumatoid arthritis: a prognostic indicator of disease activity? *J Autoimmun* 1988;1:353–361.
192. Corkill MM, et al. New immunological measures of disease activity in rheumatoid arthritis: interleukin 6 and soluble interleukin 2 receptor levels in a 6 month trial [Abstract]. *Clin Rheumatol* 1990;9:121.
193. Cush JJ, Rothlein R, Lindsley HB, et al. Increased levels of circulating intercellular adhesion molecule 1 in the sera of patients with rheumatoid arthritis. *Arthritis Rheum* 1993;36:1098–1102.
194. Hamerman D, Wood DD. Interleukin 1 enhances synovial cell hyaluronate synthesis. *Proc Soc Exp Biol Med* 1984;177:205–210.
195. Butler DM, Vitti GF, Leizer T, et al. Stimulation of the hyaluronic acid levels of human synovial fibroblasts by recombinant human tumor necrosis factor α, tumor necrosis factor β (lymphotoxin), interleukin-1a, and interleukin-b. *Arthritis Rheum* 1988;31:1281–1289.

196. Yaron I, Meyer FA, Deyer JM, et al. Some recombinant human cytokines stimulate glycosaminoglycan synthesis in human synovial fibroblast cultures and inhibit it in human articular cartilages cultures. *Arthritis Rheum* 1989;32:173–180.
197. Dahl IM, Husby G. Hyaluronic acid production *in vitro* by synovial lining cells from normal and rheumatoid joints. *Ann Rheum Dis* 1985;44:647–657.
198. Engström-Laurent A, Hallgren R. Circulating hyaluronate in rheumatoid arthritis: relationship to inflammatory activity and the effect of corticosteroid therapy. *Ann Rheum Dis* 1985;44:83–88.
199. Poole AR, Witter J, Roberts N. Inflammation and cartilage metabolism in rheumatoid arthritis. Studies of the blood markers hyaluronic acid, orosomucoid and keratan sulfate. *Arthritis Rheum* 1990;33: 790–799.
200. Engström-Laurent A, Hällgren R. Circulating hyaluronic acid levels vary with physical activity in healthy subjects and in rheumatoid arthritis patients. Relationship to synovitis mass and morning stiffness. *Arthritis Rheum* 1987;30:1333–1338.
201. Hørslev-Petersen K, Bentsen KD, Engström-Laurent A. Serum amino terminal type III procollagen peptide and serum hyaluronan in rheumatoid arthritis: relation to clinical and serological parameters of inflammation during 8 and 24 months treatment with levamisole, penicillamine or azathioprine. *Ann Rheum Dis* 1988;47:116–126.
202. Konttinen YT, Soari H, Honkanen YE. Serum baseline hyaluronate and disease activity in rheumatoid arthritis. *Clin Chim Acta* 1990; 193:39–48.
203. Paimela L, Heiskamen A, Kurki D. Serum hyaluronate level as a predictor of radiologic progression in early rheumatoid arthritis. *Arthritis Rheum* 1991;34:815–821.
204. Fex E, Eberhardt K, Saxne T. Tissue-derived macromolecules and markers of inflammation in serum in early rheumatoid arthritis: relationship to development of joint destruction in hands and feet. *Br J Rheumatol* 1997;36:1161–1165.
205. Saxne T, Wollheim FA, Pettersson H. Proteoglycan concentration in synovial fluid: predictor of future cartilage destruction in rheumatoid arthritis. *Br Med J* 1987;295:1447–1448.
206. Mansson B, Geborek P, Saxne T. Cartilage and bone macromolecules in knee joint synovial fluid in rheumatoid arthritis: relation to development of knee or hip joint destruction. *Ann Rheum Dis* 1997;56: 91–96.
207. Witter J, Roughley PJ, Webber C. The immunologic detection and characterization of cartilage proteoglycan degradation products in synovial fluids of patients with arthritis. *Arthritis Rheum* 1987;30: 519–529.
208. Poole AR, Dieppe P. Biological markers in rheumatoid arthritis. *Semin Arthritis Rheum* 1994;23:17–31.
209. Mansson B, Carey D, Alini M. Cartilage and bone metabolism in rheumatoid arthritis: differences between rapid and slow progression of disease identified by markers of cartilage metabolism. *J Clin Invest* 1995;95:1071–1077.
210. Glant TT, Mikecz K, Roughley PJ. Age-related changes in protein-related epitopes of human articular cartilage proteoglycan. *Biochem J* 1986;236:71–75.
211. Poole AR, Ionescu M, Swan A. Changes in cartilage metabolism in arthritis are reflected by altered serum and synovial fluid levels of glycosaminoglycan epitomes on fragments of the cartilage proteoglycan aggrecan. Implications for pathogenesis. *J Clin Invest* 1994; 94:25–33.
212. Forslind K, Eberhardt K, Jonnson A. Increased serum concentrations of cartilage oligomeric matrix protein. A prognostic marker in early rheumatoid arthritis. *Br J Rheumatol* 1992;31:593–598.
213. Neidhart M, Hauser N, Paulsson M, et al. Small fragments of cartilage oligomeric matrix protein in synovial fluid and serum as markers for cartilage degradation. *Br J Rheumatol* 1997;36:1151–1160.
214. Wollheim FA, Eberhardt KB, Johnson U, et al. HLA DRB1* typing and cartilage oligomeric matrix protein (COMP) as predictors of joint destruction in recent-onset rheumatoid arthritis. *Br J Rheumatol* 1997;36:847–849.
215. Black D, Marabani M, Strurrock RD. Urinary excretion of the hydroxypyridinium cross links of collagen in patients with arthritis. *Ann Rheum Dis* 1989;48:641–644.
216. Seibel MJ, Duncan A, Rubins SP, et al. Urinary hydroxypyridinium crosslinks provide indices of cartilage and bone involvement in arthritic disease. *J Rheumatol* 1989;16:964–970.
217. Uebelhart D, Gineyts E, Chapuy MC. Urinary excretion of pyridinium cross links: a new marker of bone resorption in metabolic bone disease. *Bone Miner* 1990;8:87–96.
218. Robins SP, Black D, Paterson CR. Evaluation of urinary hydroxypyridinium cross link measurements as resorption markers in metabolic bone disease. *Eur J Clin Invest* 1991;21:310–315.
219. McLaren AM, Isdale AH, Whiting PIJ. Physiological variations in the urinary excretion of pyridinium crosslinks of collagen. *Br J Rheumatol* 1993;32:307–312.
220. Peel N, al-Dehaimi A, Colwell A. Sulfasalazine may interfere with HPLC assay of urinary pyridinium crosslinks [Letter]. *Clin Chem* 1994;40:167–168.
221. Price PA, Williamson MK, Lothringer JW, et al. Origin of the vitamin K–dependent bone protein found in plasma and its clearance by kidney and bone. *J Biol Chem* 1981;256:12760–12766.
222. Gundberg CM, Markowitz MG, Mizruchi M. Osteocalcin in human serum: a circadian rhythm. *J Clin Endocrinol Metab* 1985;60:736–739.
223. Sambrook PN, Ansell BM, Foster S. Bone turnover in early rheumatoid arthritis 1. Biochemical and kinetic indexes. *Ann Rheum Dis* 1985;44:575–579.
224. Ekenstam EA, Ljuwghall S, Hallgren R. Serum osteocalcin in rheumatoid arthritis and other inflammatory arthritides: relation between inflammatory activity and the effect of glucocorticoids and remission inducing drugs. *Ann Rheum Dis* 1986;45:484–490.
225. Campion GV, Delmas PD, Dieppe PA. Serum and synovial fluid osteocalcin (bone Gla protein) levels in joint disease. *Br J Rheumatol* 1989;28:393–398.
226. Pietschmann P, Machold KP, Wowsczuk W. Serum osteocalcin concentrations in patients with rheumatoid arthritis. *Ann Rheum Dis* 1989;48:654–657.
227. Gevers G, Devos P, DeRoo U. Increased levels of osteocalcin (serum bone Gla-protein) in rheumatoid arthritis. *Br J Rheumatol* 1986;25: 260–262.
228. Saxne T, Zunio L, Heinegard D. Increased release of bone sialoprotein into synovial fluid reflects tissue destruction in rheumatoid arthritis. *Arthritis Rheum* 1995;38:82–90.
229. Marhoffer W, Schatz H, Stracke H. Serum osteocalcin levels in rheumatoid arthritis: a marker for accelerated bone turnover in late onset rheumatoid arthritis. *J Rheumatol* 1991;18:1158–1162.
230. Brennan FM, Browne KA, Green PA, et al. Reduction of serum matrix metalloproteinase 1 and matrix metalloproteinase 3 in rheumatoid arthritis patients following anti-tumour necrosis factor-alpha therapy. *Br J Rheumatol* 1997;36:643–650.
231. Ishiguro N, Ito T, Obata K, et al. Determination of stromelysin-1, 72 and 92 kDa type IV collagenase, tissue and inhibitor of metalloproteinase 1 (TIMP-1) and TIMP-2 in synovial fluid and serum from patients with rheumatoid arthritis. *J Rheumatol* 1996;23:1599–1604.
232. Kievitis JH, Goslings J, Schuit HRL. Rheumatoid arthritis and the positive LE-cell phenomenon. *Ann Rheum Dis* 1956;15:211–216.
233. Vartio T, Vaheri A, von Essen R. Fibronectin in synovial fluid and tissue in rheumatoid arthritis. *Eur J Clin Invest* 1981;11:207–212.
234. Webb J, Whaley K, MacSween R. Liver disease in rheumatoid arthritis and Sjögren's syndrome: prospective study using biochemical and serological markers of hepatic dysfunction. *Ann Rheum Dis* 1975;34: 70–81.
235. Permin H, Wiik A. The prevalence of IgE antinuclear antibodies in rheumatoid arthritis and systemic lupus erythematosus. *Acta Pathol Microbiol Scand [C]* 1978;86C:245–249.
236. Wiik A, Permin H. The prevalence and possible significance of IgD granulocyte-specific antinuclear antibodies in neutropenic and non-neutropenic cases of rheumatoid arthritis. *Acta Pathol Microbiol Scand [C]* 1978;86C:19–22.
237. Abu-Shakra M, Krup M, Slor H. Anti-Sm-RNP activity in sera of patients with rheumatic and autoimmune diseases. *Clin Rheumatol* 1990;9:346–355.
238. Nojima T, Kamata M, Matsunobu T, et al. Detection of autoantibodies in sera from patients with rheumatoid arthritis. *Ryumachi* 1994; 34:871–878.
239. Tsuzaka K, Ogasawara T, Tojo T. Relationship between autoantibodies and clinical parameters in Sjögren's syndrome. *Scand J Rheumatol* 1993;22:1–9.
240. Schellekens GA, de Jong B. Frank HJ, et al. Citrulline is an essential constituent of antigenic determinants recognized by rheumatoid arthritis-specific autoantibodies. *J Clin Invest* 1998; 101:273–281.

241. Girbal-Neuhauser E, Durieux J, Arnaud M, et al. The epitopes targeted by the rheumatoid arthritis-associated antifilaggrin autoantibodies are posttranslationally generated on various sites of (Pro) filaggrin by deimination of arginine residues. *J Immunol* 1999;162: 585–594.
242. Menard HA, Lapointe E, Rochdi MD, Zhou ZJ. Insights into rheumatoid arthritis derived from the Sa immune system. *Arthritis Res* 2000; 2:429–432.
243. Bas S, Perneger TV, Seitz M, et al. Diagnostic tests for rheumatoid arthritis:comparison of anti-cyclic citrullinated peptide antibodies, anti-keratin antibodies, and IgM rheumatoid factors. *Rheumatol* 2002;41:809–814.
244. Nienhuis RL, Mandema E. A new serum factor in patients with rheumatoid arthritis, the antiperinuclear factor. *Ann Rheum Dis* 1964;23: 302–305.
245. Janssens X, Veys EM, Verbuggen G. The diagnostic significance of the antiperinuclear factor for rheumatoid arthritis. *J Rheumatol* 1988;15:1346–1350.
246. Youinou P, LeGoff P, Dumay A. The antiperinuclear factor: I. Clinical and serologic associations. *Clin Exp Rheumatol* 1990;8:259–264.
247. Westgeest AA, Boerbooms AM, Jongmans M. Antiperinuclear factor: indicator of more severe disease in seronegative rheumatoid arthritis. *J Rheumatol* 1987;14:893–897.
248. Boerbooms AM, Westgeest AA, Reckers P. Immunogenetic heterogeneity of seronegative rheumatoid arthritis and the antiperinuclear factor. *Ann Rheum Dis* 1990;49:15–17.
249. Vincent C, Serre G, Lapeyre F. High diagnostic value in rheumatoid arthritis of antibodies to the stratum corneum of rat oesophagus epithelium, so-called "antikeratin antibodies." *Ann Rheum Dis* 1989; 48:712–722.
250. Paimela L, Gripenberg M, Kurki P. Antikeratin antibodies: diagnostic and prognostic markers for early rheumatoid arthritis. *Ann Rheum Dis* 1992;51:743–746.
251. von Essen R, Kurki P, Isomaki H. Prospect for an additional laboratory criterion for rheumatoid arthritis. *Scand J Rheumatol* 1993;22: 267–272.
252. Vincent C, Serre G, Fournig B. Natural IgG to epidermal cytokeratins vs IgG to the stratum corneum of the rat oesophagus epithelium, so-called "antikeratin antibodies," in rheumatoid arthritis and other rheumatic diseases. *J Autoimmun* 1991;4:493–505.
253. Kirstein H, Mathiesen FK. Antikeratin antibodies in rheumatoid arthritis. *Scand J Rheumatol* 1987;16:331–337.
254. Kurki P, Aho K, Palusuo T. Immunopathology of rheumatoid arthritis. *Arthritis Rheum* 1992;35:914–917.
255. Simon M, Gibral E, Sebbag M. The cytokeratin filament-aggregating protein filaggrin is the target of the so-called "antikeratin antibodies," autoantibodies specific for rheumatoid arthritis. *J Clin Invest* 1993;92:1387–1393.
256. Vincent C, deKeyser F, Masson-Bessiere C, et al. Anti-perinuclear factor compared with the so called "antikeratin" antibodies to human epidermis filaggrin, in the diagnosis of arthritides. *Ann Rheum Dis* 1999;58:42–48.
257. Hoet RM, Boerbooms AM, Areu DSM, et al. Antiperinuclear factor, a marker autoantibody for rheumatoid arthritis: colocalisation of the perinuclear factor and profilaggrin. *Ann Rheum Dis* 1991;50:611–618.
258. Sebbag M, Simon C, Vincent C, et al. The perinuclear factor and the so-called antikeratin antibodies are the same rheumatoid arthritis-specific autoantibodies. *J Clin Invest* 1995; 95: 2672–2679.
259. Aho K, Palosuo T, Lukka M, et al. Antifilaggrin antibodies in recent-onset arthritis. *Scand J Rheumatol* 1999;28:113–116.
260. Slack SL, Mannik M, Dale BA. Diagnostic value of antibodies to filaggrin in rheumatoid arthritis. *J Rheumatol* 1998;25:847–851.
261. Despres N, Boire G, Lopez-Longo FJ. The Sa system: a novel antigen-antibody system specific for rheumatoid arthritis. *J Rheumatol* 1994; 21:1027–1033.
262. Heuber W, Hassfeld W, Smolen JS, et al. Sensitivity and specificity of anti-Sa autoantibodies for rheumatoid arthritis. *Rheumatology* 1999; 38:155–159.
263. Masson-Bessiere C, Sebbag M, Girbal-Neuhauser E, et al. The major synovial targets of the rheumatoid arthritis-specific antifilaggrin autoantibodies are deiminated forms of the α-and β-chains of fibrin. *J Immunol* 2001;166:4177–4184.
264. Vossenaar ER, Nijenhuis S, Helsen MM, et al. Citrullination of synovial proteins in murine models of rheumatoid arthritis. *Arthritis Rheum* 2003;48:2489–2500.
265. Asaga H, Nakashima K, Senshu T, et al. Immunocytochemical localization of peptidylarginine deaminase in human eosinophils and neutrophils. *J Leukoc Biol* 2001;70:46–51.
266. Hill JA, Southwood S, Sette A, et al. The conversion of arginine to citrulline allows for a high-affinity peptide interaction with the rheumatoid arthritis-associated HLA-DRB1*0401 MHC class II molecule. *J Immunol* 2003;171:538–541.
267. Jansen ALMA, van der Horst-Bruinsma IE, van Schaardenburg D, et al. Rheumatoid factor and antibodies to cyclic citrullinated peptide differentiate rheumatoid arthritis from undifferentiated polyarthritis in patients with early arthritis. *J Rheumatol* 2002;29:2074–2076.
268. Rantapaa-Dahlqvist S, De Jong BA, Berglin E, et al. Antibodies against cyclic citrullinated peptide and IgA rheumatoid factor predict the development of rheumatoid arthritis. *Arthritis Rheum* 2003;48: 2741–2749.
269. Meyer O, Labarre C, Dougados M, et al. Anticitrullinated protein/peptide antibody assays in early rheumatoid arthritis for predicting five year radiographic damage. *Ann Rheum Dis* 2003;62:120–126.
270. Genevay S, Hayem G, Verpillat P, et al. An eight year prospective study of outcome prediction by antiperinuclear factor and antikeratin antibodies at onset of rheumatoid arthritis. *Ann Rheum Dis* 2002; 61:734–736.
271. Montecucco C, Caporal R. Antibodies from patients with rheumatoid arthritis and systemic lupus erythematosus recognize different epitopes of a single heterogeneous nuclear RNP core protein. Possible role of cross-reacting antikeratin antibodies. *Arthritis Rheum* 1990;33:180–186.
272. Venables PJW, Pawlowski T, Mumford PA. Reaction of antibodies to rheumatoid arthritis nuclear antigen with a synthetic peptide corresponding to part of Epstein-Barr nuclear antigen 1. *Ann Rheum Dis* 1988;47:270–279.
273. Hassfeld W, Steiner G, Grininger W. Autoantibody to the nuclear antigen RA33: a marker for early rheumatoid arthritis. *Br J Rheumatol* 1993;32:199–203.
274. Meyer O, Tanye F, Fabregas D. Anti-RA 33 antinuclear autoantibody in rheumatoid arthritis and mixed connective tissue disease: comparison with antikeratin and antiperinuclear antibodies. *Clin Exp Rheumatol* 1993;11:473–478.
275. Coremans IE, Hagen EC, Daha MR. Antilactoferrin antibodies in patients with rheumatoid arthritis are associated with vasculitis. *Arthritis Rheum* 1992;35:1466–1475.
276. Mulder AH, Horst G, van Leeuwen MA. Antineutrophil cytoplasmic antibodies in rheumatoid arthritis. Characterization and clinical correlations. *Arthritis Rheum* 1993;36:1054–1060.
277. Hauschild S, Schmitt WH, Csernok E, et al. ANCA in systemic vasculitides, collagen vascular diseases, rheumatic disorders and inflammatory bowel diseases. *Adv Exp Med Biol* 1993;336:245–251.
278. Savige JA, Danigs DJ, Gatenba PA. Anti-neutrophil cytoplasmic antibodies (ANCA): their detection and significance: report from workshops. *Pathology* 1994;26:186–193.
279. Coremans IE, Hagen EC, van der Voort EC. Autoantibodies to neutrophil cytoplasmic enzymes in Felty's syndrome. *Clin Exp Rheumatol* 1993;11:255–262.
280. Cambridge G, Williams M, Leaker B. Anti-myeloperoxidase antibodies in patients with rheumatoid arthritis: prevalence, clinical correlates, and IgG subclass. *Ann Rheum Dis* 1994;53:24–29
281. Mustila A, Korpela M, Mustonen J, et al. Perinuclear antineutrophil cytoplasmic antibody in rheumatoid arthritis: a marker of sever disease with associated nephropathy. *Arthritis Rheum* 1997;40:710–717.
282. Brimnes J, Halberg P, Jacobsen S, et al. Specificities of antineutrophil autoantibodies in patients with rheumatoid arthritis. *Clin Exp Immunol* 1997;110:250–256.
283. Coremans IE, Hagen EC, van der Woude FJ. Antilactoferrin antibodies in patients with rheumatoid arthritis are associated with vasculitis. *Adv Exp Med Biol* 1993;336:357–362.
284. Charles PJ, Maini RN. Antibodies to neutrophil cytoplasmic antigens in rheumatoid arthritis. *Adv Exp Med Biol* 1993;336:367–370.
285. Nishiya K, Oohera E, Ooishi M. Detection of antineutrophil cytoplasmic antibodies in sera from patients with rheumatoid arthritis by

indirect immunofluorescence technique. *Rinsho Byori* 1994;42:176–182.

286. Clague RB. Autoantibodies to cartilage collagens in rheumatoid arthritis. Do they perpetuate the disease or are they irrelevant? *Br J Rheumatol* 1989;28:1–5.
287. Jasin HE. Autoantibody specificities of immune complexes sequestered in articular cartilage of patients with rheumatoid arthritis and osteoarthritis. *Arthritis Rheum* 1985;28:241–248.
288. Tarkowski A, Klareskog L, Carlsten H. Secretion of antibodies to types I and II collagen by synovial tissue cells in patients with rheumatoid arthritis. *Arthritis Rheum* 1989;32:1087–1092.
289. Rudolphi U, Hohlbaum A, Lang B. The B cell repertoire of patients with rheumatoid arthritis. Frequencies and specificities of peripheral blood B cells reacting with human IgG, human collagenase, a mycobacterial heat shock protein and other antigens. *Clin Exp Immunol* 1993;92:404–411.
290. Morgan K, Buckse C, Collins I. Antibodies to type II and XI collagens: evidence for the formation of antigen specific as well as cross reacting antibodies in patients with rheumatoid arthritis. *Ann Rheum Dis* 1988;47:1008–1013.
291. Morgan K, Clauque RB, Collins I. A longitudinal study of anticollagen antibodies in patients with rheumatoid arthritis. *Arthritis Rheum* 1989;32:139–145.
292. Banerjee S, Luthra HS, Moore SB. Serum IgG anti-native type II collagen antibodies in rheumatoid arthritis: association with HLA DR4 and lack of clinical correlation. *Clin Exp Rheumatol* 1988;6:373–380.
293. Karopoulos C, Rowley MJ, Handley CJ. Intrasynovial levels of sulphated glycosaminoglycans and autoantibodies to type II collagen in rheumatoid arthritis: a correlative analysis. *Rheumatol Int* 1993;13:15–20.
294. Konstantinov K, Halberg P, Wiik A. Clinical manifestations in patients with autoantibodies specific for nuclear lamin proteins. *Clin Immunol Immunopathol* 1992;62:112–119.
295. Senecal JL, Raymond Y. Autoantibodies to major and minor nuclear lamins are not restricted to autoimmune diseases. *Clin Immunol Immunopathol* 1992;63:115–125.
296. Brito J, Biamonti G, Caporali R, et al. Autoantibodies to human nuclear lamin B2 protein. Epitope specificity in different autoimmune diseases. *J Immunol* 1994;153:2268–2277.
297. Podgorski MR, Gaulding NJ, Hall ND. Autoantibodies to lipocortin-1 are associated with impaired glucocorticoid responsiveness in rheumatoid arthritis. *J Rheumatol* 1992;19:1668–1671.
298. Sioud M, Dybward A, Jespersen L, et al. Characterization of naturally occurring autoantibodies against tumour necrosis factor-alpha (TNF-alpha): *in vitro* function and precise epitope mapping by phage epitope library. *Clin Exp Immunol* 1994;98:520–525.
299. Peichl P, Ceska M, Broell H, et al. Human neutrophil activating peptide/interleukin 8 acts as an autoantigen in rheumatoid arthritis. *Ann Rheum Dis* 1992;51:19–22.
300. Peichl P, Pursch E, Broll H, et al. Anti-IL-8 autoantibodies and complexes in rheumatoid arthritis: polyclonal activation in chronic synovial tissue inflammation. *Rheum Int* 1999;18:141–145.
301. Pignone A, Matucci-Cerinic M, Mori-Ini M. Suppression of autoantibodies to factor VIII and correction of factor VIII deficiency with a combined steroid-cyclophosphamide porcine factor VIII treatment in a patient with rheumatoid arthritis. *J Intern Med* 1992;231:617–619.
302. Ballard HS, Nyamuswa G. Life-threatening haemorrhage in a patient with rheumatoid arthritis and a lupus anticoagulant coexisting with acquired autoantibodies against factor VIII. *Br J Rheumatol* 1993;32:515–517.
303. Salih AM, Nixon NB, Dawes PT, et al. Soluble adhesion molecules and anti-endothelial cell antibodies in patients with rheumatoid arthritis complicated by peripheral neuropathy. *J Rheum* 1999;26:551–555.
304. Zurgil N, Bakimer R, Moutsopoulos HM. Antimitochondrial (pyruvate dehydrogenase) autoantibodies in autoimmune rheumatic diseases. *J Clin Immunol* 1992;12:201–209.
305. Vardi P, Brik R, Barzilai D. Frequent induction of insulin autoantibodies by D-penicillamine in patients with rheumatoid arthritis. *J Rheumatol* 1992;19:1527–1530.
306. London MG, Muirden KD, Hewitt JV. Serum cholesterol in rheumatic diseases. *BMJ* 1963;1:1380–1383.
307. Heldenberg D, Caspi D, Levtov O, et al. Serum lipids and lipoprotein concentrations in women with rheumatoid arthritis. *Clin Rheumatol* 1983;2:387–391.
308. Bausserman LL, Bernigr ON, McAdam KO. Serum amyloid A and high density lipoproteins during the acute phase response. *Eur J Clin Invest* 1988;18:619–626.
309. Sukenik S, Henkin J, Zimlichman S. Serum and synovial fluid levels of serum amyloid A protein and C-reactive protein in inflammatory and noninflammatory arthritis. *J Rheumatol* 1988;15:942–945.
310. Wallberg-Jonsson S, Dahlen G, Johnson O, et al. Lipoprotein lipase in relation to inflammatory activity in rheumatoid arthritis. *J Intern Med* 1996;240:373–380.
311. Block WD, Buchanan OH, Freyberg RH. Serum lipids in patients with rheumatoid arthritis and in patients with obstructive jaundice. *Arch Intern Med* 1941;68:18 24.
312. Haataja M, Nieminen AL, Makisara P. Prostaglandin precursors in rheumatoid arthritis. *J Rheumatol* 1982;9:91–93.
313. Hagenfeldt L, Wennmalm A. Turnover of a prostaglandin precursor, arachidonic acid, in rheumatoid arthritis. *Eur J Clin Invest* 1975;5:235–239.
314. Jeremy R, Wilkinson P. The mechanism of hypoalbuminemia in rheumatoid arthritis. *Arthritis Rheum* 1964;7:740–741.
315. Wilkinson P, Jeremy R, Brooks FO, et al. The mechanism of hypoalbuminemia in rheumatoid arthritis. *Ann Intern Med* 1965;63:109–114.
316. Ballantyne FC, Fleck A, Dick WC. Albumin metabolism in rheumatoid arthritis. *Ann Rheum Dis* 1971;30:265–270.
317. Kosaka S. β_2-glycoprotein I in rheumatoid arthritis. *Tohoku J Exp Med* 1977;122:223–228.
318. Swedlund HA, Hunder GG, Gleich GJ. Alpha-1-antitrypsin in serum and synovial fluid in rheumatoid arthritis. *Ann Rheum Dis* 1974;33:162–164.
319. Rhodes K, Scott A, Markham RG. Immunological sex differences: a study of patients with rheumatoid arthritis, their relatives and controls. *Ann Rheum Dis* 1969;28:104–120.
320. Thompson RA, Asquith P. Quantitation of exocrine IgA in human serum in health and disease. *Clin Exp Immunol* 1970;7: 491–500.
321. Pekelharing JM, Hepo E, Kamerling JP. Alterations in carbohydrate composition of serum IgG from patients with rheumatoid arthritis and from pregnant women. *Ann Rheum Dis* 1988;47:91–95.
322. Tomana M, Schrohenloher RE, Koopman WJ. Abnormal glycosylation of serum IgG from patients with chronic inflammatory diseases. *Arthritis Rheum* 1988;31:333–338.
323. Parekh RB, Roitt IM, Isenberg DA. Galactosylation of IgG associated oligosaccharides: reduction in patients with adult and juvenile onset rheumatoid arthritis and relation to disease activity. *Lancet* 1988;1:966–969.
324. Parekh R, Isenberg D, Rook G. A comparative analysis of disease-associated changes in the galactosylation of serum IgG. *J Autoimmun* 1989;2:101–114.
325. Axford JS, MacKenzie L, Lydyard DM. Reduced B-cell galactosyltransferase activity in rheumatoid arthritis. *Lancet* 1987;2:1486–1488.
326. Tsuchiya N, Endo T, Matsuta K. Effects of galactose depletion from oligosaccharide chains on immunological activities of human IgG. *J Rheumatol* 1989;16:285–290.
327. Mackechnie HL, Ogryzlo MA, Pruzanski W. Heterogeneity of IgM/IgG cryocomplexes: immunological-clinical correlation. *J Rheumatol* 1975;2:225–240.
328. Zubler RH, Nydegger U, Perrin LH. Circulating and intra-articular immune complexes in patients with rheumatoid arthritis. Correlation of ^{125}I-C1q binding activity with clinical and biological features of the disease. *J Clin Invest* 1976;57:1308–1319.
329. Petersen NE, Elmgreen J, Teisner B. Activation of classical pathway complement in chronic inflammation. Elevated levels of circulating C3d and C4d split products in rheumatoid arthritis and Crohn's disease. *Acta Med Scand* 1988;223:557–560.
330. Swaak AJG, Han H, van Rooyen A. Complement (C3) metabolism in rheumatoid arthritis in relation to the disease course. *Rheumatol Int* 1988;8:61–65.
331. Morgan BP, Daniels RH, Williams BD. Measurement of terminal complement complexes in rheumatoid arthritis. *Clin Exp Immunol* 1988;73:473–478.

332. Franco AE, Schur PH. Hypocomplementemia in rheumatoid arthritis. *Arthritis Rheum* 1971;14:231–238.
333. Hunder GG, McDuffie FC. Hypocomplementemia in rheumatoid arthritis. *Am J Med* 1973;54:461–472.
334. Mongan ES, Cass RM, Jacox RF. A study of the relation of seronegative and seropositive rheumatoid arthritis to each other and to necrotizing vasculitis. *Am J Med* 1969;47:23–35.
335. Glass D, Raum D, Gibson D. Inherited deficiency of the second component of complement. Rheumatic disease associations. *J Clin Invest* 1976;58:853–861.
336. Thompson PW, Houghton BJ, Clifford C. The source and significance of raised serum enzymes in rheumatoid arthritis. *Q J Med* 1990;76: 869–879.
337. Laffon A, Morena A, Gutierrez-Bucero A. Hepatic sinusoidal dilatation in rheumatoid arthritis. *J Clin Gastroenterol* 1989;11:653–657.
338. Barr JH Jr, Stolzer BL, Eisenbeis CH Jr. Serum glutamic oxalacetic transaminase in rheumatoid arthritis and certain rheumatoid musculoskeletal disorders. *Arthritis Rheum* 1958;1:147–150.
339. Malmquist E, Reichard H. Serum ornithine carbamoyl transferase and transaminase activity in rheumatic disease. *Acta Rheumatol Scand* 1962;8:170–182.
340. Whaley K, Goudie RB, Williamson J. Liver disease in Sjögren's syndrome and rheumatoid arthritis. *Lancet* 1970;1:861–863.
341. Lefkovits AM, Farrow IJ. The liver in rheumatoid arthritis. *Ann Rheum Dis* 1955;14:162–168.
342. Movitt ER, Davis AE. Liver biopsy in rheumatoid arthritis. *Am J Med Sci* 1953;226:516–520.
343. Lavernia CJ, Sierra RJ, Baerga L. Nutritional parameters and short term outcome in arthroplasty. *J Am Coll Nutr* 1999;18:274–278.
344. Morgan SL, Baggott JE, Vaughn WH. Supplementation with folic acid during methotrexate therapy for rheumatoid arthritis. A double-blind, placebo-controlled trial. *Ann Intern Med* 1994;121:833–841.
345. Morgan SL, Hine RJ, Vaughn WH, et al. Dietary intake and circulating vitamin levels of rheumatoid arthritis patients treated with methotrexate. *Arthritis Care Res* 1993;6:4–10.
346. Dunzi L, Cauasin F, Ramonda R, et al. Retinol binding protein, zinc and acute phase response in rheumatoid arthritis. *Clin Exp Rheumatol* 1990;8:616–617.
347. Roubenoff R, Roubenoff RA, Selhub J. Abnormal vitamin B_6 status in rheumatoid cachexia. Association with spontaneous tumor necrosis factor a production and markers of inflammation. *Arthritis Rheum* 1995;38:105–109.
348. Schumacher HR, Bernhart ZW, Gyorgy P. Vitamin B_6 levels in rheumatoid arthritis: effect of treatment. *Am J Clin Nutr* 1975;28:1200–1203.
349. Youssef AAR, Wood B, Baron DN. Serum copper: a marker of disease activity in rheumatoid arthritis. *J Clin Pathol* 1983;36:14–17.
350. Makisara P, Ruutsalo HM, Nissila M. Serum copper in rheumatoid arthritis and ankylosing spondylitis. *Ann Med Exp Biol Fenn* 1968; 46:177–178.
351. Marrella M, Morretti U, Pasqualicchio M. Plasma and total blood cell copper in rheumatoid arthritis. *Agents Actions* 1990;29:120–121.
352. Balogh Z, El-Ghobarey AF, Fell GS, et al. Plasma zinc and its relationship to clinical symptoms and drug treatment in rheumatoid arthritis. *Ann Rheum Dis* 1980;39:329–332.
353. Cimmino MA, Pang L, Cutolo M, et al. Zinc concentrations in rheumatoid and psoriatic arthritis. Are they relevant to the inflammatory process? *Scand J Rheumatol* 1986;15:403–406.
354. Pedersen LM, Christensen JM. Chromium, nickel and cadmium in biological fluids in patients with rheumatoid arthritis compared to healthy controls. *Acta Pharmacol Toxicol (Copenh)* 1986;59(suppl 7):392–395.
355. Niedermeier W, Griggs JH. Trace metal composition of synovial fluid and blood serum of patients with rheumatoid arthritis. *J Chronic Dis* 1971;23:527–536.
356. Plantin LO, Strandberg PO. Whole-blood concentrations of copper and zinc in rheumatoid arthritis studied by activation analysis. *Acta Rheumatol Scand* 1965;11:30–34.
357. Niederstadt C, Happ T, Tatsis E, et al. Glomerular and tubular proteinuria as markers of nephropathy in rheumatoid arthritis. *Rheumatology (Oxf)* 1999;38:28–33.
358. Tishler M, Caspi D, Almog Y. Increased incidence of urinary tract infection inpatients with rheumatoid arthritis and secondary Sjögren's syndrome. *Ann Rheum Dis* 1992;51:604–606.
359. Sørensen AWS. Investigations of the kidney function in rheumatoid arthritis: II. *Acta Rheumatol Scand* 1961;7:138–144.
360. Nived O, Sturfelt G, Westling H. Is serum creatinine concentration a reliable index of renal function in rheumatic diseases? *BMJ* 1983; 286:684–685.
361. Salomon MI, Gallo G, Poon TP. The kidney in rheumatoid arthritis. A study based on renal biopsies. *Nephron* 1974;12:297–310.
362. Joseph J, Sahn SA. Connective tissue disease and the pleura. *Chest* 1993;104:262–270.
363. Horler AR, Thompson M. The pleural and pulmonary complications of rheumatoid arthritis. *Ann Intern Med* 1959;50:1179–1203.
364. Walker WC, Wright V. Pulmonary lesions and rheumatoid arthritis. *Medicine* 1968;47:501–519.
365. Baggenstoss AH, Rosenberg EF. Visceral lesions associated with chronic infectious rheumatoid arthritis. *Arch Pathol* 1943;35:503–516.
366. Pritiken JD, Jensen WA, Yenokida GG. Respiratory failure due to a massive rheumatoid pleural effusion. *J Rheumatol* 1990;17:673–675.
367. Sahn SA. Pleural fluid pH in the normal state and in diseases affecting the pleural space. In: Chretien J, Bignon J, Hirsch A, eds. *The pleura in health and disease.* New York: Marcel Dekker, 1985:253–266.
368. Cech P, Matuso L, Nydegger MU. Immune complexes in pleural fluid from rheumatoid arthritis patients. *Acta Haematol* 1982;67: 220–221.
369. Glovsky MM, Louie JS, Pitts WH. Reduction of pleural fluid complement activity in patients with systemic lupus erythematosus and rheumatoid arthritis. *Clin Immunol Immunopathol* 1976;6: 31–41.
370. Salomaa ER, Viander M, Saaresranta T, et al. Complement components and their activation products in pleural fluid. *Chest* 1998;114: 723–730.
371. Halla JT, Koopman WJ, Schrohenloher RE, et al. Local synthesis of IgM and IgM rheumatoid factor in rheumatoid pleuritis. *J Rheumatol* 1983;10:204–209.
372. Nosanchuk JS, Naylor B. A unique cytologic picture in pleural fluid from patients with rheumatoid arthritis. *Am J Clin Pathol* 1967;50: 330–335.
373. Geisinger KR, Vance RP, Prater T. Rheumatoid pleural effusion: a transmission and scanning electron microscopic evaluation. *Acta Cytol* 1985;29:239–247.
374. Shinto R, Prete P. Characteristic cytology in rheumatoid pleural effusion. *Am J Med* 1988;85:587–589.
375. Boddington MM, Spriggs AI, Morton JA. Cytodiagnosis of rheumatoid pleural effusions. *J Clin Pathol* 1971;24:95–106.
376. Faurschou P, Faarup P. Granulocyte containing cytoplasmic inclusions in human tuberculous pleuritis. *Scand J Respir Dis* 1973;54: 341–346.
377. Soderblom T, Pettersson T, Nyberg P, et al. High pleural fluid hyaluronan concentrations in rheumatoid arthritis. *Eur Respir J* 1999;13:519–522.
378. Amick LD. Muscle atrophy in rheumatoid arthritis: an electrodiagnostic study. *Arthritis Rheum* 1960;3:54–63.
379. Vemireddi NK, Redford JB, PombeJara CN. Serial nerve conduction studies in carpal tunnel syndrome secondary to rheumatoid arthritis. Preliminary study. *Arch Phys Med Rehabil* 1979;60:393–396.
380. Yates DAH. Muscular changes in rheumatoid arthritis. *Ann Rheum Dis* 1963;22:342–347.
381. Toolanen G. Cutaneous sensory impairment in rheumatoid atlantoaxial subluxation assessed quantitatively by electrical stimulation. *Scand J Rheumatol* 1987;16:27–32.

CHAPTER 58

Rheumatoid Factor

S. Louis Bridges, Jr. and Anne Davidson

Rheumatoid factors (RFs) are defined as autoantibodies reactive with epitopes in the Fc portion of IgG. These autoantibodies may be of the IgM, IgA, IgG, or IgE isotype and exhibit considerable diversity with regard to fine-binding specificity. Although initially believed to be specific for rheumatoid arthritis (RA), RFs may occur in the sera of ostensibly normal individuals and patients with a variety of chronic inflammatory and infectious diseases (Table 58.1). Nevertheless, the presence of significantly elevated levels of RF in the serum identifies individuals at increased risk for developing RA. Furthermore, the presence of RF is associated with certain clinical features in individuals with RA. Circumstantial evidence favors a role for complexes of RF with IgG, particularly those complexes formed at sites of tissue involvement (e.g., synovial membranes), in the pathogenesis of RA.

TABLE 58.1. *Diseases associated with elevated serum rheumatoid factor*

Rheumatic diseases (reviewed in reference 295)
Rheumatoid arthritis
Systemic lupus erythematosus
Sjögren syndrome
Scleroderma
Polymyositis/dermatomyositis
Chronic bacterial infections
Subacute bacterial endocarditis (78,81)
Leprosy (77)
Tuberculosis (79)
Syphilis (75)
Lyme disease (311)
Viral diseases
Rubella (82)
Cytomegalovirus (85)
Infectious mononucleosis (76,84)
Influenza (83)
Acquired immunodeficiency syndrome (312)
Parasitic diseases (80)
Chronic inflammatory diseases, cause uncertain
Sarcoidosis
Periodontal disease (313)
Pulmonary interstitial disease (314)
Liver disease (315)
Mixed cryoglobulinemia (316–318)
Hyper γ-globulinemic purpura (319)

HISTORICAL PERSPECTIVE

The association between elevated serum RF and RA was first noted in the late 1930s by Waaler (1) and subsequently by Rose and colleagues (2). Originally called agglutination activating factor, the term *rheumatoid factor* was coined in 1949 by Pike et al. (3). The original assay for RF, the sheep cell agglutination test (SCAT), detects RF through its ability to augment the agglutination of sheep red blood cells sensitized with rabbit amboreceptor (anti–sheep red blood cell antibody). Although widely used, it proved to be a technically demanding procedure and was never standardized. Efforts to overcome the technical difficulties presented by the SCAT resulted in several practical modifications, including an adaptation of the passive hemagglutination procedure (4), use of IgG-coated bentonite particles (the bentonite flocculation test) (5), and the agglutination of human group-O Rh^+ red blood cells sensitized with human incomplete anti-Rh antibody (the sensitized human red cell agglutination test) (6), which are no longer in general use. At present, the latex fixation test (7), a modification of the SCAT, is widely used in clinical situations.

Reports of the association between serum RF and RA inspired many studies of RF production, specificity, and biologic and physicochemical properties in an attempt to gain insight into the pathogenesis of RA. The isolation of RF from patients with RA was problematic, however, because of the relatively small amounts of RF present in the circulation and its polyclonality. It was observed many years ago that a significant fraction of IgM paraproteins expressed in patients with cryoglobulinemia or Waldenström macroglobulinemia exhibit RF activity. In addition, large amounts of monoclonal RF proteins could be isolated from patients with these diseases. Thus, extensive study of RF from patients with paraproteinemias has been undertaken, stimulated by the belief that they were representative of RFs present in other diseases, including RA. Studies of RF from patients with cryoglobulinemia or Waldenström macroglobulinemia have yielded important insights concerning their binding specificity, biologic properties, and genetic origins and have provided a useful reference point for approaching similar questions concerning polyclonal RFs present in RA and other autoimmune diseases.

Specificity

The binding specificities of RFs associated with the rheumatic diseases have been partially delineated using a number of approaches. These include studies of binding to cleavage products of the Fc region of immunoglobulin (8), screening of overlapping peptides from the Fc region (9,10) and from cross-reactive proteins (11), and molecular mapping of the Fc region using exon exchange and site-directed mutagenesis (12). Comparison of the specificities of the RFs from patients with RA and those from normal individuals or that arise as a result of clonal B-cell expansion in patients with cryoglobulinemia or Waldenström macroglobulinemia have revealed some instructive differences.

Several allotypic and nonallotypic determinants distributed among all four subclasses of IgG have been identified for RF in RA (8) (Table 58.2). Allotypic determinants are immunogenic epitopes generated by genetic polymorphisms in the C_H2 or C_H3 domains of the Fc region. Interaction of rheumatoid factors with an allotypic determinant that is not present on self-IgG has been observed in RF-positive RA patients and may be explained by structural alterations in the Fc region that mimic the allotypic difference, perhaps induced by immune complex formation (13).

TABLE 58.2. *Localization of IgG antigens interacting with rheumatoid factors*

	Heavy-chain constant region	
Subclass	C_H2	C_H3
IgG1	Ga[a] (γ1-2-4)[b] Non-bl	Gm(a) (Glm(1)) Gm(x) (Glm(2)) Non-a
IgG2	Ga(γ1-2-4) Non-bl	Non-a
IgG3	Gm(g) (G3m(21)) Gm(bl) (G3m(5)) Non-bl	Non-a
IgG4	Ga (γ1-2-4)	γ4 Non-a

[a]Ga site may be located in the C_H2 domain or C_H2–C_H3 interface region (8,320).

[b]Alternative nomenclature.

Data from Natvig JB, Gaarder PI, Turner MW. IgG antigens of the Cgamma2 and Cgamma3 homology regions interacting with rheumatoid factors. *Clin Exp Immunol* 1972;12(2):177–184.

Modified from Koopman WJ, Schrohenloher RE. Rheumatoid factor. In: Utsinger PD, Zvaifler NJ, Ehrlich GE, eds. *Rheumatoid arthritis: etiology, diagnosis, management.* Philadelphia: JB Lippincott, 1985:217–241, with permission.

Further work using proteolytic fragments of Fc indicated that the major nonallotypic antigenic site is located in the C_H2 domain or the C_H2–C_H3 interface region of the Fc fragment (8) and overlaps with the sites recognized by staphylococcal and streptococcal Fc-binding proteins (14). This dominant nonallotypic determinant, also known as the Ga specificity, is present only on IgG1, 2, and 4. Absence of the Ga specificity on IgG3 is due in part to the presence of an arginine rather than the usual histidine at residue 435 located within the C_H2–C_H3 interface. The Ga specificity is common among RFs from normal individuals. In contrast, IgM RF synthesized by RA synovial B cells has a greater reactivity and avidity for IgG3 than for IgG1, which suggests that one or more sites on IgG3 are important antigens for RF production in RA synovium (15,16). Elevated serum RF with specificity for IgG3 may be associated with clinically severe disease in certain patient populations (17).

Molecular mapping of the antigen binding site for a panel of monoclonal RFs using chimeric Fc regions generated by exon shuffling and site-directed mutagenesis has indicated that RFs from RA patients bind a variety of discontinuous epitopes composed of amino acids in both the C_H2 and C_H3 domains (12). Analysis of reactivity of overlapping heptapeptides synthesized on plastic pins indicated a somewhat different set of amino acids in the C_H2 and C_H3 domains of IgG as important in the binding of RF, but supports the conclusion that RA-derived RFs react with discontinuous epitopes spanning both constant regions (9,10). Studies using chimeric Fc regions have further shown that RA-derived RFs have a much broader range of antigenic specificities than either RFs from normal individuals or monoclonal RFs from patients with monoclonal gammopathies, most of which display the Ga specificity.

Consistent with the broader range of antigenic specificities displayed by RFs from RA patients, these RFs have a variety of cross-reactivities. RFs from patients with RA characteristically react with IgG of various mammalian species, including rabbits, cows, and horses (18). RFs that cross-react with rabbit IgG are specific for the Ga site or closely related structures of human IgG together with the non-a allotypic antigen (19). RFs from some patients with RA also cross-react with β_2-microglobulin, the invariant chain of class I major histocompatibility complex (MHC) molecules (11). This cross-reactivity likely reflects conformational homology present between β_2-microglobulin and the constant regions of IgG, despite different primary sequences (20). Variable degrees of cross-reactivity with other nonimmunoglobulin antigens, including DNA-histone nucleoprotein (21), have also been noted.

STRUCTURAL FEATURES

In addition to IgM RF (detected by routine serologic procedures currently in clinical use), the occurrence of IgA

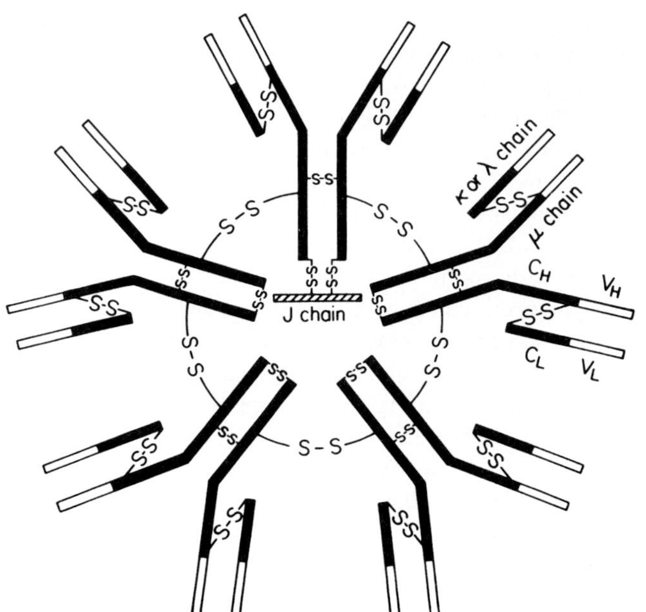

FIG. 58.1. Polypeptide chain structure of human immunoglobulin M. (Reproduced from Koopman WJ, Schrohenloher RE. Rheumatoid factor. In: Utsinger PD, Zvaifler NJ, Ehrlich GE, eds. *Rheumatoid arthritis: etiology, diagnosis, management.* Philadelphia: JB Lippincott, 1985:217–241, by permission.)

and IgG RF is well established (22–25), and there is evidence for the occurrence of IgE RF (26). Structurally, the IgM RF molecule consists of five identical subunits joined by disulfide bonds to form a pentameric structure (Fig. 58.1). Similarly, most IgA RFs in RA and Sjögren syndrome are polymeric, even though serum IgA is predominantly monomeric (27,28). Although IgG RF is exclusively monomeric, complex formation with itself and other IgG molecules can yield higher-molecular-weight species (29, 30) (Table 58.3).

A number of studies have identified structural features of the immunoglobulin V regions of RFs that are responsible for their antigenic specificity. Specificity of RFs for Fc appears to be dependent to some extent on the length and charge characteristics in the heavy-chain complementarity determining region 3 (CDR3) intervals (31). Similarly, both RF specificity and polyreactivity of B'20, a high-affinity, polyspecific RA-derived IgM RF, is dependent on its unique heavy-chain CDR3 domain (32). Nevertheless, fine specificity can be modified by residues in the light-chain complementarity determining regions (CDRs) (33).

Recent crystallographic studies of a low-avidity Ga-specific IgM RF (RF-AN) bound to IgG Fc have revealed that the epitope recognized by RF-AN includes the C_H2/C_H3 cleft region, and overlaps the binding sites of bacterial Fc-binding proteins (34). The variable region residues from RF-AN involved in recognition of the Fc region are all located at the edge of the conventional antigen-binding site and include only four of the six CDRs. The paucity of CDR residues involved in Fc binding prompts speculation that this RF may have an additional, different specificity (35). An important light-chain contact residue was generated through somatic mutation, suggesting antigen-driven selection in the production of this RF.

BIOLOGIC PROPERTIES

Substantial evidence favors the view that RF contributes to tissue injury in RA. Local production of RF in the synovium, the major site of inflammation in RA, is well documented (36–39). Moreover, RFs are prominent constituents of immune complexes in sera and synovial fluids (23,24, 40,41) and within polymorphonuclear leukocytes of patients with RA (42). RF-containing immune complexes can also be eluted from RA synovial tissue (43) and cartilage (44). Disease severity and activity in RA tend to correlate with levels of RF (45–48).

Although the evidence indicating a pathogenetic role for RFs in RA is largely indirect, several mechanisms have been implicated. Both IgM RF and IgG RF can enhance complement activation by IgG complexes (49–54). Levels of both hemolytic complement and individual complement components in rheumatoid synovial fluid are consistent with local complement consumption (55,56), as is detection of cleavage products of C3, C4, and factor B (57). The latter observation further suggests that both the alternative and classic pathways are activated. Catabolic rates of C4 and factor B in patients with RA correlate with

TABLE 58.3. *Characteristics of major human rheumatoid factors*

Immunoglobulin isotype	Molecular form	Approximate molecular weight (daltons)	Sedimentation coefficient (S)
IgM	Pentamer	950,000	19
	Complexed with IgG	1,700,000	22
IgA	Monomer	160,000	7
	Polymer	320,000 to ~1,000,000	10–20
IgG	Monomer	150,000	7
	Self-associated complexes	300,000 to ~600,000	9–14

Modified from Koopman WJ, Schrohenloher RE. Rheumatoid factor: mechanisms of production and biological significance. In: Teodorescu M, Froelich CJ, eds. *Advanced immunoassays in rheumatology.* Boca Raton, FL: CRC Press, 1994:29–50, with permission.

the concentration of serum RF, but not with the concentration of other serum antibodies (58).

Several studies have suggested that IgM-RF may significantly modify the handling of immune complexes *in vivo*. Studies in mice and rats have demonstrated that RF promotes clearance of intravenously or intraperitoneally administered immune complexes (59,60). RF was found to enhance both the attachment and ingestion of soluble heat-aggregated human IgG by human monocytes and mouse macrophages, although this effect diminished in the presence of excess RF (59). It was postulated that RF stimulates pinocytosis of soluble immune complexes by increasing their size.

RF may directly activate natural killer (NK) cells by cross-linking their Fcγ receptors, such as FcγRIII (CD16) (61). Activation of synovial fluid NK cells by RF induces secretion of interferon-γ and of tumor necrosis factor (TNF), which plays an important role in the pathogenesis of RA (62). FcγRIII is also the dominant receptor on macrophages that mediates cytokine release after exposure to RF immune complexes (63). RF also appears to down-regulate some NK cell functions. Although the frequency of NK cells in peripheral blood and synovial fluid lymphocytes from patients with RA was comparable, expression of FcγRIII was significantly lower in the latter. Additionally, the synovial fluid lymphocytes exhibited decreased functional cytotoxicity and antibody-dependent cell-mediated cytotoxicity (ADCC) compared with peripheral blood lymphocytes. Incubation of normal peripheral blood lymphocytes with either RF-positive synovial fluid from patients with RA or affinity-purified RF that also contained IgG resulted in a similar decrease in FcγRIII expression, NK cell activity, and ADCC.

In addition to secretion of RF antibody, considerable evidence indicates that RF B cells may function as important antigen-presenting cells (64). Antigen-specific B cells can bind their cognate antigen and function efficiently as antigen-presenting cells (65,66), reflecting the advantage of these cells in competing for antigen present in low concentration. By virtue of their capacity to bind and internalize antigen–IgG antibody complexes, RF B cells can present antigens contained in the immune complexes to antigen-specific T helper cells as efficiently as antigen-specific B cells (67,68). Thus, RF B cells may serve as an increasingly important focus for T-cell help during the course of a secondary immune response. These observations suggest that RF B cells migrating into the synovium of patients with RA could present a variety of complexed antigens to relevant T-helper cells, thus serving to perpetuate local immune responses and amplify synovial RF production.

Most of the information on pathogenesis of RF in RA has been derived from IgM RF and, to a lesser extent, IgG RF. The possible role of IgA RF is less clear, although it may be associated with particular disease features. Differences in the effector functions of IgA compared with IgM and IgG may influence the role of IgA-RF in tissue injury. IgA is generally considered incapable of fixing complement by the classical pathway, although it may activate the alternative pathway (69,70). Thus, the overall contribution of RF to tissue injury is likely to be related to the pattern of isotypes expressed in a particular patient or at a specific site of inflammation.

RF also has some antiinflammatory properties. RFs from patients with RA or subacute bacterial endocarditis inhibit phagocytosis by human polymorphonuclear leukocytes of staphylococci coated with human or rabbit IgG antibody (71), presumably by blocking the Fc receptor binding site. In the presence of complement, RF likely can also interfere with phagocytosis of IgG complexes via complement receptors by blocking the complement-fixing sites in the IgG molecule. Similarly, IgM-RF may actually decrease the extent of complement depletion by IgG complexes, presumably by competing for or masking the complement binding sites in the Fc regions of the IgG (72–74).

In normal individuals, RF may have important physiologic functions that help protect against infectious organisms. Its frequent association with bacterial or parasitic infections (75–81) and transient appearance following immunization with bacterial or viral antigens (82–86) argues for RF being a vital part of the host response to infectious agents. Studies demonstrating that RF can enhance complement-dependent neutralization of herpes simplex virus (87) and increase resistance to pathogenic trypanosomes in rats (88) support this concept.

MECHANISMS UNDERLYING RHEUMATOID FACTOR PRODUCTION

RFs consist of a heterogeneous population of autoantibodies reactive with a multiplicity of determinants localized to the Fc portion of IgG. As discussed above, specificities of RFs occurring in a particular disease may not be identical to those of RFs in a different disease. Observations of this nature suggested that induction of RF synthesis might involve different pathways in different clinical conditions and that elucidation of such pathways could provide helpful clues concerning disease pathogenesis.

Environmental factors such as coffee or tobacco may influence RF production. Coffee consumption was studied for association with RF in a cross-sectional survey of 6,809 subjects with no clinical evidence of arthritis (89). The number of cups of coffee drunk daily was found to be directly proportional to the prevalence of RF positivity. There have now been several studies reporting an association between smoking cigarettes and RF in RA patients (90,91) and subjects without rheumatic diseases (92). Mattey et al. (93) investigated whether the association between RF production and smoking in RA was influenced by the presence of the HLA DRB1 shared epitope. Among 371 RA patients, those who had ever smoked were significantly more likely to be RF positive than nonsmokers (odds ratio 2.2, $p < 0.0001$). Examination of the major shared epitope (SE) genotypes in this RA population by multivariate logistic regression analysis revealed that only DRB1*0401 was associated with RF positivity, and that this was independent of the influence of smoking.

B-Cell Origins of Rheumatoid Factor

It has become increasingly clear that autoantibodies can arise from a variety of different B-cell populations. "Natural" autoantibodies present in normal individuals are generally of low affinity and are encoded by immunoglobulin genes that are not somatically mutated, indicating that the B cells that produced them have matured outside the germinal center. The source of these autoantibodies is thought to be B cells that derive from the B1 or marginal zone B-cell subsets (94,95). These cells, once activated in a T cell–independent manner, undergo proliferation and class switching in extrafollicular locations and rarely undergo somatic mutation (94,95). In addition, a subset of B cells activated during the T cell–dependent response differentiate into low-affinity unmutated short-lived cells in the extrafollicular region (96). In contrast, many pathogenic autoantibodies are of the IgG class and have accumulated somatic mutations, indicating that the B cells that produced them have undergone antigen-driven germinal center maturation and have received T-cell help. Those B cells that migrate into the follicle to form a germinal center may further differentiate into memory cells or long-lived plasma cells (97).

The lack of somatic mutation, affinity maturation, and acquisition of memory of the RF response in normal individuals is consistent with limitation of the physiologic RF response to the subset of B cells that mature in the extrafollicular compartment and do not enter the germinal center. In contrast, RFs in patients with RA display characteristics of both "natural" autoantibodies and antigen-driven autoantibodies. Although some are of low affinity and are unmutated, others have class switched to the IgG isotype, have acquired mutations, and are of high affinity (98). This suggests that although there may be an expansion of T cell–independent B-cell subsets in RA, antigen selection also plays an important role in the expression of RF in RA patients.

Recent attention has been directed toward the B1 subpopulation of B cells that bears the CD5 molecule typically expressed on the surface of T lymphocytes (99). Increased numbers of CD5$^+$ (B1) B cells are present in the circulation of patients with RA (100). It is of interest that CD5$^+$ B cells obtained from healthy unimmunized individuals appear to preferentially elaborate autoantibodies, including RF (101, 102). As expected, these autoreactive antibodies exhibit low affinity and polyspecificity (103). In patients with RA, however, CD5$^+$ B cells also elaborate higher-affinity monoreactive RF (104,105). The relationship between autoantibodies synthesized by CD5$^+$ B cells *in vitro* and those expressed in autoimmune disease has not been determined.

The propensity of CD5$^+$ B cells to elaborate IgM antibodies reactive with a variety of bacterial antigens (103,106,107) has suggested that these cells may play an important role in natural immunity. Whether CD5-positive B cells constitute a distinct B cell lineage is uncertain (108). Indeed, some evidence indicates that CD5 may be an activation antigen (109). Thus, elevated CD5$^+$ B cells in RA could reflect enhanced *in vivo* B-cell activation consistent with increased expression of other activation markers such as human leukocyte antigen (HLA)-DR molecules (110).

Abundant evidence suggests that at least part of the RF response in RA patients derives from B cells that have undergone T cell–dependent and antigen-driven germinal center maturation. Molecular genetic characteristics suggestive of an oligoclonal, antigen receptor–mediated B-cell response include nonrandom utilization of immunoglobulin variable (V) domains, high levels of somatic mutation, high replacement to silent (R:S) substitution ratios in the CDRs (111), and class switching to IgG isotypes. These characteristics suggest affinity maturation of the antibody response. The most definitive proof of an antigen-driven B-cell response is the finding of clonally-related V sequences (i.e., those that are derived from the same germ line V, D, and J gene segments) that contain shared mutations, and have high affinity for antigen. RFs present in individual autoimmune MRL/lpr mice exhibit V region somatic mutation patterns and class switching most consistent with an antigen-driven response (111).

Several molecular studies of immunoglobulin V gene expression have also provided evidence of antigen-driven expansion of unselected RA synovial B cells (112–114), RF-negative RA synovial B cells (115), RF-secreting B cells from RA synovia (116–119) and peripheral blood (120), and RFs produced by circulating CD5-positive cells (B1 cells) (104). Activated helper T cells are potent stimulators of RF secretion by B cells from patients with RA (121). This finding, along with the presence of clonally-related V-gene sequences in RFs from patients with RA, suggests that RF production in RA is, at least in part, the result of a T cell-dependent B cell response and that RF producing cells in individuals with RA develop in the germinal center. However recent findings using an RF transgenic mouse suggest that RF may encounter excessive T-cell help and undergo affinity maturation in the extrafollicular region in the autoimmune prone MRL/lpr mouse (122). This may allow autoreactive B cells to escape normal regulatory mechanisms that prevail in the germinal center environment. Whether this mechanism applies in human autoimmune disease or whether it is an artifact of a transgenic system remains to be determined.

The presence of clonally related RF-secreting B cells and plasma cells in RA synovial tissue is well documented. There are two possible mechanisms by which B cells secreting clonally related RF may be present in RA synovial tissue: migration of clonally related B cells into RA synovium or generation of a T cell–dependent B-cell response within the synovial lymphocytic infiltrates. RA synovia often contain lymphoid follicles, some of which have structures similar to germinal centers, the site of affinity maturation of the B-lymphocyte response. The histologic similarities between lymphoid tissue and RA synovia, coupled with the finding of clonally related B cells raises the possibility that synovia can support function similar to that in normal secondary lymphoid organs (114,123). The local environment of the RA synovium can support differentiation of B cells into terminally differentiated plasma cells (124,125). Plasma cells are present in the synovial fluid of patients with RA and other types of arthritis, but synovial IgM RF production is typically found only in patients with RF-positive RA, suggesting that the local environment in the RA joint favors RF production (126,127). Thus, in RA, the synovial membrane, normally a delicate two- to three-cell layer thick membrane, appears to be capable of being transformed into a lymphoid organ that can produce autoantibodies, including RF.

Antigens that Elicit Rheumatoid Factor Production

The antigens that elicit an RF response in RA have not been completely delineated. Polyclonal B-cell activators, such as lipopolysaccharide (128) and the Epstein-Barr virus (129), which activate B cells nonspecifically through receptors different from the B-cell receptor (BCR), are generally effective inducers of RF production *in vitro*. In addition, RF can be induced both by T cell-independent BCR stimuli such as staphylococcal protein A (130), and by stimuli that require T-cell help, including pokeweed mitogen (131) and immune complexes. The fact that peripheral blood B lymphocytes obtained from healthy individuals can be induced to elaborate IgM RF by a wide variety of polyclonal B-cell activators (129,131) provides firm evidence that RF-programmed B cells are constituents of the naïve B-cell repertoire deriving from both T cell–independent and T cell–dependent B-cell subsets.

The nature of the specific antigens that elicit an RF response *in vivo* is still not known. One hypothesis is that the antigen is IgG itself. Initial studies in animals indicated that repeated immunization with a variety of antigens could induce expression of auto-anti-IgG antibodies (132, 133). Subsequent studies indicated that the auto-anti-IgG responses elicited following secondary immunization were indeed RF and were directed against IgG complexed to the immunizing antigen (134,135). Booster immunization with tetanus toxoid in humans is also accompanied by RF responses (136,137), presumed to be triggered by IgG-containing immune complexes generated during the secondary immune response.

It is also possible that RFs are elicited by cross-reacting antigens. Cross-reactivities of some RFs with non-IgG antigens, including DNA-histone nucleoprotein (21), nonhistone nuclear protein (138), denatured DNA (139), and nitrophenyl groups (140), have been described. These findings raise the possibility that these (or as yet unidentified) antigens could induce or perpetuate RF responses under some circumstances. For example, RF production by B cells from patients with RA can be enhanced by *Staphylococcus aureus* Cowan 1 (121) and bacterial superantigens such as staphylococcal enterotoxin D (141). RF can be produced in a T cell–independent fashion in BALB/c mice by immunization with immune complexes of vesicular stomatitis virus (VSV) coated with monoclonal IgM anti-VSV glycoprotein antibodies (142). The antigenic epitopes in VSV are regularly spaced in a rigid paracrystalline membrane, which seems to be critical for RF production (142). These data suggest a role for antigens from infectious agents in the production of RF (143).

Similarities in binding specificities of several bacterial and viral Fc-binding proteins and some RF for the $C_\gamma2$–$C_\gamma3$ interface region of IgG have been delineated (14,144,145). It has therefore been suggested that exposure to foreign Fc-binding proteins might induce RF responses by an anti-idiotype mechanism (144,146,147).

Potential Role of Altered Glycosylation of Immunoglobulin G in Rheumatoid Factor Responses

Abnormalities of IgG structure might also contribute to the induction of RF. Indeed, altered glycosylation of IgG in some patients with RA has been demonstrated convincingly (75,148). Normal IgG is a glycoprotein with N-linked oligosaccharides, two of which are invariably located in the Fc portion of the molecule at asparagine (Asn) residue 297. An increase in galactose-deficient oligosaccharide terminating in *N*-acetylglucosamine located at this residue has been observed in patients with RA (148) and may be associated with reduced levels of B-cell galactosyltransferase (149). Aging is also correlated with an increased frequency of agalactosylated oligosaccharides in IgG, but this does not explain the abnormality observed in RA (150,151).

Alterations in the oligosaccharide moiety in the Fc portion of IgG could lead to exposure of one or more epitopes, which are ordinarily masked in the more completely galactosylated molecule, with consequent induction of RF (148). On the other hand, occurrence of this abnormality of IgG in Crohn disease and ulcerative colitis (150,152,153), diseases in which RF is usually absent, argues against a role for agalactosylated IgG in the induction of RF. Moreover, binding of RF from patients with RA to IgG preparations containing abnormally elevated concentrations of agalactosylated IgG is indistinguishable from binding to normal IgG (150, 154), although evidence has been obtained for existence of a subpopulation of RF with enhanced binding to IgG that is deficient in galactose (155).

Although posttranslationally modified IgG does not appear to act as an inducing antigen for RF production, there is some evidence that immune complexes containing agalactosyl IgG may be more pathogenic than those containing normally glycosylated IgG (156), and patients with high levels of agalactosyl IgG have a more aggressive disease course (157).

Other mechanisms for alteration of IgG have been proposed. Ultraviolet irradiation of IgG has been shown to modify its cysteine, tryptophan, tyrosine, and lysine residues by free radical reactions (158). These changes are accompanied by a characteristic autofluorescence and partial aggregation. Comparable changes in IgG were produced by activated neutrophils, presumably by oxygen free radicals (i.e., superoxide anion and hydroxyl radical) released into the media. Identification of IgG monomers and aggregates with identical fluorescent properties in rheumatoid sera and synovial fluids has raised the possibility that neutrophil-derived oxygen radical–induced damage to IgG occurs *in vivo*.

Another abnormality that may occur in RA is the modification of immunoglobulin by advanced glycation end products (AGEs). This posttranslational modification can result from hyperglycemia or oxidative stress. IgM antibodies against AGE-modified IgG (IgM anti-IgG AGE) were detected in 33% to 60% of RF-positive individuals, but were not found in RF-negative individuals with RA or other rheumatic and autoimmune diseases (159).

Influence of Cytokines on Rheumatoid Factor Expression

Cytokines also likely influence induction of RF production. $CD14^+$ monocyte-lineage cells from the bone marrow of patients with RA, but not from patients with osteoarthritis, induce B cells to secrete large amounts of RF (160). Interleukin-10 (IL-10) has been shown to play an important role in spontaneous IgM RF secretion by peripheral blood B cells from patients with RA (161). Increased serum and synovial fluid levels of IL-10 have been reported in patients with RA, likely from the non–T cell population of cells (predominantly monocytes and B cells) (162). In that study, IL-10 levels correlated with serum RF titers and spontaneous IgM-RF production *in vitro*. Conversely, IL-4 has been shown to decrease both spontaneous and induced production of IgM-RF by peripheral blood lymphocytes from patients with RA (163). Monocytes also secrete the TNF-like cytokine B-lymphocyte stimulator (BlyS) (BAFF, TALL-1) that is an important B-cell survival and differentiation factor. BLyS transgenic mice have hypergammaglobulinemia, increased circulating immune complexes, and high titers of RF in the serum (164). BLyS levels are increased in the serum of RA patients. Of interest, higher levels of BLyS have been found in the synovial fluid of patients with RA than in the serum, suggesting that local BLyS production may help drive RF production in the joint (165).

Animal Studies of Tolerance

In normal individuals, a state of immune unresponsiveness to self-antigens is maintained, termed self-tolerance. B-cell tolerance may be regulated during B-cell development in bone marrow (central) or in mature B cells in secondary lymphoid organs (peripheral). In order to gain insight into RF production, several groups of investigators have studied the regulation of B cell tolerance in mice. Tighe, Carson, and colleagues have analyzed the mechanism of induction of tolerance to human IgG using transgenic mice that express a high-affinity human IgM RF that does not cross-react with mouse IgG (166). These mice express low levels of serum RF and cannot be induced to produce RF even when immunized with aggregated human IgG, suggesting that the B cells are regulated, perhaps by some cross-reactive self antigen. However, the B cells can be rescued by antigen stimulation together with T-cell help or ligation of CD40, and they can then enter the germinal center and differentiate into plasma cells. Injection of soluble deaggregated human IgG, which does not elicit T-cell help, into transgenic animals caused an antigen-specific deletion of IgM RF B cells without any evidence for anergy. The deletion was preceded by an abortive phase of partial activation (167) and was independent of the Fas/Fas ligand pathway of apoptosis (168). These studies suggest that cross-linking of the receptor of a high-affinity RF-producing B cell in the absence of T-cell help is a mechanism for regulation of these cells.

Shlomchik, Weigert, and their colleagues established a different RF transgenic mouse model, using V genes derived from either a high affinity or an intermediate affinity (AM14) anti-IgG2a RF both isolated from an autoimmune MRL/lpr mouse (169). These RFs bind only IgG2a of the "a" allotype ($IgG2a^a$) but not $IgG2a^b$. Thus, by crossing the transgenes onto an IgH^a (BALB/c) background or to a congenic IgH^b (CB.17) background, the RF-expressing B cells could be studied when they were self-specific (IgH^a) or when they were not self-specific (IgH^b). Whereas the high-affinity RF was regulated by deletion or receptor editing in IgH^a mice, the numbers of AM14 transgene-expressing B cells in peripheral lymphoid organs of IgH^a mice were similar to those of IgH^b mice. Furthermore, AM14 RF B cells could make primary immune responses, indicating that self-antigen had not induced anergy. Thus, it does not appear to be necessary to break central tolerance to generate RF of intermediate affinity, even in nonautoimmune mice (170). Interestingly, some anti-IgG2a RF B cells were clustered in the T-cell-rich inner periarteriolar lymphatic sheath of the spleen, suggesting that RF autoantibody production in MRL/lpr mice may be a mechanistically distinct process from conventional antibody production (171).

In these animal studies, it has been shown that B cells producing high-affinity RFs are regulated by central tolerance but B cells producing lower affinity RFs are below the affinity threshold for tolerance induction by this mechanism. These B cells can be activated in the presence of immune complexes and T-cell help. Some RFs generated in the course of normal immune responses derive from short-lived B cells that do not differentiate into memory cells. Under normal physiologic circumstances, RFs induced in the germinal center in the course of an immune response to a foreign antigen will be tolerized by soluble IgG or by immune complexes once T-cell help is no longer available, and they will not differentiate into memory or long-lived plasma cells. In patients with RA, an excess of T-cell help, immune complexes, stimulatory cytokines such as BLyS, and eliciting antigens may all contribute to the perpetuation of the RF response.

GENETIC ORIGIN OF RHEUMATOID FACTOR IN HEALTH AND DISEASE

Approaches used to investigate the V region diversity of polyclonal RF include serologic analysis of serum RF using monoclonal antibodies (MoAbs), which identify V region gene products (i.e., idiotypic determinants), and nucleotide sequencing of V regions of RF elaborated by cloned B-cell lines obtained from healthy controls and patients with rheumatic diseases.

Idiotypic Analysis

Because patients with RA have relatively low levels of serum RF, information concerning the structural basis of RF expression has largely come from the study of IgM paraproteins, because approximately 10% of these proteins exhibit RF activity and large amounts are present in the serum (172). The seminal work of Henry Kunkel and his colleagues (173) provided great insight into the area of cross-reactive idiotypes (CRIs) in RFs from patients with RA and paraproteinemias. Initial efforts, using polyclonal antisera directed against idiotypes (V region determinants) expressed by RF paraproteins, indicated the existence of one major and two minor idiotypic families designated Wa, Po, and Bla, respectively (174,175). Although the precise structural basis of these CRIs remains obscure, the Wa CRI appears to be a conformational antigenic determinant involving both heavy and light chain structures located in the antigen-binding site (174,176). The Wa CRI is not restricted to RFs (177).

In view of difficulties in defining cross-reactive RF idiotypic groups by means of polyclonal serologic reagents, efforts were directed toward generating MoAbs reactive with structurally defined shared idiotopes. Two of these MoAbs, 17.109 (178) and 6B6.6 (179), recognize distinct VκIII L chain idiotopes present on approximately two thirds of IgM RF paraproteins (172). Molecular studies have demonstrated that the 17.109 cross-reactive idiotype is encoded by the VκIIIb germ line gene segment humkv325 (180,181). The 6B6.6 cross-reactive idiotype is encoded by the VκIIIa germ line gene segment humkv328 (duplicated gene segments L2 and L16) (182).

Similar approaches have been taken with regard to identifying structurally defined CRIs shared by heavy-chain V regions of RF paraproteins. Monoclonal antibody G6 recognizes a V_H1 idiotope shared by a subgroup of RF, which is encoded by the germ line gene designated V1–69 (hv1263, DP-10, 51P1) (183,184). Monoclonal antibody B6 recognizes an RF-associated V_H3 cross-reactive idiotype apparently encoded by a germ line gene closely related to or identical to V3–30.b (hv3005) (183,185,186). Another subgroup of RF contains heavy chains positive for the Lc1 CRI encoded by a V_H4 gene (187). Monoclonal antibody 9G4 recognizes a conformation-dependent CRI associated with the V_H4 gene segment V4–34 (VH4.21) (188).

Cross-sectional and longitudinal data indicate that a substantial proportion (if not all) of patients with RA synthesize some RF bearing either the 17.109 or 6B6.6 VκIII CRI (179,189). However, only a small fraction (~1%) of RF in individual sera appear to express either CRI. These observations suggest that either the germ line genes humkv325 and humkv328 encode only a small proportion of RF in RA, or extensive somatic mutation leads to loss of the idiotope. The occurrence of low proportions of 17.109 or 6B6.6 CRI RF before disease onset (190), and minimal changes in levels over time (189), support the former hypothesis. Germ line genes humkv325 and humkv328 do not encode disease-specific RF, since the 17.109 and 6B6.6 CRIs have been observed in RF-positive healthy adults in a pattern comparable with that seen in RA (190). Additionally, low levels of both of these VκIII cross-reactive idiotypes are found in normal immunoglobulins (172,179).

Analysis of Immunoglobulin Heavy- and Light-Chain Variable Domains

Although serologic studies have the advantage of directly analyzing RF expressed *in vivo*, they are constrained by the small number of MoAbs recognizing structurally defined CRIs that are available. Moreover, this approach cannot distinguish between the influence of somatic mutation of a particular germ line V gene segment (with consequent loss of germ line–encoded cross-reactive idiotype) versus utilization of a different germ line gene segment. For these reasons, many investigators have turned to sequence analysis of V_H and V_L domains expressed in RF-secreting B-cell lines to provide clues to the genetic basis of RF production. Based on these studies, the highly restricted pattern of V gene segment use exhibited by paraprotein RF apparently is not shared by RF-secreting B-cell lines rescued from patients with RA. Although potential biases may be introduced by the techniques used to generate RF-secreting B cell lines (e.g., Epstein-Barr virus transformation and heterohybridization), a recent study has shown that the method for immortalizing IgM RF–producing B cells from RA patients does not influence the specificity of the RFs obtained (191).

Immunoglobulin heavy- and light-chain V domains encode the portion of an antibody responsible for antigen recognition (see Chapter 13). Although restricted V gene utilization in RFs from RA were initially reported, it became apparent as more studies were published that there is remarkable restriction in V genes used in normal immune responses. In most B-cell responses, the same V_H, Vκ, and Vλ gene segments are used repeatedly, in a nonstochastic fashion. For example, of 50 Vκ gene segments with open reading frames, 24 have been reported to be functionally rearranged and approximately 87% of these functionally rearranged sequences are derived from only 11 gene segments (192). Similarly, approximately 62% of functionally rearranged Vλ sequences are derived from 5 gene segments out of 30 functional gene segments (193). Thus, restriction in the V gene repertoires of autoantibodies such as RF is not necessarily evidence of disease-specific V gene segments.

There have been many studies of V_H and V_L gene segments utilized in RFs from B cells in synovial fluid, synovial tissue, peripheral blood, and bone marrow of individuals with RA. Although unmodified germ line sequences have been reported, the preponderance of V region sequences are mutated in patterns consistent with antigen selection.

Most of the V_H gene segments in RFs from patients with RA are derived from the larger V_H1, V_H3, and V_H4 families, although one member of the V_H7 family has been reported (186,194). Several gene segments are of particular interest because of their repeated use. The V_H1 gene segment V1–69, which encodes the G6 cross-reactive idiotype, is among the most frequently reported V_H gene segments expressed in RFs from patients with RA. The V_H3-gene segment V3–23 (VH26, 30P1) and the set of closely related V_H3 gene segments V3–30 (1.9III), V3–30.3 (56P1), and V3–30.b (hv3005) are also commonly used in RFs from patients with RA. However, a number of other V_H gene segments are capable of encoding RF activity in RA (reviewed in reference 195).

There is substantial overlap of the repertoire of V_H gene segments expressed in RFs and those used in the fetal repertoire (196), in B cells from patients with lymphoid malignancies such as chronic lymphocytic leukemia (CLL) (197), in paraproteinemias (198), in RFs from healthy immunized donors (199), and in normal adult repertoires (200–202). This overlap is likely a reflection of the finding that a much smaller number of V_H gene segments are expressed than was originally thought. In fact, of the approximately 95 potentially functional germ line V_H gene segments, only 51 have open reading frames and have been found to rearrange (203).

V_L repertoires in RFs from patients with RA are more diverse than those from patients with paraproteinemias, in which approximately two thirds of RFs use VκIII gene segments. Although VκIII gene segments humkv325, humkv328, and Vg are commonly used, members of the VκI family, the VκII family, and the single member VκIV family have also been reported (reviewed in reference 195). Analyses of Vλ expression in RFs from RA have shown frequent representation of members of the VλI and VλIII families (reviewed in reference 195). Interestingly, the germ line VλII gene segment that encodes the 8.12 cross-reactive idiotype associated with anti-DNA antibodies from patients with systemic lupus erythematosus (204) has also been found to encode RFs from patients with RA (205,206).

As with V_H gene segments, there is considerable overlap of V_L gene segments expressed in RFs from patients with RA and in antibodies from normal individuals and those with other diseases. Of the approximately 75 germ line Vκ gene segments, only 24 have been reported to be functionally rearranged; 11 gene segments have been found to account for approximately 87% of all functionally rearranged Vκ sequences reported in the literature (192). Approximately 37% of these sequences are derived from the VκIII gene segments humkv325 (20%), humkv328 (9%), and Vg (8%) (192). Thus, there appear to be factors other than utilization of germ line V_H and V_L gene segments that contribute to RF activity.

Particular structural domains of the antibody V region may be important in determining self-reactivity. The antigen-binding site is generated by the juxtaposition of the three regions of sequence hypervariability (i.e., CDR1, CDR2, and CDR3) present in both H and L chains. CDR3 is the product of V_H-D_H-J_H joining in the H chain and V_L-J_L joining in the L chain. The H and L chain CDR3s form the center of the antigen-binding site, so their length and amino acid composition can affect the antigenic specificity of the antibody. There does not appear to be preferential utilization of particular D_H or J_H gene segments in RFs, because many different D_H and J_H gene segments can be present in RFs from patients with RA (207).

The effect of mutations in the V_H-D_H-J_H join on self-reactivity was recently addressed by examining the effect of single amino acid residue changes within the H chain CDR3 region of an IgM polyreactive natural antibody, SMI, secreted by a $CD5^+$ B-cell line derived from a patient with CLL (208). SMI is encoded by the nonmutated V_H1 gene 51P1 (V1–69) and the nonmutated VκIII gene humkv325. Specificity was dramatically changed by several point mutations. These observations support the supposition that the autoantigen-binding activity of the conserved autoantibody-associated germ line V genes is associated with somatic modifications of junctional sequences in the course of immunoglobulin gene rearrangement.

In addition to somatic mutation and use of different germ line gene segments, sequence diversity in the CDR3 domain is effected by addition of non–germ line–encoded nucleotides (N regions). These nucleotides are added at the sites of D_H-J_H and V_H-D_H joining at the time of gene segment rearrangement. Two splice variants of the enzyme terminal deoxynucleotidyl transferase (TdT) mediates both N region addition, as well as exonuclease activity (209). TdT was initially thought to be active only during H chain rearrangement, but not during L chain rearrangement. However, there is substantial evidence that N-region addition occurs in Vκ-Jκ and Vλ-Jλ joins derived from B cells of normal individuals (114,210,211) and patients with RA (114,212,213). Vκ transcripts from unselected B cells of some patients with RA contain a high proportion of long CDR3 regions (11 amino acid codons) compared with normal individuals, due in part to increased N-region addition (213). Vκ domains with 11 amino acid CDR3s are found in some RFs derived from peripheral blood, synovial fluid, and synovial tissue lymphocytes from patients with RA (205,214,215). However, most κ chain–containing RFs from patients with RA contain CDR3 intervals of 8, 9, or 10 codons (216–220). Thus, 11 amino acid κ-chain CDR3s are not required for RF activity. Of note, however, studies of TdT knockout mice have shown that the frequency of RF-producing B cells is reduced due to a lower incidence of polyreactivity (221). TdT does appear to be expressed in RA synovium, as do recombination activating genes 1 and 2, which may contribute to secondary immunoglobulin rearrangements in B cells, so-called receptor revision (222,223).

DETECTION

Most procedures used to detect RF activity in clinical specimens are based on the agglutination of carrier particles, most commonly polystyrene latex or red blood cells, coated with human or rabbit IgG. These generally represent modifications of the sensitized sheep cell agglutination test (SCAT or Waaler-Rose test) (2,224) and the latex fixation test of Singer and Plotz (7), which detect primarily IgM-RF.

The latex fixation test (7), without question, represents the most significant modification of the SCAT. In this procedure, sheep red blood cells are replaced by inert particles of polystyrene latex and the rabbit amboreceptor by pooled human Cohn-fraction II IgG. Conditions were carefully selected for optimal sensitivity and reproducibility with a minimum of spontaneous agglutination. Results of analysis from patients with RA by this procedure compared favorably with those obtained by the SCAT. Sera from 71% of the patients were reactive in this assay, as compared with only 2.7% of sera from patients with other conditions (225). Simplicity and freedom from the technical difficulties associated with the SCAT resulted in rapid adoption of the latex fixation test for routine detection of RF in clinical specimens. Of note, the presence of serum RF can interfere with thyroid function tests (226) and tests for malaria (227–230).

The original latex fixation test has now been largely replaced in the clinical laboratory by RF test kits available from several manufacturers. Most use latex reagents and rapid slide agglutination tests for screening purposes or qualitative results and tube dilution procedures for quantitative results. The latex reagents, however, vary in particle size, in the presence of stabilizing agents, and in the IgG preparations used to coat the particles. Some variability of results with different commercial kits for RF may therefore be encountered (231). Use of a reference standard and reporting results in international units substantially improves agreement of test results obtained by different procedures (232,233).

For larger clinical laboratories, measurement of RF by automated rate nephelometry provides a useful alternative to the standard agglutination tests (234). The method is based on the capacity of RF to precipitate aggregated human IgG. It measures the rate of increase in light scatter from particles suspended in solution formed by interaction of RF with an aggregated IgG reagent. Results are quantitated in international units after calibration of the instrument with an appropriate reference standard. Rheumatoid factor values obtained by this method compare favorably with those by latex fixation (235,236).

An interest in improving both sensitivity and quantitative accuracy, as well as identifying RF of different isotypes, has led to development of specific immunoassays capable of measuring nanogram quantities of RF (237–239). Although not widely used for measurement of clinical samples, these procedures have been extensively applied in research. The noncompetitive solid-phase "sandwich type" assay, in which IgG (usually human) is absorbed onto wells of plastic microtest plates, has proven most useful. After reaction with a dilution of the serum or other sample to be tested, bound IgM RF or IgA RF is detected by $(Fab')_2$ fragments of the appropriate antibody labeled with an enzyme, such as alkaline phosphatase (150,179), or labeled with iodine 125 (237,238).

Measurement of IgG RF presents special problems in that both the RF activity and the antigenic sites are located on IgG molecules. Additionally, non-RF IgG present as antigen bound to IgM RF can contribute to false-positive results. Thus, most immunoassays for IgG RF use tubes or microtest wells coated with rabbit IgG (237) and often incorporate procedures to remove or destroy IgM RF (240).

CLINICAL SIGNIFICANCE OF RHEUMATOID FACTOR

Population Studies

The prevalence of RF has been determined in several defined populations. In a longitudinal study involving approximately two thirds of the population of Tecumseh, Michigan, the prevalence of a positive latex fixation test for RF (greater than 1:20 titer) was approximately 3%, with essentially identical rates observed in men and women (241). The prevalence rate of RF in this population increased with age such that nearly 9% of women and 14% of men over 70 years of age tested positively, a finding in agreement with several other studies. Prevalences of RF, however, clearly vary among different populations as established in a study of Blackfoot and Pima Indians (242).

A critical question addressed by some population-based studies concerns the significance of a positive test result for serum RF in an apparently healthy individual. That ostensibly healthy persons may exhibit a positive RF test result is well documented. Indeed, more than two thirds of those with elevated serum RF in the Tecumseh study did not exhibit manifestations of RA (241). Considerable evidence, however, does indicate that increased levels of serum RF enhance the likelihood of an individual eventually developing RA. Ball and Lawrence followed 19 asymptomatic individuals with elevated serum RF for 5 years in England, and 7 developed evidence of RA (243). Aho and colleagues examined sera from 30 individuals who developed RA during a Finnish cardiovascular disease survey and found that 12 exhibited positive tests for RF (SCAT titers ≥1:32) from 4 months to 5 years before disease diagnosis (244). del Puente and colleagues analyzed data obtained from a longitudinal study of 2,712 Pima Indians conducted over a 19-year period (245). Regular biennial examinations, including a medical history, joint examination, radiographs, and RF determination (SCAT), were performed. A convincing correlation was observed between the incidence of RA and the SCAT titer (Fig. 58.2).

More recently, Halldorsdottir et al. (246) used a cohort of 14,000 participants in an Icelandic population study to follow the stability of serum RF over time and to assess the incidence of RA in subjects with transient or persistent increase in one or more RF isotypes. The study was begun in 1967. Between 1974 and 1983, a total of 13,858 participants were evaluated for the presence of rheumatic disease and had serum stored. In 1996, 135 participants with positive RF at study entry were clinically evaluated for the diagnosis of RA, and ELISAs for IgG RF, IgM RF, and IgA RF were performed. Most of these individuals (n = 115) had RF isotypes assayed as part of a follow-up study performed in 1987. Of the 135 participants, 15 had manifestations of RA when initially seen between 1974 and 1987. About 40% of the participants who had an elevated RF of only one isotype in the original sample had become RF negative in 1996 compared with only 15% of those with increase of two or three RF isotypes ($p = 0.002$). Seven of the 120 asymptomatic RF-positive participants developed RA during the observation period, which ranged from 9 to 22 years (mean 16.5 years). None of the 36 patients who were RF negative at the follow-up visit developed RA. Only 1 of 30 subjects with a persistently elevated RF of one isotype developed RA, compared with 6 of 54 with more than one isotype (relative risk 7.5). Taken together, these results indicate that elevated serum RF levels provide a marker for increased susceptibility to developing RA.

A recent population study in Pima Indians has suggested that the occurrence of RF, as well as RA, may be declining (247). This study evaluated the relative contributions of age, secular, and birth-cohort influences on RF positivity. RF data were available on 5,345 Pima Indians born between 1886 and 1975, who were surveyed at biennial intervals between 1966 and 1995. Based on an age-period-cohort analysis, there was a decline in the proportion of positive test results for RF (titer ≥1:32). There was a clear birth-cohort effect, with the highest likelihood of RF positivity in individuals born near the end of the nineteenth century, with continuing decline in RF positivity up to the most recent birth cohort. Thus, in the Pima Indian population, environmental influences in early life may influence the likelihood of RF positivity.

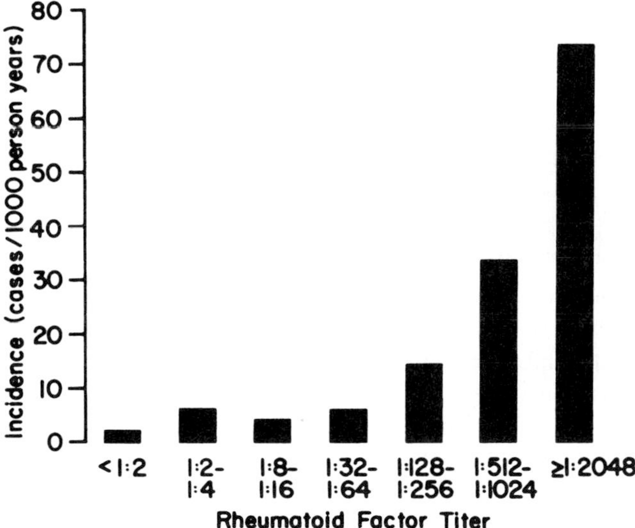

FIG. 58.2. Age- and sex-adjusted incidence of rheumatoid arthritis in the Pima Indian population analyzed relative to rheumatoid factor titer before the diagnosis of rheumatoid arthritis ($p < 0.001$, controlling for age, sex, and number of clinical criteria fulfilled). (Reproduced from del Puente A, Knowler WC, Pettitt DJ, et al. The incidence of rheumatoid arthritis is predicted by rheumatoid factor titer in a longitudinal population study. *Arthritis Rheum* 1988;31:1239–1244, by permission.)

Utility of Rheumatoid Factor in Diagnosing Rheumatoid Arthritis

The presence of serum RF by any method positive in less than 5% of normal control subjects is one of the criteria for diagnosis of RA (224). Approximately 75% of patients with RA exhibit elevated titers of serum RF when tested by conventional techniques such as the latex fixation test or SCAT. A lesser proportion of patients with other rheumatic diseases, including systemic lupus erythematosus, Sjögren syndrome, scleroderma, and polymyositis/dermatomyositis, also express elevated serum RF (Table 58.1).

RF can also be seen in normal individuals and those with a variety of chronic inflammatory or infectious diseases (Table 58.1). These RFs tend to react preferentially with human IgG, although exceptions occur. In the case of subacute bacterial endocarditis, elevated levels of RF generally disappear after treatment of the underlying infection (78). In contrast to serum RF present in nonrheumatic diseases, the RF occurring in RA sera commonly exhibits broad reactivity with both human and heterologous (e.g., rabbit) IgG.

Several studies have indicated that this broad reactivity of RF in RA reflects the presence of multiple distinct subpopulations of RF in the sera of these patients (248–250).

The presence of RF in a multitude of conditions other than RA limits the disease specificity of the test. Furthermore, the fact that serum RF is not found in all individuals with RA limits the sensitivity of the test in the diagnosis of RA. The predictive value of a test for a particular disease depends on the test's sensitivity and specificity, and the pretest probability of the disease. Based on these parameters, and on the population studies cited above, the RF assay is not a useful test for screening asymptomatic individuals and should not be ordered in this setting. Similarly, the RF assay is not often useful in patients with diffuse musculoskeletal pain and fatigue without other features of RA such as joint swelling. Such patients are most likely to have fibromyalgia or localized soft tissue rheumatism. In a study of 711 new patients referred to rheumatologists by primary care physicians, RF had been requested in 25%, while only 6% had RA (251), yielding a positive predictive value for RA of only 44%. Thus, in this patient population, the RF assay appeared to be used inappropriately, resulting in questionable clinical utility.

Using assumptions of a 1% pretest probability (based on disease prevalence in the general population), a test sensitivity of 80%, and a test specificity of 95%, Shmerling and Delbanco estimated the positive predictive value of RF (likelihood of RA based on a positive RF result) to be only 16% (252). The RF assay has also been found to have a relatively low positive predictive value for RA (24%) or for any rheumatic disease (34%) in a general hospital-based practice (253). The negative predictive value (exclusion of disease with a negative test result) was much better (89% for RA and 85% for any rheumatic disease), suggesting that the RF assay is more useful in excluding RA than in diagnosing it.

Although the RF assay may not be particularly useful in diagnosing RA or other rheumatic diseases in patients in the general population, it does have usefulness in a highly selected group of patients, namely those in a rheumatology outpatient clinic. In a study of 8,287 rheumatic disease patients, Wolfe and colleagues found a positive predictive value of 80% at the clinic prevalence rate for RA of 16.4% (254). Thus, the RF assay appears to be a useful test in the context of a rheumatology practice.

The RF assay is the most useful laboratory test in the diagnosis of RA. Because of its lack of specificity for RA, however, other diagnostic (auto)antibodies have been sought. The most well characterized of these recently appreciated antibodies are those reactive with synthetic peptides containing citrulline, a posttranslationally modified (deiminated) arginine residue that has been described in RA (reviewed in reference 255). There have been multiple studies to compare the sensitivity and specificity of these antibodies in the diagnosis of RA. These antibodies are discussed in detail elsewhere in this text.

Rheumatoid Factor in Chronic Hepatitis C Virus Infection

Hepatitis C virus (HCV) infection is a common problem worldwide. In the United States, there is an estimated prevalence rate of 1.8%, with approximately 75% of the infections (representing as many as 2.7 million people) thought to be chronic (256). The hepatitis C virus has recently been identified (257) and serologic tests for HCV infection developed. HCV has been identified as the causative agent in a large proportion of individuals with essential mixed cryoglobulinemia (258–260). Cryoglobulins from patients with HCV-associated cryoglobulinemic vasculitis often have RF activity. In addition, subjects with acute or chronic HCV often have arthralgias and may have low level serum RF. Persico et al. (261) analyzed the prevalence of RF, cryoglobulins, and cryoglobulinemic syndrome longitudinally over a 7-year period in 213 subjects with chronic hepatitis and 24 with cirrhosis. Among the chronic hepatitis patients, the prevalence of RF, cryoglobulins, and cryoglobulinemic syndrome were 2%, 0.8%, and 0%, respectively, whereas in cirrhosis patients the proportions were 4%, 8%, and 0%. Although the incidence of HCV infection has declined since the identification of the causative organism, chronic sequelae such as cirrhosis may take many years to become apparent. Despite the fact that a small proportion of individuals with chronic hepatitis have positive serum RF, the absolute number of chronic HCV patients is quite large. Thus, referral to rheumatologists for evaluation of possible RA in individuals with chronic HCV, arthralgias, and positive RF will likely be common in the coming years.

Significance of Rheumatoid Factor in Patients with Rheumatoid Arthritis

The precise serologic status of patients fulfilling criteria for RA, but lacking elevated serum RF by conventional testing ("seronegative" RA), is less clear. Occasionally, "hidden" RF can be detected in serum IgM of patients with seronegative RA after it is separated from autologous IgG (262). A substantial proportion, perhaps 50%, of patients with seronegative RA have elevated levels of serum RF when measured by sensitive assays such as radioimmunoassay or ELISA, although concentrations are significantly lower than in sera from patients with seropositive RA (238). Although these observations suggest a continuum of RF levels among patients with RA, the distinction between seropositive and seronegative RA (defined by conventional RF testing) has nonetheless proven to be of clinical significance.

Predisposition to seropositive RA is associated with inheritance of particular MHC class II HLA-DR4 or -DR1 alleles, whereas the association of DR4 with seronegative RA is generally less striking (or absent) (263–269). Although the pathogenetic mechanisms underlying the association between certain MHC alleles and seropositive RA remains to be unraveled, molecular analysis has revealed a common amino acid motif shared by disease susceptibility DR alleles in the third hypervariable region of their β chains, referred to as the shared epitope (SE) (270). The possibility that these MHC class II alleles favor enhanced responsiveness to determinants in the Fc portion of IgG cannot be excluded; however, DR4 does not associate with increased levels of RF in the sera of healthy individuals (271). On the other hand, DR4 correlates with RF expression in unaffected first-degree relatives of patients with seropositive RA, suggesting that DR4 may directly predispose to RF production (272). Further evidence supporting an association between DR4 and RF responses comes from the finding that polyclonally activated peripheral blood lymphocytes obtained from DR4-positive healthy individuals elaborate higher levels of IgM RF *in vitro* than peripheral blood lymphocytes from their DR4-negative counterparts (273).

In RA, HLA-DR4 alleles have been reported to be strongly associated with RF positivity in RA (274), whereas others have not found this to be the case (275). In a study of women with recent-onset RA, RF positivity was found more frequently among DR4-positive individuals with the shared epitope than among DR1-positive individuals with the epitope (276). This finding suggests that DR4 or genes linked to DR4, rather than the susceptibility epitope itself, is associated with RF positivity. The possibility that DR4 may also confer increased risk for more severe disease, unrelated to the presence of RF, has also been suggested by several studies (269,275,277,278). In a recent study of RF-positive patients with RA with erosive disease, individuals with two DRB1 genes containing the susceptibility epitope were more likely to have nodules, extraarticular manifestations, and joint surgery than those with a single susceptibility allele (279).

A study of early synovitis demonstrated an association between the shared epitope and radiographic erosions at 2 years disease duration in RF-negative subjects, but not in RF-positive subjects (280). Mattey et al. (281) analyzed the radiographic outcome, HLA-DRB1 genotypes, and RF status in 299 RA patients with established disease. RF-negative patients with the shared epitope had more severe radiographic findings than RF-negative patients without the shared epitope. The mean radiographic score was significantly higher in RF-positive patients than in RF-negative patients; there was no evidence of a gene dosing effect based on the number of copies of the shared epitope. Multiple regression analysis confirmed independent associations of RF positivity and presence of the shared epitope with radiographic outcome. Thus, RF most likely influences disease severity in RA through mechanisms other than those involved in the MHC/antigen presentation pathway. Potential other genetic influences on RF production include a 32–base pair deletion allele in the CC chemokine receptor 5 gene, which seems to be associated with the absence of IgM RF (282). This finding suggests that cell migration plays a role in RF production in RA.

Although there appear to be no significant qualitative histologic differences between joints of patients with RF-positive RA and those with RF-negative RA (283), seropositive and seronegative RA exhibit clinical differences. Seropositivity is associated with more aggressive articular disease, both radiographically and functionally (284–290).

Recent longitudinal and cross-sectional studies in early inflammatory arthritis have strengthened the hypothesis that RF has a role in radiographic damage. In a longitudinal study of 439 subjects with early inflammatory polyarthritis, predictors of radiographic severity at the time of the initial radiographs were found to be RF status, C-reactive protein levels, the presence of nodules, and number of swollen joints at baseline (291). After adjusting for baseline severity, a high titer of RF (>1:160) was an independent predictor of deterioration over 5 years; subjects with an initial RF at that level had a progression in their Larsen score that was 2.3 times (95% confidence interval 1.7–3.2) higher than that in the RF-negative individuals. A smaller study (292) showed that RF and, to a lesser degree, joint space narrowing score were independent predictors of radiologic progression in RA. Another study documented an odds ratio of developing new erosions during the first year of RA to be 9.7 (95% CI 1.05–89.93) in RF-positive patients compared with RF-negative individuals (293). RF was among the important predictors of radiographic damage and progression in a 3-year prospective study of 191 RA patients with disease duration of less than 1 year (294). Logistic regression analysis revealed that the only baseline values that were predictive of the 3-year radiologic scores were IgM rheumatoid factor positivity, DRB1*04 genes, pain score, and total radiologic score. Progression of joint damage was predicted by the erythrocyte sedimentation rate (ESR), IgM rheumatoid factor positivity, DRB1*04 genes, and erosions score at baseline.

In addition to more severe joint disease, patients with seropositive RA have a significantly higher frequency of extraarticular involvement (including subcutaneous nodules, vasculitis, leg ulcers, and neuropathy) than patients with seronegative RA (48,295). Furthermore, RF positivity is also one of several risk factors for increased mortality from RA (296,297). Mikuls et al. (298) found that RA was associated with significantly increased mortality in a cohort of older women (the Iowa Women's Health Study), and the association appeared to be restricted to those with RF-positive disease. Similar results were found in the analysis of excess mortality in 1,236 patients with inflammatory polyarthritis registered with the Norfolk Arthritis Register (299). RF-positive patients had an increased rate of death from all causes; the majority of the excess mortality could be attributed to cardiovascular causes.

Although disease activity tends to correlate with levels of RF (45–48), traditional outcome measures such as the number of swollen and tender joins, physician and patient global assessment, and acute phase reactants or ESR are more useful in following disease activity. Several investigators have attempted to delineate the clinical significance of changes in RF levels in patients with RA. Interpretation of these studies has generally been complicated by accompanying changes in medication. Nonsteroidal anti-inflammatory drugs (NSAIDs) were initially reported to directly suppress RF production *in vitro* and *in vivo* (300, 301). More recent studies indicate that decreases in serum RF associated with NSAID administration correlate with improvement in disease activity (302). Treatment with methotrexate and, to a lesser extent, clinical improvement, have been shown to decrease serum IgM-RF production in patients with RA (47). Suppression of spontaneous *in vitro* RF production by peripheral blood lymphocytes obtained from patients with RA following initiation of methotrexate therapy is also consistent with a direct effect of this agent on RF production (303). Taken together, these data indicate that RF levels in RA are likely influenced both by the clinical activity of the disease and the concomitant therapeutic regimen.

Although it is not performed routinely in a clinical setting, IgA RF may be a useful diagnostic and prognostic marker in RA. Elevation of both IgM RF and IgA RF appears to be relatively specific for RA because this combination is rarely found in other rheumatic diseases (304,305). Serum samples collected from nearly 14,000 randomly selected individuals were analyzed by Jonsson et al. (306) for RF isotypes, and 173 RF-positive and 156 matched RF-negative subjects were evaluated clinically. Of the 17 RF-positive individuals who were diagnosed with RA, 14 (82%) had a combined elevation of IgM and IgA RF. IgA RF is found in the sera of one third of patients with active RA and seems to be associated with a rapidly progressive course, extraarticular manifestations (307,308), and enrichment of particular circulating lymphocyte subsets ($CD5^+$ B cells and $CD4^+$/$CD45RO^+$ T cells) (309). Similarly, RA patients with IgA RF and IgM RF using rabbit IgG have significantly higher disease activity and more radiologic damage than RF negative patients (310).

REFERENCES

1. Waaler E. On the occurrence of a factor in human serum activating the specific agglutination of sheep blood corpuscles. *Acta Pathol Microbiol Scand* 1940;17:172–188.
2. Rose HM, Ragan C, Pearce E, et al. Differential agglutination of normal and sensitive sheep erythrocytes by sera of patients with rheumatoid arthritis. *Proc Soc Exp Biol Med* 1948;68:1–6.
3. Pike RM, Sulkin SE, Coggeshall HC. Serological reaction in rheumatoid arthritis. II. Concerning the nature of the factor in rheumatoid arthritis serum responsible for increased agglutination of sensitized sheep erythrocytes. *J Immunol* 1949;63:447–463.
4. Heller G, Jacobson AS, Kolodny MH, et al. The hemagglutination test for rheumatoid arthritis. II. The influence of human plasma fraction II (gamma globulin) on the reaction. *J Immunol* 1954;72:66–78.
5. Bozicevich J, Bunim JJ, Freund J, et al. Bentonite flocculation test for rheumatoid arthritis. *Proc Soc Exp Biol Med* 1958;97:180–183.
6. Waller MV, Vaughan JH. Use of anti-Rh sera for demonstrating agglutination activating factor in rheumatoid arthritis. *Proc Soc Exp Biol Med* 1956;92:198–200.
7. Singer JM, Plotz CM. The latex fixation test. I. Application to the serologic diagnosis of rheumatoid arthritis. *Am J Med* 1956;21(6):888–892.
8. Natvig JB, Gaarder PI, Turner MW. IgG antigens of the Cgamma2 and Cgamma3 homology regions interacting with rheumatoid factors. *Clin Exp Immunol* 1972;12(2):177–184.
9. Williams RC Jr, Malone CC. Rheumatoid-factor-reactive sites on C_H2 established by analysis of overlapping peptides of primary sequence. *Scand J Immunol* 1994;40(4):443–456.
10. Peterson C, Malone CC, Williams RC Jr. Rheumatoid-factor-reactive sites on CH3 established by overlapping 7-mer peptide epitope analysis. *Mol Immunol* 1995;32(1):57–75.
11. Williams RC Jr, Malone CC, Tsuchiya N. Rheumatoid factors from patients with rheumatoid arthritis react with β_2-microglobulin. *J Immunol* 1992;149:1104–1113.
12. Bonagura VR, Artandi SE, Davidson A, et al. Mapping studies reveal unique epitopes on IgG recognized by rheumatoid arthritis-derived monoclonal rheumatoid factors. *J Immunol* 1993;151:3840–3852.
13. Williams RC Jr, Malone CC, Casali P. Heteroclitic polyclonal and monoclonal anti-Gm(a) and anti-Gm(g) human rheumatoid factors react with epitopes induced in Gm(a-), Gm(g-) IgG by interaction with antigen or by nonspecific aggregation. A possible mechanism for the *in vivo* generation of rheumatoid factors. *J Immunol* 1992;149(5):1817–1824.
14. Stone GC, Sjobring U, Bjorck L, et al. The Fc binding site for streptococcal protein G is in the C gamma 2-C gamma 3 interface region of IgG and is related to the sites that bind staphylococcal protein A and human rheumatoid factors. *J Immunol* 1989;143(2):565–570.
15. Robbins DL, Skilling J, Benisek WF, et al. Estimation of the relative avidity of 19S IgM rheumatoid factor secreted by rheumatoid synovial cells for human IgG subclasses. *Arthritis Rheum* 1986;29(6):722–729.
16. Robbins DL, Benisek WF, Banjamini E, et al. Differential reactivity of rheumatoid synovial cells and serum rheumatoid factors to human immunoglobulin G subclasses 1 and 3 and their CH3 domains in rheumatoid arthritis. *Arthritis Rheum* 1987;30:489–497.
17. Tokano Y, Arai S, Hashimoto H, et al. The distinct subgroup of patients with rheumatoid arthritis shown by Ig G3-reactive rheumatoid factor. *Autoimmunity* 1989;5(1–2):107–114.
18. Butler VP Jr, Vaughan JH. Hemagglutination by rheumatoid factor of cells coated with animal gamma globulins. *Proc Soc Exp Biol Med* 1964;116:585–593.
19. Gaarder PI, Michaelsen TE. Specificity of rheumatoid factors cross-reacting with human and rabbit IgG. *Acta Pathol Microbiol Scand [B]* 1974;82(5):733–741.
20. Williams RCJ, Malone CC, Kolaskar AS, et al. Antigenic determinants reacting with rheumatoid factor: epitopes with different primary sequences share similar conformation. *Mol Immunol* 1997;34(7):543–556.
21. Aitcheson CT, Peebles C, Joslin F, et al. Characteristics of antinuclear antibodies in rheumatoid arthritis. Reactivity of rheumatoid factor with a histone-dependent nuclear antigen. *Arthritis Rheum* 1980;23(5):528–538.
22. Heimer R, Levin FM. On the distribution of rheumatoid factors among the immunoglobulins. *Immunochemistry* 1966;3(1):1–10.
23. Kunkel HG, Müller-Eberhard HJ, Fudenberg HH, et al. Gamma globulin complexes in rheumatoid arthritis and certain other conditions. *J Clin Invest* 1961;40:117–129.
24. Schrohenloher RE. Characterization of the γ-globulin complexes present in certain sera having high titers of anti-γ-globulin activity. *J Clin Invest* 1966;45(4):501–512.
25. Dunne JV, Carson DA, Spiegelberg HL, et al. IgA rheumatoid factor in the sera and saliva of patients with rheumatoid arthritis and Sjögren's syndrome. *Ann Rheum Dis* 1979;38(2):161–165.
26. Zuraw BL, O'Hair CH, Vaughan JH, et al. Immunoglobulin E-rheumatoid factor in the serum of patients with rheumatoid arthritis, asthma, and other diseases. *J Clin Invest* 1981;68(6):1610–1613.
27. Elkon KB, Delacroix DL, Gharavi AE, et al. Immunoglobulin A and polymeric IgA rheumatoid factors in systemic sicca syndrome: partial characterization. *J Immunol* 1982;129(2):576–581.
28. Schrohenloher RE, Koopman WJ, Alarcón GS. Molecular forms of IgA rheumatoid factor in serum and synovial fluid of patients with rheumatoid arthritis. *Arthritis Rheum* 1986;29(10):1194–1202.
29. Ogawa T, Tarkowski A, McGhee ML, et al. Analysis of human IgG and IgA subclass antibody-secreting cells from localized chronic inflammatory tissue. *J Immunol* 1989;142:1150–1158.
30. Pope RM, Teller DC, Mannik M. The molecular basis of self-association of IgG-Rheumatoid factors. *J Immunol* 1975;115(2):365–373.

31. Bas S, Djavad N, Schwager J, et al. Relation between the heavy chain complementarity region 3 characteristics and rheumatoid factor binding properties. *Autoimmunity* 1998;27(4):191–199.
32. Zhang M, Majid A, Bardwell P, et al. Rheumatoid factor specificity of a VH3-encoded antibody is dependent on the heavy chain CDR3 region and is independent of protein A binding. *J Immunol* 1998;161(5): 2284–2289.
33. Zhang M, Spey D, Ackerman S, et al. Rheumatoid factor idiotypic and antigenic specificity is strongly influenced by the light chain VJ junction. *J Immunol* 1996;156(9):3570–3575.
34. Corper AL, Sohi MK, Bonagura VR, et al. Structure of human IgM rheumatoid factor Fab bound to its autoantigen IgG Fc reveals a novel topology of antibody-antigen interaction. *Nat Struct Biology* 1997; 4(5):374–381.
35. Sutton BJ, Corper AL, Sohi MK, et al. The structure of a human rheumatoid factor bound to IgG Fc. *Adv Exp Med Biol* 1998;435: 41–50.
36. Smiley JD, Sachs C, Ziff M. *In vitro* synthesis of immunoglobulin by rheumatoid synovial membrane. *J Clin Invest* 1968;47:624–632.
37. Taylor-Upsahl MM, Abrahamsen TG, Natvig JB. Rheumatoid factor plaque-forming cells in rheumatoid synovial tissue. *Clin Exp Immunol* 1977;28(2):197–203.
38. Wernick RM, Lipsky PE, Marban-Arcos E, et al. IgG and IgM rheumatoid factor synthesis in rheumatoid synovial membrane cell cultures. *Arthritis Rheum* 1985;28:742–752.
39. Koopman WJ, Miller RK, Crago SS, et al. IgA rheumatoid factor: evidence for independent expression at local sites of tissue inflammation. *Ann NY Acad Sci* 1983;409:258–272.
40. Franklin EC, Holman HR, Müller-Eberhard HJ, et al. An unusual protein component of high molecular weight in the serum of certain patients with rheumatoid arthritis. *J Exp Med* 1957;105:425–438.
41. Winchester RJ, Agnello V, Kunkel HG. Gamma globulin complexes in synovial fluids of patients with rheumatoid arthritis. Partial characterization and relationship to lowered complement levels. *Clin Exp Immunol* 1970;6(5):689–706.
42. Vaughan JH, Jacox RJ, Noell P. Relation of intracytoplasmic inclusions in joint fluid leukocytes to anti-gamma-G globulins. *Arthritis Rheum* 1968;11(2):135–144.
43. Munthe E, Natvig JB. Characterization of IgG complexes in eluates from rheumatoid tissue. *Clin Exp Immunol* 1971;8(2):249–262.
44. Jasin HE. Autoantibody specificities of immune complexes sequestered in articular cartilage of patients with rheumatoid arthritis and osteoarthritis. *Arthritis Rheum* 1985;28:241–248.
45. Cats A, Hazevoet HM. Significance of positive tests for rheumatoid factor in the prognosis of rheumatoid arthritis. A follow-up study. *Ann Rheum Dis* 1970;29:254–260.
46. Allen C, Elson CJ, Scott DGI, et al. IgG antiglobulins in rheumatoid arthritis and other arthritides: relationship with clinical features and other parameters. *Ann Rheum Dis* 1981;40:127–131.
47. Alarcón GS, Schrohenloher RE, Bartolucci AA, et al. Suppression of rheumatoid factor production by methotrexate in patients with rheumatoid arthritis: evidence for differential influences of therapy and clinical status on IgM and IgA rheumatoid factor expression. *Arthritis Rheum* 1990;33:1156–1161.
48. van Zeben D, Hazes JM, Zwinderman AH, et al. Clinical significance of rheumatoid factors in early rheumatoid arthritis: results of a follow up study. *Ann Rheum Dis* 1992;51(9):1029–1035.
49. Zvaifler NJ, Schur P. Reactions of aggregated mercaptoethanol treated gamma globulin with rheumatoid factor—precipitin and complement fixation studies. *Arthritis Rheum* 1968;11(4):523–536.
50. Schmid FR, Roitt IM, Rocha MJ. Complement fixation by a two-component antibody system: immunoglobulin G and immunoglobulin M anti-globulin (rheumatoid factor). Parodoxical effect related to immunoglobulin G concentration. *J Exp Med* 1970;132(4):673–693.
51. Tesar JT, Schmid FR. Conversion of soluble immune complexes into complement-fixing aggregates by IgM-rheumatoid factor. *J Immunol* 1970;105(5):1206–1214.
52. Tanimoto K, Cooper NR, Johnson JS, et al. Complement fixation by rheumatoid factor. *J Clin Invest* 1975;55:437–445.
53. Brown PB, Nardella FA, Mannik M. Human complement activation by self-associated IgG rheumatoid factors. *Arthritis Rheum* 1982; 25(9):1101–1107.
54. Sabharwal UK, Vaughan JH, Fong S, et al. Activation of the classical pathway of complement by rheumatoid factors. Assessment by radioimmunoassay for C4. *Arthritis Rheum* 1982;25(2):161–167.
55. Pekin TJ Jr, Zvaifler NJ. Hemolytic complement in synovial fluid. *J Clin Invest* 1964;43:1372–1382.
56. Ruddy S, Austen KF. The complement system in rheumatoid synovitis. I. An analysis of complement component activities in rheumatoid synovial fluids. *Arthritis Rheum* 1970;13(6):713–723.
57. Perrin LH, Nydegger UE, Zubler RH, et al. Correlation between levels of breakdown products of C3, C4, and properdin factor B in synovial fluids from patients with rheumatoid arthritis. *Arthritis Rheum* 1977; 20(2):647–652.
58. Kaplan RA, Curd JG, Deheer DH, et al. Metabolism of C4 and factor B in rheumatoid arthritis. Relation to rheumatoid factor. *Arthritis Rheum* 1980;23(8):911–920.
59. Van Snick JL, Van RE, Markowetz B, et al. Enhancement by IgM rheumatoid factor of *in vitro* ingestion by macrophages and *in vivo* clearance of aggregated IgG or antigen-antibody complexes. *Eur J Immunol* 1978;8(4):279–285.
60. Davis JS, Torrigiani G. Effects of rheumatoid factor on *in vivo* distribution of aggregated human IgG and antigen-antibody complexes. *Proc Soc Exp Biol Med* 1967;125:772–776.
61. Hendrich C, Kuipers JG, Kolanus W, et al. Activation of CD16+ effector cells by rheumatoid factor complex. Role of natural killer cells in rheumatoid arthritis. *Arthritis Rheum* 1991;34(4):423–431.
62. Saxne T, Palladino MA Jr, Heinegard D, et al. Detection of tumor necrosis factor alpha but not tumor necrosis factor beta in rheumatoid arthritis synovial fluid and serum. *Arthritis Rheum* 1988;31(8):1041–1045.
63. Abrahams VM, Cambridge G, Lydyard PM, et al. Induction of tumor necrosis factor alpha production by adhered human monocytes: a key role for Fcgamma receptor type IIIa in rheumatoid arthritis. *Arthritis Rheum* 2000;43(3):608–616.
64. Carson DA, Chen PP, Kipps TJ. New roles for rheumatoid factor. *J Clin Invest* 1991;87:379–383.
65. Chesnut RW, Grey HM. Studies on the capacity of B cells to serve as antigen-presenting cells. *J Immunol* 1981;126(3):1075–1079.
66. Rock KL, Benacerraf B, Abbas AK. Antigen presentation by hapten-specific B lymphocytes. I. Role of surface immunoglobulin receptors. *J Exp Med* 1984;160(4):1102–1113.
67. Roosnek E, Lanzavecchia A. Efficient and selective presentation of antigen-antibody complexes by rheumatoid factor B cells. *J Exp Med* 1991;173(2):487–489.
68. Tighe H, Chen PP, Tucker R, et al. Function of B cells expressing a human immunoglobulin M rheumatoid factor autoantibody in transgenic mice. *J Exp Med* 1993;177(1):109–118.
69. Boackle RJ, Pruitt KM, Mestecky J. The interactions of human complement with interfacially aggregated preparations of human secretory IgA. *Immunochemistry* 1974;11(9):543–548.
70. Pfaffenbach G, Lamm ME, Gigli I. Activation of the guinea pig alternative complement pathway by mouse IgA immune complexes. *J Exp Med* 1982;155(1):231–247.
71. Messner RP, Laxidal T, Quie PG, et al. Serum opsonin, bacteria, and polymorphonuclear leukocyte interactions in subacute bacterial endocarditis. Anti-gamma-globulin factors and their interaction with specific opsonins. *J Clin Invest* 1968;47(5):1109–1120.
72. Bernhard GC, Cheng W, Talmage DW. The reaction of rheumatoid factor and complement with γ-globulin coated latex. *J Immunol* 1962; 88:750–762.
73. Heimer R, Levin FM, Kahn MF. Inhibition of complement fixation by human serum. II. The activity of a γ-1M globulin and rheumatoid factor in complement fixation reactions. *J Immunol* 1963;91:866–872.
74. Davis JS, IV, Bollet AJ. Protection of a complement-sensitive enzyme system by rheumatoid factor. *J Immunol* 1964;92:139–144.
75. Peltier A, Christian CL. The presence of the "rheumatoid factor" in sera from patients with syphilis. *Arthritis Rheum* 1959;2:1–7.
76. Dresner E, Trombly P. The latex-fixation reaction in nonrheumatoid diseases. *N Engl J Med* 1959;261:981–988.
77. Cathcart ES, Williams RC Jr, Ross H, et al. The relationship of the latex fixation test to the clinical and serologic manifestions of leprosy. *Am J Med* 1961;31:758–765.
78. Williams RC Jr, Kunkel HG. Rheumatoid factor, complement and conglutinin aberrations in patients with subacute bacterial endocarditis. *J Clin Invest* 1962;41(666):675.
79. Singer JM, Plotz CM, Peralta FM, et al. The presence of anti-gamma globulin factors in sera of patients with active pulmonary tuberculosis. *Ann Intern Med* 1962;56(545):552.

80. Houba V, Allison AC. M-antiglobulins (rheumatoid-factor-like globulins) and other gamma-globulins in relation to tropical parasitic infections. *Lancet* 1966;1(7442):848–852.
81. Carson DA, Bayer AS, Eisenberg RA, et al. IgG rheumatoid factor in subacute bacterial endocarditis: relationship to IgM rheumatoid factor and circulating immune complexes. *Clin Exp Immunol* 1978; 31(1):100–103.
82. Johnson RE, Hall AP. Rubella arthritis: report of cases studied by latex tests. *N Engl J Med* 1958;258:743–745.
83. Svec KH, Dingle JH. The occurrence of rheumatoid factor in association with antibody response to influenza A2 (Asian) virus. *Arthritis Rheum* 1965;8:524–529.
84. Kaplan ME. Cryoglobulinemia in infectious mononucleosis: quantitation and characterization of the cryoproteins. *J Lab Clin Med* 1968; 71(5):754–765.
85. Langenhuysen MMAC. Antibodies against g-globulin after blood transfusion and cytomegalovirus-infection. *Clin Exp Immunol* 1971; 9(3):393–398.
86. Levine PR, Axelrod DA. Rheumatoid factor isotypes following immunization. *Clin Exp Rheumatol* 1985;3(2):147–149.
87. Ashe WK, Daniels CA, Scott GS, Notkins AL. Interaction of rheumatoid factor with infectious herpes simplex virus-antibody complexes. *Science* 1971;172(979):176–177.
88. Clarkson AB Jr, Mellow GH. Rheumatoid factor-like immunoglobulin M protects previously uninfected rat pups and dams from Trypanosoma lewisi. *Science* 1981;214(4517):186–188.
89. Heliovaara M, Aho K, Knekt P, et al. Coffee consumption, rheumatoid factor, and the risk of rheumatoid arthritis. *Ann Rheum Dis* 2000; 59(8):631–635.
90. Saag KG, Cerhan JR, Kolluri S, et al. Cigarette smoking and rheumatoid arthritis severity. *Ann Rheum Dis* 1997;56(8):463–469.
91. Masdottir B, Jonsson T, Manfredsdottir V, et al. Smoking, rheumatoid factor isotypes and severity of rheumatoid arthritis. *Rheumatology (Oxford)* 2000;39(11):1202–1205.
92. Jonsson T, Thorsteinsson J, Valdimarsson H. Does smoking stimulate rheumatoid factor production in non-rheumatic individuals? *APMIS* 1998;106(10):970–974.
93. Mattey DL, Dawes PT, Clarke S, et al. Relationship among the HLA-DRB1 shared epitope, smoking, and rheumatoid factor production in rheumatoid arthritis. *Arthritis Rheum* 2002;47(4):403–407.
94. Martin F, Kearney JF. Marginal-zone B cells. *Nat Rev Immunol* 2002; 2(5):323–335.
95. Martin F, Kearney JF. B1 cells: similarities and differences with other B cell subsets. *Curr Opin Immunol* 2001;13(2):195–201.
96. MacLennan IC, Toellner KM, Cunningham AF, et al. Extrafollicular antibody responses. *Immunol Rev* 2003;194:8–18.
97. O'Connor BP, Gleeson MW, Noelle RJ, et al. The rise and fall of long-lived humoral immunity: terminal differentiation of plasma cells in health and disease. *Immunol Rev* 2003;194:61–76.
98. Sasso EH. Immunoglobulin V genes in rheumatoid arthritis. *Rheum Dis Clin North Am* 1992;18:809–836.
99. Herzenberg LA, Stall AM, Lalor PA, et al. The Ly-1 B cell lineage. *Immunol Rev* 1986;93:81–102.
100. Plater-Zyberk C, Maini RN, Lam K, et al. A rheumatoid arthritis B cell subset expresses a phenotype similar to that in chronic lymphocytic leukemia. *Arthritis Rheum* 1985;28(9):971–976.
101. Casali P, Burastero SE, Nakamura M, et al. Human lymphocytes making rheumatoid factor and antibody to ssDNA belong to Leu-1$^+$ B-cell subset. *Science* 1987;236:77–81.
102. Hardy RR, Hayakawa K, Shimizu M, et al. Rheumatoid factor secretion from human Leu-1$^+$ B cells. *Science* 1987;236(4797):81–83.
103. Nakamura M, Burastero SE, Notkins AL, et al. Human monoclonal rheumatoid factor–like antibodies from CD5 (Leu-1)$^+$ B cells are polyreactive. *J Immunol* 1988;140:4180–4186.
104. Mantovani L, Wilder RL, Casali P. Human rheumatoid B-1a (CD5$^+$B) cells make somatically hypermutated high affinity IgM rheumatoid factors. *J Immunol* 1993;151(1):473–488.
105. Burastero SE, Casali P, Wilder RL, et al. Monoreactive high affinity and polyreactive low affinity rheumatoid factors are produced by CD5$^+$ B cells from patients with rheumatoid arthritis. *J Exp Med* 1988;168:1979–1992.
106. Mercolino TJ, Arnold LW, Hawkins LA, et al. Normal mouse peritoneum contains a large population of Ly-1$^+$ (CD5) B cells that recognize phosphatidyl choline. Relationship to cells that secrete hemolytic antibody specific for autologous erythrocytes. *J Exp Med* 1988;168(2):687–698.
107. Forster I, Rajewsky K. Expansion and functional activity of Ly-1$^+$ B cells upon transfer of peritoneal cells into allotype-congenic, newborn mice. *Eur J Immunol* 1987;17(4):521–528.
108. Kearney JF. CD5$^+$ B-cell networks. *Curr Opin Immunol* 1993;5(2): 223–226.
109. Werner-Favre C, Vischer TL, Wohlwend D, et al. Cell surface antigen CD5 is a marker for activated human B cells. *Eur J Immunol* 1989; 19(7):1209–1213.
110. Cush JJ, Lipsky PE. Cellular basis for rheumatoid inflammation. *Clin Orthop Rel Res* 1991;265:9–22.
111. Shlomchik MJ, Marshak-Rothstein A, Wolfowicz CB, et al. The role of clonal selection and somatic mutation in autoimmunity. *Nature* 1987;328:805–811.
112. Lee SK, Bridges SL Jr, Kirkham PM, et al. Evidence of antigen receptor-influenced oligoclonal B lymphocyte expansion in the synovium of a patient with longstanding rheumatoid arthritis. *J Clin Invest* 1994;93:361–370.
113. Clausen BE, Bridges SL Jr, Lavelle JC, et al. Clonally-related immunoglobulin VH domains and non-random use of DH gene segments in rheumatoid arthritis synovium. *Mol Med* 1998;4:240–257.
114. Bridges SL Jr. Frequent N addition and clonal relatedness among immunoglobulin lambda light chains expressed in rheumatoid arthritis synovia and PBL, and the influence of Vlambda gene segment utilization on CDR3 length. *Mol Med* 1998;4(8):525–553.
115. Krenn V, Konig A, Hensel F, et al. Molecular analysis of rheumatoid factor (RF)-negative B cell hybridomas from rheumatoid synovial tissue: evidence for an antigen-induced stimulation with selection of high mutated IgVH and low mutated IgVL/lambda genes. *Clin Exp Immunol* 1999;115(1):168–175.
116. Randen I, Brown D, Thompson KM, et al. Clonally related IgM rheumatoid factors undergo affinity maturation in the rheumatoid synovial tissue. *J Immunol* 1992;148:3296–3301.
117. Olee T, Lu EW, Huang DF, et al. Genetic analysis of self-associating immunoglobulin G rheumatoid factors from two rheumatoid synovia implicates an antigen-driven response. *J Exp Med* 1992;175(3):831–842.
118. Ermel RW, Kenny TP, Chen PP, et al. Molecular analysis of rheumatoid factors derived from rheumatoid synovium suggests an antigen-driven response in inflamed joints. *Arthritis Rheum* 1993;36(3):380–388.
119. Ermel RW, Kenny TP, Wong A, et al. Analysis of the molecular basis of synovial rheumatoid factors in rheumatoid arthritis. *Clin Immunol Immunopathol* 1997;84(3):307–317.
120. Hakoda M, Kamatani N, Taniguchi A, et al. Generation and molecular characterisation of monoclonal IgG4 rheumatoid factor from a patient with rheumatoid arthritis. *Ann Rheum Dis* 1997;56(1):74–77.
121. Hirohata S, Inoue T, Miyamoto T. Frequency analysis of human peripheral blood B cells producing IgM-rheumatoid factor. Differential effects of stimulation with monoclonal antibodies to CD3 and *Staphylococcus aureus*. *J Immunol* 1990;145:1681–1686.
122. Citron BP, Halpern M, McCarron M, et al. Necrotizing angiitis associated with drug abuse. *N Engl J Med* 1970;283(19):1003–1011.
123. Schroder AE, Greiner A, Seyfert C, et al. Differentiation of B cells in the nonlymphoid tissue of the synovial membrane of patients with rheumatoid arthritis. *Proc Natl Acad Sci U S A* 1996;93:221–225.
124. Dechanet J, Merville P, Durand I, et al. The ability of synoviocytes to support terminal differentiation of activated B cells may explain plasma cell accumulation in rheumatoid synovium. *J Clin Invest* 1995;95:456–463.
125. Kim HJ, Krenn V, Steinhauser G, et al. Plasma cell development in synovial germinal centers in patients with rheumatoid and reactive arthritis. *J Immunol* 1999;162:3053–3062.
126. Reparon-Schuijt CC, Van Esch WJ, Van Kooten C, et al. Functional analysis of rheumatoid factor-producing B cells from the synovial fluid of rheumatoid arthritis patients. *Arthritis Rheum* 1998;41(12): 2211–2220.
127. Lettesjo H, Nordstrom E, Strom H, et al. Autoantibody patterns in synovial fluids from patients with rheumatoid arthritis or other arthritic lesions. *Scand J Immunol* 1998;48(3):293–299.
128. Dresser DW, Popham AM. Induction of an IgM anti-(bovine)-IgG response in mice by bacterial lipopolysaccharide. *Nature* 1976;264 (5586):552–554.

129. Slaughter L, Carson DA, Jensen FC, et al. *In vitro* effects of Epstein-Barr virus on peripheral blood mononuclear cells from patients with rheumatoid arthritis and normal subjects. *J Exp Med* 1978;148(5):1429–1434.
130. Dalal N, Roman S, Levinson AI. *In vitro* secretion of human IgM rheumatoid factor. Evidence for distinct rheumatoid factor populations in health and disease. *Arthritis Rheum* 1990;33(9):1340–1346.
131. Koopman WJ, Schrohenloher RE. *In vitro* synthesis of IgM rheumatoid factor by lymphocytes from healthy adults. *J Immunol* 1980;125:934–939.
132. Abruzzo JL, Christian CL. The induction of a rheumatoid factor-like substance in rabbits. *J Exp Med* 1961;114:791–806.
133. Williams RC Jr, Kunkel HG. Antibodies to rabbit γ-globulin after immunizing with various preparations of autologous γ-globulin. *Proc Soc Exp Med* 1963;112:554–561.
134. Nemazee DA, Sato VL. Induction of rheumatoid antibodies in the mouse. Regulated production of autoantibody in the secondary humoral response. *J Exp Med* 1983;158(2):529–545.
135. Nemazee DA. Immune complexes can trigger specific, T cell–dependent, autoanti-IgG antibody production in mice. *J Exp Med* 1985;161(1):242–256.
136. Welch MJ, Fong S, Vaughan J, et al. Increased frequency of rheumatoid factor precursor B lymphocytes after immunization of normal adults with tetanus toxoid. *Clin Exp Immunol* 1983;51(2):299–304.
137. Tarkowski A, Czerkinsky C, Nilsson LA. Simultaneous induction of rheumatoid factor– and antigen-specific antibody-secreting cells during the secondary immune response in man. *Clin Exp Immunol* 1985;61(2):379–387.
138. Mason JC, Venables PJ, Smith PR, et al. Characterisation of non-histone nuclear proteins cross reactive with purified rheumatoid factors. *Ann Rheum Dis* 1985;44(5):287–293.
139. Rubin RL, Balderas RS, Tan EM, et al. Multiple autoantigen binding capabilities of mouse monoclonal antibodies selected for rheumatoid factor activity. *J Exp Med* 1984;159(5):1429–1440.
140. Reininger L, Spertini F, Shibata T, et al. Rheumatoid factor autoantibody-binding site: a molecular analysis using monoclonal antibodies with dual anti-TNP and anti-IgG activities. *Eur J Immunol* 1989;19(11):2123–2130.
141. He X, Goronzy JJ, Weyand CM. The repertoire of rheumatoid factor-producing B cells in normal subjects and patients with rheumatoid arthritis. *Arthritis Rheum* 1993;36(8):1061–1069.
142. Fehr T, Bachmann MF, Bucher E, et al. Role of repetitive antigen patterns for induction of antibodies against antibodies. *J Exp Med* 1997;185(10):1785–1792.
143. Posnett DN, Edinger J. When do microbes stimulate rheumatoid factor? *J Exp Med* 1997;185(10):1721–1723.
144. Oppliger IR, Nardella FA, Stone GC, et al. Human rheumatoid factors bear the internal image of the Fc binding region of staphylococcal protein A. *J Exp Med* 1987;166(3):702–710.
145. Johansson PJ, Schroder AK, Nardella FA, et al. Interaction between herpes simplex type 1–induced Fc receptor and human and rabbit immunoglobulin G (IgG) domains. *Immunology* 1986;58(2):251–255.
146. Mouritsen S. Rheumatoid factors are anti-idiotypic antibodies against virus-induced anti-Fc receptor antibodies. A hypothesis for the induction of some rheumatoid factors. *Scand J Immunol* 1986;24(5):485–490.
147. Williams RC Jr. Rheumatoid factors: historical perspective, origins and possible role in disease. *J Rheumatol (Suppl)* 1992;32:42–45.
148. Parekh RB, Dwek RA, Sutton BJ, et al. Association of rheumatoid arthritis and primary osteoarthritis with changes in the glycosylation pattern of total serum IgG. *Nature* 1985;316(6027):452–457.
149. Axford JS, Mackenzie L, Lydyard PM, et al. Reduced B-cell galactosyltransferase activity in rheumatoid arthritis. *Lancet* 1987;2(8574):1486–1488.
150. Tomana M, Schrohenloher RE, Koopman WJ, et al. Abnormal glycosylation of serum IgG from patients with chronic inflammatory diseases. *Arthritis Rheum* 1988;31(3):333–338.
151. Parekh R, Roitt I, Isenberg D, et al. Age-related galactosylation of the N-linked oligosaccharides of human serum IgG. *J Exp Med* 1988;167(5):1731–1736.
152. Go MF, Schrohenloher RE, Tomana M. Deficient galactosylation of serum IgG in inflammatory bowel disease: correlation with disease activity. *J Clin Gastroenterol* 1994;18(1):86–87.
153. Dube R, Rook GA, Steele J, et al. Agalactosyl IgG in inflammatory bowel disease: correlation with C-reactive protein. *Gut* 1990;31(4):431–434.
154. Newkirk MM, Lemmo A, Rauch J. Importance of the IgG isotype, not the state of glycosylation, in determining human rheumatoid factor binding. *Arthritis Rheum* 1990;33(6):800–809.
155. Soltys AJ, Hay FC, Bond A, et al. The binding of synovial tissue-derived human monoclonal immunoglobulin M rheumatoid factor to immunoglobulin G preparations of differing galactose content. *Scand J Immunol* 1994;40(2):135–143.
156. Rademacher TW, Williams P, Dwek RA. Agalactosyl glycoforms of IgG autoantibodies are pathogenic. *Proc Natl Acad Sci U S A* 1994;91(13):6123–6127.
157. van Zeben D, Rook GA, Hazes JM, et al. Early agalactosylation of IgG is associated with a more progressive disease course in patients with rheumatoid arthritis: results of a follow-up study. *Br J Rheumatol* 1994;33(1):36–43.
158. Lunec J, Blake DR, McCleary SJ, et al. Self-perpetuating mechanisms of immunoglobulin G aggregation in rheumatoid inflammation. *J Clin Invest* 1985;76(6):2084–2090.
159. Ligier S, Fortin PR, Newkirk MM. A new antibody in rheumatoid arthritis targeting glycated IgG: IgM anti-IgG-AGE. *Br J Rheumatol* 1998;37(12):1307–1314.
160. Hirohata S, Yanagida T, Koda M, et al. Selective induction of IgM rheumatoid factors by CD14+ monocyte-lineage cells generated from bone marrow of patients with rheumatoid arthritis. *Arthritis Rheum* 1995;38(3):384–388.
161. Perez L, Orte J, Brieva JA. Terminal differentiation of spontaneous rheumatoid factor-secreting B cells from rheumatoid arthritis patients depends on endogenous interleukin-10. *Arthritis Rheum* 1995;38(12):1771–1776.
162. Cush JJ, Splawski JB, Thomas R, et al. Elevated interleukin-10 levels in patients with rheumatoid arthritis. *Arthritis Rheum* 1995;38(1):96–104.
163. Hidaka T, Kitani A, Hara M, et al. IL-4 down-regulates the surface expression of CD5 on B cells and inhibits spontaneous immunoglobulin and IgM-rheumatoid factor production in patients with rheumatoid arthritis. *Clin Exp Immunol* 1992;89(2):223–229.
164. Mackay F, Woodcock SA, Lawton P, et al. Mice transgenic for BAFF develop lymphocytic disorders along with autoimmune manifestations. *J Exp Med* 1999;190(11):1697–1710.
165. Tan SM, Xu D, Roschke V, et al. Local production of B lymphocyte stimulator protein and APRIL in arthritic joints of patients with inflammatory arthritis. *Arthritis Rheum* 2003;48(4):982–992.
166. Tighe H, Heaphy P, Baird S, et al. Human immunoglobulin (IgG) induced deletion of IgM rheumatoid factor B cells in transgenic mice. *J Exp Med* 1995;181(2):599–606.
167. Tighe H, Warnatz K, Brinson D, et al. Peripheral deletion of rheumatoid factor B cells after abortive activation by IgG. *Proc Natl Acad Sci U S A* 1997;94(2):646–651.
168. Warnatz K, Kyburz D, Brinson DC, et al. Rheumatoid factor B cell tolerance via autonomous Fas/FasL-independent apoptosis. *Cell Immunol* 1999;191(1):69–73.
169. Shlomchik MJ, Zharhary D, Saunders T, et al. A rheumatoid factor transgenic mouse model of autoantibody regulation. *Int Immunol* 1993;5(10):1329–1341.
170. Hannum LG, Ni D, Haberman AM, et al. A disease-related rheumatoid factor autoantibody is not tolerized in a normal mouse: implications for the origins of autoantibodies in autoimmune disease. *J Exp Med* 1996;184(4):1269–1278.
171. Jacobson BA, Rothstein TL, Marshak-Rothstein A. Unique site of IgG2a and rheumatoid factor production in MRL/lpr mice. *Immunol Rev* 1997;156:103–110.
172. Crowley JJ, Goldfien RD, Schrohenloher RE, et al. Incidence of three cross-reactive idiotypes on human rheumatoid factor paraproteins. *J Immunol* 1988;140:3411–3418.
173. Bearn AG, Dixon FJ, Benacerraf B. Henry G. Kunkel 1916–1983. An appreciation of the man and his scientific contributions and a bibliography of his research papers. *J Exp Med* 1985;161(5):869–895.
174. Kunkel HG, Agnello V, Joslin FG, et al. Cross-idiotypic specificity among monoclonal IgM proteins with anti-gamma-globulin activity. *J Exp Med* 1973;137:331–342.
175. Agnello V, Arbetter A, Ibanez de Kasep G, et al. Evidence for a subset of rheumatoid factors that cross-react with DNA-histone and have a distinct cross-idiotype. *J Exp Med* 1980;151:1514.

176. Agnello V, Barnes JL. Human rheumatoid factor crossidiotypes. I. WA and BLA are heat-labile conformational antigens requiring both heavy and light chains. *J Exp Med* 1986;164(5):1809–1814.
177. Knight GB, Agnello V, Bonagura V, et al. Human rheumatoid factor cross-idiotypes. IV. Studies on WA XId- positive IgM without rheumatoid factor activity provide evidence that the WA XId is not unique to rheumatoid factors and is distinct from the 17.109 and G6 XIds. *J Exp Med* 1993;178:1903–1911.
178. Carson DA, Fong S. A common idiotope on human rheumatoid factors identified by a hybridoma antibody. *Mol Immunol* 1983;20: 1081–1087.
179. Schrohenloher RE, Accavitti MA, Bhown AS, et al. Monoclonal antibody 6B6.6 define a cross-reactive kappa light chain idiotope on human monoclonal and polyclonal rheumatoid factors. *Arthritis Rheum* 1990;33:1870–1198.
180. Radoux V, Chen PP, Sorge JA, et al. A conserved human germline Vk gene directly encodes rheumatoid factor light chains. *J Exp Med* 1986;164:2119–2124.
181. Chen PP, Albrandt K, Kipps TJ, et al. Isolation and characterization of human VkIII germ-line genes. Implications for the molecular basis of human VkIII light chain diversity. *J Immunol* 1987;139(5):1727–1733.
182. Chen PP, Robbins DL, Jirik FR, et al. Isolation and characterization of a light chain variable region gene for human rheumatoid factors. *J Exp Med* 1987;166:1900–1905.
183. Mageed RA, Dearlove M, Goodall DM, et al. Immunogenic and antigenic epitopes of immunoglobulins. XVII—-Monoclonal antibodies reactive with common and restricted idiotopes to the heavy chain of human rheumatoid factors. *Rheumatol Int* 1986;6(4):179–183.
184. Chen PP, Liu M-F, Glass CA, et al. Characterization of two immunoglobulin VH genes that are homologous to human rheumatoid factors. *Arthritis Rheum* 1989;32:72–76.
185. Crowley JJ, Mageed RA, Silverman GJ, et al. The incidence of a new human cross-reactive idiotype linked to subgroup VHIII heavy chains. *Mol Immunol* 1990;27(1):87–94.
186. Pascual V, Randen I, Thompson K, et al. The complete nucleotide sequences of the heavy chain variable regions of six monospecific rheumatoid factors derived from Epstein-Barr virus–transformed B cells isolated from the synovial tissue of patients with rheumatoid arthritis. *J Clin Invest* 1990;86:1320–1328.
187. Silverman GJ, Schrohenloher RE, Accavitti MA, et al. Structural characterization of the second major cross-reactive idiotype group of human rheumatoid factors. Association with the VH4 gene family. *Arthritis Rheum* 1990;33(9):1347–1360.
188. Potter KN, Li Y, Pascual V, et al. Molecular characterization of a cross-reactive idiotope on human immunoglobulins utilizing the VH4–21 gene segment. *J Exp Med* 1993;178(4):1419–1428.
189. Koopman WJ, Schrohenloher RE, Carson DA. Dissociation of expression of two rheumatoid factor cross-reactive kappa L chain idiotopes in rheumatoid arthritis. *J Immunol* 1990;144:3468–3472.
190. Davidson A, Keiser HD, Del Puente A, et al. Expression of rheumatoid factor idiotypes 17.109, 6B6.6 and 4C9 in the sera of Pima Indians. *Autoimmunity* 1994;18(4):251–258.
191. Bonagura VR, Kwong T, Kenny T, et al. The specificity of synovial IgM rheumatoid factors (RF) for genetically engineered IgG antibodies is not affected by the method used to immortalize RF-producing B cells. *Scand J Immunol* 1999;49(1):106–111.
192. Cox JPL, Tomlinson IM, Winter G. A directory of human germ-line V kappa segments reveals a strong bias in their usage. *Eur J Immunol* 1994;24:827–836.
193. Ignatovich O, Tomlinson IM, Jones PT, et al. The creation of diversity in the human immunoglobulin Vl repertoire. *J Mol Biol* 1997; 268(1):69–77.
194. Fang Q, Kannapell CC, Gaskin F, et al. Human rheumatoid factors with restrictive specificity for rabbit immunoglobulin G: auto- and multi-reactivity, diverse VH gene segment usage and preferential usage of V lambda IIIb. *J Exp Med* 1994;179(5):1445–1456.
195. Bridges SL Jr. Rheumatoid factor. In: Koopman WJ, ed. *Arthritis and allied conditions.* Baltimore: Williams & Wilkins, 2000:1223–1244.
196. Schroeder HW Jr, Wang JY. Preferential utilization of conserved immunoglobulin heavy chain variable gene segments during human fetal life. *Proc Natl Acad Sci U S A* 1990;87:6146–6150.
197. Kipps TJ, Tomhave E, Pratt LF, et al. Developmentally restricted immunoglobulin heavy chain variable region gene expressed at high frequency in chronic lymphocytic leukemia. *Proc Natl Acad Sci U S A* 1989;86:5913–5917.
198. Crouzier R, Martin T, Pasquali JL. Monoclonal IgM rheumatoid factor secreted by CD5-negative B cells during mixed cryoglobulinemia. Evidence for somatic mutations and intraclonal diversity of the expressed VH region gene. *J Immunol* 1995;154(1):413–421.
199. Børretzen M, Natvig JB, Thompson KM. Heterogeneous RF structures between and within healthy individuals are not related to HLA DRB1*0401. *Mol Immunol* 1997;34(12–13):929–938.
200. Suzuki I, Pfister L, Glas A, et al. Representation of rearranged VH gene segments in the human adult antibody repertoire. *J Immunol* 1995;154:3902–3911.
201. Stewart AK, Huang C, Stollar BD, et al. High-frequency representation of a single VH gene in the expressed human B cell repertoire. *J Exp Med* 1993;177(2):409–418.
202. Stewart AK, Huang C, Long AA, et al. VH-gene representation in autoantibodies reflects the normal human B-cell repertoire. *Immunol Rev* 1992;128:101–122.
203. Cook GP, Tomlinson IM. The human immunoglobulin VH repertoire. *Immunol Today* 1995;16(5):237–242.
204. Paul E, Iliev AA, Livneh A, et al. The anti-DNA-associated idiotype 8.12 is encoded by the VIII gene family and maps to the vicinity of the L chain CDR1. *J Immunol* 1992;149:3588–3595.
205. Pascual V, Victor K, Randen I, et al. Nucleotide sequence analysis of rheumatoid factors and polyreactive antibodies derived from patients with rheumatoid arthritis reveals diverse use of VH and VL gene segments and extensive variability in CDR-3. *Scand J Immunol* 1992; 36:349–362.
206. Ezaki I, Shingu M, Hashimoto M, et al. Analysis of the genes encoding the variable regions of human IgG rheumatoid factor. *J Rheumatol* 1994;21(11):2005–2010.
207. Randen I, Thompson KM, Pascual V, et al. Rheumatoid factor V genes from patients with rheumatoid arthritis are diverse and show evidence of an antigen-driven response. *Immunol Rev* 1992;128: 49–71.
208. Martin T, Crouzier R, Weber J-C, et al. Structure-function studies on a polyreactive (natural) autoantibody: polyreactivity is dependent on somatically generated sequences in the third complementarity-determining region of the antibody heavy chain. *J Immunol* 1994; 152:5988–5996.
209. Thai TH, Purugganan MM, Roth DB, et al. Distinct and opposite diversifying activities of terminal transferase splice variants. *Nat Immunol* 2002;3(5):457–462.
210. Klein R, Jaenichen R, Zachau HG. Expressed human immunoglobulin kappa genes and their hypermutation. *Eur J Immunol* 1993;23: 3248–3262.
211. Victor KD, Capra JD. An apparently common mechanism of generating antibody diversity: length variation of the VL-JL junction. *Mol Immunol* 1994;31(1):39–46.
212. Lee SK, Bridges SL Jr, Koopman WJ, et al. The immunoglobulin kappa light chain repertoire expressed in the synovium of a patient with rheumatoid arthritis. *Arthritis Rheum* 1992;35:905–913.
213. Bridges SL Jr, Lee SK, Johnson ML, et al. Somatic mutation and CDR3 lengths of immunoglobulin κ light chains expressed in patients with rheumatoid arthritis and normal individuals. *J Clin Invest* 1995;96:831–841.
214. Martin T, Blaison G, Levallois H, et al. Molecular analysis of the VkIII-Jk junctional diversity of polyclonal rheumatoid factors during rheumatoid arthritis frequently reveals N addition. *Eur J Immunol* 1992;22:1773–1779.
215. Victor KD, Randen I, Thompson K, et al. Rheumatoid factors isolated from patients with autoimmune disorders are derived from germline genes distinct from those encoding the Wa, Po, and Bla cross reactive idiotypes. *J Clin Invest* 1991;87:1603–1613.
216. Ezaki I, Kanda H, Sakai K, et al. Restricted diversity of the variable region nucleotide sequences of the heavy and light chains of a human rheumatoid factor. *Arthritis Rheum* 1991;34:343–350.
217. Youngblood K, Fruchter L, Ding G, et al. Rheumatoid factors from the peripheral blood of two patients with rheumatoid arthritis are genetically heterogeneous and somatically mutated. *J Clin Invest* 1994; 93(2):852–861.
218. Weisbart RH, Wong AL, Noritake D, et al. The rheumatoid factor reactivity of a human IgG monoclonal autoantibody is encoded by a variant VkII L chain gene. *J Immunol* 1991;147:2795–2801.

219. Gause A, Küppers R, Mierau R. A somatically mutated VkIV gene encoding a human rheumatoid factor light chain. *Clin Exp Immunol* 1992;88:430–434.
220. Deftos M, Olee T, Carson DA, et al. Defining the genetic origins of three rheumatoid synovium-derived IgG rheumatoid factors. *J Clin Invest* 1994;93(6):2545–2553.
221. Weller S, Conde C, Knapp AM, et al. Autoantibodies in mice lacking terminal deoxynucleotidyl transferase: evidence for a role of N region addition in the polyreactivity and in the affinities of anti-DNA antibodies. *J Immunol* 1997;159(8):3890–3898.
222. Zhang Z, Bridges SL Jr. Expression of RAG and TdT and evidence of receptor revision in synovial B lymphocytes in rheumatoid arthritis [Abstract]. *Scand J Immunol* 1999;50(1):101.
223. Zhang Z, Wu X, Limbaugh BH, et al. Expression of recombination-activating genes and terminal deoxynucleotidyl transferase and secondary rearrangement of immunoglobulin kappa light chains in rheumatoid arthritis synovial tissue. *Arthritis Rheum* 2001;44(10): 2275–2284.
224. Arnett FC, Edworthy SM, Bloch DA, et al. The American Rheumatism Association 1987 revised criteria for the classification of rheumatoid arthritis. *Arthritis Rheum* 1988;31:315–324.
225. Plotz CM, Singer JM. The latex fixation test. II. Results in rheumatoid arthritis. *Am J Med* 1956;21:893–896.
226. Despres N, Grant AM. Antibody interference in thyroid assays: a potential for clinical misinformation. *Clin Chem* 1998;44(3):440–454.
227. Bartoloni A, Strohmeyer M, Sabatinelli G, et al. False positive ParaSight-F test for malaria in patients with rheumatoid factor. *Trans R Soc Trop Med Hyg* 1998;92(1):33–34.
228. Bartoloni A, Sabatinelli G, Benucci M. Performance of two rapid tests for *Plasmodium falciparum* malaria in patients with rheumatoid factors. *N Engl J Med* 1998;338(15):1075.
229. Laferi H, Kandel K, Pichler H. False positive dipstick test for malaria. *N Engl J Med* 1997;337(22):1635–1636.
230. Mishra B, Samantaray JC, Kumar A, et al. Study of false positivity of two rapid antigen detection tests for diagnosis of *Plasmodium falciparum* malaria. *J Clin Microbiol* 1999;37(4):1233.
231. Bas S, Perneger TV, Kunzle E, et al. Comparative study of different enzyme immunoassays for measurement of IgM and IgA rheumatoid factors. *Ann Rheum Dis* 2002;61(6):505–510.
232. Taylor RN, Fulford KM, Jones WL. Reduction of variation in results of rheumatoid factor tests by use of a serum reference preparation. *J Clin Microbiol* 1977;5(1):42–45.
233. Taylor RN, Fulford KM. Assessment of laboratory improvement by the Center for Disease Control Diagnostic Immunology Proficiency Testing Program. *J Clin Microbiol* 1981;13(2):356–368.
234. Finley PR, Hicks MJ, Williams RJ, et al. Rate nephelometric measurement of rheumatoid factor in serum. *Clin Chem* 1979;25(11): 1909–1914.
235. Adebajo AO, Wright JK, Cawston TE, et al. Rheumatoid factor quantitation: a comparison of ELISA and nephelometric methods. *Med Lab Sci* 1991;48(1):47–51.
236. Keshgegian AA, Straub CW, Loos EF, et al. Rheumatoid factor measured with the QM300 nephelometer: clinical sensitivity and specificity. *Clin Chem* 1994;40(6):943.
237. Hay FC, Nineham LJ, Roitt IM. Routine assay for detection of IgG and IgM antiglobulins in seronegative and seropositive rheumatoid arthritis. *BMJ* 1975;3(5977):203–204.
238. Koopman WJ, Schrohenloher RE. A sensitive radioimmunoassay for quantitation of IgM rheumatoid factor. *Arthritis Rheum* 1980;23(3): 302–308.
239. Koopman WJ, Schrohenloher RE, Solomon A. A quantitative assay for IgA rheumatoid factor. *J Immunol Meth* 1982;50(1): 89–98.
240. Wernick R, LoSpalluto JJ, Fink CW, et al. Serum IgG and IgM rheumatoid factors by solid phase radioimmunoassay. A comparison between adult and juvenile rheumatoid arthritis. *Arthritis Rheum* 1981;24(12):1501–1511.
241. Mikkelsen WM, Dodge HJ, Duff IF, et al. Estimates of the prevalence of rheumatic diseases in the population of Tecumseh, Michigan, 1959–60. *J Chronic Dis* 1967;20(6):351–369.
242. Bennett PH, Burch TA. The distribution of rheumatoid factor and rheumatoid arthritis in the families of Blackfeet and Pima Indians. *Arthritis Rheum* 1968;11(4):546–553.
243. Ball J, Lawrence JS. The relationship of rheumatoid serum factor to rheumatoid arthritis: a 5-year follow up of a population sample. *Ann Rheum Dis* 1963;22:311–318.
244. Aho K, Palosuo T, Raunio V, et al. When does rheumatoid disease start? *Arthritis Rheum* 1985;28(5):485–489.
245. Del Puente A, Knowler WC, Pettitt DJ, et al. The incidence of rheumatoid arthritis is predicted by rheumatoid factor titer in an longitudinal population study. *Arthritis Rheum* 1988;31:1239–1244.
246. Halldorsdottir HD, Jonsson T, Thorsteinsson J, et al. A prospective study on the incidence of rheumatoid arthritis among people with persistent increase of rheumatoid factor. *Ann Rheum Dis* 2000;59(2): 149–151.
247. Enzer I, Dunn G, Jacobsson L, et al. An epidemiologic study of trends in prevalence of rheumatoid factor seropositivity in Pima Indians: evidence of a decline due to both secular and birth-cohort influences. *Arthritis Rheum* 2002;46(7):1729–1734.
248. Butler VP Jr, Vaughan JH. The reaction of rheumatoid factor with animal gamma-globulins: quantitative considerations. *Immunology* 1965;8:144–159.
249. Heimer R, Schwartz ER, Freyberg RH. Different rheumatoid factors in the serum of one patient with rheumatic arthritis. *J Lab Clin Med* 1961;57:16–31.
250. Williams RC Jr, Kunkel HG. Separation of rheumatoid factors of different specificities using columns conjugated with gamma-globulin. *Arthritis Rheum* 1963;6:665–675.
251. Suarez-Almazor ME, Gonzalez-Lopez L, Gamez-Nava JI, et al. Utilization and predictive value of laboratory tests in patients referred to rheumatologists by primary care physicians. *J Rheumatol* 1998; 25(10):1980–1985.
252. Shmerling RH, Delbanco TL. The rheumatoid factor: an analysis of clinical utility. *Am J Med* 1991;91(5):528–534.
253. Shmerling RH, Delbanco TL. How useful is the rheumatoid factor? An analysis of sensitivity, specificity, and predictive value. *Arch Intern Med* 1992;152(12):2417–2420.
254. Wolfe F, Cathey MA, Roberts FK. The latex test revisited: rheumatoid factor testing in 8,287 rheumatic disease patients. *Arthritis Rheum* 1991;34:951–960.
255. Davidson A, Bridges SL Jr. Autoimmunity in rheumatoid arthritis. In: Haynes BF, Pisetsky DS, St Clair EW, eds. *RA: a textbook of rheumatoid arthritis*. Philadelphia: Lippincott Williams & Wilkins, 2003.
256. Alter MJ, Kruszon-Moran D, Nainan OV, et al. The prevalence of hepatitis C virus infection in the United States, 1988 through 1994. *N Engl J Med* 1999;341(8):556–562.
257. Choo QL, Kuo G, Weiner AJ, et al. Isolation of a cDNA clone derived from a blood-borne non-A, non- B viral hepatitis genome. *Science* 1989;244(4902):359–362.
258. Pascual M, Perrin L, Giostra E, et al. Hepatitis C virus in patients with cryoglobulinemia type II [Letter]. *J Infect Dis* 1990;162(2):569–567.
259. Ferri C, Greco F, Longombardo G, et al. Antibodies to hepatitis C virus in patients with mixed cryoglobulinemia. *Arthritis Rheum* 1991; 34(12):1606–1610.
260. Agnello V, Chung RT, Kaplan LM. A role for hepatitis C virus infection in type II cryoglobulinemia. *N Engl J Med* 1992;327(21): 1490–1495.
261. Persico M, De Marino FA, Di Giacomo RG, et al. Prevalence and incidence of cryoglobulins in hepatitis C virus-related chronic hepatitis patients: a prospective study. *Am J Gastroenterol* 2003;98(4):884–888.
262. Cracchiolo A, Bluestone R, Goldberg LS. Hidden antiglobulins in rheumatic disorders. *Clin Exp Immunol* 1970;7(5):651–655.
263. Stastny P. Association of the B-cell alloantigen DRw4 with rheumatoid arthritis. *N Engl J Med* 1978;298:869–871.
264. Schiff B, Mizrachi Y, Orgad S, et al. Association of HLA-Aw31 and HLA-DR1 with adult rheumatoid arthritis. *Ann Rheum Dis* 1982;41 (4):403–404.
265. Karr RW, Rodey GE, Lee T, et al. Association of HLA-DRw4 with rheumatoid arthritis in black and white patients. *Arthritis Rheum* 1980;23(11):1241–1245.
266. Alarcón GS, Koopman WJ, Acton RT, et al. Seronegative rheumatoid arthritis. A distinct immunogenetic disease? *Arthritis Rheum* 1982; 25(5):502–507.
267. Dobloug JH, Førre Ø, Kass E, et al. HLA antigens and rheumatoid arthritis. Association between HLA-DRw4 positivity and IgM rheumatoid factor production. *Arthritis Rheum* 1980;23(3):309–313.

268. Queiros MV, Sancho MR, Caetano JM. HLA-DR4 antigen and IgM rheumatoid factors. *J Rheumatol* 1982;9(3):370–373.
269. Olsen NJ, Callahan LF, Brooks RH, et al. Associations of HLA-DR4 with rheumatoid factor and radiographic severity in rheumatoid arthritis. *Am J Med* 1988;84(2):257–264.
270. Gregersen PK, Silver J, Winchester R. The shared epitope hypothesis: an approach to understanding the molecular genetics of susceptibility to rheumatoid arthritis. *Arthritis Rheum* 1987;30:1205–1213.
271. Gran JT, Husby G, Thorsby E. The prevalence of HLA-DR4 and HLA-DR3 in healthy persons with rheumatoid factor. *Scand J Rheumatol* 1985;14(1):79–82.
272. Silman AJ, Ollier B, Mageed RA. Rheumatoid factor detection in the unaffected first degree relatives in families with multicase rheumatoid arthritis. *J Rheumatol* 1991;18(4):512–515.
273. Olsen NJ, Stastny P, Jasin HE. High levels of *in vitro* IgM rheumatoid factor synthesis correlate with HLA-DR4 in normal individuals. *Arthritis Rheum* 1987;30(8):841–848.
274. Perdriger A, Chales G, Semana G, et al. Role of HLA-DR-DR and DR-DQ associations in the expression of extraarticular manifestations and rheumatoid factor in rheumatoid arthritis. *J Rheumatol* 1997;24(7):1272–1276.
275. Calin A, Elswood J, Klouda PT. Destructive arthritis, rheumatoid factor, and HLA-DR4. Susceptibility versus severity, a case-control study. *Arthritis Rheum* 1989;32(10):1221–1225.
276. Nelson JL, Dugowson CE, Koepsell TD, et al. Rheumatoid factor, HLA-DR4, and allelic variants of DRB1 in women with recent-onset rheumatoid arthritis. *Arthritis Rheum* 1994;37(5):673–680.
277. Jaraquemada D, Ollier W, Awad J, et al. HLA and rheumatoid arthritis: susceptibility or severity? *Dis Markers* 1986;4(1–2):43–53.
278. Walker DJ, Griffiths ID. HLA associations are with severe rheumatoid arthritis. *Dis Markers* 1986;4(1–2):121–132.
279. Weyand CM, Hicok KC, Conn DL, et al. The influence of HLA-DRB1 genes on disease severity in rheumatoid arthritis. *Ann Intern Med* 1992;117:801–806.
280. El Gabalawy HS, Goldbach-Mansky R, Smith D, et al. Association of HLA alleles and clinical features in patients with synovitis of recent onset. *Arthritis Rheum* 1999;42(8):1696–1705.
281. Mattey DL, Hassell AB, Dawes PT, et al. Independent association of rheumatoid factor and the HLA-DRB1 shared epitope with radiographic outcome in rheumatoid arthritis. *Arthritis Rheum* 2001;44(7):1529–1533.
282. Garred P, Madsen HO, Petersen J, et al. CC chemokine receptor 5 polymorphism in rheumatoid arthritis. *J Rheumatol* 1998;25(8):1462–1465.
283. Fujinami M, Sato K, Kashiwazaki S, et al. Comparable histological appearance of synovitis in seropositive and seronegative rheumatoid arthritis. *Clin Exp Rheumatol* 1997;15(1):11–17.
284. Plant MJ, Jones PW, Saklatvala J, et al. Patterns of radiological progression in early rheumatoid arthritis: results of an 8 year prospective study. *J Rheumatol* 1998;25(3):417–426.
285. Möttönen T, Paimela L, Leirisalo-Repo M, et al. Only high disease activity and positive rheumatoid factor indicate poor prognosis in patients with early rheumatoid arthritis treated with "sawtooth" strategy. *Ann Rheum Dis* 1998;57(9):533–539.
286. Wolfe F, Sharp JT. Radiographic outcome of recent-onset rheumatoid arthritis: a 19-year study of radiographic progression. *Arthritis Rheum* 1998;41(9):1571–1582.
287. Zeidler HK, Kvien TK, Hannonen P, et al. Progression of joint damage in early active severe rheumatoid arthritis during 18 months of treatment: comparison of low-dose cyclosporin and parenteral gold. *Br J Rheumatol* 1998;37(8):874–882.
288. Scott DL. Prognostic factors in early rheumatoid arthritis. *Rheumatology (Oxford)* 2000;39(suppl 1):24–29.
289. Bas S, Perneger TV, Mikhnevitch E, et al. Association of rheumatoid factors and anti-filaggrin antibodies with severity of erosions in rheumatoid arthritis. *Rheumatology (Oxford)* 2000;39(10):1082–1088.
290. Bas S, Perneger TV, Seitz M, et al. Diagnostic tests for rheumatoid arthritis: comparison of anti-cyclic citrullinated peptide antibodies, anti-keratin antibodies and IgM rheumatoid factors. *Rheumatology (Oxford)* 2002;41(7):809–814.
291. Bukhari M, Lunt M, Harrison BJ, et al. Rheumatoid factor is the major predictor of increasing severity of radiographic erosions in rheumatoid arthritis: results from the Norfolk Arthritis Register Study, a large inception cohort. *Arthritis Rheum* 2002;46(4):906–912.
292. Vittecoq O, Pouplin S, Krzanowska K, et al. Rheumatoid factor is the strongest predictor of radiological progression of rheumatoid arthritis in a three-year prospective study in community-recruited patients. *Rheumatology (Oxford)* 2003;42(8):939–946.
293. Machold KP, Stamm TA, Eberl GJ, et al. Very recent onset arthritis—clinical, laboratory, and radiological findings during the first year of disease. *J Rheumatol* 2002;29(11):2278–2287.
294. Combe B, Dougados M, Goupille P, et al. Prognostic factors for radiographic damage in early rheumatoid arthritis: a multiparameter prospective study. *Arthritis Rheum* 2001;44(8):1736–1743.
295. Koopman WJ, Schrohenloher RE. Rheumatoid factor. In: Utsinger PD, Zvaifler NJ, Ehrlich GE, ed. *Rheumatoid arthritis*. Philadelphia: JB Lippincott, 1985:217–241.
296. Jacobsson LT, Knowler WC, Pillemer S, et al. Rheumatoid arthritis and mortality. A longitudinal study in Pima Indians. *Arthritis Rheum* 1993;36(8):1045–1053.
297. van Schaardenburg D, Hazes JM, de Boer A, et al. Outcome of rheumatoid arthritis in relation to age and rheumatoid factor at diagnosis. *J Rheumatol* 1993;20(1):45–52.
298. Mikuls TR, Saag KG, Criswell LA, et al. Mortality risk associated with rheumatoid arthritis in a prospective cohort of older women: results from the Iowa Women's Health Study. *Ann Rheum Dis* 2002;61(11):994–999.
299. Goodson NJ, Wiles NJ, Lunt M, et al. Mortality in early inflammatory polyarthritis: cardiovascular mortality is increased in seropositive patients. *Arthritis Rheum* 2002;46(8):2010–2019.
300. Ceuppens JL, Rodriguez MA, Goodwin JS. Non-steroidal anti-inflammatory agent inhibit the synthesis of IgM rheumatoid factor *in vitro*. *Lancet* 1982;1(8271):528–530.
301. Goodwin JS, Ceuppens JL, Rodriguez MA. Administration of non-steroidal anti-inflammatory agents in patients with rheumatoid arthritis. Effects on indexes of cellular immune status and serum rheumatoid factor levels. *JAMA* 1983;250(18):2485–2488.
302. Cush JJ, Lipsky PE, Postlethwaite AE, et al. Correlation of serologic indicators of inflammation with effectiveness of nonsteroidal anti-inflammatory drug therapy in rheumatoid arthritis. *Arthritis Rheum* 1990;33(1):19–28.
303. Olsen NJ, Callahan LF, Pincus T. Immunologic studies of rheumatoid arthritis patients treated with methotrexate. *Arthritis Rheum* 1987;30:481–488.
304. Jonsson T, Steinsson K, Jonsson H, et al. Combined elevation of IgM and IgA rheumatoid factor has high diagnostic specificity for rheumatoid arthritis. *Rheumatol Int* 1998;18(3):119–122.
305. Swedler W, Wallman J, Froelich CJ, et al. Routine measurement of IgM, IgG, and IgA rheumatoid factors: high sensitivity, specificity, and predictive value for rheumatoid arthritis. *J Rheumatol* 1997;24(6):1037–1044.
306. Jonsson T, Thorsteinsson J, Valdimarsson H. Elevation of only one rheumatoid factor isotype is not associated with increased prevalence of rheumatoid arthritis—a population based study. *Scand J Rheumatol* 2000;29(3):190–191.
307. Pai S, Pai L, Birkenfeldt R. Correlation of serum IgA rheumatoid factor levels with disease severity in rheumatoid arthritis. *Scand J Rheumatol* 1998;27(4):252–256.
308. Jonsson T, Valdimarsson H. What about IgA rheumatoid factor in rheumatoid arthritis? *Ann Rheum Dis* 1998;57(1):63–64.
309. Arinbjarnarson S, Jonsson T, Steinsson K, et al. IgA rheumatoid factor correlates with changes in B and T lymphocyte subsets and disease manifestations in rheumatoid arthritis. *J Rheumatol* 1997;24(2):269–274.
310. Houssien DA, Jonsson T, Davies E, et al. Rheumatoid factor isotypes, disease activity and the outcome of rheumatoid arthritis: comparative effects of different antigens. *Scand J Rheumatol* 1998;27(1):46–53.
311. Kujala GA, Steere AC, Davis JS. IgM rheumatoid factor in Lyme disease: correlation with disease activity, total serum IgM, and IgM antibody to *Borrelia burgdorferi*. *J Rheumatol* 1987;14(4):772–776.
312. Jackson S, Tarkowski A, Collins JE, et al. Occurrence of polymeric IgA1 rheumatoid factor in the acquired immune deficiency syndrome. *J Clin Immunol* 1988;8(5):390–396.
313. Hirsch HZ, Tarkowski A, Koopman WJ, et al. Local production of IgA- and IgM-rheumatoid factors in adult periodontal disease. *J Clin Immunol* 1989;9(4):273–278.

314. Tomasi TB Jr, Fudenberg HH, Finby N. Possible relationship of rheumatoid factors and pulmonary disease. *Am J Med* 1962;33:243–248.
315. Bonomo L, LoSpalluto J, Ziff M. Anti-gamma globulin factors in liver disease. *Arthritis Rheum* 1963;6:104–114.
316. Kritzman J, Kunkel HG, McCarthy J, et al. Studies of a Waldenström-type macroglobulin with rheumatoid factor properties. *J Lab Clin Med* 1961;57:905–917.
317. LoSpalluto J, Dorward B, Miller W Jr, et al. Cryoglobulinemia based on interaction between a gamma macroglobulin and 7S gamma globulin. *Am J Med* 1962;32:142–147.
318. Meltzer M, Franklin EC, Elias K, et al. Cryoglobulinemia—a clinical and laboratory study. II. Cryoglobulins with rheumatoid factor activity. *Am J Med* 1966;40(6):837–856.
319. Capra JD, Winchester RJ, Kunkel HG. Hypergammaglobulinemic purpura. Studies on the unusual anti-g-globulins characteristic of the sera of these patients. *Medicine* 1971;50(2):125–138.
320. Sasso EH, Barber CV, Nardella FA, et al. Antigenic specificities of human monoclonal and polyclonal IgM rheumatoid factors. The C gamma 2-C gamma 3 interface region contains the major determinants. *J Immunol* 1988;140(9):3098–3107.

CHAPTER 59

The Evaluation and Treatment of Rheumatoid Arthritis

Nathan J. Zvaifler and Maripat Corr

Once considered barely manageable, rheumatoid arthritis (RA) is now recognized to be a treatable disease. This is usually ascribed to new, powerful biologic agents, but this improved prognosis largely results from a new paradigm for the use of conventional drugs. Numerous studies in the 1990s clearly demonstrate that early recognition of RA and rapid institution of disease-modifying antirheumatic drugs (DMARDs, also known as slow acting or second-line treatments) results in better control of disease and favorably influence its outcome. Moreover, drugs that previously were considered inadequate for treating established disease are efficacious when used in early intervention studies. Therefore, it is possible that the timing of DMARD therapy is at least as important as the agent chosen. Because this approach is a radical departure from the "wait and see" and "nothing can be done about rheumatoid arthritis" sentiments of the past, the evidence supporting this new paradigm will be reviewed before discussing individual treatments.

INTRODUCTION

In the 1960s and 1970s, most DMARDs used to treat RA were shown in double-blind multiclinical trials to be more effective than placebo (1–3). These were short-term studies, however, and when the same patients were examined years later, only about 20% were still taking the initial medication; half discontinued because of loss of efficacy, and the remainder due to drug side effects (4,5). Even when methotrexate came into widespread use, the retention rates were less than 60%. After much introspection, the failures were ascribed to the existing treatment paradigm; namely, an initial program of rest, education, physiotherapy, and salicylates, or other nonsteroidal antiinflammatory drugs (NSAIDs) for several months. Then, and only then, if the disease was still active, DMARDs were introduced stepwise, usually in 3- to 6-month trials, moving from the mildest agents (aminoquinoline antimalarials such as chloroquine or hydroxychloroquine, or sulfasalazine) to the more toxic D-penicillamine or gold compounds; and only then to the most aggressive immunosuppressive or cytotoxic drugs (cytoxan, azathioprine, or methotrexate) (6,7). Intraarticular corticosteroids were allowed for local flare-ups, but systemic administration was a last resort using only the smallest amounts possible (6).

Three suggestions were made to improve treatment. First, approximately 10% to 20% of patients have spontaneous remissions of RA. These occur mainly in the first 12 months of disease and rarely after 2 years. Perhaps early or aggressive pharmacologic interventions, at a time when a "window of therapeutic opportunity" exists, would improve the outcome of RA. Second, the pathogenesis of RA is complex, involving multiple pathways—inflammatory, immunologic, and destructive—akin to a disease like cancer. Therefore, if individual DMARDs have only limited success, perhaps synergies could be found in combinations of drugs; that is, the rheumatologist approaches RA the way an oncologist treats cancer. Third, new therapies were needed, and these should be based on an increased appreciation of the molecular mechanisms underlying RA.

Early Intervention

The first suggestion (early treatment) required a better understanding of the natural history of RA, particularly in its initial months. To learn more, early arthritis clinics were established, usually in European countries, where populations are stable, health care is nationalized, and general physicians can refer patients without loss of income. When the diagnosis of early RA simply required the recent onset of synovitis in one or more joints, then only a minority of patients, between 15% and 33%, had persistent arthritis at follow-up years later. Viral infections (particularly parvovirus B19) were the most common explanations for transient synovitis, but many cases remained undiagnosed (7,8). If inclusion criteria were limited to patients with signs and symptoms of polyarticular inflammation present for a few weeks to months, then almost half the participants had either a recognizable nonrheumatoid inflammatory joint diseases (sarcoid, spondyloarthropathy, crystal, reactive, psoriatic, or osteoarthritis) or an "undifferentiated arthritis" (7,9,10). A short duration of symptoms (between 6 weeks and 6 months), morning stiffness of less than 1 hour, fewer than three affected joint areas, a negative test for serum rheumatoid factor (RF) or the absence of erosions in joint radiographs at presentation were all features of patients who did not have, or were not likely to develop, RA. Conversely, in all early arthritis clinics there were significant numbers of patients (27%–68%) who were indistinguishable from those with established RA. They had symmetric arthritis, multiple swollen and tender joints, prolonged (hours) morning stiffness, elevated inflammatory indices [such as erythrocyte sedimentation rate (ESR) and C-reactive protein (CRP)], and most importantly, positive test results for RF. This phenotype persisted for years, confirming the reliability of establishing a diagnosis of early RA. Analysis and follow-up of these same subjects also provided strong evidence that joint damage and disability begins early and that DMARDs can improve long-term outcome and quality of life in RA (11,12).

Despite variability due to differences in techniques, selection of joints for analysis (hands and wrists vs. feet vs. large joints), discrimination of joint space narrowing from joint erosions, blinded or non-blinded observers, serial or random readings, and types of study design, serial radiographs remain the gold standard for assessing structural damage and progression of RA. Most publications on early arthritis agree that approximately 75% of patients have joint erosions detectable at presentation or they appear within 2 years from the onset of symptoms (13,14). Even more persuasive are studies using magnetic resonance imaging, ultrasonography, bone mineral densitometry, and synovial biopsies demonstrating that inflammatory changes are already present in the synovium before patients become symptomatic, and if left untreated will lead to structural damage. This represents the hypothetical window of opportunity for slowing, halting, or reversing the rheumatoid process. If true, then early institution of DMARD treatment might improve the long-term outcome of RA. This seems to be the case whether outcome is expressed as mortality, disability, quality of life, or radiographic progression (15–17).

Early therapeutic intervention might not only influence disability from joint deformity, but also enhance longevity. For instance, 622 patients with newly diagnosed RA of variable duration were evaluated 10 years after the inception of disease. The cohort of patients with early disease, who were treated aggressively with DMARDs, had the same mortality rate as a normal population (16). Heretofore, RA had always been associated with a shortened life span (18). Functional ability, which improved after treatment, remained constant throughout the follow-up period. In five other randomized, placebo-controlled trials of DMARDs in early RA, the treated groups (two hydroxychloroquine; two sulfasalazine; and one oral gold) did significantly better than controls with reduction in joint swelling, and improved functional scores and inflammation measures. Equally impressive, in five other trials of outcomes in RA patients, those treated with a DMARD early did significantly better than a matched group of patients who started the same therapeutic agent 6 to 12 months later (reviewed in references 7 and 10).

Combination Therapy

The second suggestion was that some synergy might be obtained by combining antirheumatic drugs that by themselves had only limited efficacy. This approach has precedents in the treatment of many chronic diseases, such as tuberculosis, hypertension, heart failure, and cancer. The initial studies in patients with established RA, usually comparing two DMARDs to either one alone, yielded equivocal results (19–21). Some showed a modest advantage, but this was offset by increased drug side effects. Enthusiasm for drug combinations has increased in the past decade, perhaps because these studies have included larger numbers of patients, newer treatments, or multiple drugs together. Different strategies have also been tried: two drugs given simultaneously, and continued throughout the study (parallel administration); serial use of DMARDs (sawtooth strategy); initial high doses of drugs followed by gradual reduction as disease control improves (step-down strategy); or gradual introduction of different drugs at larger doses in response to disease activity (step-up strategy) (see Chapter 33).

An early influential trial compared patients with established RA disease treated for 2 years with either methotrexate alone, or sulfasalazine plus hydroxychloroquine, or all three medications together. Follow-up results favored the combination treatment (22). In another study, 56 patients who failed at least four DMARDs, including methotrexate, were given a combination of methotrexate (15 mg/wk), cyclophosphamide (50 mg three times a week), and chloroquine (250 mg/day). Results were compared to those achieved with prior methotrexate treatment and to results in a matched group of patients who were given methotrexate for the first time. The combination group improved the most in the first year, significantly better than they had with methotrexate alone. With longer follow-up, however, those newly treated with methotrexate had a better outcome (23). Prior attempts at treating recalcitrant RA with drug combinations that included cytotoxic agents, such as cytoxan or chlorambucil, were effective in controlling joint symptoms, but were eventually discontinued because of hematologic complications or the development of neoplasms (24). A summary of all studies (through 2000) that used multiple conventional drugs together supports combination therapy, but it is not clear that any one combination or strategy is better than another (21). These improved results are probably explained by using higher doses of conventional DMARDs (e.g., weekly methotrexate at 15–20 mg rather than 7.5 mg), the availability of new agents (leflunomide, cyclosporine), and a more permissive attitude toward long-term, low-dose corticosteroids, or even very large amounts of prednisone for short periods (60 mg/day in the step-down strategy) (25).

Results obtained with combination treatments are easier to interpret in patients with early arthritis (<2 years), who have not been previously exposed to DMARDs. Most trials compare methotrexate plus one or several other DMARDs versus monotherapy. After 1 to 2 years, the combination cohort generally does better than the monotherapy group in both clinical and radiographic measurements; however, except for more frequent remissions, the overall differences are not always great or sustained (21). The addition of biologic agents to conventional DMARDs represents a significant advance in the treatment of established and recent-onset RA. These compounds are discussed in more detail below and in Chapter 32.

New Antirheumatic Therapies

In the 1990s there was a rapid expansion of drugs for treating RA. Some are adaptations of existing compounds. For instance, FK-506 is an improvement on cyclosporine A, and is equally effective. As of this writing, however, it has not been approved as an RA treatment by the U.S. Food and Drug Administration (FDA). Leflunomide, has many similarities to methotrexate. It reversibly inhibits the enzyme dihydroorotate dehydrogenase, the rate limiting step in the synthesis of pyrimidines, which impairs the progression of the cell cycle in different cells, especially activated T-lymphocytes and monocyte/macrophages. Leflunomide is effective in both early and established RA, either as monotherapy or in combinations (see Chapter 32). The most exciting new compounds, however, are agents that interfere with the action of proinflammatory cytokines, including tumor necrosis factor-α (TNF-α), interleukin-1 (IL-1), IL-6, and IL-8. These cytokines are present in the synovium and synovial fluid of RA patients along with their natural inhibitors: IL-10, transforming growth factor-β, IL-1 receptor antagonist (IL-1Ra), and soluble receptors for IL-1 and TNF-α. The prediction that reestablishing the normal balance between pro- and antiinflammatory cytokines would ameliorate RA has proven remarkably prescient. The spectacular success of monoclonal anti-TNF-α antibodies, recombinant soluble TNF receptor (TNFR), and IL-1Ra in suppressing joint inflammation and destruction (reviewed in Chapters 39 and 40) is likely just a forerunner of many other biologic therapies, which hopefully will provide long-term control of RA.

MANAGEMENT OF PATIENTS WITH RHEUMATOID ARTHRITIS

The many and often complex problems of RA patients are seldom accommodated by a single physician, even an arthritis specialist. Most often, a patient with joint complaints contacts a primary care physician, who must determine the cause of the symptoms. Having considered the possibility of RA, the primary physician is obligated to establish a firm diagnosis, document disease activity, and predict the outcome. At this point, consultation with a rheumatologist should be considered if there is either uncertainty about the diagnosis, a common problem in early RA, or there are features that portend a poor prognosis. Those with an established diagnosis of RA need education about the course their disease might take, the risk for joint damage and loss of function, available treatments and their side effects, the need for extra rest at home or at work, and advice about employment. These goals can be facilitated by the special skills of social workers, vocational counselors, and physical and occupational therapists. Continued collaboration between the rheumatologist and the referring physician is often necessary for supervision of medications, laboratory testing for potential drug toxicities, and management of concomitant medical conditions.

ASSESSING DISEASE ACTIVITY

The expression of RA varies greatly among individuals and differs in the same patient over time. Measuring these differences is necessary for evaluating treatment. Two simple sets of disease activity criteria for use in drug trials and clinical practice have been validated and are in general use (26,27) (Table 59.1). They assess different aspects of the rheumatoid process: inflammation, pain, physical disability, and health status. Articular inflammation, the most important feature of RA, is expressed as joint swelling and tenderness. Methods to quantify these changes include the total number of joints affected, area of joint involvement (small joints vs. large joints), or disease severity. For example, the American College of Rheumatology (ACR) core set evaluates 68 joints, including the distal interphalangeal (DIP) joints of the hands and the proximal interphalangeal (PIP) joints of the feet (28). These were eliminated in the European League Against Rheumatism (EULAR) core set because osteoarthritis (OA) can confound evaluation of the DIP joints, and assessment of the PIPs of the toes is difficult. Scoring just 28 joints (10 PIPs, 10 metacarpal phalangeals (MCP), 2 wrists, 2 elbows, 2 shoulders, and 2 knees) did not compromise the swollen and tender joint counts (26).

A simple visual analogue scale (VAS) is used to grade the intensity of pain in patients with RA. The subject is asked

TABLE 59.1. *Core set of variables to assess disease activity in rheumatoid arthritis*

Disease activity measure	Core sets: EULAR	Core sets: ACR
Tender joint count	28 joints scored	68 joints scored
Swollen joint count	28 joints scored	68 joints scored
Pain on visual analogue scale	X	X
Physician's global assessment of disease activity		X
Patient's global assessment of disease activity		X
Physical function	X	X
Radiographic analysis	X	X
Acute phase reactant	X	X

ACR, American College of Rheumatology; EULAR, European League Against Rheumatism; X, included.

Adapted from Van Reil PLCM. Provisional guidelines for measuring disease activity in clinical trials on rheumatoid arthritis. *Br J Rheumatol* 1992;31:793–794 (EULAR data); and Felson DT, Anderson JJ, Boers M, et al. The American College of Rheumatology preliminary core set of disease activity measures for rheumatoid arthritis clinical trials. The Committee on Outcome Measures in Rheumatoid Arthritis Clinical Trials. *Arthritis Rheum* 1993;36:729–740 (ACR data), with permission.

to indicate his or her current status by marking an X on a 0- to 10-cm horizontal scale with "no pain" at one end and "worst possible pain" at the other. A global assessment of disease activity is measured the same way; both the patient and the physician evaluating the patient answer the question "how well are you (the patient) doing today considering all the ways your arthritis affects you" by placing an X on separate 10-cm horizontal scales. A patient's function or disability is usually based on a self-reporting questionnaire. The Health Assessment Questionnaire and the Arthritis Impact Measurement Score are two popular, validated instruments sensitive to clinical changes (28,29).

Radiographs of selected involved joints should be obtained at the initial evaluation to confirm the diagnosis of RA and to assess its severity. Scoring methods developed by Sharp (30) and Larsen (31) quantify both joint space narrowing (cartilage loss) and bone erosions. The earliest structural changes often occur in the fourth and fifth metatarsalphalangeal (MTP) joints of the feet, but the hands and wrists are usually evaluated because they are more convenient to measure. Radiographic changes in large joints, like the knees, appear later in the disease and are of less utility. Reevaluation at 1- or 2-year intervals can determine whether the current treatment is influencing joint damage or only controlling inflammation, because these two parameters are not synonymous.

RESPONSE TO TREATMENT

Table 59.2 presents two commonly used instruments to evaluate treatment responses. One, developed by Paulus (32), is an arbitrary collection of relatively easy to measure variables. A 20% improvement in joint swelling and joint tenderness plus two of the other four measures discriminates between an active drug and placebo in clinical trials and is an FDA requirement for approving new DMARDs. The ACR criteria are similar to the Paulus 20% improvement criteria, except that pain and disability (measured by VAS) have been added and morning stiffness deleted. Improvement of 20% or more in five of the seven items, including joint swelling and tenderness, is significant (27).

Remission is the goal of RA therapy; unfortunately, however, there is no one definition of the term. Reasonable end

TABLE 59.2. *Response criteria based on change in disease activity*

Improvement in:	Paulus et al. (four out of six)	ACR (five out of seven, including first two)
Joint tenderness	≥20%	≥20%
Joint swelling	≥20%	≥20%
ESR	≥20%	≥20%
Physician's global assessment of disease activity	≥40%	≥20%
Patient's global assessment of disease activity	≥40%	≥20%
Morning stiffness	≥20%	
Pain		≥20%
Disability		≥20%

ACR, American College of Rheumatology; ESR, erythrocyte sedimentation rate.

Adapted from Paulus HE, Egger MJ, Ward JR, et al. Analysis of improvement in individual rheumatoid arthritis patients treated with disease-modifying antirheumatic drugs, based on the findings in patients treated with placebo. The Cooperative Systematic Studies of Rheumatic Diseases Group. *Arthritis Rheum* 1990;33:477–484; and Fries JF, Spitz P, Kraines RG, et al. Measurement of patient outcome in arthritis. *Arthritis Rheum* 1980;23:137–145 (ACR data), with permission.

points might include disappearance of symptoms of morning stiffness, fatigue, and joint pain; loss of joint tenderness, swelling, and pain on motion; and normalization of inflammatory indicators (ESR or CRP). Although these are easily determined early in RA, chronic disease deformities and damage to periarticular soft tissues complicates evaluation. Temporal considerations are also important. How long should a patient remain asymptomatic? The ACR suggests that a remission should be sustained for at least 2 consecutive months (33), but anti-TNF-α monoclonal antibodies, like infliximab, completely control disease in some patients when given intravenously every 8 weeks; yet disease actively returns rapidly with longer intervals between infusions or when the treatment is discontinued. Therefore, only normalization of disease activity in the absence of RA therapy can distinguish between disease control and disease remission. Unfortunately, this rigorous end point is rarely achieved.

THERAPEUTICS

Nonsteroidal Antiinflammatory Drugs

A number of drugs are available for control of joint inflammation. Among them are NSAIDs, intraarticular injections of long-acting glucocorticosteroids, and low doses of prednisone or prednisolone. Aspirin, although effective, requires frequent dosing in large amounts (3–5 g/day) and has a high incidence of side effects. Therefore, aspirin has been replaced by the more convenient NSAIDs. Although differing among themselves in chemical structure, these compounds share antiinflammatory, analgesic, and antipyretic properties. The designation NSAID distinguishes them from opioids, nonnarcotic analgesics, salicylates, and glucocorticoids. NSAIDs work quickly to reduce pain and inflammation, but do not affect the underlying disease process, and do not protect against cartilage loss, bone erosion, or soft tissue damage. Most are organic acids that share an ability to inhibit prostaglandin synthesis by blocking cyclooxygenase (COX) enzymes (details of COX-1 and -2 isoforms are presented in Chapter 31).

Clinical responses and toxicities to NSAIDs differ greatly among individuals. These variable responses are not explained by recognizable patient characteristics or the structure or pharmacology of the drugs. This variability, however, means that serial trials of individual NSAIDs should be used to find the best drug for each patient. Maximum approved doses should be prescribed, and if a satisfactory clinical response is not achieved after 2 to 3 weeks, another NSAID should be tried. Multiple drugs can be tested, but there is no evidence that combinations of NSAIDs are any better than full doses of a single NSAID. Nor is any one superior to another for the treatment of RA. The choice is usually dictated by the physician's prior experience, and the patient's preference. Ease of administration is important. Longer-acting NSAIDs allow once or twice daily dosing, a favorable attribute, but their slow excretion can sometimes complicate management of toxic reactions.

Although generally well tolerated, NSAIDs have a number of side effects (see Chapter 31). Gastrointestinal complaints are common, ranging from dyspepsia, to pain, to subtle blood loss, or occasionally massive bleeding, the major cause of hospitalization or death associated with NSAID use. The bleeding has been ascribed to NSAID blockade of the COX-1 isoform, which is expressed constitutively in the stomach and protects the gastric mucosa by elaborating prostaglandins. The recognition of a COX-2 isoform, which is induced in response to tissue injury, prompted the hope that blocking the COX-2 enzyme would yield compounds that are antiinflammatory without gastric toxicity, thus rendering the less specific NSAIDs obsolete. However, specific COX-2 inhibition is incomplete; gastric side effects still occur, albeit less often; and their antiinflammatory activity is no greater than conventional NSAIDs, at a much greater cost. An additional observation is the loss of gastrointestinal benefits of specific COX-2 inhibitors in patients taking low-dose aspirin for cardioprotection (34). Significant gastrointestinal bleeding is mainly limited to those RA patients with the following characteristics: over the age of 65 years; being treated for congestive heart failure; taking prednisone or anticoagulants; a history of peptic ulcer disease or prior upper GI bleeding; and possibly tobacco and alcohol use (35). Therefore, we favor prescribing maximum doses of nonspecific NSAIDs first and reserving COX-2 selective inhibitors for patients who either have risk factors for bleeding or have failed several conventional NSAIDs.

Corticosteroids

Although often maligned, corticosteroids are a mainstay of RA treatment. The question is not whether to use them; rather, it is how and when. They relieve joint inflammation; improve symptoms of stiffness, fatigue, and loss of appetite; reduce ESR and CRP levels; and increase hemoglobin values. In addition, significantly less radiographic evidence of joint damage was found at 2 years in early RA patients taking low-dose prednisone (7.5 mg/day) compared with controls (36). The adverse effects of long-term corticosteroid use are well recognized (see Chapter 34). Both morbidity and mortality are dose and time dependent. There are no precise guidelines for prescribing corticosteroids, but as a rule prednisone doses should not exceed 10 mg/day in men, 7.5 mg/day in women, and less in postmenopausal women. Women who take more than 7.5 mg/day for longer than 3 months risk bone loss and should have their bone mineral density measured regularly (see Chapter 34). Different formulations of oral steroids are no better than prednisone, although some physicians prefer prednisolone, which has an equivalent potency and side effects. The favorable response to low-dose prednisone early in RA, and the finding that when radiographic changes fail to appear in the first few years they are unlikely to develop thereafter, suggests that the benefits of corticosteroid treatment after 3 years for nonerosive RA will be offset by the increased risks for toxicity (37).

Prednisone is not meant to be used alone or in doses that completely suppress joint inflammation. In combination with other agents, however, small doses can contribute significantly to control of disease activity. Low-dose prednisone is often used in RA patients with new-onset disease while waiting for the slower-acting DMARDs to become effective. Steroids are also indicated when there is an incomplete response to DMARDs. Usually prednisone is prescribed as a single, oral, morning dose, but occasionally administering it twice daily or once in the evening yields better results, especially for minimizing morning stiffness. Every other day therapy is seldom effective in RA. Prolonged administration of prednisone results in a dependency that can be difficult to treat. Abrupt withdrawal often induces an acute flare-up of the arthritis, and, rarely, a systemic rheumatoid disease with necrotizing vasculitis and mononeuropathy develops in patients with rheumatoid nodules and strongly positive serum RF tests. Reduction of the steroid dose must be gradual, over weeks, and in small decrements (1–2.5 mg/wk) until arthritis recurs. Then it is best to return to the last dose that controlled joint symptoms and try again several weeks later. The physician must not be confused by pseudorheumatism, which reflects a relative adrenal insufficiency following a steroid dose reduction. The low-grade fever and musculoskeletal complaints of pseudorheumatism can last days to weeks and might occur with each decrease in steroid dose, but synovitis is absent. Prednisone doses of less than 5 mg/day, which approach physiologic concentrations, are well tolerated. Complete discontinuation may not be achieved, unless the RA activity is suppressed by concomitant therapy.

Large intravenous doses (pulses) of methylprednisolone have been advocated to obtain quick relief of systemic systems of RA or control flare-ups of joint disease. Infusions of 1,000 mg of methylprednisolone every other day for three doses acts rapidly and the benefits may persist, sometimes up to 3 or 4 months. However, we do not advocate this as a chronic therapy. Nor is this the only schedule, because 100 mg and 300 mg of methylprednisolone are nearly as effective as 1,000 mg; intramuscular and intravenous routes are equally effective; and there is no evidence that more than one bolus is needed (38). Moreover, it is important to avoid large corticosteroid doses before the diagnosis of RA is firmly established, because masking synovitis might result in a failure to commence appropriate DMARD treatment.

Inflammation in a single large joint is well managed by an intraarticular injection of a long acting, crystalline form of corticosteroid (see Chapter 35). Following their uptake by synovial lining cells, these compounds control local inflammation, often for many months. It is imperative, however, to obtain synovial fluid for culture at the time of joint aspiration, because septic arthritis can complicate RA, and antibiotics, rather than corticosteroids, would be required. Diffusion of the long-acting corticosteroid from the injected joint can improve distant joints and control systemic symptoms. Repeated joint injections are not advised. They are equivalent to regular intramuscular doses of corticosteroids with all the attendant complications, including osteonecrosis. Traditionally, injections of a single joint are limited to three or four per year, although this is not supported by clinical evidence.

Disease-Modifying Antirheumatic Drugs

Second-line agents, slow-acting antirheumatic drugs, remission-inducing drugs, and DMARDs are interchangeable terms. Although biologic agents are also properly designated as DMARDs, this section will be limited to conventional DMARDs. Many factors influence the choice of one or another of this class of drug: relative efficacy; speed of action; costs of medication and laboratory monitoring, and frequency of physician visits; adverse reactions; and comorbid conditions. For women, conception, pregnancy, and breast-feeding are also important considerations (discussed later in this chapter). No one DMARD treatment or combination of DMARDs is best for all RA patients. Accordingly, the recommendations we make reflect our choices, based on our experience and critique of the abundant literature on RA treatments.

Commonly used conventional DMARDs include hydroxychloroquine, sulfasalazine, methotrexate, and leflunomide. Also approved by the FDA for RA, but less frequently used, are azathioprine, minocycline, and cyclosporine A. Information on oral and injectable gold, D-penicillamine, and chloroquine, which are seldom prescribed anymore, is presented in Chapter 42.

Sulfasalazine

Patients who present with mild disease and few erosions on joint radiographs are good candidates for sulfasalazine monotherapy (39). The drug is favored in Europe because of its rapid onset of action (3–6 weeks) and low incidence of serious side effects. Treatment is begun at 500 mg twice daily for 10 to 14 days. In the absence of nausea, vomiting, photosensitivity, or skin rash the dose is increased to two tablets (1,000 mg) twice a day. If no improvement is noted after 3 months of treatment, the dose can be increased to 1,500 mg twice daily for 4 additional weeks. In patients with a modest response [20% improvement in ACR criteria (ACR20)], sulfasalazine can be continued in combination with a second DMARD. Interactions with other antirheumatic drugs are uncommon. Because of the rare complications of myelosuppression or hemolytic anemia in individuals with glucose-6-phosphate dehydrogenase enzyme deficiency, monthly blood counts are recommended for 3 months after starting the drug and every 3 to 4 months thereafter (40).

Hydroxychloroquine

Multiple double-blind, placebo-controlled trials support the efficacy of 4-amino-quinoline antimalarial drugs for the treatment of RA (1–3). Both chloroquine (250 mg/day) and hydroxychloroquine (200 mg/twice a day) can be used, but the later is favored because of a lower incidence of ocular toxicity. A shortcoming of hydroxychloroquine is its slow onset: usually 3 months before antirheumatic effects are observed, and sometimes improvement is delayed 6 to 9 months. Monotherapy is usually reserved for patients with mild disease, but because of mild and infrequent toxic reactions and the absence of drug interactions, hydroxychloroquine is included in many DMARD combinations. The most common side effects are maculopapular rashes, gastrointestinal disturbances, nonspecific neurologic complaints, and other problems relating to the drug's affinity for, and tight binding to, melanin pigments. Bleaching of the hair or eyebrows, hyperpigmentation in photoexposed areas, and increased melanin in dark-skinned people can be troublesome. A greater concern is drug deposition in the pigment of the retina, which can lead to visual impairment. This complication was recognized in the past when larger doses of chloroquine were used, but limiting the hydroxychloroquine dose to 6 mg/kg or less per day obviates the problem (41). Nevertheless, patients with macular disease should avoid hydroxychloroquine and those with chronic exposure need to be evaluated by an ophthalmologist familiar with the drug's ocular toxicity every 6 to 12 months. Retinopathy can occur in the absence of visual symptoms. With early detection, this process is reversible, but stopping the drug later will not prevent blindness. We favor sulfasalazine over hydroxychloroquine for the patient with early RA, because it works faster, but in established disease either one is satisfactory.

Methotrexate

No other DMARD enjoys the popularity of methotrexate for the treatment of RA. Original concerns about acute and long-term toxicities limited its use to patients with severe, refractory disease, but the side effects proved manageable, and multiple randomized trials demonstrated a relatively high retention rate, good disease control, and retardation of joint damage at all stages of disease (see Chapter 32). Clinical responses occur 3 to 6 weeks after reaching therapeutic levels. The beginning dose is usually 7.5 mg (three tablets) taken together on 1 day each week. Incremental increases of 2.5 mg/wk are made every 4 weeks until either maximum control of joint inflammation or symptoms of toxicity appear. Improvement usually requires doses of 15 to 20 mg/wk, but patient responses are quite variable. Stomatitis, anorexia, nausea, or diarrhea often interfere at higher doses, but these can be minimized by either adding folic acid (1–2 mg/day), giving the drug by injection, or reducing the dose. Occasionally, giving half the dose twice a week is helpful. Stopping the medication for 2 weeks sometimes eliminates the aforementioned adverse effects. Increasing doses of methotrexate are often required over time to maintain clinical improvement. Disease suppression is lost within 4 weeks of stopping the drug, but control is recaptured at the same dose 3 to 4 weeks after restarting the medication.

Drug interactions with methotrexate are more theoretical than real. Renal tubular secretion of the drug can be competitively inhibited by organic acids, including certain NSAIDs. These effects are dose related and are usually only seen with the large doses of methotrexate required for cancer chemotherapy. At the once weekly low doses used to treat RA, such interactions are rarely clinically relevant. Patients with reduced glomerular filtration, taking NSAIDs or cyclosporine A and methotrexate at doses of greater than 20 mg/wk require careful monitoring. Folic acid deficiencies can predispose to toxicity.

Side effects occur in 7% to 90% of methotrexate-treated RA patients (42). The great variability in reporting is probably explained by the mild nature of most complaints, the willingness of many patients to tolerate them rather than discontinue an effective medication, and greater experience administering the drug. Minor gastrointestinal symptoms, macrocytosis, cytopenias, alopecia, and mild skin rash are usually managed by folic acid supplements. The more significant pulmonary and hepatic toxicities are detailed in Chapter 32. Bone marrow suppression can result from renal insufficiency, serious systemic infection, and concomitant administration of trimethoprim-sulfamethoxazole. There might be an increase in opportunistic infections in RA patients treated with methotrexate. Rheumatoid nodules can appear, enlarge, or significantly increase in number in patients taking methotrexate (43). It has been suggested, without confirmation, that hydroxychloroquine can decrease the clusters of these troublesome, often painful, small nodules.

The ACR guidelines for monitoring methotrexate therapy include regular complete blood counts and liver function tests, monthly for the first 6 months and every 1 to 2 months thereafter (1). Small elevations (less than threefold) in alanine aminotransferase or aspartate aminotransferase should be followed closely and evaluated again after a dose reduction or after stopping the drug for a short period. Persistent (more than threefold) increases of hepatic enzymes warrants discontinuation of methotrexate. Issues concerning liver biopsy are discussed in Chapter 32.

Leflunomide

Leflunomide, the first pyrimidine inhibitor available for RA treatment, was shown to be superior to placebo and equivalent to either sulfasalazine or methotrexate in improving arthritis activity, functional status, and retarding radiographic evidence of joint damage in a number of recently published, well-controlled trials (44,45). Because of the drug's long half-life, the manufacturer recommends a loading dose of 100 mg/day for 3 days to achieve a steady state and then regular doses of 20 mg once a day. In our experience, using 20 mg/day from the outset decreases the troublesome side effect of diarrhea, with only a modest prolongation of the usual time to improvement (6–8 weeks). Sometimes, gastrointestinal toxicities can be controlled by reducing the dose to 10 mg/day without sacrificing clinical benefits. Elevations of liver enzyme measurements can be troublesome, sometimes requiring drug discontinuation. They are managed as described above for methotrexate and in Chapter 32. At this time, there is no evidence that methotrexate and leflunomide taken together increase the risk for hepatotoxicity, and the combination is being used successfully to treat active RA (46). Monitoring recommendations are similar to methotrexate (1). Cholestyramine enhances leflunomide excretion and is used to treat overdoses or serious toxicity, including potential for teratogenicity in pregnancy (discussed in a later section). To date, neither pulmonary side effects nor lymphoma has been associated with leflunomide use.

Other Conventional DMARDs

Several older drugs have efficacy and are approved for use in RA, but they are seldom prescribed anymore (see Chapter 42). Some, like gold compounds, have significant side effects, are less successful when taken by mouth, or are painful as intramuscular injections. D-penicillamine is no longer used because of the development of proteinuria, nephrotic syndrome, or the induction of one of several autoimmune diseases.

Occasionally, when joint disease appears intractable, immunomodulatory agents are tried (see Chapter 41). Except for methotrexate, however, immunomodulatory drugs are only used in combination with other DMARDs. The long-term complications of cyclophosphamide and chlorambucil, such as bone marrow suppression or neoplasms, limit their use in RA. Azathioprine has a mild side effect profile, and is favored by some rheumatologists, especially for lowering the prednisone dose in patients with corticosteroid dependency. Since the advent of the biologic DMARDs, we rarely prescribe cyclosporine A, primarily because of the frequent complications of hypertension and renal insufficiency.

Antibiotics

For decades, infection has been considered a possible cause of RA and anecdotal reports of the efficacy of antibiotics have been cited as evidence. However, antibiotics have multiple actions. Tetracyclines, for example, have antiinflammatory effects and inhibit certain collagenases (47). Minocycline affords some joint protection to rodents with experimental arthritis. Two controlled trials, one European and one American, found that 200 mg/day of minocycline improved (25%) joint symptoms and laboratory studies in patients with active, established RA better than placebo (48,49). More remarkable, a group of seropositive RA patients with less than 1 year of disease taking prednisone, but no previous DMARDs, were randomized to take either minocycline (200 mg/day) or hydroxychloroquine (200 mg/twice a day). At 2 years, the minocycline-treated patients achieved an ACR50 response more often (60%) than the hydroxychloroquine group (33%), and a number of patients discontinued prednisone (50). This finding supports the idea that drugs that are only modestly effective in established disease perform better in early RA. Side effects are mild and include dizziness, photosensitive skin rashes, and gastrointestinal complaints. A troublesome problem can be skin hyperpigmentation, which develops in 10% to 30% of patients who take the drug for 2 years. A recent appreciation that minocycline can reduce ischemia-induced tissue injury, inhibit production of NO_2 and the release of cytochrome C from cells, and block certain downstream caspases all point to ways that minocycline could modulate RA (51).

Biologic DMARDs

An exciting advance in the treatment of RA is agents that specifically block cytokines known to play key roles in disease pathogenesis (Chapters 39 and 40). Drugs targeting TNF-α and IL-1 are FDA approved at this time, and investigational agents that interfere with other cytokines, such as an anti-IL-6 receptor antibody, also show promise in clinical trials. The three available anti-TNF-α agents differ in structure. Adalimumab (DE27) is a recombinant human anti-TNF-α antibody, whereas infliximab is a chimeric anti-TNF-α antibody consisting of a human constant region (Fc) "grafted" onto the variable region (Fv) of the murine antibody. Etanercept, on the other hand, functions as a soluble TNF receptor that competes for TNF-α binding to the natural p75 surface receptor. It is a TNFR-p75–IgG-Fc fusion protein. Infliximab is administered by intravenous infusion at a dose of 3 mg/kg. Following infusion at 0, 2, and 4 weeks, the drug's benefits are usually maintained by infusions every 8 weeks (reviewed in Chapter 39). The manufacturers of both etanercept and adalimumab provide their drugs in prefilled and premeasured syringes for self-administered subcutaneous injection. They are easy to use, provided that the patient has sufficient manual dexterity. The recommended dose of etanercept is 25 mg twice weekly and for adalimumab is 40 mg every other week. These doses can be adjusted by increasing the amount of drug or shortening the interval between administrations.

Each of the three anti-TNF reagents will diminish the signs and symptoms of RA in a majority of patients, and in most cases they halt the progression of bone erosions (52–56). None of them, however, induces complete disease remission, and joint symptoms recur in most individuals a few weeks after the drugs are discontinued. Approximately half the patients taking anti-TNF-α drugs exhibit an ACR50 response or greater improvement. There is no explanation why some patients respond and others do not, but changing to an alternative anti-TNF-α preparation is sometimes effective.

The use of the biologic DMARDs is limited by several factors, not the least of which is their cost, which approximates $12,000 to $15,000 per annum per patient. Exposure to a foreign protein poses the risk for generating an antibody against the therapeutic modality. Theoretically there is a greater risk with antibodies that contain murine components (infliximab), but naturally occurring antiidiotypic antibodies can develop to portions of the "humanized" antibodies. Some evidence suggests that such antibodies can reduce the effectiveness of anti-TNF reagents. The concomitant use of methotrexate may decrease antiidiotypic antibody reactions (56). An unanticipated complication of treatment with anti-TNF-α drugs is the development of antinuclear and anti-DNA antibodies, and a few patients develop lupus-like symptoms (57,58). Multiple sclerosis, another autoimmune disease, can be reactivated or exacerbated. Latent demyelinated central nervous system lesions are reported to become symptomatic or become larger (59–61). Whether immune mechanisms are responsible for the increased risk for lymphoma reported in RA patients treated with the anti-TNF-α agents is unclear. A greater risk to patients from these drugs, however, is the development of severe and life-threatening infections. Infliximab, in particular, has been associated with reactivation and dissemination of tuberculosis (62,63). Before embarking on biologic DMARD treatment, patients at risk for any of the possible adverse events described above need to be excluded or treated, as is the case with a positive tuberculous skin reaction or pulmonary tuberculosis.

Although it is possible to use anti-TNF-α agents as monotherapy, they are usually more effective when given in combination with other DMARDs, especially methotrexate. Anti-TNF-α agents appear to be effective in early-onset RA (64), but because of their great cost, the uncertainties of long-term sequelae, and the improved prognosis when patients with early RA are treated quickly and aggressively with conventional DMARDs, it makes sense to save these agents for patients who have an incomplete response to more traditional DMARDs. Anti-TNF treatment appears to be safe in RA patients whose use of alcoholic beverages would limit enthusiasm for methotrexate.

Interleukin-1 is an important cytokine in animal models of arthritis and plays a pivotal role in bone and cartilage damage in RA. A recombinant form of human IL-1Ra, anakinra, is a competitive antagonist of IL-1 that engages the IL-1 receptor and antagonizes the actions of IL-1. It is less effective clinically than the anti-TNF-α agents in treating RA, but can retard the development of bone loss (65–67). IL-1Ra is administered as a 100-mg daily subcutaneous injection and can cause pain at injection sites. The risk for reactivating latent tuberculosis, predisposing to other infections, or increased incidence of lymphoma, complications that might limit anti-TNF-α agents, are not seen with IL-1Ra. Although it has been suggested that IL-1Ra and an anti-TNF-α be combined to retard bone and cartilage damage, there are no data supporting their use together and the cost can be prohibitive. Under certain circumstances and with particular risk factors present in an individual patient, IL-1Ra might be the preferred agent.

GUIDELINES FOR TREATING A PATIENT WITH EARLY RHEUMATOID ARTHRITIS

Only after the clinical suspicion of RA has been confirmed by the presence of morning stiffness lasting more than 30 minutes, swelling in three or more joints, and tenderness in the MCP or MTP joints should the physician begin antiinflammatory treatment with NSAIDs or low-dose prednisone. These are maintained while awaiting the results of laboratory investigations and radiographs of the hands and feet. A quantitative RF test with titers greater than 1:80 or 30 IU and autoantibodies to cyclic citrullinated peptides (anti CCP) supports the diagnosis of RA, and higher values predict a poor outcome. Likewise, bone erosions in radiographs and consistent twofold or greater elevation of inflammatory indices (ESR or acute-phase proteins) are each bad prognostic factors. Patients with these features require rapid institution of DMARD therapy, which is best done by either a rheumatologist or a primary physician knowledgeable about RA.

The type, sequence, and number of DMARDs is determined by disease activity, the presence of factors that predict a poor outcome, or evidence of joint damage at the time of presentation. Other considerations are the physician's preferences and patient's comorbidities. We favor an aggressive approach from the outset: combining methotrexate (7.5 mg once a week) with folate (1 mg daily), and hydroxychloroquine (200 mg twice daily) or sulfasalazine (2,000–3,000 mg/day), in addition to a baseline NSAID and/or low-dose prednisone (5.0–7.5 mg/day) and possibly a proton pump inhibitor. If there are no contraindications, the methotrexate dose is increased stepwise to 15 or 17.5 mg weekly by the third month. Failure to achieve a 50% reduction in disease activity and inflammatory indices signals a need for a further increase in the methotrexate dose (if tolerated) or the addition of a third DMARD. Currently we favor starting leflunomide at a dose of 10 mg/day with careful attention to transaminase determinations, since both drugs can be hepatotoxic. Minocycline (200 mg/day) could be an alternative. If the disease is still active (less than an ACR50 response) 3 months later, and the three DMARDs are at maximum tolerated doses, then we consider anti TNF-α agents. Others might try alternative treatments such as azathioprine, cyclosporine A, mycophenolate, or cyclophosphamide, but if cost is not a consideration, none are likely to be as effective as the anti-TNF-α agents. Gradual reductions in the doses of other drugs are indicated after the RA comes under control. There is no good advice about the rate, sequence, or choice of which DMARD to lower. Our inclination is to decrease prednisone first, if the dose exceeds 5.0 mg/day; otherwise, lowering methotrexate seems advisable. Often synovitis or inflammatory indices return when the methotrexate dose is lower than 7.5 mg/wk. Then, a return to the last dose that controlled the joint disease is indicated.

GUIDELINES FOR TREATING A PATIENT WITH ESTABLISHED RHEUMATOID ARTHRITIS

Unfortunately, rheumatologists seldom see patients with early RA. More often the disease is long standing and has not responded to one or another drug. When confronted by patients with chronic, recalcitrant RA, we devote the initial consultation to a search for factors that might account for previous failures. Is the diagnosis of RA correct? What drugs have been taken, in what doses, alone or in combination? Are there factors, including comorbid conditions, that prevent or compromise the use of certain antirheumatic therapies? Most important, are the levels of the inflammatory indices or the radiographic changes in the joints consistent with the patient's complaints? Too often, active RA is confused with a secondary fibromyalgia or chronic pain syndrome, the pseudorheumatism of prolonged use of steroids, coincidental or superimposed degenerative arthritis, or impediments resulting from joint contractures and misalignment. These will not respond to DMARD therapy.

As noted, multiple drugs are now available that effectively treat RA. Information about them is provided in this chapter and in Section III of this textbook. Here we present our approach to choosing among them and maximizing their benefits for patients with established RA. Several principles guide us:

- DMARD use in RA requires a correct diagnosis.
- DMARDs must be taken at their maximum tolerated dose.
- DMARDs should not be stopped, except for toxicity or disease remission.
- DMARDs are added rather than replaced.
- DMARD schedules that produce less than 50% improvement need to be modified.

In a patient with chronic RA who has neither taken nor discontinued DMARDs, we institute them, unless there are contraindications. The approach is similar to that for patients with a recent onset of disease, namely, adding methotrexate and hydroxychloroquine or sulfasalazine on a baseline of an NSAID and prednisone (5.0–7.5 mg/day). The dose of methotrexate is increased by 2.5 mg/wk every 4 weeks until a maximum tolerated dose is achieved. Reassessment should be performed after 3 months. If significant (>50%) improvement has not occurred, then the physician has several options. We favor adding another DMARD, either leflunomide (10–20 mg/day) or azathioprine (1.5–2.0 mg/kg/day), while continuing the methotrexate at the highest tolerated dose. Often this requires switching to subcutaneous methotrexate administration. Leflunomide, although it has more side effects, is preferred because improvement with azathioprine is slow, often taking more than 12 weeks. At this point, an inadequate therapeutic response warrants the addition of any one of the three approved anti-TNF-α reagents. With patients who are not taking methotrexate, we usually add subcutaneous injections of etanercept (25 mg twice a week). If infliximab is prescribed, then we prefer to use it in combination with methotrexate.

Alternative medications, including cyclophosphamide, cyclosporine A, and IL-1Ra, or investigational therapies, such as *Staphylococcus* protein A immunoadsorption, intravenous gamma globulin, or new biologic agents, are reserved for individuals who have failed or cannot tolerate the program described above. An antibody to an antigen on the surface of B cells (CD20) appears promising, but has not yet been approved by the FDA. Problems in individual joints, either inflammation or destruction, are managed with intraarticular injections of nonabsorbable corticosteroids or surgery, respectively.

GUIDELINES FOR TREATING A PATIENT WITH LATE-ONSET RHEUMATOID ARTHRITIS

A small cadre of elderly patients, mostly men, abruptly develop an inflammatory polyarthritis and diffuse swelling of the hands. This presentation, sometimes called "late-onset RA" has features that resemble polymyalgia rheumatica (68). These include the absence of serum RF or the HLA-DR beta-1 "susceptibility haplotype," less destructive joint disease, and an excellent response to 10 to 15 mg/day of prednisone. Aggressive DMARD treatment is seldom warranted in the absence of the usual factors that predict a poor prognosis for RA. However, if the response to prednisone is either inadequate, or toxicity ensues, or the dose cannot be lowered to safer levels by 12 weeks, then treatment with hydroxychloroquine or sulfasalazine should be used rather than moving directly to methotrexate. Because elderly patients can have underlying retinal disease, a baseline ophthalmologic examination is warranted before starting hydroxychloroquine. Older patients also have a decline in their drug clearance mechanisms and can be at higher risk for toxicities and complications of methotrexate therapy.

REPRODUCTION CONCERNS WITH DMARDs

Rheumatoid arthritis affects women of childbearing age, and some of the medications used to treat this disease can affect conception, pregnancy, fetal development, or lactation. The patient should be informed of the risks for impaired fertility and congenital malformations before prescribing certain DMARDs. Hence, pregnancy should be excluded before initiating them, and women taking these agents must use effective methods to prevent conception. If menses are delayed, the patient should be advised to notify her physician promptly. At this time there are insufficient data to recommend terminating a pregnancy. The patient should be referred to an obstetric group with expertise in high-risk neonatology to obtain appropriate prenatal testing and counseling.

Methotrexate is one of the DMARDs that requires specific mention in terms of fetal toxicity (69). Taken during pregnancy, it can result in intrauterine death, facial clefts, and distal limb anomalies (70,71). This teratogenic effect is a result of direct inhibition of dihydrofolate reductase in the fetus and is not an effect of the drug on the mother (72). Although experience in pregnancy with leflunomide is limited, it is also rated category X by the FDA based on animal data suggesting an increased risk for fetal death and teratogenicity (73). Because the drug has a very long half-life and is unpredictably eliminated, it should be stopped 3 months prior to conception or immediately if a pregnancy occurs. Cholestyramine is used to eliminate the drug (see Chapter 32). A conservative approach after leflunomide washout would be to have the woman wait for three menstrual cycles before conceiving. A man should wait for at least one spermatogenesis cycle.

Rheumatoid arthritis frequently improves during pregnancy, and drug therapy can be reduced or eliminated. NSAIDs can be used until the final 6 weeks, and low to moderate doses of corticosteroids are safe throughout pregnancy. Sulfasalazine and hydroxychloroquine can be maintained. Azathioprine is not recommended for pregnant women because there is an undefined risk for carcinogenesis and fetal neutropenia (74,75). Cyclosporine A, cytoxan, chlorambucil, leflunomide, and methotrexate are all contraindicated (reviewed in reference 76). The effects of biologic agents that block TNF-α and IL-1 are yet to be determined.

In the 3 months following pregnancy, there is often a flare-up in joint disease that requires DMARD treatment. The time to restart these medications should be dictated by the clinical activity of the disease. During lactation, some drugs enter the mother's milk and can adversely affect the baby (77). Prednisone, sulfasalazine, and hydroxychloroquine can be used cautiously, but azathioprine, gold, cytoxan, cyclosporine A, methotrexate, and TNF-α inhibitors are best avoided (reviewed in reference 76).

Reproductive concerns of male patients are often overlooked. Both methotrexate and sulfasalazine can cause male infertility, which usually reverses when the drug is discontinued (78,79). Cyclophosphamide can lower sperm counts, and there are isolated reports of congenital anomalies in infants whose fathers received the drug (80,81). Presently, there are insufficient data about effects of leflunomide on male-mediated fetal toxicity, so the manufacturer is recommending a drug elimination protocol prior to conception (see Chapter 32).

COMORBIDITIES THAT CAN INFLUENCE DECISIONS ABOUT DMARDs

Questions concerning alcohol abuse, foreign travel, tuberculosis exposure, previous drug use, blood transfusions, and concurrent and past medical conditions should be addressed before initiating DMARD therapy. Risk factors fall into four categories: occult infection (particularly tuberculosis and hepatitis), liver damage, renal dysfunction, and known malignancies. Reproductive concerns have already been discussed.

Patients with underlying liver disease from either alcohol use or viral causes are at a higher risk for methotrexate- or leflunomide-induced hepatic toxicities. Also, DMARDs can reactivate quiescent hepatitis; therefore, prescreening for hepatitis C antibody or hepatitis B surface antigen is advisable in such patients if these drugs are being considered. Besides leflunomide and methotrexate, a small number of patients with chronic hepatitis developed liver toxicity when given sulfasalazine or plaquenil. Gold administration, however, did not alter liver function in the few patients reported with chronic viral hepatitis (82). NSAIDs, either alone or in combination with methotrexate, can also increase the risk for hepatotoxicity. To date, anti-CD20 monoclonal antibody therapy is not approved for RA, but appears promising. It has been well tolerated during treatment of patients with autoimmune hemolytic anemia and hepatitis C, and appears to have less risk for exacerbating infections than the anti-TNF-α agents (83–85).

A focus on the liver is appropriate when evaluating patients for DMARD treatments; however, the kidneys are the major mechanism for drug elimination. Patients with significantly impaired renal function are poor candidates for methotrexate and leflunomide, both of which are excreted by the kidneys. Subtle renal impairment can become a significant factor in patients given NSAIDs when they are relatively volume depleted or are taking concurrent angiotensin-converting enzyme inhibitors. Patients with renal dysfunction who have fluid retention do better with steroids that lack mineralocorticoid activity, such as methylprednisolone.

When opting to use an anti-TNF agent, there are special considerations, including the potential for disseminating occult tuberculosis infection (62,63). As discussed above, it is advisable to assess the patient's history and risk for tuberculosis and to place a tuberculous skin test. Lymphomas develop more often in RA patients than in the general population. This is independent of concomitant treatment and complicates the assessment of the added risk of a particular drug. This problem is underscored by recent reports of lymphomas occurring in patients exposed to the TNF-α-blocking agents (86).

ACKNOWLEDGMENTS

We are grateful to Dr. P. Hlavin for critical review of the manuscript. This work was funded in part by grants from the National Institutes of Health.

REFERENCES

1. Guidelines for the management of rheumatoid arthritis: 2002 update. American College of Rheumatology Subcommittee on Rheumatoid Arthritis Guidelines. *Arthritis Rheum* 2002;46:328–346.
2. Wolfe F, Sharp JT. Radiographic outcome of recent-onset rheumatoid arthritis: a 19-year study of radiographic progression. *Arthritis Rheum* 1998;41:1571–1582.
3. Lipsky PE. Disease modifying drugs. In: Utsinger PD, Zvaifler NJ, Ehrlich GE, eds. *Rheumatoid arthritis,* 1st ed. Philadelphia: JB Lippincott, 1985:601–634.
4. Scott DL, Symmons DP, Coulton BL, et al. Long-term outcome of treating rheumatoid arthritis: results after 20 years. *Lancet* 1987;1: 1108–1111.
5. Wolfe F, Hawley DJ, Cathey MA. Termination of slow acting antirheumatic therapy in rheumatoid arthritis: a 14-year prospective evaluation of 1017 consecutive starts. *J Rheumatol* 1990;17:994–1002.
6. Wilske KR, Healey LA. Remodeling the pyramid—a concept whose time has come. *J Rheumatol* 1989;16:565–567.
7. Kim JM, Weisman MH. When does rheumatoid arthritis begin and why do we need to know? *Arthritis Rheum* 2000;43:473–484.
8. Harrison BJ, Symmons DP, Brennan P, et al. Natural remission in inflammatory polyarthritis: issues of definition and prediction. *Br J Rheumatol* 1996;35:1096–1100.
9. Harrison BJ, Symmons DP, Barrett EM, et al. The performance of the 1987 ARA classification criteria for rheumatoid arthritis in a population based cohort of patients with early inflammatory polyarthritis. American Rheumatism Association. *J Rheumatol* 1998;25:2324–2330.
10. Emery P, Breedveld FC, Dougados M, et al. Early referral recommendation for newly diagnosed rheumatoid arthritis: evidence based development of a clinical guide. *Ann Rheum Dis* 2002;61: 290–297.
11. Young A, Bielawska C, Corbett M, et al. A prospective study of early onset rheumatoid arthritis over fifteen years: prognostic features and outcome. *Clin Rheumatol* 1987;6:12–19.
12. Symmons DP, Jones MA, Scott DL, et al. Longterm mortality outcome in patients with rheumatoid arthritis: early presenters continue to do well. *J Rheumatol* 1998;25:1072–1077.
13. van der Heijde DM. Joint erosions and patients with early rheumatoid arthritis. *Br J Rheumatol* 1995;34:74–78.
14. Fuchs HA, Kaye JJ, Callahan LF, et al. Evidence of significant radiographic damage in rheumatoid arthritis within the first 2 years of disease. *J Rheumatol* 1989;16:585–591.
15. van der Heide A, Jacobs JW, Bijlsma JW, et al. The effectiveness of early treatment with "second-line" antirheumatic drugs. A randomized, controlled trial. *Ann Intern Med* 1996;124:699–707.
16. Kroot EJ, van Leeuwen MA, van Rijswijk MH, et al. No increased mortality in patients with rheumatoid arthritis: up to 10 years of follow up from disease onset. *Ann Rheum Dis* 2000;59:954–958.
17. Albers JM, Paimela L, Kurki P, et al. Treatment strategy, disease activity, and outcome in four cohorts of patients with early rheumatoid arthritis. *Ann Rheum Dis* 2001;60:453–458.
18. Pinals RS. Survival in rheumatoid arthritis. *Arthritis Rheum* 1987;30: 473–475.
19. Dougados M, Smolen JS. Pharmacological management of early rheumatoid arthritis—does combination therapy improve outcomes? *J Rheumatol Suppl* 2002;66:20–26.
20. Felson DT, Anderson JJ, Meenan RF. The efficacy and toxicity of combination therapy in rheumatoid arthritis. A meta-analysis. *Arthritis Rheum* 1994;37:1487–1491.
21. Goekoop YP, Allaart CF, Breedveld FC, et al. Combination therapy in rheumatoid arthritis. *Curr Opin Rheumatol* 2001;13:177–183.
22. O'Dell JR, Haire CE, Erikson N, et al. Treatment of rheumatoid arthritis with methotrexate alone, sulfasalazine and hydroxychloroquine, or a combination of all three medications. *N Engl J Med* 1996;334: 1287–1291.
23. Keyszer G, Keysser C, Keysser M. Efficacy and safety of a combination therapy of methotrexate, chloroquine and cyclophosphamide in patients with refractory rheumatoid arthritis: results of an observational study with matched-pair analysis. *Clin Rheumatol* 1999;18: 145–151.
24. Csuka M, Carrera GF, McCarty DJ. Treatment of intractable rheumatoid arthritis with combined cyclophosphamide, azathioprine, and hydroxychloroquine. A follow-up study. *JAMA* 1986;255:2315–2319.
25. Boers M, Verhoeven AC, Markusse HM, et al. Randomised comparison of combined step-down prednisolone, methotrexate and sulphasalazine with sulphasalazine alone in early rheumatoid arthritis. *Lancet* 1997;350:309–318.
26. Van Reil PLCM. Provisional guidelines for measuring disease activity in clinical trials on rheumatoid arthritis. *Br J Rheumatol* 1992;31: 793–794.
27. Felson DT, Anderson JJ, Boers M, et al. The American College of Rheumatology preliminary core set of disease activity measures for rheumatoid arthritis clinical trials. The Committee on Outcome Measures in Rheumatoid Arthritis Clinical Trials. *Arthritis Rheum* 1993;36:729–740.
28. Fries JF, Spitz P, Kraines RG, et al. Measurement of patient outcome in arthritis. *Arthritis Rheum* 1980;23:137–145.
29. Meenan RF, Gertman PM, Mason JH. Measuring health status in arthritis. The arthritis impact measurement scales. *Arthritis Rheum* 1980;23:146–152.
30. Sharp JT, Lidsky MD, Collins LC, et al. Methods of scoring the progression of radiologic changes in rheumatoid arthritis. Correlation of radiologic, clinical and laboratory abnormalities. *Arthritis Rheum* 1971;14:706–720.
31. Larsen A. How to apply Larsen score in evaluating radiographs of rheumatoid arthritis in long-term studies. *J Rheumatol* 1995;22:1974–1975.
32. Paulus HE, Egger MJ, Ward JR, et al. Analysis of improvement in individual rheumatoid arthritis patients treated with disease-modifying antirheumatic drugs, based on the findings in patients treated with placebo. The Cooperative Systematic Studies of Rheumatic Diseases Group. *Arthritis Rheum* 1990;33:477–484.
33. Pinals RS, Masi AT, Larsen RA. Preliminary criteria for clinical remission in rheumatoid arthritis. *Arthritis Rheum* 1981;24:1308–1315.
34. Silverstein FE, Faich G, Goldstein JL, et al. Gastrointestinal toxicity with celecoxib vs nonsteroidal anti-inflammatory drugs for osteoarthritis and rheumatoid arthritis: the CLASS study: a randomized controlled trial. Celecoxib Long-term Arthritis Safety Study. *JAMA* 2000;284:1247–1255.
35. Gabriel SE, Jaakkimainen L, Bombardier C. Risk for serious gastrointestinal complications related to use of nonsteroidal anti-inflammatory drugs. A meta-analysis. *Ann Intern Med* 1991;115:787–796.
36. Conn DL, Lim SS. New role for an old friend: prednisone is a disease-modifying agent in early rheumatoid arthritis. *Curr Opin Rheumatol* 2003;15:193–196.
37. Kirwan JR. Systemic low-dose glucocorticoid treatment in rheumatoid arthritis. *Rheum Dis Clin North Am* 2001;27:389–403, ix–x.
38. Smith MD, Ahern MJ, Roberts-Thomson PJ. Pulse steroid therapy in rheumatoid arthritis: can equivalent doses of oral prednisolone give similar clinical results to intravenous methylprednisolone? *Ann Rheum Dis* 1988;47:28–33.
39. Dougados M, Combe B, Cantagrel A, et al. Combination therapy in early rheumatoid arthritis: a randomised, controlled, double blind 52 week clinical trial of sulphasalazine and methotrexate compared with the single components. *Ann Rheum Dis* 1999;58:220–225.
40. Recommendations for the prevention and treatment of glucocorticoid-induced osteoporosis. American College of Rheumatology Task Force on Osteoporosis Guidelines. *Arthritis Rheum* 1996;39:1791–1801.
41. Mackenzie AH. Dose refinements in long-term therapy of rheumatoid arthritis with antimalarials. *Am J Med* 1983;75:40–45.

42. Felson DT, Anderson JJ, Meenan RF. The comparative efficacy and toxicity of second-line drugs in rheumatoid arthritis. Results of two metaanalyses. *Arthritis Rheum* 1990;33:1449–1461.
43. Kerstens PJ, Boerbooms AM, Jeurissen ME, et al. Accelerated nodulosis during low dose methotrexate therapy for rheumatoid arthritis. An analysis of ten cases. *J Rheumatol* 1992;19:867–871.
44. Emery P, Breedveld FC, Lemmel EM, et al. A comparison of the efficacy and safety of leflunomide and methotrexate for the treatment of rheumatoid arthritis. *Rheumatology (Oxford)* 2000;39:655–665.
45. Smolen JS, Kalden JR, Scott DL, et al. Efficacy and safety of leflunomide compared with placebo and sulphasalazine in active rheumatoid arthritis: a double-blind, randomised, multicentre trial. European Leflunomide Study Group. *Lancet* 1999;353:259–266.
46. Weinblatt ME, Kremer JM, Coblyn JS, et al. Pharmacokinetics, safety, and efficacy of combination treatment with methotrexate and leflunomide in patients with active rheumatoid arthritis. *Arthritis Rheum* 1999;42:1322–1328.
47. Golub LM, Ramamurthy N, McNamara TF, et al. Tetracyclines inhibit tissue collagenase activity. A new mechanism in the treatment of periodontal disease. *J Periodont Res* 1984;19:651–655.
48. Kloppenburg M, Breedveld FC, Terwiel JP, et al. Minocycline in active rheumatoid arthritis. A double-blind, placebo-controlled trial. *Arthritis Rheum* 1994;37:629–636.
49. Tilley BC, Alarcon GS, Heyse SP, et al. Minocycline in rheumatoid arthritis. A 48-week, double-blind, placebo-controlled trial. MIRA Trial Group. *Ann Intern Med* 1995;122:81–89.
50. O'Dell JR, Paulsen G, Haire CE, et al. Treatment of early seropositive rheumatoid arthritis with minocycline: four-year followup of a double-blind, placebo-controlled trial. *Arthritis Rheum* 1999;42:1691–1695.
51. Zhu S, Stavrovskaya IG, Drozda M, et al. Minocycline inhibits cytochrome c release and delays progression of amyotrophic lateral sclerosis in mice. *Nature* 2002;417:74–78.
52. Lipsky PE, van der Heijde DM, St Clair EW, et al. Infliximab and methotrexate in the treatment of rheumatoid arthritis. Anti-Tumor Necrosis Factor Trial in Rheumatoid Arthritis with Concomitant Therapy Study Group. *N Engl J Med* 2000;343:1594–1602.
53. Furst DE, Breedveld FC, Burmester GR, et al. Updated consensus statement on tumour necrosis factor blocking agents for the treatment of rheumatoid arthritis (May 2000). *Ann Rheum Dis* 2000;59:1–2.
54. Weinblatt ME, Kremer JM, Bankhurst AD, et al. A trial of etanercept, a recombinant tumor necrosis factor receptor:Fc fusion protein, in patients with rheumatoid arthritis receiving methotrexate. *N Engl J Med* 1999;340:253–259.
55. den Broeder AA, Joosten LA, Saxne T, et al. Long term anti-tumour necrosis factor alpha monotherapy in rheumatoid arthritis: effect on radiological course and prognostic value of markers of cartilage turnover and endothelial activation. *Ann Rheum Dis* 2002;61:311–318.
56. Maini R, St Clair EW, Breedveld F, et al. Infliximab (chimeric anti-tumour necrosis factor alpha monoclonal antibody) versus placebo in rheumatoid arthritis patients receiving concomitant methotrexate: a randomised phase III trial. ATTRACT Study Group. *Lancet* 1999;354:1932–1939.
57. Favalli EG, Sinigaglia L, Varenna M, et al. Drug-induced lupus following treatment with infliximab in rheumatoid arthritis. *Lupus* 2002;11:753–755.
58. Charles PJ, Smeenk RJ, De Jong J, et al. Assessment of antibodies to double-stranded DNA induced in rheumatoid arthritis patients following treatment with infliximab, a monoclonal antibody to tumor necrosis factor alpha: findings in open-label and randomized placebo-controlled trials. *Arthritis Rheum* 2000;43:2383–2390.
59. van Oosten BW, Barkhof F, Truyen L, et al. Increased MRI activity and immune activation in two multiple sclerosis patients treated with the monoclonal anti-tumor necrosis factor antibody cA2. *Neurology* 1996;47:1531–1534.
60. Mohan N, Edwards ET, Cupps TR, et al. Demyelination occurring during anti-tumor necrosis factor alpha therapy for inflammatory arthritides. *Arthritis Rheum* 2001;44:2862–2869.
61. Sicotte NL, Voskuhl RR. Onset of multiple sclerosis associated with anti-TNF therapy. *Neurology* 2001;57:1885–1888.
62. Gardam MA, Keystone EC, Menzies R, et al. Anti-tumour necrosis factor agents and tuberculosis risk: mechanisms of action and clinical management. *Lancet Infect Dis* 2003;3:148–155.
63. Keane J, Gershon S, Wise RP, et al. Tuberculosis associated with infliximab, a tumor necrosis factor alpha-neutralizing agent. *N Engl J Med* 2001;345:1098–1104.
64. Bathon JM, Martin RW, Fleischmann RM, et al. A comparison of etanercept and methotrexate in patients with early rheumatoid arthritis. *N Engl J Med* 2000;343:1586–1593.
65. Cohen S, Hurd E, Cush J, et al. Treatment of rheumatoid arthritis with anakinra, a recombinant human interleukin-1 receptor antagonist, in combination with methotrexate: results of a twenty-four-week, multicenter, randomized, double-blind, placebo-controlled trial. *Arthritis Rheum* 2002;46:614–624.
66. Bresnihan B, Alvaro-Gracia JM, Cobby M, et al. Treatment of rheumatoid arthritis with recombinant human interleukin-1 receptor antagonist. *Arthritis Rheum* 1998;41:2196–2204.
67. Jiang Y, Genant HK, Watt I, et al. A multicenter, double-blind, dose-ranging, randomized, placebo-controlled study of recombinant human interleukin-1 receptor antagonist in patients with rheumatoid arthritis: radiologic progression and correlation of Genant and Larsen scores. *Arthritis Rheum* 2000;43:1001–1009.
68. Deal CL, Meenan RF, Goldenberg DL, et al. The clinical features of elderly-onset rheumatoid arthritis. A comparison with younger-onset disease of similar duration. *Arthritis Rheum* 1985;28:987–994.
69. Milunsky A, Graef JW, Gaynor MF Jr. Methotrexate-induced congenital malformations. *J Pediatr* 1968;72:790–795.
70. Buckley LM, Bullaboy CA, Leichtman L, et al. Multiple congenital anomalies associated with weekly low-dose methotrexate treatment of the mother. *Arthritis Rheum* 1997;40:971–973.
71. Donnenfeld AE, Pastuszak A, Noah JS, et al. Methotrexate exposure prior to and during pregnancy. *Teratology* 1994;49:79–81.
72. Sutton C, McIvor RS, Vagt M, et al. Methotrexate-resistant form of dihydrofolate reductase protects transgenic murine embryos from teratogenic effects of methotrexate. *Pediatr Dev Pathol* 1998;1:503–512.
73. Brent RL. Teratogen update: reproductive risks of leflunomide (Arava); a pyrimidine synthesis inhibitor: counseling women taking leflunomide before or during pregnancy and men taking leflunomide who are contemplating fathering a child. *Teratology* 2001;63:106–112.
74. DeWitte DB, Buick MK, Cyran SE, et al. Neonatal pancytopenia and severe combined immunodeficiency associated with antenatal administration of azathioprine and prednisone. *J Pediatr* 1984;105:625–628.
75. Cote CJ, Meuwissen HJ, Pickering RJ. Effects on the neonate of prednisone and azathioprine administered to the mother during pregnancy. *J Pediatr* 1974;85:324–328.
76. Janssen NM, Genta MS. The effects of immunosuppressive and anti-inflammatory medications on fertility, pregnancy, and lactation. *Arch Intern Med* 2000;160:610–619.
77. American Academy of Pediatrics Committee on Drugs. The transfer of drugs and other chemicals into human milk. *Pediatrics* 1994;93:137–150.
78. O'Morain C, Smethurst P, Dore CJ, et al. Reversible male infertility due to sulphasalazine: studies in man and rat. *Gut* 1984;25:1078–1084.
79. Sussman A, Leonard JM. Psoriasis, methotrexate, and oligospermia. *Arch Dermatol* 1980;116:215–217.
80. Watson AR, Rance CP, Bain J. Long term effects of cyclophosphamide on testicular function. *BMJ* 1985;291:1457–1460.
81. Russell JA, Powles RL, Oliver RT. Conception and congenital abnormalities after chemotherapy of acute myelogenous leukaemia in two men. *BMJ* 1976;1:1508.
82. Mok MY, Ng WL, Yuen MF, et al. Safety of disease modifying anti-rheumatic agents in rheumatoid arthritis patients with chronic viral hepatitis. *Clin Exp Rheumatol* 2000;18:363–368.
83. Sansonno D, De Re V, Lauletta G, et al. Monoclonal antibody treatment of mixed cryoglobulinemia resistant to interferon alpha with an anti-CD20. *Blood* 2003;101:3818–3826.
84. Arzoo K, Sadeghi S, Liebman HA. Treatment of refractory antibody mediated autoimmune disorders with an anti-CD20 monoclonal antibody (rituximab). *Ann Rheum Dis* 2002;61:922–924.
85. Ahrens N, Kingreen D, Seltsam A, et al. Treatment of refractory autoimmune haemolytic anaemia with anti-CD20 (rituximab). *Br J Haematol* 2001;114:244–245.
86. Brown SL, Greene MH, Gershon SK, et al. Tumor necrosis factor antagonist therapy and lymphoma development: twenty-six cases reported to the Food and Drug Administration. *Arthritis Rheum* 2002;46:3151–3158.

SECTION VI

Other Inflammatory Arthritis Syndromes

CHAPTER 60

Seronegative Polyarthritis Including Adult Still's Disease

Jan Tore Gran and Gunnar Husby

The term *seronegative polyarthritis* encompasses a spectrum of inflammatory joint disorders characterized by persistent absence of serum rheumatoid factors (RFs) and arthritis of more than five joints. Because the absence of RF is a distinct diagnostic requisite for seronegative arthritis, the phenomenon of RF is addressed in some detail in this chapter (see also Chapter 58).

RHEUMATOID FACTORS

Immunology

RFs are antibodies with specificity directed against antigenic determinants in the Fc region of immunoglobulin G (IgG) (1). The antibodies have traditionally been detected by agglutination techniques using sheep red blood cells or latex particles to which human IgG is attached (1). The results of the tests are expressed in antibody titers that relate to the reciprocal of dilution required to eliminate reactivity. To improve sensitivity and specificity of the tests, newer techniques such as radioimmunoassays, enzyme-linked immunosorbent assays (ELISAs), and nephelometry have been developed (1). After the introduction of such techniques, it became clear that RF may be found among the IgM, IgG, IgA, and IgE classes of immunoglobulin (2).

Rheumatoid Factor in Healthy Persons

Since the discovery of RF by Waaler (3) and Rose and co-workers (4), published in 1940 and 1948, respectively, it has become apparent that these antibodies occur not only in rheumatoid arthritis (RA) but also in a variety of disorders of immunologic, infectious, and neoplastic origin (5). Population surveys and studies of blood donors have also disclosed the presence of RF among persons without detectable disease (5).

Using conventional agglutination techniques, serum RF may be found in 1% to 5% of healthy persons (5), and is usually of the IgM type (6), partially because this technique has preference for IgM antibodies. With the advent of ELISA, however, it became evident that RF can be detected and quantified in most persons (6). Thus, when employing ELISA for RF detection, it appears more appropriate to speak of "increased levels" rather than "false-positive results" in the general population (6).

The prevalence of IgM-RF among healthy persons increases with age, whereas a similar increase is not found for the IgA and IgG isotypes of RF (6). The IgM antibodies that occur in healthy subjects are further characterized by relatively low affinity for their specific IgG antigen and low titer (1). In RA, RF may be of IgM, IgG, and IgA classes and often display high affinity for IgG (7). Moreover, occurrence of serum RF in healthy subjects does not seem to be associated with the human leukocyte antigen human leukocyte antigen (HLA)-DR4 (8), which is found in increased frequency among patients with RA (9). Thus, the precise understanding of naturally occurring RFs requires further biochemical and immunologic study.

Population surveys have shown that only a small proportion of persons with RF actually suffer from RA (5). Jonsson and co-workers (2) collected blood samples from 13,858 randomly selected subjects and found that RA was present in only 19% of those with positive test results for serum RF. In a similar population-based survey (5), 11% of seropositive persons satisfied the diagnostic criteria for rheumatoid disease. Thus, in randomly selected persons, the presence of serum RF is not a good predictor of RA. This is further demonstrated by the study of Shmerling and Delbanco (10) in a teaching hospital. Analysis of 563 requests for RF revealed a positive predictive value of only 24% to 34%. Accordingly, the diagnostic value of RF tests appears largely dependent on the pretest likelihood of RA. However, Goodman and co-workers (11) suggested that if both the sheep cell agglutination test and RA latex agglutination test results are positive, there is a threefold increase in the relative risk for a patient to meet the American Rheumatism Association (ARA), now designated the American College of Rheumatology (ACR), criteria for RA (12), as compared with subjects who have only one positive test result.

There are also conflicting opinions as to whether the presence of RF in healthy persons increases the risk for developing RA at a later stage (13–19). One study found that 80% of RF-positive individuals became negative in the course of 3 years, and remained free of RA (15). Other studies have found that persistent positive test results for RF are strongly associated with the development of rheumatoid disease (14,19). It is unclear if such findings indicate a pathogenetic role of RF in RA or signify a difference between transient and persistent RF. Again, there is reason to believe that important qualitative differences between RF in healthy persons and in patients with RA exist and that the precise nature of RF occurring in healthy persons remains obscure.

RF-Positive and RF-Negative Rheumatoid Arthritis

In RA, RF has been associated with a more severe disease course and more frequent extraarticular manifestations (20–26). However, several reports have indicated a similar disease course in RA patients with and without RF (9,27–30). Thus, the pathogenic and prognostic significance of RF in RA remains an enigma. Determining the significance of RF in RA is further complicated by the fact that some patients develop RA without the presence of such antibodies. It is usually estimated that about 12% to 25% of the RA population persistently lack detectable serum RF (31). Such patients are designated seronegative RA; they are addressed in detail in this chapter.

SERONEGATIVE RHEUMATOID ARTHRITIS

General Considerations

Prevalence

The frequency of seronegative RA in the general population has not been estimated by means of longitudinal surveys of the total population at risk, and therefore remains speculative (32). If 25% of all RA patients are considered RF negative, and 1% of the total population is estimated to have RA, then the population prevalence of seronegative RA would be 0.25% (32). On the other hand, if erosions are regarded as mandatory for the diagnosis of RA, perhaps not more than 0.3% of the population suffer from RA (32). A minimum estimate of the occurrence of seronegativity of 10% (33) would yield a prevalence of seronegative erosive RA of approximately 0.03%. Thus, the population frequency of seronegative RA probably ranges from 0.03% to 0.25%, depending on the diagnostic criteria used, but it by no means represents a common rheumatic disorder. For example, in a recent community-based series of patients with RA in Finland (34), seronegative nonerosive RA was rarely detected.

Diagnostic Criteria

As the term implies, seronegative RA denotes a disease that is clinically characterized as RA but lacks detectable serum RF. Accordingly, the diagnosis of seronegative RA should be based on the 1987 ACR criteria for RA (35). For a diagnosis of RA, these criteria require the presence of at least four of seven criteria. Both in the old 1958 ARA criteria (12) and the new 1987 ACR criteria for RA (35), erosions are not requisite. Thus, any patient with symmetric polyarthritis, including the small joints of the upper extremity, associated with morning stiffness may be designated RA.

Using the ACR criteria for defining seronegative RA, however, is associated with certain problems. First, patients meeting such criteria may suffer from a variety of disorders other than RA (7). Second, the presence or absence of RF may vary in time, and seroconversion is not an infrequent phenomenon in RA (36,37). In the early stages of RA, seroconversion from positivity to negativity may occur in as many as half of the patients with clinically diagnosed RA (37), and may also occur by virtue of treatment with slow-acting antirheumatic drugs (38). Thus, at least for scientific purpose, stricter criteria for seronegative RA appear necessary.

In 1987, we suggested diagnostic criteria for seronegative RA to be used in scientific studies (9) (Table 60.1). These criteria were not meant to replace other criteria for RA but rather to be used in addition to the ACR criteria (35). According to these criteria, only patients with radiolographic joint erosions should be included; these criteria therefore appear suitable for comparing disease severity in seropositive and seronegative RA. However, if the incidence of erosive disease in RA is to be determined, such criteria are useless. The criteria also require a disease duration of at least 3 years during which time the patients have been followed closely. Such a requirement is meant to ensure clinical observations that may facilitate the recognition of other seronegative arthropathies that consequently will be excluded. During the observation period of 3 years, at least three tests for RF should be performed; persistent negative results are indicative of seronegative RA. The main purpose of the criteria for seronegative RA is to ensure reliability in studies comparing relevant clinical and laboratory manifestations in seronegative and seropositive RA. These criteria (9) have been used in subsequent studies (39,40).

The question remains whether seronegative RA represents a discrete disease entity or is a variant of rheumatoid disease. In this context, the advent of HLA typing provided a useful investigative tool for studying the relationship between seronegative and seropositive RA. Unfortunately, the studies of HLA-DR antigens in RA have yielded conflicting results (9). Some studies have found that the increased frequency of HLA-DR4 is restricted to seropositive RA (9), whereas other surveys have observed similar prevalences of DR4 in seropositive and seronegative RA (9).

An association between DR4 and seropositive RA exclusively would be consistent with a different etiopathogenesis in seronegative and seropositive RA. In this context, studies comparing the histologic appearance of synovitis in seropositive and seronegative RA found similar pathologic findings in both disease variants (41), suggesting similar pathomechanisms. An alternative explanation for the appearance of the two RA variants is that HLA-DR4 represents a prognostic factor and is associated with the spontaneous production of RF. However, no clear association between severe prognosis and DR4 has been established, even in those studies indicating an exclusive association between DR4 and seropositive RA (42). Moreover, a direct association between RF and DR4 is likewise questionable (9).

Other studies have observed a similar prevalence of DR4 in seropositive and seronegative RA (9). According to these studies, seropositive and seronegative RA are variants of the same disease, and factors other than HLAs may regulate the production of RF. In our opinion, the lack of appropriate diagnostic criteria for seronegative RA has been a major contributor to the conflicting results (9).

TABLE 60.1. *Suggested diagnostic criteria for seronegative rheumatoid arthritis (RA) (9)*

Inclusion criteria
American College of Rheumatology criteria for RA (35)
Radiographic bony erosions
Disease duration of more than 3 years
At least three negative tests for serum rheumatoid factor
Exclusion criteria
Radiographic sacroiliitis or spondylitis
Psoriasis
Symptomatic inflammatory bowel disease
Any other rheumatic disease
First-degree relatives with psoriasis, ankylosing spondylitis, reactive arthritis, or inflammatory bowel disease

Possible Explanations for the Absence of Rheumatoid Factor in Rheumatoid Arthritis

It has been suggested that some patients with seronegative RA are, in fact, seropositive, but their RF is complexed to circulating IgG and appears "hidden" (42). A given serum may thus contain RF even though it is not detectable by conventional laboratory techniques. However, other studies have failed to demonstrate hidden complement fixing IgM RF in the sera of seronegative RA (43).

Another possibility is that the patient's serum contains IgG RF without the simultaneous presence of IgM RF (40). Because IgG RF reacts poorly in conventional agglutination tests, such cases would be perceived as RF negative (40). Newer techniques have also revealed the presence of RF of an IgA or IgE isotype in some patients classified as seronegative RA (44–46). More investigations are warranted to study these possibilities further.

Other studies have indicated that seronegative RA patients may have a deficient number of B cells committed to RF synthesis, an intact regulatory network preventing the production of RF, or an active production of antiidiotypic antibodies that suppress RF production (31). Yet another explanation is that the prevalence of seronegativity in RA is far less frequent than previously anticipated (34). When seronegative RA patients are followed closely, it becomes evident that a significant number express symptoms and findings of other inflammatory rheumatic diseases (5,7,47). Polyarticular RA-like psoriatic arthritis may pose diagnostic problems (47). The skin disease may develop several years after the onset of joint disease. One of the author's patients, for many years classified as seronegative RA, developed psoriasis 42 years after the onset of arthritis. If nonerosive polyarthritis is accepted as seronegative RA, diagnosis may become even more difficult because several nonrheumatoid diseases may exhibit such findings.

A particular problem regarding RF status and drug therapy is that, as previously stated, seroconversion from seropositivity to seronegativity may occur by virtue of treatment with slow-acting antirheumatic drugs. For example, chrysotherapy has been shown to cause a significant decrease in titer of IgG RF, IgA RF (48), and IgM RF (49). If reduction or elimination of serum RF is a consequence of response to therapy, determination of seronegativity during later stages of the disease may give the false impression of less severe RA. Patients who are seronegative may be so because of response to therapy. The inclusion of such cases in various patient materials may bias the results toward an impression of favorable prognosis in seronegative RA. Conversely, the persistence of serum RF may indicate unresponsiveness to therapy and the RF regarded as pathogenetically significant. Seroconversion from positivity to negativity for RF and vice versa does not, however, seem to influence the final outcome of RA (37,50,51), but the possible impact of administration of remittive agents has not been excluded in most studies.

Clinical Manifestations of Seronegative Rheumatoid Arthritis

Demography

Age at onset and sex ratio appear similar in seropositive and seronegative RA (8). Familial aggregation of RA appears in most, but not all, studies to occur in seropositive disease but not in its seronegative counterpart (52–55).

Joint Distribution

Seropositive RA patients are often thought to have more severe involvement of the hands and feet in contrast to more frequent involvement of large lower and upper extremity joints in seronegative RA (31). However, in seronegative patients with prominent involvement of large- and medium-sized peripheral joints, it is of great importance to rule out the presence of other seronegative diseases, in particular the B27-associated diseases and psoriatic arthritis (56). A Norwegian study (8) failed to disclose significant differences between seropositive and seronegative RA with respect to joint distribution. These findings were supported by a recent British study (57) involving a cohort of 537 patients with inflammatory polyarthritis (IP) registered in The Norfolk Arthritis Register, United Kingdom, who had radiographs of hands and feet performed 5 years after the date of inclusion. A total of 212 patients (39%) had erosive disease and, overall, IP was found to be symmetric. Despite more erosions in the RF-positive group, the degree of symmetry did not differ in the RF-positive compared to the RF-negative patients with IP.

Erosions

If patients with recent onset of symmetric polyarthritis are followed prospectively during the course of several years, patients who are seropositive appear to have a significantly greater chance of developing radiographic joint erosions (57,58). According to Kaarela and co-workers (47), 99% of patients with seropositive RA ultimately will develop erosive disease. Furthermore, the incidence of spontaneous clinical remissions are much greater in the RF-negative group (59). Wolfe and co-workers (60) reported that complete resolution of manifestations occurs in more than 50% of patients with undifferentiated polyarthritis, and that latex positivity (RF) was the strongest predictor of failure to resolve subsequently. Thus, in patients with recent-onset symmetric polyarthritis, the development of erosions (58), poor functional outcome, and low incidence of clinical remission correlate significantly with the presence of detectable serum RF.

However, several surveys have not demonstrated significant differences between seropositive and seronegative RA with regard to disease severity in patients with radiographic joint erosions (9). Møttønen (61) found that the rate of development of new erosions was the same in seronegative and seropositive disease. Also, some investigators have found that the level of RF in seropositive RA patients does not influence the degree of radiographic destruction (57). The interpretation of studies comparing incidence and degree of erosions in seropositive and seronegative RA, however, is hampered by use of different criteria among different investigators (9). Indeed, the rate and degree of destruction may be similar in erosive seropositive and seronegative disease; however, when radiographic erosions are not included as an obligatory criterion for RA, the presence of RF is a good predictor of such manifestations.

Extraarticular Manifestations

Necrotizing vasculitis occurs more frequently among patients with seropositive disease (1). In addition, the concentration of RF seems to correlate with the incidence of vasculitis (23,24,26), and patients with IgG RF and IgA RF appear particularly susceptible to such extraarticular manifestations (2,62). Necrotizing vasculitis, however, has been described in seronegative RA as well (31). In general, the prevalence of vasculitis is lower in studies of patients outside of large referral centers (63).

Subcutaneous nodules are more frequent among patients with seropositive disease (21,63,64). In one study, 85% of the patients with such manifestations had detectable serum RF (65). However, nodules may be observed occasionally in seronegative patients (25). Because subcutaneous nodules are observed infrequently in joint diseases other than RA, contamination with other seronegative rheumatic diseases may bias the calculations of their frequency.

Interestingly, it has been suggested that amyloidosis occurs more frequently among patients without detectable serum RF (66), and it has been associated with the presence of HLA-B27 in patients with RA (67). It should be noted that amyloidosis occurs in diseases other than RA, particularly the HLA-B27-associated diseases, namely ankylosing spondylitis and reactive arthritis (68). Differentiating between seronegative RA and ankylosing spondylitis that exhibits persistent peripheral polyarthritis may be difficult. It is also of interest to note that the development of amyloidosis in RA has been associated with persistent high disease activity and severe disease (69). Because seropositive disease is usually regarded as the more severe variant of RA, amyloidosis would be expected to occur more frequently among patients with serum RF. Thus, the reported association between seronegativity and amyloidosis should be investigated further.

Prognosis

Seronegative RA has usually been regarded as a mild variant of seropositive RA (25,58). The majority of studies comparing seropositive and seronegative RA have claimed a more favorable prognosis for the latter (22). However, the impression of improved functional outcome in seronegative RA compared with seropositive RA, might be due to inclusion of patients without erosive disease. If erosive disease is analyzed, it has been argued that the two variants display similar prognostic outcomes (9).

Treatment

In patients with recent-onset symmetric polyarthritis, it is usually recommended that treatment should be started as soon as possible. This is particularly the case if radiographic erosions have already appeared. Most often, however, erosions develop after several months of disease. In patients with recent-onset seronegative, nonerosive disease, the rate of spontaneous remission is, as mentioned, not negligible (60). Thus, the clinician is confronted with the decision to start treatment in a patient who may, regardless of drug administration, remit spontaneously, or, alternatively, to delay the start of therapy in a patient prone to develop radiographic destruction. Owing to the lack of reliable prognostic indicators in seronegative RA, it is perhaps advisable to observe the patient for a period of 3 months before starting administration of remittive agents. If symmetric polyarthritis is still present and signs and symptoms of other disorders have not appeared, standard regimens used for seropositive RA should be initiated.

Conclusions

Patients with seronegative RA should be carefully followed to rule out other seronegative rheumatic diseases. When a definite diagnosis is established after a minimum of 3 months of observation, the patients should be treated as if suffering from seropositive RA. When radiographic erosions develop, the functional outcome is similar to its seropositive counterpart. However, subcutaneous nodules and vasculitis occur less frequently in seronegative RA.

SERONEGATIVE POLYARTHRITIS WITH PITTING EDEMA

Diagnostic accuracy in the group of patients with seronegative polyarthritis has been enhanced by the description of a subset of elderly patients suffering from arthritis and edema with favorable prognosis.

Kinsella (70) and Porsmann (71) both reported a distinct subgroup of elderly patients who had a very acute onset of disease, further characterized by rapid fluctuations, but with complete remission within a year. The disease occurred predominantly in men and often involved the large joints. Owing to favorable prognosis, the disease was termed benign RA of the elderly. Interestingly, an abrupt onset of arthritis had previously been associated with a better overall outcome (72–76).

In 1985, McCarty and co-workers (77) described eight elderly men and two women with similar disease expression. The patients presented with symmetric acute polyarthritis and flexor digitorum tenosynovitis associated with pitting edema of the dorsum of both hands and both feet. No patient had detectable serum RF, and radiographic examinations revealed no erosions. All patients went into complete and presumably permanent remission. HLA typing demonstrated HLA-B7 in six of eight tested patients. The patient material was extended to 13 patients 5 years later (78). Follow-up disclosed complete remission in all patients without relapses. A constant feature during remission was asymptomatic flexor contractures of the fingers and wrists. The relative risk for contracting such a disease if possessing HLA-B7 was 4.4. The syndrome is termed remitting seronegative, symmetric synovitis with pitting edema (RS3PE) (78).

Four additional patients were reported by Chaouat and Le Parc (79). These researchers also observed a benign disease course, because all cases remitted during a 9- to 18-month period. In a retrospective multicenter study of 27 patients (18 men and 9 women) with RS3PE (80), the mean age of the patients was 71.7 years (range 58–92 years), and the joints most frequently affected were the metacarpophalangeals, proximal interphalangeals, wrists, and shoulders. Erosions were present in only one patient.

Although the prognosis of this syndrome generally appears excellent, peripheral synovitis and pitting edema have been reported as the first manifestations of underlying malignant disease (81). Roldan and co-workers described a 63-year-old woman who presented with seronegative symmetric synovitis and pitting edema in whom non-Hodgkin's lymphoma manifested (82). Similarly, we have recently seen a 70-year-old man with explosive onset of seronegative polyarthritis and pitting edema of the hands, who concomitantly developed myelomatosis. During recent years, RS3PE has been associated with T-cell lymphoma and myelodysplastic syndrome (80), gastric carcinoma (83), and endometrial adenocarcinoma (84).

In more recent articles by Paira et al. (85), 4 of 12 patients with RS3PE had associated malignancies (two solid cancers and two hematologic). In one case, RS3PE preceded onset of the neoplastic disorder. The investigators noted that the idiopathic RS3PE cases all responded to low-dose steroids, whereas the paraneoplastic ones were resistant to such treatment.

Whether or not the syndrome represents a variant of RA among elderly patients or is a distinct disease entity is at present unknown. Awareness of this disease variant is important, however, because administration of disease-remitting agents appears unnecessary. The presence of concomitant malignant disease among elderly patients should be evaluated.

SERONEGATIVE POLYARTHRITIS IN THE ELDERLY

Much attention has been focused on seronegative polyarthritis occurring among elderly patients. Deal and co-workers (86) noted that abrupt onset of symptoms occurred somewhat more frequently among patients with elderly onset RA as compared with cases beginning prior to age 60. Elderly patients had subcutaneous nodules less frequently and, of particular interest, 52% of the patients lacked detectable serum RF. The initial clinical presentation resembled that of polymyalgia rheumatica.

The similarity between polymyalgia rheumatica and seronegative RA in elderly patients has been reported by Healey (87,88). Other investigators have also observed a frequent occurrence of peripheral arthritis in polymyalgia rheumatica (89). Thus, the possibility exists that some older patients classified as seronegative RA in fact suffered from polymyalgia rheumatica. However, the incidence of radiographic joint erosions in such patients should be studied before any firm conclusions are drawn. Polymyalgia rheumatica is infrequently associated with destructive arthritis (90), so the absence of erosions may, to some extent, favor polymyalgia rheumatica rather than seronegative RA. Among 287 patients with polymyalgia rheumatica and temporal arteritis followed prospectively in our clinic, 25% have developed peripheral arthritis, but less than 20% of these have developed polyarticular joint disease (91).

Alternatively, seronegative RA with onset at old age may represent a subgroup of RA exhibiting characteristic features such as more benign disease evolution, more abrupt onset, and less frequent extraarticular features. The study of Inoue and co-workers (92) is of interest in this respect. They noted that there was an equal sex ratio, less frequent seropositivity, and a tendency toward more involvement of larger joints among patients with older age at onset of RA. The lower prevalence of RF and the frequent large joint involvement were rather characteristic of a subset of patients who exhibited osteoarthritis before the onset of RA. Thus, acute polysynovitis, possibly related to preceding polyarticular osteoarthritis, could be an alternative differential diagnosis in seronegative RA with older age at onset.

Consequently, the presentation of seronegative polyarthritis in elderly patients should be subjected to careful clinical, laboratory, and radiographic evaluation before reaching a final diagnosis and initiating therapy. However, awareness of diseases other than RA in such patients is by no means limited to the elderly.

ADULT-ONSET STILL'S DISEASE

Definition, History, Etiopathogenesis, and Pathology

Adult-onset Still's disease (AOSD) is a clinical disease entity characterized by quotidian fever, evanescent rash, arthralgia or arthritis, leukocytosis, liver involvement, polyserositis, and an almost uniform absence of detectable serum autoantibodies. The term *AOSD* was coined by Bywaters in 1971 (93), but as pointed out by Larsson (94), an adult patient with signs and symptoms of what later became known as Still disease was reported in 1895 by Bannatyne and Wohlman (95), 1 year before the classic monograph of George Still (96).

Although subjected to numerous investigations during the past two decades, the etiopathogenesis of AOSD remains an enigma. Because the clinical picture strikingly resembles that of an infectious disorder, the majority of studies regarding etiology have focused on putative microbiologic candidates. But so far, no one has succeeded in isolating an infective agent directly from a patient's specimen, except for one case (97). However, separate case reports have associated AOSD with acquired toxoplasmosis (98), parvovirus B19 (99), Epstein-Barr virus (100), *Mycoplasma pneumoniae* (101), and *Chlamydia pneumoniae* (102), suggesting that different bacterial and viral infections may trigger or contribute to the development of AOSD (103).

At present, no single genetic factor conferring risk for contracting AOSD has been identified, and familial occurrence has not been reported (97). The finding of AOSD in only one of identical twins may also point to environmental factors rather than genetic susceptibility (104). The possible influence of hormonal factors has also been studied. Katz et al. reported a woman who had recurrent episodes of AOSD after two successive pregnancies and suggested that AOSD may be influenced by gestational status (105). Furthermore, de Miguel et al. (106) described the occurrence of AOSD during the first pregnancy in two women; in one of them, a second pregnancy was not associated with a flare-up. Two patients developed AOSD shortly after pregnancy. However, some researchers have concluded that pregnancy seems to have no effect on AOSD and, conversely, that AOSD has no influence on pregnancy, fetal growth, or infant death (107). Clearly, further studies are required before firm conclusions can be drawn. In addition, other potential risk factors in AOSD, including stress, should be subjected to further investigations (108).

No pathognomic tissue lesion has been described in AOSD, and histologic examinations of biopsy specimens from serous membranes, skin, and joints have revealed nonspecific inflammation only. However, lymph node biopsies exhibiting intense, somewhat atypical, paracortical immunoblastic hyperplasia, simulating lymphoma, may be of diagnostic value (109,110). The nodal histology differs from that of RA in which follicular B-cell reactions generally predominate (111). Although such lesions offer no explanation concerning the etiopathogenesis of AOSD, they may be useful in the diagnostic evaluation of patients with seronegative polyarthritis.

Clinical Features

The cardinal clinical features of AOSD are fever, rash, and arthritis, the most common presenting manifestation being a hectic fever of up to 40°C or more (112–114). The fever occurs especially in the evening and may be preceded by chills. In most studies (113–115), the overwhelming majority (>90%) of patients had significant fever, lasting from 8 weeks to 8 months, most often exhibiting a single daily spike (113). The fever most frequently exhibits a quotidian or, less commonly, double-quotidian spiking pattern (97).

An evanescent salmon colored or pink rash may occur in up to 97% of cases (115). It is located most often proximally on the limbs and on the trunk and may disappear spontaneously. Some researchers have noted that the rash may be induced by thermal or mechanical stimulation of the skin (97). The individual lesions consist of small pink morbilliform macules with a clear center but may also assume an urticarial or pruritic appearance. The rash may appear only during temperature spikes (113). In addition to the typical rash, persistent plaques on the face, neck, and upper and lower back may develop (116), and sometimes linear pigmentation (117) or thrombocytopenic purpura is present (118,119).

Although not always present initially (112), joint involvement may manifest as either arthralgia or arthritis and appears in approximately 90% of cases during the disease course (97,114–116). Most patients have polyarthritis, usually accompanied by several hours of morning stiffness. The inflammatory joint disease affects both small and large joints in a symmetric and nonmigratory pattern, but, unlike RA, often sparing fingers and toes (97,114–116). However, the wrist is frequently involved. The predilection for the carpometacarpal and tarsometatarsal joints is noteworthy (120,121). The disease may exhibit a characteristic evolution as carpometacarpal and intercarpal joint spaces become selectively narrowed without erosions before bony ankylosis eventually occurs. Finally, myalgias frequently accompany joint pain (113), but inflammatory myositis is rare (122).

A typical clinical feature of AOSD is pharyngitis manifesting as sore throat, which appears in approximately 48% to 92% of the patients (113,123,124). Except for slight redness, no particular clinical findings are observed.

Lymphadenopathy is seen in 44% of the patients, most commonly involving the cervical and submandibular chains, occasionally affecting the deep lymph nodes as well (113). Splenomegaly may be detected in up to 40% of cases (113) and abdominal pain in less than 10%. A few cases of serous peritonitis have also been observed (124). Involvement of the liver is frequently noted. The majority of patients most often exhibit moderate hepatomegaly and abnormal transaminase levels (113). Liver failure has been reported in several cases (97,125–127), occasionally being fatal (128).

Involvement of lungs and heart may also be observed. Pleuritis, bilateral pulmonary infiltrates, and interstitial lung disease may occur (113). Although pleural effusions and transient pulmonary infiltrates are most frequently encountered, lung involvement may become life-threatening if progressing to adult respiratory distress syndrome (129, 130). About a quarter of cases with AOSD have cardiac involvement, most often presenting as pericarditis (113). Cardiac involvement is often seen early in the course of the disease and may lead to life-threatening complications such as pericardial tamponade or constriction (114,131,132). Myocarditis (133,134) and endocarditis have also been reported (135).

Although occurring in less than 10% of patients (113), central nervous system manifestations have been reported in several cases. These include psychoorganic syndrome with complete disorientation and stupor, sensory and motor aphasia (136), brainstem hemorrhage (97,137,138), meningoencephalopathy (97,139), aseptic meningitis (140), status epilepticus and pyramidal syndrome (97), sensorineural hearing loss (141), sensorimotor peripheral neuropathy (139), cerebral hemorrhage (142), and variants of Guillain-Barré (142) syndrome.

Renal involvement most often manifests as proteinuria during febrile episodes (113). Interstitial nephritis, subacute glomerulonephritis, IgA nephropathy (97), renal amyloidosis (143–146), mesangial glomerulonephritis (147), and nephrotic syndrome (148) have been reported.

Ophthalmologic manifestations rarely occur (113), but uveitis has been reported (139).

Although AOSD cannot at present be classified as a paraneoplastic disorder, clinicians should be aware of the occurrence of AOSD as an apparent manifestation of malignant disease (149) and the development of lymphoma during the disease course (150).

Laboratory Manifestations

In AOSD, there is an inflammatory reaction with an erythrocyte sedimentation rate (ESR) often exceeding 100 mm/h and increased levels of fibrinogen, gammaglobulins, C reactive protein, and ferritin. The most striking laboratory feature is leukocytosis in the range of 1,500 to 62,000 per mm^3 with predominant polymorphonuclear leukocytosis (113). Thrombocytopenia is rare, whereas anemia is common (113).

Of diagnostic value is the occurrence of hyperferritinemia, which may be helpful in monitoring disease activity (151,152). In one study, 7 of 9 patients had serum ferritin levels of more than 4,000 ng/mL (normal 80–200) (152). In the study of Yamaguchi et al. (133), 20 of 30 patients had hyperferritinemia four times as high as normal limits. Ferritin is a multisubunit protein, abundant in the liver and heart, but also present in most other tissues. In plasma, ferritin is glycosylated (GF) and in one study (153), the combination of a GF level of less than or equal to 20% of total ferritin with ferritin above the upper limit of normal yielded a sensitivity of 70.5% and specificity of 83.2% for the diagnosis of AOSD. The combination of a GF level of less than or equal to 20% with ferritin five times normal produced a sensitivity of 43.2% and a specificity of 92.9%. This latter combination allowed an AOSD diagnosis to be ruled out in 6 of 8 control patients who met Yamaguchi's positive criteria (154).

The reason for the high ferritin levels observed in AOSD remains somewhat unclear, but as mentioned, elevated levels suggest a diagnosis of AOSD, providing other causes of acute inflammation are carefully excluded. Iron status in patients with acute-phase reactions should be evaluated by measuring concentrations of soluble transferrin receptor in serum (155).

Diagnostic Criteria

The diagnosis of AOSD remains problematic because it is based on clinical findings alone (97). In a clinical context, sustained fever, evanescent rash, and arthritis together with the exclusion of other rheumatic and infectious disorders often enable the clinician to establish a diagnosis of AOSD. For use in research and epidemiologic surveys, the criteria suggested by Yamaguchi (Table 60.2) are recommended (133). These criteria appear to exhibit the highest sensitivity (93.5%), compared with criteria suggested by others (156).

TABLE 60.2. *Yamaguchi criteria for adult-onset Still's disease (133)*

Major criteria
1. Fever of 39°C or greater for at least 1 week
2. Arthritis or arthralgia for at least 2 weeks
3. Macular or maculopapular, nonpruritic, pink rash
4. Leucocytosis of at least 10,000/mm^3 (at least 80% neutrophils)

Minor criteria
1. Pharyngitis (sore throat)
2. Lymphadenopathy and/or splenomegaly
3. Abnormalities of liver function tests
4. Tests for rheumatoid factors and antinuclear antibodies negative

Exclusions: infection, malignant disease, inflammatory rheumatic disease. Five or more criteria required, including two or more major criteria (133).

Epidemiology and Demography

AOSD is a rare disease, and no epidemiologic survey has been performed to determine its true occurrence. A retrospective study revealed a yearly incidence of 0.16 per 100,000 population (157), whereas another study found an annual incidence of 0.22 to 0.34 per 100,000 population and a prevalence of 0.73 to 1.47 per 100,000 in a population 16 years of age or older (158). Most likely, these figures represent minimum values only.

The age at onset is often between 15 and 61 years, with a median of 21 years, and more than 80% of cases begin before the age of 32 (159). Nonetheless, patients with age at onset of 72 and 75 years have been reported (160,161). Although AOSD defines a disease entity beginning in adulthood, clinicians must be aware that the condition may represent a recurrence of juvenile Still's disease in adulthood after a variable disease-free interval. The female to male ratio is about 2 to 1 (94).

Therapy

Although regularly recommended as the drug of choice, aspirin may be ineffective in as many as 88% of cases (113,159,162). If effective, rather high doses (4–6 g/d) are often required (113). On the other hand, nonsteroidal anti-inflammatory drugs should be administered early, because a significant number of patients respond favorably to these agents (163).

In the majority of cases, however, oral corticosteroids are necessary to adequately suppress disease activity, and in the vast majority of cases, 0.5 to 1.0 mg/kg/day of prednisolone will offer rapid control of acute disease manifestations (110). Relapses, which frequently occur, should be managed by intravenous methylprednisolone pulses (164).

In patients not responding to corticosteroids or developing unacceptable corticosteroid-associated side effects, methotrexate (MTX) appears to be the drug of choice (165,166). Remission is often achieved within 3 to 16 weeks after starting therapy (167), facilitating significant reduction of corticosteroid doses (168).

Patients not responding to corticosteroids and MTX represent a serious problem. In such cases, options available include gold sodium thiomalate (169), penicillamine (120), oral cyclophosphamide (170), cyclosporine A (171, 172), intravenous gammaglobulin (173), and sulphasalazine (174), but the experience with these agents is limited. The latter drug should be used with caution, because a rather high incidence of side effects has been reported in AOSD (174). In patients who do not respond to available therapy, but continue to have sustained and severe disease, autologous stem cell transplantation may be considered (175).

Recently, uncontrolled studies have appeared using tumor necrosis factor alpha inhibitors. In one such study, all six patients responded favorably to infliximab (176) and, in another study of 12 patients, 10 improved on etanercept (177). These biologic agents may replace the role of traditional disease-modifying drugs in AOSD.

Outcome and Disease Course

Predicting outcome and disease course in individual patients with AOSD is difficult. However, different patterns of disease courses may be identified rather early. Two forms of disease evolution may be distinguishable clinically: a self-limited remitting disease with or without recurrent cyclic exacerbations and persistent disease activity continuing for more than 1 year (178). Other workers (160) prefer to classify disease course in AOSD into four different patterns: monocyclic systemic disease, chronic articular polycyclic systemic disease, polycyclic systemic disease, and chronic articular monocyclic systemic disease, the latter being most prevalent. Chronic articular disease may be associated with the worst outcome (160). Polyarthritis at onset and involvement of proximal limb joints may predict chronic articular disease (162).

In one study of 11 female patients followed for 7 to 36 years, 10 had a chronic course characterized by remissions and exacerbations (179). In another study, more than one systemic flare-up was experienced by 58% of the patients (162). Despite causing disability, pain, and, in many, the need for long-term medication, patients with AOSD are resilient. Among 104 patients studied, approximately half of the patients required medication even 10 years after diagnosis (180). The levels of pain and physical disability were low compared to patients with other rheumatic diseases. Moreover, the disease did not interfere with educational attainment, occupational prestige, social functioning and support, time lost from work, or family income in most patients (180).

DIFFERENTIAL DIAGNOSES IN SERONEGATIVE POLYARTHRITIS

Several studies have emphasized the importance of excluding diagnoses other than RA in seronegative polyarthritis (1,7,9) (Table 60.3). Because a single clinical examination provides only a glimpse of the disease, longitudinal observations are usually necessary to enhance diagnostic accuracy.

The seronegative spondyloarthropathy complex (see Chapters 63 and 64) embraces a group of disorders characterized by the presence of HLA-B27 together with varying mucocutaneous, gastrointestinal tract, eye, and joint manifestations. Approximately one fourth of such patients have inflammatory peripheral joint disease, with the predominant pattern being an asymmetric oligoarthritis affecting large and medium-sized extremity joints (181). Polyarthritis is infrequently seen in patients with ankylosing spondylitis (182) (see Chapter 63). Male sex, onset of disease prior to the age of 50, and prominent back stiffness strongly favor a diagnosis of ankylosing spondylitis (182).

TABLE 60.3. *Seronegative polyarthritis: diagnoses to be considered*

- Seronegative rheumatoid arthritis
- Seronegative polysynovitis with pitting edema
- Polymyalgia rheumatica
- Seronegative spondyloarthropathies
  - Ankylosing spondylitis
  - Reactive arthritis
    - Psoriatic arthritis
    - Bowel diseases
      - Ulcerative colitis
      - Crohn's disease
      - Whipple's disease
      - Collagenous colitis
      - Celiac disease
- Connective tissue diseases
  - Systemic lupus erythematosus
  - Mixed connective tissue disease
- Crystal arthritis
  - Gout
  - Chondrocalcinosis
- Infection
  - Bacterial arthritis including Lyme disease
  - Fungal arthritis
  - Viral arthritis (especially parvovirus)
- Miscellaneous diseases
  - Hematologic disorders
  - Liver diseases
  - Endocrinopathies
  - Metabolic disorders
  - Sarcoidosis
- Degenerative joint disease
  - Osteoarthritis
  - Erosive osteoarthropathy

Reactive arthritis (see Chapter 64) is often preceded by gastrointestinal tract or urogenital manifestations (183) and is often accompanied by involvement of mucous membranes (184). The asymmetric oligoarthritis most often encountered in reactive arthritis is usually of limited duration (185). However, some patients with reactive arthritis may develop chronic disease (185).

Psoriatic arthritis should always be considered in patients with seronegative polyarthritis. The distribution of joint involvement may be strikingly similar to that seen in seronegative RA (186). Such patients may also develop radiographic erosions that can be very difficult to differentiate from those observed in rheumatoid disease (186). Careful clinical examination of the skin, including the scalp, ear canal, and fingernails and toenails may reveal lesions compatible with a diagnosis of psoriasis. A family history of psoriasis should strengthen the suspicion of psoriatic arthritis (186). Involvement of the distal interphalangeal joints also may indicate psoriatic arthritis (186). However, the clinical and laboratory picture may be identical to that of

RA, and the development of skin lesions may postdate arthritis by decades.

About 10% to 15% of patients with Crohn disease and ulcerative colitis develop arthritis confined to the peripheral joints (187) (see Chapter 66). The arthritis is usually of limited duration and not infrequently fluctuates with the activity of the gastrointestinal disease (187). However, arthritis may antedate intestinal manifestations by years and be of significant severity (187). Celiac disease is usually diagnosed in late life and occasionally is associated with polyarthritis (188). Positive test results for antigliadin and endomysial antibodies strongly suggest gluten-sensitive enteropathy, and an appropriate dietary regimen often significantly improves or abolishes the joint disease (189,190). Although rare, another gastrointestinal disease associated occasionally with arthritis is Whipple disease (191). The demonstration of intestinal lesions and microbiologic diagnosis may be difficult (192), and gastrointestinal symptoms may be delayed for several years (191).

Arthritis induced by virus infections may be accompanied by polyarthritis, but most often the joint disease is of limited duration. One exception is arthritis caused by human parvovirus B19, which occasionally may last for several months (193). The presence of erythema infectiosum and the demonstration of parvovirus-specific serum antibodies may lead to a correct diagnosis of parvovirus arthritis (Chapter 128).

The systemic connective tissue diseases often manifest symptoms and signs involving the peripheral joints. More than 80% of patients with systemic lupus erythematosus (SLE) (see Chapter 70) have joint complaints, although arthralgias and tenosynovitis are more frequent than prominent polyarthritis (194). Erosions are rare in SLE (194), but Jaccoud's arthropathy of both hands and feet may lead to misinterpretation as erosive seronegative RA, unless radiographs are performed (194). Patients with mixed connective tissue disease (see Chapter 69) also frequently develop nonerosive polyarthritis, although of rather limited severity (194). A clinical history of skin manifestations, pleuropericardial involvement, Raynaud phenomenon, photosensitivity, and central nervous system involvement may raise suspicion of a systemic connective tissue disease. Analysis of antinuclear antibodies in serum will most often help to establish a definite diagnosis.

Seronegative polyarthritis may also be the presenting manifestation of an occult malignancy (195–200). Both epithelial (201) and lymphoproliferative neoplastic diseases (202) should be carefully ruled out in patients with seronegative arthritis. If arthritis is accompanied by persisting fever, rash, fatigue, loss of weight, night sweats, gastrointestinal or respiratory symptoms, sparing of the wrists and small finger joints, and lack of response to appropriate therapeutic regimens, the possibility of coexisting cancer should be considered.

Polyarticular septic arthritis is rare, but is nevertheless sometimes overlooked with severe consequences for involved joints. Infection should always be considered in any patient presenting with arthritis of recent onset. Similarly, gout involving multiple joints is not uncommon (203). Sarcoid arthritis most often presents as an acute oligoarthritis accompanied by hilar adenopathy and erythema nodosum, but may occasionally manifest as a chronic polyarthritis (204).

Finally, the initial stages of osteoarthritis may mimic early rheumatoid disease. Erosive osteoarthropathy, exhibiting clinical synovitis and radiographic erosions, may be particularly difficult to differentiate from RA, but careful observations reveal the degenerative nature of the joint disease.

REFERENCES

1. Vaughan JH. Pathogenetic concept and origins of rheumatoid factors in rheumatoid arthritis. *Arthritis Rheum* 1993;36:1–5.
2. Jonsson T, Thorsteinsson J, Kolbeinsson A, et al. Population study of the importance of rheumatoid factor isotypes in adults. *Ann Rheum Dis* 1992;51:863–868.
3. Waaler E. On the common occurrence of a factor in serum activating the specific agglutination of sheep blood corpuscles. *Acta Pathol Microbiol Scand* 1940;17:172–188.
4. Rose HM, Ragan C, Pearce E, et al. Differential agglutination of normal and sensitized sheep erythrocytes of patients with rheumatoid arthritis. *Proc Soc Exp Biol Med* 1948;68:1–6.
5. Gran JT, Husby G, Thorsby E. The prevalence of HLA DR4 and HLA DR3 in healthy persons with rheumatoid factor. *Scand J Rheumatol* 1985;14:79–82.
6. van Schaardenburg D, Lagaay AM, Otten HG, et al. The relation between class-specific serum rheumatoid factors and age in the general population. *Br J Rheumatol* 1993;32:546–549.
7. Kaarela K, Alekberova Z, Lehtinen K, et al. Seronegative rheumatoid arthritis:a clinical study with HLA typing. *J Rheumatol* 1990;17:1125–1129.
8. Gran JT, Husby G, Thorsby E. The association between rheumatoid arthritis and the HLA antigen DR4. *Ann Rheum Dis* 1983;42:292–296.
9. Gran JT, Husby G. Seronegative rheumatoid arthritis and HLA DR4: proposal for criteria. *J Rheumatol* 1987;14:1079–1082.
10. Shmerling RH, Delbanco TL. The rheumatoid factor: an analysis of clinical utility. *Am J Med* 1991;91:528–534.
11. Goodman LA, Pisko EJ, Foster SL, et al. Analysis of combined rheumatoid factor determinations by the rheumatoid arthritis latex and sheep cell agglutination tests and the American Rheumatism Association criteria for rheumatoid arthritis. *J Rheumatol* 1987;14:234–239.
12. Ropes MV, Bennett GA, Cobb S, et al. Diagnostic criteria for rheumatoid arthritis. 1959 revision. *Bull Rheum Dis* 1958;9:175–176.
13. Ball J, Lawrence JS. The relationship of rheumatoid serum factor to rheumatoid arthritis. *Ann Rheum Dis* 1963;22:311–318.
14. Waller M, Toone EC. Normal individuals with positive tests for rheumatoid factor. *Arthritis Rheum* 1968;11:50–55.
15. Gran JT, Johannessen A, Husby G. A study of IgM rheumatoid factors in a middle-aged population of Northern Norway. *Clin Rheumatol* 1984;3:163–168.
16. del Puente A, Knowler WC, Pettitt DJ, et al. The incidence of rheumatoid arthritis is predicted by rheumatoid factor titer in a longitudinal population study. *Arthritis Rheum* 1988;31:1239–1244.
17. Thorsteinsson J, Bjørusson OJ, Kolbeinsson A, et al. A population study of RF in Iceland. *Ann Clin Res* 1975;7:183–193.
18. Cathcart EG, O'Sullivan JB. A longitudinal study of rheumatoid factors in a New England town. *Ann NY Acad Sci* 1969;168:41–51.
19. Aho K, Heliovaara M, Maatela J, et al. Rheumatoid factors antedating clinical rheumatoid arthritis. *J Rheumatol* 1991;18:1282–1284.
20. van Zeben D, Hazes JMW, Zwinderman AH, et al. Clinical significance of rheumatoid factors in early rheumatoid arthritis: results of a follow-up study. *Ann Rheum Dis* 1992;51:1029–1035.

21. Edelman J, Russell AS. A comparison of patients with seropositive and seronegative rheumatoid arthritis. *Rheumatol Int* 1983;3:47–48.
22. van der Heijde MFM, van Riel PLCM, van Rijswijk MH, et al. Influence of prognostic features on the final outcome in rheumatoid arthritis: a review of the literature. *Semin Arthritis Rheum* 1988;17: 284–292.
23. Geirsson AJ, Sturfelt G, Truedsson L. Clinical and serologic features of severe vasculitis in rheumatoid arthritis: prognostic implications. *Ann Rheum Dis* 1987;46:727–733.
24. Gordon DA, Stein JL, Broder I. The extraarticular features of rheumatoid arthritis. *Am J Med* 1973;54:445–452.
25. Cats A, Hazevoet HM. Significance of positive tests for rheumatoid factor in the prognosis of rheumatoid arthritis. *Ann Rheum Dis* 1970; 29:254–260.
26. Momgan ES, Cass RM, Jacox RF, et al. A study of the relation of seronegative and seropositive rheumatoid arthritis to each other and to necrotizing vasculitis. *Am J Med* 1969;47:23–35.
27. Amos RS, Constable TJ, Crockson RA. Rheumatoid arthritis: relation of serum C-reactive protein and erythrocyte sedimentation rates to radiographic changes. *BMJ* 1977;1:195–197.
28. Dawes PT, Fowler PD, Jackson R. Prediction of progressive joint damage in patients with rheumatoid arthritis receiving gold or penicillamine therapy. *Ann Rheum Dis* 1986;45:945–949.
29. Westedt ML, Daha MR, Baldwin WM. Serum immune complexes containing IgA appear to predict erosive arthritis in a longitudinal study in rheumatoid arthritis. *Ann Rheum Dis* 1986;45:809–815.
30. Reilly PA, Elswood J, Calin A. Therapeutic intervention in rheumatoid arthritis: a case-controlled comparison of seronegative and seropositive disease. *Br J Rheumatol* 1988;27:102–105.
31. Alarcón GS. Seronegative polyarthritis. In: *Arthritis and allied condition,* 12th ed. Philadelphia: Lea & Febiger, 1993:1013–1020.
32. Gran JT. The epidemiology of rheumatoid arthritis. *Monogr Allerg Immunol* 1987;21:162–196.
33. Calin A, Elswood J, Klouda PT. Destructive arthritis, rheumatoid factor and HLA DR4. *Arthritis Rheum* 1989;32:1221–1225.
34. Hakala M, Sajanti E, Ikaheimo I, et al. High prevalence of rheumatoid factor in community-based series of patients with rheumatoid arthritis meeting the new (1987) ARA criteria. *Scand J Rheumatol* 1998;27: 368–372.
35. Arnett FC, Edworthy SM, Bloch DA, et al. The American Rheumatism Association 1987 criteria for the classification of rheumatoid arthritis. *Arthritis Rheum* 1988;31:315–324.
36. Jones VE, Puttick AH, Cohen BJ. Rheumatoid arthritis: clinical onset, seropositivity, and a possible cause. *Arthritis Rheum* 1985;28:814–815.
37. Masi AT, Maldonado-Cocco JA, Kaplan SB, et al. Prospective study of the early course of rheumatoid arthritis in young adults: comparison of patients with and without rheumatoid factor positivity at entry and identification of variables correlating with outcome. *Semin Arthritis Rheum* 1976;5:299–326.
38. Empire Rheumatism Council. Gold therapy in rheumatoid arthritis—final report of a multicenter controlled trial. *Ann Rheum Dis* 1961;20: 315–333.
39. Watson Buchanan W, Singal DP. Seronegative rheumatoid arthritis: tell it as it is. *J Rheumatol* 1994;21:391–393.
40. Aho K, Kurki P. Seropositive versus seronegative rheumatoid arthritis—time for a new definition. *J Rheumatol* 1994;21:388–390.
41. Fujinami M, Sato K, Kashiwazaki S, et al. Comparable histological appearance of synovitis in seropositive and seronegative rheumatoid arthritis. *Clin Exp Rheumatol* 1997;15:11–17.
42. Olsen NJ, Callahan LF, Brooks RH, et al. Associations of HLA-DR4 with rheumatoid factor and radiographic severity in rheumatoid arthritis. *Am J Med* 1988;84:257–264.
43. Robbins DL, Moore TL. Lack of hidden complement fixing IgM rheumatoid factor in adult seronegative rheumatoid arthritis. *Ann Rheum Dis* 1980;39:64–67.
44. Gioud-Paquet M, Auvinet M, Raffin T. IgM rheumatoid factor (RF), IgA RF, IgE RF and IgG RF detected by ELISA in rheumatoid arthritis. *Ann Rheum Dis* 1987;46:65–71.
45. Carson DA, Pasquali JL, Tsoukas CD. Physiology and pathology of rheumatoid factors. *Springer Semin Immunopathol* 1981;4:161–179.
46. Bonagura VR, Wedgewood JF, Agostino N. Seronegative rheumatoid arthritis, rheumatoid factor cross reactive idiotype expression, and hidden rheumatoid factors. *Ann Rheum Dis* 1989;48:488–495.
47. Kaarela K, Luukkainen R, Koskimies S. How often is seropositive rheumatoid arthritis an erosive disease? An 17-year follow-up study. *J Rheumatol* 1993;20:1670–1673.
48. Rudge SR, Pound JD, Bossingham DH, et al. Class specific rheumatoid factors in rheumatoid arthritis: response to chrysotherapy and relationship to disease activity. *J Rheumatol* 1985; 12:432–436.
49. Pope RM, Lessard J, Nunnery E. Differential effects of therapeutic regimens on specific classes of rheumatoid factor. *Ann Rheum Dis* 1986;45:183–189.
50. Tuomi T, Aho K, Palosuo T, et al. Significance of rheumatoid factors in an eight-year longitudinal study of arthritis. *Rheumatol Int* 1988;8: 21–26.
51. Cats A, Hazevoet HM. Significance of positive tests for rheumatoid factor in the prognosis of rheumatoid arthritis. *Ann Rheum Dis* 1970; 29:254–260.
52. Bland JH, Brown EW. Seronegative and seropositive rheumatoid arthritis: clinical, radiological and biochemical differences. *Ann Intern Med* 1964;60:88–94.
53. Lawrence JS. Rheumatoid arthritis—nature or nurture? *Ann Rheum Dis* 1970;29:357–379.
54. Wilkinson M, Torrance WM. Clinical background of rheumatoid vascular disease. *Ann Rheum Dis* 1967;26:475–480.
55. Edelman J, Russell AS. A comparison of patients with seropositive and seronegative rheumatoid arthritis. *Rheumatol Int* 1983;3:47–48.
56. Jantti JK, Kaarela K, Lehtinen KES. Seronegative oligoarthritis: a 23-year follow-up study. *Clin Rheumatol* 2002;21:353–356.
57. Bukhari M, Lunt M, Harrison BJ, et al. Erosions in inflammatory polyarthritis are symmetrical regardless of rheumatoid factor status: results from a primary care-based inception cohort of patients. *Rheumatology* 2002;41:246–252.
58. Feigenbaum SL, Masi AT, Kaplan SB. Prognosis in rheumatoid arthritis. *Am J Med* 1979;66:377–384.
59. Ragan C, Farrington E. The clinical features of rheumatoid arthritis. *JAMA* 1962;181:663–667.
60. Wolfe F, Ross K, Hawley DJ, et al. The prognosis of rheumatoid arthritis and undifferentiated polyarthritis syndrome in the clinic: a study of 1141 patients. *J Rheumatol* 1993;20:2005–2009.
61. Møttønen TT. Prediction of erosiveness and rate of development of new erosions in early rheumatoid arthritis. *Ann Rheum Dis* 1988;47: 648–653.
62. Brik R, Lorber M, Rivkin M, et al. ELISA determined IgM and IgA rheumatoid factors in seronegative rheumatoid arthritis and psoriatic arthritis. *Clin Exp Rheumatol* 1990;8:293–296.
63. Salvarini C, Macchioni P, Mantovani W, et al. Extraarticular manifestations of rheumatoid arthritis and HLA antigens in Northern Italy. *J Rheumatol* 1992;19:242–246.
64. Panayi GS, Celinska E, Emery P, et al. Seronegative and seropositive rheumatoid arthritis: similar diseases. *Br J Rheumatol* 1987;26:172–180.
65. Wager O, Ripatti N, Laine V, et al. Clinical evaluation of the serological tests in rheumatoid arthritis. *Acta Rheum Scand* 1961;7:209–218.
66. Maury CPJ, Teppo AM, Wafin F, et al. Class-specific rheumatoid factors, DR antigens, and amyloidosis in patients with rheumatoid arthritis. *Ann Rheum Dis* 1988;47:546–552.
67. Pasternack A, Tiilikainen A. HLA-B27 in rheumatoid arthritis and amyloidosis. *Tissue Antigens* 1977;9:80–89.
68. Husby G. Amyloidosis in ankylosing spondylitis. *Scand J Rheumatol* 1980;suppl 32:67–70.
69. Husby G. Amyloidosis. *Semin Arthritis Rheum* 1992;22:67–82.
70. Kinsella RA. *Proceedings of the Interstate Postgraduate Medical Assembly of North America* 1942:13.
71. Porsman VA. *Proceedings of the Congress of European Rheumatology,* vol 2. Barcelona, Spain: Editorial Scienta 1951:479.
72. Otten HA, Westendrop Boerma F. Significance of the Waaler Rose test, streptococcal agglutination, and antistreptolysin titer in the prognosis of rheumatoid arthritis. *Ann Rheum Dis* 1959;18:24–28.
73. Bywaters EGL, Curwen M, Dresner E. Ten-year follow-up of rheumatoid arthritis. *Lancet* 1960;2:1381.
74. Fleming A, Crown JM, Corbett M. Prognostic value of early features in rheumatoid disease. *BMJ* 1976;1:1243–1245.
75. Moesmann G. Clinical features in subacute rheumatoid arthritis in old age. *Acta Rheum Scand* 1968;14:285–297.

76. Wawrzynska-Pagowska J, Brzezinska B, Brzozowska M. Observations on the symptoms and signs of "early" rheumatoid arthritis in a prospective study. *Acta Rheum Scand* 1970;16:99–105.
77. McCarty DJ, O'Duffy JD, Pearson L, et al. Remitting seronegative symmetrical synovitis with pitting oedema. RS3PE syndrome. *JAMA* 1985;254:2763–2767.
78. Russell EB, Hunter JB, Pearson L, et al. Remitting, seronegative, symmetrical synovitis with pitting edema—13 additional cases. *J Rheumatol* 1990;17:633–639.
79. Chaouat D, Le Parc JM. The syndrome of seronegative symmetrical synovitis with pitting edema (RS3 PE syndrome): a unique form of arthritis in the elderly? Report of 4 additional cases. *J Rheumatol* 1989;16:1211–1213.
80. Olive A, del Blanco J, Pons M, et al. The clinical spectrum of remitting seronegative symmetrical synovitis with pitting edema. *J Rheumatol* 1997;24:333–336.
81. Dorfman HD, Siegel HL, Perry MC, et al. Non-Hodgkin's lymphoma of the synovium simulating rheumatoid arthritis. *Arthritis Rheum* 1987;30:155–161.
82. Roldan MR, Martinez F, Roman J, et al. Non-Hodgkin's lymphoma: initial manifestation. *Ann Rheum Dis* 1993;52:85–86.
83. Tada Y, Sato H, Yoshizawa S, et al. Remitting seronegative symmetrical synovitis with pitting edema associated with gastric carcinoma. *J Rheumatol* 1997;24:974–975.
84. Olivo D, Mattace R. Concurrence of benign edematous polysynovitis in the elderly (RS3PE syndrome) and endometrial carcinoma. *Scand J Rheumatol* 1997;26:67–68.
85. Paira S, Graf C, Roverano S, et al. Remitting seronegative symmetrical synovitis with pitting edema: a study of 12 cases. *Clin Rheumatol* 2002;21:146–149.
86. Deal CL, Meenan RF, Goldenberg DL, et al. The clinical features of elderly-onset rheumatoid arthritis. *Arthritis Rheum* 1985;28:987–994.
87. Healey LA. Long-term follow-up of polymyalgia rheumatica: evidence for synovitis. *Semin Arthritis Rheum* 1984;13:322–328.
88. Healey LA, Sheets PK. The relation of polymyalgia rheumatica to rheumatoid arthritis. *J Rheumatol* 1988;15:750–752.
89. O'Duffy JD, Wahner HW, Hunder GG. Joint imaging in polymyalgia rheumatica. *Mayo Clin Proc* 1976;51:519–524.
90. Kyle V, Tudor J, Wraight EP, et al. Rarity of synovitis in polymyalgia rheumatica. *Ann Rheum Dis* 1990;49:155–157.
91. Myklebust G, Gran JT. A prospective study of 287 patients with polymyalgia rheumatica and temporal arteritis: clinical and laboratory manifestations at onset of disease and at the time of diagnosis. *Br J Rheumatol* 1996;35:1161–1168.
92. Inoue K, Shichikawa K, Nishioka J, et al. Older age at onset rheumatoid arthritis with or without osteoarthritis. *Ann Rheum Dis* 1987;46: 908–911.
93. Bywaters EGL. Still's disease in the adult. Ann Rheum Dis 1971;30: 121–133.
94. Larson EB. Adult Still's disease. *Medicine* 1984;63:82–91.
95. Bannatyne GA, Wohlmann AS. Rheumatoid arthritis: its clinical history, etiology and pathology. *Lancet* 1895;1:1120.
96. Still GF. On a form of chronic joint disease in children. *Med Chir Trans* 1897;80:47–50.
97. Ohta A, Yamaguchi M, Kaneoka H, et al. Adult Still's disease: review of 228 cases from the literature. *J Rheumatol* 1987;14:1139–1146.
98. Balleari E, Cutolo M, Accardo S. Adult-onset Still's disease associated to *Toxoplasma gondii* infection. *Clin Rheumatol* 1991;10:326–327.
99. Pouchot J, Ouakil H, Debin ML, et al. Adult Still's disease associated with acute human parvovirus B19 infection. *Lancet* 1993;341:1280–1281.
100. Schifter T, Lewinski UH. Adult onset Still's disease associated with Epstein-Barr virus infection in a 66-year old woman. *Scand J Rheumatol* 1998;27:458–460.
101. Perez C, Artola V. Adult Still's disease associated with *Mycoplasma pneumoniae* infection. *Clin Infect Dis* 2001;32:E105–E106.
102. Takeda H, Ling M, Ochi M, et al. A patient with adult Still's disease with an increased *Chlamydia pneumoniae* antibody titer. *J Infect Chemother* 2002;8:262–265.
103. Valtonen JM, Kosunen TU, Karjalainen J, et al. Serological findings in patients with acute syndromes fulfilling the proposed criteria of adult Still's disease. *Scand J Rheumatol* 1997;26:342–345.
104. Brandwein SR, Salusinsky-Sternbach M. Adult Still's disease in only one of identical twins. *J Rheumatol* 1989;16:1599–1601.
105. Katz WE, Starz TW, Winkelstein A. recurrence of adult Still's disease after pregnancy. *J Rheumatol* 1990;17:373–374.
106. de Miguel E, Cuesta M, Martin-Mola E, et al. Adult Still's disease and pregnancy. *J Rheumatol* 1992;19:498.
107. Loet XL, Daragon A, Duval C, et al. Adult onset Still's disease and pregnancy. *J Rheumatol* 1993;20:1158–1161.
108. Sampalis JS, Medsger TA, Fries JF, et al. Risk factors for adult Still's disease. *J Rheumatol* 1996;23:2049–2054.
109. Valente RM, Banks PM, Conn DL. Characterization of lymph node histology in adult Still's disease. *J Rheumatol* 1989;16:349–354.
110. Quaini F, Manganelli P, Pileri S, et al. Immunohistological characterization of lymph nodes in two cases of adult onset Still's disease. *J Rheumatol* 1991;18:1418–1423.
111. Reichert LJ, Keuning JJ, van Beek M, et al. Lymph node histology simulating T-cell lymphoma in adult-onset Still's disease. *Ann Haematol* 1992;65:53–54.
112. Esdaile JM, Tannenbaum H, Hawkins D. Adult Still's disease. *Am J Med* 1980;68:825–828.
113. Reginato AJ, Schumacher HR, Baker DG, et al. Adult onset Still's disease: experience in 23 patients and literature review with emphasis on organ failure. *Semin Arthritis Rheum* 1987;17:39–57.
114. Pouchot J, Sampalis JS, Beaudet F, et al. Adult Still's disease: Manifestations, disease course, and outcome in 62 patients. *Medicine* 1991;70:118.
115. Ohta A, Yamaguchi M, Tsunematsu T, et al. Adult Still's disease: a multicenter survey of Japanese patients. *J Rheumatol* 1990;17:1058–1063.
116. Lubbe J, Hofer M, Chavaz P, et al. Adult-onset Still's disease with persistent plaques. *Br J Dermatol* 1999;141:710–713.
117. Suzuki S, Kimura K, Aoki M, et al. Persistent plaques and linear pigmentation in adult-onset Still's disease. *Dermatology* 2001;202: 333–335.
118. Boki KA, Tsirantonaki MJ, Markakis K, et al. Thrombotic thrombocytopenic purpura in adult Still's disease. *J Rheumatol* 1996;23:385–387.
119. Diamond JR. Hemolytic uremic syndrome/thrombocytopenic purpura (HUS/TTP) complicating adult Still's disease: remission induced with intravenous immunoglobulin G. *J Nephrol* 1997;10:253–257.
120. Goldman JA, Beard MR, Casey HL. Acute febrile juvenile rheumatoid arthritis in adults: cause of polyarthritis and fever. *South Med J* 1980;73:555–563.
121. Medsger TA, Christy WC. Carpal arthritis with ankylosis in late onset Still's disease. *Arthritis Rheum* 1976;19:232.
122. Moreno-Alvarez MJ, Citera G, Maldonado-Cocco JA, et al. Adult Still's disease and inflammatory myositis. *Clin Exp Rheumatol* 1993; 11:659–661.
123. Nguyen KHY, Weisman MH. Severe throat as a presenting symptom of adult onset Still's disease: a case series and review of the literature. *J Rheumatol* 1997;24:592–597.
124. Pollet SM, Vogt PJ, Leek JC. Serous peritonitis in adult Still's syndrome. *J Rheumatol* 1990;17:98–101.
125. Takami A, Nakao S, Miyamori H, et al. Adult-onset Still's disease with submassive hepatic necrosis. *Int Med* 1995;34:89–91.
126. Janssen HL, van Laar JM, van Hoek B, et al. Severe hepatitis and pure red cell aplasia in adult Still's disease: good response to immunosuppressive therapy. *Dig Dis Sci* 1999;44:1639–1642.
127. McFarlane M, Harth M, Wall WJ. Liver transplant in adult Still's disease. *J Rheumatol* 1997;24:2038–2041.
128. Dino O, Provenzano G, Giannuoli G, et al. Fulminant hepatic failure in adult onset Still's disease. *J Rheumatol* 1996;23:784–785.
129. Cheema GS, Quismorio FP. Pulmonary involvement in adult-onset Still's disease. *Curr Opin Pulmon Med* 1999;5:305–309.
130. Iglesias J, Sathiraju S, Marik PE. Severe systemic inflammatory response syndrome with shock and ARDS resulting from Still's disease. *Chest* 1999;115:1738–1740.
131. Jamieson TW. Adult Still's disease complicated by cardiac tamponade. *JAMA* 1983;249:2065–2066.
132. Moder KG, Miller TD, Allen GL. Cardiac tamponade: an unusual feature of adult onset Still's disease. *J Rheumatol* 1995;22:180–182.
133. Yamaguchi M, Ohta A, Tsunematsu T, et al. Preliminary criteria for classification of adult Still's disease. *J Rheumatol* 1992; 19: 424–430.
134. Bank I, Marboe CC, Redberg RF, Jacobs J. Myocarditis in adult Still's disease. *Arthritis Rheum* 1985;28:452.

135. Taillan B, Fuzibet JG, Vinti H, et al. Adult onset Still's disease complicated by endocarditis with fatal evolution. *Clin Rheumatol* 1989;8:541.
136. Bruckle W, Eisenhut C, Goebel FD. Cerebral involvement in adult Still's disease. *Clin Rheumatol* 1992;11:276–279.
137. Wouters JMGW, Froeling PGA, van de Putte LBA. Adult-onset Still's disease complicated by hypercalcemia: possible relationship with rapidly destructive polyarthritis. *Ann Rheum Dis* 1985;44:345–348.
138. Garrote FJ, Marco J, Obeso G, et al. Aseptic meningitis and focal central nervous system involvement in a case of adult Still's disease. *J Rheumatol* 1993;20:765–767.
139. Denault A, Dimopoulos MA, Fitzcharles MA. Meningoencephalitis and peripheral neuropathy complicating adult Still's disease. *J Rheumatol* 1990;17:698–700.
140. Sisselman SG. Adult onset Still's disease presenting as aseptic meningitis in a young healthy female. *Del Med J* 1999;71:181–184.
141. Markuss HM, Stolk B, van der Mey AGL, et al. Sensorineural hearing loss in adult Still's disease. *Ann Rheum Dis* 1988;47:600–602.
142. Kurabayashi H, Kubota K, Tamura K, et al. Cerebral haemorrhage complicating adult-onset Still's disease. *J Int Med Res* 1996;24:492–494.
143. Harrington TM, Moran JJ, davis DE. Amyloidosis in adult Still's disease. *J Rheumatol* 1981;8:833–836.
144. Wendling D, Humbert PG, Billerey C, et al. Adult onset Still's disease and related renal amyloidosis. *Ann Rheum Dis* 1991;50:257–259.
145. Ishii T, Sasaki T, Muryoi T, et al. Systemic amyloidosis in a patient with adult onset Still's disease. *Int Med* 1993;32:50–52.
146. Oh YB, Bae SC, Jung JH, et al. Secondary renal amyloidosis in adult onset Still's disease: case report and review of the literature. *Korean J Intern Med* 2000;15:131–134.
147. Wendling D, Hory B, Blanc D. Adult Still's disease and mesangial glomerulonephritis. Report of two cases. *Clin Rheumatol* 1990;9:95–99.
148. Jassim A, Kumar N, Kelly C. Adult Still's disease with nephrotic syndrome at presentation. *Rheumatology* 1999;38:283.
149. Neishi J, Tsukada Y, Maehara T, et al. Adult Still's disease as a paraneoplastic manifestation of breast cancer. *Scand J Rheum* 2000;29:328–330.
150. Trotta F, Dovigo L, Scapoli G, et al. Immunoblastic malignant lymphoma on adult onset Still's disease. *J Rheumatol* 1993;20:1788–1792.
151. Schwarz-Eywill M, Heilig B, Bauer H, et al. Evaluation of serum ferritin as a marker for adult Still's disease activity. *Ann Rheum Dis* 1992;51:683–685.
152. van Reeth C, le Moel G, Lasne Y, et al. Serum ferritin and isoferritins are tools for diagnosis of active adult Still's disease. *J Rheumatol* 1994;21:890–895.
153. Vignes S, Le Moel G, Fautrel B, et al. Percentage of glycosylated serum ferritin remains low throughout the course of adult onset Still's disease. *Ann Rheum Dis* 2000;59:347–350.
154. Fautrel B, Le Moel G, Saint-Marcoux B, et al. Diagnostic value of ferritin and glycosylated ferritin in adult Still's disease. *J Rheumatol* 2001;28:322–329.
155. ten Kate J, Drenth JPH, Kahm MF, et al. Iron saturation of serum ferritin in patients with adult Still's disease. *J Rheumatol* 2001;28:2213–2215.
156. Masson C, le Loet X, Liote F, et al. Comparative study of 6 types of criteria in adult Still's disease. *J Rheumatol* 1996;23:495–497.
157. Magadur-Joly G, Billaud E, Barrier JH, et al. Epidemiology of adult Still's disease: estimate of the incidence by a retrospective study in west France. *Ann Rheum Dis* 1995;54:587–590.
158. Wakai K, Ohta A, Tamakoshi A, et al. Estimated prevalence and incidence of adult Still's disease: findings by a nationwide epidemiological survey in Japan. *J Epidemiol* 1997;7:221–225.
159. Cush JJ, Medsger TA, Christy WC, et al. Adult Still's disease. *Arthritis Rheum* 1987;30:186–194.
160. Uson J, Pena JM, del Arco A, et al. Still's disease in a 72- year old man. *J Rheumatol* 1993;20:1608–1609.
161. Tamura K, Kubota K, Kurabayashi H, et al. Elderly onset of adult Still's disease: report of a case. *Clin Rheumatol* 1994;13:117–118.
162. Masson C, le Loet X, Liote F, et al. Adult Still's disease. Part II. Management, outcome and prognostic factors. *Rev Rhum* 1995;62:758–765.
163. Bujak JS, Aptekar RG, Decker JL, et al. Juvenile rheumatoid arthritis presenting in the adult as fever of unknown origin. *Medicine* 1973;52:431–443.
164. Bisagni-Faure A, Job-Deslandre C, Menkes CJ. Intravenous methylprednisolone pulse therapy in Still's disease. *J Rheumatol* 1992;19:1487–1488.
165. Kraus A, Alarcon-Segovia D. Fever in adult onset Still's disease. Response to methotrexate. *J Rheumatol* 1991;18:918–920.
166. Fujii T, Akizuki M, Kameda M, et al. Methotrexate treatment in patients with adult onset Still's disease—retrospective study of 13 Japanese cases. *Ann Rheum Dis* 1997;56:144–148.
167. Aydintug AO, D'Cruz D, Cervera R, et al. Low dose methotrexate treatment in adult Still's disease. *J Rheumatol* 1992;19:431–435.
168. Fautrel B, Borget C, Rozenberg S, et al. Corticosteroid sparing effect of low dose methotrexate treatment in adult Still's disease. *J Rheumatol* 1999;26:373–378.
169. Fabricant MS, Chandor SB, Friou GJ. Still disease in adults. *JAMA* 1973;225:273–274.
170. Sato M, Takeda A, Honzu H, et al. Adult Still's disease with Sjøgren's syndrome successfully treated with intravenous pulse methylprednisolone and oral cyclophosphamide. *Int Med* 1993;32:730–732.
171. Shojania K, Chalmers A, Rangno K. Cyclosporin A in the treatment of adult Still's disease. *J Rheumatol* 1995;22:1391–1392.
172. Marchesoni A, Ceravolo GP, Battafarano N, et al. Cyclosporin A in the treatment of adult onset Still's disease. *J Rheumatol* 1997;24:1582–1587.
173. Kulke R, Koeppel M, Hey D. Treatment of adult Still's disease with intravenous immunoglobulin. *Lancet* 1996;347:337.
174. Jung JH, Jun JB, Yoo DH, et al. High toxicity of sulphasalazine in adult-onset Still's disease. *Clin Exp Rheumatol* 2000;18:245–248.
175. Lanza F, Dominici M, Govoni M, et al. Prolonged remission state of refractory adult onset Still's disease following CD34-selected autologous peripheral blood stem cell transplantation. *Bone Marrow Transplant* 2000;25:1307–1310.
176. Kraetsch HG, Antoni C, Kalden JR, et al. Successful treatment of a small cohort of patients with adult Still's disease with infliximab: first experiences. *Ann Rheum Dis* 2001;60:55–57.
177. Husni ME, Maier AL, Mease PJ, et al. Etanercept in the treatment of adult patients with Still's disease. *Arthritis Rheum* 2001;46:1171–1177.
178. Terkeltaub R, Esdaile JM, Decary F, et al. HLA-Bw35 and prognosis in adult Still's disease. *Arthritis Rheum* 1981;24:1469.
179. Elkon KB, Hughes GRV, Bywaters EGL, et al. Adult-onset Still's disease. *Arthritis Rheum* 1982;25:647–654.
180. Sampalis JS, Esdaile JM, Medsger TA, et al. A controlled study of the long-term prognosis of Adult Still's disease. *Am J Med* 1995;98:384.
181. Gran JT, Husby G. The epidemiology of ankylosing spondylitis. A review. *Semin Arthritis Rheum* 1993;22:319–334.
182. Gran JT, Husby G. Ankylosing spondylitis: a comparative study of patients found in an epidemiological study, and those admitted to a department of rheumatology. *J Rheumatol* 1984;11:788–793.
183. Calin A. Reiter's syndrome and reactive arthropathy: sex distribution. *Scand J Rheumatol* 1980;(suppl 32):41–44.
184. Calin A. Reiter's syndrome: epidemiology and immunogenetics. *Scand J Rheumatol* 1980;(suppl 32):178–173.
185. Mmki-Ikola O, Granfors K. Salmonella-triggered reactive arthritis. *Scand J Rheumatol* 1992;21:265–270.
186. Wright V. Arthropathia psoriatica—a clinical entity. *Scand J Rheumatol* 1980;suppl 32:25–30.
187. Gran JT, Husby G. Joint manifestations in gastrointestinal diseases. Part I: pathophysiological aspects, ulcerative colitis and Crohn's disease. *Dig Dis* 1992;10:274–294.
188. Bourne JT, Kumar P, Huskisson EC, et al. Arthritis in celiac disease. *Ann Rheum Dis* 1985;44:592–598.
189. Parke AL, Fagan EA, Chadwick VS, et al. Celiac disease and rheumatoid arthritis. *Ann Rheum Dis* 1984;43:378–380.
190. Pinals RS. Arthritis associated with glutensensitive enteropathy. *J Rheumatol* 1986;13:201–204.
191. Gran JT, Husby G. Joint manifestations in gastrointestinal diseases. Part II: Whipple's disease, enteric infections, intestinal bypass operations, gluten sensitive enteropathy, pseudomembranous colitis and collagenous colitis. *Dig Dis* 1992;10:295–312.
192. Relman DA, Schmidt TM, MacDermott RP, et al. Identification of the uncultured bacillus of Whipple's disease. *N Engl J Med* 1992;327:293–301.

193. Gran JT, Johnsen V, Myklebust G, et al. The variable clinical picture of arthritis induced by human parvovirus B19. *Scand J Rheumatol* 1995;24:174–179.
194. Hughes GRV. Connective tissue diseases. In: *Systemic lupus erythematosus,* 3rd ed. Oxford: Blackwell Scientific, 1987:3–71.
195. Sheon RP, Kirsner AB, Tangsintanapas P, et al. Malignancy in rheumatic disease: interrelationships. *J Am Geratr Soc* 1977;25:20–27.
196. Calabro JJ. Arthritis as an early cancer clue. *Arthritis Rheum* 1971;14:154.
197. Lansbury J. Collagen disease complicating malignancy. *Ann Rheum Dis* 1953;12:301–305.
198. Mackenzie AH, Scherbel AL. Connective tissue syndromes associated with carcinoma. *Geriatrics* 1963;18:745–753.
199. Butler RC, Thompson JM, Keat ACS. Paraneoplastic rheumatic disorders: a review. *J R Soc Med* 1987;80:168–172.
200. Wilson S, Brooks PM. Rheumatic manifestations of neoplasia. *Curr Opin Rheumatol* 1993;5:99–103.
201. Eggelmeijer F, Macfarlane JD. Polyarthritis as the presenting symptom of the occurrence and recurrence of a laryngeal carcinoma. *Ann Rheum Dis* 1992;51:556–557.
202. McDonagh JE, Clarke F, Smith SR, et al. Non-Hodgkin's lymphoma presenting as polyarthritis. *Br J Rheumatol* 1994;33:79–84.
203. Kelley WN, Fox IH, Palella TD. Gout and related disorders of purine metabolism. In: Kelley WN, Harris ED, Ruddy S, et al., eds. *Textbook of rheumatology.* Philadelphia: WB Saunders, 1989:396–1397.
204. Spilberg I, Silzbach LE, McEwen CE. The arthritis of sarcoidosis. *Arthritis Rheum* 1969;12:126.

CHAPTER 61

Juvenile Idiopathic Arthritis (Juvenile Rheumatoid Arthritis)

Robert W. Warren, Marietta M. De Guzman, Christine B. Bernal, and Maria D. Perez

Juvenile idiopathic arthritis (JIA) is a new name for an old set of diseases. JIA will presumably and eventually become the consensus term to supplant the American and European terms of *juvenile rheumatoid arthritis* (JRA) and *juvenile chronic arthritis* (JCA), respectively. JIA is a disease that is at least centuries old, although "ancient" data are scant. The remains of an adolescent with skeletal changes consistent with chronic arthritis from approximately A.D. 1000 were discovered in the Andes (1). Although recognized in the 1500s, careful descriptions of childhood arthritis did not appear until Cronil (2) and Diamant-Berger's (3) work in the 1800s. Diamant-Berger was the first to report growth disturbances associated with chronic childhood arthritis in his review of 38 cases in 1890. Nevertheless, it was the meticulous clinical documentation of Dr. George Still in 1897 that led to the perspective that arthritis in children was largely different from rheumatoid arthritis (RA) seen in adults.

Indeed, JIA is a group of idiopathic chronic diseases of childhood that affect joints and other tissues in approximately 1 in 1,000 children. Although only a minority of JIA patients still have inflammatory disease as adults, JIA often produces significant functional or emotional disability. Levinson and Wallace (4) reviewed functional outcome data and reported that about one third of patients become significantly physically disabled, and more than half have joint erosions. David and co-workers (5) reported severe disability among young adults, with a mean 20-year follow-up, in 8% with systemic, 34% with rheumatoid factor (RF)-negative polyarticular, 38% with RF-positive polyarticular, and 86% with extended pauciarticular (polyarticular course) disease. Most of the disability in the last group was secondary to ocular disease. In contrast, in a Norwegian study of 53 JIA patients after approximately 10 years of follow-up, 60% were in remission with no functional disability, only 23% had erosive joint disease, and only 8% were severely disabled (Steinbrocker III/IV) (6). JIA is associated later in life with more pain, more disability, and decreased employment, but no difference from controls in income, education, or birth rates (7). The mortality rate in the United States is less than 1% (8).

Secondary disability is also a critical issue for children with JIA and includes psychosocial concerns, such as body image, self-esteem, and dependence (9); suboptimal school achievement due to psychosocial maladjustment and increased absence (10); and family problems, including depression, work loss, separation and divorce, and financial difficulties (11). Of note, these problems do not correlate highly with the severity of arthritis; indeed, such difficulties are observed among children and families with only mild oligoarthritis (12), whereas some children and teenagers with severe polyarthritis appear to have few secondary residua.

CLASSIFICATION CRITERIA OF JIA

Preceding JIA by 25 years, criteria for JRA were established in 1973 (13) and revised in 1977 (14) as the occurrence of arthritis in a child under 16 years of age and lasting at least 6 weeks in at least one joint with no other known etiology. Arthritis was defined as swelling, or two of the following findings: heat, limited motion, tenderness, and pain on motion. JRA was subdivided into three major subgroups, based on disease onset in the first 6 months of illness: (a) systemic, characterized by spiking fevers, evanescent rash, and other extraarticular disease; (b) pauciarticular, with four

TABLE 61.1. *Juvenile idiopathic arthritis: classification of arthritis without known cause, presenting before 16 years of age, and lasting at least 6 weeks (18)*

Disease	Criteria	Exclusions	Descriptors
Systemic arthritis	Daily fever lasting at least 2 weeks, documented quotidian for at least 3 days Arthritis (which may trail fever) One or more of Evanescent, erythematous, nonfixed rash Generalized lymphadenopathy Serositis Liver and/or spleen enlargement	No specific exclusions, except emphasized importance of excluding infection and malignancy	Age at onset of arthritis Arthritis pattern in first 6 months ("onset") No arthritis Oligoarthritis Polyarthritis Arthritis pattern after 6 months ("course") No arthritis Oligoarthritis Polyarthritis Systemic features after 6 months Positive RF CRP level
Oligoarthritis	Arthritis involving 1–4 joints in first 6 months of disease, of two subcategories: Persistent: affecting no more than 4 joints during disease course Extended: affecting a total of more than 4 joints after the first 6 months of disease	Confirmed family history[a] of psoriasis Confirmed family history of HLA-B27-associated disease Positive RF HLA-B27-positive male with disease onset after 8 years of age Systemic arthritis	Age of onset Patterns of arthritis at 6 months and last clinic visit Large joints only Small joints only Limb predominance Specific joints affected symmetry Anterior uveitis (acute or chronic) Positive ANA HLA class I and II predisposing and protective alleles
Polyarthritis (rheumatoid factor negative)	Arthritis involving >4 joints in first 6 months of disease Negative RF	Positive RF Systemic arthritis	Age of onset Symmetry of arthritis Positive ANA Uveitis (acute or chronic)
Polyarthritis (rheumatoid factor positive)	Arthritis involving >4 joints in first 6 months of disease Positive RF, two tests at least 3 months apart	Negative RF Systemic arthritis	Age of onset Symmetry of arthritis Positive ANA Immunogenetics
Psoriatic arthritis	Arthritis and psoriasis, or arthritis and at least two of: Dactylitis Nail pitting or onycholysis Confirmed family history of psoriasis	Positive RF Systemic arthritis	Age at onset of arthritis/psoriasis Patterns of arthritis 6 months after disease onset, and at last clinic visit: Large joints only Small joints only Limb predominance Specific joints Symmetry Disease course Oligoarthritis Polyarthritis Positive ANA Anterior uveitis Chronic Acute HLA descriptors
Enthesitis-related arthritis	Arthritis *and* enthesitis, or arthritis *or* enthesitis with at least two of: SI tenderness and/or inflammatory spinal pain Positive HLA-B27 Confirmed family history of HLA-B27-associated disease Acute anterior uveitis Arthritis onset in a male after 8 years of age	Confirmed family history of psoriasis Systemic arthritis	Age at onset of arthritis or enthesitis Patterns of arthritis Large joints only Small joints only Limb predominance Specific joints Symmetry Disease course Oligoarthritis Polyarthritis
Other arthritis	Criteria of no other classification fulfilled, or criteria of more than one classification fulfilled	Fulfilled criteria for single classification	

[a]Confirmed family history means documentation by physician of disease in a first- or second-degree relative; in the case of psoriasis, confirmation must be made by a dermatologist.

ANA, antinuclear antibody; CRP, C-reactive protein; HLA, human leukocyte antigen; RF, rheumatoid factor; SI, sacroiliac joint.

or fewer affected joints; and (c) polyarticular, with five or more affected joints. Despite the obvious phenomenologic character of the definition of JRA, and the absence of any diagnostic test, the definition has been surprisingly effective; at 5-year follow-up, over 97% of children so identified still carried the diagnosis (15).

Nevertheless, nomenclature has become controversial in the past few years (16,17). Historically named JRA, and still commonly referred to as such in the United States, the illness has been called JCA in Europe. Although historically quite relevant, the American usage of *rheumatoid* unfortunately evokes in parents the specter of their parents and friends with adult RF-positive RA, an entity that is relevant to only about 5% of JRA patients. Of greater concern, the limited subtyping of JRA to systemic, pauciarticular, and polyarticular makes the correlation of data from different research groups across the world difficult. Finally, JRA subtyping of pauciarticular and polyarticular disease reflects the *onset* of disease, which is far less relevant than disease course and progression.

With this backdrop, a new and universal classification of JIA is slowly gaining acceptance. Fink and the International League Against Rheumatism (ILAR) Task Force (1995) developed the Santiago criteria and identified seven candidate diseases under the rubric of idiopathic childhood arthritis, each with its own set of criteria: systemic arthritis, polyarthritis (RF positive), polyarthritis (RF negative), pauciarthritis, extended pauciarthritis, arthritis with enthesitis, and psoriatic arthritis. This classification was revised as the Durban criteria for JIA in the second meeting of the Classification Task Force of the Pediatric Standing Committee of ILAR in March 1997, and published in 1998 (18). The Durban classification for JIA is presented in Table 61.1 in abbreviated form. Note that "descriptors" are not criteria for classification but characteristics that may be used to focus further clinical research for better disease delineation in the future. Indeed, evolution of these criteria is likely. As the understanding of JIA advances, fewer subvarieties will remain idiopathic.

The differences between JRA and JIA also necessitate clarification about the scope of this chapter. Though JIA includes psoriatic arthritis, the latter will not be covered in this discussion in any detail, and can be found elsewhere in this text (see Chapter 65). Similarly, the JIA classification of "arthritis with enthesitis," clearly a *forme fruste* of spondyloarthropathy, is more appropriately considered in detail in the construct of the human leukocyte antigen (HLA)-B27-associated diseases, also discussed elsewhere in this text (see Chapters 63–66). Finally, the value of the new classification of JIA is currently limited by the fact that few clinical studies have used these definitions; the great body of clinical description has utilized the classic JRA (or JCA) subtypes. Thus, this chapter will present data (e.g., concerning the epidemiology of JIA) based on the disease definitions used in the conduct of the studies themselves, so data will be presented in terms of JRA or JCA. Consequently, considerable extrapolation of study results to the new diagnostic classification is necessary.

EPIDEMIOLOGY AND ETIOLOGY

Joint pain is the chief complaint of about 1% of children seeking acute medical evaluation per year, and about 1% of these children will develop chronic arthritis (19,20). Thus, JIA is a fairly common group of diseases, occurring in over 1 in 1,000 children. However, a discussion of the epidemiology of the disease has intrinsic limitations:

1. The definition of the idiopathic arthritides of children is changing. Thus, there is no major body of literature that addresses the epidemiology of JIA as an entity.
2. The disease described is not homogeneous. Indeed, nothing but the phenomenology of the definition and the history of association holds systemic arthritis together with the other varieties of the disease.
3. Case finding in studies has been largely retrospective. Thus, because it is acknowledged that JIA, and particularly pauciarthritis, is underdiagnosed, reported prevalence and incidence figures may be low. Retrospective case acquisition may also result in limited case finding in minority populations.

Given these limitations, and to limit confusion, epidemiologic information here is given in the context of the disease definition (case finding) used in the referenced study. Thus, the prevalence of JRA has been reported to be as low as 0.16 to 0.43 per 1,000 (21,22), but is more typically reported at approximately 1 to 2 per 1,000 (23–25). However, when Manners and Diepeveen (26) mailed surveys to families in an Australian community study, they subsequently examined and found 7 (of 9 out of 2,241 12-year-olds) previously undiagnosed children with JCA. This suggests a prevalence for JCA (which includes spondyloarthropathies) of 4 per 1,000. Determining absolute, or even relative, prevalence figures for the separate categories of JIA is currently difficult, because relative prevalence has varied dramatically among reports for JRA itself, and because the categories of disease in JIA are different (psoriatic arthritis and enthesitis-related arthritis included).

Meanwhile, recent incidence figures for JRA/JCA have been more similar, ranging from 11.7 per 100,000 per year in a 1996 study from Rochester, Minnesota (27), to 35 per 100,000 per year in an East Berlin study (25). Other studies report incidence in this general range (24,28–31).

Age at onset and gender varies by JRA/JIA categories. Specifically, no peak age of onset is observed for systemic disease (32). Taken as a whole, JRA age at onset peaks at less than 4 to 5 years (24,30,33,34); in fact, more than half of all children with JRA present by 5 years of age (32).

Gender representation in JRA also varies by JRA/JIA subtype. There is no gender preference among children with systemic disease (32), but there is a female predominance of approximately 3:1 for other subtypes of JRA (32).

Most studies report overall female preponderance in JRA of 1.5- to 2-fold (24,25,30), but a recent Minnesota study reported a female:male ratio of 7:8 (27).

Ethnicity is clearly an important factor in JRA prevalence, although recent work has suggested equivalence of African-American and white frequencies in the United States (35). Schwartz and co-workers (36) found that African-American children with JRA are typically older at onset, particularly in the oligoarticular group (8.1 vs. 4.8 years of age), more likely to be RF positive, and less likely to have a positive antinuclear antibody (ANA) status and to develop uveitis. In contrast, another study concluded that African-American patients were 15 times more likely than whites to have uveitis, and that their uveitis was more severe (37). Concerns remain about referral bias. Some data have suggested lower frequencies among Chinese populations, but at least some Native American populations appear substantially more susceptible, with a 3.2-fold frequency compared with whites in a Canadian study (35). Some Native American populations are apparently much more likely to have RF-positive polyarthritis (37,38). Finally, there are reported differences by geography, with a prevalence, similar to that of the United States, in France of 0.77 to 1.0 per 1,000 (39) and Sweden (40), and a lower incidence of 0.054 per 1,000 per year reported in Costa Rica (41). Studies from Thailand (42), India (43,44) and among African-American (36) and Canadian aboriginals (45) showed more frequent positivity of IgM RF. It is unclear whether these geographic variations represent the impact of environmental factors or genetic differences among populations.

The etiology of JIA remains largely mysterious, but the different forms of JIA may well reflect an abnormal immune response to infection or other environmental stress, strongly influenced by immunogenetic factors. The immunogenetic hypothesis is discussed below. Also, a post-traumatic etiology, possibly exposing new autoantigens after injury, is consistent with the common reports, particularly for oligoarthritis, of starting after a fall (46). However, it is also plausible that the injury occurred because of pain or joint instability associated with the arthritis itself. Furthermore, stress may be relevant to the pathogenesis of JIA (47). Finally, infectious and postinfectious etiologies are plausible (48), and relatively strong data suggest that enthesitis-related arthritis is related to gram-negative organisms (49). Notably, T cells from JRA patients often react to bacterial heat shock proteins (50). In addition, a number of infectious and postinfectious conditions mimic JIA quite well. For example, chronic Lyme arthritis in children can look remarkably like oligoarthritis (51), and parvovirus-associated arthropathy can be clinically indistinguishable from systemic arthritis (52,53). Japanese children with polyarticular JRA had a higher seroprevalence of parvovirus B19 antibody than matched controls (54). Other agents associated with JRA include *Mycoplasma* (55,56), mumps (57), and rubella (58,59). However, despite these reports, and discussion about possible seasonality of onset of systemic arthritis or subsets thereof (60–62) and juvenile spondyloarthropathy (63), no infectious agent has been clearly associated with JIA (nor with JRA or JCA).

Immunopathogenesis and Immunogenetics

There have been a number of excellent, detailed reviews of the immunopathogenesis of JIA (64–69); a brief overview is presented here.

Immunologic and Serologic Features

The laboratory findings in JIA are clearly those of acute-phase reaction, particularly in the systemic arthritis subtype. The elevations in erythrocyte sedimentation rate (ESR), C-reactive protein (CRP), complement components C3 and C4, serum amyloid A (SAA)-related protein, ferritin, platelet count, and white blood cell (WBC) count have been documented in the literature. The majority of these proteins are not only synthesized by the liver, but also produced by cells such as macrophages and endothelial cells at local sites of inflammation. The ESR is an indirect measure of these acute-phase reactants and reflects a change in plasma viscosity due to an increase in the dielectric constant in molecules such as immunoglobulin and fibrinogen. CRP is an acute-phase reactant whose production appears to be under the control of interleukin-6 (IL-6). Because of the acute-phase properties of the complement components, the total hemolytic complement (CH_{50}) is also reflective of acute-phase reaction. There is also evidence of complement activation, particularly in the systemic arthritis subtype (70–75). Standard tests such as CH_{50}, C3, and C4 determinations have not correlated with clinical activity because there is increased synthesis of complement components, including C3 and C4, during inflammation and infection. When the rate of synthesis of these acute-phase reactants is greater than the rate of catabolism, complement consumption may be masked. However, complement activation product (e.g., C4a, C4d, C3a, and iC3b) assays have demonstrated complement activation in the presence of increased synthesis.

Measurements of C3 split products from serum or plasma have inconsistently shown complement activation in systemic arthritis, whereas complement activation and immune complexes have subsequently been found in all subsets of JIA and correlate with disease activity (70–75).

Cytokines and Immunopathogenesis

As our understanding of the control of synthesis of these molecules has increased, a cytokine profile has emerged, particularly in the systemic arthritis subtype. These new data on cytokine elaboration bring us closer to understanding the elusive driving force for the immunologic/inflammatory reaction in the juvenile arthritides. These findings have contributed to the treatment of juvenile arthritis with immunomodulatory agents that influence cytokine control/levels (see Chapter 62).

Efforts concentrated on the role of helper T cell subset 1 and 2 (T_H1/T_H2) pathways in the pathogenesis of JIA may help define subtypes of patients. Muller and co-workers (76) found reduced *in vitro* IL-10 production in patients with systemic JRA (after phytohemoglutinin or lipopolysaccharide stimulation), but increased IL-1 receptor antagonist (IL-1Ra) and soluble tumor necrosis factor-α (TNF-α) receptors p55 and p75. Gattorno and co-workers (77) found increased IL-12 (p40) in active versus inactive disease, which correlated with the ESR and CRP. Soluble TNF receptors p55 and p75 were also found to be markers for disease activity and correlated with the ESR and CRP (78).

Ozen and co-workers (79) found increased T_H1 synovial fluid mononuclear cells by identifying an increased interferon (IFN-γ)/IL-4 proinflammatory profile. Gattorno and colleagues (80) found that synovial fluid T cells from pauciarticular patients had heterogeneous phenotypes but produced IFN-γ in a T_H1/T_H0 pattern. These data suggest that proinflammatory and antiinflammatory cytokines modulate joint inflammation, and the ratio may determine the degree of erosive disease. Murray and co-workers (81) found IFN-γ less often in systemic disease. The combination of IL-4 and IL-10 was found more frequently in nonerosive articular disease compared with erosive articular disease. This suggested that IL-4, possibly in combination with IL-10, has an antiinflammatory or disease-restricting role.

IL-4 is generally antiinflammatory; however, it also induces soluble CD23 [the low-affinity receptor for immunoglobulin E (IgE) Fc] release in serum and increased CD23 surface expression. CD23 is involved in the induction of nitric oxide and proinflammatory IL-1, IL-6, and TNF-α. Kutukculer and Caglayan (82) found increased synovial and plasma levels of soluble CD23 in both pauciarticular and polyarticular patients compared with controls, as well as increased TNF-α and IL-6 in active disease (83). Massa and co-workers (84) also found increased soluble CD23 in systemic arthritis patients (associated with monocyte CD23 expression) and in ANA-positive pauciarticular patients (associated with B-cell CD23 expression); this was not related to disease activity. These findings imply B-cell activity and autoantibody production in pauciarticular disease and monocyte activation and inflammatory mediators in systemic arthritis.

De Benedetti and co-workers (85) have found an increase in IL-8 and monocyte chemoattractant protein-1 (MCP-1) in active systemic arthritis patients compared with the other subtypes. This correlated with increased systemic symptoms but not with the number of involved joints or level of inflammation. The levels were higher in synovial fluid than in serum and, in synovial fluid, correlated with increased WBC counts and synovial IL-6 levels (IL-6 induces endothelial cell production of IL-8 and MCP-1) (38). They also found increased IL-6 in active systemic arthritis and in the synovial fluid of systemic versus pauciarticular patients (86,87). However, there was an increase in IL-1 in pauciarticular versus systemic arthritis patients. Madson and co-workers (88) found an increase in IL-2 receptors (IL-2R) and IL-6 that correlated with active disease. They also observed that IL-1, IL-2R, and IL-6 were higher in synovial fluid than serum. In subsequent studies, Keul and co-workers (89) found an increase in soluble IL-6 receptor in the systemic arthritis patients compared with the other subtypes, and this correlated with fever. Interestingly, Fishman and co-workers (90) found a polymorphism of the IL-6 gene associated with a decrease in IL-6 levels, which may protect against systemic JRA. Based on such findings, it has been suggested by De Benedetti and Mafini that IL-6 plays a critical role in the expression of the laboratory (i.e., increases in SAA protein and ferritin) and clinical features of systemic arthritis (66). Maeno and colleagues found that IL-18 levels are elevated in patients with systemic onset JIA. Serum IL-18 levels correlated with serum ferritin levels, hepatosplenomegaly, and serositis (91).

Tselepis and colleagues (92) found that active JRA patients had decreased levels of platelet-activating factor–acetylhydrolase (PAF-AH), which inactivates PAF and may result in less antiinflammatory activity in active JRA. Overall, there seems to be a mixed T_H1/T_H2 profile in systemic arthritis, as discussed by Raziuddin and co-workers (93). Anti-CD3/CD28 stimulated increases in IL-4 and IL-10 with associated decreases in IL-2 and IFN-γ. This balance between proinflammatory and antiinflammatory cytokines may be lost in chronic inflammatory diseases such as JIA. Further studies are necessary, but current data suggest that future therapy may consist of combinations of anticytokines or recombinant cytokine receptors in order to shift the balance away from an inflammatory response in JIA.

Cellular Response and Immunopathogenesis

Studies of T cell subsets in peripheral blood of children with JIA/JRA have been inconsistent and difficult to interpret and consequently will not be considered in detail here. As in adults with RA, $CD4^+$ T cells are found in synovial tissue in patients with JRA (94). The $V_\delta1^+$ T cells predominate and are CD45RA positive (naive phenotype), whereas $V_\delta2^+$ cells demonstrate a CD45RO-positive memory phenotype (95). Murray and colleagues (96) reported higher levels of T-cell activation ($CD3^+$, IL-2R positive) in pauciarticular than polyarticular synovial tissue. Activation of $CD8^+$ versus $CD4^+$ T cells was more prominent in pauciarticular patients. Kjeldsen-Kragh and co-workers (97) demonstrated an activated T-cell receptor (TCR) δ/γ population in JRA synovial cells with a predominance of $V_\delta1^+$ cells. Zhang and co-workers (98) examined the synovial fluid Vβ TCR repertoire in JRA patients and found low proportions of clonally expanded T cells. In contrast, Sioud and colleagues (99) suggested an antigen- or superantigen-driven immune response by demonstrating oligoclonal TCR Vβ expansion in JRA synovial fluid. Thompson and colleagues

(100) examined $V_{\beta}20$ and $V_{\beta}8$ T-cell clonal expansion specific to synovial tissue as models for pauciarticular and polyarticular JRA, and suggested T-cell recognition of a limited group of antigens in these subtypes. Khalkhali-Ellis and co-workers (101) found T cells with macrophage attributes in synovial fluid of different subtypes of JRA, but this is of unknown significance.

Wouters and co-workers found that patients with oligoarticular and polyarticular JIA have increased numbers of HLA-DR-positive T cells, consistent with T-cell activation and T cells in the blood coexpressing CD57 and CD16/56, indicating terminal differentiation of $CD8^+$ T cells. By contrast, in patients with systemic JIA there was no increase in the activation or differentiation markers on T cells, but a profound decrease in circulating natural killer cells (102).

Tsokos and co-workers (103,104) found that circulating B cells are increased in patients with systemic and polyarticular JRA. Jarvis and co-workers (105) suggested that the expanded $CD5^+$ B-cell population preferentially contributes to IgM RF production in patients with polyarticular JRA. Khalkhali-Ellis and colleagues (106) exposed normal synovial fibroblasts to synovial fluid from JRA patients and demonstrated proliferation, destruction of cartilage matrix, and release of matrix metalloproteinases (MMPs). TNF-α is an activator of the transcription factor nuclear factor κB (NFκB), which appears to be up-regulated in JRA (107), indicating that this signal transduction pathway contributes to the overall inflammatory response.

Humoral Response and Immunopathogenesis

An elevation in one or all of the immunoglobulin classes that results from a polyclonal activation of B cells may account for the low-level antibody titers detected against infectious agents and autoantigens observed in some patients with JIA.

ANA positivity in JRA, as detected by immunofluorescence assays (IFAs), has approached 50% to 60% in some studies (108,109). In the standard fluorescent ANA, antibodies are detected by binding to a human epithelioid tumor cell line (HEp-2) cell substrate, with the homogeneous and speckled patterns being most common. The newer enzyme-linked immunosorbent assays (ELISAs) that utilize specific sets of antigens (e.g., Sm/RNP, SSA/SSB, SCL-70, Jo-1, anti-DNA, and sometimes histones) may not be appropriate for the assessment of JRA patients (110). The ANA in JRA patients seems to detect a different set of antigens than those identified in other autoimmune diseases, such as systemic lupus erythematosus (SLE) (111). Autoantibodies to nonhistone chromosomal protein HMG-1 and HMG-2 (112), HMG-17 (113), HeLa cell nuclear antigens of 50 and 40 kd (114), and the nuclear antigen DEK (primarily in pauciarticular patients) (115) have been identified in patients with JRA. The ANA by ELISA clearly does not identify the same patients as are identified by IFA (110,116).

Mulder and co-workers (117) identified antineutrophil cytoplasmic antibodies (against both cytoplasmic and nuclear antigens) in 35% of Dutch children with JRA compared with 5% in healthy controls. The titers appeared to be higher in active disease. Albani and co-workers (118) suggested a role for heat shock proteins (*Escherichia coli* dnaj) in the JRA immune response and showed anti-dnaj antibody titers that were higher in polyarticular than systemic or pauciarticular patients. The titers were higher in synovial fluid than serum and correlated with disease activity. Olds and Miller (119) identified antibodies to monophosphoryl lipid A in pauciarticular JRA patients, which correlated with C3 activation. These antibodies also correlated with numbers of active joints and were higher in synovial fluid than blood (120). The target epitope for these antibodies appears to be to the phosphorylated diglucosamine core of lipid A (121). This lends support to a microbial etiology for pauciarticular disease.

The prevalence of anticardiolipin antibodies in juvenile chronic arthritis, reported in a review by Ravelli and Martini (122), ranged from 7.9% to 53%. IgG and IgM antiphospholipid (aPL) antibodies to either cardiolipin or phosphatidyl serine were detected in 35% of JRA patients (109) (evenly distributed among the subtypes). Disease severity did not correlate with the presence of the aPL antibody or with the titer of the antibody. In another study, aPL antibody positivity in JRA patients was 67%, and 55% of these patients had antibodies to phospholipids other than cardiolipin (phosphatidylethanolamine, phosphatidylinositol, phosphatidic acid, phosphatidylglycerol, or phosphatidylserine) (123).

Classic rheumatoid factors (RFs) are pentameric IgM antibodies, but RFs can be of any Ig subclass. The most commonly used tests, however, detect mainly IgM RFs, and only 7% to 10% of patients with JRA are RF positive by latex fixation tests (124). Acid treatment of sera prior to testing dissociates complexes of high-affinity RFs and IgG that may otherwise mask RF activity in assays (125). These hidden 19S RFs have been found in up to 75% of JRA patients (126). ELISA (which can detect all classes of RF with modification) can detect hidden RFs in IgM fractions of serum and identify RFs in up to 35% of JRA patients (127). Walker and co-workers (128) detected IgA-RF in 58% of active polyarticular (but not systemic or pauciarticular) JRA patients, which correlated with disease severity. As is found in adult RA, the so-called major RF-cross-reactive idiotype is elevated in JRA patients, and is higher in systemic arthritis than in polyarticular or pauciarticular patients (129,130).

Circulating immune complexes (CICs) have been well documented in JIA (71,131–133) and can be measured by several assays that rely on the interaction of immune complexes with complement, antiglobulins, or with cellular receptors (e.g., C3 or Fc receptors). CICs that do not fix complement (e.g., that contain IgA or IgG4) are not detected by the complement-based or RAJI cell assays. In addition, IgM-RF inhibits the binding of complement components to immune complexes (134,135). CIC detected by Fc receptor–based assays must contain IgG. The size, composition, and solubility of CIC determines the ability to activate neutrophils, monocytes, and endothelial cells, or to generate anaphylatoxins (C3a/C5a) and elaborate cytokines. Peripheral blood mononuclear cells stimulated with high-molecular-weight CIC containing IgM RF and C3b produced larger amounts of TNF-α, IL-6, and IL-8 (proinflammatory activity) than smaller complexes (136). Clearance of immune complexes from the circulation may be impaired because IgM RF interferes with complement-mediated immune complex processing, including binding of C1q and C4b to the immune complex. As in SLE, the complement receptor-1 (CR1)-mediated clearance of immune complexes in JIA may also be impaired because the CR1 number per erythrocyte is reduced (75,137). This decrease in CR1 per erythrocyte correlated better with disease activity in JRA than with particular JRA subtypes (75).

Immunogenetics of Juvenile Arthritis

There have been a number of excellent reviews on the immunogenetics of juvenile arthritis (68,138–144). The goals for immunogenetics studies in JIA have been to identify genetic factors that influence the pattern and severity of joint disease and thus affect disease outcome. In addition to providing clues concerning the pathogenesis of the disease, the identification of these factors at the time of diagnosis would facilitate more aggressive disease-modifying interventions for subsets of patients at higher risk for a worse prognosis. A number of studies have addressed outcome in JIA (145–149), with risk factors associated with subsequent disability, including persistent polyarthritis, age at onset of less than 6 years, duration of disease greater than 1 year from onset to referral, and disability at initial presentation. The presence and gene dosage for the rheumatoid epitope and certain HLA-DR4 alleles have been shown to be relevant in predicting those patients with adult RA who are at highest risk for a worse prognosis (150,151) (see Chapter 55). The determination of HLA-DRB1 alleles early in the course of RA may identify a group in which more aggressive treatment should be initiated.

Genetic associations with JRA, specifically with HLA class II alleles, have been identified by from several centers in the United States and Europe. Problems arising from the available studies include the heterogeneity (clinically and serologically) of patients classified with the diagnosis of JRA and the fact that these studies have been performed in whites of largely northern and western European ancestry. Although previous studies make an attempt to separate the three major JRA subtypes, there exists a gray zone in which patients do not fit into clear subtypes. This is now being addressed using the new classification criteria; however, the studies to date are complicated by this problem. For example, there are patients who present with systemic features but have a polyarticular course, and those who present with four or fewer joints and subsequently follow a polyarticular course. Some patients present with systemic-onset disease but either do not have arthritis or have only a few affected joints; these patients may later turn out to have inflammatory bowel disease or experience a transient course of disease lasting 6 to 12 months, with ultimate resolution of symptoms consistent with a postinfectious reactive process. Exclusion of patients with spondyloarthropathy, enthesitis, psoriatic arthritis, and other reactive processes has not been consistent (sometimes because of the short time that a patient is followed). Also, there is difficulty in determining whether alleles such as HLA-DRB1*0801, DQA1*0401, and DQB1*0402 are more important in disease susceptibility because of the linkage disequilibrium between specific HLA class II loci as opposed to a true relationship with disease susceptibility per se. Studies in ethnic populations other than whites of northern and western European ancestry have only initially addressed these issues because such linkage is not so pronounced.

The etiology of JIA is unknown, although both genetic and environmental factors have been implicated. Family studies have shown an increased concordance in identical twins (152). Moroldo and co-workers (153) reported a greater than expected concordance for pauciarticular and polyarticular JRA between sibling pairs, but only the twin sets developed disease at approximately the same point in time. A number of reports over the years have demonstrated associations of JRA with class II genes of the major histocompatibility complex (MHC). In whites, the most consistent associations of pauciarticular JRA have been with HLA-DR5 (DR11), DR8 (DRB1*0801), and DPw2.1 (DPB1*0201) (154–158). Some studies have also demonstrated associations with HLA-DRB1*1301 (156,159), although this was not observed by others (155). HLA-DQA1*0101 has been associated with a diminished risk for chronic iridocyclitis and a heightened risk for a persistent polyarticular course, despite early pauciarticular onset JRA (159,160). Because the normal function of HLA molecules is the presentation of antigenic peptides, it has been suggested that alleles of the DQA1 locus (*0401, *0501, *0601) may be responsible for presenting arthrogenic peptides in early-onset pauciarticular JRA and that the pathogenic process involves the presentation of HLA-A2- or HLA-DPB1*0201-derived peptides presented by DQ molecules (139).

Seronegative (RF-negative) polyarticular JRA has also been associated with HLA-DR8 (DRB1*0801), as well as with HLA-DQw4 and DPw3 (DPB1*0301) (138,150,161, 162), especially in patients under 5 years of age. HLA-DRB1*1101 and *1104 and HLA-DRB1*0801, *0802, and *0804 are the implicated subtypes of HLA-DR5 (DR11) and DR8, respectively (155,162). In these studies, there was no linkage of HLA-DR5 (DR11) or DR8 haplotypes to HLA-DPB1*0201 (associated with pauciarticular JRA), or of HLA-DR8 haplotypes to HLA-DPB1*0301 (associated with seronegative polyarticular JRA). It was suggested that HLA-DRB1 and DPB1 may have different roles in JRA (because there were no unique shared sequences), and may affect outcome differently.

Seropositive (RF-positive) polyarticular JRA is associated with the same HLA-DR4 subtypes as adult RA, including HLA-DRB1*0401, DRB1*0404, and DRB1*0405 (138,162). Linkage disequilibrium between HLA-DR8 (DRB1*0801) and DQw4 (DQA1*0401, DQB1*0402) alleles has made it difficult to pinpoint which of these loci (DRB1, DQA1, DQB1) are more important in disease susceptibility, because most of the published studies involved white populations. HLA-DRB1*0801 itself is the most common HLA-DR8 subtype in northwestern and central European whites. In the African-American population, HLA-DQA1*0401 and DQB1*0402 are associated not only with HLA-DR8 but also with HLA-DR3 (DR18 or DRB1*0302) (163). HLA-DR8 is also frequently associated with HLA-DQw7 (DQA1*0401, DQB1*0301). Schwartz and colleagues (36) have described significant phenotypic differences between African-American and white patients with JRA. More recent typing data, acquired from JRA populations of different ethnicity, suggests that African Americans, Hispanics, and whites have similar genetic risk factors for JRA (164).

HLA associations with systemic JRA have been inconsistent because of the small numbers of patients and the clinical heterogeneity. These have included DR8 (165,166), DR5 (165,167), DR4 (168), and Dw7 (169). Pachman and co-workers (170) reported HLA-DRB1 allelic associations with systemic arthritis patients who evolved into a polyarticular course, but not in those patients who continued with systemic features.

Other Immune and Genetic Associations

Forero and co-workers (171) investigated the previous associations of pauciarticular disease with autoantibodies to the DEK oncogene protein (115,172) and with HLA-A*0202 (142,172). They found that peptides derived from the DEK protein can bind to HLA-A*0201, and suggested that the resulting complexes may be able to stimulate $CD8^+$ T cells in patients with pauciarticular JRA. Feichtlbauer and co-workers (173) reported that the microsatellite locus DQ CAR, located between DQA1 and DQB1, showed a significant positive association with JIA for the allele DQ CAR 121 (associated with DQA1*0501 and with DQB1*0301 corresponding to the molecule DQ7 on the cell surface). Charmley and co-workers (174) found an association between the HLA-DQA1*0101 allele and haplotypes of the TCR V_β6.1 gene in early-onset pauciarticular JRA patients. The TAP2B gene was increased in early-onset pauciarticular disease compared with controls (175). Ploski and Forre (141) have suggested that increased susceptibility to early-onset pauciarticular JRA (also to iridocyclitis) involves IL-1α, TCR V_β6.1b, and homozygosity for an LMP2 gene variant. The trimolecular complex (HLA, TCR, and antigen) differed in its relative associations between patients with JRA and adult RA (176).

Smerdel and co-workers found that D6S265*5 could be a marker for an additional susceptibility gene in JIA that is distinct from HLA-A*02, adding to the risk conferred by DQ4;DQ8 (177).

Associations have been described with late-onset pauciarticular JRA and HLA-B27. HLA-B27 typing has not been performed routinely by all pediatric rheumatologists because of low previous estimates in patients with juvenile arthritis. False-negative testing does occur by standard techniques, which is overcome by the increased sensitivity of DNA typing (178). Savolainen and co-workers (179) have reported that 27% of uncomplicated JRA patients in the Finnish population are HLA-B27 positive, whereas 44% of complicated (severe disease/worse outcome) JRA patients are HLA-B27 positive. The study population was primarily polyarticular, with fewer systemic JRA patients and very few pauciarticular patients.

DIFFERENTIAL DIAGNOSIS

This section does not develop an exhaustive roadmap for the differential diagnosis of JIA, but rather offers some insight into the complexity of the issue as well as some general directions.

Evaluation of a child with joint complaints is often a difficult challenge for a number of reasons:

1. The limited knowledge of parents about arthritis in children, perhaps limiting health care, with the common assumption that extremity pain is secondary to injury.
2. The typically limited exposure and training of pediatricians, family physicians, and adult rheumatologists about joint examination and arthritis in children.
3. The relative paucity of trained pediatric rheumatologists, with those board certified by the American Board of Pediatrics numbering 192, as of 2002.
4. The broad differential diagnosis of disease.
5. The typically minor and often transient complaints, such as the brief morning limp body habitus of the young child, i.e., the "chunky toddler," making assessment of joint swelling at least difficult by inspection, if not palpation.
6. The young child's lack of cooperation with the joint examination.
7. The lack of tests that are truly diagnostic.
8. The insensitivity of plain films and the high cost of more useful diagnostic imaging.

However, making the correct diagnosis is clearly important, so that disability from JIA and associated problems such as serositis and uveitis can be minimized. In addition, both the criteria for JIA as well as the health of the child necessitate that other etiologies of childhood arthritis be excluded, such as leukemia, inflammatory bowel disease, and septic arthritis. A nonexhaustive list, including categories of candidate illnesses with examples, is provided in Table 61.2. Pain amplification syndromes, such as reflex neurovascular dystrophy, fibromyalgia, and growing pains, are not included in the list (although important in the differential diagnosis of JIA) because they do not involve objectively verifiable arthritis. Of note, when children present urgently with arthritis without a history of recent trauma, McCarthy and colleagues (180) found that approximately 20% will have a serious bacterial infection; 20% a mechanical, noninflammatory disorder such as chondromalacia patellae; and 20% a rheumatic disease (the remainder will have viral or fungal illness, malignancy, or hematologic disorders). Thus, only a small minority of children presenting acutely with arthritis will have JIA.

TABLE 61.2. *Arthritis in children*

Rheumatologic diseases and associated conditions
Juvenile idiopathic arthritis
Dermatomyositis
Systemic lupus erythematosus
Mixed connective tissue disease
Systemic vasculitides
Henoch-Schönlein purpura
Polyarteritis nodosa
Scleroderma
Spondyloarthropathies
Juvenile ankylosing spondylitis
Inflammatory bowel disease
Psoriatic spondyloarthritis
Immunodeficiency diseases
Reactive arthritides
Rheumatic fever
Gram-negative associated diseases
Infectious arthritis
Bacterial, including staph, strep, lyme, tuberculosis
Viral
Epstein-Barr virus
Parvovirus
HIV
Rubella
Fungal
(Kawasaki disease)
Congenital musculoskeletal conditions
Lysosomal storage diseases
Chondrodysplasias and other disorders of bone and connective tissue
Neonatal-onset multisystem inflammatory disease (NOMID)
Acquired nonrheumatic musculoskeletal conditions
Traumatic arthritis
Legg-Perthes-Calvé disease
Toxic synovitis
Chondromalacia patellae
Osteochondritis dissecans
Hypertrophic pulmonary osteoarthropathy
Slipped femoral capital epiphysis
Osteoid osteoma
Hypermobility syndrome
Neoplastic diseases
Leukemia and lymphoma
Bone tumors
Ewing
Osteosarcoma
Histiocytosis
Neuroblastoma
Other diseases
Sickle cell disease
Hemophilia and other coagulopathies
Hypothyroidism
Sarcoidosis

A history of joint complaints from children should be taken seriously, because McCarthy et al. (180) found that 82% of such children have objective findings (Table 61.2). A history of joint swelling, pain, limited motion, and stiffness is important. In addition, care should be taken to detail any diffuse pain and pain or tenderness of extremities, even if not at a joint. Although the occurrence of a limp is an obvious and common concern, change or difficulty in the performance of any age-appropriate motor activities should also be investigated, such as walking, running, crawling, jumping, coloring, writing, buttoning, tying, eating, and holding a cup or spoon. Because most arthritis in children is posttraumatic or reactive, any report of injury, exposure, or infection in the preceding days to weeks is relevant. Data such as the pattern of arthritis (e.g., asymmetry, number of joints, migration) are helpful, as are the symptom duration, constancy (stable or intermittent), tempo, and responsiveness to intervention. Children with oligoarthritis are commonly asymptomatic after minutes of morning stiffness and limp. Although JIA may present with few or multiple joint involvement, children with oligoarthritis are more likely to have infectious, hematologic, or posttraumatic conditions, whereas the differential diagnosis for polyarthritis more typically includes other rheumatic, postinfectious (such as rheumatic fever), and lymphoproliferative diseases. Finally, it should be appreciated that joint pain reported by a young child is often far less than the physician-rated severity of disease on joint examination (181,182); thus, pain report is an important but sometimes insensitive indicator of JIA disease activity. It should be noted, however, that poor pain report methodology may be the problem, and use of instruments such as the Pediatric Pain Questionnaire may provide more valuable data (183). Finally, there may be associated problems that help define the cause of the child's joint complaints. Historical data concerning linear growth, weight loss or gain, gastrointestinal complaints, fever, weakness, and rash may be particularly helpful in clarifying the diagnosis.

Physical examination may also suggest a diagnosis, and attention should be directed to other systems in addition to the musculoskeletal examination. Fever in rheumatic diseases is often spiking and quotidian, as in systemic arthritis (184). Two thirds of children with rash and arthritis have rheumatic disease, and three fourths of children with fever and joint complaints have rheumatic disease or bacterial infection and almost never traumatic or other orthopedic conditions (180). As with adults, a child with acute arthritis should always be considered to have a bacterial infection until proven otherwise.

There are no diagnostic laboratory tests for JIA. The complete blood count and urinalysis, and a metabolic profile may provide information entirely consistent with—or unusual for—the diagnosis. Acute-phase reactants are inconsistently elevated in JIA, particularly in children with oligoarthritis, although they typically are quite elevated in systemic arthritis. Measurements of serum immunoglobulins and total hemolytic complement are often indicated in the evaluation of children with arthritis, because of the possibility of associated immunodeficiency. Since systemic arthritis is the cause of fever of unknown origin in only about 10% of children (185,186), extensive studies may be required to exclude diagnoses such as infection, leukemia, or inflammatory bowel disease. Such studies commonly include complete blood counts and liver function tests, bone marrow studies, chest films, abdominal ultrasonography or computed tomography (CT), bone scan, small or large bowel contrast studies, and endoscopy. Wallendal and co-workers (187) noted that lactate dehydrogenase levels are likely to be significantly higher in patients with malignancy compared to those with systemic arthritis, whereas uric acid levels were not different.

Referral patterns to the Pediatric Rheumatology Center at Texas Children's Hospital in Houston suggest that primary care physicians are using an ANA test to help determine their referral. Specifically, the great majority of children referred to rule out JRA have a positive ANA test, when in fact only about half of all JRA patients are ANA positive (188). Beyond the concern of the limited sensitivity of the test is the finding that perhaps 6% of normal children have a positive test result (188). Thus, ANA testing for the diagnosis of JIA is strongly discouraged, although it is relevant as a descriptor of disease, particularly because of the associated increased risk for uveitis in patients diagnosed with oligoarthritis.

Given that RF was shown to be present in only about 5% of children with JRA by Eichenfield and colleagues (189), it also is clearly a poor diagnostic test for the disease, although critical in the classification of JIA polyarthritis.

Diagnostic imaging plays an important role in the diagnosis of JIA, generally to help exclude other diagnoses, such as bone tumors and Legg-Calvé-Perthes disease. Lucent metaphyseal bands in the long bones of children over 2 years of age are suggestive but not diagnostic of leukemia (190). Bone scans and magnetic resonance imaging (MRI) might suggest a diagnosis of osteomyelitis. MRI might indicate that joint symptomatology is the result of intraarticular derangement. On the other hand, joint erosions on plain films at the time of diagnosis of JIA are extremely rare because a thick layer of nonossified growth cartilage lies beneath the thin articular cartilage of young children (190).

Again, even arthrocentesis does not give data diagnostic for JIA. Synovial fluid WBC counts in clinically active joints have been reported to range from 600 cells/mm^3 (191) to over 100,000 cells/mm^3 (192), although typical counts are about 10,000 cells/mm^3. Thus, synovial fluid WBC counts in JIA can be similar to those of patients with reactive arthritis, partially treated bacterial infections, and viral and fungal arthritis.

In sum, antecedent history (trauma, infection), history of morning stiffness and gelling, associated findings, documented arthritis, and arthrocentesis are often helpful in making a diagnosis of JIA, whereas ANA and RF data are typically useless. Referral to a pediatric rheumatologist should be strongly considered when chronic or severe signs and symptoms develop without a clear diagnosis. In addition, because of the large team of specialists usually required to care optimally for a child with rheumatic disease, referral is also appropriate for care management.

PRESENTATION AND COURSE

Systemic Arthritis

Ten percent to 15% of children with JRA (and presumably JIA) have systemic disease. The typical child with systemic arthritis is under 4 years of age (193,194) and previously healthy, and develops an explosive illness with high spiking fever, sometimes to 106°F, with an associated evanescent, pink rash, typically on the proximal extremities and trunk (Fig. 61.1). Lesions are often clustered, typically macular, and occasionally pruritic. The Koebner sign may be present. The rash typically disappears as fever abates, with body temperature often dropping to a subnormal range in the early morning in children treated with nonsteroidal antiinflammatory drugs (NSAIDs) (195). The rash is not diagnostic; similar exanthems can be seen with viral illnesses. Biopsies of the rash have shown only edema or mild perivascular infiltrates (196,197). Other common presenting systemic signs include fatigue, irritability, and drowsiness (198), myalgias (199), generalized adenopathy (with reactive hyperplasia on biopsy), and hepatosplenomegaly. Arthritis may occur along with these symptoms, or follow weeks to months later, making diagnosis quite difficult. Although patients with systemic arthritis are often uncomfortable, they only rarely have severe pain, a finding that should prompt consideration of malignancy (200). Many patients with systemic arthritis present with serositis; pericarditis occurs in more than 33% (201). Tamponade is a rare and life-threatening complication (202,203). Although many patients have pericarditis only at disease onset, some have recurrent attacks that last for weeks (204).

Patients with systemic arthritis commonly present with dramatic leukocytosis, typically with WBC counts of greater than 20,000; an often severe nonhemolytic anemia (e.g., hemoglobin levels <6 g/dL) with indices typical of chronic

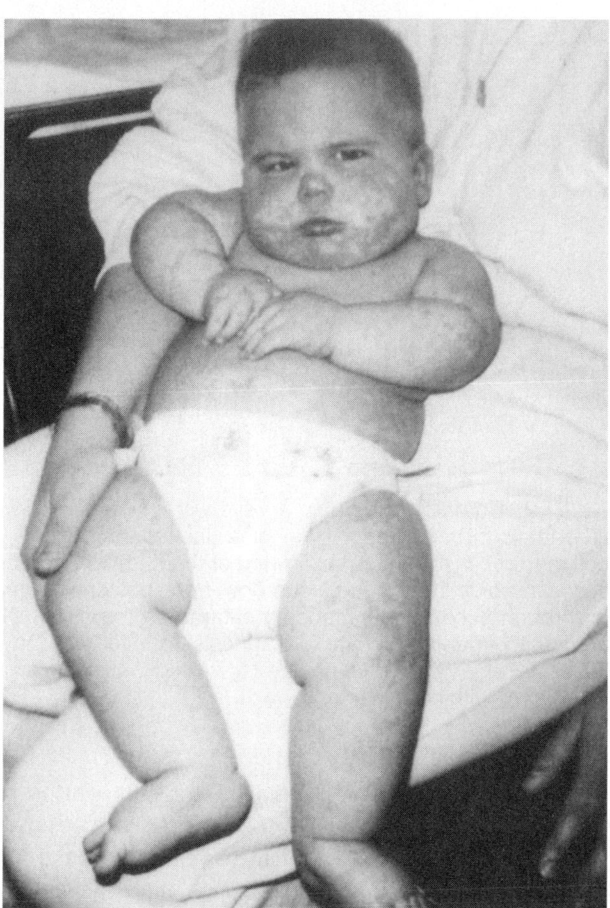

FIG. 61.1. The florid erythematous maculopapular rash of a child with systemic juvenile rheumatoid arthritis. This rash appeared with fever (daily spike to 103°F) and then faded.

disease; elevated ESR often greater than 100; and negative ANA and serum RF. Ferritin levels are often extremely high, particularly in older children (205). Platelet counts at presentation are typically elevated; a low platelet count, or even a normal platelet count in the face of a very elevated ESR, or other signs and symptoms of persistent inflammation, should be taken as prima facie evidence for either a different diagnosis (e.g. leukemia, sepsis) or systemic JRA complicated by disseminated intravascular coagulation (DIC). Mild coagulopathy in systemic arthritis is apparently common, since Bloom and co-workers (206) reported that 23 of 24 consecutive patients had elevated fibrin d-dimer levels, which correlated with fever and decreased with clinical symptomatology. However, a small fraction of patients develop macrophage activation syndrome (MAS, also called hemophagocytic syndrome or reactive hematophagocytic lymphohistiocytosis), typically but not necessarily early in their course (207,208). MAS is a life-threatening disease. Children with MAS typically became acutely ill with moderate to severe DIC (thrombocytopenia, elevated d-dimers and fibrin split products, low fibrinogen, and prolonged prothrombin time and partial thromboplastin time), a decreasing ESR, severe anemia and leukopenia, and liver dysfunction (including low albumin and elevated transaminases) (209). Bone marrow aspirate/biopsy characteristically reveals active phagocytosis by macrophages and histiocytes. MAS has also been reported in children with polyarthritis, and has been associated with Epstein-Barr virus (EBV) infection (210).

Although systemic symptoms generally resolve within a year of presentation, some patients have flare-ups of systemic signs thereafter, whereas a few others continue to have nearly continuous fever and rash. Up to 50% of systemic arthritis patients evolve into a chronic polyarthritis, and in up to 25% of patients the arthritis is erosive, particularly in the hip (211). This disease is indistinguishable clinically from polyarticular JIA. On the other hand, van der Net and co-workers (212) reported only mild disability in most children with a mean disease duration of nearly 6 years. This contrasts to a report from Taiwan in which 43% of patients with systemic JRA had a chronic arthritis, and a total of 24% had a severe destructive polyarthritis (213). Two recent comparable studies, using Kaplan-Meier curves, estimated 10-year remission rates of 37% to 38% for this JRA subset (214,215). Late relapses after prolonged disease remissions have been noted to occur in 34% of patients after a mean remission period of 9 years (216). Although the mortality rate for JRA as a whole is reported in the United States as less than 1%, the 15-year survival rate for systemic JRA has been reported as only 86% (217).

Other complications noted among patients with systemic arthritis include carditis, with reports of aortic valve regurgitation (218); hepatitis (possibly partially attributable to sensitivity to NSAIDs); anemia in nearly 40% (219); and infection and sepsis, secondary to therapy or MAS. Anemia may be secondary to iron deficiency and high IL-6 levels, interfering with iron delivery (220); to decreased erythropoietin levels (221); or to erythropoietin insensitivity. Uveitis is rare, although yearly screening is still suggested. Amyloidosis is rarely seen in the United States, but curiously is reported in about 5% of patients in Europe (222,223). Systemic growth failure is reported in children with other forms of JIA, and is common in patients with systemic disease (224,225), although catch-up growth may occur with disease control or remission. Evaluation of growth is discussed in detail below.

Oligoarthritis

Children meeting the JIA criteria for oligoarthritis, in both the persistent and extended subcategories, generally fit the old JRA criteria for type I pauciarticular JRA (226). This group comprised about 35% of all JRA patients. Children with persistent oligoarthritis continue to have arthritis in four or fewer joints, even after the first 6 months of disease, whereas children with extended oligoarthritis have more than four joints affected over time. Studies of all children with pauciarticular JRA indicate that up to 20% of that group evolve into a polyarticular course of disease (227); extrapolation would thus suggest that persistent oligoarthritis is much more common than the extended variety.

The typical child with oligoarthritis is a girl, presenting in early childhood. The disease typically begins at 1 to 4 years of age, and uncommonly after age 7 (228). Systemic signs and symptoms are absent. Arthritis typically occurs in large joints, with the knee most commonly involved initially (229). Sharma and Sherry (230) reported that other joint disease, in order of occurrence after the knees, involves ankles, fingers, toes, wrists, elbows, and hips, respectively. The occurrence of early small joint involvement suggests either extended oligoarthritis or another diagnosis (e.g., psoriatic arthritis, which is not excluded from this category because of the absence of psoriasis in the child and family at the time of diagnosis of JIA). Presentation of oligoarthritis at the hip is distinctly unusual, and should engender consideration of other diagnoses. In a recent study of pauciarthritis patients, 68% were ANA positive (230). All should be RF negative.

With no reported increased mortality risk for oligoarthritis, the principal complications are articular and periarticular damage, and chronic uveitis; these complications need have no temporal correlation (231). Although commonly perceived as having little permanent impact on the child, likely because the inflammatory phase typically ends before adulthood, Cassidy and Martel (232) reported in 1977 that 25% of children with JRA oligoarthritis had cartilage and bone destruction in the involved joints, changes that are more obvious on MRI. A more recent longitudinal study (233), noted joint erosion in 35%. In addition, contractures and local growth abnormalities occur, particularly in young patients (234) with periarticular osteoporosis or local bone overgrowth (232). The latter often leads to longer leg length on the side of the affected knee. Finally, only about 20% of patients with oligoarthritis remit within 5 years (235). These outcomes have led recently to more aggressive therapy, including long-acting intraarticular steroid injections.

Children at greatest risk for chronic anterior uveitis include young girls who are ANA positive (236) and HLA-DR5 positive (237). Two studies have shown that the overall prevalence of uveitis among oligoarthritis patients was 15% (230,238) whereas Guillaume et al. (233) noted this ophthalmologic complication in as many as 35% of 207 children followed for at least 6 years. Although uveitis is classically associated with redness of the eye, photophobia, and eye pain, children with oligoarthritis and their parents often report no symptoms, even when permanent ocular damage has occurred (239), thus leading to visual loss. Findings on routine ophthalmologic examination may include scleral redness, limbic suffusion, irregular pupil, hypopion, cataract, and decreased visual acuity. Unfortunately, many children with significant uveitis have no findings except on slit-lamp examination (Fig. 61.2). Thus, routine slit-lamp examination is suggested as frequently as every 3 months for the high-risk group, and every 6 months for polyarthritis patients (239). Despite care, 21% of patients have recurrent attacks of uveitis lasting more than 10 years (239), and 11% of children with uveitis develop visual impairment (238). Earlier studies reported far more dismal results (239), with severe visual loss in 26% of affected eyes.

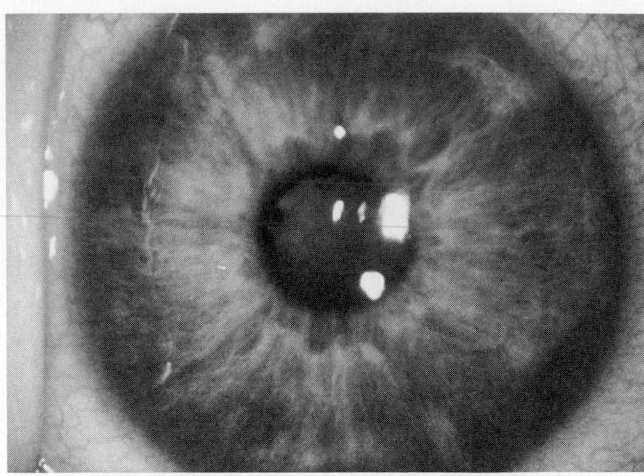

FIG. 61.2. Chronic changes in an eye with juvenile rheumatoid arthritis iritis: posterior synechiae (iris-lens adhesions at pupil margin); iris bombe (shallowing of the anterior chamber caused by blockage of aqueous flow from posterior chamber through pupil); and secondary cataract. (From Hiles DA. Slide atlas of pediatric physical diagnosis. In: Zitelli BJ, Davis HW, eds. *Pediatric ophthalmology.* New York: Gower Medical, 1987:17.15, with permission.)

Polyarthritis

Polyarthritis affects about 30% to 40% of children with JRA and perhaps the same percentage of JIA patients; approximately 75% of patients are girls, with onset peaks at 1 to 3 and 8 to 10 years of age (240). Children with either RF-positive or -negative polyarthritis typically present with mild systemic signs and symptoms, including fatigue, low-grade fever, minimal if any weight loss, and mild anemia. Uveitis is uncommon in this group, but still reported in 5% (238), and thus screening every 6 months by slit-lamp examination is recommended (239). The arthritis may be symmetric at onset, involving multiple large and small joints (Fig. 61.3), but more commonly the disease begins in a few joints, and then evolves over a few months as an additive polyarthritis. In fact, an explosive polyarthritis is more consistent with reactive disease.

Over time, involvement of the cervical spine can lead to fusion, C1–2 subluxation, and rarely to spinal cord symptomatology from impingement (Fig. 61.4). Temporomandibular joint disease is associated with micrognathia (241) secondary to local growth defects and joint destruction, and can lead to associated headache and poor glutition (242). Hip disease can also be particularly severe, and require joint replacement even before age 20.

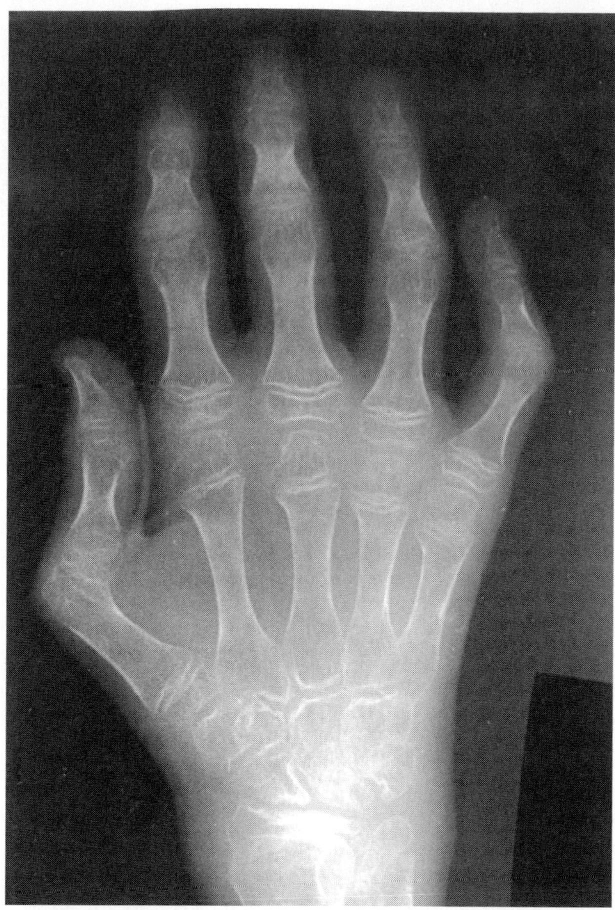

FIG. 61.3. Hand radiograph in a 9-year-old girl with juvenile rheumatoid arthritis (JRA). Note the severe osteopenia with very thin metacarpal cortices. The medullary space is relatively wide. Severe osteopenia is common in severe JRA. The carpals are also very irregular, and there are erosions in the carpals, distal radius, metacarpal-carpal joint, and metacarpophalangeal joint. There is subluxation of the first metacarpophalangeal joint and bulbous enlargement of the distal ends of both the proximal and middle phalanges. The epiphysis of the proximal phalanx of the index finger is irregular, and there is narrowing of that joint space.

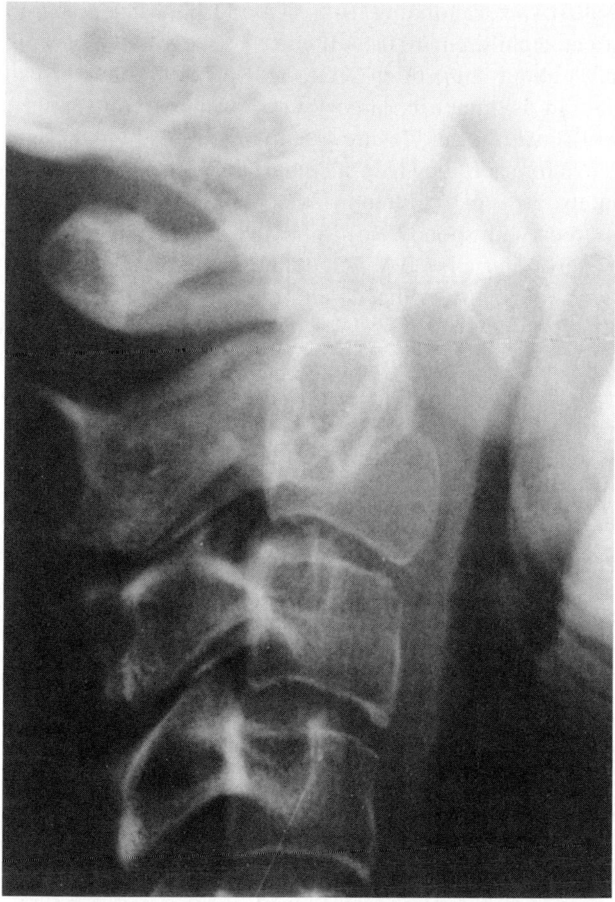

FIG. 61.4. Flexion lateral radiograph of the cervical spine showing C1–2 subluxation in a 15-year-old girl with juvenile rheumatoid arthritis. The separation between the odontoid and the anterior arch of the atlas was not apparent in films taken in the neutral position. This is an important complication because subluxation can compress the spinal cord. The normal distance between the anterior arch of the atlas and the odontoid should not exceed 5 mm. Here it was 7 mm.

Rheumatoid Factor–Negative Disease

Twenty-five percent to 35% of children with JIA have RF-negative polyarthritis. Importantly, this illness is clinically distinct from RF-positive disease; children who are RF negative are younger and they rarely become RF positive later in the course of the disease. Severe, erosive, and unremitting arthritis has been reported in approximately 15% of patients (243). Extraarticular manifestations of disease are uncommon, although rheumatoid nodules are occasionally appreciated. Approximately 25% of children with RF-negative disease are ANA positive (244). Given the clinical course and immunogenetic findings, it may well be that at least some children with extended oligoarthritis, and others with RF-negative polyarthritis, have the same disease.

Rheumatoid Factor–Positive Disease

This disease accounts for only about 5% of all children with JIA. It is apparently identical to adult RA. RF-positive polyarthritis in children is associated with an approximate 50% risk for a severe and deforming arthritis (243), with poorer functional outcome, sometimes with rheumatoid nodules (245) and vasculitis, although the latter is quite rare in children. Rheumatoid nodules in children with JIA are indistinguishable from those of adults with RA and of children with benign rheumatoid nodulosis (246). About half of patients with RF-positive polyarthritis are ANA positive.

Enthesitis-Related Arthritis

Although this condition is discussed in more detail elsewhere in this text in the context of HLA-B27-associated diseases (see Chapters 63–66), some comment is appropriate here. Enthesitis-related arthritis represents 15% to 20%

of all JIA, extrapolating from JRA and JCA data (247,248). Affected children are usually over 8 years of age, generally male (about 4:1), often HLA-B27 positive, and typically have an asymmetric, large joint, lower extremity arthritis (249). Juvenile ankylosing spondylitis (JAS), with clear evidence for sacroiliac (SI; or spinal) disease, affects approximately 20% of children with spondyloarthropathy (200). Children with spondyloarthropathies are clearly included in the new criteria for JIA, with enthesitis as a major criterion, and the recognition that SI and inflammatory spinal symptomatology may also occur.

The typical child at presentation is a teenage boy with a swollen knee. The hip may also be affected early in the course. Complaints of low back pain, particularly in the morning, difficulty sitting and standing for long periods, and poor sleep are common, as are complaints of other joint pain. Examination reveals enthesitis, particularly patellar or calcaneal. Bursal or large joint swelling is often painless. Radiographs of the SI joints are typically normal in children at presentation, but bone scans may be positive, and contrast-enhanced MRI of the SI joints may be helpful (250). Complete blood count and ESR are rarely significantly abnormal. HLA-B27 is present in about 60% of patients with spondyloarthropathy, and the great majority with JAS (200); however, as is clear from the new classification criteria, HLA-B27 neither establishes nor negates the diagnosis.

This disease may be complicated by progressive axial skeletal disease and deformity. Children with HLA-B27 and evidence for spinal limitation (positive Schober test) are at greatest risk, with nearly 20% developing definite sacroiliitis at 5 years (251). Children with JAS have a low prevalence of mild mitral or aortic regurgitation, as do adults (252). Acute anterior uveitis occurs in about 10% to 25% of children with JAS (253,254), with HLA-B27-positive children presumably at greatest risk. Finally, arthritis, initially classified as enthesitis-related arthritis may precede a diagnosis of psoriasis or inflammatory bowel disease by months to years.

Psoriatic Arthritis

Psoriatic arthritis is addressed elsewhere in this text (see Chapter 65). It should be noted, however, that arthritis precedes a diagnosis of psoriasis in 40% to 50% of children ultimately diagnosed with psoriatic arthritis (255,256).

Other Arthritis

There are children with JIA who do not fit the rules of classification, such as the occasional child with apparent enthesitis-related arthritis who later develops an erosive RF-positive polyarthritis. Similarly, there are children classified now as having persistent or extended oligoarthritis who do not meet criteria for psoriatic disease but will later develop psoriasis, and have compatible joint findings (e.g., "pencil and cup" radiologic findings of phalangeal joints sometimes seen in psoriatic arthritis).

EVALUATION OF DISEASE ACTIVITY AND PROGRESSION IN JUVENILE IDIOPATHIC ARTHRITIS PATIENTS AND POPULATIONS

Quantitative Joint Evaluations, and Functional and Quality of Life Assessment Tools

At a time when the therapeutic options for children with JIA are becoming increasingly complex, instruments that assist in the objective serial evaluation of arthritis in individual children (and populations) with JIA are very important. Instruments for this purpose include the Juvenile Arthritis Functional Status Index (257), Juvenile Arthritis Functional Assessment Scale (258), the parent- or child-completed Juvenile Arthritis Functional Assessment Report (259), and, most recently, the JRA Core Set Criteria (260,261). The latter criteria include active joint count, limitation of motion, physician and parent/patient global assessments, functional assessment, and ESR, with an improvement defined as greater than 30% improvement in at least three of six criteria with a greater than 30% worsening in no more than one criterion. Other investigators have shown that the physician and parent global assessment instruments are more sensitive to change in JCA patients than articular variables, morning stiffness, ESR, and CRP (262).

More complex instruments that provide deeper insight into functional status and child quality of life include the Functional Status II (R) Measure (263), the Childhood Health Assessment Questionnaire (CHAQ) (264), the more recently developed Childhood Health Questionnaire (265), and the Juvenile Arthritis Quality-of-Life Questionnaire (JAQQ) (266). The JAQQ may prove particularly valuable because it has been shown to be sensitive to changes observed in reported pain and physician global assessment. The Impact on Family Scale (267) is particularly useful in elucidating the effect of chronic illness on family function. All of these instruments may be used serially, but the CHAQ has not been shown to be sensitive to change for patients with oligoarticular JCA (268).

Growth and Maturation

Tracking of local growth disturbance, typically bony overgrowth near an affected joint of a growing child, is best accomplished by radiographic studies as discussed below. Systemic growth disturbances, usually resulting in short stature (269) or delayed puberty (270), are common among children with systemic arthritis and polyarthritis. Both linear height and menarche should be followed. In addition, however, there are other factors that may lead to poor or delayed growth and maturation. Nutrition evaluations are often pertinent, because protein-calorie malnutrition has been reported (271), as well as various vitamin and mineral abnormalities (272). Delayed skeletal maturation may also reflect treatment with steroids (e.g., with inhibitory effect on osteoblastic activity as indicated by serum osteocalcin) (273,274), but may also relate to endocrine abnormalities, which may also be tracked. Production of insulin-like growth factor-1 is diminished in JRA, and corrected with recombinant human growth hormone treatment, which results in a dose-dependent increase in height velocity (275, 276). Bone and cartilage growth are certainly affected by cytokines, such as TNF-α. Pepmueller and colleagues (277) found that osteocalcin and bone-derived alkaline phosphatase, both markers for bone formation, were low in JRA patients, and inversely related to disease activity. Percera and colleagues found increased urinary excretion of biochemical markers of bone turnover such as deoxypyridinoline, and hydroxyproline (278), which are measures of increased bone resorption. Bone mineral density is lower than expected in JRA patients, even among those never treated with steroids, and correlates inversely with disease severity and disability (279). Young adults who suffered from JRA as children but whose disease is inactive may attain normal bone mineral density eventually; however, if JRA remains active into adulthood, then increased risk for osteopenia and osteoprosis may occur (280).

LABORATORY STUDIES

Laboratory studies are not particularly helpful in tracking JIA disease activity and progression. There is no relationship between ANA titer or pattern, or with RF titer and disease severity. Similarly, the ESR bears only a weak relationship to clinical disease activity, except in systemic disease (281–283); CRP has similarly been reported to be of little additional value in JRA (284,285). Although common in systemic arthritis and polyarthritis, mild anemia is an insensitive indicator of joint disease activity. Serum and urine neopterin may be helpful, but remain primarily research tools.

DIAGNOSTIC IMAGING

Pediatric rheumatologists vary in their protocols, if any, for serial diagnostic imaging assessments for children with JIA. Pertinent observations include the following:

1. A small percentage of children with polyarthritis will have "dry" arthritis, that is, progressive erosive arthritis without significant joint swelling or pain. Thus, clinical indicators for radiographic study may be limited in these patients.
2. The advent of MRI has clearly demonstrated that significant articular and growth cartilage damage sometimes occurs, even in patients with oligoarthritis, when unexpected on plain films. This reflects the fact that damage to noncalcified growth cartilage, which underlies articular cartilage in growing children, cannot be visualized on plain film. If healing does not occur, such damage could result in obvious erosions as the skeleton matures.
3. MRI studies are not only expensive, but generally require at least conscious sedation of young children, with its

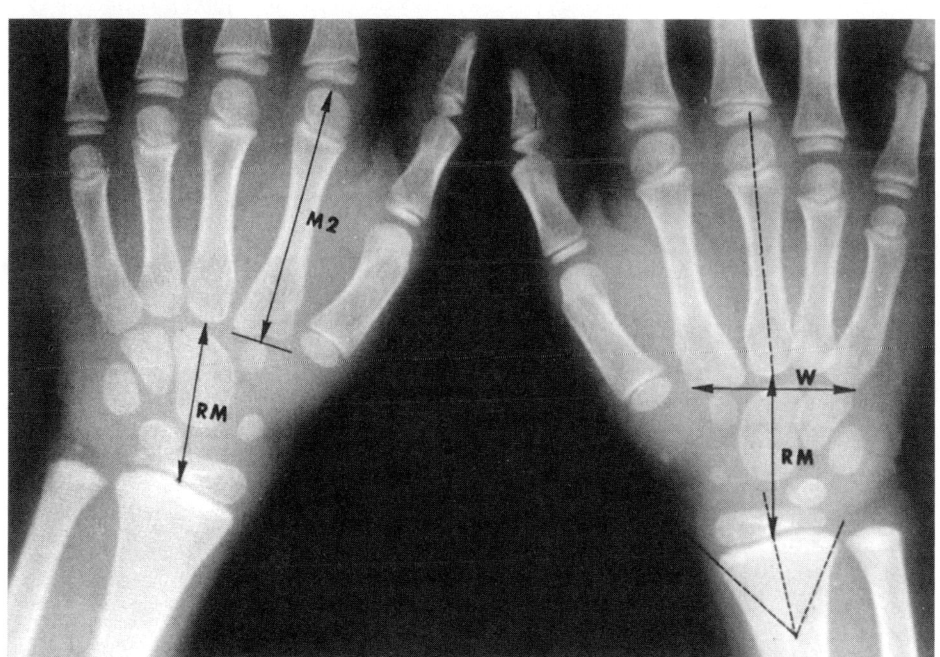

FIG. 61.5. Hand measurements used to evaluate carpal size in children. Radiometacarpal length (*RM*) is measured from the base of the third metacarpal to the middle of the radial growth plate, whereas the second metacarpal length (*M2*) is the maximum length of the second metacarpal. The RM can also be compared to the width (*W*). (From Poznanski AK, Hernandez RJ, Guire KE, et al. Carpal length in children—a useful measurement in the diagnosis of rheumatoid arthritis and some congenital malformation syndromes. *Radiology* 1978;129:661–668, with permission.)

associated risk. Thus, a thoughtful cost-benefit analysis is necessary.

4. Particularly for children with oligoarthritis, who have not historically been treated with aggressive therapies (such as methotrexate), the demonstration of destructive, and certainly progressive, joint disease might lead to the use of such therapies, and potentially better outcomes, although their use is associated with higher health risks from adverse effects of additional medication.

With these perspectives in mind, at least yearly plain films of affected and inflamed joints of children with polyarthritis and extended oligoarthritis seem reasonable. Some rheumatologists survey all joints in such patients as frequently as every 6 months. Although the intent of this discussion is not to develop a treatise on radiographic findings in JIA, particularly since radiographic study of joints is discussed in detail elsewhere in this text (see Chapter 6), there are some observations and techniques that are particularly relevant to childhood arthritis:

1. Periarticular bone size and shape should be compared with age-appropriate norms in the growing child, and compared with the unaffected side, in asymmetric joint disease. Such comparisons are particularly relevant for the hand and knee (286,287).

2. Serial assessments of carpal size and length by plain film, a technique pioneered by Poznanski and colleagues (288), is explained in Fig. 61.5, and serial data are presented for a child with JRA in Fig. 61.6. Such data indicate

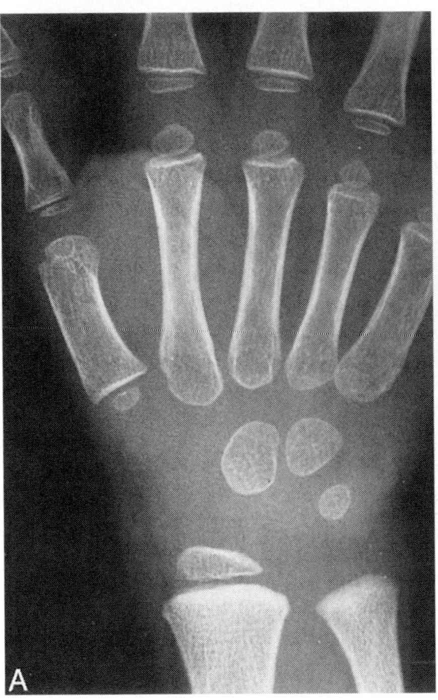

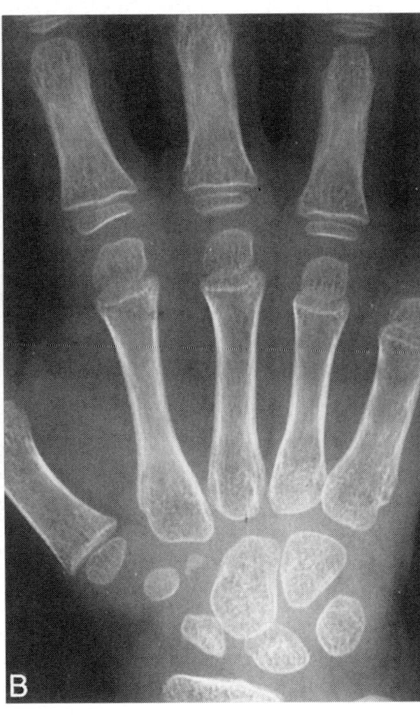

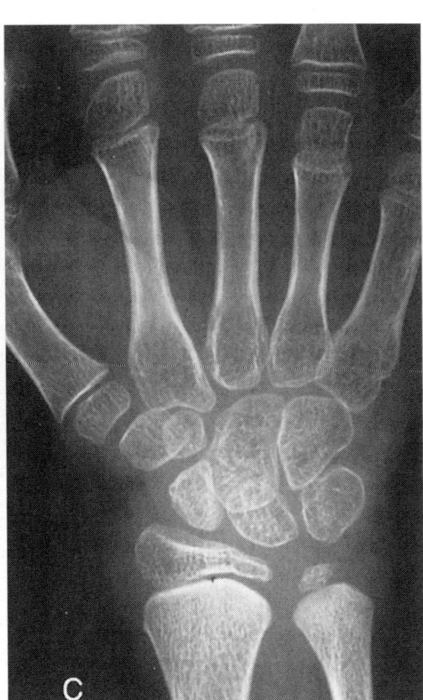

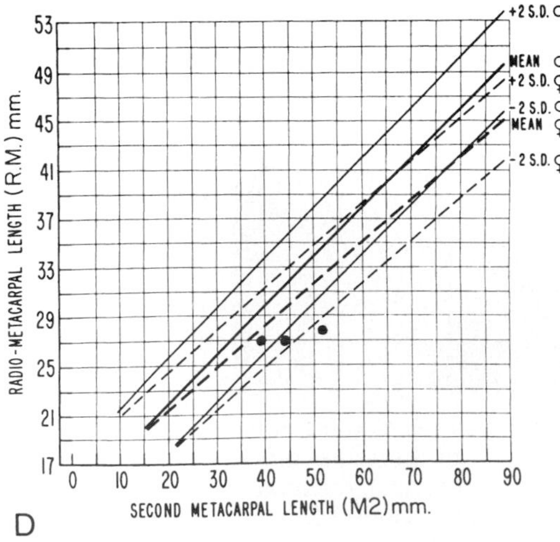

FIG. 61.6. Three consecutive films of a girl with juvenile rheumatoid arthritis at ages 2 years 3 months **(A)**, 4 years 9 months **(B)**, and 6 years 9 months **(C)**, and a chart of the normal relationship between RM and M2 for boys and girls **(D)**. There is little evidence of carpal disease in **A**; somewhat close carpals are seen in **B** and **C**. Plotted on the normal curves, the carpals clearly have not grown. On the last image the carpus is well below the 2 standard deviation line for girls. (From Poznanski AK, Conway JJ, Shkolnik A, et al. Radiological approaches in the evaluation of joint disease in children. *Rheum Dis Clin North Am* 1987;13:57–73, with permission.)

that significant erosive disease has occurred over time. Poznanski et al. (289) have also applied this technique to evaluation of knee disease.

3. Leg length discrepancy is best evaluated by CT, particularly in the face of a knee flexion contracture (290). Objective measurement of the leg length discrepancy may be plotted by observing the leg length discrepancy via CT scan every 6 months (291).

4. Serial flexion and extension views of the cervical spine to rule out atlantoaxial subluxation are commonly obtained in children with active polyarthritis (Fig. 61.4).

5. The value of serial MRI studies with contrast has been discussed above. T1-weighted MRI with fat suppression postcontrast may be particularly helpful. Inflamed synovial tissue gives a high signal with gadolinium, as opposed to normal synovium (292–294) (Figs. 61.7 and 61.8).

6. Dual-photon absorptiometry is becoming increasingly important in the ongoing evaluation of bone loss, particularly in JIA patients with systemic and polyarticular subtypes treated with steroids.

7. Ultrasonography can reveal synovial fluid that is not clinically evident, as shown by Sureda and colleagues (295) in 22% of 36 JRA patients.

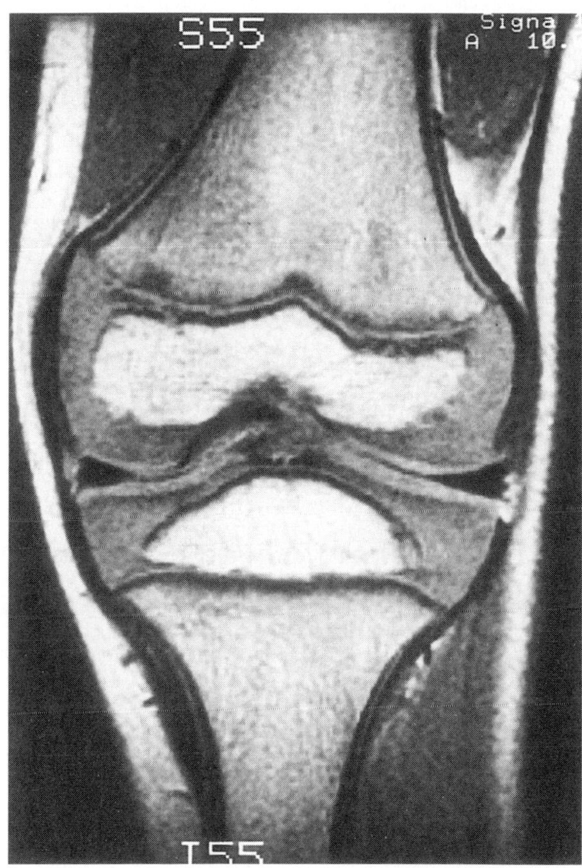

FIG. 61.7. Normal knee in a 4-year-old boy. Magnetic resonance imaging with T1 weighting. The epiphyseal centers have high signal *(white)* because they contain fatty marrow. Note the thick cartilage covering them *(gray)*. This represents the growth cartilage. This, in turn, is covered by a thin layer of articular cartilage *(lighter gray)*. The presence of the thick cartilage over the osseus portion is the reason that bony erosion is a late finding in juvenile rheumatoid arthritis, because much cartilage must be destroyed before bone is affected. The menisci are well-formed *(black triangles)*.

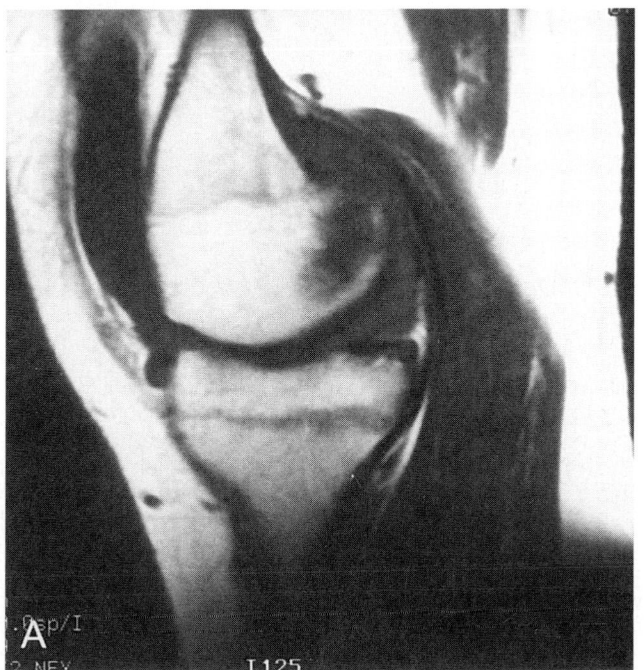

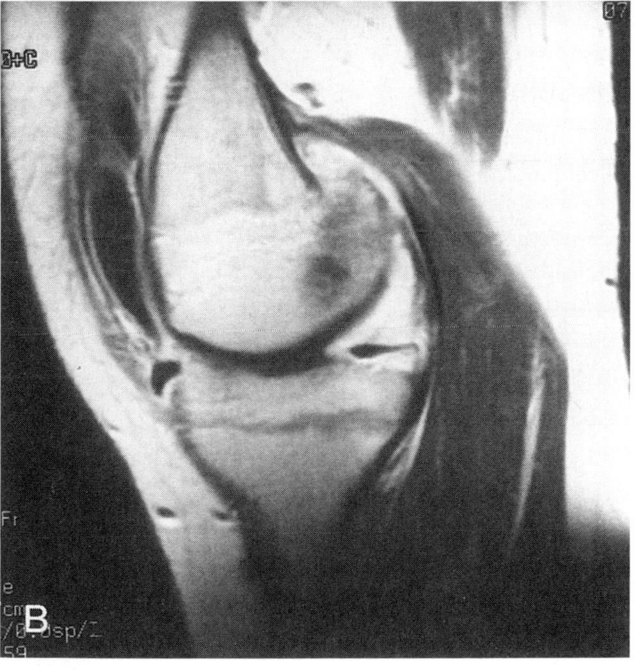

FIG. 61.8. Synovitis and synovial effusion in the knee of a 15-year-old girl with juvenile rheumatoid arthritis (JRA). **A:** A sagittal T1-weighted magnetic resonance image. **B:** T1-weighted after gadolinium injection. *Continued*

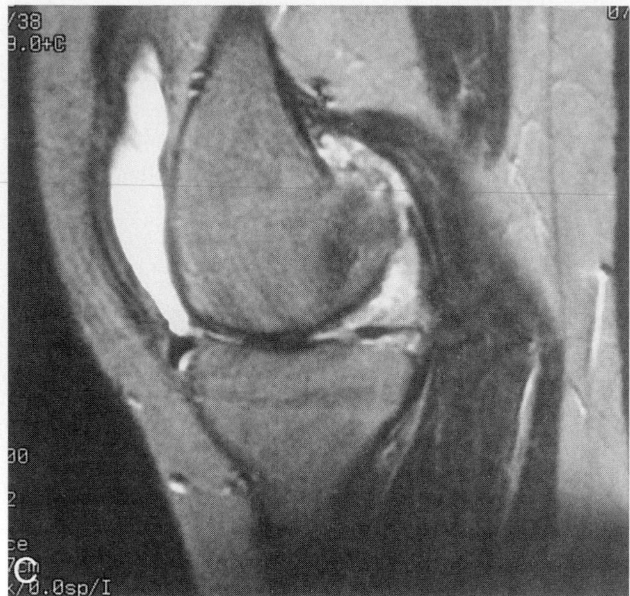

FIG. 61.8. *Continued* **C:** T2-weighted image showing high signal areas *(white)* in the suprapatellar pouch anteriorly and in the posterior part of the knee joint as well. There is some irregularity of the high signal areas, which may represent some pannus. However, it is not possible to determine which part of the high signal is fluid and which is synovitis. This distinction can be made by comparing the pre- **(A)** and post- **(B)** gadolinium images. On the postcontrast study **(B)** the hypervascular inflamed synovium is enhanced (appears *white*). There is enhancement around the joint effusion, which has a low signal *(black)* on T1 weighting, and there is inflamed synovium posteriorly. There is also enhancement around the menisci, which appear small and deformed, a common finding in JRA.

CONCLUSION

JIA (previously designated JRA in the United States) is a collection of distinct illnesses, linked principally by the phenomenology of idiopathic joint disease in children. Consequently, we can expect that focused clinical and basic research will lead to further differentiation of subcategories of JIA, and then to a clearer picture of etiology and optimal therapy. A discussion of therapy for JIA follows in Chapter 62.

ACKNOWLEDGMENTS

This work was supported in part by grants from the Gulf Coast Chapter of the Arthritis Foundation.

REFERENCES

1. Buikstra JE, Poznanski A, Cerna ML, et al. A case of juvenile rheumatoid arthritis from pre-Columbian Peru: a life in science. In: Builskra JE, ed. *Papers in honor of J. Lawrence Angel.* Kampsville, IL: Center for American Archeology, 1990:99.
2. Cronil V. Memoire sur le coincidences pathologiques du rheumatisme articulaire chronique. *C R Soc Biol (Paris)* 1864;4:2–25.
3. Diamant-Berger S. *Du rheumatisme noueux (polyarthrite deformante) che les enfants.* Paris: Lecrosnier et Babe, 1891:1–148.
4. Levinson JE, Wallace CA. Dismantling the pyramid. *J Rheumatol* 1992;19(suppl 33):6–10.
5. David J, Cooper C, Hickey L, et al. The functional and psychological outcomes of juvenile chronic arthritis in young adulthood. *Br J Rheumatol* 1994;33:876–881.
6. Flato B, Aasland A, Vinje O, et al. Outcome and predictive factors in juvenile rheumatoid arthritis and juvenile spondyloarthropathy. *J Rheumatol* 1998;25:366–375.
7. Peterson LS, Mason T, Nelson AM, et al. Psychosocial outcomes and health status of adults who have had juvenile rheumatoid arthritis. *Arthritis Rheum* 1997;40:2235–2240.
8. Baum J, Gutowska G. Death in juvenile rheumatoid arthritis. *Arthritis Rheum* 1977;20:253.
9. VanVujm IH, Hoyeraal HM, Fagertun H. Chronic family difficulties and stress life events in recent onset juvenile arthritis. *J Rheumatol* 1989;16:1088–1092.
10. Sturge C, Garralda ME, Boissin M, et al. School attendance and juvenile chronic arthritis. *Br J Rheumatol* 1997;36:1218–1223.
11. Olson DH, Sprenkle D, Russell C. Circumplex model of marital and family systems. I. Cohesion and adaptability dimensions. *Family Process* 1979;18:3–28.
12. McAnarney ER, Pless BI, Satterwhite B, et al. Psychological problems of children with chronic juvenile arthritis. *Pediatrics* 1974;53:523–528.
13. Brewer EJ, Base JC, Cassidy JT, et al. Criteria for the classification of juvenile rheumatoid arthritis. *Bull Rheum Dis* 1973;23:712–719.
14. Brewer EJ, Bass J, Cassidy JT, et al. Current proposed revision of JRA criteria. *Arthritis Rheum* 1977;20:195–199.
15. Jacobs JC. *Pediatric rheumatology for the practitioner,* 2nd ed. New York: Springer-Verlag, 1993.
16. Cassidy JT. What's in a name? Nomenclature of juvenile arthritis. A North American View. *J Rheumatol* 1993;20(suppl 40):4–8.
17. Prieur A-M, Kaufman MT, Griscelli C, et al. What's in a name? Nomenclature of juvenile arthritis. A European view. *J Rheumatol* 1993;20(suppl 40):9.
18. Petty RE, Southwood TR, Baum J, et al. Revision of the proposed classification criteria for juvenile idiopathic arthritis: Durban 1997. *J Rheumatol* 1998;10:1991–1994.
19. Towner SR, Michael CJ Jr, O'Fallon WM, et al. The epidemiology of juvenile arthritis in Rochester, Minnesota 1960–1979. *Arthritis Rheum* 1983;26:1208–1213.
20. Kunnamo I, Kallio P, Pelkonen P. Incidence of arthritis in urban Finnish children: a prospective study. *Arthritis Rheum* 1986;29:1232–1238.
21. Gewanter HL, Baum J. The frequency of juvenile arthritis. *J Rheumatol* 1989;16:556–557.
22. Cassidy JT, Nelson AM. The frequency of juvenile arthritis [Editorial]. *J Rheumatol* 1988;15:535–536.
23. Pless IB, Satterwhite B, Van Vechten D. Chronic illness in childhood: a regional survey of care. *Pediatrics* 1976;58:37–46.
24. Towner SR, Michet CJ, O'Fallon WM, et al. The epidemiology of juvenile arthritis in Rochester, Minnesota 1960–1979. *Arthritis Rheum* 1983;26:1208–1213.
25. Kiessling U, Doring E, Listing J, et al. Incidence and prevalence of juvenile chronic arthritis in East Berlin 1980–1988. *J Rheumatol* 1998;25:1837–1843.
26. Manners PJ, Diepeveen DA. Prevalence of juvenile chronic arthritis in a population of 12-year-old children in urban Australia. *Pediatrics* 1996;98:84–90.
27. Peterson LS, Mason T, Nelson AM, et al. Juvenile rheumatoid arthritis in Rochester, Minnesota 1960–1993: is the epidemiology changing? *Arthritis Rheum* 1996;39:1385–1390.
28. Anderson GB, Fasth A, Andersson J, et al. Incidence and prevalence of juvenile chronic arthritis: a population survey. *Ann Rheum Dis* 1987;46:277–281.
29. Tower SR, Michet CJ, O'Fallon WM, et al. The epidemiology of juvenile rheumatoid arthritis in Rochester, Minnesota 1960–79. *Arthritis Rheum* 1983;26:1208–1213.
30. Gare A, Fasth A, Anderson J, et al. Incidence and prevalence of juvenile chronic arthritis: a population survey. *Ann Rheum Dis* 1987;45:277.
31. Kunnamo I, Kallio P, Pelkonen P. Incidence of arthritis in urban Finnish children. *Arthritis Rheum* 1986;29:1232–1238.
32. Sullivan DB, Cassidy JT, Petty RE. Pathogenic implication of age of onset in juvenile rheumatoid arthritis. *Arthritis Rheum* 1975;18:251–255.

33. Hanson H, Kornreich HK, Bernstein B, et al. Three subtypes of juvenile rheumatoid arthritis: correlations of age at onset, sex, and serologic factors. *Arthritis Rheum* 1977;20(suppl):184.
34. Sullivan DB, Cassidy JT, Petty RE. Pathogenic implications of age of onset in juvenile rheumatoid arthritis. *Arthritis Rheum* 1975;18:251–255.
35. Lawrence RC, Hochberg MC, Kelsey JL, et al. Estimates of the prevalence of selected arthritic and musculoskeletal diseases in the United States. Report of the National Arthritis Data Workgroup. *J Rheumatol* 1989;16:427–441.
36. Schwartz MM, Simpson P, Kerr KL, et al. Juvenile rheumatoid arthritis in African Americans. *J Rheumatol* 1997;24:1826–1829.
37. Cimaz CG, Fink CW. The articular prognosis of pauciarticular onset juvenile arthritis is not influenced by the presence of uveitis. *J Rheumatol* 1996;23:257–359.
38. Romano G, Sironi M, Toniatti C, et al. Role of IL-6 and its soluble receptor in induction of chemokinins and leukocyte recruitment. *Immunity* 1997;6:315–325.
39. Prieur AM, LeGall E, Karman F. Epidemiologic survey of juvenile chronic arthritis. *Clin Exp Rheumatol* 1987;5:217–223.
40. Anderson Gäre B, Fasth A. The natural history of juvenile chronic arthritis: a population based cohort study: I. Onset and disease process. *J Rheumatol* 1995;22:295–307.
41. Arguedas O, Porras O, Fasth A. Juvenile chronic arthritis in Costa Rica: a pilot referral study. *Clin Exp Rheumatol* 1995;13:119–123.
42. Pongpanich B, Daengroongroj P. Juvenile rheumatoid arthritis: clinical characteristics in 100 Thai patients. *Clin Rheumatol* 1988;7:257–261.
43. Aggrawal A, Mistra R. Juvenile chronic arthritis in India: is it different from that seen in Western countries? *Rheumatol Int* 1994:14;53–56.
44. Haffejee IE, Raga J, Coovadia HM. Juvenile chronic arthritis in black and Indian South African children. *Sa Mediese Tydyskrif* 1984;65: 510–514.
45. Oen K, Schroeder P, Jacobson K et al. Juvenile rheumatoid arthritis in a Canadian First Nations (aboriginal) population: onset subtypes and HLA associations. *J Rheumatol* 1998;25:783–790.
46. Cassidy JT, Petty RE. *Juvenile rheumatoid arthritis. Textbook of pediatric rheumatology,* 3rd ed. Philadelphia: WB Saunders, 1995:138.
47. Heisel JS. Life changes as etiologic factors in juvenile rheumatoid arthritis. *J Psychosom Res* 1972;16:411–442.
48. Phillips PE. Evidence implicating infectious agents in rheumatoid arthritis and juvenile rheumatoid arthritis. *Clin Exp Rheumatol* 1988; 6:87–94.
49. Sieper J, Braun J, Doring E, et al. Aetiological role of bacteria associated with reactive arthritis in pauciarticular juvenile chronic arthritis. *Ann Rheum Dis* 1992;51:1208–1214.
50. Danieli MG, Markovits D, Gabrielli A, et al. Juvenile rheumatoid arthritis patients manifest immune reactivity to the mycobacterial 65-kDa heat shock protein, to its 180–188 peptide, and to a partially homologous peptide of the proteoglycan link protein. *Clin Immunol Immunopathol* 1992;64:121–128.
51. Steere AC, Gibofsky A, Pattarroyo ME, et al. Chronic Lyme arthritis: clinical and immunogenetic differentiation form rheumatoid arthritis. *Ann Intern Med* 1979;90:896–901.
52. Naides SJ, Scharosch LL, Foto F, et al. Rheumatologic manifestations of human parvovirus B19 infection in adults. Initial two-year clinical experience. *Arthritis Rheum* 1990;33:1297–1309.
53. Nocton JJ, Miller LC, Tucker LB, et al. Human parvovirus B19-associated arthritis in children. *J Pediatr* 1993;122:186–190.
54. Mimori A, Misaki Y, Hachiya T, et al. Prevalence of antihuman parvovirus B19 IgG antibodies in patients with refractory rheumatoid arthritis and polyarticular juvenile rheumatoid arthritis. *Rheumatol Int* 1994;14:87–90.
55. Cimolai N, Malleson P, Thomas E, et al. *Mycoplasma pneumoniae* associated arthropathy: confirmation of the association by determination of the anti-polypeptide IgM response. *J Rheumatol* 1989;16:1150–1152.
56. Oen K, Fast M, Postl B. Epidemiology of juvenile rheumatoid arthritis in Manitoba, Canada, 1975–92: cycles in incidence. *J Rheumatol* 1995; 22:745–750.
57. Gordon SC, Lauter CB. Mumps arthritis: a review of the literature. *Rev Infect Dis* 1984;6:338–344.
58. Grahame R, Armstrong R, Simmons N, et al. Chronic arthritis associated with the presence of intersynovial rubella virus. *Ann Rheum Dis* 1983;42:2–13.
59. Chantler JK, Tingle AJ, Petty RE. Persistent rubella virus infection associated with chronic arthritis in children. *N Engl J Med* 1985;313: 1117–1123.
60. Lindsley CB. Seasonal variation in systemic onset juvenile rheumatoid arthritis [Letter]. *Arthritis Rheum* 1987;30:838–839.
61. Feldman BM, Birdi N, Boone JE, et al. Seasonal onset of systemic-onset juvenile rheumatoid arthritis. *J Pediatr* 1996;129:513–518.
62. Uziel Y, Pomeranz A, Brik R, et al. Seasonal variation in systemic onset juvenile rheumatoid arthritis in Israel. *J Rheumatol* 1999;26(5): 1187–1189.
63. Prieur AM, Listrat V, Dougados M. Evaluation of a possible seasonal onset in juvenile arthritis from 2954 cases obtained from a multicenter European survey. *Clin Exp Rheumatol* 1994;12(suppl):124.
64. Gallagher KT, Bernstein B. Juvenile rheumatoid arthritis. *Curr Opin Rheumatol* 1999;11:372–376.
65. Moore TL. Immunopathogenesis of juvenile rheumatoid arthritis. *Curr Opin Rheumatol* 1999;11:377–383.
66. De Benedetti F, Martini A. Is systemic juvenile rheumatoid arthritis an interleukin 6 mediated disease? [Editorial]. *J Rheumatol* 1998;25: 203–207.
67. Mangge H, Schauenstein K. Cytokines in juvenile rheumatoid arthritis (JRA). *Cytokine* 1998;10:471–480.
68. Lindsley C. Juvenile rheumatoid arthritis and spondyloarthropathies. *Curr Opin Rheumatol* 1995;7:425–429.
69. Jarvis JN. Pathogenesis and mechanisms of inflammation in the childhood rheumatic diseases. *Curr Opin Rheumatol* 1998;10:459–467.
70. Miller JJ 3d, Hsu Y-P, Moss R, et al. The immunologic and clinical associations of the split products of C3 in plasma in juvenile rheumatoid arthritis. *Arthritis Rheum* 1979;22:502–507.
71. Miller JJ 3d, Osborne CL, Hsu Y-P. C1q binding in serum in juvenile rheumatoid arthritis. *J Rheumatol* 1980;7:665–670.
72. Miller JJ 3d, Olds LC, Silverman ED, et al. Different patterns of C3 and C4 activation in the varied types of juvenile arthritis. *Pediatr Res* 1986;20:1332–1337.
73. Mollnes TE, Paus A. Complement activation in synovial fluid and tissue from patients with juvenile rheumatoid arthritis. *Arthritis Rheum* 1986;29:1359–1364.
74. Jarvis JN, Pousak T, Krenz M, et al. Complement activation and immune complexes in juvenile rheumatoid arthritis. *J Rheumatol* 1993; 20:114–117.
75. Myones BL, Fuller CR, Silverman ED, et al. Evidence for complement activation in subsets of juvenile rheumatoid arthritis (JRA) and correlation with activity of disease [Abstract]. *J Rheumatol* 1986;13: 981.
76. Muller K, Herner EB, Stagg A, et al. Inflammatory cytokines and cytokine antagonists in whole blood cultures of patients with systemic juvenile chronic arthritis. *Br J Rheumatol* 1998;37:562–569.
77. Gattorno M, Picco P, Vignola S, et al. Serum interleukin 12 concentration in juvenile chronic arthritis. *Ann Rheum Dis* 1998;57:425–428.
78. Gattorno M, Picco P, Buoncompagni A, et al. Serum p55 and p75 tumour necrosis factor receptors as markers of disease activity in juvenile chronic arthritis. *Ann Rheum Dis* 1996;55:243–247.
79. Ozen S, Tucker LB, Miller LC. Identification of Th subsets in juvenile rheumatoid arthritis confirmed by intracellular cytokine staining. *J Rheumatol* 1998;25:1651–1653.
80. Gattorno M, Facchetti P, Ghiotto F, et al. Synovial fluid T cell clones from oligoarticular juvenile arthritis patients display a prevalent Th1/Th0-type pattern of cytokine secretion irrespective of immunophenotype. *Clin Exp Immunol* 1997;109:4–11.
81. Murray KJ, Grom AA, Thompson SD, et al. Contrasting cytokine profiles in the synovium of different forms of juvenile rheumatoid arthritis and juvenile spondyloarthropathy: prominence of interleukin 4 in restricted disease. *J Rheumatol* 1998;25:1388–1398.
82. Kutukculer N, Caglayan S. Plasma and synovial fluid soluble CD23 concentrations in children with juvenile chronic arthritis. *Autoimmunity* 1998;27:155–158.
83. Kutukculer N, Caglayan S, Aydogdu F. Study of pro-inflammatory (TNF-alpha, IL-1alpha, IL-6) and T-cell-derived (IL-2, IL-4) cytokines in plasma and synovial fluid of patients with juvenile chronic arthritis: correlations with clinical and laboratory parameters. *Clin Rheumatol* 1998;17:288–292.
84. Massa M, Pignatti P, Oliveri M, et al. Serum soluble CD23 levels and CD23 expression on peripheral blood mononuclear cells in juvenile chronic arthritis. *Clin Exp Rheumatol* 1998;16:611–616.

85. De Benedetti F, Pignatti P, Bernasconi S, et al. Interleukin 8 and monocyte chemoattractant protein-1 in patients with juvenile rheumatoid arthritis. Relation to onset types, disease activity, and synovial fluid leukocytes. *J Rheumatol* 1999;26:425–431.
86. De Benedetti F, Massa M, Robbioni P, et al. Correlation of serum interleukin-6 levels with joint involvement and thrombocytosis in systemic juvenile rheumatoid arthritis. *Arthritis Rheum* 1991;34: 1158–1163.
87. De Benedetti F, Pignatti P, Gerloni V, et al. Differences in synovial fluid cytokine levels between juvenile and adult rheumatoid arthritis. *J Rheumatol* 1997;24:1403–1409.
88. Madson KL, Moore TL, Lawrence JM 3rd, et al. Cytokine levels in serum and synovial fluid of patients with juvenile rheumatoid arthritis. *J Rheumatol* 1994;21:2359–2363.
89. Keul R, Heinrich PC, Muller-Newen G, et al. A possible role for soluble IL-6 receptor in the pathogenesis of systemic onset juvenile chronic arthritis. *Cytokine* 1998;10:729–734.
90. Fishman D, Faulds G, Jeffery R, et al. The effect of novel polymorphisms in the interleukin-6 (IL-6) gene on IL-6 transcription and plasma IL-6 levels, and an association with systemic-onset juvenile chronic arthritis. *J Clin Invest* 1998;102:1369–1376.
91. Maeno N, Takei S, Nomura Y, et al. High elevated serum levels of interleukin-18 in systemic juvenile idiopathic arthritis subtypes or in Kawasaki disease. *Arthritis Rheum* 2002;46(9):2539–2540.
92. Tselepis AD, Elisaf M, Besis S, et al. Association of the inflammatory state in active juvenile rheumatoid arthritis with hypo-high-density lipoproteinemia and reduced lipoprotein-associated platelet-activating factor acetylhydrolase activity. *Arthritis Rheum* 1999;42:373–383.
93. Raziuddin S, Bahabri S, Al-Dalaan A, et al. A mixed Th1/Th2 cell cytokine response predominates in systemic onset juvenile rheumatoid arthritis: immunoregulatory IL-10 function. *Clin Immunol Immunopathol* 1998;86:192–198.
94. Forre O, Thoen J, Dobloug JH, et al. Detection of T-lymphocyte subpopulation in the peripheral blood and the synovium of patients with rheumatoid arthritis and juvenile rheumatoid arthritis using monoclonal antibodies. *Scand J Immunol* 1982;15:221–226.
95. Kjeldsen-Kragh J, Quayle AJ, Vinje O, et al. A high proportion of the V delta 1+ synovial fluid gamma delta T cells in juvenile rheumatoid arthritis patients express the very early activation marker CD69, but carry the high molecular weight isoform of the leucocyte common antigen (CD45RA). *Clin Exp Immunol* 1993;91:202–206.
96. Murray KJ, Luyrink L, Grom AA, et al. Immunohistological characteristics of T cell infiltrates in different forms of childhood onset chronic arthritis. *J Rheumatol* 1996;23:2116–2124.
97. Kjeldsen-Kragh J, Quayle A, Kalvenes C, et al. T gamma delta cells in juvenile rheumatoid arthritis and rheumatoid arthritis. In the juvenile rheumatoid arthritis synovium the T gamma delta cells express activation antigens and are predominantly V delta 1+, and a significant proportion of these patients have elevated percentages of T gamma delta cells. *Scand J Immunol* 1990;32:651–659.
98. Zhang H, Phang D, Laxer RM, et al. Evolution of the T cell receptor beta repertoire from synovial fluid T cells of patients with juvenile onset rheumatoid arthritis. *J Rheumatol* 1997;24:1396–1402.
99. Sioud M, Kjeldsen-Kragh J, Suleyman S, et al. Limited heterogeneity of T cell receptor variable region gene usage in juvenile rheumatoid arthritis synovial T cells. *Eur J Immunol* 1992;22:2413–2418.
100. Thompson SD, Murray KJ, Grom AA, et al. Comparative sequence analysis of the human T cell receptor beta chain in juvenile rheumatoid arthritis and juvenile spondyloarthropathies: evidence for antigenic selection of T cells in the synovium. *Arthritis Rheum* 1998;41: 482–497.
101. Khalkhali-Ellis Z, Roodman ST, Knutsen AP, et al. Expression of macrophage markers by a population of T cells obtained from synovial fluid of a subgroup of patients with juvenile rheumatoid arthritis. *J Rheumatol* 1998;25:352–360.
102. Wouters CHP, Ceuppens JL, Stevens EAM. Different circulating lymphocyte profiles in patients with different subtypes of juvenile idiopathic arthritis. *Clin Exp Rheumatol* 2002;20:230–248.
103. Tsokos GC, Mavridis A, Inghirami G, et al. Cellular immunity in patients with systemic juvenile rheumatoid arthritis. *Clin Immunol Immunopathol* 1987;42:86–92.
104. Tsokos GC, Inghirami G, Pillemer SR, et al. Immunoregulatory aberrations in patients with polyarticular juvenile rheumatoid arthritis. *Clin Immunol Immunopathol* 1988;47:62–74.
105. Jarvis JN, Kaplan J, Fine N. Increase in CD5+ B cells in juvenile rheumatoid arthritis. *Arthritis Rheum* 1992;35:204–207.
106. Khalkhali-Ellis Z, Seftor EA, Nieva DR, et al. Induction of invasive and degradative phenotype in normal synovial fibroblasts exposed to synovial fluid from patients with juvenile rheumatoid arthritis: role of mononuclear cell population. *J Rheumatol* 1997;24:2451–2460.
107. Sioud M, Mellbye O, Forre O. Analysis of the NF-kappa B p65 subunit, Fas antigen, Fas ligand and Bcl-2-related proteins in the synovium of RA and polyarticular JRA. *Clin Exp Rheumatol* 1998;16: 125–134.
108. Osborn TG, Patel NJ, Moore TI, et al. Use of the HEp-2 cell substrate in the detection of antinuclear antibodies in juvenile rheumatoid arthritis. *Arthritis Rheum* 1984;27:1286–1289.
109. Myones BL, Anderson BD, Rivas-Chacon RF, et al. Anti-phospholipid antibodies in juvenile rheumatoid arthritis (JRA) [Abstract]. *Arthritis Rheum* 1990;33(suppl):93.
110. Fawcett PT, Rose CD, Gibney KM, et al. Use of ELISA to measure antinuclear antibodies in children with juvenile rheumatoid arthritis. *J Rheumatol* 1999;26:1822–1826.
111. Saulsbury FT. Antibody to ribonucleoprotein in pauciarticular juvenile rheumatoid arthritis. *J Rheumatol* 1988;15:295–297.
112. Wittemann B, Neuer G, Michels H, et al. Autoantibodies to nonhistone chromosomal protein HMG-1 and HMG-2 in sera of patients with juvenile rheumatoid arthritis. *Arthritis Rheum* 1990;33:1378–1383.
113. Neuer G, Bustin M, Michels H, et al. Autoantibodies to the chromosomal protein HMG-17 in juvenile rheumatoid arthritis. *Arthritis Rheum* 1992;35:472–475.
114. Haber PL, Osborn TG, Moore TL. Antinuclear antibody in juvenile rheumatoid arthritis sera reacts with 50–40 kDa antigen (s) found in HeLa nuclear extracts. *J Rheumatol* 1989;16:949–954.
115. Szer IS, Sierakowska H, Szer W. A novel autoantibody to the putative oncoprotein DEK in pauciarticular onset juvenile rheumatoid arthritis. *J Rheumatol* 1994;21:2136–2142.
116. Emlen W, O'Neill L. Clinical significance of antinuclear antibodies. Comparison of detection with immunofluorescence and enzyme-linked immunosorbent assay. *Arthritis Rheum* 1997;40:1612–1618.
117. Mulder L, van Rossum M, Horst G, et al. Antineutrophil cytoplasmic antibodies in juvenile chronic arthritis. *J Rheumatol* 1997;24:568–575.
118. Albani S, Ravelli A, Massa M, et al. Immune responses to the *Escherichia coli* dnaj heat shock protein in juvenile rheumatoid arthritis and their correlation with disease activity. *J Pediatr* 1994; 124:651–565.
119. Olds LC, Miller JJ 3d. C3 activation products correlate with antibodies to lipid A in pauciarticular juvenile arthritis. Arthritis Rheum 1990;33:520–524.
120. Miller JJ 3d, Olds LC. Antibodies to lipid A in pauciarticular juvenile arthritis: clinical studies. J Rheumatol 1992;19:959–963.
121. Miller JJ 3rd, Zhu S, Smith RL. Anti-lipid A antibodies in childhood arthritis: methods of immobilization affect quantitation and cross-reactivity measured by ELISA. *J Rheumatol* 1996;23:2125–2131.
122. Ravelli A, Martini A. Antiphospholipid antibody syndrome in pediatric patients. *Rheum Dis Clin North Am* 1997;23:657–676.
123. Marzan KA, Myones BL. Occurrence of antiphospholipid antibodies other than anticardiolipin in pediatric rheumatic diseases [Abstract]. *Arthritis Rheum* 1995;38(suppl):338.
124. Moore TL. Rheumatoid factors. *Clin Immunol Newsletter* 1998;18: 89–96.
125. Moore TL, Dorner RW, Osborn TG, et al. Hidden 19S IgM rheumatoid factors. *Semin Arthritis Rheum* 1988;18:72–75.
126. Moore TL, Dorner RW, Weiss TD, et al. Hidden 19S IgM rheumatoid factor in juvenile rheumatoid arthritis. *Pediatr Res* 1980;14:1135–1138.
127. Moore TL, Dorner RW. Rheumatoid factors. *Clin Biochim* 1993;26: 75–84.
128. Walker SM, McCurdy DK, Shaham B, et al. High prevalence of IgA rheumatoid factor in severe polyarticular-onset juvenile rheumatoid arthritis, but not in systemic-onset or pauciarticular-onset disease. *Arthritis Rheum* 1990;33:199–204.
129. Ilowite NT, Wedgwood JF, Bonagura VR. Expression of the major cross-reactive idiotype of juvenile rheumatoid arthritis. *Arthritis Rheum* 1989;32:265–270.
130. Ilowite NT, O'Reilly ME, Hatam L, et al. Expression of the rheumatoid factor cross-reactive idiotype in JRA: association with disease

onset subtype, disease activity, and disease severity. *Scand J Rheumatol* 1992;21:51–54.

131. Rossen RD, Brewer EJ, Person DA, et al. Circulating immune complexes and antinuclear antibodies in juvenile rheumatoid arthritis. *Arthritis Rheum* 1977;20:1485–1490.
132. Moran H, Ansell BM, Mowbray JF, et al. Antigen-antibody complexes in the serum of patients with juvenile chronic arthritis. *Arch Dis Child* 1979;54:120–122.
133. Jarvis JN, Taylor H, Iobidze M, et al. Complement activation and immune complexes in children with polyarticular juvenile rheumatoid arthritis: a longitudinal study. *J Rheumatol* 1994;21:1124–1127.
134. Doekes G, Schouten J, Cats A, et al. Reduction of complement activation capacity of soluble immune complexes by IgM rheumatoid factor. *Immunology* 1985;47:675–680.
135. Jarvis JN, Lockman JC, Levine RP. IgM rheumatoid factor and the inhibition of the covalent binding of C4b to IgG in immune complexes. *Clin Exp Rheum* 1993;11:135–141.
136. Jarvis JN, Wang W, Moore HT, et al. *In vitro* induction of proinflammatory cytokine secretion by juvenile rheumatoid arthritis synovial fluid immune complexes. *Arthritis Rheum* 1997;40:2039–2046.
137. Thomsen BS, Heilmann C, Jacobsen SEH, et al. Complement C3b receptors on erythrocytes in patients with juvenile rheumatoid arthritis. *Arthritis Rheum* 1987;30:967–971.
138. Vehe RK, Begovich AB, Nepom BS. HLA susceptibility genes in rheumatoid factor positive juvenile rheumatoid arthritis. *J Rheumatol* 1990;17(suppl 26):11–15.
139. Albert ED, Scholz S. Juvenile arthritis: genetic update. *Baillieres Clin Rheumatol* 1998;12:209–218.
140. Graham TB, Glass DN. Juvenile rheumatoid arthritis: ethnic differences in diagnostic types [Editorial]. *J Rheumatol* 1997;24:1677–1679.
141. Ploski R, Forre O. Non-HLA genes and susceptibility to juvenile chronic arthritis. *Clin Exp Rheumatol* 1994;12(suppl 10):15–17.
142. Fernandez-Vina M, Fink CW, Stastny P. HLA associations in juvenile arthritis. *Clin Exp Rheumatol* 1994;12:205–214.
143. Nepom B. The immunogenetics of juvenile rheumatoid arthritis. *Rheum Dis Clin North Am* 1991;17:825–842.
144. Nepom B, Glass D. Juvenile rheumatoid arthritis and HLA: report of the Park City III workshop. *J Rheumatol* 1992;19(suppl 33):70–74.
145. Hull RG. Outcome in juvenile arthritis. *Br J Rheumatol* 1988;27 (suppl I):66–71.
146. Calabro JJ, Burnstein SL, Staley HL, et al. Prognosis in juvenile rheumatoid arthritis: a fifteen-year followup of 100 patients. *Arthritis Rheum* 1977;20(suppl 2):285–290.
147. Hanson V, Kornreich H, Bernstein B, et al. Prognosis of juvenile rheumatoid arthritis. *Arthritis Rheum* 1977;20(suppl 2):279–284.
148. Wallace CA, Levinson JE. Juvenile rheumatoid arthritis: outcome and treatment for the 1990s. *Rheum Dis Clin North Am* 1991;17: 891–905.
149. Quirk ME, Young MH. The impact of JRA on children, adolescents, and their families. Current research and implications for future studies. *Arthritis Care Res* 1990;3:36–43.
150. Weyand CM, Hicok KC, Conn DL, et al. The influence of HLA-DRB1 genes on disease severity in rheumatoid arthritis. *Ann Intern Med* 1992;117:801–806.
151. Gough A, Faint J, Salmon M, et al. Genetic typing of patients with inflammatory arthritis at presentation can be used to predict outcome. *Arthritis Rheum* 1994;37:1166–1170.
152. Ansell BM. Chronic arthritis in childhood. *Ann Rheum Dis* 1978; 37:107–120.
153. Moroldo MB, Tague BL, Shear ES, et al. Juvenile rheumatoid arthritis in affected sib pairs. *Arthritis Rheum* 1997;40:1962–1966.
154. Begovich AB, Bugawan TL, Nepom BS, et al. A specific HLA-DPB allele is associated with pauciarticular juvenile rheumatoid arthritis but not adult rheumatoid arthritis. *Proc Natl Acad Sci U S A* 1989; 88:9489–9493.
155. Barron KS, Joseph A, MacLeod M, et al. DNA analysis of HLA-DR, DQ and DP genes in pauciarticular juvenile rheumatoid arthritis. *J Rheumatol* 1991;18:1723–1729.
156. Fernandez-Vina MA, Fink CW, Stastny P. HLA antigens in juvenile arthritis. Pauciarticular and polyarticular juvenile arthritis are immunogenetically distinct. *Arthritis Rheum* 1990;33:1787–1799.
157. Glass D, Litvin D, Wallace K, et al. Early onset pauciarticular juvenile rheumatoid arthritis associated with human leukocyte antigen DRw5, iritis and antinuclear antibody. *J Clin Invest* 1980;66:426–429.
158. Arnaiz-Villena A, Gomez-Reino JJ, Gamin ML, et al. DR, C4 and Bf allotypes in juvenile rheumatoid arthritis. *Arthritis Rheum* 1984;27: 1281–1285.
159. Ploski R, Vinje O, Ronningen KS, et al. HLA class II alleles and heterogeneity of juvenile rheumatoid arthritis. DRB1*0101 may define a novel subset of the disease. *Arthritis Rheum* 1993;36:465–472.
160. van Kerckhove C, Luyrink L, Taylor J, et al. HLA-DQA1*0101 haplotypes and disease outcome in early onset pauciarticular juvenile rheumatoid arthritis. *J Rheumatol* 1991;18:874–879.
161. Fernandez-Vina MA, Fink CW, Stastny P. HLA antigens in juvenile arthritis. *Arthritis Rheum* 1990;33:1787–1794.
162. Barron KS, Silverman ED, Gonzalez JC, et al. DNA analysis of HLA-DR, DQ, and DP alleles in children with polyarticular juvenile rheumatoid arthritis. *J Rheumatol* 1992;19:1611–1616.
163. Hurley CK, Gregersen PK, Gorski J, et al. The DR3 (w18), DQw4 haplotype differs from DR3 (w17), DQw2 haplotypes at multiple class II loci. *Hum Immunol* 1989;25:37–50.
164. Reveille JD, Spencer CH, Rivas-Chacon RF, et al. HLA-DRB1, DQA1, DQB1, and DPB1 alleles in children with juvenile arthritis from three ethnic groups [Abstract]. *Arthritis Rheum* 1997;40(suppl): 241.
165. Morling N, Friis J, Heilmann C, et al. HLA antigen frequencies in juvenile chronic arthritis. *Scand J Rheumatol* 1985;14:209–216.
166. Fantini F, Gerloni V, Murelli M, et al. HLA phenotypes in Italian children affected with juvenile chronic arthritis. *Clin Exp Rheumatol* 1987;5(suppl):F32.
167. Forre O, Dobloug JH, Hoyeraal HM, et al. HLA antigens in juvenile arthritis. Genetic basis for the different subtypes. *Arthritis Rheum* 1983;26:35–38.
168. Miller ML, Aaron S, Jackson J, et al. HLA gene frequencies in children and adults with systemic onset juvenile rheumatoid arthritis. *Arthritis Rheum* 1985;28:146–150.
169. Stastny P, Fink CW. Different HLA-D associations in adult and juvenile rheumatoid arthritis. *J Clin Invest* 1979;63:124–130.
170. Pachman LM, Goronzy JJ, Miller ML, et al. HLADRB1 antigens in children with symptoms of systemic onset juvenile rheumatoid arthritis (SO-JRA) [Abstract]. *Arthritis Rheum* 1997;40:S241.
171. Forero L, Zwirner NW, Fink CW, et al. Juvenile arthritis, HLA-A2 and binding of DEK oncogene-peptides. *Hum Immunol* 1998;59: 443–450.
172. Murray KJ, Szer W, Grom AA, et al. Antibodies to the 45 kDa DEK nuclear antigen in pauciarticular onset juvenile rheumatoid arthritis and iridocyclitis: selective association with MHC gene. *J Rheumatol* 1997;24:560–567.
173. Feichtlbauer P, Gomolka M, Brunnler G, et al. HLA region microsatellite polymorphisms in juvenile arthritis. *Tissue Antigens* 1998; 52:220–229.
174. Charmley P, Nepom BS, Concannon P. HLA and T cell receptor beta-chain DNA polymorphisms identify a distinct subset of patients with pauciarticular-onset juvenile rheumatoid arthritis. *Arthritis Rheum* 1994;37:695–701.
175. Donn RP, Davies EJ, Holt PL, et al. Increased frequency of TAP2B in early onset pauciarticular juvenile chronic arthritis. *Ann Rheum Dis* 1994;53:261–264.
176. Grom AA, Giannini EH, Glass DN. Juvenile rheumatoid arthritis and the trimolecular complex (HLA, T cell receptor, and antigen). Differences from rheumatoid arthritis. *Arthritis Rheum* 1994;37:601–607.
177. Smerdel A, Benedicte A, Ploski R, et al. A gene in the telomeric HLA complex distinct from HLA-A is involved in predispostion to juvenile idiopathic arthritis. *Arthritis Rheum* 2002;46(6);1614–1619.
178. Kirveskari J, Kellner H, Wuorela M, et al. False-negative serological HLA-B27 typing results may be due to altered antigenic epitopes and can be detected by polymerase chain reaction. *Br J Rheumatol* 1997; 36:185–189.
179. Savolainen HA, Lehtimaki M, Kautiainen H, et al. HLA B27: a prognostic factor in juvenile chronic arthritis. *Clin Rheumatol* 1998;17: 121–124.
180. McCarthy PL, Wasserman D, Spiesel SZ, et al. Evaluation of arthritis and arthralgia in the pediatric patient. *Clin Pediatr (Phila)* 1980;19: 183–190.
181. Scott PJ, Ansell BM, Huskisson EC. Measurement of pain in juvenile chronic polyarthritis. *Ann Rheum Dis* 1977;36:186–187.

182. Varni JW, Wilcox KT, Hanson V, et al. Chronic musculoskeletal pain and functional status in juvenile rheumatoid arthritis: an empirical model. *Pain* 1988;32:1–7.
183. Varni JW, Thompson KL, Hanson V. The Varni/Thompson pediatric pain questionnaire. I. Chronic musculoskeletal pain in juvenile rheumatoid arthritis. *Pain* 1987;28:7.
184. Callen JP. Myositis and malignancy. *Curr Opin Rheumatol* 1989;1: 468–472.
185. Pizzo PA, Lovejoy FH Jr, Smith DH. Prolonged fever in children: review of 100 cases. *Pediatrics* 1975;55:468–473.
186. Lohr JA, Hendley JO. Prolonged fever unknown origin. *Clin Pediatr* 1977;16:768–773.
187. Wallendal M, Stork L, Hollister JR. The discriminating value of serum lactate dehydrogenase levels in children with malignant neoplasms presenting as joint pain. *Arch Pediatr Adolesc Med* 1996;150: 70–73.
188. McCune WJ, Wise PT, Cassidy JT. A comparison of antibody tests in children with juvenile rheumatoid arthritis on Hep-2 cell and mouse liver substrates. *J Rheumatol* 1986;13:198.
189. Eichenfield AH, Athreya BH, Doughty RA, et al. Utility of rheumatoid factor in the diagnosis of juvenile rheumatoid arthritis. *Pediatrics* 1986;78:480–484.
190. Pachman LM, Poznanski AK. Juvenile (rheumatoid) arthritis. In: Koopman WJ, ed. *Arthritis and allied conditions: a textbook of rheumatology,* 13th ed. Baltimore: Williams & Wilkins, 1997:1162.
191. Cassidy JT, Petty RE. Juvenile rheumatoid arthritis. *Textbook of pediatric rheumatology,* 3rd ed. Philadelphia: WB Saunders, 1995: 176.
192. Baldassare AR, Chang F, Zuckner J. Markedly raised synovial fluid leukocyte counts not associated with infectious arthritis in children. *Ann Rheum Dis* 1978;37:404–409.
193. Grokoest AW, Snyder AI, Schlaeger R. *Juvenile rheumatoid arthritis.* Boston: Little, Brown, 1962.
194. Petty RE. Epidemiology of juvenile rheumatoid arthritis. In: Miller JJ III, ed. *Juvenile rheumatoid arthritis.* Littleton, MA: PSG, 1979: 135.
195. Ansell BM, Bywater EGL. Diagnosis of "probable" Still's disease and its outcome. *Ann Rheum Dis* 1962;21:253–262.
196. Calabro JJ, Marchesano JM. Rash associated with juvenile rheumatoid arthritis. *J Pediatr* 1968;72:611–619.
197. Schlesinger BE, Forsyth CC, White RHR, et al. Observations on the clinical course and treatment of one hundred cases of Still's disease. *Arch Dis Child* 1961;36:65–76.
198. Jan JE, Hill RH, Low MD. Cerebral complications in juvenile rheumatoid arthritis. *Can Med Assoc J* 1972;1073:623–625.
199. Schaller JG. The diversity of JRA. *Arthritis Rheum* 1977;20(suppl): 52–63.
200. Cabral DA, Malleson PN, Petty RE. Spondyloarthropathies of childhood. *Pediatr Clin North Am* 1995;42:1051.
201. Bernstein B, Takahashi M, Hanson V. Cardiac involvement in juvenile rheumatoid arthritis. *J Pediatr* 1985;85:313–317.
202. Brewer E. Juvenile rheumatoid arthritis-cardiac involvement. *Arthritis Rheum* 1977;20:231–236.
203. Miller JJ III. Carditis in JRA. In: Miller JJ III, ed. *Juvenile rheumatoid arthritis.* Littleton, MA: PSG, 1979:165–173.
204. Svantesson H, Bjorkhem G, Elborgh R. Cardiac involvement in juvenile rheumatoid arthritis: a follow-up study. *Acta Paediatr Scand* 1983;72:345–350.
205. Schwarz-Eywill M, Heilig B, Bauer H, et al. Evaluation of serum ferritin as a marker for adult Still's disease activity. *Ann Rheum Dis* 1992;51:683–685.
206. Bloom BJ, Tucker LB, Miller LC, et al. Fibrin d-dimer as a marker of disease activity in systemic onset juvenile rheumatoid arthritis. *J Rheumatol* 1998,25:1620–1625.
207. Morris JA, Adamson AR, Holt PJL, et al. Still's disease and the virus-associated haemophagocytic syndrome. *Ann Rheum Dis* 1985; 44:349–353.
208. Heaton DC, Moller PW. Case report: Still's disease associated with coxsackie infection and haemophagocytic syndrome. *Ann Rheum Dis* 1985;44:341–344.
209. Stephan JL, Zeller J, Hubert P, et al. Macrophage activation syndrome and rheumatic disease in childhood: a report of four new cases. *Clin Exp Rheumatol* 1993;11:451–456.
210. Davies SV, Dean JD, Wardrop CA, et al. Epstein-Barr virus–associated haemophagocytic syndrome in a patient with juvenile chronic arthritis. *Br J Rheumatol* 1994;33:495–497.
211. Ansell BM, Wood PHN. Prognosis in juvenile chronic arthritis. *Clin Rheum Dis* 1976;2:397–412.
212. van der Net J, Kuis W, Prakken ABJ, et al. Correlates of disablement in systemic onset juvenile chronic arthritis. *Scand J Rheumatol* 1997; 26:188–196.
213. Lin SJ, Huany JL, Chao HC, et al. A follow-up study of systemic-onset juvenile rheumatoid arthritis in children. *Chung Hua Min Kuo Hsiao Erh Ko I Hsueh Tsa Chih* 1999;40:176–181.
214. Minden K, Kiessling U, Listing J, et al. Prognosis of patients with juvenile chronic arthritis and juvenile spondyloarthropathy. *J Rheumatol* 2000;27:2256–2263.
215. Oen K, Malleson PA, Cabral DA, et al. Disease course and outcome of juvenile rheumatoid arthritis in a multicenter cohort. *J Rheumatol* 2002;29:1989–1999.
216. Lomater C, Gerloni V, Gattinara M, et al. Systemic onset juvenile idiopathic arthritis: a retrospective study of 80 consecutive patients followed for 10 years. *J Rheumatol* 2000;27:491–496.
217. Svantesson H, Akesson A, Eberhardt K, et al. Prognosis in juvenile rheumatoid arthritis with systemic onset. *Scand J Rheumatol* 1983; 12;139–144.
218. Heyd J, Glaser J. Early occurrence of aortic valve regurgitation in a youth with systemic-onset juvenile rheumatoid arthritis. *Am J Med* 1990;89:123–124.
219. Brewer EJ, Giannini E, Person D. *Juvenile rheumatoid arthritis,* 2nd ed. Philadelphia: WB Saunders, 1982.
220. Cazzola M, Ponchio L, de Benedetti F, et al. Defective iron supply for erythropoiesis and adequate endogenous erythropoietin production in the anemia associated with systemic-onset juvenile chronic arthritis. *Blood* 1996;87:4824–4830.
221. Hochbery MC, Arnold CM, Hogans BB, et al. Serum immunoreactive erythropoietin in rheumatoid arthritis: impaired response to anemia. *Arthritis Rheum* 1988;31:1318–1321.
222. Schnitzer TJ, Ansell BM. Amyloidosis in juvenile chronic polyarthritis. *Arthritis Rheum* 1977;20(suppl):245–252.
223. Calabro JJ. Amyloidosis and juvenile rheumatoid arthritis. *J Pediatr* 1969;75:521.
224. Bernstein BH, Stobie D, Singsen BH, et al. Growth retardation in juvenile rheumatoid arthritis (JRA). *Arthritis Rheum* 1977;20:212–216.
225. Polito C, Strano CG, Olicieri AN, et al. Growth retardation in nonsteroid treated juvenile rheumatoid arthritis. *Scand J Rheumatol* 1997;26:99–103.
226. Schaller JG. The diversity of JRA. *Arthritis Rheum* 1977;20(suppl): 52–63.
227. Prieur AM, Ansel BM, Bardfeld R, et al. Is onset type evaluated during the first three months of disease satisfactory for defining the subgroups of juvenile chronic arthritis? A EULAR cooperative study (1983–1986). *Clin Exp Rheumatol* 1990;8:321–325.
228. Sullivan DB, Cassidy JT, Petty RE. Pathogenic implications of age of onset in juvenile rheumatoid arthritis. *Arthritis Rheum* 1975;18:251–255.
229. Sherry DD, Bohnsak J, Salmonson K, et al. Painless juvenile rheumatoid arthritis. *J Pediatr* 1990;116:921–923.
230. Sharma S, Sherry DD. Joint distribution at presentation in children with pauciarthritis. *J Pediatr* 1999;134(5):642–643.
231. Rosenberg AM, Oen KG. The relationship between ocular and articular disease activity in children with juvenile rheumatoid arthritis and associated uveitis. *Arthritis Rheum* 1986;29:797–800.
232. Cassidy JT, Martel W. Juvenile rheumatoid arthritis: clinicoradiologic correlations. *Arthritis Rheum* 1977;20(suppl):207–211.
233. Guillaume S, Prieur AM, Coste J, et al. Long term outcome and prognosis in oligoarticular-onset juvenile idiopathic arthritis. *Arthritis Rheum* 2000;43:1858–1865.
234. Vostrejs M, Hollister JR. Muscle atrophy and leg length discrepancies in pauciarticular juvenile rheumatoid arthritis. *Am J Dis Child* 1988;142:343–345.
235. Cassidy JT, Levinson JE, Brewer EJ Jr. The development of classification criteria for children with juvenile rheumatoid arthritis. *Bull Rheum Dis* 1989;38:1–7.
236. Kanski JJ. Uveitis in juvenile chronic arthritis: incidence, clinical features and prognosis. *Eye* 1988;2:641–645.

237. Suciu-Foca N, Jacobs J, Godfrey M, et al. HLA-DR5 in juvenile rheumatoid arthritis confined to a few joints. *Lancet* 1980;2:40.
238. Candell Chalom E, Goldsmith DP, Koehler MA, et al. Prevalence and outcome of uveitis in a regional cohort of patients with juvenile rheumatoid arthritis. *J Rheumatol* 1997;24:2031–2034.
239. Kanski JJ. Screening for uveitis in juvenile chronic arthritis. *Br J Ophthalmol* 1989;73:225–228.
240. Sullivan DB, Cassidy JT, Petty RE. Pathogenic implications of age of onset in juvenile rheumatoid arthritis. *Arthritis Rheum* 1975;18: 251–255.
241. Forsberg M, Agerberg G, Persson M. Mandibular dysfunction in patients with juvenile rheumatoid arthritis. *J Craniomandib Disord* 1988;2:201–208.
242. Siamopopulou-Mavridou A, Asimakopoulos D, Mavridis A, et al. Middle ear function in patients with juvenile chronic arthritis. *Ann Rheum Dis* 1990;49:620–623.
243. Schaller JG. Juvenile rheumatoid arthritis. *Arthritis Rheum* 1977;20: 165–170.
244. Jacobs JC. *Pediatric rheumatology for the practitioner,* 2nd ed. New York: Springer-Verlag, 1993:276.
245. Kaye BR, Kaye RL, Bobrove A. Rheumatoid nodules. Review of the spectrum of associated conditions and proposal of a new classification, with a report of four seronegative cases. *Am J Med* 1984; 76:279–292.
246. Mesara BW, Brody GL, Oberman HA. "Pseudorheumatoid" subcutaneous nodules. *Am J Clin Pathol* 1966;45:684–691.
247. Schaller JG. The diversity of JRA. *Arthritis Rheum* 1977;20(suppl): 52–63.
248. Denardo BA, Tucker LB, Miller LC, et al. Demography of a regional pediatric rheumatology patient population. *J Rheumatol* 1994;21: 1553–1561.
249. Schaller JG. The diversity of JRA. *Arthritis Rheum* 1977;20 (suppl):53.
250. Braun J, Bollow M, Eggens U, et al. Use of dynamic magnetic resonance imaging with fast imaging in the detection of early and advanced sacroiliitis in spondyloarthropathy patients. *Arthritis Rheum* 1994;37:1039–1045.
251. Jacobs JC, Berdon ED, Johnston WE. HLA-B27-associated spondyloarthritis and enthosopathy in childhood: clinical, pathologic, and radiographic observations in 58 patients. *J Pediatr* 1982;100:521.
252. Stamato T, Laxer RM, de Freitas C, et al. Prevalence of cardiac manifestations of juvenile ankylosing spondylitis. *Am J Cardiol* 1995;75: 744–746.
253. Ansell BM. Juvenile spondylitis and related disorders. In: Moll JMH, ed. *Ankylosing spondylitis.* Edinburgh: Churchill Livingstone, 1980:120.
254. Schaller J. Ankylosing spondylitis of childhood onset. *Arthritis Rheum* 1977;20(suppl):398–401.
255. Lambert JR, Ansell BM, Stephenson E, et al. Psoriatic arthritis in childhood. *Clin Rheum Dis* 1976;2:339.
256. Shore A, Ansell BM. Juvenile psoriatic arthritis—an analysis of 60 cases. *J Pediatr* 1982;100:529–535.
257. Wright FV, Kimber JL, et al. Development of a disability measurement tool for juvenile rheumatoid arthritis—the Juvenile Arthritis Functional Status Index. *J Rheum* 1996;23(6):1066–1079.
258. Lovell DJ, Howe S, Shear E, et al. Development of a disability measurement tool for juvenile rheumatoid arthritis—the Juvenile Arthritis Functional Assessment Scale. *Arthritis Rheum* 1989;32:1390–1395.
259. Howe S, Levinson J, Shear E, et al. Development of a disability measurement tool for juvenile rheumatoid arthritis: the Juvenile Arthritis Functional Assessment Report for children and their parents. *Arthritis Rheum* 1991;34:873–880.
260. Giannini EH, Ruperto N, Ravelli A, et al. Preliminary definition of improvement in juvenile arthritis. *Arthritis Rheum* 1997;40:1202–1209
261. Ruperto N, Ravelli A, Falcini F, et al. Performance of the preliminary definition of improvement in juvenile chronic arthritis patients treated with methotrexate. *Ann Rheum Dis* 1998;57:38–41.
262. Ruperto N, Ravelli A, Falcini F, et al. Responsiveness of outcome measures in juvenile chronic arthritis. *Rheumatology* 1999;38(2): 176–180.
263. Stein REK, Jessop DJ. Functional Status II (R) Measure: a measure of child health status. *Med Care* 1990;28:1041–1055.
264. Singh G, Athreya B, Fried J, et al. Measurement of health status in children with juvenile rheumatoid arthritis. *Arthritis Rheum* 1994;37: 1761–1769.
265. Landgraf JM, Abetz L, Ware JE. *The CHQ user's manual,* 1st ed. Boston, MA: The Health Institute, New England Medical Center, 1996.
266. Duffy CM, Arsenault L, Watanabe Duffy KN, et al. The juvenile Arthritis quality of Life Questionnaire: development of a new responsive index for juvenile rheumatoid arthritis and juvenile spondyloarthritides. *J Rheumatol* 1997;24:738–746.
267. Stein REK, Riessman CK. The development of an Impact-on-Family Scale: preliminary findings. *Med Care* 1980;18:465–472.
268. Ruperto N, Ravelli A, Migliavacca D, et al. Responsiveness of clinical measures in children with oligoarticular juvenile chronic arthritis. *J Rheumatol* 1999;26(8):1827–1830.
269. White PH. Growth abnormalities in children with juvenile rheumatoid arthritis. *Clin Orthop* 1990;259:46–50.
270. Fraser PA, Hoch S, Erlandson D, et al. The timing of menarche in juvenile rheumatoid arthritis. *J Adolesc Health* 1988;9:483–487.
271. Henderson CJ, Lovell DJ, Gregg DJ. A nutritional screening test for use in children and adolescents with juvenile rheumatoid arthritis. *J Rheumatol* 1992;19:1276–1281.
272. Bacon MC, White PH, Raiten DJ, et al. Nutritional status growth in juvenile rheumatoid arthritis. *Semin Arthritis Rheum* 1990;20:97–106.
273. Peretz A, Praet JP, Bosson D, et al. Serum osteocalcin in the assessment of corticosteroid induced osteoporosis. Effect of long and short term corticosteroid treatment. *J Rheumatol* 1989;16:363–367.
274. Ou LS, See LC, Wu CJ, et al. Association between serum inflammatory cytokines and disease activity in juvenile idiopathic arthritis. *Clin Rheumatol* 2002;21(1):52–56.
275. Davies UM, Jones J, Reeve J, et al. Juvenile rheumatoid arthritis: effects of disease activity and recombinant human growth hormone on insulin-like growth factor 1, insulin-like growth factor binding proteins 1 and 3, and osteocalcin. *Arthritis Rheum* 1997;40:332–340.
276. Simin D, Touati G, Prieur AM, et al. Growth hormone treatment of short stature and metabolic dysfunction in juvenile chronic arthritis. *Acta Paediatr Suppl* 1999;88(428):100–105.
277. Pepmueller PH, Cassidy JT, Allen SH, et al. Bone mineralization and bone mineral metabolism in children with juvenile rheumatoid arthritis. *Arthritis Rheum* 1996;39:746–757.
278. Pereira RM, Falco V, Corrente JE, et al. Abnormalities in the biochemical markers of bone turnover in children with juvenile chronic arthritis. *Clin Exp Rheumatol* 1999;17(2):251–255.
279. Henderson CJ, Cawkwell GD, Specker BL, et al. Predictors of total body bone mineral density in non-corticosteroid-treated prepubertal children with juvenile rheumatoid arthritis. *Arthritis Rheum* 1997;40: 1967–1975.
280. Haugen M, Lien G, Flato B, et al. Young adults with juvenile arthritis in remission attain normal peak bone mass at the lumbar spine and forearm. *Arthritis Rheum* 2000;43(7):1504–1510.
281. Giannini EH, Brewer EJ. Poor correlation between the erythrocyte sedimentation rate and clinical activity in juvenile rheumatoid arthritis. *Clin Rheumatol* 1987;6:197–201.
282. Kunnamo I, Kallio P, Pelkonen P, et al. Clinical signs and laboratory tests in the differential diagnosis of arthritis in children. *Am J Dis Child* 1987;141:34–40.
283. Giannini EH, Brewer EJ. Poor correlation between the erythrocyte sedimentation rate and clinical activity in juvenile rheumatoid arthritis. *Clin Rheumatol* 1987;6:197–201.
284. Hussein A, Stein J, Ehrich JHH. C-reactive protein in the assessment of disease activity in juvenile rheumatoid arthritis and juvenile spondyloarthritis. *Scand J Rheumatol* 1987;16:101–105.
285. van der Net J, Kuis W, Prakken ABJ, et al. Correlates of disablement in systemic onset juvenile chronic arthritis. *Scand J Rheumatol* 1997; 26:188–196.
286. Greulich WW, Pyle SI, Todd TW. Radiographic atlas of skeletal development of the hand and wrist. Stanford, CA: Stanford University Press, 1959:1–256.
287. Pyle SI, Hoerr NL. *A radiographic standard of reference for the growing knee.* Springfield, IL: Charles C Thomas, 1969:1–135.
288. Poznanski AK, Hernandez RJ, Guire KE, et al. Carpal length in children—a useful measurement in the diagnosis of rheumatoid arthritis and some congenital malformation syndromes. *Radiology* 1978;129:661–668.

289. Poznanski AK, Roche AF, Mukherjee D, et al. Norms of the apparent width of the knee joint: useful measures in the evaluation of children with juvenile rheumatoid arthritis. *Am J Radiol* 1995;145:870.
290. Aaron A, Weinstein D, Thickman D, et al. Comparison of orthoroentgenography and computed tomography in the measurement of limb-length discrepancy. *J Bone Joint Surg Am* 1992;74(6): 897–902.
291. Eastwood DM, Cole WG. A graphic method of timing the correction of leg-length discrepancy. *J Bone Joint Surg Am* 1995;77(5):743–747.
292. Bjorkengren AG, Geborek P, Rydholm U, et al. MR imaging of the knee in acute rheumatoid arthritis. *Am J Radiol* 1990;155:329–332.
293. Konig H, Sieper J, Karl-Juergen W. Rheumatoid arthritis: evaluation of hypervascular and fibrous pannus with dynamic MR imaging enhanced with Gd-DTPA. *Radiology* 1990;176:473–477.
294. Kursunoglu-Brahme S, Riccio T, Weisman MH, et al. Rheumatoid knee: role of gadopentetate-enhanced MR imaging. *Radiology* 1990; 176:831–835.
295. Sureda D, Quiroga S, Arnal C, et al. Juvenile rheumatoid arthritis of the knee: evaluation with US. *Radiology* 1994;190:403–406.

CHAPTER 62

Treatment of Juvenile Rheumatoid Arthritis

Edward H. Giannini and Hermine I. Brunner

An appropriately designed comprehensive care management program for a child with juvenile rheumatoid arthritis (JRA) has many components, only one of which is pharmacotherapy. This statement is true regardless of the onset or type of course of JRA that the patient demonstrates. Additionally, the impact of JRA has been shown to have a variety of deleterious effects on the family of the child. Thus, consideration of the needs of the entire family, including psychosocial and financial, is essential when developing a management program. Because JRA is a chronic illness, the long-term, as well as the short-term, needs of the patient and family must be anticipated and addressed. As described in Chapter 61, an emerging consensus is that the diseases now collectively designated as JRA in the United States will be referred to as juvenile idiopathic arthritis (JIA).

TABLE 62.1. *Treatment team for the child with arthritis*

Patient
Parents, siblings, other caregivers
Physicians
Primary care physician
Pediatric rheumatologist
Other consultants (as indicated)
Orthopedic surgeon
Ophthalmologist
Dentist
Other
Allied health professionals
Nurse
Social worker
Physical therapist
Occupational therapist
Psychologist
Nutritionist
Community agencies
School
Vocational agencies

Keeping the child with JRA out of the hospital and in the mainstream of life is central to the management approach. Much of the recent effort that is described later in this chapter has been directed toward the goal of providing necessary services and therapy, which in years past required hospitalization, on an outpatient basis.

Thus, the overall management program is carried out best by a multidisciplinary team of health professionals with expertise in dealing with children and families. Team membership may vary in detail; an optimal membership team is shown in Table 62.1. The essential components include a focus on the child and family in the community setting, the provision of comprehensive care required for an optimal outcome for the child, the coordination of services by an experienced clinician, and a high degree of intrateam communication and cooperation. This construct of management has been termed family-centered, community-based, coordinated care (1). Excellent self-help books are available to help patients, families, and care providers in recognizing and meeting the needs of children and adolescents with JRA (2,3). Numerous associations and foundations provide materials and Web-based information, and hold meetings aimed at assisting patients and families of children with rheumatic diseases. These include the American Juvenile Arthritis Organization, a council of the Arthritis Foundation, the Myositis Association, and the Lupus Foundation of America.

AIM OF TREATMENT

The aim of treatment of children with JRA is to minimize the effects of inflammation. This includes control of pain, prevention of loss or restoration of range of motion, restoration of function, and the promotion of normal growth and development, thereby resulting in an acceptable quality of life.

Control of Pain

Management of chronic pain in children is a complicated and occasionally difficult problem and might receive insufficient attention in children with JRA, many of whom do not complain of pain (4). Discomfort associated with JRA is often described as aching or stiffness, becoming severe only when extensive joint damage has occurred. The nearly constant presence of painful joints has a significant negative effect on the overall well-being of the child, and his or her ability to function. Furthermore, physical therapy, although necessary, can be uncomfortable.

Prevention of Loss or Restoration of Range of Motion

Loss of range of motion accompanies joint inflammation and requires prompt attention to minimize its effects on long-term function. Extension losses are most significant, although flexion losses, especially of the elbows, wrists, metacarpophalangeal joints, hips, and knees, are also common.

Although normal physical activities should be encouraged, it is not sufficient for the child simply to "be active." An additional program of active and passive stretching is almost always necessary. The program should be prescribed by an experienced physical therapist and carried out at home by the parents. Some parents understandably have difficulty being both parent and therapist, and some children require additional visits to a physical therapist for a brief, intensive intervention and to establish a more manageable home program. The chronic nature of these disorders requires ongoing intervention that can be carried out at home with periodic revisions to the program by the physical therapist. The exercise program should be instituted early in the treatment course, once antiinflammatory medications have had an opportunity to minimize inflammation and provide analgesia. If ignored, losses of active extension can become fixed contractures, posing an even more difficult therapeutic problem. Although sufficient rest is important, it is rarely appropriate to confine the child to bed.

Restoration of Function

In designing therapy programs, especially for small children, the focus should be on areas of motion loss or muscle weakness that most significantly affect function. It is often not possible to exercise all of the joints in a reasonable time, and priorities must be established. Loss of hand function or the ability to stand or walk are of great functional importance and are priorities in physical management. Patients and their families should be instructed in joint protection guidelines in order to remain active but minimize stress on the joints.

Promotion of Normal Growth and Development

Normal physical and psychological growth and development are the foremost goals of treatment. Physical or pharmacologic therapies might have to be modified at times to accommodate these goals. Understanding the physical, psychological, and social developmental milestones and their importance to the child's lifelong well-being will help prevent overly aggressive or indulgent treatment. A child with JRA should be treated as a normal child with exceptions made as required. The child's relationships with his or her parents, siblings, other family members, schoolmates, and other members of the community should be as normal as possible.

Impairment of physical growth might occur as a result of the disease or deficient nutrition, or as a side effect of treatment with corticosteroids. Children with chronic arthritis are frequently malnourished (5,6). Restoration of adequate nutrition can have a beneficial effect on growth velocity. Growth hormone has been used to promote growth, but the cost is high, the effect moderate, and the influence on adult height unknown (7–9). With the availability of more potent antiarthritis drugs, growth failure secondary to corticosteroid use or because of long-standing active disease is less of an issue now than in the past.

Health-Related Quality of Life

Recent emphasis on patient-centered outcomes has emphasized the need to consider and measure the child's health-related quality of life (HRQOL). Easy to use, well-validated tools for the measurement of HRQOL, even in younger children, are now available. The Pediatric Quality of Life Inventory is a modular formatted instrument with generic core scales and condition-specific and treatment-related modules (10,11). Recent reviews underscore the importance of measuring HRQOL and urge clinicians to use these instruments in the routine clinic to help increase their utilization in clinical care (12).

ELEMENTS OF THE COMPREHENSIVE MANAGEMENT PROGRAM

A minimum of five aspects of care constitute the essential components of a comprehensive management program for the child with JRA: (a) physical management, (b) psychosocial care, (c) nutritional aspects, (d) pharmacologic management, and (e) a group of nonrheumatologic aspects of medical care collectively referred to as other medical aspects. Importantly, these different aspects of management must not be thought of as independent entities (i.e., one having no influence on the next). The coordination of these components is vital, and determines the success or failure of the entire program.

Physical Management

Physical and occupational therapists have a central role in the comprehensive management program of the child with JRA. These two specialists should play an active role from the time of diagnosis and be familiar with the unique problems posed by the arthritic child. Effective treatment must allow sufficient time for the development of a trusting relationship between child and therapist. In general, following the assessment of range of motion and muscle strength, the joints most in need of attention should be determined and a specific treatment program instituted.

A landmark turning point for all children with disabilities was the passage by the U.S. Congress in 1975 of the Education for All Handicapped Children's Act (Public Law 94–142) that required all public schools to provide a free appropriate public education (FAPE) for all children with disabilities who were 6 to 21 years of age. The law provided for free supportive services that are required to assist the child, including, among many others, physical and occupational therapy. A later law (Public Law 102–119) passed in 1991, the Individuals with Disabilities Education Act Amendments, provided for even more extensive services to families. These provisions have given tremendous impetus for keeping children with rheumatic diseases in the mainstream of life.

Physical Therapy

An extensive review of the methods of physical therapy appropriate for use in the child with JRA is not possible here. The reader is referred to the reference list for detailed manuals of physical therapy evaluation and treatment of the JRA patient (13–15). The goals of physical therapy treatment of the patient with JRA include (a) maintenance or increase of joint range of motion, (b) maintenance or increase of muscular strength, (c) maintenance or increase of endurance for activities of daily living, (d) decrease of pain, and (e) maintenance of neutral postural alignment.

Education of the parents and patient about the need for, and methods of, physical therapy is essential to ensure adherence with the home treatment and exercise program.

Care must be taken not to exceed the child's physical and psychological tolerance for any treatment program. Few children under the age of 5 or 6 years can tolerate an exercise program that takes more than 15 or 20 minutes twice daily. Older children are unlikely to comply with a program that takes more than 30 minutes twice daily. Games, books, and toys help to distract the child, and prolong the time available for therapy. For intensive inpatient treatment, treatment sessions of 1 hour twice daily with 1 additional hour of hydrotherapy can be accomplished. It is best to arrange the physical therapy sessions for the time of day that is most suitable for the child, often in the late morning or early afternoon. A hot shower, bath, or hydrotherapy before beginning the exercises will diminish stiffness and pain, and will facilitate optimal results. When possible, an effort should be made to schedule treatment programs around school hours to minimize loss of educational opportunities.

Occupational Therapy

An occupational therapist is required to adequately assess the child's functional capabilities, paying particular attention to age-specific activities of daily living (16). As with physical therapy, space limitations do not allow for a comprehensive review of the methods of occupational therapy specific to JRA. However, the goals of occupational therapy are closely related to those of physical therapy: (a) improve efficiency of effort (energy conservation); (b) substitute certain activities for others (joint protection); (c) increase independence by the use of assistive aids and techniques; and (d) use splints to correct or prevent deformities, correct or prevent contractures, and aid flexion and extension of involved areas.

As with physical therapy, the patient and parent must be educated early regarding the necessity of wearing splints and using the prescribed assistive devices to prevent further damage to susceptible joints and tissues.

Specific Approaches

Pain Management Strategies

Previous research supports that children with JRA have a lower pain threshold compared with healthy children (17), which could be due to central and peripheral neural sensitization (18). The intensity of pain is not only related to the degree of the underlying disease activity, but also to the ability of the child to use pain coping strategies (19). Besides disease control, cooling of inflamed joints and transcutaneous electrical stimulation are helpful. In addition, cognitive behavioral interventions can be used, such as cognitive refocusing and guided imagery to lower the conscious attention to pain. Pain control stress management techniques, such as progressive muscle relaxation and meditative breathing, have been used successfully (18).

Hydrotherapy

Warm water (96°F) provides relief from pain, and the buoyancy of the water helps children strengthen muscles and increase the range of motion of affected joints. The psychological benefit of hydrotherapy also adds to the overall effectiveness of this approach.

Passive Stretching

Passive stretching is necessary, but should be done with caution. Specific hazards include the tendency to increase subluxation of the tibia at the knee or of the carpus at the wrist, and the risk for fracture of osteoporotic bone. Lying in a prone position is useful in reducing hip flexion contractures if the pelvis is properly anchored in a neutral position.

Active Exercise

Active movement of joints with or without resistance is needed to rebuild muscle strength. Alone, however, active exercise is seldom sufficient to regain lost range. The child should be encouraged to put all involved joints through the full available active range of motion at least once daily. Observation of a decreased active range of motion can be the first clue to the worsening of disease in a particular joint.

Serial Casting

Flexion contracture at the knee or elbow, and flexion contracture or ulnar deviation at the wrist, often respond well to careful serial casting. Application of a fiberglass cast in a position of maximal extension for 2 to 5 days, followed by physical therapy and reapplication of the cast in a few more degrees of extension for additional 2 to 5 days, is useful for management of flexion contractures in which gains achieved by passive stretching by the physical therapist have reached a plateau. Serial casting protocols vary in duration due to the concern of regaining flexion. The 2- to 5-day interval has not been associated with failure to regain flexion. A well-fitted resting splint or bivalved cast should be worn at night for 3 to 6 months following the procedure to maintain the final position achieved. Occasionally, gentle manipulation of the joint under anesthetic after injection of intraarticular triamcinolone hexacetonide, followed by application of the cast in maximal extension for a 48-hour period, is needed; this procedure can be expected to be effective if adequate follow-up physical therapy is instituted.

Splinting

Resting, working, or, occasionally, dynamic splints in older children for wrists and fingers are useful for preventing and correcting deformities. Attention must be directed to a comfortable fit to ensure compliance. Splints require frequent readjustment to allow for improved position and growth, and the ongoing supervision of an occupational therapist is essential. Resting splints for wrists, knees, and, occasionally, ankles are useful for maintaining good positioning and minimizing pain associated with movement at night. It is usually easier for the child to wear one or, at most, two night splints at a time. If more are required, they should be alternated every other night. Working splints for the wrist provide support and relief from pain associated with writing or other hand functions. Alterations in writing equipment or style are also useful for the school-aged child with small joint disease of the hands.

Cervical Collars

Soft cervical collars can reduce neck pain and may be worn day or night. Hard collars might be required in the unlikely event of significant cervical instability, but are often poorly accepted by the child because of restriction of movement.

Shoes and Insoles

The selection of appropriate footwear is important for the child with lower extremity arthritis. Attention should be directed to ensuring that shoes are the correct size and have a firm heel support and cushioned soles. Custom-molded insoles, constructed of semirigid thermoplastic or soft accommodating materials, are of considerable help in dealing with foot and ankle pain and might minimize progressive deformity as the child grows. They should be made with the child in a non-weight-bearing position, with the talus in neutral position to provide support for the arch. Specific problems, such as pronation or pain in the metatarsophalangeal joints, may also be effectively managed by well-made insoles.

Lifts and Leg Length Inequalities

Overgrowth of one leg caused by inflammation of a joint (usually the knee) on that side might require the application of a lift to the sole of the shoe on the opposite leg. Uncompensated leg length inequality can produce alterations in gait and can exacerbate disease in the ankle, hip, or back. Minor discrepancies in leg length (less than ¼ inch) seldom require treatment or can be overcome by inserting a thin insole into the contralateral shoe. Even if minor, the discrepancy can cause pelvic asymmetry on standing (noted by unequal anterior superior iliac spines positions), the discrepancy should be corrected with shoe insoles in order to reduce any stress caused by the altered alignment.

Psychosocial Aspects of Management

Although most children and adolescents cope well with the social and psychosocial consequences of JRA (20,21), they are at a higher risk for overall adjustment problems (22). Children with severe and active JRA are likely to have difficulties with social acceptance (23). Thus, a child with chronic disease such as JRA might have a number of problems that require the expertise of a social worker or psychologist. The family, school, and community, as well as the child, can be negatively affected by the challenges presented by arthritis (24). Some of the most common and most significant problems are discussed here.

Child's Self-Image

In the competitive world in which most of today's children grow up, physical achievement and attractive physical appearance often assume unjustified importance (25). Both can be impaired by a disease such as chronic arthritis. More importantly, the child's confidence in his or her abilities and appearance might be fragile. Recognition of this can help the caregiver understand difficult behavior patterns, nonadherence with medical interventions, withdrawal, and depression.

School Participation

With a few exceptions, children with chronic arthritis should attend a regular school. Participation in physical education, to the limit of the child's ability, should be encouraged. Discussions with the child's classroom teacher, physical education teacher, and school nurse or counselor provide guidance that enables the school personnel to work productively with the child and parents. In older children, consideration of vocational goals and provision of work-readiness experiences are important (26).

Recreation

Ideally, the child with arthritis should participate in school and community recreation programs with other children. Recreational swimming, bicycling, and low-impact sporting activities are recommended. For a child living in a remote or isolated community, the opportunity to meet other children with similar challenges can be provided by a recreational program such as summer camp. The opportunities that such a camp presents for patient, parent, and professional education are also important (27).

Family Functioning

The unexpected development of chronic, potentially disabling disease in a young child can have devastating consequences on the functioning of the family unit, ranging from depression and guilt to divorce (28). Although most families of children with chronic arthritis function similarly to families of healthy children, mothers especially of children with JRA show increased signs of physiologic distress (29). Appropriate counseling by a social worker or psychologist can be an important facet of management of the child and family. Good family functioning is important, because it is related to the child's functioning, depression, and adjustment to the disease (30).

Patient and Parent Education

Treatment effectiveness can be enhanced by education of the patient and parent and, as needed, of other significant caregivers in the family. This can best be accomplished by ensuring the availability of an understanding, informed health professional, often a nurse, who can explain symptoms, the effects and side effects of treatment, and the necessity for follow-up by other specialists such as ophthalmologists, orthopedists, and orthodontists. This task can be facilitated by use of the written and audiovisual educational material available from the Arthritis Foundation in the United States or the Arthritis Society in Canada.

Financial Burden

Although many costs for children with long-term illness are borne by insurance plans, there are inevitably additional costs associated with the child's illness. The costs of JRA for the health system are estimated to average $7,900 annually. In addition, families of children with chronic arthritis spend at least 5% of their income on health-care expenses due to arthritis (31). This can pose a considerable burden to the family, and sometimes require the social worker's advice with respect to financial planning and use of community resources. These factors must also be considered by the physician who is prescribing medications and splints or other orthoses.

Nutritional Aspects of Management

Children with chronic inflammatory diseases are at risk for the development of complications secondary to nutritional deficiencies, including osteoporosis (32). Decreased food intake accompanies chronic diseases of many types, including JRA, owing to anorexia. Medications, such as nonsteroidal anti-inflammatory drugs (NSAIDs) and hydroxychloroquine, may aggravate the anorexia. Temporomandibular joint disease may also contribute to decreased food intake because of pain associated with chewing. It is important to ensure that the child with arthritis has a diet that is balanced in food types and sufficient in calories. Referral to a registered dietitian for comprehensive nutritional assessment and provision of nutrition education and continued support is essential for the optimal management of the child with chronic arthritis (33).

Obesity may be secondary to inactivity imposed by lower extremity arthritis, or excessive food intake secondary to glucocorticoid use. Dietary management of the overweight child is complex, and care must be taken to ensure a balanced diet even when calories are moderately restricted. Management of the weight gain associated with long-term glucocorticoid use is even more difficult. Steroids make many children ravenously hungry, and restriction of food intake may be problematic. Occasionally, sodium restriction and the judicious use of diuretics may facilitate weight loss in this group of children. Steroid-induced weight gain is usually temporary; when the prednisone dose is reduced below 4 or 5 mg per day, the cushingoid weight gain disappears. Rarely, steroid-induced hyperglycemia may require restriction of simple carbohydrates in the diet.

Failure to thrive, characterized by abnormally low rates of growth in weight and height, is a common feature of children with prolonged inflammatory disease. In such children, nutritional supplementation may be indicated to optimize growth potential. A diet consisting of small, frequent, nutrient-dense feedings may be beneficial. Nocturnal, nasogastric tube feedings have been used to improve depleted protein stores and promote growth in children with prolonged growth failure (34).

Dietary supplements of vitamins, iron, and calcium are appropriate in some children with JRA. To minimize osteoporosis associated with prolonged glucocorticoid use, it is important to provide the minimum daily recommended quantities of vitamin D (400 IU) and calcium (500 mg for 1- to 3-year-olds, 800 mg for 4- to 8-year-olds, and 1,300 mg for those over 9 years of age) (35). Supplemental iron should be considered in children with significant hypochromic anemia. Although this complication is likely to reflect the effects of inflammation, increased gastrointestinal blood loss from NSAIDs may contribute to iron deficiency.

Many children with arthritis are given unconventional dietary remedies in the mistaken belief that they are beneficial. There is no special diet for children with JRA, nor are there any special foods that prevent or cure the disease. Dietary counseling on the importance of a well-balanced diet and the avoidance of potentially harmful dietary practices should be provided. Demonstration by the rheumatology team of an active and supportive interest in the child's nutrition and growth, and forewarning parents concerning the frequency and inaccuracy of claims concerning special diets for children with arthritis usually prevent inappropriate dietary manipulations.

Pharmacologic Aspects of Management

Overview of General Approach

Pharmacologic management of patients with JRA is complex. No medication currently available is universally effective or without adverse side effects. Until recently, efficacy was generally limited to improving signs and symptoms of disease. With the advent and availability of immune response modifiers (or "biologics"), prevention (and perhaps amelioration) of structural damage to the joint is sometimes possible, and certain medications may actually alter the course of the disease. Still, treatment remains ameliorative rather than curative. Medical treatment of JRA can improve quality of life and physical function, and limit deformity and disability.

Work continues in the effort to elucidate predictor variables (demographic, clinical, genetic) that may help to identify early those patients who are likely to experience a more resistant disease course, and thus be candidates for more aggressive therapy. At present, however, it remains difficult to decide which patients should be treated with higher tier drugs before irreversible joint damage has occurred (36). There may be a window of opportunity during the early stages of disease when a favorable response to aggressive therapy is more likely. Pharmacogenomics and RNA expression assays are beginning to have an impact on elucidating those patients more or less likely to respond to a given therapy (37).

The general approach to medical treatment of JRA today no longer can be represented by the so-called therapeutic pyramid, with NSAIDs at the base and more aggressive agents at the apex (38,39). The pharmacotherapeutic approach to the child with JRA, even early in the illness, depends on the disease course and treatment preferences of the patient and their families. A general overview of approaches to each subtype of JRA is presented in Table 62.2.

General Approach to Pharmacotherapy of Pauciarticular Juvenile Rheumatoid Arthritis

Children presenting with this form of JRA are no longer, without exception, started on systemic therapy with NSAIDs. Intraarticular injections of long-acting glucocorticosteroids such as triamcinolone hexacetonide and triamcinolone acetonide may be used initially in a high proportion of patients, even among those with multiple affected joints (doses and side effects are discussed in greater detail below). Most patients experience extended periods of disease quiescence in injected joints, and many physicians repeatedly inject the same joint after the beneficial affect has waned.

Systemic therapy among pauciarticular patients typically begins with NSAIDs but may move quickly to more aggressive therapy such as methotrexate (MTX). The NSAID of first choice remains naproxen (10–20 mg/kg/day divided two to three times daily, up to 1,250 mg/day). Nabumetone is the second most popular NSAID in children, and is given as a single daily dose of 1,000 to 2,000 mg. Studies of cyclooxygenase-2 (COX-2) inhibitors are underway in pauciarticular patients, and their use is undoubtedly rapidly increasing, even before pivotal studies in children are published.

MTX remains the second-line drug of first choice and is started quickly when NSAIDs fail (39), particularly among those in whom the physician feels that progression to a polyarticular course of disease is likely. Initial dose is typically 15 mg/m^2 per week (average weekly dose 0.4 mg/kg)

TABLE 62.2. *Approach to therapeutic management of the child with juvenile rheumatoid arthritis*

Disease course	NSAIDs	Intraarticular steroids	Oral or intravenous steroids	Methotrexate	Advanced therapies (DMARDs)	Biologic agents
Pauciarticular	■	■		■		
Polyarticular	■	■	■	■	■	■
Systemic	■	■	■	■	■	■

DMARD, disease-modifying antirheumatic drug; NSAID, nonsteroidal antiinflammatory drug.

(40), with some physicians using doses as high as 30 to 40 mg/m^2 per week. In children with pauciarticular onset of disease who are only partially responsive to MTX or in whom aggressive disease is likely to develop, etanercept is now frequently given even early in the disease course. The dose is 0.4 mg/kg per subcutaneous injection (maximum 25 mg per injection) given twice a week. At present, other drugs such as sulfasalazine, leflunomide, cytotoxic agents, and biologics (other than etanercept) such as infliximab and interleukin-1 receptor antagonist (IL-1Ra), play little role in the treatment of pauciarticular disease.

General Approach to Pharmacotherapy of Polyarticular Juvenile Rheumatoid Arthritis

In patients with polyarthritis in whom the arthritis is destructive or poorly controlled by NSAIDs, a second-line medication is added early in the disease course. MTX (at doses mentioned above), or sulfasalazine (30–50 mg/kg/day) are the two drugs of choice. Unlike treatment of adult RA, triple-drug therapy, consisting of concurrent MTX, sulfasalazine, and hydroxychloroquine, plays little role in the management of poly-JRA. Etanercept is combined with MTX in a high proportion of those cases, which are only partially responsive to MTX or sulfasalazine. Brunner et al. conducted a therapeutic survey during 1999 and 2000 among nine pediatric rheumatologists who consecutively sampled 395 patients with JRA (40). Oral glucocorticosteroids were used in 19 of 191 polyarticular patients in the survey (mean dose 0.19 mg/kg/day). Intraarticular steroids are frequently used to bring inflamed joints under control while waiting for the effects of second-line agents to be realized. A host of anti–tumor necrosis factor (TNF) agents and other immune response modifiers, such as anti-IL-1Ra and CTLA4-Ig, are currently under study in poly-JRA. However, current data regarding the effectiveness and safety of these agents are, at present, largely anecdotal.

General Approach to Pharmacotherapy of Systemic Juvenile Rheumatoid Arthritis

The general approach to pharmacologic management to systemic JRA is more complex than other forms of JRA due to the multiple manifestations that may be present. NSAIDs, prednisone (including IV steroid pulses for life-threatening complications such as pericarditis), and intra-articular steroids typically are used early in the disease. The mean dose of prednisone among 50 systemically ill children was 0.38 mg/kg/day in Brunner's survey (40). MTX at doses discussed above can be initiated early. Although the first pivotal trial of etanercept in systemic JRA is still underway and results have not been reported, its use in this subtype is quite common. A host of other biologic agents are currently being investigated for their therapeutic utility in systemic JRA. These include TNF blockers, IL-1Ra, and anti-IL-6 (39,41).

The use of cyclosporine, once a mainstay of treatment of systemic JRA, has diminished rapidly in the United States with the increased use of MTX and biologics.

Specific Agents

Nonsteroidal Antiinflammatory Drugs

Common Usage. Commonly used NSAID preparations and their relevant properties are described elsewhere in this text (see Chapter 31). NSAIDs do not alter the natural history of JRA, but they do lessen stiffness and pain, and increase range of motion, thus facilitating participation in physical therapy programs. The analgesic effect of NSAIDs is rapid; the antiinflammatory effect takes longer to achieve and requires doses up to twice as large as those needed for analgesia. NSAIDs alone are sufficient to control arthritis in only about one fourth of all patients with JRA (40), and most of these are in the pauciarticular subgroup.

Pediatric trials of aspirin, fenoprofen, ketoprofen, sodium meclofenamate, pirprofen, and proquazone conducted by the Pediatric Rheumatology Collaborative Study Group (PRCSG) and employing a standard methodology concluded that the differences in effectiveness between these NSAIDs were small, although some seemed more toxic than others (42). Using data from earlier trials, the group demonstrated that about 50% of children who eventually respond favorably to an NSAID do so by 2 weeks of therapy, but that up to one fourth will not respond until about 12 weeks of therapy (43). The mean time to response is 30 days, and the likelihood of an initial response to an NSAID is independent of the type of disease onset. A later study by the PRCSG showed that liquid ibuprofen was as effective as aspirin and had a better safety profile (44).

Availability of the new selective COX-2 inhibitors undoubtedly have reduced the gastrointestinal consequences observed with older NSAIDs, particularly in adult patients (45–47). Large-scale trials of celecoxib (Celebrex, Pfizer Inc., New York, NY, U.S.A.), meloxicam (Mobic, Boehringer-Ingelheim Pharma KG, Ingelheim, Germany), and rofecoxib (Vioxx, Merck & Co., West Point, PA, U.S.A.) are currently underway in children with JRA. Preliminary data are available from a phase I/II trial of meloxicam (48). Foeldvari et al. reported on a 12-week open-label study of meloxicam at a dosage of 0.25 mg/kg once daily in 36 patients with JRA requiring NSAIDs. Thirty-one completed the study. Using the American College of Rheumatology (ACR) Pediatric 30 Criteria as the primary outcome (49), 44% improved by week 4, 62% by week 12, and 74% by week 52. Drug-related adverse events occurred in 5 patients and were mild.

Large endoscopic studies of patients with adult rheumatoid arthritis (RA) have shown conclusively that these agents produce less gastrointestinal bleeding than do the other NSAIDs, which variably inhibit both COX-1 and COX-2 (45,50). Anecdotal reports suggest that they are not without side effects (51,52), including in patients with JRA

(53). At present, these agents are considerably more expensive than conventional NSAIDs. Additionally, many of the gastrointestinal problems that concern internists are of lesser concern to the pediatrician. Thus, the ultimate usefulness of these agents in JRA remains to be determined (54).

Options. According to the survey of Brunner (40) cited above, there is a clear preference for naproxen. Of the 303 patients on NSAIDs, 55% were given naproxen. It is dosed twice daily, comes in liquid and pill forms, and has a favorable toxicity-to-efficacy profile. Its ability to produce pseudoporphyria, however, limits its usefulness in fair-skinned individuals (55). Other NSAIDs identified in the survey and the frequency with which they were given were nabumetone in 15%, COX-2 inhibitors or indomethacin in 7%, respectively, ibuprofen or tolmetin sodium in 6%, respectively, and other NSAIDs in 4%.

It would appear, then, that deciding which NSAID to use in a particular patient is partly science and mainly art. In general, NSAID effectiveness is idiosyncratic. A favorable initial response occurs in over half of patients on the first NSAID prescribed. Fifty percent of those showing inadequate response on the first NSAID will improve with another drug of the same class (56).

In clinical practice, lack of efficacy can often be traced to poor patient compliance. Starting with an NSAID that has a favorable toxicity-to-efficacy profile and can be taken on a convenient schedule in a convenient formulation is a reasonable approach. Adequate education about the need to use NSAIDs routinely must be emphasized. To be used as an antiinflammatory medication, not simply an analgesic, NSAIDs must be taken on a consistent basis. If an NSAID is not adequately effective after a 2- to 3-month trial, then an alternative NSAID can be tried (43). Acetaminophen may be used with an NSAID on an as-needed basis for fever or pain. Combining NSAIDs should be done with caution, if at all; synergy may occur in toxicity but not necessarily efficacy (56,57).

Precautions. An overview of safety monitoring of patients with JRA on NSAID therapy is provided in Table 62.3. The majority of children tolerate NSAID therapy quite well. The most common side effect of NSAID therapy is abdominal pain and anorexia. Undoubtedly, NSAIDs can cause clinically significant gastrointestinal side effects, but the risk for serious gastrointestinal injury must be weighed against the substantial potential for alleviating disease signs and symptoms (58,59). Any patient on chronic NSAID therapy should be monitored for adverse renal, hepatic, and gastrointestinal effects. Because of the occasional occurrence of interstitial nephritis and renal papillary necrosis, a routine urinalysis should be performed every 3 to 6 months. Slight elevations of serum levels of the liver enzymes aspartate aminotransferase (AST) and alanine aminotransferase (ALT) frequently occur in children receiving NSAIDs, and these serum enzymes should be measured every 3 to 6 months. Elevations in the transaminases are most common with salicylates but may be seen with other NSAIDs.

Children and parents should be aware of the signs and symptoms of gastric ulcer and gastrointestinal bleeding, which are uncommon but important side effects of NSAIDs. NSAIDs should be taken with food to minimize gastric irri-

TABLE 62.3. *Summary of monitoring of antiarthritis medications in children with juvenile rheumatoid arthritis*

Medication	Frequency of Monitoring	Laboratory Studies to Be Performed
NSAIDs	0, 1, 3 and every 6 mo	CBC and differential, ALT, AST, albumin, BUN, creatinine, UA
Adalimumab	0, 0.5, 1 and every 3 mo	CBC and differential, ESR or CRP; ANA and dsDNA every 6 mo; PPD at baseline
Anakinra	0, 0.5, 1 and every 3 mo	CBC and differential, ESR or CRP
Cyclosporin	0, 0.5, 1 and every 2 mo	CBC and differential, ESR or CRP, ALT, AST, albumin, BUN, creatinine, UA, CSA trough
Etanercept	0.05, 1 and every 3 mo	CBC and differential, ESR or CRP; ANA and dsDNA at 0 and every 6 mo; PPD at baseline
Hydroxycholoroquine	Eyes every 6 mo, laboratory studies 0, 1, and every 3 mo	CBC and differential, ALT, AST, albumin, ESR or CRP
Infliximab	With each infusion	CBC and differential, ESR or CRP; ANA and dsDNA at 0 and every 6 mo; PPD at baseline
Leflunomide	0, 0.5, 1 and every 2 mo	CBC and differential, ALT, AST, albumin, BUN, creatinine
Methotrexate	0, 0.5 and every 2 mo	CBC and differential, ALT, AST, albumin, BUN, creatinine
Prednisone	0, 1 and every 2 mo	CBC and differential, ALT, AST, albumin, BUN, creatinine, glucose, UA; lipid profile at 0 and 6 mo; if calcium and vitamin D supplementation, then urine calcium/creatinine ratio and serum calcium at 0 and every 6 mo
Sulfasalazine	0, 0.5, 1 and every 3 mo	CBC and differential, ALT, AST, albumin, BUN, UA, creatinine, ESR or CRP; immunoglobulins at 0 and every 6 mo

ALT, alanine transaminase; ANA, antinuclear antibody; AST, aspartate transaminase; BUN, blood urea nitrogen; CBC, complete blood count; CRP, C-reactive protein; dsDNA, double-stranded DNA; ESR, erythrocyte sedimentation rate; NSAIDS, nonsteroidal anti-inflammatory drugs; PPD, purified protein derivative; UA, urinalysis.

tation. Gastrointestinal protective medications such as sucralfate, antacids, or histamine (H_2) blockers are sometimes used.

NSAIDs also may have deleterious effects on coagulation and the central nervous system. Most NSAIDs increase bruising and some cause frank abnormalities in coagulation. Additionally, mood alteration and tinnitus may be produced by NSAID therapy.

There are a few contraindications: tolmetin and indomethacin in patients with cardiac dysfunction because of the hemodilution effect; aspirin in patients with asthma; and any salicylate in glucose-6-phosphate dehydrogenase (G6PD) deficiency, influenza, and varicella infections, because of the association with Reye syndrome.

Second-Line Agents

Approximately three fourths of children with JRA will not respond adequately to an NSAID alone, and treatment with a second-line drug should then be considered (60). The second-line drugs are a diverse group of medications, some of which are more toxic than NSAIDs and take longer to have an effect. These agents are often referred to as disease-modifying antirheumatic drugs (DMARDs). The term *DMARDs* formerly was considered a misnomer. With the advent of newer, more effective agents, and the use of combinations of second-line agents, disease modification now appears to be an attainable goal.

Many of the second-line agents have now undergone clinical evaluation in large-scale, double-blind, placebo-controlled trials in children with JRA. In many pediatric rheumatology clinics, MTX is the drug of choice for polyarthritis following inadequate response to NSAIDs. A general guide to monitoring of safety of the second-line agents and biologics can be found in Table 62.3.

Methotrexate. By the mid-1980s controlled trials in adults with RA had shown MTX to be very effective while maintaining an acceptable short-term safety profile (see also Chapter 32). Anecdotal reports in children with JRA were similarly encouraging. Based on these data, the PRCSG research network undertook a multinational, double-blind, placebo-controlled trial of the drug in children that demonstrated conclusively that MTX achieved greater efficacy than did placebo, and that the minimum effective dose was at least 10 mg/m^2 of body surface area per week (60). A subsequent metanalysis of randomized placebo-controlled trials of D-penicillamine (10 mg/kg/day), hydroxychloroquine (6 mg/kg/day), auranofin (0.5 mg/kg/ day), and two dose levels of MTX (5 and 10 mg/m^2/wk) concluded that only MTX (10 mg/m^2/wk) was significantly more effective than placebo. Furthermore, the higher dose of MTX produced greater effect sizes for all response variables than any other treatment studied (61). A long-term follow-up study of JRA patients who had received MTX showed that a high proportion of children were able to remain on the drug for extended periods (62). MTX is relatively safe for at least several years of treatment at a dose of 10 mg/m^2/wk (63). An extensive review in the English-language literature of all major published studies of MTX in children with JRA concluded that potential benefits greatly outweigh the risks (36). At present, MTX has become the preferred second-line agent among most practitioners. In the survey by Brunner et al. cited above, MTX was used in nearly 40% of the 395 patients surveyed (40). There is now firm evidence that MTX may actually slow or halt the progression of bony destruction in adult RA as evidenced by radiographs (64–66). It does not, however, appear to induce long-standing disease remissions. MTX absorption is highly variable, but oral absorption at doses over 10 to 30 mg/m^2 is poor (67). Both subcutaneous and intramuscular routes are equally effective for higher doses or in patients with poor absorption; however, the subcutaneous route is perhaps more convenient and less painful (68).

Preliminary reports of the clinical utility of higher dose MTX (up to 1.2 mg/kg/wk) are encouraging, and the practice of prescribing more than 10 mg/m^2/wk in the MTX-nonresponsive patient has already become widespread (67). In a recent landmark study conducted in 20 countries reported by Ruperto et al. (69), 80 patients with JRA who failed to respond to conventional doses of MTX according to the ACR Pediatric 30 were randomized to receive either medium (15 mg/m^2/wk; maximum of 20 mg/wk) or higher doses (30 mg/m^2/wk; maximum of 40 mg/wk) of MTX for 6 months. Among the 40 randomized to medium dose, 62.5% improved using the ACR Pediatric 30 (49), compared with 57.5% in the higher-dose group (p = NS). There were no significant differences in safety. Thus, doses of MTX greater than 20 mg/wk do not appear to provide added clinical benefit over lower doses.

Because MTX has a number of significant safety concerns, clinicians wish to taper or discontinue MTX as soon and as rapidly as possible. Ravelli et al. have shown that patients who have achieved remission on MTX and who are quickly discontinued from therapy (2–5 months after achieving remission) frequently relapse (70). In addition, patients who do relapse are often difficult to "recapture" with MTX therapy. These investigators concluded that MTX should be continued for about 1 year after remission is realized.

Common adverse effects of MTX include oral ulcers [which can be lessened by supplemental folic acid 1 mg/day or folinic acid 2.5–7.5 mg once weekly given 24 hours after MTX (71)], gastrointestinal disturbances, and, to a lesser extent, bone marrow suppression. Initial concerns about carcinogenesis and infertility appear to have been unwarranted, but the teratogenic properties of the drug are well recognized. Pulmonary opportunistic infections with *Pneumocystis carinii* have been reported in adult patients with RA treated with MTX (72,73).

The risk for hepatic injury was initially felt to be very high, but if alcohol intake is eliminated, other hepatotoxic drugs are minimized, and careful monitoring occurs, the risk for hepatic injury in children appears to be modest. The ACR has published guidelines for the frequency and indications for performing liver biopsy in adult RA patients given MTX (74). The appropriateness of these guidelines for children has not been subjected to large-scale studies. However, in a study of 33 percutaneous liver biopsies from 25 patients with JRA treated with MTX, Hashkes et al. found credible evidence that the adult guidelines are likely suitable for children also (75). Recommendations for routine liver biopsy after several years of treatment with no abnormalities in transaminases may be overly cautious. However, persistent elevation of the transaminases, even if only mildly elevated, is an indication for biopsy (68).

Sulfasalazine. Sulfasalazine is approved for use in children and adults with inflammatory bowel disease and in adults with RA. It currently plays a minor role in children with poly- or pauciarticular JRA and is never given to children with systemic JRA due to a relatively high rate of development of serum sickness. Brunner et al. found that only 5% of 195 children with JRA on second-line agents were given the agent (40). Unlike adult RA, it is rarely used in triple-drug therapy (sulfasalazine, hydroxychloroquine, MTX) for JRA.

A recent review by Brooks found reports in the literature of 550 JRA patients treated with the agent (76). About half of the children had pauciarticular and one third had polyarticular JRA. The agent was reported to have at least some efficacy in each of these subgroups. Intolerance and toxicity were reported to be similar to that seen in adults, with the exception of an increase of serum sickness among the systemically ill patients.

Several uncontrolled studies have suggested that sulfasalazine is a useful therapeutic agent for JRA, and a double-blind placebo-controlled, multicenter study has demonstrated its superiority compared with placebo in treating children with pauciarticular and polyarticular JRA (77). Sulfasalazine can be given at a dose of 50 mg/kg/day up to a maximum of 2 to 2.5 g/day. An effect is usually not seen before 4 to 6 weeks (77), but may not be seen for 3 months. Sulfasalazine should not be given to children with hypersensitivity to sulfa drugs or salicylates, to those with G6PD deficiency, to those with elevated liver enzymes or hematocytopenia, or to children with active systemic onset JRA. Potential toxicity to liver and bone marrow should be monitored. Nausea, vomiting, and diarrhea may occur, but are usually mild. Stevens-Johnson syndrome is rare but a potentially serious complication. Sulfasalazine may cause transient infertility in males (see Chapter 42).

Leflunomide. This agent is a novel isoxazole drug with antiproliferative and immunosuppressive properties (see Chapter 32). Numerous studies in adults with RA have shown it to be relatively safe and highly effective at daily doses of 20 mg (78). Studies are underway currently to assess leflunomide's pharmacologic properties in children. Silverman et al. reported the results of a randomized controlled trial of leflunomide (10 mg every other day after a loading dose; maximum 20 mg/day) versus MTX (0.5 mg/kg/wk up to 25 mg/wk) in 94 patients with polyarticular course JRA (79). After 16 weeks of therapy, 68% of the leflunomide group and 89% of the MTX group met the ACR Pediatric 30 definition of improvement ($p < 0.016$). Similarly, analysis of results by the Percent Improvement Index favored MTX. The researchers concluded that both agents were highly effective. A better response in the leflunomide group may have been realized with a higher dose. It was well tolerated in this group of patients and provided a therapeutic alternative to those who had failed to achieve a maximal response from MTX.

In the future this agent may become a therapeutic option in those who fail to respond or are intolerant of MTX. However, its known teratogenetic effect and long half-life will likely limit its use in JRA, at least in adolescents (80).

Hydroxychloroquine. This antimalarial medication still maintains a minor role as a second-line agent in JRA, and is given to about 10% of children on DMARDs. It has an immunomodulatory effect and inhibits collagenases (see Chapter 42). It is given at a dose of 5 to 6 mg/kg/day in a single daily dose to a maximum of 300 mg/day. Gastrointestinal absorption is highly variable, ranging from 30% to 100% (81). Onset of action takes several months, and 88% of responders will have done so by 6 months (82). The most severe side effects are dose-related retinal toxicity due to drug deposition and macular degeneration. Although the recommendations regarding ophthalmologic monitoring remain unclear (83), visual field and color vision evaluations should be obtained prior to, and every 6 to 12 months after, initiating hydroxychloroquine therapy (providing the recommended dose is not exceeded). The skin may acquire a muddy appearance due to dermal accumulation of the drug.

Thalidomide. Recently, there has been renewed interest in the use of this immunomodulatory agent in patients with systemic JRA unresponsive to conventional therapy. To date the data consist of anecdotal reports of small case series (84). This agent's safety and efficacy have not been explored in systemic JRA in legitimate clinical trials.

D-Penicillamine. A PRCSG study of D-penicillamine concluded that this drug had little or no therapeutic advantage over placebo (85). Attempts to recognize subgroups of JRA patients in whom this agent may provide therapeutic benefit were similarly unsuccessful (86). This and other studies ushered in an era during which this traditional treatment fell out of favor with many practitioners. Its role in the management of JRA is negligible.

Parenteral Gold. With the increasing acceptance of MTX as the second-line agent of first choice, the role of parenterally administered gold salts in the management of JRA has decreased dramatically in the past 15 years. Gold salts, primarily gold sodium thiomalate (Myochrysine, Merck) and aurothioglucose (Solganol, Schering Corp., Kenilworth, NJ, U.S.A.), were among the earliest effective drugs to be used to combat joint inflammation (87,88) (see Chapter 42). Although their use in arthritis was reported as early as the

1920s, there has never been a controlled, blinded trial of injectable gold in patients with JRA. Use of gold salts in treating JRA is now considered of historical interest only.

Oral Gold. An oral gold preparation, auranofin (Ridaura, Prometheus Laboratories, Inc., San Diego, CA) entered the market in the mid-1980s for treatment of adult RA. A series of studies by the PRCSG showed that oral gold was well absorbed by children with JRA and was quite safe, but that its efficacy was little more than that of placebo (89–92). It currently has no significant role in the pharmacologic management of JRA.

Intravenous Immune Globulin. Intravenous immune globulin (IVIG) has been used to treat children with systemic and polyarticular JRA. Although anecdotal reports were promising (93,94), a small controlled trial of IVIG in systemic JRA showed little benefit (95). A double-blind placebo-controlled study (96) of IVIG in polyarticular JRA showed some benefit in three fourths of the patients after treatment with 1.0 to 1.5 g of IVIG bimonthly for 2 months, then monthly for 6 months. The effect was transient, however. Considering the cost, the potential risk for disease transmission (97), and the limited efficacy, the role of IVIG in treating children with JRA is very limited. In the 1999 to 2000 survey by Brunner et al. (40), none of the 395 patients studied had received IVIG.

Cytotoxic Drugs (Azathioprine, Chlorambucil, Cyclosporine). Cytotoxic drugs are also discussed in Chapter 41. There is limited experience with the use of azathioprine in childhood arthritis. Kvien et al. reported the results of a double-blind, randomized 16-week comparison of azathioprine and placebo in 32 children with JRA taking NSAIDs and a moderate dose of prednisone (98). The differences between azathioprine and placebo were minimal, but there was a tendency for patients receiving azathioprine to exhibit some improvement. Savolainen et al. reported the longer-term outcome of 129 patients with JRA treated with azathioprine who were refractory to other agents (99). Remission was achieved in 15%, and temporary remission in 14%. Treatment was terminated due to adverse side effects in only 14%, and among these the side effects occurred within the first 2 months of treatment. The researchers concluded that the agent is useful in severe JRA with an acceptable safety profile. Whether or not the expected improvement outweighs the risks for toxicity, both immediate and long term, is difficult to assess. At present, azathioprine plays virtually no role in the treatment of any form of JRA.

The alkylating agent chlorambucil has been used for the treatment of JRA, especially when complicated by uveitis or amyloidosis (100,101). Although its use in the treatment of the eye disease has been largely discontinued, it might be required for the treatment of the extremely rare but life-threatening complication of amyloidosis (102) (see Chapter 93).

Although cyclosporine has been used to treat a range of rheumatic diseases (see Chapter 41), its use in children with JRA has been limited. Ostensen et al. (103) administered cyclosporine to children with refractory JRA. Toxicity (anemia, elevated creatinine) or inefficacy led to withdrawal of the drug in 11 of 14 patients studied. Recently, a large phase IV study of the drug was completed in the United States, South America, Mexico, and Europe (104). Three hundred thirty-nine patients, totaling 489 years of follow-up, had been treated with median doses of cyclosporine (largely Neoral, Novartis Pharmaceuticals, East Hanover, NJ, U.S.A.) 3.2 mg/kg/day for a median time of 1.3 years; 54% of the patients had systemic, 32% had polyarticular, and 14% had pauciarticular JRA. The researchers concluded that the drug is given for relatively short periods of time before discontinuation chiefly due to inefficacy. Renal complications occur in a substantial proportion of patients, although these tend to resolve quickly after discontinuation of the agent. In line with these unencouraging findings is that the use of cyclosporine worldwide has decreased dramatically with the advent and availability of the immune response modifiers.

Glucocorticosteroids

Since 1949, when Hench et al. (105) first described the clinical effect of corticosteroids in adults with RA (see Chapter 34), pediatric rheumatologists have been interested in the utility of these hormones in treating children (15). After a period of great enthusiasm for the use of cortisone and its analogues, the negative effects of such therapy became apparent (106). Prednisone and related drugs have continued to play an important role in the management of the systemic manifestations of JRA and in some patients with severe arthritis (40). Clinicians agree, however, that every attempt should be made to keep the dose, frequency, and duration of steroid administration to a minimum. If possible, prednisone should be given in the morning (rather than at night) to minimize growth suppression. If steroid use is longer than 5 or 6 days, there is a risk for suppression of the hypothalamic-pituitary-adrenal axis. For this reason, the drug must not be discontinued abruptly but should be tapered gradually over a few days (after brief use) or over several weeks (after prolonged use), since the recovery of normal adrenal responsiveness may take several months. Even gradual tapering of prednisone may be followed by a transient increase in musculoskeletal pain, an event that must be differentiated from a disease flare-up. Similar to NSAIDs, glucocorticosteroids do not alter the natural history of JRA.

Systemic Corticosteroids. High-dose intravenous hydrocortisone or methylprednisolone is sometimes of sustained benefit in the management of joint disease, but its use is usually restricted to children with life-threatening complications such as severe pericarditis, or disseminated intravascular coagulation due to macrophage activation syndrome.

Oral prednisone has a pivotal place in the management of many children with systemic-onset JRA, especially those with pericarditis and fever. Although an alternate day regimen has been advocated, it often fails to control the systemic disease. For this reason, it is usually necessary to prescribe daily or twice daily prednisone in a dose of 0.5 to 2.0 mg/kg, using the least amount of prednisone in the fewest doses per day that control the symptom or sign for which the drug was prescribed.

Oral prednisone in low dose (0.1–0.2 mg/kg/day) is often of benefit to the child with moderately well-controlled disease, but in whom night pain or incapacitating morning stiffness is the major problem. A small dose of prednisone at night may eliminate these symptoms and allow the child to function normally. Similarly, low-dose prednisone may be helpful in controlling symptoms during a flare-up of polyarticular disease, or while waiting for the onset of therapeutic effect of the DMARDs. Doses of prednisone below 0.2 mg/kg/day are not usually associated with significant cushingoid features. Growth suppression is one of the most worrisome long-term adverse effects and occurs in young children who are on prolonged glucocorticosteroid therapy in dosages equivalent to 3 mg/day of prednisone and increases substantially with higher doses (107). Treatment with growth hormone may be beneficial, especially if disease control has been achieved (8,9). Consideration should be given to the use of calcium and vitamin D supplements of children receiving long-term moderate- or high-dose corticosteroids in an effort to minimize osteoporosis (35). Significant trabecular bone loss occurs with doses that exceed 7.5 mg/day in most adults (108). The other well-recognized complications of long-term glucocorticosteroid use in adults may also occur in the child. They include immunosuppression, central nervous system effects (concentration problems, depression, psychosis), cataracts, protein wasting and myopathy. The necessity for administration of additional glucocorticosteroids at the time of surgical or other stress in the glucocorticosteroid-treated child should be recognized.

Intraarticular Glucocorticosteroids. Generally, injection of glucocorticosteroids directly into inflamed joints is of considerable benefit in the management of children with limited arthritis, particularly when treatment with NSAIDs has failed to completely control the disease, or children with limited arthritis who are intolerant to NSAIDs. Triamcinolone acetonide and triamcinolone hexacetonide result in more frequent and sustained benefit than other intraarticular preparations. A dose of triamcinolone hexacetonide of up to 20 mg per joint in small joints, and up to 40 mg per joint in large joints is appropriate. Higher doses of triamcinolone acetonide compared with those of triamcinolone hexacetonide have been suggested (109). For very young children (under 8 years of age), those in whom multiple joints are to be injected, those in whom hip joints are to be injected, or in children who are not expected to cooperate, joint injection under general anesthetic or conscious sedation is indicated. For others, the use of topical anesthetics in combination with local infiltration (1% xylocaine) often permits the procedure to be performed in the ambulatory clinic. Recently, the efficacy of topical anesthetics alone to achieve pain control during joint injections has been questioned (110). Following aspiration of the excess synovial fluid, and injection of triamcinolone (hex)acetonide, the needle track is carefully obliterated to minimize the risk for subcutaneous lipoatrophy. There is limited evidence that decreased motion and weight-bearing of the injected joint improves the therapeutic effects of joint injections. The joint can also be placed in a cast or splint for 24 to 48 hours. More recently, ultrasound-guided injections have been used to inject tendon sheaths and to improve the accurate deposition of the intraarticular glucocorticosteroid into the joint space (109).

Corticosteroids and the Treatment of Anterior Uveitis

Most children with anterior uveitis complicating JRA require topical glucocorticosteroids to control the ocular inflammation. The agents commonly used are dexamethasone 0.1%, prednisolone acetate 1.0%, and fluorometholone 0.1%. A prompt reduction in the flare-up and a reduction in the number of inflammatory cells in the anterior chamber is usually seen. Some children require subtenon's injections, however, and occasionally children with severe chronic uveitis need intravenous methylprednisolone (30 mg/kg per dose, to a maximum of 1 g per dose) given for 1 to 3 consecutive days. In addition to glucocorticosteroids, children with uveitis usually require mydriatics. More severe and persistently active uveitis should be treated with systemic NSAIDs and/or systemic MTX (111). For uveitis uncontrollable by these therapies, chlorambucil, TNF antagonists, or cyclosporine should be considered (112–114). Chelation of band keratopathy and removal of cataracts are occasionally necessary (115).

Adverse Side Effects of Glucocorticosteroids

Adverse effects of glucocorticosteroids are numerous (116). An infectious illness should be viewed seriously. Varicella infection, in particular, can be life-threatening (117). Varicella immunization should be considered for all nonimmune patients, if the disease course allows it. If immunization is not feasible, then varicella zoster immune globulin should be given to a nonimmune child on long-term steroids within 48 hours of a known exposure to chickenpox. Acyclovir given at the onset of varicella significantly decreases the disease severity during the infection, and given for 7 days, starting 7 to 9 days after an exposure, may abort varicella infection (118,119). All patients on steroids and those within 6 months of discontinuation should wear a Medi-Alert bracelet, because stress doses of steroids are needed for surgical procedures and significant illnesses.

Immune Response Modifiers (Biologics)

Rheumatology, as well as other areas such as oncology and endocrinology, are now reaping the benefits from the advances that have taken place in molecular biology and cellular immunology during the past decade (120,121) (see

Chapter 39). T-cell surface markers (CD4), T-cell receptors, human leukocyte antigen molecules, cytokines, cytokine receptors, and an array of adhesion molecules are all potential targets of specific immunomodulatory therapy. Etanercept (TNF receptor p75 Fc fusion protein) is a TNF antagonist and the first immune response modifier to be used in large numbers of children with polyarticular course JRA. Based on the studies of etanercept in children by Lovell et al. (122,123), this agent appears to be at least as effective as MTX and has an extremely good toxicity profile. Russo et al. recently reported that etanercept was capable of inducing a sustained response in one third of 19 cases of systemic JRA (124).

Other biologic therapies such as infliximab, adalimumab, and CTLA4 Ig are being investigated in children with JRA. These specifically targeted therapies hold the promise of altering disease course while avoiding the potential for substantial toxicity from other second-line agents.

Combination Therapy Using Advanced Drug Therapy

The use of various combinations of corticosteroids, conventional DMARDs, and biologics is becoming a more common approach to the management of children with severe unresponsive polyarticular or systemic arthritis, based largely on studies in adults such as those of O'Dell et al. (125). Combinations that have been used in systemic-onset JRA include intravenous methylprednisolone and cyclophosphamide (126) and MTX and pulse cyclophosphamide (127). The addition of hydroxychloroquine to MTX, with or without corticosteroids, is also used in some clinics in children with polyarticular disease, although efficacy has not been proven in placebo-controlled randomized trials. Perhaps the most frequent combination therapy in use today for aggressive JRA is MTX and etanercept. This combination may produce a synergistic therapeutic effect, as shown by Weinblatt et al. (128) in patients with adult RA. Although these and other combinations are occasionally used, they should be considered only in children with severe disease that is unresponsive to MTX or sulfasalazine alone, and only under the supervision of an experienced pediatric rheumatologist.

Nontraditional Remedies, Complementary or Alternative Medicine

It is likely that most children with chronic illness take nontraditional remedies or complementary or alternative medicine (CAM) at some time during their disease course (129). A recent study supports that at any given time during their disease course, 64% of the children with arthritis will use at least one CAM remedy and 50% of them at least 2 CAM remedies (130). Well-meaning friends and relatives sometimes inundate parents with advice about "cures" that are often available only at distant locations and often at great expense (see Chapter 43). The practitioner's anticipation of this issue is important, and frank discussion with parents and patient about the widespread use of CAM remedies can help to minimize their use. It is important to foster an atmosphere in which parents can freely discuss the use of CAM. The nurse is often the ideal health professional to deal with this problem. The medical team must be aware of all drugs that the patient is taking, both physician-prescribed and self-prescribed, in order to understand the origin of side effects. It is reasonable to permit the use of CAM provided they are not likely to be detrimental to the child's health or to interfere with the efficacy of prescribed therapy.

Nutraceuticals

During the past 10 years there has been an explosion in the availability, sales, and use of nutritional supplements. Many of these products are derived from herbs or animal tissue, and have not undergone legitimate scientific testing to establish efficacy, although most are thought to be very safe. Informal surveys of pediatric rheumatologists suggest that a high proportion of children with JRA are supplementing their physician-prescribed therapy with combinations of glucosamine hydrochloride and chondroitin sulfate. These agents are thought to possess cartilage-modifying properties. An excellent recent review of the product's current status is provided by Towheed (131). There is some evidence for the effectiveness of the combination of glucosamine hydrochloride (500 mg), chondroitin sulfate (400 mg), and manganese ascorbate (76 mg) per capsule, sold under the trade name Cosamin-DS (Nutramax Laboratories, Edgewood, MD, U.S.A.). Leffler et al. (132) conducted a 16-week randomized, double-blind crossover trial of Cosamin-DS, 3 capsules daily, in 34 men from the U.S. Navy diving and special warfare community who had chronic pain and radiographic degenerative joint disease of the knee or low back pain (the SEALS trial). Knee osteoarthritis symptoms, patient assessment of treatment, visual analogue scale for pain, and physical examination scores all improved by a statistically significant amount. There were no serious or unexpected adverse drug effects. At present, large trials of this combination agent are underway in adult RA patients, and pilot trials have begun in children with JRA.

Unfortunately, these compounds are not regulated by the U.S. Food and Drug Administration, and the quality assurance of the manufacturing process is not standard or scrutinized. Adebowale et al. (133) analyzed the contents of glucosamine and chondroitin in several marketed products to determine how much the label deviated from what was actually in the product. Deviations from the label claim ranged from 0% to more than 115%.

Conclusions Regarding Pharmacologic Management

Sweeping changes in the approach to pharmacologic management have occurred within the past 10 years. The therapeutic pyramid is considered a relic of the past and has been replaced by more aggressive treatment approaches early in the course of illness, even among those with pauciarticular disease. Salicylates, once the mainstay of therapy, now have almost no role, having been replaced by NSAIDs such as naproxen and nabumetone and, more recently, the COX-2 inhibitors. MTX has become the second-line agent of first choice and is frequently given earlier in the disease course than previously. Biologic agents, such as etanercept, are now becoming available for use in children, and promise to have a major impact on therapeutic regimens in the near future. Systemic glucocorticosteroids, although still important, are avoided as much as possible. In contrast, intraarticular corticosteroids are assuming an important place in the management of arthritis. These changes have come about because of an expanded knowledge base acquired from accumulating clinical experience and controlled trials concerning the effectiveness, safety, and tolerability of the various agents.

Problems of Compliance or Adherence with Pharmacologic Interventions

Compliance (also referred to as adherence with advice and instructions) is, at best, incomplete (134). The health professional can maximize compliance by providing comprehensive information about expected benefits and side effects of drugs and by allaying unjustified concerns about toxicity (135). Dose regimens that conform to the child's daily routine are more likely to succeed than are those that demand rigid medication ingestion at inconvenient times of the day. It might be better, for example, to have the child take the midday NSAID after school, rather than at lunchtime. Minimizing dose frequency also helps the child to comply with prescribed intake. Medication charts or compartmentalized pillboxes can also help the child remember if she or he has taken the medication prescribed that day. Home exercise programs are often subject to noncompliance, particularly if the time demands placed on the child and family are unrealistic. Noncompliance might be a greater problem in the independence-seeking adolescent than in the young child (135).

OTHER ASPECTS OF MEDICAL MANAGEMENT

Consultation with other specialists or subspecialists is essential in view of the array of possible complications and number of organs that may become involved during the JRA disease process.

The patient should be seen by an ophthalmologist at the time of diagnosis and periodically thereafter. This is true for all JRA patients, not just those with pauciarticular onset, because ocular involvement may occur in any of the disease subtypes (Table 62.4).

TABLE 62.4. *Frequency of ophthalmologic visits for children with juvenile rheumatoid arthritis (JRA) and without known iridocyclitis*[a]

	Age of Onset	
JRA Subtype at onset	<7 yr[b]	≥7 yr[c]
Pauciarticular		
+ANA	H[d]	M
−ANA	M	M
Polyarticular		
+ANA	H[d]	M
−ANA	M	M
Systemic	L	L

[a]High risk (H) indicates ophthalmologic examinations every 3 to 4 months. Medium risk (M) indicates ophthalmologic examinations every 6 months. Low risk (L) indicates ophthalmologic examinations every 12 months.

[b]All patients are considered at low risk 7 years after the onset of their arthritis and should have yearly ophthalmologic examinations indefinitely.

[c]All patients are considered at low risk 4 years after the onset of their arthritis and should have yearly ophthalmologic examinations indefinitely.

[d]All high-risk patients are considered at medium risk 4 years after the onset of their arthritis.

ANA, antinuclear antibody test.

From Section of Rheumatology and Section on Ophthalmology. Guidelines for ophthalmologic examinations in children with JRA. *Pediatrics* 1995;92:295–296, with permission.

Dental problems frequently occur in JRA. Dental caries are found with a higher incidence among children with JRA, perhaps associated with prolonged salicylate therapy. Additionally, involvement of the temporomandibular joint and the presence of micrognathia or retrognathia can have severe consequences on dentition and mastication (see Chapter 100).

Transition clinics that facilitate the transfer of care of the chronically ill adolescent from the pediatrician to the internist or other adult specialist undoubtedly fulfill an unmet need for young adults whose physical, social, educational, and career milestones have been delayed by chronic disease (136,137). It is recognized that many adult medical caregivers lack the knowledge and expertise to deal with the special medical and social problems of this group of young adults (26). For the most part, no specialized medical resources have been available for this group, and often these patients either remain dependent on pediatric care or become lost to follow-up. Transition clinics have these goals: promoting continuity of care; encouraging independence of patients so that they take increasing responsibility for their overall management; assisting in optimal adolescent development related to sexuality, psychosocial, and career planning; and providing emotional support during the transition period (136). An additional important function of the transition clinic is to enable a better understanding of the long-term consequences of disease and treatment.

Surgery

The role of orthopedic surgery in the management of the child with chronic arthritis is limited, although in adulthood, patients with childhood onset of arthritis may benefit dramatically from joint replacement once growth has been completed (138,139). Two major factors support a conservative attitude toward surgical intervention in the child: age and growth potential, and the finite life span of prosthetic devices (139,140).

Synovectomy and Soft Tissue Releases

Synovectomy has been used to treat JRA, but the evidence for its efficacy is limited (141–143). A single controlled study of the effect of synovectomy at 2 years showed improvement in pain, swelling, and activity of disease in the synovectomized joints in comparison with those treated conservatively (142). Roles reported that synovectomy of the knee and elbow was useful, particularly in the older child (144). Other studies have demonstrated that, in the long-term, benefit from synovectomy is likely small. To date, insufficient data are available to allow recommendations of this approach except in unusual circumstances.

Tenosynovectomy of the extensor or flexor tendons of the hand is occasionally necessary in the older child with polyarticular JRA in whom a proliferative tenosynovitis interferes with active range of motion of the fingers.

Range restrictions secondary to soft tissue contracture, especially at the hip, knee, and elbow, might improve following soft tissue releases (140,145). It is essential that physical therapy programs be an integral part of such therapy.

Joint Replacement

Replacement of joints is seldom indicated in the pediatric age range. However, such procedures can be of dramatic benefit in the older, fully grown teenager in whom pain or severe range restriction has become a significant problem (146,147).

Surgical Management of Temporomandibular Joint Disease

Severe micrognathia can result from bilateral temporomandibular joint arthritis, loss of mandibular condyles, shortening of the rami, and miniaturization of the body of the mandible. Surgical reconstruction can yield dramatic improvement (148,149) (see Chapter 100).

Anesthetic Considerations

The safety of surgical management of the child with JRA can be significantly compromised by difficulty in the administration of endotracheal anesthetic (150). Immobility or instability of the cervical spine, restricted opening of the jaw secondary to temporomandibular joint disease, or, rarely, cricoarytenoid joint arthritis can make intubation difficult (151). The pediatrician, surgeon, and anesthetist should all be aware of the risks. It is appropriate to obtain preoperative flexion and extension lateral radiographs of the cervical spine to detect C1–2 instability or fusion of the posterior elements. Having the patient wear a soft cervical collar to the operating room might help remind the caregiver of the potential complications of the cervical spine disease.

Bone Marrow Transplantation

Perhaps because of the success seen in other autoimmune disease, bone marrow transplantation (BMT), particularly autologous hematopoietic stem cell transplantation (AHSCT), is being considered as a new therapeutic strategy in JRA (152,153) (see Chapter 36). At present, however, protocols for AHSCT transplants in children with severe JRA are still under development. Transplantation-associated mortality in JRA, especially in children with system disease, has been found to be 10 times higher than in adults with RA (>10% vs. 1.4%) (152).

Gene Therapy

Although arthritis is a complex trait with unclear genetic linkage patterns, gene therapy has a potential role (154) (see Chapter 37). Beneficial genes may be incorporated into the synovial lining cells such that their products are secreted directly into the joint space. Candidate genes encode for antiinflammatory, immunosuppressive, and chondroprotective or chondroreparative proteins. To date, gene therapy has not been attempted in children with JRA. This exciting prospect may enter the JRA management scenario in the next several years (155), although there are likely special concerns in children compared with adults, such as the reported association of growth plate damage induced by adenoviral vectors (156).

REFERENCES

1. Brewer EJ, Giannini EH, Person DA. Appendix II. Patient's and parent's manual. Physical therapy program for parents with JRA and other rheumatic diseases. In: *Juvenile rheumatoid arthritis* 2nd ed. Philadelphia: WB Saunders, 1982:305–326.
2. Brewer EJ, Angel KC. *Parenting a child with arthritis.* Los Angeles: Lowell House, 1992.
3. Brewer EJ, Angel KC. *The arthritis source book.* Los Angeles: Lowell House, 1993.
4. Sherry DD, Bohnsack J, Salmonson K, et al. Painless juvenile rheumatoid arthritis. *J Pediatr* 1990;116:921–923.
5. Henderson CJ, Lovell DJ. Assessment of protein-energy malnutrition in children and adolescents with juvenile rheumatoid arthritis. *Arthritis Care Res* 1989;2:108–113.
6. Miller ML, Chacko JA, Young EA. Dietary deficiencies in children with juvenile rheumatoid arthritis. *Arthritis Care Res* 1989;2:22–24.
7. Bechtold S, Ripperger P, Muhlbayer D, et al. GH therapy in juvenile chronic arthritis: results of a two-year controlled study on growth and bone. *J Clin Endocrinol Metab* 2001;86:5737–5744.
8. Simon D, Lucidarme N, Prieur AM, et al. Treatment of growth failure in juvenile chronic arthritis. *Horm Res* 2002;58(suppl 1):28–32.
9. Al-Mutair A, Bahabri S, Al-Mayouf S, et al. Efficacy of recombinant human growth hormone in children with juvenile rheumatoid arthritis and growth failure. *J Pediatr Endocrinol Metab* 2000;13:899–905.

10. Varni JW, Seid M, Kurtin PS. PedsQL 4.0: reliability and validity of the Pediatric Quality of Life Inventory version 4.0 generic core scales in healthy and patient populations. *Med Care* 2001;39:800–812.
11. Varni JW, Seid M, Smith Knight T, et al. The PedsQL in pediatric rheumatology: reliability, validity, and responsiveness of the Pediatric Quality of Life Inventory Generic Core Scales and Rheumatology Module. *Arthritis Rheum* 2002;46:714–725.
12. Russak SM, Croft JD Jr, Furst DE, et al. The use of rheumatoid arthritis health-related quality of life patient questionnaires in clinical practice: lessons learned. *Arthritis Rheum* 2003;49:574–584.
13. Scull SA, Dow MB, Athreya BH. Physical and occupational therapy for children with rheumatic diseases. *Pediatr Clin North Am* 1986; 33:1053–1077.
14. Tecklin JS. *Pediatric physical therapy.* Philadelphia: Lippincott Williams & Wilkins, 1999.
15. Brewer EJ, Giannini EH, Person DA. *Juvenile rheumatoid arthritis.* Philadelphia: WB Saunders, 1982.
16. MacBain KP, Hill RH. A functional assessment for juvenile rheumatoid arthritis. *Am J Occup Ther* 1973;27:326–330.
17. Thastum M, Zachariae R, Herlin T. Pain experience and pain coping strategies in children with juvenile idiopathic arthritis. *J Rheumatol* 2001;28:1091–1098.
18. Kuis W, Heijnen CJ, Sinnema G, et al. Pain in childhood rheumatic arthritis. *Baillieres Clin Rheumatol* 1998;12:229–244.
19. Schanberg LE, Lefebvre JC, Keefe FJ, et al. Pain coping and the pain experience in children with juvenile chronic arthritis. *Pain* 1997;73: 181–189.
20. Huygen AC, Kuis W, Sinnema G. Psychological, behavioural, and social adjustment in children and adolescents with juvenile chronic arthritis. *Ann Rheum Dis* 2000;59:276–282.
21. Noll RB, Kozlowski K, Gerhardt C, et al. Social, emotional, and behavioral functioning of children with juvenile rheumatoid arthritis. *Arthritis Rheum* 2000;43:1387–1396.
22. LeBovidge JS, Lavigne JV, Donenberg GR, et al. Psychological adjustment of children and adolescents with chronic arthritis: a meta-analytic review. *J Pediatr Psychol* 2003;28:29–39.
23. Reiter-Purtill J, Gerhardt CA, Vannatta K, et al. A controlled longitudinal study of the social functioning of children with juvenile rheumatoid arthritis. *J Pediatr Psychol* 2003;28:17–28.
24. Akikusa JD, Allen RC. Reducing the impact of rheumatic diseases in childhood. *Best Pract Res Clin Rheumatol* 2002;16:333–345.
25. Miller JJ 3rd, Spitz PW, Simpson U, et al. The social function of young adults who had arthritis in childhood. *J Pediatr* 1982;100:378–82.
26. Ansell BM, Chamberlain MA. Children with chronic arthritis: the management of transition to adulthood. *Baillieres Clin Rheumatol* 1998;12:363–373.
27. Stefl ME, Shear ES, Levinson JE. Summer camps for juveniles with rheumatic disease: do they make a difference? *Arthritis Care Res* 1989;2:10–15.
28. Henoch MJ, Batson JW, Baum J. Psychosocial factors in juvenile rheumatoid arthritis. *Arthritis Rheum* 1978;21:229–233.
29. Gerhardt CA, Vannatta K, McKellop JM, et al. Comparing parental distress, family functioning, and the role of social support for caregivers with and without a child with juvenile rheumatoid arthritis. *J Pediatr Psychol* 2003;28:5–15.
30. Cuneo KM, Schiaffino KM. Adolescent self-perceptions of adjustment to childhood arthritis: the influence of disease activity, family resources, and parent adjustment. *J Adolesc Health* 2002;31:363–371.
31. Allaire SH, DeNardo BS, Szer IS, et al. The economic impacts of juvenile rheumatoid arthritis. *J Rheumatol* 1992;19:952–955.
32. McDonagh JE. Osteoporosis in juvenile idiopathic arthritis. *Curr Opin Rheumatol* 2001;13:399–404.
33. Helgeland M, Svendsen E, Forre O, et al. Dietary intake and serum concentrations of antioxidants in children with juvenile arthritis. *Clin Exp Rheumatol* 2000;18:637–641.
34. Lovell DJ, White PH. Growth and nutrition in JRA. In: Woo P, White PH, Ansell BM, eds. *Paediatric rheumatology update.* Oxford: Oxford University Press, 1990:47.
35. American Academy of Pediatrics. Calcium requirements of infants, children, and adolescents (RE 9904). *Pediatrics* 1999;104:1152–1157.
36. Giannini EH, Cassidy JT. Methotrexate in juvenile rheumatoid arthritis. Do the benefits outweigh the risks? *Drug Saf* 1993;9:325–339.
37. Rosen P, Moroldo MB, Lovell DJ, et al. Discordant phenotypes for methotrexate response in juvenile rheumatoid arthritis. Presented at the American College of Rheumatology, New Orleans, LA, 2002. Vol. 46.
38. Murray KJ, Lovell DJ. Advanced therapy for juvenile arthritis. *Best Pract Res Clin Rheumatol* 2002;16:361–378.
39. Chikanza IC. Juvenile rheumatoid arthritis: therapeutic perspectives. *Paediatr Drugs* 2002;4:335–348.
40. Brunner HI, Kim KN, Ballinger SH, et al. Current medication choices in juvenile rheumatoid arthritis II—update of a survey performed in 1993. *J Clin Rheumatol* 2001;7:295–300.
41. Lehman TJA. Clinical trials for the treatment of systemic onset juvenile rheumatoid arthritis—juvenile idiopathic arthritis. *Curr Rheumatol Rep* 2000;2:313–315.
42. Brewer EJ Jr, Giannini EH. Standard methodology for Segment I, II, and III Pediatric Rheumatology Collaborative Study Group studies. I. Design. *J Rheumatol* 1982;9:109–139.
43. Lovell DJ, Giannini EH, Brewer EJ Jr. Time course of response to nonsteroidal antiinflammatory drugs in juvenile rheumatoid arthritis. *Arthritis Rheum* 1984;27:1433–1437.
44. Giannini EH, Brewer EJ, Miller ML, et al. Ibuprofen suspension in the treatment of juvenile rheumatoid arthritis. Pediatric Rheumatology Collaborative Study Group. *J Pediatr* 1990;117:645–652.
45. Hawkey CJ. COX-2 inhibitors. *Lancet* 1999;353:307–314.
46. Ofman JJ, Maclean CH, Straus WL, et al. Meta-analysis of dyspepsia and nonsteroidal antiinflammatory drugs. *Arthritis Rheum* 2003;49: 508–518.
47. Kruger K. [Current status of COX II inhibitors in therapy of rheumatoid arthritis in comparison with conventional non-steroidal anti-inflammatory agents. Attempt at an evaluation with regard to evidence-based medicine]. *Z Rheumatol* 2001;60:481–484.
48. Foeldvari I, Burgos-Vargas R, Thon A, et al. High response rate in the phase I/II study of meloxicam in juvenile rheumatoid arthritis. *J Rheumatol* 2002;29:1079–1083.
49. Giannini EH, Ruperto N, Ravelli A, et al. Preliminary definition of improvement in juvenile arthritis. *Arthritis Rheum* 1997;40:1202–1209.
50. Goldstein JL, Silverstein FE, Agrawal NM, et al. Reduced risk of upper gastrointestinal ulcer complications with celecoxib, a novel COX-2 inhibitor. *Am J Gastroenterol* 2000;95:1681–1690.
51. Bonnel RA, Villalba ML, Karwoski CB, et al. Aseptic meningitis associated with rofecoxib. *Arch Intern Med* 2002;162:713–715.
52. Mandell BF. COX 2-selective NSAIDs: biology, promises, and concerns. *Cleve Clin J Med* 1999;66:285–292.
53. Cummins R, Wagner-Weiner L, Paller A. Pseudoporphyria induced by celecoxib in a patient with juvenile rheumatoid arthritis. *J Rheumatol* 2000;27:2938–2940.
54. Ilowite NT. Current treatment of juvenile rheumatoid arthritis. *Pediatrics* 2002;109:109–115.
55. Lang BA, Finlayson LA. Naproxen-induced pseudoporphyria in patients with juvenile rheumatoid arthritis. *J Pediatr* 1994;124:639–642.
56. Skeith KJ, Jamali F. Clinical pharmacokinetics of drugs used in juvenile arthritis. *Clin Pharmacokinet* 1991;21:129–149.
57. Roth SH. NSAID and gastropathy: a rheumatologist's review. *J Rheumatol* 1988;15:912–919.
58. Lindsley CB. Uses of nonsteroidal anti-inflammatory drugs in pediatrics. *Am J Dis Child* 1993;147:229–236.
59. Lindsley CB. Identification and treatment of nonsteroidal antiinflammatory drug-induced gastroduodenal injury in children [Reply]. *Am J Dis Child* 1993;147:1281.
60. Giannini EH, Brewer EJ, Kuzmina N, et al. Methotrexate in resistant juvenile rheumatoid arthritis. Results of the U.S.A.-U.S.S.R. double-blind, placebo-controlled trial. The Pediatric Rheumatology Collaborative Study Group and The Cooperative Children's Study Group. *N Engl J Med* 1992;326:1043–1049.
61. Giannini EH, Cassidy JT, Brewer EJ, et al. Comparative efficacy and safety of advanced drug therapy in children with juvenile rheumatoid arthritis. *Semin Arthritis Rheum* 1993;23:34–46.
62. Giannini EH, Fink NA. Low-dose methotrexate in children with JRA. Results of post-trial long-term follow-up program [Abstract]. Presented at the 57th Annual Scientific Meeting of the American College of Rheumatology, San Antonio, Texas, November 7–11, 1993. Abstracts. *Arthritis Rheum* 1993;36(suppl):54.
63. Graham LD, Myones BL, Rivas-Chacon RF, Pachman LM. Morbidity associated with long-term methotrexate therapy in juvenile rheumatoid arthritis. *J Pediatr* 1992;120:468–473.
64. Alarcon GS, Lopez-Mendez A, Walter J, et al. Radiographic evidence of disease progression in methotrexate treated and nonmethotrexate disease modifying antirheumatic drug treated rheumatoid arthritis patients: a meta-analysis. *J Rheumatol* 1992;19:1868–1873.

65. Rau R, Herborn G, Karger T, Werdier D. Retardation of radiologic progression in rheumatoid arthritis with methotrexate therapy. A controlled study. *Arthritis Rheum* 1991;34:1236–1244.
66. Jeurissen ME, Boerbooms AM, van de Putte LB, et al. Influence of methotrexate and azathioprine on radiologic progression in rheumatoid arthritis. A randomized, double-blind study. *Ann Intern Med* 1991;114:999–1004.
67. Wallace CA, Sherry DD. Preliminary report of higher dose methotrexate treatment in juvenile rheumatoid arthritis. *J Rheumatol* 1992;19:1604–1607.
68. Brooks PJ, Spruill WJ, Parish RC, et al. Pharmacokinetics of methotrexate administered by intramuscular and subcutaneous injections in patients with rheumatoid arthritis. *Arthritis Rheum* 1990;33:91–94.
69. Ruperto N, Murray K, Gerloni V, et al. A randomized trial of methotrexate (MTX) in medium versus higher doses in children with juvenile idiopathic arthritis (JIA) who failed on standard doses. *Arthritis Rheum* 2002;46 (suppl):195.
70. Ravelli A, Viola S, Ramenghi B, et al. Frequency of relapse after discontinuation of methotrexate therapy for clinical remission in juvenile rheumatoid arthritis. *J Rheumatol* 1995;22:1574–1576.
71. Ravelli A, Migliavacca D, Viola S, et al. Efficacy of folinic acid in reducing methotrexate toxicity in juvenile idiopathic arthritis. *Clin Exp Rheumatol* 1999;17:625–627.
72. Lang B, Riegel W, Peters T, et al. Low dose methotrexate therapy for rheumatoid arthritis complicated by pancytopenia and *Pneumocystis carinii* pneumonia. *J Rheumatol* 1991;18:1257–1259.
73. Stenger AA, Houtman PM. Methotrexate, pneumonitis, and infection. *Ann Rheum Dis* 1992;51:1179; author reply 1179–1180.
74. Kremer JM, Alarcon GS, Lightfoot RW Jr, et al. Methotrexate for rheumatoid arthritis. Suggested guidelines for monitoring liver toxicity. American College of Rheumatology. *Arthritis Rheum* 1994;37:316–328.
75. Hashkes PJ, Balistreri WF, Bove KE, et al. The relationship of hepatotoxic risk factors and liver histology in methotrexate therapy for juvenile rheumatoid arthritis. *J Pediatr* 1999;134:47–52.
76. Brooks CD. Sulfasalazine for the management of juvenile rheumatoid arthritis. *J Rheumatol* 2001;28:845–853.
77. van Rossum MA, Fiselier TJ, Franssen MJ, et al. Sulfasalazine in the treatment of juvenile chronic arthritis: a randomized, double-blind, placebo-controlled, multicenter study. Dutch Juvenile Chronic Arthritis Study Group. *Arthritis Rheum* 1998;41:808–816.
78. Rozman B. Clinical experience with leflunomide in rheumatoid arthritis. Leflunomide Investigators' Group. *J Rheumatol Suppl* 1998;53:27–32.
79. Silverman ED, Spiegel L, Jung LK, et al. Efficacy and safety of leflunomide (LEF) versus methotrexate (MTX) in the treatment of pediatric patients with juvenile rheumatoid arthritis (JRA). *Arthritis Rheum* 2003;48:3654 (Abstract) Szz.
80. Lyons Jones K, Johnson DL, Chambers CD. Monitoring leflunomide (Arava) as a new potential teratogen. *Teratology* 2002;65:200–202.
81. Tett SE. Clinical pharmacokinetics of slow-acting antirheumatic drugs. *Clin Pharmacokinet* 1993;25:392–407.
82. van Kerckhove C, Giannini EH, Lovell DJ. Temporal patterns of response to D-penicillamine, hydroxychloroquine, and placebo in juvenile rheumatoid arthritis patients. *Arthritis Rheum* 1988;31:1252–1258.
83. Silman A, Shipley M. Ophthalmological monitoring for hydroxychloroquine toxicity: a scientific review of available data. *Br J Rheumatol* 1997;36:599–601.
84. Lehman TJ, Striegel KH, Onel KB. Thalidomide therapy for recalcitrant systemic onset juvenile rheumatoid arthritis. *J Pediatr* 2002;140:125–127.
85. Brewer EJ, Giannini EH, Kuzmina N, et al. Penicillamine and hydroxychloroquine in the treatment of severe juvenile rheumatoid arthritis. Results of the U.S.A.-U.S.S.R. double-blind placebo-controlled trial. *N Engl J Med* 1986;314:1269–1276.
86. Giannini EH, Brewer EJ, Kuzmina N, et al. Characteristics of responders and nonresponders to slow-acting antirheumatic drugs in juvenile rheumatoid arthritis. *Arthritis Rheum* 1988;31:15–20.
87. Lande K. Die gunstige Beeinflussung schleichender Dauerinfekte durch Solganol. *Munch Med Worchenschr* 1927;74:1132–1134.
88. Forestier J. L'aurotherapie dans les rheumatismes chronique. *Bull Mem Soc Med Hop Paris* 1929;53:323–327.
89. Giannini EH, Person DA, Brewer EJ, et al. Blood and serum concentrations of gold after a single dose of auranofin in children with juvenile rheumatoid arthritis. *J Rheumatol* 1983;10:496–468.
90. Giannini EH, Brewer EJ, Person DA. Blood gold concentrations in children with juvenile rheumatoid arthritis undergoing long-term oral gold therapy. *Ann Rheum Dis* 1984;43:228–231.
91. Giannini EH, Brewer EJ Jr, Kuzmina N, et al. Auranofin in the treatment of juvenile rheumatoid arthritis. Results of the USA-USSR double-blind, placebo-controlled trial. The USA Pediatric Rheumatology Collaborative Study Group. The USSR Cooperative Children's Study Group. *Arthritis Rheum* 1990;33:466–476.
92. Giannini EH, Barron KS, Spencer CH, et al. Auranofin therapy for juvenile rheumatoid arthritis: results of the five-year open label extension trial. *J Rheumatol* 1991;18:1240–1242.
93. Silverman ED, Laxer RM, Greenwald M, et al. Intravenous gamma globulin therapy in systemic juvenile rheumatoid arthritis. *Arthritis Rheum* 1990;33:1015–1022.
94. Prieur AM, Adleff A, Debre M, et al. High dose immunoglobulin therapy in severe juvenile chronic arthritis: long-term follow-up in 16 patients. *Clin Exp Rheumatol* 1990;8:603–608.
95. Silverman ED, Cawkwell GD, Lovell DJ, et al. Intravenous immunoglobulin in the treatment of systemic juvenile rheumatoid arthritis: a randomized placebo controlled trial. Pediatric Rheumatology Collaborative Study Group. *J Rheumatol* 1994;21:2353–2358.
96. Giannini EH, Lovell DJ, Silverman ED, et al. Intravenous immunoglobulin in the treatment of polyarticular juvenile rheumatoid arthritis: a phase I/II study. Pediatric Rheumatology Collaborative Study Group. *J Rheumatol* 1996;23:919–924.
97. Bjoro K, Froland SS, Yun Z, et al. Hepatitis C infection in patients with primary hypogammaglobulinemia after treatment with contaminated immune globulin. *N Engl J Med* 1994;331:1607–11.
98. Kvien TK, Hoyeraal HM, Sandstad B. Azathioprine versus placebo in patients with juvenile rheumatoid arthritis: a single center double blind comparative study. *J Rheumatol* 1986;13:118–123.
99. Savolainen HA, Kautiainen H, Isomaki H, et al. Azathioprine in patients with juvenile chronic arthritis: a longterm followup study. *J Rheumatol* 1997;24:2444–2450.
100. Palmer RG, Kanski JJ, Ansell BM. Chlorambucil in the treatment of intractable uveitis associated with juvenile chronic arthritis. *J Rheumatol* 1985;12:967–970.
101. Ansell BM, Eghtedari A, Bywaters EG. Chlorambucil in the management of juvenile chronic polyarthritis complicated by amyloidosis. *Ann Rheum Dis* 1971;30:331.
102. Savolainen HA. Chlorambucil in severe juvenile chronic arthritis: longterm followup with special reference to amyloidosis. *Clin Exp Rheumatol* 2003;21:347.
103. Ostensen M, Hoyeraal HM, Kass E. Tolerance of cyclosporine A in children with refractory juvenile rheumatoid arthritis. *J Rheumatol* 1988;15:1536–1538.
104. Giannini EH, Ruperto N, Tomasi AL, et al. Neoral registry in polyarticular juvenile rheumatoid arthritis. *Pediatr Rheum Online J* 2003;1:63.
105. Hench P, Kendall EC, Slocumb CH, et al. The effect of a hormone of the adrenal cortex (17-hydoxy-11-dehydrocorticosterone compound E) and of pituitary adrenocorticorophic hormone on rheumatoid arthritis: preliminary report. *Proc Staff Meet Mayo Clin* 1949;24:181–197.
106. Prieur A-M. The place of corticosteroid therapy in juvenile chronic arthritis in 1992. Presented at the Proceedings of OMERACT, Conference on Outcome Measures in Rheumatoid Arthritis Clinical Trials, Maastricht, the Netherlands, April 29–May 3, 1992. *J Rheumatol* 1993;20(suppl 37):32–34.
107. Brouhard B, Travis LB. Inhibition of linear growth by alternative day steroids. *J Pediatr* 1977;91:343–348.
108. Sambrook P. Corticoid induced osteoporosis. *J Rheumatol Suppl* 1996;45:19–22.
109. Cleary AG, Murphy HD, Davidson JE. Intra-articular corticosteroid injections in juvenile idiopathic arthritis. *Arch Dis Child* 2003;88:192–196.
110. Uziel Y, Berkovitch M, Gazarian M, et al. Evaluation of eutectic lidocaine/prilocaine cream (EMLA) for steroid joint injection in children with juvenile rheumatoid arthritis: a double blind, randomized, placebo controlled trial. *J Rheumatol* 2003;30:594–596.
111. Weiss AH, Wallace CA, Sherry DD. Methotrexate for resistant chronic uveitis in children with juvenile rheumatoid arthritis. *J Pediatr* 1998;133:266–268.

112. Miserocchi E, Baltatzis S, Ekong A, et al. Efficacy and safety of chlorambucil in intractable noninfectious uveitis: the Massachusetts Eye and Ear Infirmary experience. *Ophthalmology* 2002;109:137–142.
113. Kilmartin DJ, Forrester JV, Dick AD. Cyclosporin A therapy in refractory non-infectious childhood uveitis. *Br J Ophthalmol* 1998;82: 737–742.
114. Reiff A, Takei S, Sadeghi S, et al. Etanercept therapy in children with treatment-resistant uveitis. *Arthritis Rheum* 2001;44:1411–1415.
115. Lam LA, Lowder CY, Baerveldt G, et al. Surgical management of cataracts in children with juvenile rheumatoid arthritis-associated uveitis. *Am J Ophthalmol* 2003;135:772–778.
116. Rimsza ME. Complications of corticosteroid therapy. *Am J Dis Child* 1978;132:806–810.
117. Dowell SF, Bresee JS. Severe varicella associated with steroid use. *Pediatrics* 1993;92:223–228.
118. Asano Y, Yoshikawa T, Suga S, et al. Postexposure prophylaxis of varicella in family contact by oral acyclovir. *Pediatrics* 1993;92: 219–222.
119. Suga S, Yoshikawa T, Ozaki T, et al. Effect of oral acyclovir against primary and secondary viraemia in incubation period of varicella. *Arch Dis Child* 1993;69:639–642; discussion 642–643.
120. St Clair EW, Haynes BF. The future of rheumatoid arthritis treatment. *Bull Rheum Dis* 1993;42:1–4.
121. Elliott MJ, Maini RN. New directions for biological therapy in rheumatoid arthritis. *Int Arch Allergy Immunol* 1994;104:112–125.
122. Lovell DJ, Giannini EH, Reiff A, et al. Etanercept in children with polyarticular juvenile rheumatoid arthritis. Pediatric Rheumatology Collaborative Study Group. *N Engl J Med* 2000;342:763–769.
123. Lovell D, Giannini EH, Lange M, et al. Safety and efficacy of Enbrel (etanercept) in the extended treatment of polyarticular-course JRA [Abstract]. Presented at the American College of Rheumatology Annual Scientific Meeting, Boston, Massachusetts, November 13–17, 1999. Abstracts. *Arthritis Rheum* 1999;42(suppl):117.
124. Russo RAG, Katsicas MM. Sustained response to etanercept in systemic juvenile idiopathic arthritis. American College of Rheumatology, Orlando, FL, 2003. *Arthritis Rheum* 2003;48(suppl):98.
125. O'Dell JR, Haire CE, Erikson N, et al. Treatment of rheumatoid arthritis with methotrexate alone, sulfasalazine and hydroxychloroquine, or a combination of all three medications. *N Engl J Med* 1996; 334:1287–1291.
126. Wallace CA, Sherry DD. Trial of intravenous pulse cyclophosphamide and methylprednisolone in the treatment of severe systemic-onset juvenile rheumatoid arthritis. *Arthritis Rheum* 1997;40:1852–1855.
127. Shaikov AV, Maximov AA, Speransky AI, et al. Repetitive use of pulse therapy with methylprednisolone and cyclophosphamide in addition to oral methotrexate in children with systemic juvenile rheumatoid arthritis—preliminary results of a longterm study. *J Rheumatol* 1992;19:612–616.
128. Weinblatt ME, Kremer JM, Bankhurst AD, et al. A trial of etanercept, a recombinant tumor necrosis factor receptor:Fc fusion protein, in patients with rheumatoid arthritis receiving methotrexate. *N Engl J Med* 1999;340:253–259.
129. Southwood TR, Malleson PN, Roberts-Thomson PJ, et al. Unconventional remedies used for patients with juvenile arthritis. *Pediatrics* 1990;85:150–154.
130. Hagen LE, Schneider R, Stephens D, et al. Use of complementary and alternative medicine by pediatric rheumatology patients. *Arthritis Rheum* 2003;49:3–6.
131. Towheed TE. Current status of glucosamine therapy in osteoarthritis. *Arthritis Rheum* 2003;49:601–604.
132. Leffler CT, Philippi AF, Leffler SG, et al. Glucosamine, chondroitin, and manganese ascorbate for degenerative joint disease of the knee or low back: a randomized, double-blind, placebo-controlled pilot study. *Milit Med* 1999;164:85–91.
133. Adebowale A, Cox D, Liang Z, et al. Analysis of glucosamine and chondroitin sulfate content in marketed products and the caco-2 permeability of chondroitin sulfate raw materials. *J Am Nutraceutical Assoc* 2000;3:37–44.
134. Kroll T, Barlow JH, Shaw K. Treatment adherence in juvenile rheumatoid arthritis—a review. *Scand J Rheumatol* 1999;28:10–18.
135. Kyngas H. Motivation as a crucial predictor of good compliance in adolescents with rheumatoid arthritis. *Int J Nurs Pract* 2002;8: 336–341.
136. Sathananthan R, David J. The adolescent with rheumatic disease. *Arch Dis Child* 1997;77:355–358.
137. White PH, Shear ES. Transition/job readiness for adolescents with juvenile arthritis and other chronic illness. *J Rheumatol Suppl* 1992; 33:23–27.
138. Spencer CH, Bernstein BH. Hip disease in juvenile rheumatoid arthritis. *Curr Opin Rheumatol* 2002;14:536–541.
139. Parvizi J, Lajam CM, Trousdale RT, et al. Total knee arthroplasty in young patients with juvenile rheumatoid arthritis. *J Bone Joint Surg Am* 2003;85:1090–1094.
140. McCullough CJ. Surgical management of the hip in juvenile chronic arthritis. *Br J Rheumatol* 1994;33:178–183.
141. Jacobsen ST, Levinson JE, Crawford AH. Late results of synovectomy in juvenile rheumatoid arthritis. *J Bone Joint Surg Am* 1985;67:8–15.
142. Kvien TK, Pahle JA, Hoyeraal HM, et al. Comparison of synovectomy and no synovectomy in patients with juvenile rheumatoid arthritis. A 24-month controlled study. *Scand J Rheumatol* 1987;16: 81–91.
143. Maenpaa H, Kuusela P, Lehtinen J, et al. Elbow synovectomy on patients with juvenile rheumatoid arthritis. *Clin Orthop* 2003:65–70.
144. Roles N. Synovectomy of the knee and elbow. In: Arden GP, Ansell BM, eds. *Surgical management of juvenile chronic polyarthritis.* London: Academic, 1978:75.
145. Witt JD, McCullough CJ. Anterior soft-tissue release of the hip in juvenile chronic arthritis. *J Bone Joint Surg Br* 1994;76:267–270.
146. Ruddlesdin C, Ansell BM, Arden GP, et al. Total hip replacement in children with juvenile chronic arthritis. *J Bone Joint Surg Br* 1986;68:218–222.
147. Rydholm U, Boegard T, Lidgren L. Total knee replacement in juvenile chronic arthritis. *Scand J Rheumatol* 1985;14:329–335.
148. Svensson B, Adell R. Costochondral grafts to replace mandibular condyles in juvenile chronic arthritis patients: long-term effects on facial growth. *J Craniomaxillofac Surg* 1998;26:275–285.
149. Svensson B, Feldmann G, Rindler A. Early surgical-orthodontic treatment of mandibular hypoplasia in juvenile chronic arthritis. *J Craniomaxillofac Surg* 1993;21:67–75.
150. D'Arcy E, Fell RH. Anesthesia in juvenile chronic polyarthritis. In: Arden GP, Ansell BM, ed. *Surgical management of juvenile chronic polyarthritis.* London: Academic, 1978:63.
151. Goldhagen JL. Cricoarytenoiditis as a cause of acute airway obstruction in children. *Ann Emerg Med* 1988;17:532–533.
152. Van Laar JM, Tyndall A. Intense immunosuppression and stem-cell transplantation for patients with severe rheumatic autoimmune disease: a review. *Cancer Control* 2003;10:57–65.
153. Wulffraat N, van Royen A, Bierings M, et al. Autologous haemopoietic stem-cell transplantation in four patients with refractory juvenile chronic arthritis. *Lancet* 1999;353:550–553.
154. Evans CH, Whalen JD, Ghivizzani SC, et al. Gene therapy in autoimmune diseases. *Ann Rheum Dis* 1998;57:125–127.
155. Londino AV, Rothman D, Robbins PD, et al. Gene therapy for juvenile rheumatoid arthritis? *J Rheumatol* 2000;27(suppl 58):53–55.
156. de Hooge AS, van de Loo FA, Bennink MB, et al. Growth plate damage, a feature of juvenile idiopathic arthritis, can be induced by adenoviral gene transfer of oncostatin M: a comparative study in gene-deficient mice. *Arthritis Rheum* 2003;48:1750–1761.

CHAPTER 63

Ankylosing Spondylitis

John C. Davis, Jr.

Ankylosing spondylitis (AS) is a chronic inflammatory disease of unknown etiology characterized by inflammation of spinal joints and adjacent structures that may lead to progressive and ascending bony fusion of the spine. Peripheral joints are less often affected; however, hip and shoulder joints (often considered as axial manifestaions) are involved in one third of cases. Inflammatory lesions of extraarticular organs, such as the eye and heart, may occur (1,2). AS is genetically, clinically, epidemiologically, and radiographically related to a family of diseases historically know as the seronegative spondyloarthropathies (3–5). Other members of this disease group include (a) juvenile spondylitis; (b) reactive arthritis (ReA); (c) psoriatic arthritis associated with spondylitis; (d) the arthropathies associated with inflammatory bowel disease (ulcerative colitis, and Crohn's disease); and (e) undifferentiated spondylitis in which features of two or more of these disorders occur in the same patient but do not fulfill criteria for any of the above mentioned groups. Other members of this group may include SAPHO (synovitis, acne, pustulosis, hyperostosis, and osteitis) syndrome, acne-associated arthritis, and Whipple disease. The spondyloarthropathies are entities that are pathogenetically distinct from rheumatoid arthritis (RA) and should no longer be considered a variant of RA. Features that are common among the spondyloarthropathies include (a) a predilection of spinal joint involvement, causing sacroiliitis and spondylitis; (b) peripheral arthritis, typically oligoarticular and asymmetric of the lower extremities; (c) inflammation of bony insertions for tendons and ligaments (enthesopathy), which is considered a hallmark of the disease; (d) young age at onset of symptoms; (e) negative test result for rheumatoid factor; and (f) a familial predisposition and a strong association with the major histocompatibility complex (MHC) class I molecule, human leukocyte antigen (HLA)-B27.

Several classification criteria exist for the spondyloarthropathies; however, definitive diagnosis is often delayed because of the reliance on radiographic criteria for sacroiliitis, and ongoing efforts are underway to develop diagnostic criteria that will help identify patients at earlier stages of disease. Newer imaging techniques, such as magnetic resonance imaging (MRI) and ultrasonography, may help with this process (6–9). The recent identification of anti–*Saccharomyces cerevisiae* antibody (ASCA) as the first serum marker associated with spondyloarthropathies (10) may offer an additional diagnostic tool for the high proportion of patients who have overlapping, atypical, or undifferentiated disease patterns (11).

By definition, idiopathic AS implies exclusion of the other spondyloarthropathies and is typically a disease that predominantly involves the axial skeleton. A definite diagnosis of AS is dependent on the radiographic demonstration of grade 3 or 4 sacroiliitis (Stoke Ankylosing Spondylitis Spine Score) that is unilateral or grade 2 or greater bilateral, and one or more clinical symptoms or signs, as recommended by the Modified New York Criteria (8,9) (Table 63.1). The occurrence of sacroiliitis alone, whether symptomatic or not, should not be considered solely to represent definite AS, although it may represent an early or mild form of the disease.

Until recently, therapeutic options for patients with AS have at best been able to reduce some of the symptoms of the disease. Many patients with AS have severe or progressive disease, which is responsible for significant direct and indirect socioeconomic costs. Traditional therapies including nonsteroidal antiinflammatory drugs (NSAIDs) and disease-modifying antirheumatic drugs (DMARDs), such as methotrexate and sulfasalazine, provide limited relief of symptoms. There is accumulating evidence that anti–tumor necrosis factor (anti-TNF) therapy is highly effective in AS, improving signs and symptoms of disease and quality of life, which may subsequently reduce the socioeconomic costs associated with the disease. However, further research is needed to demonstrate whether patients benefit

TABLE 63.1. *Classification criteria for ankylosing spondylitis*

Amor Classification for Spondyloarthropathies[a]
- Clinical systems/past history (score). Requires a score of ≥6 for spondyloarthropathy.
  - Lumbar/dorsal pain at night; morning stiffness (1)
  - Asymmetrical oligoarthritis (2)
  - Buttock pain (1)
  - Sausagelike toe/digit (2)
  - Heel pain/enthesopathy (2)
  - Iritis (2)
  - Nongonococcal urethritis/cervicitis <1 mo (1)
  - Acute diarrhea <1 mo (1)
  - Psoriasis, balanitis, IBD (2)
- Radiologic findings (2)
  - Sacroiliitis (bilateral grade 2 or unilateral grade >2)
- Genetic background (2)
  - HLA-B27 positive
  - Family history of AS, REA, IBD, psoriasis, or uveitis
- Response to treatment (2)
  - Clear-cut improvement (within 48 h) to NSAIDs

European Spondyloathropathy Study Group Criteria for Spondyloarthropathies[b]
1. Inflammatory spinal pain
2. Synovitis (symmetric or predominantly lower limbs)
   One or more of the following (in addition to criterion 1 or 2):
   - Alternate buttock pain
   - Sacroiliitis
   - Enthesopathy
   - Positive family history
   - Psoriasis
   - IBD
   - Urethritis/cervicitis/diarrhea <1 month prior

Modified New York Criteria[c]
- Low-back pain of ≥3 months' duration improved by exercise and not relieved by rest
- Limitation of lumbar spine in sagittal and frontal planes
- Chest expansion decreased relative to normal values for age and sex
- Bilateral sacroiliitis, grade 2–4[d]
- Unilateral sacroiliitis, grade 3–4[d]
- Definite AS if unilateral grade 3 or 4 or bilateral grade 2–4 sacroiliitis and any clinical criteria.

[a]Amor B, et al. *Rev Rhum Mal Osteoartic* 1990; 57:85–89.

[b]Dougados M, van der Linden S, Juhlin R, et al. The European Spondyloarthropathy Study Group preliminary criteria for the classification of spondyloarthropathy. *Arthritis Rheum* 1991; 34:1218–1227.

[c]van der Linden S, Valkenburg HA, Cats A. Evaluation of diagnostic criteria for ankylosing spondylitis. *Arthritis Rheum* 1984;27:361–367.

[d]Grading of radiographs: 0 = normal; 1 = suggestive; 2 = minimal sacroiliitis; 3 = moderate sacroiliitis; 4 = complete ankylosis.

AS, ankylosing spondylitis; IBD, inflammatory bowel disease; NSAID, nonsteroidal anti-inflammatory drug; ReA, reactive arthritis.

Dawes PT. Stoke ankylosing spondylitis spine score. *J Rheumatol* 1999;26:993–996.

from long-term therapy and whether radiologic progression and ankylosis can be slowed or halted.

HISTORICAL OVERVIEW

Although there is paleopathologic evidence of the existence of AS in ancient remains, most descriptions probably represent diffuse idiopathic skeletal hyperostosis (DISH) or other conditions (12). The Egyptian Pharaoh Ramses II, believed by some to represent the Pharaoh described in the biblical Exodus, appears to have had AS, based on radiographic studies conducted in the 1990s (13,14). The Irish physician Bernard Connor (15,16) provided the first pathologic description and drawing of AS in 1693, based on an ankylosed skeleton unearthed in a French cemetery. Strümpell in 1897 and Marie in 1898 (17–19) are often credited with the first clinical reports; however, earlier probable descriptions appeared in the mid-1800s (16). Krebs, Scott, and Forestier concurrently described "sacroiliitis" after spinal roentgenology evolved in the 1930s, and Robert and Forestier drew attention to the characteristic "syndesmophyte" on radiographs shortly thereafter (20,21).

Radiotherapy was successfully used by Scott in the 1920s to ease the spinal pain of AS, but later studies revealed a high incidence of subsequent leukemia, and the practice has been abandoned. Clinically useful drugs as well as salicylates and opiates became available in 1949 with the release of phenylbutazone and, in 1965, indomethacin. Clinical, epidemiologic, and family studies by Moll, Haslock, MacRae, and Wright in the 1960s and 1970s showed the interrelationships among AS, ReA, psoriatic arthritis, and enteropathic arthritis, which led to the concept of the seronegative spondyloarthropathies (3). In 1973, Brewerton et al. (22) and Schlosstein et al. (23) discovered the genetic association with HLA-B27, which subsequently solidified the classification and broadened the spectrum of the spondyloarthropathies. The genetic sequences of the cloned HLA-B27 gene and its subtypes were established in the late 1980s (24,25), and the crystal structure of the molecule with its peptide-binding groove was described in 1991 (26,27). In 1990, Hammer et al. (28) studied an HLA-B27 transgenic rat, which spontaneously developed a disease resembling the spondyloarthropathies, thereby producing the strongest evidence for the direct participation of HLA-B27 in the pathogenesis of AS. In 1994, these same investigators found that arthritis failed to develop in transgenic rats raised in a germ-free environment—emphasizing the additional requirement for pathogens in disease pathogenesis (29). Recent large genetic studies in twins and families suggest that AS is primarily a complex, multiplicative polygenic disease with a ubiquitous but essential contribution from, as yet, unidentified environmental factors. HLA-B27 appears to contribute less than 50% of the genetic risk, and other genetic regions are currently being studied (30–32).

Several studies support the idea of possible cross-reactions between bacteria (including *Klebsiella* species) and the B27 molecule. However, pathogenic hypotheses have not been fully elucidated, and many bacterial organisms have been added to the list of pathogens possibly linked to the initiation of AS.

EPIDEMIOLOGY AND GENETICS

Males appear to be affected two to three times more frequently by AS than female subjects; however, females often have atypical presentations and are underdiagnosed (33). Age at onset typically ranges from the teens to age 35 and peaks at around age 28. Approximately 15% of adult American and European cases have been found to have a childhood onset, whereas a higher proportion (40%) of juvenile-onset cases has been reported from developing countries (34).

The prevalence of AS has been best studied in white populations and varies from 0.2% in white Americans to 0.9% in white Germans to 1.4% in northern Norwegian populations (35,36). Because disease susceptibility is linked to HLA-B27 (>90% of AS cases are positive in most groups), disease prevalence tends to parallel the frequency of this genetic polymorphism in different ethnic populations, accounting for the low disease expression in Africans (37–41) and Japanese (42,43) and the high prevalences in certain Native American tribes, Inuits (44,45), and Siberian Chukotkas (46). The disease develops in approximately 20% of unrelated HLA-B27-positive white individuals (36,47). However, the strength of the association between HLA-B27 and AS varies among races. Because prevalence data on AS are not available for African Americans, estimates of approximately 25% of the frequency in whites have been based on several U.S. community studies (35).

Recent molecular studies have defined HLA-B27 as a serologic specificity encompassing 26 different alleles that encode 24 different proteins or subtypes (B*2701–B*2725; with the exception of B*2722, which was retracted in April 2002) (25,48–55). HLA-B*2705 appears to be the primordial gene from which the others evolved and is the most common allele associated with AS (90%) in American and European whites, Mexican Americans, Native Americans, Siberians, and African Americans, whereas B*2702 is found in approximately 10% of these groups and occurs more frequently in Middle Eastern and North African patients. The rare HLA-B*2703 occurs in some West African and African-American patients (48,49), contrary to earlier reports that it might not confer disease susceptibility (56). Among Chinese, Thai, and Asian Indian patients with AS, HLA-B*2704 predominates and HLA-B*2707 occurs with lower frequency. Notably, HLA-B*2706, the most common subtype in certain southeast Asian populations, does not appear to be associated with AS (57,58). Similarly, HLA-B*2709 shows a similar lack of association among Sardinians (59). The 13 most recent subtypes have not yet been studied for disease association (54).

A family history of AS can be found in 15% to 20% of cases (60). The risk for AS in an HLA-B27-positive relative of a patient with AS is approximately 20% (61), whereas almost no risk exists for HLA-B27-negative relatives. Patients with AS who are negative for HLA-B27 show similar articular manifestations as HLA-B27-positive individuals; however, they differ in that they typically have an older age at onset, absence of a family history of AS, and significantly lower frequencies of iritis and cardiac manifestations (61). Formal genetic studies of multiplex AS families have repeatedly demonstrated linkage to the MHC and HLA-B27 (32,62,63). Genome-wide studies have since confirmed the MHC on chromosome 6 to be significant in the development of AS (64,65). Concordance for the disease is 63% to 75% in monozygotic twins compared with 12.5% in all dizygotic twins and 27% in HLA-B27-positive dizygotic twins (30). MHC genes as a whole, including HLA-B27, account for only half of the susceptibility for AS; therefore, additional genetic or environmental factors are important. Another HLA-class I allele, HLA-B60, increases the risk for AS threefold in both HLA-B27-positive and HLA-B27-negative individuals (30), and additional MHC effects from the class II alleles HLA-DR1 and HLA-DR8 (66–68), and possibly class III TNF-promoter alleles (69,70), have been reported. Gene mapping studies have implicated non-B27 genes both within the MHC and elsewhere for involvement in susceptibility to AS. Recently published whole genome studies in British whites involving a total of 188 families with 255 affected sibling pairs provide strong evidence as to the loci encoding the non-MHC genetic susceptibility to AS (71). Independent support of these findings has been conveyed in a preliminary report on genome scans with microsatellite markers (32). These scans also revealed non-MHC regions overlapping with susceptibility regions suggested for psoriasis and inflammatory bowel disease (32). Genome-wide screens are underway in several other countries. More than 1,000 sibling pairs are likely to be screened over the next 5 years, providing researchers with an excellent map of genetic susceptibility to AS.

ETIOLOGY AND PATHOGENESIS

The cause of inflammation in AS is unknown; however, the fact that environmental factors are involved in the pathogenesis of AS has been firmly established by the fact that concordance is not complete between identical twins. Pathogenic hypotheses for AS have only recently been confirmed by experimental data (10,72–77). Epidemiologic studies in humans showed that outbreaks of infections with microorganisms such as *Salmonella* and *Campylobacter* were followed by joint symptoms and enthesitis in genetically susceptible individuals (72). In another study, monozygotic twins suffering from AS showed cellular hyporeactivity against *Klebsiella pneumoniae, Streptococcus pyogenes*, and *Candida albicans* compared with healthy twins (73). Although the specific role of bacteria has not been delineated in AS, many organisms have been implicated.

Klebsiella pneumoniae, a common colonizer of the gut, has been implicated as a causative microbe in a number of clinical and experimental studies (74); however, attempts to confirm these observations have been unsuccessful (78,79). *Klebsiella* shares a 6-amino-acid homology with HLA-B27, suggesting that molecular mimicry could play a role (80). One study of gene bank sequences determined that HLA-B27 shares more sequence homologies with enteric bacteria than does any other HLA-B locus allele, which suggests that this class I MHC gene might confer a considerable degree of immune tolerance to gram-negative bacteria or, alternatively, might result in an increased immunologic reaction to self (81). The hypothesis that enteric bacteria are requisites for AS is strengthened by the recent observations that HLA-B27 transgenic rats fail to develop the expected axial and peripheral arthritis, or bowel inflammation, when raised in a germ-free environment (29). Observations of occult bowel inflammation in a high percentage of AS patients (75), as well as a favorable therapeutic response to sulfasalazine, also support the possibility of an enteric pathogen.

A previous report of persistent bacterial antigens and possibly dormant, but viable, microorganisms in the peripheral joints of patients with ReA led to speculation concerning bacterial antigens and microorganisms in the spinal joints in AS (82). One study of sacroiliac joint biopsies using nested polymerase chain reaction (PCR) found no evidence of bacterial DNA from *Klebsiella* or the organisms implicated in ReA (83). Additionally, elevated serum levels of immunoglobulin A (IgA) antibodies to the causative bacteria in ReA have been reported, probably reflecting increased mucosal immunity to persisting infection (84,85). Recent searches for increased serum levels of antibodies to a variety of bacteria in AS patients have led to the discovery of the first serum marker associated with AS: ASCA. Hoffman et al. investigated whether ASCA, an important serologic marker for Crohn's disease, would be present in spondyloarthropathies because of the well-known clinical and pathologic relationships among these diseases (e.g., subclinical bowel inflammation present in many patients with AS and rheumatic manifestations common with Crohn's disease). When compared with healthy controls or patients with RA, patients with AS had significantly increased ASCA IgA levels (10). However, no differences in ASCA IgA levels were noted between HLA-B27-positive and HLA-B27-negative patients (10). Other studies conducted in HLA-B27-positive patients with AS have also shown significantly higher IgG antibody levels to *Klebsiella*, *Yersinia*, and *Salmonella* (76,77).

Several studies of synovial fluid in ReA have demonstrated that mononuclear cells proliferate specifically to the organism that triggered the arthritis, and bacteria-specific T-cell responses, both HLA class II (DR and DP) and, more recently, HLA class I (B27) restricted, have been detected (86–88). Even though examination of synovial fluid and synovial membrane specimens for bacterial DNA by PCR is increasingly used to diagnose ReA, such assays have not been standardized and are not generally available for spinal joints. Maki-Ikola et al. measured synovial fluid samples from eight patients with AS. Enzyme immunoassay and radial immunodiffusion demonstrated no clear evidence for intraarticular antibody production against three *Klebsiella pneumoniae* capsular types, *Escherichia coli*, or *Proteus mirabilis* (89). However, sacroiliac biopsies from AS patients have revealed infiltrating T cells and macrophages, as well as high levels of the cytokines TNF and transforming growth factor (TGF) (90,91).

The strong association of the HLA class I allele HLA-B27 with AS has been recognized for over 25 years; however, the pathogenic mechanism linking HLA-B27 with AS and other spondyloarthropathies remains a mystery. HLA-B27 has an unusual cell biology compared with other HLA molecules and it demonstrates an interesting ability to form heavy-chain homodimers *in vitro*. Dimerization is dependent on disulphide bonding through an unpaired cysteine at position 67. HLA-B27 homodimer formation has also been demonstrated in certain cell lines *in vivo*, and preliminary data suggest that significant numbers of T cells from patients with AS express a ligand for HLA-B27 homodimers (92). These findings have extended our understanding of the immunologic function of HLA-B27, and have led to the hypothesis that HLA-B27 heavy-chain dimerization may be involved in the pathogenesis of AS.

CLINICAL FEATURES AND DIAGNOSIS

Modes of Presentation

The three sets of classification criteria most commonly referenced for AS are the Amor, the European Spondyloarthropathy Study Group, and the Modified New York (1987) criteria (Table 63.1). Chronic low back pain and stiffness are typically the first symptoms of AS (93–99). Onset is usually insidious, and patients often cannot date when symptoms first began, or precisely localize the areas affected. Complaints of alternating pain, first in one buttock and then the other, occasionally with radiation down the posterior thigh, can be elicited from some patients and probably represent sacroiliac involvement. Often these symptoms are incorrectly ascribed to hip disease or sciatica. Because low back discomfort is such a common complaint in the population at large, much attention has been directed to differentiating inflammatory from noninflammatory back pain (93). Characteristically, inflammatory back symptoms are suggested by prominent stiffness and pain in the morning or after other periods of rest (gel phenomenon) that improve with exercise (Table 63.2). Such symptoms are most likely to reflect AS in a person under 40 years of age. Additional history suggesting AS includes back pain that forces the individual out of bed at night or is not relieved by lying down, as well as concomitant chest wall pain (94). Although symptoms of inflammatory back disease often are useful in raising the likelihood of AS, it must be emphasized that some patients with AS will have only nonspecific or even no low back complaints despite typical radiographic changes (96). Additionally, family studies of AS have demonstrated that HLA-B27-positive relatives who have typical inflammatory back symptoms (97) or chest pain (98) may not show radiographic evidence of sacroiliitis or spondylitis. Follow-up of such individuals by using serial spinal radiographs indicated that an average of 9 years may elapse before sacroiliac joints show diagnostic radiographic changes (99).

Less commonly, patients with AS may have a peripheral arthritis, typically monoarticular or oligoarticular, and often affecting one or both knees (95). Enthesitis, especially involving Achilles or plantar tendon insertions, may appear alone or with arthritis (100,101). In adult patients with predominantly this presentation, ReA should be considered. However, juvenile spondylitis or the seronegative enthesopathy and arthritis (SEA) syndrome of children, especially in males, typically presents in this fashion (102–104). Other patterns of AS onset in children have been described, including ankylosing tarsitis (105), symmetric polyarthritis, and dominant cervical spine involvement (106). There are few long-term follow-up studies of such children. It appears, however, that many of these patients eventually develop spinal symptoms and a more typical axial course (101,107). Plain sacroiliac radiographs are unreliable in detecting sacroiliitis in children; however, contrast-enhanced MRI has been reported to be more sensitive (108). The appearance of hip involvement has been correlated with early age at onset of AS and indicates a poor prognosis (109).

TABLE 63.2. *Features of inflammatory back pain*

Younger age at onset of pain (peak 26 years)
Pain and early morning stiffness of the spine
Improvement with exercise/activity
Insidious in onset
Symptoms lasting longer than 3 months
Spinal mobility and deep breathing may be restricted
Radiographic evidence of sacroiliitis or ankylosis

Physical Examination and Disease Course

The earliest abnormality on physical examination in AS is usually tenderness in the sacroiliac joints or pain in the same areas elicited by hip hyperextension. Results of the straight leg-raising test, often used to detect sciatic nerve irritation by a ruptured disc, are typically negative, and deep tendon reflexes in the lower extremities are normal (94,95). More objective findings occur with longer disease duration and include flattening of the normal lordotic curvature and restriction of movement in all planes of the lumbar spine. The Schober test of lumbar flexion is significantly reduced (<3 cm) and the patient is unable to touch fingers to floor by a considerable distance. When the disease has advanced to the thoracic spine, restricted chest expansion (<2.5 cm) due to costovertebral joint fusion is a reasonably specific sign of AS, especially in a young individual (95). Additionally, the normal kyphosis of the dorsal spine becomes accentuated, and the patient assumes a "stooped shoulder" appearance (Fig. 63.1). Cervical spine involvement, classically believed to be a late disease manifestation, may occur earlier in women. Pain and stiffness in cervical joints and surrounding muscles is followed by a decreased ability to fully extend the neck. The extent of this deformity can be measured by the occiput-to-wall distance, in which the standing patient places the back of the heels against a wall and attempts to touch the wall with the back of the head. Loss of lateral rotation also occurs, and eventually the neck may lose all motion and become fixed in a flexed position. If this deformity is extreme, forward vision may be compromised. Depending on the severity of both cervical and thoracic kyphosis, the patient may need to stand with knees voluntarily flexed to maintain a center of gravity.

Radiographic Abnormalities

Sacroiliitis, usually bilateral, is the most frequent and earliest radiographic manifestation of AS (110). The first

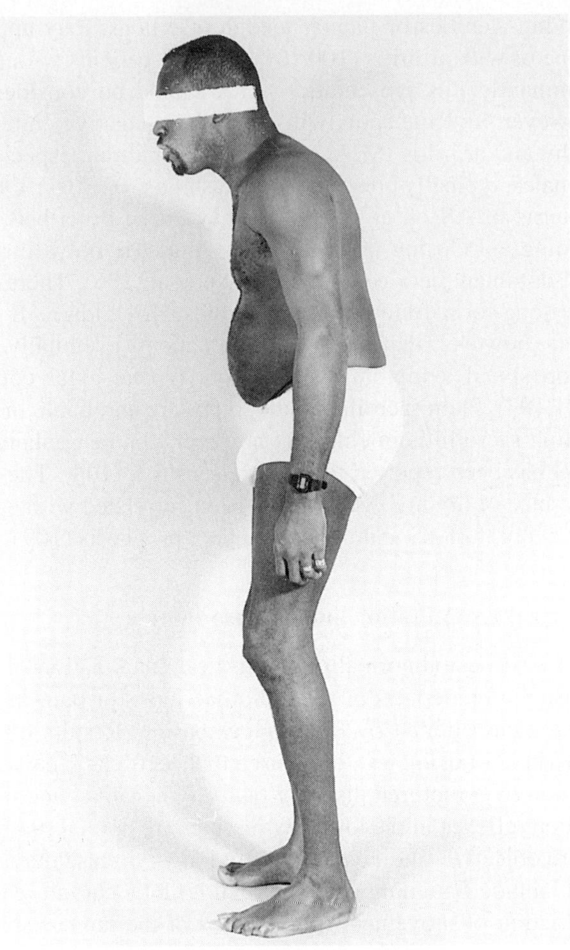

FIG. 63.1. Posture of patient with severe and advanced ankylosing spondylitis. Note loss of normal lumbar lordosis, presence of dorsal kyphosis, cervical fixation in mild flexion, and compensatory flexion of the knees.

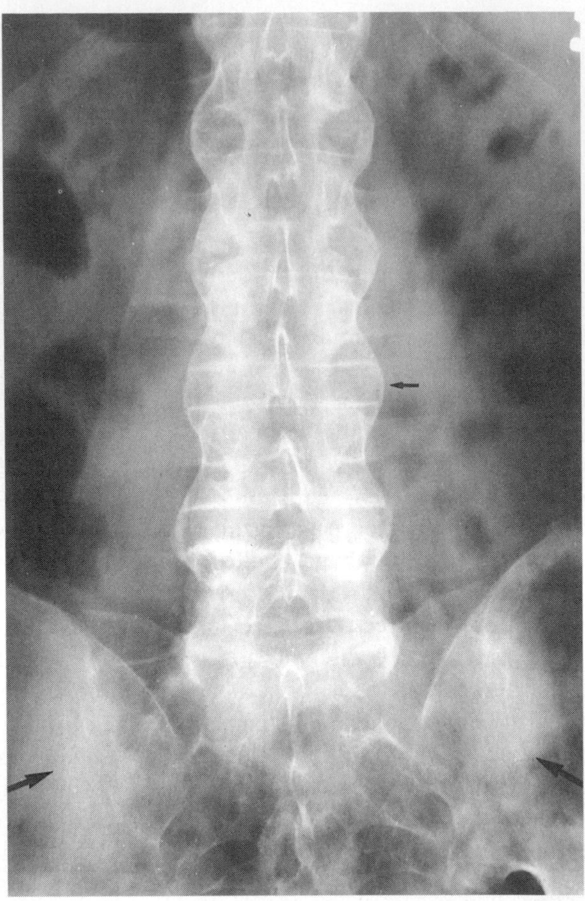

FIG. 63.2. Anteroposterior radiograph of the upper pelvis and lumbar spine. Both sacroiliac joints (*large arrows*) are fused (grade IV sacroiliitis), and there are bilateral, symmetric syndesmophytes (*small arrow*), resulting in the typical "bamboo" appearance of ankylosing spondylitis.

radiographic signs of sacroiliitis include "pseudowidening" of the joint and sclerosis at one or both joint margins (Stokes grades 1 and 2) (111), usually in the lower two thirds, which has a synovial lining. With more advanced disease, sclerosis and erosions appear at both joint margins (grade 3), and later bony fusion across the joint and loss of sclerosis occurs (grade 4; Fig. 63.2). Interpretation of sacroiliac radiographs is difficult, and there is much interobserver variation, especially in the early stages of disease (112,113).

An anteroposterior view of the pelvis is usually not an adequate means of detecting early sacroiliac disease because the normal forward tilt of the pelvis precludes a view of the entire length of the joints. Rather, radiographs of the pelvis aimed 30 degrees cephalad (Ferguson views) and oblique-angled views of each joint are usually necessary for adequate assessment. Care must be taken to disregard congenital anomalies and degenerative changes, as well as osteitis condensans ilii (110). Computed tomography (CT) has been shown to be a more sensitive technique for detecting early sacroiliitis when standard radiographs are normal (114). Newer imaging modalities such as MRI may be helpful in showing sacroiliitis in the early phase of disease (115,116). In evaluation of spinal and sacroiliac joint abnormalities, MRI, in addition to plain radiography, can visualize soft tissue abnormalities and neurologic compromise without use of intrathecal contrast (117). Bone scans are not reliable, especially in bilateral disease, because of normally high uptakes of radiolabeled tracers by the sacroiliac joints.

Bone mineral density (BMD) has been assessed by dual-energy x-ray absorptiometry in both premenopausal and postmenopausal women with AS. These studies concluded that women with AS have reduced hip BMD, when compared with age and gender-matched control (118,119). Furthermore, a cross-sectional study of 71 male and female patients confirmed that AS patients have decreased BMD values at both the spine and femur, as well as total body measurements, reflecting generalized bone loss (120).

Other pelvic abnormalities that may be detected radiographically in patients with AS include osteitis pubis (sclerosis and bony irregularities at the symphysis pubis), as well as bony erosions or "whiskering" along the margins of the ischial tuberosities, iliac crests, or proximal trochanters, indicative of enthesitis (110). The most characteristic radiographic changes of AS in the lumbar, dorsal, and cervical spine include "squaring" of the vertebral bodies due to erosions of their normally concave anterior, superior, and inferior surfaces, often appearing as "shiny corners" (Romanus lesions) (121) (Fig. 63.3). Additionally, ossification of spinal ligaments, which bridge the intervertebral discs, results in the characteristic "syndesmophytes" (Figs. 63.2 and 63.3). When many syndesmophytes are present bilaterally, the radiographic appearance is that of a "bamboo spine" (Fig. 63.2). In general, the syndesmophytes seen in AS, as well as in enteropathic spondylitis, are symmetric and bilateral and have their insertions at the upper and lower margins of adjacent vertebral bodies. In contrast, syndesmophytes occurring in ReA and psoriatic spondylitis tend to be asymmetric and have nonmarginal vertebral insertions (122,123). Zygapophyseal joints in AS also are obliterated by bony fusion. The presence of bony fusion of cervical apophyseal joints may be particularly discriminating for AS in some atypical cases described in children and women (106) (Fig. 63.4). Less commonly, erosions of upper cervical structures such as the transverse ligament or odontoid process may lead to subluxation (124), similar to that seen in RA, or even upward migration of the odontoid into the brainstem (platybasia), resulting in a neurologic catastrophe (125). Generalized spinal osteopenia is common in AS, probably due to immobility and local cytokine release (126,127), and spinal fractures, especially of the neck, may occur after minor trauma (128,129). As segments of the spine become progressively fused, pain often disappears. The appearance of renewed pain may indicate a complicating fracture, which may not be apparent on standard radiographs (130). In this circumstance, a bone scan may show increased uptake of tracer in the fracture site, which may then require further elucidation by CT (131). Another cause of renewed spinal pain, usually sharply localized and exacerbated by exercise, is spondylodiscitis (Andersson lesion), a sterile, circumscribed, destructive process involving one vertebral body and the adjacent intervertebral disc, which may mimic an infectious discitis or osteomyelitis (132,133).

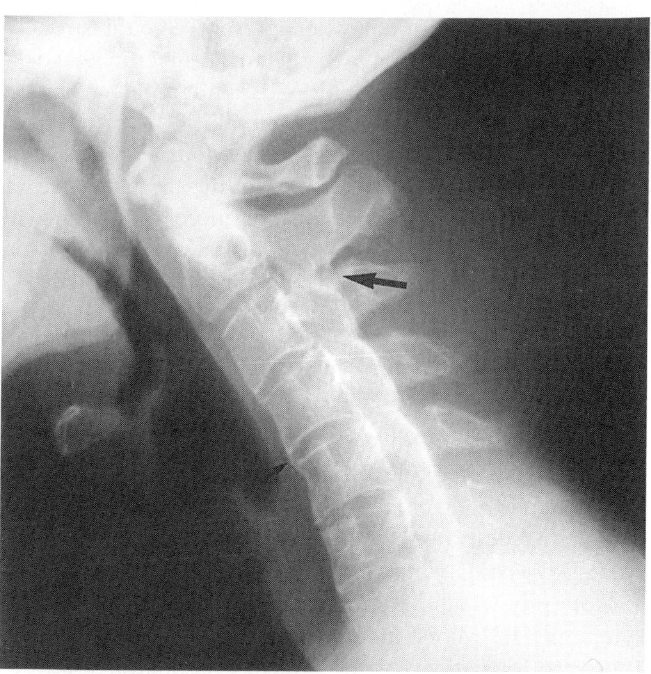

FIG. 63.4. Lateral radiograph of the cervical spine in ankylosing spondylitis. Bony fusion of apophyseal joint between C2 and C3 (*large arrow*) and all other apophyseal joints below this level also are fused. A marginal syndesmophyte is also shown (*small arrow*).

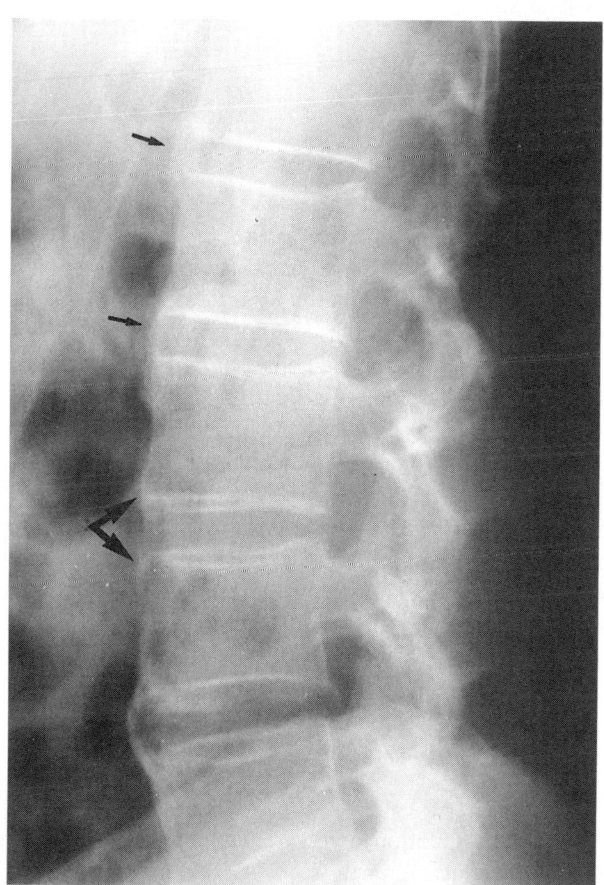

FIG. 63.3. Lateral radiograph of the lumbar spine in ankylosing spondylitis with "shiny corners" or Romanus lesions (*large arrows*) due to marginal erosions of vertebral bodies and typical marginal syndesmophytes (*small arrows*).

Involved peripheral joints may show osteopenia and erosions similar to those of RA. More often in AS, however, are findings of bony ankylosis in wrists, tarsal bones, hips, or small joints of the fingers and toes.

Differential Diagnosis

Although symptoms of inflammatory back disease, especially in young men, and the typical spinal abnormalities on physical examination, when present, should strongly suggest the diagnosis of AS, the most specific diagnostic findings are the characteristic radiographic changes. Sacroiliitis, especially when bilateral, is a virtual prerequisite for definite diagnosis. The Modified New York (9) Diagnostic Criteria for AS require the presence of radiographic sacroiliitis and one or more of the clinical symptoms or signs (Table 63.1). Bilateral radiographic sacroiliitis, when properly interpreted, has a limited differential diagnosis, with the most common causes being the spondyloarthropathies and infectious processes (Table 63.3). In a 5-year follow-up study designed to assess locally available investigations in the early diagnosis of inflammatory sacroiliitis, Eastmond et al. analyzed plain film evidence of grade 2 radiologic sacroiliitis (bilateral or unilateral) and found it to be the most reliable predictor for the development of AS (134). CT scanning and HLA-B27 testing were of no added value in this study.

More problematic are patients with characteristic spinal symptoms in whom radiographic studies are normal or equivocal, or patients with atypical presentations, including children or women, who have predominantly peripheral arthritis, enthesitis, and cervical spine symptoms. Initial radiographs of the sacroiliac regions and spine are often difficult to interpret in children, and men, in general, may have more severe radiographic changes in the lower spine and hips than women. These factors make a definitive diagnosis of AS difficult in children and women. Although CT or MRI of the sacroiliac joints may be an option in some patients, a less expensive approach may be a blood test for HLA-B27. And although diagnostic testing for HLA-B27 was discouraged in the early 1980s (135), studies conducted two decades later demonstrated its potential usefulness as an adjunct in diagnosis, especially if the patient had inflammatory back symptoms (36,136,137). The frequency of HLA-B27 is more than 90% in AS patients and approximately 8% in most healthy white populations. Thus, a "false-positive" result (HLA-B27 positivity unrelated to the patient's symptoms) would be expected to occur approximately 8% of the time, and a "false-negative" result (patient has HLA-B27-negative AS) less than 10% of the time. As with any other test, the predictive value of HLA-B27 is greatest when the physician has reason to believe that the disease is present (136). The finding of HLA-B27 is even more predictive of disease in ethnic populations in which the normal frequency of this genetic marker is low, such as African (2%) or Japanese (<1%) patients. In Native Americans and other groups with high normal background levels of HLA-B27, it is much less useful as a diagnostic aid.

TABLE 63.3. *Causes of sacroiliitis*

Spondyloarthropathies
Ankylosing spondylitis
Reactive arthritis
Psoriatic arthritis
Inflammatory bowel disease
Acne-associated arthritis or SAPHO syndrome
Intestinal bypass arthritis
Undifferentiated spondylitis
Infectious
Pyogenic infections
Tuberculosis
Brucellosis
Whipple's disease
Other
Hyperparathyroidism
Paraplegia
Sarcoidosis

SAPHO syndrome, synovitis, acne, pustulosis, hyperostosis, osteitis.

Causes other than AS for spinal pain and restriction can usually be excluded by standard radiographs. An exception may be DISH (or Forestier disease), in which prominent syndesmophytes may mimic AS. DISH, however, can usually be differentiated from AS by its later age at onset, larger and more flowing ligamentous (often referred to as "candle-wax dripping" in appearance) ossifications, and most important, the absence of sacroiliitis (110). DISH also is not associated with HLA-B27 (138). A DISH-like syndrome has been described in patients, often young, receiving long-term retinoid therapy. Again, sacroiliitis should be absent in such patients, although one case report suggests otherwise (139).

Extraarticular Manifestations

Ocular

Episodes of acute anterior uveitis or iritis occur in approximately 25% of AS patients during the course of the disease (140). Usually, one eye is affected at a time, and there are often long intervals between attacks. Typical symptoms include the sudden onset of ocular pain, redness, and photophobia. Unless inflammation is promptly suppressed, debris may accumulate in the anterior chamber, causing pupillary and lens dysfunction and blurring of vision. In some cases, the posterior chamber becomes inflamed, causing macular edema and further visual compromise. Permanent blindness is unusual but may occur in some patients, especially those not treated promptly and aggressively. Acute anterior uveitis of this type shows a strong association with HLA-B27, regardless of whether the patient has spondyloarthropathy.

Cardiac

Aortic regurgitation and variable degrees of atrioventricular or bundle-branch block occur in approximately 5% of patients with AS, usually after long-standing disease, but occasionally preceding arthritis symptoms (141). Less often, mitral regurgitation accompanies aortic disease

(142). Nearly all patients with cardiac manifestations are HLA-B27 positive. This finding has suggested an HLA-B27-associated cardiac syndrome consisting of aortic root disease and conduction abnormalities (143,144). Once the murmur of aortic regurgitation is heard, the disease follows a relentless course to heart failure, usually over several years. There is no effective therapy except for valvular replacement. Similarly, complete heart block requires implantation of a cardiac pacemaker.

Bergfeldt et al. (144) have conducted extensive clinical studies of spondylitic heart disease. Of 223 men who had pacemaker implantation for conduction disturbances, radiographic evidence of sacroiliitis was identified in 19 (8.5%), which is significantly higher than the prevalence of sacroiliitis in the general population (145). The combination of heart block and aortic insufficiency found in 91 pacemaker recipients was associated with a spondyloarthropathy in 15% to 20% and in 88% with HLA-B27 (146). Moreover, HLA-B27 was positive in 17% of 83 patients with complete heart block who had no clinical or radiographic evidence of arthritis as compared with 6% in a normal control population, a statistically significant difference (147).

The pathologic lesions responsible for spondylitic heart disease were well described by Bulkley and Roberts (148) in eight patients after autopsy. Grossly, there was dilatation and thickening of the walls of the proximal aortic root, and shortening and thickening of the aortic valve cusps. Histopathologically, the vasa vasorum were found to be surrounded by collections of plasma cells and lymphocytes, and their lumens were narrowed. The thickening of the aorta and ventricular septum was due to adventitial scarring and intimal proliferation, with a prominent fibrous "bump" located below the valvular cusps. In those cases in which heart block occurred, there was extension of this fibrosing process into the atrioventricular bundle or proximal bundle branches. Transthoracic echocardiographic studies have detected the fibrous bump or aortic valvular thickening in 31% of patients with AS who had no clinically apparent spondylitic heart disease (149,150); however, transesophageal echocardiography appears to be more sensitive in detecting aortic and mitral valve abnormalities in a higher percentage of patients (150,151). Echocardiographic examination of diastolic function has recently shown cardiac involvement in AS patients who lack clinical symptoms (152).

Pulmonary

Lung involvement in AS is unusual (153–155). Despite diminished chest expansion due to costovertebral joint fusion, patients with AS rarely have significant reductions in total lung and vital capacities because diaphragmatic function is not impaired. When it does occur, pulmonary involvement in AS consists principally of upper lobe fibrotic changes and chest wall restriction. Bilateral apical pulmonary fibrosis occurs in approximately 1% of patients with AS, usually after many years of disease, and cavitation mimicking tuberculosis occurs in one third of these patients. Rarely, colonization of these cavities by *Aspergillus* occurs, requiring consideration of antifungal therapy.

Renal

Secondary renal amyloidosis is the most common cause of renal involvement in AS (62%) followed by IgA nephropathy (30%) and mesangioproliferative glomerulonephritis (5%). Other rare causes include membranous nephropathy (1%), focal segmental glomerulosclerosis (1%), and focal proliferative glomerulonephritis (1%) (156). Secondary amyloidosis complicates the course of AS and other spondyloarthropathies in 1% to 3% of cases, and has been reported more commonly in Europe than in the United States. Proteinuria, often in the nephrotic range, is the usual presentation, and progression to renal failure is common. Abdominal fat pad or rectal biopsies for amyloid may be found in approximately 7% of unselected cases of AS, but clinically significant disease does not develop in most (157). Proteinuria, with or without renal function impairment, also may indicate the presence of IgA nephropathy, which is of considerable interest in view of elevations of serum IgA in AS patients (158). Renal dysfunction and proteinuria can result from use of NSAIDs and traditional DMARDs, such as sulfasalazine, or large amounts of analgesic use.

Neurologic

Besides cervical spine fractures and dislocations, a slowly progressive cauda equina syndrome may appear late in the disease course (159). Usual symptoms include sensory loss in lumbar and sacral dermatomes and, less often, lower extremity weakness and pain, and loss of urinary and rectal sphincter tone. MRI is the most reliable means of demonstrating the characteristic enlarged dural sacs and arachnoid diverticula and excluding other potentially surgically correctable myelopathies (160,161). There may be an increased frequency of multiple sclerosis in AS patients, but this has not been proven by definitive epidemiologic studies (162).

Gastrointestinal Tract

Asymptomatic areas of both macroscopic and microscopic inflammation in the proximal colon and terminal ileum have been demonstrated by ileocolonoscopy in up to 60% of patients with AS (79). Although of considerable pathogenetic interest, these findings did not indicate a high likelihood of developing overt Crohn's disease or ulcerative colitis. In a follow-up study, 2 to 9 years after their first ileocolonoscopy, 6.5% of the patients developed overt

Crohn's disease, although they had no clinical signs of inflammatory bowel disease at their first visit. All of these patients evolved into AS, and most of them suffered from persistent peripheral arthritis (163).

LABORATORY FEATURES

The most characteristic laboratory abnormalities are elevations of the erythrocyte sedimentation rate and other acute-phase reactants—especially C-reactive protein. Similarly, the platelet count may be slightly or moderately elevated, and there may be mild anemia, depending on the severity of the inflammatory process. Serum IgA levels are elevated in most patients, but whether these represent antibodies to causative bacteria is still being investigated. Test results for rheumatoid factors and antinuclear antibodies are negative, and serum complement levels are normal or high. HLA-B27 is positive in more than 90% of patients, and its frequency approaches 100% in those with acute anterior uveitis or spondylitic heart disease. Modest elevations of bone alkaline phosphatase and creatine kinase occur in some patients, but their significance is unclear (164).

TREATMENT

The major aims of management include (a) the pharmacologic relief of pain and stiffness; (b) a physical therapy and lifestyle modifications program aimed at preserving spinal mobility or, at least, preventing spinal deformity and disability; and (c) the prompt recognition and management of articular and extraarticular complications. It is essential that the patient be well educated in the natural history of this disease and the rationale for each treatment modality.

Pharmacologic

NSAIDs are usually necessary, at least initially, to relieve pain and stiffness before a patient can satisfactorily perform appropriate exercises. In general, aspirin is usually inadequate. Indomethacin is a popular NSAID, however other NSAIDs are commonly used, none of which have demonstrated superior efficacy in AS. The usage of indomethacin should be geared to the severity of symptoms and degree of relief attained, but nightly administration of the 75-mg sustained-release preparation may be particularly useful in preventing night pain and morning stiffness (165). Many other NSAIDs, including tolmetin, piroxicam, and diclofenac, may prove more effective in individual patients. The recent addition of selective cyclooxygenase-2 (COX-2) inhibitors, with less potential for gastrointestinal toxicity, offers additional potentially useful NSAIDs. Results of clinical studies confirm the relevant antiinflammatory effect of COX-2 inhibitors like celecoxib, with significant improvement of both pain and function in patients with AS (166). Patients taking NSAIDs require monitoring for the usual gastrointestinal and renal complications inherent to these agents.

Second-line drugs should be considered not only when a patient becomes refractory to NSAIDs or has serious NSAID-induced side effects, but also when a patient has progressive disease. Several DMARDs, such as sulfasalazine, methotrexate, gold, azathioprine, and cyclosporine, have been suggested to be effective in patients with chronic progressive AS. Multiple controlled clinical trials have demonstrated the effectiveness of sulfasalazine (usually 2–3 g daily) for AS, especially early in the disease (167–169). Such studies have shown improvement in spinal symptoms, and perhaps spinal mobility, peripheral arthritis, and, impressively, in reducing the levels of acute-phase reactants. One study demonstrated that the sulfapyridine moiety, rather than the salicylate, accounted for its therapeutic effects (170). It remains unclear, however, whether sulfasalazine improves disease through its antibiotic effect on intestinal bacteria or through other immunomodulatory or antiinflammatory properties.

Efficacy of conventional DMARDs, including methotrexate, azathioprine, and cyclophosphamide has not been established by controlled studies. Pulse high-dose methylprednisolone has proved temporarily effective in acute flare-ups (171). Long-term low-dose corticosteroids may be necessary at times, especially for refractory peripheral arthritis; however, drug-related osteoporotic effects should be considered and monitored via BMD or biochemical assay.

Newer agents under investigation for the treatment of AS include TNF inhibitors such as etanercept and infliximab; the pyrimidine inhibitor leflunomide; and the interleukin-1 inhibitor anakinra. Numerous reports have demonstrated the efficacy and safety of the TNF inhibitors—etanercept and infliximab—in patients with AS. These agents have already been approved for use in the treatment of RA. Etanercept is also indicated in psoriatic arthritis and infliximab in Crohn's disease. A 1-year placebo-controlled, multicenter trial found infliximab to be effective in active AS patients (172). Based on this one study, infliximab was approved for use in the treatment of AS in the European Union. According to the results of several larger studies, etanercept is also an effective and well-tolerated treatment for patients with AS (173,174). The findings of these trials not only confirm the unequivocal efficacy of etanercept in the treatment of patients with active AS who are receiving conventional NSAID therapy, but also show that no additional therapy with conventional DMARDs and steroids is needed to obtain the results (175). AS patients receiving etanercept have also experienced significant improvements in spinal mobility and functionality measures (174). The impressive antiinflammatory effects of the TNF inhibitors, etanercept and infliximab, have led to their use in multiple diseases besides their original indication for RA. Ongoing and future research will strive to reveal the potential of these therapeutic agents in other inflammatory disorders.

Complications that may arise with AS also require pharmacologic intervention. Acute anterior uveitis requires prompt treatment by an ophthalmologist (140). Local corticosteroid and mydriatic drops are the usual first approach. Patients with more refractory eye disease, however, may require retrobulbar injections or even systemic corticosteroids for short periods. There is no known medical treatment for the cardiac, pulmonary, and renal lesions of AS.

Physical Therapy

Formal instruction in proper posture and exercises emphasizing spinal mobility and strengthening of spinal extensors should be provided to every patient initially and reemphasized periodically. Range-of-motion exercises for the neck, shoulders, and hips, as well as deep-breathing exercises to maintain chest expansion, should also be emphasized (176,177). In 2001, a review of scientific evidence from clinical evaluations of physical therapy and exercise in AS acknowledged physiotherapy accompanied by disease education as an effective intervention (178). Swimming is an excellent modality for achieving all these goals. Canes or walkers may be necessary for patients with severe spinal kyphosis, or lower extremity arthritis. Soft cervical collars should be used by patients with neck fusion or subluxation in situations in which they are exposed to possible injury. Adaptive devices such as prism glasses may be necessary to ensure forward vision in those with severe cervical flexion, and special mirrors in automobiles may help those with decreased spinal rotation (179).

Surgical Approaches

Total hip replacement is the most common orthopedic surgical procedure needed by patients with AS, and the results are usually satisfactory (180). Occasionally, heterotopic bone formation around the implant may mimic complicating infection, and at times, new bone may encase the prosthesis and restrict motion (181). Osteotomy of the spine has been used to correct severe spinal deformity but is fraught with hazard (182). Moreover, for any surgical procedure requiring general anesthesia, intubation must be approached cautiously because of cervical spine fragility and limitation of mouth opening (183).

OUTCOME ASSESSMENT

The emergence of new treatment options in AS, resulting from recent advances in immunology, has accelerated the need for universal standards to systematically assess treatment response and indications in AS. Numerous assessment methods are currently available in AS, including laboratory measurements, metrology, radiographs, and questionnaires; however, continued work is needed to improve existing methods and to conduct meaningful clinical trials. Outcome criteria, such as those developed by the Assessment in Ankylosing Spondylitis (ASAS) Working Group, have been successfully applied in evaluating response to AS treatment. The ASAS Working Group is an international group that comprises rheumatologists, epidemiologists, patients with AS, and representatives from the pharmaceutical industry from more than 20 countries. The ASAS improvement criteria consist of four outcome domains (184) (Table 63.4).

TABLE 63.4. *Assessment in ankylosing spondylitis working group improvement criteria*

Improvement of ≥20% and absolute improvement of ≥10 units on a 0–100 scale in at least three of the following domains:
Patient global assessment (VAS global)
Pain assessment (VAS)
Function (BASFI)
Inflammation (average of least two VAS in BASDAI)
Absence of deterioration (20% worsening) in potential remaining domain(s)

BASDAI, Bath Ankylosing Spondylitis Disease Activity Index; BASFI, Bath Ankylosing Spondylitis Functional Index; VAS, visual analogue scale.

Data from Anderson JJ, Baron G, van der Heijde D, et al. Ankylosing spondylitis assessment group preliminary definition of short-term improvement in ankylosing spondylitis. *Arthritis Rheum* 2001;44:1876–1886.

ASAS improvement criteria have already been published for assessing short-term improvement with symptom-modifying antirheumatic drugs using outcome data from placebo-controlled trials of NSAIDs (185). The ASAS Working Group is currently developing response criteria for disease-controlling antirheumatic treatment based on results of studies with biologic treatments, such as etanercept and infliximab (186).

PROGNOSIS

Several long-term studies indicate that the prognosis of AS is good in the majority of patients (2,179,187,188). Only 10% to 20% become significantly disabled over long periods (20–38 years), and 85% to 90% are able to pursue full-time employment, despite progression to severe spinal restriction in approximately half of patients. A predictable pattern of disease usually emerges after the first 10 years. Hip disease, which typically begins early and in the youngest patients, is an indicator of a poor functional outcome.

Mortality from the disease itself occurs in fewer than 5% of patients, most commonly from cervical fractures and dislocations, spondylitic heart disease, and amyloid nephropathy. Malignancies are increased only in those who have received spinal irradiation, and include a five-fold increase in leukemias and a 62% excess of other cancers (187,189–191).

CONCLUSION

AS is a chronic inflammatory process that is insidious in onset and may progressively lead to spinal fusion. The pathogenesis of AS is becoming better understood, and immune-mediated mechanisms involving HLA-B27, cytokines (e.g., TNF-α), inflammatory cellular infiltrates, and genetic and environmental factors are thought to have key roles. The detection of sacroiliitis by radiography, MRI, or CT in the presence of clinical manifestations is considered diagnostic for AS. Although NSAIDs effectively relieve inflammatory symptoms and are presently first-line drug treatment, they are also associated with harmful gastrointestinal and renal side effects. For symptoms refractory to NSAIDs, second-line treatments, including corticosteroids and various DMARDs, have been used but are of limited benefit, especially for spinal symptoms and ankylosis. TNF inhibitors such as etanercept and infliximab target the inflammatory mechanisms underlying AS, and thus, may favorably alter the disease process, in addition to providing symptom relief. These new treatments offer positive effects on quality of life and long-term functional disability, potentially reducing the economic impact of the disease for society and patients (192).

REFERENCES

1. Moll JMH. *Ankylosing spondylitis.* Edinburgh: Churchill Livingston, 1980.
2. Khan MA. Ankylosing spondylitis and related spondyloarthropathies: spine: state of the art reviews. *Rheum Dis Clin North Am* 1990;4:497–688.
3. Moll JMH, Haslock I, MacRae I, et al. Associations between ankylosing spondylitis, psoriatic arthritis, Reiter's disease, the intestinal arthropathies, and Behçet's syndrome. *Medicine (Baltimore)* 1974;53: 343–364.
4. Arnett FC. The seronegative spondyloarthropathies. *Bull Rheum Dis* 1987;37:1–12.
5. Yu D, ed. Spondyloarthropathies. *Rheum Dis Clin North Am* 1998;24: 663–915.
6. Dougados M, van der Linden S, Juhlin R, et al. The European Spondyloarthropathy Study Group preliminary criteria for the classification of spondyloarthropathy. *Arthritis Rheum* 1991;34:1218–1227.
7. Kellgren JH, Jeffrey MR, Ball J. *The epidemiology of chronic rheumatism.* Oxford: Blackwell, 1963:326.
8. Gofton JP. Report from the subcommittee on diagnostic criteria for ankylosing spondylitis. In: Bennett PH, Wood PHN, eds. *Population studies of the rheumatic diseases.* New York: Excerpta Medica, 1968: 314–316.
9. van der Linden S, Valkenburg HA, Cats A. Evaluation of diagnostic criteria for ankylosing spondylitis. *Arthritis Rheum* 1984;27:361–367.
10. Hoffman IE, Demetter P, Peeters M, et al. Anti-*Saccharomyces cerevisiae* IgA antibodies are raised in ankylosing spondylitis and undifferentiated spondyloarthropathy. *Ann Rheum Dis* 2003;62:455–459.
11. Boyer GS, Templin DW, Bowler A, et al. A comparison of patients with spondyloarthropathy seen in specialty clinics with those identified in a community wide epidemiologic study: has the classic case misled us? *Arch Intern Med* 1997;157:2111–2117.
12. Rogers JM, Waldron T, Dieppe P, et al. Arthropathies in paleopathology: the basis of classification according to most probable cause. *J Archaeol Sci* 1987;14:179–193.
13. Ramses II. Magnificence on the Nile. In: Lost civilizations. Alexandria, VA: Time-Life Books, 1993:154.
14. Blumberg BS, Blumberg JL. Bernard Connor (1666–1698) and his contribution to the pathology of ankylosing spondylitis. *J Hist Med* 1958;20:349–366.
15. Arnett FC. Ankylosing spondylitis 1992: from Connor to transgenes. *J Irish Coll Phys Surg* 1993;22:207–211.
16. Strümpell A. Bemerkungen uber chronisch-ankylosierende Entzundung der Wirbelsaule und der Huftergelenks. *Dtsch Z Nervenheilk* 1897;11:338–342.
17. Strümpell A. Observations on chronic-ankylosing inflammation of the vertebrae and hip joints [English translation]. In: *Clinical orthopaedics and related research.* Philadelphia: JB Lippincott, 1971:4–6.
18. Marie P. Sur la spondylose rhizomelique. *Rev Med* 1898;18:285–315.
19. Bechterew VM. Steifigheit der wirbelsaule und ihre verkrumnung als besondere erkrankungsform. *Neurol Zentbl* 1893;12:426.
20. Forestier J. Gilbert Scott memorial oration: ankylosing spondylitis at the beginning of the century. *Rheumatism* 1964;20:28–34, 52–53.
21. Forestier J, Rotes-Querol J. *Ankylosing spondylitis: clinical considerations, roentgenology, pathologic anatomy, treatment.* Springfield, IL: Charles C Thomas, 1956.
22. Brewerton DA, Hart FD, Nichols A, et al. Ankylosing spondylitis and HL-A27. *Lancet* 1973;1:904–907.
23. Schlosstein L, Terasaki PI, Bluestone R, et al. High association of an HLA antigen, W27, with ankylosing spondylitis. *N Engl J Med* 1972;288:704–706.
24. Coppin HL, McDevitt HO. Absence of polymorphism between HLA-B27 genomic exon sequences isolated from normal donors and ankylosing spondylitis patients. *J Immunol* 1986;137:2168–2172.
25. MacLean L. HLA-B27 subtypes: implications for the spondyloarthropathies. *Ann Rheum Dis* 1992;51:929–931.
26. Madden DR, Gorga JC, Strominger JL, et al. The structure of HLA-B27 reveals nonamer self-peptides bound in an extended conformation. *Nature* 1991;353:321–325.
27. Madden DR, Gorga JC, Strominger JL, et al. The three-dimensional structure of HLA-B27 at 2.1 A resolution suggests a general mechanism for tight peptide binding to MHC. *Cell* 1992;70:1035–1048.
28. Hammer RE, Malka SD, Richardson JA, et al. Spontaneous inflammatory disease in transgenic rats expressing HLA-B27 and human beta 2m: an animal model of HLA-B27-associated human disorders. *Cell* 1990;63:1099–1112.
29. Taurog JD, Richardson JA, Croft JT, et al. The germfree state prevents development of gut and joint inflammatory disease in HLA-B27 transgenic rats. *J Exp Med* 1994;180:2359–2364.
30. Brown MA, Kennedy LG, MacGregor AJ, et al. Susceptibility to ankylosing spondylitis in twins. *Arthritis Rheum* 1997;40:1823–1828.
31. Arnett FC, Chakraborty R. Ankylosing spondylitis: the dissection of a complex genetic disease. *Arthritis Rheum* 1997;40:1746–1748.
32. Brown MA, Pile KD, Kennedy G, et al. A genome-wide screen for susceptibility loci in ankylosing spondylitis. *Arthritis Rheum* 1998;41: 588–595.
33. Will R, Edmunds L, Elswood J, et al. Is there sexual inequality in ankylosing spondylitis? A study of 498 women and 1202 men. *J Rheumatol* 1990;17:1649–1652.
34. Burgos-Vargas R, Naranjo A, Castillo J, et al. Ankylosing spondylitis in the Mexican mestizo: patterns of disease according to age at onset. *J Rheumatol* 1989;16:186–191.
35. Lawrence RC, Helmick CG, Arnett FC, et al. Estimates of the prevalence of arthritis and selected musculoskeletal disorders in the United States. *Arthritis Rheum* 1998;41:778–799.
36. Braun J, Bollow M, Remlinger G, et al. Prevalence of spondyloarthropathies in HLA-B27 positive and negative blood donors. *Arthritis Rheum* 1998;41:58–67.

37. Baum J, Ziff M. The rarity of ankylosing spondylitis in the black race. *Arthritis Rheum* 1971;14:12–18.
38. Chalmers IM. Ankylosing spondylitis in African blacks. *Arthritis Rheum* 1980;23:1366–1370.
39. Khan MA, Braun WE, Kushner I, et al. HLA B27 in ankylosing spondylitis: differences in frequency and relative risk in American Blacks and Caucasians. *J Rheumatol* 1977;4:39–43.
40. Mbayo K, Mbuyi-Muamba JM, Lurhuma AZ, et al. Low frequency of HLA-B27 and scarcity of ankylosing spondylitis in a Zairean Bantu population. *Clin Rheumatol* 1998;17:309–310.
41. Brown MA, Jepson A, Young A, et al. Ankylosing spondylitis in West Africans: evidence for a non-HLA-B27 protective effect. *Ann Rheum Dis* 1997;56:68–70.
42. Sonozaki H, Seki H, Chang S, et al. Human lymphocyte antigen, HL-A27, in Japanese patients with ankylosing spondylitis. *Tissue Antigens* 1975;5:131–136.
43. Tsujimoto M. Epidemiological research on the prevalence of ankylosing spondylitis. *Med J Osaka Univ* 1978;28:363–381.
44. Gofton JP, Chalmers A, Price GE, et al. HL-A27 and ankylosing spondylitis in B.C. Indians. *J Rheumatol* 1975;2:314–318.
45. Boyer GS, Templin DW, Cornoni-Huntley JC, et al. Prevalence of spondyloarthropathies in Alaskan Eskimos. *J Rheumatol* 1994;21:2292–2297.
46. Alexeeva L, Krylov M, Vturin V, et al. Prevalence of spondyloarthropathies and HLA-B27 in the native population of Chukotka, Russia. *J Rheumatol* 1994;21:2298–2300.
47. Braun J, Bollow M, Remlinger G, et al. Prevalence of spondylarthropathies in HLA-B27 positive and negative blood donors. *Arthritis Rheum* 1998;41:58–67.
48. Gonzalez-Roces S, Alvarez MV, Gonzalez S, et al. HLA-B27 polymorphism and worldwide susceptibility to ankylosing spondylitis. *Tissue Antigens* 1997;49:116–123.
49. Reveille J. HLA-B27 and the seronegative spondyloarthropathies. *Am J Med Sci* 1998;316:239–249.
50. Kanga U, Mehra NK, Larrea CL, et al. Seronegative spondyloarthropathies and HLA-B27 subtypes: a study in Asian Indians. *Clin Rheumatol* 1996;15:13–18.
51. Nasution AR, Mardjuadi A, Kunmartini S, et al. HLA-B27 subtypes positively and negatively associated with spondyloarthropathy. *J Rheumatol* 1997;24:1111–1114.
52. Hemmatpour SK, Dunn PP, Evans PR, et al. Functional characterization and exon 2-intron 2-exon 3 gene sequence of HLA-B*2712 as found in a British family. *Eur J Immunogenet* 1998;25:395–402.
53. Alharbi SA, Mahmoud FF, Al Awadi A, et al. Association of MHC class I with spondyloarthropathies in Kuwait. *Eur J Immunogenet* 1996;23:67–70.
54. Ball EJ, Khan MA. HLA-B27 polymorphism. *Joint Bone Spine* 2001;68:378–382.
55. Khan MA, Ball EJ. Genetic aspects of ankylosing spondylitis. *Best Pract Res Clin Rheumatol* 2002;16:675–690.
56. Hill ASV, Allsopp CEM, Kwiatkowski D, et al. HLA class I typing by PCR: HLA-B27 and an African B27 subtype. *Lancet* 1991;337:640–642.
57. Ren EC, Koh WH, Sim D, et al. Possible protective role of HLA-B*2706 for ankylosing spondylitis. *Tissue Antigens* 1997;49:67–69.
58. Garcia F, Marina A, Lopez de Castro JA. Lack of carboxyl-terminal tyrosine distinguishes the B*2706-bound peptide repertoire from those of B*2704 and other HLA-B27 subtypes associated with ankylosing spondylitis. *Tissue Antigens* 1997;40:215–221.
59. Fiorillo MT, Greco G, Maragno M, et al. The naturally occurring polymorphism Asp116–His116, differentiating the ankylosing spondylitis-associated HLA-B*2705 from the non-associated HLA-B*2709 subtype, influences peptide-specific CD8 T cell recognition. *Eur J Immunol* 1998;28:2508–2516.
60. Hochberg MC, Bias WB, Arnett FC. Family studies in HLA-B27 associated arthritis. *Medicine* 1978;57:463–473.
61. Khan MA, Kushner I, Braun WE. Comparison of clinical features of HLA-B27 positive and negative patients with ankylosing spondylitis. *Arthritis Rheum* 1977;60:909–912.
62. Rubin LA, Amos CI, Wade JA, et al. Investigating the genetic basis for ankylosing spondylitis. *Arthritis Rheum* 1994;37:1212–1220.
63. Amos CI, Wan Y, Siminovitch KA, et al. Estimating the strength of genetic effects: a comparison of maximum likelihood and transmission disequilibrium methods in the study of ankylosing spondylitis. *Hum Immunol* 1997;57:44–50.
64. Laval SH, Timms A, Edwards S, et al. Whole-genome screening in ankylosing spondylitis: evidence of non-MHC genetic-susceptibility loci. *Am J Hum Genet* 2001;68:918–926.
65. Martinez-Borra J, Gonzalez S, Lopez-Vazquez A, et al. HLA-B27 alone rather than B27-related class I haplotypes contributes to ankylosing spondylitis susceptibility. *Hum Immunol* 2000;61:131–139.
66. Maksymowych WP, Wessler A, Schmitt-Egenolf M, et al. Polymorphism in an HLA linked proteasome gene influences phenotypic expression of disease in HLA-B27 positive individuals. *J Rheumatol* 1994;21:665–669.
67. Reveille JD, Ball EJ, Khan MA. HLA-B27 and genetic predisposing factors in spondyloarthropathies. *Curr Opin Rheumatol* 2001;13:265–272.
68. Brown MA, Kennedy LG, Darke C, et al. The effect of HLA-DR genes on susceptibility to and severity of ankylosing spondylitis. *Arthritis Rheum* 1998;41:460–465.
69. Hohler T, Schaper T, Schneider PM, et al. Association of different tumor necrosis factor promoter allele frequencies with ankylosing spondylitis in HLA-B27 positive individuals. *Arthritis Rheum* 1998;41:1489–1492.
70. Kaiijzel EL, Brinkman BM, van Krugten MV, et al. Polymorphism within the tumor necrosis factor alpha (TNF) promoter region in patients with ankylosing spondylitis. *Hum Immunol* 1999;60:140–144.
71. Brown MA, Wordsworth BP, Reveille JD. Genetics of ankylosing spondylitis. *Clin Exp Rheumatol* 2002;20(6)(suppl 28):43–49.
72. Berthelot JM, Glemarec J, Guillot P, et al. New pathogenic hypotheses for spondyloarthropathies. *Joint Bone Spine* 2002;69:114–122.
73. Hohler T, Hug R, Schneider PM, et al. Ankylosing spondylitis in monozygotic twins: studies on immunological parameters. *Ann Rheum Dis* 1999;58:435–440.
74. Ebringer A. Ankylosing spondylitis is caused by *Klebsiella*. *Rheum Dis Clin North Am* 1992;18:105–121.
75. Mielants H, Veys EM, Goemaere S, et al. Gut inflammation in the spondyloarthropathies: clinical, radiologic, biologic and genetic features in relation to the type of histology: a prospective study. *J Rheumatol* 1991;18:1542–1551.
76. Dominguez-Lopez ML, Burgos Vargas R, Galicia-Serrano H, et al. IgG antibodies to enterobacteria 60 kDa heat shock proteins in the sera of HLA-B27 positive ankylosing spondylitis patients. *Scand J Rheumatol* 2002;31:260–265.
77. Tiwana H, Natt RS, Benitez-Brito R, et al. Correlation between the immune responses to collagens type I, III, IV and V and *Klebsiella pneumoniae* in patients with Crohn's disease and ankylosing spondylitis. *Rheumatology* 2001;40:15–23.
78. Russell AS, Suarez-Almazor ME. Ankylosing spondylitis is not caused by *Klebsiella*. *Rheum Dis Clin North Am* 1992;18:95–104.
79. Lahesmaa R, Skurnik M, Granfors K, et al. Molecular mimicry in the pathogenesis of spondyloarthropathies: a critical appraisal of cross-reactivity between microbial antigens and HLA-B27. *Br J Rheumatol* 1992;31:221–229.
80. Schwimmbeck PL, Yu DTY, Oldstone MBA. Autoantibodies to HLA B27 in the sera of HLA B27 patients with ankylosing spondylitis and Reiter's syndrome: molecular mimicry with *Klebsiella pneumoniae* as potential mechanism of autoimmune disease. *J Exp Med* 1987;166:173–181.
81. Scofield RH, Warren WL, Koelsch G, et al. A hypothesis for the HLA-B27 immune dysregulation in spondyloarthropathy: contributions from enteric organisms, B27 structure, peptides bound by B27, and convergent evolution. *Proc Natl Acad Sci U S A* 1993;90:9330–9334.
82. Granfors K. Do bacterial antigens cause reactive arthritis? *Rheum Dis Clin North Am* 1992;18:37–48.
83. Braun J, Tuszewski M, Ehlers S, et al. Nested polymerase chain reaction strategy simultaneously targeting DNA sequences of multiple bacterial species in inflammatory joint diseases: examination of sacroiliac and knee joint biopsies of patients with spondyloarthropathies and other arthritides. *J Rheumatol* 1998;24:1101–1105.
84. Granfors K, Toivanen A. IgA-anti-*Yersinia* antibodies in *Yersinia* triggered reactive arthritis. *Ann Rheum Dis* 1986;46:561–565.
85. Wollenhaupt HJ, Drech T, Schneider C, et al. Specific serum IgA-antibodies in *Chlamydia*-induced arthritis. *Z Rheumatol* 1989;48:86–88.
86. Hermann E. T cells in reactive arthritis. *APMIS* 1993;101:177–186.

87. Marker-Hermann E, Meyer zum Buschenfelde KH, Wildner G. HLA-B27-derived peptides as autoantigens for T lymphocytes in ankylosing spondylitis. *Arthritis Rheum* 1997;40:2047–2054.
88. Ugrinovic S, Mertz A, Wu P, et al. A single nonamer from the *Yersinia* 60-kD heat shock protein is the target of HLA-B27 restricted CTL response in *Yersinia*-induced reactive arthritis. *J Immunol* 1997;159: 5715–5723.
89. Maki-Ikola O, Penttinen M, Von Essen R, et al. IgM, IgG and IgA class enterobacterial antibodies in serum and synovial fluid in patients with ankylosing spondylitis and rheumatoid arthritis. *Br J Rheumatol* 1997;36:1051–1053.
90. Braun J, Bollow M, Neure L, et al. Use of immunohistologic and *in situ* hybridization techniques in the examination of sacroiliac joint biopsy specimens from patients with ankylosing spondylitis. *Arthritis Rheum* 1995;38:499–505.
91. Braun J, Tuszewski M, Ehlers S, et al. Nested polymerase chain reaction strategy simultaneously targeting DNA sequences of multiple bacterial species in inflammatory joint diseases. II. Examination of sacroiliac and knee joint biopsies of patients with spondyloarthropathies and other arthritides. *J Rheumatol* 1997;24:1101–1105.
92. Bowness P. HLA B27 in health and disease: a double-edged sword? *Rheumatology* 2002;41:857–868.
93. Calin A, Porta J, Fries JF, et al. Clinical history as a screening test for ankylosing spondylitis. *JAMA* 1977;237:2613–2614.
94. Blackburn WD Jr, Alarcón GS, Ball GV. Evaluation of patients with back pain of suspected inflammatory nature. *Am J Med* 1988;85: 766–770.
95. Gran JT. An epidemiologic survey of the signs and symptoms of ankylosing spondylitis. *Clin Rheum Dis* 1985;4:161–169.
96. Hochberg MC, Borenstein DG, Arnett FC. The absence of back pain in classical ankylosing spondylitis. *Johns Hopkins Med J* 1978;143: 181–183.
97. Kahn MS, van der Linden S, Kushner I, et al. Spondylitic disease without radiographic evidence of sacroiliitis in relatives of HLA-B27 positive ankylosing spondylitis patients. *Arthritis Rheum* 1985;28: 40–43.
98. van der Linden SM, Kahn MA, Rentsch HU, et al. Chest pain without radiographic sacroiliitis in relatives of patients with ankylosing spondylitis. *J Rheumatol* 1988;15:836–839.
99. Mau W, Zeidler H, Mau R, et al. Clinical features and prognosis of patients with possible ankylosing spondylitis: results of a 10 year follow-up. *J Rheumatol* 1988;15:1109–1114.
100. Ball J. The enthesopathy of ankylosing spondylitis. *Br J Rheumatol* 1983;22(suppl):25–28.
101. Olivieri I, Barozzi L, Padula A. Enthesopathy: clinical manifestations, imaging and treatment. *Baillieres Clin Rheumatol* 1998;12: 665–681.
102. Edmonds J, Morris RI, Metzger AL, et al. Follow-up study of juvenile chronic polyarthritis with particular reference to histocompatibility antigen W.27. *Ann Rheum Dis* 1974;33:289–292.
103. Jacobs JC. Spondyloarthritis and enthesopathy. *Arch Intern Med* 1983;143:103–107.
104. Rosenberg AM, Petty RE. A syndrome of seronegative enthesopathy and arthropathy in children. *Arthritis Rheum* 1982;25:1041–1047.
105. Burgos-Vargas R, Petty RE. Juvenile ankylosing spondylitis. *Rheum Dis Clin North Am* 1992;18:123–143.
106. Arnett FC, Bias WB, Stevens MB. Juvenile-onset chronic arthritis: clinical and roentgenographic features of a unique HLA-B27 subset. *Am J Med* 1980;69:369–376.
107. Burgos-Vargas R, Pacheco-Tena C, Vazquez-Mellado J. A short-term follow-up of enthesitis and arthritis in the active phase of juvenile onset spondyloarthropathies. *Clin Exp Rheumatol* 2002;20:727–731.
108. Bollow M, Braun J, Biedermann T, et al. Use of contrast-enhanced MR imaging to detect sacroiliitis in children. *Skel Radiol* 1998;27: 606–616.
109. Amor B, Santos RS, Nahal R, et al. Predictive factors for the longterm outcome of spondyloarthropathies. *J Rheumatol* 1994;21: 1883–1887.
110. Resnick D, Niwayama G. Ankylosing spondylitis. In: Resnick D, ed. *Diagnosis of bone and joint disorders*. Philadelphia: WB Saunders, 1981:1040–1102.
111. Dawes PT. Stoke Ankylosing Spondylitis Spine Score. *J Rheumatol* 1999;26:993–996.
112. Hollingsworth PN, Cheah PS, Dawkins RL, et al. Observer variation in grading sacroiliac radiographs in HLA-B27 positive individuals. *J Rheumatol* 1983;10:247–254.
113. van Tubergen A, Heuft-Dorenbosch L, Schulpen G, et al. Radiographic assessment of sacroiliitis by radiologists and rheumatologists: does training improve quality? *Ann Rheum Dis* 2003;62:519–525.
114. Fam AG, Rubenstein JD, Chin-Sang H, et al. Computed tomography in the diagnosis of early ankylosing spondylitis. *Arthritis Rheum* 1985;28:930–937.
115. Yu W, Feng F, Dion E, et al. Comparison of radiography, computed tomography and magnetic resonance imaging in the detection of sacroiliitis accompanying ankylosing spondylitis. *Skel Radiol* 1998; 27:311–320.
116. Khan MA. Thoughts concerning the early diagnosis of ankylosing spondylitis and related diseases. *Clin Exp Rheumatol* 2002;20(6) (suppl 28):6–10.
117. Oostveen JC, van de Laar MA. Magnetic resonance imaging in rheumatic disorders of the spine and sacroiliac joints. *Semin Arthritis Rheum* 2000;30:52–69.
118. Juanola X, Mateo L, Nolla JM, et al. Bone mineral density in women with ankylosing spondylitis. *J Rheumatol* 2000;27:1028–1031.
119. Speden DJ, Calin AI, Ring FJ, et al. Bone mineral density, calcaneal ultrasound, and bone turnover markers in women with ankylosing spondylitis. *J Rheumatol* 2002;29:516–521.
120. Toussirot E, Michel F, Wendling D. Bone density, ultrasound measurements and body composition in early ankylosing spondylitis. *Rheumatology (Oxford)* 2001;40:882–888.
121. Aufdermaur M. Pathogenesis of square bodies in ankylosing spondylitis. *Ann Rheum Dis* 1989;48:628–631.
122. McEwen C, DiTata D, Lingg C, et al. Ankylosing spondylitis and spondylitis accompanying ulcerative colitis, regional enteritis, psoriasis and Reiter's disease: a comparative study. *Arthritis Rheum* 1971; 14:291–318.
123. Helliwell PS, Hickling P, Wright V. Do the radiological changes of classic ankylosing spondylitis differ from the changes found in the spondylitis associated with inflammatory bowel disease, psoriasis, and reactive arthritis? *Ann Rheum Dis* 1998;57:135–140.
124. Sorin S, Askari A, Moskowitz RW. Atlantoaxial subluxation as a complication of early ankylosing spondylitis: two case reports and a review of the literature. *Arthritis Rheum* 1979;22:273–276.
125. Little H, Swinson DR, Cruickshank B. Upward subluxation of the axis in ankylosing spondylitis. *Am J Med* 1976;60:279–285.
126. Lee YS, Schlotzhauer T, Ott YSM, et al. Skeletal status of men with early and late ankylosing spondylitis. *Am J Med* 1997;103:233–241.
127. Bronson WD, Walker SE, Hillman LS, et al. Bone mineral density and biochemical markers of bone metabolism in ankylosing spondylitis. *J Rheumatol* 1998;25:929–935.
128. Murray GC, Persellin RH. Cervical fracture complicating ankylosing spondylitis: a report of eight cases and review of the literature. *Am J Med* 1981;70:1033–1041.
129. Cooper C, Carbone L, Michet CJ, et al. Fracture risk in patients with ankylosing spondylitis: a population based study. *J Rheumatol* 1994; 21:877–882.
130. Dunn N, Preston B, Jones KL. Unexplained back pain in longstanding ankylosing spondylitis. *BMJ* 1985;291:1632–1634.
131. Resnick D, Williamson S, Alazraki N. Focal spinal abnormalities on bone scans in ankylosing spondylitis: a clue to the presence of fracture or pseudarthrosis. *Clin Nucl Med* 1995;6:213–217.
132. Dihlmann W, Delling G. Disco-vertebral destructive lesions (so-called Andersson lesions) associated with ankylosing spondylitis. *Skel Radiol* 1983;3:10–16.
133. Kabaskal Y, Garrett SL, Calin A. The epidemiology of spondylodiscitis in ankylosing spondylitis, a controlled study. *Br J Rheumatol* 1996;35:660–663.
134. Eastmond CJ, Robertson EM. A prospective study of early diagnostic investigations in the diagnosis of ankylosing spondylitis. *Scott Med J* 2003;4:21–23.
135. Calin A. HLA-B27: to type or not to type? *Ann Intern Med* 1980; 92:208–211.
136. Khan MA, Khan MK. Diagnostic value of HLA-B27 testing in ankylosing spondylitis and Reiter's syndrome. *Ann Intern Med* 1982;96: 70–76.

137. Cauli A, Dessole G, Fiorillo MT, et al. Increased level of HLA-B27 expression in ankylosing spondylitis patients compared with healthy HLA-B27-positive subjects: a possible further susceptibility factor for the development of disease. *Rheumatology* 2002;41:1375–1379.
138. Yagon R, Khan MA. Confusion of roentgenographic differential diagnosis of ankylosing hyperostosis (Forestier's disease) and ankylosing spondylitis. *Spine* 1990;4:561–575.
139. Kaplan G, Haettich B. Rheumatological symptoms due to retinoids. *Baillieres Clin Rheumatol* 1991;5:77–97.
140. Rosenbaum JT. Acute anterior uveitis and spondyloarthropathies. *Rheum Dis Clin North Am* 1992;18:143–151.
141. Stewart SR, Robbins DL, Castles JJ. Acute fulminant aortic and mitral insufficiency in ankylosing spondylitis. *N Engl J Med* 1978;299: 1448–1449.
142. Roberts WC, Hollingsworth JF, Bulkley BH, et al. Combined mitral and aortic regurgitation in ankylosing spondylitis. *Am J Med* 1974; 56:237–242.
143. Lautermann D, Braun J. Ankylosing spondylitis—cardiac manifestations. *Clin Exp Rheumatol* 2002;20(6)(suppl 28):11–115.
144. Bergfeldt L. HLA-B27 associated cardiac disease. *Ann Intern Med* 1997;127:621–629.
145. Bergfeldt L, Edhag O, Vedin L, Vallin H. Ankylosing spondylitis: an important cause of severe disturbances of the cardiac conduction system. *Am J Med* 1982;73:187–191.
146. Bergfeldt L, Insulander P, Lindblom D, et al. HLA-B27: an important genetic risk factor for lone aortic regurgitation and severe conduction system abnormalities. *Am J Med* 1988;85:12–18.
147. Bergfeldt L, Moller E. Complete heart block: another HLA-B27 associated disease manifestation. *Tissue Antigens* 1983;21:385–390.
148. Bulkley BH, Roberts WC. Ankylosing spondylitis and aortic regurgitation. *Circulation* 1973;48:1014–1027.
149. LaBresh KA, Lally EV, Sharma SC, Ho G. Two-dimensional echocardiographic detection of preclinical aortic root abnormalities in rheumatoid variant diseases. *Am J Med* 1985;78:908–912.
150. Arnason JA, Patel AK, Rahko PS, Sundstrom WR. Transthoracic and transesophageal echocardiographic evaluation of the aortic root and subvalvular structures in ankylosing spondylitis. *J Rheumatol* 1996;23:120–123.
151. Roldan CA, Chavez J, Wiest PW, et al. Aortic root disease and valve disease associated with ankylosing spondylitis. *J Am Coll Cardiol* 1998;32:1397–1404.
152. Yildirir A, Aksoyek S, Calguneri M, et al. Echocardiographic evidence of cardiac involvement in ankylosing spondylitis. *Clin Rheumatol* 2002;21:129–134.
153. Boushea DK, Sundstrom WR. The pleuropulmonary manifestations of ankylosing spondylitis. *Semin Arthritis Rheum* 1989;18: 277–281.
154. Campbell AH, MacDonald CB. Upper lobe fibrosis associated with ankylosing spondylitis. *Br J Chest Dis* 1965;59:90–100.
155. Fisher LR, Cawley MID, Holgate ST. Relation between chest expansion, pulmonary function and exercise tolerance in patients with ankylosing spondylitis. *Ann Rheum Dis* 1990;9:921–925.
156. Strobel ES, Fritschka E. Renal diseases in ankylosing spondylitis: review of the literature illustrated by case reports. *Clin Rheumatol* 1998;17:524–530.
157. Gratacos J, Orellana C, Sanmarti R, et al. Secondary amyloidosis in ankylosing spondylitis: a systematic survey of 137 patients using abdominal fat aspiration. *J Rheumatol* 1997;24:912–925.
158. Lai KN, Li PKT, Hawkins B, et al. IgA nephropathy associated with ankylosing spondylitis: occurrence in women as well as in men. *Ann Rheum Dis* 1989;48:435–437.
159. Russell ML, Gordon DA, Ogryzlo MA, et al. The cauda equina syndrome of ankylosing spondylitis. *Ann Intern Med* 1973;78:551–554.
160. Sparling MJ, Bartleson JD, McLeod PA, et al. Magnetic resonance imaging of the arachnoid diverticulae associated with cauda equina syndrome in ankylosing spondylitis. *J Rheumatol* 1989;16:1335–1337.
161. Charlesworth CH, Savy LE, Stevens J, et al. MRI demonstration of arachnoiditis in cauda equina syndrome of ankylosing spondylitis. *Neuroradiology* 1996;38:462–465.
162. Hanrahan PS, Russell AS, McLean DR. Ankylosing spondylitis and multiple sclerosis: an apparent association. *J Rheumatol* 1988;15: 1512–1514.
163. Mielants H, Veys EM, Cuvelier C, et al. The evolution of spondyloarthropathies in relation to gut histology. III. Relation between gut and joint. *J Rheumatol* 1995;22:2279–2284.
164. Calin A. Raised serum creatine phosphokinase activity in ankylosing spondylitis. *Ann Rheum Dis* 1975;34:244–248.
165. Calabro JJ. Sustained-release indomethacin in the management of ankylosing spondylitis. *Am J Med* 1985;79:39–51.
166. Dougados M, Behier JM, Jolchine I, et al. Efficacy of celecoxib, a cyclooxygenase 2-specific inhibitor, in the treatment of ankylosing spondylitis: a six-week controlled study with comparison against placebo and against a conventional nonsteroidal antiinflammatory drug. *Arthritis Rheum* 2001;44:180–185.
167. Ferez MB, Tugwell P, Goldsmith CH, et al. Meta-analysis of sulfasalazine in ankylosing spondylitis. *J Rheumatol* 1990;17:1482–1486.
168. Dougados M, van der Linden S, Leirisalo-Repo M, et al. Sulfasalazine in spondyloarthropathy: a randomized, multicentre, double-blind, placebo-controlled study. *Arthritis Rheum* 1995;38: 618–627.
169. Clegg DO, Reda DJ, Weisman MH, et al. Comparison of sulfasalazine and placebo in the treatment of ankylosing spondylitis. *Arthritis Rheum* 1996;39:2004–2112.
170. Taggart A, Gardiner P, McEvoy F, et al. Which is the active moiety of sulfasalazine in ankylosing spondylitis? *Arthritis Rheum* 1996;39: 1400–1405.
171. Mintz G, Enriquez RD, Mercado U, et al. Intravenous methylprednisolone pulse therapy in severe ankylosing spondylitis. *Arthritis Rheum* 1981;24:734–736.
172. Braun J, Brandt J, Listing J, et al. Treatment of active ankylosing spondylitis with infliximab: a randomised controlled multicentre trial. *Lancet* 2002;359:1187–1193.
173. Gorman JD, Sack KE, Davis JC Jr. Treatment of ankylosing spondylitis by inhibition of tumor necrosis factor alpha. *N Engl J Med* 2002;346:1349–1356.
174. Davis JC, van der Heijde D, Braun J, et al. Recombinant human tumor necrosis factor (etanercept) for treating ankylosing spondylitis: a randomized controlled trial. *Arthritis Rheum* 2003;114: 31–37.
175. Brandt J, Khariouzov A, Listing J, et al. Six-month results of a double-blind, placebo-controlled trial of etanercept treatment in patients with active ankylosing spondylitis. *Arthritis Rheum* 2003;48: 1667–1675.
176. Kraag G, Stokes B, Groh J, et al. The effects of comprehensive home physiotherapy and supervision of patients with ankylosing spondylitis: a randomized controlled trial. *J Rheumatol* 1990;17: 229–233.
177. Santos H, Brophy S, Calin A. Exercise in ankylosing spondylitis: how much is optimum? *J Rheumatol* 1998;25:2156–2160.
178. Dagfinrud H, Hagen K. Physiotherapy interventions for ankylosing spondylitis. *Cochrane Database Syst Rev* 2001;4:CD002822.
179. Wordsworth BP, Mowat AG. A review of 100 patients with ankylosing spondylitis with particular reference to socioeconomic effects. *Br J Rheumatol* 1986;25:175–180.
180. Calin A, Elswood J. The outcome of 130 total hip replacements and 2 revisions in ankylosing spondylitis: high success rate after a mean followup of 7.5 years. *J Rheumatol* 1989;16:955–958.
181. Sundaram NA, Murphy JCM. Heterotopic bone formation following total hip arthroplasty in ankylosing spondylitis. *Clin Orthop* 1986; 207:223–226.
182. Camargo FP, Cordeiro EN, Napoli MMM. Corrective osteotomy of the spine in ankylosing spondylitis: experience with 66 cases. *Clin Orthop* 1986;208:157–167.
183. Sinclair JR, Mason RA. Ankylosing spondylitis. The case for awake intubation. *Anesthesia* 1984;39:3–11.
184. van der Heijde D, Calin A, Dougados M, et al. Selection of instruments in the core set for DC-ART, SMARD, physical therapy, and clinical record keeping in ankylosing spondylitis. Progress report of the ASAS Working Group. Assessments in Ankylosing Spondylitis. *J Rheumatol* 1999;26:951–954.
185. Anderson JJ, Baron G, van der Heijde D, et al. Ankylosing spondylitis assessment group preliminary definition of short-term improvement in ankylosing spondylitis. *Arthritis Rheum* 2001;44:1876–1886.
186. Braun J, Pham T, Sieper J, et al. International ASAS consensus statement for the clinical use of biologic agents in patients with ankylosing spondylitis (AS) in daily practice [Abstract OP0104]. Presented at EULAR, Lisbon, Portugal, 2003.

187. Gran JT, Skomsvoll JF. The outcome of ankylosing spondylitis: a study of 100 patients. *Br J Rheumatol* 1997;36:766–771.
188. Kaprove RE, Little AH, Graham DC, et al. Ankylosing spondylitis: survival in men with and without radiotherapy. *Arthritis Rheum* 1980;23:57–61.
189. Carette S, Graham D, Little H, et al. The natural disease course of ankylosing spondylitis. *Arthritis Rheum* 1983;266:186–190.
190. Smith PG, Doll R. Mortality among patients with ankylosing spondylitis after a single treatment course with x-rays. *BMJ* 1982;284:449–460.
191. Lehtinen K. Cause of death in 79 patients with ankylosing spondylitis. *J Rheumatol* 1980;9:145–147.
192. Boonen A, Severens JL. Ankylosing spondylitis: what is the cost to society, and can it be reduced? *Best Pract Res Clin Rheumatol* 2002;16:691–705.

CHAPTER 64

Reactive Arthritis

Muhammad Asim Khan and Joachim Sieper

Reactive arthritis is an acute or subacute, aseptic, nonsuppurative, inflammatory arthritis occurring in an immunologically sensitized and genetically predisposed individual secondary to a primary infectious process elsewhere in the body. Nonproliferating microbial products or antigens may be present in the joint, but there is absence of the traditional evidence of sepsis (1–11). Except for human leukocyte antigen B27 (HLA-B27), the genes responsible for both the susceptibility to and the severity of the disease have not been definitely identified (1,2,12).

The arthritis is typically asymmetric and oligoarticular, more often affecting the joints of the lower extremities, and occurs within a month of an episode of a primary infectious trigger. It is frequently associated with characteristic extraarticular features, such as urethritis, ocular inflammation (conjunctivitis or acute iritis), enthesitis (Achilles tendonitis and plantar fasciitis), dactylitis ("sausage digits"), or mucocutaneous lesions (6–11).

Several forms of arthritis can be described as "reactive" (or postinfectious), such as acute rheumatic fever, but the term "reactive arthritis" is restricted to acute arthritis that usually, but not exclusively, appears shortly after certain infections of the genitourinary or gastrointestinal tracts, and is associated with HLA-B27 (5–11). Aho et al. introduced the term "reactive arthritis" in 1976, and it has been used interchangeably with Reiter's syndrome, but the use of the latter term is generally discouraged these days (9–13). These two terms, however, are pathogenically related due to their documented or presumed postinfectious onset, and they occur more commonly in individuals inheriting HLA-B27. The term "Reiter's syndrome" has been used to refer to the classical triad of arthritis, ocular inflammation (conjunctivitis or anterior uveitis), and urethritis/cervicitis; while "incomplete Reiter syndrome" refers to the presence of only two of these features (10).

The preferred term, "reactive arthritis," is more inclusive, and encompasses both complete and incomplete Reiter's syndrome; most patients with reactive arthritis do not present with the classical triad. However, reactive arthritis may itself turn out to be a transitory term as the etiopathogenesis of this disease becomes better understood in the near future. Reactive arthritis belongs to a cluster of interrelated and overlapping chronic inflammatory rheumatic diseases, termed the "spondyloarthropathies" or "spondyloarthritides," which also includes ankylosing spondylitis, arthritis associated with psoriasis and inflammatory bowel diseases, and undifferentiated forms of these diseases (14–19). The articular inflammation often includes the entheses, which are the site of bony insertion of ligaments and tendons; the sacroiliac joints and the axial skeleton; and sometimes nonarticular structures, such as the skin, buccal or gut mucosa, eye, and aortic valve, which may also exhibit inflammatory lesions (6–10,20–22). Spondyloarthropathies, unlike rheumatoid arthritis, are strongly associated with HLA-B27, lack any association with rheumatoid factor, and therefore have often been labeled as "seronegative" (12,14,16,17) (see Chapter 61). However, the HLA-B27-association varies markedly among the different forms of spondyloarthropathies and also among racial/ethnic groups in the world (14,16,17). These diseases are more common than previously realized, and the most widely used classification criteria (European Spondyloarthropathy Study Group and Amor criteria for spondyloarthropathies) encompass the currently recognized wider disease spectrum (14–19,23) (see Chapter 61).

Numerous reactive arthritides initiated by a variety of arthritogenic organisms have been described (1–10). The initiating trigger is usually a genitourinary infection with *Chlamydia trachomatis* or an enteritis due to certain gram-negative enterobacteria, such as *Shigella, Salmonella, Yersinia*, or *Campylobacter* (Table 64.1). Genitourinary tract infection with *C. trachomatis* is the more commonly recognized initiator of reactive arthritis in developed countries and, therefore, this form of reactive arthritis ("uroarthritis")

TABLE 64.1. *Infectious organisms associated with the onset of reactive arthritis*

Enteric pathogens
Shigella flexneri, serotype 2a, 1b
Yersinia enterocolitica (serotypes 0:3, 0:8, 0:9)
Y. pseudotuberculosis
Salmonella typhimurium
S. enteritidis
S. paratyphi
S. heidelberg
S. abony
S. blocley
S. schwarzengrund
S. haifa
S. manila
S. newport
S. bovismorbificans
Campylobacter jejuni
C. fetus
Clostridium difficile
Vibrio parahaemolyticus
Urogenital pathogens
Chlamydia trachomatis
C. psittaci
? *Ureaplasma urealyticum*
Others
BCG intravesical injection for inoperable bladder cancer
C. pneumoniae

BCG, bacillus Calmette-Guérin

generally occurs in a young population that is sexually active. Gastrointestinal infections with enterobacteria, on the other hand, are the more common triggers of reactive arthritis ("enteroarthritis") in the developing parts of the world, affecting both young and old. Urethritis and cervicitis can accompany arthritis after acute bacterial diarrhea; and, conversely, the genital lesions (such as circinate balanitis) can occur in postenteritic reactive arthritis.

HISTORICAL OVERVIEW

Hans Reiter, in 1916, published a paper describing a Prussian officer with urethritis, conjunctivitis, and arthritis after an episode of bloody diarrhea (24). He named the illness "spirochaetosis arthritica" based on the microscopic identification of a spirochete. In the same year, Fiessinger and Leroy described a similar patient with a postdysenteric "oculo-urethro-synovial syndrome" (7–9). However, there are earlier descriptions of a similar syndrome. For example, in 1775 Senter described the plight of three young soldiers in the American Revolutionary War who developed an acute, severe inflammatory polyarthritis within 21 days of an acute diarrheal illness (7). In 1776 Stoll provided the first description of postdysenteric illness manifesting the classical triad of arthritis, conjunctivitis, and urethritis (7). Christopher Columbus may have had reactive arthritis when he developed postdysenteric fever, with recurrent ocular inflammation and arthritis, in 1494. It was severe enough to result in disability and intermittent visual impairment, and he died at age 55 with "crippling arthritis." (25). Paronen, in 1948, and Noer, in 1963, conclusively linked epidemic *Shigella* dysentery with the onset of reactive arthritis (26,27).

The postvenereal association was noted as early as the sixteenth century, when van Forest, and later Matiniere in the seventeenth century, recognized arthritis as a complication of urethritis (9). The sixteenth century Renaissance artist, Benvenuto Cellini, may have had reactive arthritis, as he described in his autobiography his symptoms of postvenereal ocular inflammation and generalized rash, followed later by a chronic arthropathy and low back pain (28). The postvenereal association of the triad of arthritis, conjunctivitis, and urethritis was reported in five patients by Benjamin Brodie in 1818 (7–9).

EPIDEMIOLOGY

Epidemiologic estimates of the prevalence and incidence of reactive arthritis are limited because of (a) the lack of consensus regarding classification or diagnostic criteria, (b) the nomadic nature of a young target population, (c) the underreporting of venereal disease, and (d) the gross underrecognition of milder cases (1–9,16,17,23,29,30). Several proposals for classification criteria for reactive arthritis have been made since the American Rheumatism Association definition of reactive arthritis as an episode of peripheral arthritis of more than 1 month's duration occurring in association with urethritis or cervicitis (11,31–33). There are no generally accepted diagnostic criteria; a working definition was proposed at the Third International Workshop on Reactive Arthritis in 1996 (34) (Tables 64.2A and B).

The relative incidence of postenteritic and postvenereal or idiopathic reactive arthritis is highly variable and depends on the geographic locale, age group, and environ-

TABLE 64.2A. *A proposed working definition (diagnostic criteria) for reactive arthritis as suggested by the Third International Workshop on Reactive Arthritis*

Typical peripheral arthritis
Predominantly of lower limbs, asymmetric oligoarthritis

Plus

Evidence of preceding infection
(a) Where clear clinical diarrhea or urethritis within weeks: Laboratory confirmation is desirable but not essential
(b) Where no clear clinical infection: Laboratory confirmation of infection is essential

Exclusion criteria
Patients with other known causes of mono-/oligoarthritis

(From Kingsley G, Sieper J. Third International Workshop on Reactive Arthritis. *Ann Rheum Dis* 1996;55:564–584.)

TABLE 64.2B. *Laboratory tests used for the diagnosis of preceding infection in the diagnostic work-up in patients with assumed reactive arthritis, as suggested by the Third International Workshop on Reactive Arthritis*

Stool culture
Helpful if positive; stool culture in absence of diarrhea rarely positive
Urethral culture or urethral/urine PCR
These tests should be used and are helpful, with and without symptomatic preceding urethritis/cervicitis
Serology
IgG plus IgA or plus IgM specific for single bacteria can be used in the diagnostic work-up
PCR for chlamydial DNA in the joint
A good test where available

(From Kingsley G, Sieper J. Third International Workshop on Reactive Arthritis. *Ann Rheum Dis* 1996;55:564–565.)

mental and socioeconomic conditions. Genitourinary tract infection with *C. trachomatis* is the more commonly recognized initiator of reactive arthritis in developed countries, while infections with enterobacteria are the more common triggers in the developing parts of the world. The spectrum of triggering infections, however, seems to be changing because *Yersinia*-associated arthritis is becoming relatively less common in Europe, whereas arthritis in association with *Campylobacter* or *Salmonella* infections seems to be increasing (3,4,17,35–38).

Reactive arthritis occurs at a frequency of 1% to 4% after nongonococcal urethritis secondary to *C. trachomatis*. It is 5 to 6 times more common in males than females, and most commonly affects young individuals who are sexually promiscuous, with peak onset during the third decade of life (1–9,39). The disease in women may be underdiagnosed because they may not have genitourinary symptoms, and their disease expression is usually less severe. Although a patient with postvenereal reactive arthritis may have concomitant gonococcal urethritis, this infection does not seem to trigger reactive arthritis, and the same may be true of urogenital infection with *Ureaplasma urealyticum* (see Chapter 124).

A recent study in Scotland showed that on routine medical examination 9.8% of healthy asymptomatic young male military recruits (mostly between the ages of 16–22) were infected with *Chlamydia*, and 88% of these individuals were asymptomatic, a figure much higher than the usually cited 50% (40). The remaining 12% had minor symptoms so that they had not felt the need to report to staff during medical examination. Epidemiologic data from military populations have suggested that reactive arthritis may be the most common cause of inflammatory arthritis among soldiers. However, in the post-AIDS era a significant decrease in reactive arthritis has been reported in a study of the Greek Army, and over the same time periods a significant decrease in parallel in the number of nongonococcal and gonococcal urogenital infections was also observed (41). The prevalence of dysentery had remained unchanged, and the observed decline of reactive arthritis was attributed to the promotion of condom use through a campaign against HIV-AIDS that was initiated in 1984. The occurrence of *Chlamydia*-induced reactive arthritis in a high risk group can also be curtailed by early eradication of *Chlamydia* infection by effective treatment (42).

The frequency of reactive arthritis after enteritis varies between 0 and 15%, can occur at all ages, and equally affects both men and women (1–9). This marked variation is likely to be due to genetic and socioeconomic differences in various populations, and the triggering microbe's marked variation (even within same genus and species) in its ability to infect and survive inside the host (which might influence its arthritogenicity) (1–9). The frequency of reactive arthritis in unselected populations after enteric infections with *Salmonella, Shigella,* and *Yersinia* has been reported to be between 1% and 4%. However, studies of epidemic dysentery secondary to arthritogenic bacterial strains suggest that reactive arthritis develops in 2% to 6% of infected individuals, and up to 20% of those who possess HLA-B27 (8,9,24). The postenteritic form of reactive arthritis may occur sporadically or as a sequel to epidemic outbreaks of bacterial enteritis. In 1963, a naval vessel carrying 1,276 men was the site of epidemic *Shigella* dysentery that affected 602 sailors, and nine of them subsequently developed reactive arthritis (29).

The age adjusted incidence rate for reactive arthritis between 1950 and 1980 among male subjects younger than 50 years in Rochester (Olmstead County), Minnesota, was reported to be 3.5 cases per 100,000 men (43). Similarly, a 2-year survey of reactive arthritis in Oslo, Norway, reported a minimal incidence rate of 4.6 and 5.0 cases per 100,000 for reactive arthritis caused by *Chlamydia* and enterobacteria (*Salmonella, Yersinia, Campylobacter*), respectively (44). However, in Finland the annual incidence of arthritis after urogenital or bowel infection is 30 per 100,000 adults (8,9).

Reactive arthritis can occur following intravesical injection of bacillus Calmette-Guérin (BCG) into bladder cancer (that is surgically nonresectable), but not with BCG vaccination that is used in some countries to decrease the risk of tuberculosis (45,46). These reactive arthritis patients have inflammatory peripheral arthritis, back pain, and dactylitis, and 50% to 70% possess HLA-B27. The enteric pathogen *Clostridium difficile* can also trigger reactive arthritis after pseudomembranous colitis, and nearly 50% of these patients possess HLA-B27 (47). Respiratory tract infections caused by *Chlamydia pneumoniae* have also been reported to trigger reactive arthritis, but only in a few patients (48,49).

CLINICAL FEATURES

A detailed clinical history taking and physical examination may be needed to reveal the antecedent infectious event and to detect the presence of associated extraarticular clinical features that may suggest the diagnosis of reactive arthritis (1–9,50). The temporal sequence, along with the presence of serological evidence of preceding microbial infection, or microbial products (but not replicating microbes) in the involved joints, indicate that the patient's arthritis is triggered by an infectious process (50). An identifiable infectious trigger may not be apparent in up to one-fourth of all cases, and the precise triggering organism may remain unknown, partly because the triggering infectious process subsides before the onset of arthritis, or because the patient may seek medical help late in the disease course.

Onset

The earliest manifestation of reactive arthritis is usually the occurrence of one or more of the extraarticular features, and arthritis is usually the most prominent, although often the last to appear. But it usually occurs within 4 weeks of the triggering event, often when the symptoms of genitourinary and ocular inflammation are subsiding or have resolved (6–9). Involvement of the *genitourinary system* may result in dysuria with or without urethral discharge, prostatitis in men, and cervicitis/vaginitis in women. The precipitating episode of diarrhea is often mild, but it can be severe or prolonged. Patients with *Shigella*-induced enteritis can have bloody diarrhea, and those with *Yersinia*-induced enteritis often have mild recurrent abdominal symptoms. The abdominal pain may be confused with acute appendicitis or salpingitis. Symptoms due to ocular inflammation consist of conjunctivitis and, much less commonly, acute anterior uveitis. Constitutional symptoms are common at the outset of the disease but are usually mild. Fever, if present, is low grade, but some patients can have prominent fever that may suggest an underlying septic process. Additional systemic manifestations of inflammation, including morning stiffness, malaise, fatigue. anorexia, weight loss, myalgia, and arthralgia may be present.

Arthritis

The arthritis is typically acute, asymmetric and additive inflammatory oligoarthritis. At the onset, the involvement of the joints of the lower extremity (knees, ankles, and toes) is most common (1–10), and is often responsive to anti-inflammatory drugs (Figs. 64.1 and 64.2). The acute onset, especially when monoarticular, can sometimes be confused with septic or gouty arthritis because of the intensity and pattern of articular presentation. The arthritis may progress in an additive and often asymmetric fashion to involve the joints of the upper extremities and the axial spine, but occurrence of arthritis limited to the upper extremity is extremely uncommon. It can affect shoulders, elbows, and wrists. Inflammation of the digits *(dactylitis)* typically leads to diffuse swelling, the so-called "sausage digit" that results from inflammatory changes affecting the joint capsule, tendon sheath, entheses, periarticular structures, or periosteal bone (51). Rarely, there is widespread polyarthritis that may resemble rheumatoid arthritis, and some patients may become bedridden. In such patients, however, the diagnosis of reactive arthritis is suggested by the evolution, the asymmetric pattern of joint involvement, the associated enthesitis and extraarticular features, the clinical course, and the absence of serum rheumatoid factor.

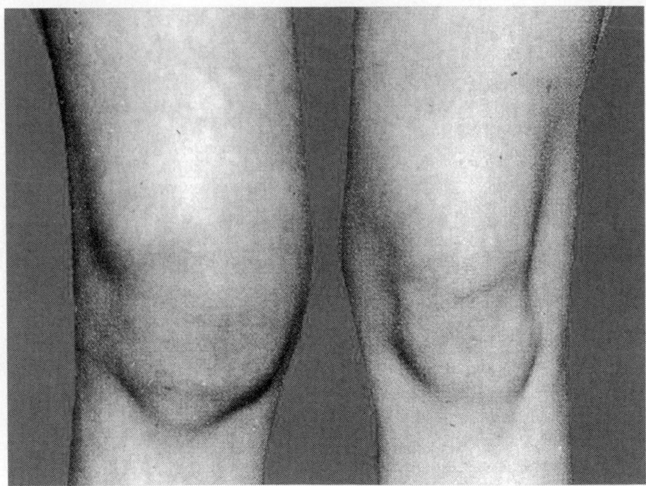

FIG. 64.1. Unilateral painful knee effusion is a common clinical presentation in patients with acute reactive arthritis.

The arthritis of the extremities on average involves 5 joints, and resolves in 3 to 6 months, although some patients may continue to have mild musculoskeletal symptoms for more than 1 year (1–10). Although frequently self-limiting,

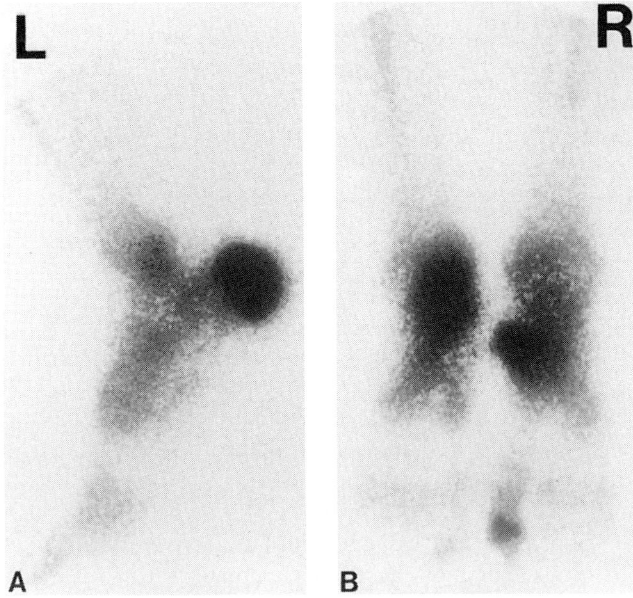

FIG. 64.2. A 30-year-old man with reactive arthritis with painful ankles and heels. Isotopic uptake on technetium-99m–phosphate scintigraphy indicates enthesitis of the left calcaneus **(A)** and right navicular, with synovitis of the right first interphalangeal joint **(B)**.

reactive arthritis can have the potential for chronicity or recurrences, and can result in damage to the involved peripheral or axial joints (Fig. 64.3). There may be symptomatic evidence of axial involvement (sacroiliitis or spondylitis) in close to 50% of patients, presenting as inflammatory low back pain and stiffness, alternating buttock pain, and sometimes associated sacroiliac or spinal tenderness. Recurrent episodes of arthritis may appear in up to 15% of cases, and are more common in patients with *Chlamydia*-induced reactive arthritis, but it is unclear whether this results from persistence of infection or reinfection with *Chlamydia*. Approximately 15% to 30% of patients develop chronic or recurrent arthritis, sacroiliitis, or progress to ankylosing spondylitis in later years. These patients are mostly those who have a positive family history for spondyloarthropathy, or are positive for HLA-B27. Some of these patients have disabling and destructive arthritis or recalcitrant enthesitis.

Enthesitis

Enthesitis is one of the most distinctive musculoskeletal manifestations of the spondyloarthropathies, and refers to inflammation at the sites of tendinous or ligamentous insertions onto bone (18–20). It is observed in up to 70% of patients with reactive arthritis, and most often manifests as tenderness and sometimes pain, with or without swelling at the entheses. The most characteristic and clinically helpful site of involvement is at the insertion of the posterior and inferior surfaces of the calcaneum (Achilles tendon and plantar fascia insertions, respectively), which can result in painful heels and difficulty on walking (Fig. 64.2). Other common sites include spinal processes, ischium, iliac crest, greater femoral trochanter, tibial tubercle, and the digits (dactylitis). There can also be associated tendinitis or tenosynovitis.

Mucocutaneous Involvement

Inflammation of the mucosal surface of the genitourinary tract can result in urethritis/cystitis and cervicitis/vaginitis. The symptoms can be mild or transient, acute or subacute, and some patients have a sterile, mucoid, or mucopurulent discharge (52). The genitourinary symptoms are often seen early in the disease, regardless of whether the syndrome is associated with a postdysenteric or postvenereal trigger, but show a tendency to relapse. Genital lesions can occur in some patients; they often start as vesicles that may evolve into shallow ulcerations or plaques. They occur on the urethral meatus, the glans or the shaft of the penis, may precede the onset of joint symptoms, usually show a characteristic serpiginous border, and are called *circinate balanitis* (9). They are nearly always painless, unless secondarily infected, and heal without leaving a scar. In uncircumcised patients, the foreskin has to be retracted to detect the lesions on the glans and, in circumcised patients, the lesions tend to become dry and form crusts or plaques. Prostatitis and cystitis can occur in some patients. Cervicitis in women

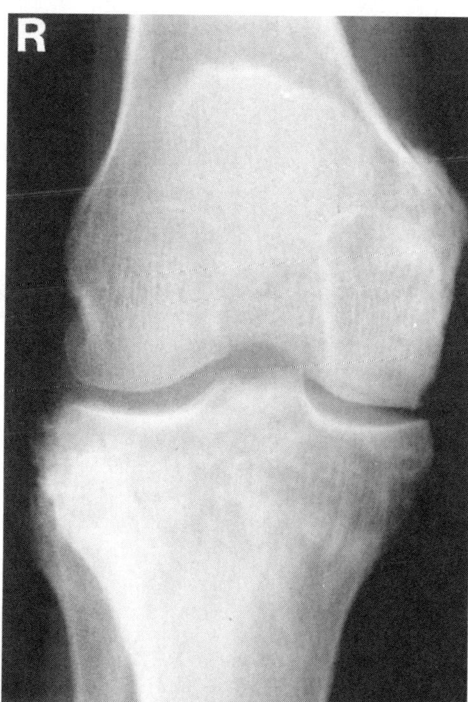

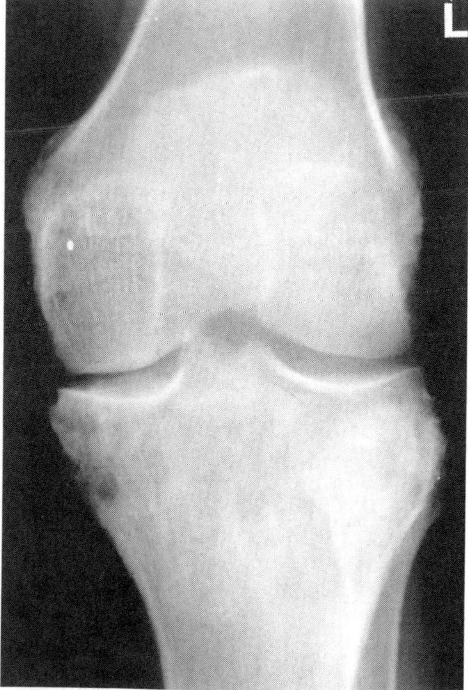

FIG. 64.3. Radiographs depict marginal erosions with adjacent reactive bone, condylar periostitis, and normal juxtaarticular mineralization in a 27-year-old man with reactive arthritis.

is often asymptomatic, requiring pelvic examination for its detection. Salpingitis can also occur. The occurrence of circinate lesions over the external genitalia (*circinate vulvitis*) is very rare (53).

Keratoderma blennorrhagicum is a painless, papulosquamous hyperkeratotic cutaneous eruption frequently found on the soles of the feet (Fig. 64.4). It can also occur on the toes, fingers, and palms, and rarely on the scrotum, penis, trunk, and scalp. It is often referred to *pustulosis palmoplantaris* when present on the palms of the hands and the soles of the feet. The lesion starts as a painless vesicle with clear liquid and with an erythematous base that progresses to become maculopapular and later hyperkeratotic. These skin lesions are frequently indistinguishable either clinically or histopathologically from pustular psoriasis (see Chapter 65). Patients have been reported with overlapping features of reactive arthritis and psoriatic arthritis, suggesting a shared etiopathogenic mechanism in some patients. Nail changes can also occur, more often in those who develop chronic arthritis, and include yellowish or grayish discoloration, thickening, ridging, or subungual hyperkeratosis (onycholysis), but nail pitting is rarely seen (54). Other less common mucocutaneous features include painless shallow buccal mucosal ulcerations or shiny patches that can be an early and transient manifestation. It should be emphasized that the psoriasiform lesions over the external genitalia (circinate balanitis and circinate vulvitis) do not directly relate to the presence of genitourinary infection and, conversely, sterile urethritis can accompany arthritis after acute bacterial diarrhea (9,52,53,55). Lesions can resolve spontaneously without leaving a scar, but may recur. Erythema nodosum can sometimes be seen, primarily as a feature of *Yersinia*-induced enteritis.

Ocular Inflammation

Conjunctivitis is the most common ocular manifestation. It is often an early clinical finding, and is seen in one-third of patients with the postvenereal form of the disease, but is relatively more common among patients with postenteritic (especially *Shigella*) reactive arthritis. Symptoms and signs of conjunctivitis are usually bilateral, mild, and transient. Conjunctivitis usually accompanies or occurs within several days of onset of urethritis, and lasts for days

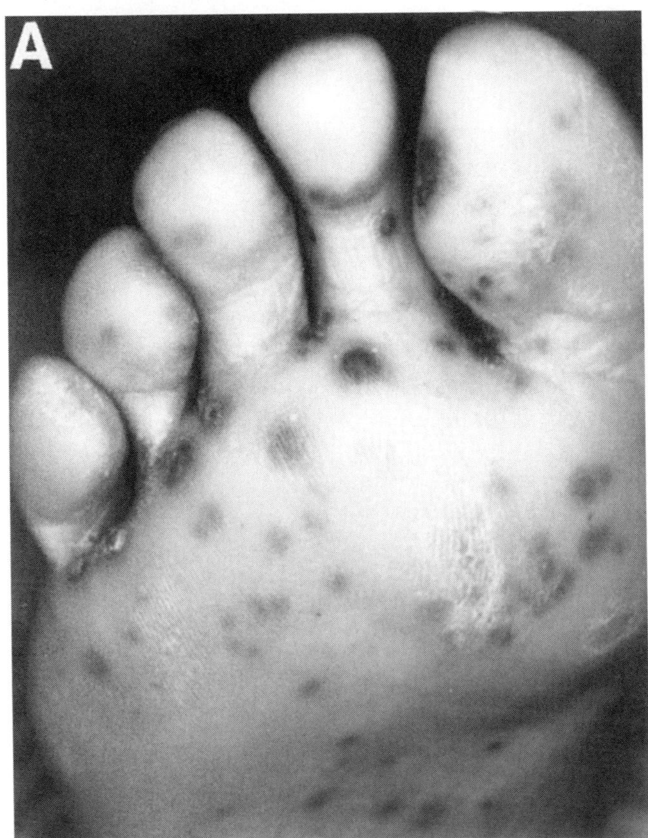

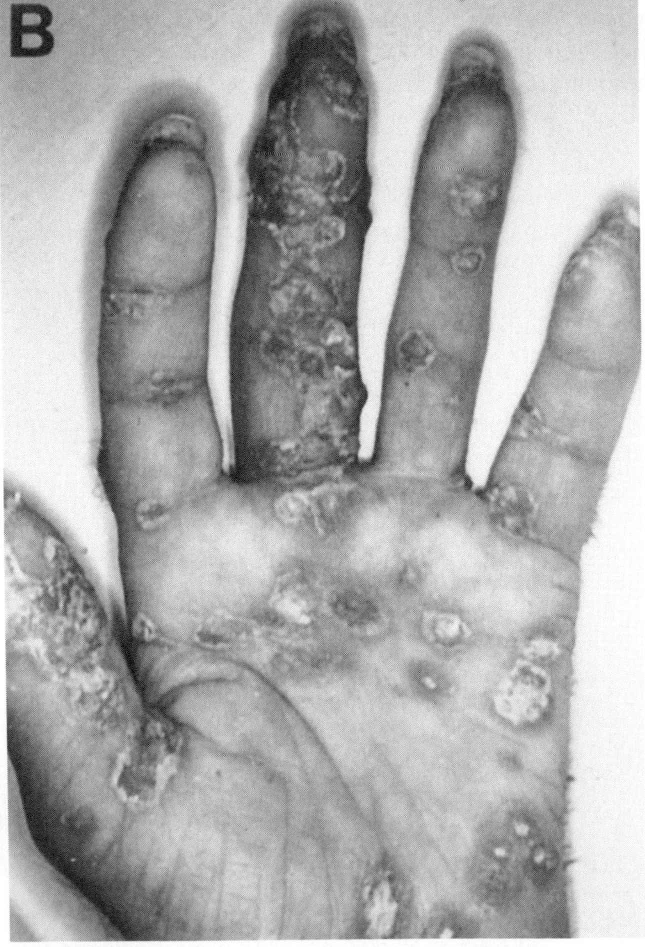

FIG. 64.4. A: Early lesions of keratoderma blennorrhagicum on the sole in reactive arthritis. **B**: Chronic lesions on the palm and digits in reactive arthritis.

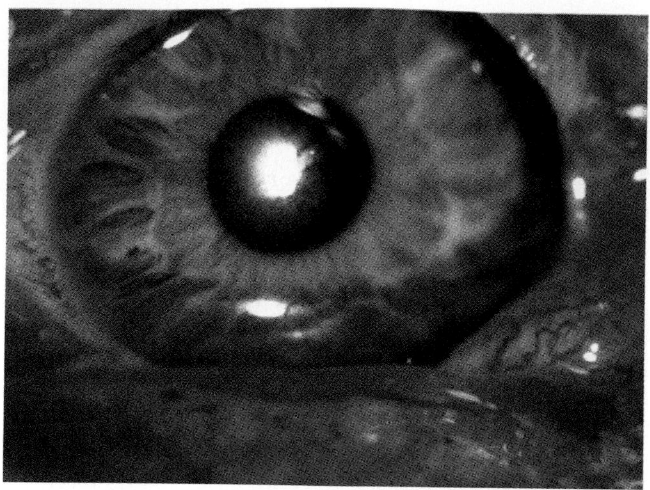

FIG. 64.5. Severe ocular inflammation in a patient with reactive arthritis. The inflammation is usually mild affecting when the conjunctiva, but some patients can have acute anterior uveitis.

rather than weeks, but it can be recurrent or severe (Fig. 64.5). It is usually painless (but can cause burning and irritation), and often nonpurulent. The conjunctival redness, if mild, can easily be overlooked unless the palpebral conjunctiva is examined, and the patient should be asked about recent crusting of the eyelids, especially in the morning, which suggests subtle conjunctivitis (8–10).

Between 10% and 20% of patients with reactive arthritis, especially those who possess HLA-B27, may experience one or more episodes of acute anterior uveitis, and it can be an independent event in some patients due to the shared susceptibility to both reactive arthritis and uveitis attributable to the presence of HLA-B27. It usually results in unilateral eye pain, redness, lacrimation, photophobia, and some blurring of vision, but responds well to treatment. However, some patients may develop more persistent inflammation of the uveal tract that may pursue a chronic or relapsing course, or bilateral uveitis can occur. The inflammation may, on rare occasions, affect even the posterior uveal tract or cause keratitis. Uveitis may be a presenting manifestation or occur at any time in the course of the disease, and can be recurrent and involve either eye (56,57). In a study of 236 consecutive patients with uveitis seen in an ophthalmology clinic, spondyloarthropathy was found to be the underlying cause in 13% (7.2% with reactive arthritis and 5.5% with ankylosing spondylitis) (57). In this subset of patients, the uveitis was associated with the presence of HLA-B27, uniformly acute in onset, unilateral, anterior in location, and responded well to treatment.

Other Features

Cardiac involvement in reactive arthritis is rare, and is usually a late manifestation mostly seen among patients with severe long-standing disease. This can result in asymptomatic cardiac conduction disturbances such as a prolonged PR interval and nonspecific ST-segment alterations on electrocardiogram, complete heart block, inflammation of the ascending aorta and aortic regurgitation, or pericarditis/myocarditis (7–9,58). Urinary abnormalities, such as proteinuria and microscopic hematuria, are sometimes detected on routine urinalysis, with or without impairment of renal function. There is rarely occurrence of secondary amyloidosis in patients with severe persistent disease (59). Serositis, pulmonary infiltrates, and central nervous system involvement have rarely been reported. Apart from the known association of enteritis with reactive arthritis, gastrointestinal inflammation may occur as part of the reactive arthritis itself, and therefore gastrointestinal symptoms and inflammatory lesions can occur in association with a postvenereal trigger (60,61) (see Chapter 66).

PATHOLOGY

Synovitis results in inflammatory synovial fluid (cell count can range from 5,000 to 50,000 mm^3) that exhibits a predominance of polymorphonuclear leukocytes. There is no local complement consumption (8–10). The histology of inflammatory synovitis is nonspecific (edema, vascular changes, and infiltration of lymphocytes, polymorpho nuclear leukocytes, and plasma cells) and not unique to reactive arthritis. Unlike rheumatoid synovitis, extensive pannus formation is rare. Moreover, the inflammatory process is generally nonerosive. Bone erosions are uncommon and observed only in patients with persistent inflammation. Other pathologic findings that are characteristic of reactive arthritis and related spondyloarthropathies include inflammation (infiltration of macrophages and lymphocytes) at the bony insertion of ligaments and tendons (enthesitis), bone resorption and remodeling resulting from subchondral osseous hyperplasia, and periosteal new bone formation (1–8,18–21). This can lead to excessive production of heterotopic bone at sites of inflammation in some patients. Other causes of enthesopathy are listed in Table 64.3.

The cutaneous lesions show infiltration with inflammatory cells including lymphocytes and plasma cells, as well as parakeratosis, acanthosis, and thickening of the horny layer, similar to those observed in psoriasis. The urogenital mucosal lesions have similar histology but lack keratosis. There is subclinical inflammation in the terminal ileum and colon in some patients, regardless of the presence or absence of HLA-B27, clinical manifestations, or treatment with nonsteroidal antiinflammatory drugs (NSAIDs). Histology of these lesions can resemble those associated with bacterial enteritis ("acute" lesions), or show "chronic" changes similar to those observed in patients with Crohn's disease. Acute histopathology is most often associated with enteropathic reactive arthritis, while chronic lesions are more commonly observed in patients with ankylosing spondylitis or Crohn's disease (60,61) (see Chapter 66).

TABLE 64.3. *Causes of enthesopathy*

Inflammatory
Ankylosing spondylitis
Reactive arthritis/Reiter's syndrome
Psoriatic arthritis
Enteropathic arthritis/Inflammatory bowel disease
Juvenile spondyloarthropathy/Late-onset pauciarticular juvenile arthritis
Undifferentiated spondyloarthropathy
Miscellaneous: Lyme disease, Leprosy
Mechanical/degenerative
Trauma
Osteoarthritis
Metabolic/endocrine
Diffuse idiopathic skeletal hyperostosis (Forestier disease)
Acromegaly
Fluorosis
Retinoid therapy
Hypoparathyroidism
Hyperparathyroidism
POEMS syndrome
X-linked hypophosphatemia

POEMS, polyneuropathy, organomegaly, endocrinopathy, M-protein, and skin changes.

Even patients with postvenereal reactive arthritis can develop intestinal pathology, although this is milder and less frequent. The degree of intestinal inflammation has been noted to closely parallel the patient's clinical status and response to therapy with NSAIDs and sulfasalazine.

ETIOPATHOGENESIS

The clinical and epidemiologic data strongly implicate interplay between microbial antigens and the genetic predisposition of the host in determining disease susceptibility and possibly chronicity. How these elements interact to cause an immunologically mediated reactive arthropathy is currently uncertain (1–4). The association of reactive arthritis with HLA-B27, and studies of HLA-B27 transgenic rats have clearly established the critical role of HLA-B27 and environmental/infectious triggers in the development of reactive arthritis (62,63). These rats develop features of reactive arthritis, including gut inflammation and psoriasiform skin and nail changes. The gut inflammation and arthritis do not develop in these rats if they are born and bred in a germ-free environment, although they still develop skin and nail pathology. The rats rapidly develop gut inflammation and arthritis on removal from the sterile environment and this inflammatory disease can be partially prevented by antibiotic treatment.

The demonstration of microbial antigens within the inflamed synovium suggests that reactive arthritis may be related to the persistence of microbial antigens (Figs. 64.6 and 64.7). *Yersinia enterocolitica* for instance, is taken up by

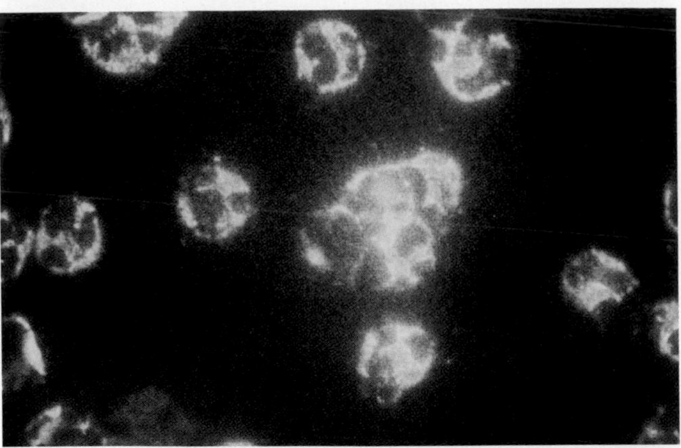

FIG. 64.6. Detection of intracellular *Yersinia enterocolitica* in the synovial fluid of a patient with acute *Yersinia*-induced reactive arthritis by immunofluorescence. (From Granfors K, Jalkanen S, von Essen R, et al. *Yersinia* antigens in synovial fluid cells from patients with reactive arthritis. *N Engl J Med* 1989;320:216–221, with permission.)

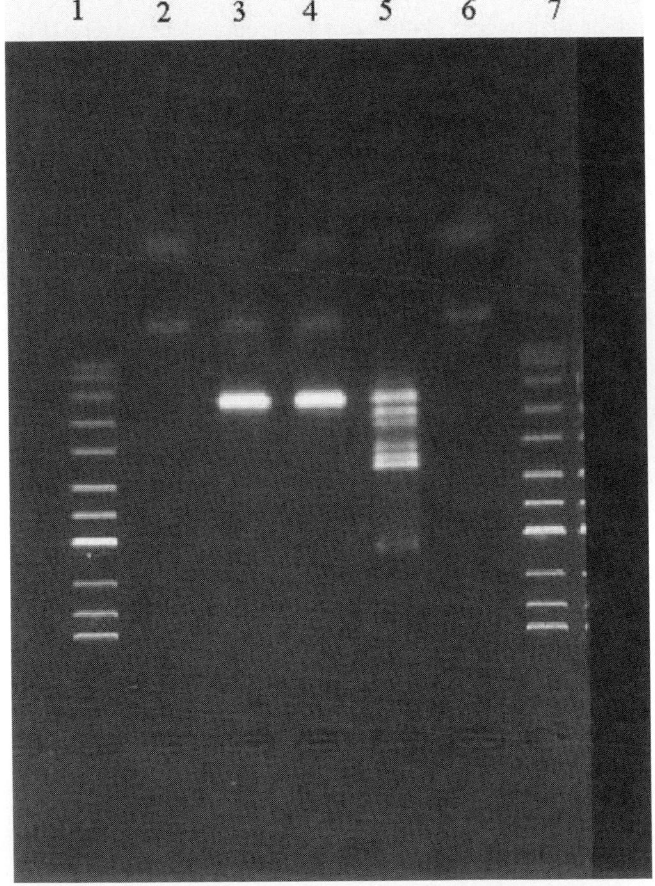

FIG. 64.7. Detection of *Chlamydia trachomatis* in the synovial fluid of two patients with reactive arthritis by polymerase chain reaction (PCR) (**Lanes 4 and 5**). **Lane 1 and 7:** Molecular weight markers. **Lanes 2 and 6:** Negative controls. **Lane 3:** Positive control, using purified *C. trachomatis* elementary bodies. A major outer membrane protein (MOMP)–specific nested PCR was employed. (Courtesy of Freise J, Schnarr S, Kuipers J. Hannover, Germany.)

M cells in Peyer patches through an interaction between invasin, a bacterial protein, and host β_1-integrin (1–4,64). *Yersinia* can use phagocytes as a carrier, can surmount endothelial barriers, and can reach synovial tissues via the bloodstream. Lymph nodes seem to act as a reservoir for *Yersinia* in a rat model in which the live microbe or its specific DNA fragments were undetected in the synovial tissue, but the lymph nodes were positive for *Yersinia* even after several months, and this was accompanied by a strong and long-lasting antibody response (65).

Reactive arthritis seems to result when *Yersinia*-derived arthritogenic epitopes are presented by phagocytes in the synovium to T cells because T-cell responses to HLA-B27 restricted peptide epitopes from the 60 kDa heat shock protein and the *Yersinia* urease β-subunit have been detected in the joint (66). Taken together, these results suggest that it is likely that *Yersinia* can persist outside the joint in lymph nodes or the mucosa, and that bacterial antigens reach the joint via monocytic cells. A similar mechanism has been suggested for *Salmonella*-induced reactive arthritis, and synovial persistence of bacterial lipopolysaccharide (LPS) has been demonstrated (67), but it is very difficult to detect *Salmonella* DNA in the joint (68).

In contrast to the enterobacteria, *C. trachomatis* is an obligate intracellular pathogen that primarily resides in epithelial cells but can infect other cell types as well (e.g., macrophages and nonprofessional phagocytic cells) (1–4, 69). *C. trachomatis* has a complicated life cycle including an infectious (elementary bodies) stage outside of the cell and a noninfectious (reticular bodies) stage inside of the cell. It replicates inside host cells and its antigens seem to be processed, both by the class I and the class II major histocompatibility complex (MHC) pathway, to be presented to CD4+ and CD8+ T cells (70,71). *C. trachomatis* can persist for a long time in the body, and traces of chlamydial RNA and DNA have been detected by polymerase chain reaction (PCR) in the joint (69). However, despite many attempts, no chlamydial organisms have been cultured from the inflamed joints of patients with reactive arthritis (69). A possible imbalance of cytokines such as tumor necrosis factor-α (TNF-α) and interleukin-10 (IL-10) may support the persistence of *Chlamydia* and other bacteria *in vivo* (72).

Role of HLA-B27

Because the main function of HLA class I molecules is to present peptide antigens to cytotoxic T cells, it has been proposed that the antigen-presenting properties of HLA-B27 could be crucial in the pathogenesis of reactive arthritis and related spondyloarthropathies.

Arthritogenic Peptide Hypothesis

The most favored theory for the association between HLA-B27 and spondyloarthropathies is the "*arthritogenic peptide hypothesis.*" It suggests that some HLA-B27 subtypes, due to their unique amino-acid residues, bind specific arthritogenic peptides that are recognized by CD8+ T cells (73) (Fig. 64.8). Furthermore, in response to these bacterial peptides, autoreactive T cells recognizing antigens with sufficient structural similarity between bacteria and self might become activated by self peptides, such as those in the joint or spine. This hypothesis is supported by several direct and indirect observations.

One major supporting argument comes from studies in humans showing the differential association of some of the HLA-B27 subtypes with ankylosing spondylitis (74–77). While B*2705, B*2702, B*2704, and B*2707 are strongly associated with the disease, the HLA-B27 subtypes B*2709 in Sardinians (Italy) and B*2706 in Southeast Asians seem to lack this association. Most interestingly, B*2709 differs from the disease-associated B*2705 by only one amino-acid substitution (change of aspartic acid (Asp) 116 to histidine (His) 116). B*2706 differs from the disease-associated B*2704 subtype by only two amino acid substitutions (change of His^{114} to Asp^{114} and of Asp^{116} to tyrosine 116) (74,77). These differences are all located in the peptide-binding groove. Therefore, it has been hypothesized that B*2706 and B*2709, the two subtypes that are not disease-associated, do not present arthritogenic peptides, in contrast to the disease-associated subtypes.

The possibly crucial role of arthritogenic peptides for disease pathogenesis is also supported by studies of HLA-B27 transgenic rats expressing an HLA-B27 restricted influenza–derived peptide with high affinity to HLA-B27 (78). These HLA-B27 transgenic rats have a significantly lower incidence of arthritis than HLA-B27 transgenic rats expressing an unrelated peptide, suggesting that the unknown arthritogenic bacterial peptide(s) is (are) competing with the influenza peptide for HLA-B27 binding. The concept that microbial peptides with sufficient structural similarity to self peptides can activate potentially autoreactive T cells by cross-reactivity in the periphery has been proposed as a possible mechanism for triggering autoimmunity (79,80). An oligoclonal expansion of CD8+ T cells has been reported in spondyloarthropathy patients (81,82). The synovial fluid derived from different HLA-B27+ patients suffering from reactive arthritis and triggered by different bacteria revealed an astonishingly high homology of T-cell receptors. These results lead to the suggestion that similar antigens are recognized by these oligoclonally expanded CD8+ T cells, and this suggests the possibility that under certain conditions specific arthritogenic peptide(s) might indeed be produced and presented to the host immune system.

It was long-time dogma that bacterial-derived peptides could not be presented to MHC class I molecules because they could not gain access to the class I pathway, with some exceptions such as *Listeria*. It has now become clear that even peptides from proteins that originate via the extracellular environment of a cell can induce a CD8+ T-cell response against obligate intracellular bacteria (83,84). This

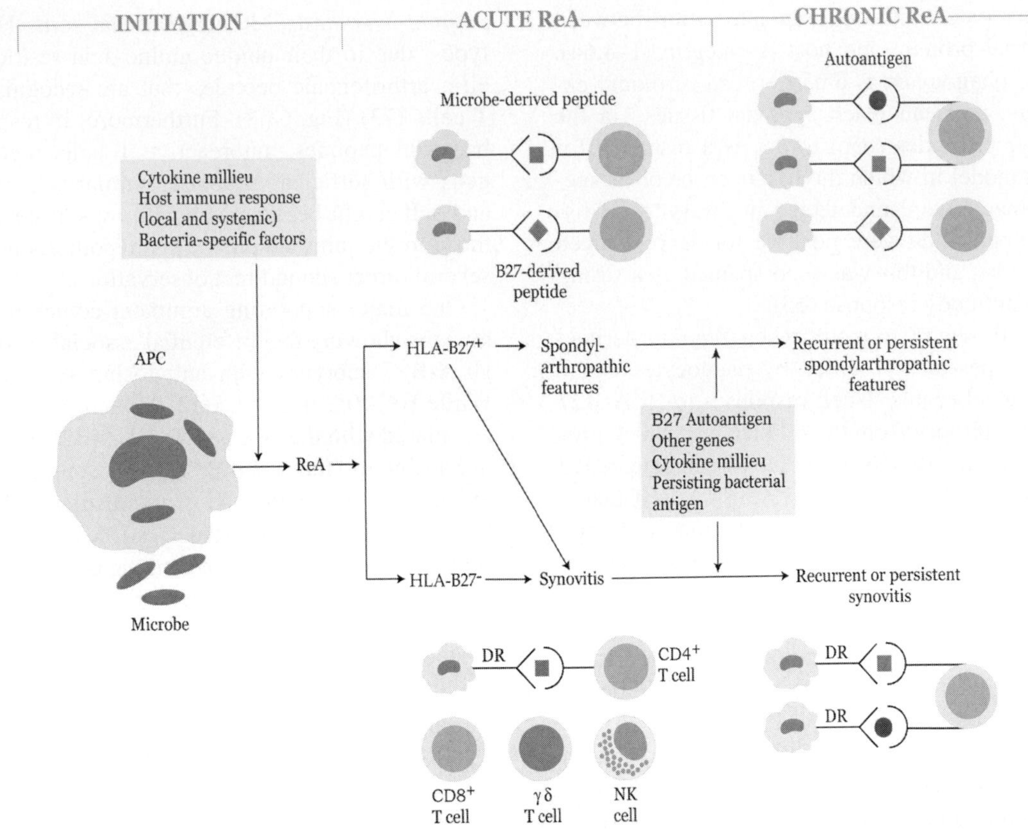

FIG. 64.8. Hypothesis for the pathogenesis of reactive arthritis. Exposure to microbes leads to synovitis of peripheral joints in HLA-B27–positive and HLA-B27–negative patients, while specific spondyloarthropathic features (such as sacroiliitis, enthesitis, and iritis) occur predominantly in HLA-B27–positive patients. In synovitis, a CD4+ response to persisting bacterial antigen seems to be of great importance while, for spondyloarthropathic features (and also for chronic synovitis in HLA-B27–positive patients), other mechanisms may be more relevant. *APC,* antigen-presenting cell; *NK,* natural killer; *ReA,* reactive arthritis. (From Sieper J, Kingsley J. Recent advances in the pathogenesis of reactive arthritis. *Immunol Today* 1996;17:160–163, with permission.)

has been demonstrated for *C. trachomatis*, and enterobacteria such as *Yersinia* or *Salmonella* (85–87). An HLA-B27–restricted CD8+ T-cell response to peptides derived from several chlamydial proteins in patients with *Chlamydia*-induced reactive arthritis has also been observed (88). However, it is of interest that in the HLA-B27 transgenic rat model for spondyloarthropathy, CD8 α/β T cells are not essential to the pathogenesis of arthritis or colitis (78,89).

An HLA-B27 self-derived dodecamer peptide (from the intracytoplasmic tail of the HLA-B27 molecule) has been reported that is a natural ligand of three of the disease-associated HLA-B27 subtypes (HLA-B*2702, HLA-B*2704, and HLA-B*2705) (90). Most interestingly, this peptide is not a natural ligand of HLA-B*2706 and HLA-B*2709, the two subtypes not associated with ankylosing spondylitis, and shows a striking homology to a peptide-sequence derived from the DNA-primase from *C. trachomatis*. Induction of breakdown of cytotoxic T lymphocyte (CTL) tolerance to self HLA-B27 by exposure to *C. trachomatis* has also been proposed to have some pathogenic role (91). It has been suggested that the exposure to *Chlamydia* may activate previously quiescent autoreactive T cells recognizing an HLA-B27 self-derived peptide, even if there is no sequence homology with the bacterial peptide.

Other Hypotheses

An interesting concept, the "HLA-B27 misfolding hypothesis," states that HLA-B27 itself is directly involved in the pathologic process of spondyloarthropathies because the molecule can exist in a misfolded state and form a novel β_2-microglobulin–free heavy chain homodimer (92–94). HLA-B27 misfolding is associated with aberrant intermolecular disulfide bond formation (dimerization) in the endoplasmic reticulum. This homodimer formation could be facilitated by unpaired free cysteine residues at position 67 (Cys 67) of the HLA-B27 heavy chain α_1 helix.

A "multi-hit" model proposes that immune activation at disease sites in reactive arthritis and related spondyloarthropathies results from an additive effect of arthritogenic microbial products (including LPS), HLA-B27, and other genetic factors, as well as biomechanical factors (Fig. 64.8) (22).

DIAGNOSIS

The typical joint pattern is an asymmetric arthritis without radiographic changes, predominantly of the lower limbs, which presents in the majority of patients as a mono- or oligoarthritis. Since patients with such a joint pattern constitute up to 50% of the patients in early arthritis clinics, reactive arthritis is an important differential diagnosis in daily clinical practice (7–10,30,55,95). The clinical triad of arthritis, urethritis/cervicitis, and conjunctivitis/iritis is observed in only up to one-third of patients with reactive arthritis because a large number of patients, despite careful evaluation, do not have documented genitourinary, enteric, or ocular symptoms. But such patients can often be identified on the basis of an acute, additive oligoarthritis that is accompanied by other clinically helpful features such as inflammatory back pain (due to sacroiliitis/spondylitis), dactylitis, enthesitis (plantar fasciitis, Achilles tendinitis), and mucocutaneous lesions (shallow painless buccal mucosal lesions, keratoderma blennorrhagica, balanitis, or onycholysis without nail pitting). For example, in a study of patients with *Salmonella*-induced reactive arthritis, only 13% patients had eye inflammation, but 44% had inflammatory back pain and 20% had enthesitis (96).

Reactive arthritis must be distinguished from other forms of acute arthritis, such as septic arthritis (especially gonococcal arthritis), crystal-induced arthritis, erythema nodosum, acute sarcoidosis (Löfgren syndrome), acute rheumatic fever, Lyme arthritis, and seronegative rheumatoid arthritis on clinical grounds and after appropriate laboratory tests and synovial fluid analyses. Laboratory results are consistent with an inflammatory process; there are moderate to marked elevations of the erythrocyte sedimentation rate and C-reactive protein, and there may be thrombocytosis, leukocytosis, and a mild normochromic, normocytic anemia. (7–10,95). There is no association with rheumatoid factor and antinuclear antibodies. Some patients with severe uncontrolled disease may show mild to moderate elevations of hepatic enzymes indicative of hepatocellular inflammation rather than cholestasis. The strong association with HLA-B27 and its clinical use is discussed later in this chapter. An association with antineutrophil cytoplasmic antibodies against lactoferrin or myeloperoxidase has been suggested, but its clinical use needs further study (97).

The synovial fluid white blood cell count in patients with reactive arthritis can range from 5,000 to 50,000 mm^3, and compared with the serum, the synovial fluid glucose level is not reduced significantly, as it is in septic arthritis (8–10). No microbes are seen on Gram stain and cultures are negative. The synovial fluid may occasionally contain the so-called "Reiter's cells," which are large mononuclear cells containing several ingested polymorphonuclear leukocytes, which in turn contain inclusion bodies that may represent microbial antigens.

A careful history, identification of extraarticular features, appropriate use of serologic testing, response to therapy, and sometimes a prolonged follow-up may be needed in some patients before a conclusive diagnosis can be made (8–10). Distinction from psoriatic arthritis or enteropathic arthritis can sometimes be difficult. Difficulties in diagnosis are due to the fact that at the moment there is no single diagnostic test, and most patients with reactive arthritis do not manifest the classical triad (29,98).

The American College of Rheumatology (ACR) has proposed less stringent criteria that require the presence of peripheral arthritis of more than 1 month's duration, occurring in association with urethritis/cervicitis (10,11). These criteria exhibit a sensitivity of 84.3% and a specificity of 98.2% when used to distinguish patients with reactive arthritis from those with psoriatic arthritis, seronegative rheumatoid arthritis, gonococcal arthritis, or ankylosing spondylitis. However, they have not been generally accepted, largely because a substantial number of patients at the outset of their disease may not meet these criteria, and such "unclassified" patients may be more numerous than those who fulfill the criteria. A working definition of reactive arthritis was proposed at the Third International Workshop on Reactive Arthritis in 1996 (Tables 64.2A and B) (34), but generally accepted validated diagnostic criteria are urgently needed (29–33). The European Spondyloarthropathy Study Group (ESSG) criteria (18) and the Amor criteria (19,33), which have been proposed as classification criteria to encompass the wider spectrum of the spondyloarthropathies, have been misused as diagnostic criteria.

These and other criteria used for the diagnosis of reactive arthritis relied nearly exclusively on clinical indicators of a preceding symptomatic infection such as urethritis/cervicitis or on symptoms characteristic for the whole group of spondyloarthropathies, such as enthesitis (29). However, none of these criteria has been accepted unequivocally by the clinical and scientific community. It is likely that in a substantial proportion of reactive arthritis patients the preceding infection is asymptomatic or associated only with minor symptoms. This form of arthritis is currently labeled as undifferentiated arthritis/ oligoarthritis. Alternative nosologic terms, such as *incomplete Reiter syndrome, undifferentiated spondyloarthropathy, sexually acquired reactive arthritis* (SARA), or the *BASE syndrome* (HLA-B27, arthritis, sacroiliitis, and extraarticular inflammation) have been used to classify some of the patients with inflammatory arthritis, who often possess HLA-B27 but fail to meet the ACR criteria for reactive arthritis (10,14–17, 51,98–100). The clinical use and validity of such terminology has not been tested.

It has recently been suggested to apply a combination of tests and clinical symptoms in order to make the diagnosis of reactive arthritis (50,101). For example, one may need clinical evidence of a preceding infection plus a positive serology or identification of a bacterium by serology or culture/PCR/ligand chain reaction plus a positive test for HLA-B27 (Figs. 64.9 and 64.10). The tests used for the identification of triggering bacteria are only useful if applied by physicians familiar with the clinical picture of reactive arthritis, and with the differential diagnosis of rheumatic diseases. None of the tests is useful if the clinical picture is not suggestive of reactive arthritis and if other diagnoses have not been excluded. Except in some selected patients, none of the tests or the clinical symptoms alone gives a posttest probability strong enough to make a definite diagnosis of reactive arthritis. This is especially true for serology and for HLA-B27 testing, and also for the spondyloarthropathy-specific symptoms such as enthesitis, which are of little value if used alone. An exception to this might be a positive PCR result for the detection of *Chlamydia* in the symptomatic joint.

Calculation of Posttest Probabilities for the Diagnosis of Reactive Arthritis

Application of most tests is generally best if the pretest probability is relatively high, ideally between 40% and 60% (102). If the pretest probability is low, however, even a positive test result does not convincingly support the target diagnosis. Thus, in a patient with a joint pattern noncharacteristic for reactive arthritis, such as symmetric polyarthritis of the hands affecting proximal interphalangeal (PIP) and metacarpal phalangeal (MCP) joints, the diagnosis of reactive arthritis is highly unlikely. The pretest probability therefore is low and any further test for the possibility of reactive arthritis is unwise. Conversely, a relatively high pretest probability of reactive arthritis because of a characteristic joint pattern can be further increased by clinical preselection that involves exclusion of other diseases in the differential diagnosis, such as gout, Löfgren syndrome, or Lyme arthritis (50,101).

Laboratory tests for the identification of the triggering bacterium are available and are increasingly used in a diagnostic workup for reactive arthritis (101). For the physician, an estimation about the likelihood that a diagnosis can be made if a test result is positive is of great interest. This posttest probability of the disease in the presence of a positive test result strongly depends on the expected likelihood of the disease before applying the test and on the sensitivity and the specificity of the test used (50,101,102).

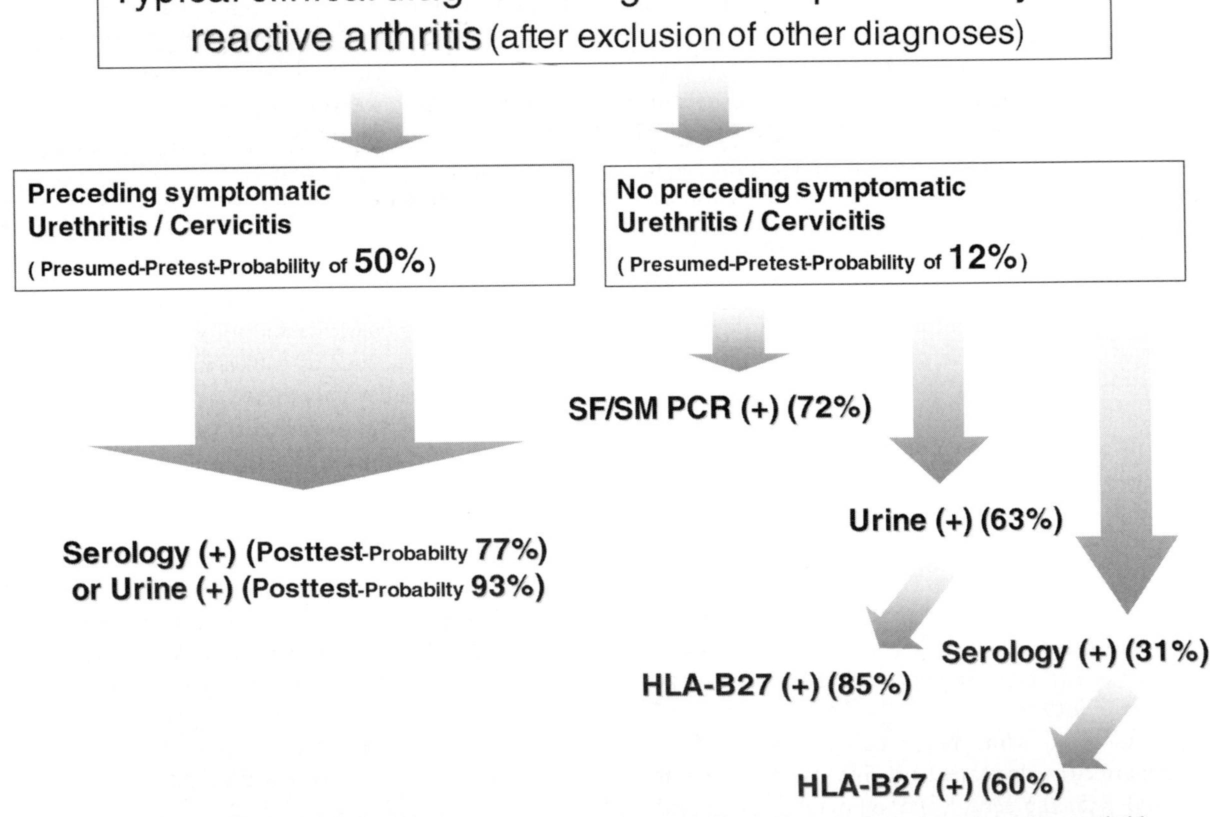

FIG. 64.9. The clinical approach (algorithm) for the diagnosis of *Chlamydia*-induced reactive arthritis and calculated posttest probability in case of a positive test or a combination of tests. (For more details see Sieper J, Rudwaleit M, Braun J, et al. Typical clinical diagnostic algorithm for diagnosing reactive arthritis: role of clinical setting in the value of serologic and microbiologic assays. *Arthritis Rheum* 2002;46:319–327.)

Typical clinical picture of post-enteritic reactive arthritis
(after exclusion of other diagnoses)

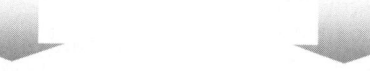

Preceding Symptomatic Enteritis
(Presumed **Pretest**-Probabilty of **30%**)

No Preceding Symptomatic Enteritis
(Presumed **Pretest**-Probabilty of **12%**)

Serology (+)
(Posttest-Probabilty 80%)

Stool culture (+)
(Posttest-Probabilty 68%)

Serology (+)
(Posttest-Probabilty 56%)

HLA-B27 (+)
(Posttest-Probabilty 80%)

FIG. 64.10. The clinical approach (algorithm) for the diagnosis of *Yersinia*-or *Salmonella*-induced reactive arthritis and calculated posttest probability in case of a positive test or a combination of tests. (For more details see Sieper J, Rudwaleit M, Braun J, et al. Diagnosing reactive arthritis: role of clinical setting in the value of serologic and microbiologic assays. *Arthritis Rheum* 2002;46:319–327.)

Many of the data on pretest probability, as well as specificity (proportion of patients without the disease with a negative test result) and sensitivity (proportion of patients with the disease with a positive test result) of tests for patients with reactive arthritis are available (50,101). Figures 64.9 and 64.10 indicate the posttest probabilities in the case of a positive test or a combination of positive tests under circumstances in which other diagnoses were excluded, and this is further differentiated according to whether a preceding symptomatic infection is present or not (50,101).

Identification of Bacteria Triggering Reactive Arthritis

Isolation of a microbial trigger after reactive arthritis has developed is an unusual event, especially in the postenteritic form of the disease, but serologic evidence of an antecedent *Chlamydia* or *Yersinia* infection is frequently present in individuals with reactive arthritis related to these organisms. The prevalence of infections with these bacteria certainly differs between countries and even between areas in the same country and might also change over time. Therefore, the examples given below have to be adjusted to the local conditions. *C. trachomatis*, *Yersinia,* and *Salmonella* are the most relevant pathogens triggering reactive arthritis in developed countries, and most information is available for these bacteria.

Stool cultures are needed for detecting enteric infection by disease-triggering bacteria, but a negative result does not exclude the diagnosis of reactive arthritis or its enteric trigger when there is a history of diarrhea. It is not uncommon for the stool cultures to become negative by the time patients seek medical help for arthritis. In acute *Yersinia*-induced reactive arthritis, IgG plus IgA antibacterial antibodies can be detected in almost all patients and IgA antibodies can still be detectable in more than 80% of patients after a year. In acute *Salmonella* infections, an LPS-based enzyme immunoassay (EIA), using commercially available LPS of *Salmonella typhimurium* and *Salmonella enteritidis*, has a sensitivity of about 92% compared with 64% for the Widal (hemagglutination) test (103). However, several months after the infection, the EIA can still be positive (IgG plus IgA or IgM) in about 92%, but the Widal drops to 16%.

The use of serology for the diagnosis of infections with *C. trachomatis* is hampered by a relatively high prevalence of positive antibody titers among controls and by a possible cross-reactivity with antibodies directed against *Chlamydia pneumoniae* (104). Antibody titers should be elevated at least 2 standard deviations above that of a control population. Antibodies of the IgG subclass alone do not necessarily reflect a recent infection because they can be elevated for months after an infection, whereas IgM- and IgA-antibodies reflect an acute or persistent infection. However, these antibodies can also be positive in a control population with a high infection rate, resulting in reduced specificity of this test.

The whole *C. trachomatis* or *Chlamydia*-specific major outer membrane protein (MOMP) or LPS has been used as antigens (50). The specificity and sensitivity of currently available tests has been estimated not to be higher than 78% and 73%, respectively, which is used for the calculations in Figure 64.9. The sensitivity of these tests seems to be limited possibly because *C. trachomatis* is an obligatory intracellular pathogen that is countered predominantly by a cellular immune response. Tests based on chlamydial LPS have a high sensitivity but cannot differentiate between *C. trachomatis* and *C. pneumoniae* infections (105). Therefore, using *C. trachomatis*–specific peptides from the MOMP one can differentiate between the chlamydial species or even serovars.

The search for *C. trachomatis* in the urogenital tract (in the first portion of the morning urine by PCR or ligand chain reaction) seems to be an acceptable and relatively easy diagnostic approach with a result comparable to urogenital swab analysis. Additional molecular biology techniques include the use of reverse transcriptase (RT)-PCR for highly unstable bacterial rRNA-transcripts to identify viable bacteria in the synovial fluid and synovial tissue samples. Only small amounts of synovial fluid or synovial membrane are necessary for such a test (105,106). The PCR technology is not very sensitive for peripheral blood (105). The method of synovial sample preparation significantly influences the sensitivity of the subsequent PCR. Different sample preparations and PCR applications have been developed for *C. trachomatis* but their standardization is urgently needed.

In patients with undifferentiated arthritis but with a joint pattern compatible with reactive arthritis, chlamydial DNA has been detected by PCR (Fig. 64.7) in about 30% of cases. However, the specificity of this test is not 100% because chlamydial DNA has also sometimes been found in control groups (such as patients with rheumatoid arthritis or healthy individuals) (101). The sensitivity of the test is also limited, especially in some early cases of typical *Chlamydia*-induced arthritis where no chlamydial DNA has been found, possibly because of an effective cellular immune response. Therefore, a sensitivity of only 80% is used. Thus, a positive PCR in the case of a 12% pretest probability results in a 73% posttest probability of reactive arthritis (Fig. 64.9), but it can be as high as 90% if a pretest probability of 30% is assumed. It has to be stressed that there is no agreement at the moment on the optimum technique to detect *Chlamydia* by PCR. Furthermore, none of the commercially available tests is sensitive enough to detect chlamydial DNA reliably in synovial fluid when compared with the amplification methods such as nested PCR.

Yersinia and probably also *Salmonella* can persist *in vivo* as indicated by elevated IgA or IgM titers and by the detection of these pathogens in the peripheral blood for months and even years (35,107–109). However, DNA of these bacteria is only rarely detected inside the joint, and it has been suggested that mucosa and lymph nodes might serve as a reservoir for *Yersinia* and *Salmonella*. Therefore, a *Salmonella*- or *Yersinia*-specific PCR for joint material does not currently play a clinically helpful role in the diagnosis of reactive arthritis (Fig. 64.10).

HLA-B27 and Spondyloarthropathy-Specific Features in the Diagnosis of Reactive Arthritis

An association between reactive arthritis and HLA-B27 was described more than 30 years ago, based mainly on patients seen at hospitals and, therefore, mostly consisted of those with more severe disease (12). In more recent studies based on epidemics or on community investigations, the HLA-B27 association is not higher than 50%, and is even weaker among many racial/ethnic groups, including African Americans. To conservatively calculate the clinical use of HLA-B27 testing in whites as an aid to diagnosis, one can use a specificity of 85%; it implies that HLA-B27 is present in 15% in the control population. The reasons are that HLA-B27–positivity in control patients with other arthritides may be slightly above the background 8% prevalence, and that the prevalence of HLA-B27 among populations of Nordic and Eastern European descent can reach 15% (110).

As an illustrative example, an HLA-B27 test is ordered in a clinical state of uncertainty where a pretest probability of reactive arthritis was 40% (for example, a patient with an isolated oligoarticular, asymmetric arthritis in the lower limb, in whom other diagnoses have been excluded). If the HLA-B27 test result is positive in this patient, a posttest probability of reactive arthritis comes out to be only 69%. However, the combination of HLA-B27 testing with the detection of *C. trachomatis* in the urogenital tract, or with a positive serologic test for a known arthritogenic trigger, can further increase the probability for the diagnosis of reactive arthritis in such a patient (See Fig. 64.9).

MUSCULOSKELETAL IMAGING

Radiographic abnormalities can be observed in up to 70% of patients with chronic reactive arthritis, and may be characterized by soft tissue swelling (especially sausage digits), periosteal reactive new bone formation, joint space narrowing, juxtaarticular osteopenia, and less commonly by bony erosions in the small joints of the feet, hands, knees, and sacroiliac joints (111,112) (Figs. 64.2, 64.3, 64.11 and 64.12). The bony erosions tend to be marginal or central in position and may be accompanied by adjacent bony proliferation, which tends to obscure erosive margins. Presence of enthesitis is suggested radiographically and by ultrasonography by the development of erosions and reactive new bone formation at these sites. Bony proliferation in reactive arthritis usually develops in one of several sites including the periosteum, with a linear or fluffy appearance adjacent to cortical margins, especially along the shafts of the metacarpals, metatarsals, phalanges, distal femur, and malleolar regions. Similar changes at the entheses, especially calcaneum, ischium, and femoral trochanters, result in a poorly defined or

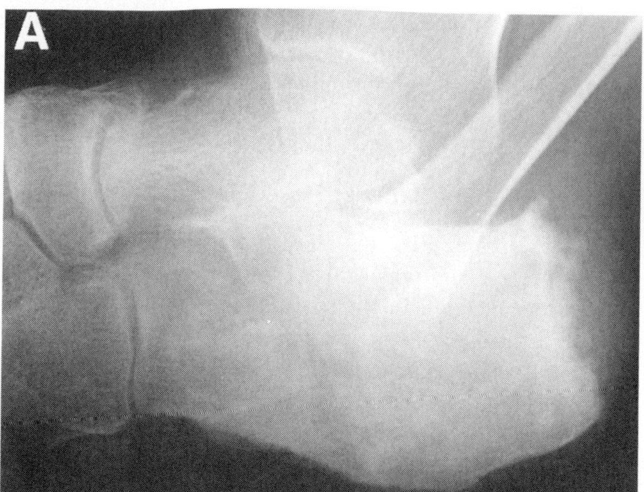

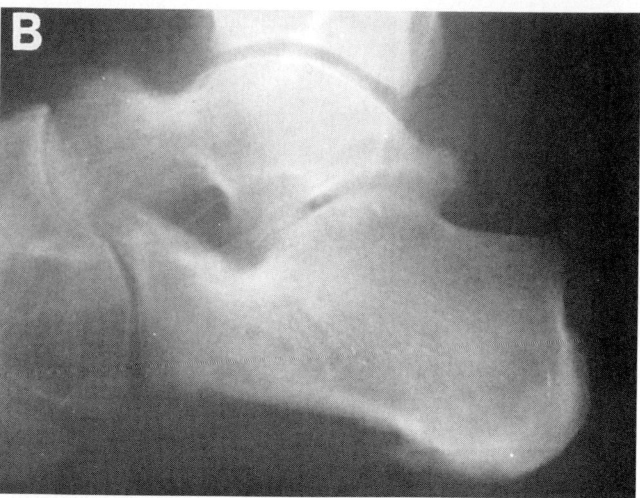

FIG. 64.11 Enthesitis involving the os calcis with **(A)** erosive changes at the insertions of the Achilles tendon and **(B)** at the plantar aponeurosis. There is "fluffy" reactive bone formation at the insertion of the plantar aponeurosis.

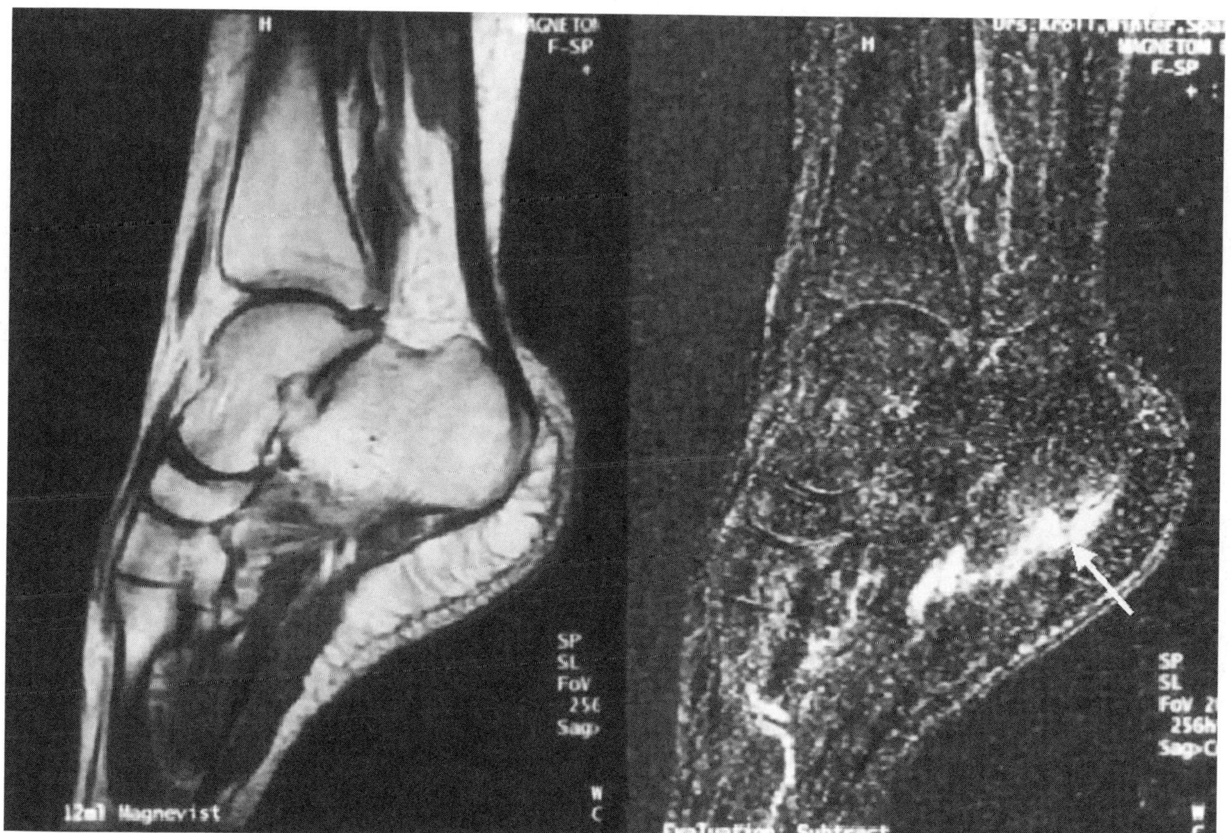

FIG. 64.12. Enthesitis of the plantar fascia as detected by gadolinium-enhanced magnetic resonant imaging, and is better demonstrated by subsequent subtraction imaging, as shown on the right by the arrow. (From Braun J, Khan MA, Sieper J. Enthesitis and ankylosis in spondyloarthropathy: what is the target of the immune response. *Ann Rheum Dis* 2000;59:985–994, with permission.)

fluffy osseous appearance. Calcaneal abnormalities appear as erosive changes on the posterior and plantar surfaces, sometimes associated with spurs at the plantar aponeurosis insertion and thickening of the Achilles tendon (Fig. 64.13). Spondyloarthropathy-specific features such as enthesitis have been suggested to be of use in the diagnosis of reactive arthritis, but the presence of arthritis plus enthesitis per se is not helpful in making a diagnosis of reactive arthritis because it has less than 30% sensitivity and the entheses may also be involved in other conditions (101). The ESSG observed that enthesitis has 80% specificity, because approximately 20% of the control patients without spondyloarthropathy had enthesitis (18). On using these values, the observed increase from a pretest probability of 40% to a posttest probability of 50% is quite small.

Radiologic involvement of the axial skeleton results in sacroiliitis, most commonly involving the lower synovium-lined portion, and its incidence increases with chronicity and duration of disease (111,112). For example, up to 50% of individuals with chronic reactive arthritis may show radiographic evidence of sacroiliitis. Although bilateral sacroiliac involvement is common, it tends to be unilateral or asymmetric at early stages of reactive arthritis. Initially, erosions are most evident on the iliac side of the synovial portion of the joint. These progress to "pseudowidening" with eventual bony proliferation, sclerosis, and ankylosis.

When compared with ankylosing spondylitis, axial abnormalities in reactive arthritis are less common and less extensive. It is uncommon to observe squaring of vertebral bodies and involvement of the cervical spine and hip joints (111–113). Whereas the spondylitis of ankylosing spondylitis is an ascending process, isolated involvement of the thoracic or lumbar spine may be the initial radiographic finding in the spine in reactive arthritis. Asymmetry and skip lesions involving the spine are common. Axial disease often manifests as paravertebral ossifications and comma-shaped nonmarginal syndesmophytes that are often unilateral or asymmetric and tend to spare the anterior surface of the spine. Similar findings can occur in patients with psoriatic spondylitis, and they typically affect the lower three thoracic and upper three lumbar vertebrae (111–113). It has been estimated that about 20% of HLA-B27+ reactive arthritis patients progress to ankylosing spondylitis after more than 10 years.

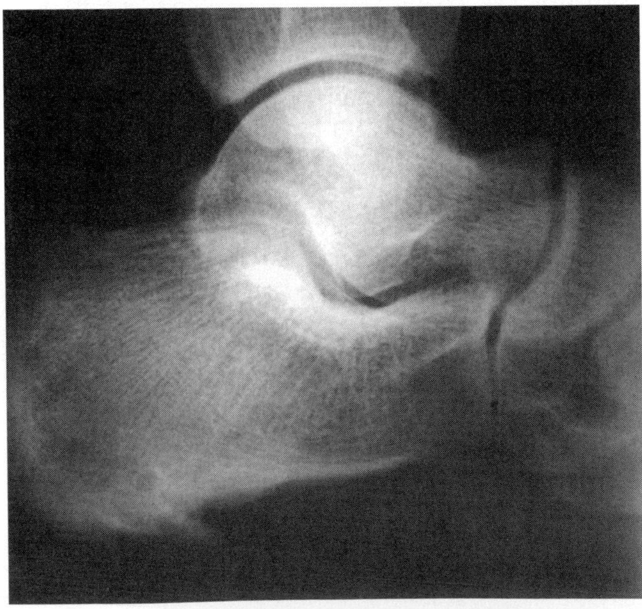

FIG. 64.13. Calcaneal spur in a patient with reactive arthritis.

The radiographic abnormalities are often more striking in the lower extremities (toes, calcaneus, tarsus, ankle, knee, and sacroiliac joints), and tend to be asymmetric (111,112). Tendinous and ligamentous calcification has also been observed in reactive arthritis, especially in the collateral ligaments of the knee, and in the metacarpophalangeal and interphalangeal joints. Radiographic involvement of the upper extremity is uncommon in reactive arthritis and may occur as focal or asymmetric oligoarticular involvement without resultant deformity. Bony ankylosis of peripheral joints is rarely observed. Erosions or reactive bone formation may occur in the sternoclavicular and manubriosternal joint and symphysis pubis.

Ultrasound can be useful in detecting tendinitis/enthesitis. Scintigraphy can detect enthesitis that may not be apparent by physical examination, and can also detect early sacroiliac involvement, especially when unilateral or asymmetric, in the absence of radiographic abnormalities. However, scintigraphy has low specificity. Computed tomography (CT) can be helpful in detecting sacroiliac involvement when radiographs are equivocal. Magnetic resonance imaging (MRI), with or without gadolinium enhancement, and subtraction imaging has been used with increasing frequency because of its superior ability to identify abnormalities of synovium, cartilage, tendon, and entheses (Fig. 64.12) (111, 112,114, 115). When compared with CT and scintigraphy, MRI, with or without gadolinium enhancement, is most sensitive at detecting sacroiliitis.

CLINICAL COURSE

The prognosis and course of individual patients with reactive arthritis and related spondyloarthropathies is varied and unpredictable (3,7–10,17,116–118). Disparate reports of clinical course and relapse rates of reactive arthritis may be confounded by inadequate disease definition and classification of these patients, inconsistent follow-up, selection bias, differences in postdysenteric and postvenereal forms of the disease, and differences in race/ethnic/genetic factors. Despite the potential for chronicity, several prospective longitudinal studies have shown that patients with reactive arthritis maintain a higher level of continued employment than do individuals with other inflammatory arthritides (119). Approximately 15% to 30% of patients develop chronic or recurrent arthritis, or sacroiliitis, or progress to ankylosing spondylitis in later years. These patients are mostly those who are severely affected, have a positive family history for spondyloarthropathy, or are positive for HLA-B27 (116). Severe disability occurs in fewer than 15% of patients and is frequently secondary to unrelenting lower extremity arthritis and enthesitis/dactylitis, aggressive axial involvement, or visual impairment. Death is rare and in the past it was usually attributed to cardiac complications or amyloidosis (59).

HIV-ASSOCIATED REACTIVE ARTHRITIS

Prospective studies of HIV-positive and HIV-negative populations, and data from Africa, have provided support for a role of HIV infection in the occurrence of reactive arthritis and other articular manifestations (120–124). HIV-associated reactive arthritis was first described in 1987 in the United States, when a group of patients were reported with both AIDS and severe arthritis or an illness resembling typical reactive arthritis, psoriatic arthritis, or undifferentiated spondyloarthropathy (120). The most common manifestations are arthralgia and arthritis; the latter was especially aggressive, and in many patients it had developed after they had become profoundly immunosuppressed. HLA-B27 was present in the majority of the white patients. More than one-third of patients demonstrate an antecedent enteric or urogenital infection. However, the widespread use of highly effective anti-retroviral therapy in developed countries has now markedly decreased the prevalence and expression of reactive arthritis among the HIV-infected population.

The arthritis evolves in two main patterns: an additive, asymmetric polyarthritis, or an intermittent oligoarthritis that most commonly affects the lower extremities. Dactylitis, conjunctivitis, urethritis, recalcitrant enthesitis, and plantar fasciitis can also occur and sometimes predominate. There are recent reports of aseptic necrosis. Early reports from developed countries reported asymmetric oligoarthritis to be the usual pattern, but polyarticular involvement is now observed more frequently in African countries (115–119). The arthritis differs from classical reactive arthritis in terms of its greater severity and chronicity, and a relatively poor response to conventional drug therapy. However, efficacy of infliximab treatment has been reported in an HIV-positive patient with severe reactive arthritis (125). Although the occurrence of sacroiliitis has sometimes been observed, axial spinal ankylosis is not observed and acute anterior uveitis is rare. Patients are prone to bone and joint infections when their CD4+ T-cell count becomes markedly diminished (see Chapter 129). HIV testing is not warranted in all patients suspected of having reactive arthritis, but it may be considered in those with reactive arthritis and psoriatic arthritis who are engaged in high-risk behavior or situations.

In sub-Saharan Africa, due to the very high prevalence of HIV infection and lack of widespread use of highly effective anti-retroviral therapy, many patients are now being seen with associated reactive arthritis, psoriasis, psoriatic arthritis, and related spondyloarthropathies. This is all the more remarkable given the almost complete absence of HLA-B27 in Bantu populations of Africa, and spondyloarthropathies used to be extremely rare among them (117–119). For example, the prevalence of spondyloarthropathies in Lusaka, the capital of Zambia, has now been calculated to be approximately 180 per 100,000 in HIV-infected individuals; this is 12 times higher than in the population unaffected with HIV.

THERAPY

Treatment should be directed at relief of pain, suppression of inflammation, maintenance of function, optimal joint protection, and, when appropriate, eradication of infection (3,4,7–9,115,126,127). NSAIDs form the basis of therapy and they should be used regularly in full therapeutic antiinflammatory dose over an extended period of time. The patient should be advised against using the NSAIDs occasionally or only for their analgesic effect. Joint aspiration and intraarticular corticosteroid administration of triamcinolone hexacetonide may help to obtain prompt and prolonged relief from severe or persistent synovitis, only after septic arthritis has been excluded. The differential diagnosis from septic arthritis may sometimes be difficult and short hospitalization may be needed for patients with severe arthritis. Antibiotic treatment should be initiated if true joint infection is not excluded. Joint rest and even temporary splinting may be needed in severe cases to alleviate pain, but should be used sparingly because it may result in muscle wasting. Physical therapy is valuable during convalescence to regain muscle strength and full range of joint motion. A comfortable pair of shoes and shoe inserts to alter weight bearing may help the patient with painful feet. Prolonged NSAID therapy is indicated as long as clinical and laboratory evidence of ongoing inflammation is present. Patient education is a priority as it is likely to improve compliance and enhance active participation of the patient in the therapeutic program. Appropriate use of exercises that include joint stretching, muscle strengthening, and range of motion exercises to maintain function and to alleviate discomfort on walking should be emphasized. Inactivity and immobilization should be discouraged.

In a very severe case of acute reactive arthritis where the patient is either intolerant or has not responded to multiple attempts at conventional NSAID therapy, or the newer cyclooxygenase-2 (COX-2) inhibitors, and many joints are affected, a short course of oral corticosteroids may be needed, tapering down the dose according to improvement. It is advisable to avoid prolonged therapy because systemic corticosteroids are relatively ineffective in the routine management of patients with reactive arthritis (126,131). Nonetheless, locally administered corticosteroids (such as topical use for severe ocular inflammation, and intraarticular, perilesional, or enthesial injections) may be important adjuncts in the management of some patients. Use of high-dose intravenous "pulse" corticosteroids has not been studied in reactive arthritis.

Antirheumatic "disease-modifying" drugs can be tried in some patients with persistent polyarthritis. Sulfasalazine is the best-studied second-line treatment for reactive arthritis and randomized, controlled trials have indicated the drug's minimal to moderate efficacy in the treatment of peripheral arthritis, but it is not effective for axial disease and enthesitis (126–131). It has been shown to correct the subclinical intestinal inflammation often associated with spondyloarthropathies. Methotrexate appears to be effective for treatment of persistent peripheral arthritis (132,133) and azathioprine was shown to be effective in a placebo-controlled crossover trial in a very small number of patients (134). Skin lesions are treated either with topical corticosteroids or keratinolytic agents such as salicylic acid ointment. In severe cases, retinoids or methotrexate may be used. Acute anterior uveitis must be diagnosed and treated promptly to prevent synechiae and other resultant complications.

Antimicrobial Therapy

Antibiotic treatment of the triggering infection is only recommended if the presence of infection can still be identified after the onset of arthritis (135). For example, in *Yersinia* infections, the aim of such antibiotic therapy is to minimize the spread of infection within the family. However, a cautious approach should be exercised because antibiotic treatment may prolong the carrier state in some forms of enteritis and short-term antibiotic treatment does not influence the course of postenteritic reactive arthritis (136). It is obvious that once the trigger has been pulled, the chain of events takes its course anyway. But early treatment of patients with urogenital chlamydial infection in high endemic areas does reduce relapses of reactive arthritis (42, 137). A retrospective study in Greenland found that early vigorous antibiotic treatment of chlamydial urethritis (with either tetracycline or erythromycin) resulting in eradication of *Chlamydia*, curtailed the occurrence of chronic or recurrent *Chlamydia*-induced reactive arthritis (42).

Given the persistence of reactive arthritis-associated bacteria such as *C. trachomatis* and *Yersinia in vivo*, it has been an obvious question whether prolonged antibiotic therapy is effective in the treatment of chronic reactive arthritis (138–141). However, there is no clear benefit of long-term antibiotic ciprofloxacin treatment in patients with reactive arthritis and undifferentiated oligoarthritis (138). In contrast to these results, a recent follow-up study of patients, who 4 to 7 years previously had been treated with a 3-month course of either ciprofloxacin or placebo, indicated that the HLA-B27+ subgroup of patients with reactive arthritis might benefit in the long run from ciprofloxacin therapy (139). However, these promising findings from a small study need to be confirmed in future larger studies (140,141).

Anti-Tumor Necrosis Factor Therapy

Anti-tumor necrosis factor (TNF) therapy with infliximab or etanercept has been found to be very effective in treating spondyloarthropathies, including severe reactive arthritis, and intractable enthesitis (127,142–150). Short-term effectiveness and safety of anti–TNF-α therapy in reactive and unclassified arthritis has been reported, but controlled studies and long-term follow-up is needed. Infliximab, but not etanercept, is also effective in Crohn disease (147,150). There is a case report of anti–TNF-α treatment for nephrotic syndrome in a patient with juvenile inflammatory bowel disease–associated spondyloarthropathy, complicated with amyloidosis and glomerulonephritis (151). Consensus statements are being developed to establish criteria to be used in deciding which patient with spondyloarthropathy may need this treatment and how to evaluate the therapeutic response (152,153).

For HIV-associated reactive arthritis, initial therapy with NSAIDs is advised, but for those with unrelenting arthritis or enthesitis who fail to respond completely, there are anecdotal reports of efficacy of therapy with sulfasalazine, etretinate, and anti–TNF-α therapy (125,154–157). The use of high-dose corticosteroids, methotrexate, and other cytotoxic agents carries the risk of precipitating more severe immunosuppression. Anti retroviral therapies may improve the cutaneous manifestations of reactive arthritis.

REFERENCES

1. Sieper J, Braun J, Kingsley GH. Report on the Fourth International Workshop on Reactive Arthritis. *Arthritis Rheum* 2000;43:720.
2. Granfors K, Märker-Hermann E, De Keyser P, et al. The cutting edge of spondyloarthropathy research in the millennium. *Arthritis Rheum* 2002;46:606.
3. Flores D, Marquez J, Garza M, Espinoza LR. Reactive arthritis: newer developments. *Rheum Dis Clin North Am* 2003;29:37–59.
4. Gaston H, Lillicrap MS. Arthritis associated with *enteric* infection. *Best Pract Res Clin Rheumatol* 2003;17:219–229.
5. Keat A. Reactive arthritis or post-infective arthritis? *Best Pract Res Clin Rheumatol* 2002;16:507–522.
6. Amor B. Reiter's syndrome: diagnosis and clinical features. *Rheum Dis Clin North Am* 1998;24:677–695.
7. Cush JJ, Lipsky PE. Reiter's syndrome and reactive arthritis. In: Koopman WJ, ed. *Arthritis and allied conditions: a textbook of rheumatology*, 14th ed. Baltimore: Williams & Wilkins, 2000.
8. Toivanen A, Toivanen P, eds. *Reactive arthritis*. Boca Raton, FL: CRC Press, 1988.
9. Toivanen A. Reactive arthritis: clinical features and treatment. In: Hochberg M, Silman A, Smolen J, et al., eds. *Rheumatology*, 3rd ed. St. Louis: Mosby, 2003:1233–1240.
10. Arnett FC. Incomplete Reiter's syndrome; clinical comparison with classical triad. *Ann Rheum Dis* 1979;38[Suppl 1]:73–78.
11. Willkens RF, Arnett FC, Bitter T, et al. Reiter's syndrome; evaluation of preliminary criteria for definite disease. *Arthritis Rheum* 1981;24: 844–849.
12. Brewerton DA, Caffrey M, Nicholls A, et al. Reiter's disease and HL-A 27. *Lancet* 1973;3:996–998.

13. Wallace DJ, Weisman MH. The physician Hans Reiter as prisoner of war in Nuremberg: a contextual review of his interrogations (1945–1947) *Arthritis Rheum* 2003;32:208–230.
14. Khan MA. Update on spondyloarthropathies. *Ann Intern Med* 2002; 136:896–907.
15. Khan MA, van der Linden SM. A wider spectrum of spondyloarthropathies. *Semin Arthritis Rheum* 1990;20:107–113.
16. Calin A, Taurog J, eds. *The spondylarthritides*. Oxford, UK: Oxford University Press, 1998.
17. van der Linden S, Pascual E, eds. Spondyloarthropathies. *Best Pract Res Clin Rheumatol* 2002;16:495–705.
18. Dougados M, van der Linden S, Juhlin R, et al. The European Spondyloarthropathy Study Group preliminary criteria for the classification of spondyloarthropathy. *Arthritis Rheum* 1991;34:1218–1227.
19. Amor B, Dougados M, Mijiyawa M, et al. Criteria for the classification of spondyloarthropathies. *Rev Rheum Mal Osteoartic* 1990;57:85–89.
20. Braun J, Khan MA, Sieper J. Entheses and enthesopathy: what is the target of the immune response. *Ann Rheum Dis* 2000;59:985–994.
21. François RJ, Braun J, Khan MA. Entheses and enthesitis: a histopathological review and relevance to spondyloarthropathies. *Curr Opin Rheumatol* 2001;13:255–264.
22. McGonagle D, Marzo-Ortega H, Benjamin M, et al. Conference summary: report on the Second International Enthesitis Workshop. *Arthritis Rheum* 2003;48:896–905.
23. Braun J, Bollow M, Remlinger G, et al. Prevalence of spondyloarthropathies in HLA-B27 positive and negative donors. *Arthritis Rheum* 1998;41:58–67.
24. Reiter H. Uber eine bisher unerkannte spirochaeteninfektion (spirochaetosis arthritica). *Dtsch Med Wochenschr* 1916;42:1535–1536.
25. Weissmann G. They all laughed at Christopher Columbus. *Hosp Pract* 1986;21:29–41.
26. Paronen I. Reiter's disease: a study of 344 cases observed in Finland. *Acta Med Scand* 1948;131[212 Suppl]:1–112.
27. Noer HR. An experimental epidemic of Reiter's syndrome. *JAMA* 1966;198:693–698.
28. Anderson B. Did Benvenuto Cellini (1500–1571) have Reiter's disease? *Sex Transm Dis* 1989;16:47–48.
29. Sieper J, Braun J. Problems and advances in the diagnosis of reactive arthritis [Editorial] *J Rheumatol* 1999;26:1222–1224.
30. Khan MA. Thoughts concerning the early diagnosis of ankylosing spondylitis and related diseases. *Clin Exp Rheumatol* 2002;20[Suppl 28]:S6–S10.
31. Pacheco-Tena C, Burgos-Vargas R, Vasquez-Mellado J, et al. A proposal for the classification of patients for clinical and experimental studies on reactive arthritis. *J Rheumatol* 1999;26:1338–1346.
32. Hölsemann JL, Zeidler H. Diagnostic evaluation of classification criteria for rheumatoid arthritis and reactive arthritis in an early synovitis outpatient clinic. *Ann Rheum Dis* 1999,58:278–280.
33. Amor B, Dougados M, Listrat V, *et al.* Are classification criteria for spondyloarthropathy useful as diagnostic criteria? *Rev Rheum* (English ed) 1995;6:10–15.
34. Kingsley G, Sieper J. Third International Workshop on Reactive Arthritis. 23–26 September 1995, Berlin, Germany. Report and abstracts. *Ann Rheum Dis* 1996;55:564–584.
35. Leirisalo-Repo M, Hannu T, Mattila L. Microbial factors in spondyloarthropathies: insights from population studies. *Curr Opin Rheumatol* 2003;15:408–412.
36. Soderlin MK, Kautianen H, Puolakkainen M, et al. Infections preceding early arthritis in southern Sweden: a prospective population-based study. *J Rheumatol* 2003;30: 459–464.
37. Hannu T, Mattila L, Nuorti JP, et al. Reactive arthritis after an outbreak of *Yersinia pseudotuberculosis* serotype O:3 infection *Ann Rheum Dis* 2003;62:866–869.
38. Sinha R, Aggarwal A, Prasad K, et al. Sporadic enteric reactive arthritis and undifferentiated spondyloarthropathy: evidence for involvement of *Salmonella typhimurium*. *J Rheumatol* 2003;30:105–113.
39. Rich E, Hook EW, Alarcon GS, et al. Reactive arthritis in patients attending an urban sexually transmitted diseases clinic. *Arthritis Rheum* 1996;39:1172–1177.
40. McKay L, Clery H, Carrick-Anderson K, et al. Genital *Chlamydia trachomatis* infection in a subgroup of young men in the UK. *Lancet* 2003;361:1792.
41. Iliopoulos A, Karras D, Ioakimidis D, et al. Changes in the epidemiology of Reiter's syndrome (reactive arthritis) in the post-AIDS era? An analysis of cases appearing in the Greek Army. *J Rheumatol* 1995;22: 252–254.
42. Bardin T, Enel C, Cornelis F, et al. Antibiotic treatment of venereal disease and Reiter's syndrome in a Greenland population. *Arthritis Rheum* 1992;35:190–194.
43. Michet CJ, Machado EB, Ballard DJ, et al. Epidemiology of Reiter's syndrome in Rochester, Minnesota: 1950–1980. *Arthritis Rheum* 1988; 31:428–431.
44. Kvien TK, Glennass A, Melby K, et al. Reactive arthritis: incidence, triggering agents and clinical presentation. *J Rheumatol* 1994;21:115–122.
45. Clavel G, Grados F, Cayrolle G, et al. Polyarthritis following intravesical BCG immunotherapy: report of a case and review of 26 cases in the literature. *Rev Rheum* (English ed) 1999;66:115–118.
46. Schwartzenberg JM, Smith DD, Lindsley HB. Bacillus Calmette-Guerin associated arthropathy mimicking undifferentiated spondyloarthropathy. *J Rheumatol* 1999;26:933–935.
47. Cope A, Anderson J, Wilkins E. *Clostridium difficile* toxin-induced reactive arthritis in a patient with chronic Reiter's syndrome. *Eur J Clin Microbiol Infect Dis* 1992;11:40–43.
48. Gran JT, Hjetland R, Andreassen AH. Pneumonia, myocarditis and reactive arthritis due to *Chlamydia pneumoniae. Scand J Rheumatol* 1993;22:43–44.
49. Braun J, Laitko S, Treharne J, et al. Chlamydia pneumoniae: a new causative agent of reactive arthritis and undifferentiated oligoarthritis. *Ann Rheum Dis* 1994;53:100–105.
50. Sieper J, Rudwaleit M, Braun J, et al. Diagnosing reactive arthritis. Role of clinical setting in the value of serologic and microbiologic assays. *Arthritis Rheum* 2002;46:319–327.
51. Padula A, Scarano E, Giasi V, et al. Juvenile onset isolated HLA-B27-associated dactylitis. *Semin Arthritis Rheum* 2003;32(5):341–342.
52. Keat AC. Does a sterile urethritis occur in Reiter's syndrome secondary to gastrointestinal infection? *Rheumatology* 1992;31:106.
53. Thambar IV, Dunlop R, Thin RN, et al. Circinate vulvitis in Reiter's syndrome. *Sex Transm Infect* 1977;53:260–262.
54. Ingram GJ, Scher RK. Reiter's syndrome with nail involvement: is it psoriasis? *Cutis* 1985;36:37–40.
55. Keat A. Reiter's syndrome and reactive arthritis. *N Engl J Med* 1983; 309:1606–1615.
56. Banares A, Hernandez-Garcia C, Fernandex-Gutierrez, et al. Eye involvement in the spondyloarthropathies. *Rheum Dis Clin North Am* 1998;24:771–784.
57. Rosenbaum JT. Characterization of uveitis associated with spondyloarthropathies. *J Rheumatol* 1989;16:792–796.
58. Paulus, HE, Pearson CM, Pitts W. Aortic insufficiency in 5 patients with Reiter's syndrome: a detailed clinical and pathological study. *Am J Med* 1972;53:464–472.
59. Wakefield D, Charlesworth J, Pussell B, et al. Reiter's syndrome and amyloidosis. *Rheumatology* 1987;26:156–158.
60. de Keyser F, Baeten D, Van Den BF, et al. Gut inflammation and spondyloarthropathies. *Curr Rheumatol Rep.* 2002;4:525–532.
61. Cuvelier C, Barbatis C, Mielants H, et al. Histopathology of intestinal inflammation related to reactive arthritis. *Gut* 1987;28:394–401.
62. Hammer RE, Maika SD, Richardson JA, et al. Spontaneous inflammatory disease in transgenic rats expressing HLA-B27 and human B2m: an animal model of HLA-B27-associated human disorders. *Cell* 1990; 63:1099–1112.
63. Taurog JD, Richardson JA, Croft JT, et al. The germfree state prevents development of gut and joint inflammatory disease in HLA-B27 transgenic rats. *J Exp Med* 1994;180:2359–2364.
64. Granfors K, Jalkanen S, von Essen R, et al. *Yersinia* antigens in synovial fluid cells from patients with reactive arthritis. *N Engl J Med* 1989;320: 216.
65. Merilhati-Palo R, Gripenberg-Lerche C, Soderstrom K, et al. Long term followup of SHR rats with experimental *Yersinia* associated arthritis. *Ann Rheum Dis* 1992;51:91–96.
66. Mertz AK, Daser A, Skurnik M, et al. The evolutionary conserved ribosomal protein L23 and the cationic urease beta-subunit of *Yersinia enterocolitica* O:3 belong to the immunodominant antigens in *Yersinia*-triggered reactive arthritis: implications for autoimmunity. *Mol Med* 1997;1:44.
67. Granfors K, Jalkanen S, Lindberg AA, et al. *Salmonella* lipopolysaccharide in synovial cells from patients with reactive arthritis. *Lancet* 1990;335:685.

68. Nikkari S, Rantakokko K, Ekman P, et al. *Salmonella*-triggered reactive arthritis: use of polymerase chain reaction, immunocytochemical staining, and gas chromatography-mass spectrometry in the detection of bacterial components from synovial fluid. *Arthritis Rheum* 1998; 41:1054.
69. Inman RD, Whittum-Hudson JA, Schumacher HR, et al. *Chlamydia* and associated arthritis. *Curr Opin Rheumatol* 2000;12:254.
70. Thiel A, Wu P, Lauster R, et al. Analysis of the antigen specific T cell response in reactive arthritis by flow cytometry. *Arthritis Rheum* 2000; 43:2834.
71. Kuon W, Lauster R, Böttcher U, et al. Recognition of chlamydial antigen by HLA-B27-restrictd cytotoxic T cells in HLA-B*2705 transgenic CBA (H-2^k) mice. *Arthritis Rheum* 1997;40:945.
72. Braun J, Yin Z, Spiller I, et al. A low TNFα-secretion of peripheral blood mononuclear cells but no other T helper 1 or 2 cytokine correlates with chronicity in reactive arthritis. *Arthritis Rheum* 1999;42: 2039.
73. Benjamin R, Parham P. Guilty by association: HLA-B27 and ankylosing spondylitis. *Immunol Today* 1990;11:137.
74. Fiorillo MT, Greco G, Maragno M, et al. The naturally occurring polymorphism Asp116–His116, differentiating the ankylosing spondylitis–associated HLA-B*2705 from the non-associated HLA-B*2709 subtype, influences peptide-specific CD8 T cell recognition. *Eur J Immunol* 1998;28:2508.
75. Feltkamp TE, Mardjuadi A, Huang F, et al. Spondyloarthropathies in eastern Asia. *Curr Opin Rheumatol.* 2001;13:285–290.
76. Khan MA. HLA-B27 polymorphism and association with disease [Editorial]. *J Rheumatol* 2000;27:1110.
77. Khan MA, Ball EJ. Ankylosing spondylitis and genetic aspects. *Best Pract Res Clin Rheumatol* 2002;16:675–690.
78. Taurog JD, Maika SD, Satumtira N, et al. Inflammatory disease in HLA-B27 in transgenic rats. *Immunol Rev*. 1999;169:209.
79. Wucherpfennig KW. Mechanisms for the induction of autoimmunity by infectious agents. *J Clin Invest* 2001;108:1097.
80. Prinz I, Zerrahn J, Kaufmann SH, et al. Promiscuous peptide recognition of an autoreactive CD8(+) cell clone is responsible for autoimmune intestinal pathology. *J Autoimmun* 2002;18:281.
81. Duchmann R, Lambert C, May E, et al. CD4+ and CD8+ clonal T cell expansions indicate a role in antigens in ankylosing spondylitis; a study in HLA-B27+ monozygotic twins. *Clin Exp Immunol* 2001;123: 315.
82. May E, Märker-Hermann, Wittig BM, et al. Identical T cell expansion in the colon mucosa and the synovium of a patient with enterogenic spondyloarthropathy. *Gastroenterology* 2000;119:1745.
83. Pfeifer JD, Wick MJ, Roberts L, et al. Phagocytic processing of bacterial antigens for class I MHC presentation to cells. *Nature* 1993;361: 359.
84. Rock KL. A new foreign policy. MHC class I molecules monitor the outside world. *Immunol Today* 1996;17:131.
85. Loomis WP, Starnbach MN. T cell responses to *Chlamydia trachomatis*. *Curr Opin Microbiol* 2002;5:87.
86. Ugrinovic S, Mertz A, Wu P, et al. A single nonamer from the *Yersinia* 60-kDa heat shock protein is the target of HLA-B27-restricted CTL response in *Yersinia*-induced reactive arthritis. *J Immunol* 1997;159: 5715.
87. Maksymowych WP, Ikawa T, Yamaguchi A, et al. Invasion by *Salmonella typhimurium* induces increased expression of the LMP, MECL, and PA28 proteasome genes and changes in the peptide repertoire of HLA-B27. *Infect Immun* 1998;66:4624.
88. Kuon W, Holzhütter HG, Appel A, et al. Identification of HLA-B27-restricted peptides from the *Chlamydia trachomatis* proteome with possible relevance to HLA-B27-associated diseases. *J Immunol* 2001; 167:4738.
89. May E, Dorris ML, Satumtira N, et al. CD8 alpha beta T cells are not essential to the pathogenesis of arthritis or colitis in HLA-B27 transgenic rats. *J Immunol* 2003;170:1099 – 1105.
90. Ramos M, Alvarez I, Sesma L, et al. Molecular mimicry of an HLA-B27-derived HLA-B27 ligand of arthritis-linked subtypes with chlamydial proteins. *J Biol Chem* 277:37573, 2002.
91. Popov I, Dela Cruz CS, Barber B, et al. Breakdown of CTL tolerance to self HLA-B*2705 induced by exposure to *Chlamydia trachomatis*. *J Immunol* 169:4033, 2002.
92. McMichael A, Bowness P. HLA-B27: natural function and pathogenic role in spondyloarthritis. *Arthritis Res* 2002;4[Suppl 3]:153.
93. Colbert RA. HLA-B27 misfolding: a solution to the spondyloarthropathy conundrum? *Mol Med Today* 2000;6:224.
94. Bird LA, Peh CA, Kollnberger S, et al. Lymphoblastoid cells express HLA-B27 homodimers both intracellularly and at the cell surface following endosomal recycling. *Eur J Immunol* 2003;33:748–759.
95. Hughes RA, Keat AC. Reiter's syndrome and reactive arthritis: a current view. *Semin Arthritis Rheum* 1994;24:190–210.
96. Mattila L, Leirisalo-Repo M, Pelkonen P, et al. Reactive arthritis following an outbreak of *Salmonella bovismorbificans* infection. *J Infect* 1998;36:289–295.
97. Stoffel MP, Csernok E, Gross WL. Are antineutrophil cytoplasmic antibodies of immunodiagnostic value in reactive arthritis? *J Rheumatol* 1996;23:1670–1672.
98. Thomson GT, Inman RD. Diagnostic conundra in the spondyloarthropathies: towards a base for revised nosology. *J Rheumatol* 1990; 17:426–429.
99. Dubost JJ, Soubrier M, Ristori JM, et al. Late-onset spondyloarthropathy mimicking reflex sympathetic dystrophy syndrome. *Joint Bone Spine* 2003;70(3):226–229.
100. Toivainen P, Toivanen A. Two forms of reactive arthritis? *Ann Rheum Dis* 1999,58:737–741.
101. Rudwaleit M, van der Heijde D, Khan MA, et al. How to diagnose axial spondyloarthropathy early? *Ann Rheum Dis* 2004;63:535–543.
102. Khan MA, Khan MK. Diagnostic value of HLA-B27 testing in ankylosing spondylitis and Reiter's syndrome. *Ann Intern Med* 1982;96: 70–76.
103. Isomaki O, Vuento R, Granfors K. Serological diagnosis of salmonella infections by enzyme immunoassay. *Lancet* 1989;1:1411–1414.
104. Bas S, Vischer TL. *Chlamydia trachomatis* antibody detection and diagnosis of reactive arthritis. *Br J Rheumatol* 1998;37:1054–1059.
105. Kuipers JG, Jurgens-Saathoff B, Bialowons A, et al. Detection of *Chlamydia trachomatis* in peripheral blood leukocytes of reactive arthritis patients by polymerase chain reaction. *Arthritis Rheum* 1998; 41:1894–1895.
106. Kuipers JG, Nietfeld L, Dreses-Werringloer U, et al. Optimised sample preparation of synovial fluid for detection of *Chlamydia trachomatis* DNA by polymerase chain reaction. *Ann Rheum Dis* 1999;58:103–108.
107. Wuorela M, Granfors K. Infectious agents as triggers of reactive arthritis. *Am J Med Sci* 1998;316:264–270.
108. Nikkari S, Rantakokko K, Edman P, et al. *Salmonella*-triggered reactive arthritis: use of polymerase chain reaction, immunocytochemical staining, and gas chromatography-mass spectroscopy in the detection of bacterial components from synovial fluid. *Arthritis Rheum* 1999; 42:84–89.
109. Yu D Kuipers JG. Role of bacteria and HLA-B27 in the pathogenesis of reactive arthritis. *Rheum Dis Clin North Am* 2003;29(1): 21–36.
110. Khan MA. HLA-B27 and its subtypes in world populations. *Curr Opin Rheumatol* 1995;7:263–269.
111. Klecker RJ, Weissman BN. Imaging features of psoriatic arthritis and Reiter's syndrome. *Semin Musculoskelet Radiol* 2003;7(2): 115–126.
112. Braun J, Bollow M, Sieper J. Radiologic diagnosis and pathology of the spondyloarthropathies. *Rheum Dis Clin North Am* 1998;24:697–735.
113. Helliwell PS, Hickling P, Wright V. Do the radiological changes of classic ankylosing spondylitis differ from the changes found in the spondylitis associated with inflammatory bowel disease, psoriasis and reactive arthritis. *Ann Rheum Dis* 1998;57:135–140.
114. Khan MA. Ankylosing spondylitis: clinical features. In: Hochberg M, Silman A, Smolen J, ed. *Rheumatology*, 3rd ed. London: Mosby: A Division of Harcourt Health Sciences Ltd., 2003:1161–1181.
115. Khan MA. Spondyloarthropathies. In: Hunder G, ed. *Atlas of rheumatology*, 4th ed. Philadelphia: Current Medicine, 2004 (*in press*).
116. Amor B, Silva Santos R, Nahal R, et al. Predictive factors for the long-term outcome of spondyloarthropathies. *J Rheumatol* 1994;21: 1883–1887.
117. MA Brown, Brophy S, Bradbury L, et al. Identification of major loci controlling clinical manifestations of ankylosing spondylitis. *Arthritis Rheum* 2003;48(8):2234–2239.
118. MF Doran, S Brophy, K MacKay, et al. Predictors of long-term outcome in ankylosing spondylitis. *J Rheumatol* 2003;30(2):316–320.

119. Kaarela K, Lehtinen K, Luukkainen R. Work capacity of patients with inflammatory joint diseases: an eight year follow-up study. *Scand J Rheumatol* 1987;16:403–406.
120. Winchester R, Bernstein DH, Fischer HD, et al. The co-occurrence of Reiter's syndrome and acquired immunodeficiency. *Ann Intern Med* 1987;106:19–26.
121. Vassilopoulos D, Calabrese LH. Rheumatic aspects of human immunodeficiency virus infection and other immunodeficient states. In: Hochberg M, Silman A, Smolen J, eds. *Rheumatology*, 3rd ed. St. Louis: Mosby, 2003:1115–1129.
122. Mody GM, Parke FA, Reveille JD. Articular manifestations of human immunodeficiency virus infection. *Best Pract Res Clin Rheumatol* 2003;17:265–287.
123. Njobvu P, McGill P, Kerr H, et al. Spondyloarthropathy and human immunodeficiency virus infection in Zambia. *J Rheumatol* 1998;25: 1553–1559.
124. Mijiyawa M, Oniankitan O, Khan MA. Spondyloarthropathies in sub-Saharan Africa. *Curr Opin Rheumatol* 2000;12:263–268.
125. Gaylis N. Infliximab in the treatment of an HIV positive patient with Reiter's syndrome. *J Rheumatol* 2003;30:407–411.
126. Amor B, Dougados M, Khan MA, et al. Management of refractory ankylosing spondylitis and related spondyloarthropathies. *Rheum Dis Clin North Am* 1995;21:117–128.
127. Braun J, van der Heijde D. Novel approaches in the treatment of ankylosing spondylitis and other spondyloarthritides. *Expert Opin Investig Drugs* 2003;12:1097–1109.
128. Clegg DO, Reda DJ, Weisman MH, et al. Comparison of sulfasalazine and placebo in the treatment of reactive arthritis (Reiter's syndrome): a Department of Veterans Affairs Cooperative Study. *Arthritis Rheum* 1996;39:2021–2027.
129. Clegg DO, Reda DJ, Abdellatif M. Comparison of sulfasalazine and placebo for the treatment of axial and peripheral articular manifestations of the seronegative spondyloarthropathies. *Semin Arthritis Rheum* 1999;42:2325–2329.
130. Egsmose C, Hansen TM, Andersen LS, et al. Limited effect of sulphasalazine treatment in reactive arthritis: a randomised double blind placebo controlled trial. *Ann Rheum Dis* 1997;56:32–36.
131. Leirisalo-Repo M. Prognosis, course of disease, and treatment of the spondyloarthropathies. *Rheum Dis Clin North Am* 1998;24:737–751.
132. Owen ET, Cohen ML. Methotrexate and Reiter's disease. *Ann Rheum Dis* 1979;38:48–50.
133. Creemers MCW, van Riel PLCM, Franssen MJAM, et al. Second-line treatment in seronegative spondyloarthropathies. *Semin Arthritis Rheum* 1994;24:71–81.
134. Calin A. A placebo-controlled, crossover study of azathioprine in Reiter's syndrome. *Ann Rheum Dis* 1986;45:653–655.
135. Sieper J, Braun J. Treatment of reactive arthritis with antibiotics. *Br J Rheumatol* 1998;37:717–720.
136. Locht H, Kihlstrom E, Lindstrom FD. Reactive arthritis after salmonella among medical doctors: study of an outbreak. *J Rheumatol* 1993;20:845–848.
137. Carlin EM, Keats AC; World Health Organization. European guidelines for the management of sexually acquired reactive arthritis. *Int J STD AIDS* 2001;12[Suppl 3]:94–102.
138. Sieper J, Fendler C, Laitko S, et al. No benefit of long-term ciprofloxacin treatment in patients with reactive arthritis and undifferentiated oligoarthritis: a three month, multicenter, double-blind, randomized, placebo controlled study. *Arthritis Rheum* 1999;42:1386–1396.
139. Yli-Kerttula T, Luukkainen R, Yli-Kerttula U, et al. Effect of a three-month course of ciprofloxacin on the outcome of reactive arthritis. *Ann Rheum Dis* 2000;59:565–570.
140. Lauhio A, Leirisalo-Repo M, Lähdeuirta J, et al. Double-blind, placebo-controlled study of three-month treatment with lymecycline in reactive arthritis, with special reference to chlamydia arthritis. *Arthritis Rheum* 1991;34:6–14.
141. Yli-Kerttula T, Luukkainen R, Yli-Kerttula U, et al. Effect of a 3 month course of ciprofloxacin on the late prognosis of reactive arthritis. *Ann Rheum Dis* 2003;62:880–884.
142. Oili KS, Niinisalo H, Korpilahde T, et al. Treatment of reactive arthritis with infliximab. *Scand J Rheumatol* 2003;32(2):122–124.
143. Meader R, Hsia E, Kitumnuaypong T, et al. TNF involvement and anti-TNF therapy of reactive and unclassified arthritis. *Clin Exp Rheumatol* 2002;20[Suppl 28]: S130–S134.
144. Mease PJ. Disease-modifying antirheumatic drug therapy for spondyloarthropathies: advances in treatment. *Curr Opin Rheumatol* 2003; 15(3):205–212.
145. Rosenbaum JT, Smith JR. Anti-TNF therapy for eye involvement in spondyloarthropathy. *Clin Exp Rheumatol* 2002;20[6 Suppl 28]: S143–S145.
146. Meador R, Hsia E, Kitumnuaypong T, et al. TNF involvement and anti-TNF therapy of reactive and unclassified arthritis. *Clin Exp Rheumatol* 2002;20[6 Suppl 28]:S130–S134.
147. Braun J, Brandt J, Listing J, et al. Biologic therapies in the spondyloarthritis: new opportunities, new challenges. *Curr Opin Rheumatol* 2003;15(4):394–407.
148. J Braun, J Brandt, J Listing, et al. Long-term efficacy and safety of infliximab in the treatment of ankylosing spondylitis: an open, observational, extension study of a three-month, randomized, placebo-controlled trial. *Arthritis Rheum* 2003;48(8):2224–2233.
149. J Brandt, Khariouzov A, Listing J, et al. Six-month results of a double-blind, placebo-controlled trial of etanercept treatment in patients with active ankylosing spondylitis. *Arthritis Rheum* 2003;48 (6):1667–1675.
150. Marzo-Ortega H, McGonagle D, O'Connor P, et al. Efficacy of etanercept for treatment of Crohn's related spondyloarthritis but not colitis. *Ann Rheum Dis* 2003;62:74–76.
151. Verschueren P, Lensen F, Lerut E, et al. Benefit of anti-TNF-α treatment for nephrotic syndrome in a patient with juvenile inflammatory bowel disease associated spondyloarthropathy complicated with amyloidosis and glomerulonephritis. *Ann Rheum Dis* 2003;62:368–369.
152. Braun J, Pham T, Sieper J, et al. International ASAS consensus statement for the use of anti-tumour necrosis factor agents in patients with ankylosing spondylitis. *Ann Rheum Dis* 2003;62:817–824.
153. Pham T, van der Heijde D, Calin A, et al. Initiation of biological agents in patients with ankylosing spondylitis: results of a Delphi study by the ASAS Group. *Ann Rheum Dis* 2003;62:812–816.
154. Youssef PP, Vertouch JV, Jones PD. Successful treatment of human immunodeficiency virus-associated Reiter's syndrome with sulfasalazine. *Arthritis Rheum* 1992;35:723–724.
155. Disla E, Rhim HR, Reddy A, et al. Improvement in CD4 lymphocyte count in HIV-Reiter's syndrome after treatment with sulfasalazine. *J Rheumatol* 1994;21:662–664.
156. Louthrenoo W. Successful treatment of severe Reiter's syndrome associated with human immunodeficiency virus infection with etretinate: report of 2 cases. *J Rheumatol* 1993;20:1243–1246.
157. Williams HC, Du Vivier AWP. Etretinate and AIDS-related Reiter's disease. *Br J Dermatol* 1991;124:389–293.

CHAPTER 65

Psoriatic Arthritis

Robert M. Bennett

Psoriasis is a chronic autoimmune skin disease that afflicts about 2% of Caucasians. Some 10% to 40% of patients with psoriasis develop a chronic inflammatory arthritis. Psoriatic arthritis (PSA) has a superficial resemblance to rheumatoid arthritis (RA), but is considered to be clinically and genetically distinct, with a different pathogenesis. Historically, the association between psoriasis and arthritis was first noted by Alibert (1) in 1818; he mentioned "affections arthritiques or rheumatismales" under a subheading of "Lepre squammeuse," which appeared in a discourse on skin diseases. The term *psoriatic arthritis* (psoriasis arthritique) was first used by the French dermatologist, Pierre Bazin, in 1860 (2). A detailed description of psoriasis-associated arthritis was provided in the doctoral thesis of Charles Bourdillon in 1888 (3). In the late nineteenth and early twentieth centuries, however, there was no general consensus that PSA was a discrete entity; many writers considered the association to be a coincidental occurrence of RA and psoriasis.

In the 1920s, there were several case reports championing the concept of PSA (4). It was not until an association of rheumatoid factor and RA was described in 1948 that a clearer classification became possible (5). The observation that the majority of patients with an erosive arthritis and psoriasis were seronegative (6), coupled with the introduction of criteria for the diagnosis of RA (7), provided a new impetus for reexamining the concept of PSA. Baker (6) noted that seronegative polyarthritis was associated with psoriasis in 20% of patients; in comparison, only 1.2% of patients with seropositive arthritis had psoriasis. This suggested that the prevalence of psoriasis was increased 10-fold when associated with seronegative arthritis. A strong association between psoriasis and arthritis had been noted in family studies. Moll and Wright (8) studied 310 first- or second-degree relatives of 108 patients with PSA. Twenty-one percent of the relatives had psoriasis alone, 11% had a seronegative arthritis, 7.4% had sacroiliitis or spondylitis, and 1.8% had erosive polyarthritis. Compared with 83 spousal controls, the prevalence of seronegative arthritis was significantly increased; the prevalence of erosive polyarthritis was similar in the two groups (1.8%). These data indicate an 80% to 90% chance of inheritability in a first-degree relative of a patient with PSA. The strikingly divergent effects of human immunodeficiency virus (HIV) infection on the course of PSA, compared with RA, have provided the most compelling evidence that these are two distinctively different rheumatic diseases (see "Pathogenesis" below).

JOINT PATHOLOGY

Psoriasis is an inflammatory skin disorder with a proliferative component (scale production). The inflammation is due to an accumulation of neutrophils and activated $CD8^+$ T lymphocytes in the epidermis with an infiltration of $CD4^+$ T lymphocytes in the dermis (9). It is postulated that $CD8^+$ T cells are triggered by an unknown antigen(s) and secrete various cytokines that (a) cause a proliferation of keratinocytes, and (b) stimulate an inflammatory infiltrate (10). In this respect, it is of interest that there is a preponderance of $CD8^+$ T cells in the synovial fluid in PSA and a reversal of the CD4/CD8 ratio in comparison to RA (11). The joint findings in PSA are a juxtaposition of synovitis and an enthesitis. Entheses are the attachment sites where ligaments and tendons merge with bone (12). In PSA this attachment becomes inflamed and enlarged (enthesitis). McGonagle et al. (13,14) proposed that an enthesitis is the primary lesion in PSA. Although mechanical microtrauma at an enthesis can cause inflammatory changes, the possession of the human leukocyte antigen (HLA)-B27 gene is associated with the presence of bone edema at the site of the fascial insertion (15). The synovial histology in PSA is similar to RA as regards the degree of synovial proliferation, type of mononuclear cell infiltration, and extent of angiogenesis

(16); however the synovial vascular pattern is different in that PSA is characterized by predominantly tortuous/bushy vessels whereas the vessels in RA tend to be straight and branching (17).

Bone resorption and formation is a distinctive feature of a subset of PSA patients. As this occurs in relation to sites of disease activity it seems likely to involve an inflammation-induced dysregulation of osteoclast and osteoblast activity. Osteoclast development is controlled by a tumor necrosis factor (TNF) superfamily receptor-ligand pair known as receptor activator of nuclear-factor-kappa B (RANK) and its ligand (RANKL). A natural inhibitor of this system is a soluble receptor called osteoprotegerin, which competes with RANK for binding to RANKL. It has recently been found that there is a marked increase in osteoclast precursors (OCPs) in the blood of PSA patients (18). It is hypothesized that these OCPs arise from TNF-α-activated peripheral blood mononuclear cells (PBMCs) that have migrated into the inflamed synovium and subchondral bone (possibly as a result of mechanically induced tissue microtrauma at the enthesis). At these sites they are exposed to unopposed RANKL and TNF-α. This leads to both osteoclastogenesis at the erosion front and in subchondral bone.

PATHOGENESIS

The pathogenesis of PSA involves an interplay of genetic, immunologic, and environmental factors (19). Although occasional pedigrees have been described with a Mendelian pattern of inheritance, most pedigrees cannot be explained on the basis of a single gene and are presumed to be inherited on a multifactorial basis. Seventy percent of monozygotic twins with psoriasis are concordant for the disease (20). On the other hand, there is a report of discordance for PSA in monozygotic twins who have been followed up for 40 years (21). The carefully controlled study of more than 100 families by Moll and Wright (8) indicated that the first-degree relatives of PSA patients are nearly 50-fold more likely to develop PSA than the general population. Furthermore, spousal controls were not predisposed to develop PSA, suggesting that if environmental factors play a role in pathogenesis, they must act on a permissive genetic background.

When compared with the strong association of RA with HLA-DR4, and of ankylosing spondylitis (AS) and reactive arthritis with HLA-B27, the HLA associations with PSA have been less clear. The strongest genetic association with PSA appears to be Cw*0602 (OR 7.33) and MICA-A9 (OR 3.57) (22).

A genotype analysis of 100 PSA patients from 39 families, revealed a paternal transmission associated with chromosome 16q (paternal LOD score 4.19 versus maternal LOD score 1.03) (23).

Comparing early onset (before age 40) with late onset PSA, there is an increased family history of psoriasis and PSA and an increased prevalence of HLA-Cw*0602 (21% versus 11%) and B-17 (22% versus 5%) in patients with early onset disease (24). An interesting second lineage of evolutionarily conserved MHC class genes, the MIC genes, has evolved in parallel with human class 1 genes (25). They have a high degree of sequence homology with the classic major histocompatability complex (MHC)-1 genes. The MIC-A gene has 20 alleles, and the MIC-B gene has 11 alleles (26,27). The MICA-002 allele has been reported to have a higher frequency in (relative risk [[RR]], 3.2), and especially in the polyarticular form (RR, 9.35), compared with skin psoriasis (28). This susceptibility is independent of linkage dysequilibrium with Cw*0602 and suggests that the MICA-002 allele may be a candidate gene for the development of PSA. Most studies have shown an association of HLA-B27 with sacroiliitis and axial involvement, and there also seems to be a similar association with HLA-B39 (22). Another difference between RA and PSA is that the prevalence of the HLA-DRB1 shared epitope is not increased in PSA patients (24).

There is an association of HIV infection with severe PSA (29–36). The aggressive nature of PSA in patients with HIV infection suggests a distinctly different pathogenesis in comparison to RA. As HIV infection preferentially depletes T-helper cells ($CD4^+$), it is to be anticipated that diseases dependent on these cells will be ameliorated; such is the case for RA and systemic lupus erythematosus (SLE) (37,38). This experiment of nature points to an interaction of class I HLA molecules and $CD8^+$ T cells (and possibly γδ T cells) as being fundamental to the pathogenesis of PSA (29,35). The association of PSA with HIV infection is convincing evidence for its being distinct from RA. Class II HLA molecules also may be relevant to the initiation of PSA, as it has been reported to develop in patients being treated with intramuscular interferon-γ (a potent inducer of class II MHC expression) (39).

Keratinocyte growth is abnormal in psoriasis; these cells normally take 3 weeks to double, whereas in psoriatic plaque, they take only 3 days (40). Dermal fibroblasts secrete a stimulatory factor that drives keratinocyte turnover. Transforming growth factor-β (TGF-β) is a candidate for this role, as it is overexpressed in the psoriatic epidermis and has potent angiogenic properties (41). Proliferative changes may result from an overexpression of c-myc (a protooncogene that up-regulates the response of cells to growth signals) (42). TNF-α appears to play a role in skin psoriasis, with serum levels and monocyte production being elevated in active disease and improved by successful treatment (43). A TNF-α gene mutation at position −238 was found in 32% of patients with early onset PSA compared with 7% of controls (44).

HLA-DR expression on keratinocyte suspensions, obtained from suction blisters of active psoriatic plaques, was increased in 70% of 38 patients. Sixteen of these patients had typical PSA (45). Significantly, PSA did not develop in any of the 15 patients who lacked HLA-DR expression on keratinocytes. It was proposed that keratinocytes may process exogenous (e.g., bacterial, virus) or endogenous antigens and activate T cells directly. Another potential portal of entry for exogenous antigens is the gut. Schatteman (46) found that 30% of patients with axial involvement had evidence of gut inflammation compared with 20% with oligoarticular disease and 0% of patients with polyarticular disease. These findings are consonant with the notion that PSA may be a reactive arthritis to bowel or psoriatic plaque flora (47). Possible triggering antigens include streptococcal cell-wall proteins (48) and staphylococcal superantigens (49). If there were a specific antigen involved in the immunopathogenesis of PSA, an oligoclonality of the T-cell receptor among synovial T cells would be expected. In one case study, such an oligoclonality was demonstrated (50). In contrast, in a flow cytometry study of synoviocyte T cell–receptor-β chain expression, oligoclonal expansion was not seen (51).

The distinct clinical features of PSA compared with RA may be the result of a differential expression of cytokines at the enthesis versus the synovium (14). RA patients have higher levels of synovial fluid interleukin-6 (IL-6) and IL-8 than patients with PSA and osteoarthritis (OA), whereas PSA subjects had higher levels of IL-13 than RA patients (52). Analysis of T cells in synovial fluid has revealed a reversal of the CD4:CD8 ratio in PSA compared to RA (0.7 versus 1.1), with activated (HLA-DR$^+$) and mature (CD45RO$^+$) CD8$^+$ T cells predominating (53). Proinflammatory cytokines such as TNF-α appear to be central to the disease, because TNF-α blockade has been shown to effectively improve clinical outcome in PSA and joint erosions and accelerated progression of erosive disease in early PSA have been associated with TNF-α −308 and TNF-β +252 polymorphisms (54). Activated T cells have been shown to produce cytokines such as interferon-γ and RANKL, which stimulate osteoclastogenesis. The activation of T cells in patients with PSA has been ascribed to the "arthritogenic peptide" theory. This postulates that a currently unknown peptide fragment interacts with HLA-B27 on the surface of antigen-presenting cells and that this HLA-peptide complex stimulates cytotoxic CD8$^+$ lymphocytes (55). It is thought that the "unknown" peptide is probably of bacterial origin as several bacteria have been associated with spondyloarthropathies (*Salmonella, Shigella, Yersinia,* and *Campylobacter* in reactive arthritis, and *Chlamydia* and *Streptococcus* in the case of guttate psoriasis).

The dual role of T cells in immunobiology and skeletal biology provides a possible link between HLA-B27, proinflammatory cytokines, and bone cells in PSA (56). McGonagle has proposed the following hypothesis to link enthesopathy to the HLA-B27 gene. The normal enthesis is a site of increased biomechanical stress. In both mechanically induced and an inflammatory enthesopathy, there are varying degrees of microtrauma in the underlying bone. When this occurs in mechanically induced plantar fasciitis or in non–B27-related spondyloarthropathies, the degree of bone pathology is usually limited. However, in B27-positive subjects with spondyloarthropathy, these bone changes trigger an autoimmune response to a native protein in either the fibrocartilage adjacent to the bone or the bone itself (15).

CLINICAL FEATURES

In most cases, the diagnosis of PSA is readily made on the basis of characteristic findings that occur in combination (Table 65.1).

Prevalence

A review of community-based research suggests an incidence rate for PSA of about 6/100,000 per annum, and a prevalence of about 1/1,000 (57). PSA is found in about 15% of patients attending early arthritis clinics (58).

Age at Onset

Whereas uncomplicated psoriasis usually appears in the second and third decades, the onset of associated arthritis is commonly delayed by some two decades (59). A juvenile onset of PSA is well recognized; the age at onset is usually between 9 and 12 years (60,61). There appears to be a bimodality of age at onset, with a stronger familial tendency, a history of antecedent skin lesions, and fewer actively inflamed joints in the early onset group.

Sex Ratio

The reported male/female ratio in PSA has varied widely in different surveys. Data pooled from 10 different studies indicated a male-to-female ratio of 1:1.04 (8); this contrasts with the approximately 3:1 female preponderance in seropositive RA.

Patterns of Onset and Distribution

In the majority of patients, there is a lag of approximately two decades between the onset of psoriasis and the evolution

TABLE 65.1. *Clinical features of psoriatic arthritis in patients from two centers*

Features (%)	Jones et al. (84)	Veale et al. (86)
Oligoarticular	22	43
Polyarticular	63	33
Predominant DIP	1	16
Spondyloarthropathy	6	2
Arthritis mutilans	4	2
SAPHO	1	2
Nail involvement	67	57
Monoarthritis	4	NG
Back pain	NG	44

DIP, distal interphalangeal; SAPHO, synovitis, acne, pustulosis, hyperostosis, and osteitis; NG, not given.

of PSA. Biondi-Oriente et al. (62) studied 647 patients with psoriasis; PSA developed in 138 of these patients. Psoriasis antedated the arthritis in 68% of patients and followed it in 21% (62); an isochronous onset occurred in 11%. There is a well-recognized association between trauma to a joint and a flare of PSA in that same joint (63–68). An explosive onset of severe skin disease and arthritis, or a dramatic change in the severity of skin disease with an associated arthritis, is a clue to an associated HIV infection (29,30,34–36).

PSA is readily recognized on presentation as an oligoarticular arthritis with predominant involvement of distal interphalangeal (DIP) joints and flexor tenosynovitis; this is not the most common presentation (69). Several large surveys have indicated that an oligoarticular distribution occurs in only 16% to 30% of patients, whereas a polyarticular pattern is seen in 40% to 60% (70,71).

Two recent studies, each with 100 patients, found somewhat different patterns of presentation (Table 65.1). Five clinical patterns of PSA are recognized:

Group 1: Predominant involvement of DIP joints. As an isolated finding in the absence of other joint involvement, DIP changes in PSA occur in only about 8% to 16% of patients.

Group 2: Arthritis mutilans. Arthritis mutilans is due to osteolysis of the phalanges and metacarpals. It occurs in about 5% of patients and is often associated with sacroiliitis. The designation of arthritis mutilans is usually applied to the hands (Fig. 65.1), but a similar involvement may occur in the feet.

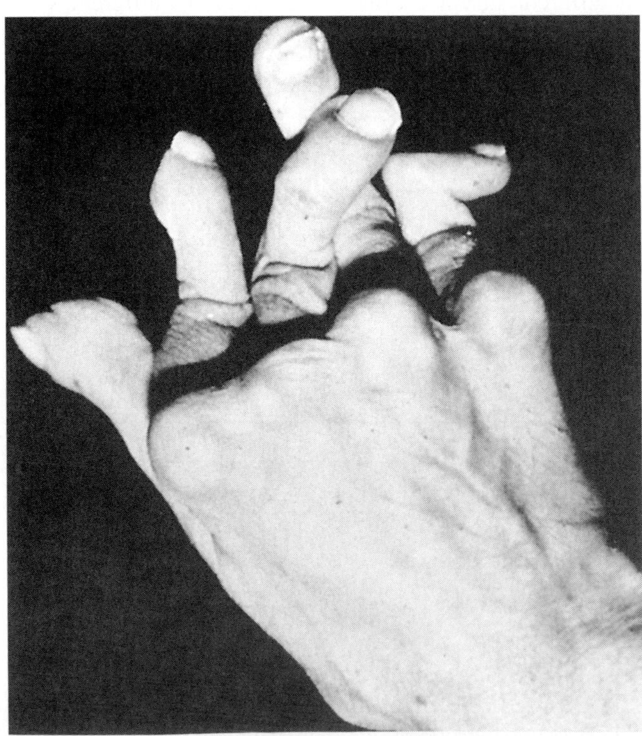

FIG. 65.1. Severe resorptive arthropathy resulting in arthritis mutilans.

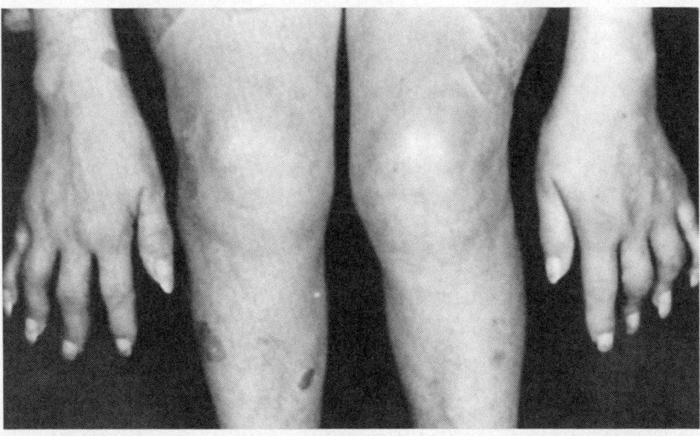

FIG. 65.2. Asymmetric polyarthritis resembling rheumatoid arthritis in a patient with psoriasis.

Group 3: Symmetric polyarthritis. The presentation with symmetric polyarthritis is similar to that of RA, and several studies have noted this to be the most common pattern of joint involvement in psoriasis (Fig. 65.2). Compared with RA, there is a higher frequency of DIP involvement and a tendency for bony ankylosis of the DIP and proximal interphalangeal (PIP) joints, leading to claw deformities of the hands (Fig. 65.3).

Group 4: Oligoarticular arthritis. This is the most characteristic pattern of joint involvement in psoriasis. It is an asymmetric arthritis usually involving scattered DIP, PIP, metacarpophalangeal (MCP), and metatarsophalangeal (MTP) joints. Involvement of an MCP and PIP joint with an associated flexor tenosynovitis is a common occurrence, seen as a "sausage" digit (Fig. 65.4). This pattern of joint involvement is seen in approximately 15% to 40% of patients.

Group 5: Axial involvement. Both sacroiliitis and spondylitis are associated with PSA; however, this is seldom the presenting complaint and usually occurs after several years of peripheral joint disease (72–74). Unlike AS, there is a ten-

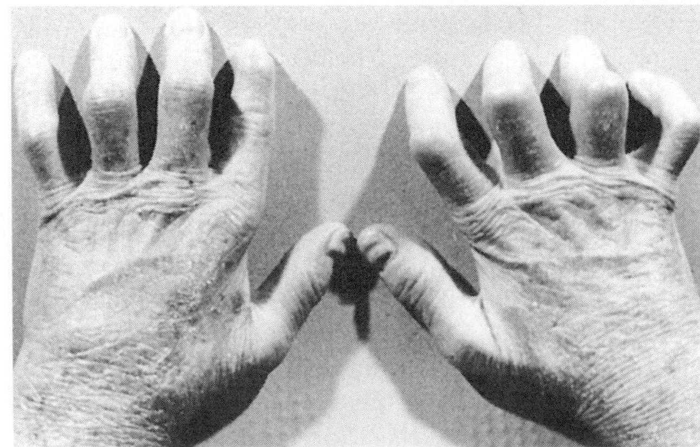

FIG. 65.3. Long-standing psoriatic arthritis with a symmetric distribution. This patient had a "claw deformity" due to bony ankylosis of the proximal and distal interphalangeal joints.

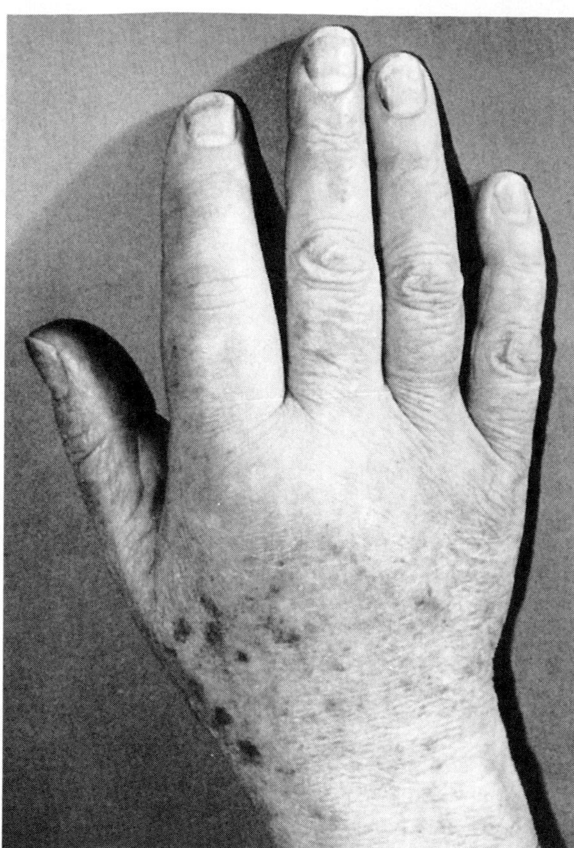

FIG. 65.4. Psoriatic arthritis involving the metacarpophalangeal and proximal interphalangeal joints of the index finger with an associated flexor tenosynovitis. This combination gives rise to the "sausage" digit.

dency for the sacroiliac involvement to be asymmetric and to have a predilection for atypical syndesmophytes that affect random segments of the spine. A spondylitis-like picture occurs in 20% to 40% of patients with PSA (71). In comparison with classic AS, psoriatic patients often display discordance between the occurrence of sacroiliitis and spondylitis. Lambert and Wright (75) found spondylitis in 40% of 130 patients with PSA, but only 21% had sacroiliitis. Sixty percent of patients with syndesmophytes had normal sacroiliac joints, and they had no more symptoms or signs of spinal disease than did those with normal spinal radiographs. Axial involvement occurred mostly in men (male/female ratio, 6:1), and the onset of psoriasis was somewhat later in life.

Gladman et al. (76) compared PSA spondyloarthropathy and classic AS. Patients with AS had more symptoms of inflammatory back and neck pain and a greater limitation of lumbar and cervical spine motion. Radiologically, they had more grade IV sacroiliitis and classic syndesmophytes. Salvarani et al. (77) described two major forms of cervical spine involvement in psoriatic spondyloarthropathy: (a) an inflammatory erosive-subluxing presentation resembling RA occurred in 26% of patients, of whom 53% had subaxial subluxations; and (b) an AS-like picture that occurred in 44%. There was no sacroiliac joint involvement in 36% (all in this latter group were $B27^-$). Predictors of an inflammatory RA presentation included HLA-B39, HLA-DR4, and radiocarpal erosions. Cervical spine involvement may rarely cause neurologic compromise—in one case, a patient with both atlantoaxial subluxation and multiple subaxial subluxations developed neurologic compromise at several levels and required surgery (78).

Psoriatic Arthritis and Trauma

The observation that PSA is sometimes closely associated with trauma to the involved joint continues to be reported (63–67). Scarpa et al. (68) reviewed the occurrence of environmental triggers in 138 patients with PSA and compared them with 138 patients with RA. Specific triggering events were described in 9% of PSA patients but only in 1% of RA patients. The initiating events in PSA were operations (four patients); trauma (three patients); abortions (three patients); and one patient each with myocardial infarction, thrombophlebitis, and drug toxicity. Two small series described the occurrence of PSA in association with reflex sympathetic dystrophy (67,79). Finger dactylitis and pitting edema over the dorsum of the hand has been reported after contusive trauma to the hand in a patient with long-standing *psoriasis sine arthritis* (80).

Pregnancy and Hormonal Issues

The effects of pregnancy and menopause were studied in relation to the expression of PSA in 33 patients (81); 33% had onset of arthritis within 3 months after delivery, and 15% had a perimenopausal flare. Ostensen (82) noted that PSA either improved or remitted in 80% of pregnancies, with a postpartum flare noted in 70%. An interesting case study reported cyclic flares of PSA associated with menstruation (83); there was a marked improvement in symptoms and joint count when estrogen production was suppressed.

Skin and Nail Findings

Skin lesions usually antedate the appearance of PSA by one to two decades. Biondi et al. (62) reported the following patterns of psoriasis in association with PSA: vulgaris, 85%; eruptive, 11%; erythrodermic, 2.5%; and pustular, 1.2%. The evolution of mild skin disease to a widespread erythrodermic pattern with an associated flare in arthritis may represent a clue to an associated HIV infection. In a minority of patients, in which the arthritis appears first, it is difficult to make a definitive diagnosis of PSA. Indeed verification of the correct diagnosis is apparent only retrospectively. In the assessment of such patients, it is important to search carefully for the psoriatic lesions in hidden areas (e.g., scalp, perineum, natal cleft, or umbilicus). When attempting to ascertain the presence of minimal psoriasis,

TABLE 65.2. *Criteria for diagnosis of borderline psoriasis*

1. Psoriasis of the scalp must be palpable
2. Presumed scalp psoriasis, simulating dandruff, must exhibit normal skin between plaques
3. In the presence of eczema or seborrheic states, lesions other than classic plaques cannot be accepted as psoriasis
4. Toenail lesions alone cannot be accepted as evidence of psoriasis
5. In the absence of psoriasis elsewhere, only classic nail changes (i.e., pitting, onycholysis, and discoloration of the lateral nail edge) can be accepted as unequivocal psoriasis. In such cases, fungal infection should be excluded by microscopy and culture
6. Flexural lesions can be accepted only if they have the classic appearance of a psoriatic plaque. In such cases, microscopy of scrapings must be done to exclude Tinea or Candida infection
7. Pustular lesions of the palms and soles are not acceptable unless accompanied by classic skin or nail lesions elsewhere

there are several pitfalls to be avoided, and it is useful to bear in mind the criteria laid down by Baker (6) (Table 65.2).

Nail involvement is often a useful clue in diagnosing PSA. Jones et al. (84) found psoriatic nail changes in 63% of PSA patients compared with 37% of patients with psoriasis alone. In those patients in whom arthritis preceded skin lesions, 88% were noted to have psoriatic nail changes. In another study, nails were involved in 86.5% of patients with PSA (85). The most common findings are pitting in the fingernails and subungual hyperkeratosis in the toenails. Other types of nail involvement include onycholysis (Fig. 65.5), transverse ridges, leukonychia, and crumbling. There is a moderate correlation between DIP involvement and nail changes (86). Interestingly, the presence of nail lesions has been reported as favoring a better prognosis (87). Abnormal nail findings are

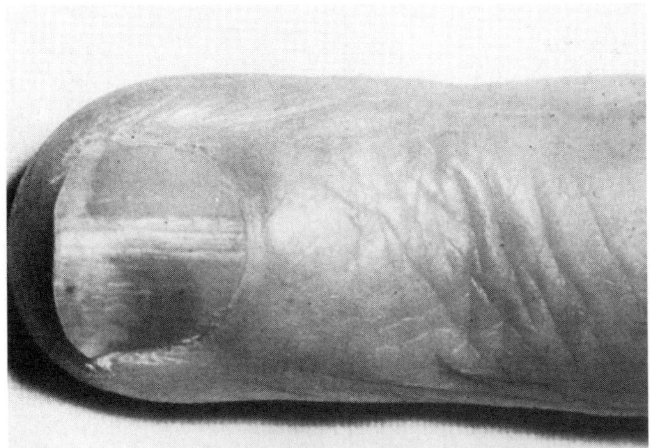

FIG. 65.5. Onycholysis plus psoriasis of the nail bed in a patient who had an oligoarticular pattern of arthritis.

not specific for psoriasis, and the differential diagnosis includes fungal and bacterial infections, alopecia areata, lichen planus, and trauma. Fungal infections that frequently cause hyperkeratosis and onycholysis are *Trichophyton rubrum* and *T. mentagrophytes*. When in doubt, nail clippings should be examined for fungus by using potassium hydroxide preparations and cultures. It is important to note that healthy individuals often have a few nail pits, but these are usually shallow and more irregular than those found in psoriatic patients. Wright and Moll (88) stated that 20 pits are suggestive of PSA, and more than 60 are diagnostic.

Unusual Syndromes Associated with Psoriatic Arthritis

Several interrelated syndromes have been associated with PSA (Table 65.3). The synovitis, acne, pustulosis, hyperostosis, and osteitis syndrome (SAPHO) is increasingly being recognized as an association with PSA (89–92). Such patients often have an anterior chest wall syndrome or unexplained bone pain. Chest computed tomography (CT) shows involvement of the sternoclavicular joint, often in association with sternocostoclavicular hyperostosis (Fig. 65.6). Long bones may be involved and be misdiagnosed as osteomyelitis or Ewing sarcoma. Joint involvement is seen as an acute pseudoinfectious arthritis, unresponsive to antibiotics, which may be rapidly destructive. This syndrome was initially described in association with acne conglobata; however, the most frequently associated skin condition is palmoplantar pustulosis. Other associations include psoriasis, Crohn disease, ulcerative colitis, various manifestations of severe acne, and even dissecting cellulitis.

Palmoplantar pustulosis may occur as part of the SAPHO syndrome or alone. In isolated cases, the predominant complaint is chest wall pain due to chronic inflammation of bone and entheses related to the sternum, manubriosternum, and clavicle (92,93).

Spondylodiscitis is found in about 30% of patients with SAPHO, and more rarely in association with palmoplantar pustulosis, psoriasis *sine* joint involvement, and chronic multifocal recurrent osteomyelitis (94). The discitis is due to noninfectious disc inflammation with an associated enthesitis. Symptoms relate predominantly to chest wall pain.

Psoriatic onychopachydermoperiostitis refers to a noninfectious thickening of the skin overlying the terminal phalanx of the first toe (95). Only minimal evidence of psoriasis or PSA may be present.

TABLE 65.3. *Unusual syndromes associated with psoriatic arthritis*

SAPHO (synovitis, acne, pustulosis, hyperostosis, and osteitis)
Spondylodiscitis
Palmar plantar pustulosis
Psoriatic onychopachydermoperiostitis
Chronic multifocal recurrent osteomyelitis

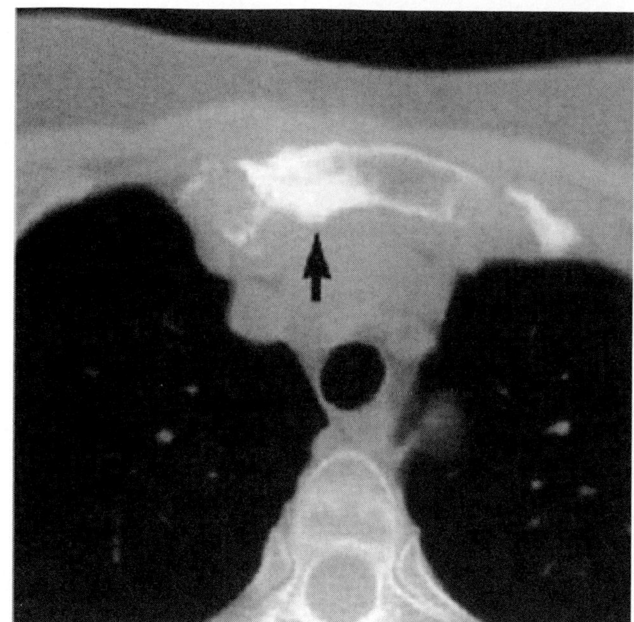

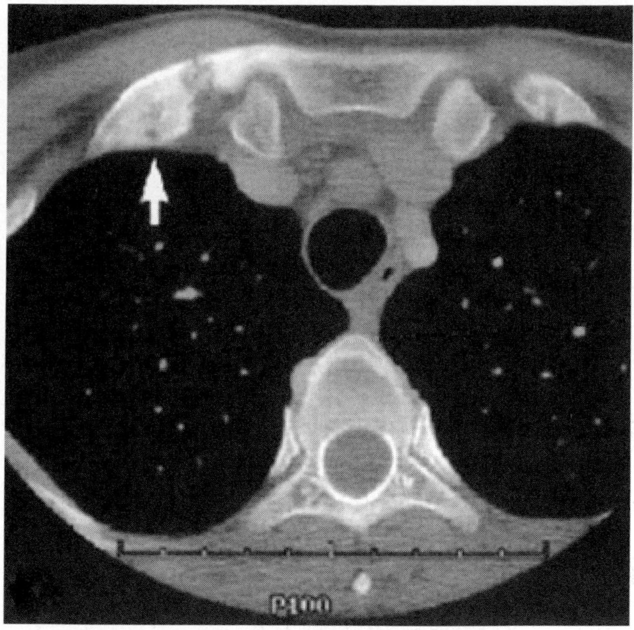

FIG. 65.6. Radiologic findings in SAPHO (synovitis, acne, pustulosis, hyperostosis, and osteitis). **A:** Computed tomography (CT) of chest showing an expanded and sclerotic manubrium. **B:** CT chest showing an expanded and sclerotic first rib with lytic areas and overlying soft tissue swelling. (From Van Doornum S, Barraclough D, McColl G, Wicks I. SAPHO: rare or just not recognized? *Semin Arthritis Rheum* 2000;30(1):70—77, with permission.)

Chronic multifocal recurrent osteomyelitis is a noninfectious bone lesion that typically involves the clavicles and long bones. Symptomatically these patients have intermittent fever with local swelling and pain (96). Radiographs suggest infectious osteomyelitis. Associated features may include palmoplantar pustulosis and psoriasis (97,98).

Extraarticular Associations

In contradistinction to RA, vasculitis and its clinical correlates are not seen in PSA. Inflammatory eye disease occurs in about 30% of patients with PSA. The diagnoses made in one report were conjunctivitis, 19.6%; iritis, 7.1%; episcleritis, 1.8%; and keratoconjunctivitis sicca, 2.7% (99). Of those patients with iritis, 43% had sacroiliitis and 40% were positive for HLA-B27, whereas tests for antinuclear antibodies (ANA) were negative in all patients with iritis (99). A small number of patients with PSA have a chronic bilateral uveitis that is predominantly posterior and may be refractory to therapy (100). This presentation is mainly seen in HLA-B27$^+$ males and may be the presenting feature of the PSA.

One study described an increased prevalence (11%) of renal involvement in PSA; the major features were hematuria, proteinuria, or cylindruria (101). A Swedish study suggested that renal involvement is more common than previously thought; that is, if it is specifically evaluated by appropriate testing (102). Out of 33 patients with PSA, 23.3% had renal abnormalities as defined by creatinine clearance below the lower cutoff of normal distribution or urinary excretion of albumin more than 25 mg/24 hours. Those with renal involvement tended to have increased serum β_2-microglobulin and acute phase elevations (erythrocyte sedimentation rate [ESR] and C-reactive protein [CRP]).

Mitral valve prolapse was reported in 14 (56%) of 25 patients with PSA compared with only 6.4% of psoriatic patients without arthritis (103); aortic regurgitation also has been noted (104). A well-documented, but inexplicable, association with myopathy has been described (105). An occasional association with Sjögren syndrome (SS) has been described (106,107). Collins et al. (108) studied 36 patients with PSA and compared them with patients with psoriasis alone; they found that patients with arthritis had a reduced stimulated salivary flow rate and one patient had definite SS. A more recent study using the European criteria for SS reported that 31.7% of women with various spondyloarthropathies, compared to 2.9% of controls, had SS (109). A positive ANA was found in 50% of patients and HLA-B27 was present in 84.6% of the patients with SS.

Single case reports have described amyloidosis (110), immunoglobulin A (IgA) nephropathy with an interstitial pneumonia (111), and pyoderma gangrenosum (112). Upper or lower distal extremity swelling (usually unilateral) with pitting edema was reported to be more common in PSA than in RA (21% versus 5%). The swelling was due to tenosynovitis and was the presenting feature in 20% of patients subsequently diagnosed with PSA (113).

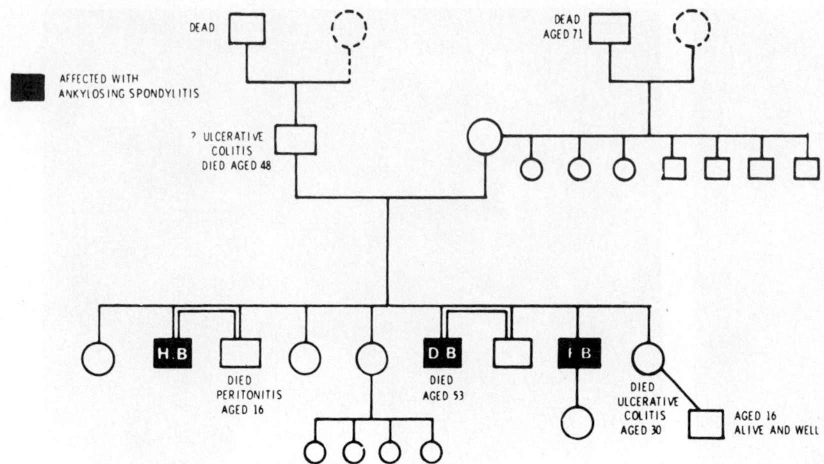

FIG. 65.7. Family study in which psoriasis, ulcerative colitis, and ankylosing spondylitis showed a "clustering" phenomenon. Patients DB and FB have psoriasis in addition to ankylosing spondylitis.

Fibromyalgia is probably a common association with PSA, as in other rheumatic disorders; in one study global ratings of patient satisfaction with health were associated with American College of Rheumatology (ACR) functional class and number of fibromyalgia tender points rather than with traditional clinical measures of inflammation and damage (114).

Disease Interrelations

The seronegative arthritides often display common features, the most frequent being sacroiliitis, spondylitis, and ocular inflammation in the setting of HLA-B27 positivity. Because HLA-B27 is strongly associated with an inherited susceptibility to both sacroiliitis and iritis, these common features may be manifestations of a shared genetic background rather than "specific complications" per se. Conditions described or associated with PSA include ulcerative colitis (115), AS (116,117), Crohn's disease (115), reactive arthritis (118), and Behçet's syndrome (119). Sometimes a striking familial clustering of these diseases is seen, as shown in Fig. 65.7; in this family, psoriasis, ulcerative colitis, and AS were grouped together over two generations (116).

LABORATORY FINDINGS

Other than the finding of a negative rheumatoid factor (RF), there are no laboratory tests that aid in the diagnosis of either psoriasis or PSA (120). Positive tests for RF in psoriatic patients with coexistent erosive arthritis most likely reflect the concurrent presence of RA and psoriasis. Analysis of synovial fluid usually reveals an inflammatory picture with elevated leukocytes (predominantly neutrophils). The occasional occurrence of ANA in patients with PSA has a prevalence comparable to that of the normal population. Circulating immune complexes have been detected in up to 50% of patients with both psoriasis and PSA; one report indicates that these are predominantly of the IgA isotype (121). Hyperuricemia occurs in 10% to 20% of patients and has been related to the severity of the skin disease (122). Presumably, this reflects increased nucleoprotein catabolism due to rapid cell turnover, although Lambert and Wright (123) suggest that elevated uric acid levels in PSA are a complication of therapy rather than disease-related.

IMAGING

Radiographs of patients with PSA exhibit several discriminatory features in comparison to RA. Marginal erosions often have proliferative new bone formation, and there may be joint fusion, acroosteolysis, and periostitis (69). In contradistinction to RA, bone density in PSA is usually preserved (124). This tendency to less bone loss has been confirmed by both neutron activation analysis of calcium turnover (125) and osteocalcin levels (126). Technetium-99m Dicarroxy Propane Diphosonate (DPD) and F18-fluorodeoxyglucose-positron emission tomography (FDG PET) scanning can be useful for obtaining an overall assessment of bone involvement in PSA and may identify unsuspected SAPHO (127). Technetium-labeled IgG scanning has been reported to be useful in delineating early joint involvement in PSA (128). Magnetic resonance imaging (MRI) appears to be especially useful in demonstrating enthesopathy, osteitis, and bone marrow edema (129,130) (Fig 65.8). Distinctive radiographic features of PSA include asymmetric oligoarticular distribution, relative absence of oligoarticular osteopenia, involvement of the DIP joints, and involvement of the sacroiliac joints (131,132). Less common findings include (a) erosion of terminal phalangeal tufts (acroosteolysis) (Fig. 65.8); (b) whittling of phalanges and of metacarpal and metatarsal joints (Fig. 65.9); (c) cupping of the proximal portion of the phalanges (Fig. 65.9); (d) bony ankylosis (Fig. 65.10); (e) destruction of isolated small joints (Fig. 65.11); (f) predilection for DIP and PIP joints with relative sparing of MCP and MTP

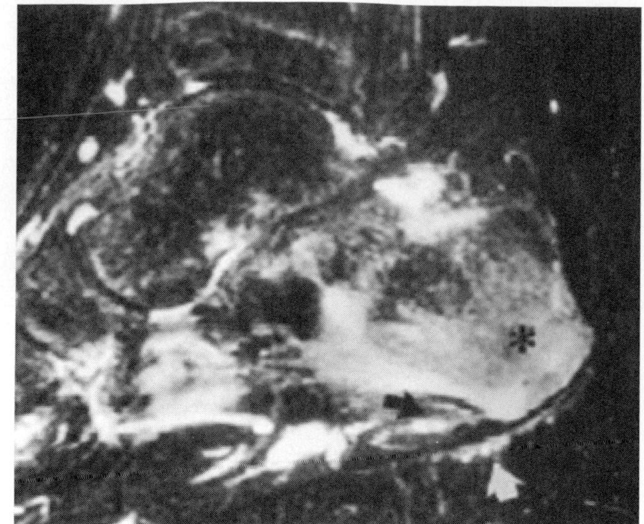

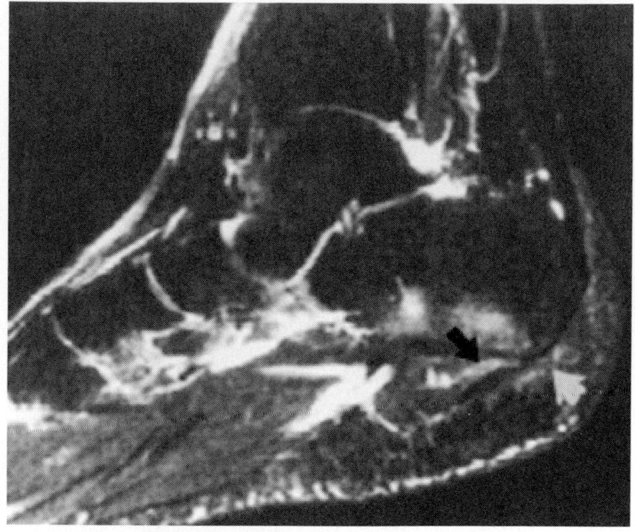

FIG. 65.8. Magnetic resonance images of the heel using T2 fat-supressed sagittal sequences in two patients with acute plantar fasciitis. **A:** HLA-B27–positive patient with spondylarthropathy (SpA), showing severe bone edema in the calcaneum (*). There is also soft tissue edema in the superficial (*white arrow*) and deep (*black arrow*) soft tissues surrounding the insertion of the plantar fascia. **B:** HLA-B27–negative patient with mechanically induced plantar fasciitis, showing soft tissue edema in the superficial (*white arrow*) and deep (*black arrow*) soft tissues surrounding the insertion of the plantar fascia, but less extensive than that in the SpA patient. The extent of bone edema in these patients was comparable to that seen in HLA-B27–negative patients with SpA. (From McGonagle D, Marzo-Ortega H, O'Connor P, et al. The role of biomechanical factors and HLA-B27 in magnetic resonance imaging-determined bone changes in plantar fascia enthesopathy. *Arthritis Rheum* 2002; 46(2):489–493, with permission.)

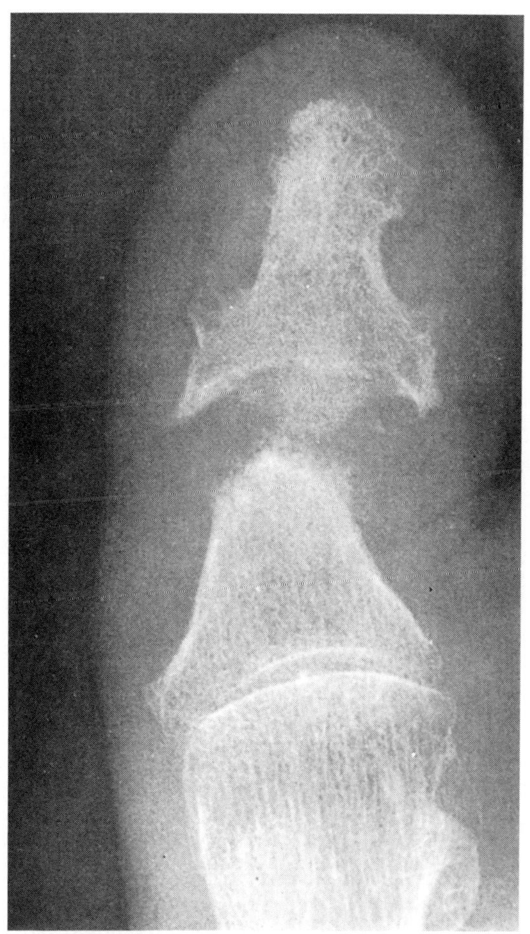

FIG. 65.9. "Whittling" of the middle phalanx and expansion of the base of the distal phalanx—the "pencil-in-cup" deformity.

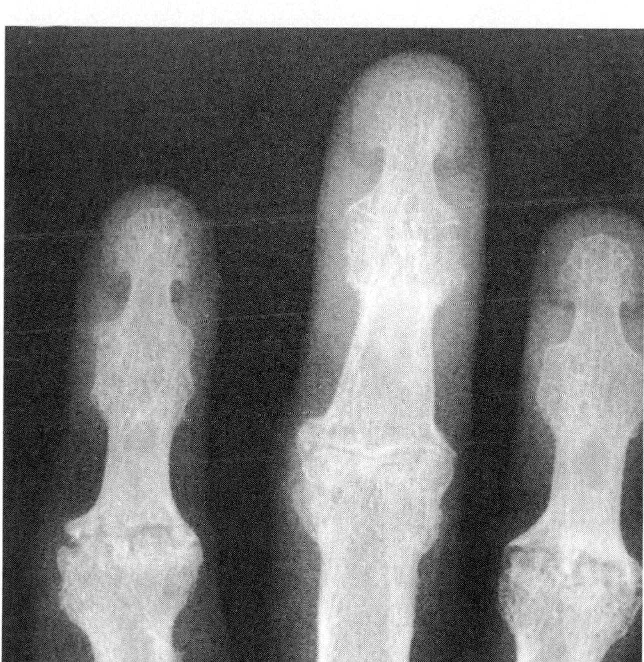

FIG. 65.10. Bony ankylosis of distal interphalangeal joints in a patient with psoriatic arthritis.

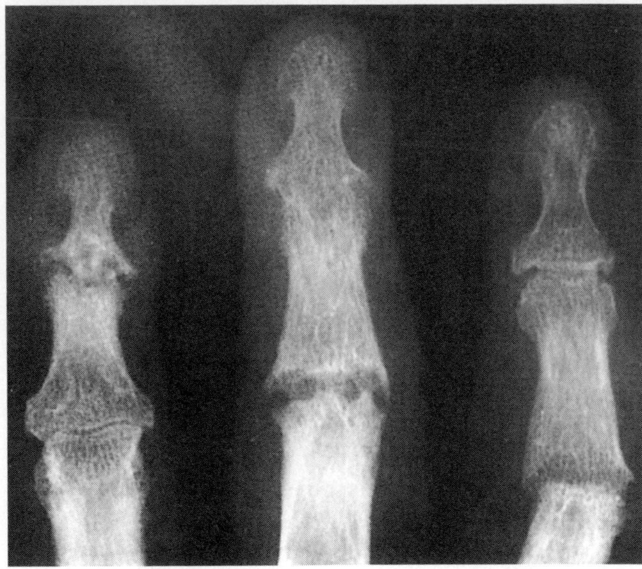

FIG. 65.11. Complete destruction of middle proximal interphalangeal joint. Also note bony ankylosis of corresponding distal interphalangeal joint.

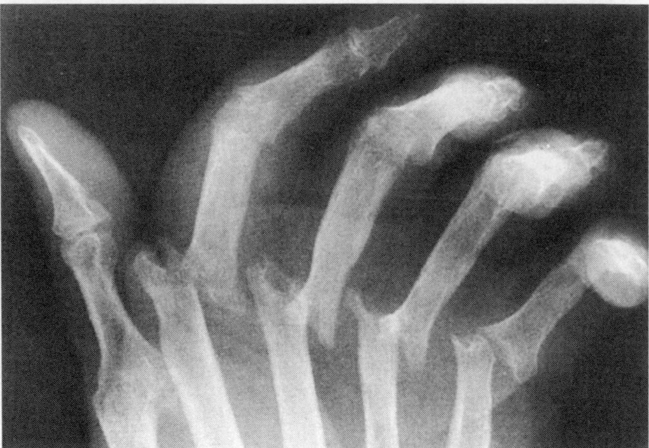

FIG. 65.13. Osteolysis of bones of metacarpophalangeal joints with resulting subluxations.

joints (Figs. 65.12 and 64.13); (g) osteolysis of bones (arthritis mutilans), particularly the metatarsals (Fig. 65.14); and (h) relative lack of osteoporosis when compared with a similar degree of joint involvement in RA. Findings in the axial skeleton include (a) paravertebral ossification (133)—this is not unique to psoriasis, as it is seen in senile ankylosing hyperostosis, diffuse idiopathic skeletal hyperostosis (DISH), paraplegia, fluorosis, hypoparathyroidism, familial hypophosphatemia, and hereditary/familial articular and vascular calcification; (b) atypical syndesmophytes—often present without sacroiliitis (75) (Fig. 65.15); (c) asymmet-

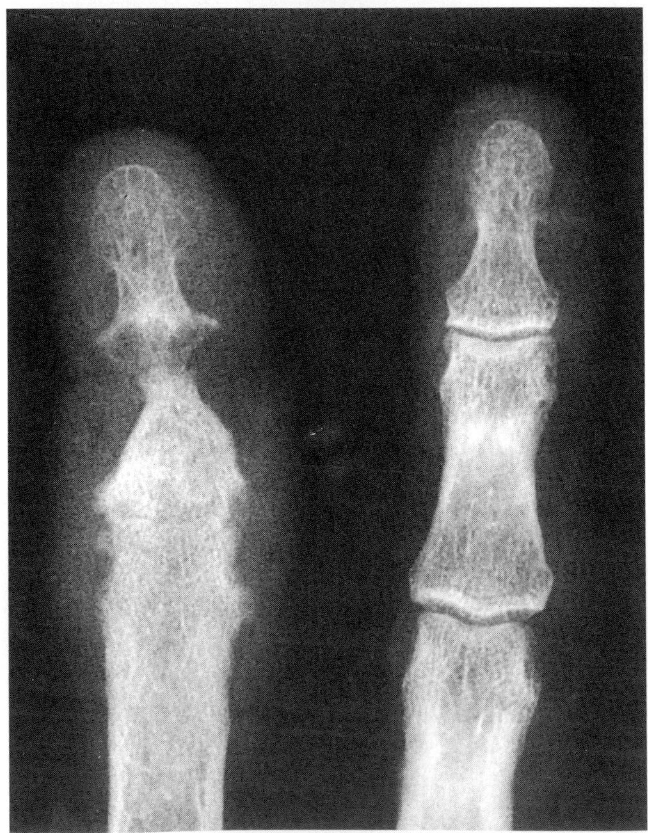

FIG. 65.12. Destructive arthritis of an isolated distal interphalangeal joint with osteolysis of the proximal phalanx.

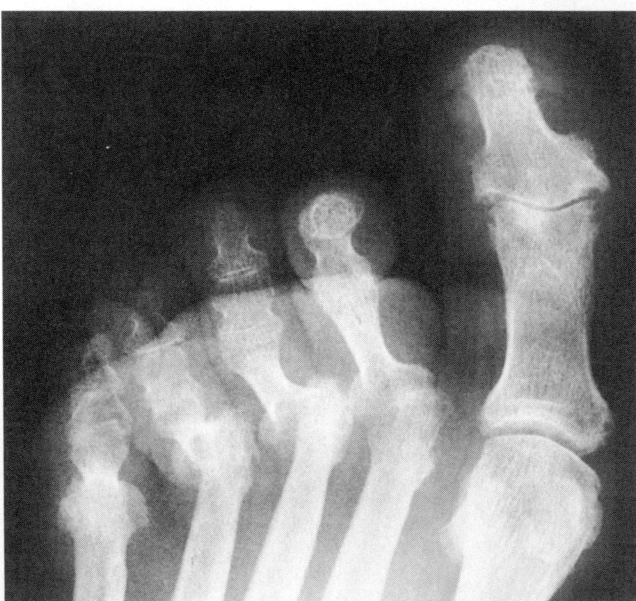

FIG. 65.14. Prominent metatarsophalangeal joint involvement with subluxation and cupping of the base of the proximal phalanges. The big toe distal interphalangeal joint shows characteristic marginal erosions.

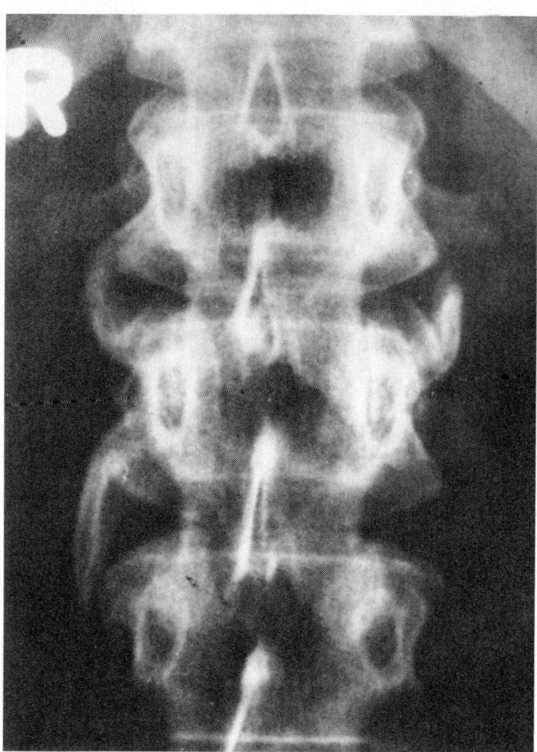

FIG. 65.15. Psoriatic arthritis with axial involvement. The patient was HLA-B27+ and had no radiologic evidence of sacroiliitis, but atypical syndesmophytes are observed.

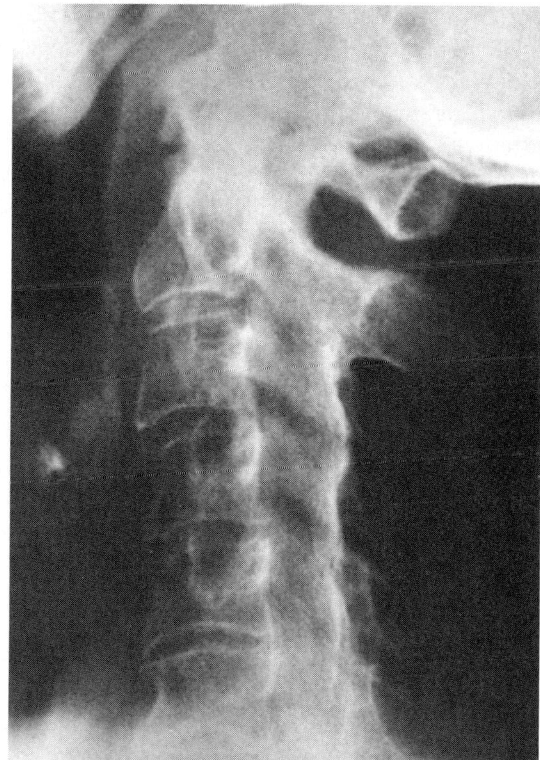

FIG. 65.16. Ankylosis of cervical apophyseal joints in a patient with psoriatic spondylitis in association with bilateral sacroiliitis.

ric sacroiliitis (134); (d) solid fusion of thoracic vertebrae (135); (e) rarity of the typical bamboo spine of AS (135); (f) a tendency for cervical spine disease to exhibit intervertebral disc-space narrowing and ankylosis (Fig. 65.16); and (g) apophyseal sclerosis and interspinous or anterior ligamentous calcification (131). Upper cervical spine disease occurs with both atlantoaxial fusion and subluxation (136–138). Involvement of the upper cervical spine can be associated with either ankylosis or with atlantoaxial subluxation as observed in RA (136–139). Temporomandibular joint involvement with condylar erosions and condylar osteolysis is a well-recognized feature of the disease (94, 140), and ultrasound imaging is a useful tool in its evaluation (141).

DIFFERENTIAL DIAGNOSIS

A diagnosis of PSA is usually obvious in a patient with inflammatory arthritis occurring in association with unequivocal psoriasis (Table 65.4). Problems arise when evidence for psoriasis is lacking or ambiguous; in such cases, it is useful to follow the guidelines for the diagnosis of borderline psoriasis (Table 65.2). Seborrheic dermatitis resembles scalp psoriasis, whereas fungal infections may mimic psoriatic nail involvement. Nail pitting alone lacks specificity in differentiating between psoriasis and other conditions such as exfoliative dermatitis and eczema. Isolated nail pitting is a normal occurrence; 20 fingernail pits suggests psoriasis, and more than 60 pits are virtually never found in the absence of psoriasis (88). Keratoderma blennorrhagicum, as seen in reactive arthritis, is indistinguishable both clinically and histologically from pustular psoriasis. Because mild conjunctivitis may occur in psoriasis, it cannot be relied on to differentiate reactive arthritis from PSA (99). Primary OA bears a superficial resemblance to DIP involvement in PSA; in such instances, the presence of Heberden and Bouchard nodes and involvement of the first carpometacarpal joint may help establish a diagnosis

TABLE 65.4. *Clinical characteristics suggestive of psoriatic arthritis*

Involvement of DIP joints in absence of primary osteoarthritis
Asymmetric joint involvement
Absence of rheumatoid factor and subcutaneous nodules
Flexor tenosynovitis and "sausage" digits
A family history of psoriatic arthritis
Significant nail pitting (>20 pits)
Axial radiographs showing one or more of the following: sacroiliitis, syndesmophytes (often "atypical"), and paravertebral ossification
Peripheral radiographs showing an erosive arthritis with a relative lack of osteopenia; in particular, DIP erosions with expansion of the base of the terminal phalanx and terminal phalangeal osteolysis

of OA. Erosive OA may be mistaken for PSA, but in typical cases, the "mouse ear" radiologic findings of psoriatic involvement are readily distinguished from the "gull wing" appearance of OA. Acute-onset PSA, involving the knee and first toe, may resemble gout; in such cases, joint aspiration for the detection of urate crystals is advised. Occasionally both gout and pseudogout occur in association with well-defined PSA. PSA may flare after trauma to a joint. Persistence of a "traumatic arthritis," in association with an inflammatory joint fluid, should suggest that the patient may have early PSA (6,63).

JUVENILE PSORIATIC ARTHRITIS

There is a bimodality in age of onset of PSA (24). Patients with childhood onset, when followed into adulthood, have a stronger genetic component, a more frequent history of antecedent skin lesions, and fewer actively inflamed joints than the late-onset group.

Biondi-Oriente et al. (142) reported PSA in only 1% of 425 cases of psoriasis starting in childhood. Koo et al. (143) reported a 1.6% prevalence of PSA in 664 Hungarian children with juvenile chronic arthritis. Southwood et al. (61) proposed criteria for the definition of juvenile PSA. Definite juvenile PSA was defined as arthritis with a typical psoriatic rash, plus at least three of four of these minor criteria: dactylitis, nail pitting, psoriasis-like rash, or family history of psoriasis. Probable juvenile PSA was defined as arthritis plus two of the minor criteria. Sills (144) reported that the female-to-male ratio in juvenile PSA is about 3:2, in contradistinction to the 1:1 ratio in adults.

The mean age of onset for both juvenile psoriasis and PSA is 9 to 12 years, with the arthritis antedating the skin changes in 50% of patients. The onset tends to be more acute than in adults, with a monoarticular onset in about one-third of cases. In another study, the onset of PSA was usually pauciarticular but progressed to a polyarticular course in 66% of patients (20). A sausage digit was the presenting feature in 12% of children and occurred at some stage in 23%.

Another distinction from adult PSA is the occurrence of hip involvement in 30% to 40% of children, sometimes requiring bilateral hip arthroplasty (60). Chronic anterior uveitis was found in 17% of children with PSA and was accompanied by ANA in 63%. In another study, iridocyclitis was found in 8% of children (60); patients with this presentation had an earlier onset (mean, 4 years), most were girls, and they tended to fare poorly. The association of juvenile arthritis and a positive ANA may result in an initial misdiagnosis of pauciarticular juvenile rheumatoid arthritis (JRA). The overall outcome for most patients with juvenile PSA is difficult to ascertain from the current literature. One report suggests a relatively benign course (144). Shore and Ansell (60), however, observed a more severe course, with 35% requiring systemic corticosteroids, and 25% requiring remitting drugs such as gold, penicillamine, or azathioprine.

In some children pauciarticular JRA is difficult to differentiate from juvenile psoriatic PSA. One study found that the odds of a patient with oligoarticular juvenile PSA having small joint disease or wrist disease within 6 months of disease onset was much higher than in patients with oligoarticular JRA (145).

PROGNOSIS

For most patients, PSA is a nuisance rather than a significant cause of persistent dysfunction (146,147). In a 10-year follow-up of 227 patients, only 5% developed a deforming arthritis, and 97 lost less than a year from work (148). However, Gladman et al. (70) have challenged the concept that PSA is generally benign. In a study of 220 patients with PSA, they found a 40% incidence of deforming erosive arthropathy, with 17% of patients having five or more deformed joints. Stage III and IV radiographic changes occurred in 28% and 14% of patients, respectively. Eleven percent of patients had class III or IV functional impairment. On the other hand, the same authors have reported remissions in PSA. In 391 patients with PSA, 69 individuals sustained an average remission of 2.6 years. Male sex, fewer actively inflamed and damaged joints, and better functional class at presentation to clinic were associated with remission (149).

A follow-up study of combined clinical (inflamed joint count, damaged joint count, presence of back involvement, and arthritis mutilans) and radiographic changes in 88 PSA patients found that 49% and 77% showed deterioration at 1 and 5 years, respectively (150). In another follow-up, there was a significant increase in the number of joints involved after 5 years (median 6 versus 11, $p < .001$) and Health Assessment Questionnaire scores (median 0.375 versus 0.5, $p < .001$). The median rate of joint progression was 0.42 peripheral joints per year (range 0–7.2) with the highest involvement in the first year of arthritis (median 4.0 joints/year) (151). A polyarticular onset (five or more swollen joints) of PSA appears to be an independent risk factor which predicts the progression to erosive and deforming disease (152).

Wong et al. (153) documented 53 deaths in a group of 428 patients with PSA. Cardiorespiratory disease accounted for 48% of deaths and cancer accounted for 17%. Prognostic indicators for death were an ESR greater than 15 mm/hour, radiologic evidence of joint destruction, and a history of prior medications for psoriasis. A large study from the Rochester Epidemiology Project did not associate PSA with increased mortality (153a). Other rare problems associated with morbidity are the development of aortic valve incompetence (104) or atrioventricular conduction defects; these complications usually are seen in association with spondylitis. There has been recent interest regarding the effects of coping strategies and learned helplessness in chronic disease as possible predictors of functional outcome. A comparison of patients with RA and PSA found that mood and coping strategies correlated with concurrent functional status and were not predictors of future function (154).

MANAGEMENT

Patients with PSA have to bear the burden of two chronic and currently incurable diseases. Patients with PSA have a similar impairment in their quality of life as patients with RA and report more role limitations due to emotional problems and bodily pain. An important general principle in managing patients with chronic disease is the establishment of a productive dialogue that allows the patient to express fears and obtain enlightened answers. One can be optimistic that most patients with PSA will follow a relatively benign course without serious systemic complications; however, such a generalization is of little solace to patients in whom arthritis mutilans is developing.

Mild Disease

The general principles espoused in the treatment of patients with RA (see Chapter 59) are pertinent to the management of patients with PSA. Many patients with mild disease need only antiinflammatory doses of a nonsteroidal antiinflammatory drug (NSAID). Flares that usually only affect one or two joints, can be effectively treated with local corticosteroid injections. The least soluble preparation, triamcinolone hexacetonide (Aristospan) is the drug of choice because systemic absorption is minimized and the local effect is maximized. A relative contraindication to joint injections is the presence of psoriatic lesions in the overlying skin (155); these are often colonized with staphylococci and streptococci, and at least one case of pyogenic arthritis has been described after intraarticular injections through a psoriatic plaque (88). Leukotrienes have been implicated in the pathogenesis of the skin disease. Thus, it is theoretically possible that strong cyclooxygenase inhibitors may exacerbate the skin lesions by diversion of arachidonic acid metabolites to the lipoxygenase pathway. A flare of skin lesions has occasionally been noted after treatment with indomethacin, phenylbutazone, and oxyphenbutazone (156). Little information exists concerning the role of diet in management of PSA; however, polyunsaturated ethylester lipids (as are commonly found in fish) have been reported to provide a useful adjuvant to the standard therapy (157).

Progressive Disease

At tertiary referral centers, polyarticular joint involvement has been noted in 30% to 60% of patients with PSA and arthritis mutilans occurs in about 5%. Compared with RA, there have been few controlled trials of disease-modifying agents in PSA. Most studies have not adequately separated the response of patients with relatively mild oligoarticular disease from those with polyarticular destructive disease (158).

There is a general agreement that systemic corticosteroids should be avoided in PSA; this advice is not based on their lack of efficacy, but rather on the exacerbation of the skin lesions observed with attempted tapering (159).

Many of the "classic" disease-modifying agents used in the treatment of RA also are used in the treatment of PSA.

Specific Therapeutic Agents

Antimalarials

Antimalarials have been used with enthusiasm by some investigators; one study claimed a 75% response rate to hydroxychloroquine in a dose of 200 to 400 mg/day (160). Gladman et al. (161) reported that 75% of patients taking chloroquine had a greater than 30% reduction in active joint inflammation over a 6-month period compared with 58% of controls. Six patients taking chloroquine had a flare of their psoriasis (but there was no exfoliative dermatitis), and six of the controls experienced a flare of their skin disease.

Gold Salts

Several reports suggested that chrysotherapy is of benefit in PSA. In one study of intramuscular gold, significant improvement occurred in 71% of patients with PSA compared with 60% of patients with RA (162). Treatment with gold sodium thiomalate (GST) and methotrexate (MTX) has been reported to have more toxicities in PSA patients than in RA patients. In a head to head comparison of gold and MTX, the MTX group experienced more benefit (163).

Sulfasalazine

Sulfasalazine has been used in the treatment of PSA with varied results (164–166). A common problem with sulfasalazine is hypersensitivity to the sulfonamide component. McCarthy and Coughlan (167) described a desensitization technique with a 33% success rate in nine patients. Clegg et al. (168) found no significant difference in efficacy between sulfasalazine (2,000 mg/day) and placebo in a 36-week study. Rahman et al. (169) reported a similar failure of sulfasalazine in a 24-month study and noted a 38% dropout rate due to side effects.

Methotrexate

There is a general consensus that cytotoxic agents are of benefit in destructive PSA. The most widely studied and commonly used agent is MTX (170). In 1964, a double-blind study of 21 patients demonstrated that high-dose MTX (3 intramuscular doses of MTX of (1–3 mg/kg) at 10-day intervals) was effective in suppressing both skin and joint manifestations; however, there was a 30% incidence of adverse effects (171). Dermatologists have been especially concerned with MTX-induced liver injury in the treatment of *psoriasis sine arthritis* and have recommended periodic liver biopsies. However, Espinoza et al. (172) found no progression on repeated liver biopsies in 40 patients with PSA and suggested that routine biopsies were not necessary. Fifteen cases of MTX-induced pancytopenia with two deaths were analyzed (173). Risk factors for cytopenia were (a) an elevated creatinine, (b) increasing mean corpuscular volume (MCV), and (c) concomitant therapy with trimethoprim–sulfamethoxazole.

Cyclosporin A

Cyclosporin A (CSA) has been used in patients with severe PSA that is refractory to other treatments (174,175). Salvarani et al. (176) found that 7 of 12 PSA patients had a greater than 50% reduction in active joints, as well as skin improvement; responders exhibited decreased serum levels of the soluble IL-2 receptor (sIL-2R). The efficacy and tolerability of CSA was compared with symptomatic therapy (ST) alone and sulfasalazine (SSZ) (177). Overall, CSA was more efficacious than either SSZ or ST in terms of pain relief, swollen joint count, tender joint count, total Arthritis Impact Measurement Scale score, the ACR 50% and ACR 70% scores, and patient global assessment. The Psoriasis Severity Index was significantly lower in the CSA than in the ST and SSZ groups. The most common adverse event in the CSA group was mild, reversible kidney dysfunction.

Anti-TNF Agents

Etanercept

Etanercept is a soluble TNF-receptor (TNFR) antagonist consisting of two p75 (TNFR) domains fused to the Fc portion of human immunoglobulin. In a 12-week randomized, double-blind, placebo-controlled study, etanercept (25 mg twice-weekly subcutaneous injections) or placebo was evaluated in 60 patients with PSA and psoriasis (178).

The percent of patients achieving an ACR 20%, ACR 50%, and ACR 70% response was 73%, 50% and 13%, respectively, compared to 13%, 3%, and 0% in the placebo group. A median improvement in skin disease activity in the etanercept group was 46% versus 9% in the placebo group (179). In a 6-month open-label extension of this study, the original placebo patients achieved responses to etanercept comparable to the group originally randomized to the active drug. Furthermore, efficacy was maintained in the original group; many patients decreased or discontinued concomitant prednisone or MTX.

Infliximab

Infliximab is a chimeric (murine/human) monoclonal antibody that binds to TNF and thereby inhibits its binding to its receptor. It has also been used with impressive results in the management of PSA. In a 54-week, open-label study, 10 patients received intravenous infliximab (5 mg/kg; weeks 0, 2, and 6 with individualized dosing after week 10). There was a 20% improvement according to the ACR criteria in all patients at week 2; 8 patients improved 70% (ACR 70%) at week 10, and 6 patients maintained a 70% response out to week 54. MRIs at week 10 revealed an 82.5% mean reduction in inflammation compared to baseline. There were no significant adverse events, including severe infections or infusion reactions (180). Two smaller studies have reported similar results (181,182). In the latter study, a reduction in synovial thickness, vascularity, and infiltration with neutrophils/macrophages paralleled the beneficial effect of infliximab.

Alefacept

Alefacept [a lymphocyte function antigen (LFA)-3/human IgG1 fusion protein] is a recently introduced biologic agent that blocks LFA-3 interaction with CD2 and thus dampens T-cell responses. In an open-label study, 11 patients with active PSA were treated with alefacept for 12 weeks and followed clinically with the Disease Activity Score (DAS), synovial biopsies, and T-cell subsets in peripheral blood. There was a reduction in arthritis activity (55% achieved the DAS response criteria), the extent of skin psoriasis, and serum levels of acute-phase reactants. Clinical improvement was associated with a reduction in the number of macrophages and T-effector cells in the synovium (183).

Interleukin-10 (IL-10)

A 28-day double-blind, placebo-controlled study of IL-10 in PSA evaluated clinical disease and synovial/skin biopsies, peripheral blood leukocytes, and MRIs (184). A modest but significant clinical improvement in skin, but not articular, DAS was observed. Overall, there was a modulation of immune responses related to changes in endothelial activation and leukocyte recruitment/effector function.

Other Issues

Severe bone pain may present a problem in some PSA patients; in such cases a diagnosis of SAPHO syndrome should be considered (185) as there are several reports of successful treatment with either pamidronate (186) or infliximab (187,188).

A caveat to the treatment of PSA with cytotoxic agents is the use of these agents in HIV-positive patients. Maurer et al. (189) reported on three HIV-positive patients with PSA treated with MTX; one developed an opportunistic infection.

Surgery

Indications for surgical interventions in PSA are similar to those for RA. Zangger et al. (190) reported a 7% prevalence of joint surgery over a 13-year follow-up in PSA patients. The most common operations were hip and knee replacements followed by MCP arthroplasty and finger or wrist fusion. Wound infection resulting from the skin colonization with pathogenic bacteria is of concern (155); there is an occasional anecdotal report of an infected prosthesis (191). However, it has been shown that the standard procedure for preoperative skin preparation is as effective in sterilizing psoriatic plaques as in uninvolved skin (192). In a review of hand surgery in PSA, two of the most useful procedures were found to be MCP joint arthroplasties and fusion of fixed flexion contractures of the PIP and DIP joints in positions of maximal function (193). There is an increasing awareness that the temporomandibular joint may be involved in PSA and have been described (194).

REFERENCES

1. Alibert JL. *Precis theorique et pratique sur les maladies de la peau.* Paris: Caille et Ravier, 1818.
2. Bazin P. *Theoriques et cliniques sur les affections cutanees de nature arthritique et arthreux.* Paris: Monograph, Delahaye, 1860:154–161.
3. Bourdillon C. *These de Paris* 1888;298.
4. Hench PS. Arthropathia psoriatica—presentation of a case. *Proc Mayo Clin* 1927;2:80–92.
5. Rose HM, Ragan C, Pearce E, et al. Differential agglutination of normal and sensitized sheep erythrocytes by sera of patients with RA. *Proc Soc Exp Biol Med* 1948;68:1–6.
6. Baker H. Epidemiological aspects of psoriasis and arthritis. *Br J Dermatol* 1966;78:249–261
7. Ropes MW, Bennett EA, Cobb S, et al. Diagnostic criteria for RA. *Bull Rheum Dis* 1959;9:175–176.
8. Moll JM, Wright V. Familial occurrence of psoriatic arthritis. *Ann Rheum Dis* 1973;32:181–201.
9. Prens E, Debets R, Hegmans J. T lymphocytes in psoriasis. *Clin Dermatol* 1995;13:115–129.
10. Nestle FO, Turka LA, Nickoloff BJ. Characterization of dermal dendritic cells in psoriasis: autostimulation of T lymphocytes and induction of Th1 type cytokines. *J Clin Invest* 1994;94:202–209.
11. Costello P, Fiter J, O'Farrelly C, et al. Predominance of CD8+ T lymphocytes in psoriatic arthritis. *J Rheumatol* 1999;26:1117–1124.
12. Resnick D, Niwayama G. Entheses and enthesopathy: anatomical, pathological, and radiological correlation. *Radiology* 1983;146:1–9.
13. McGonagle D, Gibbon W, Emery P. Classification of inflammatory arthritis by enthesitis. *Lancet* 1998;352:1137–1140.
14. McGonagle D, Conaghan PG, Emery P. Psoriatic arthritis: a unified concept twenty years on. *Arthritis Rheum* 1999;42:1080–1086.
15. McGonagle D, Marzo-Ortega H, O'Connor P, et al. The role of biomechanical factors and HLA-B27 in magnetic resonance imaging-determined bone changes in plantar fascia enthesopathy. *Arthritis Rheum* 2002;46(2):489–493.
16. Ceponis A, Konttinen YT, Imai S. Synovial lining, endothelial and inflammatory mononuclear cell proliferation in synovial membranes in psoriatic and reactive arthritis: a comparative quantitative morphometric study. *Br J Rheumatol* 1998;37:170–178.
17. Reece RJ, Canete JD, Parsons WJ, et al. Distinct vascular patterns of early synovitis in psoriatic, reactive, and rheumatoid arthritis. *Arthritis Rheum* 1999;42(7):1481–1484.
18. Ritchlin CT, Haas-Smith SA, Li P, et al. Mechanisms of TNF-alpha-and RANKL-mediated osteoclastogenesis and bone resorption in psoriatic arthritis. *J Clin Invest* 2003;111(6):821–831.
19. Gladman DD. Psoriatic arthritis: recent advances in pathogenesis and treatment. *Rheum Dis Clin North Am* 1992;18:247–256.
20. Garber EM, Nall ML, Watson W. Natural history of psoriasis in 61 twin pairs. *Arch Dermatol* 1974;109:207–211.
21. Gottlieb M, Calin A. Discordance for psoriatic arthropathy in monozygotic twins. *Arthritis Rheum* 1979;22:805–806.
22. Gonzalez S, Martinez-Borra J, Lopez-Vazquez A, et al. MICA rather than MICB, TNFA, or HLA-DRB1 is associated with susceptibility to psoriatic arthritis. *J Rheumatol* 2002;29(5):973–978.
23. Karason A, Gudjonsson JE, Upmanyu R, et al. A susceptibility gene for psoriatic arthritis maps to chromosome 16q: evidence for imprinting. *Am J Hum Genet* 2003;72(1):125–131.
24. Korendowych E, Dixey J, Cox B, et al. The influence of the HLA-DRB1 rheumatoid arthritis shared epitope on the clinical characteristics and radiological outcome of psoriatic arthritis. *J Rheumatol* 2003; 30(1):96–101.
25. Espinoza LR, van Solingen R, Cuellar ML, et al. Insights into the pathogenesis of psoriasis and psoriatic arthritis. *Am J Med Sci* 1998; 316:271–276.
26. Riegert P, Wanner V, Bahram S. Genomics, isoforms, expression, and phylogeny of the MHC class I-related MR1 gene. *J Immunol* 1998; 161:4066–4077.
27. Ando H, Mizuki N, Ota M, et al. Allelic variants of the human MHC class I chain-related B gene (MICB). *Immunogenetics* 1997;46:499–508.
28. Gonzalez S, Martinez-Borra J, Torre-Alonso JC, et al. The MICA-A9 triplet repeat polymorphism in the transmembrane region confers additional susceptibility to the development of psoriatic arthritis and is independent of the association of Cw*0602 in psoriasis. *Arthritis Rheum* 1999;42:1010–1016.
29. Winchester R, Brancato L, Itescu S, et al. Implications from the occurrence of Reiter's syndrome and related disorders in association with advanced HIV infection. *Scand J Rheumatol* 1988;74:89–93.
30. Berman A, Espinoza LR, Aguillar JL, et al. Rheumatic manifestations of human immunodeficiency virus infection. *Am J Med* 1988;85: 59–64.
31. Espinoza LR, Jara LJ, Espinoza CG, et al. There is an association between human immunodeficiency virus infection and spondyloarthropathies. *Rheum Dis Clin North Am* 1992;18:257–266.
32. Espinoza LR, Berman A, Vasey FB, et al. Psoriatic arthritis and acquired immunodeficiency syndrome. *Arthritis Rheum* 1988;31:1034–1040.
33. Reveille JD, Conant MA, Duvic M. Human immunodeficiency virus-associated psoriasis, psoriatic arthritis, and Reiter's syndrome: a disease continuum. *Arthritis Rheum* 1990;33:1574–1578.
34. Duvic M, Johnson TM, Rapini RP, et al. Acquired immunodeficiency syndrome-associated psoriasis and Reiter's syndrome. *Arch Dermatol* 1987;123:1622–1632.
35. Brancato L, Itescu S, Skovron ML, et al. Aspects of the spectrum, prevalence and disease susceptibility determinants of Reiter's syndrome and related disorders associated with HIV infection. *Rheumatol Int* 1989;9:137–141.
36. Johnson TM, Duvic M, Rapini RP, et al. AIDS exacerbates psoriasis. *N Engl J Med* 1985;313:1415.
37. Bijlsma JW, Derksen RW, Huber-Bruning O, et al. Does AIDS "cure" rheumatoid arthritis? *Ann Rheum Dis* 1988;47:350–351.
38. Furie R, Kaell A, Petrucci R, et al. Systemic lupus erythematosus complicated by infection with human immunodeficiency virus. *Arthritis Rheum* 1988;31[Suppl]:56.
39. O'Connell PG, Gerber LH, Digiovanna JJ, et al. Arthritis in patients with psoriasis treated with gamma-interferon. *J Rheumatol* 1992;19: 80–82.
40. Payne CMER. Psoriatic science. *Br Med J* 1987;295:1158–1160.
41. Elder JT, Fisher GJ, Lindquist PB, et al. Overexpression of transforming growth factor alpha in psoriatic epidermis. *Science* 1989;243:811–813.
42. Osterland CK, Wilkinson RD, St Louis EA. Expression of c-myc protein in skin and synovium in psoriasis and psoriatic arthritis. *Clin Exp Rheumatol* 1990;8:145–150.
43. Mizutani H, Ohmoto Y, Mizutani T, et al. Role of increased production of monocytes TNF-alpha, IL-1beta and IL-6 in psoriasis: relation to focal infection, disease activity and responses to treatments. *J Dermatol Sci* 1997;14:145–153.
44. Hohler T, Kruger A, Schneider PM, et al. A TNF-alpha promoter polymorphism is associated with juvenile onset psoriasis and psoriatic arthritis. *J Invest Dermatol* 1997;109:562–565.
45. Gottlieb AB, Fu SM, Carter DM, et al. Marked increase in the frequency of psoriatic arthritis in psoriasis patients with HLA-DR+ keratinocytes. *Arthritis Rheum* 1987;30:901–907.

46. Schatteman L, Mielants H, Veys EM, et al. Gut inflammation in psoriatic arthritis: a prospective ileocolonoscopic study. *J Rheumatol* 1995; 22:680–683.
47. Vasey FB, Seleznick MJ, Fenske NA, et al. New signposts on the road to understanding psoriatic arthritis. *J Rheumatol* 1989;16:1405–1407.
48. Lapadula G, Iannone F, Covelli M, et al. Anti-enterobacteria antibodies in psoriatic arthritis. *Clin Exp Rheumatol* 1992;10:461–466.
49. Yamamoto T, Katayama I, Nishioka K. Peripheral blood mononuclear cell proliferative response against staphylococcal superantigens in patients with psoriasis arthropathy. *Eur J Dermatol* 1999;9:17–21.
50. Lu Y, Kim BS, Pope RM. Clonal heterogeneity of synovial fluid T lymphocytes in inflammatory synovitis. *Clin Immunol Immunopathol* 1992; 63:28–33.
51. Focherini MC, Uguccioni M, Cattini L, et al. T cell receptor beta chain gene usage in rheumatoid arthritis. *Boll Soc Ital Biol Sper* 1993; 69:93–97.
52. Spadaro A, Rinaldi T, Riccieri V, et al. Interleukin 13 in synovial fluid and serum of patients with psoriatic arthritis. *Ann Rheum Dis* 2002;61 (2):174–176.
53. Costello P, Bresnihan B, O'Farrelly C, et al. Predominance of CD8+ T lymphocytes in psoriatic arthritis. *J Rheumatol* 1999; 26(5):1117–1124
54. Balding J, Kane D, Livingstone W, et al. Cytokine gene polymorphisms: association with psoriatic arthritis susceptibility and severity. *Arthritis Rheum* 2003;48(5):1408–1413.
55. Fearon U, Veale DJ. Pathogenesis of psoriatic arthritis. *Clin Exp Dermatol* 2001;26(4):333–337.
56. Huang W, Schwarz EM. Mechanisms of bone resorption and new bone formation in spondyloarthropathies. *Curr Rheumatol Rep* 2002;4(6): 513–517.
57. Taylor WJ. Epidemiology of psoriatic arthritis. *Curr Opin Rheumatol* 2002;14(2):98–103.
58. Veale D, FitzGerald O. Psoriatic arthritis. *Best Pract Res Clin Rheumatol* 2002;16(4):523–535.
59. Lombolt G. *Psoriasis: prevalence, spontaneous course, and genetics: a census study on the prevalence of skin disease in the Faroe Islands*. Copenhagen: GEC Gad, 1963.
60. Shore A, Ansell BM. Juvenile psoriatic arthritis: an analysis of 60 cases. *J Pediatr* 1982;100:529–535.
61. Southwood TR, Petty RE, Malleson PN, et al. Psoriatic arthritis in children. *Arthritis Rheum* 1989;32:1007–1013.
62. Biondi-Oriente C, Scarpa R, Pucino A, et al. Psoriasis and psoriatic arthritis: dermatological and rheumatological co-operative clinical report. *Acta Derm Venereol Suppl* (Stockh) 1989;146:69–71.
63. Langevitz P, Buskila D, Gladman DD. Psoriatic arthritis precipitated by physical trauma. *J Rheumatol* 1990;17:695–697.
64. Doury P. Psoriatic arthritis with physical trauma. *J Rheumatol* 1993; 20:1629.
65. Olivieri I, Gemignani G, Christou C, et al. Trauma and seronegative spondyloarthropathy: report of two more cases of peripheral arthritis precipitated by physical injury. *Ann Rheum Dis* 1989;48:520–521.
66. Olivieri I, Gherardi S, Bini C, et al. Trauma and seronegative spondyloarthropathy: rapid joint destruction in peripheral arthritis triggered by physical injury. *Ann Rheum Dis* 1988;47:73–76.
67. Pages M, Lassoued S, Fournie B, et al. Psoriatic arthritis precipitated by physical trauma: destructive arthritis or associated with reflex sympathetic dystrophy? *J Rheumatol* 1992;19:185–186.
68. Scarpa R, della Valle G, Del Puente A, et al. Physical trauma triggers psoriasis in a patient with undifferentiated seronegative spondyloarthropathy. *Clin Exp Rheumatol* 1992;10:100–102.
69. Helliwell P, Marchesoni A, Peters M, et al. A re-evaluation of the osteoarticular manifestations of psoriasis. *Br J Rheumatol* 1991;30:339–345.
70. Gladman DD, Shuckett R, Russell ML, et al. Psoriatic arthritis (PSA): an analysis of 220 patients. *Q J Med* 1987;62:127–141.
71. Scarpa R, Oriente P, Pucino A, et al. Psoriatic arthritis in psoriatic patients. *Br J Rheumatol* 1984;23:246–250.
72. O'Donnell BF, O'Loughlin S, Codd MB, et al. HLA typing in Irish psoriatics. *Ir Med J* 1993;86:65–68.
73. Troughton PR, Morgan AW. Laboratory findings and pathology of psoriatic arthritis. *Baillieres Clin Rheumatol* 1994;8:439–463.
74. Mullen RH, Farber EM. Some thoughts on psoriatic arthritis. *Cutis* 1985;36:388–390.
75. Lambert JR, Wright V. Psoriatic spondylitis: a clinical and radiological description of the spine in psoriatic arthritis. *Q J Med* 1977;46:411–425.
76. Gladman DD, Brubacher B, Buskila D, et al. Differences in the expression of spondyloarthropathy: a comparison between ankylosing spondylitis and psoriatic arthritis. *Clin Invest Med* 1993;16:1–7.
77. Salvarani C, Macchioni P, Cremonesi T, et al. The cervical spine in patients with psoriatic arthritis: a clinical, radiological and immunogenetic study. *Ann Rheum Dis* 1992;51:73–77.
78. Spadaro A, Riccieri V, Sili Scavalli A, et al. Multiple cervical cord compressions in psoriatic arthritis. *Clin Rheumatol* 1992;11:51–54.
79. Sandorfi N, Freundlich B. Psoriatic and seronegative inflammatory arthropathy associated with a traumatic onset: 4 cases and a review of the literature. *J Rheumatol* 1997;24:187–192.
80. Padula A, Belsito F, Barozzi L, et al. Isolated tenosynovitis associated with psoriasis triggered by physical injury. *Clin Exp Rheumatol* 1999;17(1):103–104.
81. McHugh NJ, Laurent MR. The effect of pregnancy on the onset of psoriatic arthritis. *Br J Rheumatol* 1989;28:50–52.
82. Ostensen M. The effect of pregnancy on ankylosing spondylitis, psoriatic arthritis, and juvenile rheumatoid arthritis. *Am J Reprod Immunol* 1992;28:235–237.
83. Stevens HP, Ostlere LS, Black CM, et al. Cyclical psoriatic arthritis responding to anti-oestrogen therapy. *Br J Dermatol* 1993;129:458–460.
84. Jones SM, Armas JB, Cohen MG, et al. Psoriatic arthritis: outcome of disease subsets and relationship of joint disease to nail and skin disease. *Br J Rheumatol* 1994;33:834–839.
85. Lavaroni G, Kokelj F, Pauluzzi P, et al. The nails in psoriatic arthritis. *Acta Derm Venereol Suppl* (Stockh) 1994;186:113.
86. Veale D, Rogers S, Fitzgerald O. Classification of clinical subsets in psoriatic arthritis. *Br J Rheumatol* 1994;33:133–138.
87. Gladman DD, Farewell VT, Wong K, et al. Mortality studies in psoriatic arthritis: results from a single outpatient center. II. Prognostic indicators for death. *Arthritis Rheum* 1998;41:1103–1110.
88. Wright V, Moll JMH. *Seronegative polyarthritis*. Amsterdam: North Holland, 1976.
89. Kahn MF, Khan MA. The SAPHO syndrome. *Baillieres Clin Rheumatol* 1994;8:333–362.
90. Kahn MF. Psoriatic arthritis and synovitis, acne, pustulosis, hyperostosis, and osteitis syndrome. *Curr Opin Rheumatol* 1993;5:428–435.
91. Jurik AG. Seronegative anterior chest wall syndromes: a study of the findings and course at radiography. *Acta Radiol Suppl* 1992;381:1–42.
92. Earwaker JW, Cotten A. SAPHO: syndrome or concept? Imaging findings. *Skeletal Radiol* 2003;32(6):311–327.
93. Sonozaki H, Mitsui H, Miyanaga Y, et al. Clinical features of 53 cases with pustulotic arthro-osteitis. *Ann Rheum Dis* 1981;40:547–553.
94. Toussirot E, Dupond JL, Wendling D. Spondylodiscitis in SAPHO syndrome: a series of eight cases. *Ann Rheum Dis* 1997;56:52–58.
95. Boisseau-Garsaud AM, Beylot-Barry M, Doutre MS, et al. Psoriatic onycho-pachydermo-periostitis: a variant of psoriatic distal interphalangeal arthritis? *Arch Dermatol* 1996;132:176–180.
96. Schuster T, Bielek J, Dietz HG, et al. Chronic recurrent multifocal osteomyelitis (CRMO). *Eur J Pediatr Surg* 1996;6:45–51.
97. Carr AJ, Cole WG, Roberton DM, Chow CW. Chronic multifocal osteomyelitis. *J Bone Joint Surg Br* 1993;75:582–591.
98. Helliwell P, Marchesoni A, Peters M, et al. A re-evaluation of the osteoarticular manifestations of psoriasis. *Br J Rheumatol* 1991;30: 339–345.
99. Lambert JR, Wright V. Eye inflammation in psoriatic arthritis. *Ann Rheum Dis* 1976;35:354–356.
100. Paiva ES, Macaluso DC, Edwards A, et al. Characterisation of uveitis in patients with psoriatic arthritis. *Ann Rheum Dis* 2000;59(1):67–70.
101. Omdal R, Husby G. Renal affection in patients with ankylosing spondylitis and psoriatic arthritis. *Clin Rheumatol* 1987;6:74–79.
102. Alenius GM, Stegmayr BG, Dahlqvist SR. Renal abnormalities in a population of patients with psoriatic arthritis. *Scand J Rheumatol* 2001;30(5):271–274.
103. Pines A, Ehrenfeld M, Fisman EZ, et al. Mitral valve prolapse in psoriatic arthritis. *Arch Intern Med* 1986;146:1371–1373.
104. Muna WF, Roller DH, Craft J, et al. Psoriatic arthritis and aortic regurgitation. *JAMA* 1980;244:363–365.
105. Thomson GT, Johnston JL, Baragar FD, et al. Psoriatic arthritis and myopathy. *J Rheumatol* 1990;17:395–398.
106. Rodriguez de la Serna A, Casas Gasso F, Diaz Lopez C, et al. Association of Sjögren's syndrome with psoriatic arthritis. *Can Med Assoc J* 1984;131:1329–1332.

107. Whaley K, Chisholm DM, Williamson J, et al. Sjögren's syndrome in psoriatic arthritis, ankylosing spondylitis and Reiter's syndrome. *Acta Rheumatol Scand* 1971;17:105–114.
108. Collins P, Rogers S, Jackson J, et al. Psoriasis, psoriatic arthritis and the possible association with Sjögren's syndrome. *Br J Dermatol* 1992;126:242–245.
109. Scotto dF, Grilo RM, Vergne P, et al. Is the relationship between spondyloarthropathy and Sjogren's syndrome in women coincidental? A study of 13 cases. *Joint Bone Spine* 2002; 69(4):383–387.
110. Saxena S, Verma K, Bhuyan UN,. Amyloidosis complicating psoriatic arthropathy. *J Assoc Physicians India* 1992;40:609–610.
111. Hiki Y, Kokubo T, Horii A, et al. A case of severe IgA nephropathy associated with psoriatic arthritis and idiopathic interstitial pneumonia. *Acta Pathol Jpn* 1993;43:522–528.
112. Smith DL, White CR Jr. Pyoderma gangrenosum in association with psoriatic arthritis. *Arthritis Rheum* 1994;37:1258–1260.
113. Cantini F, Salvarani C, Olivieri I, et al. Distal extremity swelling with pitting edema in psoriatic arthritis: a case-control study. *Clin Exp Rheumatol* 2001;19(3):291–296.
114. Long JA, Husted JA, Gladman DD, et al. The relationship between patient satisfaction with health and clinical measures of function and disease status in patients with psoriatic arthritis. *J Rheumatol* 2000; 27(4):958–966.
115. Ansell BM, Wigley RAD. Arthritis manifestations in regional enteritis. *Ann Rheum Dis* 1964;23:64–72.
116. Bennett RM. Familial spondylitis. *Proc R Soc Lond Biol* 1971;64: 663–664.
117. Moll JM, Haslock I, Macrae IF, et al. Associations between ankylosing spondylitis, psoriatic arthritis, Reiter's disease, the intestinal arthropathies, and Behçet's syndrome. *Medicine* (Baltimore) 1974; 53:343–364.
118. Trentham DE, Kammer GM, McCune WJ, et al. Autoimmunity to collagen: a shared feature of psoriatic and rheumatoid arthritis. *Arthritis Rheum* 1981;24:1363–1369.
119. Mason RM, Barnes GC. Behçet's syndrome with arthritis. *Ann Rheum Dis* 1969;28:95–103.
120. Partsch G. Laboratory features of psoriatic arthritis. *Z Rheumatol* 1987;46:220–226.
121. Hall RP, Gerber LH, Lawley TJ. IgA-containing immune complexes in patients with psoriatic arthritis. *Clin Exp Rheumatol* 1984;2:221–225.
122. Taccari E, Gigante MC, Sorgi ML, et al. Serum uric acid levels in psoriatic arthritis. *Scand J Rheumatol* 1985;14:94.
123. Lambert JR, Wright V. Serum uric acid levels in psoriatic arthritis. *Ann Rheum Dis* 1977;36:264–267.
124. Porter GG. Plain radiology and other imaging techniques. *Baillieres Clin Rheumatol* 1994;8:465–482.
125. Reid DM, Kennedy NS, Nicoll J, et al. Total and peripheral bone mass in patients with psoriatic arthritis and rheumatoid arthritis. *Clin Rheumatol* 1986;5:372–378.
126. Magaro M, Altomonte L, Mirone L, et al. Serum osteocalcin as an index of bone turnover in active rheumatoid arthritis and in active psoriatic arthritis. *Clin Rheumatol* 1989;8:494–498.
127. Pichler R, Weiglein K, Schmekal B, et al. Bone scintigraphy using Tc-99m DPD and F18-FDG in a patient with SAPHO syndrome. *Scand J Rheumatol* 2003;32(1):58–60.
128. Stoeger A, Mur E, Penz-Schneeweiss D, et al. Technetium-99m human immunoglobulin scintigraphy in psoriatic arthropathy: first results. *Eur J Nucl Med* 1994;21:342–344.
129. McGonagle D, Gibbon W, O'Connor P, et al. Characteristic magnetic resonance imaging entheseal changes of knee synovitis in spondylarthropathy. *Arthritis Rheum* 1998;41:694–700.
130. Jevtic V, Watt I, Rozman B, et al. Distinctive radiological features of small hand joints in rheumatoid arthritis and seronegative spondyloarthritis demonstrated by contrast-enhanced (Gd-DTPA) magnetic resonance imaging. *Skeletal Radiol* 1995;24:351–355.
131. Gold RH, Bassett LW, Seeger LL. The other arthritides: roentgenologic features of osteoarthritis, erosive osteoarthritis, ankylosing spondylitis, psoriatic arthritis, Reiter's disease, multicentric reticulohistiocytosis, and progressive systemic sclerosis. *Radiol Clin North Am* 1988;26:1195–1212.
132. Sherman M. Psoriatic arthritis: observations on the clinical, roentgenographic and radiological changes. *J Bone Joint Surg Am* 1952; 34:831–852.
133. Bywaters EGL, Dixon ASJ. Paravertebral ossification in psoriatic arthritis. *Ann Rheum Dis* 1965;24:313–331.
134. Jajic I. Radiological changes in the sacro-iliac joints and spine of patients with psoriatic arthritis and psoriasis. *Ann Rheum Dis* 1968; 27:1–6.
135. Leonard DG, O'Duffy JD, Rogers RS. Prospective analysis of psoriatic arthritis in patients hospitalized for psoriasis. *Mayo Clin Proc* 1978;53:511–518.
136. Dzioba RB, Benjamin J. Spontaneous atlantoaxial fusion in psoriatic arthritis: a case report. *Spine* 1985;10:102–103.
137. Blau RH, Kaufman RL. Erosive and subluxing cervical spine disease in patients with psoriatic arthritis. *J Rheumatol* 1987;14:111–1117.
138. Lee ST, Lui TN. Psoriatic arthritis with C-1-C-2 subluxation as a neurosurgical complication. *Surg Neurol* 1986;26:428–430.
139. Laiho K, Kauppi M. The cervical spine in patients with psoriatic arthritis. *Ann Rheum Dis* 2002;61(7):650–652.
140. Kononen M. Radiographic changes in the condyle of the temporomandibular joint in psoriatic arthritis. *Acta Radiol* 1987;28:185–188.
141. Melchiorre D, Calderazzi A, Maddali BS, et al. A comparison of ultrasonography and magnetic resonance imaging in the evaluation of temporomandibular joint involvement in rheumatoid arthritis and psoriatic arthritis. *Rheumatology* (Oxford) 2003;42(5):673–676.
142. Biondi-Oriente C, Scarpa R, Oriente P. Prevalence and clinical features of juvenile psoriatic arthritis in 425 psoriatic patients. *Acta Derm Venereol Suppl* (Stockh) 1994;186:109–110.
143. Koo E, Balogh Z, Gomor B. Juvenile psoriatic arthritis. *Clin Rheumatol* 1991;10:245–249.
144. Sills EM. Psoriatic arthritis in childhood. *Johns Hopkins Med J* 1980; 146:49–53.
145. Huemer C, Malleson PN, Cabral DA, et al. Patterns of joint involvement at onset differentiate oligoarticular juvenile psoriatic arthritis from pauciarticular juvenile rheumatoid arthritis. *J Rheumatol* 2002; 29(7):1531–1535.
146. Coulton BL, Thomson K, Symmons DP, et al. Outcome in patients hospitalised for psoriatic arthritis. *Clin Rheumatol* 1989;8:261–265.
147. Anonymous. Prognosis of psoriatic arthritis [Editorial]. *Lancet* 1988; 2:375–376.
148. Roberts ME, Wright V, Hill AG, et al. Psoriatic arthritis: follow-up study. *Ann Rheum Dis* 1976;35:206–212.
149. Gladman DD, Hing EN, Schentag CT, et al. Remission in psoriatic arthritis. *J Rheumatol* 2001;28(5):1045–1048.
150. Khan M, Gladman DD. Clinical and radiological changes during psoriatic arthritis disease progression. *J Rheumatol* 2003;30(5):1022–1026.
151. McHugh NJ, Balachrishnan C, Jones SM. Progression of peripheral joint disease in psoriatic arthritis: a 5-yr prospective study. *Rheumatology* (Oxford) 2003.
152. Queiro-Silva R, Torre-Alonso JC, Tinture-Eguren T, et al. A polyarticular onset predicts erosive and deforming disease in psoriatic arthritis. *Ann Rheum Dis* 2003; 62(1):68–70.
153. Wong K, Gladman DD, Husted J, et al. Mortality studies in psoriatic arthritis: results from a single outpatient clinic. I. Causes and risk of death. *Arthritis Rheum* 1997;40:1868–1872.
153a. Shbeeb M, Uramoto KM, Gibson LE, et al. The epidemiology of psoriatic arthritis in Olmsted County, Minnesota, USA, 1982–1991. *J Rheumatol* 2000;27(5):1247–1250.
154. Husted JA, Gladman DD, Farewell VT, et al. Health-related quality of life of patients with psoriatic arthritis: a comparison with patients with rheumatoid arthritis. *Arthritis Rheum* 2001;45(2):151–158.
155. Noble WC, Sarin JA. Carriage of *Staphylococcus aureus* in psoriasis. *Br Med J* 1968;1:417–418.
156. Katayama H, Kawad A. Exacerbation of psoriasis induced by indomethacin. *J Dermatol* 1981;8:323.
157. Lassus A, Dahlgren AL, Halpern MJ, et al. Effects of dietary supplementation with polyunsaturated ethyl ester lipids (Angiosan) in patients with psoriasis and psoriatic arthritis. *J Intern Med Res* 1990; 18:68–73.
158. Daunt AO, Cox NL, Robertson JC, et al. Indices of disease activity in psoriatic arthritis. *J R Soc Med* 1987;80:556–558.
159. Kammer GM, Soter NA, Gibson DJ, et al. Psoriatic arthritis: a clinical, immunologic and HLA study of 100 patients. *Semin Arthritis Rheum* 1979;9:75–97.
160. Sayers ME, Mazanec DJ. Use of antimalarial drugs for the treatment of psoriatic arthritis. *Am J Med* 1992;93:474–475.

161. Gladman DD, Blake R, Brubacher B, et al. Chloroquine therapy in psoriatic arthritis. *J Rheumatol* 1992;19:1724–1726.
162. Dorwart BB, Gall EP, Schumacher HR, et al. Chrysotherapy in psoriatic arthritis: efficacy and toxicity compared to rheumatoid arthritis. *Arthritis Rheum* 1978;21:513–515.
163. Lacaille D, Stein HB, Raboud J, et al. Long-term therapy of psoriatic arthritis: intramuscular gold or methotrexate? *J Rheumatol* 2000;27 (8):1922–1927.
164. Farr M, Kitas GD, Waterhouse L, et al. Sulphasalazine in psoriatic arthritis: a double-blind placebo-controlled study. *Br J Rheumatol* 1990;29:46–49.
165. Fraser SM, Hopkins R, Hunter JA, et al. Sulphasalazine in the management of psoriatic arthritis. *Br J Rheumatol* 1993;32:923–925.
166. Newman ED, Perruquet JL, Harrington TM. Sulfasalazine therapy in psoriatic arthritis: clinical and immunologic response. *J Rheumatol* 1991;18:1379–1382.
167. McCarthy C, Coughlan R. Sulphasalazine desensitisation in patients with arthritis. *Ir J Med Sci* 1994;163:238–239.
168. Clegg DO, Reda DJ, Mejias E, et al. Comparison of sulfasalazine and placebo in the treatment of psoriatic arthritis: a Department of Veterans Affairs Cooperative Study. *Arthritis Rheum* 1996;39:2013–2020.
169. Rahman P, Gladman DD, Cook RJ, et al. The use of sulfasalazine in psoriatic arthritis: a clinic experience. *J Rheumatol* 1998;25:1957–1961.
170. Cuellar ML, Espinoza LR. Methotrexate use in psoriasis and psoriatic arthritis. *Rheum Dis Clin North Am* 1997;23:797–809.
171. Black RL, O'Brien WM, Van Scott EJ, et al. Methotrexate therapy in psoriatic arthritis. *JAMA* 1964;189:743–747.
172. Espinoza LR, Zakraoui L, Espinoza CG, et al. Psoriatic arthritis: clinical response and side effects to methotrexate therapy. *J Rheumatol* 1992;19:872–877.
173. al-Awadhi A, Dale P, McKendry RJ. Pancytopenia associated with low dose methotrexate therapy: a regional survey. *J Rheumatol* 1993; 20:1121–1125.
174. Kokelj F, Lavaroni G, Stinco G. Psoriatic arthritis treated with cyclosporin A. *Allerg Immunol* (Paris) 1992;24:393–394.
175. Salvarani C, Macchioni P, Boiardi L, et al. Low dose cyclosporin A in psoriatic arthritis: relation between soluble interleukin 2 receptors and response to therapy. *J Rheumatol* 1992;19:74–79.
176. Sarzi-Puttini P, Cazzola M, Panni B, et al. Long-term safety and efficacy of low-dose cyclosporin A in severe psoriatic arthritis. *Rheumatol Int* 2002;21(6):234–238.
177. Spadaro A, Riccieri V, Sili-Scavalli A, et al. Comparison of cyclosporin A and methotrexate in the treatment of psoriatic arthritis: a one-year prospective study. *Clin Exp Rheumatol* 1995;13:589–593.
178. Mease PJ, Goffe BS, Metz J, et al. Etanercept in the treatment of psoriatic arthritis and psoriasis: a randomised trial. *Lancet* 2000;356 (9227):385–390.
179. Mease P. Psoriatic arthritis: the role of TNF inhibition and the effect of its inhibition with etanercept. *Clin Exp Rheumatol* 2002;20[6 Suppl 28]:S116–S121.
180. Antoni C, Dechant C, Hanns-Martin Lorenz PD, et al. Open-label study of infliximab treatment for psoriatic arthritis: clinical and magnetic resonance imaging measurements of reduction of inflammation. *Arthritis Rheum* 2002;47(5):506–512.
181. Cauza E, Spak M, Cauza K, et al. Treatment of psoriatic arthritis and psoriasis vulgaris with the tumor necrosis factor inhibitor infliximab. *Rheumatol Int* 2002;22(6):227–232.
182. Baeten D, Kruithof E, Van den BF, et al. Immunomodulatory effects of anti-tumor necrosis factor alpha therapy on synovium in spondylarthropathy: histologic findings in eight patients from an open-label pilot study. *Arthritis Rheum* 2001;44(1):186–195.
183. Kraan MC, van Kuijk AW, Dinant HJ, et al. Alefacept treatment in psoriatic arthritis: reduction of the effector T cell population in peripheral blood and synovial tissue is associated with improvement of clinical signs of arthritis. *Arthritis Rheum* 2002;46(10):2776–2784.
184. McInnes IB, Illei GG, Danning CL, et al. IL-10 improves skin disease and modulates endothelial activation and leukocyte effector function in patients with psoriatic arthritis. *J Immunol* 2001;167(7): 4075–4082.
185. Van Doornum S, Barraclough D, McColl G, et al. SAPHO: rare or just not recognized? *Semin Arthritis Rheum* 2000;30(1):70–77.
186. Courtney PA, Hosking DJ, Fairbairn KJ, et al. Treatment of SAPHO with pamidronate. *Rheumatology* (Oxford) 2002;41(10):1196–1198.
187. Wagner AD, Andresen J, Jendro MC, et al. Sustained response to tumor necrosis factor alpha-blocking agents in two patients with SAPHO syndrome. *Arthritis Rheum* 2002;46(7):1965–1968.
188. Olivieri I, Padula A, Ciancio G, et al. Successful treatment of SAPHO syndrome with infliximab: report of two cases. *Ann Rheum Dis* 2002; 61(4):375–376.
189. Maurer TA, Zackheim HS, Tuffanelli L, et al. The use of methotrexate for treatment of psoriasis in patients with HIV infection. *J Am Acad Dermatol* 1994;31:372–375.
190. Zangger P, Gladman DD, Bogoch ER. Musculoskeletal surgery in psoriatic arthritis. *J Rheumatol* 1998;25:725–729.
191. Kummerle K, Wessinghage D, Schweikert CH. Risk of alloplastic replacements in degenerative and inflammatory diseases of joints. *Acta Orthop Belg* 1971;37:541—548.
192. Lynfield YL, Ostroff G, Abraham J. Bacteria, skin sterilization and wound healing in psoriasis. *N Y J Med* 1972;72:1247–1250.
193. Belsky MR, Feldon P, Millender LH, et al. Hand involvement in psoriatic arthritis. *J Hand Surg* 1982;7:203–207.
194. Kononen M. Craniomandibular disorders in psoriatic arthritis: a radiographic and clinical study. *Proc Finn Dent Soc* 1987;83[Suppl 8–10]:1–45.

CHAPTER 66

Enteropathic Arthritis

Herman Mielants, Dominique Baeten, Filip De Keyser, and Eric M. Veys

Inflammatory joint disease is generally considered an enteropathic arthritis if the gastrointestinal tract is directly involved in the pathogenesis. A wide spectrum of other rheumatic diseases may be accompanied by gastrointestinal manifestations or intestinal complications, but not all of these diseases can be classified as enteropathic arthritides. The most common enteropathic arthritides belong to the spondyloarthropathies (1). This group of diseases is characterized by the absence of rheumatoid factor and the presence of sacroiliitis (with or without spondylitis), inflammatory peripheral arthritis (generally pauciarticular and asymmetric in distribution), and ligament and tendon involvement (enthesopathy). Other features include clinical overlap of the different spondyloarthropathies, familial aggregation, and strong association with human leukocyte antigen-B27 (HLA-B27). Syndromes within this spectrum include ankylosing spondylitis, reactive arthritis (urogenital or enterogenic), psoriatic arthritis, the late-onset pauciarticular subtype of juvenile chronic arthritis (JCA), idiopathic inflammatory bowel disease (IBD), Crohn's disease and ulcerative colitis, and the undifferentiated spondyloarthropathies.

The inclusion of IBD in this group of diseases emphasizes the relation between gut inflammation and joint inflammation. This relation is corroborated by ileocolonoscopic evidence of subclinical gut inflammation in other forms of spondyloarthropathy (1). Other gut diseases, such as celiac disease and intestinal bypass surgery, also are occasionally accompanied by joint inflammation, but these are not considered to be spondyloarthropathies.

CLINICAL ENTITIES

Idiopathic Inflammatory Bowel Disease

Crohn's disease and ulcerative colitis are discussed together because they have comparable rheumatologic and other associated features that cannot be easily differentiated.

Epidemiology

The prevalence of ulcerative colitis ranges from 50 to 100 individuals per 100,000 in the general population. The disease seems to be more frequent in whites than in nonwhites, and more frequent in the Jewish population than any other. The prevalence of Crohn's disease has increased during the last few decades to about 75 per 100,000. In a screening study for colorectal cancer involving 37,000 individuals without intestinal symptoms (2), the combined prevalence of ulcerative colitis and Crohn's disease was 56 per 100,000, whereas the prevalence of symptomatic IBD is estimated as 90 to 150 per 100,000. Ongoing epidemiologic studies suggest that the true prevalence may have been underestimated by 27% to 35%. These studies also suggest the existence of patients with subclinical IBD. Arthritis is the most common extraintestinal manifestation of IBD and appears in 2% to 20% of patients with either ulcerative colitis or Crohn's disease. However, the occurrence of peripheral arthritis is more frequent in patients with colonic involvement and more extensive bowel disease.

Intestinal Symptoms

Crohn's disease is characterized by the classic triad of abdominal pain, weight loss, and diarrhea. Disease onset may be insidious, and progression, subclinical. Abdominal pain is frequent but not severe. Weight loss in the range of 10% to 20% of body weight is common, as are low-grade fever and general debility. At a later stage, fistulae and abscesses may appear. Diarrhea and intestinal blood loss are the most common abdominal manifestations of ulcerative colitis. Diarrhea is almost always present, whereas fever and weight loss are less common. In ulcerative colitis, the mucosa is diffusely involved. The lesions (including superficial ulcerations, edema, friability, and microabscesses) are confined to the colonic mucosa. In Crohn's disease, the lesions may occur in the entire gastrointestinal tract, although the terminal ileum and colon are preferentially involved. The lesions are usually ulcerative, but their distribution is patchy. They can occur superficially as in ulcerative colitis, but frequently are transmural and granulomatous. Aphthoid ulceration, pseudopyloric metaplasia, and sarcoidlike granulomas are virtually pathognomonic findings. Sometimes it is difficult to distinguish between ulcerative colitis and Crohn's disease. In the presence of isolated colonic involvement, the histologic appearance may be comparable.

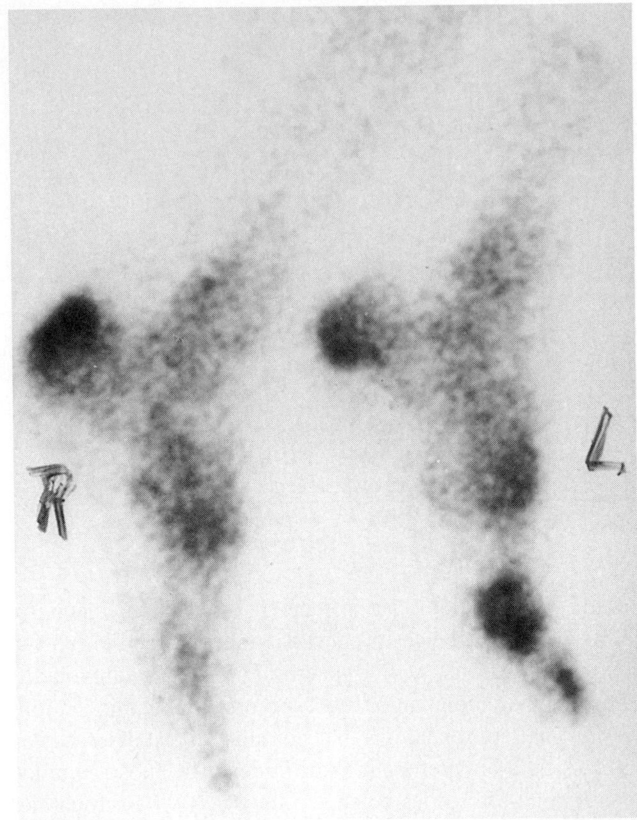

FIG. 66.1. In a spondyloarthritic patient, technetium-99m Methyleendiphosphanate (DMP) scan discloses inflammatory enthesopathies of the feet including insertion of Achilles tendon of the right foot and plantar fascia of the left foot.

Peripheral Arthritis

The frequency of peripheral arthritis in IBD ranges from 10% to 22% of patients (1,3,4), with a higher prevalence in Crohn's disease (5). In an extensive retrospective study in the Oxford Inflammatory Bowel Disease clinic (6) involving 1,459 patients with IBD, arthritis was described in 6% of patients with ulcerative colitis and 10% of patients with Crohn's disease. In a study from the gastrointestinal clinic in Ghent (7), synovitis was seen in 10% of IBD patients and enthesitis in 7%, but 29% of the patients reported a history of swollen joints. The discrepancy in prevalence can be correlated with the subspecialty clinic attended by the patient, because in a rheumatologic clinic, articular involvement was described in 68% of patients with ulcerative colitis (8). The prevalence of arthritis in IBD increases with the duration of the gut disease, going from 12% to 30% in a 20-year follow-up (9).

The sex ratio in IBD is equal, and peak age is between 25 and 44 years. In both diseases, the arthritis is pauciarticular, generally asymmetric, and frequently transient and migratory. Large and small joints, predominantly of the lower limbs, are involved. The arthritis usually is nondestructive, self-limiting, and many attacks subside within 4 to 6 weeks (10). Recurrences are common. Sausagelike fingers and toes may occur (dactylitis). Enthesopathies, especially inflammation of the Achilles tendon or of the insertion of the plantar fascia, are known manifestations (Fig. 66.1) and also may involve the knee or other sites, occuring in about 10% of the patients (11). Clubbing and, rarely, periostitis may occur in Crohn's disease. The peripheral arthritis becomes chronic in some cases and destructive lesions of small joints and hips may occur.

In about 40% of the cases of Crohn's disease with actual articular symptoms during the disease course, intestinal symptoms coincide with the joint manifestations and in 40% they antedate them (11), but the articular symptoms may precede the intestinal symptoms in about 20% of the cases by years (10,11). In some cases of spondyloarthropathies, Crohn's disease remains subclinical, with joint and tendon inflammation being the only clinical manifestations (12). In a prospective study of 123 patients with spondyloarthropathy 8 (6%) patients developed Crohn's disease 2 to 9 years after the appearance of joint symptoms (13). In ulcerative colitis, there is a more distinct temporal relation between attacks of arthritis and flares of bowel disease. Surgical removal of diseased colon can induce remission of peripheral arthritis. In Crohn's disease, colonic involvement increases the susceptibility to peripheral arthritis, but surgical removal has little effect on the joint disease (14).

In the Oxford study (6), enteropathic peripheral arthropathy without axial involvement was subdivided into pauciarticular large joint arthropathy and symmetric polyarthropathy. In the pauciarticular type, joint symptoms were mostly acute and self-limiting. The arthritis coincided with relapses of IBD, and the disease was strongly associated with extraintestinal manifestations such as erythema nodosum and uveitis. Interestingly, in 31% of these patients, arthropathies developed up to 3 years before diagnosis of IBD. The polyarticular joint symptoms persisted for months to years, ran a course independent of IBD, and were not associated with other extraintestinal manifestations except uveitis. This polyarticular type of joint involvement is rather uncommon (11) and in a prospective population-based study of 521 IBD patients, no patients fulfilled the clinical picture of this type of arthropathy (10).

Axial Involvement

Axial involvement occurs in both diseases. The true prevalence of sacroiliitis in IBD is unclear because the onset frequently is insidious. Prevalence rates of 10% to 20% for sacroiliitis and 7% to 12% for spondylitis have been reported, although the actual figures are probably higher because of the existence of subclinical axial involvement. Using computed tomography scans, sacroiliitis was detected in 45% of patients with Crohn's disease with low back pain, most of them were not recognized in classic radiographs (15). In a study from an IBD clinic (7), 30% of the patients with IBD had inflammatory low back pain, and 33% had a Shober Index of less than 3 cm. One-third of the patients had stage II unilateral or bilateral sacroiliitis, and in 18% of the patients, the sacroiliitis was asymptomatic; the prevalence of asymptomatic sacroiliitis was found to be 24% in another study (16).

Spondyloarthropathy fulfilling the European Spondyloarthropathy Study Group (ESSG) criteria (17) could be diagnosed in 35% of the patients, and ankylosing spondylitis could be diagnosed in 10%. These frequencies are probably underestimated because patients with IBD attending the rheumatologic clinic were excluded. In a population-based cohort of 202 IBD patients in Italy and the Netherlands (11), these figures were 18% and 3%, respectively. A higher prevalence of spondyloarthropathy (28%) was found in patients with ulcerative colitis followed up in an Italian gastrointestinal unit (18).

In review studies of ankylosing spondylitis, IBD occurred in between 4% (19) and 6% (20) of patients. Although it is generally accepted that men are more likely to develop ankylosing spondylitis than are women, in these studies the male-to-female ratio of patients with IBD and ankylosing spondylitis was 1:1, which is different from the ratio in uncomplicated ankylosing spondylitis (3:1). However, women with IBD and ankylosing spondylitis were shown to have a younger age at onset of ankylosing spondylitis and more severe disease than male patients with IBD (especially when IBD and ankylosing spondylitis are present in other members of the family). In general, joint disease was more severe, as defined by the intake of nonsteroidal antiinflammatory drugs and decrease of spinal mobility, in patients with combined IBD and ankylosing spondylitis than in those with uncomplicated ankylosing spondylitis (21).

However, the clinical picture may be indistinguishable from that of uncomplicated ankylosing spondylitis. The patient complains of low back pain, thoracic or cervical pain, buttock pain, and chest pain. Limitation of lumbar or cervical motion and reduced chest expansion are characteristic clinical signs. Peripheral arthritis may be present. The onset of axial involvement does not parallel that of bowel disease, but frequently precedes it (3,21). The course also is totally independent of the course of the intestinal disease. Bowel surgery does not alter the course of associated sacroiliitis or spondylitis.

In a prospective clinical study, essentially all the patients with spondyloarthropathy in whom Crohn's disease occurred after 2 to 9 years developed axial involvement and fulfilled criteria for ankylosing spondylitis (13).

Extraintestinal and Extraarticular Features

A variety of cutaneous, mucosal, serosal, and ocular manifestations occur in IBD (Table 66.1). Skin lesions are observed in 10% to 25% of patients. Erythema nodosum parallels the activity of bowel disease, tends to occur in patients with active peripheral arthritis, and is probably a disease-related manifestation (22). Pyoderma gangrenosum is a more severe but less common extraarticular manifestation, which is not related to the activity of the bowel and joint disease. Leg ulcers and thrombophlebitis also may occur.

Ocular manifestations, especially anterior uveitis, frequently accompany IBD (3% to 11%). Uveitis in patients with associated spondyloarthropathy is often acute in onset,

TABLE 66.1. *Extraintestinal manifestations of Crohn's disease and ulcerative colitis*

Extraintestinal manifestations	IBD (%)[a]	Related to intestinal manifestations
Peripheral arthritis	11–20	+
Pauciarticular	7	+
Polyarticular	4.5	–
Clubbing/periostitis	2	–
Enthesitis	7–15	+
Inflammatory low-back pain	10–30	–
Sacroiliitis	10–35	–
Spondylitis	2–10	–
Erythema nodosum	3–7	+
Pyoderma gangrenosum	2	–
Uveitis	6–13	±
Aphthous ulceration	?	+
Amyloidosis	1 (25 ?)	+
Nephrolithiasis	3	–
Primary sclerosing cholangitis	?	–
Diagnosis spondyloarthropathy	35	
Diagnosis ankylosing spondylitis	10	

IBD, inflammatory bowel disease.
[a]Prevalence (%) of different extraintestinal manifestations in Crohn's disease and ulcerative colitis and their relation with the intestinal manifestations (the prevalence of amyloidosis in Crohn's disease between parenthesis was found in a postmortem study).

unilateral, and transient, but recurrences are common (23). It generally spares the choroid and retina; however, in uncomplicated IBD lesions are frequently bilateral, insidious in onset, and chronic in duration (24). Granulomatous uveitis is rare but may be present in Crohn's disease. Acute anterior uveitis is associated with the occurrence of axial involvement and the presence of HLA-B27. Conjunctivitis and episcleritis also have been observed. In an ileocolonoscopic study involving patients with acute uveitis, inflammatory gut lesions were found in 66% (25), predominating in patients with acute anterior uveitis and associated spondyloarthopathy. Aphthous ulcerations, mainly affecting the buccal mucosa and tongue, are common in Crohn's disease and can parallel disease activity. Amyloidosis is a well-recognized cause of death in Crohn's disease. The incidence in clinical series is approximately 1% (26), but postmortem studies have revealed evidence of amyloid in 25% of patients with Crohn's disease. Nephrolithiasis has been reported in 6% of patients with Crohn's disease and 3% of patients with ulcerative colitis.

Laboratory and Radiologic Findings

There are no diagnostic laboratory tests for the arthritis or spondylitis of IBD. Elevated serum acute-phase reactants (especially C-reactive protein), thrombocytosis (especially in Crohn's disease), and hypochromic anemia due to chronic blood loss or chronic inflammation are common findings. Rheumatoid factor is absent.

Anti-*Saccharomyces cerevisiae* antibodies (ASCA) are considered to be an important marker for Crohn's disease, though their pathologic role is not yet clear (27). Recently ASCA immunoglobulin A (IgA) levels were found to be significantly higher in spondyloarthropathies, more specifically in ankylosing spondylitis than healthy controls and patients with rheumatoid arthritis (RA) (28), suggesting that this serum marker could identify those with spondyloarthropathy at risk for developing ankylosing spondylitis.

Synovial fluid analysis is consistent with an inflammatory arthritis with leukocyte counts ranging from 1,500 to 50,000/mm^3, predominantly neutrophils. Synovial histology reveals only nonspecific inflammation, although granulomas have been described.

Radiographs of the peripheral joints generally do not exhibit erosions. Erosive lesions, mainly of the metacarpophalangeal and metatarsal joints, occasionally have been described, differing from RA only by their pauciarticular and asymmetric distribution.

Destructive lesions of the hip have been reported and related to Crohn's disease–like lesions on gut biopsy in undifferentiated spondyloarthropathies (29). The axial joint involvement of IBD is indistinguishable from that of uncomplicated ankylosing spondylitis, although the frequency of asymmetric sacroiliitis is probably higher (30). Enthesopathies do not differ radiologically from those seen in the spondyloarthropathies.

Genetics and HLA-B27

Substantial evidence favors a genetic cause for IBD. Familial aggregation of Crohn's disease and ulcerative colitis has been amply documented. Both diseases are believed to be genetically linked, because both occur within the same families, but neither disease has been associated with HLA antigens in family studies. IBD complicated by peripheral arthritis is not associated with HLA-B27. Sacroiliitis and spondylitis in IBD are associated with HLA-B27, but to a lesser degree than is uncomplicated ankylosing spondylitis (33% vs. 71%). Interestingly, ankylosing spondylitis patients lacking the HLA-B27 antigen are at a higher risk of developing IBD than are HLA-B27$^+$ ankylosing spondylitis patients (31,32). On the other hand, more than 50% of subjects who have HLA-B27 in combination with Crohn's disease will develop ankylosing spondylitis (33).

HLA-BW62 occurs in a high proportion of spondyloarthropathy patients with Crohn's diseaselike lesions on gut biopsy (34), as well as in patients with proven Crohn's disease. The B27-B44 phenotype also placed patients at a high risk of developing both Crohn's disease and ankylosing spondylitis (35). In the Oxford study, pauciarticular joint involvement was associated with HLA-B27 (27% vs. 7% in controls), HLA-B35 (32% vs. 15%), and especially DRB1*0103 (33% vs. 3%), whereas the polyarticular form was associated only with HLA-B44 (62% vs. 30%) (36). The Ghent study demonstrated that the presence of the shared epitope segregates with synovitis in patients with IBD without sacroiliitis (7).

Recently, two independently working groups, reported on the correlations between mutations in the NOD 2 (CARD 15) gene, a host defense gene located on chromosome 16, and increased susceptibility for Crohn's disease (37,38). NOD2 encodes an intracellular protein whose expression is restricted to monocytes/macrophages, with infrequent expression detected in lymphocytes; it has binding affinity for bacterial liposaccharides and other bacterial components and helps to control the inflammatory response they induce. The protein is involved in nuclear factor (NF)-κB activation and apoptosis through two N-terminal caspase recruitment domains (hence the term *CARD*) (39). The prevalence of this mutation in Crohn's disease is about 30% (37,38,40). The linkage of CARD 15 variants has been related to clinical phenotypes such as younger age at onset, preferential involvement of small bowel (41,42), or fibrostenosing disease (43). No association was found with extraintestinal manifestations.

Different investigators have studied the association of CARD 15/NOD 2 variants in patients with spondyloarthropathy and found no increased prevalence, concluding that these variants do not affect the risk of developing primary ankylosing spondylitis (44–46). By studying spondyloarthropathy patients who 15 years earlier underwent ileocolonoscopy (31), prevalence of CARD 15 mutations in the subgroup of patients previously demonstrating chronic gut inflammation (42%) was similar to patients with uncomplicated Crohn's disease (48%) and significantly higher than controls (47). In spondyloarthropathy patients with chronic inflammation, 15% will develop Crohn's disease. Spondyloarthropathy patients harboring CARD 15 mutations might be at a higher risk for evolution to Crohn's disease.

Therapy

The treatment of peripheral arthritis and spondylitis in patients with IBD is the same as in ankylosing spondylitis. Nonsteroidal antiinflammatory drugs (NSAIDs; see Chapter 31) are the first choice, although they may cause an exacerbation of intestinal symptoms in ulcerative colitis. Intraarticular corticosteroid injections may be beneficial in monarticular flares. Sulfasalazine (see Chapter 42), which has been successfully used to treat colonic inflammation in ulcerative colitis and Crohn's disease, has been found to be effective in the treatment of the peripheral arthritis accompanying the spondyloarthropathies (48), especially if intestinal inflammation is present (49). It may also have a favorable effect on the peripheral arthritis of IBD. Although frequently inducing a clinical remission in spondyloarthropathies, sulfasalazine does not prevent the development of IBD (49). Oral corticosteroids may reduce peripheral synovitis, but have no effect on axial symptoms. Their systematic use is justified only if they are required to control the bowel disease. Gold, D-penicillamine, and antimalarial drugs are ineffective. Low-dose methotrexate (MTX), successfully used in the treatment of RA and in some cases of refractory IBD (50), has not yet been proven effective in joint inflammation associated with Crohn's disease or ulcerative colitis.

It has been demonstrated that treatment with a single infusion of chimeric monoclonal antibody cA2 directed against tumor necrosis factor (TNF)-α (infliximab) was highly effective in the short-term treatment of intestinal involvement in treatment-resistant Crohn's disease (51), even resulting in the closure of enterocutaneous fistulae (52). Moreover, the results of the Crohn's disease clinical trial evaluating infliximab in a new long-term treatment regimen (ACCENT) study showed that maintenance therapy with infliximab in moderate to severe Crohn's disease prolonged the response and remission of the disease (53, 54). In an open pilot study (55), a significant improvement in articular and axial symptoms, together with a remission of gut inflammation, was observed in four patients with Crohn's disease with associated spondyloarthropathy (Fig. 66.2), suggesting that resistant joint and axial manifestations in Crohn's disease might respond to the administration of infliximab.

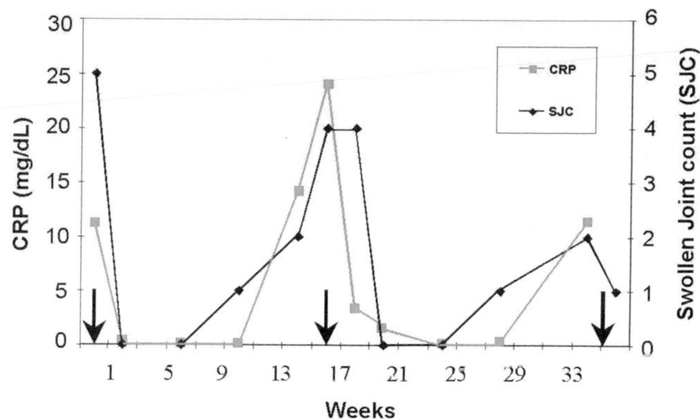

FIG. 66.2. Treatment of Crohn's disease associated spondyloarthropathy with infliximab. *Arrows* indicate infusions of infliximab.

ENTEROGENIC REACTIVE ARTHRITIS

Reactive arthritis can be defined as joint inflammation initiated by infectious agents, in which the causative microorganism cannot be isolated from the joint. Immunofluorescence and molecular biology techniques have demonstrated microbial antigens of arthritogenic gastrointestinal pathogens (*Yersinia* and *Salmonella*) in the synovial fluid and membrane of patients with reactive arthritis (56). *Salmonella* (57) and *Yersinia* (58) DNA have been detected by polymerase chain reaction in reactive arthritis joints. The reactive arthritides are considered to be spondyloarthropathies because of the typical pattern of peripheral joint involvement, the possible occurrence of enthesopathies and sacroiliitis, and the increased prevalence of HLA-B27. In prospective studies, it has been demonstrated that patients with *Yersinia*-induced arthritis can develop Crohn's disease (31).

Arthritogenic Gastrointestinal Pathogens

Salmonella typhimurium, Shigella flexneri, Yersinia enterocolitica (especially serotype 3), *Y. pseudotuberculosis,* and *Campylobacter jejuni* are the most common gastrointestinal pathogens capable of initiating peripheral arthritis. With regard to *Shigella*, only *S. flexneri,* and not *S. sonnei,* has been implicated as a causative agent of reactive arthritis, suggesting that the "arthritogenic" factor may not be a universal feature of a given family of pathogens.

The high frequency of infectious enteritis, especially of *Yersinia* infections, the fact that the gastrointestinal symptoms preceding the arthritis often are minimal, and the fact that fecal cultures can be negative at the moment of the appearance of the arthritis, render the definite diagnosis of enterogenic reactive arthritis difficult.

Clinical Symptoms

Peripheral Arthritis

The onset of arthritis usually occurs within 6 to 14 days after the onset of diarrhea, but can occur up to 3 months later. The duration of diarrhea is strongly correlated with the occurrence of joint symptoms (59). The duration of the articular episode is approximately 4 months (60). The arthritis is mainly monoarticular or pauciarticular and asymmetric, and affects the lower limbs predominantly. In nearly 30% of patients, multiple episodes of arthritis occur, and in 5% to 20%, the arthritis becomes chronic. Chronic spondyloarthropathy was found in 13% of patients with reactive *Salmonella*-induced arthritis (61). In some cases, recurrence is caused by another enterogenic or urogenic infection.

Synovial fluid analysis reveals mild to marked inflammation: the white blood cell count ranges from 4,000 to 120,000 cells/mm^3, with predominantly polymorphonuclear cells.

Enthesopathy usually involves the calcaneum, and dactylitis (sausage digits or toes), due to tenosynovitis of a digital tendon sheath, may occur.

Radiographic lesions of the peripheral joints are rare, but, if present, are identical to those seen in association with IBD. In the course of the disease, some patients complain of buttock pain. Radiographic evidence of sacroiliitis has been described in 6% to 9% of the patients, generally in those with chronic or recurrent peripheral arthritis.

Gastrointestinal Symptoms and Associated Features

Fever and diarrhea generally precede the arthritis by 1 to 2 weeks, although this interval can be longer, and is sometimes more than 3 months. Diarrhea can be absent, and there is no relation between the severity of the gut symptoms and either the development of articular episodes or the severity of joint symptoms.

Conjunctivitis occurs in 30% of the patients. Urogenital symptoms, mainly urethritis or balanitis, complete the picture initially described as Reiter's syndrome.

Acute anterior uveitis occurs mainly in HLA-B27$^+$ patients, but appears to be independent and not related in time to the triggering infectious episode. Mouth ulcers and erythema nodosum have been reported after *Yersinia* infection. Keratodermia blennorrhagicum, described in the entity of urogenic reactive arthritis, does not occur in enterogenic forms.

Relation to HLA-B27

As in the other spondyloarthropathies, the prevalence of HLA-B27 is increased in reactive arthritis, including those forms induced by enterogenic agents. The reported prevalence of HLA-B27 ranges between 60% and 80%. Inflammatory low back pain and sacroiliitis are more frequent in HLA-B27$^+$ patients (61).

Treatment

NSAIDs are effective in the treatment of reactive arthritis, as are intraarticular injections of corticosteroids. In open studies, sulfasalazine has been claimed effective for patients with reactive arthritis, and these data have been confirmed in a controlled study (62).

Short-term conventional antimicrobial therapy has no effect on the joint symptoms and does not modify the course of ongoing disease. In a 3-month double-blind study of ciprofloxacin in the treatment of chronic reactive arthritis, a significant improvement in clinical parameters, although not significantly different from placebo, was demonstrated (63). Because *Yersinia* can be harbored in gut mucosa and lymphoid tissue (64), long-term antibiotic treatment should be considered. In an animal model in which *Yersinia* was injected, arthritis could also be prevented if antibiotics were administered less than 5 days after the inoculation (65).

OTHER FORMS OF SPONDYLOARTHROPATHIES

The gut obviously plays a role in the pathogenesis of IBD, enterogenic reactive arthritis, and Whipple disease. However, subclinical gut inflammation has been demonstrated in virtually all forms of spondyloarthropathies. Numerous ileocolonoscopic studies have demonstrated a high prevalence of gut inflammation in patients with ankylosing spondylitis (1,31), other forms of reactive arthritis, and undifferentiated spondyloarthropathies (1,31): in other words, in patients with clinical, laboratory, radiologic, and genetic features of the spondyloarthropathies, but who cannot be classified into one of the distinct clinical entities. Recent studies have demonstrated gut inflammation in some forms of juvenile chronic arthritis (JCA), notably in the pauciarticular late-onset form, which is frequently associated with HLA-B27 and considered to be a form of spondyloarthropathy (66). Inflammatory gut lesions were found in nine of twelve children with this type of JCA. In the follow-up, in six of these patients, ankylosing spondylitis developed; all had gut inflammation at the first examination. In two of these patients, Crohn's disease developed.

In acute anterior uveitis, chronic inflammatory gut lesions were found in 66% of cases (25). The histology of the lesions and the patchy distribution resembled Crohn's disease, suggesting that the gut is involved in the pathogenesis of acute anterior uveitis.

In psoriatic arthritis, gut inflammation was demonstrated only in the pauciarticular and axial forms, considered to be spondyloarthropathies, and not in the polyarticular form (67).

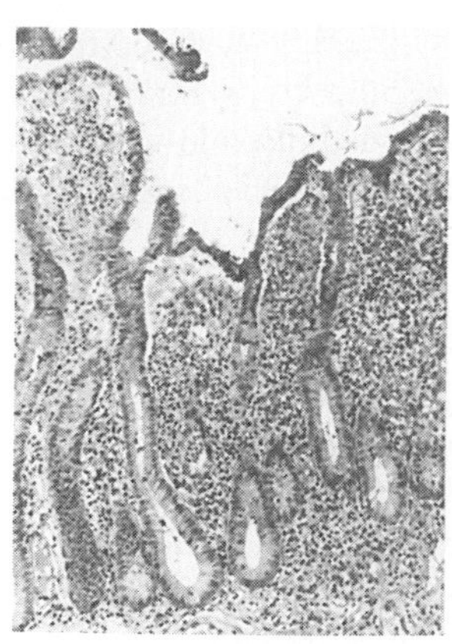
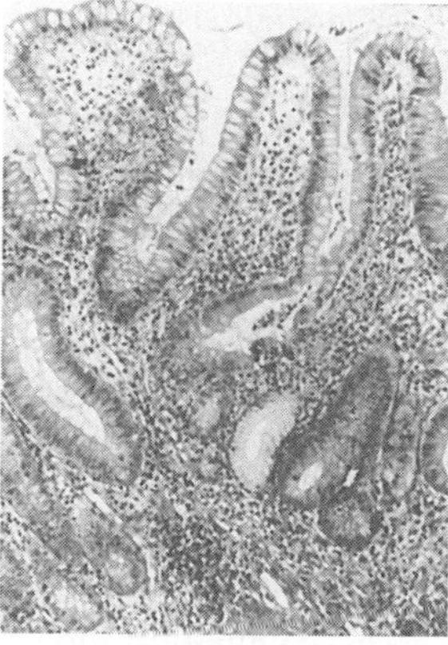

FIG. 66.3. Left: Acute ileitis with preserved villus and crypt architecture. The lamina propria is infiltrated by polymorphonuclear cells, lymphocytes, and plasma cells. The villus epithelium is regenerating (hematoxylin and eosin stain, original magnification ×124). **Right:** Chronic ileitis with irregular, blunt villi. The crypts are distorted and feature pseudopyloric metaplasia. The lamina propria contains a mainly lymphoplasmocytic infiltrate, and there is a basal lymphoid follicle (hematoxylin and eosin stain, original magnification ×124).

The histologic lesions are subdivided into "acute lesions" resembling acute bacterial enteritis and "chronic lesions" resembling the pathology of chronic idiopathic IBD (Fig. 66.3). The clinical, laboratory, and radiographic disease manifestations in patients with chronic lesions resemble the features of IBD and ankylosing spondylitis, whereas patients with acute lesions exhibit clinical features of enterogenic reactive arthritis (68).

Subclinical Gut Inflammation

Obviously, some patients with spondyloarthropathy can be considered to have enteropathic arthritides, although most have no clinical intestinal symptoms. Studies on the evolution of disease in these patients have demonstrated that most patients with normal histology or acute intestinal lesions exhibited transient arthritis, whereas the majority of those with chronic intestinal lesions had persistent inflammatory joint symptoms; about 6% of these patients developed Crohn's disease (31). Serial ileocolonoscopic studies (69) demonstrated that the remission of the rheumatic disease was always associated with the disappearance of the gut inflammation, whereas half of the patients with joint inflammation harbored persistent gut inflammation; 40% of the latter developed IBD. These findings underline the close relation between gut and joint inflammation in the spondyloarthropathies. This close relation was confirmed in human HLA-B27 transgenic rats, which in germ-free conditions did not develop joint or gut inflammation (70).

Consequently, some patients with spondyloarthropathy may have a form of subclinical Crohn's disease in which the joint symptoms are the only clinical expression.

Genetics

The prevalence of HLA-B27 in undifferentiated spondyloarthropathies is similar to that found in the reactive arthritides. Family studies of proven cases of Crohn's disease and ankylosing spondylitis have revealed a familial aggregation of subclinical gut inflammation (1).

Therapy

NSAIDs are the treatment of choice. Because of the presence of subclinical gut inflammation, administration of sulfasalazine is justified in spondyloarthropathy that is refractory to NSAIDs. The beneficial effect of sulfasalazine has been demonstrated not only in ankylosing spondylitis (48,71), but also in reactive arthritis, psoriatic arthritis (72), undifferentiated spondyloarthropathies (73), late-onset pauciarticular JCA (74), and acute anterior uveitis (75). Finally anti–TNF-α blockade with infliximab has demonstrated effectiveness in different forms of spondyloarthropathy. An open pilot study demonstrated the efficacy of infliximab in different subtypes of spondyloarthropathy (76). Using a dosage of 5 mg/kg every 14 weeks, the intravenous administration of infliximab induced a sustained significant decrease of all symptoms on retreatment over a 1-year period, although recurrence of symptoms frequently was observed beginning at 6 weeks prior to the following infusion (77). This indicated that the dosing interval of 14 weeks was too long and it was therefore decreased to 8 weeks. A double-blind placebo controlled monocentric study of 40 patients with spondyloarthropathy (78) confirmed the beneficial effects of infliximab on peripheral arthritis, axial involvement, enthesitis, and inflammatory serum parameters. Another double-blind placebo controlled study in ankylosing spondylitis (79) confirmed the efficacy of this treatment in this disease for which no disease-modifying drugs were previously available.

NONSTEROIDAL ANTIINFLAMMATORY DRUGS AND THE GUT

NSAIDs can induce subclinical intestinal abnormalities including increased intestinal loss of protein and blood (80); even bowel ulcerations have been demonstrated (81) (see Chapter 31). In some cases, strictures of the small intestine have been associated with prolonged use of NSAIDs (82). NSAID-induced intestinal blood loss can be reduced by sulfasalazine treatment (83). However, NSAID-related changes are more common in the proximal parts of the jejunum and ileum than in the terminal ileum and colon (80). Virtually all ileocolonoscopic studies in patients with spondyloarthropathy have demonstrated the absence of any association between gut lesions and the use of NSAIDs (1). The inflammatory findings in terminal ileum and colon of patients with spondyloarthropathies cannot be explained by the use of NSAIDs. In the large intestine, NSAIDs, however, may provoke relapse of quiescent IBD, especially in ulcerative colitis (84), and those prone to relapses do so within a few days after receiving these drugs. Use of NSAIDs may be associated with an increased risk of emergency admission to the hospital for colitis caused by IBD, particularly among patients with no previous history (85).

It is now clear that NSAIDs do not act only through cyclooxygenase (COX) inhibition, but also have different targets such as NFκB and peroxisome proliferation–activated receptor (PPAR)-γ (86). Although the new selective COX-2 inhibitors have a proven benefit in preventing gastric lesions, it is not clear if these drugs have the same protective effect on the colon, since COX-2 inhibition might have a detrimental role in ulcer healing (87).

WHIPPLE'S DISEASE

Whipple's disease is a multisystem disorder characterized in its fully expressed form by steatorrhea and severe weight loss (which are the main intestinal symptoms), fever, arthritis, serositis, lymphadenopathy, leukocytosis, and often thrombocytosis.

Whipple's disease occurs most often in men (90%) and in middle-aged individuals, and the joint symptoms may antedate the intestinal complaints by more than 5 years. Arthritis flares are not related temporally to exacerbations of intestinal symptoms. Arthralgias are a common finding. The arthritis is polyarticular, symmetric, and usually transient, but may become chronic. Synovial effusions contain between 4,000 and 100,000 leukocytes/mm^3, consisting mainly of polymorphonuclear cells.

Radiolographic lesions are rare. The incidence of sacroiliitis and spondylitis is controversial, as well as the relation with HLA-B27. A variety of ophthalmologic and neurologic syndromes may occur, including anterior and posterior uveitis, vitritis, ocular palsies, and progressive encephalopathy.

Joint manifestations in Whipple's disease are probably a form of enterogenic arthritis, caused by an infection of the intestine. Characteristic periodic acid–Schiff (PAS) staining deposits are found in the macrophages of the small intestine and in the mesenteric nodes. These cells also contain rod-shaped free bacilli best seen by electron microscopy (88). These bacilliform bodies are considered to be the etiologic agent, because they disappear when the patients are successfully treated with antibiotics. Synovial histologic studies suggest that the joint also can be directly invaded by the causative organism. A unique 1,321-base pair bacterial 16S ribosomal RNA sequence was amplified from duodenal tissue of 5 patients with Whipple's disease, but not from duodenal tissue of 10 patients without the disorder (89). Phylogenetic analysis showed the bacterium to be a gram-positive actinomycete, which was designated *Tropheryma whippelii*. The polymerase chain reaction for this sequence now provides a specific test for the disease.

A correct diagnosis is important, because the condition responds well to appropriate antibiotic therapy. In patients with severe illness, parenteral therapy with ceftriaxone (2 g/day) is advocated. Long-term therapy for more than 1 year with trimethoprim–sulfamethoxazole (160/800 g orally twice daily) or 1 g/day tetracycline is necessary (90).

Intestinal Bypass Arthritis

Intestinal bypass surgery (jejunocolostomy or jejunoileostomy), which has been a popular treatment for morbid obesity, may give rise to an arthritis-dermatitis syndrome that is sometimes associated with renal, hepatic, and hematologic disorders. Polyarthritis develops in 20% to 80% of the cases. Symptoms appear 2 to 30 months after surgery. The arthritis is polyarticular, symmetric, and migratory, affecting both upper and lower limb joints. Chronic arthritis develops in one-fourth of the patients. The duration of the arthritis is unpredictable, and there is no relation between the joint symptoms and abnormal bowel movements.

Radiographic deformities or erosions are not seen. Sacroiliac and spine involvement, although uncommon, has been described. In 66% to 80% of the patients, a variety of dermatologic abnormalities occur. Erythema nodosum, maculae progressing to papules and vesiculopustules, urticaria, and nodular dermatitis have been reported. Other associated features are Raynaud phenomenon, paresthesias, pericarditis, pleuritis, glomerulonephritis, retinal vasculitis, and superficial thrombophlebitis.

The pathogenesis involves bacterial overgrowth and mucosal alterations in the blind loop. The disease seems to be immune-mediated; cryoprecipitates and other circulating complexes containing immunoglobulins, complement, bacterial antibodies, and antigens are found in the serum (91). Bacterial overgrowth in the blind loop could be responsible for a substantial increase of antigenic stimulation. Acute symmetric polyarthritis involving the peripheral and axial skeleton has been described 1 week to 2 years after a restorative proctocolectomy with an ileal porch and anastomosis for ulcerative colitis (92). In these cases, the dissemination of immune complexes resulting from the increased absorption of bacterial antigens due to the bacterial overgrowth was considered pathogenic.

NSAIDs are usually sufficient to control the arthritis. Oral antibiotics, such as tetracycline, clindamycin, or metronidazole given intermittently or continuously, can reduce the symptoms through a reduction of bacterial overgrowth.

Only surgical reanastomosis of the bypassed segment of the intestine gives complete resolution of all symptoms and may be necessary in refractory cases.

OTHER DISEASES ASSOCIATED WITH GASTROINTESTINAL AND JOINT INVOLVEMENT

Celiac Disease

Celiac disease (gluten-sensitivity enteropathy) is known to be associated with abnormal intestinal permeability. Many disorders, including dermatitis herpetiformis, hyposplenism, and autoimmune disorders, have been related to this disease.

Celiac disease can be divided into three types: (a) one in which diarrhea (usually steatorrhea) is the main feature; (b) one with constitutional disturbances such as lassitude, weight loss, and malaise; and (c) one with varied extraintestinal findings such as neuropathy and osteomalacia. Bowel symptoms are absent in 50% of the patients, especially in types (b) and (c). Arthritis may occur in the three different types of celiac disease.

The distribution of the arthritis varies but is usually polyarticular and symmetric, involving predominantly the large joints (hips, knees, and shoulders). Radiographic changes are rare.

In a clinical review of 200 patients with celiac disease (93), arthritis was present in 26% of the patients. Peripheral arthritis was present in 19 patients, axial involvement in 15, and both in 18 patients. Patients on a regular diet had significantly more joint or axial manifestations than did patients on a gluten-free diet. Conversely, there is a striking response of the joint manifestations to a gluten-free diet (94), although rechallenge does not provoke arthritis.

Vasculitis Syndromes

These syndromes include a number of autoimmune diseases in which the gut is not primarily involved, although inflammation of the abdominal (usually mesenteric) arteries with secondary vasculitic lesions in the gut mucosal and submucosal layers may occur.

Henoch-Schönlein Purpura

This disease, which occurs mainly in children, is a form of hypersensitivity vasculitis. The disease is characterized by the triad of nonthrombocytopenic purpura, arthritis, and abdominal pain. The characteristic skin lesions are palpable purpura, representing leukoclastic venulitis. Arthritis, involving predominantly the lower limbs, is transient. Gastrointestinal symptoms include severe cramping and colicky abdominal pain that are sometimes associated with gastrointestinal hemorrhage. Rarely, protein-losing enteropathy and even perforation may occur. There is no direct temporal relation between articular and intestinal symptoms. Mild renal involvement, consisting of glomerulitis with microscopic hematuria, occurs in 50% of the cases. The disease usually remits spontaneously within a week, but recurrences are common before complete remission is achieved.

Rheumatoid Arthritis

The initial pathologic change in RA is believed to occur in small blood vessels. The most important extraarticular complications of RA are due to an inflammatory vascular disease, giving rise to digital arteritis, peripheral neuropathy, and visceral arteritis.

Intestinal involvement, due to partial infarction of intestinal arteries, causes abdominal pain, which at first is intermittent, but is continuous later. This can lead to intestinal bleeding or perforation. There is no direct relation with the joint manifestations, but most RA patients with this complication have high rheumatoid factor titers, and subcutaneous nodules are common. The prognosis is very poor, and the outcome is frequently fatal.

Systemic Lupus Erythematosus

The most common intestinal manifestation of systemic lupus erythematosus is abdominal pain, which may be accompanied by nausea and less often by diarrhea. In most patients, abdominal pain occurs in association with evidence of disease activity in other systems. Abdominal pain is usually colicky and not related to joint manifestations. The symptoms are caused mainly by mesenteric arteritis, and colonic perforations may occur.

Polyarteritis Nodosa

This disease is characterized by panmural necrotizing inflammatory lesions in small and medium-sized muscular arteries. On angiography of the celiac trunk and the abdominal arteries, characteristic saccular or fusiform aneurysms and narrowing of arteries can be found, which are of diagnostic importance. Gastrointestinal involvement, mainly abdominal pain, is seen in 50% of the patients. Nausea, vomiting, diarrhea, icterus, ulceration with bleeding, infarction, or perforation are other possible manifestations. Infarction and perforation are usually fatal.

Scleroderma

Scleroderma is a systemic disease characterized by excessive deposition of collagen and other connective tissue components in the skin and multiple internal organs. Gastrointestinal involvement is common in this disease and is characterized mainly by a motility dysfunction of the entire gastrointestinal tract.

Reduced oral aperture, loss of lamina dura with loosening of the teeth, and severe esophageal dysfunction with dysphagia are features of upper gastrointestinal tract involvement.

Characteristically, hypomotility with atony, marked dilatation, and functional ileus are present in the small intestine and the colon. Abdominal cramps, malabsorption, and constipation, sometimes alternating with diarrhea, are the clinical manifestations. The disturbed intestinal motility leads to stasis and secondary bacterial overgrowth.

The pathology consists of normal mucosa with mild villous atrophy, infiltrations of the lamina propria by lymphocytes and plasma cells, fibrous thickening of the submucosa, and thickening of the walls of small arteries and arterioles.

Almost unique to systemic sclerosis is the development of wide-mouthed, often square pseudodiverticula along the antimesenteric border of the transverse and descending colon.

Miscellaneous Rheumatic Diseases

Behçet Disease

Behçet disease is characterized by the presence of buccal, ocular, genital, and skin ulcerations accompanied by arthritis. The disease is associated with HLA-B51 (95). It resembles features of the spondyloarthropathies (because sacroiliitis and spondylitis may be present) and IBD. Virtually all features of Behçet disease can be present in Crohn's disease of the colon. Diarrhea, abdominal pain, and colonic ulceration, rarely with perforation, are possible clinical manifestations. Intestinal involvement is seen in 60% of Japanese patients with Behçet (96), predominantly localized to the ileocecal region, and can be difficult to differentiate from Crohn's disease because rectovaginal fistulae and perianal ulceration also occur. In Western countries, however, symptomatic IBD in Behçet is uncommon (97) and controversy exists as to whether these cases represent true involvement of the colon by Behçet disease, or merely coincidental IBD.

Amyloidosis

Primary amyloidosis, or amyloidosis secondary to chronic inflammatory diseases, may cause gastrointestinal manifestations, including obstruction, ulceration, malabsorption, hemorrhage, protein loss, and diarrhea. At a later stage, potentially fatal gastrointestinal bleeding may occur. These manifestations may occur through direct infiltration with amyloid or through infiltration of the autonomic nervous system.

Familial Mediterranean Fever

Familial Mediterranean fever is a genetic disorder, inherited as an autosomal-recessive disorder with complete penetrance. The characteristic symptoms include intermittent fever, recurrent abdominal pain, and joint inflammation. The abdominal crises resemble acute peritonitis, lasting from 12 to 24 hours. Serous fluid may accumulate in the abdominal cavity, and intestinal obstruction may occur.

The arthritis occurs together with, or independent of, the other manifestations and is generally asymmetric, involving predominantly the lower limbs. Attacks can persist for 2 or 3 weeks. Amyloidosis is a frequent complication.

Collagenous Colitis

This condition consists of intermittent watery diarrhea without bleeding. Ten percent of the patients have arthritis. On biopsy, linear deposition of hyaline material, 1- to 100-mm thick, principally consisting of collagen type III, is found in the subepithelium of the colon. The pathogenesis is unknown.

PATHOGENETIC CONSIDERATIONS

As indicated by the clinical picture of IBD, enterogenic reactive arthritis, and other forms of spondyloarthropathy, the pathogenesis of enteropathic arthritis involves abnormal immune activation in the gut followed by inflammation of the peripheral joints and other target organs. Both microorganisms and a predisposing genetic context are likely to be crucial players in this process, as illustrated in animal models. Therefore, a better understanding of the normal and pathologic immunobiology of the gut (including the barrier defense mechanisms such as gut permeability and the IgA cycle, the innate immune system, and the adaptive immune system) and the joint might shed light on the relation between joint and gut inflammation in the spondyloarthropathies.

Animal Models Illustrating the Relation between the Gut and Joints: Influence of Microorganisms and Genetic Factors

Covalent complexes of peptidoglycan and polysaccharides, the primary structural components of bacteria cell walls, can induce acute and chronic arthritis after local or systemic injection in laboratory animals (98–102). A transient arthritis was produced by bacteria from a patient with Crohn's disease (101) and by bacteria from gram-positive normal enteric flora (100–102). Oral challenge with methylated bovine serum albumin (mBSA) produced a flare in mice with unilateral chronic mBSA antigen–induced arthritis (103). A peripheral arthritis was induced in pigs by feeding them a protein-rich diet, resulting in an abnormal intestinal microbial flora, with increased numbers of *Clostridia perfringens* and increased antibody titers to this organism (104).

It was hypothesized that a primary enteric infection with mucosal and mesenteric lymph node invasion could lead to systemic circulation of bacterial peptidoglycan and polysaccharide complexes, thereby inducing arthritis. Alternatively, increased permeability due to intestinal inflammation, as in IBD or in undifferentiated spondyloarthropathy, could lead to increased mucosal absorption and systemic distribution of arthritogenic bacterial cell wall polymers from the normal enteric microflora, resulting in the initiation and perpetuation of arthritis. Recently more attention has been directed toward a naturally occurring joint disease in mice, ankylosing enthesopathy (ANKENT). The prevalence of ANKENT is dependent on genetic background, sex, age, and environment. It ranges from 1% to 30% in normal mice, depending on the strain (105). Relevant to this disease, transgenic mice bearing human B27 were constructed; this manipulation increased the risk of the mice developing ANKENT, but, as in humans, most B27^{+} mice remained healthy. Thus, the B27 gene only increases the relative risk for ANKENT (106). Several double transgenic B27 and human β_2-microglobulin rat lines have been generated (107). Rats from two of the transgenic lines (LEW 21–4H and 33–3) spontaneously developed a multiorgan inflammatory disease analogous to the human disorders related to HLA-B27 and involving the gastrointestinal tract, peripheral and axial joints, male genital tract, skin, nails, and heart. Susceptibility to disease was clearly related to gene copy number and the level of expression of B27 (108). The most prevalent site of inflammation in the transgenic rats appeared to be the gastrointestinal tract, suggesting that the events initiating the disease process occur in the gastrointestinal tract. The disease manifestations can be reproducibly transferred to healthy rats, either transgenic or nontransgenic, by bone marrow or fetal liver cells (108). T cells, however, also are critical because athymic transgenic rats fail to develop the disease.

The role of bacteria in triggering the disease in B27 rats has been addressed by maintaining the animals in a germ-free environment. Under these conditions, the B27 lines remain free from joint and gut disease, but may have skin and genital lesions (70).

Gut inflammation also occurs in the HLA-B27 transgenic mice. Introduction of a human β_2 microglobulin transgene in these mice was necessary to achieve stable expression of the HLA molecule at the cell surface. Although these mice have a functional HLA-B27 product, B27 transgenic mice usually remain healthy. One group found diminished clearance of *Yersinia enterocolitica* after intestinal infection in B27 transgenic mice compared with mice transgenic for another human class I locus (A2) or nontransgenic mice (109). Foci of gut inflammation, as well as minimal sterile joint synovitis, were described only in the B27 transgenic mice.

Since these animal models seem to confirm that interaction of microorganisms with the gut immune system in a well-defined genetic context may be the key factors in enteropathic arthritis, we will review the different elements of the gastrointestinal immune system.

Barrier Defense Mechanisms: Gut Permeability and IgA Cycle

Normal gut permeability is regulated by an intact layer of gut epithelial cells, which is maintained by different types of homophilic adhesion molecules including E-cadherin (discussed later in the chapter). Altered gut permeability could permit luminal antigens to be absorbed through the mucosa and the lamina propria (110), thereby eliciting various systemic immunologic responses and inflammatory reactions in different tissues (111). Such increased permeability could be induced by different drugs, the disease itself, or perhaps by genetic determinants. Disturbed permeability might not be associated with inflammatory symptoms in the absence of the necessary antigens or in the absence of a sufficient immunologic response.

Increased gut permeability has been demonstrated in patients with IBD (112,113) and in their asymptomatic relatives (114), suggesting that it could be a primary etiologic factor. It also has been described in other forms of spondyloarthropathy, such as that associated with *Yersinia* infections (115) or ankylosing spondylitis (116,117). In spondyloarthropathy patients, gut permeability was significantly more disturbed in patients with chronic gut inflammation than in those with acute gut inflammation (118). In the former group, gut inflammation was related to more severe joint inflammation and destruction. This suggests that the transgression of the mucosal barrier was more continuous. A study performed in patients with ankylosing spondylitis and their first-degree relatives demonstrated increased small intestinal permeability compared with that in controls, in both patients and first-degree relatives (119).

Gut permeability is disturbed by the intake of drugs such as NSAIDs and corticosteroids, irrespective of the disease for which they are prescribed (110,120,121). Because histopathologic gut abnormalities were found only in patients with spondyloarthropathies, however, and not in those with other inflammatory joint disorders, even though antiinflammatory drugs had been given for both conditions, it is still possible that increased gut permeability plays a primary role in the pathogenesis of spondyloarthropathies. This is illustrated by two experiments. First, bypassing the epithelial barrier and injecting a cell-wall extract derived from luminal bacteria directly into the bowel wall induces a chronic, relapsing disease very similar to Crohn's disease and arthritis (122). Second, simply interfering with the function of E-cadherin, an important mediator of adhesion interactions between cells along the crypt villus axis, induces inflammation similar to Crohn's disease (123,124). The latter observations suggest that genetically induced increases in paracellular permeability might promote IBD. Of interest, an up-regulation of E-cadherin and its associated catenins was demonstrated in clinically overt IBD wih a decreased expression in ulcer-associated epithelium (125). Similarly, in spondyloarthropathy, an increased expression of the proteins of the E-cadherin/catenin complex in acute and chronic subclinical gut inflammation was described (126).

Another important barrier between the luminal microorganisms and their antigens and the gastrointestinal immune system is the presence of IgA antibodies in the gut lumen. Approximately 70% to 80% of all immunoglobulin-producing cells in the human body are located in the gut-associated lymphoid tissue (GALT), which includes organized structures such as the Peyer patches (PPs) (Figs. 66.4, 66.5), the submucosal and mesenteric lymph nodes, and lymphoid and nonlymphoid cells of nonepithelial origin dispersed throughout the gut in the epithelial layer and the lamina propria (127–129). Most of these immunoglobulin-producing cells (70% to 90%) are IgA immunocytes (plasma cells and plasma blasts). Immunocytes adjacent to exocrine

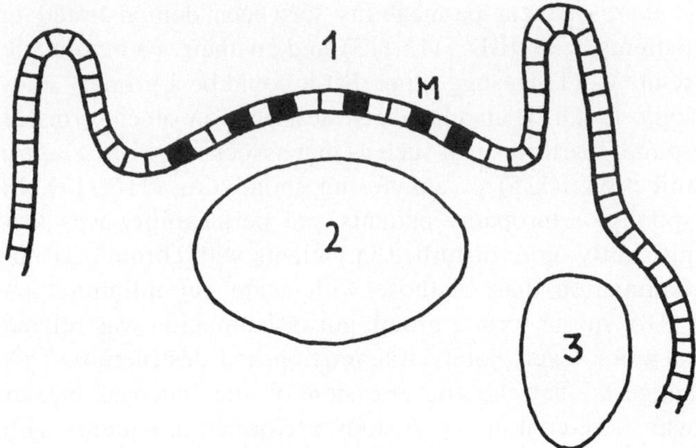

FIG. 66.4. The Peyer patches (PPs) have long been considered as the mammalian bursa equivalents, but more recent immunofluorescence studies have provided evidence of T-cell localization in PPs before B-cell follicle formation. PPs contain three major components: the dome (*1*), the thymic dependent area (*2*), and the follicle (*3*). The dome epithelium contains the columnar absorptive cells, next to a few goblet cells, and the membranous cells (*M*). The thymic-dependent area, in which T-helper cells predominate, is located at the transition between the dome and the villi and is in close connection with lymphatics and high endothelial venules; underlying the dome, the follicle, which is separated from the epithelial layer by a mixed population of lymphocytes, macrophages, and lymphoblasts, consists essentially of B cells, of which a high percentage bear surface immunoglobulin A in the germinal center. Germinal center B cells are actively dividing, and this tissue also contains dendritic cells and macrophages.

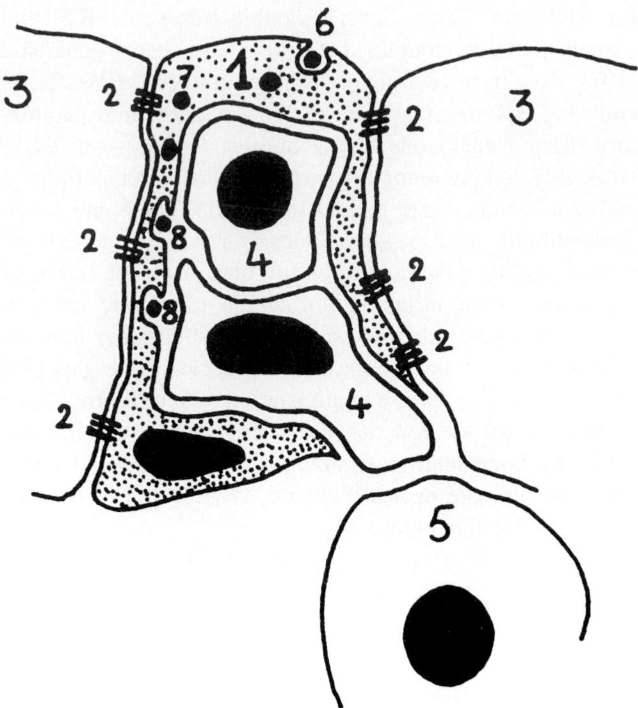

FIG. 66.5. The M cells (*1*) possess a basal nucleus with irregular contour and exhibit characteristic interdigitations (*2*) with other columnar cells. Between the M cells and the columnar cells (*3*), interspersed lymphoid cells (*4*) are observed, which occasionally are in close apposition to the cell membrane of the M cells. They form pseudopods that insert into lacunae formed in the plasma membrane of the M cells. Phagocytic macrophages (*5*) also are present under the lymphoid elements. M cells are constantly HLA-DR negative and contain abundant pinocytic vesicles (*6, 7*) suggesting a role of these cells in the transport of antigen, without processing, from the gut lumen to underlying antigen-presenting cells. They deliver antigenic macromolecules or microorganisms (*8*) to underlying mononuclear cells, resulting in the initiation of an immune response.

glands produce mainly dimeric or higher polymeric IgA (pIgA), containing, in addition to the monomeric IgAs, a disulfide-linked polypeptide designated "joining" chain (J chain) (130). The transport of dimeric IgA is mediated by a secretory component synthesized by the rough endoplasmic reticulum of epithelial cells. After terminal glycosylation in the Golgi complex, transmembranous expression of secretory component occurs at the basolateral cell surface. Dimeric IgA containing J chain is fixed on the transmembrane secretory component by two disulfide bridges involving one heavy chain of one of the IgA subunits. After endocytosis and transcytosis, the secretory IgA (SIgA) is released into the lumen (131–133).

Antigen absorption in the gut is affected by secretory antibodies. If this mechanism is inadequate, the internal environment requires protection against ensuing harmful systemic immune reactions (e.g., IgG, IgE, and T cell–mediated delayed hypersensitivity responses). A common term, *oral tolerance,* is used for the suppressive mechanisms. Administration of antigen by the oral route stimulates CD4$^+$ T cell–helper activity for IgA responses in the PPs, producing a simultaneous stimulation of CD8$^+$ suppressor T cells specific for the IgG class, which migrate from the PPs to the spleen, where they mediate suppression of systemic responses (134). Direct injection of the antigen into the PPs does not induce oral tolerance (135). The cellular elements involved in these suppressive mechanisms are still not fully delineated. The following events are postulated to down-regulate the delayed-type hypersensitivity and systemic IgG and IgE responses, while maintaining the local IgA response in healthy individuals. The epithelial cells or specialized mucosal macrophages process antigens and present them to CD8$^+$ suppressor cells, which generate suppressive regulatory signals (136). The CD4$^+$ helper cells are of little assistance to IgG- and IgE-producing B cells. In contrast, signals coming from a contrasuppressor CD8$^+$ subset intervene in the stimulation of those CD4$^+$ cells that up-regulate IgA-bearing immunocytes. In diseased individuals, interruption of the epithelial layer is accompanied by abnormal stimulation of antigen-presenting cells, resulting in enhanced DR expression on epithelial cells, and consequently, overstimulation of CD4$^+$ cells. This, in turn, leads to increased production of SIgA, and excessive IgG responses and delayed-type hypersensitivity.

Thus, if in the normal situation the luminal IgA is sufficient to provide a first line of defense against microorganisms, it is likely that increased gut permeability with higher antigen stimulation leads to a strong activation of Ig production. If overstimulation initially activates the "first line of defense" (inductive sites—i.e., the secretory immune responses); in contrast, accelerated luminal antigen presentation through a break in the epithelial layer, together with cytokines released from activated monocytes, might activate the "second line of defense" (effector sites—i.e., a systemic type of reaction aimed at elimination of the massive antigen penetration into the mucosa). But this second-line defense mechanism, which promotes immune elimination and limits dissemination of antigen, might disturb normal mucosal immunologic homeostasis by enrolling B cells of the systemic immune system. The postulated switch from secretory local immunity to a systemic type of local immune reaction could have opposing consequences: the local down-regulation of J chain in the IgA immunocytes could shift the production of polymeric IgA to monomers, jeopardizing secretory immunity (128,137,138). The disproportionate increase of IgG-producing cells could favor further inflammation and tissue damage through complement activation and arming of killer cells, and cause autoimmune responses locally and in target organs at a distance (e.g., joints).

Several studies have focused on IgA and other immunoglobulins in IBD and spondyloarthropathy. IgG-, IgA-, and IgM-producing cells in the gut are increased in both IBD and spondyloarthropathy with chronic inflammatory gut lesions, and are paralleled by an increase in serum concentration of these three immuoglobulin isotypes (139,140,141). More recently, ASCA or antibodies directed against the cell wall mannan of *Saccharomyces cerevisiae*, commonly known as baker's or brewer's yeast, were detected in the serum of Crohn's disease patients (27,142). Although their pathologic role is not yet clear, ASCA is a useful tool to discriminate between Crohn's disease and ulcerative colitis and has been associated with distinct clinical subtypes of Crohn's disease, especially small bowel involvement (143–146). Similarly, ASCA IgA are also elevated in ankylosing spondylitis and undifferentiated spondloarthopathy (28). However, the fact that the IgG levels were not elevated fits in the concept that spondyloarthropathy is a model for early immune alterations of the gut in IBD.

The Innate Immune System

When microbial antigens from the gut lumen escape the primary defense mechanisms described above, they will come in direct contact with the immune system and lead eventually to immune-mediated tissue inflammation. Two different pathways can contribute to this process: antigen-uptake and presentation by antigen-presenting cells to T lymphocytes (or the so-called adaptive immunity) or direct stimulation of inflammatory cells such as monocytes, macrophages, and neutrophils, but also intestinal epithelial cells (the so-called innate immune system).

These cells recognize microbial pathogen-associated molecular patterns (or PAMPs) through their toll-like receptors (TLRs) and initiate a rapid and quite nonspecific innate immune response. After binding of bacterial lipoproteins (TLR2), endotoxins (TLR4), flagellin (TLR5), or bacterial CpG dinucleotides (TLR9), the TLRs in association with the adaptor molecule MyD88 initiate a signaling cascade resulting in the activation of NFκB, and the induction of oxidative stress, and the production of inflammatory cytokines.

Although these mechanisms have not yet been studied thoroughly in IBD and spondyloarthropathy, there is preliminary evidence of an abnormal expression of TLR on gastrointestinal epithelial cells in IBD (147). On the other hand, there are numerous studies indicating an abnormal balance between pro- and antiinflammatory monocyte/macrophage-derived cytokines in IBD and spondyloarthropathy, especially TNF-α and interleukin (IL)-10.

TNF-α is produced predominantly by monocytes and macrophages and, to a lesser extent, by activated T cells. It acts on a broad spectrum of target cells. TNF-α induces macrophages to produce IL-1, IL-8, and IL-12. Endothelium responds to TNF-α with enhanced expression of adhesion molecules, thus leading to increased cell infiltration. Fibroblasts constitute another TNF-α target, responding with IL-6 secretion, which itself induces an acute-phase response, as well as increased synthesis of metalloproteinases and decreased production of matrix molecules. In addition, TNF-α alters epithelial permeability, thus compromising the gut barrier function. Several data suggest an imbalance between pro- and antiinflammatory cytokines in the gut mucosa in patients with Crohn's disease (148). Increased serum levels and stool concentrations of TNF-α and an elevated number of TNF-α-secreting mucosal cells in patients with Crohn's disease strongly suggest TNF-α as a key mediator of inflammation in this disease, and thus as an important target molecule.

IBDs may be associated with a decreased production of cytokines suppressing macrophage and T-cell function, including IL-10. Several data indicate that IL-10 is required for maintenance of immune homeostasis in the gut. Especially interesting is the observation that IL-10–deficient mice develop enteritis (149) and that IL-10 supplementation is effective in suppressing this inflammation. In addition, IL-10 is efficacious in the treatment of gut inflammation in another model of bowel inflammation, rabbit immune complex–induced colitis (induction of colitis by rectal instillation of formalin followed by intravenous infusion of heat-aggregated rabbit immunoglobulin) (150).

Data regarding the role of IL-10 in patients with spondyloarthropathy are scarce. Claudepierre et al. (151) reported IL-10 plasma levels to be correlated with disease activity in patients with spondyloarthropathy, in particular with duration of morning stiffness, pain, and C-reactive protein levels. Simon et al. (152) observed that synovial fluid–derived T-cell clones, from patients with chlamydial reactive arthritis, express IL-10 mRNA. IL-10 also was shown to be produced by psoriatic synovium (153). It is not possible now to define the role of IL-10 in the development of spondyloarthropathy. One may consider a feedback response aimed at controlling inflammation. Another interpretation might be that IL-10, given its immunosuppressive role, favors the persistence of bacterial antigens, which could provoke or perpetuate inflammation.

Besides an altered balance between pro- and antiinflammatory cytokines, there is also evidence of an altered presence and phenotype of monocytes/macrophages in the gut mucosa of IBD and spondyloarthropathy patients. HLA-DR–expressing CD68$^+$ macrophages are found in human GALT immediately below the follicle-associated epithelium (154–156). A recent study indicates that these cells are increased in the gut of patients with spondyloarthropathy, even before macro- or microscopic inflammation occurs (157).

Moreover, a particular subset of macrophages expressing the scavenger receptor (CD163) are selectively increased in Crohn's disease and in noninflamed gut mucosa of patients with spondyloarthropathy, emphasizing that even histologically normal intestine exhibits subclinical immune alterations in spondyloarthropathy (158). Functional analysis of the CD163 macrophages suggests that they could contribute to the synovial inflammation by two different mechanisms. First, they express high levels of HLA-DR and induce a greater allogeneic T-cell response than CD163-negative macrophages, possibly playing a role in the local reactivation of memory T cells by presenting either persisting bacterial antigens, cross-reacting antigens derived from cartilage, or HLA-B27 heavy chains (158,159). Second, they can produce large amounts of the proinflammatory cytokine TNF-α but not of the antiinflammatory cytokine IL-10 (158), which could disturb the local inflammatory balance.

From a clinical perspective, the major impact of TNF-α blockade on Crohn's disease (but not ulcerative colitis) and spondyloarthropathy supports the concept that an alteration of the innate immune system, by an inappropriately high and sustained inflammatory response of macrophages and other cells to microbial compounds, plays an important role in the pathogenesis of these diseases.

The Adaptive Immune System

Besides the innate immune system, luminal antigens are likely to induce an adaptive immune response in the gut through uptake and processing of antigens by antigen-presenting cells, followed by presentation to infiltrating lymphocytes. Therefore, antigen presentation, influx and outflux of lymphocytes mediated by specific adhesion molecules, and the functional outcome (Th1 vs. Th2 cytokines) are all of interest in the pathogenesis of enteropathic arthritis.

Antigen Uptake, Processing, and Presentation

Luminal particles are preferentially taken up through specialized areas of the follicle-associated epithelium, the so-called M cells (154) (Fig. 66.6). These unique bell-shaped cells, which sample antigens nonspecifically and by receptor-mediated uptake, can apparently function as antigen-processing cells. However, major histocompatibility complex (MHC) class II expression is low on M cells (155). The M-cell pockets that represent putative sites of initial antigen encounter contain only occasional CD68$^+$ or CD11c$^+$ antigen-presenting cells, but are packed with B and T cells. The dominant CD4$^+$ T-cell subset generally belongs to the CD45RO$^+$ memory phenotype. In striking contrast, most (80% to 90%) of the ordinary intraepithelial lymphocytes in the remaining follicle-associated epithelium and small intestinal villus epithelium consist of the CD8$^+$ phenotype (160). The most likely cells to mediate MHC class II interactions with T cells in the M-cell pockets are the predominating (66%) memory B cells that lack surface IgD (sIgD) and usually express HLA-DR (Fig. 66.7). This interaction may lead to IL-2 secretion and promote T-cell survival and proliferation. A different result might be obtained if naive B cells, which lack the necessary costimulatory molecules, capture antigens in competition with a much smaller number of antigen-presenting cells in the M-cell areas. One possible outcome could be the induction of T-cell anergy and, hence, tolerance. Moreover, engagement of the alternative high-affinity CD28-homologue B7 receptor, CTLA-4, which is expressed transiently on activated T cells, might provide negative signals, possibly leading to apoptosis, anergy, and down-regulation of T helper-1 or T helper-2–type cytokines (which might cause immune deviation) (161,162). The suppressive function of CTLA-4 might be particularly important for high-dose tolerance induction (163).

In reactive arthritis, the causative antigens are likely derived from the triggering organisms (*Yersinia enterocolitica, Salmonella typhimurium, Shigella flexneri,* or *Campylobacter*), which can be cultured from the stool early in the disease. The presence of serum IgA antibodies to plasmid-encoded secreted proteins and the persistence of *Yersinia* in the gut or gut lymphoid tissue (68,164) suggest an impaired elimination of these antigens from the gut wall. Enteric infectious agents, bacterial overgrowth, or a local mucin defect (165) might initiate increased epithelial permeability, abrogation of oral tolerance, and immunologic stimulation, followed by enhanced delayed hypersensitivity and systemic IgG response. Molecular mimicry between bacterial antigens and HLA-B27 has been suggested to play a role in the pathogenesis of reactive arthritides. *Klebsiella pneumoniae* nitrogenase shares a hexapeptide (QTDRED) with the

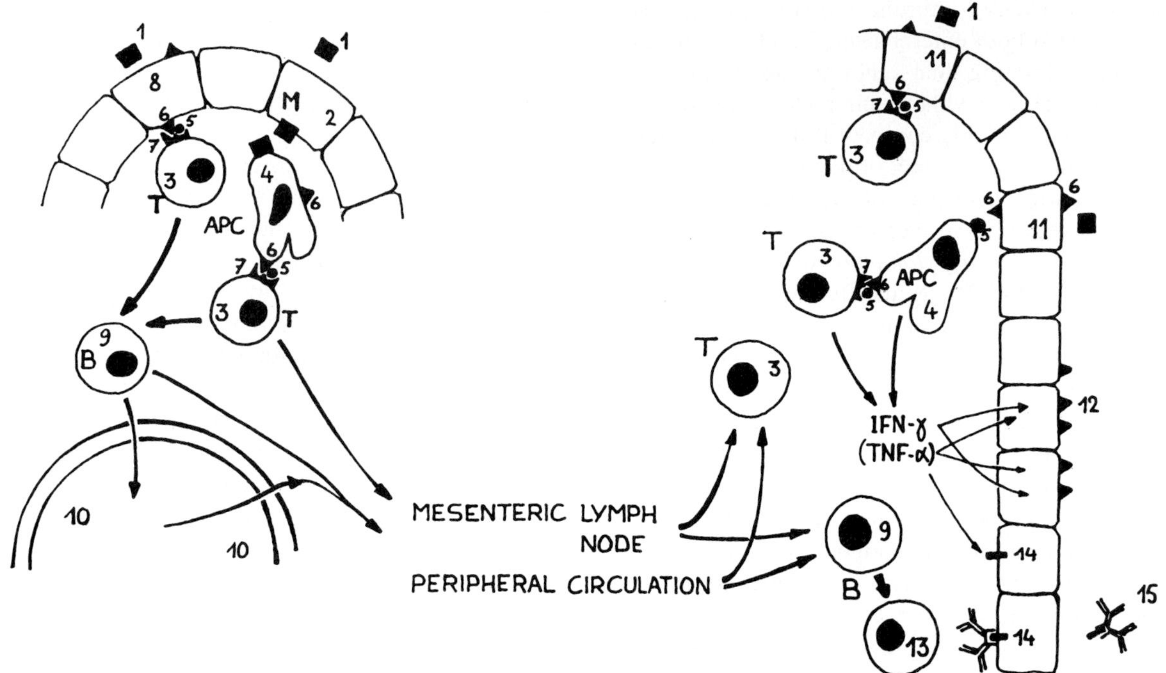

FIG. 66.6. Interactions between gut epithelium, lymphoid cells, and accessory cells can be summarized as follows: antigenic material (*1*) in the lumen of the gut is transported by the M cells (*2*) into Peyer patches (PPs) and is presented to the T cells (*3*) by subepithelial HLA-DR+ dendritic cells after processing by macrophages (*4*). If the antigen is processed in the gut lumen, HLA-DR+ enterocytes (*8*) can directly present it to T cells. A T cell stimulated by the HLA-DR+ enterocyte induces B-cell (*9*) differentiation, which is switched to immunoglobulin A (IgA) expression. Antigen presentation by dendritic cells in the follicle induces T-cell activation and B-cell differentiation in the germinal centers (*10*); through mesenteric lymph nodes and peripheral blood circulation, these cells undergo a migration to secretory tissues. At the secretory site, HLA-DR+ enterocytes (*11*) are responsible for antigen uptake and presentation, and for T-cell stimulation at that place. Interferon (IFN)-γ and tumor necrosis factor (TNF)-α, released by activated lymphocytes (IFN-γ) and macrophages (TNF-α), enhance local epithelial HLA-DR expression (*12*), and induce terminal B-cell differentiation (*13*). They also increase the membranous expression of secretory chain (SC) (*14*), and in this way, the release of dimeric IgA (*15*) in the secretion (*5*, processed antigen; *6*, DR molecule; *7*, T-cell receptor).

HLA-B27.5 molecule (166). *Yersinia* adhesin A (Yad A) shares a linear tetrapeptide (TRDE) with the B27 molecule (between amino acids 70 and 78 in the variable region of the α_1-helix) (167), and OmpH of *Salmonella typhimurium* shares five amino acids in a nonlinear fashion in the same site of the B27 molecule (168). Furthermore, it has been shown that isolates of *Shigella flexneri* that cause enteric infection and reactive arthritis carry a 2-Mol plasmid, pHS-2, which encodes a B27 mimetic peptide (a five-amino-acid peptide that is homologous with the polymorphic region of the HLA-B27 α_1 domain) (169). Molecular mimicry exists within these molecules, but its role in the pathogenesis of reactive arthritis is unclear (170).

In some cases, the triggering bacterium can be identified by means of an antigen-specific proliferative response of T cells. Usually several intracellular antigens are recognized by CD4+ T cells. More specific information about antigenic specificity has been obtained by investigating T-cell clones. Immunodominant 60-kd heat-shock protein of reactive arthritis triggering bacteria has been found to be a target antigen for cellular immune responses (171). In a patient with

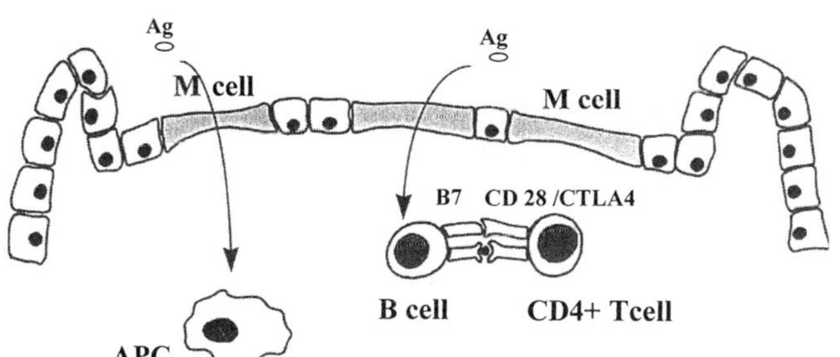

FIG. 66.7. Luminal antigens are preferentially taken up by mucosal associated-lymphoid tissue (MALT) through M cells and are taken up for processing in the lamina propria by classic macrophages or B cells. Within the M-cell pockets, memory B cells are the most likely cells to mediate major histocompatibility complex (MHC) class II interactions with T cells. These cells also express the costimulatory molecule B7. The outcome of this B cell–T cell interaction may very much depend on the T-cell ligand that binds B7. B7/CD28 interaction induces T-cell activation. Alternatively, engagement of B7 with CTLA-4, which is expressed transiently on activated T cells, might provide negative signals (anergy or apoptosis). If naive B cells, which lack costimulatory molecules like B7, capture antigens, T-cell anergy is the predicted outcome.

Yersinia-triggered reactive arthritis, a clone also was isolated that recognized both enterobacterial and human heat-shock protein, suggesting that autoimmune mechanisms may also play a role (172). Other immunodominant proteins of *Yersinia* include the highly conserved ribosomal proteins L2 and L23 and the 19-kd subunit of the urease of *Yersinia*.

Whereas the antigens responsible for reactive arthritis are probably derived from species of infecting *Salmonella, Shigella, Yersinia,* and *Campylobacter*, in spondyloarthropathies associated with IBD or undifferentiated spondyloarthropathies, the responsible antigen or group of antigens remains unresolved. Nonetheless, the aberrant DR expression on epithelial cells (173,174) is likely related to an increased antigen processing and presentation role, resulting in an overstimulation of $CD4^+$ cells in the lamina propria (175–178). The increased expression of DR by macrophages in the lamina propria might be involved in abrogation of oral tolerance to luminal antigens (179). Expression of DR antigens by the epithelium might mediate an enhanced uptake and presentation of luminal antigens, resulting in stimulation of help, rather than suppression. The number of M cells, which are scarce in normal ileum, was found to be increased (≤24% of follicle-associated epithelial cells) in the inflamed mucosa of patients with spondyloarthropathy. These M cells showed a thin rim of cytoplasm covering groups of lymphocytes. In chronic inflammatory lesions, necrotic M cells, rupture of M cells, and lymphocytes entering the gut lumen were observed (180). The rupture of M cells at the top of the lymphoid follicles leads to interruption of the gut epithelial lining and allows luminal contents to have access to the lymphoid tissue, and could be responsible for an exponential increase of local antigen stimulation.

Lymphocyte Migration and Receptors Mediating Lymphocyte Homing to the Gut

After uptake and processing, luminal antigens are presented to lymphocytes present in the gut mucosa. The process of lymphocyte trafficking into and out of the gut is regulated mainly by receptors that belong to a group of molecules referred to as adhesion molecules, which constitute the molecular basis for cell–cell as well as cell–matrix interactions (181–184). These receptors not only regulate cell migration, but also may regulate important functional activities of the cell when engaged. Tissue-specific vascular adhesion molecules are often referred to as "vascular addressins." Their lymphocyte counterreceptors are known as "homing receptors."

Alpha-4-Beta-7 and Its Ligands

The $\alpha_4\beta_7$ integrin is known to be expressed on some lymphocytes that preferentially "home" to the gut (185). $\alpha_4\beta_7$ can act as a receptor for vascular cell adhesion molecule-1 (VCAM-1) and fibronectin (186), both of which are induced during inflammation. It was shown that $\alpha_4\beta_7$ also serves as a ligand for the mucosal vascular addressin CAM-1 (MadCAM-1) (187–189). This is a 58- to 66-kd glycoprotein, expressed selectively on mucosal lymphoid organ high endothelial venules (HEVs) and on gut lamina propria venules (187).

Lymphocyte binding to HEVs of PPs involves the mucosal vascular addressin, MadCAM-1 (190,191). Indeed, antibodies to the latter addressin block lymphocyte interactions with HEVs *in vitro* and lymphocyte homing into PP HEVs *in vivo*. This addressin also is involved in directing lymphocyte traffic into the lamina propria of the small and large intestine wall, the lactating mammary gland, and the inflamed pancreas.

The anti-$\alpha_4\beta_7$ monoclonal antibody Act-1, which does not inhibit adhesion of $\alpha_4\beta_7$ to VCAM-1 (185,186), does inhibit adhesion to MadCAM-1 (188), suggesting that the $\alpha_4\beta_7$-binding site for VCAM-1 and MadCAM-1 are not identical.

The β_7 chain also can associate with another a chain, designated α_E. This integrin is expressed predominantly on lymphocytes residing in intestinal sites and seems to be involved in their interaction with epithelial cells (192). $\alpha_4\beta_7$ is expressed on the surface of more than 95% of intraepithelial lymphocytes located in the intestine, but fewer than 2% of peripheral blood T cells (193). This receptor also is expressed on intraepithelial lymphocytes in the mammary glands. During *in vitro* culture of intestinal intraepithelial lymphocytes, expression of the marker decreases significantly. Exposure to transforming growth factor-β (TGF-β) dramatically increases $\alpha_4\beta_7$ expression (194,195).

Intraepithelial lymphocytes are predominantly CD4-$CD8^+$ (196) and use a restricted repertoire of T cell–receptor V region segments (197). The majority of human intraepithelial lymphocytes express T-cell receptors. A small population, however, carries the gd receptor. They express a different profile of integrins than peripheral blood T cells; $\alpha_4\beta_7$ is a prominent integrin selectively expressed on intestinal intraepithelial lymphocytes. Intestinal intraepithelial lymphocytes are localized *in vivo* to the basolateral surface of polarized epithelial cells. Because the epithelium contains no vascular structures, it is reasonable to suppose that mucosal lymphocytes go through a series of adhesive interactions at different sites to migrate to or localize in the epithelium. These steps include adherence to the endothelial cells of blood vessels within the mucosal site (lamina propria), and migration across the endothelium into the surrounding tissues toward the epithelium, where they adhere to the basolateral surface of epithelial cells.

To identify a specific adhesion molecule on epithelial cells that might mediate adhesion to intraepithelial lymphocytes, Cepek et al. (198) immunized mice with a mucosal epithelial cell line known to support divalent cation-dependent intraepithelial lymphocyte adhesion. The resultant hybridoma culture supernatants were screened for the ability to inhibit adhesion of intraepithelial lymphocytes to epithelial cells. One efficient inhibitor stained the basolateral surface of intestinal epithelial cells. Biochemical characterization of the corresponding antigen revealed that it was epithelial cadherin

(E-cadherin). E-cadherin, a member of the cadherin family, is a single-chain transmembrane polypeptide. The extracellular portion usually consists of five homologous domains of about 110 residues. The short cytoplasmic tail interacts with the cytoskeleton by means of proteins called *catenins*. The adhesive function of cadherins is primarily localized in the first amino-terminal domain. This domain was shown by Overduin et al. (199) to have a structure with remarkable similarity to the immunoglobulin fold (although there is no sequence homology). Calcium binding induces a conformational change at the adhesion face. E-cadherin classically functions in homophilic (cadherin/cadherin) interactions (200). As intraepithelial lymphocytes are negative for E-cadherin expression, there is a lack of substrate for homophilic interaction between intraepithelial lymphocytes and epithelial cells, and the cadherin-mediated interaction is therefore heterophilic (through E-cadherin and $\alpha_E\beta_7$).

Another adhesion molecule of particular interest is vascular adhesion protein-1 (VAP-1), a nonclassic inflammation-inducible endothelial molecule involved in leukocyte-subtype–specific rolling under physiologic shear. Molecularly, VAP-1 belongs to a special class of cell surface amino oxidases. The enzymatic reaction itself and the biologically active end products can potentially regulate the adhesive status of the vessel wall. Thus, VAP-1 is an ectoenzyme that has interrelated adhesive and enzymatic functions in regulating physiologic trafficking and inflammation (201).

VAP-1 is prominently expressed on synovial vessels in inflamed synovium (202). Salmi and Jalkanen isolated gut-derived leukocytes from patients with Crohn's disease and ulcerative colitis (203). Using function-blocking monoclonal antibodies and *in vitro* frozen section adhesion assays, these investigators studied whether these cells bind to synovial vessels and which molecules mediate the interaction. The results showed that mucosal leukocytes from inflamed bowel bind well to venules in synovial membrane. Small intestinal lymphocytes adhered to synovial vessels using multiple homing receptors and their corresponding endothelial ligands. Of these, only intercellular CAM (ICAM)-1 significantly supported binding of immunoblasts. In contrast, P-selectin glycoprotein ligand-1-interaction with P-selectin accounted for practically all synovial adherence of mucosal macrophages. In addition, blocking of VAP-1 significantly inhibited binding of all such leukocyte subsets to joint vessels. Thus, different leukocyte populations derived from inflamed gut bind avidly to synovial vessels using a distinct repertoire of adhesion molecules, suggesting that their recirculation may contribute to the development of arthritis in IBDs.

Role of T-Cell Cytokines in Gut Homeostasis and Inflammation

Activation of epithelial and lamina propria T cells by luminal antigens or other stimuli can result in different functional outcomes. The T lymphocytes can undergo apoptosis (deletion), be anergized, or programmed to produce cytokines. The T-cell cytokines can be classified as Th1 cytokines (interferon-γ, IL-2, TNF-α) and Th2 cytokines (IL-4, IL-5, IL-13). There are numerous reports on the Th1/Th2 cytokine profiles in peripheral blood and gut mucosa of patients with Crohn's disease, but the data are often conflicting. This may be related to the technical approaches used, since techniques such as ELISA, ELISPOT, and RT-PCR largely ignore the cellular source of the measured cytokine. In contrast, the detection of intracellular cytokines by flow cytometry assures the cellular origin of the cytokines, but one cannot exclude that the stimulation *in vitro* does not reflect the physiologic behavior of the T cells *in situ*. Although Crohn's disease is generally considered as a Th1-mediated disease, recent studies using flow cytometry indicated a relative decrease of the production of Th1 cytokines in both peripheral blood lymphocytes and colonic lamina propria lymphocytes in Crohn's disease compared to healthy controls (204,205).

Interestingly, similar observations were made in spondyloarthropathy. Using the same approach as for Crohn's disease, it was demonstrated that mucosal lymphocytes from the gut of spondyloarthropathy patients also expressed an impaired Th1 profile, although more than half of the patients had no clinical or histologic signs of gut inflammation (206). Low secretion of interferon (IFN)-γ, IL-2, or TNF-α and an increase in IL-10 production by T cells was also reported in peripheral blood of patients with reactive arthritis (207), ankylosing spondylitis (208), and other types of spondyloarthropathy (209) compared to both healthy controls and patients with RA. Taken together, these studies indicate that there is an impaired Th1/Th2 balance in both the gut of patients with Crohn's disease and spondyloarthropathy. Thus, functional characterization of T cells in spondyloarthropathy highlights again the similarity between gut inflammation in spondyloarthropathy and Crohn's disease. Moreover, these findings are consistent with the concept that a defective Th1 response, especially at the mucosal site, may impair immune defense against intracellular bacteria and thereby contribute to a decreased immune tolerance against bacterial antigens. This is believed to be a crucial trigger for inflammation or autoimmunity in reactive arthritis, but also probably in other types of spondyloarthropathy and in Crohn's disease. Illustrating this theory, it was demonstrated that low secretion of TNF-α, but not other T-cell cytokines, correlated with chronicity in reactive arthritis (210).

IMMUNOBIOLOGY OF THE JOINT

Whereas the gut plays an essential role in the pathogenesis of enterogenic arthritis, the disease is clinically characterized by synovial inflammation of peripheral and axial joints. In order to clarify the clinical and pathogenic relationship between the gut and the joint, it is of importance to have a better understanding of the normal immunohistology of the synovial membrane, the global immunopathology of gut-associated arthritis, and the relationship between specific alterations of the innate and adaptive immune system in gut and joint of patients with spondyloarthropathy.

The Normal Synovial Membrane

The normal synovial membrane consists of two compartments: the synovial lining layer and the sublining. The lining layer, situated at the luminal surface, is the interface between the synovial membrane and the joint cavity (211). It plays a role in the production of synovial fluid components, the absorption of fluid and substances from the joint space, and blood/synovial fluid exchanges (212). Histologically, it is composed of one or two cell layers of synovial intimal cells, called synoviocytes. Two types of synoviocytes have been identified (213,214). The type A or "macrophage-like" synoviocytes are derived from monocytic cells of the bone marrow and can be considered as resident CD68$^+$ macrophages. Accordingly, they possess the capacity to phagocytize and to present antigens in an MHC class II context. The type B or "fibroblast-like" synoviocytes are of mesenchymal origin (215). They have a prominent, rough, endoplasmatic reticulum and show high uridine diphosphoglucose dehydrogenase activity (216, 217), indicating the synthesis of matrix molecules such as hyaluran, collagens, and fibronectin (218). In contrast to other fibroblasts, they express decay accelerating factor (DAF, CD55) and VCAM-1, which can interact with CD97 and $\alpha 4\beta 1$ (VLA-4) expressed on type A synoviocytes (219,220). The two cell types are imbedded in a specialized extracellular matrix (221). Beneath the synovial lining, but not separated from it by a basal membrane, lies the sublining layer, which consists of loose connective tissue with scattered blood vessels and relatively few cells, mainly fibroblasts, macrophages, and fat cells.

The Synovial Membrane in Spondyloarthropathy

In inflammatory diseases of the joint, the synovial membrane exhibits a number of characteristic alterations, including increased vascularity with activation of the endothelial cells (increased expression of adhesion molecules), increased infiltration with predominantly mononuclear cells (lymphocytes and macrophages), and thickening of the synovial lining layer eventually leading to the formation of a so-called pannus which can attach to and invade articular cartilage and bone. Recent studies have provided a more detailed insight in the specific alterations observed in spondyloarthropathy synovitis. A first striking characteristic is that the macro- and microscopic hypervascularization, which is a general hallmark of synovitis, is even more pronounced in spondyloarthropathy than in RA (222–225). Several factors implicated in this process were recently identified in spondyloarthropathy synovium: vascular endothelial growth factor (VEGF), angiopoietins, TGF-β, and matrix metalloproteinase (MMP)-9 (226,227). These factors as well as the neovascularization marker $\alpha V\beta 3$ integrin might be interesting therapeutic targets in spondyloarthropathy. The endothelium of the synovial blood vessels is highly activated as illustrated by the expression of ICAM-1, and Platelet endothelial cell adhesion molecule (PECAM). Interestingly, the expression of E-selectin appears to be lower in spondyloarthropathy than in RA, which could contribute to infiltration with different subsets of inflammatory cells.

As to the inflammatory infiltration of spondyloarthropathy synovium, it is essentially composed of lymphocytes and macrophages. The number of infiltrating CD3$^+$ T cells, CD4$^+$ T cells, and CD20$^+$ B cells is slightly lower in spondyloarthropathy than in RA (224). Similarly, there are fewer lymphoid aggregates which is paralleled by a relative scarcity of follicular dendritic cells in spondyloarthropathy synovium (158). The global number of CD68$^+$ macrophages is similar or even lower than in inflamed RA synovial tissue, possibly related to the spondyloarthropathy subtype (224,225,228,229).

Immune Linkages Between Gut and Synovium in Spondyloarthropathy

Considering the specific luminal and microbial antigens and the alterations of the adaptive and innate immune system in the gut, much effort has been directed toward the identification of similar mechanisms in the joints of patients with enteropathic arthritis.

As to the triggering antigens, early in the disease the triggering organisms (*Yersinia enterocolitica, Salmonella typhimurium, Shigella flexneri,* or *Campylobacter*) can be cultured from the stool, but culture of the joint has been repeatedly unsuccessful. Bacterial antigens from *Yersinia* and *Salmonella* were demonstrated in the synovial fluid and the synovial membrane of patients with enterogenic reactive arthritis (56, 230–232). Only stable bacterial degradation products, not whole bacteria, are present at the site of inflammation in *Yersinia*-triggered reactive arthritis, because no *Yersinia* chromosomal DNA could be detected (231).

It is noteworthy that microorganisms that trigger reactive arthritis share three important features: they infect mucosal surfaces, they express lipopolysaccharides on their outer membrane, and they are intracellular organisms (233). It was shown that synovial mononuclear cells from patients with reactive arthritis proliferate specifically to the triggering bacterial agent *in vitro* (234). It also was demonstrated that the proliferation was inhibited by cyclosporine and by monoclonal antibodies to MHC class II antigens, suggesting it was attributable to MHC class II–restricted T cells (235). Indeed, most of the T-cell clones from synovial fluid of patients with reactive arthritis are CD4$^+$, MHC class II—restricted, and of the T helper–1 type (236,237). However, the known association of reactive arthritis with the MHC class I gene, B27, suggests that antigenic peptides should be presented for recognition by $CD8^+$ T cells. Furthermore, the organisms associated with reactive arthritis are intracellular pathogens, whereas MHC class II molecules present exogenous antigen peptides that have been endocytosed by host antigen-presenting cells (236). These arguments prompted investigation of the local synovial $CD8^+$ T-cell population. It has been suggested that bacteria-specific cytotoxic T lymphocytes might provide the link between the initiating agent and the cellular immune response. Isolation of a large number of $CD8^+$ T lymphocyte clones, derived from the synovial fluid of patients with spondyloarthropathy, allow identification of three B27-restricted CTL clones with specificity for *Yersinia* and *Salmonella* (238). Further analysis of a large panel of T-cell clones will shed more light on the role of B27 in the presentation of arthritogenic peptides. The fact that, unlike other class I molecules, HLA-B27 molecules devoid of bound antigenic peptides (i.e., empty) can be found on the cell surface (239) may be important in relation to molecular mimicry theory.

Based on the demonstration of synovial T-cell clones with specificity for gastrointestinal pathogens and on the absence of these pathogens in the joint, it was postulated that T cells could specifically recirculate from the gut to the joints in enteropathic arthritis. This process is most likely regulated by specific adhesion molecules present both in the gut and the synovium. Gut-derived lymphocytes from patients with IBD were demonstrated to be able to bind to synovial vessels using multiple homing receptors and their corresponding endothelial ligands, including VAP-1 (203). As mentioned previously, another set of important adhesion molecules in the gut are the β7 integrins. Analyzing the spondyloarthropathy joint, there is also a differential expression of the integrins $\alpha_E\beta7$ and $\alpha4\beta7$ on synovium-derived T-cell lines in spondyloarthropathy, while one of the ligands of $\alpha4\beta7$, VCAM-1, is highly expressed in spondyloarthropathy synovium (240,241). Further support for the recirculation hypothesis has been suggested by the identification of identical T-cell expansions in the colon mucosa and the synovium of a patient with enterogenic spondyloarthropathy (242).

Beside similarities in antigen-specificity and adhesion molecule expression, T cells in the gut and the synovium of patients with spondyloarthropathy also showed similar functional profiles. Indeed, analysis of synovial fluid T cells and synovial membrane specimens in spondyloarthropathy confirmed that the decreased Th1 (interferon-γ)/Th2 (IL-4) ratio also extended to the joint of spondyloarthropathy patients (243,244).

Whereas all these data suggest that the linkage between gut and synovium in enteropathic arthritis is essentially mediated by the adaptive immune system, recent evidence also supports the concept of shared abnormalities of the innate immune system between gut and joint, including the abnormal expression of macrophage scavenger receptors. The macrophage receptor with collagenous structure (MARCO), which plays a role in the defense against gram-negative bacteria, is up-regulated on PBMC of patients developing reactive arthritis but is low in the synovial compartment in spondyloarthropathy compared to RA, thus suggesting a defective host defense mechanism in the spondyloarthropathy joint (245). On the other hand, the previously mentioned scavenger receptor CD163 was not only increased in the gut of patients with Crohn's disease and spondyloarthropathy (illustrating again the relationship between both diseases, but also the fact that alterations of the innate immune system may be early phenomena in the inflammation cascade); the same subset of macrophages was also demonstrated to be selectively increased in spondyloarthropathy synovium compared to RA synovium and thus appeared to be another candidate for a role in the gut–synovium axis (158). As in the gut, alterations of the macrophage population and function in the joint may contribute to the pathogenesis of the disease in different ways: defective clearance of bacteria, presentation of autoantigens to T cells, and alteration of the balance between pro- and antiinflammatory cytokines. The latter is supported by the influence of IL-10.G microsatellites on the development of reactive arthritis (246), the effect of recombinant human IL-10 in psoriatic arthritis (247), the demonstration of TNF-α in the sacroiliac joint of ankylosing spondylitis patients and in synovium of psoriatic arthritis patients (248,249), and the impressive effect of TNF-α blockade not only on clinical manifestations of spondyloarthropathy, but also on the immunopathology of the synovial membrane (209,241), suggesting that these phenomena may be secondary to abnormalities in the macrophage-derived cytokine balance.

CONCLUSIONS

Better insights into the pathogenesis of enteropathic arthritis confirm the biologic and immunologic relationship between Crohn's disease and spondyloarthropathy on the one hand, and between gut and joint inflammation in these diseases on the other hand. Whereas T cells and their cytokines are still believed to play a role in this concept, recent evidence points mainly to alterations of the innate immune system and, more precisely, macrophages and their products. These data are consistent with the hypothesis that the combination of an impaired bacterial clearance and an uncontrolled inflammatory response in genetically susceptible hosts can lead to a breakdown of normal immunologic tolerance and to a pathogenic cellular immune response to specific bacterial species, thereby inducing inflammation in the gut and the joint. Down-regulating the uncontrolled inflammatory response by TNF-α blockade has proven to be a very effective clinical strategy in spondyloarthropathy, but one may raise concerns as to the consequences of impairment of host defense and increased risk for major infections in these patients. Therefore, further exploration of the pathogenesis of these diseases is mandatory to develop alternative strategies to restore the balance between pro- and antiinflammatory cytokines without affecting the normal immune response against bacteria.

REFERENCES

1. Mielants H, Veys EM. Enteropathic arthritis. In: Koopman WJ, ed. *Arthritis and allied conditions*. 14th ed. Philadelphia: Lippincott Williams & Wilkins, 2001:1362–1382.
2. Mayberry JF, Ballantyne KC, Hardcastle JD, et al. Epidemiological study of asymptomatic inflammatory bowel disease: the identification of cases during a screening programme for colorectal cancer. *Gut* 1989;30:481–483.
3. Palm O, Moum B, Ongre A, et al. Prevalence of ankylosing spondylitis and other spondylarthropathies among patients with inflammatory bowel disease: a population study (the IBSEN study). *J Rheum* 2002; 29:511–515.
4. Salvarini C, Fornaciari G, Beltrami M, et al. Musculoskeletal manifestations in inflammatory bowel disease. *Eur J Int Med* 2000:11:210–214.
5. Gravallese EM, Kantrowitz FG. Arthritic manifestations of inflammatory bowel disease. *Am J Gastroenterol* 1988;83:703–709.
6. Orchard TR, Wordsworth BP, Jewell DP. Peripheral arthropathies in inflammatory bowel disease: their articular distribution and natural history. *Gut* 1998;42:387–391.
7. De Vlam K, De Vos M, Mielants H, et al. Spondyloarthropathy in inflammatory bowel disease: prevalence and HLA association. *J Rheumatol* 2000;27:2860–2865.
8. Scarpa R, Del Puente A, D'Arienzo A, et al. The arthritis of ulcerative colitis: clinical and genetic aspects. *J Rheumatol* 1992;19:373–377.
9. Veloso FT, Carvalho J, Magro F. Immune-related systhemic manifestations of inflammatory bowel disease—a prospective study of 792 patients. *J Clin Gastroenterol* 1996;23:29–34.
10. Palm O, Moum B, Jahnsen J, et al. The prevalence and incidence of peripheral arthritis in patients with inflammatory bowel disease, a prospective population based study (the IBSEN study). *Rheumatology* 2001;40:1256–1261.
11. Salvarini C, Vlachonikolis IG, Van Der Heijde DM, et al. Musculoskeletal manifestations in a population based cohort of inflammatory bowel disease patients. *Scand J Gastroenterol* 2001;12:1307–1313.
12. Mielants H, Veys EM. The gut in the spondyloarthropathies. *J Rheumatol* 1990;17:7–10.
13. Mielants H, Veys EM, Cuvelier C, et al. The evolution of spondylarthropathies in relation to gut histology. Part I: clinical aspects. *J Rheumatol* 1995;22:2266–2272.
14. Isdale A, Wright V. Seronegative arthritis and the bowel: the gut and rheumatic diseases. *Baillieres Clin Rheumatol* 1989;3:285–301.
15. Steer S, Jones H, Hibbert J, et al. Low back pain, sacroiliitis and the relationship with HLA-B27 in Crohn's disease. *J Rheum* 2003;30: 518–522.
16. Queiro R, Maiz J, Intxaosti J, et al. Subclinical sacroiliitis in inflammatory bowel disease: a clinical and follow-up study. *Clin Rheum* 2000;19:445–449.
17. Dougados M, Van Der Linden J, Juhlin R, et al., for The European Spondyloarthropathy Study Group. The European Spondyloarthropathy Study Group preliminary criteria for the classification of spondyloarthropathy. *Arthritis Rheum* 1991;34:1218–1226.
18. Bardazzi G, Mannoni A, D'Albasio G, et al. Spondyloarthritis in patients with ulcerative colitis. *Ital J Gastroenterol* 1997;29:520–524.
19. Kennedy GL, Will R, Calin A. Sex ratio in the spondyloarthropathies and its relationship to phenotypic expression, mode of inheritance and age at onset. *J Rheumatol* 1993;20:1900–1904.
20. Edmonds L, Elswood J, Kennedy GL, et al. Primary ankylosing spondylitis in psoriatic and enteropathic spondyloarthropathies: a controlled analysis. *J Rheumatol* 1991;19:696–698.
21. Brophy S, Pavy S, Lewis P, et al. Inflammatory eye, skin and bowel disease in spondyloarthritis: genetic, phenotypic and enviromental factors. *J Rheum* 2001;28: 2667–2673.
22. Schorr-Lesnick B, Brandt LJ. Selected rheumatologic and dermatologic manifestations of inflammatory bowel disease. *Am J Gastroenterol* 1988;83:216–223.
23. Rosenbaum T. Characterization of uveitis associated with spondyloarthritis. *J Rheumatol* 1989;16:792–796.
24. Lyons JL, Rosenbaum JT. Uveitis associated with inflammatory bowel disease compared with uveitis associated with spondylarthropathy. *Arch Ophtalmol* 1997;115:61–64.
25. Banares AA, Jover JA, Fernandez-Gutiérrez B, et al. Bowel inflammation in anterior uveitis and spondyloarthropathy. *J Rheumatol* 1995; 22:1112–1117.
26. Greenstein AJ, Janowitz HD, Sachar DB. The extraintestinal complications of Crohn's disease and ulcerative colitis: a study of 700 patients. *Medicine* 1976;55:401–412.
27. Main J, Mckenzie H, Yeaman GR, et al. Antibody to *Saccharomyces cerevisiae* (baker's yeast) in Crohn's disease. *BMJ* 1988;297:1105–1106.
28. Hoffman IEA, Demetter P, Peeters M, et al. Anti-*Saccharomyces cerevisiae* IgA antibodies are raised in ankylosing spondylitis and undifferentiated spondylarthropathy. *Ann Rheum Dis* 2003;62:455–459.
29. Mielants H, Veys EM, Goethals K, et al. Destructive hip lesions in seronegative spondyloarthropathies: relation to gut inflammation. *J Rheumatol* 1990;17:335–340.
30. Helliwell PS, Hickling P, Wright V. Do the radiological changes of classic ankylosing spondylitis differ from the changes found in the spondylitis associated with inflammatory bowel disease, psoriasis and reactive arthritis? *Ann Rheum Dis* 1998;57:135–140.
31. Mielants H, Veys EM, Cuvelier C, et al. The evolution of spondyloarthropathies in relation to gut histology. Part II: histological aspects. *J Rheumatol* 1995;22:2273–2278.
32. Dekker-Saeys AJ, Keat ACS. Follow-up study of ankylosing spondylitis over a period of 12 years. *Scand J Rheumatol* 1990;[Suppl 57]: 120–121.
33. Russell AS, Percy JS, Schlaut JS, et al. Transplantation antigens in patients with Crohn's disease: the linkage of associated ankylosing spondylitis with HLA-W27. *Am J Dig Dis* 1995;20:359–361.
34. Mielants H, Veys EM, Joos R, et al. HLA-antigens in seronegative spondyloarthropathies: reactive arthritis and arthritis in ankylosing spondylitis: relation to gut inflammation. *J Rheumatol* 1987;14:466–471.
35. Purman J, Zeidler H, Bertrams J, et al. HLA antigens in ankylosing spondylitis associated with Crohn's disease: increased frequency of the HLA phenotype B27, B44. *J Rheumatol* 1988;15:1658–1661.
36. Orchard TR, Thiyagraja S, Welsh KI, et al. Clinical phenotype is related to HLA genotype in the peripheral arthropathy of inflammatory bowel disease. *Gastroenterology* 2000;118:274–279.
37. Hugot JP, Chamaillard M, Zouali H, et al. Association of NOD 2 leucine-reach repeat variants with susceptibility to Crohn's disease. *Nature* 2001 ;411:599–603.
38. Ogura Y, Bonen DK, Inohara N, et al. A frameshift mutation in NOD 2 associated with susceptibility to Crohn's disease. *Nature* 2001;411: 603–606.
39. Ogura Y, Inohara N, Benito A et al. NOD 2, a NOD 1/Apaf. 1 family member that is restricted to monocytes and activates NF-Kappa B. *J Biol Chem* 2001;276:4812–4818.
40. Hampe J, Cuthbert A, Croucher PJ, et al. Association between insertion mutation in NOD 2 gene and Crohn's disease in German and British populations. *Lancet* 2001;357:1925–1928.
41. Lesage S, Zouali H, Cezard JP, et al. CARD 15/NOD 2 mutational analysis and fenotype-phenotype correlation in 612 patients with inflammatory bowel disease. *Am J Hum Genet* 2002;70:845–857.
42. Ahmad T, Armuzzi A, Bunce M, et al. The molecular classification of the clinical manifestations of Crohn's disease. *Gastroenterology* 2002;122:854–866.
43. Abreu MT, Taylor KD, Lin YC, et al. Mutations in NOD 2 are associated with fibrostenosing disease in patients with Crohn's disease. *Gastroenterology* 2002;123: 679–688.
44. Micelli-Richard C, Zouali H, Lesage S, et al. CARD 15/NOD 2 analysis in spondylarthropathy. *Arthritis Rheum* 2002;46:1405–1406.
45. Crane AM, Bradbury L, Van Heel DA, et al. Role of NOD 2 variants in spondylarthritis. *Arthritis Rheum* 2002 46:1629–1633.
46. Ferreros-Vidal I, Amarelo J, Barros F, et al. Lack of association of ankylosing spondylitis with the most common NOD 2 susceptibility alleles to Crohn's disease. *J Rheumatol* 2003;30:102–104.
47. Peeters H, Vander Cruyssen B, Laukens D, et al. Radiologic sacroiliitis, a hallmark of spondylitis is linked with CARD15 gene polymorphisms in patients with Crohn's disease. *Ann Rheum Dis* 2004 (in press).

48. Nissila M, Lethinen K, Leirisalo-Repo M, et al. Sulphasalazine in the treatment of ankylosing spondylitis. *Arthritis Rheum* 1988;31:1111–1116.
49. Mielants H, Veys EM, Cuvelier C, et al. Course of gut inflammation in spondyloarthropathies and therapeutic consequences. *Baillieres Clin Rheumatol* 1996;10:147–164.
50. Baron TH, Truss CD, Elson CD. Low-dose oral MTX in refractory inflammatory bowel disease. *Dig Dis Sci* 1993;38:1551–1553.
51. Targan SR, Hanauer SB, Van Deventer SJH, et al. A short-time study of chimeric monoclonal antibody cA2 to tumor necrosis factor a for Crohn's disease: Crohn's Disease cA2 Study Group. *N Engl J Med* 1997;337:1029–1035.
52. Present D, Mayer L, Van Deventer SJH, et al. Anti-TNF-alpha chimeric antibody (cA2) is effective in the treatment of the fistulae of Crohn's disease: a multicenter randomized, double-blind, placebo-controlled study. *Am J Gastroenterol* 1997;92:1746(abst 648).
53. Rutgeerts P, D'Haens G, Targan S, et al. Efficacy and safety of retreatment with anti-tumor necrosis factor antibody (infliximab) to maintain remission in Crohn's disease. *Gastroenterology* 1999;117:761–769.
54. Keating GM, Perry CM. Infliximab: an update review of its use in Crohn's disease and rheumatoid arthritis. *Bio Drugs* 2002;16:111–148.
55. Van Den Bosch F, Kruithof E, De Vos M, et al. Crohn's disease associated with spondyloarthropathy: effect of TNF α blockade with infliximab on articular symptoms. *Lancet* 2000;25(356):1821–1822.
56. Granfors K, Jalkanen S, Von Essen R, et al. *Yersinia* antigens in synovial fluid cells from patients with reactive arthritis. *N Engl J Med* 1989;320:216–221.
57. Nikkari S, Möttönen T, Saario R et al. Demonstration of *Salmonella* DNA in the synovial fluid in reactive arthritis. *Arthritis Rheum* 1996;39:S185.
58. Wilkinson NZ, Ward ME, Kingsley GH. Detection of bacteria in rheumatoid and reactive arthritis synovial fluid using a kingdom-specific polymerase chain reaction: evidence in support of a role for bacteria in the pathogenesis of inflammatory arthritis. *Arthritis Rheum* 1997;40:S270.
59. Locht H, Mølbak K, Krogfelt KA. High frequency of reactive joint symptoms after outbreak of *Salmonella enteritidis*. *J Rheum* 2002;29:767–771.
60. Keat AE. Reiter's syndrome and reactive arthritis in perspective. *N Engl J Med* 1983;309:1606–1615.
61. Leirisalo-Repo M, Hannu T, Lehtinen A, et al. Long term prognosis of reactive salmonella arthritis. *Ann Rheum Dis* 1997;56:516–520.
62. Clegg DO, Reda DJ, Weiseman MH, et al. Comparison of sulfasalazine and placebo in the treatment of reactive arthritis (Reiter's syndrome). *Arthritis Rheum* 1996;39:2021–2027.
63. Toivanen A, Yli-Kerttula T, Luukkainen R, et al. Effect of antimicrobial treatment on chronic reactive arthritis. *Clin Exp Rheumatol* 1993;11:301–307.
64. De Koning J, Heeseman J, Hoogkamp-Korstanje JAA, et al. *Yersinia* in intestinal biopsy specimens from patients with seronegative spondyloarthropathy: correlation with specific serum IgA antibodies. *J Infect Dis* 1989;159:109–112.
65. Zhang Y, Toivanen A, Toivanen P. Experimental *Yersinia*-triggered reactive arthritis: effect of a 3 week course of ciprofloxacin. *Br J Rheumatol* 1997;36:541–546.
66. Mielants H, Veys EM, Cuvelier C, et al. Gut inflammation in children with late onset pauci-articular juvenile chronic arthritis and evolution to adult spondyloarthropathy: a prospective study. *J Rheumatol* 1993;20:1567–1572.
67. Schatteman L, Mielants H, Veys EM, et al. Gut inflammation in psoriatic arthritis: a prospective ileocolonoscopic study. *J Rheumatol* 1995;22:680–683.
68. Mielants H, Veys EM, Goemaere S, et al. Gut inflammation in the spondylarthropathies: clinical, radiological, biological and genetic features in relation to the type of histology: a prospective study. *J Rheumatol* 1991;18:1542–1551.
69. Mielants H, Veys EM, Cuvelier C, et al. The evolution of spondylarthropathies in relation to gut histology. III. Relation between gut and joint. *J Rheumatol* 1995;22:2279–2284.
70. Taurog JD, Richardson JA, Croft JAT, et al. The germfree state prevents development of gut and joint inflammatory disease in HLA-B27 transgenic rats. *J Exp Med* 1994;180:2359–2364.
71. Clegg DO, Reda DJ, Weiseman MH, et al. Comparison of sulfasalazine and placebo in the treatment of ankylosing spondylitis. *Arthritis Rheum* 1996;39:2004–2012.
72. Clegg DO, Reda DJ, Weiseman MH, et al. Comparison of sulfasalazine and placebo in the treatment of psoriatic arthritis. *Arthritis Rheum* 1996;39:2013–2020.
73. Dougados M, Maetzel A, Mijiyawa M, et al. Evaluation of sulphasalazine in the treatment of spondylarthropathies. *Ann Rheum Dis* 1992;51:955–958.
74. Joos R, Veys EM, Mielants H, et al. Sulphasalazine treatment in juvenile chronic arthritis: an open study. *J Rheumatol* 1991;18:880–884.
75. Breitbant A, Bauer H, Krastell H, et al. Sulfasalazine in recurrent anterior uveitis: a new therapeutical strategy. *Arthritis Rheum* 1993;36 [Suppl]:S225(abst).
76. Van Den Bosch F, Kruithof E, Baeten D, et al. Effects of a loading dose regimen of three infusions of chimeric monoclonal antibody to tumor necrosis factor alpha (infliximab) in spondyloarthropathy: an open pilot study. *Ann Rheum Dis* 2000;59:428–433.
77. Kruithof E, Van Den Bosch F, Baeten D, et al. Repeated infusions of infliximab a chimeric anti-TNF alpha monoclonal antibody in patients with active spondylarthropathy: one year follow-up. *Ann Rheum Dis* 2002;61:207–212.
78. Van Den Bosch F, Kruithof E, Baeten D. Randomized double-blind comparison of chimeric monoclonal antibody to tumor necrosis factor alpha (infliximab) versus placebo in active spondyloarthropathy. *Arthritis Rheum* 2002;46:755–765.
79. Braun J, Brandt J, Listing I, et al. Treatment of active ankylosing spondylitis with infliximab: a randomised controlled multicentre trial. *Lancet* 2002;359:1187–1193.
80. Bjarnason I, Hayllar J, Mac Pherson AT, et al. Side-effects of non-steroidal anti-inflammatory drugs on the small and large intestine in man. *Gastroenterology* 1993;104:1832–1847.
81. Morris AJ, Madhock R, Sturrock RD, et al. Enteroscopic diagnosis of small bowel ulceration in patients receiving non-steroidal anti-inflammatory drugs. *Lancet* 1991;337:520.
82. Allison MC, Howatson AG, Torrance CJ, et al. Gastrointestinal damage associated with the use of non-steroidal anti-inflammatory drugs. *N Engl J Med* 1992;327:749–754.
83. Hayllar J, Smith T, MacPherson A, et al. Non-steroidal anti-inflammatory drug-induced small intestinal inflammation and blood loss. *Arthritis Rheum* 1994;37:1146–1150.
84. Rampton DS, McNek NL, Sarner M. Analgesic ingestion and other factors preceding relapse in ulcerative colitis. *Gut* 1993;24:187–189.
85. Evans JMM, McMahon AD, Murray FE, et al. Non-steroidal anti-inflammatory drugs are associated with emergency admission to hospital for colitis due to inflammatory bowel disease. *Gut* 1997;40:619–622.
86. Cipolla G, Crema F, Sacco S, et al. Nonsteroidal anti-inflammatory drugs and inflammatory bowel disease: current perspectives. *Pharmacol Res* 2002;46:1–6.
87. Smale S, Natt RS, Orchard TR, et al. Inflammatory bowel disease and spondylarthropathy. *Arthritis Rheum* 2001;44:2728–2736.
88. Fleming J, Russel H, Wiesnek D, et al. Whipple's disease: clinical, biochemical and histopathologic features and assessment of treatment in 29 patients. *Mayo Clin Proc* 1988;63:539–551.
89. Relman DA, Schmidt TM, MacDermott RP, et al. Identification of the uncultured bacillus of Whipple's disease. *N Engl J Med* 1992;327:293–301.
90. Marth T, Raoult D. Whipple's disease. *Lancet* 2003;361:239–246.
91. Clegg DO, Zone JJ, Samuelson CD, et al. Circulating immune complexes containing secretory IgA in jejunoileal bypass disease. *Ann Rheum Dis* 1985;44:239–244.
92. Axon JMC, Hawley PR, Huskisson EC. Ileal porch arthritis. *Br J Rheumatol* 1993;32:586–588.
93. Lubrano E, Ciacci C, Ames PRJ, et al. The arthritis of coeliac disease: prevalence and pattern in 200 adult patients. *Br J Rheumatol* 1996;35:1314–1318.
94. Bourne JT, Kumar P, Huskisson E. Arthritis and celiac disease. *Ann Rheum Dis* 1985;44:592–598.
95. Kaklamani VG, Vaiopoulos G, Kaklamanis PC. Behçet's disease. *Semin Arthritis Rheum* 1998;27:197–217.
96. Kasahara Y, Tanaka S, Nishimo M, et al. Intestinal involvement in Behçet's disease: review of 136 surgical cases in the Japanese literature. *Dis Colon Rectum* 1981;24:103–106.

97. Yurdakul S, Tuzuner N, Yurdakul I, et al. Gastrointestinal involvement in Behçet's syndrome: a controlled study. *Ann Rheum Dis* 1996; 55:208–210.
98. Inman RE. Arthritis and enteritis: an interface of protean manifestations [Editorial]. *J Rheumatol* 1987;4:406–410.
99. Lehman JJA, Allen JB, Plotz PH, et al. Polyarthritis in rats following the systemic injection of *Lactobacillus casei* cell walls in aquarous suspension. *Arthritis Rheum* 1983;26:1259–1265.
100. Stimpson SA, Brown RR, Anderig K, et al. Arthropathic properties of cell wall polymers from normal flora bacteria. *Infect Immun* 1986; 51:240–249.
101. Severijnen AJ, Hazenberg MP, Van De Merwe JP. Induction of chronic arthritis in rats by cell wall fragments of anaerobic coccoid rods isolated from the faecal flora of patients with Crohn's disease. *Digestion* 1988;39:118–125.
102. Severijnen AJ, Van Kleef R, Hazenberg P, et al. Cell wall fragments from major residents of the human intestinal flora induce chronic arthritis in rats. *J Rheumatol* 1989;16:1061–1068.
103. Leus JW, Van Den Berg WR, Van De Putte LA. Flare-up of antigen-induced arthritis in mice after challenge with oral antigen. *Clin Exp Immunol* 1984;58:364–371.
104. Mansson I, Norberg R, Olhagen B, et al. Arthritis in pigs induced by dietary factor: microbiological, clinical and histological studies. *Clin Exp Immunol* 1971;9:677–693.
105. Ivanyi P, Eulderink F, Van Alphe VL, et al. Joint disease in B27 transgenic mice. In: Lipsky P, Taurog JD, eds. *HLA-B27+ spondylarthropathies*. New York: Elsevier, 1991:71–83.
106. Ivanyi P. B27 transgenic mice and disease. *J Rheumatol* 1990;87 [Suppl]:97.
107. Hammer RE, Maika SD, Richardson JA, et al. Spontaneous inflammatory disease in transgenic rats expressing HLA-B27 and human b2m: an animal model of HLA-B27-associated human disorders. *Cell* 1990;63:109–112.
108. Breban H, Hammer RE, Richardson JA, et al. Susceptibility to HLA-B27 associated inflammatory disease in rats resides in bone marrow derived cells. *Arthritis Rheum* 1992;35:S57.
109. Ismail N, Chamberlain J, Inman R. Persistence and dissemination of *Yersinia enterocolitica* (Ye) 0:8 after intragastric challenge in B27-transgenic mice. *Arthritis Rheum* 1994;37:S211.
110. Bjarnasson I, Williams P, So A, et al. Intestinal permeability and inflammation in rheumatoid arthritis: effects of non-steroidal anti-inflammatory drugs. *Lancet* 1984;2:1171–1193.
111. Katz KD, Hollander D. Intestinal mucosal permeability and rheumatological diseases. *Baillieres Clin Rheumatol* 1989;3:271–284.
112. Jenkins RT, Jones DB, Goodacre RL, et al. Reversibility of increased intestinal permeability to ^{51}Cr EDTA in patients with gastrointestinal inflammatory diseases. *Am J Gastroenterol* 1987;82:1159–1164.
113. Bjarnasson I, O'Moran C, Levi J, et al. Absorption of ^{51}Chromium-labelled ethylenediamide tetraacetate in inflammatory bowel diseases. *Gastroenterology* 1983;85:318–327.
114. Hollander D, Vadheim C, Brettholz E, et al. Increased intestinal permeability in patients with Crohn's disease and their relatives. *Ann Intern Med* 1986;105:853–885.
115. Serrander R, Magnusson KE, Kihlstrom E. Acute *Yersinia* infections in man increase permeability for low molecular polyethylene glycols. *Scand J Infect Dis* 1986;18:409–413.
116. Smith MD, Gibson RA, Brooks PM. Abnormal bowel permeability in ankylosing spondylitis and rheumatoid arthritis. *J Rheumatol* 1985;12:299–305.
117. Wendling G, Bidet A, Guidet M. Intestinal permeability in ankylosing spondylitis. *J Rheumatol* 1990;17:114–115.
118. Mielants H, De Vos M, Goemaere S, et al. Intestinal mucosal permeability in inflammatory rheumatic diseases. Part II: role of disease. *J Rheumatol* 1991;18:394–400.
119. Vaile JH, Meddings JB, Yacyshyn BR, et al. Bowel permeability and CD45RO expression on circulating CD20^{+} B cells in patients with ankylosing spondylitis and their relatives. *J Rheumatol* 1999; 26:128–135.
120. Bjarnasson I, Zanelli C, Smith T, et al. Non-steroidal anti-inflammatory drug-induced intestinal inflammation in humans. *Gastroenterology* 1987;93:450–454.
121. Mielants H, Goemaere S, De Vos M, et al. Intestinal mucosal permeability in inflammatory rheumatic diseases. Part I: role of antiinflammatory drugs. *J Rheumatol* 1991;8:389–393.
122. Yamada T, Sartor RB, Marshall S, et al. Mucosal injury and inflammation in a model of chronic granulomatous colitis in rats. *Gastroenterology* 1993;104:759–771.
123. Hermiston ML, Gordon JI. Inflammatory bowel disease and adenoma in mice expressing a dominant negative N-cadherin. *Science* 1995;270:1203–1207.
124. Hermiston ML, Gordon JI. In vivo analysis of cadherin function in the mouse intestinal epithelium: essential roles in adhesion, maintenance of differentiation, and regulation of programmed cell death. *J Cell Biol* 1995;129:489–506.
125. Demetter P, De Vos M, Van Damme N, et al. Focal upregulation of E-cadherin-catenin complex in inflamed bowel mucosa but reduced expressio in ulcer-associated lineage. *Am J Clin Pathol* 2000;114: 364–370.
126. Demetter P, Baeten D, De Keyser F, et al. Subclinical gut inflammation in spondyloarthropathy patients is associated with upregulation of the E-cadherin/catenin complex. *Ann Rheum Dis* 2000;59:211–216.
127. Brandtzaeg P, Bjerke K. Human Peyer's patches: lympho-epithelial relationships and characteristics of immunoglobulin-producing cells. *Immunol Invest* 1989;18:29–45.
128. Bjerke K, Brandtzaeg P, Fausa O. T cell distribution is different in follicle-associated epithelium of human Peyer's patches and villous epithelium. *Clin Exp Immunol* 1988;74:270–275.
129. Turesson I. Distribution of immunoglobulin-containing cells in human bone marrow and lymphoid tissues. *Acta Med Scand* 1976; 199:293–304.
130. Brandtzaeg P, Korsrud FR. Significance of different J chain profiles in human tissues: generation of IgA and IgM with binding site for secretory component is related to the J chain expressing capacity of the total local immunocyte population, including IgG and IgD producing cells, and depends on the clinical state of the tissue. *Clin Exp Immunol* 1984;58:709–718.
131. Brandtzaeg P. Role of J chain and secretory component in receptor mediated glandular and hepatic transport of immunoglobulins in man. *Scand J Immunol* 1985;22:111–116.
132. Mestecky J, McGhee JR. Immunoglobulin A (IgA): molecular and cellular interactions involved in IgA biosynthesis and immune response. *Adv Immunol* 1987;40:153–245.
133. Brandtzaeg P, Halstensen TS, Kett K, et al. Immunobiology and immunopathology of human gut mucosa: humoral immunity and intraepithelial lymphocytes. *Gastroenterology* 1989;97:1562–1584.
134. James SP. Cellular immune mechanisms in the pathogenesis of Crohn's disease. *In Vivo* 1988;2:1–8.
135. Dunkley ML, Husband AJ. Distribution and functional characteristics of antigen-specific helper T cells arising after Peyer's patch immunization. *Immunology* 1987;61:475–482.
136. Modlin RL, Brenner MB, Krangel MS, et al. T-cell receptors of human suppressor cells. *Nature* 1987;329:541–545.
137. Kett K, Brandtzaeg P, Fausa O. J-chain expression is more prominent in immunoglobulin A2 than in immunoglobulin A1 colonic immunocytes and is decreased in both subclasses associated with inflammatory bowel disease. *Gastroenterology* 1988;94:1419–1425.
138. MacDermott RP, Nash GS, Bertovich MJ, et al. Altered patterns of secretion of monomeric IgA and IgA subclass 1 by intestinal mononuclear cells in inflammatory bowel disease. *Gastroenterology* 1986; 91:379–385.
139. Cuvelier C, Mielants H, De Vos M, et al. Immunoglobulin containing cells in terminal ileum and colorectum of patients with arthritis related gut inflammation. *Gut* 1988;29:916–925.
140. Mayer L, Eisenhardt D. Defect in immunoregulatory intestinal epithelial cells in inflammatory bowel disease. In: MacDermot RP, ed. *Inflammatory bowel disease: current status and future approach*. Amsterdam: Exerpta Medica, 1988:9–16.
141. Veys EM, Van Laere M. Serum IgG, IgM and IgA levels in ankylosing spondylitis. *Ann Rheum Dis* 1973;32:493–498.
142. Sendid B, Colombel F, Jacquinot PM, et al. Specific antibody response to oligomannosidic epitopes in Crohn's disease. *Clin Diagn Lab Immunol* 1996;3:219–226.
143. McKenzie H, Main J, Pennington CR, et al. Antibody to selected strains of *Saccharomyces cerevisiae* (baker's and brewer's yeast) and *Candida albicans* in Crohn's disease. Gut 1990;31:536–538.
144. Quinton J-F, Sendid B, Reumaux D, et al. Anti-*Saccharomyces cerevisiae* mannan antibodies combined with anti-neutrophil cytoplas-

matic autoantibodies in inflammatory bowel disease: prevalence and diagnostic role. *Gut* 1998;42:788–791.

145. Hoffenberg EJ, Fidanza S, Sauaia A. Serologic testing for inflammatory bowel disease. *J Pediatr* 1999;134:447–452.
146. Peeters M, Jossens S, Vermeire S, et al. Diagnostic value of anti-*Saccharomyces cerevisiae* and anti-neutrophil cytoplasmic autoantibodies in inflamatory bowel disease. *Am J Gastroenterol* 2001;96: 730–734.
147. Cario E, Podolsky DK. Differntial alteration in intestinal epithelial cell expression of toll-like receptor 3 (TLR3) and TLR4 in inflammatory bowel disease. *Infect Immun* 2000;68:7010–7017.
148. Fiocchi C. Inflammatory bowel disease: etiology and pathogenesis. *Gastroenterology* 1998;115:182–205.
149. Kuhn R, Lohler J, Rennick D, et al. Interleukin-10-deficient mice develop chronic enterocolitis. *Cell* 1993;75:263–274.
150. Grool TA, Van Dullemen H, Meenan J, et al. Anti-inflammatory effect of Interleukin-10 in rabbit immune complex-induced colitis. *Scand J Gastroenterol* 1998;33:754–758.
151. Claudepierre P, Rymer JC, Chevalier X. IL-10 plasma levels correlate with disease activity in spondyloarthropathy [Letter]. *J Rheumatol* 1997;24:1659–1661.
152. Simon AK, Seipelt E, Wu P, et al. Analysis of cytokine profiles in synovial T cell clones from chlamydial reactive arthritis patients: predominance of the Th1 subset. *Clin Exp Immunol* 1993;94:122–126.
153. Ritchlin C, Haas-Smith S, Looney J. Production, tissue distribution and function of IL-10 in psoriatic synovium. *Arthritis Rheum* 1996; 39:S163.
154. Brandtzaeg P, Valnes K, Scott H, et al. The human gastrointestinal secretory immune system in health and disease. *Scand J Gastroenterol* 1985;[Suppl 114]:17–38.
155. Bjerke K, Brandtzaeg P. Lack of relation between expression of HLA-DR and secretory component (SC) in follicle-associated epithelium of human Peyer's patches. *Clin Exp Immunol* 1988;71:502–507.
156. Bjerke K, Halstensen TS, Jahnsen F, et al. Distribution of macrophages and granulocytes expressing L1 protein (calprotectin) in human Peyer's patches compared with normal ileal lamina propria and mesenteric lymph nodes. *Gut* 1993;34:1357–1363.
157. Demetter P, Van Huysse JA, De Keyser F, et al. Increase in lymphoid follicles and leucocyte adhesion molecules emphasizes a role for the gut in spondyloarthropathy pathogenesis. *J Pathol* 2002;198:517–522.
158. Baeten D, Demetter P, Cuvelier CA, et al. Macrophages expressing the scavenger receptor CD163: a link between immune alterations of the gut and synovial inflammation in spondyloarthropathy. *J Pathol* 2002; 196:343–350.
159. Sanchez C, Domenech N, Vazquez J, et al. The porcine 2A10 antigen is homologous to human CD163 and related to macrophage differentiation. *J Immunol* 1999;162:5230–5237.
160. Bjerke K, Brandtzaeg P, Fausa O. T cell distribution is different in follicle-associated epithelium of human Peyer's patches and villous epithelium. *Clin Exp Immunol* 1988;74:270–275.
161. Boise LH, Noel PJ, Thompson CB. CD28 and apoptosis. *Curr Opin Immunol* 1995;7:620–625.
162. Saito T. Negative regulation of T cell activation. *Curr Opin Immunol* 1998;10:313–321.
163. Samoilova EB, Horton JL, Zhang H, et al. CTLA-4 is required for the induction of high dose oral tolerance. *Int Immunol* 1998;10:491–498.
164. Hoogkamp-Korstanje JAA, de Koning J, Heeseman J. Persistence of *Yersinia enterocolitica* in man. *Infection* 1988;16:81–85.
165. Podolsky DK. Glycoproteins in inflammatory bowel disease. In: Jarnerot G, ed. *Inflammatory bowel disease*. New York: Raven Press, 1987:53–65.
166. De Vries DD, Dekker-Saeys AJ, Gyodi E, et al. Absence of autoantibodies to peptides shared by HLA-B27.5 and *Klebsiella pneumoniae* nitrogenase in serum samples from HLA-B27 positive patients with ankylosing spondylitis and Reiter's syndrome. *Ann Rheum Dis* 1992; 51:783–789.
167. Lahesmaa R, Skurnik M, Vaara M, et al. Molecular mimicry between HLA-B27 and *Yersinia, Salmonella, Shigella* and *Klebsiella* within the same region of HLA a1-helix. *Clin Exp Immunol* 1991;86:399–404.
168. Hoski P, Rhen M, Kantele J, et al. Isolation, cloning, and primary structure of a cationic 16-kDa outer membrane protein of *Salmonella typhimurium*. *J Biol Chem* 1989;264:18973–18975.
169. Stieglitz H, Lipsky P. Association between reactive arthritis and antecedent infection with *Shigella flexneri* carrying a 2-Md plasmid and encoding an HLA-B27 mimetic epitope. *Arthritis Rheum* 1993; 36:1387–1391.
170. Schwimbeck P, Yu DTY, Oldstone MBA. Autoantibodies to HLA-B27 in the sera of HLA-B27 patients with ankylosing spondylitis and Reiter's syndrome. *J Exp Med* 1987;166:173–181.
171. Probst P, Hermann E, Meyer zum Büschenfelde K-M, et al. Multiclonal synovial T cell response to *Yersinia enterocolitica* in reactive arthritis. *J Infect Dis* 1993;167:385–391.
172. Hermann E, Lohse AW, Van der Zee R, et al. Synovial fluid-derived *Yersinia*-reactive T cells responding to human 65kDa heat-shock protein and heat stressed antigen-presenting cells. *Eur J Immunol* 1991;21:2139–2143.
173. Zinberg J, Vecchi M, Sakamaki S, et al. Intestinal tissue associated antigens in the pathogenesis of inflammatory bowel disease. In: Jarnerot G, ed. *Inflammatory bowel disease*. New York: Raven Press, 1987:67–76.
174. Cuvelier C, Mielants H, De Vos M, et al. Major histocompatibility class II antigen (HLA-DR) expression by ileal epithelial cells in patients with seronegative spondylarthropathies. *Gut* 1990;31:545–549.
175. Selby WS, Janossy G, Mason DY, et al. Expression of HLA-DR antigens by colonic epithelium in inflammatory bowel disease. *Clin Exp Immunol* 1983;53:614–618.
176. McDonald GB, Jewell DP. Class II antigen (HLA-DR) expression by intestinal epithelial cells in inflammatory diseases of colon. *J Clin Pathol* 1987;40:312–317.
177. Rognum TO, Brandtzaeg P, Elgjo K, et al. Heterogeneous epithelial expression of class II (HLA-DR) determinants and secretory component related to dysplasia in ulcerative colitis. *Br J Cancer* 1987;56: 419–424.
178. Fais S, Pallone F, Squarcia O, et al. HLA-DR antigens on colonic epithelial cells in inflammatory bowel disease: I. Relation to the state of activation of lamina propria lymphocytes and to the epithelial expression of other surface markers. *Clin Exp Immunol* 1987;68: 605–612.
179. Selby WS, Poulter LW, Hobbs S, et al. Heterogeneity of HLA-DR positive histiocytes in human intestinal lamina propria: a combined histochemical and immunohistological analysis. *J Clin Pathol* 1983; 36:379–384.
180. Cuvelier CA, Quatacker J, Mielants H, et al. M-cells are damaged and increased in number in inflamed human ileal mucosa. *Histopathology* 1994;24:417–426.
181. Picker LJ. Lymphocyte homing. *Curr Opin Immunol* 1992;4:227–286.
182. Picker LJ. Control of lymphocyte homing. *Curr Opin Immunol* 1994; 6:394–406.
183. Bevilacqua MP. Endothelial-leukocyte adhesion molecules. *Annu Rev Immunol* 1993;11:767–804.
184. Adams DH, Shaw S. Leucocyte-endothelial interactions and regulation of leucocyte migration. *Lancet* 1994;343:831–836.
185. Schweighoffer T, Tanaka Y, Tidswell M, et al. Selective expression of integrin $\alpha_4\beta_7$ on a subset of human CD4$^+$ memory T cells with hallmarks of gut tropism. *J Immunol* 1993;151:717–729.
186. Postigo AA, Sanchez-Mateos P, Lazarovits AI, et al. $\alpha_4\beta_7$ integrin mediates B cell binding to fibronectin and vascular adhesion molecule-1: expression and function of α_4 integrins on human B lymphocytes. *J Immunol* 1993;151:2471–2483.
187. Berlin C, Berg EL, Briskin MJ, et al. $\alpha_4\beta_7$ integrin mediates lymphocyte binding to the mucosal vascular addressin MadCAM-1. *Cell* 1993;74:185–195.
188. Erle DJ, Briskin MJ, Butcher EC. Expression and function of the MadCAM-1 receptor on human leukocytes. *J Immunol* 1994;153: 517–528.
189. Hamman A, Andrew DP, Jablonski-Westrich D, et al. Role of α-integrins in lymphocyte homing to mucosal tissues *in vivo*. *J Immunol* 1994;152:3282–3293.
190. Streeter PR, Berg EL, Rouse BTN, et al. A tissue-specific endothelial cell molecule involved in lymphocyte homing. *Nature* 1988;331: 41–46.
191. Briskin MJ, McEvoy LM, Butcher EC. MadCAM-1 has homology to immunoglobulin and mucin-like adhesion receptors and to IgA1. *Nature* 1993;363:461–464.

192. Cepek KL, Parker CM, Madara JL, et al. Integrin $a_E b_7$ mediates adhesion of T lymphocytes to epithelial cells. *J Immunol* 1993;150:3459–3470.
193. Cerf-Bensussan N, Jarry A, Brousse N, et al. A monoclonal antibody (HML-1) defining a novel membrane molecule present on human intestinal lymphocytes. *Eur J Immunol* 1987;17:1279.
194. Barnard JA, Beauchamp RD, Coffey RJ, et al. Regulation of intestinal epithelial cell growth by transforming growth factor type β. *Proc Natl Acad Sci U S A* 1989;86:1578–1582.
195. Koyama SY, Podolsky DK. Differential expression of transforming growth factor α and β in intestinal epithelial cells. *J Clin Invest* 1989;83:1768–1773.
196. Brandtzaeg P, Sollic LM, Thrane PS, et al. Lymphoepithelial interactions in the mucosal immune system. *Gut* 1988;29:1116.
197. Van Kerckhove C, Russell GJ, Deusch K, et al. Oligoclonality of human intestinal intraepithelial T cells. *J Exp Med* 1992;175:57–63.
198. Cepek KL, Shaw SK, Parker CM, et al. Adhesion between epithelial cells and T lymphocytes mediated by E-cadherin and $\alpha_E\beta_7$ integrin. *Nature* 1994;372:190–193.
199. Overduin M, Harvey TS, Bagby S, et al. Solution structure of the epithelial cadherin domain responsible for selective cell adhesion. *Science* 1995;267:386–389.
200. Geiger B, Ayalon O. Cadherins. *Annu Rev Cell Biol* 1992;8:307–332.
201. Salmi M, Jalkanen S. VAP-1: an adhesin and and enzyme. *Trends Immunol* 2001;22:211–216.
202. Salmi M, Rajala P, Jalkanen S. Homing of mucosal leukocytes to joints. Distinct endothelial ligands in synovium mediate leukocyte-subtype specific adhesion. *J Clin Invest* 1997;99:2165–2175.
203. Salmi M, Jalkanen S. Human leukocyte subpopulations from inflamed gut bind to joint vasculature using distinct sets of adhesion molecules. *J Immunol* 2001;166:4650–4657.
204. Mack DR, Beedle S, Warren J, et al. Peripheral blood intracellular cytokine analysis in children newly diagnosed with inflammatory bowel disease. *Pediatr Res* 2002;51:328–332.
205. Van Damme N, De Keyser F, Demetter P, et al. The proportion of Th1 cells, which prevail in gut mucosa, is decreased in inflammatory bowel syndrome. *Clin Exp Immunol* 2001;125:383–390.
206. Van Damme N, De Vos M, Baeten D, et al. Flow cytometric analysis of gut mucosal lymphocytes supports an impaired Th1 cytokine profile in spondyloarthropathy. *Ann Rheum Dis* 2001;60:495–499.
207. Yin Z, Braun J, Neure L, et al. Crucial role of interleukin-10/interleukin-12 balance in the regulation of the type 2 T helper cytokine response in reactive arthritis. *Arthritis Rheum* 1997;40:1788–97.
208. Rudwaleit M, Siegert S, Yin Z, et al. Low T cell production of TNF_{alpha} and IFN_{gamma} in ankylosing spondylitis: its relation to HLA-B27 and influence of the TNF-308 gene polymorphism. *Ann Rheum Dis* 2001;60:36–42.
209. Baeten D, Van Damme N, Van den Bosch F, et al. Impaired Th1 cytokine production in spondyloarthropathy is restored by anti-TNF_{alpha}. *Ann Rheum Dis* 2001;60:750–755.
210. Braun J, Yin Z, Spiller I, et al. Low secretion of tumor necrosis factor alpha, but no other Th1 or Th2 cytokines, by peripheral blood mononuclear cells correlates with chronicity in reactive arthritis. *Arthritis Rheum* 1999;42:2039–2044.
211. Iwanaga T, Shikichi M, Kitamura H, et al. Morphology and functional roles of synoviocytes in the joint. *Arch Histol Cytol* 2000;63:17–31.
212. Hendersen B. The contribution made by cytochemistry to the study of the metabolism of the normal and rheumatoid synovial lining cell (synoviocyte). *Histochem J* 1982;14:527–544.
213. Graabaek PM. Characteristics of the two types of synoviocytes in rat synovial membrane. An ultrastructural study. *Lab Invest* 1984;50:690–702.
214. Palmer DG, Selvendran Y, Allen C, et al. Features of synovial membrane identified with monoclonal antibodies. *Clin Exp Immunol* 1985;59:529–38.
215. Barland P, Novikoll AB, Hamerman D. Electron microscopy of the human synovial membrane. J Cell Biol 1982;14:207–220.
216. Edwards JC. The nature and origins of synovium: experimental approaches to the study of synoviocyte differentiation. *J Anat* 1994;184:493–501.
217. Wilkinson LS, Pitsillides AA, Worrall JG, et al. Light microscopic characterization of the fibroblast-like synovial intimal cell (synoviocyte). *Arthritis Rheum* 1992;35:1179–1184.
218. Mapp PI, Revell PA. Fibronectin production by synovial intimal cells. *Rheumatol Int* 1985;5:229–237.
219. Hamann J, Wishaup JO, Van Lier RAW, et al. Expression of the activation antigen CD97 and its ligand CD55 in rheumatoid synovial tissue. *Arthritis Rheum* 1999;42:650–658.
220. Morales Ducret J, Wayner E, Elices MJ, et al. Alpha 4/beta 1 integrin (VLA-4) ligands in arthritis. Vascular cell adhesion molecule-1 expression in synovium and on fibroblast-like synoviocytes. *J Immunol* 1992;149:1424–1431.
221. Revell PA, Al-Saffar N, Fish S, et al. Extracellular matrix of the synovial intimal cell layer. *Ann Rheum Dis* 1995;54:404–407.
222. Ceponis A, Konttinen YT, Mac Kevicius Z, et al. Aberrant vascularity and von Willebrand factor distribution in inflamed synovial membrane. *J Rheumatol* 1996;23:1880–1886.
223. Reece RJ, Canete JD, Parsons WJ, et al. Distinct vascular patterns of early synovitis in psoriatic, reactive, and rheumatoid arthritis. *Arthritis Rheum* 1999;42:1481–1484.
224. Baeten D, Demetter P, Cuvelier C, et al. Comparative study of the synovial histology in rheumatoid arthritis, spondyloarthropathy, and osteoarthritis: influence of disease duration and activity. *Ann Rheum Dis* 2000;59:945–953.
225. Veale D, Yanni G, Branes L, et al. Reduced synovial macrophage numbers, ELAM-1 expression, and lining layer hyperplasia in psoriatic arthritis as compared with rheumatoid arthritis. *Arthritis Rheum* 1993;36:893–900.
226. Fraser A, Fearon U, Reece R, et al. Matrix metalloproteinase 9, apoptosis, and vascular morphology in early arthritis. *Arthritis Rheum* 2001;44:2024–2028.
227. Fearon U, Griosios K, Fraser A, et al. Angiopoietins, growth factors, and vascular morphology in early arthritis. *J Rheumatol* 2003;30:260–268.
228. Kraan MC, Haringman JJ, Post WJ, et al. Immunohistological analysis of synovial tissue for differential diagnosis in early arthritis. *Rheumatology* 1999;38:1074–1080.
229. Smeets TJM, Dolhain RJEM, Breedveld FC, et al. Analysis of the cellular infiltrates and expression of cytokines in synovial tissue of patients with rheumatoid arthritis and reactive arthritis. *J Pathol* 1998;88:84–90.
230. Lahesmaa-Rantala R, Granfors K, Isomaki H, et al. *Yersinia* specific immune complexes in the synovial fluid of patients with *Yersinia* triggered reactive arthritis. *Ann Rheum Dis* 1987;46:510–514.
231. Hammer M, Zeidler H, Klisma S, et al. *Yersinia enterocolitica* in the synovial membrane of patients with *Yersinia*-induced arthritis. *Arthritis Rheum* 1990;33:1795–1800.
232. Nikkari S, Merilahti-Palo R, Saaro R, et al. *Yersinia*-triggered reactive arthritis: use of polymerase chain reaction and immunocytochemical staining in the detection of bacterial components from synovial specimens. *Arthritis Rheum* 1992;35:682–687.
233. Mäki-Ikola O, Granfors K. *Salmonella* triggered reactive arthritis. *Lancet* 1992;339:1096–1098.
234. Ford DK, Schuller M. Synovial lymphocyte responses to microbial agents differentiate the arthritis of enteric reactive arthritis from the arthritis of inflammatory bowel disease. *J Rheumatol* 1988;15:1239–1242.
235. Gaston JSH, Life PF, Granfors K, et al. Synovial T lymphocyte recognition of organisms that trigger reactive arthritis. *Clin Exp Immunol* 1989;76:348–353.
236. Hassel AB, Pilling D, Reynolds D, et al. MHC restriction of synovial fluid lymphocytes responses to the triggering organism in reactive arthritis: absence of a class I-restricted response. *Clin Exp Immunol* 1992;83:442–447.
237. Lahesmaa R, Yssel H, Batsford S, et al. *Yersinia enterocolitica* activates a T helper type-1 like T cell subset in reactive arthritis. *J Immunol* 1992;148:3079–3085.
238. Hermann E, Yu DTY, Meyer zum Büschenfelde KH, et al. HLA-B27 restricted CD8 T cells derived from synovial fluids of patients with reactive arthritis and ankylosing spondylitis. *Lancet* 1993;342:646–650.
239. Benjamin RJ, Madrigal JA, Parham P. Peptide binding to empty HLA-B27 molecules of viable human cells. *Nature* 1991;351:74–77.
240. Elewaut D, De Keyser F, Van den Bosch F, et al. Enrichment of T cells carrying $_{beta}7$ integrins in inflamed synovial tissue from patients with early spondyloarthropathy, compared to rheumatoid arthritis. *J Rheumatol* 1998;25:1932–1937.

241. Baeten D, Kruithof E, Van den Bosch F, et al. Immunomodulatory effects of anti-tumor necrosis factor alpha therapy on synovium in spondyloarthropathy: histologic findings in eight patients from an open-label pilot study. *Arthritis Rheum* 2001;44:186–195.
242. May E, Marker-Hermann E, Wittig BM, et al. Identical T-cell expansions in the colon mucosa and the synovium of a patient with enterogenic spondyloarthropathy. Gastroenterology 2000;119: 1745–1755.
243. Yin Z, Siegert S, Neure L, et al. The elevated ratio of interferon gamma-/interleukin-4-positive T cells found in synovial fluid and synovial membrane of rheumatoid arthritis patients can be changed by interleukin-4 but not by interleukin-10 or transforming growth factor beta. *Rheumatology* 1999;38:1058–1067.
244. Canete JD, Martinez SE, Farres J, et al. Differential Th1/Th2 cytokine patterns in chronic arthritis: interferon gamma is highly expressed in synovium of rheumatoid arthritis compared with seronegative spondyloarthropathies. *Ann Rheum Dis* 2000;59:263–268.
245. Seta N, Granfors K, Sahly H, et al. Expression of host defense scavenger receptors in spondyloarthropathy. *Arthritis Rheum* 2001;44: 931–939.
246. Kaluza W, Leirisalo-Repo M, Marker-Hermann E, et al. IL10.G microsatellites mark promoter haplotypes associated with protection against the development of reactive arthritis in Finnish patients. *Arthritis Rheum* 2001;44:1209–1214.
247. McInnes IB, Illei GG, Danning CL, et al. IL-10 improves skin disease and modulates endothelial activation and leucocyte effector functions in patients with psoriatic arthritis. *J Immunol* 2001;167:4075–4082.
248. Braun J, Bollow M, Neure L, et al. Use of immunohistologic and *in situ* hybridization techniques in the examination of sacroiliac joint biopsy specimens from patients with ankylosing spondylitis. *Arthritis Rheum* 1995;38:499–505.
249. Danning CL, Illei GG, Hitchon C, et al. Macrophage-derived cytokine and nuclear factor $_{kappa}$B p65 expression in synovial membrane and skin of patients with psoriatic arthritis. *Arthritis Rheum* 2000; 43:1244–1256.

CHAPTER 67

The Liver in Arthritis and Rheumatic Disease

Alexander P. Ruggieri

The rheumatologist encounters clinical issues involving the liver in several general clinical arenas. These are summarized and classified in Table 67.1. While many of the classical rheumatic diseases managed by rheumatologists, such as rheumatoid arthritis (RA), can have subtle hepatic manifestations, significant hepatic-related clinical features are usually uncommon and insignificant in these disorders. Exceptions include polymyalgia rheumatica (PMR) associated with giant cell arteritis (1–5) and Still's disease (6–10).

Liver function abnormalities can be detected in approximately 20% of patients with PMR and giant cell arteritis. The serologic picture is that of a mild hepatitic or cholestatic reaction with predominant elevation of alkaline phosphatase. Hyperbilirubinemia is rare. The pathogenesis of the liver enzyme elevation is unknown but generally resolves in response to corticosteroid therapy administered for the underlying disease and significant liver impairment does not occur.

Still's disease both in adult and pediatric (systemic juvenile rheumatoid arthritis) forms can have significant hepatic involvement characterized by hepatitis, hepatomegaly with portal hypertension and ascites, and marked transaminase elevations, which contribute to the morbidity and mortality of the disease. Acute fulminant liver failure (11) occurs that may be unresponsive to conventional therapy, thus requiring liver transplantation (12).

Significant musculoskeletal manifestations can occur in a variety of primary liver disorders. Among these diseases, the various bone and articular findings can be prominent and problematic. These include symmetric inflammatory arthritis occurring in autoimmune or immune complex associated liver disorders (hepatitis C–related cryoglobulinemia, autoimmune hepatitis, primary biliary cirrhosis), crystal-induced arthritis associated with chondrocalcinosis (Wilson's disease, hemochromatosis), osteoarthritis (metabolic syndrome and steatohepatitis) (13–15), hypertrophic osteoarthropathy and Dupuytren's tendon contractures (Fig. 67.1) associated with end-stage liver diseases from any source (16,17), and osteoporosis associated with disordered vitamin D metabolism (18,19) in advanced liver diseases. Many of these liver disorder–related arthropathies and osteopathies respond to treatments for the underlying liver disease. Many of them will remit after liver transplantation (16). Sarcoidosis is a systemic inflammatory disorder which can result in mixed hepatic and articular clinical features. This disorder and several other metabolic disorders (Wilson's disease, hemochromatosis), which are associated with both liver and

TABLE 67.1. *Classification of clinical areas involving the liver in rheumatology*

1. Classic rheumatic diseases with hepatic manifestations
   a. polymyalgia rheumatica
   b. Still's disease
2. Hepatic diseases with immunologically mediated extrahepatic manifestations
   a. acute and chronic infection with hepatotropic viruses (hepatitis B, hepatitis C)
   b. mixed cryoglobulinemia
3. Autoimmune liver diseases
   a. autoimmune hepatitis
   b. primary biliary cirrhosis
   c. sclerosing cholangitis
   d. sarcoidosis
4. Antirheumatic drugs with hepatotoxic effects
5. Metabolic disorders with hepatic and articular manifestations
   a. Wilson's disease
   b. hemochromatosis
   c. steatohepatitis, insulin resistance, and osteoarthritis (the "metabolic syndrome")
6. Musculoskeletal findings in end stage liver disease
   a. hypertrophic osteoarthropathy
   b. Dupuytren's contracture
   c. osteoporosis

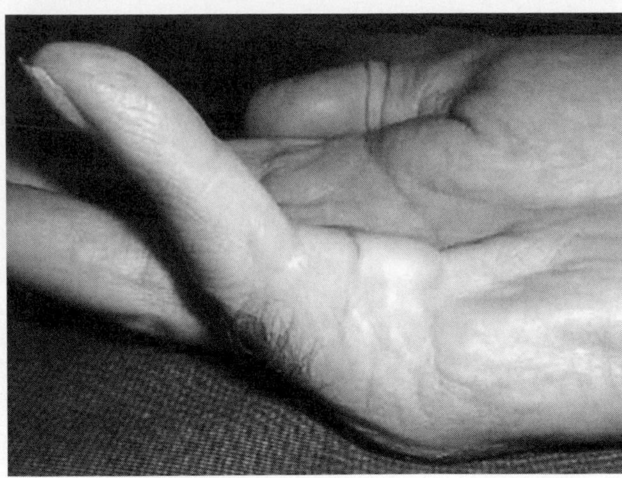
A

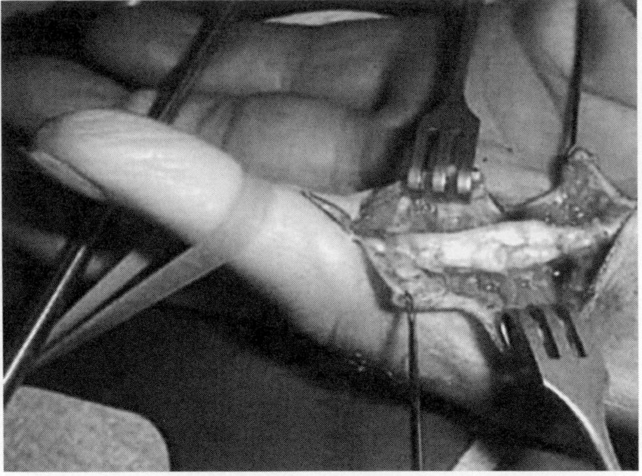
B

FIG. 67.1. A: Dupuytren's contracture of the palmar flexor tendons. **B:** Surgical dissection showing thickening and contracture of the tendon and its surrounding aponeurosis.

articular findings, are covered elsewhere in this text (Chapters 94 and 120).

IMMUNOLOGICALLY MEDIATED EXTRAHEPATIC RHEUMATIC MANIFESTATIONS OF HEPATIC DISEASES

The Hepatotropic Viral Infections

Hepatitis C

Rheumatic manifestations frequently occur in hepatitis C virus (HCV) infection (20). These include fatigue, arthralgias, myalgias, arthritis, sicca symptoms, and autoantibody expression. Generally, transmission is bloodborne. The vigorous screening of blood donors has left intravenous drug abuse as the major risk factor for acquiring the infection. While education and stringent control of blood donor programs have resulted in decline in the incidence from a peak of more than 250,000 in the early 1980s to less than 40,000 new cases per year today in the U.S., globally it is anticipated that the vast majority of infected individuals have yet to be diagnosed. Because early acute illness (21) associated with acute HCV infection is transient, mild, or asymptomatic, it is often the rheumatologist, while evaluating these extrahepatic rheumatic-type manifestations in the setting of unexplained serum elevations in liver transaminase levels, who will make the diagnosis of the chronic infected state. In these settings, the diagnosis is confirmed by HCV antibody detection using immunoassay and recombinant immunoblot assay, simultaneously with HCV ribonucleic acid (RNA) measurement in the serum by polymerase chain reaction, branched DNA assay, or transcription-mediated amplification.

The most clinically striking extrahepatic manifestations of hepatitis C infection are those of systemic vasculitis (22), most frequently involving small vessels of the skin, nerves, and kidney, and resulting in clinical presentations such as palpable purpura, skin ulceration, stocking glove axonal sensory neuropathy, mononeuritis multiplex, membranoproliferative glomerulonephritis, sicca complex, and polyarthritis. Vasculitis associated with chronic HCV infection seems to be almost always associated with the presence of cryoglobulins and is believed to be mediated through the same mechanisms underlying mixed cryoglobulinemia vasculitis (MCV). Indeed, in the last 10 years, many studies have demonstrated that infection with HCV virus is involved in the pathogenesis of most cases of mixed cryoglobulinemia vasculitis (23). There are no reports of HCV-related vasculitis occurring without detectable circulating cryoglobulins. However, published series of patients with chronic HCV indicate an overall low prevalence of significant detectable cryoglobulins and in those who are positive, a low rate of emergence of clinically significant vasculitis (24–26). When present, cryoglobulinemic vasculitis in chronic HCV infection tends to most often involve type II cryoglobulins [monoclonal immunoglobulin M (IgM) rheumatoid factor associated with polyclonal immunoglobulins] with cryocrits greater than 3% (27).

The relationship between the severity of liver disease and the extent of vasculitis varies: patients may be asymptomatic carriers of cryoglobulins but may have chronic hepatitis according to usual criteria; in some cases, cryoglobulinemic patients may have little or no active liver disease with normal alanine amino transferase and mild liver lesions at liver biopsy; patients may have severe manifestations of MCV; and, finally, in other patients there may be active liver disease and MCV-related symptoms both present (28).

Prior to widespread appreciation of the etiologic role of HCV infection in cryoglobulinemic vasculitis and the availability of antiviral therapy, many cases of HCV cryoglobulinemic vasculitis were treated solely with immunosuppressant drugs (corticosteroids, cyclophosphamide, and plasmapheresis alone or in combination) with variable success (29,30). The introduction of interferon-alpha (IFN-α) and ribavirin has raised expectations and hopes for success in reducing the progression to cirrhosis and the incidence of hepatocellular carcinoma, and in managing the extrahepatic manifestations of chronic HCV infection. Compiled data from several studies (22) support an expected clinical response rate of 75% in patients considered to have mild or moderate disease. Renal and neurologic manifestations usually are the most refractory to response, often indicating irreversible end organ damage. Response rates and relapse rates correlate with virologic load reduction (31). Cumulative observations and reports to date support the view that combination therapy with IFN-α and ribavirin should be considered as a principal initial therapeutic strategy for chronic HCV-associated cryoglobulinemic vasculitis and that virus elimination almost always leads to elimination of the clinical burden of cryoglobulinemic vasculitis. This assertion should be tempered by the understanding that antiviral therapy, while potentially successful, may often be inadequate and associated with significant use limiting side effects or lead to exacerbations of vasculitis manifestations (32–34). Decisions to use immunosuppressive therapy are complicated not only by questions related to efficacy but also concerns about amplification of the underlying HCV infection with acceleration of the disease. While corticosteroid therapy has been shown to result in increased viremia (35,36), retrospective review of one series of patients with HCV-associated cryoglobulinemic glomerulonephritis indicated no acute liver damage or accelerated end-stage hepatic outcomes associated with combinations of corticosteroids, cyclophosphamide, and plasmapheresis (37).

Hepatitis B

In its only known natural reservoir (humans), hepatitis B virus (HBV) in the acute or chronically infected state can cause an array of rheumatic-type symptoms. As with hepatitis C, hematogenous spread is the principal route of infectivity, but transmission by fecal–oral route and perinatal transmission can occur as well.

The most common rheumatic presentation occurring during the acute phase of infection is the "arthritis–dermatitis" syndrome (38), consisting of an urticarial, petechial, or maculopapular eruption and a symmetric polyarthritis involving the small joints in a symmetric fashion. The presence of hepatitis B surface antigen and evidence of complement consumption in synovial and dermal tissue supports an immune complex–mediated pathogenesis (39). As the acute infection resolves so does the syndrome and it rarely lasts more than a few weeks. Many patients never enter an icteric phase and, unless abnormal liver functions are noted, the true etiology may be missed. Full recovery is the rule as the acute infection resolves and can be treated with simple nonsteroidal antiinflammatory drugs (NSAIDs).

Chronic HBV infection rarely is accompanied by immune complex phenomenon (40,41) ranging from mild leukocytoclastic (42) or urticarial vasculitis (43) to full-blown polyarteritis nodosa (44–47), microscopic polyangiitis (48), and membranous glomerulopathy (49). There have also been isolated reports of vasculitis induced by hepatitis B vaccination (50,51). Use of traditional immunosuppressive therapy to manage immune complex–mediated extrahepatic manifestations of chronic HBV has always raised concerns of worsening or reactivation of the underlying HBV infection (52). Three drugs are available currently for the treatment of chronic hepatitis B that can be used concurrently with immunosuppressive therapy (53). These are IFN-α, lamivudine, and adefovir dipivoxil (54). IFN-α has been used in the treatment of chronic hepatitis B infection for many years and has been used to manage extrahepatic vasculitic manifestations of the disease (55,56). It exerts its antiviral effect by inhibiting synthesis of viral DNA and by activating antiviral enzymes. IFN-α also amplifies the cellular immune response against hepatocytes infected with HBV by increasing expression of class I histocompatibility antigens and by simulating the activity of helper T lymphocytes and natural killer cells. Lamivudine, a nucleoside analogue, directly inhibits HBV DNA polymerase, has shown rapid antiviral effects, and has been successful in combination with immunosuppressive therapy (57–59). The disadvantage to lamivudine is a high rate of viral resistance with continued use of the drug. A new agent, adefovir dipivoxil, a nucleotide analogue that inhibits the HBV polymerase, is effective in lamivudine-resistant HBV infection.

HEPATIC TOXIC EFFECTS OF ANTIRHEUMATIC DRUG THERAPIES

The liver plays a major physiological role in detoxification and metabolism of many external nonphysiological chemicals and agents and, in that role, is susceptible to injury from a variety of mechanisms. Among the chemical agents used as drugs in the management of arthritis and rheumatic disease, all carry some potential for idiosyncratic liver injury in any given patient. The discussion below focuses on a limited set of pharmacologic agents worthy of special concern with respect to liver toxicity either because of specific experience documenting such or because the frequency and volume of their use makes what might otherwise be rare hepatic effects a more pressing concern.

Methotrexate

Methotrexate (MTX) has been an important therapeutic agent in rheumatic disease management, particularly rheumatoid and psoriatic arthritis. Among the potentially serious adverse effects of MTX therapy warranting disclosure to patients and purposeful monitoring is hepatocellular injury. MTX therapy in the setting of rheumatic diseases can lead to hepatic fibrosis, cirrhosis, and liver failure (60). Transaminase elevations commonly occur during the course of MTX and can fluctuate in and out of the normal range. Significant correlation between hepatic aspartate aminotransferase (AST) levels and progression of histologic deterioration in patients with RA receiving chronic weekly MTX has been demonstrated (61). Histologic evidence of hepatic fibrosis can develop in as many as half of patients treated with MTX over time and severity correlates with obesity, alcohol intake, age, presence of diabetes, and duration of therapy (62). The spectrum of pathologic changes that can be seen are nonspecific, consisting of fatty change, nuclear pleomorphism, hepatocyte necrosis, portal chronic inflammatory infiltrates, fibrosis, and cirrhosis. Many of the histopathologic changes seen in MTX-induced liver damage are identical to those seen in nonalcoholic steatosis and steatohepatitis (63). The mechanism of liver injury is poorly understood; intracellular accumulation of MTX polyglutamate and consequent folate depletion are suspected to play a role (64).

Prior adverse experiences with MTX-induced hepatotoxicity in other disorders prompted the development of guidelines for the use and monitoring of MTX in the treatment of RA, which were published in 1994 (65). Since the issuance of these guidelines, the positive prospective experiences of some with long-term use of MTX in RA has prompted calls for less stringent revisions of the guidelines (66). Cogent arguments against relaxation of established guidelines have been made as well (67). Use of the current monitoring guidelines in making decisions regarding liver biopsy has been shown to be efficacious and cost effective in identifying those in whom liver biopsy is necessary (68). Given the known hepatotoxic effects of MTX especially in psoriatic arthritis, the increasing complexity and numbers of medications with hepatotoxic potential (statins, anticonvulsants, antidepressants, NSAIDs (69)) that might be used concurrently with MTX, the high prevalence in many populations of obesity and steatohepatitis (70) which can potentially enhance MTX hepatotoxicity, and the success in preventing serious MTX-induced liver injury when the guidelines have been effectively applied, there seems to be little basis for relaxation of current MTX monitoring guidelines. Heightened concern for hepatotoxicity of MTX is warranted in patients with advanced age, duration of MTX therapy extending beyond 3 years, concurrent obesity, hypertriglyceridemia, diabetes, psoriasis, and chronic alcohol use.

Serum transaminase elevations are common during MTX use, can fluctuate in and out of the normal range, and are usually associated with reversible liver injury. Persistent transaminase elevations are associated with more permanent hepatic architecture changes. Progressive decline in serum albumin, especially in association with unexplained thrombocytopenia, portends clinically significant hepatic fibrosis.

No reliable conclusion can be made regarding the presence and extent of hepatic injury on the basis of serum tests alone. Liver biopsy remains the gold standard for this determination (71). Interpretation of liver histology from biopsy specimens obtained from patients taking MTX relies on the Roenigk grading system (72). Grade I represents normal findings except possibly for the presence of fatty change. Grade 2 includes fatty change together with severe spotty hepatocellular necrosis. Grade 3A includes findings of mild portal fibrosis, while grade 3B represents piecemeal necrosis or moderate to severe septal fibrosis with portal to portal or portal triad to central vein bridging fibrosis. Grade 4 represents complete loss of normal hepatic architecture with fibrosis, cirrhosis, and nodular regeneration.

Guidelines for monitoring liver toxicity due to MTX in patients receiving the drug for RA have been published (65) and endorsed by the American College of Rheumatology. Adherence to the guidelines demands a pretreatment evaluation to include aspartate aminotransferase (AST), alanine aminotransferase (ALT), alkaline phosphatase, albumin, bilirubin, hepatitis B and C serologic studies, complete blood counts, and serum creatinine. Pretreatment liver biopsy is recommended for patients with unexplained abnormalities in the above-mentioned studies or in patients with habitual alcohol consumption. If the above pretreatment studies are normal, MTX administration can proceed while monitoring the AST, ALT, and albumin every 4 to 8 weeks. If over a 12-month period 5 of 9 AST determinations are abnormal to any degree outside the normal range (or 6 abnormals out of 12 monthly determinations), a liver biopsy is recommended before continuing MTX. If the liver biopsy results demonstrate Roenigk grade 3B or 4, then MTX should be discontinued. For a Roenigk grade 3A or less, MTX can be resumed again while observing liver function tests as described above. MTX should be discontinued in anyone who refuses to comply with these guidelines or who uses alcohol habitually. Concurrent folic acid supplementation has been shown to reduce the risk of transaminase elevations and discontinuation rates in RA patients taking MTX (73).

Leflunomide

Leflunomide exerts an immunomodulatory effect by preventing proliferation of activated lymphocytes through inhibition of dihydroorotate dehydrogenase, a critical step in *de novo* pyrimidine synthesis (74). Hepatic transaminase elevation was among the more common side effects seen in clinical trials (75). While early controlled studies demonstrated acceptable efficacy and safety profiles in patients with RA (76,77) and in transplantation patients (78), isolated reports of serious hepatic failure events (79,80) have led some to urge recommendations that the agent be withdrawn from Food and Drug Administration–approved clinical uses (81). These recommendations have been rejected to date after further review. Leflunomide has been used in combination with MTX with no apparent amplification of hepatic injury risk in term-limited studies (82); however, there has been at least one report of micronodular cirrhosis in a patient using concurrent MTX and leflunomide therapy despite adherence to close monitoring based on accepted MTX monitoring guidelines (80). Serious unexpected hepatic toxicity can occur with leflunomide and currently there are no formally adopted or clinically vetted guidelines for monitoring for hepatic injury other than those provided by the manufacturer.

Nonsteroidal Antiinflammatory Drugs

Although NSAIDs are among the most frequently prescribed drugs, hepatotoxic effects are relatively rare and are overshadowed by more conspicuous side effects on the upper gastrointestinal tract. Because of the widespread use of these agents, often driven by intense marketing and fanfare when new NSAIDs are introduced for clinical use, the potential for hepatic effects can be underappreciated and can lead to isolated catastrophic events resulting in abrupt withdrawal of the drugs from clinical use, as exemplified by bromfenac (83–86). As one might expect from the large variety of NSAIDs and their divergent chemical structures, the types and frequency of reported hepatic injury are variable. Hepatic injury can occur through cholestatic, oxidative stress, or hypersensitivity mechanisms. Among selective cyclooxygenase (COX)-2 inhibitors, there have been several reports of hepatic injury due to celecoxib (87–90). Rofecoxib has not been implicated in liver injury to date. Evidence supports a possible role for preexisting sulfonamide allergy and risk of liver toxicity from celecoxib (91).

Acetaminophen

Acetaminophen has no antiinflammatory properties, but is an often recommended analgesic for arthritis pain. Acetaminophen hepatotoxicity has been recognized for decades and is currently the most common cause of drug-induced liver disease (92). Hepatocyte damage is the result of glutathione depletion, leading to the accumulation of toxic metabolites. Prolonged fasting, concurrent alcohol consumption, underlying liver disease, and drug doses exceeding 4 g/day are major risk factors for this complication.

Infliximab

Infliximab is an engineered biologic licensed for use in Crohn's disease and RA. It is a chimeric monoclonal antibody to tumor necrosis factor (TNF)-α and represents a new class of highly targeted biologically active protein molecules with little if any metabolic overhead and, as such, carries little expectation of organ-specific toxicity. Hepatotoxicity was not observed in premarketing trials (93,94). Two reports of liver injury have emerged attributed to infliximab. One patient with Crohn's disease developed severe cholestasis with resolution requiring 2 months (95). Another patient with long-standing RA developed acute hepatitis (96). This patient also developed a positive antinuclear antibody (ANA) and high levels of anti-double stranded DNA. Neither of these patients experienced permanent injury or fatality. Paradoxically, TNF-α has emerged as a key factor in various aspects of liver disorders (97,98), particularly steatohepatitis where it mediates not only the early stages of fatty liver disease, but also the transition to more advanced states of liver damage.

AUTOIMMUNE LIVER DISEASES

Autoimmune Hepatitis

Waldenström is credited with the making the first observation of the clinical entity characterized by acneiform rash, spider angiomas, amenorrhea, and marked hypergammaglobulinemia that today is designated "autoimmune hepatitis" (99). Initially this entity was thought to be the result of chronic viral infection, but the appearance of serologic markers of autoimmunity in patients led to appreciation of the role of loss of immunologic tolerance in the pathogenesis of inflammatory destruction of hepatic architecture and introduction of the terms "lupoid hepatitis" and "autoimmune chronic active hepatitis" to describe the condition. Clinical trials demonstrating the success of corticosteroids and azathioprine in controlling clinical features validated this notion (100). The frequent use of percutaneous liver biopsy in evaluation of these patients led to the appreciation of a morphologic spectrum ranging from lymphoplasmacytic infiltration within the portal tracts to extension of this process causing disruption of the limiting plate with "piecemeal necrosis" and varying degrees of bridging necrosis and fibrosis (101). The terms "chronic persistent hepatitis" and "chronic active hepatitis" were used to define the two extreme ends of this morphologic spectrum.

The recognition that the morphologic features of chronic persistent and chronic active hepatitis could be seen in a wide range of acute and chronic liver disorders, the absence of consistent transaminase elevation patterns that distinguishes autoimmune hepatitis, the variable clinical progression, and the identification of numerous serologic autoimmune markers in the disorder have prompted two international expert panel workgroups to address proper definitions, nomenclature, and clinical classification criteria (102,103). The result of this consensus effort was the formal abandonment of the terms "chronic persistent," "chronic active," and "lupoid hepatitis." The term "autoimmune hepatitis" was formally adopted to represent "an unresolving, predominantly periportal hepatitis usually with hypergammaglobulinemia and tissue autoantibodies, which is responsive to immunosuppressive therapy in most cases" (104). Because no features of autoimmune hepatitis were recognized to be pathognomonic, the consensus effort also emphasized the importance of exclusion of liver disorders with established etiologies before assigning the diagnosis.

The final consensus report of the International Autoimmune Hepatitis Group catalogued some of the more prominent clinical, epidemiologic, biochemical, immunologic, and histologic features of the disorder (105). Clinically, patients can present with an insidious illness or signs of acute severe hepatic failure. Frequent symptoms include lethargy, fatigue, malaise, nausea, weight loss, abdominal pain, skin rash, arthralgias, and myalgias. Physical findings can be those of hepatic failure and include hepatosplenomegaly, ascites, jaundice, peripheral edema, and, rarely, encephalopathy. Some patients present with signs of cirrhosis. Concurrent autoimmune disorders can be present, the most common of which are RA and autoimmune thyroid disease. Many patients are discovered during routine health screens at a time when they are minimally symptomatic with mild constitutional symptoms. The typical biochemical profile shows a "hepatitic" pattern with elevations in serum transaminase and bilirubin concentrations and typically normal alkaline phosphatase levels. Hypergammaglobulinemia is an almost universal finding due to elevations in the IgG isotype. Variation in the degree and pattern of biochemical abnormalities can be considerable and low or near normal values do not exclude a diagnosis of autoimmune hepatitis.

Serologic evidence of circulating autoantibodies is evident in the vast majority of patients with ANA and anti–smooth muscle antibodies (SMA) accounting for the majority. Seronegativity for these antibodies does not necessarily exclude the diagnosis as some patients will seroconvert in time. A small proportion of patients will be seropositive for type 1 liver–kidney microsomal (anti-LKM1) antibodies that react with the cytochrome isoenzyme P450 2D6 (106). Seropositivity for anti-LKM1 usually occurs in the absence of ANA and SMA and, because of its relative high specificity for autoimmune hepatitis, anti-LKM1 should be checked before excluding a diagnosis merely on the basis of absence of more commonly encountered autoantibodies (107). Circulating anti-LKM1 antibodies have been postulated to account for some reported cases of antimitochondrial antibody positivity in certain cases of autoimmune hepatitis, a serologic finding otherwise highly specific for primary biliary cirrhosis (108).

A widely recognized feature of autoimmune hepatitis is a high degree of responsiveness to prednisone alone or in combination with azathioprine. Several trials have demonstrated the effectiveness of these agents in improving clinical, histologic, and laboratory features of the disease (109–111). Combination therapy helps to achieve therapeutic effectiveness at the lowest possible dose of corticosteroid in order to minimize corticosteroid-induced side effects. Remission can be achieved in almost all patients with 10- to 20-year survival rates in excess of 80% at all histologic grades and levels of severity (112,113). The same general principles used to guide corticosteroid use in other rheumatic diseases apply for their use in autoimmune hepatitis. Vitamin D supplementation may be particularly important in controlling the osteoporosis-related effects of corticosteroids in autoimmune hepatitis because of the role of the liver in generating active forms of this vitamin (114). It should be noted that genes responsible for encoding thiopurine methyltransferase (TPMT), an enzyme that determines the metabolism of azathioprine, are highly polymorphic (115) and such polymorphisms can result in variable sensitivity, toxicity, and efficacy of a given dose in patients. Measurement of TPMT activity can help guide dosing and toxicity monitoring decisions (116). While many patients can achieve remission, others may often require indefinite treatment (62). When conventional approaches with corticosteroids and azathioprine fail, other novel immunosuppressive agents have shown potential promise. These include tacrolimus, mycophenolate mofetil, budesonide, deflazacort, and ursodeoxycholic acid (UDCA) (117). Liver transplantation is an option for refractory cases and has been successfully applied in autoimmune hepatitis (118). The actuarial 10-year survival after transplantation in autoimmune hepatitis is 75% and autoantibodies and hypergammaglobulinemia may disappear. Recurrence of autoimmune hepatitis has been noted in as many as 17% of patients and can be effectively managed with conventional immunosuppressive treatments (119).

Primary Biliary Cirrhosis

When the target of an autoimmune or inflammatory process involves the intralobular bile ducts of the liver, ensuing destruction can lead to loss of the exocrine integrity of the bile duct system, the accumulation of bile secretions exerting toxic effects through the detergent effects of constituent bile acids, cholestasis, secondary hepatocyte damage, cirrhosis, and liver failure. This pathologic sequence is exactly that seen in primary biliary cirrhosis (PBC), a condition whose characteristic pathologic lesion stems from a persistent T lymphocyte–mediated attack on intralobular bile duct epithelial cells. The characteristic serologic marker of PBC is antimitochondrial antibodies (120,121). The majority of patients with PBC will demonstrate positive antimitochondrial antibodies, but 5% to 10% of patients with typical features of PBC do not have detectable antimitochondrial antibodies. Their condition is referred to as antimitochondrial antibody-negative primary biliary cirrhosis or "autoimmune cholangitis" and is characterized by similar clinical, laboratory and histologic abnormalities, clinical course, and survival as antimitochondrial antibody positive patients (122). The targets of these antibodies are mitochondrial antigens normally present on the inner mitochondrial membrane, but are aberrantly expressed in the apical region of the bile duct epithelial cells in patients with PBC (123,124). The mitochondrial antigens responsible for loss of immune tolerance in PBC have been characterized as belonging to the E2 subunit of a related group of enzymes involved in energy metabolism with pyruvate dehydrogenase

(PDH) activity known as branched chain keto-acid dehydrogenase and ketoglutaric dehydrogenase (125). A nine-amino acid sequence in the PDH E2 subunit has been identified as the major antigenic target in PBC (126).

Observations including:

(a) the ability of this peptide to induce the proliferation of specific, major histocompatibility class I–restricted $CD8^+$ cytotoxic T lymphocytes from the majority of human leukocyte antigen (HLA)-A* 0201 PBC patients
(b) the relative high frequency of T lymphocytes recognizing this peptide in liver tissue in PBC patients
(c) the blunted, peptide-specific, $CD8^+$ T lymphocytotoxicity observed in peripheral blood monocytes derived from HLA-A* 0201 PBC patients challenged with a modified version of this peptide epitope containing an alanine substitution at position 5 (127,128)

all support a major autoantigenic role for this peptide sequence and the potential for modification of autoreactive PDH peptides as an immunomodulatory treatment for PBC.

Fatigue and pruritus are the most common presenting symptoms of PBC. It is not uncommon for the diagnosis to be made in asymptomatic individuals after routine screening of liver function studies. While most patients are diagnosed earlier, recent studies suggest the natural history of PBC is not changing (129). Median survival has generally been observed to be about 9 years. Mortality has been shown to be 3 times higher than age- and sex-matched individuals with as high as 42% of deaths related to complications of liver failure. UDCA, a choleretic agent, has been shown to slow progression to cirrhosis and can improve histologic and biochemical features and clinical symptoms, and extend the time to transplantation. It has not been shown to reduce the incidence of liver failure or affect mortality (130). Immunosuppressive therapy has not been shown to have a consistent clinically measurable salutary effect. While several studies have suggested a beneficial role for MTX (131), colchicine (132,133), and mofetil mycophenolate (134), these findings have not been consistently supported. Liver transplantation has been successful for advanced disease, but cholestasis can recur in the allograft (135,136). A recent study pointed to the potential role of *Chlamydia pneumoniae* as an etiologic agent, raising the possibility of a role for antibiotic therapy (137).

Primary Sclerosing Cholangitis

Primary sclerosing cholangitis (PSC) is a chronic cholestatic liver disease characterized by fibrosing inflammation and obliteration of intra- or extrahepatic bile ducts. The disease is one of the most common cholestatic diseases in adults and is diagnosed with increasing frequency. It has been reported in association with ulcerative colitis (138,139), systemic sclerosis (140), and autoimmune thyroid disease (141). Aside from viral hepatitis and alcoholic liver disease, PSC is one of the most common indications for liver transplantation (142). Patients with PSC have an increased incidence of bile duct carcinomas, and those with ulcerative colitis also have an increased incidence of colonic carcinomas. In end-stage disease, liver transplantation is the treatment of choice. Immunosuppressive treatment has little effect.

UDCA, which has been shown to improve liver histology and survival in patients with primary biliary cirrhosis, has a beneficial effect in PSC, provided that patients who develop major duct stenoses are treated endoscopically. The aim is to treat patients as early as possible to prevent progression to the advanced stages of the disease. During treatment with UDCA, stenoses of major ducts may develop, and early endoscopic dilation is highly effective. Because UDCA treatment improves but does not cure cholestatic liver diseases, permanent treatment seems to be necessary. Such prolonged treatment with UDCA may be recommended because, until now, no side effects have been reported. In patients with end-stage disease, UDCA is not effective and liver transplantation is indicated (143).

MUSCULOSKELETAL FINDINGS IN ADVANCED STAGE LIVER DISEASE

Hypertrophic osteoarthropathy is a clinical constellation involving clubbing of the fingertips together with painful inflammatory arthritis of the distal interphalangeal joints of the digits and pain in the diaphyses of the long bones. The triad of clubbing, arthritis, and periostitis has been associated with a number of conditions, most notably thoracic and extrathoracic malignancies, but also, relevant to this discussion, hepatic neoplasms and cirrhosis from any cause. Radiographic abnormalities are distinctive with hypertrophic bone similar to that seen in osteoarthritis and periosteal elevation along the diaphyses of long bones. Management can be difficult. Transplantation often results in resolution (16,144,145).

Dupuytren's contracture is a fibrosing condition affecting the aponeurosis of the palmar flexor tendons (Figure 67.1A). It can be associated with many conditions such as diabetes and ovarian cancer, but is often seen in patients with hepatobiliary malignancies and in cirrhosis of the liver. Treatments, other than therapy of the underlying condition, include local corticosteroid injections and reconstructive surgery (Figure 67.1B).

REFERENCES

1. Kyle V. Laboratory investigations including liver in polymyalgia rheumatica/giant cell arteritis. *Baillieres Clin Rheumatol* 1991;5(3): 475–484.
2. Kyle V, Wraight EP, Hazleman BL. Liver scan abnormalities in polymyalgia rheumatica/giant cell arteritis. *Clin Rheumatol* 1991;10(3): 294–297.
3. Kosolcharoen P, Magnin GE. Liver dysfunction and polymyalgia rheumatica. A case report. *J Rheumatol* 1976;3(1):50–53.
4. Long R, James O. Polymyalgia rheumatica and liver disease. *Lancet* 1974;1(7847):77–79.

5. von Knorring J, Wassatjerna C. Liver involvement in polymyalgia rheumatica. *Scand J Rheumatol* 1976;5(4):197–204.
6. Gallo M, Calvanese A, Oscuro F, et al. [Acute hepatitis in a patient with adult onset Still disease]. *Clin Ter* 1997;148(4):183–187.
7. Esdaile JM, Tannenbaum H, Lough J, Hawkins D. Hepatic abnormalities in adult onset Still's disease. *J Rheumatol* 1979;6(6):673–679.
8. Dino O, Provenzano G, Giannuoli G, et al. Fulminant hepatic failure in adult onset Still's disease. *J Rheumatol* 1996;23(4):784–785.
9. Arber N, Weinberger A, Fadila R, et al. Adult onset Still's disease. *Clin Rheumatol* 1989;8(3):339–344.
10. Tesser JR, Pisko EJ, Hartz JW, et al. Chronic liver disease and Still's disease. *Arthritis Rheum* 1982;25(5):579–582.
11. Ott SJ, Baron A, Berghaus T, et al. Liver failure in adult Still's disease during corticosteroid treatment. *Eur J Gastroenterol Hepatol* 2003; 15(1):87–90.
12. McFarlane M, Harth M, Wall WJ. Liver transplant in adult Still's disease. *J Rheumatol* 1997;24(10):2038–2041.
13. Cerulli J, Malone M. Outcomes of pharmacological and surgical treatment for obesity. *Pharmacoeconomics* 1998;14(3):269–283.
14. Rosenbloom AL, Silverstein JH. Connective tissue and joint disease in diabetes mellitus. *Endocrinol Metab Clin North Am* 1996;25(2): 473–483.
15. Spector TD, MacGregor AJ. The St. Thomas' UK Adult Twin Registry. *Twin Res* 2002;5(5):440–443.
16. Taillandier J, Alemanni M, Samuel D, et al. Hepatic hypertrophic osteoarthropathy: the value of liver transplantation. *Clin Exp Rheumatol* 1998;16(1):80–81.
17. Pitt P, Mowat A, Williams R, et al. Hepatic hypertrophic osteoarthropathy and liver transplantation. *Ann Rheum Dis* 1994;53(5): 338–340.
18. Holick MF. Vitamin D: a millennium perspective. *J Cell Biochem* 2003;88(2):296–307.
19. Carey E, Balan V. Metabolic bone disease in patients with liver disease. *Curr Gastroenterol Rep* 2003;5(1):71–77.
20. Vassilopoulos D, Calabrese LH. Rheumatic manifestations of hepatitis C infection. *Curr Rheumatol Rep* 2003;5(3):200–204.
21. Farrell GC. Drugs and steatohepatitis. *Semin Liver Dis* 2002;22(2): 185–194.
22. Vassilopoulos D, Calabrese LH. Hepatitis C virus infection and vasculitis: implications of antiviral and immunosuppressive therapies. *Arthritis Rheum* 2002;46(3):585–597.
23. Cacoub P, Costedoat-Chalumeau N, Lidove O, et al. Cryoglobulinemia vasculitis. *Curr Opin Rheumatol* 2002;14(1):29–35.
24. Persico M, De Marino FA, Di Giacomo Russo G, et al. Prevalence and incidence of cryoglobulins in hepatitis C virus-related chronic hepatitis patients: a prospective study. *Am J Gastroenterol* 2003;98(4):884–888.
25. Cacoub P, Poynard T, Ghillani P, et al. Extrahepatic manifestations of chronic hepatitis C. MULTIVIRC Group. Multidepartment Virus C. *Arthritis Rheum* 1999;42(10):2204–2212.
26. Cicardi M, Cesana B, Del Ninno E, et al. Prevalence and risk factors for the presence of serum cryoglobulins in patients with chronic hepatitis C. *J Viral Hepat* 2000;7(2):138–143.
27. Donada C, Crucitti A, Donadon V, et al. Systemic manifestations and liver disease in patients with chronic hepatitis C and type II or III mixed cryoglobulinaemia. *J Viral Hepat* 1998;5(3):179–185.
28. Lunel F, Musset L. Mixed cryoglobulinemia and hepatitis C virus infection. *Minerva Med* 2001;92(1):35–42.
29. Dispenzieri A, Gorevic PD. Cryoglobulinemia. *Hematol Oncol Clin North Am* 1999;13(6):1315–1349.
30. Gorevic PD, Kassab HJ, Levo Y, et al. Mixed cryoglobulinemia: clinical aspects and long-term follow-up of 40 patients. *Am J Med* 1980; 69(2):287–308.
31. Hadziyannis SJ, Vassilopoulos D. Complex management issues: management of HCV in the atypical patient. *Baillieres Best Pract Res Clin Gastroenterol* 2000;14(2):277–291.
32. Cid MC, Hernandez-Rodriguez J, Robert J, et al. Interferon-alpha may exacerbate cryoglobulinemia-related ischemic manifestations: an adverse effect potentially related to its anti-angiogenic activity. *Arthritis Rheum* 1999;42(5):1051–1055.
33. Gordon AC, Edgar JD, Finch RG. Acute exacerbation of vasculitis during interferon-alpha therapy for hepatitis C-associated cryoglobulinaemia. *J Infect* 1998;36(2):229–230.
34. Harle JR, Disdier P, Pelletier J, et al. Dramatic worsening of hepatitis C virus-related cryoglobulinemia subsequent to treatment with interferon alfa. *JAMA* 1995;274(2):126.
35. Fong TL, Valinluck B, Govindarajan S, et al. Short-term prednisone therapy affects aminotransferase activity and hepatitis C virus RNA levels in chronic hepatitis C. *Gastroenterology* 1994;107(1):196–199.
36. Magrin S, Craxi A, Fabiano C, et al. Hepatitis C viremia in chronic liver disease: relationship to interferon-alpha or corticosteroid treatment. *Hepatology* 1994;19(2):273–279.
37. D'Amico G. Renal involvement in hepatitis C infection: cryoglobulinemic glomerulonephritis. *Kidney Int* 1998;54(2):650–671.
38. Duffy J, Lidsky MD, Sharp JT, et al. Polyarthritis, polyarteritis and hepatitis B. *Medicine* (Baltimore) 1976;55(1):19–37.
39. Schumacher HR, Gall EP. Arthritis in acute hepatitis and chronic active hepatitis. Pathology of the synovial membrane with evidence for the presence of Australia antigen in synovial membranes. *Am J Med* 1974;57(4):655–664.
40. Sergent JS. Extrahepatic manifestations of hepatitis B infection. *Bull Rheum Dis* 1983;33(6):1–6.
41. Dienstag JL. Hepatitis B as an immune complex disease. *Semin Liver Dis* 1981;1(1):45–57.
42. Bonkovsky HL, Liang TJ, Hasegawa K, et al. Chronic leukocytoclastic vasculitis complicating HBV infection. Possible role of mutant forms of HBV in pathogenesis and persistence of disease. *J Clin Gastroenterol* 1995;21(1):42–47.
43. Greaves M. Chronic urticaria. *J Allergy Clin Immunol* 2000;105(4): 664–672.
44. Balkaran BN, Teelucksingh S, Singh VR. Hepatitis B-associated polyarteritis nodosa and hypertensive encephalopathy. *West Indian Med J* 2000;49(2):170–171.
45. Guo X, Gopalan R, Ugbarugba S, et al. Hepatitis B-related polyarteritis nodosa complicated by pulmonary hemorrhage. *Chest* 2001;119(5): 1608–1610.
46. Czaja AJ. Extrahepatic immunologic features of chronic viral hepatitis. *Dig Dis* 1997;15(3):125–144.
47. Menon Y, Singh R, Cuchacovich R, et al. Pulmonary involvement in hepatitis B-related polyarteritis nodosa. *Chest* 2002;122(4):1497–1498.
48. Lhote F, Cohen P, Genereau T, et al. Microscopic polyangiitis: clinical aspects and treatment. *Ann Med Interne* (Paris) 1996;147(3):165–177.
49. Mouthon L, Deblois P, Sauvaget F, et al. Hepatitis B virus-related polyarteritis nodosa and membranous nephropathy. *Am J Nephrol* 1995;15(3):266–269.
50. Zaas A, Scheel P, Venbrux A, et al. Large artery vasculitis following recombinant hepatitis B vaccination: 2 cases. *J Rheumatol* 2001; 28(5):1116–1120.
51. Saadoun D, Cacoub P, Mahoux D, et al. [Postvaccine vasculitis: a report of three cases]. *Rev Med Interne* 2001;22(2):172–176.
52. Shibolet O, Ilan Y, Gillis S, et al. Lamivudine therapy for prevention of immunosuppressive-induced hepatitis B virus reactivation in hepatitis B surface antigen carriers. *Blood* 2002;100(2):391–396.
53. Hoofnagle JH, di Bisceglie AM. The treatment of chronic viral hepatitis. *N Engl J Med* 1997;336(5):347–356.
54. Marcellin P, Boyer N. Chronic viral hepatitis. *Best Pract Res Clin Gastroenterol* 2003;17(2):259–275.
55. Wartelle-Bladou C, Lafon J, Trepo C, et al. Successful combination therapy of polyarteritis nodosa associated with a pre-core promoter mutant hepatitis B virus infection. *J Hepatol* 2001;34(5):774–779.
56. Willson RA. Extrahepatic manifestations of chronic viral hepatitis. *Am J Gastroenterol* 1997;92(1):3–17.
57. Stecevic V, Pevzner MM, Gordon SC. Successful treatment of hepatitis B-associated vasculitis with lamivudine. *J Clin Gastroenterol* 2003;36(5):451.
58. Maclachlan D, Battegay M, Jacob AL, et al. Successful treatment of hepatitis B-associated polyarteritis nodosa with a combination of lamivudine and conventional immunosuppressive therapy: a case report. *Rheumatology* (Oxford) 2000;39(1):106–108.
59. Lau CF, Hui PK, Chan WM, et al. Hepatitis B associated fulminant polyarteritis nodosa: successful treatment with pulse cyclophosphamide, prednisolone and lamivudine following emergency surgery. *Eur J Gastroenterol Hepatol* 2002;14(5):563–566.
60. Gilbert SC, Klintmalm G, Menter A, et al. Methotrexate-induced cirrhosis requiring liver transplantation in three patients with psoriasis. A

word of caution in light of the expanding use of this 'steroid-sparing' agent. *Arch Intern Med* 1990;150(4):889–891.
61. Kremer JM, Furst DE, Weinblatt ME, et al. Significant changes in serum AST across hepatic histological biopsy grades: prospective analysis of 3 cohorts receiving methotrexate therapy for rheumatoid arthritis. *J Rheumatol* 1996;23(3):459–461.
62. Kremer JM, Lee RG, Tolman KG. Liver histology in rheumatoid arthritis patients receiving long-term methotrexate therapy. A prospective study with baseline and sequential biopsy samples. *Arthritis Rheum* 1989;32(2):121–127.
63. Langman G, Hall PM, Todd G. Role of non-alcoholic steatohepatitis in methotrexate-induced liver injury. *J Gastroenterol Hepatol* 2001; 16(12):1395–1401.
64. Kevat S, Ahern M, Hall P. Hepatotoxicity of methotrexate in rheumatic diseases. *Med Toxicol Adverse Drug Exp* 1988;3(3):197–208.
65. Kremer JM, Alarcon GS, Lightfoot RW, Jr, et al. Methotrexate for rheumatoid arthritis. Suggested guidelines for monitoring liver toxicity. American College of Rheumatology. *Arthritis Rheum* 1994;37(3): 316–328.
66. Yazici Y, Erkan D, Paget SA. Monitoring methotrexate hepatic toxicity in rheumatoid arthritis: is it time to update the guidelines? *J Rheumatol* 2002;29(8):1586–1589.
67. Kremer JM. Not yet time to change the guidelines for monitoring methotrexate liver toxicity: they have served us well. *J Rheumatol* 2002;29(8):1590–1592.
68. Erickson AR, Reddy V, Vogelgesang SA, West SG. Usefulness of the American College of Rheumatology recommendations for liver biopsy in methotrexate-treated rheumatoid arthritis patients. *Arthritis Rheum* 1995;38(8):1115–1119.
69. Chitturi S, George J. Hepatotoxicity of commonly used drugs: non-steroidal anti-inflammatory drugs, antihypertensives, antidiabetic agents, anticonvulsants, lipid-lowering agents, psychotropic drugs. *Semin Liver Dis* 2002;22(2):169–183.
70. Angulo P. Nonalcoholic fatty liver disease. *N Engl J Med* 2002;346 (16):1221–1231.
71. Bravo AA, Sheth SG, Chopra S. Liver biopsy. *N Engl J Med* 2001; 344(7):495–500.
72. Roenigk HH Jr, Auerbach R, Maibach HI, et al. Methotrexate guidelines—revised. *J Am Acad Dermatol* 1982;6(2):145–155.
73. van Ede AE, Laan RF, Rood MJ, et al. Effect of folic or folinic acid supplementation on the toxicity and efficacy of methotrexate in rheumatoid arthritis: a forty-eight week, multicenter, randomized, double-blind, placebo-controlled study. *Arthritis Rheum* 2001;44(7):1515–1524.
74. Fox RI. Mechanism of action of leflunomide in rheumatoid arthritis. *J Rheumatol Suppl* 1998;53:20–26.
75. Hewitson PJ, Debroe S, McBride A, et al. Leflunomide and rheumatoid arthritis: a systematic review of effectiveness, safety and cost implications. *J Clin Pharm Ther* 2000;25(4):295–302.
76. Cohen S, Cannon GW, Schiff M, et al. Two-year, blinded, randomized, controlled trial of treatment of active rheumatoid arthritis with leflunomide compared with methotrexate. Utilization of Leflunomide in the Treatment of Rheumatoid Arthritis Trial Investigator Group. *Arthritis Rheum* 2001;44(9):1984–1992.
77. Emery P, Breedveld FC, Lemmel EM, et al. A comparison of the efficacy and safety of leflunomide and methotrexate for the treatment of rheumatoid arthritis. *Rheumatology* (Oxford) 2000;39(6):655–665.
78. Williams JW, Mital D, Chong A, et al. Experiences with leflunomide in solid organ transplantation. *Transplantation* 2002;73(3):358–366.
79. Legras A, Bergemer-Fouquet AM, Jonville-Bera AP. Fatal hepatitis with leflunomide and itraconazole. *Am J Med* 2002;113(4):352–353.
80. Weinblatt ME, Dixon JA, Falchuk KR. Serious liver disease in a patient receiving methotrexate and leflunomide. *Arthritis Rheum* 2000; 43(11):2609–2611.
81. Moynihan R. FDA officials argue over safety of new arthritis drug. *BMJ* 2003;326(7389):565.
82. Mroczkowski PJ, Weinblatt ME, Kremer JM. Methotrexate and leflunomide combination therapy for patients with active rheumatoid arthritis. *Clin Exp Rheumatol* 1999;17[6 Suppl 18]:S66–S68.
83. Rabkin JM, Smith MJ, Orloff SL, et al. Fatal fulminant hepatitis associated with bromfenac use. *Ann Pharmacother* 1999;33(9):945–947.
84. Moses PL, Schroeder B, Alkhatib O, et al. Severe hepatotoxicity associated with bromfenac sodium. *Am J Gastroenterol* 1999;94(5): 1393–1396.
85. Hunter EB, Johnston PE, Tanner G, et al. Bromfenac (Duract)-associated hepatic failure requiring liver transplantation. *Am J Gastroenterol* 1999;94(8):2299–2301.
86. Fontana RJ, McCashland TM, Benner KG, et al. Acute liver failure associated with prolonged use of bromfenac leading to liver transplantation. The Acute Liver Failure Study Group. *Liver Transpl Surg* 1999;5(6):480–484.
87. Alegria P, Lebre L, Chagas C. Celecoxib-induced cholestatic hepatotoxicity in a patient with cirrhosis. *Ann Intern Med* 2002;137(1):75.
88. Maddrey WC, Maurath CJ, Verburg KM, et al. The hepatic safety and tolerability of the novel cyclooxygenase-2 inhibitor celecoxib. *Am J Ther* 2000;7(3):153–158.
89. Mohammed F, Smith AD. Cholestatic hepatitis in association with celecoxib. Classification of drug associated liver dysfunction is questionable. *BMJ* 2002;325(7357):220; author reply 220.
90. Nachimuthu S, Volfinzon L, Gopal L. Acute hepatocellular and cholestatic injury in a patient taking celecoxib. *Postgrad Med J* 2001;77 (910):548–550.
91. Wiholm BE. Identification of sulfonamide-like adverse drug reactions to celecoxib in the World Health Organization database. *Curr Med Res Opin* 2001;17(3):210–216.
92. Acetaminophen is main cause of acute liver failure. *Health News* 2003;9(2):6.
93. Hanauer SB. Review article: safety of infliximab in clinical trials. *Aliment Pharmacol Ther* 1999;13[Suppl 4]:16–22; discussion 38.
94. Rutgeerts P, D'Haens G, Targan S, et al. Efficacy and safety of retreatment with anti-tumor necrosis factor antibody (infliximab) to maintain remission in Crohn's disease. *Gastroenterology* 1999;117(4):761–769.
95. Menghini VV, Arora AS. Infliximab-associated reversible cholestatic liver disease. *Mayo Clin Proc* 2001;76(1):84–86.
96. Saleem G, Li SC, MacPherson BR, et al. Hepatitis with interface inflammation and IgG, IgM, and IgA anti-double-stranded DNA antibodies following infliximab therapy: comment on the article by Charles et al. *Arthritis Rheum* 2001;44(8):1966–1968.
97. Tilg H. Cytokines and liver diseases. *Can J Gastroenterol* 2001;15 (10):661–668.
98. Tilg H, Diehl AM. Cytokines in alcoholic and nonalcoholic steatohepatitis. *N Engl J Med* 2000;343(20):1467–1476.
99. Mackay IR, Toh BH. Autoimmune hepatitis: the way we were, the way we are today and the way we hope to be. *Autoimmunity* 2002; 35(5):293–305.
100. Heneghan MA, McFarlane IG. Current and novel immunosuppressive therapy for autoimmune hepatitis. *Hepatology* 2002;35(1):7–13.
101. Popper H, Paronetto F, Schaffner F. Immune processes in the pathogenesis of liver disease. *Ann N Y Acad Sci* 1965;124(2):781–799.
102. Desmet VJ, Gerber M, Hoofnagle JH, et al. Classification of chronic hepatitis: diagnosis, grading and staging. *Hepatology* 1994;19(6): 1513–1520.
103. Johnson PJ, McFarlane IG. Meeting report: International Autoimmune Hepatitis Group. *Hepatology* 1993;18(4):998–1005.
104. Terminology of chronic hepatitis. International Working Party. *Am J Gastroenterol* 1995;90(2):181–189.
105. Alvarez F, Berg PA, Bianchi FB, et al. International Autoimmune Hepatitis Group Report: review of criteria for diagnosis of autoimmune hepatitis. *J Hepatol* 1999;31(5):929–938.
106. Manns MP, Griffin KJ, Sullivan KF, et al. LKM-1 autoantibodies recognize a short linear sequence in P450IID6, a cytochrome P-450 monooxygenase. *J Clin Invest* 1991;88(4):1370–1378.
107. Duchini A, McHutchison JG, Pockros PJ. LKM-positive autoimmune hepatitis in the western United States: a case series. *Am J Gastroenterol* 2000;95(11):3238–3241.
108. Gregorio GV, Portmann B, Mowat AP, et al. A 12-year-old girl with antimitochondrial antibody-positive autoimmune hepatitis. *J Hepatol* 1997;27(4):751–754.
109. Cook GC, Mulligan R, Sherlock S. Controlled prospective trial of corticosteroid therapy in active chronic hepatitis. *Q J Med* 1971;40 (158):159–185.
110. Murray-Lyon IM, Stern RB, Williams R. Controlled trial of prednisone and azathioprine in active chronic hepatitis. *Lancet* 1973;1 (7806):735–737.

111. Soloway RD, Summerskill WH, Baggenstoss AH, et al. Clinical, biochemical, and histological remission of severe chronic active liver disease: a controlled study of treatments and early prognosis. *Gastroenterology* 1972;63(5):820–833.
112. Roberts SK, Therneau TM, Czaja AJ. Prognosis of histological cirrhosis in type 1 autoimmune hepatitis. *Gastroenterology* 1996;110(3):848–857.
113. Davis GL, Czaja AJ, Ludwig J. Development and prognosis of histologic cirrhosis in corticosteroid-treated hepatitis B surface antigen-negative chronic active hepatitis. *Gastroenterology* 1984;87(6):1222–1227.
114. Schalm SW, Ammon HV, Summerskill WH. Failure of customary treatment in chronic active liver disease: causes and management. *Ann Clin Res* 1976;8(3):221–227.
115. Krynetski EY, Tai HL, Yates CR, et al. Genetic polymorphism of thiopurine S-methyltransferase: clinical importance and molecular mechanisms. *Pharmacogenetics* 1996;6(4):279–290.
116. Stolk JN, Boerbooms AM, de Abreu RA, et al. Reduced thiopurine methyltransferase activity and development of side effects of azathioprine treatment in patients with rheumatoid arthritis. *Arthritis Rheum* 1998;41(10):1858–1866.
117. Czaja AJ. Treatment of autoimmune hepatitis. *Semin Liver Dis* 2002;22(4):365–378.
118. Sanchez-Urdazpal L, Czaja AJ, van Hoek B, et al. Prognostic features and role of liver transplantation in severe corticosteroid-treated autoimmune chronic active hepatitis. *Hepatology* 1992;15(2):215–221.
119. Gonzalez-Koch A, Czaja AJ, Carpenter HA, et al. Recurrent autoimmune hepatitis after orthotopic liver transplantation. *Liver Transpl* 2001;7(4):302–310.
120. Surh CD, Danner DJ, Ahmed A, et al. Reactivity of primary biliary cirrhosis sera with a human fetal liver cDNA clone of branched-chain alpha-keto acid dehydrogenase dihydrolipoamide acyltransferase, the 52 kD mitochondrial autoantigen. *Hepatology* 1989;9(1):63–68.
121. Gershwin ME, Mackay IR, Sturgess A, et al. Identification and specificity of a cDNA encoding the 70 kd mitochondrial antigen recognized in primary biliary cirrhosis. *J Immunol* 1987;138(10):3525–3531.
122. Gisbert JP, Jones EA, Pajares JM, et al. Review article: is there an optimal therapeutic regimen for antimitochondrial antibody-negative primary biliary cirrhosis (autoimmune cholangitis)? *Aliment Pharmacol Ther* 2003;17(1):17–27.
123. Berg PA, Klein R. Mitochondrial antigen/antibody systems in primary biliary cirrhosis: revisited. *Liver* 1995;15(6):281–292.
124. Berg PA, Doniach D, Roitt IM. Mitochondrial antibodies in primary biliary cirrhosis. I. Localization of the antigen to mitochondrial membranes. *J Exp Med* 1967;126(2):277–290.
125. Migliaccio C, Van de Water J, Ansari AA, et al. Heterogeneous response of antimitochondrial autoantibodies and bile duct apical staining monoclonal antibodies to pyruvate dehydrogenase complex E2: the molecule versus the mimic. *Hepatology* 2001;33(4):792–801.
126. Kita H, Lian ZX, Van de Water J, et al. Identification of HLA-A2-restricted CD8 (+) cytotoxic T cell responses in primary biliary cirrhosis: T cell activation is augmented by immune complexes cross-presented by dendritic cells. *J Exp Med* 2002;195(1):113–123.
127. Kita H, Matsumura S, He XS, et al. Analysis of TCR antagonism and molecular mimicry of an HLA-A0201-restricted CTL epitope in primary biliary cirrhosis. *Hepatology* 2002;36(4 Pt 1):918–926.
128. Kita H, Matsumura S, He XS, et al. Quantitative and functional analysis of PDC-E2-specific autoreactive cytotoxic T lymphocytes in primary biliary cirrhosis. *J Clin Invest* 2002;109(9):1231–1240.
129. Prince M, Chetwynd A, Newman W, et al. Survival and symptom progression in a geographically based cohort of patients with primary biliary cirrhosis: follow-up for up to 28 years. *Gastroenterology* 2002;123(4):1044–1051.
130. Heathcote EJ. Management of primary biliary cirrhosis. The American Association for the Study of Liver Diseases practice guidelines. *Hepatology* 2000;31(4):1005–1013.
131. Bonis PA, Kaplan MM. Low-dose methotrexate in primary biliary cirrhosis. *Gastroenterology* 1999;117(6):1510–1513.
132. Lee YM, Kaplan MM. Efficacy of colchicine in patients with primary biliary cirrhosis poorly responsive to ursodiol and methotrexate. *Am J Gastroenterol* 2003;98(1):205–208.
133. Kaplan MM, Schmid C, Provenzale D, et al. A prospective trial of colchicine and methotrexate in the treatment of primary biliary cirrhosis. *Gastroenterology* 1999;117(5):1173–1180.
134. Jones EA. Rationale for trials of long-term mycophenolate mofetil therapy for primary biliary cirrhosis. *Hepatology* 2002;35(2):258–262.
135. Khettry U, Anand N, Faul PN, et al. Liver transplantation for primary biliary cirrhosis: a long-term pathologic study. *Liver Transpl* 2003;9(1):87–96.
136. Kurdow R, Marks HG, Kraemer-Hansen H, et al. Recurrence of primary biliary cirrhosis after orthotopic liver transplantation. *Hepatogastroenterology* 2003;50(50):322–325.
137. Kaplan MM. Primary biliary cirrhosis: past, present, and future. *Gastroenterology* 2002;123(4):1392–1394.
138. Nakayama M, Tsuji H, Shimono J, et al. Primary biliary cirrhosis associated with ulcerative colitis. *Fukuoka Igaku Zasshi* 2001;92(10):354–359.
139. Koulentaki M, Koutroubakis IE, Petinaki E, et al. Ulcerative colitis associated with primary biliary cirrhosis. *Dig Dis Sci* 1999;44(10):1953–1956.
140. Fraile G, Rodriguez-Garcia JL, Moreno A. Primary sclerosing cholangitis associated with systemic sclerosis. *Postgrad Med J* 1991;67(784):189–192.
141. Janssen HL, Smelt AH, van Hoek B. Graves' hyperthyroidism in a patient with primary sclerosing cholangitis. Coincidence or combined pathogenesis? *Eur J Gastroenterol Hepatol* 1998;10(3):269–271.
142. Zein CO, Lindor KD. Primary sclerosing cholangitis. *Semin Gastrointest Dis* 2001;12(2):103–112.
143. Stiehl A, Benz C, Sauer P. Primary sclerosing cholangitis. *Can J Gastroenterol* 2000;14(4):311–315.
144. Vickers C, Herbert A, Neuberger J, et al. Improvement in hypertrophic hepatic osteoarthropathy after liver transplantation. *Lancet* 1988;2(8617):968.
145. Cunnane G, O'Byrne AM, Hegarty J, et al. Hepatic hypertrophic osteoarthropathy and liver transplantation. *Ann Rheum Dis* 1994;53(12):840.

CHAPTER 68

Intermittent and Periodic Arthritis Syndromes

Daniel L. Kastner and Ivona Aksentijevich

Physicians have been fascinated with the concept of periodically recurring diseases since antiquity, when Galen related the periods of fevers with the phases of the moon (1). With the advance of medical science, many of the disorders that the ancients tied to celestial cycles have now been explained on the basis of human or microbial physiology. Nevertheless, by 1951 there remained a number of recurring disorders of unknown etiology that were grouped together by Reimann (2) under the rubric of "periodic disease," with the suggestion that their periodicity might derive from a common etiology. Among Reimann's periodic diseases are several of the recurring arthropathies to be discussed in this chapter. All of these diseases are characterized by a clinical course of exacerbations and remissions, although it is now clear that for most of these disorders clocklike periodicity is the exception rather than the rule.

With the benefit of over 50 years of additional scrutiny, great strides have been made in understanding the molecular and cellular underpinnings of the recurrent arthropathies. Perhaps most noteworthy has been the recognition of several Mendelian autoinflammatory syndromes that may present with intermittent arthritis or arthralgia (Table 68.1), and the subsequent identification of the causative genes and the proteins they encode (reviewed in reference 3). As will

TABLE 68.1. *Differential diagnosis of intermittent arthritis*

Mendelian autoinflammatory diseases
- Hereditary recurrent fever syndromes
  - Familial Mediterranean fever (FMF), OMIM 249100[a]
  - The cryopyrinopathies
    - Familial cold autoinflammatory syndrome (FCAS), OMIM 120100
    - Muckle-Wells syndrome (MWS), OMIM 191100
      - Neonatal onset multisystem inflammatory disease (NOMID), also known as chronic infantile neurologic cutaneous and arthropathy (CINCA) syndrome, OMIM 607115
  - Tumor necrosis factor (TNF) receptor-associated periodic syndrome (TRAPS), OMIM 142680
  - Hyperimmunoglobulinemia D syndrome (HIDS), OMIM 260920
- Other Mendelian autoinflammatory syndromes
  - Syndrome of pyogenic arthritis with pyoderma gangrenosum and acne (PAPA), OMIM 604416

Idiopathic intermittent arthropathies
- Intermittent hydrarthrosis
- Eosinophilic synovitis
- Palindromic rheumatism
- Tietze syndrome

Crystalline arthropathies
- Gout
- Calcium pyrophosphate crystal deposition disease

Enteropathic arthritides
- Inflammatory bowel disease
- Intestinal bypass arthropathy
- Celiac disease
- Whipple's disease

Hemoglobinopathies: sickle-cell disease

Hyperlipidemias: types II and IV

Infectious diseases
- Lyme
- Parvovirus

Reactive arthritis

Recurrent osteomyelitis syndromes
- Chronic recurrent multifocal osteomyelitis (CRMO)
- Synovitis, acne, pustulosis, hyperostosis, and osteitis (SAPHO)

Relapsing polychondritis

Spondyloarthropathies
- Ankylosing spondylitis
- Psoriatic arthritis

Storage diseases: Gaucher's disease

Systemic vasculitis: Behçet's disease

[a]The six-digit OMIM number refers to Online Mendelian Inheritance in Man, a continually updated catalogue of genetic disorders available at: *www.nlm.nih.gov/omim/*.

be discussed, these discoveries have vindicated Riemann's concept of common or related etiologies, with three hereditary recurrent fever syndromes caused by mutations in a single protein, denoted cryopyrin (or NALP3) (4–8), and a fourth periodic fever (familial Mediterranean fever, or FMF) caused by mutations in pyrin (alternatively, marenostrin) (9,10), which shares a critical functional domain with cryopyrin. Yet another of these Mendelian disorders, the syndrome of pyogenic arthritis with pyoderma gangrenosum and acne (PAPA), is caused by mutations in a protein that binds pyrin (11). Moreover, both PAPA syndrome and all of the known hereditary recurrent fevers appear to be disturbances in proinflammatory cytokine regulation. Not surprisingly, at a molecular and cellular level there is evidence for subclinical disease even when patients with these conditions are asymptomatic, with the episodic flares representing the exacerbations that rise above the threshold of clinical detection.

A second group of idiopathic intermittent arthropathies that are not Mendelian disorders, including intermittent hydrarthrosis, eosinophilic synovitis, palindromic rheumatism, and Tietze syndrome is also discussed. Each is defined solely on the basis of clinical criteria, and may represent multiple pathophysiologic processes with convergent clinical expression. An important goal of the next several years will be to explore the molecular and cellular basis of these disorders, as well as understanding the patients with conditions resembling the Mendelian autoinflammatory diseases but with no identifiable genetic mutations.

When approaching the patient with a recurring arthropathy, it is important to remember that the joint may be the end organ in a wide variety of episodic systemic illnesses, as shown in Table 68.1. While the hereditary autoinflammatory diseases and the idiopathic intermittent arthropathies are the focus of the current chapter, these conditions fit into a much broader context of recurring arthropathies that are listed in the lower half of Table 68.1. Recognition of this fact is important not only in reaching the correct diagnosis in any given patient, but in our continuation of the Reimannian search for unifying cellular and molecular mechanisms in the broad spectrum of recurring human disease.

MENDELIAN AUTOINFLAMMATORY DISEASES

The systemic autoinflammatory diseases are a group of disorders characterized by seemingly unprovoked inflammation and notable for the relative paucity of high-titer autoantibodies or antigen-specific T cells (3,12,13). This latter feature distinguishes autoinflammatory illnesses from the diseases usually classified as autoimmune, such as systemic lupus erythematosus and rheumatoid arthritis (RA), in which the adaptive immune response plays a more prominent role. While the pathogenesis of a number of autoinflammatory conditions, such as chronic recurrent multifocal osteomyelitis (CRMO) and inflammatory bowel disease, is complex and only incompletely understood, several of these disorders have been shown to be caused by mutations in specific genes controlling the innate immune response. These include the aforementioned PAPA syndrome and six conditions that are often grouped together as the hereditary periodic (or recurrent) fever syndromes (14–16, Table 68.1) and that present with self-limited episodes of fever and localized inflammation, sometimes affecting the joints.

The molecular genetic causes of the Mendelian autoinflammatory diseases discussed in this chapter are summarized in Table 68.2, and typical pedigrees illustrating the inheritance of these disorders are shown in Figure 68.1. FMF and the hyperimmunoglobulinemia D syndrome (HIDS) are inherited as autosomal-recessive traits (17,18), while the tumor necrosis factor receptor-associated periodic syndrome (TRAPS), familial cold autoinflammatory syndrome (FCAS; also known as familial cold urticaria, or FCU), Muckle-Wells syndrome (MWS), and PAPA syndrome are dominantly inherited (12,19–22). The neonatal-onset multisystem inflammatory disease [NOMID; also known as the chronic infantile neurologic cutaneous and arthropathy (CINCA) syndrome] usually arises as a *de novo* mutation with diminished reproductive fitness (7,8), with dominant transmission documented in only a few cases (7).

Although these illnesses have probably existed for many generations, their description as unique nosologic entities has been a relatively recent development. In 1940 a large family with cold-induced episodes of fever, urticarial rash, and arthralgia—most likely the first report of FCAS—was published (19), and shortly thereafter FMF was first described as a distinct disorder (23). Muckle and Wells reported their eponymous syndrome of fever, urticarial rash, limb pain, deafness, and amyloidosis in 1962 (21), and the remaining three hereditary periodic fever syndromes were first described in the early 1980s (24–27). PAPA syndrome was only first reported as a clinical entity in 1997 (22).

The Human Genome Project has catalyzed the discovery of four different genes underlying the hereditary recurrent fever syndromes. *MEFV,* the gene mutated in FMF, was identified in 1997 (9,10). It encodes pyrin, a previously unknown regulator of inflammation that has subsequently been shown to define a large family of proteins that regulate inflammation and apoptosis (28–34). In early 1999, mutations in the 55 kDa tumor necrosis factor (TNF) receptor, *TNFRSF1A,* were identified in several families with dominantly inherited periodic fever syndromes (12), establishing TRAPS as the first human disease shown to be caused by mutations in TNF receptors. Several months later two independent groups reported mutations in the gene encoding mevalonate kinase, a key enzyme in cholesterol and isoprenoid synthesis, in HIDS (35,36), a discovery that was quite unexpected and is still not completely understood. In 2001 the process came full circle with the discovery of mu-

TABLE 68.2. *Mendelian autoinflammatory diseases with intermittent articular manifestations*

Disease	Inheritance (chromosome)	Gene	Protein	Possible pathogenesis
Familial Mediterranean fever (FMF)	Recessive (16p13.3)	*MEFV*	Pyrin (marenostrin)	Increased interleukin (IL)-1β activation, impaired leukocyte apoptosis, increased nuclear factor (NF)-κB activation
Familial cold autoinflammatory syndrome (FCAS)	Dominant (1q44)	*CIAS1/NALP3/ PYPAF1*	Cryopyrin (NALP3)	Increased IL-1β and NF-κB activation
Muckle-Wells syndrome (MWS)	Dominant *(1q44)*	*CIAS1/NALP3/ PYPAF1*	Cryopyrin (NALP3)	Increased IL-1β and NF-κB activation
Neonatal-onset multisystem inflammatory disease (NOMID) or chronic infantile neurologic cutaneous and arthropathy (CINCA) syndrome	Dominant/ *de novo (1q44)*	*CIAS1/NALP3/ PYPAF1*	Cryopyrin (NALP3)	Increased IL-1β and NF-κB activation
Tumor necrosis factor receptor-associated periodic syndrome (TRAPS)	Dominant (12p13)	*TNFRSF1A*	55 kDa TNF receptor (p55, CD120a)	Impaired ectodomain cleavage of p55 receptors, probably other additional mechanisms
Hyperimmunoglobulinemia D syndrome (HIDS)	Recessive (12q24)	*MVK*	Mevalonate kinase	Temperature-dependent mevalonate kinase enzyme activity causes a deficiency in isoprenoid compounds, leading to increased IL-1β secretion
Pyogenic arthritis with pyoderma gangrenosum and acne (PAPA)	Dominant (15q24)	*PSTPIP1/ CD2BP1*	Proline serine threonine phosphatase interacting protein 1 *or* CD2 binding protein 1	Mutations cause increased PSTPIP1 binding to pyrin, leading to increased IL-1β secretion

tations in cryopyrin, a pyrin family member, in FCAS and MWS (4), and the following year cryopyrin mutations were established in about half of patients with NOMID/CINCA (7,8).

These deeper mechanistic insights have also permitted the recognition of etiologic connections among clinical syndromes, an example of which is the newly established relationship between FMF and PAPA syndrome. Although both FMF and PAPA syndrome are autoinflammatory diseases of the skin and joints, the causal linkage between these conditions was not recognized until PAPA syndrome was found to be caused by mutations in proline serine threonine phosphatase interacting protein 1 (PSTPIP1; also known as CD2 binding protein-1 [CD2BP1]) (37), and PSTPIP1/CD2BP1 was shown to be a pyrin-binding protein (11). Moreover, the web of related or interacting proteins and the corresponding clinical disorders extends well beyond the genes and diseases discussed in this chapter. For example, cryopyrin shares homology in two protein domains with NOD2/CARD15, which is mutated both in Crohn disease (38,39) and Blau syndrome (40), a rare Mendelian disorder with granulomatous inflammation of the skin, eyes, and joints. It is likely that the tools of genomics and proteomics will reveal even wider networks of disease relationships, with all of the attendant opportunities for improved diagnosis and targeted approaches to therapy.

Familial Mediterranean Fever

Although genetic evidence suggests that FMF has existed at least since biblical times, the first case report was probably the 1908 description of a 16-year-old Jewish girl suffering from recurrent episodes of fever, leukocytosis, and abdominal pain (41). The first documentation that this represented a new clinical entity came in 1945, when Siegal (23) discussed 10 cases of "benign paroxysmal peritonitis." Subsequently this disorder has been described under a variety of names, including recurrent polyserositis (42), recurrent hereditary polyserositis (43), periodic disease (44), and FMF (45,46).

Of these names, FMF enjoys the widest currency, and conveys several salient clinical features. However, it should not be overinterpreted. Because FMF is recessively inherited (Fig. 68.1), a positive family history of FMF is not required to make the clinical diagnosis and, in fact, a family history can be elicited in only about half the cases of FMF (45,47). "Mediterranean" was originally applied to this disorder because most early Israeli patients were Sephardic Jews who

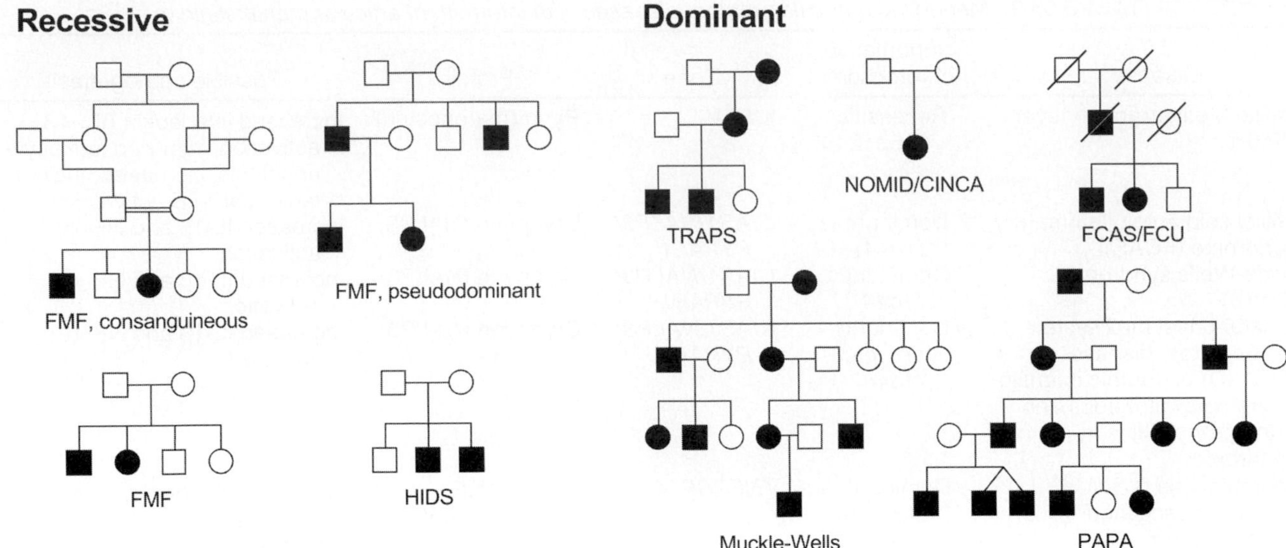

FIG. 68.1. Typical pedigrees of families with the Mendelian autoinflammatory diseases. **Left:** Familial Mediterranean fever (FMF) and the hyperimmunoglobulinemia D syndrome (HIDS) are inherited as autosomal-recessive traits. Under this mode of inheritance, two mutant alleles are required for clinical disease. In families in which two unaffected parents marry, on average one-fourth of the offspring would be affected. Particularly in FMF families of Middle Eastern descent, there may be a history of consanguinity, as illustrated by the first-cousin marriage at the upper left. In the FMF family with pseudodominance, there is the appearance of parent-to-child transmission of disease, as would be seen with a dominant mode of inheritance. However, in many cases this can be explained by the fact that the unaffected parent (in this case, the mother) is an asymptomatic carrier. **Right:** The tumor necrosis factor receptor–associated periodic syndrome (TRAPS), the neonatal-onset multisystem inflammatory disease (NOMID; also known as chronic infantile neurologic, cutaneous, and arthropathy syndrome, CINCA), familial cold autoinflammatory syndrome (FCAS; also known as familial cold urticaria, FCU), Muckle-Wells syndrome (MWS), and the syndrome of pyogenic arthritis with pyoderma gangrenosum and acne (PAPA) are all inherited as autosomal-dominant traits. Under this mode of inheritance, only one mutant allele is required for clinical disease. An affected parent would be expected to pass on the disease on average to half of his or her offspring. Particularly in TRAPS, variability in penetrance can sometimes lead to the observation of affected offspring with a parent who carries the mutated allele but has mild symptoms or perhaps no symptoms at all. The presence of father-to-son transmission distinguishes autosomal-dominant inheritance from X-linked inheritance. In NOMID/CINCA, mutations usually arise *de novo*, but are often not transmitted because of the severity of the NOMID/CINCA phenotype.

had emigrated from North Africa and Turkey (45,46). FMF has also long been recognized to be common among Armenians (47), Turks (48,49), and Arabs (43,50), and recent molecular analyses indicate that it is also relatively frequent among Italians (51–53), Greeks (54,55), and other Mediterranean populations (56,57). However, there are patients meeting both clinical and molecular genetic criteria for FMF who have no known Mediterranean ancestry (58,59). Finally, it should be noted that although fever is invariably observed in this condition when it is sought, some FMF patients are unaware of any temperature elevation during their attacks.

Clinical Features

Attacks

FMF is characterized by acute attacks of fever and localized inflammation, usually involving the peritoneum, pleura, joints, or skin (Fig. 68.2, Table 68.3). The first attacks of FMF usually begin in childhood or adolescence. It is not uncommon for FMF to present in infancy, although it is usually not at first suspected, especially in nations with low disease prevalence. Most large series report that 80% to 90% of FMF patients have their first attack by age 20 (46,47,50). Prior to the availability of genetic testing, FMF was seldom reported with an onset after the age of 40 (60) and, in fact, the diagnosis was considered questionable under these circumstances. DNA testing has now facilitated the recognition of late-onset disease, but patients presenting after the age of 40 still comprise only a small minority of cases, usually manifesting relatively mild disease (61).

In typical FMF attacks, there may be a prodromal period of a few hours, during which time some patients experience chills. Attacks generally last from 12 to 72 hours, with those involving the joints tending to be somewhat longer. The degree of temperature elevation varies from patient to patient

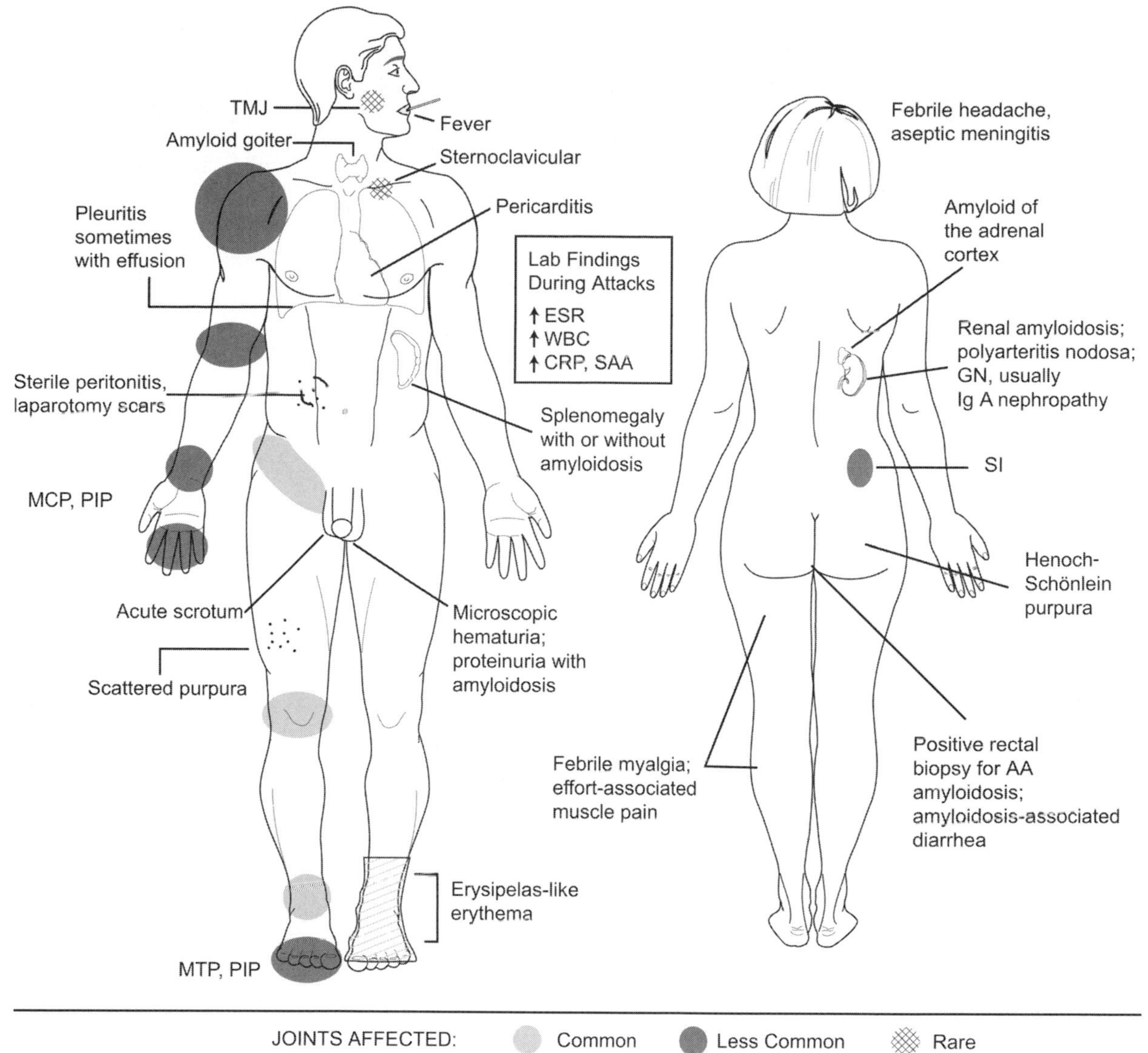

FIG. 68.2. Clinical features of familial Mediterranean fever. Illustration of a particular feature on the male or female figure is not intended to imply a gender-related risk.

and from one attack to the next. Occasionally in children, fever may be the sole presenting symptom (50,62), although other manifestations develop with time. Between attacks, patients are asymptomatic. The interval between attacks may range from days to months, and the frequency of attacks can fluctuate with time. Moreover, the type of attack (abdominal, pleural, arthritic) may vary from one episode to the next. In some patients attacks may be precipitated by strenuous physical activity or emotional stress.

The frequency of FMF attacks may also be affected by gender-specific factors. Overall, approximately 60% of reported cases occur in males. Consistent with the possibility that female sex hormones may influence FMF, some women with FMF note an increased frequency of attacks with menses (63), and remissions may occur during pregnancy (46,47).

Approximately 95% of FMF patients experience an abdominal attack some time during their illness, and about half present with abdominal pain as their first manifestation (46). The intensity of the peritoneal attack varies from mild distention to peritonitis. Severe episodes may begin with a dull ache, but the pain worsens within hours. Discomfort may be localized to one quadrant of the abdomen, or generalized. Because of peritoneal inflammation, peristalsis slows or stops, so that constipation is much more common than diarrhea. In the more severe attacks, patients may have board-like abdominal rigidity with generalized direct and rebound tenderness, and air–fluid levels on upright films of the abdomen. Contrast-enhanced computed tomography (CT) of the abdomen may demonstrate engorged mesenteric vessels with thickened mesenteric folds, mesenteric lymphadenopathy, splenomegaly, or small amounts of ascites (64). If a

TABLE 68.3. *Clinical features of the hereditary recurrent fever syndromes*

Clinical feature	FMF	FCAS/FCU	MWS	NOMID/CINCA	TRAPS	HIDS
Ethnicity	Jewish, Armenian, Arab, Turkish, Italian	Mostly European	Northern European	Any ethnic group	Any ethnic group	Dutch, French, other European
Duration of episodes	1–3 d	Usually < 24 h	24–48 h	Nearly continuous, with exacerbations	Often > 1 wk	3–7 d
Abdominal symptoms	Mild pain—peritonitis; constipation > diarrhea	Nausea with attacks	Sometimes abdominal pain	Uncommon	Mild pain—peritonitis; diarrhea or constipation	Severe pain, vomiting; diarrhea > constipation; peritonitis uncommon
Pleurisy	Frequent	Not seen	Rare	Rare	Frequent	Rare
Pericarditis	Small effusions, rarely symptomatic	Not seen	None reported	None reported	Rare	None reported
Scrotal pain	Usually prepubertal boys	Not seen	None reported	None reported	Can occur	Rare
Arthropathy	Intermittent monoarthritis; sacroiliitis; rarely protracted nonaxial arthritis	Debilitating polyarthralgia with attacks	Intermittent arthralgia, large-joint oligoarticular arthritis	Epiphyseal/patellar overgrowth, periosteal elevation, intermittent or chronic arthritis	Arthralgia, large-joint nondestructive arthritis	Arthralgia, symmetric nondestructive polyarthritis
Myalgia	Effort-associated myalgia common; febrile myalgia rare	Common	Common	Can be present	Common; migratory and often associated with severe stiffness	Uncommon
Cutaneous	Erysipeloid erythema	Urticarial rash provoked by cold exposure	Urticarial rash	Urticarial rash	Migratory erysipelas-like rash most common	Erythematous macules and papules on limbs and trunk, urticaria
Ocular	Uncommon	Conjunctivitis	Conjunctivitis, episcleritis, optic disc edema	Conjunctivitis, uveitis, papilledema, progressive blindness	Conjunctivitis, periorbital edema; rarely uveitis	Uncommon
Neurologic	Aseptic meningitis rare	Headache	Sensorineural deafness	Headache, chronic meningitis, mental retardation, deafness	Uncommon	Headache
Lymph/Spleen	Splenomegaly > lymphadenopathy	Not seen	Not prominent	Hepatosplenomegaly, adenopathy with flares	Splenomegaly > lymphadenopathy	Cervical adenopathy with attacks
Vasculitis	Henoch-Schönlein purpura (HSP), polyarteritis nodosa, febrile myalgia, possibly Behçet's disease	None reported	None reported	Has been reported	HSP, lymphocytic vasculitis reported	Cutaneous vasculitis common; rarely, HSP
Amyloidosis	Risk varies with *MEFV, SAA1* genotypes, gender, environmental factors	Uncommon	Reported in ~25% of cases	Develops in a minority of patients who reach adulthood	~10% of cases, with cysteine mutations at higher risk	None reported
Treatment	Colchicine prophylaxis; steroids for protracted febrile myalgia	NSAIDs; anakinra investigational	NSAIDs, prednisone; anakinra investigational	Anakinra investigational	NSAIDs in mild cases; steroids for acute attacks; etanercept prophylaxis	Arthritis may respond to NSAIDs or steroids; statins, etanercept investigational

FCAS, familial cold autoinflammatory syndrome; FMF, familial Mediterranean fever; HIDS, hyperimmunoglobulinemia D syndrome; MWS, Muckle-Wells syndrome; NOMID/CINCA, neonatal-onset multisystem inflammatory disease, chronic infantile neurologic cutaneous and arthropathy syndrome; NSAIDs, nonsteroidal antiinflammatory drugs; TRAPS, tumor necrosis factor receptor-associated periodic syndrome.

laparotomy is performed, a small amount of sterile exudate rich in polymorphonuclear leukocytes is found, but frank ascites is extremely rare. If the patient is simply observed, the pain dissipates within 24 hours and totally resolves within 72 hours. Repeated abdominal attacks of FMF may occasionally lead to the development of peritoneal adhesions, and there have been case reports of peritoneal mesothelioma as a possible late complication (65,66), but this is very rare.

Pleural attacks have been reported in 25% to 50% of Jewish (46), Arab (43), and Turkish (67) patients; the percentage may be higher in Armenians (47). Pleural attacks run a similar time course to the abdominal attacks. Pain is usually unilateral. Breath sounds may be diminished, and a friction rub may be present. A small effusion may be present on roentgenograms, and occasionally atelectasis has been reported (68). Recurrent attacks sometimes lead to pleural thickening (69). Pleural mesothelioma is an extremely rare complication (70).

Arthralgia and arthritis are both common in FMF (50, 71–73). The frequency of arthritis in North African Jewish FMF patients is about 75% (73,74), while about half that percentage are affected among Iraqi Jews (74), Arabs (43, 50,75), Turks (49,67), and Armenian Americans (47). Recent data from most (76–78), although not all (67), large series associate homozygosity for the M694V *MEFV* mutation with the predilection to develop arthritis, and thus the population frequencies of this genotype may account for the aforementioned differences.

Arthritis may be the presenting symptom in FMF, especially in children. Arthritic attacks are most commonly acute, but in the precolchicine era protracted episodes occurred in about 5% of FMF patients with arthritis (79); they are still sometimes reported (73,75,80). The acute arthritis of FMF is usually monoarticular, most frequently involving the knee, ankle, and hip (Fig. 68.2). Less common patterns of arthritis described in children include simultaneous symmetric two-joint involvement, polyarticular symmetric arthritis, oligoarticular migratory asymmetric arthritis, and involvement of the small joints of the hand (72,80). Acute monoarticular arthritic attacks are abrupt in onset, often accompanied by excruciating pain. They may have a similar time course to the peritoneal and pleural attacks, but sometimes last as long as a month. Fever may only be present at the beginning of the synovial attack. Effusions are usually present, but erythema and warmth may be unimpressive. Synovial fluid often contains large numbers of polymorphonuclear leukocytes (Fig. 68.3A); the mucin clot is good, viscosity is poor, and cultures are sterile. Aside from soft tissue swelling and sometimes mild osteoporosis, roentgenographic changes are usually not present during the acute attack.

Protracted arthritis begins as an acute attack, but marked effusions persist, sometimes for several months (79). The knee and hip are most commonly affected in protracted episodes, accounting for about three-fourths of the cases in one large series (79). During the course of a protracted attack, the patient may develop synovitis in a second joint. Patients with protracted arthritis often develop marked muscle atrophy because movement exacerbates joint pain. Most episodes of protracted arthritis subside within months, with hip involvement tending to last the longest. Radiographic findings include severe juxtaarticular osteoporosis, lytic erosions, and osteonecrosis of the femoral head. Juxtaarticular sclerosis and joint-space narrowing sometimes occur with resolution of the protracted arthritis. Pathologic fractures of the femur may also occur upon resumption of weight bearing after protracted knee arthritis. Overall, in about two-thirds of the episodes of protracted arthritis there is complete functional recovery.

The prognosis is worst in the hip, where about 80% of cases develop residual incapacity due to osteoarthritis or osteonecrosis. Repeated joint aspiration may reduce the frequency of the latter complication. With total hip replacement surgery there is a high frequency of aseptic loosening (33% at an average of 7 years). For this reason, cementless hip prostheses have been recommended in FMF patients requiring this surgery (81). In FMF patients with chronic knee effusions refractory to arthrocentesis and corticosteroid injection, early chemical or arthroscopic synovectomy may obviate the need for open synovectomy (82,83).

Chronic inflammation of the sacroiliac joints (Fig. 68.3B) also appears to occur more commonly in FMF patients than in the general population (84–86). This may present as an isolated radiographic finding, or with symptoms of low back pain. Affected individuals are usually not human leukocyte antigen (HLA)-B27$^+$. When present, sacroiliitis can occur with or without other involvement of the spine, peripheral arthritis, or enthesitis. The sacroiliitis of FMF can arise despite daily colchicine treatment, and may require additional treatment with nonsteroidal antiinflammatory drugs (NSAIDs) or second-line agents (86).

Nonuremic pericarditis is rare in FMF, although it has been reported, sometimes even complicated by tamponade (87). An echocardiographic study of randomly selected American FMF patients revealed pericardial abnormalities, which usually did not correlate with symptoms, in more than one-fourth (88), although a more recent echocardiographic study reported a much lower frequency of pericardial effusions during attacks of FMF (89). A retrospective analysis of 3,976 Israeli FMF patients identified one or more episodes of clinical pericarditis over 20 years in 27 patients (90), with no serious sequelae.

The most characteristic cutaneous lesion in FMF is erysipelas-like erythema (Fig. 68.3C), which is regarded by many experts as highly specific (91,92). The observed frequency of this lesion varies widely among published series, ranging from 3% to 46% (43,46,93), and may be related to the M694V homozygous genotype (93). These lesions may occur alone with fever or may accompany an episode of arthritis, and may be provoked by prolonged walking. They usually occur below the knee, on the anterior aspect of the leg, or on the dorsum of the foot, either

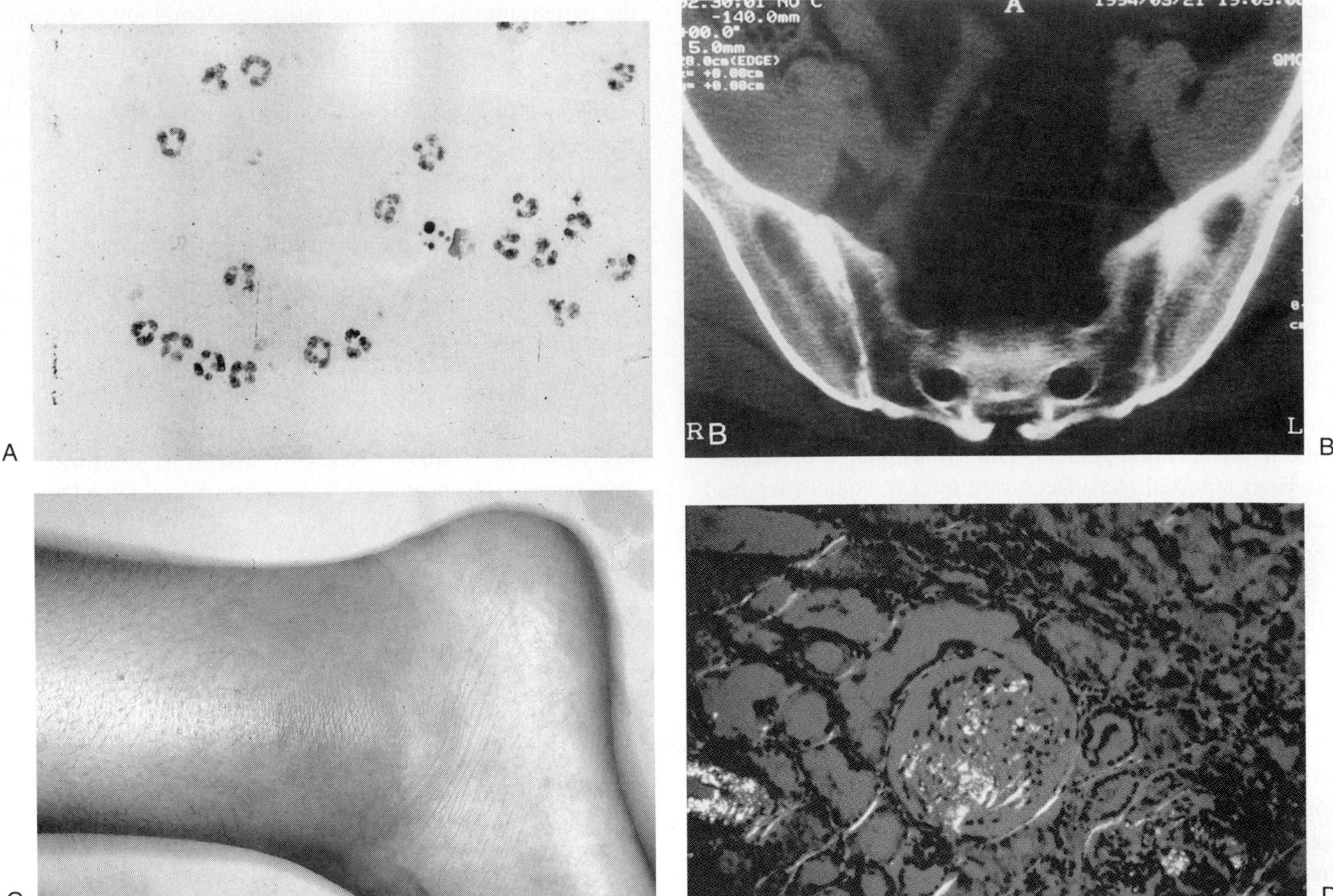

FIG. 68.3. Clinical features of familial Mediterranean fever (FMF). **A:** Smear of synovial fluid from the knee of an Israeli patient with FMF, during an attack. (From Kastner DL. Familial Mediterranean fever: the genetics of inflammation. *Hosp Pract* 1998;33:131–158, with permission.) **B:** Computed tomography scan demonstrating sclerosis of the sacroiliac joints in a FMF patient. (Courtesy of Drs. Avi Livneh and Pnina Langevitz, Sheba Medical Center.) **C:** Erysipelas-like erythema in a patient with FMF. (From Azizi E, Fisher BK. Cutaneous manifestations of familial Mediterranean fever. *Arch Dermatol* 1976; 112:364–366, with permission.) **D:** Amyloid deposition in the kidney of an FMF patient. The patient later developed end stage renal disease and underwent renal transplantation. Congo red staining, with polarization, demonstrating amyloid in two glomeruli and a vessel. (Courtesy of Dr. James E. Balow, National Institutes of Health, Bethesda, MD.)

unilaterally or symmetrically. They appear as sharply demarcated, erythematous, warm, tender, swollen areas of 10 to 15 cm in diameter. Histologically, there is a mixed perivascular cellular infiltrate of polymorphonuclear leukocytes, histiocytes, and lymphocytes; immunofluorescence demonstrates C3 deposits in the capillary walls (92). Henoch-Schönlein purpura occurs in about 5% of children with FMF (46,62,94), and a recent study demonstrated an increased frequency of individuals with two *MEFV* mutations among Israeli children with idiopathic Henoch-Schönlein purpura (95). Episodic scattered purpuric lesions, appearing on the face, trunk, or extremities, are also more frequently observed in children (96). Other nonspecific cutaneous manifestations have also been reported (91,96).

A small percentage of prepubertal boys with FMF develop episodes of unilateral acute scrotum, and in some this is the first manifestation of FMF (97–100). Patients present with the gradual onset (>12 hours) of pain, scrotal swelling, and edema, accompanied by tenderness and swelling of the involved groin. Scrotal exploration usually reveals only inflammation of the tunica vaginalis (an embryologic remnant of the peritoneal membrane), although testicular torsion can occur. In cases in which color Doppler ultrasound or testicular radionuclide scintigraphy do not demonstrate decreased perfusion, conservative management may be appropriate.

Febrile myalgia is another uncommon type of FMF attack (101,102). Brief attacks may last 2 to 3 days, while protracted febrile myalgia may last up to 6 weeks. In the latter case, patients have fever, excruciating muscle pain, abdominal pain, arthritis, diarrhea, and/or purpura. During these episodes, the creatine kinase is normal, the erythrocyte sedimentation rate (ESR) is accelerated, and the electromyogram shows a nonspecific myopathy. More commonly, FMF patients, especially children, develop transient myalgias related to vigorous exertion. These latter episodes are often accompanied by low grade fever and can last from a few hours to 3 days. Spontaneous myalgia (without fever) can also occur in FMF patients, and usually lasts for a few hours (102).

Laboratory findings during FMF attacks (103) include leukocytosis and an accelerated ESR. Several acute-phase proteins, including C-reactive protein (CRP), serum amyloid A (SAA), fibrinogen, haptoglobin, C3, and C4, are also elevated. Depending on the timing of phlebotomy, it may take observation of more than one attack to document these changes. FMF patients also may have transient albuminuria and microscopic hematuria during attacks. Rarely, hyperbilirubinemia is noted during attacks (104).

The Intercritical Period

The usual clinical presentation of FMF is one of episodic illness punctuated by periods during which the patient feels quite well. Between attacks, FMF patients have no residual pain, except in the case of protracted arthritis discussed above. Very rarely, FMF patients may have what appear to be almost continuous symptoms, which are sometimes explained as very frequent episodes with little or no interval from one to the next. Rare patients have also developed adhesions and intestinal obstruction from repeated attacks (105). It is not unusual for physical examination to reveal splenomegaly, even in the absence of amyloidosis, especially in children (62).

Laboratory findings in many FMF patients are consistent with persistent subclinical inflammation, even when they are completely symptom-free. These include an accelerated ESR, and increased levels of SAA and CRP (106–108). Between attacks, FMF patients may also have mild anemia, persistently elevated fibrinogen levels, and moderate elevations in serum immunoglobulins (103). The expression of messenger RNA (mRNA) for proinflammatory cytokines in circulating leukocytes from asymptomatic FMF patients is also increased, relative to healthy controls (109).

Amyloidosis

The most serious manifestation of FMF is the development of systemic amyloidosis. This results from the deposition of SAA in a number of organs, most commonly the kidneys, adrenals, intestine, spleen, lung, and testes (46). The major clinical consequence of amyloidosis in FMF is the development of the nephrotic syndrome and, eventually, uremia. Some patients also manifest intestinal malabsorption. Despite massive infiltration of the adrenals, patients are rarely Addisonian. With the advent of dialysis and renal transplantation, amyloid deposition can now also be seen in organs where it was previously rare, such as the liver, thyroid, and heart (110,111). In contrast to other forms of amyloidosis, the amyloidosis of FMF is not associated with neuropathy or arthropathy.

Not all FMF patients develop amyloidosis, but most patients who experience this complication do so by age 40. Rarely, patients may present with amyloid nephropathy before their first FMF attack (phenotype II) (46,112), an observation that is much more understandable in light of recent data that SAA levels may be elevated even when FMF patients are asymptomatic (106–108). Before the initiation of colchicine prophylaxis, very high frequencies of amyloidosis were reported among some populations, especially North African Jews and Turks (46,48).

The overall incidence of amyloidosis in FMF has diminished markedly in the last 30 years, due to the increased recognition and earlier diagnosis of FMF, the widespread use of colchicine, and perhaps other improvements in general medical care that reduce the SAA load during intercurrent illnesses. It is therefore difficult to provide accurate figures with regard to the current risk of amyloidosis among untreated individuals, especially in Western countries, but the potential for amyloidosis remains an important consideration in the care of patients with FMF. There is an extensive literature relating the risk of amyloidosis in FMF to ethnic background. Among Jews, the frequency of FMF amyloidosis is highest in those of North African ancestry, intermediate in Iraqi Jews, and low in Ashkenazi (Eastern European) Jews (74,113,114). A very high incidence of amyloidosis was initially reported in Turkish patients (48), but current estimates are lower (67). Amyloidosis is even less common in Arabs (43,50,115), and seldom seen among Armenian Americans (47).

Genotype–phenotype studies conducted after the cloning of *MEFV* suggest that some of the foregoing observations may be correlated with specific FMF genotypes. Most notably, among Armenians, Arabs, and Jews the risk of amyloidosis is increased among individuals homozygous for the M694V mutation (76–78,115–121). The M694I and V727A-E148Q complex allele may also increase the risk of amyloidosis in these populations, although the numbers of cases are smaller (78,119,120). In several studies from Turkey, no specific *MEFV* mutation has been associated with amyloidosis (67,122–125), although the risk is increased among Turkish patients with a family history of this complication (125,126). It should be emphasized that, even in populations in which the M694V association does hold, amyloidosis also can occur in association with other genotypes, although less frequently. Other genetically determined factors that may increase amyloid risk include male gender and the *SAA1* α/α genotype (121,127,128). Polymorphisms at the major histocompatibility complex class I chain–related gene A (MICA) have been associated with an earlier age of onset and more frequent attacks of FMF

(129), but the effect on susceptibility to amyloidosis is not yet known.

Nongenetic factors may also play a role in determining amyloid risk. For example, the incidence of amyloidosis among Armenian Americans, even before the availability of colchicine, was much lower than among Armenians in Armenia, for whom the risk is still quite high (47,76,118, 130). Female FMF patients with amyloidosis who become pregnant may experience deterioration in renal function (131), especially if their 24-hour urine protein exceeds 2 g at conception.

Since albuminuria is an early finding in FMF amyloidosis, patients should undergo periodic urinalyses, especially those who are at high risk. In the face of persistent proteinuria, the diagnosis of amyloid can be confirmed by the characteristic apple-green appearance of a biopsy specimen stained with Congo red and viewed under polarized light (Fig. 68.3D). In one large series (132), the sensitivity of renal biopsy for detecting amyloidosis in FMF was 88%, followed by rectal biopsy at 75%, liver biopsy at 48%, and gingival biopsy at 19%. Many physicians prefer the rectal biopsy because it is relatively noninvasive. The sensitivity of bone marrow biopsy in a more recent small series (133) was found to be 80%, and the sensitivity of testicular biopsy is about 87% (134). Abdominal fat aspiration has a low sensitivity to detect amyloidosis in FMF (135).

Due, in part, to poor vascular access and hemodynamic instability, patients who progress to end-stage renal disease have a lower survival rate on hemodialysis than age-matched dialysis patients (136–140). The frequency of acute attacks of FMF is sometimes reduced on hemodialysis (141). Although some centers report lower patient and graft survival rates in FMF than in other renal diseases (142), other recent series demonstrate similar patient and graft survival rates (143–145). Early transplantation is preferred (143). Daily colchicine is required to prevent amyloid deposition in the graft (discussed later in the chapter) (146), but even patients maintained on this regimen can develop late amyloid accumulation in other organs, such as the gastrointestinal tract, thyroid, and heart (110,111,142). It is important to note that cyclosporine-based anti-rejection therapy can lead to colchicine toxicity (147–149), probably because cyclosporine inhibits the multidrug resistance (MDR1) transport system, which is necessary for hepatic and renal excretion of colchicine (149–153). Moreover, a recent series demonstrated that in FMF patients cyclosporine-based immunosuppressive regimens were associated with detrimental effects on long-term renal graft function and survival, relative to an azathioprine/prednisone-based regime (154).

Other Features

Vasculitis is more common among FMF patients than in the general population (155–157). As noted previously, about 5% of children with FMF develop Henoch-Schönlein purpura (46,62,94). There have also been several reports of polyarteritis nodosa (PAN) with FMF (155–162). Compared with other PAN patients, those with FMF present at a younger age, are more likely to have perirenal hematoma, and have a better overall prognosis (162). Overlap syndromes of classic PAN with microscopic polyarteritis are also more common in FMF (162). Both PAN and typical FMF attacks may present with abdominal pain and fever; the persistence of symptoms and the presence of hypertension, thrombocytosis, or nephritis should alert the physician to the possibility of PAN. Protracted febrile myalgia is yet a third presentation of vasculitis in FMF (101,157,163). Renal involvement can sometimes be seen, and in one FMF family, PAN and protracted febrile myalgia have been reported in siblings (157).

Besides amyloidosis and vasculitis, various types of glomerulonephritis (GN) have also been reported in FMF (164–168). These include postinfectious GN, diffuse mesangial proliferative GN with immunoglobulin A (IgA) or IgM deposits, and type II (immune complex) rapidly progressive GN. A recent review of the literature demonstrated a total of 21 patients with biopsy-proven GN (168), but it is likely that this represents an underestimate of the true frequency.

There have also been a small number of reports of neurologic findings in FMF (169–174). These include increased protein and pleiocytosis in the cerebrospinal fluid, with or without meningeal irritation, and various electroencephalogram (EEG) abnormalities. More commonly, patients experience fever-associated headaches, and children may have febrile convulsions. The possibility of central nervous system involvement in FMF takes on new significance in light of the prominent neurologic findings, including aseptic meningitis, in patients with mutations in cryopyrin, a protein structurally and functionally related to the FMF protein (4–8).

Finally, within the last 5 years new associations have been proposed between FMF and several other inflammatory diseases. Most notably, there is a growing body of literature on a possible relationship between FMF and Behçet disease (175–179). If confirmed, Behçet disease would be the fourth type of vasculitis associated with FMF. Bearing in mind the difficulties in establishing a relationship between two diseases that are both common in the Middle East, the data suggest a complicated and possibly synergistic interaction between susceptibility genes for these two disorders. Two recent studies also indicate an increased incidence of inflammatory bowel disease among patients with FMF (180,181). Taken together, these data suggest that *MEFV* mutations may contribute to a much broader spectrum of inflammatory phenotypes than is usually associated with FMF.

Genetics

In the 1960s, segregation analysis in Israeli families manifesting the classic features of FMF (serositis, arthritis, rash, and/or amyloidosis) established this disease as a single-gene recessive disorder with incomplete penetrance (i.e., some individuals with the appropriate genotype might not develop clinical disease) (17,46). Parent-to-child transmission of FMF, when observed, has been explained by pseudodominance (Fig. 68.1), in which one parent is affected and the other is an asymptomatic carrier (52,76). Identical twins are concordant for FMF, although there are differences in the type and severity of attacks (182). Given the predominance of males in the large early series (43,46,47), penetrance in females is thought to be less than in males, although it is possible that confusion of abdominal attacks with gynecologic symptoms and underreporting in females for cultural reasons may also contribute to the skewed gender ratio. Consistent with the recessive mode of inheritance, a history of consanguinity (Fig. 68.1) can sometimes be elicited, especially in families from the Middle East.

Prior to the identification of *MEFV*, FMF had been reported most frequently among Armenians, Turks, Arabs, Iraqi Jews, and Sephardic Jews. The latter group is descended from the Jewish population that left Spain after the Inquisition in 1492, settling along the Mediterranean coast of North Africa, Turkey, the Balkans, and the Middle East. Population-based estimates of FMF prevalence and family studies indicated FMF carrier frequencies of between 1:5 and 1:16 in non-Ashkenazi (North African and Iraqi) Jewish and Armenian populations (183–185). These figures are extraordinarily high, suggesting a carrier advantage for heterozygotes, as is seen, for example, for hemoglobin mutations in areas endemic for malaria (186).

Because functional, hypothesis-driven approaches to identify the FMF gene were not productive, a positional cloning strategy was ultimately used. In 1992, genetic linkage studies placed the FMF susceptibility locus on the distal short arm of chromosome 16 (187), and the candidate chromosomal interval for *MEFV* was subsequently narrowed by analyses of genetic recombinations in families (188) and conserved haplotypes in populations (189–192). Eventually, all of the genes within a much-refined interval were systematically screened for disease-associated mutations, leading in 1997 to the identification of *MEFV* (9,10). Mutations in this novel gene were found in absolute association with FMF carrier chromosomes in two large, independent sets of well-characterized FMF families and ethnically matched controls, and there were no disease-associated variants in any of the other genes in the relevant chromosomal interval. Moreover, the gene identified is expressed predominantly in granulocytes (9), the major cell type involved in the inflammatory attacks of FMF.

MEFV consists of 10 exons (Fig. 68.4) covering approximately 15 kilobases (kb) of genomic DNA on chromosome 16p13.3. The gene encodes a 3.7-kb transcript, the protein product of which is 781 amino acids in length (9). This protein has been variously named *pyrin* (9) to connote its relationship to fever, or *marenostrin* (10) after the Latin name for the Mediterranean, *Mare nostrum* (our sea). When first cloned, the N-terminal half of pyrin was quite unique

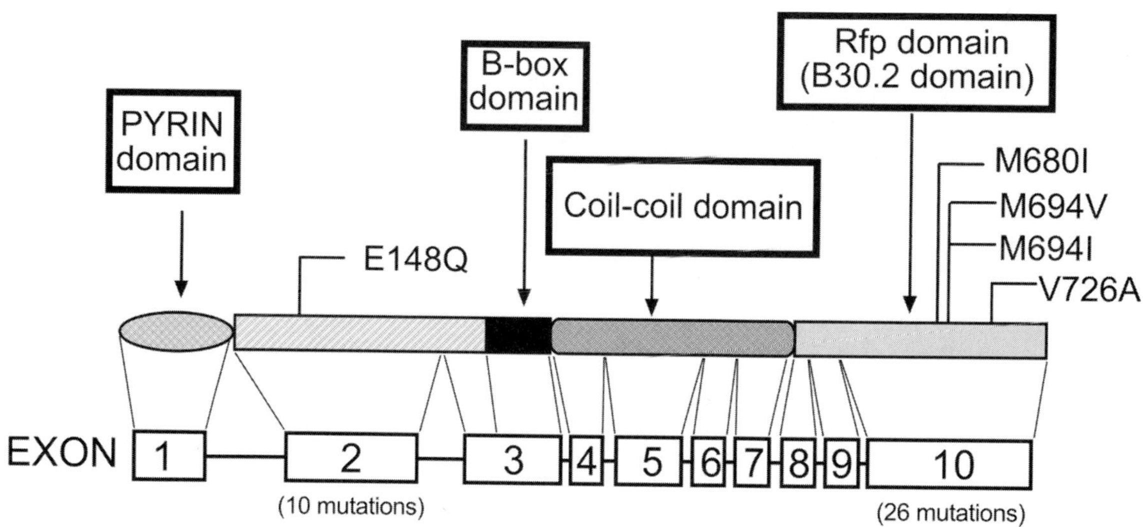

FIG. 68.4. Schematic diagram of the coding region of *MEFV*, the gene causing familial Mediterranean fever (FMF), and the corresponding domain structure and disease-associated mutations of pyrin (also known as marenostrin), the encoded protein. As depicted in the lower part of the figure, *MEFV* consists of 10 exons. Of the 43 mutations described at the time of this writing (go to *the website available at: fmf.igh.cnrs.fr/infevers/* for an updated listing), 10 are in exon 2 and 26 are in exon 10. Exon 1 encodes an N-terminal 92 amino acid PYRIN domain that permits cognate interactions with other proteins involved in the regulation of inflammation and apoptosis. The B-box zinc-finger domain (amino acids 375–407), the coiled-coil domain (amino acids 408–594), and the B30.2 domain (amino acids 598–774) are found as a cassette in a number of other proteins, and may be involved in protein-protein interactions. The approximate locations of five major missense mutations causing FMF are also indicated.

relative to other proteins in the sequence databases, but the first 92 amino acids are now known to define a motif (the PYRIN domain) found in a number of proteins that have subsequently been cloned (28–34). As will subsequently be described in greater detail below, the PYRIN domain facilitates the interactions among proteins involved in the regulation of cytokine activation and apoptosis. The C-terminal half of pyrin contains a B-box zinc-finger (residues 375–407), an α-helical (coiled-coil) domain (residues 408–594), and a B30.2 (ret finger protein, or rfp) domain (residues 598–774). Both the B-box and coiled-coil mediate multimerization when found in other proteins (193). The B30.2 domain is found in intracellular, transmembrane, and secreted proteins, and may also be involved in protein/protein interactions (194–197).

All four of the disease-associated mutations initially described in *MEFV* are single-nucleotide substitutions in exon 10 that cause conservative amino-acid substitutions in the B30.2 domain of pyrin (9,10; Fig. 68.4). Two of these mutations affect residue 694, leading to the substitution of valine or isoleucine for the normal methionine (and designated M694V and M694I, respectively). A third mutation also leads to the substitution of isoleucine for methionine at residue 680 (M680I), while the fourth causes the substitution of alanine for valine at residue 726 (V726A). M694V is observed across a number of ethnic groups, and is by far the predominant mutation in North African Jews. Nevertheless, based on microsatellite and intragenic single nucleotide haplotypes, it is likely that all modern-day carriers of this mutation are descended from a common founder. Since this mutation and the associated haplotype are observed in populations that have been separate since biblical times, the historical data suggest that the mutation is at least 2,000 years old (Fig. 68.5). Although the ethnic distribution is somewhat different, the V726A mutation is also broadly distributed and associated with a single ancestral haplotype, again suggesting a common ancient founder (distinct from the M694V founder).

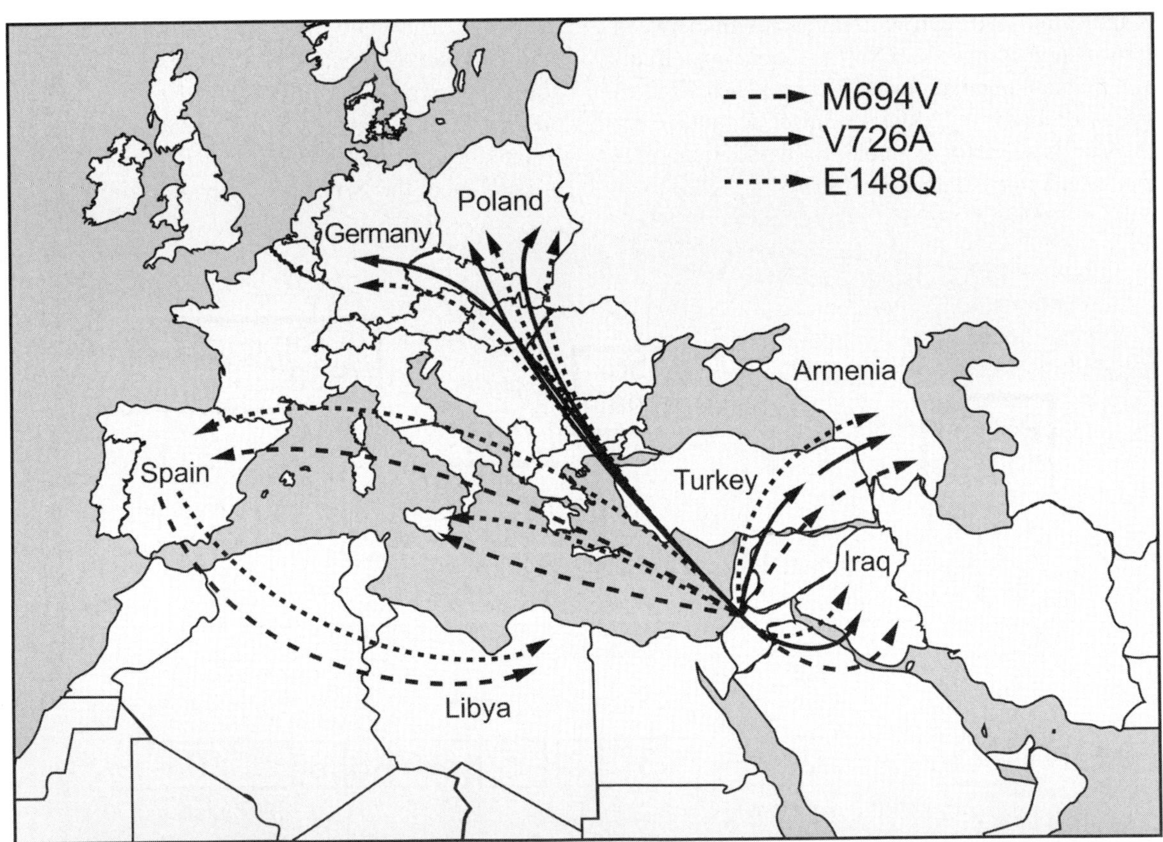

FIG. 68.5. Historical spread of three major mutations in *MEFV*, the gene causing familial Mediterranean fever, deduced from analyses of carrier haplotypes in affected populations. The M694V mutation presumably arose in the Middle East in biblical times, and was then carried first to the Iberian peninsula by Jewish settlers, and then to North Africa with the Sephardic Jewish expulsion of 1492. This mutation, with the associated haplotype, is seen in Iraqi Jews, Armenians, and southern Italians, as well as other ethnic groups. The V726A mutation and associated haplotype spread to some of the same populations, as well as the Ashkenazi Jewish population of Eastern Europe and the Druze population in the Middle East. The E148Q mutation and associated haplotype is widely distributed. (Adapted from Kastner DL. Familial Mediterranean fever: the genetics of inflammation. *Hosp Pract* 1998;33:131–158.)

As of the time of this writing, a total of 43 mutations have been described (198; available on the Internet at *fmf.igh.cnrs.fr/infevers/*), 38 of which are single nucleotide substitutions leading to an amino-acid change. Three of the remaining five mutations are short, in-frame deletions. Only two mutations, a frame-shift in exon 2 and a nonsense mutation in exon 10, would be predicted to truncate the pyrin protein. It is possible that the continued presence of the pyrin protein, albeit mutated, is necessary for the FMF phenotype, and that the known missense mutations result in subtle structural changes in pyrin that create an easily perturbed equilibrium predisposing to intermittent exacerbations (9). Twenty-six (60%) of the currently known mutations reside in exon 10. Four distinct mutations have been identified at residue 694, and another three distinct mutations at residue 680. Ten mutations have been identified in exon 2, two affecting residue 148. The only exon 2 variant to be seen in substantial numbers of patients is the substitution of glutamine for glutamic acid at residue 148 (E148Q). Like M694V and V726A, E148Q is seen in several different Mediterranean populations, and haplotype data suggest a third major ancient founder (52). Recent data also suggest a high frequency of E148Q among Indian and Chinese populations (199).

Because E148Q homozygotes are much less frequent in FMF cohorts than would be predicted from the frequency of E148Q carriers, some have suggested that this variant is not pathogenic (200,201). On the other hand, a small number of E148Q homozygotes with clinical FMF have been described (202), and E148Q is sometimes the only identifiable mutation in *trans* with an exon 10 mutation in patients with moderate to severe FMF (51,52,119,203). Moreover, E148Q can sometimes be seen in *cis* with certain exon 10 mutations in so-called complex alleles, and at least in some cases the phenotype associated with the E148Q complex allele is more severe than the phenotype associated with the exon 10 mutation alone (78). E148Q has also been associated with a greater risk of amyloidosis in patients with other rheumatic diseases, and is seen in patients with a broad spectrum of inflammatory phenotypes (199). For all of these reasons, E148Q is likely to be more than just a benign polymorphism, although it does appear to be the mildest and least penetrant of the *MEFV* mutations.

At the other end of the spectrum is the M694V mutation. As noted previously, Jewish, Armenian, and Arab patients who are homozygous for this mutation are at increased risk for developing systemic amyloidosis (76–78,115–121), although this appears not to be the case in the Turkish population (67,122–125). M694V homozygotes may also be at increased risk for an early age of onset, more frequent attacks, arthritis, and erysipeloid erythema (76–78,93,204). Some studies also indicate that the M694I mutation and the V726A-E148Q complex allele confer increased risk for amyloidosis (78,119,120).

Identification of the gene for FMF has broadened both the ethnic distribution and the clinical spectrum of FMF. Genetic testing has permitted the recognition of milder disease, often with less frequent attacks, among a number of ethnic groups, most notably Ashkenazi Jews and Italians, not previously thought to be high-risk populations (51–53,205–207). Not surprisingly, milder mutations such as E148Q and V726A are more common than M694V in these populations.

As has been the case for a number of Mendelian genetic disorders, population surveys indicate that the penetrance of FMF is lower than expected. Direct screening for mutations has demonstrated carrier frequencies of at least 20% among North African, Iraqi, and Ashkenazi Jews, Arabs, Turks, and Armenians (205–209). A carrier rate of 20% predicts a mutation frequency of 10% and a disease frequency of 1% in the population. The measured incidence of FMF, where it is known (183), is less than half of the estimated population frequency, suggesting that there are substantial numbers of people with two mutations in *MEFV* but without clinical symptoms. Recent family studies have confirmed this prediction (210,211), and contrast with the much stronger relationship between *MEFV* genotype and disease in the families analyzed in FMF positional cloning studies (9,10). Those original families were specifically chosen for disease severity, unambiguous diagnoses, and sibships with multiple affected individuals, all factors that would favor the cosegregation of putative modifier alleles tending to increase the penetrance of *MEFV* mutations.

Moreover, while there are individuals with two mutations and no symptoms, it is also clear that the presence of a single *MEFV* mutation may confer at least a biochemical, and sometimes a clinical, effect. There is now ample evidence that individuals bearing one *MEFV* mutation exhibit an increased acute-phase response (212–214), even though they do not usually meet clinical criteria for FMF. This inflammatory phenotype in heterozygotes may confer a selective advantage that accounts for the high frequency of several different *MEFV* mutations in Mediterranean populations. In addition, most large series indicate that a substantial fraction (up to 30%) of patients with clinical FMF have only one demonstrable mutation (52,76,120,123,215–217), even when the entire coding region is sequenced (217). Although noncoding mutations remain a possibility, they would not explain the divergence from Hardy-Weinberg equilibrium that has recently been described (217). Finally, two different rare *MEFV* variants, the deletion of codon 694 (δM694) and the M694I-E148Q complex allele, have been convincingly associated with the dominant transmission of typical FMF (218). Taken together, these data strongly suggest that a simple, single-gene recessive model does not completely describe either the current clinical picture of FMF or the broader spectrum of *MEFV*-associated phenotypes.

This problem awaits resolution through the identification of modifier genes or additional loci that can independently confer the FMF phenotype. As noted previously, alleles at MICA appear to have a modifier effect on FMF severity

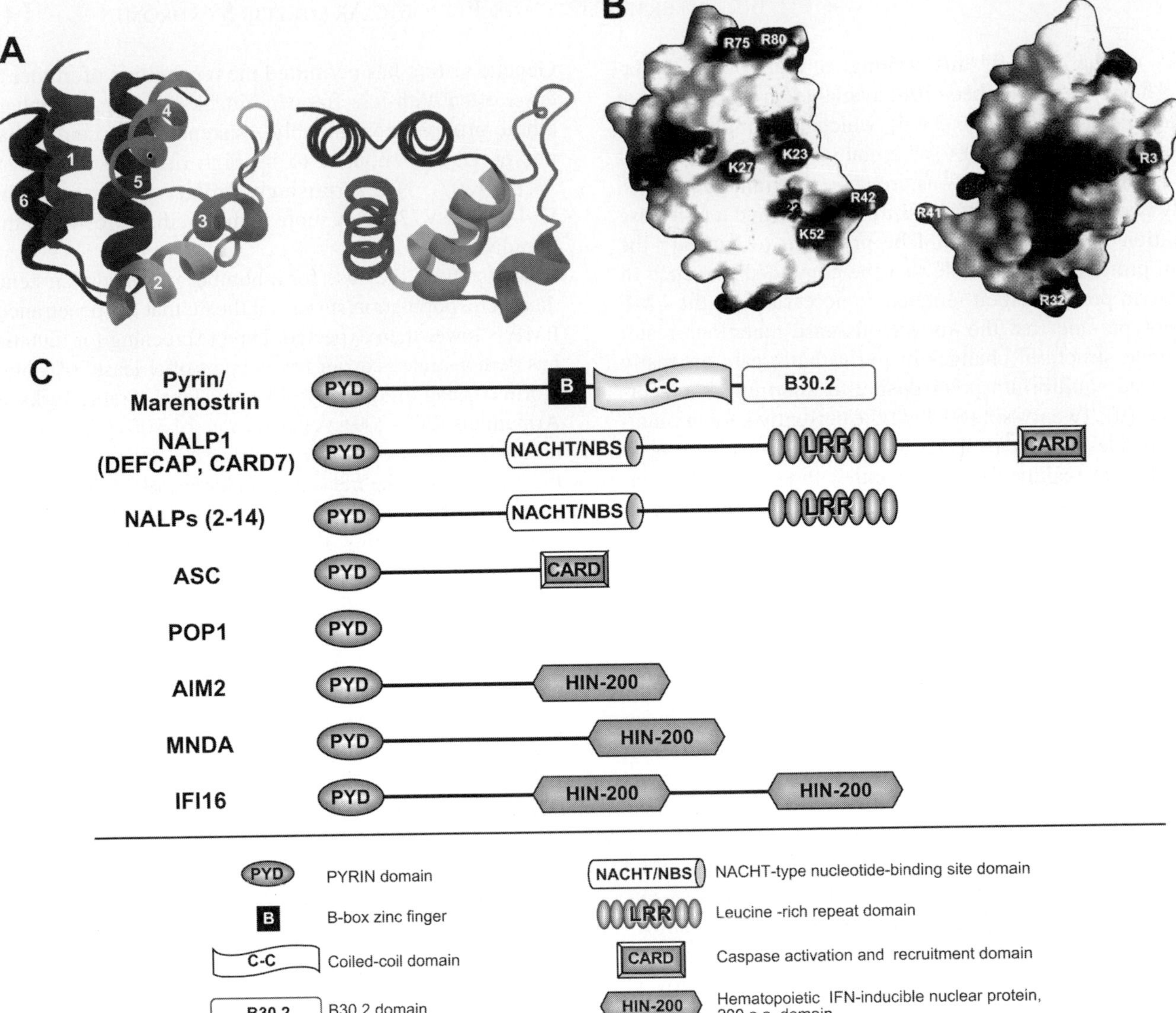

FIG. 68.6. The PYRIN domain. **A:** Ribbon diagram of the predicted three-dimensional structure of a human PYRIN domain, showing six α-helices arranged in the death-domain fold structure that is also observed in death domains, death effector domains, and caspase activation and recruitment domains (CARD). The views on the left and right differ by a 90 degree rotation about a horizontal axis. The structure depicted is computationally predicted from human ASC (apoptosis-associated specklike protein with a CARD). (Adapted from Liepinsh E, Barbals R, Dahl E, et al. The death-domain fold of the ASC PYRIN domain, presenting a basis for PYRIN/PYRIN recognition. *J Mol Biol* 2003;332:1155–1163.) **B:** Computationally predicted electrostatic surface charge distributions of oppositely charged faces of the respective PYRIN domains of pyrin (**left**) and ASC (**right**). Regions of high negative charge are shown in *red;* regions of high positive charge are shown in *blue*. Interactions between the positively charged face of pyrin's PYRIN domain with the negatively charged face of ASC's PYRIN domain may explain how these proteins bind one another. (Adapted from Richards N, Schaner P, Diaz A, et al. Interaction between pyrin and the apoptotic speck protein (ASC) modulates ASC-induced apoptosis. *J Biol Chem* 2001;276:39320–39329.) **C:** Structure of human proteins with an N-terminal PYRIN domain. Pyrin is the only known member of this family with a C-terminal cassette comprised of a B-box, coiled-coil, and B30.2 domain. The NALP family of proteins is so-named because each member has (at least) a NACHT domain [domain present in neuronal apoptosis inhibitor protein (NAIP), the major histocompatibility complex class II transactivator (CIITA), HET-E (incompatibility locus protein from *Podospora anserina*), and TP1 (mammalian telomerase-associated proteins)], a Leucine-rich repeat (LRR) domain, and a PYRIN domain. The NACHT domain contains a nucleotide binding site (NBS), which may play a regulatory role, while the LRRs are 20–29-residue sequence motifs that are also found in toll-like receptors and can bind bacterial-derived substances. NALP1, but not NALPs 2–14, has a C-terminal CARD. NALP3 is the same as cryopyrin, which is mutated in familial cold autoinflammatory syndrome (FCAS), Muckle-Wells syndrome (MWS), and neonatal-onset multisystem inflammatory disease (NOMID). POP1 (PYRIN-only protein 1) contains only a PYRIN domain. AIM2 (absent in melanoma 2), MNDA (myeloid cell nuclear differentiation antigen), and IFI16 (interferon-γ-inducible protein 16) are hematopoietic interferon-inducible transcriptional regulators.

(129), and there are other modifiers for amyloidosis susceptibility (121,127,128). There is also increasing speculation that there may be at least one additional FMF gene besides *MEFV*. The evidence for this includes the existence of Turkish FMF families unlinked to chromosome 16p (219) and a recent mathematical analysis of *MEFV* mutations in the Armenian enclave of Karabakh (217). Bearing in mind the caveat that the frequency of mutation-negative patients is, to a point, inversely related to the thoroughness of the genetic analysis, there are at least a few patients with clinical FMF but no identifiable mutations at every major center. Perhaps most notable is the large percentage of FMF patients on the Mediterranean island of Mallorca without demonstrable *MEFV* mutations (220). It is possible that evolutionary pressures that select for *MEFV* mutations in the Mediterranean basin may also select for mutations in other genes encoding proteins in the same or related inflammatory pathways.

Pathophysiology

As noted previously, the recognition of a 92 amino-acid motif at the N-terminus of the pyrin/marenostrin protein (Fig. 68.4) has provided critical insight into the function of pyrin in normal physiology and the possible mechanism of inflammatory attacks in FMF. This N-terminal domain, which has variously been denoted the PYRIN domain, PYD, PAAD, or DAPIN, is a 6-α-helix motif (Fig. 68.6A) that is structurally similar to death domains, death effector domains, and caspase-recruitment domains (CARDs) (28–32,221–226). The three-dimensional conformation of all four of these domains permits homotypic protein/protein interactions. Thus, proteins with death domains can interact with proteins bearing certain other death domains, proteins with death effector domains can interact with proteins bearing certain other death effector domains, and so on. The PYRIN domain of pyrin specifically interacts with the PYRIN domain of another protein called ASC (apoptosis-associated specklike protein with a CARD), a bipartite adaptor that is comprised of an N-terminal PYRIN domain and a C-terminal CARD (222,227–230). As depicted in Figure 68.6B, it is likely that pyrin binds ASC through electrostatic charge interactions on the opposite faces of their respective PYRIN domains (222). Variants of the PYRIN domain are also found in at least 19 other proteins in the human genome, many of which are implicated in the control of inflammation (Fig. 68.6C).

The interaction of pyrin with ASC places pyrin upstream in several pathways regulating interleukin-1β (IL-1β) secretion, nuclear factor κB (NF-κB) activation, and apoptosis. ASC not only binds pyrin through cognate PYRIN domain interactions, but also oligomerizes with caspase-1 (IL-1β converting enzyme, or ICE) through CARD–CARD binding (Fig. 68.7) (230–234). The interaction of ASC with ICE leads to the autocatalytic activation of ICE and the consequent cleavage of the 31 kDa precursor form of IL-1β into its biologically active 17 kDa fragment, a potent mediator of fever and inflammation. The interaction of pyrin with ASC appears to be a key regulatory step in the ASC–caspase-1–IL-1β cascade, and pyrin-deficient animals exhibit exaggerated responses to endotoxin through this pathway (230). Pyrin also plays a role in the regulation of leukocyte apoptosis, probably through ASC and caspase-8 (222,228–230), and modulates NF-κB activation, perhaps because of the action of ASC on the inhibitor of NF-κB (IκB) kinase complex (229,235).

Pyrin is expressed predominantly in neutrophils, the major cell type found in FMF inflammatory exudates, and in eosinophils and cytokine-activated monocytes (236,237). Modest reductions in *MEFV* message have been reported in peripheral blood leukocytes from patients with FMF (238). *MEFV* message is also inducible by IL-1β in cultures of synovial and peritoneal fibroblasts (239), an observation that could account for the predilection for serosal and synovial inflammation in FMF. Although the precise molecular mechanism of FMF-associated mutations remains to be elucidated, it is likely that these pyrin variants lead to accentuated innate immune responses, as are seen in pyrin-deficient mice (230). Moreover, the heightened sensitivity of these mice to endotoxin suggests a paradigm in which transient bacteremias might provoke exaggerated inflammatory responses to what would ordinarily be innocuous events. Such a defect in homeostasis might also extend to stress hormone-induced IL-1β production, and provide a mechanism for the oft-reported association of physical or psychological stress with febrile episodes in FMF.

When it was first identified, pyrin was hypothesized to be a transcription factor, largely because of its homology with other known transcription factors and the computational deduction of two overlapping nuclear targeting signals (9). However, subsequent transfection experiments have placed full-length pyrin in the cytoplasm, associated with the cytoskeleton (240,241). A relatively rare splice variant lacking exon 2 does concentrate in the nucleus (242), but the physiologic role of this variant, or other potential cleavage products of pyrin, remains to be established.

Besides the elevation in acute-phase reactants that is seen during and, to a lesser extent, between attacks, there are a number of other immunologic abnormalities that have been observed in patients with FMF, and may represent events downstream of the effects of pyrin on IL-1β secretion, NF-κB activation, and apoptosis. Serum levels of TNF-α, IL-6, IL-8, soluble IL-2 receptor, and soluble p55 and p75 TNF receptors, but not IL-10, are significantly increased during FMF attacks (243–247), and patients have been noted to have elevated serum levels of TNF-α, even in the attack-free state (248). By intracellular cytokine staining and flow cytometry, the percentage of interferon (IFN)-γ^+ T helper (Th) 1 cells is increased in asymptomatic FMF patients, and to an even greater degree during attacks, relative to healthy controls; numbers of IL-4^+ Th2 cells in the peripheral blood of FMF patients are not different from controls (249). Peripheral blood leukocyte mRNA levels

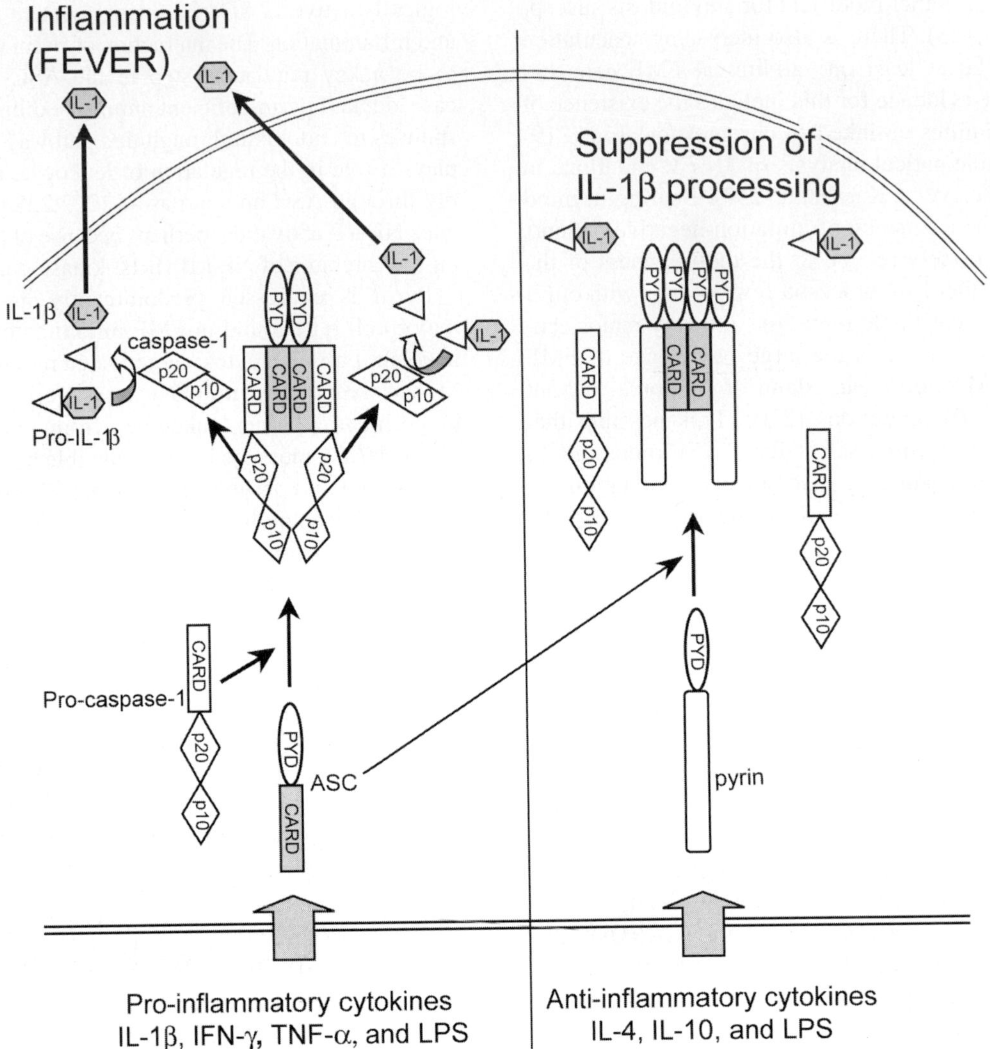

FIG. 68.7. Proposed role of pyrin in regulating ASC-mediated caspase-1 activation. **Left:** Lipopolysaccharide (LPS) and proinflammatory cytokines induce ASC [apoptosis-associated specklike protein with a caspase activation and recruitment domain (CARD)], which binds pro-caspase-1 [the inactive precursor of caspase-1, or interleukin-1β converting enzyme (ICE)] through cognate CARD-CARD interactions and leads to caspase-1 oligomerization and autocatalysis. Active p10/p20 subunits cleave pro-interleukin (IL)-1β to mature IL-1β, leading to fever and inflammation. **Right:** LPS and antiinflammatory cytokines can induce pyrin, which binds ASC through homotypic PYRIN domain interactions, sequestering ASC and blocking its interaction with caspase-1. *CARD*, caspase activation and recruitment domain; *PYD*, PYRIN domain. (From Chae JJ, Komarow HD, Cheng J, et al. Targeted disruption of pyrin, the FMF protein, causes heightened sensitivity to endotoxin and a defect in macrophage apoptosis. *Mol Cell* 2003;11:591–604, with permission.)

for several proinflammatory cytokines, including TNF-α, IL-1β, IL-6, and IL-8, are also increased in attack-free FMF patients (109). Nevertheless, it is rare to see positive antinuclear antibodies, rheumatoid factors, anticardiolipin antibodies, or antibodies against double-stranded DNA (dsDNA), Sm, RNP, SSA/Ro, SSB/La, or neutrophil cytoplasmic antigens (250–253).

Granulocyte and monocyte function have not been studied systematically since the positional cloning of *MEFV.* Although several very early studies of granulocytes in FMF failed to demonstrate abnormalities (254,255), a number of subtle functional differences have been noted. Neutrophils, but not monocytes, from asymptomatic patients exhibit an increased oxidative metabolic burst in response to *N*-formyl-methionyl-leucyl-phenylalanine (256). FMF neutrophils also release more lysozyme in response to high temperatures than control cells (257). Eosinophilic cationic protein, a marker for eosinophil activity and turnover, is elevated in the blood of patients during their attacks (258). Although neutrophils from patients with FMF have not been noted to have an increased chemotactic response to endotoxin (259) or to skin abrasion (254), they do exhibit increased spontaneous migration using an agarose migration technique (260).

Prior to the positional cloning of *MEFV*, studies of serosal fluids from patients and healthy controls suggested a deficiency of a putative inhibitor of the fifth component of complement in FMF (261,262). Comparison of the sequence of *MEFV* with peptide sequences of the partially purified inhibitor did not produce a match, and the gene encoding the inhibitor has not been cloned. It has therefore been difficult to conclusively establish or refute such a mechanism in the pathophysiology of FMF. Abnormalities in plasma and urine catecholamines had also been observed in the pre-*MEFV* era (263–265), but as of this writing no causal linkage has been established between these observations and what is currently known of the biology of pyrin.

Diagnosis

Prior to the identification of *MEFV*, the diagnosis of FMF was, of necessity, made purely on clinical grounds. Several sets of criteria had been proposed (46,266–268), with the Tel-Hashomer criteria the most widely cited (268). All four criteria sets concur that the cardinal features of the disease are short (12 hours to 3 days), recurrent (3 or more) episodes of fever (rectal temperature > 38°C) with painful manifestations in the abdomen, chest, joints, or skin, in the absence of any other demonstrable causative factors. The Tel-Hashomer criteria set recognizes milder attacks, exertional leg pain, and a favorable response to colchicine as minor criteria, and a positive family history, age of onset less than 20 years, appropriate ethnicity, parental consanguinity, an acute-phase response during attacks, episodic proteinuria/hematuria, and an unproductive laparotomy as supportive criteria. The diagnosis can then be made with appropriate combinations of major, minor, or supportive criteria (268).

The Tel-Hashomer clinical criteria for FMF perform very well, with sensitivities and specificities greater than 95%, in populations in which the frequency of FMF is high, the attacks are relatively severe, and physicians are experienced. There are no data on the sensitivity and specificity of these criteria sets in Western nations, where the disease frequency is lower, the attacks may be significantly milder (because of a different spectrum of mutations), and most physicians have little or no experience in recognizing a "typical" attack. Moreover, in Western countries the frequency of other periodic fevers, such as TRAPS and HIDS, may approach or even exceed the frequency of FMF. For all of these reasons the clinical criteria established in the Middle East are unlikely to perform as well in Western countries, even though they may provide important clinical guidance in the diagnostic workup.

Therefore, genetic testing has assumed a major adjunctive role, particularly in the U.S. and Western Europe. Based on the foregoing discussion of the genetics of FMF, it is clear that DNA diagnostic testing must also be interpreted with caution. Of course, everything is straightforward when genetic testing reveals two *MEFV* mutations, in *trans,* in a patient clinically suspected of having FMF, or when genetic testing reveals no mutations in a patient in whom the diagnosis is thought to be unlikely. Genetic testing may also be helpful in assessing the risk of amyloidosis in patients with clinically unambiguous FMF. However, as was noted previously, even in countries where FMF is relatively common and, in centers where testing is state-of-the-art, as many as one third of patients meeting clinical criteria for FMF have only one demonstrable *MEFV* mutation, and a (usually) small percentage of patients with clinical FMF will be found to have no *MEFV* mutations. These observations may be explained by the presence of *MEFV* mutations that are not currently screened (e.g., in the promoter or deep within introns), by a second FMF locus, or by the possibility that under some circumstances one mutation may be sufficient to produce symptoms. In such cases where genetic testing for FMF fails to resolve clinical uncertainty, considerations include a therapeutic trial of colchicine and assessment for other hereditary periodic fever syndromes (Table 68.3).

There are several other points to bear in mind when interpreting the results of genetic testing for FMF. Most diagnostic laboratories do not routinely screen the whole coding region of *MEFV*, but instead either sequence all of exon 10 (where the majority of FMF-associated mutations have been found) and then screen for specific common mutations (such as E148Q) outside of exon 10, or perform only directed testing for specific mutations, both within and outside of exon 10, without sequencing. The latter approach will only detect the specific mutations being assayed, and will even miss other mutations at the same residue. For example, a mutation-specific assay for M694V cannot detect M694I, M694L, or δM694. Most centers test at least for M694V, V726A, and E148Q, but may not test for mutations that are particularly common among certain ethnic groups, such as M694I among Arabs (10), R761H in Iranians and Armenians (57), and F479L in Greeks (54).

Even when two mutations are identified, it is important to bear in mind that some mutations, particularly E148Q, can occur in *cis* with others (52,57), and therefore studies of other family members may be necessary to distinguish, for example, between a single V726A-E148Q complex allele, versus V726A and E148Q on opposite chromosomes. Except in this setting, screening of asymptomatic family members is generally not performed, since the discovery of two *MEFV* mutations may adversely affect insurability in individuals who may never develop symptoms of FMF. There is still no consensus on presymptomatic screening in families with FMF and a strong history of amyloidosis (269), and, for medical ethics reasons, the role, if any, of prenatal diagnosis is extremely controversial.

To date there are neither protein-based tests nor assays for *MEFV* expression or function that would aid in the diagnosis, although recent advances raise this possibility. In the early 1980s a metaraminol infusion test was proposed for the diagnosis of FMF (263), but this test is not widely used because of concerns regarding its safety (270,271). Elevated levels of dopamine β-hydroxylase were also reported (264) but have not been verified (272–274).

One of the most important factors in making the diagnosis of FMF is a suitable index of suspicion. Important clinical features that help distinguish FMF from the other hereditary periodic fevers are summarized in Table 68.3. The differential diagnosis in a particular case is specific to the type of attack (peritoneal, joint, etc.). Since most FMF presents before age 20, acute appendicitis may be an important consideration; the spontaneous resolution of fever is often the first evidence for FMF. Usually the diagnosis requires observation over time, unless the patient has already had several documented attacks when he or she presents. Porphyria can present with intermittent abdominal pain and fever, but can be recognized by the presence of hypertension during attacks, dominant inheritance, and elevated porphyrins in the urine (275). Hereditary angioedema can cause intermittent abdominal pain, but does not usually cause fever. It is also inherited as autosomal dominant, and C1 esterase inhibitor levels are reduced (276,277). In children, another major consideration is distinguishing FMF from systemic-onset juvenile chronic arthritis (see Chapter 61). Important points to consider include the characteristic evanescent rash of juvenile chronic arthritis (which is not seen in FMF), the pattern of fever (intermittent quotidian pattern in juvenile chronic arthritis versus 1- to 3-day episodes in FMF), the pattern of arthritis (chronic polyarthritis in juvenile chronic arthritis versus intermittent monoarthritis in FMF), and the presence of lymphadenopathy (much more common in juvenile chronic arthritis than FMF). The syndrome of periodic fever, aphthous stomatitis, pharyngitis, and cervical adenitis (278) can also sometimes be confused with FMF in the pediatric population. In adults presenting with monoarticular arthritis, joint aspiration for crystals and bacterial culture may aid in the diagnosis. In women presenting with abdominal pain, especially if there is menstrual variation in symptoms, gynecologic evaluation may be required to rule out endometriosis and pelvic inflammatory disease.

Treatment

Goldfinger is generally credited with first suggesting the prophylactic use of colchicine in FMF in 1972 (279). Three large randomized placebo-controlled studies published in 1974 established the efficacy of continuous daily colchicine (1–2 mg/day) in preventing the attacks of FMF (280–282). Overall, about three-fourths of patients experience a near-complete remission on colchicine, and close to 95% note a marked improvement (many patients do not experience the full therapeutic effect of colchicine unless they take 1.2–1.8 mg/day). Colchicine is also effective in preventing the amyloidosis of FMF. In a study of 960 Israeli patients who did not have proteinuria at entry, life-table analysis showed a cumulative rate of proteinuria of 2% after 11 years in 906 patients who complied with a regimen of 1 to 2 mg of colchicine/day, versus 49% after 9 years in 54 patients who admitted noncompliance (283). Continuous colchicine is usually preferable to intermittent therapy because of its efficacy in preventing amyloidosis, even though intermittent therapy may sometimes be effective in aborting attacks (284).

Colchicine is also beneficial for FMF patients who already have proteinuria (285–287). Chances of stabilization or improvement of proteinuria are greatest if the initial serum creatinine is less than 1.5 mg/dL and the dose of colchicine is greater than 1.5 mg/day (284). Tubulointerstitial injury at presentation and noncompliance are poor prognostic factors (287). Daily doses of colchicine of 1.5 mg or more are also needed to prevent graft amyloidosis in FMF patients who have received a kidney transplant (146). The combination of cyclosporine and colchicine should be avoided when possible in transplant patients because cyclosporine inhibits the MDR1 transport system necessary for hepatic and renal excretion of colchicine (149–153).

Although colchicine is also effective in treating mesangial proliferative nephritis in FMF (166), it is not sufficient in treating rapidly progressive glomerulonephritis (167) or polyarteritis nodosa (158–162). In these latter two conditions, cyclophosphamide and high-dose steroids are usually necessary. Henoch-Schönlein purpura and protracted febrile myalgia (101,102) in FMF may also require steroid therapy.

The mechanism by which colchicine prevents or ameliorates the attacks of FMF is incompletely understood. It is well-established that colchicine interacts with microtubules (288) and is concentrated in granulocytes (289), perhaps because of a lack of the *MDR1*-encoded P-glycoprotein membrane pump in this cell type (290,291). It is intriguing to note that pyrin itself is expressed predominantly in neutrophils and associates with microtubules (9,236,241), although a direct functional connection with colchicine remains to be established. Colchicine also inhibits neutrophil/endothelial interactions by its effects on E-selectin distribution on endothelial cells and L-selectin expression on neutrophils (292), thereby inhibiting neutrophil chemotaxis (254,259), and reduces circulating cytokine levels in FMF patients (248).

The most likely mechanism by which colchicine prevents or reverses amyloidosis in FMF is through its effects on the underlying inflammatory process. Based on the observation of "phenotype II" FMF patients who develop amyloidosis before experiencing febrile attacks, there has been speculation that the amyloidosis of FMF is a disease manifestation distinct from the acute attacks (293), and therefore that colchicine may prevent amyloidosis independently of its effect on inflammation. However, it now appears that phenotype II can be explained by the well-documented elevation in acute-phase reactants, including SAA, that occurs in FMF patients even between attacks, and colchicine has been shown to control this subclinical inflammation (106–108). Moreover, further evidence against a role for colchicine in blocking amyloid deposition (rather than SAA production) comes from patients with TRAPS, whose inflammatory attacks are generally not controlled by colchicine, and who may develop amyloidosis even while receiving full prophylactic doses (294,295). Current data from patients with a number of inflammatory conditions indicate that amyloid deposits are in a state of dynamic equilibrium, and that intensive antiinflammatory treatments tailored to the underlying disorder (keeping the SAA concentration below 10 mg/L) are associated with regression (296,297). Targeted strategies aimed at depleting other components of amyloid deposits, such as serum amyloid P (298), may eventually provide an alternative treatment for established amyloidosis in FMF and other autoinflammatory disorders.

The most frequent toxicity of colchicine is diarrhea, but this can often be minimized by initiating therapy with gradually increasing doses. Jejunal biopsies of FMF patients on long-term colchicine show relatively minor histologic effects (299). Nevertheless, colchicine induces significant lactose intolerance in some patients and a lactose-free diet is sometimes helpful in controlling the gastrointestinal side effects of colchicine (300). Rarely, colchicine may impair corneal wound healing after ocular surgery (301–303), although it is currently not recommended to discontinue colchicine before any surgery, ophthalmologic or otherwise (303).

Colchicine is metabolized in the liver, undergoes enterohepatic recirculation, and is excreted in the urine; dose adjustments may be necessary in patients with either kidney or liver disease (304,305). A small number of FMF patients on colchicine may develop mild, reversible increases in serum aminotransferases. Because colchicine is metabolized in the liver by the cytochrome P (CYP) 3A4 isoform of the CYP-450 system, a number of drug interactions are possible (305). Among the agents that can lead to increased colchicine levels through this mechanism are cimetidine (305), ketoconazole (305), erythromycin (306), and simvastatin, lovastatin, and atorvastatin (but not fluvastatin or pravastatin) (307). Grapefruit juice can also inhibit CYP 3A4, leading to increased colchicine blood levels (305). The risk of toxicity from any of these interactions is magnified in the setting of hepatic or renal insufficiency.

Colchicine can cause a reversible myopathy and neuropathy, characterized by elevated creatine kinase levels, seen primarily in older adult patients with impaired renal function or in patients with renal failure (308,309). Nevertheless, colchicine myoneuropathy has been observed in rare patients with normal renal function, including children (310–312). Colchicine doses in children must be carefully titrated to efficacy and toxicity, bearing in mind that in children under the age of 5 years the dose adjusted to body surface area (but not the total dose) is greater than in older children (313). Despite these caveats, colchicine is generally safe in children, and in fact has had a major impact on correcting the growth delay formerly seen in children with frequent FMF attacks (314).

The potential effect of colchicine on female reproductive function is a frequent source of concern among FMF patients. Untreated, FMF itself can adversely impact female fertility in a number of ways. Repeated abdominal attacks may cause peritoneal adhesions and consequent tubal obstruction, amyloidosis may impair ovulatory function, and acute peritoneal attacks may induce abortion or early delivery in pregnancies that do occur (315,316). Regular colchicine prophylaxis has markedly reduced the incidence of adhesions and amyloidosis, and, if taken during pregnancy, reduces the frequency of acute abdominal attacks. The miscarriage rate in FMF has been reduced from 25% to 30% in the precolchicine era to a current rate close to that in the general population (315). In a series of 225 completed pregnancies in 116 women with FMF, there was no increase in pregnancy complications among women taking colchicine before or during pregnancy (317). The rate of trisomy 21 in the offspring of women taking colchicine is estimated to be about twice that expected among age-matched controls, and for this reason amniocentesis is usually advised for women who were taking colchicine at the time of conception (315,317), although the need for this procedure has recently been questioned (316,318). Successful *in vitro* fertilization has been reported in a woman with FMF receiving colchicine (319). Although small concentrations of drug are detectable in the breast milk of lactating women with FMF taking colchicine, breast-feeding is considered safe (320).

Colchicine-associated male infertility was observed in one small series (321), but more recent analyses suggest that male infertility in FMF is more likely to be the result of amyloidosis than colchicine toxicity (322–325). Although it is possible that colchicine taken by the father at the time of conception could increase the risk of chromosomal abnormalities, a recent prospective study did not demonstrate such an effect (315), leading some to reconsider the recommendation of amniocentesis in this setting.

The risk of serious colchicine toxicity is much increased when intravenous doses are given to patients already receiving oral colchicine (326–329). In the most extreme cases, this may lead to multiple organ failure and death. Therefore, in cases in which FMF patients have acute attacks despite colchicine therapy, supplemental intravenous colchicine should not be given to abort the attack. Instead, therapy should be supportive, avoiding narcotic analgesics. A recent small open-label pilot study (329a) showed promising results when a small dose of intravenous colchicine was administered weekly to FMF patients who had frequent attacks despite maximal doses of oral colchicine, but this approach should still be considered investigational. The only usual indication for intravenous colchicine is in the perioperative period, if a patient is unable to take medication by mouth, with appropriate adjustments for bioavailability (305).

FMF patients on colchicine may develop abdominal pain, either because of "breakthrough" attacks or because of another intraabdominal process. The physician must be alert to these latter possibilities, especially if the patient describes the episode as atypical for FMF. Elective appendectomy is usually not performed in FMF patients except in the rare cases where frequent abdominal attacks occur despite colchicine treatment (330,331).

Therapeutic options for FMF patients poorly responsive to colchicine, or who cannot tolerate a therapeutic dose, are limited. In some cases IFN-α, given by subcutaneous injection with the earliest signs of an attack, may be useful adjunctive therapy (332,333). Allogeneic bone marrow transplantation has recently been proposed as a treatment for refractory FMF (334), but many experts currently regard the risk–benefit ratio as unacceptable (335). Given the recent findings regarding the role of pyrin in cytokine regulation, targeted biologic therapies are a potentially fertile area of investigation.

The Cryopyrinopathies

The cryopyrinopathies are a group of three clinical disorders that are all caused by dominantly inherited mutations in *CIAS1* (for cold-induced autoinflammatory syndrome-1), a gene that encodes a PYRIN domain–containing protein called cryopyrin (4). Three other names, *PYPAF1* (336), *NALP3* (6), and *CATERPILLER 1.1* (337), have also been used to denote this gene and its protein product. The cryopyrinopathies include the familial cold autoinflammatory syndrome (FCAS)/familial cold urticaria (FCU), Muckle-Wells syndrome (MWS), and the neonatal onset multisystem inflammatory disease (NOMID)/chronic infantile neurologic cutaneous and articular (CINCA) syndrome (4–8). Although these illnesses have been described as distinct nosologic entities, all three can present with fevers, urticarial skin rash, varying degrees of arthralgia/arthritis, neutrophil-mediated inflammation, and an intense acute-phase response.

The severity of joint and neurosensory involvement and the frequency of amyloidosis help to distinguish among the cryopyrinopathies. In general, patients with FCAS/FCU have the least severe clinical phenotype, with MWS intermediate, and NOMID/CINCA the most severe. FCAS/FCU has a very clear cold-induced episodic quality (20,338), while NOMID/CINCA presents with nearly continuous clinical symptoms that fluctuate in severity (24,25,339, 340). As will be discussed below, there is considerable blurring of the clinical boundaries between FCAS/FCU and MWS, and between MWS and NOMID/CINCA, and there are certain *CIAS1* mutations that have been associated with both FCAS/FCU and MWS (4–6,341), and others that have been associated with both MWS and NOMID/CINCA (5,7,8,341–343). Thus, the cryopyrinopathies represent a spectrum of autoinflammatory disease that is caused by mutations in a single gene, probably influenced by a number of as yet undefined genetic and environmental modifiers. Reflecting this etiologic concept, the cryopyrin-associated autoinflammatory disorders will be discussed here as a group.

Clinical Features

Familial Cold Autoinflammatory Syndrome/Familial Cold Urticaria

FCAS/FCU is characterized by cold-induced episodes of fever, urticarial rash, arthralgia, and conjunctivitis (20, 338). Other associated symptoms include chills, profuse sweating, drowsiness, headache, extreme thirst, and nausea. Generalized cold exposure is the usual trigger for the inflammatory episodes of FCAS/FCU, whereas localized exposure to cold objects or drinking cold liquids does not usually induce attacks. In one large study, the mean duration of cold exposure required to evoke an attack was 52 minutes, with a range of 5 minutes to 3 hours (338). The lag time from the beginning of cold exposure to the onset of symptoms averaged 2.5 hours, and the average length of attacks was about 12 hours. Longer, colder exposures generally provoke more severe episodes, and a common setting for attacks is cold, damp, windy weather. In some individuals, symptoms may occur on an almost daily basis, tending to be worse in the evening and to resolve by the morning. Symptoms usually begin within the first 6 months of life.

The rash of FCAS/FCU often starts on the face or extremities and then becomes generalized. It can present as petechiae, erythematous patches, or confluent erythematous plaques (20). In contrast to acquired cold urticaria, in which serum histamine levels are increased and there are mast cells present in the lesions, serum histamine levels are normal and mast cells are not seen in increased numbers in biopsies of FCAS/FCU skin lesions (338). Biopsies obtained after cold challenge instead show neutrophil efflux from vessels and progressive microvascular damage, including endothelial cell swelling, smudging, vacuolization, and luminal narrowing (344). For these reasons FCAS/FCU is not a true form of urticaria, and hence the proposal to replace *familial cold urticaria* with *familial cold autoinflammatory syndrome* (4, 338). Other older synonyms include familial polymorphous cold eruption and cold hypersensitivity.

Patients with FCAS/FCU commonly complain of polyarthralgia with their attacks, most frequently involving the hands, knees, and ankles, with the feet, wrists, and elbows also sometimes affected. Some patients may also develop a nonerosive deforming arthropathy similar to the postrheumatic fever arthropathy of Jaccoud (345). On examination these patients have reducible deformities of the metacarpophalangeal and proximal interphalangeal joints, sometimes with ulnar deviation.

Watering, blurred vision, and ocular pain sometimes accompany the conjunctivitis of FCAS/FCU, but periorbital edema has not been reported. Laboratory features of the attacks include polymorphonuclear leukocytosis, an accelerated ESR, and elevations in CRP and SAA. In a survey of 45 affected individuals from 6 American families, amyloidosis occurred in only 1 woman, late in life (338). At least 4 of her ancestors also had late-onset renal disease, but her monozygotic twin did not.

Muckle-Wells Syndrome

MWS was first described in a Derbyshire family with dominantly inherited, episodic "aguey bouts" comprised of (a) chills, rigors, and a general sense of malaise; (b) aching and stabbing pains in the distal limbs and larger joints; and (c) a generalized urticaria-like rash (21). Members of this propositus family also developed progressive bilateral sensorineural deafness, beginning in childhood, and amyloid nephropathy.

Since the initial description of this family in 1962, there have been a number of other families and sporadic cases of this syndrome reported in the literature. In a review of 78 cases in 1979 (346), 66 (85%) had typical recurring "aguey bouts," 58 (74%) had hearing loss, and 27 (35%) had nephropathy, 13 of whom had biopsy-proven amyloidosis. Most of the published cases are of Northern European ancestry.

In contrast with FCAS/FCU, the attacks of MWS have been associated with both hot and cold temperatures (21, 347), and have sometimes been related to emotional stress (21). The episodes of MWS are also somewhat longer than in FCAS/FCU, lasting in the range of 24 to 48 hours (21, 346,348). These episodes may begin as early as the first day of life, and most patients experience their first attack by adolescence. In addition to constitutional symptoms, limb pain, and rash, some patients experience abdominal pain, conjunctivitis, or episcleritis (347,348) with their attacks. Laboratory findings include leukocytosis and elevated acute-phase reactants.

Figure 68.8A shows the typical urticaria-like rash of MWS. As is the case for FCAS/FCU, the rash appears not to be true urticaria, with biopsies showing a perivascular and interstitial infiltrate of neutrophils and lymphocytes in the papillary dermis (349). Vasculitis is not present. Although arthralgia is more common than frank arthritis in MWS, both intermittent oligoarticular synovitis and a more persistent pyogenic arthritis have been reported (347,350), usually affecting the knees, ankles, or wrists. Bilateral pes cavus has also been noted in some patients (21).

Figure 68.8B depicts bilateral audiograms from a 23-year-old patient with MWS. Sensorineural hearing loss was first noted in this patient at about age 8, affecting primarily high frequency perception. The etiology of hearing loss in MWS is unknown. Postmortem examinations of patients in the original MWS family demonstrated no evidence of amyloidosis in the inner ear, but the organ of Corti and the vestibular sensory epithelium were absent, and there was ossification of the basilar membrane and atrophy of the cochlear nerve (21). An inflammatory etiology is possible but, as yet, has not been established.

The amyloidosis of MWS is of the AA type, affecting the kidneys, spleen, adrenals, thyroid, and testes (350). As previously noted, only about one-third of patients with MWS develop this complication, and, when it does occur, amyloidosis usually presents in adulthood.

Neonatal Onset Multisystem Inflammatory Disease/Chronic Infantile Neurologic, Cutaneous, and Articular Syndrome

NOMID/CINCA is the most severe of the cryopyrinopathies, presenting with an urticarial rash similar to that seen in FCAS/FCU and MWS, but also manifesting central nervous system involvement and a highly characteristic and sometimes disabling arthropathy (24,25,339,340). Symptoms are often present in infancy. Some patients develop systemic AA amyloidosis, although precise figures are not available. About 20% of patients die, mainly from infection or neurologic complications, before reaching adulthood (339,351).

The rash of NOMID/CINCA is often seen within the first few days of life, and usually within the first 6 months. Once it develops, the rash may wax and wane, but it is nearly always present. The rash is migratory and usually nonpruritic, but itching can develop when it worsens with fever or sunlight (351). Histologically, the epidermis is normal, with mild inflammation in the dermis and a mostly polymorphonuclear perivascular infiltrate (340).

The neurosensory manifestations of NOMID/CINCA can vary substantially in severity. Headache is common, and smaller percentages of patients may develop seizures, hypotonia, or hemiplegia (340). Some children with NOMID/CINCA perform well academically, while others have learning disabilities and still others are mentally retarded. The majority of patients have evidence of aseptic meningitis, with increased cerebrospinal fluid (CSF) pressure, pleiocytosis (predominantly polymorphonuclear leukocytes), and elevated CSF protein (352). EEG abnormalities are also common (351). Imaging studies may demonstrate mild ventricular dilatation, cerebral atrophy, prominent sulci, and, in older patients, calcification of the falx cerebri and dura (340).

As in MWS, progressive high-frequency sensorineural hearing loss often occurs in NOMID/CINCA (352). Ocular changes are also common, and include conjunctivitis, anterior uveitis, and posterior segment abnormalities. Chronic anterior uveitis was present in about half of the patients in a recent large series (353). Optic disk changes were observed in over 80% of the same series, and included optic disk edema, pseudopapilledema, and optic atrophy (353). Visual impairment and even blindness may develop.

The articular manifestations of NOMID/CINCA can be seen in early childhood, but are not usually present at birth. As is the case for the neurosensory involvement, there is a great deal of patient-to-patient variability in the joint findings (339,340,351). At the mild end of the spectrum, some

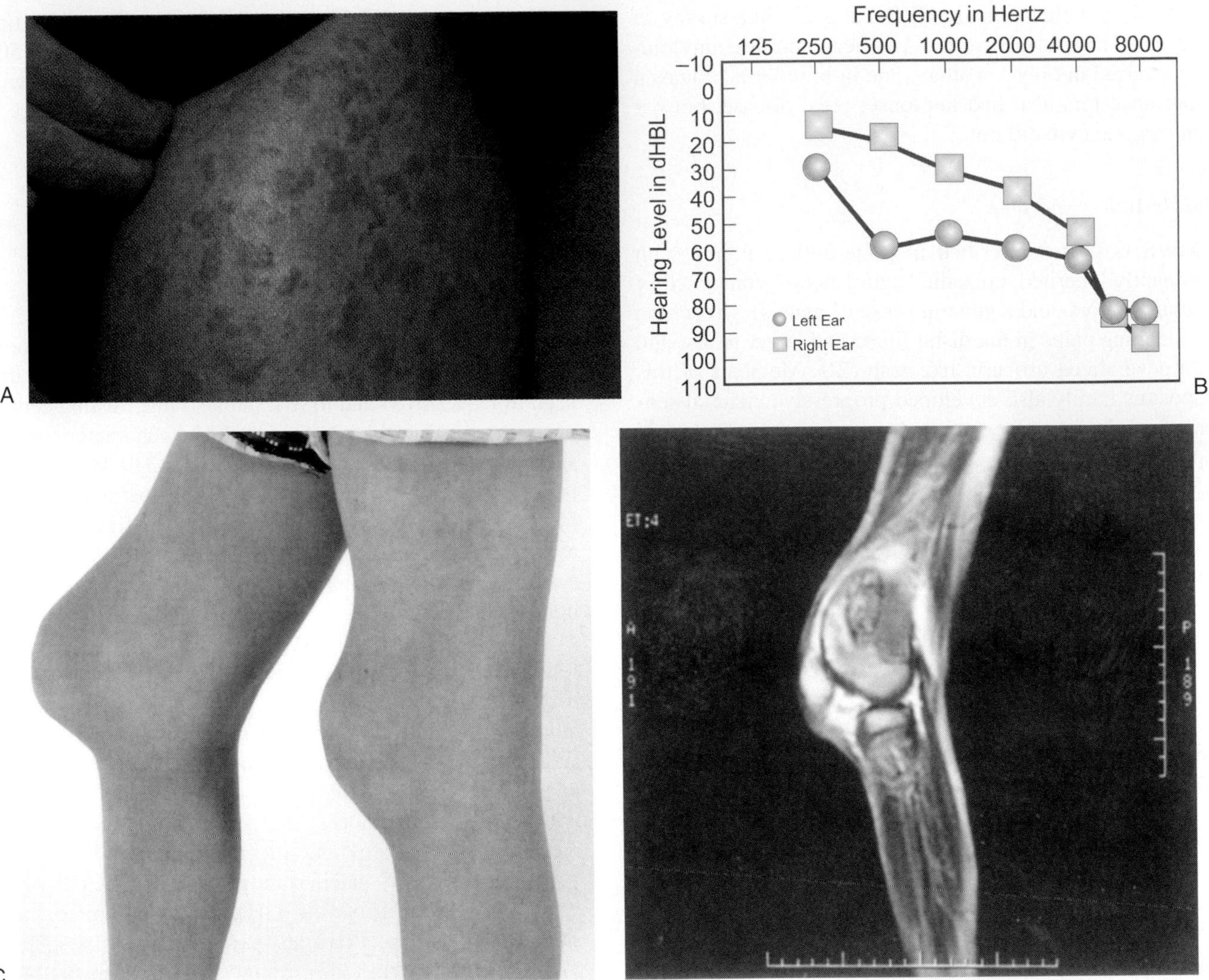

FIG. 68.8. Clinical features of the cryopyrin-associated disorders. **A:** Urticarial rash in a patient with Muckle-Wells syndrome. **B:** Audiograms from the same patient, demonstrating bilateral high-frequency hearing loss. Bone conduction was the same as air conduction (not shown), documenting the sensorineural nature of the hearing impairment. **C:** Patellar overgrowth and knee contractures in a patient with neonatal-onset multisystem inflammatory disease (NOMID)/chronic infantile neurologic, cutaneous, and articular (CINCA) syndrome. **D.** Magnetic resonance image of the right knee of the same patient, demonstrating the absence of significant synovial enhancement and the presence of epiphyseal and patellar bony overgrowth. (Panels **C** and **D** from Aksentijevich I, Nowak M, Mallah M, et al. De novo *CIAS1* mutations, cytokine activation, and evidence for genetic heterogeneity in patients with neonatal-onset multisystem inflammatory disease (NOMID). A new member of the expanding family of pyrin-associated autoinflammatory diseases. *Arthritis Rheum* 2002;46:3340–3348, with permission.)

patients experience arthralgia with mild swelling but no radiographic changes. At the other end of the continuum, about half of the patients exhibit a severe symmetric arthropathy within the first year of life, which can involve the knees, ankles, elbows, wrists, hands, or feet (but rarely the shoulders, hips, or cervical spine). These children develop bony deformities, as seen in the knees of the patient in Figure 68.8C, resulting from epiphyseal and growth cartilage overgrowth. Synovial proliferation is much less common, although sterile effusions are sometimes seen, probably as a local reaction to epiphyseal disturbances. Progressive contractures, particularly of the knees, can also occur (Fig. 68.8C).

Radiographically, in patients with the more severe form of arthropathy, premature patellar ossification and overgrowth is common (339,340,351,352,354). The epiphyses of the long bones, particularly the proximal ends of both tibias, can be enlarged with irregular ossification that gives a "breadcrumb" (*en mie de pain*) appearance. Flaring of the metaphyses is also seen, with marked irregularity of epiphyseal plates of the femur, radius, and tibia, and consequent premature growth plate closure and shortening of the long bones (339). As shown in the magnetic resonance image in Figure 68.8D, these changes occur in the absence of significant synovial proliferation. Synovial biopsy, when performed, demonstrates mild inflammation with perivascular neutrophilic, eosinophilic, and mast cell infiltration, but without a proliferative pannus (355). Skull films demonstrate increased cranial volume, frontal bosselation, and delayed closure of the anterior fontanelle.

Other frequent clinical findings in NOMID/CINCA include fever, lymphadenopathy, and hepatosplenomegaly (339,340,351,352). Vasculitis, thrombosis, and amyloidosis are potentially life-threatening complications. Laboratory findings include leukocytosis with a predominance of polymorphonuclear leukocytes and eosinophils, anemia of chronic disease, thrombocytosis, and a brisk acute-phase response. As is the case for FCAS/FCU and MWS, high-titer autoantibodies are not usually seen in NOMID/CINCA.

Clinical Overlap Syndromes

Although the cryopyrinopathies have been described as three distinct clinical entities, there are patients and families that suggest a more continuous spectrum of phenotypes. For example, a North Indian family with a documented *CIAS1* mutation manifests episodes of chills, fever, urticarial rash, and arthralgia upon exposure to cold, as would be seen in FCAS/FCU, but also includes several members with amyloidosis, a finding more typical of MWS (6,356). Periorbital edema, a feature not recognized in either FCAS/FCU or MWS, was also observed in several members of this family.

Similarly, there are cases that blur the boundary between MWS and NOMID/CINCA. In some cases, patients who were diagnosed with MWS early in life because of the typical inflammatory attacks ("aguey bouts") and sensorineural hearing loss are later found to have clinical manifestations more typical of NOMID/CINCA (342,349). At present there are no examples of overlap cases or families between FCAS/FCU and NOMID/CINCA, but the issue has not been examined carefully enough with lumbar punctures and imaging studies to be totally certain.

Genetics

Within a period of 6 months in late 1999 and early 2000, independent linkage studies placed the susceptibility loci for both MWS (348) and FCAS/FCU (357) on the distal portion of the long arm of chromosome 1. Several months later, the susceptibility locus for the North Indian family with the FCAS/FCU–MWS overlap syndrome was mapped to the same chromosomal region (356), suggesting that all three conditions might be allelic disorders of the same gene.

Additional genetic markers on chromosome 1 were used to narrow the region of interest from approximately 10 million base pairs of DNA to a more manageable critical region of about 1 million base pairs, and a map of exons and expressed genes was then constructed. By late 2001, Hoffman et al. had identified one large (1,753 base pair) exon with four disease-associated missense substitutions, three in FCAS/FCU families and one in a MWS family (4). This exon was found to be the third of a nine-exon gene they named *CIAS1,* with a potential 1,034 amino-acid product. Because of alternative splicing at the 3′ end of the mRNA (removing exons 4 and 6 from the mature transcript), the predicted protein is 920 amino acids in length. Like *MEFV,* the gene causing FMF, this gene is expressed predominantly in peripheral blood leukocytes, and encodes an N-terminal PYRIN domain (4). To connote its relationship both to cold exposure and to fever, the protein was named "cryopyrin." By the end of 2002, mutations in this gene had also been described in NOMID/CINCA and in the North Indian FCAS/FCU–MWS overlap syndrome (6–8).

Figure 68-9 is a schematic representation of the genomic structure of *CIAS1* and the corresponding domains of the cryopyrin protein. In addition to the N-terminal PYRIN domain, residues 217–533 comprise a nucleotide binding site (NBS) domain of the NACHT subfamily [358; so named because it is present in the neuronal apoptosis inhibitor protein (NAIP), the major histocompatibility complex class II transactivator (CIITA), HET-E (incompatibility locus protein from *Podospora anserina*), and TP1 (mammalian telomerase-associated proteins)], and residues 697–920 constitute a 7-element leucine-rich repeat (LRR) domain. This arrangement of PYRIN, NACHT, and LRR domains is found in a family of 14 human NALP (NACHT, LRR, PYRIN) proteins (34; Fig. 68.6). The NACHT–LRR combination (without the PYRIN domain) is also found in NOD2/CARD15, the gene mutated in both Crohn disease (38,39) and Blau syndrome (40), as well as the family of cytosolic resistance (R) proteins that mediate plant resistance to a variety of bacteria, viruses, and fungi (359).

As was noted in the discussion of the pyrin protein, PYRIN domains are found in a number of proteins involved in the regulation of inflammation and apoptosis, and are involved in cognate interactions with other proteins with PYRIN domains. The NACHT domain contains seven distinct motifs, including an adenosine triphosphatase (ATPase)-specific P-loop and a Mg^{++}-binding site, and is thought to regulate oligomerization (34,358). The LRRs of a number of proteins, including NOD2 and the Toll-like receptors, mediate interactions with the so-called pathogen-associated molecular patterns (PAMPs) found on many microbes (34,360–362).

Figure 68.9 also depicts the locations of the 29 known disease-associated *CIAS1* mutations (4–8,341–343,363). It is remarkable that all of the currently known mutations are found in exon 3, affecting the NACHT domain or the immediately flanking region of the cryopyrin protein. All 29 mutations represent missense changes, suggesting that more drastic mutations that result in a truncated or absent protein product may either lead to a different phenotype or

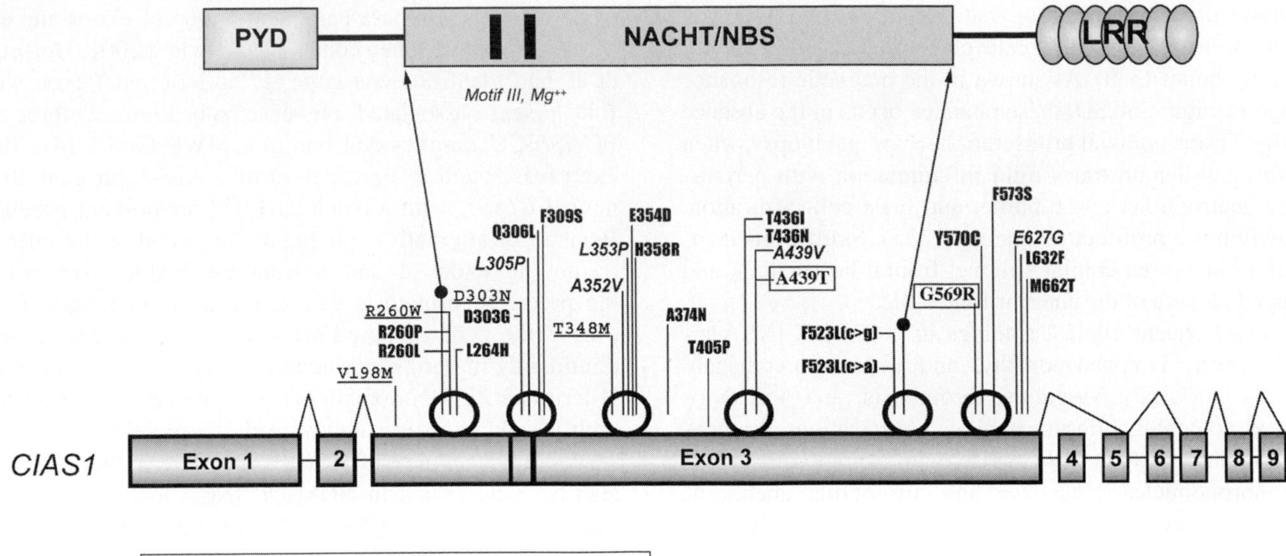

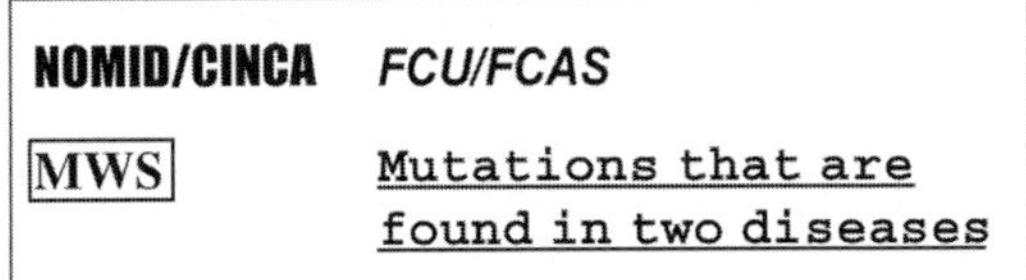

FIG. 68.9. Disease-associated mutations in the *CIAS1* gene, which encodes cryopyrin. The exon-intron structure of *CIAS1* is depicted in the lower part of the figure. Note that all 29 of the mutations that have been described to date in the literature are in exon 3, which encodes the NACHT/NBS domain, and that these mutations are grouped in 6 clusters. At the protein level, 22 of the 29 mutations are located within the NACHT/NBS domain of cryopyrin (depicted in the upper part of the figure), and 7 mutations are found in the immediately flanking region. Mutations depicted in **bold** have been observed in the neonatal-onset multisystem inflammatory disease (NOMID)/chronic infantile neurologic, cutaneous, and articular (CINCA) syndrome; mutations in *italics* have been observed in familial cold autoinflammatory syndrome (FCAS)/familial cold urticaria (FCU); *boxed* mutations have been observed in Muckle-Wells syndrome (MWS). Underlined mutations have been observed in more than one clinical condition: V198M and R260W in FCAS/FCU and MWS, and D303N and T348M in NOMID/CINCA and MWS. *PYD*, PYRIN domain; *LRR*, leucine-rich repeat domain.

be incompatible with life. A similar predilection for missense changes has been observed for *MEFV* and, in fact, the other periodic fever genes *(TNFRSF1A* and *MVK)* as well, suggesting that such changes may predispose to intermittent or fluctuating symptoms by somehow creating an unstable equilibrium.

It is also noteworthy that most of the known mutations are found in relatively small clusters, and in fact there are multiple "hits" at residues 260, 303, 436, 439, and 523. Although the crystal structure of cryopyrin is not yet known, computational modeling suggests that many of the mutations in the NACHT domain are located along the nucleotide-binding cleft or in a prolongation of the cleft in the three-dimensional structure, in regions involved in the "sensing" of the nucleotide-binding state (341). It is interesting to note that a comparison of the predicted three-dimensional structure of cryopyrin with that of NOD2/CARD15 indicates that the R260W mutation of cryopyrin and the Blau syndrome–associated R334W mutation of NOD2/CARD15 induce the same amino-acid change at a homologous, structurally conserved residue (364,365).

Limited genotype/phenotype correlations can also be observed. The Y570C, F309S, and F523L mutations have all been associated with severe disease (8,341), while the L353P mutation has been noted in four different North American families with FCAS/FCU, associated with a common ancestral founder haplotype (363). V198M and R260W have both been associated with two different disorders, FCAS/FCU and MWS, at the milder end of the severity spectrum (4–6,341), while D303N and T348M have been associated with MWS and NOMID/CINCA, at the more severe end of the spectrum (5,7,8,341–343). Nevertheless, even within individual clusters of mutations, there can be great phenotypic variability. For example, D303G/N, Q306L, and F309S are all associated with the severe end of the phenotypic spectrum, while L305P, in the same cluster, is found in FCAS/FCU.

Pathophysiology

Current concepts of the pathogenesis of the cryopyrinopathies revolve around our understanding of the modular domain structure of the cryopyrin protein. As is the case for the homologous domain in the FMF protein, the PYRIN domain of cryopyrin has been shown to interact specifically with the cognate domain in ASC (229,336,366). In various transfection systems, cryopyrin has been shown to regulate IL-1β secretion (232,234), NF-κB activation (229,235,336, 337,366), and apoptosis (229), and under some experimental conditions pyrin and cryopyrin appear to have mutually antagonistic effects (229).

The LRR of cryopyrin may exert an autoinhibitory effect, since NALP deletion mutations lacking the LRR are constitutively activated (233). This has given rise to the proposed pathophysiologic mechanism (34) shown in Figure 68.10. In this model, under baseline conditions the binding of the LRR to the NACHT domain inhibits the oligomerization of cryopyrin and consequent formation of multimeric complexes with ASC, which lead to the activation of IL-1β. Introduction of a hypothetical proinflammatory factor X, perhaps a bacterial protein, leads to a factor X/LRR interaction and subsequent release of the autoinhibitory effect of the LRR. In patients with NACHT domain mutations, the LRR/NACHT interaction may be less stable, perhaps allowing other perturbations, such as cold temperature, to release the autoinhibition and permit cryopyrin to activate the downstream cascade of inflammatory events. By this model, the interaction of wild-type cryopyrin with ASC leads to IL-1β maturation, with NACHT domain mutations leading to a gain of function. This contrasts

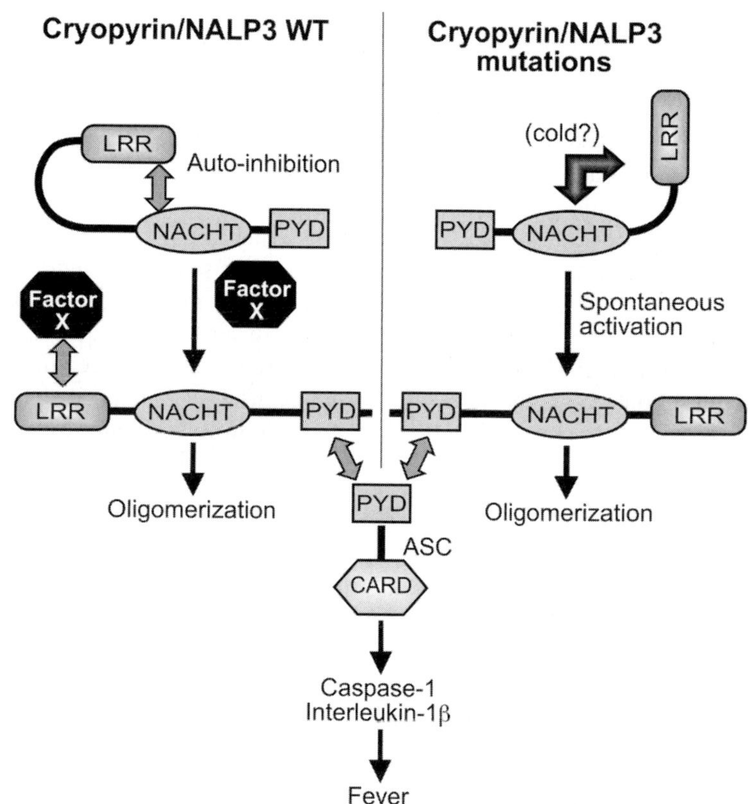

FIG. 68.10. Proposed role of the cryopyrin/NALP3 protein in interleukin (IL)-1β activation. **Left:** In unstimulated cells, the activity of cryopyrin/NALP3 is thought to be inhibited through the binding of the leucine-rich repeats (LRRs) to the NACHT domain, thereby inhibiting oligomerization and ASC binding. This autoinhibition is relieved through interactions with an unknown "factor X," thereby leading to oligomerization of cryopyrin/NALP3 and formation of macromolecular complexes with ASC. Such macromolecular complexes result in caspase-1 activation and IL-1β maturation, and consequently fever and inflammation. The effect of wild-type cryopyrin is therefore opposite to that hypothesized for pyrin in Figure 68.7. **Right:** Mutations found in the NACHT domain of cryopyrin/NALP3 in patients with autoinflammatory diseases might weaken the interaction between the LRRs and the remainder of the cryopyrin/NALP3 protein, resulting in decreased autoinhibition. Spontaneous activation might occur, resulting in inflammatory attacks. *PYD*, PYRIN domain; *LRR*, leucine-rich repeat domain; *CARD*, caspase activation and recruitment domain; *NACHT*, domain present in neuronal apoptosis inhibitor protein (NAIP), the major histocompatibility complex class II transactivator (CIITA), HET-E (incompatibility locus protein from *Podospora anserina*), and TP1 (mammalian telomerase-associated proteins); *ASC*, apoptosis-associated specklike protein with a CARD. (Adapted from Tschopp J, Martinon F, Burns K. NALPs: A novel protein family involved in inflammation. *Nature Rev Mol Cell Biol* 2003;4:95–104.)

with the model proposed for pyrin (Fig. 68.7), in which the interaction of wild-type pyrin with ASC inhibits IL-1β activation, with FMF-associated mutations leading to a loss of function. These two models are consistent with the respective dominant and recessive inheritance of autoinflammatory phenotypes for cryopyrin and pyrin, and with the aforementioned antagonism between the effects of these two proteins in transfection systems.

Based on this model, one would predict that IL-1β, NF-κB, and the regulation of apoptosis might each play a central role in the pathogenesis of the cryopyrinopathies. In a single patient with NOMID/CINCA, IL-1β precursor protein was found to be constitutively produced on Western analysis (8), but a systematic evaluation of the effect of cryopyrin mutations on IL-1β processing has not yet been published. The finding of high levels of *CIAS1* message in polymorphonuclear leukocytes and cultured chondrocytes has led to the suggestion that disease-associated mutations impair apoptosis in these cell types (7), but this hypothesis has not yet been tested. Other observations that may represent downstream effects of *CIAS1* mutations include the disease-associated fluctuation in serum IL-6 levels in two patients with MWS (367), and the increased expression of the activation marker CD10 on neutrophils from patients with NOMID/CINCA (368).

Diagnosis

Recurring fevers, early onset of urticaria-like skin rash, and elevated acute-phase proteins should raise the clinical suspicion of one of the cryopyrinopathies. Features that are helpful in distinguishing these conditions from the other hereditary periodic fever syndromes are listed in Table 68.3. As is the case for FMF, the diagnosis of FCAS/FCU, MWS, and NOMID/CINCA often involves a combination of clinical and molecular genetic data.

Using *CIAS1* mutational analysis as a tool in validation, a set of clinical criteria has recently been proposed for FCAS/FCU (20,338). The six criteria include: (a) recurrent intermittent episodes of fever and rash that primarily follow natural or experimental generalized cold exposure; (b) autosomal-dominant pattern of inheritance; (c) age of onset less than 6 months of age; (d) duration of most attacks less than 24 hours; (e) presence of conjunctivitis associated with attacks; and (f) absence of deafness, periorbital edema, lymphadenopathy, or serositis. In a large, genetically characterized FCAS/FCU family with 36 affected individuals and 37 unaffected individuals, using a threshold of four positive criteria led to a complete correlation with the known genotypes (20). It is not known how many, if any, individuals in the general population meet four of these criteria but do not have a demonstrable *CIAS1* mutation.

Besides the other cryopyrinopathies, the major differential diagnostic consideration in FCAS/FCU is distinguishing this condition from acquired cold urticaria (ACU). Among the distinctive features of the latter syndrome are an onset in adulthood, sporadic inheritance pattern, spontaneous remission within months to years, induction of symptoms with localized cold exposure (such as placing an ice cube on the skin), the presence of true urticaria with tissue mast cells and increased serum histamine, and, in some patients, the presence of angioedema, wheezing, or hypotension (338).

The cardinal clinical features of MWS include the typical "aguey bouts," as described previously, sensorineural hearing loss, and systemic amyloidosis (346). A systematic set of clinical criteria of the sort described for FCAS/FCU has not been formulated. Nevertheless, even taking the classic descriptions as the guideline, it is not known how many patients have clinical MWS without identifiable *CIAS1* mutations, although a few such patients are known to exist.

The clinical diagnosis of NOMID/CINCA is usually made based on the presence of episodic fever, early-onset urticarial rash, chronic meningitis, and arthropathy that can range from transient flares to marked deformity (339, 340,341). Based on the current literature, only about half of patients diagnosed with NOMID/CINCA by physicians familiar with the condition have identifiable mutations in *CIAS1* (7,8,341).

Physicians interested in molecular genetic testing should also be aware of certain technical issues, as well as the questions of sensitivity and specificity already noted. First, although the research papers describing *CIAS1* mutations in these disorders have generally screened the entire coding sequence for mutations, commercial diagnostic laboratories may focus only on exon 3, since this is where all of the currently known mutations are located. Although this strategy is likely to have a relatively high (but still unknown) sensitivity, it is possible that some mutations could be missed. Second, as is the case with most genes, single-nucleotide polymorphisms have also been identified in *CIAS1*, and thus any newly identified sequence variants should be screened on control populations before inferring a possible causal connection (363). As for FMF and all of the other Mendelian autoinflammatory disorders discussed in this chapter, a frequently updated database of mutations and polymorphisms for the cryopyrinopathies can be found on the Internet at *fmf.igh.cnrs.fr/infevers/*.

Treatment

Prior to the identification of *CIAS1* mutations in these disorders, there were no proven treatments for any of these three conditions. In FCAS/FCU, antihistamines are predictably ineffective in most patients (369), as is colchicine (338). NSAIDs have been used with modest effect to treat the arthralgia of FCAS/FCU, and high-dose corticosteroids are effective in some cases, but carry unacceptable side effects. Anabolic steroids (370) and gold salts have been helpful in a few patients. Colchicine (348) and high-dose steroids have been used to treat the attacks of MWS in some patients, with variable effects.

Attempts to treat NOMID/CINCA have also been disappointing (339,340). NSAIDs may palliate pain but are ineffective in attenuating inflammation. High-dose corticosteroids may have antipyretic and analgesic effects, but do not have significant effects on the cutaneous system, central nervous system, or joint manifestations. Cytotoxic agents have also been ineffective, and may have the potential to induce malignancy in these patients (24,371). Physical therapy and splinting does play an important role in preventing contractures.

Based on the discovery of mutations in *CIAS1* and the consequent pathophysiologic insights, there has been great interest in targeted biologic therapies, particularly aimed at the IL-1 pathway. A recent pilot study demonstrated rapid and dramatic effects, both on symptoms and acute-phase reactants, in two mutation–positive patients treated with the IL-1 receptor antagonist anakinra (372). Both of these patients harbored the R260W mutation, one with MWS and the other with the FCAS/FCU–MWS overlap syndrome. It will be important to replicate these results in a larger experience, and to test the efficacy of this strategy in patients with the more severe phenotype of NOMID/CINCA. Although perhaps less direct, other anticytokine therapies may also have a role in these disorders (373).

Tumor Necrosis Factor Receptor-Associated Periodic Syndrome

Besides MWS and FCAS/FCU, which present with a relatively distinctive rash, there remained, prior to 1999, a group of dominantly inherited, ethnically diverse periodic fever syndromes clinically more similar to FMF, most of which had been described in case reports of single families. The most thoroughly studied of these families was a large kindred of Irish/Scottish ancestry with a condition that had been termed familial Hibernian fever (26,374). A large Australian pedigree of Scottish ancestry was noted to have a similar condition (375), but this was called benign autosomal-dominant familial periodic fever because it was unclear that this family had the same condition as the first. Smaller families of Swedish (376), German (377,378), Finnish (379), Dutch (380), Austrian (381), mixed Irish/English/German (382,383), and Puerto Rican (383) ancestry had also been reported. While relatively prolonged (>1 week) attacks and poor responsiveness to colchicine were common themes, there were a number of clinical differences among these families, most notably the presence or absence of amyloidosis and the types of skin rash. In light of this ethnic diversity and clinical heterogeneity, it was not clear whether these dominantly inherited periodic fevers represented one or more mutations in a single locus, or mutations in several genes.

The first evidence that one genetic locus might account for a significant subset of these autosomal-dominant families came in 1998, when linkage studies placed the susceptibility loci for familial Hibernian fever and benign autosomal-dominant familial periodic fever in the same region of chromosome 12p13 (375,384). This interval harbors a number of plausible candidate genes, including CD4, LAG-3, and CD27 (all of which encode T-lymphocyte signaling molecules), the genes for the complement components C1r and C1s, and *TNFRSF1A*, the gene encoding the 55-kDa receptor for TNF-α (also known as p55, CD120a, and TNFR1). Within one year, six different *TNFRSF1A* mutations were reported in a series of seven families with dominantly inherited periodic fevers (12), including the Irish/Scottish familial Hibernian fever family, the Australian family of Scottish ancestry, the Finnish family, and the family of mixed Irish/English/German ancestry, all noted above. Another family with a *TNFRSF1A* mutation was of French-Canadian ancestry. Systemic amyloidosis was observed in at least one member of four of the seven families.

The term *TNF receptor-associated periodic syndrome* (TRAPS) was proposed as a nomenclature that would unify families of disparate ethnic backgrounds and clinical phenotypes sharing this common pathogenesis, while historical terms such as *familial Hibernian fever* could be retained to denote individual variants or for clinical diagnosis. The term *autosomal-dominant recurrent fever* (ADRF) has been proposed to include TRAPS, as well as other dominantly inherited periodic fevers not caused by mutations in *TNFRSF1A* (385).

The 5 years since the initial description of TRAPS as a distinct nosologic entity have witnessed major strides in our understanding of this condition. TRAPS is now recognized as the second most common hereditary periodic fever syndrome, behind FMF, and, as of this writing, 32 disease-associated *TNFRSF1A* mutations have been published (12, 386–397). Moreover, certain TRAPS-associated *TNFRSF1A* variants have recently been observed in association with other inflammatory disorders (388,393,398), underscoring the importance of the TNF pathway in the regulation of innate immunity in humans.

Clinical Features

As is the case for the other hereditary recurrent fever syndromes, TRAPS is manifested by episodes of fever and localized inflammation. Several of the important clinical features of TRAPS are listed and contrasted with the other hereditary recurrent fever syndromes in Table 68.3. Consistent with the original rationale for the TRAPS nomenclature, patients have been described from a wide range of ethnic groups, including those in which FMF (388,392,393) and HIDS (387,389,391,393,395) are common, as well as in African-American (388) and East Asian (395,399) populations. In general, the attacks of TRAPS tend to be longer than those associated with any of the other hereditary recurrent fever syndromes, although there is a great degree of variability, with some patients experiencing episodes similar in duration to FMF (393), and others manifesting attacks

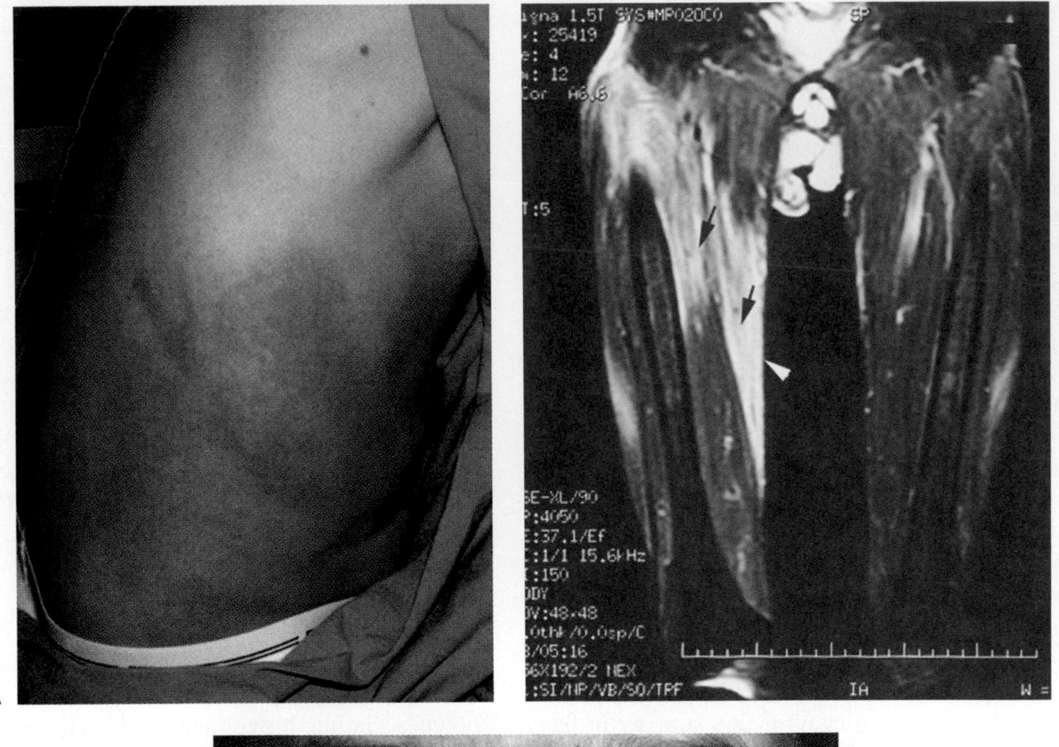

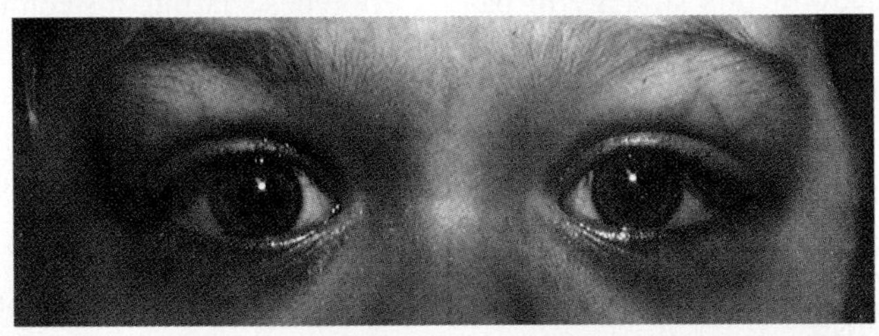

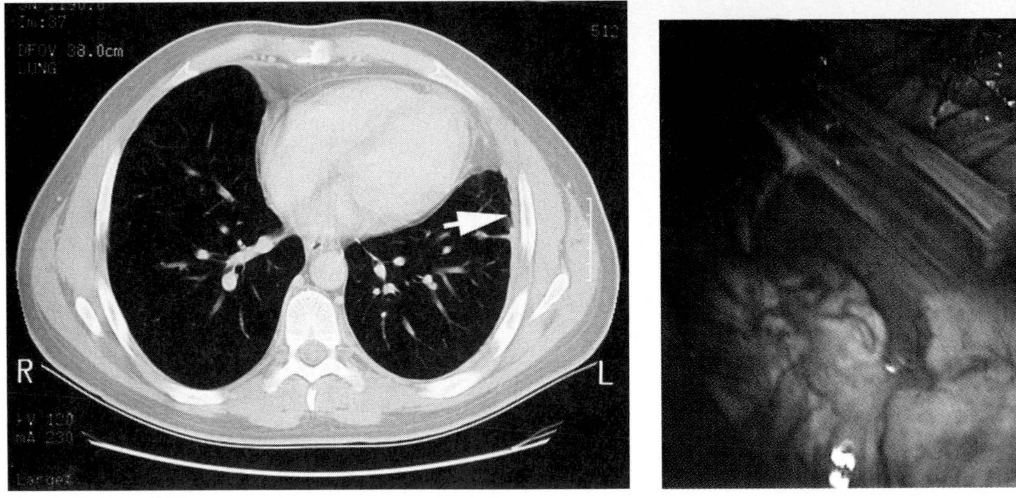

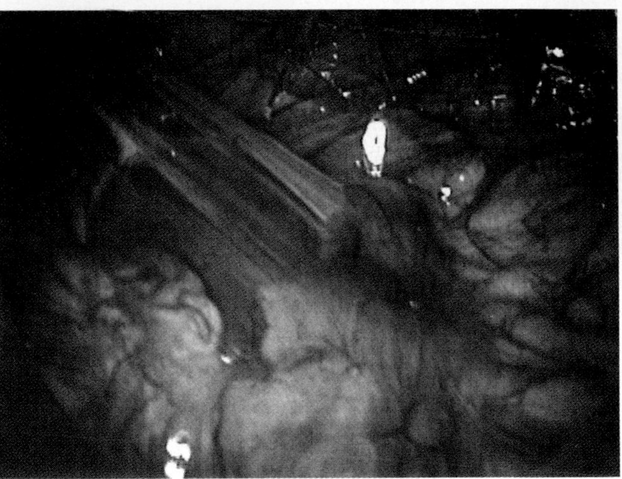

FIG. 68.11. Clinical features of the tumor necrosis factor (TNF) receptor-associated periodic syndrome (TRAPS). **A:** Migratory erythema on the flank of a patient with the T50M *TNFRSF1A* mutation. **B:** Sagittal view of the proximal thighs of a second patient with the T50M *TNFRSF1A* mutation using STIR magnetic resonance imaging, demonstrating edematous changes within muscle compartments, intraseptal regions (*black arrows*), and extending to the skin (*white arrowhead*). **C:** Bilateral periorbital edema in a 4-year-old girl with the H22Y mutation. **D:** Computed tomography with intravenous contrast of the chest from a third patient with the T50M *TNFRSF1A* mutation during active pleuritic symptoms, demonstrating an area of pleural thickening on the left chest wall (*arrow*). **E:** Peritoneal adhesions demonstrated during laparoscopic surgery in the same patient as in Panel C. (Panels A, B, and D from Hull KM, Drewe E, Aksentijevich I, et al. The TNF receptor-associated periodic syndrome (TRAPS). Emerging concepts of an autoinflammatory disorder. *Medicine (Baltimore)* 2002;81:349–368, with permission. Panel C from Toro JR, Aksentijevich I, Hull KM, et al. Tumor necrosis factor receptor-associated periodic syndrome: a novel syndrome with cutaneous manifestations. *Arch Dermatol* 2000;136:1487–1494, with permission.)

lasting more than 1 month at a time, or that are almost continuous (374).

The cutaneous manifestations of TRAPS can be quite distinctive (294,400). Perhaps the most characteristic rash is a migratory macular area of erythema, ranging in size from 1 to 28 cm, that can occur on the torso (Fig. 68.11A) or can migrate distally on an arm or a leg. Such lesions are tender and warm and blanch with pressure. Other cutaneous manifestations include annular patches and generalized serpiginous patches and plaques (294,400). Histologic examination usually demonstrates superficial and deep perivascular mononuclear infiltrates (400); less commonly a low-grade lymphocytic vasculitis may also be seen (374).

Migratory erythematous lesions on the limbs are often accompanied by myalgia in the underlying muscle groups. Magnetic resonance imaging demonstrates inflammatory changes extending into the muscle compartments (Fig. 68.11B). In one such case a full-thickness muscle biopsy demonstrated normal myofibrils but a severely destructive monocytic fasciitis (401). In another case lymphocytic vasculitis of the muscle was noted (402).

Ocular involvement is quite common in TRAPS, occurring in 90% of a recent series of 50 mutation-positive patients (294). Periorbital edema (Fig. 68.11C) was observed in 78% of those with ocular manifestations, and conjunctivitis was observed in almost 90%. Rarely, uveitis may also occur.

In addition to the clinical manifestations described above, which may be somewhat distinctive for TRAPS among the hereditary recurrent fevers, TRAPS patients commonly develop episodes of serositis. Over 90% of patients experience attacks of abdominal pain, which, like FMF, may present with findings of an acute abdomen. Pleurisy is also common, occurring in about half of patients, and sometimes is associated with findings on plain roentgenograms or CT (Fig. 68.11D). Pericarditis, although uncommon, may occur (393). Repeated serosal attacks can sometimes lead to adhesions, as illustrated in Figure 68.11E.

Arthralgia is more common during TRAPS attacks than frank arthritis. When it does occur, the arthritis of TRAPS is usually monoarticular and nonerosive, affecting mainly the hips, knees, or ankles. Tenosynovitis of the flexor and extensor tendons of the hands and feet has also been observed (294).

As is the case for FMF, male patients with TRAPS sometimes present with acute scrotal inflammation, probably due to inflammation of the tunica vaginalis. It is also interesting to note that 8 of 10 affected males in the original familial Hibernian fever family had inguinal hernias, compared with 1 of 21 unaffected male family members (374).

Local trauma and mild infections sometimes provoke attacks in TRAPS. Other frequently mentioned inciting factors include psychological stress and physical exertion. As is the case in FMF, pregnancy is sometimes associated with a remission or amelioration of attacks (374,396,403).

Patients with TRAPS mount a vigorous acute-phase response during their attacks, including a marked leukocytosis and thrombocytosis, an accelerated ESR, and elevated levels of CRP, SAA, fibrinogen, haptoglobin, and C3 complement. As is the case for both FMF and HIDS, IgA is frequently polyclonally increased. IgD levels are usually normal, but can be modestly elevated (391,393). A minority of patients have positive antinuclear antibodies, and low-titer anticardiolipin antibodies are also sometimes observed.

As noted, systemic amyloidosis has been found in at least one member of four of the seven families first reported with this condition. As is the case for FMF, the amyloidosis of TRAPS is of the AA type (295,389,390), and can cause renal or hepatic failure (294). As additional patients have been ascertained, more accurate estimates of the frequency of amyloidosis have been possible. In a series of 100 patients published in 2001 (388), 14 had this complication. With over twice that number of patients now reported in the literature, current estimates of the risk of amyloidosis in TRAPS are about 10%.

Genetics

The susceptibility gene for TRAPS was initially mapped to chromosome 12p13 (375,384), and was subsequently found to be *TNFRSF1A*, the gene encoding the 55-kDa receptor for the proinflammatory cytokine TNF-α (12). This receptor is found on a wide variety of cell types, and belongs to a family of proteins with repeating cysteine-rich extracellular domains (404–406; Fig. 68.12). A second, structurally related 75 kDa TNF receptor (variously denoted TNFRSF1B, p75, TNFR2, or CD120b) is expressed predominantly on leukocytes and endothelial cells and is encoded on chromosome 1p (407), and to date has not been associated with autoinflammatory disease. The TNFRSF1A protein has four extracellular cysteine-rich domains, a transmembrane domain, and an intracellular death domain. Five of the first six mutations identified (12) were single nucleotide substitutions leading to missense changes in highly conserved extracellular cysteines, thus disrupting the stability of the extracellular domains by preventing the formation of disulfide bonds. The sixth of these mutations, a threonine to methionine substitution adjacent to an extracellular cysteine, disrupts a conserved intrachain hydrogen bond. The dominant inheritance of TRAPS is likely to be due to the fact that signaling is induced through homotrimerization of this receptor (408), with structural modifications of even one of the three receptor molecules in the complex possibly disrupting necessary interactions.

At the time of this writing, there were a total of 32 published mutations (12,386–397), 15 of which involve substitutions at cysteine residues that disrupt conserved extracellular disulfide bonds (Fig. 68.12). Five cysteine residues are "hot spots" with more than one documented mutation. One mutation involves a splice site in intron 3, resulting in a transcript encoding four additional extracellular amino acids (388), and another mutation causes a single

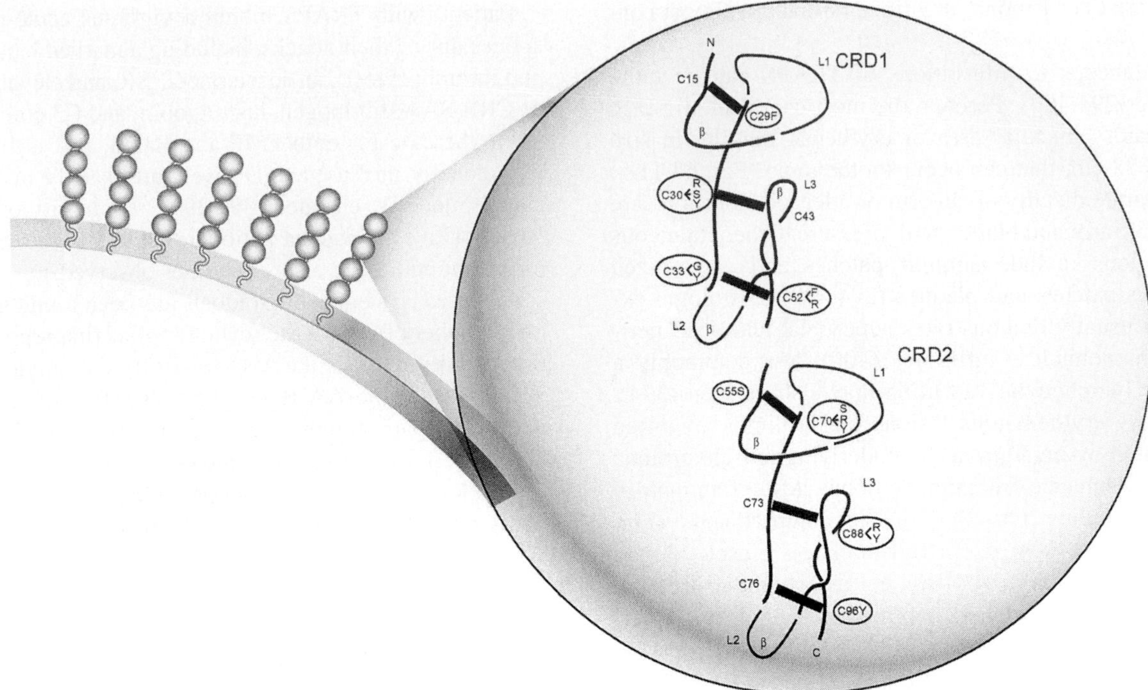

FIG. 68.12. *TNFRSF1A* mutations in the tumor necrosis factor (TNF) receptor-associated periodic syndrome (TRAPS). Representation of the crystallographically determined structure of the TNFRSF1A protein extracellular cysteine-rich domains (CRDs) 1 and 2. The three disulfide bonds of CRD1 and CRD2 are depicted by thick black bars. Only the 15 mutations resulting in substitutions at cysteine residues (of the 32 currently published mutations) are shown. Note that 8 of the 12 possible cysteine residues participating in disulfide bonds have been shown to be affected, and that multiple mutations have been identified at C30, C33, C52, C70, and C88. The β-turn positions indicated by "β"-loop domains are denoted as "L1–L3." (Adapted from Hull KM, Drewe E, Aksentijevich I, et al. The TNF receptor-associated periodic syndrome (TRAPS). Emerging concepts of an autoinflammatory disorder. *Medicine (Baltimore)* 2002;81:349–368, with permission.)

amino acid deletion (395). The remaining 15 mutations are single nucleotide changes leading to substitutions at noncysteine residues in the extracellular domains of TNFRSF1A. The two most common TRAPS mutations, R92Q and T50M, both fall into this latter group of noncysteine mutations, and the residues affected (R92 and T50) are both mutational "hot spots" at which other mutations (R92P, T50K) have also been reported. Thirty of the 32 mutations are in exons 2–4, and 30 of the 32 mutations are in the first two cysteine-rich domains (the two most distal to the membrane). One mutation is in the third cysteine-rich domain, and one encodes a substitution close to the membrane (I170N), near the site of metalloprotease-mediated ectodomain cleavage (discussed later in the chapter).

Although analysis of the first reported families suggested a penetrance of over 90% (12), a more complex picture has emerged with additional data. Two substitutions, R92Q and P46L, have been observed in about 1% of the Caucasian (388) and African-American and Arab populations (388,392,393), and appear to be low-penetrance mutations. R92Q has been observed at increased frequency in an early arthritis clinic (388) and in association with atherosclerosis (398), but does not seem to affect the severity of RA (409). In one patient the P46L mutation has been associated with Crohn disease and amyloidosis (393). Overall, the penetrance of cysteine mutations appears to be higher than the penetrance on noncysteine substitutions (388). Cysteine mutations may also be associated with a higher risk of amyloidosis (388), although it is important to note that this complication has been observed in patients with noncysteine mutations as well (388, 393,395).

In several large series, there are both families and isolated individuals who have a TRAPS-like illness but do not have mutations in the coding region of *TNFRSF1A* (388,393,395). Such data suggest that there may be additional loci that cause the TRAPS phenotype.

Pathophysiology

There are a number of possible mechanisms by which mutations in the p55 TNF receptor could cause an autoinflammatory disorder. In the initial description of TRAPS (12), data were presented against the possibility that the

C52F mutation increases the affinity of the receptor for its ligand, or that this mutation leads to constitutive activation. This latter mechanism has been observed for certain other cytokine receptors when the disruption of intrachain disulfide bonds permits the formation of interchain disulfide bonds, leading to receptor aggregation and ligand-independent activation (410). Alternatively, evidence was presented that leukocytes from patients with the C52F mutation have a defect in the activation-induced ectodomain cleavage of the p55 TNF receptor (12) (Fig. 68.13). Normally, proinflammatory stimuli induce metalloproteases that promote the shedding of the extracellular domains of both the p55 and p75 TNF receptors (411,412). This cleavage may contribute to the clearance of these receptors from the membrane, thereby preventing repeated signaling, and producing a pool of soluble receptors that may attenuate the inflammatory response by competing with membrane-bound receptors for ligand (413).

In patients with the C52F mutation, there was very little clearance of the p55 TNF receptor from the cell surface upon activation, and markedly reduced release of p55 into the supernatants, relative to controls. In contrast, activation-induced shedding of the p75 TNF receptor was normal. Consistent with these observations, granulocytes and monocytes from these patients expressed very high levels of membrane p55 TNF receptor, and soluble levels of p55 in the blood were inappropriately low. Since all but one of the documented mutations in the p55 protein are remote from the asparagine 172–valine 173 site where receptor cleavage actually occurs, the inhibition of cleavage is presumably due to the structural aberrations caused by disrupting extracellular disulfide bonds.

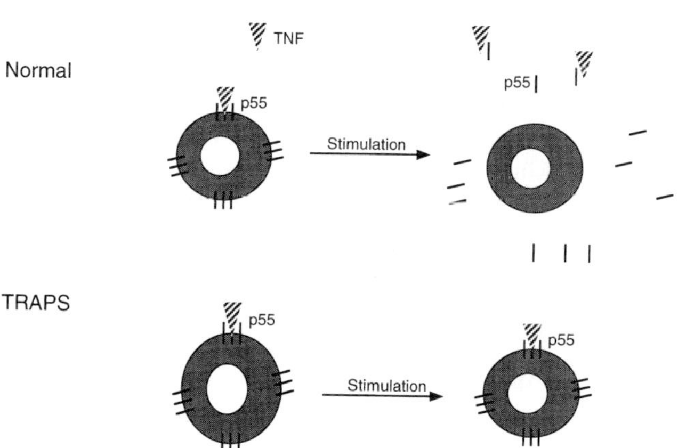

FIG. 68.13. Impaired shedding of mutant p55 tumor necrosis factor (TNF) receptors. In normal physiology, stimulation with proinflammatory cytokines leads to cleavage of p55 TNF receptors by metalloproteases, thereby preventing repeated signaling, and producing a pool of soluble receptors that may attenuate the inflammatory response by competing with membrane-bound receptors. In many, but not all, patients with the TNF receptor-associated periodic syndrome (TRAPS), normal receptor shedding does not occur.

Subsequently, p55 receptor shedding has been studied in a total of 15 TRAPS-associated mutations. Impaired receptor shedding has been observed by flow cytometry in 9, including H22Y, C30S, C33G, P46L, T50M, T50K, C52F, F112I, and I170N (which is very close to the cleavage site), but not in T37I, ΔD42, C52R, the splice mutation, N65I, or R92Q (12,388,394,395). Moreover, impaired ectodomain cleavage does not seem to correlate with disease severity. Inappropriately low soluble serum p55 levels are seen in a broader spectrum of patients (395). These data suggest that there must be additional mechanisms by which *TNFRSF1A* mutations cause autoinflammatory disease. Possibilities include effects on ligand-binding, on ligand-independent receptor association (414), and on the relative balance of signaling through p55 and p75 TNF receptors.

As previously noted, there are a number of downstream effects of these mutations, with marked elevations in acute-phase proteins. In addition, IL-6 levels have been noted to be increased during febrile attacks (415).

Diagnosis

As with the other two hereditary periodic fever syndromes, the cornerstone of diagnosis is a clinical index of suspicion. Table 68.3 compares TRAPS with FMF, HIDS, FCAS/FCU, MWS, and NOMID/CINCA. TRAPS can be distinguished from systemic-onset juvenile chronic arthritis and adult-onset Still disease by virtue of fever pattern, the clinical course of the arthritis, and the cutaneous manifestations.

Although there are several clinical features that may strongly suggest the diagnosis, the gold standard is the identification of *TNFRSF1A* mutations. Current experience suggests a broadening clinical spectrum with the identification of new mutations, and therefore it is likely that some new diagnoses will be unexpected, at least until the full clinical range is described. Conversely, there are at least a small number of families, and a larger number of sporadic cases, that clinically resemble TRAPS but do not have identifiable *TNFRSF1A* mutations (388,393,395).

The percentage of patients with suspected TRAPS who are mutation-positive depends greatly on the characteristics of the patient base and the experience of the clinician, but is below 20% in major referral centers (388,393,395). Moreover, the distribution of soluble serum p55 levels among mutation-negative suspected TRAPS patients can be high, normal, or low; soluble p55 levels for mutation-positive patients are usually low, but can be "pseudonormalized" with inflammatory attacks or renal insufficiency (395).

As is the case for the other hereditary recurrent fever syndromes, TRAPS patients who are mutation-positive often ask whether other asymptomatic family members should undergo genetic screening. In some cases, detailed interviews with allegedly asymptomatic relatives raise a sufficient index of suspicion to warrant testing, and testing may also be advisable in families with a strong history of TRAPS-associated amyloidosis. However, for those cases where the suspicion is low and there is no history of amyloidosis, the desire to know should be balanced against the possibility of finding a mutation with reduced penetrance, and the potential impact that a genetic variant of uncertain significance would have on insurability. It should also be noted that several cases of *de novo TNFRSF1A* mutations have been described in the literature (392,395).

A number of practical issues should also be addressed in connection with genetic testing. First, it is unfortunately the case that two different numbering systems are used to denote *TNFRSF1A* mutations. The convention used throughout this chapter, and in most published reports (12,386–395,397), begins the numbering of residues at the leucine that follows the cleavage of the signal peptide. The alternate numbering system, which includes the signal peptide, results in designations that are 29 *greater* than those reported here. For example, the mutation that is denoted R92Q here would be called R121Q in the alternate system. Second, whenever potential new mutations are reported, one should be aware of the possibility that the substitution is a benign polymorphism. This issue should be addressed with mutational screens of ethnically matched controls. For a frequently updated source of both mutations and polymorphisms in *TNFRSF1A,* the reader is referred to the INFEVERS website at *fmf.igh.cnrs.fr/infevers/.*

Prognosis and Treatment

The prognosis of TRAPS is largely dependent on whether a patient develops amyloidosis. As previously noted, the most recent data indicate that the overall risk of amyloidosis in TRAPS is about 10%. The risk may be somewhat higher among patients with cysteine mutations (388), although it is important to remember that the risk is not zero for the noncysteine mutations (388,393,395). A positive family history for amyloidosis may also be a risk factor.

Prior to the discovery of *TNFRSF1A* mutations, many patients with TRAPS were treated with colchicine because of the similarities with FMF. Daily colchicine prevents neither the acute attacks nor the amyloidosis of TRAPS (294,295). NSAIDs can be used in mild attacks, with corticosteroids reserved for more severe cases. Patients respond within hours to the latter therapy, but symptoms may not completely resolve, and, over time, serious toxicities may develop.

Based on the intrinsic role of the TNF-α pathway in TRAPS, there has been considerable interest in biologic interventions that target this pathway. The largest experience to date is with etanercept, the recombinant p75 TNFR:Fc fusion protein. Pilot studies using etanercept at the usual adult dose for RA (25 mg subcutaneously twice weekly), or at the pediatric dose for juvenile RA (0.4 mg/kg subcutaneously twice weekly), have demonstrated a favorable effect on both clinical and laboratory parameters (13,294,416,417). In a series of seven patients, five corticosteroid-responsive patients with the C33Y mutation demonstrated reductions in steroid requirements and acute-phase reactants while on twice weekly etanercept (418), while responses in two steroid refractory patients with the R92Q mutation were less convincing. Preliminary results from an open-label series of 15 patients with a broader spectrum of mutations demonstrated significant dose-dependent reductions in symptoms, in the use of other antiinflammatory medications, and in acute-phase reactants (419). Parameters were compared between 3-month baseline, twice-weekly treatment, thrice-weekly treatment, and washout phases.

For TRAPS patients with relatively infrequent episodes, intermittent etanercept dosing has been tried with beneficial effects (391,397). Such a regimen might not have an impact on amyloid deposition, if this were a major concern. The effect of twice or thrice weekly etanercept on amyloid deposition may depend on the magnitude of SAA elevations in the blood. One patient with the C33Y mutation and nephrotic proteinuria experienced a marked reduction (but not a normalization) in proteinuria within 3 months of beginning twice weekly etanercept, with evidence of regression of amyloidosis by radionuclide serum amyloid P-scanning within 7 months of beginning treatment (420). On the other hand, a patient with the C52F mutation and a strong family history of amyloidosis developed nephrotic range proteinuria despite a dramatic symptomatic response to etanercept (421). The latter observation suggests that monitoring of SAA levels, or radionuclide scanning, may be important in titrating therapy in TRAPS patients at especially high risk of developing amyloidosis.

Hyperimmunoglobulinemia D Syndrome

In 1984 van der Meer and colleagues (27) first described the hyperimmunoglobulinemia D with periodic fever syndrome (HIDS) in six patients of Dutch ancestry. During the subsequent 15 years a great deal was learned about the clinical and immunologic features of this disorder, and by 1999 a registry of 144 patients had been established (422). That same year, two groups independently reported the somewhat surprising discovery that mutations in *MVK*, the gene encoding the cholesterol biosynthetic enzyme mevalonate kinase, cause HIDS (35,36,423). The ramifications of this finding are likely to extend far beyond the family of systemic autoinflammatory disorders to provide important insights into the pathogenesis and treatment of inflammation in a much broader setting.

Clinical Features

HIDS is contrasted with the other hereditary periodic fever syndromes in Table 68.3. To date, about half of reported HIDS patients are of Dutch ancestry; most of the remainder are from Europe (preponderantly from the northern part of France), although cases have been reported from Japan, Turkey, and the United States (15,424–427). HIDS presents in early childhood, with a median age of onset of 6 months (422,424). The gender ratio of HIDS patients is about 1:1 (422). Patients experience recurrent high fevers, often heralded by chills and headache, that gradually decrease after 3 to 7 days. There is considerable variability in the intervals between attacks, but the usual is every 4 to 8 weeks. Provocative factors include childhood immunizations, trauma, surgery, menses, and minor infections. The frequency of attacks tends to be highest during childhood and adolescence (15).

Abdominal pain occurs frequently with attacks. Peritoneal irritation is much less common than in FMF, although it can occur, and may lead to adhesions (424). Diarrhea is more likely than constipation, and vomiting is also a frequent manifestation. Arthralgia is often present during attacks, and about 70% of patients develop a nondestructive arthritis, usually associated with the febrile episodes (424,428–430). As in FMF, arthritis is seen with greater frequency in younger patients, tends to affect the large joints, and is characterized by a large influx of polymorphonuclear leukocytes into the synovial space. Unlike FMF, HIDS arthritis frequently occurs with abdominal pain and is often polyarticular; protracted HIDS arthritis has not been observed.

Cutaneous lesions are very common during the attacks of HIDS (424,431). Often there are widespread, occasionally painful, erythematous macules 0.5 to 2 cm in diameter, with the larger lesions developing an annular appearance. Unlike the erysipeloid erythema of FMF, there is no predilection for the lower legs, and unlike the erythematous patches of TRAPS, the lesions of HIDS are not usually migratory. Sometimes the rash of HIDS can manifest as a diffuse erythematous macular and papular eruption, even affecting the palms and soles, as illustrated in Figure 68.14. Other cutaneous manifestations of HIDS include erythematous papules and nodules, urticaria, and a morbilliform rash. Histologic examination shows varying degrees of cutaneous vasculitis, with perivascular inflammatory cells; immunofluorescence may show deposits of IgD, IgM, or C3. Henoch-Schönlein purpura (428) and erythema elevatum diutinum (a chronic benign variant of cutaneous necrotizing vasculitis) (426) have also been reported in children with HIDS. Aphthous ulcers of the mouth and vagina have also been observed in HIDS.

Pleurisy and pericarditis have not been observed in HIDS. One patient with recurrent scrotal involvement was recently reported (432). There are no published cases of amyloidosis in HIDS (15), although it has been found in the mother and maternal uncle of one patient (424). In contrast with the other hereditary periodic fevers, HIDS is characterized by diffuse tender lymphadenopathy, most prominent in the neck during attacks. Severe headache is also common during attacks (424), although there are no data regarding cerebrospinal fluid or imaging studies in these patients. Splenomegaly is also observed during febrile episodes in about 50% of children.

Patients with HIDS often exhibit accelerated ESRs, leukocytosis, elevated CRP levels, and sometimes transient hematuria during attacks (15,424,433). Before the identification of *MVK* as the causative gene, the observation of polyclonally elevated IgD levels (>100 U/mL, or >14.1 mg/dL) on two occasions at least 1 month apart (424) was thought to be definitive for the diagnosis. The recent identification of mutation-positive patients with typical clinical findings without elevated IgD levels (35,432–434) has brought this latter point into question. There is no correlation between the IgD level and the frequency or intensity of attacks. IgA levels, primarily of the IgA1 subclass, are also frequently elevated in HIDS patients (424,433,435,436). During attacks, elevated levels of mevalonic acid can usually be detected in the urine (35,36,437,438).

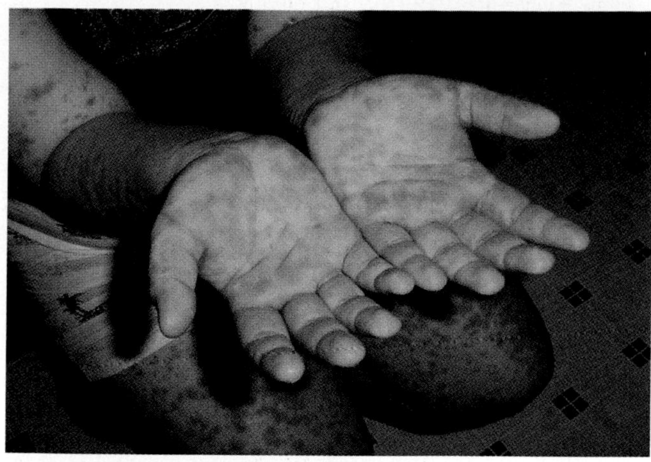

FIG. 68.14. Diffuse erythematous macular and papular rash in a patient with hyperimmunoglobulinemia D syndrome. This patient, of mixed Albanian and Irish ancestry, was found to have the V377I mutation and a mutation resulting in the deletion of exon 3 in the mevalonate kinase cDNA. (From Takada K, Aksentijevich I, Mahadevan V, et al. Favorable preliminary experience with etanercept in two patients with the hyperimmunoglobulinemia D and periodic fever syndrome. *Arthritis Rheum* 2003;48:2645–2651, with permission.)

Genetics

HIDS is inherited as a single-gene, autosomal-recessive trait with nearly complete penetrance (18,422). Linkage studies in affected families excluded a susceptibility locus in the *MEFV* region of chromosome 16p (18,439), as well as in the immunoglobulin heavy chain region of chromosome 14q (18).

The susceptibility gene for HIDS was identified by two independent groups who used very different strategies. One group specializing in metabolic diseases made the fortuitous observation that a patient with the clinical picture of HIDS, but without elevated IgD levels, had abnormal levels of mevalonic acid in the urine during febrile crises (35). Urine studies of two other patients with more typical HIDS yielded similar results; mutational screening of *MVK* in four patients produced three different missense substitutions (proline for histidine at residue 20, H20P; threonine for isoleucine at residue 268, I268T; and isoleucine for valine at residue 377, V377I). Biochemical assays of skin fibroblasts from patients harboring these mutations demonstrated 1% to 3% of the mevalonate kinase enzymatic activity found in control fibroblasts.

The second group performed linkage analysis in families with HIDS to localize the causative gene to chromosome 12q24 (36), which contains *MVK*. Mutations in *MVK* that lead to complete deficiency of enzymatic activity were already known to be associated with periodic fevers, lymphadenopathy, arthralgia, rash, and abdominal distress, as might be seen in HIDS, but such patients also manifest several other features, including cataracts, mental retardation, hypotonia, and failure to thrive (440–442). Reasoning that the hyperimmunoglobulinemia D syndrome might be the result of less severe mutations, this group screened 16 families for *MVK* mutations. In addition to the I268T and V377I mutations already noted, a missense mutation substituting leucine for proline at residue 165 (P165L), a 92 base pair (bp) deletion at the 5′ end of the gene, and the absence of expression of one allele, were also described. Biochemical studies demonstrated low levels of enzymatic activity in patients' fibroblasts, and increased urinary excretion of mevalonic acid during febrile attacks.

MVK is an 11-exon gene (443,444) on chromosome 12q, encoding a 396 amino-acid protein (445). Since the initial identification of *MVK* mutations as the cause of HIDS, more than 20 mutations have been published (432,434, 443,444,446,447), and, as is the case for FMF, the cryopyrinopathies, and TRAPS, updated lists of *MVK* mutations and polymorphisms are maintained at the INFEVERS website at: *fmf.igh.cnrs.fr/infevers/*. HIDS-associated mutations are distributed throughout the coding sequence, while the phenotypically much more severe mutations associated with mevalonic aciduria are clustered around the sequences encoding enzymatically active sites in the protein.

A very high percentage of patients with HIDS have at least one copy of the V377I *MVK* mutation. Recent population studies indicate that carriers for this mutation share a common DNA haplotype, suggesting an ancestral relationship (448). Approximately 0.6% of the population in the Netherlands are carriers for this mutation (448,449). A recent analysis of the distribution of this variant among individuals carrying *MVK* mutations indicated a marked underrepresentation of homozygotes for V377I in HIDS (449), suggesting that homozygotes for this mutation may exhibit a much milder phenotype than individuals with other combinations of mutations, or perhaps no disease phenotype at all.

Pathophysiology

Mevalonate kinase is a homodimeric peroxisomal enzyme that catalyzes the conversion of mevalonic acid to 5-phosphomevalonic acid (Fig. 68.15) in the synthesis of sterols (cholesterol, steroid hormones, vitamin D, and bile salts) and nonsterol isoprene compounds (423,450,451). The latter compounds are involved in a wide variety of cellular functions, including electron transport (ubiquinones and heme A), protein glycosylation (dolichols), protein synthesis (isopentene tRNA), and prenylation of adenine transduction proteins (farnesylated and geranylated proteins). This latter process is important to the function of several intermediates of signal transduction, including the Ras, Rho/Rac, and Rab families of small GTP binding proteins (452).

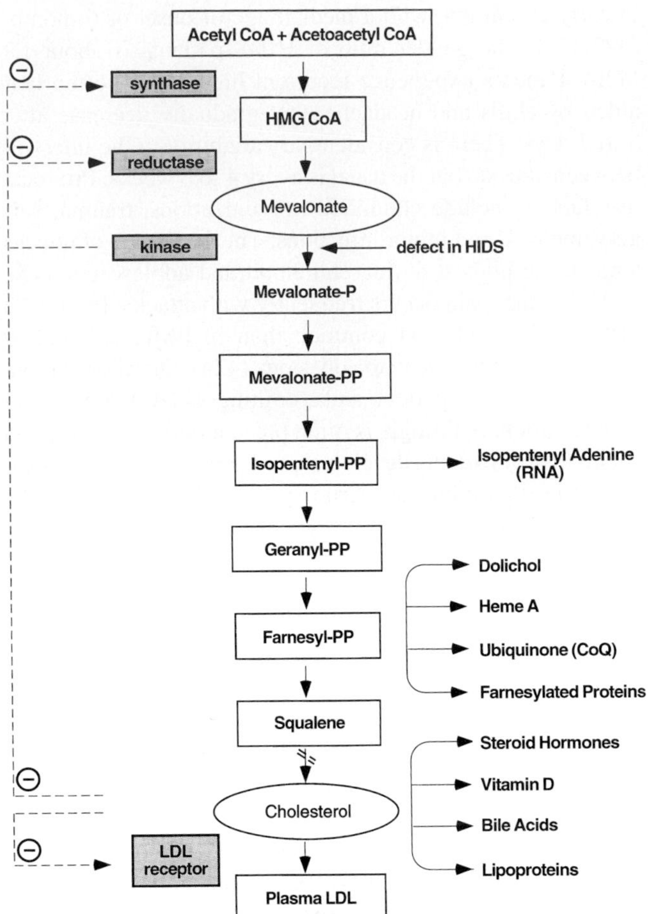

FIG. 68.15. The mevalonate pathway. Patients with the hyperimmunoglobulinemia D syndrome have mutations in the mevalonate kinase gene, leaving 1% to 3% residual enzymatic activity. Patients with mevalonic aciduria have more profound loss-of-function mutations.

The mutations associated with HIDS lead to markedly reduced, but not absent, mevalonate kinase enzyme activity (35,36). Decreased mevalonate kinase activity leads to induction of 3-hydroxy-3-methylglutaryl (HMG)–CoA reductase (453), the enzyme immediately preceding mevalonate kinase in the pathway, accumulation of mevalonate, and a consequent increase in urinary levels of this compound (Fig. 68.16). Recent comparisons of cell lines harboring wild-type or V377I mutant mevalonate kinase indicate that the mutant enzyme functions best at 30°C, and that the residual

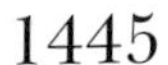

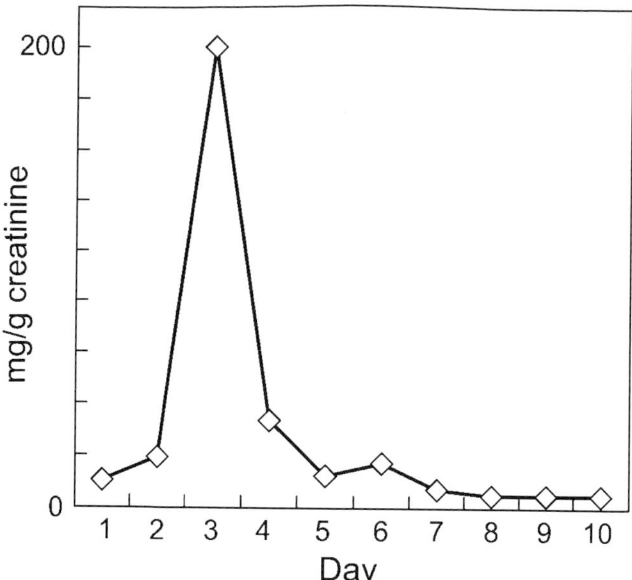

FIG. 68.16. Urinary mevalonate levels during an attack of the hyperimmunoglobulinemia D syndrome. Daily measurements of the urinary mevalonate in the same patient depicted in Figure 68.14 revealed elevated baseline levels and a significant spike during a typical febrile attack (normal range mean ± SD, 0.40 ± 0.18 mg/g creatinine). (From Takada K, Aksentijevich I, Mahadevan V, et al. Favorable preliminary experience with etanercept in two patients with the hyperimmunoglobulinemia D and periodic fever syndrome. *Arthritis Rheum* 2003;48: 2645–2651, with permission.)

activity present at 37°C is markedly diminished at 39°C (454). This observation may explain the frequently noted association of HIDS attacks with childhood immunizations and upper respiratory infections, as well as the spikes in urinary mevalonate that coincide with attacks (Fig. 68.16).

It is unlikely that febrile attacks are triggered or exacerbated by the increased mevalonate blood mevalonate levels, since two patients with mevalonic aciduria developed febrile attacks when treated with the HMG–CoA reductase inhibitor lovastatin (441). It is also unlikely that cholesterol deficiency is the cause of HIDS, since the serum cholesterol levels in patients are only slightly diminished (422), and there is little clinical similarity with other disorders of the mevalonate pathway, such as the Smith-Lemli-Opitz syndrome, in which cholesterol deficiency is important to the pathogenesis (423,442).

Although the connection between the mevalonate pathway and IgD remains somewhat obscure, there are data indicating that elevated IgD in the serum contributes to the pathogenesis of the autoinflammatory syndrome by potentiating the release of proinflammatory cytokines (455). Nevertheless, as noted earlier, rare patients have the clinical features of HIDS and mutations in *MVK* with normal serum IgD levels. Other points against an essential role for IgD elevations in this disorder include (a) febrile attacks may precede IgD elevation; (b) the frequency and intensity of attacks do not correlate with IgD levels; (c) IgD levels do not fluctuate with attacks; and (d) IgD-containing immune complexes are present in the sera of patients with elevated IgD, regardless of whether they have HIDS (424,435).

Other immunologic abnormalities noted during attacks include substantial elevations of serum IL-6, IFN-γ and soluble type-II phospholipase A_2, as well as modest elevations of TNF-α. Circulating IL-1 receptor antagonist and soluble p55 and p75 TNF receptors are also increased during attacks, but serum IL-1α, IL-1β, and IL-10 are not (456). During attacks urinary levels of neopterin and leukotriene E_4 are also elevated (457,458). Moreover, unstimulated peripheral blood mononuclear cells from patients with HIDS release more IL-1β, IL-6, and TNF-α than controls, and supernatants from patients' mononuclear cells induce mRNA for acute-phase proteins in Hep3B cells (459).

It is possible that the excessive production of proinflammatory cytokines by HIDS mononuclear cells may be tied to deficiencies in isoprenoids normally synthesized through the mevalonate pathway. In an *in vitro* model system, antigen-stimulated IL-1β secretion was accentuated in HIDS mononuclear cells, an effect that was accentuated by lovastatin and reduced by mevalonate, farnesol, and geranylgeraniol (460). Although not examined in this study, it is possible that the small GTP binding proteins, which undergo prenylation, may be the link between the mevalonate pathway and the febrile attacks of HIDS.

Diagnosis

Although the identification of mutations in *MVK* has opened the door to DNA testing, it has also uncovered new complexities. Prior to the discovery of the underlying gene, the diagnosis was, of necessity, made by documenting elevations in serum IgD levels (>100 IU/mL, or >14.1 mg/dL) on two occasions at least one month apart, with a compatible clinical history. In many cases, a diagnosis of HIDS made in this way agrees with genetic testing, or with the demonstration of increased levels of urinary mevalonate during febrile episodes, and such cases are now sometimes referred to as "classic-type HIDS" (461).

However, in a recent series, about one-fourth of patients meeting clinical criteria for HIDS were mutation-negative, prompting the designation "variant-type HIDS" (461). In this study, classic-type HIDS patients had lower mevalonate kinase activity, higher serum IgD levels, and more symptoms with their attacks than patients with the variant type. Moreover, as previously noted, there are a small number of patients with genetic and biochemical disease who have normal serum IgD levels (35,432–434). Some authors have suggested that patients with genetic/biochemical disease should be denoted "Dutch-type periodic fever," regardless of their IgD levels (433). Given a suitable index of suspicion of HIDS, it is reasonable to take the combined approach of measuring serum IgD levels and undertaking either genetic or biochemical testing. Many DNA diagnostic laboratories perform an initial screen for the two most common HIDS mutations, V377I and I268T, before undertaking more extensive sequencing.

There are a number of conditions associated with elevated serum IgD levels that do not manifest the clinical features of HIDS. These include IgD multiple myeloma, Hodgkin disease, cigarette smoking, diabetes mellitus, pregnancy, hyperimmunoglobulinemia E syndrome, ataxia telangiectasia, acquired immunodeficiency syndrome and other immunodeficiency disorders, and recurrent infections (e.g., tuberculosis and aspergillosis) (424,435,462). Features that help distinguish mevalonic aciduria from HIDS include almost absent levels of mevalonate kinase activity, short stature, ataxia, and ocular involvement (463).

Key clinical differences between HIDS and FMF, FCAS/FCU, MWS, NOMID/CINCA, and TRAPS are summarized in Table 68.3. It bears emphasis that the serum IgD level may not be a useful discriminator in an individual case, since a small percentage of patients with the other two hereditary periodic fever syndromes will also have elevated levels (391,393,439,464). In children it is important to distinguish HIDS from systemic-onset juvenile chronic arthritis (Still disease). In addition to the differential diagnostic considerations discussed for juvenile chronic arthritis and FMF, the presence of pleurisy or pericarditis favors juvenile chronic arthritis over HIDS.

Prognosis and Treatment

HIDS does not seem to have a major effect on longevity (422,424). Attacks tend to be more severe during childhood, and to ameliorate after adolescence (422). Despite the similarity with FMF, most patients do not respond to colchicine, although a few may. Variable results have also been observed with cyclosporine, intravenous immunoglobulin, and corticosteroids. Articular manifestations may respond either to NSAIDs or corticosteroids. Although lovastatin has precipitated exacerbations in classic mevalonic aciduria (441), preliminary experience with this class of drugs has been encouraging (422), and randomized trials are now underway.

Given recent findings regarding cytokine abnormalities in HIDS, there is considerable interest in therapies that target these inflammatory mediators. A small trial of thalidomide, an inhibitor of TNF-α production, IFN-γ secretion, and leukocyte chemotaxis, resulted in nonsignificant decreases in the CRP and SAA, without an effect on the attack rate (465). In contrast, a pilot study of etanercept in two mutation-positive patients demonstrated dramatic effects on symptoms (434). To date there are no published studies on IL-1 inhibition in HIDS.

Pyogenic Arthritis with Pyoderma Gangrenosum and Acne

Although not usually categorized as one of the hereditary recurrent fevers, PAPA syndrome is included in this discussion for several reasons. Clinically, PAPA syndrome can present with fever as well as recurrent episodes of pyogenic arthritis, but without evidence of autoantibodies or antigen-specific T cells, and therefore falls under the rubric of the autoinflammatory recurrent arthritic syndromes discussed in this chapter. Genetically, it is inherited as an autosomal-dominant trait, like all of the hereditary recurrent fever syndromes. The underlying gene has recently been shown to encode a protein that interacts with pyrin, the prototypic hereditary periodic fever protein.

PAPA syndrome was first described in a large family seen at the Mayo Clinic (22), and 3 years later was independently described as familial recurrent arthritis by a group in Dallas (466). Both families manifested an episodic, mono- or pauciarticular, nonaxial destructive arthritis beginning in childhood. The elbows, shoulders, knees, and ankles were most often affected; some episodes occurred after minor trauma. Similar to FMF, synovial fluid was purulent, but cultures were uniformly negative. Synovial biopsy in a patient from the second family demonstrated a polymorphonuclear infiltrate, without evidence of immunoglobulin or complement deposits by immunofluorescence. Unlike the usual case with FMF, the arthritis often led to periosteal proliferation and, in some cases, ankylosis. Articular manifestations usually preceded the cutaneous manifestations.

Skin disease in PAPA syndrome tends to develop around the time of puberty. Figure 68.17A illustrates pyoderma gangrenosum covering nearly the entire forearm in a teenage boy. As is the case for PAPA-associated arthritis, pyoderma gangrenosum is sometimes induced by trauma, and may evolve from an erythematous pustule to a necrotic ulcer within days. Histologically, there is an intense infiltrate of polymorphonuclear leukocytes, without evidence of vasculitis. Severe cystic acne, usually localized to the face, chest, or back (Fig. 68.17B), is also common. Both lesions are extremely painful, often necessitating the use of narcotic analgesics. Some patients also manifest the phenomenon of pathergy, with sterile abscess formation at the site of injections or phlebotomy.

Other possibly related clinical manifestations that were not observed in all members of the Mayo Clinic family included adult-onset insulin-dependent diabetes mellitus, membranous glomerulonephritis, and cytopenias induced by sulfonamides. During inflammatory flares, laboratory findings in all affected individuals of both families included leukocytosis, a brisk acute-phase response, and anemia of chronic disease. Investigation of serum immunoglobulins, complement, rheumatoid factor, antinuclear antibodies, and anticardiolipin antibodies were uniformly normal/negative in the two families.

Genetic studies established linkage to the long arm of chromosome 15 in both families (466,467). Within two years, two different missense mutations in the gene encoding CD2-binding protein 1 (CD2BP1), or proline serine threonine phosphatase interacting protein (PSTPIP1), were identified in the respective families (37). CD2BP1/PST-

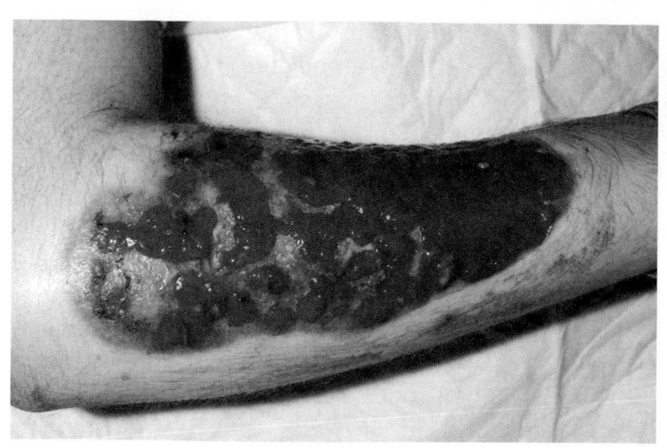

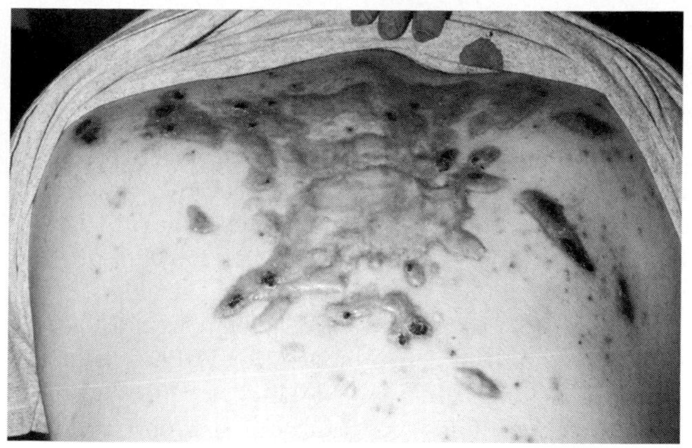

FIG. 68.17. Clinical features of the syndrome of pyogenic arthritis with pyoderma gangrenosum and acne (PAPA). **A:** Pyoderma gangrenosum on the right forearm of a patient with PAPA syndrome and the A230T mutation in proline serine threonine phosphatase interacting protein 1 (PSTPIP1)/CD2 binding-protein 1 (CD2BP1). **B:** Severe cystic acne in the same patient depicted in Panel A.

PIP1 is expressed predominantly in hematopoietic tissue and the lung (468,469), and is the mammalian homologue of a yeast protein involved in the organization of the cytoskeleton (470).

Subsequent experiments have demonstrated that CD2BP1/PSTPIP1 interacts with pyrin, the protein mutated in FMF (11). Both PAPA-associated mutants show increased levels of tyrosine phosphorylation and, consequently, increased binding to pyrin, relative to wild-type. Consistent with the hypothesis that these mutations exert a dominant negative effect on the cytokine-regulatory effects of pyrin, peripheral blood leukocytes from a clinically active PAPA patient showed markedly increased IL-1β production, and cell lines transfected with both PAPA-associated mutants also demonstrated increased IL-1β production, relative to wild-type. Figure 68-18 illustrates the proposed mechanism by which the PAPA mutations may interfere with the function of pyrin.

The differential diagnosis of pyoderma gangrenosum subsumes a number of systemic diseases, including inflammatory bowel disease, monoclonal gammopathies, hematologic

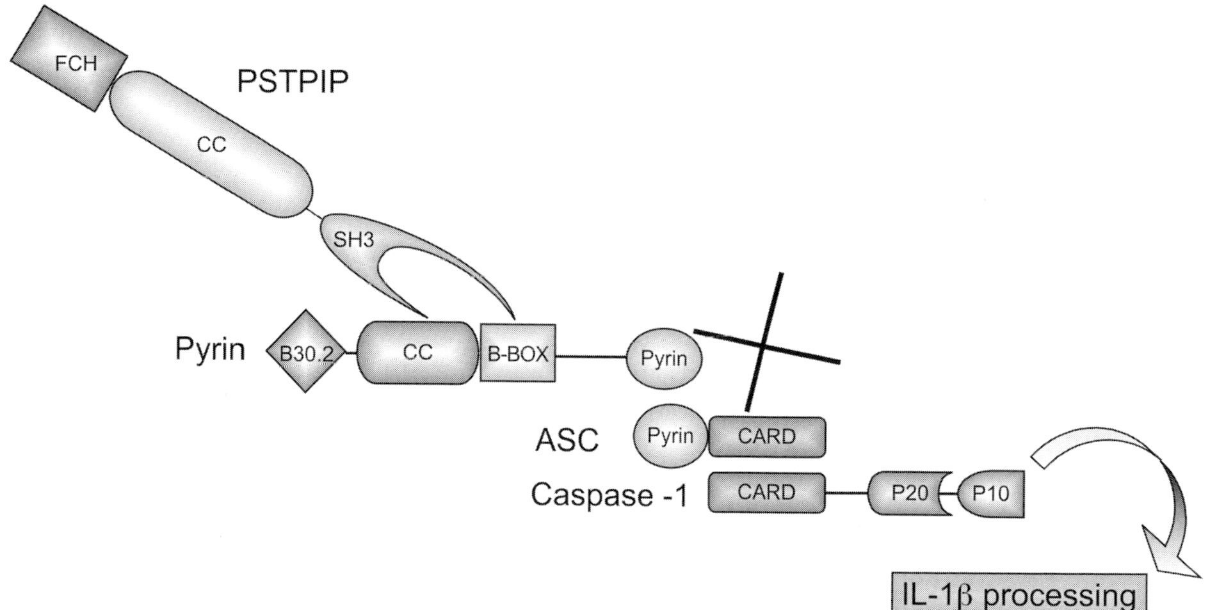

FIG. 68.18. Proposed mechanism of mutations in the syndrome of pyogenic arthritis with pyoderma gangrenosum and acne (PAPA). As shown in Figure 68.7, pyrin regulates the activation of interleukin (IL)-1β through ASC and caspase-1. PAPA-associated mutations in proline serine threonine phosphatase interacting protein 1 (PSTPIP1) cause increased affinity of PSTPIP1 for pyrin. This may contribute to the clinical phenotype of PAPA by sequestering pyrin, thus shifting the regulatory balance in favor of increased IL-1β processing, as has been observed in pyrin-deficient mice. ASC, apoptosis-associated specklike-protein with a CARD; CARD, caspase activation and recruitment domains.

malignancies, chronic active hepatitis, primary biliary cirrhosis, paroxysmal nocturnal hemoglobinuria, systemic lupus erythematosus, and the antiphospholipid antibody syndrome (471). Pyoderma gangrenosum can also be associated with a number of arthritides, including seropositive RA, the arthritis of inflammatory bowel disease, Behçet disease, psoriatic arthritis, and the SAPHO syndrome (synovitis, acne, pustulosis, hyperostosis, osteitis). Although the clinical picture of PAPA syndrome is rather distinctive, genetic testing may facilitate the correct diagnosis in ambiguous cases.

To date the most effective therapy for PAPA syndrome has been the early institution of high-dose corticosteroids (22,466). Affected joints may require aspiration, injection with corticosteroids, or open drainage. Local wound care is extremely important in the treatment of pyoderma gangrenosum, and pain management is often a central issue in caring for these patients. In light of the recent data linking PAPA syndrome to the pyrin pathway, biologic therapies targeted at IL-1 may be an attractive area for clinical investigation.

IDIOPATHIC INTERMITTENT ARTHROPATHIES

In contrast with the hereditary periodic fever syndromes and PAPA syndrome, which are all systemic diseases with arthritic manifestations, the idiopathic intermittent arthropathies (Table 68.4) are disorders that appear to involve primarily the joints and adjacent structures. Familial clustering has been occasionally observed in palindromic rheumatism and intermittent hydrarthrosis, but the predisposing genes remain to be defined. Clinical heterogeneity, in part due to the lack of uniform diagnostic criteria, may also hamper our ability to understand this group of disorders.

Palindromic Rheumatism

Palindromic rheumatism was first described by Hench and Rosenberg (472) in 1944. As originally defined, palindromic rheumatism refers to the occurrence of multiple afebrile attacks of arthritis or periarthritis (inflammation of soft tissue adjacent to the joints) with pain, swelling, and redness. Attacks were described as developing suddenly, usually affecting a single joint, and lasting hours to days. Recurrences could occur over irregularly spaced intervals. Despite these inflammatory episodes, no residual disability developed, and roentgenograms were normal. In the tradition of Hippocrates, who had used the adjective "palindromic" in connection with rashes and abscesses, these authors chose the term *palindromic rheumatism* to emphasize its recurring nature.

Additional clinical features (473), including the frequency with which various joints are affected, are summarized in Figure 68.19. Periarticular swelling occurs in the subcutaneous tissues near the joints, may be accompanied by arthritis or develop independently, is usually tender, and is usually 2 to 4 cm in diameter. Small, sometimes painful subcutaneous nodules can also develop near the elbows, knees, or wrists, but especially on the fingers. These can be precipitated by pressure on the affected area. Both the periarticular swelling and nodules are usually transient.

In some cases, there is a mild to moderate acceleration in the ESR during attacks (472–475). Rheumatoid factor is positive in about half of patients with palindromic rheuma-

TABLE 68.4. *The idiopathic intermittent arthropathies*

	Attacks	Affected joints	Disease associations	Prognosis	Treatment
Palindromic rheumatism	~2 d; monoarticular arthritis or periarticular soft tissue inflammation; irregular intervals	MCPs, PIPs, wrists, shoulders, MTPs, ankles	Rheumatoid arthritis	~50% have persistent palindromic rheumatism; ~33% develop rheumatoid arthritis	Gold salts, antimalarials, D-penicillamine
Intermittent hydrarthrosis	3–5 d; monoarticular; large effusions	Primarily knees; sometimes hip, ankle, elbow	Menses	Attacks at predictable intervals; sometimes spontaneous remissions	NSAIDs, intraarticular steroids, synovectomy
Eosinophilic synovitis	1–2 wks; monoarthritis triggered by trauma	Knee, MTP	Allergy, dermatographism	Self-limited episodes; benign prognosis	Symptomatic
Tietze's syndrome	Episodes last wks to mos	Costosternal, costochondral, sternoclavicular	Trauma, respiratory infections	Good	Local heat, NSAIDs, local injection of anesthetic, corticosteroids

MCP, metacarpal phalangeal joint; MTP, metatarsal phalangeal joint; NSAIDs, nonsteroidal antiinflammatory drugs; PIP, proximal interphalangeal joint.

Proposed diagnostic criteria

- History of brief, sudden-onset recurrent attacks of arthritis (usually monoarticular) or of soft tissue inflammation
- Direct observation of one attack by a physician
- >5 attacks in the last 2 years
- <2 joints involved in different attacks
- Negative roentgenograms
- Exclusion of other recurrent monoarthritides, gout, chrondrocalcinosis, intermittent hydrarthrosis, FMF

Clinical features

- Usually monoarticular attacks
- Often excruciating joint pain
- Most attacks last <2 days
- Paraarticular inflammation
- Small nodules on tendons in hands, fingers, thumb pads
- Overall, M:F ≈ 1
- Mean age of onset ≈ 45

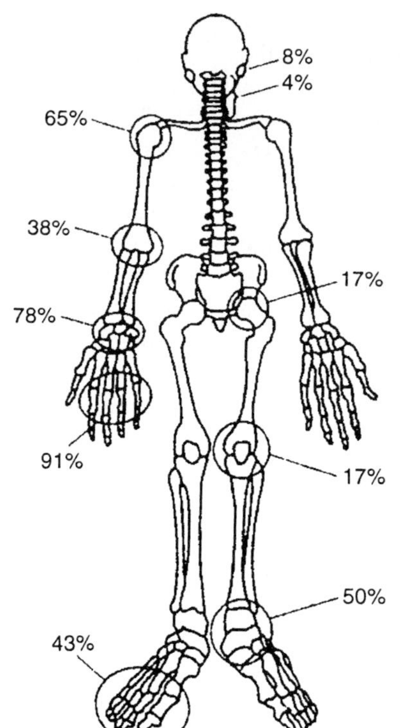

Laboratory findings

- ESR ↑ during attacks
- About 50% RF positive
- ANA negative
- Synovial fluid → 150–12,700 WBC
- About 50% anti-CCP positive

Prognosis

- 48% persistent PR
- 33% develop RA
- 15% remission
- 4% develop other diseases

Treatment

- No large controlled studies
- NSAIDS for relief of joint pain
- Varying results with:
  Injectable gold
  D-penicillamine
  Antimalarials
- Other agents that are sometimes effective:
  Sulfasalazine
  Colchicine
  Dapsone
  Chlorambucil

FIG. 68.19. Clinical and laboratory features of palindromic rheumatism. Diagnostic criteria are adapted from references 473 and 480. Percentages of joint involvement are based on a review of experience with 227 patients (473); figures on prognosis are based on a compilation of data on 653 patients (473).

tism (473). The percentages are higher in those patients who go on to develop RA (475,476), and conversion to seropositivity sometimes foreshadows the clinical transition. Antibodies to cyclic citrullinated peptide and keratin are found in about half of patients with palindromic rheumatism (477). The value of these antibodies in predicting progression to RA among these patients is currently unknown. Other laboratory studies, including antinuclear antibodies and complement determinations, are usually unremarkable (473,475). Synovial biopsy early in an attack demonstrates an influx of inflammatory cells, particularly polymorphonuclear leukocytes (472). As the attack subsides, these inflammatory cells are cleared and there is a transient period of fibroblast proliferation.

In light of the fact that some patients with palindromic rheumatism eventually develop RA, and given the HLA-DR1 and HLA-DR4 associations in the latter disease, there have been a number of analyses of HLA antigens in palindromic rheumatism. A compilation of several large series in the early 1990s failed to demonstrate a strong association between DR1 or DR4 and palindromic rheumatism (473). However, molecular DNA typing in a more recent series of 147 patients with palindromic rheumatism, 149 patients with RA, and 149 ethnically matched controls came to a different conclusion (478). There was a significant increase in the prevalence of the shared epitope DRB-0401 and DRB-0404 alleles in palindromic rheumatism (65%) relative to controls (39%), and homozygosity for shared epitope alleles was a significant independent risk factor for progression to chronicity. Occasional families have been reported in which there are multiple cases of palindromic rheumatism, or in which one member has palindromic rheumatism and a second has RA (474). Particularly interesting is a Finnish report of two HLA-identical ($DR4^+$) brothers who developed palindromic rheumatism; the younger brother went on to erosive RA after 3 years, while the older brother remained palindromic over a period of 12 years (479).

Given the paucity of laboratory clues to the diagnosis of palindromic rheumatism, various sets of clinical criteria have been formulated. Most of these, including those listed in Figure 68.19, are based on the proposal of Pasero and Barbieri (480), but do not require a negative rheumatoid factor or normal acute-phase reactants. Even adhering to such criteria, it is likely that this diagnosis includes a heterogeneous group of disorders. A review of longitudinal data on 653 cases of palindromic rheumatism indicated that 33% eventually develop RA, while 4% develop other disorders ranging from Wegener granulomatosis to Whipple disease (473). A more recent retrospective analysis of 127 patients with palindromic rheumatism identified a subset with a positive rheumatoid factor and early involvement of the wrist and proximal interphalangeal joints as having the highest risk of progression to RA or other connective tissue diseases (481). The even more recent aforementioned study of HLA typing indicates a probable independent role for the shared epitope, but not several cytokine polymorphisms, in progression (478). There is substantial variability in the reported prevalence of palindromic rheumatism from different centers, but the highest estimates are 20-fold less than the prevalence of RA (480).

Perhaps because of the overlap between palindromic rheumatism and RA, agents such as injectable gold (473, 474,476) and antimalarials (482) have been used with some success. Nevertheless, there have been no large controlled studies regarding the treatment of this disorder, and the occurrence of spontaneous remissions undoubtedly further clouds the picture.

Intermittent Hydrarthrosis

Among all of the periodic arthritides described in this chapter, intermittent hydrarthrosis (also called periodic benign synovitis) most often exhibits true periodicity. In 1910, Sir Archibald Garrod wrote, "Intervals between the successive attacks are, as a rule, so regular that the patients can foretell with accuracy the day, and sometimes even the hour, when a recurrence is to be expected, and can make their arrangements accordingly" (483). A later review of 47 cases seen at the Mayo Clinic indicated that, although early in the course of intermittent hydrarthrosis periodicity might not be apparent, most patients eventually establish a very reproducible rhythm of attacks (484). A given pattern of periodicity may last for years (the most frequent interval observed in the Mayo Clinic series was every 14 days), but occasionally the interval changes during the course of the illness.

The clinical picture is that of recurrent pain, limitation of motion, and swelling, usually affecting a single joint. Occasionally, more than one joint can be involved. In some patients, two or more joints may alternate swelling, with the same interval between attacks for each joint. In most cases, each attack lasts 3 to 5 days. Although there are often massive effusions, there is little redness or warmth over the affected joint, and fever is not common (484).

Some authors have described this condition as one that occurs most often in young women, but a review of 101 cases indicated a relatively even gender ratio, with most cases beginning between the ages of 20 and 50 (485). Nevertheless, there are certainly cases in which attacks begin with menarche, coincide with menses, or remit during pregnancy or after menopause (484). There are no good data on the prevalence of intermittent hydrarthrosis; at the Mayo Clinic 47 cases were identified over a 24-year period.

Attacks are notable for the absence of an acute-phase response (484). The ESR, leukocyte count, and hematocrit are normal during attacks. Despite numerous attacks involving a single joint, roentgenograms remain normal. Synovial fluid is mildly inflammatory, with polymorphonuclear leukocytes predominating early and mononuclear cells most abundant late in the attack. Synovial biopsies may demonstrate edema, hyperemia, variable inflammatory infiltrates, and villous synovial projections (484).

The pathogenesis of intermittent hydrarthrosis is unknown. As noted above, in women there may be a definite connection with hormonal changes. In one case, elevated levels of synovial fluid histamine were documented (486). Reimann and Angelides (487) described a 5-generation family with 23 members affected with intermittent hydrarthrosis. However, it should be noted that many of the affected individuals in this family presented very early in life, and that the familial occurrence of intermittent hydrarthrosis is uncommon.

Because of its rarity, there are no large series addressing the treatment of intermittent hydrarthrosis. Spontaneous remissions of several years, sometimes followed by relapses, have been reported (484). Depending on the severity of attacks, NSAIDs can sometimes be beneficial. Recently, two patients were reported to have responded to low-dose colchicine (488). Intraarticular steroids sometimes induce attack-free intervals of several months (484, 486). In particularly severe cases, surgical synovectomy may induce remission (484). In one case, synovectomy of the right knee was associated with a remission. Seventeen years later, attacks began in the left knee, and were also successfully treated with synovectomy. Refractory cases have also been treated with intraarticular radioactive gold (489).

Eosinophilic Synovitis

Eosinophilic synovitis refers to an entity first described in 1986, in which individuals with a personal or family history of allergy develop acute, painless monoarthritis after minor trauma (490). Swelling develops rapidly, usually over 12 to 24 hours, and lasts 1 to 2 weeks. Although effusions are often large, there is little associated heat, erythema, or pain. The knee is the most frequently affected joint (490,491).

As is the case for intermittent hydrarthrosis, the white count and ESR are usually normal during attacks. The peripheral eosinophil count is also normal, but some patients have elevated IgE levels. One of the original seven patients had an antinuclear antibody present at a titer of 1:160.

Synovial fluids show mildly elevated leukocyte counts, with 16% to 52% eosinophils in the initial series. The synovial fluid during attacks is translucent to opaque, with poor viscosity and poor mucin clot formation. Wet preparations of synovial fluid show Charcot-Leyden crystals, bipyramidal, hexagonal-shaped protein crystals formed by intracellular lipases in eosinophils. Slight pressure on the coverslip and overnight incubation at 4°C favor the identification of these crystals. With the resolution of the attack, synovial eosinophilia resolves.

By screening for Charcot-Leyden crystals, about 0.5% of synovial fluids are eosinophilic (490). Other disorders associated with synovial eosinophilia (492) include RA, psoriatic arthritis, rheumatic fever, parasitic arthritides, infectious arthritides such as tuberculous arthritis and Lyme disease, and the hypereosinophilic syndrome. Synovial eosinophilia may also be observed in metastatic adenocarcinoma (493) and after arthrography (494).

Features that set patients with eosinophilic synovitis apart from those with other causes of synovial eosinophilia include an allergic history in the patient or family, and the presence of dermatographism (490). Allergic symptoms do not accompany the attacks of arthritis. The authors of the original description of this disorder speculated that synovial trauma nonimmunologically triggers mast cell degranulation, thus attracting eosinophils and producing an effusion that is analogous to dermatographism. The longer duration of swelling in the joint compared with the skin may be due to anatomic differences in resorption.

Eosinophilic synovitis appears to be a self-limited condition requiring only symptomatic therapy. It is apparently rare, but exact prevalence figures are not available.

Tietze Syndrome

Tietze syndrome, first described by the surgeon Alexander Tietze (495) in 1921, refers to the painful, nonsuppurative swelling of the costosternal, costochondral, or sternoclavicular joints in the absence of other possible causes (496). This syndrome often has a course of exacerbations lasting weeks to months, followed by remissions, although less frequently protracted swelling may occur (497). There are no serious sequelae. Tietze syndrome is much less common than costochondritis, in which there is costochondral pain but no swelling (496).

In some cases, trauma or respiratory infections have been associated with the onset of symptoms (497,498). Pain can be severe, occurring both at rest and with exertion. Tietze syndrome is often exacerbated by coughing, deep inspiration, or bending, and emotional stress sometimes intensifies the pain. The average age of onset is about 30 years, but there is a substantial range (496), and a series of eight children has been reported (499). Men and women are affected equally. Most frequently, patients have isolated single lesions at the second or third costal cartilages; swelling can be several centimeters in diameter. The right and left sides are affected with equal frequency. The overlying skin is freely movable and not erythematous, although there may be local warmth.

Laboratory studies, including the white count and ESR, are normal (497). Roentgenograms occasionally demonstrate increased calcification at the affected sites, but are otherwise normal (496). A tomographic study of 13 patients with Tietze syndrome showed three with anatomic variants of the sternum, and two others with marginal osteophytes at the affected sternocostal joint (500). CT may demonstrate enlargement of the cartilage, ventral angulation of the cartilage, or normal anatomy (501). Imaging with gallium 67 sometimes shows accumulation of radioactivity in the lesions (502). Biopsies of lesions are normal or show a number of nonspecific findings, such as calcareous deposits, fibroblast nodules, and fibrotic changes and ossification (496).

It should be noted that a number of other conditions can cause costochondral swelling (496). These include septic lesions, RA, ankylosing spondylitis, psoriatic arthritis, synovitis-acne-pustulosis-hyperostosis-osteitis (SAPHO), gout, tumors (503,504), and condensing osteitis. These cannot be considered to be causes of Tietze syndrome, since the definition requires that there be no other explanations for the swelling. However, it is entirely possible that some cases that would previously have been classified as Tietze syndrome now fit into one of these other categories.

Excluding these other conditions, mechanical factors may be important in the pathogenesis of Tietze syndrome. The prognosis is good. Treatment consists of reassurance, local heat, NSAIDs, and the local injection of anesthetic and corticosteroids (496). When coughing is an aggravating factor, an Ace bandage can be applied to the chest wall, although care must be taken not to restrict respiratory movement, particularly in older individuals.

REFERENCES

1. Anonymous. Periodic diseases [Editorial]. *Lancet* 1948;1:565–566.
2. Reimann, HA. Periodic disease. *Medicine* (Baltimore) 1951;30:219–245.
3. Hull KM, Shoham N, Chae JJ, et al. The expanding spectrum of systemic autoinflammatory disorders and their rheumatic manifestations. *Curr Opin Rheumatol* 2003;15:61–69.
4. Hoffman HM, Mueller JL, Broide DH, et al. Mutation of a new gene encoding a putative pyrin-like protein causes familial cold autoinflammatory syndrome and Muckle-Wells syndrome. *Nature Genet.* 2001; 29:301–305.
5. Dodé C, le Dû N, Cuisset L, et al. New mutations of *CIAS1* that are responsible for Muckle-Wells syndrome and familial cold urticaria: a novel mutation underlies both syndromes. *Am J Hum Genet* 2002;70: 1498–1506.
6. Aganna E, Martinon F, Hawkins PN, et al. Association of mutations in the *NALP3/CIAS1/PYPAF1* gene with a broad phenotype including recurrent fever, cold sensitivity, sensorineural deafness, and AA amyloidosis. *Arthritis Rheum* 2002;46:2445–2452.
7. Feldmann J, Prieur A-M, Quartier P, et al. Chronic infantile neurological cutaneous and articular syndrome is caused by mutations in *CIAS1*, a gene highly expressed in polymorphonuclear cells and chondrocytes. *Am J Hum Genet* 2002;71:198–203.
8. Aksentijevich I, Nowak M, Mallah M, et al. De novo *CIAS1* mutations, cytokine activation, and evidence for genetic heterogeneity in patients with neonatal-onset multisystem inflammatory disease (NOMID). A new member of the expanding family of pyrin-associated autoinflammatory disease. *Arthritis Rheum* 2002;46:3340–3348.
9. International FMF Consortium. Ancient missense mutations in a new member of the *RoRet* gene family are likely to cause familial Mediterranean fever. *Cell* 1997;90:797–807.
10. French FMF Consortium. A candidate gene for familial Mediterranean fever. *Nature Genet* 1997;17:25–31.
11. Shoham NG, Centola M, Mansfield E, et al. Pyrin binds the PSTPIP1/CD2BP1 protein, defining familial Mediterranean fever and PAPA syndrome as disorders in the same pathway. *Proc Natl Acad Sci USA* 2003; 100:13501–13506.
12. McDermott MF, Aksentijevich I, Galon J, et al. Germline mutations in the extracellular domains of the 55 kDa TNF receptor, TNFR1, define

a family of dominantly inherited autoinflammatory syndromes. *Cell* 1999;97:133–144.
13. Galon J, Aksentijevich I, McDermott MF, et al. *TNFRSF1A* mutations and autoinflammatory syndromes. *Curr Opin Immunol* 2000;12:479–486.
14. Delpech M, Grateau G. Genetically determined recurrent fevers. *Curr Opin Immunol* 2001;13:539–542.
15. Drenth JP, van der Meer, JW. Hereditary periodic fever. *N Engl J Med* 2001;345:1748–1757.
16. McDermott MF. Genetic clues to understanding periodic fevers, and possible therapies. *Trends Mol Med* 2002:8:550–554.
17. Sohar E, Pras M, Heller J, et al. Genetics of familial Mediterranean fever. *Arch Intern Med* 1962;110:109–118.
18. Drenth JP, Mariman EC, van der Velde-Visser SD, et al. International Hyper-IgD Study Group. Location of the gene causing hyperimmunoglobulinemia D and periodic fever syndrome differs from that for familial Mediterranean fever. *Hum Genet* 1994;94:616–620.
19. Kile RM, Rusk HA. A case of cold urticaria with an unusual family history. *JAMA* 1940;114:1067–1068.
20. Johnstone RF, Dolen WK, Hoffman HM. A large kindred with familial cold autoinflammatory syndrome. *Ann Allergy Asthma Immunol* 2003; 90:233–237.
21. Muckle TJ, Wells M. Urticaria, deafness, and amyloidosis: a new heredo-familial syndrome. *Q J Med* 1962;31:235–248.
22. Lindor NM, Arsenault TM, Solomon H, et al. A new autosomal dominant disorder of pyogenic sterile arthritis, pyoderma gangrenosum, and acne: PAPA syndrome. *Mayo Clin Proc* 1997;72:611–615.
23. Siegal S. Benign paroxysmal peritonitis. *Ann Intern Med* 1945;23: 1–21.
24. Prieur A-M, Griscelli C. Arthropathy with rash, chronic meningitis, eye lesions, and mental retardation. *J Pediatr* 1981;99:79–93.
25. Hassink SG, Goldsmith DP. Neonatal onset multisystem inflammatory disease. *Arthritis Rheum* 1983;26:668–673.
26. Williamson LM, Hull D, Mehta R, et al. Familial Hibernian fever. *Q J Med* 1982;51:469–480.
27. van der Meer JW, Vossen JM, Radl J, et al. Hyperimmunoglobulinaemia D and periodic fever: a new syndrome. *Lancet* 1984;1:1087–1090.
28. Bertin J, DiStefano PS. The PYRIN domain: a novel motif found in apoptosis and inflammation proteins. *Cell Death Differ* 2000;7:1273–1274.
29. Martinon F, Hofmann K, Tschopp J. The pyrin domain: a possible member of the death domain-fold family implicated in apoptosis and inflammation. *Curr Biol* 2001:11:R118–120.
30. Staub E, Dahl E, Rosenthal A. The DAPIN family: a novel domain links apoptotic and interferon response proteins. *Trends Biochem Sci* 2001;26:83–85.
31. Pawlowski K, Pio F, Chu Z, et al. PAAD—a new protein domain associated with apoptosis, cancer and autoimmune diseases. *Trends Biochem Sci* 2001;26:85–87.
32. Kastner DL, O'Shea JJ. A fever gene comes in from the cold. *Nature Genet* 2001;29:241–242.
33. Harton JA, Linhoff MW, Zhang J, et al. Cutting edge: CATERPILLER: a large family of mammalian genes containing CARD, pyrin, nucleotide-binding, and leucine-rich repeat domains. *J Immunol* 2002;169:4088–4093.
34. Tschopp J, Martinon F, Burns K. NALPs: a novel protein family involved in inflammation. *Nature Rev Mol Cell Biol* 2003;4:95–104.
35. Houten SM, Kuis W, Duran M, et al. Mutations in *MVK*, encoding mevalonate kinase, cause hyperimmunoglobulinemia D and periodic fever syndrome. *Nature Genet* 1999;22:175–177.
36. Drenth JP, Cuisset L, Grateau G, et al. Mutations in the gene encoding mevalonate kinase cause hyper-IgD and periodic fever syndrome. *Nature Genet* 1999;22:178–181.
37. Wise CA, Gillum JD, Seidman CE, et al. Mutations in CD2BP1 disrupt binding to PTP PEST and are responsible for PAPA syndrome, an autoinflammatory disorder. *Hum Mol Genet* 2002;11:961–969.
38. Hugot JP, Chamaillard M, Zouali H, et al. Association of NOD2 leucine-rich repeat variants with susceptibility to Crohn's disease. *Nature* 2001;411:599–603.
39. Ogura Y, Bonen DK, Inohara N, et al. A frameshift mutation in NOD2 associated with susceptibility to Crohn's disease. *Nature* 2001;411: 603–606.
40. Miceli-Richard C, Lesage S, Rybojad M, et al. CARD15 mutations in Blau syndrome. *Nature Genet* 2001:29:19–20.
41. Janeway TC, Mosenthal HO. An unusual paroxysmal syndrome, probably allied to recurrent vomiting, with a study of the nitrogen metabolism. *Trans Assoc Am Physicians* 1908;23:504–518.
42. Ehrenfeld EN, Eliakim M, Rachmilewitz M. Recurrent polyserositis (familial Mediterranean fever; periodic disease). A report of fifty-five cases. *Am J Med* 1961;31:107–123.
43. Barakat MH, Karnik AM, Majeed HW, et al. Familial Mediterranean fever (recurrent hereditary polyserositis) in Arabs. A study of 175 patients and review of the literature. *Q J Med* 1986;60:837–847.
44. Mamou H, Cattan R. La maladie périodique (sur 14 cas personnels dont 8 compliqués de néphropathies). *Semin Hop Paris* 1952;28: 1062–1070.
45. Heller H, Sohar E, Sherf L. Familial Mediterranean fever. *Arch Intern Med* 1958;102:50–71.
46. Sohar E, Gafni J, Pras M, et al. Familial Mediterranean fever. A survey of 470 cases and review of the literature. *Am J Med* 1967;43:227–253.
47. Schwabe AD, Peters RS. Familial Mediterranean fever in Armenians. Analysis of 100 cases. *Medicine* (Baltimore) 1974;53:453–462.
48. Ozdemir AI, Sokmen C. Familial Mediterranean fever among the Turkish people. *Am J Gastroenterol* 1969;51:311–316.
49. Ozen S, Karaaslan Y, Ozdemir O, et al. Prevalence of juvenile chronic arthritis and familial Mediterranean fever in Turkey: a field study. *J Rheumatol* 1998;25:2445–2449.
50. Majeed HA, Rawashdeh M, El-Shanti H, et al. Familial Mediterranean fever in children: the expanded clinical profile. *Q J Med* 1999;92: 309–318.
51. Samuels J, Aksentijevich I, Torosyan Y, et al. Familial Mediterranean fever at the millennium: clinical spectrum, ancient mutations, and a survey of 100 American referrals to the National Institutes of Health. *Medicine* (Baltimore) 1998;77:268–297.
52. Aksentijevich I, Torosyan Y, Samuels J, et al. Mutation and haplotype studies of familial Mediterranean fever reveal new ancestral relationships and evidence for a high carrier frequency with reduced penetrance in the Ashkenazi Jewish population. *Am J Hum Genet* 1999; 64:949–962.
53. La Regina M, Nucera G, Diaco M, et al. Familial Mediterranean fever is no longer a rare disease in Italy. *Eur J Hum Genet* 2003;11:50–56.
54. Deltas CC, Mean R, Rosou E, et al. Familial Mediterranean fever (FMF) mutations occur frequently in the Greek-Cypriot population of Cyprus. *Genetic Test* 2002;6:15–21.
55. Konstantopoulos K, Kanta A, Deltas C, et al. Familial Mediterranean fever associated with pyrin mutations in Greece. *Ann Rheum Dis* 2003;62:479–481.
56. Dodé C, Pêcheux C, Cazeneuve C, et al. Mutations in the *MEFV* gene in a large series of patients with a clinical diagnosis of familial Mediterranean fever. *Am J Med Genet* 2000;92:241–246.
57. Touitou I. The spectrum of familial Mediterranean fever (FMF) mutations. *Eur J Hum Genet* 2001;9:473–483.
58. Tomiyama N, Oshiro S, Higashiuesato Y, et al. End-stage renal disease associated with familial Mediterranean fever. *Intern Med* 2002;41: 221–224.
59. Shinozaki K, Agematsu K, Yasui K, et al. Familial Mediterranean fever in 2 Japanese families. *J Rheumatol* 2002;29:1324–1325.
60. Rozenbaum M, Rosner I. The clinical features of familial Mediterranean fever of elderly onset. *Clin Exp Rheumatol* 1994;12:347–348.
61. Tamir N, Langevitz P, Zemer D, et al. Late-onset familial Mediterranean fever (FMF): a subset with distinct clinical, demographic, and molecular genetic characteristics. *Am J Med Genet* 1999;87:30–35.
62. Gedalia A, Adar A, Gorodischer R. Familial Mediterranean fever in children. *J Rheumatol* 1992;19[Suppl 35]:1–9.
63. Ben-Chetrit E, Ben-Chetrit A. Familial Mediterranean fever and menstruation. *BJOG* 2001;108:403–407.
64. Zissin R, Rathaus V, Gayer G, et al. CT findings in patients with familial Mediterranean fever during an acute abdominal attack. *Br J Radiol* 2003;76:22–25.
65. Gentiloni N, Febbraro S, Barone C, et al. Peritoneal mesothelioma in recurrent familial peritonitis. *J Clin Gastroenterol* 1997;24:276–279.
66. Belange G, Gompel H, Chaouat Y, et al. Malignant peritoneal mesothelioma occurring in periodic disease: apropos of a case. *Rev Med Interne* 1998;19:427–430.
67. Yalçinkaya F, Çakar N, Misirlioglu M, et al. Genotype-phenotype correlation in a large group of Turkish patients with familial Mediterranean fever: evidence for mutation-independent amyloidosis. *Rheumatology* (Oxford) 2000;39:67–72.

68. Brauman A, Gilboa Y. Recurrent pulmonary atelectasis as a manifestation of familial Mediterranean fever. *Arch Intern Med* 1987;147: 378–379.
69. Livneh A, Langevitz P, Pras M. Pulmonary associations in familial Mediterranean fever. *Curr Opin Pulm Med* 1999;5:326–331.
70. Lidar M, Pras M, Langevitz P, et al. Thoracic and lung involvement in familial Mediterranean fever (FMF). *Clin Chest Med* 2002;23:505–511.
71. Heller H, Gafni J, Michaeli D, et al. The arthritis of familial Mediterranean fever (FMF). *Arthritis Rheum* 1966;9:1–17.
72. Majeed HA, Rawashdeh M. The clinical patterns of arthritis in children with familial Mediterranean fever. *Q J Med* 1997;90:37–43.
73. Brik R, Shnawi M, Kasinetz L, et al. The musculoskeletal manifestations of familial Mediterranean fever in children genetically diagnosed with the disease. *Arthritis Rheum* 2001;44:1416–1419.
74. Pras E, Livneh A, Balow JE Jr, et al. Clinical differences between north African and Iraqi Jews with familial Mediterranean fever. *Am J Med Genet* 1998;75:216–219.
75. Uthman I, Hajj-Ali RA, Arayssi T, et al. Arthritis in familial Mediterranean fever. *Rheumatol Int* 2001;20:145–148.
76. Cazeneuve C, Sarkisian T, Pécheux C, et al. *MEFV*-gene analysis in Armenian patients with familial Mediterranean fever: diagnostic value and unfavorable renal prognosis of the M694V homozygous genotype–genetic and therapeutic implications. *Am J Hum Genet* 1999;65: 88–97.
77. Brik R, Shinawi M, Kepten I, et al. Familial Mediterranean fever: clinical and genetic characterization in a mixed pediatric population of Jewish and Arab patients. *Pediatrics* 1999:103:e70.
78. Gershoni-Baruch R, Brik R, Shinawi M, et al. The differential contribution of MEFV mutant alleles to the clinical profile of familial Mediterranean fever. *Eur J Hum Genet* 2002;10:145–149.
79. Sneh E, Pras M, Michaeli D, et al. Protracted arthritis in familial Mediterranean fever. *Rheumatol Rehabil* 1977;16:102–106.
80. Ince E, Çakar N, Tekin M, et al. Arthritis in children with familial Mediterranean fever. *Rheumatol Int* 2002;21:213–217.
81. Salai M, Langevitz P, Blankstein A, et al. Total hip replacement in familial Mediterranean fever. *Bull Hosp Jt Dis* 1993;53:25–28.
82. Salai M, Zemer D, Segal E, et al. Chronic massive knee effusion in familial Mediterranean fever. *Semin Arthritis Rheum* 1997;27:169–172.
83. Yalçinkaya Y, Tekin M, Tümer N, et al. Protracted arthritis of familial Mediterranean fever (an unusual complication). *Br J Rheumatol* 1997; 36:1228–1230.
84. Brodey PA, Wolff SM. Radiographic changes in the sacroiliac joints in familial Mediterranean fever. *Radiology* 1975;114:331–333.
85. Lehman TJ, Hanson V, Kornreich H, et al. HLA-B27–negative sacroiliitis: a manifestation of familial Mediterranean fever in childhood. *Pediatrics* 1978;61:423–426.
86. Langevitz P, Livneh A, Zemer D, et al. Seronegative spondyloarthropathy in familial Mediterranean fever. *Semin Arthritis Rheum* 1997;27:67–72.
87. Zimand S, Tauber T, Hegesch T, et al. Familial Mediterranean fever presenting with massive cardiac tamponade. *Clin Exp Rheumatol* 1994;12:67–69.
88. Dabestani A, Noble LM, Child JS, et al. Pericardial disease in familial Mediterranean fever. An echocardiographic study. *Chest* 1982;81: 592–595.
89. Tutar E, Yalçinkaya F, Øzkaya N, et al. Incidence of pericardial effusion during attacks of familial Mediterranean fever. *Heart* 2003;89: 1257–1258.
90. Kees S, Langevitz P, Zemer D, et al. Attacks of pericarditis as a manifestation of familial Mediterranean fever. *Q J Med* 1997;90:643–647.
91. Azizi E, Fisher BK. Cutaneous manifestations of familial Mediterranean fever. *Arch Dermatol* 1976;112:364–366.
92. Barzilai A, Langevitz P, Goldberg I, et al. Erysipelas-like erythema of familial Mediterranean fever: clinicopathologic correlation. *J Am Acad Dermatol* 2000;42:791–795.
93. Koné Paut I, Dubuc M, Sportouch J, et al. Phenotype-genotype correlation in 91 patients with familial Mediterranean fever reveals a high frequency of cutaneomucous features. *Rheumatology* (Oxford) 2000; 39:1275–1279.
94. Rawashdeh MO, Majeed HA. Familial Mediterranean fever in Arab children: the high prevalence and gene frequency. *Eur J Pediatr* 1996; 155:540–544.
95. Gershoni-Baruch R, Broza Y, Brik R. Prevalence and significance of mutations in the familial Mediterranean fever gene in Henoch-Schönlein purpura. *J Pediatr* 2003;143:658–661.
96. Majeed HA, Quabazard Z, Hijazi Z, et al. The cutaneous manifestations in children with familial Mediterranean fever (recurrent hereditary polyserositis). A six-year study. *Q J Med* 1990;75:607–616.
97. Eshel G, Vinograd I, Barr J, et al. Acute scrotal pain complicating familial Mediterranean fever in children. *Br J Surg* 1994;81: 894–896.
98. Livneh A, Madgar I, Langevitz P, et al. Recurrent episodes of acute scrotum with ischemic testicular necrosis in a patient with familial Mediterranean fever. *J Urol* 1994;151:431–432.
99. Majeed HA, Ghandour K, Shahin HM. The acute scrotum in Arab children with familial Mediterranean fever. *Pediatr Surg Int* 2000; 16:72–74.
100. Lausch E, Fisch M, Beetz R. Familial Mediterranean fever as an unusual cause of acute scrotum. *J Urol* 2001;165:1262–1263.
101. Langevitz P, Zemer D, Livneh A, et al. Protracted febrile myalgia in patients with familial Mediterranean fever. *J Rheumatol* 1994;21: 1708–1709.
102. Majeed HA, Al-Qudah AK, Qubain H, et al. The clinical patterns of myalgia in children with familial Mediterranean fever. *Semin Arthritis Rheum* 2000;30:138–143.
103. Eliakim M, Levy M, Ehrenfeld M. *Recurrent polyserositis (familial Mediterranean fever, periodic disease)*. Amsterdam: Elsevier: North-Holland, 1981:87–95.
104. Majeed HA, Halabi I, Al-Taleb O. Recurrent hyperbilirubinaemia, a feature of familial Mediterranean fever: report of a child and review of the literature. *Ann Trop Paediatr* 1998;18:13–15.
105. Ciftci AO, Tanyel FC, Buyukpamukcu N, et al. Adhesive small bowel obstruction caused by familial Mediterranean fever: the incidence and outcome. *J Pediatr Surg* 1995;30:577–579.
106. Tunça M, Kirkali G, Soytürk M, et al. Acute phase response and evolution of familial Mediterranean fever. *Lancet* 1999;353:1415.
107. Korkmaz C, Øzdogan H, Kasapçopur, et al. Acute phase response in familial Mediterranean fever. *Ann Rheum Dis* 2002;61:79–81.
108. Duzova A, Bakkaloglu A, Besbas N, et al. Role of A-SAA in monitoring subclinical inflammation and in colchicine dosage in familial Mediterranean fever. *Clin Exp Rheumatol* 2003;21:509–514.
109. Notarnicola C, Didelot MN, Seguret F, et al. Enhanced cytokine mRNA levels in attack-free patients with familial Mediterranean fever. *Genes Immun* 2002;3:43–45.
110. Yildiz A, Akkaya V, Kiliçaslan, et al. Cardiac and intestinal amyloidosis in a renal transplant recipient with familial Mediterranean fever. *J Nephrol* 2001;14:125–127.
111. Altiparmak MR, Pamuk ÖN, Pamuk GE, et al. Amyloid goitre in familial Mediterranean fever: report on three patients and review of the literature. *Clin Rheumatol* 2002;21:497–500.
112. Kutlay S, Yilmaz E, Koytak ES, et al. A case of familial Mediterranean fever with amyloidosis as the first manifestation. *Am J Kidney Dis* 2001;38:E34.
113. Pras M, Bronshpigel N, Zemer D, et al. Variable incidence of amyloidosis in familial Mediterranean fever among different ethnic groups. *Johns Hopkins Med J* 1982;150:22–26.
114. Meyerhoff J. Familial Mediterranean fever: report of a large family, review of the literature, and discussion of the frequency of amyloidosis. *Medicine* (Baltimore) 1980;59:66–77.
115. Majeed HA, El-Shanti H, Al-Khateeb MS, et al. Genotype/phenotype correlations in Arab patients with familial Mediterranean fever. *Semin Arthritis Rheum* 2002;31:371–376.
116. Livneh A, Langevitz P, Shinar Y, et al. *MEFV* mutation analysis in patients suffering from amyloidosis of familial Mediterranean fever. *Amyloid* 1999;6:1–6.
117. Shohat M, Magal N, Shohat T, et al. Phenotype-genotype correlation in familial Mediterranean fever: evidence for an association between Met694Val and amyloidosis. *Eur J Hum Genet* 1999;7: 287–292.
118. Mimouni A, Magal N, Stoffman N, et al. Familial Mediterranean fever: effects of genotype and ethnicity on inflammatory attacks and amyloidosis. *Pediatrics* 2000;105:e70.
119. Ben-Chetrit E, Backenroth R. Amyloidosis induced, end stage renal disease in patients with familial Mediterranean fever is highly associated with point mutations in the MEFV gene. *Ann Rheum Dis* 2001; 60:146–149.

120. Mansour I, Delague V, Cazeneuve C, et al. Familial Mediterranean fever in Lebanon: mutation spectrum, evidence for cases in Maronites, Greek Orthodoxes, Greek Catholics, Syriacs and Chiites and for an association between amyloidosis and M694V and M694I mutations. *Eur J Hum Genet* 2001;9:51–55.
121. Gershoni-Baruch R, Brik R, Zacks N, et al. The contribution of genotypes at the MEFV and SAA1 loci to amyloidosis and disease severity in patients with familial Mediterranean fever. *Arthritis Rheum* 2003;48:1149–1155.
122. Yalçinkaya F, Akar N, Misirlioglu M. Familial Mediterranean fever—amyloidosis and the Val726Ala mutation. *N Engl J Med* 1998;338:993–994.
123. Akar N, Misiroglu M, Yalçinkaya F, et al. MEFV mutations in Turkish patients suffering from familial Mediterranean fever. *Hum Mutat* 2000;15:118–119.
124. Tekin M, Yalçinkaya F, Çakar N, et al. MEFV mutations in multiplex families with familial Mediterranean fever: is a particular genotype necessary for amyloidosis? *Clin Genet* 2000;57:430–434.
125. Yalçinkaya F, Tekin M, Çakar N, et al. Familial Mediterranean fever and systemic amyloidosis in untreated Turkish patients. *Q J Med* 2000;93:681–684.
126. Saatçi Ů, Ozen S, Özdemir S, et al. Familial Mediterranean fever in children: report of a large series and discussion of the risk and prognostic factors of amyloidosis. *Eur J Pediatr* 1997;156:619–623.
127. Cazeneuve C, Ajrapetyan H, Papin S, et al. Identification of *MEFV*-independent modifying genetic factors for familial Mediterranean fever. *Am J Hum Genet* 2000;67:1136–1143.
128. Akar N, Hasipek M, Akar E, et al. Serum amyloid A1 and tumor necrosis factor-alpha alleles in Turkish familial Mediterranean fever patients with and without amyloidosis. *Amyloid* 2003;10:12–16.
129. Touitou I, Picot M-C, Domingo C, et al. The MICA region determines the first modifier locus in familial Mediterranean fever. *Arthritis Rheum* 2001;44:163–169.
130. Aivasian AA, Savgorodniaia AM, Abramian MK, et al. Immunogenesis of periodic disease. *Klin Med* (Mosk) 1977;55:41–97.
131. Livneh A, Cabili S, Zemer D, et al. Effect of pregnancy on renal function in amyloidosis of familial Mediterranean fever. *J Rheumatol* 1993;20:1519–1523.
132. Blum A, Sohar E. The diagnosis of amyloidosis. Ancillary procedures. *Lancet* 1962;1:721–724.
133. Sungur C, Sungur A, Ruacan S, et al. Diagnostic value of bone marrow biopsy in patients with renal disease secondary to familial Mediterranean fever. *Kidney Int* 1993;44:834–836.
134. Özdemir BH, Özdemir OG, Özdemir FN, et al. Value of testis biopsy in the diagnosis of systemic amyloidosis. *Urology* 2002;59:201–205.
135. Tishler M, Pras M, Yaron M. Abdominal fat tissue aspirate in amyloidosis of familial Mediterranean fever. *Clin Exp Rheumatol* 1988;6:395–397.
136. Eliahou HE, Iaina A, Reisin E, et al. Probability of survival in hypertensive and nonhypertensive patients on maintenance hemodialysis. *Isr J Med Sci* 1977;13:33–38.
137. Jacob ET, Bar-Nathan N, Shapira Z, et al. Renal transplantation in the amyloidosis of familial Mediterranean fever. *Arch Intern Med* 1979;139:1135–1138.
138. Pras M, Gafni J, Jacob ET, et al. Recent advances in familial Mediterranean fever. *Adv Nephrol* 1984;13:261–270.
139. Martinez-Vea A, Garcia C, Carreras M, et al. End-stage renal disease in systemic amyloidosis: clinical course and outcome on dialysis. *Am J Nephrol* 1990;10:283–289.
140. Sever MS, Turkmen A, Sahin S, et al. Renal transplantation in amyloidosis secondary to familial Mediterranean fever. *Transplant Proc* 2001;33:3392–3393.
141. Rubinger D, Friedlaender MM, Popovtzer MM. Amelioration of familial Mediterranean fever during hemodialysis. *N Engl J Med* 1979;301:142–144.
142. Turkmen A, Yildiz A, Erkoc R, et al. Transplantation in renal amyloidosis. *Clin Transplant* 1998;12:375–378.
143. Shmueli D, Lustig S, Nakache R, et al. Renal transplantation in patients with amyloidosis due to familial Mediterranean fever. *Transplant Proc* 1992;24:1783–1784.
144. Kilicturgay S, Tokyay R, Arslan G, et al. The results of transplantation of patients with amyloid nephropathy. *Transplant Proc* 1992;24:1788–1789.
145. Sherif AM, Refaie AF, Sobh MA, et al. Long-term outcome of live donor kidney transplantation for renal amyloidosis. *Am J Kidney Dis* 2003;42:370–375.
146. Livneh A, Zemer D, Siegal B, et al. Colchicine prevents kidney transplant amyloidosis in familial Mediterranean fever. *Nephron* 1992;60:418–422.
147. Siegal B, Zemer D, Pras M. Cyclosporine and familial Mediterranean fever amyloidosis. *Transplantation* 1986;41:793–794.
148. Yussim A, Bar-Nathan N, Lustig S, et al. Gastrointestinal, hepatorenal, and neuromuscular toxicity caused by cyclosporine-colchicine interaction in renal transplantation. *Transplant Proc* 1994;26:2825–2826.
149. Gruberg L, Har-Zahav Y, Agranat O, et al. Acute myopathy induced by colchicine in a cyclosporine treated heart transplant recipient: possible role of the multidrug resistance transporter. *Transplant Proc* 1999;31:2157–2158.
150. Minetti EE, Minetti L. Multiple organ failure in a kidney transplant patient receiving both colchicine and cyclosporine. *J Nephrol* 2003;16:421–425.
151. Speeg KV, Maldonado AL, Liaci J, et al. Effect of cyclosporine on colchicine secretion by the kidney multidrug transporter studied *in vivo*. *J Pharmacol Exp Ther* 1992;261:50–55.
152. Speeg KV, Maldonado AL. Effect of cyclosporine on colchicine partitioning in the rat liver. *Cancer Chemother Pharmacol* 1993;32:434–436.
153. Simkin PA, Gardner GC. Colchicine use in cyclosporine treated transplant recipients: how little is too much? *J Rheumatol* 2000;27:1334–1337.
154. Shabtai M, Ben-Haim M, Zemer D, et al. Detrimental effects of cyclosporin A on long-term graft survival in familial Mediterranean fever renal allograft recipients: experience of two transplantation centers. *Isr Med Assoc J* 2002;4[11 Suppl]:935–939.
155. Ozdogan H, Arisoy N, Kasapìapur O, et al. Vasculitis in familial Mediterranean fever. *J Rheumatol* 1997;24:323–327.
156. Ozen S. New interest in an old disease: familial Mediterranean fever. *Clin Exp Rheumatol* 1999;17:745–749.
157. Tekin M, Yalçinkaya F, Tümer, et al. Familial Mediterranean fever—renal involvement by diseases other than amyloid. *Nephrol Dial Transplant* 1999;14:475–479.
158. Sachs D, Langevitz P, Morag B, et al. Polyarteritis nodosa and familial Mediterranean fever. *Br J Rheumatol* 1987;26:139–141.
159. Glikson M, Galun E, Schlesinger M, et al. Polyarteritis nodosa and familial Mediterranean fever: a report of 2 cases and review of the literature. *J Rheumatol* 1989;16:536–539.
160. Schlesinger M, Oren S, Fano M, et al. Perirenal and renal subcapsular haematoma as presenting symptoms of polyarteritis nodosa. *Postgrad Med J* 1989;65:681–683.
161. Tinaztepe K, Güçer S, Bakkaloglu A, et al. Familial Mediterranean fever and polyarteritis nodosa: experience of five paediatric cases. A causal relationship or coincidence? *Eur J Pediatr* 1997;156:505–506.
162. Ozen S, Ben-Chetrit E, Bakkaloglu A, et al. Polyarteritis nodosa in patients with familial Mediterranean fever: a concomitant disease or a feature of FMF? *Semin Arthritis Rheum* 2001;30:281–287.
163. Sidi G, Shinar Y, Livneh A, et al. Protracted febrile myalgia of familial Mediterranean fever. Mutation analysis and clinical correlations. *Scand J Rheumatol* 2000;29:174–176.
164. Said R, Hamzeh Y, Said S, et al. Spectrum of renal involvement in familial Mediterranean fever. *Kidney Int* 1992;41:414–419.
165. Eliakim M, Rachmilewitz M, Rosenmann E, et al. Renal manifestations in recurrent polyserositis (familial Mediterranean fever). *Isr J Med Sci* 1970;6:228–245.
166. Said R, Nasrallah N, Hamzah Y, et al. IgA nephropathy in patients with familial Mediterranean fever. *Am J Nephrol* 1988;8:417–420.
167. Said R, Hamzeh Y, Tarawneh M, et al. Rapid progressive glomerulonephritis in patients with familial Mediterranean fever. *Am J Kidney Dis* 1989;14:412–416.
168. Akpolat T, Akpolat I, Karagoz F, et al. Familial Mediterranean fever and glomerulonephritis and review of the literature. *Rheumatol Int* 2004;24:43–45.
169. Priest RJ, Nixon RK. Familial recurring polyserositis: a disease entity. *Ann Intern Med* 1959;51:1253–1274.
170. Eliakim M, Bental E. Recurrent polyserositis ("periodic disease"): electroencephalographic changes. *Arch Intern Med* 1961;108:91–99.

171. Vilaseca J, Tor J, Guardia J, et al. Periodic meningitis and familial Mediterranean fever. *Arch Intern Med* 1982;142:378–379.
172. Schwabe AD. Meningitis in familial Mediterranean fever. *Am J Med* 1988:85:715–717.
173. Barakat MH, Mustafa HT, Shakir RA. Mollaret's meningitis. A variant of recurrent hereditary polyserositis, both provoked by metaraminol. *Arch Neurol* 1988;45:926–927.
174. Gedalia A, Zamir S. Neurologic manifestations in familial Mediterranean fever. *Pediatr Neurol* 1993;9:301–302.
175. Schwartz T, Langevitz P, Zemer D, et al. Behçet's disease in familial Mediterranean fever: characterization of the association between the two diseases. *Semin Arthritis Rheum* 2000;29:286–295.
176. Touitou I, Magne X, Molinari N, et al. *MEFV* mutations in Behçet's disease. *Hum Mutat* 2000;16:271–272.
177. Livneh A, Aksentijevich I, Langevitz P, et al. A single mutated *MEFV* allele in Israeli patients suffering from familial Mediterranean fever and Behçet's disease (FMF-BD). *Eur J Hum Genet* 2001;9:191–196.
178. Akpolat T, Yilmaz E, Akpolat I, et al. Amyloidosis in Behçet's disease and familial Mediterranean fever. *Rheumatology* (Oxford) 2002; 41:592–593.
179. Ben-Chetrit E, Cohen R, Chajek-Shaul T. Familial Mediterranean fever and Behçet's disease—are they associated? *J Rheumatol* 2002; 29:530–534.
180. Cattan D, Notarnicola C, Molinari N, et al. Inflammatory bowel disease in non-Ashkenazi Jews with familial Mediterranean fever. *Lancet* 2000;355:378–379.
181. Fidder HH, Chowers Y, Lidar M, et al. Crohn disease in patients with familial Mediterranean fever. *Medicine* (Baltimore) 2002;81:411–416.
182. Shohat M, Livneh A, Zemer D, et al. Twin studies in familial Mediterranean fever. *Am J Med Genet* 1992;44:179–182.
183. Yuval Y, Hemo-Zisser M, Zemer D, et al. Dominant inheritance in two families with familial Mediterranean fever (FMF). *Am J Med Genet* 1995;57:455–457.
184. Rogers DB, Shohat M, Petersen GM, et al. Familial Mediterranean fever in Armenians: autosomal recessive inheritance with high gene frequency. *Am J Med Genet* 1989;34:168–172.
185. Daniels M, Shohat T, Brenner-Ullman A, et al. Familial Mediterranean fever: high gene frequency among the non-Ashkenazi and Ashkenazic Jewish populations in Israel. *Am J Med Genet* 1995;55: 311–314.
186. Weatherall DJ, Miller LH, Baruch DI, et al. Malaria and the red cell. *Hematology (Am Soc Hematol Educ Program)* 2002;35–57.
187. Pras E, Aksentijevich I, Gruberg L, et al. Mapping of a gene causing familial Mediterranean fever to the short arm of chromosome 16. *N Engl J Med* 1992;326:1509–1513.
188. Aksentijevich I, Pras E, Gruberg L, et al. Refined mapping of the gene causing familial Mediterranean fever by linkage and homozygosity studies. *Am J Hum Genet* 1993;53:451–461.
189. Aksentijevich I, Pras E, Gruberg L, et al. Familial Mediterranean fever in Moroccan Jews: demonstration of a founder effect by extended haplotype analysis. *Am J Hum Genet* 1993;53:644–651.
190. Levy EN, Shen Y, Kupelian A, et al. Linkage disequilibrium mapping places the gene causing familial Mediterranean fever close to *D16S246*. *Am J Hum Genet* 1996;58:523–534.
191. French FMF Consortium. Localization of the familial Mediterranean fever gene (FMF) to a 250-kb interval in non-Ashkenazi Jewish founder haplotypes. *Am J Hum Genet* 1996;59:603–612.
192. Balow JE Jr, Shelton DA, Orsborn A, et al. A high-resolution genetic map of the familial Mediterranean fever candidate region allows identification of haplotype-sharing among ethnic groups. *Genomics* 1997;44:280–291.
193. Centola M, Aksentijevich I, Kastner DL. The hereditary periodic fever syndromes: molecular analysis of a new family of inflammatory diseases. *Hum Mol Genet* 1998;7:1581–1588.
194. Henry J, Mather IH, McDermott MF, et al. B30.2-like domain proteins: update and new insights into a rapidly expanding family of proteins. *Mol Biol Evol* 1998;15:1696–1705.
195. Rhodes DA, Stammers M, Malcherek G, et al. The cluster of *BTN* genes in the extended major histocompatibility complex. *Genomics* 2001;71:351–362.
196. Meyer M, Gaudieri S, Rhodes DA, et al. Cluster of TRIM genes in the human MHC class I region sharing the B30.2 domain. *Tissue Antigens* 2003;61:63–71.
197. Kimura F, Suzu S, Nakamura Y, et al. Cloning and characterization of a novel RING-B-box-coiled-coil protein with apoptotic function. *J Biol Chem* 2003;278:25046–25054.
198. Sarrauste de Menthiére C, Terriére S, Pugnére D, et al. INFEVERS: the registry for FMF and hereditary inflammatory disorders mutations. *Nucleic Acids Res* 2003;31:282–285.
199. Booth DR, Lachmann HJ, Gillmore JD, et al. Prevalence and significance of the familial Mediterranean fever gene mutation encoding pyrin Q148. *Q J Med* 2001;94:527–531.
200. Ben-Chetrit E, Lerer I, Malamud E, et al. The E148Q mutation in the MEFV gene: is it a disease-causing mutation or a sequence variant? *Hum Mutat* 2000;15:385–386.
201. Tchernitchko D, Legendre M, Cazeneuve C, et al. The E148Q *MEFV* allele is not implicated in the development of familial Mediterranean fever. *Hum Mutat* 2003;22:339–340.
202. Ozen S, Besbas N, Bakkaloglu A, et al. Pyrin Q148 mutation and familial Mediterranean fever. *Q J Med* 2002;95:332–333.
203. Akar N, Akar E, Yalçinkaya F. E148Q of the MEFV gene causes amyloidosis in familial Mediterranean fever patients. *Pediatrics* 2001; 108:215.
204. Dewalle M, Domingo C, Rozenbaum M, et al. Phenotype-genotype correlation in Jewish patients suffering from familial Mediterranean fever. *Eur J Hum Genet* 1998;6:95–97.
205. Stoffman N, Magal N, Shohat T, et al. Higher than expected carrier rates for familial Mediterranean fever in various Jewish ethnic groups. *Eur J Hum Genet* 2000;8:307–310.
206. Kogan A, Shinar Y, Lidar M, et al. Common *MEFV* mutations among Jewish ethnic groups in Israel: high frequency of carrier and phenotype III states and absence of a perceptible biological advantage of the carrier state. *Am J Med Genet* 2001;102:272–276.
207. Gershoni-Baruch R, Shinawi M, Leah K, et al. Familial Mediterranean fever: prevalence, penetrance and genetic drift. *Eur J Hum Genet* 2001;9:634–637.
208. Yilmaz E, Ozen S, Balci B, et al. Mutation frequency of familial Mediterranean fever and evidence for a high carrier rate in the Turkish population. *Eur J Hum Genet* 2001;9:553–555.
209. Torosyan Y, Aksentijevich I, Sarkisian T, et al. A population-based survey reveals an extremely high FMF carrier frequency in Armenia, suggesting heterozygote advantage. *Am J Hum Genet* 1999;65[Suppl]: 2266.
210. Gershoni-Baruch R, Shinawi M, Shamaly H, et al. Familial Mediterranean fever: the segregation of four different mutations in 13 individuals from one inbred family: genotype-phenotype correlation and intrafamilial variability. *Am J Med Genet* 2002;109: 198–201.
211. Tunça M, Akar S, Hawkins PN, et al. The significance of paired MEFV mutations in individuals without symptoms of familial Mediterranean fever. *Eur J Hum Genet* 2002;10:786–789.
212. Tunça M, Kirkali G, Soytürk M, et al. Acute phase response and evolution of familial Mediterranean fever. *Lancet* 1999;353:1415.
213. Poland DC, Drenth JP, Rabinovitz E, et al. Specific glycosylation of α_1-acid glycoprotein characteristics patients with familial Mediterranean fever and obligatory carriers of MEFV. *Ann Rheum Dis* 2001; 60:777–780.
214. Ozen S, Bakkaloglu A, Yilmaz E, et al. Mutations in the gene for familial Mediterranean fever: do they predispose to inflammation? *J Rheumatol* 2003;30:2014–2018.
215. Medlej-Hashim M, Rawashdeh M, Chouery E, et al. Genetic screening of fourteen mutations in Jordanian familial Mediterranean fever patients. *Hum Mutat* 2000;15:384.
216. Padeh S, Shinar Y, Pras E, et al. Clinical and diagnostic value of genetic testing in 216 Israeli children with familial Mediterranean fever. *J Rheumatol* 2003;30:185–190.
217. Cazeneuve C, Hovannesyan Z, Geneviève D, et al. Familial Mediterranean fever among patients from Karabakh and the diagnostic value of *MEFV* gene analysis in all classically affected populations. *Arthritis Rheum* 2003;48:2324–2331.
218. Booth DR, Gillmor JD, Lachmann HJ, et al. The genetic basis of autosomal dominant familial Mediterranean fever. *Q J Med* 2000;93: 217–221.
219. Akarsu AN, Saatçi Ü, Ozen S, et al. Genetic linkage study of familial Mediterranean fever (FMF) to 16p13.3 and evidence for genetic heterogeneity in the Turkish population. *J Med Genet* 1997;34:573–578.

220. Domingo C, Touitou I, Bayou A, et al. Familial Mediterranean fever in the 'Chuetas' of Mallorca: a question of Jewish origin or genetic heterogeneity. *Eur J Hum Genet* 2000;8:242–246.
221. Fairbrother WJ, Gordon NC, Humke EW, et al. The PYRIN domain: a member of the death domain-fold superfamily. *Protein Sci* 2001; 10:1911–1918.
222. Richards N, Schaner P, Diaz A, et al. Interaction between pyrin and the apoptotic speck protein (ASC) modulates ASC-induced apoptosis. *J Biol Chem* 2001;276:39320–39329.
223. Liu T, Rojas A, Ye Y, et al. Homology modeling provides insights into the binding mode of the PAAD/DAPIN/pyrin domain, a fourth member of the CARD/DD/DED domain family. *Protein Sci* 2003;12: 1872–1881.
224. Liepinsh E, Barbals R, Dahl E, et al. The death-domain fold of the ASC PYRIN domain, presenting a basis for PYRIN/PYRIN recognition. *J Mol Biol* 2003;332:1155–1163.
225. Hiller S, Kohl A, Fiorito F, et al. NMR structure of the apoptosis- and inflammation-related NALP pyrin domain. *Structure* 2003;11:1199–1205.
226. Eliezer D. Folding pyrin into the family. *Structure* 2003;11:1190–1191.
227. Masumoto J, Taniguchi S, Ayukawa K, et al. ASC, a novel 22 kDa protein, aggregates during apoptosis of human promyelocytic leukemia HL-60 cells. *J Biol Chem* 1999;274:33835–33838.
228. Masumoto J, Dowds TA, Schaner P, et al. ASC is an activating adaptor for NF-κB and caspase-8-dependent apoptosis. *Biochem Biophys Res Commun* 2003;303:69–73.
229. Dowds TA, Masumoto J, Chen FF, et al. Regulation of cryopyrin/ Pypaf1 signaling by pyrin, the familial Mediterranean fever gene product. *Biochem Biophys Res Commun* 2003;302:575–580.
230. Chae JJ, Komarow HD, Cheng J, et al. Targeted disruption of pyrin, the FMF protein, causes heightened sensitivity to endotoxin and a defect in macrophage apoptosis. *Mol Cell* 2003;11:591–604.
231. Srinivasula SM, Poyet J-L, Razmara M, et al. The PYRIN-CARD protein ASC is an activating adaptor for caspase-1. *J Biol Chem* 2002;277:21119–21122.
232. Wang L, Manji GA, Grenier JM, et al. PYPAF7, a novel PYRIN-containing Apaf1-like protein that regulates activation of NF-κB and caspase-1-dependent cytokine processing. *J Biol Chem* 2002;277: 29874–29880.
233. Martinon F, Burns K, Tschopp J. The inflammasome: a molecular platform triggering activation of inflammatory caspases and processing of proIL-1β. *Mol Cell* 2002;10:417–426.
234. Stehlik C, Lee HS, Dorfleutner A, et al. Apoptosis-associated speck-like protein containing a caspase recruitment domain is a regulator of procaspase-1 activation. *J Immunol* 2003;171:6154–6163.
235. Stehlik C, Fiorentino L, Dorfleutner A, et al. The PAAD/PYRIN-family protein ASC is a dual regulator of a conserved step in nuclear factor κB activation pathways. *J Exp Med* 2002;196:1605–1615.
236. Centola M, Wood G, Frucht DM, et al. The gene for familial Mediterranean fever, *MEFV,* is expressed in early leukocyte development and is regulated in response to inflammatory mediators. *Blood* 2000; 95:3223–3231.
237. Papin S, Cazeneuve C, Duquesnoy P, et al. The TNFα-dependent activation of the human Mediterranean fever (MEFV) promoter is mediated by a synergistic interaction between C/EBPβ and NFκB p65. *J Biol Chem* 2003;278;48839–48847.
238. Notarnicola C, Didelot M-N, Koné-Paut I, et al. Reduced MEFV messenger RNA expression in patients with familial Mediterranean fever. *Arthritis Rheum* 2002;46:2785–2793.
239. Matzner Y, Abedat S, Shapiro E, et al. Expression of the familial Mediterranean fever gene and activity of the C5a inhibitor in human primary fibroblast cultures. *Blood* 2000;96:727–731.
240. Tidow N, Chen X, Müller C, et al. Hematopoietic-specific expression of *MEFV,* the gene mutated in familial Mediterranean fever, and subcellular localization of its corresponding protein, pyrin. *Blood* 2000; 95:1451–1455.
241. Mansfield E, Chae JJ, Komarow HD, et al. The familial Mediterranean fever protein, pyrin, associates with microtubules and colocalizes with actin filaments. *Blood* 2001;98:851–859.
242. Papin S, Duquesnoy P, Cazeneuve C, et al. Alternative splicing at the *MEFV* locus involved in familial Mediterranean fever regulates translocation of the marenostrin/pyrin protein to the nucleus. *Hum Mol Genet* 2000;9:3001–3009.
243. Erken E, Günesaçar R, Ozbek S, et al. Serum soluble interleukin-2 receptor levels in familial Mediterranean fever. *Ann Rheum Dis* 1996;55:852–855.
244. Gang N, Drenth JP, Langevitz P, et al. Activation of the cytokine network in familial Mediterranean fever. *J Rheumatol* 1999;26:890–897.
245. Direskeneli H, Özdogan H, Korkmaz C, et al. Serum soluble intercellular adhesion molecule 1 and interleukin 8 levels in familial Mediterranean fever. *J Rheumatol* 1999;26:1983–1986.
246. Baykal Y, Saglam K, Yilmaz MI, et al. Serum sIL-2r, IL-6, IL-10, and TNF-α level in familial Mediterranean fever patients. *Clin Rheumatol* 2003;22:99–101.
247. Akcan Y, Bayraktar Y, Arslan S, et al. The importance of serial measurements of cytokine levels for the evaluation of their role in pathogenesis in familial Mediterranean fever. *Eur J Med Res* 2003;8:304–306.
248. Kiraz S, Ertenli I, Arici M, et al. Effects of colchicine on inflammatory cytokines and selectins in familial Mediterranean fever. *Clin Exp Rheumatol* 1998;16:721–724.
249. Aypar E, Ozen S, Okur H, et al. Th1 polarization in familial Mediterranean fever. *J Rheumatol* 2003;30:2011–2013.
250. Ben-Chetrit E, Levy M. Autoantibodies in familial Mediterranean fever (recurrent polyserositis). *Br J Rheumatol* 1990;29:459–461.
251. Swissa M, Schul V, Korish S, et al. Determination of autoantibodies in patients with familial Mediterranean fever and their first degree relatives. *J Rheumatol* 1991;18:606–608.
252. Rozenbaum M, Rosner I. Familial Mediterranean fever is not associated with the antiphospholipid syndrome. *Clin Exp Rheumatol* 1993; 11:578–579.
253. Rozenbaum M, Rosner I, Naschitz Y, et al. Absence of antineutrophil cytoplasmic autoantibodies in familial Mediterranean fever. *J Rheumatol* 1995;22:376–377.
254. Dinarello CA, Chusid MJ, Fauci AS, et al. Effect of prophylactic colchicine therapy on leukocyte function in patients with familial Mediterranean fever. *Arthritis Rheum* 1976;19:618–622.
255. Bar-Eli M, Wilson L, Peters RS, et al. Microtubules in PMNs from patients with familial Mediterranean fever. *Am J Med Sci* 1982;284: 2–7.
256. Anton PA, Targan SR, Vigna SR, et al. Enhanced neutrophil chemiluminescence in familial Mediterranean fever. *J Clin Immunol* 1988;8: 148–156.
257. Bar-Eli M, Territo MC, Peters RS, et al. A neutrophil lysozyme leak in patients with familial Mediterranean fever. *Am J Hematol* 1981; 11:387–395.
258. Konca K, Erken E, Ydrysoglu S. Increased serum eosinophil cationic protein levels in familial Mediterranean fever. *J Rheumatol* 1998;25: 1865–1867.
259. Bar-Eli M, Ehrenfeld M, Levy M, et al. Leukocyte chemotaxis in recurrent polyserositis (familial Mediterranean fever). *Am J Med Sci* 1981;281:15–18.
260. Disdier P, Fossat C, Veit V, et al. Hyperactive polymorphonuclear leukocytes migration in patients with familial Mediterranean fever. *Clin Rheumatol* 1996; 15:517–518.
261. Matzner Y, Brzezinski A. C5a-inhibitor deficiency in peritoneal fluids from patients with familial Mediterranean fever. *N Engl J Med* 1984;311:287–290.
262. Ayesh SK, Azar Y, Barghouti II, et al. Purification and characterization of a C5a-inactivating enzyme from human peritoneal fluid. *Blood* 1995;85:3503–3509.
263. Barakat MH, El-Khawad AO, Gumaa KA, et al. Metaraminol provocative test: a specific diagnostic test for familial Mediterranean fever. *Lancet* 1984;1:656–657.
264. Barakat MH, Gumaa KA, Malhas LN, et al. Plasma dopamine beta-hydroxylase: rapid diagnostic test for recurrent hereditary polyserositis. *Lancet* 1988;2:1280–1283.
265. Barakat MH, Malhas LN, Gumaa KK. Catecholamine metabolism in recurrent hereditary polyserositis. Pathogenesis of acute inflammation: the retention-leakage hypothesis. *Biomed Pharmacother* 1989; 43:763–769.
266. Livneh A, Langevitz P, Zemer D, et al. Criteria for the diagnosis of familial Mediterranean fever. *Arthritis Rheum* 1997;40:1879–1885.

267. Schwabe AD, Terasaki PI, Barnett EV, et al. Familial Mediterranean fever. Recent advances in pathogenesis and management. *West J Med* 1977;127:15–23.
268. Eliakim M, Levy M, Ehrenfeld M. *Recurrent polyserositis (familial Mediterranean fever, periodic disease)*. Amsterdam: Elsevier/North-Holland, 1981:16.
269. Ben-Chetrit E, Sagi M. Genetic counselling in familial Mediterranean fever: has the time come? *Rheumatology* 2001;40:606–609.
270. Cattan D, Dervichian M, Courillon A, et al. Metaraminol provocation test for familial Mediterranean fever. *Lancet* 1984;1:1130–1131.
271. Buades J, Bassa A, Altás J, et al. The metaraminol test and adverse cardiac effects. *Ann Intern Med* 1989;111:259–260.
272. Ben-Chetrit E, Gutman A, Levy M. Dopamine-β-hydroxylase activity in familial Mediterranean fever. *Lancet* 1990;335:176.
273. Broadbent PG, Raynes JG, McAdam KPWJ, et al. Recurrent hereditary polyserositis. *Br Med J* 1991;302:349–350.
274. Courillon-Mallet A, Cauet N, Dervichian M, et al. Plasma dopamine beta-hydroxylase activity in familial Mediterranean fever. *Isr J Med Sci* 1992;28:427–429.
275. Cox TM. The porphyrias. In: Warrell DA, Cox TM, Firth JD, et al., eds. *Oxford Textbook of Medicine*, 4th ed. Oxford: Oxford University Press, 2003:2.61–2.73.
276. Weinstock LB, Kothari T, Sharma RN, et al. Recurrent abdominal pain as the sole manifestation of hereditary angioedema in multiple family members. *Gastroenterology* 1987;93:1116–1118.
277. Kaplan AP. Urticaria and angioedema. In: Middleton E Jr, Ellis EF, Yunginger JW, et al., eds. *Allergy: principles and practice*, 5th ed. St. Louis: Mosby, 1998:1104–1122.
278. Thomas KT, Feder HM, Lawton AR, et al. Periodic fever syndrome in children. *J Pediatr* 1999;135:15–21.
279. Goldfinger SE. Colchicine for familial Mediterranean fever. *N Engl J Med* 1972;287:1302.
280. Zemer D, Revach M, Pras M, et al. A controlled trial of colchicine in preventing attacks of familial Mediterranean fever. *N Engl J Med* 1974;291:932–934.
281. Dinarello CA, Wolff SM, Goldfinger SE, et al. Colchicine therapy for familial Mediterranean fever. A double-blind trial. *N Engl J Med* 1974;291:934–937.
282. Goldstein RC, Schwabe AD. Prophylactic colchicine therapy for familial Mediterranean fever. A controlled, double-blind study. *Ann Intern Med* 1974;81:792–794.
283. Zemer D, Pras M, Sohar E, et al. Colchicine in the prevention and treatment of the amyloidosis of familial Mediterranean fever. *N Engl J Med* 1986;314:1001–1005.
284. Wright DG, Wolff SM, Fauci AS, et al. Efficacy of intermittent colchicine therapy in familial Mediterranean fever. *Ann Intern Med* 1977;86:162–165.
285. Livneh A, Zemer D, Langevitz P, et al. Colchicine treatment of AA amyloidosis of familial Mediterranean fever. An analysis of factors affecting outcome. *Arthritis Rheum* 1994;37:1804–1811.
286. Simsek B, Islek I, Simsek T, et al. Regression of nephrotic syndrome due to amyloidosis secondary to familial Mediterranean fever following colchicine treatment. *Nephrol Dial Transplant* 2000;15:281–282.
287. Öner A, Erdogan O, Demircin G, et al. Efficacy of colchicine therapy for amyloid nephropathy of familial Mediterranean fever. *Pediatr Nephrol* 2003;18:521–526.
288. Hastie SB. Interactions of colchicine with tubulin. *Pharmacol Ther* 1991;51:377–401.
289. Chappey ON, Niel N, Wautier JL, et al. Colchicine disposition in human leukocytes after single and multiple oral administration. *Clin Pharmacol Ther* 1993;54:360–367.
290. Ben-Chetrit E, Levy M. Does the lack of the P-glycoprotein efflux pump in neutrophils explain the efficacy of colchicine in familial Mediterranean fever and other inflammatory diseases? *Med Hypotheses* 1998;51:377–380.
291. Ben-Chetrit E, Levy M. Familial Mediterranean fever. *Lancet* 1998;351:659–664.
292. Cronstein BN, Molad Y, Reibman J, et al. Colchicine alters the quantitative and qualitative display of selectins on endothelial cells and neutrophils. *J Clin Invest* 1995;96:994–1002.
293. Heller H, Sohar E, Gafni J, et al. Amyloidosis in familial Mediterranean fever. An independent genetically determined character. *Arch Intern Med* 1961;107:539–550.
294. Hull KM, Drewe E, Aksentijevich I, et al. The TNF receptor-associated periodic syndrome (TRAPS). Emerging concepts of an autoinflammatory disorder. *Medicine* (Baltimore) 2002;81:349–368.
295. Dodé C, Hazenberg BPC, Pêcheux C, et al. Mutational spectrum in the *MEFV* and *TNFRSF1A* genes in patients suffering from AA amyloidosis and recurrent inflammatory attacks. *Nephrol Dial Transplant* 2002;17:1212–1217.
296. Gillmore JD, Lovat LB, Persey MR, et al. Amyloid load and clinical outcome in AA amyloidosis in relation to circulating concentration of serum amyloid A protein. *Lancet* 2001;358:24–29.
297. Cunnane G. Amyloid proteins in pathogenesis of AA amyloidosis. *Lancet* 2001;358:4–5.
298. Pepys MB, Herbert J, Hutchinson WL, et al. Targeted pharmacological depletion of serum amyloid P component for treatment of human amyloidosis. *Nature* 2002;417:254–259.
299. Hart J, Lewin KJ, Peters RS, et al. Effect of long-term colchicine therapy on jejunal mucosa. *Dig Dis Sci* 1993;38:2017–2021.
300. Fradkin A, Yahav J, Zemer D, et al. Colchicine-induced lactose malabsorption in patients with familial Mediterranean fever. *Isr J Med Sci* 1995;31:616–620.
301. Alster Y, Varssano D, Loewenstein A, et al. Delay of corneal wound healing in patients treated with colchicine. *Ophthalmology* 1997;104:118–119.
302. Leibovitch I, Alster Y, Scherrmann JM, et al. Colchicine in tear fluid of treated patients with familial Mediterranean fever. *Cornea* 2003;22:191–193.
303. Leibovitch I, Alster Y, Lazar M, et al. Corneal wound healing in a patient treated with colchicine for familial Mediterranean fever. *Rheumatology* 2003;42:1021–1022.
304. Ben-Chetrit E, Scherrmann J-M, Zylber-Katz E, et al. Colchicine disposition in patients with familial Mediterranean fever and renal impairment. *J Rheumatol* 1994;21:710–713.
305. Ben-Chetrit E, Levy M. Colchicine: 1998 update. *Semin Arthritis Rheum* 1998;28:48–59.
306. Caraco Y, Putterman C, Rahamimov R, et al. Acute colchicine intoxication— possible role of erythromycin administration. *J Rheumatol* 1992;19:494–496.
307. Hsu W-C, Chen W-H, Chang M-T, et al. Colchicine-induced acute myopathy in a patient with concomitant use of simvastatin. *Clin Neuropharmacol* 2002;25:266–268.
308. Kuncl RW, Duncan G, Watson D, et al. Colchicine myopathy and neuropathy. *N Engl J Med* 1987;316:1562–1568.
309. Altiparmak MR, Pamuk ON, Pamuk GE, et al. Colchicine neuromyopathy: a report of six cases. *Clin Exp Rheumatol* 2002;20[4 Suppl 26]:S13–16.
310. Harel L, Mukamel M, Amir J, et al. Colchicine-induced myoneuropathy in childhood. *Eur J Pediatr* 1998;157:853–855.
311. Kissin EY, Corbo JC, Farraye FA, et al. Colchicine myopathy in a patient with familial Mediterranean fever and normal renal function. *Arthritis Rheum* 2003;49:614–616.
312. Sayarlioglu M, Sayarlioglu H, Ozen S, et al. Colchicine-induced myopathy in a teenager with familial Mediterranean fever. *Ann Pharmacother* 2003;37:1821–1824.
313. Özkaya N, Yalçinkaya F. Colchicine treatment in children with familial Mediterranean fever. *Clin Rheumatol* 2003;22:314–317.
314. Zemer D, Livneh A, Danon YL, et al. Long-term colchicine treatment in children with familial Mediterranean fever. *Arthritis Rheum* 1991;34:973–977.
315. Ben-Chetrit E, Levy M. Reproductive system in familial Mediterranean fever: an overview. *Ann Rheum Dis* 2003;62:916–919.
316. Mijatovic V, Hompes PG, Wouters MG. Familial Mediterranean fever and its implications for fertility and pregnancy. *Eur J Obstet Gynecol Reprod Biol* 2003;108:171–176.
317. Rabinovitch O, Zemer D, Kukia E, et al. Colchicine treatment in conception and pregnancy: two hundred thirty-one pregnancies in patients with familial Mediterranean fever. *Am J Reprod Immunol* 1992;28:245–246.
318. Michael O, Goldman RD, Koren G, et al. Safety of colchicine therapy during pregnancy. *Can Fam Physician* 2003;49:967–969.
319. Ditkoff EC, Sauer MV. Successful pregnancy in a familial Mediterranean fever patient following assisted reproduction. *J Assist Reprod Genet* 1996;13:684–685.

320. Ben-Chetrit E, Scherrmann J-M, Levy M. Colchicine in breast milk of patients with familial Mediterranean fever. *Arthritis Rheum* 1996; 39:1213–1217.
321. Ehrenfeld M, Levy M, Margalioth EJ, et al. The effects of long-term colchicine therapy on male fertility in patients with familial Mediterranean fever. *Andrologia* 1986;18:420–426.
322. Ben Chetrit E, Backenroth R, Haimov-Kochman R, et al. Azoospermia in familial Mediterranean fever patients: the role of colchicine and amyloidosis. *Ann Rheum Dis* 1998;57:259–260.
323. Haimov-Kochman R, Ben-Chetrit E. The effect of colchicine treatment on sperm production and function: a review. *Hum Reprod* 1998; 13:360–362.
324. Kastrop P, Kimmel I, Bancsi L, et al. The effect of colchicine treatment on spermatozoa: a cytogenetic approach. *J Assist Reprod Genet* 1999;16:504–507.
325. Haimov-Kochman R, Prus D, Ben-Chetrit E. Azoospermia due to testicular amyloidosis in a patient with familial Mediterranean fever. *Hum Reprod* 2001;16:1218–1220.
326. Putterman C, Ben-Chetrit E, Caraco Y, et al. Colchicine intoxication: clinical pharmacology, risk factors, features, and management. *Semin Arthritis Rheum* 1991;21:143–155.
327. Simons RJ, Kingma DW. Fatal colchicine toxicity. *Am J Med* 1989; 86:356–357.
328. Wallace SL, Singer JZ. Review: systemic toxicity associated with the intravenous administration of colchicine. Guidelines for use. *J Rheumatol* 1988;15:495–499.
329. Bonnel RA, Villalba ML, Karwoski CB, et al. Deaths associated with inappropriate intravenous colchicine administration. *J Emerg Med* 2002;22:385–387.
329a. Lidar M, Kedem R, Langevitz P, et al. Intravenous colchicine for treatment of patients with familial Mediterranean fever unresponsive to oral colchicine. *J Rheumatol* 2003;30:2620–2623.
330. Reissman P, Durst AL, Rivkind A, et al. Elective laparoscopic appendectomy in patients with familial Mediterranean fever. *World J Surg* 1994;18:139–141.
331. Schwabe AD. Invited commentary. *World J Surg* 1994;18:141–142.
332. Tankurt E, Tunça M, Akbaylar H, et al. Resolving familial Mediterranean fever attacks with interferon alpha. *Br J Rheumatol* 1996;35: 1188–1189.
333. Tunça M, Tankurt E, Akpinar HA, et al. The efficacy of interferon alpha on colchicine-resistant familial Mediterranean fever attacks: a pilot study. *Br J Rheumatol* 1997;36:1005–1008.
334. Milledge J, Shaw PJ, Mansour A, et al. Allogeneic bone marrow transplantation: cure for familial Mediterranean fever. *Blood* 2002; 100:774–777.
335. Touitou I, Ben-Chetrit E, Gershoni-Baruch R, et al. Allogenic bone marrow transplantation: not a treatment yet for familial Mediterranean fever. *Blood* 2003;102:409.
336. Manji GA, Wang L, Geddes BJ, et al. PYPAF1, a PYRIN-containing Apaf1-like protein that assembles with ASC and regulates activation of NF-κB. *J Biol Chem* 2002;277:11570–11575.
337. O'Connor W Jr, Harton JA, Zhu X, et al. Cutting edge: CIAS1/cryopyrin/PYPAF1/NALP3/CATERPILLER 1.1 is an inducible inflammatory mediator with NF-κB suppressive properties. *J Immunol* 2003;171:6329–6333.
338. Hoffman HM, Wanderer AA, Broide DH. Familial cold autoinflammatory syndrome: phenotype and genotype of an autosomal dominant periodic fever. *J Allergy Clin Immunol* 2001;108:615–620.
339. Hashkes PJ, Lovell DJ. Recognition of infantile-onset multisystem inflammatory disease as a unique entity. *J Pediatr* 1997;130:513–515.
340. Prieur AM. A recently recognised chronic inflammatory disease of early onset characterized by the triad of rash, central nervous system involvement and arthropathy. *Clin Exp Rheumatol* 2001;19:103–106.
341. Neven B, Callebaut I, Prieur A-M, et al. Molecular basis of the spectral expression of *CIAS1* mutations associated with phagocytic cell-mediated auto-inflammatory disorders (CINCA/NOMID, MWS, FCU). *Blood* 2004;103:2809–2815.
342. Granel B, Philip N, Serratrice J, et al. *CIAS1* mutation in a patient with overlap between Muckle-Wells and chronic infantile neurological cutaneous and articular syndromes. *Dermatology* 2003;206:257–259.
343. Rösen-Wolff A, Quietzsch J, Schröder H, et al. Two German CINCA (NOMID) patients with different clinical severity and response to anti-inflammatory treatment. *Eur J Haematol* 2003;71:215–219.
344. Tonnesen MG, Clark RAF, Siegal SL, et al. Cyclic endothelial cell injury and chronic blood vessel wall alterations in familial cold urticaria. *Clin Res* 1985;33:690(abst).
345. Commerford PJ, Meyers OL. Arthropathy associated with familial cold urticaria. *S Afr Med J* 1977;51:105–108.
346. Muckle TJ. The 'Muckle-Wells' syndrome. *Br J Dermatol* 1979;100: 87–92.
347. Watts RA, Nicholls A, Scott DG. The arthropathy of the Muckle-Wells syndrome. *Br J Rheumatol* 1994;33:1184–1187.
348. Cuisset L, Drenth JP, Berthelot J-M, et al. Genetic linkage of the Muckle-Wells syndrome to chromosome 1q44. *Am J Hum Genet* 1999;65:1054–1059.
349. Lieberman A, Grossman ME, Silvers DN. Muckle-Wells syndrome: case report and review of cutaneous pathology. *J Am Acad Dermatol* 1998;39:290–291.
350. Schwartz RE, Dralle H, Linke RP, et al. Amyloid goiter and arthritides after kidney transplantation in a patient with systemic amyloidosis and Muckle-Wells syndrome. *Am J Clin Pathol* 1989;92:821–825.
351. Prieur A-M, Griscelli C, Lampert F, et al. A chronic, infantile, neurological, cutaneous and articular (CINCA) syndrome. A specific entity analysed in 30 patients. *Scand J Rheumatol* 1987;66[Suppl]:57–68.
352. Torbiak RP, Dent PB, Cockshott WP. NOMID—a neonatal syndrome of multisystem inflammation. *Skeletal Radiol* 1989;18:359–364.
353. Dollfus H, Häfner R, Hofmann HM, et al. Chronic infantile neurological cutaneous and articular/neonatal onset multisystem inflammatory disease syndrome. Ocular manifestations in a recently recognized chronic inflammatory disease of childhood. *Arch Ophthalmol* 2000;118:1386–1392.
354. Kaufman RA, Lovell DJ. Infantile-onset multisystem inflammatory disease: radiologic findings. *Radiology* 1986;160:741–746.
355. Yarom A, Rennebohm RM, Levinson JE. Infantile multisystem inflammatory disease: a specific syndrome? *J Pediatr* 1985;106:390–396.
356. McDermott MF, Aganna E, Hitman GA, et al. An autosomal dominant periodic fever associated with AA amyloidosis in a north Indian family maps to distal chromosome 1q. *Arthritis Rheum* 2000;43: 2034–2040.
357. Hoffman HM, Wright FA, Broide DH, et al. Identification of a locus on chromosome 1q44 for familial cold urticaria. *Am J Hum Genet* 2000;66:1693–1698.
358. Koonin EV, Aravind L. The NACHT family—a new group of predicted NTPases implicated in apoptosis and MHC transcription activation. *Trends Biol Sci* 2000;25:223–224.
359. Dangl JL, Jones, JD. Plant pathogens and integrated defence responses to infection. *Nature* 2001;411:826–833.
360. Inohara N, Ogura Y, Nuñez G. Nods: a family of cytosolic proteins that regulate the host response to pathogens. *Curr Opin Microbiol* 2002;5:76–80.
361. Chamaillard M, Girardin SE, Viala J, et al. NODS, NALPS, and NAIP: intracellular regulators of bacterial-induced inflammation. *Cell Microbiol* 2003;5:581–592.
362. Girardin SE, Boneca IG, Viala J, et al. NOD2 is a general sensor of peptidoglycan through muramyl dipeptide (MDP) detection. *J Biol Chem* 2003;278:8869–8872.
363. Hoffman HM, Gregory SG, Mueller JL, et al. Finstructure mapping of *CIAS1:* identification of an ancestral haplotype and a common FCAS mutation, L353P. *Hum Genet* 2003;112:209–216.
364. Albrecht M, Lengauer T, Schreiber S. Disease-associated variants of PYPAF1 and NOD2 result in similar alterations of conserved sequence. *Bioinformatics* 2003;19:2171–2175.
365. Albrecht M, Domingues FS, Schreiber S, et al. Structural localization of disease-associated sequence variations in the NACHT and LRR domains of PYPAF1 and NOD2. *FEBS Lett* 2003;554:520–528.
366. Gumucio DL, Diaz A, Schaner P, et al. Fire and ICE: The role of pyrin domain-containing proteins in inflammation and apoptosis. *Clin Exp Rheumatol* 2002;20[Suppl 26]:S45–S53.
367. Gerbig AW, Dahinden CA, Mullis P, et al. Circadian elevation of IL-6 levels in Muckle-Wells syndrome: a disorder of the neuroimmune axis? *Q J Med* 1998;91:489–492.
368. Leone V, Presani G, Perticarari S, et al. Chronic infantile neurological cutaneous articular syndrome: CD10 over-expression in neutrophils is a possible key to the pathogenesis of the disease. *Eur J Pediatr* 2003;162:669–673.

369. Zip CM, Ross JB, Greaves MW, et al. Familial cold urticaria. *Clin Exp Dermatol* 1993;18:338–341.
370. Ormerod AD, Smart L, Reid TM, et al. Familial cold urticaria. Investigation of a family and response to stanozolol. *Arch Dermatol* 1993;129:343–346.
371. DeCunto CL, Liberatore DI, San Roman JL, et al. Infantile-onset multisystem inflammatory disease: a differential diagnosis of systemic juvenile rheumatoid arthritis. *J Pediatr* 1997;130:551–556.
372. Hawkins PN, Lachmann HJ, McDermott MF. Interleukin-1-receptor antagonist in the Muckle-Wells syndrome. *N Engl J Med* 2003;348:2583–2584.
373. Federico G, Rigante D, Pugliese AL, et al. Etanercept induces improvement of arthropathy in chronic infantile neurological cutaneous articular (CINCA) syndrome. *Scand J Rheumatol* 2003;32:312–314.
374. McDermott EM, Smillie DM, Powell RJ. Clinical spectrum of familial Hibernian fever: a 14-year follow-up study of the index case and extended family. *Mayo Clin Proc* 1997;72:806–817.
375. Mulley J, Saar K, Hewitt G, et al. Gene localization for an autosomal dominant familial periodic fever to 12p13. *Am J Hum Genet* 1998;62:884–889.
376. Bergman F, Warmenius S. Familial perireticular amyloidosis in a Swedish family. *Am J Med* 1968;45:601–606.
377. Gertz MA, Petitt RM, Perrault J, et al. Autosomal dominant familial Mediterranean fever-like syndrome with amyloidosis. *Mayo Clin Proc* 1987;62:1095–1100.
378. Hawle H, Winckelmann G, Kortsik CS. Familiares Mittelmeerfieber in einer deutschen Familie. [Familial Mediterranean fever in a German family.] *Dtsch Med Wochenschr* 1989;114:665–668.
379. Karenko L, Pettersson T, Roberts P. Autosomal dominant "Mediterranean fever" in a Finnish family. *J Intern Med* 1992;232:365–369.
380. Zweers EJ, Erkelens DW. Een Nederlandse familie met familiale mediterrane koorts. [A Dutch family with familial Mediterranean fever.] *Ned Tijdschr Geneeskd* 1993;137:1570–1573.
381. Mache CJ, Goriup U, Fischel-Ghodsian N, et al. Autosomal dominant familial Mediterranean fever-like syndrome. *Eur J Pediatr* 1996;155:787–790.
382. Gadallah MF, Vasquez F, Abreo F, et al. A 38-year-old man with nephrotic syndrome, episodic fever, and abdominal pain. *J La State Med Soc* 1995;147:493–499.
383. Zaks N, Kastner DL. Clinical syndromes resembling familial Mediterranean fever. In: Sohar E, Gafni J, Pras M, eds. *Familial Mediterranean fever.* First international conference. London and Tel Aviv: Freund, 1997:211–215.
384. McDermott MF, Ogunkolade BW, McDermott EM, et al. Linkage of familial Hibernian fever to chromosome 12p13. *Am J Hum Genet* 1998;62:1446–1451.
385. Grateau G, Drenth JP, Delpech M. Hereditary fevers. *Curr Opin Rheumatol* 1999;11:75–78.
386. Dodé C, Papo T, Fieschi, et al. A novel missense mutation (C30S) in the gene encoding tumor necrosis factor receptor 1 linked to autosomal-dominant recurrent fever with localized myositis in a French family. *Arthritis Rheum* 2000;43:1535–1542.
387. Aganna E, Aksentijevich I, Hitman G, et al. Tumor necrosis factor receptor-associated periodic syndrome (TRAPS) in a Dutch family: evidence for a *TNFRSF1A* mutation with reduced penetrance. *Eur J Hum Genet* 2001;9:63–66.
388. Aksentijevich I, Galon J, Soares M, et al. The tumor-necrosis-factor receptor–associated periodic syndrome: new mutations in *TNFRSF1A,* ancestral origins, genotype-phenotype studies, and evidence for further genetic heterogeneity of periodic fevers. *Am J Hum Genet* 2001;69:301–314.
389. Jadoul M, Dodé C, Cosyns J-P, et al. Autosomal-dominant periodic fever with AA amyloidosis: novel mutation in tumor necrosis factor receptor 1 gene. *Kidney Int* 2001;59:1677–1682.
390. Simon A, Dodé C, van der Meer J, et al. Familial periodic fever and amyloidosis due to a new mutation in the *TNFRSF1A* gene. *Am J Med* 2001;110:313–316.
391. Simon A, van Deuren M, Tighe PJ, et al. Genetic analysis as a valuable key to diagnosis and treatment of periodic fever. *Arch Intern Med* 2001;161:2491–2493.
392. Aganna E, Zeharia A, Hitman GA, et al. An Israeli Arab patient with a de novo *TNFRSF1A* mutation causing tumor necrosis factor receptor–associated periodic syndrome. *Arthritis Rheum* 2002;46:245–249.
393. Dodé C, André M, Bienvenu T, et al. The enlarging clinical, genetic, and population spectrum of tumor necrosis factor receptor–associated periodic syndrome. *Arthritis Rheum* 2002;46:2181–2188.
394. Nevala H, Karenko L, Stjernberg S, et al. A novel mutation in the third extracellular domain of the tumor necrosis factor receptor 1 in a Finnish family with autosomal-dominant recurrent fever. *Arthritis Rheum* 2002;46:1061–1066.
395. Aganna E, Hammond L, Hawkins PN, et al. Heterogeneity among patients with tumor necrosis factor receptor–associated periodic syndrome phenotypes. *Arthritis Rheum* 2003;48:2632–2644.
396. Kriegel MA, Hüffmeier U, Scherb E, et al. Tumor necrosis factor receptor–associated periodic syndrome characterized by a mutation affecting the cleavage site of the receptor: implications for pathogenesis. *Arthritis Rheum* 2003;48:2386–2388.
397. Weyhreter H, Schwartz M, Kristensen TD, et al. A new mutation causing autosomal dominant periodic fever syndrome in a Danish family. *J Pediatr* 2003;142:191–193.
398. Poirier O, Nicaud V, Gariepy J, et al. Polymorphism R92Q of the tumour necrosis factor receptor 1 gene is associated with myocardial infarction and carotid intima-media thickness—the ECTIM, AXA, EVA, and GENIC studies. *Eur J Hum Genet* 2004;12:213–219.
399. Kusuhara K, Nomura A, Nakao F, et al. Tumor necrosis factor receptor-associated periodic syndrome with a novel mutation in the *TNFRSF1A* gene in a Japanese family. *Eur J Pediatr* 2004;163:30–32.
400. Toro JR, Aksentijevich I, Hull K, et al. Tumor necrosis factor receptor–associated periodic syndrome. A novel syndrome with cutaneous manifestations. *Arch Dermatol* 2000;136:1487–1494.
401. Hull KM, Wong K, Wood GM, et al. Monocytic fasciitis. A newly recognized clinical feature of tumor necrosis factor receptor dysfunction. *Arthritis Rheum* 2002;46:2189–2194.
402. Drewe E, Lanyon PC, Powell RJ. Emerging clinical spectrum of tumor necrosis factor receptor–associated periodic syndrome: comment on the articles by Hull et al and Dodé et al. *Arthritis Rheum* 2003;48:1768–1769.
403. Rösen Wolff A, Kreth H-W, Hofmann S, et al. Periodic fever (TRAPS) caused by mutations in the TNFα receptor 1 (*TNFRSF1A*) gene of three German patients. *Eur J Haematol* 2001;67:105–109.
404. Loetscher H, Pan Y-CE, Lahm H-W, et al. Molecular cloning and expression of the human 55 kd tumor necrosis factor receptor. *Cell* 1990;61:351–359.
405. Schall TJ, Lewis M, Koller KJ, et al. Molecular cloning and expression of a receptor for human tumor necrosis factor. *Cell* 1990;61:361–370.
406. Bazzoni F, Beutler B. The tumor necrosis factor ligand and receptor families. *N Engl J Med* 1996;334:1717–1725.
407. Smith CA, Davis T, Anderson D, et al. A receptor for tumor necrosis factor defines an unusual family of cellular and viral proteins. *Science* 1990;248:1019–1023.
408. Engelmann H, Holtmann H, Brakebusch C, et al. Antibodies to a soluble form of a tumor necrosis factor (TNF) receptor have TNF-like activity. *J Biol Chem* 1990;265:14497–14504.
409. Glossop JR, Nixon NB, Dawes PT, et al. No association of polymorphisms in the tumor necrosis factor receptor I and receptor II genes with disease severity in rheumatoid arthritis. *J Rheumatol* 2003;30:1406–1409.
410. Watowich SS, Yoshimura A, Longmore GD, et al. Homo-dimerization and constitutive activation of the erythropoietin receptor. *Proc Natl Acad Sci U S A* 1992;89:2140–2144.
411. Reddy P, Slack JL, Davis R, et al. Functional analysis of the domain structure of tumor necrosis factor-α converting enzyme. *J Biol Chem* 2000:275:14608–14614.
412. Chui X, Hawari F, Alsaaty S, et al. Identification of ARTS-1 as a novel TNFR1-binding protein that promotes TNFR1 ectodomain shedding. *J Clin Invest* 2002;110:515–526.
413. Engelmann H, Aderka D, Rubinstein M, et al. A tumor necrosis factor-binding protein purified to homogeneity from human urine protects cells from tumor necrosis factor toxicity. *J Biol Chem* 1989;264:11974–11980.
414. Chan FK, Chun HJ, Zheng L, et al. A domain in TNF receptors that mediates ligand independent receptor assembly and signaling. *Science* 2000;288:2351–2354.
415. McDermott EM, Powell RJ. Circulating cytokine concentrations in familial Hibernian fever. In: Sohar E, Gafni J, Pras M, eds. *Familial*

Mediterranean fever. First international conference. London and Tel Aviv: Freund, 1997:189–192.

416. Kastner DL, Aksentijevich I, Galon J, et al. TNF receptor associated periodic syndromes (TRAPS): novel TNFR1 mutations and early experience with etanercept therapy. *Arthritis Rheum* 1999;42:S117 (abst).
417. Nigrovic PA, Sundel RP. Treatment of TRAPS with etanercept: use in pediatrics. *Clin Exp Rheumatol* 2001;19:484–485.
418. Drewe E, McDermott EM, Powell PT, et al. Prospective study of anti-tumour necrosis factor receptor superfamily 1B fusion protein, and case study of anti-tumour necrosis factor receptor superfamily 1A fusion protein, in tumour necrosis factor receptor associated periodic syndrome (TRAPS): clinical and laboratory findings in a series of seven patients. *Rheumatology* 2003;42:235–239.
419. Hull KM, Aksentijevich I, Singh H, et al. Efficacy of etanercept for the treatment of patients with TNF receptor-associated periodic syndrome (TRAPS). *Arthritis Rheum* 2002;46:S378(abst).
420. Drewe E, McDermott EM, Powell RJ. Treatment of the nephrotic syndrome with etanercept in patients with the tumor necrosis factor receptor–associated periodic syndrome. *N Engl J Med* 2000;343: 1044–1045.
421. Hull KM, Kastner DL, Balow JE. Hereditary periodic fever. *N Engl J Med* 2002;346:1415.
422. Simon A, Drenth JP. Genes associated with periodic fevers highlighted at Dutch workshop. *Lancet* 1999;354:2141. [Further details of this workshop can be found on the Internet at *http://hids.net.*]
423. Valle D. You give me fever. *Nature Genet* 1999;22:121–122.
424. Drenth JP, Haagsma CJ, van der Meer JW, International Hyper-IgD Study Group. Hyperimmunoglobulinemia D and periodic fever syndrome. The clinical spectrum in a series of 50 patients. *Medicine* (Baltimore) 1994;73:133–144.
425. Topaloglu R, Saatçi Ü. Hyperimmunoglobulinaemia D and periodic fever mimicking familial Mediterranean fever in the Mediterranean. *Postgrad Med J* 1991;67:490–491.
426. Miyagawa S, Kitamura W, Morita K, et al. Association of hyperimmunoglobulinaemia D syndrome with erythema elevatum diutinum. *Br J Dermatol* 1993;128:572–574.
427. Grose C, Schnetzer JR, Ferrante A, et al. Children with hyperimmunoglobulinemia D and periodic fever syndrome. *Pediatr Infect Dis J* 1996;15:72–77.
428. Haraldsson A, Weemaes CM, deBoer AW, et al. Immunological studies in the hyper-immunoglobulin D syndrome. *J Clin Immunol* 1992; 12:424–428.
429. Loeliger AE, Kruize AA, Bijilsma JW, et al. Arthritis in hyperimmunoglobulinaemia D. *Ann Rheum Dis* 1993;52:81.
430. Drenth JP, Prieur AM. Occurrence of arthritis in hyperimmunoglobulinaemia D. *Ann Rheum Dis* 1993;52:765–766.
431. Drenth JP, Boom BW, Toonstra J, et al., International Hyper-IgD Study Group. Cutaneous manifestations and histologic findings in the hyperimmunoglobulinemia D syndrome. *Arch Dermatol* 1994; 130:59–65.
432. Saulsbury FT. Hyperimmunoglobulinemia D and periodic fever syndrome (HIDS) in a child with normal serum IgD, but increased serum IgA concentration. *J Pediatr* 2003;143:127–129.
433. Frenkel J, Houten SM, Waterham HR, et al. Mevalonate kinase deficiency and Dutch type periodic fever. *Clin Exp Rheumatol* 2000;18: 525–532.
434. Takada K, Aksentijevich I, Mahadevan V, et al. Favorable preliminary experience with etanercept in two patients with the hyperimmunoglobulinemia D and periodic fever syndrome. *Arthritis Rheum* 2003;48:2645–2651.
435. Hiemstra I, Vossen JM, van der Meer JW, et al. Clinical and immunological studies in patients with an increased serum IgD level. *J Clin Immunol* 1989;9:393–400.
436. Klasen IS, Göertz JH, van de Wiel AS, et al. Hyper-immunoglobulin A in the hyperimmunoglobulinemia D syndrome. *Clin Diagn Lab Immunol* 2001;8:58–61.
437. Frenkel J, Houten SM, Waterham HR, et al. Clinical and molecular variability in childhood periodic fever with hyperimmunoglobulinaemia D. *Rheumatology* 2001;40:579–584.
438. Kelley RI, Takada K, Aksentijevich I. Hereditary periodic fever. *N Engl J Med* 2002;346:1416.
439. Livneh A, Drenth JP, Klasen IS, et al. Familial Mediterranean fever and hyperimmunoglobulinemia D syndrome: two diseases with distinct clinical, serologic, and genetic features. *J Rheumatol* 1997;24: 1558–1563.
440. Hoffmann G, Gibson KM, Brandt IK, et al. Mevalonic aciduria—an inborn error of cholesterol and nonsterol isoprene biosynthesis. *N Engl J Med* 1986;314:1610–1614.
441. Hoffmann GF, Charpentier C, Mayatepek E, et al. Clinical and biochemical phenotype in 11 patients with mevalonic aciduria. *Pediatrics* 1993;91:915–921.
442. Kelley RI. Inborn errors of cholesterol biosynthesis. *Adv Pediatr* 2000;47:1–53.
443. Houten SM, Koster J, Romeijn G-J, et al. Organization of the mevalonate kinase (*MVK*) gene and identification of novel mutations causing mevalonic aciduria and hyperimmunoglobulinemia D and periodic fever syndrome. *Eur J Hum Genet* 2001;9:253–259.
444. Cuisset L, Drenth JP, Simon A, et al. Molecular analysis of *MVK* mutations and enzymatic activity in hyper-IgD and periodic fever syndrome. *Eur J Hum Genet* 2001;9:260–266.
445. Schafer BL, Bishop RW, Kratunis VJ, et al. Molecular cloning of human mevalonate kinase and identification of a missense mutation in the genetic disease mevalonic aciduria. *J Biol Chem* 1992;267: 13229–13238.
446. Houten SM, Wanders RJ, Waterham HR. Biochemical and genetic aspects of mevalonate kinase and its deficiency. *Biochim Biophys Acta* 2000;1529:19–32.
447. Arkwright PD, McDermott MF, Houten SM, et al. Hyper IgD syndrome (HIDS) associated with *in vitro* evidence of defective monocyte TNFRSF1A shedding and partial response to TNF receptor blockade with etanercept. *Clin Exp Immunol* 2002;130:484–488.
448. Simon A, Mariman EC, van der Meer JW, et al. A founder effect in the hyperimmunoglobulinemia D and periodic fever syndrome. *Am J Med* 2003;114:148–152.
449. Houten SM, van Woerden CS, Wijburg FA, et al. Carrier frequency of the V377I (1129G>A) *MVK* mutation, associated with hyper-IgD and periodic fever syndrome, in the Netherlands. *Eur J Hum Genet* 2002;11:196–200.
450. Goldstein JL, Brown MS. Regulation of the mevalonate pathway. *Nature* 1990;343:425–430.
451. Brown MS, Goldstein JL. The SREBP pathway: regulation of cholesterol metabolism by proteolysis of a membrane-bound transcription factor. *Cell* 1997;89:331–340.
452. Sinensky M. Recent advances in the study of prenylated proteins. *Biochim Biophys Acta* 2000;1484:3115–3124.
453. Houten SM, Schneiders MS, Wanders RJ, et al. Regulation of isoprenoid/cholesterol biosynthesis in cells from mevalonate kinase-deficient patients. *J Biol Chem* 2003;278:5736–5743.
454. Houten SM, Frenkel J, Rijkers GT, et al. Temperature dependence of mutant mevalonate kinase activity as a pathogenic factor in hyper-IgD and periodic fever syndrome. *Hum Mol Genet* 2002;11:3115–3124.
455. Drenth JP, Goertz J, Daha MR, et al. Immunoglobulin D enhances the release of tumor necrosis factor-alpha, and interleukin-1 beta as well as interleukin-1 receptor antagonist from human mononuclear cells. *Immunology* 1996;88:355–62.
456. Drenth JP, van Deuren M, van der Ven-Jongekrijg J, et al. Cytokine activation during attacks of the hyperimmunoglobulinemia D and periodic fever syndrome. *Blood* 1995;85:3586–3593.
457. Drenth JP, Powell RJ, Brown NS, et al. Interferon-γ and urine neopterin in attacks of the hyperimmunoglobulinemia D and periodic fever syndrome. *Eur J Clin Invest* 1995;25:683–686.
458. Frenkel J, Willemsen MA, Weemaes CM, et al. Increased urinary leukotriene E_4 during febrile attacks in the hyperimmunoglobulinaemia D and periodic fever syndrome. *Arch Dis Child* 2001;85: 158–159.
459. Drenth JP, van der Meer JW, Kushner I. Unstimulated peripheral blood mononuclear cells from patients with the hyper-IgD syndrome produce cytokines capable of potent induction of C-reactive protein and serum amyloid A in Hep3B cells. *J Immunol* 1996;157:400–404.
460. Frenkel J, Rijkers GT, Mandey SH, et al. Lack of isoprenoid products raises *ex vivo* interleukin-1β secretion in hyperimmunoglobulinemia D and periodic fever syndrome. *Arthritis Rheum* 2002;46:2794–2803.
461. Simon A, Cuisset L, Vincent M-F, et al. Molecular analysis of the mevalonate kinase gene in a cohort of patients with the hyper-IgD and periodic fever syndrome: its application as a diagnostic tool. *Ann Intern Med* 2001;135:338–343.

462. Boom BW, Daha MR, Vermeer B-J, et al. IgD immune complex vasculitis in a patient with hyperimmunoglobulinemia D and periodic fever. *Arch Dermatol* 1990;126:1621–1624.
463. Prietsch V, Mayatepek E, Krastel H, et al. Mevalonate kinase deficiency: enlarging the clinical and biochemical spectrum. *Pediatrics* 2003;111:258–261.
464. Medlej-Hashim M, Petit I, Adib S, et al. Familial Mediterranean fever: association of elevated IgD plasma levels with specific MEFV mutations. *Eur J Hum Genet* 2001;9:849–854.
465. Drenth JP, Vonk AG, Simon A, et al. Limited efficacy of thalidomide in the treatment of febrile attacks of the hyper-IgD and periodic fever syndrome: a randomized, double-blind, placebo-controlled trial. *J Pharmacol Exp Ther* 2001;298:1221–1226.
466. Wise CA, Bennett LB, Pascual V, et al. Localization of the gene for familial recurrent arthritis. *Arthritis Rheum* 2000;43:2041–2045.
467. Yeon HB, Lindo NM, Seidman JG, et al. Pyogenic arthritis, pyoderma gangrenosum, and acne syndrome maps to chromosome 15q. *Am J Hum Genet* 2000;66:1443–1448.
468. Spencer S, Dowbenko D, Cheng J, et al. PSTPIP: a tyrosine phosphorylated cleavage furrow–associated protein that is a substrate for a PEST tyrosine phosphatase. *J Cell Biol* 1997;138:845–860.
469. Li J, Nishizawa K, An W, et al. A cdc15-like adaptor protein (CD2BP1) interacts with the CD2 cytoplasmic domain and regulates CD2-triggered adhesion. *EMBO J* 1998;17:7320–7336.
470. Fankhauser C, Reymond A, Cerutti L, et al. The S. pombe cdc15 gene is a key element in the reorganization of F-actin at mitosis. *Cell* 1995;82:435–444.
471. Wolff K, Stingl G. Pyoderma gangrenosum. In: Freedberg IM, Eisen AZ, Wolff K, et al, eds. *Fitzpatrick's dermatology in general medicine,* 6th ed. New York: McGraw-Hill, 2003:1140–1148.
472. Hench PS, Rosenberg EF. Palindromic rheumatism. A "new," oft recurring disease of joints (arthritis, periarthritis, para-arthritis) apparently producing no articular residues. Report of thirty-four cases; its relation to "angioneural arthrosis," "allergic rheumatism" and rheumatoid arthritis. *Arch Intern Med* 1944;73:293–321.
473. Guerne PA, Weisman MH. Palindromic rheumatism: part of or apart from the spectrum of rheumatoid arthritis. *Am J Med* 1992;93:451–460.
474. Mattingly S. Palindromic rheumatism. *Ann Rheum Dis* 1966;25:307–317.
475. Wajed MA, Brown DL, Currey HL. Palindromic rheumatism. Clinical and serum complement study. *Ann Rheum Dis* 1977;36:56–61.
476. Hannonen P, Müttünen T, Oka M. Palindromic rheumatism. A clinical survey of sixty patients. *Scand J Rheumatol* 1987;16:413–420.
477. Salvador G, Gomez A, Viñas O, et al. Prevalence and clinical significance of anti-cyclic citrullinated peptide and antikeratin antibodies in palindromic rheumatism. An abortive form of rheumatoid arthritis? *Rheumatology* 2003;42:972–975.
478. Maksymowych WP, Suarez-Almazor ME, Buenviaje H, et al. HLA and cytokine gene polymorphisms in relation to occurrence of palindromic rheumatism and its progression to rheumatoid arthritis. *J Rheumatol* 2002;29:2319–2326.
479. Hannonen P, Hakola M, Oka M. Palindromic rheumatism in two nonidentical brothers with identical HLA including DR4. *Ann Rheum Dis* 1985;44:202–204.
480. Pasero G, Barbieri P. Palindromic rheumatism: you just have to think about it! *Clin Exp Rheumatol* 1986;4:197–199.
481. Gonzalez-Lopez L, Gamez-Nava JI, Jhangri GS, et al. Prognostic factors for the development of rheumatoid arthritis and other connective tissue diseases in patients with palindromic rheumatism. *J Rheumatol* 1999;26:540–545.
482. Gonzalez-Lopez L, Gamez-Nava JI, Jhangri G, et al. Decreased progression to rheumatoid arthritis or other connective tissue diseases in patients with palindromic rheumatism treated with antimalarials. *J Rheumatol* 2000;27:41–46.
483. Garrod AE. Concerning intermittent hydrarthrosis. *Q J Med* 1910;3:207–220.
484. Weiner AD. Periodic benign synovitis. Idiopathic intermittent hydrarthrosis. *J Bone Joint Surg* 1956;38A:1039–1055.
485. Mattingly S. Intermittent hydrarthrosis. *Br Med J* 1957;32:139–143.
486. Malone DG, Wilder RL. Participation of synovial mast cells in intermittent hydrarthrosis. *Arthritis Rheum* 1989;32:357–358.
487. Reimann HA, Angelides AP. Periodic arthralgia in twenty-three members of five generations of a family. *JAMA* 1951;146:713–716.
488. Queiro-Silva R, Tinturé-Eguren T, L<aaopez-Lagunas I. Successful therapy with low-dose colchicine in intermittent hydrarthrosis. *Rheumatology* 2003;42:391–392.
489. Topp JR, Cross EG, Fam AG. Treatment of persistent knee effusions with intra-articular radioactive gold. *Can Med Assoc J* 1975;112:1085–1089.
490. Brown JP, Rola-Pleszczynski M, Mänard H-A. Eosinophilic synovitis: clinical observations on a newly recognized subset of patients with dermatographism. *Arthritis Rheum* 1986;29:1147–1151.
491. Atanes A, Fernandez V, Nunez R, et al. Idiopathic eosinophilic synovitis. Case report and review of the literature. *Scand J Rheumatol* 1996;25:183–185.
492. Kay J, Eichenfield AH, Athreya BH, et al. Synovial fluid eosinophilia in Lyme disease. *Arthritis Rheum* 1988;31:1384–1389.
493. Goldenberg DL, Kelley W, Gibbons RB. Metastatic adenocarcinoma of synovium presenting as an acute arthritis. Diagnosed by closed synovial biopsy. *Arthritis Rheum* 1975;18:107–110.
494. Hasselbacher P, Schumacher HR. Synovial fluid eosinophilia following arthrography. *J Rheumatol* 1978;5:173–176.
495. Tietze A. Über eine eigenartige Häufung von Fällen mit Dystrophie der Rippenknorpel. *Berlin Klin Wochenschr* 1921; 58:829–831.
496. Aeschlimann A, Kahn MF. Tietze's syndrome: a critical review. *Clin Exp Rheumatol* 1990;8:407–412.
497. Levey GS, Calabro JJ. Tietze's syndrome: report of two cases and review of the literature. *Arthritis Rheum* 1962;5:261–269.
498. Jurik AG, Graudal H. Sternocostal joint swelling—clinical Tietze's syndrome. Report of sixteen cases and review of the literature. *Scand J Rheumatol* 1988;17:33–42.
499. Mukamel M, Kornreich L, Horev G, et al. Tietze's syndrome in children and infants. *J Pediatr* 1997;131:774–775.
500. Jurik AG, Justesen T, Graudal H. Radiographic findings in patients with clinical Tietze syndrome. *Skeletal Radiol* 1987;16:517–523.
501. Edelstein G, Levitt RG, Slaker DP, et al. Computed tomography of Tietze syndrome. *J Comput Assist Tomogr* 1984;8:20–23.
502. Honda N, Machida K, Mamiya T, et al. Scintigraphic and CT findings of Tietze's syndrome: report of a case and review of the literature. *Clin Nucl Med* 1989;14:606–609.
503. Thongngarm T, Lemos LB, Lawhon N, et al. Malignant tumor with chest wall pain mimicking Tietze's syndrome. *Clin Rheumatol* 2001; 20:276–278.
504. Fioravanti A, Tofi C, Volterrani L, et al. Malignant lymphoma presenting as Tietze's syndrome. *Arthritis Rheum* 2002;47:229–230.

Subject Index

Page numbers followed by the letter *f* refer to figures; those followed by the letter *t* refer to tabular material.

D

H

L

P